Vaccines

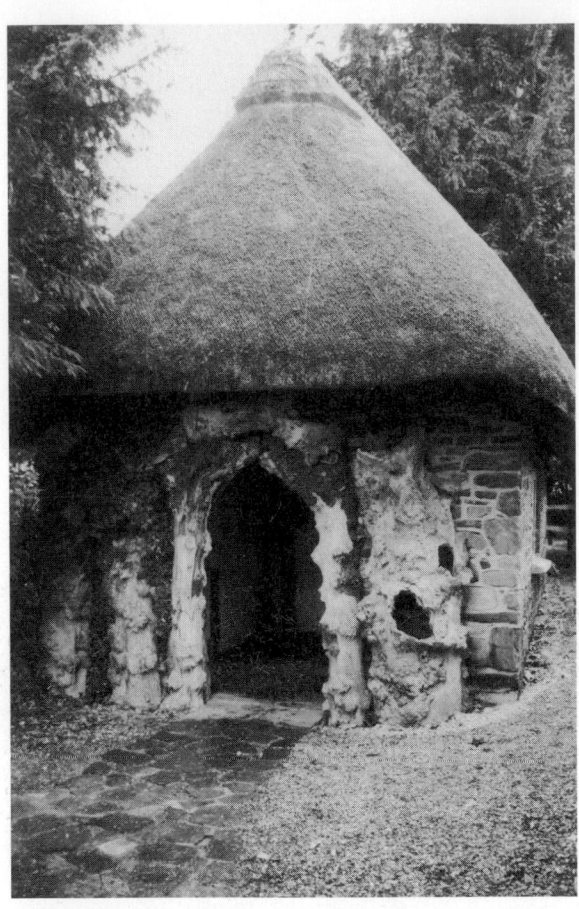

"Vaccination cottage" near the home of Edward Jenner in Berkeley, England, where he administered smallpox vaccine to thousands of the rural poor. (Photo by Stanley A. Plotkin.)

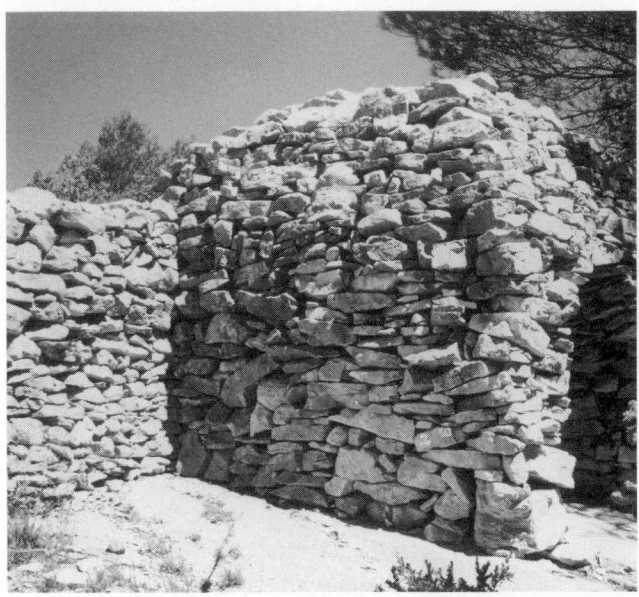

Part of a 20-km wall erected in 1720 in Provence to prevent people escaping a plague epidemic in Marseilles from spreading disease. The photo shows a guardhouse. (Photo by Stanley A. Plotkin.)

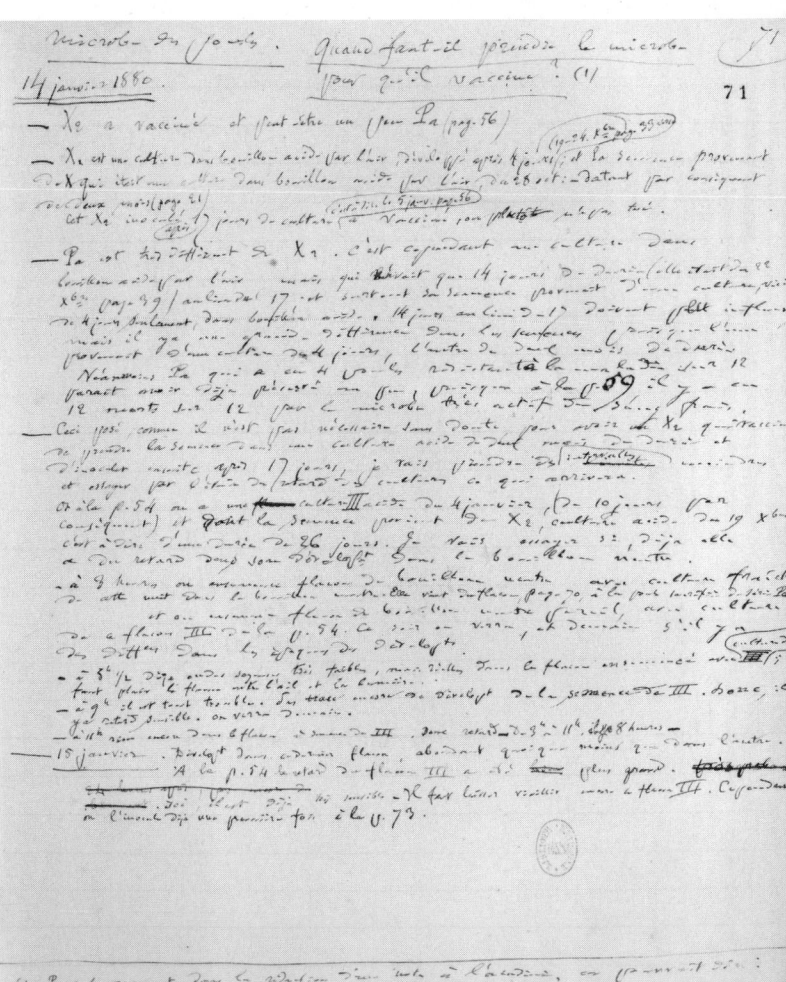

71

A page from the notebook of Louis Pasteur recording the first evidence of protection by a vaccine made in the laboratory, in this case a vaccine against *Pasturella multocida*-caused diarrhea in chickens. (Courtesy of the Bibliothèque Natioanle, Paris.)

FOURTH • EDITION
Vaccines

Stanley A. Plotkin, M.D.

Emeritus Professor of Pediatrics, University of Pennsylvania
Emeritus Professor, Wistar Institute
Adjunct Professor of International Health, Johns Hopkins University
Former Chief, Division of Infectious Diseases
  The Children's Hospital
  Philadelphia, Pennsylvania
Former Medical and Scientific Director, Mérieux Connaught, Paris, France
Medical and Scientific Consultant, Aventis Pasteur

Walter A. Orenstein, M.D.

Assistant Surgeon General, United States Public Health Service
Director, National Immunization Program
Centers for Disease Control and Prevention
Atlanta, Georgia

with assistance of

Paul A. Offit, M.D.

Chief, Section of Infectious Diseases
Professor of Pediatrics
The University of Pennsylvania School of Medicine
Henle Professor of Immunologic and Infectious Diseases
The Children's Hospital
Philadelphia, Pennsylvania

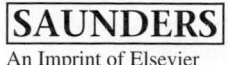
SAUNDERS
An Imprint of Elsevier

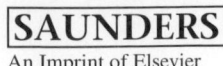

An Imprint of Elsevier

The Curtis Center
Independence Square West
Philadelphia, Pennsylvania 19106

NOTICE

Infectious Disease is an ever-changing field. Standard safety precautions must be followed, but as new research and clinical experience broaden our knowledge, changes in treatment and drug therapy may become necessary or appropriate. Readers are advised to check the most current product information provided by the manufacturer of each drug to be administered to verify the recommended dose, the method and duration of administration, and contraindications. It is the responsibility of the licensed prescriber, relying on experience and knowledge of the patient, to determine dosages and the best treatment for each individual patient. Neither the publisher nor the author assumes any liability for any injury and/or damage to persons or property arising from this publication.

The Publisher

Library of Congress Cataloging-in-Publication Data

Library of Congress Cataloging-in-Publication Data
Vaccines/[edited by] Stanley A. Plotkin, Walter A. Orenstein, with assistance of Paul
A. Offit – 4th ed.
   p.; cm.
   Includes bibliographical references and index.
   ISBN 0-7216-9688-0
   1. Vaccines. I. Plotkin, Stanley A., II. Orenstein, Walter A.
   [DNLM: 1. Vaccines. 2. Immunization Programs. 3. Vaccination. QW 805 V1163 2004]
   QR 189.V268 2004
   615'.372– dc21

Printed in The United States of America

Last digit is the print number: 9   8   7   6   5   4   3   2

Acknowledgments

This book could not have been accomplished without the dedicated work of Ms. Grace Fries, my assistant. I also thank Jean-Jacques Bertrand and Dave Williams of Aventis Pasteur for their indulgence during the time necessary to create this edition.

S.A.P.

Many thanks to Mrs. Gayle Hickman for her assistance in preparing, revising, and tracking submission of manuscripts. All this was accomplished while continuing her regular full-time duties in the National Immunization Program (NIP). I also want to thank the staff of NIP who continued to provide national leadership in the control of vaccine-preventable diseases so I would have the opportunity to work on this book.

W.A.O.

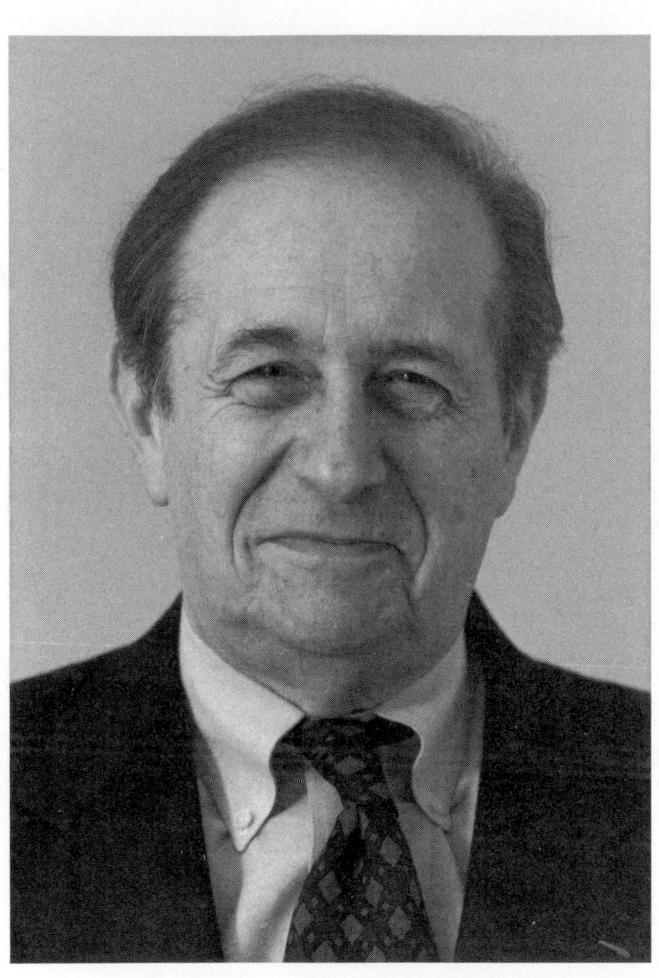

Stanley A. Plotkin, M.D.

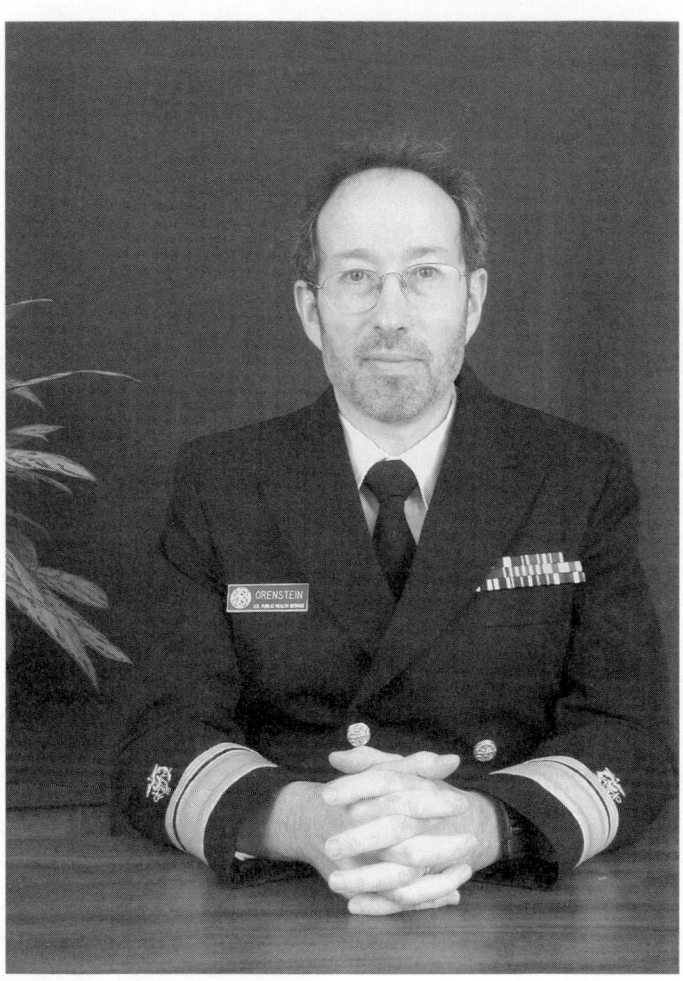

Walter A. Orenstein, M.D.

To Susan, the love of my life.
S.A.P.

To my loving wife, Diane, and our children, Eleza and
Evan, whose support has made my life's work possible.
W.A.O.

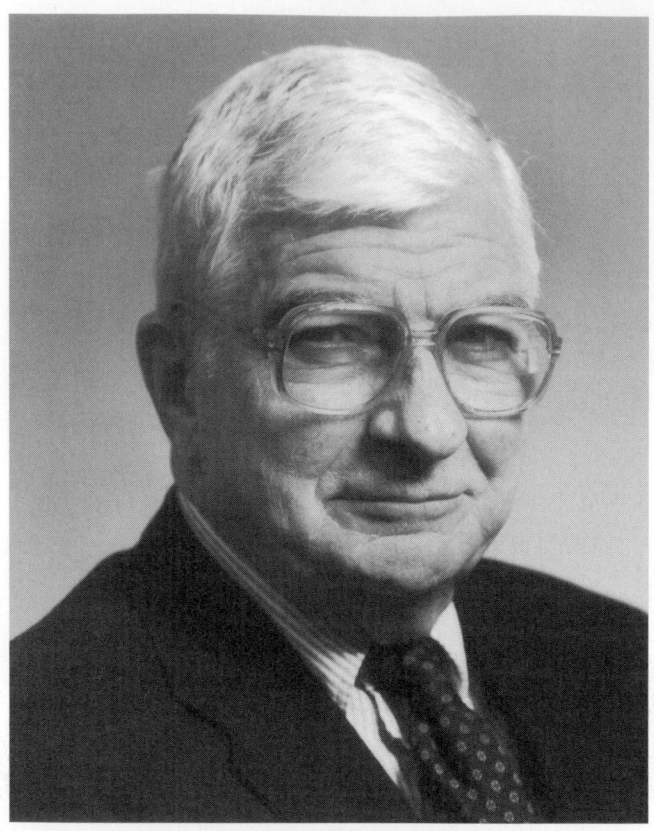

Edward A. "Ted" Mortimer, Jr., M.D.
March 22, 1922–July 20, 2002

Ted Mortimer was the coeditor of the first and second editions of *Vaccines* in 1988 and 1994. Ted had an illustrious career in pediatrics, epidemiology, and vaccinology spanning five decades. He was Assistant Director and Associate Director of the Department of Pediatrics at Cleveland Metropolitan General Hospital, Cleveland, Ohio, from 1952 to 1966, and following this was the first Professor and Chairman, Department of Pediatrics, at the University of New Mexico School of Medicine, Albuquerque, New Mexico, from 1966 to 1975.

In 1975, Dr. Mortimer became the Elisabeth Severance Prentiss Professor and Chairman, Department of Epidemiology and Community Health, as well as Professor of Pediatrics at Case Western Reserve University School of Medicine, Cleveland, Ohio. He served in these roles for 10 years. He subsequently was Vice Chairman of the Department of Epidemiology and Biostatistics from 1985 to 1992 and Professor Emeritus in that department from 1992 until his death in July 2002.

Ted was a recognized expert on vaccines. He served as a member or consultant to the Committee on Infectious Diseases of the American Academy of Pediatrics (AAP) from 1966 through 1982. In 1977, he was a member of the AAP Task Force on Immunization Policy. From 1978 through 1995, Ted served as a full member or liaison member of the Advisory Committee on Immunization Practices (ACIP) of the U.S. Department of Health and Human Resources. From 1987 to 1991, Ted was a member of the Consultative Group on Vaccine Development for the Agency for International Development and a panel member on Standard Bacterial Vaccines and Toxoids for the Bureau of Biologics, Food and Drug Administration, from 1973 to 1980.

Ted's early research related to group A streptococcal infections and rheumatic fever and the epidemiology of *Staphylococcus aureus* infections. In 1962, he and Martha Lepow were the first to observe the association of varicella and salicylates in Reye's syndrome.

Ted focused on vaccines and vaccine issues in the 1970s, and in this regard he authored or coauthored many significant publications. His main interest was pertussis, and he was an early innovator in the epidemiologic approach to the study of vaccine effectiveness as well as adverse events attributed to vaccines. He was an early leader in the demonstration that vaccination benefits exceeded even perceived risks of immunization. He emphasized that temporal associations between immunization and adverse events were not necessarily cause-and-effect relationships. One Mortimer slide to make the point was as follows: "Some people who go outside after a rainstorm and see frogs believe it rained frogs."

The revised ACIP statement on DTP immunization drafted by Ted and two others in 1990 was a bold step forward, and it clearly indicated correctly that there was no evidence that this vaccine caused either sudden infant death syndrome or brain damage. Ted was a thorn in the side of plaintiff lawyers in DTP vaccine litigations, and he was extensively criticized by members of the antivaccine community. However, his efforts and belief in sound epidemiologic data contributed to extensive progress relating to pertussis immunization during the last two decades.

I had the opportunity to work closely with Ted on numerous projects since 1977. In spite of intense criticism directed at him by people who believed that pertussis vaccine caused both death and brain damage, he remained steadfast in his search for scientific truth. He was never afraid to present his point of view even when it was unpopular, and, in spite of aggressive attacks against him, he maintained his incredible sense of humor. Working with me in Japan as consultants to the Lederle acellular pertussis vaccine project, Ted was the leader in our interactions with the Japanese experts, and his wisdom and humor often carried the day.

Ted's scientific and sensible approach to vaccines will be missed.

James D. Cherry

Contributors

Gordon Ada D.Sc.
John Curtin School of Medical Research, Australian
National University, Canberra, Australia.
The Immunology of Vaccination

William L. Atkinson M.D., M.P.H.
Medical Epidemiologist, National Immunization Program,
Centers for Disease Control and Prevention, Atlanta,
Georgia.
General Immunization Practices

Elizabeth Day Barnett M.D.
Associate Professor of Pediatrics, Boston University
School of Medicine, Director, International Clinic, Boston
Medical Center, Boston, Massachusetts.
Vaccines for International Travel

P. Noel Barrett Ph.D.
Vice President, Research and Development, Baxter
Vaccines Biomedical Research Center, Vienna, Austria.
Tick-Borne Encephalitis virus Vaccine

Eileen M. Barry Ph.D.
Assistant Professor of Medicine, University of Maryland,
Baltimore, Maryland.
Diarrheal Disease Vaccines

Norman W. Baylor Ph.D.
Associate Director for Policy, Office of Vaccines Research
and Review, Center for Biologics Evaluation and Research,
Food and Drug Administration, Rockville, Maryland.
Regulation and Testing of Vaccines

Beth P. Bell M.D., M.P.H.
Chief, Epidemiology Branch, Division of Viral Hepatitis,
National Center for Infectious Diseases, Centers for
Disease Control and Prevention, Atlanta, Georgia.
Hepatits A Vaccine

Robert B. Belshe M.D.
Professor of Medicine and Pediatrics and Molecular
Biology, St. Louis University, St. Louis, Missouri.
Influenza Vaccine—Live

Jeffrey M. Bethony Ph.D.
Assistant Professor, Department of Microbiology and
Tropical Medicine, The George Washington University
Washington, D.C.
Parasitic Disease Vaccines

Julian Bilous M.B.Ch.B., M.T.H.
Coordinator, Expanded Programme on Immunization,
Vaccines and Biologicals Department,
World Health Organization, Geneva,
Switzerland.
Immunization in Developing Countries

Steven B. Black M.D.
Associate Clinical Professor, Pediatrics,
University of California, San Francisco,
California; Co-Director, Kaiser
Permamente Vaccine Center, Oakland,
California.
Pneumococcal Conjugate Vaccine

Hugues H. Bogaerts M.D., F.F.P.M.
Vice President Worldwide Medical,
GlaxoSmithKline Biologicals,
Rixensart, Belgium;
Invited Lecturer, Catholic University of Louvain,
Belgium.
Combination Vaccines

Luciana L. Borio M.D.
Clinical Fellow, Department of Medicine, Division of
Infectious Diseases, Johns Hopkins
University School of Medicine, Baltimore,
Maryland.
Smallpox and Vaccinia

Ray Borrow Ph.D.
Head of Vaccine Evaluation Department, Manchester
Medical Microbiology Partnership, Manchester Royal
Infirmary, Manchester, UK.
Meningococcal Vaccines

Philip S. Brachman M.D.
Professor, Department of International Health, Rollins
School of Public Health, Emory University, Atlanta,
Georgia.
Anthrax Vaccine

Carolyn B. Bridges M.D.
Medical Epidemiologist, Influenza Branch,
Division of Viral and Rickettsial Diseases,
National Center for Infectious Diseases,
Centers for Disease Control and Prevention,
Atlanta, Georgia.
Influenza Vaccine—Inactivated

Robert T. Chen M.D., M.A.
Chief, Immunization Safety Branch, Epidemiology and
Surveillance Division, National Immunization Program,
Centers for Disease Control and Prevention, Atlanta,
Georgia.
Safety of Immunizations

H. Fred Clark Ph.D., D.V.M.
Research Professor of Pediatrics, School of Medicine,
University of Pennsylvania, Philadelphia,
Pennsylvania.
Rotavirus Vaccines

Stephen L. Cochi M.D., M.P.H.
Associate Director for Global Immunization and Director,
Global Immunization Division,
National Immunization Program, Centers for Disease
Control and Prevention, Atlanta, Georgia.
*Immunization in Developing Countries; Poliovirus
Vaccine—Live*

Nancy J. Cox Ph.D.
Chief, Influenza Branch, National Center for Infectious
Diseases
Centers for Disease Control and Prevention, Atlanta,
Georgia.
Influenza Vaccine—Inactivated

Felicity T. Cutts M.B.Ch.B., M.Sc., M.D.
Honorary Professor of Epidemiology, LSHTM, London,
England; Director, Pneumococcal Vaccine Trial,
Medical Research Council, The Gambia.
Immunization in Developing Countries

Robert S. Daum M.D., C.M.
Professor of Pediatrics, Biological Sciences Collegiate
Division, Committee on Microiology and Committee on
Molecular Medicine; Section Chief, Pediatric Infectious
Diseases, Department of Pediatrics, University of Chicago,
Chicago, Illinois.
Staphylococcus Vaccine

Robert L. Davis M.D., M.P.H.
Associate Professor, Pediatrics and Epidemiology,
University of Washington, Seattle, Washington.
Safety of Immunizations

Michael D. Decker M.D., M.P.H.
Adjunct Professor of Preventive Medicine and Medicine
(Infectious Diseases), Vanderbilt University School of
Medicine, Nashville, Tennessee; Vice President,
Science and Medical Affairs, Aventis Pasteur, Swiftwater,
Pennsylvania.
Pertussis Vaccine; Combination Vaccine

David T. Dennis M.D., M.P.H., D.C.M.T.
Teaching Affiliate, Department Microbiology, Colorado
State University; Guest Researcher, Division of Vector-
Borne Infectious Diseases,
National Center for Infectious Diseases, Centers for
Disease Control and Prevention, Fort Collins, Colorado
Plague

Friedrich Dorner Ph.D.
Professor, University for Veterinary Medicine and
University for Agricultural Sciences; President,
Global Research and Development,
Member of the Board of Directors,
Baxter AG and Baxter
Vaccines AG, Vienna, Austria.
Tick-Borne Encephalitis Virus Vaccine

R. Gordon Douglas M.D.
Adjunct Professor of Medicine, Cornell University
Medical College, Ithaca, New York; Director of Strategic
Planning, Vaccine Research Center, NIAID, National
Institutes of Health, Bethesda, Maryland; Chairman,
Board of Directors, Vical Inc., San Diego, California.
The Vaccine Industry

Filip Dubovsky M.D., M.P.H., F.A.A.P.
Preventive Medicine Resident, Johns Hopkins
University, Fellow in Infectious Diseases and Tropical
Pediatrics, University of Maryland,
Baltimore, Maryland; Chief Scientific Officer, Malaria
Vaccine Initiative, PATH, Rockville, Maryland.
Malaria Vaccine

Gary B. Ebbert Ph.D.
Head of Global Operations, King Pharmaceuticals, Bristol,
Tennessee.
Vaccine Manufacturing

Kathryn M. Edwards M.D.
Professor of Pediatrics, Vanderbilt University
School of Medicine; Vice Chair for Clinical
Research, Department of Pediatrics,
Vanderbilt Children's Hospital, Nashville,
Tennessee.
Pertussis Vaccines

William Egan Ph.D.
Deputy Director, Office of Vaccines Research
and Review, National Institutes of Health,
Bethesda, Maryland.
*Vaccine Additives and Manufacturing Residuals in the
United States—Licensed Vaccines*

Ronald W. Ellis Ph.D.
Senior Vice President, Research and Development and
General Manager, Shire Biologics, Inc., Northborough,
Massachusetts.
Technologies for Making New Vaccines

Juhani Eskola M.D., Ph.D.
Senior Vice President, Medical, Aventis
Pasteur, Lyon, France.
Pneumococcal Conjugate Vaccine

Geoffrey Evans M.D.
Medical Director, Division of
Vaccine Injury and Compensation, Research Director,
U.S. Department of Health and Human Services,
Office of the General Council, Public Health Division,
Rockville, Maryland.
Legal Issues

Ian M. Feavers Ph.D.
Principal Scientist, Division of Bacteriology, National Institute for Biological Standards and Control (NIBSC), Potters Bar, Hertfordshire, UK.
Meningococcal Vaccines

David S. Fedson M.D.
Former Director, Medical Affairs Europe, Aventis Pasteur MSD, Lyon, France.
Pneumococcal Polysaccharide Vaccine

Stephen M. Feinstone M.D.
Chief, Laboratory of Hepatitis Viruses, Center for Biologics Evaluation and Research, Food and Drug Administration, Bethesda, Maryland.
Hepatitis A Vaccine

Paul E. M. Fine V.M.D., Ph.D.
Professor of Communicable Disease Epidemiology, London School of Hygiene and Tropical Medicine, London, UK.
Community Immunity

Theresa M. Finn Ph.D.
Scientific Reviewer, Division of Vaccines and Related Products Applications, Office of Vaccines Research and Review, Center for Biologics Research and Review, Food and Drug Administration, Bethesda, Maryland.
Vaccine Additives and Manufacturing Residuals in United States—Licensed Vaccines

Arthur M. Friedlander M.D.
Adjunct Professor of Medicine, School of Medicine, Uniformed Services University of the Health Sciences, Bethesda, Maryland; Senior Medical Scientist, U.S. Army Medical Research Institute of Infectious Diseases, Frederick, Maryland.
Anthrax Vaccine

Keiji Fukuda M.D., M.P.H.
Assistant Clinical Professor, Department of Community and Preventive Medicine, Emory University School of Medicine; Chief, Epidemiology Section, Influenza Branch, National Center for Infectious Diseases, Centers for Disease Control and Prevention, Atlanta, Georgia.
Influenza Vaccine—Inactivated

Charlotte A. Gaydos Ph.D., M.P.H.
Associate Professor, Division of Infectious Diseases, Department of Medicine, Johns Hopkins University, Baltimore, Maryland.
Adenovirus Vaccine

Joel C. Gaydos M.D., M.P.H.
Adjunct Professor, George Washington University, Washington, D.C., Adjunct Professor, Uniformed Services University, Bethesda, Maryland; Director, Public Health Practices, Department of Defense Global Emerging Infections Surveillance and Response System, Walter Reed Army Institute of Research, Silver Spring, Maryland.
Adenovirus Vaccine

Anne A. Gershon M.D.
Professor of Pediatrics, Columbia University College of Physicians and Surgeons; Attending Physician, Children's Hospital of New York, New York, New York.
Varicella Vaccine

Marc P. Girard D.Sc., D.V.M.
Director-General, Fondation Mérieux, Lyon, France.
Human Immunodeficiency Virus

Roger I. Glass Ph.D., M.D., M.P.M.
Adjunct Professor, Department of International Health, Rollins School of Public Health, Emory University; Research Professor, Department of Pediatrics, Emory University School of Medicine; Chief, Viral Gastroenteritis Section, Centers for Disease Control and Prevention, Atlanta, Georgia.
Rotavirus Vaccines

John D. Grabenstein R.Ph., Ph.D.
Deputy Director for Military Vaccines, Army Surgeon General's Office, Falls Church, Virginia.
Anthrax Vaccine

Dan M. Granoff M.D.
Senior Scientist, Children's Hospital Oakland Research Institute, Oakland, California.
Meningococcal Vaccines

Anne G. Gregerson B.A.
University of Chicago Children's Hospital, Pediatric Infectious Diseases, Chicago, Illinois.
Staphylococcus Vaccines

Charles J. Hackett Ph.D.
Chief, Molecular and Structural Immunology Section, Basic Immunology Branch, Division of Allergy, Immunology, and Transplantation, National Institute of Allergy and Infectious Diseases, National Institutes of Health, Bethesda, Maryland.
Safety of Multiple Antigen Administration

Neal A. Halsey M.D.
Professor, Department of International Health, Director, Institute for Vaccine Safety, Johns Hopkins Bloomberg School of Public Health; Professor, Department of Pediatrics, Department of Medicine, Johns Hopkins University, School of Medicine, Baltimore, Maryland.
Vaccination of Human Immunodeficiency Virus-Infected Persons; Measles Vaccine

Scott B. Halstead M.D.
Adjunct Professor, Department of Preventive Medicine and Biometrics, Uniformed Services University of the Health Sciences, Bethesda, Maryland.
Japanese Encephalitis Vaccines

Deborah Harris J.D. (deceased)
Senior Attorney, U.S. Department of Health and Human
Services, Office of the General Counsel, Public Health
Division, Rockville, Maryland.
Legal Issues

Stanley L. Hem Ph.D.
Professor of Physical Pharmacy, Purdue University, West
Lafayette, Indiana.
Immunologic Adjuvants

Donald A. Henderson M.D., M.P.H.
Founding Director, Hopkins Center for Civilian
Biodefencse Strategies,
University Distinguished Service Professor,
The Johns Hopkins University, Baltimore,
Maryland.
Smallpox and Vaccinia

Alan R. Hinman M.D., M.P.H.
Adjunct Professor, Epidemiology and International
Health, Rollins School of Public Health, Emory
University, Atlanta, Georgia; Principal Investigator, All
Kids Count, Task Force for Child Survival and
Development, Decatur, Georgia.
*Immunization in the United States; Cost-Benefit and
Cost-Effectiveness Analysis of Vaccine Policy*

Peter J. Hotez Ph.D., M.D.
Professor and Chair, Department of Microbiology and
Tropical Medicine, The George Washington University,
Washington, D.C.
Parasitic Disease Vaccines

Mark A. Kane M.D., M.P.H.
Director, Children's Vaccine Program at Program for
Appropriate Technology in Health (PATH), Seattle,
Washington.
Hepatitis B Vaccine

Ruth A. Karron M.D.
Associate Professor, International Health, Bloomberg
School of Public Health; Joint Appointment, Pediatrics,
School of Medicine, Johns Hopkins University, Baltimore,
Maryland.
Respiratory Syncytial Virus Vaccine

Olen M. Kew Ph.D.
Chief, Molecular Virology Section, Respiratory and
Enteric Viruses Branch, Division of Viral and Rickettsial
Diseases, National Center for Infectious Diseases,
Centers for Disease Control and Prevention, Atlanta,
Georgia.
Poliovirus Vaccine—Live

Hilary Koprowski M.D.
Professor, Department of Microbiology and Immunology;
Head, Center of Neurovirology,
Thomas Jefferson University; President,
Biotechnology Foundation Laboratories, Philadelphia,
Pennsylvania.
Rabies Vaccine

Wayne C. Koff Ph.D.
Senior Vice President, Research and Development,
International Aids Vaccine Initiative,
New York, New York.
Human Immunodeficiency Virus

Phyllis E. Kozarsky M.D.
Professor of Medicine, Infectious Diseases; Director,
Tropical and Travel Medicine, Emory University School of
Medicine, Atlanta, Georgia.
Vaccines for International Travel

J. Michael Lane M.D., M.P.H.
Emeritus Professor, Preventive Medicine,
Emory University School of Medicine,
Atlanta, Georgia.
Smallpox and Vaccinia

Dennis R. Lang Ph.D.
Deputy Director, DERT, National Institute of
Environmental Health Sciences, National Institutes of
Health, Research Triangle Park, North Carolina.
Cholera Vaccines

Roland A. Levandowski M.D.
Medical Officer, Division of Viral Products, Center for
Biologics Evaluation and Research, Bethesda, Maryland.
Influenza Vaccine—Inactivated

Emily Marcus Levine J.D.
Senior Attorney, U.S. Department of Health and Human
Services, Office of the General Counsel, Public Health
Division, Rockville, Maryland.
Legal Issues

Myron M. Levine M.D., D.T.P.H.
Professor and Director, Division of Geographic Medicine,
Department of Medicine; Professor and Director, Division
of Infectious Diseases and Tropical Pediatrics, Department
of Pediatrics; Director, Center for Vaccine Development,
University of Maryland School of Medicine, Baltimore,
Maryland.
Typhoid Fever Vaccines

Per Ljungman M.D., Ph.D.
Head, Department of Hematology; Professor, Head,
Sections of Hematology, Department of Medicine,
Huddinge University Hospital, Stockholm, Sweden.
Vaccination in the Immunocompromised Host

Douglas R. Lowy M.D.
Chief, Laboratory of Cellular Oncology,
National Cancer Institute, National Institutes of Health,
Bethesda, Maryland.
*Human Papillomavirus Vaccine for Cervical Cancer
Prevention*

H. F. Maassab Ph.D.
Professor Emeritus Department of Epidemiology, School of
Public Health, University of Michigan, Ann Arbor,
Michigan.
Influenza Vaccine—Live

Frank Mahoney M. D., M. P. H.
Captain, U.S. Public Health Service; Head, Disease
Surveillance Program, U.S. Naval Medical Research Unit
No. 3, Cairo, Egypt.
Hepatitis B Vaccine

Harold S. Margolis M.D.
Director, Division of Viral Hepatitis, National Center for
Infectious Diseases, Centers for Disease Control and
Prevention, Atlanta, Georgia.
Hepatits B Vaccine

Eugene D. Mascolo B.S.
Aventis Pasteur, Swiftwater, Pennsylvania.
Vaccine Manufacturing

Eric E. Mast M. D., M. P. H.
Medical Epidemiologist, Division of Viral Hepatitis,
National Center for Infectious Diseases, Centers for
Disease Control and Prevention, Atlanta, Georgia.
Hepatitis B Vaccine

Timothy D. Mastro M.D.
Deputy Director, Global AIDS Program, Centers for
Disease Control and Prevention, Atlanta, Georgia.
Human Immunodeficiency Virus

Paul M. Mendelman M.D.
Consulting Professor of Pediatrics, Stanford University
School of Medicine, Stanford, California; Vice
President and Group Leader, Infectious Diseases and
Vaccines, MedImmune Vaccines, Inc., Mountainview,
California.
Influenza Vaccine—Live

Karen Midthun M.D.
Director, Office of Vaccines Research and Review, Center
for Biologics Evaluation and Review, Food and Drug
Administration, Rockville, Maryland.
Regulation and Testing of Vaccines

Mark A. Miller M.D.
Associate Director for Research; Director, Division of
International Epidemiology and Population Studies,
Fogarty International Center, National Institutes of
Health, Bethesda, Maryland.
*Cost-Benefit and Cost-Effectiveness Analysis
of Vaccine Policy*

Thomas P. Monath M.D.
Adjunct Professor, Harvard School of Public Health,
Boston, Massachusetts; Chief Scientific Officer, Acambis,
Inc., Cambridge, Massachusetts.
Yellow Fever Vaccine

William J. Moss M.D., M.P.H.
Assistant Research Professor, Bloomberg School of Public
Health, Johns Hopkins University, Baltimore,
Maryland.
*Vaccination of Human Immunodeficiency Virus-Infected
Persons*

Trudy V. Murphy M.D.
Medical Epidemiologist, Epidemiology and Surveillance
Divison, National Immunization Program, Centers for
Disease Control and Prevention, Atlanta, Georgia.
Tetanus Toxoid

Daniel M. Musher M.D.
Professor of Medicine; Professor of Molecular
Virology and Microbiology, Baylor College of Medicine;
Chief of Infectious Diseases, Veterans Affairs Medical
Center, Houston, Texas.
Pneumococcal Polysaccharide Vaccine

James P. Nataro M.D., Ph.D.
Professor of Pediatrics, Medicine, and Microbiology and
Immunology, Center for Vaccine Development,
University of Mayland School of Medicine, Baltimore,
Maryland.
Diarrheal Disease Vaccines

Paul A. Offit M.D.
Professor of Pediatrics, The University of Pennsylvania
School of Medicine; Chief, Division of Infectious Diseases,
The Children's Hospital of Philadelphia, Philadelphia,
Pennsylvania.
Safety of Multiple Antigen Administration; Rotavirus Vaccine

Jean-Marc J. Olivé M.D., M.P.H.
World Health Organization,
Representative in the Philippines, Manila, Philippines.
Immunization in Europe

Walter A. Orenstein M.D.
Assistant Surgeon General, United States Public Health
Service
Director, National Immunization Program
Centers for Disease Control and Prevention
Atlanta, Georgia.
Tetanus Toxoid; Immunization in the United States

Mark Papania M.D., M.P.H.
Chief, Measles Elimination Activity, National
Immunization Program, Centers for
Disease Control and Prevention,
Atlanta, Georgia.
Measles Vaccine

Georges Peter M.D.
Professor and Vice Chair for Faculty Affairs, Department
of Pediatrics, Brown Medical School; Director, Division of
Pediatric Infectious Diseases, Rhode Island Hospital,
Providence, Rhode Island.
General Immunization Practices

Larry K. Pickering M.D., F.A.A.P.
Professor of Pediatrics, Department of Pediatrics,
Emory University School of Medicine; Senior Advisor to
the Director, National Immunization Program,
Centers for Disease Control and Prevention, Atlanta,
Georgia.
General Immunization Practices

Phillip R. Pittman M.D., M.P.H.
Senior Medical Scientist, USAMRIID, Fort Detrick, Maryland.
Miscellaneous Limited-Use Vaccines

Stanley A. Plotkin M.D.
Emeritus Professor of Pediatrics, University of Pennsylvania, Philadelphia, Pennsylvania; Emeritus Professor, Wistar Institute; Medical and Scientific Consultant, Aventis Pasteur; Former Medical and Scientific Director, Pasteur Mérieux Connaught, Marnes-la-Coquette, France; Former Chief, Division of Infectious Diseases, The Children's Hospital of Philadelphia, Philadelphia, Pennsylvania.
A Short History of Vaccination; Mumps Vaccine; Poliovirus Vaccine—Inactivated; Rubella Vaccines; Miscellaneous Limited-Use Vaccines; Rabies Vaccine; Tick-Borne Encephalitis Virus Vaccine; Cytomegalovirus Vaccine

Susan L. Plotkin M.S.L.S.
A Short History of Vaccination

N. Regina Rabinovich
Malaria Vaccine Initiative, PATH, Rockville, Maryland.
Malaria Vaccine

Susan Reef M.D.
National Immunization Program, Centers for Disease Control and Prevention, Atlanta, Georgia.
Rubella Vaccine

Frederick C. Robbins M.D.
Professor Emeritus, Department of Epidemiology and Biostatistics, School of Medicine, Case Western University, Euclid, Ohio.
The History of Polio Vaccine Development

Lance E. Rodewald M.D.
Director, Immunization Services Division, National Immunization Program, Centers for Disease Control and Prevention, Atlanta, Georgia.
Immunization in the United States

Martha H. Roper M.D., M.P.H., D.T.M.H.
Medical Epidemiologist, Epidemiology and Surveillance Division, National Immunization Program, Centers for Disease Control and Prevention, Atlanta, Georgia.
Tetanus Toxoid

Charles E. Rupprecht V.M.D., Ph.D.
Chief, Rabies Section, Centers for Disease Control and Prevention, Atlanta, Georgia.
Rabies Vaccine

William A. Rutala Ph.D., M.P.H.
Professor of Medicine, Adult Infectious Disease Division, Department of Epidemiology, University of North Carolina School of Medicine, Chapel Hill, North Carolina.
Vaccines for Health Care Workers

David A. Sack MD
Professor, Bloomberg School of Public Health, Johns Hopkins University, Baltimore, Maryland; Director, ICDDRR, Centre for Health and Population Research, Dhaka, Bangladesh.
Cholera Vaccines

David M. Salisbury M.D., F.R.C.P., F.R.C.P.C.H., F.F.P.H.M.
Head of Immunisation and Infectious Disease, Department of Health, London, UK.
Immunization in Europe

John T. Schiller Ph.D.
Section Chief, Laboratory of Cellular Oncology, National Cancer Institute, National Institutes of Health, Bethesda, Maryland.
Human Papillomavirus Vaccine for Cervical Cancer Prevention

Jane Seward M.B.B.S., M.P.H.
Chief, Varicella Activity, Viral Vaccine Preventable Diseases Branch, National Immunization Program, Centers for Disease Control and Prevention, Atlanta, Georgia.
Varicella Vaccine

Kristine M. Sheedy Ph.D.
Health Communications Specialist, National Immunization Program, Centers for Disease Control and Prevention, Atlanta, Georgia.
Safety of Immunizations

Henry Shinefield M.D.
Co-Director of Kaiser Permanente Study Center, Clinical Professor of Pediatrics and Dermatology, University of California, San Francisco.
Pneumococcal Conjugate Vaccine

Devender Singh-Sandhu Ph.D.
Senior Research Scientist, Aventis Pasteur, Limited, Toronto, Canada.
Poxviruses as Immunization Vehicles

Kim Connelly Smith M.D., M.P.H.
Associate Professor, Community and General Pediatrics, University of Texas-Houston Medical School; Medical Director, The Children's Tuberculosis Clinics, Lyndon B. Johnson Hospital, Memorial Hermann Children's Hospital, Houston, Texas.
Bacille Calmette-Guérin Vaccine

Jeffrey R. Starke M.D.
Professor of Pediatrics, Baylor College of Medicine; Chief of Pediatrics, Director, Children's Tuberculosis Clinic, Ben Taub General Hospital, Houston, Texas.
Bacille Calmette-Guérin Vaccine

Allen C. Steere M.D.
Professor of Medicine, Harvard Medical School; Director, Rheumatology, Massachusetts General Hospital, Boston, Massachusetts.
Lyme Disease Vaccine

Robert Steffen M.D.
Professor of Travel Medicine, University of Zurich; Director, World Health Organization Collaborating Center for Travellers' Health Zurich, Switzerland.
Vaccines for International Travel

Peter M. Strebel M.B.Ch.B., M.P.H
Chief, Global Measles Branch, Global Immunization
Division, National Immunization Program, Centers for
Disease Control and Prevention, Atlanta, Georgia.
Measles Vaccines

Roland W. Sutter M.D., M.P.H., T.M.
Medical Officer, World Health Organization, Geneva,
Switzerland.
Poliovirus Vaccine—Live

Michiaki Takahashi M.D.
Emeritus Professor, Osaka University, Suita City; Director,
The Research Foundation for Microbial Diseases of Osaka
University, Suita City, Osaka, Japan.
Varicella Vaccine

James Tartaglia Ph.D.
Aventis Pasteur, Toronto, Canada.
Poxviruses as Immunization Vehicles

Richard W. Titball D.Sc., Ph.D.
Professor, London School of Hygiene and Tropical
Medicine, University of London and University of
Plymouth, UK; Group Leader Microbiology, Defence
Science and Technology Laboratory Porton Down,
Salisbury, Wiltshire, UK.
Plague

Theodore F. Tsai M.D., M.P.H.
Senior Director, Vaccine, Clinical Affairs, Wyeth
Pharmaceuticals, St. Davids, Pennsylvania.
Poliovirus Vaccine—Inactivated
Japanese Encephalitis Vaccines

Emmanuel Vidor M.D.
Clinical Development, Medical Department, Aventis
Pasteur, Lyon, France.
Poliovirus Vaccine—Inactivated

Charles R. Vitek M.D., M.P.H.
Medical Epidemiologist, HIV Vaccine Section,
Epidemiology Branch, Division of HIV/AIDS
Prevention National Center for HIV, STD, and TB
Prevention-Surveillance and Epidemiology, Centers for
Disease Control and Prevention, Atlanta, Georgia.
Diphtheria Toxoid

Frederick R. Vogel Ph.D.
Project Leader, Research and Development, Aventis
Pasteur, Marcy l'Etoile, France.
Immunologic Adjuvants

Joel I. Ward M.D.
Director, Center for Vaccine Research, UCLA School of
Medicine, Harbor-UCLA
Medical Center, Torrance, California.
Haemophilus influenzae Vaccine

Richard L. Ward Ph.D.
Professor, Department of Pediatrics, Children's Hospital
Medical Center, Cincinnati, Ohio.
Rotavirus Vaccines

Steven G. F. Wassilak M.D.
Medical Officer, Polio Eradication Vaccine-Preventable
Diseases and Immunization Programme, World Health
Organization Regional Office for Europe, Copenhagen,
Denmark.
Tetanus Toxoid

John C. Watson M.D., M.P.H.
Captain, U.S. Public Health Service; Medical
Epidemiologist, Parasitic Diseases
Epidemiology Branch, Division of Parasitic
Diseases, National Center for Infectious Diseases, Centers
for Disease Control and Prevention,
Atlanta, Georgia.
General Immunization Practices

David J. Weber M.D., M.P.H.
Professor of Medicine, Pediatrics and Epidemiology,
Schools of Medicine and Public Health, University of
North Carolina at Chapel Hill; Medical Director,
Departments of Hospital Epidemiology and Occupational
Health Services, University of North Carolina Health Care
System, Chapel Hill, North Carolina.
Vaccines for Health Care Workers

Jay D. Wenger M.D.
Project Manager, National Polio Surveillance Project,
New Delhi, India.
Haemophilus influenzae Vaccine

Melinda Wharton M.D., M.P.H.
Director, Epidemiology and Surveillance Division,
National Immunization Program, Centers for Disease
Control and Prevention, Atlanta, Georgia.
Diphtheria Toxoid

E. Diane Williamson Ph.D.
Group Leader, Microbiology, Defence Science and
Technology Laboratory, Porton Down, Salisbury Wilts,
UK.
Plague

Preface

The 4 years since the publication of the last edition have been the best of times and the worst of times for vaccination. New strategies to produce vaccines based on our ever-increasing ability to manipulate genes and proteins are pouring forth from academic laboratories. Moreover, during that period, older technologies have brought to licensure (in some countries) a conjugated pneumococcal polysaccharide vaccine, a conjugated meningococcal group C vaccine, an intranasal live, attenuated influenza vaccine, and multiple combined pediatric vaccines based on acellular pertussis components.

On the negative side, we have seen the licensure and then recall of a rotavirus vaccine as a result of an unforeseen adverse reaction, and the recognition that mutated oral poliovirus vaccine strains can cause not only sporadic cases of paralytic disease but also epidemics.

And what shall we say about bioterrorism? On the one hand, the terrorist attacks brought vaccines to the center of attention and reversed a tendency in the lay public to think that infectious diseases were no longer important. On the other hand, the concept that eradication of an infectious agent leads to cessation of the need for vaccines against that agent may have received a fatal blow when it was realized that, absent vaccination, many organisms become potential weapons.

Overall, the recent past has seen a growing focus on vaccine safety. Given that vaccines are administered to almost all healthy children and adults in many countries, rare but serious illnesses that would have occurred anyway will coincidentally follow vaccination. Some will link these events as cause and effect and will argue that the causal link must be accepted unless there is strong contrary evidence. This puts a substantial burden on the vaccine community, rather than on those making the accusation, to gather evidence. Accumulation of evidence takes time and, even when accumulated, the evidence may never be sufficient to convince vaccine critics. The legacy of unfounded skepticism can be low vaccine coverage and a return to epidemic disease. Nevertheless, the goal must be to acquire valid scientific data that are acceptable to the vast majority of the public. Most well-conducted scientific studies have not supported the idea that vaccines cause rare serious adverse events. For example, several large case-control studies provided evidence against a causal association of multiple sclerosis with hepatitis B vaccination, and a large body of virologic and epidemiologic information counters the association of autism with measles, mumps, rubella (MMR) vaccination. Thus it is essential to deal with concerns about vaccine safety—openly, explicitly, and scientifically—performing research as appropriate and putting vaccine risks and benefits into proper perspective.

However, the greater problem in the 21st century will be the provision of modern vaccines to the large parts of the world desperately in need of them. Even if, by the waving of some magical wand, all countries could afford to obtain vaccines for their people, there would be an insufficient supply. The number of vaccine manufacturers worldwide is limited, and many are parts of large pharmaceutical firms. Vaccine divisions must compete with the larger drug divisions to obtain resources to continue to produce vaccines and to develop new ones. Recent disruptions in the U.S. vaccine supply indicate its fragility and demonstrate the need to assure that vaccine producers have incentives to enter and remain in markets, to continue production of older needed vaccines, and to assure adequate investments in upgrading plants to meet "state of the art" requirements for Good Manufacturing Practices. Modern vaccines are costly to develop and to make, and the idea that they should cost pennies is not only wrong, but also counterproductive to their availability. To bring new and better vaccines to market to address more infectious disease burdens, there must be adequate financial rewards to vaccine producers. Yet people at all economic levels are demanding the protection afforded by vaccination. A financing system is needed, worldwide, to assure access to vaccines for all persons, rich or poor, while also assuring continued manufacturer participation in vaccine production.

Thus all of us—vaccine developers, producers, public health practitioners, and government officials—have our work cut out: to make sure that every person in the world who needs a vaccine receives it. Although this is a daunting task, we should take it up with joy, as the result will be diminished human misery.

Stanley A. Plotkin
Walter A. Orenstein

Contents

VACCINES FOR SPECIAL CIRCUMSTANCES

SELECTED VACCINES OF THE FUTURE

Chapter 1

A Short History of Vaccination

SUSAN L. PLOTKIN • STANLEY A. PLOTKIN

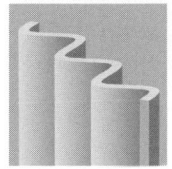

Vaccination as a deliberate attempt to protect humans against disease has a long history, although only in the 20th century did the practice flower into the routine vaccination of large populations. During the past 200 years, since the time of Edward Jenner (Fig. 1–1), vaccination has controlled the following 10 major diseases, at least in parts of the world: smallpox, diphtheria, tetanus, yellow fever, pertussis, *Haemophilus influenzae* type b disease, poliomyelitis, measles, mumps, and rubella. In the case of smallpox, the dream of eradication has been fulfilled, because this disease—at least naturally occurring disease—has disappeared from the world.[1] Poliomyelitis is targeted by the World Health Organization for eradication by the year 2005. Vaccinations against influenza, hepatitis A, hepatitis B, varicella, pneumococcal and meningococcal infections have made major headway against those diseases, although much remains to be done.

The impact of vaccination on the health of the world's peoples is hard to exaggerate. With the exception of safe water, no other modality, not even antibiotics, has had such a major effect on mortality reduction and population growth.

Early Developments

Attempts to vaccinate did not begin with Edward Jenner. In the seventh century, some Indian Buddhists drank snake venom in an attempt to become immune to its effect. They may have been inducing toxoid-like immunity.[2] Writings citing the use of inoculation and variolation in 10th-century China[3–5] make interesting reading but apparently cannot be verified.[6] There is, however, 18th-century documentation of variolation in China with reference to its use in the late 17th century. A Chinese medical text printed in 1742, *The Golden Mirror of Medicine*, listed four forms of inoculation against smallpox practiced in China at least since 1695: (1) the nose plugged with powdered scabs laid on cotton wool, (2) powdered scabs blown into the nose, (3) the undergarments of an infected child put on a healthy child for several days, and (4) a piece of cotton smeared with the contents of a vesicle and stuffed into the nose.[3,6] Another text on Chinese medicine, published a century before Jenner's work, stated that white cow fleas were used for smallpox prevention.[4] The fleas were ground into powder and made into pills, which may have been the first attempt at an oral vaccine.

Variolation, the introduction of dried pus from smallpox pustules into the skin of the patient, was practiced at regular intervals by the Brahmin caste of Hindus in India in the 16th century. Some claim that a description of variolation can be found in the *Atharva Veda* (a pre-Hindu Indian religious text circa 1000 BC), but this is probably exaggerated enthusiasm.[7] Vaccination for smallpox with cowpox did not

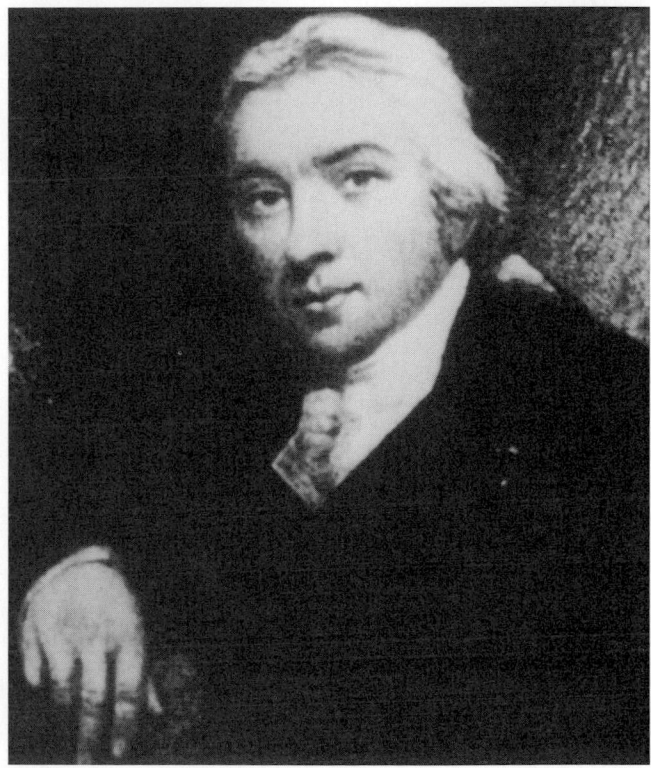

FIGURE 1–1 ▪ Edward Jenner. (Photo courtesy of the Institute of the History of Medicine, The Johns Hopkins University, Baltimore, MD.)

begin to be used in India until after Jenner's discovery, although, when "vaccination" arrived in India, attempts were made to alter some Indian religious documents to make it appear to be an earlier Indian practice.[7]

Similarly, in the mid-18th century, several treatises were written on inoculation against measles, and the Scottish physician Francis Home actively inoculated humans against measles and published the results of his work.[8-10]

Variolation was introduced into England by Lady Mary Wortley Montagu in 1721, when she returned from Constantinople, where she had observed Muslims use the technique. Although the treatment was often effective, results were erratic, and 2% to 3% of those treated died of smallpox contracted from the variolation itself.[11] Indeed, despite the risk, George Washington insisted that new recruits to the Continental Army undergo inoculation against smallpox, to which the Americans were highly susceptible, whereas the great majority of their English enemies were immune from early childhood exposure.[12] Voltaire lauded the inoculation of Circassian women in his "Persian Letters." Thus, although the precise origin of variolation remains unknown, it appears to have developed somewhere in Central Asia in the early part of the second millennium and then spread east to China and west to Turkey and Europe. In 1774 in Yetminster, England (Dorset County), a cattle breeder named Benjamin Jesty, himself immune to smallpox after contracting cowpox from his herd, deliberately inoculated his wife and two children with cowpox to avoid a smallpox epidemic. His experiment succeeded; the two children remained immune even 15 years later, when they were deliberately inoculated with smallpox.[11]

Despite these antecedents, Edward Jenner's work with cowpox vaccination holds title to the first scientific attempt to control an infectious disease by means other than transmitting the disease.[13]

Cowpox was not a widespread infection. It appeared sporadically in certain rural counties of England. Thus the local wisdom that those who contracted cowpox "did not take the smallpox" was not widely known. Jenner took this village folklore and experimented with it. Eventually, he proved that cowpox could be passed directly from one infected person to another, thereby providing "large-scale" inoculation without depending on the sporadic outbreaks of natural cowpox. When Jenner published his work *Variolae Vaccinae* in 1798, he brought to the attention of the entire medical community the merits of inoculation with the relatively obscure animal disease cowpox to prevent one of humankind's deadliest scourges. Years after his own successful experiments had been published and his reputation secured, Jenner acknowledged Jesty's early work.

During the 87 years that elapsed between Jenner's *Variolae Vaccinae* treatise and Louis Pasteur's (Fig. 1–2) first human vaccination against rabies (1885), the ideas of attenuation and virulence were developing, and the necessity of revaccination was discussed.[14] By 1810, Jenner realized that immunity against smallpox was not lifelong, but he did not know why.[11] The concept of *passages* of the immunizing agent (transmission from one human or animal to another) was well formed. In 1836, Edward Ballard discussed the problems of choosing new strains of cowpox for

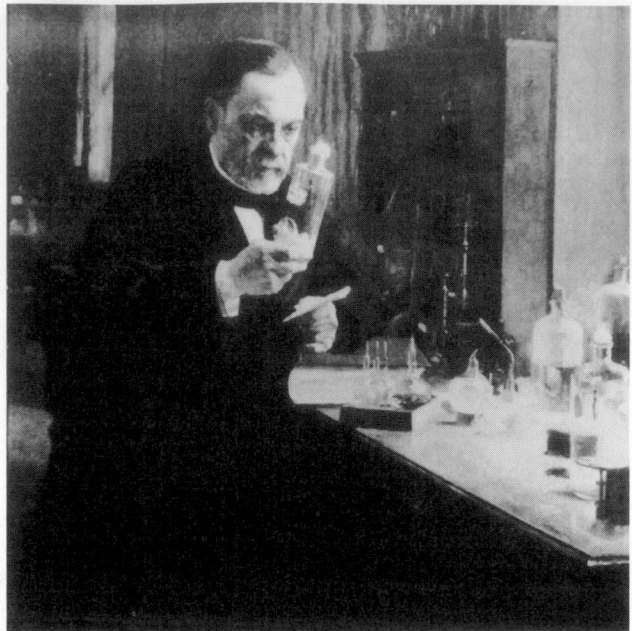

FIGURE 1–2 ■ Louis Pasteur. (Photo courtesy of the Pasteur Institute, Paris.)

vaccination because the old strains were too weak from so many passages. He recommended that the lymph (vesicle fluid) be passed back through a calf to regain strength.[15]

The "lymph" obtained from the cow soon came under scrutiny.[16] Concern had long been expressed that other diseases, such as syphilis, were occasionally transmitted along with the vaccinia virus. Around 1850, German scientists began to use glycerin to kill bacteria and also to preserve the lymph.[17] That process made possible a ready supply of a stable vaccine of consistent potency.[11]

Pasteur's work on the attenuation of the chicken cholera bacterium in the late 1870s was the first major advance after Jenner's *Variolae Vaccinae*. Pasteur drew on concepts that had been developing for at least 40 years: attenuation; modification through passage; renewed virulence; and, most important, the need to replace person-to-person (or animal-to-animal) vaccination with something safer, more consistent, and less likely to transmit other diseases.

In the summer of 1879, Pasteur left a chicken cholera culture (*Pasteurella multocida*), exposed to air over a long holiday. On his return, he noticed that the culture, weakened by exposure to air, provided immunity against a challenge with virulent organisms. He was quick to perceive that the principle was the same as Jenner's (i.e., using a weakened form of a microbe to provide immunity), although attenuation had been achieved in a different manner.[17] Pasteur thought it might be preferable to use a weakened form of chicken cholera itself to prevent the disease, rather than a related organism as in Jenner's use of vaccinia to prevent smallpox. A weakened form would be less likely to transmit other diseases. Publication of his results to the Academy of Sciences in 1880 generated considerable interest.[18] Pasteur's chicken cholera vaccine harkened back to Lady Montagu's variolation technique, which had used a weakened form of smallpox to inoculate against smallpox. Therefore, the modern concept of vaccination, involving the development of vaccines in the laboratory and using the same agent that caused the disease, was really introduced with Pasteur's chicken cholera vaccine, 5 years before the famous vaccination of Joseph Meister against rabies.

Pasteur's research on anthrax began in 1877 and overlapped with his work on chicken cholera. In 1876, Robert Koch had demonstrated the anthrax bacillus and described its capability to survive indefinitely in the form of spores.[19] Although Casimir Davaine had seen the bacillus in 1850, and had even postulated it as the cause of anthrax,[20,21] Koch was the first to obtain pure cultures of anthrax bacillus. He transmitted it to several laboratory animals and proved that there was a causal relationship between this bacillus and the disease anthrax.

Pasteur was aware of Davaine's and Koch's work, as well as that of a veterinarian named Henri Toussaint.[22] Indeed, he was in a neck-and-neck competition with Toussaint to find an anthrax vaccine. The first public controlled experiment of anthrax vaccination took place at Pouilly-le-Fort on May 5, 1881.[23] It was initiated by Pasteur in an effort to silence his many critics, who doubted that vaccination could be done systematically. Pasteur inoculated 24 sheep, one goat, and six cows with attenuated anthrax bacilli. On May 17, these same animals were inoculated again with more virulent but still attenuated anthrax bacilli. At the same time, 24 sheep, one goat, and four cows were kept as controls and given no inoculations. On May 31, both groups were inoculated with virulent anthrax, from spores that Pasteur had kept in his laboratory since 1877.

By June 2, 21 of the nonvaccinated sheep and the nonvaccinated goat were dead. Two more nonvaccinated sheep died before the spectators' eyes, and the last one succumbed before the day's end. All the vaccinated sheep, the vaccinated goat, and the six cows remained healthy. (The nonvaccinated cows did not die but showed clear evidence of having contracted anthrax. Their size perhaps had saved them.) At the end of this experiment, the triumphant Pasteur wrote that he had shown that humans could now have vaccines, cultivatable at will by a method that could be generalized.

It has since been documented that Pasteur's results with chicken cholera and anthrax were not as clear cut as was previously thought. It appears that Pasteur deliberately withheld critical data in his communications to the Academie de Medicine.[24-26] However, this in no way detracts from the significance of his findings, which proved that one could "create" standardized, reproducible vaccines at will. Pasteur's experiments with chicken cholera and anthrax[23] announced to the world that a new, scientific era in vaccination had begun.

By the time the rabies vaccine was first administered to humans in 1885,[27] the general public as well as the scientific community was well aware of the "new vaccination," but only in relation to animals. When Joseph Meister and Jean Baptiste Jupille were vaccinated against rabies, there was a vociferous outcry. The thought of deliberately introducing a deadly agent—in any form—into a human being was met with horror and outrage. The concept of attenuation did not appease the general public or many in the medical community; those cases of rabies that occurred in vaccinees were attributed to the vaccine and were viewed as medical murders. Even Émile Roux, one of Pasteur's staunchest allies and a collaborator in the rabies experiments, was appalled at the vaccination of Joseph Meister,

which he thought was unjustified by the experiments conducted up to that point. An examination of Pasteur's laboratory notebooks indicates that Roux was right to object.[25] These same notebooks also tell us that, before vaccinating Joseph Meister, Pasteur had vaccinated two other people who had little chance of survival after having been seriously bitten by rabid animals. One of the two had died.[25] Roux, although he was a physician, did not give the injections to Joseph Meister. He left Pasteur's laboratory in protest and did not return for many months.[25,28] The fact that hundreds of people were saved from rabies—many more than those who allegedly died from vaccination—did not lessen the opposition to rabies vaccination in humans. After all, 45 years earlier, variolation had been made a felony in England because it introduced the actual virus into human beings.[11]

The next major step in vaccine development took place in the United States shortly after Pasteur's administration of the chemically attenuated rabies vaccine. It involved a new concept that was equally important: killed vaccines. In 1886, Daniel Elmer Salmon and Theobald Smith (Fig. 1–3) published their work on a killed hog cholera "virus" vaccine.[29,30] The virus, killed by heat, immunized pigeons against the disease. The vaccine that they developed was actually a bacterial vaccine against a cholera-like salmonellosis,[31] but the term *virus* in the latter half of the 19th century did not have the specific meaning it has today. These events show that the ideas of live and killed vaccines developed almost simultaneously. The seminal work of Salmon and Smith bore fruit for humans 15 years later, when killed vaccines were developed for typhoid, cholera, and plague.

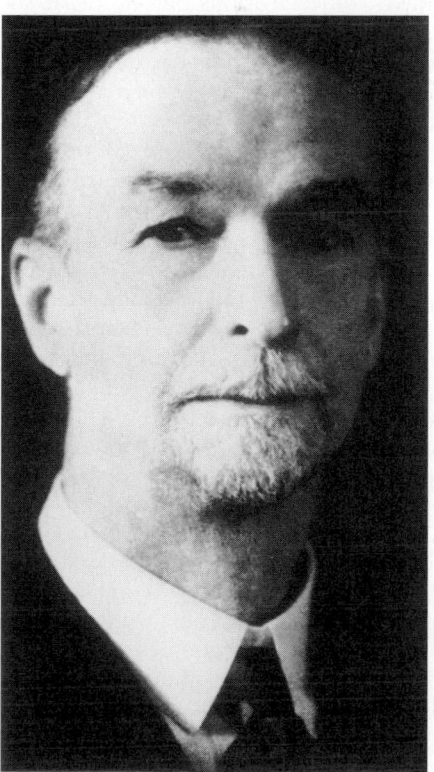

FIGURE 1–3 ■ Theobald Smith. (From Cohen B [ed]. Chronicles of the Society of American Bacteriologists, 1899–1950. Washington, D.C. American Society for Microbiology, 1950, p 36, with permission.)

In 1888, Salmon read a paper to the American Association for the Advancement of Science defending their (Salmon and Smith's) priority in developing the first killed vaccine.[32] Ironically, their competitors were Charles Chamberland and Roux from Pasteur's laboratory, who had published on the same topic in December 1887,[33] 16 months after Salmon and Smith's original paper. The Institut Pasteur had just been established in 1887; Pasteur was at the height of his fame and worldwide prestige. Not surprisingly, Salmon and Smith, who were working for the U.S. Department of Agriculture at the time of their discovery, saw their claim lost in the aura surrounding Pasteur and his associates. Thus, even 100 years ago, the Institut Pasteur and the U.S. government were involved in disputations over discovery rights—similar to the late 20th-century controversy over the discovery of the human immunodeficiency virus.

In parallel with the focused research on vaccines, important work on immunity was also being pursued at the end of the 19th century. Elie Metchnikoff, another Pasteur protégé, first published his theory of cellular immunity in 1884.[11,34] He named those body cells that ingested and destroyed invading microorganisms and other foreign bodies phagocytes. Although he did not appreciate the role of serum and plasma in immunity at this early date, his work was truly pioneering, and for this he shared the Nobel Prize with Paul Ehrlich in 1908 for research in immunity.

Ehrlich's receptor theory of immunity was an equally strong contribution to vaccine development. When he developed this theory in 1897, it was used mainly to explain toxin-antitoxin interactions. However, as the theory gradually expanded to meet various objections, it soon became one of the cornerstones of 20th-century immunology.[35] Ehrlich's other major contribution during this period was to point out the difference between active and passive immunity.[11,36]

At the end of the 19th century, we begin to see the practical results of the creative period of the 1870s and 1880s in the development of killed vaccines for typhoid, plague, and cholera. Richard Pfeiffer and Wilhelm Kolle in Germany and Almroth Wright in England worked independently on killed typhoid vaccines.[37–40] To this day, the debate continues as to exactly who inoculated the first human with killed typhoid vaccine. In truth, all three individuals deserve credit, because it is now clear that several groups were working on typhoid vaccine at that time.[41]

Shibasaburo Kitasato and Alexandre Yersin, each working independently, in 1894 discovered the causative bacillus of the plague, Pasteurella pestis.[11,42,43] With Albert Calmette and Amédée Borelle, Yersin went on to develop a killed vaccine for animals,[44] but it was Waldemar Haffkine who was given the task of developing a vaccine against human plague.[45,46] He was in India working on cholera vaccine, but, when bubonic plague developed in Bombay, he switched to studies of plague immunization. Haffkine was the first to be injected with his new killed plague vaccine. More than 8000 people were then vaccinated within a few weeks. For a while, Haffkine was considered a hero. However, subsequent evaluation of the vaccine by the Indian Plague Commission and the Mulkowal incident of 1902, when 19 people died from contaminated vaccine, resulted in the removal of Haffkine from his post by the Indian government. His scientific career and reputation were severely damaged; he never fully recovered from the incident and retired early from science at age 55 years. Later, with the wisdom of hindsight, the Indian government renamed the Plague Research Laboratory where he had worked as The Haffkine Institute. Perhaps as important as his development of the plague vaccine was Haffkine's contribution to the literature on the proper way to conduct clinical trials.[47]

John Snow had shown from 1848 to 1849 that cholera was transmitted by contaminated water,[48] although he did not know the identity of the contaminant. That answer was supplied by Robert Koch, when he isolated Vibrio cholerae as the causal organism in 1883.[49] Early attempts at a vaccine were made by Jaime Ferrán, a pupil of Pasteur, and by Haffkine. Both used live cultures, and both vaccines were given up because of severe reactions.[11] Kolle developed a heat-killed cholera vaccine in 1896.[50,51] He grew the vibrios in agar, suspended them in saline solution, heated them at 50°C for a few minutes (later changed to 56°C for 1 hour), and then added 0.5% phenol.

Thus, at the very beginning of the 20th century, there were two human virus vaccines: Jenner's original variola vaccine and Pasteur's rabies vaccine (both live). Three human bacterial vaccines also existed, for typhoid, cholera, and plague (all killed). The 19th century's end also saw the end of the use of arm-to-arm lymph inoculation as a vehicle for smallpox vaccine. This technique was replaced by glycerinated calf lymph in 1898.[11] The majority of the fundamental concepts of vaccinology had been introduced by the end of the 19th century; the work of the early 20th century would bring refinements to these theoretical underpinnings. Not until the advent of cell culture would the field again become so dramatically fertile (Table 1–1).

Early 20th Century

After the introduction of typhoid vaccines, Almroth Wright proceeded with a field trial among 4000 volunteers from the Indian Army that gave encouraging results. He proposed mass immunization of British troops during the Boer War (1899), but, because of opposition by influential people, he was able to vaccinate only 14,000 volunteers. In fact, opposition ran so high that consignments of vaccine were dumped overboard from transport ships in Southampton. The result was catastrophic: more than 58,000 cases of typhoid and 9000 deaths in the British Army.[38] A bitter battle over the merits of the vaccine took place in the British Medical Journal between Wright and the statistician Karl Pearson. The scientific community itself was divided on the value of vaccination; one could expect no more from the general public. Ultimately, the War Board initiated a broad-based trial that showed the overwhelming effectiveness of the vaccine. Wright was then knighted. By the time World War I broke out, general vaccination was conducted in the British Army, although it was still not mandatory.[38,52]

Roux and Yersin had demonstrated in 1888 that the diphtheria bacillus produced a powerful toxin.[11,53] Two years later, Emil von Behring and Kitasato, following up on preliminary work by Karl Fraenkel, published results that

TABLE 1–1 ▪ Outline of the Development of Human Vaccines

Live, Attenuated	Killed Whole Organism	Protein or Polysaccharide	Genetically Engineered
18TH CENTURY			
Smallpox (1798)			
19TH CENTURY			
Rabies (1885)	Typhoid (1896) Cholera (1896) Plague (1897)		
EARLY 20TH CENTURY			
Tuberculosis (1927) (Bacille Calmette-Guérin) Yellow fever (1935)	Pertussis (1926) (whole cell) Influenza (1936) Rickettsia (1938) (typhus)	Diphtheria (1923)[*] Tetanus (1927)[*]	
AFTER WORLD WAR II			
Polio (oral) Measles Mumps	Polio (injected) Rabies (cell culture) Japanese encephalitis	Pneumococcus[†] Meningococcus[†] *Haemophilus influenzae* PRP[†]	Hepatitis B recombinant (yeast or mamallian cell derived) Acellular pertussis (some components)
Rubella Adenovirus Typhoid (salmonella Ty21a) Varicella Rotavirus (reassortants) Cold-Adapted Influenza (CAIV)	Tick-borne encephalitis Hepatitis A Cholera	Pneumococcal conjugate[‡] Meningococcal conjugate[‡] *H. influenzae* PRP-conjugate[‡] Hepatitis B (plasma derived)[*] Typhoid (Vi)[†] Acellular pertussis[*] Anthrax[§]	Lyme (*Escherichia coli* recombinant)

[*]Purified proteins.
[§]Extracted proteins from whole organisms.
[†]Capsular polysaccharides.
[‡]Capsular polysaccharides conjugated to carrier proteins.
PRP, polyribosylribitol phosphate.

showed the presence of powerful antitoxins in the serum of animals previously infected with low doses of diphtheria bacilli.[54,55] The antitoxin neutralized diphtheria toxin in culture. Further experiments showed that the antitoxin provided protection in animals against challenge with the diphtheria bacillus itself. Progress occurred so rapidly after von Behring's discovery that the first child was treated with diphtheria antitoxin just 1 year later, in December 1891. Shortly thereafter, commercial production of diphtheria antitoxin began.

In the early 20th century, the chemical inactivation of diphtheria and other bacterial toxins led to the development of the first toxoids: diphtheria and tetanus. Here also Theobald Smith played a significant role. In 1907, he determined that "toxoids" provided immunity in guinea pigs. In 1909, reporting on long-lasting immunity against diphtheria in guinea pigs immunized with toxoid, he suggested that the method of making toxoids "invites further regard to its ultimate applicability to the human body."[31,56]

In 1923, Alexander Glenny and Barbara Hopkins showed that diphtheria toxin could be transformed into a toxoid by formalin.[57] The discovery came about when the containers in which the batches of diphtheria toxin were kept were cleaned with formalin (they were too large to be autoclaved). The residual formalin in the vats rendered the batch of toxin so weak that 1000 times the normal dose did

not kill the guinea pigs. Although using this "toxoid" was certainly safer than using toxin, it could be administered only in conjunction with antitoxin. In that same year, Gaston Ramon developed a diphtheria toxoid that could be used on its own (i.e., without antitoxin) by adding formalin and incubating the mixture at 37°C for several weeks.[58]

Ramon and Christian Zoeller went on to use a tetanus toxoid developed in the same manner for the first human vaccinations against tetanus in 1926.[59,60]

The vaccine against tuberculosis, Bacille Calmette-Guérin (BCG), was the first live vaccine for humans to be produced since Pasteur's rabies vaccine in 1885. Albert Calmette was a Pasteur protégé and founder of the Pasteur Institutes at Lille and in Indochina.[11] In 1906, Calmette and Camille Guérin started subculturing a strain of mycobacteria obtained from a bovine, which they perhaps thought was the tubercle bacillus. After 13 years of attenuation by 230 passages in beef bile, this strain eventually became the BCG strain. Clinical trials in children began in 1921, and the vaccine became available for human use in 1927.[11,61–65]

In 1931, E. W. Goodpasture introduced the use of the chorioallantoic membrane of the fertile hen's egg as a medium for growing viruses.[28,66] This technique represented a major advance, because until then human viruses could be grown only in animals such as ferrets and mice. Ferrets were very expensive, and mouse brain could produce allergic brain encephalitis. The chick embryo proved to be a cheaper and safer medium for the cultivation of viruses. S. Monkton Copeman had made an earlier attempt to use hens' eggs to grow a virus. In the Milroy Lectures for 1898, he mentioned conducting such an experiment while studying the relationship between vaccinia and variola, but he had little success at that time.[67]

Yellow fever virus was isolated in 1927 by two independent groups: researchers at the Rockefeller Foundation working in Nigeria, who isolated the Asibi strain,[68–70] and those at the Pasteur Institute in Senegal, who isolated the French strain.[71,72]

The French strain was given to various research groups for study.[72] In 1928, A. W. Sellards at the Harvard Medical School began collaborative research on the French strain with Jean Laigret at the Pasteur Institute in Senegal. Max Theiler, working for Sellards, developed an animal model to study the virus.[73] Using mouse brain tissue as a medium, others were able to "fix" the neurovirulence of the strain,[74] which then was used as a vaccine. Theiler left Harvard after this work to join the Rockefeller Institute. The French strain yellow fever vaccine that resulted from Theiler's work at Harvard was a live vaccine derived from mouse brain passage.[75] It was used first in humans without immune serum by Sellards and Laigret in 1932.[76] However, owing to the strain's passage through mouse brain tissue, the neurovirulence of the French strain presented grave dangers.

The Rockefeller group attempted to develop a more attenuated vaccine, using the Asibi strain. Theiler then developed the 17D strain from Asibi in fertile hen's egg membrane per Goodpasture's method. Although not as potent as the French strain, the 17D strain was much safer.[28,72,77–79] The French strain certainly saved many lives, especially in French West Africa, where it was used extensively. It remained in production (in modified form) until 1982; however, safety concerns about the use of mouse brain tissue overrode its proven efficacy, and 17D won out as the vaccine strain of choice.[72]

Wilson Smith, Christopher Andrewes, and Patrick Laidlaw isolated influenza A virus in ferrets in 1933.[80] Frank Horsfall, Alice Chenoweth, and colleagues developed a live virus vaccine in mouse lung tissue in 1936.[81,82] Chenoweth claimed that it became inactivated or nonreplicating when it was administered parenterally.[82,83] That same year, 1936, saw the development of two influenza A vaccines in embryonated eggs, one (live) by Wilson Smith[84] and the other (killed) by Thomas Francis and Thomas Magill.[85,86] Even though these two vaccines were considered safer because they were developed in embryonated eggs, Chenoweth's mouse lung vaccine had a higher virus yield and was the first to demonstrate true protection in humans, albeit transient.

In 1937, Anatol Smorodintsev and colleagues in the Soviet Union reported on the administration of the Wilson Smith strain to humans, using dosages that were lethal when given to mice.[87] This vaccine is considered to be the first live human influenza virus vaccine, and, although it would not receive a passing grade by today's standards (20% of vaccinees developed febrile influenza), it absolutely demonstrated the role of the virus in the development of influenza.[83,88]

Once rickettsiae were discovered by Charles Nicolle in 1909 to be the cause of typhus, many attempts were made to develop vaccines against these organisms.[11] The first truly successful vaccine was developed in 1938 by Herald Cox,[89] who used the yolk sac of the chick embryo to grow *Rickettsia rickettsii*. Although Cox worked on Rocky Mountain spotted fever, once he found a method to cultivate the rickettsia, killed vaccines for typhus and Q fever quickly followed. There was a heavy demand for the typhus vaccine during World War II.[11,90,91]

Jules Bordet and Octave Gengou first observed the causal agent of pertussis in 1900 and cultivated it by 1907.[11] The production and testing of several vaccines were attempted without formal trials. Thorvald Madsen later carried out the first controlled clinical trials of a pertussis vaccine (i.e., whole killed organisms) on the Faeroe Islands from 1923 to 1924 and again in 1929.[92,93] During the 1923 to 1924 epidemic, Madsen reported that the vaccine did not prevent disease but greatly reduced mortality and the severity of illness among vaccinated individuals. By the 1929 epidemic, the vaccine had been considerably improved.[94] Several whole-cell pertussis vaccines were in use by the late 1940s.[95,96]

After World War II

The golden age of vaccine development began in 1949 with virus propagation in stationary cell culture. Goodpasture's method using chick embryo membrane was successful, but most searches for improved techniques centered around the flask culture technique of Maitland and Maitland.[11,31] They grew vaccinia virus in sterile cultures of minced chicken kidney in media composed of chicken serum and mineral salts. George Gey improved the virus yield of this method by continually rolling the tubes and thus increasing the oxygenation of the cells.[31]

John Enders, Thomas Weller, and Fred Robbins took up research on cell culture at Boston Children's Hospital in the late 1940s. After using cultures of the Maitland type, they decided to try to grow viruses in human cells using fibroblasts grown from the skin and muscle tissue of infants who had died soon after birth. Their first success was to grow Lansing type II poliovirus in human cell culture.[97] The ability to grow human viruses outside a living host, in a relatively easy and safe manner, led to an explosion of creativity in vaccinology that continues unabated (see Table 1–1).

Live Virus Vaccines

The first live polio vaccine, developed with a variant virus strain grown in mice, was tested in humans in 1950 by Hilary Koprowski.[98] The first licensed product developed using the cell culture technique of Enders, Weller, and Robbins was the trivalent, formalin-inactivated polio vaccine of Jonas Salk, licensed in 1955.[99] About 6 years later, live poliovirus vaccines grown in monkey kidney cell culture by Albert Sabin came into wide use.[100] Thanks to the use of these vaccines, polio has been eradicated from the Western Hemisphere, and the World Health Organization has targeted the year 2005 to efface the disease from the entire world.

During the late 1950s, Samuel Katz, Enders, and colleagues developed the Edmonston strain of measles vaccine, grown in chick embryo cell culture,[101] which was attenuated further by Anton Schwarz[102] and Maurice Hilleman and colleagues.[103] Hilleman also attenuated the Jeryl Lynn strain of mumps virus in the hen's egg and obtained licensure in 1967.[104] Passage in cell culture was used to attenuate rubella virus, and by 1970 several strains had been developed by Harry Meyer and Paul Parkman[105]; Abel Prinzie, Constant Huygelen, and colleagues[106]; and Stanley Plotkin.[107] The last strain (Wistar-RA27/3), grown in human fibroblasts, is now the sole rubella vaccine in wide use.

The adenoviruses remained unidentified until the second half of the 20th century, when the virus was recovered from adenoids that had been surgically removed.[108] The group of viruses was subsequently named "adenoviruses" by a committee headed by Enders.[109] Formalin-inactivated whole-virus vaccines were made against types 4 and 7 and were licensed for military use. In the early 1960s, the adenovirus seed stock was discovered to be contaminated with simian virus 40 (SV40),[110] and, when attempts to eliminate SV40 failed, the vaccine was withdrawn in 1963.[111]

Attenuated live adenovirus vaccine studies continued, using HEK cells, and subsequently human diploid cell strains, thus eliminating the SV40 problem. An enteric-coated vaccine tablet was produced for types 4, 7, and 21[112-116]; the vaccine received licensure, again only for use in the military. Wyeth was the sole producer of adenovirus vaccine; they ceased production in 1996, primarily because of regulatory issues and lack of interest by the military. Not unexpectedly, within a few years outbreaks of adenovirus respiratory diseases began to reoccur in military recruits. After several years of searching for another manufacturer, the U.S. Army signed a contract with a small vaccine company to produce adenovirus vaccine.

The live attenuated Oka strain of varicella vaccine was developed in the 1970s by Michiaki Takahashi[117,118] and underwent extensive clinical trials before being licensed in Japan and several European countries.[119,120] After a long and convoluted development, licensure was obtained in the United States in 1995.[121] It is now recommended for all healthy individuals older than 1 year, and coverage is increasing.[122] Studies are underway to determine if the vaccine will prevent or ameliorate zoster (shingles) in older adults.

Frank Burnet and D. R. Bull had shown in the 1940s that live, attenuated influenza virus could be produced in embryonated eggs but also that the virus mutated rapidly. Therefore, the vaccines that were produced were not consistently attenuated and often produced disease.[123,124] By the 1960s, a live vaccine that was safe for adults was obtained,[125,126] but it could not be used in children, who became febrile.[127] Work on live virus vaccine was interrupted in favor of the annually administered killed influenza vaccine, which has consistently proved to be safe and effective but with no lasting local or cellular immunity.

Newer vaccine design technologies in the 1990s, including reassortment, reverse genetics, and cold adaptation, have again made it possible to develop live, attenuated influenza vaccines that may confer long-term immunity and obviate the need for injections.

Three attenuated master strains were developed for live influenza vaccines: host-range (hr), temperature-sensitive (ts), and cold-adapted (ca) mutants. Only the cold-adapted influenza vaccine (CAIV) developed by Hunein Maassab has reached licensure.[128] Other strains were abandoned because of inconsistent attenuation, instability, and, occasionally, reversion to virulence.[129] Cold-adapted strains allow the vaccine virus to grow in the relative coolness of the subject's nasal passages (32°C) but not in warmer internal organs, particularly the lungs (37°C).[130] CAIV is administered by nasal spray and is a good example of the advantages of reassortant technology. Each year a new influenza vaccine can be made by reassorting the six internal genes from Maassab's master strains with the genes coding for the hemagglutinin and neuraminidase surface glycoproteins of circulating wild strains of influenza viruses.[129,131] The vaccine has been shown to be at least as effective as the killed vaccine and may offer longer and broader immunity.[129,132-136] It has the advantage of easy administration and may offer significant cross-protection against antigenically drifted wild strains.

An orally administered live rotavirus reassortant vaccine was licensed for use in the United States in September 1998.[137] The vaccine consisted of a mixture of type 3 monkey virus and reassortants derived from types 1, 2, and 4 of human rotavirus and 10 genes derived from the same monkey virus.[138,139] Within 10 months of licensure, cases of intussusception among vaccine recipients were reported to the Vaccine Adverse Event Reporting System.[140-142] The Advisory Committee on Immunization Practices determined that intussusception occurred with significantly increased frequency within the first 2 weeks after vaccination. The vaccine was formally withdrawn from the market in November 1999.[143]

A large literature of "post-mortem" analysis of what went wrong now exists, because rotavirus is a significant worldwide problem and a vaccine is desperately needed.[144-146] Fortunately, several other candidate rotavirus vaccines are in advanced human trials.

Live Bacterial Vaccine

Subsequent to the early work on killed typhoid vaccine, a variety of heat-phenol–killed or acetone-killed, parenteral typhoid vaccines became available.[147-150] All were subject to high rates of adverse reactions and were never considered quite satisfactory. An important advance was made by René Germanier and E. Fürer when they developed an attenuated strain of the Gal E mutant Ty21a of *Salmonella typhi*.[151] Based on the results from preliminary vaccine studies in a volunteer group in the United States,[152] large trials were conducted successfully in Egypt[153] and in Chile.[154,155] Protection rates varied; however, there were few adverse reactions, and oral formulation of this vaccine made it less expensive to produce and distribute.[156,157]

Whole Virus Vaccines

As mentioned above, the first whole-virus vaccine produced by the tissue culture revolution was the Salk inactivated polio vaccine.

The adaptation of rabies virus to human diploid cell culture permitted the development of a potent inactivated rabies vaccine by Koprowski, Tadeusz Wiktor, and associates.[158] Since then, many other cell culture rabies vaccines have been developed, including a vaccinia-recombinant rabies vaccine for veterinary use.[159]

The development of a Japanese encephalitis vaccine was attempted during World War II,[160] but the current vaccine, consisting of formalin-inactivated whole virus harvested from mouse brain, was developed in Japan in 1965.[161] It was put into use almost immediately to vaccinate Japanese children, although few data regarding its efficacy had been published.

After two Americans who had traveled in Asia died from Japanese encephalitis, the U.S. Department of Defense conducted a vaccine trial in northern Thailand,[162] which showed an efficacy of 91%. A bivalent live vaccine was developed using both the Nakayama-NIH strain (from the original vaccine) and the Beijing-1 strain, in order to provide immunity to strains from different geographical areas. Japanese encephalitis vaccine has been available for distribution in the United States and other countries since that trial.[162–164] X. Y. Yu and co-workers have developed an inactivated vaccine and a live, attenuated vaccine against Japanese encephalitis, each in primary hamster kidney cells.[165–169] Both of these vaccines are manufactured and available for use only in the People's Republic of China.

A vaccine against hepatitis A virus (HAV) remained elusive until relatively recently. In 1979, Paul Provost and Hilleman[170] were able to grow HAV in cell culture, thus opening the path for the development of a vaccine. Provost and co-workers developed the first inactivated HAV vaccine in 1986[171]; however, the cell culture used to produce the HAV antigen was not suitable for use in humans. Formaldehyde-inactivated, whole-virion HAV vaccines grown in human fibroblasts were later developed and licensed.[172,173]

The first killed tick-borne encephalitis (TBE) vaccine, produced in mouse brain, was developed in the Soviet Union in 1937, shortly after the virus had been identified and the tick vector verified.[174,175] In the 1960s, based on the work of R. Benda and L. Danes,[176,177] E. N. Levkovich in the Soviet Union[178] and C. Kunz in Austria[179] each used chick embryo cell culture to develop less reactogenic, formalin-inactivated vaccines. A subunit vaccine was developed by Heinz, Kunz, and Fauma in 1980[180] and appears to be effective against different isolates of the TBE virus that all share a homologous envelope glycoprotein.[181–183] Since the collapse of the Soviet Union and the opening of Eastern Europe, the geographical range of TBE has been shown to be large. A second inactivated TBE vaccine (Chiron Behring) was licensed in Germany in 1991.[184]

Vaccines Based on Bacterial Proteins, Polysaccharides, and Protein-Conjugated Polysaccharides

Whole-cell pertussis vaccine caused a number of adverse reactions. By 1975, after two Japanese infants were thought to have died because of pertussis vaccination, public rejection of the vaccine reached such proportions that the Japanese Ministry of Health suspended its use. An astronomical increase in the incidence of pertussis followed: 206 reported cases in 1971 grew to 13,105 cases by 1979.[185] This increase in turn led to the development of an acellular per-

tussis vaccine based on the isolated main protective antigens of *Bordetella pertussis*: toxin and filamentous hemagglutinin.[185–187] Other components contained in the vaccine may also be important. Acellular pertussis vaccines that are less reactogenic than whole-cell pertussis vaccine have been licensed for use in Japan since 1981 and were licensed in the United States in 1996 for children 2 months and older.[188]

Modern work on a human anthrax vaccine began in the second half of the 20th century. The vaccine, named Anthrax Vaccine Adsorbed (AVA), contains the extracted proteins from anthrax bacilli, in particular the protein called "Protective Antigen" that forms part of the toxin. These were obtained from sterile filtrates of an attenuated, unencapsulated, nonproteolytic strain of *Bacillus anthracis*.[189–191] A randomized field study on a similar anthrax vaccine developed by Merck took place from 1955 to 1959 at four mills that processed raw goat hair destined for the suit manufacturing industry.[192,193] Production was later transferred to the Michigan Biologic Products Institute, which in 1998 became BioPort. AVA was relicensed in 2002.

Human anthrax had not been viewed as a serious problem in the late 20th century. Worldwide there were fewer than 2000 cases annually, mostly cutaneous, in the 1980s and 1990s.[194] The bioterrorism in the fall of 2001, when highly refined anthrax spores were sent through the U.S. postal system, changed that perception. Much attention is now being given to assuring the availability and safety of the supply of anthrax vaccine for both the military and the general public.[195] Research has been accelerated to find a new-generation anthrax vaccine based on Protective Antigen that will require fewer injections to attain full immunity.

During the 1970s and 1980s, several bacterial vaccines consisting of purified capsular polysaccharides were developed. These included meningococcal group A and C vaccines, developed by Malcolm Artenstein,[196] Emil Gotschlich,[197] and associates. Meningococcal vaccines had been attempted in the 1940s but failed.[198] Modern work on humoral immunity to meningococcal disease got underway at the Walter Reed Hospital in 1966 and ultimately resulted in the development of capsular polysaccharide vaccines against meningococcal groups A and C.[196,197,199–201]

By the early 1970s, group C meningococcal polysaccharide vaccine was routinely administered to U.S. army recruits and had virtually eliminated the disease within the military.[198] However, the vaccine did not provide immunity to children younger than 2 years of age, and the duration of immunity was uncertain. Additional boosters resulted in reduced immune responses.[202,203]

The pneumococcal polysaccharide vaccine was developed by Robert Austrian and associates.[204] It took less than 20 years from the time pneumococcus was first isolated (in 1880, by Pasteur and George Sternberg simultaneously)[205,206] to discover the multiplicity of pneumococcal serotypes and thus appreciate the complexity of developing a vaccine against it. A killed, whole-cell pneumococcal vaccine was made by Almroth Wright in 1911 and tested in South African gold mine workers, but eventually the vaccine was abandoned.[207,208] By the late 1940s, extensive work on capsular polysaccharides resulted in a multivalent capsular polysaccharide pneumococcal vaccine (4-valent and later 6-valent).[209–211] However, antibiotics were so successful that the vaccine fell by the wayside.

Austrian and Jerome Gold pointed out the continued severity of pneumococcal disease despite the introduction of antibiotics.[212] A modern capsular polysaccharide pneumococcal vaccine was subsequently developed for adults by Austrian, initially with 14 antigens (in 1977) and later increased to 23 antigens (in 1983).[204,206]

The first-generation *H. influenzae* type b vaccine was developed by Porter Anderson,[213] Rachel Schneerson,[214] and associates. In the 1920s and 1930s, Margaret Pittman had determined that, of the six different polysaccharides of *H. influenzae*, organisms encapsulated with type b caused the largest proportion of serious disease in children. She identified the composition of the capsule as a polymer of ribosylribitol phosphate, now called polyribosylribitol phosphate (PRP).[215] In the 1970s, several teams began research and efficacy studies on an *H. influenzae* type b vaccine, primarily in Finland and North Carolina.[213,214,216–218] This work ultimately culminated in the 1985 licensure of the PRP vaccine.[219] However, the vaccine was not effective for children younger than 18 months—those most at risk for bacterial meningitis—and it had limited efficacy in older children. Vaccines against *H. influenzae* type b bacteria advanced rapidly to a second and third generation.

As Avery and Goebel had shown (in relation to pneumococcus) that the immunogenicity of a capsular polysaccharide could be increased by binding it to a carrier protein,[220,221] Schneerson and Robbins linked PRP to diphtheria toxoid and developed the first conjugate polysaccharide vaccine.[222] This vaccine had improved immunogenicity and efficacy and was licensed in 1987 for children older than 15 months. Younger children still remained at risk, but three more immunogenic conjugates soon followed, using nontoxic diphtheria toxoid (HbOC) derived from a mutant strain, an outer membrane protein of *Neisseria meningitidis* (PRP-OMP), or tetanus toxoid.[219,222]

Several group A and/or group C meningococcal conjugates were developed, conjugated to either a diphtheria or a tetanus toxoid; they provide longer-term immunity than the polysaccharide vaccine, as well as immunity to those younger than 2 years of age.[202,203,223–226] The group C conjugate was licensed in the United Kingdom in 1999 and immediately placed in the universal immunization schedule in November of that same year.[223] Despite extensive postlicensure studies,[203,224–226] the conjugate vaccine has not been licensed in the United States as of this writing.

Although the pneumococcal polysaccharide vaccine was effective in adults, it did not protect children younger than 2 years of age, among whom more than 80% of invasive pneumococcal disease occurs, so protein conjugation technology was applied to develop a vaccine that would protect this important group.[227] A heptavalent pneumococcal conjugate vaccine (conjugated to a nontoxic mutant of diphtheria) was produced by Wyeth Lederle, extensively tested by Steven Black and associates, and found to be safe, efficacious, and immunogenic in children younger than 2 years, those most at risk.[228,229] The vaccine was licensed in the United States in February 2000.[230,231] A 1-year postlicensure follow-up study by Black and associates demonstrated a dramatic reduction in age-specific invasive pneumococcal

disease incidence attributable to the use of the pneumococcal conjugate vaccine.[232]

A purified Vi polysaccharide component vaccine against typhoid was developed by J. Landy, M. E. Webster, and colleagues[233–235] and later improved on by K. H. Wong and associates[236] and John Robbins and J. B. Robbins.[237]

Recombinant Protein Vaccines

The discovery that the particles of hepatitis B surface antigen (HBsAg) found in infected people are immunogenic and protective but noninfectious[238–240] provided the basis for efforts to purify these particles from the blood of chronic carriers. Hilleman and colleagues succeeded in licensing a plasma-derived vaccine in the United States in 1981.[241] Although the vaccine was safe and effective,[242] the acquired immunodeficiency syndrome epidemic arrived at about the same time as licensure of the vaccine; products made from the derivatives of human blood came to be considered potentially dangerous. Despite rigorous safety testing and many inactivation processes to kill any foreign agent in the vaccine, the manufacturer could not overcome the reluctance of the public and physicians to use a product that had even a remote risk of containing the human immunodeficiency virus. Also, because the vaccine depended on human serum, sources of antigen were limited.

These obstacles prompted the formulation of the first recombinant vaccine, which was licensed in 1986. Development was accomplished by cloning the gene for HBsAg in yeast (*Saccharomyces cerevisiae*) and in mammalian cells. HBsAg was produced by the cells and then made into vaccine through adsorption on an alum adjuvant.[243–246] In yeast, the surface antigen aggregated into particles very similar to the extensively purified surface region antigen from the plasma-derived vaccine.[247] Initial trials and subsequent studies have shown the recombinant vaccine to be as effective as the plasma-derived vaccine.[245,248,249] In addition, because it is derived from a gene, it does not bear the stigma of possible contamination with undetected foreign agents.

Lyme disease was first recognized in the United States in 1975, and within a quarter century it became the most frequently diagnosed vector-borne disease in the country.[250–253] Named after the town of Lyme, Connecticut, where it was first isolated, it was referred to as "Lyme arthritis" until 1982, when, because there was a constellation of illnesses associated with the infection, the name was changed to Lyme disease.[254] The spirochete causing the disease in the United States was identified by Burgdorfer in 1982[255] and subsequently named *Borrelia burgdorferi*. Personal protection, spraying, and antibiotics[256–259] did not stem the rising tide of Lyme infection.

Two vaccine candidates were put into extensive clinical trials.[260–264] Each was based on a recombinant *Escherichia coli* strain containing the gene for outer surface protein (OspA) of the American Lyme strain.[251] The vaccine produced by GlaxoSmithKline was approved by the FDA in 1999 and recommended for use in persons ages 15 to 70 who lived or worked in endemic areas of infection.[253]

Despite the extensive clinical trials and postlicensure surveillance, the vaccine was not well accepted because of a tepid recommendation from the CDC, the alternative of antibiotic treatment after infection, and the need for booster doses. Equally important, a series of class action and individual lawsuits were brought against the manufacturer claiming that the vaccine causes chronic arthritis and other autoimmune problems, although the evidence for vaccine-induced arthritis is absent.[252] In April 2002, GlaxoSmith Kline withdrew the vaccine from the market because of lack of demand.

Bioterrorism and Vaccines

Both anthrax (see above) and smallpox, ancient scourges of mankind, have returned to the front pages after the terrorist attacks late in 2001.

The possible possession of smallpox virus by terrorists and the inability to account for all of Russia's cache of smallpox virus has led to the urgent production of a stockpile of the classic smallpox vaccine and the call for development of new vaccines. Thus the two goals of eradicating smallpox virus and eliminating vaccination with vaccinia virus may be frustrated at the last moment.

Aside from smallpox and anthrax, the threat of bioterrorism will lead to renewed research on vaccines against plague, tularemia, hemorrhagic fevers, and other pathogens.

Vaccines are needed more than ever before. The majority of vaccines now being developed use new technologies because they appear to offer greater safety (the ability to eliminate unwanted and often unknown contaminants). The focus is on subunit (purified protein or polysaccharide), genetically engineered, or vectored antigens because the target pathogens are intracellular and difficult to immunize against. However, older methods such as attenuation and inactivation continue to yield new vaccines.

The early 21st century may well mirror the 40 years after Pasteur's momentous and controversial rabies trial; public reaction will compel scientists to find ever more ingenious and secure ways to protect humans against disease. At the beginning of this chapter, the positive impact of vaccination on the health of the world's population was emphasized. During the 21st century, vaccines may take on the additional role of major defensive weapons. Even with all of the uncertainties, the new technologies guarantee that the golden age of vaccinology will turn to platinum.

REFERENCES

1. Global Commission for the Certification of Smallpox Eradication. The Achievement of the Global Eradication of Smallpox. Geneva, World Health Organization, 1979.
2. deBary WT (ed). The Buddhist Tradition in India, China and Japan. New York, Vintage Books, 1972.
3. Hume EH. The Chinese Way in Medicine. Baltimore, Johns Hopkins University Press, 1940.
4. Wong KC, Wu LT. History of Chinese Medicine. Tientsin, China, Tientsin Press, 1932.
5. Huard PA, Wong K. Chinese Medicine. New York, McGraw-Hill, 1968.
6. Leung AK. Variolation and vaccination in late imperial China, ca 1570–1911. In Plotkin SA, Fantini B (eds). Vaccinia, Vaccination, Vaccinology: Jenner, Pasteur, and Their Successors. Paris, Elsevier, 1996, pp 65–71.
7. Major RH. A History of Medicine. Springfield, IL, Charles C Thomas, 1954.
8. Huygelen C. The long prehistory of modern measles vaccination. In Plotkin SA, Fantini B (eds). Vaccinia, Vaccination, Vaccinology:
Jenner, Pasteur, and Their Successors. Paris, Elsevier, 1996, pp 257–263.
9. Plotkin SA. Vaccination against measles in the 18th century. Clin Pediatr (Phila) 6:312–315, 1967.
10. Enders JF. Francis Home and his experimental approach to medicine. Bull Hist Med 38:101–112, 1964.
11. Parish HJ. A History of Immunization. London, E & S Livingstone, 1965.
12. Fenn EA. Pox Americana: The Great Smallpox Epidemic of 1775–82. New York: Hill and Wang, 2001.
13. Jenner E. An Inquiry into the Causes and Effects of the Variolae Vaccinae. London, Low, 1798.
14. DuMesnil O. Nécessité de la révaccination des ouvriers venants prendre du travail à Paris. Ann Hyg Paris 3(suppl)1:444, 1879.
15. Ballard E. On Vaccination, Its Value and Alleged Dangers. London, Longmans, 1868.
16. Dudgeon JA. Development of smallpox vaccine in England in the eighteenth and nineteenth centuries. Br Med J 1:1367–1372, 1963.
17. Copeman SM. Vaccination, Its Natural History and Pathology. London, Macmillan, 1899.
18. Pasteur L. De l'atténuation du virus du choléra des poules. C R Acad Sci Paris 91:673–680, 1880.
19. Koch R. The aetiology of anthrax based on the ontogeny of the anthrax bacillus. Med Classics 2:787, 1937. (Original publication: Beitr Biol Pflanz 2:277, 1877.)
20. Davaine C. Researches into infusoria of the blood in the disease known as sang de rate. In Nicolle J (ed). Louis Pasteur: A Master of Scientific Enquiry. London, Hutchinson, 1961, pp 172–178.
21. Besredka A. Local Immunisation [Plotz H, English trans]. London, Ballière, 1927.
22. Toussaint H. Sur quelques points relatifs à l'immunité charbonneuse. C R Acad Sci Paris 93:163, 1881.
23. Pasteur L, Chamberland C-E, Roux E. Sur la vaccination charbonneuse. C R Acad Sci Paris 92:1378–1383, 1881.
24. Cadeddu A. Pasteur et le choléra des Poules: révision critique d'un récit historique. Hist Phil Life Sci 7:87–104, 1985.
25. Geison GL. The Private Science of Louis Pasteur. Princeton, NJ, Princeton University Press, 1995.
26. Cadeddu A. Pasteur et la vaccination contre le charbon: une analyse historique et critique. Hist Phil Life Sci 9:255–276, 1987.
27. Pasteur L. Méthode pour prévenir la rage après morsure. C R Acad Sci Paris 101:765–772, 1885.
28. Williams G. Virus Hunters. London, Hutchinson, 1960.
29. Salmon DE, Smith T. On a new method of producing immunity from contagious diseases. Am Vet Rev 10:63–69, 1886.
30. Salmon DE. The theory of immunity from contagious diseases. Proc Am Assoc Adv Sci 35:262–266, 1886.
31. Chase A. Magic Shots: A Human and Scientific Account of the Long and Continuing Struggle to Eradicate Infectious Diseases by Vaccination. New York, William Morrow & Co, 1982.
32. Salmon DE. Discovery of the production of immunity from contagious diseases by chemical substances formed during bacterial multiplication. Proc Am Assoc Adv Sci 37:275–280, 1888.
33. Roux E, Chamberland C-E. Immunité contre la septicémie conferée par des substances solubles. Ann Inst Pasteur Paris 1:561–572, 1887.
34. Metchnikoff E. Immunity in the Infective Diseases [English trans]. Cambridge, UK, Cambridge University Press, 1905.
35. Ehrlich P. Die Werthbemessung des diphtherie Heil-serum und deren theoretische Grundlagen. Klin Jahrb Jena 6:299–326, 1897.
36. Ehrlich P. On immunity with special reference to cell life. [From Proc R Soc, 1900.] In Himmelweit F (ed). The Collected Papers of Paul Ehrlich. Vol. 2. London, Pergamon Press, 1957, pp 178–195.
37. Kolle W, Hetsch H. Experimental Bacteriology [Eyre J (ed); Erikson D, trans 7th German ed]. London, Allen and Unwin, 1929.
38. Colebrook L. Almroth Wright: Provocative Doctor and Thinker. London, Heinemann, 1954.
39. Wright AE, Semple D. Remarks on vaccination against typhoid fever. Br Med J 1:256–259, 1897.
40. Pfeiffer R, Kolle W. Experimentelle Untersuchungen zur Frage der Schutzimpfung des Menschen gegen Typhus adbdominalis. Dtsch Med Wochenschr 22:735–737, 1896.
41. Sansonetti PJ. Vaccination against typhoid fever: a century of research. End of the beginning or beginning of the end? In Plotkin SA, Fantini B (eds). Vaccinia, Vaccination, Vaccinology: Jenner, Pasteur, and Their Successors. Paris, Elsevier, 1996, pp 115–120.

42. Kitasato S. The bacillus of bubonic plague. Lancet 2:428–430, 1894.

43. Yersin A. La peste bubonique à Hong Kong. Ann Inst Pasteur Paris 8:662–667, 1894.

44. Yersin A, Calmette A, Borrel A. La peste bubonique: deuxième note. Ann Inst Pasteur Paris 9:589–592, 1895.

45. Haffkine WM. Remarks on the plague prophylactic fluid. Br Med J 1:1461, 1897.

46. Haffkine WM. Protective inoculation against plague and cholera [editorial]. Br Med J 1:35–36, 1899.

47. Löwy I. Producing a trustworthy knowledge: early field trials of anticholera vaccines in India. In Plotkin SA, Fantini B (eds). Vaccinia, Vaccination, Vaccinology: Jenner, Pasteur, and Their Successors. Paris, Elsevier, 1996, pp 121–126.

48. Snow J. Snow on Cholera; Being a Reprint of Two Papers, Together with a Bibliographic Memoir by B. W. Richardson. New York, Commonwealth Fund, 1936.

49. Koch R. Der Seitens des Dr. Koch an den Staatssecretari des Innern Herrn Staatsminster von Boetticher Excellenz erstettete Bericht von Alexandrie, 17 September 1883. Dtsch Med Wochenschr 9:615, 743–744, 1883.

50. Kolle W. Zur aktiven Immunisierung der Menschen gegen Cholera. Zentralbl Bakteriol Abt Jena 19:97–104, 1896.

51. Kolle W. Die aktive Immunisierung der Menschen gegen Cholera, nach Haffkine's Verfahren in Indien ausgefuhrt. Zentralbl Bakteriol Abt Jena 19:217–221, 1896.

52. Fleming A, Petrie GF. Recent Advances in Vaccine and Serum Therapy. Philadelphia, Blakiston, 1934.

53. Roux E, Yersin A. Contribution à l'étude de la diphtérie. Ann Inst Pasteur Paris 2:629–661, 1888.

54. von Behring E, Kitasato S. Über das Zustandekommen der Diphtherie—Immunität und der Tetanus—Immunität bie Tieren. Dtsch Med Wochenschr 16:1113–1114, 1890.

55. von Behring E. Untersuchungen über das Zustandekommen der Diphtherie—Immunität bei Tieren. Dtsch Med Wochenschr 16:1145–1148, 1890.

56. Smith T. Degree and duration of passive immunity to diphtheria toxin transmitted by immunized female guinea-pigs to their immediate offspring. J Med Res 16:359–379, 1907.

57. Glenny AT, Hopkins BE. Diphtheria toxoid as an immunising agent. Br J Exp Pathol 4:283–288, 1923.

58. Ramon G. Sur le pouvoir floculant et sur les propriétés immunisantes d'une toxine diphtérique rendue anatoxique (anatoxine). C R Acad Sci Paris 177:1338–1340, 1923.

59. Ramon G, Zoeller C. De la valeur antigénique de l'anatoxine tétanique chez l'homme. C R Acad Sci Paris 182:245–247, 1926.

60. Ramon G, Zoeller C. L'anatoxine tétanique et l'immunisation active de l'homme vis-à-vis du tétanos. Ann Inst Pasteur Paris 41:803–833, 1927.

61. Calmette A, Guérin C. Origine intestinale de la tuberculose pulmonaire et mécanism de l'infection tuberculose: 2ème et 3ème memoires. Ann Inst Pasteur Paris 20:353–363, 609–624, 1906.

62. Calmette A, Guérin C, Breton M. Contribution à l'étude de la tuberculose expérimentale du cobaye (infection et essais de vaccination par la voie digestive). Ann Inst Pasteur Paris 21:401–416, 1907.

63. Calmette A, Guérin C. Contribution à l'étude de l'immunité antituberculose chez les bovidés. Ann Inst Pasteur Paris 28:329–337, 1914.

64. Calmette A. La Vaccination Préventive Contre la Tuberculose par le B.C.G. Paris, Masson, 1927.

65. Calmette A. L'Infection Bacillaire et la Tuberculose (4th ed). Paris, Masson, 1936.

66. Woodruff AM, Goodpasture EW. The susceptibility of the chorioallantoic membrane of chick embryos to infection with the fowl-pox virus. Am J Pathol 7:209–222, 1931.

67. Wilkinson L. The development of the virus concept as reflected in corpora of studies on individual pathogens. 5. Smallpox and the evolution of ideas on acute (viral) infections. Med Hist 23:1–28, 1979.

68. Warren AJ. Landmarks in the conquest of yellow fever. In Strode G (ed). Yellow Fever. New York, McGraw-Hill, 1951, pp 5–37.

69. Stokes A, Bauer JH, Hudson NP. Transmission of yellow fever to Macacus rhesus, preliminary note. JAMA 90:253–254, 1928.

70. Sawyer WA, Lloyd WDM, Kitchen SF. Preservation of yellow fever virus. J Exp Med 50:1–13, 1929.

71. Mathis C, Sellards AW, Laigret J. Sensibilité du Macacus rhesus au virus de la fièvre jaune. C R Acad Sci Paris 186:604–606, 1928.

72. Monath TP. Yellow fever vaccines: the success of empiricism, pitfalls of application, and transition to molecular vaccinology. In Plotkin SA, Fantini B (eds). Vaccinia, Vaccination, Vaccinology: Jenner, Pasteur, and Their Successors. Paris, Elsevier, 1996, pp 157–182.

73. Theiler M. Susceptibility of white mice to virus of yellow fever. Science 71:367, 1930.

74. Lloyd W, Penna HA, Mahaffy AF. Yellow fever virus encephalitis in rodents. Am J Hyg 18:323–344, 1933.

75. Sawyer WA, Kitchen SF, Lloyd W. Vaccination of humans against yellow fever with immune serum and virus fixed for mice. Proc Soc Exp Biol Med 29:62–64, 1931.

76. Sellards AW, Laigret J. Vaccination de l'homme contre la fièvre jaune. C R Acad Sci Paris 194:1609–1611, 1932.

77. Theiler M, Smith HH. The use of yellow fever virus by in vitro cultivation for human immunization. J Exp Med 65:787–800, 1937.

78. Lloyd W, Theiler M, Ricci NI. Modification of virulence of yellow fever virus by cultivation in tissues in vitro. Trans R Soc Trop Med Hyg 29:481–529, 1936.

79. Theiler M, Smith HH. Effect of prolonged cultivation in vitro upon pathogenicity of yellow fever virus. J Exp Med 65:767–786, 1937.

80. Smith W, Andrewes CH, Laidlaw PP. A virus obtained from influenza patients. Lancet 2:66–68, 1933.

81. Horsfall FL Jr, Lennette EH, Rickard ER, Hirst GK. Studies on the efficacy of a complex vaccine against influenza A. Public Health Rep 56:1863–1875, 1941.

82. Chenoweth A, Waltz AD, Stokes J Jr, Gladen RG. Active immunization with the viruses of human and swine influenza. Am J Dis Child 52:757, 1936.

83. Kilbourne ED. A race with evolution—a history of influenza vaccines. In Plotkin SA, Fantini B (eds). Vaccinia, Vaccination, Vaccinology: Jenner, Pasteur, and Their Successors. Paris, Elsevier, 1996, pp 183–188.

84. Smith W. The complement-fixation reaction in influenza. Lancet 2:1256–1259, 1936.

85. Francis T Jr, Magill TP. Vaccination of human subjects with virus of human influenza. Proc Soc Exp Biol Med 33:604–606, 1936.

86. Francis T Jr, Magill TP. The antibody response of human subjects vaccinated with the virus of human influenza. J Exp Med 65:251–259, 1937.

87. Smorodintsev AA, Tushinsky MD, Drobyshevskaya AI, Korovin AA. Investigation on volunteers infected with the influenza virus. Am J Med Sci 194:159–170, 1937.

88. Kilbourne ED. A history of influenza virology. In Koprowski H, Oldstone MBA (eds). Microbe Hunters—Then and Now. Bloomington, IL, Medi-Ed Press, 1996, pp 187–204.

89. Cox HR. Use of yolk sac of developing chick embryo as medium for growing rickettsiae of Rocky Mountain spotted fever and typhus groups. Public Health Rep 53:2241–2247, 1938.

90. Weindling P. Victory with vaccines: the problem of typhus vaccines during World War II. In Plotkin SA, Fantini B (eds). Vaccinia, Vaccination, Vaccinology: Jenner, Pasteur, and Their Successors. Paris, Elsevier, 1996, pp 341–347.

91. Harden VK. Rocky Mountain Spotted Fever: History of a Twentieth-Century Disease. Baltimore, Johns Hopkins University Press, 1990.

92. Madsen T. Whooping cough: its bacteriology, diagnosis, prevention and treatment. Boston Med Surg J 192:50–60, 1925.

93. Madsen G. Vaccination against whooping cough. JAMA 101:187–188, 1933.

94. Granström M. The history of pertussis vaccination: from whole-cell to subunit vaccines. In Plotkin SA, Fantini B (eds). Vaccinia, Vaccination, Vaccinology: Jenner, Pasteur, and Their Successors. Paris, Elsevier, 1996, pp 107–114.

95. Burnette WN, Mar VL, Bartley TD, et al. The molecular engineering of pertussis toxoid. Dev Biol Stand 73:75–79, 1991.

96. Lapin JH. Whooping Cough. Springfield, IL, Charles C Thomas, 1943.

97. Enders JF, Weller TH, Robbins FC. Cultivation of the Lansing strain of poliomyelitis virus in cultures of various human embryonic tissues. Science 109:85–87, 1949.

98. Koprowski H, Jervis GA, Norton TW. Immune responses in human volunteers upon oral administration of a rodent-adapted strain of poliomyclitis virus. Am J Hyg 55:108–126, 1952.

99. Salk JE, Krech U, Youngner JS, et al. Formaldehyde treatment and safety testing of experimental poliomyelitis vaccines. Am J Public Health 44:563–570, 1954.

100. Sabin AB, Hennessen WA, Winsser J. Studies on variants of poliomyelitis virus. I. Experimental segregation and properties of avirulent variants of three immunological types. J Exp Med 99:551–576, 1954.

101. Katz SL, Kempe CH, Black FL, et al. Studies on an attenuated measles virus vaccine. VIII. General summary and evaluation of results of vaccine. N Engl J Med 263:180–184, 1960.

102. Schwarz AJF. Preliminary tests of a highly attenuated measles vaccine. Am J Dis Child 103:386–389, 1962.

103. Hilleman MR, Buynak EB, Weibel RE, et al. Development and evaluation of the Moraten measles virus vaccine. JAMA 206:587–590, 1968.

104. Hilleman MR, Buynak EB, Weibel RE, Stokes J Jr. Live attenuated mumps-virus vaccine. N Engl J Med 278:227–232, 1968.

105. Meyer HM, Parkman PD. Rubella vaccination: a review of practical experience. JAMA 215:613–619, 1971.

106. Prinzie A, Huygelen C, Gold J, et al. Experimental live attenuated rubella virus vaccine: clinical evaluation of Cendehill strain. Am J Dis Child 118:172–177, 1969.

107. Plotkin SA, Farquhar JD, Katz M, Buser F. Attenuation of RA27/3 rubella virus in WI-38 human diploid cells. Am J Dis Child 118:178–185, 1969.

108. Rowe WP, Huebner RJ, Gilmore LK. Isolation of a cytopathogenic agent from human adenoids undergoing spontaneous degeneration in tissue culture. Proc Soc Exp Biol Med 84:570–573, 1953.

109. Enders JF, Bell JA, Dingle JH, et al. Adenoviruses: group name proposed for new respiratory-tract viruses. Science 124:119–120, 1956.

110. Rubin BA, Rorke LB. Adenovirus vaccines. In Plotkin SA, Mortimer EA (eds). Vaccines. Philadelphia, WB Saunders, 1988, pp 492–512.

111. Top JHR. Control of adenovirus acute respiratory disease in U.S. Army trainees. Yale J Biol Med 48:185–195, 1975.

112. Top FH Jr, Buescher EL, Bancroft WH, et al. Immunization with live types 7 and 4 adenovirus vaccines. II. Antibody response and protective effect against acute respiratory disease due to adenovirus type 7. J Infect Dis 124:155–160, 1971.

113. Top FH Jr, Dudding BA, Russell PK. Control of respiratory disease in recruits with types 4 and 7 adenovirus vaccines. Am J Epidemiol 84:141–146, 1971.

114. Top FH Jr, Grossman RA, Bartelloni PJ. Immunization with live types 7 and 4 adenovirus vaccines. I. Safety, infectivity, and potency of adenovirus type 7 vaccine in humans. J Infect Dis 124:148–154, 1971.

115. Couch RB, Chanock RM, Cate TR. Immunization with types 4 and 7 adenovirus by selective infection of the intestinal tract. Am Rev Respir Dis 88:394–403, 1963.

116. Chanock RM, Ludwig W, Huebner RJ, et al. Immunization by selective infection with type 4 adenovirus grown in human diploid tissue culture. I. Safety and lack of oncogenicity and test for potency in volunteers. JAMA 195:445–452, 1966.

117. Takahashi M, Otsuka T, Okuno Y, et al. Live vaccine used to prevent the spread of varicella in children in hospitals. Lancet 2:1288–1290, 1974.

118. Takahashi M, Okuno Y, Otsuka T, et al. Development of a live attenuated varicella vaccine. Biken J 18:25–33, 1975.

119. Weibel RE, Neff BJ, Kuter B, et al. Live attenuated varicella virus vaccine efficacy trial in healthy children. N Engl J Med 310:1409–1415, 1984.

120. Arbeter AM, Starr SE, Weibel R, Plotkin SA. Live attenuated varicella vaccine: immunization of healthy children with the OKA strain. J Pediatr 100:886–893, 1982.

121. Krause P, Klinman DM. Efficacy, immunogenicity, safety, and use of live attenuated chickenpox vaccine. J Pediatr 127:518–525, 1995.

122. Gershon AA. Live-attenuated varicella vaccine. Infect Dis Clin North Am 15:65–81, 2001.

123. Burnet FM, Bull DR. Changes in influenza virus associated with adaptation to passage in chick embryos. Aust J Exp Biol Med Sci 21:55–69, 1943.

124. Beare AS, Bynoe ML, Tyrrell DAJ. Investigation into the attenuation of influenza viruses by serial passage. Br Med J 4:482, 1968.

125. Minor TE, Dick EC, Dick RC, Inhorn SL. Attenuated influenza A vaccine (Alice) in an adult population: vaccine-related illness, serum and nasal antibody production and intrafamily transmission. J Clin Microbiol 2:403, 1975.

126. Zaky DA, Douglas RG Jr, Betts RF, et al. Safety and efficacy of "Alice" influenza virus vaccine in normal healthy adults. J Infect Dis 133:669–675, 1976.

127. Hall CB, Douglas RG, Fralonardo SA. Live attenuated influenza virus vaccine trial in children. Pediatrics 56:991–998, 1975.

128. Maassab HF, DeBorde DC. Development and characterization of cold-adapted viruses for use as live virus vaccines. Vaccine 3:355–369, 1985.

129. Maassab HF, Herlocker ML, Bryant ML. Live influenza virus vaccine. In Plotkin SA, Orenstein WA (eds). Vaccines (3rd ed). Philadelphia, WB Saunders, 1999, pp 909–927.

130. Abramson JS. Intranasal cold-adapted, live, attenuated influenza vaccine. Pediatr Infect Dis J 18:1103–1104, 1999.

131. Mendelman PM, Cordova J, Cho I. Safety, efficacy and effectiveness of the influenza virus vaccine, trivalent, types A and B, live, cold-adapted (CAIV-T) in healthy children and healthy adults. Vaccine 19:2221–2226, 2001.

132. Edwards KM, Dupont WD, Westrich MK, et al. A randomized controlled trial of cold-adapted and inactivated vaccines for the prevention of influenza A disease. J Infect Dis 169:68–76, 1994.

133. Belshe RB, Mendelman PM, Treanor J, et al. The efficacy of live attenuated, cold-adapted, trivalent, intranasal influenza virus vaccine in children. N Engl J Med 338:1405–1412, 1998.

134. Piedra PA, Glezen P. Influenza in children: epidemiology, immunity and vaccines. Semin Pediatr Infect Dis 2:140–146, 1991.

135. Longini IM Jr, Halloran ME, Nizam A, et al. Estimation of the efficacy of live, attenuated influenza vaccine from a two-year, multicenter vaccine trial: implications for influenza epidemic control. Vaccine 18:1902–1909, 2000.

136. Belshe RB, Gruber WC, Mendelman PM, et al. Correlates of immune protection induced by live, attenuated, cold-adapted, trivalent, intranasal influenza virus vaccine. J Infect Dis 181:1133–1137, 2000.

137. Rotavirus vaccine for the prevention of rotavirus gastroenteritis among children: Recommendations of the Advisory Committee on Immunization Practices (ACIP). MMWR 48(RR-2):1–20, 1999.

138. Midthun K, Greenberg HB, Hoshino Y, et al. Reassortant rotaviruses as potential live rotavirus vaccine candidates. J Virol 53:949–954, 1985.

139. Clark HF, Glass RI, Offit PA. Rotavirus vaccines. In Plotkin SA, Orenstein WA (eds). Vaccines (3rd ed). Philadelphia, WB Saunders, 1999, pp 987–1005.

140. Intussusception among recipients of rotavirus vaccine—United States, 1998–1999. MMWR 48(27): 577–581, 1999.

141. Barnes G. Intussusception and rotavirus vaccine. J Pediatr Gastroenterol Nutr 29:375, 1999.

142. Suzuki H, Katsushima N, Konno T. Rotavirus vaccine put on hold. Lancet 354:1390, 1999.

143. Withdrawal of rotavirus vaccine recommendation. MMWR 48(43):1007, 1999.

144. Dennehy PH, Bresee JS. Rotavirus vaccine and intussusception: where do we go from here? Infect Dis Clin North Am 15:189–207, 2001.

145. Matson DO. A different perspective on a rotavirus vaccine. Vaccine 19:2763, 2001.

146. Rennels MB. The rotavirus vaccine story: a clinical investigator's view. Pediatrics 106:123–125, 2000.

147. Yugoslav Typhoid Commission. A controlled field trial of the effectiveness of acetone-dried and inactivated and heat-phenol–inactivated typhoid vaccines in Yugoslavia. Bull World Health Organ 30:623–630, 1964.

148. Ashcroft MT, Singh B, Nicholson CC, et al. A seven-year field trial of two typhoid vaccines in Guyana. Lancet 2:1056–1059, 1967.

149. Polish Typhoid Commission. Controlled field trials and laboratory studies on the effectiveness of typhoid vaccines in Poland 1961–64. Bull World Health Organ 34:211–222, 1966.

150. Hejfec LB, Samin LV, Lejtman MZ, et al. A controlled field trial and laboratory study of five typhoid vaccines in the USSR. Bull World Health Organ 34:321–339, 1966.

151. Germanier R, Fürer E. Isolation and characterization of Gal E mutant Ty21a of Salmonella typhi: A candidate for a live, oral typhoid vaccine. J Infect Dis 131:553–558, 1975.

152. Gilman RH, Hornick RB, Woodward WE, et al. Immunity in typhoid fever: evaluation of Ty21a—an epimeraseless mutant of S. typhi as a live oral vaccine. J Infect Dis 136:717–723, 1977.

153. Wahdan MH, Série C, Cerisier Y, et al. A controlled field trial of live *Salmonella typhi* strain Ty21a oral vaccine against typhoid: three-year results. J Infect Dis 145:292–295, 1982.
154. Levine MM, Black RE, Ferreccio C, et al. Large-scale field trial of Ty21a live oral typhoid vaccine in enteric-coated capsule formulation. Lancet 1:1049–1052, 1987.
155. Hackett J. Salmonella-based vaccines. Vaccine 8:5–11, 1990.
156. Black RE. Efficacy of one or two doses of Ty21a *Salmonella typhi* vaccine in enteric-coated capsules in a controlled field trial. Vaccine 8:81–84, 1990.
157. Ferreccio C, Levine M, Rodriguez H, et al. Comparative efficacy of two, three and four doses of Ty21a live oral typhoid vaccine in enteric-coated capsules: a field trial in an endemic area. J Infect Dis 159:766–769, 1989.
158. Wiktor TJ, Fernandez MV, Koprowski H. Cultivation of rabies virus in human diploid cell strain WI-38. J Immunol 93:353–366, 1964.
159. Wiktor TJ, MacFarlane RI, Reagen KJ, et al. Protection from rabies by vaccinia virus recombinant containing the rabies virus glycoprotein gene. Proc Natl Acad Sci U S A 81:7194–7198, 1984.
160. Sabin AB. Encephalitis. *In* Coates JB Jr, Hoff EC, Hoff PM (eds). Preventive Medicine in WWII. Vol. 7. Washington, DC, Office of the Surgeon General, Department of the Army, 1964, pp 9–21.
161. Takaku K, Yamshita T, Osanai T, et al. Japanese encephalitis purified vaccine. Biken J 11:25–39, 1968.
162. Hoke CH, Nisalak A, Sangawhipa N, et al. Protection against Japanese encephalitis by inactivated vaccines. N Engl J Med 319:608–614, 1988.
163. Poland JD, Cropp CB, Craven RB, et al. Evaluation of the potency and safety of inactivated Japanese encephalitis vaccine in US inhabitants. J Infect Dis 161:878–882, 1990.
164. Centers for Disease Control. Japanese encephalitis with special reference to the low risk for travelers to the 1988 Olympics to be held in Korea. Advisory Memorandum No. 93. Atlanta, GA, Centers for Disease Control, 1988.
165. Gu PW, Ding ZF. Inactivated Japanese encephalitis (JE) vaccine made from hamster cell culture [review]. Jpn Encephalitis Hemorrhagic Fever Renal Syndrome Bull 2:15–26, 1987.
166. Yu YX, Wu PF, Ao J, et al. Selection of a better immunogenic and highly attenuated live vaccine virus strain of JE. I. Some biological characteristics of SA 14-14-2 mutant. Chin J Microbiol Immunol 1:77–84, 1981.
167. Ao J, Yu Y, Tang YS, et al. Selection of a better immunogenic and highly attenuated live vaccine strain of Japanese encephalitis. II. Safety and immunogenicity of live JBE vaccine SA14-14-2 observed in inoculated children. Chin J Microbiol Immunol 3(4):245–248, 1983.
168. Xin YY, Ming ZG, Peng GY, et al. Safety of a live-attenuated Japanese encephalitis virus vaccine (SA14-14-2) for children. Am J Trop Med Hyg 39:214–217, 1988.
169. Huang CH. Studies of Japanese encephalitis in China. Adv Virus Res 27:71–101, 1982.
170. Provost PJ, Hilleman MR. Propagation of human hepatitis A virus in cell culture in vitro. Proc Soc Exp Biol Med 160:213–221, 1979.
171. Provost PJ, Hughes JV, Miller WJ, et al. An inactivated hepatitis A vaccine of cell culture origin. J Med Virol 19:23–31, 1986.
172. Wiedermann M, Ambrosch F, Kollaritsch H, et al. Safety and immunogenicity of an inactivated hepatitis A candidate vaccine in healthy adult volunteers. Vaccine 8:581–584, 1990.
173. André FE, Hondt d'E, Delem AD, Safary A. Clinical assessment of the safety and efficacy of an inactivated hepatitis-A vaccine—rationale and summary of findings. Vaccine 10:S160–S168, 1992.
174. Smorodinstev AA, Kagan UV, Levkovich EN, et al. Experimenteller und epidemiologischer Beitrag zur aktiven Immunisierung gegen die Frülin-Sommer-Zecken-Encephalitis. Arch Ges Virusforsch 3:1, 1941.
175. Smorodinstev AA. Tick-borne spring-summer encephalitis. Prog Med Virol 1:210–247, 1958.
176. Benda R, Danes L. Study of the possibility of preparing a vaccine against tick-borne encephalitis, using tissue culture methods. V. Experimental data for the evaluation of the efficiency of formol treated vaccines in laboratory animals. Acta Virol 5:37, 1961.
177. Benda R, Danes L. Evaluation of the immunogenic efficiency of tick-borne encephalitis virus vaccine. *In* Libikova H (ed). Biology of Viruses of the Tick-Borne Encephalitis Complex. Prague, Czechoslovak Academy of Sciences, 1962, p 245.
178. Levkovich EN. Experimental and epidemiological bases of the specific prophylaxis of tick-borne encephalitis. *In* Livikova H (ed). Biology of Viruses of the Tick-Borne Encephalitis Complex. Prague, Czechoslovak Academy of Sciences, 1962, p 317.
179. Kunz C. Aktiv und passive Immunoprophylaxe der Frühsommer-Meningoencephalitis (FSME). Arzneim Forsch 28:1806, 1962.
180. Heinz FX, Kunz C, Fauma H. Preparation of a highly purified vaccine against tick-borne encephalitis by continuous flow zonal ultracentrifugation. J Med Virol 6:213–222, 1980.
181. Heinz FX, Kunz C. Homogeneity of the structural glycoprotein from European isolates of tick-borne encephalitis virus: comparison with other flaviviruses. J Gen Virol 57:263–274, 1981.
182. Heinz FX, Berger R, Tuma W, et al. A topological and functional model of epitopes on the structural glycoprotein of tick-borne encephalitis virus defined by monoclonal antibodies. Virology 126:525–537, 1983.
183. Stephenson JR, Lee JM, Wilton-Smith PD. Antigenic variation among members of the tick-borne encephalitis complex. J Gen Virol 65:81–89, 1984.
184. Barrett PN, Dorner F, Plotkin SA. Tick-borne encephalitis vaccine. *In* Plotkin SA, Orenstein WA (eds). Vaccines (3rd ed). Philadelphia, WB Saunders, 1999, pp 767–780.
185. Sato Y, Izumiya K, Sato H, et al. Role of antibody to leukocytosis-promoting factor hemagglutinin and to filamentous hemagglutinin in immunity to pertussis. Infect Immun 31:1223–1231, 1981.
186. Sato Y, Kimura M, Fukimi H. Development of a pertussis component vaccine in Japan. Lancet 1:122–126, 1984.
187. Kimura M, Hikino N. Results with a new DTP vaccine in Japan. Dev Biol Stand 61:545–561, 1985.
188. Edwards KM, Decker MD, Mortimer EA Jr. Pertussis vaccine. *In* Plotkin SA, Orenstein WA (eds). Vaccines (3rd ed). Philadelphia, WB Saunders, 1999, pp 293–344.
189. Ivins BE, Essell JW Jr, Jemski J, et al. Immunization studies with attenuated strains of *Bacillus anthracis*. Infect Immun 52:454–458, 1986.
190. Ivins BE, Welkos SL. Recent advances in the development of an improved human anthrax vaccine. Eur J Epidemiol 4:12–19, 1988.
191. Little SF, Knudson GB. Comparative efficacy of *Bacillus anthracis* live spore vaccine and protective antigen vaccine against anthrax in the guinea pig. Infect Immun 63:509–512, 1986.
192. Brachman PS, Gold H, Plotkin S, et al. Field evaluation of a human anthrax vaccine. Am J Pub Health 52:632–645, 1962.
193. Plotkin SA, Brachman PS, Utell M, et al. An epidemic of inhalation anthrax, the first in the twentieth century. Am J Med 29:992–1001, 1960.
194. Brachman PS, Friedlander AM. Anthrax. *In* Plotkin SA, Orenstein WA (eds). Vaccines (3rd ed). Philadelphia, WB Saunders, 1999, pp 629–637.
195. Institute of Medicine. The Anthrax Vaccine: Is It Safe? Does It Work? Washington, DC, National Academy Press, 2002.
196. Artenstein MS, Gold R, Zimmerly JG, et al. Prevention of meningococcal disease by group C polysaccharide vaccine. N Engl J Med 282:417–420, 1970.
197. Gotschlich EC, Liu TY, Artenstein MS. Human immunity to the meningococcus. III. Preparation and immunochemical properties of the group A, group B and group C meningococcal polysaccharides. J Exp Med 129:1349–1365, 1969.
198. Lepow ML, Perkins BA, Hughes PA, Poolman JT. Meningococcal vaccines. *In* Plotkin SA, Orenstein WA (eds). Vaccines (3rd ed). Philadelphia, WB Saunders, 1999, pp 711–727.
199. Goldschneider I, Gotschlich EC, Artenstein MS. Human immunity to the meningococcus. I. The role of humoral immunity. J Exp Med 129:1307–1326, 1969.
200. Goldschneider I, Gotschlich ED, Artenstein MS. Human immunity to the meningococcus. II. The development of natural immunity. J Exp Med 129:1327–1348, 1969.
201. Gotschlich ED, Goldschneider I, Artenstein MS. Human immunity to the meningococcus. V. The effect of immunization with meningococcal group C polysaccharide on the carrier state. J Exp Med 129:1385–1395, 1969.
202. Richmond P, Kaczmarski E, Borrow R, et al. Meningococcal C polysaccharide vaccine induces immunologic hyporesponsiveness in adults that is overcome by meningococcal C conjugate vaccine. J Infect Dis 181:761–762, 2000.

203. Choo S, Zuckerman J, Goilav C, et al. Immunogenicity and reactogenicity of a group C meningococcal conjugate vaccine compared with a group A+C meningococcal polysaccharide vaccine in adolescents in a randomised observer-blind controlled trial. Vaccine 18:2686–2692, 2000.

204. Austrian R, Douglas RM, Schiffman G, et al. Prevention of pneumococcal pneumonia by vaccination. Trans Assoc Am Physicians 89:184–192, 1976.

205. Fedson DS, Musher DM, Eskola J. Pneumococcal vaccine. *In* Plotkin SA, Orenstein WA (eds). Vaccines (3rd ed). Philadelphia, WB Saunders, 1999, pp 553–607.

206. Austrian R. Bacterial polysaccharide vaccines. *In* Plotkin SA, Fantini B (eds). Vaccinia, Vaccination, Vaccinology: Jenner, Pasteur, and Their Successors. Paris, Elsevier, 1996, pp 127–133.

207. Wright AE, Parry Morgan W, Colebrook L, Dodgson RW. Observations on prophylactic inoculation against pneumococcus infections and on the results which have been achieved by it. Lancet 1:1–10, 87–95, 1914.

208. Maynard GD. Memorandum on Rand Mines pneumococcic vaccine experiment. Med J S Afr 9:91–95, 1913.

209. McCarty M. A retrospective look: how we identified the pneumococcal transforming substance as DNA. J Exp Med 179:385–394, 1994.

210. Lederberg J. The transformation of genetics by DNA: an anniversary celebration of Avery, MacLeod and McCarty (1944). Genetics 136:423–426, 1994.

211. Avery OT, MacLeod CM, McCarty M. Studies on the chemical nature of the substance inducing transformation of pneumococcal types: induction of transformation by a desoxyribonucleic acid fraction isolated from pneumococcus type III [re-publication of a 1944 paper]. Mol Med 1:344–365, 1995.

212. Austrian R, Gold J. Pneumococcal bacteremia with special reference to bacteremic pneumococcal pneumonia. Ann Intern Med 60:759–776, 1964.

213. Anderson P, Peter G, Johnston RB Jr, et al. Immunization of humans with polyribophosphate, the capsular antigen of *Haemophilus influenzae* type b. J Clin Invest 51:39–44, 1972.

214. Schneerson R, Rodrigues LP, Parke JC Jr, et al. Immunity to disease caused by *H. influenzae* type b. II. Specificity and some biologic characteristics of "natural," infection-acquired, and immunization-induced antibodies to the capsular polysaccharide of *H. influenzae* type b. J Immunol 107:1081–1089, 1971.

215. Robbins JB, Schneerson R, Pittman M. *Haemophilus influenzae* type b infections. *In* Germanier R (ed). Bacterial Vaccines. Orlando, FL, Academic Press, 1984, pp 289–316.

216. Peltola H, Kayhty H, Sivonen A, et al. *Haemophilus influenzae* type b capsular polysaccharide vaccine in children: a double-blind field study of 100,000 vaccinees 3 months to 5 years of age in Finland. Pediatrics 60:730–737, 1977.

217. Peltola H, Kayhty H, Virtanen M, et al. Prevention of *Haemophilus influenzae* type b bacteremic infections with the capsular polysaccharide vaccine. N Engl J Med 310:1561–1566, 1984.

218. Parke JC Jr, Schneerson R, Robbins JB, et al. Interim report of a controlled field trial of immunization with capsular polysaccharides *of Haemophilus influenzae* type b and group C *Neisseria meningitidis* in Mecklenburg County, North Carolina. J Infect Dis 136:S51–S57, 1977.

219. Ward J. Prevention of invasive *Haemophilus influenzae* type b disease: lessons from vaccine efficacy trials. Vaccine 9(suppl):S17–S24, 1991.

220. Avery OT, Goebel WF. Chemical-immunological studies on conjugated carbohydrate-proteins. II. Immunological specificity of synthetic sugar-protein antigens. J Exp Med 50:533–542, 1929.

221. Goebel WF. Studies on antibacterial immunity induced by artificial antigens. I. Immunity to experimental pneumococcal infection with an antigen containing cellobiuronic acid. J Exp Med 69:353–364, 1939.

222. Schneerson R, Barrera O, Sutton A, Robbins JB. Preparation, characterization and immunogenicity of *Haemophilus influenzae* type b polysaccharide-protein conjugates. J Exp Med 152:361–376, 1980.

223. Lakshman R, Jones I, Walker D, et al. Safety of a new conjugate meningococcal C vaccine in infants. Arch Dis Child 85:391–397, 2001.

224. Bramley JC, Hall T, Finn A, et al. Safety and immunogenicity of three lots of meningococcal serogroup C conjugate vaccine administered at 2, 3, and 4 months of age. Vaccine 19:2924–2931, 2001.

225. English M, MacLennan JM, Bowen-Morris JM, et al. A randomised, double-blind, controlled trial of the immunogenicity and tolerability of a meningococcal group C conjugate vaccine in young British infants. Vaccine 19:1232–1238, 2001.

226. Richmond R, Borrow R, Goldblatt D, et al. Ability of 3 different meningococcal C conjugate vaccines to induce immunologic memory after a single dose in UK toddlers. J Infect Dis 183:160–163, 2001.

227. Eskola J, Antilla M. Pneumococcal conjugate vaccines. Pediatr Infect Dis J 18:543–551, 1999.

228. Black SB, Shinefield HR, Fireman B, et al. Efficacy, safety and immunogenicity of heptavalent pneumococcal conjugate vaccine in children. Pediatr Infect Dis J 19:187–195, 2000.

229. Klein JO. The pneumococcal conjugate vaccine arrives: a big win for kids. Pediatr Infect Dis J 19:181–182, 2000.

230. American Academy of Pediatrics, Committee on Infectious Diseases. Policy Statement: Recommendations for the prevention of pneumococcal infections, including the use of pneumococcal conjugate vaccine (Prevnar), pneumococcal polysaccharide vaccine, and antibiotic prophylaxis. Pediatrics 106:362–366, 2000.

231. Overturf GD, for the Committee on Infectious Diseases. Technical Report: Prevention of pneumococcal infections, including the use of pneumococcal conjugate and polysaccharide vaccines and antibiotic prophylaxis. Pediatrics 106:367–376, 2000.

232. Black SB, Shinefield HR, Hansen J, et al. Postlicensure evaluation of the effectiveness of seven valent pneumococcal conjugate vaccine. Pediatr Infect Dis J 20:1105–1107, 2001.

233. Landy J. Studies of Vi antigen. VI. Immunization of human beings with purified Vi antigen. Am J Hyg 50:52–62, 1954.

234. Landy M, Gaines S, Seal JP, et al. Antibody responses of man to three types of antityphoid immunizing agents. Am J Public Health 44:1572–1579, 1954.

235. Webster ME, Landy M, Freeman ME. Studies on Vi antigen. II. Purification of Vi antigen from *Escherichia coli* 5396/38. J Immunol 69:135–142, 1952.

236. Wong KH, Feeley JC, Northrup RS, et al. Vi antigen from *Salmonella typhosa* and immunity against typhoid fever. I. Isolation and immunologic properties in animals. Infect Immun 9:348–353, 1974.

237. Robbins JD, Robbins JB. Reexamination of the protective role of the capsular polysaccharide Vi antigen of *Salmonella typhi*. J Infect Dis 150:436–439, 1984.

238. Prince AM. An antigen detected in the blood during the incubation period of serum hepatitis. Proc Natl Acad Sci U S A 60:814, 1968.

239. Krugman S, Giles JP, Hammond J. Infectious hepatitis: evidence for two distinctive clinical, epidemiological, and immunological types of infection. JAMA 200:365–373, 1967.

240. Krugman S, Giles JP, Hammond J. Viral hepatitis, type B (MS-2 strain): studies on active immunization. JAMA 217:41–45, 1971.

241. Hilleman MR, Bertland VA, Bunyak EB, et al. Clinical and laboratory studies of HBsAg vaccine. *In* Vyas GN, Cohen SN, Schmid R (eds). Viral Hepatitis. Philadelphia, Franklin Institute Press, 1978, pp 525–527.

242. Krugman S. The newly licensed hepatitis B vaccine: characteristics and indications for use. JAMA 247:2012–2015, 1982.

243. Valenzuela P, Medina A, Rutter WJ, et al. Synthesis and assembly of hepatitis B virus surface antigen particles in yeast. Nature 298:347–350, 1982.

244. McAleer WJ, Buynak EB, Maigetter RZ, et al. Human hepatitis B vaccine from recombinant yeast. Nature 307:178–180, 1984.

245. Skolnick EM, McLean AA, West DJ, et al. Clinical evaluation in healthy adults of a hepatitis B vaccine made by recombinant DNA. JAMA 251:2812–2815, 1984.

246. Michel M-L, Pontisso P, Sobczak E, et al. Synthesis in animal cells of hepatitis B surface antigen particles carrying a receptor for polymerized human serum albumin. Proc Natl Acad Sci U S A 81:7708–7712, 1984.

247. Emini EA, Ellis RW, Miller WJ, et al. Production and immunological analysis of recombinant hepatitis B vaccine. J Infect 13(suppl A):3–9, 1986.

248. Scheiermann N, Gesemann M, Mauer C, et al. Persistence of antibodies after immunization with a recombinant yeast-derived hepatitis B vaccine following two different schedules. Vaccine 8(suppl):S44–S46, 1990.

249. Andreá FE. Overview of a 5-year clinical experience with a yeast-derived hepatitis B vaccine. Vaccine 8(suppl):S74–S78, 1990.

250. Poland GA, Jacobson RM. The prevention of Lyme disease with vaccine. Vaccine 19:2303–2308, 2001.
251. Evans J, Fikrig E. Lyme disease vaccine. *In* Plotkin SA, Orenstein WA (eds). Vaccines (3rd ed). Philadelphia, WB Saunders, 1999, pp 968–982.
252. Rahn DW. Lyme vaccine: issues and controversies. Infect Dis Clin North Am 15:171–187, 2001.
253. Availability of Lyme disease vaccine. MMWR 48(2): 35–36, 43, 1999.
254. Steere AC, Malawista SE, Craft JE, et al. Lyme disease: First International Symposium. Yale J Biol Med 57:445–713, 1984.
255. Burgdorfer W, Barbour AG, Hayes SF, et al. Lyme disease—a tick-borne spirochetosis? Science 216:1317–1319, 1982.
256. Rahn DW, Malawista SE. Lyme disease: recommendations for diagnosis and treatment. Ann Intern Med 114:472–481, 1991.
257. Steere AC, Malawista SE, Newman JH, et al. Antibiotic therapy in Lyme disease. Ann Intern Med 93:108, 1980.
258. Steere AC, Pachner A, Malawista SE. Successful treatment of neurologic abnormalities of Lyme disease with high-dose intravenous penicillin. Ann Intern Med 99:767–772, 1983.
259. Rahn DW, Malawista SE. Treatment of Lyme disease. *In* Rogers DE, Bone RC, Cline MJ, et al (eds). Yearbook of Medicine. St. Louis, CV Mosby, 1994, pp 21–36.
260. Telford SR, Fikrig E. Progress towards a vaccine for Lyme disease. Clin Immunother 4:49–60, 1995.
261. Hoecke CV, Comberbach M, De Grave D, et al. Evaluation of the safety, reactogenicity and immunologenicity of three recombinant outer surface protein (OspA) Lyme vaccines in healthy adults. Vaccine 14:1620–1626, 1996.
262. Hoecke CV, Lebacq E, Beran J, et al. Alternative vaccination schedules (0, 1, and 6 months versus 0, 1, and 12 months) for a recombinant OspA Lyme disease vaccine. Clin Infect Dis 28:1260–1264, 1994.
263. Sigal LH, Zahradnik JM, Levin P, et al. Vaccine consisting of recombinant *Borrelia burgdorferi* outer-surface protein A to prevent Lyme disease. N Engl J Med 339:216–222, 1998.
264. Steere AC, Sikand VK, Meurice F, et al. Vaccination against Lyme disease with recombinant *Borrelia burgdorferi* outer-surface lipoprotein A with adjuvant. N Engl J Med 339:209–215, 1998.

Chapter 2

The History of Polio Vaccine Development

FREDERICK C. ROBBINS

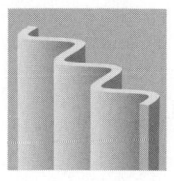

Poliomyelitis viruses probably have been prevalent as infectious agents of humans from the time that humans gathered together in villages and groups large enough to facilitate the person-to-person spread of infectious agents. Paralytic disease, however, was not recognized to be a significant problem until late in the 19th century, when epidemics began to appear in northern Europe.[1] Heine provided one of the first descriptions of the clinical disease as we now know it.[2] The earliest and best description of an epidemic of any size is that of Medin from Stockholm in 1887.[3] From that time on, seasonal (summer and early fall in the Northern Hemisphere) epidemics of increasing severity occurred in the industrialized countries. The average age of patients also rose, with concomitant increases in the severity of disease and its mortality.[4] By 1953, the incidence of paralytic poliomyelitis in the United States was more than 20 per 100,000 population. Although this rate was not particularly high compared with that of other diseases such as measles, much public concern was generated by polio because of its mysterious seasonal incidence (an attribute that is still not adequately explained), its disfiguring nature, and its propensity for paralyzing the respiratory muscles. Paralyzed patients often required artificial assistance to breathe, usually through the use of that cumbersome and fearsome instrument, the "iron lung," or Drinker respirator.

Pre–Tissue Culture Era

Not long after polio had been recognized as an epidemic disease, Landsteiner and Popper were able to reproduce the disease in monkeys by intraperitoneal inoculation of a filtrate of central nervous system tissue from a fatal case.[5,6] Although this discovery was of great importance, the monkey was not an experimental animal that lent itself well to the kind of research necessary to elucidate the characteristics and epidemiology of the poliovirus or to develop preventive measures. In 1939, Armstrong succeeded in adapting the Lansing strain of poliovirus to rodents, which made it possible to expand the scope of experimentation.[7] However, the usefulness of the rodent-adapted virus was limited because it was a single type, later found to be type 2. Many years later, Li and Schaeffer were able to adapt a type 1 strain to mice.[8]

In the 40-year interval from the isolation of the poliovirus in monkeys to the development of tissue culture techniques, considerable progress was made in understanding poliomyelitis.[4] Evidence was presented to suggest that the virus multiplied in the gastrointestinal tract and that infection could be transferred by the fecal–oral route.[9,10] Monkeys were shown to develop immunity to challenge with active virus, and various efforts were made to prepare experimental vaccines. The starting material was central nervous system tissue from infected monkeys that had been treated in a variety of ways. Although some success was reported, the experiments were inconsistent, and the results were disappointing overall.[11,12] In spite of the ambiguous animal data, in 1936 two investigators independently conducted field trials of vaccines prepared from monkey spinal cord, using children and some adults as subjects. Brodie and Park[13] used a formalin-treated preparation, whereas Kolmer[14] treated the spinal cord suspension with ricinoleate to "attenuate" the virus. Kolmer assumed that it was necessary to use live virus to achieve immunity.

By modern standards, these trials were ill conceived. The scientific base was woefully inadequate to justify human trials. Appropriate tests for safety and efficacy were lacking, and, indeed, there seems to have been little concern for the known risk attendant with the injection of central nervous system tissue. Furthermore, it was not yet known whether there was more than one type of poliovirus, and there was no readily available means to diagnose infection. Thousands of subjects received these vaccines, some of whom developed paralysis soon after inoculation, often in the inoculated limb. These findings raised the specter of persistence of live virulent virus in the vaccine, and the trials were terminated.[15–17]

Another abortive attempt to prevent polio was by chemical treatment of the nasal mucosa, with the purpose of blocking viral invasion. Picric acid, sodium alum, and zinc sulfate were instilled into the nose. This rather bizarre procedure was based on the observation that certain species of monkeys could be infected by the nasopharyngeal route and that prior treatment with the aforementioned chemicals seemed to interfere with infection. Trials in humans were not promising, and this technique was soon abandoned.[18,19]

In the effort to develop better methods for propagating the virus, various investigators[19] tried tissue culture without success, except for Sabin and Olitsky, who in 1936 reported the growth of poliovirus in cultures of human embryonic brain tissue.[20] However, they had no success with cells from non–nervous system tissues. These results tended to strengthen the idea that poliovirus was a strict neurotrope, in spite of the evidence that it was present in the nasopharynx and intestine in vivo.

Burnet and Jackson, from the Walter and Eliza Hall Institute of Melbourne, Australia, mentioned in a paper published in 1940 that they had had suggestive success in propagating a local strain of poliovirus (Mars) in cultures of human fetal pharyngeal and intestinal tissues.[21] Unfortunately, they did not pursue these findings; otherwise, the vaccine might have been available almost a decade earlier. The techniques employed by Burnet and Jackson were not significantly different from those of Sabin. The discrepancy in results most likely can be attributed to differences in the viral strains employed, as is discussed subsequently.

A large-scale cooperative experiment in monkeys, reported in 1949, demonstrated conclusively that there were three, and only three, immunologically distinct strains of poliovirus; this was crucial information in compounding a fully protective vaccine.[22–25] Using children in a field trial of human serum γ-globulin as a prophylactic against polio, Hammon and colleagues demonstrated a significant level of protection against paralytic disease.[26] This finding—that relatively low levels of antibody could prevent invasion of the central nervous system—provided encouragement to those who were developing a means of active immunization. An excellent analysis of the pathogenesis of poliomyelitis and the implication for the success of preventive measures was published by Bodian in 1952 and is still applicable today.[27]

Tissue Culture Era

Although much had been learned about polio and its causative virus, there was no optimism in 1949 about the possibility of developing a practical means of preventing polio with the techniques at hand.[28,29] That same year, however, Enders and colleagues (Fig. 2–1) published the paper in *Science* that described the successful cultivation of the Lansing strain of poliovirus in cultures of human non–nervous system tissues,[30] which provided the breakthrough that was so eagerly sought. There is no ready explanation as to why these experiments succeeded whereas those of Sabin and Olitsky did not. The principal technical difference was that, in Enders's laboratory, the cultures were maintained for a longer time, with periodic changes of nutrient medium; the availability of antibiotics that were incorporated in the medium made this possible. Sabin did go back to the original virus (MV strain) used in the 1936 experiments and found it to be noncytopathic for monkey kidney cells.[31] The implication is that, after many passages in monkey brain, it had lost its capacity to infect non–nervous system cells.

Poliovirus was soon found to propagate in cells from a variety of tissues from both humans and nonhuman primates.[32–37] The monkey kidney became the preferred source of tissue for much subsequent work, including the growth of virus for vaccine production. Because the virus was released into the tissue culture medium, the cell-free fluid component of the culture made an excellent source of virus, relatively free of extraneous proteinaceous material, from which the inactivated vaccine was prepared.

It was noted early in the course of poliovirus cultivation that infected cells were rapidly destroyed,[38] and this "cytopathic" effect was exploited as an indicator of viral replication. Thus a single test tube, flask, or, later, well in a plastic plate could be used as the equivalent of an experimental animal. With some technical modifications, one could use tissue cultures for virus titration, antibody quantification, virus isolation from clinical specimens, and antigenic typing of virus isolates.[39–45] These relatively simple techniques greatly facilitated the development and testing of vaccines.

Dulbecco, adapting a technique that he had developed for producing plaques in monolayers of chick embryo cells

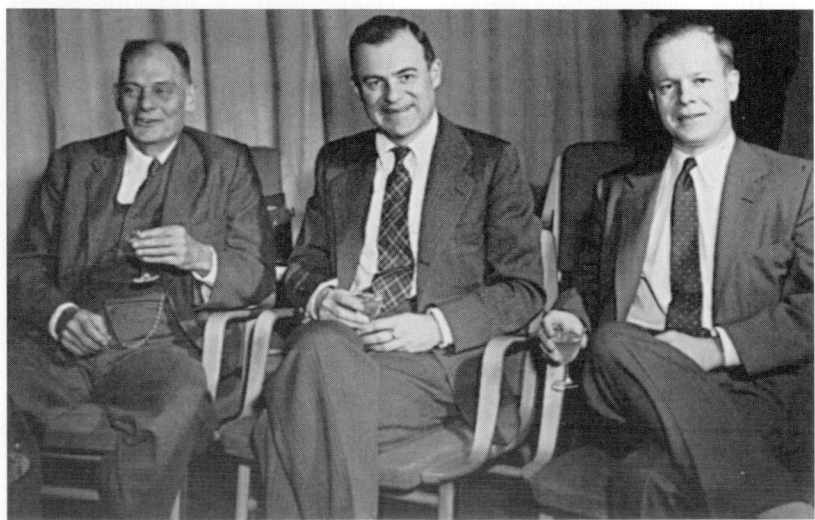

FIGURE 2–1 ■ John Enders, Frederick Robbins, and Thomas Weller in Stockholm, 1954.

in culture with western equine encephalitis and Newcastle disease viruses,[46] was able to do the same with polioviruses.[47] He prepared monolayers from suspensions of monkey kidney cells prepared by trypsinization. The plaquing techniques placed the study of poliovirus and other animal viruses on a quantitative basis comparable to the technique that had proved to be fruitful with bacteriophages. The ability to establish clones from single virus particles was invaluable in the development of lines of poliovirus suitable for use as live, attenuated vaccines.

Trypsin had been used for preparing cells for transfer from plasma clot cultures since first described by Rous and Jones in 1916.[48] However, only after Dulbecco's work did trypsinization become widely used as the standard method of preparing cell suspensions for viral propagation in tissue cultures.[49] Homogeneous suspensions of kidney cells prepared by trypsinization proved to be a more practical source of cells than HeLa cells, which had been used by some investigators for tissue culture titration of poliovirus or its antibody.[50-54]

Although it was only after the observations of Enders, Robbins, and Weller that techniques based on the cytopathic effect of viruses on cells in tissue culture became widely used, many investigators had previously observed various kinds of effects of viruses on cells in tissue culture.[19] Sanders and Alexander isolated directly in tissue cultures a virus from cases of keratoconjunctivitis.[55] Huang performed titrations of western equine encephalitis virus and antibody to this virus, using cytopathology as the indicator of virus growth.[56] He also employed the interference phenomenon to titrate noncytopathic viruses (St. Louis encephalitis and Jungeblut-Sanders mouse viruses) in culture,[57] foreshadowing the techniques later employed for rubella virus. Huang also used pH change as an indicator of virus growth.[58] By incorporating sulfadiazine in the medium for bacteriostasis, Sanders and Huang were able to use tissue cultures in field studies.[59] Thus the work of Huang and associates anticipated many of the practical applications of tissue cultures that were to prove valuable in the work with poliovirus and, later, with many other viruses.

With the availability of tissue culture techniques making a vaccine against poliomyelitis a realistic possibility, a number of laboratories began work toward this end. Salk and colleagues chose to pursue a formalin-inactivated vaccine, whereas Milzer and associates[60] pursued ultraviolet irradiation as a means of inactivation. Cox, Koprowski, and Sabin took the approach of a live attenuated vaccine.[61-64]

Inactivated Vaccines

Milzer, Wolf, and colleagues pursued the ultraviolet irradiation–inactivated vaccine to the point of demonstrating immunogenicity in humans,[60,65] but it was never adopted for general use.

Work on the formalinized vaccine proceeded apace in Salk's laboratory. Using virus grown in tissue cultures of monkey kidney as starting material, Salk and his colleagues determined the formalin inactivation curve; performed safety and immunogenicity studies in animals; and, by 1953, had performed preliminary studies in humans.[66-69] Salk supported the hypothesis that, once the host had been primed

with an adequate dose of antigen, the booster response would occur on challenge with inactive antigen or live virus.[70] On live virus challenge, antibody would be elaborated rapidly enough to prevent viremia and thus paralysis. Although viremia had been demonstrated in monkeys,[27] it was some time later that it was demonstrated in humans.[71,72] In April 1953, a letter signed by Rivers and the members of the Vaccine Advisory Committee of the National Foundation for Infantile Paralysis was published in the *Journal of the American Medical Association*, suggesting some steps that should be taken before the inactivated vaccine could be considered for a large-scale field trial.[73,74] By early 1954, the data were considered sufficient to warrant conducting such a trial, and the decision was made to proceed.

Francis of the University of Michigan School of Public Health was director of the project, which was the largest experiment of its kind up to that time.[75] Trial participants included a total of 1,829,916 children in communities from all parts of the United States, and several from Canada and Finland. The experiment involved both observed controls and, in some areas, placebo controls. The results were presented on April 12, 1955. The conclusions were that the vaccine was safe and effective at a level of approximately 70% and that effectiveness could be correlated with potency, as measured by antibody response in children. On the basis of the evidence from the trial and the data presented by the manufacturers, the products of six producers were licensed within a few days after the announcement of the field trial results.

The Cutter Episode

Interest in the vaccine was high, and many communities organized specific programs, which obtained widespread coverage. However, not long after the vaccine had become generally available, cases of paralytic disease were reported in recipients.[76-78] Because the interval between vaccination and onset of disease corresponded to the incubation period of polio, and because the paralysis usually occurred in the inoculated limb, it was suspected that these cases were caused by residual active virus in the vaccine. Epidemiologic investigation revealed that almost all the cases occurred in children who had received vaccine made by the same manufacturer—Cutter. On further investigation, it was established that certain lots of the Cutter vaccine were particularly implicated.

The Public Health Service immediately suspended vaccination, recalled the Cutter vaccine, and launched an intensive investigation, including a careful review of the regulations governing the manufacture of vaccine and the techniques employed by the companies.[79] Active virus was isolated from a number of vaccine lots. As a result, new requirements were introduced for safety testing along with a filtration step. With these relatively modest changes, the problem was solved, and no untoward reactions from the inactivated vaccine have since been observed.

Cutter produced the smallest amount of vaccine of any of the manufacturers, and the products of the other companies proved to be safe. Nonetheless, 260 cases of poliomyelitis were identified as being caused by the Cutter vaccine. Of these, 94 were in vaccinees, 126 were in family contacts, and 40 were in community contacts. Of the 260 cases, 192 were paralytic;

there were no deaths. Surprisingly, the "Cutter incident" did not shake public confidence in the vaccine, and when vaccination was resumed, it was well accepted. The outcome might have been very different if the product of just one other manufacturer had proved to be unsafe.

One important outcome of the Cutter incident was the creation of the surveillance unit at the Centers for Disease Control (now the Centers for Disease Control and Prevention [CDC]), which has maintained excellent scrutiny of polio and other vaccination programs.

With the resumption of vaccination in the United States and many other countries, the impact on the incidence of disease soon became evident.[80,81]

Live, Attenuated Vaccines

The use of attenuated forms of organisms for the induction of active immunity dates back at least to Jenner's use of the cowpox virus to immunize against smallpox. Pasteur reduced the virulence of rabies virus by the desiccation of infected spinal cords, and bacille Calmette-Guérin was attenuated by passage in an unfavorable medium. However, the first demonstration of attenuation of a virus in tissue culture was that of Lloyd and Theiler and their associates[82,83] with the yellow fever virus. The attenuated virus that resulted from prolonged passage in cultures of chick embryo tissue proved to be a safe and effective immunizing agent in humans.

The idea of attenuated poliovirus vaccines as opposed to killed vaccines appealed to many investigators, because it was presumed that an active infection most nearly reproduced the natural situation and could be expected to give longer-lasting immunity and greater resistance of the bowel to reinfection.

It was demonstrated in Enders's laboratory that the polioviruses lost virulence for the central nervous system on passage in non–nervous system tissues.[45] The characteristics of strains suitable as vaccines would need to include the following:

1. The capacity to parasitize the gut and induce neutralizing antibody
2. An inability to infect the central nervous system and thus cause disease
3. Genetic stability such that the strains would not revert to neurovirulence after multiplication in the human host (but see the comments below in the sections on *Disease Associated with the Oral Vaccine* and *Eradication*).

The approaches were, of necessity, empirical and involved passage of virus in rodents, various types of tissue culture, and a combination of the two.[61-64,84-86] The first published report on the use of a live, attenuated poliovirus in a human appeared in 1952 from Koprowski and co-workers.[61] They used virus attenuated by passage through cotton rats.

Three groups in the United States were the principal investigators working to develop a live, attenuated polio vaccine. They were Cox at Lederle, Koprowski and associates at the Wistar Institute in Philadelphia, and Sabin in Cincinnati. Cox and Koprowski were working with strains of the same origin, whereas Sabin developed his own set of mutant viruses. During the 1950s, much work was conducted to test the immunogenicity and safety of the vaccine strains in the laboratory. An important point at issue was the genetic

stability of the vaccine strains—would they revert to virulence after multiplying in the human host? Unfortunately, few in vitro markers of virulence, such as growth at higher temperature, were available, and these were not particularly precise. The most definitive test for neurovirulence was considered to be inoculation of monkeys intracerebrally or directly into the spinal cord. Although expensive and requiring expert interpretation, the monkey test was adopted as the definitive test for neurovirulence by the regulatory agencies. The literature from this period on attenuated vaccine viruses is voluminous, and no effort is made to provide a comprehensive bibliography here. However, a number of international conferences on poliomyelitis were held, some dealing specifically with the oral attenuated vaccines, and a perusal of the findings from these conferences can provide one with a reasonably complete picture of the development of the vaccines and their early use.[87-94]

Field trials of increasingly large size were conducted with the various candidate strains in different parts of the world. It was difficult to conduct large-scale trials in the United States because the Salk vaccine had been licensed and was being used widely; therefore, only a few trials were conducted there.[95-97] Originally, the different types of vaccines were fed separately because some degree of interference occurred among them. However, it was later found that, by adjusting the amounts, virus interference could be overcome to a large extent; a trivalent vaccine thereby became possible. In 1957, a World Health Organization (WHO) committee recommended that field trials be conducted with Sabin's strains.[92] The first large-scale trial of these strains occurred in 1958. In Singapore, 200,000 children received type 2 vaccine in an effort to abort, through interference, a type 1 epidemic. The vaccine virus did indeed appear to interfere with the wild virus and to be safe. In the same year, Sabin provided Professor Chumakov of Moscow a supply of his attenuated virus strains, which were used for early field trials and as seed for the manufacture of vaccine in what was then the Union of Soviet Socialist Republics (USSR). The Soviets moved rapidly. In just over a year, approximately 15 million people were vaccinated without any recorded untoward event and with evident effectiveness. By 1960, about 100 million people in the USSR and Eastern European countries had received the three individual types of Sabin vaccine separately.[98,99] This large success was presented as evidence to support an application for licensure in the United States of the Sabin live poliovirus vaccine. Dr. Dorothy Horstmann was asked to visit the USSR and Eastern European countries to evaluate the program and the reliability of the data. Her report in 1959 was favorable,[100] and, in part on the basis of her evaluation, the vaccine was licensed in 1960. Thus, within just over 10 years from the time that tissue culture techniques were first described, two effective and safe vaccines against poliomyelitis were available for general use.

Role of the National Foundation for Infantile Paralysis

An important element in the developments leading up to the achievement of poliovirus vaccines was the National

Foundation for Infantile Paralysis. The foundation was established in 1938 as a goal-oriented voluntary organization. Its principal goal was to prevent polio, and thus a significant proportion of the money raised by voluntary contributions was used to support virus research and fellowships for investigators. The scientific program was led by Dr. Thomas Rivers, who enlisted as advisers the most knowledgeable individuals from the scientific community. Benison's book, *An Oral History Memoir*,[16] gives an interesting account of the conduct of the research effort. Once a vaccine became a possibility, the foundation supported the developmental work by Salk and Sabin and financed the large-scale field trial of the inactivated vaccine. The way in which this program was conducted effectively illustrates how biomedical research can function in solving a practical problem. The first need is to establish a knowledge base, which is derived from basic explorations. Only when the scientific base has been laid can the practical goal—in this instance, the vaccine—be successfully pursued.[101]

The Simian Virus 40 Episode

In 1960, Sweet and Hilleman described the isolation of a virus that caused a typical vacuolation in cells from cynomolgus monkeys; the virus had been isolated from cultures of rhesus monkey kidney cells.[102] This virus, simian virus 40 (SV40), was found to cause an inapparent infection in rhesus monkeys in nature. It remained latent in the kidney cells until activated in tissue culture and could be detected only by testing in cultured cells from a susceptible species. It was found to be a contaminant of many lots of both inactivated and live vaccines. SV40's inactivation curve with formaldehyde was such that some active virus might survive an exposure that was fully adequate to inactivate poliovirus.[103]

Once the presence of the contaminating virus was recognized, proper measures were taken to ensure its exclusion from the vaccine. However, this finding did cause a great deal of concern, because SV40 was a DNA virus of the papovavirus family and had been shown to cause cancer in several species of animals and to transform cells in culture.[104,105] Evidence was presented that some people who received contaminated poliovirus vaccines orally or parenterally developed antibodies to SV40,[106–108] and that virus occasionally was isolated from the feces of recipients of oral poliovirus vaccine (OPV).[109] Similar findings were obtained with volunteer subjects who had received SV40 by the respiratory route.[110] In some populations, antibodies to SV40 were present in sera collected before poliovirus vaccines had been available, suggesting that the antibodies were evoked by natural infection with related viruses.[111,112]

Two epidemiologic approaches have been taken in assessing whether SV40-contaminated vaccine causes any deleterious effects in recipients. Fraumeni and associates compared the causes of mortality, particularly from cancer, between populations that presumably had received SV40-contaminated vaccine and those that had not.[113] No differences of any kind were found. In addition, during an observation period of 17 to 19 years, prospective surveillance of a cohort of approximately 1077 infants who received contaminated OPV in the first days of life and 150

who received inactivated (killed) poliovirus vaccine (IPV) that contained SV40 intramuscularly revealed no excessive incidence of cancer or mortality from any other cause.[114,115] These findings, although not absolute proof of the benignity of SV40 in humans, are reassuring, and it seems highly unlikely that SV40 is carcinogenic or otherwise pathogenic for humans. However, the experience with SV40 has clearly demonstrated one of the problems associated with the use of primary cell cultures to produce vaccines and biologics for use in humans.

Killed Poliovirus Vaccine Versus Oral Poliovirus Vaccine

The new availability of the live (OPV) vaccine prompted a comparison with the IPV already in use. The principal points raised were the following:

1. IPV had been used widely for approximately 6 years and had proved to be safe and effective.
2. OPV was less expensive and much simpler to administer. Thus it was more suitable than IPV for mass campaigns and programs directed at difficult-to-reach populations, because IPV had to be administered by injection with a four-dose schedule.
3. The principal disadvantage of OPV was its relative lability, compared with that of IPV, at temperatures above freezing. There was also concern that it would not be effective in the presence of an enterovirus infection.
4. Early evidence indicated that, whereas both vaccines gave satisfactory protection against paralytic disease, the active infection of the bowel that occurred with OPV resulted in resistance to reinfection more similar to that resulting from natural infection. Conversely, IPV seemed to produce little resistance to intestinal infection.[116,117] Thus OPV could be expected to be more effective than IPV in interrupting the spread of the virus within the community. A side benefit of OPV was thought to be the spread of the vaccine virus from vaccinees to susceptible contacts, thus amplifying its effect.[118–121]
5. In spite of the 1954 field trial's evidence of the effectiveness of IPV, there was some concern that outbreaks of paralytic disease were still occurring between 1955, when IPV was licensed, and 1961, when OPV became available. Thus some questions were raised about the true effectiveness of IPV as it was produced and used in the United States; indeed, Berkovich and colleagues[122] presented evidence that the 1959 epidemic of polio in Boston was likely caused by the use of low-potency vaccine.

In 1962, Luther Terry, the Surgeon General of the U.S. Public Health Service, issued Public Health Service recommendations for the use of poliomyelitis vaccine for the 1962 poliomyelitis season.[123] The relative advantages of OPV and the IPV were enumerated, but neither vaccine was recommended to the exclusion of the other. However, OPV was soon being given almost exclusively in the United States. By 1964, the Committee on the Control of Infectious Diseases of the American Academy of

Pediatrics[124] expressed a clear preference for OPV: "Evaluation of the virtues and limitations of killed and live polio vaccines reveals a clearcut superiority of the OPV from the point of view of ease of administration, immunogenic effect, protective capacity, and potential for the eradication of poliomyelitis."

As already indicated, the USSR had previously determined to use OPV exclusively, and most countries did the same. However, Sweden, Finland, and the Netherlands chose to administer only IPV and thus provided an interesting population with which to compare the effectiveness of IPV and OPV. In the early years of OPV use, monotypic vaccines were used in sequence—vaccines 1, 3, and 2 at 6-week or 2-month intervals, followed 6 months later by a dose of trivalent vaccine. Later, the trivalent vaccine was found to be adequate, and a simplified regimen was adopted in the United States: three doses of trivalent vaccine at 2-month intervals beginning at 2 months of age, given simultaneously with the first inoculation of the diphtheria and tetanus toxoids and pertussis (DTP) vaccine. A fourth dose of trivalent OPV approximately 1 year later completed the series, and a fifth dose was administered on entry to school.[125]

In those countries that have been able to achieve a high level of immunization, whether with OPV or IPV, paralytic poliomyelitis has become almost unknown. This group encompasses most of the industrialized countries. Among less developed countries, Cuba and Costa Rica[126] appear to have achieved eradication. In the United States, the fall in incidence of paralytic polio that had begun with the introduction of IPV in 1955 continued at much the same rate after 1963, when OPV became the predominant vaccine in use. By 1969, only about a dozen cases were recorded in the entire country, and this average has continued up to the present, except that in more recent years all the cases have been vaccine associated. A total of 69 cases were reported from 1978 to 1983. Fifty-one cases were classified as vaccine associated, six of which occurred in immunodeficient children.[127] Furthermore, only one case of infection caused by a wild strain (nonvaccine) of poliovirus has been identified since 1980.

Disease Associated with the Oral Poliovirus Vaccine

Although OPV has been highly effective, its benefits have been achieved at some cost, namely, vaccine-associated cases of paralysis. Largely because of the excellent surveillance system that had been set up by the CDC, it was recognized soon after OPV became used on a large scale that cases of paralytic disease were occurring in vaccinees and their intimate contacts. Given the time of year when these cases occurred, the temporal association with vaccination, and the fact that the virus isolated from the cases had the characteristics of vaccine strains, there was a strong presumption that these cases of paralytic disease were caused by the vaccine virus.[128–130] As more data have accumulated, it is clear that only rarely do either vaccinees or contacts contract paralytic polio from the vaccine virus. A small proportion of these patients are immunodeficient, but most have no detectable immunologic or other abnormality that

might enhance their susceptibility to infection. It also has been shown that some normal vaccinees develop viremia, usually owing to type 2 virus, although this viremia does not seem to be associated with paralytic disease.[131–133]

In a 10-year multinational study conducted under the auspices of the WHO, it was found that vaccine-associated cases developed in all countries but that there was considerable variation in incidence, with a few countries having notably higher rates than others[134–136]; no reason for this variation was identified. Type 3 virus was isolated most often from cases in vaccinees, and type 2 from contact cases. From the data of the WHO study and additional data gathered in the United States by the CDC, rough estimates of the risk of paralysis to vaccinees and contacts can be made. Based on the number of doses of vaccine distributed, the risk to recipients and contacts is well below one case per 1 million doses. However, the risk from the first dose (one case per 500,000 doses administered for recipients and contacts) is considerably higher than that from subsequent doses (one case per 13 million doses). Thus, OPV does pose a small risk to recipients of the vaccine and their nonimmune intimate contacts, most of whom are adults. Obviously, the risk to contacts should be further reduced as the level of immunity in the community is increased. In most circumstances, the risk-benefit ratio is acceptable. However, in countries such as the United States, in which vaccine-associated cases account for all the indigenous cases of paralytic polio, even though few, consideration led to changing the policy so as to use IPV for primary immunization, which, as far as we know, carries no risk.[137–140] The pertinence of this consideration was enhanced by a number of developments.

Workers at the Rijks Institut voor de Volksgezardheid in Bilthoven, the Netherlands, developed a more potent and more highly purified IPV[141] that requires only two doses—possibly one—for primary immunization.[142] Furthermore, polio vaccine can be successfully combined with DTP vaccine, as well as other antigens, greatly simplifying the use of IPV.[143]

Data from those countries that have used only IPV[144–147] indicate unequivocally that poliomyelitis has been controlled and that the virus can no longer be recovered from the environment. In each instance, the percentage of the population immunized has been very high (approximately 90%), and herd immunity seems to have been achieved. It has been hypothesized that, in societies in which fecal–oral spread is limited, the principal route of spread is from close contact, and pharyngeal virus is the most important source of infection. Infection of the pharyngeal cells is suppressed much more readily by circulating antibody than is infection of the lower bowel, which is relatively insensitive to antibody and where high titers are required to show any demonstrable effect.[147,148] Even in highly immunized populations, however, small outbreaks of paralytic poliomyelitis resulting from wild viruses have occurred in groups of people who were not immunized. This type of outbreak occurred in the Netherlands among a religious sect that rejected vaccination.

In 1984, there was a small outbreak of type 3 polio in Finland.[149,150] There had been no poliomyelitis in Finland for 20 years when, in October 1984, a few cases of clinical disease occurred. Type 3 virus of wild type was isolated from all the patients, 45% of 86 intimate contacts, and 15% of 700 well children in the vicinity. The same virus also was isolated from sewage at a number of sites in the country. Nine cases of paralysis and one of meningoencephalitis were reported. All but two of the patients had been immunized, and the one fatality, a 17-year-old male adolescent, had received five doses of IPV. In attempting to explain the re-establishment of wild poliovirus in a highly immunized population that had been virus free for many years, three factors were identified as possible contributing causes:

1. The vaccine that had been in use was found to be of marginal potency for type 3 virus.
2. There had been a drop in the percentage of infants and young children receiving vaccine.
3. There was a minor antigenic difference between the circulating wild virus and the virus in the vaccine.

It is probable that the most important factor was the poor potency of the vaccine, although the other factors may have played some role.

In response to the evidence of widespread infection, 1.5 million children younger than 19 years were given a dose of IPV, and, in a mass campaign shortly thereafter, a dose of OPV was administered to approximately 94% of the entire population of 4.5 million. At present, the country is once again polio free, and the regular use of a more potent IPV has been resumed.

The Finnish experience is instructive in several ways. First, it emphasizes the value of an effective surveillance program. Second, it indicates that attention should be paid to monitoring the potency of the vaccines being used and again illustrates the relationship among vaccine potency, antibody response, and protection. However, it does not appear to support the hypothesis that prior experience with the antigen, even in the absence of detectable antibody, primes the immune system so that response to infection will be rapid enough to prevent disease. Third, even in the relatively small, homogeneous country of Finland, with its well-organized health care delivery system, there was some decrease in the percentage of vaccinated children in the population. This suggests that, as one might expect, with the disappearance of a disease for 20 years or more, it becomes more difficult to motivate both the public and the health providers to sustain immunization against a threat that seems purely theoretical. Finally, it is reassuring that, in spite of considerable seeding of the population with a virulent strain of poliovirus, only a few cases of paralytic disease occurred; presumably, the high level of immunity in the community kept it in check.

Another experience that has been instructive is the 1982 epidemic of paralytic polio in Taiwan.[151] This epidemic, in which there were 1031 recorded cases of paralytic disease (and an overall attack rate of 5.8 per 100,000), was the largest outbreak in the history of Taiwan. The outbreak occurred although there had been only the occasional case of paralytic polio since 1975. Routine immunization with OPV had been conducted since 1967, and approximately 80% of infants had received at least two doses of trivalent OPV. Thus the level of immunization was quite high, comparable with that in most of the industrialized countries. Approximately 66% of the cases had received no vaccine, and 19% had received only one dose. The evidence indicated that the epidemic was due primarily to a pool of non-immunized susceptible people rather than to a failure of the vaccine. Indeed, vaccine efficacy was calculated to be 82% for one dose and more than 95% for two or more doses.

This experience reinforces the observation that polio can occur in nonimmunized susceptible people even when there is a high overall rate of vaccination. In spite of the widespread use of OPV for a number of years, spread from vaccinees to nonvaccinated susceptible people seems not to have been an important factor in supplementing immunity in the population. This result tends to conform with the observation of Fox and colleagues[119] that, whereas vaccine strains disseminate readily to susceptible people within the family, spread to less intimate contacts is limited. It has also raised the question as to whether OPV induces intestinal immunity that is as effective and long lasting as is generally believed.[152,153]

Polio in Developing Countries

Poliomyelitis presents a special problem in developing countries, particularly those in the tropical zone. It is only recently that poliomyelitis has been recognized as a significant problem in these countries. With careful surveillance and the conducting of lameness surveys, a considerable reservoir of paralytic disease in children has been detected.[154,155] Indeed, the incidence of crippling disease in those countries in which surveys were done was found to be as high as in industrialized countries before vaccine was available. Epidemiologically, the disease occurs in young children, and there is no seasonal peak.

It was expected that OPV would be the ideal vaccine in Third World countries.[156] Experience in Cuba and Costa Rica, in particular, indicated a high level of effectiveness, and paralytic disease has virtually disappeared.[126] However, in other developing countries, particularly those in the tropical zone, experience has not been so satisfactory. The problem is due in part to the lability of the vaccine (i.e., exposure to high temperatures leads to inactivation), so that the vaccine must be kept refrigerated at all times. This is not always easy to guarantee in tropical, underdeveloped countries. Even when the so-called *cold chain* has been well managed, however, the live vaccines have proved to be less effective in these environments than anticipated; the exact reason for this is not known. Speculation has included the possibility of (1) interference by other enteroviruses that tend to be prevalent in these populations, (2) interference in some nonspecific way owing to diarrhea that is common in infants in these countries, and (3) antibody in the breast milk. Although there does seem to be a difference in effectiveness in the tropical countries, in those situations in which the active vaccine has been delivered to a large proportion of the population, satisfactory control of the disease has been possible. Thus the problem seems to be as much logistical as it is scientific.

Most of the successful programs in tropical or developing countries have employed the technique of mass vaccination campaigns. Sabin has been the principal proponent of this approach, and there is no question that, when the logistics are well handled, this technique can be highly effective.[157-160] However, legitimate concern has been expressed that such targeted campaigns can absorb resources to the detriment of a broader sustained health care program based on primary care, which few would disagree is the ultimate goal. In many countries, unfortunately, this goal is not realizable in the near future, and targeted campaigns ideally should be used to further this goal rather than retard it.

With the production of the more potent IPV, there has been increased interest in its use in developing and tropical countries.[161,162] IPV is more heat stable, has antibody response as good as or better than OPV, and has no untoward effects. In spite of these advantages, however, it still must be given parenterally, which requires needles and syringes. Jet injectors might overcome this need, but they present major problems of maintenance in the field. It may be that some prepackaged system (e.g., Ezeject), such as was developed by Hilleman and associates[163] for measles, will help solve the delivery problem. However, there are still the matters of cost and the safe disposal of used syringes.

Thus, for use in developing and tropical countries, both OPV and IPV have advantages and disadvantages. OPV is inexpensive, easy to administer, and ideally suited for use in mass campaigns and in situations lacking adequately trained health professionals. However, it is less effective in tropical climates for unknown reasons, and its sensitivity to heat makes it difficult to transport and store. It is doubtful that the greater intestinal immunity conferred by OPV, or its somewhat limited capacity to spread to unvaccinated people, is a major factor in its favor in the tropical environment.

IPV is more stable, seems to be fully effective in the tropics, and, with the development of more potent vaccines, requires no more doses than does OPV. However, it is still much more expensive than OPV and, because it must be injected, requires a more sophisticated delivery system.

Regardless of which vaccine is used, it would seem that, if paralytic polio is to be controlled in tropical countries, a high rate of immunization (80% to 90%) in young infants must be achieved and maintained. The need for sustaining a high level of immunity in infants and young children is probably greater in the tropical zone, where viral dissemination occurs year round, than in the temperate zone, where dissemination is seasonal.[164] This immunity level demands political commitment and adequate infrastructure, both of which are often lacking.

Molecular Biology of Poliomyelitis and Implications for the Future

Rapid advances in molecular biology have made it possible to learn more about the structure of the poliovirus and its genome. This information offers the prospect of manipulating virulence; preparing more stable, inexpensive, and safe vaccines; and accurately characterizing viral strains.[165–167]

Results of studies on the structure of the viral particle have shown that populations of virions are made up of infective particles—designated as D particles—and noninfective, or empty, particles—designated as C particles. These two types of particles are similar antigenically but have detectable differences that may be related to tertiary structure. The viral capsid is composed of 60 copies of each

of four polypeptides (V_1, V_2, V_3, and V_4) that surround the single-stranded RNA genome of about 7450 nucleotides.[168]

A key observation that set the stage for exploration of the molecular biology of poliovirus was that of Racaniello and Baltimore,[169] who were able to prepare DNA complementary to the poliovirus RNA and to show that this DNA was infectious when introduced into mammalian cells. This finding has made possible genetic manipulation that was otherwise impossible.

The base sequence of poliovirus RNA and complementary DNA has been established. Progress has been rapid in determining the relationship between the genomic location and the polypeptide structure, including the identity of certain epitopes and their position on the genome; this information makes it possible to produce the specific peptides using cloning techniques. Purified or synthetic peptides are rarely very antigenic in themselves and require some form of adjuvant. Wimmer and colleagues, however, have shown that two relatively small peptides (VP1) derived from the polypeptides of type 1 poliovirus were capable of priming an animal so that a broad antibody response was obtained on reimmunization.[170] It is also possible to consider construction of a strain of poliovirus possessing the key epitopes of the three types.[167]

Rapid progress is being made in defining the molecular basis for virulence or the lack of it. Although the construction of stable avirulent strains is far from possible now, it is a reasonable goal. Avirulent types 1 and 2 have more base substitutions compared with wild strains than does type 3, which may explain the greater genetic instability of the type 3 virus.

At a less sophisticated level, the treatment of poliovirus RNA with ribonuclease T_1 produces a variety of oligonucleotides that, when separated by two-dimensional electrophoresis, give a "fingerprint" that is characteristic for each viral strain.[171] This technique makes possible what is referred to as *molecular epidemiology*, by which the source of viral isolates can be defined with comparative ease. Vaccine strains can be distinguished from wild strains, and a particular virus can be tracked. This technique was used with the agent that infected people belonging to a religious sect in the Netherlands who transmitted it to contacts in Canada and the United States. With the use of oligonucleotide fingerprinting, the infectious agent was shown to be the same virus strain. The polymerase chain reaction is another means of rapid, accurate characterization of virus strain.

Thus, aside from their innate scientific interest, studies of the molecular biology of the poliovirus offer the prospect of practical outcomes, such as cheaper, more stable, and more effective vaccines, as well as new tools for epidemiologic investigations and diagnosis.

Eradication of Poliomyelitis

From the experiences in many countries, it is evident that paralytic disease caused by wild poliovirus can be eliminated. Elimination may be achieved with either IPV or OPV, provided that a high level of immunization is obtained and maintained in the population. With the present OPV strains, rare cases of paralysis resulting from the vaccine viruses will continue to occur in vaccinees and their contacts. With the available OPV, then, it does not appear that paralytic disease caused by polioviruses can be totally eliminated. However, it has been pointed out that this elimination has been achieved with the sole use of IPV or a combined regimen, such as was used in Denmark.[172]

If we define *control* of poliomyelitis as a reduction of poliovirus-induced paralytic disease to very low levels, such as exist in the United States, we can consider this level of control to have been achieved in most of the industrialized countries and in some developing countries. However, *eradication*, defined as an absence of the causative agent from the environment, has seldom been accomplished for any length of time. Even when eradication has been demonstrated, as in Finland, where for many years polioviruses could not be isolated from sewage samples, infection and disease can occur from wild viruses introduced from the outside; such infection can occur even when only a small group of susceptible people remains in the population. Thus, as long as wild polioviruses exist in the world, it will be necessary to maintain consistently high levels of immunization to control or eradicate poliomyelitis in a country or region.

Obviously, if worldwide eradication of polioviruses could be accomplished, as was done successfully with smallpox, it would no longer be necessary to continue vaccination. In reviewing whether diseases other than smallpox might be eradicated, Stetten[173] cited polio as a possibility, and it was considered further at the 1980 International Conference on the Eradication of Infectious Diseases.[174]

Certain features make the global eradication of poliomyelitis technically feasible.[175–177] These features include the following:

1. Immunity can be provided by two excellent vaccines, and viral transmission can be interrupted.
2. There is no animal reservoir.
3. There are only three immunologic types of virus.
4. OPV is inexpensive and easy to administer in mass campaigns.
5. It is expected that the more potent IPV will require fewer doses for primary immunization and will be less expensive than OPV.

The features of polio that militate against its easy eradication are as follows:

1. IPV is relatively inefficient in preventing the spread of virus.
2. Poliovirus is contagious, particularly by the fecal–oral route.
3. The use of OPV in tropical countries has had peculiar problems.
4. Eradication efforts are complicated by the technical issues concerning administration of the vaccine, such as monitoring a cold chain, particularly for OPV; the need to give IPV by injection; and cost factors, particularly for IPV.
5. Recent evidence has indicated that the polioviruses are subject to recombination with other enteroviruses leading to persistent circulation of strains that have reverted to neurovirulence. The most dramatic example is the experience in the island of Hispaniola, which includes the countries of Haiti and the Dominican Republic. There had been no confirmed

cases of paralytic polio in either country since 1989. In the years 2000 and 2001 a small outbreak of paralytic polio was confirmed. The virus was found to be a Type 1 but was demonstrably different genetically from the vaccine virus or the wild type and is referred to as Vaccine Derived Polio Virus (VDPV). The outbreak was controlled by saturating the area with OPV. The finding emphasizes the need to maintain a high level of immunity in the population if OPV is being used.[177a]

6. Probably most important is whether, in many countries, the political will exists that is so necessary for a successful effort to be undertaken. There is continual tension between those who favor mass campaigns and those who emphasize the value of incorporating vaccination into primary care programs and consider mass campaigns as distracting and as diverting resources from the development of ongoing basic health services.
7. Verification of success will be more difficult than was the case with smallpox. Inapparent infection occurs often (100 to 1000 people are infected for each paralytic case), requiring the use of methods such as sewage sampling and population surveys to demonstrate the absence of wild viruses. Furthermore, a number of other viruses and conditions can mimic paralytic poliomyelitis.[178–180] A particularly dramatic example of this was the 1982 epidemic of enterovirus 71 infection in Bulgaria, in which there were more than 700 nonparalytic cases, with 149 cases of paralysis and 44 deaths.[181] These cases could be distinguished from poliomyelitis only by virus isolation and antibody determination.

At the 1984 International Symposium on Poliomyelitis Control, it was concluded that, whereas global eradication of poliomyelitis was probably technically feasible, a realistic goal for the near future should be the control of paralytic disease, with eradication in certain countries or regions.[182]

In spite of the difficulties that were anticipated, the Pan-American Health Organization in 1985 began a major campaign to eradicate poliovirus from the Western Hemisphere. Support from the countries of the region has been remarkably strong, and various organizations have contributed resources, including Rotary International, which has provided considerable support in money and volunteer workers.

The program has required skilled management and organization, and a remarkable spirit of cooperation has been generated. Regional laboratories have been set up, surveillance systems organized, and volunteer participation enlisted. To a great extent, countries have relied on mass campaigns with oral vaccine. When suspicious cases have occurred in an area, house-to-house programs have been conducted to saturate the area. One of the most difficult problems has been to differentiate poliomyelitis cases from paralysis due to other causes. This process requires conducting a careful clinical evaluation, obtaining adequate specimens, and transporting these specimens to a laboratory in good time.[183] Another problem that has had to be solved is distinguishing between wild viruses and vaccine strains, the latter being widely disseminated in the environment.

Molecular biologic techniques such as polymerase chain reaction have been developed at the CDC and are highly sensitive and discriminating. The program has been remarkably successful, and most countries of the Americas have had no cases of infection caused by wild poliovirus for periods of years. The last case was diagnosed in Peru in September 1991, although compatible cases still occur in which polio cannot be ruled out.

Following these efforts, the problem then became that of proving that eradication had been achieved. An international commission for certification was established similar to the one that was created during the smallpox campaign. The commission stipulated certain criteria that must be met for certification to be proven[184]:

1. No cases of poliomyelitis caused by a wild virus for 3 years within the hemisphere
2. A satisfactory surveillance system, including adequate diagnostic procedures to distinguish poliovirus infection from other causes of acute flaccid paralysis
3. Environmental surveys (e.g., sewage, stool surveys) that demonstrate the absence of wild poliovirus

In 1994, the International Commission for Certification of Poliomyelitis Eradication in the Americas met to review the individual country reports. No cases caused by wild virus had occurred since the one in 1991. It was found that environmental surveys were not very useful but that the large number of specimens tested from suspect cases and their contacts, all of which were negative, provided adequate data. The commission concluded that the evidence was sufficient to declare that eradication had been achieved in the Western Hemisphere.[185]

The experience in the Americas has been instrumental in the WHO Assembly's initiation of a program of global eradication.[186] Eradication will not be an easy task; it would be expedited were a heat-stable vaccine available. Thus the development of such a vaccine has been given priority by international bodies. In spite of the absence of a more stable vaccine, the global eradication of polio is proceeding remarkably well. There is reason to believe that eradication has been achieved in China, and mass immunization days are being conducted in many countries in Eastern Europe, Asia, and Africa. The WHO set a goal of global eradication by the year 2000. This was not achieved, but there is reason to believe that it can occur within 5+ years. (A summary of the status of the global program as of 1997 was reviewed in a special issue of the *Journal of Infectious Diseases*.[187]) Only when global eradication has been achieved will it be possible to cease routine vaccination—the eventual goal—and to relegate poliomyelitis and its causative virus to history. The CDC has published a statement indicating that type 2 poliovirus is no longer circulating globally.

A surprising event occurred in July 2000 through February 2001 on the island of Hispaniola, where 17 cases of paralytic polio caused by poliovirus were identified, 3 in Haiti and 14 in the Dominican Republic. The last case of wild polio infection was in 1989. The causative agent was type 1 poliovirus, but, on genotyping, it was found to be closely related to the vaccine virus and more distantly related to wild virus. It is referred to as vaccine-derived virus or a mutant. It is presumed that, because of the low level of immunization of this population, the vaccine virus

was able to circulate, thus leading to mutation. The outbreak was controlled by an intensive campaign of vaccination. This experience emphasizes the importance of maintaining a high level of immunity in the population.

Although not published, evidence has been presented that a vaccine-derived type 2 mutant circulated for a number of years in Egypt and may have been present in China and Israel.

Vaccination Regimens

As has previously been indicated, different vaccines and different regimens are used in different countries. Much of the world uses OPV (i.e., trivalent oral polio vaccine) exclusively, whereas Sweden, Finland, France, and the Netherlands use only IPV, in most instances combined with DPT or with diphtheria and tetanus toxoids (DT). Certain countries in Africa, particularly the French-speaking countries, are also using IPV. Denmark employs IPV for primary immunization combined with DT, followed by three doses of OPV. Some countries use mass campaigns once or twice a year; in Brazil, for example, there is a 2-day period twice a year when every young child, regardless of previous history, is immunized. Neither the vaccine nor the regimen adopted seems to be critical, provided that adequate coverage is achieved.

In 1988, the Evaluation of Poliomyelitis Vaccine Policy Options Committee of the Institute of Medicine of the National Academy of Sciences[188] recommended that primary immunization in the United States should be with combined DPT-IPV, to be followed later by a dose of OPV. This recommendation was made because the only poliovirus-induced paralysis since 1980 was caused by the vaccine virus. This regimen should prevent most vaccine cases and still provide intestinal immunity.[189] More recently, the recommendation has been made to use only IPV unless there is a specific situation for OPV. If there is no history of immunization or if the history is unknown, three doses of IPV 1 month apart can be given to the contact, and the child can receive the first dose of OPV simultaneously with the third IPV dose.

Although such a procedure is prudent, it has been stressed repeatedly that immunization of the adult should not be allowed to interfere with immunization of the infant. Only parents or others having comparable intimate contact with the infant are at risk, and mothers are at greater risk than fathers. Although such advice is not always mentioned in official recommendations, it would probably be wise to advise the contacts to wash their hands, particularly after changing diapers, and to educate them about properly disposing of soiled diapers.

Although there is still much to be done before eradication of wild polioviruses is achieved, consideration is already being given to how we should proceed when it is accomplished. Of course, the key issue is when or if vaccination should be terminated. A number of issues must be considered.

OPV should no longer be used after eradication since it causes a rare case of paralytic disease and can be transmitted to the susceptible contacts. Furthermore, immunodeficient persons may excrete the vaccine virus for long periods of time (years) and as has been seen on several occasions may mutate to become more like the wild virus. As long as OPV is in use it is important that a high level of immunity be maintained in the population (≥80%) in order to inhibit circulation of OPV or the vaccine-derived polio virus (VDPV). With the cessation of OPV, vaccination should be continued with IPV. Unfortunately, it is difficult to determine how long IPV should be continued because we are not sure about the frequency of long-term excretors nor how long excretion persists in such persons.

Another issue that has to be considered when eradication is achieved is laboratory containment of wild virus. Specimens of wild polioviruses exist in laboratories throughout the world. Although poliovirus is not the ideal agent for bio warfare, it could cause trouble if a wild strain escaped from a laboratory when most of the population was non-immune. WHO has requested countries to take a census of those labs that harbor specimens of wild poliovirus and to assure that proper precautions are taken to prevent escape.[190,191,192]

Because practices are subject to change, one should be aware of the sources of information about current recommendations of the various official or quasi-official bodies. One such source is the package insert prepared by the vaccine manufacturer and approved by the Food and Drug Administration. Another is the American Academy of Pediatrics' *Red Book: Report of the Committee on Infectious Diseases*, which is revised every few years. The recommendations of the Advisory Committee on Immunization Practices serve as the basis for decisions by most governmental agencies and are usually in agreement with the *Red Book*. These recommendations are published in the *Morbidity and Mortality Weekly Report* of the CDC. Finally, there is the *Guide for Adult Immunization* of the American College of Physicians.

REFERENCES

1. Hutchin EF. Historical summary. *In* Poliomyelitis: A Survey Made Possible by a Grant from the International Committee for the Study of Infantile Paralysis. Baltimore, Williams & Wilkins, 1932, pp 1–22.
2. Heine J. Beobachtungen Über Lahmungs zustande der unteren Extremitatien und deren Behandlung. Stuttgart, Kohler, 1840.
3. Medin O. Über eine Epidemic von spinaler Kinderlahmung. Verh Int Med Kongr 2(6):37, 1891.
4. Paul JR. Poliomyelitis. *In* Clinical Epidemiology. Chicago, University of Chicago Press, 1966, pp 177–195.
5. Landsteiner K, Popper E. Mikroscopische Preparate von einem menschlichen and zwei Affenruckenmarken. Klin Wochenschr 21:1830, 1908.
6. Landsteiner K, Popper E. Übertragung der Poliomyelitis acuta auf Affen. Z Immunitaetsforsch Exp Ther 2:377, 1909.
7. Armstrong C. The experimental transmission of poliomyelitis to the eastern cotton rat. Public Health Rep 54:1719, 1939.
8. Li CP, Schaeffer M. Adaptation of type 1 poliomyelitis virus to mice. Proc Soc Exp Biol Med 82:477, 1953.
9. Melnick JL, Horstmann DM. Active immunity to poliomyelitis in chimpanzees following subclinical infection. J Exp Med 85:287, 1947.
10. Howe HA, Bodian D, Morgan IM. Subclinical poliomyelitis in the chimpanzee and its relation to alimentary reinfection. Am J Hyg 51:85, 1950.
11. Rivers TM. Immunity in virus diseases with particular reference to poliomyelitis. Am J Public Health 26:136, 1936.
12. Hammon WMcD. Possibilities of specific prevention and treatment of poliomyelitis. Pediatrics 6:696, 1950.
13. Brodie M, Park WH. Active immunization against poliomyelitis. Am J Public Health 26:119, 1936.
14. Kolmer JA. Vaccination against acute anterior poliomyelitis. Am J Public Health 26:126, 1936.
15. Leake JP. Poliomyelitis following vaccination against this disease. JAMA 105:2152, 1935.
16. Benison S. Tom Rivers: reflections on a life in medicine and science. *In* Benison S (ed). An Oral History Memoir. Cambridge, MA, MIT Press, 1967, pp 184–190.
17. Rivers TM. Discussion of papers on poliomyelitis by William M. Park, MD, and Maurice Brodie, MD, and John A. Kolmer, MD, October 1938. *In* Benison S (ed). An Oral History Memoir. Cambridge, MA, MIT Press, 1967, pp 599–601.
18. Van Rooyen CF, Rhodes AJ. Virus Diseases of Man. London, Oxford University Press, 1940.
19. Robbins FC, Enders JF. Tissue culture techniques in the study of animal viruses. Am J Med Sci 220:316, 1950.
20. Sabin AB, Olitsky PK. Cultivation of poliomyelitis virus in vitro in human embryonic nervous tissue. Proc Soc Exp Biol Med 31:357, 1936.
21. Burnet FM, Jackson AV. Poliomyelitis 4. The spread of poliomyelitis virus in cynomolgus monkeys with particular reference to infection by the pharyngeal-intestinal route. Aust J Exp Biol Med Sci 18:361, 1940.
22. Bodian D. Differentiation of types of poliomyelitis viruses. I. Reinfection experiments in monkeys (second attacks). Am J Hyg 49:200, 1949.
23. Morgan IM. Differentiation of types of poliomyelitis viruses. II. By reciprocal vaccination-immunity. Am J Hyg 49:225, 1949.
24. Bodian D, Morgan IM, Howe HA. Differentiation of types of poliomyelitis viruses. III. The grouping of fourteen strains into three basic immunological types. Am J Hyg 49:234, 1949.
25. Kessel JF, Pait CF. Immunologic groups of poliomyelitis viruses. Am J Hyg 51:76, 1950.
26. Hammon WM, Coriell LL, Wehrle PF, Stokes J. Evaluation of Red Cross gamma globulin as a prophylactic agent for poliomyelitis. 4. Final report of results based on clinical diagnoses. JAMA 151:1272, 1953.
27. Bodian D. A reconsideration of the pathogenesis of poliomyelitis. Am J Hyg 55:414, 1952.
28. Hammon WMcD. Immunity in poliomyelitis. Bacteriol Rev 13:135, 1949.
29. Burnet FM. Some aspects of the epidemiology of poliomyelitis. Proc R Aust Coll Physicians 4:95, 1949.
30. Enders JF, Weller TH, Robbins FC. Cultivation of the Lansing strain of poliomyelitis virus in cultures of various human embryonic tissues. Science 109:85, 1949.
31. Sabin AB. Non-cytopathic variants of poliomyelitis viruses and resistance to superinfection in tissue culture. Science 120:357, 1954.
32. Weller TH, Robbins FC, Enders JF. Cultivation of poliomyelitis virus in cultures of human foreskin and embryonic tissues. Proc Soc Exp Biol Med 72:153, 1949.
33. Weller TH, Enders JF, Robbins FC, Stoddard MB. Studies on the cultivation of poliomyelitis viruses in tissue culture. I. The propagation of poliomyelitis viruses in suspended cell cultures of various human tissues. J Immunol 69:645, 1952.
34. Robbins FC, Weller TH, Enders JF. Studies on the cultivation of poliomyelitis viruses in tissue culture. II. The propagation of poliomyelitis viruses in roller-tube cultures of various human tissues. J Immunol 69:673, 1952.
35. Smith WM, Chambers VC, Evans CA. Growth of neurotropic viruses in extraneural tissues: preliminary report on propagation of poliomyelitis virus [Lansing and Hof strains] in cultures of human testicular tissue. Northwest Med 49:368, 1950.
36. Syverton JT, Scherer WF, Butorac G. Propagation of poliomyelitis virus in cultures of monkey and human testicular tissues. Proc Soc Exp Biol Med 77:23, 1951.
37. Smith WM, Chambers VC, Evans CA. Growth of neurotropic viruses in extraneural tissues. IV. Poliomyelitis virus in human testicular tissue in vitro. Proc Soc Exp Biol Med 76:696, 1951.
38. Robbins FC, Enders JF, Weller TH. Cytopathogenic effect of poliomyelitis viruses in vitro on human embryonic tissues. Proc Soc Exp Biol Med 75:370, 1950.
39. Robbins FC, Enders JF, Weller TH, Florentino GL. Studies on the cultivation of poliomyelitis viruses in tissue culture. V. The direct isolation and serologic identification of virus strains in tissue culture from patients with nonparalytic and paralytic poliomyelitis. Am J Hyg 54:286, 1951.
40. Ledinko N, Riordan JT, Melnick JL. Multiplication of poliomyelitis viruses in tissue cultures of monkey testes. I. Growth curves of type 1

(Brunhilde) and type 2 (Lansing) strains and description of a quantitative neutralization test. Am J Hyg 55:323, 1952.

41. Riordan JT, Ledinko N, Melnick JL. Multiplication of poliomyelitis viruses in tissue cultures of monkey testes. II. Direct isolation and typing of strains from human stools and spinal cords in roller tubes. Am J Hyg 55:339, 1952.

42. Youngner JS, Ward EN, Salk JE. Studies on poliomyelitis viruses in cultures of monkey testicular tissue. I. Propagation of virus in roller tubes. Am J Hyg 55:291, 1952.

43. Youngner JS, Ward EN, Salk JE. Studies on poliomyelitis viruses in cultures of monkey testicular tissue. II. Differences among strains in tissue culture infectivity with preliminary data on the quantitative estimation of virus and antibody. Am J Hyg 55:301, 1952.

44. Youngner JS, Lewis LJ, Ward EN, Salk JE. Studies on poliomyelitis viruses in cultures of monkey testicular tissue. III. Isolation and immunologic identification of poliomyelitis viruses from fecal specimens by means of roller-tube cultures. Am J Hyg 55:347, 1952.

45. Enders JF, Robbins FC, Weller TH. The cultivation of the poliomyelitis viruses in tissue culture. Les Prix Nobel 1954. Stockholm, The Nobel Foundation, 1955.

46. Dulbecco R. Production of plaques in monolayer tissue cultures by single particles of an animal virus. Proc Natl Acad Sci U S A 38:747, 1952.

47. Dulbecco R, Vogt M. Plaque formation and isolation of pure lines with poliomyelitis viruses. J Exp Med 99:167, 1954.

48. Rous P, Jones FS. A method for obtaining suspensions of living cells from the fixed tissue, and for the plating out of individual cells. J Exp Med 23:549, 1916.

49. Melnick JL. Tissue culture techniques and their application to original isolation, growth, and assay of poliomyelitis and orphan viruses. Ann N Y Acad Sci 61:754, 1955.

50. Youngner JS. Monolayer tissue cultures. I. Preparation and standardization of suspensions of trypsin-dispersed monkey kidney cells. Proc Soc Exp Biol Med 85:202, 1954.

51. Youngner JS. Monolayer tissue cultures. II. Poliomyelitis virus assay in roller-tube cultures of trypsin-dispersed monkey kidney. Proc Soc Exp Biol Med 85:527, 1954.

52. Salk JE, Youngner JS, Ward EN. Use of color change of phenol red as the indicator in titrating poliomyelitis or its antibody in a tissue culture system. Am J Hyg 60:214, 1954.

53. Lipton MM, Steigman AJ. A simple colorimetric test for poliomyelitis virus and antibody. Proc Soc Exp Biol Med 88:114, 1955.

54. Robertson HE, Brunner KT, Syverton JT. Propagation in vitro of poliomyelitis viruses. VII. pH change of HeLa cell cultures for assay. Proc Soc Exp Biol Med 88:119, 1955.

55. Sanders M, Alexander RC. Epidemic keratoconjunctivitis. I. Isolation and identification of a filterable virus. J Exp Med 77:71, 1943.

56. Huang CH. Further studies on the titration of the western strain of equine encephalomyelitis virus in tissue culture. J Exp Med 78:111, 1943.

57. Huang CH. Titration of St. Louis encephalitis virus and Jungeblut-Sanders mouse virus in tissue culture. Proc Soc Exp Biol Med 54:158, 1943.

58. Huang CH. A visible method for titration and neutralization of viruses on the basis of pH changes in tissue cultures. Proc Soc Exp Biol Med 54:160, 1943.

59. Sanders M, Huang CH. Tissue cultures for virus investigations in the field. Am J Public Health 34:461, 1944.

60. Milzer A, Levinson SO, Shaughnessy HJ, et al. Immunogenicity studies in human subjects of trivalent tissue culture poliomyelitis vaccine inactivated by ultraviolet irradiation. Am J Public Health 44:26, 1954.

61. Koprowski H, Jervis GA, Norton TW. Immune responses in human volunteers upon oral administration of a rodent adapted strain of poliomyelitis virus. Am J Hyg 55:108, 1952.

62. Sabin AB, Hennessen WA, Winsser J. Studies on variants of poliomyelitis virus: experimental segregation and properties of avirulent variants of three immunologic types. J Exp Med 99:551, 1954.

63. Sabin AB. Immunity in poliomyelitis with special reference to vaccination. WHO Monogr Ser 26:297, 1955.

64. Sabin AB. Characteristics and genetic potentialities of experimentally produced and naturally occurring variants of poliomyelitis virus. Ann N Y Acad Sci 61:924, 1955.

65. Wolf AM, Shaughnessy HJ, Church RE, et al. Immunogenicity, in children, of ultraviolet-treated poliomyelitis vaccine. JAMA 161:775, 1956.

66. Salk JE, Bennett BL, Lewis LJ, et al. Studies in human subjects on active immunization against poliomyelitis. I. A preliminary report of experiments in progress. JAMA 151:1081, 1953.

67. Salk JE. Recent studies in immunization against poliomyelitis. Pediatrics 12:471, 1953.

68. Salk JE, Bennett BL, Lewis LJ, et al. Studies in human subjects on active immunization against poliomyelitis. II. A practical means of inducing and maintaining antibody formation. Am J Public Health 44:994, 1954.

69. Salk JE, Krech U, Youngner JS, et al. Formaldehyde treatment and safety testing of experimental poliomyelitis vaccines. Am J Public Health 44:563, 1954.

70. Salk JE. A concept of the mechanism of immunity for preventing paralyses in poliomyelitis. Ann N Y Acad Sci 61:1023, 1955.

71. Bodian D, Paffenbarger RS. Poliomyelitis infection in households: frequency of viremia and specific antibody response. Am J Hyg 60:83, 1954.

72. Horstmann DM, McCollum RW, Mascola AD. Viremia in human poliomyelitis. J Exp Med 99:355, 1954.

73. Rivers TM. Vaccine for poliomyelitis [correspondence]. JAMA 151:1224, 1953.

74. Research on a vaccine for the prevention of poliomyelitis [editorial]. JAMA 151:1198, 1953.

75. Francis T, Napier JA, Voight RB, et al. Evaluation of the 1954 Field Trial of Poliomyelitis Vaccine: Final Report. Ann Arbor, Poliomyelitis Vaccine Evaluation Center, Department of Epidemiology, School of Public Health, University of Michigan, 1957.

76. Nathanson N, Langmuir AD. The Cutter incident: poliomyelitis following formaldehyde-inactivated poliovirus vaccination in the United States during the spring of 1955. I. Background. Am J Hyg 78:16, 1963.

77. Nathanson N, Langmuir AD. The Cutter incident: poliomyelitis following formaldehyde-inactivated poliovirus vaccination in the United States during the spring of 1955. II. Relationship of poliomyelitis to Cutter vaccine. Am J Hyg 78:29, 1963.

78. Nathanson N, Langmuir AD. The Cutter incident: poliomyelitis following formaldehyde-inactivated poliovirus vaccination in the United States during the spring of 1955. III. Comparison of the clinical character of vaccinated and contact cases occurring after use of high-rate lots of Cutter vaccine. Am J Hyg 78:61, 1963.

79. U.S. Public Health Service Technical Report on Salk Poliomyelitis Vaccine. Rockville, MD, Public Health Service, 1955.

80. Langmuir AD. Results obtained by means of vaccine composed of inactivated viruses. In Poliomyelitis: Proceedings of the Fourth International Poliomyelitis Conference. Philadelphia, JB Lippincott, 1958, p 86.

81. Langmuir AD. Inactivated virus vaccines: protective efficacy. In Poliomyelitis: Proceedings of the Fifth International Poliomyelitis Conference. Philadelphia, JB Lippincott, 1961, p 105.

82. Lloyd W, Theiler M, Ricci NI. Modification of the virulence of yellow fever virus by cultivation in tissue in vitro. Trans R Soc Trop Med Hyg 29:481, 1936.

83. Theiler M, Smith HH. The effect of prolonged cultivation in vitro upon the pathogenicity of yellow fever virus. J Exp Med 65:767, 1937.

84. Melnick JL. Variations in poliomyelitis virus on serial passage through tissue culture. Cold Spring Harb Symp Quant Biol 18:278, 1953.

85. Roca-Garcia M, Jervis GA. Experimentally produced poliomyelitis variant in chick embryo. Ann N Y Acad Sci 61:911, 1955.

86. Li CP, Schaeffer M, Nelson DB. Experimentally produced variants of poliomyelitis virus combining in vivo and in vitro techniques. Ann N Y Acad Sci 61:902, 1955.

87. Poliomyelitis: Proceedings of the First International Poliomyelitis Congress. Philadelphia, JB Lippincott, 1948.

88. Poliomyelitis: Proceedings of the Second International Poliomyelitis Congress. Philadelphia, JB Lippincott, 1951.

89. Poliomyelitis: Proceedings of the Third International Poliomyelitis Congress. Philadelphia, JD Lippincott, 1954.

90. Poliomyelitis: Proceedings of the Fourth International Poliomyelitis Congress. Philadelphia, JB Lippincott, 1957.

91. Poliomyelitis: Proceedings of the Fifth International Poliomyelitis Congress. Philadelphia, JB Lippincott, 1961.

92. Live Poliovirus Vaccines: Proceedings of the First International Conference on Live Poliovirus Vaccines. Washington, DC, Pan-American Health Organization, 1959.

93. Live Poliovirus Vaccines: Proceedings of the Second International Conference on Live Poliovirus Vaccines. Washington, DC, Pan-American Health Organization, 1960.

94. Oral Live Poliovirus Vaccine: Proceedings of the Fourth Scientific Conference of the Institute of Poliomyelitis and Virus Encephalitis and the International Symposium on Live Poliovirus Vaccine. Moscow, Academy of Medical Sciences of the USSR, 1961.

95. Sabin AB. Immunization of chimpanzees and human beings with avirulent strains of poliomyelitis virus. Ann N Y Acad Sci 61:1050, 1955.

96. Koprowski H. Historical aspects of the development of live virus vaccine in poliomyelitis. Br Med J 2:5192, 1960.

97. Cabasso VJ, Jervis GA, Moyer AW, et al. Cumulative testing experience with consecutive lots of oral poliomyelitis vaccine. Br Med J 1:373, 1960.

98. Benison S. International medical cooperation: Dr. Albert Sabin, live poliovirus vaccine and the Soviets. Bull Hist Med 56:460, 1982.

99. Sabin AB. Role of my cooperation with Soviet scientists in the conquest of polio: some lessons and challenges. The 23rd Cosmos Club Award. Washington, DC, 1986.

100. Horstmann D. Report on live poliovirus vaccination in the Union of Soviet Socialist Republics, Poland and Czechoslovakia, August–October 1959. New Haven, CT, Yale University Press, 1960, pp 1–122.

101. Shannon JA. National Institutes of Health: present and potential contribution to application of biomedical knowledge. Research in the Service of Man: Biomedical Knowledge, Development and Use. US Senate, 90th Congress, 1st Session, Document No. 55, 1967.

102. Sweet BH, Hilleman MR. The vacuolating virus, SV_{40}. Proc Soc Exp Biol Med 105:420, 1960.

103. Gerber P, Hottle GA, Grubbs RE. Inactivation of vacuolating virus (SV_{40}) by formaldehyde. Proc Soc Exp Biol Med 108:205, 1961.

104. Eddy BE. Simian virus (SV_{40}): An oncogenic virus. Prog Exp Tumor Res 4:1, 1964.

105. Schein HM, Enders JF. Transformation induced by simian virus 40 in human renal cell cultures. I. Morphology and growth characteristics. Proc Natl Acad Sci U S A 48:1164, 1962.

106. Gerber P. Patterns of antibodies to SV_{40} in children following the last booster with inactivated poliomyelitis vaccines. Proc Soc Exp Biol Med 125:1284, 1967.

107. Shah KV. Evidence for an SV_{40}-related papovavirus infection of man. Am J Epidemiol 95:199, 1972.

108. Shah K, Nathanson N. Human exposure to SV_{40}: review and comment. Am J Epidemiol 103:1, 1976.

109. Melnick JL, Stinebaugh S. Excretion of vacuolating SV_{40} virus (papovavirus group) after ingestion as a contaminant of oral poliovaccine. Proc Soc Exp Biol Med 109:965, 1962.

110. Morris JA, Johnson KM, Aulisio CG, et al. Clinical and serologic responses in volunteers given vacuolating virus [SV_{40}] by respiratory route. Proc Soc Exp Biol Med 108:56, 1961.

111. Geissler F, Scherneek S, Prokoph H, et al. SV_{40} in human brain tumors: risk factor or passenger? In Giraldo G, Beth E (eds). The Role of Viruses in Human Cancer. Vol. 2. New York, Elsevier, 1984, pp 265–279.

112. Geissler E, Konzer P, Scherneek S, Zimmerman W. Sera collected before introduction of contaminated polio vaccine contain antibodies against SV_{40}. Acta Virol 29:420, 1985.

113. Fraumeni JF, Ederer F, Miller RW. An evaluation of the carcinogenicity of simian virus 40 in man. JAMA 185:713, 1963.

114. Fraumeni JF, Stark CR, Gold E, Lepow ML. Simian virus 40 in polio vaccine: follow-up of newborn recipients. Science 167:59, 1970.

115. Mortimer EA Jr, Lepow ML, Gold E, et al. Long-term follow-up of persons inadvertently inoculated with SV_{40} as neonates. N Engl J Med 305:1517, 1981.

116. Fox JP. Epidemiology of poliomyelitis in populations before and after vaccination with inactivated viruses. In Poliomyelitis: Proceedings of the Fourth International Poliomyelitis Conference. Philadelphia, JB Lippincott, 1958, pp 136–149.

117. Sabin AB. Present status of attenuated live virus poliomyelitis vaccine. JAMA 162:1589, 1956.

118. Horstmann DM, Wiederman JC, Paul JR. Attenuated type 1 poliovirus vaccine: its capacity to infect and to spread from vaccinees within an institutional population. JAMA 170:1, 1959.

119. Fox JP, LeBlanc DR, Gelfand HM, et al. Spread of a vaccine strain of poliovirus in southern Louisiana communities. In Proceedings of the Second International Conference on Live Poliovirus Vaccines. Washington, DC, Pan-American Health Organization, 1960.

120. Kimball AC, Barr RN, Bauer H, et al. Minnesota studies with oral poliomyelitis vaccine: community spread of orally administered attenuated poliovirus vaccine strains. In Proceedings of the Second International Conference on Live Poliovirus Vaccines. Washington, DC, Pan-American Health Organization, 1960.

121. Paul JR. Poliomyelitis immunization—1963. Med Clin North Am 47:1219, 1963.

122. Berkovich S, Pickering JE, Kibrick S. Paralytic poliomyelitis in Massachusetts, 1959: a study of the disease in a well vaccinated population. N Engl J Med 264:1323, 1961.

123. U.S. Public Health Service. Interim document gives advice on use of Salk and Sabin vaccines. JAMA 180:23, 1962.

124. Red Book: Report of the Committee on Infectious Diseases (14th ed). Elk Grove Village, IL, American Academy of Pediatrics, 1964.

125. Red Book: Report of the Committee on Infectious Diseases (20th ed). Elk Grove Village, IL, American Academy of Pediatrics, 1986.

126. Assaad F, Ljungars-Esteves K. World overview of poliomyelitis: regional patterns and trends. Rev Infect Dis 6(suppl 2):S302, 1984.

127. Kim-Farley RJ, Bart KJ, Schonberger LB, et al. Poliomyelitis in the USA: virtual elimination of disease caused by wild virus. Lancet 2:1315, 1984.

128. Henderson DA, Witte JJ, Morris L, et al. Paralytic disease associated with oral polio vaccines. JAMA 190:41, 1964.

129. Report of the Special Advisory Committee on Oral Poliomyelitis Vaccines to the Surgeon General of the Public Health Service: oral poliomyelitis vaccines. JAMA 190:49, 1964.

130. Sabin AB. Commentary on oral poliomyelitis vaccines. JAMA 190:164, 1964.

131. McKay HW, Fodor AR, Kokko UP. Viremia following the administration of live poliovirus vaccines. Am J Public Health 53:274, 1963.

132. Horstmann DM, Opton EM, Klemperer R, et al. Viremia in infants vaccinated with oral poliovirus vaccine (Sabin). Am J Hyg 79:47, 1964.

133. Melnick JL, Proctor RO, Ocampo AR, et al. Free and bound virus in serum after administration of oral poliovirus vaccine. Am J Epidemiol 84:329, 1966.

134. World Health Organization Consultative Group. The relationship between acute persisting spinal paralysis and poliomyelitis vaccine (oral): results of a WHO enquiry. Bull World Health Organ 53:319, 1976.

135. World Health Organization Consultative Group. The relationship between acute persisting spinal paralysis and poliomyelitis vaccine—results of a ten-year inquiry. Bull World Health Organ 60:231, 1982.

136. Division of Immunization, Centers for Disease Control. Risks of oral polio vaccine. Paper presented at the meeting of the Advisory Committee on Immunization Practices, Atlanta, GA, October 24, 1985.

137. Salk D. Eradication of poliomyelitis in the United States. I. Live virus vaccine–associated and wild poliovirus disease. Rev Infect Dis 2:228, 1980.

138. Salk D. Eradication of poliomyelitis in the United States. II. Experience with killed poliovirus vaccine. Rev Infect Dis 2:243, 1980.

139. Salk D. Eradication of poliomyelitis in the United States. III. Poliovaccines—practical considerations. Rev Infect Dis 2:258, 1980.

140. Fox JP. Eradication of poliomyelitis in the United States: a commentary on the Salk review. Rev Infect Dis 2:277, 1980.

141. Van Wezel AL, Van Steenis G, van der Marel P, Osterhaus ADME. Inactivated poliovirus vaccine: current production methods and new developments. Rev Infect Dis 6(suppl 2):S335, 1984.

142. McBean AM, Thoms ML, Johnson RH, et al. A comparison of the serologic responses to oral and injectable trivalent poliovirus vaccines. Rev Infect Dis 6(suppl 2):S552, 1984.

143. Cohen H, Nagel J. Two injections of diphtheria-tetanus-pertussis polio vaccine as the backbone of a simplified immunization schedule in developing countries. Rev Infect Dis 6(suppl 2):S350, 1984.

144. Bijkerk H. Surveillance and control of poliomyelitis in the Netherlands. Rev Infect Dis 6(suppl 2):S451, 1984.

145. Lapinleimu K. Elimination of poliomyelitis in Finland. Rev Infect Dis 6(suppl 2):S457, 1984.

146. Bottiger M. Long-term immunity following vaccination with killed poliovirus vaccine in Sweden, a country with no circulating poliovirus. Rev Infect Dis 6(suppl 2):S548, 1984.

147. Fox JP. Modes of action of poliovirus vaccines and relation to resulting immunity. Rev Infect Dis 6(suppl 2):S352, 1984.

148. Chin TDY. Immunity induced by inactivated poliovirus vaccine and excretion of virus. Rev Infect Dis 6(suppl 2):S369, 1984.

149. Poliomyelitis—Finland. MMWR 34:5–6, 1985.

150. Update: Poliomyelitis outbreak—Finland. 1984–1985. MMWR 35:82–86, 1986.

151. Kim-Farley RJ, Rutherford G, Lichfield P, et al. Outbreak of paralytic poliomyelitis, Taiwan. Lancet 2:1322, 1984.

152. John TJ. Poliomyelitis in Taiwan: lessons for developing countries [letter to the editor]. Lancet 1:872, 1985.

153. Division of Immunization, Centers for Disease Control. Community spread of poliovaccine virus. Paper presented at the meeting of the Advisory Committee on Immunization Practices, Atlanta, GA, October 24, 1985.

154. Bernier RH. Some observations on lameness surveys. Rev Infect Dis 6(suppl 2):S371, 1984.

155. Heymann DL. House-to-house and school lameness surveys in Cameroon: a comparison of two methods for estimating the prevalence and annual incidence of paralytic poliomyelitis. Rev Infect Dis 6(suppl 2):S376, 1984.

156. Cruz RR. Cuba: mass polio vaccination program, 1962–1982. Rev Infect Dis 6(suppl 2):S408, 1984.

157. Sabin A. Vaccination against poliomyelitis in economically underdeveloped countries. Bull World Health Organ 58:141, 1980.

158. Montefiore DG. Problems of poliomyelitis immunization in countries with warm climates. In Proceedings of the International Conference on the Application of Vaccines Against Viral, Rickettsial, and Bacterial Diseases of Man (Pan-American Health Organization Scientific Publication No. 226). Washington, DC, Pan-American Health Organization/World Health Organization, 1970.

159. Sabin AB. Strategy for rapid elimination and continuing control of poliomyelitis and other vaccine preventable diseases of children in developing countries. BMJ 292:531, 1986.

160. Robbins FC, Nightingale EO. Selective primary health care: strategies for control of disease in the developing world. IX. Poliomyelitis. Rev Infect Dis 5:957, 1983.

161. Salk J. One-dose immunization against paralytic poliomyelitis using noninfectious vaccine. Rev Infect Dis 6(suppl 2):S444, 1984.

162. Stoeckel P, Schlumberger M, Parent G, et al. Use of killed poliovirus vaccine in a routine immunization program in West Africa. Rev Infect Dis 6(suppl 2):S463, 1984.

163. Hilleman MR, McAteer WJ, McLean AA, et al. Stabilized measles vaccine in a novel single-dose delivery system: a practical reality for the worldwide elimination of measles. Rev Infect Dis 5:511, 1983.

164. Nathanson N. Epidemiologic aspects of poliomyelitis eradication. Rev Infect Dis 6(suppl 2):S308, 1984.

165. Almond JW, Stanway G, Cann AJ, et al. New poliovirus vaccines: a molecular approach. Vaccine 2:179, 1984.

166. Baltimore D. Picornaviruses are no longer black boxes. Science 229:1366, 1985.

167. Minor PD, Schild GC, Cann AJ, et al. Studies on the molecular aspects of antigenic structure and virulence of poliovirus. Ann Inst Pasteur Paris 137:107, 1986.

168. Hogle JM, Chow M, Filman DJ. Three-dimensional structure of poliovirus at 2.9 Å resolution. Science 229:1358, 1985.

169. Racaniello VR, Baltimore D. Cloned poliovirus complementary DNA is infectious in mammalian cells. Science 214:916, 1981.

170. Wimmer E, Emini EA, Jameson BA. Peptide priming of poliovirus neutralizing antibody response. Rev Infect Dis 6(suppl 2):S505, 1984.

171. Kow OM, Nottay BK. Molecular epidemiology of polioviruses. Rev Infect Dis 6(suppl 2):S499, 1984.

172. Von Magnus H, Petersen I. Vaccination with inactivated poliovirus vaccine and oral poliovirus vaccine in Denmark. Rev Infect Dis 6(suppl 2):S471, 1984.

173. Stetten D. Eradication [editorial]. Science 210:1203, 1980.

174. Report on the International Conference on the Eradication of Infectious Diseases: can infectious diseases be eradicated? Rev Infect Dis 4:912, 1982.

175. Yekutiel P. Lessons from the big eradication campaigns. World Health Forum 2:465, 1981.

176. Chin J. Can poliomyelitis be eliminated? Rev Infect Dis 6(suppl 2):S581, 1984.

177. Melnick JL. Towards the eradication of poliomyelitis. In La Maza LM, Peterson EM (eds). Symposium on Medical Virology: Proceedings of the 1981 International Symposium on Medical Virology, Anaheim, CA. New York, Elsevier Biomedical, 1982, pp 261–299.

177a. Kew O, Morris-Glasgow V, Landaverde M, et al. Outbreak of poliomyelitis in Hispaniola associated with circulating Type 1 vaccine-derived; derived poliovirus. Science 296, 2002.

178. Sabin AB. Paralytic poliomyelitis: old dogmas and new perspectives. Rev Infect Dis 3:543, 1981.

179. Gear JHS. Non-polio causes of polio-like paralytic syndromes. Rev Infect Dis 6(suppl 2):S379, 1984.

180. Grist NR, Bell EJ. Paralytic poliomyelitis and non-polio enteroviruses: studies in Scotland. Rev Infect Dis 6(suppl 2):S385, 1984.

181. Melnick JL. Enterovirus type 71 infections: a varied clinical pattern sometimes mimicking paralytic poliomyelitis. Rev Infect Dis 6(suppl 2):S387, 1984.

182. Robbins FC. International Symposium on Poliomyelitis Control: summary and recommendations. Rev Infect Dis 6(suppl 2):S596, 1984.

183. Andrus JK, de Quadros CA, Olive JM. The surveillance challenge: final stages of eradication of poliomyelitis in the Americas. MMWR 41:21, 1992.

184. First Meeting of the International Commission for Certification of Poliomyelitis Eradication in the Americas. 9th Technical Advisory Group Meeting on Vaccine-Preventive Diseases. International Commission for Certification of Poliomyelitis Eradication in the Americas, Washington, DC, 1990.

185. Robbins FC, de Quadros CA. Certification of the eradication of indigenous transmission of wild poliovirus in the Americas. J Infect Dis 175(suppl 1):S281, 1997.

186. Wright PF, Kim-Farley RJ, de Quadros CA, et al. Strategies for the global eradication of poliomyelitis by the year 2000. N Engl J Med 325:1774, 1991.

187. Cochi SL, Hull HF, Sutter RW, et al. Global poliomyelitis eradication initiative: status report. J Infect Dis 175(suppl 1), 1997.

188. Report of a study: an evaluation of poliomyelitis vaccine policy options. Washington, DC, National Academy of Sciences, Institute of Medicine, 1988, pp 1–50.

189. Poliomyelitis prevention in the United States: introduction of a sequential vaccination schedule of inactivated poliovirus vaccine followed by oral poliovirus vaccine. Recommendations of the Advisory Committee on Immunization Practices (ACIP). MMWR 46:1–25.

190. Global Polio Eradication Initiative Polio Endgame briefing pack 2002. Geneva World Health Organization. Pamphlet updates available at www.polioeradication.org.

191. Henderson DA. Countering the past eradication threat of smallpox and polio. Clin Infect Dis 34:79–83, 2002.

192. Vastag B. At polio's end game strategies differ. JAMA 286(22):2797, 2001.

Chapter 3

The Immunology of Vaccination

GORDON ADA

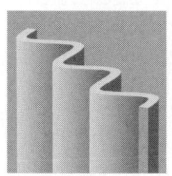

Many of the most successful vaccines that have been in general use for decades were developed without any or with only a slight knowledge of the way the mammalian immune system operates and how that system can be manipulated to achieve different responses. In developing a live, attenuated viral vaccine, for example, the essential criteria were that the product would be safe but effective at protecting against clinical disease if the vaccinees were later exposed to the wild-type agent. The need was very great. For example, exposure to measles caused great morbidity and mortality in a naive population.[1]

Two features characterize many of the agents for which current, successful viral and bacterial vaccines have been developed:

1. The agent causes an acute infection (e.g., many viral and all extracellular bacterial infections); or, if the agent fails to rapidly cause death, the host's immune response cleared the infection within approximately 1 week.
2. The agent is antigenically stable; or, if there are different serotypes in the field (e.g., measles and the three subtypes of poliovirus), each remains essentially antigenically stable.

The major exception is influenza virus, for which a new vaccine with antigenic properties closely matching the prevailing circulating strains is made each year. For the former agents, the main requirement of a vaccine is to induce the formation of an antibody of sufficiently high titer to neutralize the infectivity of almost all of the wild-type agents. The small proportion of wild-type agents that escape neutralization by antibody most likely will cause only a subclinical infection. This feature of infectious agents led to the demonstration—with poliovirus vaccines, for example[2]—that a vaccine preparation would be successful if it induced in a recipient a certain titer of specific antibody. In such situations, a subunit or hapten-carrier conjugate containing the antigenic moiety that possesses major neutralizing epitopes also would likely be successful if its immunogenicity were sufficiently high.

The pressure to better understand the immune mechanisms involved in preventing or controlling an infection increases considerably when one is faced with the need to develop vaccines against agents that naturally cause persistent or chronic infections. This includes parasites such as plasmodia, some bacteria such as *Chlamydia* species, and viruses such as human immunodeficiency virus (HIV), which are subject to substantial antigenic variation. To a significant extent, such a need coincides with a much-increased understanding of the properties and functions of components of the mammalian immune system, so that more immunologists are now involved in the general area of vaccinology.

This chapter briefly outlines our current understanding of the adaptive immune system, new approaches to manipulating different components of that system, and the major requirements expected of a vaccine if it is to be effective. A more detailed account can be found elsewhere.[3]

The Nature of the Mammalian Immune System

Two systems contribute to mammalian immunity—the innate (nonspecific, nonadaptive) and the acquired (specific, adaptive) systems. Both are necessary for survival in nature. The former consists of a series of specialized cells, such as macrophages, neutrophils, natural killer (NK) cells, dendritic cells (DCs), and different products, such as the cytokines; α-, β-, and γ-interferons (IFNs); chemokines; and larger proteins such as the C-reactive proteins and those of the complement cascade.[4] Components of the innate system may be activated within minutes or hours after an infection is initiated. This rapid response is a necessary requirement of the innate immune system, because it generally takes several days (sometimes much longer) for components of the adaptive system to acquire effector function. It was previously thought that the innate and adaptive systems were quite distinct, but it is now realized that they are intimately connected. Thus, γ-IFN, a critical cytokine, used to be called *immune interferon* because it was thought to be made only by effector T cells, but it is now known to be made also by NK cells. Another example is the classical and alternative complement pathways that share the later effector functions, but differ in that antigen–antibody complexes are recognized in the former, whereas a pathogen surface is recognized in the latter. Most importantly, macrophages and especially DCs are the most effective cells at presenting antigen (antigen-presenting cells [APCs]) to cells (lymphocytes) of the adaptive immune system. Their properties are described in more detail later in the chapter.

Adaptive Immune System

This system, which developed later during evolution than the innate system, differs from the latter in two critical properties—great specificity and memory, both of which are the exclusive hallmarks of one cell type, the lymphocyte. Because the practice of vaccination depends utterly on these properties, the remainder of this chapter outlines our current knowledge of important features of the adaptive immune system.

The Two Classes of Lymphocytes

Humoral Response

Immunoglobulin (Ig) receptors on B lymphocytes recognize and interact with epitopes of antigens. The complex is endocytosed and then processed within the cell, thereby completing a first step that leads to activation and differentiation processes involved in the formation of a plasma cell. Plasma cells produce and secrete different subclasses of antibodies (IgM, IgG, IgA, IgE) with specificities very similar to those of the IgM and IgD receptors on the cell surface. Once secreted, the antibodies circulate around the body and hence act independently of the plasma cell. The epitopes recognized may be a linear peptide or carbohydrate sequence or, quite frequently, a shape (about 25 × 25 Å) formed by adjacent sequences within a molecule or by adjacent molecules; this latter structure is called a discontinuous epitope. Both types of epitopes may have strict three-dimensional conformations, and even mutations outside the epitope can modify its conformation.[5,6]

Cell-Mediated Immune Response

Responses mediated by T (thymus-derived) lymphocytes are referred to as *cell-mediated*, even though many are mediated by secreted factors called cytokines (many also are called interleukins [ILs] and referred to by IL numbers). In contrast to hormones, cytokines almost invariably act over very short distances. Many cells, including B cells, express receptors for cytokines and chemokines, but T cells are both major producers of and responders to these factors. T cells are a more diverse group than B cells and express three different classes of receptors: (1) the specific T-cell receptor (TCR) that is composed of two chains, usually α and β, and recognizes processed antigen that is presented by the APC; (2) a receptor that is specific for the co-stimulator molecule usually expressed by the APC; and (3) receptors recognizing different cytokines and chemokines.

The two main classes of T cells express either the CD4 or the CD8 differentiation antigens, which function as accessory molecules to the TCR. CD4+ T cells and CD8+ T cells are said to be class II or class I major histocompatibility complex (MHC)–restricted cells, respectively, because they recognize antigenic peptides complexed with class II

MHC or class I MHC molecules at the surface of the APC. A major role of CD4+ T cells is to provide help for B cells to make antibody; hence they are called T-helper (Th) cells. In both humans and mice, there are two subsets of Th cells—Th1 and Th2 cells—that are distinguished by the profiles of the cytokines produced and their effector functions (Table 3–1). In addition to the role of Th2 cells in the production of cytokines, the interaction of the CD40 ligand on the Th2 cell with CD40 antigen on the B cell is required to initiate the switching of IgM production to IgG, IgA, or IgE production. In contrast, a major function of CD8+ T cells is to recognize and lyse infected target cells, hence they are called cytotoxic T lymphocytes (CTLs). This function of CTLs was first demonstrated with virus-infected cells but is also seen with cells infected with bacteria or parasites. CTLs secrete a panel of cytokines that resemble those secreted by Th1 cells, so that CTLs and Th1 cells are referred to as *type 1 cells*, and Th2 cells as *type 2 cells*. More recently, there has been evidence, at least from in vitro work, that CD8+ T cells convert to a form resembling Th2 cells after exposure to the cytokine IL-4, which is secreted by Th2 cells. These two subsets of CD8+ T cells are now called cytotoxic T-cell populations types 1 and 2 (Tc1 and Tc2) to bring the nomenclature into line with CD4+ T cell subsets.[7]

Cytokines (including interleukins) have a central role in influencing immune responses. Table 3–1 indicates the patterns mainly of interleukins secreted by the different T cells with $\alpha\beta$ chain receptors and the influence this has on the type of antibody produced by B cells. (A second group of T cells with $\gamma\delta$ chain receptors is described later.) Two cytokines especially have a dominant effect, IL-4 in switching

TABLE 3–1 ■ Cytokines Secreted by and Effector Activities of T-Lymphocyte Subsets, and Their Influence on Ig Isotypes Produced by B Cells (Helper Activities)

	CD4+ T cells		CD8+ T cells	
	Th1	Th2	Tc1	Tc2
Cytokines secreted				
IL-2	+	−	+	−
IL-3	+	−	−	−
IL-4	−	+	−	+
IL-5	−	+	−	+
IL-6	−	+	−	?
IL-10	−	+	−	?
IL-13	−	+	−	?
TNF-α	+	+	−	−
TNF-β	+	−	+	−
IFN-γ	+	−	+	−
Effector activity				
Cytotoxicity[*]	−	−	+	−
DTH	+	−	+/−	−
Helper activity				
Ig produced by B cells	IgG2a[†] IgG1[‡]	IgG1[†], IgA[†] IgE[‡]	−	+

[*]Class I MHC-restricted cytotoxic activity of primary (uncultured) cells.
[†]In mice.
[‡]In humans.
DTH, delayed-type hypersensitivity; IFN, interferon; IL, interleukin, cytokine; TNF, tumor necrosis factor.

a Th1 response to a Th2 response (see later), and IL-12, together with IL-18 (both secreted by activated APCs), inducing strong Th1 responses. The influence of IL-2, IL-4, and IL-12, as components of new candidate vaccines, is being currently assessed in clinical trials and is discussed later. Overexpression of IL-4, IL-9, and IL-13, which may occur in strong Th2 responses, can lead to chronic allergic inflammation.[8] In contrast, overexpression of some Th1-type cytokines—IL-2, IL-7, IL-10, and tumor necrosis factor-α (TNF-α) (or in some cases, their receptors)—is associated with autoimmune conditions, such as inflammatory bowel disease. Underexpression of TNFα and the TCR for transforming growth factor (TGF-β) can lead to systemic lupus erythematosus.[9]

T cells play a central role in immune responses. Because they are the first component of the adaptive system to achieve effector activity after infection, they must be able to circulate freely within the lymphoid system and reach sites of inflammation.

Antigen-Presenting Cells

Whereas the B-cell receptors (IgD and IgM, but principally the latter) often directly recognize a foreign antigen (which may vary from a portion of a protein to protein aggregates), the TCR recognizes an antigen that has been "processed" within an APC. Peptides derived from foreign antigens bind to a self-antigen, the MHC protein, to form a complex that is expressed at the cell surface. Generally, but not invariably, noninfectious material (e.g., a protein) will enter a cell via the endosomal/lysosomal pathway. After this material is degraded in lysosomes, an appropriate peptide forms a complex with a class II MHC molecule, and this is expressed at the cell surface. In contrast, if an infectious agent enters the cytoplasm of the APC and replicates, some newly synthesized foreign protein (as well as self-proteins) is degraded to peptides that may associate with a class I MHC molecule, and the complex will be expressed at the cell surface. The separation of these pathways is not absolute. A protein may fuse with the cell membrane or some protein may escape from a lysosome such that, in either case, the protein enters the cytoplasmic pathway and a CD8$^+$ T-cell response can occur. Furthermore, a number of adjuvant preparations are now available that promote a CD8$^+$ T-cell response to an antigen preparation that otherwise would not induce such a response, as is described later. A second crucial property of an APC is to express a co-stimulator molecule for which a receptor is present on the naive T cell. Without this second signal, a naive T cell is not activated and dies (apoptosis).

Figures 3–1 and 3–2 outline the major cellular interactions that lead, respectively, to T-cell and B-cell activation and differentiation to become effector cells. The formation of Tc2 cells is not illustrated in Figure 3–1 because there is doubt about the exact pathway in vivo.

Cells that express high levels of MHC and co-stimulator molecules are often referred to as *professional* APCs. Though macrophages may act as APCs, and B cells present antigen to activated or memory T cells, the major APCs are the different DCs (including Langerhans' cells). These were originally called *veiled cells* because of the extensive folding of the plasma membrane. A major role of these cells is to recognize "danger" in the form of compounds that are common to many bacteria, such as lipopolysaccharides. Some danger signals are recognized by special receptors, called toll-like receptors (TLRs), on DCs. Bacterial DNA, unlike vertebrate DNA, has a high content of unmethylated CpG motifs,[10] and these are recognized as indicating danger by the receptor TLR9 on DCs.[11] Absorption of the DNA-receptor complex activates the DC, and, as it begins to mature, the foreign DNA is transcribed and translated, and the antigens processed. Immature DCs express the chemokine receptors CCR-1, -3, and -5, which bind the corresponding chemokines found in areas that can become inflamed following an infection. Once a DC is activated, expression of these receptors is down-regulated, allowing cell maturation and expression of CD40 and of different chemokine receptors—CCR-4 but especially CCR-7—to occur. This switch facilitates passage of the DCs via afferent lymph vessels to the draining lymph node, where the corresponding chemokines occur.[12] Once in the T-cell–rich area of the node, the MHC–peptide complex expressed on the DC membrane is recognized by the antigen-specific receptors, CD40 by theCD40 ligand and the receptor for the co-stimulator molecules on appropriate immunocompetent naive or memory T cells.[4] The T cells are activated and some migrate to the site of inflammation. This sequence of events is illustrated in Figure 3–3. As is discussed later, immunizing with bacterial DNA containing segments of vertebrate DNA coding for foreign antigens is a very effective way of priming the adaptive immune response to foreign antigens.

Responses of Lymphocytes During an Infection

Immunocompetent, naive T cells are long lived because of frequent contact with MHC–self-peptide complexes and exposure to IL-7. There may be no more than a few thousand lymphocytes with a TCR of the same, individual specificity. Because some infectious agents replicate rapidly, the adaptive response also should be rapid. During an acute infection in mice, such as an influenza virus infection in the lung, some virus is carried to the draining lymph nodes via DCs. At least for CD8 T cells, there can be three to four divisions per day so that by day 5 to 6, when maximum levels of these cells are found, there may have been more than 1000-fold expansion in number of the responding cells.[13] During differentiation and acquisition of cytotoxic activity, the cells down-regulate expression of CCR-7 so they can exit the draining node and travel to the site of inflammation, in this case, the infected lung. The sequence of appearance of regulatory and effector T cells in the lung is first CD4$^+$ T cells and then CD8$^+$ T cells, the latter being first seen at about day 3 to 4.[14] The decrease in lung virus titers begins at days 5 to 8 (depending on the size of the infecting dose), coinciding with the increase in CTL activity in the lung. CTL activity is no longer detected about 3 days after infectious virus disappears (days 10 to 12) because, either when the need is past or possessing a short half-life, 90% or more of the CTLs die, and the remainder turn into memory cells.[13,15] These persist for many months in the presence of IL-15 and in the absence of specific antigen, possibly for the life of the mouse.[16] Under the influence

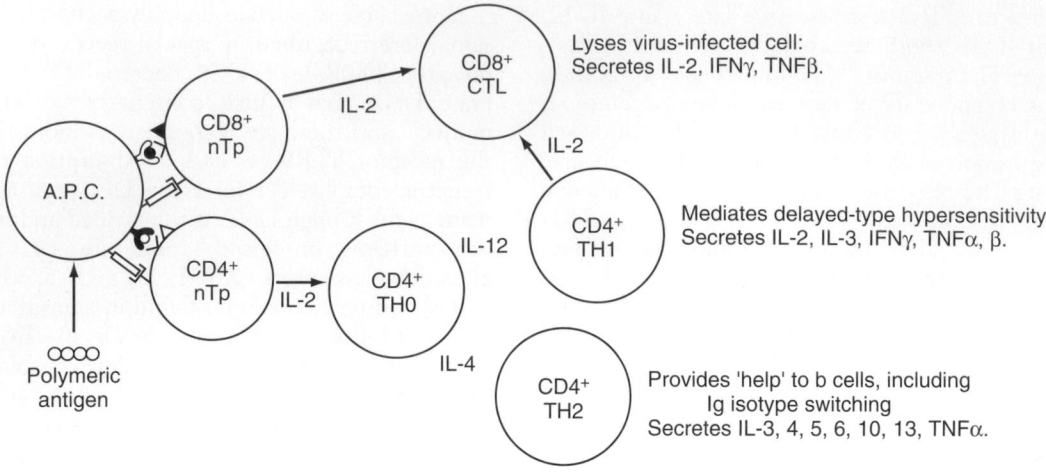

Lyses virus-infected cell:
Secretes IL-2, IFNγ, TNFβ.

Mediates delayed-type hypersensitivity
Secretes IL-2, IL-3, IFNγ, TNFα, β.

Provides 'help' to b cells, including
Ig isotype switching
Secretes IL-3, 4, 5, 6, 10, 13, TNFα.

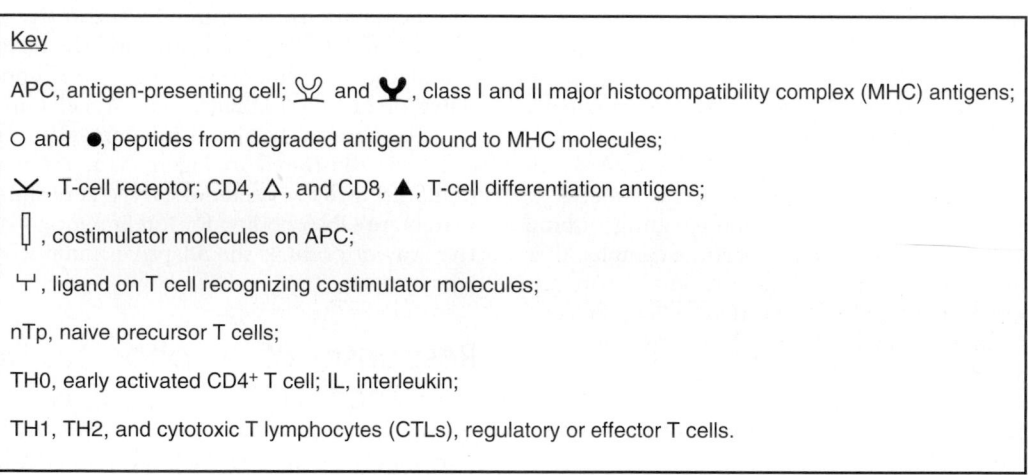

Key

APC, antigen-presenting cell; ⋎ and ⋏, class I and II major histocompatibility complex (MHC) antigens;

○ and ●, peptides from degraded antigen bound to MHC molecules;

⋎, T-cell receptor; CD4, △, and CD8, ▲, T-cell differentiation antigens;

⫿, costimulator molecules on APC;

⊔, ligand on T cell recognizing costimulator molecules;

nTp, naive precursor T cells;

TH0, early activated CD4⁺ T cell; IL, interleukin;

TH1, TH2, and cytotoxic T lymphocytes (CTLs), regulatory or effector T cells.

FIGURE 3–1 ▪ Antigen presentation and T-cell activation. (From Ada G. Vaccines. *In* Nathanson N [ed]. Viral Pathogenesis. Philadelphia, Lippincott–Raven, 1997, pp 371–399, with permission.)

of IL-15, there is up-regulation of expression of markers such as CD44.[17]

Antibody-secreting cells (ASCs) producing first IgM are found in the infected lung at about day 6; some days later, IgG and IgA ASCs then appear,[14] but infectious virus has been cleared before there are really significant numbers of the latter cells. The IgG, IgA, and IgE receptors on maturing B cells undergo affinity maturation while in the lymphoid follicles (see Fig. 3–3). Antigen, in the form of antigen–antibody complexes attached to complement receptors on the surface of follicular dendritic cells (FDCs), facilitates the selection of those cells with the highest affinity receptors for differentiation into plasma cells or memory B cells. ASCs are present for at least 18 months, although in gradually decreasing numbers. Maximum levels of specific B memory cells are found at about 3 months. In mice, ASCs formed early in an immune response to an infection have a short half-life, whereas ASCs formed later survive and continue to secrete antibody for extended periods (>1 year).[18] Thus it may not be necessary for antigen to persist on FDCs for extended periods (many years) in order to maintain continuing production of antibody. Such a system

seems sensible because the early production of short-lived cells allows the benefits of affinity maturation to be utilized, and the later production of long-lived cells is economical. If the secret of this "switch" (from short to very long life) could be found, it might be possible to obtain long-lived antibody production to some vaccines, with fewer injections.

The pattern of antibody production seen following immunization with thymus-dependent (protein) antigens is similar to that described following an infection. Thus, in rats, *Salmonella* flagella induce first IgM followed by long-lived production of IgG, whereas the monomer, flagellin, induces only IgG production. In contrast, B lymphocytes responding to a thymus-independent antigen, such as a polysaccharide with repeating epitopes, produce mainly (>90%) IgM, which neither undergoes affinity maturation nor induces memory. Though low levels of IgG and IgA also may be formed,[19] the sequence of events that result in the IgM-secreting cells switching to IgG or IgA production is not yet clear. It may involve CD40 on the B cells reacting with its ligand on other cells and the presence of interleukins such as IL-4 and IL-10.

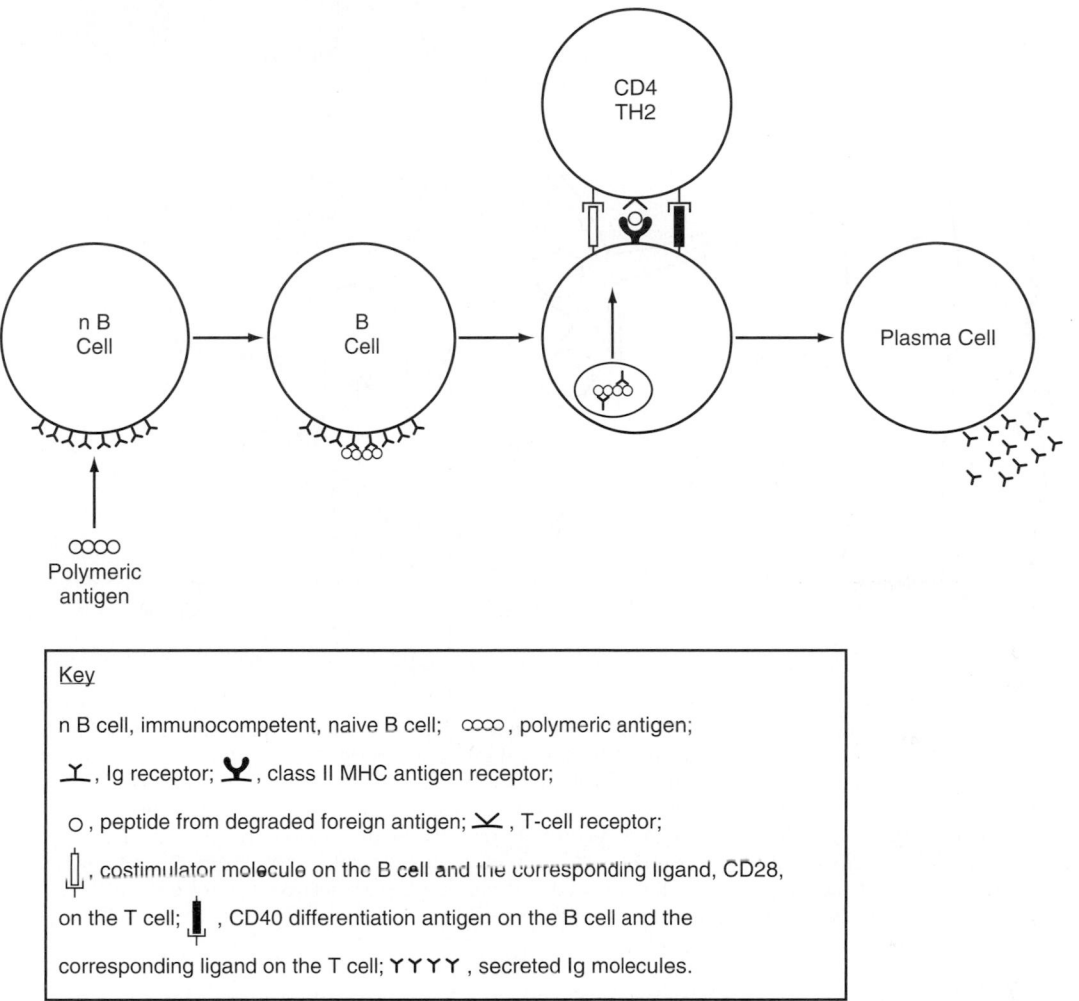

Key

n B cell, immunocompetent, naive B cell;   oooo , polymeric antigen;

 Y , Ig receptor; Y , class II MHC antigen receptor;

 o , peptide from degraded foreign antigen; X , T-cell receptor;

 , costimulator molecule on the B cell and the corresponding ligand, CD28,

on the T cell;   , CD40 differentiation antigen on the B cell and the

corresponding ligand on the T cell; Y Y Y Y , secreted Ig molecules.

FIGURE 3–2 ▪ Antigen presentation and B-cell activation. (From Ada G. Vaccines. *In* Nathanson N [ed]. Viral Pathogenesis. Philadelphia, Lippincott–Raven, 1997, pp 371–399, with permission.)

In the case of human HIV-1 infections, CTLs are found in the blood at the time of viremia[20,21] which may occur a few weeks after exposure to the virus. The increasing CTL activity again coincides with decreasing viremia. Thereafter, in most infected individuals, effector CTLs are present in the blood for some years. This quite unusual occurrence is thought to result from the intense CTL response in the lymphoid tissues, where a high rate of viral replication occurs. Neutralizing antibody often is found shortly after viremia occurs; in some cases, however, such antibody may not be detected for months after the initiation of infection.[20] This observation is consistent with the murine influenza result noted above, suggesting that, in a naive host, CTL formation is the major response for controlling and sometimes clearing a viral infection.[21,22] As an HIV infection progresses to clinical disease, the CTLs become dysfunctional, losing the ability to produce IL-2 and TNF-α. This can happen in chimeric simian/human immunodeficiency virus–infected rhesus monkeys. Prevaccination, which prevents progression to disease, preserves the functional ability of the CTLs.[23]

The Role of Different Immune Responses

Table 3–2 summarizes the roles of different components of the immune response in preventing, controlling, and clearing an infectious agent. There are two types of infections—extracellular and intracellular. In the former, specific antibody is crucially important in preventing infection and at all subsequent stages. Cytokines secreted by CD4+ Th1 cells help to activate phagocytic cells such as macrophages and thereby facilitate the uptake and destruction of the agent, either as such or complexed with antibody. Theoretically, at least, CTLs are unlikely to be formed nor would they be expected to have a role in such situations. The remainder of this section provides evidence to support the assessment in Table 3–2.

Intracellular Infections: The Role of Antibody

Neutralization of the infectivity of the challenge agent is a critical role for specific antibody. If some infectious agent escapes neutralization and replicates in host cells,

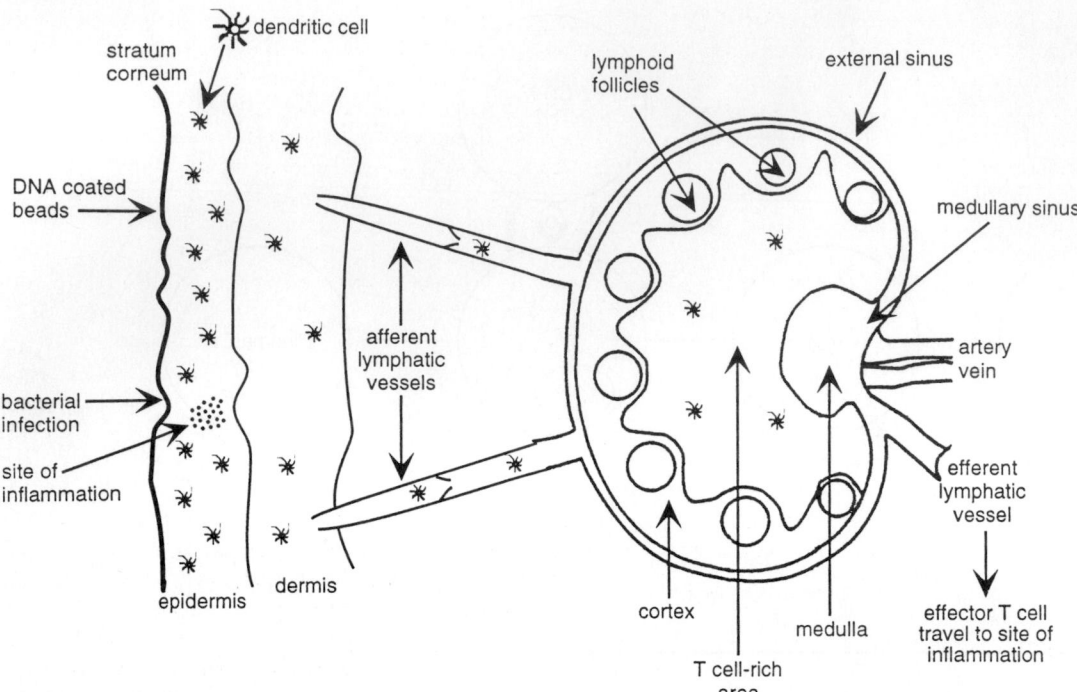

FIGURE 3–3 ▪ Presentation of antigen by dendritic (Langerhans') cells to T lymphocytes in the draining lymph node. An infection can occur via the skin (or a mucosal surface) or antigen can be introduced into the body via these surfaces (e.g., via DNA-coated gold beads using a gene gun, or by transcutaneous immunization, in which an antigen and adjuvant is applied to washed skin using a patch[115]). The foreign antigens may react with the dendritic (Langerhans') cells in the epidermis, and this can result in their activation. The expression of different chemokine receptors allows the cells to migrate via the afferent lymphatic vessels to the draining lymphoid tissue. During this passage, the cells mature, process the antigens, express the MHC–foreign peptides complex at their surface, and finally interact with T lymphocytes in the T cell–rich area of the lymph node. The activated T lymphocytes, with delayed-type hypersensitivity or cytotoxic function, may then migrate back to the site of inflammation resulting from the infection.

antibody may neutralize any progeny agent (e.g., prevent or limit viremia) and destroy infected cells through antibody-dependent cellular cytotoxicity and complement-mediated lysis.[24] There are reports of model systems where antibody has cleared an intracellular infection. Certain monoclonal antibodies (MAbs) to the fusion protein of respiratory syncytial virus (RSV) were found to clear an infection in mice.[25] These antibodies may have been endocytosed into an infected cell and thus prevented viral formation. It also has been shown that a preparation of anti-RSV Fab, made by the technique of combinatorial libraries expressed on phages, cleared the virus infection when instilled intranasally into the lungs of infected mice daily for 3 days.[26] In another example, MAbs or hyperimmune serum specific for Sindbis virus were able to clear the virus from infected neurons in mice with severe combined immunodeficiency disease (SCID).[27] SCID mice infected with a low dose of egg-grown influenza virus that caused delayed death (occurring at about 18 days) were protected from death if transfused with specific antibody.[28] Though these examples are of considerable interest in demonstrating a potential use for high-titer antibodies, they are atypical. There are many examples of an intracellular infection persisting in the presence of high titers of specific antibody.

Does specific antibody ever completely prevent an infection, and thus induce so-called sterilizing immunity? Probably not, but we do not know. The difficulty of finding a correct answer is indicated by experiments of Ramphal

and colleagues. When mice were transfused with high-titer anti-influenza IgG and then infected by intranasal inoculation of virus of the correct specificity, only the surface epithelial cells became infected—the mice had tracheitis.[29] However, when the mice were transfused with high-titer

TABLE 3–2 ▪ Functions of Lymphocyte Subsets Following Vaccination of Mice Against Extracellular (Bacteria) or Intracellular (Viruses, Bacteria) Infections

Type of response	Stages of Infectious Process[*]		
	Prevent	Reduce	Clear/Control
Extracellular infection			
Antibody[†]	+++	+++	+++
CD4+ Th1	–	++	++
CD8+ Tc1	–	–	–
Intracellular infection			
Antibody[†]	+++	++	+/–
CD4+ Th1			
Bacterial infections	–	+++	+++
Viral infections	–	++	+
CD8+ Tc1 (CTLs)	–	+++	+++
CD8+ Tc2	–		
	Suppresses CTL activity		

[*]+++, very important; ++, important, +, less important.
[†]CD4+ Th2 cells help B cells to produce IgG, IgA, and IgE antibodies.

polymerized IgA (which is converted to secretory IgA (sIgA) on passage through the surface epithelial cells into the airways) and then inoculated with virus, most (but *not* all) mice were protected and showed no sign of infection when the surface layer of cells in the lung air passages was examined in detail.[30] Subsequent experiments showed that the protection was due to the sIgA.[31]

If a vaccine-induced neutralizing antibody titer is sufficiently high and closely matches the viral antigen specificity, nearly all of the challenge virus should be neutralized; if this occurs, the vaccine may not need to additionally induce a strong type 1 T-cell response to control the minor infection caused by any escaped virus. A vaccine that induces the generation of type 1 effector T cells assumes greater relevance and importance as (1) the specificity of vaccine-induced neutralizing antibody increasingly diverges from the antigenic specificity of the challenge virus, and (2) naive susceptible cells are infected by intimate contact with virus-producing cells (e.g., the formation of syncytia).

Intracellular Infections: The Role of Type 1 T-Cell Responses

The role of type 1 T-cell responses in viral and other intracellular infections is discussed sequentially. In viral infections, the evidence favoring a dominant role for CTLs has been reviewed[32]; the information is summarized in Table 3–3.[33–43] Overall, the findings reported in this table support the dominant role of CTLs in controlling and frequently clearing viral infections.

It is difficult to find data in support of a dominant role for CD4+ Th1 cells in viral infections. In one special situation, the zosteriform spread model of a herpesvirus type 2 infection in mice, Th1 cells were clearly protective against the cutaneous infection.[44] In contrast, CTLs mediated protection when the infection spread to the nervous system.[45] Especially in in vitro experiments, Th1 cells facilitate a CTL response; however, there are now a number of reports confirming that, in knockout (KO) mice lacking CD4+ T cells, quite strong CTL responses can be generated to some viral infections.[46,47] In one report it was shown with a persistent viral infection (herpesvirus in CD4+ T cell KO mice) that a strong CTL response was induced but that, over time, the CTL response in the KO mice decreased markedly compared with the response in control mice.[47] The authors suggested that an effect like this might operate in those HIV-1 infections that progress to acquired immunodeficiency syndrome.

In bacterial and other infections, the picture appears to be less clear cut. In murine listeriosis, CTLs specific for a single nonamer peptide determinant of the bacterial protein listeriolysin are protective in vivo.[48] Furthermore, it has since been shown that specific immune CD8+ T cells, but not immune CD4+ T cells, lyse *Listeria monocytogenes*–infected hepatocytes in a class I MHC-restricted fashion.[49] In contrast, depletion of CD4+ T cells in mice infected with bacille Calmette-Guérin (BCG; attenuated *Mycobacterium bovis*), using specific antiserum to deplete both cell types, resulted in a large increase in the numbers of bacteria, whereas depletion of CD8+ T cells apparently had little effect on the course of infection.[50] Other work using cell transfer also pointed to the importance of CD4+ T cells in controlling infection of mice with virulent *Mycobacterium tuberculosis*, though a role for CD8+ T cells was not ruled out.[51] However, later work using β_2-microglobulin (β_2m) KO mice (which cannot make functional CD8+ T cells) showed that CTLs were very important in controlling a virulent *M. tuberculosis* infection but not important for controlling a BCG infection.[52] In a separate study in mice, both CD4+ type 1 cells and CTLs were found to have a protective role in BCG infections,[53] with the former possibly being highly effective in containing the organism in granulomas. When mice were infected with mouse-passaged *M. tuberculosis*, $\gamma\delta$ T cells were found to have a protective role in the early stages of infection.[54]

TABLE 3–3 ■ Summary of Evidence Supporting a Dominant Role for CTLs in Control and Clearance of Many Viral Infections

GENERAL ARGUMENTS
1. Clearance of many viral infections is associated with the induction of a CTL response prior to the appearance of neutralizing antibody.
2. Nearly all mammalian cell types express class I MHC antigens. Exceptions include gametes, neurons, red blood cells, cells of the trophoblast.
3. CTLs secrete potent cytokines with antiviral and macrophage-activating activities, such as IFN-γ and TNF-α, and chemokines.
4. Infected cells become susceptible to lysis by CTLs long before viral progeny are made.

MORE DIRECT EVIDENCE
1. Transfer of specific effector CTLs into an MHC-compatible host clears established infections in a specific organ or protects from death. In humans, CTLs have been shown to reconstitute specific CMV[33,34] and Epstein-Barr virus[35] immunity after allogeneic bone marrow transplants.
2. Using lymphocytic choriomeningitis virus (LCMV), a noncytopathic virus, in infections of mice, CTLs have been shown to lyse infected cells in vivo[37] as well as in vitro. Similarly, virus-specific CTLs transferred to transgenic mice expressing the hepatitis B surface antigen caused apoptosis of the hepatocytes.[37] The cytotoxicity of LCMV-specific CTLs is greatly impaired in perforin-deficient mice.[38]
3. In the case of HIV-1 infections, there are four situations in which virus- and serum antibody negative individuals who were exposed to HIV have HIV-specific CTL activity: in babies born of infected mothers,[39,40] in long-term seronegative partners of infected people,[41] in long-time African prostitutes,[42] and in some health care workers exposed once to HIV.[43]

Reviewed by Ada and McElrath.[32]

Francisella tularensis infections cause the lethal disease tularemia.[55] An attenuated live vaccine strain (LVS) is highly virulent for mice when given intraperitoneally but much less so when given intradermally. Using CD8[+] T cell KO mice and CD4[+] T-cell–negative mice, it was found that either cell class was sufficient to resolve a sublethal intradermal LVS infection and subsequently to protect against a lethal challenge of these bacteria.[56] This suggested that (1) although one cell type may have a stronger role than the other at different times during the infection or with different levels of infection, both were important; and (2) γδ T cells also had a more subtle but a still significant role to play in protection.

Chlamydia trachomatis is an obligate intracellular bacterium responsible for causing trachoma and genital infections. In a study in an endemic area, the blood of children and adults with the human leukocyte antigen (HLA) B8 or B35 haplotype was tested for the presence of CTLs reacting with nonapeptides from the major outer membrane and heat shock proteins of the chlamydia. Although the number of positives was not very high, CTL responses were observed only in children resolving a current infection and in adults lacking scarring of the conjunctiva, suggesting that these cells may be important in resolving a natural infection.[57]

The effect of genetic disruptions in mice on the progress of protozoal infections has been reviewed,[58] but there are too few examples to draw clear conclusions as yet. Using β_2m KO mice, for example, no difference was found with infection by *Plasmodium* species or *Leishmania major*, whereas the infection with *Trypanosoma cruzi* was exacerbated. It had been shown earlier that CD8[+] T cells were important in protection in *Toxoplasma gondii*–infected normal mice.

Regional Immunity

The area of the mucosa is far greater than that of the skin, and, with the exception of the female vagina, it is generally well endowed with draining lymphoid tissues. The main routes leading to infection are the gut, the rectum, the genitourinary tract, the respiratory tract, and the eye. Studies over many years led to the concept[59] of a common mucosal system whereby infection at one mucosal site could result in protection at that and at other mucosal sites. For example, the adenovirus vaccine is administered orally and protection is afforded against a respiratory infection. There is much yet to be learned about this system, however. For reasons as yet unclear, immunization via the respiratory tract rather than the oral route appears to be more effective at affording some protection in the female genital tract.

The mucosal immune system has several characteristic features (reviewed by Lamm[60]). Foremost is the formation and secretion into the lumen of sIgA, of which, in humans, there are two classes: sIgA1 and sIgA2. Dimeric IgA, secreted from plasma cells, binds to a polymeric Ig receptor (pIgR) on the basolateral surface of the epithelial cells that line the mucous membrane. The complex is endocytosed and the external domain of the pIgR is split off at the apical surface of the cells. The remaining portion, now termed the *secretory component*, remains attached to IgA to form sIgA, which is secreted into the mucosal lumen. sIgA is the first line of defense because it binds to antigens and to microbes and their toxins, and helps to prevent especially viruses from attaching to or penetrating the mucosal surface.[30,31] This function is enhanced by the resistance of sIgA to many proteases, though sIgA1 is particularly susceptible to some bacterial proteases.

There is increasing evidence from in vitro studies with Sendai and influenza viruses[61,62] that IgA in transit through an epithelial cell can contact and effectively neutralize a virus that may infect those cells; this function is supported by several in vivo studies. There is additional evidence that the complexes so formed may be discharged into the lumen. In this particular circumstance, it has been suggested that IgA should be able to synergize with cell-mediated immune responses in controlling an intracellular infection.[60]

Two other aspects deserve brief comment. Oral administration of soluble antigens, in contrast to particulate preparations, often leads to antibody tolerance. This is in part a safety response against antigens in food. Second, mucosal antibody responses are usually much shorter than serum antibody responses for reasons that are not clear. The ability to prolong mucosal antibody responses would add further to the attractions of oral and respiratory immunization routes.

A diverse group of cells, the intraepithelial lymphocytes, are composed largely of CD8[+] T cells. Some have the usual $\alpha\beta$ TCRs, but others have $\gamma\delta$ TCRs. Some are cytotoxic, and one of their roles may be to destroy infected epithelial cells. Antiviral CD8[+] CTLs with $\alpha\beta$ TCRs have been found in the vaginal mucosa of simian immunodeficiency virus–infected monkeys[63] and in cytobrush specimens from the cervices of HIV-infected women.[64] Cells with $\gamma\delta$ TCRs are increasingly seen to have diverse functions. One group—Vγ2Vδ2T cells, found only in primates—recognize nonpeptide antigens secreted by some bacteria and parasites (e.g., polysaccharides) and rapidly mediate resistance to the infection.[65]

Commentary on the Roles of Different T-Cell Subsets in Intracellular Infections

It has become abundantly clear that varying results can be obtained using KO mice to elucidate the roles of different T cells. In CD8[+] T cell–deficient mice, compensatory mechanisms such as greater activity of NK cells or primary CD4[+] T cells displaying cytotoxic activity can contribute to controlling an infection. Nevertheless, a pattern most clearly seen with viral infections is beginning to emerge. There is significantly impaired clearance of lymphocytic choriomeningitis virus,[38] Theiler's virus,[66] and ectromelia virus[67] in CD8[+] T cell–deficient mice. In contrast, such mice have survived infection with influenza virus (in SCID mice[28,68]), vaccinia virus (in nu⁻/nu⁻ mice[69,70]), and Sendai virus.[71] A notable difference among these findings is that the former (i.e., lymphocytic choriomeningitis, Theiler's, and ectromelia viruses) are natural mouse pathogens, whereas influenza and vaccinia virus are not. The Sendai virus case is of special interest because it behaves like a mouse pathogen. In Sendai virus–infected β_2m KO mice, there is delayed clearance but many mice survive. However, in such situations in mice, the primary CD4[+] T cells can become cytotoxic. Because the virus mainly infects the lung epithelial cells, which are class II MHC positive, the "unnaturally" cytotoxic CD4$^+$ T cells "take over" the role of CD8$^+$ CTLs. In regard to the bacteria, CD8$^+$ T cells are also very important in *Listeria* infections and in virulent *Mycobacterium* infections, but they are less important in infections with the attenuated BCG strain. Thus, in some situations, CD4$^+$ type 1 cells can contribute significantly to protection.

This review illustrates one important message. Vaccines for human use are made to protect against natural human pathogens. Therefore, if there is reason for a vaccine to stimulate a type 1 T-cell response (as discussed earlier), the decision should be to choose a protocol for vaccine development that induces specific CD8$^+$ in addition to a CD4$^+$ type 1 T-cell response. Conditions for stimulating a CD8$^+$ CTL response usually also stimulate a type 1 CD4$^+$ T-cell response, whereas protocols for stimulating the latter response do not always induce a CTL response.

Pathogenesis of Infections and Vaccine Requirements

The interpretations expressed in Table 3–2 concerning the relative roles of different responses—antibody versus type 1 T cells—in the control of an intracellular infection represent an "average" situation. The pathogenesis of a particular infection could influence the relative intensity of the responses that a vaccine to control that infection should induce. Three different situations are possible:

1. Poliovirus infects the gut mucosa, and the viral progeny is mainly secreted into the gut. Oral poliovirus vaccine (OPV) induces IgM and IgG as well as sIgA; however, it is the sIgA that not only greatly limits the initial infection but also neutralizes much of the viral progeny. The IgM and IgG induced by OPV and inactivated poliovirus vaccine prevent the viremia that can occur in some cases and that might otherwise result in infection of nerve cells. The importance of the antibody response is indicated by the ratings given in Table 3–4. Similarly, with diphtheria and tetanus, the overwhelming need is for the vaccines to induce sufficiently high levels of antibody to "neutralize" the secreted toxins.
2. In the case of measles, mumps, and perhaps to a lesser extent rubella, the initial infection leads to a primary viremia. After infections at other sites, a secondary viremia may follow. Because the viremias do not

appear to be cell associated, it is important for a vaccine to induce a strong antibody response as well as a type 1 T-cell response to limit production of virus at both the primary and secondary sites. (This is the basis of the ratings given in Table 3–4.)
3. If, after the initial infection, viral progeny become largely (although not necessarily entirely) cell associated, being passed from cell to cell, then a desirable vaccine is one that induces a strong type 1 T-cell response to contain and clear a subsequent infection. Pox and rabies viral infections are in this category (see Table 3–4). Similarly, after exposure to M. *tuberculosis*, infected cells transport the organisms from the lung to other sites in the body, where fibrosis and encapsulation can occur. Here again, a vaccine that induces a strong type 1 T-cell response is important (Table 3–4), as illustrated by the discussion in the earlier section.

Immunologic Memory

The most effective vaccines induce strong immunologic memory; however, especially in the case of T cells, this has been one of the more difficult areas in which to elucidate mechanisms. Some aspects of this topic have been reviewed.[72]

B-Cell Memory

Memory B cells are formed in the germinal centers (GCs) of lymphoid tissue. Foreign antigen, as antigen–antibody complexes and in the presence of complement (C'), attach via C' receptors to the surface of FDCs. A rapidly dividing B cell, the centrocyte, in the GC undergoes somatic hypermutation. Subsequently, cells with Ig receptors of higher affinity are selected by the retained antigen to undergo further differentiation. Some of these become ASCs, such as plasma cells, most of which migrate to the bone marrow. Others become memory B cells, which circulate around the body. When these cells return to antigen-containing lymphoid tissue, the cycle of differentiation may begin again, resulting in the production of more antibodies. Even intact viral particles (e.g., HIV-1[73]) may attach to FDCs in this way, thereby assisting in the production of antibody that binds with high affinity to the intact virus, some of which would therefore be expected to neutralize infectivity (especially viral) effectively.

Memory B cells, in contrast to naive, immunocompetent cells and because they have earlier interacted with Th cells, express receptors of other subtypes—IgA, IgG, or IgE. There is some evidence that they express less of another B cell marker.[3]

The purpose of a boosting dose of antigen is to induce the differentiation of existing B memory cells to form ASCs, to induce the formation of additional B memory cells, and to increase or replenish the antigen depot in the GCs. This would enhance the recruitment of cells from the total memory B-cell pool. An early experiment[74] demonstrated the importance of the size of the antigen dose. Groups of rats were immunized with 10-fold graded doses of

TABLE 3–4 ■ Relative Roles of Antibody or Type 1 T Cells in Control of Some Infections for Which Vaccines Are Available

Disease Agent	Antibody*	Type 1 T Cell*
Poliovirus, *Clostridium tetani*, *Corynebacterium diphtheriae*	+++	+
Measles, mumps, rabies viruses	++	++
Pox, CMV, and EBV viruses; *Mycobacterium tuberculosis*	+	+++

*+++ very important; ++, important; +, less important.
CMV, cytomegalovirus; EBV, Epstein-Barr virus.

Salmonella flagella, varying from 100 pg to 10 µg in amount. This antigen is polymeric, resists degradation, and induces long-lasting antibody production. Six weeks later, each group of rats was challenged with a dose of flagella varying from 1 ng to 10 µg. Antibody titers were subsequently measured at different times. The answer was clear cut: An anamnestic response was not seen until the boosting dose of antigen was at least as high as the priming dose.

Some forms of immunization may be more effective at priming rather than boosting. Mice immunized with a DNA preparation of influenza virus hemagglutinin were boosted 4 weeks later with a fowlpox virus–hemagglutinin construct. Three weeks later, anti-hemagglutinin antibody titers were measured: Mice immunized with 10 or 100 µg of DNA before the challenge had antibody titers 25- to 50-fold higher than controls.[75] It may be that antigens that persist in a depot with adjuvant or on FDCs (e.g., polymers) are more effective than soluble, monomeric antigens at priming an immune response. Priming with DNA is of special interest and is further discussed later.

T-Cell Memory

Less is known about the development of memory T cells, but there are significant differences in this respect between B and T cells. As mentioned previously, there is a rapid expansion of responding T cells during an acute infection, but, once the infection is cleared, most effector cells die. In contrast, memory cells survive. Unlike the B-cell receptor, there is no somatic hypermutation to increase the affinity of the TCR during this expansion phase. Instead, there is a marked increase in avidity,[76] presumably as a result of a clustering together of TCRs (possibly in the same way that IgM has a higher avidity than IgG). Also, it is now generally recognized that persistence of specific antigen is not required for long-term CTL memory to occur,[3,77] and it is therefore not surprising that memory T cell formation does not seem to be limited to any particular site. There is no surface marker that unequivocally distinguishes memory from naive T cells.[78] Some evidence indicates that one TCR marker, an isoform of the CD45 molecule, is expressed at higher levels[17] on memory cells. This pattern has made it more difficult to distinguish clearly between activated, effector, and memory T cells.

To properly discharge their role, it is critical, especially for memory T cells, that they migrate freely around the body. It was early shown that chronic thoracic duct drainage would remove virtually all T cells but only some B cells from a mouse (reviewed by Sprent[79]).

One important property of memory T cells is that the requirements for stimulation to become effector cells are less stringent than those for naive T cells.[80] For example, memory T cells can be stimulated by APCs that do not express the co-stimulator molecule.[77] Furthermore, naive T cells require from 6 to greater than 30 hours of stimulation by APCs to become fully activated, whereas memory T cells are activated within 2 hours.[81] The net result is that a memory T-cell response has shortened kinetics and is also likely to be a stronger response. For example, CTLs to a primary influenza virus (e.g., H_1N_1) infection are first detected about 4 days[82] later in the lungs of mice infected intranasally with the virus, and reach peak levels at 6 to 7 days. If mice receive a priming dose of influenza virus (H_2N_2) some weeks before challenge with H_1N_1 virus, CTLs are found 1 to 2 days earlier and reach higher levels more rapidly than in the primary response.[82] This time difference may not seem large but could be critical in the case of a virus, such as influenza, that has an 8- to 10-hour replication cycle. For a marked boosting effect such as this to occur, a sufficient quantity of the challenge virus must avoid neutralization by pre-existing antibody to initiate a substantial infection. Antibodies to the H_1N_1 and H_2N_2 influenza viruses do not cross-neutralize.

Currently, a topic of great interest is what determines whether a naive cell differentiates into an effector cell or a memory cell.[81] One possibility is that a memory T cell is a naive cell that has been only partly activated by exposure to the APC. A greater knowledge of this pathway could influence future vaccine design.

Immunomodulation

Alum, first used in the 1940s, is still the only adjuvant regularly used in human vaccination. For many years, however, there have been great efforts to develop more effective preparations, especially by pharmaceutical companies.

It is convenient to separate the actions of adjuvants into three types[3,83]:

1. The formation of a depot of antigen primarily at the site of application and from which the antigen is released over a period of time that can be varied
2. The activation and maturation of APCs, particularly dendritic cells and macrophages, resulting in the expression of different chemokine receptors, and thus allowing different patterns of migration
3. An increased synthesis and secretion of enhancing factors, such as cytokines and chemokines, that act principally but not only on cells of the immune system, especially T and B lymphocytes.

In addition to achieving these goals, an adjuvant must be safe, it should with reasonable specificity target particular cells of the immune system, and it should be stable and affordable. By the nature of their role simply as immunomodulators, the development of preparations that fulfill all of these criteria is a time-consuming and expensive task. Table 3–5 describes in general terms a variety of materials used as adjuvants and gives a general statement about their activities. Not surprisingly, initial studies usually have been in murine systems because it is much more expensive to carry out experiments with primates and especially clinical trials. Preparations that showed promise in murine systems have sometimes given less encouraging results in primates or humans.

Alum has been by far the most common adjuvant used in humans. MF59, an oil-in-water emulsion containing squalene, has been well tolerated and has enhanced antibody production to antigens from HIV-1, herpesvirus, and influenza.[84]

A major recent advance has been the recognition that some cells of the innate immune system, especially APCs such as DCs, have receptors that recognize products that are common to some infectious agents, especially different bacteria, such as lipopolysaccharide and monophosphoryl lipid A.[85] The presence of such products signifies danger to the innate system. Interaction of the product (ligand) with the

TABLE 3–5 ■ Materials with Adjuvant Activity and Possible Sites of Action

Activities	Materials
Delayed release of antigen	Depot formers: water-in-oil, oil-in-water emulsion; controlled release devices; carriers (e.g., alum)
Mobilization of T-cell help	Proteins as carriers: polyclonal activators of T cells, PPD, polyA/poly U
Modulation of Ig receptors on B cells	B-cell mitogens: antigen polymerizing factors
Localization of antigens in T-dependent areas	Hydrophobic antigens: addition of lipid tail to proteins
Stimulation of APCs	MDP derivatives: LPS, lipid A, bacterial DNA (with CpG motives)
Facilitation of cell–cell interaction	Surface-acting materials (e.g., saponin, lysolethicin, Quil A, liposomes, pluronic polymers)
Focusing of antigen on cells with Fc receptors	Activators of alternate pathway of complement, inulin, zymozan, endotoxin

APCs, antigen-presenting cells; LPS, lipopolysaccharide; MPD, muramyl dipeptide; PPD, purified protein derivatives.
Modified from Ada G, Ramsay A. Vaccines, Vaccination and the Immune Response. Philadelphia, Lippincott–Raven, 1997.

appropriate receptor initiates the process of DC activation and maturation, and this leads in turn to a very strong T-cell response. Bacterial DNA is of special interest because, unlike mammalian DNA, it contains unmethylated CpG motifs that are recognized as foreign (i.e., dangerous) by DCs.[86] These bacterial products enhance both systemic and mucosal responses, and CpG DNA is claimed to induce stronger immune responses with less toxicity than other adjuvants.[87] To judge from recent work,[88,89] CpG DNA will be increasingly used as an adjuvant.

Selective Induction of Different Immune Responses

Adjuvants stimulate the production of certain cytokines, and some of these, at least in the mouse, can influence the production of different immunoglobulin isotypes (reviewed in Ada and Ramsay[3]). For example, IL-6 stimulates mucosal IgA as well as IgG responses. Two cytokines in particular, IL-4 and IL-12, have been shown to dominate the overall immune response: IL-4 induces a type 2 T-cell response characterized by strong Ig responses. However, when introduced early into the response to an infectious agent, by using a chimeric live vector containing DNA coding for IL-4, the subsequent CTL response[90] was greatly decreased. Infection of mice genetically resistant to ectromelia with IL-4–expressing ectromelia virus caused high mortality rates. Even mice preimmunized with the resistant strain and infected with the IL-4–expressing ectromelia showed a significant level of mortality.[91]

In contrast, transfer of IL-12 favors a type 1 T-cell response. In one report, a single subcutaneous injection of recombinant IL-12 of rhesus monkeys 2 days before challenge with P. cynomolgi sporozoites protected all of seven monkeys.[92] Protection was associated with high levels of IFN-γ that may have contributed to the elimination of infected hepatocytes. In another example, coadministration of a DNA preparation to induce an anti–HIV-1 response in mice together with DNA coding for IL-12 resulted in a "dramatic increase" in the specific CTL response.[93] This approach would need to be monitored carefully, because there are other reports showing that administration of IL-12 can lead to unwanted effects. For example, IL-12 has been shown to exacerbate O. volvulus antigen-mediated corneal pathology by enhancing chemokine expression and recruitment of inflammatory cells.[94]

An estimate of the effectiveness of different preparations of viruses and bacteria or viral antigens and of some immunomodulators at inducing CTL responses is presented in Table 3–6.[90,91,93,95–110] Attenuated preparations of viruses or bacteria that induce an acute infection generally have been highly effective at generating CTL responses. They are also effective when used as vectors of other antigens. Currently, DNA seems to be at least as effective as attenuated infectious agents at inducing CTL responses.[95] Inclusion of DNA coding for many antigens into the vector or into the DNA construct should give a broader response. The responses to inactivated whole virus may vary. γ-Irradiated but not ultraviolet-inactivated influenza A virus induces a strong, cross-reactive influenza A CTL response.[97,98] Feline immunodeficiency virus, inactivated with paraformaldehyde and administered with threonyl muramyl dipeptide and Syntox Adjuvant Formulation-Microfluidized (SAF-M), induced strong and long-lasting CTL responses. When used as a vaccine in cats, the protective immunity observed was associated with CTL activity.[99] Table 3–6 also indicates that, although alum preferentially induces a strong antibody response, there are now a variety of preparations or methods of antigen formulation that may induce medium to strong CTL responses. A comparison of a number of different delivery systems for the induction of CTL responses[111] showed that the three most immunogenic systems were bacterial DNA, recombinant Ty virus-like particles, and a recombinant attenuated vaccinia virus preparation (Ankara). Adsorbing the chimeric bacterial DNA onto cationic poly(lactide-co-glycolide) microparticles (which are biodegradable and biocompatible) greatly improved antibody and, to a lesser extent, CTL responses.[112]

The "Prime/Boost" Approach for Inducing Strong Immune Responses

Following the earlier demonstration of greatly improved antibody production using a prime (chimeric DNA)/boost (chimeric live vector) vaccination sequence, this approach has now been extended to generate remarkably high levels of CTL activity in mice and monkeys (reviewed by Ada[96]). Recombinant bacterial DNA has proved to be very effective for priming, and recombinant poxviruses (Ankara, fowl) or adenoviruses, or modified IL-2, are used for the booster immunization. In the absence of neutralizing antibodies, the enhanced CTL responses cleared HIV-1, simian

TABLE 3–6 ■ Selective Induction of Cytotoxic T-Cell Responses

Preparation	CTL Induction*	Reference
Viruses, bacteria		
Live, attenuated viruses, bacteria	+++	
Recombinant, live attenuated viruses, bacteria	++	
Bacterial DNA as immunogen	+++	95
Prime with chimeric bacterial DNA, boost with recombinant live vector	++++	96
Inactivated (ultraviolet irradiation) whole virus†	–	97
Inactivated (γ-irradiation) whole virus†	++	98
Inactivated whole virus with adjuvants‡	++	99
Immunomodulators		
Alum	–	100
IL-4	–	90, 91
IL-12	+++	93
Lipid-associated antigens	++	101–105
Liposomes, FCA, FIA, QS21, lipopeptides		
Particulate antigens	++	106–109
ISCOMs, antigens on beads or aggregated, lipid-encapsulated antigen; virus-like particles		
Oxidative conjugation to mannan	+++	110

*+++, high levels; ++, medium levels; –, little, if any, generated.
†Influenza virus inactivated by ultraviolet or γ-irradiation.
‡Feline immunodeficiency virus, inactivated with paraformaldehyde and administered with threonyl muramyl dipeptide and syntax adjuvant formulation-microfluidized.
FCA, Freund's complete adjuvant; FIA, Freund's incomplete adjuvant; QS21, derived from saponin; ISCOMs, immunostimulating complexes.

immunodeficiency virus, and Ebola virus infections and prevented disease in monkeys, as well as malaria in mice. Where tested, priming with the chimeric pox virus and boosting with DNA was much less efficient.

The ability to generate strong type 1 T-cell responses, and the exciting information accruing following the sequencing of the genomes of important bacterial and parasitic human pathogens are very important developments. They offer the prospect of developing vaccines that will clear rather than prevent infections by those agents that to date have resisted vaccine development based on generating strong antibody responses.

Requirements for Successful Vaccination

The requirements for successful vaccination can be described as follows (modified from Ada and Ramsay[3]):

1. The activation of APCs, involving the processing of antigens by the lysosomal or cytoplasmic pathways, the expression of co-stimulatory factors and chemokine receptors at the cell surface, and the secretion of certain cytokines.
2. The activation, replication, and differentiation of T and B lymphocytes leading to the generation of large pools of memory cells of both types.
3. The incorporation of sufficient B cell epitopes to generate strong neutralizing antibody responses, and of T-cell determinants that bind with high affinity to at least the major regional HLA haplotypes so that the complex is recognized by the T-cell receptor.

4. The long-term persistence of conformationally intact antigen, preferably as aggregates complexed with antibody and held at the surface of FDCs in lymphoid tissues. This allows the continuing production of cells that secrete antibody of increasingly higher affinity, and of memory B cells.

There are two further considerations with regard to point 3. Sometimes one or a few T-cell determinants in an antigen may be dominant in the sense that other determinants are recognized less well—the concept of *immunodominance*. The infectious agents may escape control by CTLs if these determinants are in a variable region of the antigen. In this situation, attempts should be made to induce responses to less dominant determinants in conserved regions of the antigen.[113] Second, because of a phenomenon called *cross-tolerance*, all individuals expressing an MHC antigen of a given specificity may not respond to a determinant that is known to bind strongly to that molecule.[114] This again stresses the need for a vaccine to contain several T-cell determinants. These aspects and the evidence favoring the interpretation proposed in point 4 are discussed in greater detail elsewhere.[3]

Acknowledgment

The author would like to thank Stanley Plotkin for helpful comments on drafts of this chapter.

REFERENCES

1. Panum PL. Observations made during the epidemic of measles on the Faroe Islands in the year 1846. Med Classics 3:839–886, 1939.

2. Salk J, Drucker JA, Malvy D. Noninfectious poliovirus vaccine. *In* Plotkin SA, Mortimer ER (eds). Vaccines (2nd ed). Philadelphia, WB Saunders, 1994, pp 205–228.

3. Ada G, Ramsay A. Vaccines, Vaccination and the Immune Response. New York, Lippincott–Raven, 1997.

4. Medzhitov R, Janeway C. Innate immunity. N Engl J Med 343:338–344, 2000.

5. Nara PL, Smit L, Dunlop N, et al. Emergence of viruses resistant to neutralization by V3 specific antibodies in experimental human immunodeficiency virus type IIIB infection of chimpanzees. J Virol 64:3779–3791, 1990.

6. Parry N, Fox G, Rowlands D, et al. Structural and serological evidence for a novel method of antigenic variation in foot and mouth disease virus. Nature 347:569–572, 1990.

7. Croft M, Carter L, Swain SL, Dutton RW. Generation of polarized antigen-specific CD8 effector populations: reciprocal action of inter-leukins (IL)-4 and IL-12 in promoting type 2 instead of type 1 cytokine profiles. J Exp Med 180:1715–1725, 1994.

8. Kay AB. Allergy and allergic diseases. N Engl J Med 344:30–37, 109–113, 2000.

9. Davidson A, Diamond B. Autoimmune diseases. N Engl J Med 345:340–350, 2001.

10. Krieg AM, Wagner H. Causing a commotion in the blood: immunotherapy progresses from bacteria to bacterial DNA. Immunol Today 21:521–526, 2001.

11. Modlin RL. A toll for DNA vaccines. Nature 408:659–660, 2000.

12. Sato K, Kawasaki H, Nagayama H, et al. Signalling events following chemokine receptor ligation in human dendritic cells at different developmental stages. Int Immunol 13:167–179, 2001.

13. Sprent J, Tough DF. T cell death and memory. Science 293:245–248, 2001.

14. Ada GL, Jones PD. The immune response to influenza infection. Cont Top Microbiol Immunol 128:1–54, 1986.

15. Mullbacher A, Flynn, K. Aspects of cytotoxic T cell memory. Immunol Rev 150:113–128, 1996.

16. Waldmann TA, Tagaya Y. The multifaceted regulation of interleukin-15 expression and the role of this cytokine in NK cell differentiation and host response to intracellular pathogens. Annu Rev Immunol 17:19–49, 1999.

17. Imagawa DT, Lee MH, Wolinsky SM, et al. Human immunodeficiency virus type 1 infection in homosexual men who remain seronegative for prolonged periods. N Engl J Med 320:1458–1462, 1989.

18. Slifka MK, Antia R, Whitmire JK, Ahmed R. Humoral immunity due to long-lived plasma cells. Immunity 8:363–372, 1998.

19. Rodrigo M-J, Miravitlles M, Cruz M-J, et al. Characterization of specific immunoglobulin G (IgG) and its subclasses (IgG1 and IgG2) against the 23-valent pneumococcal vaccine in a healthy adult population: proposal for response criteria. Clin Diagn Lab Immunol 4:168–172, 1997.

20. Borrow P, Lewicki H, Hahn B, et al. Virus-specific CD8+ cytotoxic T lymphocyte activity associated with control of viremia in primary human immunodeficiency virus type-1 infection. Virology 68:6103–6110, 1994.

21. Koup RA, Safrit JT, Cao Y, et al. Temporal association of cellular immune responses with the initial control of viremia in primary human immunodeficiency virus type-1 syndrome. J Virol 68:4650–4655, 1994.

22. Zhang X, Sun S, Hwang I, et al. Potent and selective stimulation of memory phenotype C8+ T cells in vivo by IL-15. Immunity 8:591–597, 1998.

23. McKay PF, Schmitz JE, Barouch DH, et al. Vaccine protection against functional CTL abnormalities in the simian human immunodeficiency virus-infected rhesus monkeys. J Immunol 168:332–337, 2002.

24. Plotkin SA. Immunologic correlates of protection induced by vaccination. Pediatr Infect Dis 20:63–75, 2001.

25. Taylor G. The role of antibody in controlling and/or clearing virus infections. *In* Ada GL (ed). Strategies in Vaccine Design. Austin, TX, RG Landes, 1994, pp 17–34.

26. Chanock RM, Crowe JE, Murphy BR, Burton DR. Human monoclonal antibody Fab fragments cloned from combinatorial libraries: potential usefulness in prevention and/or treatment of major human viral disease. Infect Agents Dis 2:118–131, 1993.

27. Griffin DE, Levine B, Tyor WB, Irani DN. The immune response in viral encephalovirus. Semin Immunol 4:111–119, 1992.

28. Scherle PA, Palladino G, Gerhardt W. Mice can recover from pulmonary influenza virus infection in the absence of class I-restricted cytotoxic T cells. J Immunol 148:212–221, 1992.

29. Ramphal R, Cogliano RB, Shands JW, Small PA. Serum antibody prevents lethal murine influenza pneumonitis but not tracheitis. Infect Immun 29:992–996, 1979.

30. Renegar KB, Small PA. Passive transfer of local immunity to influenza virus infection by IgA antibody. J Immunol 146:1972–1978, 1991.

31. Renegar KB, Small PA. Immunoglobulin A mediates murine anti-influenza virus immunity. J Virol 65:2146–2148, 1992.

32. Ada GL, McElrath MJ. HIV-vaccine induced cytotoxic T cell response: potential role in vaccine efficacy. AIDS Res Hum Retroviruses 13:243–248, 1996.

33. Riddell SR, Watanabe KS, Goodrich JM, et al. Restoration of viral immunity in immunodeficient humans by the adoptive transfer of T cell clones. Science 257:238–241, 1992.

34. Walter EA, Greenberg PD, Gilbert MJ, et al. Reconstitution of cellular immunity against cytomegalovirus in recipients of allogeneic bone marrow by transfer of T cell clones from the donor. N Engl J Med 33:1038–1044, 1995.

35. Rooney CM, Smith CA, Ng CY, et al. Use of gene-modified virus-specific T lymphocytes to control Epstein-Barr virus-related lymphoproliferation. Lancet 345:9–13, 1995.

36. Kyburz D, Speiser DE, Battegay M, et al. Lysis of infected cells in vivo by anti-viral cytotoxic T cells demonstrated by release of cell internal viral proteins. Eur J Immunol 23:1540–1545, 1993.

37. Ando K, Guidotti LC, Wirth S, et al. Class I-restricted cytotoxic T lymphocytes are directly cytopathic for their target cells in vivo. J Immunol 152:3245–3253, 1994.

38. Kagi D, Ledermann B, Burki K, et al. Cytotoxicity mediated by T cells and natural killer cells is greatly impaired in perforin-deficient mice. Nature 369:31–36, 1994.

39. Rowland-Jones S, Sutton J, Ariyoshi K, et al. HIV-specific CTL activity in an HIV-exposed but uninfected infant. Lancet 341:860–861, 1993.

40. Cheynier R, Langlade-Demoyen P, Marescot M, et al. CTL responses in the PBMC of children born to HIV-infected mothers. Eur J Immunol 22:2211–2217, 1992.

41. Langlade-Demoyen P, Ngo-Giang-Huong N, Ferchat F, Oksenhendler E. Human immunodeficiency virus (HIV) nef-specific cytotoxic T lymphocytes in non-infected heterosexual contacts of HIV-infected patients. J Clin Invest 93:1293–1297, 1994.

42. Rowland-Jones S, Sutton J, Ariyoshi K, et al. HIV-specific cytotoxic T cells in HIV-exposed but uninfected Gambian women. Nat Med 1:59–64, 1995.

43. Pinto LA, Sullivan J, Berzofsky JA, et al. Env-specific cytotoxic T lymphocytes in HIV seronegative health care workers occupationally exposed to HIV-contaminated body fluids. J Clin Invest 96:867–876, 1995.

44. Simmons A, Nash AA. Zosteriform spread of herpes simplex virus as a model of recrudescence and its use to investigate the role of immune cells in the prevention of recurrent disease. J Virol 52:816–821, 1984.

45. Simmons A, Tscharke DC. Anti-CD8 impairs clearance of herpes simplex virus from the nervous system: implications for the fate of virally infected neurones. J Exp Med 175:1337–1344, 1992.

46. Liu Y, Mullbacher A. Activated B cells can deliver help for the in vitro generation of antiviral cytotoxic T cells. Proc Natl Acad Sci U S A 86:4629–4633, 1989.

47. Cardin RD, Brooks JW, Sarawar SR, Doherty PC. Progressive loss of CD8+ T cell-mediated control of a γ-herpesvirus in the absence of CD4+ T cells. J Exp Med 184:863–871, 1996.

48. Harty JT, Bevan MJ. T cells specific for a single nonamer epitope of *Listeria monocytogenes* are protective in vivo. J Exp Med 175:1531–1538, 1992.

49. Jiang X, Gregory SH, Wing EJ. Immune CD8+ T lymphocytes lyse *Listeria monocytogenes*-infected hepatocytes by a classical class I-restricted mechanism. J Immunol 158:287–293, 1997.

50. Pedrazzini T, Hug K, Louis JA. Importance of L3T4+ and Lyt-2+ cells in the immunologic control of infection with *Mycobacterium bovis* strain bacillus Calmette-Guérin in mice. J Immunol 139:2032–2037, 1987.

51. Leveton C, Barnass S, Champion B, et al. T cell mediated protection of mice against virulent *Mycobacterium tuberculosis*. Infect Immun 57:390–395, 1989.

52. Flynn JL, Goldstein MM, Triebold KJ, et al. Major histocompatibility class I-restricted T cells are required for resistance to *Mycobacterium tuberculosis* infection. Proc Natl Acad Sci U S A 89:12013–12017, 1993.

53. Ladel CH, Daugelat S, Kaufmann SHE. Immune response to *Mycobacterium bovis* bacille Calmette Guérin infection in major histocompatibility complex class I- and II-deficient knock-out mice:

contribution of CD4 and CD8 T cells to acquired resistance. Eur J Immunol 25:377–384, 1995.

54. Ladel CH, Blum C, Dreher A, et al. Protective role of γ/δ T cells and α/β T cells in tuberculosis. Eur J Immunol 25:2877–2881, 1995.

55. Tarnvic A. Nature of protective immunity to *Francisella tularensis*. Rev Infect Dis 11:440–450, 1989.

56. Yee D, Rhinehart-Jones TR, Elkins KL. Loss of either CD4+ or CD8+ T cells does not affect the magnitude of protective immunity to an intracellular pathogen, *Francisella tularensis* strain LVS. J Immunol 157:5042–5048, 1996.

57. Holland MJ, Conway DJ, Blanchard TJ, et al. Synthetic peptides based on *Chlamydia trachomatis* antigens identify cytotoxic T lymphocyte responses in subjects from trachoma-endemic populations. Clin Exp Immunol 107:44–49, 1997.

58. Arnoldi J, Kaufmann SHE. The contribution of CD8+ cytolytic T cells to the control of bacterial and parasitic infections. *In* Ada GL (ed). Strategies in Vaccine Design. Austin, TX, RG Landes, 1994, pp 83–98.

59. Rudzik O, Clancy RL, Percy DYE, et al. Repopulation with IgA-containing cells of bronchial and intestinal lamina propria after transfer of homologous Peyer's patches and bronchial lymphocytes. J Immunol 114:1599–1604, 1975.

60. Lamm ME. Interaction of antigens and antibodies at mucosal surfaces. Annu Rev Microbiol 51:311–340, 1997.

61. Mazanec MB, Coudret CL, Fletcher DR. Intracellular neutralization of influenza virus by IgA anti-HA monoclonal antibodies. J Virol 69:1339–1343, 1995.

62. Mazanec MB, Kaetzel CS, Lamm ME, et al. Intracellular neutralization of virus by immunoglobulin A antibodies. Proc Natl Acad Sci U S A 89:6901–6905, 1992.

63. Lohman BL, Miller CJ, McChesney MB. Antiviral cytotoxic T lymphocytes in vaginal mucosa of simian immunodeficiency virus-infected rhesus macaques. J Immunol 155:5855–5860, 1995.

64. Musey L, Hu Y, Eckert L, et al. HIV induces cytotoxic T lymphocytes in the cervix of infected women. J Exp Med 185:293–303, 1997.

65. Wang L, Kamath A, Das H, et al. Antibacterial effect of human $V\gamma 2V\delta 2$ T cells in vivo. J Clin Invest 108:1349–1357, 2001.

66. Fiette L, Aubert C, Brahie M, Rossi CP. Theiler's virus infection of beta 2-microglobulin-deficient mice. J Virol 67:589–592, 1993.

67. Karupiah G. Type 1 and type 2 cytokines in antiviral defense. Vet Immunol Immunopathol 63:105–109, 1998.

68. Eichelberger M, Allan W, Zijlstra M, et al. Clearance of influenza virus respiratory infection in mice lacking class I major histocompatibility complex-restricted CD8+ T cells. J Exp Med 174:875–880, 1991.

69. Ramshaw IA, Andrew ME, Phillips SM, et al. Recovery of immunodeficient mice from a vaccinia virus/IL-2 recombinant infection. Nature 329:545–547, 1987.

70. Spriggs MK, Koller BH, Sato T, et al. B2 microglobulin–CD8+ T cell-deficient mice survive inoculation with high doses of vaccinia viruses and exhibit altered IgG responses. Proc Natl Acad Sci U S A 89:6070–6074, 1992.

71. Hou S, Doherty PC, Zijlstra M, et al. Delayed clearance of Sendai virus in mice lacking class I MHC-restricted CD8+ T cells. J Immunol 149:1319–1325, 1992.

72. Doherty PC, Ahmed R. Memory to viruses. *In* Nathanson N (ed). Viral Pathogenesis. Philadelphia, Lippincott–Raven, 1997, pp 141–162.

73. Heath SL, Tew John G, Tew J Grant, et al. Follicular dendritic cells and human immunodeficiency virus infectivity. Nature 377:740–744, 1995.

74. Nossal GJV, Austin CM, Ada GL. Antigens in immunity. VII. Analysis of immunological memory. Immunology 9:333–348, 1965.

75. Leong KH, Ramsay AJ, Morin MJ, et al. Generation of enhanced immune responses by consecutive immunization with DNA and recombinant fowlpox virus. *In* Brown F, Chanock R, Ginsberg H, Norrby E (eds). Vaccines 95. Cold Spring Harbor, NY, Cold Spring Harbor Laboratory Press, 1995, pp 327–331.

76. Slifka MK, Whitton JL. Functional avidity maturation of CD8+ T cells without selection of higher affinity TCR. Nat Immunol 2:711–717, 2001.

77. Mullbacher A, Flynn K. Aspects of cytotoxic T cell memory. Immunol Rev 150:113–128, 1996.

78. Jacob J, Baltimore D. Modelling T-cell memory by genetic marking of memory T cells in vivo. Nature 399:593–597, 1999.

79. Sprent J. Circulating T and B lymphocytes in the mouse. 1. Migratory properties. Cell Immunol 7:10–39, 1973.

80. Byrne JA, Butler JL, Cooper MD. Differential activation requirements for virgin and memory T cells. J Immunol 141:3249–3257, 1988.

81. Lanzavecchia A, Sallusto F. Regulation of T cell immunity by dendritic cells. Cell 106:263–266, 2001.

82. Yap KL, Ada GL. The recovery of mice from influenza A virus infection: adoptive transfer of immunity with influenza virus-specific cytotoxic T cells recognizing a common virion antigen. Scand J Immunol 8:413–420, 1978.

83. Chedid L. Adjuvants of immunity. Ann Immunol Inst Pasteur 136D: 283–291, 1985.

84. Podda A. The adjuvanted influenza vaccines with novel adjuvants: experience with the MF59-adjuvanted vaccine. Vaccine 19:2673–2680, 2001.

85. Baldridge JR, Yorgensen Y, Ward JR, Ulrich JT. Monophosphoryl lipid A enhances mucosal and systemic immunity to vaccine antigens following intranasal administration. Vaccine 18:2416–2425, 2000.

86. Wagner H. Toll meets bacterial CpG DNA. Immunity 14:499–502, 2001.

87. Weeratna RD, McCluskie MJ, Xu Y, Davis HL. CpG DNA induces stronger immune responses with less toxicity than other adjuvants. Vaccine 18:1755–1762, 2000.

88. Miconnet I, Koenig S, Speiser D, et al. CpG are efficient adjuvants for specific CTL induction against tumor antigen-derived peptide. J Immunol 168:1212–1218, 2002.

89. Verthelyi D, Kenney RT, Seder RA, et al. CpG oligodeoxynucleotides as vaccine adjuvants in primates. J Immunol 168:1659–1663, 2002.

90. Sharma DP, Ramsay AJ, Maguire DJ, et al. Interleukin-4 mediates down regulation of antiviral cytokine expression and cytotoxic T lymphocyte responses and exacerbates vaccinia virus infection in vivo. J Virol 70:7103–7107, 1996.

91. Jackson RJ, Ramsay AJ, Christensen CD, et al. Expression of mouse interleukin-4 by a recombinant ectromelia virus suppresses cytolytic lymphocyte responses and overcomes genetic resistance to mousepox. J Virol 75:1205–1210, 2001.

92. Hoffman SL, Crutcher FM, Puri SK, et al. Sterile protection of monkeys against malaria after administration of interleukin-12. Nat Med 3:80–83, 1997.

93. Kim JJ, Ayavoo V, Bagarazzi ML, et al. In vivo engineering of a cellular immune response by coadministration of IL-12 expression vector with a DNA immunogen. J Immunol 158:816–826, 1997.

94. Pearlman E, Lass JH, Bardenstein DS, et al. IL-12 exacerbates helminth-mediated corneal pathology by augmenting inflammatory cell recruitment and chemokine expression. J Immunol 158:827–833, 1997.

95. McDonnell WM, Askari FK. Molecular medicine: DNA vaccines. N Engl J Med 334:42–45, 1995.

96. Ada G. Advances in immunology: vaccines and vaccination. N Engl J Med 345:1042–1053, 2001.

97. Braciale TJ, Yap KL. Role of viral infectivity in the induction of influenza virus-specific cytotoxic T cells. J Exp Med 147:1236–1252, 1978.

98. Mullbacher A, Ada GL, Tha Hla R. Gamma-irradiated influenza A virus can prime for a cross-reactive and cross-protective immune response against influenza A virus. Immunol Cell Biol 66:153–158, 1988.

99. Flynn JN, Keating P, Hosie MJ, et al. Env-specific CTL predominate in cats protected from feline immunodeficiency virus infection by vaccination. J Immunol 157:3658–3665, 1996.

100. Bomford R. Relative adjuvant efficacy of AL(OH)$_3$ and saponin is related to the immunogenicity of the antigen. Int Arch Allergy Appl Immunol 75:280–281, 1984.

101. Gupta RK, Relyveld EH, Lindblad EB, et al. Adjuvants—a balance between toxicity and adjuvanticity. Vaccine 11:293–306, 1993.

102. Yong K, Ying L, Kapp JA. Ovalbumin injected with complete Freund's adjuvant stimulates cytolytic responses. Eur J Immunol 25:549–553, 1995.

103. Blum-Tirouvanziam U, Beghdadi-Rais C, Roggero MA, et al. Elicitation of specific cytotoxic T cells by immunization with malaria soluble synthetic soluble peptides. J Immunol 153: 4134–4137, 1994.

104. Hancock GE, Speelman DJ, Frenchick PJ, et al. Formulation of the purified fusion protein of respiratory syncytial virus with the saponin QS21 induces protective immune responses in Balb/c mice that are similar to those generated by experimental infection. Vaccine 13:391–400, 1995.

105. Sauzet JP, Deprez B, Martinon F, et al. Long-lasting anti-viral cytotoxic T lymphocytes induced in vivo with chimeric-multirestricted lipopeptides. Vaccine 13:1339–1345, 1995.

106. Jones PD, Tha Hla R, Morein B, Ada GL. Cellular immune response in the murine lung to local immunization with influenza A virus glycoproteins in micelles and ISCOMS. Scand J Immunol 27:645–652, 1988.

107. Kovacsovics-Bankowski M, Clark K, Benacceraf B, Rock KL. Efficient major histocompatibility complex class I presentation of exogenous antigen upon phagocytosis by macrophages. Proc Natl Acad Sci U S A 90:4942–4996, 1993.

108. Bachmann MF, Kundig TM, Freer G, et al. Induction of protective cytotoxic T cells with viral proteins. Eur J Immunol 24:2228–2236, 1994.

109. Zhou F, Rouse BT, Huang L. Induction of cytotoxic T lymphocytes in vivo with protein entrapped in membranous vehicles. J Immunol 149:1599–1604, 1992.

110. Apostolopoulos V, Loveland BE, Pietersz GA, McKenzie IFC. CTL in mice immunized with human mucin 1 are MHC restricted. J Immunol 155:5089–5094, 1995.

111. Allsopp CEM, Plebanski M, Gilbert S, et al. Comparison of numerous delivery systems for the induction of cytolytic T lymphocytes. Eur J Immunol 26:1951–1959, 1996.

112. O'Hagan D, Singh M, Ugozzoli M, et al. Induction of potent immune responses by cationic microparticles with adsorbed human immunodeficiency virus DNA vaccines. J Virol 75:9037–9043, 2001.

113. Good MF. Harnessing cytotoxic T lymphocytes for vaccine design. Lancet 345:1003–1007, 1995.

114. Hill AB, Mullbacher A, Blanden RV. Ir genes, peripheral cross-tolerance and immunodominance in MHC class I-restricted T-cell responses: an old quagmire revisited. Immunol Rev 133:75–92, 1993.

115. Glenn GM, Taylor DN, Li X, et al. Transcutaneous immunization: a human vaccine delivery strategy using a patch. Nat Med 6:1403–1407, 2000.

Chapter 4

The Vaccine Industry

R. GORDON DOUGLAS

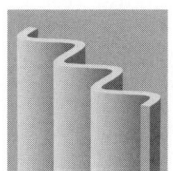

The vaccine industry is composed of companies that receive their revenue chiefly from sales of vaccine products or expectations thereof, and that are engaged in any of the following activities: research, development, manufacture, sales, marketing, and distribution of vaccines. The vaccine industry is relatively small but growing. Sales in 1999 were estimated to be $6 billion US worldwide.[1] Although components of the vaccine industry are found worldwide—in 50 countries according to the World Health Organization—the large vaccine companies with annual sales of vaccine products of $1 billion or greater who are engaged in all the above activities are concentrated in the United States and Europe.

The United States has been extraordinarily successful in vaccine research and development (R&D).[2,3] In the past 25 years, more than two thirds of all new vaccines approved worldwide have been developed in the United States. Eighteen new vaccines were approved between 1980 and 1996.[4,5] This success results from a "delicate fabric of public and private collaboration" that evolved in response to scientific, public health, and economic forces during the past 50 years.[6] This "delicate fabric" is a network of independent industrial, governmental, and academic partners engaged in vaccine R&D. It is not controlled by a single authority. Each component makes independent decisions based on its own interests. It is important that policy makers be aware of this independence and interdependence.

Vaccine development is difficult, complex, and costly and includes both clinical and process components. Clinical development involves studies of the effects of vaccines on patients for safety and efficacy, and process development involves investigations of manufacturing techniques required to transfer laboratory procedures to mass production with consistency and safety. Because the essential components of the final product for most vaccines cannot be measured with chemical precision, to assure consistency biologic manufacturing processes are controlled by assessing product components at multiple stages of the manufacturing cycle, thus requiring development of multiple analytic assays that must be validated. In process development, multiple tasks must be completed in a timely fashion; some can be done simultaneously, whereas others must follow sequentially. Any change in the manufacturing process may result in a change in the end product, and thus a different vaccine. Therefore, improvements in manufacturing processes cannot be undertaken once a Phase III trial is begun. As a result of these factors, vaccine development requires strong management systems and controls, and clinical and process development tasks must be closely coordinated. Investigator-initiated research, which has been so successful for National Institutes of Health (NIH)–funded basic research, will not work for development. In addition, process development may be as costly as clinical development. As development proceeds toward licensure, costs escalate as clinical studies become larger, manufacturing scales up, and facilities must be built. Postlicensure studies of safety and efficacy of vaccines are essential and represent a large additional cost.

Manufacturing plants are very expensive, ranging from US $50 to $200 million depending on the size (dose requirements) and manufacturing complexity. With few exceptions, each vaccine requires a different plant because of unique manufacturing requirements. Some processes are scalable, such as bacterial or yeast fermentation, so that increasing the size of the manufacturing unit (i.e., fermenter) somewhat will greatly increase the yield; unit cost will decrease with volume increase. Other manufacturing processes, particularly those dependent on viral growth in cell cultures, are not scalable. Additional plants must be built to increase the yield, so unit costs do not appreciably decrease with volume increases. The commitment to build a plant must be made early (4 to 5 years before expected licensure) in order to expedite product to the market. Otherwise a gap of 1 to 5 years between licensure and launch of product to the market will occur. Such decisions pose large financial risks if the product in development fails, and, in any case, require easy access to large amounts of capital, an attribute of large pharmaceutical companies.

Estimates of the cost of development of a new drug or vaccine have risen from $231 million US in 1991 to $802 million US in 2001.[7,8] These estimates take into account all costs, including R&D costs on products that fail, postlicensure clinical studies, and improvements in manufacturing processes. Approximately 50% of the cost is tangible, and the remainder is the cost of capital. These numbers have been debated (others estimate $100 to $200 million US[8]);

however, the higher estimates have been validated in two ways. First, the number of new vaccines brought to licensure annually by a company or the industry is very small, and is related to R&D expenditures of $600 to $800 million US. Thus, if a company spent $100 million annually for vaccine R&D, one might expect one new product every 6 to 8 years, and this appears to hold true. Second, biotechnology companies that are focused on one vaccine and have successfully brought it to market have spent $500 to $700 million on R&D (e.g., Aviron/Medimmune).

Role of Partners

In order to understand the predominant role of industry in the development of vaccines, one must examine its role in relation to those of its partners. The relative contributions of the various partners to the "delicate fabric" of vaccine R&D is shown in Table 4–1. Several branches of the U.S. government play major roles in vaccine R&D. The NIH is the major funder via intra- and extramural (largely academic) programs of fundamental research (e.g., recombinant DNA technology or T-cell memory studies, which may lead to new vaccine concepts) and directed research on pathogens and specific vaccine concepts to yield candidate vaccines. The NIH, through its vaccine trials networks, has recently increased its role in clinical development domestically and internationally.

The Food and Drug Administration (FDA) is the agency responsible for licensing new pharmaceutical products. The FDA establishes standards for manufacturing processes, facilities, and pre- and postlicensing clinical studies to ensure that licensed vaccines are safe and effective. These standards have a profound impact on the nature and direction of vaccine development and its costs. In addition, the FDA maintains a strong research base internally, so that it is better positioned to evaluate data from various studies.

The Centers for Disease Control and Prevention (CDC) conducts epidemiologic studies, defines the magnitude of the public health impact of disease, and performs surveillance needed to identify risk factors. Its primary role in vaccine R&D is to establish public health priorities for vaccine development, and to be the primary government agency responsible for postlicensure studies of safety and efficacy, usually conducted in conjunction with a large company. Through the Advisory Committee on Immunization Practices, it recommends usage of vaccines, and it is responsible for most of the public purchases (approximately 55% of all childhood vaccines in the United States), thus giving the CDC a major role in determining the demand and potential profit associated with vaccines. Professional organizations such as the American Academy of Pediatrics and the American College of Physicians also make recommendations for vaccine usage.

The U.S. Department of Defense (DOD) performs targeted vaccine research and development to help it perform its mission of protecting young adults serving in the military against infectious disease before their deployment outside the United States. Thus the DOD assesses the risk of encounters with various infectious diseases in specific theaters of current or potential operations. It directs its research to these targets if vaccines are not available in the private sector. The resulting vaccines may benefit U.S. travelers and residents of endemic areas as well. In addition to R&D activities, the DOD has limited manufacturing capacity to produce pilot lots of investigational vaccines, but much of this work is done in cooperation with large and small companies. A plan for a government-owned, contractor-operated vaccine manufacturing facility has been approved recently that, when operational, will greatly increase the DOD's manufacturing capacity.

The U.S. Agency for International Development (USAID) supports limited targeted R&D related to those vaccines that potentially will have the greatest impact on children under the age of 5 years in developing countries.

Nongovernmental organizations are playing an increasing role. Recently, the Bill and Melinda Gates Foundation has provided three organizations, the International AIDS Vaccine Initiative, the Malaria Vaccine Initiative, and the Sequella Global Tuberculosis Foundation, with significant funding for development of vaccines that would have the greatest impact on diseases of developing countries.

TABLE 4–1 ▪ U.S. Network Partners' Relative Contributions to Vaccine Research and Development*

	Research		Development			
	Basic/Related	Targeted	Process	Clinical	Manufacture	Postlicensure Studies
NIH	+++	+++		++		
CDC						++
FDA		+	+	+		+
DOD	+	+	+	+		+
USAID		+		+		
Large company	+	+++	+++	+++	+++	+++
Small company	+	+++	±	±	±	
Academia	+++	+++		+++		
NGOs		+		+		

*Relative contribution: +++, major; ++, intermediate; +, minor; ±, varies by company.
NIH, National Institutes of Health; CDC, Centers for Disease Control and Prevention; FDA, Food and Drug Administration; DOD, U.S. Department of Defense; USAID, U.S. Agency for International Development; NGOs, nongovernmental organizations.
Adapted from Marcuse EK, Braiman J, Douglas RG, et al, for the National Vaccine Advisory Committee. United States vaccine research: a delicate fabric of political and private collaboration. Reproduced with permission from Pediatrics 100:1015–1020, 1997.

The role of large, full-service vaccine companies (Table 4–2) is predominantly in development. They engage in some limited basic research, significant amounts of targeted research regarding specific organisms, and the preponderance of activity in clinical and process development. Expertise in process development and biologic engineering resides almost exclusively in such companies; there is no other resource for such development. Clinical development that will satisfy FDA standards is also done mostly by the large companies, funneled through academia and commercial research organizations.

Role of Small Companies

Many small organizations, often referred to as biotechnology companies, are engaged in vaccine research. They often are started by a university scientist with an idea. He or she convinces one or more venture capitalists to support the early research. Such organizations will have 10 to 50 employees, almost all of whom are engaged in research. No or limited capacity exists in process development, manufacturing, distribution, sales, or marketing. If research results are favorable, several additional rounds of venture funding may be undertaken; when certain milestones are reached, such as an investigational new drug (IND) filing, starting a Phase III clinical study, and/or proof of concept in Phase II clinical trials, stock may be issued to be publicly traded (initial public offering, or IPO), resulting in availability of more funds for R&D. As studies progress, capacity in process engineering, clinical studies, and manufacturing must be built. Such companies can fail at any stage, and often do. Poor laboratory results will preclude additional venture or public funding. Because of the large hurdle of adding new capacities and expertise, many companies in later stage development will opt for strategies other than "go it alone." Partnering with large, full-scale companies by out-licensing development rights on a given product, and contracting for process development and/or manufacturing, are common alternative strategies.

Although 60 or so small companies claim engagement in vaccine research and development, only about a dozen or so consider it a major activity, and only a very few, such as Chiron or Medimmune, have made it to the market or close to the market on their own (see Table 4–2). More have licensed their idea to larger companies that have then completed development, yielding new vaccines such as those for hepatitis B and *Haemophilus influenzae* type B. The greatest contributions of the biotechnology companies have been the introduction of multiple ideas into early vaccine development, and testing them to determine if they should be rejected or carried forward. These small companies are dependent on several factors for their success: (1) a vibrant basic research environment that allows for creation of new ideas, an environment that exists in well-funded (NIH) academic research programs; (2) a strong venture capital community that views vaccine companies as being as potentially financially rewarding as other investment opportunities; and (3) strong patent laws providing the intellectual property protection that is essential for venture and public funding of a research idea.

TABLE 4–2 ■ Vaccine Companies Worldwide

Name of Company	Location
LARGE FULL-SCALE COMPANIES*	
Aventis (Aventis Pasteur division)	France/Germany
Chiron (Chiron Vaccines division)	Italy
GlaxoSmithKline (GSK-Biologicals division)	U.K.
Merck & Co. (Merck Vaccine division)	U.S.
Wyeth (Wyeth–Lederle Vaccines division)	U.S.
SMALLER VACCINE COMPANIES†	
Baxter (Baxter Vaccines division)	Austria
Berna Products	Switzerland
Bioport	U.S.
CSL	Australia
Medimmune	U.S.
Powderject	U.K.
Serum Institute of India	India
BIOTECH VACCINE COMPANIES‡	
Acambis PLC	U.K.
Avant Immunotherapeutics	U.S.
Bavarian Nordic	Germany
Cantab Pharmaceuticals	U.K.
Cell Tech Pharma	U.K.
Corixa	U.S.
Genzyme Transgenics	U.S.
ID Biomedical	U.S.
NABI	U.S.
Rhein Biotech	The Netherlands
Vaxgen	U.S.
Vical Incorporated	U.S.
REGIONAL VACCINE COMPANIES§	
Biologico – Sidus	Argentina
Solvay	Belgium
Biolab Sanus Farma	Brazil
Butantan Institute	
Bio Manguinhos	
Intervax	Bulgaria
Kang Tai	China
NVSI of China	
Shanghai Biological Institute	
Center for Genetic Engineering and Biotechnology	Cuba
Statens Serum Institute	Denmark
Organon Teknika	France
Enpharma	Germany
Kohl Pharma	
MTK Pharma	
Robert Koch Institute	
Sachsciche Seruumwerke	
Western Pharma	
Biological E.	
Shanta Biotech	
Bio Farma	Indonesia
Kedrion	Italy
Biken	Japan
Chibaken Kessei	
Denka Seiken	
Japan BCG	
Kaketsuken	
Meiji	
Takeda Takuhin Kog	
Boryung Biopharma	Korea
Cheil Jedang	

Continued

such as varicella, rotavirus, and pneumococcal conjugate vaccine. Large companies believe that vaccines should be priced according to value to society: reduction in health care costs, reduction in related costs, relief from pain and suffering, and/or prevention of death. Such prices far exceed manufacturing costs, but are essential to produce the revenue stream that allows vaccines to be competitive with other products in large pharmaceutical companies for R&D and manufacturing resources, and to create a business potential competitive with other industries in the eyes of venture capitalists.

A vigorous large-company vaccine industry is dependent on several factors: (1) a rich research environment, sponsored largely by the NIH and mostly carried out in academia, as the source for new creative ideas; (2) strong patent laws and protection of intellectual property; and (3) freedom to price products at fair levels related to the value of a product to society. Although the first two of these factors have been consistently present in recent years, downward pressure on price is a major threat to current companies and a disincentive to new companies. Freedom to price vaccines is restricted to the private market. Less than one half of the vaccines for children sold in the United States are sold in the private market; the rest are sold to federal or state governments at reduced prices. Controls are even greater in Western Europe and Japan, and internationally there is strong downward pressure on prices as one moves from well developed to less developed regions of the world.

In addition to partial price controls, a result of public purchase of the majority of vaccines, the vaccine industry is intensely regulated. It cannot sell its product until the product is approved by the FDA; each batch must be released by the FDA; and the usage of the product, and its market size, is largely determined by the CDC. Thus the vaccine industry does not operate in a free-market environment, and its behavior reflects these constraints.

The vaccine industry has contracted since 1967, when 26 different companies held vaccine licenses in the United States. In 1980, 17 companies held vaccine licenses; by 1993, of the 17 companies holding licenses, 6 had not held licenses in 1980, and 6 companies that had held licenses in 1980 no longer did.[5,9,10] In 2002, only 12 companies held vaccine licenses.[4] Some of this contraction is due to consolidation and building of larger, stronger companies (e.g., the merger of Lederle Laboratories, Inc. and Wyeth Laboratories, Inc.), but some is due to departure from the vaccine business (e.g., Eli Lilly & Co., E. R. Squibb & Sons). Because the pharmaceutical industry has grown in number and size in this same time period, it is apparent that vaccine business is less attractive to large companies than pharmaceutical business.

Doses Versus Dollars

Estimates of the total worldwide vaccine market revenue are $6 billion US. The top five western suppliers (see Table 4–2)[1] account for approximately 80% of these sales, or $4.8 billion US; the remainder come from regional vaccine com-

panies, the largest of which are located in middle-income countries such as India and Brazil (Table 4–2). In contrast, the same top five western companies supply only approximately 52% of the doses, or 2.8 million of 5.4 billion doses worldwide, with the remainder coming from regional vaccine companies. The majority of the top companies' dose volume consists of polio vaccine; if that is deleted (as it will be when polio eradication is achieved), their supply volume drops to 20% of worldwide volume. Volume output from U.S.-based large companies is much less than from those based in Europe; again, much of this difference is due to polio vaccine supply.

Vaccines for Unmet Needs: Role of the Vaccine Industry

To involve companies in development and manufacturing of vaccines to meet needs such as biodefense or health needs of poorer countries, incentives must be established to convince large companies that they should develop and manufacture such products. Such incentives might take the form of guaranteed purchase of certain volumes of a vaccine if specified standards are met, direct contracting by a government agency, or some other publicly funded mechanism. Companies may be willing to engage in such work; indeed, they may already have donated or sold vaccine at very low prices to poorer countries. However, such practices alone will not solve the enormity of the health problems worldwide. Without special incentives, it is unrealistic to expect companies to engage in R&D on diseases that only, or predominantly, affect the poorer regions of the world.[10]

REFERENCES

1. Whitehead P. Mercer Management Consulting New York, N.Y. Report to GAVI/The Vaccine Fund, 2002.
2. Warren KS. New scientific opportunities and old obstacles in vaccine development. Proc Natl Acad Sci U S A 83:9275–9277, 1986.
3. Halsted SB, Gellin BG. Immunizing children: can one shot do it all? *In* Medical and Health Annual 1994. Chicago, Encyclopedia Britannica, 1994.
4. Cohen J. Public health: U.S. vaccine supply falls seriously short. Science 295:1998–2001, 2002.
5. Peter G, des Vignes-Kendrick M, Eickhoff TC, et al. Lessons learned from a review of the development of selected vaccines. National Vaccine Advisory Committee. Pediatrics 104(4 pt 1):942–950, 1999.
6. Marcuse EK, Braiman J, Douglas RG, et al, for the National Vaccine Advisory Committee. United States vaccine research: a delicate fabric of political and private collaboration. Pediatrics 100:1015–1020, 1997.
7. Gregerson J. Vaccine development: the long road from initial idea to product licensure. *In* Levine MM, Woodrow GC, Kaspe JB, Cobon GS (eds). New Generation Vaccines. New York, Marcel Dekker, 1987, pp 1165–1183.
8. DiMasi J, Hansen R, Grabowski H. Cost of new drug development. SCRIP 2702:15, 2001.
9. Mercer Management Consulting. Testimony on vaccine policy before the U. S. House of Representatives Committee on Commerce, June 15, 1995.
10. Sing M, William MK. Supplying vaccines: an overview of the market and regulatory content. *In* Pauley M, Robinson CA, Sepe SJ, et al (eds). Supplying Vaccine: An Economic Analysis of Critical Issues. Amsterdam, IOS Press/Ohmsha, 1995, pp 45–99.

Chapter 5

Vaccine Manufacturing

GARY B. EBBERT • EUGENE D. MASCOLO

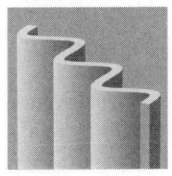

More than 1 billion doses of human vaccines are manufactured annually worldwide,[1-4] and "manufacturers continue to seek ways to improve current vaccines for existing clinical indications and to develop new immunogens for both pediatric and adult use."[2]

The success of a vaccine in preventing disease depends on several factors, including the quality of the immunizing agent, how it is handled, and its use by clinicians. This chapter focuses on the production of a quality immunizing agent.[3-6]

In the United States, vaccines are regulated as biologic products. "The Food and Drug Administration's (FDA) Center for Biologics Evaluation and Research (CBER) is responsible for regulating vaccines in the United States. Current authority for the regulation of vaccines resides primarily in Section 351 of the Public Health Service Act and specific sections of the Federal Food, Drug and Cosmetic Act."[7,8] Section 351 of the Public Health Service Act gives the federal government the authority to license biologic products as well as the establishments where they are produced.[9] "Vaccines undergo a rigorous review of laboratory, nonclinical, and clinical data to ensure the safety, efficacy, purity, and potency of these products. Vaccines approved for marketing may also be required to undergo additional studies to further evaluate the vaccine and often to address specific questions about the vaccine's safety, effectiveness, or possible side effects."[10]

New vaccines are subjected to a well-defined regulatory process for approval. The approval process consists of three principal elements[11]:

1. Testing for safety and effectiveness through nonclinical and clinical studies.
2. Preparing and submitting data and other related information for the investigational new drug application (IND).
3. Review of the submissions by the FDA.

When a manufacturer satisfies the pretesting requirements and demonstrates that the vaccine is sufficiently safe to be used in initial clinical trials, the manufacturer prepares and submits an IND application to the FDA.[11]

Investigational New Drug Application

The manufacturer or sponsor must submit an IND application to the FDA. The IND application describes the vaccine, its method of manufacture, and the quality control (QC) tests for release. Also included is information about the vaccine's safety and ability to elicit a protective immune response (immunogenicity) in animal testing, as well as the proposed clinical protocol for studies in humans.

Premarketing (prelicensure) vaccine clinical trials are usually done in three phases[9,11,12]:

Phase I—These are the initial safety and immunogenicity studies performed involving a small number of subjects (usually < 20).

Phase II—These are dose-ranging studies and involve a larger subject group of hundreds of individuals (typically 50 to several hundred).

Phase III—These studies involve several hundred to several thousand subjects and provide more extensive information on effectiveness and safety.

These trials may be conducted at several sites and may include both controlled and uncontrolled studies. The type and amount of clinical testing vary. Clinical vaccine development time averages 5 years but can range from 2 to 10 years.[11]

At any stage of the studies, the FDA may request additional information or studies or may halt the current clinical studies if data raise concerns about either safety or effectiveness.[13]

If all three phases of clinical development are successful, the manufacturer may submit a Biologics License Application (BLA).[8] Since the enactment of the FDA Modernization Act of 1997, only the BLA is required, and the licensing procedure has been simplified. The prelicensing inspection provides most of the information that was previously obtained from the Establishment License Application.[9] The BLA must provide the FDA reviewer team (medical officers, microbiologists, chemists, biostatisticians, and so on) with the necessary efficacy and safety information to make a risk/benefit assessment. During this stage, the proposed manufacturing facility undergoes a prelicensing inspection.[13,14]

After the FDA's review of a license application, the manufacturer and the FDA may present their findings to the Vaccines and Related Biological Products Advisory Committee (VRBPAC). This is a non-FDA expert committee that consists of scientists, physicians, biostatisticians, and a consumer representative. The committee gives the FDA advice on the safety and efficacy of the vaccine.[13]

Regulations also require adequate product labeling for health care providers to understand the vaccine's proper use and its potential benefits and risks so that they may safely deliver the vaccine to the public.[8]

Even after the vaccine and the manufacturing processes are approved, the FDA continues to oversee the production of vaccines. Monitoring of the product and of production activities continues as long as the manufacturer holds a license for the product. This includes periodic inspections of the manufacturing facilities. The FDA may require manufacturers to submit their own test results of potency, safety, and purity for each vaccine lot. In addition, manufacturers may be required to submit an annual report for certain changes made to the approved application.[15,16]

Because all potential adverse events cannot be anticipated, many vaccines undergo Phase IV studies. These consist of formal studies on a vaccine once it is on the market. The Vaccine Adverse Event Reporting System (VAERS) enables the government to identify any problems after the product is on the market.[9,13,17,18] Reports to the VAERS are welcome from all those who have a concern, including patients, parents, health care providers, pharmacists, and vaccine manufacturers.[10,19]

Product Development

Vaccine development involves the process of taking a new antigen or immunogen identified in the research process and developing this substance into a final vaccine that can be evaluated through preclinical and clinical studies to determine the safety and efficacy of the resultant vaccine. During this process, the product's components, in-process materials, final product specifications, and manufacturing process are defined. The manufacturing scale used during development is usually significantly smaller than that used in the final manufacturing process. Phase I, and sometimes Phase II, clinical trial vaccines are typically produced in product development, but it is usually anticipated that at least one of the three or more consistency lots used for Phase III clinical trials will be manufactured at full-scale production volume. The product manufactured during the development phase is manufactured according to current good manufacturing practices (cGMPs).[20]

Good Clinical Practices

In addition to determining which clinical studies are necessary, the FDA sets minimum standards for conducting these tests. The FDA does this through a set of regulations called good clinical practices (GCPs). In general, the GCPs outline the responsibilities of people who are involved in a clinical trial, including the manufacturer or sponsor, the investigator, the monitor, and the institutional review board (IRB).[21]

The manufacturer or sponsor is responsible for selecting qualified investigators and providing them with the information they need to properly conduct an investigation. The sponsor ensures that the investigation is monitored and conducted in accordance with the general investigational plan and protocols in the IND application. The sponsor is also responsible for maintaining an effective IND application and keeping the FDA and investigators informed of any significant new adverse effects or risks related to the product.[21]

The IRB's function is to see that risks to clinical subjects are minimized and that the subjects are adequately informed about the clinical trial and its implications for their treatment. The IRB consists of at least five people, each member having the professional competence to review research activities. At least one board member must have a primary interest other than science, such as law, ethics, or religion.

Current Good Manufacturing Practices

According to federal regulations, manufacturing means all the steps in the propagation or manufacture and preparation of products and includes, but is not limited to, filling, testing, labeling, packaging, and storage by the manufacturer.[22] The BLA can only be approved after examination of the product and after the determination that the product complies with standards established in the BLA.[23] The product must be available for inspection during all phases of manufacturing.[24] The BLA can be issued only after inspection of the establishment(s) listed in the BLA and after the determination that the establishment complies with the standards established in the BLA and the requirements prescribed in the applicable regulations.[25]

Federal regulations set forth detailed cGMPs that provide methods to ensure that the product meets safety requirements, and that the product has the inherent identity, strength, quality, and purity characteristics. These regulations include provisions for the following:

- Quality control
- Personnel qualifications and responsibilities
- Building and facilities—design, construction, and maintenance
- Equipment—design, construction, cleaning, and maintenance
- Components and product containers and closures
- Production and process controls
- Packaging and labeling control
- Holding and distribution
- Laboratory controls
- Records and reports
- Returned and salvaged products

The cGMPs are detailed in Sections 210 through 226 and Section 600 of the Code of Federal Regulations (CFR).[26,27]

Examples of Vaccine Production

Live Vaccine (Oral Polio)

Poliovirus live oral trivalent vaccine is a mixture of three types of attenuated polioviruses (Sabin) prepared in *Macaca* or *Cercopithecus* monkey kidney cell cultures: type 1 (LS-c, 2ab/KP$_2$), type 2 (P712, Ch, 2ab/KP$_2$), and type 3 (Leon 12a,b/KP$_3$).[28]

The cells are grown in Eagle's basal medium, consisting of Earle's balanced salt solution containing amino acids, antibiotics, and calf serum. After cell growth, the medium is removed and inoculated with one of the attenuated polioviruses suspended in the same medium without calf serum. The resulting monovalent virus is pooled, tested, and filtered before being used for trivalent vaccine formulation.

Each human dose of the live oral trivalent vaccine is constituted to have infectivity titers in the final container material of $10^{6.0}$ to $10^{7.0}$ for type 1, $10^{5.1}$ to $10^{6.1}$ for type 2, and $10^{5.8}$ to $10^{6.8}$ for type 3 when assayed in Hep-2 cells. The final vaccine is a sterile suspension of poliovirus types 1, 2, and 3, unpreserved, normally containing antibiotics and stabilizers.[29,30]

Criteria for Qualification of the Seed Virus

Each seed virus used in vaccine manufacturing is prepared from an acceptable strain in monkey kidney cell cultures. The seed virus must be demonstrated to be free of extraneous microbial agents except for unavoidable bacteriophage.[31] (There is a possibility that bacteriophage may be present in the medium, with a possible source being the calf serum, a component of the medium used for cell growth.) In addition, the neurovirulence of each of the first five consecutive monovalent virus pools (MVPs) prepared from the seed virus must meet the neurovirulence requirements.[32]

Manufacture of Live Poliovirus

The working seed virus (WSV) in vaccine manufacturing is prepared in a seed lot system from a master virus seed (MVS) lot.[33] A WVS consists of material having the same composition and origin, with a specific lot number and date of manufacture, and is usually one passage removed from the MVS. Both the MVS and the WSV are qualified for use during the licensing process.[34] Virus in the final vaccine should represent no more than five tissue culture passages from the original strain.[35]

Kidneys are processed separately for each monkey. The resulting viral fluid is identified as a separate monovalent harvest and is kept separate from other monovalent harvests until all samples for testing are taken.[36] Before inoculation with the seed virus, and at least 3 days after complete formation of the tissue sheet, the tissue culture growth in vessels derived from each pair of kidneys is examined microscopically for cell degeneration. If such evidence is observed, the tissue cultures from that pair of kidneys must not be used for vaccine manufacturing.[37]

The tissue found free of cell degeneration is tested for further evidence of freedom from demonstrable, viable, microbial agents. If these tests indicate the presence of any viable microbial agent in the monkey kidney production vessels, the viral harvest from these tissue cultures is not used for poliovirus vaccine manufacture.[38]

CONTROL VESSELS

At least 25% of the cell suspension from each pair of kidneys is set aside and used to establish control cultures, which must be examined microscopically for cell degenera-

tion for an additional 14 days. The culture fluids from such controls must be tested both at the time of the virus harvest and at the end of the observation period. In the culture systems just described, the control cell sheet is also examined for the presence of hemadsorbing viruses by the addition of guinea pig red blood cells.[39] At least 80% of the control vessels must be free of cell degeneration at the end of the observation period to qualify the kidneys for poliovirus vaccine manufacture. If any extraneous agent is present at the time of virus harvest, the virus harvest from that tissue culture preparation is not used for poliovirus vaccine manufacture. If any tests or observations demonstrate the presence of any microbial agent known to be capable of producing human disease, the virus grown in each tissue culture preparation is not used for vaccine production.[40]

INCUBATION

The temperature of the kidney tissue production vessels after inoculation with the virus is held at 33°C to 35°C during the course of virus propagation.[41] Virus grown at higher temperatures selects for virulence; therefore, the indicated incubation temperatures must be adhered to strictly.

VIRUS HARVESTS

Virus harvests are conducted no later than 72 hours after virus inoculation. Virus harvested from kidney tissue from one monkey may be tested separately, or samples of viral harvest from more than one pair of kidneys may be combined, identified, and tested as an MVP. The samples are withdrawn immediately after harvesting.[42]

Additional tests for safety are conducted on the MVP. The pools must demonstrate no viable microbial agents except for unavoidable bacteriophage and the intended attenuated live poliovirus. The vaccine is tested for the absence of other infectious agents, including polioviruses of other types or strains.[43] After the harvest and removal of samples for safety testing, the pool is sterile filtered, yielding a sterile MVP.[44] The sterile-filtered MVP is then tested for potency.

POTENCY TESTING

Concentrations of living virus in each MVP are expressed as infectivity titer per milliliter for cell cultures, using the live, attenuated reference poliovirus of the same type as a control. Titration of the MVP is not a valid test unless the titration of the reference virus, when tested in parallel, is within $\pm 0.5 \log_{10}$ of its established titer.[45]

NEUROVIRULENCE TESTING

After the MVP is sterile filtered, a neurovirulence test is performed in *Macaca* monkeys.[46] In this test, the absence of neurovirulence of the MVP is confirmed after intraspinal inoculation in monkeys shown not to have neutralizing antibodies.[47] As a control, monkeys are separately inoculated with a reference attenuated poliovirus. The MVP may be used for poliovirus vaccines if a comparative analysis of the test results demonstrates that the numerical value (quantified neuropathology results) assigned for neurovirulence of the MVP is equal to or less than that of the corresponding type of reference attenuated poliovirus.[48] "If the numerical value assigned for neurovirulence of the MVP is greater than that of the Reference Attenuated Poliovirus, the MVP is acceptable if the difference between these two values is not greater than that calculated by a mathematical method that is expected to reject vaccines with neurovirulence identical to the reference at a frequency of not less than 1 in 100 when one group of monkeys is inoculated. When two or three groups are injected with the same MVP under test, the frequency of rejection shall not be less than five in 100 and 10 in 100, respectively. If the difference in numerical values is greater than that calculated, irrespective of which reference preparation was used in the test, the MVP is unacceptable and not used for manufacturing."[49]

ADDITIONAL TESTS FOR SAFETY

Before Filtration. Tests are performed on the MVP before filtration to demonstrate the absence of microbial agents, except for unavoidable bacteriophage and the intended live, attenuated poliovirus. The vaccine is tested for the absence of other infectious agents, including poliovirus of other types or strains. These tests include the following[50,51]:

1. Inoculation of rabbits
2. Inoculation of adult mice
3. Inoculation of suckling mice
4. Inoculation of guinea pigs
5. Inoculation of monkey kidney tissue cultures
6. Inoculation of human cell cultures
7. Inoculation of rabbit kidney tissue culture
8. Tests for in vitro markers

After Filtration. In addition to the required neurovirulence tests, the following safety tests are performed on each MVP after the filtration process[52]:

1. In vitro marker tests
2. Final container sterility test, if needed

GENERAL REQUIREMENTS

Each MVP must (1) be manufactured by the same procedure, (2) meet the criteria for neurovirulence for monkeys,[53] (3) meet the criteria of in vitro markers,[54] and (4) be released for further manufacturing by the director of the CBER.[55]

SAMPLES AND PROTOCOLS

The following materials must be submitted to the director of the CBER: a protocol that consists of a summary of the history of manufacture of each MVP,[56] including any test results requested by the director of the CBER; 20 mL of MVP before filtration[57]; and 40 mL of MVP after filtration.[58]

Formulation

The trivalent poliovirus vaccine is formulated from MVPs consisting of the three types of attenuated polioviruses. The human dose of trivalent poliovirus vaccine must be constituted to have infectivity titers in the final container material of $10^{6.0}$ to $10^{7.0}$ for type 1, $10^{5.1}$ to $10^{6.1}$ for type 2, and $10^{5.8}$ to $10^{6.8}$ for type 3 when assayed in Hep-2 cells.[59]

GENERAL REQUIREMENTS

No lot of trivalent vaccine may be released by the manufacturer unless each MVP has met all the requirements and has been released by the CBER for further manufacturing.[60]

LABELING

The final container label must bear a statement indicating that liquid vaccine may not be used for more than 7 days after the container is opened.[61]

SAMPLES AND PROTOCOLS

For each trivalent vaccine, the following materials must be submitted in accordance with instructions from the director of the CBER[62]:

1. A protocol that consists of a summary of the history of manufacture of each trivalent lot, including any test results requested by the director of the CBER[63]
2. A 20-mL sample of the MVP before filtration[64]
3. A 40-mL sample of the MVP after filtration[65]
4. A total of at least 50 single doses of the trivalent vaccine[66]

The final vaccine is a sterile suspension of polioviruses types 1, 2, and 3, unpreserved, normally containing antibiotics and stabilizers.

Combination Vaccine

A combination vaccine consists of two or more live organisms, inactivated organisms, or purified antigens combined by the manufacturer or mixed immediately before administration.[67] A combination vaccine is intended to prevent multiple diseases or prevent one disease caused by different strains or serotypes of the same organism. "Vectored vaccines and conjugated vaccines are combination vaccines if the prevention of the disease caused by the vector organism or the carrier moiety is to be one of the combination's indications."[67]

Regulatory Requirements

Regulations that pertain to biologic products also apply to combination vaccines. The CFR section on permissible combinations (Title 21, Section 610.17) states that licensed products may not be combined with other licensed or unlicensed products unless a license is obtained for the combined product.

Manufacturing Issues for Combination Vaccines

Combining monovalent vaccines may result in a combination that is less safe or effective than is desired. For example, the components of inactivated vaccines may adversely affect one or more of the active components. This occurred when whole-cell pertussis vaccine and inactivated poliovirus vaccine were combined, resulting in a combination with decreased pertussis potency.[67]

When live vaccines are combined, immunologic interference has been observed between vaccine viruses or virus subtypes. "Consequently, the combined components stimulated weaker immune responses than did viruses administered separately. Component cross-reactivity could also occur with a combination of live vaccines where recombinational events may allow attenuated organisms to be reconstituted to virulent forms."[67] The CBER advises that the combination should be characterized and its components assessed through a battery of physicochemical, biochemical, and biologic assays.

The CBER also recommends conducting preclinical animal studies to determine the consequences of combination on potency and immunogenicity. The manufacturer must evaluate some of the physical characteristics, including the combination vaccine's resuspension, and ensure container and closure suitability. If the combination vaccine's volume is too large or its concentration is too high to be safely administered, the manufacturer may pursue the possibility of dose reduction for some or all of its components. The effects of such changes should be assessed before clinical trials.[67]

Killed Virus (Influenza)

"Influenza Virus Vaccine, USP, for intramuscular use is a sterile suspension prepared from influenza viruses propagated in chicken embryos. This vaccine is the primary method for preventing influenza and its more severe complications."[68]

This vaccine contains two strains of influenza A viruses (H1N1 and H3N2) and a single influenza B virus. The two type A viruses are identified by their subtypes of hemagglutinin (HA) and neuraminidase (NA). The HA and NA glycoproteins of influenza A virus comprise the major surface proteins and the principle immunizing antigens of the virus. "These proteins are inserted into the viral envelopes as spike-like projections in a ratio of about 4:1."[69]

The trivalent subunit vaccine is the predominant influenza vaccine used today. This vaccine is produced from viral strains that are identified early each year by the World Health Organization, the Centers for Disease Control and Prevention (CDC), and the CBER. For U.S.-licensed manufacturers, the viral strains are normally acquired from the CBER or the CDC. These viral strains are used to prepare the inoculums for vaccine production.

The substrate most commonly used by producers of influenza vaccine is the 11-day-old embryonated chicken egg. A monovalent virus (suspension) is received from either the CBER or the CDC. The monovalent virus suspension is passed in eggs. The inoculated eggs are incubated for a specific time and temperature regimen under controlled relative humidity and then harvested. The harvested allantoic fluids, which contain the live virus, are tested for infectivity, titer, specificity, and sterility. These fluids are then stored wet frozen at extremely low temperatures to maintain the stability of the monovalent seed virus (MSV).[70] This MSV is also certified by the CBER.

The MSV is then used to prepare the inoculum for influenza vaccine production. Ampules of the MSV are diluted to the desired titer. The diluted viral suspension representing the MSV is then tested for the same characteristics as those listed above.[70] The certified MSV is then used to inoculate a relatively large quantity of eggs. The egg inoculation process involves instilling a small volume of the monovalent viral suspension directly into the egg's allantoic fluid. Some manufacturers include antibiotics in the inoculum to control allantoic fluid bioburden levels.[71] The large quantity of inoculated eggs are then incubated for a predetermined time, temperature, and relative humidity, depending on the viral strain, during which time the virus propagates to relatively high infectivity titers. Viral yields vary considerably from strain to strain.

After completion of the incubation process, the eggs are inspected to determine their viability and integrity. During this process, any of the eggs determined to be cracked, dead, or flawed are discarded. After inspection, the inoculated eggs are refrigerated to facilitate harvesting of the allantoic fluid. This fluid, which contains a high concentration of the live virus, is then harvested from the eggs, collected, and held under refrigeration for further processing.[68,71]

The harvested virus is concentrated, purified, and then inactivated with formaldehyde, or, depending on the vaccine manufacturer,[71] the virus-containing fluids are inactivated with formaldehyde before concentration. Fluid containing the formaldehyde may be further clarified and held under a predetermined temperature and time regimen to completely inactivate the virus; the regimen used may vary depending on the viral strain.[68]

The viral antigens are concentrated and refined by column chromatography or purified in a linear sucrose density gradient solution using a continuous-flow centrifuge.[68,71]

Disruption and inactivation of the virus to smaller subunit particles is accomplished in some influenza vaccines by adding tri(n)butylphosphate and polysorbate 80, USP, to the column eluting fluids. The recovered subvirion (split-virus) suspension is freed of substantial portions of the disrupting agents by resin treatments and of other undesirable materials by dialysis through membranes of controlled pore size.[71]

Other influenza vaccines contain virus disrupted by the use of polyethylene glycol p-isoctylphenyl ether (Triton X-100®; Rohm and Haas) to produce a "split-antigen."[72] In this case, the split antigen is then further purified by chemical means and suspended in sodium phosphate–buffered isotonic sodium chloride solution. The resultant final monovalent split-virus concentrate may contain a preservative and stabilizer, depending on the specific product design.[68]

Depending on the product design and the processing steps involved in the manufacturing of an inactivated monovalent influenza split-virus concentrate, several in-process tests may be incorporated. Before the concentrate is sterilized via filtration, a prefiltration bioburden assay may be performed to determine the total microbial population of the concentrate and its challenge to the sterilizing filter. The final concentrate is normally tested for sterility, virus inactivation, potency, endotoxin, protein content, stabilizer concentration, residuals (including antibiotics, detergents, inactivating agents, and so on), pH, sodium chloride concentration, identity, and preservative concentration, if present.

Concentrates of the same strain can be pooled and tested per the testing regimen listed above or they can be held as a single concentrate. For U.S.-licensed products, manufacturers and the CBER test the concentrates or concentrate pools for potency. The CBER evaluates the test results and assigns the final potency value. The final trivalent inactivated subunit vaccine is then formulated according to the approved vaccine formula. The resulting trivalent bulk vaccine contains not less than 15 μg HA per stain per 0.5-mL dose. The viral antigen content has been standardized by immunodiffusion tests, according to current U.S. Public Health Service requirements. Therefore, each 0.5-mL dose contains a total of at least 45 μg HA.[68,71] Thimerosal is also included as a preservative at a concentration of 1:10,000. Antibiotics, when used in the influenza vaccine manufacturing process, are reported as not detectable by assay procedures in the final product.[71] One manufacturer uses a stabilizer, gelatin, at a concentration of 0.05%.[71]

The final trivalent bulk vaccine is then tested for potency, sterility, sodium chloride concentration, residuals (including antibiotics, detergents, inactivating agents, and so on), protein concentration, preservative concentration, pH, virus inactivation, stabilizer concentration, endotoxin, and the like, depending on the product license. The safety test is conducted on the final container. [The general safety test for inactivated influenza vaccine is specified in 21 CFR Section 610.11a, "Inactivated Influenza Vaccine General Safety Test."[72] This regulation specifies that 5 mL of inactivated influenza vaccine can be injected either subcutaneously or intraperitoneally into each of at least two guinea pigs through the test period. Repeat tests are allowed, and specific criteria for these tests are specified in 21 CFR Section 610.11.[73] Additionally, 0.5 mL of the vaccine must be injected intraperitoneally into each of at least two mice. The test is satisfactory if all animals (guinea pigs and mice) survive the test period, they do not exhibit any unexpected response, and they do not lose weight. Also, Section 610.11a specifies that the endotoxin content of the vaccine must be less than or equal to a reference preparation provided by the FDA.[72]]

If the bulk vaccine meets the QC and CBER release criteria, the final containers are aseptically filled with vaccine and closed. These containers are 100% inspected for particulates and other defects, labeled, packaged, and stored under refrigeration. The final containers are tested for general safety, pyrogen, sterility, identity, and other quality attributes, depending on the specific product formulation.[72,74–76] Only after the filled containers are tested for the attributes required by the license and also meet quality assurance/QC and CBER release criteria is the product released for distribution.

A conceptual manufacturing flow diagram for killed influenza virus is presented in Figure 5–1.

Haemophilus B Conjugate Vaccine

Haemophilus b conjugate vaccine is instrumental in preventing Haemophilus influenzae type b (Hib), a leading cause of serious systemic bacterial disease in young children worldwide. Hib is also the most frequent cause of bacterial meningitis in the same population. "The mortality rate from Hib meningitis is about 5%. In addition, up to 35% of survivors develop neurologic sequelae, including seizures, deafness, and mental retardation. Other invasive diseases caused by Hib include cellulitis, epiglottitis, sepsis, pneumonia, septic arthritis, osteomyelitis, and pericarditis."[77] Antibody to the polyribosylribitol phosphate (PRP) capsule of Hib is the primary contributor to serum bactericidal activity, and increasing levels of antibody are associated with decreasing risk of invasive Hib disease.[78]

In the 1970s, polysaccharide vaccines derived from PRP were being used in the hope that these vaccines would be able to elicit a response that produced bactericidal serum These vaccines were shown to be 90% effective, but only in children ages 2 years and older and only for a short period

of time. In the 1980s, the conjugate vaccine approach was investigated based on findings of Goebel and Avery that a T-independent antigen could be changed to a T-dependent antigen by conjugation to a protein carrier.[79] The unconjugated protein is typically removed from the protein-polysaccharide conjugate using either gel filtration chromatography or ultrafiltration.[80,81]

The conjugate vaccines differ by protein carrier, polysaccharide size, and method of chemical conjugation, including use of a spacer (a linking moiety) between the PRP and the protein carrier.[78]

From Table 5–1, it can be seen that every conjugate vaccine included differs somewhat in product design. Each of these vaccines includes a different carrier protein. Some include different sizes of the polysaccharide and different linkages as defined by their conjugation chemistry. Also, the final formulation of these vaccines is different as well. One is lyophilized, two contain 10 μg of the purified capsular polysaccharide, and one contains 7.5 and another 25 μg of the same. Other components of each vaccine formulation vary as well.

Because of design differences between the Haemophilus b conjugate vaccines listed in Table 5–1, one can expect that differences also exist in the manufacturing and testing processes used for these products. Conceptually, each of the products listed in Table 5–1 requires pure cultures of Hib to start the manufacturing process. These seed cultures are tested for identity, purity, and titer.[70] The pure cultures are passed further to verify purity and to increase titer before being used to inoculate a complex, semisynthetic or chemically defined fermentation medium.[77,81,82] The fermenter is incubated for a specified time/temperature regimen. After completion of the incubation process, the resultant fermenter culture is usually sampled and tested for titer, purity, pH, and the like. The PRP isolated from Hib is purified and sized (where required) by various methods. Some of these methods include ethanol fractionation, enzyme digestion, phenol extraction, and diafiltration.[77] Oligosaccharides can be purified and sized by diafiltrations through a series of ultrafiltration membranes.[82] Several steps are involved in the purification and sizing process depending on the specific product design. In-process testing is used to verify that each step in the purification and polysaccharide sizing process is functioning as designed, in a consistent, reproducible manner. The resultant purified, sized PRP concentrate is tested for various quality attributes. Some of these tests could include polysaccharide, ribose, moisture, endotoxin, protein, phosphorus, and nucleic acid contents; identity; molecular size; sterility; residuals; and purity.

Most of the processed polysaccharide preparations are partially depolymerized either before or during the chemical modification. Some of the methods that can be used to chemically modify the purified polysaccharides are as follows[82]:

1. The polysaccharide is reacted with cyanogen bromide to introduce groups that react with spacer molecules or with the carrier protein. Ultrafiltration is used to remove excess reactants from the polysaccharide.
2. Periodate oxidation of purified polysaccharide is used to generate free aldehyde groups on low-molecular-weight polysaccharides containing 15 to 30 repeat units.

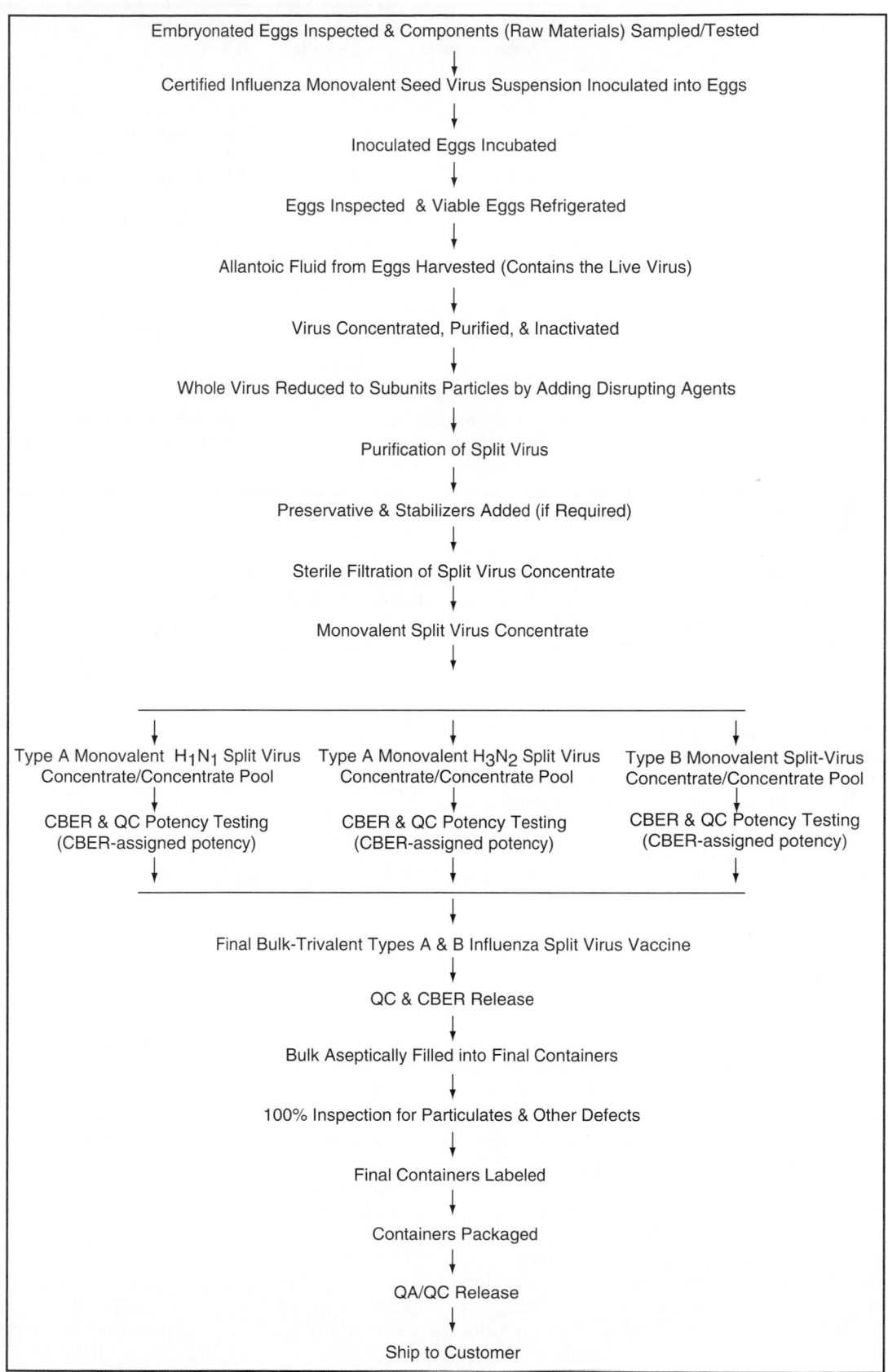

FIGURE 5–1 ▪ Conceptual manufacturing flow diagram for influenza virus vaccine.

TABLE 5–1 ▪ *Haemophilus* b Conjugate Vaccines

Vaccine[78]	Manufacturer	Polysaccharide Size	Protein Carrier	Linkage	Final Vaccine (0.5-mL dose)
ActHIB[81]	Aventis Pasteur	Large	Tetanus Toxoid	Spacer	Lyophilized, 10 µg of purified capsular polysaccharide conjugated to 24 µg of inactivated tetanus toxoid & 8.5% sucrose reconstituted with 0.4% saline
ProHIBiT[82]	Connaught Labs, Inc.	Medium	Diphtheria Toxoid	Spacer	25 µg of purified capsular polysaccharide & 18 µg of diphtheria toxoid protein in sodium phosphate–buffered isotonic sodium chloride solution, including preservative thimerosal at 1:10,000
HibTITER[83]	Lederle-Praxis	Small	CRM$_{197}$ mutant *Corynebacterium diphtheriae* protein	No spacer	10 µg of purified *Haemophilus* b saccharide, ~25 µg CRM$_{197}$ protein; multidose vials contain thimerosal at 1:10,000 as preservative
Liquid PedvaxHIB[77]	Merck & Co.	Medium	*Neisseria meningitidis* outer membrane protein complex (OMPC)	Spacer	7.5 µg of *Haemophilus* b PRP, 125 µg of *N. meningitidis* OMPC & 225 µg of amorphous aluminum hydroxyphosphate sulfate in 0.9% sodium chloride

3. The polysaccharide is reacted with carbonyldiimidazole and butanediamine to form a reactive intermediate with a terminal amino group. This group is acylated to form the final derivitized polysaccharide.

4. Adipic acid dihydrazide is covalently bound to the polysaccharide through cyanogen bromide activation of the polysaccharide.

The polysaccharides chemically modified via each of these methods should be assessed for the number of functional groups introduced for use in the conjugation reaction.[82] A functional group is an arrangement of atoms that displays a characteristic reactivity pattern [i.e., alcohol (–OH), acyl group (RCO$^-$), amino (NH$_3$), and so on].[83]

A gel filtration method and the size distribution of the size-reduced polysaccharide are specified for each type of conjugate vaccine to ensure reproducibility of the conjugation process.[82]

The protein carrier for each of the products currently licensed in the United States is unique to each *Haemophilus* b conjugate vaccine. The protein carriers for each of these products are listed in Table 5–1. Liquid PedvaxHIB® (Merck & Co., Inc.) uses the outer membrane protein complex (OMPC) from *Neisseria meningitidis* serogroup B. This bacterium is grown in a complex fermentation medium. The OMPC from *N. meningitidis* is purified by detergent extraction, ultracentrifugation, diafiltration, and sterile filtration.[77]

The carrier protein for HibTITER® (Lederle-Praxis) is identified as Diphtheria CRM$_{197}$. CRM$_{197}$ is a nontoxic variant of diphtheria toxin isolated from cultures of *Corynebacterium diphtheriae* c7 (B$_{197}$) grown in a casamino acids and yeast extract–based medium that is ultrafiltered before use. CRM$_{197}$ is purified through ultrafiltration, ammonium sulfate precipitation, and ion-exchange chromatography to high purity.[82]

The protein carriers for ActHIB™ (Aventis Pasteur) and ProHIBiT® (Connaught Labs, Inc.)[84] are tetanus and diphtheria toxoids, respectively. The tetanus toxoid is prepared by extraction, ammonium sulfate purification, and formalin inactivation of the toxin from cultures of *Clostridium tetani* (Harvard strain) grown in a modified Mueller-Miller medium. The toxoid is filter sterilized before the conjugation process.[81] The *C. diphtheriae* culture is also grown in a modified Mueller-Miller medium. The diphtheria toxin is detoxified with formalin and purified by serial ammonium sulfate fractionations and diafiltration.[85]

Significant in-process testing is conducted to verify the quality attributes of the resultant carrier protein. Some of these tests may include protein content, sterility, endotoxin, safety, nucleic acids, purity, potency, and residuals, depending on the specific protein carrier.[82,86]

Processing of Carrier Protein

Reactive functional groups or "spacers" in some processes are introduced into the carrier protein before conjugation to the polysaccharide. When this approach is used, the degree of "substitution" of the protein should be monitored for consistency.[82] The degree of substitution refers to the number of functional groups incorporated into the protein.

Protein activation methods that have been used include[87]

1. The introduction into diphtheria toxoid of a specified concentration of "spacer groups" reactive with activated polysaccharide.

2. The addition of thiol groups to the OMPC of *N. meningitidis* group B.

Conjugation of PRP to Carrier Protein

The PRP-diphtheria conjugate and the PRP-tetanus conjugate both include a six-carbon adipic spacer that links the diphtheria toxoid and tetanus toxoid carrier proteins, respectively, to the PRP. The PRP-OMPC conjugate includes a bigeneric spacer meningococcal outer membrane carrier protein conjugated to the PRP. In the PRP-CRM$_{197}$ conjugation process, the carrier protein is coupled directly by reductive amination to the oligosaccharides prepared by cleaving the PRP with periodate to give fragments with free aldehyde termini.

Conjugates

The conjugation methods discussed above require multistep processes. Both the method and the control procedures used to ensure the reproducibility, stability, and safety of the conjugate must be established.[82,88]

It is possible that residual unreacted functional groups potentially capable of reacting in vivo may be present. After the conjugation process, the process must be validated to demonstrate that it does not produce conjugate vaccines containing such groups. Any remaining groups should be made unreactive by using capping agents.

The *Haemophilus* b conjugate vaccine is purified via various steps (ultrafiltration, gel filtration, sterile filtration, and so on), depending on the specific product design. After completion of the purification process, the conjugate is tested to assess consistency of manufacture. The following QC tests may be applicable for the conjugate, depending on the product design: residuals, free polysaccharide, polysaccharide content, protein content, polysaccharide-to-protein ratio, molecular size, absence of blood groups, sterility, preservative, endotoxin/pyrogen, and free protein.[82,86]

Haemophilus b conjugate vaccines are formulated into final bulk vaccines. The conjugates may be pooled and diluted to vaccine strength. Adjuvants, preservatives, and other formulation ingredients are added at this time. The final bulk vaccine is stored at refrigeration temperature until QC testing and CBER release is obtained. (Freeze-dried conjugates are released by the CBER in the final container.) The final bulk vaccine is generally tested for the following quality attributes by the manufacturer's QC department: sterility, preservatives, polysaccharide content, identity, protein content, protein-to-polysaccharide ratio, and adjuvant. If the final bulk vaccine meets all the QC release criteria, a sample and a protocol are submitted to the CBER for review. On notice of release from the CBER, the final bulk vaccine is ready for aseptic filling. The final container is then tested for the following by the manufacturer's QC department: sterility, identity, safety, polysaccharide content, moisture content (freeze-dried products), pyrogen content, adjuvant content, and preservative content.[82,86,88]

Hepatitis B Vaccine Manufacturing

History

"The basis for the development of inactivated hepatitis B vaccine [HBV] stemmed from (1) the discovery of Australia antigen, (2) its subsequent identification as HBsAg, and (3) the demonstration that heat-inactivated serum containing HBV and [hepatitis B surface antigen] HBsAg was not infectious, but was immunogenic and partially protective against subsequent exposure to HBV. The detection of anti-HBs in the serum of the recipients of the heat-inactivated preparation indicated that the noninfectious HBsAg particle was the immunizing antigen needed for vaccine production."[89]

The hepatitis B vaccine licensed by Merck & Co., Inc., in the United States in November 1981 was a subunit vaccine. For this vaccine, the plasma was derived from human

hepatitis B chronic carriers. "In such individuals, a substantial quantity of HBsAg, the major viral envelope protein, is not incorporated into virions in infected liver cells. Rather, this excess HBsAg is assembled with cellular lipids into non-infectious lipoprotein spheres about 22 nm in diameter. After secretion from cells, these particles circulate in plasma at levels up to 0.5 mg/mL."[89] For this vaccine, the HBsAg particles were purified from the plasma.[89,90] Three separate vaccine inactivation steps were used to ensure that the product did not contain adventitious viruses (i.e., human immunodeficiency virus [HIV]).[91]

The vaccine derived from this processing consisted of 20 μg surface antigen per dose with 0.5 mg Al^{3+}(alum) per milliliter and thimerosal. "The worldwide use of many millions of doses of inactivated hepatitis B vaccine has confirmed its safety. No serious side effects have been observed to be related to the vaccine."[91] There is no evidence to suggest an association between hepatitis B vaccine and HIV infection. However, despite the excellent safety profile of the vaccine, acceptance has been less than anticipated. Furthermore, the human source for HBsAg has become limited for the production of sufficient quantities of vaccine. Therefore, a second-generation recombinant-derived hepatitis B vaccine was needed.[90]

Recombinant Vaccine

In July 1986, a recombinant hepatitis B vaccine (Recombivax HB®; Merck Sharp & Dohme) was licensed in the United States. To produce this vaccine, the HBsAg or "S" gene was inserted into an expression vector that was capable of directing the synthesis of large quantities of HBsAg in *Saccharomyces cerevisiae*. For Recombivax HB, the gene for the adw subtype of HBsAg was used. Analysis of the HBsAg particles expressed by and purified from the yeast cells has been demonstrated to be equivalent to the HBsAg derived from the plasma of the blood of hepatitis B chronic carriers.[89,91,92]

Manufacturing

The recombinant *S. cerevisiae* cells expressing HBsAg are grown in stirred tank fermenters. The medium used in this process is a complex fermentation medium that consists of an extract of yeast, soy peptone, dextrose, amino acids, and mineral salts. In-process testing is conducted on the fermentation product to determine the percentage of host cells with the expression construct.[9] At the end of the fermentation process, the HBsAg is harvested by lysing the yeast cells. It is separated by hydrophobic interaction and size-exclusion chromatography. The resulting HBsAg is assembled into 22-nm–diameter lipoprotein particles. The HBsAg is purified to greater than 99% for protein by a series of physical and chemical methods. The purified protein is treated in phosphate buffer with formaldehyde, sterile filtered, and then co-precipitated with alum (potassium aluminum sulfate) to form bulk vaccine adjuvanted with amorphous aluminum hydroxyphosphate sulfate. The vaccine contains no detectable yeast DNA but may contain not more than 1% yeast protein.[9,90,91] In GlaxoSmithKline's hepatitis B vaccine (recombinant) (Engerix-B®), the surface antigen expressed in *S. cerevisiae* cells is purified by several physiochemical steps and formulated as a suspension of the antigen absorbed on aluminum hydroxide. The procedures used to manufacture Engerix-B result in a product that contains no more than 5% yeast protein. No substances of human origin are used in its manufacture.[92] Vaccines against hepatitis B prepared from recombinant yeast cultures are noninfectious[92] and are free of association with human blood or blood products.[91]

"Each lot of hepatitis B vaccine is tested for safety, in mice and guinea pigs, and for sterility."[91] QC product testing for purity and identity includes numerous chemical, biochemical, and physical assays on the final product to assure thorough characterization and lot-to-lot consistency. Quantitative immunoassays using monoclonal antibodies can be used to measure the presence of high levels of key epitopes on the yeast-derived HBsAg. A mouse potency assay is also used to measure the immunogenicity of hepatitis B vaccines. The effective dose capable of seroconverting 50% of the mice (ED_{50}) is calculated.[90]

Recombivax HB [hepatitis B vaccine (recombinant)] is a sterile suspension for intramuscular injection. It is supplied in four formulations: pediatric, adolescent/high-risk infant, adult, and dialysis.

Formulations that include a preservative contain thimerosal, a mercury derivative, at 1:20,000 or 50 µg/mL. All formulations contain approximately 0.5 mg of aluminum (provided as amorphous aluminum hydroxyphosphate sulfate) per milliliter of vaccine.[91]

Engerix-B is a sterile suspension for intramuscular administration. It is supplied in two formulations: pediatric/adolescent (without a preservative) and adult (with thimerosal as the preservative).

The QC testing requirements for the release of recombinant hepatitis B vaccine are summarized in Table 5–2.

Because recombinant hepatitis B vaccine is extensively characterized, there has been an exception granted for one vaccine in that lot-by-lot release by the CBER is not required. This particular vaccine, in addition to being extensively characterized, had to demonstrate a "track record" of continued safety, purity, and potency in order to qualify for this exemption.[9,93]

Formulation Components

Preservatives

Preservatives are added to vaccines only when there is a risk of contamination, such as when the vaccine is prepared in multidose vials. If single-dose containers are used, preserva-

tives can be avoided. Vaccines currently licensed in the United States may be preserved using either thimerosal, 2-phenoxyethanol and formaldehyde, phenol, benzethonium chloride (phemerol), or 2-phenoxyethanol. For a combination vaccine, the preservative in one monovalent vaccine can affect the potency of the other vaccine. Thimerosal has been shown to adversely affect the potency of the inactivated poliovirus vaccine combination with diphtheria and tetanus toxoids and adsorbed pertussis vaccine.[67]

Although thimerosal, an inorganic mercury compound containing ethylmercury, has been successfully and safely used as a vaccine preservative since the 1930s, recent concerns regarding neurologic disorders that might be associated with it have resulted in a reduction in usage. Ethylmercury differs from methylmercury, an organic mercury compound and known neurotoxin. Methylmercury has been extensively studied and constitutes a major health concern because of its propensity to accumulate in seafood. Generally, the most significant finding with the use of thimerosal is minor reactions, as evidenced by redness and swelling at the injection site.

To date, federal standards that deal with limits for mercury have been based on research and data accumulated on methylmercury. In 1997, as part of the Food and Drug Modernization Act (FDAMA), the FDA undertook a review of the use and impact of thimerosal in vaccines.[94] This review concluded that, although there were no safety-related issues associated with vaccines that contained thimerosal as a preservative, under certain conditions, the amount of mercury administered exceeded Environmental Protection Agency standards for methylmercury intake. Since then, additional research has been initiated through the support of the National Institute of Allergy and Infectious Diseases and the National Institutes of Environmental Health Sciences.[95]

Although findings to date have failed to conclusively demonstrate a causal relationship between vaccines preserved with thimerosal and certain neurodevelopmental disorders,[96] the vaccine industry, in conjunction with the FDA, has reduced or eliminated thimerosal from most vaccines. To date, these changes have resulted in a greater than 98% reduction in the mercury exposure that 6-month-old children likely experience as a result of required immunizations.[97]

Whether or not a preservative is used, the manufacturer still needs to evaluate the vaccine for potency and reversion to toxicity for each of the active components. The manufacturer should also determine the levels of constituents or antimicrobials remaining in the vaccine and conduct studies on the preservative's ability to prevent contamination of the product.

Stabilizers

Vaccine stability is essential in being able to reliably deliver a safe, effective product to key target populations. In many areas of the globe, "cold chains" are either nonexistent or can be easily compromised. Therefore, these areas require vaccines with high thermal stability.

It is believed that the instability of vaccines can be attributed, at least in part, to the loss of antigenic properties or, as in the case of live viral vaccines, to the loss of infectivity. Work has been heavily focused on those factors that

TABLE 5–2 ■ Testing Requirements for the Release of Recombinant Hepatitis B Vaccine

Type of Test[67]	Stage of Production
Plasmid retention	Fermentation product
Purity and identity	Bulk-adsorbed product or nonadsorbed bulk product
Sterility	Final bulk product
Sterility	Final container
General safety	Final container
Pyrogen	Final container
Purity	Final container
Potency	Final container

influence the structural and conformational integrity of vaccine epitopes, such as temperature and pH. Each vaccine category (i.e., live, attenuated; inactivated viral or bacterial antigens; toxoids; or antitoxins) presents different challenges to the scientist. Bacterial vaccines, for example, can demonstrate instability because of the hydrolysis and aggregation of protein and carbohydrate molecules.

Research and development efforts in the global vaccine community have been focused heavily on developing oral polio vaccines with increased thermal stability in addition to improving other globally important vaccines. The stabilizer of choice for oral polio vaccine remains $MgCl_2$. Molar $MgSO_4$ has been demonstrated to stabilize viruses such as respiratory syncytial virus and measles virus. Other vaccines, such as the yellow fever vaccine, have been stabilized effectively through the use of lactose-sorbitol and sorbitol-gelatin combinations.

Bovine Spongiform Encephalopathy

Bovine spongiform encephalopathy (BSE) was first diagnosed in 1986 in Great Britain, with approximately 95% of all reported cases having been found in the United Kingdom. Because of growing concerns regarding the potential risks of using materials of bovine origin sourced from countries associated with BSE, manufacturers are developing alternative stabilizers and nutritional supplements sourced from acceptable countries.[98,99] The vaccine manufacturing process has used a variety of animal-derived materials, including amino acids, glycerol, detergents, gelatin, enzymes, blood, and milk. The FDA's latest revision to their guidance "Points to Consider in the Characterization of Cell Lines Used to Produce Biologics" recommends that manufacturers provide information on cell culture history, isolation, media used, identity, and adventitious agent testing of biologic product cell lines.[100] Working bacterial and viral seeds developed using components derived from countries where BSE is known to occur need to be re-derived using acceptable components. Master seeds are currently not under the same requirements. The U.S. Department of Agriculture maintains a close, worldwide surveillance program with a published list of unacceptable countries for component sourcing.[101]

Formulation, Filling, Packaging, and Distribution of Vaccines

Because of the thermal lability of vaccines, terminal sterilization using dry or moist heat is generally not feasible. Even the application of terminal filtration using sterilizing-grade filters is limited at times because of the characteristics and composition of the vaccine antigens, adjuvants, stabilizers, or excipients used. These factors demand the exertion of high levels of control over the environment, equipment, facilities, people, procedures, and components used during the various phases of vaccine manufacturing operations.

Formulation Phase

Formulation consists of combining all components that constitute the final vaccine and uniformly mixing them in a single vessel (Fig. 5–2). Operations are conducted in a highly controlled environment with employees wearing special protective clothing to avoid any adventitious contamination of the critical work area. Control monitoring of the environment and critical surfaces are conducted during operations. QC testing at this stage usually consists of safety, potency, purity, sterility, and other assays specific to the product.

Filling and Packaging Phase

During this phase, individual, scrupulously cleaned, depyrogenated single- or multiple-dose containers are filled with vaccine and sealed with sterile stoppers or plungers (Fig. 5–3). If the vaccine is to be freeze dried, the vial stoppers are inserted only partially to allow moisture to escape during the lyophilization process, and the vials are moved to a special lyophilization chamber. All vials receive outer caps over the stopper to secure them. To preclude the introduction of extraneous viable and nonviable contamination, all filling operations must take place in a highly controlled environment where people, equipment, and components need to be introduced into the critical area in a controlled manner. After filling, all containers are inspected using semiautomated or automated equipment designed to detect any minute cosmetic and physical defects. As with the formulation phase of the vaccine manufacturing operation, extensive control monitoring of the environment and critical surfaces is conducted during operations. QC testing at this stage also consists of safety, potency, purity, sterility, and other assays that may be specific to the product.

Labeling is applied, followed by packaging one or more containers into suitable cartons.

During the 1990s, specially designed chambers known as isolator filling lines were developed that allow extremely high levels of control over the critical filling environment. These isolators were patterned after similar, smaller devices that have been in use for sterility testing for about 20 years. Isolators provide total separation between dissimilar environments and are capable of achieving interior operational

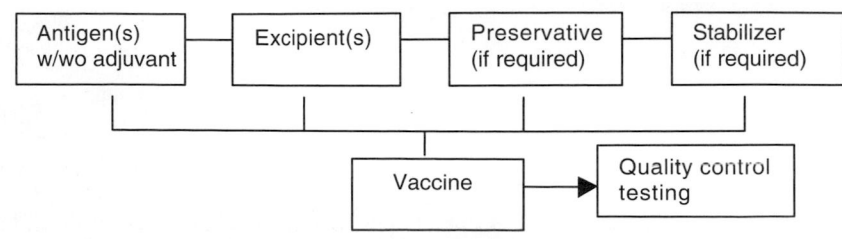

FIGURE 5–2 ■ Algorithm of the vaccine formulation phase.

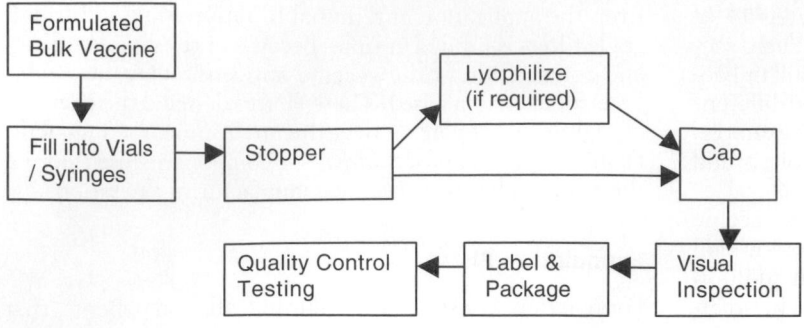

FIGURE 5–3 ■ Algorithm of the filling and packaging phase.

sterility assurance levels (SALs) of 10^6 (i.e., one chance in a million of introducing a microorganism into a final container), thus approximating the levels achieved via classical terminal heat sterilization. In comparison, conventional clean rooms and filling lines normally operate with SALs of 10^3. Isolators do not exchange air directly with the surrounding environment but rather filter the air through high-efficiency particulate air (HEPA) or ultra-low particulate air (ULPA) filters. The interior of the isolator is rendered sterile through the use of chemical sterilants with or without heat. All materials entering the isolator do so through sterilizing tunnels or special air locks. Isolators generally are equipped with Clean in Place (CIP) and in some instances Sterilize in Place (SIP) technology. Access to the isolator is through sealed glove ports that separate operational personnel from the critical interior environment.[102] An example of a typical isolator filling line is the MAFS® Mini Aseptic Filling System (Bosch Packaging Technology) (Fig. 5–4).

Distribution, Storage, and Stability of Vaccines

Vaccine efficacy can be adversely affected by improper distribution and storage conditions. The sensitivity of vaccines

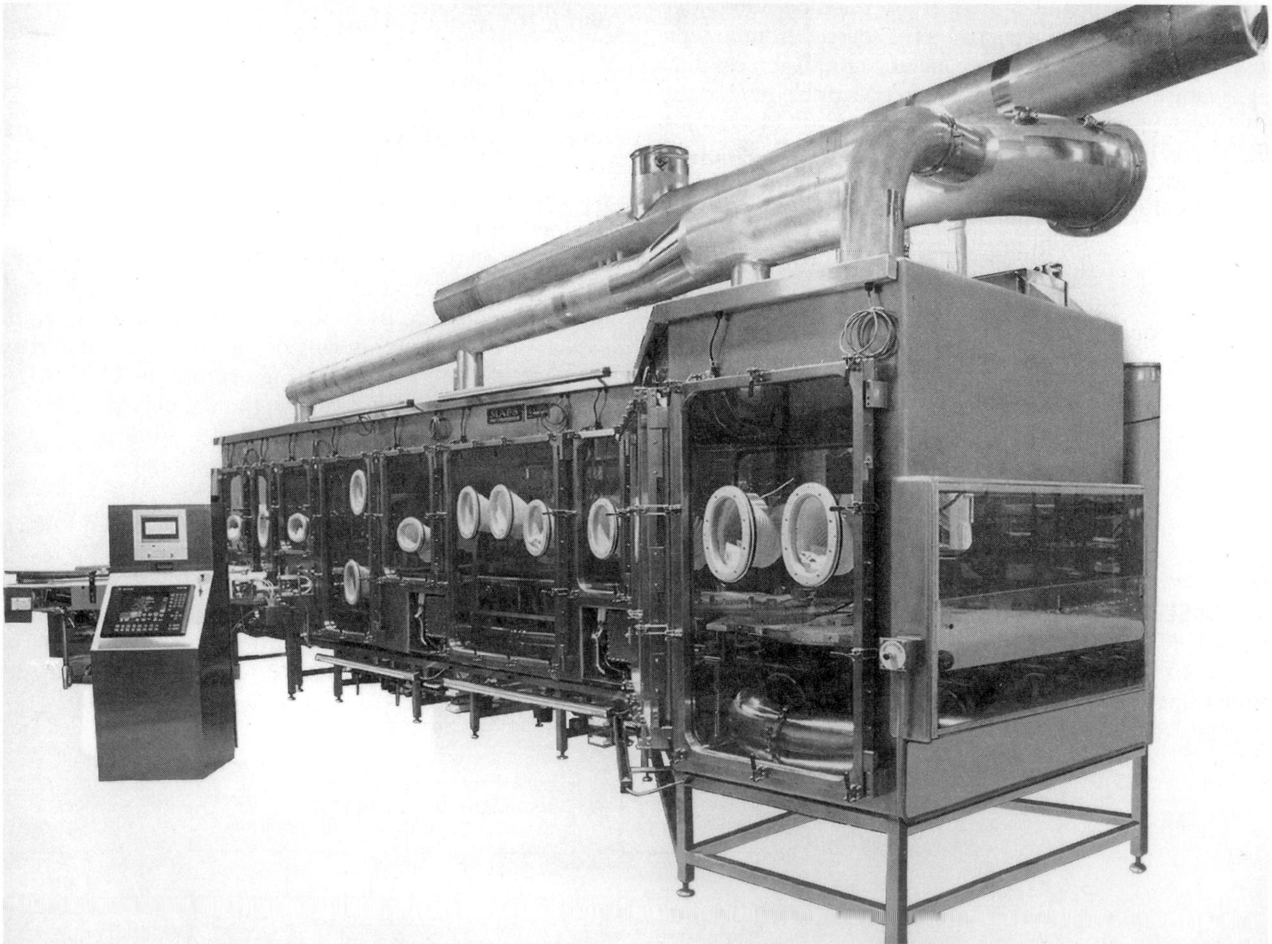

FIGURE 5–4 ■ MAFS® Mini Aseptic Filling System. (Photo courtesy of Bosch Packaging Technology, Inc., Minneapolis, MN.)

to adverse environmental conditions, particularly temperature extremes, varies depending on their composition. Live, attenuated vaccines tend to be more susceptible than killed vaccines and toxoids.[1] The addition of stabilizers or lyophilization, when feasible, tends to improve the thermal resistance of vaccines.

Stability

Although recommended storage conditions for many vaccines have been detailed,[103] the vaccine manufacturers are responsible for developing data before and after licensing that demonstrate the stability of their vaccines under recommended storage conditions. Generally, these programs provide data to support the development of new products intended for clinical use, routine support of currently marketed products, expiration date extension, and supporting distribution conditions.[104,105] Accelerated studies conducted at elevated temperatures are commonly applied to better understand the impact of transient temperature excursions on the vaccine. Manufacturers are required to assure that products under their control are maintained under appropriate conditions so that the identity, strength, quality, and purity of the products are not affected.[106]

Distribution

Currently only a limited number of vaccines are required by federal regulation to have specified shipping temperatures.[104] Although most vaccine manufacturers use insulated containers and other precautions for the brief (usually 24 to 72 hours) shipping time, occasional, unanticipated temperature excursions may occur that could have a detrimental impact on the shipped product. Before accepting any vaccine shipment, users should look for any evidence of improper transportation conditions, including excessive transport time and possible adverse ambient temperature conditions.[1]

Storage and Use

Vaccines should be stored under conditions recommended by the product's labeling. Particular care should be taken in clinics, where refrigerators may contain freezer compartments inside of the primary refrigeration section, to be certain that vaccines are not stored too close to the freezer compartment. Monitoring the interior temperature of refrigerators and freezers is critical. If accurate recording charts are not available, then the use of an accurate maximum and minimum thermometer is recommended.

Before use, vaccines should be examined for any unusual physical changes that may signal that the vial may have been subjected to extreme conditions. Although irreversible damage to a vaccine by breaking its "cold chain" during storage or shipping is not always readily evident, examination of the primary container before use should be routine. In some instances, vaccine degradation is evidenced by unusual color, failure to resuspend, or unusual precipitate.

REFERENCES

1. Casto DT, Brunell PA. Safe handling of vaccines. Pediatrics 87:108–112, 1991.
2. Mathieu M (ed). Biologics Development: A Regulatory Overview (2nd ed). Waltham, MA, Parexel International Corporation, 1997, pp 123–124.
3. Peter G. Childhood immunizations. N Engl J Med 327:1794–1800, 1992.
4. Mitchell VS, Philipose NM, Sanford JP (eds). The Children's Vaccine Initiative: Achieving the Vision. Washington, DC, Institute of Medicine, National Academy Press, 1993.
5. Parkman PD, Hardegree MC. Regulation and testing of vaccines. In Plotkin SA, Mortimer EA Jr (eds). Vaccines (2nd ed). Philadelphia, WB Saunders, 1994, pp 889–901.
6. Hinman AR, Orenstein WA. Public health considerations. In Plotkin SA, Mortimer EA Jr (eds). Vaccines (2nd ed). Philadelphia, WB Saunders, 1994, pp 903–932.
7. Centers for Disease Control and Prevention, National Vaccine Program Office. Vaccine Fact Sheets, 2001, p 1. Available at: www.cdc.gov/od/nvpo/fs_tableII_doc2.htm
8. Code of Federal Regulations, Title 21, Sec. 601.2(a). Washington, DC, Office of the Federal Register, National Archives & Records Administration, April 1, 2001.
9. Parkman PD, Hardegree MC. Regulation and testing of vaccines. In Plotkin SA, Mortimer EA Jr (eds). Vaccines (3rd ed). Philadelphia, WB Saunders, 1999, pp 1131–1143.
10. Center for Biologics Evaluation and Research. Vaccines, February 20, 2002. Available at: www.fda.gov/cber/vaccines.htm
11. Mathieu M. The new drug approval process: a primer. In New Drug Development: A Regulatory Overview. Cambridge, MA, Parexel International Corporation, 1990, pp 1–12.
12. Code of Federal Regulations, Title 21, Part 312. Washington, DC, Office of the Federal Register, National Archives & Records Administration, 1997.
13. Center for Biologics Evaluation and Research. Vaccine Product Approval Process, 2001. Available at: www.fda.gov/cber/vaccine/vacappr.htm
14. Code of Federal Regulations, Title 21, Sec. 601.12. Washington, DC, Office of the Federal Register, National Archives & Records Administration, April 1, 2001.
15. Code of Federal Regulations, Title 21, Sec. 601.12(d). Washington, DC, Office of the Federal Register, National Archives & Records Administration, April 1, 2001.
16. Guidance for Industry: Reports on the Status of Postmarketing Studies—Implementation of Section 130 of the Food & Drug Administration Modernization Act of 1997. Rockville, MD, U.S. Food and Drug Administration, April 2001, pp 6, 7.
17. National Vaccine Advisory Committee. United States vaccine research: a delicate fabric of public and private collaboration. Pediatrics 100:1015–1020, 1997.
18. Stehlin I. How FDA works to ensure vaccine safety. FDA Consumer Magazine, March 30 (2):1996.
19. Centers for Disease Control and Prevention. National Immunization Program, February 20, 2002. Available at: www.cdc.gov/nip
20. Mathieu M. Clinical testing of new drugs. In New Drug Development: A Regulatory Overview. Cambridge, MA, Parexel International Corporation, 1990, pp 83–104.
21. Mathieu M. Good clinical practices. In New Drug Development: A Regulatory Overview. Cambridge, MA, Parexel International Corporation, 1990, pp 105–118.
22. Code of Federal Regulations, Title 21, Sec. 600.3(u). Washington, DC, Office of the Federal Register, National Archives & Records Administration, April 1, 2001.
23. Code of Federal Regulations, Title 21, Sec. 601.20(a). Washington, DC, Office of the Federal Register, National Archives & Records Administration, April 1, 2001.
24. Code of Federal Regulations, Title 21, Sec. 601.20(b-2). Washington, DC, Office of the Federal Register, National Archives & Records Administration, April 1, 2001.
25. Code of Federal Regulations, Title 21, Sec. 601.20(d). Washington, DC, Office of the Federal Register, National Archives & Records Administration, April 1, 2001.
26. Code of Federal Regulations, Title 21, Secs. 211–226. Washington, DC, Office of the Federal Register, National Archives & Records Administration, April 1, 2001.
27. Code of Federal Regulations, Title 21, Sec. 600. Washington, DC, Office of the Federal Register, National Archives & Records Administration, April 1, 2001.
28. Code of Federal Regulations, Title 21, Sec. 630.10(a). Washington, DC, Office of the Federal Register, National Archives & Records Administration, April 1, 1996.
29. Code of Federal Regulations, Title 21, Sec. 630.12(a). Washington, DC, Office of the Federal Register, National Archives & Records Administration, April 1, 1996.

30. Code of Federal Regulations, Title 21, Sec. 630.10(c). Washington, DC, Office of the Federal Register, National Archives & Records Administration, April 1, 1996.
31. Code of Federal Regulations, Title 21, Sec. 630.11(c-1). Washington, DC, Office of the Federal Register, National Archives & Records Administration, April 1, 1996.
32. Code of Federal Regulations, Title 21, Sec. 630.11(c-2). Washington, DC, Office of the Federal Register, National Archives & Records Administration, April 1, 1996.
33. Code of Federal Regulations, Title 21, Sec. 630.11(c-4). Washington, DC, Office of the Federal Register, National Archives & Records Administration, April 1, 1996.
34. FDA Form 2438, Program 7345.002, Chapter 45 (Vaccines and Allergenic Products), Part III. Rockville, MD, U.S. Food and Drug Administration, May 1984, p 4.
35. Code of Federal Regulations, Title 21, Sec. 630.13(a). Washington, DC, Office of the Federal Register, National Archives & Records Administration, April 1, 1996.
36. Code of Federal Regulations, Title 21, Sec. 630.13(b-2). Washington, DC, Office of the Federal Register, National Archives & Records Administration, April 1, 1996.
37. Code of Federal Regulations, Title 21, Sec. 630.13(b-3). Washington, DC, Office of the Federal Register, National Archives & Records Administration, April 1, 1996.
38. Code of Federal Regulations, Title 21, Sec. 630.13(b-3). Washington, DC, Office of the Federal Register, National Archives & Records Administration, April 1, 1996.
39. Code of Federal Regulations, Title 21, Sec. 630.13(b-4). Washington, DC, Office of the Federal Register, National Archives & Records Administration, April 1, 1996.
40. Code of Federal Regulations, Title 21, Sec. 630.13(b-5). Washington, DC, Office of the Federal Register, National Archives & Records Administration, April 1, 1996.
41. Code of Federal Regulations, Title 21, Sec. 630.13(b-6). Washington, DC, Office of the Federal Register, National Archives & Records Administration, April 1, 1996.
42. Code of Federal Regulations, Title 21, Sec. 630.13(b-7). Washington, DC, Office of the Federal Register, National Archives & Records Administration, April 1, 1996.
43. Code of Federal Regulations, Title 21, Sec. 630.18(a). Washington, DC, Office of the Federal Register, National Archives & Records Administration, April 1, 1996.
44. Code of Federal Regulations, Title 21, Sec. 630.13(b-8). Washington, DC, Office of the Federal Register, National Archives & Records Administration, April 1, 1996.
45. Code of Federal Regulations, Title 21, Sec. 630.15(a). Washington, DC, Office of the Federal Register, National Archives & Records Administration, April 1, 1996.
46. Code of Federal Regulations, Title 21, Sec. 630.16(a,b). Washington, DC, Office of the Federal Register, National Archives & Records Administration, April 1, 1996.
47. Code of Federal Regulations, Title 21, Sec. 630(b). Washington, DC, Office of the Federal Register, National Archives & Records Administration, April 1, 1996.
48. Code of Federal Regulations, Title 21, Sec. 630.16(b-2). Washington, DC, Office of the Federal Register, National Archives & Records Administration, April 1, 1996.
49. Code of Federal Regulations, Title 21, Sec. 630.16(b-2). Washington, DC, Office of the Federal Register, National Archives & Records Administration, April 1, 1996.
50. Code of Federal Regulations, Title 21, Sec. 630.18(a). Washington, DC, Office of the Federal Register, National Archives & Records Administration, April 1, 1996.
51. Code of Federal Regulations, Title 21, Sec. 630.18(a-1 to a-7). Washington, DC, Office of the Federal Register, National Archives & Records Administration, April 1, 1996.
52. Code of Federal Regulations, Title 21, Sec. 630.18(b,c). Washington, DC, Office of the Federal Register, National Archives & Records Administration, April 1, 1996.
53. Code of Federal Regulations, Title 21, Sec. 630.19(a-2). Washington, DC, Office of the Federal Register, National Archives & Records Administration, April 1, 1996.
54. Code of Federal Regulations, Title 21, Sec. 630.9(a-3). Washington, DC, Office of the Federal Register, National Archives & Records Administration, April 1, 1996.
55. Code of Federal Regulations, Title 21, Sec. 630.19(a-4). Washington, DC, Office of the Federal Register, National Archives & Records Administration, April 1, 1996.
56. Code of Federal Regulations, Title 21, Sec. 630.19(c-1). Washington, DC, Office of the Federal Register, National Archives & Records Administration, April 1, 1996.
57. Code of Federal Regulations, Title 21, Sec. 630.19(c-2). Washington, DC, Office of the Federal Register, National Archives & Records Administration, April 1, 1996.
58. Code of Federal Regulations, Title 21, Sec. 630.19(c-3). Washington, DC, Office of the Federal Register, National Archives & Records Administration, April 1, 1996.
59. Code of Federal Regulations, Title 21, Sec. 630.15 (b). Washington, DC, Office of the Federal Register, National Archives & Records Administration, April 1, 1996.
60. Code of Federal Regulations, Title 21, Sec. 630.19 (1-4). Washington, DC, Office of the Federal Register, National Archives & Records Administration, April 1, 1996.
61. Code of Federal Regulations, Title 21, Sec. 630.19 (b). Washington, DC, Office of the Federal Register, National Archives & Records Administration, April 1, 1996.
62. Code of Federal Regulations, Title 21, Sec. 630.19 (c). Washington, DC, Office of the Federal Register, National Archives & Records Administration, April 1, 1996.
63. Code of Federal Regulations, Title 21, Sec. 630.19 (c-1). Washington, DC, Office of the Federal Register, National Archives & Records Administration, April 1, 1996.
64. Code of Federal Regulations, Title 21, Sec. 630.19 (c-3). Washington, DC, Office of the Federal Register, National Archives & Records Administration, April 1, 1996.
65. Code of Federal Regulations, Title 21, Sec. 630.19 (c-3). Washington, DC, Office of the Federal Register, National Archives & Records Administration, April 1, 1996.
66. Code of Federal Regulations, Title 21, Sec. 630.19 (c-4). Washington, DC, Office of the Federal Register, National Archives & Records Administration, April 1, 1996.
67. Guidance for Industry for the Evaluation of Combination Vaccines for Preventable Diseases: Production, Testing, and Clinical Studies. Rockville, MD, Center for Biologics Evaluation and Research, 1997, pp 1–4.
68. Product Information: Fluzone®: Influenza Virus Vaccine Trivalent Types A and B (Zonal Purified, Subvirion) 2001-2002 Formula for 6 Months and Older. Swiftwater, PA, Aventis Pasteur, Inc, April 2001.
69. Kilbourne ED, Johansson BE, Grajower B. Independent and disparate evolution in nature of influenza A virus hemagglutinin and neuraminidase glycoproteins. Proc Natl Acad Sci U S A 87:786–790, 1990.
70. Code of Federal Regulations, Title 21, Sec. 610.18. Washington, DC, Office of the Federal Register, National Archives & Records Administration, April 1, 2001.
71. Product Information: FluShield®: Influenza Virus Vaccine, Trivalent Types A and B (Purified Subvirion) 2001–2002 Formula. Marietta, PA, Wyeth Laboratories, July 17, 2001.
72. Code of Federal Regulations, Title 21, Sec. 610.11(a). Washington, DC, Office of the Federal Register, National Archives & Records Administration, April 1, 2001.
73. Code of Federal Regulations, Title 21, Sec. 610.11. Washington, DC, Office of the Federal Register, National Archives & Records Administration, April 1, 2001.
74. Code of Federal Regulations, Title 21, Sec. 610.12. Washington, DC, Office of the Federal Register, National Archives & Records Administration, April 1, 2001.
75. Code of Federal Regulations, Title 21, Sec. 610.14. Washington, DC, Office of the Federal Register, National Archives & Records Administration, April 1, 2001.
76. Code of Federal Regulations, Title 21, Sec. 610.13(b). Washington, DC, Office of the Federal Register, National Archives & Records Administration, April 1, 2001.
77. Product Information: Liquid PedvaxHIB®: Haemophilus b Conjugate Vaccine (Meningococcal Protein Conjugate). West Point, PA, Merck & Co, Inc, January 2001.
78. Haemophilus b conjugate vaccines for prevention of Haemophilus influenza type b disease among infants and children two months of age and older: Recommendations of the ACIP. MMWR 40(RR01):1, 7, 1991.

79. Knopf P, de Groot A. Development of vaccines to infectious diseases: *Haemophilus influenza* type b, p 3 of 4. Retrieved on January 26, 2000: *www.brown.edu/course/Bio-160/Projects1999/bmenin/haeinfl.html*

80. Lees A. Immunology abstract: Rapid and low cost processing of conjugate vaccines to remove unconjugated protein, January 23, 2002. Retrieved on 23 January, 2002: *www.usuhs.mil/med/researchlees. html*

81. Product Information: ActHIB™: *Haemophilus* b Conjugate Vaccine (Tetanus Toxoid Conjugate). Swiftwater, PA, Aventis Pasteur, Inc, September 2000.

82. Requirements for *Haemophilus* type b conjugate vaccines (Requirements for Biological Substances No. 46). World Health Organ Tech Rep Ser 814:22–29, 1991.

83. Newton TA. An introduction to organic chemistry, March 18, 2002, p 1. Available at: *www.usm.maine.edu/~newton/Chy251_253/Lectures/Introduction.html*

84. Product Information: Tetanus and Diphtheria Toxoids Adsorbed for Adult Use. Swiftwater, PA, Aventis Pasteur, Inc, June 1996.

85. Code of Federal Regulations, Title 21, Secs. 610.10–610.15. Washington, DC, Office of the Federal Register, National Archives & Records Administration, April 1, 2001.

86. Anderson PW. New and improved vaccines against *Haemophilus influenza* type b infections. *In* Woodrow FC, Levin MM (eds). New Generation Vaccines. Rochester, NY, University of Rochester School of Medicine and Dentistry, 1990, pp 349–355.

87. Ellis RW. New and improved vaccines against hepatitis. *In* Woodrow FC, Levin MM (eds). New Generation Vaccines. Rochester, NY, University of Rochester School of Medicine and Dentistry, 1990, pp 439–444.

88. Krugman S. Hepatitis B vaccine. *In* Plotkin SA, Mortimer EA Jr (eds). Vaccines. Philadelphia, WB Saunders, 1988, pp 458–473.

89. Hepatitis B vaccine: evidence confirming lack of AIDS transmission. MMWR 33(49):685–687, 1984.

90. Mahoney FJ, Kane M. Hepatitis B vaccine. *In:* Plotkins SA, Orenstein WA (eds). Vaccines (3rd ed). Philadelphia, WB Saunders, 1999, pp 158–182.

91. Product Information: Recombivax HB®: Hepatitis B Vaccine (Recombinant). West Point, PA, Merck & Co, Inc, May 2001, pp 1–14.

92. Prescribing Information: Engerix-B®: Hepatitis B Vaccine (Recombinant). Philadelphia, GlaxoSmithKline, December 2000.

93. Points to Consider on Plasmid DNA Vaccines for Preventive Infectious Disease Indications. FDA Cyberfax Info System: TX/RX No. 6045. May 7, 1997.

94. Center for Biologics Evaluation and Research. Thimerosal in Vaccines, January 29, 2002. Available at: *www.fda.gov/cber/vaccine/thimerosal.htm*

95. Centers for Disease Control and Prevention. Mercury and Vaccines, January 29, 2002. Available at: *www.cdc.gov/nip/vacsafe/concerns/thimerosal/default.htm*

96. Centers for Disease Control and Prevention. Mercury & Thimerosal, January 29, 2002. Available at: *www.cdc.gov/nip/vacsafe/concerns/thimerosal/faqs-mercury.htm*

97. Centers for Disease Control and Prevention. Availability of Thimerosal-free Vaccines, January 29, 2002. Available at: *www.cdc.gov/nip/vacsafe/concerns/thimerosal/faqs-availfree.htm*

98. New approaches to stabilization of vaccines potency: developments in biological standardization. World Health Organization/International Association of Biological Standardization Symposium on Progress on the Stability of Vaccines, Vol. 87, Geneva; May 29–31, 1995.

99. Assessment of risk of bovine spongiform encephalopathy in pharmaceutical products. Pharmaceutical Research and Manufactures of *America BSE Committee*. Available at www.fda.gov/ohrms/dockets/ac/00/backgrd/3635b1c_1_Summary.pdf.

100. Points to Consider in the Characterization of Cell Lines Used to Produce Biologics. Rockville, MD, Center for Biologics Evaluation and Research, May 17, 1993.

101. USDA List of Countries Where BSE Exists. Rockville, MD, Department of Health & Human Services, May 1996.

102. Bosch Packaging Technology, Inc. Minneapolis, MN. FDA Isolator Technology Conference, Irvine, CA, October 16–17, 2000.

103. Code of Federal Regulations, Title 21, Sec. 615. Washington, DC, Office of the Federal Register, National Archives & Records Administration, April 1, 2001.

104. Code of Federal Regulations, Title 21, Sec. 211.166. Washington, DC, Office of the Federal Register, National Archives & Records Administration, April 1, 2001.

105. Draft Guidelines for Industry: Stability testing drug substances and drug products. Rockville, MD, Center for Drug Evaluation and Research and Center for Biologics Evaluation and Research, June 1998.

106. Code of Federal Regulations, Title 21, Sec. 211.142. Washington, DC, Office of the Federal Register, National Archives & Records Administration, April 1, 2001.

Chapter 6

Immunologic Adjuvants

FREDERICK R. VOGEL • STANLEY L. HEM

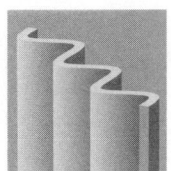

Immunologic adjuvants are agents incorporated into vaccine formulations to enhance the immunogenicity of the vaccine antigens. The immunogenicity of a vaccine is defined as its ability to evoke an immune response in the vaccinated individual. Ramon serendipitously discovered the concept of using adjuvants to nonspecifically enhance immune response to vaccine antigens in 1925 while he was producing diphtheria antitoxin in horses.[1] He observed that horses that had spontaneously developed abscesses at the injection site, which he attributed to "banal germs of the skin," produced serum with greater antitoxin titers. Ramon conducted experiments in which he induced sterile abscesses in the horses by injecting common substances such as breadcrumbs and tapioca mixed with diphtheria or tetanus toxoid antigen. The mixture of antigen particularly with tapioca enhanced antitoxin responses over antigen given alone.[2] The term *adjuvant*, which Ramon coined, is derived from the Latin word *adjuvare*, meaning to help or aid.

In 1926 Glenny and colleagues[3] discovered the adjuvant effects of aluminum salts. These adjuvants, commonly referred to as "alum adjuvants," are the only adjuvants presently used in vaccines licensed in the United States and are a main focus of this chapter.

Early vaccines were composed of whole killed bacteria, attenuated or inactivated viruses, or bacterial toxoids. These vaccines were less pure than vaccines produced using modern methods of purification. However, these less purified vaccines often contained "intrinsic adjuvants" that included minute concentrations of active exotoxins or endotoxins. The intrinsic adjuvanticity of these vaccines enhanced immune responses to them and could be exploited to increase the immunogenicity of other antigens delivered with them. The combination of whole-cell pertussis vaccine with diphtheria toxoid was shown by Greenberg and Fleming[4] to increase antibody responses to the toxoid antigen.

More recently, advances in the fields of protein purification and recombinant DNA technology have led to the development of more highly purified and defined antigens for use in human vaccines. However, the purification of vaccine antigens often has resulted in the elimination of intrinsic adjuvant properties, which can have the unwanted effect of lowering the immunogenicity of the highly purified antigens. At the same time, the number of vaccines that are now available and recommended during the first years of life[5] creates a need for developing combination vaccines. Combination vaccines are composed of antigens from multiple strains of the same infectious agent or different infectious agents that are administered together. Combination vaccines are designed to reduce the number of individual injections needed to accomplish the recommended childhood immunization series. The protective immune response generated to the multiple antigens contained in a combination vaccine should be equivalent to the response to each antigen if delivered separately. The use of immunologic adjuvants to enhance the immunogenicity of highly purified subunit vaccines and combination vaccines is a promising strategy to improve protective immune responses to these vaccines.

Classification of Immunologic Adjuvants

Many natural and synthetic substances that have been shown to possess adjuvant activities have been tested in experimental vaccine models in animals and in humans.[6] Table 6–1 shows a classification based on physical and chemical properties of adjuvants that have been evaluated for human candidate vaccines. This chapter is limited to a review of examples of three types of adjuvants presently incorporated in licensed vaccine formulations or with extensive clinical experience: (1) mineral salt adjuvants; (2) MF59, an emulsion-based adjuvant employed in an influenza vaccine licensed in Europe; and (3) monophosphoryl lipid A, a microbial adjuvant with extensive clinical experience presently in human candidate vaccines under development. Table 6–2 lists examples of the types of licensed vaccines formulated with immunologic adjuvants.

Adjuvant Mechanisms of Action

Understanding of the human immune system has advanced significantly during the past 20 years. Adjuvant researchers are applying much of this new knowledge to elucidating the mechanisms of adjuvant action. Adjuvants function

TABLE 6–1 ■ Types of Immunologic Adjuvants

Type of Adjuvant	General Examples	Specific Examples/References
Mineral salt	Aluminum hydroxide/phosphate ("alum adjuvants")	69,70
	Calcium phosphate	71
Microbial	Muramyl dipeptide (MDP)	72
	Bacterial exotoxins	Cholera toxin (CT)[7]
		Escherichia coli–labile toxin (LT)[11]
	Endotoxin-based adjuvants	Monophosphoryl lipid A (MPL®)[73]
	Bacterial DNA	CpG oligonucleotides[74]
Particulate	Biodegradable polymer microspheres	75
	Immune-stimulating complexes (ISCOMs)	76
	Liposomes	77
Oil-emulsion and surfactant-based adjuvants	Freund's incomplete adjuvant	78
	Microfluidized emulsions	MF59[62]
		SAF[79]
	Saponins	80
		QS-21[81]
Synthetic	Muramyl peptide derivatives	Murabutide[82]
		Threony-MDP[83]
	Nonionic block copolymers	L121[80]
	Polyphosphazene (PCPP)	84
	Synthetic polynucleotides	Poly A:U, poly I:C[85]
Cytokines	IL-2, IL-12, GM-CSF, IFN-γ	21,22
Genetic	Cytokine genes or genes encoding co-stimulatory molecules delivered as plasmid DNA	IL-12, IL-2, IFN-γ, CD40L[86,87]

through three basic mechanisms: (1) effects on antigen delivery and presentation, (2) induction of immunomodulatory cytokines, and (3) effects on antigen-presenting cells (APCs).

Adjuvant Effects on Antigen Delivery and Presentation

The original mechanism of action attributed to adjuvants was the so-called depot effect, in which mineral salt or emulsion-based adjuvants (e.g., Freund's adjuvant) associate with antigen and effectively increase its biologic and immunologic "half-life" at the site of injection. Although this mechanism does play a role, this explanation of adjuvant activity has proved too simplistic by itself, and it has

been refined to include the improved delivery of antigen to APCs and to the secondary lymphoid organs. The immunogenicity of synthetic peptides and other soluble antigens that otherwise would be rapidly cleared from the injection site without sufficient delivery to the draining lymph nodes can be improved using mineral salt or emulsion-based adjuvants.

Particulate adjuvants, including some liposomes and microspheres, also can be used to protect antigens from proteolytic destruction in the stomach, allowing orally administered antigens to pass into the small intestines for delivery to the gut-associated lymphoid system. Adjuvants can also target antigen to APCs (macrophages and dendritic cells). In addition, adjuvants such as the cholera toxin B subunit (CTB)[7] and *Ulex europaeus* agglutinin 1 (UEA1)[8] can

TABLE 6–2 ■ Types of Licensed Vaccines Containing Adjuvants

Vaccine	Trade Name*	Adjuvant
Diphtheria and tetanus vaccine (DT)	Diphtheria and Tetanus Toxoids Adsorbed USP (1)	Aluminum potassium sulfate
DT + acellular pertussis (DTaP)	Tripedia® (1)	Aluminum potassium sulfate
Haemophilus influenzae type B (Hib)	Liquid PedvaxHIB® (2)	Aluminum hydroxyphosphate sulfate
DTaP + Hib	TriHIBit® (1)	Aluminum potassium sulfate
Hepatitis B (recombinant)	Recombivax HB® (2)	Aluminum hydroxyphosphate sulfate
Hepatitis B + Hib	COMVAX™ (2)	Aluminum hydroxyphosphate sulfate
Hepatitis A	Havrix® (3)	Aluminum hydroxide
Hepatitis A + hepatitis B	Twinrix® (3)	Aluminum phosphate/aluminumoxide hydrated
Pneumococcal conjugate vaccine	Prevnar™ (4)	Aluminum phosphate
Influenza vaccine	Fluad™ (5)†	MF59

*Manufacturers: 1, Aventis Pasteur; 2, Merck & Co.; 3, GlaxoSmithKline; 4, Wyeth; 5, Chiron.
†Licensed in Europe.

deliver antigen to M cells of the Peyer's patches. ADP-ribosylating exotoxins such as cholera toxin (CT) and *Escherichia coli* heat-labile enterotoxin (LT) have also been employed to facilitate nasal,[9] oral,[10] and transcutaneous[11] immunization.

Adjuvants can also enhance antigen presentation. Phagocytosis by macrophages of particulate adjuvants consisting of synthetic beads with surface-conjugated antigen, or liposomes containing encapsulated antigen and lipid A, results in antigen release into the cytoplasm. Antigen delivered to the cytoplasm by these particulate adjuvants is treated as endogenous antigen produced intracellularly during viral replication. The antigen is then processed through the major histocompatibility complex (MHC) class I presentation pathway, and this can lead to induction of cytotoxic T lymphocytes (CTLs).[12,13] Ingestion of liposomal lipid A by macrophages has also been shown to enhance (MHC) class II presentation of the liposome-encapsulated antigen by macrophages.[14]

Induction of Immunomodulatory Cytokines by Adjuvants

Adjuvants can induce the production of various cytokines and chemokines, which then act directly or indirectly on helper lymphocyte subsets to modulate immune responses. T-helper (Th) subsets have been defined by the cytokines they produce. Th1 cells are defined as helper T cells that produce interferon-γ (IFN-γ) and interleukin 2 (IL-2), while Th2 helper cells produce IL-4, IL-5, and IL-10. The Th1 versus Th2 paradigm, although continually undergoing evolution and refinement, has given adjuvant researchers a reference point to classify the activity of various immunologic adjuvants that act primarily through the induction of immunomodulatory cytokines.[15] In mice, adjuvants that enhance Th1-like responses, evidenced by delayed-type hypersensitivity (DTH) reactions, also elicit immunoglobulin (IgG_{2a}) antibody subclass responses. Adjuvants such as CT and aluminum salt adjuvants can bias the immune response toward Th2-like responses, predominantly enhancing antibody production, including that of IgA or IgE. IgE-mediated allergies are associated with Th2 responses to allergens.

The ability to elicit and maintain Th1-biased immune responses is a common goal for the development of both prophylactic vaccines against infectious diseases[16] and therapeutic vaccines designed to combat allergies.[17]

CpG Oligodeoxynucleotides

One of the most promising classes of new adjuvants is the immunostimulatory sequences in bacterial DNA. These are short sequences of DNA containing unmethylated cytosine and guanine dinucleotides, so-called CpG motifs. They trigger B-cell activation and induce cytokine secretion, leading to a Th1 response. CpG oligodeoxynucleotides (CpG ODN) work as adjuvants for both systemic and mucosally administered antigens.[18,19]

The use of CpG adjuvants to preferentially induce Th1 over Th2 responses and potentially to "redirect" immune responses that have a natural Th2 bias has also been studied. Weeratna et al. compared immune responses generated in young (<1 week) or adult (6 to 8 weeks) mice primed

with hepatitis B surface antigen (HBsAg) formulated with either alum or CpG ODN adjuvant. CpG ODN resulted in Th1-biased responses, whereas alum induced Th2-biased responses in both the young and adult animals. Mice primed with alum and later boosted with CpG ODN exhibited a Th1-biased response, whereas mice primed with CpG ODN and boosted with alum-adjuvanted HBsAg maintained their initial Th1 bias. These results suggested to the authors that CpG ODN could redirect a Th2-biased immune response toward a Th1 response in this HBsAg model.[20] Alternatively, the secondary immunization with CpG ODN may have elicited a de novo Th1-biased response to the HBsAg.

Cytokine Adjuvants

Several cytokines have been used as experimental vaccine adjuvants, including IL-2 and IFN-γ.[21,22] IL-12 is a recently characterized cytokine that may play a pivotal role in the adjuvant activities of several microbial adjuvants. The adjuvant activity of IL-12 has been demonstrated in a leishmaniasis vaccine in mice. Immunization of BALB/c mice with *Leishmania major* antigens and IL-12 induced leishmania-specific CD4+ Th1 cells and conferred protection against infection with *L. major*. Immunization of control animals with antigen alone elicited Th2 responses that were not protective.[23] The use of microbial adjuvants that induce the endogenous production of IL-12 may be preferable over the use of the preformed cytokine itself as an adjuvant for human prophylactic vaccines. A clinical study has shown that 1- or 4-fμg doses of recombinant IL-12 injected concomitantly with a pneumococcal polysaccharide vaccine induced dose-dependent fever and flu-like symptoms in human subjects.[24]

Cytokine mixtures, including granulocyte-macrophage colony-stimulating factor (GM-CSF), tumor necrosis factor-α (TNF-α), and IL-12 emulsified with incomplete Freund's adjuvant (IFA), have also been employed to steer the immune response in a desired direction.[25] In these studies, the investigators demonstrated that in BALB/c mice, GM-CSF acted in synergy with IL-12 to produce CTL responses and suppression of the Th2 cytokines IL-4 and IL-10 when delivered with human immunodeficiency virus type 1 [HIV-1] peptide antigens in IFA.

Adjuvant Effects on Antigen-Presenting Cells

Adjuvant researchers have begun to study the effect of adjuvants on APCs, and in particular the dendritic cell. Dupuis and his co-investigators demonstrated that fluorescein-labeled gD2 antigen from type 2 herpes simplex virus (HSV-2) formulated in MF59, an emulsion-based adjuvant, was internalized by dendritic cells after intramuscular injection in mice.[26] The maturation of dendritic cells bearing antigen is required for optimal presentation of antigen and induction of immune responses through stimulation of T cells.[27] Adjuvants that induce dendritic cell maturation enhance immune responses through T-cell activation.

Ahonen et al. demonstrated that the synthetic adjuvant R-848 (Resiquimod), previously shown to induce IL-12 and IFN-α secretion, induces the maturation of human monocyte-derived dendritic cells. Maturation of dendritic cells was demonstrated through the induction of cell surface expression of CD83 and increased cell surface expression of CD80, CD86, CD40, and human leukocyte antigen (HLA)-DR. R-848 also induced cytokine and chemokine secretion from dendritic cells. R-848 was shown to enhance dendritic cell antigen-presenting functions, as measured by increased T-cell proliferation and T-cell cytokine secretion in both allogeneic and autologous T-cell systems.[28] Understanding the ability of adjuvants to increase both antigen uptake by and maturation of these cells is critical to the use of adjuvants as selective immunopotentiators in vaccine design.

Adjuvant Safety

The benefits of incorporating a particular adjuvant into vaccine formulations to enhance immunogenicity must be balanced against the potential risk of inducing adverse reactions by the inclusion of the adjuvant. Local adverse reactions that have been reported with adjuvanted vaccines include inflammation at the injection site, the induction of granulomas, or the formation of sterile abscesses.[29] Systemic reactions to adjuvants have been studied in laboratory animals. In animal models, systemic reactions observed include fever, adjuvant arthritis, and anterior chamber uveitis.[30] However, retrospective analyses of previous human cohorts, including a large group of soldiers immunized with an influenza vaccine formulated with IFA, suggest that animal models do not always accurately predict adjuvant reactivity in humans.[31] Adverse reactions seen in clinical trials are generally limited to pain at the injection site, malaise, and fever. Such reactions may be due to synergy between the adjuvant and biologically active vaccine antigens such as bacterial exotoxins or endotoxins. These combinations might promote, through the induction of pro-inflammatory cytokines, reactions that would not be seen with more inert antigens combined with the same adjuvant.

Therefore, although extensive preclinical toxicity studies may have been performed separately on both the adjuvant and the antigen to be incorporated into a candidate vaccine, a final safety evaluation of the exact vaccine formulation slated for Phase I clinical testing should be conducted. This evaluation should be conducted in a small animal species in which the antigen has been found to be immunogenic and that can be reproducibly immunized via the same route anticipated for use in humans. The dose and frequency of administration of the vaccine also should meet or exceed those anticipated to be employed in the clinical trial. An adjuvant safety and immunogenicity test, conducted in rabbits, was designed by a collaborative effort between the Center for Biologics Evaluation and Research, the Food and Drug Administration, and the National Institute of Allergy and Infectious Diseases.[32] The development of similar standardized safety testing for adjuvanted vaccines delivered by routes other than percutaneous injection is presently under study.

Aluminum Salt Adjuvants

Aluminum-containing adjuvants have historically served as immunopotentiators in vaccines and continue to be the most widely used adjuvants. Several aluminum compounds are used and are known as aluminum hydroxide adjuvant, aluminum phosphate adjuvant, and alum. All three of these commonly used names are scientific misnomers. The structure and properties of these adjuvants, their clearance following intramuscular or subcutaneous administration, the mechanisms by which they adsorb antigens, the elution of the adsorbed antigen by interstitial fluid, and the mechanisms by which they stimulate the immune response are discussed here.

Structure and Properties

Aluminum hydroxide adjuvant is not crystalline aluminum hydroxide, or $Al(OH)_3$, but rather crystalline aluminum oxyhydroxide (AlOOH).[33] This difference is important because crystalline aluminum hydroxide has a low surface area (approximately 20 to 50 m^2/g) and is a poor adsorbent. Crystalline aluminum oxyhydroxide has a surface area of approximately 500 m^2/g,[34] which makes it an excellent adsorbent. This high surface area is due to its morphology. The primary particles are fibers having dimensions of approximately $5 \times 2 \times 200$ nm (Fig. 6–1 *left*).

The crystalline nature of aluminum hydroxide adjuvant is an important property because it allows identification based on x-ray diffraction bands at 6.46, 3.18, 2.35, 1.86, 1.44, and 1.31 Å.[33] The x-ray diffraction pattern also serves as an indirect measure of surface area. The sharpness of the x-ray diffraction bands is characterized by the width of the band at half-height (WHH). The WHH is directly related to the adsorptive capacity of aluminum hydroxide adjuvant for bovine serum albumin.[35]

Aluminum oxyhydroxide is a stoichiometric compound. Thus the surface is composed of Al–OH and Al–O–Al groups. The Al–OH surface groups can either accept a proton, resulting in a positive surface charge, or donate a proton, resulting in a negative surface charge. As seen in Figure 6–2, the isoelectric point (iep) of Al–OH is 11.4. Thus, aluminum hydroxide adjuvant exhibits a positive surface charge at pH 7.4, the pH of interstitial fluid. Aluminum hydroxide adjuvant is soluble in acidic media (below pH 4) and in basic media (above pH 10) (Fig. 6–3 *bottom*). It is also soluble at neutral pH in solutions of α-hydroxy acids such as citric acid.[36,37]

Aluminum phosphate adjuvant is chemically amorphous aluminum hydroxyphosphate in which some of the hydroxyl groups of aluminum hydroxide are replaced by phosphate groups.[33] It is not a stoichiometric compound, because the degree of substitution of phosphate for hydroxyl varies widely depending on the method of preparation. Phosphate plays an important role because it sterically prevents the development of order and keeps the adjuvant amorphous. The disordered, amorphous state is responsible for the high surface area and high adsorptive capacity. As seen in Figure 6–1 (*right*), the primary particle has a plate-like morphology with a diameter of approximately 50 nm.

The surface of aluminum phosphate adjuvant is composed of Al–OH and Al–OPO$_3$ groups. The iep varies from 9.4 to 4.5 depending on the degree of phosphate substitution.[38] Commercial aluminum phosphate adjuvants have iep values in the 4.5 to 5.5 range. Thus commercial aluminum phosphate adjuvants are negatively charged at pH

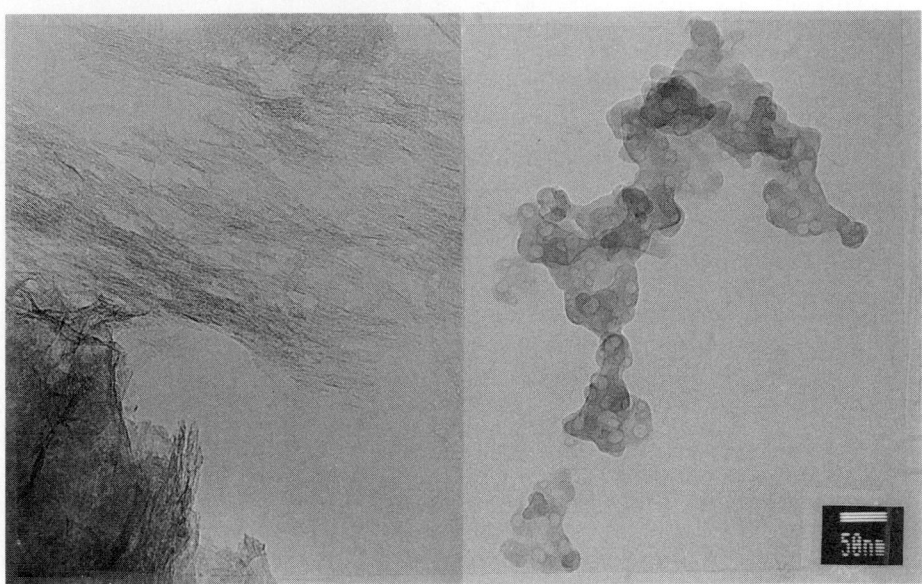

FIGURE 6–1 ■ Transmission electron photomicrograph of aluminum hydroxide adjuvant (*left*) and aluminum phosphate (*right*). (From Shirodkar S, Hutchinson RL, Perry DL, et al. Aluminum compounds used as adjuvants in vaccines. Pharm Res 7(12):1282–1288, 1990, with permission.)

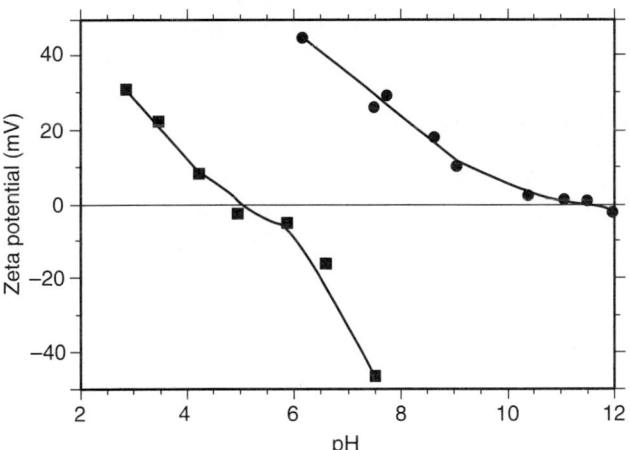

FIGURE 6–2 ■ Isoelectric points of aluminum hydroxide adjuvant (●) and aluminum phosphate adjuvant (■). (From Rinella JV Jr., White JL, Hem SL. Effect of pH on the elution of model antigens from aluminum-containing adjuvants. J Colloid Interface Sci 205:161–165, 1998, with permission.)

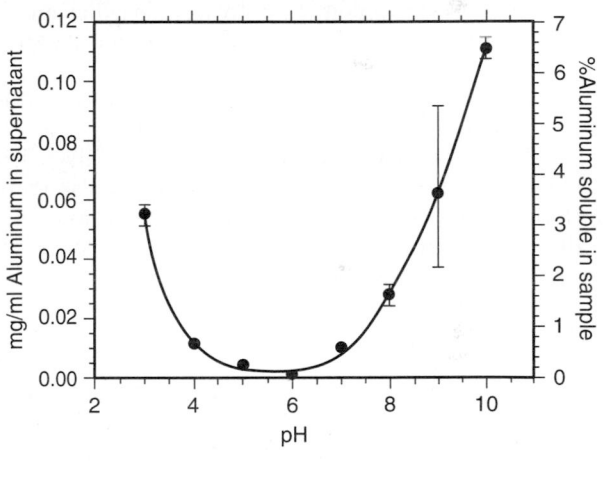

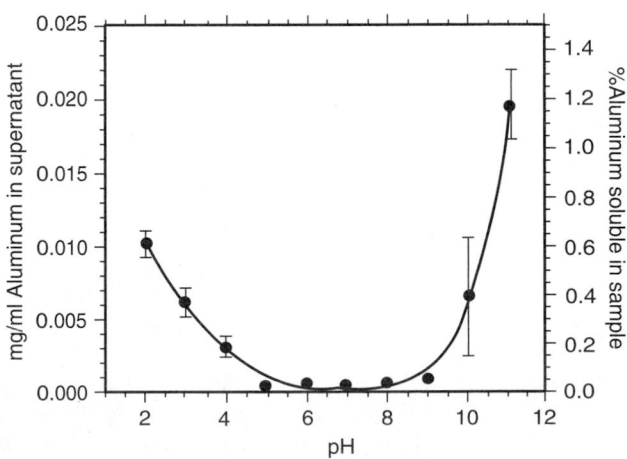

FIGURE 6–3 ■ Effect of pH on the solubility of aluminum phosphate adjuvant (*top*) and aluminum hydroxide adjuvant (*bottom*) after a 45-minute exposure period. The error bars represent 95% confidence intervals of the mean. (From Rinella JV Jr., White JL, Hem SL. Effect of pH on the elution of model antigens from aluminum-containing adjuvants. J Colloid Interface Sci 205: 161–165, 1998, with permission.)

7.4 (see Fig. 6–2). Aluminum phosphate adjuvants are soluble in acidic media (< pH 4), in basic media (> pH 8) (see Fig. 6–3 *top*), and at neutral pH in solutions of citric acid.[36,37] Aluminum phosphate adjuvant is generally more soluble than aluminum hydroxide adjuvant because of its amorphous structure.

Alum, which is water soluble, is chemically aluminum potassium sulfate, $AlK(SO_4)_2$. It is used in many industries as a source of aluminum cations. The earliest vaccines containing aluminum adjuvants were prepared by in situ precipitation. A solution of alum was mixed with a solution of the antigen dissolved in a phosphate buffer. The aluminum-antigen solution was titrated with a base such as ammonium hydroxide or sodium hydroxide, which precipitated the aluminum. It is common practice to refer to the adjuvant produced by in situ precipitation as alum. The precipitate is chemically amorphous aluminum hydroxyphosphate and has composition and properties similar to those of aluminum phosphate adjuvant.[33,39]

The techniques that can be used to characterize aluminum-containing adjuvants have been reviewed by White and Hem.[40]

Clearance of Aluminum Salt Adjuvants

Many millions of doses of vaccines containing aluminum adjuvants have been administered since their immunopotentiation property was recognized in 1926.[3] The vaccines are usually administered by intramuscular or subcutaneous injection. Thus they come in contact with interstitial fluid.

Interstitial fluid contains three α-hydroxycarboxylic acids: citric acid, lactic acid, and malic acid. α-Hydroxycarboxylic acids are good chelators of aluminum and thus solubilize the aluminum adjuvants. The total concentration of these three acids has been estimated at 2.7 mEq/L.[37] In vitro dissolution studies have shown that aluminum hydroxide and aluminum phosphate adjuvants dissolve in a solution containing 2.7 mEq/L of citric acid at pH 7.4.[41] The crystalline aluminum hydroxide adjuvant dissolves more slowly than amorphous aluminum phosphate adjuvant.

The absorption and clearance of aluminum-containing adjuvants was studied in rabbits using adjuvants labeled with ^{26}Al.[42] ^{26}Al does not occur naturally. Thus any ^{26}Al in the blood, urine, or tissues following intramuscular administration is from the dissolution of the adjuvant in interstitial fluid. ^{26}Al can be accurately quantified by accelerator mass spectrometry.

Figure 6–4 shows the ^{26}Al blood level curve following intramuscular administration of ^{26}Al-labeled aluminum hydroxide and aluminum phosphate adjuvants. ^{26}Al was found in the blood at the first sampling point (1 hour) for both adjuvants. Thus dissolution of aluminum-containing adjuvants begins on administration. The area under the blood level curves indicated that 17% of the aluminum hydroxide and 51% of the aluminum phosphate adjuvant had dissolved in interstitial fluid and had been absorbed into the blood in 28 days.[42]

Adsorption Mechanisms

The major mechanisms responsible for the adsorption of antigens are electrostatic attraction, hydrophobic forces, and ligand exchange. Electrostatic attraction is probably the most frequently utilized adsorption mechanism.

Electrostatic attraction can be optimized by determining the iep of the antigen and then selecting an adjuvant that will have the opposite surface charge at the desired pH. For example, at pH 7.4 aluminum hydroxide adjuvant (iep = 11.4) adsorbs albumin (iep = 4.8) but does not adsorb lysozyme (iep = 11.0). In contrast, aluminum phosphate adjuvant (iep = 4.0) adsorbs lysozyme but not albumin at pH 7.4.[43]

The iep of aluminum hydroxide adjuvant can be modified by exposure to phosphate anion. An experimental malaria antigen, R32tet32 (iep = 12.8), was not adsorbed by aluminum hydroxide adjuvant.[44] However, adsorption occurred when the vaccine was formulated with a phosphate buffer. Some of the phosphate anions displaced hydroxyls from the surface of the aluminum hydroxide adjuvant, reduced the iep, and led to electrostatic attraction.

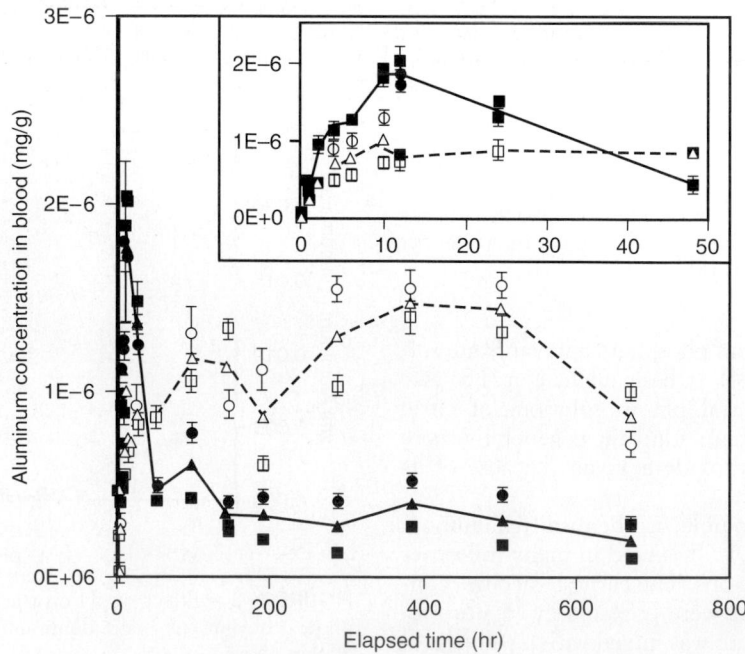

FIGURE 6–4 ■ Blood concentration profile after intramuscular administration of ^{26}Al labeled aluminum hydroxide adjuvant (■, rabbit 1, ●, rabbit 2; ▲, mean) or aluminum phosphate adjuvant (□, rabbit 3; ○, rabbit 4; △, mean). The *solid line* represents aluminum hydroxide adjuvant and the *dashed line* represents aluminum phosphate adjuvant. (From Flarend RE, Hem SL, White JL, et al. In vivo absorption of aluminum-containing vaccine adjuvants using ^{26}Al. Vaccine 15:1314–1318, 1997, with permission.)

Care must be taken in selecting a buffer for an aluminum hydroxide adjuvant–containing vaccine. Electrostatic attraction for an acidic antigen may be reduced or even reversed if a phosphate buffer is used. Acetate and TRIS are examples of buffers that do not alter the iep of aluminum hydroxide adjuvant.[33]

Aluminum hydroxide adjuvant can also be pretreated to lower the iep and optimize electrostatic adsorption of basic antigens.[45] Figure 6–5 (*bottom*) shows that lysozyme (iep = 11.0) was adsorbed by aluminum hydroxide adjuvant (iep = 11.4) at pH 7.4 when the adjuvant was pretreated with phosphate anion. The electrophoretic mobility of untreated aluminum hydroxide adjuvant was +2 μm cm/V s. Pretreatment with four concentrations of phosphate anion reduced the iep to 7.9, 5.8, 5.1, and 4.6. No adsorption occurred when the electrophoretic mobility of the aluminum hydroxide adjuvant was positive. The adsorptive capacity increased as the surface charge became more negative.

The ionic strength of the vaccine is important when adsorption is due to electrostatic attraction. The adsorptive capacity of lysozyme (iep = 11) by aluminum phosphate adjuvant (iep = 5.0) at pH 7.4 was reduced from 0.66 mg lysozyme per milligram aluminum to zero as the concentration of sodium chloride in the formulation was increased from 0.06 to 0.25 M.[46] The ionic strength of the vaccine should be kept as low as possible when the antigen is adsorbed by electrostatic attraction.

Hydrophobic forces also contribute to the adsorption of antigens by aluminum-containing adjuvants. The contribution of hydrophobic attractive forces can be determined by observing the effect of ethylene glycol on adsorption.[46] Ethylene glycol stabilizes the hydration layer of proteins, which renders hydrophobic interactions thermodynamically unfavorable. The addition of ethylene glycol to a bovine serum albumin–aluminum hydroxide model vaccine does not affect the adsorptive capacity, indicating that hydrophobic interactions do not contribute to the adsorption. However, the adsorption of lysozyme by aluminum phosphate adjuvant is reduced by the addition of ethylene glycol, indicating that hydrophobic interactions play a role in the adsorption of lysozyme.

The adsorption of phosphate by hydroxylated mineral surfaces occurs by ligand exchange. Phosphate anions bind directly to surface aluminum by replacing hydroxyl groups. This is the strongest adsorption force. The effects of ligand exchange are seen in the adsorption of ovalbumin. Ovalbumin is a phosphoglycoprotein having a molecular mass of 45,000 Da and an iep of 4.6. It contains up to two accessible phosphate groups.[47] The adsorption of ovalbumin by the series of aluminum hydroxide adjuvants pretreated with phosphate as described earlier was studied. Figure 6–5 (*top*) shows that the greatest adsorptive capacity of negatively charged ovalbumin occurs when the aluminum hydroxide adjuvant is positively charged. However, significant adsorption (0.25 mg ovalbumin per milligram aluminum) occurred even when the surface charge of the aluminum hydroxide adjuvant was strongly negative. Ligand exchange by the phosphate groups is a strong enough adsorption force to overcome the electrostatic repulsive force.

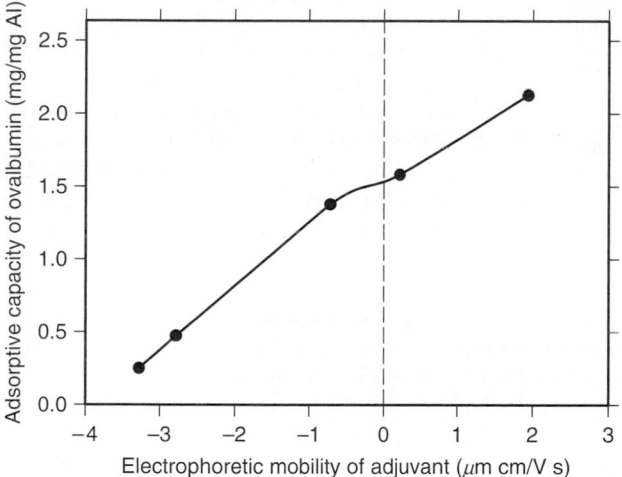

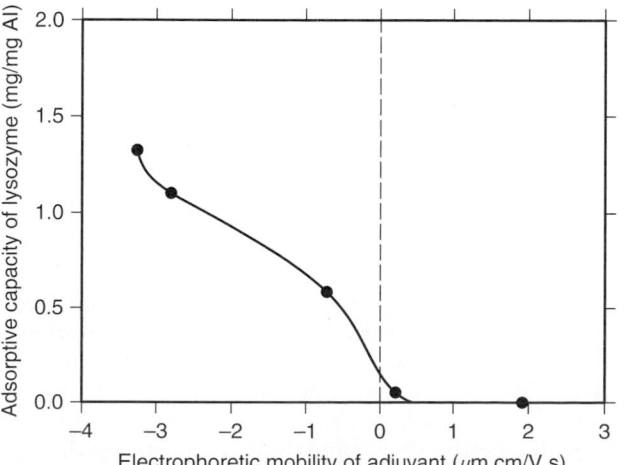

FIGURE 6–5 ■ Effect of surface charge of phosphate-treated aluminum hydroxide adjuvant on the adsorptive capacity of ovalbumin at pH 7.4 and 25°C. (From Chang M-F, White JL, Nail SL, Hem SL. Role of the electrostatic attractive force in the adsorption of proteins by aluminum hydroxide adjuvant. PDA J Pharm Sci Technol 51(1):25–29, 1997, with permission.)

Desorption in Interstitial Fluid

Vaccines come in contact with interstitial fluid following intramuscular or subcutaneous administration. The composition of interstitial fluid is very different from the formulation of the vaccine. In vitro studies have identified several components of interstitial fluid, including phosphate,[48] citrate,[37] and fibrinogen,[49] all of which cause rapid elution of previously adsorbed antigens. Lysozyme was almost completely eluted from aluminum phosphate adjuvant after exposure to sheep interstitial fluid for 15 minutes.[47] Under similar conditions, ovalbumin was almost completely eluted from aluminum hydroxide adjuvant in 4 hours.

Three lysozyme–aluminum adjuvant vaccines were prepared containing the same amount of lysozyme. However, the surface charge was modified by pretreatment with phosphate to produce adsorption of 3%, 35%, or 85% of the lysozyme. When the three vaccines were diluted with sheep interstitial fluid, the degree of adsorption in all three vaccines changed to 40%. Each vaccine exhibited immunopotentiation in rabbits compared to a solution of lysozyme. However, each vaccine produced the same antibody titer. It was concluded that the potentiation of the immune response by aluminum-containing adjuvants correlates with the degree of adsorption of the antigen in interstitial fluid following administration rather than with the degree of adsorption in the vaccine formulation.[50]

Mechanisms of Action

It is surprising that there is no consensus regarding the mechanisms by which aluminum-containing adjuvants potentiate the immune response. Three potential mechanisms are frequently cited to explain how aluminum-containing adjuvants increase antibody production: the depot mechanism, the inflammation mechanism, and the promotion of uptake of antigens by APCs[51]:

1. The depot mechanism postulates that the aluminum-containing adjuvant and the adsorbed antigen remain at the site of injection. The antigen is released slowly to stimulate the production of antibodies.
2. The inflammation mechanism is based on the hypothesis that aluminum-containing adjuvants cause inflammation at the site of injection. APCs are rapidly attracted to the site of inflammation. Because the antigen is also present at the site of injection, APCs encounter a high concentration of antigen.
3. It has also been proposed that adsorption of antigen to aluminum-containing adjuvants converts the soluble antigen to a particulate form. APCs can take up particulate matter by phagocytosis. Thus antigen, which remains adsorbed, is taken into macrophages and dendritic cells.

It is likely that all three proposed mechanisms contribute to the immunopotentiation produced by aluminum-containing adjuvants. On administration, the very small particles of aluminum-containing adjuvants cause inflammation at the site of injection. APCs are recruited to the site of inflammation. APCs such as macrophages and dendritic cells can take up antigen that is present in interstitial fluid by pinocytosis. Thus even antigens that are rapidly desorbed from the adjuvant particles enter APCs. It is likely that the concentration of desorbed antigen in the vicinity of the adjuvant particles is higher than would be the case if a solution of antigen was administered. Thus the aluminum adjuvant acts to produce a high concentration of antigen in interstitial fluid in the microenvironment of the APCs. Antigen that remains adsorbed to the adjuvant particles and the adjuvant particles are taken into the APCs by phagocytosis. Thus, aluminum-containing adjuvants produce a high concentration of antigen within APCs, which results in immunopotentiation.

Macrophagic Myofasciitis

Focal histologic lesions were observed in patients with diffuse muscular symptoms that included persistent myalgias, arthralgias, and persistent fatigue. In the approximately 130 cases studied, these lesions were identified as macrophagic myofasciitis (MMF).[52] Intracytoplasmic inclusions in the infiltrating macrophages have been identified as containing aluminum by electron microscopy, microanalysis, and atomic adsorption spectroscopy. The presence of aluminum in the deltoid muscle biopsies suggested to Gherardi et al. that the source of the aluminum was aluminum hydroxide adjuvant.[52] However, no relationship between the presence of aluminum and MMF and the clinical symptoms has been established to date. The Vaccine Safety Advisory Committee of the World Heath Organization reviewed MMF at a meeting of the committee in 1999. The committee found that there was no basis for recommending a change in vaccination practices involving vaccine selection, schedule, delivery practices, or information regarding aluminum-containing vaccines. The committee recommended that "research studies be undertaken to evaluate the clinical, epidemiological and basic science aspects of MMF."[53] The FDA, while recognizing the desirability of new adjuvants, has confirmed its support of aluminum salts in vaccines.[53a]

MF59 Adjuvant

MF59 is an oil-in-water microfluidized emulsion composed of stable droplets (250 nm) of the metabolizable oil squalene (4.3% w/v) and two surfactants, polyoxyethylene sorbitan monooleate (Tween 80; 0.5% w/v) and sorbitan trioleate (Span-85; 0.5% w/v). Chiron Vaccines developed MF59 to be a human vaccine adjuvant with higher potency than aluminum hydroxide and equally low toxicity. MF59 was initially developed as a vehicle for an additional muramyl peptide adjuvant, MTP-PE, but was found to possess marked adjuvant properties itself. MF59 is used in Fluad™ (Chiron Vaccines, Sienna, Italy), an influenza vaccine recently licensed in Europe. The immunogenicity and protective efficacy of influenza vaccine with and without the adjuvant MF59 initially was determined in mice. The addition of MF59 significantly increased the antibody response to the influenza antigens over a wide dose range. Equivalent antibody titers were seen using 50- to 200-fold less antigen concentrations when combined with MF59 as compared with vaccine alone.[54]

A clinical trial to evaluate the safety and tolerability of this influenza vaccine compared with a conventional nonadjuvanted influenza vaccine was conducted in elderly ambulatory patients. Volunteers were vaccinated with one dose of either vaccine each year for 3 consecutive years; 92 volunteers received at least one dose, 74 received two doses, and 67 received all three doses. The objective of these studies was to evaluate the safety of repetitive injections of the adjuvanted vaccine in elderly subjects. There were no reports of any vaccine-related serious adverse events or of safety concerns related to study vaccines after the first, second, or third immunization. The adjuvanted vaccine induced more local reactions than the conventional vaccine; however, the reactions were normally mild and limited to the first 2 to 3 days after immunization. No statistically significant difference between groups in systemic postimmunization reactions was reported except for a mild, transient malaise after the first immunization. Compared with the first immunization, no increase in postimmunization reactions was seen after the second and third immunizations.[55]

The safety and immunogenicity of Fluad was evaluated in elderly people and in volunteers with underlying chronic diseases. Data from a clinical database of more than 10,000 elderly people immunized with various influenza vaccines demonstrated that, although common postimmunization reactions were seen more frequently in recipients of the MF59-adjuvanted vaccine, it was well tolerated, including when used to re-immunize in successive influenza seasons. Fluad elicited higher immune responses with statistically significant increases of postimmunization geometric mean titers and seroconversion and seroprotection rates compared with nonadjuvanted influenza vaccines. This effect was most marked for the A/H3N2 and the B strains. The higher immunogenicity of the MF59-adjuvanted vaccine was maintained after subsequent immunizations. The highest adjuvant effect was seen in subjects with low preimmunization titers and in those affected by chronic underlying diseases.[56]

The safety and adjuvanticity of MF59-adjuvanted vaccines has been tested in toddlers and infants with recombinant HIV and cytomegalovirus (CMV) vaccines. Borkowsky et al. reported that an MF59-adjuvanted HIV-1 SF-2 gp120 vaccine elicited higher cell-mediated immune responses as measured by lymphoproliferation than an alum-adjuvanted HIV-1 MN gp120 vaccine in infants born to HIV-1-infected mothers. In these studies, the neonates were immunized with either vaccine at birth, 2 weeks, 2 months, and 5 months.[57] Both the MF59-adjuvanted and alum-adjuvanted recombinant HIV-1 gp120 subunit vaccine were demonstrated to be safe and well tolerated in neonates.[58] MF59-adjuvanted HIV-1 gp120 vaccine administered at birth and 2, 8, and 20 weeks of age was also shown to induce gp120 antibody responses in infants born to HIV-1-infected mothers.[59] Immune responses of young children to an MF59-adjuvanted CMV vaccine were higher than those observed in adults after immunization or after natural CMV infection.[60]

The ability of MF59 to enhance the immunogenicity of polysaccharide-protein conjugate vaccines was investigated in infant baboons. Baboons 1 to 4 months of age were immunized intramuscularly with *Neisseria meningitidis* group C and *Haemophilus influenzae* type b oligosaccharide-CRM$_{197}$ conjugate vaccines. The lyophilized vaccines were reconstituted with phosphate-buffered saline, aluminum hydroxide adjuvant, or MF59. Each animal was given three injections of the respective formulations, with one injection every 4 weeks. Four weeks after each immunization, the MF59 group had up to 7-fold higher geometric mean anticapsular antibody titers than the aluminum hydroxide adjuvant group and 5- to 10-fold higher *N. meningitidis* group C bactericidal antibody titers.[61]

MF59 is a safe, practical, and potent adjuvant for use with human vaccines, with more than 5 million doses distributed. The formulation is easily manufactured, may be sterilized by filtration, and is both compatible and efficacious with all antigens tested to date. MF59 has been shown both in animal models and in humans to be a potent stimulator of cellular and humoral responses to subunit antigens. Toxicology studies in animal models and Phase I through IV studies in humans have demonstrated the safety of MF59 with HSV, HIV, and influenza vaccines.[62]

Monophosphoryl Lipid A (MPL®) Adjuvant

Johnson et al. discovered the adjuvant effect of the lipopolysaccharide (LPS) endotoxin from gram-negative bacteria in 1956.[63] Since then, a goal of adjuvant researchers has been to identify molecules that would retain the powerful immunopotentiating effect of native LPS or its adjuvant-active moiety lipid A but that would be devoid of the pyrogenicity and toxic effects that preclude the use of native molecules as adjuvants for human vaccines.

MPL adjuvant (Corixa, Inc.) is monophosphoryl lipid A prepared from the LPS of a heptoseless mutant (R595) of *Salmonella minnesota*. MPL differs from the native lipid A portion of LPS by the absence of an acid-labile phosphate group and a base-labile acyl group. MPL retains the immunomodulating activity of LPS but exhibits greatly reduced toxicity. MPL has undergone extensive preclinical testing, has been clinically evaluated as an immunologic adjuvant in more than 10,000 volunteers, and is a component of a cancer vaccine, Melacine® (Corixa Inc./Schering Plough), which is currently licensed in Canada.

A recombinant HBsAg vaccine was formulated with an adjuvant system termed SBAS4, which was composed of a combination of an aluminum salt adjuvant and MPL. In a clinical study, this vaccine formulation was assessed in 27 healthy adult volunteers using the commercial aluminum-adjuvanted hepatitis vaccine Engerix-B® (GlaxoSmithKline) as the control. The two vaccine formulations showed similar reactogenicity profiles after three doses given at birth and 1 and 6 months. Local reactions observed were mild, the most frequently cited being soreness at the site of injection. Seroprotection was achieved after two doses in all subjects given the MPL-adjuvanted vaccine, while the control vaccine induced seroprotection after the third dose. Higher anti-HBsAg antibody titers were observed after the second and third doses in the group that received MPL adjuvant. In addition, cellular immunity as measured by HBsAg-specific lymphoproliferation was stronger in the MPL-adjuvanted group than with Engerix-B.[64]

Because of its safety and extensive clinical evaluation, MPL is a strong candidate for use as an adjuvant for human preventive and therapeutic vaccines against infectious and neoplastic diseases. Vaccine antigens tested with MPL include recombinant proteins, polysaccharide conjugates, allergens, and tumor antigens. MPL also has been shown to enhance immune responses generated by plasmid DNA vaccines.[65]

Mechanism of Action

MPL activates APCs, leading to the release of a cascade of immunomodulatory cytokines including IL-12, IL-1, TNF-α, and GM-CSF. The interactions with APCs result in enhanced phagocytosis and increased expression of MHC molecules. MPL also stimulates the production of IL-2 and IFN-γ characteristic of Th1 cell responses.[66,67] The Th1 immune response elicited by MPL induces cell-mediated immunity and complement-fixing antibodies.[17]

Synthetic acylated monosaccharide molecules structurally related to lipid A are presently under development and testing by Corixa, Inc. These synthetic compounds are referred to as aminoalkyl glucosaminide phosphates (AGPs), with adjuvant activities similar to MPL. AGPs enhance Th1 responses and are effective when administered nasally as well as parenterally. Mucosal immunization with AGPs results in enhanced IgG and IgA responses as well as cell-mediated immunity.[68]

Future Adjuvant Research and Development

In conclusion, although aluminum salt adjuvants will continue in the future as the mainstay of adjuvants employed in licensed vaccines worldwide, greater emphasis by vaccine manufacturers now is being placed on the discovery, development, and testing of new adjuvants for use with modern vaccines. The ability to select from a palate of thoroughly accepted adjuvants would allow vaccine formulators greater flexibility in the rational design of vaccines. Appropriate use of safe and effective adjuvants would likely allow for significant reduction in the amount of antigen required per dose of vaccine, creating the ability to produce greater quantities of vaccines, thus expanding the protective coverage of a target population using existing manufacturing capacity. Adjuvants will also aid in the development of novel vaccine delivery systems and routes of administration, such as transcutaneous or mucosal vaccine delivery, leading to improved vaccine compliance, increased efficacy, and the reduction of manufacturing and distribution costs.

REFERENCES

1. Ramon G. Sur l'aumentation anormale de l'antitoxine chez les chevaux producteurs de sérum antidiphtérique. Bull Soc Centr Med Vet 101:227–234, 1925.
2. Ramon G. Procédés pour accroitre la production des antitoxines. Ann Inst Pasteur (Paris) 40:1–10, 1926.
3. Glenny A, Pope C, Waddington H, Wallace U. The antigenic value of toxoid precipitated by potassium alum. J Pathol Bacteriol 29:31–40, 1926.
4. Greenberg J, Fleming D. Increased efficiency of diphtheria toxoid when combined with pertussis vaccine. Can J Public Health 38:279–282, 1947.
5. Recommended childhood immunization schedule—United States, 2002. MMWR 51:31–33, 2002.
6. Vogel FR, Powell MF. A compendium of vaccine adjuvants and excipients. In Powell MF, Newman MJ (eds). Vaccine Design: The Subunit and Adjuvant Approach. New York, Plenum Press, 1995, pp 141–248.
7. Holmgren J, Lycke N, Czerkinsky C. Cholera toxin and cholera B subunit as oral-mucosal adjuvant and antigen vector systems. Vaccine 11:1179–1184, 1993.
8. Clark MA, Blair H, Liang L, et al. Targeting polymerised liposome vaccine carriers to intestinal M cells. Vaccine 20:208–217, 2001.
9. Hagiwara Y, Iwasaki T, Asanuma H, et al. Effects of intranasal administration of cholera toxin (or Escherichia coli heat-labile enterotoxin) B subunits supplemented with a trace amount of the holotoxin on the brain. Vaccine 19:1652–1660, 2001.
10. McGhee JR, Xu-Amano J, Miller CJ, et al. The common mucosal immune system: from basic principles to enteric vaccines with relevance for the female reproductive tract. Reprod Fertil Dev 6:369–379, 1994.
11. Scharton-Kersten T, Yu J, Vassell R, et al. Transcutaneous immunization with bacterial ADP-ribosylating exotoxins, subunits, and unrelated adjuvants. Infect Immun 68:5306–5313, 2000.
12. Rock KL. A new foreign policy: MHC class I molecules monitor the outside world. Immunol Today 17:131–137, 1996.
13. Rao M, Alving CR. Delivery of lipids and liposomal proteins to the cytoplasm and Golgi of antigen-presenting cells. Adv Drug Deliv Rev 41:171–188, 2000.
14. Verma JN, Rao M, Amselem S, et al. Adjuvant effects of liposomes containing lipid A: enhancement of liposomal antigen presentation and recruitment of macrophages. Infect Immun 60:2438–2444, 1992.
15. Moingeon P, Haensler J, Lindberg A. Towards the rational design of Th1 adjuvants. Vaccine 19:4363–4372, 2001.
16. Neuzil KM, Johnson JE, Tang YW, et al. Adjuvants influence the quantitative and qualitative immune response in BALB/c mice immunized with respiratory syncytial virus FG subunit vaccine. Vaccine 15:525–532, 1997.
17. Baldridge JR, Yorgensen Y, Ward JR, Ulrich JT. Monophosphoryl lipid A enhances mucosal and systemic immunity to vaccine antigens following intranasal administration. Vaccine 18:2416–2425, 2000.
18. McCluskie MJ, Davis HL. CpG as mucosal adjuvant. Vaccine 18:231–237, 2000.
19. Weeratna RD, McCluskie MJ, Xu Y, Davis HL. CpG DNA induces stronger immune responses with less toxicity than other adjuvants. Vaccine 18:1755–1762, 2000.
20. Weeratna RD, Brazolot MC, McCluskie MJ, Davis HL. CpG ODN can re-direct the Th bias of established Th2 immune responses in adult and young mice. FEMS Immunol Med Microbiol 32:65–71, 2001.
21. Banyer JL, Hamilton NH, Ramshaw IA, Ramsay AJ. Cytokines in innate and adaptive immunity. Rev Immunogenet 2:359–373, 2000.
22. Nohria A, Rubin RH. Cytokines as potential vaccine adjuvants. Biotherapy 7:261–269, 1994.
23. Scott P, Trinchieri G. IL-12 as an adjuvant for cell-mediated immunity. Semin Immunol 9:285–291, 1997.
24. Hedlund J, Langer B, Konradsen HB, Ortqvist A. Negligible adjuvant effect for antibody responses and frequent adverse events associated with IL-12 treatment in humans vaccinated with pneumococcal polysaccharide. Vaccine 20:164–169, 2001.
25. Ahlers JD, Dunlop N, Alling DW, et al. Cytokine-in-adjuvant steering of the immune response phenotype to HIV-1 vaccine constructs: granulocyte-macrophage colony-stimulating factor and TNF-alpha synergize with IL-12 to enhance induction of cytotoxic T lymphocytes. J Immunol 158:3947–3958, 1997.
26. Dupuis M, Murphy TJ, Higgins D, et al. Dendritic cells internalize vaccine adjuvant after intramuscular injection. Cell Immunol 186:18–27, 1998.
27. Bancheereau J, Steinman RM. Dendritic cells and the control of immunity. Nature 392:245–252, 1998.
28. Ahonen CL, Gibson SJ, Smith RM, et al. Dendritic cell maturation and subsequent enhanced T-cell stimulation induced with the novel synthetic immune response modifier R-848. Cell Immunol 197:62–72, 1999.
29. Bernier RH, Frank JAJ, Nolan TFJ. Abscesses complicating DTP vaccination. Am J Dis Child 135:826–828, 1981.
30. Allison AC, Byars NE. Immunological adjuvants: desirable properties and side-effects. Mol Immunol 28:279–284, 1991.
31. Page WF, Norman JE, Benenson AS. Long-term follow-up of army recruits immunized with Freund's incomplete adjuvanted vaccine. Vaccine Res 2:141–149, 1993.
32. Goldenthal KL, Cavagnaro JA, Alving CR, Vogel FR. Safety evaluation of vaccine adjuvants. National Cooperative Vaccine Development Working Group. AIDS Res Hum Retroviruses 9:S45–S49, 1993.
33. Shirodkar S, Hutchinson RL, Perry DL, et al. Aluminum compounds used as adjuvants in vaccines. Pharm Res 7:1282–1288, 1990.
34. Johnston CT, Wang S-L, Hem SL. Measuring the surface area of aluminum hydroxide adjuvant. J Pharm Sci 91:1702–1706, 2002.
35. Masood H, White JL, Hem SL. Relationship between protein adsorptive capacity and the X-ray diffraction pattern of aluminium hydroxide adjuvants. Vaccine 12:187–189, 1994.
36. Rinella JV Jr., White JL, Hem SL. Effect of pH on the elution of model antigens from aluminum-containing adjuvants. J Colloid Interface Sci 205:161–165, 1998.
37. Seeber SJ, White JL, Hem SL. Solubilization of aluminum-containing adjuvants by constituents of interstitial fluid. J Parenter Sci Technol 45:156–159, 1991.
38. Liu J-C, Feldkamp JR, White JL, Hem SL. Adsorption of phosphate by aluminum hydroxycarbonate. J Pharm Sci 73:1355–1358, 1984.
39. Hem KJ, Dandashli EA, White JL, Hem SL. Accessibility of antigen in vaccines produced by in situ alum precipitation. Vaccine Res 5:189–191, 1996.
40. White JL, Hem SL. Characterization of aluminum-containing adjuvants. In Brown F, Corbel M, Griffiths E (eds). Physico-Chemical Procedures for the Characterization of Vaccines. Basel, Karger 2000, pp 217–228.

41. Hem SL. Elimination of aluminum adjuvants. Vaccine 20(suppl 3):S40–S43, 2002.

42. Flarend RE, Hem SL, White JL, et al. In vivo absorption of aluminum-containing vaccine adjuvants using 26Al. Vaccine 15:1314–1318, 1997.

43. Seeber SJ, White JL, Hem SL. Predicting the adsorption of proteins by aluminum-containing adjuvants. Vaccine 9:201–203, 1991.

44. Callahan PM, Shorter AL, Hem SL. The importance of surface charge in the optimization of antigen-adjuvant interactions. Pharm Res 8:851–858, 1991.

45. Chang M-F, White JL, Nail SL, Hem SL. Role of the electrostatic attractive force in the adsorption of proteins by aluminum hydroxide adjuvant. PDA J Pharm Sci Technol 51:25–29, 1997.

46. al-Shakhshir RH, Regnier FE, White JL, Hem SL. Contribution of electrostatic and hydrophobic interactions to the adsorption of proteins by aluminum-containing adjuvants. Vaccine 13:41–44, 1995.

47. Shi Y, HogenEsch H, Hem SL. Change in the degree of adsorption of proteins by aluminum-containing adjuvants following exposure to interstitial fluid: freshly prepared and aged model vaccines. Vaccine 20:80–85, 2001.

48. Rinella JV Jr., White JL, Hem SL. Effect of anions on model aluminum-adjuvant-containing vaccines. J Colloid Interface Sci 172:121–130, 1995.

49. Heimlich JM, Regnier FE, White JL, Hem SL. The in vitro displacement of adsorbed model antigens from aluminum-containing adjuvants by interstitial proteins. Vaccine 17:2873–2881, 1999.

50. Chang M, Shi Y, Nail SL, et al. Degree of antigen adsorption in the vaccine or interstitial fluid and its effect on the antibody response in rabbits. Vaccine 19:2884–2889, 2001.

51. Gupta RK, Rost BE, Relyveld E, Siber GR. Adjuvant properties of aluminum and calcium compounds. In Powell MF, Newman MJ (eds). Vaccine Design: The Subunit and Adjuvant Approach. New York, Plenum Press, 1995, pp 237–238.

52. Gherardi RK, Coquet M, Cherin P, et al. Macrophagic myofasciitis lesions assess long-term persistence of vaccine-derived aluminum hydroxide in muscle. Brain 124:1821–1831, 2001.

52a. Brenner A. Macrophagic Myofasciitis: a summary of Dr. Gheradt's presentations. Vaccine 20:55–56, 2002.

53. WHO Vaccine Safety Advisory Committee. Macrophagic myofasciitis and aluminum-containing vaccines. Wkly Epidemiol Rec 41:338–340, 1999.

53a. Baylor NW, Egan W, Richman P. Aluminum salts in vaccines —US perspective. Vaccine 20:518–523, 2002.

54. Cataldo DM, van Nest G. The adjuvant MF59 increases the immunogenicity and protective efficacy of subunit influenza vaccine in mice. Vaccine 15:1710–1715, 1997.

55. Minutello M, Senatore F, Cecchinelli G, et al. Safety and immunogenicity of an inactivated subunit influenza virus vaccine combined with MF59 adjuvant emulsion in elderly subjects, immunized for three consecutive influenza seasons. Vaccine 17:99–104, 1999.

56. Podda A. The adjuvanted influenza vaccines with novel adjuvants: experience with the MF59-adjuvanted vaccine. Vaccine 19:2673–2680, 2001.

57. Borkowsky W, Wara D, Fenton T, et al. Lymphoproliferative responses to recombinant HIV-1 envelope antigens in neonates and infants receiving gp120 vaccines. AIDS Clinical Trial Group 230 Collaborators. J Infect Dis 181:890–896, 2000.

58. Cunningham CK, Wara DW, Kang M, et al. Safety of 2 recombinant human immunodeficiency virus type 1 (HIV-1) envelope vaccines in neonates born to HIV-1-infected women. Clin Infect Dis 32:801–807, 2001.

59. McFarland EJ, Borkowsky W, Fenton T, et al. Human immunodeficiency virus type 1 (HIV-1) gp120-specific antibodies in neonates receiving an HIV-1 recombinant gp120 vaccine. J Infect Dis 184:1331–1335, 2001.

60. Mitchell DK, Holmes SJ, Burke RL, et al. Immunogenicity of a recombinant human cytomegalovirus gB vaccine in seronegative toddlers. Pediatr Infect Dis J 21:133–138, 2002.

61. Granoff DM, McHugh YE, Raff HV, et al. MF59 adjuvant enhances antibody responses of infant baboons immunized with Haemophilus influenzae type b and Neisseria meningitidis group C oligosaccharide CRM197 conjugate vaccine. Infect Immun 65:1710–1715, 1997.

62. Ott G, Barchfeld GL, Chernoff D, et al. MF59: design and evaluation of a safe and potent adjuvant for human vaccines. Pharm Biotechnol 6:277–296, 1995.

63. Johnson AG, Gaines S, Landy M. Studies on the theta antigen of Salmonella typhosa. V. Enhancement of antibody to protein antigens by purified lipopolysaccharide. J Exp Med 103:225, 1956.

64. Thoelen S, Van Damme P, Mathei C, et al. Safety and immunogenicity of a hepatitis B vaccine formulated with a novel adjuvant system. Vaccine 16:708–714, 1998.

65. Lodmell DL, Ray NB, Ulrich JT, Ewalt LC. DNA vaccination of mice against rabies virus: effects of the route of vaccination and the adjuvant monophosphoryl lipid A (MPL). Vaccine 18:1059–1066, 2000.

66. De Becker G, Moulin V, Pajak B, et al. The adjuvant monophosphoryl lipid A increases the function of antigen-presenting cells. Int Immunol 12:807–815, 2000.

67. Salkowski CA, Detore GR, Vogel SN. Lipopolysaccharide and monophosphoryl lipid A differentially regulate interleukin-12, gamma interferon, and interleukin-10 mRNA production in murine macrophages. Infect Immun 65:3239–3247, 1997.

68. Baldridge JR. A synthetic adjuvant, RC-529, moves into the clinic [abstr]. Abstracts of the 3rd Meeting on Novel Adjuvants in or Close to Human Clinical Testing. Annecy, France 2002.

69. Aggerbeck H, Heron I. Adjuvanticity of aluminum hydroxide and calcium phosphate in diphtheria-tetanus vaccines—I. Vaccine 13:1360–1365, 1995.

70. Hem SL, White JL. Structure and properties of aluminum-containing adjuvants. Pharm Biotechnol 6:249–276, 1995.

71. Relyveld EH. Preparation and use of calcium phosphate adsorbed vaccines. Dev Biol Stand 65:131–136, 1986.

72. Chedid L, Audibert F, Jolivet M. Role of muramyl peptides for the enhancement of synthetic vaccines. Dev Biol Stand 63:133–140, 1986.

73. Ulrich JT, Myers KR. Monophosphoryl lipid A as an adjuvant: past experiences and new directions. Pharm Biotechnol 6:495–524, 1995.

74. Corral RS, Petray PB. CpG DNA as a Th1-promoting adjuvant in immunization against Trypanosoma cruzi. Vaccine 19:234–242, 2000.

75. Gupta RK, Chang AC, Siber GR. Biodegradable polymer microspheres as vaccine adjuvants and delivery systems. Dev Biol Stand 92:63–78, 1998.

76. Morein B, Bengtsson KL. Immunomodulation by iscoms, immune stimulating complexes. Methods 19:94–102, 1999.

77. Wassef NM, Alving CR, Richards RL. Liposomes as carriers for vaccines. Immunomethods 4:217–222, 1994.

78. Jensen FC, Savary JR, Diveley JP, Chang JC. Adjuvant activity of incomplete Freund's adjuvant. Adv Drug Deliv Rev 32:173–186, 1998.

79. Allison AC, Byars NE. Syntex adjuvant formulation. Res Immunol 143:519–525, 1992.

80. Allison AC. Squalene and squalane emulsions as adjuvants. Methods 19:87–93, 1999.

81. Kensil CR. Saponins as vaccine adjuvants. Crit Rev Ther Drug Carrier Syst 13:1–55, 1996.

82. Lederer E. New developments in the field of synthetic muramyl peptides, especially as adjuvants for synthetic vaccines. Drugs Exp Clin Res 12:429–440, 1986.

83. Allison AC. Immunological adjuvants and their modes of action. Arch Immunol Ther Exp (Warsz) 45:141–147, 1997.

84. Payne LG, Jenkins SA, Andrianov A, Roberts BE. Water-soluble phosphazene polymers for parenteral and mucosal vaccine delivery. Pharm Biotechnol 6:473–493, 1995.

85. Johnson AG. Molecular adjuvants and immunomodulators: new approaches to immunization. Clin Microbiol Rev 7:277–289, 1994.

86. Kim JJ, Yang J, Manson KH, Weiner DB. Modulation of antigen-specific cellular immune responses to DNA vaccination in rhesus macaques through the use of IL-2, IFN-gamma, or IL-4 gene adjuvants. Vaccine 19:2496–2505, 2001.

87. Iwasaki A, Stiernholm BJ, Chan AK, et al. Enhanced CTL responses mediated by plasmid DNA immunogens encoding costimulatory molecules and cytokines. J Immunol 158:4591–4601, 1997.

Chapter 7

Vaccine Additives and Manufacturing Residuals in United States– Licensed Vaccines

THERESA M. FINN • WILLIAM EGAN

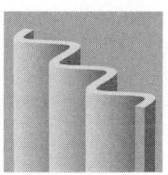

In addition to one or more *immunogens*,* a vaccine contains, or may contain, any of several added substances—for example, an adjuvant or a preservative. Residual components from the manufacturing process also will be present in the vaccine in varying amounts. This chapter addresses the type and amounts of additives that are present in vaccines, the rationale for their inclusion, and the federal regulations that address these additives. Additionally, residual materials from the manufacturing process that are present in the final formulation of the vaccine, as well as relevant federal regulations regarding these residuals, are discussed. Finally, albeit to a limited extent, several issues and concerns that currently pertain to the use of, or presence of, some of these additives and residuals are examined. This chapter focuses on U.S.-licensed vaccines; other, non-U.S.-licensed, vaccines may contain the same types of additives and residuals, although the amounts that may be present in any given vaccine may differ.

For the purposes of this chapter, *additives* refer to those materials that are added to the immunogen by the manufacturer for a specific purpose. Additives include adjuvants, preservatives (i.e., antimicrobial agents), and stabilizers, as well as materials that are added to affect pH and isotonicity. In addition to additives, vaccines will contain residuals that remain from the licensed manufacturing process. The *final formulation* of immunogen plus additives

and residuals defines the specific vaccine. Some information regarding additives and residuals is considered to be trade secret and thus confidential, and cannot be discussed in this chapter.

Vaccine manufacturing includes in-process and release tests, along with their respective specifications, for the allowable quantity of additives and certain residuals that may be present in the vaccine. These tests and accompanying specifications are detailed in the product license; some of these specifications may be provided in the vaccine's package insert. A manufacturer may not remove, change, or adjust the quantity of an additive, or change the manufacturing process, without submitting a license supplement to the FDA describing that change (along with the data supporting the change) and obtaining approval of that change in the licensed vaccine. Food and Drug Administration (FDA) regulations (in Title 21 of the Code of Federal Regulations [21 CFR]) define the use and labeling of preservatives and adjuvants, and these regulations are described, as appropriate, in this chapter. FDA regulations address whether the use of, and quantity of, additives and residuals should be disclosed on the vaccine label (21 CFR § 610.61); specifically,

> The following shall appear on the label affixed to each package containing a product:
> . . .(e) The preservative used and its concentration; . . .
> . . .(l) Known sensitizing substances, or reference to an enclosed circular containing appropriate information;
> (m) The type and calculated amount of antibiotics added during manufacture;
> (n) The inactive ingredients when a safety factor, or reference to an enclosed circular containing appropriate information;
> (o) The adjuvant, if present;
> (p) The source of the product when a factor in safe administration;

---

*An *immunogen* is a preparation consisting of all or a portion of a disease causing organism, or the nucleic acid that encodes one or more of the proteins from that organism, or all or a portion of a human tissue, and is administered to an individual to induce an immune response to the immunogen for the treatment or prevention of a disease or condition.

(q) The identity of each microorganism used in manufacture, and, where applicable, the production medium and method of inactivation

Vaccine Additives

Preservatives

Preservatives are added to vaccine formulations to prevent the growth of bacteria or fungi that inadvertently may be introduced into the vaccine during use. In some cases, preservatives are used during the manufacturing process (e.g., in buffers and column washes) to prevent microbial growth. Improvements in manufacturing technology, however, have decreased this need for the addition of preservatives to control bioburden during the manufacturing process. The CFR requires that, with certain defined exceptions, preservatives must be added to multidose vials of vaccines. Tragic consequences have followed the use of multidose vials that did not contain a preservative and have served, in part, as the impetus for this requirement (for a discussion of a number of the incidents related to the lack of preservatives in vaccines, see Wilson[1]). Specifically, 21 CFR § 610.15(a) states that

> *Products in multiple-dose containers shall contain a preservative, except that a preservative need not be added to Yellow Fever Vaccine; Polio-virus Vaccine Live Oral; viral vaccines labeled for use with the jet injector; dried vaccines when the accompanying diluent contains a preservative; or to an Allergenic Product in 50 percent or more volume in volume (v/v) glycerin.*

This regulation also requires that the preservative used:

> *[S]hall be sufficiently nontoxic so that the amount present in the recommended dose of the product will not be toxic to the recipient, and in the combination used it shall not denature the specific substances in the product to result in a decrease below the minimum acceptable potency within the dating period when stored at the recommended temperature.*

The CFR does not, however, provide a definition of a preservative. A definition of a preservative (antimicrobial effectiveness) that has been used by the FDA for vaccines and other biologicals is found in the U.S. Pharmacopoeia (USP).[2] This is a functional definition wherein the final formulation of the vaccine, including the preservative, is challenged with specified quantities of the following organisms: *Candida albicans, Aspergillus niger, Escherichia coli, Staphylococcus aureus,* and *Pseudomonas aeruginosa.* The test sample (preservative containing vaccine plus the microorganism) is incubated at 20° to 25°C and the number of viable microorganisms is determined on days 7, 14, 21, and 28. A preservative is deemed acceptable if (1) bacteria are reduced to less than 0.1% of the challenge dose by day 14; (2) yeasts and molds remain at or below the level of the initial inoculum on days 7 and 14; and (3) on day 28, the number of organisms is at, or below, the day 14 level. An acceptable preservative therefore must be able to kill more than 99.9% of the added bacteria by day 14 and not permit their subsequent regrowth through day 28 and, additionally, does not permit the growth of yeast and mold over the 28-day test

period. It is important to note that the antimicrobial agent, by itself, is not tested; it is only the final formulation that is tested.

Preservatives cannot completely eliminate the risk of bacterial or fungal contamination of vaccines; moreover, they do not address any potential viral contamination. The scientific literature contains reports[3,4] (see also Wilson[1]) of bacterial contamination of vaccines despite the presence of a preservative, emphasizing the need for meticulous attention to technique in withdrawing vaccines from multiuse vials. At present, only four preservatives are used in U.S.-licensed vaccines: phenol, benzethonium chloride, 2-phenoxyethanol, and thimerosal (termed *thiomersal* in some other countries).

Thimerosal is the most commonly used preservative in vaccines worldwide; however, it is not compatible with all vaccine formulations. For example, it has been known for a number of years that thimerosal has a deleterious effect on the potency of inactivated poliovirus vaccine (IPV).[5,6] (Indeed, it is unlikely that any single preservative will be compatible with all vaccine formulations at the amounts necessary to meet the requirements of the USP antimicrobial effectiveness test—or that of other official pharmacopoeias.) An alternate preservative is necessary for IPV. 2-Phenoxyethanol, a preservative that is used in other products,[7] has been found to be compatible with various IPV vaccine formulations; it is used as a preservative in both of the currently U.S.-licensed vaccines (IPOL® [Aventis Pasteur] and Poliovax® [Aventis Pasteur; Poliovax® is not currently marketed in the Unites States]). Additionally, two of the currently licensed diphtheria and tetanus toxoids and acellular pertussis (DTaP) vaccines, DAPTACEL™ (Aventis Pasteur) and Infanrix® (GlaxoSmithKline), utilize 2-phenoxyethanol as a preservative.

Phenol currently is used in three U.S.-licensed vaccines, the polysaccharide vaccines: Pneumovax® 23 (a 23-valent pneumococcal polysaccharide vaccine from Merck & Co), TYPHIM Vi® (*Salmonella typhi* capsular polysaccharide from Aventis Pasteur); and Dryvax® (the smallpox vaccine from Wyeth); each of these vaccines contains 0.25% phenol as a preservative. According to the National Institutes of Health (NIH) Minimum Requirements, phenolic compounds (such as phenol or the various creosols) are not permitted as preservatives in diphtheria and tetanus toxoid–containing products[8,9] This requirement is also reflected in other regulations or requirements, such as those of the World Health Organization (WHO).[10] It has been reported[11] that phenol damages diphtheria toxoid, "so that its immunizing power falls rapidly." Benzethonium chloride is currently used in only one U.S.-licensed vaccine, Anthrax Vaccine Adsorbed (Biothrax™), manufactured by BioPort.

In recent years, considerable controversy has surrounded the use of thimerosal, an organomercurial, in vaccines. Although allergic responses to thimerosal have been described,[12] a more recent controversy has centered on the hypothesis that exposure to thimerosal, a derivative of ethyl mercury, may be causally linked to autism and other neurodevelopmental disorders in children. The various guidelines for mercury exposure, ranging from 0.1 µg/kg body weight/day[13] to 0.47 µg/kg body weight/day,[14] have been developed based on epidemiologic and laboratory studies of methyl mercury. In 2001, the Immunization Safety Review Committee of the National Academy of Science's Institute of Medicine (IOM) reviewed the issues surrounding thimerosal and vaccines and concluded that the evidence was inadequate to either accept or reject a causal relationship between thimerosal exposure from childhood vaccines and the neurodevelopmental disorders of autism, attention deficit hyperactivity disorder, and speech or language delay. Although the existing scientific data did not establish any causal link between thimerosal exposure and the investigated neurodevelopmental disorders, the IOM nevertheless recommended that thimerosal-containing vaccines not be used in infants.[15] Again, although there are no clear data regarding a potential link between thimerosal and neurodevelopmental disorders, the U.S. Public Health Service (PHS), first in July 1999[16] and again in June 2000,[17] recommended that thimerosal be removed from pediatric vaccines as expeditiously as possible. The July 1999 PHS statement was issued jointly with the American Academy of Pediatrics; the June 2000 PHS statement was issued jointly with the American Academy of Pediatricians, the American Academy of Family Physicians, and the Advisory Committee on Immunization Practices. Letters from the Center for Biologics Evaluation and Research (CBER) of the FDA, in 1999[18] and again in 2000,[19] to the various vaccine manufacturers noted that the removal of thimerosal from vaccines was merited and requested manufacturers' timelines for thimerosal removal or submission of an explanation as to why thimerosal removal was not currently feasible. The European Agency for the Evaluation of Medicinal Products (EMEA) has also noted, as a precautionary measure, "that, although there is no evidence of harm caused by the level of exposure from vaccines, it would be prudent to promote the general use of vaccines without thiomersal and other mercury-containing preservatives."[20]

At present, all of the U.S.-licensed, routinely recommended, pediatric vaccines (hepatitis B, DTaP, *Haemophilus influenzae* type b, IPV, pneumococcal conjugate vaccine, measles-mumps-rubella [MMR], and varicella) that are being manufactured are either thimerosal free or contain only trace amounts of thimerosal (<1 μg of mercury per dose) as a residual from the manufacturing process (Table 7–1). The currently used varicella, MMR, IPV, and pneumococcal conjugate vaccines have always been thimerosal free. Two influenza virus vaccines (Fluvirin® from Evans Vaccine and Fluzone® from Aventis Pasteur) are currently available in presentations that contain only trace amounts of thimerosal (< 1 μg of mercury per dose); both manufacturers simultaneously market formulations that contain thimerosal as a preservative. Finally, a pediatric presentation of the diphtheria and tetanus toxoid vaccine (DT) is available from Aventis Pasteur in a presentation containing only a trace of thimerosal as a manufacturing residual.

Adjuvants

Adjuvants are materials that enhance and direct the immune response. They are discussed in detail in Chapter 6. Vaccine adjuvants are not licensed separately; rather, the adjuvant is a constituent of the licensed vaccine and it is the vaccine formulation, *in toto*, that is tested in clinical trials and is licensed (*vide supra*). As a consequence,

an adjuvant cannot be added or removed or the amount in a licensed vaccine changed without submitting a supplement to the vaccine license and obtaining approval from the FDA. At present, only the various aluminum salts—aluminum hydroxide, aluminum phosphate, alum (potassium aluminum sulfate), or mixed aluminum salts—are utilized in U.S.-licensed vaccines. Despite their worldwide use for over 50 years, surprisingly little is known about the mechanism whereby the aluminum salts function as adjuvants (see, e.g., HogenEsch[21]). There is no *a priori* reason why other vaccine adjuvants could not be used in future U.S.-licensed vaccines; indeed, a number of non–aluminum-based adjuvants are included in various vaccines being studied under the Investigational New Drug process. Data supporting the need for an adjuvant, and the safety of the vaccine containing the new adjuvant, are needed.

The specific aluminum salt (hydroxide, phosphate, sulfate, or mixed) and the quantity of aluminum that is contained in a number of commonly used vaccines are presented in Table 7–1. (The aluminum content that is listed for some vaccines noted in Table 7–1 represents the upper limit of the specification; the vaccine may routinely contain less aluminum.) Currently, live vaccines do not contain an adjuvant. By regulation (21 CFR § 610.15(a)), the aluminum content of a vaccine cannot exceed 0.85 mg of aluminum per dose if the level is assayed, or 1.14 mg/dose if determined by calculation based on the amount of the aluminum compound that is added. To harmonize with WHO recommendations, this regulation was amended in 1981 to permit up to 1.25 mg of aluminum per dose. However, the higher amount was permitted only "provided that data demonstrating that the amount of aluminum used is safe and necessary to produce the intended effect are submitted to and approved by the Director, Center for Biologics Evaluation and Research" (21 CFR § 610.15(a)).

Concerns have been raised in recent years about the use of aluminum in vaccines and potential adverse outcomes that may be associated with its use at the levels that exist in individual vaccines and through the additive effects of multiple vaccinations. These concerns about the use of aluminum in vaccines prompted a workshop that was sponsored by the National Vaccine Program Office (NVPO) in May 2000. The general use of aluminum salts in vaccines[22] and aluminum toxicokinetics[23] were reviewed during the workshop.

A specific safety issue discussed at this workshop was a histologic entity termed *macrophagic myofasciitis* (MMF). MMF has been described in several subjects who received vaccines containing aluminum hydroxide as an adjuvant. It has been hypothesized that the development of this histologic entity may be the result of a persistent vaccination granuloma that serves as a stimulus for the development of a systemic syndrome.[24] MMF as a histologic entity, its association with a clinical syndrome, and its potential relationship to vaccines were discussed at the NVPO workshop.[25] In their overall summary of the workshop, Eickhoff and Meyers[26] noted that, although the MMF histologic lesions are likely caused by aluminum-containing vaccines, the relationship between these lesions and the systemic symptoms of some patients has yet to be established. They also noted that, "Based on 70 years of experience, the use of salts

TABLE 7–1 ■ Preservatives, Adjuvants, and Inactivation Residues Noted in the Labeling of Selected U.S.-Licensed Vaccines

Vaccine	Trade Name[*]	Preservative (amount/dose) and µg Hg/Dose (If Noted)	Adjuvant and Aluminum Content/Dose	Inactivation Residues (Amount/dose If Noted)
		BACTERIAL VACCINES		
Td (adult)	None/API	Thimerosal (50 µg)	Alum [KAl (SO$_4$)$_2$] Al: ≤ 0.28 mg	Formaldehyde (%NN)
	None/MassDPH	Thimerosal (17 µg)	AlPO$_4$ Al: 0.45 mg	Formaldehyde (<0.1 mg)
DTaP	DAPTACEL™	2-Phenoxyethanol (3.3 mg)	AlPO$_4$ Al: 0.33 mg	Formaldehyde (≤0.1 mg) Gluteraldehyde (<50 ng)
	Infanrix®	2-Phenoxyethanol (2.5 mg)	Al(OH)$_3$ Al:≤ 0.625 mg	Formaldehyde (≤0.1 mg) Gluteraldehyde (%NN)
	Tripedia®	Single dose: none Multidose: thimerosal (50 µg) 25 µg Hg	alum: KAl(SO$_4$)$_2$ Al: ≤ 0.170 mg	Formaldehyde (≤0.1 mg)
		VIRAL VACCINES		
Hepatitis A	Havrix® 0.5-mL pediatric dose	2-Phenoxyethanol (2.5 mg)	Al (OH)$_3$ Al: 0.25 mg/dose	Formalin (≤0.05 mg)
	1.0-mL adult dose	2-Phenoxyethanol (5 mg)	Al(OH)$_3$ Al: 0.5 mg/1-mL dose	Formalin (≤0.1 mg/1 mL dose)
	VAQTA® 0.5-mL pediatric dose	None	Al(OH)$_3$ Al: 0.225 mg/dose	Formaldehyde (<0.4 µg)
	1.0-mL adult dose	None	Al(OH)$_3$ Al: 0.45 mg/1-mL dose	Formaldehyde (<0.8 µg/1 mL dose) β-Propiolactone (<LOD)
Influenza	Fluvirin® (2001–2002) (single-dose vial)	None ≤ 0.98 µg Hg (residual from manufacturing)	None	
	FluShield® (2001–2002) (multi-dose vial)	Thimerosal (50 µg) 25 µg Hg	None	Formaldehyde (%NN)
	Fluzone®† (2001–2002) (multi-dose vial)	Thimerosal 25 µg Hg	None	Formaldehyde (%NN)
Japanese encephalitis virus	JE-Vax (1-mL dose)†	Thimerosal (70 µg/1-mL dose)	None	Formaldehyde (<100 µg/1-mL dose)
Polio	Poliovax®†	2-Phenoxyethanol (2.5 mg) and 27 ppm formaldehyde	None	Formaldehyde (27 ppm)
	IPOL®	2-Phenoxyethanol (2.5 mg) and formaldehyde (≤ 100 µg)	None	Formaldehyde ≤ 0.1 mg
Rabies‡	Imovax® (1-mL dose) (lyophilized)	None	None	β-Propiolactone (%NN)
	RabAvert® (1-mL dose) (lyophilized)	None	None	β-Propiolactone (%NN)
	None/BioPort (1-mL dose)	Thimerosal (100 µg/1 mL dose)	≤ 2 mg AlPO$_4$/1 mL dose	β-Propiolactone (%NN)

*Dose is 0.5 mL except where noted.
†Stabilizers used: Fluzone: 0.05% gelatin, 250 µg/mL; JE-Vax: gelatin 0.5 µg/mL dose; Poliovax: human serum albumin, 2.5 mg/dose.
‡Stabilizers used: see Table 7–2.
API, Aventis Pasteur, Inc.; < LOD, below the limit of detection; MassDPH, Massachusetts Department of Public Health Biologic Lab; %NN, amount in final container not noted on labeling.

of aluminum as adjuvants in vaccines has proven safe and effective." However, they also identified the need for more pharmacokinetic and bimetal (mercury and aluminum) toxicologic studies.

Stabilizers

Various "stabilizers" are added to vaccines. Stabilizers are materials that help to protect the vaccine from adverse conditions such as the freeze-drying process (for those vaccines that are freeze-dried) or heat. For freeze-dried (lyophilized) preparations of vaccines, it is additionally necessary to add materials that provide a bulk matrix for the vaccine. The amount of an immunogen that is contained in a vaccine can be extremely small, on the order of tens of micrograms or less. If sufficient amounts of various materials were not added to the vaccine prior to lyophilization, the vaccine would not be readily observable and would undoubtedly adhere to the vial wall. As an illustration of this latter point, ActHIB® (Aventis Pasteur), a polysaccharide conjugate vaccine, contains only approximately 10 µg of purified polysaccharide conjugated to 24 µg of tetanus toxoid. The viral mass for the live viral vaccines is even smaller, just fractions of a microgram per dose (deriving from about 10^3 to 10^5 viral particles per dose). Thus there is a need to provide a matrix for containing these vaccines during freeze-drying.

The types of material that are added to vaccines as stabilizers include sugars (such as sucrose and lactose), amino acids (such as glycine or the monosodium salt of glutamic acid), and proteins (such as human serum albumin [HSA] or gelatin). The stabilizers that are used for a number of common vaccines are listed in Table 7–2.

Added proteins are of concern for two main reasons. The first concern arises from the potential for animal- and human-derived protein to contain one or more adventitious agents. The second concern arises from the potential for animal- or human-derived protein to elicit an allergic reaction in susceptible individuals. The two animal- or human-derived proteins that are used as stabilizers in U.S.-licensed vaccines are HSA and gelatin. The FDA requires that, if HSA is used in vaccine manufacture, only U.S.-licensed HSA may be used. Additionally, an FDA guidance recommends that the following statement appear in the Warnings section of the package insert for HSA-containing products[27]:

> This product contains albumin, a derivative of human blood. Based on effective donor screening and product manufacturing processes, it carries an extremely remote risk for transmission of viral diseases. Although there is a theoretical risk for transmission of Creutzfeldt-Jakob disease (CJD), no cases of transmission of CJD or viral disease have ever been identified that were associated with the use of albumin.

For HSA produced as a recombinant DNA protein, this warning would not be required (because it would not be derived from blood), nor would it be necessary for the albumin to be separately licensed by the FDA.

Gelatin or processed gelatin is also used as a stabilizer. Gelatin may be bovine or porcine derived. Despite the use of a harsh manufacturing procedure (extremes of heat and pH) in the production of gelatin, there is a concern, nonetheless, for the presence of the bovine spongiform encephalopathy (BSE) agent in bovine-derived material.

Thus, any bovine-derived gelatin that is added to vaccines, or used in the vaccine manufacturing process, must be sourced from a non-BSE country (*vide infra*).[28] A second concern for gelatin relates to allergic responses. Allergic responses to gelatin, although rare, have been documented in the literature.[29–31] It has been hypothesized that use of partially hydrolyzed gelatin, which contained a small amount of high-molecular-weight gelatin as a stablizer, contributed to an increase in the incidence of allergic reactions following use of Japanese vaccines stabilized with gelatin.[31,32] Nakayama and Aizawa noted that a change to modified porcine gelatin, together with discontinuation of the use of gelatin-containing DTaP vaccines, may have contributed to a decrease in the incidence of allergic reactions following administration of monovalent measles and mumps vaccine in Japan.[32] An allergic response to gelatin is a contraindication to receiving gelatin-containing vaccines.

Various buffers (e.g., phosphate buffer) are also used in vaccines to maintain a particular pH range, and salts (e.g., NaCl) may be added to achieve isotonicity.

Manufacturing Residuals

In principle, any and all of the materials that are used in the manufacturing process may be present in the final vaccine formulation. For the purposes of this chapter, materials that are present in the final vaccine formulation that derive from the manufacturing process are termed *residuals*. Various steps in the manufacturing process may remove or reduce the amounts of many of these residuals. However, for various vaccines, either an acceptable technology to remove these manufacturing residuals may not exist or there may be no perceived need (safety or potential for an adverse effect on efficacy) for their removal. As a general principle, it is not possible to remove a particular substance completely, nor is it possible to demonstrate that a particular substance has been completely removed. For many substances, the residual amount may be below the limits of detection by current analytic technologies, and may, for practical reasons, be considered "absent."

Bacterial and viral inactivation substances must be noted in the package labeling [21 CFR § 610.61(q)]. Residual bacterial or cellular culture components, such as antibiotics, that are used during manufacture, as well as sensitizing substances (generally proteins) and other inactive ingredients when considered a safety factor, also must be noted in the labeling [21 CFR § 610.61 (l)(m)(n)]. There may be some overlap between these categories; however, they are grouped in this manner for convenience and to aid a discussion of these materials as they are affected by current regulations. Residual bacterial or cell culture components may be included in these categories, but other residuals, such as DNA and endotoxin, are not required to be noted in labeling.

Inactivation Residuals

Various agents may be used to inactivate bacteria and viruses or to detoxify bacterial toxins. As examples, the tetanus and diphtheria toxins are treated with formaldehyde to produce

TABLE 7-2 ■ Vaccine Stabilizers, Manufacturing Residuals, and Cell Lines Noted in Labeling of Selected U.S.-Licensed Vaccines

Vaccine	Trade Name*	Stabilizers per Single Dose	Manufacturing Residuals (Except Inactivating Agents) per Dose	Cell Line
LIVE BACTERIAL VACCINES				
BCG	Mycobax® 0.1-mL adult dose 0.05-mL infant dose	MSG, %NN	NN	N/A
Typhoid	Vivotif Berna® 1 capsule	Sucrose, 26–130 mg Ascorbic acid, 1–5 mg Amino acid mix, 1.4–7 mg Lactose, 100–180 mg Magnesium stearate, 3.6–4.4 mg	NN	N/A
LIVE VIRAL VACCINES				
Measles, mumps, and rubella	M-M-R® II	Sorbitol, 14.5 mg Gelatin, 14.5 mg Sucrose, 1.9 mg HSA, 0.3 mg Phosphate Glutamate	Media components Neomycin, ~25 µg FBS, <1 ppm	Chick embryo cell culture WI-38 cells
Varicella	Varivax®	Sucrose, 25 mg MSG, 0.5 mg Gelatin, 12.5 mg KPO$_4$—monobasic, 0.08 mg NaPO$_4$—dibasic, 0.45 mg	MRC-5 DNA and protein KCl, 0.08 mg NaPO$_4$—monobasic, trace EDTA, trace Neomycin, trace FBS, trace	MRC-5
Yellow fever	YF-Vax®	Gelatin and sorbitol	NN	Chick embyos
INACTIVATED VIRAL VACCINES				
Rabies	Imovax® (1-mL dose)	None	Albumin, <100 mg Neomycin sulfate, <150 µg Phenol red, <20 µg	MRC-5
	RabAvert® (1-mL dose)	Polygeline, <12 mg Potassium glutamate, <1 mg	Na-EDTA, <0.3 mg Ovalbumin, <3 ng, Neomycin, <1 µg Chlortetracycline, <20 ng, Amphotericin B, <2 ng	Chicken fibroblasts
POLYSACCARIDE AND CONJUGATE VACCINES				
Haemophilus b conjugate vaccine	ActHIB®	Sucrose, 42.5 mg	NN	N/A
Meningococcal polysaccaride groups A, C, Y, W-135	Menomune®-A/C/Y/ W-135	Lactose, 2.5–5 mg	NN	N/A

*Dose of 0.5 mL except where noted.

HSA, human serum albumin; MSG, monosodium glutamate; N/A, not applicable (i.e., only applies to viral vaccines); NN = none noted in product labeling; %NN = amount in final container not noted on product labeling.

the diphtheria and tetanus toxoid vaccines; viruses, such as the polio or rabies viruses, may be inactivated (rendered incapable of forming progeny viruses) with formaldehyde or β-propiolactone, respectively, to produce the inactivated viral vaccines. Other inactivating agents, such as glutaraldehyde or hydrogen peroxide, have been used. The goal of these chemical treatments is to inactivate the bacterium or virus or remove a toxin activity while still preserving the antigenicity of the product against the homologous organism or toxin. Following inactivation, a virus or bacterium may be processed further to furnish particular antigens. For example, after inactivation, the influenza viruses are "split" by various chemical treatments (e.g., tri-*n*-butyl phosphate) in order that more purified vaccines can be produced.

Formaldehyde has a long and extensive history of use in the preparation of bacterial and viral vaccines. For example, formaldehyde was used by Ramon in 1923 to detoxify diphtheria—yielding a diphtheria toxoid vaccine termed an *anatoxine* by Ramon.[33] Requirements for the use of formaldehyde and the permitted residual amount of formaldehyde that is allowed for diphtheria toxoid are provided in the NIH Minimum Requirements.[8] Similar NIH Minimum Requirements exist for tetanus toxoid.[9] These documents note that residual-free formaldehyde in the finished product should not be in excess of 0.02% (i.e., 0.1 mg for a 0.5-mL vaccine dose). Formaldehyde also is used to inactivate viruses (e.g., the polio and influenza viruses) when preparing vaccines. The amount of residual formaldehyde that is present or allowed in these and various other U.S.-licensed vaccines is provided in Table 7–1; as for the diphtheria and tetanus toxoids, the amount does not exceed 0.02%.

Inactivating agents other than formaldehyde have been used in various U.S.-licensed vaccines and include glutaraldehyde, which has been used to inactivate pertussis toxin in two acellular pertussis vaccines, DAPTACEL™ and Infanrix®; and β-propiolactone, which has been used in the inactivation of an influenza virus vaccine, Fluvirin® and the three U.S.-licensed rabies vaccines, RabAvert® (Chiron Behring), Imovax® (Aventis Pasteur), and Rabies Vaccine Adsorbed (BioPort) (Rabies Vaccine Adsorbed is not currently available). Hydrogen peroxide is used by North American Vaccines/Baxter to inactivate pertussis toxin for inclusion in their DTaP vaccine, Certiva™ (Certiva™ is no longer marketed in the United States).

A concern has been voiced over the presence of residual formaldehyde in vaccines. This concern stems from the known toxic effects of formaldehyde as well as its carcinogenicity potential. The U.S. Environmental Protection Agency (EPA) has established a Reference Dose (RfD) for formaldehyde through the oral route.[34] The RfD is defined by the EPA as "an estimate (with uncertainty spanning perhaps an order of magnitude) of a daily exposure to the human population (including sensitive subgroups) that is likely to be without an appreciable risk of deleterious effects during a lifetime."[35] The RfD refers to noncancer effects. The RfD for formaldehyde (oral administration) is 0.2 mg/kg of body weight per day.[34] The amount of residual formaldehyde in vaccines, which are administered infrequently, not daily, is below this level.

Formaldehyde has been further classified by the EPA as a "probable human carcinogen of medium carcinogenic haz-

ard" (the EPA's B1 classification).[34] The bulk of the carcinogenicity studies on formaldehyde have focused on chronic respiratory exposure because this is the primary route of industrial and routine household exposure. There are fewer data regarding ingested or parenteral exposure to formaldehyde, and the EPA has not developed a risk estimate for either oral or parenteral exposure.[34] Data regarding carcinogenicity studies may be found in documents from the EPA[34] and the International Agency for Research on Cancer.[36]

One point regarding formaldehyde should be made; formaldehyde is naturally present in the human body as the result of various biochemical processes.[36,37] The steady state level of formaldehyde in the bloodstream of humans is approximately 2.6 mg/L.[38] The amount of formaldehyde that is naturally, continuously present in the blood of humans, or turned over in a particular day, is in excess of the amount that is present as a vaccine residual.

Residual Cell Culture Materials

Antibiotics

The CFR permits the addition of antibiotics (with the exception of penicillin) in viral vaccine manufacture (21 CFR § 610.15 (c)). Antibiotics that have been used include streptomycin, polymyxin B, neomycin, and gentamicin. Although a manufacturer need not specifically test for these antibiotics in the final container, the calculated amount of residual antibiotics (based on dilutions of the amount that was added) must be noted on the packaging carton (21 CFR § 610.61(m)). The amount of residual antibiotics in several U.S.-licensed vaccines can be found in Table 7–2.

Sensitizing Substances

The CFR's labeling regulations (21 CFR § 610.61(l)) provide that "[k]nown sensitizing substances" should be listed on the product label. Further, 21 CFR § 610.15(b) states that "[e]xtraneous protein known to be capable of producing allergenic effects in human subjects shall not be added to a final virus medium of cell culture produced vaccines intended for injection." These regulations address the possibility that animal-derived proteins present in the final formulation of a vaccine can cause allergic reactions in some vaccine recipients. (Other sensitizing substances, such as preservatives and stabilizers, are addressed in other sections of these regulations.) Animal-derived materials are used extensively in vaccine manufacturing—particularly in viral cultures. When viral vaccines are grown in embryonated chicken eggs (influenza and yellow fever vaccines) or chick embryo fibroblast cell culture (measles or mumps virus vaccines), the label will state that residual chicken proteins may be present in the final formulation and, in addition, may state the amount of residual avian proteins in the final formulation (see Table 7–2). The label also will urge caution when vaccinating a person with such known allergies.

The two U.S.-licensed hepatitis B vaccines, Engerix-B® (GlaxoSmithKline) and Recombivax HB® (Merck & Co), are recombinant DNA–derived proteins and are produced in yeast; their package inserts note that residual yeast protein may be present (Engerix-B® contains not more than 5% and Recombivax HB® not more than 1% yeast protein).

Inactive Ingredients

Although the Food, Drug & Cosmetic Act (Sec. 502(e)(1)(A)(iii)) states that all inactive ingredients should be noted in labeling; it also states that this requirement is not necessary if trade secret information would be disclosed. However, the CFR does state that an inactive ingredient should be listed in the labeling if the ingredient's presence is considered a safety factor (21 CFR 610.61(n)). In some cases, even in the absence of any evidence that a particular material might pose a safety factor, manufacturers have elected to disclose the presence of residual materials such as detergents, solvents, and chelating agents (see Table 7–1 for a list of inactive ingredients in vaccines). In addition, many manufacturers will provide a brief summary of manufacturing methods, including the reagents used in various steps, such as precipitation (ammonium sulfate) or bacterial culture (e.g., an antifoam agent such as polydimethylsiloxane). Many of these substances are removed or markedly reduced in subsequent manufacturing steps.

Bacterial and Cellular Residuals

For bacterial vaccines, in addition to the desired antigen(s), manufacturing residuals may include various bacterial cell constituents. Naturally, whole-cell vaccines—such as the previously used whole-cell pertussis vaccine—will contain high levels of these components. At present, no parenteral whole-cell bacterial vaccine is in use in the United States (an oral, live, attenuated bacterial vaccine, Typhoid Vaccine Live Oral Ty21a [Swiss Serum and Vaccine Institute/Berna Products], is in use).

Vaccines derived from gram-negative bacteria may contain lipopolysaccharide (LPS), commonly termed *endotoxin*, a component of the bacterium's outer membrane. Stimulation of the innate immune system by LPS can produce an inflammatory response that can result in fever, shock, and death.[39] There are differences among the LPS structures from different organisms and, consequently, their respective response potential. There are currently two tests that may be used to detect LPS in biological products, the limulus amebocyte lysate (LAL) test and the rabbit pyrogen test. The LAL test is the one that is used most commonly at this time. The lysate from the amebocytes of the horseshoe crab, *Limulus polyphemus*, clots in the presence of LPS and forms the basis for this test.[40,41] The limulus lysate that is used to test for bacterial endotoxin in U.S.-licensed vaccines (and other FDA-regulated biological products) is itself a U.S.-licensed product. Prior to the development and acceptance of the LAL test, manufacturers performed the rabbit pyrogenicity test. The rabbit pyrogenicity test is still an acceptable test for endotoxin. The amount of endotoxin remaining in a final vaccine formulation will be dependent on a number of factors, including the purification steps that are used in vaccine production. Although endotoxin testing of antigens derived from gram-negative bacteria is performed during the manufacturing process, and there may be a release specification for this test, the labeling may not contain this information. Two of the DTaP vaccine labels (those for Infanrix® [GlaxoSmithKline] and Tripedia® [Aventis Pasteur]) include the amount of endotoxin contributed by the inactivated pertussis components (<5 Endotoxin Units/dose and <50 Endotoxin Units/dose, respectively).

Residual bacterial protein may be present in the final vaccine formulation of bacterial vaccines. The consequence of this residual protein can vary; its presence may be neutral or harmful. For example, it has been recognized for many years that the presence of residual protein may contribute to increased reactogenicity of diphtheria toxoid.[42,43] However, it has also been believed that any such protein contributed to the immunogenicity of the vaccine.[44]

Polysaccharide, conjugated polysaccharide, and purified protein vaccines undergo a number of purification steps that reduce the amount of residual bacterial protein. However, these purification steps may not totally eliminate cellular or media protein components. During development of the product, a number of assessments of purity will have been performed—such as silver staining or immunoblot of polyacrylamide gel electrophoresis (PAGE) gels. Following licensure, purity and quality of the vaccine antigen is often assessed by sodium dodecyl sulfate–PAGE as a release test. However, there is a limit to the sensitivity of these methods. This limitation is illustrated in publications of the National Institute of Allergy and Infectious Disease–sponsored multicenter acellular pertussis trial. These publications[45,46] show that some children vaccinated with a fourth and fifth dose of Tripedia® (DTaP; a two-component pertussis vaccine containing PT and FHA), following previous doses of Tripedia or a fourth dose of Tripedia® following a primary series with whole-cell pertussis vaccine, had a booster response to pertactin and fimbriae, suggesting that there was sufficient antigen in Tripedia® to stimulate an immune response.

Cell substrates used in viral vaccine manufacture include two diploid cell strains of human origin (MRC-5 and WI-38); the simian-derived, continuous cell line (Vero cells); the simian-derived diploid cell strain (FRhL cells); and chick embryo and chick embryo fibroblasts. Residual protein from these cell lines will be present to varying degrees in the vaccines produced from them. There is a particular concern, as noted previously, for residual egg proteins in sensitive individuals. The U.S.-licensed Japanese encephalitis vaccine, JE-VAX® (Aventis Pasteur), is produced in mouse brains.

Residual cellular DNA from primary and diploid cells, as well as from bacterial cells, may be present in the final vaccine formulation, and this DNA is not considered to pose any risk. Residual DNA from continuous cell lines, such as Vero cells, has been considered by a WHO study group.[47] The WHO Expert Committee on Biological Standardization assessed the risk of a transformational event as negligible and concluded that levels of up to 10 ng/dose of injected product are acceptable.[47] This limit was a revision of an earlier, more conservative limit (≤ 100 pg per parenteral dose) proposed by the 1986 WHO Expert Committee.[48] In revising this limit, the 1997 Expert Committee considered data from human and animal experience. This included data from nonhuman primates showing that milligram amounts of DNA containing an activated oncogene from human tumor cells had not caused a tumor during 10 years of evaluation; consideration that human blood contains substantial amounts of DNA in plasma, and consideration that contaminating DNA in a biological product would likely be in small fragments unlikely to encode a functional gene.[47] The committee concluded that continuous-cell-line DNA could be considered a contaminant rather than a significant risk factor requiring removal to extremely low levels, hence the revised limit of 10 ng/dose. Manufacturers do not necessarily need to demonstrate that each lot meets this specification through specific testing on each lot; they may be able to validate that the purification process can remove DNA to this level, or below. This limit of 10 ng of residual DNA per dose does not apply to products derived from microorganisms, diploid cell strains, or primary animal cells, or to oral vaccines made with continuous cell lines.[47] At present, the only U.S.-licensed vaccine that is produced in a continuous cell line is IPV (IPOL®); this vaccine is produced in Vero cells and contains less than 10 pg of DNA per dose.[49]

Adventitious Agents

Use of animal-derived materials, such as gelatin, fetal calf serum, or primary animal-derived cells, in vaccine manufacture raises concerns relating to the potential presence of adventitious contaminants. Regulations (21 CFR § 610.18) require that cultures used in the manufacture of products be free from extraneous organisms and that cell lines should be tested for the presence of detectable microbial agents. A 1993 FDA guidance document[50] stated that master cell banks should be tested for adventitious agents and that animal-derived materials should be free from contaminants and adventitious agents, including viruses and the agent of BSE. Manufacturers are required to perform such testing as necessary and to ensure that the certification provided with any raw material is adequate (e.g., documentation that bovine-derived gelatin is not sourced from a BSE-affected or BSE-risk country[28]). Adventitious agent testing is described in detail in U.S.[50] and international[51,52] guidance documents. The use of polymerase chain reaction–based reverse transcriptase assays to test for adventitious retroviruses is addressed in a CBER letter to manufacturers.[53] The testing that has been carried out for adventitious agents is not described in the product labeling. However, the manufacturing method, including the cell lines and culture media that are used, are described.

TRANSMISSIBLE SPONGIFORM ENCEPHALOPATHY AGENTS

The lack of sensitive, specific, or readily accessible premortem diagnostic test for transmissible spongiform encephalopathies (TSEs), such as BSE or CJD, limits surveillance and the ability to test for contamination of products for these agents. Diagnosis of a TSE disease is definitively confirmed by post-mortem examination of brain tissue. However, even this examination is limited in sensitivity because, at earlier stages of disease, the TSE agent may be present in undetectably low concentrations. Because of these limits on testing, potential contamination of animal-derived materials with TSE agents is controlled through restricted sourcing. Manufacturers of U.S.-licensed vaccines are required to ensure that bovine-derived materials are sourced from a country that is not on the U.S. Department of Agriculture (USDA) list of countries that either have BSE or are at risk for BSE. The list of such countries is maintained by the USDA[54] (see 9 CFR § 94.18) and is updated as necessary.

In 2000, it was discovered that some manufacturers of U.S.-licensed vaccines had not followed FDA recommendations with regard to the sourcing of bovine materials from BSE-free countries. A joint session of the FDA's Transmissible Spongiform Encephalopathy Advisory Committee and the Vaccines and Related Biological Products Advisory Committee recommended that, in the future, bovine-derived materials used to make working cell and seed banks and in routine production be replaced with material from the countries not on the USDA list. The committees determined that the risk of contamination of the existing master cell or seed banks was so remote that they did not warrant rederivation. The advisory committees also recommended that the public be informed of affected vaccines. Thus, since December 2000, the CBER has maintained a list of affected vaccines on its Web site.[55]

Summary

A final container vaccine will contain materials in addition to the active immunogen. These materials will include those added by the manufacturer to effect a specific purpose—such as stabilizers and adjuvants. They also include residual materials from the manufacturing process. Although not all of the results of all final release and in-process testing are contained in the labeling that accompanies a product, the CFR does specify which information should be included. Package inserts also contain information on manufacturing methods and growth conditions.

REFERENCES

1. Wilson GS. The Hazards of Immunization. New York, The Athlone Press, 1967, pp 75–84.
2. United States Pharmacopoeia (24th ed). Rockville, MD, United States Pharmacopoeia, 1999, pp 1809–1813.
3. Bernier RH, Frank JA, Nolan TF. Abscesses complicating DTP vaccination. Am J Dis Child 135:826–828, 1981.
4. Simon PA, Chen RT, Elliot JA, Schwartz B. Outbreak of pyogenic abscesses after diphtheria and tetanus toxoids and pertussis vaccine. Pediatr Infect Dis J 12:368–371, 1993.
5. Davisson EO, Powell HM, MacFarlane JO, et al. The preservation of poliomyelitis vaccine with stabilized merthiolate. J Lab Clin Med 47:8–19, 1956.
6. Sawyer LA, McInnis J, Patel A, et al. Deleterious effect of thimerosal on the potency of inactivated poliovirus vaccine. Vaccine 12:851–856, 1994.
7. Poudrier JK. Final report on the safety assessment of phenoxyethanol. J Am Coll Toxicol 9:259–277, 1990.
8. NIH Minimum Requirements: Diphtheria Toxoid (4th rev). Bethesda, MD, National Institutes of Health, March 1, 1947.
9. NIH Minimum Requirements: Tetanus Toxoid (4th rev). Bethesda, MD, National Institutes of Health, December 15, 1952.
10. WHO Expert Committee on Biological Standardization. Requirements for diphtheria, tetanus, pertussis, and combined vaccines. World Health Organ Tech Rep Ser 800, 1990.
11. Barre M, Glenny AT, Pope CG, Lingood FV. Preparation of alum-precipitated toxoid for use as an immunizing agent. Lancet 241:301, 1941.
12. Cox NH, Forsyth A. Thimerosal allergy and vaccination reactions. Contact Dermatitis 18:229–233, 1988.
13. Mahaffey KR, Rice G, Swartout J. An Assessment of Exposure to Mercury in the United States: Mercury Study Report to Congress (Document EPA-452/R097-006). Washington, DC, U.S. Environmental Protection Agency, 1997.
14. World Health Organization. Trace Elements and Human Nutrition and Health. Geneva, World Health Organization, 1996, p 209.
15. Stratton K, Gable A, McCormick MC (eds). Immunization Safety Review: Thimerosal-Containing Vaccines and Neurodevelopmental Disorders. Washington, DC, National Academy Press, 2001.

16. Recommendations regarding the use of vaccines that contain thimerosal as preservative. MMWR 48:996–998, 1999.

17. Notice to readers: summary of the joint statement on thimerosal in vaccines. MMWR 49:622–631, 2000.

18. Center for Biologics Evaluation and Research. Letter to manufacturers regarding plans for continued use of thimerosal as a vaccine preservative, July 1, 1999. Available at *www.fda.gov/cber/ltr/thim070199.htm*

19. Center for Biologics Evaluation and Research. Letter to manufacturers regarding plans for continued use of thimerosal as a vaccine preservative—update, May 31, 2000. Available at *www.fda.gov/cber/ltr/thim053100.htm*

20. EMEA Public Statement on Thiomersal Containing Medicinal Products (Doc Ref EMEA/20962/99). London, European Agency for the Evaluation of Medicinal Products, July 8, 1999.

21. HogenEsch H. Mechanisms of stimulation of the immune response by aluminum adjuvants. Vaccine 20(suppl):S34–S39, 2002.

22. Baylor NW, Egan W, Richman P. Aluminum salts in vaccines—US perspective. Vaccine 20:S18–S23, 2002. (Corrigendum Vaccine 20:3428, 2002)

23. Keith LS, Jones DE, Chou CHJ. Aluminum toxicokinetics regarding infant diet and vaccinations. Vaccine 20(suppl):S13–S17, 2002.

24. Gherardi RK, Coquet M, Cherin P, et al. Macrophagic myofasciitis: an emerging entity. Groupe d'Etudes et Recherche sur les Maladies Musculaires Acquises et Dysimmunitaires (GERMMAD) de l'Association Francaise contre les Myopathies (AFM). Lancet 352:347–352, 1998.

25. Brenner M. Macrophagic myofasciitis: a summary of Dr. Gherardi's presentations. Vaccine 20(suppl):S5–S6, 2002.

26. Eickhoff TC, Myers M. Conference Report. Workshop summary: aluminum in vaccines. Vaccine 20(suppl):S1–S4, 2002.

27. U.S. Food and Drug Administration. Guidance for Industry—Revised preventive measures to reduce the possible risk of transmission of Creutzfeldt-Jakob Disease (CJD) and variant Creutzfeldt-Jakob Disease (vCJD) by blood and blood products, 2002. Available at *www.fda.gov/cber/bse/bse.htm*

28. U.S. Food and Drug Administration. Guidance for Industry—The sourcing and processing of gelatin to reduce the potential risk posed by bovine spongiform encephalopathy (BSE) in FDA-regulated products for human use, 1997. Available at *www.fda.gov/opacom/more-choices/industry/guidance/gelguide.htm*

29. Sakaguchi M, Inouye S. IgE sensitization to gelatin: the probable role of gelatin containing diphtheria-tetanus-acellular pertussis (DTaP) vaccines. Vaccine 18:2055–2058, 2000.

30. Georgitis JW, Fasano MB. Allergenic components of vaccines and avoidance of vaccine-related adverse events. Curr Allergy Rep 1:11–17, 2001.

31. Pool V, Braun MM, Kelso JM, et al and the VAERS Team. Prevalence of anti-gelatin IgE antibodies in people with anaphylaxis after measles-mumps-rubella vaccine in the United States. Pediatrics, 110:e71, 2002; see also *www.pediatrics.org/cgi/contents/full/110/6/e71*

32. Nakayama T, Aizawa C. Change in gelatin content of vaccines associated with reduction in reports of allergic reactions. J Allergy Clin Immunol 106:591–592, 2000.

33. Ramon G. Sur le pouvoir floculant et sur les proprietes immunisants d'une toxine diphtherique rendue anatoxique (anatoxine). C R Acad Sci 177:1338–1340, 1923.

34. U.S. Environmental Protection Agency, Integrated Risk Information System. Formaldehyde (CASRN 50-00-0). Available at *www.epa.gov/iris/subst/0419.htm*

35. U.S. Environmental Protection Agency, Office of Air Quality Planning and Standards. Residual risk: Report to Congress, March 4, 1999 (EPA-453/R-99-001). Available at *www.epa.gov/ttn/oarpg/t3/reports/risk_rep.pdf*

36. IARC Monograph on the Evaluation of Carcinogenic Risks to Humans. Vol. 62. Wood Dust and Formaldehyde. Washington, DC, International Agency for Research on Cancer, 1995.

37. Heck Hd'A, Casanova M, Starr TB. Formaldehyde toxicity—new understanding. CRC Crit Rev Toxicol 20:397–426, 1990.

38. Heck Hd'A, Casanova-Schmitz M, Dodd PB, et al. Formaldehyde (CH₂O) concentrations in the blood of humans and Fischer-344 rats exposed to CH₂O under controlled conditions. Am Ind Hyg Assoc J 46:1–3, 1985.

39. Triantafilou M, Triantafilou K. Lipopolysaccharide recognition: CD14, TLRs and the LPS-activation cluster. Trends Immunol 23:301–304, 2002.

40. William KL. Endotoxins, Pyrogens, LAL Testing, and Depyrogenation (2nd ed). New York, Marcel Dekker, 2001.

41. TenCate JW, Bueller HR, Sturk A, Levin J (eds). Bacterial Endotoxins: Structure, Biomedical Significance, and Detection with the Limulus Amebocyte Lysate Test. New York, Alan R. Liss, 1985.

42. Pappenheimer AM Jr, Lawrence HS. Immunization of adults with diphtheria toxoid II. An analysis of the pseudoreactions to the Schick test. Am J Hyg 47:233–241, 1948

43. Relyveld EH, Bizzini B, Gupta RK. Rational approaches to reduce adverse reactions in man to vaccines containing tetanus and diphtheria toxoids. Vaccine 16:1016–1023, 1998.

44. Holt LB. Developments in Diphtheria Prophylaxis. London, William Heineman Medical Books, 1950.

45. Pichichero ME, deLoria MA, Rennels MB, et al. A safety and immunogenicity comparison of 12 acellular pertussis vaccines and one whole-cell pertussis vaccine given as a fourth dose in 15- to 20-month-old children. Pediatrics 100:772–788, 1997.

46. Pichicero ME, Edwards KM, Anderson EL, et al. Safety and immunogenicity of six acellular pertussis vaccines and one whole-cell pertussis vaccine given as a fifth dose in four- to six-year-old children. Pediatrics 105:E11, 2000.

47. WHO Expert Committee on Biological Standardization. Requirements for the use of animal cells as in vitro substrates for the production of biologicals (Requirements for Biological Substances No. 50). WHO Tech Rep Ser 878, 1998.

48. WHO Expert Committee on Biological Standardization. Requirements for continuous cell lines used for biological production. WHO Tech Rep Ser 745, 1987.

49. Montagnon BJ, Vincent-Falquet JC. Experience with the vero cell line. Dev Biol Stand 93:119–123, 1998.

50. Center for Biologics Evaluation and Research. Points to consider in the characterization of cell lines used to produce biologicals, May 17, 1993. Available at *www.fda.gov/cber/gdlns/ptccells.htm*

51. ICH Harmonized Tripartite Guideline Q5A: Quality of biotechnological products: viral safety evaluation of biotechnology products derived from cell lines of human or animal origin. Fed Reg 63(185):51074 1998.

52. ICH Harmonized Tripartite Guideline Q5D: Derivation and characterization of cell substrates used for production of biotechnological/biological products. Fed Reg 63(182):50244–50249, 1998.

53. Center for Biologics Evaluation and Research. Letter to viral vaccine IND sponsors—use of PCR-based reverse transcriptase assay, December 14, 1998. Available at *www.fda.gov/cber/ltr/viral121498.htm*

54. U.S. Department of Agriculture Veterinary Services National Center for Import-Export Products Program. List of USDA-recognized animal health status of countries/areas regarding specific livestock or poultry diseases, October 2, 2002. Available at *www.aphis.usda.gov/NCIE/country.html*

55. Center for Biologics Evaluation and Research. Bovine spongiform encephalopathy (BSE). Available at *www.fda.gov/cber/bse/bse.htm*

Chapter 8

General Immunization Practices

WILLIAM L. ATKINSON • LARRY K. PICKERING •
JOHN C. WATSON • GEORGES PETER

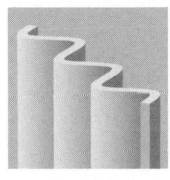 Recommendations for immunization practices are based on scientific knowledge of vaccine characteristics, the principles of immunization, the epidemiology of specific diseases, and host characteristics. In addition, the experience and judgment of public health officials and specialists in clinical and preventive medicine play a key role in developing recommendations that maximize the benefits and minimize the risks and costs associated with immunization. General guidelines for immunization practices are based on evidence and expert opinion of the benefits, costs, and risks of vaccinations as they apply to the current epidemiology of disease and use of vaccines in the United States. However, many of the principles are universal and are applicable to other countries where different public health infrastructures may exist.

Vaccine Storage and Handling

Vaccines must be properly shipped, stored, and handled to avoid loss of their biologic activities. Recommended storage and handling requirements for each vaccine are given in each manufacturer's product label.[1] Correct shipping, storage, and handling practices also are published in the recommendations of the major vaccine policy-making committees, such as the Advisory Committee on Immunization Practices (ACIP) of the United States Public Health Service, the Centers for Disease Control and Prevention and the American Academy of Pediatrics (AAP) (see Chapter 53).[2-5] Failure to adhere to these requirements can result in loss of vaccine potency, leading to an inadequate immune response in the vaccinee. Visible evidence of altered vaccine integrity may not be present. The manufacturer should be contacted when questions arise about the correct handling of a vaccine. New vaccines or new formulations of an existing vaccine may have different shipping, storage, and handling requirements. Table 8–1 gives recommended storage practices for the most commonly used vaccines in the United States.

Exposure to either higher or lower temperatures than recommended can inactivate a vaccine (see Table 8–1). For example, live virus vaccines such as oral poliovirus vaccine (OPV) and varicella are sensitive to temperatures above freezing and should be kept frozen until just before administration. Measles-mumps-rubella (MMR) vaccine and yellow fever vaccine should be kept frozen, although storage below 8°C (46°F) and below 5°C (41°F), respectively, is acceptable.[3,6] However, vaccines composed of purified antigens or inactivated microorganisms, such as hepatitis A, hepatitis B, *Haemophilus influenzae* type b (Hib), and influenza, can lose their potency if frozen and therefore should be kept at 2° to 8°C (36° to 46°F) and never frozen.[3,4] Diluents should not be frozen, and may be kept at room or refrigerator temperature.[3,4] Maintenance of a "cold chain" from vaccine production to use helps ensure vaccine potency at the time of administration. Temperature monitoring and control is important for storage and handling of all vaccines, particularly during transport and field use. Temperatures should be monitored regularly (at least twice a day), preferably using a thermometer that records current, maximum, and minimum temperatures. Whereas maintenance of cold and freezing temperatures is a problem in tropical climates, data suggest that inappropriate freezing of inactivated vaccines is a problem in maintaining vaccine stability in cold and temperate climates.[7] Kendal and associates[7] have suggested methods for packing and shipping vaccines based on tests conducted under representative conditions within the United States. Shipping containers should be sturdy and the correct size for the amount of vaccine to be shipped. Appropriate insulation (e.g., panels and boxes of polystyrene, isocyanurate, or polyurethane) and cold source (e.g., dry ice, gel packs, or bottles with frozen liquid) should be used to maintain the recommended temperature. Loose fillers do not provide reliable temperature insulation.

Vaccines should not be reconstituted until immediately before use. If not administered within the time interval

TABLE 8–1 ■ Recommended Storage Conditions for Commonly Used Vaccines*

Vaccine	Recommended Temperature	Duration of Stability†	Normal Appearance
Diphtheria and tetanus toxoids and acellular pertussis vaccine, adsorbed (DTaP)	2–8°C. Do not freeze. As little as 24 h at <2°C or >25°C may cause antigens to fall from suspension and be difficult to resuspend.	Not more than 18 mo from the time of issue from manufacturer's cold storage	Markedly turbid and whitish suspension. If product contains clumps of material that cannot be resuspended with vigorous shaking, it should *not* be used.
Diphtheria and tetanus toxoids and whole-cell pertussis vaccine, adsorbed (DTP)	2–8°C. Do not freeze. As little as 24 h at <2°C or >25°C may cause antigens to fall from suspension and be difficult to resuspend.	Not more than 18 mo from the time of issue from manufacturer's cold storage	Markedly turbid and whitish suspension. If product contains clumps of material that cannot be resuspended with vigorous shaking, it should *not* be used.
Diphtheria toxoid, adsorbed	2–8°C. Do not freeze.	Not more than 2 yr from the time of issue from manufacturer's cold storage	Turbid and white, slightly gray, or slightly pink suspension
Haemophilus b conjugate vaccine: HbOC (diphtheria CRM$_{197}$ protein conjugate)	2–8°C. Do not freeze.	Not more than 2 yr from date of issue from manufacturer's cold storage	Clear, colorless liquid
Haemophilus b conjugate vaccine: PRP-D (diphtheria toxoid conjugate)	2–8°C. Do not freeze.	Not more than 2 yr from date of issue from manufacturer's cold storage	Clear, colorless liquid
Haemophilus b conjugate vaccine: PRP-OMP (meningococcal protein conjugate)	*Lyophilized formulation:* 2–8°C. Do not freeze formulation or diluent.	Not more than 2 yr from date of issue from manufacturer's cold storage	
	Reconstituted formulation: 2–8°C. Do not freeze.	Discard reconstituted vials if not used within 24 h	*Reconstituted:* after agitation, slightly opaque, white suspension
Haemophilus b conjugate vaccine: PRP-T (tetanus toxoid conjugate)	*Lyophilized formulation:* 2–8°C. Do not freeze formulation or diluent. May be reconstituted with DTP produced by Connaught Laboratories.	Not more than 2 yr from date of issue from manufacturer's cold storage	
	Reconstituted formulation: 2–8°C. Do not freeze.	Vaccine should be used immediately when reconstituted	*Reconstituted:* clear and colorless
Hepatitis A virus vaccine, inactivated	2–8°C. Do not freeze. Do not use if product has been frozen.	2 yr, if kept refrigerated	Opaque, white suspension
Hepatitis B virus vaccine, inactivated (recombinant)	2–8°C. Storage outside this temperature range may reduce potency. Freezing substantially reduces potency.	2 yr from date of issue from manufacturer's cold storage	After thorough agitation, a slightly opaque, white suspension
Influenza virus vaccine (subvirion)	2–8°C. Freezing destroys potency.	Vaccine is recommended only during the year for which it is manufactured; antigenic composition differs annually	Clear, colorless liquid
Measles-mumps-rubella virus (MMR) vaccine, live	*Lyophilized formulation:* 2–8°C, but may be frozen. Protect from light, which may inactivate virus.		*Reconstituted:* clean, yellow solution
	Diluent: store at room temperature or refrigerated, do not freeze.		
	Reconstituted formulation: 2–8°C. Protect from light, which may inactivate virus.	Discard reconstituted vial if not used within 8 h	
Measles virus vaccine, live	See MMR	See MMR	See MMR
Mumps virus vaccine, live	See MMR	See MMR	See MMR
Rubella virus vaccine, live	See MMR	See MMR	See MMR
Pneumococcal conjugate vaccine, polyvalent	2–8°C. Do not freeze.		
Pneumococcal polysaccharide vaccine, polyvalent	2–8°C. Freezing destroys potency.	See expiration date on vial	Clear, colorless, or slightly opalescent liquid

Continued

TABLE 8–1 ■ Recommended Storage Conditions for Commonly Used Vaccines*—cont'd

Vaccine	Recommended Temperature	Duration of Stability†	Normal Appearance
Poliovirus vaccine, inactivated (IPV)	2–8°C. Do not freeze.	Not more than 1 yr from date of issue from manufacturer's cold storage	Clear, colorless suspension. Vaccine that contains particulate matter, develops turbidity, or changes in color should *not* be used.
Poliovirus vaccine, live, oral (OPV)	Must be stored at <0°C. Because of sorbitol in the vaccine, it will remain fluid at temperatures above −14°C. Refreezing the thawed product is acceptable (maximum of 10 thaw–freeze cycles), if the temperature never exceeds 8°C, and the cumulative thawing time is <24 h.	Not more than 1 yr from date of issue from manufacturer's cold storage	Clear solution, usually red or pink, from the phenol red (pH indicator) it contains; may have a yellow color if shipment was packed with dry ice. Color changes that occur during storage or thawing are unimportant, provided the solution remains clear.
Tetanus and diphtheria toxoids, absorbed (DT and Td)	2–8°C. Do not freeze.	Not more than 2 yr from the time of issue from manufacturer's cold storage	Markedly turbid and white suspension. If product contains clumps of material that cannot be resuspended with vigorous shaking, it should *not* be used.
Varicella virus vaccine‡	*Lyophilized formulation:* keep frozen, at temperature of −15°C or colder. Protect from light.	Lyophilized formulation: 18 mo	*Lyophilized formulation:* whitish powder
	Diluent: store at room temperature or refrigerated. *Reconstituted formulation:* use immediately; do not store.	Discard reconstituted vial if not used within 30 min	*Reconstituted formulation:* clear, colorless to pale yellow liquid
	For temporary storage, unreconstituted vaccine may be stored at 2–8°C for a maximum of 72 h.	Discard if not used within 72 h (do not refreeze)	

*For recently licensed combination vaccines, see package inserts; instructions may be different from those for products listed in the table. Also, any changes in the formulation of currently available immunizing agents may alter their appearance, stability, and storage requirements.
†Questions regarding the stability of biologics subjected to potentially harmful environmental conditions should be addressed to the manufacturer of the product in question.
‡For questions concerning stability, contact the manufacturer by calling 1-800-9-VARIVAX.
From American Academy of Pediatrics. Active immunization. *In* Pickering L (ed). 2000 Red Book: Report of the Committee on Infectious Diseases (25th ed). Elk Grove Village, IL, American Academy of Pediatrics, 2000, pp 10–13, with permission.

recommended by the manufacturer, reconstituted vaccine should be discarded.[3] With the exception of OPV, live virus vaccines should not be refrozen after thawing (see Table 8–1). Certain vaccines (e.g., MMR and varicella) also must be protected from light to prevent inactivation of the vaccine virus.

The majority of vaccines have a similar appearance after they are drawn into a syringe. Instances in which the wrong vaccine inadvertently was administered often are attributable to the practice of prefilling syringes or drawing doses of a vaccine into multiple syringes before their immediate need.[5] The routine practice of prefilling syringes should be discouraged because of the potential for such administration errors. To prevent errors, vaccine doses should not be drawn into a syringe until immediately before administration. In certain circumstances where a single vaccine type is used (e.g., in advance of a community influenza vaccination campaign), filling multiple syringes before their immediate use can be considered. Care should be taken to ensure that the cold chain is maintained until the vaccine is administered. When the syringes are filled, the type of vaccine, lot number, and date of filling must be carefully labeled on each syringe, and the doses should be administered as soon as possible after filling.

Certain vaccines are distributed in multidose vials. When opened, the remaining doses from partially used multidose vials can be administered until the expiration date printed on the vial or vaccine packaging, provided that the vial has been stored correctly and that the vaccine is not visibly contaminated.[5]

Administration of Vaccines

Complete and accurate records documenting the administration of all vaccines should be maintained by both health care providers who administer vaccines and vaccine recipients (or their parents). For each immunization, the following information should be recorded: (1) date of vaccination; (2) product administered, manufacturer, lot number, and expiration date; (3) site and route of administration; and (4) name, address, and title of health care provider administering the vaccine.

Infection Control and Sterile Injection Technique

Infection resulting from administration of vaccines is unlikely if appropriate precautions are taken. Hands should be washed with soap and water or cleansed with an alcohol-based waterless antiseptic hand rub before each patient contact to reduce the risk of bacterial contamination and transmission of infection between recipients and health care personnel. In general, the use of protective gloves is not necessary when administering vaccines unless the health care worker will have contact with potentially infectious body fluids or has open lesions on the hands.[2,5]

Failure to follow relevant infection control guidelines can result in transmission of blood-borne pathogens or bacterial infection and abscess formation. Contamination of an injection site can occur from bacteria on the skin at the site of injection. To prevent such contamination, skin at the injection site should be prepared with isopropyl alcohol (70%) or another disinfecting agent and allowed to dry before injection.[8] Transmission of pathogens also can occur if needles, syringes, vaccines, or other equipment used to administer vaccines becomes contaminated. To prevent such contamination, syringes and needles must be sterile. A separate needle and syringe should be used for each injection. Disposable needles and syringes should be discarded after a single use in a labeled, puncture-proof container to prevent inadvertent needle-stick injury or reuse. Because recapping and removing a used needle from a syringe can result in injury to the user, needles should not be recapped after use.[2] The needle and syringe should be discarded as a single unit without removing the needle from the syringe. Single-use disposable needles and syringes should not be sterilized and reused.

If only reusable (i.e., nondisposable) needles and syringes are available, they must be thoroughly cleaned and sterilized after each injection to prevent transmission of blood-borne or other pathogens between patients. Reusable syringes are usually glass rather than plastic. Because of its inert characteristics, glass can be cleaned and sterilized more easily than plastic. Because hypodermic needles enter deep tissues, great care must be taken to ensure that all contaminants are removed from the needle and syringe.[8,9] Liquid germicides alone are insufficient for needle sterilization because of the restricted access of the chemical agent to the narrow lumen of the needle.[9] Strict adherence to the recommended time and temperature for the sterilization procedure used must be observed.[8]

Route of Administration

One or more routes of administration (e.g., intramuscular, subcutaneous, intradermal, intranasal, or oral) are recommended for each vaccine and are listed both in the manufacturer's product label and in published recommendations of immunization advisory committees (Table 8–2).[2,5] These routes usually are determined during prelicensure vaccine studies and are based on vaccine composition and immunogenicity. Vaccines should be administered in sites where they elicit the desired immune response and where the likelihood of local tissue, neural, or vascular injury is minimal.[2] To avoid unnecessary local and systemic adverse events and to ensure the appropriate immune response, persons administering vaccines should not deviate from the recommended route of administration in the product label unless specific data can be cited to justify an alternative route. A route of administration or anatomic site of injection different from that recommended can result in an inadequate immune response. For example, the immunogenicity of hepatitis B vaccine and rabies vaccine is substantially lower when the gluteal instead of the deltoid vaccination site is used.[10,11] The reduced immunogenicity is presumably due to inadvertent injection into subcutaneous or deep fatty tissue rather than muscle.[12,13]

Deep intramuscular injection generally is recommended for adjuvant-containing vaccines because subcutaneous or intradermal administration can cause marked local irritation, induration, skin discoloration, inflammation, and granuloma formation.[2,5] However, subcutaneous injection can lessen the risk of local neurovascular injury and is recommended for vaccines that are less reactogenic and immunogenic when administered by this route, such as live virus vaccines. Intradermal administration is preferred for live bacille Calmette-Guérin (BCG) vaccine.[14]

Although some persons experienced in administering vaccines advocate aspiration (i.e., the syringe plunger is pulled back before injection), particularly before intramuscular injection, no data exist to document the necessity for this procedure. If the person administering the vaccine prefers to aspirate prior to injection, and if aspiration results in blood in the needle hub, the needle should be withdrawn and a new site should be selected.

Subcutaneous Injections

Vaccines recommended for subcutaneous injection usually are administered into the thigh of infants less than 12 months old and the upper, outer triceps area of persons 12 months of age and older. Subcutaneous injections also can be administered into the upper, outer triceps area of an infant, if necessary. A 5/8-inch, 23- to 25-gauge needle is recommended in most situations.[2,5] The needle is inserted into the tissues below the dermal layer of the skin. To avoid administering the vaccine into a muscle, the skin and subcutaneous tissue should be held gently between the thumb and fingers to raise these tissues from the muscle layer. The needle is inserted into the resulting skinfold at an approximately 45-degree angle.[2]

Intramuscular Injections

Selection of the site of injection and needle size is based on the volume of vaccine to be administered, the thickness of the overlying subcutaneous tissue, the size of the muscle, and the desired depth below the muscle surface into which the material is to be injected. For most intramuscular injections, the quadriceps muscle mass in the anterolateral aspect of the upper thigh and the deltoid muscle of the upper arm are the preferred vaccination sites.[2,5]

The quadriceps muscle mass in the anterolateral thigh is most commonly used for intramuscular injection in infants,

TABLE 8–2 ■ Licensed Vaccines and Toxoids Available in the United States, by Type and Recommended Routes of Administration

Vaccine	Type	Route
Anthrax	Inactivated bacteria	Subcutaneous
BCG (bacille Calmette-Guérin)	Live bacteria	Percutaneous (intradermal)
Diphtheria-tetanus-pertussis (DTP)	Toxoids; inactivated whole bacteria	Intramuscular
Diphtheria–tetanus–acellular pertussis (DTaP)	Toxoids; inactivated bacterial components	Intramuscular
Hepatitis A	Inactivated virus	Intramuscular
Hepatitis B	Recombinant viral antigen	Intramuscular
DTaP-Hepatitis B-IPV	Toxoids; inactivated bacterial components; recombinant viral antigen; inactivated virus	Intramuscular
Hepatitis A-hepatitis B	Inactivated virus; recombinant viral antigen	Intramuscular
Haemophilus influenzae type b conjugate (Hib)	Bacterial polysaccharide conjugated to protein	Intramuscular
Hib-DTaP	Bacterial polysaccharide conjugated to protein; toxoids; inactivated bacterial components	Intramuscular
Hib–hepatitis B	Bacterial polysaccharide conjugated to protein; recombinant viral antigen	Intramuscular
Influenza	Inactivated viral components	Intramuscular
Japanese encephalitis	Inactivated virus	Subcutaneous
Measles	Live virus	Subcutaneous
Measles-mumps-rubella (MMR)	Live virus	Subcutaneous
Meningococcal	Bacterial polysaccharide (serotypes A/C/Y/W-135)	Subcutaneous
Mumps	Live virus	Subcutaneous
Pneumococcal conjugate	Bacterial polysaccharide conjugated to protein	Intramuscular
Pneumococcal polysaccharide	Bacterial polysaccharide (23 serotypes)	Intramuscular; subcutaneous
Poliovirus, inactivated (IPV)	Inactivated virus	Subcutaneous
Poliovirus, oral (OPV)	Live virus	Oral
Rabies	Inactivated virus	Intramuscular
Rubella	Live virus	Subcutaneous
Tetanus	Toxoid (inactivated toxin)	Intramuscular
Tetanus-diphtheria (Td or DT)*	Toxoids (inactivated toxins)	Intramuscular
Typhoid		
Live oral/Ty21a	Live bacteria	Oral
Vi polysaccharide	Capsular polysaccharide	Intramuscular
Vaccinia (small pox)	Live virus	Intradermal (scarification)
Varicella	Live virus	Subcutaneous
Yellow fever	Live virus	Subcutaneous

*Td, tetanus and diphtheria toxoids for use in persons 7 years of age and older; DT, tetanus and diphtheria toxoids for use in children younger than 7 years.

whereas the deltoid muscle of the upper arm is the usual recommended site for older children and adults.[12] After a child begins to walk, the upper arm is the preferred site.[12,15] By this age, the child's deltoid muscle is usually large enough to be used for intramuscular injection. Although the anterolateral thigh is also an acceptable site, intramuscular injection into the thighs of 18-month-old children has been reported to cause transient limping.[12,16,17]

Because of the potential risk of injury to the sciatic nerve, the gluteal region is not recommended for routine vaccination.[2,5,18] This recommendation is based primarily on reported cases of sciatic nerve injury resulting from injection of antibiotics or antiserum into the gluteus.[12,19-24] No reports of direct nerve injury resulting from gluteal injection of current childhood vaccines have been published.[25-27]

When injections are given in the gluteal site, care must be taken to avoid nerve injury. The central region of the buttocks should be avoided. The needle should be inserted into the upper, outer quadrant and directed anteriorly (i.e., not caudally or perpendicular to the skin surface). The ventrogluteal site (i.e., the center of the triangle bounded by the

anterior superior iliac spine, the tubercle of the iliac crest, and the upper border of the greater trochanter of the femur) can also be used and is free of major neurovascular structures.[12] Because of the large volume that must be injected and the large muscle mass, the gluteal site often is used for passive immunization with immune globulin preparations.[2,18]

A 22- to 25-gauge needle is appropriate for intramuscular administration of most vaccines. The ideal needle length may depend on the vaccination technique.[28] One technique for intramuscular injections consists of gently bunching the muscle in the free hand while the needle is inserted perpendicular to the skin.[28] A second technique consists of using the thumb and index finger to stretch the skin flat over the injection site while inserting the needle perpendicular to the skin and injecting the vaccine.[28,29]

The subcutaneous tissue and muscle layer thickness of the anterolateral thigh and deltoid region have been determined by ultrasonography.[28,30,31] On the basis of the resulting data, a 5/8-inch (16-mm) needle used according to the second technique described above is estimated to be adequate for intramuscular injection in the thigh of infants and toddlers and in the deltoid of toddlers.[28] However, using the "bunching" technique described above, a 7/8- to 1-inch (22- to 25-mm) needle would be necessary for adequate intramuscular penetration of the thigh of a 4-month-old infant and of the thigh and deltoid of toddlers and older children.[2,5,28,30]

For adolescents and adults, the ideal needle length for intramuscular injection depends on the weight and sex of the vaccinee. Poland et al.[31] reported that women have a greater deltoid fat pad thickness by ultrasonography and a greater deltoid skinfold thickness than men of an equal body mass index. These authors recommended a 1-inch (25-mm) needle for men for all weight ranges studied (e.g., 59 to 118 kg); a 5/8-inch (16-mm) needle is indicated for women weighing less than 60 kg, a 1-inch (25-mm) needle is sufficient for women weighing 60 to 90 kg, and a 1½-inch (38-mm) needle is recommended for women weighing more than 90 kg. The ACIP recommends a 1- to 1½-inch needle for all persons 18 years of age or older.[5]

BLEEDING DISORDERS

Persons with bleeding disorders such as hemophilia and persons receiving anticoagulant therapy can be at increased risk for bleeding after intramuscular injection. When vaccines recommended for intramuscular injection are indicated, vaccination can be scheduled shortly after administration of clotting factor replacement or similar therapy.[5] A 23-gauge or smaller needle can be used, and firm pressure without rubbing should be applied to the injection site for several minutes.[32] Alternatively, vaccines recommended for intramuscular injection could be administered subcutaneously to persons with a bleeding disorder if the immune response and clinical reaction to these vaccines are expected to be comparable by either route of injection.[2] An example is Hib conjugate vaccine.[33–35]

Intradermal Injections

The deltoid region of the upper arm or the volar surface of the forearm is used for most intradermal injections.[2,5,18] A 3/8- to 3/4-inch, 25- to 27-gauge needle is recommended. The needle is inserted into the epidermis at an angle parallel to the long axis of the forearm. Care should be taken that the needle is inserted such that the entire bevel penetrates the skin and the injected solution raises a small bleb, thus demonstrating intradermal rather than subcutaneous injection of the vaccine. Because the amount of injected antigen is small, inadvertent subcutaneous injection may result in a suboptimal immunologic response.[2,5,18] BCG vaccine usually is administered near the middle of the upper arm, over the insertion of the deltoid muscle.[36]

Smallpox (vaccinia) vaccine is administered by the intradermal route using multiple punctures with a unique bifurcated needle held perpendicular to the skin (see Chapter 9). A successful vaccination results in a pustular lesion ("Jennerian pustule") at the vaccination site 6 to 8 days after primary vaccination. The skin reaction following revaccination may be less pronounced, with more rapid progression and healing, than that after primary vaccination.[37,38]

Oral Administration

For vaccines given orally, the vaccine must be swallowed and retained. If a patient spits out, fails to swallow, or regurgitates a vaccine immediately after administration, the dose should be repeated.[2,39] Vomiting within 10 minutes is also a reason to readminister the dose of vaccine. If a second dose of the vaccine also is not retained, the dose should be readministered at a later date.[2,5,39]

Needle-Shielding/Needle-Free Devices

Blood-borne diseases (e.g., hepatitis B and C and human immunodeficiency virus [HIV]) are occupational hazards for health care workers. In November 2000, to reduce the incidence of needle-stick injuries among health care workers and the consequent risk for blood-borne diseases acquired from patients, the Needlestick Safety and Prevention Act was signed into law in the United States. The act directs the U.S. Occupational Safety and Health Administration (OSHA) to strengthen its existing blood-borne pathogen standards. Those standards were revised and became effective in April 2001.[40] These federal regulations require the use of safer injection devices, such as needle-shielding devices or needle-free injectors, for parenteral vaccination in all clinical settings when such devices are appropriate, commercially available, and capable of achieving the intended clinical purpose. The rules also require that records be kept documenting the occurrence of injuries caused by medical sharps (except in workplaces with fewer than 10 employees) and that nonmanagerial employees be involved in the evaluation and selection of safer devices to be procured.

Needle-shielding or needle-free devices that might satisfy the occupational safety regulations for administering parenteral injections are available in the United States and are listed at multiple websites.[41–44] Additional information regarding implementation and enforcement of these regulations is available at the OSHA website at *www.osha-slc.gov/needlesticks*.

Jet Injectors

Jet injectors (JIs) are needle-free devices that drive liquid medication through a nozzle orifice, creating a narrow stream under high pressure that penetrates skin to deliver a drug or vaccine into intradermal, subcutaneous, or intramuscular tissues.[45,46] Increasing attention to JI technology as an alternative to conventional needle injection has resulted from efforts to reduce the frequency of needle-stick injuries to health care workers[40] and to overcome the improper reuse and other drawbacks of needles and syringes in economically developing countries.[41,47,48] JIs have been reported safe and effective in administering different live and inactivated vaccines for viral and bacterial diseases.[41] The immune responses generated are usually equivalent to, and occasionally greater than, those induced by needle injection. However, local reactions or injury, such as redness, induration, pain, blood, and ecchymosis at the injection site, can be more frequent for vaccines delivered by JIs compared with needle injection.[41,46] Multiple-use nozzle JIs have been used most frequently during mass vaccination campaigns and by the military to vaccinate large numbers of persons in a short interval.[49–52]

The multiple-use nozzle of some JIs can become contaminated with blood or other infectious agents during use, which could result in person-to-person transmission of blood-borne pathogens.[53–56] The multiple-use nozzle JI that has been used most widely in the United States (Ped-O-Jet; Keystone Industries, Cherry Hill, NJ) has not been implicated in such transmission of blood-borne pathogens.[57,58] However, an outbreak of hepatitis B attributed to noncompliant use of another multiple-use nozzle JI produced in the United States has been reported.[59,60]

The potential risk of disease transmission associated with multiple-use nozzle JIs is greatest when vaccinating groups or populations in which the prevalence of hepatitis B virus, HIV, or other blood-borne pathogens is likely to be high because of behavioral or other risk factors.[61,62] Brito et al.[62] estimated the theoretical risk of patient-to-patient transmission of hepatitis B virus from use of a contaminated JI to be as high as 1 in 388 to 1 in 3367 injections in a population with a prevalence of chronic carriage of hepatitis B virus as high as 15%.

The potential risk of disease transmission can be minimized by effective training of health care workers on the proper care and use of JIs and, if contamination with blood or other body fluid is evident, by changing the injector tip or removing the JI from use until the nozzle is properly sterilized. Swabbing the injector nozzle tip with alcohol or acetone between injections is recommended to reduce the risk of blood-borne disease transmission.[63] However, results from one in vitro study of transmission of hepatitis B surface antigen (HBsAg) suggested that mechanical cleaning of a contaminated JI tip with a cotton ball moistened with acetone may reduce but not eliminate the potential risk of blood-borne disease transmission.[60]

Despite the potential risks, multiple-use nozzle JIs may be helpful for the rapid vaccination of large numbers of persons with the same vaccine when the use of needles and syringes is not practical. Public health authorities must assess whether the public health benefit from using a JI outweighs any potential risk of blood-borne disease transmission.[5] Because of the risks, the World Health Organization no longer encourages the use of multiple-use nozzle JIs for mass vaccination campaigns.[64]

Unlike multiple-use nozzle JIs, those that employ a single-use disposable nozzle reduce the potential risk of blood-borne disease transmission both from vaccinee to vaccinee and from vaccinee to the person administering vaccine.[46,64,65]

Alleviation of Pain and Discomfort Associated with Vaccination

Several methods have been reported to reduce the pain and discomfort associated with vaccination injection, but they have not been tested widely.[46] Pretreatment with topical lidocaine-prilocaine emulsion cream or patch can decrease the pain of diphtheria and tetanus toxoids and pertussis (DTP) vaccination among infants by causing superficial anesthesia.[66–68] Preliminary evidence indicates that this product does not interfere with the immune response to MMR.[67] This cream is not approved by the U.S. Food and Drug Administration for use in infants younger than 1 month of age or in infants younger than 12 months of age who are receiving treatment with methemoglobin-inducing agents because of a lack of safety data in neonates and concern about possible development of methemoglobinemia.[66,69] Acquired methemoglobinemia is induced by oxidizing agents, particularly chlorates and inorganic and organic nitrites, or by exposure to certain drugs or their metabolites.[70]

Acetaminophen often is given to children to reduce the discomfort and fever associated with vaccination.[71] However, acetaminophen can cause formation of methemoglobin and, thus, may interact with lidocaine-prilocaine cream if given concurrently.[66] Ibuprofen or another nonsteroidal analgesic can be used, if necessary.

A topical refrigerant spray can reduce the short-term pain associated with injections and can be as effective as lidocaine-prilocaine cream.[72–74] Oral administration of sweet-tasting fluid just before injection may cause a calming or analgesic effect in some infants.[75] Distraction techniques such as listening to music or "blowing away pain" also may help children cope with the discomfort associated with vaccination.[76,77]

The Z-track method of injection also may decrease the pain associated with intramuscular injection.[2] Traction is applied to the skin and subcutaneous tissues prior to insertion of the needle and is released after injection.

Ages for Administration of Immunobiologics

Recommendations for the age and timing of vaccination are based on multiple considerations and may vary in different countries. Optimal response to a vaccine depends on a number of factors, including the nature of the vaccine and the age and immune status of the recipient. Recommendations for the age at which vaccines are administered are influenced by age-specific risks for disease, age-specific risks for complications, ability of persons of a certain age to respond to the vaccine, and potential interference with the immune response by passively transferred maternal antibody or previously administered antibody-containing blood products. Vaccines are usually recommended for members of the youngest age group at risk for experiencing the disease for whom efficacy and safety have been demonstrated. These principles are exemplified by the following examples.

The optimal timing for administration of measles vaccine depends on both the rate of disappearance of passively acquired maternal antibody and the risk of exposure to measles virus. At birth and in the first 6 months of life, most infants have passive immunity to measles because of transplacentally acquired maternal measles antibodies. These antibodies interfere with the immune response to live virus measles vaccine by limiting vaccine virus replication. In many developing countries, where measles is highly endemic and frequently affects infants, routine measles vaccination is recommended at age 9 months[78] (see Chapter 55). However, in the United States, where measles is less common and usually does not occur in infants, measles vaccine is recommended routinely at age 12 to 15 months.[2,79]

Another example is the recommended age of pertussis vaccination. Early infancy is the time of greatest risk of serious complications from naturally occurring pertussis, but infants who are younger than 1 month do not respond as well immunologically to pertussis vaccine as older infants do.[80-83] Initiation of routine immunization with pertussis vaccine is recommended at age 2 months.[84,85] This scheduling represents a compromise between factors affecting the immune response and the epidemiology of the disease necessitating early protection against pertussis.[82,86,87]

Vaccination too early in life also may affect the immune response to subsequent doses of vaccine. For example, neonatal administration of diphtheria and tetanus toxoids (DT) may result in suppression of antibody responses to subsequent doses of Hib conjugate vaccines covalently linked to forms of those toxoids.[88] When children who receive measles vaccine before the age of 1 year are revaccinated, they develop vaccine-induced immunity against disease but may have a somewhat diminished antibody response compared with children vaccinated initially after their first birthday.[89,90]

The recommended routine childhood immunization schedule for infants, children, and adolescents for the United States is revised annually, and is approved by the ACIP, the AAP, and the American Academy of Family Physicians. A vaccine schedule for adults is now available for routine use as well as for immunocompromised and high-risk persons.[91] Recent U.S. vaccination schedules are given in Figures 8-1 and 8-2.[92,93] The most current vaccination schedules are available from the National Immunization Program of the Centers for Disease Control and Prevention website at *www.cdc.gov/nip*. The recommended and minimum ages and recommended and minimum acceptable intervals between doses of vaccines commonly used in the United States are listed in Table 8-3. Other vaccination schedules are discussed in Chapters 53 through 55.

Spacing of Vaccine Doses

Spacing of Multiple Doses of the Same Vaccine

Although administration of one dose of some vaccines may induce a protective antibody response, most vaccines require administration of multiple doses in a primary series for development of immunity. Examples of the former are rubella, yellow fever, and hepatitis A vaccines; examples of the latter are poliovirus, hepatitis B, and pertussis vaccines. In addition, periodic revaccination ("booster doses") with certain vaccines may be necessary to maintain immunity. Examples are typhoid vaccines and tetanus and diphtheria toxoids.

Because of immunologic memory, longer than routinely recommended intervals between doses do not impair the immunologic response to live and inactivated vaccines that require more than one dose to achieve primary immunity. Similarly, delayed administration of recommended booster doses does not adversely affect the antibody response to such doses.[2,5] Thus the interruption of a recommended primary series or an extended lapse between booster doses does not necessitate re-initiation of the entire vaccination series. For example, lengthening the interval between two doses of inactivated poliovirus vaccine (IPV) may increase the antibody response to the second dose.[94,95] In the case of oral typhoid (Ty21a) vaccine, an exception has been proposed. Specifically, if the primary vaccination series is interrupted for longer than 3 weeks, the primary series should be started again (see Chapter 39). A practical question arises when a person fails to complete the full course of immunization with 3-4 doses of Ty21a. Does one need to simply complete the number of doses or must one complete the full schedule? A definitive answer is not available. However, as a rule of thumb, if less than three weeks have passed since the last dose, one may continue to complete the immunization with the missing doses. If more than three weeks have passed, the full series of this well-tolerated vaccine should be administered.

Vaccination providers should strive to adhere as closely as possible to recommended childhood immunization schedules. Clinical studies confirm that recommended ages and intervals between doses of multidose antigens provide optimal protection or have the best evidence of efficacy. Table 8-3 lists recommended intervals between doses of commonly used vaccines.

In certain circumstances, administering doses of a multidose vaccine at shorter than the recommended intervals might be necessary. Examples include when a person is behind schedule and needs to be brought up-to-date as quickly as possible, or in cases of impending international travel. In these situations, an accelerated schedule with intervals between doses shorter than those recommended for routine vaccination can be used. Although the effectiveness of all accelerated schedules has not been evaluated in clinical trials, immune responses with accelerated intervals are likely to induce adequate protection.[5] Accelerated, or minimum, intervals and ages that can be used for scheduling catch-up vaccinations are listed in Table 8-3.

Vaccine doses generally should not be administered at intervals less than these minimum intervals or earlier than the minimum age. Administration of doses of a vaccine at intervals less than the minimum intervals or earlier than the minimum age may result in a reduced immune response with diminished vaccine efficacy and should be avoided.[2,5] Multiple doses of some live vaccines are recommended to stimulate an immune response to different types of the same virus, such as poliovirus types 1, 2, and 3, or to induce immunity in persons who failed to mount an immune response to an earlier dose of vaccine, such as measles.[39,79] These multiple doses constitute a primary vaccination series and are not "booster doses."

Spacing of Different Vaccines

Guidelines for spacing the administration of different vaccines are given in Table 8-4. Inactivated vaccines do not interfere with the immune response to other inactivated vaccines or to live vaccines. An inactivated vaccine can be administered either simultaneously or at any time before or after a different inactivated vaccine or live vaccine.

The possibility that two doses of the same or different live virus vaccines administered within too short an interval

Recommended Childhood and Adolescent Immunization Schedule -- United States, 2003

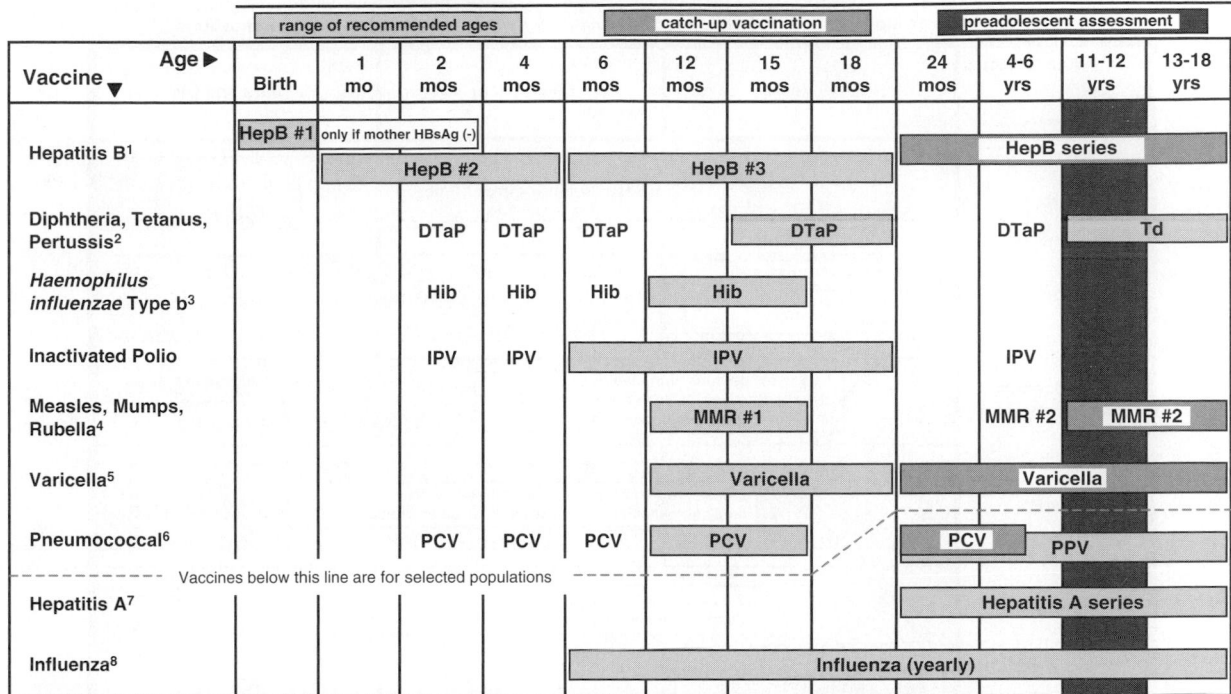

This schedule indicates the recommended ages for routine administration of currently licensed childhood vaccines, as of December 1, 2002, for children through age 18 years. Any dose not given at the recommended age should be given at any subsequent visit when indicated and feasible. ▢ Indicates age groups that warrant special effort to administer those vaccines not previously given. Additional vaccines may be licensed and recommended during the year. Licensed combination vaccines may be used whenever any components of the combination are indicated and the vaccine's other components are not contraindicated. Providers should consult the manufacturers' package inserts for detailed recommendations.

1. Hepatitis B vaccine (HepB). All infants should receive the first dose of hepatitis B vaccine soon after birth and before hospital discharge; the first dose may also be given by age 2 months if the infant's mother is HBsAg-negative. Only monovalent HepB can be used for the birth dose. Monovalent or combination vaccine containing HepB may be used to complete the series. Four doses of vaccine may be administered when a birth dose is given. The second dose should be given at least 4 weeks after the first dose, except for combination vaccines which cannot be administered before age 6 weeks. The third dose should be given at least 16 weeks after the first dose and at least 8 weeks after the second dose. The last dose in the vaccination series (third or fourth dose) should not be administered before age 6 months.

Infants born to HBsAg-positive mothers should receive HepB and 0.5 mL Hepatitis B Immune Globulin (HBIG) within 12 hours of birth at separate sites. The second dose is recommended at age 1-2 months. The last dose in the vaccination series should not be administered before age 6 months. These infants should be tested for HBsAg and anti-HBs at 9-15 months of age.

Infants born to mothers whose HBsAg status is unknown should receive the first dose of the HepB series within 12 hours of birth. Maternal blood should be drawn as soon as possible to determine the mother's HBsAg status; if the HBsAg test is positive, the infant should receive HBIG as soon as possible (no later than age 1 week). The second dose is recommended at age 1-2 months. The last dose in the vaccination series should not be administered before age 6 months.

2. Diphtheria and tetanus toxoids and acellular pertussis vaccine (DTaP). The fourth dose of DTaP may be administered as early as age 12 months, provided 6 months have elapsed since the third dose and the child is unlikely to return at age 15-18 months. **Tetanus and diphtheria toxoids (Td)** is recommended at age 11-12 years if at least 5 years have elapsed since the last dose of tetanus and diphtheria toxoid-containing vaccine. Subsequent routine Td boosters are recommended every 10 years.

3. Haemophilus influenzae type b (Hib) conjugate vaccine. Three Hib conjugate vaccines are licensed for infant use. If PRP-OMP (PedvaxHIB® or ComVax® [Merck]) is administered at ages 2 and 4 months, a dose at age 6 months is not required. DTaP/Hib combination products should not be used for primary immunization in infants at ages 2, 4 or 6 months, but can be used as boosters following any Hib vaccine.

4. Measles, mumps, and rubella vaccine (MMR). The second dose of MMR is recommended routinely at age 4-6 years but may be administered during any visit, provided at least 4 weeks have elapsed since the first dose and that both doses are administered beginning at or after age 12 months. Those who have not previously received the second dose should complete the schedule by the 11-12 year old visit.

5. Varicella vaccine. Varicella vaccine is recommended at any visit at or after age 12 months for susceptible children, i.e. those who lack a reliable history of chickenpox. Susceptible persons aged ≥13 years should receive two doses, given at least 4 weeks apart.

6. Pneumococcal vaccine. The heptavalent **pneumococcal conjugate vaccine (PCV)** is recommended for all children age 2-23 months. It is also recommended for certain children age 24-59 months. **Pneumococcal polysaccharide vaccine (PPV)** is recommended in addition to PCV for certain high-risk groups. See MMWR 2000;49(RR-9);1-38.

7. Hepatitis A vaccine. Hepatitis A vaccine is recommended for children and adolescents in selected states and regions, and for certain high-risk groups; consult your local public health authority. Children and adolescents in these states, regions, and high risk groups who have not been immunized against hepatitis A can begin the hepatitis A vaccination series during any visit. The two doses in the series should be administered at least 6 months apart. See MMWR 1999;48(RR-12);1-37.

8. Influenza vaccine. Influenza vaccine is recommended annually for children age ≥6 months with certain risk factors (including but not limited to asthma, cardiac disease, sickle cell disease, HIV, diabetes, and household members of persons in groups at high risk; see MMWR 2002;51(RR-3);1-31), and can be administered to all others wishing to obtain immunity. In addition, healthy children age 6-23 months are encouraged to receive influenza vaccine if feasible because children in this age group are at substantially increased risk for influenza-related hospitalizations. Children aged ≤12 years should receive vaccine in a dosage appropriate for their age (0.25 mL if age 6-35 months or 0.5 mL if aged ≥3 years). Children aged ≤8 years who are receiving influenza vaccine for the first time should receive two doses separated by at least 4 weeks.

For additional information about vaccines, including precautions and contraindications for immunization and vaccine shortages, please visit the National Immunization Program Website at www.cdc.gov/nip or call the National Immunization Information Hotline at 800-232-2522 (English) or 800-232-0233 (Spanish).

Approved by the Advisory Committee on Immunization Practices (www.cdc.gov/nip/acip),the American Academy of Pediatrics (www.aap.org), and the American Academy of Family Physicians (www.aafp.org).

FIGURE 8-1 ▪ Recommended childhood immunization schedule, United States, 2002.

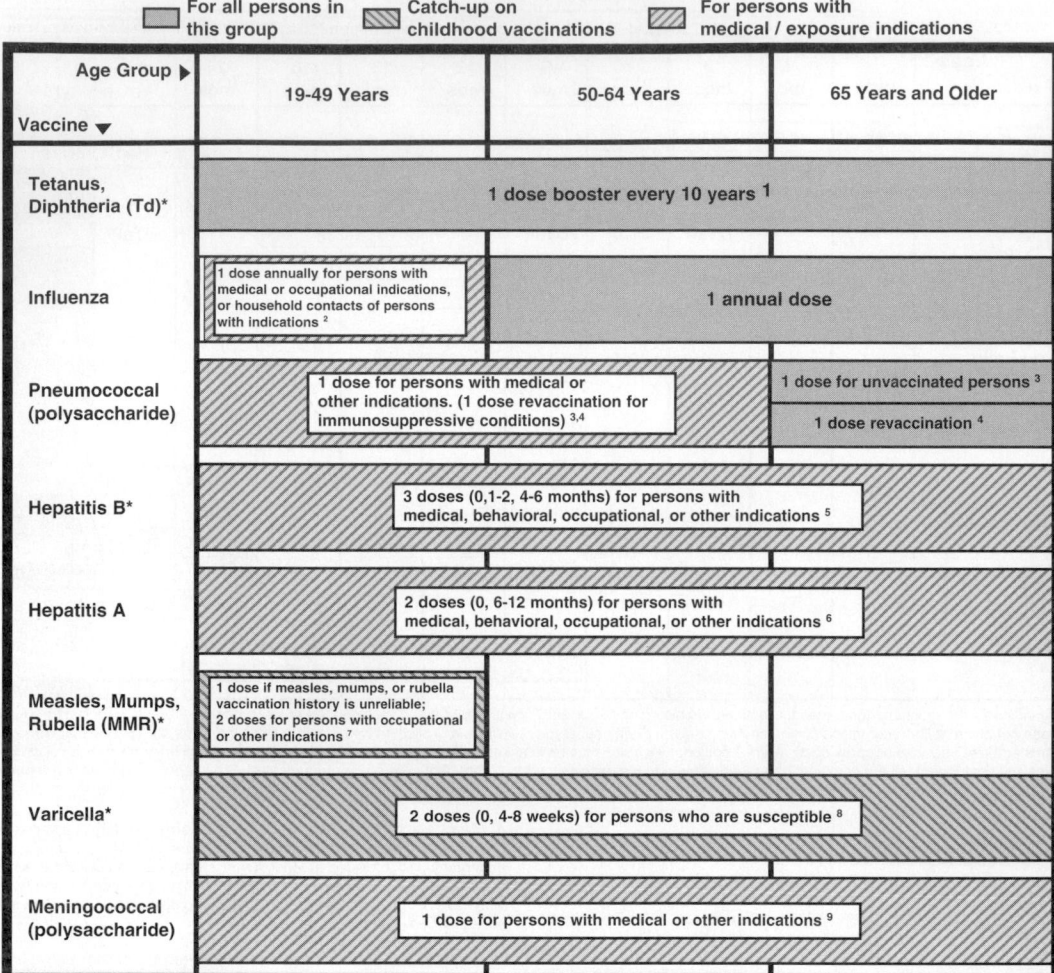

Recommended Adult Immunization Schedule, United States, 2002-2003

| For all persons in this group | Catch-up on childhood vaccinations | For persons with medical / exposure indications |

Age Group ▶ / Vaccine ▼	19-49 Years	50-64 Years	65 Years and Older
Tetanus, Diphtheria (Td)*	1 dose booster every 10 years [1]		
Influenza	1 dose annually for persons with medical or occupational indications, or household contacts of persons with indications [2]	1 annual dose	
Pneumococcal (polysaccharide)	1 dose for persons with medical or other indications. (1 dose revaccination for immunosuppressive conditions) [3,4]		1 dose for unvaccinated persons [3] / 1 dose revaccination [4]
Hepatitis B*	3 doses (0,1-2, 4-6 months) for persons with medical, behavioral, occupational, or other indications [5]		
Hepatitis A	2 doses (0, 6-12 months) for persons with medical, behavioral, occupational, or other indications [6]		
Measles, Mumps, Rubella (MMR)*	1 dose if measles, mumps, or rubella vaccination history is unreliable; 2 doses for persons with occupational or other indications [7]		
Varicella*	2 doses (0, 4-8 weeks) for persons who are susceptible [8]		
Meningococcal (polysaccharide)	1 dose for persons with medical or other indications [9]		

See Footnotes for Recommended Adult Immunization Schedule, United States, 2002-2003 on back cover.

*Covered by the Vaccine Injury Compensation Program. For information on how to file a claim call 800-338-2382. Please also visit www.hrsa.osp.gov/vicp To file a claim for vaccine injury write: U.S. Court of Federal Claims, 717 Madison Place, N.W.,Washington D.C. 20005. 202 219-9657.

This schedule indicates the recommended age groups for routine administration of currently licensed vaccines for persons 19 years of age and older. Licensed combination vaccines may be used whenever any components of the combination are indicated and the vaccine's other components are not contraindicated. Providers should consult the manufacturers' package inserts for detailed recommendations.

Report all clinically significant post-vaccination reactions to the Vaccine Adverse Event Reporting System (VAERS). Reporting forms and instructions on filing a VAERS report are available by calling 800-822-7967 or from the VAERS website at www.vaers.org.

For additional information about the vaccines listed above and contraindications for immunization, visit the National Immunization Program Website at www.cdc.gov/nip/ or call the National Immunization Hotline at 800-232-2522 (English) or 800-232-0233 (Spanish).

Approved by the Advisory Committee on Immunization Practices (ACIP), and accepted by the American College of Obstetricians and Gynecologists (ACOG) and the American Academy of Family Physicians (AAFP)

Footnotes for Recommended Adult Immunization Schedule, United States, 2002-2003

1. **Tetanus and diphtheria (Td)**—A primary series for adults is 3 doses: the first 2 doses given at least 4 weeks apart and the 3rd dose, 6-12 months after the second. Administer 1 dose if the person had received the primary series and the last vaccination was 10 years ago or longer. MMWR 1991; 40 (RR-10): 1-21.The ACP Task Force on Adult Immunization supports a second option: a single Td booster at age 50 years for persons who have completed the full pediatric series, including the teenage/young adult booster. Guide for Adult Immunization. 3rd ed.ACP 1994: 20.
2. **Influenza vaccination**—Medical indications: chronic disorders of the cardiovascular or pulmonary systems including asthma; chronic metabolic diseases including diabetes mellitus, renal dysfunction, hemoglobinopathies, immunosuppression (including immunosuppression caused by medications or by human immunodeficiency virus [HIV]), requiring regular medical follow-up or hospitalization during the preceding year; women who will be in the second or third trimester of pregnancy during the influenza season. Occupational indications: health-care workers.Other indications: residents of nursing homes and other long-term care facilities; persons likely to transmit influenza to persons at high-risk (in-home care givers to persons with medical indications, household contacts and out-of-home caregivers of children birth to 23 months of age, or children with asthma or other indicator conditions for influenza vaccination, household members and care givers of elderly and adults with high-risk conditions; and anyone who wishes to be vaccinated. MMWR 2002; 51 (RR-3): 1-31.
3. **Pneumococcal polysaccharide vaccination**—Medical indications: chronic disorders of the pulmonary system (excluding asthma), cardiovascular diseases, diabetes mellitus, chronic liver diseases including liver disease as a result of alcohol abuse (e.g., cirrhosis), chronic renal failure or nephrotic syndrome, functional or anatomic asplenia (e.g., sickle cell disease or splenectomy), immunosuppressive conditions (e.g., congenital immunodeficiency, HIV infection, leukemia, lymphoma, multiple myeloma, Hodgkins

disease, generalized malignancy, organ or bone marrow transplantation), chemotherapy with alkylating agents, anti-metabolites, or long-term systemic corticosteroids. Geographic/other indications: Alaskan Natives and certain American Indian populations. Other indications: residents of nursing homes and other long-term care facilities. MMWR 1997; 47 (RR-8): 1-24.
4. **Revaccination with pneumococcal polysaccharide vaccine**—One time revaccination after 5 years for persons with chronic renal failure or nephrotic syndrome, functional or anatomic asplenia (e.g., sickle cell disease or splenectomy), immunosuppressive conditions (e.g., congenital immunodeficiency, HIV infection, leukemia, lymphoma, multiple myeloma, Hodgkins disease, generalized malignancy, organ or bone marrow transplantation), chemotherapy with alkylating agents, antimetabolites, or long-term systemic corticosteroids. For persons 65 and older, one-time revaccination if they were vaccinated 5 or more years previously and were aged less than 65 years at the time of primary vaccination. MMWR 1997; 47 (RR-8): 1-24.
5. **Hepatitis B vaccination**—Medical indications: hemodialysis patients, patients who receive clotting-factor concentrates. Occupational indications: health-care workers and public-safety workers who have exposure to blood in the workplace, persons in training in schools of medicine, dentistry, nursing, laboratory technology, and other allied health professions.Behavioral indications: injecting drug users, persons with more than one sex partner in the previous 6 months, persons with a recently acquired sexually-transmitted disease (STD), all clients in STD clinics, men who have sex with men.Other indications: household contacts and sex partners of persons with chronic HBV infection, clients and staff of institutions for the developmentally disabled, international travelers who will be in countries with high or intermediate prevalence of chronic HBV infection for more than 6 months, inmates of correctional facilities. MMWR 1991; 40 (RR-13): 1-25. (www.cdc.gov/travel/diseases/hbv.htm)

FIGURE 8–2 ■ Recommended adult immunization schedule, United States, 2002.

Recommended Immunizations for Adults with Medical Conditions, United States, 2002-2003

| ▨ | For all persons in this group | ▨ | Catch-up on childhood vaccinations | ▨ | For persons with medical / exposure indications | ■ | Contraindicated |

Medical Conditions ▼ Vaccine ▶	Tetanus-Diphtheria (Td)*	Influenza	Pneumo-coccal (polysacch-aride)	Hepatitis B*	Hepatitis A	Measles, Mumps, Rubella (MMR)*	Varicella*
Pregnancy		A					
Diabetes, heart disease, chronic pulmonary disease, chronic liver disease, including chronic alcoholism		B	C		D		
Congenital immunodeficiency, leukemia, lymphoma, generalized malignancy, therapy with alkylating agents, antimetabolites, radiation large amounts of corticosteroids			E				F
Renal failure / end stage renal disease, recipients of hemodialysis or clotting factor concentrates			E	G			
Asplenia including elective splenectomy and terminal complement component deficiencies			E, H, I				
HIV infection			E, J			K	

A. If pregnancy is at 2nd or 3rd trimester during influenza season.

B. Although chronic liver disease and alcoholism are not indicator conditions for influenza vaccination, give 1 dose annually if the patient is ≥ 50 years, has other indications for influenza vaccine, or if the patient requests vaccination.

C. Asthma is an indicator condition for influenza but not for pneumococcal vaccination.

D. For all persons with chronic liver disease.

E. Revaccinate once after 5 years or more have elapsed since initial vaccination.
F. Persons with impaired humoral but not cellular immunity may be vaccinated.
MMWR 1999; 48 (RR-06): 1-5.

6. Hepatitis A vaccination—For the combined HepA-HepB vaccine use 3 doses at 0, 1, 6 months. Medical indications: persons with clotting-factor disorders or chronic liver disease. Behavioral indications: men who have sex with men, users of injecting and noninjecting illegal drugs. Occupational indications: persons working with HAV-infected primates or with HAV in a research laboratory setting. Other indications: persons traveling to or working in countries that have high or intermediate endemicity of hepatitis A. *MMWR* 1999; 48 (RR-12): 1-37. (www.cdc.gov/travel/diseases/hav.htm)
7. Measles, Mumps, Rubella vaccination (MMR)—Measles component: Adults born before 1957 may be considered immune to measles. Adults born in or after 1957 should receive at least one dose of MMR unless they have a medical contraindication, documentation of at least one dose or other acceptable evidence of immunity. A second dose of MMR is recommended for adults who:
  • are recently exposed to measles or in an outbreak setting
  • were previously vaccinated with killed measles vaccine
  • were vaccinated with an unknown vaccine between 1963 and 1967
  • are students in post-secondary educational institutions
  • work in health care facilities
  • plan to travel internationally
Mumps component: 1 dose of MMR should be adequate for protection. Rubella component: Give 1 dose of MMR to women whose rubella vaccination history is unreliable and counsel women to avoid becoming pregnant for 4 weeks after vaccination. For women of child-bearing age, regardless of birth year, routinely determine rubella immunity and counsel women regarding congenital rubella syndrome. Do not vaccinate pregnant women or those planning to become pregnant in the next 4 weeks. If pregnant and susceptible, vaccinate as early in postpartum period as possible. *MMWR* 1998; 47 (RR-8): 1-57.

G. Hemodialysis patients:Use special formulation of vaccine (40 ug/mL) or two 1.0 mL 20 ug doses given at one site.Vaccinate early in the course of renal disease. Assess antibody titers to hep B surface antigen (anti-HBs) levels annually. Administer additional doses if anti-HBs levels decline to <10 milliinternational units (mIU)/ mL.

H. Also administer meningococcal vaccine.

I. Elective splenectomy: vaccinate at least 2 weeks before surgery.

J. Vaccinate as close to diagnosis as possible when CD4 cell counts are highest.

K. Withhold MMR or other measles containing vaccines from HIV-infected persons with evidence of severe immunosuppression. *MMWR* 1996; 45: 603-606, *MMWR* 1992; 41 (RR-17): 1-19.

8. Varicella vaccination—Recommended for all persons who do not have reliable clinical history of varicella infection, or serological evidence of varicella zoster virus (VZV) infection; health-care workers and family contacts of immunocompromised persons, those who live or work in environments where transmission is likely (e.g., teachers of young children, day care employees, and residents and staff members in institutional settings), persons who live or work in environments where VZV transmission can occur (e.g., college students, inmates and staff members of correctional institutions, and military personnel), adolescents and adults living in households with children, women who are not pregnant but who may become pregnant in the future, international travelers who are not immune to infection. Note: Greater than 90% of U.S. born adults are immune to VZV. Do not vaccinate pregnant women or those planning to become pregnant in the next 4 weeks. If pregnant and susceptible, vaccinate as early in postpartum period as possible. *MMWR* 1996; 45 (RR-11): 1-36, *MMWR* 1999; 48 (RR-6): 1-5.
9. Meningococcal vaccine (quadrivalent polysaccharide for serogroups A, C, Y, and W-135)—Consider vaccination for persons with medical indications: adults with terminal complement component deficiencies, with anatomic or functional asplenia. Other indications: travelers to countries in which disease is hyperendemic or epidemic ("meningitis belt" of sub-Saharan Africa, Mecca, Saudi Arabia for Hajj). Revaccination at 3-5 years may be indicated for persons at high risk for infection (e.g., persons residing in areas in which disease is epidemic). Counsel college freshmen, especially those who live in dormitories, regarding meningococcal disease and the vaccine so that they can make an educated decision about receiving the vaccination. *MMWR* 2000; 49 (RR-7): 1-20. Note: The AAFP recommends that colleges should take the lead on providing education on meningococcal infection and vaccination and offer it to those who are interested. Physicians need not initiate discussion of the meningococcal quadravalent polysaccharide vaccine as part of routine medical care.

FIGURE 8–2 ■ Cont'd.

TABLE 8–3 ■ Recommended and Minimum Ages and Intervals Between Doses of Vaccines Commonly Used in the United States*†

Vaccine and Dose Number	Recommended Age for This Dose	Minimum Age for This Dose	Recommended Interval to Next Dose	Minimum Interval to Next Dose
Hepatitis B				
Hep B1‡	Birth–2 mo	Birth	1–4 mo	4 wk
Hep B2	1–4 mo	4 wk	2–17 mo	8 wk
Hep B3§	6–18 mo	6 mo	—	—
Diphtheria and tetanus toxoids and acellular pertussis (DTaP)				
DTaP1	2 mo	6 wk	2 mo	4 wk
DTaP2	4 mo	10 wk	2 mo	4 wk
DTaP3	6 mo	14 wk	6–12 mo	6 mo
DTaP4	15–18 mo	12 mo	3 yr	6 mo
DTaP5	4–6 yr	4 yr	—	—
Haemophilus influenzae type b (Hib)‡,**				
Hib1	2 mo	6 wk	2 mo	4 wk
Hib2	4 mo	10 wk	2 mo	4 wk
Hib3¶	6 mo	14 wk	6–9 mo	8 wk
Hib4	12–15 mo	12 mo	—	—
Poliovirus vaccine (PV)—oral (live) or injected (inactivated)				
PV1	2 mo	6 wk	2 mo	4 wk
PV2	4 mo	10 wk	2–14 mo	4 wk
PV3	6–18 mo	14 wk	3.5 yr	4 wk
PV4	4–6 yr	18 wk	—	—
Pneumococcal conjugate vaccine (PCV)‖				
PCV1	2 mo	6 wk	2 mo	4 wk
PCV2	4 mo	10 wk	2 mo	4 wk
PCV3	6 mo	14 wk	6 mo	8 wk
PCV4	12–15 mo	12 mo	—	—
Measles, mumps, and rubella (MMR)				
MMR1	12–15 mo**	12 mo	3–5 yr	4 wk
MMR2	4–6 yr	13 mo	—	—
Varicella††	12–18 mo	12 mo	4 wk††	4 wk‡‡
Hepatitis A				
Hep A1	≥2 yr	2 yr	6–18 mo	6 mo
Hep A2	≥30 mo	30 mo	—	—
Influenza‡‡	—	6 mo	1 mo	4 wk
Pneumococcal polysaccharide (PPV)				
PPV1	—	2 yr	5 yr§§	5 yr
PPV2	—	7 yr§§	—	—

*Age and interval recommendations for vaccines may be different outside the United States.

†Combination vaccines are available. Using licensed combination vaccines is preferred over separate injections of their equivalent component vaccines. When administering combination vaccines, the minimum age for administration is the oldest age for any of the individual components; the minimum interval between doses is equal to the greatest interval of any of the individual antigens.

‡A combination hepatitis B–Hib vaccine is available (Comvax, manufactured by Merck Vaccine Division). This vaccine should not be administered to infants less than 6 weeks of age because of the Hib component.

§Hepatitis B3 should be administered 8 weeks or more after hepatitis B2 and 16 weeks after hepatitis B1, and it should not be administered before age 6 months.

‖For Hib and PCV, children receiving the first dose of vaccine at age 7 months, or older require fewer doses to complete the series (see Chapters 14 and 22).

¶For a regimen of only polyribosylribitol phosphate–meningococcal outer membrane protein (PRP-OMP; PedvaxHib, manufactured by Merck Vaccine Division), a dose administered at age 6 months is not required.

**During a measles outbreak, if cases are occurring among infants less than 12 months of age, measles vaccination of infants 6 months and older can be undertaken as an outbreak control measure. However, doses administered at less than 12 months of age should not be counted as part of the series in the United States.

††Children ages 12 months to 13 years require only one dose of varicella vaccine. Persons 13 years or older should receive two doses separated by 4 or more weeks.

‡‡Two doses of inactivated influenza vaccine are recommended for children ages 6 months to 9 years who are receiving the vaccine for the first time. Children ages 6 months to 9 years who have previously received influenza vaccine and persons 9 years or older require only one dose per influenza season.

§§A second dose of PPV are recommended for persons at highest risk for serious pneumococcal infection and those who are likely to have a rapid decline in pneumococcal antibody concentration. Revaccination 3 years after the previous dose can be considered for children at highest risk for severe pneumococcal infection who would be less than 10 years of age at the time of revaccination (see Chapter 22).

TABLE 8–4 ■ Guidelines for Spacing the Administration of Inactivated and Live Antigens

Antigen Combination	Recommended Minimum Interval Between Doses
≥2 inactivated	None; can be administered simultaneously or at any interval between doses
Inactivated and live	None; can be administered simultaneously or at any interval between doses
≥2 live parenteral*	4-week minimum interval if not administered simultaneously

*Live oral vaccines (e.g., Ty21a typhoid vaccine, oral polio vaccine) can be administered simultaneously or at any interval before or after inactivated or live parenteral vaccines.

may inhibit the immunologic response to the second dose is based on evidence from both animal and human studies. Petralli et al.[96,97] reported that the immune response to smallpox vaccination was affected by prior administration of live, attenuated measles vaccine. Interferon produced in response to the initial dose of measles virus vaccine has been postulated to inhibit replication of vaccinia virus in the subsequent vaccine dose. In a study in two U.S. health maintenance organizations, persons who received varicella vaccine less than 30 days after MMR vaccination had an increased risk of varicella vaccine failure (i.e., varicella disease in a vaccinated person) of 2.5-fold compared with persons who received varicella vaccine before or 30 days or more after MMR.[98] In contrast, Stefano et al., in a 1999 study, determined that the response to yellow fever vaccine is not affected by monovalent measles vaccine administered 1 to 27 days earlier.[99] No evidence indicates that live virus vaccines administered orally interfere with live virus vaccines administered parenterally or orally.

To minimize the potential risk for interference, parenterally administered live virus vaccines not administered on the same day should be administered 4 weeks or more apart whenever possible. If parenterally administered live virus vaccines are separated by less than 4 weeks, readministration of the live virus vaccine given second should be considered.[5] Yellow fever vaccine can be administered at any time after single-antigen measles vaccine. Oral and parenteral live virus vaccines can be administered simultaneously or at any interval before or after each other, if indicated.[5]

Too-frequent administration of some inactivated vaccines, such as tetanus toxoid, can result in increased rates of reactions in some vaccinees.[2,5,100] Such reactions probably result from formation of circulating antigen-antibody complexes.[2,101–104]

Simultaneous Administration of Different Vaccines

Simultaneous administration of all indicated vaccines is an essential component of childhood vaccination programs.[2,5] Simultaneous administration of different vaccines is particularly important when return of the recipient for further vaccination is uncertain, when imminent exposure to several vaccine-preventable diseases is expected, or when preparing for international travel on short notice.

Unless specifically licensed for injection in the same syringe, different vaccines administered simultaneously should be injected separately and at different anatomic sites. If both upper and lower limbs must be used for simultaneous administration of different vaccines, the anterolateral thigh is often chosen for intramuscular injections and

the deltoid region for subcutaneous injections. If more than one injection must be administered in a single limb of an infant or young child, the thigh usually is preferred because of its large muscle mass. The distance separating two injections in the same limb should be sufficient (e.g., 1 to 2 inches) to minimize the chance of overlapping local reactions.[15,16] In general, different vaccines, including live virus products, can be administered simultaneously without reducing their safety and effectiveness[105] (see Table 8–4). Studies of cortisol concentration and behavioral responses of infants to vaccination indicate that responses are similar in infants who receive two injections during one visit and those who receive a single injection, suggesting that a second injection does not increase stress.[106,107]

Whereas simultaneous administration of vaccines associated with frequent local or systemic reactions could result in accentuation of these reactions, increased severity or incidence of adverse reactions has not been observed after simultaneous administration of the most widely used vaccines.[5] Similarly, simultaneous administration of vaccines generally does not cause immunologic interference.[105] An exception is concurrent administration of yellow fever and cholera vaccines.[108,109]

Interference by Immune Globulins

Passively acquired antibodies can interfere with the immune response to certain vaccines, both live and inactivated, and to toxoids. The result can be either the absence of seroconversion or a blunting of the immune response with lower final antibody concentrations in the vaccinee. Passively acquired antibody, however, does not affect the immune response to all vaccines.

Interference with Live Virus Vaccines

To elicit an adequate immune response, live vaccine virus must replicate within the recipient. The probable mechanism by which passively acquired immune globulin blunts the immune response is neutralization of vaccine virus, resulting in inhibition of viral replication and insufficient antigenic mass.[110] For example, persisting transplacentally acquired maternal measles antibodies inhibit the response to live measles vaccine in infants for as long as 12 months and perhaps longer.[111–113] The age to which inhibition persists has been correlated with concentrations of maternal or cord blood antibodies.[114–116] Rubella vaccine virus may be less susceptible than measles vaccine virus to these transplacentally acquired maternal antibodies.[117]

Intramuscular or intravenous administration of immune globulin–containing preparations (e.g., serum immune globulin, hyperimmune globulins, intravenous immune globulin, and blood) before or simultaneous with certain vaccines also can affect the immune response to live virus vaccines. When partially attenuated Edmonston B measles vaccine, which is no longer available in the United States, was administered concurrently with measles immune globulin in an effort to reduce the incidence of adverse events associated with this vaccine, the rate of seroconversion was not affected but the geometric mean titer of serum measles antibody was diminished.[118–120] In a study of an investigational bacterial polysaccharide immune globulin (BPIG), children had a reduced immune response to live measles vaccine for as long as 5 months after receipt of BPIG.[121] The measles antibody seroconversion rate and geometric mean titer were lower among children who received BPIG compared with children who received placebo. Blunting of the immune response to live rubella vaccine also occurred after receipt of BPIG but was less marked and of shorter duration.[121]

Although passively acquired antibodies can interfere with the response to rubella vaccine, the low dose of anti-Rh(D) globulin administered to postpartum women has not been demonstrated to inhibit the immune response to RA27/3 strain rubella vaccine.[122] Parenterally administered immune globulin preparations also do not appear to adversely affect the immune response to yellow fever vaccine.[123] Although high concentrations of passively acquired antibodies may reduce the serum antibody response to live poliovirus vaccine, they have little effect on replication of vaccine virus and development of gastrointestinal tract immunity.[82,123–125] Data are insufficient to determine the extent to which passively acquired antibodies interfere with the immune response to other live viral or bacterial vaccines, such as varicella, mumps, and typhoid (Ty21a strain).[126] A humanized mouse monoclonal antibody product (palivizumab) is available for prevention of respiratory syncytial virus infection among infants and young children. This product contains only antibody to respiratory syncytial virus; hence, it will not interfere with immune response to live vaccines.[127]

Interference with Inactivated and Component Vaccines

Interference with current inactivated and component vaccines is less marked than with live vaccines and requires exposure to large doses of passively acquired antibodies.[82,125,128, 129] The mechanism by which passively acquired antibodies interfere with the immunologic response to inactivated and toxoid vaccines is not clear. Moderate doses of parenterally administered immune globulins have not inhibited development of a protective immune response to DTP, tetanus toxoid, hepatitis B vaccines, Hib conjugate vaccines, and rabies vaccines.[129–131] Although the concurrent administration of inactivated hepatitis A vaccine and immune globulin can result in lower serum antibody concentrations than if vaccine alone is administered, seroconversion rates have not been diminished.[132–134] In another study, infants with high concentrations of passively acquired maternal antibody to hepatitis A virus had lower serum antibody concentrations after receipt of hepatitis A vaccine but had seroconversion rates similar to those of vaccinated infants without maternal antibodies.[135] Further studies have been undertaken to determine if these findings are of clinical significance.

The manufacturer of Respiratory Syncytial Virus Immune Globulin, Intravenous (RSV-IGIV) suggests that an additional dose of certain vaccines (i.e., diphtheria and tetanus toxoids and acellular pertussis [DTaP] vaccine; DTP; Hib; and OPV) may be necessary to ensure a protective immune response from these vaccines in recipients of RSV-IGIV.[136] However, currently available data are inconclusive and do not support this recommendation.[137] The humanized mouse monoclonal antibody product (palivizumab) does not interfere with the immune response to inactivated vaccines.[127]

Recommendations for Spacing Administration of Vaccines and Immune Globulins

Interference of immune globulins with the immune response to vaccines is dose related and, therefore, more likely to occur and to persist for a longer period after receipt of larger doses of immune globulins.[121,138] The recommended interval between administration of immune globulin preparations and vaccines is based on the following considerations: (1) whether evidence suggests interference between immune globulin and the vaccine; (2) the dose of the immune globulin administered; and (3) the expected half-life of immunoglobulin G. Recommended intervals between administration of immune globulin preparations and various live and killed vaccines are listed in Tables 8–5 and 8–6.

In the United States, inactivated and component (subunit) vaccines may be administered simultaneously with or at any time before or after receipt of an immune globulin preparation.[2,5,18] The vaccine and immune globulin preparation should be administered at different sites, and the standard recommended doses of the corresponding vaccines should be given.[2,5] Supplemental doses are not indicated.

Recommendations for administration of live virus vaccines vary on the basis of the aforementioned considerations. After receipt of an immune globulin preparation or other blood product, measles vaccine should be deferred during the intervals listed in Table 8–6.[125,139] Human blood and immune globulin preparations also contain rubella, mumps, and varicella antibodies. High doses of passively acquired antibodies can inhibit the immune response to live rubella vaccine for as long as 3 months.[121,140] The effect of immune globulin preparations on the response to live mumps and live varicella vaccines has not been defined. To reduce the possibility of interference, postponement of administration of rubella, mumps, and varicella vaccines for the intervals indicated in Table 8–6 is prudent.[5]

Immune globulin preparations administered too soon after vaccination with MMR or varicella vaccines can interfere with the immune response. Therefore, if administration of an immune globulin preparation becomes necessary less than 2 weeks after receipt of MMR, its component vaccines, or varicella vaccine, readministration of the vaccine is recommended after the appropriate interval listed in Tables 8–5 and 8–6, unless serologic testing indicates that a

TABLE 8–5 ■ Guidelines for Spacing the Administration of Antibody-Containing Products* and Vaccines

SIMULTANEOUS ADMINISTRATION	
Immunobiologic Combination	Recommended Minimum Interval Between Doses
Antibody-containing product and inactivated antigen	None; can be administered simultaneously at different sites or at any time between doses
Antibody-containing product and live antigen	Generally should not be administered simultaneously[†] If simultaneous administration of measles-containing vaccine is unavoidable, administer at different sites and revaccinate or test for seroconversion after the recommended interval indicated in Table 8–6

NONSIMULTANEOUS ADMINISTRATION		
Immunobiologic Administered		Recommended Minimum Interval Between Administration of Antibody-Containing Product and Vaccine Antigen
First	Second	
Antibody-containing product	Inactivated antigen	None
Inactivated antigen	Antibody-containing product	None
Antibody-containing product	Live antigen	Dose related[†‡]
Live antigen	Antibody-containing product	2 wk

*Blood products containing substantial amounts of immunoglobulin, including intramuscular and intravenous immune globulin, specific hyperimmune globulin (e.g, hepatitis B immune globulin, tetanus immune globulin, varicella-zoster immune globulin, and rabies immune globulin), whole blood, packed red cells, plasma, and platelet products.
[†]Yellow fever, oral poliovirus vaccine, and oral Ty21a typhoid vaccines are exceptions to these recommendations. These live, attenuated vaccines can be administered at any time before, after, or simultaneously with an antibody-containing product without substantially decreasing the antibody response.
[‡]The duration of interference of antibody-containing products with the immune response to the measles component of measles-containing vaccine is dose related (see Table 8–6). High doses of passively acquired antibody can inhibit the immune response to live rubella vaccine for up to 3 months. The effect of antibody-containing products on the response to live mumps and varicella vaccines has not been determined.

protective antibody response has already occurred.[5] For example, if whole blood is administered less than 14 days after receipt of varicella vaccine, the vaccine should be readministered at least 6 months after the whole blood unless serologic testing indicates an adequate immune response to the initial dose of varicella vaccine.

Because the immune responses to OPV and yellow fever vaccines have not been demonstrated to be adversely affected by immune globulin preparations, these vaccines can be administered at any time in relation to the receipt of immune globulin preparations.[123] Live oral typhoid (Ty21a) vaccine also is recommended for administration irrespective of the receipt of immune globulin preparations.[5,141]

Interchangeability of Vaccines of Different Manufacturers

Combination and monovalent vaccines against the same diseases with similar antigens and produced by the same manufacturer are considered interchangeable in most situations.[2,5] However, supporting data on the safety, immunogenicity, and efficacy of using comparable vaccines from different manufacturers for different doses of a vaccination series frequently are limited or unavailable. When the same vaccine cannot be used to complete an immunization series, similar vaccines produced by different manufacturers or produced by the same manufacturer in different countries generally have been considered acceptable to complete the immunization series provided each vaccine is given according to licensed recommendations.[2,5]

Some diseases have serologic correlates of immunity that can be used to evaluate vaccine interchangeability. For example, in studies in which one or more doses of hepatitis B vaccine produced by one manufacturer were followed by doses from another manufacturer, the immune response was comparable to that resulting from use of a single vaccine type.[142,143] Whereas Hib conjugate vaccines differ in antigen composition, interchangeability of different products has been validated on the basis of the accepted serologic correlate of immunity against Hib invasive disease.[144-146]

Determination of vaccine interchangeability is more difficult for diseases without serologic correlates of immunity. For example, in the absence of such a correlate for *Bordetella pertussis* infection, the interchangeability of acellular pertussis vaccines is difficult to assess. Available data from one study indicate that, for the first three doses of the DTaP series, one or two doses of Tripedia (manufactured by Aventis Pasteur) followed by Infanrix (manufactured by GlaxoSmithKline) for the remaining doses(s) is comparable to three doses of Tripedia with regard to immunogenicity, as measured by antibodies to diphtheria, tetanus, and pertussis toxoids and filamentous hemagglutinin.[147] However, in the absence of a clear serologic correlate of protection for pertussis, the relevance of these immunogenicity data for protection against pertussis is unknown. Thus, when feasible, acellular pertussis vaccine from the same manufacturer is preferred for the entire primary vaccination series. Nevertheless, either of these two products can be used to continue or complete the series if this regimen is not feasible.[2,148] Data are not available regarding interchangeability of DAPTACEL (approved in May 2002 and manufactured by Aventis Pasteur Limited) with Tripedia or Infanrix.

TABLE 8–6 ▪ Suggested Intervals Between Administration of Antibody-Containing Products for Various Indications and Vaccines Containing Live Measles Vaccine*†

Product/Indication	Dose (mg IgG/kg Body Weight)*	Recommended Interval (mo) Before Measles Vaccination
Respiratory syncytial virus immune globulin (IG) monoclonal antibody (Synagis)‡	15 mg/kg intramuscularly (IM)	None
Tetanus IG	250 units (10 mg IgG/kg) IM	3
Hepatitis A IG		
Contact prophylaxis	0.02 mL/kg (3.3 mg IgG/kg) IM	3
International travel	0.06 mL/kg (10 mg IgG/kg) IM	3
Hepatitis B IG	0.06 mL/kg (10 mg IgG/kg) IM	3
Rabies IG	20 IU/kg (22 mg IgG/kg) IM	4
Varicella IG	125 units/10 kg (20–40 mg IgG/kg) IM, maximum 625 units	5
Measles IG		
Standard (i.e., nonimmunocompromised) contact	0.25 mL/kg (40 mg IgG/kg) IM	5
Immunocompromised contact	0.50 mL/kg (80 mg IgG/kg) IM	6
Blood transfusion		
Red blood cells (RBCs), washed	10 mL/kg (negligible IgG/kg) intravenously (IV)	None
RBCs, adenine-saline added	10 mL/kg (10 mg IgG/kg) IV	3
Packed RBCs (hematocrit 65%)§	10 mL/kg (60 mg IgG/kg) IV	6
Whole blood (hematocrit 35%–50%)§	10 mL/kg (80–100 mg IgG/kg) IV	6
Plasma/platelet products	10 mL/kg (160 mg IgG/kg) IV	7
Cytomegalovirus intravenous immune globulin (IGIV)	150 mg/kg maximum	6
Respiratory syncytial virus IGIV	750 mg/kg	9
IGIV		
Replacement therapy for immune deficiencies ‖	300–400 mg/kg IV‖	8
Immune thrombocytopenic purpura	400 mg/kg IV	8
Immune thrombocytopenic purpura	1000 mg/kg IV	10
Kawasaki disease	2 g/kg IV	11

*This table is not intended for determining the correct indications and dosages for using antibody-containing products. Unvaccinated persons might not be fully protected against measles during the entire recommended interval, and additional doses of immune globulin or measles vaccine might be indicated after measles exposure. Concentrations of measles antibody in an immune globulin preparation can vary by manufacturer's lot. Rates of antibody clearance after receipt of an immune globulin preparation might vary also. Recommended intervals are extrapolated from an estimated half-life of 30 days for passively acquired antibody and an observed interference with the immune response to measles vaccine of 5 months after a dose of 80 mg IgG/kg.

†High doses of passively acquired antibody can inhibit the immune response to live rubella vaccine for up to 3 months. The effect of antibody-containing products on the response to live mumps and varicella vaccines has not been determined.

‡Contains antibody only to respiratory syncytial virus.

§Assumes a serum IgG concentration of 16 mg/mL.

‖Measles and varicella vaccination is recommended for children with asymptomatic or mildly symptomatic human immunodeficiency virus (HIV) infection but is contraindicated for persons with severe immunosuppression from HIV or any other immunosuppressive disorder.

However, any of these products can be used to complete the DTaP series if the product(s) administered for earlier doses are unknown or unavailable.

Hypersensitivity to Vaccine Components

Types of Reactions

Hypersensitivity reactions after vaccination can be local or systemic, and can vary in severity from mild discomfort at the site of vaccination to severe anaphylaxis. Onset can be either immediate or delayed. Serious allergic reactions are rare. Whether a specific hypersensitivity reaction is caused by a vaccine component or an unrelated environmental allergen can be difficult to determine. However, symptoms occurring immediately after vaccination that are suggestive of an anaphylactic reaction generally contraindicate further administration of that vaccine to the recipient.[2,5]

Urticaria and anaphylactic reactions have been reported after administration of DTP, diphtheria and tetanus toxoids (DT, Td), and tetanus toxoid.[149–151] Whereas immunoglobulin E–type antibodies to tetanus and diphtheria antigens have been identified in some patients with these symptoms, transient urticaria-like rashes are not a contraindication to subsequent vaccination because they are unlikely to be anaphylactic unless they appear within minutes after vaccination.[2,151–153] A serum sickness–type reaction caused by circulating complexes of vaccine antigen and previously acquired antibody is the probable cause of these reactions, and subsequent vaccination is unlikely to result in the necessary ratio of antigen to antibody concentration to form immune complexes.[151,154]

Tetanus toxoid is contraindicated in persons who experienced an immediate anaphylactic reaction to tetanus toxoid–containing vaccine, unless the person can be desensitized to the toxoid.[2] Because of the importance of tetanus immunization and the uncertainty about which vaccine component might be the cause of the reaction, the patient may be referred to an allergist for evaluation and possible desensitization.[151,155–158] On occasion, a history of a prior allergic reaction to tetanus vaccine may refer to a reaction to tetanus antitoxin of equine origin given for tetanus prophylaxis before human-derived tetanus immune globulin became available in the 1960s. Thus, before use of tetanus toxoid is discontinued because of an alleged episode of anaphylaxis, skin testing and possible desensitization should be considered.[155,156]

Local or systemic reactions, such as redness and soreness at the vaccination site and fever, have been associated with receipt of DTP, plague, cholera, and inactivated whole-cell typhoid vaccines.[104,159–163] Such reactions usually are caused by a toxin in the vaccine rather than by hypersensitivity to a specific component.

With some vaccines, such as Japanese encephalitis, immediate or delayed onset of generalized urticaria and angioedema that can progress to respiratory distress and hypotension has been reported after vaccination.[164–166] The pathogenesis of these reactions is not known.

Vaccine Components Causing Hypersensitivity

Proteins

Egg protein is a constituent of vaccines prepared with use of embryonated chicken eggs, such as influenza and yellow fever vaccines. On rare occasions, these vaccines can induce anaphylaxis or other immediate hypersensitivity reactions, and these reactions are sometimes attributed to egg protein antigen.[2,5,167–170] As a result, these vaccines are contraindicated in persons with a history of anaphylactic reactions to egg ingestion unless desensitization has been successfully completed.[2,5,167,168,170,171] For example, persons needing yellow fever vaccine who have a history of systemic anaphylaxis-like symptoms after egg ingestion can be skin tested with yellow fever vaccine before vaccination and desensitized if necessary.[2,5,167] Although possible, skin testing and desensitization with influenza vaccine often are precluded by the risk of reactions, the need for yearly vaccination, and the availability of chemoprophylaxis with antiviral agents active against influenza virus.[2,168,171,172]

Measles and mumps vaccines are produced in chick embryo fibroblast cell culture. Persons with hypersensitivity to eggs are at low risk for anaphylactic reactions to these vaccines, and skin testing with vaccine is not predictive of allergic reaction after immunization.[2,173–175] Therefore, neither skin testing nor administration of gradually increasing doses of vaccine is required when these vaccines are administered to persons who are allergic to eggs.[2,79,139,176]

Live virus vaccines, such as measles, mumps, rubella, yellow fever, and varicella, contain gelatin as a stabilizer. Persons with a history of allergy to gelatin have experienced on rare occasions an anaphylactic reaction after vaccination with such a vaccine.[177–179] Skin testing of persons with a history of systemic anaphylaxis-like symptoms after gelatin ingestion may be useful to identify those at risk for severe hypersensitivity reactions to vaccination, but no protocol for such testing or desensitization has been published. Because gelatin used as a vaccine stabilizer may be of porcine origin, whereas ingested food gelatin may be of bovine origin, the absence of a history of allergy to gelatin-containing foods does not eliminate the possibility of a gelatin-mediated reaction to vaccine.

Approximately 6% of persons who receive a booster dose of human diploid rabies vaccine develop a serum sickness–type illness.[180,181] This reaction is thought to be caused by sensitization to human albumin that has been altered chemically by a virus-inactivating agent used in the production of the vaccine.[2,182]

Latex

Latex is liquid sap from the commercial rubber tree. Latex contains naturally occurring impurities (e.g., plant proteins and peptides), which are believed to be responsible for allergic reactions. Latex is processed to form natural rubber latex and dry natural rubber. Dry natural rubber and natural rubber latex might contain the same plant impurities as latex but in lesser amounts. Natural rubber latex is used to produce medical gloves, catheters, and other products, whereas dry natural rubber is used in syringe plungers, vial stoppers, and injection ports on intravascular tubing. Synthetic rubber and synthetic latex also are used in medical gloves, syringe plungers, and vial stoppers, but they do not contain natural rubber or natural latex, or the impurities linked to allergic reactions.

The most common type of latex sensitivity is contact-type (type 4) allergy, usually as a result of prolonged contact with latex-containing gloves.[183] Although injection procedure–associated latex allergies among patients with diabetes mellitus have been described,[184–186] allergic reactions, including anaphylaxis, after vaccination procedures are rare. Only one report of an allergic reaction after administering hepatitis B vaccine in a patient with known severe allergy (anaphylaxis) to latex has been published.[187]

If a person reports a severe (anaphylactic) allergy to latex, vaccines supplied in vials or syringes that contain natural rubber should not be administered, unless the benefit of vaccination outweighs the risk of an allergic reaction to the vaccine. For latex allergies other than anaphylactic allergies, such as a history of contact allergy to latex gloves, vaccines supplied in vials or syringes that contain dry natural rubber or natural rubber latex can be administered.[5]

Antibiotics

Live virus vaccines frequently contain trace amounts of one or more antibiotics, such as neomycin, streptomycin, and polymyxin B. Vaccine contents are listed in the manufacturer's product label for each vaccine. The most common allergic response to neomycin is a delayed-type (cell-mediated) local contact dermatitis consisting of an erythematous, pruritic papule that occurs 48 to 96 hours after vaccine administration.[2,5,188] Such delayed-type reactions are not contraindications for vaccination.[2,5,188,189] However, persons who have experienced an anaphylactic reaction to neomycin or to another antibiotic vaccine constituent should not receive vaccines containing that antibiotic.[2,5,190,191]

No vaccines currently licensed in the United States contain penicillin or penicillin derivatives.

Thimerosal

Thimerosal is an organic mercurial compound in use since the 1930s and added to certain immunobiologic products as a preservative. A joint statement issued by the U.S. Public Health Service and the AAP in 1999[192] established the goal of removing thimerosal as soon as possible from vaccines routinely recommended for infants. Although no evidence exists of any harm caused by low concentrations of thimerosal in vaccines, and the risk was only theoretical,[193] this goal was established as a precautionary measure.

The potential health effects of mercury exposure of any type and the elimination of mercury from vaccines was considered to be a feasible means of reducing an infant's total exposure to mercury in a world where other environmental sources of exposure, such as certain foods or air, are more difficult or impossible to eliminate. Since mid-2001, vaccines produced in the United States that are recommended routinely for children have been manufactured without thimerosal as a preservative and contain either no thimerosal or only trace amounts. Thimerosal as a preservative is present in certain other vaccines. Examples are Td, DT, one of two adult hepatitis B vaccines, influenza vaccine, and Japanese encephalitis vaccine. Formulations of influenza vaccine with a reduced concentration of thimerosal or no thimerosal as a preservative are now available in the U.S..

Receiving thimerosal-containing vaccines has been postulated to lead to induction of allergy in some persons.[194-196] However, there is limited scientific evidence for this assertion. Hypersensitivity to thimerosal usually consists of local delayed-type hypersensitivity reactions.[197-199] Thimerosal elicits positive delayed-type hypersensitivity patch tests in 1% to 18% of persons tested, but these tests have limited or no clinical relevance.[200,201] The majority of patients do not experience reactions to thimerosal administered as a component of vaccines even when patch or intradermal tests for thimerosal indicate hypersensitivity.[197,201] A localized or delayed-type hypersensitivity reaction to thimerosal is not a contraindication to receipt of a vaccine that contains thimerosal.[2,5,198,202]

Management of Acute Vaccine Adverse Reactions

Although rare after vaccination, the immediate onset and life-threatening nature of an anaphylactic reaction require that personnel and facilities providing vaccination be capable of providing initial care for suspected anaphylaxis. Epinephrine and equipment for maintaining an airway should be available for immediate use.

Anaphylaxis usually begins within several minutes of administration of vaccine. Rapid recognition and initiation of treatment are required to prevent possible progression to cardiovascular collapse. If flushing, facial edema, urticaria, itching, swelling of the mouth or throat, wheezing, difficulty breathing, or other signs of anaphylaxis occur, the patient should be placed in a recumbent position with the legs elevated. Aqueous epinephrine (1:1000) should be administered intramuscularly or subcutaneously, and can be repeated within 10 to 20 minutes.[203] A dose of diphen-hydramine hydrochloride may shorten the reaction, but it will have little immediate effect. Maintenance of any airway and oxygen administration may be necessary. Arrangements should be made for immediate transfer to an emergency facility for further evaluation and treatment. All patients should be observed for at least 12 hours after the onset of symptoms.[203]

Postvaccination syncope, unrelated to allergy, also can occur, most commonly among adolescents and young adults. In a report of 697 cases of syncope after vaccination, six patients suffered skull fractures, cerebral bleeding, or cerebral contusion from falls.[204] Nearly 90% of the cases of syncope in this series occurred within 15 minutes or less of vaccination, and 98% of cases occurred within 30 minutes. Because of the small risk of an anaphylactic reaction and the unrelated risk of postvaccination syncope, the AAP recommends observation for 15 to 20 minutes after immunization whenever possible.[2] If syncope develops, patients should be observed until the symptoms resolve.

Special Considerations

Vaccination of Preterm Infants

The immune response to vaccination is a function of postnatal rather than of gestational age.[205-207] Transplacentally acquired maternal antibody is present in lower concentrations and thus persists for a shorter interval in preterm infants than in gestationally mature infants.[206,208-210] Because premature infants have less transplacentally acquired maternal antibody, inhibition of the immune response in premature infants may be less than that in full-term infants.[206,211]

DTP, OPV, IPV, and Hib vaccines generally are immunogenic and safe for preterm infants when vaccination is initiated at the same chronologic age (i.e., approximately 2 months) and administered according to the same routine schedule as for full-term infants.[212-219] However, some studies also suggest that the immune response to certain vaccines may be impaired when vaccination of extremely premature infants or those of very low birth weight is initiated at the usual time.[215,216,219-223] For example, D'Angio et al.[215] reported that a similar proportion of extremely premature infants (i.e., less than 29 weeks' gestation and birth weight less than 1000 g) and full-term infants had protective antibody concentrations to tetanus toxoid, Hib, and poliovirus serotypes 1 and 2 after a vaccination series of three doses of DTP and Hib vaccines and two doses of poliovirus vaccine (i.e., IPV followed by OPV) initiated at a chronologic age of 2 months. However, the preterm infants were less likely to have detectable antibody to poliovirus serotype 3. Protective antibody titers against diphtheria, tetanus, Hib polyribosylribitol phosphate (PRP), and poliovirus serotypes 1 and 2 were still present when the children were retested at 3 to 4 years of age. However, in the follow-up study, a lower proportion of premature infants had anti-PRP antibody titers greater than 1.0 μg/mL than did full-term infants (50% vs. 88%, respectively).[224] Munoz et al.[225] also reported that, after administration of Hib vaccine at 2 and 4 months' postnatal age, the geometric mean concentration of serum Hib antibody was significantly lower among infants with a gestational age less than 28 weeks than in other infants.

Lau et al. reported that the seroconversion rate to hepatitis B vaccine was lower in preterm infants weighing less than 2000 g who were vaccinated soon after birth than in preterm infants vaccinated at a later age or term infants vaccinated shortly after birth.[222] Other investigators have observed a diminished immune response to hepatitis B vaccine among premature infants of lower gestational ages (e.g., less than 33 weeks) or of lower birth weights (e.g., less than 2000 g).[218,225–227] However, by chronologic age 1 month, all premature infants, regardless of initial birth weight or gestational age, are as likely to respond as adequately as older and larger infants.[227–229] Premature infants born to HbsAG-positive women must receive immunoprophylaxis with hepatitis B vaccine and hepititis B immune globulin (HBIG) within 12 hours after birth.[230,231] If these infants weigh less than 2,000 g at birth, the initial vaccine dose should not be counted toward completion of the hepititis B vaccine series, and three additional doses of hepatitis B vacine should be administered, beginning when the infant is age 1 month.[5] For preterm infants born to mothers not tested for HbsAg during pregnancy, the maternal HbsAg status should be determined as soon as possible after delivery and the infant should recive hepititis B vaccine within 12 hours after birth. If these infants weigh less than 2,000 g at birth, HBIG (0.5 mL) should also be given if the mother's HbsAg test result is not available within the initial 12 hours of birth, because of the potentially reduced immunogenicity of vaccine in these infants. In addition, the initial vaccine dose should not be counted towards completion of the hepatitis B vaccine series, and three additional doses of hepatitis B vaccine should be administered, beginning when the infant is age 1 month. The optimal timing of the first dose of hepatitis B vaccine for premature infants of HBsAg-negative mothers with a birth weight of less than 2000 g has not been determined. However, these infants can receive the first dose of the hepatitis B vaccine series at a chronologic age of 1 month. Premature infants discharged from the hospital before a chronologic age of 1 month can receive hepatitis B vaccine at discharge, if they are medically stable and have gained weight consistently.[5]

Several studies suggest that the incidence of adverse events after vaccination of preterm infants is the same as or lower than that of full-term infants vaccinated at the same chronologic age.[212,215,216] A temporal association between receipt of DTP and Hib vaccine and a transient increase or recurrence of apnea in premature infants has been reported, although the significance of this finding is unclear.[232]

In summary, infants who are born prematurely should be immunized at the same postnatal chronologic age and according to the same recommended schedule as full-term infants.[5,231] The one exception, as previously discussed, is hepatitis B vaccine. The recommended standard dose of each vaccine should be administered; divided or reduced doses are not indicated.[5,231,232–235] A preterm infant who is still hospitalized at age 2 months can receive the vaccines routinely scheduled at that age. However, in those countries in which IPV is used, although OPV is the polio vaccine of choice, IPV may be considered for hospitalized infants. Because poliovirus vaccine strains are excreted after receipt of OPV, IPV will decrease the risk of transmission of vaccine viruses in the hospital.[39,231]

Breast-Feeding and Immunization

Neither inactivated nor live virus vaccines administered to a lactating mother or infant who is breast-feeding have adverse consequences.[2,5] Because inactivated and component vaccines do not multiply within the body, they pose no special risk for lactating mothers or their infants. Lactating mothers also may safely receive live virus vaccines, such as yellow fever, MMR, OPV, varicella, and rubella, without interruption of their breast-feeding schedule.[5,79,231,236] Although vaccines that contain attenuated live viruses or bacteria replicate within the vaccine recipient, most live vaccine strains are not known to be secreted in human milk. An exception is attenuated rubella vaccine virus, which has been detected in human milk and recovered from the nasopharynxes and throats of some breast-fed infants after maternal immunization.[237,238] In one study, transient seroconversion to rubella virus without evidence of clinical disease was noted in 25% of the breast-fed infants.[237]

Breast-feeding of infants does not adversely affect their development of a protective immune response and is not a contraindication for any vaccine.[5,236,239–244] The antibody responses to the components of DTP and Hib conjugate vaccines are not inhibited by breast-feeding.[82,245,246] Vaccination of breast-fed infants results in protective immunity, although doses of OPV administered to these infants during the first 3 days of life may be somewhat less effective than doses administered to older breast-fed infants and infants who are not breast-fed.[82,240,241,243,247,248] Breast-fed infants who acquired rubella vaccine virus and rubella-specific antibodies from human milk have a normal immune response to rubella vaccine administered at 15 to 18 months of age.[242]

Compared with infants who are formula fed, breast-fed infants may have an enhanced immune response to certain oral and parenteral vaccines, such as conjugate Hib vaccine, OPV, and DT.[246,249–251] However, the significance of such an effect is unclear.

Oral rhesus rotavirus vaccine is a possible exception to the lack of inhibition by breast-feeding of the immune response to vaccines. Meta-analyses of studies using a single dose of various rhesus rotavirus vaccines concluded that the immune response to these vaccines was reduced in breast-fed infants.[252,253] However, the potential inhibitory effect is largely overcome by administration of three doses of vaccine, and no significant decrease in the protective efficacy of rhesus rotavirus vaccine was observed in breast-fed compared with non–breast-fed infants.[254,255]

Vaccination During Pregnancy

Risk to a developing fetus from vaccination of the mother during pregnancy is primarily theoretical. No evidence exists of risk from vaccinating pregnant women with inactivated virus or bacterial vaccines or toxoids.[256,257] Benefits of vaccinating pregnant women usually outweigh potential risks when the likelihood of disease exposure is high, when infection would pose a risk to the mother or fetus, and when the vaccine is unlikely to cause harm. Table 8–7 lists vaccines that are indicated and contraindicated during

TABLE 8–7 ■ Vaccination During Pregnancy

Vaccine	Type	Indications for Vaccination During Pregnancy
LIVE VIRUS		
Measles-mumps-rubella	Live, attenuated virus	Contraindicated
Poliomyelitis	Trivalent live, attenuated virus (oral poliovirus vaccine)	Persons at substantial risk of exposure to polio
Varicella	Live, attenuated virus	Contraindicated
Yellow fever	Live, attenuated virus	Contraindicated, except if exposure to yellow fever virus is unavoidable
LIVE BACTERIAL		
Typhoid	Live, attenuated bacteria (Ty21a)	Should reflect actual risks of disease and probable benefits of vaccine
INACTIVATED VIRUS		
Hepatitis A	Inactivated virus	Data on safety in pregnancy are not available; should weigh the theoretical risk of vaccination against the risk of disease
Hepatitis B	Recombinant-produced, purified hepatitis B surface antigen	Pregnancy is not a contraindication
Influenza	Inactivated type A and type B virus components	Recommended both for women who will be in the second or third trimester during influenza season and for patients with serious underlying disease; consult health authorities for current recommendations
Japanese encephalitis	Inactivated virus	Should reflect actual risks of disease and probable benefits of vaccine
Poliomyelitis	Inactivated virus (inactivated poliovirus vaccine)	Persons at substantial risk of exposure to polio
Rabies	Inactivated virus	Substantial risk of exposure
INACTIVATED BACTERIAL		
Haemophilus influenzae type b conjugate	Polysaccharide-protein	Only for high-risk persons
Meningococcal	Polysaccharide	Only in unusual outbreak situations
Pneumococcal	Polysaccharide	Only for high-risk persons
Typhoid	Polysaccharide	Should reflect actual risks of disease and probable benefits of exposure
TOXOIDS		
Tetanus-diphtheria	Combined tetanus-diphtheria toxoids, adult formulation (Td)	Lack of primary series, or no booster within last 10 yr (5 yr, if other than clean minor wounds)
OTHER		
Immune globulins, pooled or hyperimmune	Immune globulin or specific globulin preparations	Exposure or anticipated exposure to measles, hepatitis A, hepatitis B, rabies, tetanus

pregnancy. No known risk exists for the fetus from passive immunization of pregnant women with immune globulin preparations.

Use of Live Vaccines

Live vaccines contain attenuated viruses or bacteria that multiply within the vaccine recipient. Because some of the diseases they prevent, such as rubella or varicella, are known to have teratogenic or other serious effects on the fetus, live virus vaccines usually are contraindicated during pregnancy.[5,231,239] All pregnant women should be evaluated for immunity to rubella.[79,258] Women susceptible to rubella should be vaccinated immediately after delivery.

Pregnancy should be avoided for 4 weeks after the receipt of parenteral live virus vaccines, by which time antibody production usually has occurred and vaccine-virus viremia is expected to have ceased.[79,236,259] Routine pregnancy testing of women of child-bearing age before administering a live virus vaccine is not recommended.[5,79] The ACIP recommends that the clinician should ask if a woman is pregnant or attempting to become pregnant, not administer live virus vaccines if a woman states that she is pregnant or attempting to become pregnant, explain the potential risk for the fetus to the woman who states that she is not pregnant, and then administer the indicated live virus vaccine.[5,79] Both OPV and yellow fever vaccine can be administered to pregnant women who are nonimmune and at substantial risk of imminent exposure to infection, such as from impending international travel.[5,231,260]

Despite precautions, some pregnant women may be inadvertently vaccinated with a live virus vaccine, or a woman may become pregnant soon after receiving a live virus vaccine. Available data have not demonstrated any serious risk to the mother or fetus.[259,261–269] Because of the existing safety data and because the risk to the fetus is largely theoretical, administration of a live vaccine during pregnancy is not a reason to consider interruption of the pregnancy.[79,236] A Varicella Vaccination in Pregnancy Registry, like that which documented the apparent safety of inadvertent rubella vaccination during pregnancy, has been established to monitor prospectively maternal-fetal outcomes in pregnant women inadvertently vaccinated with varicella vaccine (U.S. telephone: 1-800-986-8999).[231,236]

Use of Inactivated Vaccines

Inactivated and component vaccines pose no special risk during pregnancy because they do not multiply within the body. Although one study reported an association between administration of IPV during pregnancy and malignant neoplasms of neural origin in offspring,[270] this finding has not been confirmed by other investigators, and IPV can be administered to a pregnant woman who requires immediate protection against poliomyelitis.[5,231,260] Other inactivated and component vaccines and toxoids are not known to be deleterious when they are administered during pregnancy and are sometimes indicated to prevent infection with possible serious outcomes for both mother and fetus.

Hepatitis B vaccine is recommended for pregnant women at risk for hepatitis B virus infection.[230] Hepatitis A, pneumococcal polysaccharide, and meningococcal polysaccharide vaccines should be considered for women at increased risk for those infections.[271–273]

Healthy women in the second and third trimesters of pregnancy have been demonstrated to be at increased risk for hospitalization from influenza.[274] Therefore, routine influenza vaccination is recommended for healthy women who will be beyond the first trimester of pregnancy (i.e., ≥14 weeks of gestation) during influenza season (usually December through March in the United States).[168] Women who have medical conditions that increase their risk for complications of influenza should be vaccinated before the influenza season, regardless of the stage of pregnancy.

In some cases, vaccination during pregnancy is intended to protect the fetus or newborn infant from infection. For example, neonatal tetanus remains common in many developing countries where women are not adequately immunized before pregnancy and childbirth and protection of the newborn infant from neonatal tetanus is dependent on placental transfer of maternal antibody from an immune mother.[275,276] Widespread vaccination of pregnant women in such areas has demonstrated the safety and efficacy of administering tetanus toxoid during pregnancy to prevent neonatal tetanus.[277] In the United States, administration of Td is recommended for pregnant women who have not completed a primary vaccination series or who need a booster dose.[5,155,239]

Some physicians prefer to wait until the second or third trimester of pregnancy to administer inactivated or component vaccines or toxoids.[239] However, no increased risk to the mother or fetus from vaccination during the first trimester has been demonstrated, and vaccination in some cases may be indicated before the second or third trimester. Examples include influenza, hepatitis B, and Td vaccines.[5,168,230,231,239]

Vaccination of Household Contacts

Administration of both live and inactivated vaccines to household members does not present a known hazard to pregnant women. Although transmission of varicella vaccine virus from a 12-month-old infant to his pregnant mother has been reported, no virus was detected in fetal tissue after an elective abortion.[278] Pregnancy of a mother is not a contraindication to administration of varicella vaccine, or any other vaccine in the childhood immunization schedule, to her child.[236,279]

Vaccines Received Outside the United States

The ability of a clinician to determine that a person is protected on the basis of country of origin and his or her records alone is limited. Only written documentation should be accepted as evidence of prior vaccination. Written records are more likely to predict protection if the vaccines, dates of administration, intervals between doses, and the person's age at the time of immunization are comparable to the current U.S. recommendations.[5] Although vaccines with inadequate potency have been produced in other countries,[280,281] the majority of vaccines used worldwide are produced with adequate quality control standards and are potent.

The number of American families adopting children from outside the United States has increased substantially in recent years.[282] Adopted children's birth countries often have immunization schedules that differ from the recommended childhood immunization schedule in the United States. Differences between that schedule and those used in other countries include the vaccines administered, the recommended ages of administration, and the number and timing of doses (see Chapter 55). The ACIP has published guidelines for assessing and vaccinating international adoptees.[5] Children adopted in the United States from other countries should receive vaccines according to U.S.-recommended schedules.

Data are inconclusive regarding the extent to which an internationally adopted child's immunization record reflects the child's protection. A child's record might indicate administration of MMR vaccine when only single-antigen measles vaccine was administered. A study of children adopted from the People's Republic of China, Russia, and Eastern Europe determined that only 39% (range 17% to 88% by country) of children with documentation of more than three doses of DTP before adoption had protective serologic concentrations of diphtheria and tetanus antitoxin.[283] This raised questions about whether the vaccines received were potent, or whether the immunization records purporting to show receipt of at least three doses were an accurate reflection of the true number of doses actually received. However, antibody testing was performed by a hemagglutination assay, which may underestimate protection and cannot directly be compared with antitoxin concentration measured by other tests.[284] A second study measured antibody to diphtheria and tetanus toxins among 51 children who had records of having received two or more doses of DTP. The majority of the children were from Russia, Eastern Europe, and Asian countries, and 78% had received all their vaccine doses in an orphanage. Ninety-four percent had evidence of protection against diphtheria (enzyme immunoassay [EIA] >0.1 IU/mL). A total of 84% had protection against tetanus (EIA >0.5 IU/mL). Among children without protective tetanus antitoxin concentration, all except one had records of three or more doses of vaccine, and the majority of nonprotective concentrations were categorized as indeterminate (EIA = 0.05 to 0.49 IU/mL).[285] Reasons for the discrepant findings in these two studies probably relate to different laboratory methodologies; the study using a hemagglutination assay might have underestimated the number of children who were protected. Additional studies using standardized methodologies are needed.

If a question exists regarding whether vaccines administered outside the United States were immunogenic, several approaches may be considered. Repeating the vaccinations as age-appropriate is an acceptable option; this usually is safe and avoids the need to obtain and interpret serologic tests.[5] If avoiding unnecessary injections is desired, judicious use of serologic testing can be helpful in determining which immunizations are needed, particularly for DTP/DTaP vaccine. Although no established serologic correlates exist for protection against pertussis, diphtheria and tetanus antitoxin levels may be used as surrogates to assess whether doses listed on the immunization record were actually received or were potent.[85]

Vaccination providers can revaccinate a child with DTaP vaccine without regard to recorded doses. However, increased rates of moderate to severe local adverse reactions after the fourth and fifth doses of DTP or DTaP have been reported.[148] If a revaccination option is adopted and a severe local reaction occurs, serologic testing for specific immunoglobulin G (IgG) antibody to tetanus and diphtheria toxins can be performed before administering additional doses. Protective concentrations indicate that further doses are unnecessary, and subsequent vaccination should occur as age appropriate.

Instead of revaccinating a child with DTaP when there is a question about the validity of a record that indicates receipt of three or more doses of DTP or DTaP, serologic testing for specific IgG antibody to both diphtheria and tetanus toxin can be obtained. If a protective concentration is present, recorded doses can be considered valid, and the vaccination series should be completed as age appropriate. Indeterminate antibody concentration might indicate immunologic memory but waning antibody. Serology can be repeated after a booster dose if the vaccination provider wishes to avoid revaccination with a complete series.[5]

A third alternative for a child with a record of three or more prior doses of DTP or DTaP, where there is concern about the validity of the record, is to administer a single booster dose, followed by serologic testing after 1 month for specific IgG antibody to both diphtheria and tetanus toxins. If a protective concentration is obtained, the recorded doses can be considered valid and the vaccination series completed as age appropriate. Children with indeterminate concentration after a booster dose should be revaccinated with a complete series.[5]

Serologic testing for HBsAg is recommended for international adoptees. Children determined to be HBsAg positive should be monitored for development of liver disease.[231] Household members of HBsAg-positive children should be vaccinated. A child whose records indicate receipt of three or more doses of vaccine can be considered protected, and additional doses are not needed if at least one dose was administered at or after 6 months of age. Children who received their last hepatitis B vaccine dose at less than 6 months of age should receive an additional dose at 6 months of age or older.[5] Those who have received fewer than three doses should complete the series at the recommended intervals and ages (see Table 8–3).

Vaccination of Persons with a Personal or Family History of Seizures

Infants and young children with either a personal history of seizures or a parent or sibling with a history of seizures are at increased risk for seizures after receipt of whole-cell pertussis or MMR (or monovalent measles) vaccine.[79,286,287] In most cases, these seizures are brief, self-limited, and associated with fever. Studies have not established a causal association between these seizures and residual seizure disorders or permanent neurologic sequelae.[288,289] Because acellular pertussis vaccines are associated less frequently with fever than are whole-cell pertussis vaccines, DTaP vaccine is preferred for immunizing children in the United States against pertussis.[85,148]

Because neurologic disorders such as epilepsy or degenerative disorders marked by loss of developmental milestones often become manifest during infancy, pertussis vaccination may coincide with onset or recognition of such disorders and cause confusion about the etiologic role of the vaccine. For infants with a personal history of a seizure, delaying pertussis vaccination is recommended until a progressive neurologic disorder is excluded or the cause of the seizure has been established.[87,231] Acetaminophen or ibuprofen can be administered at the time of pertussis vaccination and every 4 hours for 24 hours thereafter to reduce the possibility of postvaccination fever.[85] Because measles vaccine is administered at an age when a child's neurologic status is likely to already have been established, deferring measles immunization of a child with a personal history of a seizure is not recommended.[79,231]

Pertussis and measles vaccinations are not contraindicated in persons with a family history of seizures. Even though children with a parent or sibling who has had a seizure are themselves at increased risk for a seizure, the benefits of administering pertussis and measles vaccine to children with a family history of convulsions substantially outweigh the small risks because the seizures are usually febrile in origin, generally have a benign outcome, and are not likely to be confused with manifestations of a previously unrecognized neurologic disorder.[79,85,231,288,289]

Vaccination During Acute Illness

The decision to administer or delay vaccination because of an intercurrent or recent acute illness depends on evaluation of the etiology of the disease and the severity of symptoms.[2,5] Mild illness, either febrile (≥38°C) or afebrile, is not a contraindication to vaccination.[2,5] Although one study reported a lower rate of seroconversion to the measles but not to the rubella or mumps components of MMR vaccine in children with evidence of a recent or current upper respiratory tract infection compared with children without this history,[290] a difference in seroconversion to measles vaccine in healthy children compared with children who are ill has not been found in other studies.[114,291–295]

Acute minor illnesses, such as upper respiratory tract infection, diarrhea, and acute otitis media, are common during infancy and childhood.[296] Postponing vaccination in children with minor febrile or afebrile illness constitutes a missed opportunity to protect a child from disease, can contribute to outbreaks of vaccine-preventable disease, and can significantly impede efforts to immunize infants and young children on schedule.[297–300] Every opportunity should be used to provide indicated vaccines and to avoid missed opportunities in persons who may not return for medical care and administration of recommended vaccines.[2,5,301] The potential benefit of preventing disease by timely vaccination far outweighs any small possible risk of vaccine failure.

Vaccination usually is deferred in persons who have moderate or severe illness. A person with signs or symptoms of moderate or severe illness at the scheduled time of vaccination should be requested to return as soon as the illness improves so that vaccines can be administered at the recommended ages. Waiting until after a person has recovered from the acute phase of a moderate or severe illness avoids superimposing a reaction to vaccination on the underlying illness or mistakenly attributing a manifestation of the underlying illness to the vaccine.[2,5]

Contraindications to and Precautions Regarding Vaccination

Vaccine contraindications and precautions are described in the manufacturer's product labeling and in the recommendations for the use of vaccines developed by national advisory committees such as the ACIP and the Committee on Infectious Diseases of the AAP. In the United States, the content of the product label is regulated by the Food and Drug Administration on the basis of specific studies required of the manufacturer to prove the safety and efficacy of a specific product. Most recommendations of vaccine advisory committees are the same as those in the product label. However, differences sometimes exist because of advisory committees' assessments of the risks and benefits of a given recommendation, their goal to make immunization as practical as possible, and their responsibility to develop recommendations for the use of vaccines in circumstances in which specific safety and efficacy data may be limited but for which physicians, nurses, and public health officials need guidance. For example, the manufacturer's product label recommends that women vaccinated with live varicella virus vaccine avoid becoming pregnant for

3 months, whereas the ACIP and AAP advise waiting only 1 month.[1,236,302] Similarly, the AAP and ACIP advise that pregnancy should not be considered a contraindication to hepatitis B vaccination, whereas the manufacturer's product label states that hepatitis B vaccine should be administered to pregnant women if it is indicated.[1,230,303]

A contraindication indicates that a vaccine should not be administered. In contrast, a precaution specifies a situation in which vaccine may be indicated if the benefit of vaccination to the individual patient is judged to outweigh the risk.[5] Contraindications and precautions may be generic and apply to all vaccines, or they may be specific to one or more vaccines (Table 8–8). The following two guidelines apply to all vaccines: (1) an anaphylactic reaction to a vaccine or vaccine constituent contraindicates further use of that vaccine or vaccines containing that constituent (see *Vaccine Components Causing Hypersensitivity*), and (2) moderate or severe acute illness, regardless of the absence or presence of fever, is a precaution to vaccination (see *Vaccination During Acute Illness*).

Immunosuppression resulting from underlying disease or therapy is a contraindication for receipt of most live vaccines.[5,79,231] Exceptions are measles and varicella vaccines, which are recommended for HIV-infected persons who are not severely immunosuppressed.[79,231,304,305] Corticosteroid therapy can suppress the immune system of an otherwise healthy person, although the minimal dose and duration of therapy necessary to cause immunosuppression are not well defined. Underlying disease, concurrent therapies, and the frequency and route of administration of corticosteroids also can affect immunosuppression. Steroid therapy does not usually contraindicate administration of live vaccines when given in low to moderate doses administered daily or on alternate days, physiologic maintenance doses, or doses administered topically, by aerosol, or by local (e.g., intra-articular) injection.[5,79,231] In most cases, persons receiving high doses of systemic corticosteroids (i.e., at least 2 mg/kg per day, or 20 mg/day of prednisone or its equivalent) for less than 14 days can receive live vaccines immediately after discontinuation of therapy.[2,5] However, live vaccines usually are not administered to persons who have received high doses of systemic corticosteroids for 14 days or more until at least 1 month after cessation of steroid therapy.[5,231]

Live vaccines usually are contraindicated for pregnant women because of a theoretical risk to the fetus (see *Vaccination During Pregnancy*). However, the small theoretical risk from administration of a live vaccine to a pregnant woman is sometimes far outweighed by the risk of contracting a disease with serious consequences for mother and fetus.

Health care providers sometimes inappropriately consider a condition to be a contraindication or precaution to vaccination.[2,5] Withholding vaccine in such instances results in a missed opportunity to administer needed vaccine. A concise summary of appropriate and inappropriate contraindications, as of February 2002, is given in Table 8–8, adapted from the national *Standards for Pediatric Immunization Practices* (see Chapter 53).

TABLE 8–8 ■ Guide to Contraindications to and Precautions Regarding Commonly Used Vaccines*

Vaccine	True Contraindications and Precautions*	Untrue (Vaccines Can Be Administered)
General for all vaccines, including diphtheria and tetanus toxoids and whole-cell/acellular pertussis vaccine (DTP/DTaP); pediatric diphtheria-tetanus toxoid (DT); adult tetanus-diphtheria toxoid (Td); live (OPV) or inactivated (IPV) poliovirus vaccine; measles-mumps-rubella vaccine (MMR); *Haemophilus influenzae* type b vaccine (Hib); hepatitis A vaccine; hepatitis B vaccine; varicella vaccine; pneumococcal conjugate vaccine (PCV); influenza vaccine; and pneumococcal poly-saccharide vaccine (PPV)	*Contraindications* Serious allergic reaction (e.g., anaphylaxis) after a previous vaccine dose Serious allergic reaction (e.g., anaphylaxis) to a vaccine component *Precautions*† Moderate or severe acute illness with or without fever	Mild acute illness with or without low-grade fever Mild to moderate local reaction (i.e., swelling, redness, soreness); low-grade or moderate fever after previous dose Lack of previous physical examination in well-appearing infant or child Current antimicrobial therapy Convalescent phase of illness Premature birth (hepatitis B vaccine might be an exception in certain circumstances)‡ Recent exposure to an infectious disease History of penicillin allergy, other nonvaccine allergies, relatives with allergies, receiving allergen extract immunotherapy
DTP/DTaP	*Contraindications* Severe allergic reaction after a previous dose or to a vaccine component Encephalopathy (e.g., coma, decreased level of consciousness; prolonged seizures) within 7 days of administration of previous dose of DTP or DTaP Progressive neurologic disorder, including infantile spasms, uncontrolled epilepsy, progressive encephalopathy: defer DTP/DTaP until neurologic status is clarified and stabilized *Precautions*† Fever of >40.5°C ≤48 h after vaccination with a previous dose of DTP/DTaP Collapse or shock-like state (i.e., hypotonic hyporesponsive episode) ≤48 h after receiving a previous dose of DTP/DTaP Seizure within 3 days of receiving a previous dose of DTP/DTaP§ Persistent, inconsolable crying lasting ≥3 h ≤48 h after receiving a previous dose of DTP/DTaP Moderate or severe acute illness with or without fever	Temperature of <40.5°C, fussiness or mild drowsiness after a previous dose of DTP/DTaP Family history of seizures§ Family history of sudden infant death syndrome Family history of an adverse event after DTP/DTaP administration Stable neurologic conditions (e.g., cerebral palsy, well-controlled convulsions, developmental delay)
DT, Td	*Contraindication* Severe allergic reaction after a previous dose or to a vaccine component *Precautions*† Guillain-Barré syndrome ≤6 wk after previous dose of tetanus toxoid–containing vaccine Moderate or severe acute illness with or without fever	—
IPV	*Contraindication* Severe allergic reaction to previous dose or vaccine component *Precautions*† Pregnancy Moderate or severe acute illness with or without fever	—
OPV	*Contraindications* Severe allergic reaction to previous dose or vaccine component Infection with human immunodeficiency virus (HIV) or a household contact with HIV infection	Breast-feeding Current antimicrobial therapy Mild diarrhea

Continued

TABLE 8–8 ■ Guide to Contraindications to and Precautions Regarding Commonly Used Vaccines*—cont'd

Vaccine	True Contraindications and Precautions*	Untrue (Vaccines Can Be Administered)
	Known immunodeficiency (hematologic and solid tumors; congenital immunodeficiency; long-term immunosuppressive therapy) Immunodeficient household contact *Precautions*† Pregnancy Moderate or severe acute illness with or without fever	
MMR‖	*Contraindications* Severe allergic reaction after a previous dose or to a vaccine component (e.g., gelatin) Pregnancy Known severe immunodeficiency (e.g., hematologic and solid tumors; congenital immunodeficiency; long-term immunosuppressive therapy¶ or severely symptomatic HIV infection) *Precautions*† Recent (≤11 mo) receipt of antibody-containing blood product (specific interval depends on product; see text and Table 8–6) History of thrombocytopenia or thrombocytopenic purpura Moderate or severe acute illness with or without fever	Positive tuberculin (TB) skin test Simultaneous TB skin testing** Breast-feeding Pregnancy of recipient's mother or other close or household contact Recipient is child-bearing-age female Immunodeficient family member or household contact Asymptomatic or mildly symptomatic HIV infection Allergy to eggs
Hib	*Contraindications* Severe allergic reaction after a previous dose or to a vaccine component Age <6 wk *Precaution*† Moderate or severe acute illness with or without fever	—
Hepatitis B	*Contraindication* Severe allergic reaction after a previous dose or to a vaccine component *Precautions*† Infant weighing <2000 g‡ Moderate or severe acute illness with or without fever	Pregnancy Autoimmune disease (e.g., systemic lupus erythematosis or rheumatoid arthritis)
Hepatitis A	*Contraindication* Severe allergic reaction after a previous dose or to a vaccine component *Precautions*† Pregnancy Moderate or severe acute illness with or without fever	—
Varicella‖	*Contraindications* Severe allergic reaction after a previous dose or to a vaccine component Substantial suppression of cellular immunity Pregnancy *Precautions*† Recent (<11 mo) receipt of antibody-containing blood product (specific interval depends on product; see text and Table 8–6) Moderate or severe acute illness with or without fever	Pregnancy of recipient's mother or other close or household contact Immunodeficient family member or household contact†† Asymptomatic or mildly symptomatic HIV infection Humoral immunodeficiency (e.g., agammaglobulinemia)
PCV	*Contraindication* Severe allergic reaction after a previous dose or to a vaccine component *Precaution*† Moderate or severe acute illness with or without fever	—
Influenza	*Contraindication* Severe allergic reaction to previous dose or vaccine component, including egg protein *Precaution*† Moderate or severe acute illness with or without fever	Nonsevere (e.g., contact) allergy to latex or thimerosal Concurrent administration of coumadin or aminophylline

Continued

TABLE 8–8 ■ Guide to Contraindications to and Precautions Regarding Commonly Used Vaccines*—cont'd

Vaccine	True Contraindications and Precautions*	Untrue (Vaccines Can Be Administered)
PPV	*Contraindication* Severe allergic reaction after a previous dose or to a vaccine component *Precaution*† Moderate or severe acute illness with or without fever	—

*This information is based on the recommendations of the Advisory Committee on Immunization Practices (ACIP), and of the Committee on Infectious Diseases of the American Academy of Pediatrics (AAP). Sometimes these recommendations vary from those in the manufacturer's product label. For more detailed information, health care providers should consult the published recommendations of the ACIP, AAP, the American Academy of Family Physicians (AAFP), and the manufacturer's product label.

†Events or conditions listed as precautions should be reviewed carefully. Benefits and risks of administering a specific vaccine to a person under these circumstances should be considered. If the risk from the vaccine is believed to outweigh the benefit, the vaccine should not be administered. If the benefit of vaccination is believed to outweigh the risk, the vaccine should be administered. Whether and when to administer DTP/DTaP to children with proven or suspected underlying neurologic disorders should be decided on a case-by-case basis.

‡Hepatitis B vaccination should be deferred for infants weighing less than 2000 g if the mother is documented to be hepatitis B surface antigen (HbsAg) negative at the time of the infant's birth. Vaccination can commence at chronologic age 1 month. For infants born to HbsAg-positive women, hepatitis B immune globulin and hepatitis B vaccine should be administered at or soon after birth regardless of weight.

§Acetaminophen or other appropriate antipyretic can be administered to children with a personal or family history of seizures at the time of DTaP vaccination and every 4 to 6 hours for 24 hours thereafter to reduce the possibility of postvaccination fever.

‖MMR and varicella vaccines can be administered on the same day. If not administered on the same day, these vaccines should be separated by 28 or more days.

¶Substantially immunosuppressive steroid dose is considered to be 2 or more weeks of daily receipt of 20 mg, or 2 mg/kg body weight, of prednisone or equivalent.

**Measles vaccination can suppress tuberculin reactivity temporarily. Measles-containing vaccine can be administered on the same day as tuberculin skin testing. If testing cannot be performed until after the day of MMR vaccination, the test should be postponed for 4 or more weeks after the vaccine. If an urgent need exists to skin test, do so with the understanding that reactivity might be reduced by the vaccine.

††If a vaccinee experiences a presumed vaccine-related rash 7 to 25 days after vaccination, he or she should avoid direct contact with immunocompromised persons for the duration of the rash.

REFERENCES

1. Physicians' Desk Reference. Montvale, NJ, Medical Economics Company, 2002.
2. American Academy of Pediatrics. Active immunization. *In* Pickering L (ed). 2003 Red Book: Report of the Committee on Infectious Diseases (26th ed). Elk Grove Village, IL, American Academy of Pediatrics, 2003, pp 7–53.
3. Vaccine Management: Recommendations for Handling and Storage of Selected Biologicals. Atlanta, Centers for Disease Control and Prevention, 1996.
4. Galazka A, Milstien J, Zaffran M. Thermostability of Vaccines (WHO/GPV/98.07). Geneva, World Health Organization, 1998.
5. Centers for Disease Control and Prevention. General recommendations on immunization: recommendations of the Advisory Committee on Immunization Practices (ACIP). MMWR 51(RR-2):1–35, 2002.
6. Centers for Disease Control. Yellow fever vaccine: recommendations of the Immunization Practices Advisory Committee (ACIP). MMWR 39(RR-6):1–6, 1990.
7. Kendal AP, Synder R, Garrison PJ. Validation of cold chain procedures suitable for distribution of vaccines by public health programs in the USA. Vaccine 15:1459–1465, 1997.
8. Fulginiti VA. Practical aspects of immunization practice. *In* Fulginiti VA (ed). Immunization in Clinical Practice. Philadelphia, JB Lippincott, 1982, pp 49–55.
9. Widmer AF, Frey R. Decontamination, disinfection and sterilization. *In* Manual of Clinical Microbiology (7th ed). Washington, DC, American Society for Microbiology, 1999, pp 138–164.
10. Shaw FE Jr, Guess HA, Roets JM, et al. Effect of anatomic injection site, age, and smoking on the immune response to hepatitis B vaccination. Vaccine 7:425–430, 1989.
11. Fishbein DB, Sawyer LA, Reid-Sanden FL, Weir EH. Administration of human diploid-cell rabies vaccine in the gluteal area [letter]. N Engl J Med 318:124–125, 1988.
12. Bergeson PS, Singer SA, Kaplan AM. Intramuscular injections in children. Pediatrics 70:944–948, 1982.
13. Lachman E. Applied anatomy of intragluteal injections. Am Surg 29:236–241, 1963.
14. Centers for Disease Control and Prevention. The role of BCG vaccine in the prevention and control of tuberculosis in the United States: a joint statement by the Advisory Council for the Elimination of Tuberculosis and the Advisory Committee on Immunization Practices. MMWR 45(RR-4):1–18, 1996.
15. Scheifele D, Bjornson G, Barreto L, et al. Controlled trial of *Haemophilus influenzae* type B diphtheria toxoid conjugate combined with diphtheria, tetanus and pertussis vaccines, in 18-month-old children, including comparison of arm versus thigh injection. Vaccine 10:455–460, 1992.
16. Ipp MM, Gold R, Goldbach M, et al. Adverse reactions to diphtheria, tetanus, pertussis-polio vaccination at 18 months of age: effect of injection site and needle length. Pediatrics 83:679–682, 1989.
17. Bergeson PS. Immunizations in the deltoid region [letter]. Pediatrics 85:134–135, 1990.
18. American College of Physicians Task Force on Adult Immunization and Infectious Diseases Society of America. General recommendations for adult immunization. *In* Guide for Adult Immunization (3rd ed). Philadelphia, American College of Physicians, 1994, pp 1–11.
19. Gilles FH, French JH. Postinjection sciatic nerve palsies in infants and children. J Pediatr 58:195–204, 1961.
20. Combes MA, Clark WK, Gregory CF, James JA. Sciatic nerve injury in infants: recognition and prevention of impairment resulting from intragluteal injections. JAMA 173:1336–1339, 1960.
21. Curtiss PH, Tucker HJ. Sciatic palsy in premature infants: a report and follow-up study of ten cases. JAMA 174:1586–1588, 1960.
22. Brandt PA, Smith ME, Ashburn SS, Graves J. IM injections in children. Am J Nurs 72:1402–1406, 1972.
23. Gilles FH, Matson DD. Sciatic nerve injury following misplaced gluteal injections. J Pediatr 76:247–254, 1970.

24. Clark K, Williams PE Jr, Willis W, McGavran WL. Injection injury of the sciatic nerve. Clin Neurosurg 17:111–125, 1969.

25. MacDonald NE, Marcuse EK. Neurologic injury after vaccination: buttocks as injection site [letter]. Can Med Assoc J 150:326, 1994.

26. Marcuse EK, MacDonald NE. Neurologic injury after vaccination in buttocks [letter]. Can Med Assoc J 155:374, 1996.

27. Marcuse EK, MacDonald NE. Vaccine injury—no reports [letter]. Pediatrics 99:144, 1997.

28. Grosswasser J, Kahn A, Bouche B, et al. Needle length and injection technique for efficient intramuscular vaccine delivery in infants and children evaluated through an ultrasonographic determination of subcutaneous and muscle layer thickness. Pediatrics 100:400–403, 1997.

29. World Health Organization. Module 3: When and how to give vaccines. *In* Immunization in Practice—A Guide for Health Workers Who Give Vaccines (EPI/PHW/84/3 Rev 1). Geneva, World Health Organization, 1984.

30. Hick JF, Charbonneau JW, Brackke DM. Optimum needle length for diphtheria-tetanus-pertussis inoculation of infants. Pediatrics 84:136–137, 1989.

31. Poland GA, Borrud A, Jacobson RM. Determination of deltoid fat pad thickness: implications for needle length in adult immunization. JAMA 277:1709–1711, 1997.

32. Evans DIK, Shaw A. Safety of intramuscular injection of hepatitis B vaccine in haemophiliacs. Br Med J 300(67):1694–1695, 1990.

33. Kristensen K. Antibody response to a *Haemophilus influenzae* type b polysaccharide tetanus toxoid conjugate vaccine in splenectomized children and adolescents. Scand J Infect Dis 24:629–632, 1992.

34. Granoff DM, Suarez BK, Pandey JP, Shackelford PG. Genes associated with the G2m(23) immunoglobulin allotype regulate the IgG subclass responses to *Haemophilus influenzae* type b polysaccharide vaccine. J Infect Dis 157:1142–1149, 1988.

35. *Haemophilus influenzae* B immunization. Drug Ther Bull 31:1–2, 1993.

36. Tuberculosis: BCG immunisation. *In* Salisbury DM, Begg NT (eds). 1996 Immunisation Against Infectious Disease. London, Her Majesty's Stationery Office, 1996, pp 219–241.

37. Centers for Disease Control and Prevention. Vaccinia (smallpox) vaccine: recommendations of the Advisory Committee on Immunization Practices (ACIP). MMWR 50(RR-10):1–25, 2001.

38. Breman JG, Henderson DA. Diagnosis and management of smallpox. N Engl J Med 346:1300–1308, 2002.

39. Centers for Disease Control and Prevention. Poliomyelitis prevention in the United States: introduction of a sequential vaccination schedule of inactivated poliovirus vaccine followed by oral poliovirus vaccine. MMWR 46(RR-3):1–25, 1997.

40. Occupational Safety and Health Administration. Occupational exposure to bloodborne pathogens; needlestick and other sharps injuries; final rule (29 CFR Part 1910). Fed Reg 66:5318–25, 2001. Available at *www.osha-slc.gov/FedReg_osha_pdf/FED20010118A.pdf*.

41. Centers for Disease Control and Prevention. Needle-free injection technology. Atlanta, National Immunization Program, 2001. Available at *www.cdc.gov/nip/dev/jetinject.htm*

42. International Health Care Worker Safety Center. List of safety-engineered sharp devices and other products designed to prevent occupational exposures to bloodborne pathogens. Charlottesville, University of Virginia, 2001. Available at *www.med.virginia.edu/medcntr/centers/epinet/safetydevice.html*

43. California Department of Health Services. California list of needleless systems and needles with engineered sharps injury protection. Sacramento, California Department of Health Services, 2001. Available at *www.dhs.cahwnet.gov/ohb/SHARPS/disclaim.htm*

44. National Alliance for the Primary Prevention of Sharps Injuries (NAPPSI). The NAPPSI primary and secondary prevention needlestick safety device list & notification to clinicians on sharps injury protection. Carlsbad, CA, NAPPSI, 2001. Available at *www.nappsi.org/safety.shtml*

45. Hingson RA, Davis HS, Rosen M. Historical development of jet injection and envisioned uses in mass immunization and mass therapy based upon two decades' experience. Mil Med 128:516–524, 1963.

46. Reis EC, Jacobson RM, Tarbell S, Weniger BG. Taking the sting out of shots: control of vaccination-associated pain and adverse reactions. Pediatr Ann 27:375–385, 1998.

47. Simonsen L, Kane A, Lloyd J, et al. Unsafe injections in the developing world and transmission of bloodborne pathogens: a review. Bull World Health Organ 77:789–800, 1999.

48. Kane A, Lloyd J, Zaffran M, et al. Transmission of hepatitis B, hepatitis C and human immunodeficiency viruses through unsafe injections in the developing world: model-based regional estimates. Bull World Health Organ 77:801–807, 1999.

49. Spiegel A, Greindl Y, Lippeveld T, et al. Effect of two meningococcal vaccination strategies during the epidemic in N'Djamena, Chad, in 1988. Bull World Health Organ 71:311–315, 1993.

50. Hoke CH Jr, Egan JE, Sjogren MH, et al. Administration of hepatitis A vaccine to a military population by needle and jet injector and with hepatitis B vaccine. J Infect Dis 171(suppl 1):S53–S60, 1995.

51. Nuefield PD, Katz L. Comparative evaluation of three jet injectors for mass immunization. Can J Public Health 68:513–516, 1977.

52. Warren J, Ziherl FA, Kish AW, Ziherl LA. Large-scale administration of vaccines by means of an automatic jet injection syringe. JAMA 157:633–637, 1955.

53. Brink PRG, van Loon AM, Trommelen JCM, et al. Virus transmission by subcutaneous jet injection. J Med Microbiol 20:393–397, 1985.

54. Stanfield JP, Bracken PM, Waddell KM, Gall D. Diphtheria-tetanus-pertussis immunization by intradermal jet injection. Br Med J 2:197–199, 1972.

55. Rosenthal SR. Transference of blood by various inoculation devices. Am Rev Respir Dis 96:815–819, 1967.

56. Zachoval R, Deinhardt F, Gurtler L, et al. Risk of virus transmission by jet injection [letter]. Lancet 1:189, 1988.

57. Abb J, Deinhardt F, Eisenburg J. The risk of transmission of hepatitis B virus using jet injection in inoculation. J Infect Dis 144:179, 1981.

58. Robertson JS. Jet injectors and infection. Public Health 101:147–148, 1987.

59. Canter J, MacKey K, Good LS, et al. An outbreak of hepatitis B associated with jet injections in a weight reduction clinic. Arch Intern Med 150:1923–1927, 1990.

60. Centers for Disease Control. Hepatitis B associated with jet gun injection—California. MMWR 35:446–447, 1986.

61. Aylward B, Kane M, McNair-Scott R, Hu DH. Model-based estimates of the risk of human immunodeficiency virus and hepatitis B virus transmission through unsafe injections. Int J Epidemiol 24:446–452, 1995.

62. Brito GS, Chen RT, Stefano CA, et al. The risk of transmission of HIV and other blood borne diseases via jet injectors during immunization mass campaigns in Brazil [abstr PC0132]. *In* Abstracts from the Tenth International Conference on AIDS, Yokohama, Japan, August 7–12, 1994.

63. Aylward B, Lloyd J, Zaffran M, et al. Reducing the risk of unsafe injections in immunization programmes: financial and operational implications of various injection technologies. Bull World Health Organ 73:531–540, 1995.

64. Zaffran M, Lloyd J, Clements J, Stilwell B. A Drive to Safer Injections (WHOGPVSAGE.97/WP.05, 1997). Geneva, World Health Organization, 1997.

65. Parent du Chatelet I, Lang J, Schlumberger M, et al. Clinical immunogenicity and tolerance studies of liquid vaccines delivered by jet-injector and a new single-use cartridge (Imule): comparison with standard syringe injection. Vaccine 15:449–458, 1997.

66. Taddio A, Nulman I, Goldbach M, et al. Use of lidocaine-prilocaine cream for vaccination pain in infants. J Pediatr 124:643–648, 1994.

67. Halperin SA, McGrath P, Smith B, Houston T. Lidocaine-prilocaine patch decreases the pain associated with subcutaneous administration of measles-mumps-rubella vaccine but does not adversely affect the antibody response. J Pediatr 136:789–794, 2000.

68. Uhari M. A eutectic mixture of lidocaine and prilocaine for alleviating vaccination pain in infants. Pediatrics 92:719–721, 1993.

69. Jakobson B, Nilsson A. Methemoglobinemia associated with a prilocaine-lidocaine cream and trimethoprim-sulphamethoxazole: a case report. Acta Anaesthesiol Scand 29:453–455, 1985.

70. Mansouri A, Lurie AA. Concise review: methemoglobinemia. Am J Hematol 42:7–12, 1993.

71. Lewis K, Cherry JD, Sachs MH, et al. The effect of prophylactic acetaminophen administration on reactions to DTP vaccination. Am J Dis Child 142:62–65, 1988.

72. Abbott K, Fowler-Kerry S. The use of a topical refrigerant anesthetic to reduce injection pain in children. J Pain Symptom Manage 10:584–590, 1995.

73. Maikler VE. Effects of a skin refrigerant/anesthetic and age on the pain responses of infants receiving immunizations. Res Nurs Health 14:397–403, 1991.

74. Reis E, Holubkov R. Vapocoolant spray is equally effective as EMLA cream in reducing immunization pain in school-aged children. Pediatrics 100:E5, 1997. Available at *www.pediatrics.org/cgi/content/full/100/6/e5*

75. Allen KD, White DD, Walburn JN. Sucrose as an analgesic agent for infants during immunization injections. Arch Pediatr Adolesc Med 150:270–274, 1996.

76. French GM, Painter EC, Coury DL. Blowing away shot pain: a technique for pain management during immunization. Pediatrics 93:384–388, 1994.

77. Fowler-Kerry S, Lander JR. Management of injection pain in children. Pain 30:169–175, 1987.

78. World Health Organization. Measles Vaccine. Available at *www.who.int/vaccines/en/measles.shtml*.

79. Centers for Disease Control and Prevention. Measles, mumps, and rubella vaccine use and strategies for elimination of measles, rubella, and congenital rubella syndrome and control of mumps: recommendations of the Advisory Committee on Immunization Practices (ACIP). MMWR 47(RR-8):1–57, 1998.

80. Evans DG, Smith JWG. Response of the young infant to active immunization. Br Med Bull 19:225–229, 1963.

81. Orenstein WA, Weisfeld JS, Halsey NA. Diphtheria and tetanus toxoids and pertussis vaccine, combined. *In* Halsey NA, de Quadros CA (eds). Recent Advances in Immunization: A Bibliographic Review (PAHO Scientific Publication No. 451). Washington, DC, Pan-American Health Organization, 1983, pp 30–51.

82. Halsey N, Galazka A. The efficacy of DPT and oral poliomyelitis immunization schedules initiated from birth to 12 weeks of age. Bull World Health Organ 63:1151–1169, 1985.

83. Wilkins J, Chan LS, Wehrle PF. Age and dose interval as factors in agglutinin formation to pertussis vaccine. Vaccine 5:49–54, 1987.

84. American Academy of Pediatrics. Pertussis. *In* Pickering L (ed). 2003 Red Book: Report of the Committee on Infectious Diseases (26th ed). Elk Grove Village, IL, American Academy of Pediatrics, 2003, pp 472–486.

85. Centers for Disease Control and Prevention. Pertussis vaccination: use of acellular pertussis vaccines among infants and young children. Recommendations of the Advisory Committee on Immunization Practices (ACIP). MMWR Morb Mortal Wkly Rep 1997;46(RR-7):1–25.

86. Galazka AM. Module 4: Pertussis. *In* The Immunologic Basis for Immunization Series. Global Programme for Vaccines and Immunization, Expanded Programme on Immunization. Geneva, World Health Organization, 1993, pp 1–20.

87. Funkhouser AW, Wassilak SG, Orenstein WA, et al. Estimated effects of a delay in the recommended vaccination schedule for diphtheria and tetanus toxoids and pertussis vaccine. JAMA 257:1341–1346, 1987.

88. Lieberman JM, Greenberg DP, Wong VK, et al. Effect of neonatal immunization with diphtheria and tetanus toxoids on antibody responses to *Haemophilus influenzae* type b conjugate vaccines. J Pediatr 126:198–205, 1995.

89. Murphy MD, Brunell PA, Lievens AW, et al. Effect of early immunization on antibody response to reimmunization with measles vaccine as demonstrated by enzyme-linked immunosorbent assay (ELISA). Pediatrics 74:90–93, 1984.

90. McGraw TT. Reimmunization following early immunization with measles vaccine: a prospective study. Pediatrics 77:45–48, 1986.

91. Centers for Disease Control and Prevention. Recommended adult immunization schedule—United States, 2002–2003. MMWR 51:904–908, 2002.

92. American Academy of Pediatrics, Committee on Infectious Diseases. Recommended childhood immunization schedule—United States, January–December 2002. Pediatrics 101:154–157, 1998.

93. Centers for Disease Control and Prevention. Recommended childhood immunization schedule—United States, 2002. MMWR 51:31–33, 2002.

94. McBean AM, Thoms ML, Albrecht P, et al. Serologic response to oral polio vaccine and enhanced-potency inactivated polio vaccines. Am J Epidemiol 128:615–628, 1988.

95. Salk J. One-dose immunization against paralytic poliomyelitis using a noninfectious vaccine. Rev Infect Dis 6(suppl 2):S444–S450, 1984.

96. Petralli JK, Merigan TC, Wilbur JR. Circulating interferon after measles vaccination. N Engl J Med 273:198–201, 1965.

97. Petralli JK, Merigan TC, Wilbur JR. Action of endogenous interferon against vaccinia infection in children. Lancet 2:401–405, 1965.

98. Centers for Disease Control and Prevention. Simultaneous administration of varicella vaccine and other recommended childhood vaccines—United States, 1995–1999. MMWR 50:1058–1061, 2001.

99. Stefano I, Sato HK, Pannuti CS, et al. Recent immunization against measles does not interfere with the sero-response to yellow fever vaccine. Vaccine 17:1042–1046, 1999.

100. Myers MG, Beckman CW, Vosdingh RA, Hankins WA. Primary immunization with tetanus and diphtheria toxoids: reaction rate and immunogenicity in older children and adults. JAMA 248:2478–2480, 1982.

101. Eisen AH, Cohen JJ, Rose B. Reaction to tetanus toxoid: report of a case with immunologic studies. N Engl J Med 269:1408–1411, 1963.

102. Schneider CH. Reactions to tetanus toxoid: a report of five cases. Med J Aust 1:303–305, 1964.

103. Edsall G, Elliot MW, Peebles TC, Eldred MC. Excessive use of tetanus toxoid boosters. JAMA 202:111–113, 1967.

104. Levine L, Edsall G. Tetanus toxoid: what determines reaction proneness? J Infect Dis 144:376, 1981.

105. King GE, Hadler SC. Simultaneous administration of childhood vaccines: an important public health policy that is safe and efficacious. Pediatr Infect Dis J 13:394–407, 1994.

106. Ramsay DS, Lewis M. Developmental change in infant cortisol and behavioral response to inoculation. Child Dev 65:1491–1502, 1994.

107. Lewis M, Ramsay DS, Suomi SJ. Validating current immunization practice with young infants. Pediatrics 90:771–773, 1992.

108. Felsenfeld O, Wolf RH, Gyr K, et al. Simultaneous vaccination against cholera and yellow fever. Lancet 1:457–458, 1973.

109. Gateff C. Influence de la vaccination anticholerique sur l'immunisation antiamarile associee. Bull Soc Pathol Exot 66:258–266, 1973.

110. Black FL. Measles active and passive immunity in a worldwide perspective. Prog Med Virol 36:1–33, 1989.

111. Albrecht P, Ennis FA, Saltzman EJ, Krugman S. Persistence of maternal antibody in infants beyond 12 months: mechanism of measles vaccine failure. J Pediatr 91:715–718, 1977.

112. Wilkins J, Wehrle PF. Additional evidence against measles vaccine administration to infants less than 12 months of age: altered immune response following active/passive immunization. J Pediatr 94:865–869, 1979.

113. Linnemann CC, Dine MS, Bloom JE, Schiff GM. Measles antibody in previously immunized children: the need for revaccination. Am J Dis Child 124:53–57, 1972.

114. Halsey NA, Boulos R, Mode F, et al. Response to measles vaccine in Haitian infants 6 to 12 months old: influence of maternal antibodies, malnutrition, and concurrent illnesses. N Engl J Med 313:544–577, 1985.

115. Black FL, Berman LL, Borgono JM, et al. Geographic variation in infant loss of maternal measles antibody and in prevalence of rubella antibody. Am J Epidemiol 124:442–452, 1986.

116. Dagan R, Slater PE, Duvdevani P, et al. Decay of maternally derived measles antibody in a highly vaccinated population in southern Israel. Pediatr Infect Dis J 14:965–969, 1995.

117. Immunization of man against rubella: discussion on sessions III and IV. Am J Dis Child 118:307–321, 1969.

118. Krugman S, Giles JP, Jacobs AM, Friedman H. Studies with a further attenuated live measles-virus vaccine. Pediatrics 31:914–928, 1963.

119. Lingham S, Miller CL, Clarke M, Pateman J. Antibody response and clinical reactions in children given measles vaccine with immunoglobulin. Br Med J (Clin Res Ed) 292:1044–1045, 1986.

120. Benson PF, Butler NR, Goffe AP, et al. Vaccination of infants with living attenuated measles vaccine (Edmonston strain) with and without gamma-globulin. Br Med J 2:851–853, 1964.

121. Siber GR, Werner BC, Halsey NA, et al. Interference of immune globulin with measles and rubella immunization. J Pediatr 122:204–211, 1993.

122. Black NA, Parsons A, Kurtz JB, et al. Postpartum rubella immunization: a controlled trial of two vaccines. Lancet 2:990–992, 1983.

123. Kaplan JE, Nelson DB, Schonberger LB, et al. The effect of immune globulin on the response to trivalent oral poliovirus and yellow fever vaccinations. Bull World Health Organ 62:585–590, 1984.

124. Simoes EAF, Padmini B, Steinhoff MC, et al. Antibody response of infants to two doses of inactivated poliovirus vaccine of enhanced potency. Am J Dis Child 139:977–980, 1985.

125. American Academy of Pediatrics, Committee on Infectious Diseases. Recommended timing of routine measles immunization for children who have recently received immune globulin preparations. Pediatrics 93:682–685, 1994.
126. Sato H, Albrecht P, Reynolds DW, et al. Transfer of measles, mumps, and rubella antibodies from mother to infant: its effect on measles, mumps, and rubella immunization. Am J Dis Child 133:1240–1243, 1979.
127. American Academy of Pediatrics. Respiratory syncytial virus. In Pickering L (ed). 2003 Red Book: Report of the Committee on Infectious Diseases (26th ed). Elk Grove Village, IL, American Academy of Pediatrics, 2003, pp 523–528.
128. Siber GR, Snydman DR. Use of immune globulin in the prevention and treatment of infections. Curr Clin Top Infect Dis 12:208–256, 1992.
129. Habig WH, Tankersley DL. Tetanus. In Cryz SJ (ed). Vaccines and Immunotherapy. New York, Pergamon Press, 1991, pp 13–19.
130. Plotkin SA, Rupprecht CE, Koprowski H. Rabies vaccine. In Plotkin SA, Orenstein WA (eds). Vaccines (3rd ed). Philadelphia, WB Saunders, 1999, pp 743–766.
131. Letson GW, Santosham M, Reid R, et al. Comparison of active and combined passive/active immunization of Navajo children against Haemophilus influenzae type b. Pediatr Infect Dis J 7:747–752, 1988.
132. Leentvaar-Kuijpers A, Coutinho RA, Brulein V, Safary A. Simultaneous passive and active immunization against hepatitis A. Vaccine 10(suppl 1):S138–S141, 1992.
133. Wagner G, Lavanchy D, Darioli R, et al. Simultaneous active and passive immunization against hepatitis A studied in a population of travelers. Vaccine 11:1027–1032, 1993.
134. Green MS, Cohen D, Lerman Y, et al. Depression of the immune response to an inactivated hepatitis A vaccine administered concomitantly with immune globulin. J Infect Dis 168:740–743, 1993.
135. Shapiro CN, Letson GW, Huehn D, et al. Effect of maternal antibody on immunogenicity of hepatitis A vaccine in infants [abstr H61]. In Program and Abstracts of the 35th Interscience Conference on Antimicrobial Agents and Chemotherapy (ICAAC), San Francisco, September 17–20, 1995.
136. Product Information: RespiGam Respiratory Syncytial Virus Immune Globulin Intravenous (Human). Gaithersburg, MD, Medimmune, 1996.
137. American Academy of Pediatrics. Respiratory syncytial virus immune globulin intravenous: indications for use. Pediatrics 99:645–650, 1997.
138. Mason W, Takahashi M, Schneider T. Persisting passively acquired measles antibody following gamma globulin therapy for Kawasaki disease and response to live virus vaccination [abstr 311]. In Program and Abstracts of the 32nd meeting of the Interscience Conference on Antimicrobial Agents and Chemotherapy, Los Angeles, October 11–14, 1992.
139. American Academy of Pediatrics. Measles. In Pickering L (ed). 2003 Red Book: Report of the Committee on Infectious Diseases (26th ed). Elk Grove Village, IL, American Academy of Pediatrics, 2003, pp 419–429.
140. American Academy of Pediatrics. Rubella. In Pickering L (ed). 2003 Red Book: Report of the Committee on Infectious Diseases (26th ed). Elk Grove Village, IL, American Academy of Pediatrics, 2003, pp 536–541.
141. Centers for Disease Control and Prevention. Typhoid immunization—recommendations of the Advisory Committee on Immunization Practices (ACIP). MMWR 43(RR-14):1–7, 1994.
142. Bush LM, Moonsammy GI, Boscia JA. Evaluation of initiating a hepatitis B vaccination schedule with one vaccine and completing it with another. Vaccine 9:807–809, 1991.
143. Chan CY, Lee SD, Tsai YT, Lo KJ. Booster response to recombinant yeast-derived hepatitis B vaccine in vaccinees whose anti-HBs responses were initially elicited by a plasma-derived vaccine. Vaccine 9:765–767, 1991.
144. Anderson EL, Decker MD, Englund JA, et al. Interchangeability of conjugated Haemophilus influenzae type b vaccines in infants. JAMA 273:849–853, 1995.
145. Bewley KM, Schwab JG, Ballanco GA, Daum RS. Interchangeability of Haemophilus influenzae type b vaccines in the primary series: evaluation of a two-dose mixed regimen. Pediatrics 98:898–904, 1996.
146. Greenberg DP, Lieberman JM, Marcy SM, et al. Enhanced antibody response in infants given different sequences of heterogeneous Haemophilus influenzae type b conjugate vaccines. J Pediatr 126:206–211, 1995.
147. Greenberg DP, Pickering LK, Senders SD, et al. Interchangeability of 2 diphtheria-tetanus-acellular pertussis vaccines in infancy. Pediatrics 109:666–672, 2002.
148. Centers for Disease Control and Prevention. Use of diphtheria toxoid-tetanus toxoid-acellular pertussis vaccine as a five-dose series: supplemental recommendations of the Advisory Committee on Immunization Practices (ACIP). MMWR 49(RR-13):1–8, 2000.
149. Zaloga GP, Chernow B. Life-threatening anaphylactic reactions to tetanus toxoid. Ann Allergy 49:107–108, 1982.
150. Institute of Medicine. Evidence concerning pertussis vaccines and other illnesses and conditions. In Howson CP, Howe CJ, Fineberg HV (eds). Adverse Effects of Pertussis and Rubella Vaccines. Washington, DC, Institute of Medicine, 1991, pp 144–186.
151. Mortimer EA, Sorensen RU. Urticaria following administration of diphtheria–tetanus toxoids–pertussis vaccine [letter]. Pediatr Infect Dis J 6:876–877, 1987.
152. Matuhasi T, Ikegami H. Elevation of levels of IgE antibody to tetanus toxin in individuals vaccinated with diphtheria-pertussis-tetanus vaccine. J Infect Dis 146:290, 1982.
153. Nagel J, Svec D, Waters T, Fireman P. IgE synthesis in man. I. Development of specific IgE antibodies after immunization with tetanus-diphtheria (Td) toxoids. J Immunol 118:334–341, 1977.
154. Lewis K, Jordan SC, Cherry JD, et al. Petechiae and urticaria after DTP vaccination: detection of circulating immune complexes containing vaccine-specific antigens. J Pediatr 109:1009–1012, 1986.
155. American Academy of Pediatrics. Tetanus. In Pickering L (ed). 2003 Red Book: Report of the Committee on Infectious Diseases (26th ed). Elk Grove Village, IL, American Academy of Pediatrics, 2003, pp 611–616.
156. Jacobs RL, Lowe RS, Lanier BQ. Adverse reactions to tetanus toxoid. JAMA 247:40–42, 1982.
157. Mansfield LE, Ting S, Rawls DO, Frederick R. Systemic reactions during cutaneous testing for tetanus toxoid hypersensitivity. Ann Allergy 57:135–137, 1986.
158. Facktor MA, Bernstein RA, Fireman P. Hypersensitivity to tetanus toxoid. J Allergy Clin Immunol 52:1–12, 1973.
159. Sisk CW, Lewis CE. Reactions to tetanus-diphtheria toxoid (adult). Arch Environ Health 11:34–36, 1965.
160. Beneson AS, Joseph PR, Oseasohn RO. Cholera vaccine field trials in East Pakistan. 1. Reaction and antigenicity studies. Bull World Health Organ 38:347–357, 1968.
161. Marshall JD Jr, Bartelloni PJ, Cavanaugh DC, et al. Plague immunization. II. Relation of adverse clinical reactions to multiple immunizations with killed vaccine. J Infect Dis 129(suppl): S19–S25, 1974.
162. Hejfec LB, Salmin LV, Lejtman MZ, et al. A controlled field trial and laboratory study of five typhoid vaccines in the USSR. Bull World Health Organ 34:321–339, 1966.
163. Ashcroft MT, Ritchie JM, Nicholson CC. Controlled field trial in British Guiana school children of heat-killed-phenolized and acetone-killed lyophilized typhoid vaccines. Am J Hyg 79:196–206, 1964.
164. Robinson HC, Russell ML, Csokonay WM. Japanese encephalitis vaccine and adverse effects among travelers. Can Dis Wkly Rep 17:173–177, 1991.
165. Anderson MM, Ronne T. Side effects with Japanese encephalitis vaccine. Lancet 337:1044, 1991.
166. Ruff TA, Eisen D, Fuller A, Kass R. Adverse reactions to Japanese encephalitis vaccine. Lancet 338:881–882, 1991.
167. Harvey RE, Posey WC, Jacobs RL. The predictive value of egg skin tests and yellow fever vaccine skin tests in egg-sensitive individuals [abstr 213]. J Allergy Clin Immunol 63:196–197, 1979.
168. Centers for Disease Control and Prevention. Prevention and control of influenza: recommendations of the Advisory Committee on Immunization Practices. MMWR 51(RR-3):1–31, 2002.
169. Yamane N, Uemura H. Serological examination of IgE- and IgG-specific antibodies to egg protein during influenza virus immunization. Epidemiol Infect 100:291–299, 1988.
170. Bierman CW, Shapiro GG, Pierson WE, et al. Safety of influenza vaccination in allergic children. J Infect Dis 136:S652–S655, 1977.
171. Murphy KR, Strunk RC. Safe administration of influenza vaccine in asthmatic children sensitive to egg proteins. J Pediatr 106:931–933, 1985.

172. American Academy of Pediatrics. Influenza. *In* Pickering L (ed). 2003 Red Book: Report of the Committee on Infectious Diseases (26th ed). Elk Grove Village, IL, American Academy of Pediatrics, 2003, pp 382–391.

173. Fasano MB, Wood RA, Cooke SK, Sampson HA. Egg hypersensitivity and adverse reactions to measles, mumps, and rubella vaccine. J Pediatr 120:978–981, 1992.

174. Kemp A, Van Asperen P, Mukhi A. Measles immunization in children with clinical reactions to egg protein. Am J Dis Child 144:33–35, 1990.

175. James JM, Burks AW, Roberson PK, Sampson HA. Safe administration of measles vaccine to children allergic to eggs. N Engl J Med 332:1262–1266, 1995.

176. American Academy of Pediatrics. Mumps. *In* Pickering L (ed). 2003 Red Book: Report of the Committee on Infectious Diseases (26th ed). Elk Grove Village, IL, American Academy of Pediatrics, 2003, pp 439–443.

177. Kelso JM, Jones RT, Yunginger JW. Anaphylaxis to measles, mumps, and rubella vaccine mediated by IgE to gelatin. J Allergy Infect Dis 91:867–872, 1993.

178. Sakaguchi M, Ogura H, Inouye S. IgE antibody to gelatin in children with immediate-type reactions to measles and mumps vaccines. J Allergy Infect Dis 96:563–565, 1995.

179. Sakaguchi M, Nakayama T, Inouye S. Food allergy to gelatin in children with systemic immediate-type reactions, including anaphylaxis, to vaccines. J Allergy Infect Dis 98:1058–1061, 1996.

180. Centers for Disease Control. Systemic allergic reactions following immunization with human diploid cell rabies vaccine. MMWR 33:185–188, 1984.

181. Dreeson DW, Bernard KW, Parker RA, et al. Immune complex–like disease in 23 persons following a booster dose of rabies human diploid cell vaccine. Vaccine 4:45–49, 1986.

182. Anderson MC, Baer H, Frazier DJ, Quinnan JV. The role of specific IgE and beta-propiolactone in reactions resulting from booster doses of human diploid cell rabies vaccine. J Allergy Clin Immunol 80:861–868, 1987.

183. Slater JE. Latex allergy. J Allergy Clin Immunol 94:139–149, 1994.

184. Towse A, O'Brien M, Twarog FJ, et al. Local reaction secondary to insulin injection: a potential role for latex antigens in insulin vials and syringes [short reports]. Diabetes Care 18:1195–1197, 1995.

185. Bastyr EJ. Latex allergen allergic reactions [letter]. Diabetes Care 19:546, 1996.

186. MacCracken J, Stenger P, Jackson T. Latex allergy in diabetic patients: a call for latex-free insulin tops [letter]. Diabetes Care 19:184, 1996.

187. Lear JT, English JSC. Anaphylaxis after hepatitis B vaccination [letter]. Lancet 345:1249, 1995.

188. Rietschel RL, Bernier R. Neomycin sensitivity and the MMR vaccine [letter]. JAMA 245:571, 1981.

189. Elliman D, Dhanraj B. Safe MMR vaccination despite neomycin allergy [letter]. Lancet 337:365, 1991.

190. Kwittken PL, Rosen S, Sweinberg SK. MMR vaccine and neomycin allergy [letter]. Am J Dis Child 147:128–129, 1993.

191. Goh CL. Anaphylaxis from topical neomycin and bacitracin. Aust J Dermatol 27:125–126, 1986.

192. Centers for Disease Control and Prevention. Thimerosal in vaccines: a joint statement of the American Academy of Pediatrics and the Public Health Service. MMWR 48:563–565, 1999.

193. Ball LK, Ball R, Pratt RD. Assessment of thimerosal use in childhood vaccines. Pediatrics 107:1147–1154, 2001.

194. Rietschel RL, Adams RM. Reactions to thimerosal in hepatitis B vaccines. Dermatol Clin 8:161–164, 1990.

195. Noel I, Galloway A, Ive FA. Hypersensitivity to thimerosal in hepatitis B vaccine [letter]. Lancet 338:705, 1991.

196. Forstrom L, Hannulksela M, Kousa M, Lehmuskallio E. Merthiolate hypersensitivity and vaccination. Contact Dermatitis 6:241–245, 1980.

197. Aberer W. Vaccination despite thimerosal sensitivity. Contact Dermatitis 24:6–10, 1991.

198. Kirkland LR. Ocular sensitivity to thimerosal: a problem with hepatitis B vaccine? South Med J 83:497–499, 1990.

199. Cox NH, Forsyth A. Thiomersal allergy and vaccination reactions. Contact Dermatitis 18:229–233, 1988.

200. Möller H. All these positive tests to thimerosal. Contact Dermatitis 31:209–213, 1994.

201. Wantke F, Demmer CM, Götz M, Jarisch R. Contact dermatitis from thimerosal: 2 years' experience with ethylmercuric chloride in patch testing thimerosal-sensitive patients. Contact Dermatitis 30:115–118, 1994.

202. Reisman RE. Delayed hypersensitivity to merthiolate preservative. J Allergy 43:245–248, 1969.

203. American Academy of Pediatrics. Passive immunization. *In* Pickering L (ed). 2003 Red Book: Report of the Committee on Infectious Diseases (26th ed). Elk Grove Village, IL, American Academy of Pediatrics, 2003, pp 53–66.

204. Braun MM, Patriarca PA, Ellenberg SS. Syncope after immunization. Arch Pediatr Adolesc Med 151:255–259, 1997.

205. Rothberg RM. Immunoglobulin and specific antibody synthesis during the first weeks of life of premature infants. J Pediatr 75:391–399, 1969.

206. Bernbaum J, Anolik R, Polin RA, Douglas SD. Development of the premature infant's host defense system and its relationship to routine immunization. Clin Perinatol 11:73–84, 1984.

207. Wara DW, Barrett DJ. Cell-mediated immunity in the newborn: clinical aspects. Pediatrics 64(suppl):822–828, 1979.

208. Evans HE, Akpata SO, Glass L. Serum immunoglobulin levels in premature and full-term infants. Am J Clin Pathol 56:416–418, 1971.

209. Whitelaw A, Parkin J. Development of immunity. Br Med Bull 44:1037–1051, 1988.

210. Hyvarinen M, Zeltzer P, Oh W, Stiehm ER. Influence of gestational age on the newborn serum levels of alpha$_1$-fetoglobulin, IgG globulin and albumin. J Pediatr 82:430–437, 1973.

211. Linder N, Yaron M, Handsher R, et al. Early immunization with inactivated poliovirus vaccine in premature infants. J Pediatr 127:128–130, 1995.

212. Koblin BA, Townsend TR, Munoz A, et al. Response of preterm infants to diphtheria-tetanus-pertussis vaccine. Pediatr Infect Dis J 7:704–711, 1988.

213. Smolen P, Bland R, Heiligenstein E, et al. Antibody response to oral polio vaccine in premature infants. J Pediatr 103:917–919, 1983.

214. Conway S, James J, Balfour A, Smithells R. Immunization of the preterm baby. J Infect 27:143–150, 1993.

215. D'Angio CT, Maniscalco WM, Pinchichero ME. Immunologic response of extremely premature infants to tetanus, *Haemophilus influenzae*, and polio immunizations. Pediatrics 96:18–22, 1995.

216. Pullan CR, Hull D. Routine immunization of preterm infants. Arch Dis Child 64:1438–1441, 1989.

217. Linder N, Yaron M, Handsher R, et al: Early immunization with inactivated poliovirus vaccine in premature infants. J Pediatr 127:128–130, 1995.

218. Chirico G, Belloni C, Gasparoni A, et al. Hepatitis B immunization in infants from HbsAg negative mothers. Pediatrics 92:717–719, 1993.

219. Kristensen K, Gyhrs A, Lausen B, et al. Antibody response to *Haemophilus influenzae* type b capsular polysaccharide conjugated to tetanus toxoid in preterm infants. Pediatr Infect Dis J 15:525–529, 1996.

220. O'Shea TM, Dillard RG, Gillis DC, Abramson JS. Low rate of response to enhanced inactivated polio vaccine in preterm infants with chronic illness. Clin Res Reg Affairs 10:49–57, 1993.

221. Washburn LK, O'Shea TM, Gillis DC, et al. Response to *Haemophilus influenzae* type b conjugate vaccine in chronically ill premature infants. J Pediatr 123:791–794, 1993.

222. Lau Y, Tam AYC, Ng KW, et al. Response of preterm infants to hepatitis B vaccine. J Pediatr 121:962–965, 1992.

223. Munoz A, Salvador A, Brodsky NL, et al. Antibody response of low birth weight infants to *Haemophilus influenzae* type b polyribosylribitol phosphate–outer membrane protein conjugate vaccine. Pediatrics 96:216–219, 1995.

224. Khalak R, Pichichero ME, D'Angio CT. Three-year follow-up of vaccine response in extremely preterm infants. Pediatrics 101:597–603, 1998.

225. Chawareewong S, Jirapongsa A, Lokaphadhana K. Immune response to hepatitis B vaccine in premature neonates. Southeast Asian J Trop Med Public Health 22:39–40, 1991.

226. Losonsky GA, Stephens I, Mahoney F, et al. Preliminary results evaluating the immunogenicity of hepatitis B vaccination of premature infants starting in the first week of life [abstr 1752]. Pediatr Res 31:293a, 1995.

227. Patel DM, Butler J, Feldman S, et al. Immunogenicity of hepatitis B vaccine in healthy very low birth weight infants. J Pediatr 131:641–643, 1997.

228. Kim SC, Chung EK, Hodinka RL, et al. Immunogenicity of hepatitis B vaccine in preterm infants. Pediatrics 99:534–536, 1997.

229. Losonsky GA, Wasserman SS, Stephens I, et al. Hepatitis B vaccination of premature infants: a reassessment of current recommendations for delayed immunization. Pediatrics 103:E14, 1999.

230. Centers for Disease Control. Hepatitis B virus: a comprehensive strategy for eliminating transmission in the United States through universal childhood vaccination. Recommendations of the Immunization Practices Advisory Committee (ACIP). MMWR 40(RR-13):1–25, 1991.

231. American Academy of Pediatrics. Immunization in special clinical circumstances. In Pickering L (ed). 2003 Red Book: Report of the Committee on Infectious Diseases (26th ed). Elk Grove Village, IL, American Academy of Pediatrics, 2003, pp 66–98.

232. Sanchez PJ, Laptook AR, Fisher L, et al. Apnea after immunization of preterm infants. J Pediatr 130:746–751, 1997.

233. Bernbaum J, Daft A, Samuelson J, Polin RA. Half-dose immunization for diphtheria, tetanus, pertussis: response of pre-term infants. Pediatrics 83:471–476, 1989.

234. Bernbaum J, Polin RA. Re: Half-dose immunization for diphtheria, tetanus, pertussis [letter]. Pediatrics 86:144–145, 1990.

235. Plotkin SA. Re: Half-dose immunization for diphtheria, tetanus, pertussis [letter]. Pediatrics 86:145, 1990.

236. Centers for Disease Control and Prevention. Prevention of varicella: recommendations of the Advisory Committee on Immunization Practices (ACIP). MMWR 45(RR-11):1–36, 1996.

237. Losonsky GA, Fishaut JM, Strussenberg J, Ogra PL. Effect of immunization against rubella on lactation products. II. Maternal-neonatal interactions. J Infect Dis 145:661–666, 1982.

238. Losonsky GA, Fishaut JM, Strussenberg J, Ogra PL. Effect of immunization against rubella on lactation products. I. Development and characterization of specific immunologic reactivity in breast milk. J Infect Dis 145:654–660, 1982.

239. American College of Physicians Task Force on Adult Immunization and Infectious Diseases Society of America. Immunizations for special groups of patients. In Guide for Adult Immunization (3rd ed). Philadelphia, American College of Physicians, 1994, pp 25–41.

240. Kim-Farley R, Brink E. Orenstein W, Bart K. Vaccination and breast-feeding [letter]. JAMA 248:2451–2452, 1982.

241. Patriarca PA, Wright PF, John TJ. Factors affecting the immunogenicity of oral polio vaccine in developing countries: review. Rev Infect Dis 13:926–939, 1991.

242. Krogh V, Duffy LC, Wong D, et al. Postpartum immunization with rubella virus vaccine and antibody response in breast-feeding infants. J Lab Clin Med 113:695–699, 1989.

243. John TJ, Devaranjan LV, Luther L, Vijayarathnam P. Effect of breast-feeding on seroresponse of infants to oral poliovirus vaccination. Pediatrics 57:47–53, 1976.

244. Agarwal A, Sharma D, Kumari S, Khare S. Antibody response to three doses of standard and double dose of trivalent oral poliovaccine. Indian Pediatr 28:1141–1145, 1991.

245. Stephens S, Kennedy CR, Lakhani PK, Brenner MK. In vivo immune responses of breast- and bottle-fed infants to tetanus toxoid antigen and to normal gut flora. Acta Paediatr Scand 73:426–432, 1984.

246. Pabst HF, Spady DW. Effect of breast-feeding on antibody response to conjugate vaccine. Lancet 336:269–270, 1990.

247. Katz M, Plotkin S. Oral polio immunization of the newborn infant: a possible method for overcoming interference by ingested antibodies. J Pediatr 73:267–270, 1968.

248. Deforest A, Parker PB, DiLiberti JH, et al. The effect of breast-feeding on the antibody response in infants to trivalent oral poliovirus vaccine. J Pediatr 83:93–95, 1973

249. Hahn-Zoric M, Fulconis F, Minoli I, et al. Antibody responses to parenteral and oral vaccines are impaired by conventional and low protein formulas as compared to breast-feeding. Acta Paediatr Scand 79:1137–1142, 1990.

250. Pabst HF, Godel J, Grace M, et al. Effect of breast-feeding on immune response to BCG vaccination. Lancet 1:295–297, 1989.

251. Pickering LK, Granoff DM, Erickson JR, et al. Modulation of the immune system by human milk and infant formula containing nucleotides. Pediatrics 101:242–249, 1998.

252. Pichichero ME. Effect of breast-feeding on oral rhesus rotavirus vaccine seroconversions: a meta-analysis. J Infect Dis 162:753–755, 1990.

253. Glass RI, Ing DJ, Stoll BJ, Ing RT. Immune response to rotavirus vaccines among breast-fed and non–breast-fed children. In Mestecky J (ed). Immunology of Milk and the Neonate. New York, Plenum Publishing, 1991, pp 249–253.

254. Rennels MB. Influence of breast-feeding and oral poliovirus vaccine on the immunogenicity and efficacy of rotavirus vaccines. J Infect Dis 174(suppl 1):S107–S111, 1996.

255. Rennels MB, Wasserman SS, Glass RI, Keane VA. Comparison of immunogenicity and efficacy of rhesus rotavirus reassortment vaccines in breast-fed and non-breast-fed children. Pediatrics 96:1132–1136, 1995.

256. Koren G, Pastuszak A, Ito S. Drugs in pregnancy. N Engl J Med 338:1128–1137, 1998.

257. Grabenstein JD. Vaccines and antibodies in relation to pregnancy and lactation. Hosp Pharmacy 34:949–960, 1999.

258. Centers for Disease Control and Prevention. Control and prevention of rubella: evaluation and management of suspected outbreaks, rubella in pregnant women, and surveillance for congenital rubella syndrome. MMWR 50(RR-12):1–24, 2001.

259. Centers for Disease Control and Prevention. Revised ACIP recommendation for avoiding pregnancy after receiving a rubella-containing vaccine. MMWR 50:1117, 2001.

260. Centers for Disease Control and Prevention. Poliomyelitis prevention in the United States: updated recommendations of the Advisory Committee on Immunization Practices (ACIP). MMWR 49(RR-5):1–22, 2000.

261. Centers for Disease Control. Rubella vaccination during pregnancy—United States, 1971–1988. MMWR 38:289–293, 1989.

262. Sheppard S, Smithells RW, Dickson A, Holzel H. Rubella vaccination and pregnancy: preliminary report of a national survey. Br Med J (Clin Res Ed) 292:727, 1986.

263. Enders G. Rubella antibody titers in vaccinated and nonvaccinated women and results of vaccination during pregnancy. Rev Infect Dis 7(suppl 1):S103–S107, 1985.

264. Redd SC, Markowitz LE, Katz SL. Measles vaccine. In Plotkin SA, Orenstein WA Jr (eds). Vaccines (3rd ed). Philadelphia, WB Saunders, 1999, pp 222–266.

265. Plotkin SA, Wharton M. Mumps vaccine. In Plotkin SA, Orenstein WA Jr (eds). Vaccines (3rd ed). Philadelphia, WB Saunders, 1999, pp 267–292.

266. Harjulehto-Mervaala T, Aro T, Hiilesmaa VK, et al. Oral polio vaccination during pregnancy: lack of impact on fetal development and perinatal outcome. Clin Infect Dis 18:414–420, 1994.

267. Nasidi A, Monath TP, Vandenberg J, et al. Yellow fever vaccination and pregnancy: a four-year prospective study. Trans R Soc Trop Med Hyg 87:337–339, 1993.

268. Tsai TF, Paul R, Lynberg MC, Letson GW. Congenital yellow fever virus infection after immunization in pregnancy. J Infect Dis 168:1520–1523, 1993.

269. Shields KE, Galil K, Seward J, et al. Varicella vaccine exposure during pregnancy: data from the first 5 years of the pregnancy registry. Obstet Gynecol 98:14–19, 2001.

270. Heinonen OP, Shapiro S, Monson RR, et al. Immunization during pregnancy against poliomyelitis and influenza in relation to childhood malignancy. Int J Epidemiol 2:229–235, 1973.

271. Centers for Disease Control and Prevention. Prevention of pneumococcal disease: recommendations of the Advisory Committee on Immunization Practices (ACIP). MMWR 46(RR-8):1–24, 1997.

272. Centers for Disease Control and Prevention. Prevention of hepatitis A through active or passive immunization: recommendations of the Advisory Committee on Immunization Practices (ACIP). MMWR 48(RR-12):1–37, 1999.

273. Centers for Disease Control and Prevention. Prevention and control of meningococcal disease and college students: recommendations of the Advisory Committee on Immunization Practices (ACIP). MMWR 49(RR-7):1–20, 2000.

274. Neuzil KM, Reed GW, Mitchel EF, et al. Impact of influenza on acute cardiopulmonary hospitalizations in pregnant women. Am J Epidemiol 148:1094–1102, 1998.

275. Prevots DR. Neonatal tetanus. Bull World Health Organ 76(suppl 2):135–136, 1998.

276. World Health Organization. Neonatal Tetanus: Progress Towards the Global Elimination of Neonatal Tetanus, 1990–1997. Available at *www.who.int/vaccines-diseases/diseases/NeonatalTetanus.shtml*

277. Expanded Programme on Immunization, Global Advisory Group. Issues in Neonatal Tetanus Control. Geneva, World Health Organization, 1987.

278. Salzman MB, Sharrar RG, Steinberg S, LaRussa P. Transmission of varicella-vaccine virus from a healthy 12-month-old child to his pregnant mother. J Pediatr 131:151–154, 1997.

279. Long SS. Toddler-to-mother transmission of varicella-vaccine virus: how bad is that? J Pediatr 131:10–12, 1997.

280. Hlady WG, Bennett JV, Samadi AR, et al. Neonatal tetanus in rural Bangladesh: risk factors and toxoid efficacy. Am J Public Health 82:1365–1369, 1992.

281. de Quadros CA, Andrus JK, Olive J-M, de Macedo CG. Polio eradication from the Western Hemisphere. Annu Rev Public Health 13:239–252, 1992.

282. U.S. Department of State. International adoptions. Washington, DC, U.S. Department of State, 2001. Available at *www.travel.state.gov/adopt.html*

283. Hostetter MK, Johnson DE. Immunization status of adoptees from China, Russia, and Eastern Europe [abstr 851]. In Proceedings of the 1998 Pediatric Academic Societies Annual Meeting, New Orleans, May 5, 1998.

284. Kriz B, Burian V, Sladky K, et al. Comparison of titration results of diphtheric antitoxic antibody obtained by means of Jensen's method and the method of tissue cultures and haemagglutination. J Hyg Epidemiol Microbiol Immunol 22:485–493, 1978.

285. Staat MA, Daniels D. Immunization verification in internationally adopted children [abstract]. Pediatr Res 49(4):468a, 2001.

286. Centers for Disease Control. Diphtheria, tetanus, and pertussis: recommendations for vaccine use and other preventive measures. Recommendations of the Immunization Practices Advisory Committee (ACIP). MMWR 40(RR-10):1–28, 1991.

287. Livengood JR, Mullen JR, White JW, et al. Family history of convulsions and use of pertussis vaccine. J Pediatr 115:527–531, 1989.

288. Institute of Medicine. Pertussis vaccines and evidence concerning pertussis vaccines and central nervous system disorders, including infantile spasms, hypsarrhythmia, aseptic meningitis, and encephalopathy. In Howson CP, Howe CJ, Fineberg HV (eds). Adverse Effects of Pertussis and Rubella Vaccines. Washington, DC, National Academy Press, 1991, pp 65–124.

289. Institute of Medicine. Measles and mumps vaccines. In Stratton KR, Howe CJ, Johnston RB Jr (eds). Adverse Events Associated with Childhood Vaccines: Evidence Bearing on Causality. Washington, DC, National Academy Press, 1994, pp 118–186.

290. Krober MS, Stracener CE, Bass JW. Decreased measles antibody response after measles-mumps-rubella vaccine in infants with colds. JAMA 265:2095–2096, 1991.

291. King GE, Markowitz LE, Heath J, et al. Antibody response to measles-mumps-rubella vaccine of children with mild illness at the time of vaccination. JAMA 275:704–707, 1996.

292. Ndikuyeze A, Munoz A, Stewart S, et al. Immunogenicity and safety of measles vaccine in ill African children. Int J Epidemiol 17:448–455, 1988.

293. Atkinson W, Markowitz L, Baughman A, et al. Serologic response to measles vaccination among ill children [abstr 422]. In Program and Abstracts of the 32nd Interscience Conference on Antimicrobial Agents and Chemotherapy, Anaheim, CA, October 11–14, 1992.

294. Dennehy PH, Saracen CL, Peter G. Seroconversion rates to combined measles-mumps-rubella-varicella (MMRV) vaccine of children with upper respiratory tract infection. Pediatrics 94:514–516, 1994.

295. Ratnam S, West R, Gadag V. Measles and rubella antibody response after measles-mumps-rubella vaccination in children with afebrile upper respiratory tract infection. J Pediatr 127:432–434, 1995.

296. Wald ER, Dashefsky B, Byers C, et al. Frequency and severity of infections in day care. J Pediatr 112:540–546, 1988.

297. Hutchins SS, Escolan J, Markowitz LE, et al. Measles outbreak among unvaccinated preschool-aged children: opportunities missed by health care providers to administer measles vaccine. Pediatrics 83:369–374, 1989.

298. Farizo KM, Stehr-Green PA, Markowitz LE, Patriarca PA. Vaccination levels and missed opportunities for measles vaccination: a record audit in a public pediatric clinic. Pediatrics 89:589–592, 1992.

299. Lewis T, Osborn LM, Lewis K, et al. Influence of parental knowledge and opinions on 12-month diphtheria, tetanus, and pertussis vaccination rates. Am J Dis Child 142:283–286, 1988.

300. McConnochie KM, Roghmann KJ. Immunization opportunities missed among urban poor children. Pediatrics 89:1019–1026, 1992.

301. Centers for Disease Control and Prevention. Standards for pediatric immunization practices. MMWR 42(RR-5):1–13, 1993.

302. American Academy of Pediatrics. Varicella-zoster infections. In Pickering L (ed). 2003 Red Book: Report of the Committee on Infectious Diseases (26th ed). Elk Grove Village, IL, American Academy of Pediatrics, 2003, pp 672–686.

303. American Academy of Pediatrics. Hepatitis B. In Pickering L (ed). 2003 Red Book: Report of the Committee on Infectious Diseases (26th ed). Elk Grove Village, IL, American Academy of Pediatrics, 2003, pp 318–336.

304. Centers for Disease Control and Prevention. Measles pneumonitis following measles-mumps-rubella vaccination of a patient with HIV infection, 1993. MMWR 45:603–606, 1996.

305. Centers for Disease Control and Prevention. Prevention of varicella: update recommendations of the Advisory Committee on Immunization Practices (ACIP). MMWR 48(RR-6):1–5, 1999.

Chapter 9

Smallpox and Vaccinia

DONALD A. HENDERSON • LUCIANA L. BORIO • J. MICHAEL LANE

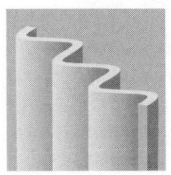 Smallpox eradication was certified by the World Health Assembly on May 8, 1980.[1] This was an event that many hoped would consign smallpox to history. Over the past 10 years, however, clear evidence has emerged that scientists in the Soviet Union had developed methods by which smallpox could be used as a strategic weapon on intercontinental ballistic missiles,[2] and manufacturing facilities had been constructed that were capable of producing the virus in ton quantities. As was learned, other studies in Soviet laboratories, especially the VECTOR laboratory in Novosibirsk, pursued the possible use of recombinant products of smallpox virus as biologic weapons. These activities, still partially cloaked in secrecy, coupled with the migration of former Soviet scientists to laboratories in other countries such as Iran, Iraq, and North Korea, have raised the specter of smallpox being used as a biologic weapon.

The release of an aerosol of smallpox virus and its subsequent spread is recognized, rightly, as posing the possibility of an international catastrophe. Accordingly, the United States and a number of other countries have begun to contract for the delivery of new stocks of smallpox vaccine and to plan for an appropriate emergency response should smallpox recur. They are working with the World Health Organization (WHO) to devise means for coping with smallpox wherever it might recur in recognition of the fact that an outbreak anywhere threatens all countries. The interest in smallpox as a disease and in its prevention has risen sharply, and so this chapter has been expanded.

History

Smallpox, an exanthematous viral disease, was once prevalent throughout the world, existing as an endemic infection wherever concentrations of population were sufficient to sustain transmission. Outbreaks of variola major, the only known variety until the end of the 19th century, resulted in case-fatality rates of 30% or more among unvaccinated persons. Most of those who survived had distinctive residual facial pockmarks, and some were blind. A less severe variety, variola minor (known also as alastrim), produced a milder illness with case-fatality rates of 1% or less. Variola minor was first described in South Africa late in the 19th century by de Korte[3] and in the United States in 1897 by Chapin.[4] It eventually became the prevalent variety throughout the United States, parts of South America, Europe, and some areas of eastern and southern Africa.[5]

There is no animal reservoir of smallpox and no long-term human carrier state. Thus the virus must spread continuously from human to human to survive. Historians speculate that it emerged sometime after the first agricultural settlements, about 10,000 BC.[6] The first certain evidence of smallpox in the ancient world comes from mummified remains of the 18th Egyptian dynasty (1580 to 1350 BC) and of the better known Ramses V (1157 BC).[7] Written descriptions of the disease did not appear until the 4th century AD in China[8] and the 10th century in southwestern Asia.[9]

Smallpox was probably carried from northeastern Africa to India by Egyptian traders during the first millennium BC,[5] where it became established as an endemic infection. Whether smallpox persisted in Africa is uncertain. Epidemics of disease are described in the Bible and in Greek and Roman literature, but descriptions of clinical signs are sparse. Only one of these epidemics can be identified possibly as being smallpox.[8] It occurred in Athens beginning in 430 BC and was described by Thucydides. There is no original Greek or Latin word for smallpox, despite its distinctive rash. Smallpox spread with increasing frequency from the populated endemic areas of Asia and perhaps Africa into less populous areas of these continents and into Europe, becoming established as an endemic infection when populations increased sufficiently in number.[10]

The name *variola* was first used during the sixth century by Bishop Marius of Avenches (Switzerland). The term is derived from the Latin *varius* (spotted) or *varus* (pimple).[11] Although Marius provided no clinical description of the disease concerned, there is little doubt that smallpox was endemic in parts of Europe by this time.[8] In the Anglo-Saxon world, by the 10th century, the word *poc* or *pocca*, a bag or pouch, described an exanthematous disease, possibly smallpox, and English accounts began to use the word *pockes*. When syphilis appeared in Europe in the late 15th century, writers began to use the prefix *small* to distinguish variola, the smallpox, from syphilis, the great pox.[12]

Smallpox began to be imported into the Western Hemisphere in the early 16th century. Catastrophic epidemics followed that literally decimated Amerindian tribes and resulted in the collapse of both the Aztec and Incan empires.[6] Central and southern Africa probably became endemic for smallpox about this time or soon thereafter.

The impact of smallpox on history and human affairs was profound.[8] Deities to smallpox became a part of the cultures of India, China, and parts of Africa. In Europe, by the end of the 18th century, an estimated 400,000 persons died annually from smallpox, and survivors accounted for one third of all cases of blindness. During the 18th century, five reigning European monarchs died of smallpox, and the Austrian Hapsburg line of succession shifted four times in four generations.

A method for protection against naturally acquired smallpox infection appears to have been discovered in India sometime before AD 1000.[13,14] There it became the practice to deliberately inoculate, either into the skin or by nasal insufflation, scabs or pustular material from lesions of patients. This practice (now called variolation) resulted in an illness usually less severe than that acquired naturally by inhalation of droplets. From India, variolation spread to China, western Asia, Africa, and finally, in the early 18th century, to Europe and North America.[15] Case-fatality rates associated with variolation were one tenth as great or less as when infection was naturally acquired, but those infected were capable of transmitting smallpox to others.[16] After cowpox (an orthopoxvirus closely related to variola virus) began to be used as a protective vaccine, the practice of variolation diminished. As recently as the 1960s and 1970s, however, variolation was performed among remote populations in parts of Ethiopia, western Africa, Afghanistan, and Pakistan.[5]

In 1796, Edward Jenner (Fig. 9–1) demonstrated that material could be taken from a human pustular lesion caused by cowpox virus and inoculated into the skin of another person, producing a similar localized and limited infection.[17] He showed that an inoculated individual was protected from infection with smallpox after recovery. He called the material *vaccine*, from the Latin *vacca*, meaning cow, and the process *vaccination*. Pasteur,[18] in recognition of Jenner's discovery, later broadened the term to denote preventive inoculation with other agents. Jenner's discovery was immediately recognized for its significance. Within 5 years, his paper had been translated into six other languages,[19] and vaccine had begun to be employed widely in many countries of Europe. Within a decade it had been transported to countries throughout the world. The chronicles of the de Balmis expedition of 1803 to 1806 vividly describe the transport of the vaccine by sea to Spanish colonies in the Americas and Asia by arm-to-arm vaccination of orphaned children.[20,21]

As the 19th century progressed, the initial wave of enthusiasm for vaccination subsided. Difficulties were experienced in sustaining the virus through arm-to-arm inoculation. Occasionally syphilis, leprosy, and other infections were transmitted in the process.[22,23] Although vaccination material, dried on threads or ivory points, was transported over long distances, it was often noninfectious on receipt.

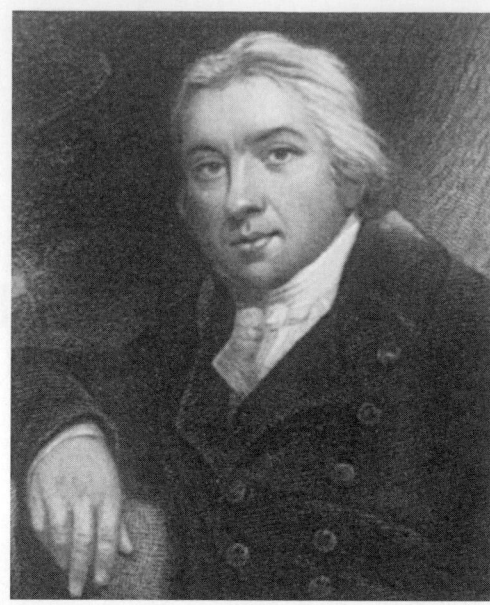

FIGURE 9–1 ■ Edward Jenner (1749–1823) demonstrated that a person inoculated and infected with cowpox was protected against smallpox. The procedure, which he called vaccination, represented the first use of a vaccine in the prevention of disease. (Courtesy of the Institute of the History of Medicine, The Johns Hopkins University, Baltimore, MD.)

When fresh material was sought, problems occurred in finding cows or horses with infections caused by cowpox or a related orthopoxvirus.[24] In some areas, significant opposition occurred among religious leaders and antivaccinationist societies who opposed the principle of infecting humans with an animal disease.[25] Confidence in vaccination was also diminished by the occurrence of smallpox in patients who had previously been successfully vaccinated. Jenner had forcefully contended that protection was lifelong, similar to immunity following natural smallpox, but it became apparent that this was not so. The need for revaccination was demonstrated early in the century,[26] but it was not widely accepted until many decades later.

Growth of vaccinia on the flank of a calf offered the prospect for provision of an adequate and safer supply of vaccine material. This approach was employed in Italy as early as 1805,[27] but appears to have been unknown elsewhere until it was widely publicized at a medical congress in 1864.[28] Thereafter, the practice gradually spread to other countries, although arm-to-arm vaccination in England continued until it was finally banned in 1898.[29] With an assured source of vaccinia, the numbers of vaccinations in Europe increased, and the incidence of smallpox in the more industrialized countries diminished. However, most of Europe did not become smallpox free until after World War I, and transmission was not stopped throughout Europe and North America until after World War II.

In tropical and semitropical areas, and in less developed countries, smallpox continued largely unabated until the middle of the 20th century. These countries experienced continuing difficulties in sustaining the virus through arm-to-arm inoculation. After calves began to be used for vaccine production, the harvested vaccine remained viable for only a few days at ambient tropical temperatures, thus limiting its widespread application. The only control programs that were notably successful were in Indonesia and certain French colonies, which began using specially prepared and more stable air-dried[30] or freeze-dried[31] vaccine in the 1920s.

In the late 1940s, Collier perfected a commercially feasible process for large-scale production of a stable freeze-dried vaccine.[32] This offered vastly better possibilities for smallpox control. Recognizing the value of heat-stable vaccine, the Pan American Sanitary Organization[33] decided to undertake a hemisphere-wide eradication program in 1950, and by 1967 smallpox had been eliminated from all countries of the Americas except Brazil. In 1958, Dr. Victor Zhdanov, Vice Minister of Health of the Union of Soviet Socialist Republics (USSR), proposed to the World Health Assembly that a global smallpox eradication program be undertaken,[34] and this was so decided the following year.[35] Some progress was made during the period from 1959 to 1966, but the results overall were disappointing. Finally, in 1966, the World Health Assembly decided to intensify the eradication program by providing additional funds specifically for this effort.[36]

During 1967, the year the Intensified Global Eradication Program began, an estimated 10 to 15 million smallpox cases[1] occurred in the 31 countries in which the disease was endemic. The eradication campaign was based on a twofold strategy: (1) mass vaccination campaigns in each country, using vaccine of ensured potency and stability, that would reach at least 80% of the population (a coverage level that would be assessed by independent teams); and (2) special programs to detect and contain cases and outbreaks.[37] Full implementation of the latter strategy, called "surveillance and containment," greatly accelerated eradication. Numerous problems had to be surmounted, including deficient organization and supervision in national health services, epidemic smallpox among refugees fleeing areas stricken by civil war and famine, shortages of funds and vaccine, and a host of problems posed by difficult terrain, climate, and cultural beliefs.[38-40] Despite these problems, steady progress was made and, on October 26, 1977, the last known naturally occurring case of smallpox occurred in Merka, Somalia.[41] Two further cases occurred in 1978 as a result of a laboratory infection in Birmingham, England,[42] but these were the last. An extensively illustrated volume entitled *Smallpox and Its Eradication*[5] provides a detailed account of the eradication campaign, and an overall account of progress in smallpox control throughout history. It also gives a description of the virology, the clinical features, and the pathogenesis of the disease. Complementing this text is a historical record of smallpox, *The Greatest Killer: Smallpox in History*, by Hopkins (originally issued in 1983 under the title *Princes and Peasants*).[8] Detailed accounts of national programs are provided in books dealing with those in India,[43,44] Bangladesh,[45] Ethiopia,[46] and Somalia.[47]

Background

Clinical Description

Smallpox is caused by either of two closely related viruses, variola major and variola minor, that can only be distinguished by polymerase chain reaction (PCR) analysis. Clinically they are indistinguishable except for the fact that variola minor cases experience fewer systemic symptoms, less extensive rash, little persistent scarring, and fewer fatalities. The disease has an incubation period of about 12 days, with a range of 7 to 17 days. A 2- to 3-day prodrome of high fever, malaise, and prostration with headache and backache is followed by the development of a maculopapular rash (Fig. 9–2). The rash appears first on the mucosa of the mouth and pharynx, the face, and the forearms and then spreads to the legs and trunk. Within 1 to 2 days, the rash becomes vesicular and then pustular. The pustules are characteristically round, tense, and deeply embedded in the dermis. Crusts begin to form about the eighth or ninth day. When they separate, they leave pigment-free skin and frequently pitted scars. The eruption is characteristically more extensive on the face, arms, and legs (Fig. 9–3), and lesions often are found on the palms and soles. Death usually occurs late in the first week or during the second week of the illness, and is probably due to the effects of an overwhelming viremia.[48] Cases of smallpox among pregnant women occasionally result in spontaneous abortion of the fetus or a stillborn infant with evidence of lesions on the skin.[5]

A WHO classification scheme for smallpox[49] describes five different types: (1) ordinary, (2) flat (also known as

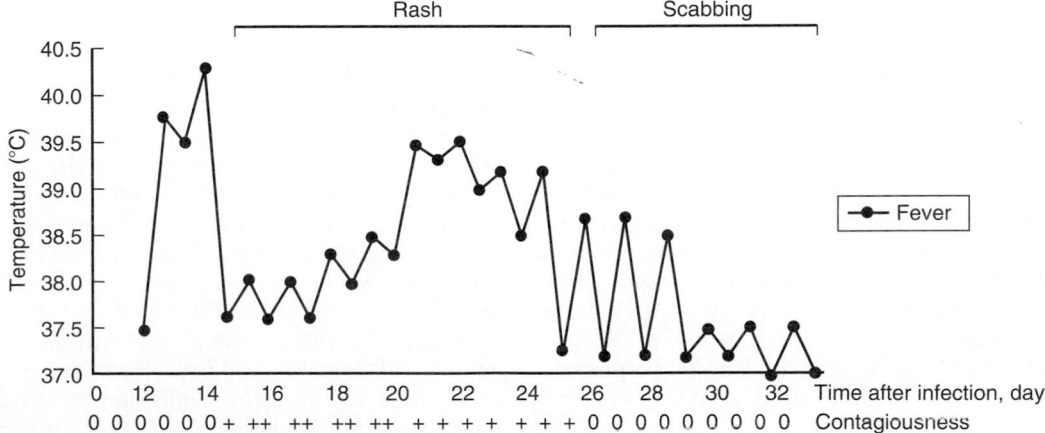

FIGURE 9–2 ■ Typical temperature chart of a patient with smallpox infection, showing the approximate time of appearance and evolution of the rash, and the period in which the patient is contagious after acquisition of infection. (Adapted from Henderson DA, Inglesby TV, Bartlett JG, et al. Smallpox as a biological weapon: medical and public health management. JAMA 281:2127–2137, 1999.)

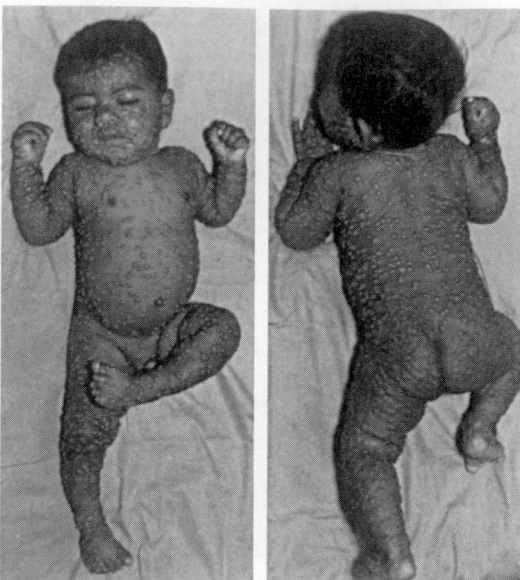

FIGURE 9–3 ■ A typical case of variola major about 7 days after the onset of rash. (From the World Health Organization Smallpox Recognition Card, courtesy of the World Health Organization, Geneva, Switzerland.)

"malignant"), (3) hemorrhagic, (4) vaccine modified, and (5) variola *sine eruptione*. Utilizing this classification scheme, Rao analyzed the frequency and case-fatality rates of vaccinated and unvaccinated cases in Madras, India.[50] Among those not previously vaccinated, the vast majority of variola major cases (approximately 89%) were of the *"ordinary"* type, and carried a fatality rate of approximately 30%. "*Flat*" smallpox accounted for 6.7% of cases, and had an associated mortality of 96%. "*Hemorrhagic*" cases accounted for 2.4% of cases. They were more common in pregnant women; 96% died. Extensive bleeding into the skin and the gastrointestinal tract preceded death. Cases "*modified*" by prior vaccination had many fewer lesions and, in Rao's series, accounted for 2.1% of the cases and resulted in no deaths. The rash in such persons was usually more scant and atypical, and the evolution of lesions more rapid. Variola *sine eruptione* (without rash) occurred in highly immune individuals who had laboratory evidence of infection but were not infectious for others.

Virology

Variola virus belongs to the genus *Orthopoxvirus*, family Poxviridae, which includes vaccinia, monkeypox, cowpox, camelpox, and ectromelia (mousepox).[51] All species exhibit extensive serologic cross-reactivity, both in in vitro tests and in experimental animals. The poxvirus genome, the largest of all virions, is a brick-shaped structure with a diameter of about 200 nm, consisting of a single molecule of a double-stranded DNA. It differs from most other DNA viruses in that it multiplies in the cytoplasm rather than in the nucleus of susceptible cells.

The orthopoxviruses grow and produce a cytoplasmic effect in cultured cells derived from many species,[52,53] although they generally grow best in cells from humans and other primates. The four that infect humans (variola, vaccinia, cowpox, and monkeypox viruses) cannot be differentiated readily from one another in most cell cultures. For

diagnostic purposes, therefore, they are customarily grown on the chorioallantoic membrane of 10- to 12-day-old chick embryos, on which they produce pocks characteristic of their species.[54] Newer PCR techniques have been developed recently that permit their differentiation (see *Diagnosis* below).

Pathogenesis

Smallpox generally follows the progression in the host described by Fenner et al. for ectromelia.[5] Natural smallpox infection occurs by implantation of variola virus on the respiratory mucosa. The virus is usually transmitted as virions in droplets expressed from nasal and oropharyngeal secretions. Higher concentrations of virus are believed to be expelled by patients with the hemorrhagic and malignant forms of the disease. When cough is present, the virus can be expelled as a fine-particle aerosol,[55] but cough is not a typical symptom of ordinary smallpox. After migration to and multiplication in regional lymph nodes, an asymptomatic viremia develops about the third or fourth day, followed by multiplication of virus in the spleen, bone marrow, and lymph nodes. A secondary viremia occurs some 8 to 10 days later, accompanied by high fever and toxemia. The virus, contained in leukocytes, then localizes in small blood vessels of the dermis and beneath the oral and pharyngeal mucosa, where it subsequently infects adjacent cells. In the skin, this process causes the characteristic maculopapular lesions that then evolve into vesicular and pustular lesions. Lesions are more extensive on the face and extremities, perhaps because the virus grows most readily at temperatures slightly below 37°C. Lesions in the mouth and pharynx ulcerate quickly because of the absence of a stratum corneum, releasing large amounts of virus into the saliva about the time the cutaneous rash first becomes visible. Virus titers in saliva are highest during the first week of rash, corresponding with the period during which patients are most contagious.

Hemagglutinin-inhibiting (HI) and neutralizing antibodies can be detected beginning about the sixth day of illness or, on average, about 18 days after infection, and complement-fixing (CF) antibodies approximately 2 days later.[56,57] Neutralizing antibodies are long lasting. HI antibodies decline to low levels within 5 years, and CF antibodies rarely persist for longer than 6 months. Little is known about the development of cell-mediated immunity following smallpox, but it probably plays a significant part in immunity.

Vaccinia-induced antibody responses are more rapid. They can be detected as early as the 10th day[58] after primary vaccination and within a week after revaccination. Evidence of cell-mediated immunity also occurs about the eighth or ninth day.[5] This accelerated response is associated with complete or partial protection from smallpox infection in persons vaccinated within 3 or 4 days after exposure.

Except for the lesions in the skin and mucous membranes and reticulum cell hyperplasia, other organs are seldom involved in variola infection. Secondary bacterial infection is not common. Death, when it occurs, probably results from the toxemia associated with circulating immune complexes and soluble variola antigens.[10,59] Encephalitis sometimes ensues that is indistinguishable from the acute postinfectious perivascular demyelination observed as a complication of infection with vaccinia, measles, and varicella.

As patients recover, the scabs separate and the characteristic pitted scarring gradually develops (Fig. 9–4). The scars are most evident on the face and result from the destruction of sebaceous glands followed by shrinking of granulation tissue and fibrosis. Approximately 75% to 80% of persons who recover have persistent scarring for life.[5]

Diagnosis

In endemic areas or when smallpox was known to be circulating, most cases could be diagnosed readily by the presence of a prodromal febrile illness, the appearance of a typical deep-seated rash, the centrifugal distribution of lesions, and the fact that all lesions were at the same stage of development on any given area of the body. The infrequent hemorrhagic cases were often initially misdiagnosed as meningococcemia, acute leukemia, or drug toxicity. Their diagnosis often was assisted by examination of patients who were the source of their infection or to whom they had transmitted disease. Varicella was by far the most frequent disease confused with smallpox. Smallpox patients who had previously been vaccinated, and those with variola minor, sometimes exhibited a sparse and atypical rash with minimal systemic symptoms that resembled varicella. Severe cases of varicella in adults with extensive rash were also sometimes mistaken for smallpox.[60] For this reason, the Centers for Disease Control and Prevention (CDC) has produced and distributed a chart with an algorithm to assist in the differential diagnosis of acute febrile illness associated with rash.[61]

A suspected case of smallpox must be reported immediately to the appropriate local, state, or territorial health department and, through them, to the CDC and the WHO. The diagnosis of a suspected poxvirus infection is approached by first ruling out varicella using direct immunofluorescence methods and/or PCR for varicella zoster and herpes simplex viruses. If these tests are negative, the presence of poxvirus DNA can be rapidly established by PCR testing and by electron microscopic examination of vesicular or pustular fluid or scabs. These methods are available at the CDC, the U.S. Army Medical Research Institute of Infectious Diseases, and designated member laboratories of the national Laboratory Response Network. Consultation with the CDC will determine which tests should be done at which location. Specimens that are required include vesicular or pustular material (scraped or swabbed from the base of a lesion), punch biopsies, scabs, or venous blood. Detailed specimen collection guidelines are available from the CDC.[62] Only personnel immunized against smallpox within the past 3 years, or personnel wearing appropriate respiratory and barrier protective equipment, should collect specimens from suspected patients.

Differentiation between variola, vaccinia, and monkeypox is usually apparent from the patient's history of possible exposure and the characteristics of growth of the virus on the chorioallantoic membrane of chick embryos. PCR techniques for rapid identification and differentiation of orthopoxviruses have been developed and are reliable when used on banked laboratory specimens. Their sensitivity and specificity using fresh material obtained from smallpox patients is unknown.[63]

Recovered patients exhibit high titers of neutralizing, HI, and CF orthopoxvirus antibodies. However, identification of which of the orthopoxvirus species was the responsible agent for a past infection is difficult by laboratory means alone, although cross-absorption studies can be helpful. Characteristic residual facial scars are useful in documenting prior cases of variola major,[64] although some will fade over decades. Persistent scars are too infrequent to be of value in identifying recovered cases of variola minor.[65]

Epidemiology

Transmission of Naturally Occurring Variola Major

Transmission of variola virus, with few exceptions, resulted from droplets expressed from the oral, nasal, or pharyngeal mucosa of an overtly ill patient that were inhaled by susceptible persons in close contact with the patient. Such transmission was possible from the time of onset of rash and was most frequent during the first week of the exanthem. Spread was generally through large droplets and, thus, was not widely dispersed.[5,66] Downie et al. analyzed the immediate environment of smallpox patients in a hospital in Madras.[66] They held a fluid impinger, which screened out particles larger than 18 microns, by patients' oral cavities for 10 to 15 minutes as the patients talked and coughed, and compared the isolation rates of variola virus from the impinger to those of settling plates placed below air samplers under the same conditions. The recovery rate of variola virus from the impinger was only about 11% compared to the recovery rate in the settling plates of 40%. These data suggested that virus was rarely found in small, airborne nuclei, and commonly found in large droplets.

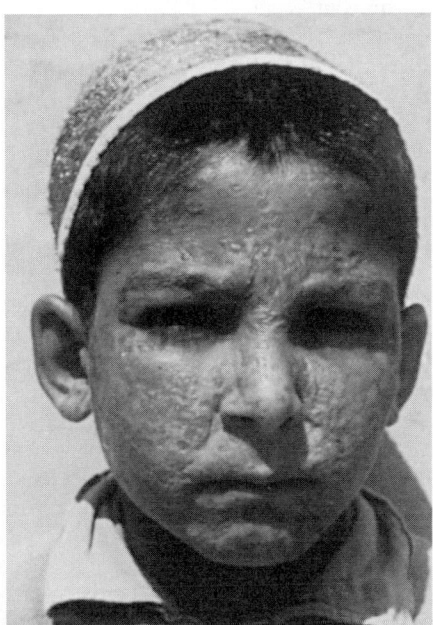

FIGURE 9–4 ■ An Afghani boy with characteristic residual facial scars after smallpox. (Courtesy of the World Health Organization, Geneva, Switzerland.)

Virus also was present in scabs that had separated from the skin lesions of convalescing patients,[67] but epidemiologic evidence showed that infected scabs played a negligible role in transmission of infection, presumably because the virus was tightly bound in its fibrin matrix. It was standard practice during the global eradication program to isolate patients until all scabs had separated from the skin, even though little transmission occurred after scabs had formed.

Airborne infection over longer distances was uncommon, although two outbreaks within hospitals demonstrated this to be possible.[55,68] They probably resulted from true small-droplet nuclei dispersal. In the outbreak that occurred in a hospital in Meschede, Germany, in 1970, a patient initially presumed to have typhoid fever (and cared for under contact isolation precautions) gave rise to 19 other cases of smallpox.[55] Dissemination in this outbreak was favored by low relative humidity, prevailing air currents within the hospital building, and the presence of cough in the patient. Although cough is not a typical finding of ordinary smallpox, in this instance it would have facilitated viral aerosolization.

Instances occurred in which a patient spread the disease to large numbers of contacts, but these were infrequent. In an outbreak in Yugoslavia in 1972, a patient with hemorrhagic smallpox was misdiagnosed as having a severe allergic reaction to penicillin. He was hospitalized because of the development of hemorrhagic disease. In all, he infected 38 health care workers and patients before dying. In another episode, a woman who had vaccine-modified smallpox spread disease to 16 others. She was a neighborhood matriarch who was visited by many friends and neighbors in her community during her illness, and had prolonged face-to-face conversations with many.[5,69]

Infection of persons such as mortuary workers who handled dead bodies, and laundry workers who handled linen from patients, has also been repeatedly documented.[10,70] However, various older accounts that purport to document transmission over great distances on other fomites, such as carpets, letters, and cotton rags, are suspect because the virus does not survive for long periods at customary ambient temperatures.[71]

Another method of transmission, the ancient practice of variolation (inoculation into the skin of material from pustules or scabs from patients), continued in a number of remote areas until August 1976 and was responsible for many cases in Afghanistan and Ethiopia. Those individuals so inoculated often developed extensive rash and transmitted infection to susceptible contacts by droplet infection.[5]

Uncertainty exists as to how contagious smallpox might be following an introduction in today's population. Mathematical modelers have used a wide variety of measures of R0, the average number of contacts that each infected patient would infect in the course of an epidemic. R0 values for smallpox transmission in the general population (exclusive of transmission in health care settings) would most likely be, on average, less than 3.0, although possibly higher than this in winter and much lower in summer when heat and humidity are high. The values of R0 are substantially lower than for other diseases, such as measles, for which the estimated R0 is 12 to 18.[72] However, R0 values increase substantially when hospital-based transmission is considered.[72] Investigation in Europe between 1950 and 1973 indicated that Ro values may increase to 10 to 12 when hospital-based transmission is included.

Geographic Scope and Epidemiologic Characteristics

Smallpox was once worldwide in scope, persisting as endemic disease in areas where susceptible populations were sufficiently large to permit year-round transmission. In remote or isolated areas, epidemics occurred when the disease was introduced, but, because infection results in durable immunity, transmission ceased when the number of susceptible contacts diminished to low numbers. Before vaccination was introduced, almost everyone either died from the disease or became immune.

After vaccination became available, its use followed a common pattern. At first, vaccination was practiced most extensively among middle- and upper-income groups in or near cities where the vaccine was produced, and in more prosperous countries. Thus, during the 20th century, the incidence of smallpox was highest in the developing countries in rural areas and among lower socioeconomic groups in urban areas.

The seasonal pattern of smallpox was similar to that of varicella, measles, meningococcal meningitis, and other epidemic respiratory diseases. Its incidence was highest during winter and spring. This seasonal peak was consonant with the observation that the duration of survival of an orthopoxvirus in the aerosolized form is inversely proportional to temperature and humidity.[73] Seasonal variation undoubtedly was amplified in many countries by social events, such as the congregation of large numbers of people at festivals and marriage parties during the dry season, and the seasonal movement of nomads. Where there was less variation in temperature and humidity, as in equatorial areas of Indonesia and the Democratic Republic of Congo (formerly Zaire), there was less fluctuation in incidence throughout the year.

There were also longer-term temporal trends in incidence in the endemic areas, with major epidemics at intervals of 4 to 7 years.[5,74] These long-term peaks presumably related to accumulation of susceptible persons, and may have been influenced by events such as famine and civil war, which caused extensive refugee movements and widespread dissemination of the virus.

The age distribution of smallpox cases depended on the immunity of the population, whether the immunity was acquired by vaccination or by infection. Because the disease is less infectious than other childhood diseases such as measles, cases regularly occurred among adults. As recently as 1974 to 1975 in India, where vaccination was widely practiced and smallpox was endemic, adults constituted 21% of a carefully documented series of 23,546 patients; 2%, or 412, of these patients were older than 50 years (Table 9–1). In western Africa between 1967 and 1969, most cases occurred in rural villages, and the age distribution of cases approximated the age profile of the population.[75] Men and women were equally affected in all endemic countries.

The severe Asian form of variola major customarily had overall case-fatality rates of about 20%, but they ranged from 40% to 50% for those younger than 1 year and were

TABLE 9–1 ■ India: Cases of Smallpox, Deaths, and Case-Fatality Rates, by Age Group, 1974 to 1975

Age Group (yr)	Number of Cases (% Distribution by Age)	Number of Deaths	Case-Fatality Rate (%)
<1	1373(6)	597	43.5
1–4	5867(25)	1436	24.5
5–9	5875(25)	783	13.3
10–19	5542(23)	432	7.8
≥20	4889(21)	855	17.5
Total	23,546(100)	4103	17.4

From Basu RN, Jesek Z, Ward NA. The eradication of smallpox from India. *In* History of International Public Health No. 2. New Delhi, World Health Organization South-East Asia Regional Office, 1979, p 59.

customarily about 30% among the unvaccinated. Variola major in Africa was a somewhat milder disease, with age-standardized case-fatality rates of about 10% to 15%. Variola minor, which after 1967 was present only in Brazil and southern and eastern Africa, resulted in case-fatality rates of 1% or less.

Within the household, smallpox was as infectious as chickenpox but less infectious than measles.[76–78] With few exceptions, however, smallpox spread less widely and rapidly than these diseases. This finding can be accounted for by the fact that transmission of variola virus did not occur until the onset of rash, as attested by numerous epidemiologic observations. By then, most patients already were confined to bed because of the high fever and malaise of the prodromal illness; secondary cases usually were restricted to the few who came in contact with patients in the household or hospital. For this reason, smallpox outbreaks tended to be clustered in a segment of a town or village and in localized areas of a province or district.[79–82] In endemic areas, a given case of smallpox seldom resulted in more than two to five cases in a subsequent generation, most of whom were relatives or friends.

On the Indian subcontinent, where variola major was prevalent, studies in affected villages showed that secondary household or compound attack rates usually ranged from an average of two to five or more patients per infected case during the seasonal increase of incidence to well under one patient per infected case during the late spring and summer.[81,83–86] One study showed a higher attack rate among people in continuous attendance to cases (27%), compared to those who lived in the compound but left periodically for work (6%).[85] Note, however, that these studies were conducted in villages where there was substantial immunity from previous smallpox infection and vaccination, a factor that serves to retard transmission.

Most outbreaks could be contained successfully by isolating patients and, through vaccination, building a containment barrier of immune persons around patients and those to whom they were most likely to transmit disease (sometimes referred to as "ring vaccination"). In practice, efforts were made to vaccinate all household and close contacts of patients as soon as possible, and, in turn, to vaccinate their household contacts so that, if the contacts did develop smallpox, they would be less likely to spread infection further. In developing countries, the extension of vaccination to a village or local area of a town or city often proved useful. This approach was possible, in part, because vaccination, administered even as late as 2 to 3 days after

exposure to an infected patient, could prevent disease. Vaccination as late as the fourth or fifth day could substantially modify the disease to a more attenuated form.

Analysis of outbreaks following importation of smallpox into Europe after 1950 provide some insight as to how smallpox might spread after a deliberate introduction today. Thirteen of 49 importations yielded no further cases. Seventeen resulted in only one or two subsequent generations of cases. Forty-six outbreaks of smallpox resulted in 854 cases. Fully 430 of these 854 patients acquired smallpox in the hospital, either as health care workers, patients, or visitors. Non–health care workers who got the disease were largely family members or other intimate contacts.[5,8]

The Significance of Smallpox as a Public Health Problem

During recent centuries, smallpox was the most universally feared of all diseases. It could occur and spread in any country; case-fatality rates were altered little by therapy. Virtually all nations made efforts to prevent it. It was not dependent on a vector, and thus could occur in any season. Better sanitation and improved economic conditions helped control diseases such as cholera and typhoid, but such measures had little influence on smallpox.

Jenner's discovery of a protective inoculation was understandably lauded and, although it conferred a high level of protection for a number of years, it was recognized that revaccination was necessary. It was generally believed that vaccination immunity began to wane after 3 to 5 years, but no country was able to sustain a vaccination program that ensured that everyone in the population was fully protected at all times. Thus all countries feared possible smallpox importations and subsequent spread. Through the mid-1970s, international sanitary regulations required travelers to all countries to present certificates attesting to the fact that they had been successfully vaccinated within the preceding 3 years. Even countries that were free of smallpox continued national vaccination programs, at least of children and those in the military, in the belief that this practice would serve to impede the spread of disease if it were introduced. When importations occurred, they were frequently accompanied by public hysteria and a demand for mass vaccination.

The costs of preventive measures for smallpox were substantial. Sencer and Axnick[87] documented activities and expenditures for smallpox control in the United States during 1968, nearly 20 years after its last case of smallpox. In all, 14.2 million persons were vaccinated that year, of which 5.6 million were primary vaccinations and 8.6 million were revaccinations. Because of vaccine complications, 238 required hospitalization, 9 died, and 4 were permanently disabled. The total costs to the country, including the costs of quarantine services, were estimated to be $150 million. Other countries, such as the United Kingdom and the Federal Republic of Germany, maintained special hospitals to be opened to receive patients when imported cases of smallpox occurred. When importations occurred, national authorities frequently took extreme measures. For instance, in Yugoslavia in 1972, the entire population was vaccinated, borders were closed to commerce, and thousands who had possibly been exposed were isolated in hotels co-opted for this purpose.[88]

Although the concern was great, importations of smallpox into industrialized Europe, North America, and Japan were relatively infrequent after 1958. There were only 49 documented importations between 1949 and 1971,[89] with none after 1973.[5] Most importations resulted from improperly vaccinated visitors returning from Bangladesh, India, and Pakistan, although importations from Africa and South America also occurred.

Countries in the endemic regions of the world experienced more frequent importations because travelers and nomads moved freely across long open borders, and reinfected countries that had become smallpox free. Relative to the extent and numbers of travelers, however, importations were comparatively few. This reflected the fact that smallpox outbreaks tended to remain localized, with transmission to relatives or friends in adjacent houses or villages. Travelers were usually adults immune to smallpox as a result of past infections or immunizations. Those who traveled long distances by plane were the more affluent and thus better vaccinated, with less contact with the lower socioeconomic groups and rural peoples, among whom most cases occurred.

Smallpox as a Bioterrorism Weapon

The first documented use of smallpox as a biologic weapon was by British forces during the French and Indian Wars (1754 to 1767). During that time, British soldiers were ordered to distribute smallpox-infected blankets to Indians.[90] Major epidemics subsequently occurred. Military actions during the ensuing years of the American Revolution likewise served to spread smallpox among the colonial troops. No subsequent use of smallpox as a weapon is known. Undoubtedly, this resulted, in substantial part, from increasingly widespread vaccination and a decrease in vulnerability to the disease.

Coincident with the declaration in 1980 that smallpox had been eradicated,[5] The World Health Assembly recommended that all countries cease smallpox vaccination. All complied, and vaccine production facilities closed. Population immunity has steadily waned since that time, leaving an increasingly vulnerable population. In the years that followed eradication, the WHO recommended that all diagnostic and research laboratories either destroy their stocks of smallpox virus or transfer them to one of two designated reference laboratories, at the CDC in the United States or the Research Institute of Viral Preparations in Moscow, Russian Federation. All countries reported voluntary compliance. Later, it was found that the Russians moved their smallpox samples to one of their previous biologic weapons development facilities in Siberia, known as VECTOR.[91]

During the 1980s, leadership in the Soviet Union, having identified smallpox to be one of the best potential bioweapons, began an extensive program of research and development focused on smallpox. Much of this work was conducted at VECTOR. Manufacturing facilities were built and a large stockpile produced. The program, concealed in the biotechnology and pharmaceutical industries, had the capacity to produce upwards of 20 tons of smallpox virus annually for use in bombs and intercontinental ballistic missiles.[2,92] Extensive research programs sought to develop optimal dissemination and delivery systems, and to maximize the virus viability during and after dissemination.[92]

During recent years, funds for the Russian laboratories have decreased and half or more of the scientists have left their positions, some going to other countries. Whether they have taken samples of smallpox virus with them is unknown. Countries such as North Korea, Libya, and Syria are now suspected of being engaged in offensive biologic weapons development,[93] although there is no definite proof that they possess smallpox virus. In 1995, Iraq admitted to the United Nations Special Commission that it possessed an extensive program of research, testing, and weaponization of biologic weapons.[94] Among the agents being tested in this program was camelpox.[95] Although there is no evidence that camelpox causes disease in humans,[96] there are concerns that it may be used as a surrogate virus for smallpox research and development.

Variola virus may be lyophilized and is relatively stable as an aerosol.[73] The infectious dose, as suggested from the epidemiology of a hospital outbreak in which aerosol spread was documented,[55] may be only a few virions. Thus it is believed that smallpox could be effectively disseminated through aerosolization. This seems far more likely than the media speculation that "fanatics" may infect themselves and circulate freely in densely populated areas or areas of high mobility, such as airports. This scenario is improbable because patients infected with smallpox are very ill from the time the prodromal phase ensues, and generally unable to circulate widely.

If an attack were to occur, diagnosis may be delayed because of a lack of familiarity of most physicians with this eradicated disease. However, awareness is rapidly growing among physicians. There are several educational outreach efforts underway. This heightened index of suspicion is corroborated by the increasing number of health care workers reporting cases of "febrile illnesses associated with rash" to the CDC in 2002 (Dr. Julie Gerberding, personal communication, 2002).

Since the terrorist events of September 11, 2001, the federal government has procured a large stock of vaccine to meet the needs of the nation in the event of an outbreak of smallpox.[97] As of the end of 2002, more than 300 million doses were in stock. In 2002, the CDC released a guidance plan to public health agencies detailing the necessary steps to be taken to contain an outbreak of smallpox, including the mass immunization of the entire population in a timely fashion, if need arises.[98] A deliberate release of smallpox remains a low-likelihood, but a high-consequence event.

Active Immunization

Vaccine Strains

Strains of Vaccine and Their Passage

Many strains of vaccinia, known by different names, have been used by different producers during this and the past century, but little is known about their origins or passage histories. Characterization of strains is further complicated by the fact that a seed lot system for vaccine production was not used until the 1960s. Thus even those strains with common names and ancestors have different passage histories, having been passed sequentially through a variety of vaccinifers, such as cows, sheep, and water buffalo, with periodic passages through rabbits, horses, and even humans. Indicative of the ignorance of vaccine technology until recent decades is a statement of the Ministry of Health of Great Britain, which, in 1928,[99] advised that seed lymph could be obtained from (1) "smallpox direct"; (2) cowpox; (3) horsepox, sheep-pox, or goatpox; and (4) vaccinia in the human body.

Jenner is believed to have used cowpox in vaccination, but the vaccinia virus strains used most recently are a different species of orthopoxvirus with distinctive DNA maps that are similar to each other but different from both cowpox and variola. That the vaccinia strains are not mutants of variola virus seems certain,[100] but where the present vaccinia species arose is unknown. It may have arisen either as a hybrid of cowpox and another orthopoxvirus or through thousands of serial passages under artificial conditions of culture. It is also possible that the species represents a laboratory survivor of a now naturally extinct species of orthopoxvirus.[101]

In 1958, a WHO Study Group first recommended that a seed lot system be employed in vaccine manufacture. Beginning in 1967, an increasing number of vaccine producers, encouraged by the WHO, began to use one of two strains. Most common was the Lister strain from the Lister Institute in England, which was propagated as seed virus by the National Public Health Institute of the Netherlands for distribution by the WHO. The second strain was the New York City Board of Health strain (NYCBOH), propagated by Wyeth Laboratories, Radnor, PA. Two of the largest countries, China and India, used other strains called, respectively, the Temple of Heaven strain and the Patwadanger strain.

Further Attenuated Vaccine Strains

The relative risks and benefits of vaccination have changed with the eradication of smallpox. During the eradication campaign, strains that were stable and produced high "take" rates (resulting in solid immunity) were needed. Concern now has shifted to developing strains that have lower pathogenicity. Modern understanding of the genetics of vaccinia, and the ability to manipulate the genome, suggest that such strains may be developed. Such attenuated strains might be used to provide primary protection as a one- or two-dose schedule, or to protect against the adverse effects of vaccinia when given as the initial vaccination of a two-step process (utilizing the well-tested NYCBOH or Lister strains as the second step). Much of the work on such strains is reviewed in Chapter 49.

During the 1930s, vaccinia strains began to be attenuated by serial passages in an effort to diminish the incidence of serious adverse events.[5] The first was the Rivers strain, which was derived from the NYCBOH strain.[102] Three principal variants were developed that had been passed repeatedly through rabbit testes, chick embryo explants, and chorioallantoic membranes of embryonated hens' eggs.[103] Rivers and colleagues[104,105] showed that the "second revived strain" produced less severe reactions in rabbits and humans than did the NYCBOH strain, especially if it was inoculated intradermally. This strain, administered with 2 mL of vaccinia immune globulin (VIG), was used for primary vaccination of 60,000 Dutch army recruits by van der Noordaa and colleagues.[106] One mild case of postvaccinal encephalitis occurred, but this was a lower incidence than the Dutch Army experienced after administration of other strains. The resultant neutralizing antibody titers were lower than those usually observed, which called into question the level of protection provided against smallpox. The strain was not further employed.

Another variant of the Rivers vaccine, the CVI-78 strain, also produced less severe local reactions. Kempe and his colleagues used it to vaccinate children with eczema,[107] but it did not seem likely to provide adequate protection against smallpox.[108] A large-scale comparative trial sponsored by the National Institutes of Health[109,110] showed that the CVI-78 strain was 10-fold less infectious than the Lister and NYCBOH strains, and produced smaller skin lesions and fewer febrile responses. However, 70% of children failed to develop neutralizing antibody, and, even after challenge vaccination with the NYCBOH strain, 25% still did not respond with neutralizing antibody.

Another attenuated vaccine, the modified vaccinia virus Ankara (MVA) strain, was produced by a German research group[111] through more than 500 passages in chick embryo fibroblast cells.[112,113] During passage, multiple deletions occurred and it became much more host range restricted. Laboratory studies demonstrated unimpaired MVA gene expression in human cells and a block in virion morphogenesis.[114] The ability to achieve a high expression of recombinant genes despite abortive replication is a significant characteristic of this mutant virus.[115] Studies presently are being conducted by the National Institute of Allergy and Infectious Diseases comparing antibody responses of those persons receiving two intramuscular doses of a high-titer MVA strain with those receiving one dose of MVA vaccine followed by vaccination with the NYCBOH strain (Dr. Carole Heilman, personal communication, 2002).

Another attenuated strain, LC 16m8, was produced by Hashizume in the 1970s by repeated passage of Lister-strain vaccinia at low temperature in rabbit kidney cells.[116-118] This strain produced HI and neutralizing antibodies in humans, and, in a field trial of 50,000 children, produced markedly less severe reactions than other strains.[119] Further studies employing this strain are planned by Japanese investigators (Dr. Isao Arita, personal communication, 2002) and by Francis and his colleagues at the U.S. company Vaxgen (Dr. Donald Francis, personal communication, 2002).

Another attenuated strain, NYVAC, stemmed from the recognition that 50 or more of the nearly 200 genes of vaccinia virus are dispensable for replication in tissue culture cells, and that deletion of some of these genes reduced virulence in animal models.[120–122] In all, 18 genes were deleted from the Copenhagen strain of vaccinia virus to produce this strain.[123] Several studies indicate that NYVAC has potential for a human vaccine, perhaps to be used as would the nonreplicating MVA strain.[124,125]

A significant problem in developing attenuated strains is that assessment of their efficacy will be impossible to assess with certainty. Because of the absence of human smallpox cases, a determination of efficacy under the conditions of a natural challenge is not possible; in addition, there is no suitable animal model of variola virus infection, and surrogate serologic measures of protection are unknown. The evaluation of efficacy thus will have to rely on comparison of serologic responses with those induced by the NYCBOH or Lister strains and challenge of vaccinated monkeys with aerosols of monkeypox virus.

Dosage and Route

Jenner realized that the skin had to be abraded to produce a successful vaccination. Over the years, a number of methods were developed to break open the skin and introduce the virus. Early vaccine preparations undoubtedly had variable titers, and fairly vigorous techniques sometimes were used to enhance the chance of successful vaccination. A variety of knives, needles, and scalpels were used to scarify the skin. Some techniques, most notably the rotary lancets used in India, Pakistan, and Bangladesh, were painful and caused significant lesions even in the absence of viral replication. In the United States, during the 1920s, Leake[126] vigorously promoted a multiple pressure technique, in which virus was pressed into the skin by multiple firm pressures with the blunt side of a needle. He emphasized the importance that blood not be drawn, believing that bleeding might wash out the virus. In practice, it proved difficult to strike the proper balance between vaccinating too vigorously, thus drawing blood, and vaccinating too gently, thus failing to implant the virus.

In the early days of the worldwide eradication campaign, specially adapted jet-injector guns were employed to accelerate mass vaccination efforts, particularly in West Africa and Brazil. The guns proved to be cumbersome and expensive to maintain, and not well adapted to house-to-house vaccination methods employed by surveillance and containment teams. They were abandoned in favor of the bifurcated needle, which was invented in 1965 by Dr. Benjamin Rubin of Wyeth Laboratories.

Presently, vaccine is inoculated intradermally with a bifurcated needle. No alcohol, acetone, or other skin preparation should be used. The vaccine should have a titer of not less than 10^8 pock-forming units per milliliter by assay on the chorioallantoic membranes of 12-day-old chick embryos. Approximately 0.0025 mL of vaccine adheres by capillary action between the tines of the bifurcated needle when it is dipped into the vaccine. The needle is positioned vertically to the skin surface, usually the lateral surface of the upper arm (Fig. 9–5), with the heel of the hand resting on the arm. Fifteen rapid strokes are made sufficiently forcefully so that a trace of blood appears at the vaccination site within 20 to 30 seconds. Good technique produces virtually 100% "takes" in vaccinia-naïve individuals.

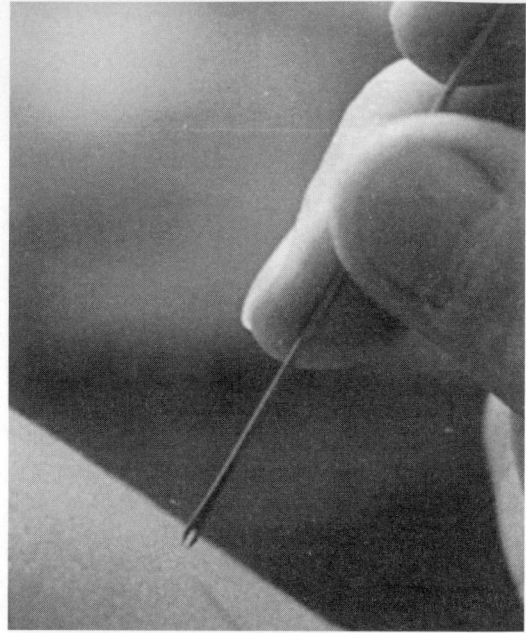

FIGURE 9–5 ▪ The bifurcated needle positioned to begin multiple-puncture vaccination. (Courtesy of the World Health Organization, Geneva, Switzerland.)

Site Care

The vaccination site should be covered until the scab forms. A loose gauze dressing during the 2 to 3 weeks in which virus is shed from the site[32] prevents clothing from being soiled and the accidental abrasion of the lesion. More occlusive dressings, even if semipermeable, may cause maceration of the skin and the development of satellite lesions.[127] Studies of the optimal site care to prevent the spread of vaccinia and to avoid excessive local reaction (such as skin maceration) are in progress. The Advisory Committee on Immunization Practices (ACIP) of the CDC recommends that recently vaccinated non–health care workers cover the site with a loose gauze bandage and adhere to strict hand hygiene after contact with the vaccinated site. Bathing is acceptable, but the site should be kept dry otherwise. A separate towel should be used to dry the vaccinated site until a scab forms.[128] For recently vaccinated health care workers, the ACIP recommends avoidance of contact with high-risk patients, if possible, until the scab separates. If contact is unavoidable, meticulous hand hygiene and a dressing comprising gauze (or a similar absorbent material) covered with a semiocclusive dressing, or a product that combines an absorbent base with an overlying semipermeable layer, are recommended during direct patient care until the scab separates.[128,129] The ACIP does not believe that health care workers need to be placed on administrative leave after being vaccinated unless they develop extensive skin lesions, which would preclude adherence with the infection control precautions described above.

Production of Vaccine

Most vaccine was grown on the skin of a calf, sheep, or water buffalo and harvested after sacrifice of the animal. The vaccine usually was purified by the addition of fluorocarbon and differential centrifugation, and its bacterial content was reduced by the addition of phenol. Peptone was added as a stabilizing agent, and the vaccine was freeze dried. Because of its source, calfskin vaccine inevitably contained some bacteria but, when properly prepared, the number of bacteria was 10 organisms/mL or less. Microbiologic examination was required to confirm that none were human pathogens. For reconstitution of the vaccine for multiple puncture vaccination, a solution of 50% (volume per volume) glycerin in McIlvaine solution was used. The vaccine in its freeze-dried form was required to retain a potency of not less than 10^8 pock-forming units per milliliter after incubation at 37°C for 1 month.

During the 1960s and 1970s, laboratories in Brazil, New Zealand, Sweden, and the United States (Texas State Health Department) harvested vaccinia virus from the chorioallantoic membranes of chick embryos, a simple process that permits production of a bacteria-free vaccine. However, vaccine from this source proved difficult to produce in a satisfactory thermostabile, freeze-dried form and, as far as is known, only Sweden produced vaccine in eggs that were free of avian leukosis virus.

Vaccinia virus grown in tissue culture initially proved difficult to produce as a thermostabile, freeze-dried product but, in the 1970s Hekker and colleagues[130] eventually achieved good results using Lister-strain vaccinia virus grown primarily in rabbit kidney cells. In field trials, the vaccine was comparable to vaccine grown on calf skin,[131,132] but, because of the impending conclusion of the smallpox eradication program, the WHO made no effort to introduce the method for use in other laboratories.

Because of the eradication of smallpox and the cessation of routine vaccination, the number of production laboratories diminished from 76 in 1977 to 11 in 1985, and, by 2000, the only one remaining was a laboratory in Chiba, Japan (since closed), that produced small amounts of the attenuated vaccine LC 16m8 for use in protecting laboratory staff working with orthopoxviruses. However, increasing concern about the possible use of smallpox as a biologic weapon caused the United States, in September 2000, to contract with an American-based company, Acambis, to develop for licensure and to produce 40 million doses of freeze-dried, tissue-culture vaccine utilizing the NYCBOH strain cells. The contract called for the company to sustain production capability for 20 years. A second contract, issued in November 2001, provided for the production of an additional 155 million doses of the NYCBOH strain in Vero cells through a joint effort by Acambis and Baxter Laboratories. A Danish-based company, Bavarian Nordic, recently has begun production of Lister-strain vaccinia in chick embryo fibroblast tissue cell culture and contemplates the possible production of MVA vaccine for use as a first dose in a vaccination schedule to be followed by vaccination with the conventional Lister strain. Other countries, including Brazil, the Netherlands, Japan, and Russia, have indicated an interest in vaccine production using either tissue culture production methods or traditional calfskin growth.

Storage Conditions

Freeze-dried smallpox vaccine is the most stable of the currently available vaccines. The vaccine can be preserved indefinitely at −20°C, and most batches can be preserved for many months to years at 4°C. International standards require that the vaccine in its freeze-dried form maintain full potency when it is incubated at 37°C for 1 month. Studies of vaccine produced at the Lister Institute demonstrated that it retained full potency for 64 weeks when incubated at temperatures of up to 45°C, and for 104 weeks at 37°C.[133] Not all vaccines are this stable, but assay of vaccines produced in India and the former USSR and retrieved from the field revealed batches of vaccine that met potency standards after 6 to 9 months of exposure at high ambient summer temperatures. After reconstitution, the vaccine is much more sensitive to temperature and exposure to direct light. During the eradication program, unused reconstituted vaccine was routinely discarded at the end of each day, but in fact it will remain potent for a much longer time. Studies of reconstituted NYCBOH strain vaccine, grown in calves, showed that vaccine retained satisfactory potency for 1 month when subjected to alternate 12-hour cycles of 4°C and 25°C temperatures, much like temperature conditions to which the vaccine might be subjected in a clinic today (Dr. Karen Midthun, personal communication, 2002).

Results of Vaccination

Successful primary vaccination results in virus proliferation in the basal cells of the epidermis, producing the typical Jennerian vesicle (Fig. 9–6). A papule with surrounding erythema develops in 3 to 5 days, rapidly becoming a vesicle and later a pustule. It reaches its maximum size after 8 to 10 days. A scab forms that separates at 14 to 21 days, leaving a typical vaccination scar. A low-grade fever usually accompanies the development of the pustule, and swelling and tenderness of the draining lymph nodes is often observed. When European vaccine was used, viremia occasionally occurred between the 3rd and 10th days,[134] and the virus was sometimes isolated from tonsillar swabs.[135] Efforts by Kempe in the 1960s to grow virus from the blood of NYCBOH strain recipients postvaccination were unsuccessful (Dr. Michael Lane, personal communication, 2002).

In a trial to assess clinical responses to Wyeth's Dryvax (NYCBOH strain), initial vaccination was successful in 665 of 680 subjects (97.8%). The frequency and severity of systemic signs and symptoms are shown in Table 9–2. The most frequent symptoms were pain at the vaccination site, muscle aches, and fatigue. Although slight elevations in temperature were common, overt fever (>38.3°C) occurred only in 3.3% of subjects, prior to the 10th day after vaccination in the vast majority. In all, 14% of subjects developed rashes at other than the vaccination site, usually pustular or vesicular, affecting the chest and back, with spontaneous resolution in all. A total of 36% of subjects were sufficiently debilitated from the vaccine to have trouble sleeping, or miss at least 1 day of work, school, or recreational activities.[136]

An individual's response to revaccination depends on the person's degree of immunity. In highly immune individuals, erythema typically develops within 24 to 48 hours as a classical delayed hypersensitivity reaction. Benenson[137] showed that this reaction could be elicited with both live and inactivated vaccine in previously vaccinated patients.

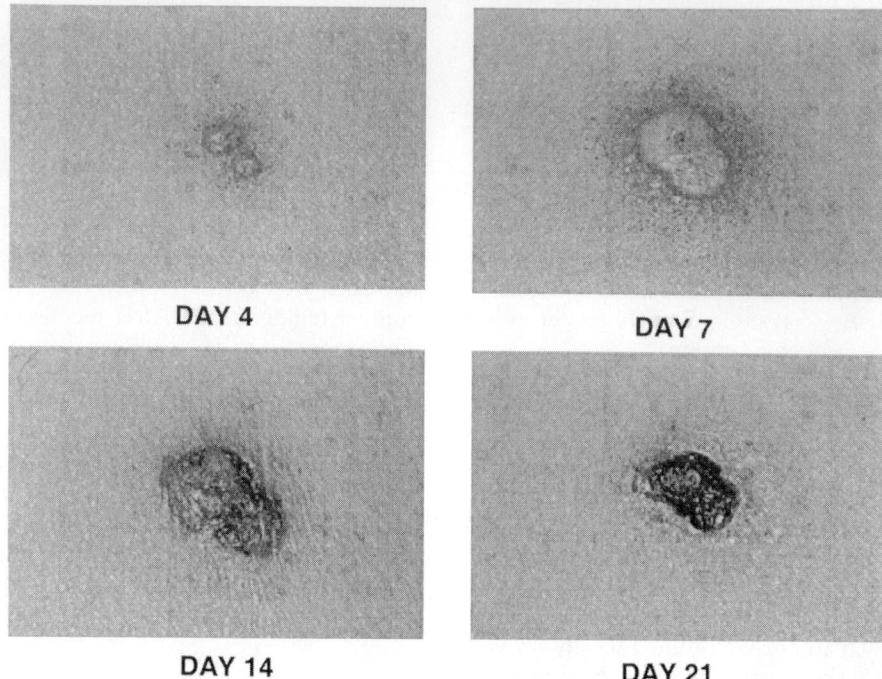

DAY 4   **DAY 7**

DAY 14   **DAY 21**

FIGURE 9–6 ■ Normal reaction evolution after primary vaccination. (From Centers for Disease Control and Prevention. Vaccinia (smallpox) vaccine: recommendations of the Advisory Committee on Immunization Practices (ACIP), 2001. MMWR 50(RR-10):1–25, 2001.)

Persons with some residual cell-mediated immunity, but not enough to inhibit viral replication, develop erythema and a pustule at the site that evolves more rapidly than a primary vaccination reaction. If this is present at 6 to 8 days, it is considered to be evidence of virus proliferation and is termed a *major reaction*. It should be noted that those individuals with substantial immunity may experience no more than a hypersensitivity reaction. Because it is impossible to distinguish clinically between a hypersensitivity reaction resulting from the use of impotent vaccine or poor vaccination technique, and a similar reaction resulting from a high level of immunity, the WHO Expert Committee on Smallpox[49] recommended that such a response be termed an *equivocal reaction*. Persons with equivocal reactions should be revaccinated with vaccine of known high potency using a vigorous technique.

After primary vaccination, neutralizing and HI antibodies develop about the 10th day and are present in almost all persons by the end of 2 weeks; CF antibodies develop in less than half of vacinees.[58] Because the antibody response after primary vaccination usually occurs 4 to 8 days earlier than the response after naturally acquired smallpox infection,[138] primary vaccination, even after exposure, can modify or abort the disease. Such data as are available indicate the likelihood of substantial protection against disease even when vaccination takes place as much as 2 to 3 days after infection, and at least partial protection against a fatal outcome when administered as late as 4 to 5 days after infection occurs. Neutralizing antibodies are the most persistent and may be detected for 20 years or more; HI and CF antibodies, however, usually are not detectable beyond 6 months. Antibody response after revaccination is more rapid, usually within 7 days, and antibody titers are gener-

ally higher. However, some persons who exhibit a substantial rise in neutralizing antibody titer after revaccination fail to exhibit a rise in either HI or CF antibody levels.

Little is known about the cell-mediated immunity that is induced, although Pincus and Flick[139] demonstrated the beginning development of delayed hypersensitivity, an index of cell-mediated immunity, as early as 2 days after vaccination. In a trial designed to evaluate the immunogenicity of undiluted and diluted smallpox vaccine in primary vaccinees, the development of a vesicle after vaccination correlated with the development of vaccinia virus–specific cytotoxic T-cell responses.[140] Interestingly, there was a dose-response effect in that higher doses of vaccine produced a stronger cytotoxic T-cell response. Conversely, the absence of a primary skin vesicle after primary vaccination was associated with the lack of T-cell or B-cell responses.

Protection Afforded by Vaccination

Reliable data about the efficacy and durability of protection afforded by vaccination are sparse. Before 1967, revaccination every 3 to 10 years was considered essential to ensure protection. This practice was based on early data largely from the United Kingdom, such as those provided by Hanna,[141] and on more recent data from India.[50] These studies compared the frequency of smallpox cases among those with and without vaccination scars. However, the vaccine in use in the populations studied was far lower in titer than that used after 1967, and most of the vaccine was heavily contaminated with bacteria. In India, the vaccination instrument used was the rotary lancet, which frequently produced localized sepsis and an apparent scar even

TABLE 9–2 ■ Frequency and Severity of Systemic Signs and Symptoms of Vaccinia Virus Replication and Pain Among All the Subjects with Vesicle Formation After the First Vaccination[*]

	Number of Subjects (Percent)				
Variable	Days 0–6 (N = 665)	Days 7–9 (N = 665)	Days 10–12 (N = 665)	Days 13–14 (N = 665)	Days 15 and Beyond (N = 205)[†]
Oral temperature[‡]					
≥37.7°C (100°F)	15 (2.3)	59 (8.9)	35 (5.3)	4 (0.6)	2 (1.0)
≥38.3°C (101°F)	6 (0.9)	20 (3.0)	19 (2.9)	2 (0.3)	0
≥38.8°C (102°F)	2 (0.3)	5 (0.8)	2 (0.3)	0	0
Headache					
None	371 (55.8)	395 (59.4)	412 (62.0)	559 (84.1)	173 (84.4)
Mild	194 (29.2)	178 (26.8)	161 (24.2)	76 (11.4)	21 (10.2)
Moderate	86 (12.9)	78 (11.7)	75 (11.3)	25 (3.8)	8 (3.9)
Severe	14 (2.1)	14 (2.1)	17 (2.6)	5 (0.8)	0
Muscle aches					
None	400 (60.2)	330 (49.6)	381 (57.3)	603 (90.7)	191 (93.2)
Mild	204 (30.7)	198 (29.8)	176 (26.5)	52 (7.8)	10 (4.9)
Moderate	55 (8.3)	120 (18.0)	94 (14.1)	7 (1.1)	1 (0.5)
Severe	6 (0.9)	17 (2.6)	14 (2.1)	3 (0.5)	0
Chills					
None	575 (86.5)	547 (82.3)	562 (84.5)	653 (98.2)	199 (97.1)
Mild	68 (10.2)	75 (11.3)	59 (8.9)	8 (1.2)	2 (1.0)
Moderate	16 (2.4)	31 (4.7)	34 (5.1)	2 (0.3)	0
Severe	6 (0.9)	12 (1.8)	10 (1.5)	2 (0.3)	0
Nausea					
None	560 (84.2)	572 (86.0)	586 (88.1)	640 (96.2)	195 (95.1)
Mild	77 (11.6)	67 (10.1)	52 (7.8)	17 (2.6)	4 (2.0)
Moderate	20 (3.0)	19 (2.9)	21 (3.2)	6 (0.9)	2 (1.0)
Severe	8 (1.2)	7 (1.1)	6 (0.9)	2 (0.3)	1 (0.5)
Fatigue					
None	314 (47.2)	348 (52.3)	380 (57.1)	549 (82.6)	166 (81.0)
Mild	246 (37.0)	186 (28.0)	184 (27.7)	88 (13.2)	32 (15.6)
Moderate	89 (13.4)	114 (17.1)	84 (12.6)	21 (3.2)	6 (2.9)
Severe	16 (2.4)	17 (2.6)	17 (2.6)	7 (1.1)	0
Rash at sites other than vaccination site					
None	643 (96.7)	628 (94.4)	598 (89.9)	631 (94.9)	182 (88.8)
Mild	17 (2.6)	31 (4.7)	51 (7.7)	31 (4.7)	16 (7.8)
Moderate	5 (0.8)	5 (0.8)	12 (1.8)	3 (0.5)	1 (0.5)
Severe	0	1 (0.2)	4 (0.6)	0	2 (1.0)
Pain at vaccination site					
None	301 (45.3)	156 (23.5)	155 (23.3)	488 (73.4)	157 (76.6)
Mild	311 (46.8)	284 (42.7)	307 (46.2)	163 (24.5)	44 (21.5)
Moderate	51 (7.7)	212 (31.9)	181 (27.2)	14 (2.1)	2 (1.0)
Severe	2 (0.3)	13 (2.0)	22 (3.3)	0	0

[*]There were no significant differences among the groups, with the exception that the group given undiluted vaccine had a higher incidence of muscle aches on days 0 through 6 (P = 0.01 by the Kruskal–Wallis test) and a higher incidence of local pain on days 10 through 12 (P = 0.0037 by the Kruskal–Wallis test) than did the other two groups. Mild symptoms were easily tolerated; moderate symptoms were bothersome but did not preclude the performance of routine activities; severe symptoms precluded the performance of routine activities.
[†]Data were missing for some of the 205 subjects who reported data after these obtained from the 14-day diary card.
[‡]The temperatures are nested.
From Frey SE, Couch RB, Tacket CO, et al. Clinical responses to undiluted and diluted smallpox vaccine. N Engl J Med 346:1265–1274, 2002, with permission. Copyright © 2002, Massachusetts Medical Society. All Rights Reserved.

when only the diluent was applied. The estimates of protection after successful vaccination in these studies are probably understated.

From studies conducted since 1967, it is probable that vaccinial immunity is more durable than most investigators believed, especially in endemic areas. The evidence is indirect, however, because there are no serologic indices that are known to correlate with protection. Unfortunately, resistance to intradermal inoculation with vaccinia virus has been mistakenly equated by some with resistance to variola virus acquired by droplet inhalation. With the available higher titer vaccines, studies show that major reactions can be induced in persons successfully vaccinated as recently as 3 to 6 months before and, indeed, in more than 10% of those who experienced smallpox only 1 year previously.[142] Because natural infection effectively confers permanent immunity, it is apparent that the ability of vaccinia virus to proliferate in the basal cells of the dermis correlates poorly with the level of protection afforded against natural infection.

In most countries, 90% or more of cases occurred among individuals without vaccination scars. This finding led to surveys in the endemic countries that disclosed vaccine efficacy ratios of 80% or more among those vaccinated 20 years previously. Heiner and colleagues[78] showed that this protection could not be attributed solely to the vaccine. They discovered that previously vaccinated persons often developed noncontagious inapparent infections (termed *variola sine eruptione*) with substantial increases in antibody levels. Immunity in the endemic countries was thus a composite of past experiences with both vaccinia and variola infections.

Data from countries where smallpox was introduced after an absence of many years provide insufficient information to permit a calculation of vaccine efficacy ratios, but they do suggest that vaccinia provides long-term protection against a fatal outcome.[89] Among 680 cases of variola major occurring after importations of smallpox into Europe, the case-fatality rate was 52% among those who had never been vaccinated, 1.4% among those vaccinated up to 10 years before exposure, 7% among those vaccinated 10 to 20 years before exposure, and 11.1% among those vaccinated more than 20 years before.[89]

Correlates of Protection

What aspects of the immune response following vaccination are required to protect an individual from smallpox infection are not perfectly understood, but likely involve a combination of both humoral and cellular immunity. Neutralizing antibodies develop in almost all primary vaccinees by the end of 2 weeks and can persist for 30 years or more.[143] However, the titer of neutralizing antibody required to protect against smallpox is unknown. Titers of neutralizing antibodies measured in primary vaccinees at 1 year were only 23.7% of the titers measured on day 28 after vaccination.[140] Much of the available data on persistence of these antibodies comes from revaccinees who may have had one or more subclinical infections.

Cell-mediated immunity to vaccinia may develop as early as 2 days after primary immunization, and may be long lived. Demkowitz and colleagues found evidence of T-cell activity against vaccinia as much as 50 years after vaccination among individuals who had lived only in nonendemic areas,[144] and Frelinger and Garba reported T-cell activity in persons vaccinated more than 35 years previously.[145] The development of a vesicle after primary vaccination correlated with the development of cytotoxic T-cell responses in a recent trial.[140] Although there was no significant difference in the magnitude of the cytotoxic T-cell response between the group that received undiluted vaccine and the group that received a 1:10 diluted vaccine, the group that received 1:100 diluted vaccine had a considerably lower cytotoxic T-cell response despite vesicle formation after immunization. Furthermore, production of vaccinia virus–specific interferon-γ in peripheral blood monocytes was greatest in those who received undiluted vaccine, and

smallest in those who received 1:100 diluted vaccine, irrespective of vesicle formation. What, if any, correlation exists between T-cell activity and immunity to a naturally occurring challenge is also unknown.

These data and epidemiologic observations suggest the following about the probable protection afforded against acquiring smallpox and against the occurrence of fatal outcomes:

1. Patients who survive smallpox are fully protected for life from experiencing the disease a second time.
2. Persons who have had a primary vaccination and who have experienced a subclinical smallpox infection (variola *sine eruptione*) are likewise protected for life.
3. Persons who have had a primary vaccination and one or more successful revaccinations, even if more than 30 years ago, probably sustain substantial protection against a fatal outcome and some protection against acquiring the disease. It must be noted, however, that a "successful" revaccination requires that the vaccination has been properly performed so that the individual has experienced a "major" reaction (see under *Results of Vaccination* above). Because of the practice in the United States of vaccinating less vigorously so as not to draw blood, it is quite possible that many of the revaccinations administered in the United States were not successful.
4. Persons who have a primary revaccination only will have reasonably complete protection against acquiring smallpox for at least 3 to 5 years, but protection steadily wanes and is probably minimal to nil after 30 years. Protection against a fatal outcome of smallpox, however, may persist for a longer time and may, indeed, for some, extend beyond 30 years.

Simultaneous Administration with Other Antigens

Smallpox vaccine can be administered at the same time as a number of other antigens, usually at a different site, with levels of safety and efficacy comparable to those observed when the vaccines are given separately. Simultaneous administration of oral poliovirus and smallpox vaccines became a routine practice in many countries beginning in the 1960s.[146,147] Smallpox and bacille Calmette-Guérin (BCG) vaccines began to be administered to newborns in Hong Kong in the 1960s.[148] This became a common practice in many African countries in the late 1960s. Yellow fever and smallpox vaccines were mixed and administered successfully in many French-speaking areas of western Africa,[149] and measles and smallpox vaccines were simultaneously administered throughout western Africa from 1967 to 1972.[150] Mixing of smallpox, yellow fever, and measles vaccines for inoculation by jet injection resulted in a diminished immune response to yellow fever vaccine,[151] but responses were satisfactory when different sites of inoculation were used. Ruben and colleagues[152] extended the studies to the simultaneous administration by jet injection, but at different sites, of smallpox, yellow fever, measles, and diphtheria-tetanus-pertussis (DTP) vaccines. They found that systemic reactions were no more frequent or severe than those that occur after measles or smallpox vaccination alone, although there was a diminished immune response to measles. This last observation was not confirmed in subsequent studies. From these and other observations, Foege and Foster[153] concluded that it was safe and efficacious to administer simultaneously all the vaccines (oral poliovirus, DTP, measles, and BCG) then employed in the WHO Expanded Programme of Immunisation, as well as smallpox and yellow fever vaccines. The ACIP recommends that varicella and smallpox vaccines be administered at least 4 weeks apart[129] because, if postvaccination skin lesions occur following the concomitant administration of these two vaccines, it may not be possible to determine which vaccine was responsible and to provide appropriate care.

Complications of Vaccination

Skin Reactions

Vacinees may develop a variety of skin rashes after vaccination. Most are benign, but two can be life threatening: eczema vaccinatum and progressive vaccinia (Tables 9–3 and 9–4).

Eczema vaccinatum (Fig. 9–7A) follows vaccination (or accidental implantation from vaccinated contacts) of individuals with active or quiescent atopic dermatitis (including eczema). Either concurrently with or shortly after the development of the local vaccinial lesion, or after an incubation period of about 5 days in an unvaccinated eczematous contact, a vaccinial eruption occurs at sites that are eczematous or that had previously been so. The areas become intensely inflamed, and the eruption sometimes spreads to normal skin. Constitutional symptoms are usually severe, with high temperature and generalized lymphadenopathy. The patients may lose fluid and electrolytes through exudation. Deaths are uncommon if the condition is properly treated, but those that do occur are usually in young children with severe eczema who acquire vaccinia through contact.

Progressive vaccinia (sometimes called vaccinia necrosum, vaccinia gangrenosa, or disseminated vaccinia) (Fig. 9–7B) is the most severe complication of vaccination, and affects immunodeficient persons. These include, among others, those with agammaglobulinemia, defective cell-mediated immunity, and immune deficiency associated with tumors of the reticuloendothelial system or from the use of immunosuppressive drugs. In the 1960s, this population was composed mostly of those with agammaglobulinemia or chronic lymphocytic leukemia. Today, patients with serious immunosuppression from human immunodeficiency virus (HIV) or organ transplantation would comprise most of this at-risk population. In such patients, the vaccinia lesion fails to heal and usually does not show the cardinal signs of inflammation. Secondary lesions sometimes appear elsewhere on the body and then gradually spread. VIG, as well as methisazone (N-methylisatin β-thiosemicarbazone), are reported to have been partially effective in treatment.[154] Data are sparse, however, and methisazone is no longer available for use. Cidofovir, an antiviral agent licensed in 1996 for the treatment of cytomegalovirus retinitis in acquired immunodeficiency syndrome (AIDS) patients, shows in vitro activity against orthopoxviruses, and may prevent disease in animal models when given shortly before or at the time of vaccinia infection,[155] but has not yet been shown to have therapeutic value in treating an established infection of any orthopoxvirus. Ribavirin, another antiviral drug with in vitro activity against vaccinia, was used successfully with VIG in the treatment of one patient with progressive vaccinia.[156]

Generalized vaccinia (Fig. 9–7C) occurs in immunocompetent individuals from the systemic spread of vaccinia from

TABLE 9–3 ■ Complications of Smallpox Vaccination in the United States, 1968

Vaccination Status and Age (yr)	Estimated Number of Vaccinations	Number of Reported Cases (Deaths)					
		Postvaccinal Encephalitis	Progressive Vaccinia	Eczema Vaccinatum	Generalized Vaccinia	Accidental Infection	Other
Primary vaccinations							
<1	614,000	4 (3)	—	5	43	7	10
1–4	2,733,000	6	1	31	47	91	40
5–9	1,553,000	5 (1)	1 (1)	11	20	32	8
10–19	406,000	—	1 (1)	3	5	3	1
≥20	288,000	1	2	7	13	4	5
Unknown		—	—	1	3	5	2
Total	5,594,000	16 (4)	5 (2)	58	131	142	66
Revaccinations							
<1	—	—	—	—	—	—	—
1–4	478,000	—	—	1	—	1	1
5–9	1,643,000	—	1 (1)	4	1	3	2
10–19	2,657,000	—	1	3	—	—	—
≥20	3,796,000	—	4 (1)	—	9	3	6
Total	8,574,000	—	6 (2)	8	10	7	9
Unvaccinated contacts		—	—	60 (1)	2	44	8
Total	14,168,000	16 (4)	11 (4)	126 (1)	143	193	83

From Lane JM, Ruben FL, Neff JM, Millar JD. Complications of smallpox vaccination, 1968: national surveillance in the United States. N Engl J Med 281:1201–1208, 1969, with permission.

TABLE 9–4 ■ Complications per 1 Million Smallpox Vaccinations in the United States During 1968

Vaccination Status and Age (yr)	Postvaccinal Encephalitis	Progressive Vaccinia	Eczema Vaccinatum	Generalized Vaccinia	Accidental Infection	Other
Primary vaccination						
1	6.5	—	8.1	70.0	11.4	16.3
1–4	2.2	*	11.3	17.2	33.3	14.6
5–9	3.2	*	7.1	12.9	20.6	5.2
10–19	—	*	*	12.3	*	*
≥20	*	*	24.3	45.1	13.9	17.4
Total	2.9	0.9	10.4	23.4	25.4	11.8
Revaccination						
1	—	—	—	—	—	—
1–4	—	—	*	—	*	*
5–9	—	*	2.4	*	*	*
10–19	—	*	*	—	—	—
≥20	—	1.1	—	2.4	*	1.6
Total	—	0.7	0.9	1.2	0.8	1.0

*Fewer than four cases; rate not computed.

From Lane JM, Ruben FL, Neff JM, Millar JD. Complications of smallpox vaccination, 1968: national surveillance in the United States. N Engl J Med 281:1201–1208, 1969, with permission.

the vaccination site. It is a benign reaction in which one to many lesions develop within 6 to 9 days after vaccination at locations other than the vaccination site. The evolution of these lesions follows the same temporal course as that of the vaccination lesion itself. Although patients may experience high fever and malaise, an uneventful recovery without the need for specific therapy is the norm.

Accidental implantation (or inoculation) of vaccinia virus occurs when virus from the primary site is transferred to other parts of the body (or to other individuals). Accidental implantation is the most common adverse event following vaccination, and occurs most frequently in young children who cannot refrain from scratching the itchy vaccination site and then scratching other areas of the body. The most common sites for implantation are the vulva, perineum, and eyelids (Fig. 9–7D). Lesions resulting from accidental implantation usually heal without therapy at the same time as the primary site lesion. Occasionally, implantation of the eyelids leads to *vaccinia keratitis*. In the only large series available, 6% of patients with ocular implantation had corneal involvement.[157]

Although VIG frequently was given to patients with ocular vaccinia in the hope that it would reduce inflammation, VIG is contraindicated in patients with corneal lesions because antibody-antigen precipitates corneal scars and blindness.[158] *Erythema multiforme* (Fig. 9–7E) is the term used to identify several types of benign skin rashes that require only symptomatic therapy. Rarely, bullous lesions of Stevens-Johnson syndrome develop, requiring aggressive supportive and even steroid therapy. *Bacterial infection* (Fig. 9–7F) of the site, usually secondary to staphylococcus and/or streptococcus, was common when vaccine was contaminated with bacteria on calfskin. With improved methods, such infections ceased to occur. Pyogenic infection may be difficult to distinguish from normal but vigorous primary takes. Such infections require antimicrobial therapy for resolution.

Postvaccinal Encephalopathy and Encephalitis

Among those without known contraindications to vaccination, postvaccinal encephalopathy and encephalitis are the most serious adverse events. The incidence of these

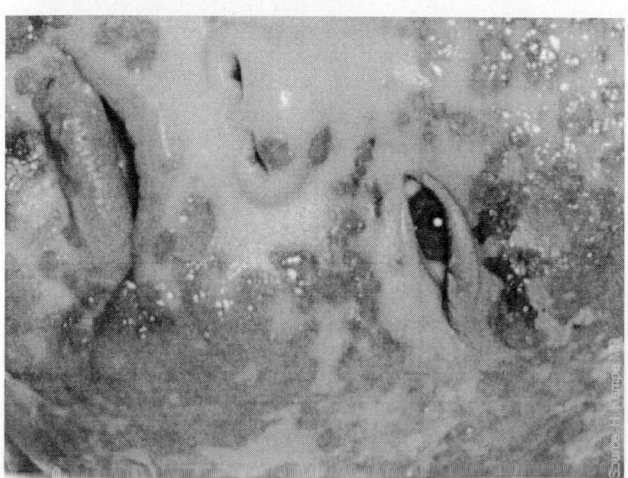

FIGURE 9–7 ■ Complications of vaccination. A, Eczema vaccinatum.

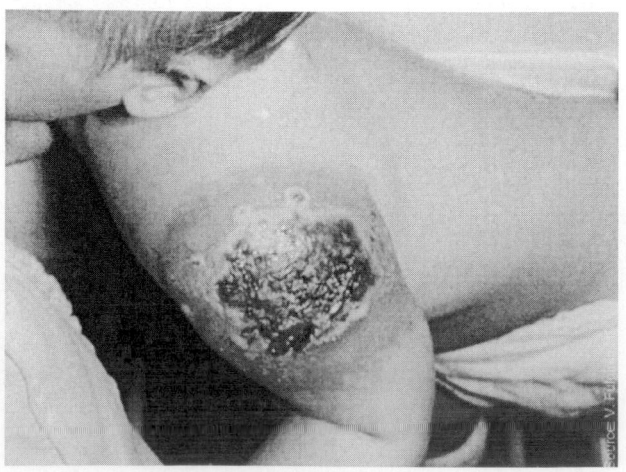

FIGURE 9–7 ■ B, Progressive vaccinia.

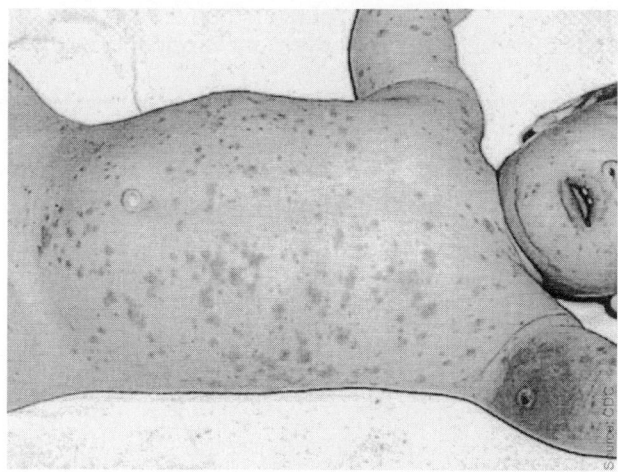

FIGURE 9–7 ■ C, Generalized vaccinia.

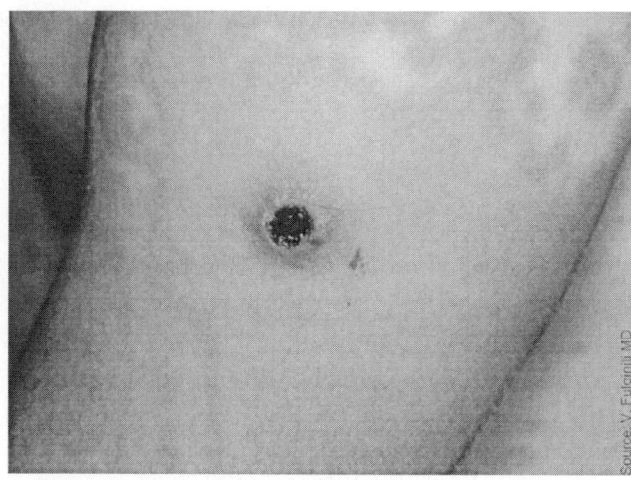

FIGURE 9–7 ■ E, Erythema multiforme.

complications was substantially higher in Europe, where more reactogenic strains were in common use in the 1950s and early 1960s,[159] than in the United States, where the NYCBOH strain was employed. DeVries distinguished two pathologic forms[160]: encephalopathy primarily in children younger than 2 years, and encephalitis or encephalomyelitis in older persons. Postvaccinal encephalopathy is characterized by general hyperemia of the brain, lymphocytic infiltration of the meninges, widespread degenerative changes in ganglion cells, and perivascular hemorrhage. Symptoms are severe and begin abruptly within 6 to 10 days after vaccination,[161] with fever and convulsions, usually followed by hemiplegia and aphasia. Death, when it occurs, follows within a few days. Recovery is seldom complete; the patient is left with mental impairment and some degree of paralysis. Postvaccinal encephalitis is characterized by perivenous demyelination and microglial proliferation, and primarily afflicts persons older than 2 years. It is similar to the form of postviral encephalitis observed after vaccination against rabies or after measles infection. Illness usually begins between 8 and 15 days after vaccination and

is accompanied by fever, vomiting, headache, malaise, and anorexia followed by disorientation and drowsiness and sometimes convulsions and coma. Death occurs in 10% to 35% of cases, usually within a week. Some survivors have residual paralysis or mental impairment. Paralysis, when it is present, tends to be of the upper motor neuron type. Among those patients who recover fully, symptoms and signs resolve within 2 weeks.[162–169]

Many reports document the frequency of cases of postvaccinal encephalopathy and encephalitis in Europe and the United States. The rates are difficult to compare because of differing criteria for diagnosis and variability in the completeness of reporting (Table 9–5). The incidence rates reported from the Netherlands, Germany, and Austria were higher than those in the United Kingdom, which in turn appeared to be marginally higher than those found in the United States.[170–172] Whatever the criteria and methods, differences between the rates appeared to be real. This fact caused a number of countries, during the 1960s, to begin using the Lister strain, then in use in the United Kingdom. A dramatic reduction in the incidence of post-

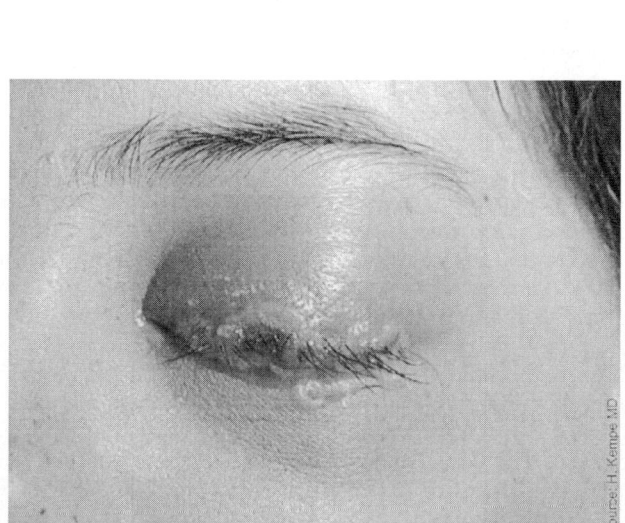

FIGURE 9–7 ■ D, Accidental implantation of vaccinia virus on the eyelids.

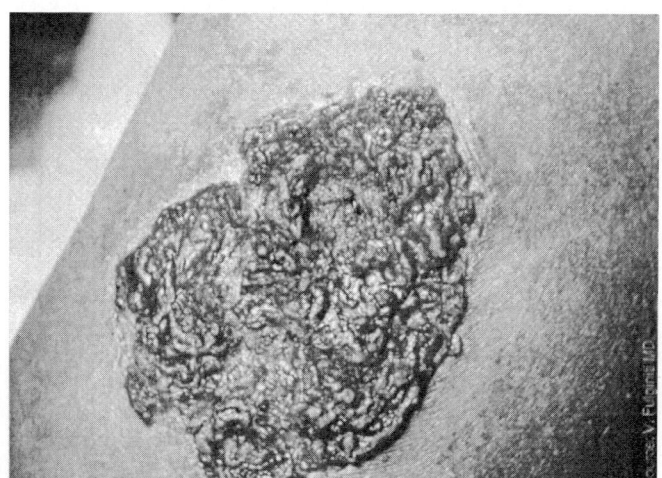

FIGURE 9–7 ■ F, Bacterial superinfection of the vaccinated site. (A and D courtesy of Dr. H. Kempe; B, E, and F courtesy of Dr. V. Fulginiti; C courtesy of the Centers for Disease Control and Prevention.)

TABLE 9–5 ■ Incidence of Postvaccinal Encephalopathy (in Infants Younger Than 2 Years) and Postvaccinal Encephalomyelitis (in Persons Older Than 2 Years) After Primary Vaccination, in Various Countries and at Various Times

Country and Investigator	Encephalopathy (age <2 yr)	
	Number of Cases	Number of Vaccinations
Austria 1948–1953 (Berger and Puntigam,[161] 1954)	6	58,438
England and Wales 1951–1960 (Conybeare,[162] 1964)	40	2,960,406
Germany		
Bavaria 1945–1953 (Herrlich,[163] 1954)	51	1,008,000
Dusseldorf 1948 (Stuart,[164] 1947; Femmer,[165] 1948)	0	28,768
Hamburg 1939–1958 (Seeleman,[166] 1960)	34	367,390
Netherlands		
1924–1928 (van den Berg,[167] 1946)	6	155,730
1940–1943 (Stuart,[164] 1947)	22	441,294
1959–1963 (Polak,[160] 1973)	34	1,033,000
1964–1971 (Polak,[160] 1973)	16	1,495,000
United States 1968		
National survey (Lane et al,[168] 1969)	4	614,000*
10-state survey (Lane et al,[171] 1970)	3	71,000*

*Age younger than 1 year.
†Age 1 year or older.
From Fenner F, Henderson DA, Arita I, et al. Smallpox and Its Eradication. Geneva, World Health Organization, 1988, p 307,[5] with permission.

vaccinal encephalitis subsequently occurred.[162,173] The incidence in the Netherlands between 1964 and 1971 appeared to approach that in the United States; 10 of the 16 cases were fatal, however, compared with only 4 of 16 cases reported in the United States in 1968. These differences are not statistically significant, but the results are consistent with other observations that suggest that the NYCBOH strain may be somewhat less pathogenic than the Lister strain.

No single laboratory test correlates with strain virulence, but Marrenikova and colleagues,[174] using the results of a series of studies in mice and rats, provided a broad classification of a number of strains as follows: (1) least pathogenic: NYCBOH and EM-63 (a derivative of this strain); (2) moderately pathogenic: Lister, Berne, and Patwadanger (from India); and (3) highly pathogenic, Denmark, Tashkent (an older Russian strain), and Ikeda (an older Japanese strain).

Unusual Adverse Events

Congenital vaccinia is rare, having been documented on fewer than 20 occasions.[175] Vaccination during pregnancy does not appear to result in an increase in the incidence of abortions or stillbirths.[176–178] No studies have implicated vaccinia virus as a teratogen.[179] The development of a malignant skin tumor, such as a melanoma, in the vaccination scar many years later is a rare occurrence.[180] Vaccinial osteomyelitis occasionally has been recorded and sometimes confirmed by recovery of vaccinia virus.[181]

Myopericarditis

In March 2003, following the reinstitution of smallpox vaccination of U.S. military personnel, 35 cases of myocarditis were reported among approximately 450,000 of those who had received primary vaccinations (approximately one in 12,000 primary vaccinees), whereas no cases occurred among those who had been previously vaccinated (Dr. John Grabenstein, personal communication). The cases experienced fever, fatigue and myalgia, accompanied by chest pain, beginning between 7 and 12 days post-vaccination. Electrocardiograms showed ST-segment changes and an increase in circulating cardiac enzymes, consistent with myopericarditis. Except for one individual who developed severe heart failure, the patients were generally able to be discharged back to active duty within 7 to 10 days. Occasional cases of myopericarditis after smallpox vaccination had been reported in the past but whether they were associated causally or temporally was often unclear as myopericarditis has been recognized to occur not uncommonly in association with a number of viral infections.[182] The number of cases occurring this year over a comparatively brief time span post-vaccination strongly suggests that, in the past, few adults received primary vaccinations and seldom in groups. Follow-up studies are in progress but the current vaccination program is being continued.

Other Types of Heart Disease

Among health care workers who were vaccinated in the United States, several heart-related incidents were reported through the monitoring system: cases of angina, myocardial infarction and myopericarditis. These events were detected by a sensitive system designed to monitor adverse events of all types and in no way do the reports imply that they are caused by the vaccine. Many of those afflicted had known heart dis-

Cases per Million	Encephalomyelitis (age >2 yr)		
	Number of Cases	Number of Vaccinations	Cases per Million
103	26	21,323	1219
14	26	859,963	30
51	17	140,800	121
0	14	67,068	209
93	12	26,713	449
39	127	548,420	232
50	56	160,775	348
33	—	—	—
11	—	—	—
7	12	4,980,000†	2
42	5	579,000†	9

ease or significant risk factors and most, if not all, were coincidental occurrences in time. Further studies are in progress.

Meanwhile, the CDC, on the advice of ACIP, recommended that people with known heart disease or those who have three or more risk factors for heart disease (such as hypertension, hyperlipidemia, diabetes mellitus, tobacco use, or a first-degree relative with premature cardiac disease) defer being vaccinated for the present.[183] Should they be at immediate risk of acquiring smallpox, however, vaccination should be performed.

Contact Vaccinia

Contact vaccinia may occur from the accidental mechanical transfer of vaccinia virus from recently vaccinated person to close contacts. Primary vaccination lesions shed vaccinia from about the third day until a scab forms.[184] Several population-wide studies of contact vaccinia have been performed, and these have been reviewed by Neff and colleagues.[185] Two of the studies dealt with the incidence of contact transmission during the course of emergency vaccination campaigns in the United States and Great Britain. During the 1947 New York City outbreak of smallpox, 5 to 6 million persons were vaccinated using the NYCBOH strain. In all, 28 persons developed eczema vaccinatum as a result of close contact with a vaccine recipient, and two of them died.[186] During the 1962 smallpox outbreak in Great Britain, at least 3,250,000 persons were vaccinated utilizing the Lister strain vaccine. There were 185 cases of eczema vaccinatum, of whom 89 resulted from contact with a vaccine recipient; seven with contact vaccinia died.[187]

National surveys to assess the frequency of complications were conducted in 1963 and 1968 by, respectively, Neff and his colleagues, and Lane and his colleagues. Both used several methods to detect possible cases, but most reports consisted of individuals who had received VIG for the treatment of complications. The two surveys yielded very similar results: the rates for the respective years were 8.7 and 10.7 cases of contact eczema vaccinatum per million primary vaccines. The incidence of accidental infection resulting from contact was somewhat lower than that for eczema vaccinatum. In all, three deaths were recorded among 114 persons with eczema vaccinatum acquired by contact. There were no cases of progressive vaccinia or postvaccinal encephalitis resulting from transfer of vaccinia virus to contacts (Table 9–6).

In statewide surveys in 1963 and 1968,[173,188] physicians were individually contacted and asked to report cases. The rates for contact eczema vaccinatum were approximately double those derived from the national surveys. It was thought that the higher rates reflected more complete reporting, especially of less severe complications.

Neff et al., in their review, noted that contact vaccinia required very close contact, seldom occurred outside the home, and rarely occurred as a result of hospital contact. Those transmitting vaccinia were predominantly children. During the 1960s, it occurred comparatively infrequently, at the rate of only 2 to 6 per 100,000 primary vaccinations.[185]

Data from the 1960s are informative but provide only limited insight as to what might be anticipated as a result of large-scale vaccination today, especially of adults. During the 1960s, most persons were vaccinated at about 1 year of age or before school entry. Not surprisingly, most cases of contact vaccinia resulted from transfer of vaccinia from young children to other children or adults in the household. Most adults who were being vaccinated had had a primary vaccination, and most would have experienced a vaccinial lesion that would be much less pronounced than a primary take and would shed less virus. There are now, as well, a proportionately larger number of persons who are at higher risk

TABLE 9–6 ▪ Summary of 1960s Data on Risk of Transmission of Vaccinia by Contacts*

Source	No. of Primary Vaccinations	Cases (Deaths) Eczema Vaccinatum Vaccinated	Cases (Deaths) Eczema Vaccinatum Contact
England and Wales[185] 1962	3 250 000	48 (4)[†]	89 (7)[†]
United States,[170] 1963	6 239 000	54 (0)	54 (2)
United States,[168] 1968	5 594 000	58 (0)	60 (1)
United States,[172] 1963	298 000	24	5
United States,[169] 1968	650 000	25	13

*— indicate data not reported.
[†]Based on 137 cases with full information on age, sex, and source of infection.
[‡]The rate of accidental infection in a pediatric clinic was found to be equal to 1 case per 170 primary vaccinations.[186]
From Neff JM, Lane M, Fulginiti VA, Henderson DA. Contact vaccinia—transmission of vaccinia from smallpox vaccination. JAMA 288:1901–1905, 2002,[185] with permission. Copyrighted 2002, American Medical Association.

of experiencing complications. The prevalence of atopic dermatitis in the current population is considerably higher,[189–191] as is the prevalence of serious immunodeficiency in the population because of HIV,[192] organ transplantation,[193] cancer chemotherapy,[194] and the availability of corticosteroid and immunomodulatory therapy for a range of prevalent inflammatory and musculoskeletal diseases.[195]

Vaccinia Immune Globulin

VIG is an immune serum globulin preparation made from the plasma of recently vaccinated donors. It contains a high titer of neutralizing antibody. The first use of VIG was by Kempe at the University of Colorado, who prepared VIG for use at his center for treatment of adverse events following vaccination.[196] Because adverse events were rare, controlled clinical trials to measure the efficacy of VIG were never performed. Historical controls and the opinion of expert clinicians suggest that VIG is effective, however, in the treatment of cutaneous complications.

Progressive vaccinia was universally fatal before the introduction of VIG.[196] After VIG was introduced, the case-fatality rate dropped to about 25% to 50%, although data may be confounded in that other interventions were often simultaneously employed, such as antiviral agents, transfusions of blood from recently vaccinated donors, and surgical débridement.[197] Severe eczema vaccinatum in the pre-VIG era had a case-fatality rate of 8% to 30%.[187,196] After the institution of VIG, the case-fatality rate fell to 1% or less.[172]

Note that VIG is contraindicated in patients whose ocular vaccinia is complicated by keratitis; in rabbits such therapy causes corneal scarring presumably from precipitation of antigen-antibody complexes.[160] Kempe and his colleagues used VIG to treat patients with variola major in Madras, and used it in prophylaxis of some contacts of patients.[198] Marrenikova also conducted a small trial. These trials sug-

gest there might be some reduction in incidence and severity of smallpox, but the trials were too small and inadequately controlled to draw conclusion.[5] Because of the cost and difficulties in preparing and administering VIG, further studies were not pursued.

VIG is now in short supply, and is available only under an Investigational New Drug application, held by the CDC. The recommended dose is an intramuscular injection of 0.6 mL/kg of body weight; severely ill patients may require repeated doses. Quantities of VIG sufficient for treatment of complications are being prepared; the new supplies will be an intravenous formulation to facilitate administration.[97]

Indications for Vaccination

In endemic countries, which consisted of most of the world until after World War I, vaccination was recommended for everyone, with revaccination to occur every 3 to 10 years. The only exceptions were infants, for whom primary vaccination customarily was delayed until they were 3 to 12 months of age, mainly because frequent vaccination failures occurred at an earlier age. As higher titer vaccines became available in the 1920s, French and then German physicians showed that a high proportion of successful vaccinations could be achieved at birth, and, in some hospitals, this became routine practice.[199] At least one city in the United States, Detroit, mandated neonatal vaccination in the mid-1920s.[200]

As time passed and smallpox incidence declined, smallpox-free countries began to delay primary vaccination until children were older. This resulted in part from the demonstration that maternal antibody inhibited virus proliferation[202] and in part from the belief that older children could better handle the fever and systemic symptoms of vaccinial infection. Vaccination at a later age was also less likely to be associated mistakenly with other events, such as sudden infant death syndrome, which might be temporally but not

SMALLPOX AND VACCINIA 143

Cases per Million Primary Vaccinations					
Accidental Infection		Eczema Vaccinatum		Accidental Infection	
Vaccinated	Contact	Vaccinated	Contact	Vaccinated	Contact
NATIONAL SURVEYS					
—	—	14.8	27.4	—	—
85	22	8.7	8.7	13.6	3.5
142	44	10.4	10.7	25.4	7.9
STATE SURVEYS					
—	—	80.5	16.8	—	—
344	29	38.5	20.0	529.2‡	44.6

causally related. Some European countries recommended that vaccination be delayed until the second year of life to avoid the possible erroneous attribution to vaccinia of cases of encephalopathy resulting from other causes.[162] The United States started vaccinating at 12 months of age when studies suggested a higher frequency of postvaccinal encephalitis among infants vaccinated at 9 to 12 months than among children vaccinated between 1 and 4 years of age.[170] No studies were subsequently performed to show that complications became less frequent after these changes in policy.

Vaccination practices in the developing countries tended to parallel those in Europe and North America. By 1967, most countries, even those with endemic smallpox, delayed vaccination until the child was 3 to 9 months of age. Notable exceptions included Hong Kong,[148] where neonatal vaccination had been traditional at least since World War II, and Madras, India,[50] where neonatal vaccination had been introduced in the late 1950s. During the late 1960s, vaccines that met international standards of potency consistently produced high levels of vaccination takes in newborns. Newborn vaccination became widely recommended, although not all countries followed the practice. There are no adequate studies that compare the efficacy and durability of immunity provided at birth with that provided at older ages, nor are there data that permit a comparison of the relative frequency of vaccination complications at infancy and older ages.

Primary vaccination was provided for adults if required, although there were concerns that adults might have a higher incidence of postvaccinal encephalitis and other serious complications. Earlier European data suggested this to be the case,[159] although studies conducted in the United States did not confirm it.[170,172] A review of U.S. military medical records between 1946 and 1962, conducted by the CDC, found no cases of central nervous system complications among an estimated 2 million recruits given primary vaccinations. The differences between European and U.S. studies probably reflect differences in the pathogenicity of different strains.

Routine vaccination ceased in all countries in the early 1980s, although a number of countries continued for a number of years to provide vaccination to military forces in case variola virus were to be used as a biologic warfare agent. Otherwise, vaccination, until recently, has been recommended only for those working in laboratories and animal handlers working in facilities where orthopoxviruses are used.[128]

Recommendations for wider use of the vaccine are now under review in the United States and some other countries because of the threat of use of smallpox as a biologic weapon. By the end of 2002, the United States had acquired sufficient vaccine to permit, if necessary, vaccination of the entire country. Because of the substantial risks associated with vaccination, this was not considered to be desirable unless the risk of release of smallpox virus was substantial. As additional vaccine has become available, it has been possible to consider several options for its use in addition to use during an emergency and for laboratory workers engaged in work with orthopoxviruses. The ACIP recommended that vaccination be undertaken to protect those deemed to be at highest risk should an outbreak occur.[202] These would include "smallpox public health response teams" at federal and state levels who would be expected to investigate cases, as well as "smallpox health care teams" composed of health care workers in acute care hospitals who would be expected to provide 24-hour care for acutely ill smallpox patients in hospitals. In this plan, every acute care hospital would have the opportunity to establish "smallpox health care teams," comprising emergency room, intensive care unit, and general medical unit staff; selected medical house staff from a variety of disciplines; medical subspecialists; infection control professionals; respiratory therapists; radiology technicians; security personnel; and housekeeping staff. It is estimated that some 500,000 persons would be eligible. By vaccinating these groups, experience in vaccination would be gained by those who would be responsible both for vaccinating larger numbers should an outbreak occur and for caring for those with complications of vaccination. At the same time, military personnel considered to be at special risk are being vaccinated. When individuals at highest risk have been vaccinated, attention will be directed to other groups at special risk, such as emergency first responders (police, fire, and emergency medical personnel), postal workers, and others.

When studies of the new tissue culture vaccines have been completed, the vaccine will be made available to those requesting it albeit, it will be recommended that they not be vaccinated unless the risk or actuality of a smallpox release warrants it.

Meanwhile, a number of other countries in Europe, Asia, and Latin America are contracting for supplies of vaccine and new vaccine production facilities are being prepared. The WHO is exploring mechanisms and resources to deal with an outbreak of smallpox wherever it might occur. It would now appear that there can never be a final chapter to the eradication of smallpox. Eternal vigilance and the availability of vaccine will be requirements far into the distant future.

Contraindications to Vaccination

The WHO recognized no contraindications to vaccination in areas that were endemic for smallpox for two reasons. First, the risk associated with smallpox infection was significantly greater than the risk of complications. Second, most vaccinations were performed by individuals without medical training who could not be expected to recognize conditions such as eczema, or to identify patients with immune deficiency syndromes. The WHO recommended that only patients who were extremely sick not be vaccinated because their subsequent death might be attributed mistakenly to vaccination.

In nonendemic areas, several conditions were and currently are accepted as contraindications. These include immune deficiency, central nervous system, and skin disorders and pregnancy.

Immune Deficiency Disorders

Primary or acquired immune deficiency disorders include agammaglobulinemia, hypogammaglobulinemia, a variety of neoplasms, and AIDS. Persons with such disorders are at substantial risk of developing the frequently fatal progressive vaccinia and should not be vaccinated. The ACIP does not require mandatory HIV testing prior to smallpox vaccination, but recommends that HIV testing should be readily available to those who wish to be tested or those with risk factors for HIV infection.[129] It is not known whether persons infected with HIV with higher CD4 cell counts could be safely immunized, although this is probable. The vaccine is also contraindicated for those on immunosuppressive drugs for the treatment of cancer or for organ transplant maintenance, or on systemic steroid therapy (≤ 2 mg/kg/day or ≤ 20 mg/day for longer than 14 days).[203]

Eczema, Atopic Dermatitis, and Other Skin Disorders

Individuals with active or a past history of eczema or atopic dermatitis, irrespective of disease severity, are at special risk of developing eczema vaccinatum after they or their close contacts are vaccinated.[129] Family members with eczema are at risk from contact spread of vaccinia virus, so either the healthy vaccinee or the eczematous family member should live apart until the lesion has fully scabbed over. Other skin conditions that may be of concern, if extensive, are acne, burns, impetigo, varicella zoster, herpes, psoriasis, open or surgical incision wounds, Darier's disease, and contact dermatitis. It is best for vaccination to be deferred until the condition is resolved. If vaccine is administered, patients should be counseled in ways to prevent the transfer of vaccinia from the primary site to the affected area.[129]

Disorders of the Central Nervous System

Some countries considered disorders of the central nervous system in potential vaccinees to be contraindications to vaccination. It was hoped that this might decrease the risk of postvaccinal encephalitis, but there is no evidence that this diminished the risk.

Pregnancy

Pregnant women are not vaccinated on the general principle that immunization of any sort should be avoided during pregnancy, and because of the very low risk of fetal vaccinia. The ACIP does not recommend routine pregnancy testing of women of child-bearing age prior to smallpox vaccination, but does recommend the exclusion of women who are pregnant or intend to become pregnant within a 4-week period following vaccination.[129] Because fetal vaccinia appears to be an extraordinarily rare complication, inadvertent vaccination of a pregnant woman is not a reason to terminate pregnancy.

Other Contraindications

Vaccine is contraindicated in those who have a history of hypersensitivity to vaccine components (such as polymyxin B sulfate, streptomycin sulfate, chlortetracycline hydrochloride, and neomycin sulfate).[206] Because persons with certain inflammatory eye disorders (that predispose to itching or rubbing the eye) might be more likely to autoinoculate their eyes following vaccination, it may be best to avoid vaccinating them.

Some authorities recommended withholding vaccination from patients suffering from various serious acute or chronic illnesses, hypothesizing that the response to vaccination might be abnormal. There is no evidence for this occurrence except that leprosy patients sometimes developed erythema nodosum leprosum or neuritis after primary vaccination.[207,208] In endemic areas, however, leprosy patients were vaccinated because the risk of smallpox substantially outweighed the risk of adverse events.

Public Health Considerations

Epidemiologic Effects of Vaccination

United States

Smallpox vaccination in the United States began in 1800, but its routine widespread use did not occur until the 1900s. Waterhouse performed the first vaccinations in Boston in July 1800 using material provided by Jenner.[209] President Thomas Jefferson actively promoted vaccination.[210] Because propagation of the virus was primarily dependent on arm-to-arm transfer of material from a successful vaccinee to others, vaccination was practiced sporadically. Epidemics of variola major continued to occur at intervals, depending on population density and frequency of importations.

Toward the end of the 19th century in the United States, vaccinia virus began to be propagated on the flank of a calf, making vaccine more readily and widely available. By 1897, smallpox had largely been eliminated,[4] the result of vaccination and outbreak control. That summer, however, an outbreak of variola minor occurred in Pensacola, Florida. Within 4 years, this variety of smallpox had spread across the country.[211] The origin of this strain is unknown. However, a similarly mild strain of smallpox, called Kaffir pox, had begun to circulate widely in South Africa in the early 1890s. What, if any, connection there was between these two foci of variola minor is unknown.

Although outbreaks of variola major continued to occur until about 1927, most 20th-century cases of smallpox in the United States were caused by variola minor. Because the disease was mild and the case-fatality rate was less than 1%, interest in vaccination waned. To control the disease, public health authorities sought to compel vaccination as a requirement for school entry, an action upheld by the Supreme Court.[212,213] However, antivaccinationist sentiment and antipathy toward compulsory measures prevailed in many states, most of which did not pass legislation or prohibited compulsory vaccination. Reported cases of smallpox declined from 102,791 in 1921 to 30,151 in 1931. Between 1932 and 1939, 5000 to 15,000 cases were reported annually, with 23 to 52 deaths. During the following decade, reported cases steadily diminished, with the last occurring in 1949. This progress occurred in the absence of any nationally coordinated smallpox control effort, and little is known about the extent of vaccination immunity in the country during the 1940s, or about the epidemiology of smallpox. Leake[126] attributed improved smallpox control and its eventual elimination to the wider availability of refrigeration and, consequently, better preservation of the vaccine. Routine vaccination continued in the United States until 1972 as a protection in case smallpox was imported, and was enforced in most states by compelling vaccination for school entry. In the early 1960s, many importations of smallpox occurred in Europe; almost half of all subsequent cases occurred as a result of contact in hospitals. Accordingly, beginning in the 1960s, the CDC urged the routine vaccination of hospital staff, but few hospitals complied. After the global eradication of smallpox, distribution of vaccine was restricted to the military, and to the few laboratories that were working with orthopoxviruses.

Other Industrialized Countries

Through the 1800s, other industrialized countries had experiences with vaccination similar to that in the United States. After the initial surge of enthusiasm for vaccination in the early 1800s, vaccination was less uniformly and extensively practiced in most countries until near the close of the century, when the vaccinia virus began to be propagated on calves. By 1900, a number of countries in northern Europe had become smallpox free. By 1914, the incidence in most countries had decreased to comparatively low levels. Even so, during the period from 1910 to 1914, Russia reported 200,000 deaths, and nearly 25,000 deaths were recorded in other European countries.[214,215] World War I led to a resurgence of smallpox in Russia, and it spread from there to many other countries. During the 1920s, vaccination programs led to the interruption of smallpox transmission in many European countries. By the mid-1930s, smallpox occurred only after importations except in Spain and Portugal, where endemic smallpox persisted until 1948 and 1953, respectively.

Of the other major industrialized countries, Canada interrupted transmission of smallpox in the early 1940s and Japan about 1950. Vaccination continued in all the industrialized countries, as it did in the United States, until the mid- to late 1970s as a protection in case smallpox was reintroduced. Australia and New Zealand were two notable exceptions. These countries, protected by distance and strict quarantine measures, never vaccinated widely but also never became endemic for smallpox.

Eradication from the World

The first commitment to smallpox eradication was made in 1950 by the Pan American Sanitary Organization, which decided that year on a hemisphere-wide effort.[216] Freeze-dried vaccine produced by an improved commercial process[32] was employed in mass vaccination campaigns, which during the succeeding decade eliminated smallpox from all countries except Argentina, Brazil, Colombia, and Ecuador.

In 1958, the Soviet Union proposed to the World Health Assembly that the WHO undertake a global eradication program[34]; a proposal was agreed on in 1959.[35] During the succeeding 7 years, a number of countries embarked on mass vaccination campaigns, and several, including China, eliminated the disease (Fig. 9–8). Overall, however, progress was disappointing, especially in Africa and in the Indian subcontinent. Few countries voluntarily contributed resources, and the WHO, then preoccupied with a costly and disappointing global malaria eradication program, provided few of its own resources and little support.

Frustrated by lack of progress in the program, although skeptical about the feasibility of the concept of eradication itself, the World Health Assembly in 1966 decided, finally, to provide to the WHO a special allocation of $2.4 million annually for an intensified global smallpox eradication effort.[36] It expressed hope that the task might be accomplished within a 10-year period, that is, by December 1976.[38]

In the intensified program, the strategy emphasized two principles that ultimately proved to be critical to its success. The first was to ensure, through the use of international vaccine testing centers, that all vaccine in the program met accepted standards and, likewise, to ensure, through the concurrent sample surveys, that satisfactory vaccination coverage had been achieved and that the vaccinations had been successful. The second principle was the identification of the absence of cases as the program's principal objective and the need to measure progress not in terms of number of vaccinations performed, as had been the practice, but in terms of a declining incidence of smallpox. This principle required the development of an effective case notification system and focused attention on measures to reduce incidence.

Provision of adequate supplies of fully potent vaccine was a critical initial problem.[217,218] Early surveys revealed that not more than 10% of the vaccine being produced in or provided to endemic countries met accepted international standards. Laboratories in Canada and the Netherlands agreed to test samples of all vaccine to be used in the program, manufacturers collaborated in developing a detailed production manual, and consultants and equipment were provided to vaccine production laboratories in endemic countries. Donations of vaccine, primarily from the Soviet Union and the United States, met initial needs. By 1973, more than 80% of all vaccine for the program was produced in the developing countries.

During 1967, the first year of the program, 44 countries, 31 of which were endemic, reported 217,218 cases of smallpox. The endemic countries were Brazil, most countries of Africa south of the Sahara, and five countries in Asia: Afghanistan, India, Indonesia, Nepal, and Pakistan (see Fig. 9–8). Later surveys revealed that only about 1% of all cases were being reported. Thus it is estimated that between 10 and 15 million cases occurred that year in countries with a total population of about 1.2 billion.

Vaccination technique and results improved. The WHO encouraged abandonment of traditional methods of vaccination by scarification or rotary lancet. Jet injectors were introduced in 1967 for programs in Brazil and western and central Africa. One year later, the bifurcated needle, developed by Wyeth Laboratories, proved to be extremely effective in multiple-puncture vaccinations, inexpensive, and easy to use.[219] By 1969, bifurcated needles were in use in all countries. Vaccination with the bifurcated needle required only one fourth as much vaccine, even illiterate village volunteers required less than an hour's training in its proper use, and workers could vaccinate as many as 1000 persons per day.

Vaccination programs were developed or strengthened in all endemic and neighboring countries, the last of them beginning in 1971. Although the strategy also called for the improvement of national reporting systems and containment of outbreaks by special teams, such activities were slow to begin. It quickly became apparent, however, that these activities, referred to as the surveillance-containment strategy, could serve to interrupt smallpox transmission

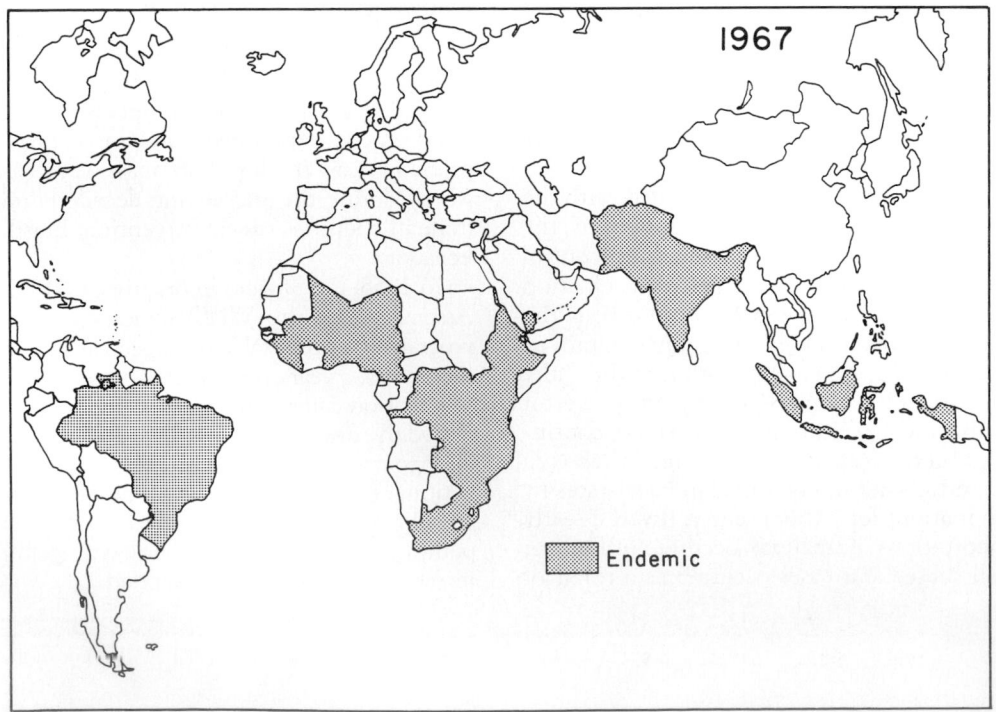

FIGURE 9–8 ■ Countries with endemic smallpox in 1967 when the intensified program was initiated.

more easily and quickly than anyone had imagined, even where vaccinial immunity was low.[82,83,220]

With increasingly greater emphasis on surveillance-containment activities, endemic smallpox steadily receded (Fig. 9–9; see also Fig. 9–8). It was eliminated from 20 countries of western and central Africa by 1970,[75] from Brazil in 1971, from Indonesia in 1972, and from the entire continent of Asia in 1975. Ethiopia stopped transmission in 1976 and Somalia on October 26, 1977. The last naturally occurring case of smallpox developed less than 1 year after the originally projected 10-year target date.

WHO-organized international commissions visited each of the endemic countries and areas to confirm the fact of eradication. In May 1980, the World Health Assembly, acting on the recommendation of a WHO Global Commission, announced that worldwide eradication had been achieved and recommended that routine smallpox vaccination be discontinued (Fig. 9–10).[1] The WHO established an international stockpile of vaccine in the event it should ever again be required, and encouraged laboratories to destroy their stocks of variola virus. As of 1997, official repositories of variola virus remained in only two research laboratories—one in the United States and one in Russia.

The overall cost of the program was about $300 million, of which $100 million represented international assistance. The savings, as a result of cessation of vaccination and quarantine measures, has been estimated to be in excess of $1 billion annually.[5]

Surveillance–Containment

The strategy of surveillance and containment proved highly effective in controlling the spread of smallpox throughout the global eradication program, whether in villages or in major cities.[5] It is the strategy that is given priority for the control of an outbreak should one occur in this country, whether or not large-scale vaccination is also undertaken. The reason for this and the concept are straightforward—to detect cases as quickly as possible, to isolate them, and to vaccinate all individuals who have been in contact with the cases since the time they became ill and those to whom the contacts might transmit infection if they become ill. The method originally was called "ring vaccination" by Dixon,[10] a term that some have erroneously interpreted to mean a geographic ring when, in fact, it means erecting a barrier of immune persons around the case and his or her contacts (Fig. 9–11).

The surveillance–containment strategy worked as well as it did because of a number of quite unique clinical and epidemiologic features of smallpox. First is the fact that smallpox virus, to sustain itself, must pass from one individual to another, each of whom experiences a clinically obvious infection with rash. There are no persons with subclinical infection who can spread the disease unnoticed, and there is no animal reservoir. It is a simple matter to identify where smallpox is at any time and to know how and by whom it has been spread. An outbreak may be envisaged

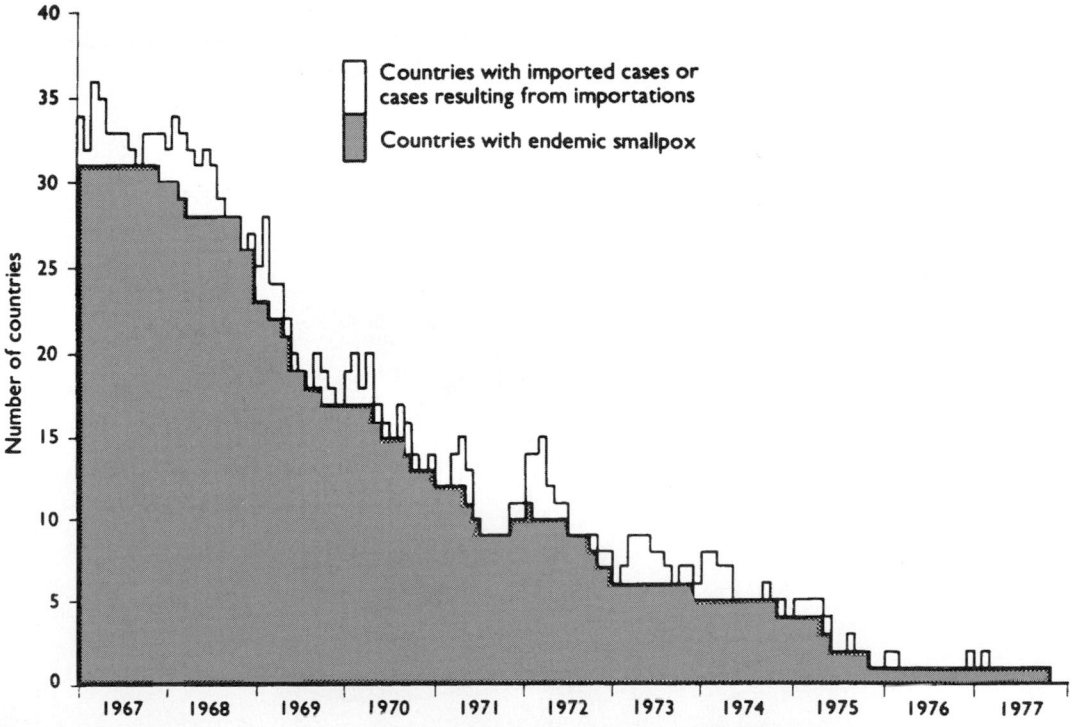

FIGURE 9–9 ■ Number of countries experiencing smallpox each year from 1967 to 1978. (From Fenner F, Henderson DA, Arita I, et al. Smallpox and Its Eradication. Geneva, World Health Organization, 1988, pp 517–538, with permission.)

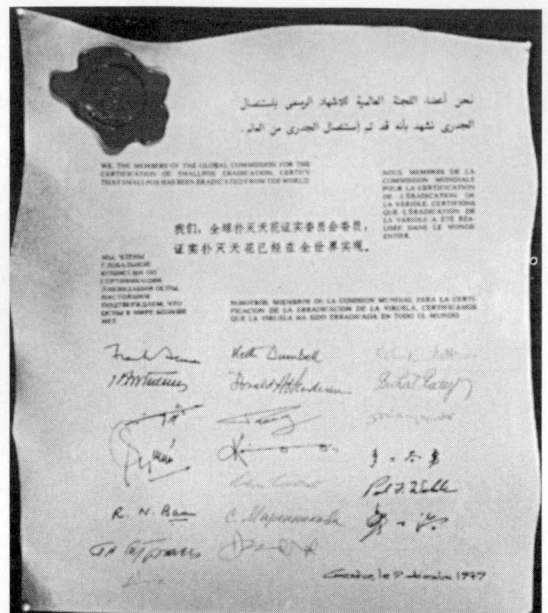

FIGURE 9–10 ■ Document signed on December 9, 1979, by members of the World Health Organization Global Commission, certifying that smallpox had been eradicated. (From Fenner F, Henderson DA, Arita I, et al. Smallpox and Its Eradication. Geneva, World Health Organization, 1988, frontispiece, with permission.)

as a continuing chain of cases with control measures being directed at breaking the chain.

Second is the fact that the individual is able to transmit infection only from the time of onset of rash until scabs form. Although a patient normally experiences a 10- to 12-day asymptomatic incubation period after he or she is infected, he or she cannot transmit virus during this period. Thus, although an infected patient may contact all

manner of persons during the incubation period, he or she will not infect them. Next, the infected patient experiences a 2- to 3-day prodromal period before rash develops. With variola major, the Asian form of smallpox and the one of concern, patients during the prodromal phase experience a very high fever and serious systemic symptoms and take to bed. Even though they are very ill, they still cannot transmit infection to others until skin and oropharyngeal lesions begin to develop and the virus begins to shed into the oropharynx. Not surprisingly, most patients are successful in transmitting smallpox only to household members and to those with whom they have contact in the hospital.

The strategy of containment, therefore, is to identify contacts of the patient *since he or she first became ill* and to vaccinate them. Usually, the numbers of such contacts are comparatively few and do not include such persons as fellow passengers on trains or subways or fellow workers in an office complex. If vaccination is done within the first few days after their exposure, smallpox may be prevented or, at least, a fatal outcome may be avoided. To whom are the contacts likely to transmit disease? Members of their own households or those whom they expose in hospitals. Thus the strategy calls for vaccinating household members of contacts.

Hospital contacts are likewise of major importance. They include not only hospital staff but also other patients and visitors. Most person-to-person contact results from droplets expressed by the patient from the mouth in the course of speaking. Those patients and visitors who are most likely to become infected are those who come within 6 feet of the patient. Such individuals must be identified as soon as possible and vaccinated.

It is important to note that patients who are severely ill with malignant or hemorrhagic smallpox and who may be coughing pose a special risk. Such patients constitute only a small percentage of those who develop smallpox, but they are capable of generating fine-particle aerosols that can drift over very long distances within a building. Should such

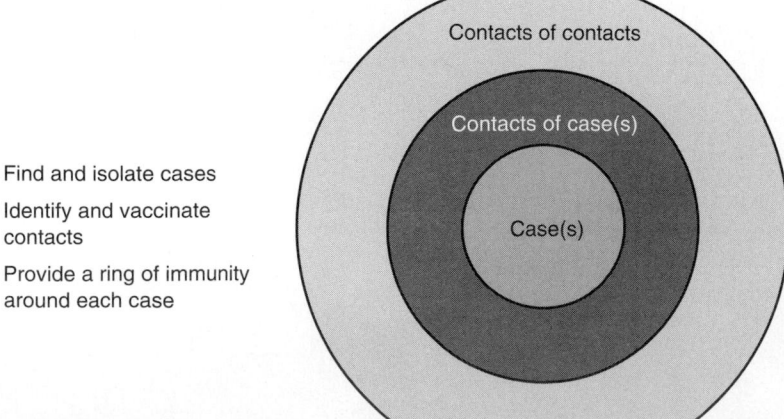

- Find and isolate cases
- Identify and vaccinate contacts
- Provide a ring of immunity around each case

FIGURE 9–11 ■ Schematic representation of the "surveillance and containment" strategy used to control outbreaks of smallpox, in which cases are isolated, contacts are identified and isolated, and a ring of immunity is created around each case by vaccinating contacts of contacts as well.

cases be admitted to a hospital without special infection control precautions, large numbers throughout the hospital might need to be vaccinated.

Destruction of the Virus

With the eradication of smallpox, the WHO recommended that all laboratories either destroy their stocks of variola or transfer them to one of two designated reference laboratories (WHO Collaborating Centres on Smallpox and other Poxvirus Infections), at the CDC in Atlanta, Georgia, or the Research Institute of Viral Preparations in Moscow, Russian Federation.[221] All countries reported voluntary compliance with WHO recommendations.[222]

From 1980, when the World Health Assembly declared that eradication had been achieved, many countries questioned repeatedly whether it might not be prudent to destroy the known remaining laboratory stocks of variola virus to provide added assurance that the virus might not accidentally or even deliberately be released into an unprotected world. This was considered in 1986 by a WHO *Ad Hoc* Committee on Orthopoxvirus Infections, which recommended a broader consultation with the international community and unanimously recommended destruction of the virus if no serious objections were raised.[223] Meanwhile, in preparation for possible destruction, a library of cloned DNA restriction fragments of selected strains was prepared, and later the genomes of a number of prototype strains were fully or partially sequenced.[224] In 1990, the *Ad Hoc* Committee on Orthopoxvirus Infections proposed a deadline for destruction of the virus of December 31, 1993.[225] Arguments were advanced both supporting[224] and objecting to[226] destruction of the virus stocks. Arguments against destruction stemmed from concerns that it would prohibit significant advances in understanding the pathogenesis of variola virus, and that destruction of the two known repositories would not guarantee that forgotten or hidden stocks of virus would not be preserved elsewhere.[225] Arguments for destruction of the virus stemmed from concerns that an unintentional release of virus in an increasingly susceptible global population would lead to a serious outbreak, that all should be done to ensure that smallpox never again would afflict humankind, and that the available cloned DNA fragments and sequence information of several strains of variola would allow scientific inquiry into the virus and an understanding of its properties.

In 1993, five distinguished scientific organizations, both national and international, were asked to formally consider the question of destruction. Each replied, in writing, that it supported destruction of the virus. In 1994, the question again was reviewed in depth by the WHO *Ad Hoc* Committee, which again recommended to the WHO Director General that the considerations, on balance, strongly favored destruction of the virus.[225] The proposed date for the destruction of the remaining stocks of variola virus was June 30, 1995.[225] The recommendations were to be submitted for consideration at the World Health Assembly in May 1995. However, the executive board of the WHO postponed voting on the issue because of opposition on the part of some members of the WHO Committee, specifically, the United States, Russia, and the

United Kingdom.[227] In 1996, the World Health Assembly finally decided that destruction of the virus should take place and set the date for June 30, 1999. As the date approached, objections again were raised by the members, who asserted that the virus was needed to develop antiviral drugs and more attenuated vaccines. The 1999 WHO Assembly recommended temporary retention of the virus up to, but no later than, 2002.[221] It asked the Director General to appoint an oversight committee that would review and approve all research that was to be undertaken and would assure that all necessary safety precautions would be taken.

In May 2002, the World Health Assembly once again recommended that the virus be retained; no new date has been set for its destruction. Research programs using the virus are continuing at the CDC and at the VECTOR Institute in Novosibirsk.[228]

REFERENCES

1. World Health Organization. Global Commission for the Certification of Smallpox Eradication. The global eradication of smallpox: final report of the Global Commission for the Certification of Smallpox Eradication, Geneva, December 1979. Geneva, World Health Organization, 1980.
2. Alibek K, Handelman S. Biohazard. New York, Random House, 1999.
3. De Korte W E. Amaas, or kaffir milk-pox. Lancet 1:1273–1276, 1904.
4. Chapin, C.V. Variation in type of infectious disease as shown by the history of smallpox in the United States 1895–1912. J Infect Dis 13:171–196, 1913.
5. Fenner F, Henderson DA., Arita I, et al. Smallpox and Its Eradication. Geneva, World Health Organization, 1988.
6. McNeill WH. Plagues and Peoples. Garden City, N.Y., Anchor Press, 1976.
7. Ruffer MA. Pathological note on the royal mummies of the Cairo Museum. *In* Studies in the Paleopathology of Egypt, RL Moodie, Editor. Chicago, University of Chicago University Press, 1921, pp 175–176.
8. Hopkins DR. The Greatest Killer: Smallpox in History. Chicago, University of Chicago Press, 2002.
9. Rhazes (Al-Razi, Abu Bakr Muhammad ibn Zakariya). De Variolis et Morbillis Commentarius. Londini, G Bowyer, 1766. English translation: Med Class 4:22–84, 1939.
10. Dixon CW. Smallpox. London, Churchill, 1962.
11. Moore JC. The History of the Small Pox. London, Longman Hurst Rees Orme and Brown, 1815.
12. Creighton CA. History of Epidemics in Britain. London, Cass, 1965.
13. Macgowan DJ. Report on the Health of Wenchow for the Half-Year Ended 31 March 1884. China, Imperial Maritime Customs Medical Reports 27:9–18, 1884.
14. Needham J. China and the Origins of Immunology. Centre of Asian Studies Occasional Papers and Monographs, No. 41. Hong Kong, Centre of Asian Studies University of Hong Kong, 1980.
15. Miller G. Putting Lady Mary in her place: a discussion of historical causation. Bull Hist Med 55:2–16, 1981.
16. Miller G. The Adoption of Inoculation for Smallpox in England and France. Philadelphia, University of Pennsylvania Press, 1957.
17. Jenner E. An Inquiry into the Causes and Effects of the Variolae Vaccinae: A Disease Discovered in Some of the Western Counties of England, Particularly Gloucestershire, and Known by the Name of the Cow Pox. Birmingham, AL, Classics of Medicine Library, 1978.
18. Pasteur L. Vaccination in relation to chicken-cholera and splenic fever. Transactions of the International Medical Congress, Seventh Session; London; August 29, 1881, 1:85–90. *In* Oeuvres de Pasteur Râeunies. Vol. 6, Reproduced in Vallery-Radot Pasteur, Editor. Paris, Masson et Cie, 1933, pp 370–378.
19. LeFanu W. A Bio-bibliography of Edward Jenner 1749–1823. London, Harvey & Blythe, 1951.
20. del Castillo FF. Los Viajes de Don Francisco Xavier de Balmis. Mexico, Galas de Mexico, 1960.

21. Bowers J Z. The Fielding H. Garrison Lecture: The odyssey of smallpox vaccination. Bull Hist Med 55:17–33, 1981.

22. Nott JC. Smallpox epidemic in Mobile during the winter of 1865–1866. Nashville J Med Surg 2:372–380, 1867.

23. Creighton C. The Natural History of Cow-Pox and Vaccinal Syphilis. London, Cassell, 1887.

24. Baxby D. The origins of vaccinia virus. J Infect Dis 136:453–45, 1977.

25. Burroughs Wellcome and Company. The History of Inoculation and Vaccination for the Prevention and Treatment of Disease; Lecture Memoranda, American Medical Association, 1913. London, Burroughs Wellcome & Co., 1913.

26. Edwardes EJ. A Concise History of Small-Pox and Vaccination in Europe. London, H. K. Lewis, 1902.

27. Galbiati G. Memoria Sulla Inoculazione Vaccina coll'Umore Ricavato Immediatemen dall Vacca Precedentemente Inoculata. Napoli, 1810.

28. Lyon, Congres Medical de. Compterendu des travaux et des discussions. Gazette Med Lyon 19:449–471, 1864.

29. Dudgeon J A. Development of smallpox vaccine in England in the eighteenth and nineteenth centuries. BMJ 1:1367–1372, 1963.

30. Otten L. Trockenlymphe. Z Hyg Infektionskrankh 107:677–696, 1927.

31. Fasquelle R, Fasquelle A. A propos de l'histoire de la lutte contre la variole dans les pays d'Afrique francophone. Bull Soc Pathol Exot Filiales 64:734–756, 1971.

32. Collier L H. The development of a stable smallpox vaccine. J Hyg 53:76–101, 1955.

33. Pan American Sanitary Organization. Pan-American Health Organization. Final Reports of the First, Second and Third Meetings of the Directing Council. No. 247. Pan American Sanitary Organization, Washington, D.C., 1950.

34. World Health Organization. Eradication of Smallpox. Official Records of the World Health Organization. No. 87. World Health Organization, Geneva, 1958.

35. World Health Organization. Smallpox Eradication. Official Records of the World Health Organization. No. 95. World Health Organization, Geneva, 1959.

36. World Health Organization. Official Records of the World Health Organization. No. 152. World Health Organization, Geneva, 1966.

37. World Health Organization. Handbook for Smallpox Eradication in Endemic Areas. Geneva, World Health Organization, 1967.

38. Henderson DA. The eradication of smallpox. Sci Am 235:25–33, 1976.

39. Henderson DA. A discussion on technologies for rural health. Smallpox eradication. Proc R Soc Lond B Biol Sci 199:83–97, 1977.

40. Henderson DA. The deliberate extinction of a species. Proc Am Philos Soc 126:461–471, 1982.

41. Deria A, Jezek Z, Markvart K, et al. The world's last endemic case of smallpox: surveillance and containment measures. Bull World Health Organ 58:279–83, 1980.

42. Shooter RA. Report of the Investigation into the Cause of the 1978 Birmingham Smallpox Occurrence. Her Majesty's Stationery Office, London, 1980.

43. Basu RN, Jezek Z, Ward N A. The eradication of smallpox from India. In History of International Public Health No. 2. New Delhi, World Health Organization, South-East Asia Regional Office, 1979.

44. Brilliant L B. The management of smallpox eradication in India. Ann Arbor, University of Michigan Press, 1985.

45. Joarder A K, Tarantola D, Tulloch J. The eradication of smallpox from Bangladesh. New Delhi, World Health Organization South-East Asia Regional Office, 1980.

46. Yemane T, Wickett J, and the International Commission for the Certification of Smallpox Eradication. Smallpox Eradication in Ethiopia: Report to the International Commission for the Certification of Smallpox Eradication. Geneva, Global Smallpox Eradication Programme World Health Organization; Smallpox Eradication Programme Ministry of Health Ethiopia, 1979.

47. Jezek Z, Al Aghbari M, Hatfield R, et al. Smallpox Eradication in Somalia. World Health Organization Eastern Mediterranean Regional Office and Ministry of Health, Somali Democratic Republic, Alexandria, 1981.

48. Martin DB. The cause of death in smallpox: an examination of the pathology record. Mil Med 167:546 551, 2002.

49. WHO Expert Committee on Smallpox. First report. WHO Technical Report Series No. 283. World Health Organization, Geneva, 1964.

50. Rao A R. Smallpox. Bombay, Kothari Book Depot, 1972.

51. Nakano J H. Human poxvirus diseases. In Laboratory Diagnosis of Viral Infections, E H Lennette, Editor. New York, Dekker, 1985, pp 401–423.

52. Hahon, N. Cytopathogenicity and propagation of variola virus in tissue culture. J Immunol 81:426–432, 1958.

53. Pirsch J B, Mika L A, Purlson E H. Growth characteristics of variola virus in tissue culture. J Infect Dis 113:170–178, 1963.

54. World Health Organization. Guide to the Laboratory Diagnosis of Smallpox for Smallpox Eradication Programmes. Geneva, World Health Organization, 1969.

55. Wehrle P F, Posch J, Richter K H, Henderson D A. An airborne outbreak of smallpox in a German hospital and its significance with respect to other recent outbreaks in Europe. Bull World Health Organ 43:669–79, 1970.

56. Downie A W, Saint Vincent L, Rao A R, Kempe C H. Antibody response following smallpox vaccination and revaccination. J Hyg (Lond) 67:603–608, 1969.

57. Downie A W, Saint Vincent L, Goldstein L, et al. Antibody response in non-haemorrhagic smallpox patients. J Hyg (Lond) 67:609–618, 1969.

58. McCarthy K, Downie A W, Bradley W H. The antibody response in man following infection with viruses of the pox group. II. Antibody response following vaccination. J Hyg 56:466–478, 1958.

59. Downie A W, McCarthy K, Macdonald A, et al. Virus and virus antigen in the blood of smallpox patients. Their significance in early diagnosis and prognosis. Lancet 2:164–166, 1953.

60. White E. Chickenpox in Kerala. Indian J Public Health 22:141–151, 1978.

61. Centers for Disease Control and Prevention. Evaluating patients for smallpox: acute generalized vesicular or pustular rash illness protocol. 2002. http://www.bt.cdc.gov/agent/smallpox/diagnosis/pdf/spox-poster-full.pdf. accessed 09/24/02.

62. Centers for Disease Control and Prevention. Guide D. Specimen Collection Guidelines. 2002. http://www.bt.cdc.gov/agent/smallpox/lab-testing/index.asp. accessed 10/4/02.

63. Ropp S L, Jin Q, Knight J C, et al. PCR strategy for identification and differentiation of small pox and other orthopoxviruses. J Clin Microbiol 33:2069–2076, 1995.

64. Jezek Z, Basu R N, Arya Z S. Problem of persistence of facial pock marks among smallpox patients. Indian J Public Health 22:95–101, 1978.

65. Jezek Z, Hardjotanojo W. Residual skin changes in patients who have recovered from variola minor. Bull World Health Organ 58:139–140, 1980.

66. Downie A W, Meiklejohn M, St Vincent L, et al. The recovery of smallpox virus from patients and their environment in a smallpox hospital. Bull World Health Organ 33:615–122, 1965.

67. Mitra A C, Sarkar J K, Mukherjee M K. Virus content of smallpox scabs. Bull World Health Organ 51:106–107, 1974.

68. Anders W, Posch J Die Pockenausbrucke 1961/62 in Nordrhein-Westfalen. Bundesgesundheitbl 17:265–269, 1962.

69. Smallpox in Yugoslavia. Med J Aust 1:1063–1064, 1972.

70. Hopkins D R, Lane J M, Cummings E C, Millar J D. Two funeral-associated smallpox outbreaks in Sierra Leone. Am J Epidemiol 94:341–347, 1971.

71. Huq F. Effect of temperature and relative humidity on variola virus in crusts. Bull World Health Organ 54:710–712, 1976.

72. Gani R, Leach S. Transmission potential of smallpox in contemporary populations. Nature 414:748–751, 2001.

73. Harper G J. Airborne micro-organisms: survival tests with four viruses. J Hyg 59:479–486, 1961.

74. Rogers L. Smallpox and vaccination in British India during the last seventy years. Proc R Soc Lond 38:135–139, 1944.

75. Foege W H, Millar J D, Henderson D A. Smallpox eradication in West and Central Africa. Bull World Health Organ 52:209–222, 1975.

76. Hope Simpson RE. Infectiousness of communicable diseases in the household (measles, chickenpox and mumps). Lancet 2:549–554, 1952.

77. Carvalho Filho E S de, Morris L, Lavigne de Lemos A, et al. Smallpox eradication in Brazil, 1967–1969. Bull World Health Organ 43:797–808, 1970.

78. Heiner, G. G., Fatima, N., Daniel, R. W., et al. A study of inapparent infection in smallpox. Am J Epidemiol 94:252–268, 1971.

79. Henderson, R. H., Yekpe, M. Smallpox transmission in southern Dahomey: a study of a village outbreak. Am J Epidemiol 90:423–420, 1969.

80. Thomas DB, McCormack WM, Arita, I, et al. Endemic smallpox in rural East Pakistan. I. Methodology, clinical and epidemiologic characteristics of cases, and intervillage transmission. Am J Epidemiol 93:361–72, 1971.

81. Thomas DB, Arita, I, McCormack WM, et al. Endemic smallpox in rural East Pakistan. II. Intervillage transmission and infectiousness. Am J Epidemiol 93:373–383, 1971.

82. Thomas DB, Mack TM, Ali A, Muzaffar Khan M. Epidemiology of smallpox in West Pakistan. 3. Outbreak detection and interlocality transmission. Am J Epidemiol 95:178–89, 1972.

83. Mack TM, Thomas DB, Ali A, Muzaffar Khan M. Epidemiology of smallpox in West Pakistan. I. Acquired immunity and the distribution of disease. Am J Epidemiol 95:157–168, 1972.

84. Rao AR, Jacob ES, Kamalakshi S, et al. Epidemiological studies in smallpox. a study of intrafamilial transmission in a series of 254 infected families. Indian J Med Res 56:1826–1854, 1968.

85. Heiner GG, Fatima N, McCrumb FR, Jr. A study of intrafamilial transmission of smallpox. Am J Epidemiol 94:316–326, 1971.

86. Sommer A. Foster SO. The 1972 smallpox outbreak in Khulna Municipality, Bangladesh. I. Methodology and epidemiologic findings. Am J Epidemiol 99:291–302, 1974.

87. Sencer DJ, Axnick NW. Cost-benefit analysis. International Symposium on Vaccination Against Communicable Diseases. Symposia Series in Immunobiological Standardization 22:37–46, 1973.

88. Stojkovic L, Birtasevic B, Borjanovic S, et al (eds). Variola u Jugoslaviji 1972 Godine. Ljubljana, CCP Delo, 1974.

89. Mack TM. Smallpox in Europe, 1950–1971. J Infect Dis 125:161–169, 1972.

90. Fenn EA. Pox Americana: the great smallpox epidemic of 1775–1782. New York, Hill and Wang, 2001.

91. Miller J, Engelberg S, Broad WJ. Germs: Biological Weapons and America's Secret War. Waterville, ME, G.K. Hall, 2002.

92. Davis C J. Nuclear blindness: an overview of the biological weapons programs of the former Soviet Union and Iraq.PG - 509–512. Emerg Infect Dis 5, 1999.

93. Monterey Institute of International Studies. Chemical and Biological Weapons: Possession and Programs Past and Present 2001. http://cns.miis.edu/research/cbw/possess.htm. Accessed 10/16/2002.

94. United Nations, United Nations Special Commission (UNSCOM). Report of the Executive Chairman on the Activities of the Special Commission Established by the Secretary-General Pursuant to Paragraph 9 (b) (i) of Resolution 687 (1991). 1998. http://www.un.org/Depts/unscom/sres98-332.htm.Accessed 10/16/2002.

95. Zilinskas RA. Iraq's biological weapons. the past as future? JAMA 278:418–424, 1997.

96. Jezek Z, Kriz B, Rothbauer V. Camelpox and its risk to the human population. J Hyg Epidemiol Microbiol Immunol 27:29–42, 1983.

97. LeDuc JW, Damon I, Relman DA, et al. Smallpox research activities: U.S. interagency collaboration, 2001. Emerg Infect Dis 8:743–745, 2002.

98. Centers for Disease Control and Prevention. Smallpox Vaccination Clinic Guide. 2002. http://www.bt.cdc.gov/agent/smallpox/vaccination/pdf/smallpox-vax-clinic-guide.pdf. Accessed 09/24/02.

99. United Kingdom, Ministry of Health. Report of the Committee on Vaccination. His Majesty's Stationery Office, London, 1928.

100. Herrlich A, Mayer A, Mahnel H, Munz E. Experimental studies on transofrmation of the variola virus into the vaccinia virus. Arch Gesamte Virusforsch 12:579–599, 1963.

101. Baxby D. Jenner's Smallpox Vaccine: The Riddle of Vaccinia Virus and Its Origin. London, Heinemann Educational Books, 1981.

102. Rivers TM. Cultivation of vaccine virus for Jennerian prophylaxis in man. J Exp Med 54:453–461, 1931.

103. Barker LF. Further attenuated vaccinia virus: a possible alternative for primary immunization. In Sixth Annual Immunization Conference. Atlanta, GA, March 11-13, 1969, pp 55.

104. Rivers TM, Ward SM. Jennerian prophylaxis by mean of intradermal injections of cultured vaccine virus. J Exp Med 62:549–560, 1935.

105. Rivers TM, Ward SM, Baird RD. Amount and duration of immunity induced by intradermal inoculation of cultured vaccine virus. J Exp Med 69.857–866, 1939.

106. van der Noordaa J, Dekking F, Posthuma J, Beunders BJ. Primary vaccination with an attenuated strain of vaccinia virus. Arch Gesamte Virusforsch 22:210–214, 1967.

107. Kempe CH, Fulginiti V, Minamitani M, Shinefield H. Smallpox vaccination of eczema patients with a strain of attenuated live vaccinia (CVI-78). Pediatrics 42:980–985, 1968.

108. Tint H. The rationale for elective prevaccination with attenuated vaccine (CV-178) in preventing some vaccination complications. In International Symposium on Smallpox Vaccine. Symposia Series in Immunobiological Standardization 19:281–292, 1973.

109. Galasso GJ, Mattheis MJ, Cherry JD, et al. Clinical and serologic study of four smallpox vaccines comparing variations of dose and route of administration. summary. J Infect Dis 135:183–186, 1977.

110. McIntosh KA comparative study of four smallpox vaccines in children. In Vaccinia Viruses as Vectors for Vaccine Antigens: Proceedings of the Workshop on Vaccinia Viruses as Vectors for Vaccine Antigens, held November 13-14, 1984, in Chevy Chase, Maryland, U.S.A, G.V. Quinnan, Editor. New York, Elsevier, 1985, pp 77–84.

111. Hochstein-Mintzel V, Hanichen T, Huber HC, Stickl H. An attenuated strain of vaccinia virus (MVA): successful intramuscular immunization against vaccinia and variola (author's transl). Zentralbl Bakteriol [Orig A] 230:283–297, 1975.

112. Mayr A, Hochstein-Mintzel V, Stickl H. Abstammung, Eigenschaften und Verwendung des attenuierten Vaccinia-stammes MVA. Infection 3:6–14, 1975.

113. Stickl H, Hochstein-Mintzel V, Mayr A, et al. MVA vaccination against smallpox: clinical tests with an attenuated live vaccinia virus strain (MVA) (author's transl). Dtsch Med Wochenschr 99:2386–2392, 1974.

114. Sutter G, Moss B. Nonreplicating vaccinia vector efficiently expresses recombinant genes. Proc Natl Acad Sci U S A 89:10847–10851, 1992.

115. Sutter G, Wyatt LS, Foley PL, et al. A recombinant vector derived from the host range-restricted and highly attenuated MVA strain of vaccinia virus stimulates protective immunity in mice to influenza virus. Vaccine 12:1032–1040, 1994.

116. Hashizume SA new attenuated strain of vaccinia virus, LC 16m8: basic information [in Japanese]. J Clin Virol 3:229–235, 1975.

117. Hashizume S, Yoshizawa H, Morita M, and Suzuki K. Properties of attenuated mutant of vaccinia virus, LC 16m8, derived from Lister strain. In Vaccinia Viruses as Vectors for Vaccine Antigens: Proceedings of the Workshop on Vaccinia Viruses as Vectors for Vaccine Antigens, held November 13–14, 1984, in Chevy Chase, Maryland, U.S.A, G.V. Quinnan, Editor. New York, Elsevier, 1985, pp 87–99.

118. Kato S. Low neurovirulent variant of Lister strain of vaccinia virus. In Vaccinia Viruses as Vectors for Vaccine Antigens: Proceedings of the Workshop on Vaccinia Viruses as Vectors for Vaccine Antigens, held November 13–14, 1984, in Chevy Chase, Maryland, U.S.A, G.V. Quinnan, Editor. New York, Elsevier, 1985, pp 85–86.

119. Japan Ministry of Health. Report of Committee on Smallpox Vaccination [in Japanese]. J Clin Virol 3:269–278, 1975.

120. Buller RM, Smith GL, Cremer K., et al. Decreased virulence of recombinant vaccinia virus expression vectors is associated with a thymidine kinase-negative phenotype. Nature 317:813–815, 1985.

121. Lee MS, Roos JM, McGuigan LC, et al. Molecular attenuation of vaccinia virus: mutant generation and animal characterization. J Virol 66:2617–2630, 1992.

122. Buller RM, Palumbo GJ. Poxvirus pathogenesis. Microbiol Rev 55:80–122, 1991.

123. Tartaglia J, Perkus ME, Taylor J, et al. NYVAC: a highly attenuated strain of vaccinia virus. Virology 188:217–232, 1992.

124. Konishi E, Pincus S, Paoletti E, et al. A highly attenuated host range-restricted vaccinia virus strain, NYVAC, encoding the prM, E, and NS1 genes of Japanese encephalitis virus prevents JEV viremia in swine. Virology 190:454–458, 1992.

125. Stephensen CB, Welter J, Thaker SR, et al. Canine distemper virus (CDV) infection of ferrets as a model for testing Morbillivirus vaccine strategies: NYVAC- and ALVAC-based CDV recombinants protect against symptomatic infection. J Virol 71:1506–1513, 1997.

126. Leake JP. Questions and answers on smallpox vaccination. Public Health Rep 42:221–238, 1927.

127. McClain DJ, Harrison S, Yeager CL, et al. Immunologic responses to vaccinia vaccines administered by different parenteral routes. J Infect Dis 175:756–763, 1997.

128. Centers for Disease Control and Prevention. Vaccinia (smallpox) vaccine: recommendations of the Immunization Practices Advisory Committee (ACIP), 2001. MMWR Recomm Rep 50:1–25, 2001.

129. Centers for Disease Control and Prevention. Summary of October 2002 ACIP Smallpox Vaccination Recommendations, 2002. http://www.bt.cdc.gov/agent/smallpox/vaccination/acip-recs-oct2002.asp. Accessed 11/27/02.

130. Hekker AC, Bos JM, and Smith LA stable freeze-dried smallpox vaccine made in monolayer cultures of primary rabbit kidney cells. J Biol Stand 1: 21–32, 1973.

131. Hekker AC, Huisman J, Polak MF, et al. Field work with a stable freeze-dried vaccine prepared in monolayaers of rabbit kidney cells. *In* International Symposium on Smallpox Vaccine. Symposia Series in Immunobiological Standardization 19:187–195, 1973.

132. Hekker AC, Bos JM, Rai NK, et al. Large-scale use of freeze-dried smallpox vaccine prepared in primary cultures of rabbit kidney cells. Bull World Health Organ 54:279–284, 1976.

133. Cross RM, Kaplan C, McClean D. The heat resistance of dried smallpox vaccine. Lancet 1:446–448, 1957.

134. Blattner RJ, Norman J.O, Heyes F.M, Aksu I. Antibody response to cutaneous inoculation with vaccinia virus: viremia and viruria in vaccination children. J Pediatr 64:839–852, 1964.

135. Gins HA, Hackenthal H, Kamentzewa N. Experimentelle Untersuchungen u ber die Generalisierung des Vaccine-Virus beim Menschen und Versuchstier. Z Hyg Infektionskrankh 110:429–441, 1929.

136. Frey SE, Couch RB, Tacket CO, et al. Clinical responses to undiluted and diluted smallpox vaccine. N Engl J Med 346:1265–1274, 2002.

137. Benenson AS. Immediate (so-called immune) reaction to smallpox vaccination. JAMA 143:1238–1249, 1950.

138. Downie AW, McCarthy K. The antibody response in man following infection with viruses of the pox group. III. Antibody response in smallpox. J Hyg 56:479–487, 1958.

139. Pincus WB, Flick JA. The role of hypersensitivity in the pathogenesis of vaccinia virus infection in humans. J Pediatr 62:57–62, 1963.

140. Frey SE, Newman FK, Cruz J, et al. Dose-related effects of smallpox vaccine. N Engl J Med 346:1275–1280, 2002.

141. Hanna W. Studies in Smallpox and Vaccination. Bristol, Wright, 1913.

142. Zikmund V, Das N, Krishnayengar R, Kameswara Rao, B. Contribution to the problem of challenge vaccination. observations on vaccination of cured smallpox cases in India in 1971, 1972, and 1973. Indian J Public Health 22:102–106, 1978.

143. el-Ad B, Roth Y, Winder A, et al. The persistence of neutralizing antibodies after revaccination against smallpox. J Infect Dis 161:446–448, 1990.

144. Demkowicz WE, Jr, Littaua RA, Wang J, Ennis FA. Human cytotoxic T-cell memory: long-lived responses to vaccinia virus. J Virol 70:2627–2631, 1996.

145. Frelinger JA. and Garba ML. Responses to smallpox vaccine. N Engl J Med 347:689–690, 2002.

146. Winter PA; Mason JH; Kuhr E; et al. Combined immunization against poliomyelitis, diphtheria, whooping cough, tetanus and smallpox. S Afr Med J 37:513–515, 1963.

147. Karchmer A. W, Friedman JP, Casey HL, et al. Simultaneous administration of live virus vaccines. measles, mumps, poliomyelitis, and smallpox. Am J Dis Child 121:382–388, 1971.

148. Lin HT. A study of the effect of simultaneous vaccination with BCG and smallpox vaccine in newborn infants. Bull World Health Organ 33:321–336, 1965.

149. Meers PD. Further observations on 17D-yellow fever vaccination by scarification, with and without simultaneous smallpox vaccination. Trans R Soc Trop Med Hyg 54:493–501, 1960.

150. Breman JG, Coffi E, Bomba-Ire R, et al. Evaluation of a measles-smallpox vaccination campaign by a sero-epidemiologic method. Am J Epidemiol 102:564–571, 1975.

151. Meyer HM. Jr, Hostetler DD. Jr, Bernheim BC, et al. Response of Volta children to jet inoculation of combined live measles, smallpox and yellow fever vaccines. Bull World Health Organ 30:783–794, 1964.

152. Ruben FL, Smith EA, Foster SO, et al. Simultaneous administration of smallpox, measles, yellow fever, and diphtheria-pertussis-tetanus antigens to Nigerian children. Bull World Health Organ 48:175–181, 1973.

153. Foege WH. Foster SO. Multiple antigen vaccine strategies in developing countries. Am J Trop Med Hyg 23:685–689, 1974.

154. Brainerd HD, Hanna L, Jawetz E. Methisazone in progressive vaccinia. N Engl J Med 276:620–622, 1967.

155. De Clercq E. Cidofovir in the treatment of poxvirus infections. Antiviral Res 55:1–13, 2002.

156. Kesson AM, Ferguson JK, Rawlinson WD, Cunningham AL. Progressive vaccinia treated with ribavirin and vaccinia immune globulin. Clin Infect Dis 25:911–914, 1997.

157. Ruben FL. Lane JM. Ocular vaccinia. an epidemiologic analysis of 348 cases. Arch Ophthalmol 84:45–48, 1970.

158. Fulginiti VA, Winograd LA, Jackson M, Ellis P. Therapy of experimental vaccinal keratitis. effect of idoxuridine and VIG. Arch Ophthalmol 74:539–544, 1965.

159. Wilson GS. The Hazards of Immunization. London, Athlone P., 1967.

160. Vries E. de. Postvaccinial Perivenous Encephalitis. A Pathological Anatomical Study on the Place of Postvaccinial Perivenous Encephalitis in the Group Encephalitides (the Disease of Turnbull-Lucksch-Bastiaanse). Amsterdam, Elsevier, 1960.

161. Weber G. Lange J. Zur Variationsbreite der "Inkubationszeiten" postvakzinaler zerebraler Erkrankungen. Dtsch Med Wochenschr 86:1461–1468, 1961.

162. Polak MF. Complications of smallpox vaccination in the Netherlands, 1959-1970. *In* International Symposium on Smallpox Vaccine. Symposia Series in Immunobiological Standardization 19:235–242, 1973.

163. Berger K. Puntigam, FU ber die Erkrankungshaufigkeit verschiedener Altersklassen von Erstimpflingen an postvakzinaler Enzephalitis nachsubcutaner Pockenschutzimpfung. Wien Med 104:487–492, 1954.

164. Conybeare ET. Illnesses attributed to smallpox vaccination, 1951-1960. Part II. Illnesses reported as affecting the central nervous system. Monthly Bulletin of the Ministry of Health and the Public Health Laboratory Service 23:150–159, 1964.

165. Herrlich A. Probleme der Pocken und Pockenschutzimpfung. Munch Med Wochenschr 96:529–533, 1954.

166. Stuart G. Memorandum on postvaccinal encephalitis. Bull World Health Organ 1:36–53, 1947–1948.

167. Femmer J. Cited by Wilson GS. Hazards of Immunization. London, Athlone, 1967.

168. Seeleman K. Zerebrale Komplikationen nach Pock-enschutzimpfungen mit besonderer Berucksichtigung der Alterdisposition in Hamburg 1936 bis 1958. Dtsch Med Wochenschr 85:1081–1089, 1960.

169. van den Berg CA. L'encephalite post- vaccinale aux Pays-Bas. Bull Office Intern Hyg Publique 38:847–848, 1946.

170. Lane JM, Ruben FL, Neff JM, and Millar JD. Complications of smallpox vaccination, 1968. N Engl J Med 281:1201–1208, 1969.

171. Lane JM, Ruben FL, Neff JM, Millar JD. Complications of smallpox vaccination, 1968: results of ten statewide surveys. J Infect Dis 122:303–309, 1970.

172. Neff JM Lane JM Pert JH, et al. Complications of smallpox vaccination. I. National survey in the United States, 1963. N Engl J Med 276:125–132, 1967.

173. Berger K, Heinrich W. Decrease in postvaccinal deaths in Austria after introducing a less pathogenic virus strain. *In* International Symposium on Smallpox Vaccine. Symposia Series in Immunobiological Standardization 19:199–203, 1973.

174. Marrenikova SS, Chimishkyan KL, Maltseva NN, et al. Characteristics of virus strains for production of smallpox vaccines. *In* Proceedings of the Symposium on Smallpox. Zagreb: Yugoslav Academy of Sciences and Arts, 1969, pp 65–79.

175. Communicable Disease Center. Manual of Operations: West and Central Africa Smallpox Eradication/Measles Control Program. Atlanta, Centers for Disease Control, 1966.

176. Bellows MT, Hyman MR, Merritt KK, et al. Effect of smallpox vaccination on outcome of pregnancy. Public Health Rep 64:319–323, 1949.

177. Abramowitz LJ. Vaccination and virus diseases during pregnancy. S Afr Med J 31:13, 1957.

178. Bourke GJ; Whitney RJ. Smallpox vaccination in pregnancy; a prospective study. BMJ 5364:1544–1546, 1964.

179. Tondury G, Foukas M. Die Gefahrdung des menschlichen Keimlings durch Pockenimpfung in Graviditate. Pathol Microbiol 27:602–623, 1964.

180. Marmelzat WL. Malignant tumors in smallpox vaccination scars: a report of 24 cases. Arch Dermatol 97:400–406, 1968.

181. Sewall S. Vaccinia osteomyelitis. report of a case with isolation of the vaccinia virus. Bull Hosp Jt Dis 10:59–63, 1949.

182. Karjalainen J, Heikkila J, Nieminen MS et al. Etiology of mild acute infectious myocarditis. Acta Med Scand 213: 65–73, 1983.

183. Centers for Disease Control and Prevention. Interim smallpox fact sheet: Smallpox Vaccine and Heart Problems. *http://www.bt.cdc.gov/agent/smallpox/vaccination/heartproblems.asp*. Accessed April 14, 2002.

184. Cooney EL, Collier AC, Greenberg PD, et al. Safety of and immunological response to a recombinant vaccinia virus vaccine expressing HIV envelope glycoprotein. Lancet 337:567–572, 1991.

185. Neff JM Lan M, Fulginiti VA, Henderson DA. Contact vaccinia-transmission of vaccinia from smallpox vaccination. JAMA 288:1901–1905, 2002.

186. Greenberg M. Complication of vaccination against smallpox. Am J Dis Children 76:492–502, 1948.

187. Copeman PW M, Wallace HJ. Eczema vaccinatum. BMJ 2:906–908, 1964.

188. Neff JM, Drachman RH. Complications of smallpox vaccination, 1968 surveillance in a comprehensive care clinic. Pediatrics 50:481–483, 1972.

189. Raimer SS. Managing pediatric atopic dermatitis. Clin Pediatr (Phila) 39:1–14, 2000.

190. Habbick BF, Pizzichini MM, Taylor B, et al. Prevalence of asthma, rhinitis and eczema among children in 2 Canadian cities: the International Study of Asthma and Allergies in Childhood. CMAJ 160:1824–1828, 1999.

191. Laughter D, Istvan JA, Tofte SJ, Hanifin JM. The prevalence of atopic dermatitis in Oregon schoolchildren. J Am Acad Dermatol 43:649–655, 2000.

192. Centers for Disease Control and Prevention. HIV/AIDS Surveillance Report. 2002. *http://www.cdc.gov/hiv/stats/hasr1302.htm.*Accessed 09/26/02.

193. (UNOS), United Network for Organ Sharing. All recipients: age at time of transplant. 2002. *http://www.unos.org/.*Accessed 09/26/02.

194. National Cancer Institute. CanQues. 2002. *http://srab.cancer.gov/Prevalence/canques.html*. Accessed 09/26/02.

195. Lawrence RC, Helmick CG, Arnett FC, et al. Estimates of the prevalence of arthritis and selected musculoskeletal disorders in the United States. Arthritis Rheum 41:778–799, 1998.

196. Kempe CH. Studies on smallpox and complications of smallpox vaccination. Pediatrics 26:176–189, 1960.

197. Fulginiti V, Kempe CH, Hathaway WE, et al. Progressive vaccinia in immunologic deficient individuals. In Immunologic deficiency diseases in man. Birth Defects Original Article Series, D. Bergsma and R.A. Good, eds. New York, National Foundation-March of Dimes, 1968, pp 129–145.

198. Kempe CH, Bowles C, Meikeljohn G, et al. The use of vaccinia hyperimmune gamma-globulin in the prophylaxis of smallpox. Bull World Health Organ 25:41–48, 1961.

199. Urner JA. Some observations of the vaccination of pregnant women and newborn infants. Am J Obstet Gynecol 13:70–76, 1927.

200. Lieberman BL. Vaccination of pregnant women and newborn infants. Am J Obstet Gynecol 14:217–220, 1927.

201. Donnally HH and Nicholson MM. A study of vaccination in five hundred newborn infants. JAMA 103:1269–1275, 1934.

202. Centers for Disease Control and Prevention. Draft Supplemental Recommendations of the ACIP: Use of Smallpox (Vaccinia) Vaccine, June 2002. *http://www.bt.cdc.gov/agent/smallpox/vaccination/acip-guidelines.asp*. Accessed 10/15/02.

203. Mukherjee MK, Sarkar JK, Mitra AC. Pattern of intrafamilial transmission of smallpox in Calcutta, India. Bull World Health Organ 51:219–225, 1974.

204. Bicknell WJ. The case for voluntary smallpox vaccination. N Engl J Med 346:1323–1325, 2002.

205. DeRugy V and Pena CV. Responding to the threat of smallpox bioterrorism. Policy Analysis 434:1–16, 2002.

206. Centers for Disease Control and Prevention. Smallpox Vaccination and Adverse Events Training Module 2002. *http://www.bt.cdc.gov/training/smallpoxvaccine/reactions/default.htm*. Accessed 11/27/02.

207. Webster IM. The response of leprosy patients to smallpox vaccine. West Afr Med J 8:322–324, 1959.

208. Browne SG, Davis EM. Reaction in leprosy precipitated by smallpox vaccination. Lepr Rev 33:252–254, 1962.

209. Blake JB. Benjamin Waterhouse and the Introduction of Vaccination; A Reappraisal. Philadelphia, University of Pennsylvania Press, 1957.

210. Halsey RH. How the President, Thomas Jefferson, and Doctor Benjamin Waterhouse Established Vaccination as a Public Health Procedure. History of Medicine Series, No. 5. New York, New York Academy of Medicine, 1936.

211. Chapin CV, Smith J. Permanency of the mild type of smallpox. J Preventive Med 6:273–320, 1932.

212. Vaughan, VC. Smallpox before and after Edward Jenner. Hygeia 1:205–211, 1923.

213. Woodward SB, Feemster RF. The relation of smallpox morbidity to vaccination laws. N Engl J Med 208:317–318, 1933.

214. Low RB. The Incidence of Small-pox Throughout the World in Recent Years. Reports to the Local Government Board on Public Health and Medical Subjects NS No. 117. London, His Majesty's Stationery Office, 1918.

215. Henneberg G. The distribution of smallpox in Europe 1919-1948. In World Atlas of Epidemic Diseases, Part II, E. Rodenwaldt and H.H.J. Jusatz, Editors. Hamburg, Falk- Verlag, 1952, pp 3 v. (loose-leaf).

216. Rodrigues BA. Smallpox eradication in the Americas. Bull Pan Am Health Organ 9:53–68, 1975.

217. Arita I. The control of vaccine quality in the smallpox eradication programme. In International Symposium on Smallpox Vaccine. Symposia Series in Immunobiological Standardization 19:79–87, 1973.

218. Arita I and Henderson DA. Freeze-dried vaccine for the smallpox eradication programme. In Proceedings of the Symposium on Smallpox. Zagreb: Yogoslav Academy of Sciences and Arts, 1969, pp 39–50.

219. Henderson DA, Arita I, Shafa E. Studies of the Bifurcated Needle and Recommendations for Its Use. Unpublished document. Geneva, World Health Organization, 1969.

220. Foege WH, Millar JD, Lane JM. Selective epidemiologic control in smallpox eradication. Am J Epidemiol 94:311–315, 1971.

221. World Health Organization. Smallpox eradication. destruction of variola virus stocks. Wkly Epidemiol Rec 74:188–191, 1999.

222. Tucker JB. Scourge: The Once and Future Threat of Smallpox. New York, Atlantic Monthly Press, 2001.

223. World Health Organization. Report of the WHO Ad Hoc Committee on Orthopoxvirus Infections. Wkly Epidemiol Rec 6:289, 1986.

224. Mahy BW, Almond JW, Berns KI, et al. The remaining stocks of smallpox virus should be destroyed. Science 262:1223–1224, 1993.

225. World Health Organization. Report of the Ad Hoc Committee on Orthopoxvirus Infections. Exectutive Board Report EB/95/33 dated October 10, 1994.

226. Roizman B, Joklik W, Fields B, Moss B. The destruction of smallpox virus stocks in national repositories: a grave mistake and a bad precedent. Infect Agents Dis 3:215–217, 1994.

227. Marwick C. Smallpox virus destruction delayed yet again. JAMA 273:446, 1995.

228. Stone R. Smallpox research. world health body fires starting gun. Science 296:1383, 2002.

Chapter 10

Vaccination in the Immunocompromised Host

PER LJUNGMAN

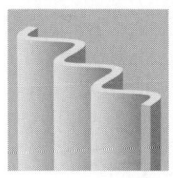

Over the past 30 years, the number of patients who are immunocompromised has increased rapidly. These patients can be immunocompromised by, for example, the immunosuppression given after solid organ transplantation or hematopoietic stem cell transplantation (SCT), or increased intensity of therapy for malignancies with intensified chemotherapy protocols or with protocols resulting in T-cell suppression. Infections have been major obstacles for successful transplantation. In transplant patients, the highest risk for infection usually is early after the transplant. However, many of these patients remain immunosuppressed as a result of either the interaction between the graft and the host, as in graft-versus-host disease (GVHD) after allogeneic SCT, or by the immunosuppressive therapy given to prevent graft rejection.

Immunizations of immunocompromised individuals are important from two points of view. Obviously, the need to protect the patient against serious infections is the primary goal. However, the public health point of view is also significant because it is important not to have an increasing number of individuals vulnerable to serious infectious agents (e.g., poliovirus). Both aspects require an analysis of risks and benefits for the individual patient.

Another potentially important issue is whether and how to vaccinate hospital staff or family members. Vaccination of these individuals could confer benefit, for example, by reducing the potential for exposing immunocompromised patients to such infections as influenza. However, there is also the potential for causing harm by spreading a vaccine strain of a virus to the patient; thus individuals caring for or living with an immunocompromised patient should not be vaccinated with an oral poliovirus vaccine that might cause a secondary infection in the patient.[1]

Patients with Cancer

Cancer chemo- and radiotherapy has been intensified substantially during the past decade. Because findings from studies of the results of immunization in patients undergoing such therapy are old, they might not represent the true situation today. In particular, very few studies of immunity and vaccination have been published regarding adult solid tumor patients undergoing active anticancer therapy. Furthermore, many of the studies involve mixed study populations frequently not specified as to type of cancer and intensity of given therapy. Most studies have concentrated on patients with hematologic malignancies, so the discussion in the remainder of this section refers mostly to leukemia and lymphoma patients unless otherwise stated. A summary of the recommendations is shown in Table 10–1.

Killed Vaccines

Pneumococcal Vaccine

Pneumococci are important causes of infection in patients with hematologic malignancies. Patients with Hodgkin's disease are frequently splenectomized as a part of their diagnosis and therapy, which makes this group especially vulnerable to disseminated pneumococcal infections. Several studies have been performed using the pneumococcal polysaccharide-based vaccines in patients with cancer. In children with leukemia, the 14-valent vaccine gave suboptimal antibody responses.[2] Similar results were found with the 23-valent vaccine in patients with multiple myeloma, among whom less than 40% obtained "protective" antibody levels after vaccination.[3] The response in patients with Hodgkin's disease varies with the time relative to therapy at which the immunization is performed. Patients who have immunizations performed after chemo- and/or radiotherapy have a severe impairment of the antibody response.[4,5] In contrast, a good response can be obtained if immunizations are performed before therapy is initiated.[6,7] The response in children with Hodgkin's disease is poorer if immunizations were performed after splenectomy.[8] However, antibody responses can be elicited in splenectomized patients with non-Hodgkin's lymphomas and Hodgkin's disease,[9] although the response is impaired for several years after treatment of Hodgkin's disease.[7] Patients with carcinoma of the head or neck had poor

TABLE 10–1 ■ Recommendations for Immunizations in Cancer Patients

Vaccine	Recommendation	Comments
Pneumococci	Yes	Lymphoma patients. Preferably before initiation of chemotherapy. If given during chemotherapy, revaccination should be considered after cessation.
Conjugated Hib	Yes	Children with cancer; patients with Hodgkin's disease. Preferably before initiation of chemotherapy.
Influenza	Yes	Seasonal to all cancer patients. Two doses give better immune response.
Varicella	Yes	Seronegative children and young adults in remission from malignant disease. Not during active chemo- or radiotherapy.
Measles	Individual consideration	Depending on the local epidemiologic situation. Not during active chemo- or radiotherapy.

antibody responses when immunizations were performed early after radiotherapy.[10] Chan et al. showed that priming with a 7-valent conjugated pneumococcal vaccine could improve the response to the 23-valent polysaccharide vaccine in patients with previously treated Hodgkin's disease.[11] The recently licensed conjugate vaccines might improve the responses in patients with cancer. However, repeated doses, as used in healthy infants, are probably necessary. Molrine et al. showed that a single dose of a pneumococcal conjugate vaccine gave suboptimal responses in patients who had been treated for Hodgkin's disease.[12]

Immunization of patients with lymphoma against pneumococcal infections is recommended as early as possible after diagnosis and before chemo- and/or radiotherapy is initiated.

Haemophilus influenzae Type b Vaccine

Severe infections in cancer patients with *Haemophilus influenzae* type b (Hib) are less common than pneumococcal infections. However, children with leukemia are at a greater than sixfold increased risk for Hib infection compared to normal children.[13] Immunization with a conjugated Hib vaccine results in lower antibody responses than in normal children, and a booster dose is ineffective. Longer duration and intensity of antileukemic chemotherapy were associated with a poor response to immunization.[13,14] Children undergoing therapy for solid tumors also have lower than normal responses to vaccination with an Hib vaccine.[15] Immunization with a conjugated Hib vaccine is indicated in children with cancer, preferably early during anticancer chemotherapy.

Very limited data are available regarding the risk for severe Hib infections and the response to vaccination in adult patients with cancer. Patients with multiple myeloma had antibody responses comparable to those of normal healthy adults.[3] Molrine et al. showed that 99% of patients with Hodgkin's disease in whom therapy had been discontinued responded to vaccination.[12] Jurlander et al. showed in a randomized study that a histamine type 2 blocker, ranitidine, was able to improve the response to immunization with a conjugated Hib vaccine.[16]

Influenza Vaccine

Influenza vaccination is recommended in immunocompromised patients.[17] The morbidity and mortality of influenza vary in different types of cancer patients, with the most severe consequences occurring in acute leukemia patients undergoing induction chemotherapy.[18] The morbidity in adult patients with other types of hematologic malignancies and in patients with solid tumors is probably lower, although good epidemiologic data are lacking.[19] However, many of these patients are elderly and are likely also to have other diseases, strengthening the indication for vaccination. Kempe et al. reported that children with cancer were more likely to develop influenza, but their symptoms had a duration similar to that of healthy controls and, although the size of the study was small, there were few clinical complications.[20]

Results of two studies of influenza vaccination in children with acute lymphoblastic leukemia show that the proportion of children reaching "protective" antibody levels varied between 45% and 100% for the different influenza subtypes in the vaccines, with the poorest results for the influenza A (H1N1) subtype.[21,22] It has been reported that an antibody titer protective in healthy controls failed to prevent influenza in 24% of children with cancer, but the possibility that the severity of the infection was reduced in the cases of vaccine failure cannot be excluded.[20]

The data regarding vaccination efficacy in adult patients with solid tumors are limited. In a study of lung cancer patients, the vaccination response was similar to that of healthy controls.[23] Similarly, the humoral response was adequate in a group of women with breast cancer.[24] In contrast, most published studies show that adult patients with hematologic malignancies respond poorly to vaccination. In a study including patients with multiple myeloma, the response rate to one dose of vaccine was only 19%.[3] In another study including patients with chronic lymphocytic leukemia, 63% had an antibody response that was retained at 30 and 60 days after vaccination. However, patients with low immunoglobulin G (IgG) levels responded poorly.[25] The rate of response also might vary with the influenza subtypes in the vaccine. Brydak and Calbecka, in a small study including a mixed group of patients with hematologic malignancies, showed response rates of 10% for influenza A (H1N1), 35% for influenza A (H3N2), and 70% for influenza B.[26] One way to improve the results is to give repeated doses of vaccine. Adults with lymphoma receiving a two-dose schedule showed responses of approximately

30% after one dose and approximately 45% after two doses of vaccine.[27]

Although influenza immunization is recommended in cancer patients, it must be recognized that the protective effectiveness is likely to be low in the patients who are at highest risk of severe complication. Thus other preventive strategies are needed. Elting et al. reported that most influenza infections in acute leukemia patients undergoing chemotherapy were nosocomially acquired, and immunizations of family members and hospital staff should therefore be considered.[18]

Tetanus Toxoid, Diphtheria Toxoid, and Inactivated Poliovirus Vaccine

The protection against tetanus, diphtheria, and poliovirus is frequently low in cancer patients undergoing chemotherapy. Hammarström et al. haves shown that 41% of non-transplanted acute leukemia patients were not protected against tetanus.[28] Risk factors for loss of immunity were acute lymphoblastic versus acute myelogenous leukemia, more advanced disease, and increasing age. Lymphoma patients are also likely to have deficient immunity. In children treated for cancer, the immunities against tetanus, diphtheria, and poliovirus were lower than what would be expected in an age-matched population.[29,30] In contrast, Nordoy et al. reported that treatment of low-grade non-Hodgkin's lymphoma patients with radioimmunotherapy did not influence specific immunity to tetanus.[31]

Immunity to tetanus toxoid, diphtheria toxoid, and poliovirus is frequently deficient in cancer patients, and immunizations should be considered in these individuals. The responses to diphtheria toxoid and tetanus toxoid vaccinations in adult cancer patients have not been systematically studied. However, in children undergoing maintenance chemotherapy, the vaccination responses were similar to those of healthy individuals.[29]

To my knowledge, only one small study has been published regarding efficacy of an inactivated poliovirus vaccine in leukemia patients. Stenvik et al. reported on 14 children with leukemia who were given a booster dose of vaccine, with 12 of 14 responding.[32] No data exist regarding the vaccination of adults with cancer. Despite the absence of data, it seems logical to recommend an investigation of poliovirus immunity and booster immunization for cancer patients traveling to areas of the world that are still endemic for poliovirus. The oral poliovirus vaccine can induce paralytic disease in immunocompromised patients and should not be used.[33] Furthermore, the vaccine strain might be transferred from healthy family members, so the use of an inactivated vaccine when relatives are immunized is recommended. Finally, live poliovirus vaccine also should be avoided in health care workers caring for severely immunocompromised patients.[1]

Other Bacterial Infections

Vaccinations could be considered against pertussis and meningococci, although no studies have been published in patients with cancer regarding the frequency or severity of these infections. Rautonen et al. showed similar responses to vaccination with a meningococcal vaccine in children with acute leukemia compared to normal children. However, the study was performed in the early 1980s, when the antileukemic regimen was less intensive than currently used protocols.[34]

Hepatitis B Virus

Hepatitis B virus (HBV) infection is a major cause of morbidity in many parts of the world. Severe primary HBV infections are rare in cancer patients. Nevertheless, immunization of patients against HBV might be indicated in countries where the prevalence of HBV is high. The currently available vaccines are plasma derived or produced through DNA recombinant technology.

In contrast to the situation for other vaccines, several studies have been performed regarding the efficacy of HBV vaccination. The results are summarized in Table 10–2. All studies cited in the table report results in children, and to my knowledge no study has reported results in adults with cancer or hematologic malignancy.

Live Vaccines

Varicella Virus Vaccine

Primary varicella infections cause high mortality in children with cancer. The existing vaccine is live, attenuated, and based on the Oka strain.[35] The vaccine was shown to be effective and safe in children with leukemia who were in remission.[36] The seroconversion rate was 88% after one dose and 98% after one to two doses. The rate of varicella infection in vaccines was 8%; all infected children had mild disease.[36] The frequency of side effects from the vaccine is low, and breakthrough vaccine disease can be treated effectively with acyclovir.[36,37] The immunity is stable over at least 5 years after immunization. The risk for herpes zoster after vaccination is lower compared to that in patients who had natural varicella disease.[38,39] In a small randomized study, varicella vaccine was given to children with newly diagnosed cancer before starting chemotherapy. There was a high rate of seroconversion and no severe side effects were found, but the number of included patients was low.[40]

Household exposure to varicella is associated with more severe varicella disease in secondary cases. An option would then be to immunize healthy seronegative family members when the child with cancer is undergoing intensive therapy and a live vaccine cannot be given. Diaz et al. showed that the vaccine virus cannot be isolated from oropharyngeal secretions of the immunized siblings.[41] None of the children with cancer showed clinical or serologic evidence of vaccine virus transmission. However, vaccine virus may be present in vesicular rashes, and transmission can rarely occur though with mild or no consequences. Immunization with the varicella vaccine is indicated in seronegative patients with cancer when the cancer chemotherapy schedule allows immunization.

TABLE 10–2 ▪ Results of HBV recombinant vaccine studies in children with malignancies

Diagnoses	Vaccine	On/off therapy	No. of patients	Vaccine dose
Leukemia[1]	Emgerix B	Maintenance	50	20 µg
	GenHevac	Maintenance	44	20 µg
ALL[2]	Emgerix B	Induction	94	20 µg < 10ys
				40 µg > 10ys
ALL[3]	Emgerix B	Induction	111	20 µg < 10ys
				40 µg > 10ys
Lymphoma[4]	GenHevac	Induction	23	40 µg
Solid tumors[4]	GenHevac	Induction	47	40 µg
Leukemia[4]	GenHevac	Maintenance	48	40 µg
Leukemia/lymphoma[5]	Emgerix B	No	36	20 µg < 10ys
		Maintenance	18	40 µg > 10ys
Leukemia[6]	Emgerix B	On	64	20 µg
		Off	58	

[1] Yetgin S, Tunc B, Koc A, Toksoy HB, Ceyhan M, Kanra G. Two booster dose hepatitis B virus vaccination in patients with leukemia. Leuk Res 25(8):647–649, 2001.

[2] Goyal S, Pai SK, Kelkar R, Advani SH. Hepatitis B vaccination in acute lymphoblastic leukemia. Leuk Res 22(2):193–195, 1998.

[3] Somjee S, Pai S, Kelkar R, Advani S. Hepatitis B vaccination in children with acute lymphoblastic leukemia: results of an intensified immunization schedule. Leuk Res 23(4):365–367, 1999.

Measles

Measles is still an important infectious agent in some countries, and infections in patients with cancer have a high rate of mortality. Kaplan et al. reviewed 27 published cases, among whom 20 (74%) developed pneumonitis and 8 (30%) died.[42] There was a tendency toward lower mortality in previously vaccinated patients.

Immunization with the live, attenuated vaccine has been contraindicated because of the risk of severe side effects in cancer patients undergoing chemotherapy, but this vaccine can be given at 3 months after cessation of cancer therapy. It might also be important to investigate the immune status in family members and, if necessary, immunize, for example, siblings. Measles immunization is not recommended in patients with cancer. However, immunization with the measles vaccine can be considered in cancer patients not receiving active cancer chemotherapy in epidemiologic situations when the risk for measles is increased.

Other Live Vaccines

Very limited data exist on immunization with mumps, rubella, or Bacille Calmette-Guèrin (BCG) vaccine in cancer patients. However, the use of these vaccines is not recommended during active cancer therapy.

Bone Marrow and Peripheral Stem Cell Transplantation Patients

In allogeneic SCT recipients, four components combine in the production of the immunodeficient state of the patient: (1) the immunosuppressive activity of the primary disease and treatment, (2) the high doses of chemo- and radiotherapy used to eradicate the host's immune system, (3) the immunologic reactivity between the graft and the host, and (4) the immunosuppressive therapy given after transplantation. In autologous bone marrow transplantation (BMT) recipients, only the first two components have to be con-

sidered. A summary of recommendations for these positions is shown in Table 10–3.

Allogeneic Bone Marrow Transplantation

After an allogeneic BMT, the immune system of the recipient is replaced by the immune system of the donor. Immunity to infectious agents is transferred by the graft and can be detected in the patient early after the BMT.[43–50] The transferred immunity is usually of a finite duration, and over time an increasing number of patients become susceptible to infections with, for example, tetanus,[45,51] poliovirus,[52,53] and measles.[54] The immune status of the donor is important for the short-term transfer of immunity and can be boosted by immunizing the donor before the transplant.[47,55–57]

The transplantation period can be divided into three distinct phases, each with its unique combination of risks and benefits of immunization. The early post-transplant phase is characterized by neutropenia, and the characteristic infections are caused by bacteria and fungi for which immunization is unlikely to be effective. During the intermediate post-transplant phase, the most common severe infections are caused by cytomegalovirus (CMV), varicella-zoster virus (VZV), Streptococcus pneumoniae, and H. influenzae. The risk for infections is strongly influenced by the presence of GVHD. The pattern of infections is similar during the late phase after BMT. However, long-term protection against other infectious agents such as tetanus, diphtheria, poliovirus, and measles also should be considered. Several studies have shown a loss of immunity to tetanus, poliovirus, and diphtheria during an extended follow-up after BMT.[51–53,58]

Killed Vaccines

PNEUMOCOCCAL VACCINE

Pneumococcal infections are significant causes of morbidity and mortality after allogeneic BMT. The risk for severe infections is increased in patients with chronic GVHD.[59–61] Immunization with the currently available pneumococcal

No. of doses	Schedule	Booster?	Seroconversion rate
3	0, 1, 6 m	12 m	32.1%
3	0, 1, 2 m	6 m	38.6%
3	0, 1, 2 m	12 m	19.5% (10.5% protected)
5	0, 1, 2, 3, 4 m	12 m	29.7% (18.9% protective)
3	0, 1, 2 m	12 m	48% after 3; 74% after 4 doses
3	0, 1, 2 m	12 m	77% after 3; 94.4% after 4 doses
3	0, 1, 2 m	12 m	88% after 3; 90% after 4 doses
4	0, 1, 2, 6 m		88%
3	0, 1, 2 m	6 m	26%
			88%

[4] Meral A, Sevinir B, Gunay U. Efficacy of immunization against hepatitis B virus infection in children with cancer. Med Pediatr Oncol 35(1):47–51, 2000.

[5] Rokicka-Milewska R, Jackowska T, Sopylo B, Kacperska E, Seyfried H. Active immunization of children with leukemias and lymphomas against infection by hepatitis B virus. Acta Paediatr Jpn 35(5): 400–403, 1993.

[6] Polychronopoulou-Androulakaki S, Panagiotou JP, Kostaridou S, Kyratzopoulou A, Haidas S. Immune response of immunocompromised children with malignancies to a recombinant hepatitis B vaccine. Pediatr Hematol Oncol 13(5):425–431, 1996

vaccines can elicit antibody responses 6 to 12 months after BMT in patients without GVHD but has been ineffective in eliciting adequate immune responses in patients with chronic GVHD.[56,62–65] In particular, the specific IgG2 responses have been poor.[65,66] Children given pneumococcal polysaccharide vaccines had short-lived responses and low avidity,[67] in contrast to adults, in whom the avidity was good.[68] However, in adults the opsonophagocytic activity was poor against pneumococcal subtype 19F.[69] The immune response was not significantly improved by two doses of pneumococcal vaccine as compared to one dose.[56] In a study in which donors were immunized against pneumococci and recipients immunized with the same vaccines after the transplantation, the recipients' immune response against pneumococci was not improved when they were immunized at 12 and 24 months after BMT.[70] Thus, responses to vaccination with polysaccharide vaccines are suboptimal in many patients.

The new conjugated vaccines also might improve immunization results in patients with chronic GVHD; preliminary results support this hypothesis (V. Hammarström and P. Ljungman, unpublished data). Molrine et al. performed a randomized study comparing pretransplant vaccination of patients and their donors with the heptavalent conjugated vaccine or no vaccination pretransplant. All patients thereafter received three doses of the vaccine at 3, 6, and 12 months after transplantation. The majority of patients (72% to 100% for different serotypes) developed protective

TABLE 10–3 ■ Recommendations for Immunizations in Stem Cell Transplant Patients

Vaccine	Recommendation	Comments
Tetanus toxoid + diphtheria toxoid (DT)	Yes	Three doses (DT) starting at 6–12 months after transplantation
Influenza	Yes	Seasonal, beginning at 6–12 months after transplantation
Inactivated poliovirus	Yes	Three doses starting at 6–12 months after transplantation. OPV is contraindicated.
Conjugated Hib	Yes	Two to three doses starting at 6–12 months after transplantation
Pneumococcal polysaccharide vaccine	Yes	One or two doses started at 6–12 months after transplantation
Pneumococcal conjugate vaccine	Individual consideration	Children, patients with chronic GVHD
Hepatitis B	Regional	In countries where vaccination is recommended to the general population. Three doses started at 6–12 months.
Measles	Individual consideration	Not before 24 months after BMT; not to be given in patients with GVHD disease
Rubella	Individual consideration	Females with pregnancy potential
Varicella	Individual consideration	Seronegative patients, not before 24 months after BMT; not to be given in patients with GVHD

BMT, bone marrow transplantation; GVHD, graft-versus-host disease; OPV, oral poliovirus vaccine.
Adapted from recommendations of the European Group for Blood and Marrow Transplantation (1999)[73] and the Centers for Disease Control and Prevention (2000).[72]

antibody levels at 12 months after SCT.[71] There was also an improved response (67% vs. 36%) to the first dose when compared to the polysaccharide vaccine. Other randomized studies are ongoing.

Despite the poor responses to vaccination in some patients, current recommendations are to vaccinate all allogeneic SCT patients with the polysaccharide vaccine.[72-74] These are likely to change when more data on the conjugate vaccine become available. The degree of protection against invasive pneumococcal disease from the vaccine will depend on the circulating serotypes in the community because only seven serotypes are included in the vaccine. However, it seems logical today to vaccinate patients who do not respond to the polysaccharide vaccine, young children, and patients with chronic GVHD with the heptavalent conjugate vaccine. It is possible that immune response to the polysaccharide vaccine can be improved if it is given after the conjugate vaccine, and this can be considered.

HAEMOPHILUS INFLUENZAE TYPE B VACCINE

Haemophilus influenzae is also an important cause of infection in allogeneic BMT recipients. In contrast to the situation with pneumococci, immunization with Hib can elicit protective immune responses.[56,62,75] However, it has been reported that time after transplantation is important for the immune response to Hib vaccine in transplanted children.[76] A good immune response could be elicited when the donor was immunized before transplantation and the recipient at 3 months after transplantation.[70] Immunization with an Hib vaccine is indicated for all allogeneic BMT recipients.[72-74]

INFLUENZA VACCINE

Influenza A and B infections can be severe and life threatening in SCT recipients.[19,77-79] Severe infections frequently occur early after SCT when immunizations are ineffective. Whether a pretransplant immunization of the marrow donor and/or recipient would be protective has not been studied. Another option for protecting patients early after SCT would be to reduce the risk of the patient's contracting influenza by immunizing family members and hospital staff, thereby reducing the risk for transmission of the infection to the patient.[72] The time after SCT is important for vaccine efficacy, with patients vaccinated later after SCT having better responses.[80,81] Adding granulocyte-macrophage colony-stimulating factor (GM-CSF) to influenza vaccine resulted in some minor improvements in the response to influenza B vaccine.[81] Influenza vaccination is recommended for all allogeneic SCT recipients.[72,73]

HEPATITIS B VIRUS VACCINE

Severe HBV infections are rare after SCT unless an HBV-positive donor is used for a seronegative recipient. Nevertheless, immunization of patients against HBV in countries where the prevalence of HBV is high might be indicated. Immunization early after SCT is likely to be ineffective unless the donor is immunized. The immunization of the marrow donor allows a transfer of immunity to the recipient.[55,57] A transferred donor immunity can be long lasting in at least 50% of patients.[82] Whether this transferred immunity can prevent an infection in the recipient is presently unknown. Recent case reports further suggest that transfer of immunity from an HBV-immune donor can clear the virus from an HBV antigen and DNA–positive recipient.[83,84] Further studies are needed to assess the usefulness of donor vaccination as immune therapy against HBV. Vaccination is recommended after allogeneic SCT.[72,73]

TETANUS TOXOID, DIPHTHERIA TOXOID, AND INACTIVATED POLIOVIRUS VACCINES

Most BMT patients will lose immunity to tetanus toxoid, diphtheria toxoid, and poliovirus during extended follow-up. Several studies of immunization with these vaccines have been published.[51-53] A new primary schedule with repeated doses of these vaccines is needed to obtain stable protective immunity.[51-53] The inactivated poliovirus vaccine should be used to prevent a vaccine-induced paralytic disease. In most of the published studies, the immunization programs were initiated approximately 1 year after SCT. However, it has been shown that good and lasting immune responses could be obtained when immunizations were started at 6 months after SCT.[85] Gerritsen et al. immunized children before BMT followed by revaccination as early as 6 weeks after BMT. Thirty percent of the patients responded to early immunization.[86] The vaccination of allogeneic SCT recipients with three doses of tetanus toxoid, diphtheria toxoid, and inactivated poliovirus vaccine is recommended.[72-74]

Pertussis vaccination after bone marrow transplantation has not been studied, but in young patients, it would appear rational to include an acellular pertussis vaccine with diphtheria and tetanus vaccines.[262]

OTHER KILLED VACCINES

Vaccination with meningococcal polysaccharide vaccine can elicit good responses in SCT recipients against both serogroups A and C.[87] Meningococcal vaccination is not routinely recommended after allogeneic SCT.[72]

Live, Attenuated Vaccines

VARICELLA VACCINE

Primary VZV infections can be very severe after allogeneic transplantation. The existing vaccine is live and attenuated and therefore cannot be used early in the post-transplant period. A seronegative patient should probably be immunized before transplantation providing that enough time can elapse from the vaccination to the transplant procedure. This strategy has not been tested in a clinical study; however, children with acute leukemia who have been immunized with the varicella vaccine have certainly subsequently undergone allogeneic SCT. There are no data available concerning the use of the VZV vaccine after BMT to prevent primary or reactivated VZV infection. It would probably be important to prevent primary VZV infections in seronegative BMT recipients. Because there are effective antiviral agents against VZV, the potential risk from the vaccine virus is probably low. Patients with GVHD and ongoing immunosuppression should not be immunized. A high proportion of BMT patients develop herpes zoster that occasionally becomes severe. Redman et al. used heat-inactivated varicella vaccine and showed no reduction in the risk of developing herpes zoster but a reduced severity of the herpes zoster in the immunized group.[88] A recent study was done by the same group in which patients undergoing autologous stem cell transplantation for lymphomas received heat-inactivated varicella vaccine in four doses: within 30 days of vaccination, and 30, 60, and 90 days after vaccination. During the 12 months post-transplant, the rate of zoster was 13% in vaccinees and 33% in unactivated patients, giving an efficacy of 61%.[88a] However, live varicella vaccination is contraindicated after allogeneic SCT.[72]

CYTOMEGALOVIRUS VACCINE

CMV is one of the most important pathogens encountered by patients after BMT. The currently available vaccine—a live, attenuated virus based on the Towne strain[89]—has not been tested in BMT recipients. Other vaccines based on new vaccine technology, such as subcomponent vaccines and vaccines using other virus vectors, are currently in early clinical development.

MEASLES VACCINE

Most BMT patients will become seronegative to measles during an extended follow-up.[90,91] There are documented cases of fatal measles in BMT recipients.[42] However, during an outbreak in Brazil, only one of eight patients with measles developed interstitial pneumonia, and all survived.[91] Immunization can only be considered in allogeneic BMT patients without chronic GVHD or ongoing immunosuppression. Existing data in such patients indicate that measles vaccine can be given without severe side effects at 2 years after BMT.[92] Earlier vaccination is being evaluated at present.[91]

OTHER LIVE VACCINES

Other vaccines that can be considered in allogeneic SCT recipients are those for rubella, BCG, mumps, and yellow fever. These vaccines are live and attenuated, and the possible benefits must be weighed against the risk for side effects. Rubella vaccine could be indicated in female patients who have retained the potential for becoming pregnant. Existing data indicate that rubella vaccine can be given without severe side effects at 2 years after BMT in patients without chronic GVHD or ongoing immunosuppression.[92] The same risks exist with the vaccine against mumps. The risk for severe infections with mumps virus in BMT recipients is likely to be very low, although a case report of a fatal infection has been published.[93] Yellow fever is a life-threatening infection primarily occurring in South America and southern and central Africa. Rio et al. have presented three patients who were immunized at 5 years after BMT without severe side effects.[94] Immunization could be considered in patients who must visit areas where yellow fever is endemic. The BCG vaccine can cause severe infections in patients with depressed T-cell function and is not recommended in BMT recipients.

Autologous Stem Cell Transplantation

In autologous SCT recipients, there is obviously no immunologic disparity between the graft and the host. The immune regeneration is faster than after allogeneic SCT in most patients and even more so after peripheral SCT. Autologous SCT patients are usually not prone to severe infections that are preventable by immunization during the early phase after transplant. However, several studies have shown that autologous transplant recipients will also lose protective immunity to tetanus, poliovirus, and measles during a long-term follow-up.[53,95-98] There is no difference in the capacity to retain immunity against tetanus between autologous BMT and autologous peripheral blood SCT recipients despite the fact that peripheral blood stem cell grafts contain a larger number of B cells.[97]

Killed Vaccines

INFLUENZA VACCINE

Influenza virus immunization is recommended from 6 months after autologous SCT.[77] However, the response to vaccination is likely to be suboptimal early after transplantation.[80,81] In one study, no patient responded if the immunization was performed earlier than 6 months after autologous BMT,[80] and, in a study that added GM-CSF to influenza vaccination, an antibody response was elicited in less than half of the patients vaccinated during the first year after SCT.[81]

PNEUMOCOCCAL VACCINE AND CONJUGATED HIB VACCINE

Autologous SCT patients are less prone than allogeneic patients to develop severe infections with Hib or pneumococci. Most infections occur early after the transplantation when the response to immunization is poor. Vaccination of all autologous SCT patients with pneumococcal polysaccharide vaccine and Hib vaccine is recommended by the Centers for Disease Control and Prevention,[72] whereas the European Group for Blood and Marrow Transplantation recommends vaccination of subgroups of autologous SCT recipients.[73]

The response to a single dose of pneumococcal vaccine is poor regardless of the stem cell source,[56,99] and remains decreased compared to controls for several years after transplantation for lymphoma.[98] There is no advantage to vaccinating patients before the stem cell harvest with pneumococcal polysaccharide-based vaccine.[70] The immune response might be improved by immunizing the patient before the stem cell harvest. Immunization with a conjugated Hib vaccine before the harvest followed by immunization at 3, 6, 12, and 24 months after autologous BMT improved antibody titers over those present after the dose given at 3 months after the transplantation.[100]

TETANUS TOXOID, DIPHTHERIA TOXOID, AND POLIOVIRUS VACCINE

Autologous BMT recipients have an increased risk compared to the normal population to lose protective immunity to poliovirus,[96,98] diphtheria,[98] and tetanus.[97] Reimmunization with repeated doses of inactivated poliovirus vaccine, diphtheria toxoid, and tetanus toxoid effectively restores protective immunity in autologous SCT recipients.[53,96,98,99,101] There was no difference in response in autologous BMT and peripheral blood stem cell graft recipients.[99] The immune response early after the autologous BMT can be improved by immunizing the patient before the stem cell harvest followed by tetanus toxoid given repeatedly after the autologous BMT.[100] Immunization with tetanus toxoid, diphtheria toxoid, and inactivated poliovirus is recommended after autologous SCT.[72–74]

Live, Attenuated Vaccines

MEASLES VACCINE

Children who have been immunized to measles before autologous BMT frequently become seronegative during follow-up, but adults who experienced natural measles disease before autologous BMT usually remain immune to measles during a follow-up of 3 years after transplant.[95] The risk for side effects after immunization seems to be low.[95] Measles vaccination is recommended for autologous SCT recipients but not earlier than 24 months after SCT.[72] However, because of the lower risk to lose specific immunity in adults, determination of the antibody level and vaccination of only seronegative patients could be considered.[73]

VARICELLA-ZOSTER VIRUS VACCINE

No studies have been done with the varicella vaccine specifically in seronegative autologous SCT patients. However, there is no real difference in the immune status between autologous SCT patients and children with acute leukemia in remission, and therefore vaccination can be considered in seronegative autologous SCT recipients. A small study showed seroconversion and no severe side effects in seronegative SCT recipients.[102] Based on lack of information, varicella vaccination is not recommended after autologous SCT.[72]

Solid Organ Transplant Recipients

The need for immunization in solid organ transplant recipients can arise from three factors, each causing a suppression of the immune system: the immunosuppressive activity of the underlying disease (e.g., chronic renal failure), rejection of the organ graft, and the immunosuppressive therapy given after the transplantation. Immunizations can be given either before solid organ transplantation, with the aim of preventing infections occurring during the early post-transplant phase, or after the transplantation, with the aim of preventing late infections. A summary of the recommendations is shown in Table 10–4.

Killed Vaccines

Hepatitis B Virus Vaccine

HBV might be transferred to a solid organ transplant recipient either by an HBV-positive organ graft or through blood transfusions. HBV vaccination is recommended in HBV-negative patients before the transplantation because there is an increased risk of severe HBV infections in transplant patients. However, the efficacy of HBV vaccine was low in patients on hemodialysis[103,104] and in patients with end-stage liver disease waiting for liver transplantation.[105,106] Response rates and antibody levels were lower than in healthy controls. Different schedules have been used in attempts to improve the response to vaccinations, including accelerated dose schedules and double-strength doses.[107–110] The seroconversion rates in the different studies varied from 31% to 62%. Factors associated with better responses were young age,[107] children with biliary atresia,[111] a milder

TABLE 10–4 ▪ Recommendations for Immunizations in Solid Organ Transplant Recipients

Vaccine	Recommendation Before Transplantation*	Recommendation After Transplantation*	Comments
KILLED VACCINES			
Conjugated Hib	1		Children
Hepatitis A virus	1	Depending on serostatus	Adults and children; liver transplantation
Influenza	2	2	Adults and children
Hepatitis B virus	2	Depending on serostatus	Seronegative adults and children
Pneumococci	2	2	Adults and children
Poliovirus	2	Depending on serostatus	Complete primary schedule before transplantation (children)
Tetanus and diphtheria toxoid	2	1	Complete primary schedule before transplantation (children)
			Booster dose before transplantation (adults)
LIVE VACCINES			
MMR	2	Contraindicated	Complete primary schedule before transplantation (children)
Varicella	2	Not recommended (see text)	Before transplantation in seronegative patients

*Recommendations: 1, strongly recommended for all patients (benefit >> risk); 2, recommended (benefit > risk).
Adapted from Avery RK, Ljungman P. Prophylactic measures in the solid-organ recipient before transplantation. Clin Infect Dis 33(suppl 1):S15–S21, 2001.

grade of liver disease,[107] and specific human leukocyte antigen types.[107] Besides poor responses to vaccination, the antibody levels decreased rapidly after liver transplantation so that up to 35% of the patients who had seroconverted became seronegative after liver transplantation.[107,108] Despite the less than optimal responses, pretransplant immunization is recommended.[112]

The efficacy of HBV vaccination was reported as being low after solid organ transplantation, with response rates between 5% and 15%.[113,114] Reports suggest that pediatric liver transplant patients can achieve good vaccination responses (70% seroconversion[115]). The type of immunosuppression also influences the vaccination response in that patients receiving triple immunosuppression (cyclosporine, corticosteroids, and azathioprine) responded less well than patients receiving cyclosporine only.[115] HBV vaccinations as protection against reactivation in patients transplanted for HBV-induced cirrhosis have been used in two studies giving different results. Sanches-Fueyo et al. reported good results with this strategy using a double dose of HBV vaccine,[116] whereas Angelico et al. reported poor results with a similar strategy.[117]

Hepatitis A Virus

Hepatitis A virus (HAV) can cause decompensation and death in patients with chronic liver disease. Therefore, vaccination can be an important protective strategy. Patients with chronic liver or renal disease awaiting transplantation are able to respond to an HAV vaccination, although the results are not as good as in normal individuals.[118] Vaccination results after liver or renal transplantation are poorer compared to those in healthy individuals,[119,120] and antibody levels decrease more rapidly.[120]

Influenza

Influenza can cause severe infections in renal transplant patients.[19,77] The reported results of immunization vary with the age of the patients. Adult patients have poorer antibody responses to influenza vaccinations than do immune-competent controls after renal transplantation,[121,122] liver transplantation,[123,124] and heart transplantation.[125,126] In contrast, studies have shown normal responses to influenza immunization in children after renal transplantation.[127–129] Vaccination is safe and does not cause graft rejection.[126,130–132] Immunization is recommended for solid organ transplant recipients.[17,112]

Pneumococci and Hib

Immunizations against *S. pneumoniae* and *H. influenzae* can be considered for patients and in particular for children waiting for a solid organ transplantation.[133,134] The Hib vaccine was reported to be similarly effective in renal transplant recipients and controls.[135] There have been conflicting reports regarding the efficacy of the 23-valent polysaccharide pneumococcal vaccine after transplantation. In some studies it was reported to be similar to that in healthy controls after liver transplantation,[136] heart transplantation,[125,136] and renal transplantation.[137] In other studies, the antibody responses were reported to be suppressed after heart transplantation[138] and liver transplantation.[139] Furthermore, it was reported that antibody levels declined faster than in controls.[139] No study has reported results with the pneumococcal conjugate vaccines.

Tetanus and Diphtheria Toxoid

Impaired vaccination responses have been reported to tetanus and diphtheria toxoid in dialysis patients. One year and 5 years after vaccination, 35% and 32%, respectively, of patients were protected against diphtheria.[140] Sixty-five percent of patients were protected against tetanus at 12 months after transplantation.[140] In children who had undergone renal transplantation, immunity to diphtheria was found in 38% and to tetanus in 90%.[141] Thus immunity to tetanus seemed to be more durable than immunity to diphtheria. A combined booster vaccination gave protective antibody levels to diphtheria in 95% of patients, but at 12 months only 76% remained protected.[141] All patients became protected against tetanus, with antibody levels comparable to those reached in normal children.

Pertussis vaccination after solid organ transplantation has not been studied, but continuation of basic immunization with an acellular vaccine (in combination with diphtheria and tetanus vaccines) is recommended starting 6 to 12 months later.[141a]

Other Killed Vaccines

A study performed in heart transplant patients reported lower vaccine response to tick-borne encephalitis vaccine compared to healthy controls.[142] No studies have been performed in solid organ transplant patients with acellular pertussis vaccine or meningococcal vaccine. However, the risks with these vaccines are negligible, and vaccination could be considered in certain epidemiologic situations, in particular for children and young adults.

Live, Attenuated Vaccines

Immunization with live vaccines has not been recommended after solid organ transplantation because of the risk of vaccine-associated complications. However, vaccination before the transplantation could protect from later severe infectious complications and might be considered.

Varicella Vaccine

VZV can cause severe and potentially fatal disease in patients after organ transplantation. It is important to consider the vaccination of seronegative patients awaiting organ transplantation. Varicella vaccine given to uremic children awaiting renal transplantation was shown to be safe and reduced the post-transplant risk for varicella in pre-vaccination seronegative patients.[143] A follow-up study showed that the protection was long lasting, with 42% of the patients still having antibodies at more than 10 years after immunization. Furthermore, the risk for varicella was lower and the disease was significantly less severe in immunized than in nonimmunized patients.[144] Similar results were seen in a study of children with chronic liver disease awaiting transplantation, with a vaccination efficacy of 100% and no severe vaccine-associated side effects.[145] A small study of varicella vaccination in children with renal transplants showed a good serologic response and no severe side effects.[146] However, further studies are needed.

Cytomegalovirus

CMV is an important pathogen in patients after solid organ transplantation. A live, attenuated virus vaccine based on the Towne strain has been in use until recently.

Randomized studies have shown a reduction in the severity of CMV disease and a reduction in graft rejection primarily in seronegative recipients getting organs from seropositive donors.[89,147] However, antiviral chemoprophylaxis is effective for prevention of CMV disease, and the vaccine is not currently available for general use. Ongoing work with new CMV vaccines may change this situation in the future.

Measles, Mumps, and Rubella

Measles-mumps-rubella vaccinations have been given to infants awaiting renal transplantation with good responses to vaccination: 88% of the patients developed immunity to all three components of the vaccine.[148] Analyzing the components separately, 89% developed immunity to measles, 88% to mumps, and 100% to rubella.

Children with Congenital Immune Deficiencies

Many different types of congenital immune deficiencies exist with differing defects of the immune system. Both B-cell and T-cell defects can influence the effectiveness of immunization, and there is an increased risk for side effects with live and attenuated vaccines. Therefore, immunizations with live, attenuated vaccines such as measles, mumps, rubella, varicella, smallpox, and BCG should be avoided in children with congenital T-cell immune deficiencies.[149] However, not infrequently the immune deficiency is diagnosed based on an abnormal response to the BCG vaccination.[150] Live poliovirus vaccine should be avoided in all children with congenital immune deficiencies, particularly B cell deficiency, because vaccine-associated polio or prolonged excretion of vaccine virus may occur (see Chapter 25). Moreover, an alternative killed vaccine exists. It is also important to use inactivated poliovirus vaccine in family members of children with congenital immune deficiencies.[149] Children with milder forms of congenital immune defects, such as those with only slightly decreased CD4+ cell numbers, might be vaccinated with live vaccines based on experience from human immunodeficiency virus–infected children. Immune globulin therapy may negatively influence the response to varicella and measles vaccination. Children with complement deficiencies can be given all routinely used vaccines,[149] and should receive meningococcal vaccine. Children with problems in phagocytic function should not receive BCG, but should receive annual influenza vaccination.

Killed vaccines are safe but might be ineffective in children with congenital B-cell deficiencies. Whereas oral poliovirus vaccine is contraindicated, other live virus vaccines, such as measles and varicella, should be considered. Children with partial antibody production capacity, such as those with IgG subclass deficiencies and immunoglobulin A deficiency, should be given routine killed vaccines such as tetanus toxoid, diphtheria toxoid, pertussis, Hib, and pneumococcal vaccine. Vaccine-induced antibody levels might decrease quicker than in healthy children, and revaccinations might be considered. Although no data exist in this population, it seems logical to use the conjugated pneumococcal vaccine in

this group of children. Yearly influenza vaccination is also recommended.

Patients with Rheumatologic Disorders

Killed Vaccines

Vaccinations of patients with rheumatologic diseases must be considered from two viewpoints: the response to vaccination during immunosuppressive therapy with corticosteroids or other agents and the risk for flare-up of the disease. There have been reports of development of rheumatic diseases closely associated with previous vaccinations.[151,152] In patients with established systemic lupus erythematosus (SLE), existing data support the safety of influenza vaccine, and no more flare-ups were seen in the vaccinated patients than in the control patients.[153–155] Similarly, vaccinations with pneumococcal polysaccharide,[156–158] tetanus toxoid, and Hib were shown to be safe in patients with SLE.[158]

The immunogenicity of influenza vaccine has been studied in patients with SLE. Most patients are able to respond, although the responses tend to be lower in patients compared to controls[154,155,159] and correlated to steroid therapy.[154] Children with rheumatologic diseases respond well to influenza vaccination.[160] Vaccinations with pneumococcal polysaccharide were shown to be effective in patients with rheumatoid arthritis and SLE.[156–158] Elkayam et al. showed, however, that 20% to 33% of patients failed to respond to at least one of the analyzed serotypes.[157] Battafarano et al. showed that patients on active immunosuppressive therapy had lower responses than patients who did not receive active immunosuppression.[158] This study also analyzed responses in SLE patients to tetanus toxoid and Hib. The responses were 90% to tetanus toxoid and 88% to Hib.[158]

Live Vaccines

Live vaccines are not recommended in patients with rheumatoid diseases treated with immunosuppressive therapy;[161] however, children given physiologic maintenance doses of corticosteroids can receive live vaccines during corticosteroid therapy.[149]

REFERENCES

1. Zuckerman M, Brink N, Kyi M, Tedder R. Exposure of immunocompromised individuals to health-care workers immunised with oral poliovaccine [letter]. Lancet 343:985–986, 1994.
2. Feldman S, Malone W, Wilbur R, Schiffman G. Pneumococcal vaccination in children with leukemia. Med Pediatr Oncol 13:69–72, 1985.
3. Robertson JD, Nagesh K, Jowitt SN, et al. Immunogenicity of vaccination against influenza, Streptococcus pneumoniae and Haemophilus influenzae type B in patients with multiple myeloma. Br J Cancer 82:1261–1265, 2000.
4. Levine A, Overturf G, Field R, et al. Use and efficacy of pneumococcal vaccine in patients with Hodgkin's disease. Blood 54:1171–1175, 1979.
5. Siber G, Weitzman S, Aisenberg A, et al. Impaired antibody response to pneumococcal vaccine after treatment for Hodgkin's disease. N Engl J Med 299:442–448, 1978.
6. Addiego JJ, Ammann A, Schiffman G, et al. Response to pneumococcal polysaccharide vaccine in patients with untreated Hodgkin's disease. Lancet 2:450–452, 1980.

7. Frederiksen B, Specht L, Henrichsen J, et al. Antibody response to pneumococcal vaccine in patients with early stage Hodgkin's disease. Eur J Haematol 43:45–49, 1989.
8. Donaldson S, Vosti K, Berberich F, et al. Response to pneumococcal vaccine among children with Hodgkin's disease. Rev Infect Dis 3:S133–S143, 1981.
9. Grimfors G, Söderqvist M, Holm G, et al. A longitudinal study of class and subclass antibody response to pneumococcal vaccination in splenectomized individuals with special reference to patients with Hodgkin's disease. Eur J Haematol 45:101–108, 1990.
10. Ammann A, Schiffman G, Addiego J, et al. Immunization of immunosuppressed patients with pneumococcal polysaccharide vaccine. Rev Infect Dis 3:S160–S167, 1981.
11. Chan C, Molrine D, George S, et al. Pneumococcal conjugate vaccine primes for antibody responses to polysaccharide pneumococcal vaccine after treatment for Hodgkin's disease. J Infect Dis 173:256–258, 1996.
12. Molrine DC, George S, Tarbell N, et al. Antibody responses to polysaccharide and polysaccharide-conjugate vaccines after treatment of Hodgkin disease. Ann Intern Med 123:828–834, 1995.
13. Feldman S, Gigliotti F, Shenep J, et al. Risk of *Haemophilus influenzae* type b disease in children with cancer and response of immunocompromised leukemic children to a conjugate vaccine. J Infect Dis 161:926–931, 1990.
14. Ridgway D, Wolff L, Deforest A. Immunization response varies with intensity of acute lymphoblastic leukemia therapy. Am J Dis Child 145:887–891, 1991.
15. Shenep J, Fledman S, Gigliotti F, et al. Response of immunocompromised children with solid tumors to a conjugate vaccine for *Haemophilus influenzae* type b. J Pediatr 125:581–584, 1994.
16. Jurlander J, de Nully Brown P, Skov P, et al. Improved vaccination response during ranitidine treatment, and increased plasma histamine concentrations in patients with B cell chronic lymphocytic leukemia. Leukemia 9:1902–1909, 1995.
17. Prevention and control of influenza: recommendations of the Advisory Committee on Immunization Practices (ACIP). MMWR Morb Mortal Wkly Rep 48:1–28, 1999.
18. Elting LS, Whimbey E, Lo W, et al. Epidemiology of influenza A virus infection in patients with acute or chronic leukemia. Support Care Cancer 3:198–202, 1995.
19. Ljungman P, Andersson J, Aschan J, et al. Influenza A in immunocompromised patients. Clin Infect Dis 17:244–247, 1993.
20. Kempe A, Hall C, MacDonald N, et al. Influenza in children with cancer. J Pediatr 115:33–39, 1989.
21. Brydak LB, Rokicka-Milewska R, Machala M, et al. Immunogenicity of subunit trivalent influenza vaccine in children with acute lymphoblastic leukemia. Pediatr Infect Dis J 17:125–129, 1998.
22. Brydak LB, Rokicka-Milewska R, Jackowska T, et al. Kinetics of humoral response in children with acute lymphoblastic leukemia immunized with influenza vaccine in 1993 in Poland. Leuk Lymphoma 26:163–169, 1997.
23. Anderson H, Petrie K, Berrisford C, et al. Seroconversion after influenza vaccination in patients with lung cancer. Br J Cancer 80:219–220, 1999.
24. Brydak LB, Guzy J, Starzyk J, et al. Humoral immune response after vaccination against influenza in patients with breast cancer. Support Care Cancer 9:65–68, 2001.
25. Gribabis DA, Panayiotidis P, Boussiotis VA, et al. Influenza virus vaccine in B-cell chronic lymphocytic leukaemia patients. Acta Haematol 91:115–118, 1994.
26. Brydak LB, Calbecka M. Immunogenicity of influenza vaccine in patients with hemato-oncological disorders. Leuk Lymphoma 32:369–374, 1999.
27. Lo W, Whimbey E, Elting L, et al. Antibody response to a two-dose influenza vaccine regimen in adult lymphoma patients on chemotherapy. Eur J Clin Microbiol Infect Dis 12:778–782, 1993.
28. Hammarström V, Pauksen K, Svensson H, et al. Tetanus immunity in patients with hematological malignancies Supp Care Cancer 1998;6:469–472.
29. van de Does-van der Berg A, Hermans J, Nagel J, van Steenis G. Immunity to diphtheria, pertussis, tetanus, and poliomyelitis in children with acute lymphocytic leukemia after cessation of chemotherapy. Pediatrics 67:222–229, 1981.
30. von der Hardt K, Jungert J, Beck J, Heininger U. Humoral immunity against diphtheria, tetanus and poliomyelitis after antineoplastic therapy in children and adolescents—a retrospective analysis. Vaccine 18:2999–3004, 2000.
31. Nordoy T, Kolstad A, Tuck M, et al. Radioimmunotherapy with iodine-131 tositumonab in patients with low-grade non-Hodgkin's B-cell lymphoma does not induce loss of acquired humoral immunity against common antigens. Clin Immunol 100:40–48, 2001.
32. Stenvik M, Hovi L, Siimes M, et al. Antipolio prophylaxis of immunocompromised children during a nationwide oral poliovaccine campaign. Pediatr Infect Dis J 6:1106–1110, 1987.
33. Löffel M, Meienberg O, Diem P, Mombelli G. Vaccine poliomyelitis in an adult undergoing chemotherapy for non-Hodgkin's lymphoma. Schweiz Med Wochenschr 112:419–421, 1982.
34. Rautonen J, Siimes MA, Lundstrom U, et al. Vaccination of children during treatment for leukemia. Acta Paediatr Scand 75:579–585, 1986.
35. Takahashi M, Okuno Y, Otsuka T, et al. Development of a live attenuated varicella vaccine. Biken J 18:25–33, 1975.
36. Gershon A, Steinberg S. Persistence of immunity to varicella in children with leukemia immunized with live attenuated varicella vaccine. N Engl J Med 320:892–897, 1989.
37. Brunell P, Geiser C, Novelli V, et al. Varicella-like illness caused by live varicella vaccine in children with acute lymphocytic leukemia. Pediatrics 79:922–927, 1987.
38. Lawrence R, Gershon A, Holzman R, Steinberg S. The risk for zoster after varicella vaccination in children with leukemia. N Engl J Med 318:543–548, 1988.
39. Hardy I, Gershon A, Steinberg S, LaRussa P. The incidence of zoster after immunization with live attenuated varicella vaccine: a study in children with leukemia. Varicella Vaccine Collaborative Group. N Engl J Med 325:1545–1550, 1991.
40. Cristofani L, Weinberg A, Peixoto V, et al. Administration of live attenuated varicella vaccine to children with cancer before starting chemotherapy. Vaccine 9:873–876, 1991.
41. Diaz P, Au D, Smith S, Amylon M, et al. Lack of transmission of the live attenuated varicella vaccine virus to immunocompromised children after immunization of their siblings. Pediatrics 87:166–170, 1991.
42. Kaplan L, Daum R, Smaron M, McCarthy C. Severe measles in immunocompromised patients. JAMA 267:1237–1241, 1992.
43. Lum L. The kinetics of immune reconstitution after human marrow transplantation. Blood 69:369–380, 1987.
44. Lum L, Seigneuret M, Storb R. The transfer of antigen-specific humoral immunity from marrow donors to marrow recipients. J Clin Immunol 6:389–396, 1986.
45. Lum L, Noges J, Beatty P, et al. Transfer of specific immunity in marrow recipients given HLA-mismatched, T cell-depleted, or HLA-identical marrow grafts. Bone Marrow Transplant 3:399–406, 1988.
46. Lum L, Munn N, Schanfield M, Storb R. The detection of specific antibody formation to recall antigens after human bone marrow transplantation. Blood 67:582–587, 1986.
47. Saxon A, Mitsuyaso R, Stevens R, et al. Transfer of specific immune responses after bone marrow transplantation. J Clin Invest 78:959–967, 1986.
48. Wahren B, Gahrton G, Linde A, et al. Transfer and persistence of viral antibody-producing cells in bone marrow transplantation. J Infect Dis 150:358–365, 1984.
49. Witherspoon R, Storb R, Ochs H, et al. Recovery of antibody production in human allogeneic marrow graft recipients: influence of time posttransplantation, the presence or absence of chronic graft-versus-host disease, and antithymocyte globulin treatment. Blood 58:360–368, 1981.
50. Witherspoon R, Matthews D, Storb R, et al. Recovery of in vivo cellular immunity after human marrow grafting: influence of time post-grafting and acute graft-versus-host disease. Transplantation 37:145–150, 1984.
51. Ljungman P, Wiklund HM, Duraj V, et al. Response to tetanus toxoid immunization after allogeneic bone marrow transplantation. J Infect Dis 162:496–500, 1990.
52. Ljungman P, Duraj V, Magnius L. Response to immunization against polio after allogeneic marrow transplantation. Bone Marrow Transplant 7:89–93, 1991.
53. Engelhard D, Handsher R, Naparstek E, et al. Immune responses to polio vaccination in bone marrow transplant recipients. Bone Marrow Transplant 8:295–300, 1991.
54. Ljungman P, Lewensohn-Fuchs I, Hammarström V, et al. Long-term immunity to measles, mumps, and rubella after allogeneic bone marrow transplantation. Blood 84:657–663, 1994.

55. Ilan Y, Nagler A, Adler R, et al. Adoptive transfer of immunity to hepatitis B virus after T cell-depleted allogeneic bone marrow transplantation. Hepatology 18:246–252, 1993.
56. Guinan EC, Molrine DC, Antin JH, et al. Polysaccharide conjugate vaccine responses in bone marrow transplant patients. Transplantation 57:677–684, 1994.
57. Wimperis J, Brenner M, Prentice H, et al. Transfer of a functioning humoral immune system in transplantation of T-lymphocyte-depleted bone marrow. Lancet 1:339–343, 1986.
58. Lum L. Effects of acute and chronic GVHD on immune recovery after BMT. In Burakoff SJ, Dees HJ, Ferrera J, et al. (eds). Graft-vs-Host Disease. New York, Marcel Dekker, 1990, pp 369–380.
59. Cordonnier C, Bernaudin JF, Bierling P, et al. Pulmonary complications occurring after allogeneic bone marrow transplantation: a study of 130 consecutive transplanted patients. Cancer 58:1047–1054, 1986.
60. Aucouturier P, Barra A, Intrator L, et al. Long lasting IgG subclass and antibacterial polysaccharide antibody deficiency after allogeneic bone marrow transplantation. Blood 70:779–785, 1987.
61. Winston DJ, Schiffman G, Wang DC, et al. Pneumococcal infections after human bone-marrow transplantation. Ann Intern Med 91:835–841, 1979.
62. Parkkali T, Kayhty H, Ruutu T, et al. A comparison of early and late vaccination with Haemophilus influenzae type B conjugate and pneumococcal polysaccharide vaccines after allogeneic BMT. Bone Marrow Transplant 18:961–967, 1996.
63. Avanzini M, Carra A, Maccario R, et al. Antibody response to pneumococcal vaccine in children receiving bone marrow transplantation. J Clin Immunol 15:137–144, 1995.
64. Barra A, Cordonnier C, Preziosi MP, et al. Immunogenicity of Haemophilus influenzae type b conjugate vaccine in allogeneic bone marrow recipients. J Infect Dis 166:1021–1028, 1992.
65. Hammarström V, Pauksen K, Azinge J, et al. The influence of graft versus host reaction on the response to pneumococcal vaccination in bone marrow transplant patients. J Support Care Cancer 1:195–199, 1993.
66. Lortan J, Vellodi A, Jurges E, Hugh-Jones K. Class- and subclass-specific pneumococcal antibody levels and response to immunization after bone marrow transplantation. Clin Exp Immunol 88:512–519, 1992.
67. Spoulou V, Victoratos P, Ioannidis JP, Grafakos S. Kinetics of antibody concentration and avidity for the assessment of immune response to pneumococcal vaccine among children with bone marrow transplants. J Infect Dis 182:965–969, 2000.
68. Parkkali T, Kayhty H, Anttila M, et al. IgG subclasses and avidity of antibodies to polysaccharide antigens in allogeneic BMT recipients after vaccination with pneumococcal polysaccharide and Haemophilus influenzae type b conjugate vaccines. Bone Marrow Transplant 24:671–678, 1999.
69. Parkkali T, Vakevainen M, Kayhty H, et al. Opsonophagocytic activity against Streptococcus pneumoniae type 19F in allogeneic BMT recipients before and after vaccination with pneumococcal polysaccharide vaccine. Bone Marrow Transplant 27:207–211, 2001.
70. Molrine D, Guinan E, Antin J, et al. Donor immunization with Haemophilus influenzae type B (HIB)-conjugate vaccine in allogeneic bone marrow transplantation. Blood 87:3012–3018, 1996.
71. Molrine D, Antin J, Guinan E, et al. Pneumococcal conjugate vaccine (PCV) elicits protective responses in allogeneic bone marrow transplant (BMT) recipients [abstr 2035]. Abstracts of the meeting of the Interscience Conference on Antimicrobial Agents and Chemotherapy, Chicago, 2001.
72. Guidelines for preventing opportunistic infections among hematopoietic stem cell transplant recipients: recommendations of CDC, the Infectious Disease Society of America, and the American Society of Blood and Marrow Transplantation. Morb Mortal Wkly Rep 49:1–125, 2000.
73. Ljungman P. Immunization of transplant recipients. Bone Marrow Transplant 23:635–636, 1999.
74. Ljungman P, Cordonnier C, de Bock R, et al. Immunisations after bone marrow transplantation: results of a European survey and recommendations from the Infectious Diseases Working Party of the European Group for Blood and Marrow Transplantation. Bone Marrow Transplant 15:455–460, 1995.
75. Barra A, Cordonnier C, Preziosi M, et al. Immunogenicity of Haemophilus influenzae type b conjugate vaccine in allogeneic bone marrow recipients. J Infect Dis 166:1021–1028, 1992.
76. Avanzini MA, Carra AM, Maccario R, et al. Immunization with Haemophilus influenzae type b conjugate vaccine in children given bone marrow transplantation: comparison with healthy age-matched controls. J Clin Immunol 18:193–201, 1998.
77. Aschan J, Ringdén O, Ljungman P, et al. Influenza B in transplant patients. Scand J Infect Dis 21:349–350, 1989.
78. Whimbey E, Elting LS, Couch RB, et al. Influenza A virus infections among hospitalized adult bone marrow transplant recipients. Bone Marrow Transplant 13:437–440, 1994.
79. Ljungman P, Ward KN, Crooks BN, et al. Respiratory virus infections after stem cell transplantation: a prospective study from the Infectious Diseases Working Party of the European Group for Blood and Marrow Transplantation. Bone Marrow Transplant 28:479–484, 2001.
80. Engelhard D, Nagler A, Hardan I, et al. Antibody response to a two-dose regimen of influenza vaccine in allogeneic T cell-depleted and autologous BMT recipients. Bone Marrow Transplant 11:1–5, 1993.
81. Pauksen K, Linde A, Hammarstrom V, et. Granulocyte-macrophage colony-stimulating factor as immunomodulating factor together with influenza vaccination in stem cell transplant patients. Clin Infect Dis 30:342–348, 2000.
82. Ilan Y, Nagler A, Zeira E, et al. Maintenance of immune memory to the hepatitis B envelope protein following adoptive transfer of immunity in bone marrow transplant recipients. Bone Marrow Transplant 26:633–638, 2000.
83. Brugger S, Oesterreicher C, Hofmann H, et al. Hepatitis B virus clearance by transplantation of bone marrow from hepatitis B immunized donor. Lancet 349:996–997, 1997.
84. Ilan Y, Nagler A, Adler R, et al. Ablation of persistent hepatitis B by bone marrow transplantation from a hepatitis B-immune donor. Gastroenterology 104:1818–1821, 1993.
85. Parkkali T, Ölander R-M, Ruutu T, et al. A randomized comparison between early and late vaccination with tetanus toxoid vaccine after allogeneic BMT. Bone Marrow Transplant 19:933–938, 1997.
86. Gerritsen E, Van Tol M, Van't Veer M, et al. Clonal dysregulation of the antibody response to tetanus-toxoid after bone marrow transplantation. Blood 84:4374–4382, 1994.
86a. Edwards KM, Gruber WC. Immunization in hematopoietic cell transplantation. Pediatr Pathol Molec Med 2000; 19:133–148.
87. Parkkali T, Kayhty H, Lehtonen H, et al. Tetravalent meningococcal polysaccharide vaccine is immunogenic in adult allogeneic BMT recipients. Bone Marrow Transplant 27:79–84, 2001.
88. Redman R, Nader S, Zerboni L, et al. Early reconstitution of immunity and decreased severity of herpes zoster in bone marrow transplant recipients immunized with inactivated varicella vaccine. J Infect Dis 178:578–585, 1997.
88a. Hata A, Asanuma H, Rinki M, et al. Use of an inactivated varicella vaccine in recipients of hematopoietic-cell transplants. N Eng J Med 347:26–34, 2002.
89. Plotkin SA, Starr SE, Friedman HM, et al. Effect of Towne live virus vaccine on cytomegalovirus disease after renal transplant: a controlled trial. Ann Intern Med 114:525–531, 1991.
90. Ljungman P, Levensohn-Fuchs I, Hammarström V, et al. Long-term immunity to measles, mumps and rubella after allogeneic bone marrow transplantation. Blood 84:657–664, 1994.
91. Machado CM, Goncalves FB, Pannuti CS, et al. Measles in bone marrow transplant recipients during an outbreak in Sao Paulo, Brazil. Blood 99:83–87, 2002.
92. Ljungman P, Fridell E, Lönnqvist B, et al. Efficacy and safety of vaccination of marrow transplant recipients with a live attenuated measles, mumps, and rubella vaccine. J Infect Dis 159:610–615, 1989.
93. Bakshi N, Lawson J, Hanson R, et al. Fatal mumps meningoencephalitis in a child with severe combined immunodeficiency after bone marrow transplantation. J Child Neurol 11:159–162, 1996.
94. Rio B, Marjanovic Z, Lévy V, et al. Vaccination for yellow fever after bone marrow transplantation. Bone Marrow Transplant 17 (suppl 1):95, 1996.
95. Pauksen K, Duraj V, Ljungman P, et al. Immunity to and immunization against measles, rubella and mumps in patients after autologous bone marrow transplantation. Bone Marrow Transplant 9:427–432, 1992.
96. Pauksen K, Hammarström V, Ljungman P, et al. Immunity to poliovirus and immunization with inactivated poliovaccine after autologous bone marrow transplantation. Clin Infect Dis 18:547–552, 1994.
97. Hammarström V, Pauksen K, Björkstrand B, et al. Tetanus immunity in autologous bone marrow and blood stem cell transplant patients. Bone Marrow Transplant 22:67–72, 1998.

98. Nordoy T, Husebekk A, Aaberge IS, et al. Humoral immunity to viral and bacterial antigens in lymphoma patients 4–10 years after high-dose therapy with ABMT: serological responses to revaccinations according to EBMT guidelines. Bone Marrow Transplant 28:681–687, 2001.

99. Gandhi MK, Egner W, Sizer L, et al. Antibody responses to vaccinations given within the first two years after transplant are similar between autologous peripheral blood stem cell and bone marrow transplant recipients. Bone Marrow Transplant 28:775–781, 2001.

100. Molrine D, Guinan E, Antin J, et al. *Haemophilus influenzae* type b (HIB)-conjugate immunization before bone marrow harvest in autologous bone marrow transplantation. Bone Marrow Transplant 17:1149–1155, 1996.

101. Hammarström V, Ljungman P. Unpublished data.

102. Sauerbrei A, Prager J, Hengst U, et al. Varicella vaccination in children after bone marrow transplantation. Bone Marrow Transplant 20:381–383, 1997.

103. Crosnier J, Junges P, Courouce A-M, et al. Randomized placebo-controlled trial of hepatitis B surface antigen vaccine in French haemodialysis units. II. Haemodialysis patients. Lancet 2:797–800, 1981.

104. Stevens C, Alter H, Taylor P, et al. Hepatitis B virus vaccine in patients receiving hemodialysis: immunogenicity and efficacy. N Engl J Med 311:496–501, 1984.

105. Van Thiel D, el-Ashmawy L, Love K, et al. Response to hepatitis B vaccination by liver transplant candidates. Dig Dis Sci 37:1245–1249, 1992.

106. Villeneuve E, Vincelette J, Villeneuve JP. Ineffectiveness of hepatitis B vaccination in cirrhotic patients waiting for liver transplantation. Can J Gastroenterol 14(suppl B):59B–62B, 2000.

107. Arslan M, Wiesner RH, Sievers C, et al. Double-dose accelerated hepatitis B vaccine in patients with end-stage liver disease. Liver Transplant 7:314–320, 2001.

108. Horlander JC, Boyle N, Manam R, et al. Vaccination against hepatitis B in patients with chronic liver disease awaiting liver transplantation. Am J Med Sci 318:304–307, 1999.

109. Dominguez M, Barcena R, Garcia M, et al. Vaccination against hepatitis B virus in cirrhotic patients on liver transplant waiting list. Liver Transplant 6:440–442, 2000.

110. Engler SH, Sauer PW, Golling M, et al. Immunogenicity of two accelerated hepatitis B vaccination protocols in liver transplant candidates. Eur J Gastroenterol Hepatol 13:363–367, 2001.

111. Sokal E, Ulla L, Otte J. Hepatitis B vaccine response before and after transplantation in 55 extrahepatic biliary atresia children. Dig Dis Sci 37:1250–1252, 1992.

112. Avery RK, Ljungman P. Prophylactic measures in the solid-organ recipient before transplantation. Clin Infect Dis 33(suppl 1):S15–S21, 2001.

113. Wagner D, Wagenbreth I, Stachan-Kunstyr R, Flik J. Failure of vaccination against hepatitis B with Gen H-B-Vax-D in immunosuppressed heart transplant patients. J Infect Dis 166:1021–1028, 1992.

114. Wagner D, Wagenbroth J, Stachan-Kunstyr R, et al. Hepatitis B vaccination of immunosuppressed heart transplant recipients with the vaccine Hepa Gene 3 containing pre-S1, pre-S2, and S gene products. Clin Invest 72:240–352, 1994.

115. Duca P, Del Pont JM, D'Agostino D. Successful immune response to a recombinant hepatitis B vaccine in children after liver transplantation. J Pediatr Gastroenterol Nutr 32:168–170, 2001.

116. Sanchez-Fueyo A, Rimola A, Grande L, et al. Hepatitis B immunoglobulin discontinuation followed by hepatitis B virus vaccination: a new strategy in the prophylaxis of hepatitis B virus recurrence after liver transplantation. Hepatology 31:496–501, 2000.

117. Angelico M, Di Paolo D, Trinito MO, et al. Failure of a reinforced triple course of hepatitis B vaccination in patients transplanted for HBV-related cirrhosis. Hepatology 35:176–181, 2002.

118. Dumot JA, Barnes DS, Younossi Z, et al. Immunogenicity of hepatitis A vaccine in decompensated liver disease. Am J Gastroenterol 94:1601–1604, 1999.

119. Arslan M, Wiesner RH, Poterucha JJ, Zein NN. Safety and efficacy of hepatitis A vaccination in liver transplantation recipients. Transplantation 72:272–276, 2001.

120. Gunther M, Stark K, Neuhaus R, et al. Rapid decline of antibodies after hepatitis A immunization in liver and renal transplant recipients. Transplantation 71:477–479, 2001.

121. Sanchez-Fructuoso AI, Prats D, Naranjo P, et al. Influenza virus immunization effectivity in kidney transplant patients subjected to two different triple-drug therapy immunosuppression protocols: mycophenolate versus azathioprine. Transplantation 69:436–439, 2000.

122. Versluis D, Beyer W, Masurel N, et al. Impairment of the immune response to influenza vaccination in renal transplant recipients by cyclosporine, but not azathioprine. Transplantation 42:376–379, 1986.

123. Duchini A, Hendry RM, Nyberg LM, et al. Immune response to influenza vaccine in adult liver transplant recipients. Liver Transplant 7:311–313, 2001.

124. Soesman NM, Rimmelzwaan GF, Nieuwkoop NJ, et al. Efficacy of influenza vaccination in adult liver transplant recipients. J Med Virol 61:85–93, 2000.

125. Dengler TJ, Strnad N, Buhring I, et al. Differential immune response to influenza and pneumococcal vaccination in immunosuppressed patients after heart transplantation. Transplantation 66:1340–1347, 1998.

126. Fraund S, Wagner D, Pethig K, et al. Influenza vaccination in heart transplant recipients. J Heart Lung Transplant 18:220–225, 1999.

127. Edvardsson VO, Flynn JT, Deforest A, et al. Effective immunization against influenza in pediatric renal transplant recipients. Clin Transplant 10:556–560, 1996.

128. Furth S, Neu A, McColley S, et al. Immune response to influenza vaccination in children with renal disease. Pediatr Nephrol 9:566–568, 1995.

129. Mauch TJ, Bratton S, Myers T, et al. Influenza B virus infection in pediatric solid organ transplant recipients. Pediatrics 94:225–229, 1994.

130. Blumberg EA, Fitzpatrick J, Stutman PC, et al. Safety of influenza vaccine in heart transplant recipients. J Heart Lung Transplant 17:1075–1080, 1998.

131. Burbach G, Bienzle U, Stark K, et al. Influenza vaccination in liver transplant recipients. Transplantation 67:753–755, 1999.

132. Kimball P, Verbeke S, Flattery M, et al. Influenza vaccination does not promote cellular or humoral activation among heart transplant recipients. Transplantation 69:2449–2451, 2000.

133. Linnemann CJ, First M, Schiffman G. Response to pneumococcal vaccine in renal transplant and hemodialysis patients. Arch Intern Med 141:1637–1640, 1981.

134. Furth S, Neu A, Case B, et al. Pneumococcal polysaccharide vaccine in children with chronic renal disease: a prospective study of antibody response and duration. J Pediatr 128:99–101, 1996.

135. Sever MS, Yildiz A, Eraksoy H, et al. Immune response to *Haemophilus influenzae* type B vaccination in renal transplant recipients with well-functioning allografts. Nephron 81:55–59, 1999.

136. Dengler T, Strnad N, Zimmermann R, et al. Pneumococcal vaccination after heart and liver transplantation: immune responses in immunosuppressed patients and in healthy controls. Dtsch Med Wochenschr 121:1519–1525, 1996.

137. Kazancioglu R, Sever MS, Yuksel-Onel D, et al. Immunization of renal transplant recipients with pneumococcal polysaccharide vaccine. Clin Transplant 14:61–65, 2000.

138. Blumberg EA, Brozena SC, Stutman P, et al. Immunogenicity of pneumococcal vaccine in heart transplant recipients. Clin Infect Dis 32:307–310, 2001.

139. McCashland TM, Preheim LC, Gentry MJ. Pneumococcal vaccine response in cirrhosis and liver transplantation. J Infect Dis 181:757–760, 2000.

140. Kruger S, Muller-Steinhardt M, Kirchner H, Kreft B. A 5-year follow-up on antibody response after diphtheria and tetanus vaccination in hemodialysis patients. Am J Kidney Dis 38:1264–1270, 2001.

141. Enke BU, Bokenkamp A, Offner G, et al. Response to diphtheria and tetanus booster vaccination in pediatric renal transplant recipients. Transplantation 64:237–241, 1997.

141a. Burroughs M, Moscona A. Immunization of pediatric solid organ transplant candidates and recipients. Clin Infect Dis 2000; 30:857–869.

142. Dengler TJ, Zimmermann R, Meyer J, et al. Vaccination against tick-borne encephalitis under therapeutic immunosuppression: reduced efficacy in heart transplant recipients. Vaccine 17:867–874, 1999.

143. Broyer M, Boudailliez B. Varicella vaccine in children with chronic renal insufficiency. Postgrad Med J 61(suppl 4):103–106, 1985.

144. Broyer M, Tete M, Guest G, et al. Varicella and zoster in children after kidney transplantation: long-term results of vaccination. Pediatrics 99:35–39, 1997.

145. Nithichaiyo C, Chongsrisawat V, Hutagalung Y, et al. Immunogenicity and adverse effects of live attenuated varicella vaccine (Oka-strain) in children with chronic liver disease. Asian Pac J Allergy Immunol 19:101–105, 2001.

146. Zamora I, Simon J, Da Silva M, Piqueras A. Attenuated varicella virus vaccine in children with renal transplants. Pediatr Nephrol 8:190–192, 1994.

147. Plotkin SA, Higgins R, Kurtz JB, et al. Multicenter trial of Towne strain attenuated virus vaccine in seronegative renal transplant recipients. Transplantation 58:1176–1178, 1994.

148. Flynn JT, Frisch K, Kershaw DB, et al. Response to early measles-mumps-rubella vaccination in infants with chronic renal failure and/or receiving peritoneal dialysis. Adv Perit Dial 15:269–272, 1999.

149. Pickering LK (ed). Immunization in special clinical circumstances. *In* 2000 Red Book Report of the Committee on Infectious Diseases (25th ed). Elk Grove Village, IL, American Academy of Pediatrics, 2000.

150. Casanova J, Blanche S, Emile J, et al. Idiopathic disseminated bacillus Calmette-Guérin infection: a French national retrospective study. Pediatrics 98:774–778, 1996.

151. Machida H, Nishitani M. Drug susceptibilities of isolates of varicella-zoster virus in a clinical study of oral brovavir. Microbiol Immunol 34:407–411, 1990.

152. Older SA, Battafarano DF, Enzenauer RJ, Krieg AM. Can immunization precipitate connective tissue disease? Report of five cases of systemic lupus erythematosus and review of the literature. Semin Arthritis Rheum 29:131–139, 1999.

153. Abu-Shakra M, Zalmanson S, Neumann L, et al. Influenza virus vaccination of patients with systemic lupus erythematosus: effects on disease activity. J Rheumatol 27:1681–1685, 2000.

154. Herron A, Dettleff G, Hixon B, et al. Influenza vaccination in patients with rheumatic diseases: safety and efficacy. JAMA 242:53–56, 1979.

155. Williams GW, Steinberg AD, Reinertsen JL, et al. Influenza immunization in systemic lupus erythematosus: a double-blind trial. Ann Intern Med 88:729–734, 1978.

156. Klippel JH, Karsh J, Stahl NI, et al. A controlled study of pneumococcal polysaccharide vaccine in systemic lupus erythematosus. Arthritis Rheum 22:1321–1325, 1979.

157. Elkayam O, Paran D, Caspi D, et al. Immunogenicity and safety of pneumococcal vaccination in patients with rheumatoid arthritis or systemic lupus erythematosus. Clin Infect Dis 34:147–153, 2002.

158. Battafarano DF, Battafarano NJ, Larsen L, et al. Antigen-specific antibody responses in lupus patients following immunization. Arthritis Rheum 41:1828–1834, 1998.

159. Louie JS, Nies KM, Shoji KT, et al. Clinical and antibody responses after influenza immunization in systemic lupus erythematosus. Ann Intern Med 88:790–792, 1978.

160. Kanakoudi-Tsakalidou F, Trachana M, Pratsidou-Gertsi P, et al. Influenza vaccination in children with chronic rheumatic diseases and long-term immunosuppressive therapy. Clin Exp Rheumatol 19:589–594, 2001.

161. Ioannou Y, Isenberg DA. Immunisation of patients with systemic lupus erythematosus: the current state of play. Lupus 8:497–501, 1999.

Chapter 11

Vaccination of Human Immunodeficiency Virus–Infected Persons

WILLIAM J. MOSS • NEAL A. HALSEY

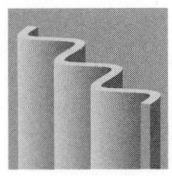 In the absence of appropriate antiretro-viral therapy, human immunodeficiency virus (HIV) infection results in a progressive decline in CD4$^+$ T-lymphocytes, decreased ability to mount protective responses to new antigenic stimuli, loss of prior immunity, and increased risk of complications from infections. As with other causes of serious immune suppression, HIV infection can impair the effectiveness of vaccines and increase the risk of serious adverse events from live vaccines. Fewer HIV-infected children and adults develop protective antibody titers after vaccination than do HIV-uninfected persons. The magnitude of the antibody response often is correlated with the level of immune suppression as measured by the CD4$^+$ T-lymphocyte cell count. In general, HIV-infected adults with CD4$^+$ T-lymphocyte counts less than 200 cells/mm^3 and HIV-infected children with CD4$^+$ T-lymphocyte percentages less than 15 have poor serologic responses to vaccines. Of those who develop an initial antibody response following vaccination, antibody titers frequently wane at a faster rate in HIV-infected persons than in HIV-uninfected persons. Live viral and bacterial vaccines pose an increased risk to HIV-infected persons because of the potential for disease caused by uncontrolled replication of the vaccine strain; this risk increases with severe immune suppression. T-lymphocyte proliferation induced by vaccination can transiently increase plasma HIV RNA levels, but an effect of vaccination on HIV disease progression has not been found in most studies.

Vaccination is generally safe and effective early in infancy before HIV infection causes significant immune suppression. The rate of progression to clinically apparent immune suppression is variable and depends on factors relating to the host and to the virus. Accordingly, the safety and effectiveness of vaccines in HIV-infected children vary with age at vaccination and immune status of the HIV-infected child. Partial or protective immunity against the agents usually persists until immune suppression has become severe, although antibody titers to some antigens (measles virus, tetanus toxoid, and hepatitis B virus) may wane with lesser degrees of immune suppression. In older HIV-infected children and adults, the immune response to primary immunization may be impaired.

Readers should also consult chapters on individual vaccines.

Guidelines for Use of Vaccines in Human Immunodeficiency Virus–Infected Persons

Guidelines for vaccination of HIV-infected persons take into consideration the risks of vaccination, the risks of exposure to diseases, and the risks of complications from the diseases.[1,2] The World Health Organization recommends administering all routinely recommended vaccines for asymptomatic children and adults.[2] For symptomatic persons with HIV infection, bacille Calmette-Guérin (BCG) and yellow fever vaccines are not recommended because of the potential for increased risk of complications. All other vaccines are recommended for HIV-infected persons regardless of symptoms. In settings where the risk from exposure to disease may be less, and testing for immunologic status and alternatives to live vaccines are available, more specific recommendations have been made by advisory committees such as the Advisory Committee on Immunization Practices and the Committee on Infectious Diseases of the American Academy of Pediatrics (Table 11–1).

Nonreplicating Vaccines

Diphtheria and Tetanus Toxoids and Pertussis Vaccine

Following primary immunization in infancy, 40% to 100% of HIV-infected children respond to tetanus and diphtheria

TABLE 11–1 ■ WHO/UNICEF and ACIP Recommendations for Immunization of HIV-Infected Children and Adults[1,2]

Vaccine	Asymptomatic HIV Infection	Symptomatic HIV Infection	Comments
		WHO/UNICEF	
BCG	Recommended	Not recommended	Administered at birth
DTP	Recommended	Recommended	
OPV	Recommended	Recommended	IPV may be used if symptomatic
Measles	Recommended	Recommended	Administered at 6 and 9 mo
Hepatitis B	Recommended	Recommended	As for HIV-uninfected children
Yellow fever	Recommended	Not recommended	Until safety is further evaluated
Tetanus toxoid	Recommended	Recommended	5 doses

Vaccine	Children with HIV infection or AIDS	Adults with HIV Infection or AIDS	Comments
		ACIP	
DTP	Recommended	Not applicable	
OPV	Contraindicated	Contraindicated	
IPV	Recommended	Use if indicated	
MMR	Recommended/considered	Recommended/considered	Not if severe immune suppression (CD4 percent <15)
Hib	Recommended	Considered	Consider risk of disease in adults
Hepatitis B	Recommended	Recommended	
Pneumococcal	Recommended	Recommended	
Meningococcal		Use if indicated	
Influenza	Recommended	Recommended	Not for infants <6 mo of age
Td		Recommended	
BCG	Contraindicated	Contraindicated	
Yellow fever	Contraindicated	Contraindicated	Consider if exposure is unavoidable
Vaccinia	Contraindicated	Contraindicated	
Anthrax	Use if indicated	Use if indicated	
Plague	Use if indicated	Use if indicated	

ACIP, Advisory Committee on Immunization Practices; BCG, bacille Calmette-Guérin vaccine; DTP, diphtheria and tetanus toxoids and pertussis vaccine; Hib, *Haemophilus influenzae* type b vaccine; IPV = inactivated poliovirus vaccine; MMR, measles-mumps-rubella vaccine; OPV, oral poliovirus vaccine; Td, tetanus-diphtheria toxoid; UNICEF = United Nations International Children's Emergency Fund; WHO, World Health Organization.

toxoids by developing protective concentrations of diphtheria and tetanus antitoxins (Table 11–2). Data on the immunogenicity of pertussis vaccines are more limited and interpretation more difficult because serologic correlates of protection have not been identified. The limited data suggest that the proportion of children who seroconvert and the geometric mean antibody titers to pertussis toxin are lower in HIV-infected children compared to healthy controls.[13] However, there is no evidence that HIV-infected children have higher vaccine failure rates than HIV-uninfected children following diphtheria, tetanus, or pertussis immunization.[14]

Hepatitis B Vaccine

Serologic response rates have varied, but only 25% to 50% of HIV-infected children developed protective antibody following hepatitis B vaccination in most studies (Table 11–3). As with tetanus and diphtheria toxoids, response rates in younger children are higher than in adults, and responses correlated with CD4+ T-lymphocyte cell counts in some studies. Attempts to overcome the decreased response by administering higher doses or extra doses of hepatitis B vaccine have not been promising in children,[18,20] although, in a study of 20 HIV-infected adults, 7 of the 9 individuals who failed to respond to the initial three-dose series developed a protective antibody response

after three additional doses of hepatitis B vaccine.[27] HIV-infected children and adults who respond to hepatitis B vaccine have a more rapid decline in antibody titer than do uninfected persons. For example, only 42% of HIV-infected children who seroconverted after a primary three-dose series (10 μg/dose) of hepatitis B vaccine, or after an additional 20-μg dose in those who did not respond to the primary series, had protective antibody titers 13 to 18 months later.[21] Although in immunologically normal persons loss of detectable antibody after developing protective concentrations of antibody ($\geq$10 mIU) does not mean loss of protection against disease, some HIV-infected adults who were exposed to hepatitis B several years after developing those responses have developed surface antigenemia, clinical disease, and persistent hepatitis B surface antigen carriage.[28]

Hepatitis A Vaccine

As with hepatitis B vaccine, HIV-infected adults are less likely to develop a protective antibody response following vaccination against hepatitis A, and have lower antibody titers than do HIV-uninfected persons. Approximately 90% of immunologically normal adults and 95% to 100% of children over 2 years of age develop protective antibodies 1 month after a single dose of hepatitis A vaccine, but only 70% to 90% of HIV-infected adults seroconverted following two to three doses of hepatitis A vaccine.[29–31]

TABLE 11-2 ■ Immunogenicity of Diphtheria and Tetanus Toxoids and Pertussis Vaccines in HIV-Infected Children and Adults

Vaccine	Ref.	Country	No. of Subjects	Age	% of HIV-Infected Persons Developing Protective Antibody Titers
TETANUS TOXOID					
	3	USA	5	2–6 yr	40%; titers lower than in controls
	4	France	13	1–24 mo	62%; lower titers in children with opportunistic infections
	5	Italy	17	18–84 mo	77%; titers lower than in controls
	6	France	25	Adults	77%; no difference in GMT titer from controls
	7	Switzerland	10	Adults	increase in GMT; correlated with CD4 cell counts
	8	Netherlands	47	Adults	84%; correlated with CD4 cell count
	9	Chile	26	Adults	23%; decline in antibody titers at 1 yr
DTP					
	10	USA	17	11–90 mo	60% to tetanus; 18% to diphtheria; CMI in some children without protective antibody titers
	11	USA	37	<4 yr	91% to tetanus; 76% to diphtheria; better responses early in life
	12	Zaire	48	<4 mo	96% to tetanus; 71% to diphtheria; titers lower than in controls
ACELLULAR PERTUSSIS					
	13	Italy	12	6–107 mo	75%; titers lower than in controls; correlated with CD4 cell count

CMI, cell-mediated immunity; DTP, diphtheria and tetanus toxoids and pertussis vaccine; GMT, geometric mean antibody titer.

Influenza Virus Vaccine

Limited data suggest that influenza vaccine is effective in preventing symptomatic influenza infection in many HIV-infected adults. Influenza vaccine was most effective in HIV-infected persons with CD4+ T-lymphocyte counts greater than 100 cells/mm^3 during an outbreak at a residential facility in New York City.[32] In persons with severe immune suppression, a second dose of influenza vaccine did not result in greater immunogenicity.[33,34] Nevertheless, in a randomized, placebo-controlled trial, none of 55 HIV-infected adults who received influenza vaccine, as compared to 10 of 47 who received saline, developed laboratory-confirmed symptomatic influenza.[35]

Polysaccharide and Polysaccharide-Protein Conjugate Vaccines

In the absence of acquired immunodeficiency syndrome (AIDS) or profoundly diminished CD4+ T-lymphocyte cell counts, 37% to 86% of HIV-infected children developed protective antibody responses following three doses of *Haemophilus influenzae* type b conjugate vaccines, but the geometric mean titers were lower than in HIV-uninfected persons of similar ages.[36-40] Antibody concentrations wane more rapidly in HIV-infected children, but booster doses of vaccine induce rapid increases in antibody, suggesting retention of immunologic memory in some HIV-infected children.[41] In one study of 48 HIV-infected children, antibody titers decreased to below 1 μg/mL in 43% of HIV-infected children 1 year after vaccination, compared to only 11% of HIV-uninfected children.[38]

No data are available regarding the response to meningococcal polysaccharide vaccine in HIV-infected children or adults, but the response to 23-valent pneumococcal polysaccharide vaccine is poorer than in HIV-uninfected persons. The antibody response to a glycoprotein conjugate pneumococcal vaccine was better than that of the polysaccharide vaccine in HIV-infected persons, except for those adults with CD4+ T-lymphocyte counts less than 200 cells/mm^3.[42,43] Because polysaccharides are processed as T-independent antigens, the immune response is not affected by HIV-induced impairment of the immune system as much as with T-dependent antigens. However, the antibody response to specific pneumococcal polysaccharide serotypes varies, with some serotypes eliciting poor antibody responses in HIV-infected persons with CD4+ T-lymphocyte counts less than 200 cells/mm^3.[44] In HIV-infected Ugandan adults, the 23-valent polysaccharide pneumococcal vaccine was found to be ineffective in preventing first episodes of invasive pneumococcal disease.[45]

Safety of Nonreplicating Vaccines

Nonreplicating vaccines are not associated with increased risks of complications in immunocompromised persons. However, a study of HIV-infected Ugandan adults found an increased incidence of pneumonia in recipients of 23-valent pneumococcal polysaccharide vaccine as compared to unvaccinated HIV-infected adults.[45] The authors hypothesized that immunization may result in destruction of polysaccharide-responsive B-cell clones, but no specific data to support this hypothesis were provided.

TABLE 11–3 ■ Immunogenicity of Hepatitis B Vaccines in HIV-Infected Children and Adults

Ref.	Country	Vaccine and Dose	No. of Subjects	Age	% of HIV-Infected Persons Developing Protective Antibody Titers
15	Italy	Engerix-B (20 µg)	18	2 newborns 16 children	78%; titers lower than in controls; no correlation with CD4 cell count; poor response to booster dose
16	USA	<11 yr: Engerix-B (10 µg) or Recombivax HB (2.5 µg) >11 yr: Engerix-B (20 µg) or Recombivax HB (5 µg)	24	5–115 mo	25%; correlated with CD4 cell count
17	USA	Recombivax HB (2.5 µg)	17	1 day to 4 mo	35%; no correlation with CD4 cell count
18	Italy	Engerix-B (20 µg)	5	2–6 mo	20%
19	Spain	Engerix-B (10 µg)	17	10 neonates 7 children: 1–63 mo	41%; no correlation with CD4 cell count
20	USA	Booster doses <11 yr: Engerix-B (20 µg) >11 yr: Engerix-B (40 µg)	14*	21–30 mo	14%; 0 of 7 developed antibody response after 2nd booster dose
21	Italy	Engerix-B (10 µg)	20	1–102 mo	45%; not correlated with CD4 cell count; 73% of 11 responded to booster (20 µg)
22	USA	Plasma-derived	16	Adults	56%; titers lower than in controls
23	Belgium	Recombinant	32	Adults	28%; titers lower than in controls
24	Spain	Recombinant	21	Adults	24%; titers lower than in controls
25	UK	Engerix-B (20 µg)	12	Adults	17%; poor response to additional dose
26	Australia	Plasma-derived or recombinant	14	Adults	43%
27	France	Genhevac B (20 µg)	20	Adults	55% after 3 injections; 78% of 9 nonresponders after 3 additional doses

*Follow-up study of children previously reported by Rutstein et al.[17]

Live Bacteria Vaccines

Bacille Calmette-Guérin Vaccine

The tuberculin skin test is the only practical tool for determining the response to BCG vaccination, but the diameter of the skin test following immunization is not a good predictor of protection against Mycobacterium tuberculosis disease.[46] In Rwanda, only 37% of HIV-infected infants developed a skin test response greater than 6 mm in diameter after BCG vaccination, as compared with 57% of HIV-uninfected infants born to HIV-infected women and 70% of infants born to HIV-uninfected women.[47]

Protection conferred by BCG vaccination against tuberculous meningitis and miliary tuberculosis in HIV-uninfected populations has varied widely, most likely as a result of differences in BCG strains and study methodology, but a recent meta-analysis has estimated an overall protection of approximately 80%.[48] Studies of tuberculosis in adults who were vaccinated with BCG in infancy have not shown clear protective benefit.[49,50] Thus these variable data from normal populations are inadequate to make definitive conclusions about the effectiveness of BCG for protection against tuberculosis in HIV-infected children or adults.

BCG causes local ulcers and regional lymphadenitis in normal hosts at rates varying from 4 to 30 per 1000 vaccinated infants depending on the vaccine strain, technique of administration, and vaccine dose.[51] There are several reports of regional lymphadenitis, poorly healing ulcers, and fistulas developing in HIV-infected infants (Table 11–4). Administration of BCG vaccine to HIV-infected children in the first month of life is associated with relatively low rates of complications because immune suppression takes several months to develop. In direct comparisons, the rates

of these complications have been similar in HIV-infected and HIV-uninfected infants, but the lymphadenitis in HIV-infected children has been more severe.

More than 28 cases of disseminated BCG have been reported in many HIV-infected children and adults (Table 11–4).[65] Disseminated disease usually occurs several months to years after vaccination, but was reported in one 30-year-old with HIV infection who was vaccinated at birth.[66] Disseminated BCG infection is more likely to occur when the vaccine is administered to individuals with clinical AIDS or advanced immune suppression. Reactivation of latent BCG organisms can occur with progressive immune suppression, causing regional or disseminated disease.[60] In one study, however, no cases of disseminated BCG were found among 155 adult patients with AIDS who had received BCG in infancy and whose blood was cultured for mycobacteria.[50]

Live Virus Vaccines

Oral Poliovirus Vaccine

The proportion of HIV-infected children who responded to three doses of polio vaccine was greater than 90% in most studies (Table 11–5). In the Democratic Republic of Congo (formerly Zaire), 97% of HIV-infected children developed protective antibody titers to poliovirus types 1, 2, and 3 after three doses of oral poliovirus vaccine (OPV).[12] However, this study was conducted when there was widespread circulation of wild-type polioviruses that could have contributed to the high percentage of children with antibody. No direct estimates of polio vaccine efficacy have been conducted in HIV-infected children. However, wild-type polioviruses

TABLE 11–4 ■ Adverse Events Associated with BCG Vaccination in HIV-Infected Children

Reference	Country	Study Population	Adverse Events
4	France	18 HIV-infected	Disseminated BCG in 3 (17%)
52	Uganda	54 children born to HIV-infected women	No complications
53	France	67 HIV-infected	BCG lymphadenitis in 7 (10%)
54	Canada	1 HIV-infected	Disseminated BCG in a 2-month-old girl
55	Belgium	1 HIV-infected	Disseminated BCG in a 4-month-old boy from Zaire
56	Zambia	42 HIV-infected	BCG lymphadenitis in 1 (3%)
57	Switzerland	1 HIV-infected	Disseminated BCG in an 8-month-old girl from Argentina
58	Congo	21 HIV-infected	BCG lymphadenitis in 5 (24%)
47	Rwanda	37 HIV-infected	BCG lymphadenitis in 2 (5%)
59	Zaire	21 HIV-infected	No complications
12	Zaire	48 HIV-infected 640 HIV-uninfected	Lymphadenitis in 5% HIV-infected and 3.5% HIV-uninfected Fistulas in 5% HIV-infected and 6–8% HIV-uninfected
60	France	68 HIV-infected	4 with BCG lymphadenitis, 3 with fistula, 2 with disseminated BCG (13%)
61	Haiti	13 HIV-infected	BCG lymphadenitis, ulceration, or abscess in 4 (31%); double dose of BCG
62	USA	1 HIV-infected	BCG bacteremia in a 3-year-old HIV-infected Brazilian girl
63	Australia	1 HIV-infected	BCG lymphadenitis
64	Thailand	26 HIV-infected	No complications

have been successfully eliminated from several countries with high prevalence rates of HIV infection.

The risk of vaccine-associated paralytic poliomyelitis (VAPP) is increased in persons with primary B-cell immunodeficiency disorders.[72] Nevertheless, more than 1000 HIV-infected children received at least one dose of OPV without complications in the United States before it was known that they or their mothers were HIV infected, and several thousand HIV-infected children in other countries have been vaccinated. Only two HIV-infected children have been reported with VAPP following receipt of OPV (Table 11–5): one 2-year-old, HIV-infected Romanian girl[70] and one child in Zimbabwe.[71] In Romania, the rate of VAPP in all children was approximately 10-fold higher than the estimated one case per 2.5 million doses administered in the United States and Europe, most likely related to simultaneous administration of multiple injections.[73] Thus, HIV infection in these two children with VAPP could be chance associations and not evidence of an increased risk associated with HIV infection. If the risk of VAPP is increased in HIV-infected persons, the attributable risk is very low.

Measles Vaccine

The antibody response to measles vaccine is impaired in HIV-infected persons (Table 11–6).[74] In three prospective studies, approximately one quarter to one third of HIV-infected children responded to a single dose of standard-titer measles vaccine.[77] In a study of HIV-seropositive children in Zaire, 65% had protective titers of measles antibody 3 months after measles vaccination, at 9 months of age, although only 36% of 11 symptomatic children seroconverted compared with 77% of 26 asymptomatic children.[75] The response to a second dose of vaccine was variable, but generally poor, in five studies.[77] In cross-sectional studies, the study populations varied widely in age at immunization, number of vaccine doses received, time since immunization, type of measles antibody assay used,

TABLE 11–5 ■ Immunogenicity and Safety of Poliovirus Vaccines in HIV-Infected Children

Ref.	Country	Vaccine*	No. of Subjects	Age	Safety	% of HIV-Infected Persons Developing Protective Antibody Titers After ≥ 3 Doses
4	France	OPV	15	1–24 mo	No adverse events	40% to type 2; 33% to types 1 and 3
67	USA	OPV	23	1–180 mo	No adverse events	91%; lower titers with advanced disease
68	USA	OPV	180	1–132 mo	No adverse events	Immunogenicity not studied
69	Italy	IPV	9	4–42 mo	No adverse events	100% to types 1 and 2; 88% to type 3
5	Italy	OPV and/or IPV	12	18–84 mo	No adverse events	100% to type 2; 92% to types 1 and 3; decrease in titers over 2 yr in 4 children studied
12	Zaire	OPV	48	<4 mo	No adverse events	97%; titers lower than controls
70	Romania	OPV	1	26 mo	Flaccid paralysis, vaccine-strain poliovirus type 2 in stool	Lacked protective antibody titers to all three types despite receipt of four doses of OPV
71	Zimbabwe	OPV	1	4 yr	Paralysis of right leg 2 wk after second OPV	Lacked antibodies to polioviruses types 1 and 3 despite having received OPV during first year of life

*IPV, inactivated polio vaccine; OPV, oral polio vaccine.

TABLE 11–6 ▪ Prospective Studies of the Immunogenicity of Measles Vaccine in HIV-Infected Children

Reference	Country	Number of Children	Age	Response to Primary Immunization	Response to Repeat Immunization
75	Zaire	37	21 mo	36% of 11 symptomatic 77% of 26 asymptomatic	
76	USA	8	11–41 mo	25%	n.a.
77*	USA	35	12–194 mo	37%	0%
78	USA	2	n.a.	n.a.	50%
79	USA	4	22–121 mo	n.a.	0%
80	USA	11	72–120 mo	n.a.	36%
81	USA	7	31–120 mo	n.a.	14%
82	Thailand	16	9 mo	57%	n.a.

*Four children received repeat immunization.
n.a., information not available.

and degree of immunosuppression at the time of assessment. In children, the prevalence of measles antibody after vaccination varied from 17% to 100%, with a median of 60%.[74] The majority of HIV-infected adults, however, were already seropositive.[83,84] An association between lack of measles-specific antibodies after vaccination and low CD4+ T-lymphocyte count (<600 cells/mm^3) was documented in one prospective study[77] and two cross-sectional studies.[81,85] In Ugandan children, poor antibody response to measles vaccine was associated with stunting but not with HIV infection.[86] HIV-infected children appear to have a more rapid decline in measles antibody as compared to HIV-uninfected children,[81] with a median time to loss of enzyme immunoassay–detectable antibody of 30 months in one study of 17 HIV-infected children.[85]

Placental transfer of maternal antibodies, including antibody to measles, may be impaired in HIV-infected women.[87–90] The lower amounts of maternal antibody correlated with an improved response of their infants to measles vaccine administered at 6 months of age; and less immunosuppression at 6 to 9 months of age may contribute to higher response rates than at 12 to 15 months of age.[90]

Prospective studies revealed no increased risk of adverse events in the few weeks following immunization with standard- and high-titer measles vaccines for HIV-infected children as compared to uninfected children.[74] A retrospective survey conducted by the New York City Department of Health found no complications following measles immunization of HIV-infected children.[68] No evidence of persistent measles vaccine virus excretion was found in 10 HIV-infected children immunized with measles-mumps-rubella (MMR) vaccine.[79] Only one serious adverse event has been reported following administration of measles vaccine to an HIV-infected person.[91,92] A 20-year-old HIV-infected man, who had a very low CD4+ T-lymphocyte cell count at the time he received a second dose of MMR vaccine, developed cough and progressive pulmonary infiltrates 10 months after immunization. An open lung biopsy showed giant cell pneumonitis, and measles vaccine virus was identified in the lung tissue. He died several months later from the progressive pneumonitis. A British HIV-infected child with a CD4+ T-lymphocyte cell count of 340/μL who received MMR vaccine developed rash disease and interstitial pneumonia, from which

he recovered. Vaccine-strain measles genome was present in his blood.[93]

Mumps and Rubella Vaccines

In many countries, mumps and rubella vaccines are administered in combination with measles vaccine. Limited data suggest that HIV-infected persons are as likely to develop protective antibody titers to mumps and rubella vaccines as HIV-uninfected persons.[78,94–96] In one study, antibodies to mumps were present in seven, and antibodies to rubella in all eight, vaccinated HIV-infected children.[95] In another study, no difference was observed in the proportion of HIV-infected and uninfected children who responded to rubella vaccine, although the median antibody titer was lower in HIV-infected children.[78] No cases of measles, mumps, or rubella were observed in vaccinated HIV-infected children followed in the European Collaborative Study,[14] and no serious adverse events resulting from mumps or rubella vaccines have been reported in HIV-infected persons.

Varicella Virus Vaccine

Varicella in HIV-infected children is more severe than in uninfected children, and HIV-infected children and adults are at increased risk of developing herpes zoster following varicella infection. Varicella vaccine was safe and immunogenic, as determined by antibody and lymphocyte proliferation assay responses, in mildly symptomatic American HIV-infected children (Centers for Disease Control and Prevention [CDC] stage N1 or A1).[97] However, disseminated vaccine-strain varicella was reported in an HIV-infected child with a CD4+ T-lymphocyte count of only 8 cells/mm^3.[98] Given the potential severity of varicella and herpes zoster in HIV-infected children and the potential risks of live varicella vaccine, the American Academy of Pediatrics recommends that varicella vaccine be considered for HIV-infected children in CDC class I (CD4+ T-lymphocyte percentage of 25 or more) with mild or no signs or symptoms.[99]

Yellow Fever Virus Vaccine

Limited data suggest that HIV-infected children respond poorly to yellow fever vaccine, but seroconversion rates were high in HIV-infected adults who were not severely immuno-compromised.[100] Only 3 (17%) of 18 HIV-infected children developed an antibody response to yellow fever vaccine compared to 74% of 57 HIV-uninfected children.[101] No data are available on the protection against disease following yellow fever vaccination of HIV-infected persons.

Few severe complications have been reported as a result of inadvertent immunization of immunocompromised individuals with yellow fever vaccine, but experience is limited. Fatal myeloencephalitis caused by yellow fever vaccine was reported in a 53-year-old HIV-infected man in Thailand,[102] although no adverse events were observed following yellow fever vaccination of two other HIV-infected adults.[103] Seven normal adults with a severe yellow fever–like illness (six of the cases fatal) were reported with evidence of vaccine virus in affected tissues, but none had evidence of HIV infection.[104]

Live, Attenuated Influenza Virus Vaccine

The trivalent, cold-adapted, live, attenuated influenza vaccine was shown to be safe in small studies of 57 HIV-infected adults[105] and 24 HIV-infected children.[106] After 2 doses of vaccine, 77% of the HIV-infected children and 83% of the control children had a fourfold or greater rise in influenza antibody in response to at least one of the three vaccine strains.[106] Few HIV-infected adults had a seroresponse to the live, attenuated influenza vaccine, although only a few recipients were susceptible to the vaccine strains before vaccination.[105]

Vaccines Against Agents of Bioterrorism

Little or no information is available on the safety, immunogenicity, or effectiveness of vaccines against agents of bioterrorism (smallpox, anthrax, tularemia, plague) in HIV-infected persons. Vaccinia vaccine is contraindicated in HIV-infected persons, although plague and anthrax vaccines should be used if indicated.[1] Disseminated vaccinia was reported in an HIV-infected military recruit,[107] subsequently, officials estimated that more than 300 HIV-infected recruits had received smallpox vaccine. Other serious complications would be expected in HIV-infected persons if vaccination against smallpox were conducted in large populations.

Effect of Vaccination on Human Immunodeficiency Virus Disease Progression

Activation of T-lymphocytes following immunization could potentially augment HIV replication and result in more rapid progression of HIV disease. Several studies, but not all,[108] have described transient elevations of HIV RNA plasma levels lasting several days following immunization with tetanus toxoid[109] and influenza,[110–114] pneumococcal,[115,116] and hepatitis B[27,117] vaccines. None of these investigations has found prolonged elevation of HIV RNA viral load, decreased CD4+ T-lymphocyte cell counts, or accelerated HIV disease progression following immunization.

Although the transient rise in HIV viral load following administration of tetanus toxoid to pregnant women could theoretically affect the risk of maternal–infant HIV transmission, an increased risk of transmission is unlikely if vaccination occurs at least 4 weeks prior to delivery.

Effect of Antiretroviral Therapy on Immune Responses to Vaccines

Immune restoration can follow antiretroviral therapy in HIV-infected adults and children,[118] and several studies have found enhanced responses to vaccination among HIV-infected persons receiving effective, highly active antiretroviral therapy (HAART). Repeat vaccination with MMR vaccine was more likely to result in an antibody response in children receiving HAART than in children receiving non-HAART antiretroviral therapy.[119] In an uncontrolled study, 48% of 31 HIV-infected adults developed a fourfold increase in antibody titers to tetanus toxoid, and 73% developed antibodies to hepatitis A vaccine, after receiving antiretroviral therapy for at least 48 weeks.[120] Deferring vaccination in HIV-infected persons with advanced immunosuppression until HIV replication is controlled by HAART should result in improved responses to vaccination.

REFERENCES

1. Centers for Disease Control and Prevention. Recommendations of the Advisory Committee on Immunization Practices (ACIP): Use of vaccines and immune globulins in persons with altered immunocompetence. MMWR 42(RR-4):1–18, 1994.
2. Global Programme for Vaccines and Immunization, Expanded Programme on Immunization. Immunization Policy (WHO Document WHO/EPI/GEN/95.03, 25–27). Geneva, World Health Organization, 1996.
3. Bernstein LJ, Ochs HD, Wedgwood RJ, Rubinstein A. Defective humoral immunity in pediatric acquired immune deficiency syndrome. J Pediatr 107:352–357, 1985.
4. Blanche S, Le Deist F, Fischer A, et al. Longitudinal study of 18 children with perinatal LAV/HTLV III infection: attempt at prognostic evaluation. J Pediatr 109:965–970, 1986.
5. Barbi M, Biffi MR, Binda S, et al. Immunization in children with HIV seropositivity at birth: antibody response to polio vaccine and tetanus toxoid. AIDS 6:1465–1469, 1992.
6. Ballet JJ, Sulcebe G, Couderc LJ, et al. Impaired anti-pneumococcal antibody response in patients with AIDS-related persistent generalized lymphadenopathy. Clin Exp Immunol 68:479–487, 1987.
7. Opravil M, Fierz W, Matter L, et al. Poor antibody response after tetanus and pneumococcal vaccination in immunocompromised, HIV-infected patients. Clin Exp Immunol 84:185–189, 1991.
8. Kroon FP, van Dissel JT, de Jong JC, van Furth R. Antibody response to influenza, tetanus, and pneumococcal vaccines in HIV-seropositive individuals in relation to the number of CD4+ lymphocytes. AIDS 8:469–476, 1994.
9. Talesnik E, Vial PA, Labarca J, et al. Time course of antibody response to tetanus toxoid and pneumococcal capsular polysaccharides in patients infected with HIV. J Acquir Immune Defic Syndr Hum Retrovirol 19:471–477, 1998.
10. Borkowsky W, Steele CJ, Grubman S, et al. Antibody responses to bacterial toxoids in children infected with human immunodeficiency virus. J Pediatr 110:563–566, 1987.
11. Borkowsky W, Rigaud M, Krasinski K, et al. Cell-mediated and humoral immune responses in children infected with human immunodeficiency virus during the first four years of life. J Pediatr 120:371–375, 1992.
12. Ryder RW, Oxtoby MJ, Mvula M, et al. Safety and immunogenicity of bacille Calmette-Guerin, diphtheria-tetanus-pertussis, and oral polio vaccines in newborn children in Zaire infected with human immunodeficiency virus type 1. J Pediatr 122:697–702, 1993.

13. De Martino M, Podda A, Galli L, et al. Acellular pertussis vaccine in children with perinatal human immunodeficiency virus-type 1 infection. Vaccine 15:1235–1238, 1997.

14. Dunn DT, Newell ML, Peckham CS, Vanden Eijden VS. Routine vaccination and vaccine-preventable infections in children born to human immunodeficiency virus-infected mothers. European Collaborative Study. Acta Paediatr 87:458–459, 1998.

15. Zuin G, Principi N, Tornaghi R, et al. Impaired response to hepatitis B vaccine in HIV infected children. Vaccine 10:857–860, 1992.

16. Diamant EP, Schechter CB, Hodes DS, Peters VB. Immunogenicity of hepatitis B vaccine in human immunodeficiency virus infected children. Pediatr Infect Dis J 12:877–878, 1993.

17. Rutstein RM, Rudy B, Codispoti C, Watson B. Response to hepatitis B immunization by infants exposed to HIV. AIDS 8:1281–1284, 1994.

18. Zuccotti GV, Riva E, Flumine P, et al. Hepatitis B vaccination in infants of mothers infected with human immunodeficiency virus. J Pediatr 125:70–72, 1994.

19. Arrazola MP, de Juanes JR, Ramos JT, et al. Hepatitis B vaccination in infants of mothers infected with human immunodeficiency virus. J Med Virol 45:339–341, 1995.

20. Choudhury SA, Peters VB. Responses to hepatitis B vaccine boosters in human immunodeficiency virus-infected children. Pediatr Infect Dis J 14:65–67, 1995.

21. Scolfaro C, Fiammengo P, Balbo L, et al. Hepatitis B vaccination in HIV-1 infected children: double efficacy doubling the paediatric dose. AIDS 10:1169–1170, 1996.

22. Collier AC, Corey L, Murphy VL, Handsfield HH. Antibody to human immunodeficiency virus (HIV) and suboptimal response to hepatitis B vaccination. Ann Intern Med 109:101–105, 1988.

23. Keet IPM, van Doornum G, Safary A, Coutinho RA. Insufficient response to hepatitis B vaccination in HIV-positive homosexual men. AIDS 6:509–510, 1992.

24. Bruguera M, Cremades M, Salinas R, et al. Impaired response to recombinant hepatitis B vaccine in HIV-infected persons. J Clin Gastroenterol 14:27–30, 1992.

25. Tayal SC, Sankar KN. Impaired response to recombinant hepatitis B vaccine in asymptomatic HIV-infected individuals. AIDS 8:558–559, 1994.

26. Wong EKL, Bodsworth NJ, Slade MA, et al. Response to hepatitis B vaccination in a primary care setting: influence of HIV infection, CD4+ lymphocyte count and vaccination schedule. Int J STD AIDS 7:490–494, 1996.

27. Rey D, Krantz V, Partisani M, et al. Increasing the number of hepatitis B vaccine injections augments anti-HBs response rate in HIV-infected patients: effects on HIV-1 viral load. Vaccine 18:1161–1165, 2000.

28. Halder SC, Judson FN, O'Malley PM, et al. Outcome of hepatitis B virus infection in homosexual men and its relation to prior human immunodeficiency virus infection. J Infect Dis 163:454–459, 1991.

29. Hess G, Clemens R, Bienzle U, et al. Immunogenicity and safety of an inactivated hepatitis A vaccine in anti-HIV positive and negative homosexual men. J Med Virol 46:40–42, 1995.

30. Tilzey AJ, Palmer SJ, Harrington C, O'Doherty MJ. Hepatitis A vaccine responses in HIV-positive persons with haemophilia. Vaccine 14:1039–1041, 1996.

31. Neilsen GA, Bodsworth NJ, Watts N. Response to hepatitis A vaccination in human immunodeficiency virus infected and -uninfected homosexual men. J Infect Dis 176:1064–1067, 1997.

32. Fine AD, Bridges CB, De Guzman AM, et al. Influenza A among patients with human immunodeficiency virus: an outbreak of infection at a residential facility in New York City. Clin Infect Dis 32:1784–1791, 2001.

33. Kroon FP, van Dissel JP, de Jong JC, et al. Antibody response after influenza vaccination in HIV-infected individuals: a consecutive 3-year study. Vaccine 18:3040–3049, 2000.

34. Miotti PG, Nelson KE, Dallabetta GA, et al. The influence of HIV infection on antibody responses to a two-dose regimen of influenza vaccine. JAMA 262:779–783, 1989.

35. Tasker SA, Treanor JJ, Paxton WB, Wallace MR. Efficacy of influenza vaccination in HIV-infected persons: a randomized, double-blind, placebo-controlled trial. Ann Intern Med 131:430–433, 1999.

36. Peters VB, Sood SK. Immunity to Haemophilus influenzae type b polysaccharide capsule in children with human immunodeficiency virus infection immunized with a single dose of Haemophilus vaccine. J Pediatr 125:74–77, 1994.

37. Gibb D, Spoulou V, Giacomelli A, et al. Antibody responses to Haemophilus influenzae type b and Streptococcus pneumoniae vaccines in children with human immunodeficiency virus infection. Pediatr Infect Dis J 14:129–135, 1995.

38. Gibb D, Giacomelli A, Masters J, et al. Persistence of antibody responses to Haemophilus influenzae type b polysaccharide conjugate vaccine in children with vertically acquired human immunodeficiency virus infection. Pediatr Infect Dis J 15:1097–1101, 1996.

39. Rutstein RM, Rudy BJ, Cnaan A. Response of human immunodeficiency virus-exposed and -infected infants to Haemophilus influenzae type b conjugate vaccine. Arch Pediatr Adolesc Med 150:838–841, 1996.

40. Read JS, Frasch CE, Rich K, et al. The immunogenicity of Haemophilus influenzae type b conjugate vaccines in children born to human immunodeficiency virus-infected women. Pediatr Infect Dis J 17:391–397, 1998.

41. Peters VB, Sood SK. Immunity to Haemophilus influenzae type b after reimmunization with oligosaccharide CRM_{197} conjugate vaccine in children with human immunodeficiency virus infection. Pediatr Infect Dis J 16:711–713, 1997.

42. Ahmed F, Steinhoff MC, Rodreguez-Barradas MC, et al. Effect of human immunodeficiency virus type 1 infection on the antibody response to a glycoprotein conjugate pneumococcal vaccine: results from a randomized trial. J Infect Dis 173:83–90, 1996.

43. King JC, Vink PE, Farley JJ, et al. Comparison of the safety and immunogenicity of a pneumococcal conjugate with a licensed polysaccharide vaccine in human immunodeficiency virus and non-human immunodeficiency virus-infected children. Pediatr Infect Dis J 15:192–196, 1996.

44. Kroon FP, van Dissel JT, Ravensbergen E, et al. Antibodies against pneumococcal polysaccharides after vaccination in HIV-infected individuals: 5-year follow-up of antibody concentrations. Vaccine 18:524–530, 2000.

45. French N, Nakiyingi J, Carpenter LM, et al. 23-Valent pneumococcal polysaccharide vaccine in HIV-1-infected Ugandan adults: double-blind, randomised and placebo controlled trial. Lancet 355: 2106–2111, 2000.

46. Comstock GW. Does the protective effect of neonatal BCG vaccination correlate with vaccine-induced tuberculin reactions? Am J Respir Crit Care Med 154:263–264, 1996.

47. Msellati P, Dabis F, Lepage P HD, et al. BCG vaccination and pediatric HIV infection—Rwanda, 1988–1990. MMWR 40:833–836, 1991.

48. Colditz GA, Brewer TF, Berkey CS, et al. Efficacy of BCG vaccine in the prevention of tuberculosis: meta-analysis of the published literature. JAMA 271:698–702, 1994.

49. Allen S, Batungwanayo J, Kelinkowske K, et al. Two year incidence of tuberculosis in cohorts of HIV-infected and uninfected urban Rwandan women. Am Rev Respir Dis 146:1439–1444, 1992.

50. Marsh BJ, von Reyn CF, Edwards J, et al. The risks and benefits of childhood bacille Calmette-Guerin immunization among adults with AIDS. AIDS 11:669–672, 1997.

51. Lotte A, Wasz-Hockert P, Poisson N, et al. BCG complications: estimates of the risks among vaccinated subjects and statistical analysis of their main characteristics. Adv Tuberc Res 21:107–193, 1984.

52. Carswell M. BCG immunization in the children of HIV-positive mothers [letter]. AIDS 1:258, 1987.

53. Bregere P. BCG vaccination and AIDS. Bull Int Union Tuberc Lung Dis 63:40–41, 1988.

54. Houde C, Dery P. Mycobacterium bovis sepsis in an infant with human immunodeficiency virus infection. Pediatr Infect Dis J 7:810–811, 1988.

55. Ninane J, Grymonprez A, Burtonboy G, et al. Disseminated BCG in HIV infection. Arch Dis Child 63:1268–1269, 1988.

56. Hira SK, Kamanga J, Bhat GJ, et al. Perinatal transmission of HIV-1 in Zambia. BMJ 299:1250–1252, 1989.

57. Ten Dam HG. BCG vaccination and HIV infection. Bull Int Union Tuberc Lung Dis 65:38–39, 1990.

58. Lallemant Le Coeur S, Lallemant M, Cheynier D, et al. Bacillus Calmette-Guerin immunization in infants born to HIV-seropositive mothers. AIDS 5:195–199, 1991.

59. Green SD, Nganga A, Cutting WA, Davies AG. BCG immunization in children born to HIV positive mothers [letter]. Lancet 340:799, 1992.

60. Besnard M, Sauvion S, Offredo C, et al. Bacillus Calmette-Guerin infection after vaccination of human immunodeficiency virus-infected children. Pediatr Infect Dis J 12:993–997, 1993.

61. O'Brien KL, Ruff AJ, Louis MA, et al. *Bacillus* Calmette-Guerin complications in children born to HIV-1-infected women with a review of the literature. Pediatrics 95:414–418, 1995.

62. Edwards KM, Kernodle DS. Possible hazards of routine *Bacillus* Calmette-Guerin immunization in human immunodeficiency virus-infected children. Pediatr Infect Dis J 15:836–838, 1996.

63. Sharp MJ, Mallon DFJ. Regional *Bacillus* Calmette-Guerin lymphadenitis after initiating antiretroviral therapy in an infant with human immunodeficiency virus type 1 infection. Pediatr Infect Dis J 17:660–662, 1999.

64. Thaithumyanon P, Thisyakorn U, Punnahitananda S, et al. Safety and immunogenicity of *Bacillus* Calmette-Guerin vaccine in children born to HIV-infected women. Southeast Asian J Trop Med Pub Health 31:482–486, 2000.

65. Talbot EA, Perkins MD, Silva SFM, Frothingham R. Disseminated bacille Calmette-Guerin disease after vaccination: case report and review. Clin Infect Dis 24:1139–1146, 1997.

66. Armbruster C, Junker W, Vetter N, Jaksch G. Disseminated bacille Calmette-Guerin infection in an AIDS patient 30 years after BCG vaccination [letter]. J Infect Dis 162:1216, 1990.

67. Krasinski K, Borkowsky W. Response to polio vaccination in children infected with human immunodeficiency virus [abstract]. Pediatr Res 21:328A, 1987.

68. McLaughlin M, Thomas P, Onorato I, et al. Live virus vaccines in human immunodeficiency virus infected children: a retrospective survey. Pediatrics 82:229–233, 1988.

69. Barbi M, Bardare M, Luraschi C, et al. Antibody response to inactivated polio vaccine (E-IPV) in children born to HIV positive mothers. Eur J Epidemiol 8:211–216, 1992.

70. Ion-Nedelcu N, Dobrescu A, Strebel PM, Sutter RW. Vaccine-associated paralytic poliomyelitis and HIV infection. Lancet 343:51–52, 1994.

71. Chitsike I, van Furth R. Paralytic poliomyelitis associated with live oral poliomyelitis vaccine in child with HIV infection in Zimbabwe: case report. BMJ 318:841-843, 1999.

72. Sutter RW, Prevots DR. Vaccine-associated paralytic poliomyelitis among immunodeficient persons. Infect Med 11:426–438, 1994.

73. Strebel PM, Aubert-Combiescu A, Ion-Nedelcu N, et al. Paralytic poliomyelitis in Romania, 1984–1992: evidence for a high risk of vaccine-associated disease and reintroduction of wild-virus infection. Am J Epidemiol 140:1111–1124, 1994.

74. Moss WJ, Cutts F, Griffin DE. Implications of the human immunodeficiency virus epidemic for control and eradication of measles. Clin Infect Dis 29:106–112, 1999.

75. Oxtoby MJ, Ryder R, Mvula M, et al. Patterns of immunity to measles among African children infected with human immunodeficiency virus. Presented at the Epidemic Intelligence Service Conference, Atlanta, Georgia. April 3–5, 1989.

76. Krasinski K, Borkowsky W. Measles and measles immunity in children infected with human immunodeficiency virus. JAMA 261:2512–2516, 1989.

77. Palumbo P, Hoyt L, Demasio K, et al. Population-based study of measles and measles immunization in human immunodeficiency virus-infected children. Pediatr Infect Dis J 11:1008–1014, 1992.

78. Brena AE, Cooper ER, Cabral HJ, Pelton SI. Antibody response to measles and rubella vaccine by children with HIV infection. J Acquir Immune Defic Syndr 6:1125–1129, 1993.

79. Frenkel LM, Nielsen H, Garakian A, Cherry JD. A search for persistent measles, mumps and rubella vaccine virus in children with human immunodeficiency type-1 infection. Arch Pediatr Adolesc Med 148:57–60, 1994.

80. Brunell PA, Vimal V, Sandhu M, et al. Abnormalities of measles antibody response in human immunodeficiency virus type 1 (HIV-1) infection. J Acquir Immune Defic Syndr Hum Retrovirol 10:540–548, 1995.

81. Arpadi SM, Markowitz LE, Baughman AL, et al. Measles antibody in vaccinated human immunodeficiency virus type 1-infected children. Pediatrics 97:653–657, 1996.

82. Thaithumyanon P, Punnahitananda S, Thisyakorn U, et al. Immune responses to measles immunization and the impacts on HIV-infected children. Southeast Asian J Trop Med Pub Health 31:658–662, 2000.

83. Wallace MR, Hooper DG, Graves SJ, Malone JL. Measles seroprevalence and vaccine response in HIV-infected adults. Vaccine 12:1222–1224, 1994.

84. Kemper CA, Gangar M, Arias G, et al. The prevalence of measles antibody in human immunodeficiency virus-infected patients in Northern California. J Infect Dis 178:1177–1180, 1998.

85. Al-Attar I, Reisman J, Muehlmann M, McIntosh K. Decline of measles antibody titers after immunization in human immunodeficiency virus-infected children. Pediatr Infect Dis J 14:149–151, 1995.

86. Waibale P, Bowlin SJ, Mortimer EA, Whalen C. The effect of human immunodeficiency virus-1 infection and stunting on measles immunoglobulin-G levels in children vaccinated against measles in Uganda. Int J Epidemiol 28:341–346, 1999.

87. Embree JE, Datta P, Stackiw W, et al. Increased risk of early measles in infants of human immunodeficiency virus type 1-seropositive mothers. J Infect Dis 165:262–267, 1992.

88. Lepage P, Dabis F, Msellati P, et al. Safety and immunogenicity of high-dose Edmonston-Zagreb measles vaccine in children with HIV-1 infection: a cohort study in Kigali, Rwanda. Am J Dis Child 146:550–555, 1992.

89. Cutts FT, Mandala K, St. Louis M, et al. Immunogenicity of high-titer Edmonston-Zagreb measles vaccine in HIV-infected children in Kinshasa, Zaire. J Infect Dis 167:1418–1421, 1993.

90. Rudy BJ, Rutstein RM, Pinto-Martin J. Response to measles immunization in children infected with human immunodeficiency virus. J Pediatr 125:72–74, 1994.

91. Centers for Disease Control and Prevention. Measles pneumonitis following measles-mumps-rubella vaccination of a patient with HIV infection, 1993. MMWR 45:603–606, 1996.

92. Angel JB, Walpita P, Lerch RA, et al. Vaccine-associated measles pneumonitis in an adult with AIDS. Ann Intern Med 129:104–106, 1998.

93. Goon P, Cohen B, Jin L, et al. MMR vaccine in HIV-infected children—potential hazards? Vaccine 19:3816–3819, 2001.

94. Hilgartner MW, Maeder MA, Mahoney EM, et al. Response to measles, mumps, and rubella revaccination among HIV-positive and HIV-negative children and adolescents with hemophilia. Hemophilia Growth and Development Study. Am J Hematol 66:92–98, 2001.

95. Molyneaux PJ, Mok JYQ, Burns SM, Yap PL. Measles, mumps, and rubella immunisation in children at risk of infection with human immunodeficiency virus. J Infect 27:151–153, 1993.

96. Sprauer MA, Markowitz LE, Nicholson JKA, et al. Response of human immunodeficiency virus-infected adults to measles-rubella vaccination. J Acquir Immune Defic Syndr 6:1013–1016, 1993.

97. Levin MJ, Gershon AA, Weinberg A, et al. Immunization of HIV-infected children with varicella vaccine. J Pediatr 139:305–310, 2001.

98. Kramer JM, LaRussa P, Tsai WC, et al. Disseminated vaccine strain varicella as the acquired immunodeficiency syndrome-defining illness in a previously undiagnosed child. Pediatrics 108:e39, 2001.

99. American Academy of Pediatrics. Varicella-zoster infections. *In* Pickering LK (ed). 2000 Red Book: Report of the Committee on Infectious Diseases (25th ed). Elk Grove Village, IL, American Academy of Pediatrics, 2000, pp 624–638.

100. Goujon C, Touin M, Feuillie V, et al. Good tolerance and efficacy of yellow fever vaccine among carriers of human immunodeficiency virus [abstract]. J Travel Med 2:145, 1995.

101. Sibailly TS, Wiktor SZ, Tsai TF, et al. Poor antibody response to yellow fever vaccination in children infected with human immunodeficiency virus type 1. Pediatr Infect Dis J 16:1177–1179, 1997.

102. Kengsakul K, Sathirapongsasuti K, Punyagupta S. Fatal myeloencephalitis following yellow fever vaccination in a case with HIV infection. J Med Assoc Thai 85:131–134, 2002.

103. Receveur MC, Thiebaut R, Vedy S, et al. Yellow fever vaccination of human immunodeficiency virus-infected patients: report of 2 cases. Clin Infect Dis 31:E7–E8, 2002.

104. Marianneau P, Georges-Courbot M, Deubel V. Rarity of adverse effects after 17D yellow-fever vaccination. Lancet 358:84–85, 2001.

105. King JC Jr, Treanor J, Fast PE, et al. Comparison of the safety, vaccine virus shedding, and immunogenicity of influenza virus vaccine, trivalent, types A and B, live cold-adapted, administered to human immunodeficiency virus (HIV)-infected and non-HIV-infected adults. J Infect Dis 181:725–728, 2000.

106. King JC, Fast PE, Zangwill KM, et al. Safety, vaccine virus shedding and immunogenicity of trivalent, cold-adapted, live attenuated influenza vaccine administered to human immunodeficiency virus-infected and noninfected children. Pediatr Infect Dis J 20:1124–1131, 2001.

107. Redfield RR, Wright DC, James WD, et al. Disseminated vaccinia in a military recruit with human immunodeficiency virus (HIV) disease. N Engl J Med 316:673–676, 1987.

108. Glesby MJ, Hoover DR, Farzadegan H, et al. The effect of influenza vaccination on human immunodeficiency virus type 1 load: a randomized, double-blind, placebo-controlled study. J Infect Dis 174:1332–1336, 1996.

109. Stanley SK, Ostrowski MA, Justement JS, et al. Effect of immunization with a common recall antigen on viral expression in patients infected with human immunodeficiency virus type 1. N Engl J Med 334:1222–1230, 1996.

110. Ho DD. HIV-1 viraemia and influenza. Lancet 339:1549, 1992.

111. Staprans SI, Hamilton BL, Follansbee SE, et al. Activation of virus replication after vaccination of HIV-1-infected individuals. J Exp Med 182:1727–1737, 1995.

112. O'Brien WA, Grovit-Ferbas K, Namazi A, et al. Human immunodeficiency virus-type 1 replication can be increased in peripheral blood of seropositive patients after influenza vaccination. Blood 86:1082–1089, 1995.

113. Ramilo O, Hicks PJ, Borvak J, et al. T cell activation and human immunodeficiency virus replication after influenza immunization of infected children. Pediatr Infect Dis J 15:197–203, 1996.

114. Tasker SA, O'Brien WA, Treanor JJ, et al. Effects of influenza vaccination in HIV-infected adults: a double-blind, placebo-controlled trial. Vaccine 16:1039–1042, 1998.

115. Brichacek B, Swindells S, Janoff EN, et al. Increased plasma human immunodeficiency virus type 1 burden following antigenic challenge with pneumococcal vaccine. J Infect Dis 174:1191–1199, 1996.

116. Keller M, Deveikis A, Cutillar-Garcia M, et al. Pneumococcal and influenza immunization and human immunodeficiency virus load in children. Pediatr Infect Dis J 19:613–618, 2000.

117. Cheeseman SH, Davaro RE, Ellision RT. Hepatitis B vaccination and plasma HIV-1 RNA. N Engl J Med 334:1272, 1996.

118. Cooney EL. Clinical indicators of immune restoration following highly active antiretroviral therapy. Clin Infect Dis 34:224–233, 2002.

119. Berkelhamer S, Borock E, Elsen C, et al. Effect of highly active antiretroviral therapy on the serological response to additional measles vaccinations in human immunodeficiency virus-infected children. Clin Infect Dis 32:1090–1094, 2001.

120. Valdez H, Smith KY, Landay A, et al. Response to immunization with recall and neoantigens after prolonged administration of an HIV-1 protease inhibitor-containing regimen. AIDS 14:11–21, 2000.

Chapter 12

Bacille Calmette-Guérin Vaccine

KIM CONNELLY SMITH • JEFFREY R. STARKE

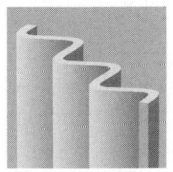

The bacille Calmette-Guérin (BCG) vaccines are the oldest of the vaccines currently used throughout the world.[1] They have been given to 4 billion people and have been used routinely since the 1960s in almost all countries of the world, with the exception of a few industrialized countries. The United States and the Netherlands are the only countries that have never routinely recommended BCG vaccination.[2] Yet, despite their widespread use, tuberculosis remains the single pathogen responsible for the most deaths and disease in the world.[3,4] It is estimated that one third of the world's current population is infected with *Mycobacterium tuberculosis* and that 8 million cases of disease and 2 to 3 million deaths can be attributed to this organism annually.[4-6] Although most technologically advanced countries have managed to essentially control—although not eradicate—tuberculosis, the incidence of disease and infection is increasing in many poorer areas of the world. The economic and social consequences of tuberculosis in these developing countries are enormous, and only in the past decade have they been fully recognized by governments, the World Bank, and the World Health Organization (WHO).[7]

There probably is no other widely used vaccine that is as controversial as BCG. Its effects in extremely large randomized, controlled, and case-control studies have been widely disparate, in some cases demonstrating a great degree of protection and in others offering no benefit. However, trials of BCG vaccines have provided some of the best and most complete information on tuberculosis in human populations and have played an important role in the development of vaccine trial methodology.[8] The BCG history contains aspects of folklore and superstition that often supersede facts in discussion and public health policy.[9] Many of the difficulties in evaluating the effectiveness of BCG vaccines are intrinsic to the pathogenic and immunologic events in the host that develop in response to infection with M. *tuberculosis*. The lack of reliable laboratory or serologic markers for immunity

to mycobacteria has hampered efforts to determine how BCG affects the host and what level of protection it provides, and has limited studies of its efficacy to animal models of disease and field trials in humans.[10] Advances in understanding the human immune response to tuberculosis and promising work in the development of new serologic tests will be important for future vaccine development.[11]

Many industrialized countries have decreased their use of BCG vaccination as tuberculosis rates have fallen. However, two developments in the clinical expression of tuberculosis have prompted a renewed interest in BCG vaccination in developed countries, especially within health care settings.[12,13] First, the interaction between tuberculosis and infection with the human immunodeficiency virus (HIV) has been noted. People with untreated HIV infection who were previously infected with M. *tuberculosis* develop tuberculosis disease at a rate of 5% to 10% per year, compared with the lifetime risk of 5% to 10% in immunocompetent adults.[14] The interaction of these infections was partly responsible for the resurgence of tuberculosis in the United States during the late 1980s and early 1990s. The safety and efficacy of BCG vaccination in adults and children with HIV infection are not yet well established.[15,16] Second, outbreaks of tuberculosis caused by strains resistant to both isoniazid and rifampin have occurred in many countries.[17,18] The focal points of many outbreaks have been HIV-infected patients and their health care providers.[19,20] Because no known chemotherapy regimen can prevent the progression of latent tuberculosis infection to tuberculosis disease in people infected with multidrug-resistant M. *tuberculosis*, some experts have suggested that a BCG vaccine should be used in carefully selected high-risk settings in the United States.[21]

Human Tuberculosis: A Brief History

Tuberculosis was probably the leading cause of death in Europe and the United States in recorded history.[22] The earliest known cases of tuberculosis were discovered in ancient Egyptian mummies, who suffered from tuberculosis of the spine, dating back to 4000 to 2000 BC.[23] Pulmonary tuberculosis was known in the time of Hippocrates as *phthisis*, which is derived from the Greek for "wasting away." The incidence of tuberculosis increased dramatically in Europe until the beginning of the 19th century, when rates peaked at 700 cases per 100,000 persons annually, then declined.

As industrialization, urbanization, and the accompanying social trends extended beyond Europe to the United States, tuberculosis followed. In the mid-19th century, annual tuberculosis mortality rates in eastern cities of the United States averaged 400 per 100,000 population. With improving socioeconomic conditions, the mortality rate fell to 200 per 100,000 around 1900 and to 26 per 100,000 by 1950.[24] These rates fell long before the availability of chemotherapy and without the use of BCG vaccine. It has long been recognized that stress in the forms of war, famine, population displacement, and crowded living and working conditions favors the spread of tuberculosis among humans and that periods of improvement in societal conditions favor its rapid decline. The influence of these and other societal conditions on tuberculosis case rates must be considered in BCG vaccine trials, which, by necessity, take place over a prolonged time.

In 1882, Koch identified the tubercle bacillus as the cause of human tuberculosis. The discovery that tuberculosis was an infectious disease led to the development of four basic disease control strategies.[22] First, the lack of effective treatment led to the creation of the sanatorium movement in 1854 in Europe and, in 1882, by Trudeau in the United States.[25] The measures used included exposure to fresh air and sunlight, community participation, and ordinances to improve sanitation and housing. The second development was the application of pasteurization to cow's milk, which virtually eliminated human disease caused by *Mycobacterium bovis*. The third development was the creation of BCG vaccines.[5] The final development was the discovery of antituberculosis drugs, which could cure established disease and prevent progression of latent tuberculosis infection to disease; the discovery of these drugs effectively closed the doors of sanatoria. In the United States, the combined use of curative chemotherapy and contact investigation for persons with infectious tuberculosis has been the cornerstone of tuberculosis control for the past four decades.

Background

Clinical Description

The terminology used for the stages of tuberculosis can be confusing, but it follows the pathophysiology closely.[26] *Latent tuberculosis infection* (LTBI) is the preclinical stage of infection with M. *tuberculosis*. The result of the tuberculin skin test is positive, but findings on chest radiography are basically normal, and there are no signs or symptoms of illness. *Tuberculosis disease* occurs when clinical manifestations of pulmonary or extrapulmonary tuberculosis become apparent, either on the chest radiograph or in clinical signs and symptoms. The word *tuberculosis* usually refers to the disease. The time interval between the establishment of

LTBI and the onset of disease may be several weeks or many decades. This variable, long-term period of dormant infection is one factor that makes BCG vaccine trials so difficult to perform and interpret.

The majority of adults and children who acquire primary infection with M. *tuberculosis* develop no signs or symptoms at any time, because the infection is held dormant by the host's immune system. On occasion, the initiation of infection is marked by several days of low-grade fever and mild cough that are indistinguishable from the symptoms of a viral respiratory infection.

When pulmonary tuberculosis disease occurs, the clinical presentation varies markedly by age. The physical signs and symptoms of primary intrathoracic tuberculosis in children are usually surprisingly meager considering the degree of radiographic changes that are often seen.[27]

Young infants and adolescents are more likely to have significant clinical findings than are older children.[25,28] Many children with pulmonary tuberculosis have no symptoms or physical findings; they are discovered only by contact tracing of an adult with infectious tuberculosis.[29] Nonproductive cough, mild dyspnea, and low-grade fever are the most common symptoms in infants. Other systemic complaints, such as night sweats, anorexia, and decreased activity (malaise), are less common. Pulmonary physical signs are even less common. Some infants and children with bronchial obstruction that is caused by inflamed hilar or peritracheal lymph nodes eroding through the bronchial wall develop signs of air trapping, such as localized wheezing or decreased breath sounds. These may be accompanied by tachypnea or frank respiratory distress.

Reactivation pulmonary tuberculosis occurs most often in adolescents and adults and has a wide spectrum of clinical manifestations. Often, until the disease is moderately or far advanced, symptoms are minimal and are usually attributed to other causes such as bronchitis or "smoker's cough."[30] The most common constitutional symptoms are low-grade fever, night sweats, malaise, irritability, fatigue, weakness, and weight loss.[31,32] The patient initially may experience mild cough, but the respiratory symptoms become more pronounced with the development of caseous necrosis and the liquefaction of lung tissue. At this time, sputum production is usually apparent, often accompanied by mild hemoptysis. Chest pain may be localized and have a pleuritic quality. Dyspnea usually indicates either extensive disease or some form of bronchial obstruction. Physical findings are usually less prominent than would be expected given the degree of radiographic change. Fine rales may be heard over the area of involvement, and egophony will occasionally be heard over a large cavity.

Although reactivation pulmonary tuberculosis may involve any lung segment, the disease occurs in the apical or posterior segment of the upper lobes or the superior segment of the lower lobes in 95% of cases.[31,33,34] The typical pattern is airspace consolidation of a patchy or confluent nature. Cavitation is fairly common in adults with reactivation disease, but lymph node enlargement is rarely seen in the immunocompetent host. As the lesions become chronic, they become more sharply delineated and irregular in contour. The development of fibrosis leads to volume loss in the involved lung. The combination of patchy pneumonitis, fibrosis, and calcification is strongly suggestive of tuberculosis. Older adults are more prone to having unusual radiographic manifestations of tuberculosis, including lower lung field disease.[35]

Adults with HIV infection who develop pulmonary tuberculosis often have a clinical and radiographic presentation that differs from that of the classical disease.[36-38] The earlier tuberculosis develops with concomitant HIV infection, the more "usual" is its clinical presentation, whereas a later presentation often has atypical features.[39] The primary symptoms are usually nonspecific, including fever, cough, malaise, and weight loss. However, with advanced HIV infection, the radiographic presentation of tuberculosis often includes hilar or mediastinal adenopathy and diffuse or miliary pulmonary infiltrates, but an absence of cavitation.[40,41] Lower lung field involvement and endobronchial tuberculosis are much more common in patients with HIV infection.[42] Disseminated or extrapulmonary tuberculosis occurs in more than half of the patients.[39,43]

Extrapulmonary manifestations of disease occur in approximately 15% of immunocompetent adults and 25% of children with tuberculosis.[44] Virtually any organ of the body can be involved. Superficial lymph node disease in the cervical or supraclavicular regions is the most common manifestation, accounting for 67% of the cases of extrapulmonary tuberculosis in children. The affected nodes are typically enlarged and firm and are not tender but are fixed to underlying or overlying tissues.[45] Pleural tuberculosis accounts for almost one quarter of the cases of extrapulmonary tuberculosis, but it is uncommon in children and rare in infants. Other common sites of tuberculosis are the genitourinary system, the bones and joints, the peritoneum, and the pericardium.

Two forms of tuberculosis are rapidly life threatening: disseminated or miliary disease and meningitis. The early clinical manifestations of miliary tuberculosis are protean, depending on the load of disseminated organisms and in which tissues they lodge. Lesions are usually largest in the lungs, spleen, liver, and bone marrow. The onset of clinical disease may be explosive, the patient becoming gravely ill during several days.[46] More often, the onset is insidious. Early systemic signs include malaise, anorexia, weight loss, and low-grade fever. Within several weeks, hepatosplenomegaly and generalized lymphadenopathy develop in about half of the patients. The lungs become filled with tubercles, accompanied by the onset of dyspnea, cough, rales, or wheezing. Signs or symptoms of meningitis or peritonitis are found in 20% to 40% of patients with advanced disease. Early diagnosis is often difficult because the signs and symptoms are nonspecific, classical radiographic findings are absent, and 40% of patients have a negative tuberculin skin test reaction. If untreated, the disease usually becomes fatal.

Central nervous system tuberculosis is the most serious complication, being uniformly fatal if effective treatment is not given.[47,48] The meningeal exudate usually concentrates near the brain stem and may infiltrate the cortical or meningeal blood vessels, producing inflammation, obstruction, and subsequent infarction of the cerebral cortex. The brain stem inflammation accounts for the frequent involvement of cranial nerves III, VI, and VII, and it interferes with the normal flow of cerebrospinal fluid, which leads to hydrocephalus. The clinical progression of tuberculous meningitis may be rapid over several days but more commonly occurs in several weeks. The first stage is characterized by nonspecific symptoms such as fever, headache, malaise, irritability, and drowsiness. The second stage often begins abruptly with lethargy, nuchal rigidity, seizures, vomiting, hypertonia, and focal neurologic findings. The third stage is marked by coma, hemiplegia, deterioration in vital signs, and, eventually, death. The prognosis of tuberculous meningitis correlates closely with the clinical stage of illness at the time that antituberculosis chemotherapy is started. Particularly in developing countries, the diagnosis is often delayed by the lack of available diagnostic tests, and death or profound handicap is a common outcome.

Bacteriology

In 1882, Robert Koch discovered the Koch bacillus—the etiologic agent of human tuberculosis—now known as M. tuberculosis. All members of the genus Mycobacterium share the property of acid-fastness, which is related to the complex cell wall structure that contains derivatives of mycolic acid. Each species of mycobacteria has a unique pattern of mycolic acids that can be distinguished by high-performance liquid chromatography.[49] Several species of mycobacteria with similar growth characteristics and biochemical reactions are classified together into the M. tuberculosis complex. Three species—M. tuberculosis, M. africanum, and M. ulcerans—are primarily human pathogens. M. bovis, the fourth member of this complex, causes tuberculosis primarily in cattle and other animals but can cause disease in humans who have extensive contact with infected animals or who drink animal milk laden with the organism. Veterinary control programs have all but eliminated M. bovis disease in the United States, but human infection still occurs in some countries with less stringent controls.[50]

Although nontuberculous mycobacteria were discovered shortly after Koch's discovery of the tubercle bacillus, they were not recognized as human pathogens until the 1940s, about 20 years after the first use of BCG.[51] Currently, more than 55 species of these nontuberculous or environmental mycobacteria have been described, of which about half can be pathogenic in humans.[52] Many species of nontuberculous mycobacteria are present in soil, ground water, or aerosols throughout the world, with higher concentrations being present nearer the equator. The most ubiquitous species are those of the M. avium-intracellulare complex. Although disease rates resulting from these environmental mycobacteria are low, they probably have other immunologic effects on humans that are of significance in the prevention and control of tuberculosis. Their interactions with the effects of BCG vaccine are probably important and may explain some of the variability in reported clinical trials.

Pathogenesis as It Relates to Prevention

The primary complex of tuberculosis consists of local disease at the portal of entry—which is the lung in more than 95% of cases—and at the regional lymph nodes that drain the area of the primary focus. Tubercle bacilli within inhaled particles larger than 10 μm are usually caught by the mucociliary mechanisms of the bronchial tree and expelled. Smaller particles are inhaled beyond the clearance mechanisms.[53] The number of organisms required to establish infection is unknown, but it is likely that only several organisms are necessary. Most of the bacilli are ingested and killed, but, in animal models, approximately 10% of the organisms survive.[54] These tubercle bacilli multiply first in the alveoli and alveolar ducts. They also multiply within macrophages and are released when these cells die. The released bacilli chemotactically attract inactivated monocytes and lymphocytes from the bloodstream, creating the formation of an early primary tubercle.[55]

After several weeks of infection, great numbers of tubercle bacilli grow symbiotically within inactivated macrophages. The onset of delayed hypersensitivity and cell-mediated immunity greatly alters the pathogenic picture. The "incubation period" between the time the tubercle bacilli enter the body and the development of cutaneous hypersensitivity is usually between 2 and 12 weeks, most often between 3 and 8 weeks. At this time, the tissue reaction intensifies, and the primary complex may temporarily become visible on the chest radiograph. Caseous necrosis and eventual encapsulation of the primary complex usually occur. During the development of the primary complex and the accelerated caseation brought on by the development of delayed hypersensitivity, tubercle bacilli spread from the primary complex to many parts of the body through the blood stream and lymphatics. The tissues most commonly seeded are the liver, spleen, meninges, lymph nodes, kidneys, bone, and apices of the lungs. When this dissemination involves large numbers of bacilli in a susceptible host, disseminated tuberculosis follows. More commonly, small numbers of disseminated bacilli leave microscopic foci in these tissues, which may be the origin of either extrapulmonary tuberculosis or reactivation, adult-type pulmonary tuberculosis that occurs in some individuals.

Tuberculosis disease that occurs more than a year after infection is thought to be caused mainly by endogenous regrowth of persisting bacilli that remain from the primary infection and subclinical dissemination.[56] In some individuals, a temporary decline in the ability of their cell-mediated immunity to keep persisting bacilli dormant leads to massive replication of organisms and reactivation disease. In developed countries with low rates of tuberculosis, disease caused by exogenous reinfection from another person is rare.[57,58] In countries in which tuberculosis rates remain high, exogenous reinfection may be a more common cause of disease. The reactivation form of pulmonary disease has also been called secondary, postprimary, or adult-type tuberculosis. This is the most infectious form of tuberculosis. The most common manifestation of reactivation tuberculosis is an infiltrate or cavity in the apex of the lung. Extrapulmonary forms of tuberculosis, including meningitis, can arise as reactivation disease, but dissemination during reactivation is rare among immunocompetent hosts.

If young children with tuberculosis infection do not suffer primary disease, their risk of developing reactivation tuberculosis later in life is low. Conversely, older children and adolescents rarely develop disease as a complication of the primary infection but have a higher risk of developing reactivation disease as an adolescent or adult. The timing of infection must be taken into account when vaccine efficacy is being determined, and vaccine effects on the occurrence of both primary and reactivation disease must be considered separately because vaccination may prevent one form but not the other.

The immunologic reactions to M. tuberculosis are a critical determinant of clinical expression of infection and vaccine efficacy. Unfortunately, the exact immunologic mechanisms that characterize human resistance to M. tuberculosis remain undetermined. Two important host responses are (1) delayed-type hypersensitivity, which kills bacilli-laden inactivated macrophages, resulting in tissue damage; and, (2) a cell-mediated or macrophage-activating response, which amplifies the ability of macrophages to kill the bacilli they ingest.[59] Although both processes are associated with tuberculin reactivity and are transferable by lymphocytes, there is strong evidence that they are mediated by different mechanisms.[60,61]

One component of immunity to M. tuberculosis is the activation of macrophages by cytokines derived from T-helper (Th) cells. It also appears likely that cytolytic activity is involved in protection by facilitating destruction of immunologically effete, bacilli-laden cells, enabling immunocompetent activated macrophages to rephagocytose bacilli.[61,62] In addition, there is evidence that apoptosis facilitates killing of intracellular bacilli, whereas simple necrosis does not.[63]

An important emerging concept is that differences in the maturation pathways of Th cells may help explain why some mycobacterial challenges do not result in protection as a result of macrophage activation or cytolytic activity.[64] Th cells follow two distinct maturation pathways, resulting in Th1 and Th2 cells. The cell types can be identified by the cytokines they secrete or induce: Th1 cells produce interleukin-2 and interferon-γ, whereas Th2 cells produce or induce interleukin-4, -6, and -10. Cytokines associated with one pathway may inhibit the other, leading to a locked-in immune response.[65] Certain antigenic challenges may "imprint" the immune system with a predisposition to mount either a Th1 or Th2 response to future challenges with the same or a similar antigen.[66]

It appears that progressive tuberculosis is usually associated with a Th2 or a mixed Th1 and Th2 T-cell response, whereas a pure Th1 response mediates protection.[67,68] In the presence of Th1 cytokines, tumor necrosis factor (TNF) facilitates macrophage activation and granuloma formation. However, some factor produced or induced by a Th2 response renders tissues sensitive to destruction by TNF, explaining, in part, the gross tissue necrosis most often seen in reactivation pulmonary tuberculosis.[69,70] Obviously, genetic control over the responses is also important.

It appears that, in tuberculosis, the immune system is a "two-edged sword" capable of inflicting damage to either the invader or the host.[61] An effective vaccine should induce or boost protective immune responses (Th1) but not those that cause tissue necrosis (Th2). One explanation for the marked variation in the efficacy of BCG vaccines is the differing effect of sensitization of the population by saprophytic mycobacteria in the environment. A study in mice demonstrated that prior exposure to environmental mycobacteria (especially M. avim) resulted in an immune response that blocked multiplication of BCG after vaccination and inhibited induction of a protective immune response.[70a] In some regions or populations, an initial Th1 response may be produced by this sensitization that can be boosted by a BCG vaccine, whereas, in others, an induced Th2 response may be boosted, with possible adverse effects.[61] It has been postulated that BCG vaccination of persons already infected with M. tuberculosis may actually promote reactivation of tuberculosis soon after vaccination by enhancing previously weak Th2 mechanisms.[71] In many countries, BCG vaccines are given to newborns before sensitization by environmental mycobacteria can occur. Again, genetic influences or maturational differences in the development of Th-cell pathways could explain different responses to and efficacy of BCG vaccination. The specific cellular and cytokine responses to BCG vaccination in infants remain unstudied.

Diagnosis

In looking at field trials of BCG vaccines, it is critically important to consider the diagnostic techniques used to define subsequent cases of tuberculosis within the study population. In most poor countries, the only diagnostic test is an acid-fast smear of the sputum; mycobacterial cultures and radiography are not available. The limitations of current diagnostic techniques are especially important in considering childhood or extrapulmonary tuberculosis.

Tuberculin Skin Test

A positive reaction to a tuberculin skin test is the hallmark of latent infection with M. tuberculosis. When tuberculin reactivity is due to infection by the tubercle bacillus, it usually remains for the individual's lifetime, even after chemotherapy is taken.[72,73] The "gold standard" test is the Mantoux test, the intradermal injection of purified protein derivative (PPD) by use of a needle and syringe. Although experienced health care workers usually demonstrate good interobserver agreement on results, inexperienced observers frequently report results inaccurately.[74]

Unfortunately, 10% of adults and children with tuberculosis disease have anergy for tuberculin.[75,76] A variety of host-related factors such as young or old age, poor nutrition, immunosuppression by disease or drugs, viral infections (particularly measles, varicella, and influenza), and overwhelming tuberculosis can lower tuberculin reactivity.[77] Many patients co-infected with HIV and M. tuberculosis have anergy for tuberculin with or without anergy to other skin test antigens.[78]

False-positive reactions to tuberculin also occur. Recent exposure to environmental mycobacteria can result in cross-sensitization and a false-positive reaction to a Mantoux test.[79] A study of U.S. naval recruits in the 1950s and 1960s showed that up to 70% of young adults from certain geographic regions (southeastern United States) had some sensitization to mycobacterial antigens.[80] The reactions to tuberculin PPD in these individuals were usually transient and produced an induration of less than 12 mm, although larger reactions occurred.

The interpretation of the Mantoux tuberculin skin test reaction should be influenced by the purpose for which the test was given and by the consequences of false classification. The appropriate cutoff size indicating a positive reaction varies with the person being tested and with related epidemiologic factors.[81] The Centers for Disease Control

and Prevention, the American Academy of Pediatrics, and the American Thoracic Society recommend varying cutoff points for a positive reaction by the risk of tuberculosis infection (Table 12–1). For adults and children at the highest risk for tuberculosis, a reactive area of 5 mm is classified as positive. For other groups at high risk for tuberculosis (Table 12–2), a reactive area of 10 mm is positive. In some locales in which tuberculosis is rare, the cutoff may be increased to 15 mm for individuals with no other risk factors for tuberculosis infection or disease.

Bacille Calmette-Guérin Vaccines and the Tuberculin Skin Test

The various BCG vaccines have an effect on the results of the tuberculin skin test. Unfortunately, the effect is variable, and no reliable method can distinguish tuberculin reactions caused by BCG vaccination from those caused by infection with M. tuberculosis. In various studies with different populations and characteristics, the proportion of previously BCG-vaccinated individuals with significant skin test reactions has ranged from 0% to 90%.[82–88] The size of the skin test reaction after BCG vaccination varies with the strain and dose of the vaccine,[85,89] the route of administration,[88,90] the age of the individual,[84,87,91] the nutritional status

TABLE 12–1 ■ Size of Induration That Determines a Positive Mantoux Tuberculin Skin Test Reaction

≥5 mm	≥10 mm	≥15 mm
Contacts of infectious cases	Other groups at high risk listed in Table 12–2	No risk factors
An abnormal finding on chest radiography		
Human immunodeficiency virus infection or other immunosuppression		
Clinical illness suggestive of tuberculosis		

TABLE 12–2 ■ High-Risk Groups for Tuberculosis in Technologically Advanced Countries

INCREASED RISK OF EXPOSURE TO AN INFECTIOUS ADULT
Foreign-born persons from high-prevalence countries
Poor and medically indigent, especially city residents
Users of intravenous and other street drugs
Residents (present and former) of correctional institutions
Residents of nursing homes
Homeless persons
Health care workers in high-risk settings

INCREASED RISK OF DISEASE OCCURRING AFTER INFECTION
Persons who have co-infection with the human immunodeficiency virus
Persons who have other medical risk factors (e.g., diabetes mellitus, silicosis, carcinoma, gastrectomy)
Persons undergoing immunosuppressive therapies
Persons who are malnourished
Infants and the extreme elderly

of the individual, the number of years since vaccination[84,87,91] and the frequency of skin testing.[92] Some studies have found that the size of the skin test reaction increases with repeated BCG vaccination,[93] whereas others have found no such correlation.[94]

In a large number of studies of children who received BCG vaccine, the mean reaction to a tuberculin skin test ranged from 0 to 19 mm, although many experts believe that reactions larger than 10 to 15 mm after vaccination are unusual. Several studies have shown that the intensity of tuberculin reactivity after BCG vaccination is similar among siblings and correlates most highly among twins, indicating a likely degree of genetic control over the response.[95,96] Tuberculin reactivity then wanes rapidly during the next few years. Lifschitz[84] found that approximately 50% of infants given BCG vaccine shortly after birth were tuberculin negative at 6 months of age, and almost all children were tuberculin negative at 1 year after vaccination. A study among West African infants found that BCG vaccination prior to 1 month of age was associated with more anergy to tuberculin skin testing than vaccination after 1 month of age.[96a] A similar study found that only 18% of Sri Lankan children vaccinated with BCG at birth had significant reactions at 1 year of age, and none was significant at 5 years of age.[97] A study from Canada investigated older children and adults who had received BCG vaccine by the scarification method on the lower back either in infancy or as older children.[83] Among children with a mean age of 11 years at skin testing, 4.9% vaccinated in infancy had a positive tuberculin reaction compared with 12.5% of those vaccinated as older children. Among young adults with a mean age of 23 years at skin testing, 10.3% vaccinated in infancy had a positive skin test result compared with 25.5% of those vaccinated as older children. A similar study found that only 16% of U.S. naval recruits who had received BCG vaccine 8 to 15 years previously had a positive tuberculin skin test reaction at 10 mm or more.[86]

Interpretation of the tuberculin skin test in individuals previously vaccinated with BCG may be complicated by the booster phenomenon. The booster effect is the increase in reaction size to skin testing caused by repetitive testing in a person sensitized to mycobacterial antigens.[98,99] This phenomenon is presumably caused by stimulation of a waned immunologic response to mycobacterial antigens. Studies from Chile have shown that skin test reactions can be boosted significantly in both children and adults who previously received BCG vaccine.[100,101] Boosting is an important cause of "positive" tuberculin skin test reactions among health care workers who previously received a BCG vaccine.[102] Repetition of the skin test in a short period of time (less than 1 year) should be avoided in persons with previous BCG vaccination, or apparent conversions of the reaction from negative to positive may be created.

Severe reactions to a tuberculin skin test are extremely rare in individuals who have previously received BCG and are not infected with M. tuberculosis. Prior BCG vaccination is never a contraindication for tuberculin testing. A reaction to a skin test measuring 10 mm or more in an individual who has been vaccinated with BCG more than 3 years previously usually indicates infection with M. tuberculosis, especially if the individual has lived in an area of the world that has a high prevalence of tuberculosis. Menzies

and Vissandjee[83] found that a significant tuberculin reaction among individuals who received BCG vaccine after infancy had a positive predictive value for infection with M. tuberculosis of 17% among a Canadian-born population and 78% among recent immigrants from an area endemic for tuberculosis. The probability that a skin test reaction has resulted from infection by M. tuberculosis increases (1) as the size of the reaction increases, (2) when a patient is a contact of a person with infectious tuberculosis, (3) if the person is in a high-risk group for tuberculosis, (4) when the patient's country of origin has a high prevalence of tuberculosis, and (5) as the length of time between vaccination and tuberculin testing increases.[94]

Microbiologic Diagnosis

The most important laboratory test for the diagnosis of tuberculosis is the mycobacterial culture. Unfortunately, in many poor regions of the world where tuberculosis case rates are high, cultures are not available. The best culture specimen is freshly expectorated sputum, from which M. tuberculosis can be isolated in about 80% of cases of pulmonary tuberculosis in adults.[30] Most children with pulmonary tuberculosis cannot produce sputum. For them, the best culture material is an early morning gastric aspirate. Unfortunately, the yield from these cultures is less than 50%.[103] The yield from bronchoscopy cultures in children is usually lower than the yield from properly obtained gastric aspirate cultures.[104] The culture yield from body fluids or tissues of patients with various forms of extrapulmonary tuberculosis varies from 30% to 60%. The difficulty in microbiologically confirming the diagnosis of pulmonary tuberculosis in children and of extrapulmonary tuberculosis is a limiting factor of many BCG vaccine efficacy trials.

The most rapid and widely available procedure to detect mycobacteria is microscopic observation with use of acid-fast stains of body fluids or tissues. The most common procedures used for acid-fast staining are the carbolfuchsin methods (Ziehl-Neelsen and Kinyoun stains) and the fluorochrome method (auramine-rhodamine dyes). Fluorochrome methods are more sensitive than carbolfuchsin techniques, but at least 10^4 acid-fast bacilli per milliliter of specimen are required for detection with either method. An acid-fast stain of sputum can identify 40% to 75% of adults with pulmonary tuberculosis.[105,106] Although environmental mycobacteria can be present in sputum and create a false-positive smear, the specificity of the acid-fast smear of sputum is high, especially in locales in which tuberculosis is prevalent.[107] Unfortunately, the sensitivity of acid-fast smears of gastric aspirates from children is low, usually below 10% even in highly endemic areas.

The technique of polymerase chain reaction, which can amplify mycobacterial DNA from a specimen, has a specificity in adults of nearly 100% and a sensitivity similar to that of mycobacterial cultures, but results are available in 72 hours rather than the 3 to 6 weeks often required for conventional cultures.[108,109] The polymerase chain reaction is less useful for diagnosing pulmonary tuberculosis in children because the sensitivity is only 60% and the specificity can be unacceptably low.[110,111] A more recent study comparing an in-house polymerase chain reaction, Amplicor (Roche Diagnostics, Basel, Switzerland), acid-fast smears, and standard mycobacterial culture with clinical diagnosis in children found a sensitivity of 60% and a specificity of 97% for the polymerase chain reaction.[112]

The development of new accurate serologic tests for tuberculosis antigens and urine-based tests for glycolipids for the detection of tuberculosis disease or LTBI is greatly anticipated.[113–116] Better diagnostic tests are needed and will be an important advance in the clinical care of patients as well as tools for vaccine research. Currently the sensitivity, specificity, and positive predictive value of these tests remain low, making them poor diagnostic tools for disease confirmation at this time.[117,118] One test to measure serum interferon concentration as an assay for detection of cell-mediated immunity to tuberculosis is commercially available in Australia.[119] Once established and reliable, these tests may become important in clinical trials for new tuberculosis vaccines, solving many of the methodologic problems encountered with previous BCG vaccine trials. To test vaccine efficacy, patients in past studies had to be followed for signs of clinical tuberculosis over many years because no serologic test for tuberculosis immunity, infection, or disease was available. Once these diagnostic methods become fully developed, future tuberculosis vaccine trials will have better tools for measuring vaccine efficacy.

Clinical Diagnosis

In both developed and poorer nations, the majority of cases of pediatric tuberculosis are diagnosed on clinical grounds with the use of one of several scoring systems based on symptoms, signs, and, when available, radiographic findings.[120] Although helpful, these systems have low sensitivity and specificity. One major unaddressed problem in virtually all reported BCG trials in children is the lack of uniformity of case definitions of pediatric tuberculosis; many study authors did not report a standardized case definition, and some variation of results among trials probably can be attributed to lack of standardization— exactly what was the vaccine preventing or not preventing?

Treatment and Prevention with Antibiotics

Since antituberculosis medications were developed, starting in the 1940s and continuing through the 1960s, tuberculosis has been treatable and preventable. Guidelines for treatment are published by a number of expert groups in the United States, including the American Thoracic Society,[121,122] the American Academy of Pediatrics,[123] and the Centers for Disease Control and Prevention.[124] Most developed countries have their own published guidelines for tuberculosis treatment.[125] For developing countries, the WHO has published guidelines for national programs for tuberculosis treatment and control.[126] In general, tuberculosis disease should be treated with three or four drugs—isoniazid, rifampin, pyrazinamide, and ethambutol or streptomycin—for 2 months, followed by 4 months of isoniazid and rifampin. The choice of three versus four drugs depends on the prevalence of drug resistance in the community and the individual patient's risk of drug resistance. Four drugs usually are recommended for adults with pulmonary tuberculosis until culture and susceptibility results are available. For fully susceptible M. *tuberculosis*, a combination of isoniazid, rifampin, and pyrazinamide is the treatment of choice. Treatment for disseminated tuberculosis, complicated extrapulmonary disease, and multidrug-resistant tuberculosis usually requires more medications, longer treatment, and expert consultation. Adherence to therapy is essential for successful treatment, prevention of relapse, and prevention of drug resistance; therefore, directly observed therapy has become standard treatment in the United States as well as many other parts of the world.

Latent tuberculosis infection and disease are preventable with chemotherapy or chemoprophylaxis. Recommendations for treating exposure and infection vary by the patient's age, risk factors, and medical condition. For LTBI with no evidence of disease, 6 to 9 months of isoniazid has been shown to be efficacious in preventing the development of disease. Treatment of LTBI in adults of any age is recommended for individuals with medical conditions carrying increased risk for progression to disease, such as immunosuppressive disorders; persons with documented recent tuberculin skin test conversion; or individuals with radiographic evidence of previous disease. Prophylactic therapy with isoniazid for close contacts to persons with active pulmonary tuberculosis has been found effective in preventing infection and rapid progression to disease. Isoniazid chemoprophylaxis is recommended in exposed children 4 years of age and younger because there is a higher risk of progression to disease following infection in this age group. Also, disease in young children is more likely to be disseminated and rapid in onset, sometimes before tuberculin skin test conversion. Once infection has been excluded by a negative skin test reaction 3 months after exposure, isoniazid can be discontinued, as long as exposure has been terminated by separation or treatment of the adult source case.

Public health practices of tuberculosis control such as timely contact investigation, treatment of infected contacts, and prophylaxis for young children exposed to tuberculosis, are effective in preventing future cases. In developing countries where resources are limited, funds for medications or for public health investigation services may not be available. Tuberculosis remains one of the leading infectious public health problems worldwide, despite the availability of treatment and technology to eliminate the disease. The lack of adequate resources to control the overwhelming problem of tuberculosis, in part, explains the continued reliance on BCG vaccine in developing countries.

Transmission

Tuberculosis is a highly contagious infection. From 25% to 50% of close contacts of an active case will be infected, and transmission is common in families, schools, and hospitals. The high contagiousness is related to the production of small particle droplets when a patient coughs, and to the low dose required to infect.[126a]

Epidemiology

Developing Countries

Figure 12–1 compares the estimated numbers of tuberculosis cases by regions of the world in 1995, 1999, and 2005.[4] Rates of infection and disease are highest throughout Asia and Africa. In developing countries, the majority of disease is seen among young children and young adults. Despite widespread use of BCG vaccination, disease incidence rates have increased in every region of the world except established market economies (Fig. 12–1). It is estimated that slightly more than 300,000 annual cases are associated with HIV infection. In Africa, HIV-related tuberculosis has boosted the overall incidence of tuberculosis by 20%.[5] Many of these figures are estimates based on models of

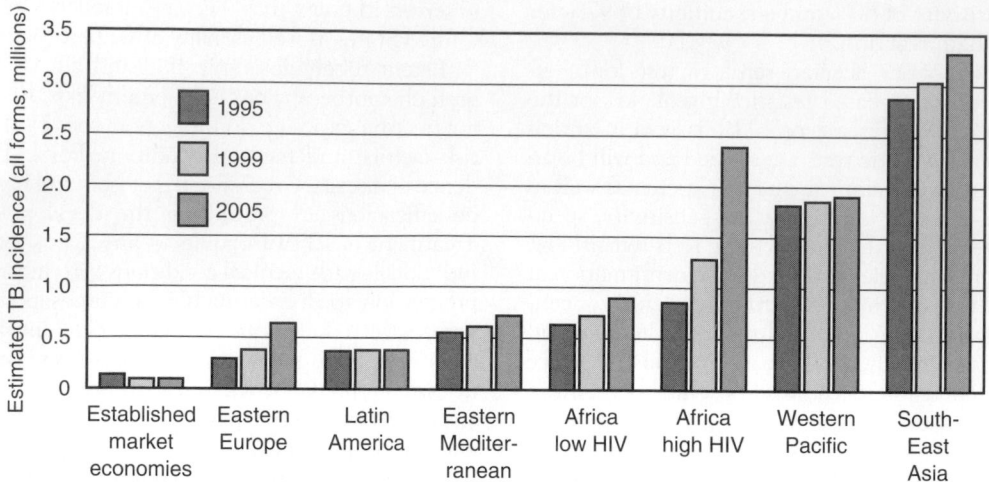

FIGURE 12–1 ■ Estimated numbers of tuberculosis cases by region of the world—1995, 1999, 2005. (From World Health Organization. Global Tuberculosis Control: WHO Report 2001 ((WHO/CDDS/TB/2001.287). Available at *www.who.int/gtb/publications/globerep01/PDF/GTBR2001whoannexes.pdf* Accessed May, 2002).

infectivity, because reported cases represent only a fraction of actual cases.[127] In developing nations, one third to one half of all individuals are infected with M. *tuberculosis*, despite widespread BCG vaccination programs.[5] The average annual incidence of new infection is 1% to 5%, and infection incidence rates are highest among young adults and children. The risk of new infection in these high-prevalence countries is fairly uniform across the population.

Developed Countries

Developed countries, including the United States, experienced a steady decline in tuberculosis case rates from the 1920s to the mid-1980s except among high-risk individuals. In the United States, the annual number of tuberculosis cases increased about 20% between 1984 and 1992.[128] Some of this increase has been linked to the concurrent HIV epidemic, but the immigration of persons at high risk for tuberculosis, the decline in public health services in some communities, and transmission of M. *tuberculosis* in congregate settings (jails, hospitals, nursing homes, shelters) have also contributed to the relative resurgence of tuberculosis. By the year 2000, a total of 16,377 cases were reported in the United States, a 7% decrease from 1999 and a 39% decrease from 1992. During this time period, rates decreased in all groups except immigrants from high-risk countries. Similar trends have been noted in other developed countries, including a national survey in England and Wales in 1998 that found that over 50% of patients with tuberculosis were born outside these countries, 39% in India and 13% in Africa.[129] Of foreign-born persons with tuberculosis, the majority are identified within the first 5 years after immigration.[130]

The peak age of tuberculosis disease varies in different population groups and countries. In most Western countries, tuberculosis infection and disease rates among whites are highest in adults older than 50 years. However, among ethnic and racial minorities, who usually experience infection and disease rates that are substantially higher than those found in whites, the majority of infections and cases occur among young adults and children.[131] In Europe and North America, tuberculosis case rates are high among foreign-born immigrants from countries with a high prevalence of tuberculosis.

Certain environments in Western countries tend to contain large numbers of persons at high risk for tuberculosis. This disease occurs disproportionately among individuals who are poor, are undernourished, have poor access to health care, and live in crowded conditions. Tuberculosis case rates are 10 to 40 times higher within some prisons,[132] nursing homes,[133] homeless populations,[134] and migrant camps[135] than in the general community. However, a recent study in Leeds, United Kingdom, found ethnicity to be the leading risk factor for tuberculosis, independent of lower socioeconomic conditions.[136] Inherited susceptibility to tuberculosis may contribute to variation among different ethnic groups as well. In some areas, health care workers are at risk because of a high likelihood of exposure to infectious patients and improper infection control practices within hospitals and other health care institutions.[137]

Significance as a Public Health Problem

The significance of tuberculosis as a public health problem is self-evident. Tuberculosis remains among the leading causes of morbidity and mortality throughout the world despite the availability of cheap and effective curative therapy, effective preventive therapy, and the use of BCG vaccine in 4 to 5 billion individuals. There is more tuberculosis afflicting humankind now than at any time in history, with 8.42 million cases estimated globally by the WHO in 1999, an increase from 7.96 million cases in 1997.[4] The World Bank calculated that tuberculosis causes about 26% of all avoidable adult deaths in developing countries.[138] Multidrug–resistant tuberculosis is on the rise, with current global rates at 1% to 2% of all cases, but in some areas the problem is much greater. The effects of multidrug–resistant tuberculosis on efforts to control or eliminate the disease will likely become an even bigger problem in the future.

If current trends continue, 10.2 million new cases are predicted in 2005, with 3.4 million in Africa and 3.2 million in Southeast Asia.[4] The inability to control tuberculosis throughout the world represents the most colossal failure of public health services in human history.

Active Immunization with Bacille Calmette-Guérin

History of BCG Vaccine Development

Initial Approaches That Were Abandoned

Organisms other than M. *bovis* have been considered candidates for vaccination of humans against tuberculosis through the years. A killed tubercle bacilli vaccine was studied in the 1930s and was found to have a protective efficacy of about 50% against disease in humans.[139] Avirulent environmental mycobacteria also have been evaluated as vaccine candidates against tuberculosis in humans, with little success. The vole bacillus and BCG are the only vaccines that have been considered seriously for human use.[140]

The live, attenuated BCG vaccine strain was first given orally to infants in Paris in 1921.[141] The peroral vaccine was used in France and other countries. In 1928, the League of Nations announced a declaration of safety for oral BCG vaccine. Unfortunately, from 1929 to 1930, 72 of 250 perorally vaccinated children in Lübeck, Germany, died of tuberculosis caused by laboratory contamination of an oral BCG preparation by virulent tubercle bacilli.[142] Despite this tragedy, BCG vaccination progressed, and new methods of administration were introduced—intradermal in 1927, multiple puncture in 1939, and scarification in 1947.[2]

Description of BCG Vaccine

A brief history of the development of BCG vaccine is summarized in Table 12–3. Two French scientists—Calmette, a physician, and Guérin, a veterinarian—began their studies on a tuberculosis vaccine in 1908.[143] The strain they selected for study was M. *bovis* from a cow with tuberculous mastitis. The isolate was cultured in a medium that contained glycerol, potato slices, and beef bile, the last to prevent contamination with M. *tuberculosis*. The organism was painstakingly subcultured every 3 weeks for 13 years, for a total of 231 cycles. The genotypic changes that resulted at various stages cannot be determined because none of the original cultures or subcultures were preserved. This long process was marked by a loss of virulence first for calves and then for guinea pigs. Phenotypic changes in the organism occurred as well, with colonies changing from rough, dry, and granular to viscous, moist, and smooth. Genotypic analysis suggests that the RD1 region of the M. *tuberculosis* genome, which codes for 9 proteins, is missing in BCG.[143a]

In 1948, the First International BCG Congress in Paris stated that BCG vaccine was effective and safe (despite the total lack of reported controlled trials or case-control studies). After World War II, the WHO and the United Nations International Children's Emergency Fund (UNICEF) organized campaigns to promote vaccination

TABLE 12–3 ■ A Brief History of Bacille Calmette-Guérin Vaccine

1902	First isolation of *Mycobacterium bovis*
1908–1921	BCG developed from serial passage of *Nocardia* strain
1921	First human BCG vaccination
1928	League of Nations adopts BCG as standard vaccine
1929–1930	Lübeck disaster: 72 children die from oral BCG preparation contaminated with virulent strain
1939	Multiple puncture technique
1947	Scarification technique introduced
1948	First International BCG Congress concluded that BCG is effective; more than 10 million vaccinations carried out
1948–1974	WHO and UNICEF campaigns; 1.5 billion vaccinations carried out
1948–1997	Yearly increase of BCG vaccination estimated from 50 million to almost 100 million

BCG, bacille Calmette-Guérin; UNICEF, United Nations International Children's Emergency Fund; WHO, World Health Organization.
Adapted from Lugosi L. Theoretical and methodological aspects of BCG vaccine from the discovery of Calmette and Guérin to molecular biology: a review. Tuber Lung Dis 73:252–261, 1992.

with BCG in several countries. The seed lot system for BCG was established in 1956,[143] and the WHO developed requirements for freeze-dried BCG vaccine in 1966.[144] Rates of BCG vaccination increased dramatically; by the end of 1974, more than 1.5 billion individuals had received the vaccine.

From 1974 to the present, BCG vaccination has been included in the WHO Expanded Programme on Immunization to strengthen the fight against infectious diseases among children in developing countries. Approximately 100 million children receive a BCG vaccine each year, expanding the total number of individuals who have received BCG to more than 4 billion.

Different Strains and Their Relationship

The original strain of M. *bovis* used to make BCG was maintained by serial passage at the Pasteur Institute, until it was lost or discarded. Before its loss, it was distributed to dozens of laboratories in many countries. Each laboratory produced its own BCG and maintained it by serial passage. It became apparent that serial subculturing on various media under the different conditions maintained by the different laboratories resulted in the production of many daughter BCG strains that differed widely in colony morphology, growth characteristics, biochemical activity, ability to cause delayed hypersensitivity, and animal virulence[145–152] (Table 12–4). The patterns of large restriction fragments created by digestion of BCG DNA vary and can be used to accurately identify specific BCG substrains.[153] In an attempt to standardize production and vaccine characteristics, the production laboratories adopted a seed lot system in the mid-1950s. In the 1960s, the WHO recommended the stabilization of the biologic characteristics of the daughter strains by lyophilization and storage of the samples at low temperature.[154]

Interlaboratory studies showed unequivocally that the strains in use today vary widely in many characteristics (see Table 12–4).[155,156] Some investigators have suggested grouping BCG substrains by certain properties.[157] Group 1

TABLE 12–4 ■ Comparison of Some of the Major BCG Vaccine Strains

Vaccine Strain[158]	Other Names	Year Obtained[158]	Strength	IS6110 RFLP[160] (Copies)	MPT64 Protein[158] (Present)	Culturable Particles per Dose[144]	Number of Manufacturers[174]	Complications Reported
Russia	Moscow	1924		2	+	Unknown	2	Disseminated BCG and osteitis
Moreau	Brazil	1925		2	+	Unknown	3	
Japan	Tokyo 172	1925	Weak	2	+	3,000,000	2	Fewer complications
Sweden	Gotheburg	1926		1	+	Unknown		Osteitis
Birkhaug		1927		1	+	Unknown		
Danish	Copenhagen 1131	1931	Strong	1	–	150,000–300,000	13	Increased complications
Prague	Czechoslovakian	1947 (from Danish)		1		Unknown		
Glaxo 1077		1954 (from Danish)	Weak	1		200,000–1,000,000	2	Fewer complications
Tice	Chicago	1934		1		200,000–800,000	1	
Frappier	Montreal	1937		1		200,000–3,200,000		
Connaught	Toronto	1948 (from Frappier)		1		Unknown		
Phipps		1938		1	–	Unknown		
Pasteur 1173 P2		Lyophilized in 1961	Strong	1	–	37,500–500,000	5	Increased complications

(Brazilian, Japanese, Swedish, and Russian) strains have secreted antigens, methoxymycolates, and two copies of the insertion sequence 6110, except for the Swedish strain, which has 1 copy of IS6110.[158] Group 2 (Dakar, Danish, Dutch, British, Pasteur, and Tice) strains have no secreted antigens or methoxymycolates and have only one copy of IS 6110 (see Table 12–4). Laboratory studies and observations in humans have shown that some BCG strains can be called "strong" (Pasteur 1173 P2, Danish 1331), whereas others are "weak" (Glaxo 1077 and Tokyo 172). The strong strains are more immunogenic in various animal models, inducing a greater degree of cutaneous hypersensitivity and better protection from tuberculosis than weaker strains.[159] Other measures of immunity, such as local granuloma formation and residual virulence, are more apparent after vaccination with the strong strains.[149,155] In the guinea pig model of tuberculosis, which is probably the closest to the pathophysiology of tuberculosis in humans, the stronger strains provide better protection.

Genomic evaluation of BCG strains has identified genetic changes over many years, including polymorphisms, duplications, and deletions.[160] Behr outlined a genealogy of BCG vaccine strains based on historical data and suggested a timeline for specific polymorphisms and deletions from the original and daughter strains.[158] There is no question that daughter BCG strains differ from each other and from the original BCG strain. The possible consequences on vaccine efficacy and/or adverse effects are not known. The differences that have evolved following years of serial passage make it difficult to compare BCG strains.

It is difficult to demonstrate that one strain of BCG is clearly superior to another in the protection of humans against tuberculosis.[161] Results of BCG vaccination in case-control studies in children and in contacts of cases whose smears were positive suggest that the protection against tuberculosis differs among the major BCG strains. The WHO has estimated that immediate protection from severe forms of tuberculosis in children is about 60% to 80% for the Glaxo 1077 strain and 60% to 95% for the Tokyo 172 strain.[162] The protection against less severe forms of tuberculosis is 24% to 50% for the Glaxo 1077 strain, 39% to 53% for the Tokyo 172 strain, and 70% to 75% for the Pasteur 1173 P2 strain. Other studies from Hong Kong and Korea also have shown that the protection for children afforded by the Pasteur strain is higher than that of the Glaxo strain.[144] A problem with the interpretation of these data is that childhood tuberculosis is much more difficult to diagnose or confirm than disease in adults, and milder forms of tuberculosis in children may have gone unnoticed in these trials. Differences in populations and environmental conditions also may have affected results of the vaccine trials.

The incidence of side effects with BCG vaccination also differs between strong and weak strains.[163] The strong strains have been associated with a higher rate of lymphadenitis and osteitis, especially among neonates.[164–167] Reduction of the vaccination dose of the strong strains also reduces the incidence of lymphadenitis, probably with little effect on immediate vaccine efficacy.

It is apparent that there is no worldwide consensus about which strain of BCG is optimal for general use. The use of a weaker strain is tempting for both vaccine producers and users, because immediate results without side effects ensure few problems initially.[154] It also appears that various BCG strains have lost efficacy over time with serial passage.[168] It has been postulated that investigators have selected BCG strains by their desire to maximize tuberculin reactivity and minimize adenitis, which may actually create strains that are the inverse of an ideal vaccine. Local customs, history, and tradition have affected vaccine policy in many countries as much as vaccine efficacy and rates of adverse reactions. The past and continued use of both strong and weak vaccine strains makes interpretation and comparison of clinical trials extremely difficult.

Constituents of BCG Vaccine

The biochemical composition of BCG vaccines varies widely, even among preparations derived from the same parent strain. For example, MPB70, a unique BCG-specific antigen that elicits a delayed hypersensitivity reaction in guinea pigs sensitized with viable BCG cells, constitutes up to 10% of the total protein content of the culture medium of the Tokyo strain but only trace amounts of protein in other strains.[144,169] The content of mycoside B, which is associated with colony morphology, varies with the production method.[170] It is not known how variations in these and other products in BCG vaccines correlate with the protective efficacy of or adverse reactions to BCG vaccine.[144]

The Tice strain of BCG vaccine was developed at the University of Illinois from a strain originated at the Pasteur Institute. The BCG organism is grown in a medium containing glycerin, asparagine, citric acid, potassium phosphate, magnesium sulfate, and iron ammonium citrate. Lactose is added to the final preparation prior to freeze-drying. No preservatives are added.[171]

Reconstituted vaccines contain both live bacilli that have pleomorphic coccal and bacillary forms and dead bacilli killed during lyophilization and reconstitution.[172] Studies conducted by the WHO have shown a wide range of culturable bacilli per dose of vaccine from various manufacturers (see Table 12–4). The vaccines with relatively low numbers of bacilli per dose are the strong, more reactogenic strains.

Manufacture of BCG Vaccine

Seed lots are lyophilized bacilli that are part of the original harvest of the various BCG strains. In most laboratories, the bacilli are grown in liquid Sauton medium as a pedicle, the classical surface-grown culture. The organisms can be grown dispersed throughout the liquid media, which produces a slightly different colony morphology.[173] An early harvest of bacilli after 6 to 9 days of growth is essential for good survival of organisms after lyophilization. Even with these controls, the daughter strains are not homogeneous but contain more than one colony type; the proportion of these types in a vaccine can be altered profoundly by culture conditions.[145,170] After filtering and pressing, the semidry mycobacterial mass is homogenized at controlled temperatures, diluted, and then freeze-dried. A stabilizer is added to the preparation. Vaccine stabilized with monosodium glutamate may be more difficult to reconstitute, whereas the presence of albumin may lead to the foaming of the product during reconstitution.[144]

Producers

There are 40 or more manufacturers of BCG vaccine throughout the world. UNICEF purchases an estimated 25% to 30% of the world's BCG supply for distribution to developing countries, the majority of which is produced by Pasteur-Mérieux-Connaught, Evans-Medeva, and the Japan BCG Laboratory. A number of other manufacturers within countries produce vaccine for local use.[174]

Starting in the mid-1970s, an international system for the production and quality control of BCG vaccines was centered at the WHO. Seed lots of the various BCG strains that had previously been subjected to laboratory testing and clinical efficacy studies were maintained by the WHO and the State Serum Institute in Copenhagen, which performed the following tasks[144]: (1) provided technical assistance to national BCG laboratories at the request of the WHO, (2) provided training in BCG production and quality control, (3) distributed reference and seed lots of BCG vaccine, (4) tested candidate BCG vaccines from providers, and (5) tested samples from BCG lots supplied to national immunization programs through UNICEF. This system used by the WHO and coordinated by the Danish State Serum Institute was ended in 1997. Quality control of BCG vaccines is now the responsibility of individual manufacturers, overseen by independent National Regulatory Authorities in the country of manufacture. Many countries do not have fully functional national control authorities; therefore the quality of BCG vaccine remains doubtful or unknown in many areas.[174]

The WHO provides an updated list of "UN Prequalified BCG Vaccines," including the name and address of manufacturers or distributors.[175]

Preparations Available

The various strains of BCG generally are known by the name of the country or laboratory in which they are kept. Although many different strains are in use, four main strains account for more than 90% of the vaccines currently in use worldwide:

1. The French (Pasteur) strain 1173 P2, used in France and by 14 other countries for their production of vaccine[176]
2. The Danish strain 1331
3. The Glaxo strain 1077, derived from the Danish strain 1331 but differing from it substantially in biologic characteristics[145,156,177] (the English "Evans" vaccine and the French "Mérieux" vaccine are the Glaxo 1077 strain)
4. The Tokyo strain 172, selected for its high resistance to lyophilization

Other commonly used strains include the Moreau (Brazil), Montreal (Canada), Russia (former Soviet Union), and Tice (United States).

Currently in the United States there are two licensed BCG vaccines: (1) the Tice strain, derived from the Pasteur strain 1173 P2, developed at the University of Illinois and manufactured by Organon Teknika Corporation (Durham, NC); and (2) the Theracys strain, derived from the Montreal strain and manufactured by Connaught Laboratories (Willowdale, Ontario).

Dosage and Route of Administration

Most countries use the intradermal route of administration using a syringe and needle. Japan and South Africa employ percutaneous administration with a multipuncture device. The last country to discontinue oral administration of BCG vaccine was Brazil in 1973. It is generally accepted that the most accurate method of BCG vaccination is intradermal injection with use of a syringe and needle, because the dose can be measured precisely and the administration can be controlled. Although many body sites can be used for vaccination, the most common site is the deltoid region of the arm. Unfortunately, intradermal injection can be difficult in newborns, especially if a large number of infants require vaccine fairly rapidly. The rate of local reactions, including ulcers and lymphadenitis, is higher with the intradermal method than with any other when other characteristics of the vaccine are controlled.[154] The intradermal method is relatively expensive, and, in many poor countries, the needles and syringes are frequently reused, with the resulting danger of transmission of hepatitis viruses or HIV. Despite these problems, the intradermal method remains widely used throughout the world and is recommended by the WHO and UNICEF.

Other methods of administration were developed to address the problems created by intradermal administration. Subcutaneous injection gives adequate results in terms of induced tuberculin sensitivity but frequently produces abscesses and unsightly, retracted scars.[178] Other techniques, such as scarification, jet injection, and use of bifurcated needles, have yielded highly variable and, in some cases, inadequate results.[178–180] The advantages of using these alternative techniques are a lower local complication rate and a choice of using a single-dose unit, which avoids cross-contamination among vaccine recipients. The multiple puncture technique was developed in the 1940s, with good early success.[181–183] The Tice vaccine in the United States uses a multipuncture technique. A multipuncture technique has been used for more than 40 years in Japan, with good apparent success and a low rate of adverse reactions.[154] There have been no conclusive reported trials that compared the various techniques of BCG administration for protection against subsequent tuberculosis, although local complication rates are generally lowest with multipuncture devices.

The recommended dosage of BCG vaccine differs by vaccine strain and age of the recipient. Most manufacturers recommend a 0.05-mL dose for infants and a 0.1-mL dose for children and adults. For each strain, the dosage is adjusted to maximize the protective effect and minimize the local reactions. The two factors that determine these results are the total mass of organisms and the viable bacilli count in the vaccine.

Vaccine Stability

For established BCG vaccines, repeated measurements of tuberculin sensitivity and lesion size as well as various in vitro tests on cultured BCG bacilli are used to verify that the vaccine lots are being reproduced satisfactorily.[144] In addition, the WHO suggests to the national programs that any change in manufacturing procedure be accompanied by field trials in tuberculin-negative humans to determine the optimal content of BCG bacilli. It is required that manufacturers conduct such studies in children on at least one batch of vaccine per year.

Several in vitro tests are used to verify consistency of BCG vaccines. A test for the number of viable bacilli is carried out by either colony growth in media or measurements of bioluminescence that are proportional to the adenosine triphosphate content of the vaccine. Growth in media is subject to considerable laboratory variability, and conditions must be controlled firmly. The viability of the vaccine is calculated by comparing the total bacterial mass as determined by dry weight or opacity with the count of viable bacilli. In general, the extent of the local reaction to BCG vaccination is proportional to the total bacterial mass, whereas the level of tuberculin sensitivity induced by the vaccine is related to the number of viable particles.[144] The thermal stability of each lot of BCG is tested. The WHO requires that the number of viable particles present after 28 days of incubation at 37°C must not be less than 20% of that in samples stored at 4°C. Differences in thermal stability can be attributed to the growth characteristics of the strain and the preparation, packaging, and storage of the lyophilized vaccine.[156,184]

Other routine quality control procedures carried out by most production laboratories include a test of identity, a test for contamination, and a test for safety in guinea pigs.

Results of Vaccination

Immune Responses to Bacille Calmette-Guérin Vaccine

The exact immune response elicited by BCG vaccination and the mechanism of action within the host are not well understood. Some information can be gleaned from field trials and autopsy studies in humans and protection studies in various animal models of tuberculosis.

Most of the major field trials and case-control trials of BCG vaccines have demonstrated that they afford a higher level of protection against the most serious forms of tuberculosis—such as meningitis and disseminated disease—than against the more moderate forms of disease.[185,186] These observations have led to the hypothesis that the protective effect of BCG derives from its interference with the hematogenous spread of bacilli from the primary focus. That is, BCG vaccination does not prevent infection with M. tuberculosis but helps the host to retard the growth of organisms at the primary site of infection and prevent massive lymphohematogenous dissemination. This hypothesis is supported by autopsy studies in humans that have shown that virtually all infections with M. tuberculosis lead to the development of pulmonary foci irrespective of the BCG vaccination status of the individual.[187]

Experiments using animal models of tuberculosis have supported the results found in humans.[10] Studies in guinea pigs and mice inoculated with tubercle bacilli by the respiratory, intravenous, or subcutaneous routes have shown that tubercle bacilli multiply for several days equally well in BCG-vaccinated and unvaccinated animals.[188–190] In the guinea pig model, the number of tubercle bacilli recovered from the lung, spleen, and lymph nodes increases at the same rate in both vaccinated and unvaccinated animals until the 14th day after infection, when replication rates fall off in the vaccinated animals.[191] The obvious implication from these studies is that BCG vaccination does not result in the permanent creation of activated macrophages within the lung.[192,193]

Studies of the immunologic events that occur within the human host after BCG vaccination are almost totally lacking. Animal studies examining the immune responses to BCG in relation to infection with M. tuberculosis have been surprisingly infrequent.[10] From some of these studies, several broad conclusions can be made with some confidence:

1. Protective immunity cannot be transferred with serum, indicating the lack of importance of antibodies in immunity.
2. Protection can be transferred with T lymphocytes, with the characteristics of the lymphocyte subpopulation required depending on the length of the interval after vaccination.[194,195]
3. The immune response in animals with strong resistance to tuberculosis does not differ from that in susceptible animals until days after infection, implying that macrophages are not activated in an immune animal.
4. The production of hydrogen peroxide and superoxide anion by activated macrophages is enhanced in animals that have been vaccinated with BCG, leading to a greater bactericidal effect against M. tuberculosis.[196]

There has been much debate concerning which epitopes of BCG induce protective immunity. It has been assumed that species-specific antigens afford protection against tuberculosis, but recent evidence suggests that this notion is incorrect. Several studies have shown that BCG vaccine affords protection against Mycobacterium leprae infection that is as great as or even greater than that against tuberculosis.[197–199] The only epitopes shared by M. tuberculosis and M. leprae are common to all mycobacteria. There is also some epidemiologic evidence that BCG protects children from lymphadenitis caused by nontuberculous mycobacteria, especially those of the M. avium complex.[200,201] It is likely that efficacy of BCG and other mycobacterial vaccines may depend on the manner in which common antigens are presented and the innate reactivity of the host immune system.[61]

Vaccination with BCG may actually act as an adjuvant for other vaccines given during the neonatal period.[201a]

Correlates of Protection

A major difficulty in studying tuberculosis and BCG immunization is the lack of an accurate immunoassay that correlates with resistance to infection. There is no serologic test for protective immunity after tuberculosis infection or BCG vaccination. Although most infectious diseases and commonly used vaccines cause a measurable serologic response for an average known duration, BCG and tuberculosis do not.[196] The immunology is complicated, and development of an assay has been hampered by the lack of understanding of the protective response and the inability to identify specific antigens that stimulate immunity. Cellular immunity has been shown to play the major role in protection, but the specific antigenic determinants and the mechanisms involved in this response are not known. Although

M. tuberculosis and BCG share many common antigens, it is unclear whether they share the specific antigenic determinants of immunity.

Given our incomplete understanding of tuberculosis immunology, we are left with imperfect indicators of immunity. Tuberculin skin test conversion has long been used as evidence of mycobacterial infection or as a sign of adequate response to BCG vaccine. Many public health programs practice repeated vaccination until individuals become tuberculin positive, believing that reactivity indicates effective protection. The relationship between postvaccination delayed hypersensitivity and protective immunity is a controversial issue, with no clear relationship established.[202] Neither the presence nor the size of postvaccination tuberculin skin test reactions reliably predicts the degree of protection afforded by BCG.[203,204] Animal studies evaluating this question have observed the following[10]: (1) no direct relationship between the size of the skin test reaction and the degree of acquired resistance was found, (2) some vaccinated animals whose skin test results remained negative were protected, and (3) tuberculin testing boosted a waning tuberculin reaction but did not boost a waning protective response. In humans, results of the Medical Research Council's BCG trial in Great Britain demonstrated a high level of protection against tuberculosis and showed that the degree of tuberculin sensitivity was independent of the degree of protection conferred by vaccination.[202] Other studies, such as the Chingleput trial in southern India, demonstrated poor protective efficacy yet had high levels of vaccine-induced tuberculin sensitivity.[205,206] Other researchers have suggested a "two-pathway" theory, proposing that BCG vaccination may trigger either protective (Lister type) or antagonistic (tuberculin or Koch type) reactions, with the most protective vaccines producing little or no tuberculin-sensitizing reactions because the two pathways are competitive.[207–210] Although the skin test reaction indicates a response of the immune system to mycobacterial infection or BCG vaccination in animals and humans, how this reaction is related to protective immunity remains unsettled. Most experts conclude that immunity and the presence of tuberculin sensitivity are related in some way but are not identical.

Advances in technology have resulted in the identification of several important proteins, antigens, and cell-mediated mechanisms related to M. tuberculosis infection and response to BCG vaccination. There has been much interest in the area of Th-cell cytokine response, the production of interferon-γ, and its possible relationship to protective immunity against tuberculosis.[211,211a] Cytotoxic lymphocytes that lyse infected macrophages also may be important in protection.[212,213] A number of antigens found in M. tuberculosis, including AG85, MPT64, ESAT-6, and CFP10, have been identified and studied as possible tools for diagnostic tests.[214] Cross-reactivity of these antigens has made it difficult to distinguish among BCG, M. tuberculosis, and environmental mycobacteria in some cases. A whole blood assay, the Quanti-FERON-TB test (CSL, Melbourne, Australia), that measures interferon-γ is commercially available in Australia and tests for latent tuberculosis infection. This assay may have advantages over the tuberculin skin test.[215] New breakthroughs in technology are on the horizon that should improve the diagnostic tools available and will be important in future vaccine trials.

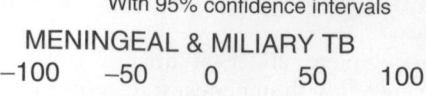

BCG vaccine efficacy (%)
With 95% confidence intervals

Asterisks (*) denote studies of
pulmonary disease in children

MENINGEAL & MILIARY TB

−100   −50   0   50   100

Study Location	Ref	Study Type	Vaccine Strain	Total Cases
Native Americana (Mil TB)	235	CT	Phipps	10
England (Both)	236	CT	Copenhagen	10
Argentina (Both)	221	CC	Mixed	18
Sao Paulo, Brazil (TBM)	186	CC	Moreau	68
Balo Horizonte, Brazil (TBM)	222	CC	Moreau	45
Indonesia (Both)	280	CC	Japan / Pasteur	15

PULMONARY TB

Study Location	Ref	Study Type	Vaccine Strain	Total Cases
England	236	CT	Copenhagen	203
Native Americans, USA	235	CT	Phipps	249
Puerto Rico	237	CT	Park	295
Mandanapalle, India	238	CT	Madras	80
USA (Georgia & Alabama)	242	CT	Tice	60
Chingleput, India	206	CT	Copen/Pasteur	533
USA (Muscogee Co, Georgia)	240	CT	Tice	7
Cameroon	278	CC	Pasteur	213
Argentina*	221	CC	Mixed	131
Indonesia*	280	CC	Japan/Pasteur	66
Kenya	230	CC	Glaxo	126
Colombia*	282	CC	Copenhagen	178

TB (VARIOUS)

Study Location	Ref	Study Type	Vaccine Strain	Total Cases
Chicago, USA	234	CT	Tice	75
Togo*	279	HH	Glaxo	175
Thailand*	257	HH	Pasteur	218
Papua New Guinea*	266	CC	?	114

LEPROSY

Study Location	Ref	Study Type	Vaccine Strain	Total Cases
Uganda	224	CT	Glaxo	242
Papua New Guinea	223	CT	Japan	283
Chingleput, India	229	CT	Copen/Pasteur	6219
Burma	226	CT	Glaxo	1494
Kenya	230	CC	Glaxo	69
Myanmar	225	CC	Mixed	245
Karonga, Malawi	228	COH	Glaxo	137
Vietnam	227	CC	Mixed	177

FIGURE 12–2 ■ Estimates of BCG vaccine efficacy against different forms of tuberculosis and leprosy, from clinical trials (CT), case control (CC), cohort (COH), and household (HH) studies. (Adapted from Fine PEM, Carneiro IAM, Milstien JB, Clements CJ. Issues Relating to the Use of BCG in Immunization Programmes: A Discussion Document. Geneva, World Health Organization, Department of Vaccines and Biologicals, 1999.)

Efficacy and Effectiveness of Bacille Calmette-Guérin Vaccine

The true effectiveness of BCG vaccine has been debated for decades. Large clinical trials conducted from the 1930s through the 1970s yielded wide-ranging and conflicting results, demonstrating efficacy ranging from 0% to 80% (Fig. 12–2). The most recent trial, in Chingleput, India, designed with hopes of settling the question of BCG's efficacy once and for all, had discouraging results and methodologic difficulties that only served to continue the argument.[205,206] Experts have offered a number of explanations for the variation in results among trials, but no one theory has been proved.[178,216–220] In recent years, researchers have studied BCG efficacy using case-control, cohort, household contact, and meta-analysis study designs, but conclusions still diverge. Even with years of study and discussion, the question "Does BCG work?" cannot be answered definitively.

Despite problems and uncertainties, BCG has enjoyed great success in one aspect—its widespread use. It is difficult to evaluate the success of the various national BCG vaccination programs for a number of reasons. Many of these programs were instituted during times of social, economic, and public health improvements that may have effected a decrease in tuberculosis independent of BCG vaccination efforts. Most of the individuals vaccinated during the early programs are only now reaching the age at which tuberculosis is most important as a public health problem,[202] and the effects of BCG on them may not yet be apparent.

Despite the controversy, there are two areas in which BCG vaccine has shown consistent benefits: protection against disseminated tuberculosis disease[221,222] and protection against leprosy.[223–228] Various studies, including controlled trials, case-control studies, and meta-analyses, have demonstrated high levels of protection against miliary tuberculosis and tuberculous meningitis, especially among vaccinated infants (see Fig. 12–2). It is generally accepted that BCG vaccine is most efficacious in preventing severe childhood disease. BCG vaccines also appear to have good efficacy against leprosy (see Fig. 12–2) and likely have contributed toward lower rates worldwide.[229–230]

Major Controlled Field Trials of BCG Vaccine

Figure 12–2 displays the estimates of efficacy from the major BCG field trials—case-control, cohort, and household contact studies.[174] Comparing the major controlled trials is difficult because they differed in a number of important aspects, including eligibility criteria, methods of disease surveillance, diagnostic criteria, vaccine strain and administration, and environmental factors. Comstock[231] has published a comprehensive comparison of the major BCG vaccine studies. Extensive discussion comparing the controlled trials also is reviewed in previous editions of this textbook.[232,233]

The randomized controlled trial is the ideal study design to address vaccine efficacy, but several considerations have complicated the evaluation of BCG vaccine with use of this method. First, the lack of a serologic test for immunity precludes laboratory determination of protection, requiring long-term clinical observation of a large population. Second, the low incidence of tuberculosis and long incubation period for disease mean that huge study groups must be observed for long periods at great cost. Third, there is no gold standard for diagnosis of tuberculosis disease other than acid-fast stain and mycobacterial culture, which can have low sensitivity, especially among children. Also, many of these trials were conducted in developing countries in which resources for diagnosis, vaccination, follow-up, and tracking were inadequate. These challenges as well as the lack of understanding of the immunology involved in protection against tuberculosis make the design and execution of clinical trials extremely difficult.

The controlled trials shown in Figure 12–2 can be grouped into three categories: those showing excellent, moderate, or poor to no protection. Three of the clinical trials demonstrated excellent protection for pulmonary and various forms of tuberculosis.[234–236] The first was conducted among North American Indians in the 1930s. The estimated efficacy in this trial was 80% with good statistical precision, calculated by subsequent investigators.[216] The second study was also conducted in the 1930s, in Chicago, among infants living in high-risk areas. The protective efficacy was 75% with good statistical precision. The third

trial, which demonstrated excellent protection, was initiated in 1950 among British schoolchildren and showed 75% efficacy. These three clinical trials had two characteristics in common. First, they were conducted in northern geographic areas with a low prevalence of environmental mycobacteria. Second, the methodology and statistical precision of these three trials have been judged to be superior compared with those of the other major BCG trials.[216]

Two clinical trials of BCG efficacy demonstrated moderate protective efficacy. The first was sponsored by the U.S. Public Health Service and conducted in Puerto Rico starting in 1949.[237] There were 73 cases of tuberculosis among the control subjects and 93 in the vaccinated group, resulting in an efficacy of 29%. The second study showing moderate protection was carried out in southern India (Madanapalle) and enrolled patients between 1950 and 1955.[238] The efficacy was originally estimated at 60%, but, after 15 years of follow-up, the protective effect had decreased to 20% with wide confidence intervals.[239] The methodology of both of these trials had many potential biases and inadequate statistical precision.[216] Both were conducted in areas with a high prevalence of environmental mycobacteria.

Three clinical trials demonstrated poor protection or no protective effect of BCG vaccination. The first was conducted in Muscogee County, Georgia, beginning in 1947.[240,241] Three cases of tuberculosis occurred in the control group and five in the vaccinated group, resulting in a negative protective efficacy and wide confidence intervals. The second study was carried out in Georgia and Alabama beginning in 1950.[242] There were 32 cases of tuberculosis in the control group and 26 cases in the BCG group, resulting in a protective efficacy of 6% with wide confidence intervals. Both of the trials in Georgia and Alabama were conducted in areas with a high prevalence of environmental mycobacteria. Both trials had potential problems with methodology, including a lack of random allocation of subjects, who were assigned by birth year, and passive follow-up surveillance for cases.

The largest BCG field trial ever conducted was cosponsored by the Indian Council of Medical Research, the WHO, and the U.S. Public Health Service. Intake began in 1968 in the Chingleput district of southern India and involved 260,000 participants from a population of 360,000.[205,206] Children younger than 1 month were excluded, but all others were eligible regardless of age or skin test reaction. Participants were randomly divided into six groups, four to receive two different doses of two types of lyophilized vaccine and two groups to receive placebo. Ten years of follow-up were planned at 2.5-year intervals, using skin tests and chest radiographs. Sputum smears and cultures were to be collected if radiographs showed evidence of tuberculosis. Unfortunately, the follow-up varied among groups depending on size of the intake skin test reaction, age, and perception of risk. Chest radiographs were not obtained for persons younger than 10 years, and only those patients with symptoms or with previous radiographs that were suggestive of tuberculosis had repeated studies at follow-up in some of the surveys. Evaluation of inter-reader variation of radiographic interpretation found low agreement. Readers agreed in only 40% to 47% of radiographic categories ranging from most severe to probable or possible tuberculosis.[206] Bacteriologic confirmation of cases diagnosed by radiography was obtained for only 22% of cases. Because of the wide range of disagreement in interpretation of chest radiographs and low yield of culture confirmation, radiographic diagnosis of tuberculosis was deemed unsatisfactory, and cases were defined only on the basis of sputum cultures that were positive for M. *tuberculosis*. Potential bias in the Chingleput study included both surveillance and diagnostic testing because of the method of follow-up. Cases among young children were probably missed because they did not routinely receive radiographs unless they were symptomatic, and symptoms are often subtle or absent in this age group. Also, case definition based on positive sputum culture is known to have poor yield in children, with only 40% to 50% testing positive under the best of circumstances. It is also noteworthy that the study was conducted in a geographic area in which environmental mycobacteria are endemic. The first results were published in 1979, after 7.5 years of follow-up. Neither of the two vaccines studied, in full or reduced dosage, showed any evidence of protection against pulmonary tuberculosis compared with that of placebo. Thus the world's largest BCG field trial served only to create more uncertainties rather than to resolve issues about the efficacy of BCG.

Possible Factors Creating Variation in Field Trials of BCG

The protection demonstrated in the major controlled BCG field trials ranged from none to 80%. It is unclear why such a wide range of results has been found in these trials, and a number of theories attempting to explain these differences have been developed (Table 12–5). Some believe that this issue cannot be answered until we have a better understanding of the immune response to tuberculosis and BCG vaccine. It is unlikely that a single explanation can account for the variation among trials.

TRIAL METHODOLOGY

Substantial variation in the quality of the methodology used in the BCG trials may have affected the outcomes. It is easy to understand the heterogeneity of methods used because the trials were conducted between 1935 and 1975 in nine

TABLE 12–5 ■ Theories Explaining Different Outcomes in Controlled Trials of Bacille Calmette-Guérin Vaccine

Trial methodology
  Subject assignment
  Diagnostic surveillance
  Case definition
  Statistical precision
Variations in vaccine
  Strain
  Administration
  Potency
  Dose
Environmental mycobacteria
  Protective effect
  Vaccine interference
Regional difference in strains of *Mycobacterium tuberculosis*
Exogenous reinfection versus endogenous reactivation

different geographic areas in three different countries, and they were directed by a number of different investigators and organizations. Further difficulties in carrying out these trials included the large number of subjects and the long duration of follow-up that was required as well as the lack of resources in some of the regions in which the studies were conducted. Double-blind methods could not be used because BCG vaccination often leaves a cutaneous scar, making it difficult to conceal the vaccination status of subjects. Subject assignment, method of case definition, diagnostic surveillance, and statistical precision are all important aspects of study design that may affect outcome and introduce bias. The role of methodologic and statistical variation among the eight major BCG trials has been critically evaluated. Some authors argue that methodologic differences may have biased some of the trials and account for the variability in outcomes,[216] whereas others believe that none of the defects in methods could have appreciably affected the results.[220,231] Unfortunately, none of the trials was conducted using all the standards of ideal experimental design.

Methodologic problems leading to bias may arise if assignment of patients is not randomized. Vaccine assignment should be based on characteristics that are unrelated to tuberculosis susceptibility, such as the patient's registration number. Vaccine recipients and control subjects should have an equal distribution of known risk factors for tuberculosis, such as age, socioeconomic status, medical conditions, and exposure. These safeguards are essential in ensuring the choice of unbiased study groups. Three of the controlled trials had methodologic problems with subject assignment, including the Chicago, Madanapalle, and Chingleput trials. All of the controlled trials used different eligibility criteria, such as age, tuberculin sensitivity, and risk of exposure, making it difficult to compare the data.

Most of the trials revealed inconsistencies and problems with the methods of case surveillance and diagnosis. A difficult challenge in studying tuberculosis is the lack of a sensitive, objective, and reliable gold standard for case diagnosis. Clearly, any patient with culture-proven tuberculosis is a case. The problems with mycobacterial cultures include low sensitivity in some populations, especially in children, and their long incubation period. Because culture may not be a sensitive diagnostic test, a combination of epidemiologic, historical, physical, radiographic, and laboratory findings must be considered for diagnosis. Clinical symptoms alone may be misleading in both adults and children because early cases may be asymptomatic. Results from some British trials showed that more than half the cases of tuberculosis were found during radiographic screening in asymptomatic patients.[139] Also, tuberculin skin test status was used as part of the diagnostic criteria for case finding in some of the trials. Because BCG vaccine can cause a positive result on a tuberculin skin test, cases may have been overestimated among the vaccinees, leading to an underestimation of the efficacy of the vaccine. Unequal surveillance of study groups may have led to underestimation or overestimation of disease. Both groups should have been observed equally to elicit symptoms and physical or radiographic findings that might have indicated tuberculosis. Diagnostic tests should have been ordered with use of the same criteria in both the vaccinated and control groups to ensure equal testing.

Five of the controlled trials had methodologic problems with surveillance and diagnostic testing. The Georgia, Puerto Rico, and Georgia–Alabama trials had no scheduled follow-up procedures, no blinded diagnostic review of radiographs, and no report of the frequencies and indications for chest radiographs. The Madanapalle and Chingleput trials also had flaws in diagnostic follow-up. Early in the Madanapalle trial, patients were observed actively and equally, and reviews were performed in a blinded fashion. With time, these safeguards were abandoned. In the Chingleput trial, the study population was actively observed, but the level of follow-up for children and tuberculin-negative patients is unclear. Cases were defined on the basis of sputum cultures that were positive for M. tuberculosis even though most children with tuberculosis do not produce sputum. Children younger than 10 years did not receive radiographs at intake, although all ages were included for vaccination, which may have led to inclusion of children who had disease at the time of enrollment. Adult patients may have been misclassified as well by the omission of radiographs, because follow-up radiographs were obtained only for patients with symptoms or a history of previously abnormal films. Radiographic blinding and reader verification were used in the Chingleput trial, but low agreement and poor correlation made these data useless in case definition.

In addition, statistical precision, which is based on the number of patients enrolled and the incidence of disease in the study population, is an important consideration in evaluating the accuracy of the results. The confidence interval estimates the precision of the results and is the range within which the true magnitude of effect lies 95% of the time. The statistical accuracy of the BCG trials has been compared in a number of publications and is illustrated in Figure 12–2.[216,243] Three trials had narrow confidence intervals, indicating high statistical precision, including the North American Indian study, the British study, and the Chicago study. These trials also reported the highest protective efficacy and demonstrated the least biased methodology. The other five trials had wide confidence intervals, indicating poor precision, and lower reported protective efficacy. The poor precision of these trials failed to exclude the possibility of higher protective efficacy.

VARIATIONS IN VACCINES

At least six different vaccines were used in the BCG controlled trials. Fresh vaccine was used in all of the studies except the Chingleput trial, which used freeze-dried preparations. Some field trials have used different vaccines within the same trial and demonstrated equal efficacy. The Chingleput and some British studies used two different vaccines. British BCG and vole vaccine from Copenhagen Laboratory were used in a British trial and demonstrated a similar protective efficacy of 77% after 20 years of follow-up.[236] The Chingleput trial also used Copenhagen BCG as well as Madras BCG vaccine. Although the results of the Indian study were different from those of the British trial, the two vaccines had similar results within the Chingleput trial.[205,206] In these examples, different vaccines have shown similar results when they are compared within the same trial and study populations.

Some vaccine strains have yielded inconsistent results among trials.[13] The Copenhagen BCG vaccine, used in the general population of southern India[238] and British schoolchildren,[236] demonstrated extremely variable efficacy between trials—0% in the Chingleput study compared with 77% in the British study. Three studies conducted in North America—the Chicago, Georgia, and Georgia–Alabama studies—used the Tice BCG vaccine yet found variable efficacy of 75%, 0%, and 14%, respectively.[235,240,242,243] Live BCG vaccine strains have changed over time, yet the trends in efficacy of BCG vaccination have not increased or decreased during almost 60 years of use.[219] On the basis of available information, definite conclusions cannot be drawn about the protective effect of the different BCG vaccines, although it is unlikely that a difference among vaccines is the only explanation for the variable results among trials.

ENVIRONMENTAL MYCOBACTERIA

The interaction between environmental mycobacteria and BCG vaccination has been considered a possible cause for variation in results among BCG trials.[218,220,244,245] Exposure to environmental mycobacteria may lead to low-grade tuberculin sensitivity, which may be associated with immunity against tuberculosis. Sensitization to environmental mycobacteria has been shown to have specific geographic patterns of distribution, occurring primarily in the tropical and subtropical regions of the world. Europe and northern parts of North America have a low prevalence of environmental mycobacteria sensitivity. In southern areas of the United States and India, skin test surveys indicate a high level of sensitization to environmental mycobacteria. Three of the controlled trials were conducted in geographic areas in which the prevalence of environmental mycobacteria is low, and these studies demonstrated the highest vaccine efficacy. Conversely, the five trials conducted in the southern United States and southern India, where the prevalence of environmental mycobacteria is high, demonstrated low vaccine efficacy. If sensitization to environmental mycobacteria induced any protective effect against tuberculosis, it could be more difficult to demonstrate a protective effect for a second agent, in this case BCG vaccine.

Evidence in animal and human studies indicates that sensitization to environmental mycobacteria provides protection against tuberculosis similar to that provided by BCG. A study of navy recruits in the United States found that those with low-grade tuberculin sensitivity had about half the incidence of tuberculosis of those with negative tuberculin skin test reactions, suggesting that sensitization to environmental mycobacteria provided some protective effect.[246] Animal studies have shown that infection with some environmental mycobacteria can induce as much protection against tuberculosis as BCG can.[247,248] In contrast, some environmental mycobacteria can block induction of immunity to TB by BCG.[248a] In addition, administration of BCG to guinea pigs previously infected with environmental mycobacteria did not boost their level of protection against tuberculosis. Obviously, sensitization to environmental mycobacteria does not provide a high level of protection against tuberculosis, because the disease continues to be prevalent in some areas with high environmental mycobacteria exposure, such as the Chingleput area of India. Some investigators have suggested that exposure to environmental mycobacteria might interfere with the response to BCG vaccination.[244,245]

HOST FACTORS

Variation in clinical trials conducted in different populations has led to the hypothesis that genetic or nutritional factors might influence the immune response. Evidence from animal research suggests that genetic factors may determine the host's response to BCG vaccines.[54,249–252] It is possible that vaccine efficacy may be lower in certain human populations owing to genetic, rather than environmental, factors. Some animal research has demonstrated that nutritional deficiencies can lower the immunologic response to BCG vaccination.[253–255] However, studies in humans have found no evidence to support this concept.[242,256,257] Interestingly, helminthic infections may reduce skin test positivity after BCG through induction of Th2 type cytokines.[257a]

REGIONAL DIFFERENCES IN MYCOBACTERIUM TUBERCULOSIS STRAINS

The theory that BCG vaccine did not protect against the regional strain of tuberculosis has been raised in respect to the Chingleput trial. The endemic strain of tuberculosis in that area is known as the south Indian variant, notable for its relatively low virulence in guinea pigs. However, studies in guinea pigs demonstrated that the Copenhagen BCG vaccine, used in the Chingleput trial, induced a high level of protection against the south Indian variant strain as well as other strains of M. tuberculosis.[258] Relatively new techniques that identify strains of tuberculosis by DNA fingerprinting may facilitate future studies of strain-related differences.

EXOGENOUS REINFECTION VERSUS ENDOGENOUS REACTIVATION

BCG vaccination does not prevent infection with M. tuberculosis but may prevent dissemination of disease. Also, in persons infected with M. tuberculosis, subsequent vaccination with BCG does not augment the level of immune response. Studies in guinea pigs demonstrated that previous infection with M. tuberculosis does not prevent reinfection with another strain in the lungs but does prevent dissemination of the second strain.[259] The majority of tuberculosis disease in adults in developed countries, such as the United States, is thought to arise from endogenous reactivation of organisms harbored within a previously infected host, as opposed to exogenous reinfection from contact with an infectious source case.[260] However, in areas in which the prevalence of tuberculosis is high, such as in many developing countries, exogenous reinfection may play a more significant role in disease transmission. Epidemiologic studies of British and Eskimo populations have suggested that the declining incidence of tuberculosis disease observed in all ages, including those who were previously infected, reflects a decrease in frequency of exogenous reinfection.[261]

Distinguishing between endogenous and exogenous infection is difficult without special laboratory techniques to distinguish the different strains of M. tuberculosis, and sensitive techniques, such as restriction fragment length polymorphism, have become available only in the past few years.[262,263] It is difficult to estimate the effect of exogenous reinfection on previously reported clinical trials, although this issue could be addressed with currently available technology.

Other Evidence of Effectiveness: Case-Control, Contact, and Meta-Analysis Studies

The cost, extensive length of follow-up, and large numbers of subjects needed to conduct a large, randomized clinical trial,

as well as the lack of consensus reached in previous studies, have led to the use of alternative methods for evaluating the efficacy of BCG vaccine.[264] In the 1980s, the WHO initiated a global study to evaluate programs in developing countries using a standardized case-contact protocol that evaluated children who were household contacts of cases with infectious disease. These children were evaluated by use of the WHO clinical scoring system and were observed during 3 months for development of tuberculosis disease. These methods as well as case-control and cohort studies, have yielded results similar to those of the major controlled trials, with efficacy ranging from 0% to more than 80% (see Fig. 12–2).[185,265,266]

Case-control and contact studies have the advantage of being fast and less expensive, but the potential for bias is increased. In retrospective studies, vaccine is not randomly allocated, so there is potential for confounding factors that may affect the outcome. Socioeconomic status is a potential confounding variable because persons with higher socioeconomic status are more likely to have access to and to use both preventive (vaccination) and curative health care and usually have a lower risk of exposure to tuberculosis. Studies that compare BCG scar rates in children who have tuberculosis with BCG scar rates within the community preclude analysis of many important potential confounding variables. Another disadvantage of retrospective studies is the decreased validity of historical information regarding vaccination status. Misclassification of vaccination status is less of a problem in BCG studies owing to the lasting scar formation that occurs in 90% to 95% of patients. Problems may arise if other marks are mistaken for BCG scars or if the vaccination does not leave a scar. Another consideration is the criteria for diagnosis of disease, especially in children. Safeguards to control for these potential problems must be strict in retrospective studies to avoid biased results. The quality of the case-control and cohort studies of BCG vaccine has varied from excellent to poor.

Findings from the case-control and cohort studies in children vary markedly, with a high level of protection of 70% or more found in many studies.[185,186,267–273] One study, looking at the efficacy of neonatal BCG vaccine over 20 years, found 82% protection in children younger than 15 years, 67% protection in the 15- to 24-year-old group, and 20% protection in persons 25 to 34 years of age, indicating better protection in younger age groups and waning immunity over time.[207] Most of the case-control and cohort studies have observed moderate protection of 30% to 66%.[257,274–281] Few studies have shown efficacy less than 20%.[282–284] Studies that separately evaluated meningitis or miliary disease demonstrated that BCG offers good protection against these more serious forms of tuberculosis in young children.[185,186,285–288] These findings are consistent with the theory that BCG protects against hematogenous spread but not against establishment of infection.

Understanding that there are limitations and potential biases in these retrospective studies, the best available information suggests that BCG provides some measure of protection to a substantial proportion of vaccinated infants and children living in places in which the risk of tuberculosis is high, and that protection is highest against tuberculous meningitis and disseminated disease.

The technique of meta-analysis, in which results of similar studies with the same hypothesis are combined to increase the number of study subjects and improve interpretation of results, has been used to evaluate BCG vaccine.[286-288] Of course, one must question the validity of these analyses considering the grossly varied conditions of and variables within the trials. Investigators at the London School of Hygiene and Tropical Medicine found 10 randomized controlled trials and 8 case-control studies that met criteria for adequate methodology.[286] For meningeal and miliary disease, the protective effect was 86% in randomized controlled trials and 75% in case-control studies. For pulmonary tuberculosis, the degree of heterogeneity among studies precluded calculation of a summary estimate of protective efficacy. In other words, the findings were too divergent to simply average the results.

Investigators at the Harvard School of Public Health[288] found 15 prospective trials and 12 case-control studies that met their criteria for adequacy in study design and controls against potential bias. In the prospective trials, the protective effect of BCG for tuberculosis disease was 51%. Among the case-control studies, protection by BCG was 50%. Analysis of eight studies involving only populations vaccinated as infants revealed a protective effect of 55% against tuberculosis among infant recipients of BCG. Seven trials reporting deaths from tuberculosis showed a BCG protective effect of 71%. The protective effect against tuberculous meningitis (five studies) was 64%, and protection against disseminated disease (three studies) was 72%.

The Harvard study used a random-effects regression model to examine variation in BCG efficacy among 13 prospective trials. Investigators found that the rate of tuberculosis in the unvaccinated group and the geographic latitude accounted for 85% of the between-study variance. Among the seven prospective trials that enrolled patients randomly, the estimated protective effect was 85% for BCG vaccination at birth, 73% for vaccination at age 10 years, and 50% for vaccination at 20 years of age. However, for the entire meta-analysis, mean age at vaccination accounted for less than 6% of the between-study variance ($P > 0.20$). Different strains of BCG were not consistently associated with more or less favorable results in the trials. Different BCG preparations and strains used in the same population gave similar levels of protection, whereas genetically identical BCG vaccines gave different levels of protection in different populations. The duration of protection from a single BCG vaccination and the role of booster doses could not be assessed owing to the inadequacy of the data.

The Harvard group also published a meta-analysis evaluating the efficacy of BCG vaccination of newborns and infants.[287,288] Five prospective trials and 11 case-control studies met the study criteria and were included in the analysis. The overall protective efficacy against all forms of tuberculosis for those vaccinated at birth or during infancy was 50% on average. Protection against death was 65%, meningitis 64%, and disseminated tuberculosis 78%.

In summary, there is no question that BCG vaccination has worked well in some situations but poorly in others. Because only a small fraction of the cases in the general population of contagious, smear-positive adult pulmonary tuberculosis are potentially preventable by BCG vaccination, BCG has had essentially no effect on the ultimate control of tuberculosis. The best use of BCG appears to be for the prevention of life-threatening forms of tuberculosis such as meningitis and disseminated disease in infants and young children. Vaccination with BCG remains the standard for tuberculosis prevention in most countries because it is available, is inexpensive, and requires only one encounter with the patient; in addition, it rarely causes serious complications, and systems for early diagnosis and effective treatment of tuberculosis are lacking in many areas of the world.

Duration of Immunity

The duration of immunity after BCG vaccination is not known. Estimates are based on data from clinical trials and case-control studies because there is no serologic test to measure immunity to tuberculosis or the immune response after BCG vaccination. A case-control study by al-Kassimi and colleagues[207] compared BCG vaccine status in 537 cases of tuberculosis with 5756 normal control subjects. All subjects were vaccinated in the neonatal period, and protection was estimated by age group or years after vaccination. The study found decreasing protection with increasing age, demonstrating a waning immunity 20 years after vaccination. A more recent study found no consistent evidence of sustained protection against pulmonary tuberculosis lasting more than 15 years.[289] Experts speculate that protection declines over time and is probably nonexistent 10 to 20 years after vaccination.

Postexposure Prophylaxis and Therapeutic Vaccination

Prophylactic therapy with isoniazid or other antituberculosis medications following exposure to contagious tuberculosis may prevent progression to active disease and should be considered in high-risk groups under certain conditions. Recommendations vary between countries depending on public health considerations, including BCG vaccination practices as well as the need to prioritize limited resources in developing countries.

Many developed countries recommend chemoprophylaxis for certain high-risk groups following exposure to tuberculosis. The American Academy of Pediatrics Committee on Infectious Diseases recommends isoniazid prophylaxis for contacts with impaired immunity and all household contacts younger than 4 years of age following significant exposure to contagious tuberculosis.[290] Initial evaluation should include a tuberculin skin test to exclude pre-existing latent infection and a chest radiograph to exclude clinical disease. Prophylaxis may be discontinued after a follow-up negative tuberculin skin test has excluded development of latent infection, usually 3 months after the last contact with the index case. Isoniazid prophylaxis is recommended unless the isolate from the source case is isoniazid resistant, in which case rifampin may be substituted. If the isolate is resistant to both isoniazid and rifampin, prophylaxis with at least two drugs to which the isolate is sensitive and consultation with an expert in treating multidrug-resistant tuberculosis should be considered. In the United Kingdom, chemoprophylaxis is recommended for children younger than 2 years of age in contact with contagious tuberculosis, with follow-up tuberculin skin testing at 6 weeks.[291]

Recommendations regarding postexposure vaccination with BCG vary between countries. Some countries are in transition from routine vaccination of all children to selective vaccination of high-risk groups, including tuberculosis contacts. In the United Kingdom, BCG vaccination is recommended for unvaccinated contacts with negative tuberculin skin tests.[291]

Safety of Bacille Calmette-Guérin Vaccine

For more than 70 years, BCG vaccines have been administered safely to billions of individuals throughout the world. Complications are rare, but the rate varies depending on the skill and method of administration; the type, strength, and dose of the vaccine; and the age and immune status of the vaccinee.[292,293] Women and older vaccinees are in general more likely to develop local reactions and abscesses, and vaccination at less than 6 months of age is better tolerated than after that age.[293a]

Common Adverse Events

Localized adverse effects are common after BCG vaccination, but serious long-term complications are rare (Table 12–6). Ninety percent to 95% of patients vaccinated with BCG develop a local reaction followed by healing and scar formation within 3 months. Individuals with latent tuberculosis infection often have an accelerated response to BCG vaccine characterized by induration within 1 to 2 days and scab formation and healing within 10 to 15 days. A study in healthy tuberculin-negative adults vaccinated with BCG found that all patients developed a local reaction with erythema, induration, and tenderness at the vaccination site; 75% developed muscle soreness; and 70% had local ulceration with drainage.[294] Only 2% developed tender regional adenopathy. A lasting cutaneous scar develops in most patients, although the likelihood is lower following vaccination in early infancy.[295]

Local ulceration and regional lymphadenitis are the most common complications, following cutaneous reactions, occurring in less than 1% of immunocompetent recipients who receive intradermal administration.[296] Local cutaneous lesions and lymphadenitis usually occur within a few weeks to months after vaccination, but symptoms may be delayed

for months in immunocompetent persons and for years in immunocompromised hosts.[297] Axillary, cervical, and supraclavicular nodes are usually involved on the ipsilateral side of vaccination. Certain BCG strains, especially the Tokyo strain and the Moreau strain in Brazil, rarely are associated with lymphadenitis, whereas the French (Pasteur) strain gives rise to a higher incidence.[292,298,299] Outbreaks of lymphadenitis after vaccination with BCG in certain countries or regions frequently have followed the introduction of a new BCG strain into the vaccination program.[300,301] It is likely that an altered technique of administration has contributed to some of these outbreaks. A study in 291 Haitian infants reported an outbreak of complications after administration of 2.0 to 2.5 times the recommended dose of BCG vaccine.[302] The complications were mild to moderate, with only a small increased risk of complications among HIV-infected children. There is no evidence that children who experience local complications are more likely to have immune deficits or to have enhanced or diminished protection against tuberculosis.[301] The risk of suppurative lymphadenitis is greater among newborns than among older infants and children, especially when a full dose of vaccine is given; therefore, the WHO recommends using a reduced dose in children younger than 30 days.

The treatment of local adenitis as a complication of BCG vaccination is controversial and ranges from observation to surgical drainage to the administration of antituberculosis drugs to a combination of surgical management and medications.[303] Nonsuppurative lymph nodes usually improve spontaneously, although resolution may take several months.[304] The WHO recommends drainage and direct instillation of an antituberculosis drug into the lesion for adherent or fistulated lymph nodes.[305] Several studies have shown that some children with lymphadenitis respond to a course of isoniazid or erythromycin of several weeks' or months' duration.[306-308] However, a comparative study of 120 patients treated for 6 months showed that regimens of isoniazid, isoniazid plus rifampin, and erythromycin did not produce different results; that medical therapy was little better than observation; and that the rate of spontaneous drainage of the lymph nodes was higher among isoniazid-treated children than among the control subjects.[268] A recent meta-analysis regarding the treatment of BCG-related adenitis found the literature lacking but, based on available studies, concluded that treatment with oral erythromycin or antituberculosis drugs did not reduce the frequency of suppuration.[309]

Rare Adverse Events

Other complications of vaccination with BCG are much less frequent. The mean risk of osteitis after BCG vaccination has varied from 0.01 per million in Japan to 300 per million in Finland.[292,310-313] As with lymphadenitis, osteitis rates have, on occasion, increased dramatically after introduction of a new vaccine strain into a region or country. Generalized BCG infection is extremely rare in immunocompetent patients.[314-318] A few autopsy studies of children who died of unrelated causes have demonstrated granulomas in various organs of vaccinated infants with apparently intact immune systems, suggesting that generalized nonfatal dissemination may occur in normal hosts.[316,319,320] Treatment of rare complications, including lupus vulgaris, erythema nodosum, iritis, osteomyelitis, and disseminated

TABLE 12–6 ■ Age-Specific Estimated Risks for Complications After Administration of Bacille Calmette-Guérin Vaccine

Complication	Incidence per 1 Million Vaccinations	
	Age <1 yr	Age 1–20 yr
Local subcutaneous abscess, regional lymphadenopathy	387	25
Musculoskeletal lesions	0.39–0.89	0.06
Multiple lymphadenitis, nonfatal disseminated lesions	0.31–0.39	0.36
Fatal disseminated lesions	0.19–1.56	0.06–0.72

From Lotte A, Wasz-Hockert O, Poisson N, et al. Second IUATLD study on complications induced by intradermal BCG-vaccination. Bull Int Union Tuberc 63:47–59, 1988, with permission.

BCG disease, should include systemic antituberculosis medications, but pyrazinamide should not be included because all strains of BCG are resistant to this drug.[174,321]

Some experts have raised questions about a possible increased risk of certain types of cancer, especially lymphomas, among BCG-vaccinated individuals compared with unvaccinated persons.[220,231] Another study proposed the possibility that BCG vaccination in newborns reduces certain childhood cancers, although the effect was small and the power was insufficient.[322] More studies may be indicated to evaluate these questions.

Adverse Events in Immunosuppressed Individuals

Fatal disseminated BCG disease has been reported at a rate of 0.19 to 1.56 cases per 1 million vaccinated,[296] with most cases occurring in patients with severe defects in cell-mediated immunity, such as chronic granulomatous disease, severe combined immunodeficiency, malnutrition, cancer, complete DiGeorge syndrome, interferon-γ receptor deficiency, or HIV infection.[320,323–329] A report of five patients from four Tunisian families with disseminated neonatal BCG infection describes profound deficiency of in vitro interferon-γ production. All five patients were found to have various interleukin-12 gene mutations affecting interferon-γ production.[330]

The safety of BCG vaccine in children and adults who are infected with HIV is unknown. Disseminated BCG infection has been described in an HIV-infected adult 30 years after he received BCG.[331] There have been other reports of disseminated BCG disease in infants and adults with HIV infection.[297,324,326,332–334] Data derived soon after BCG vaccination from Zaire,[15,335] Uganda,[336] Rwanda,[337] the Congo,[338] and Thailand[339] did not indicate an increased risk of serious adverse effects of BCG vaccination in infants of mothers infected with HIV. Long-term follow-up evaluations of these and other high-risk infants are not yet available. However, one French study showed that 9 of 68 HIV-infected children given BCG vaccine developed complications: 7 had large satellite adenopathy with or without skin fistulas, and 2 developed disseminated lesions.[340]

The efficacy of BCG vaccine in HIV-infected infants is completely unknown. One study in Ethiopian children suggested that BCG vaccine may be less protective against tuberculosis in HIV-infected children.[341] Currently, the WHO recommends giving BCG vaccine to asymptomatic HIV-infected infants who live in high-risk areas for tuberculosis. BCG is not recommended for symptomatic HIV-infected infants or for persons known to be or suspected of being HIV-infected if they are at minimal risk for infection with M. tuberculosis.[342] In reality, the lack of available HIV serodiagnosis in many regions of the world means that in some areas large numbers of HIV-infected infants and children are receiving BCG. Long-term studies of these children will be exceedingly important.

Risk of Spread to Contacts

Ulceration and drainage at the vaccination site may occur following BCG vaccination. Viable mycobacteria have been cultured from ulcerated sites for up to 2 months after vaccination, raising the question of potential spread to contacts.[343,344] It would be unusual for organisms from ulcerated sites to become airborne, which may explain the lack of reported cases of person-to-person transmission of BCG in the literature.

Indications for Bacille Calmette-Guérin Vaccine

There is a wide disparity among nations concerning vaccine schedules.[174] The official recommendation of the WHO is a single dose given in infancy. However, only three prospective community trials have evaluated the efficacy of BCG vaccine given at birth.[345] Studies of lymphocyte blastogenesis in response to PPD have shown much higher rates of immunogenic sensitization in children if BCG vaccination is delayed from the first week to 9 months of life.[345] However, even low-birth-weight newborns develop lymphocyte proliferation and interleukin-2 production in response to a BCG vaccine.[346] Another study of preterm infants vaccinated at 34 to 35 weeks 'gestation compared to infants receiving delayed vaccination at 38 to 40 weeks' gestation showed no differences in tuberculin reactivity, scar formation, or immune response.[347]

The national policy in the United Kingdom is that a single dose of BCG vaccine be offered to all children between 10 and 14 years of age, as well as to certain groups at higher risk of exposure to tuberculosis.[348–351] This policy was initiated in 1957 to deliver vaccination prior to leaving school and before entering the higher incidence period associated with young adulthood. Some areas of the UK are discontinuing this policy and moving to selective vaccination of higher risk populations, including tuberculin-negative contacts, health care workers, and younger children from immigrant populations.[291]

Many countries give the first dose of BCG in infancy and then give repeated vaccinations throughout childhood.[174] In some nations, repeated vaccination is universal; in others, it is based on either the lack of tuberculin sensitivity or the absence of a typical scar. Unfortunately, absence of a scar after BCG vaccination does not correlate with lack of tuberculin sensitivity or any specific immunologic parameter. It is reasonable that the recommended schedules would vary with the local epidemiology of tuberculosis; age groups at highest risk of disease (young children versus adolescents or young adults) could be targeted for vaccination. However, these schedule differences reflect variation among countries in both the local epidemiology of tuberculosis and the opinions concerning the mechanism and duration of protection imparted by BCG. It must be concluded that the optimal age for administration and schedule (single vs. multiple doses) has not been firmly established because adequate comparative trials have not been reported.

The United States and the Netherlands have never recommended routine BCG vaccination. Some other countries, including Sweden in 1975[352] and Czechoslovakia in 1986,[353] adopted this policy as well. All of these countries license BCG vaccine for individual use in special high-risk situations, such as children exposed to multidrug-resistant tuberculosis with no options for prophylaxis or separation from the exposure.

The International Union against Tuberculosis and Lung Disease (IUATLD) has suggested criteria to consider for countries when shifting from routine universal BCG vaccination to selective vaccination of high-risk groups.[354] The IUATLD recommends that BCG be discontinued only if

(1) an efficient notification system is in place, and either (2) the average annual notification rate of smear-positive pulmonary tuberculosis is less than 5 per 100,000; or (3) the average annual notification rate of tuberculous meningitis in children under 5 years of age is less than 1 in 10 million population over the previous 5 years; or (4) the average annual risk of tuberculosis infection is less than 0.1%. As tuberculosis rates continue to decline in developed countries, trends may continue to limit BCG vaccination to selective use and to discontinue universal immunization programs.[174]

It is known that BCG vaccine has some efficacy against leprosy, and some countries, including Brazil, Cuba, and Venezuela, now recommend BCG vaccination for contacts of leprosy patients.[174] According to the WHO, widespread BCG vaccination may have contributed to the decline of leprosy in certain populations.[355,356]

Recommendations for Use of Bacille Calmette-Guérin in the United States

In the United States, surveillance, contact investigation, prophylaxis, and treatment for latent tuberculosis infection are practiced, and BCG vaccination is considered only in limited special circumstances involving unavoidable continued exposure and failure to employ other methods of control. The Centers for Disease Control and Prevention's Advisory Council for the Elimination of Tuberculosis and Advisory Committee on Immunization Practices have published guidelines for the use of BCG vaccination in young children and health care workers.[357] In the United States, BCG immunization should be considered only for persons with a negative tuberculin skin test who are not infected with HIV, have continual exposure to multidrug-resistant tuberculosis, and cannot be removed from the exposure; or for children with continual exposure to contagious tuberculosis who cannot be removed from the exposure or treated with antituberculosis therapy. BCG vaccination also may be considered for health care workers in special high-risk settings where other tuberculosis control measures have failed.[11] One study, using a computer simulation model, suggests the use of BCG vaccination to decrease tuberculosis among homeless populations.[358]

The emergence of multidrug-resistant strains of M. tuberculosis and subsequent nosocomial outbreaks in hospitals in some areas of the United States have led to consideration of the use of BCG vaccine for the prevention and control of tuberculosis among health care workers. Health care facilities at high risk are limited to a few geographic areas of the United States with high rates of multidrug-resistant tuberculosis in the population. In general, health care workers should be protected by infection control techniques, screening, and treatment of latent tuberculosis infection. Even in high-risk settings, BCG should not be the major method of control or protection because it has unknown efficacy; does not protect unvaccinated patients or visitors; and confuses skin test, surveillance, and preventive treatment measures. Vaccination with BCG should be considered for health care workers only in areas that have a high risk of transmission of multidrug-resistant tuberculosis in which aggressive infection control measures have been implemented and have failed.[357] Even in these circum-

stances, the uncertain efficacy of BCG vaccines may make other control measures such as chemotherapy preferable to vaccination alone.

The most frequent indication for use of BCG in the United States today, which is unrelated to tuberculosis, is the treatment of bladder cancer by intravesicular administration, in which the vaccine has a nonspecific immunostimulant effect.

Contraindications to Vaccination with Bacille Calmette-Guérin

Guidelines for contraindications for BCG vaccination vary among developing countries and industrialized nations, reflective of the different resources and capabilities within health services. In developed countries, BCG vaccine is contraindicated for persons with impaired immunity, including (1) patients with HIV infection, congenital immunodeficiency, leukemia, lymphoma, or generalized malignant disease; (2) patients on suppressive corticosteroids, alkylating agents, antimetabolites, or radiation; or (3) patients who are pregnant.[357] Persons in groups at high risk for HIV infection should be administered BCG with caution.

In contrast, the WHO guideline lists symptomatic HIV infection or acquired immunodeficiency syndrome as a contraindication for BCG vaccination, while asymptomatic HIV infection is not a contraindication.[359] Because poorer areas do not have the resources or capability to test for HIV, many HIV-infected infants are vaccinated at birth. Most studies of these infants found no significant increase in adverse reactions compared to non–HIV-infected infants vaccinated with BCG.[174]

Future Vaccines for Tuberculosis

Tuberculosis will be eliminated only if new, more effective vaccines are developed.[360] Modern molecular genetics and biotechnology techniques should be applied rapidly to this problem. Because almost 2 billion people in the world already are infected with M. tuberculosis, vaccine research should address both preventing infection and halting progression of established infection to tuberculosis disease.

The varying effect of BCG vaccines may be, in part, due to our imperfect understanding of the determinants of protective immunity against tuberculosis. The significant antigens of M. tuberculosis are poorly defined and difficult to produce owing to the complex structure and chemistry of the mycobacterial cell wall. Our basic science knowledge of antigens, immune responses, and mediators must be expanded.

Because genetic factors may influence the response to BCG, environmental mycobacteria, and infection with M. tuberculosis, molecular genetics studies in animals and humans should be broadened. Animal studies have revealed that genetically determined susceptibility to mycobacteria infection in mice is regulated by a gene called Bcg, Ity, or Lsh. Bcg gene, which has been identified and characterized, codes for a membrane transport protein called Nramp.[361] The actual function of Nramp is not yet understood, but it appears to influence susceptibility to tuberculosis disease. Mapping of the genome sequence of M. *tuberculosis* has been completed and should bring new light to potential vaccine development.[362]

Innovative new approaches in tuberculosis vaccine development have emerged, including (1) plasmid DNA vector-based vaccines, which deliver genes encoding antigens (Ag 85 or hsp60) by use of vectors; (2) recombinant and mutant BCG vaccines, which use BCG as the delivery vehicle with improvements; (3) subunit vaccines, which use individual mycobacterial protein antigens to produce an immune response; and (4) attenuated M. *tuberculosis* vaccines, which lack the genes essential for virulence and contain the genes needed for protection.[363,364] All of these new strategies appear promising, and perhaps one of these techniques or a combination thereof will yield an effective new vaccine against tuberculosis. In the United Kingdom, a clinical trial in humans comparing a new tuberculosis vaccine (MVA85A) with BCG is planned to begin, with future large-scale trials planned in Africa.[365]

Major field trials for BCG or any new tuberculosis vaccine will be a tremendous challenge given the necessary scope, duration, and expense of adequate trials. There is a pressing need for identification of some correlate of natural and vaccine-derived protective immunity, based on either an animal model or a measure of immune response in humans. Current animal models are inadequate, and human markers of protective immunity have not been determined. Tuberculin sensitivity after vaccination is not an adequate "assay." Some advances have been made in diagnostic tests for tuberculosis, but these methods are still being developed and tested.[11,112] A reliable serologic test for latent tuberculosis infection and tuberculosis disease would make vaccine trials more feasible by requiring a shorter duration. Continued research on operational variables such as the age of optimal vaccination and the role of booster vaccinations is needed. Finally, data on the safety and efficacy of BCG vaccines in HIV-infected children and adults should be sought vigorously.

Public Health Considerations

For a number of reasons it is impossible to estimate the impact of the BCG vaccines on global tuberculosis. First, the widely divergent results of the BCG vaccine trials make it difficult to estimate vaccine efficacy. Second, the reported epidemiologic data on tuberculosis in the developing world is incomplete. Third, the vaccine is primarily administered to infants and children, whereas the worldwide burden of tuberculosis is mainly seen as pulmonary disease in adults. Fourth, tuberculosis increased in many countries during the 1980s and 1990s as a result of HIV as well as other factors unrelated to BCG vaccination. All of these issues make it difficult or impossible to estimate the effects of BCG vaccination programs on the epidemiology of tuberculosis.[174]

For most infectious diseases, the expectation is that the availability of a potent vaccine can lead to the elimination of the disease from human populations, if an effective global program can be developed and implemented. Clearly, the BCG vaccines have not led to the elimination of tubercu-

losis from any country in the world. The distribution of these vaccines to 4 billion people has had almost no effect on the worldwide epidemiology of tuberculosis.[3] However, it is likely that millions of cases of meningeal and disseminated tuberculosis in children have been prevented by its widespread use. Rates of leprosy, especially in Africa, also have been reduced by the use of BCG vaccination.

Some of the confusion about the current role of BCG vaccines in the control of tuberculosis has occurred because the original intent for its use has been forgotten. In most developing countries, BCG was introduced as an emergency measure because it was the only inexpensive tuberculosis control measure that could be applied on a national scale.[156] With the advent of effective and inexpensive chemotherapy, a two-pronged approach to tuberculosis control became possible, consisting of (1) case finding and treatment and (2) BCG vaccination.[5,7,178] Prior receipt of BCG vaccination and chemotherapy of persons with reactive tuberculin skin test responses who have been close contacts of known cases are not mutually exclusive; this dual approach would prevent many cases of life-threatening disease in children and future cases of infectious reactivation disease. However, in developing countries, the impact of the current level of case finding and treatment programs on tuberculosis in young children may be small. Most transmission to children occurs before the adult source case is identified, and the short incubation period for meningeal and disseminated tuberculosis means that the time for intervention with the child has already passed.[366–368] The lack of sensitive diagnostic techniques for confirming tuberculosis in children often precludes early effective treatment of their disease. Under such conditions, only effective vaccination of children can be expected to reduce the development of disease in children in a significant manner. Because the source of tuberculosis transmission to children in developing countries is usually within their household, a delay in vaccination after birth, although perhaps leading to a more vigorous and long-lasting immune response, may fail to prevent cases of childhood tuberculosis if a family member who has the disease is present.[178]

Vaccination of children with BCG probably will not prevent the majority of infectious pulmonary tuberculosis cases among adults in a population because the protection afforded by BCG appears to be of limited duration.[3] However, almost nothing is known about the efficacy for a short period of time of various BCG vaccines given to adults who have not been infected previously with M. *tuberculosis*. In developed countries, protecting high-risk adults, such as those who work with patients who have multidrug-resistant tuberculosis, is becoming a critical need when chemotherapy cannot be relied on. It is also completely unknown whether "booster" immunizations with BCG can maintain or even enhance protection against tuberculosis. It is remarkable that these basic questions about the effectiveness of BCG vaccine have never been answered or even addressed, despite the administration of more than 4 billion doses of vaccine.

The WHO has recommended that a single dose of BCG vaccine be given to newborns in developing countries with a high prevalence rate of infectious tuberculosis. This dosage schedule will have an economic impact and a short-term impact on mortality, although it will not contribute significantly to the control of tuberculosis. The United Kingdom adopted the strategy of a single dose of BCG in adolescence because the majority of cases were occurring in adolescents and young adults, and few occurred among infants and children. However, the optimal vaccine strain of BCG, the dosing schedule, the route of administration, and the age of the recipient have not been established firmly.

Many technologically advanced countries that have experienced great declines in the rate of tuberculosis have either already discontinued or are considering discontinuing BCG vaccination.[349,350,369] In the United Kingdom and Sweden, cessation of a generalized BCG vaccination program has led to a slight increase in childhood and adolescent cases of tuberculosis. However, in both areas, the majority of subsequent childhood cases have been from high-risk immigrant communities whose members lived previously in regions with high rates of tuberculosis. Fairly circumscribed groups such as these could be selectively targeted for BCG immunization or be subjected to increased surveillance and case-finding efforts.

The worldwide epidemic of HIV infection has had a profound effect on the epidemiology of tuberculosis and may have an impact on the optimal use of BCG. The safety and efficacy of BCG in HIV-infected children are really unknown at present. Epidemiology and autopsy studies will be particularly useful in establishing the role of mass BCG vaccination in developing countries at a time when the number of persons with acquired immunodeficiency syndrome is increasing.[16]

REFERENCES

1. Starke JR. Bacille Calmette-Guérin vaccine. Semin Pediatr Infect Dis 2:153–158, 1991.
2. Lugosi L. Theoretical and methodological aspects of BCG vaccine from the discovery of Calmette and Guérin to molecular biology: a review. Tuber Lung Dis 73:252–261, 1992.
3. Styblo K. Overview and epidemiologic assessment of the current global tuberculosis situation with an emphasis on control in developing countries. Rev Infect Dis 11(suppl 2):S339–S346, 1989.
4. World Health Organization. Global Tuberculosis Control: WHO Report 2001 (WHO/CDS/TB/2001.287). Geneva, World Health Organization, 2001.
5. Sudre P, ten Dam G, Kochi A. Tuberculosis: a global overview of the situation today. Bull World Health Organ 70:149–159, 1992.
6. Raviglione MC, Snider DE Jr, Kochi A. Global epidemiology of tuberculosis: morbidity and mortality of a worldwide epidemic. JAMA 273:220–226, 1995.
7. Kochi A. The global tuberculosis situation and the new control strategy of the World Health Organization. Tubercle 72:1–6, 1991.
8. Comstock GW. The International Tuberculosis Campaign: a pioneering venture in mass vaccination and research. Clin Infect Dis 19:528–540, 1994.
9. Fine PEM. Bacille Calmette-Guérin vaccines: a rough guide. Clin Infect Dis 20:11–14, 1995.
10. Smith DW. Protective effect of BCG in experimental tuberculosis. Adv Tuberc Res 22:1–97, 1985.
11. Schluger NW. Changing approaches to the diagnosis of tuberculosis. Am J Respir Crit Care Med 164:2020–2024, 2001.
12. Stevens JP, Daniel TM. Bacille Calmette-Guérin immunization of health care workers exposed to multidrug-resistant tuberculosis: a decision analysis. Tuber Lung Dis 77:315–321, 1996.
13. Brewer TF, Colditz GA. Bacille Calmette-Guérin vaccination for the prevention of tuberculosis in healthcare workers. Clin Infect Dis 20:136–142, 1995.
14. Selwyn PA, Hartel D, Lewis VA, et al. A prospective study of the risk of tuberculosis among intravenous drug users with human immunodeficiency virus infection. N Engl J Med 320:545–550, 1989.
15. Ryder RW, Oxtoby MJ, Mvula M, et al. Safety and immunogenicity of bacille Calmette-Guérin, diphtheria-tetanus-pertussis, and oral polio vaccines in newborn children in Zaire infected with human immunodeficiency virus type 1. J Pediatr 122:697–702, 1993.
16. Braun MM, Cauthen G. Relationship of the human immunodeficiency virus epidemic to pediatric tuberculosis and bacillus Calmette-Guérin immunization. Pediatr Infect Dis J 11:220–227, 1992.
17. Bloch AB, Cauthen GM, Onorato IM, et al. Nationwide survey of drug-resistant tuberculosis in the United States. JAMA 271:665–671, 1994.
18. Dye C, Espinal MA, Watt CJ, et al. Worldwide incidence of multidrug-resistant tuberculosis. J Infect Dis 185:1197–1202, 2002.
19. Dooley SW, Villarino ME, Lawrence M, et al. Nosocomial transmission of tuberculosis in a hospital unit for HIV-infected patients. JAMA 267:2632–2635, 1992.
20. Pearson ML, Jereb JA, Frieden TR, et al. Nosocomial transmission of multidrug-resistant Mycobacterium tuberculosis: a risk to patients and healthcare workers. Ann Intern Med 117:191–196, 1992.
21. Taylor R. Saranac: America's Magic Mountain. Boston, Houghton-Mifflin, 1986.
22. Bloom BR, Murray CJL. Tuberculosis: commentary on a reemergent killer. Science 257:1055–1064, 1992.
23. Morse D, Brothwell DR, Ucko PJ. Tuberculosis in ancient Egypt. Am Rev Respir Dis 90:524–541, 1964.
24. Starke JR, Smith MHD. Tuberculosis. In Feigin RD, Cherry JD (eds). Textbook of Pediatric Infectious Diseases (4th ed). Philadelphia, WB Saunders, 1998, pp 1196–1239.
25. Nemir RL. Perspectives in adolescent tuberculosis: three decades of experience. Pediatrics 78:399–404, 1986.
26. Starke JR, Correa AG. Management of mycobacterial infection and disease in children. Pediatr Infect Dis J 14:455–470, 1995.
27. Smith MHD. Tuberculosis in children and adolescents. Clin Chest Med 10:381–395, 1989.
28. Vallejo JG, Ong LT, Starke JR. Clinical features, diagnosis and treatment of tuberculosis in infants. Pediatrics 94:1–7, 1994.
29. Perry S, Starke JR. Adherence to prescribed treatment and public health aspects of tuberculosis in children. Semin Pediatr Infect Dis 4:291–298, 1993.
30. Rossman MD, Mayock RL. Pulmonary tuberculosis. In Schlossberg D (ed). Clinical Topics in Infectious Disease: Tuberculosis. New York, Springer-Verlag, 1988, pp 61–70.
31. Khan MA, Kovnat DM, Bachus B, et al. Clinical and roentgenographic spectrum of pulmonary tuberculosis in the adult. Am J Med 62:31–38, 1977.
32. Alvarez S, Shell C, Berk SL. Pulmonary tuberculosis in elderly men. Am J Med 82:602–606, 1987.
33. Gordin FM, Slutkin G, Schecter G, et al. Presumptive diagnosis and treatment of pulmonary tuberculosis based on radiographic findings. Am Rev Respir Dis 139:1090–1093, 1989.
34. Palmer PES. Pulmonary tuberculosis: usual and unusual radiographic presentations. Semin Roentgenol 14:204–242, 1979.
35. Chang SC, Lee PY, Perng RP. Lower lung field tuberculosis. Chest 91:230–232, 1987.
36. Barnes PF, Bloch AB, Davidson PT, et al. Tuberculosis in patients with human immunodeficiency virus infection. N Engl J Med 324:1644–1650, 1991.
37. Jones BE, Young SMM, Antoniskis D, et al. Relationship of the manifestations of tuberculosis to CD4 cell counts in patients with human immunodeficiency virus infection. Am Rev Respir Dis 148:1292–1297, 1993.
38. Markowitz N, Hansen N, Hopewell PC, et al. Incidence of tuberculosis in the United States among HIV-infected patients. Ann Intern Med 126:123–132, 1997.
39. Hopewell PC. Tuberculosis in persons with human immunodeficiency virus infection: clinical and public health aspects. Semin Respir Crit Care Med 18:471–484, 1997.
40. Pitchenik AE, Rubinson HA. The radiographic appearance of tuberculosis in patients with the acquired immune deficiency syndrome (AIDS) and pre-AIDS. Am Rev Respir Dis 131:393–396, 1985.
41. Long R, Maycher B, Scalcini M, Manfreda J. The chest roentgenogram in pulmonary tuberculosis patients seropositive for human immunodeficiency virus type 1. Chest 99:123–127, 1991.
42. Wasser LS, Shaw GW, Talvera W. Endobronchial tuberculosis in the acquired immunodeficiency syndrome. Chest 94:1240–1244, 1988.

43. Shafter RW, Kim DS, Weiss JP, et al. Extrapulmonary tuberculosis in patients with human immunodeficiency virus infection. Medicine (Baltimore) 70:384–397, 1991.

44. Rieder HL, Snider DE Jr, Cauthen GM. Extrapulmonary tuberculosis in the United States. Am Rev Respir Dis 141:347–351, 1990.

45. Schuitt KE, Powell DA. Mycobacterial lymphadenitis in childhood. Am J Dis Child 132:675–677, 1978.

46. Hussey G, Chisolm T, Kibel M. Miliary tuberculosis in children: a review of 94 cases. Pediatr Infect Dis J 10:832–836, 1991.

47. Doerr CA, Starke Jr, Ong LT. Clinical and public health aspects of tuberculous meningitis in children. J Pediatr 127:27–33, 1995.

48. Molavi A, Le Frock JL. Tuberculous meningitis. Med Clin North Am 69:315–331, 1985.

49. Floyd MM, Silcox VA, Jones WD Jr, et al. Separation of Mycobacterium bovis BCG from Mycobacterium tuberculosis and Mycobacterium bovis by using high-performance liquid chromatography of mycolic acids. J Clin Microbiol 30:1327–1330, 1992.

50. Sauret J, Jolis R, Ausina V, et al. Human tuberculosis due to Mycobacterium bovis: report of 10 cases. Tuber Lung Dis 73:388–391, 1992.

51. Feldman WH, Davis R, Moses HE, et al. An unusual mycobacterium isolated from sputum of a man suffering from pulmonary disease of long duration. Am Rev Tuberc 48:82–93, 1943.

52. Wyne L. The atypical mycobacteria: recognition and disease association. Crit Rev Microbiol 12:184–222, 1986.

53. Riley RL. The J. Burns Amberson lecture: Aerial dissemination of pulmonary tuberculosis. Am Rev Tuberc Pulm Dis 76:931–941, 1957.

54. Lurie MB. Resistance to Tuberculosis: Experimental Studies in Native and Acquired Defensive Mechanisms. Cambridge, MA, Harvard University Press, 1964.

55. Dannenberg AM Jr. Immune mechanisms in the pathogenesis of pulmonary tuberculosis. Rev Infect Dis 11(suppl 2):S369–S378, 1989.

56. Stead WW. Pathogenesis of a first episode of chronic pulmonary tuberculosis in man: recrudescence of residual of the primary infection or exogenous reinfection? Am Rev Respir Dis 95:729–745, 1967.

57. Raleigh JW, Weichelhausen R. Exogenous reinfection with Mycobacterium tuberculosis confirmed by phage typing. Am Rev Respir Dis 108:639–642, 1973.

58. Nardell E, McInnis B, Thomas B, et al. Exogenous reinfection with tuberculosis in a shelter for the homeless. N Engl J Med 315:1570–1575, 1986.

59. Dannenberg AM Jr. Delayed-type hypersensitivity and cell-mediated immunity in the pathogenesis of tuberculosis. Immunol Today 12:228–236, 1991.

60. Orme IM. Characteristics and specificity of acquired immunologic memory to Mycobacterium tuberculosis. J Immunol 140:3589–3593, 1988.

61. Grange JM. Vaccination against tuberculosis: past problems and future hopes. Semin Respir Crit Care Med 18:459–470, 1997.

62. Orme IM, Flynn JL, Bloom BR. The role of CD8+ T cells in immunity to tuberculosis. Trends Microbiol 1:77–78, 1995.

63. Molloy A, Laochumroonvorapong P, Kaplan G. Apoptosis, but not necrosis, of infected monocytes is coupled with killing of intracellular bacillus Calmette-Guérin. J Exp Med 180:1499–1509, 1995.

64. Orme IM, Anderson P, Boom WH. T cell response to Mycobacterium tuberculosis. J Infect Dis 167:1481–1497, 1993.

65. Mosmann TR. Regulation of immune response by T cells with different cytokine secretor phenotypes: role of a new cytokine, cytokine synthesis inhibitory factor (IL-10). Int Arch Allergy Appl Immunol 94:110–115, 1991.

66. Bretscher PA. A strategy to improve the efficacy of vaccination against tuberculosis and leprosy. Immunol Today 13:342–345, 1992.

67. Surcel HM, Troyer-Blomberg M, Paulie S, et al. Th1/Th2 profiles in tuberculosis based on proliferation and cytokine response of blood lymphocytes to mycobacterial antigens. Immunology 81:171–176, 1994.

68. Schauf V, Rom WN, Smith KA, et al. Cytokine gene activation and modified responsiveness to interleukin-2 in the blood of tuberculosis patients. J Infect Dis 168:1056–1059, 1993.

69. Rook GAW, Hernandez-Pando R. The pathogenesis of tuberculosis. Am Rev Microbiol 50:259–284, 1996.

70. Hernandez-Pando R, Rook GAW. The role of TNF in T cell–mediated inflammation depends on the Th1/Th2 cytokine balance. Immunology 82:591–595, 1994.

70a. Brandt L, Cunha JF, Olsen AW, et al. Failure of the Mycobacterium bovis BCG vaccine: some species of environmental mycobacteria block mulitplication of BCG and induction of protective immunity with tuberculosis. Infec Immun 70:672–678, 2002.

71. Springett VH, Sutherland I. A re-examination of the variations in the efficacy of BCG vaccination against tuberculosis in clinical trials. Tuber Lung Dis 75:227–233, 1994.

72. Hsu KHK. Tuberculin reaction in children treated with isoniazid. Am J Dis Child 137:1090–1092, 1983.

73. Hardy JB. Persistence of hypersensitivity to old tuberculin following primary tuberculosis in childhood: a long-term study. Am J Public Health 36:1417–1426, 1946.

74. Howard TP, Soloman DA. Reading the tuberculin skin test: who, when and how? Arch Intern Med 148:2457–2459, 1988.

75. Steiner P, Rao M, Victoria MS, et al. Persistently negative tuberculin reactions: their presence among children culture-positive for Mycobacterium tuberculosis. Am J Dis Child 134:747–750, 1980.

76. Kent DC, Schwartz R. Active pulmonary tuberculosis with negative tuberculin skin reactions. Am Rev Respir Dis 95:411–418, 1967.

77. American Thoracic Society. Diagnostic standards and classification of tuberculosis. Am Rev Respir Dis 142:725–735, 1990.

78. Huebner RE, Schein MF, Bass JB Jr. The tuberculin skin test. Clin Infect Dis 17:968–975, 1993.

79. O'Brien RJ, Geiter LJ, Snider DE Jr, et al. The epidemiology of nontuberculous mycobacterial diseases in the United States. Am Rev Respir Dis 135:1007–1014, 1987.

80. Edwards LB, Acquaviva FA, Livesay VT, et al. An atlas of sensitivity to tuberculin, PPD-B and histoplasmin in the United States. Am Rev Respir Dis 99:1–99, 1969.

81. American Thoracic Society and the Centers for Disease Control and Prevention. Diagnostic standards and classification of tuberculosis in adults and children. Am J Respir Crit Care Med 161:1376–1395, 2000.

82. Nemir RL, Teichner A. Management of tuberculin reactions in children and adolescents previously vaccinated with BCG. Pediatr Infect Dis J 2:446–451, 1983.

83. Menzies R, Vissandjee B. Effect of bacille Calmette-Guérin vaccination on tuberculin reactivity. Am Rev Respir Dis 145:621–625, 1992.

84. Lifschitz M. The value of the tuberculin skin test as a screening test for tuberculosis among BCG-vaccinated children. Pediatrics 36:624–627, 1965.

85. Horwitz O, Bunch-Christensen K. Correlation between tuberculin sensitivity after 2 months and 5 years among BCG-vaccinated subjects. Bull World Health Organ 47:49–58, 1972.

86. Comstock GW, Edwards LB, Nabangxang H. Tuberculin sensitivity eight to fifteen years after BCG vaccination. Am Rev Respir Dis 103:572–575, 1971.

87. Margus JH, Khassis Y. The tuberculin sensitivity in BCG vaccinated infants and children in Israel. Acta Tuberc Pneumonol Scand 46:113–122, 1965.

88. Landi S, Ashley MJ, Grzybowski S. Tuberculin sensitivity following the intradermal and multiple puncture methods of BCG vaccination. Can Med Assoc J 97:222–225, 1967.

89. Ashley MJ, Siebenmann CO. Tuberculin skin sensitivity following BCG vaccination with vaccines of high and low viable counts. Can Med Assoc J 97:1335–1338, 1967.

90. Kemp EB, Belshe RB, Hoft DF. Immune responses stimulated by percutaneous and intradermal bacille Calmette-Guérin. J Infect Dis 174:113–119, 1996.

91. Joncas JH, Robitaille R, Gauthier T. Interpretation of the PPD skin test in BCG-vaccinated children. Can Med Assoc J 113:127–128, 1975.

92. Magnus K, Edwards LB. The effect of repeated tuberculin testing on post-vaccination allergy. Lancet 1:643–644, 1955.

93. Ildirim I, Hacimustafaoglu M, Ediz B. Correlation of tuberculin induration with the number of bacillus Calmette-Guérin vaccines. Pediatr Infect Dis J 14:1060–1063, 1995.

94. Young TK, Mirdad S. Determinants of tuberculin sensitivity in a child population covered by mass BCG vaccination. Tuber Lung Dis 73:94–100, 1992.

95. Sepulveda RL, Heiba IM, Navarrete C, et al. Tuberculin reactivity after newborn BCG immunization in mono- and dizygotic twins. Tuber Lung Dis 75:138–143, 1994.

96. Sepulveda RL, Heiba IM, King A, et al. Evaluation of tuberculin reactivity in BCG-immunized siblings. Am J Respir Crit Care Med 149:620–624, 1994.

96a. Garly ML, Bale C, Martins CL, et al. BCG vaccination among West African infants is associated with less anergy to tuberculin and diphtheria-tetanus antigens. Vaccine 20: 468–474, 2002.

97. Karalliede S, Katugha LP, Uragoda CG. The tuberculin response of Sri Lankan children after BCG vaccination at birth. Tubercle 68:33–38, 1987.

98. Thompson NJ, Glassroth JL, Snider DE, et al. The booster phenomenon in serial tuberculin testing. Am Rev Respir Dis 119:587–597, 1979.

99. Bass JB Jr, Serio RA. The use of repeat skin tests to eliminate the booster phenomenon in serial tuberculin testing. Am Rev Respir Dis 123:394–396, 1982.

100. Sepulveda RL, Burr C, Ferrer X, et al. Booster effect of tuberculin testing in healthy 6-year-old school children vaccinated with bacillus Calmette-Guérin at birth in Santiago, Chile. Pediatr Infect Dis J 7:578–581, 1988.

101. Sepulveda RL, Ferrer X, Latrach C, et al. The influence of Calmette-Guérin bacillus immunization on the booster effect of tuberculin testing in healthy young adults. Am Rev Respir Dis 142:24–28, 1990.

102. Horowitz HW, Luciano BB, Kadel JR, et al. Tuberculin skin test conversion in hospital employees vaccinated with bacille Calmette-Guérin: recent Mycobacterium tuberculosis infection or booster effect? Am J Infect Control 23:181–187, 1995.

103. Starke JR, Taylor-Watts K. Tuberculosis in the pediatric population of Houston, Texas. Pediatrics 84:28–35, 1989.

104. Abadco DL, Steiner P. Gastric lavage is better than bronchoalveolar lavage for isolation of Mycobacterium tuberculosis in childhood pulmonary tuberculosis. Pediatr Infect Dis J 11:735–738, 1992.

105. Strumpf IJ, Tsang AY, Sayne JW. Reevaluation of sputum staining for the diagnosis of pulmonary tuberculosis. Am Rev Respir Dis 119:599–602, 1979.

106. Lipsky BA, Gates J, Tenover FC, et al. Factors affecting the clinical value of microscopy for acid-fast bacilli. Rev Infect Dis 6:214–222, 1984.

107. Gordin F, Slutkin G. The validity of acid-fast smears in the diagnosis of pulmonary tuberculosis. Arch Pathol Lab Med 114:1025–1027, 1990.

108. Eisenach KD, Sifford MD, Cane MD, et al. Detection of Mycobacterium tuberculosis in sputum samples using a polymerase chain reaction. Am Rev Respir Dis 144:1160–1163, 1991.

109. Noordhock A, Kolk A, Bjune G, et al. Sensitivity and specificity of polymerase chain reaction for detection of Mycobacterium tuberculosis: a blind comparison study among seven laboratories. J Clin Microbiol 32:277–284, 1994.

110. Pierre C, Oliver C, Lecoissier D, et al. Diagnosis of primary tuberculosis in children by amplification and detection of mycobacterial DNA. Am Rev Respir Dis 147:420–424, 1993.

111. Smith KC, Starke JR, Eisenach K, et al. Detection of Mycobacterium tuberculosis in clinical specimens from children using a polymerase chain reaction. Pediatrics 97:155–160, 1996.

112. Gomez-Pastrana D, Torronteras R, Caro P, et al. Comparison of Amplicor, in-house polymerase chain reaction, and conventional culture for the diagnosis of tuberculosis in children. Clin Infect Dis 32:17–22, 2001.

113. Julian E, Cama M, Martinez P, Luquin M. An ELISA for five glycolipids from the cell wall of Mycobacterium tuberculosis: Tween 20 interference in the assay. J Immunol Methods 252:21–30, 2001.

114. Singh KK, Zhang X, Patibandla AS, et al. Antigens of Mycobacterium tuberculosis expressed during preclinical tuberculosis: serological immunodominance of proteins with repetitive amino acid sequences. Infect Immun 69:4185–4191, 2001.

115. Tessema TA, Hamasur B, Bjune G, et al. Diagnostic evaluation of urinary lipoarabinomannan at an Ethiopian tuberculosis center. Scand J Infect Dis 33:279–284, 2001.

116. Hamasur B, Bruchfeld J, Haile M, et al. Rapid diagnosis of tuberculosis by detection of mycobacterial lipoarabinomannan in urine. J Microbiol Meth 45:41–52, 2001.

117. Pottumarthy S, Wells VC, Morris AJ. A comparison of seven tests for serological diagnosis of tuberculosis. J Clin Microbiol 38:2227–2231, 2000.

118. Al Zahrani K, Al Jahdali H, Poirier L, et al. Accuracy and utility of commercially available amplification and serologic tests for the diagnosis of minimal pulmonary tuberculosis. Am J Respir Crit Care Med 162:1323–1329, 2000.

119. Mazurek GH, LoBue PA, Daley CL, et al. Comparison of a whole-blood interferon [gamma] assay with tuberculin skin testing for detecting latent Mycobacterium tuberculosis infection. JAMA 286:1740–1747, 2001.

120. Migliori AB, Borghesi A, Rossnigo P, et al. Proposal for an improved score method for the diagnosis of pulmonary tuberculosis in childhood in developing countries. Tuber Lung Dis 73:145–149, 1992.

121. American Thoracic Society. Treatment of tuberculosis and tuberculosis infection in adults and children. Am J Respir Crit Care Med 149:1359–1374, 1994.

122. American Thoracic Society and the Centers for Disease Control and Prevention. Targeted tuberculin testing and treatment of latent tuberculosis infection. Am J Respir Crit Care Med 161(suppl):S221–S247, 2000.

123. American Academy of Pediatrics. Tuberculosis. In Pickering LK (ed). 2000 Red Book: Report of the Committee on Infectious Diseases (25th ed). Elk Grove Village, IL, American Academy of Pediatrics, 2000, pp 593–613.

124. Centers for Disease Control and Prevention. Core Curriculum on Tuberculosis: What a Clinician Should Know (4th ed). Atlanta, Centers for Disease Control and Prevention, 2000.

125. Joint Tuberculosis Committee of the British Thoracic Society. Chemotherapy and management of tuberculosis in the United Kingdom: recommendations 1998. Thorax 53:536–548, 1998.

126. World Health Organization. Treatment of Tuberculosis: Guidelines for National Programmes (2nd ed). Geneva, World Health Organization, Global Tuberculosis Programme, 1997.

126a. Musher DM. How contagious are common respiratory tract infections? N Eng J Med 348(13):1256–1266,2003.

127. Styblo K. The relationship between the risk of tuberculous infection and the risk of developing infectious tuberculosis. Bull Int Union Tuberc 60:117–119, 1985.

128. Cantwell MF, Snider DE Jr, Cauthen GM, et al. Epidemiology of tuberculosis in the United States, 1985 through 1992. JAMA 272:535–539, 1994.

129. Rose AMC, Watson JM, Graham C, et al. Tuberculosis at the end of the 20th century in England and Wales: results of a national survey in 1998. Thorax 56:173–179, 2001.

130. McKenna MT, McCray E, Onorato IM. The epidemiology of tuberculosis among foreign-born persons in the United States, 1986 to 1993. N Engl J Med 332:1071–1076, 1995.

131. Ussery XT, Valway SE, McKenna M, et al. Epidemiology of tuberculosis among children in the United States: 1985 to 1994. Pediatr Infect Dis J 15:697–704, 1996.

132. Braun MM, Truman BI, Maguire B, et al. Increasing incidence of tuberculosis in a prison inmate population: association with HIV infection. JAMA 261:393–397, 1989.

133. Stead WW. Special problems in tuberculosis. Clin Chest Med 10:397–405, 1989.

134. McAdam JM, Brickner PW, Scharer LL, et al. The spectrum of tuberculosis in a New York City men's shelter clinic (1982–1988). Chest 97:798–805, 1990.

135. Ciesielski SD, Seed JR, Esposito DH, et al. The epidemiology of tuberculosis among North Carolina migrant farm workers. JAMA 265:1715–1719, 1991.

136. Parslow R, El-Shimy NA, Cundall BC, McKinney PA. Tuberculosis, deprivation, and ethnicity in Leeds, UK, 1982–1997. Arch Dis Child 84:109–113, 2001.

137. Centers for Disease Control and Prevention. Nosocomial transmission of multidrug-resistant tuberculosis among HIV-infected persons—Florida and New York, 1988–1991. MMWR 40:585–591, 1991.

138. World Bank. World Development Report: 1993. Washington, DC, The World Bank, 1993.

139. Wells CS, Flahiff EW, Smith HH. Results obtained in man with the use of a vaccine of heat-killed tubercle bacilli. Am J Hyg 40:116–126, 1944.

140. Great Britain Medical Research Council. BCG and vole bacillus vaccines in the prevention of tuberculosis in adolescence and early life. Br Med J 2:379–396, 1959.

141. Weill-Halle B. Oral vaccination. *In* Rosenthal SR (ed). BCG Vaccination Against Tuberculosis. Boston, Little, Brown, 1957, pp 175–182.

142. Luelmo F. BCG vaccination. Am Rev Respir Dis 125(suppl):70–72, 1982.

143. International Union Against Tuberculosis. Phenotypes of BCG vaccines seed lot strains: results of an international cooperative study. Tubercle 59:139–142, 1978.

143a Lewis KN, Liao R, Guinn KM, et al. Deletion of RD1 from *Myobacterium tuberculosis* mimics bacille Calmette–Guérin attenuation. J Infect Dis 187(1)117–123, 2003.

144. Milstien JB, Gibson JJ. Quality control of BCG vaccine by WHO: a review of factors that may influence vaccine effectiveness and safety. Bull World Health Organ 68:93–108, 1990.

145. Osborn TW. Changes in BCG strains. Tubercle 64:1–13, 1983.

146. Jensen KA. Practice of the Calmette vaccination. Acta Tuberc Scand 20:1–45, 1946.

147. Jacox RF, Meade GM. Variation in the duration of tuberculin skin sensitivity produced by two strains of BCG. Am Rev Tuberc 60:541–546, 1949.

148. Dubos RJ, Pierce CH, Schaefer WB. Antituberculous immunity induced in mice by vaccination with living cultures of attenuated tubercle bacilli. J Exp Med 9:207–220, 1953.

149. Dubos RJ, Pierce CH. Differential characteristics in vitro and in vivo of several substrains of BCG. I. Multiplication and survival in vitro. Am Rev Tuberc Pulm Dis 74:655–666, 1956.

150. Pierce CH, Dubos RJ. Differential characteristics in vitro and in vivo of several substrains of BCG. II. Morphologic characteristics in vitro and in vivo. Am Rev Tuberc Pulm Dis 74:667–682, 1956.

151. Pierce CH, Dubos RJ, Schaefer WB. Differential characteristics in vitro and in vivo of several substrains of BCG. III. Multiplication and survival in vivo. Am Rev Tuberc Pulm Dis 74:683–698, 1956.

152. Dubos RJ, Pierce CH. Differential characteristics in vitro and in vivo of several substrains of BCG. IV. Immunizing effectiveness. Am Rev Tuberc Pulm Dis 74:699–717, 1956.

153. Zhang Y, Wallace RJ Jr, Mazurek GH. Genetic differences between BCG substrains. Tuber Lung Dis 76:43–50, 1995.

154. Gheorghiu M. The present and future role of BCG vaccine in tuberculosis control. Biologicals 18:135–141, 1990.

155. Sekuis VM, Freudenstein H, Sirks JL. Report on results of a collaborative assay of BCG vaccines organized by the International Association of Biological Standardization. J Biol Stand 5:85–109, 1977.

156. Gheorghiu M, Lagrange PH. Viability, heat stability and immunogenicity of four BCG vaccines prepared from four different BCG strains. Ann Immunol 134C:124–147, 1983.

157. Formukong NG, Dale JN, Osborn TW, et al. Use of gene probes based on the insertion sequence IS986 to differentiate between BCG vaccine strains. J Appl Bacteriol 72:126–133, 1992.

158. Behr MA. BCG—different strains, different vaccines? Lancet Infect Dis 2:86–92, 2002.

159. Smith D, Harding C, Chan J, et al. Potency of 10 BCG vaccines organized by the IABS. J Biol Stand 7:179–197, 1979.

160. Behr MA. Correlation between BCG genomics and protective efficacy. Scand J Infect Dis 33:249–252, 2001.

161. Comstock GW. Identification of an effective vaccine against tuberculosis. Am Rev Respir Dis 138:479–480, 1988.

162. Tuberculosis Control Program and Expanded Programme on Immunization. Efficacy of infant BCG immunization. Wkly Epidemiol Rec 28:216–218, 1986.

163. Pollock TM. BCG vaccination in man. Tubercle 40:339–412, 1959.

164. Lehman HG, Englehardt H, Freudenstein H, et al. BCG vaccination of neonates, infants, school children and adolescents. II. Safety of vaccine with strain 1331 Copenhagen. Dev Biol Stand 43:133–136, 1979.

165. Expanded Programme on Immunization/Biologicals Unit. Lymphadenitis associated with BCG immunization. Wkly Epidemiol Rec 63:381–388, 1988.

166. Expanded Programme on Immunization/Biologicals Unit. BCG-associated lymphadenitis in infants. Wkly Epidemiol Rec 30:231–232, 1989.

167. Kroger L, Brander E, Korppi M, et al. Osteitis after newborn vaccination with three different bacillus Calmette-Guérin vaccines: twenty-nine years of experience. Pediatr Infect Dis J 12:113–116, 1994.

168. Behr MA, Small PM. Declining efficacy of BCG strains over time? A new hypothesis for an old controversy [abstract]. Am J Respir Crit Care Med 155:A222, 1997.

169. Harboe M, Nagel S. MPB70, a unique antigen of *Mycobacterium bovis* BCG. Am Rev Respir Dis 129:444–452, 1984.

170. Abou-Zeid C, Rook GAW, Mannikin DE, et al. Effect of the method of preparation of bacille Calmette-Guérin vaccine on the properties of four daughter strains. J Appl Bacteriol 63:449–453, 1987.

171. TICE® BCG: BCG Live Available at *www.pdr.net* (Accessed June 3, 2002.)

172. Devadoss PO, Klegerman ME, Groves MJ. A scanning electron microscope study of mycobacterial developmental stages in commercial BCG vaccines. Curr Microbiol 22:247–252, 1991.

173. Gheorghiu M. The stability and immunogenicity of a dispersed-grown freeze-dried Pasteur BCG vaccine. J Biol Stand 15:15–26, 1988.

174. Fine PEM, Carneiro IAM, Milstien JB, Clements CJ. Issues Relating to the Use of BCG in Immunization Programmes: A Discussion Document. Geneva, World Health Organization, Department of Vaccines and Biologicals, 1999.

175. World Health Organization, Department of Vaccines, Immunization and Biologicals. UN Prequalified BCG Vaccines. Available at *www.who.int/vaccines-access/vaccines/Vaccine_Quality/UN_Prequalified/unbcgproducers.html* (Accessed June 6, 2002.)

176. Gheorghiu M, Augier J, Lagrange PH. Maintenance and control of the French BCG strain 1173P2 (primary and secondary seed lots). Bull Inst Pasteur 81:281–288, 1983.

177. Galbraith NS, Hall C. Comparative trials of British BCG vaccine double strength, and Danish BCG vaccine with standard strength British BCG vaccine. Tubercle 55:283–289, 1974.

178. ten Dam HG. Research on BCG vaccination. Adv Tuberc Res 21:79–106, 1984.

179. ten Dam HG, Fillastre C, Conge C, et al. The use of jet injectors in BCG vaccination. Bull World Health Organ 43:707–720, 1970.

180. Darmanger AM, Nekzad SM, Kuis M, et al. BCG vaccination by bifurcated needle in a pilot BCG vaccination programme. Bull World Health Organ 55:49–61, 1977.

181. Birkhaug K. An experimental and clinical investigation of a percutaneous (Rosenthal) method of BCG vaccination. Nord Med 10:1224–1231, 1941.

182. Briggs IL, Smith C. BCG vaccination by the multiple puncture method in northern Rhodesia. Tubercle 38:107–111, 1957.

183. Griffith AH. BCG vaccination by multiple puncture. Lancet 1:1170–1172, 1959.

184. Stainer DW, Landi S. Stability of BCG vaccines. Dev Biol Stand 58:119–125, 1986.

185. Smith PG. Case-control studies of the efficacy of BCG against tuberculosis. *In* International Union Against Tuberculosis. Proceedings of the XXVIth IUAT World Conference on Tuberculosis and Respiratory Diseases. Singapore, Japan, Professional Postgraduate Services International, 1987, pp 73–79.

186. Filho VW, de Castilho EA, Rodrigues LC, et al. Effectiveness of BCG vaccination against tuberculous meningitis: a case-control study in Sao Paulo, Brazil. Bull World Health Organ 68:69–74, 1990.

187. Sutherland I, Lindgren I. The protective effect of BCG vaccination as indicated by autopsy studies. Tubercle 60:225–231, 1979.

188. Smith DW, Harding G, Chan J, et al. Potency of 10 BCG vaccines as evaluated by their influence on the bacillemic phase of experimental airborne tuberculosis in guinea pigs. J Biol Stand 7:179–197, 1979.

189. Jensen KA, Bindsleu G, Holm J. Experimental studies on the development of tuberculous infection in allergic and non-allergic animals. I. Development of tuberculous infection in the lungs after inhalation of virulent tubercle bacilli. Acta Tuberc Scand 9:27–46, 1935.

190. Levy FM, Conge GA, Pasquier JF, et al. The effect of BCG-vaccination on the fate of virulent tubercle bacilli in mice. Am Rev Respir Dis 84:28–36, 1961.

191. Smith DW, McMurray DN, Wiegeshaus EH, et al. Host-parasite relationship in experimental airborne tuberculosis. IV. Early events in the course of infection in vaccinated and nonvaccinated guinea pigs. Am Rev Respir Dis 102:937–949, 1970.

192. Dannenberg AM. Cellular hypersensitivity and cellular immunity in the pathogenesis of tuberculosis: specificity, systemic and local nature, and associated macrophage enzymes. Bacteriol Rev 32:85–102, 1968.

193. Ho RS, Fok JS, Harding GE, et al. Host-parasite relationships in experimental airborne tuberculosis. VII. Fate of *Mycobacterium tuberculosis* in primary lung lesions and in primary lesion free lung

tissue infected as a result of bacillemia. J Infect Dis 138:237–241, 1978.

194. Morrison NE, Collins FM. Restoration of T-cell responsiveness by thymosin: development of antituberculosis resistance in BCG-infected animals. Infect Immun 13:554–563, 1976.

195. Lefford MJ, McGregor DD, Mackaness DB. Immune response to *Mycobacterium tuberculosis* in rats. Infect Immun 8:182–189, 1973.

196. Workshop report. Summary, conclusions, and recommendations from the International Workshop on Research Towards Global Control and Prevention of Tuberculosis: with an emphasis on vaccine development. J Infect Dis 158:248–253, 1988.

197. Browne JAK, Stone MM, Sutherland I. BCG vaccination of children against leprosy in Uganda: first results. Br Med J 1:7–14, 1966.

198. Ponninghaus JM, Fine PEM, Sterne JAC, et al. Efficacy of BCG vaccine against leprosy and tuberculosis in Northern Malawi. Lancet 339:636–639, 1992.

199. Karonga Prevention Trial Group. Randomized controlled trial of single BCG, repeated BCG, or combined BCG and killed *Mycobacterium leprae* vaccine for prevention of leprosy and tuberculosis. Lancet 348:17–24, 1996.

200. Trnka L, Dankova D, Svandova E. Six years' experience with the discontinuation of BCG vaccine. 4. Protective effect of BCG against *Mycobacterium avium-intracellulare* complex. Tuber Lung Dis 75:348–352, 1994.

201. Romanus V, Svensson A, Hollander HO. The impact of changing BCG coverage on tuberculosis in Swedish children between 1969 and 1989. Tuber Lung Dis 73:150–161, 1992.

201a. Ota MO, Vekemans J, Schlegel–Haueter SE, et al. Influence of *Myobacterium bovis* bacillus Calmette-Guérin on antibody and cytokine responses to human neonatal vaccination. J Immunol 168(2):919–925, 2002.

202. Fine PEM. The BCG story: lessons from the past and implications for the future. Rev Infect Dis 11(suppl 2):S353–S359, 1989.

203. Fine PEM, Ponnighaus JM, Maine NP. The relationship between delayed type hypersensitivity and protective immunity induced by mycobacterial vaccines in man. Lepr Rev 57(suppl 12):S274–S283, 1986.

204. Fine PEM, Sterne JAC, Ponnighaus JM, et al. Delayed type hypersensitivity, mycobacterial vaccines and protective immunity. Lancet 344:1245–1249, 1994.

205. Tuberculosis Prevention Trial. Trial of BCG vaccines in South India for tuberculosis prevention: first report. Bull World Health Organ 57:819–827, 1979.

206. Tripathy SP. Fifteen-year follow-up of the Indian BCG prevention trial. Bull Int Union Tuberc Lung Dis 62:69–73, 1987.

207. al-Kassimi FA, al-Hajjaj MS, al-Orainey IO, et al. Does the protective effect of neonatal BCG correlate with vaccine-induced tuberculin reaction? Am J Respir Crit Care Med 152:1575–1578, 1995.

208. Grange JM. Environmental mycobacteria and BCG vaccination. Tubercle 67:1–4, 1986.

209. Pithie AD, Rahelu M, Kumararatne DS, et al. Generation of cytolytic T cells in individuals infected with *Mycobacterium tuberculosis* and vaccinated with BCG. Thorax 47:695–701, 1992.

210. Fine PEM. Leprosy and tuberculosis: an epidemiological comparison. Tubercle 65:137–153, 1984.

211. Schluger NW, Rom WN. The host immune response to tuberculosis. Am J ResTpir Crit Care Med 157:679–691, 1998.

211a. Klunner T, Bartels T, Vordermeier M, Burger R, Schafer H. Immune reactions of CD4–and CD8– positive T cell subpopulations in spleen and lymph nodes of guinea pigs after vaccination with bacillus Calmette–Guérin. Vaccine 19(15–16):1968–1977, 2001.

212. Serbina NV, Liu C-C, Scanga CA, Flynn JL. CD8+ CTL from lungs of *Mycobacteria tuberculosis*-infected mice express perforin *in vivo* and lyse infected macrophages. J Immunol 165:353–363, 2000.

213. Stenger S, Modlin RL. Cytotoxic T cell responses to intracellular pathogens. Curr Opin Immunol 10:471–477, 1998.

214. Andersen P, Munk ME, Pollock JM, Doherty TM. Specific immune-based diagnosis of tuberculosis. Lancet 356:1099–1104, 2000.

215. Mazurek GH, LoBue PA, Daley CL, et al. Comparison of a whole-blood interferon gamma assay with tuberculin skin testing for detecting latent *Mycobacterium tuberculosis* infection. JAMA 286:1740–1747, 2001.

216. Clemens JD, Chuong JJH, Feinstein AR. The BCG controversy: a methodological and statistical reappraisal. JAMA 249:2362 2360 1983.

217. Fine PEM, Rodrigues LC. Modern vaccines: mycobacterial diseases. Lancet 335:1016–1020, 1990.

218. Wilson ME, Fineberg HV, Colditz GA. Geographic latitude and the efficacy of bacillus Calmette-Guérin vaccine. Clin Infect Dis 20:982–991, 1995.

219. Brewer TF, Colditz GA. Relationship between bacille Calmette-Guérin (BCG) strains and the efficacy of BCG vaccine in the prevention of tuberculosis. Clin Infect Dis 20:126–135, 1995.

220. Fine PEM. Variation in protection by BCG: implications of and for heterologous immunity. Lancet 346:1339–1345, 1995.

221. Miceli I, de Kantor IN, Colaiacovo D, et al. Evaluation of the effectiveness of BCG vaccination using the case-control method in Buenos Aires, Argentina. Int J Epidemiol 17:629–634, 1988.

222. Camargos PAM, Guimaraes MDC, Antunes CMF. Risk assessment for acquiring meningitis tuberculosis among children not vaccinated with BCG: a case control study. Int J Epidemiol 17:193–197, 1988.

223. Bagshawe A, Scott GC, Russell DA, et al. BCG vaccination in leprosy: final results of the trial in Karimui, Papua New Guinea. Bull World Health Organ 67:389–399, 1989.

224. Stanley SJ, Howland C, Stone MM, Sutherland I. BCG vaccination of children against leprosy in Uganda: final results. J Hyg (Camb) 87:235–248, 1981.

225. Bertolli J, Pangi C, Frerichs R, Halloran ME. A case-control study of the effectiveness of BCG vaccine for preventing leprosy in Yangon, Myanmar. Int J Epidemiol 26:888–895, 1997.

226. Lwin K, Sundaresan T, Gyi MM, et al. BCG vaccination of children against leprosy: fourteen year findings of the trial in Burma. Bull World Health Organ 63:1069–1078, 1985.

227. Thuc NV, Abel L, Lap VC, et al. Protective effect of BCG against leprosy and its subtypes: a case control study in Southern Viet Nam. Int J Lepr 62:532–538, 1994.

228. Ponnighaus JM, Fine PEM, Sterne JAC, et al. Efficacy of BCG against leprosy and tuberculosis in Northern Malawi. Lancet 339:636–639, 1992.

229. Tripathy SP. The case for BCG. Ann Natl Acad Med Sci 19:11–21, 1983.

230. Orege PA, Fine PEM, Lucas SB, et al. Case control study of BCG vaccination as a risk factor for leprosy and tuberculosis in Western Kenya. Int J Lepr 61:542–549, 1993.

231. Comstock GW. Field trials of tuberculosis vaccines: how could we have done them better? Control Clin Trials 15:247–276, 1994.

232. Starke JR, Connelly KK. Bacille Calmette-Guérin (BCG) vaccine. *In* Vaccines (2nd ed). Philadelphia, WB Saunders, 1994, pp 439–473.

233. Smith KC, Starke JR. Bacille Calmette-Guérin (BCG) vaccine. *In* Vaccines (3rd ed). Philadelphia, WB Saunders, 1999, pp 111–139.

234. Stein SC, Aronson JD. The occurrence of pulmonary lesions in BCG-vaccinated and unvaccinated persons. Am Rev Tuberc 68:695–712, 1953.

235. Rosenthal SR, Loewinsohn E, Graham ML, et al. BCG vaccination against tuberculosis in Chicago: a twenty-year study statistically analyzed. Pediatrics 28:622–641, 1961.

236. Hart PD, Sutherland I. BCG and vole bacillus vaccines in the prevention of tuberculosis in adolescence and early adult life. Final report to the Medical Research Council. Br Med J 2:293–295, 1977.

237. Palmer CE, Shaw LW, Comstock GW. Community trials of BCG vaccination. Am Rev Tuberc Pulm Dis 77:877–907, 1958.[AU3]

238. Frimodt-Moller J, Thomas J, Parthasanathy R. Observations on the protective effect of BCG vaccination in a south Indian rural population. Bull World Health Organ 30:545–574, 1964.

239. Frimodt-Moller J, Acharyulu G, Pillai K. Observations on the protective effect of BCG vaccination in a south Indian rural population: fourth report. Bull Int Union Tuberc 48:40–52, 1973.

240. Comstock G, Shaw L. Controlled trial of BCG vaccination in a school population. Public Health Rep 75:583–594, 1960.

241. Comstock G, Webster R. Tuberculosis studies in Muscogee County, Georgia: VII. A 20 year evaluation of BCG vaccination in a school population. Am Rev Respir Dis 100:839–845, 1969.

242. Comstock G, Palmer C. Long-term results of BCG vaccination in the southern United States. Am Rev Respir Dis 93:171–183, 1966.

243. Comstock GW. Identification of an effective vaccine against tuberculosis. Am Rev Respir Dis 138:479–480, 1988.

244. Stanford JL, Shield MJ, Rook GAW. How environmental mycobacteria may predetermine the protective efficacy of BCG. Tubercle 62:55–62, 1981.

245. Rook GAW, Bahr GM, Stanford JL. The effect of two distinct forms of cell-mediated response to mycobacteria on the protective efficacy of BCG. Tubercle 62:63–68, 1981.

246. Edwards LB, Palmer CE. Identification of the tuberculous-infected by skin tests. Ann N Y Acad Sci 154:140–148, 1968.

247. Palmer CE, Hopwood L. Effect of previous infection with unclassified mycobacteria on survival of guinea pigs challenged with virulent tubercle bacilli. Bull Int Union Tuberc 32:389–391, 1962.

248. Edwards ML, Goodrich JM, Muller D, et al. Infection with *Mycobacterium avium-intracellulare* and the protective effects of bacilli Calmette-Guérin. J Infect Dis 145:733–741, 1982.

248a Brandt L, Feino Cunha J, Weinreich Olsen A, et al. Failure of the *Mycobacterium bovis* BCG vaccine: some species of environmental mycobacteria block multiplication of BCG and induction of protective immunity to tuberculosis. Infect Immun 70(2):672–678, 2002.

249. Fine PEM. Immunogenetics of susceptibility to leprosy, tuberculosis and leishmaniasis: an epidemiological perspective. Int J Lepr 49:437–454, 1981.

250. Schurr E, Buschman E, Gros P, et al. Genetic aspects of mycobacterial infections in mouse and man. *In* Melchers F (ed). Progress in Immunology. Vol. VII. New York, Springer-Verlag, 1990, pp 994–1001.

251. Skamene E. Genetic control of susceptibility to mycobacterial infections. Rev Infect Dis 11(suppl 2):S394–S399, 1989.

252. Vidal SM, Malo D, Vogan K, et al. Natural resistance to infection with intracellular parasites: isolation of a candidate for *Bcg*. Cell 73:469–485, 1993.

253. Dubos R. Acquired immunity to tuberculosis. Am Rev Respir Dis 90:505–515, 1964.

254. Cohen MK, Bartow RA, Mintzer CL, et al. Effect of diet and genetics on *Mycobacterium bovis* BCG vaccine efficacy in inbred guinea pigs. Infect Immun 55:314–319, 1987.

255. McMurray DN, Kimball MS, Tetzlaff CL, et al. Effects of protein deprivation and BCG vaccination on alveolar macrophage function in pulmonary tuberculosis. Am Rev Respir Dis 133:1081–1085, 1986.

256. D'Arcy Hart P, Sutherland I. Acquired immunity to tuberculosis. Am Rev Respir Dis 91:939, 1965.

257. Padungchan S, Konjanart S, Kasiratta S, et al. The effectiveness of BCG vaccination of the newborn against childhood tuberculosis in Bangkok. Bull World Health Organ 64:247–258, 1986.

257a.Malhotra I, Mungai P, Wamachi A, et al. Helminth– and bacillus Calmette-Guérin; induced immunity in children sensitized in utero to filariasis and schistosomiasis. J Immunol 162(11): 6843–6848, 1999.

258. Hank JA, Chan JK, Edwards ML, et al. Influence of the virulence of *Mycobacterium tuberculosis* on protection induced by bacilli Calmette-Guérin in guinea pigs. J Infect Dis 143:734–738, 1981.

259. Ziegler JE, Edwards ML, Smith DW. Exogenous reinfection in experimental airborne tuberculosis. Tubercle 66:121–128, 1985.

260. Stead WW. The pathogenesis of pulmonary tuberculosis among older persons. Am Rev Respir Dis 91:811–822, 1965.

261. Styblo K. Recent advances in epidemiological research in tuberculosis. Adv Tuberc Res 20:1–63, 1980.

262. Eisenach KD, Crawford JT, Bates JH. Genetic relatedness among strains of the *Mycobacterium tuberculosis* complex. Am Rev Respir Dis 133:1065–1068, 1986.

263. Daley CL, Small PM, Schecter GF, et al. An outbreak of tuberculosis with accelerated progression among persons infected with the human immunodeficiency virus: an analysis using restriction-fragment-length polymorphisms. N Engl J Med 326:231–235, 1992.

264. Smith PG. Retrospective assessment of the effectiveness of BCG vaccination against tuberculosis using the case-control method. Tubercle 62:23–35, 1982.

265. Fine PEM. BCG vaccination against tuberculosis and leprosy. Br Med Bull 44:693–703, 1988.

266. Murtagh K. Efficacy of BCG [letter]. Lancet 1:423, 1980.

267. Chavalittamrong B, Chearskul S, Tuchinda M. Protective value of BCG vaccination in children in Bangkok, Thailand. Pediatr Pulmonol 2:202–205, 1986.

268. Micheli I, de Kantor IN, Colaiacovo D, et al. Evaluation of the effectiveness of BCG vaccination using the case-control method in Buenos Aires, Argentina. Int J Epidemiol 17:629–634, 1988.

269. Sirinavin S, Chotpitayasunondh T, Suwanjutha S, et al. Protective efficacy of neonatal bacillus Calmette-Guérin vaccination against tuberculosis. Pediatr Infect Dis J 10:359–365, 1991.

270. Effectiveness of BCG vaccination in Great Britain in 1978: a report from the research committee of the British Thoracic Association. Br J Dis Chest 74:215–227, 1980.

271. Ferguson RG, Simes AB. BCG vaccination of Indian infants in Saskatchewan. Tubercle 30:5–11, 1949.

272. Curtis HM, Leck I, Bamford FN. Incidence of childhood tuberculosis after neonatal BCG vaccination. Lancet 1:145–148, 1984.

273. Shannon A, Kelly P, Lucey M, et al. Isoniazid resistant tuberculosis in a school outbreak: the protective effect of BCG. Eur Respir J 4:778–782, 1991.

274. Rodriques LC, Gill ON, Smith PG. BCG vaccination in the first year of life protects children of Indian subcontinent ethnic origin against tuberculosis in England. J Epidemiol Community Health 45:78–80, 1991.

275. Packe GE, Innes JA. Protective effect of BCG vaccination in infant Asians: a case-control study. Arch Dis Child 63:277–281, 1988.

276. Houston S, Fanning A, Soskolne CL, et al. The effectiveness of bacillus Calmette-Guérin (BCG) vaccination against tuberculosis: a case-control study in treaty Indians, Alberta, Canada. Am J Epidemiol 131:340–347, 1990.

277. Young TK, Hershfield ES. A case-control study to evaluate the effectiveness of mass neonatal BCG vaccination among Canadian Indians. Am J Public Health 76:783–786, 1986.

278. Blin P, Delolme HG, Heyraud JD, et al. Evaluation of the protective effect of BCG vaccination by a case-control study in Yaounde, Cameroon. Tubercle 67:283–288, 1986.

279. Tidjani O, Amendome A, ten Dam HG. The protective effect of BCG vaccination of the newborn against childhood tuberculosis in an African community. Tubercle 67:269–281, 1986.

280. Putrali J, Sutrisna B, Rahayoe N, et al. A case-control study of effectiveness of BCG vaccination in children in Jakarta, Indonesia. *In* Proceedings of the Eastern Regional Tuberculosis Conference of IUAT, Jakarta, Indonesia, November 20–25, 1983, pp 194–200.

281. Patel A, Schofield F, Siskind V, et al. Case-control evaluation of a school-age BCG vaccination programme in subtropical Australia. Bull World Health Organ 69:425–433, 1991.

282. Shapiro C, Cook N, Evans D, et al. A case-control study of BCG and childhood tuberculosis in Cali, Colombia. Int J Epidemiol 14:441–446, 1985.

283. Smith PG. Evaluating interventions against tropical diseases. Int J Epidemiol 16:159–166, 1987.

284. Sepulveda RL, Parcha C, Sorensen RU. Case-control study of the efficacy of BCG immunization against pulmonary tuberculosis in young adults in Santiago, Chile. Tuber Lung Dis 73:372–377, 1992.

285. Thilothammal N, Kirshnamurthy PV, Runyan DK, et al. Does BCG vaccine prevent tuberculous meningitis? Arch Dis Child 74:144–147, 1996.

286. Rodriques LC, Diwan VK, Wheeler JG. Protective effect of BCG against tuberculous meningitis and miliary tuberculosis: a meta-analysis. Int J Epidemiol 22:1154–1158, 1993.

287. Colditz GA, Berkey CS, Mosteller F, et al. The efficacy of bacillus Calmette-Guérin vaccination of newborns and infants in the prevention of tuberculosis: meta-analyses of the published literature. Pediatrics 96:29–35, 1995.

288. Colditz GA, Brewer TF, Berkey CS, et al. Efficacy of BCG vaccine in the prevention of tuberculosis: meta-analysis of the published literature. JAMA 271:698–702, 1994.

289. Sterne JAC, Rodrigues LC, Guedes IN. Does the efficacy of BCG decline with time since vaccination? Int J Tuberc Lung Dis 2:200–207, 1998.

290. American Academy of Pediatrics. Tuberculosis. *In* Pickering LK (ed). 2000 Red Book: Report of the Committee on Infectious Diseases (25th ed). Elk Grove Village, IL, American Academy of Pediatrics, 2000, pp 611–612.

291. Joint Tuberculosis Committee of the British Thoracic Society. Control and prevention of tuberculosis in the United Kingdom: code of practice 2000. Thorax 55:887–901, 2000.

292. Lotte A, Wasz-Hockert O, Poisson N, et al. BCG complications: estimates of the risks among vaccinated subjects and statistical analysis of their main characteristics. Adv Tuberc Res 21:107–193, 1984.

293. Victoria MS, Shah BR. Bacillus Calmette-Guérin lymphadenitis: a case report and review of the literature. Pediatr Infect Dis J 4:295–296, 1985.

293a. Turnbull FM, McIntyre PB, Achat HM, et al. National study of adverse reactions after vaccination with bacille Calmette–Guérin. Clin Infect Dis 34(4): 447–453, 2002.

294. Brewer MA, Edwards KM, Palmer PS, Hinson HP. Bacille Calmette-Guérin immunization in normal healthy adults. J Infect Dis 170:476–479, 1994.

295. Fine PEM, Ponnighaus JM, Maine N. The distribution and implications of BCG scars, with particular reference to a population in Northern Malawi. Bull World Health Organ 67:35–42, 1989.

296. Lotte A, Wasz-Hockert O, Poisson N, et al. Second IUATLD study on complications induced by intradermal BCG-vaccination. Bull Int Union Tuberc 63:47–59, 1988.

297. Reynes J, Perez C, Lamaury I, et al. Bacille Calmette-Guérin adenitis 30 years after immunization in a patient with AIDS [letter]. J Infect Dis 160:727, 1989.

298. Gheorghiu M. Potency and suppurative adenitis in BCG vaccination. Dev Biol Stand 41:79–84, 1978.

299. Muzy de Souza GR, Sant'Anna CC, Lapane Silva JR, et al. Intradermal BCG vaccination complications—analysis of 51 cases. Tubercle 64:23–27, 1983.

300. Helmick CG, D'Souza AJ, Goddard N. An outbreak of severe BCG axillary lymphadenitis in Saint Lucia, 1982–83. West Indies Med J 35:12–17, 1986.

301. Praveen KN, Smikle MF, Prabhakar P, et al. Outbreak of bacillus Calmette-Guérin–associated lymphadenitis and abscesses in Jamaican children. Pediatr Infect Dis J 9:890–893, 1990.

302. O'Brien KL, Ruff AJ, Louis MA, et al. Bacillus Calmette-Guérin complications in children born to HIV-1–infected women with a review of the literature. Pediatrics 95:414–418, 1995.

303. Caglayan S, Yegin O, Kayean K, et al. Is medical therapy effective for regional lymphadenitis following BCG vaccination? Am J Dis Child 141:1213–1214, 1987.

304. Oguz F, Mujgan S, Alper G, et al. Treatment of bacillus Calmette-Guérin–associated lymphadenitis. Pediatr Infect Dis J 11:887–888, 1992.

305. World Health Organization. BCG Vaccination of the Newborn: Rationale and Guidelines for Country Programs. Geneva, World Health Organization, 1986.

306. Hanley SP, Gumb J, MacFarlane JT. Comparison of erythromycin and isoniazid in treatment of adverse reactions to BCG vaccination. Br Med J (Clin Res Ed) 290:970, 1985.

307. Murphy PM, Mayers DL, Brock NF, Wagner KF. Cure of bacille Calmette-Guérin vaccination abscess with erythromycin. Rev Infect Dis 11:335–337, 1989.

308. Power JT, Stewart IC, Ross JD. Erythromycin in the management of troublesome BCG lesions. Br J Dis Chest 78:192–193, 1984.

309. Goraya JS, Virdi VS. Treatment of Calmette-Guérin bacillus adenitis: a metaanalysis. Pediatr Infect Dis J 20:632–634, 2001.

310. Kroger L, Korppi M, Brander E, et al. Osteitis caused by bacillus Calmette-Guérin vaccination: a retrospective analysis of 222 cases. J Infect Dis 172:574–576, 1995.

311. Bergdahl S, Fellander M, Robertson B. BCG osteomyelitis: experience in the Stockholm region over the years 1961–1974. J Bone Joint Surg Br 58:212–216, 1976.

312. Vanicek H. Complications after initial BCG vaccination in a 5-year period in the East Bohemia region. Cesk Pediatr 43:23–26, 1988.

313. Bottiger M. Osteitis and other complications caused by generalized BCGitis. Acta Paediatr Scand 71:471–478, 1982.

314. Rouillon A, Waaler H. BCG vaccination and epidemiological situation: a decision making approach to the use of BCG. Adv Tuberc Res 19:64–126, 1976.

315. Pedersen FK, Engbaek HC, Hertz H, Vergmann B. Fatal BCG infection in an immunocompetent girl. Acta Paediatr Scand 67:519–523, 1978.

316. Trevenen CL, Pagtakhan RD. Disseminated tuberculoid lesions in infants following BCG. Can Med J 15:502–504, 1982.

317. Lachaux A, Descos B, Mertani A, et al. Infection generalisée a BCG d'evolution favorable chez un nourrisson de 3 mois sans deficit immunitaire reconnu. Arch Fr Pediatr 43:807–809, 1986.

318. Tardieu M, Truffot-Pernot C, Carriere JP, et al. Tuberculosis meningitis due to BCG in two previously healthy children. Lancet 1:440–441, 1988.

319. Gormsen H. On the occurrence of epithelioid cell granulomas in the organs of BCG vaccinated human beings. Acta Pathol Microbiol Scand 39(suppl 111):117–120, 1956.

320. Casanova JL, Blanche S, Emile JF, et al. Idiopathic disseminated bacille Calmette-Guérin infection: a French national retrospective study. Pediatrics 98:774–778, 1996.

321. Konno K, Feldmann FM, McDermott W. Pyrazinamide susceptibility and amidase activity of tubercle bacilli. Am Rev Respir Dis 95:461–469, 1967.

322. Von Kries R, Grunert VP, Kaletsch U, et al. Prevention of childhood leukemia by BCG vaccination in newborns? A population-based case-control study in Lower Saxony, Germany. Pediatr Hematol Oncol 17:541–550, 2000.

323. Gonzalez B, Moreno S, Burdach R, et al. Clinical presentation of bacillus Calmette-Guérin infections in patients with immunodeficiency syndromes. Pediatr Infect Dis J 8:201–206, 1989.

324. Boudes P, Sobel A, Deforges L. Disseminated Mycobacterium bovis infection from BCG vaccination and HIV infection [letter]. JAMA 262:2386, 1989.

325. Kobayashi Y, Komazawa Y, Kobayshi M, et al. Presumed BCG infection in a boy with chronic granulomatous disease. Clin Pediatr 23:586–589, 1984.

326. Houde C, Dery P. Mycobacterium bovis sepsis in an infant with human immunodeficiency virus infection. Pediatr Infect Dis J 11:810–811, 1988.

327. Sicevic S. Generalized BCG tuberculosis with fatal course in two sisters. Acta Paediatr Scand 61:178–184, 1972.

328. Talbot EA, Perkins MD, Silva SFM, et al. Disseminated bacille Calmette-Guérin disease after vaccination: case report and review. Clin Infect Dis 24:1139–1146, 1997.

329. Jouanguy E, Altare F, Lamhamedi S, et al. Interferon-gamma-receptor deficiency in an infant with fatal bacille Calmette-Guérin infection. N Engl J Med 335:1956–1961, 1996.

330. Elloumi-Zghal H, Barbouche MR, Chemli J, et al. Clinical and genetic heterogeneity of inherited autosomal recessive susceptibility to disseminated Mycobacterium bovis bacilli Calmette-Guérin infection. J Infect Dis 185:1468–1475, 2002.

331. Armbruster C, Junker W, Vetter N, Jaksch G. Disseminated bacille Calmette-Guérin infection in an AIDS patient 30 years after BCG vaccination [letter]. J Infect Dis 162:1216, 1990.

332. Ninane J, Grymonprez A, Burtonboy G, et al. Disseminated BCG in HIV infection. Arch Dis Child 63:1268–1269, 1988.

333. Centers for Disease Control and Prevention. Disseminated Mycobacterium bovis infection from BCG vaccination of a patient with acquired immunodeficiency syndrome. MMWR 34:227–228, 1985.

334. Edwards K, Kernodle DS. Possible hazards of routine bacillus Calmette-Guérin immunization in human immunodeficiency virus–infected children. Pediatr Infect Dis J 15:836–838, 1996.

335. Colebunders RL, Izaley L, Musampu M, et al. BCG vaccine abscesses are unrelated to HIV infection [letter]. JAMA 259:352, 1988.

336. Carswell M. BCG immunization in the children of HIV-positive mothers. AIDS 1:258, 1987.

337. Dabis F, Lepage P, Nsengumuremyi F, et al. Infection par le virus V1HI et vaccination de routine de l'enfant: une etude cohorte à Kigali, Rwanda—surveillance des effets indésirables de la vaccination [abstr C29]. In Proceedings of the Conference Internationale, Les Implications du SIDA pour la Mère et l'Enfant, Paris, 1989.

338. Lallemant–Le Coeur S, Cheynier D, Lallemant M, et al. Complications loco-régionales de la vaccination par le BCG chez des enfants nés de mères positive pour anti-HIV1: etude cas-témoins à Brazzaville [abstr WG03]. In Proceedings of the Fifth International Conference on AIDS, Montreal, 1989. Ottawa, Canada, International Development Research Center, 1989, p 982.

339. Thaithumyanon P, Thisyakorn U, Punnahitananda S, et al. Safety and immunogenicity of bacillus Calmette-Guérin vaccine in children born to HIV-1 infected women. Southeast Asian J Trop Med Public Health 31:482–486, 2000.

340. Besnard M, Sauvion S, Offredo C, et al. Bacillus Calmette-Guérin infection after vaccination of human immunodeficiency virus–infected children. Pediatr Infect Dis J 12:993–997, 1993.

341. Palme IB, Gudetta B, Degefu H, et al. Risk factors for human immunodeficiency virus infection in Ethiopian children with tuberculosis. Pediatr Infect Dis J 20:1066–1072, 2001.

342. Special Program on AIDS and Expanded Programme on Immunization. Consultation on human immunodeficiency virus (HIV) and routine childhood immunization. Wkly Epidemiol Rec 62:297–304, 1987.

343. Hoft DF, Leonardi C, Milligan T, et al. Clinical reactogenicity of intradermal bacilli Calmette-Guérin vaccination. Clin Infect Dis 28:785–790, 1999.

344. Brewer MA, Edwards KM, Palmer PS, Hinson HP. Bacilli Calmette-Guérin immunization in normal healthy adults. J Infect Dis 170:476–479, 1994.

345. ten Dam HG, Hitze KL. Does BCG vaccination protect the newborn and young infants? Bull World Health Organ 58:37–41, 1980.

346. Ferreira AA, Bunn-Moreno MM, Sant'Anna CC, et al. BCG vaccination in low birth weight newborns: analysis of lymphocyte proliferation, Il-2 generation and intradermal reaction to PPD. Tuber Lung Dis 77:476–481, 1996.

347. Thayyil-Sudhan S, Kumar A, Singh M, et al. Safety and effectiveness of BCG vaccination in preterm babies. Arch Dis Child Fetal Neonatal Ed 81:F64–F66, 1999.

348. Hart PD. Efficacy and applicability of mass BCG vaccination in tuberculosis control. Br Med J 1:587–592, 1967.

349. Sutherland I, Springett VH. The effects of the scheme for BCG vaccination of school children in England and Wales and the consequences of discontinuing the scheme at various dates. J Epidemiol Community Health 43:15–24, 1989.

350. Springett VH, Sutherland I. BCG vaccination of school children in England and Wales. Thorax 45:83–88, 1990.

351. United Kingdom Health Departments. Immunisation Against Infectious Diseases. London: Her Majesty's Stationery Office, 1996, pp 1–290.

352. Romanus V, Svensson A, Hallander HO. The impact of changing BCG coverage on tuberculosis incidence in Swedish-born children between 1969 and 1989. Tuberc Lung Dis 73:150–161, 1992.

353. Trnka L, Dankova D, Svandova E. Six years' experience with the discontinuation of BCG vaccination. Tuberc Lung Dis 74:167–172, 1993.

354. International Union Against Tuberculosis and Lung Disease. Criteria for discontinuation of vaccination programmes using Bacille Calmette Guérin (BCG) in countries with a low prevalence of tuberculosis. Tuber Lung Dis 75:179–181, 1994.

355. WHO Expert Committee on Leprosy Seventh Report. WHO Tech Rep Ser No 874, 1998.

356. World Health Organization. BCG in immunization programmes. Wkly Epidemiol Rec 76:33–40, 2001.

357. Centers for Disease Control and Prevention. The role of BCG vaccine in the prevention and control of tuberculosis in the United States: a joint statement by the Advisory Committee for the Elimination of Tuberculosis and the Advisory Committee on Immunization Practices. MMWR 45(RR-4):1–18, 1996.

358. Brewer TF, Heymann SJ, Krumplitsch SM, et al. Strategies to decrease tuberculosis in US homeless populations: a computer simulation model. JAMA 286:834–842, 2001.

359. Global Programme for Vaccines and Immunization. Immunization Policy. Geneva: World Health Organ, 1996, pp 1–51.

360. Kaufmann SHE. Vaccines against tuberculosis: the impact of modern biotechnology. Scand J Infect Dis 75(suppl):54–59, 1990.

361. Harboe M, Andersen P, Colston MJ, et al, for the European Commission COST/STC Initiative. Report of the expert panel IX. Vaccines against tuberculosis. Vaccine 14:701–716, 1996.

362. Cole ST, Brosch R, Parkhill J, et al. Deciphering the biology of Mycobacterium tuberculosis from the complete genome sequence. Nature 395:537–544, 1998.

363. Orme IM. Progress in the development of new vaccines against tuberculosis. Int J Tuber Lung Dis 1:95–100, 1997.

364. Orme IM, McMurray DN, Belisle JT. Tuberculosis vaccine development: recent progress. Trends Microbiol 9:115–118, 2001.

365. Paterson R. Human trials start for new tuberculosis vaccine. Lancet Infect Dis 1:291, 2001.

366. Briggs B, Illingworth RS, Lorber J. The human source of tuberculous infection in children. Lancet 1:263–266, 1956.

367. Andrews RH, Devadatta S, Fox W, et al. Prevalence of tuberculosis among close family contacts of tuberculous patients in south India, and influence of segregation of the patient on the early attack rate. Bull World Health Organ 23:463–510, 1963.

368. Ramakrishnan CV, Andrews RH, Devadatta S, et al. Prevalence and early attack rate of tuberculosis among close family contacts of tuberculous patients in south India under domiciliary treatment with isoniazid plus PAS or isoniazid alone. Bull World Health Organ 25:361–407, 1964.

369. Romanus V. Tuberculosis in bacillus Calmette-Guérin–immunized and unimmunized children in Sweden: a ten year evaluation following the cessation of general bacillus Calmette-Guérin immunization of the newborn in 1975. Pediatr Infect Dis J 6:272–280, 1987.

Chapter 13

Diphtheria Toxoid

MELINDA WHARTON • CHARLES R. VITEK

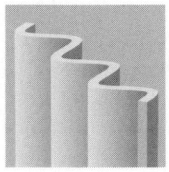

Diphtheria is an acute communicable upper respiratory illness caused by *Corynebacterium diphtheriae*, a gram-positive bacillus. The illness is characterized by a membranous inflammation of the upper respiratory tract, usually of the pharynx but sometimes of the posterior nasal passages, larynx, and trachea, and by widespread damage to other organs, primarily the myocardium and peripheral nerves. Extensive membranes and organ damage are caused by local and systemic action of a potent exotoxin produced by some strains of *C. diphtheriae*. A cutaneous form of diphtheria also occurs.

Historical descriptions of diphtheria-like illness (throat membrane, neck swelling, frequent suffocation) appear in ancient literature. The earliest historical recording is that of Hippocrates in the 5th century BC. Egyptian writings from circa 1550 BC describe a throat condition associated with cyanosis and temporary paralysis usually affecting children.[1] Subsequent detailed descriptions of the clinical picture of the disease were provided by Aretaeus in the second century AD and Aëtius in the sixth century.[2–4] However, translations of the descriptions by the two physicians indicate that diphtheria was not distinguished from other infections with somewhat similar manifestations, including Ludwig's angina and streptococcal tonsillitis, for the obvious reason that a definitive diagnostic method was unavailable. Aëtius termed the illness *Egyptian and Syrian ulcers*, indicating that it had probably been known in those two areas previously and reflecting the uncharitable tendency of the Greeks (among others) to blame pestilence on others, particularly the Egyptians. Although the disease has had many different names in various languages over the centuries, the term *diphtheria* is said to be derived from the Greek word for "leather" or "tanned skin," even though the disease was not so named until many years later.[2,4]

Only isolated reports of the disease appeared until the 17th century, during which time devastating outbreaks occurred in Spain and were described in detail by several writers.[3] Indeed, in Spanish history, 1613 is known as the Year of Diphtheria (Año de Los Garrotillos).[2] Successive outbreaks occurred in southwestern Europe approximately every 12 years through the 18th century. The earliest definitive description of diphtheria in America was that of Samuel Bard in New York in 1771, although outbreaks had previously been noted in the American colonies.[2,3,5] In the early 19th century, Bretonneau clearly delineated the clinical picture of diphtheria, convincingly argued for its communicability, successfully pioneered tracheostomy as treatment, and gave the disease its name.[2,3] A fascinating account of the horrors of diphtheria in childhood has been provided by Holt.[6]

In the second half of the 19th century, increasingly severe epidemics swept many parts of Europe and the large cities of the United States, and many efforts were made by researchers in the new field of bacteriology to identify the causative agent.[4] Progress was impeded by primitive methods for isolation of bacteria and the plethora of other organisms found in the pharynx, including streptococci. However, in 1883, Klebs first described the characteristic organisms in stained preparations of diphtheritic membranes, and Loeffler reported the successful growth of these organisms in culture a year later.[3] During the next 7 years, numerous investigators confirmed these observations and described the pathogenicity of the organism for guinea pigs.

In 1888, Roux and Yersin found that sterile broth filtrates of cultures of the organism, when injected into animals, produced death in a manner similar to that which occurred when virulent organisms were injected, thus demonstrating the presence of a potent exotoxin. Within the next few years, Behring produced antisera in guinea pigs by the injection of sublethal or inactivated broth cultures into these animals. These antisera were shown by Behring to prevent death in nonimmune animals that were challenged with virulent organisms.[2,3] Behring named this preparation *antitoxin*. For his discovery, he received the Nobel Prize in 1901, after which he changed his name to von Behring.

Within a few years, the production and use of equine diphtheria antiserum was widespread. The concept of active immunization began with Theobald Smith in 1907, who noted that long-lasting immunity to diphtheria could be produced in guinea pigs by the injection of mixtures of diphtheria toxin and antitoxin and suggested that these mixtures might do the same for humans. Following successful immunization of children by von Behring with toxin-antitoxin mixtures, immunization programs began in selected European and American cities. However, these immunizations, although usually effective, were not free of adverse reactions. In 1913, Schick introduced a skin test for immunity that consists of the injection of a small, measured amount of diphtheria toxin; in immune persons, circulating antibody neutralizes the toxin, and no local lesion is observed.[2] The Schick skin test was widely used to distinguish immune individuals and target immunization to those susceptible. In the early 1920s, Ramon showed that diphtheria toxin, when treated with heat and formalin, lost its toxic properties but retained its ability to produce serologic protection against the disease. Thus the current immunizing preparation, diphtheria toxoid, came into being.[7]

Background

Clinical Description

Classical diphtheria has an insidious onset after an incubation period of 1 to 5 days (rarely longer). The gradual onset of diphtheria is in contrast to the usually sudden, almost explosive manifestations of streptococcal pharyngitis. Symptoms of diphtheria are initially nonspecific and mild; throughout the course of the disease, fever does not usually exceed 38.5°C (101.3°F). Other early symptoms in children include diminished activity and some irritability. At the very onset of symptoms, the pharynx is injected on examination but no membrane is present. About a day after onset, small patches of exudate appear in the pharynx. Within 2 or 3 days, the patches of exudate spread and become confluent and may form a membrane that covers the entire pharynx, including the tonsillar areas, soft palate, and uvula. This membrane becomes grayish, thick, and firmly adherent. Efforts to dislodge the membrane result in bleeding. Anterior cervical lymph nodes become markedly enlarged and tender. In a proportion of patients, the lymph node swelling is associated with considerable inflammation and edema of the surrounding soft tissues, giving rise to the so-called bull neck appearance, which is associated with a higher morbidity and mortality. Although fever is rarely high, the patient characteristically appears toxic and displays a rapid, thready pulse. In untreated patients, the membrane begins to soften about a week after onset and gradually sloughs off, usually in pieces but sometimes as a single unit. As the membrane detaches, acute systemic symptoms, such as fever, begin to disappear.

Although pharyngeal diphtheria is by far the most common form of disease seen in unimmunized populations, other skin or mucosal sites may be involved. Laryngeal diphtheria occurs in 25% of cases; in three fourths of these instances, the pharynx is also involved. Isolated nasal diphtheria is uncommon (about 2% of cases). Cutaneous, aural, vaginal, and conjunctival diphtheria together account for about 2% of cases and are often secondary to nasopharyngeal infection. Although diphtheria can spread extensively in the respiratory tract or skin, deep tissue invasion or systemic spread of organisms is extremely rare.

Laryngeal diphtheria may occur at any age but is particularly prone to occur in children younger than 4 years. It is marked by insidious onset with gradually increasing hoarseness and stridor. Fever is usually slight. The diagnosis is often missed or delayed when the pharynx is not simultaneously involved. Laryngeal diphtheria is associated with greater morbidity and mortality as a result of airway obstruction and to more toxin absorption from the extensive membrane.

Cutaneous diphtheria is an indolent skin infection that often occurs at sites of burns or other wounds and may act as a source of respiratory infection in others.[8] It is more common in warmer climates and in environments of poverty, overcrowding, and poor hygiene.[9] Although sufficient diphtheria toxin is absorbed from skin lesions to frequently produce immunity, systemic complications are uncommon with cutaneous diphtheria. In warmer climates, the high incidence of cutaneous diphtheria appears to have played a major role in producing immunity in the population in the absence of high rates of respiratory diphtheria.

Complications

The impact of diphtheria is largely measured by complications attributable to the local disease and to the effect of absorbed toxin on other organs. The major threat from laryngeal diphtheria is respiratory obstruction (croup). In the past, life-endangering obstruction was managed by the insertion of a small tube through the glottis, which was left in place for 4 days or more; intubation required considerable skill and experience.[10] Intubation was subsequently replaced by tracheostomy. Even with a tracheostomy tube in place, fatal acute respiratory obstruction occasionally occurs when a portion of a laryngeal membrane is dislodged and aspirated. The membrane may extend down into the tracheobronchial tree, resulting in pneumonia and expiratory respiratory obstruction. Because of edema of the upper respiratory tract, pharyngeal and nasal diphtheria are frequently associated with secondary otitis media and sinusitis.

The majority of deaths from diphtheria are due to the effects of absorbed diphtheria toxin on various organs; severe complications from toxin absorption include acute systemic toxicity, myocarditis, and neurologic complications, primarily peripheral neuritis. The risk of complications is directly proportional to the extent of local disease, presumably because of increased production and absorption of the toxin in larger membranes. In addition, the frequency of these various complications appears to vary considerably among epidemics, for which no clear explanation is available. In the past, it was erroneously believed that the severity of the disease could be related to strains of the organism that were morphologically different on culture, being designated gravis, intermedius, and mitis.[11,12] A possible explanation for variation in reported frequency of complications is the effect of therapy with diphtheria antitoxin, as well as differences in susceptibility among affected populations.

Severe acute systemic toxicity with myocardial involvement usually occurs between the third and seventh day of the illness; many investigators classify this complication as early myocarditis.[13] Others, however, believe that the effects on the myocardium are only part of diffuse systemic toxicity, including fever, purpura, peripheral circulatory collapse, restlessness, somnolence, and disturbances of carbohydrate metabolism.[14,15] This so-called early myocarditis is usually fatal. Late myocarditis usually presents in the second or third week of illness at a time when the local symptoms of diphtheria in the respiratory tract are resolving and the patient is otherwise improving.

In either early or late myocarditis, a wide variety of clinical and electrocardiographic findings may be noted.[14] Tachycardia, distant heart sounds, and a weak pulse may be observed. Electrocardiography most often shows conduction changes and alterations in T waves. Supraventricular and ventricular ectopic rhythms are common in severe diphtheria, even in the absence of evidence of heart failure.[16] The earlier the electrocardiographic changes appear, the worse is the prognosis. Complete heart block frequently occurs and is usually fatal; ventricular pacing may not improve survival.[17] Echocardiograms show decreased contractility and ventricular dilation proportional to the severity of the clinical carditis; a left ventricular ejection fraction less than 35% is associated with an increased risk of death.[18,19] Although electro- and echocardiograms return to normal in most survivors, residual changes can be seen in some survivors of severe carditis up to several years after illness.[16,18]

Neurologic complications of diphtheria are primarily toxic peripheral neuropathies and occur in approximately 15% to 20% of cases.[20,21] The manifestations are more motor than sensory and usually begin 2 to 8 weeks after onset of the illness. In severe cases, palatal paralysis with consequent nasal voice and nasal regurgitation of ingested fluids may occur during the acute membranous phase, particularly with extensive pharyngeal disease, and are believed to be attributable to local effects of the toxin. With milder disease, palatal paralysis is common as late as the third week. Symmetric peripheral neuritis of the lower extremities is a frequent neurologic complication, usually occurring 3 to 10 weeks after onset of the infection. Diaphragmatic paralysis occasionally occurs, usually a month or more after onset, and may require mechanical respiratory support. Ocular paralysis, involving either the extraocular muscles or those of accommodation, sometimes appears, usually 5 or 6 weeks after onset. Fortunately, functional recovery from these neuropathies is the rule even in severe disease.[22]

Invasive disease due to C. diphtheriae occurs rarely, most commonly as a result of nontoxigenic strains. Bacteremia, endocarditis, osteomyelitis, and arthritis have been reported.[23–27]

Biology of the Organism and Pathogenesis of Infection

Corynebacterium diphtheriae is a slender gram-positive bacillus, usually with one end being wider, thus giving the often-described club-shaped appearance. On culture, particularly under suboptimal conditions, characteristic bands or granules appear. On smear, the organisms often have a "pick-up sticks" relationship, assuming parallel (palisade-like), V- or L-type patterns. The organisms are resistant to environmental changes, such as freezing and drying. There are four biotypes of C. diphtheriae (gravis, mitis, belfanti, and intermedius), which historically were identified by colonial morphology and biochemical differences; however, in practice, only the intermedius biotype can be distinguished reliably by colonial morphology.[28] No consistent differences are found in severity of disease caused by different biotypes.

Identified features of C. diphtheriae that are important in the pathogenesis of the disease in humans comprise certain cell wall antigens and in particular the organism's exotoxin. The cell wall contains a heat-stable O antigen, which is found in all corynebacteria. The cell wall also contains K antigens, which are heat-labile proteins that differ among strains of C. diphtheriae and therefore permit categorization of the organism into a number of types.[29] The K antigens play two roles in relation to humans: first, they appear to be important in the establishment of infection; and second, they produce local type-specific immunity. Lack of immunity to K antigens appears to be responsible for the fact that local upper respiratory tract diphtheria can occur with non–toxin-producing organisms, and toxin-producing organisms may infect persons with ample serum antitoxin levels, but neither of these instances is associated with systemic manifestations, even though a faucial membrane is produced.[30] Another factor responsible for the local invasiveness of the organism is the so-called cord factor, which is a toxic glycolipid. This glycolipid has been shown to disrupt mitochondria, depress cell respiration, and interfere with oxidative phosphorylation.[31] The term cord factor is derived from a similar substance found in Mycobacterium tuberculosis that results in the growth of the organism in serpentine coils. Undoubtedly, there are other factors as well that help C. diphtheriae establish residence and provide nutritional substrates.

Diphtheria Toxin

The exotoxin produced by C. diphtheriae is by far the most important pathogenetic factor. The extensive study of the biology of diphtheria toxin has pioneered many biomedical developments over the past century. The basic biology of diphtheria toxin, including its production and actions, has become reasonably well understood, although some gaps remain.[32,33]

The ability to produce toxin in strains of C. diphtheriae results from a nonlytic infection by one of a series of related bacteriophages containing a genetic sequence encoding the toxin. The phage integrates into specific sites present in C. diphtheriae and other Corynebacterium species. The presence of the phage is thought to confer a survival advantage to the bacterium by increasing the probability of transmission in a susceptible population; transmission may be facilitated by local tissue damage resulting from the toxin.[34,35] The sequence of diphtheria toxin has been demonstrated to be highly conserved in C. diphtheriae strains, suggesting that immunologically important differences among the toxins produced by different strains are unlikely to occur.[36] Once integrated, the tox gene is part of a multiple bacterial gene operon; other bacterial gene products in this operon are involved in the liberation and uptake of host iron.[37] The entire operon is under the control of a repressor gene, dtxR, which in the presence of iron binds to and inhibits the tox gene; toxin is produced only under low iron conditions.[38]

Diphtheria toxin is a polypeptide with a molecular weight of about 58,000. The toxin is secreted as a proenzyme, requiring enzymatic cleavage into two fragments (fragments A and B) to become active. Fragment B is responsible for attachment to and penetration of the host cell. Although nontoxic by itself, fragment B appears to be the antigen responsible for clinical immunity. The receptor domain of fragment B binds to a cell surface receptor, heparin-binding epidermal growth factor precursor,[39] with

CD9 as a co-receptor.[40] After receptor-mediated endocytosis and penetration of the cell,[41] fragments A and B are detached. The released fragment A is the toxic moiety and acts by inhibiting protein synthesis, resulting in cell death.[35] Unless cell penetration occurs, fragment A is inactive. Differences in the tissue distribution of the receptor and co-receptors may account for the differential effects of diphtheria toxin on different organs.[42,43]

The ability of *tox* gene containing bacteriophages to infect nontoxigenic strains of C. *diphtheriae* provides a potential explanation for the fact that, during outbreaks of diphtheria, both toxin-producing and non–toxin-producing strains of the organism may be isolated on culture surveys. Some evidence suggests that the introduction of a toxin-producing strain of C. *diphtheriae* into a community occasionally may initiate an outbreak by transfer of phage to nontoxigenic strains of the organism carried in the respiratory tracts of community inhabitants, rather than a new strain being the responsible agent.[44]

On mucous membranes, the toxin causes local cellular destruction, and the accumulated debris and fibrin result in the characteristic membrane. More important, absorbed toxin is responsible for remote manifestations affecting various organs, including the myocardium, nervous system, kidneys, and others. Because the lethality of diphtheria is almost entirely determined by the organism's toxin, clinical immunity depends primarily on the presence of antibodies to the toxin. In the presence of small amounts of formaldehyde, diphtheria toxin loses its attachment and enzymatic activities while retaining its immunogenicity, thus becoming a toxoid. This process is the basis of active immunization against diphtheria.

Protective Levels of Antitoxin

Several lines of evidence suggest that persons with diphtheria antitoxin levels of less than 0.01 IU/mL should be considered susceptible. Ipsen reports results of studies in which rabbits were administered antitoxin and then challenged with intravenously administered diphtheria toxin; rabbits with a serum level of 0.01 IU/mL were almost completely protected from death with the standard lethal dose.[45] However, higher doses of toxin required higher serum antitoxin levels for equivalent protection. On the basis of studies of diphtheria antitoxin levels early in the course of disease, persons with diphtheria antitoxin levels of less than 0.01 IU/mL appear to be highly susceptible to disease.[45,46] Probably no level of circulating antitoxin confers absolute protection; Ipsen[45] reported two cases of fatal diphtheria in patients with antitoxin levels above 30 IU/mL the day after onset of symptoms. Historically, clinical diphtheria was rare among individuals with a negative Schick test; the minimal serum antitoxin level associated with a negative Schick test was approximately 0.005 IU/mL.[47] Overall, the data allow some general conclusions regarding protective levels in most circumstances. An antitoxin level of 0.01 IU/mL is the lowest level giving some degree of protection, and 0.1 IU/mL is considered a protective level of circulating antitoxin. Levels of 1.0 IU/mL and above are associated with long-term protection.[48]

Several laboratory assays for diphtheria antitoxin are available. Vero cell neutralization assays are highly accurate but technically cumbersome and are available only in a few research laboratories.[49] Enzyme immunoassays (EIAs) are widely available but technically less demanding; these assays generally correlate with results from neutralization assays at concentrations greater than 0.01 IU/mL.[50] Several assays that are more accurate than standard EIAs but technically less demanding than Vero cell neutralization have been developed recently.[51,52]

Other Agents Producing Diphtheria Toxin

Some strains of two other closely related *Corynebacterium* species, C. *ulcerans* and C. *pseudotuberculosis*, have been demonstrated to produce diphtheria toxin,[53] and nontoxigenic strains can be converted to toxigenic strains by infection with β-corynebacteriophage.[54] Disease indistinguishable from that caused by toxigenic strains of C. *diphtheriae* has been associated with C. *ulcerans* infection.[55–57]

Diagnosis

Physicians need to be aware of the signs and symptoms that suggest diphtheria because diphtheria remains a threat despite its rarity in the United States. High levels of circulation of toxigenic strains of C. *diphtheriae* continue in some developing countries, and some circulation persists in many countries of the former Soviet Union after a large recent epidemic, while limited foci persist in some highly developed countries.

Usually the disease appears as membranous pharyngitis; a patient with confluent pharyngeal exudate should be suspected of having diphtheria until proven otherwise. The onset is usually gradual over the course of 1 to 2 days, and is associated with only moderate fever. Although certain clinical characteristics of membranous pharyngitis caused by diphtheria, such as the color, adherence, and odor of the membrane, can be recognized as being different from other forms of exudative pharyngitis by experienced clinicians, very few physicians in the United States currently have the experience required to base a differential diagnosis on the clinical appearance of the lesion.

Because laryngeal diphtheria usually occurs concomitantly with pharyngeal involvement, membranous pharyngitis with stridor should be considered to be diphtheria until proven otherwise. However, about a quarter of all cases of laryngeal diphtheria do not display a pharyngeal lesion and therefore may be readily misdiagnosed. The differential diagnosis includes epiglottitis caused by *Haemophilus influenzae* type b (Hib), spasmodic croup, the presence of a foreign body, and viral laryngotracheitis. There should be little confusion regarding the first three because the onset and clinical characteristics of each are well known and are different from diphtheritic croup, which ordinarily is associated with gradual onset and steady progression through hoarseness to stridor during a period of 2 or 3 days. Viral laryngotracheobronchitis may be more difficult to differentiate, and, if diphtheria is suspected for epidemiologic or other reasons, laryngoscopy is indicated.

Nasal diphtheria may be difficult to distinguish from many other causes of nasal discharge and accordingly is most likely to be suspected if the patient has been exposed to diphtheria, such as during an outbreak. Suspicion should be heightened if a serosanguineous discharge is present and if the upper lip is ulcerated, which also occurs with streptococcal infections. Any cutaneous or mucous membrane lesions at other sites should be considered suspicious if a membrane is noted.

The complications and mortality of diphtheria are inversely related to the promptness of diagnosis and treatment. Thus it is critical that the diagnosis be considered, appropriate clinical specimens be obtained, and a decision made regarding administration of antitoxin as early as possible in the course of illness. In instances in which diphtheria is suspected, treatment for the disease should be initiated immediately after bacteriologic specimens are obtained, without waiting for results. Delay, even for a few hours, may increase the risk of complications and death.

Swabs for culture should be obtained under direct visualization, preferably from the edge or beneath the edge of the membrane. Swabs should be inoculated promptly onto tellurite-containing media and onto blood agar.[58] Directly stained smears are usually grossly misleading even in experienced hands and should not be used. Cultures should be incubated promptly and interpreted by an experienced microbiologist. Because not all C. diphtheriae recovered on culture are toxigenic, testing for toxin production must be carried out by the Elek immunoprecipitation test or by cutaneous testing in guinea pigs.[58,59] In addition, the diphtheria toxin gene can be detected by polymerase chain reaction (PCR),[60–63] which can be performed directly on clinical specimens.[64]

Several approaches to typing of strains of C. diphtheriae as an adjunct to epidemiologic investigations have been developed. During the 1960s, Saragea and Maximescu[65] developed a system of phage typing and demonstrated considerable diversity of circulating strains in different countries. Subsequently, the utility of molecular typing methods was demonstrated in analysis of outbreak-related strains in Sweden[66] and the United States.[67] More recently, ribotyping,[68] pulsed-field gel electrophoresis,[68] and multilocus enzyme electrophoresis[69] have been used for molecular subtyping, as has PCR–single-strand conformation polymorphism (SSCP) analysis.[70] A rapid ribotyping method using PCR-SSCP has been described.[71]

Epidemiology

Active immunization of children with diphtheria toxoid has markedly altered the epidemiology of diphtheria, reducing diphtheria to extremely low levels in both developed countries and many developing countries. However, diphtheria continues to produce substantial childhood morbidity and mortality in developing countries with incompletely implemented childhood immunization programs.[72]

Humans are the only natural host for C. diphtheriae. Transmission is person to person, most likely by intimate respiratory and physical contact. The organism is reasonably hardy and has been isolated from the environment of persons infected with C. diphtheriae.[73–76] Nonetheless, the occurrence of indirect transmission by airborne droplet nuclei, dust, or fomites has not been established. Evidence of outbreaks caused by contaminated milk and milk products has been reported.[13,77] Cutaneous lesions appear to be important in transmission in warm climates or under conditions of poor hygiene.[8]

Historically, peaks in incidence were observed approximately every 10 years or so. Because of these secular trends, doubts were expressed about the efficacy of developments in prevention and treatment during the first half of the 20th century because the apparent effects of immunization might simply have reflected the natural epidemiology of the disease[78]; these doubts no longer exist.

In temperate climates, diphtheria occurs year-round but most often during colder months, probably because of the close contact of children indoors. In tropical climates, cutaneous diphtheria is more common and is unrelated to season. Preschool and school-age children are most often affected by respiratory diphtheria. Diphtheria was rare in infants younger than 6 months, presumably because of the presence of maternal antibody, and rare among adults, especially those living in urban areas, as a result of acquired immunity. Although no differences in diphtheria incidence were noted by gender in the prevaccine era, an increased risk of diphtheria among women was reported in several outbreaks among adults in the 1940s and subsequently.[79–82]

In the past, in the absence of immunization, most persons acquired immunity to diphtheria as measured by the Schick test without experiencing clinical diphtheria. This situation is in contrast to that with pertussis, measles, rubella, and mumps, diseases that every child was expected to experience before protective vaccines became available, but is somewhat analogous to patterns of natural immunity that are acquired against polioviruses and Hib, to which most persons developed clinical and serologic immunity without experiencing overt disease. Transplacental antitoxic immunity to diphtheria is present at birth in most infants but declines to nonprotective levels during the second 6 months of life. Thereafter, the proportion of immune children (Schick negative) in unimmunized populations gradually increases to 75% or more, presumably owing to subclinical infection with the organism, perhaps repeated infection.[83]

In the 21st century, it is difficult to comprehend what a major cause of morbidity and mortality diphtheria was in the past. For the United States before 1900, the best data are from Massachusetts; during the years 1860 to 1897, death rates from diphtheria ranged between 46 and 196 per 100,000 population annually, with a median of 78.[84] For 8 of those years, mortality exceeded 130 per 100,000, and the proportion of total deaths attributable to diphtheria annually ranged between 3% and 10% from 1860 to 1897. By 1900, a considerable fall in death rates had occurred, and the death rate continued to decline from 40 to 15 per 100,000 for the next 20 years, presumably owing to the therapeutic use of diphtheria antitoxin and, perhaps, other measures such as intubation. However, even in 1900, more than half as many deaths from diphtheria were recorded in the United States as from cancer.[84] Several interesting and readable histories of diphtheria in the late 19th and early 20th centuries have been published.[10,85]

Excellent data on morbidity, mortality, and case-fatality rates for diphtheria are available for the Province of Ontario for 1880 to 1940 and for several Canadian cities for some of those years.[86] Mortality from diphtheria exceeded 50 per 100,000 population in most years prior to the advent of diphtheria antitoxin. Mortality subsequently declined to approximately 15 per 100,000 by World War I, although morbidity rates did not decline. With the widespread use of diphtheria toxoid beginning in the late 1920s in Canada, the disease nearly disappeared. In contrast, national diphtheria immunization campaigns did not take place in Britain until the early 1940s.[87]

Since the introduction of vaccination with diphtheria toxoid, a number of diphtheria outbreaks have occurred in industrial countries. During World War II, a major outbreak spread throughout western Europe; well above 1 million cases were reported.[88,89] During World War II, outbreaks linked to Europe occurred in North America as well. A major outbreak that affected nearly 1% of the population of Halifax, Nova Scotia, during the winter of 1940 to 1941 was linked to disease imported by Norwegian sailors.[90] An outbreak occurred in Alabama in 1943 among German prisoners of war.[91]

Diphtheria Since the 1950s

By the late 1950s, diphtheria was markedly reduced in the United States, but disease continued to occur in some geographic areas. To better understand the epidemiology of diphtheria, the Diphtheria Surveillance Unit was begun in 1958 at the Communicable Diseases Center (later to become the Centers for Disease Control and Prevention). During the period 1959 to 1970, 5048 cases of diphtheria were reported in the United States, with the highest incidence rates reported in the southeast, south central, and northern plains states. Incidence rates were 20-fold higher for Native Americans and 7-fold higher for blacks compared with whites.[92] There were at least 10 outbreaks of more than 15 cases during the period, including outbreaks in Austin and San Antonio, Texas, between 1967 and 1970.[93,94]

During the following decade, diphtheria incidence continued to decline (Fig. 13–1); during the period 1971 to 1981, 853 noncutaneous and 435 cutaneous cases were reported in the United States. Incidence rates exceeded 1 per million population in South Dakota, New Mexico, Alaska, Washington, Arizona, and Montana, and incidence rates were 100-fold greater for Native Americans than for whites and blacks. There were seven outbreaks with 15 or more cases.[95] From 1972 to 1982, a large outbreak of predominantly cutaneous diphtheria occurred among residents of Skid Road in Seattle, Washington.[67,96] The Seattle outbreak and most of the other outbreaks from 1969 to 1980 were caused by toxigenic strains of the intermedius biotype, which had previously been uncommon; clonality of these strains was suggested by molecular epidemiologic studies of strains from outbreaks in Seattle[67] and the southwestern states.[97]

During the period 1980 to 1999, only 48 cases of respiratory diphtheria were reported in the United States.[98,99] The abrupt decline was partially due to cutaneous diphtheria ceasing to be nationally notifiable in 1980. However, improved childhood immunization in Mexico and other developing countries as part of the Expanded Programme on Immunization (EPI) beginning in the late 1970s is likely to have contributed to improved diphtheria control in the United States by reducing importations of toxigenic strains. In the mid-1990s, with so little disease reported in the United States, it seemed likely that toxigenic strains of C. diphtheriae were no longer circulating in this country.[98] However, in 1996, surveillance revealed widespread circulation of the organism in one northern Plains Indian community.[100] Similarly, although recognized cases of diphtheria remain rare, endemic transmission of C. diphtheriae has been documented in some native communities in Canada.[101–103] Strains from the United States and Canada were assayed by ribotyping and multilocus enzyme electrophoresis and found to be closely related to strains from the same areas during the 1970s and 1980s, suggesting ongoing endemic circulation.[100,104] Circulation has also been reported among the aboriginal population in central Australia.[105] The common denominator in these communities is likely to be poverty, crowding, and poor hygiene.

Although diphtheria has become a rare disease in most developed countries, a major epidemic of diphtheria began in the Russian Federation in 1990 and subsequently spread throughout the countries of the former Soviet Union (Fig. 13–2), with more than 157,000 cases and 5000 deaths reported between 1990 and 1998.[106] A compendium summarizing the knowledge gained from this outbreak has been published.[107] Although the causes of the epidemic remain uncertain, contributing factors included inadequate population immunity among children and adults, delayed recogni-

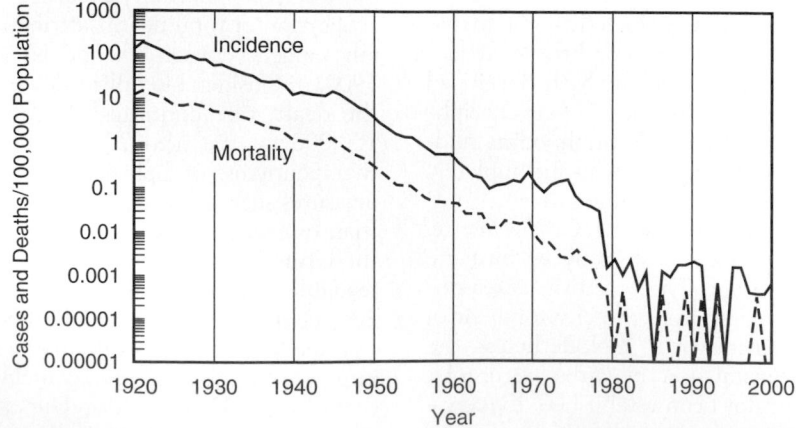

FIGURE 13 1 ■ Diphtheria incidence and mortality rates in the United States, 1920 to 2001. Years in which no deaths or cases were reported are plotted with an incidence rate of 0.00001 per 100,000 population. (Data from Centers for Disease Control and Prevention, Atlanta, Georgia.)

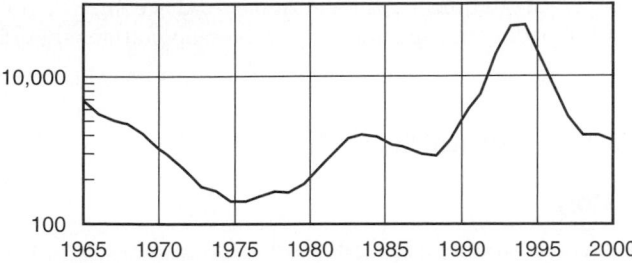

FIGURE 13–2 ■ Reported cases of diphtheria, by year, Soviet Union (1965 to 1990) and newly independent states of the former Soviet Union (1991 to 2001).

tion and public health response, and social conditions that facilitated spread once the outbreak began.[106] In the Russian Federation, the emergence of an epidemic clone of *C. diphtheriae* biotype *gravis* was demonstrated.[69] The epidemic clone was present in Russia as early as 1985, and strains of this clonal group have been retrospectively identified in different geographic areas of Russia during 1985 to 1987.[108] Many cases were due to biotype *mitis* strains as well, especially in the new independent states of Central Asia, suggesting that microbial factors alone cannot account for the epidemic.[109] The epidemic peaked in 1994 to 1995 and subsequently was brought under control by increasing immunization coverage with diphtheria toxoid among both children and adults (see additional discussion in *Results of Immunization* below).[106]

In developing countries, the implementation of the EPI program has led to dramatic falls in the global number of reported cases of diphtheria since 1980; however, marked disparities remain in reported rates between countries. Some countries have achieved control of diphtheria comparable to that in highly developed countries. In many others, disease rates have fallen dramatically but sporadic outbreaks occur, while some countries continue to have evidence of widespread circulation of toxigenic strains.[110–112]

The precise microbial events responsible for the transmission of diphtheria remain unclear. However, the molecular epidemiologic data showing clonal identity of bacteria in large numbers of infected people in the outbreaks in Seattle,[67] Sweden,[66] and Russia[69] strongly suggest that direct spread of toxigenic bacteria from one individual to another is a major factor in large epidemics. As mentioned above, the transfer of bacteriophages governing toxin production from an infected person to carriers of nontoxigenic strains also may play a role. Although no animal reservoir exists for *C. diphtheriae*, *C. ulcerans* may carry the β-corynebacteriophage that encodes diphtheria toxin,[113] and an animal reservoir does exist for this organism[114,115]—and thus for the bacteriophage. Given the worldwide ubiquity of carriage of *C. diphtheriae* and the bacteriophages implicated in toxin production, prospects for eradication of diphtheria currently seem remote. Continuing active immunization with diphtheria toxoid is the key to the control of diphtheria.

Passive Immunization

The history of the development of diphtheria antitoxin has been reviewed in detail by Andrewes and colleagues.[3] In brief, Roux and Yersin in 1888 reported their observation that bacteria-free filtrates of broth cultures of *C. diphtheriae*,

when injected into animals, produced all of the manifestations of diphtheria except for the membranous local lesions.[116] In rapid succession, other advances followed; von Behring showed that inactivated cultures of the organism injected into animals ultimately rendered them protected against living cultures, at first not recognizing the fact that the organisms themselves were unnecessary for immunity.[117] Ultimately, von Behring demonstrated the transfer of protection from an immunized animal to another by serum. Diphtheria antitoxin was first given to a child in 1891, and antitoxin was commercially produced in Germany in 1892. The use of horses for the production of antitoxin began in 1894. Worthy of note is the fact that the lack of regulated standards for the production of equine diphtheria antitoxin, which resulted in the release of contaminated antisera and the inevitable appearance of charlatans who prepared and sold similar-appearing colored water, contributed to the development of the legislated predecessors of the present Center for Biologics Evaluation and Research of the U.S. Food and Drug Administration (FDA).[118,119]

Equine diphtheria antitoxin is prepared by hyperimmunizing horses with diphtheria toxoid and toxin.[119] To diminish reactivity from horse serum, current preparations are semipurified by techniques that concentrate immunoglobulin G and remove as much extraneous protein as possible. There must be at least 500 units of antitoxin per milliliter, and sterility is attained by microfiltration. A cresol derivative is added as a preservative.

Diphtheria antitoxin is used for the treatment of diphtheria and occasionally, in the past, for prevention in exposed persons. Its therapeutic efficacy is well established, although it is in no way a substitute for prior active immunization with diphtheria toxoid. No antiserum or hyperimmune globulin of human origin is currently available.

As of January 6, 1997, licensed diphtheria antitoxin with a valid expiration date was no longer available in the United States, and no manufacturer proposed to produce it. However, for treatment of the disease in the United States, the Centers for Disease Control and Prevention has a supply of antitoxin that can be distributed for treatment under an investigational new drug protocol.[120] This antitoxin is comparable to the prior U.S. product and may be requested by calling 1-404-639-8255 during working hours or 1-404-639-2889 at night and on weekends.

A novel approach to passive immunity may be the development of recombinant modified diphtheria toxin receptor molecules to bind diphtheria toxin.[121]

Postexposure Use of Antitoxin and Toxoid

The value of antitoxin in prophylaxis is dubious. Theoretically, it should be useful in preventing the establishment of infection in exposed, susceptible persons because the toxin plays a role in local invasiveness. However, there is no acceptable clinical evidence of prophylactic efficacy; all that exist are anecdotes and small, uncontrolled series of experiments.[3] Even if it were effective, antitoxin would be of little use in controlling community outbreaks because asymptomatic carriers, rather than persons with overt disease, are usually the major source of transmission.[122] For these reasons, antitoxin is not recommended for exposed, susceptible persons, particularly in view of the high rates of subsequent serum sickness and occasional anaphylaxis. The preferred treatment for exposed, unimmunized, asymptomatic persons is to obtain a throat culture, begin immunization with a preparation containing diphtheria toxoid that is appropriate for age, and institute prophylaxis with erythromycin or penicillin for 7 days, during which time the patient must be kept under surveillance.[123]

Treatment of Diphtheria

Many studies have demonstrated the efficacy of therapy with antitoxin in reducing mortality from diphtheria primarily by preventing cardiovascular toxicity.[4,124] However, only a single controlled therapeutic trial is discussed in the literature.[125,126] This nonblinded trial consisted of treating all patients admitted on alternate days with antitoxin and comparing their outcomes with those of patients admitted on nontreatment days. Eight (3.3%) of 242 patients treated with antitoxin died, compared with 30 (12.2%) of 245 control subjects.

In addition, many observations of the direct relationship between mortality and day of disease when antitoxin was administered provide ample evidence of its efficacy. For example, among 3558 patients observed by Ker,[124] 320 cases of paralysis occurred. There was a strong direct relationship between the frequency of postdiphtheritic paralysis and the number of days between onset of illness and administration of antitoxin. Only 4.8% of 1168 patients developed paralysis when antitoxin was administered no later than the second day of illness, in contrast to 12.1% of 1375 patients who received antitoxin on the fourth day of the disease or later.

Antitoxin is given intramuscularly or intravenously; many authorities prefer the intravenous route for at least part of the dose because a therapeutic blood level can be reached more rapidly.[127] The entire therapeutic dose should be administered at one time, and the amount of antitoxin recommended varies between 20,000 and 120,000 units. Larger amounts are recommended for persons with extensive local lesions, because the amount of toxin produced depends on the size of the membrane. Furthermore, the longer the interval since onset, the higher should be the dose of antitoxin. Unfortunately, toxin that has already entered host cells is not affected by antitoxin.

Although diphtheria antitoxin is the mainstay of diphtheria therapy, penicillin or, alternatively, erythromycin should be given to hasten clearance of the organism.[123] Treatment should be continued until at least two consecutive daily cultures fail to demonstrate C. diphtheriae. Before the development of antibiotic therapy, convalescent carriage of toxigenic organisms was a major problem. Up to 50% and 25% of patients continued to harbor the organism 2 and 4 weeks after onset, respectively. As late as 2 months after onset, reported carriage rates varied between 1% and 8%.[3] Long-term convalescent carriers were often subjected to tonsillectomy, probably with some effect.[128]

Although treatment with penicillin or erythromycin has no apparent effect on the clinical course of the disease, in most instances the organism can no longer be recovered on culture within a week; subsequent convalescent carriage is thus uncommon. Patients who continue to harbor the organism after treatment with either penicillin or erythromycin should receive an additional 10-day course of oral erythromycin, and specimens for follow-up cultures should be obtained.[123]

Active Immunization

History

Subsequent to the investigations that led to the discovery of diphtheria toxin and the development of antitoxin in the 19th century, the development of current diphtheria toxoid was facilitated almost entirely by three important advances. The first of these was the discovery that balanced mixtures of toxin and antitoxin successfully immunized both animals and humans after injection.[129,130] However, a preparation designed to provide active immunity against diphtheria would be of little utility unless some means of assessing the presence of such immunity were available. Fortunately, a reasonably simple and fairly accurate skin test (the Schick test) was developed almost simultaneously.[131] The third innovative step was the development of diphtheria toxoid a decade later.[7]

The combination preparation, toxin-antitoxin, was rapidly accepted as an active immunizing agent. It was widely used in the United States beginning in 1914 and was found to protect approximately 85% of recipients.[132] There is little question that the toxin-antitoxin preparation developed by von Behring created active immunity against diphtheria, in spite of the absence of well-controlled studies, on the basis of the results of Schick testing and clinical observation.[3]

The Schick test consists of the intradermal injection of a minute amount of diphtheria toxin. The test result is ordinarily read after 48 hours; erythema and induration of 1 cm or more indicates susceptibility to diphtheria. Unfortunately, the results of the test are not that simple to interpret. Extraneous proteins in Schick test materials often produce false-positive reactions, and, accordingly, a simultaneous injection of the same material, treated with heat to destroy the toxin, is required to assess sensitivity to extraneous proteins. Excellent descriptions of the Schick test and its interpretation are available in older texts.[3,133] Because the correlation between results of the Schick test and clinical immunity to diphtheria is reasonable, although not perfect, the test served for many years as an acceptable surrogate for clinical immunity to diphtheria.

The third major innovation was the development of diphtheria toxoid.[7] Ramon treated diphtheria toxin with small amounts of formalin and found that the product retained most of its immunizing capacity while losing its toxic properties. Ramon dubbed this preparation anatoxine; this name has since been replaced with the term toxoid. For primary immunization, the toxin-antitoxin preparation was gradually replaced by toxoid in the United States and Canada during the next 15 years and elsewhere thereafter. In 1926, Glenny and co-workers[134] found that alum-precipitated toxoid was more immunogenic, and, by the mid-1940s, diphtheria toxoid was combined with tetanus toxoid and pertussis vaccine as diphtheria and tetanus toxoids and whole-cell pertussis vaccine (DTP). Adsorption of all three onto an aluminum salt followed shortly thereafter. It is clear that the immunogenicity of diphtheria toxoid, as well as that of tetanus toxoid, is enhanced by the adjuvant effects of both pertussis vaccine and the aluminum salt.[135–137] In recent years, diphtheria and tetanus toxoids with acellular pertussis components (DTaP) have been licensed, and various other combinations of DTaP with Hib vaccine, inactivated poliovirus vaccine, and hepatitis B vaccine have been developed.[138]

Current Production

At present, diphtheria toxoid is produced worldwide in a standard fashion; in the United States, production and testing procedures are specified in the Code of Federal Regulations. Specifically, a strain of C. *diphtheriae* that is known to produce large amounts of toxin is grown in a liquid medium conducive to toxin production. After appropriate incubation, sterilization is achieved by centrifugation and filtration. After ascertainment of potency, the filtrate is incubated with formalin for conversion of toxin to toxoid. The product is then further purified and concentrated to achieve the necessary dosage. It is adsorbed onto an aluminum salt, usually aluminum phosphate. Appropriate tests for potency, toxicity, and sterility are conducted both by the manufacturer and by the FDA. Potency worldwide is ascertained by determining the content of flocculating units (Lf) in established fashion; 1 Lf is the amount of toxoid that flocculates 1 unit of a standard reference diphtheria antitoxin.

Currently in the United States, diphtheria toxoid is available in combination with tetanus toxoid and in combination with tetanus toxoid and acellular pertussis vaccine as well as in other combination vaccines including DTaP. The product is available only in adsorbed form.

As of November 2002, DTaP vaccines from three manufacturers are licensed for use in infants in the United States: Tripedia (manufactured and distributed by Aventis Pasteur Inc.); Infanrix (manufactured by GlaxoSmithKline Biologicals and distributed by GlaxoSmithKline); and DAPTACEL (manufactured by Aventis Pasteur Ltd., and distributed by Aventis Pasteur Inc). One DTaP product combined with conjugated Hib vaccine is currently licensed (Aventis Pasteur Inc.) for use as the fourth dose in the DTaP and Hib vaccine series, and a combined DTaP, hepatitis B vaccine, and inactivated polio vaccine (GlaxoSmithKline) is available for use at 2, 4, and 6 months of age. The amounts of diphtheria toxoid in the DTaP vaccines currently licensed in the United States range from 6.7 to 25 Lf/0.5-mL dose. They provide levels of serum antitoxin considerably lower than those after receipt of whole-cell DTP, probably reflecting the adjuvant effect of the whole-cell pertussis component.[139,140] However, the lower antitoxin levels induced by vaccination with DTaP are probably of no clinical consequence, being manyfold higher than protective levels.[138] For routine immunization of children, five doses are recommended (at 2, 4, 6, and 15 to 18 months and at school entry before the seventh birthday). The fourth dose should be administered at least 6 months after the third dose.[141]

DTaP is ordinarily not given to children younger than 6 weeks because responses to pertussis vaccine in the young infant are suboptimal; responses to tetanus and diphtheria toxoids, however, are satisfactory in such young infants regardless of the presence of maternally derived serum antibody and without induction of immunologic tolerance.[142]

The optimal age for immunization of premature infants cannot be stated with confidence, although one small study indicates that satisfactory responses are achieved by initiating the usual DTP series at 2 months of age regardless of pregnancy duration.[143] Follow-up of a small group of children born at less than 29 weeks' gestation suggests lower diphtheria antibody levels at age 7, following a five-dose series, compared to children born at term.[144] There is evidence that high titers of transplacental antibody to diphtheria toxin inhibit serologic responses to the first two doses of diphtheria toxoid in infants, but, after the third dose (administered in the Swedish schedule at 12 months of age), the effect is no longer evident.[145]

Diphtheria and Tetanus Toxoids, Adsorbed, for Pediatric Use (DT) is recommended for the primary immunization of children younger than 7 years in whom pertussis vaccine is contraindicated. DT contains 10 to 12 Lf of diphtheria toxoid; infants who begin the series before 1 year of age should receive DT at 2, 4, 6, and 15 to 18 months of age. Satisfactory responses are obtained even in the absence of the adjuvant effect of pertussis vaccine.[146,147] For unimmunized children 1 to 7 years of age, two doses 2 months apart and a third dose 6 to 12 months later constitute primary immunization.[148]

Tetanus and Diphtheria Toxoids, Adsorbed, for Adult Use (Td) contains approximately the same amount of tetanus toxoid as do DTP and DT, but the amount of diphtheria toxoid is reduced to no more than 2 Lf/dose. This reduction minimizes reactivity in persons who may have been sensitized previously to diphtheria toxoid and is sufficient to provoke satisfactory anamnestic responses in previously immunized persons.[149] In addition, in previously unimmunized older children and adults, Td is satisfactory for primary immunization[150,151] when administered as a three-dose series, with the second dose given 4 to 8 weeks after the first dose and the third dose 6 to 12 months after the second dose.[148] Td should be administered approximately every 10 years after the completion of childhood immunization. Although Td is slightly more reactive than tetanus toxoid alone,[152] it is preferable to monovalent tetanus toxoid for prophylaxis of tetanus after wounds to maintain satisfactory population immunity against diphtheria. In the United States, DT and Td are distributed by Aventis Pasteur Inc. Monovalent diphtheria toxoid is no longer available in the United States.

Limited data regarding simultaneous administration of the first three doses of DTaP with other childhood vaccines indicate no interference with response to the diphtheria toxoid component. Data are available regarding administration of DTaP with other vaccines recommended at the same time as the fourth and fifth doses of the diphtheria, tetanus, and pertussis series (i.e., Hib conjugate vaccine, oral poliovirus vaccine, measles-mumps-rubella vaccine, and varicella vaccine) and regarding administration of whole-cell DTP (all doses in the series) with these vaccines.[140,153] DTaP may be administered simultaneously with hepatitis B vaccine, Hib vaccine, inactivated poliovirus vaccine, and pneumococcal conjugate vaccine to infants at ages 2, 4, or 6 months.

Preparations containing diphtheria toxoid should always be injected intramuscularly, not subcutaneously. As with tetanus toxoid and pertussis vaccine, prolonging the interval between doses does not require restarting the series; indeed, immunity achieved after longer intervals between doses than those recommended is at least as good as that following the regular schedule, although the subject may be unprotected in the interim. Preparations containing diphtheria toxoid should be stored at usual refrigerator temperatures but not frozen.

In other countries, DTP is administered according to alternative schedules (see Chapters 54 and 55). According to the recommended schedule for the World Health Organization's EPI, DTP is administered at 6, 10, and 14 weeks without additional doses. In a number of European countries, two doses of DTP or DTaP are administered early in the first year of life, followed by a third dose late in the first year or early in the second year of life. Recommendations regarding subsequent boosters vary by country. In response to the recent epidemic of diphtheria in the former Soviet Union, booster doses have been recommended or reinstated in a number of countries outside the former Soviet Union. Adult formulations of diphtheria and tetanus toxoids and acellular pertussis vaccines are licensed in some countries but are not yet available in the United States.

For information on constituents and stability of diphtheria toxoid, see Chapter 27 (Tetanus Toxoid).

Results of Immunization

No controlled clinical trial, acceptable by today's scientific standards, of the efficacy of the toxoid in preventing diphtheria has ever been conducted for three reasons. First, given the serious nature of the disease and the clear perception of benefit first from the toxin-antitoxin combination and subsequently from the toxoid, its value seemed obvious to early investigators. Second, the development of surrogate approaches to assessing immunity (the Schick test and serologic methods) made such trials unnecessary. Third, the early appearance of strong presumptive evidence that the toxin-antitoxin preparation and the toxoid were effective made such trials unethical.

In spite of the lack of a controlled clinical trial, ample evidence exists that diphtheria toxoid prevents clinical disease in the majority of recipients and controls the disease from the public health standpoint. First is the nearly complete disappearance of the disease in countries in which immunization has been widely employed. Second is the fact that, during outbreaks of diphtheria, rates of disease are negligible among immunized persons. Third, when partially or, rarely, fully immunized individuals acquire diphtheria, the disease is milder and complications are fewer. Fourth, a good correlation has been established between clinical protection and the presence of serum antibody to the toxin, whether resulting from disease or from immunization.

After three doses of diphtheria toxoid, virtually all infants develop diphtheria titers greater than 0.01 IU/mL.[154] Geometric mean titers vary among vaccine preparations, with some DTaP products producing significantly lower geometric mean titers than those observed after vaccination with DTP[139]; however, these differences are unlikely to be clinically significant. High maternal antibody titers suppress, but do not prevent, adequate responses of infants to two doses of vaccine, and after the third dose the suppressive

effect is gone.[154a] When the toxoid is used for primary immunization of adults, data suggest that virtually all adults develop diphtheria antitoxin titers greater than 0.01 IU/mL after administration of three doses of diphtheria toxoid and that most develop titers greater than 0.1 IU/mL.[150]

Vaccination with protein conjugate vaccines containing either diphtheria toxoid or mutant diphtheria toxin (CRM_{197}) may result in a booster response to the carrier protein.[155] Lack of baseline immunity to diphtheria may result in poor antibody responses to vaccines conjugated to CRM_{197}.[156]

Before the World Health Organization's EPI began, it was estimated that close to a million cases of diphtheria occurred annually in the Third World, with 50,000 to 60,000 deaths.[157] From 1980 to 2000, reported cases of diphtheria globally decreased from 97,811 to 9593; with control of the outbreak in the former Soviet Union, almost 80% of cases worldwide in 2000 were reported from the African and Southeast Asian regions (Fig. 13–3).[158] Under the EPI, the goal was to achieve 90% or more immunization of 1-year-old children by the year 2000; by 2000, it was estimated that the proportion who had received three doses of diphtheria toxoid in combination with tetanus toxoid and pertussis vaccine had risen from negligible levels in the early 1970s to 81% worldwide, with Africa being the lowest at approximately 55%.[159]

Effectiveness in Epidemiologic Studies

Although in most outbreaks of diphtheria the prevalence of prior immunization in persons who escape the disease is not known, a few studies have sufficient data to allow estimates of the degree of protection offered by the toxoid. Some evidence of the protective efficacy of diphtheria toxoid is provided by observations during the Halifax epidemic.[90] During the course of this outbreak, an intense effort was made to administer diphtheria toxoid to previously unimmunized individuals, and comparisons of the subsequent incidence of diphtheria in these children were made with the incidence in the unimmunized population during the next few months. Among those immunized, the monthly incidence of diphtheria fell to 24.5 per 100,000 population, about one seventh of the rate of 168.9 per 100,000 in the unimmunized during that same period. In Britain in 1943, the rate of clinical diphtheria among the unimmunized was 3.5 times that among the immunized, and mortality was 25-fold greater.[89] In an outbreak in Elgin, Texas, in 1970, only 2 of 205 fully immunized, exposed elementary schoolchildren acquired the disease.[160] In contrast, among 97 children who had received inadequate or no immunization, a 13% attack rate occurred.

In a household study during a diphtheria outbreak in San Antonio, Texas, in 1970, vaccine efficacy was estimated at only 54%.[94] However, because index cases were included and denominators of exposed individuals were unknown, the data are difficult to interpret. Furthermore, any differences in attack rates between immunized and nonimmunized individuals might have been blunted by the institution of antibiotic therapy in all members of the household on recognition of a case. Thus the apparent efficacy of 54% is probably low. In an outbreak in Yemen, the protective efficacy of diphtheria toxoid was determined to be 87% by the case-control method.[77]

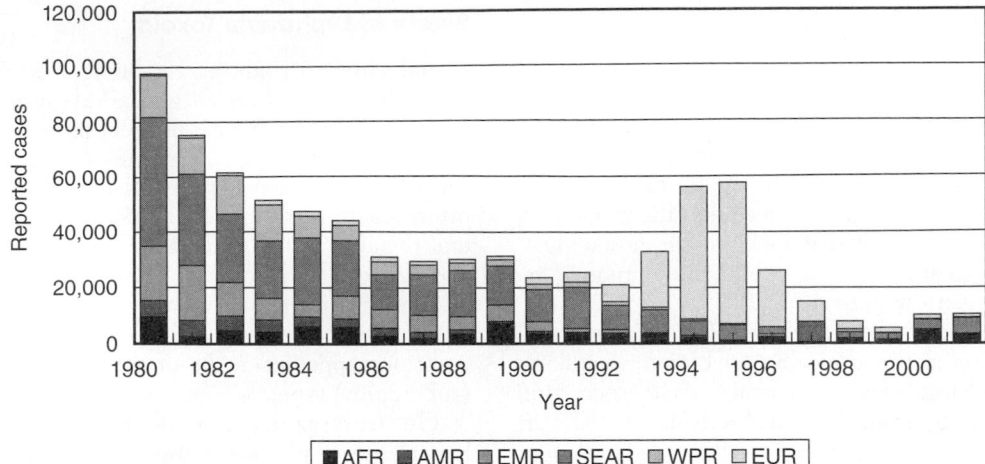

FIGURE 13–3 ■ Reported cases of diphtheria, by year and region, 1980 to 2001. AFR, African Region; AMR, American Region; EMR, Eastern Mediterranean Region; SEAR, Southeast Asia Region; WPR, Western Pacific Region; EUR, European Region. (From World Health Organization, Department of Vaccines and Biologicals. Vaccine-Preventable Diseases: Monitoring System. 2001 Global Summary. Geneva, World Health Organization, 2001, with permission.)

The effectiveness of Russian-manufactured diphtheria toxoid was evaluated in several case-control studies during the recent epidemic in the former Soviet Union. Three or more doses of diphtheria toxoid were demonstrated to be highly effective in prevention of diphtheria among children younger than 15 years in a preliminary study in Ukraine in 1992 and a subsequent study performed in Moscow in 1993. In Ukraine, the effectiveness of three or more doses was 98.2% (95% confidence interval, 90.3% to 99.9%).[161] In Moscow, the effectiveness of three or more doses was 96.9% (95% CI, 94.3% to 98.4%), increasing to 99.0% for five or more doses (95% CI, 97.7% to 99.6%).[162] In addition, administration of a booster dose of diphtheria toxoid within 2 years was shown to decrease risk of diphtheria among children 6 to 8 years of age compared with those who had received the last dose 3 to 4 or 5 to 7 years previously.[163] Among adults in the Russian Federation, the effectiveness of three or more doses compared to no doses was 70% (95% CI, 10% to 90%).[164] Similarly, recent vaccination also was found to be highly effective among adults in Ukraine.[165]

Thus it appears that the protective efficacy of diphtheria toxoid, as measured by incidence of the disease in immunized and unimmunized individuals during outbreaks, is high although not 100%. However, most reports indicate that the disease in previously immunized individuals is milder and less likely to be fatal.[95,160,166–168] In Britain in 1943, case-fatality rates in unimmunized children were more than sevenfold greater than rates in those who had been immunized (6.4% vs. 0.9%).[89] The failure to protect 100% of individuals on exposure indicates the importance of herd immunity in the disappearance of diphtheria from developed countries.[169]

Because the only immunologic effect predicted for diphtheria toxoid is induction of diphtheria antitoxin, no impact of vaccination would be expected on carriage of nontoxigenic corynebacteria. However, researchers in Italy identified 93 carriers of *Corynebacterium* species (no isolates of *C. diphtheriae* were found); 80 of the 93 carriers had diphtheria antitoxin levels of less than 0.01 IU/mL, whereas only 45 of 407 noncolonized persons had nonprotective titers, a difference that was highly significant. There was good correlation between diphtheria antitoxin concentra-

tion and the concentrations of antibodies to other corynebacterial cell wall antigens. These findings are consistent with induction of corynebacterial immunity by vaccination, which could result from impurities in some formulations of diphtheria antitoxin.[170] The epidemiologic significance and the generalizability of these observations have not been established.

Duration of Immunity

Serologic studies in Europe and the United States have demonstrated that many adults in these countries remain susceptible to diphtheria.[171–178] Differences in seroprevalence among countries reflect the varied immunization schedules among countries and for different time periods in the same nation, the effect of immunization during military service, and the unknown effects of natural exposure to toxigenic *C. diphtheriae*.[172] Although there is some variability among countries, studies of diphtheria seroprevalence frequently have demonstrated low levels of immunity among older adults. A serologic study in England and Wales showed that only 29% of adults age 60 years and older had diphtheria antitoxin titers of 0.01 IU/mL or greater.[176] A similar pattern of susceptibility is seen among elderly persons in other countries of Western Europe.[172] Some studies also demonstrated less susceptibility among males; in some countries, this may reflect immunization during military service.[172]

In spite of the relatively low levels of immunity among adults in many countries, diphtheria has remained well controlled in most countries with effective childhood immunization programs. Historically it has been thought that 70% or more of a childhood population must be immune to diphtheria to prevent major community outbreaks[179]; the herd immunity threshold has been estimated at 80% to 85%, based on the average age of infection in the prevaccine era.[180] Whether an epidemic of a given infectious disease occurs is influenced by a number of factors other than the proportion of susceptible persons in the population, including the age distribution of immune and susceptible persons, the extent of mixing of individuals and subgroups in the community, and the infectivity and routes of transmission of the organism.[169] In countries with high rates of childhood immunization against diphtheria, it may well be that epidemics do not occur among adults, up to half of whom may be susceptible, because the reservoir of disease in the childhood population has been eliminated and because the strains of C. *diphtheriae* circulating in the community are less likely to be toxigenic. Nonetheless, although there is disagreement, the proportion of susceptible adults is of sufficient concern that most authorities recommend maintenance of diphtheria immunity by periodic reinforcement with use of Td.[181]

These concerns have been heightened by the recent epidemic of diphtheria in the former Soviet Union. A striking feature of this epidemic was the proportion of cases occurring among adults, varying from 38% in Azerbaijan to 82% in Latvia and Lithuania in 1994.[182] Before 1986, the last dose of diphtheria toxoid was routinely administered at 14 to 16 years of age in the Soviet Union; in response to an increase in reported cases of diphtheria in the early 1980s, targeted vaccination of certain occupational groups was initiated, but routine use of booster vaccinations among adults was not recommended. Immunogenicity studies in Russia, Ukraine, the Baltic States, and Georgia demonstrated that some adults failed to develop a booster response to a single dose of diphtheria toxoid, suggesting that they may never have received an effective primary series in childhood.[183–187] Childhood immunization coverage was low in some regions in the late 1980s and early 1990s, in part because of an extensive list of contraindications to vaccination,[188] and this undoubtedly contributed to the epidemic.[189] For control of the epidemic, the World Health Organization recommended identification, isolation, and appropriate treatment of all cases; prevention of secondary cases by optimum management of close contacts of cases; and rapidly increasing population immunity by sustaining high coverage among children with four doses of DTP in all districts and administering a single dose of an age-appropriate formulation of diphtheria toxoid to the entire population.[182] By 1997, all countries had made significant progress in immunization of children and adults; the declines in disease incidence were most dramatic in countries that had achieved high coverage.[106]

Although the factors that allowed this epidemic to occur are not completely understood, it is apparent that, under the right combination of conditions, epidemic diphtheria can occur in industrialized countries. Notably, the outbreak occurred in spite of high vaccine coverage with a primary series among school-age children. Many of the cases occurred among adults. A large proportion of the population of adults, although seronegative, were previously primed by prior immunization or infection with toxigenic C. *diphtheriae*, as evidenced by development of protective titers after a single booster dose of toxoid. Although the immunization histories of the adult cases were difficult to ascertain, the overall population data suggest that many probably had been immune but lost immunity over time. With implementation of booster vaccination for all age groups, the outbreak came under control. The experience of this massive epidemic strongly suggests that sustaining high immunization coverage with a primary series of diphtheria toxoid among infants and administering booster doses at school entry and subsequently throughout life are important for maintenance of population immunity.

Safety of Diphtheria Toxoid

Initial efforts to administer booster doses of diphtheria toxoid to older children and adults more than 40 years ago were associated with unacceptably high rates of local and systemic reactions, sometimes sufficient to incapacitate the individual for several days.[190] Such individuals often reacted strongly on Schick testing to both the test and the control material; if the physician failed to include the control, such an individual would be deemed to be strongly Schick positive and therefore be given a booster dose of toxoid, usually with unpleasant results. These reactions appeared to be of the delayed hypersensitivity (tuberculin) type.

One early approach to this problem was to try to identify hypersensitive persons by the so-called Moloney test, which consisted of the injection of a small amount of diphtheria toxoid intradermally.[191] Local reactivity was interpreted as predictive of moderate to severe sensitivity to the toxoid and therefore deemed to be a contraindication; the test is no longer recommended and rarely, if ever, used. The solution to the problem of hyperreactivity to diphtheria toxoid lay in three measures.[192] These were enhanced purification of the toxoid to remove extraneous proteins,[193–195] adsorption of the toxoid onto an aluminum salt,[196] and reduction of the amount of diphtheria toxoid per inoculation to 1 to 2 Lf, an amount shown to be sufficient as a booster dose in a number of studies.[194,197] Aluminum salts as adjuvants also enhance antibody production.[137] These and similar developments led to current recommendations for periodic reinforcement of diphtheria immunity in older children and adults.[181] Furthermore, it has been shown that older children and adults respond satisfactorily to primary immunization with Td,[150,151] and even the elderly respond well to small doses of diphtheria toxoid.[198,199] However, children of preschool age develop significantly lower titers of antibody after low-dose diphtheria vaccine of the adult type than after the standard pediatric dose, and thus should receive the latter.[199a]

Almost all physicians are aware of the importance of tetanus prophylaxis for wounds. Fewer, however, are cognizant of the potential public health benefit from including a concomitant diphtheria booster when a tetanus booster is indicated for an injury. The use of Td, rather than monovalent tetanus toxoid, should be standard operating procedure in emergency departments, physicians' offices, and other situations in which tetanus-prone wounds are treated.[181,200,201] There are essentially no indications for monovalent tetanus toxoid at present in the United States or elsewhere.

Extensive data on adverse reactions after administration of currently available preparations of Diphtheria Toxoid, Adsorbed, are not available because the toxoid is usually administered in combination with tetanus toxoid and, in children, with pertussis vaccine as well. When it is given in combination with pertussis vaccine, local reactions often are ascribed to the pertussis-containing component. In several large clinical trials, the reactogenicity of DT was compared with that of DTaP for primary vaccination of infants. In general, the frequency of reported common systemic symptoms (i.e., temperature of 38°C or higher, crying for 1 hour or longer, irritability, drowsiness, loss of appetite, vomiting) and local reactions (i.e., redness, swelling, tenderness) after vaccination with DT or DTaP was comparable.[202–205] In clinical trials in Sweden and Italy, DT vaccines containing 15 or 25 Lf of diphtheria toxoid and 3.75 or 10 Lf of tetanus toxoid, respectively, were given to more than 7000 infants. The frequency of temperature of 38°C or higher after any vaccine dose was 35% in the Swedish trial and 9% in the Italian study. Other common systemic symptoms occurred with similar frequency in the two studies: crying for 1 hour or longer in 5% and 6%, irritability in 67% and 55%, drowsiness in 54% and 43%, loss of appetite in 22% and 26%, and vomiting in 15% and 9%. Redness and tenderness after any vaccine dose was reported in 42% and 22%, respectively, of infants in the Swedish trial, and in 19% and 9%, respectively, in the Italian trial; the frequency of marked redness or swelling was substantially lower in both studies, with redness and swelling of 2 cm or more reported in only 4% and 6%, respectively, of infants in the Swedish trial.[202,203,206] The frequency of adverse reactions after DT increased with increasing dose number.[204,205]

Available data suggest that both diphtheria and tetanus toxoids contribute to the reactogenicity of Td and DT. Among Swedish medical personnel with a history of receipt of previous primary immunization in childhood, adverse events (i.e., local tenderness and swelling >5 cm or general discomfort) were reported by 11% of those who received 2.5 Lf of diphtheria toxoid, compared with 20% of those who received 2.5 Lf of diphtheria toxoid combined with 0.75 Lf of tetanus toxoid, documenting the additive effects of the two toxoids.[207] Data from several controlled studies suggest that fever and local reactions are more common after administration of Td than after tetanus toxoid.[152,208]

In some populations, large numbers of previously primed persons develop local reactions and fever in response to diphtheria toxoid, even at low doses. In a small study of Israeli military recruits who had been previously vaccinated in childhood, mild to moderate pain at the injection site was reported by 38% and severe pain by 20% after receipt of a booster dose of 2 Lf diphtheria toxoid without tetanus toxoid; limitation of abduction was reported by 8%. Systemic symptoms of mild to moderate or severe weakness were reported by 24% and 9%, respectively, and fever of 38°C or higher was reported by a single subject (<1%).[209] Similarly, a booster dose of 1.5 Lf was administered to 215 university students with prevaccination diphtheria antitoxin levels of less than 0.1 IU/mL. Eight percent reported tenderness at the injection site, and 13% reported pain with abduction, which was marked in 2% of subjects; none had erythema or swelling noted on examination.[210]

With current formulations of diphtheria toxoid, the frequency of reported adverse events varies by prior vaccination history, prevaccination diphtheria antitoxin level, and dose of diphtheria toxoid administered. Among 123 persons 30 to 70 years of age with diphtheria antitoxin levels of 0.05 IU/mL or less, adverse events after vaccination were more severe among those who received 12 Lf of diphtheria toxoid as a booster, compared with those who received doses of 5 Lf or 2 Lf, supporting the recommendation to administer reduced doses of diphtheria toxoid to adults. All vaccines were administered without tetanus toxoid.[211] A second study in military recruits 18 to 25 years of age, most of whom had documentation of receipt of a complete primary vaccination series in childhood, also showed no differences in adverse events between doses of 5 Lf and 2 Lf of diphtheria toxoid combined with tetanus toxoid.[212]

Use of adsorbed vaccine for primary immunization has been reported to result in higher rates of local adverse reactions after subsequent booster vaccination. A higher incidence of local reactions after booster vaccination with DT was observed among Swedish schoolchildren who received adsorbed DT for primary immunization in infancy compared with those who had received nonadsorbed fluid DTP. Seventy-three percent of children who had been primed with DT reported redness, 56% swelling, and 47% itching, compared with 23%, 15%, and 21%, respectively, among those who had received DTP.[213] In contrast, local reactions did not differ among children who had received adsorbed DT for the primary series and then were boosted with either adsorbed or nonadsorbed DT.[214,215]

The potential for anaphylaxis exists with any protein antigen, but such has not been attributed to diphtheria toxoid. Curiously, the British National Childhood Encephalopathy Study, designed to examine the incidence of brain damage after the administration of pertussis vaccine, showed a slight although statistically insignificant excess of acute encephalopathy in the first 7 days after a dose of DT.[216] It is likely, however, that this excess is attributable to the induction of inevitable manifestations of pre-existing central nervous system disorders by the systemic effects of DT, as was observed with infantile spasms.[217]

Local reactions after administration of diphtheria toxoid (alone or in combination with tetanus toxoid or tetanus toxoid and pertussis vaccine) are common but usually minor; severe reactions are rare. Diphtheria toxoid is one of the safest vaccines in current use, and the benefit-to-risk ratio is therefore high.

Precautions and Contraindications

There are few contraindications to use of diphtheria toxoid. Neurologic reactions or severe hypersensitivity reactions following a previous dose are considered contraindications to further doses.[148] Local side effects alone do not preclude continued use. Vaccination of persons with severe, febrile illness generally should be deferred until recovery, but mild illnesses with or without fever should not preclude vaccination.

Some diphtheria toxoid products are packaged in containers (vials or syringes) containing latex rubber. If a person reports a severe anaphylactic allergy to latex, vaccines supplied in vials or syringes that contain natural rubber should not be administered, unless the benefit of vaccination outweighs the risk of an allergic reaction to the vaccine. For latex allergies other than anaphylactic allergies (e.g., a history of contact allergy to latex gloves), vaccines supplied in vials or syringes that contain natural rubber or natural rubber latex can be administered.[218]

Persons with a bleeding disorder or receiving anticoagulant therapy may receive indicated vaccinations by the intramuscular route if, in the opinion of a physician familiar with the patient's bleeding risk, the vaccine can be administered with reasonable safety by this route. A fine needle (≤23 gauge) should be used for the injection and firm pressure applied to the site, without rubbing, for 2 or more minutes. The patient or family should be instructed concerning the risk for hematoma from the injection.[218]

Unresolved Problems

Immunity to the exotoxin prevents the systemic manifestations of diphtheria, which are responsible for almost all of the morbidity and mortality from the disease. However, nontoxigenic strains rarely produce local disease or invasive disease; infrequent instances of local disease may occur with toxigenic strains in persons with ample serologic immunity. For this reason, there has been some interest in better defining the organism's somatic antigens and their relationship to infection in humans.[219] It is also assumed that reactivity to diphtheria toxoid, usually only a nuisance but with the potential to be serious, stems largely from extraneous proteins present in the toxoid. This reactivity limits the amount of antigen that can be administered at one time, thus requiring that several doses be administered for protection. Alternatives in the future may include vaccination by the oral[220] or nasal[221] routes or use of a highly purified, less reactive antigen[222,223] or carrier systems[224,225] for diphtheria toxoid that would require fewer injections. Such products would be particularly useful in the developing world, where severe limitations in health care personnel and financial resources are major barriers.

Active immunization against diphtheria with use of current preparations represents a remarkable triumph of preventive medicine. Nonetheless, during the 1990s, a massive epidemic of diphtheria occurred in the countries of the former Soviet Union, with more than 140,000 cases reported. To prevent future epidemics, a high level of population immunity must be maintained among children, adolescents, and adults.

REFERENCES

1. Zink A, Reischl U, Wolf H, et al. Corynebacterium in ancient Egypt. Med History 45:267–272, 2001.
2. Holmes WH. Diphtheria: History. In Bacillary and Rickettsial Infections. New York, Macmillan, 1940, pp 291–305.
3. Andrewes FW, Bulloch W, Douglas SR, et al. Diphtheria: Its Bacteriology, Pathology and Immunology. London, His Majesty's Stationery Office, 1923.
4. English PC. Diphtheria and theories of infectious disease. Pediatrics 76:1–9, 1985.
5. Caulfield E. A true history of the terrible epidemic vulgarly called the throat distemper: which occurred in His Majesty's New England colonies between the years 1735 and 1740. Yale J Biol Med 11:226–272, 1939.
6. Holt LE. Diphtheria. In Holt LE (ed). The Diseases of Infancy and Childhood. New York, D Appleton & Company, 1897, pp 951–1001.
7. Ramon G. Sur le pouvoir floculant et sur les proprietes immunisantes d'une toxin diphterique rendue anatoxine (anatoxine). C R Acad Sci 177:1338–1340, 1923.
8. Belsey MA, Sinclair M, Roder MR, LeBlanc DR. Corynebacterium diphtheriae skin infections in Alabama and Louisiana: a factor in the epidemiology of diphtheria. N Engl J Med 280:135–141, 1969.
9. Höfler W. Cutaneous diphtheria. Int J Dermatol 30:845–847, 1991.
10. Metaxas Quiroga VA. Diphtheria and medical therapy in late 19th century New York City. N Y State J Med 90:256–262, 1990.
11. Anderson JS, Happold FC, McLeod JW, Thomson JG. On the existence of two forms of diphtheria bacillus—B. diphtheriae gravis and B. diphtheriae mitis—and a new medium for their differentiation and for the bacteriological diagnosis of diphtheria. J Pathol Bacteriol 34:667–681, 1931.
12. Robinson DT, Marshall FN. Investigations on the gravis, mitis, and intermediate types of C. diphtheriae and their clinical significance. J Pathol Bacteriol 38:73–89, 1934.
13. Diphtheria. In Top FH (ed). Communicable and Infectious Diseases (4th ed). St. Louis, CV Mosby, 1960, pp 198–213.
14. Leete HM. The heart in diphtheria. Lancet 1:136–139, 1938.
15. Wesselhoeft C. Communicable diseases: cardiovascular disease in diphtheria. N Engl J Med 223:57–66, 1940.
16. Bethell DB, Dung NM, Loan HT, et al. Prognostic value of electrocardiographic monitoring of patients with severe diphtheria. Clin Infect Dis 20:1259–1265, 1995.
17. Stockins BA, Lanas FT, Saavedra JG, Opazo JA. Prognosis in patients with diphtheritic myocarditis and bradyarrhythmias: assessment of results of ventricular pacing. Br Heart J 72:190–191, 1994.
18. Loukoushkina EF, Bobko PV, Kolbasova EV, et al. The clinical picture and diagnosis of diphtheritic carditis in children. Eur J Pediatr 145:528–533, 1998.
19. Ordian AM, Iushchuk ND, Karetkina GN, et al. Clinical and prognostic significance of disturbed global and regional contractility of left ventricle in diphtheria myocarditis [in Russian]. Klin Med 78:20–23, 2000.
20. Ford FR. Diseases of the Nervous System in Infancy, Childhood and Adolescence (6th ed). Springfield, IL, Charles C Thomas, 1973, pp 716–721.
21. Longina I, Donaghy M. Diphtheritic polyneuropathy: a clinical study and comparison with Guillain-Barré syndrome. J Neurol Neurosurg Psychiatry 67:433–438, 1999.
22. Piradov MA, Pirogov VN, Popova LM, Avdunina IA. Diphtheritic polyneuropathy: clinical analysis of severe forms. Arch Neurol 58:1438–1442, 2001.
23. Afghani B, Stutman HR. Bacterial arthritis caused by Corynebacterium diphtheriae. Pediatr Infect Dis J 12:881–882, 1993.
24. Zuber PLF, Gruner E, Altwegg M, von Graevenitz A. Invasive infection with nontoxigenic Corynebacterium diphtheriae among drug users [letter]. Lancet 339:1359, 1992.
25. Poilane I, Fawaz F, Nathanson M, et al. Corynebacterium diphtheriae osteomyelitis in an immunocompetent child: a case report. Eur J Pediatr 154:381–383, 1995.
26. Patey O, Bimet F, Riegal P, et al for the Coryne Study Group. Clinical and molecular study of Corynebacterium diphtheriae systemic infections in France. J Clin Microbiol 35:441–445, 1997.
27. Reacher M, Ramsay M, White J, et al. Nontoxigenic Corynebacterium diphtheriae: an emerging pathogen in England and Wales? Emerg Infect Dis 6:640–645, 2000.
28. Funke G, von Graevenitz A, Clarridge JE, Bernard KA. Clinical microbiology of coryneform bacteria. Clin Microbiol Rev 10:125–159, 1997.
29. Lautrop H. Studies on the antigenic structure of Corynebacterium diphtheriae. Acta Pathol Microbiol Scand 27:443–447, 1950.
30. Edward DGF, Allison VD. Diphtheria in the immunized with observations on a diphtheria-like disease associated with non-toxigenic strains of Corynebacterium diphtheriae. J Hyg 49:205–219, 1951.
31. Kato M. Action of a toxic glycolipid of Corynebacterium diphtheriae on mitochondrial structure and function. J Bacteriol 101:709–716, 1970.
32. Collier RJ. Understanding the mode of action of diphtheria toxin: a perspective on progress during the 20th century. Toxicon 39:1793–1803, 2001.
33. Holmes RK. Biology and molecular epidemiology of diphtheria toxin and the tox gene. J Infect Dis 181(suppl 1):S156–S167, 2000.
34. Pappenheimer AM, Gill DM. Diphtheria. Science 182:353–358, 1973.
35. Collier RJ. Diphtheria toxin: mode of action and structure. Bacteriol Rev 39:54–85, 1975.
36. Nakao H, Mazurova IK, Glushkevich T, Popovic T. Analysis of heterogeneity of Corynebacterium diphtheriae toxin gene, tox and its regulatory element, dtxR, by direct sequencing. Res Microbiol 148:45–54, 1997.
37. Schmitt MP. Utilization of host iron sources by Corynebacterium diphtheriae: identification of a gene whose product is homologous to eukaryotic heme oxygenases and is required for the acquisition of iron from heme and hemoglobin. J Bacteriol 179:838–845, 1997.
38. Tao X, Schiering N, Zeng H, et al. Iron, DtxR, and the regulation of diphtheria toxin expression. Mol Microbiol 14:191–197, 1994.
39. Naglich JG, Metherall JE, Russell DW, Eidels L. Expression cloning of a diphtheria toxin receptor: identity with a heparin-binding EGF-like growth factor precursor. Cell 69:1051–1061, 1992.
40. Cha J-H, Brooke JS, Ivey KN, Eidels L. Cell surface monkey CD9 antigen is a coreceptor that increases diphtheria toxin sensitivity and diphtheria toxin receptor affinity. J Biol Chem 275:6901–6907, 2000.
41. Morris RE, Gerstein AS, Bonventre PF, Saelinger CB. Receptor-mediated entry of diphtheria toxin into monkey kidney (Vero) cells: electron microscopic evaluation. Infect Immun 50:721–727, 1985.

42. Vaughan TJ, Pascall JC, Brown KD. Tissue distribution of mRNA for heparin-binding epidermal growth factor. Biochem J 287:681–684, 1992.

43. Nakamura Y, Handa K, Iwamoto R, et al. Immunohistochemical distribution of CD9, heparin binding epidermal growth factor-like growth factor, and integrin $\alpha 3\alpha 1$ in normal human tissues. J Histochem Cytochem 49:439–444, 2001.

44. Pappenheimer AM Jr, Murphy JR. Studies on the molecular epidemiology of diphtheria. Lancet 2:923–926, 1983.

45. Ipsen J. Circulating antitoxin at the onset of diphtheria in 425 patients. J Immunol 54:325–347, 1946.

46. Björkholm B, Böttiger M, Christensen B, Hagberg L. Antitoxin antibody levels and the outcome of illness during an outbreak of diphtheria among alcoholics. Scand J Infect Dis 18:235–239, 1986.

47. Pappenheimer AM. The Schick test, 1913–1958. Int Arch Allergy Appl Immunol 12:35–41, 1958.

48. Efstratiou A, Maple PAC. Laboratory Diagnosis of Diphtheria. Copenhagen, World Health Organization, Expanded Programme on Immunization in the European Region, 1994.

49. Miyamura K, Nishio S, Ito A, et al. Micro cell culture method for determination of diphtheria toxin and antitoxin titres using VERO cells. I. Studies on factors affecting the toxin and antitoxin titration. J Biol Stand 2:189–201, 1974.

50. Melville-Smith M, Balfour A. Estimation of Corynebacterium diphtheriae antitoxin in human sera: a comparison of an enzyme-linked immunosorbent assay with the toxin neutralization test. J Med Microbiol 25:279–283, 1988.

51. Walory J, Grzesiowski P, Hryniewicz W. Comparison of four serological methods for the detection of diphtheria antitoxin. J Immunol Methods 245:55–65, 2000.

52. von Hunolstein C, Aggerbeck H, Andrews N, et al. European seroepidemiology network: standardization of the results of diphtheria antitoxin assays. Vaccine 18:3287–3296, 2000.

53. Wong TP, Groman N. Production of diphtheria toxin by selected isolates of Corynebacterium ulcerans and Corynebacterium pseudotuberculosis. Infect Immun 43:1114–1116, 1984.

54. Maximescu P, Oprisan A, Pop A, Potorac F. Further studies on Corynebacterium species capable of producing diphtheria toxin (C. diphtheriae, C. ulcerans, C. ovis). J Gen Microbiol 82:49–56, 1974.

55. Meers PD. A case of classical diphtheria, and other infections due to Corynebacterium ulcerans. J Infect 1:139–142, 1979.

56. Hust MH, Metzler B, Schubert U, et al. Toxische Diphtherie durch Corynebacterium ulcerans. Dtsch Med Wochenschr 119:548–553, 1994.

57. Centers for Disease Control and Prevention. Respiratory diphtheria caused by Corynebacterium ulcerans—Terre Haute, Indiana, 1996. MMWR 46:330–332, 1997.

58. Efstratiou A, Engler KH, Mazurova IK, et al. Current approaches to the laboratory diagnosis of diphtheria. J Infect Dis 181(suppl 1):S138–S145, 2000.

59. Engler KH, Glushkevich T, Mazurova IK, et al. A modified Elek test for detection of toxigenic corynebacteria in the diagnostic laboratory. J Clin Microbiol 35:495–498, 1997.

60. Pallen MJ. Rapid screening for toxigenic Corynebacterium diphtheriae by the polymerase chain reaction. J Clin Pathol 44:1025–1026, 1991.

61. Hauser D, Popoff MR, Kiredjian M, et al. Polymerase chain reaction assay for diagnosis of potentially toxigenic Corynebacterium diphtheriae strains: correlation with ADP-ribosylation activity assay. J Clin Microbiol 31:2720–2723, 1993.

62. Aravena-Romaán M, Bowman R, O'Neill G. Polymerase chain reaction for detection of toxigenic Corynebacterium diphtheriae. Pathology 27:71–73, 1995.

63. Mikhailovich VM, Melnikov VG, Mazurova IK, et al. Application of PCR for detection of toxigenic Corynebacterium diphtheriae strains isolated during the Russian diphtheria epidemic, 1990 through 1994. J Clin Microbiol 33:3061–3063, 1995.

64. Nakao H, Popovic T. Development of a direct PCR assay for detection of the diphtheria toxin gene. J Clin Microbiol 35:1651–1655, 1997.

65. Saragea A, Maximescu P. Phage typing of Corynebacterium diphtheriae. Bull World Health Organ 35:681–689, 1966.

66. Rappuoli R, Perugini M, Falsen E. Molecular epidemiology of the 1984–1986 outbreak of diphtheria in Sweden. N Engl J Med 318: 12–14, 1988.

67. Coyle MB, Groman NB, Russell JQ, et al. The molecular epidemiology of three biotypes of Corynebacterium diphtheriae in the Seattle outbreak, 1972–1982. J Infect Dis 159:670–679, 1989.

68. De Zoysa A, Efstratiou A, George RC, et al. Molecular epidemiology of Corynebacterium diphtheriae from northwestern Russia and surrounding countries studied by using ribotyping and pulsed-field gel electrophoresis. J Clin Microbiol 33:1080–1083, 1995.

69. Popovic T, Kombarova SY, Reeves MW, et al. Molecular epidemiology of diphtheria in Russia, 1985–1994. J Infect Dis 174:1064–1072, 1996.

70. Nakao H, Pruckler JM, Mazurova IK, et al. Heterogeneity of diphtheria toxin gene, tox, and its regulatory element, dxtR, in Corynebacterium diphtheriae strains causing epidemic diphtheria in Russia and Ukraine. J Clin Microbiol 34:1711–1716, 1996.

71. Nakao H, Popovic T. Development of a rapid ribotyping method for Corynebacterium diphtheriae by using PCR single-strand conformation polymorphism: comparison with standard ribotyping. J Microbiol Methods 31:127–134, 1998.

72. Galazka AM, Robertson SE. Diphtheria: changing patterns in the developing world and the industrialized world. Eur J Epidemiol 11:107–117, 1995.

73. Wright HD, Shone HR, Tucker JR. Cross infection in diphtheria wards. J Pathol Bacteriol 52:111–128, 1941.

74. Crosbie WE, Wright HD. Diphtheria bacilli in floor dust. Lancet 1:656–659, 1941.

75. Belsey MA. Isolation of Corynebacterium diphtheriae in the environment of skin carriers. Am J Epidemiol 91:294–299, 1970.

76. Larsson P, Brinkhoff B, Larsson L. Corynebacterium diphtheriae in the environment of carriers and patients. J Hosp Infect 10:282–286, 1987.

77. Jones EE, Kim-Farley RJ, Algunaid M, et al. Diphtheria: a possible foodborne outbreak in Hodeida, Yemen Arab Republic. Bull World Health Organ 63:287–293, 1985.

78. Seckel HPG. Prevention of diphtheria. Am J Dis Child 58:512–526, 1939.

79. Mortensen V. Occurrence of diphtheria in recent years, with a special view to the influence of the antidiphtheric vaccination. Acta Med Scand 125:283–293, 1946.

80. Walker JV. Age and sex distribution of diphtheria in Oldenburg, Germany. Lancet 1:422–423, 1947.

81. Madsen S. II. Diphtheria immunization. Dan Med Bull 3:116–121, 1956.

82. Vitek CR, Brisgalov SP, Bragina VY, et al. Epidemiology of epidemic diphtheria in three regions, Russia, 1994–1996. Eur J Epidemiol 15:75–83, 1999.

83. Burnet M, White DO. Natural History of Infectious Disease (4th ed). London, Cambridge University Press, 1972, pp 193–201.

84. U.S. Bureau of the Census. Historical Statistics of the United States, Colonial Times to 1970, Bicentennial Edition, Part 1. Washington, DC, US Department of Congress, 1975, pp 58, 63.

85. Hammonds EM. Childhood's Deadly Scourge: The Campaign to Control Diphtheria in New York City, 1880–1930. Baltimore, Johns Hopkins University Press, 1999.

86. McKinnon NE. Diphtheria prevented. In Cruickshank R (ed). Control of the Common Fevers. London, The Lancet Ltd, 1942, pp 41–56.

87. Lewis J. The prevention of diphtheria in Canada and Britain 1914–1945. J Social Hist 20:163–176, 1986.

88. Stowman K. Diphtheria pandemic recedes. UN World Health Organ 1:60–67, 1947.

89. Stuart G. A note on diphtheria incidence in certain countries. Br Med J 2:613–615, 1945.

90. Wheeler SM, Morton AR. Epidemiological observations in the Halifax epidemic. Am J Public Health 32:947–956, 1942.

91. Fleck S, Kellam JW, Klippen AJ. Diphtheria among German prisoners of war. Bull US Army Med Dept 74:80–89, 1944.

92. Brooks GF, Bennett JV, Feldman RA. Diphtheria in the United States, 1959–1970. J Infect Dis 129:172–178, 1974.

93. Zalma VM, Older JJ, Brooks GF. The Austin, Texas, diphtheria outbreak: clinical and epidemiological aspects. JAMA 211:2125–2129, 1970.

94. Marcuse EK, Grand MG. Epidemiology of diphtheria in San Antonio, Texas, 1970. JAMA 224:305–310, 1973.

95. Chen RT, Broome CV, Weinstein RA, et al. Diphtheria in the United States, 1971–1981. Am J Public Health 75:1393–1397, 1985.

96. Harnisch JP, Tronca E, Nolan CM, et al. Diphtheria among urban alcoholic adults: a decade of experience in Seattle. Ann Intern Med 111:71–82, 1989.

97. McCloskey RV, Saragea A, Maximescu P. Phage typing in diphtheria outbreaks in the southwestern United States, 1968–1971. J Infect Dis 126:196–199, 1972.

98. Bisgard KM, Hardy IRB, Popovic T, et al. Respiratory diphtheria in the United States, 1980–1995. Am J Public Health 88:787–791, 1998.

99. Centers for Disease Control and Prevention. Summary of notifiable diseases, United States, 1999. MMWR 48:33, 1999.

100. Centers for Disease Control and Prevention. Toxigenic Corynebacterium diphtheriae—northern plains Indian community, August–October 1996. MMWR 46:506–510, 1997.

101. Young TK. Endemicity of diphtheria in an Indian population in northwestern Ontario. Can J Public Health 75:310–313, 1984.

102. Wilson CR, Casson RI, Wherrett B, Fraser N. Toxigenic diphtheria in two isolated northern communities. Arctic Med Res Suppl: 346–347, 1991.

103. Cahoon FE, Brown S, Jamieson F. Corynebacterium diphtheriae—toxigenic isolations from northeastern Ontario [abstract K-171]. In Abstracts of the 37th Interscience Conference on Antimicrobial Agents and Chemotherapy, Toronto, Ontario, Canada, September 28–October 1, 1997.

104. Marston CK, Jamieson F, Cahoon F, et al. Persistence of a distinct Corynebacterium diphtheriae clonal group within two communities in the United States and Canada where diphtheria is endemic. J Clin Microbiol 39:1586–1590, 2001.

105. Patel M, Morey F, Butcher A, et al. The frequent isolation of toxigenic and non-toxigenic Corynebacterium diphtheriae at Alice Springs Hospital. Commun Dis Intell 18:310–311, 1994.

106. Dittmann S, Wharton M, Vitek C, et al. Successful control of epidemic diphtheria in the states of the former Union of Soviet Socialist Republics: lessons learned. J Infect Dis 181(suppl 1):S10–S22, 2000.

107. Wharton M, Dittmann S, Strebel PM, Mortimer EA (eds). Control of Epidemic Diphtheria in the Newly Independent States of the Former Soviet Union. J Infect Dis 181(suppl 1):S1–S248, 2000.

108. Skogen V, Cherkasova VV, Maksimova N, et al. Molecular characterization of Corynebacterium diphtheriae isolates, Russian 1957–1987. Emerg Infect Dis 8:516–518, 2002.

109. Wharton M, Hardy IRB, Vitek C, et al. Epidemic diphtheria in the newly independent states of the former Soviet Union. In Scheld WM, Armstrong D, Hughes JM (eds). Emerging Infections. Vol. I. Washington, DC, ASM Press, 1998, pp 165–176.

110. Tharmaphornpilas P, Yoocharoan P, Prempree P, et al. Diphtheria in Thailand in the 1990s. J Infect Dis 184:1035–1040, 2001.

111. Singh J, Ichhpujani RL, Prabha S, et al. Immunity to diphtheria in women of childbearing age in Delhi in 1994: evidence of continued Corynebacterium diphtheriae circulation. Southeast Asian J Trop Med Public Health 27:274–278, 1996.

112. Lodha R, Dash NR, Kapil A, et al. Diphtheria in urban slums in north India. Lancet 355:204, 2000.

113. Groman N, Schiller J, Russell J. Corynebacterium ulcerans and Corynebacterium pseudotuberculosis responses to DNA probes derived from corynephage and Corynebacterium diphtheriae. Infect Immun 45:511–517, 1984.

114. Hart RJC. Corynebacterium ulcerans in humans and cattle in North Devon. J Hyg (Camb) 92:161–164, 1984.

115. Bostock AD, Gilbert FR, Lewis D, Smith DCM. Corynebacterium ulcerans infection associated with untreated milk. J Infect 9:286–288, 1984.

116. Roux E, Yersin A. Contribution à l'étude de la diphthérie. Ann Inst Pasteur 2:629–664, 1888.

117. Behring E. Untersuchungen über das Zustandekommen der Diphtherie-Immunität bei Thieren. Dtsch Med Wochenschr 16:1145, 1890.

118. Kondratas RA. Death helped write the biologics law. FDA Consum 16:23–25, 1982.

119. U.S. Food and Drug Administration. Biological products; bacterial vaccines and toxoids; implementation of efficacy review. Diphtheria antitoxin. Fed Reg 50:51079–51082, 1985.

120. Centers for Disease Control and Prevention. Notice to Readers. Availability of diphtheria antitoxin through an investigational new drug protocol. MMWR 46:380, 1997.

121. Cha J-H, Brooke JS, Chang MY, Eidels L. Receptor-based antidote for diphtheria. Infect Immun 70:2344–2350, 2002.

122. Dowling HF. Diphtheria as a model. JAMA 226:550–553, 1973.

123. Farizo KM, Strebel PM, Chen RT, et al. Fatal respiratory disease due to Corynebacterium diphtheriae: case report and review of guidelines for management, investigation, and control. Clin Infect Dis 16:59–68, 1993.

124. Ker CB. Infectious Diseases, A Practical Textbook (3rd ed). London, Oxford University Press, 1929.

125. Fibiger J. Om Serumbehandling of Difteri. Hosp-Tid 4.R. 6:309, 337, 1898.

126. Hróbjartsson A, Gøtzche PC, Gluud C. The controlled clinical trial turns 100 years: Fibiger's trial of serum treatment of diphtheria. BMJ 317:1243–1245, 1998.

127. Tasman A, Minkenhof JE, Vink HH, et al. Importance of intravenous injection of diphtheria antiserum. Lancet 1:1299–1304, 1958.

128. Weaver GH. Diphtheria carriers. JAMA 76:831–835, 1921.

129. Smith T. Active immunity produced by so-called balanced or neutral mixtures of diphtheria toxin and antitoxin. J Exp Med 11:241–256, 1909.

130. von Behring E. Über ein neues Diphtheries Schutzmittel. Dtsch Med Wochenschr 39:873–876, 1913.

131. Schick B. Die Diphtherietoxin-Hauktreation des Menschen als Vorprobe der prophylaktischen Diphtherieheilseruminjektion. Munch Med Wochenschr 60:2608–2610, 1913.

132. Park WH. Duration of immunity against diphtheria achieved by various methods. JAMA 109:1681–1684, 1937.

133. Diphtheria. In Harries EHR, Mitman M. Clinical Practice in Infectious Diseases (3rd ed). Baltimore, Williams & Wilkins, 1947, pp 168–223.

134. Glenny AT, Pope CG, Waddington H, Wallace U. Immunological notes. XIII. The antigenic value of toxoid precipitated by potassium alum. J Pathol Bacteriol 29:38–39, 1926.

135. Greenberg L, Fleming DS. The immunizing efficacy of diphtheria toxoid when combined with various antigens. Can J Public Health 39:131–135, 1948.

136. Spiller V, Barnes JM, Holt LB, Cullington DE. Immunization against whooping-cough: combined v. separate inoculations. Br Med J 2:639–642, 1955.

137. Aprile MA, Wardlaw AC. Aluminum compounds as adjuvants for vaccines and toxoids in man: a review. Can J Public Health 57:343–354, 1966.

138. Edwards KM, Decker MD. Combination vaccines consisting of acellular pertussis vaccines. Pediatr Infect Dis J 16(suppl):S97–S102, 1997.

139. Edwards KM, Meade BD, Decker MD, et al. Comparison of 13 acellular pertussis vaccines: overview and serologic response. Pediatrics 96:548–557, 1995.

140. Miller E, Waight P, Laurichesse H, et al. Immunogenicity and reactogenicity of acellular diphtheria/tetanus/pertussis vaccines given as a pre-school booster: effect of simultaneous administration of MMR. Vaccine 19:3904–3911, 2001.

141. Centers for Disease Control and Prevention. Pertussis vaccination: use of acellular pertussis vaccines among infants and young children. Recommendations of the Advisory Committee on Immunization Practices (ACIP). MMWR 46(RR-7):1–25, 1997.

142. Dengrove J, Lee EJ, Heiner DC, et al. IgG and IgG subclass specific antibody responses to diphtheria and tetanus toxoids in newborns and infants given DTP immunization. Pediatr Res 20:735–739, 1986.

143. Bernbaum JC, Daft A, Anolik R, et al. Response of preterm infants to diphtheria-tetanus-pertussis immunization. J Pediatr 107:184–188, 1985.

144. Kirmani KI, Lofthus G, Pichichero ME, et al. Seven-year follow-up of vaccine response in extremely premature infants. Pediatrics 109:498–504, 2002.

145. Bjorkholm B, Granström M, Taranger J, et al. Influence of high titers of maternal antibody on the serologic response of infants to diphtheria vaccination at three, five and twelve months of age. Pediatr Infect Dis J 148:846–850, 1995.

146. Barkin AM, Pichichero ME, Samuelson JS, Barkin SZ. Pediatric diphtheria and tetanus toxoids vaccine: clinical and immunologic response when administered as the primary series. J Pediatr 106:779–781, 1985.

147. Pichichero ME, Barkin RM, Samuelson JS. Pediatric diphtheria and tetanus toxoids-adsorbed vaccine: immune response to the first booster following the diphtheria and tetanus toxoids vaccine primary series. Pediatr Infect Dis 5:428–430, 1986.

148. Centers for Disease Control and Prevention. Diphtheria, tetanus, and pertussis: recommendations for vaccine use and other preventive measures. Recommendations of the Immunization Practices Advisory Committee (ACIP). MMWR 40(RR-10):1–28, 1991.

149. Galazka AM, Robertson SE. Immunization against diphtheria with special emphasis on immunization of adults. Vaccine 14:845–857, 1996.

150. Myers MG, Beckman CW, Vosdingh RA, Hankins WA. Primary immunization with tetanus and diphtheria toxoids: reaction rates and immunogenicity in older children and adults. JAMA 248:2478–2480, 1982.

151. Feery BJ, Benenson AS, Forsyth JRL, et al. Diphtheria immunization in adolescents and adults with reduced doses of adsorbed diphtheria toxoid. Med J Aust 1:128–130, 1981.

152. Macko MB, Powell CE. Comparison of the morbidity of tetanus toxoid boosters with tetanus-diphtheria toxoid boosters. Ann Emerg Med 14:33–35, 1985.

153. King GE, Hadler SC. Simultaneous administration of childhood vaccines: an important public health policy that is safe and efficacious. Pediatr Infect Dis J 13:394–407, 1994.

154. Orenstein WA, Weisfeld JS, Halsey NA. Diphtheria and tetanus toxoids and pertussis vaccine, combined. In Halsey NA, de Quadros CA (eds). Recent Advances in Immunization: A Bibliographic Review. Washington, DC, Pan-American Health Organization, 1983, pp 30–51.

154a. Bjorkholm B, Granstrom M, Taranger J, et al. Influence of high titers of maternal antibody on the serologic response of infants to diphtheria vaccination at three, five, and twelve months of age. Pediatr Infect Dis J 14: 846–850, 1995.

155. Olander R-M, Wuorimaa T, Käyhty H, et al. Booster response to the tetanus and diphtheria toxoid carriers of 11-valent pneumococcal conjugate vaccine in adults and toddlers. Vaccine 20:336–341, 2002.

156. Shelly MA, Pichichero ME, Treanor JJ. Low baseline antibody level of diphtheria is associated with poor response to conjugated pneumococcal vaccine in adults. Scand J Infect Dis 33:542–544, 2001.

157. Walsh JA, Warren KS. Selective primary health care: an interim strategy for disease control in developing countries [special article]. N Engl J Med 301:967–974, 1979.

158. World Health Organization, Department of Vaccines, Immunizations, and Biologicals. Vaccine Preventable Diseases Monitoring System: Incidence Time Series. Available at www.who.int/vaccines-surveillance/StatsAndGraphs.htm

159. World Health Organization, Department of Vaccines and Biologicals. Vaccine-Preventable Diseases: Monitoring System. 2001 Global Summary. Geneva, World Health Organization, 2001.

160. Miller LW, Older JJ, Drake J, Zimmerman S. Diphtheria immunization: effect on carriers and the control of outbreaks. Am J Dis Child 123:197–199, 1972.

161. Chen RT, Hardy IRB, Rhodes PH, et al. Ukraine, 1992: first assessment of diphtheria vaccine effectiveness during the recent resurgence of diphtheria in the former Soviet Union. J Infect Dis 181(suppl 1):S178–S183, 2000.

162. Bisgard KM, Rhodes P, Hardy IRB, et al. Diphtheria toxoid vaccine effectiveness: a case-control study in Russia. J Infect Dis 181(suppl 1):S184–S187, 2000.

163. Vitek C, Brennan M, Gotway C, et al. Risk of diphtheria among schoolchildren in the Russian Federation in relation to time since last vaccination. Lancet 353:355–358, 1999.

164. Brennan M, Vitek C, Strebel P, et al. How many doses of diphtheria toxoid are required for protection of adults? Results of a case-control study among 40- to 49-year-old adults in the Russian Federation. J Infect Dis 181(suppl 1):S193–S196, 2000.

165. Tsu V, Tyshchenko DK. Case-control evaluation of an adult diphtheria immunization program. J Infect Dis 181(suppl 1):S188–S192, 2000.

166. Naiditch MJ, Bower AG. Diphtheria: a study of 1,433 cases observed during a ten-year period at Los Angeles County Hospital. Am J Med 17:229–245, 1954.

167. Brooks GF, Bennett JV, Feldman RA. Diphtheria in the United States, 1959–1970. J Infect Dis 129:172–178, 1974.

168. Narkevich MI, Tymchakovskaia LM. Specific features of the spread of diphtheria in Russia in the presence of mass immunization of children. Zh Mikrobiol Epidemiol Immunobiol Mar–Apr:25–29, 1996.

169. Fox JP, Elveback L, Scott W, et al. Herd immunity: basic concept and relevance to public health immunization practices. Am J Epidemiol 94:179–189, 1971.

170. Bergamini M, Fabrizi P, Pagani S, et al. Evidence of increased carriage of Corynebacterium spp. in healthy individuals with low anti-body titres against diphtheria toxoid. Epidemiol Infect 125:105–112, 2000.

171. Marlovits S, Stocker R, Efstratiou A, et al. Seroprevalence of diphtheria immunity among injured adults in Austria. Vaccine 19:1061–1067, 2001.

172. Edmunds WJ, Pebody RG, Aggerback H, et al. The sero-epidemiology of diphtheria in Western Europe. Epidemiol Infect 125:113–125, 2000.

173. Maple PA, Efstratiou A, George RC, et al. Diphtheria immunity in UK blood donors. Lancet 345:963–965, 1995.

174. Rappuoli R, Podda A, Giovannoni F, et al. Absence of protective immunity against diphtheria in a large proportion of young adults. Vaccine 11:576–577, 1993.

175. Walory J, Grzesiowski J, Hryniewicz W. The seroprevalence of diphtheria immunity in healthy population in Poland. Epidemiol Infect 126:225–230, 2001.

176. Maple PAC, Jones CS, Wall EC, et al. Immunity to diphtheria and tetanus in England and Wales. Vaccine 19:167–173, 2001.

177. McQuillan GM, Kruszon-Moran D, Deforest A, et al. Serologic immunity to diphtheria and tetanus in the United States. Ann Intern Med 136:660–666, 2002.

178. Christenson B, Hellström U, Sylvan SPE, et al. Impact of a vaccination campaign on adult immunity to diphtheria. Vaccine 19:1133–1140, 2001.

179. Howard P, Riley HD. An outbreak of diphtheria in eastern Oklahoma. J Oklahoma State Med Assoc 59:520–527, 1966.

180. Anderson RM. The concept of herd immunity and the design of community-based immunization programmes. Vaccine 10:928–935, 1992.

181. Centers for Disease Control. Update on adult immunization: recommendations of the Immunization Practices Advisory Committee (ACIP). MMWR 40(RR-12):1–94, 1991.

182. Hardy IRB, Dittmann S, Sutter RW. Current situation and control strategies for resurgence of diphtheria in newly independent states of the former Soviet Union. Lancet 347:1739–1744, 1996.

183. Maksimova NM, Sukhorukova NL, Kostyuchenko GI, et al. Specific prophylaxis of diphtheria in adults in the focus of diphtheria infection. Zh Mikrobiol Epidemiol Immunobiol Aug:36–40, 1987.

184. Golaz A, Hardy IB, Glushkevich TG, et al. Evaluation of a single dose of diphtheria-tetanus toxoids among adults in Odessa, Ukraine, 1995: immunogenicity and adverse reactions. J Infect Dis 181(suppl 1):S203–S207, 2000.

185. Sutter RW, Hardy IR, Kozlova IA, et al. Immunogenicity of tetanus-diphtheria toxoids (Td) among Ukrainian adults: implications for diphtheria control in the newly independent states of the former Soviet Union. J Infect Dis 181(suppl 1):S197–S202, 2000.

186. Rønne T, Valentelis R, Tarum S, et al. Immune response to diphtheria booster vaccine in the Baltic States. J Infect Dis 181(suppl 1):S213–S219, 2000.

187. Khetsuriani N, Music S, Deforest A, Sutter RW. Evaluation of a single dose of diphtheria toxoid among adults in the Republic of Georgia, 1995: immunogenicity and adverse reactions. J Infect Dis 181(suppl 1):S208–S212, 2000.

188. Tatochenko V, Mitjushin IL. Contraindications to vaccination in the Russian Federation. J Infect Dis 181(suppl 1):S228–S231, 2000.

189. Galazka AM, Robertson SE, Oblapenko GP. Resurgence of diphtheria. Eur J Epidemiol 11:95–105, 1995.

190. Edsall G. Immunization of adults against diphtheria and tetanus. Am J Hyg 42:393–400, 1952.

191. Moloney PJ, Fraser CJ. Immunization with diphtheria toxoid (anatoxine Ramon). Am J Public Health 17:1027–1030, 1927.

192. Edsall G, Altman JS, Gaspar AJ. Combined tetanus-diphtheria immunization of adults: use of small doses of diphtheria toxoid. Am J Public Health 44:1537–1545, 1954.

193. Pappenheimer AM Jr, Edsall G, Lawrence HS, et al. Study of reactions following administration of crude and purified diphtheria toxoid in an adult population. Am J Hyg 52:353–370, 1950.

194. Volk VK, Gottshall RY, Anderson HD, et al. Antibody response to booster dose of diphtheria and tetanus toxoids: reactions in institutionalized adults and non-institutionalized children and young adults. Public Health Rep 78:161–164, 1963.

195. Smith JWG. Diphtheria and tetanus toxoids. Br Med Bull 25:177–182, 1969.

196. James G, Longshore WA Jr, Hendry JL. Diphtheria immunization studies of students in an urban high school. Am J Hyg 53:178–261, 1951.

197. Edsall G, Banton HJ, Wheeler RE. The antigenicity of single, graded doses of purified diphtheria toxoid in man. Am J Hyg 53:283–295, 1951.

198. Ruben FL, Nagel J, Fireman P. Antitoxin responses in the elderly to tetanus-diphtheria (Td) immunization. Am J Epidemiol 108: 145–149, 1978.

199. Carson PJ, Nichol K, O'Brien J, et al. Immune function and vaccine responses in healthy advanced elderly patients. Arch Intern Med 160:2017–2024, 2000.

199a. Ciofi degli Atti ML, Salmaso S, Colter B, et al. Reactogenicity and immunogenicity of adult versus paediatric diphtheria and tetanus booster dose at 6 years of age. Vaccine 20: 74–79, 2002.

200. Levin PL. Diphtheria immunization: desirability of combined tetanus and diphtheria injection in wound management. Postgrad Med 79:139–140, 1986.

201. Golaz A, Hardy IR, Strebel P, et al. Epidemic diphtheria in the newly independent states of the former Soviet Union: implication for diphtheria control in the United States. J Infect Dis 181(suppl 1): S237–S243.

202. Greco D, Salmaso S, Mastrantonio P, et al for the Progetto Pertosse Working Group. A controlled trial of two acellular vaccines and one whole-cell vaccine against pertussis. N Engl J Med 334:341–348, 1996.

203. Gustafsson L, Hallander HO, Olin P, et al. A controlled trial of a two-component acellular, a five-component acellular, and a whole-cell pertussis vaccine. N Engl J Med 334:349–355, 1996.

204. Trollfors B, Taranger J, Lagergard T, et al. A placebo-controlled trial of a pertussis-toxoid vaccine. N Engl J Med 333:1045–1050, 1995.

205. Schmitt-Grohé S, Stehr K, Cherry JD, et al for the Pertussis Vaccine Study Group. Minor adverse events in a comparative efficacy trial in Germany in infants receiving either the Lederle/Takeda acellular pertussis component DTP (DTaP) vaccine, the Lederle whole-cell component DTP (DTP) or DT vaccine. Dev Biol Stand 89:113–118, 1997.

206. Tozzi AE, Olin P. Common side effects in the Italian and Stockholm I trials. Dev Biol Stand 89:105–108, 1997.

207. Björkholm B, Wahl FYI, Granström M, Hagberg L. Immune status and booster effects of low doses of diphtheria toxoid in Swedish medical personnel. Scand J Infect Dis 21:429–434, 1989.

208. Wassilak SGF, Orenstein WA, Sutter RW. Tetanus toxoid. In Plotkin SA, Mortimer EA (eds). Vaccines (2nd ed). Philadelphia, WB Saunders, 1994, p 76.

209. Nathum E, Lerman Y, Cohen D, et al. The immune response to booster vaccination against diphtheria toxin at age 18–21 years. Isr J Med Sci 30:600–603, 1994.

210. Mortimer J, Melville-Smith M, Sheffield F. Diphtheria vaccine for adults. Lancet 2:1182–1183, 1986.

211. Simonsen O, Kjeldsen K, Vendborg H-A, Heron I. Revaccination of adults against diphtheria I: responses and reactions to different doses of diphtheria toxoid in 30–70-year-old persons with low serum antitoxin levels. Acta Pathol Microbiol Immunol Scand C 94:213–218, 1986.

212. Simonsen O, Klaerke M, Klaerke A, et al. Revaccination of adults against diphtheria II: combined diphtheria and tetanus revaccination with different doses of diphtheria toxoid 20 years after primary vaccination. Acta Pathol Microbiol Immunol Scand C 94:219–225, 1986.

213. Blennow M, Granström M, Strandell A. Adverse reactions after diphtheria-tetanus booster in 10-year-old schoolchildren in relation to the type of vaccine given for the primary vaccination. Vaccine 12:427–430, 1994.

214. Mark A, Granström M. The role of aluminum for adverse reactions and immunogenicity of diphtheria-tetanus booster vaccine. Acta Paediatr 83:159–163, 1994.

215. Mark A, Granström B, Granström M. Immunoglobulin E responses to diphtheria and tetanus toxoids after booster with aluminum-absorbed and fluid DT-vaccines. Vaccine 13:669–673, 1995.

216. Alderslade R, Bellman MH, Rawson NSB, et al. The National Childhood Encephalopathy Study. In Whooping Cough: Reports from the Committee on the Safety of Medicines and the Joint Committee on Vaccination and Immunisation. London, Department of Health and Social Security, Her Majesty's Stationery Office, 1981, pp 79–154.

217. Bellman MH, Ross EM, Miller DL. Infantile spasms and pertussis immunisation. Lancet 1:1031–1034, 1983.

218. Centers for Disease Control and Prevention. General recommendations on immunization: recommendations of the Advisory Committee Immunization Practices (ACIP) and the American Academy of Family Physicians. MMWR 51(RR-2):1–35, 2002.

219. U.S. Food and Drug Administration. Biological products; bacterial vaccines and toxoids; implementation of efficacy review. Generic statement on diphtheria toxoid. Fed Reg 50:51013–51016, 1985.

220. Mirchamsy H, Hamedi M, Fateh G, Sassani A. Oral immunization against diphtheria and tetanus infections by fluid diphtheria and tetanus toxoids. Vaccine 12:1167–1172, 1994.

221. Aggerbeck H, Gizurarson S, Wantizin J, Heron I. Intranasal booster vaccination against diphtheria and tetanus in man. Vaccine 15:307–316, 1997.

222. Robbins FC, Robbins JB. Current status and prospects for some improved and new bacterial vaccines. Annu Rev Public Health 7:105–125, 1986.

223. Frech C, Hilbert AK, Hartmann G, et al. Physicochemical analysis of purified diphtheria toxoids: is toxoided then purified the same as purified then toxoided? Dev Biol 103:205–215, 2000.

224. Diwan M, Misra A, Khar RK, Talwar GP. Long-term high immune response to diphtheria toxoid in rodents with diphtheria toxoid conjugated to dextran as a single contact point delivery system. Vaccine 15:1867–1871, 1997.

225. Higaki M, Azechi Y, Takase T, et al. Collagen minipellet as a controlled release delivery system for tetanus and diphtheria toxoid. Vaccine 19:3091–3096, 2001.

Chapter 14

Haemophilus influenzae Vaccine

JAY D. WENGER • JOEL I. WARD

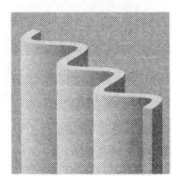

Haemophilus influenzae is a respiratory pathogen that causes a wide spectrum of human infections. These range from asymptomatic colonization of the upper respiratory tract (i.e., carriage); to infections that extend from colonized mucosal surfaces to cause otitis media, bronchitis, conjunctivitis, sinusitis and some pneumonias; to invasive infections, such as bacteremia, septic arthritis, epiglottitis, pneumonia, empyema, and meningitis. Before the availability of *Haemophilus influenzae* type b (Hib) conjugate vaccines, *H. influenzae* was the leading cause of bacterial meningitis in the United States, and in most countries worldwide, resulting in substantial morbidity and mortality.[1,2] The introduction of Hib conjugate vaccines in many countries for routine immunization of infants has nearly eliminated invasive Hib disease in those countries.

Background

History

The organism was first described in 1892 by Robert Pfeiffer, who isolated it from the lung and sputum of patients with pneumonia during the 1889–1892 pandemic of influenza. He proposed that the organism was the cause of influenza, and it was initially known as the Pfeiffer influenza bacillus.[3] The bacteria were difficult to grow on routine culture media, until it was understood that supplementation with factors X (hemin) and V (nicotinamide adenine dinucleotide [NAD]) were required for its growth. By the turn of the century, the organism had been recovered from the blood and cerebrospinal fluid (CSF) of young children with meningitis. Ambiguity remained about the etiologic role of the Pfeiffer bacillus as the cause of influenza until its etiologic role was seriously questioned during the influenza pandemic of 1918 when it became clear that it was a constituent of the normal bacterial flora of the human upper respiratory tract and not the cause of influenza. In 1920, Winslow and associates[4] renamed the organism *Haemophilus influenzae* to emphasize its requirement for blood-derived factors (X and V) for growth (*haemophilus* meaning "blood-loving") and to acknowledge its historical association with influenza. In 1933, the viral etiology of influenza was discovered, which eliminated remaining confusion about *H. influenzae* and influenza virus. Unfortunately this association still causes confusion for laypersons trying to distinguish between influenza and *H. influenzae* vaccines.

Our understanding of the microbiology and immunology of infections caused by *H. influenzae* was greatly enhanced by the pioneering work of Margaret Pittman (Fig. 14–1) in the early 1930s,[5-7] which led to the development of treatment and prevention modalities. Paralleling earlier research on the pneumococcus, she defined two major categories of *H. influenzae*: (1) encapsulated and (2) unencapsulated strains. Among the encapsulated strains, she characterized six distinct serotypes (designated a through f), which now are known to differ biochemically in the composition of their polysaccharide capsules. She observed that encapsulated type b strains were recovered primarily from blood and CSF of young patients with meningitis, and that unencapsulated strains and other *H. influenzae* serotypes were recovered primarily from respiratory tract secretions. Furthermore, she demonstrated that antibody to Hib capsule conferred type-specific protection against lethal infection in rabbits. This observation led to the later defintion of risk factors for the disease,[8-10] and to the use of antiserum as the first treatment for disease, prepared by immunization with formalin-killed Hib, in horses and later in rabbits. Prior to this, Hib meningitis and other forms of invasive Hib disease were almost always fatal. However, it was not until the late 1930s that treatment of children with meningitis using both Hib antiserum and sulfonamides substantially reduced case fatality rates.[11-13]

In 1933, Fothergill and Wright[14] described the age-related epidemiology of *H. influenzae* meningitis that affected children younger than 5 years, and noted a correlation between the risk of disease and the absence of bactericidal antibodies. Later it was shown that the major antibody contributing to the protective activity of bactericidal serum was antibody to type b capsule.[15-17] These observations suggested that naturally acquired type b anticapsular antibody

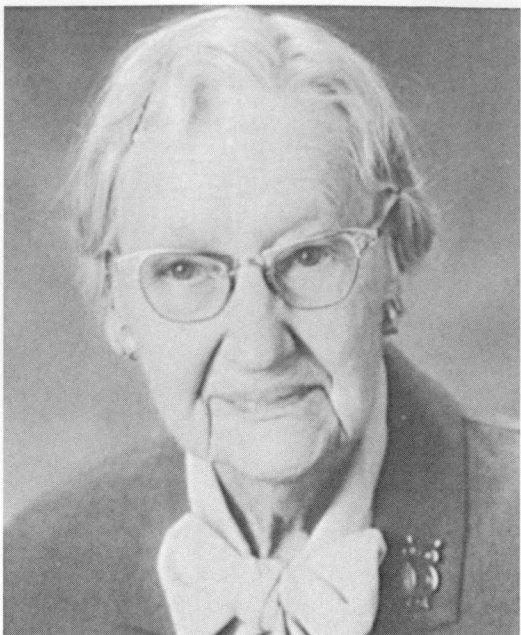

FIGURE 14–1 ▪ Margaret Pittman.

protects, and this remains the underlying premise for attempts to stimulate protective immunity with polysaccharide and polysaccharide-protein conjugate vaccines.

During much of the past 50 years, with the advent of effective antibiotics for *H. influenzae*, attention was focused on treatment rather than prevention of disease. The appreciation that the morbidity and mortality of disease could never be completely eliminated by treatment, even with prompt diagnosis and use of highly effective antibiotics and other therapies, gave further impetus to the development of Hib vaccines. The first vaccine was the purified type b polysaccharide vaccine, which was followed by the more immunogenic polysaccharide-protein conjugate vaccines. Each of the Hib vaccines is reviewed in this chapter.

Clinical Presentations

On the basis of pathogenesis, severity, and microbiologic distinction, three clinical categories of *H. influenzae* infections can be characterized. The majority of *H. influenzae* infections involve asymptomatic infection or colonization of the upper respiratory tract. The remainder extend from colonization to cause mucosal or invasive disease.

The most common clinical infections involve mucosal infections, such as otitis media, sinusitis, and bronchitis (Table 14–1). Although mucosal infections occur frequently, they rarely result in bacteremia (except in neonates or immunocompromised individuals) and therefore are rarely life threatening. The microbiologic hallmark of mucosal infections is that they are caused by the same bacteria that normally colonize the oropharynx, usually unencapsulated strains of *H. influenzae*.[18] Extension of these organisms from colonized respiratory tract passages to contiguous body sites is enhanced by the compromise of normal defense mechanisms, such as the presence of eustachian tube reflux, obstruction, foreign bodies, smoking damage to

the bronchopulmonary epithelium, antecedent viral infection, or selected immune deficiencies.

Particularly important are invasive infections that are characterized by the dissemination of bacteria, almost always type b *H. influenzae*, from the nasopharynx to the blood-stream and subsequently to other body sites. The most serious manifestation of invasive type b disease is meningitis, which accounts for about half of all recognized cases.[19–22] Even with early diagnosis and the availability of effective antimicrobial therapy, about 5% to 10% of children with Hib meningitis die.[23] Neurologic sequelae of varying severity are relatively common after Hib meningitis, occurring in 15% to 30% of survivors.[24–31] Neurologic handicaps include hearing loss, language disorders or delay, mental retardation, learning disabilities, motor abnormalities, and seizures.

The clinical distinction of invasive and mucosal disease is not absolute, inasmuch as type b strains can cause otitis media or sinusitis.[32] Likewise, other serotypes (especially type a) and nontypable strains occasionally cause bacteremia and meningitis. A notable example is neonatal sepsis or meningitis caused by nontypable strains, presumably acquired from the flora of the mother's genital tract.[33–35]

Pneumonia is caused by type b and non–type b strains. Reports from Africa and Papua New Guinea suggest that both type b and non–type b *H. influenzae* are important causes of severe acute lower respiratory tract infections in developing countries.[36–40] *Haemophilus influenzae* type b pneumonia can be associated with bacteremia, empyema, or pericarditis. Patterns recognized by radiologic examination include lobar, bronchial, and interstitial infiltrates that are useless for an etiologic diagnosis.

Although not absolute, the clinical distinction between invasive and mucosal disease is useful because there are many diagnostic, therapeutic, and prophylactic implications related to the two types of infection. The vaccines available to control *H. influenzae* disease all have the type b polysaccharide as the primary immunogen and are therefore intended to prevent only Hib disease. These vaccines have little or no impact on infections caused by non–type b strains. Likewise, antigen detection tests are type b specific. Therefore, this chapter concerns itself with the prevention of invasive Hib disease.

Microbiology

Haemophilus influenzae is a small gram-negative coccobacillus that in clinical specimens can appear filamentous or

TABLE 14–1 ▪ **Spectrum of *Haemophilus influenzae* Disease**

INVASIVE DISEASE (95% DUE TO TYPE B STRAINS)		
Meningitis	Pneumonia	Empyema
Bacteremia	Septic arthritis	Osteomyelitis
Epiglottitis	Pericarditis	Cellulitis
	Abscesses	

MUCOSAL DISEASE (PREDOMINANTLY DUE TO NONTYPABLE STRAINS)		
Otitis media	Bronchitis	Pneumonia
Sinusitis	Conjunctivitis	Urinary tract infection

pleomorphic, especially when obtained from patients who have received antibiotics. It is a nonmotile, non–spore-forming, facultative anaerobe that requires two accessory factors for *in vitro* growth. The X factor, needed for aerobic growth, is a heat-stable, iron-containing protoporphyrin that is essential for activity of the electron transport chain. The heat-labile V factor is the coenzyme, NAD. Both factors are present within erythrocytes and are released by mild heat or enzyme lysis of the red blood cells, which, if carefully done, permits growth on chocolate agar. The requirement of these factors for growth remains the primary basis for the laboratory differentiation of *H. influenzae* from other *Haemophilus* species; the organism grows in almost any enriched liquid or solid medium supplemented with X and V factors. Although it is not mandatory for growth, some strains grow better in 5% to 10% carbon dioxide. After overnight incubation on an enriched medium, colonies appear that are 0.5 to 1.5 mm in diameter and rough or granular in appearance. Encapsulated strains usually produce slightly larger colonies that are mucoid or glistening. Fermentation reactions and other metabolic activities are variable and therefore are not particularly useful for identification. However, a biotyping scheme, based on the metabolism of indole, urea, and ornithine decarboxylase activity, has been used to subtype strains.[41] Other genetically distinguishable characteristics useful in analysis of genetic relatedness include outer membrane proteins, cytoplasmic enzymes that have distinguishing isoenzyme patterns on electrophoresis, plasmids that differ by DNA analysis, and pulsed-gel electrophoresis of constitutive DNA.[42]

Several surface structures of *H. influenzae* appear to be important determinants of the organism's pathogenicity. As with many invasive pathogens, its outermost structure is a polysaccharide capsule that is antiphagocytic to white cells. The type b capsule is of clinical and immunologic importance inasmuch as type b organisms account for 95% of all strains that cause invasive disease (bacteremia and meningitis).[2,19–22,43] This polysaccharide consists of a repeating polymer of ribosyl and ribitol phosphate (polyribosylribitol phosphate [PRP]), which has a 1-to-1 linkage (Fig. 14–2). The other capsular serotypes are composed of hexose rather than pentose sugars, and only occasionally cause invasive disease. Strains without capsules frequently cause infections of the respiratory tract and adjacent structures, but rarely cause bacteremic infections.

Other important components of the *H. influenzae* cell envelope include lipopolysaccharide (endotoxin) and a number of proteins and lipids in the outer membrane. Some membrane proteins participate in cell transport (porins) and others are adhesins; the functions of still others remain undefined. Pili or fimbriae are protein filaments extending from the outer membrane that appear to mediate attachment of the organism to epithelial cells.[44] Their expression appears to be reversible, and the importance of these structures in the pathogenesis of disease is unknown.

Another important microbiologic feature of *H. influenzae* has been the development of antibiotic resistance. Resistance to a wide variety of antibiotics (e.g., sulfonamides, aminoglycosides, trimethoprim-sulfamethoxazole, erythromycin, tetracycline, penicillin) has been described, but these antibiotics are not essential for therapy. Of greater

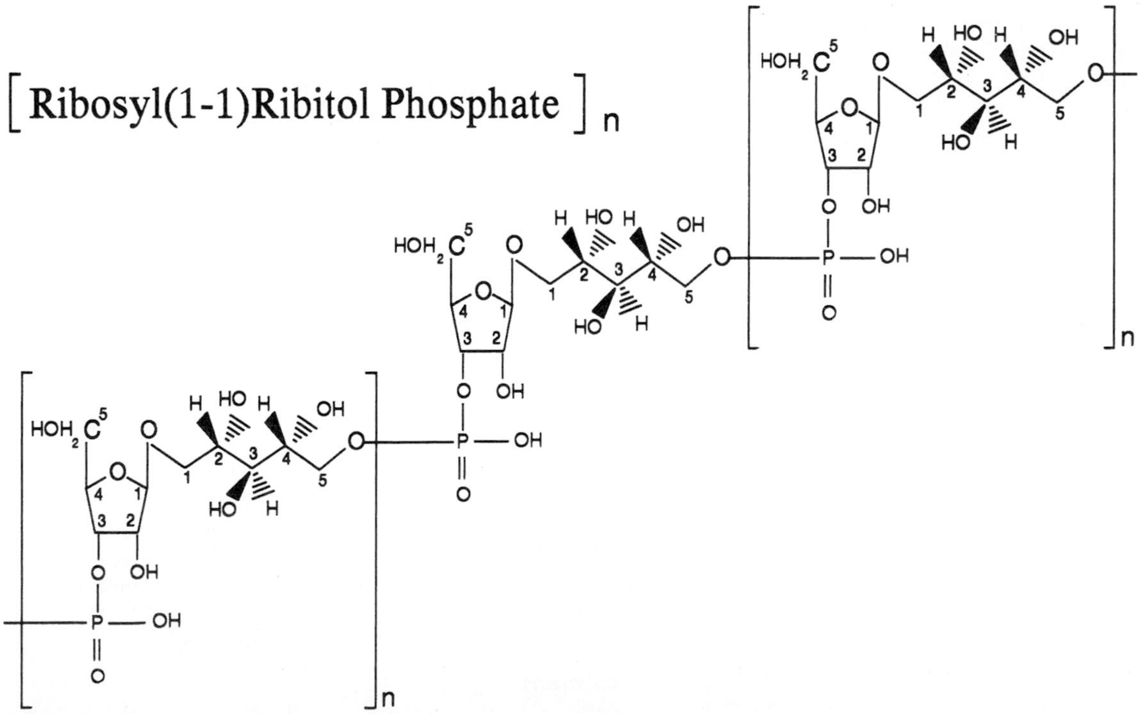

FIGURE 14–2 ▪ Repeating unit structure of *Haemophilus influenzae* type b capsular polysaccharide, shown in its protonated form: → 3) β-D Rib *f*–(1 → 1)–D-Ribol-5–(PO₂H →. (Adapted from Zon G, Robbins JD. ³¹P- and ¹³C-NMR–spectral and chemical characterization of the end-group and repeating-unit components of oligosaccharides derived by acid hydrolysis of *Haemophilus influenzae* type b capsular polysaccharide. Carbohydr Res 114:103–121, 1983.)

importance, first noted in the mid-1970s, has been resistance to ampicillin,[45–51] a primary therapeutic agent. Ampicillin resistance has been recognized worldwide,[52–57] and the mechanism of resistance usually involves plasmid-mediated β-lactamase enzyme production.[58] Resistance to chloramphenicol can be mediated by the enzyme chloramphenicol acetyltransferase,[59,60] and such strains are increasingly prevalent in some areas of the world.[53,56,60–64] Third-generation cephalosporins, in particular ceftriaxone and cefotaxime, are currently the mainstays in therapy for invasive disease.[65] Concerns about the potential for the development of resistance to these highly effective agents emphasize the need for means to prevent disease.

Pathogenesis of Disease

To develop Hib disease, an individual must experience a series of events, beginning with exposure to the organism and acquisition of infection (colonization of the mucosal membranes). Nearly all individuals are colonized with nontypable strains, and 1% to 5% of unimmunized persons carry type b strains asymptomatically.

Unfortunately, most of the factors that influence the efficiency of transmission and the ability of the organism to establish colonization are poorly understood.[66,67] Carriage rates are lowest in adults and young infants and highest in preschool-age children, presumably because of the presence or absence of immunity. In a prospective longitudinal study conducted at a day care center in Dallas, Texas, where no invasive infections occurred, the average prevalence of colonization with Hib was 10%.[68] During the 18 months of study, 71% of the children ages 18 to 35 months and 48% of the children ages 36 to 71 months were at some time colonized. Carriage rates can be as high as 58% to 91% in households or day care centers in which a case of invasive disease occurs.[69–73] Likewise, within families in which there was a case of invasive disease, colonization rates of 60% to 70% among siblings and 20% in parents have been observed.[72–74] It is not clear whether the high carriage rates in these exposed, semiclosed populations are the cause or the result of disease.[67,75–81] Close contact among exposed individuals, as occurs in families or day care centers, increases the potential for transmission, and both larger families and attendance at large day care centers increases the risk of colonization and disease.

Despite a low point prevalence of pharyngeal carriage (1% to 5%), most young children prior to immunization become colonized with Hib during the first 2 to 5 years of life[75,76,78–80,82] and consequently develop specific immunity.[17,81,83–87] Type b strains may persist in the nasopharynx for months[67,68,80] and often are not eliminated by treatment with antimicrobial agents that do not penetrate into respiratory secretions.[83,88,89]

The relationship between the carriage of type b organisms and the subsequent development of disease and immunity is not well understood. Two factors that may increase the potential for colonization and the risk of invasive disease are the size of the bacterial inoculum[90] and the presence of a concomitant viral infection.[91,92] Invasive Hib disease involves the bacteremic dissemination of the organism from the respiratory tract to distant body sites.[93,94] As studied in animals, the initial stage of invasive infection involves attachment to respiratory epithelium and penetration through the mucosa, leading to bacteremia.[93–96] The organisms appear to enter the vascular system by breaking down the tight junctions between cells and invading intercellularly.[90] Local inflammation of the nasopharyngeal tissues is generally absent.[93] The bacteremia is initially low grade, but steadily increases over hours.[93,97] The dynamics between bacterial proliferation and clearance are influenced by antibody, complement, and the reticuloendothelial system, which together determine the magnitude of the bacteremia.[98–100] The type b polysaccharide capsule is antiphagocytic and therefore is a major determinant of the organism's invasiveness. The role of other bacterial virulence factors (e.g., attachment factors, toxins) in the pathogenesis of invasive disease, as well as that of the immune factors that mitigate infection, is not well understood.

As the bacterial concentration in blood mounts, metastatic seeding occurs, especially to the meninges and to other sites including the lungs, pleura, joint synovium, and pericardium.[93] After a critical bacterial concentration in blood is exceeded, Hib organisms enter the central nervous system via the choroid plexus.[93] Inflammation of the choroid plexus is a uniform feature of meningitis. Organisms then disseminate in the CSF and reach the arachnoid villi and leptomeninges, blocking the return of CSF and thereby increasing bacterial density as well as CSF pressure.[101] In general, the magnitude of bacteremia and the density of organisms in the CSF correlate with the severity of clinical illness.[102,103]

Diagnosis

In a patient with an appropriate clinical presentation, the diagnosis of H. influenzae infection would be a positive Gram's stain from an appropriate sterile body site or isolation of the organism from an infected focus (e.g., CSF, pleural fluid, sputum, or blood). The specimens must be processed immediately and appropriately because Hib has several growth requirements, as previously described. Selective media that suppress the growth of gram-positive organisms may increase the recovery of H. influenzae from upper respiratory tract specimens.[49,104]

Other laboratory techniques are available that may assist in the microbiologic diagnosis, including rapid antigen detection and polymerase chain reaction. Such techniques are useful in the context of a patient whose cultures are sterile because of prior antibiotic therapy or to confirm the clinical diagnosis before bacterial growth occurs. The three most commonly used techniques for antigen detection are latex particle agglutination, countercurrent immunoelectrophoresis, and coagglutination. False-positive results can be due to nonspecific agglutination (i.e., rheumatoid factors) or antigenic cross-reactivity with other organisms; false-positive results also may occur in the urine of children with nasopharyngeal carriage of the organism or, more commonly, for several days after immunization with Hib PRP or conjugate vaccine.[105,106]

Treatment

Treatment of Hib bacteremia and other invasive infections requires antimicrobial therapy that will (1) penetrate the blood-brain barrier to achieve bactericidal concentrations, (2) be of adequate duration to sterilize the primary and potential secondary foci, and (3) cover the antibiotic susceptibility patterns of local invasive isolates. Resistance to several antimicrobials, including ampicillin, chloramphenicol, trimethoprim-sulfamethoxazole, rifampin, and certain second-generation cephalosporins in Hib has been increasing in several parts of the world.[57]

For proven or suspected Hib meningitis, cefotaxime or ceftriaxone is recommended until the antibiotic susceptibility of the organism is known or an alternative diagnosis is established.[65] Cefuroxime is not considered adequate for treatment of H. influenzae meningitis in that delayed sterilization may be at least twofold more common than with therapy with ampicillin, chloramphenicol, or the third-generation cephalosporins.[107,108] Also, ampicillin, formerly a mainstay of therapy for this infection, should not be used alone to empirically treat infections caused by Hib because up to 50% of Hib isolates in the United States are resistant.[57] Young children with occult Hib bacteremia need to be carefully re-evaluated because a large proportion of such patients who are initially clinically well may develop focal disease.[109,110] The duration of therapy is determined by the type of infection and the clinical response. If meningitis can be ruled out and susceptibility determined, then there is a broader spectrum of antibiotics to use.

Equally important in the overall management of a child with invasive Hib disease is adjunctive treatments. For Hib meningitis, several studies have shown that treatment with dexamethasone moderates the inflammatory cascade and decreases the likelihood of hearing loss. The recommended dose is 0.6 mg/kg per day given every 6 hours for 4 days, with the first dose given just before or with the first antibiotic dose.[111] Management of the child with meningitis requires continuing careful evaluations and treatments for complications such as the development of shock, inappropriate secretion of antidiuretic hormone, seizures, and subdural empyema, and for drainage of secondary foci of infection (joints, pleural cavity, pericardium, other abscesses).

Epidemiology

Invasive Hib disease has been a leading infectious disease problem of children worldwide.[2,112] Before the availability of vaccines, an estimated 20,000 to 25,000 persons developed invasive Hib disease annually in the United States, resulting in an estimated cumulative risk for Hib disease of one episode in every 200 children over their first 5 years of life.[23,113] Until 1992, when conjugate vaccines were used routinely for young infants in the United States, Hib was the most common cause of bacterial meningitis.[1,2] For comparison, before the availability of Hib vaccines, the incidence and mortality of Hib disease in the United States were similar to those for paralytic poliomyelitis during its peak epidemic year (1954), before the availability of poliovirus vaccines.

Humans are the only natural host for H. influenzae, and transmission occurs person-to-person through respiratory droplets or contact with respiratory secretions. There is limited evidence that contaminated fomites play a role in transmission.[114] The organism can be carried in the upper respiratory tract for prolonged periods, and disease in a susceptible person usually occurs after many transmission cycles. Owing to this asymptomatic carriage, it has not been possible to define an incubation period or pattern of transmission in endemic settings. Colonization of the birth canal and newborns also occurs.

Incidence of Disease

Invasive Hib disease occurs endemically, and community-wide epidemics have not been described. Eighty-five percent of all invasive Hib disease occurs in children younger than 5 years, so incidence data for invasive Hib disease are for this age group.[115,116]

Although invasive Hib disease is not reliably reported nationally or internationally, a number of population-based studies[2,117–130] conducted before widespread use of the vaccine made it possible to define the incidence (Table 14–2), epidemiologic characteristics, and clinical spectrum of endemic Hib disease in the United States. Differences in the methods and rigor of case-finding efforts might explain, in part, the variability in observed incidence, as could differences in microbiology, exposure, or host susceptibility. The isolation of Hib from a sterile body site is the basis for case detection, but not all infected children have cultures performed, or cultures may be negative owing to prior

TABLE 14–2 ■ Age-Specific Incidence* of Invasive Hib Disease from United States Population-Based Studies, 1976 to 1984

Age (mo)	Meningitis Only		All Invasive Disease		Cumulative Percentage of Disease
	Median	Range	Median	Range	
0–5	101	59–141	148	98–197	10–15
6–11	179	143–279	275	218–452	37–43
12–17	146	88–184	223	123–248	60–61
18–23	62	20–64	92	57–107	64–68
24–35	31	18–39	50	37–70	75–78
36–47	17	5–26	31	7–39	80–83
48–59	4	2–16	11	7–41	84–86
≥60[†]	0.2	0.1–0.2	1.3	1.2–2.4	100

*Cases per 100,000 population per year. Range of point estimates from five studies, including Alaska, 1980–1982 (excluding Eskimos, Native Americans); Atlanta, 1983–1984; Fresno County, 1976–1978; Dallas, 1982–1984; and Minnesota, 1982–1984.
[†]Cumulative percentage and incidence data for ages 60 months or older are based on studies from Alaska, Atlanta, and Fresno County, where active surveillance for all age groups was conducted.

antimicrobial therapy. For these and other reasons, even the most carefully conducted surveillance studies inevitably underestimate the true incidence of disease.

Population-based studies of the incidence of *H. influenzae* disease also have been conducted outside of the United States (Table 14–3). Many of these studies were performed in industrialized nations and show an incidence of *H. influenzae* disease that is approximately one third to two thirds that in the United States. In Sweden,[131–134] Finland,[131,135,136] the Netherlands,[137] and Australia,[138] Hib was the most common cause of bacterial meningitis. It also ranked as the leading cause of bacterial meningitis in Canada, which had a disease incidence similar to that in the United States.[139,140] In other parts of Europe, including the United Kingdom,[141,142] and in some developing countries, meningococcal meningitis was reported to be a more common etiology of meningitis. Population-based incidence data for developing countries are limited, but

H. influenzae also appears to rank as the leading cause of bacterial meningitis in most of these countries.[143–149]

Investigators in Australia reported an exceptionally high rate of invasive Hib disease among Aboriginal children in central Australia.[138,150,151] Populations with similar high risk include Navajo Indians, Alaskan Natives (Indian and Eskimo), and Apache, Yakima, Athabascan, and Canadian Indians.[127,152–158]

Most studies in Africa show rates of meningitis and invasive disease similar to those in the United States, while data from South America and the Middle East demonstrate rates of disease similar to those found in Western Europe. A study in Niger gave a rate of Hib meningitis of over 200 per 100,000 infants less than 1 year old.[159] Hib disease is also prevalent in The Gambia.[160] Peltola[161] has emphasized the heavy burden of Hib disease in Africa.

It has been difficult to adequately document the true incidence of invasive Hib disease in Asia. Many studies of

TABLE 14–3 ■ Incidence of Invasive Hib Disease, Selected Population-Based Studies Outside the United States

Location	Dates	Meningitis <1 yr	Meningitis <5 yr	All Invasive Infections <1 yr	All Invasive Infections <5 yr	Reference
AFRICA						
Senegal	1970–1979	132	36			146
The Gambia	1985–1987	297	60			144
South Africa	1991–1992					
Blacks		210	50			515
Whites		103	25			507
Niger	1981–1996	211	51			159
ASIA						
Hong Kong	1986–1990					164
Chinese					2.3	
Vietnamese					42.7	
China	1990–1992		9.9			163
Philippines	1994–1996		95			166
Singapore	1990–1995				3.3	162
AUSTRALASIA						
Australia	1985–1988					138
Aborigines			159		529	
Non-Aborigines			53		92	
New Zealand	1975–1981		27		41	513
EUROPE						
Scandinavia	1974–1984	43	26	62	41	131
France	1975–1981		15		24	496
England	1985–1988		24		33	386
MIDDLE EAST						
Qatar	1987–1989		16			499
UAE	1996–1997		31			516
Israel	1988–1990		18		34	514
THE AMERICAS						
Canada	1981–1984					139
Native		126	35			
Nonnative		70	26			
Inuit		2333	530			
Chile	1985–1987	47	15			497
Brazil	1997–1998		30			493b
Dominica	1998–1999		13			149

hospitalized patients with presumed bacterial meningitis throughout Asia (Indonesia, Singapore,[162] China,[163] Hong Kong,[164] the Philippines,[165,166] Taiwan,[167] Thailand, India,[168] Vietnam, Korea, and Japan[169]) consistently show Hib to be the leading cause of bacterial meningitis in children, but these studies all have shown a surprisingly high rate of negative bacterial cultures. The few population-based studies conducted (such as those from Hong Kong and from Hefei, China) show incidence rates approximately one tenth of those observed in North America and Europe before vaccines were in use. Multiple factors may have minimized the detection of invasive Hib disease, including (1) less clinical suspicion and evaluation of Hib disease, (2) widespread antibiotic use before hospitalization and obtaining cultures (often greater than 90%), (3) rarity of obtaining blood and CSF cultures, (4) few population-based studies with active surveillance, (5) microbiologic methods suboptimal for culturing Hib, (6) insufficient use of antigen detection methods to make a microbiologic diagnosis in antibiotic-treated individuals, and (7) Hib vaccine use in the private sector. However, the bulk of studies from Asia, including preliminary reports from studies initiated in the late 1990s developed to address some of the above issues, suggest substantially lower rates of Hib meningitis in some Asian populations. It is clear that Hib disease occurs worldwide, but with variable disease incidence and epidemiologic characteristics.

Seasonality

A bimodal seasonal pattern has been observed in most studies in the United States, with a peak occurring between September and December, a decline in cases in January and February, and a second peak appearing between March and May.[1,52,127,170] In contrast, the peak incidence of both pneumococcal and meningococcal meningitis is between January and March.[1,2] The reason for these observations is unknown, but may be related to the seasonality of births, geography, or the seasonal school attendance of older siblings who then introduce Hib into the household. Seasonality of Hib meningitis varies globally. For example, in a population-based study in Niger, no significant seasonality was noted for Hib, whereas both meningococcal and pneumococcal meningitis exhibited clear seasonal patterns.[159]

Risk Factors

Age

The most important epidemiologic feature of invasive Hib disease is its age-related risk, a feature that has been appreciated for almost a century.[14] The age-related incidence of Hib disease has been evaluated with similar methods in several population-based surveillance studies[117,124,127] (see Table 14–2). Invasive disease is relatively uncommon in infants younger than 6 months (<15% of cases), presumably because of reduced exposure, transplacental acquisition of maternal antibody, and protection conferred by breastfeeding. Risk is usually highest between the ages of 6 and 12 months. As shown in Tables 14–2 and 14–3, the proportion of disease varies by age in different populations, which emphasizes the need to vaccinate young infants as early as

possible. Different infections also have a characteristic age of occurrence.[20,127] In most U.S. populations, the peak incidence of meningitis occurs in children 6 to 9 months of age and declines markedly after 2 years of age.[119–121,130] Hib cellulitis tends to occur during the first year of life, whereas epiglottitis generally occurs in children older than 2 years.

In populations with a high incidence of disease, such as Native Americans or Aborigines, the age-specific incidence is shifted to younger ages.[127,152–154,158] Among Native Americans in southwestern Alaska, the incidence of Hib disease peaks in infants 4 to 6 months of age,[127] and similar early peaks of meningitis are observed in Navajo Indian (4 to 5 months) and Apache Indian (4 to 6 months) children.[152,154] The age shift is even more dramatic in The Gambia, where 83% of meningitis cases occur in children younger than 1 year.[144,172] This age distribution contrasts with that in U.S., Canadian, and European populations, where half of invasive disease occurs in children older than 12 months, and in Finland, where there was an even older spectrum of disease occurrence.[22]

Meningitis accounts for a small proportion of episodes in adults; pneumonia is more common.[173] Most adults who develop invasive H. influenzae disease have an underlying condition such as chronic obstructive pulmonary disease, human immunodeficiency virus (HIV) infection, alcoholism, pregnancy, or malignant disease. About half of the invasive disease in older individuals is due to Hib, with the remainder caused by other serotypes or nontypable strains.[172,173]

Gender

Although most studies show approximately equal rates of disease in boys and girls, several population-based studies[2,117,127] and national surveillance data from passively reported cases of meningitis[1] find attack rates to be 1.2-fold to 1.5-fold higher in boys than in girls.

Race and Ethnicity

The incidence of H. influenzae type b meningitis has been shown consistently to be two to four times higher for black than for white children younger than 5 years in the United States.[2,118–120,123,128,129,174] The incidence of all invasive Hib disease is 1.6-fold to 4-fold higher in blacks than in whites.[117] High incidence of invasive Hib disease also has been described in Native Americans[127,152–154,156–158,175] and in some Hispanics,[118] although studies in Dallas and Los Angeles found no difference in the incidence of Hib disease between white and Hispanic children.[124,174] The hypothesis that racial or ethnic differences in incidence of Hib disease could be due to genetically determined differences in susceptibility is unproven, because of confounding social and economic variables that are associated both with race and ethnicity and with disease risk. In a study in Atlanta,[117] there was no increased risk in blacks, compared with that in whites, once the independent effects of household crowding, day care, and family income on risk were accounted for by multivariate analysis.

Socioeconomic Factors

The interplay of factors that affect exposure to Hib as well as host susceptibility appears to determine the overall risk of invasive Hib disease.[9] Socioeconomic factors that increase the risk of Hib disease include large household size,[175–179] crowding,[82] day care attendance, vaccine access, and increased population density. Socioeconomic factors that are considered surrogates include low family income[2,119,120,128,129] and low parental education level.[119,129,178] Lack of access to vaccination is a particularly important socioeconomic factor that influences susceptibility, especially in the era of Hib conjugate vaccines.[180]

Risk in Day Care Settings

Population-based studies have found that children who attend day care are at significantly higher risk for invasive Hib disease than are children who do not attend day care.[117,122,125] One study estimated that up to 50% of all invasive Hib disease may be attributable to day care attendance.[117]

Other Risk Factors

The risk of developing invasive Hib disease is the consequence of the complex interaction of a variety of factors, including (1) exposure, (2) microbiologic characteristics of the organism, (3) susceptibility of the host,[130] and (4) immunization status. Some exposure factors, such as household crowding and day care attendance, reflect increased exposure to Hib bacteria, whereas other factors influence susceptibility. Several case-control studies reveal that breast-feeding is associated with reduced risk of invasive Hib disease in infants younger than 6 months.[117,122,180–183] Although the mechanism for protection is unknown, it may be the result of immune or nutritional factors present in human milk.[184–186] Several hematologic and immunologic disorders are associated with increased risk for Hib disease. These include HIV infection,[187–189] sickle cell anemia,[190–192] asplenia or splenectomy,[193] antibody[194,195] and complement[196,197] deficiency syndromes, and malignant neoplasms, especially Hodgkin's disease during periods of chemotherapy.[198–200] Reduced reticuloendothelial clearance of bacteria in blood by macrophages in the spleen and liver may be involved. Clearly, complement and antibody are needed to clear bacteremia and to sustain bactericidal activity in blood. There is some evidence in experimental animal models[201,202] and in children[91,92] that respiratory viral infections increase susceptibility to Hib meningitis. Antecedent or concurrent viral respiratory infection could alter mucosal immunity or bacterial flora, thereby increasing host susceptibility to invasive Hib disease.

Selected genetic markers (e.g., human leukocyte antigen, immunoglobulin allotypes) have been associated with an increased risk of invasive Hib disease.[177,203–212] However, the results of several of these studies have conflicted. Such studies are limited by potential confounding in that other known risk factors for disease were not independently evaluated. In addition, lack of control for multiple comparisons may have increased the likelihood that a statistically significant result would be found by chance. Furthermore, even in high-risk Alaskan Eskimos, in whom some genetic factors have been associated with disease risk (eg., uridine monophosphate kinase 3), the majority of patients who developed Hib disease do not possess the genetic marker and the degree of ethnic admixture does not correlate with disease risk.[208,212] Therefore, it remains to be determined whether genetic factors play a significant role in risk of disease.

Secondary Transmission

Although the contagiousness of invasive Hib disease is limited, small outbreaks and direct secondary transmission of disease can occur. *Secondary* disease (that occurring after contact with a child with invasive Hib disease) should be distinguished from endemic disease, which occurs after contact with an asymptomatic carrier of Hib. Instances of direct secondary transmission of Hib disease have been reported since 1909,[213] but only since 1978 has the risk of secondary Hib disease for contacts of a case been assessed, particularly in those younger than 2 years.[70,214,215]

A number of studies have estimated the risk of secondary disease in household contacts in the 30 days after onset of disease in an index case.[70,74,84,216–218] The overall attack rate for contacts was 0.3%, representing a risk about 600-fold higher than the age-adjusted risk in the general population.[217] However, attack rates varied significantly by age; the attack rate was more than 6% in contacts younger than 1 year, 3.3% in children younger than 2 years, 1.6% in children 24 to 47 months of age, 0.06% for children 4 to 5 years of age, and 0% for those 6 years of age or older. Among household contacts, 64% of secondary cases occurred within the first week after disease onset in the index patient, 20% during the second week, and 16% during the third and fourth weeks.[219] Thus the risk of secondary disease in the household setting is confined almost exclusively to children younger than 4 years (especially those younger than 2 years) and is concentrated in the first 2 weeks after onset of disease in the index case.

Five studies estimated the risk for day care classroom contacts of a case during the 30- to 60-day period after onset of disease in the index case.[84,218,220–222] Three of the studies demonstrated a substantial risk—1.7% to 3.2%—for contacts younger than 24 months,[84,218,222] which is comparable to that of household contacts of a similar age. However, two other studies failed to demonstrate any increased risk for secondary disease in day care contacts.[220,221] There is no obvious explanation for the disparate findings, although there can be considerable variation in the risk of secondary Hib disease over time, by degree of exposure, in different day care settings, and perhaps by geographic region.[10,219,223,224]

Transmission of secondary Hib disease in chronic care institutions for children also has been reported,[88,225] as has nosocomial transmission among the elderly in a nursing home setting.[226] Only one instance of secondary transmission in children in an acute care hospital has been reported.[227] The lack of reports of hospital-acquired disease, despite the large number of Hib cases that occurred yearly before routine immunization of infants, suggests that the risk of nosocomial transmission in acute care hospitals is low.

Chemoprophylaxis prevents secondary risk of Hib disease by reducing colonization and transmission to a nonimmunized child. The importance of chemoprophylaxis as a public health measure has decreased substantially since widespread use of Hib conjugate vaccines in infant immunization programs. Antimicrobials that are effective in the treatment of invasive Hib disease, such as ampicillin,[67] cephalosporins, and chloramphenicol,[89] may not eliminate the carrier state because they are not concentrated in upper airway secretions. Rifampin, which achieves high concentrations in respiratory secretions,[228,229] is the most effective antimicrobial agent for eradicating Hib nasopharyngeal carriage. Rifampin in a dosage of 20 mg/kg once daily (maximum daily dose 600 mg) for 4 days eradicates Hib carriage in 95% or more of household[84,216,230] or day care[70,84,88,231–233] contacts of an index case. Shorter or lower dose regimens of rifampin are less successful.[84,234–237] The fluoroquinolone antibiotics, such as ciprofloxacin, also may be effective,[238] although they have not been evaluated and are not usually indicated for children.

Immunology

Resistance to Hib infection depends on the successful integration of a variety of host defenses, including (1) mucosal factors that prevent the organism from attaching to and penetrating the respiratory epithelium; (2) activation of the alternative and classical complement pathways, which leads to killing of the organism and other inflammatory responses; (3) production of specific antibodies; (4) phagocytosis and killing by macrophages and polymorphonuclear cells in tissues, blood, and the reticuloendothelial organs (e.g., the spleen); and (5) cell-mediated immunity. It is difficult to assess the role of each of these immunologic mechanisms independently or to determine which mechanisms are most important in the host's defense. Although antibodies are not the sole defense against bacteremia, this has been the focus of vaccine research (i.e., to induce antibodies that are bactericidal, opsonophagocytic, and ultimately protective).

Anticapsular Antibody

Initially antibodies were assessed by measuring agglutinin and bactericidal titers of serum. In 1933, Fothergill and Wright[14] suggested that bactericidal activity was responsible for immunity to Hib meningitis and that acquisition of this antibody correlated inversely with the age of the individual. Maternally acquired antibody, present in infants younger than 6 months, and the natural acquisition of antibodies by children between 2 and 5 years of age were proposed as the explanation for the observed high incidence of Hib disease in children between 6 months and 2 years of age. The goal of vaccine development has been to find means to actively induce immunity by 6 months of age and thereby eliminate this window of age-related susceptibility.

Although antibodies to several surface antigens of *H. influenzae* play a role in conferring immunity,[15–17,239–245] antibody to the type b capsular polysaccharide appears to be of primary importance.[246] By 5 years of age, most children have naturally acquired anticapsular antibody that appears to provide protection,[5,17,86,246] although natural exposure also induces antibodies to outer membrane proteins, lipopolysaccharides, and other surface antigens of the bacteria that contribute to natural immunity. The evidence that anticapsular antibody protects humans from invasive Hib disease is considerable; it activates complement,[247–252] it is opsonophagocytic,[253,254] it is bactericidal,[14,16,253,255–258] and it protects animals from lethal Hib challenge.[201,259,260] Moreover, passive prophylaxis with serum preparations containing anticapsular antibody protects animals, agamma-

globulinemic patients,[5,194,246] and high-risk Apache children from invasive Hib disease.[261] In the preantibiotic era, the administration of immune sera was also an effective therapy for Hib disease.[7,12,13] However, the most compelling evidence for the protective efficacy of PRP antibody is the clinical protection achieved in older children vaccinated with purified PRP vaccine[136] and, more recently, in younger infants immunized with Hib conjugate vaccines.

Whether induced by natural infection or vaccination, anticapsular antibody responses are markedly influenced by the age of the individual. In young infants, immunization with PRP vaccine induces antibody infrequently and poorly; young children respond a little better, but older children and adults demonstrate reasonably good antibody responses.[262–265] Even invasive Hib disease does not reliably evoke an antibody response in young infants. Antibody to the type b capsule also develops after exposure to other bacteria that have immunologically cross-reactive antigens.[266,267] The level of antibody induced is influenced by the type of exposure, the age of the individual, the duration of the exposure, and the rate of antigen clearance.

Protective Levels of Anticapsular Antibodies

Although a precise minimal level of anti-PRP antibody that is protective has not been established, data from passive protection of agammaglobulinemic children, challenge experiments in infant rats, and studies of naturally acquired antibody levels in healthy individuals of various ages suggest that the minimum serum concentration of anti-PRP antibody that provides protection ranges from 0.05 μg/mL in animals[268] to 0.15 to 1.00 μg/mL in humans.[5,269–271] A serum level of 0.15 μg/ml is generally considered to indicate a positive response to conjugated vaccine. Moreover, in the Finnish PRP vaccine field trial, an antibody level of higher than 1.0 μg/mL 1 month after immunization correlated with clinical protection for a minimum of 1 year.[136,269,271] Such estimates are crude and do not take into account the different qualitative or functional properties of different immunoglobulin isotypes and immunoglobulin (Ig) G subclasses or the contribution of antibodies to other Hib antigens. Also, because vaccine-induced antibody levels decline over time, a given peak level may not predict truly long-term protection.[269–271] In addition, these antibody levels might not be readily extrapolated to immunogenicity evaluated soon after immunization or to studies with different Hib conjugate vaccines.

Class- and Subclass-Specific Antibody

A few studies have shown variable immunoglobulin isotype and IgG subclass responses to PRP polysaccharide after natural Hib exposure, disease, and immunization. Several investigations have shown that IgG, IgM, and IgA antibodies to PRP are induced by infection and vaccination.[268,272–274] Most individuals respond with IgG antibodies after PRP immunization, although some children have predominantly IgA or IgM responses.[273] The functional characteristics of these antibodies have been studied. Schreiber and associates[268] showed that IgG antibody is bactericidal, is opsonic for polymorphonuclear neutrophil leukocytes in the presence of complement, and protects animals. IgM antibody is equally protective and more bactericidal than IgG in the presence of complement, but it opsonizes poorly.

IgA antibody is not bactericidal, opsonic, or protective for animals. Some investigators have hypothesized that IgA-specific antibody blocks the activity of other more functional antibodies and may thereby reduce immunity.[273,275–277]

Data from experiments in mice and humans suggest that polysaccharide antigens induce restricted IgG subclass responses.[278–281] The findings of increased susceptibility to Hib disease in patients who are deficient in IgG subclasses (predominantly IgG2 and IgG4 deficiencies)[281–285] and the low levels of IgG2 in children younger than 2 years[286] suggest differences in the role of subclass-specific anticapsular antibodies. In adults, natural exposure or immunization with PRP vaccine results in a predominantly IgG2 subclass response.[287,288] Children develop IgG1 and IgG2 antibodies after immunization with PRP, but IgG1 antibodies predominate after immunization with Hib conjugate vaccines.[288,289] After invasive disease, there is a significant IgG4 response.[287] However, the subclass response in individuals of different ages after different exposures has not yet been studied definitively.

T Cells

Most of our understanding of the interactions of B cells, T cells, and antigen-presenting cells (e.g., macrophages) derives from extensive research in mice.[246,279–282,290,291] On the basis of T cell involvement in antibody production, antigens can be classified as T-dependent (thymus-dependent) or T-independent immunogens (Table 14–4). Most protein antigens induce helper T cell influence over antibody synthesis and are therefore considered T dependent. These antigens are first recognized and processed by macrophages and then presented to both T and B cells. The activated T cells induce proliferation and differentiation of specific antigen-reactive B-cell subpopulations. They also retain the memory necessary for subsequent booster responses.[280] Through the release of specific cytokines, helper T cells regulate (1) the magnitude of the immune response, especially in young infants; (2) the switch in immunoglobulin classes (IgM to IgG); and (3) the functional activity of antibody (avidity); as well as (4) memory capacity.

Polysaccharides consist of repeating oligosaccharide units, which are relatively primitive antigenic units that elicit weak immune responses involving minimal T-cell influences.[280] T-independent antigens elicit antibody responses primarily by direct stimulation of B cells. In general, polysaccharide vaccines have T-independent type 2 immunologic characteristics: (1) delayed ontogeny of immune responsiveness in the young, (2) limited and variable quantitative immune responses, (3) restricted isotype (predominantly IgM) and IgG subclass responses, and (4) lack of booster or anamnestic response with secondary antigenic challenge.

The quest for an Hib vaccine that is immunogenic and protects young infants involved attempts to convert the capsular polysaccharide (PRP) antigen from a T-independent to a T-dependent antigen, employing the carrier-hapten principles first defined by Landsteiner[292] in the first half of this century. To achieve this aim, PRP, which can be considered to be a hapten, is covalently linked to a T-dependent immunogen, a protein carrier, to form a conjugate vaccine. Studies with one conjugate vaccine showed that the response induced was of the mixed Th1/Th2 variety, ensuring the production of specific T cell memory.[293]

Genetic Factors

Some studies have shown associations between immune responses to PRP vaccine and genetically determined factors, such as red blood cell antigens, human leukocyte antigen, or immunoglobulin allotypes.[8,203–206,208,210,294] However, it is difficult to know whether these associations have clinical relevance, because many factors influence immunogenicity, and it is difficult to control for all these in case-control studies. Furthermore, it is not known if the antibody differences, although statistically significant, are clinically important. No single genetic relationship regulating susceptibility or immune responses to polysaccharide antigens has been convincingly demonstrated. Fortunately, the responses to the polysaccharide-protein conjugate vaccines do not appear to be so variable.

Mucosal Immunity

The role of mucosal immunity in killing Hib bacteria or inhibiting adherence to or penetration of the mucosa is poorly understood, although there have been studies of secretory IgA antibody to the type b capsule.[277,295–298] Moreover, Hib strains produce an IgA protease that can inactivate mucosal antibody.[299] The observation of reduced carriage of Hib in children given Hib conjugate vaccines,[300–303] as well as production of IgG-secretory IgA

TABLE 14–4 ■ Immunologic Features of Thymus-Dependent and Thymus-Independent Antigens

	Thymus Dependent	Thymus Independent	
		Type 1	Type 2
Ontogeny of response	Present at birth	Early	3–18 mo after birth in humans
Responses in *xid* mice	Yes	Yes	No
Memory (booster)	Yes	No	
Affinity	Matures with immunization to high		Low, no maturation
Adjuvant	Enhances response		No effect on response
Class, subclass, and combining site	Heterogeneous (IgG)		Usually restricted (IgM)

IgG, immunoglobulin G; IgM, immunoglobulin M.
Adapted from Stein KE. Thymus-independent and thymus-dependent responses to polysaccharide antigens. J Infect Dis 165(suppl 1):S49–S52, 1992.

in saliva after vaccination,[304] suggest that mucosal immunity may be important in reducing transmission of disease.

Several case-control studies have demonstrated that breast-feeding confers passive protection against invasive Hib disease.[117,122,180–182] However, breast-feeding does not ensure protection, and the mechanism for this benefit is not understood. Breast milk may provide infants with immune or nutritional factors that reduce the acquisition, attachment, or invasion of Hib organisms.[184,295]

Complement and Phagocytosis

The importance of complement in host defense against Hib is evidenced by the elimination of the bactericidal activity of serum by heat,[247–252] by the susceptibility of complement-depleted animals to Hib disease,[250,252] and by the increased susceptibility to Hib disease of patients who have specific congenital complement deficiencies, such as C2, C3, C4, and C9 deficiencies.[197,252]

Although the interaction between bacteria, antibody, and complement is complex, it is clear that complement plays an important role in host defense. Hib bacteria are capable of activating both the classical and alternative complement pathways, thereby initiating opsonophagocytosis and cell killing as well as eliciting other inflammatory responses.[252] Whereas the alternative pathway is probably most important early in the course of infection in a nonimmune host, the antibody-dependent classical complement pathway is more likely to predominate as a defense mechanism when there is humoral immunity.[252] Activation of the terminal complement components mediates the bactericidal activity of serum. Although the type b capsule is a poor activator of the alternative complement pathway, antibody to the capsule activates both the classical and alternative pathways.[251] Both encapsulated and unencapsulated organisms activate complement, underscoring the importance of noncapsular antigens in providing host defense. Other cell wall antigens activate the alternative pathway and antibody to these antigens activates the classical pathway.[247–252] Thus antibodies to both capsular and noncapsular antigens activate the complement system, primarily through the classical pathway.

Opsonization leading to phagocytosis and killing of Hib bacteria is an important element of host defense. Impairment of phagocytic function or reduction in the numbers of phagocytes results in increased susceptibility to disease, as does the loss of the spleen or impairment of its function (e.g., hemoglobinopathies).[190–193,198,199,253] The opsonic activity of serum is greatly influenced by the roles of complement and antibody. It appears that opsonization and phagocytosis of Hib are dependent on (1) IgG binding, (2) antibody activation of the classical complement pathway with deposition of C3b on the bacterial surface, and (3) direct bacterial activation of the alternative complement pathway. Relatively little is known about direct cell-mediated killing of Hib bacteria.[305]

Passive Immunization

Antibody to the type b polysaccharide is the immunologic basis for both active and passive immunization against

Hib. Although active immunization is clearly preferred for the control of Hib disease, before the availability of effective vaccines, passive prophylaxis was employed as a means of providing protection for selected high-risk groups. Passive prophylaxis was considered in high-risk settings (1) to prevent secondary disease in households, day care centers, or institutions; (2) for selected racial groups (Eskimos or Native Americans) whose members were at high risk for disease soon after birth; (3) for functionally asplenic patients (patients with sickle cell disease or splenectomized patients); and (4) for immunocompromised patients. Some also have considered maternal immunization a way to provide immunity to newborns and young infants at high risk.

A human hyperimmune globulin called bacterial polysaccharide immune globulin (BPIG) was prepared at the Massachusetts Biologic Laboratory[306–308] from the plasma of adult donors immunized with Hib, meningococcal, and pneumococcal polysaccharide vaccines. The preparation contained approximately 17 times the amount of PRP antibody found in standard immune serum globulin and provided enhanced levels of antibody to selected meningococcal and pneumococcal serotypes. Pharmacologic studies showed that high levels of antibody (about 1 µg/mL) could be achieved within 4 days after an intramuscular injection (0.5 mL/kg), and levels considered to be protective against Hib disease persisted for as long as 4 months.[309]

Significant protective efficacy against invasive Hib disease was demonstrated in Apache children who were given three doses during the first year of life.[261] The hyperimmune globulin was particularly useful in protecting young infants before an age at which they respond to vaccines, but protection lasted for only 2 to 4 months after each dose, which means that repeated administrations were necessary. A combined passive-active immunization schedule was also used in high-risk Navajo Indian infants who received simultaneous immunization with BPIG and an Hib conjugate vaccine at 2 months of age, followed by doses of vaccine at 4 and 6 months of age.[310] Infants who received concurrent passive immunization with BPIG had significantly higher anticapsular antibody concentrations at 4 months of age than did control children who received vaccine alone, and appeared to respond to second and third doses of conjugate vaccine similarly to the control children.

Another approach to passive prophylaxis for very high-risk young infants is to immunize pregnant women so that their newborns might acquire higher levels of transplacental antibody, thereby protecting them during early infancy.[311–313] In one study,[314] pregnant women were immunized with an Hib vaccine at 32 to 36 weeks' gestation. Infants of mothers who were given an Hib conjugate vaccine had high antibody levels at birth, and approximately 75% of infants were estimated to maintain protective levels of antibody through 6 months of age. This strategy has potential as an adjunct to active immunization of infants for those with high disease risk early in life, but disadvantages include questions about the safety and acceptability of vaccinating pregnant women and the inability to immunize women who do not receive prenatal care.

Active Immunization

Polyribosylribitol Phosphate Polysaccharide Vaccine

The first vaccine available for the prevention of Hib disease was the purified PRP polysaccharide vaccine licensed in the United States in April 1985 for use in children 18 to 60 months of age (Table 14–5). This vaccine is now of historical significance, because its role has been supplanted by the development and licensure of PRP-protein conjugate vaccines. The PRP vaccine was composed of an aqueous solution of the native capsular polysaccharide, PRP (see Fig. 14–2), which was extracted and purified from the supernatant of Hib broth cultures.[315–318] This vaccine is no longer available, but the lessons learned from it were important.

The immune response of children to PRP polysaccharide vaccine is strikingly age related. Young infants respond infrequently and with low antibody levels,[262,264,319] but the immune responses improve with age. Less than 45% of 12- to 17-month-old children achieve antibody levels higher than 1 µg/mL,[136,262] compared with approximately 50% to 75% of children 18 to 23 months of age[136,262,269,319] and 90% of 24- to 35-month-old children. The duration of PRP vaccine–induced antibody is also age dependent. Mean antibody titers in children vaccinated at 18 to 23 months of age fall substantially in the months after immunization,[262] and antibody levels 1.5 years later are not significantly higher than those in unvaccinated control subjects. In children 24 to 35 months old, significantly elevated mean antibody titers persist for at least 1.5 years, but not for 3.5 years. Among children who were vaccinated at 3 to 4 years of age, the mean serum antibody levels remained significantly higher than levels in unvaccinated control subjects for at least 3.5 years.[262] Although the duration of the antibody response has not been precisely defined, it is doubtful that protective immunity is maintained beyond 2 to 3 years without repeated exposure to the antigen.[320,321]

The immune response to PRP vaccine is considered to be T-cell independent and induces the production of IgG, IgM, and IgA antibodies. There is no booster response with subsequent doses, and a disproportionate amount of antibody appears to be of IgM type.[5,268,272,273,322] Differences in functional activity suggest that IgM antibody may be less active than IgG antibody, persist for shorter periods, and be less avid.[5,268,323] These studies suggest that PRP vaccine induces a relatively immature immune response, which may help explain the less than optimal protection demonstrated in clinical use.

Purified capsular polysaccharide vaccines are among the safest of all vaccines. Nearly 10 million doses of PRP vaccine were distributed in the United States between 1985 and 1989, and no association was established between the vaccine and serious reactions.[324] Minor reactions, such as fever and local reactions, were relatively uncommon, occurring in about 5% of vaccinees. The only significant concerns about safety were anecdotal reports of Hib disease that occurred within 1 week of PRP vaccination.[325–333] A statistically significant association of disease with vaccination was found in only one study,[328] whereas no increased risk of early disease was found in two others.[325,326]

These reports led some to believe that the PRP vaccine antigen absorbed out low levels of antibodies, but few, if any, immunized children of this age have pre-existing antibodies. Also, an epidemiologic analysis[330] of each of 12 cases from different studies[325–329] of Hib disease that occurred within 1 week of immunization indicated that most children were black, attended day care facilities, had recent exposure to Hib disease, or were thought to have increased susceptibility to disease (e.g., sickle cell disease, Down syndrome, recurrent Hib disease). All of these factors suggested that the affected children were not comparable to those in the general population and that the increased relative risk was due to confounding factors.

TABLE 14–5 ■ Hib Vaccines

Vaccine	Company	Trade Name	Date Licensed	Age Group (mo)
PRP	Praxis	b-CAPSA 1*	April 1985	24–59
	Connaught	Hib-VAX*		18–24
	Lederle	Hib-IMUNE*		
PRP-D	Connaught	ProHIBiT	December 1987	18–59
			December 1989	15–59
HbOC	Lederle/Praxis	HibTITER	December 1988	18–59
			December 1989	15–59
			October 1990	2, 4, 6, and 12–15
HbOC-DTP	Lederle/Praxis	TETRAMUNE	March 1993	2, 4, 6, and 15–18
PRP-OMP	Merck & Co.	PedvaxHIB	December 1989	15–59
			December 1990	2, 4, and 12–15
PRP-T	Pasteur Mérieux/Connaught	ActHIB	March 1993	2, 4, 6, and 12–15
	Pasteur Mérieux/SmithKline Beecham	OmniHIB	March 1993	2, 4, 6, and 12–15
DTaP–PRP-T	Connaught/Mérieux	TriHIBit	September 1996	15–18
PRP-OMP–Hep B	Merck & Co.	Comvax	October 1996	2, 4, 12–18

*No longer available.
DTaP, diphtheria and tetanus toxoids and acellular pertussis; DTP, diphtheria and tetanus toxoids and whole-cell pertussis; HbOC, Haemophilus b oligosaccharide conjugate; Hep B, hepatitis B; PRP, polyribosylribitol phosphate; PRP-D, PRP–diphtheria toxoid conjugate; PRP-OMP, PRP–outer membrane protein conjugate; PRP-T, PRP–tetanus toxoid conjugate.

TABLE 14–6 ■ Efficacy of PRP Vaccine in Case-Control Studies

Study Site	Time Period	Protective Efficacy*	95% Confidence Interval
Multicenter[†325]	1985–1987	~88%	74% to 96%
Connecticut and Pittsburgh, PA[341]	1988–1990	~82%	38% to 94%
Centers for Disease Control[‡327]	1986	~70%	17% to 89%
Kaiser Permanente, northern California[329]	1985–1987	~62%	−44% to 90%
Centers for Disease Control[§326]	1986	~45%	−1% to 70%
Massachusetts[341]	1988–1990	~18%	−487% to 89%
Minnesota[339]	1988–1989	−6%	−184% to 60%
Minnesota[328]	1985–1987	−55%	−238% to 29%
Los Angeles County, CA[340]	1988–1989	−58%	−309% to 39%

*Estimates of efficacy adjusted for confounders as reported.
†Conducted in Connecticut; Pittsburgh, PA; and Dallas, TX.
‡Subjects did not attend day care and were from the same areas as reported by Harrison et al.[327]
§Subjects attended day care centers. Children as young as 18.5 months were included. Subjects were from New Jersey, Los Angeles, Tennessee, Missouri, Washington, and Oklahoma.
PRP, polyribosylribitol phosphate.

There were two large-scale prospective clinical trials of the protective efficacy of Hib polysaccharide vaccine. One was conducted in Mecklenburg County, North Carolina, in which children 2 months to 5 years of age received the vaccine in a double-blind fashion.[334] Although the statistical power of this study was inadequate to assess the vaccine's efficacy accurately, it was clear that there was no substantial protective benefit for children younger than 2 years. In a large-scale randomized clinical trial conducted in Finland,[136,335] more than 98,000 children ages 3 to 71 months received either Hib polysaccharide vaccine or meningococcal group A polysaccharide vaccine in a double-blind fashion (children younger than 18 months of age received a second dose of vaccine 3 months after the first dose). There was no protective efficacy for children younger than 18 months. By contrast, for children ages 18 to 71 months at the time of immunization, the protective efficacy of PRP vaccine was 90% (95% confidence interval [CI], 56% to 96%). There has been concern about this post hoc analysis because the age at which the vaccine provided protection was not sharply defined.

In April 1985, the U.S. Food and Drug Administration (FDA) licensed Hib polysaccharide vaccine, and a single dose was recommended for all children at 24 months of age.[336,337] Although this age was beyond the period of highest risk for Hib disease, this strategy was implemented as an interim measure in an effort to reduce the incidence of disease in children by 11% to 24%, the proportion of disease that occurred in children 2 to 5 years of age. Soon thereafter, frequent reports of vaccine failures appeared, and questions arose about the vaccine's true efficacy.[338] A subsequent analysis of the data from the Finnish PRP trial revealed that the estimate of the protective efficacy of PRP vaccine for children 24 to 36 months of age (the ages at which routine immunization of U.S. children was recommended) was 80%, and the 95% CI ranged from 7% to 95%.[330]

Case-control studies (Table 14–6) were conducted to assess the effectiveness of PRP vaccine, and widely conflicting results in different geographic areas were observed.[330–333] A particularly low estimate of efficacy was reported from

TABLE 14–7 ■ Characteristics of Hib Conjugate Vaccines

Properties	PRP-D	HbOC	PRP-OMP	PRP-T
Polysaccharide				
Polymer size	Medium (heat size)	Small (periodate oxidized)	Medium (native)	Large (native)
Content	25 mg	10 mg	15 mg	10 mg
Protein Carrier	Diphtheria toxoid	CRM$_{197}$	Mening group B OMP	Tetanus toxoid
Content	18 mg	20 mg	250 mg	20 mg
Linkage	Protein	PS	Protein and PS	PS
Activation reactants	ADH	Periodate	N-ABC (PS)	ADH
	CNBr (protein)	Cyanoborohydrate	N-AHC (protein)	CNB (PS)
				Carbodiimide HCl
Linkages	Amide/protein	Secondary amino	Amide/protein	Amide/protein
	Iminocarbamate/PS		Carbamate/PS	Iminocarbamate/PS
			Thioester/spacer	
Spacer	6-carbon	None	Bigeneric	6-carbon
			1. N-ABC (linked to PS)	
			2. N-AHC (linked to protein)	

ADH, adipic dihydrazide: the completed reaction cleaves both hydrazide moieties, leaving a six-carbon linkage; CNBr, cyanogen bromide; N-ABC, N-acetylbutylcarbamate; N-AHC, N-acetylhomocysteine; CRM$_{197}$, diphtheria toxin mutant protein; HbOC, *Haemophilus* b oligosaccharide conjugate; mening group B OMP, *Neisseria meningitidis* group B outer membrane protein; PRP, polyribosylribitol phosphate; PRP-D, PRP–diphtheria toxoid conjugate; PRP-OMP, PRP–outer membrane protein conjugate; PRP-T, PRP–tetanus toxoid conjugate; PS, polysaccharide.

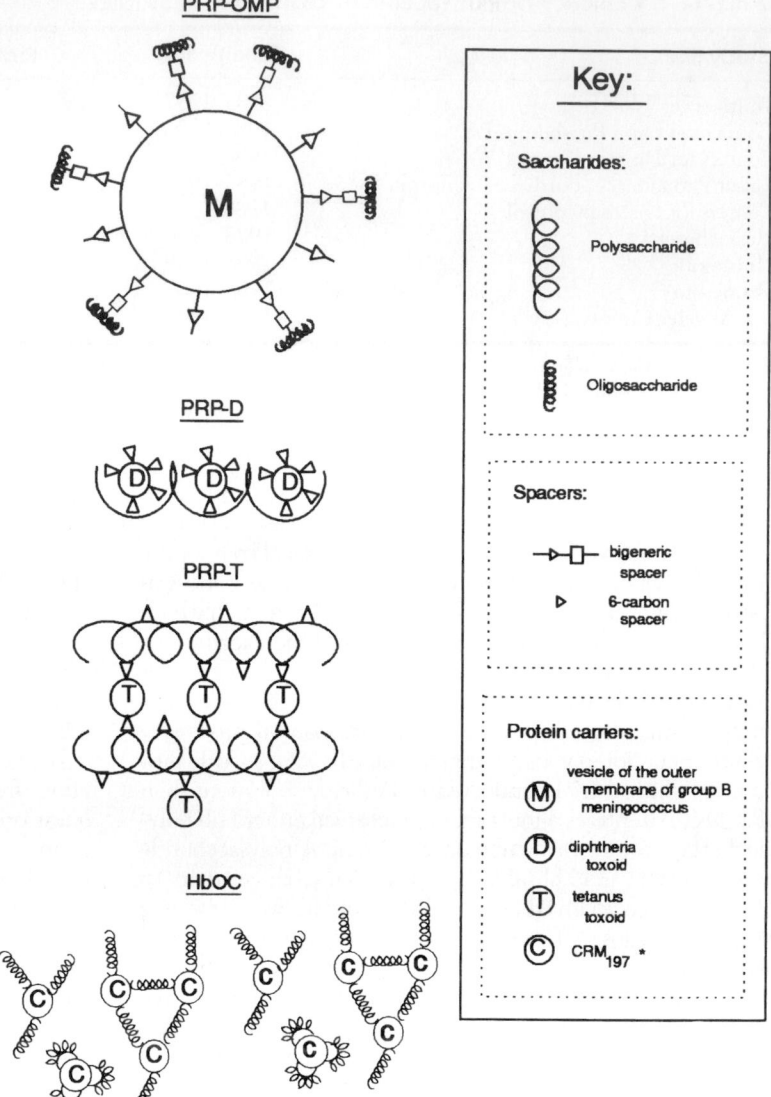

FIGURE 14–3 ■ Configurations of polyribosylribitol phosphate (PRP)–protein conjugate vaccines. *CRM$_{197}$, diphtheria toxin mutant protein; HbOC, *Haemophilus* b oligosaccharide conjugate; OMP, outer membrane protein; PRP-D, PRP–diphtheria toxoid conjugate; PRP-T, PRP–tetanus toxoid conjugate.

Minnesota[339] and Southern California.[340] Another study conducted in Connecticut, Pittsburgh, and Dallas, found the vaccine to be highly efficacious (91%, 92%, and 81% at each of these sites, respectively).[325] The results from these studies were replicated in subsequent studies at the same sites.[327,341] The reasons for these disparate case-control findings were never adequately explained.

Haemophilus influenzae Type b Conjugate Vaccines

The limited immunogenicity of the polysaccharide PRP vaccine in infants and young children led to the development of the Hib protein conjugate vaccines. These vaccines employ the carrier-hapten principles of antigen presentation first defined by Landsteiner in 1924.[292] In 1929, the first successful bacterial polysaccharide conjugate vaccine was synthesized by Avery and Goebel.[342,343] However, it was more than 50 years later that Schneerson and colleagues,[344] Gordon,[345] Anderson,[346] Tai and associates,[347] and others developed PRP polysaccharide conjugate vaccines. Basic to all conjugate vaccines is the use of an immunogenic carrier protein that is recognized by T cells and macrophages and stimulates T-

dependent (thymus-dependent) immunity. The protein carrier is covalently linked (conjugated) to the PRP polysaccharide, which, in principle, confers the immunologic responsiveness of the protein carrier on the polysaccharide hapten.

As discussed in the *Immunology* section, conjugate vaccines elicit an immune response that is characterized by activation of helper T cells. The immune response induced by T-dependent antigens is both quantitatively and qualitatively different from the response induced by T-independent antigens (e.g., PRP): (1) it is quantitatively enhanced, particularly in younger children; (2) repeated administrations elicit booster responses; (3) the immune response matures as evidenced by a predominance of IgG antibody; and (4) prior or concomitant administration of the carrier protein enhances the immune response (carrier priming).

Four Hib conjugate vaccines (see Tables 14–5 and 14–7) were developed and underwent extensive clinical evaluations. The vaccines (Fig. 14–3) all employ the same polysaccharide hapten (PRP), but otherwise differ in the size of the polysaccharide, the protein carrier, and the type of linkage as well as the type of immune response induced. Each of the conjugate vaccines is reviewed.

PRP–Diphtheria Toxoid Conjugate Vaccine

COMPOSITION

No longer available commercially in the United States, PRP–diphtheria toxoid conjugate (PRP-D) vaccine was developed by Schneerson and Robbins and their colleagues[344,348] and was later modified and produced commercially by Connaught Laboratories (ProHIBIT; Aventis Pasteur, Swiftwater, PA). It contained medium-sized lengths of polysaccharide (heat sized) that were linked to a diphtheria toxoid carrier by a six-carbon spacer. Other vaccine characteristics are listed in Table 14–7.

IMMUNOGENICITY

PRP-D was evaluated extensively in adults and children of all ages. As with PRP, the response to PRP-D in children varied by age, but PRP-D induced higher antibody levels in all ages than did PRP. In adults, a single vaccine dose elicited high levels of antibody (geometric mean titer [GMT] 200 mg/mL). In older children and adults, there were no major differences in immunogenicity between PRP-D and other Hib conjugate vaccines.[349] In children 15 months of age and older, high antibody concentrations also were achieved with a single dose, and booster doses were not required to provide lasting protection.[349,350] Similarly, when PRP-D was given as a booster dose to children 15 months of age who had been previously immunized with one of the other three Hib conjugate vaccines as infants, it induced a booster response at least as good as that induced with the primary vaccine.[351,352] PRP-D also elicited a booster response in children 9 to 15 months of age (unlike plain PRP vaccine), and two doses of PRP-D achieved antibody levels greater than 1 mg/mL in all subjects.[353] These antibody levels fell in the following year, leaving a little more than half of vaccine recipients with antibody levels greater than 1 mg/mL.

In infants younger than 6 months of age, three doses of PRP-D were required and immune responses were limited and much less than that induced by the other three Hib conjugate vaccines (Table 14–8). The antibody response to a first dose in infants 2 months of age was not measurable, and only a few infants responded after a second dose at 4 months of age. Yet even after a third dose at 6 months of age, less than half of all infants developed antibody levels greater than 1 μg/mL.[354–356] With the decline of these meager antibody levels in the ensuing 3 to 12 months, most children had levels of antibody not thought to be protective during the period of greatest disease risk.

SAFETY

Millions of doses of PRP-D were administered in the United States and Europe between 1988 and 1990 without reports of serious adverse consequences. Less than 2% of children 18 months of age and older developed fever with the administration of PRP-D.[357] Local reactions at the injection site were also infrequent and mild. Although an early anecdotal report associated three cases of Guillain-Barré syndrome with PRP-D administration in children 18 to 60 months of age,[358] subsequent evaluations could not confirm an association.[359]

EFFICACY

Before the 1987 licensure of PRP-D in the United States for children 18 months of age and older, its efficacy had not been evaluated. Subsequently, several case-control studies determined that a single dose of vaccine was 74% to 96% efficacious in preventing disease in older children.[339–341,360–362]

For young infants, two clinical efficacy trials yielded disparate protective efficacy results. In Finland,[363,364] more than 100,000 infants were enrolled in an open, randomized trial in which infants received study vaccine at 3, 4, 6, and 14 to 18 months of age. The protective efficacy of the PRP-D vaccine after three doses was 94% (95% CI, 83% to

TABLE 14–8 ■ Comparative Immunogenicity of Different Hib Conjugate Vaccines in Infants

Study	Immunization Age at	Vaccine	Antibody Levels (mg/mL) at Age					
			4 Mo		6 Mo		7 Mo	
			GMT	% >1	GMT	% >1	GMT	% >1
Vanderbilt[356]	(2, 4, 6)	PRP-D	0.06		0.08		0.28	29
		HbOC	0.09		0.13		3.08	75
		PRP-OMP	0.83		0.84	50	1.14	55
		PRP-T	0.05		0.30		3.64	83
U.S. multicenter[100]	(2, 4, 6)	HbOC	0.11		0.45	23	6.31	90
		PRP-OMP	2.69		4.00	85	5.21	88
		PRP-T	0.19	80	1.25	56	6.37	97
Finland[419]	(4, 6) 0	PRP-D			0.10	6	0.63	32
		HbOC			0.09	0	4.32	78
		PRP-T			0.82	50	6.10	96
Alaskan Native*[373]	(2, 4, 6)	PRP-D	0.04	2	0.06	11	0.55	45
		HbOC	0.07	0	0.59	43	13.72	94
		PRP-OMP†	1.37	57	2.71	79		
		PRP-T	0.08	3	0.51	41	4.38	75

*Enrollment in this study was sequential by vaccine availability. Other studies were randomized trials.
†Only two doses of PRP-OMP administered at 2 and 4 months of age.
　HbOC, *Haemophilus* b oligosaccharide conjugate; GMT, geometric mean titer; PRP, polyribosylribitol phosphate; PRP-D, PRP–diphtheria toxoid conjugate; PRP-OMP, PRP–outer membrane protein conjugate; PRP-T, PRP–tetanus toxoid conjugate.

98%), and the calculated efficacy after four doses was 100% (95% CI, 82% to 100%). In contrast, a randomized, double-blind, placebo-controlled trial conducted in Alaskan Native infants found no evidence of protection in that high-risk population.[365] More than 2100 infants were enrolled in the study and were vaccinated with PRP-D or saline placebo at approximately 2, 4, and 6 months of age. Even after three doses of vaccine, the protective efficacy was estimated to be only 43% (95% CI, −43% to 78%).[365] The discrepancy between the results of the two studies has not been fully explained, although it may be due to the higher rates of early infections in Alaskan infants. The poor efficacy seen in the Alaskan Native infants paralleled its poor immunogenicity in these infants, and there was little, if any, difference in the immunogenicity of PRP-D between Finnish and Alaskan infants.

RECOMMENDATIONS

Although PRP-D was used in toddlers in the United States and in infants in some European countries, it was not licensed for use in U.S. young infants because of concerns about its limited immunogenicity, its failure to protect high-risk infants, and the availability of more immunogenic vaccines.

Haemophilus b Oligosaccharide Conjugate Vaccine

COMPOSITION

Haemophilus b oligosaccharide conjugate (HbOC) vaccine was developed by Porter Anderson at the University of Rochester; it is manufactured, licensed, and distributed by Wyeth Laboratories (Pearl River, NY; HibTITER). HbOC differs significantly from other Hib conjugate vaccines. It consists of short oligosaccharides of approximately 20 PRP repeat units that are covalently linked, without a spacer, to the protein carrier CRM_{197}, which is a nontoxic variant of diphtheria toxin (see Table 14–7). It is a well-defined aqueous preparation without adjuvants or antibiotics and is available as a monovalent product and previously as a combined vaccine with diphtheria-tetanus–whole-cell pertussis (DTP) vaccine. The dose is 0.5 mL by intramuscular injection.

IMMUNOGENICITY

As with other Hib conjugate vaccines, a single dose of HbOC is highly immunogenic in children 18 to 24 months of age and older.[349,366–368] In young infants, immunogenicity is age dependent, and two or three doses are required. An initial dose at 2 months of age does not induce an antibody response, but a significant number of infants respond to a second dose at 4 months of age. After a third dose at 6 months, high antibody levels are achieved in nearly all infants[356,369,370] (see Table 14–8). Interestingly, antibody levels in Finland induced after two doses at 4 and 6 months of age appear to be similar to those induced by three doses given at 2, 4, and 6 months of age.[371,372] The antibody levels induced by three doses of HbOC are greater than the levels induced by PRP-D or PRP–outer membrane protein conjugate vaccine (PRP-OMP) and are roughly equivalent to those of PRP–tetanus toxoid conjugate (PRP-T).[356,373] Pre-existing maternally acquired antibody does not affect the immune response to HbOC.[310,374] Antibody persists for at least a year in most infants, but a booster is recommended between 12 and 15 months of age. Antibodies induced by

HbOC are predominantly IgG1[289,368] and are bactericidal.[370] Furthermore, children deficient in IgG2[375,376] or IgA,[375,377] children with sickle cell disease[378–380] or prior Hib disease,[381] and men infected with HIV[382] have good responses to HbOC. Diphtheria antibodies also increase significantly after a dose of HbOC,[368,383] and withholding DTP from young infants significantly inhibits the immune response to HbOC,[384,385] indicating the importance of prior exposure to the carrier protein (carrier priming) in inducing an immune response to conjugate vaccines.

SAFETY

Experience with the administration of several million doses of HbOC supports a conclusion that the vaccine is safe. Local reactions, such as erythema or tenderness, occur significantly less often after vaccination with HbOC (2%) than with DTP (19%).[386] No serious reactions have been reported with HbOC. The immunogenicity and safety profile of a combined HbOC-DTP vaccine was comparable to that of the vaccines coadministered at separate injection sites.[387,388]

EFFICACY

Two prospective studies showed that two or three doses of HbOC administered in the first 6 months of life provided a high degree of protective efficacy. In an unblinded, quasi-randomized study involving more than 60,000 infants in the Northern California Kaiser Permanente Health Plan,[389] HbOC was administered to 20,800 infants at 2, 4, and 6 months of age. Overall, only three cases of invasive Hib disease occurred in the vaccinated group compared with 22 cases in the unimmunized population (Table 14–9). All three cases in the HbOC group occurred in children who had received only one immunization. In this study, the vaccine provided no real protection after a single dose but was extremely effective after three doses, with a calculated efficacy of 100% (95% CI, 68% to 100%). The limited duration of follow-up between the second and third doses precluded an accurate assessment of the vaccine's efficacy after only two doses. Long-term follow-up in the Northern California Kaiser Permanente Health Plan confirms HbOC's efficacy.[390] The vaccine also was evaluated in Finland, where beginning in 1988 infants were randomized to receive either HbOC or PRP-D at 4, 6, and 14 to 18 months of age. During the subsequent 2 years, more than 50,000 infants were immunized with HbOC. Only 3 cases of invasive Hib disease occurred in children vaccinated with HbOC compared with 11 cases in recipients of PRP-D (P = 0.04). One case occurred after a single HbOC dose and two cases after the second dose.[391]

RECOMMENDATIONS

In October 1990, HbOC became the first Hib conjugate vaccine to be licensed in the United States for use in infants at 2, 4, and 6 months of age, with a booster dose at 12 to 15 months of age (Table 14–10).[392] In March 1993, a combined HbOC-DTP vaccine was licensed in the United States on the basis of its safety and its immunogenicity profile,[219,393] but it is not distributed in the United States because of the availability of acellular pertussis vaccines, which cannot be combined with this Hib conjugate.

TABLE 14-9 ■ Efficacy Trial of HbOC in Northern Californian Infants

Dose	Mean Age (mo)	Episodes of Hib Disease/ Subject-Years		Protective Efficacy	95% Confidence Interval
		Vaccinees	Comparison Group*		
Post 1	2.6	3/6553	2/NP	26%	−166% to 80%
Post 2	4.9	0/5512	7/NP	100%	47% to 100%
Post 3	7.2	0/12,949	12/11,335	100%	68% to 100%
Post any	1.4–2.4	3/25,014	21/26,962	84%	60% to 100%

*The comparison group consists of concurrent children at the Kaiser Permanente study clinics who refused or were never offered HbOC vaccine. Because no placebo or alternative vaccine was administered to these control subjects, the number of cases of *Haemophilus influenzae* type b disease and subject-years of follow-up that are used for comparison with the vaccinated groups are estimated on the basis of their ages and periods of follow-up. HbOC, *Haemophilus* b oligosaccharide conjugate vaccine; Hib, *Haemophilus influenzae* type b; NP, not presented in the published manuscript of the trial.

PRP–Outer Membrane Protein Conjugate Vaccine

COMPOSITION

PRP-OMP vaccine was developed and is marketed by Merck & Co. (West Point, PA; PedvaxHIB). PRP-OMP differs markedly in both composition and immunogenicity from the other Hib conjugate vaccines. It links medium lengths of PRP by a bigeneric spacer molecule to protein components of outer membrane vesicles of a strain of serogroup B *Neisseria meningitidis* (see Table 14–7). The vesicles are visible by light microscopy and contain lipopolysaccharides, outer membrane proteins, and other undefined constituents of the outer membrane of this gram-negative bacterium. The vaccine is a lyophilized preparation that is reconstituted just before administration in an aqueous buffer with aluminum adjuvant. The dose is 0.5mL by intramuscular injection.

IMMUNOGENICITY

PRP-OMP induces an immune response that is less age dependent than the response to the other Hib conjugate vaccines. Most adults and children respond to a single vaccine dose by producing high levels of antibody. A booster response is seen in older children who are given a repeated dose of PRP-OMP or PRP polysaccharide vaccine,[394] although a clear booster response is not seen in young infants with a second or third dose in a primary series.

PRP-OMP is unique among the Hib conjugate vaccines in its ability to induce a strong antibody response in young infants with the first dose. In young infants 6 weeks of age

TABLE 14–10 ■ Recommended Vaccination Schedules in the United States for Hib Conjugate Vaccines

ROUTINE SCHEDULE				
Vaccine	2 mo	4 mo	6 mo	12–15 mo
HbOC*	Dose 1	Dose 2	Dose 3	Booster[†]
PRP-T	Dose 1	Dose 2	Dose 3	Booster[†]
PRP-OMP[‡]	Dose 1	Dose 2		Booster[†]

"CATCH-UP" SCHEDULE			
Vaccine	Age at First Dose (mo)	Primary Series (Doses)	Booster[§] (mo)
HbOC[§] or PRP-T	2–6	3[‡]	12–15
	7–11	2[‡]	12–18
	12–14	1[‡]	15
	15–59	1	
PRP-OMP[‖]	2–6	2[‡]	12–15
	7–11	2[‡]	12–18
	12–14	1	15
	15–59	1	
PRP-D	12–14	1	12–15
	15–59	1	

*Or HbOC-DTP combined vaccine when both HbOC and DTP are due.
[†]Any licensed *Haemophilus influenzae* b conjugate vaccine is acceptable for the booster dose.
[‡]Or PRP-OMP–hepatitis B combined vaccine when both PRP-OMP and hepatitis B are due.
[§]At least 2 months after previous dose.
[‖]At least 2 months between doses.
HbOC, *Haemophilus* b oligosaccharide conjugate; PRP, polyribosylribitol phosphate; PRP-D, PRP–diphtheria toxoid conjugate; PRP-OMP, PRP–outer membrane protein conjugate; PRP-T, PRP–tetanus toxoid conjugate.

and older, a single injection of PRP-OMP induces a good antibody response (see Table 14–8), and 15% to 80% of infants achieve titers greater than 1 mg/mL.[395-400] A second dose at 4 months of age increases the proportion of infants with an immune response, although a small percentage of infants (less than 6%) fail to respond to two doses of PRP-OMP.[398,401] PRP-OMP does not elicit a classical booster response in most infants, but the titers achieved after two doses of PRP-OMP vaccine are higher than those achieved after two doses of HbOC, PRP-D, or PRP-T vaccines.[356,373,400] A third dose at 6 months of age does not boost levels or the proportion of responders,[374] and therefore only a two-dose primary series has been recommended for infants.

An additional concern regarding this vaccine relates to the decay of antibody levels between 4 and 12 months of age. Because the peak antibody levels are lower than those achieved after a primary series of HbOC or PRP-T vaccines, and are achieved at an earlier age, the period of time with high antibody titers is less with PRP-OMP vaccine. To compensate, a booster dose was recommended at 12 months of age, earlier than for the other two infant vaccines. Admittedly, it is not clear what antibody level must be maintained to ensure protection, and it is possible that the initial response (i.e., priming) is as important as the level of antibody. However, a late vaccine failure in the Navajo efficacy trial in a child with an initial antibody response[402] suggests that maintaining high levels is an important determinant of protection. About one fourth of vaccine recipients have levels less than 0.15 mg/mL a year after completing their primary immunization series.[403] Nevertheless, in postlicensure experience vaccine failures do not appear to be occurring.

In postlicensure studies, PRP-OMP was evaluated in newborns as a possible means to provide earlier protection for high-risk populations.[404] Surprisingly, the antibody levels achieved with three doses given at birth and at 2 and 6 months of age were markedly depressed throughout the first year of life, suggesting immune tolerance if the vaccine is given too early in life. It is not recommended to administer the vaccine before 6 to 8 weeks of age.

As with other Hib conjugate vaccines, responses to PRP-OMP are not affected by maternally acquired or passively administered antibody.[374] It is also immunogenic in high-risk individuals who had poor responses to PRP vaccine.[405] The antibody induced by PRP-OMP is primarily IgG1[289,397,406] and is opsonophagocytic[407] and bactericidal.[394,397] Functional studies of the antibodies indicate that they are of lower avidity than those elicited by HbOC or PRP-T.[408] Some have concluded that PRP-OMP's immune profile suggests that it has T-independent type 1 immune characteristics (see Table 14–4).[409] Immunization results in increases in antibody to the carrier, but there is no evidence for the possible protective efficacy of these antibodies to group B pathogen.

After licensure, a problem arose with the discovery that selected lots of PRP-OMP were significantly less immunogenic than expected. Sixteen lots, representing approximately 23% of the lots distributed between August 1990 and May 1992, elicited lower than expected antibody levels in young children. The reason for the temporarily impaired immunogenicity was not determined definitively, but may have been associated with incomplete conjugation of the PRP.[410]

SAFETY

Although PRP-OMP contains trace amounts of meningococcal endotoxin, local and systemic reactions are less than those that occur with DTP and range from 3% to 15%.[395,397-399,401,411,412] An earlier study showed higher rates of local and febrile reactions but also showed reduced rate of reactions with the addition of aluminum phosphate adjuvant. Presumably this slows the release of reactogenic components. More serious adverse reactions, specifically seizures, hospitalizations, early-onset Hib disease, and sudden infant death syndrome, have not been associated with PRP-OMP vaccination.

EFFICACY

PRP-OMP was evaluated in a randomized, double-blind, placebo-controlled trial in a high-risk Navajo Indian population.[402] More than 5000 infants were enrolled in the study and were vaccinated with PRP-OMP or placebo at approximately 2 and 4 months of age. Only 1 case of invasive Hib disease occurred in an immunized child compared with 22 cases in the placebo group, yielding an overall efficacy of 95% (95% CI, 72% to 99%) (Table 14–11). The one vaccine failure occurred at 15½ months of age in a child who had received two doses of vaccine. Consistent with its immunologic profile, the vaccine appeared to provide protection after a single dose because no cases of Hib disease occurred between the first and second injection in the vaccinated group; eight cases occurred in the placebo group. Late follow-up in this population revealed a second vaccine failure, a 7-month-old child who had received a single vaccine dose at 6 weeks of age.[413] Subsequently, PRP-OMP vaccine proved to be effective in eliminating Hib disease in participants in the Southern California Kaiser Permanente Health Plan.[414]

RECOMMENDATIONS

Previously licensed in the United States in December 1989 for use in children 15 months of age and older, PRP-OMP vaccine was licensed for use in infants in December 1990.[392] It is recommended for administration at 2 and 4 months of age with a booster dose at 12 to 15 months of age (see Table 14–10). These recommendations are different from those for HbOC and PRP-T vaccines, which require more doses. More recently, a hepatitis B–PedvaxHIB combination vaccine (Comvax) has been licensed and used to reduce the number of injections required to immunize infants (see Chapter 29).

PRP–Tetanus Toxoid Conjugate Vaccine

COMPOSITION

PRP-T was among the first PRP-protein conjugate vaccines developed at the National Institutes of Health by Schneerson and associates.[344,348] It is now manufactured by Aventis Pasteur (Lyon, France; ActHIB) and by GlaxoSmithKline (Rixensart, Belgium; OmniHIB). The vaccine contains large polysaccharide polymers that are extracted from culture supernatants and linked by a six-carbon spacer to tetanus toxoid carrier (see Table 14–7). The process of conjugation is similar to that of PRP-D and results in many cross-linkages and a complex three-dimensional structure. For reasons of maintaining potency over time, it is prepared lyophilized and is reconstituted just before administration with aqueous

TABLE 14–11 ■ Efficacy Trial of PRP-OMP in Navajo Infants

Dose	Approximate Age (mo)	Episodes of Hib Disease/ Number of Subjects		Protective Efficacy	95% Confidence Interval
		Vaccinees	Placebo Recipients		
Post 1	2	0/2588	8/2602	100%	41%–100%
Post 2	4	1/1913	14/1929	93%	53%–98%
Post any*	2–16	1/2588	22/2602	95%	72%–99%

*A second vaccine failure was subsequently reported in a 7-month-old child who had received a single vaccine dose at 8 weeks of age.
Hib, *Haemophilus influenzae* type b; PRP-OMP, polyribosylribitol phosphate–outer membrane protein conjugate vaccine.
From Santosham M, Wolff M, Reid R, et al. The efficacy in Navajo infants of a conjugate vaccine consisting of *Haemophilus influenzae* type b polysaccharide and *Neisseria meningitidis* outer-membrane protein complex. N Engl J Med 324:1767–1772, 1991. Reprinted with permission from The New England Journal of Medicine, 1991.

buffer without adjuvants or antibiotics. The dose is 0.5 mL by intramuscular injection.

IMMUNOGENICITY

The pattern of immune response to PRP-T is similar to that of HbOC. A single dose of the vaccine is highly immunogenic in adults[415] and in older children.[416] In young infants administered a first dose between 2 and 4 months of age, no response is seen in most instances. One or two additional doses can be given at 2-month intervals to induce high antibody concentrations in even the youngest infants.[356,373,400,417–420] After a second and third dose, 70% to 100% and 98% to 100% respond, respectively.[421] Some comparative immunogenicity studies show this vaccine to be the most immunogenic vaccine after three doses,[356,400] although it is not clear that these differences result in improved protective efficacy. Geometric mean anti-PRP antibody concentrations of 5 to 10 μg/mL generally are achieved after a three-dose primary series, and good antibody levels usually persist a year after immunization.[422]

As with other Hib conjugate vaccines, the antibodies induced are primarily IgG1.[423] PRP-T is immunogenic in high-risk individuals, such as those who have had bone marrow transplantation,[424] children with sickle cell anemia thalassemia or malignant neoplasms,[425,426] children with HIV infection,[428] and those who have had invasive Hib disease.[425]

SAFETY

In studies of safety and immunogenicity, the vaccine was administered to more than 115,000 children without serious side effects.[421] In children 18 to 23 months of age, local reactions were more frequent after vaccination with PRP-T than with PRP,[416] occurring in as many as 32% of recipients. These were thought to be due to Arthus-like reactions in older children who had pre-existing high levels of tetanus immunity. In infants, only 7% to 15% had reactions.[421,422] None of the reactions was serious, and they were less likely to occur with subsequent doses. Temperature higher than 38°C occurs after 4.7% to 10.0% of PRP-T administrations, and this rate is less than that after vaccination with DTP, which is usually given concurrently.

A study of the relationship between Hib and sudden infant death syndrome showed no association.[427]

There is some discrepancy in the data about the simultaneous administration of PRP-T and DTP, especially when they are mixed in the same syringe. Some studies show an interference in immune response to other antigens[429] or to PRP,[430] although the possible clinical significance of these findings is unclear.

EFFICACY

PRP-T was evaluated for its protective efficacy in four randomized, double-blind trials in infants in the United States,[421] The Gambia,[431] and Chile.[432] Two of the trials in the United States were discontinued before completion because of national recommendations to use Hib conjugate vaccines for all U.S. infants. In one trial in North Carolina, with more than 2000 randomized subjects, two cases of Hib disease occurred among control subjects, whereas none occurred among PRP-T vaccinees. In another trial in the Southern California Kaiser Permanente Health Plan with more than 10,000 subjects, three cases of Hib disease occurred among control subjects, whereas none occurred among PRP-T vaccinees.[420] These results suggested, but did not prove, that the vaccine is protective.

In the Gambian trial,[431] more than 42,000 infants received either PRP-T mixed with DTP or DTP alone at 2, 3, and 4 months of age (Table 14–12). One case of Hib disease occurred in a vaccinee compared with 19 cases among control subjects, yielding a protective efficacy of 95% (95% CI, 67% to 100%) against invasive Hib disease, a 100% protective efficacy against Hib pneumonia (95% CI, 55% to 100%), and a 21% decrease in radiologically confirmed pneumonia of all types in vaccinees compared with control subjects. PRP-T also proved to be effective in a British trial in which the vaccine was administered at 2, 3, and 4 months of age,[433,434] and in Southern California and Chilean trials when given to infants at 2, 4, and 6 months of age. Subsequent evaluation of data from Chile showed a 25% reduction in cases of disease clinically consistent with bacterial pneumonia among children receiving PRP-T vaccine.[432,435]

In addition to these studies, a nationwide immunization program with PRP-T vaccine was implemented in Finland in January 1990.[436] All infants are given doses of PRP-T at 4 and 6 months of age and a booster dose at 14 to 18 months of age. During the first 22 months of the immunization program (January 1990 to October 1991), approximately 97,000 infants were immunized with two doses of PRP-T. Two cases of invasive Hib disease occurred in vaccinees but only after one dose. No infant receiving two or more doses of the PRP-T vaccine in any study has had invasive Hib disease,[421] and this was in marked contrast to the previous experience with other Hib conjugates in Finland.

RECOMMENDATIONS

PRP-T was the last of the four Hib conjugate vaccines to complete clinical testing. In March 1993, it was licensed in the United States for use in infants.[219,393] It is recommended for use in the United States at 2, 4, and 6 months of age with a booster dose at 12 to 15 months (see Table 14–10). In November 1993, the FDA approved the reconstitution of PRP-T with DTP vaccine to allow simultaneous administration in a single injection whenever both vaccines are indicated,[437] but this vaccine is no longer in use in the United States because of the practice of use of acellular pertussis vaccines, which appear not to be compatible with PRP-T when given in the same syringe.

Additional Considerations Regarding Hib Conjugate Vaccines: Comparative Immunogenicity Studies

Comparing the immunogenicity of different vaccines between different studies should be done with caution. Apparent differences in immunogenicity between studies may be due to differences in study design, such as age of immunization, timing of postvaccination phlebotomies, differences in vaccine lots, differences in the laboratory methods used to measure antibody,[438] or differences in the statistical methods used to calculate mean levels and other analyses. Several studies have compared the immunogenicity of the different Hib conjugate vaccines in trials with standardized vaccine schedules using uniform laboratory and statistical methods.[356,373,400,419] Data from these four studies are summarized in Table 14–8. The data highlight some of the problems associated with comparisons of vaccine immunogenicity, because there are some significant differences in results between different studies.

Some conclusions can be drawn concerning immune responses by age and dose in infants. PRP-OMP is the only vaccine that induces a good immune response with an initial dose in infants immunized between 2 and 4 months of age, and a consistent and high level of antibody following a second primary dose at 4 months of age. One study suggested that PRP-OMP may induce immune tolerance if the first dose is administered at birth. Also, there is no boost induced between the second and third doses when administered to infants in the first 6 months of life.

The other Hib conjugate vaccines (HbOC and PRP-T, and previously PRP-D) rarely show a response with the first dose and require a series of two or three doses in young infants to achieve consistent high levels. The immune responses after two doses of HbOC or PRP-T in infants are variable and often undetectable. Therefore, a third primary dose is required to achieve good antibody levels in infants; however, after three doses, the levels achieved are higher than those achieved with PRP-OMP after two or three doses. PRP-D is clearly the least immunogenic of the four vaccines. Finally, the level of maternal antibody does not influence the ultimate immune response (data not shown).

Although these studies help to define the pattern of the immune response seen with each of the vaccines, they do not clearly indicate the "best" vaccine or schedule because antibody levels alone are not the only determinants of protection. Because PRP-OMP is the only vaccine that induces an antibody response in 2-month-old infants after a single dose, it is most advantageous for use in populations with incomplete immunizations and for high-risk infants at younger ages (i.e., before 6 months of age). HbOC and PRP-T produce higher and more sustained antibody levels after completion of the primary immunization series; the duration of antibody levels appears to relate to peak level achieved.

There have not been any prospective comparative vaccine efficacy trials, except for a sequential comparison of PRP-D and HbOC in Finland, in which HbOC was shown to provide better protection.[439] Each of the three vaccines licensed in the United States for use in infants (HbOC, PRP-OMP, PRP-T) appears to be highly efficacious. Postlicensure case-control and cohort studies could potentially clarify differences in efficacy, but the precision of these estimates are limited by the proportion of children receiving the different vaccines, and, at this point, none of the postlicensure studies has identified important differences.

Schedules of Primary Immunization

Differences in the epidemiology of Hib disease and in public health practices have led to the adoption of several dif-

TABLE 14–12 ■ Cases of Confirmed Invasive Hib Disease by Vaccination Status and Diagnosis in the Gambia

Doses	Pneumonia*		Meningitis		Other		All	
	PRP-T	Control	PRP-T	Control	PRP-T	Control	PRP-T	Control
0	0	1	3	1	0	0	3	2
1	2	4	3	4	0	1	5	9
2	0	5	0	4	1	1	1	10
3	0	5	1	12	0	2	1	19
Total	2	15	7	21	1	4	10	40
2 or 3	0	10	1	16	1	3	2	29

*Children with pneumonia that occurred in association with proven *Haemophilus influenzae* type b meningitis were classified as meningitis.
PRP-T, polyribosylribitol phosphate–tetanus toxoid conjugate.
Data from Mulholland K, Hilton S, Adegbola R, et al. Randomised trial of *Haemophilus influenzae* type b–tetanus protein conjugate vaccine [corrected] for prevention of pneumonia and meningitis in Gambian infants [see comments]. Lancet 349:1191–1197, 1997.

ferent national schedules of immunization. In countries where the peak of Hib disease occurs in the second 6 months of life, three doses are given before 6 months of age. The United States, Canada, and Belgium are among the countries using a 2-, 4-, and 6-months schedule. To conform to the schedule of DTP administration, France and the United Kingdom recommend Hib vaccine at 2, 3, and 4 months of age. A more compressed schedule (6, 10, and 14 weeks) has been adopted in some developing countries where considerable Hib disease may occur before 6 months of age. In contrast, in the Scandinavian countries, in which the peak of Hib disease occurs after 1 year of age, a two-dose schedule in the first year of life (5 and 7 months) followed by a booster third dose early in the second year of life is used.

Immunogenicity is influenced by the schedule used, with intervals of 2 months between doses giving better responses than intervals of 1 month. The mean titers of antibody are directly correlated with increasing age at administration of the first dose of Hib vaccine.[421]

A unique schedule was developed for high-risk Alaskan Native infants, who receive an initial dose of PRP-OMP vaccine at 2 months of age followed by PRP-T or HbOC at 4 and 6 months of age along with a further booster at 12 months of age. This mixed-sequence schedule was developed because disease was occurring in the first 4 to 6 months of life, before the immunization series could be completed. Presumably this schedule results in the youngest age of onset of protection and the highest titers over childhood years.[440] Since using this schedule, Hib disease has been completely eliminated in a population that previously had the highest known disease incidence.

Booster Immunizations and Duration of Immunity

Because antibody levels decline over time after completion of the primary immunization series in infants, a booster dose is recommended at 12 to 15 months of age in most countries. This booster dose elicits a brisk antibody response. Immunization with the Hib conjugate vaccines during infancy primes the immune system so that a booster immunization with PRP-D[351] or plain polysaccharide vaccine,[441] which is not very immunogenic in unprimed 12- to 15-month-old children, elicits a strong anamnestic response. The duration of immunity after a primary series varies with the age of the child and the vaccine. In several studies, more than 75% of infants had antibody levels above 1 μg/mL 3 to 5 years after the primary series with PRP-T or HbOC vaccine,[442-445] compared with less than 50% of infants who received the PRP-OMP vaccine.[443,446] The relative importance of absolute antibody levels versus immunologic priming regarding maintenance of long-lasting immunity is not clear. It is possible, if not likely, that a child's T cells are primed by Hib conjugate vaccine. The absolute antibody titer maintained may be secondary because the secondary immune response in a primed child with natural exposure is immediate.

It is unclear whether a single booster immunization during the second year of life is sufficient for lifelong immunity, or even whether a booster dose is necessary at all.[447] The United Kingdom has pursued a policy of not providing a Hib booster in the second year of life, which assumes long-term protection after three doses of PRP-T given at 2, 3,

and 4 months of age. At a mean age of 4.5 years, 92% of a group of previously vaccinated children retained anti-Hib antibodies, with a GMT of 0.89 μg/mL. In addition, Hib pharyngeal carriage was still low.[448] The British experience has been reviewed by Heath and colleagues, who identified 96 true vaccine failures during a 6-year period. Vaccine effectiveness declined slightly with time since vaccination: 99.4% in infants ages 5 to 11 months compared with 97.3% in infants ages 12 to 71 months.[449] More recent data from the United Kingdom suggest a recrudescence of Hib within the 1–4-year-old age group, lending support to the idea that a booster in the second year of life is needed for maximal suppression of disease.[450] Continuing follow-up should show whether efficacy wanes and whether Hib disease will become a problem in older children not given a booster. However, it should be noted that intensive postintroduction follow-up for periods of over 10 years since introduction of routine Hib immunization in many countries has shown no increase in Hib disease incidence in older children.

Carrier Priming

Some studies have shown that an optimal response to immunization with conjugate vaccines requires prior or concomitant exposure to the carrier protein (carrier priming). Withholding diphtheria and tetanus toxoids (DT) immunization in rhesus monkeys[384] and human infants[385] reduced the immune response to HbOC but not to PRP-OMP. It has been suggested that administration of the carrier protein before immunization with Hib conjugate vaccines may prime T cells for an enhanced immune response to the subsequent immunization. The effect of carrier priming on the immune response is dependent on many variables,[385] and preliminary results from two studies show the complexity of the issue. Administration of DT at 1 month of age enhanced antibody responses to HbOC and PRP-T given at 2, 4, and 6 months of age in one study,[451] but a similar study with DT given at birth did not show enhancement of the immune response.[452] In fact, immune responses to HbOC were suppressed in infants primed with DT at birth.

Pregnancy

A study conducted in an American Indian population demonstrated that vaccination of pregnant women increased antibody in their infants when measured at birth and at two months of age.[453] However, after immunization of the infants at two and four months of age with PRP-OMP vaccine, titers were lower than in control infants. However, this suppression did not appear important, and the vaccination of pregnant women may be useful in populations with very early Hib disease.

Vaccination Failures

Several groups have studied infants who develop Hib disease despite vaccination.[454-456] Some failures were attributed to B cell deficiencies, and it was notable that many patients responded with low antibody levels to infection, suggesting a more subtle immunologic defect. In addition, Hib antibody avidity was notably lower in vaccine failures than in control patients.

Prematurity causes lower responses to Hib vaccine, with subsequent increased risk of failure.[457]

Serotype Replacement

Thus far, it does not appear that the other capsular serotypes of *H. influenzae* are replacing type b. However, a report from Brazil[458] suggesting an increase in type a disease after introduction of Hib vaccine indicates the need for continued vigilance.

Hib Combination Vaccines

To reduce the number of injections necessary to vaccinate young infants, various formulations combining Hib conjugate vaccines with other routine immunogens have been developed and evaluated. Licensed, predominantly in Europe and Canada, but not the in United States, are combination vaccines with whole-cell pertussis, including DTP–PRP-T, DTP–inactivated poliovirus vaccine (IPV)–PRP-T, DTP–hepatitis B–PRP-T, and PRP-OMP–hepatitis B. In some cases, the combination vaccines are packaged as a liquid mixture in a mixed vial, whereas in others, especially PRP-T–containing combinations, a diluent (either saline or DTP vaccine) is used to reconstitute a separate vial of lyophilized PRP-T for subsequent injection in a single syringe.

Because the schedule for most Hib conjugate vaccines is identical to that for DTP, the first generation of combination vaccines included whole-cell pertussis. In general, these combination vaccines proved to be safe and were no more reactogenic than their component vaccines given separately. The available data suggest that immunization with combined whole-cell DTP/IPV/Hib can be performed without decreases in the proportion of children reaching protective levels of anti-PRP antibodies.[465,466] However, reduced immunogenicity to one or more components of some combinations (especially antibodies to pertussis components) when given as a mixture raised concern in some early studies.[459] Subsequent studies, including surveillance for whooping cough, did not provide any evidence for reduced immunogenicity or effectiveness of these vaccines.[460] Thus, the first generation of combination vaccines with Hib conjugates and DTP were immunogenic, with levels of PRP and pertussis antibodies essentially equivalent to those achieved with separate administration of the antigens.

In contrast to the whole-cell pertussis combinations, substantially lower Hib immunogenicity was observed in several studies of different diphtheria-tetanus–acellular pertussis (DTaP)–based Hib combinations. Many DTaP-Hib conjugate preparations have shown reduced anti-PRP antibody levels compared with separate administration of the same antigens. Although in general the levels of anticapsular antibody are in the low range of responses observed when the antigens are administered separately, some studies showed high proportions of nonresponders even after two and three doses of vaccine.[450] For example, Rennels et al. noted that anti-PRP antibody levels in children given separately administered IPV were substantially lower than those in children immunized with oral poliovirus vaccine (OPV).[467] In this case, children receiving DTaP/Hib and OPV had a GMT of 3.2 µg/mL, with 78% reaching 1 µg/mL, compared with a GMT of 1.2 µg/mL and 53% reaching 1 µg/mL in those receiving IPV separately. In contrast, Gylca et al. found similar GMTs and proportions of children with 0.15 or 1.0 µg/mL anti-PRP antibody among those given either DTaP/hepatitis B/IPV or DTP/IPV/Hib.[468] The reason for decreased antibody levels noted in some studies[469] are unclear, but the variation in results suggests that these differences are vaccine specific. It should be noted that the Hib immune responses with different DTaP–PRP-T combinations were variable.[461] Reasons for decreased immunogenicity of Hib in DTaP combinations are not entirely clear, but may involve (1) direct physical interference between different antigens when mixed; (2) epitope-specific suppression; and (3) variation in adjuvants with different preparations.[459,462] Regardless of cause, the reduced immunogenicity might not reflect a reduced effectiveness of Hib conjugate vaccination programs. This is based primarily on data suggesting that, in spite of reduced antibody levels after primary series with combination vaccines, these vaccines induce immune memory. This was demonstrated in a series of studies using Hib conjugates or Hib polysaccharides for the boosters at 12 to 18 months.[463] Moreover, the levels achieved with combination vaccines may exceed those shown to be protective when using less immunogenic Hib conjugates.[464] Data also have shown that, when corrected for total antibody level, functional activity of anti-PRP antibodies (avidity, or opsonophagocytic activity) did not differ by mode of vaccine administration (separate, or as a combined vaccine with DTaP).[459] Long-term surveillance of Hib disease in Europe and Canada, where Hib combination vaccines are routinely used, is important to provide confirmatory information on their efficacy.

Mixed Administration

The availability in many countries of more than one type of Hib vaccine has generated concern that administration of different vaccines to the same child might reduce immunogenicity or effectiveness. In fact, several studies have shown that Hib vaccine conjugates are interchangeable, in that primary antibody responses remained excellent and booster responses were not impaired in the schedules that were studied.[470–473] In high-risk populations with early onset of disease, initial immunization is given at 2 months of age with PRP-OMP and later doses administered are HbOC or PRP-T, thus optimizing immune response with each dose.

Indications

Hib conjugate vaccines are indicated for every infant starting at the age of 6 weeks to 2 months in those areas of the world where the incidence of Hib disease is significant. At this stage of our knowledge, that includes all areas of the world except possibly some countries in Asia, notably China.

Contraindications and Precautions

There are no contraindications unique to Hib conjugate vaccines. Vaccination should not be initiated before 6 weeks of age, especially for PRP-OMP. PRP-OMP vaccine may induce tolerance if given too soon after birth. A full description of contraindications has been published by the American Academy of Pediatrics[474] and the U.S. Public Health Service.[219] Because they are "killed" vaccines, all

Hib vaccines may be given to immunocompromised individuals or other high-risk individuals, although immunogenicity may be suboptimal and protective efficacy has not been specifically demonstrated in these groups.

There have been rare reports of serious reactions such as urticaria, erythema multiforme, seizures, renal failure, and Guillain-Barré syndrome,[358] but a causal effect has not been established. In particular, seizures and sudden infant death syndrome do not appear to be more common in vaccinees than in control subjects.[325]

Stability

Hib conjugate vaccines are relatively stable, and manufacturers recommend storage for up to 2 years at 2° to 8°C. This applies to both the liquid (HbOC, PRP-OMP, combinations) and lyophilized (PRP-T) preparations. The recommendation for storage of lyophilized Hib at 2° to 8°C is primarily to ensure that the accompanying diluent is not frozen. Liquid Hib vaccine should never be frozen.

Hib vaccine in multidose vials contains thiomersal as a preservative. Although liquid Hib vaccines are stable for at least 2 years, most manufacturers have only evaluated stability of reconstituted lyophilized Hib (in liquid form after reconstitution) for up to 24 hours.

Public Health Considerations

Impact of *Haemophilus influenzae* Type b Conjugate Vaccines on Disease and Carriage of the Organism

The effectiveness and public health impact of Hib conjugate vaccines on disease was demonstrated during the 1980s and early 1990s in industrialized countries in North America[413,414,475-478] and Europe.[436,479] Since that time, additional information has become available from routine immunization programs in the developing world, including South America, the Middle East, Africa, and the Pacific Islands. Routine immunization with Hib conjugate vaccines has resulted in dramatic decreases in the incidence of disease in the targeted populations. In general, the fall in incidence of disease has exceeded that predicted on the basis of the estimated proportion of the population that is completely immunized, suggesting an element of herd immunity. In addition, in populations where Hib conjugate vaccines were used in older children, a significant fall in incidence of disease was observed among immunized infants.

Shown in Figures 14-4 through 14-7 are the experiences in four carefully studied populations using different Hib conjugate vaccine(s). In Finland,[436,480] three different vaccines were used in sequence, and high immunization levels were achieved (see Fig. 14-4). PRP-D vaccine, in use between 1987 and 1989, proved to be effective in eliminating the majority of all Hib disease. Subsequently, the use of HbOC and PRP-T vaccine proved to be even more effective, and the routine immunization of Finnish infants has virtually eliminated Hib disease among children younger than 5 years, making Finland the first population to essentially eliminate Hib disease. Some disease continues to occur in adults and in infants younger than 4 months. With

the introduction of Hib conjugate vaccines, similar changes in incidence of disease have occurred in other European countries, such as Iceland,[481] the United Kingdom, Germany, France, Italy, and Switzerland.

In the United States, the Northern California Kaiser Permanente Health Plan has used HbOC vaccine exclusively[390] (see Fig. 14-5). Hib disease has been eliminated, with the exception of a rare case in an unimmunized child or a few cases in children with incomplete immunizations. Between 1987 and 1990, PRP-D and subsequently PRP-OMP vaccines were used in older children in the Southern California Kaiser Permanente Health Plan (see Fig. 14-6).[414] Since 1990, PRP-OMP vaccine has been used almost exclusively. There were a few PRP-D failures and only two PRP-OMP failures; Hib disease was essentially eliminated even before age-appropriate immunization levels were completely achieved. Similar control of disease has been achieved with use of PRP-OMP vaccine in Alaska and Navajo Native American populations.[413,482] Moreover, Alaskans more than 10 years old had a reduced incidence of Hib disease, although they were not themselves vaccinated, indicating a herd immunity effect.[483]

In Los Angeles County,[414] Minnesota and Dallas,[476] and selected other U.S. populations under surveillance by the Centers for Disease Control and Prevention (see Fig. 14-7),[468] similar but less complete disease eradication has been achieved. In these areas, both HbOC and PRP-OMP vaccine were used in varying proportions over time, and complete immunization has yet to be achieved. In Los Angeles, it is estimated that initially only 50% of children

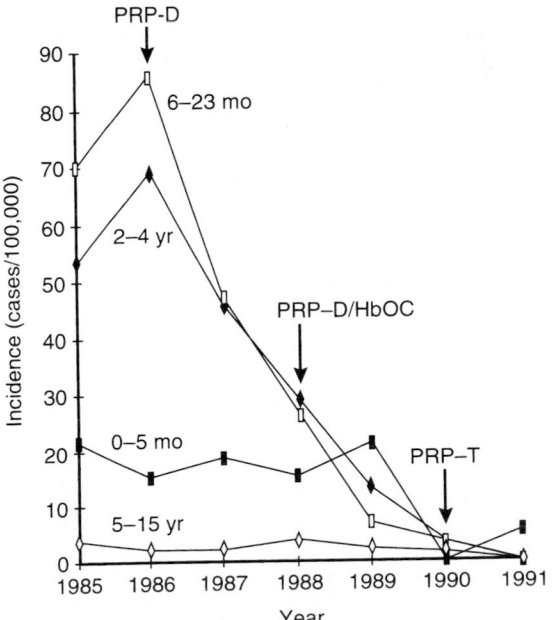

FIGURE 14-4 ■ Eradication of *Haemophilus influenzae* type b disease in Finland. Half of the population received PRP-D vaccine between 1986 and 1988. HbOC, *Haemophilus* b oligosaccharide conjugate; PRP, polyribosylribitol phosphate; PRP-D, PRP–diphtheria toxoid conjugate; PRP-T, PRP–tetanus toxoid conjugate. (From Peltola H, Kilpi T, Anttila M. Rapid disappearance of *Haemophilus influenzae* type b meningitis after routine childhood immunisation with conjugate vaccines. Lancet 340:592–594, 1992, with permission. © The Lancet Ltd., 1992.)

received three doses of HbOC or two doses of PRP-OMP vaccine by 12 months of age. Despite the early incomplete immunization of children, dramatic decreases in the incidence of disease in Los Angeles occurred. Canada also has seen a sharp reduction in Hib disease.[484]

Other examples of the efficacy of Hib conjugate vaccines abound. Some have been given in the sections above concerning the efficacy of individual conjugates. In Sweden, Hib epiglottitis decreased from an incidence of 20.9 per 100,000 children less than 5 years old in 1987 to 0.9 per 100,000 in 1996.[485] In Northern Australia, Hib vaccination showed an effectiveness of 97.5%.[486] In Uruguay, there was a spectacular reduction in incidence from 15.6 to 0.03 cases per 100,000 children under 5 years of age.[487] Data from Israel showed an effectiveness of 94.9% for invasive Hib disease and 96.6% for meningitis.[488] Success also was reported from Saudi Arabia.[489] Finally, in The Gambia, the annual incidence of Hib meningitis fell from 200 per 100,000 before vaccination to 21 per 100,000 after vaccination.[490]

The impressive effectiveness of Hib conjugate vaccines in preventing disease is due to priming of immune response in young infants and to its impact on decreasing transmission (herd immunity). Three different examples of herd immunity are provided by the experience in the United States, Norway, and Spain. Figure 14–8 shows the impact of conjugate vaccine introduction in the United States.[477] The first conjugate vaccine licensed was initially used for a period of about 2 years only in children older than 18 months of age. During this time, however, the incidence of disease declined by at least 40% in children 12 months of age and younger—children who were not themselves immunized. Thus immunization of the older individuals indirectly benefited younger children, presumably through reduction of transmission. It is also worth noting that coverage in the older age group was no higher than 60%. In Norway, a routine infant vaccination program was accompanied by a catch-up program for children through 4 years of age.[491] The disease rate in children older than 5 plummeted immediately after immunization with Hib conjugate vaccines. The rapid fall in disease incidence before all older children were immunized, as well as in the unimmunized infants, again suggests a herd effect on transmission. Data from the Valencia region in Spain show that, even with

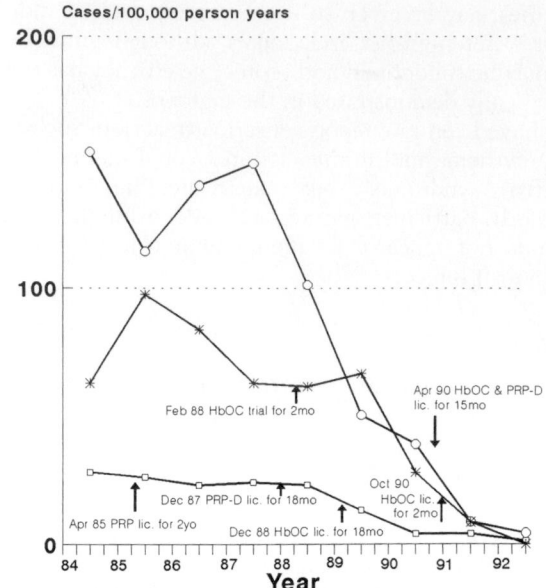

♦ 0 - 6 mo. old **⊶ 7 - 18 mo. old** **⊶ 19 - 60 mo.**

FIGURE 14–5 ■ Incidence of *Haemophilus influenzae* type b disease in the Kaiser Permanente Medical Care Program in Northern California, January 1984 to December 1992. HbOC, *Haemophilus* b oligosaccharide conjugate; mo, months old; PRP, polyribosyl-ribitol phosphate; PRP-D, PRP–diphtheria toxoid conjugate; yo, years old. (From Black SB, Shinefield HR. Immunization with oligosaccharide conjugate *Haemophilus influenzae* type b [HbOC] vaccine on a large health maintenance organization population: extended follow-up and impact on *Haemophilus influenzae* disease epidemiology. Pediatr Infect Dis J 11:610–613, 1992, with permission. © Williams & Wilkins, 1992.)

vaccination in the private sector only and relatively low coverage, a major decrease in Hib disease occurred in the whole population.[492] Rates of invasive Hib disease fell by 78% when vaccination coverage of the 0- to 5-year-old cohort was only 44%. By the end of the following year, when the vaccine was introduced as a routine immunization, disease had fallen by 91%, with vaccination coverage with three doses of Hib conjugate vaccine at only 60%.

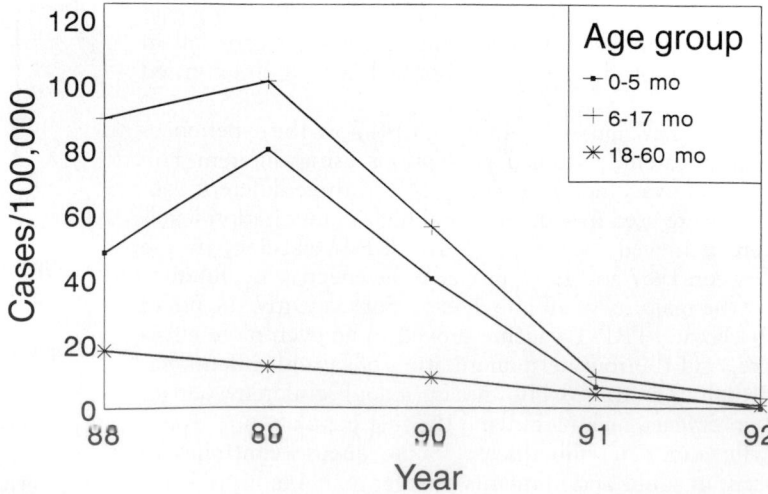

FIGURE 14–6 ■ Incidence of *Haemophilus influenzae* type b disease in the Southern California Kaiser Permanente Health Plan. (From Vadheim CM, Greenberg DP, Friksen E, et al. Eradication of *Haemophilus influenzae* type b disease in Southern California. Arch Pediatr Adolesc Med 148:51–56, 1994, with permission.)

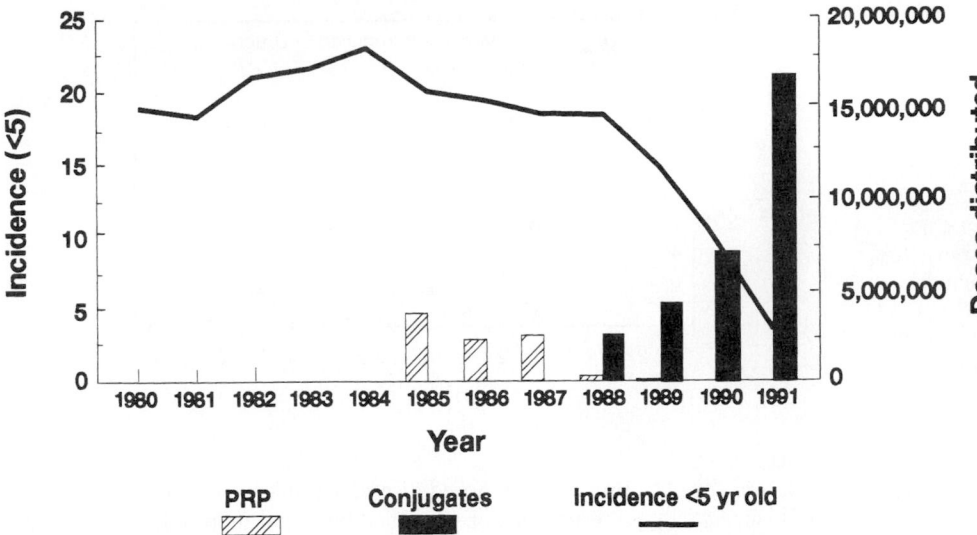

FIGURE 14–7 ■ *Haemophilus influenzae* vaccine doses sold or distributed and incidence of *H. influenzae* meningitis in children younger than 5 years in the United States, 1980 to 1991. PRP, polyribosylribitol phosphate vaccine. (Data from the National Bacterial Meningitis Reporting System [20 continuously reporting states], 1980 to 1991.)

Each of these experiences illustrates the importance of herd immunity.

Reduction in disease appears to occur more completely when a catch-up campaign is instituted at the same time routine immunization of infants is initiated, compared to programs that do not perform catch-up campaigns. A typical response to a combined infant immunization program and catch-up campaign was seen in Norway when disease declined by more than 80% during the second year of the program. In contrast, countries that introduced the vaccine only to the new birth cohort and did not simultaneously immunize older children experienced slower declines in disease. An example of this difference in impact can be seen by comparing the experience of Uruguay, which included a catch-up campaign, and Chile, which did not (Fig. 14–9). In both countries, cases declined by more than 90% compared to baseline, but it took somewhat longer for Chile to reach this goal.[493] The additive disease reduction effect of catch-up campaigns is a function not only of immunization of additional children at risk (albeit lower risk than infants), but also of reduction of carriage in an age group likely to transmit the organism to younger siblings. In deciding whether to implement a catch-up campaign, consideration must be given to the gain in disease prevented relative to the increased cost of the vaccine and delivery operations.

Widespread vaccination against type b has not so far caused problems. Strains recovered from vaccinated children are indistinguishable from those recovered from unvaccinated children.[493a] An increase in the incidence of *Haemophilus influenzae* group a was reported in Salvador, Brazil after application of Hib vaccine, but the increase was small and has not been replicated elsewhere[493b]

The benefit of Hib conjugate vaccines for individuals is clear, but, as a result of population immunity (herd immunity effects), there is also reduced transmission within the population, and therefore protection is afforded to even unimmunized individuals.

Effect on Hib Carriage

As noted previously, a major contributor to herd immunity is reduction of nasopharyngeal carriage noted first in countries in which the vaccine was first introduced.[300–303]

Substantial reduction in carriage also has been confirmed in developing countries following immunization with Hib conjugate vaccines. In The Gambia, carriage in children 1 to 2 years of age who received an Hib conjugate vaccine was 4.4% (95% CI, 3.8 to 5.7) compared with 11% (95% CI, 8.9 to 13) in children who received only DTP (a 60% reduction).[494] It should be noted, however, that in some settings carriage has not been eliminated by routine immunization of infants. Data from Alaskan Native populations showed carriage rates in Alaskan Native villagers as high as 9% before and after immunization, suggesting that the organism maintained transmission.[495] In this circumstance, when the immunization program switched from one Hib conjugate vaccine to a sequence of two different conjugate vaccines, high levels of antibody were induced earlier in life and the incidence of Hib disease fell. Comparison of two communities in Brazil, one vaccinated and the other not, also confirmed an effect on carriage.[496]

Precisely how Hib conjugate immunization reduces oropharyngeal carriage is not clear. High levels of IgG and IgA anti-PRP antibody transudate into mucosal secretions. It is not clear if this impact is from decreased acquisition or

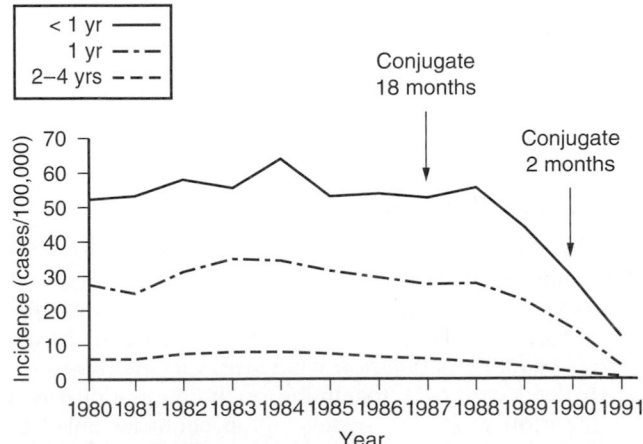

FIGURE 14–8 ■ Decline of *Haemophilus influenzae* type b disease in the United States as shown in national passive surveillance data. *Solid thick line* shows incidence of *Haemophilus* meningitis per 100,000 children less than 12 months of age, *short and long dashed line* shows rate in children 12 to 23 months of age, and *dashed line* shows rate in children 2 to 4 years of age. *Arrows* denote year of introduction of Hib conjugate vaccines for specific age groups.

FIGURE 14–9 ▪ Decline of Hib meningitis in Chile and Uruguay. Decline was somewhat more rapid in Uruguay, which included a catch-up campaign, than in Chile, which did not, but disease was reduced to negligible levels in both countries within 2 years of introduction.

decreased duration of carriage. Additional work on the immunology and microbiology of transmission and carriage is needed to clarify this issue.

The impact of Hib conjugate vaccine on carriage and disease raises the prospect of eliminating Hib disease worldwide. In populations that have implemented routine immunization, the disease incidence has been reduced drastically, but not necessarily to zero. Only Iceland has completely eliminated Hib disease, beginning 3 years after introduction of the vaccine, and lasting 8 years at the time of writing.

The United States has a goal of eliminating Hib cases in children less than 5 years of age by the year 2010.[497] Although major strides have been made toward this goal, the rate of decline of Hib disease has leveled off. An evaluation of cases from 1991 to 1994 (after the major vaccine-induced decline in Hib disease occurred) found that remaining cases were more likely to be from crowded and single-mother households, and undervaccination was associated with several markers for lower socioeconomic status.[179] Evaluation of a cluster of Hib cases in 1999 to 2000 identified an undervaccinated population.[512] In addition, persistent carriage and higher post–vaccination era rates of disease have been identified in Alaskan Native populations. It is clear that attaining the elimination goal will at least require intensified efforts to vaccinate underserved communities, as well as monitoring serotypes and analysis of ongoing surveillance data to identify underserved populations, vaccine failures, and overall effectiveness of the current strategy.

International Public Health Considerations

Obstacles to Global Use of the Vaccine

By 1995, the Hib vaccine was part of the routine national infant immunization program in fewer than 30 countries, primarily in North America, Western Europe, Australia, and New Zealand. Despite the dramatic decreases in disease in every pediatric population where the vaccine was introduced, the Expanded Programme on Immunisation-based immunization programs in developing countries failed to introduce the vaccine due to a number of factors.[493,498,499]

Perception of disease burden is a critical factor in deciding to use Hib vaccines in routine immunization programs, especially in developing countries where cost is an inhibiting factor. Recognition of Hib presents a substantial challenge in that (1) Hib is not associated with a specific,

clinically diagnosed disease syndrome (e.g., there are multiple etiologies of presumed bacterial meningitis and, except for the rare occurrence of epiglottitis, there is no specific clinical syndrome associated with Hib); (2) the disease syndromes with which it is associated are more popularly associated with other bacteria (i.e., N. meningitidis for meningitis, the pneumococcus for pneumonia); (3) antibiotics in most developing countries are given presumptively without obtaining diagnostic cultures; and (4) careful attention to specimen collection and laboratory technique is required for identification. In many developing countries, CSF and blood cultures are not obtained and Hib is not cultured in routine medical practice. As a consequence, physicians as well as the general population rarely diagnose and are not aware of Hib diseases.

In such populations, surveillance to assess disease burden is difficult or impossible to perform retrospectively. Because of difficulties in diagnosing Hib pneumonia, the primary marker of Hib disease burden has been meningitis. The number of studies in the developing world with optimal design for this purpose (population-based, laboratory-based prospective meningitis surveillance studies) is limited.[505–509] As noted above, available studies yield a picture in which rate of disease varies geographically. Published rates in North America and Africa generally range from 40 to 60 cases per 100,000 children less than 5 years old per year. In Europe, South America, and the Middle East, rates are usually in the range of 15 to 40 per 100,000 children less than 5 years. In Eastern Europe and the Asian mainland, rates of meningitis are usually less than 15 per 100,000, and often less than 5 per 100,000. The reasons for these apparent differences are unclear, and concern about the low rates in Asia in the mid-1990s led to a series of additional studies with increased attention to epidemiologic and laboratory parameters that could explain an underestimate of disease burden. Unpublished reports from these studies suggest, however, that rates on the Asian mainland are low (about 10 cases of meningitis per 100,000 children less than 5).

Although Hib conjugate vaccines were introduced in most industrialized countries because of a desire to reduce the burden of meningitis and other invasive disease, several studies suggest that Hib pneumonia may be the most important disease manifestation in developing countries. Vaccine efficacy studies in The Gambia and Chile suggest that Hib conjugate vaccine prevents 20% to 25% of pneumonia in children with a chest x-ray pattern consistent with bacterial pneumonia.[431,435] In these areas, three to five cases of Hib pneumonia were prevented for every case of Hib meningitis. Thus, in contrast to the industrialized world, where pneumonia in infants is not a major public health concern, the main public health benefit of Hib vaccines in developing countries may be prevention of pneumonia. This is especially relevant in countries with high infant mortality rates, in which pneumonia is often the single most common cause of death in children less than 5 years.

Efforts to better understand Hib disease burden in the developing world have led to development and publication of World Health Organization (WHO) guidelines for prospective, laboratory-based surveillance for Hib disease.[510] In addition, a tool for rapid assessment of Hib burden that generates estimates of combined meningitis and pneumonia burden from retrospective laboratory data and routine health statistics has been developed for use in developing countries.[511] Finally, a number of networks of laboratories have been developed to identify and report bacterial meningitis, including those in Asia, Latin America, Africa, and India.

Closely linked with the question of disease burden is the issue of cost of the vaccine to developing countries. Until recently, most developing countries included six vaccines (for measles, polio, bacille Calmette-Guérin, and DTP) in their routine infant programs. These countries can buy the complete primary immunization series for all six vaccines for a total of $1.00 per child. The most recent United Nations International Children's Emergency Fund price for Hib conjugate vaccines was $2.20 per dose, or nearly $7.00 per child for a primary series of Hib vaccine. Thus introduction of Hib conjugate vaccine may increase the cost of immunizations by a factor of 7. The necessity of committing this relatively massive amount of financial resource to a single disease prevention program has been a major constraint to the introduction of Hib vaccine into the developing world. By the year 2000, nearly 50% of countries with a gross national product per capita of $6,000 or above had introduced the vaccine, compared with less than 5% of the poorest countries, clear evidence of the impact of cost on introduction of the vaccine.

The inequity of the current system has drawn the attention of major donors and development partners, and was a major impetus to the formation of the Global Alliance for Vaccines and Immunization (GAVI) and the associated Vaccine Fund. Through the GAVI mechanism, countries have been offered subsidies for Hib and hepatitis B vaccines for a period of 5 years, after which it is hoped that the countries will be able to find additional ways to sustain an expanded program. By 2002, 10 of the poorest countries in the world have been approved for Hib vaccine through this program. It is hoped that, as the global supply of Hib conjugate vaccine expands, prices will decline. However, concerns about sustainability remain, and the cost of securing supplies of Hib conjugate vaccine remains a major stumbling block to wider implementation.

Immunization programs in developing countries have major challenges to overcome: paying for vaccine, achieving high coverage rates, obtaining consistent vaccine supplies, maintaining adequate transportation and cold chain storage, and training staff. Introduction of a new antigen into the immunization program necessarily requires changes, and often increased responsibilities for training, management, and monitoring. In programs that are already struggling to maintain themselves, the introduction of new vaccines is often viewed as an unnecessary burden. Concerns about whether new vaccines could be introduced successfully into developing countries have led to a number of approaches. It is recommended that, before introduction of new vaccines, a review of the current system be undertaken, with specific attention to those areas that will require alteration for the introduction. These may include storage and cold chain capacity and quality assessment, as well as preparations of training guidelines; evaluation of additional material needs, including injection safety equipment; and an assessment of what record-keeping materials require revision. Guidelines for introduction of Hib vaccine have been developed by the WHO that provide guidance for this process.[500] It is also obvious that, in developing countries, simplicity of presentation is very important. Thus new vaccines in combinations that do not require additional injections, and ideally do not require reconstitution, would be favored.

Future Adaptations for Broad Global Use

As outlined above, most of the early studies on Hib vaccines were performed with two- or three-dose primary series in the first 6 months of life, followed by a booster dose between 12 and 18 months. In contrast, introduction of Hib vaccine into much of the developing world is occurring without a booster dose, largely because of (1) cost, (2) high dropout rates in routine immunization program such that coverage with a booster dose would be very low, and (3) the age distribution of Hib disease, with most disease in children less than 1 year of age. The experience in the United Kingdom showing considerable effectiveness without a booster dose is particularly relevant, as are reports of effectiveness in The Gambia, where Hib disease has been reduced by over 90% with a three-dose primary schedule that does not include a booster dose.[490] However, continued surveillance to evaluate long-term impact with and without booster doses is critical.

The high cost of the vaccine for children in developing countries led some countries to evaluate the potential use of reduced dosages or schedules of vaccine. Lagos et al. evaluated both reduced number of doses in Chilean children and one-half and one-third doses of PRP-T and HbOC.[432a] Infants receiving a series of doses with one half or one third the usual amount of antigen had antibody responses as high as those receiving full doses, although the response to reduced doses of HbOC was lower. Nicol et al. demonstrated that one-tenth doses of PRP-T yielded a proportion of children with seroconversions and GMTs similar to those receiving full doses.[501] This presentation is particularly appealing operationally because it involved diluting a single-dose vial of lyophilized Hib with a 10-dose vial of DPT (both commercially available), and administering a standard 0.5-mL volume of the combination. Studies such as these raise the prospect of drastically reducing cost of Hib vaccine to developing countries. A number of issues must be addressed, however, before widespread use of reduced-dose schedules is adopted, the most important of which involve interaction with industry and regulatory bodies on licensing and recommendations for use.

Various vaccines and immunization strategies have been employed in different populations. This has been dictated by differences in licensure or availability of vaccines, differences in epidemiology, varying childhood immunization schedules, cost, and perceptions of disease burden. Initially, in industrialized countries, a primary series of two or three doses of Hib conjugate in infancy was recommended, followed by a single booster dose in the second year of life. Some countries included a catch-up campaign for older children, usually one dose given to children 1 to 4 years of age. More recently, as developing countries have introduced the vaccine, they have done so without catch-up campaigns. At the time of publication, approximately 90 countries had introduced Hib vaccine into their routine immunization program, a substantial increase from 1995 (Fig. 14–10).

Conclusions

Despite the availability of several Hib conjugate vaccines, reduction in cost, and the widespread success of Hib vaccines in controlling Hib disease in vaccinated populations, several critical issues remain concerning their use. Critical information on the clinical burden and epidemiology of disease in several areas of the world is still needed. Several recent studies performed in Eastern Europe and Asia show Hib as the major cause of bacterial meningitis, confirming its relative importance as a meningitis pathogen, but also show relatively low rates for all Hib disease. Although concern has been expressed about study methodology and laboratory methods for detection of Hib, these data suggest that prioritization of Hib vaccine use will vary by region. In addition, studies in The Gambia[431] and Chile[435] suggest that Hib vaccine significantly reduces the incidence of pneumonia, which is of potentially great importance to

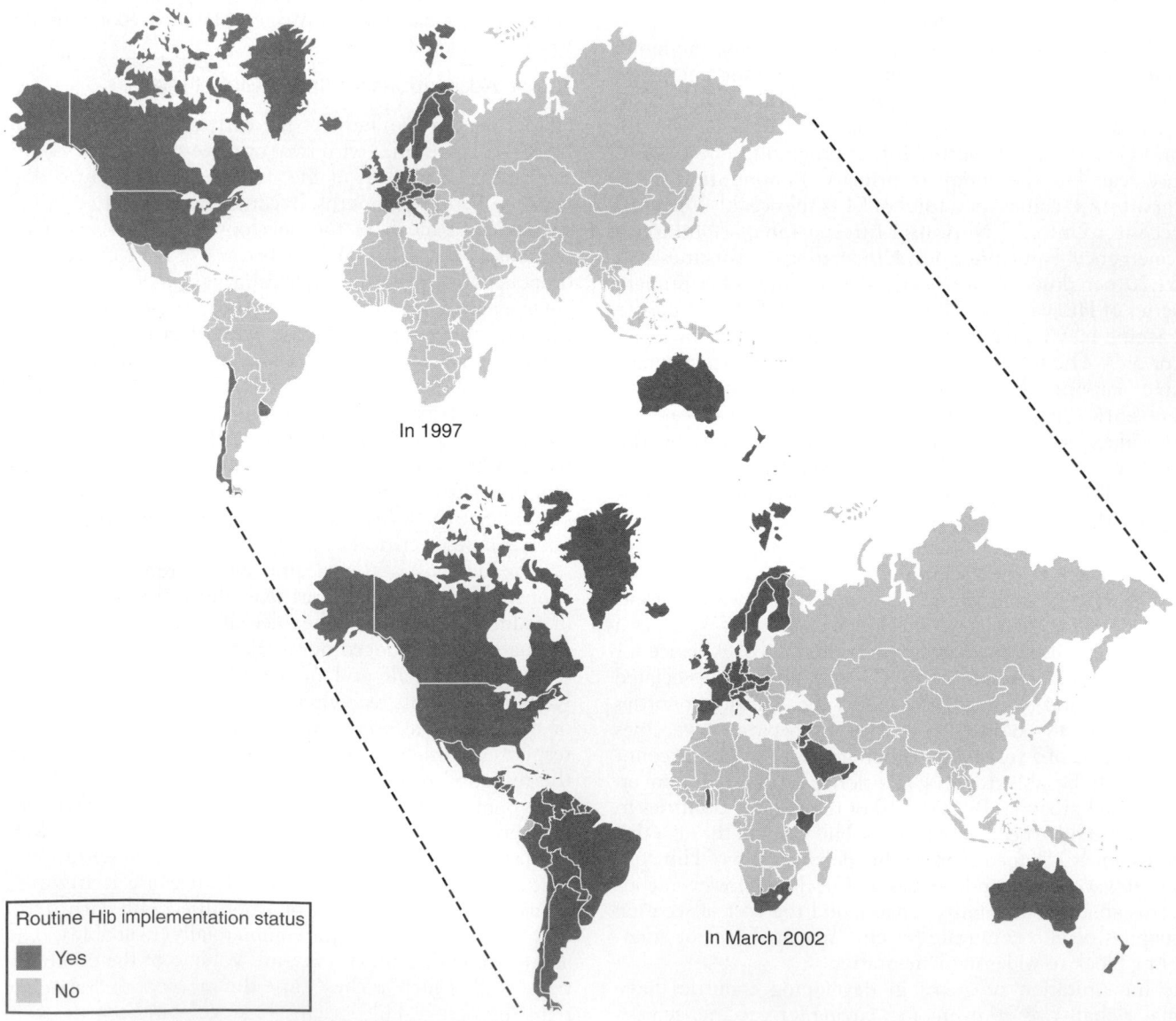

In 1997

In March 2002

Routine Hib implementation status
- ■ Yes
- ■ No

FIGURE 14–10 ■ Global progress in introduction of Hib conjugate vaccines. *Inset* shows countries that had introduced Hib conjugate vaccine into routine national immunization programs by mid-1997. Full figure shows countries that had introduced the vaccine by March 2002.

developing countries. Prioritization of Hib vaccine for introduction into developing countries must weigh cost as well as benefits for prevention of meningitis, pneumonia, and other Hib diseases.

Should the recommended schedules for each vaccine be altered to optimize protection? Several studies have suggested that alternative vaccine schedules (such as receiving the first dose at birth[502]) do not compromise immunogenicity. Others have shown that an initial dose of PRP-OMP at 2 months of age followed by subsequent doses of HbOC or PRP-T at 4 and 6 months provides enhanced immunogenicity after the third dose compared with vaccination with three doses of the same vaccine.[470,472] Could one induce earlier or greater immune responses with HbOC or PRP-T vaccine by the prior administration of diphtheria or tetanus toxoids so as to prime for the carrier proteins of these vaccines, through maternal immunization with subsequent transplacental transfer of antibody, as shown in one study,[503] or perhaps through subcutaneous rather than intramuscular injection?[504] Are current recommendations for booster immunization in the second year of life needed to ensure lifelong protection?

The immunologic determinants of protection are particularly important to delineate, as they are relevant to evaluating the protective efficacy of Hib and other conjugate vaccines, especially when detailed efficacy data may not be available. There are prospects for the construction of new polysaccharide-protein conjugate vaccines against other encapsulated bacterial pathogens or with protein carriers that may provide protection against all H. influenzae. Research in developmental immunology might explain why young infants and children are so uniquely susceptible to infection with encapsulated bacteria between 6 months and 2 years of age.

The differences in mucosal immunity induced by Hib conjugate vaccines[304] may be particularly relevant, because infection of mucosal membranes is undoubtedly the first step in the pathogenesis of disease. If the vaccines effectively eliminate carriage, as suggested by some studies,[300-303] or otherwise impede transmission of the organism, then there will be population-wide benefits in reduced disease risk, even for those who are not immunized.

Decades of clinical and laboratory work, begun more than 100 years ago, have led to the development of effective vaccines and the near-elimination of Hib disease in many countries. Before this effort, Hib was one of the most important bacterial pathogens of childhood. Amazingly, the degree of disease control has exceeded expectations, and is better than levels of immunization coverage and measured efficacy would have predicted. Unfortunately, Hib conjugate vaccines are not used in many of the most heavily affected countries in the world, leaving most of the world's children still at risk. The WHO has recently raised evaluation and control of Hib disease to high priority.

Although many unanswered questions remain, Hib disease has joined a growing list of major pediatric diseases now preventable by routine immunization. Hib conjugate vaccine technology has been the prototype for vaccines to prevent disease caused by other important encapsulated bacteria, such as the pneumococcus, meningococcus, and group B streptococcus. The lessons learned in the quest to eliminate Hib disease have important implications for the prevention of these and other bacterial diseases.

REFERENCES

1. Schlech WF, Ward JI, Band JD, et al. Bacterial meningitis in the United States, 1978 through 1981. The National Bacterial Meningitis Surveillance Study. JAMA 253:1749–1754, 1985.
2. Wenger JD, Hightower AW, Facklam RR, et al. Bacterial meningitis in the United States, 1986: report of a multistate surveillance study. The Bacterial Meningitis Study Group. J Infect Dis 162:1316–1323, 1990.
3. Santosham M, Kallman CH, Neff JM, Moxon ER. Absence of increasing incidence of meningitis caused by Haemophilus influenzae type b. J Infect Dis 140:1009–1012, 1979.
4. Winslow CE, Broadhurst J, Buchanan RE, et al. The families and genera of the bacteria: final report of the Committee of the Society of American Bacteriologists on Characterization and Classification of Bacterial Types. J Bacteriol 5:191–229, 1920.
5. Robbins JB, Parke JC Jr, Schneerson R, Whisnant JK. Quantitative measurement of "natural" and immunization-induced Haemophilus influenzae type b capsular polysaccharide antibodies. Pediatr Res 7:103–110, 1973.
6. Pittman M. Variation and type specificity in the bacterial species Haemophilus influenzae. J Exp Med 53:471–495, 1931.
7. Pittman M. The action of type-specific Haemophilus influenzae antiserum. J Exp Med 58:683–706, 1933.
8. Granoff DM, Shackelford PG, Pandey JP, Boies EG. Antibody responses to Haemophilus influenzae type b polysaccharide vaccine in relation to Km(1) and G2m(23) immunoglobulin allotypes. J Infect Dis 154:257–264, 1986.
9. Takala AK, Clements DA. Socioeconomic risk factors for invasive Haemophilus influenzae type b disease. J Infect Dis 165(suppl 1):S11–S15, 1992.
10. Marks MI, Dorchester WL. Secondary rates of Haemophilus influenzae type b disease among day care contacts. J Pediatr 111:305–306, 1987.
11. Alexander HE, Leidy G, MacPherson C. Production of types a, b, c, d, e, and f Haemophilus influenzae antibody for diagnostic and therapeutic purposes. J Immunol 54:207–211, 1946.
12. Alexander HE, Heidelberger M, Leidy G. The protective or curative element in type b Haemophilus influenzae rabbit serum. Yale J Biol Med 16:425–440, 1944.
13. Alexander HE. Experimental basis for treatment of Haemophilus influenzae infections. Am J Dis Child 66:160–171, 1943.
14. Fothergill LD, Wright J. Influenzal meningitis: the relation of age incidence to the bactericidal power of blood against the causal organism. J Immunol 24:273–284, 1933.
15. Johnston RB Jr, Anderson P, Rosen FS, Smith DH. Characterization of human immunity to polyribophosphate, the capsular antigen of Haemophilus influenzae, type b. Clin Immunol Immunopathol 1:234–240, 1973.
16. Anderson P, Johnston RB Jr, Smith DH. Human serum activities against Haemophilus influenzae, type b. J Clin Invest 51:31–38, 1972.
17. Schneerson R, Rodrigues LP, Parke JC Jr, Robbins JB. Immunity to disease caused by Haemophilus influenzae type b. II. Specificity and some biologic characteristics of "natural," infection-acquired, and immunization-induced antibodies to the capsular polysaccharide of Haemophilus influenzae type b. J Immunol 107:1081–1089, 1971.
18. Turk DC. Clinical importance of Haemophilus influenzae—1981. In Sell SH, Wright PF (eds). Haemophilus influenzae. New York, Elsevier Science Publishing, 1982, pp 3–9.
19. Todd JK, Bruhn FW. Severe Haemophilus influenzae infections. Am J Dis Child 129:607–611, 1975.
20. Dajani AS, Asmar BI, Thirumoorthi MC. Systemic Haemophilus influenzae disease: an overview. J Pediatr 94:355–364, 1979.
21. Granoff DM, Basden M. Haemophilus influenzae infections in Fresno County, California: a prospective study of the effects of age, race, and contact with a case on incidence of disease. J Infect Dis 141:40–46, 1980.
22. Peltola H, Virtanen M. Systemic Haemophilus influenzae infection in Finland. Clin Pediatr 23:275–280, 1984.

23. Cochi SL, Broome CV, Hightower AW. Immunization of U.S. children with *Haemophilus influenzae* type b polysaccharide vaccine: a cost-effectiveness model of strategy assessment. JAMA 253:521–529, 1985.

24. Taylor HG, Michaels RH, Mazur PM, et al. Intellectual, neuropsychological, and achievement outcomes in children six to eight years after recovery from *Haemophilus influenzae* meningitis. Pediatrics 74:198–205, 1984.

25. Feigin RD, Stechenberg BW, Chang MJ, et al. Prospective evaluation of treatment of *Haemophilus influenzae* meningitis. J Pediatr 88(4 pt 1):542–548, 1976.

26. Sell SHW, Merrill RE, Doyne EO, Zimsky EP. Long-term sequelae of *Haemophilus influenzae* meningitis. Pediatrics 49:206–217, 1972.

27. Sproles ET 3d, Azerrad J, Williamson C, Merrill RE. Meningitis due to *Haemophilus influenzae*: long-term sequelae. J Pediatr 75:782–788, 1969.

28. Dodge PR, Swartz MN. Bacterial meningitis—a review of selected aspects. II. Special neurologic problems, postmeningitis complications and clinicopathological correlations. N Engl J Med 272:1003–1010, 1965.

29. Ferry PC, Culbetson JL, Cooper JA. Sequence of *Haemophilus influenzae* meningitis. In Sell SH, Wright PF (eds). *Haemophilus influenzae*. New York, Elsevier Science Publishing, 1982, pp 111–117.

30. Pomeroy SL, Holmes SJ, Dodge PR, Feigin RD. Seizures and other neurologic sequelae of bacterial meningitis in children. N Engl J Med 323:1651–1657, 1990.

31. Taylor HG, Mills EL, Ciampi A, et al. The sequelae of *Haemophilus influenzae* meningitis in school-age children. N Engl J Med 323:1657–1663, 1990.

32. Harding AL, Anderson P, Howie VM, et al. *Haemophilus influenzae* isolated from otitis media. In Sell SH, Karzon DT (eds). *Haemophilus influenzae*. Nashville, TN, Vanderbilt University Press, 1973, pp 21–27.

33. Wallace RJ Jr, Baker CJ, Quinones FJ, et al. Nontypable *Haemophilus influenzae* (biotype 4) as a neonatal, maternal, and genital pathogen. Rev Infect Dis 5:123–136, 1983.

34. Campognone P, Singer DB. Neonatal sepsis due to nontypable *Haemophilus influenzae*. Am J Dis Child 140:117–121, 1986.

35. Falla TJ, Dobson SR, Crook DW, et al. Population-based study of nontypable *Haemophilus influenzae* invasive disease in children and neonates. Lancet 341:851–854, 1993.

36. Greenwood B. Epidemiology of acute lower respiratory tract infections, especially those due to *Haemophilus influenzae* type b, in The Gambia, West Africa. J Infect Dis 165(suppl 1):S26–S28, 1992.

37. Lehmann D. Epidemiology of acute respiratory tract infections, especially those due to *Haemophilus influenzae*, in Papua New Guinean children. J Infect Dis 165(suppl 1):S20–S25, 1992.

38. Shann F, Gratten M, Germer S, et al. Aetiology of pneumonia in children in Goroka Hospital, Papua New Guinea. Lancet 2:537–541, 1984.

39. Wall RA, Corrah PT, Mabey DC, Greenwood BM. The etiology of lobar pneumonia in The Gambia. Bull World Health Organ 64:553–558, 1986.

40. Shann F. Etiology of severe pneumonia in children in developing countries. Pediatr Infect Dis 5:247–252, 1986.

41. Campos JM. *Haemophilus*. In Murray PR (ed). Manual of Clinical Microbiology (6th ed). Washington, DC, ASM Press, 1995, pp 556–565.

42. Musser JM, Kroll JS, Moxon ER, Selander RK. Evolutionary genetics of the encapsulated strains of *Haemophilus influenzae*. Proc Natl Acad Sci U S A 85:7758–7762, 1988.

43. Mason EO Jr, Kaplan SL, Lamberth LB, et al. Serotype and ampicillin susceptibility of *Haemophilus influenzae* causing systemic infections in children: 3 years of experience. J Clin Microbiol 15:543–546, 1982.

44. van Ham SM, van Alphen L, Mooi FR. Fimbria-mediated adherence and hemagglutination of *Haemophilus influenzae*. J Infect Dis 165(suppl 1):S97–S99, 1992.

45. Centers for Disease Control. Ampicillin-resistant *Haemophilus influenzae* meningitis—Maryland, Georgia. MMWR 23:77–78, 1974.

46. Centers for Disease Control. Ampicillin-resistant *Haemophilus influenzae*—Texas. MMWR 23:99, 1974.

47. Tomeh MO, Starr SE, McGowan JE Jr, et al. Ampicillin-resistant *Haemophilus influenzae* type b infection. JAMA 229:295–297, 1974.

48. Khan W, Ross S, Rodriguez W, et al. *Haemophilus influenzae* type b resistant to ampicillin: a report of two cases. JAMA 229:298–301, 1974.

49. Schiffer MS, MacLowry J, Schneerson R, et al. Clinical, bacteriological, and immunological characterisation of ampicillin-resistant *Haemophilus influenzae* type b. Lancet 2:257–259, 1974.

50. American Academy of Pediatrics Committee on Infectious Diseases. Ampicillin-resistant strains of *Haemophilus influenzae* type B. Pediatrics 55:145–146, 1975.

51. Jacobson JA, McCormick JB, Hayes P, et al. Epidemiologic characteristics of infections caused by ampicillin-resistant *Haemophilus influenzae*. Pediatrics 58:388–391, 1976.

52. Istre GR, Conner JS, Glode MP, Hopkins RS. Increasing ampicillin-resistance rates in *Haemophilus influenzae* meningitis. Am J Dis Child 138:366–369, 1984.

53. Campos J, Garcia-Tornel S, Sanfeliu I. Susceptibility studies of multiply resistant *Haemophilus influenzae* isolated from pediatric patients and contacts. Antimicrob Agents Chemother 25:706–709, 1984.

54. Meyrovitch J, Frand M, Altman G, et al. Ampicillin-resistant *Haemophilus influenzae* type B infections in hospitalized pediatric patients. Isr J Med Sci 20:519–521, 1984.

55. Doern GV, Jorgensen JH, Thornsberry C, Preston DA. Prevalence of antimicrobial resistance among clinical isolates of *Haemophilus influenzae*: a collaborative study. Diagn Microbiol Infect Dis 4:95–107, 1986.

56. Campos J, Garcia-Tornel S, Gairi JM, Fabregues I. Multiply resistant *Haemophilus influenzae* type b causing meningitis: comparative clinical and laboratory study. J Pediatr 108:897–902, 1986.

57. Jorgensen JH. Update on mechanisms and prevalence of antimicrobial resistance in *Haemophilus influenzae* [see comments]. Clin Infect Dis 14:1119–1123, 1992.

58. Smith AL. Antibiotic resistance in *Haemophilus influenzae*. Pediatr Infect Dis 2:352–355, 1983.

59. Roberts MC, Swenson CD, Owens LM, Smith AL. Characterization of chloramphenicol-resistant *Haemophilus influenzae*. Antimicrob Agents Chemother 18:610–615, 1980.

60. Mendelman PM, Doroshow CA, Gandy SL, et al. Plasmid-mediated resistance in multiply resistant *Haemophilus influenzae* type b causing meningitis: molecular characterization of one strain and review of the literature. J Infect Dis 150:30–39, 1984.

61. Centers for Disease Control. Ampicillin and chloramphenicol resistance in systemic *Haemophilus influenzae* disease. MMWR 33:35–37, 1984.

62. Kenny JF, Isburg CD, Michaels RH. Meningitis due to *Haemophilus influenzae* type b resistant to both ampicillin and chloramphenicol. Pediatrics 66:14–16, 1980.

63. Uchiyama N, Greene GR, Kitts DB, Thrupp LD. Meningitis due to *Haemophilus influenzae* type b resistant to ampicillin and chloramphenicol. J Pediatr 97:421–424, 1980.

64. Simasathien S, Duangmani C, Echeverria P. *Haemophilus influenzae* type b resistant to ampicillin and chloramphenicol in an orphanage in Thailand. Lancet 2:1214–1217, 1980.

65. Feigin RD, McCracken GH Jr, Klein JO. Diagnosis and management of meningitis. Pediatr Infect Dis J 11:785–814, 1992.

66. Moxon ER. The carrier state: *Haemophilus influenzae*. J Antimicrob Chemother 18(suppl A):17–24, 1986.

67. Michaels RH, Norden CW. Pharyngeal colonization with *Haemophilus influenzae* type b: a longitudinal study of families with a child with meningitis or epiglottitis due to *H. influenzae* type b. J Infect Dis 136:222–228, 1977.

68. Murphy TV, Granoff D, Chrane DF, et al. Pharyngeal colonization with *Haemophilus influenzae* type b in children in a day care center without invasive disease. J Pediatr 106:712–716, 1985.

69. Ginsburg CM, McCracken GH Jr, Rae S, Parke JC Jr. *Haemophilus influenzae* type b disease: incidence in a day-care center. JAMA 238:604–607, 1977.

70. Granoff DM, Gilsdorf J, Gessert C, Basden M. *Haemophilus influenzae* type b disease in a day care center: eradication of carrier state by rifampin. Pediatrics 63:397–401, 1979.

71. Barenkamp SJ, Granoff DM, Munson RS Jr. Outer-membrane protein subtypes of *Haemophilus influenzae* type b and spread of disease in day-care centers. J Infect Dis 144:210–217, 1981.

72. Li KI, Dashefsky B, Wald ER. *Haemophilus influenzae* type b colonization in household contacts of infected and colonized children enrolled in day care. Pediatrics 78:15–20, 1986.

73. Ward JI, Gorman G, Phillips C, Fraser DW. *Haemophilus influenzae* type b disease in a day-care center: report of an outbreak. J Pediatr 92:713–717, 1978.

74. Campbell LR, Zedd AJ, Michaels RH. Household spread of infection due to *Haemophilus influenzae* type b. Pediatrics 66:115–117, 1980.

75. Michaels RH, Poziviak CS, Stonebraker FE, Norden CW. Factors affecting pharyngeal *Haemophilus influenzae* type b colonization rates in children. J Clin Microbiol 4:413–417, 1976.

76. Masters PL, Brumfitt W, Mendez RL, Likar M. Bacterial flora of the upper respiratory tract in Paddington families. Br Med J 1:1200–1205, 1958.

77. Dawson B, Zinnermann K. Incidence and type distribution of capsulated *Haemophilus influenzae* strains. Br Med J 1:740–742, 1952.

78. Mpairwe Y. Observations on the nasopharyngeal carriage of *Haemophilus influenzae* type b in children in Kampala, Uganda. J Hyg 68:337–341, 1970.

79. Turk DC. Naso-pharyngeal carriage of *Haemophilus influenzae* type B. J Hyg 61:247–256, 1963.

80. Lerman SJ, Kucera JC, Brunken JM. Nasopharyngeal carriage of antibiotic-resistant *Haemophilus influenzae* in healthy children. Pediatrics 64:287–291, 1979.

81. Hall DB, Lum MK, Knutson LR, et al. Pharyngeal carriage and acquisition of anticapsular antibody to *Haemophilus influenzae* type b in a high-risk population in southwestern Alaska. Am J Epidemiol 126:1190–1197, 1987.

82. Michaels RH, Stonebraker FE, Robbins JB. Use of antiserum agar for detection of *Haemophilus influenzae* type b in the pharynx. Pediatr Res 9:513–516, 1975.

83. Alpert G, Campos JM, Smith DR, et al. Incidence and persistence of *Haemophilus influenzae* type b upper airway colonization in patients with meningitis. J Pediatr 107:555–557, 1985.

84. Band JD, Fraser DW, Ajello G. Prevention of *Haemophilus influenzae* type b disease. JAMA 251:2381–2386, 1984.

85. Granoff DM, Munson RS Jr. Prospects for prevention of *Haemophilus influenzae* type b disease by immunization. J Infect Dis 153:448–461, 1986.

86. Greenfield S, Peter G, Howie VM, et al. Acquisition of type-specific antibodies to *Haemophilus influenzae* type b. J Pediatr 80:204–208, 1972.

87. Stephenson WP, Doern G, Gantz N, et al. Pharyngeal carriage rates of *Haemophilus influenzae*, type b and non-b, and prevalence of ampicillin-resistant *Haemophilus influenzae* among healthy day-care children in central Massachusetts. Am J Epidemiol 122:868–875, 1985.

88. Shapiro ED, Wald ER. Efficacy of rifampin in eliminating pharyngeal carriage of *Haemophilus influenzae* type b. Pediatrics 66:5–8, 1980.

89. Shapiro ED. Persistent pharyngeal colonization with *Haemophilus influenzae* type b after intravenous chloramphenicol therapy. Pediatrics 67:435–437, 1981.

90. Stephens DS, Farley MM. Pathogenic events during infection of the human nasopharynx with *Neisseria meningitidis* and *Haemophilus influenzae*. Rev Infect Dis 13:22–33, 1991.

91. Krasinski K, Nelson JD, Butler S, et al. Possible association of mycoplasma and viral respiratory infections with bacterial meningitis. Am J Epidemiol 125:499–508, 1987.

92. Takala AK, Meurman O, Kleemola M, et al. Preceding respiratory infection predisposing for primary and secondary invasive *Haemophilus influenzae* type b disease. Pediatr Infect Dis J 12:189–195, 1993.

93. Smith AL, Daum RS, Scheifele DW. Pathogenesis of *Haemophilus influenzae* meningitis. *In* Sell SH, Wright PF (eds). *Haemophilus influenzae*. New York, Elsevier Science Publishing, 1982, pp 89–109.

94. Moxon ER. Molecular basis of invasive *Haemophilus influenzae* type b disease. J Infect Dis 165(suppl 1):S77–S81, 1992.

95. Moxon ER, Smith AL, Averill DR, Smith DH. *Haemophilus influenzae* meningitis in infant rats after intranasal inoculation. J Infect Dis 129:154–162, 1974.

96. Ostrow PT, Moxon ER, Vernon N, Kapko R. Pathogenesis of bacterial meningitis: studies on the route of meningeal invasion following *Haemophilus influenzae* inoculation of infant rats. Lab Invest 40:678–685, 1979.

97. Gregorius FK, Johnson BL Jr, Stern WE, Brown WJ. Pathogenesis of hematogenous bacterial meningitis in rabbits. J Neurosurg 45:561–567, 1976.

98. Weller PF, Smith AL, Smith DH, Anderson P. Role of immunity in the clearance of bacteremia due to *Haemophilus influenzae*. J Infect Dis 138:427–436, 1978.

99. Weller PF, Smith AL, Anderson P, Smith DH. The role of encapsulation and host age in the clearance of *Haemophilus influenzae* bacteremia. J Infect Dis 135:34–41, 1977.

100. Rubin LG, Moxon ER. Pathogenesis of bloodstream invasion with *Haemophilus influenzae* type b. Infect Immun 41:280–294, 1983.

101. Scheld WM, Park TS, Dacey RG, et al. Clearance of bacteria from cerebrospinal fluid to blood in experimental meningitis. Infect Immun 24:102–105, 1979.

102. Feldman WE, Ginsburg CM, McCracken GH Jr, et al. Relation of concentrations of *Haemophilus influenzae* type b in cerebrospinal fluid to late sequelae of patients with meningitis. J Pediatr 100:209–212, 1982.

103. Feldman WE. Relation of concentrations of bacteria and bacterial antigen in cerebrospinal fluid to prognosis in patients with bacterial meningitis. N Engl J Med 296:433–435, 1977.

104. Chapin KC, Doern GV. Selective media for recovery of *Haemophilus influenzae* from specimens contaminated with upper respiratory tract microbial flora. J Clin Microbiol 17:1163–1165, 1983.

105. Rothstein EP, Madore DV, Girone JA, et al. Comparison of antigenuria after immunization with three *Haemophilus influenzae* type b conjugate vaccines. Pediatr Infect Dis J 10:311–314, 1991.

106. Spinola SM, Sheaffer CI, Philbrick KB, Gilligan PH. Antigenuria after *Haemophilus influenzae* type b polysaccharide immunization: a prospective study. J Pediatr 109:835–838, 1986.

107. Jacobs RF, Wright MW, Deskin RL, Bradsher RW. Delayed sterilization of *Haemophilus influenzae* type b meningitis with twice-daily ceftriaxone. JAMA 259:392–394, 1988.

108. Sirinavin S, Chiemchanya S, Visudhipan P, Lolekha S. Cefuroxime treatment of bacterial meningitis in infants and children. Antimicrob Agents Chemother 25:273–275, 1984.

109. Korones DN, Marshall GS, Shapiro ED. Outcome of children with occult bacteremia caused by *Haemophilus influenzae* type b. Pediatr Infect Dis J 11:516–520, 1992.

110. Cortese MM, Goepp J, Almeido-Hill J, et al. Children with *Haemophilus influenzae* bacteremia initially treated as outpatients: outcome in 85 American Indian children. Pediatr Infect Dis J 11:521–525, 1992.

111. Prober CG. The role of steroids in the management of children with bacterial meningitis. Pediatrics 95:29–31, 1995.

112. Institute of Medicine. Prospects for immunizing against *Haemophilus influenzae* type b. *In* New Vaccine Development: Establishing Priorities. Washington, DC, National Academy Press, 1985, pp 235–251.

113. Cochi SL, Broome CV. Vaccine prevention of *Haemophilus influenzae* type b disease: past, present and future. Pediatr Infect Dis 5:12–19, 1986.

114. Murphy TV, Clements JF, Petroni M, et al. *Haemophilus influenzae* type b in respiratory secretions. Pediatr Infect Dis J 8:148–151, 1989.

115. Makela PH, Takala AK, Peltola H, Eskola J. Epidemiology of invasive *Haemophilus influenzae* type b disease. J Infect Dis 165(suppl 1):S2–S6, 1992.

116. Shapiro ED, Ward JI. The epidemiology and prevention of disease caused by *Haemophilus influenzae* type b. Epidemiol Rev 13:113–142, 1991.

117. Cochi SL, Fleming DW, Hightower AW, et al. Primary invasive *Haemophilus influenzae* type b disease: a population-based assessment of risk factors. J Pediatr 108:887–896, 1986.

118. Baraff LJ, Wehrle PF. Epidemiology of pediatric meningitis: Los Angeles County, 1975 [abstract]. Pediatr Res 11:434, 1977.

119. Fraser DW, Henke CE, Feldman RA. Changing patterns of bacterial meningitis in Olmsted County, Minnesota, 1935–1970. J Infect Dis 128:300–307, 1973.

120. Fraser DW, Geil CC, Feldman RA. Bacterial meningitis in Bernalillo County, New Mexico: a comparison with three other American populations. Am J Epidemiol 100:29–34, 1974.

121. Fraser DW, Mitchell JE, Silverman LP, Feldman RA. Undiagnosed bacterial meningitis in Vermont children. Am J Epidemiol 102:394–399, 1975.

122. Istre GR, Conner JS, Broome CV, et al. Risk factors for primary invasive *Haemophilus influenzae* disease: increased risk from day care attendance and school-aged household members. J Pediatr 106:190–195, 1985.

123. Parke JC Jr, Schneerson R, Robbins JB. The attack rate, age incidence, racial distribution, and case fatality rate of *Haemophilus influenzae* type b meningitis in Mecklenburg County, North Carolina. J Pediatr 81:765–769, 1972.

124. Murphy TV, Osterholm MT, Pierson LM, et al. Prospective surveillance of *Haemophilus influenzae* type b disease in Dallas County, Texas, and in Minnesota. Pediatrics 79:173–180, 1987. [erratum appears in Pediatrics 79:863, 1987]

125. Redmond SR, Pichichero ME. *Haemophilus influenzae* type b disease: an epidemiologic study with special reference to day-care centers. JAMA 252:2581–2584, 1984.

126. Smith EW Jr, Haynes RE. Changing incidence of *Haemophilus influenzae* meningitis. Pediatrics 50:723–727, 1972.

127. Ward JI, Lum MK, Hall DB, et al. Invasive *Haemophilus influenzae* type b disease in Alaska: background epidemiology for a vaccine efficacy trial. J Infect Dis 153:17–26, 1986.

128. Tarr PI, Peter G. Demographic factors in the epidemiology of *Haemophilus influenzae* meningitis in young children. J Pediatr 92:884–888, 1978.

129. Floyd RF, Federspiel CF, Schaffner W. Bacterial meningitis in urban and rural Tennessee. Am J Epidemiol 99:395–407, 1974.

130. Fraser DW. *Haemophilus influenzae* in the community and in the home. *In* Sell SH, Wright PF (eds). *Haemophilus influenzae*. New York, Elsevier Science Publishing, 1982, pp 11–22.

131. Peltola H, Rod TO, Jonsdottir K, et al. Life-threatening *Haemophilus influenzae* infections in Scandinavia: a five-country analysis of the incidence and the main clinical and bacteriologic characteristics. Rev Infect Dis 12:708–715, 1990.

132. Claesson B, Trollfors B, Jodal U, Rosenhall U. Incidence and prognosis of *Haemophilus influenzae* meningitis in children in a Swedish region. Pediatr Infect Dis 3:35–39, 1984.

133. Salwen KM, Vikerfors T, Olcen P. Increased incidence of childhood bacterial meningitis: a 25-year study in a defined population in Sweden. Scand J Infect Dis 19:1–11, 1987.

134. Trollfors B, Claesson BA, Strangert K, Taranger J. *Haemophilus influenzae* meningitis in Sweden, 1981–1983. Arch Dis Child 62:1220–1223, 1987.

135. Valmari P, Kataja M, Peltola H. Invasive *Haemophilus influenzae* and meningococcal infections in Finland: a climatic, epidemiologic and clinical approach. Scand J Infect Dis 19:19–27, 1987.

136. Peltola H, Kayhty H, Virtanen M, Makela PH. Prevention of *Haemophilus influenzae* type b bacteremic infection with the capsular polysaccharide vaccine. N Engl J Med 310:1561–1566, 1984.

137. Spanjaard L, Bol P, Ekker W, Zanen HC. The incidence of bacterial meningitis in the Netherlands—a comparison of three registration systems, 1977–1982. J Infect 11:259–268, 1985.

138. Hanna JN. The epidemiology of invasive *Haemophilus influenzae* infections in children under five years of age in the Northern Territory: a three-year study [see comments]. Med J Aust 152:234–236, 1990.

139. Hammond GW, Rutherford BE, Malazdrewicz R, et al. *Haemophilus influenzae* meningitis in Manitoba and the Keewatin District, NWT: potential for mass vaccination. CMAJ 139:743–747, 1988.

140. Varaghese P. *Haemophilus influenzae* infection in Canada, 1969–1985. Can Dis Wkly Rep 12:37–43, 1986.

141. Broughton SJ, Warren RE. A review of *Haemophilus influenzae* infections in Cambridge, 1975–1981. J Infect 9:30–42, 1984.

142. Davey PG, Cruikshank JK, McManus IC, et al. Bacterial meningitis—ten years' experience. J Hyg 88:383–401, 1982.

143. Cadoz M, Prince-David M, Diop Mar I, Denis F. Epidemiology and prognosis of *Haemophilus influenzae* meningitis in Africa (901 cases) [in French]. Pathol Biol 31:128–133, 1983.

144. Bijlmer HA, van Alphen L, Greenwood BM, et al. The epidemiology of *Haemophilus influenzae* meningitis in children under five years of age in The Gambia, West Africa. J Infect Dis 161:1210–1215, 1990.

145. Wright PF. Approaches to prevent acute bacterial meningitis in developing countries. Bull World Health Organ 67:479–486, 1989.

146. Cadoz M, Denis F, Diop Mar I. An epidemiological study of purulent meningitis cases admitted to hospital in Dakar, 1970–1979 [in French]. Bull World Health Organ 59:575–584, 1981.

147. Bijlmer HA. World-wide epidemiology of *Haemophilus influenzae* meningitis: industrialized versus non-industrialized countries. Vaccine 9(suppl):S5–S9, 1991.

148. Clements DA, Booy R, Dagan R, McManus IC, et al. Comparison of the epidemiology and cost of *Haemophilus influenzae* type b disease in five western countries. Pediatr Infect Dis J 12:362–367, 1993. [erratum appears in Pediatr Infect Dis J 12:570, 1993]

149. Gomez E, Peguero M, Sanchez J, et al. Population-based surveillance for bacterial meningitis in the Dominican Republic: implications for control by vaccination. Epidemiol Infect 125:549–554, 2000.

150. Hanna JN, Wild BE. Bacterial meningitis in children under five years of age in Western Australia. Med J Aust 155:160–164, 1991.

151. Hansman D, Hanna J, Morey F. High prevalence of invasive *Haemophilus influenzae* disease in central Australia, 1986 [letter]. Lancet 2:927, 1986.

152. Losonsky GA, Santosham M, Sehgal VM, et al. *Haemophilus influenzae* disease in the White Mountain Apaches: molecular epidemiology of a high-risk population. Pediatr Infect Dis 3:539–547, 1984.

153. Coulehan JL, Michaels RH, Williams KE, et al. Bacterial meningitis in Navajo Indians. Public Health Rep 91:464–468, 1976.

154. Coulehan JL, Michaels RH, Hallowell C, et al. Epidemiology of *Haemophilus influenzae* type B disease among Navajo Indians. Public Health Rep 99:404–409, 1984.

155. Ostroy PR. Bacterial meningitis in Washington state. West J Med 131:339–343, 1979.

156. Wotton KA, Stiver HG, Hildes JA. Meningitis in the central Arctic: a 4-year experience. Can Med Assoc J 124:887–890, 1981.

157. Gilsdorf JR. Bacterial meningitis in southwestern Alaska. Am J Epidemiol 106:388–391, 1977.

158. Ward JI, Margolis HS, Lum MK, et al. *Haemophilus influenzae* disease in Alaskan Eskimos: characteristics of a population with an unusual incidence of invasive disease. Lancet 1:1281–1285, 1982.

159. Campagne G, Schuchat A, Djibo S, et al. Epidemiology of bacterial meningitis in Niamey, Niger, 1981–1996. Bull World Health Organ 77:499–508, 1999.

160. Adegbola RA, Mulholland EK, Falade AG, et al. *Haemophilus influenzae* type b disease in the western region of The Gambia: background surveillance for a vaccine efficacy trial. Ann Trop Paediatr 16:103–111, 1996.

161. Peltola H. Burden of meningitis and other severe bacterial infections of children in Africa: implications for prevention. Clin Infect Dis 32:64–75, 2001.

162. Lee YS, Kumarasinghe G, Chow C, et al. Invasive *Haemophilus influenzae* type b infections in Singapore children: a hospital-based study. J Pediatr Child Health 36:125–127, 2000.

163. Yonghong Y, Zhigua L, Xuzhuang S, et al. Acute bacterial meningitis in children in Hefea, China 1990–1992. Chinese Medical J 109:385–388, 1996.

164. Lau YL, Low LCK, Yung R, et al. Invasive *Haemophilus influenzae* type b infections in children hospitalized in Hom Kong 1986–1990. Acta Paediatr 84:173–176, 1995.

165. Limcangco MR, Salole EG, Armour CL. Epidemiology of *Haemophilus influenzae* type b meningitis in Manila, Philippines, 1994 to 1996. Pediatr Infect Dis J 19:7–11, 2000.

166. Lupisan SP, Herva E, Nohynek H, et al. Incidence of invasive *Haemophilus influenzae* type b infections in Filipino children. Pediatr Infect Dis J 19:1020–1022, 2000.

167. Hsueh PR, Wu JJ, Hsiue TR. Invasive *Streptococcus pneumoniae* infection associated with rapidly fatal outcome in Taiwan. J Formos Med Assoc 95:364–371, 1996.

168. Invasive Bacterial Infections Surveillance (IBIS) Group of the International Clinical Epidemiology Network. Are *Haemophilus influenzae* infections a significant problem in India? A prospective study and review. Clin Infect Dis 34:949–957, 2002.

169. Nakano T, Ihara T, Kamiya H, et al. Incidence of *Haemophilus influenzae* type b meningitis in Mie prefecture, Japan. Pediatr Int 43:323–324, 2001.

170. Broome CV, Schlech WF III. Recent developments in the epidemiology of bacterial meningitis. *In* Sande MA, Smith A, Root RD (eds). Bacterial Meningitis. Edinburgh, Churchill Livingstone, 1985, pp 1–10.

171. Bijlmer HA, van Alphen L. A prospective, population-based study of *Haemophilus influenzae* type b meningitis in The Gambia and the possible consequences. J Infect Dis 165(suppl 1):S29–S32, 1992.

172. Farley MM, Stephens DS, Brachman PS Jr, et al. Invasive *Haemophilus influenzae* disease in adults: a prospective, population-based surveillance. CDC Meningitis Surveillance Group [see comments]. Ann Intern Med 116:806–812, 1992.

173. Takala AK, Eskola J, van Alphen L. Spectrum of invasive *Haemophilus influenzae* type b disease in adults. Arch Intern Med 150:2573–2576, 1990.

174. Vadheim CM, Greenberg DP, Bordenave N, et al. Risk factors for invasive *Haemophilus influenzae* type b in Los Angeles County children 18–60 months of age. Am J Epidemiol 136:221–235, 1992.

175. Yost GC, Kaplan AM, Bustamante R, et al. Bacterial meningitis in Arizona American Indian children. Am J Dis Child 140:943–946, 1986.

176. Ounsted C. *Haemophilus influenzae* meningitis: a possible ecological factor. Lancet 1:161–162, 1950.

177. Granoff DM, Boies EG, Squires JE, et al. Histocompatibility leukocyte antigen and erythrocyte MNS specificities in patients with

meningitis or epiglottitis due to *Haemophilus influenzae* type b. J Infect Dis 149:373–377, 1984.

178. Michaels RH, Schultz WF. The frequency of *Haemophilus influenzae* infections: analysis of racial and environmental factors. *In* Sell SH, Karzon DT (eds). *Haemophilus influenzae*. Nashville, TN, Vanderbilt University Press, 1973, pp 243–250.

179. Jafari HS, Adams WG, Robinson KA, et al. Efficacy of *Haemophilus influenzae* type b conjugate vaccines and persistence of disease in disadvantaged populations. The *Haemophilus influenzae* Study Group. Am J Public Health 89:364–368, 1999.

180. Lum MK, Ward JI, Bender TR. Protective influence of breast feeding on the risk of developing invasive *Haemophilus influenzae* type b disease [abstract]. Pediatr Res 16(pt 2):436, 1982.

181. Takala AK, Eskola J, Palmgren J, et al. Risk factors of invasive *Haemophilus influenzae* type b disease among children in Finland. J Pediatr 115(5 pt 1):694–701, 1989.

182. Petersen GM, Silimperi DR, Chiu CY, Ward JI. Effects of age, breast feeding, and household structure on *Haemophilus influenzae* type b disease risk and antibody acquisition in Alaskan Eskimos. Am J Epidemiol 134:1212–1221, 1991.

183. Silfverdal SA, Bodin L, Hugosson S, et al. Protective effect of breast-feeding on invasive *Haemophilus influenzae* infection: a case-control study in Swedish preschool children. Int J Epidemiol 26:443–450, 1997.

184. Goldman AS. The immune system of human milk: antimicrobial, anti-inflammatory and immunomodulating properties. Pediatr Infect Dis J 12:664–671, 1993.

185. Pichichero ME, Sommerfelt AE, Steinhoff MC, Insel RA. Breast milk antibody to the capsular polysaccharide of *Haemophilus influenzae* type b. J Infect Dis 142:694–698, 1980.

186. Insel RA, Amstey M, Pichichero ME. Postimmunization antibody to the *Haemophilus influenzae* type b capsule in breast milk. J Infect Dis 152:407–408, 1985.

187. Casadevall A, Dobroszycki J, Small C, Pirofski LA. *Haemophilus influenzae* type b bacteremia in adults with AIDS and at risk for AIDS [see comments]. Am J Med 92:587–590, 1992.

188. Schlamm HT, Yancovitz SR. *Haemophilus influenzae* pneumonia in young adults with AIDS, ARC, or risk of AIDS. Am J Med 86:11–14, 1989.

189. Steinhart R, Reingold AL, Taylor F, et al. Invasive *Haemophilus influenzae* infections in men with HIV infection. JAMA 268:3350–3352, 1992.

190. Ward J, Smith AL. *Haemophilus influenzae* bacteremia in children with sickle cell disease. J Pediatr 88:261–263, 1976.

191. Powars D, Overturf G, Turner E. Is there an increased risk of *Haemophilus influenzae* septicemia in children with sickle cell anemia? Pediatrics 71:927–931, 1983.

192. Zarkowsky HS, Gallagher D, Gill FM, et al. Bacteremia in sickle hemoglobinopathies. J Pediatr 109:579–585, 1986.

193. Chilcote RR, Baehner RL, Hammond D. Septicemia and meningitis in children splenectomized for Hodgkin's disease. N Engl J Med 295:798–800, 1976.

194. Rosen FS, Janeway CA. The gamma globulins. 3. The antibody deficiency syndromes. N Engl J Med 275:769–775, 1966.

195. Farrand RJ. Recurrent haemophilus septicaemia and immunoglobulin deficiency. Arch Dis Child 45:582–584, 1970.

196. Figueroa JE, Densen P. Infectious diseases associated with complement deficiencies. Clin Microbiol Rev 4:359–395, 1991.

197. Ross SC, Densen P. Complement deficiency states and infection: epidemiology, pathogenesis and consequences of neisserial and other infections in an immune deficiency. Medicine (Baltimore) 63:243–273, 1984.

198. Siber GR. Bacteremias due to *Haemophilus influenzae* and *Streptococcus pneumoniae*: their occurrence and course in children with cancer. Am J Dis Child 134:668–672, 1980.

199. Bartlett AV, Zusman J, Daum RS. Unusual presentations of *Haemophilus influenzae* infections in immunocompromised patients. J Pediatr 102:55–58, 1983.

200. Weitzman S, Aisenberg AC. Fulminant sepsis after the successful treatment of Hodgkin's disease. Am J Med 62:47–50, 1977.

201. Myerowitz RL, Norden CW. Immunology of the infant rat experimental model of *Haemophilus influenzae* type b meningitis. Infect Immun 16:218–225, 1977.

202. Michaels RH, Myerowitz RL, Klaw R. Potentiation of experimental meningitis due to *Haemophilus influenzae* by influenza A virus. J Infect Dis 135:641–645, 1977.

203. Granoff DM, Suarez BK, Pandey JP, Shackelford PG. Genes associated with the G2m(23) immunoglobulin allotype regulate the IgG subclass responses to *Haemophilus influenzae* type b polysaccharide vaccine. J Infect Dis 157:1142–1149, 1988.

204. Lenoir AA, Pandey JP, Granoff DM. Antibody responses of black children to *Haemophilus influenzae* type b polysaccharide–*Neisseria meningitidis* outer-membrane protein conjugate vaccine in relation to the Km(1) allotype. J Infect Dis 157:1242–1245, 1988.

205. Whisnant JK, Rogentine GN, Mann DL, Robbins JB. Human cell-surface structures related to *Haemophilus influenzae* type b disease. Lancet 2:895–898, 1971.

206. Whisnant JK, Rogentine GN, Gralnick MA, et al. Host factors and antibody response in *Haemophilus influenzae* type b meningitis and epiglottitis. J Infect Dis 133:448–455, 1976.

207. Tejani A, Mahadevan R, Dobias B, et al. Occurrence of HLA types in *H. influenzae* type b disease. Tissue Antigens 17:205–211, 1981.

208. Petersen GM, Silimperi DR, Rotter JI, et al. Genetic factors in *Haemophilus influenzae* type b disease susceptibility and antibody acquisition. J Pediatr 110:228–233, 1987.

209. Granoff DM, Pandey JP, Boies E, et al. Response to immunization with *Haemophilus influenzae* type b polysaccharide-pertussis vaccine and risk of *Haemophilus* meningitis in children with the Km(1) immunoglobulin allotype. J Clin Invest 74:1708–1714, 1984.

210. Ambrosino DM, Schiffman G, Gotschlich EC, et al. Correlation between G2m(n) immunoglobulin allotype and human antibody response and susceptibility to polysaccharide encapsulated bacteria. J Clin Invest 75:1935–1942, 1985.

211. Granoff DM, Boies E, Squires J, et al. Interactive effect of genes associated with immunoglobulin allotypes and HLA specificities on susceptibility to *Haemophilus influenzae* disease. J Immunogenet 11(3–4):181–188, 1984.

212. Petersen GM, Silimperi DR, Scott EM, et al. Uridine monophosphate kinase 3: a genetic marker for susceptibility to *Haemophilus influenzae* type b disease. Lancet 2:417–419, 1985.

213. David DJ. Influenzal meningitis. Arch Intern Med 4:323–329, 1909.

214. Centers for Disease Control. Prevention of secondary cases of *Haemophilus influenzae* type b disease. 31:672–680, 1982.

215. Centers for Disease Control. Update: prevention of *Haemophilus influenzae* type b disease. MMWR 37:13–16, 1988.

216. Glode MP, Daum RS, Halsey NA, et al. Rifampin alone and in combination with trimethoprim in chemoprophylaxis for infections due to *Haemophilus influenzae* type b. Rev Infect Dis 5(suppl 3):S549–S555, 1983.

217. Ward JI, Fraser DW, Baraff LJ, Plikaytis BD. *Haemophilus influenzae* meningitis: a national study of secondary spread in household contacts. N Engl J Med 301:122–126, 1979.

218. Fleming DW, Leibenhaut MH, Albanes D, et al. Secondary *Haemophilus influenzae* type b in day-care facilities: risk factors and prevention. JAMA 254:509–514, 1985.

219. Centers for Disease Control and Prevention. Recommendations for use of *Haemophilus influenzae* conjugate vaccines and a combined diphtheria, tetanus, pertussis, and *Haemophilus* b vaccine: recommendations of the Advisory Committee on Immunization Practices (ACIP). MMWR 42(RR-13):1–15, 1993.

220. Osterholm MT, Pierson LM, White KE, et al. The risk of subsequent transmission of *Haemophilus influenzae* type b disease among children in day care: results of a two-year statewide prospective surveillance and contact survey. N Engl J Med 316:1–5, 1987.

221. Murphy TV, Clements JF, Breedlove JA, et al. Risk of subsequent disease among day-care contacts of patients with systemic *Haemophilus influenzae* type b disease. N Engl J Med 316:5–10, 1987.

222. Makintubee S, Istre GR, Ward JI. Transmission of invasive *Haemophilus influenzae* type b disease in day care settings. J Pediatr 111:180–186, 1987.

223. Broome CV, Mortimer EA, Katz SL, et al. Use of chemoprophylaxis to prevent the spread of *Haemophilus influenzae* B in day-care facilities. N Engl J Med 316:1226–1228, 1987.

224. Dashefsky B, Wald E, Li K. Management of contacts of children in day care with invasive *Haemophilus influenzae* type b disease. Pediatrics 78:939–941, 1986.

225. Bachrach S. An outbreak of *Haemophilus influenzae* type b bacteraemia in an intermediate care hospital for children. J Hosp Infect 11:121–126, 1988.

226. Smith PF, Stricof RL, Shayegani M, Morse DL. Cluster of *Haemophilus influenzae* type b infections in adults. JAMA 260:1446–1449, 1988.

227. Barton LL, Granoff DM, Barenkamp SJ. Nosocomial spread of *Haemophilus influenzae* type b infection documented by outer membrane protein subtype analysis. J Pediatr 102:820–824, 1983.

228. Devine LF, Johnson DP, Hagerman CR, et al. Rifampin: levels in serum and saliva and effect on the meningococcal carrier state. JAMA 214:1055–1059, 1970.

229. McCracken GH Jr, Ginsburg CM, Zweighaft TC, Clahsen J. Pharmacokinetics of rifampin in infants and children: relevance to prophylaxis against *Haemophilus influenzae* type b disease. Pediatrics 66:17–21, 1980.

230. Glode MP, Daum RS, Goldmann DA, et al. *Haemophilus influenzae* type B meningitis: a contagious disease of children. Br Med J 280:899–901, 1980.

231. Campos J, Garcia-Tornel S, Roca J, Iriondo M. Rifampin for eradicating carriage of multiply resistant *Haemophilus influenzae* type b. Pediatr Infect Dis J 6:719–721, 1987.

232. Cox F, Trincher R, Rissing JP, et al. Rifampin prophylaxis for contacts of *Haemophilus influenzae* type b disease. JAMA 245:1043–1045, 1981.

233. Gessert C, Granoff DM, Gilsdorf J. Comparison of rifampin and ampicillin in day care center contacts of *Haemophilus influenzae* type b disease. Pediatrics 66:1–4, 1980.

234. Daum RS, Glode MP, Goldmann DA, et al. Rifampin chemoprophylaxis for household contacts of patients with invasive infections due to *Haemophilus influenzae* type b. J Pediatr 98:485–491, 1981.

235. Glode MP, Daum RS, Boies EG, et al. Effect of rifampin chemoprophylaxis on carriage eradication and new acquisition of *Haemophilus influenzae* type b in contacts. Pediatrics 76:537–542, 1985.

236. Yogev R, Lander HB, Davis AT. Effect of rifampin on nasopharyngeal carriage of *Haemophilus influenzae* type b. J Pediatr 94:840–841, 1979.

237. Yogev R, Melick C, Kabat K. Nasopharyngeal carriage of *Haemophilus influenzae* type b: attempted eradication by cefaclor or rifampin. Pediatrics 67:430–433, 1981.

238. Darouiche R, Perkins B, Musher D, et al. Levels of rifampin and ciprofloxacin in nasal secretions: correlation with MIC90 and eradication of nasopharyngeal carriage of bacteria. J Infect Dis 162:1124–1127, 1990.

239. Hansen EJ, Frisch CF, Johnston KH. Detection of antibody-accessible proteins on the cell surface of *Haemophilus influenzae* type b. Infect Immun 33:950–953, 1981.

240. Gotoff SP. On the surface of *Haemophilus influenzae*. J Infect Dis 143:747–748, 1981.

241. Loeb MR, Smith DH. Human antibody response to individual outer membrane proteins of *Haemophilus influenzae* type b. Infect Immun 37:1032–1036, 1982.

242. Inzana TJ, Anderson P. Serum factor-dependent resistance of *Haemophilus influenzae* type b to antibody to lipopolysaccharide. J Infect Dis 151:869–877, 1985.

243. Shenep JL, Munson RS Jr, Granoff DM. Human antibody responses to lipopolysaccharide after meningitis due to *Haemophilus influenzae* type b. J Infect Dis 145:181–190, 1982.

244. Anderson P, Flesher A, Shaw S, et al. Phenotypic and genetic variation in the susceptibility of *Haemophilus influenzae* type b to antibodies to somatic antigens. J Clin Invest 65:885–891, 1980.

245. Lagergard T, Nylen O, Sandberg T, Trollfors B. Antibody responses to capsular polysaccharide, lipopolysaccharide, and outer membrane in adults infected with *Haemophilus influenzae* type b. J Clin Microbiol 20:1154–1158, 1984.

246. Robbins JB, Schneerson R, Pittman M. *Haemophilus influenzae* type b infections. *In* Germanier R (ed). Bacterial Vaccines. Orlando, FL, Academic Press, 1984, pp 290–313.

247. Tosi MF, Kaplan SL, Mason EO, et al. Generation of chemotactic activity in serum by *Haemophilus influenzae* type b. Infect Immun 43:593–599, 1984.

248. Tarr PI, Hosea SW, Brown EJ, et al. The requirement of specific anticapsular IgG for killing of *Haemophilus influenzae* by the alternative pathway of complement activation. J Immunol 128:1772–1775, 1982.

249. Quinn PH, Crosson FJ Jr, Winkelstein JA, Moxon ER. Activation of the alternative complement pathway by *Haemophilus influenzae* type b. Infect Immun 16:400–402, 1977.

250. Crosson FJ Jr, Winkelstein JA, Moxon ER. Participation of complement in the nonimmune host defense against experimental *Haemophilus influenzae* type b septicemia and meningitis. Infect Immun 14:882–887, 1976.

251. Steele NP, Munson RS Jr, Granoff DM, et al. Antibody-dependent alternative pathway killing of *Haemophilus influenzae* type b. Infect Immun 44:452–458, 1984.

252. Winkelstein JA, Moxon ER. The role of complement in the host's defense against *Haemophilus influenzae*. J Infect Dis 165(suppl 1):S62–S65, 1992.

253. Newman SL, Waldo B, Johnston RB Jr. Separation of serum bactericidal and opsonizing activities for *Haemophilus influenzae* type b. Infect Immun 8:488–490, 1973.

254. Hayashi K, Lee DA, Quie PG. Chemiluminescent response of polymorphonuclear leukocytes to *Streptococcus pneumoniae* and *Haemophilus influenzae* in suspension and adhered to glass. Infect Immun 52:397–400, 1986.

255. Norden CW. Prevalence of bactericidal antibodies to *Haemophilus influenzae*, type b. J Infect Dis 130:489–494, 1974.

256. Feigin RD, Richmond D, Hosler DW, Shackelford PG. Reassessment of the role of bactericidal antibody in *Haemophilus influenzae* infection. Am J Med Sci 262:338–346, 1971.

257. Dahlberg-Lagergard T. Target antigens for bactericidal and opsonizing antibodies to *Haemophilus influenzae*. Acta Pathol Microbiol Immunol Scand [C] 90:209–216, 1982.

258. Stull TL, Jacobs RF, Haas JE, et al. Human serum bactericidal activity against *Haemophilus influenzae* type b. J Gen Microbiol 130(pt 3):665–672, 1984.

259. Lee CJ, Malik FG, Robbins JB. The regulation of the immune response of mice to *Haemophilus influenzae* type b capsular polysaccharide. Immunology 34:149–156, 1978.

260. Schneerson R, Robbins JB. Age-related susceptibility to *Haemophilus influenzae* type b disease in rabbits. Infect Immun 4:397–401, 1971.

261. Santosham M, Reid R, Ambrosino DM, et al. Prevention of *Haemophilus influenzae* type b infections in high-risk infants treated with bacterial polysaccharide immune globulin. N Engl J Med 317:923–929, 1987.

262. Kayhty H, Karanko V, Peltola H, Makela PH. Serum antibodies after vaccination with *Haemophilus influenzae* type b capsular polysaccharide and responses to reimmunization: no evidence of immunologic tolerance or memory. Pediatrics 74:857–865, 1984.

263. Anderson P, Smith DH, Ingram DL, et al. Antibody of polyribophate of *Haemophilus influenzae* type b in infants and children: effect of immunization with polyribophosphate. J Infect Dis 136(suppl):S57–S62, 1977.

264. Smith DH, Peter G, Ingram DL, et al. Responses of children immunized with the capsular polysaccharide of *Haemophilus influenzae*, type b. Pediatrics 52:637–644, 1973.

265. Anderson P, Peter G, Johnston RB Jr, et al. Immunization of humans with polyribophosphate, the capsular antigen of *Haemophilus influenzae*, type b. J Clin Invest 51:39–44, 1972.

266. Robbins JB, Schneerson R, Glode MP, et al. Cross-reactive antigens and immunity to diseases caused by encapsulated bacteria. J Allergy Clin Immunol 56:141–151, 1975.

267. Schneerson R, Robbins JB. Induction of serum *Haemophilus influenzae* type b capsular antibodies in adult volunteers fed cross-reacting *Escherichia coli* O75:K100:H5. N Engl J Med 292:1093–1096, 1975.

268. Schreiber JR, Barrus V, Cates KL, Siber GR. Functional characterization of human IgG, IgM, and IgA antibody directed to the capsule of *Haemophilus influenzae* type b. J Infect Dis 153:8–16, 1986.

269. Kayhty H, Peltola H, Karanko V, Makela PH. The protective level of serum antibodies to the capsular polysaccharide of *Haemophilus influenzae* type b. J Infect Dis 147:1100, 1983.

270. Anderson P. The protective level of serum antibodies to the capsular polysaccharide of *Haemophilus influenzae* type b [letter]. J Infect Dis 149:1034–1035, 1984.

271. Smith DH, Hann S, Howie VM. Studies on the prevalence of antibodies to *Haemophilus influenzae* type b. *In* Sell SH, Karzon DT (eds). *Haemophilus influenzae*. Nashville, TN, Vanderbilt University Press, 1973, pp 175–185.

272. Kayhty H, Jousimies-Somer H, Peltola H, Maketa PH. Antibody response to capsular polysaccharides of groups A and C *Neisseria meningitidis* and *Haemophilus influenzae* type b during bacteremic disease. J Infect Dis 143:32–41, 1981.

273. Kayhty H, Schneerson R, Sutton A. Class-specific antibody response to *Haemophilus influenzae* type b capsular polysaccharide vaccine. J Infect Dis 148:767, 1983.

274. Kaplan SL, Mason EO Jr, Johnson G, et al. Enzyme-linked immunosorbent assay for detection of capsular antibodies against *Haemophilus influenzae* type b: comparison with radioimmunoassay. J Clin Microbiol 18:1201–1204, 1983.

275. Griffiss JM, Bertram MA. Immunoepidemiology of meningococcal disease in military recruits. II. Blocking of serum bactericidal activity by circulating IgA early in the course of invasive disease. J Infect Dis 136:733–739, 1977.

276. Musher DM, Goree A, Baughn RE, Birdsall HH. Immunoglobulin A from bronchopulmonary secretions blocks bactericidal and opsonizing effects of antibody to nontypable *Haemophilus influenzae*. Infect Immun 45:36–40, 1984.

277. Rosales SV, Lascolea LJ Jr, Ogra PL. Development of respiratory mucosal tolerance during *Haemophilus influenzae* type b infection in infancy. J Immunol 132:1517–1521, 1984.

278. Beuvery EC, van Rossum F, Nagel J. Comparison of the induction of immunoglobulin M and G antibodies in mice with purified pneumococcal type 3 and meningococcal group C polysaccharides and their protein conjugates. Infect Immun 37:15–22, 1982.

279. Riesen WF, Skvaril F, Braun DG. Natural infection of man with group A streptococci: levels; restriction in class, subclass, and type; and clonal appearance of polysaccharide-group-specific antibodies. Scand J Immunol 5:383–390, 1976.

280. Barrett DJ. Human immune responses to polysaccharide antigens: an analysis of bacterial polysaccharide vaccines in infants. Adv Pediatr 32:139–158, 1985.

281. Jennings HJ. Capsular polysaccharides as human vaccines. Adv Carbohydr Chem Biochem 41:155–208, 1983.

282. Oxelius VA, Berkel AI, Hanson LA. IgG2 deficiency in ataxia-telangiectasia. N Engl J Med 306:515–517, 1982.

283. Oxelius VA. Quantitative and qualitative investigations of serum IgG subclasses in immunodeficiency diseases. Clin Exp Immunol 36:112–116, 1979.

284. Oxelius VA. Chronic infections in a family with hereditary deficiency of IgG2 and IgG4. Clin Exp Immunol 17:19–27, 1974.

285. Schur PH, Borel H, Gelfand EW, et al. Selective gamma-g globulin deficiencies in patients with recurrent pyogenic infections. N Engl J Med 283:631–634, 1970.

286. Shackelford PG, Granoff DM, Nahm MH, et al. Relation of age, race, and allotype to immunoglobulin subclass concentrations. Pediatr Res 19:846 849, 1985.

287. Ramadas K, Petersen GM, Heiner DC, Ward JI. Class and subclass antibodies to *Haemophilus influenzae* type b capsule: comparison of invasive disease and natural exposure. Infect Immun 53:486–490, 1986.

288. Shackelford PG, Granoff DM, Nelson SJ, et al. Subclass distribution of human antibodies to *Haemophilus influenzae* type b capsular polysaccharide. J Immunol 138:587–592, 1987.

289. Ambrosino DM, Sood SK, Lee MC, et al. IgG1, IgG2, and IgM responses to two *Haemophilus influenzae* type b conjugate vaccines in young infants. Pediatr Infect Dis J 11:855–859, 1992.

290. Huber BT. B cell differentiation antigens as probes for functional B cell subsets. Immunol Rev 64:57–79, 1982.

291. Davie JM. Antipolysaccharide immunity in man and animals. *In* Sell SH, Wright PF (eds). *Haemophilus influenzae*. New York, Elsevier Science Publishing, 1982, pp 129–134.

292. Landsteiner K. The Specificity of Serologic Reactions. Cambridge, MA, Harvard University Press, 1945. (Reprinted by Dover Publications, New York, 1962.)

293. Kamboj KK, King CL, Greenspan NS, et al. Immunization with *Haemophilus influenzae* type b-CRM(197) conjugate vaccine elicits a mixed Th1 and Th2 CD(4+) T cell cytokine response that correlates with the isotype of antipolysaccharide antibody. J Infect Dis 184:931–935, 2001.

294. Pandey JP, Fudenberg HH, Virella G, et al. Association between immunoglobulin allotypes and immune responses to *Haemophilus influenzae* and *Meningococcus* polysaccharides. Lancet 1:190–192, 1979.

295. Andersson B, Porras O, Hanson LA, et al. Inhibition of attachment of *Streptococcus pneumoniae* and *Haemophilus influenzae* by human milk and receptor oligosaccharides. J Infect Dis 153:232–237, 1986.

296. Pichichero ME, Insel RA. Relationship between naturally occurring human mucosal and serum antibody to the capsular polysaccharide of *Haemophilus influenzae* type b. J Infect Dis 146:243–248, 1982.

297. Pichichero ME, Hall CB, Insel RA. A mucosal antibody response following systemic *Haemophilus influenzae* type b infection in children. J Clin Invest 67:1482–1489, 1981.

298. Pichichero ME, Insel RA. Mucosal antibody response to parenteral vaccination with *Haemophilus influenzae* type b capsule. J Allergy Clin Immunol 72(5 pt 1):481–486, 1983.

299. Mulks MH, Kornfeld SJ, Frangione B, Plaut AG. Relationship between the specificity of IgA proteases and serotypes in *Haemophilus influenzae*. J Infect Dis 146:266–274, 1982.

300. Takala AK, Eskola J, Leinonen M, et al. Reduction of oropharyngeal carriage of *Haemophilus influenzae* type b (Hib) in children immunized with an Hib conjugate vaccine. J Infect Dis 164:982–986, 1991.

301. Murphy TV, Pastor P, Medley F, et al. Decreased *Haemophilus* colonization in children vaccinated with *Haemophilus influenzae* type b conjugate vaccine. J Pediatr 122:517–523, 1993.

302. Takala AK, Santosham M, Almeido-Hill J, et al. Vaccination with *Haemophilus influenzae* type b meningococcal protein conjugate vaccine reduces oropharyngeal carriage of *Haemophilus influenzae* type b among American Indian children. Pediatr Infect Dis J 12:593–599, 1993.

303. Mohle-Boetani JC, Ajello G, Breneman E, et al. Carriage of *Haemophilus influenzae* type b in children after widespread vaccination with conjugate *Haemophilus influenzae* type b vaccines. Pediatr Infect Dis J 12:589–593, 1993.

304. Kauppi M, Eskola J, Kayhty H. Anti-capsular polysaccharide antibody concentrations in saliva after immunization with *Haemophilus influenzae* type b conjugate vaccines. Pediatr Infect Dis J 14:286–294, 1995.

305. Drexhage HA, van de Plassche EM, Kokje M, Leezenberg HA. Abnormalities in cell-mediated immune functions to *Haemophilus influenzae* chronic purulent infections of the upper respiratory tract. Clin Immunol Immunopathol 28:218–228, 1983.

306. Siber GR, Ambrosino DM, McIver J, et al. Preparation of human hyperimmune globulin to *Haemophilus influenzae* type b, *Streptococcus pneumoniae*, and *Neisseria meningitidis*. Infect Immun 45:248–254, 1984.

307. Ambrosino D, Schreiber JR, Daum RS, Siber GR. Efficacy of human hyperimmune globulin in prevention of *Haemophilus influenzae* type b disease in infant rats. Infect Immun 39:709–714, 1983.

308. Siber GR, Thompson C, Reid GR, et al. Evaluation of bacterial polysaccharide immune globulin for the treatment or prevention of *Haemophilus influenzae* type b and pneumococcal disease. J Infect Dis 165(suppl 1):S129–S133, 1992.

309. Ambrosino DM, Landesman SH, Gorham CC, Siber GR. Passive immunization against disease due to *Haemophilus influenzae* type b: concentrations of antibody to capsular polysaccharide in high-risk children. J Infect Dis 153:1–7, 1986.

310. Letson GW, Santosham M, Reid R, et al. Comparison of active and combined passive/active immunization of Navajo children against *Haemophilus influenzae* type b. Pediatr Infect Dis J 7:747–752, 1988.

311. de Andrade Carvalho A, Giampaglia CM, Kimura H. Maternal and infant antibody response to meningococcal vaccination in pregnancy. Lancet 2:809–811, 1977.

312. Amstey MS, Insel R, Munoz J, Pichichero M. Fetal-neonatal passive immunization against *Haemophilus influenzae* type b. Am J Obstet Gynecol 153:607–611, 1985.

313. Glezen WP, Englund JA, Siber GR, et al. Maternal immunization with the capsular polysaccharide vaccine for *Haemophilus influenzae* type b. J Infect Dis 165(suppl 1):S134–S136, 1992.

314. Englund JA, Glezen WP, Turner C, et al. Maternal immunization with PRP and PRP-conjugate vaccines for passive protection of infants [abstr 68]. *In* Program and Abstracts of the 31st Interscience Conference on Antimicrobial Agents and Chemotherapy, Chicago, September 29–October 2, 1991.

315. Rodrigues LP, Schneerson R, Robbins JB. Immunity to *Haemophilus influenzae* type b. I. The isolation, and some physicochemical, serologic and biologic properties of the capsular polysaccharide of *Haemophilus influenzae* type b. J Immunol 107:1071–1080, 1971.

316. Argaman M, Liu TY, Robbins JB. Polyribitol-phosphate: an antigen of four gram-positive bacteria cross-reactive with the capsular polysaccharide of *Haemophilus influenzae* type b. J Immunol 112:649–655, 1974.

317. Crisel RM, Baker RS, Dorman DE. Capsular polymer of *Haemophilus influenzae* type b. I. Structural characterization of the capsular polymer of strain Eagan. J Biol Chem 250:4926–4930, 1975.

318. Anderson P, Pichichero ME, Insel RA. Immunization of 2-month-old infants with protein-coupled oligosaccharides derived from the capsule of *Haemophilus influenzae* type b. J Pediatr 107:346–351, 1985.

319. Makela PH, Peltola H, Kayhty H, et al. Polysaccharide vaccines of group A *Neisseria meningitidis* and *Haemophilus influenzae* type b: a field trial in Finland. J Infect Dis 136(suppl):S43–S50, 1977.

320. Daum RS, Granoff DM. A vaccine against *Haemophilus influenzae* type b. Pediatr Infect Dis 4:355–357, 1985.

321. Ward JI. Is *Haemophilus influenzae* type b disease preventable? JAMA 253:554–556, 1985.

322. Insel RA, Anderson P, Pichichero ME. Anticapsular antibody to *Haemophilus influenzae* type b. *In* Sell SH, Wright PF (eds). *Haemophilus influenzae*. New York, Elsevier Science Publishing, 1982, pp 155–168.

323. Deveikis A, Ward J, Kim KS. Functional activities of human antibody induced by the capsular polysaccharide or polysaccharide-conjugate vaccines against *Haemophilus influenzae* type b. Vaccine 6:14–18, 1988.

324. Milstien JB, Gross TP, Kuritsky JN. Adverse reactions reported following receipt of *Haemophilus influenzae* type b vaccine: an analysis after 1 year of marketing. Pediatrics 80:270–274, 1987.

325. Shapiro ED, Murphy TV, Wald ER, Brady CA. The protective efficacy of *Haemophilus* b polysaccharide vaccine. JAMA 260:1419–1422, 1988.

326. Harrison LH, Broome CV, Hightower AW, et al. A day care–based study of the efficacy of *Haemophilus* b polysaccharide vaccine. JAMA 260:1413–1418, 1988.

327. Harrison LH, Broome CV, Hightower AW. *Haemophilus influenzae* type b polysaccharide vaccine: an efficacy study. *Haemophilus* Vaccine Efficacy Study Group. Pediatrics 84:255–261, 1989.

328. Osterholm MT, Rambeck JH, White KE, et al. Lack of efficacy of *Haemophilus* b polysaccharide vaccine in Minnesota. JAMA 260:1423–1428, 1988.

329. Black SB, Shinefield HR, Hiatt RA, Fireman BH. Efficacy of *Haemophilus influenzae* type b capsular polysaccharide vaccine. Pediatr Infect Dis J 7:149–156, 1988.

330. Ward JI, Broome CV, Harrison LH, et al. *Haemophilus influenzae* type b vaccines: lessons for the future. Pediatrics 81:886–893, 1988.

331. Daum RS, Marcuse EK, Giebink GS, et al. *Haemophilus influenzae* type b vaccines: lessons from the past. Pediatrics 81:893–897, 1988.

332. Murphy TV. *Haemophilus* b polysaccharide vaccine: need for continuing assessment. Pediatr Infect Dis J 6:701–703, 1987.

333. Granoff DM, Osterholm MT. Safety and efficacy of *Haemophilus influenzae* type b polysaccharide vaccine. Pediatrics 80:590–592, 1987.

334. Parke JC Jr, Schneerson R, Robbins JB, Schlesselman JJ. Interim report of a controlled field trial of immunization with capsular polysaccharides of *Haemophilus influenzae* type b and group C *Neisseria meningitidis* in Mecklenburg County, North Carolina (March 1974–March 1976). J Infect Dis 136(suppl):S51–S56, 1977.

335. Peltola H, Kayhty H, Sivonen A, Makela H. *Haemophilus influenzae* type b capsular polysaccharide vaccine in children: a double-blind field study of 100,000 vaccinees 3 months to 5 years of age in Finland. Pediatrics 60:730–737, 1977.

336. Committee on Infectious Diseases. *Haemophilus* type b polysaccharide vaccine. Pediatrics 76:322–324, 1985.

337. Immunization Practices Advisory Committee. Polysaccharide vaccine for prevention of *Haemophilus influenzae* type b disease. MMWR 34:201–205, 1985.

338. Granoff DM, Shackelford PG, Suarez BK, et al. *Haemophilus influenzae* type b disease in children vaccinated with type b polysaccharide vaccine. N Engl J Med 315:1584–1590, 1986.

339. Osterholm MT, Jacobs JL, White KE, et al. Efficacy of *Haemophilus influenzae* b plain polysaccharide (PRP) vaccine and conjugate vaccine (PRP-D) in Minnesota [abstr 449A]. *In* Program and Abstracts of the 30th Interscience Conference on Antimicrobial Agents and Chemotherapy, Atlanta, October 21–24, 1990.

340. Greenberg DP, Vadheim CM, Bordenave N, et al. Protective efficacy of *Haemophilus influenzae* type b polysaccharide and conjugate vaccines in children 18 months of age and older. JAMA 265:987–992, 1991.

341. Loughlin AM, Marchant CD, Lett S, Shapiro ED. Efficacy of *Haemophilus influenzae* type b vaccines in Massachusetts children 18 to 59 months of age. Pediatr Infect Dis J 11:374–379, 1992.

342. Avery OT, Goebel WF. Chemo-immunological studies on conjugated carbohydrate-proteins. II. Immunological specificity of synthetic sugar-protein antigen. J Exp Med 50:533–550, 1929.

343. Goebel WF, Avery OT. Chemo-immunological studies on conjugated and carbohydrate-proteins. I. The synthesis of p-aminophenol B-glucoside, p-aminophenol B-galactoside, and their coupling with serum globulin. J Exp Med 50:521–531, 1929.

344. Schneerson R, Barrera O, Sutton A, Robbins JB. Preparation, characterization, and immunogenicity of *Haemophilus influenzae* type b polysaccharide-protein conjugates. J Exp Med 152:361–376, 1980.

345. Gordon LK. Characterization of a hapten-carrier conjugate vaccine: H. *influenzae*–diphtheria conjugate vaccine. *In* Chanock RM, Lerner RA (eds). Modern Approaches to Vaccines. Cold Spring Harbor, NY, Cold Spring Harbor Laboratory Press, 1984, pp 393–396.

346. Anderson P. Antibody responses to *Haemophilus influenzae* type b and diphtheria toxin induced by conjugates of oligosaccharides of the type b capsule with the nontoxic protein CRM_{197}. Infect Immun 39:233–238, 1983.

347. Tai JY, Vella PP, McLean AA, et al. *Haemophilus influenzae* type b polysaccharide-protein conjugate vaccine. Proc Soc Exp Biol Med 184:154–161, 1987.

348. Chu C, Schneerson R, Robbins JB, Rastogi SC. Further studies on the immunogenicity of *Haemophilus influenzae* type b and pneumococcal type 6A polysaccharide-protein conjugates. Infect Immun 40:245–256, 1983.

349. Holmes SJ, Murphy TV, Anderson RS, et al. Immunogenicity of four *Haemophilus influenzae* type b conjugate vaccines in 17- to 19-month-old children. J Pediatr 118:364–371, 1991.

350. Berkowitz CD, Ward JI, Meier K, et al. Safety and immunogenicity of *Haemophilus influenzae* type b polysaccharide and polysaccharide diphtheria toxoid conjugate vaccines in children 15 to 24 months of age. J Pediatr 110:509–514, 1987.

351. Decker MD, Edwards KM, Bradley R, Palmer P. Responses of children to booster immunization with their primary conjugate *Haemophilus influenzae* type b vaccine or with polyribosylribitol phosphate conjugated with diphtheria toxoid. J Pediatr 122:410–413, 1993.

352. Lepow M, Randolph M, Cimma R, et al. Persistence of antibody and response to booster dose of *Haemophilus influenzae* type b polysaccharide diphtheria toxoid conjugate vaccine in infants immunized at 9 to 15 months of age. J Pediatr 108:882–886, 1986.

353. Lepow ML, Samuelson JS, Gordon LK. Safety and immunogenicity of *Haemophilus influenzae* type b polysaccharide–diphtheria toxoid conjugate vaccine in infants 9 to 15 months of age. J Pediatr 106:185–189, 1985.

354. Kayhty H, Eskola J, Peltola H, et al. Immunogenicity in infants of a vaccine composed of *Haemophilus influenzae* type b capsular polysaccharide mixed with DPT or conjugated to diphtheria toxoid. J Infect Dis 155:100–106, 1987.

355. Eskola J, Kayhty H, Peltola H, et al. Antibody levels achieved in infants by course of *Haemophilus influenzae* type b polysaccharide/diphtheria toxoid conjugate vaccine. Lancet 1:1184–1186, 1985.

356. Decker MD, Edwards KM, Bradley R, Palmer P. Comparative trial in infants of four conjugate *Haemophilus influenzae* type b vaccines [see comments]. J Pediatr 120(2 pt 1):184–189, 1992.

357. Vadheim CM, Greenberg DP, Marcy SM, et al. Safety evaluation of PRP-D *Haemophilus influenzae* type b conjugate vaccine in children immunized at 18 months of age and older: follow-up study of 30,000 children. Pediatr Infect Dis J 9:555–561, 1990.

358. D'Cruz OF, Shapiro ED, Spiegelman KN, et al. Acute inflammatory demyelinating polyradiculoneuropathy (Guillain-Barré syndrome) after immunization with *Haemophilus influenzae* type b conjugate vaccine [see comments]. J Pediatr 115(5 pt 1):743–746, 1989.

359. Gross TP, Hayes SW. *Haemophilus* conjugate vaccine and Guillain-Barré syndrome [letter; comment]. J Pediatr 118:161, 1991.

360. Frasch CE, Hiner EE, Gross TP. *Haemophilus* b disease after vaccination with *Haemophilus* b polysaccharide or conjugate vaccine. Am J Dis Child 145:1379–1382, 1991.

361. Nelson WL, Granoff DM. Protective efficacy of *Haemophilus influenzae* type b polysaccharide–diphtheria toxoid conjugate vaccine. Am J Dis Child 144:292–295, 1990.

362. Wenger JD, Pierce R, Deaver KA, et al. Efficacy of *Haemophilus influenzae* type b polysaccharide–diphtheria toxoid conjugate vaccine in U.S. children aged 18–59 months. *Haemophilus influenzae* Vaccine Efficacy Study Group. Lancet 338:395–398, 1991.

363. Eskola J, Kayhty H, Takala AK, et al. A randomized, prospective field trial of a conjugate vaccine in the protection of infants and young children against invasive *Haemophilus influenzae* type b disease [see comments]. N Engl J Med 323:1381–1387, 1990.

364. Eskola J, Peltola H, Takala AK, et al. Efficacy of *Haemophilus influenzae* type b polysaccharide–diphtheria toxoid conjugate vaccine in infancy. N Engl J Med 317:717–722, 1987.

365. Ward J, Brenneman G, Letson GW, Heyward WL. Limited efficacy of a *Haemophilus influenzae* type b conjugate vaccine in Alaska Native infants. The Alaska *H. influenzae* Vaccine Study Group [see comments]. N Engl J Med 323:1393–1401, 1990.

366. Madore DV, Johnson CL, Phipps DC, et al. Safety and immunogenicity of *Haemophilus influenzae* type b oligosaccharide–CRM$_{197}$ conjugate vaccine in infants aged 15 to 23 months. Pediatrics 86:527–534, 1990.

367. Turner RB, Cimino CO, Sullivan BJ. Prospective comparison of the immune response of infants to three *Haemophilus influenzae* type b vaccines [see comments]. Pediatr Infect Dis J 10:108–112, 1991.

368. Seppala I, Sarvas H, Makela O, et al. Human antibody responses to two conjugate vaccines of *Haemophilus influenzae* type B saccharides and diphtheria toxin. Scand J Immunol 28:471–479, 1988.

369. Rowe JE, Messinger IK, Schwendeman CA, Popejoy LA. Three-dose vaccination of infants under 8 months of age with a conjugate *Haemophilus influenzae* type B vaccine. Mil Med 155:483–486, 1990.

370. Madore DV, Johnson CL, Phipps DC, et al. Safety and immunologic response to *Haemophilus influenzae* type b oligosaccharide-CRM$_{197}$ conjugate vaccine in 1- to 6-month-old infants. Pediatrics 85:331–337, 1990.

371. Kayhty H, Peltola H, Eskola J, et al. Immunogenicity of *Haemophilus influenzae* oligosaccharide-protein and polysaccharide-protein conjugate vaccination of children at 4, 6, and 14 months of age. Pediatrics 84:995–999, 1989.

372. Makela PH, Eskola J, Peltola H, et al. Clinical experience with *Haemophilus influenzae* type b conjugate vaccines. Pediatrics 85(4 pt 2):651–653, 1990.

373. Bulkow LR, Wainwright RB, Letson GW, et al. Comparative immunogenicity of four *Haemophilus influenzae* type b conjugate vaccines in Alaska Native infants. Pediatr Infect Dis J 12:484–492, 1993.

374. Ward JI, Chiu CY, Wainwright RB, et al. Lack of suppressive effect of preexisting antibody on immune responses to 5 *Haemophilus influenzae* type b conjugate vaccines in young Alaskan infants [abstr 64]. In Program and Abstracts of the 30th Interscience Conference on Antimicrobial Agents and Chemotherapy, Atlanta, October 21–24, 1990.

375. Insel RA, Anderson PW. Response to oligosaccharide-protein conjugate vaccine against *Haemophilus influenzae* type b in two patients with IgG2 deficiency unresponsive to capsular polysaccharide vaccine. N Engl J Med 315:499–503, 1986.

376. Schneider LC, Insel RA, Howie G, et al. Response to a *Haemophilus influenzae* type b diphtheria CRM$_{197}$ conjugate vaccine in children with a defect of antibody production to *Haemophilus influenzae* type b polysaccharide. J Allergy Clin Immunol 85:948–953, 1990.

377. Anderson P, Insel RA. Prospects for overcoming maturational and genetic barriers to the human antibody response to the capsular polysaccharide of *Haemophilus influenzae* type b. Vaccine 6:188–191, 1988.

378. Gigliotti F, Feldman S, Wang WC, et al. Immunization of young infants with sickle cell disease with a *Haemophilus influenzae* type b saccharide–diphtheria CRM$_{197}$ protein conjugate vaccine. J Pediatr 114:1006–1010, 1989.

379. Gigliotti F, Feldman S, Wang WC, et al. Serologic follow-up of children with sickle cell disease immunized with a *Haemophilus influenzae* type b conjugate vaccine during early infancy. J Pediatr 118:917–919, 1991.

380. Rubin LG, Voulalas D, Carmody L. Immunogenicity of *Haemophilus influenzae* type b conjugate vaccine in children with sickle cell disease. Am J Dis Child 146:340–342, 1992.

381. Edwards KM, Decker MD, Porch CR, et al. Immunization after invasive *Haemophilus influenzae* type b disease: serologic response to a conjugate vaccine. Am J Dis Child 143:31–33, 1989.

382. Steinhoff MC, Auerbach BS, Nelson KE, et al. Antibody responses to *Haemophilus influenzae* type b vaccines in men with human immunodeficiency virus infection [see comments]. N Engl J Med 325:1837–1842, 1991.

383. Anderson PW, Pichichero ME, Insel RA, et al. Vaccines consisting of periodate-cleaved oligosaccharides from the capsule of *Haemophilus influenzae* type b coupled to a protein carrier: structural and temporal requirements for priming in the human infant. J Immunol 137:1181–1186, 1986.

384. Vella PP, Ellis RW. Immunogenicity of *Haemophilus influenzae* type b conjugate vaccines in infant rhesus monkeys. Pediatr Res 29:10–13, 1991.

385. Granoff DM, Rathore MH, Holmes SJ, et al. Effect of immunity to the carrier protein on antibody responses to *Haemophilus influenzae* type b conjugate vaccines. Vaccine 11(suppl 1):S46–S51, 1993.

386. Tudor-Williams G, Frankland J, Isaacs D, et al. *Haemophilus influenzae* type b conjugate vaccine trial in Oxford: implications for the United Kingdom. Arch Dis Child 64:520–524, 1989.

387. Paradiso PR, Hogerman DA, Madore DV, et al. Safety and immunogenicity of a combined diphtheria, tetanus, pertussis and *Haemophilus influenzae* type b vaccine in young infants. Pediatrics 92:827–832, 1993.

388. Black SB, Shinefield HR, Ray P, et al. Safety of combined oligosaccharide conjugate *Haemophilus influenzae* type b (HbOC) and whole cell diphtheria–tetanus toxoids–pertussis vaccine in infancy. The Kaiser Permanente Pediatric Vaccine Study Group. Pediatr Infect Dis J 12:981–985, 1993.

389. Black SB, Shinefield HR, Fireman B, et al. Efficacy in infancy of oligosaccharide conjugate *Haemophilus influenzae* type b (HbOC) vaccine in a United States population of 61,080 children. The Northern California Kaiser Permanente Vaccine Study Center Pediatrics Group [see comments]. Pediatr Infect Dis J 10:97–104, 1991.

390. Black SB, Shinefield HR. Immunization with oligosaccharide conjugate *Haemophilus influenzae* type b (HbOC) vaccine on a large health maintenance organization population: extended follow-up and impact on *Haemophilus influenzae* disease epidemiology. Pediatr Infect Dis J 11:610–613, 1992.

391. Eskola J, Peltola H, Takala A. Protective efficacy of the *Haemophilus influenzae* type b conjugate vaccine HbOC in Finnish infants [abstr 60]. In Program and Abstracts of the 30th Interscience Conference on Antimicrobial Agents and Chemotherapy, Atlanta, October 21–24, 1990.

392. Centers for Disease Control. *Haemophilus* b conjugate vaccines for prevention of *Haemophilus influenzae* type b disease among infants and children two months of age and older: recommendations of the Advisory Committee on Immunization Practices (ACIP). MMWR 40(RR-1):1–7, 1991.

393. American Academy of Pediatrics Committee on Infectious Diseases. *Haemophilus influenzae* type b conjugate vaccines: recommendations for immunization with recently and previously licensed vaccines. Pediatrics 92:480–488, 1993.

394. Weinberg GA, Einhorn MS, Lenoir AA, et al. Immunologic priming to capsular polysaccharide in infants immunized with *Haemophilus influenzae* type b polysaccharide–*Neisseria meningitidis* outer membrane protein conjugate vaccine. J Pediatr 111:22–27, 1987.

395. Ahonkhai VI, Lukacs LJ, Jonas LC, Calandra GB. Clinical experience with PedvaxHIB, a conjugate vaccine of *Haemophilus influenzae* type b polysaccharide–*Neisseria meningitidis* outer membrane protein. Vaccine 9(suppl):S38–S41, 1991.

396. Vella PP, Staub JM, Armstrong J, et al. Immunogenicity of a new *Haemophilus influenzae* type b conjugate vaccine (meningococcal protein conjugate) (PedvaxHIB). Pediatrics 85(4 pt 2):668–675, 1990.

397. Ahonkhai VI, Lukacs LJ, Jonas LC, et al. *Haemophilus influenzae* type b conjugate vaccine (meningococcal protein conjugate) (PedvaxHIB): clinical evaluation. Pediatrics 85(4 pt 2):676–681, 1990.

398. Shapiro ED, Capobianco LA, Berg AT, Zitt MQ. The immunogenicity of *Haemophilus influenzae* type B polysaccharide–*Neisseria meningitidis* group B outer membrane protein complex vaccine in infants and young children. J Infect Dis 160:1064–1067, 1989.

399. Campbell H, Byass P, Ahonkhai VI, et al. Serologic responses to an *Haemophilus influenzae* type b polysaccharide–*Neisseria meningitidis* outer membrane protein conjugate vaccine in very young Gambian infants. Pediatrics 86:102–107, 1990.

400. Granoff DM, Anderson EL, Osterholm MT, et al. Differences in the immunogenicity of three *Haemophilus influenzae* type b conjugate vaccines in infants. J Pediatr 121:187–194, 1992.

401. Yogev R, Arditi M, Chadwick EG, et al. *Haemophilus influenzae* type b conjugate vaccine (meningococcal protein conjugate): immunogenicity and safety at various doses. Pediatrics 85(4 pt 2):690–693, 1990.

402. Santosham M, Wolff M, Reid R, et al. The efficacy in Navajo infants of a conjugate vaccine consisting of *Haemophilus influenzae* type b polysaccharide and *Neisseria meningitidis* outer-membrane protein complex. N Engl J Med 324:1767–1772, 1991.

403. Sood SK, Ballanco GA, Daum RS. Duration of serum anticapsular antibody after a two-dose regimen of a *Haemophilus influenzae* type b polysaccharide–*Neisseria meningitidis* outer membrane protein conjugate vaccine and anamnestic response after a third dose. J Pediatr 119:652–654, 1991.

404. Ward JI, Bulkow L, Wainwright R, Chang S. Immune tolerance and lack of booster responses to *Haemophilus influenzae* (Hib) conjugate vaccination in infants immunized beginning at birth [abstr 984]. *In* Program and Abstracts of the 32nd Interscience Conference on Antimicrobial Agents and Chemotherapy, Anaheim, CA, October 11–14, 1992.

405. Weinberg GA, Granoff DM. Immunogenicity of *Haemophilus influenzae* type b polysaccharide-protein conjugate vaccines in children with conditions associated with impaired antibody responses to type b polysaccharide vaccine. Pediatrics 85(4 pt 2):654–661, 1990.

406. Granoff DM, Weinberg GA, Shackelford PG. IgG subclass response to immunization with *Haemophilus influenzae* type b polysaccharide–outer membrane protein conjugate vaccine. Pediatr Res 24:180–185, 1988.

407. Gray BM. Opsonophagocidal activity in sera from infants and children immunized with *Haemophilus influenzae* type b conjugate vaccine (meningococcal protein conjugate). Pediatrics 85(4 pt 2):694–697, 1990.

408. Schlesinger Y, Granoff DM. Avidity and bactericidal activity of antibody elicited by different *Haemophilus influenzae* type b conjugate vaccines. The Vaccine Study Group. JAMA 267:1489–1494, 1992.

409. Stein KE. Thymus-independent and thymus-dependent responses to polysaccharide antigens. J Infect Dis 165(suppl 1):S49–S52, 1992.

410. Advisory Committee on Immunization Practices. Update: report of PedvaxHIB lots with questionable immunogenicity. MMWR 41:878–879, 1992.

411. Santosham M, Hill J, Wolff M, et al. Safety and immunogenicity of a *Haemophilus influenzae* type b conjugate vaccine in a high-risk American Indian population [see comments]. Pediatr Infect Dis J 10:113–117, 1991. [erratum appears in Pediatr Infect Dis J 10:369, 1991]

412. Dashefsky B, Wald E, Guerra N, Byers C. Safety, tolerability, and immunogenicity of concurrent administration of *Haemophilus influenzae* type b conjugate vaccine (meningococcal protein conjugate) with either measles-mumps-rubella vaccine or diphtheria-tetanus-pertussis and oral poliovirus vaccines in 14- to 23-month-old infants. Pediatrics 85(4 pt 2):682–689, 1990.

413. Santosham M, Rivin B, Wolff M, et al. Prevention of *Haemophilus influenzae* type b infections in Apache and Navajo children. J Infect Dis 165(suppl 1):S144–S151, 1992.

414. Vadheim CM, Greenberg DP, Eriksen E, et al. Eradication of *Haemophilus influenzae* type b disease in southern California. Kaiser-UCLA Vaccine Study Group. Arch Pediatr Adolesc Med 148:51–56, 1994.

415. Schneerson R, Robbins JB, Parke JC Jr, et al. Quantitative and qualitative analyses of serum antibodies elicited in adults by *Haemophilus influenzae* type b and pneumococcus type 6A capsular polysaccharide–tetanus toxoid conjugates. Infect Immun 52:519–528, 1986.

416. Claesson BA, Trollfors B, Lagergard T, et al. Clinical and immunologic responses to the capsular polysaccharide of *Haemophilus influenzae* type b alone or conjugated to tetanus toxoid in 18- to 23-month-old children. J Pediatr 112:695–702, 1988.

417. Claesson BA, Schneerson R, Robbins JB, et al. Protective levels of serum antibodies stimulated in infants by two injections of *Haemophilus influenzae* type b capsular polysaccharide–tetanus toxoid conjugate. J Pediatr 114:97–100, 1989.

418. Holmes SJ, Fritzell B, Guito KP, et al. Immunogenicity of *Haemophilus influenzae* type b polysaccharide–tetanus toxoid conjugate vaccine in infants. Am J Dis Child 147:832–836, 1993.

419. Kayhty H, Eskola J, Peltola H, et al. Antibody responses to four *Haemophilus influenzae* type b conjugate vaccines. Am J Dis Child 145:223–227, 1991.

420. Vadheim CM, Greenberg DP, Partridge S, et al. Effectiveness and safety of an *Haemophilus influenzae* type b conjugate vaccine (PRP-T) in young infants. Kaiser-UCLA Vaccine Study Group. Pediatrics 92:272–279, 1993.

421. Fritzell B, Plotkin S. Efficacy and safety of a *Haemophilus influenzae* type b capsular polysaccharide–tetanus protein conjugate vaccine. J Pediatr 121:355–362, 1992.

422. Parke JC Jr, Schneerson R, Reimer C, et al. Clinical and immunologic responses to *Haemophilus influenzae* type b–tetanus toxoid conjugate vaccine in infants injected at 3, 5, 7, and 18 months of age. J Pediatr 118:184–190, 1991.

423. Claesson BA, Schneerson R, Lagergard T, et al. Persistence of serum antibodies elicited by *Haemophilus influenzae* type b–tetanus toxoid conjugate vaccine in infants vaccinated at 3, 5, and 12 months of age. Pediatr Infect Dis J 10:560–564, 1991.

424. Barra A, Cordonnier C, Preziosi MP, et al. Immunogenicity of *Haemophilus influenzae* type b conjugate vaccine in allogeneic bone marrow recipients. J Infect Dis 166:1021–1028, 1992.

425. Kaplan SL, Duckett T, Mahoney DH Jr, et al. Immunogenicity of *Haemophilus influenzae* type b polysaccharide–tetanus protein conjugate vaccine in children with sickle hemoglobinopathy or malignancies, and after systemic *Haemophilus influenzae* type b infection. J Pediatr 120:367–370, 1992.

426. Climaz R, Mensi C, D'Angelo E, et al. Safety and immunogenicity of a conjugate vaccine against *Haemophilus influenzae* type b in splenectomized and nonsplenectomized patients with Cooley anemia. J Infect Dis 183:1819–1821, 2001.

427. Jonville-Béra AP, Autret-Leca E, Barbeillon F, Llado JP. Relation entre vaccination par diphtérie tétanos coqueluche ± *Haemophilus influenzae* b et mort subite du nourrisson avant trois mois: étude cas-témoin. Arch Pediatr 8:1272–1273, 2001.

428. Gibb D, Spoulou V, Giacomelli A, et al. Antibody responses to *Haemophilus influenzae* type b and *Streptococcus pneumoniae* vaccines in children with human immunodeficiency virus infection. Pediatr Infect Dis J 14:129–135, 1995.

429. Clemens JD, Ferreccio C, Levine MM, et al. Impact of *Haemophilus influenzae* type b polysaccharide–tetanus protein conjugate vaccine on responses to concurrently administered diphtheria-tetanus-pertussis vaccine [see comments]. JAMA 267:673–678, 1992.

430. Ferreccio C, Clemens J, Avendano A, et al. The clinical and immunologic response of Chilean infants to *Haemophilus influenzae* type b polysaccharide–tetanus protein conjugate vaccine coadministered in the same syringe with diphtheria–tetanus toxoids–pertussis vaccine at two, four, and six months of age. Pediatr Infect Dis J 10:764–771, 1991.

431. Mulholland K, Hilton S, Adegbola R, et al. Randomised trial of *Haemophilus influenzae* type b–tetanus protein conjugate vaccine [corrected] for prevention of pneumonia and meningitis in Gambian infants [see comments]. Lancet 349:1191–1197, 1997. [erratum appears in Lancet 350:524, 1997]

432. Lagos R, Horwitz I, Toro J, et al. Large-scale, postlicensure, selective vaccination of Chilean infants with PRP-T conjugate vaccine: practicality and effectiveness in preventing invasive *Haemophilus influenzae* type b infections. Pediatr Infect Dis J 15:216–222, 1996.

432a. Lagos R, Valenzuela MT, Levine OS, et al. Economization of vaccination against *Haemophilus influenzae* type b: a randomized trial of immunogenicity of fractional dose and two-dose regimens. Lancet 351:1472–1476, 1998.

433. Booy R, Moxon ER, MacFarlane JA, et al. Efficacy of *Haemophilus influenzae* type b conjugate vaccine in Oxford region [letter]. Lancet 340:847, 1992.

434. Booy R, Hodgson S, Carpenter L, et al. Efficacy of *Haemophilus influenzae* type b conjugate vaccine PRP-T [see comments]. Lancet 344:362–366, 1994.

435. Levine OS, Lagos R, Munoz A, et al. Defining the burden of pneumonia in children preventable by vaccination against *Haemophilus influenzae* type b. Pediatr Infect Dis J 18:1060–1064, 1999.

436. Peltola H, Kilpi T, Anttila M. Rapid disappearance of *Haemophilus influenzae* type b meningitis after routine childhood immunisation with conjugate vaccines. Lancet 340:592–594, 1992.

437. Centers for Disease Control and Prevention. Food and Drug Administration approval of use of *Haemophilus influenzae* type b conjugate vaccine reconstituted with diphtheria-tetanus-pertussis vaccine for infants and children. MMWR 42:964–965, 1993.

438. Ward JI, Greenberg DP, Anderson PW, et al. Variable quantitation of *Haemophilus influenzae* type b anticapsular antibody by radioantigen binding assay. J Clin Microbiol 26:72–78, 1988.

439. Peltola H, Eskola J, Kayhty H, et al. Clinical efficacy of the PRP-D vs HbOC conjugate vaccines against *Haemophilus influenzae* type b (Hib) [abstr 975]. *In* Program and Abstracts of the 32nd Interscience Conference on Antimicrobial Agents and Chemotherapy, Anaheim, CA, October 11–14, 1992.

440. Singleton R, Bulkow LR, Levine OS, et al. Experience with the prevention of invasive *Haemophilus influenzae* type b disease by vaccination in Alaska: the impact of persistent oropharyngeal carriage [see comments]. J Pediatr 137:313–320, 2000.

441. Granoff DM, Holmes SJ, Osterholm MT, et al. Induction of immunologic memory in infants primed with *Haemophilus influenzae* type b conjugate vaccines. J Infect Dis 168:663–671, 1993.

442. Carlsson RM, Claesson BA, Lagergard T, Kayhty H. Serum antibodies against *Haemophilus influenzae* type b and tetanus at 2.5 years of age: a follow-up of 2 different regimens of infant vaccination. Scand J Infect Dis 28:519–523, 1996.

443. Kurikka S, Kayhty H, Saarinen L, et al. Immunologic priming by one dose of *Haemophilus influenzae* type b conjugate vaccine in infancy. J Infect Dis 172:1268–1272, 1995.

444. Rothstein EP, Madore DV, Long SS. Antibody persistence four years after primary immunization of infants and toddlers with *Haemophilus influenzae* type b CRM_{197} conjugate vaccine. J Pediatr 119:655–657, 1991.

445. Scheifele DW, Halperin SA, Guasparini R, et al. Extended follow-up of antibody levels and antigen responsiveness after 2 *Haemophilus influenzae* type b conjugate vaccines. J Pediatr 135(2 pt 1):240–245, 1999.

446. Calandra GB, Lukacs LJ, Jonas LC, et al. Anti-PRP antibody levels after a primary series of PRP-OMPC and persistence of antibody titres following primary and booster doses. Vaccine 11(suppl 1):S58–S62, 1993.

447. Lucas AH, Granoff DM. Imperfect memory and the development of *Haemophilus influenzae* type B disease. Pediatr Infect Dis J 20:235–239, 2001.

448. Heath PT, Bowen-Morris J, Griffiths D, et al. Antibody persistence and *Haemophilus influenzae* type b carriage after infant immunisation with PRP-T. Arch Dis Child 77:488–492, 1997.

449. Heath PT, Booy R, Azzopardi HJ, et al. Antibody concentration and clinical protection after Hib conjugate vaccination in the United Kingdom. JAMA 284:2334–2340, 2000.

450. Garner D, Weston V. Effectiveness of vaccination for *Haemophilus influenzae* type b. Lancet 361:360–361 and 395–396, 2002.

451. Granoff DM, Holmes SJ, Belshe RB, et al. Effect of carrier protein priming on antibody responses to *Haemophilus influenzae* type b conjugate vaccines in infants. JAMA 272:1116–1121, 1994.

452. Lieberman JM, Greenberg DP, Wong VK, et al. Effect of neonatal immunization with diphtheria and tetanus toxoids on antibody responses to *Haemophilus influenzae* type b conjugate vaccines. J Pediatr 126:198–205, 1995.

453. Santosham M, Englund JA, McInnes P, et al. Safety and antibody persistence following *Haemophilus influenzae* type b conjugate or pneumococcal polysaccharide vaccines given before pregnancy in women of childbearing age and their infants. Pediatr Infect Dis J 20:931–940, 2001.

454. Holmes SJ, Granoff DM. The biology of *Haemophilus influenzae* type b vaccination failure. J Infect Dis 165(Suppl 1):S121–128, 1992.

455. Heath PT, Booy R, Griffiths H, et al. Clinical immunological risk factors associated with *Haemophilus influenzae* type b conjugate vaccine failure in childhood. Clin Infect Dis J 31:973–980, 2000.

456. Breukels MA, Jol-vasn der Zijde EM, van Tol JD, Rijkers GT. Concentration and avidity of anti-*haemophilus influenzae* type b (Hib) antibodies in serum samples obtained from patients for whom Hib vaccination failed. Clin Infect Dis J 34:191–197, 2002.

457. Heath PT, Booy R, McVernon J, et al. Hib vaccination in infants born prematurely. Arch Dis Child 88:206–210, 2003.

458. Ribeiro GS, Reis JN, Cordeiro SM, et al. Prevention of *Haemophilus influenzae* type b (Hib) meningitis a emergence of serotype replacement with type a strains after introduction of Hib immunization in Brazil. J Infect Dis 187:109–116, 2003.

459. Eskola J, Ward J, Dagan R, et al. Combined vaccination of *Haemophilus influenzae* type b conjugate and diphtheria-tetanus-pertussis containing acellular pertussis. Lancet 354:2063–2068, 1999.

460. Schmitt HJ, von Kries R, Hassenpflug B, et al. *Haemophilus influenzae* type b disease: impact and effectiveness of diphtheria–tetanus toxoids–acellular pertussis (–inactivated poliovirus)/*H. influenzae* type b combination vaccines. Pediatr Infect Dis J 20:767–774, 2001.

461. Lee CY, Thipphawong J, Huang LM, et al. An evaluation of the safety and immunogenicity of a five-component acellular pertussis, diphtheria, and tetanus toxoid vaccine (DTaP) when combined with a *Haemophilus influenzae* type b–tetanus conjugate vaccine (PRP-T) in Taiwanese infants. Pediatrics 103:25–30, 1999.

462. Ball LK, Falk LA, Horne AD, Finn TM. Evaluating the immune response to combination vaccines. Clin Infect Dis 33(suppl 4):S299–S305, 2001.

463. Goldblatt D, Richmond P, Millard E, et al. The induction of immunologic memory after vaccination with *Haemophilus influenzae* type b conjugate and acellular pertussis–containing diphtheria, tetanus, and pertussis vaccine combination [see comments]. J Infect Dis 180:538–541, 1999.

464. Granoff DM. Assessing efficacy of *Haemophilus influenzae* type b combination vaccines. Clin Infect Dis 33(suppl 4):S278–S287, 2001.

465. Dagan R, Botujansky C, Watemberg N, et al. Safety and immunogenicity in young infants of *Haemophilus* b–tetanus protein conjugate vaccine, mixed in the same syringe with diphtheria-tetanus-pertussis–enhanced inactivated poliovirus vaccine. Pediatr Infect Dis J 13:356–362, 1994.

466. Araujo OO, Forleo-Neto E, Vespa GN, et al. Associated or combined vaccination of Brazilian infants with a conjugate *Haemophilus influenzae* type b (Hib) vaccine, a diphtheria-tetanus–whole-cell pertussis vaccine and IPV or OPV elicits protective levels of antibodies against Hib. Vaccine 19:367–375, 2000.

467. Rennels MB, Englund JA, Bernstein DI, et al. Diminution of the anti-polyribosylribitol phosphate response to a combined diphtheria-tetanus–acellular pertussis/*Haemophilus influenzae* type b vaccine by concurrent inactivated poliovirus vaccination. Pediatr Infect Dis J 19:417–423, 2000.

468. Gylca R, Gylca V, Benes O, et al. A new DTPa-HBV-IPV vaccine co-administered with Hib, compared to a commercially available DTPw-IPV/Hib vaccine co-administered with HBV, given at 6, 10, and 14 weeks following HBV at birth. Vaccine 19:825–833, 2000.

469. Nolan T, Hogg G, Darcy MA, et al. A combined liquid Hib (PRP-OMPC), hepatitis B, diphtheria, tetanus and whole-cell pertussis vaccine: controlled studies of immunogenicity and reactogenicity. Vaccine 19:2127–2137, 2001.

470. Anderson EL, Decker MD, Englund JA, et al. Interchangeability of conjugated *Haemophilus influenzae* type b vaccines in infants [see comments]. JAMA 273:849–853, 1995.

471. Scheifele D, Law B, Mitchell L, Ochnio J. Study of booster doses of two *Haemophilus influenzae* type b conjugate vaccines including their interchangeability. Vaccine 14:1399–1406, 1996.

472. Kovel A, Wald ER, Guerra N, et al. Safety and immunogenicity of acellular diphtheria–tetanus-pertussis and *Haemophilus* conjugate vaccines given in combination or at separate injection sites. J Pediatr 120:84–87, 1992.

473. Bewley KM, Schwab JG, Ballanco GA, Daum RS. Interchangeability of *Haemophilus influenzae* type b vaccines in the primary series: evaluation of a two-dose mixed regimen. Pediatrics 98:898–904, 1996.

474. American Academy of Pediatrics. *Haemophilus influenzae* infections. In Pickering LK (ed). 2000 Red Book: Report of the Committee on Infectious Diseases (25th ed). Elk Grove Village, IL, American Academy of Pediatrics, 2000, pp 262–272.

475. Broadhurst LE, Erickson RL, Kelley PW. Decreases in invasive *Haemophilus influenzae* diseases in U.S. Army children, 1984 through 1991 [see comments]. JAMA 269:227–231, 1993.

476. Murphy TV, White KE, Pastor P, et al. Declining incidence of *Haemophilus influenzae* type b disease since introduction of vaccination [see comments]. JAMA 269:246–248, 1993.

477. Adams WG, Deaver KA, Cochi SL, et al. Decline of childhood *Haemophilus influenzae* type b (Hib) disease in the Hib vaccine era [see comments]. JAMA 269:221–226, 1993.

478. Scheifele DW. Recent trends in pediatric *Haemophilus influenzae* type B infections in Canada. Immunization Monitoring Program, Active (IMPACT) of the Canadian Paediatric Society and the Laboratory Centre for Disease Control. CMAJ 154:1041–1047, 1996. [erratum appears in CMAJ 154:1319, 1996]

479. Teare EL, Fairley CK, White J, Begg NT. Efficacy of Hib vaccine. Lancet 344:828–829, 1994.

480. Eskola J, Peltola H, Kayhty H, et al. Finnish efficacy trials with *Haemophilus influenzae* type b vaccines. J Infect Dis 165(suppl 1):S137–S138, 1992.

481. Jonsdottir KE, Steingrimsson O, Olafsson O. Immunisation of infants in Iceland against *Haemophilus influenzae* type b. Lancet 340:252–253, 1992.

482. Moulton LH, Chung S, Croll J, et al. Estimation of the indirect effect of *Haemophilus influenzae* type b conjugate vaccine in an American Indian population. Int J Epidemiol 29:753–756, 2000.

483. Perdue DG, Bulkow LR, Gellin BG, et al. Invasive *Haemophilus influenzae* disease in Alaskan residents aged 10 years and older before and after infant vaccination programs. JAMA 283:3089–3094, 2000.

484. Scheifele D, Halperin S, Vaudry W, et al. Historic low *Haemophilus influenzae* type B case tally—Canada 2000. Can Commun Dis Rep 27:149–150, 2001.

485. Garpenholt O, Hugosson S, Fredlund H, et al. Epiglottitis in Sweden before and after introduction of vaccination against *Haemophilus influenzae* type b. Pediatr Infect Dis J 18:490–493, 1999.

486. Markey P, Krause V, Boslego JW, et al. The effectiveness of *Haemophilus influenzae* type b conjugate vaccines in a high-risk population measured using immunization register data. Epidemiol Infect 126:31–36, 2001.

487. Ruocco G, Curto S, Savio M, et al. Vaccination against *Haemophilus influenzae* type b in Uruguay: experience and impact [in Spanish]. Pan Am J Public Health 5(3):197–199, 1999.

488. Dagan R, Fraser D, Roitman M, et al. Effectiveness of a nationwide infant immunization program against *Haemophilus influenzae* b. The Israeli Pediatric Bacteremia and Meningitis Group. Vaccine 17:134–141, 1999.

489. Almuneef M, Alshaalan M, Memish Z, Alalola S. Bacterial meningitis in Saudi Arabia: the impact of *Haemophilus influenzae* type b vaccination. J Chemother 13(suppl 1):34–39, 2001.

490. Adegbola RA, Usen SO, Weber M, et al. *Haemophilus influenzae* type b meningitis in The Gambia after introduction of a conjugate vaccine. Lancet 354:1091–1092, 1999.

491. Peltola H, Aavitsland P, Hansen KG, et al. Perspective: a five-country analysis of the impact of four different *Haemophilus influenzae* type b conjugates and vaccination strategies in Scandinavia. J Infect Dis 179:223–229, 1999.

492. Diez-Domingo J, Pereiro I, Morant A, et al for the Group for the Study of Invasive Diseases. Impact of non-routine vaccination on the incidence of invasive *Haemophilus influenzae* type b (Hib) disease: experience in the autonomous region of Valencia, Spain. J Infect 42:257–260, 2001.

493. Landaverde M, Di Fabio JL, Ruocco G, et al. Introduction of a conjugate vaccine against Hib in Chile and Uruguay [in Spanish]. Pan Am J Public Health 5(3):200–206, 1999.

493a.Lucher LA, Reeves M, Hennessy T, et al. Reemergence, in Southwestern Alaska, of invasive *Haemophilus influenzae* type b disease due to strains indistinguishable from those isolated from vaccinated children. J Infect Dis 186:958–965, 2002.

493b. Ribeiro GS, Reis JN, Cordeiro SM, et al. Prevention of *Haemophilus influenzae* type b (Hib) meningitis and emergence of serotype replacement with type a strains after introduction of Hib immunization in Brazil. J Infect Dis 187:1109–1116, 2003.

494. Adegbola RA, Mulholland EK, Secka O, et al. Vaccination with a *Haemophilus influenzae* type b conjugate vaccine reduces oropharyngeal carriage of *H. influenzae* type b among Gambian children. J Infect Dis 177:1758–1761, 1998.

495. Galil K, Singleton R, Levine OS, et al. Reemergence of invasive *Haemophilus influenzae* type b disease in a well-vaccinated population in remote Alaska [see comments]. J Infect Dis 179:101–106, 1999.

496. Forleo-Neto E, de Oliveira CF, Maluf EM, et al. Decreased point prevalence of *Haemophilus influenzae* type b (Hib) oropharyngeal colonization by mass immunization of Brazilian children less than 5 years old with Hib polyribosylribitol phosphate polysaccharide–tetanus toxoid conjugate vaccine in combination with diphtheria–tetanus toxoids–pertussis vaccine. J Infect Dis 180:1153–1158, 1999.

497. Centers for Disease Control and Prevention. Progress toward elimination of *Haemophilus influenzae* type b invasive disease among infants and children—United States, 1998–2000. MMWR 51:234–237, 2002.

498. Wenger JD, DiFabio J, Landaverde JM, et al. Introduction of Hib conjugate vaccines in the non-industrialized world: experience in four "newly adopting" countries. Vaccine 18:736–742, 1999.

499. Peltola H. Worldwide *Haemophilus influenzae* type b disease at the beginning of the 21st century: global analysis of the disease burden 25 years after the use of the polysaccharide vaccine and a decade after the advent of conjugates. Clin Microbiol Rev 13:302–317, 2000.

500. World Health Organization. Introduction of *Haemophilus influenzae* Type b Vaccine into Immunization Programs (WHO/V&B 00.05). Geneva, World Health Organization, 2000.

501. Nicol M, Huebner R, Mothupi R, et al. *Haemophilus influenzae* type b conjugate vaccine diluted tenfold in diphtheria-tetanus–whole cell pertussis vaccine: a randomized trial. Pediatr Infect Dis J 21:138–141, 2002.

502. Kurikka S, Kayhty H, Peltola H, et al. Neonatal immunization: response to *Haemophilus influenzae* type b–tetanus toxoid conjugate vaccine. Pediatrics 95:815–822, 1995.

503. Englund JA, Glezen WP, Turner C, et al. Transplacental antibody transfer following maternal immunization with polysaccharide and conjugate *Haemophilus influenzae* type b vaccines. J Infect Dis 171:99–105, 1995.

504. Carlsson RM, Claesson BA, Iwarson S, et al. Antibodies against *Haemophilus influenzae* type b and tetanus in infants after subcutaneous vaccination with PRP-T/diphtheria, or PRP-OMP/diphtheria-tetanus vaccines. Pediatr Infect Dis J 13:27–33, 1994.

505. Livatowski A, Boucher J, Guyot C, et al. Epidemiology of *Haemophilus influenzae* type b infections (excluding meningitis) in two French departments [in French]. Arch Fr Pediatr 46:181–185, 1989.

506. Ferreccio C, Ortiz E, Astroza L, et al. A population-based retrospective assessment of the disease burden resulting from invasive *Haemophilus influenzae* in infants and young children in Santiago, Chile. Pediatr Infect Dis J 9:488–494, 1990.

507. Hussey G, Hitchcock J, Schaaf H, et al. Epidemiology of invasive *Haemophilus influenzae* infections in Cape Town, South Africa. Annals of Tropical Paediatrics 14:97–103, 1994.

508. Weiss DPL, Coplan P, Guess H. Epidemiology of bacterial meningitis among children in Brazil 1997–1998. Rev Saúde Pública 35(3):249–255, 2001.

509. Novelli VM, El Baba F, Lewis RG, Bissell PS. *Haemophilus influenza* type b disease in Arab Gulf states. Pediatr Infect Dis J 8:886–887, 1989.

510. World Health Organization. Generic protocol for population based surveillance of *Haemophilus influenzae* type b. (WHO/VRD/GEN/95.05) Geneva, World Health Organization, 1995.

511. World Health Organization. Estimating the local burden of *Haemophilus influenzae* type b (Hib) disease preventable by vaccination: a rapid assessment tool. (WHO/V&B/01.27) Geneva, World Health Organization, 2001.

512. Fry AM, Lurie P, Gidley M, Schmink S, et al. *Haemophilus influenzae* type b (Hib) disease among Amish children in Pennsylvania: reasons for persistent disease. Pediatrics 108:e60, 2001.

513. Voss L, Lennon D, Gillies M. *Haemophilus influenzae* type b disease in Aukland chilren. NZ Med J 102:149–151, 1989.

514. Dagan R. The Israeli Pediatric Bacteremia Meningitis Group. A two-year prospective, nation wide study to determine the epidemiology and impact of invasive childhood *Haemophilus influenzae* type b infection in Israel. Clin Infect Dis 15:720–725, 1992.

515. Hussey G, Schaaf H, Hanslo D, et al. Epidemiology of post-neonatal bacterial meningitis in Cape Town children. S Afr Med J 87:51–56, 1997

516. Uduman SA, Devadas K, Mathew T, et al. Childhood bacterial meningitis: the experience of Al Anin Hospital in the Eastern region of UAE. Emirates Med J 12:227–233, 1994.

Chapter 15

Hepatitis A Vaccine

BETH P. BELL • STEPHEN M. FEINSTONE

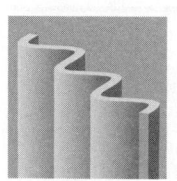

History

Although episodes of jaundice have been known since the time of Hippocrates, the earliest outbreaks that on epidemiologic grounds seem likely to have been hepatitis A occurred in Europe in the 17th and 18th centuries.[1] Early this century, Cockayne concluded that sporadic and epidemic forms of jaundice were probably manifestations of the same disease,[2] and McDonald postulated that a virus might be involved.[3] Hepatitis has been a military problem for centuries, and major outbreaks occurred among British, French, German, and Romanian troops in World War I and among German, French, American Commonwealth, and Axis troops in World War II.

The first hard data that hepatitis A was an enterically transmitted viral infection were obtained during World War II from a series of studies among experimentally infected volunteers. In a classical series of experiments, Havens[4] and Neefe and colleagues[5] were able to show that volunteers who had developed infectious hepatitis were protected from subsequent challenge with the same virus and with infectious material obtained from a separate outbreak. It was soon demonstrated that intramuscular injection of pooled normal human immune globulin could prevent or attenuate the disease.[4,6] These findings had important applications, and the practice was rapidly adopted. During an epidemic in 1945 in the Mediterranean arena, more than 2700 American soldiers were immunized. The value of this approach was rapidly apparent by an 86% reduction in the incidence of disease among immunized troops.[7]

Subsequently, when it became apparent that infectious hepatitis was clearly distinct from serum hepatitis in both mode of transmission and etiology, MacCallum suggested that the diseases be known as hepatitis A and B, replacing the terms *infectious hepatitis* (hepatitis A) and *homologous serum hepatitis* (hepatitis B). This suggestion was adopted in 1952 by the World Health Organization's First Expert Committee on Viral Hepatitis but not widely accepted by physicians and virologists until the early 1970s.

By the end of World War II, volunteer studies had clearly established that infectious hepatitis was enterically trans-

mitted and was caused by a filterable agent—presumably a virus—that was relatively heat stable but could be inactivated by chlorine.[5] The disease appeared to be caused by a single agent, seemed to be associated with lifelong immunity, and was preventable by administration of normal immune globulin. In the 1950s, these data were expanded and refined by a further series of studies conducted by Krugman and colleagues[8] at the Willowbrook State School in New York and by Melnick and Boggs[9] and their colleagues at the Joliet prison in Illinois. Fecal samples collected from the latter studies were critical in the subsequent identification of the etiologic agent of the disease by electron microscopy.[10]

Why the Disease Is Important

Hepatitis A virus (HAV) infects more than 80% of the population of many developing countries by late adolescence, and also is common in developed countries.[11,12] In the United States, hepatitis A has remained one of the most frequently reported vaccine-preventable diseases, despite the licensure of hepatitis A vaccines in 1995.[13]

Background

Clinical Description

Numerous studies have been conducted to define the incubation period of hepatitis A after natural or experimental infection in children or adults. Although disease has been seen as early as 15 days and as late as 50 days after exposure, the mean incubation period is about 28 days.[5,14,15] The average incubation period has been reported to be shorter among patients who acquired HAV infection by parenteral transmission from contaminated blood products and among nonhuman primates infected parenterally compared with those infected orally.[16–18]

Infection with HAV, as evidenced by the detection of HAV-specific immunoglobulin M (IgM) antibody in serum, may produce a wide spectrum of outcomes ranging from inapparent (asymptomatic, without elevation of serum aminotransferase levels), to subclinical (asymptomatic, with elevation of serum aminotransferase levels), to clinically evident (with symptoms). Symptoms typical of acute hepatitis include jaundice and dark urine, but symptomatic hepatitis A without jaundice also occurs.

The frequency of symptoms with HAV infection is strongly influenced by age. Children are less likely to have symptomatic infection when compared to adults; 50% to 90% of infections acquired before the age of 5 years are asymptomatic, but 70% to 95% of infected adults will have symptoms.[19-22] Jaundice is rare among young children but will occur in the majority of adults with hepatitis A.[21,22]

The clinical symptoms of acute hepatitis A in an individual patient are indistinguishable from those caused by other forms of viral hepatitis. The onset of the prodromal period, particularly in older children and adults, can be quite abrupt, and is characterized by increasing fatigue, malaise, anorexia, fever, myalgias, dull abdominal pain, nausea, and vomiting. Pediatric patients may have diarrhea or, less commonly, upper respiratory symptoms.[23,24] If present, typical symptoms of hepatitis, beginning with darkening of the urine and followed by jaundice and pale-colored stools, will appear after a period of several days to a week. In addition to jaundice and scleral icterus, physical findings may include hepatomegaly and tenderness.

The duration of illness varies, but most patients feel better within several weeks. In a large 1989 Shanghai outbreak, 90% of a subset of 8647 hospitalized patients observed carefully had recovered completely in 4 months, and all had recovered in 1 year.[14] Relapse, consisting of renewed symptoms, elevated liver function test results, and detection of virus in stools, has been found in up to 10% of cases, but recovery is universal.[25,26,27] Infection with HAV does not cause chronic infection.

A cholestatic form of hepatitis A has been reported in which patients experience persistent jaundice, usually accompanied by itching.[25,28,29] Other atypical clinical manifestations and complications, including immunologic, neurologic, hematologic, and renal extrahepatic manifestations, are rare (Table 15-1).[25,29-46]

Fulminant hepatitis A, the most severe form of the disease, is rare. The case-fatality rate, obtained from case series of hospitalized patients, has been estimated to be 0.14%.[47] In the 1988 Shanghai epidemic that involved primarily adolescents and young adults, there were 47 deaths (0.015%) recorded among the 310,746 diagnosed cases.[14] However, the case-fatality rate during a community-wide

TABLE 15-1 ■ Atypical Clinical Manifestations and Complications of Hepatitis A Virus Infection

Relapsing hepatitis A[25,29]
Fulminant hepatitis A[25,47,48,155,156]
Extrahepatic manifestations
  Transient rash or arthralgias[25,30]
  Papular acrodermatitis of childhood[31]
  Cutaneous vasculitis[32-34]
  Cryoglobulinemia[29,32,33]
  Guillain-Barré syndrome[35,39]
  Other neurologic syndromes (e.g., myeloradiculopathy, mononeuritis, vertigo, meningoencephalitis)[35-38]
  Renal syndromes (acute renal failure, nephrotic syndrome, acute glomerulonephritis)[40-42,48]
  Pancreatitis[43,48]
  Aplastic anemia and thrombocytopenia[44,46]
Cholestatic hepatitis A[25,28,48]
Hepatitis A triggering autoimmune hepatitis[25,45,48]

outbreak in the United States was approximately 0.3%.[48] Based on all reported cases of hepatitis A in the United States, the case-fatality rate from fulminant hepatitis A is approximately 0.33% (Table 15-2). Host factors reported to be associated with an increased risk of fulminant hepatitis include older age[49,50] and underlying chronic liver disease.[51-56]

Virology

HAV is a member of the *Picornaviridae* family, which includes both the enteroviruses and rhinoviruses of humans. Because of several unique features, HAV has been placed into its own genus, *Hepatavirus*.[57-63] There are four recognized human genotypes of HAV based on primary sequence variability, but there is only one known serotype.[64,65] Many strains of HAV have been described on the basis of different growth characteristics, nucleotide sequence, or geographic origin.[66-68] Polyclonal and monoclonal antibodies directed against the major antigenic determinant appear to be capable of detecting strains of HAV isolated in different parts of the world, suggesting that there is only one serotype.[69-71]

HAV is a nonenveloped, 27- to 28-nm-diameter spherical virus (Fig. 15-1) with a surface structure that suggests icosahedral symmetry, though fine resolution of the virus structure by x-ray crystallography has not yet been achieved.[10] Mature HAV virions purified from feces

TABLE 15-2 ■ Age-Specific Mortality Caused by Hepatitis A

Age Group (yr)	No. of Cases (%)	No. of Deaths (%)	Case Fatality per 1000
<5	6165 (5.3)	9 (2.4)	1.5
5-14	22,548 (19.5)	1 (0.3)	0.004
15-29	49,642 (43)	28 (7.3)	0.57
30-49	26,961 (23.3)	67 (17.6)	2.5
>49	10,235 (8.8)	276 (27.4)	27
Total	115,551	381	3.3

Data from the Centers for Disease Control and Prevention, Viral Hepatitis Surveillance Program, 1983-1989, Atlanta, GA.

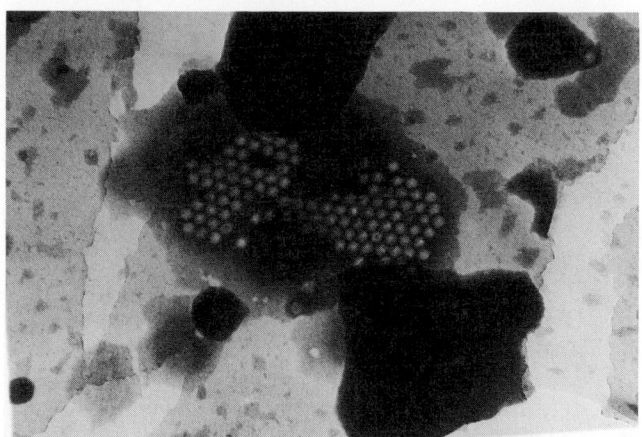

FIGURE 15–1 ■ Electron micrograph of purified hepatitis A virus particles. Magnification × 125,000.

collected from infected humans or chimpanzees band at 1.32 to 1.34 g/cm³ in CsCl and sediment at approximately 160 S.[72-74] A lower density fraction often can be detected that bands at about 1.27 g/cm³ in CsCl and sediments at 70 to 80 S and consists primarily of empty capsids. In addition, a high-density fraction (1.4 g/cm³) that may represent particles with a more open virion structure (allowing increased penetration and binding of CsCl into the viral particle) also may be found. These high-density particles have been shown to contain HAV RNA but tend to be less stable than mature virions.[74-76]

Resistance to Physical and Chemical Agents

HAV is more resistant to heat than other picornaviruses, and may be incompletely inactivated (depending on the conditions) by exposure to 60°C for 10 to 12 hours.[77,78] Complete inactivation in food requires heating to more than 85°C for at least 1 minute.[79,80] HAV may survive for days to weeks in shellfish, water, soil, or marine sediment.[81] Outbreaks of hepatitis A have been reported following ingestion of steamed shellfish, suggesting that the internal temperature achieved by steaming sometimes may be insufficient to destroy the virus.[82] HAV can be reliably inactivated by autoclaving (121°C for 30 minutes).[83]

The virus is resistant to most organic solvents and detergents as well as pH as low as 3.[75,83] HAV can be inactivated by many common disinfecting chemicals, including hypochlorite (bleach) and quaternary ammonium formulations containing 23% HCl, found in many toilet bowl cleaners.[83] Currently licensed vaccines are inactivated by 1:4000 formalin at room temperature for at least 15 days in order to exceed complete inactivation by at least threefold.

Molecular Structure

The HAV genome is composed of single-stranded linear RNA of 7478 nucleotides (strain HM175) and a molecular weight of approximately 2.25 × 10⁶.[61,84,85] The genomic RNA has positive polarity and a relatively long 5′ untranslated region (UTR) of 735 nucleotides typical of picornaviruses, followed by a single long open reading frame of approximately 6681 nucleotides coding for a polyprotein of 2227 amino acids, in turn followed by a short 3′ UTR ending with a virus-coded poly(A) tail. Sequence analysis of

the HAV genome reveals that its gene order is also characteristic of picornaviruses, with the structural genes coded by the 5′ one third of the open reading frame and the nonstructural proteins coded by the remainder. Although HAV is similar to the other picornaviruses in physical and molecular structure, it has little similarity to other picornaviruses at the nucleotide or amino acid sequence level.

As with other picornaviruses, the 5′ end of the genome does not have a cap structure but instead has a small, covalently bound, virus-coded protein termed VPg.[86] This 5′ UTR has predicted secondary structure similar to other picornavirus UTRs and includes an internal ribosomal entry site for cap-independent translation.[87,88] Translation begins at one of two in-frame AUG codons at nucleotide position 735 or 741, which initiates a single long open reading frame of 6681 nucleotides that encodes a potential polyprotein of 2227 amino acid residues in length.[89,90] Following a translation terminator sequence, the genome ends with a 3′ noncoding region of 63 nucleotides that is followed by a poly(A) tail of varying lengths typical of picornavirus genomes. The polyprotein of picornaviruses has been divided arbitrarily into three parts, termed P1, P2, and P3. The four capsid proteins are coded by the first 2373 nucleotides (P1) and the nonstructural proteins by the remainder (P2 and P3). The gene order and protein function of HAV is similar to the other picornaviruses. There are differences in the details of the protein cleavages, and HAV has only one known viral protease, protein 3C, which is responsible for all the cleavages except the final maturation cleavage of the capsid protein, VP0, into VP4 and VP2.[91-94]

The predicted VP4 molecule has never been experimentally shown to be a part of the virion particle and, at just 23 amino acids, is about one third the size of VP4 proteins of other picornaviruses. In addition, VP4s of picornaviruses are myristylated at the N-terminus after cleavage of the initial methionine or a leader peptide.[93,95] Although a potential myristylation site could be revealed in the HAV VP4 by cleavage of the first four amino acids, mutations of this myristylation site have no effect on virus replication, and it is assumed to be not active.[96]

The 2A protein of poliovirus has proteinase activity and makes the VP1/2A cleavage. However the 2A protein of HAV has no known function, and the VP1/2A cleavage seems to be performed by the major viral protease, 3C.[91] Mutants in which the central portion of 2A were deleted produced small foci in cell culture but remained virulent in marmosets.[97] The 2B and 2C proteins are believed to be involved in replication. Mutations leading to cell culture adaptation and attenuation in animals also have been mapped to these regions.[99] The protein 3AB is the precursor to VPg. Protein 3C is the virion protease, which is responsible for all the proteolytic cleavages of the HAV polyprotein except for the VP0 cleavage.[91,92,100] Protein 3D is the viral RNA–dependent RNA polymerase responsible for the replication of the genomic RNA.

Antigenic Composition

Although a variety of genotypes of HAV have been identified based on genomic sequence analysis, there appears to be only one serotype throughout the world.[64,65,69] Individuals who were infected by HAV in one part of the world are not susceptible to reinfection by virus in another part of the world, and immune globulins prepared in a variety of developed countries appear to protect travelers from disease irrespective of their destination. Vaccines prepared from virus isolates from Australia or Costa Rica induce antibody that protects worldwide.[101,102] The HAV genotypes I and III are the most genetically diverse viruses identified. A genotype I virus, HM175, and a genotype III virus, PA21, which differed by 16.8% in their nucleotide sequence in the structural protein coding region, were shown to have no significant antigenic differences in a criss-cross neutralization assay.[64,103] In addition, both viruses reacted nearly identically with a panel of 18 monoclonal antibodies.[103]

Stapleton and colleagues have made an extensive analysis of the antigenic composition of the HAV capsid through binding studies of neutralizing monoclonal antibodies and analysis of neutralization escape mutants.[104] They have shown that neutralization epitopes of HAV are contained primarily within predicted loop regions on the structural proteins VP1 and VP3. However, neutralizing monoclonal antibodies do not recognize either oligopeptides predicted to contain neutralization epitopes or denatured individual viral capsid proteins, and antibodies raised against synthetic oligopeptides do not neutralize or even bind to whole virus, which suggests that these neutralization epitopes are conformational and not linear. Binding competition assays of neutralizing monoclonal antibodies have indicated that the neutralization epitopes are contained within a closely related antigenic site.[104]

Cellular Replication

Details of HAV replication have been incompletely elucidated due to its relatively inefficient growth in vitro. Like other picornaviruses, HAV is believed to bind to the cell through a specific cellular receptor inserted into the plasma membrane. A mucin-like glycoprotein was identified in African green monkey kidney cells as an HAV cellular attachment molecule and termed *hepatitis A virus cellular receptor-1* (havcr-1). Binding of HAV to cells that express havcr-1 can be blocked by a specific monoclonal antibody to the receptor, and the complementary DNA (cDNA) coding for havcr-1 can be transfected into nonpermissive cells, rendering permissiveness for virus binding, entry, and translation. However, complete virus replication has not been demonstrated, indicating other internal blocks to replication.[105] The cys-rich immunoglobin-like region of havcr-1 is sufficient for binding of HAV. Soluble forms of havcr-1 containing the cys-rich region plus the mucin-like region neutralize and uncoat HAV, whereas forms containing only the cys-rich region do not uncoat HAV (Silberstein et al., unpublished), suggesting that the mucin-like region either provides the scaffolding for the correct presentation of the cys-rich region or interacts itself with the viral particle.

The human homologue of the monkey receptor also has been identified and shown to be functional.[106] Although the natural function of havcr-1 is unknown, the human havcr-1 has been identified in virtually all human tissues and organs that have been studied, including the liver. However, the havcr-1 message was most abundant in kidney and testes. Clearly, expression of havcr-1 does not account for tissue tropism of HAV.

Mouse genes that share homology with havcr-1, designated TIM-1, -2, and -3, have been implicated in the determination of the T-helper (Th) cell response.[107,108] Polymorphisms of the TIMs influence the differentiation of Th0 into Th1 and Th2 cells and the development of atopy in congenic mice. One group of researchers have reported an inverse association between HAV infection and atopy in humans[109,110] suggesting that human havcr-1 also could play a role in T-cell differentiation in humans.

Replication of HAV is intimately related to the cytoplasmic membranes. Intracellular virus is seen only within membrane-bound vesicles, whereas enteroviruses can be seen free in the cytoplasm. These vesicles might be released directly from the cell because virus-laden vesicles have been observed both in cell culture supernatants and in intestinal contents.[111–113]

Many HAV strains have been isolated in cell culture directly from clinical material, though the procedure may take several weeks or even months.[64] Until recently, only epithelial or fibroblast cells of primate origin had been conclusively shown to support the growth of HAV.[67,114–116] However, certain porcine, guinea pig, and dolphin cells can support the replication of HAV.[117] HAV tends to grow more slowly and generate lower yields than other picornaviruses.[67,130] The virus is largely cell associated, does not usually produce a cytopathic effect, and readily leads to persistently infected cell lines. Rapidly replicating variants of HAV have been selected that induce cytopathic effects in some cell lines.[118,119]

Cell culture of HAV has been used to alter the phenotype of the virus, primarily for growth characteristics and attenuation of virulence. Attenuated strains of HAV have been selected by multiple tissue culture passages, and cold adaptation has been achieved by passage at reduced temperature.[120,122] Some of the mutations responsible for these altered phenotypes have been determined by molecular cloning and sequencing of the mutant and comparing its sequence with the parental strain. Mutations within the 5′ UTR and mutations within the 2B and 2C coding regions of HAV RNA have been shown to enhance virus replication in vitro.[99,123]

Host Range

HAV is known to infect humans and great apes and some species of monkeys. The most extensively characterized models are the chimpanzee and two New World monkeys, tamarins and aotus (owl) monkeys.[124,126,127] The presence of antibodies in some primate species at the time of capture may indicate that there is a reservoir of infection in nature or that these antibodies may represent cross-reactive antibodies with monkey viruses. There are several reports of isolation of human HAV-related viruses from monkeys.[64,124,127] Several of these isolates have been shown to have significant sequence variation and minor antigenic differences with human HAV. Though transmission of HAV to primate handlers is well documented, it has not yet been determined if these monkey isolates are true simian hepatitis A viruses or human viruses that have infected monkey colonies, where they have persisted and adapted. Limited HAV replication has been demonstrated in guinea pigs.[128] Although HAV may be transferred to nonhuman primates and even lower order animals, it is unlikely that any of these species serves as a reservoir for HAV in the environment and is then a source of human infections.[64,124,129]

Pathogenesis as It Relates to Prevention

HAV is generally transmitted by the fecal-oral route, and this acid-resistant virus probably can survive passage through the stomach. However, it has been shown in experimental animals that oral infectivity is much lower than intravenous infectivity. One oral infectious dose was equivalent to $10^{4.5}$ intravenous doses in both tamarins and chimpanzees.[18] The primary site of HAV replication is in the liver, although there are also experimental data in chimpanzees that HAV may replicate in the oropharynx.[131] The virus has been identified by immunofluorescence in the epithelial cells of the intestinal crypts of both the jejunum and ileum of experimentally infected monkeys.[131,132] A viremic stage has been detected beginning up to 2 weeks before the onset of clinical illness and persisting for a variable period after symptoms begin in both humans and experimentally infected primates.[133–136] Although it is possible that other organs would be seeded by the viremia, HAV, like many other picornaviruses, appears to be organ specific, and the only recognized pathologic process in hepatitis A is restricted to the liver. Virus is shed from infected liver cells into the hepatic sinusoids and the bile canaliculi, passes into the intestine, and is excreted in the feces, where it may be found in high titers early in the infection.[137–139]

Because HAV is generally not cytopathic in cell culture, the pathologic findings in both experimental animals and humans show little hepatocyte damage at the peak of viral replication. Immune mechanisms, in particular cell-mediated immune responses, have been postulated to explain the hepatic injury.[140,141] In contrast, circulating antibodies are probably more important in limiting spread of virus to uninfected liver cells, which, in combination with specific T cells and interferon, is responsible for termination of the infection.[141–143]

Although liver damage occurs at the same time that circulating antibodies become detectable, studies failed to prove that the pathologic process is antibody dependent.

Whereas circulating immune complexes containing HAV and mostly HAV-specific IgM antibody has been found during infection, immunoglobulin and complement deposits were not found at the sites of liver cell damage, and resolution of disease occurred at a time when antibody levels were rising and hepatitis A antigen still could be detected in the liver.[16] Although circulating antibody limits the spread of virus and prevents reinfection, it appears to have no role in liver damage.

Immunity

Because second infections with HAV are unknown, it is assumed that immunity to the disease persists for life. In some endemic areas where exposure to the virus is common, the mean antibody levels in the population decline in older age groups, suggesting that antibody to HAV (anti-HAV) confers complete protection against reinfection.

It is known that passive immunization with immune globulin can provide complete protection against infection, indicating that serum antibody alone is sufficient to prevent infection.[144] It has been difficult to judge the effect of mucosal immunity because antibody in saliva or feces either is not detected or is present at very low levels.[145,146]

Not all aspects of the pathogenesis of HAV are understood, but it is clear that, after ingestion, the virus replicates briefly in the alimentary track without pathologic change and then is transported to the liver, possibly through the portal circulation. The liver is the major site of replication and is the source of virus that is shed into the bile and excreted in the feces. Liver cell damage is probably mediated by cytotoxic lymphocytes.

Diagnosis

Because hepatitis A is indistinguishable from other forms of acute viral hepatitis on clinical grounds, the diagnosis requires serologic detection of specific antibody responses to HAV and is confirmed by detection of HAV-specific IgM in a single acute-phase serum sample (Table 15–3).[147-149]

TABLE 15–3 ▪ Available Tests for Hepatitis A Virus and Antibody to HAV

Tests	Uses
Anti-HAV/total antibody (RIA/ELISA)*	Determine immunity/susceptibility before vaccination
	Epidemiologic studies
Anti-HAV/Ig M-specific (RIA/ELISA)*	Primary test for diagnosis of current or recent infection
	Research use, particularly for characterizing types of antibody induced by vaccination
Neutralizing antibody (radioimmunofocus inhibition [RIFIT]; HAV antigen reduction assay [HAVARNA])	Very labor intensive; not widely available or well standardized
Viral culture (cell culture)	Research use only because virus grows slowly on initial isolation
HAV antigen (RIA/ELISA)	Research use for detecting virus in various specimens (i.e., cell culture)
HAV RNA (nucleic acid testing/PCR)	Research applications
	Epidemiologic studies and outbreak investigations
	Environmental studies
Liver biopsy (light or fluorescent microscopy)	Research with animal inoculations
	Rare diagnostic dilemma or unusual clinical presentation
	Biopsy not indicated for most hepatitis A cases

HAV, hepatitis A virus; ELISA, enzyme-linked immunosorbent assay; IgM, immunoglobulin M; PCR, polymerase chain reaction; RIA, radioimmunoassay.
*Only ELISAs are currently commercially available

HAV-specific IgM antibody appears early in the course of the illness, is usually present at the time the patient seeks medical attention, and declines to undetectable levels within 6 months. Their presence in the serum is regarded as evidence of current or recent infection[150] (Fig. 15–2). Biochemical evidence of hepatitis consists of elevated levels of serum bilirubin and serum hepatic enzymes, including alanine aminotransferase (ALT), aspartate aminotransferase (AST), alkaline phosphatase, and gamma-glutamyltranspeptidase. Elevations in AST and ALT occur most consistently, and may precede the appearance of symptoms by a week or more (see Fig. 15–2). Except for patients with relapsing or cholestatic hepatitis A, serum bilirubin and aminotransferase levels usually return to normal by 2 to 3 months after illness onset.[26]

Other tests are rarely used for diagnosis of HAV infection (see Table 15–3). Viral detection assays generally have not been useful because wild-type HAV is extremely difficult to isolate in cell culture, usually requiring weeks or months. Because virus shedding peaks before the onset of clinical illness, antigen detection systems usually are insufficiently sensitive to detect HAV in stool samples. Polymerase chain reaction (PCR) techniques have been useful in certain clinical, epidemiologic, and environmental studies and potentially could be used on clinical samples, but the difficulty and expense of performing these tests as well as the ease, accuracy, and sensitivity of the serologic tests, preclude the necessity of these types of specialized assays outside of research settings.[151–153]

Commercially available serologic tests that measure the total anti-HAV are not helpful for diagnosis of acute illness because patients with distant past exposures maintain IgG-class antibody against HAV for their lifetimes. The total antibody assays are used most often in epidemiologic investigations or in determining susceptibility to HAV infection.

Treatment

No specific therapy is available for hepatitis A, and management is supportive. Most physicians do not recommend activity restriction because studies have failed to demonstrate an impact on the course of illness. Similarly, it has been customary to recommend against vigorous exercise and to encourage abstinence from alcohol, although there are few objective data that demonstrate a benefit. Medications, particularly those metabolized by the liver or that are potentially hepatotoxic, should be used with caution because the half-life may be prolonged. Hospitalization may be necessary for patients who become dehydrated from vomiting or who develop fulminant hepatitis.

Hepatitis A is occasionally complicated by cholestasis. A brief course of corticosteroids has been reported to shorten the course and reduce symptoms, primarily itching, but recovery is universal even without treatment.[29] Transplantation may be indicated in some cases of fulminant hepatitis, but because survival without transplantation is relatively high and no single factor is predictive of poor outcome, it has been difficult to establish criteria for choosing transplantation candidates.[30,154–156] Persistent HAV infection has been demonstrated in some transplant recipients, but whether this affects survival is unknown.[157]

Epidemiology

Modes of Transmission

HAV replicates in the liver, is excreted in bile, and is found in highest concentrations in stool.[158] Because of the high concentration of HAV in the stool of infected persons, fecal excretion of HAV is the primary source of virus. The highest concentrations in stool occur during the 2-week period before jaundice develops or liver enzymes become elevated, followed by a rapid decline after the appearance of jaundice (see Fig. 15–2).[10,158,159] Shedding of HAV may continue for longer periods in infected infants and children than in adults. With the use of PCR techniques, HAV RNA has been detected in stools of infected newborns for up to 6 months after infection.[160] Excretion in older children and adults has been demonstrated 1 to 3 months after clinical illness.[101,136,160] Although chronic shedding of HAV does not occur, the virus has been detected in stool during relapsing illness.[27]

During the period of viremia, which begins during the prodrome and extends through the period of liver enzyme elevation (see Fig. 15–2), HAV concentrations are several orders of magnitude lower than in stool.[135,136,161,162] However, in experiments conducted in nonhuman primates, HAV was several orders of magnitude more infectious when administered by the intravenous compared with the oral route, and animals were successfully infected with low concentrations of HAV administered by the intravenous route.[18] Although HAV occasionally may be detected in saliva in experimentally infected animals,[135] transmission by saliva has not been demonstrated.

Because enzyme immunoassays and PCR may detect defective as well as infectious viral particles, the detection of HAV antigen in the stool by enzyme immunoassays or HAV RNA in the serum or stool by PCR cannot delineate whether an infected person is infectious. It is likely that the period of infectivity is shorter than the period during which HAV RNA is detectable. Although infectivity of stools has been demonstrated in experimental studies 14 to 21 days before to 8 days after onset of jaundice, data from epidemiologic studies

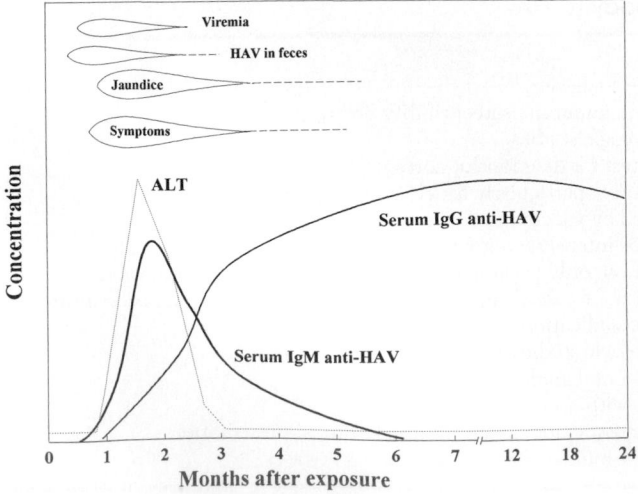

FIGURE 15–2 ■ The clinical, virologic, and serologic events after hepatitis A virus (HAV) infection. ALT, alanine aminotransferase.

suggest that peak infectivity occurs during the 2 weeks before the onset of symptoms.[133] For practical purposes, both children and adults with hepatitis A can be assumed to be noninfectious 1 week after jaundice appears.

Person to Person

Person-to-person transmission by the fecal-oral route is the predominant means of HAV transmission in the United States and throughout the world.[11,163] Most transmission occurs among close contacts, particularly in households and extended family settings.[164] Young children have the highest rates of infection and are often the source of infection for others, because infections in this age group are often asymptomatic and standards of hygiene are generally lower among young children compared to adults.[164-166]

Food-borne and Waterborne

HAV can remain infectious in the environment,[167] allowing for common-source outbreaks and sporadic cases to occur from exposure to fecally contaminated food or water. Many uncooked foods have been implicated, but even cooked foods can transmit HAV if the cooking is inadequate to kill the virus or if the food is contaminated after cooking, as commonly occurs in outbreaks associated with infected food handlers.[168-170] Contaminated shellfish were responsible for a large outbreak in Shanghai, China, in 1998, and have been implicated as the source of cases in Italy, but have rarely been associated with outbreaks in the United States in recent years.[171-174] Waterborne outbreaks of hepatitis A are uncommon in developed countries.

Blood-borne

Transfusion-related hepatitis A is rare because HAV does not result in chronic infection, and, in the developed world, blood donors have been screened for many years for elevated aminotransferase levels. However, transmission by transfusion of blood or blood derivatives collected from donors during the viremic phase of their infection has been reported, including outbreaks in Europe and the United States among patients who received factor VIII and factor IX concentrates prepared using solvent-detergent treatment to inactivate lipid-containing viruses.[162,175-177] HAV is resistant to solvent-detergent treatment, and contamination presumably occurred from plasma donors with hepatitis A who donated during the incubation period.

Since 2002, nucleic acid amplification tests such as PCR have been applied to the screening of blood for transfusion and source plasma used for the manufacture of plasma-derived products. These assays have sufficient sensitivity to remove most units of blood or plasma that contain HAV.[178]

Vertical

Two published case reports describe intrauterine transmission of HAV during the first trimester, resulting in fetal meconium peritonitis.[179,180] After delivery, both infants were found to have a perforated ileum. The risk of transmission from pregnant women who develop hepatitis A in the third trimester of pregnancy to newborns appears to be low.[181] However, newborns who acquire infection in this manner are usually asymptomatic, and an outbreak among hospital staff related to exposure to such an infant has been reported.[182]

Worldwide Disease Patterns

Hepatitis A occurs worldwide, but major geographic differences exist in endemicity and resulting epidemiologic features (Fig. 15–3). The degree of endemicity is closely related to hygienic and sanitary conditions and other

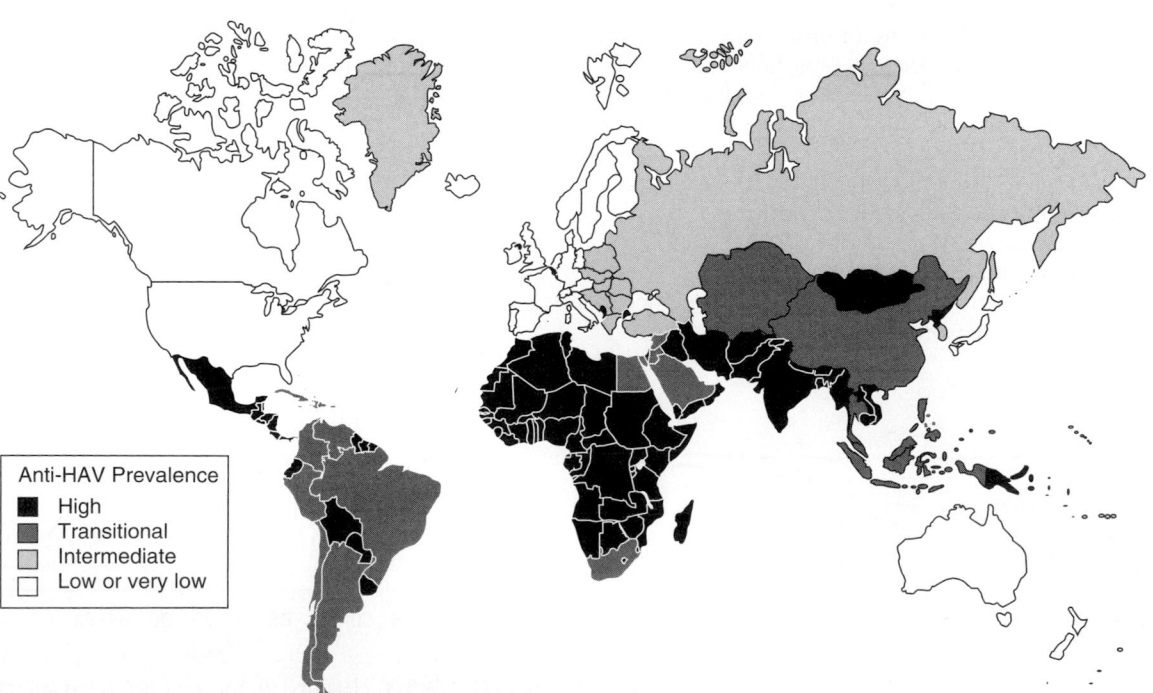

Anti-HAV Prevalence
■ High
▨ Transitional
▨ Intermediate
□ Low or very low

FIGURE 15–3 ■ World map indicating patterns of endemicity of hepatitis A virus (HAV) infection (generalized from available data). Anti-HAV, antibody to HAV. The anti-HAV prevalence patterns of high, intermediate, low, and very low endemicity are shown in Figure 15–4.

indicators of the level of development. Under conditions of overcrowding, especially when there is limited access to clean water and inadequate disposal of human feces, HAV infects most people early in life, when infection is rarely clinically apparent (Fig. 15–4). Where high standards of hygiene and sanitation apply, most children reach adult life without encountering the virus. Distinct patterns of HAV infection can be described, each with characteristic age-specific profiles of anti-HAV prevalence and hepatitis A incidence and prevailing environmental (hygienic and sanitary) and socioeconomic conditions (Fig. 15–4).[11,12]

In areas of high endemicity, represented by the least developed countries (i.e., parts of Africa, Asia, and Central and South America), poor socioeconomic conditions allow HAV to spread readily (see Fig. 15–3). Infection is nearly universal in early childhood, when asymptomatic infection predominates, and essentially the entire population is infected before reaching adolescence, as demonstrated by the age-specific prevalence of anti-HAV (see Fig. 15–4).[183,184] Susceptible adults in these areas are at high risk of infection and disease, but reported disease rates are generally low and outbreaks rare because of the high prevalence of immunity in the population. High endemicity patterns also may be seen in some ethnic or geographic groups within highly developed countries, such as aboriginal children in the north of Australia.[185]

In areas of moderate endemicity, HAV is not transmitted as readily because of better sanitary and living conditions, and the predominant age of infection is older than in areas of high endemicity (see Figs. 15–3 and 15–4).[186] Paradoxically, the overall incidence and average age of reported cases are often higher than in highly endemic areas because high levels of virus circulate in a population that includes many susceptible older children, adolescents, and young adults, who are likely to develop symptoms with HAV infection.[187] Large common-source food- and water-associated outbreaks occur because of the relatively high rate of virus transmission and large number of susceptible persons, especially among those of higher socioeconomic level. Such an outbreak occurred in Shanghai in 1988, with over 300,000 cases associated with consumption of clams harvested from water contaminated with human sewage.[188] Nevertheless, person-to-person transmission in community-wide epidemics continues to account for much of the disease in these countries.

Shifts in age-specific prevalence patterns that reflect a transition from high to intermediate endemicity are occurring in many parts of the world (see Fig. 15–3). A feature of this transitional pattern is striking variations in hepatitis A epidemiology between countries, and within countries and cities, with some areas displaying a pattern typical of high endemicity and others a pattern of intermediate endemicity.[11,189–198] Considerable hepatitis A–related morbidity and associated costs occur with this transition, even in developing countries.[199,200] For example, hepatitis A was the etiology of the fulminant hepatitis of two thirds of children presenting to two hospitals in Argentina during a 15-year period, and, in one of these hospitals performing liver transplantations, one third of liver transplantations among children were for fulminant hepatitis A.[199]

In the United States, Canada, Western Europe, and other developed countries, the endemicity of HAV infection is low (see Figs. 15–3 and 15–4). Relatively fewer children are infected, the incidence of disease is generally low, and disease often occurs in the context of community-wide and child care center outbreaks.[163,201–204] A cyclic pattern of disease incidence with peaks every 5 to 10 years has been noted in some developed countries with temperate climates. Population-based seroprevalence surveys show a gradual increase in the prevalence of anti-HAV with increasing age, primarily reflecting declining incidence, changing endemicity, and resultant lower childhood infection rates over time (see Fig. 15–4). Some countries (e.g., Scandinavia) have very low endemicity, with most cases occurring in defined risk groups such as travelers returning from areas of high or intermediate endemicity and users of injection drugs.[205]

Epidemiology in the United States

Hepatitis A is one of the most frequently reported infectious diseases in the United States that is now preventable by vaccination (see Fig. 15–5). In 1997, 30,021 cases were reported to the Centers for Disease Control and Prevention (CDC).[206] National surveillance systems collect data on symptomatic cases, and incidence models indicate that the majority of infections are not detected. One such analysis

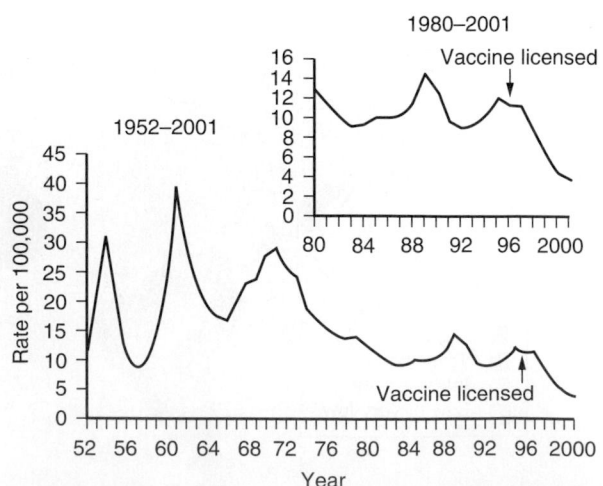

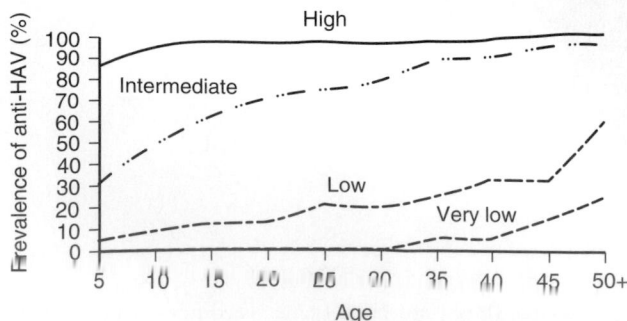

FIGURE 15–4 ■ Patterns of hepatitis A virus infection worldwide.

FIGURE 15–5 ■ Hepatitis A incidence, United States, 1952 to 2001. (Data from the Centers for Disease Control and Prevention, National Notifiable Diseases Surveillance System, Atlanta, GA. Data for 2001 are provisional.)

estimated an average of 271,000 infections per year during 1980 to 1999, 10.4 times the reported number of cases.[166]

Variation by Age and Race/Ethnicity

Historically, the highest hepatitis A rates were reported among children 5 to 14 years of age, with approximately one third of cases occurring among children younger than 15 years of age.[207] Because many young children have unrecognized asymptomatic infection, they also likely represent a major reservoir for HAV transmission. Incidence models indicate that more than half of HAV infections occur among children less than 10 years old, the majority of which are in children from birth to 4 years old.[166] Among racial/ethnic groups, before the use of hepatitis A vaccine, rates among Native Americans and Alaska Natives were more than 10 times the rate in other racial/ethnic groups, and rates among Hispanics were approximately three times higher than among non-Hispanics.[208]

Results of the Third National Health and Nutrition Examination Survey, conducted during 1988 to 1994, indicated that about one third of the U.S. population had serologic evidence of prior HAV infection.[13] Anti-HAV prevalence was related directly to age, ranging from 9% among children 6 to 11 years of age to 75% among persons older than 70 years of age, and was related inversely to income. Anti-HAV prevalence was highest among Mexican-Americans (70%), compared with non-Hispanic blacks (39%) and whites (23%).

Geographic Variation

Analysis of national surveillance data shows striking regional variation in hepatitis A incidence, with the highest rates and majority of cases consistently occurring in a limited number of states and counties concentrated in the western and southwestern United States (Fig. 15–6). Despite year-to-year fluctuations, rates in these areas consistently remained above the national average. Cases among residents of the 11 states, representing 22% of the U.S. population, in which the average annual hepatitis A incidence was 20 cases per 100,000 or greater during 1987 to 1997 (twice the national average of about 10 per 100,000) accounted for an average of 50% of reported cases (Table 15–4). An additional 18% of cases were among residents of states with average annual rates above the national average but less than twice the national average during this time (Table 15–4).

Potential Sources of Infection

Based on data from disease surveillance systems, the most commonly reported potential source of infection is household or sexual contact with a person who has hepatitis A (15% to 25% of reported cases).[163,207] Approximately 10%

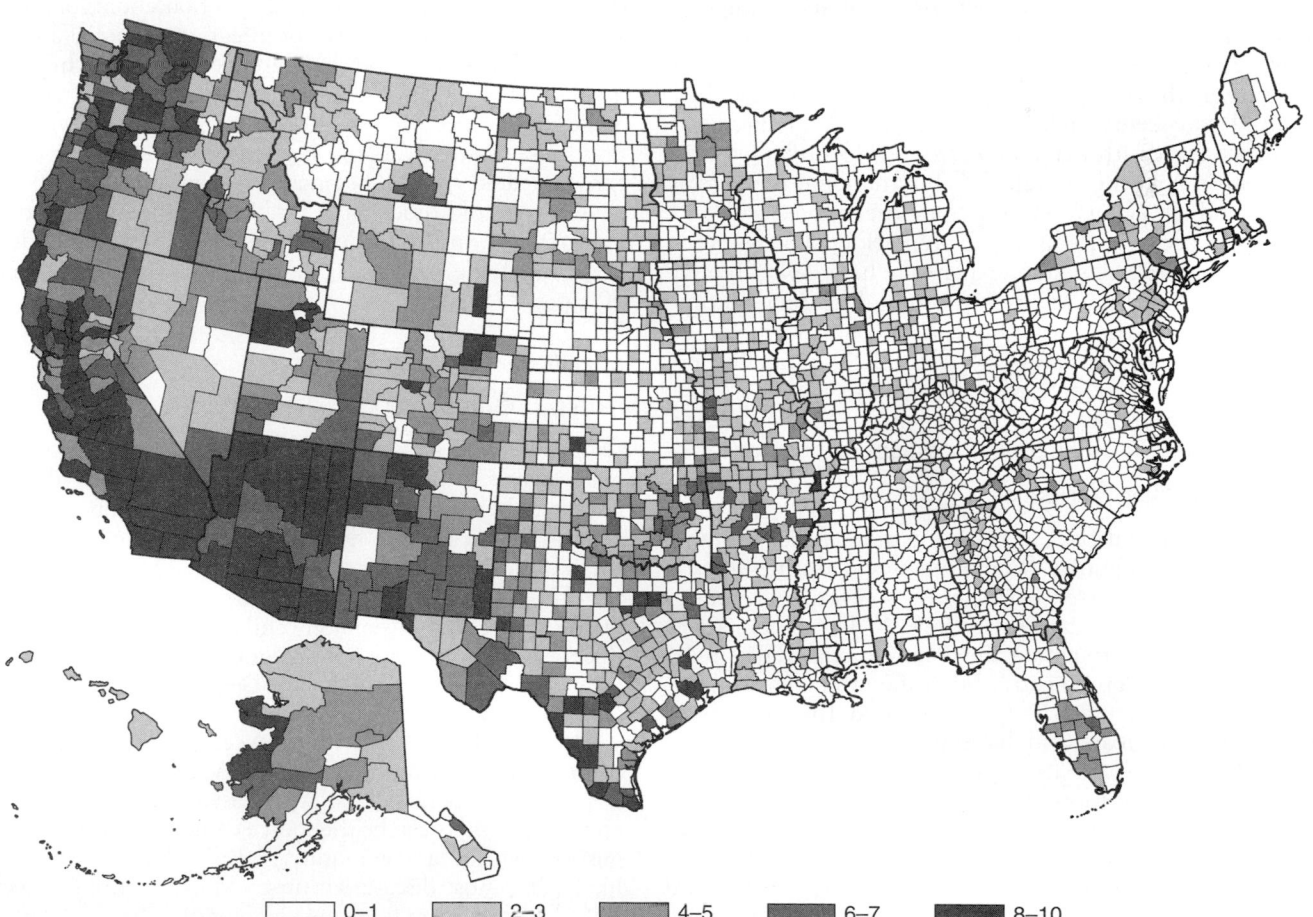

0–1   2–3   4–5   6–7   8–10

FIGURE 15–6 ■ Number of years that reported hepatitis A incidence exceeded 10 cases per 100,000, by county, 1987 through 1997. (Note: Ten cases per 100,000 was approximately the national average during 1987 to 1997.)

TABLE 15–4 ▪ Occurrence of Hepatitis A in States with Average Reported Incidence of 10 or More Cases per 100,000 Population, 1987 to 1997*

State	Rate (per 100,000)[†]	Cumulative Average Number of Cases/Year[‡]	Cumulative % Cases	Cumulative % Population[§]
Arizona	48	1852	7	2
Alaska	45	2137	8	2
Oregon	40	3297	12	3
New Mexico	40	3916	14	4
Utah	33	4519	16	5
Washington	30	6007	21	7
Oklahoma	24	6786	24	8
South Dakota	24	6953	25	8
Idaho	21	7172	26	9
Nevada	21	7449	27	10
California	20	13,706	50	22
Missouri	19	14,706	54	24
Texas	16	17,587	64	31
Colorado	16	18,138	56	33
Arkansas	14	18,483	67	34
Montana	11	18,576	68	34
Wyoming	11	18,627	68	34

*The overall U.S. rate during 1987 to 1997 was 10.8 per 100,000 population.
[†]Children living in areas (states, counties, communities) where the rate was 20 cases or more per 100,000 population should be routinely vaccinated. Children living in areas where the rate was 10 cases or more per 100,000 population, but less than 20 cases per 100,000 population, should be considered for routine vaccination.
[‡]Approximately 37% of cases were among persons under age 20 years.
[§]1997 estimates from U.S. Census data.

to 15% of reported cases occur among children and employees of child care centers and members of their households. However, this may overestimate disease truly attributable to exposure in these settings because these cases are ascribed to child care center–related contact without requiring a known contact with hepatitis A or even identifying a case of hepatitis A in the center.[163,207] International travel (5% to 7%) and suspected food- or waterborne outbreaks (2% to 5%) each account for a small proportion of cases.[202,207] Cyclic outbreaks occur among men who have sex with men and users of injecting and noninjecting drugs, and, during outbreak years, this exposure can account for 10% of nationally reported cases[163,209–212] (CDC, unpublished data). Nearly 50% of patients with hepatitis A do not have a recognized source of infection,[207] but may be contacts of persons, especially children, with asymptomatic infection.

Community-Wide Epidemics

Most cases of hepatitis A in the United States occur in the context of community-wide epidemics, during which infection is transmitted from person to person in households and extended family settings.[163] These epidemics generally spread throughout the community, and no single risk factor or risk group can be identified that can account for the majority of cases.[163] Once initiated, they often persist for several years and have proved difficult to control,[213] even when attempts were made to rapidly vaccinate some portion of the population.[214,215] Children play an important role in sustaining HAV transmission during these epidemics. During community-wide outbreaks, serologic studies of members of households with an adult case without an identified source have found that 25% to 40% of contacts less than 6 years old had serologic evidence of recent HAV infection[164] (CDC, unpublished

data). In one of these studies, 52% of households of adults without an identified source of infection included a child less than 6 years old, and the presence of a young child was associated with household transmission of HAV.[164] Transmission occurred in 80% of households in which a child less than 6 years old resided or was regularly cared for, compared to 42% of households without a child less than 6 years old (odds ratio 5.6 [95% confidence interval, 1.4 to 26.6]). In this study, transmission chains were identified involving as many as six generations and more than 20 cases.

Specific Groups and Settings

CHILD CARE CENTERS, SCHOOLS, AND INSTITUTIONS

Outbreaks in child care centers have been recognized for many decades. They rarely occur in centers that do not have children in diapers and are more common in larger centers.[21,216] Both poor hygiene among these children and the need for staff to handle and change diapers contribute to spread. As has been recognized since the 1970s, outbreaks can be sustained among children with asymptomatic infection, and often are not recognized until adult contacts (usually parents) become ill.[21,217] Despite the occurrence of outbreaks when HAV is introduced into a child care center, studies of child care center employees do not show a significantly increased prevalence of HAV infection compared with control populations.[218] Occasionally, outbreaks in child care centers can be the source of more extensive transmission within a community.[216,218,219,220] However, it is likely that most disease within child care centers reflects disease transmission from the community.

Hepatitis A cases among children in schools usually reflect disease that has been acquired in the community.

However, multiple cases among children within a school may indicate a common-source outbreak.[153] Historically, HAV infection was endemic in institutions for the developmentally disabled, but with smaller facilities and improved conditions, the incidence and prevalence of infection have decreased and outbreaks rarely are reported in the United States.[221]

USERS OF ILLICIT DRUGS

During the two past decades, outbreaks have been reported with increasing frequency among illicit drug users in North America, Australia, and Europe.[211,212,222–224] In the United States, these outbreaks, particularly in the past decade, frequently have involved users of injected and noninjected methamphetamine, who may account for up to 30% of reported cases in these communities during outbreaks.[163,212,224] Cross-sectional serologic surveys have demonstrated that injection drug users have higher prevalence of anti-HAV than the general U.S. population.[225,226] Transmission among injection drug users probably occurs through both percutaneous and fecal-oral routes.[224]

MEN WHO HAVE SEX WITH MEN

Hepatitis A outbreaks among men who have sex with men have been reported frequently, most recently in urban areas in the United States, Canada, England, and Australia, and may occur in the context of an outbreak in the larger community.[163,209,210,227–229] Seroprevalence surveys have not consistently demonstrated an elevated prevalence of anti-HAV compared to a general population of similar age.[226,230] Some studies conducted during outbreaks and seroprevalence surveys among men who have sex with men have identified specific sex practices associated with illness, whereas others have not demonstrated such associations.[209,226,228]

TRANSFUSIONS AND OTHER HEALTH CARE SETTINGS

Transfusion-related hepatitis A is rare. The risk of infection in patients with hemophilia is not known, but results of one serologic survey of hemophiliac patients suggest they may be at increased risk,[231] and outbreaks have been reported in Europe and the United States among patients who received factor VIII and factor IX concentrates.[176,232] Outbreaks also have been reported in neonatal intensive care units following transmission to hospital staff from a neonate with asymptomatic HAV infection acquired from a blood transfusion.[160,233,234] Transmission also was reported in association with an experimental treatment with lymphocytes incubated in serum from a donor with HAV infection.[235]

Nosocomial transmission from adult patients to health care workers is rare because most patients with hepatitis A are hospitalized after the onset of jaundice, when infectivity is low,[159] but has been reported in association with fecal incontinence of the patient.[236,237] Health care workers have not been found to have an increased prevalence of anti-HAV compared with control populations in serologic surveys conducted in the United States.[238]

INTERNATIONAL TRAVEL

Hepatitis A is a common infection among persons from developed countries who travel to regions with high, transitional, or intermediate endemicity (see Fig. 15–3).[239–241]

In prospective studies of American and European travelers, the risk of infection for those who did not receive immune globulin was found to be 3 to 5 per 1000 per month of stay, of the same order of magnitude as that for malaria, 10 to 100 times greater than for typhoid, and 1000 times greater than for cholera.[242,243] The risk may be higher among travelers staying in areas with poor hygienic conditions,[244] varies according to the region and the length of stay, and appears to be increased even among travelers who reported observing protective measures and staying in urban areas or luxury hotels (CDC, unpublished data). In the United States, approximately 5% to 7% of reported cases occur in persons with a history of recent international travel; children account for approximately one third of these cases[207] (CDC, unpublished data). Travelers who acquire hepatitis A during their trip also may transmit the virus to others on their return.[245]

FOOD-BORNE AND WATERBORNE

Food-borne hepatitis A outbreaks are recognized relatively infrequently in the United States. They are most commonly associated with contamination of food during preparation by a food handler with HAV infection.[168,169,246,247] Implicated foods include those not cooked after handling, such as sandwiches and salads, as well as partially cooked foods.[248–251] Food contaminated before retail distribution, such as lettuce or fruits contaminated at the growing or processing stage, increasingly has been recognized as the source of hepatitis A outbreaks.[153,171,252–255] Waterborne hepatitis A outbreaks are rare and related to sewage contamination or inadequate treatment of water.[256–258]

Although results of some serologic surveys conducted among sewage workers in Europe indicated a possible elevated risk of HAV infection, findings have not been consistent.[259–261] In published reports of three serologic surveys conducted among U.S. sewage workers and appropriate comparison populations, no substantial or consistent increase in prevalence of anti-HAV was found among sewage workers.[262–264] No work-related instances of HAV transmission have been reported among sewage workers in the United States.

Passive Immunization

Until the licensure of hepatitis A vaccines, immune globulin was the mainstay of prevention of hepatitis A for people who either were likely to be exposed or had recently been exposed. This product has proven useful for prevention of hepatitis A in travelers, Peace Corps volunteers, military personnel, and individuals recently in close contact with a person with hepatitis A, and to control outbreaks in child care centers.[144,220,265,266] For example, the rate of HAV infections among Peace Corps volunteers dropped from 1.6 to 2.1 cases per 100 per year to 0.1 to 0.3 cases per 100 per year after the institution of a mandatory program of immune globulin every 4 months.[266]

In general, when administered before exposure or within 2 weeks after exposure, immune globulin is more than 85% effective in preventing hepatitis A.[267–269] Its efficacy was first demonstrated during an outbreak in a summer camp in 1944, when 3 (6%) of 53 immune globulin recipients developed hepatitis compared to 125 (45%) of the 278 persons who did not receive it, an 87% reduction in the attack rate.[269] Similar reductions in hepatitis attack rates were observed among adults in the military and children in institutional settings who received immune globulin. The lowest effective dose and duration of protection were defined in studies that compared various immune globulin doses, conducted during the 1950s and 1960s at the Willowbrook State School and other settings where hepatitis was common.[267–272] Whether immune globulin completely prevents infection or leads to asymptomatic infection and the development of persistent anti-HAV (passive-active immunity) probably is related to the amount of time that has elapsed between exposure and immune globulin administration.[24,270] However, immune globulin has not been successful in controlling community-wide hepatitis A outbreaks, owing at least in part to the transient nature of protection and the frequency of unrecognized infection.[213]

Immune globulin is a sterile solution of antibodies prepared by a serial cold ethanol precipitation procedure from large pools of plasma, collected from tens of thousands of donors, that has tested negative for hepatitis B surface antigen, antibody to human immunodeficiency virus (HIV), and antibody to hepatitis C virus.[273] This precipitation procedure has been shown to inactivate hepatitis B virus and HIV.[272] Since 1995, immune globulin prepared in the United States has been required to be negative for hepatitis C virus RNA by PCR amplification or to be produced using a method that ensures additional virus inactivation. Because the prevalence of antibody to HAV in the population has been declining, there is a concern that antibody levels against HAV in immune globulin preparations might drop below effective levels. Although in the United States there is no standard for anti-HAV levels in immune globulin preparations, at this time there is no evidence of reduced efficacy of immune globulin.[274]

Immune globulin is recommended for postexposure prophylaxis in selected settings (Table 15–6). Household and sexual contacts of patients with hepatitis A should receive immune globulin as soon as possible but no later than 2 weeks after exposure.[13] Casual contacts, such as school classmates or co-workers, who have not had close physical contact usually do not require immune globulin prophylaxis. Aggressive use of immune globulin is indicated to control

hepatitis A outbreaks in child care centers where a child or employee is diagnosed with hepatitis A[13,217] and in other settings (e.g., hospitals, facilities for developmentally disabled persons) when outbreaks occur.[13] When a food handler is identified with hepatitis A, immune globulin should be administered to other food handlers at the food establishment and under limited circumstances to patrons.[13,168] Once cases are identified that are associated with a food service establishment, it generally is too late to administer immune globulin to patrons because the 2-week postexposure period during which immune globulin is effective will have passed.

Immune globulin also may be used for pre-exposure prophylaxis for persons who are traveling to countries with high, transitional, or intermediate hepatitis A endemicity (see Fig. 15–3), particularly those departing within 2 to 4 weeks, instead of or in addition to hepatitis A vaccine (Table 15–5).[13] Immune globulin should be given to travelers younger than 2 years of age, because hepatitis A vaccine is not licensed for children in this age group, to prevent the rare severe cases that occur and transmission to others after returning from abroad.[13] Economic analysis studies have shown that, in general, hepatitis A vaccine becomes more cost effective than immune globulin as the number of expected trips during a 10-year period involving exposure to HAV or the duration of each trip increases.[275,276] Immune globulin is also recommended for pre-exposure prophylaxis for anyone with known allergy to the vaccine or a component.

The usual dose of immune globulin for prophylaxis pre-exposure is a single intramuscular injection of 0.02 or 0.06 mL/kg (see Table 15–5). The lower dose is adequate to provide protection for up to 3 months and the higher dose is effective for up to 5 months.[274] Readministration every 5 months is necessary for extended trips, and hepatitis A vaccine, if not contraindicated, is probably a better choice for such travelers. Intramuscular preparations of immune globulin should never be given intravenously, and the intravenous preparations of immune globulin are not intended for hepatitis A prevention and are formulated at a lower globulin concentration.

Serious adverse events from immune globulin are rare. Because anaphylaxis has been reported after repeated administration to persons with immunoglobulin A deficiency, these persons should not receive IG.[277] Pregnancy or lactation is not a contraindication to immune globulin

TABLE 15–5 ■ Recommendations for Hepatitis A Pre-exposure Immunoprophylaxis

Age (yr)	Exposure Duration	Recommended Prophylaxis
<2	Short term (<3 mo)	IG 0.02 mL/kg
	3–5 mo	IG 0.06 mL/kg
	>5 mo	IG 0.06 mL/kg repeated every 5 mo
>2	Short or long term	Hepatitis A vaccine
		Hepatitis A vaccine and IG (0.02 mL/kg) if exposure is expected in less than 2–4 weeks
		Substitute IG as above if vaccine is contraindicated or refused

IG, immune globulin.

TABLE 15–6 ■ Recommendations for Hepatitis A Postexposure Prophylaxis

Time Since Exposure	Future Exposure Likely or Other Indication for Vaccination*	Recommended Prophylaxis
< 2 wk	No	IG 0.02 mL/kg
	Yes	IG 0.02 mL/kg and initiate hepatitis A vaccine series[†]
> 2 wk	No	None
	Yes	Initiate hepatitis A vaccine series[+]

*See Table 15–8.
[†]Children less than 2 years of age (for whom vaccine is not licensed) and persons with a contraindication to vaccination should receive IG 0.06 mL/kg, repeated every 5 months during exposure.
IG, immune globulin.

administration. For infants and pregnant women, a preparation that does not include thimerosal is preferable.

Active Immunization

History of Vaccine Development

Active immunization with hepatitis A vaccines was developed in a manner similar to that for poliovirus vaccines. As for poliovirus, the initial breakthrough came with the in vitro cultivation of HAV in cell lines suitable for vaccine production.[114] Formalin-inactivated, cell culture–produced whole-virus vaccines have now been approved in much of the world.[278,279]

The CR326 and the HM175 strains were found to be highly attenuated in humans and have been tested as live, attenuated vaccine candidates in primates and to a limited extent in humans.[280–283] For both strains, an inoculum of greater than 10^6 tissue culture infective doses was required to induce an antibody response in volunteers. That the vaccines infected volunteers was never proved because the only evidence was seroconversion, which could have been induced by the antigenic mass contained in the inoculum rather than new antigen produced by replication. The H2 strain has been used in clinical studies in China.[122,284]

The entire nucleotide sequences of both the wild type and the vaccine variant of HM175 have been determined.[85,89] A full-length, infectious cDNA clone of the cell culture–adapted virus was made,[285,286] and the mutations responsible for cell culture adaptation and attenuation were determined by the molecular construction of chimeric viruses.[99,123,286] It was found that substitutions and deletions in the 5 noncoding region and substitutions in the 2B/2C coding regions are highly important for cell culture adaptation and attenuation of virulence. However, mutations throughout the genome contributed to improved in vitro replication.[287] It may be difficult to develop a live vaccine that is both adequately immunogenic and attenuated because the properties of replication and pathogenesis may be closely linked.

Description of Current Vaccines and History of Development

Two inactivated hepatitis A vaccines, Havrix (GlaxoSmithKline, Philadelphia) and VAQTA (Merck & Co., Inc., West Point, PA), have been approved for use in the United States and throughout much of the world.[278,279] Two other vaccines are licensed in Europe, Canada, and selected other countries.[288,289] VAQTA is based on the CR326F strain, initially isolated from Costa Rica and the first strain to be successfully cultivated in vitro.[114] CR326F initially was isolated in a fetal rhesus kidney cell line, FRhK6. After 15 passages, it was transferred to MRC-5 cells for an additional 28 passages.[279] Havrix is based on strain HM175 of HAV, isolated from stool of a patient in a family outbreak in Australia.[290] It was originally adapted to cell culture by a series of 30 passages in primary green monkey kidney cells followed by adaptation to human embryonic lung diploid fibroblasts (MRC-5 cells).[278]

Aventis Pasteur (Lyon, France) licensed a hepatitis A vaccine in Europe, Canada, and other areas called AVAXIM, based on the GBM strain of HAV. This strain was isolated and propagated on primary human kidney cell culture for 10 passages, followed by adaptation to human diploid fibroblast cells during 20 passages.[291–293] Inoculation of chimpanzees showed that the strain had been attenuated by passage.[294] The vaccine is produced in the MRC-5 human diploid fibroblast cell strain and is processed in a way similar to the U.S.-licensed vaccines.[288]

A vaccine developed at the Swiss Serum Institute, called Epaxal, is licensed by Berna Biotech Ltd (Bern, Switzerland) in most countries in Europe and Canada and many countries in South America and other parts of the world.[289,295] The strain of HAV used in the vaccine is RG-SB, harvested from disrupted MRC-5 cells and inactivated by formalin. The liposome adjuvant, immunopotentiating, reconstituted influenza virosomes (IRIV), is composed of phosphatidylcholine, phosphatidylethanolamine, and hemagglutinin from an H_1N_1 strain of influenza virus. It is hypothesized that IRIVs may stimulate both humoral and cellular immunity by binding to macrophages and other cells primed by influenza virus.[296]

Constituents

All available inactivated vaccines include HAV antigen, but the units by which the antigen content is expressed are different for each vaccine (see below). Owing to the different assays used and the lack of an accepted standard, it is not possible to compare the antigen content of the various vaccines. Havrix, VAQTA, and AVAXIM contain aluminum hydroxide (alum) as an adjuvant. Epaxal uses liposomes as the adjuvant. Havrix and AVAXIM are formulated using 2-phenoxyethanol as a preservative; the other vaccines are formulated without preservatives. No antibiotics are present in any of the vaccines. Hepatitis A viral particles are concentrated and purified during the manufacture of all of the vaccines. Differences in the content of nonvirion proteins exist between the vaccines, but these differences have not been found to be clinically relevant.

Manufacture

All inactivated hepatitis A vaccines are produced in similar ways, with only details of the manufacturing process differing. Most vaccines are grown in MRC-5 cell culture and harvested by cell lysis. The HAV in Havrix is concentrated and purified by sterile filtration, ultrafiltration, and column chromatography. The virus is then inactivated by 250 µg formaldehyde/mL for 15 days at 37°C. The purified/inactivated virus is adsorbed on aluminum hydroxide (alum) as an adjuvant, and each mL contains approximately 0.5 mg of aluminum as aluminum hydroxide. The vaccine potency (per dose) is expressed as enzyme-linked immunosorbent assay (ELISA) units (EL.U.), as defined by a standard. Phenoxyethanol at 5 mg/mL is added as a preservative. No antibiotics are present in the vaccine.[278]

VAQTA is grown in MRC-5 cells, extracted by organic solvents, concentrated by precipitation in polyethylene glycol, purified by chromatography, inactivated by 100 µg formaldehyde/mL for 20 days at 37°C, and adsorbed on alum. The antigen content is expressed as units (U) of HAV antigen. It contains approximately 0.45 mg/mL of aluminum as alum, and contains no preservatives or antibiotics.[279]

Formalin inactivation conditions have been set empirically by determining the killing kinetics, extrapolating the curve to the zero intercept where 100% inactivation is theoretically achieved, and exceeding that time by a factor of three. Inactivation is monitored throughout the process, and steps are employed to avoid aggregation of the virus. Because HAV grows slowly in cell culture without cytopathic effect, completeness of inactivation is difficult to prove. Inactivation of these vaccines has been demonstrated by serial blind passages designed to amplify a low level of residual live virus to the point that it would be immunologically detectable. An additional margin of safety is achieved in both Havrix and VAQTA by the use of HAV strains that are highly attenuated in humans.

Preparations

Both inactivated hepatitis A vaccines licensed in the United States are available in pediatric and adult formulations (Table 15–7). AVAXIM is available for individuals older than 15 years, and a pediatric formulation has been studied in clinical trials and is available on a limited basis.[297,298] Epaxal is available for individuals older than 2 years. A combination inactivated hepatitis A and recombinant hepatitis B vaccine (Twinrix; GlaxoSmithKline) is available in the United States for persons 18 years old and older; a pediatric formulation is available in Europe, Canada, and other parts of the world.[299,300]

Dosage and Route

The pediatric dosage of Havrix, licensed in the United States for individuals 2 through 18 years of age, is 720 EL.U. (0.5 mL), to be administered in two intramuscular injections at time 0 and 6 to 12 months later (see Table 15–7). For adults, two doses of 1440 EL.U. each (1.0 mL) are administered as intramuscular injections, with the second dose given 6 to 12 months after the first. VAQTA is also licensed in two formulations, each given in a two-dose series (Table 15–7). The pediatric formulation, for children 2 to 18 years old, is 25 U (0.5 mL), and the adult formulation is 50 U (1.0 mL). For children, the second dose can be given at 6 to 18 months after the first dose, and for adults, 6 to 12 months after the first dose.

AVAXIM is administered as two intramuscular injections of 0.5 mL each, containing 160 antigen units (defined by a standard) in the adult formulation and 80 antigen units in the pediatric formulation, with the second dose given 6 to 12 months after the first (see Table 15–7).[301]

The dose of Epaxal for adults and children over 2 years old is 24 international units (IU) of inactivated hepatitis A virus, associated with 10 µg of influenza hemagglutinin and 100 µg of phospholipids.[302] The recommended schedule is two doses at time 0 and 6 to 12 months (see Table 15–7).

The adult formulation of the combination vaccine, Twinrix, includes 720 EL.U. of the hepatitis A component and 20 µg of the hepatitis B component in 1.0 mL, 0.45 mg of aluminum in the form of aluminum phosphate and alum as adjuvants, and 5.0 mg of 2-phenoxyethanol as a preservative, and is administered in a three-dose series.[303] The vaccine's performance appears to be equivalent to that of each of the single antigen vaccines administered separately.[304,305]

TABLE 15–7 ■ Recommended Doses and Schedules for Inactivated Hepatitis A Vaccines

Age (yr)	Vaccine*	Dose	Volume (mL)	No. of Doses	Schedule (mo)†
2–18	Havrix®	720 EL.U.	0.5	2	0, 6–12
	VAQTA®	25 U	0.5	2	0, 6–18
≥19	Havrix®	1440 EL.U.	1.0	2	0, 6–12
	VAQTA®	50 U	1.0	2	0, 6–12
>15	AVAXIM®	160 antigen units	0.5	2	0, 6–12
<16	AVAXIM®	80 antigen units	0.5	2	0, 6–12
≥2	Epaxal	24 IU	0.5	2	0, 6–12

*Havrix is manufactured from HAV strain HM175 by GlaxoSmithKline; VAQTA is manufactured from HAV strain CR326F′ by Merck & Co, Inc.; and AVAXIM® is manufactured by Aventis Pasteur Inc. from HAV strain GBM.
†Zero months represents timing of initial dose; subsequent numbers represent months after the initial dose.

Results of a number of studies indicate that the response of adults administered hepatitis A vaccine according to a schedule that mixed the two currently U.S. licensed vaccines was equivalent to that of adults vaccinated according to the licensed schedules.[306,307] Based on limited data, the response to a second dose delayed for a median of 35 months (range 24 to 66 months) appears to be equivalent to that of the licensed schedules.[308] Schedules with shorter intervals between doses have not been studied using the currently licensed formulations. Among persons vaccinated according to a three-dose schedule, all study subjects seroconverted but the peak antibody concentrations were lower among persons vaccinated at months 0, 1, and 2 compared with persons who were vaccinated according to a schedule with a longer time interval between the second and third dose.[309,310]

Vaccine Stability

The vaccines should be stored at 2° to 8°C, and Havrix and VAQTA have been shown to retain potency when kept for at least 2 years under those conditions.[278,311,312] Freezing destroys the vaccine, causing aggregation of the alum particles. Any vaccine that inadvertently was frozen should be discarded. HAV is a stable virus, and studies have shown that the reactogenicity and immunogenicity of Havrix after storage at 98.6°F (37°C) for 1 week, and the stability profile of VAQTA when stored at this temperature for more than 12 months did not differ from those of vaccines stored at the recommended temperature.[13,313]

Results of Vaccination

Immunogenicity of Vaccine

Antibody

In extensive studies in children and adults, the inactivated hepatitis A vaccines available in the United States have been found to be highly immunogenic. The concentration of antibody after vaccination varies with the dose and schedule of the vaccine. However, after a single dose of vaccine, antibody concentrations are higher than those produced by doses of immune globulin known to be protective. A second dose 6 to 18 months later results in a boosted antibody concentration, but the final concentration is generally lower than concentrations measured after natural infection. (Fig. 15–7).[314–317] In general, by 4 weeks after one dose of vaccine, 95% to 100% of children 2 years of age or older and adults respond with concentrations of antibody considered to be protective; the boost in antibody concentration following the second dose is likely important for long-term protection.[318–324] HAV-specific IgM antibody occasionally can be detected by standard assays, primarily if measured soon (i.e., 2 to 3 weeks) after vaccination.[288,314,325] (CDC, unpublished data).

Studies in children younger than 2 years of age suggest that the vaccine is safe, and that it is immunogenic for those who do not have passively transferred antibody from previous maternal HAV infection.[326–328] In studies of infants who received hepatitis A vaccine according to a number of

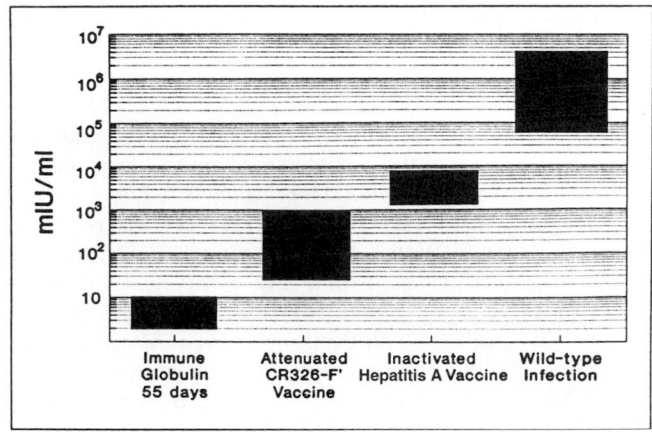

FIGURE 15–7 ▪ Comparative levels of antibody to HAV after administration of immune globulin, one dose of an attenuated hepatitis A vaccine, two doses of an inactivated hepatitis A vaccine, and natural infection. The detection limits of the HAVAB assay are approximately 100 mIU/mL. (From Lemon SM. Hepatitis A virus: current concepts of the molecular virology, immunology and approaches to vaccine development. Rev Med Virol 2:73–87, 1992, with permission.)

different schedules, those with passively transferred maternal antibody at the time of vaccination responded, but final antibody concentrations were approximately one third to one tenth those of infants who did not have passively transferred antibody and were vaccinated according to the same schedule.[327–330] The clinical significance, if any, of these lower antibody concentrations is unknown. One study found that all infants vaccinated in the presence of passively transferred maternal antibody at ages 2, 4, and 6 months responded to a booster dose 6 months later with an anamnestic response, suggesting that they had been primed by the primary series.[329] However, in another small study, two of six children who had lost detectable antibody did not have an anamnestic response to a booster dose administered approximately 6 years after receiving the primary vaccine series in infancy in the presence of passively transferred antibody.[331] The majority of infants born to anti-HAV–positive mothers have lost detectable antibody by 12 to 15 months of age,[332–334] and studies are underway to determine a dosage and schedule of hepatitis A vaccine for use in the first 2 years of life.

Conditions that may result in reduced immunogenicity include HIV infection, chronic liver disease, and older age. In two published reports of hepatitis A vaccination of men with HIV infection, approximately 75% had protective antibody concentrations after completing the vaccination series, and final antibody concentrations were considerably lower than those among HIV-negative persons.[335,336] Among HIV-infected men, higher CD4+ T-lymphocyte count at baseline was associated with response to vaccination.[335] Among persons with chronic liver disease, seroprotection rates were similar to those observed among healthy adults, but the final antibody concentrations were substantially lower.[337,338] Limited data suggest that the final antibody concentrations achieved among persons over 40 years may be somewhat lower than among younger individuals, but response rates were similar.[310,321,339,340] Other factors, such as smoking and obesity, have not been evaluated for the currently licensed formulations.

Correlates of Protection

When interpreting the results of immunogenicity studies, it is important to understand that the absolute lower limit of antibody needed to prevent HAV infection has not been determined. Anti-HAV concentrations are measured in comparison to a World Health Organization reference immunoglobulin reagent and are expressed in milli–International Units per milliliter (mIU/mL). The concentrations of antibody achieved after passive transfer by immune globulin or active induction by vaccination are 10- to 100-fold lower than those produced in response to natural infection (see Fig. 15–7). Concentrations of 10 to 20 mIU/mL, achieved about 1 to 2 months after administration of immune globulin, are known to protect against hepatitis A. Results of in vitro studies using cell culture–derived HAV indicate that even antibody concentrations less than 20 mIU/mL can be neutralizing.[341] Because no absolute protective level has been defined, generally the lower limit of detection of the particular assay being used has been considered to be the protective level. Clinical studies of Havrix have used levels greater than 20 or 33 mIU/mL, as measured using enzyme immunoassays; studies of VAQTA have used levels greater than 10 mIU/mL as measured with a modified radioimmunoassay (HAVAB).[102,318,329]

Some studies have indicated that concentrations of antibody above the defined protective concentration can be measured as early as 2 weeks after one dose.[296,315,342] However, distinct differences between the antibody induced by vaccine and the antibody detected in people who received immune globulin (which should be similar to antibody induced by infection) can be identified when results using different assays are compared.[343,344] In one study, with similar radioimmunoassay (HAVAB) titers, adult immune globulin recipients had higher neutralization titers as measured by a radioimmunofocus inhibition test (RIFIT) and an antigen reduction assay (HAVARNA), but negligible radioimmunoprecipitation titers, compared to a group of vaccinated children when measured 4 weeks after receiving one dose of vaccine.[343] In another study, the neutralizing geometric mean antibody titers of persons who received immune globulin with hepatitis A vaccine were five times higher compared to those who received hepatitis A vaccine alone, when measured 4 weeks after administration using the RIFIT assay.[344] However, it has also been shown that immune globulin prepared from the serum of vaccinees could protect a chimpanzee from HAV challenge when the titer of antibody achieved in the chimpanzee was similar to that found in humans receiving immune globulin prophylaxis.[345]

When neutralizing antibody appears after vaccination is not clear from published reports, owing to differences among assays, dosages of vaccine, and when antibody measurements were obtained. In one study, depending on the assay, 42% to 100% of children vaccinated with the currently licensed formulation had neutralizing antibody when measured 1 month after a single vaccine dose.[343] In another study, approximately two thirds of adults vaccinated with a lower dosage than the currently licensed formulation were positive for neutralizing antibody 4 weeks after one dose, and virtually all were positive 2 weeks after a second dose, given 1 month after the first.[344] In a third study, 84% of adults vaccinated with one dose of the liposomal vaccine had neutralizing antibody 2 weeks later.[296]

Herd Immunity

The demonstrated effectiveness of limited hepatitis A vaccination in interrupting outbreaks and reducing overall disease incidence (see *Efficacy and Effectiveness of Vaccine* and *Epidemiologic Effects of Vaccination* below) suggests that considerable herd immunity is achieved.[215,346–348] For example, a 94% decline in the number of reported hepatitis A cases occurred following vaccination of approximately two thirds of children in one California county during a 5-year-long demonstration project.[215]

Efficacy and Effectiveness of Vaccine

All current evidence indicates that hepatitis A vaccines are highly efficacious in preventing clinically apparent disease. In one study, 1037 healthy seronegative children 2 to 16 years of age in a community with high hepatitis A rates and periodic outbreaks received either a single dose of formalin-inactivated vaccine derived from strain CR326F, or placebo. No cases of hepatitis A occurred in the vaccinated group beginning 17 days after vaccination. In the placebo group, 34 cases of hepatitis A were observed, yielding an estimated 100% vaccine efficacy, with a lower bound of the 95% confidence interval of 87%.[349] In a large field trial of approximately 40,000 Thai children 1 to 16 years of age, the efficacy of inactivated vaccine (HM175 strain) was 94% (95% confidence interval, 79% to 99%) after two doses (360 EL.U. per dose) administered 1 month apart.[101]

A number of studies and demonstration projects have evaluated the effectiveness of hepatitis A vaccines in controlling and preventing hepatitis A in communities. In areas with the highest hepatitis A rates,[350,351] such as in Native American and Alaska Native communities, vaccination of the majority of children, and in some cases adolescents and young adults, resulted in a rapid decline in disease incidence, and, with ongoing routine vaccination of children, the reduction in disease incidence has been sustained.[346,347,349] In larger, more heterogeneous communities with lower but consistently elevated hepatitis A rates, interrupting ongoing community-wide epidemics by vaccinating children has proven difficult.[214,215] First-dose coverage generally has been low (20% to 45%), and the impact of vaccination often has been limited to vaccinated age groups, which may not represent the majority of cases. In contrast, results of a demonstration project in California of ongoing, routine vaccination of children, conducted during 1995 to 2000, suggest that this strategy can reduce hepatitis A incidence markedly over time (see *Public Health Considerations* below).[215]

Duration of Immunity

Antibody has been shown to persist in vaccinated adults and children for at least 5 to 8 years after vaccination.[352–355] In one follow-up study of infants, two thirds of those who did not have passively transferred maternal antibody at the time of vaccination had detectable anti-HAV 6 years later.[331] It is estimated from mathematical models using data from adults that protective levels of antibody following completion of the vaccination series could persist for 20 years or longer.[353-355] Whether other mechanisms (e.g., cellular memory) also contribute to long-term protection is unknown. Because the average incubation period for hepatitis A is 4 weeks and the anamnestic responses observed after the second vaccine dose are rapid and robust, it has been suggested that vaccinees who have seroconverted will be protected even if their antibody levels have fallen below protective levels. For example, in the follow-up study of infants who did not have passively transferred maternal antibody at the time of the primary series, all of those who had lost detectable antibody at the time of follow-up had an anamnestic response to a booster dose.[331] The Monroe community in which VAQTA was tested has had no cases in vaccinees during nine years after the trial, and cases in the unvaccinated have also disappeared in recent years.[355a] Additional long-term follow-up studies are needed to evaluate the long-term protective efficacy of hepatitis A vaccine and determine the need for booster doses.

Postexposure Prophylaxis with Vaccine

Several lines of evidence suggest that hepatitis A vaccine may have some efficacy when administered after exposure to HAV, but definitive studies have not yet been conducted. Hepatitis A vaccine administered soon after exposure prevented infection in a chimpanzee model.[356] Only one small randomized trial in humans has been completed. Among persons ages 1 to 40 years who were household contacts of hospitalized hepatitis A cases, hepatitis A vaccine was found to be 79% efficacious compared to no treatment in preventing infection when given within 8 days of symptom onset of the index case.[357] However, the confidence interval was wide (7% to 95%), and the study did not include a comparison group that received passive postexposure prophylaxis with immune globulin.[358] Because of the demonstrated high efficacy of immune globulin when administered after exposure to HAV, it continues to be recommended by most U.S. advisory groups for postexposure prophylaxis.[13,359]

Adverse Events

Common

Local injection site reactions (pain, tenderness, or erythema) that are mild and transient have been reported in as many as 21% of children and 56% of adults vaccinated. Systemic reactions that include fatigue, fever, diarrhea, and vomiting occur in less than 5% of vaccinees. Headache has been associated with vaccination in up to 16% of adults and 2% to 9% of children.[101,288,296,301-303,311,312,324,360,361]

Rare

Through 1998, more than 6.5 million doses, including more than 2.3 million pediatric doses, were administered to the U.S. civilian population, and more than 65 million doses had been administered worldwide.[13] Rare adverse events reported postmarketing include syncope, jaundice, erythema multiforme, anaphylaxis, brachial plexus neuropathy, transverse myelitis, encephalopathy, and others.[311,312]

No serious adverse events among children or adults have been identified that could be definitively ascribed to hepatitis A vaccine.[361,362] For events for which incidence rates are available, such as Guillain-Barré syndrome, reported rates were not higher than reported background rates.[13]

In Immunosuppressed Persons

The available hepatitis A vaccines are inactivated, and, based on limited data, administration to immunosuppressed persons does not appear to be associated with a greater risk of adverse events compared to persons with normal immune systems.[336,363] No data are available regarding the safety of live, attenuated vaccines in immunosuppressed persons.

Spread to Contacts

The inactivated vaccines do not pose a risk of spread to contacts because they do not contain viable HAV.

Indications

Recommendations for use of hepatitis A vaccine were first issued by the Advisory Committee on Immunization Practices of the U.S. Public Health Service, the American Academy of Pediatrics, and other groups in 1996, and were updated in 1999 (Table 15-8).[13,208,359] Inactivated hepatitis A vaccine is indicated for susceptible persons 2 years of age or older at increased risk of hepatitis A, and for any person wishing to obtain immunity.

Prevaccination serologic testing may be considered to reduce costs by not vaccinating persons with prior immunity, such as older adolescents and adults in certain population groups with a high prevalence of infection (e.g., persons born in areas of high hepatitis A endemicity), but should take into account the cost of testing, vaccine cost, and the likelihood that the person will return for vaccination.[364] Prevaccination testing of children is generally not cost effective. Vaccination of immune people is not harmful. Postvaccination testing is not indicated because of the high rate of vaccine response. Furthermore, testing methods that can detect the low anti-HAV antibody concentrations generated by immunization are not licensed for use in the United States.

Children Living in Areas with Consistently Elevated Hepatitis A Rates

Children living in areas where rates of hepatitis A have been consistently elevated should be routinely vaccinated, beginning at or after 2 years of age (see Fig. 15-6 and Tables 15-4 and 15-8). Various vaccination strategies can be used, including vaccinating one or more single-age cohorts of children or adolescents, vaccination of children in selected settings (e.g., day care), or vaccination of children and adolescents over a wide range of ages in a variety of settings, such as when they seek health care for other purposes.

Persons at Increased Risk of Hepatitis A or Severe Consequences

Vaccination of persons at increased risk of hepatitis A is indicated, including travelers to countries where hepatitis A is endemic (see Fig. 15-3), adolescent and adult men who have sex with men, persons who use illegal drugs, persons who work with HAV in research settings, and persons who have clotting factor disorders.[13] Vaccine is also recommended

TABLE 15–8 ■ Recommendations for Routine Pre-exposure Use of Hepatitis A Vaccine*

Group	Comments
Children living in communities with consistently elevated hepatitis A rates	Includes Alaska, Arizona, California, Idaho, Nevada, New Mexico, Oklahoma, Oregon, South Dakota, Utah, Washington, and selected areas in other states[†‡]
International travelers[§]	Immune globulin may be given in addition to or instead of vaccine; children <2 years old should receive immune globulin
Men who have sex with men	Includes adolescents
Illicit drug users	Includes adolescents
Persons with chronic liver disease	Increased risk of fulminant hepatitis A with HAV infection
Persons receiving clotting factor concentrates	
Persons who work with HAV in research laboratory settings	

*Hepatitis A vaccine is not licensed for children less than 2 years old.
†Where the average reported hepatitis A incidence during 1987 to 1997 was 20 cases or more per 100,000 population (approximately twice the national average).
‡Routine vaccination should also be considered for children living in Arkansas, Colorado, Missouri, Montana, Texas, Wyoming, and selected areas in other states where the average reported incidence during 1987 to 1997 was 10 or more cases per 100,000 population but less than 20 cases per 100,000 population.
§Persons traveling to Canada, western Europe, Japan, Australia, or New Zealand are at no greater risk than in the United States.
From CDC: Prevention of hepatitis A through active or passive immunization c: recommendations of the Advisory Committee on Immunization Practices (ACIP). MMWR 48(RR-12):1–37, 1999.

for persons with chronic liver disease because of the high case-fatality rate among these persons if they acquire hepatitis A (Table 15–8).[52]

Community-Wide Outbreaks

There has been considerable interest in using hepatitis A vaccine to control ongoing community-wide epidemics. Implementation of routine vaccination of children, which is recommended for most areas that include communities that experience these outbreaks, will prevent such outbreaks in the future. Because of logistical difficulties, accelerated vaccination as an additional measure to control outbreaks should be undertaken with caution.[13] Efforts are probably better directed toward sustained routine vaccination of children to maintain high levels of immunity and prevent future epidemics.

Other Groups and Settings

Although hepatitis A outbreaks occur in child care centers, their frequency is not high enough to warrant routine vaccination of attendees or staff to prevent them, and there is little experience using vaccine to control outbreaks when they occur.[365] When outbreaks are recognized, aggressive use of immune globulin is effective in limiting transmission.[21] In areas where routine vaccination of children is recommended, previously unvaccinated children can be vaccinated when they receive postexposure prophylaxis with immune globulin.[13] In addition, child care center attendees can be a readily accessible target population for ongoing routine vaccination programs.

The frequency of outbreaks in hospitals, institutions, and schools is not high enough to warrant routine vaccination of persons in these settings, and there are no data with respect to using vaccine to control outbreaks in these settings. Although persons who work as food handlers are not at increased risk of hepatitis A because of their occupation, they may transmit HAV to others when they contract hepatitis A.[246] To reduce the frequency of evaluations of food handlers with hepatitis A and the need for postexpo-

sure prophylaxis of patrons, public health officials in some jurisdictions have instituted measures to promote hepatitis A vaccination of food handlers.[366] However, because transmission from infected food handlers accounts for a very small proportion of cases nationwide, vaccination of food handlers is not likely to affect overall disease incidence, and has not been found to be cost effective.[367]

Contraindications and Precautions

The inactivated hepatitis A vaccines should not be used in persons with a history of a severe reaction to a prior dose of hepatitis A vaccine or allergy or hypersensitivity to the vaccine or any of its components. The safety of the inactivated hepatitis A vaccines in pregnancy has not been determined. Because the vaccine is produced from inactivated HAV, the theoretical risk to the fetus is likely to be low.

Concomitant Use with Other Vaccines

Several studies have evaluated administration of inactivated hepatitis A vaccine concomitantly with immune globulin to produce both immediate and long-term immunity.[368–371] The proportion of persons who respond to vaccination was not reduced by coadministration of immune globulin. However, the antibody concentrations elicited were lower than when vaccine alone was given. For example, in one study, 1 month after completion of the vaccine series, the geometric mean antibody concentration among persons who received a dose of immune globulin (0.06 mL/kg) with the first dose of vaccine was 4872.3 mIU/mL (range 3716.2 to 6388.2 mIU/mL) compared to 6497.8 mIU/mL (range 5110.9 to 8261.0 mIU/mL) among persons who received vaccine alone.[371] Because the concentrations induced by vaccination far exceed that needed for protection, these reductions are not considered clinically significant. The use of hepatitis A vaccine with other vaccines that might be used for travelers has been studied among adults. There was no effect on either the immunogenicity or reactogenicity of hepatitis A vaccine administered concurrently with diphtheria, polio (oral and inactivated), tetanus, hepatitis B, yellow fever, typhoid (oral and intramuscular), cholera, Japanese encephalitis, or rabies vaccines.[372–376] In one study among infants, simultaneous administration of hepatitis A vaccine did not affect the immunogenicity or reactogenicity of diphtheria-tetanus–acellular pertussis, inactivated polio, and *Haemophilus influenzae* type b vaccines.[329]

Future Vaccines

Live, attenuated vaccines have been tested in humans and were shown to be safe when given orally or parenterally. Unfortunately, the vaccines studied to date replicate poorly in humans and do not induce a satisfactory immune response when given orally. Therefore these vaccines do not have significant advantages over inactivated vaccines.[281,282]

Cohen and colleagues have assembled a full-length infectious cDNA and transcribed from the cDNA a full-length RNA that, on transfection into permissive cells, results in complete HAV replication.[285] Many of the mutations responsible for cell culture adaptation and attenuation have now been identified, although to date a virus with the ideal characteristics of in vitro growth combined with attenuation and immunogenicity in humans has not been produced.[99,123,286]

The important neutralizing epitopes of HAV appear to be conformational, and immunization with synthetic peptides or expressed capsid proteins has not induced an effective neutralizing antibody response.[377] Stapleton and colleagues have taken the approach of expressing the entire open reading frame of the HAV genome in recombinant vaccinia virus or baculovirus expression systems.[378–380] Complete or partial capsid assembly seems to occur in cells infected with this recombinant vaccinia, and antibodies raised to these purified HAV synthetic capsids are neutralizing in vitro and protective in animals. Although the immunizing effect of such a vaccine might not be greater than that of inactivated vaccines, the reduced production costs could make it an attractive alternative.

Public Health Considerations

Epidemiologic Effects of Vaccination

Communities with the Highest Hepatitis A Rates

Hepatitis A epidemics typically occur every 5 to 10 years in these communities.[346] Few cases occur among persons over 15 years old; seroprevalence data indicate that 30% to 40% of children acquire infection by 5 years of age, and almost all persons have been infected by young adulthood.[350,351,381,382] Demonstration projects conducted soon after hepatitis A vaccines became available showed that routine vaccination of children living in these communities was feasible, and that, when relatively high vaccination coverage was achieved and sustained, ongoing epidemics were interrupted, and a reduction in disease incidence was sustained.[346,347] For example, a 1992–1993 community-wide epidemic among Alaska Natives in one rural area was ended

within 4 to 8 weeks of vaccinating approximately 80% of children and young adults.[347]

Following publication in 1996 of recommendations for routine vaccination of children in these areas to prevent such outbreaks, surveys indicated vaccination coverage of 50% to 80% among preschool and school-age Native American and Alaska Native children, suggesting that recommendations were being implemented.[383] More recently, national surveillance data demonstrated a dramatic decrease in hepatitis A incidence in these populations (Fig. 15–8). By 2000, hepatitis A incidence among Native Americans and Alaska Natives had declined by 97% compared to the beginning of the decade, and was lower than the overall U.S. rate.[383] A decline of this magnitude has not been observed in the previous 30 years of surveillance, and suggests a fundamental alteration in hepatitis A epidemiology in Native American and Alaska Native communities.

Communities with Consistently Elevated Rates (see Tables 15–4 and 15–8)

Experience to date using hepatitis A vaccine to vaccinate children routinely suggests that considerable reductions in morbidity can be achieved with fairly modest vaccination coverage.[215] National hepatitis A rates have been declining precipitously over the past several years; the 2001 overall rate of 3.8 per 100,000 is a historic low (Fig. 15–9; see also Fig. 15–5). Pediatric vaccine doses purchased in the public sector by the 17 states covered by the recommendations has risen since the recommendations were made, from approximately 500,000 doses in 1998 to over 2.5 million in 2000, accounting for 95% of all public sector hepatitis A vaccine purchased in 2000 (CDC, unpublished data). Compared to the average 1987 to 1997 rate of 22.4 per 100,000, the provisional 2001 rate in these states has declined by approximately 80% to 4.2 per 100,000, compared to a 39% decrease from 5.6 to 3.4 per 100,000 elsewhere.[384] Rates have declined most dramatically among children 2 to 18 years old. The precipitous decrease in hepatitis A rates in states where vaccine purchase was greatest likely reflects, at least in part, the impact of routine vaccination of children. However, because hepatitis A incidence is cyclic, additional years of data are needed to verify that low rates are sustained and attributable to vaccination, and for a definitive

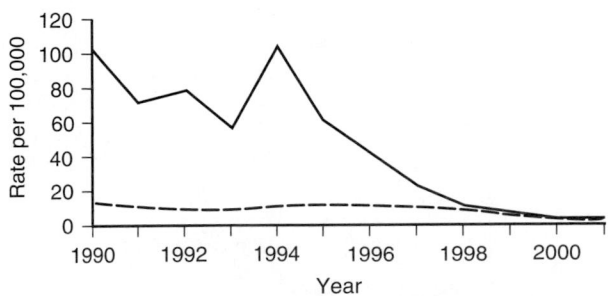

FIGURE 15–8 ■ Hepatitis A incidence, United States and Native Americans and Alaska Natives, 1990 through 2001. The *solid line* represents the rate among Native Americans and Alaska Natives; the *dashed line* represents the overall U.S. rate. (Data from the Centers for Disease Control and Prevention, National Notifiable Diseases Surveillance System, Atlanta, GA. Data for 2001 are provisional.)

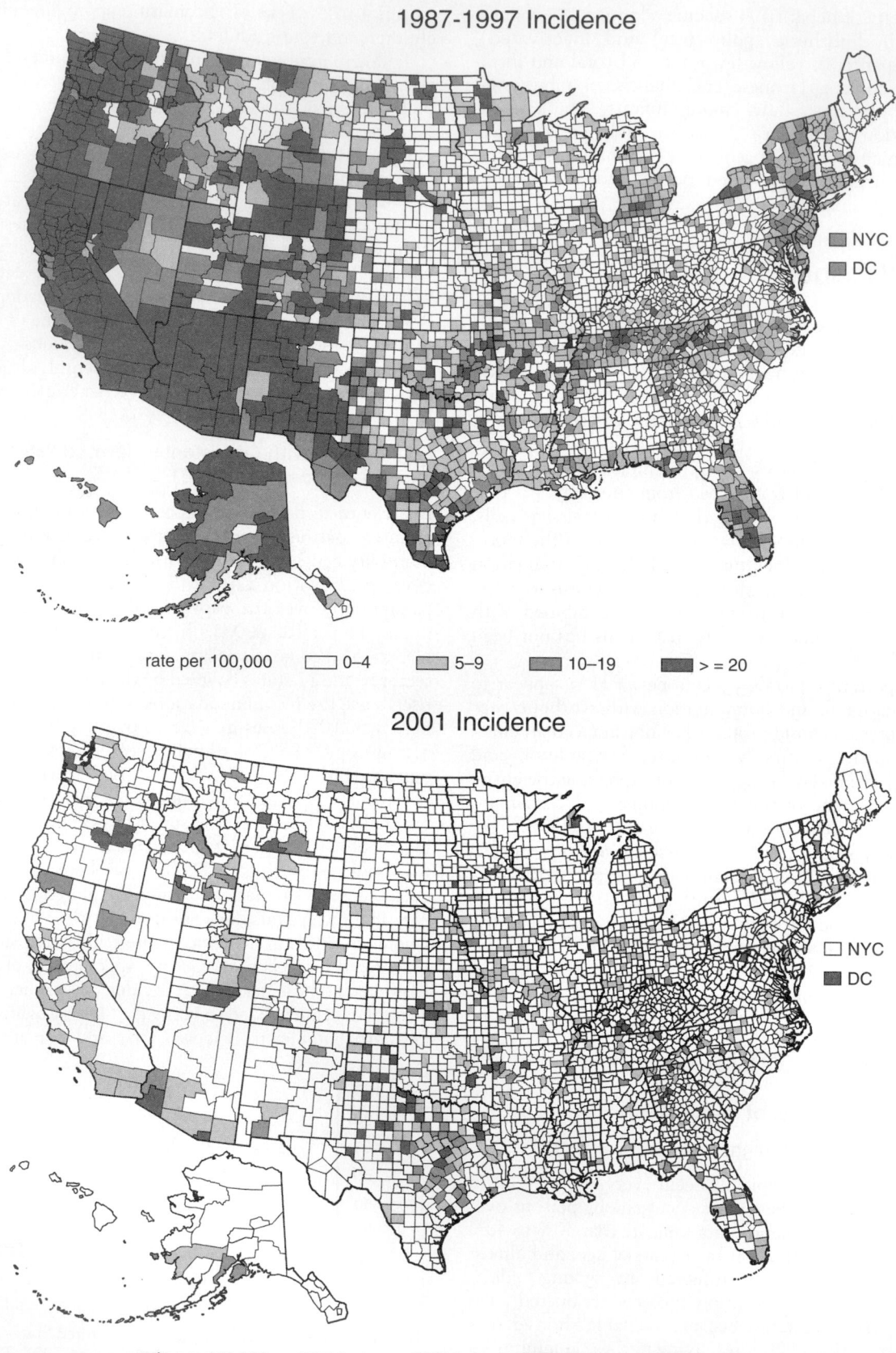

FIGURE 15–9 ■ Hepatitis A incidence rates by county, United States, 1987 to 1997 (*top*) and 2001 (*bottom*). (Data from the Centers for Disease Control and Prevention, National Notifiable Diseases Surveillance System, Atlanta, GA. Data for 2001 are provisional.)

determination of the overall impact of this strategy of routine childhood vaccination in selected, higher incidence areas.

Results of the longest demonstration project of routine hepatitis A vaccination of children in Butte County, California, a community with consistently elevated rates, preview the potential long-term impact.[215] During the 5 years before the demonstration project, Butte County's average annual hepatitis A incidence rate was 47.9 per 100,000, and ranged from a high of 122.5 to 11.8 per 100,000. From 1995 to 2000, children 2 years of age or older were offered hepatitis A vaccine without charge, and 66% of the almost 45,000 eligible children received at least one dose. The number of reported cases declined 94%, and the four cases reported in 2000 was the lowest number ever reported in the county since hepatitis surveillance began in 1966. Butte County's 2000 incidence rate of 1.9 per 100,000 was the lowest of any California county.

Disease Burden and Economic Considerations

Throughout the 1980s and early 1990s in the United States, approximately 25,000 to 35,000 hepatitis A cases were reported annually to the CDC, and incidence models suggest that the number of infections was at least 10 times higher.[166,207] With the availability of hepatitis A vaccine, hepatitis A has become one of the most frequently reported vaccine-preventable diseases.[385] The CDC estimates that approximately 100 deaths per year occur from acute liver failure because of hepatitis A, but other studies have estimated as many as 255 deaths per year.[13,386] Between 11% and 22% of persons with hepatitis A are hospitalized, and adults who become ill lose an average of 27 days of work.[13,208] Annual costs are estimated at $300 to $489 million in 1997 dollars.[13,386] One analysis indicated that hepatitis A vaccination of young children or adolescents in states with the highest disease rates would be cost saving from the societal perspective, and from the health system perspective would cost approximately $13,000 per year of life saved, comparable to other recommended vaccinations.[387,388]

Disease Control Strategies

The strategy of widespread routine vaccination of children has the potential to achieve a sustained reduction in the overall incidence of hepatitis A in the United States, by preventing infection among individuals in age groups that account for at least one third of cases and eliminating a major source of infection for others. However, to date hepatitis A vaccines cannot be readily incorporated into the routine infant schedule because they are not licensed for children less than 2 years old. Therefore, based on distinct features of hepatitis A epidemiology and experience gathered from demonstration projects and other research, a novel vaccination strategy was developed, involving incremental implementation of routine childhood hepatitis A vaccination.

The initial recommendations, published in 1996 soon after vaccines became available in the United States, called for routine vaccination of children living in communities with the highest hepatitis A rates (e.g., Native American and Alaska Native communities).[208] Although these recommendations apparently were effective in reducing disease rates in communities covered by them, implementation had little impact on overall disease incidence nationwide because only a small proportion of nationally reported cases occurred among persons and in communities covered by the recommendations. Building on the evidence from surveillance data that areas with consistently elevated hepatitis A rates could be identified that had contributed the majority of cases to the current national disease burden (see Fig. 15–6 and Table 15–4), in 1999 the recommendation for routine vaccination of children was extended to include those living in states, counties, and communities with consistently elevated hepatitis A rates (see Tables 15–4 and 15–8).[13]

At present, hepatitis A vaccination is generally not indicated in developing countries, particularly those with highest endemicity where infection in early childhood is nearly universal and disease is uncommon (see Fig. 15–4). Although vaccination strategies could be devised that are directed at areas within transitional or intermediate-endemicity countries (see Fig. 15–3) where a sizeable proportion of adults are likely to be susceptible, such as urban areas with good water and sanitation facilities, the relative cost effectiveness of hepatitis A vaccination compared with other major public health priorities has not been evaluated. However, the global disease burden associated with hepatitis A will increase in the coming years, particularly in these areas, as a larger proportion of the population remains susceptible to HAV infection into adolescence and adulthood because of continuing improvements in standards of living and sanitary and hygienic conditions.[11] If vaccine was available at a low cost and vaccination was shown to be cost effective, some countries in which a considerable susceptible adolescent and adult population has developed might find it useful to include hepatitis A in their vaccination programs.

Eradication or Elimination

In the United States, vaccination of successive cohorts of children should eventually result in a sustained reduction in disease incidence nationwide, providing the opportunity to eliminate HAV transmission. To achieve this goal, vaccination of young children nationwide will be needed. Advances in hepatitis A vaccine development, such as the availability of a vaccine that can be used in the first 2 years of life and of combination vaccines that include hepatitis A vaccine, would facilitate this effort. Additional information on the safety of the vaccine will also be important.

HAV has been considered as a target for eradication, but international bodies have not made this recommendation, primarily because of considerations of cost and feasibility.[389] At present, the disease can best be controlled by improving living conditions in the developing world and the wise application of the existing vaccines in other areas.

REFERENCES

1. Bachman L. Infectious hepatitis in Europe. In Rodenwalt E. (ed). World Atlas of Epidemic Diseases. Hamburg, Falk-Verlag, 1952.
2. Cockayne EA. Catarrhal jaundice, sporadic and epidemic, and its relations to acute yellow atrophy of the liver. Q J Med 6:1–29, 1912.

3. McDonald S. Acute yellow atrophy of the liver. Edinburgh Med J 1:83, 1908.
4. Havens W Jr. Immunity in experimentally induced infectious hepatitis. J Exp Med 84:403, 1946.
5. Neefe JR, Gellis SS, Stokes J Jr. Homologous serum hepatitis and infectious (epidemic) hepatitis: studies in volunteers bearing on immunological and other characteristics of the etiological agents. Am J Med 1:9, 1946.
6. Havens W Jr, Paul J. Prevention of infectious hepatitis with gamma globulin. JAMA 129:270–272, 1997.
7. Gellis SS, Stokes J Jr, Brother GM. The use of immune globulin (gamma globulin) in infectious (epidemic) hepatitis in the Mediterranean theatre of operations. JAMA 128:1062, 1945.
8. Ward R, Krugman S, Giles JP. Infectious hepatitis: studies of its natural history and prevention. N Engl J Med 258:407, 1958.
9. Melnick JL, Boggs JD. Human volunteer and tissue culture studies of viral hepatitis. Can Med Assoc J 106:Suppl 7, 1972.
10. Feinstone SM, Kapikian AZ, Purceli RH. Hepatitis A: detection by immune electron microscopy of a viruslike antigen associated with acute illness. Science 182:1026–1028, 1973.
11. Bell BP. Global epidemiology of hepatitis A: implications for control strategies. In Margolis HS, Alter MJ, Liang JT, Dienstag JL (eds). Viral Hepatitis and Liver Disease. London, International Medical Press, 2002, pp 9–14.
12. Hadler SC. Global impact of hepatitis A virus infection: changing patterns. In Hollinger FB, Lemon SM, Margolis HS (eds). Viral Hepatitis and Liver Disease. Baltimore, Williams & Wilkins, 1991, pp 14–20.
13. Centers for Disease Control and Prevention. Prevention of hepatitis A through active or passive immunization: recommendations of the Advisory Committee on Immunization Practices (ACIP). MMWR 48(RR-12):1-37, 1999.
14. Yao G. Clinical spectrum and natural history of viral hepatitis A in a 1988 Shanghai epidemic. In Hollinger FB, Lemon SM, Margolis HS (eds). Viral Hepatitis and Liver Disease. Baltimore, Williams & Wilkins, 1991, pp 76–78.
15. Krugman S, Giles JP, Hammond J. Infectious hepatitis: evidence for two distinctive clinical, epidemiological, and immunological types of infection. JAMA 200:365–373, 1967.
16. Margolis HS, Nainan OV. Identification of virus components in circulating immune complexes isolated during hepatitis A virus infection. Hepatology 11:31–37, 1990.
17. Sherertz RJ, Russell BA, Reuman PD. Transmission of hepatitis A by transfusion of blood products. Arch Intern Med 144:1579–1580, 1984.
18. Purcell RH, Wong DC, Shapiro M. Relative infectivity of hepatitis A virus by the oral and intravenous routes in 2 species of nonhuman primates. J Infect Dis 185:1668–1771, 2002.
19. Skinhoj P, Gluud C, Ramsoe K. Traveller's hepatitis: origin and characteristics of cases in Copenhagen 1976–1978. Scand J Infect Dis 13:1–4, 1981.
20. Gingrich GA, Hadler SC, Elder HA, et al. Serologic investigation of an outbreak of hepatitis A in a rural day-care center. Am J Public Health 73:1190–1193, 1983.
21. Hadler SC, Webster HM, Erben JJ, et al. Hepatitis A in day-care centers: a community-wide assessment. N Engl J Med 302:1222–1227, 1980.
22. Lednar WM, Lemon SM, Kirkpatrick JW, et al. Frequency of illness associated with epidemic hepatitis A virus infections in adults. Am J Epidemiol 122:226–233, 1985.
23. Fishman LN, Jonas MM, Lavine JE. Update on viral hepatitis in children. Pediatr Clin North Am 43:57–74, 1996.
24. Lemon SM. Type A viral hepatitis: new developments in an old disease. N Engl J Med 313:1059–1067, 1985.
25. Tong MJ, El Farra NS, Grew MI. Clinical manifestations of hepatitis A: recent experience in a community teaching hospital. J Infect Dis 171(suppl 1):S15–S18, 1995.
26. Koff RS. Clinical manifestations and diagnosis of hepatitis A virus infection. Vaccine 10(suppl 1):S15–S17, 1992.
27. Sjogren MH, Tanno H, Fay O, et al. Hepatitis A virus in stool during clinical relapse. Ann Intern Med 106:221–226, 1987.
28. Gordon SC, Reddy KR, Schiff L, et al. Prolonged intrahepatic cholestasis secondary to acute hepatitis A. Ann Intern Med 101:635–637, 1984.
29. Schiff ER. Atypical clinical manifestations of hepatitis A. Vaccine 10(suppl 1):S18–S20, 1992.
30. Gimson AE, White YS, Eddleston AL, et al. Clinical and prognostic differences in fulminant hepatitis type A, B, and non-A, non-B. Gut 24:1194–1198, 1983.
31. Sagi EF, Linder N, Shouval D. Papular acrodermatitis of childhood associated with hepatitis A virus infection. Pediatr Dermatol 3:31–33, 1985.
32. Inman RD, Hodge M, Johnston ME, et al. Arthritis, vasculitis, and cryoglobulinemia associated with relapsing hepatitis A virus infection. Ann Intern Med 105:700–703, 1986.
33. Ilan Y, Hillman M, Oren R, et al. Vasculitis and cryoglobulinemia associated with persisting cholestatic hepatitis A virus infection. Am J Gastroenterol 85:586–587, 1990.
34. Dan M, Yaniv R. Cholestatic hepatitis, cutaneous vasculitis, and vascular deposits of immunoglobulin M and complement associated with hepatitis A virus infection. Am J Med 89:103–104, 1990.
35. Tabor E. Guillain-Barré syndrome and other neurologic syndromes in hepatitis A, B, and non-A, non-B. J Med Virol 21:207–216, 1987.
36. Tabor E. Clinical presentation of hepatitis A. In Gerety RJ (ed). Hepatitis A. New York, Academic Press, 2002, pp 47–53.
37. Pelletier G, Elghozi D, Trepo C, et al. Mononeuritis in acute viral hepatitis. Digestion 32:53–56, 1985.
38. Bosch VV, Dowling PC, Cook SD. Hepatitis A virus immunoglobulin M antibody in acute neurological disease. Ann Neurol 14:685–687, 1983.
39. Azuri J, Lerman-Sagie T, Mizrahi A, et al. Guillain-Barré syndrome following serological evidence of hepatitis A in a child. Eur J Pediatr 158:341–342, 1999.
40. Aydin A, Mikla S, Ficicioglu C, et al. Nephrotic syndrome associated with hepatitis A virus infection. Pediatr Infect Dis J 18:391, 1999.
41. Demircin G, Oner A, Tinaztepe K, et al. Acute glomerulonephritis in hepatitis A virus infection. J Pediatr Gastroenterol Nutr 27:86–89, 1998.
42. Jamil SM, Massry SG. Acute anuric renal failure in nonfulminant hepatitis A infection. Am J Nephrol 18:329–332, 1998.
43. Mishra A, Saigal S, Gupta R, et al. Acute pancreatitis associated with viral hepatitis: a report of six cases with review of literature. Am J Gastroenterol 94:2292–2295, 1999.
44. Maiga MY, Oberti F, Rifflet H, et al. Hematologic manifestations related to hepatitis A virus: 3 cases. Gastroenterol Clin Biol 21:327–330, 1997.
45. Vento S, Garofano T, Di Perri G, et al. Identification of hepatitis A virus as a trigger for autoimmune chronic hepatitis type 1 in susceptible individuals. Lancet 337:1183–1187, 1991.
46. Ertem D, Acar Y, Arat C, et al. Thrombotic and thrombocytopenic complications secondary to hepatitis A infection in children. Am J Gastroenterol 94:3653–3655, 1999.
47. McNeil M, Hoy JF, Richards MJ, et al. Aetiology of fatal viral hepatitis in Melbourne: a retrospective study. Med J Aust 141:637–640, 1984.
48. Willner IR, Uhl MD, Howard SC, et al. Serious hepatitis A: an analysis of patients hospitalized during an urban epidemic in the United States. Ann Intern Med 128:111–114, 1998.
49. Kumashiro R, Sata M, Suzuki H. Clinical study of acute hepatitis type A in patients older than 50 years. Acta Hepatol Jpn 29:457–462, 1988.
50. Gust ID, Feinstone SM. History. In Gust ID, Feinstone SM (eds). Hepatitis. Boca Raton, FL, CRC Press, 1988, pp 1–19.
51. Akriviadis EA, Redeker AG. Fulminant hepatitis A in intravenous drug users with chronic liver disease. Ann Intern Med 110:838–839, 1989.
52. Bell BP. Hepatitis A and hepatitis B vaccination of patients with chronic liver disease. Acta Gastroenterol Belg 63:359–365, 2000.
53. Datta D, Williams I, Culver DH, et al. Association between deaths due to hepatitis A and chronic liver disease, United States, 1981–1997. Antiviral Ther 5(suppl 1):79, 2000.
54. Keeffe EB. Is hepatitis A more severe in patients with chronic hepatitis B and other chronic liver diseases? Am J Gastroenterol 90:201–205, 1995.
55. Lemon SM, Shapiro CN. The value of immunization against hepatitis A. Infect Agents Dis 3:38–49, 1994.
56. Vento S, Garofano T, Renzini C, et al. Fulminant hepatitis associated with hepatitis A virus superinfection in patients with chronic hepatitis C. N Engl J Med 338:286–290, 1998.
57. Franki RIB, Fauquet CM, Knudson DL. Classification and nomenclature of viruses: the fifth report of the International Committee on the Taxonomy of Viruses. Arch Virol Suppl 2:1, 1993.

58. Melnick JL. Classification of hepatitis A virus as enterovirus type 72 and of hepatitis B virus as hepadnavirus type 1. Intervirology 18:105–106, 1982.

59. Gust ID, Burrell CJ, Coulepis AG, et al. Taxonomic classification of human hepatitis B virus. Intervirology 25:14–29, 1986.

60. Gust ID, Coulepis AG, Feinstone SM. Taxonomic classification of hepatitis A virus. Intervirology 20:1–7, 1983.

61. Ticehurst JR. Hepatitis A virus: clones, cultures, and vaccines. Semin Liver Dis 6:46–55, 1986.

62. Cohen JI. Hepatitis A virus: insights from molecular biology. Hepatology 9:889–895, 1989.

63. Melnick JL. Properties and classification of hepatitis A virus. Vaccine 10(suppl 1):S24–S26, 1992.

64. Lemon SM, Jansen RW, Brown EA. Genetic, antigenic and biological differences between strains of hepatitis A virus. Vaccine 10(suppl 1): S40–S44, 1992.

65. Robertson BH, Jansen RW, Khanna B, et al. Genetic relatedness of hepatitis A virus strains recovered from different geographical regions. J Gen Virol 73(pt 6):1365–1377, 1992.

66. Weitz M, Siegl G. Variation among hepatitis A virus strains. I. Genomic variation detected by T1 oligonucleotide mapping. Virus Res 4:53–67, 1985.

67. Siegl G, deChastonay J, Kronauer G. Propagation and assay of hepatitis A virus in vitro. J Virol Methods 9:53–67, 1984.

68. Bradley DW, Schable CA, McCaustland KA, et al. Hepatitis A virus: growth characteristics of in vivo and in vitro propagated wild and attenuated virus strains. J Med Virol 14:373–386, 1984.

69. Lemon SM, Binn LN. Antigenic relatedness of two strains of hepatitis A virus determined by cross-neutralization. Infect Immun 42:418–420, 1983.

70. Lemon SM, Chao SF, Jansen RW, et al. Genomic heterogeneity among human and nonhuman strains of hepatitis A virus. J Virol 61:735–742, 1987.

71. Stapleton JT, Jansen R, Lemon SM. Neutralizing antibody to hepatitis A virus in immune serum globulin and in the sera of human recipients of immune serum globulin. Gastroenterology 89:637–642, 1985.

72. Siegl G, Frosner GG. Characterization and classification of virus particles associated with hepatitis A. I. Size, density, and sedimentation. J Virol 26:40–47, 1978.

73. Siegl G, Frosner GG, Gauss-Muller V, et al. The physicochemical properties of infectious hepatitis A virions. J Gen Virol 57:331–341, 1981.

74. Bradley DW, Fields HA, McCaustland KA, et al. Biochemical and biophysical characterization of light and heavy density hepatitis A virus particles: evidence HAV is an RNA virus. J Med Virol 2:175–187, 1978.

75. Siegl G, Weitz M, Kronauer G. Stability of hepatitis A virus. Intervirology 22:218–226, 1984.

76. Lemon SM, Jansen RW, Newbold JE. Infectious hepatitis A virus particles produced in cell culture consist of three distinct types with different buoyant densities in CsCl. J Virol 54:78–85, 1985.

77. Nissen E, Konig P, Feinstone SM, et al. Inactivation of hepatitis A and other enteroviruses during heat treatment (pasteurization). Biologicals 24:339–341, 1996.

78. Murphy P, Nowak T, Lemon SM, et al. Inactivation of hepatitis A virus by heat treatment in aqueous solution. J Med Virol 41:61–64, 1993.

79. Parry JV, Mortimer PP. Heat sensitivity of hepatitis A virus determined by a simple tissue culture method. J Med Virol 14:277–283, 1984.

80. Favero MS, Bond WW. Disinfection and sterilization. In Zuckerman AJ, Thomas HC (eds). Viral Hepatitis: Scientific Basis and Clinical Management. New York, Churchill Livingston, 1993, pp 565–575.

81. Sobsey MD. Survival and persistence of hepatitis A virus in environmental samples. In Zuckerman AJ (ed). Viral Hepatitis and Liver Disease. New York, Alan R. Liss, 1988, pp 121–124.

82. Millard J, Appleton H, Parry JV. Studies on heat inactivation of hepatitis A virus with special reference to shellfish. Part 1. Procedures for infection and recovery of virus from laboratory-maintained cockles. Epidemiol Infect 98:397, 1987.

83. Peterson DA, Hurley TR, Hoff JC, et al. Effect of chlorine treatment on infectivity of hepatitis A virus. Appl Environ Microbiol 45:223–227, 1983.

84. Ticehurst JR, Racaniello VR, Baroudy BM, et al. Molecular cloning and characterization of hepatitis A virus cDNA. Proc Natl Acad Sci U S A 80:5885–5889, 1983.

85. Cohen JI, Ticehurst JR, Purcell RH, et al. Complete nucleotide sequence of wild-type hepatitis A virus: comparison with different strains of hepatitis A virus and other picornaviruses. J Virol 61:50–59, 1987.

86. Weitz M, Baroudy BM, Maloy WL, et al. Detection of a genome-linked protein (VPg) of hepatitis A virus and its comparison with other picornaviral VPgs. J Virol 60:124–130, 1986.

87. Brown EA, Zajac AJ, Lemon SM. In vitro characterization of an internal ribosomal entry site (IRES) present within the 5′ nontranslated region of hepatitis A virus RNA: comparison with the IRES of encephalomyocarditis virus. J Virol 68:1066–1074, 1994.

88. Glass MJ, Jia XY, Summers DF. Identification of the hepatitis A virus internal ribosome entry site: in vivo and in vitro analysis of bicistronic RNAs containing the HAV 5′ noncoding region. Virology 193:842–852, 1993.

89. Cohen JI, Rosenblum B, Ticehurst JR, et al. Complete nucleotide sequence of an attenuated hepatitis A virus: comparison with wild-type virus. Proc Natl Acad Sci U S A 84:2497–2501, 1987.

90. Summers DF, Ehrenfeld E. Host antibody response to viral structural and nonstructural proteins after hepatitis A virus infection. J Infect Dis 165:273–280, 1992.

91. Schultheiss T, Kusov YY, Gauss-Muller V. Proteinase 3C of hepatitis A virus (HAV) cleaves the HAV polyprotein P2-P3 at all sites including VP1/2A and 2A/2B. Virology 198:275–281, 1994.

92. Schultheiss T, Sommergruber W, Kusov Y. Cleavage specificity of purified recombinant hepatitis A virus 3c proteinase on natural substrates. J Virol 69:1727–1733, 1995.

93. Jia XY, Summers DF, Ehrenfeld E. Primary cleavage of the HAV capsid protein precursor in the middle of the proposed 2A coding region. Virology 193:515–519, 1993.

94. Siegl G. Replication of hepatitis A virus and processing of proteins. Vaccine 10(suppl 1):S32–S35, 1992.

95. Kusov YY, Kazachkov YA, Dzagurov GK, et al. Identification of precursors of structural proteins VP1 and VP2 of hepatitis A virus. J Med Virol 37:220–227, 1992.

96. Tesar M, Jia XY, Summers DF, et al. Analysis of a potential myristoylation site in hepatitis A virus capsid protein VP4. Virology 194:616–626, 1993.

97. Harmon SA, Emerson SU, Huang YK, et al. Hepatitis A viruses with deletions in the 2A gene are infectious in cultured cells and marmosets. J Virol 69:5576–5581, 1995.

98. Nigro G, Taliani G, Bartmann U, et al. Hepatitis in children with thalassemia major. Arch Virol Suppl 4:265–267, 1992.

99. Funkhouser AW, Purcell RH, D'Hondt E, et al. Attenuated hepatitis A virus: genetic determinants of adaptation to growth in MRC-5 cells. J Virol 68:148–157, 1994.

100. Jia XY, Ehrenfeld E, Summers DF. Proteolytic activity of hepatitis A virus 3C protein. J Virol 65:2595–2600, 1991.

101. Innis BL, Snitbhan R, Kunasol P, et al. Protection against hepatitis A by an inactivated vaccine. JAMA 271:1328–1334, 1994.

102. Nalin DR, Kuter BJ, Brown L, et al. Worldwide experience with the CR326F-derived inactivated hepatitis A virus vaccine in pediatric and adult populations: an overview. J Hepatol 18(suppl 2):S51–S55, 1993.

103. Brown EA, Jansen RW, Lemon SM. Characterization of a simian hepatitis A virus (HAV): antigenic and genetic comparison with human HAV. J Virol 63:4932–4937, 1989.

104. Stapleton JT, Lemon SM. Neutralization escape mutants define a dominant immunogenic neutralization site on hepatitis A virus. J Virol 61:491–498, 1987.

105. Kaplan G, Totsuka A, Thompson P, et al. Identification of a surface glycoprotein on African green monkey kidney cells as a receptor for hepatitis A virus. EMBO J 15:4282–4296, 1996.

106. Feigelstock D, Thompson P, Mattoo P, et al. The human homolog of HAVcr-1 codes for a hepatitis A virus cellular receptor. J Virol 72:6621–6628, 1998.

107. McIntire JJ, Umetsu SE, Akbari O, et al. Identification of Tapr (an airway hyperreactivity regularity locus) and the linked Tim gene family. Nature Immunol 2:1096, 2001.

108. Monney L, Sabatos CA, Gaglia JL, et al. Th-1 specific cell surface protein Tim-3 regulates macrophage activation and severity of an autoimmune disease. Nature 415:536–541, 2002.

109. Matricardi PM, Rosmini F, Ferrigno L, et al. Cross sectional retrospective study of prevalence of atopy among Italian military students with antibodies against hepatitis A virus. Br Med J 314:987–988, 1987.

110. Matricardi PM, Franzinelli F, Franco A, et al. Sibship size, birth order, and atopy in 11,371 Italian young men. J Allergy Clin Immunol 101:439–444, 1998.
111. Asher LV, Binn LN, Marchwicki RH. Demonstration of hepatitis A virus in cell culture by electron microscopy with immunoperoxidase staining. J Virol Methods 15:323–328, 1987.
112. Shimizu YK, Shikata T, Beninger PR, et al. Detection of hepatitis A antigen in human liver. Infect Immun 36:320–324, 1982.
113. Shimizu YK, Mathiesen LR, Lorenz D, et al. Localization of hepatitis A antigen in liver tissue by peroxidase-conjugated antibody method: light and electron microscopic studies. J Immunol 121:1671–1679, 1978.
114. Provost PJ, Hilleman MR. Propagation of human hepatitis A virus in cell culture in vitro. Proc Soc Exp Biol Med 160:213–221, 1979.
115. Daemer RJ, Feinstone SM, Gust ID, et al. Propagation of human hepatitis A virus in African green monkey kidney cell culture: primary isolation and serial passage. Infect Immun 32:388–393, 1981.
116. Frosner GG, Deinhardt F, Scheid R. Propagation of human hepatitis A virus in a hepatoma cell culture line. Infection 7:303–305, 1979.
117. Dotzauer A, Feinstone SM, Kaplan G. Susceptibility of nonprimate cell lines to hepatitis A virus infection. J Virol 68:6064–6068, 1994.
118. Cromeans T, Fields HA, Sobsey MD. Replication kinetics and cytopathic effect of hepatitis A virus. J Gen Virol 70(pt 8):2051–2062, 1989.
119. Cromeans T, Sobsey MD, Fields HA. Development of a plaque assay for a cytopathic, rapidly replicating isolate of hepatitis A virus. J Med Virol 22:45–56, 1987.
120. Provost PJ, Bishop RP, Gerety RJ, et al. New findings in live, attenuated hepatitis A vaccine development. J Med Virol 20:165–175, 1986.
121. Talukder MA, Waller DK, Nixon P, et al. Prevalence of antibody to hepatitis A virus in a Saudi Arabian hospital population. J Infect Dis 148:1167, 1983.
122. Mao JS. Development of live, attenuated hepatitis A vaccine (H2-strain). Vaccine 8:523–524, 1990.
123. Cohen JI, Rosenblum B, Feinstone SM, et al. Attenuation and cell culture adaptation of hepatitis A virus (HAV): a genetic analysis with HAV cDNA. J Virol 63:5364–5370, 1989.
124. Balayan MS. Natural hosts of hepatitis A virus. Vaccine 10(suppl 1):S27–S31, 1992.
125. Rakela J, Mosley JW. Fecal excretion of hepatitis A virus in humans. J Infect Dis 135:933–938, 1977.
126. Maynard JE, Lorenz D, Bradley DW, et al. Review of infectivity studies in nonhuman primates with virus-like particles associated with MS-1 hepatitis. Am J Med Sci 270:81–85, 1975.
127. LeDuc JW, Lemon SM, Keenan CM, et al. Experimental infection of the New World owl monkey (Aotus trivirgatus) with hepatitis A virus. Infect Immun 40:766–772, 1983.
128. Hornei B, Kammerer R, Moubayed P. Experimental hepatitis A virus infection in guinea pigs. J Med Virol 64:402–409, 2001.
129. Dienstag JL, Davenport FM, McCollum RW, et al. Nonhuman primate-associated viral hepatitis type A: serologic evidence of hepatitis A virus infection. JAMA 236:462–464, 1976.
130. Anderson DA, Locarnini SA, Coulepis AG, et al. Restrictive events in the replication of hepatitis A virus in vitro. Intervirology 24:26–32, 1985.
131. Asher LV, Binn LN, Mensing TL, et al. Pathogenesis of hepatitis A in orally inoculated owl monkeys (Aotus trivirgatus). J Med Virol 47:260–268, 1995.
132. Karayiannis P, Jowett T, Enticott M, et al. Hepatitis A virus replication in tamarins and host immune response in relation to pathogenesis of liver cell damage. J Med Virol 18:261–276, 1986.
133. Krugman S, Ward R, Giles JP. Infectious hepatitis: detection of virus during the incubation period and in clinically inapparent infection. N Engl J Med 261:729–734, 1959.
134. Yotsuyanagi H, Iino S, Koike K, et al. Duration of viremia in human hepatitis A viral infection as determined by polymerase chain reaction. J Med Virol 40:35–38, 1993.
135. Cohen JI, Feinstone S, Purcell RH. Hepatitis A virus infection in a chimpanzee: duration of viremia and detection of virus in saliva and throat swabs. J Infect Dis 160:887–890, 1989.
136. Bower WA, Nainan OV, Han X, et al. Duration of viremia in hepatitis A virus infection. J Infect Dis 182:12–17, 2000.

137. Schulman AN, Dienstag JL, Jackson DR, et al. Hepatitis A antigen particles in liver, bile, and stool of chimpanzees. J Infect Dis 134:80–84, 1976.
138. Krawczynski KK, Bradley DW, Murphy BL, et al. Pathogenetic aspects of hepatitis A virus infection in enterally inoculated marmosets. Am J Clin Pathol 76:698–706, 1981.
139. Bradley DW, Hollinger FB, Hornbeck CL, Maynard JE. Isolation and characterization of hepatitis A virus. Am J Clin Pathol 65:876–889, 1976.
140. Vallbracht A, Fleischer B. Immune pathogenesis of hepatitis A. Arch Virol Suppl 4:3–4, 1992.
141. Kurane I, Binn LN, Bancroft WH, Ennis FA. Human lymphocyte responses to hepatitis A virus-infected cells: interferon production and lysis of infected cells. J Immunol 135:2140–2144, 1985.
142. Davis GL, Hoofnagle JH, Waggoner JG. Acute type A hepatitis during chronic hepatitis B virus infection: association of depressed hepatitis B virus replication with appearance of endogenous alpha interferon. J Med Virol 14:141–147, 1984.
143. Zachoval R, Abb J, Zachoval V, et al. Circulating interferon in patients with acute hepatitis A. J Infect Dis 153:1174–1175, 1986.
144. Winokur PL, Stapleton JT. Immunoglobulin prophylaxis for hepatitis A. Clin Infect Dis 14:580–586, 1992.
145. Stapleton JT. Host immune response to hepatitis A virus. J Infect Dis 171(suppl 1):S9–S14, 1995.
146. Stapleton JT, Lange DK, LeDuc JW, et al. The role of secretory immunity in hepatitis A virus infection. J Infect Dis 163:7–11, 1991.
147. Locarnini SA, Coulepis AG, Stratton AM, et al. Solid-phase enzyme-linked immunosorbent assay for detection of hepatitis A-specific immunoglobulin M. J Clin Microbiol 9:459–465, 1979.
148. Hansson BG, Calhoun JK, Wong DC, et al. Serodiagnosis of viral hepatitis A by a solid-phase radioimmunoassay specific for IgM antibodies. Scand J Infect Dis 13:5–9, 1981.
149. Duermeyer W, Wielaard F, van der Veen, J. A new principle for the detection of specific IgM antibodies applied in an ELISA for hepatitis A. J Med Virol 4:25–32, 1979.
150. Kao HW, Ashcavai M, Redeker AG. The persistence of hepatitis A IgM antibody after acute clinical hepatitis A. Hepatology 4:933–936, 1984.
151. Jansen RW, Siegl G, Lemon SM. Molecular epidemiology of human hepatitis A virus defined by an antigen-capture polymerase chain reaction method. Proc Natl Acad Sci U S A 87:2867–2871, 1990.
152. Purcell RH, Mannucci PM, Gdovin S, et al. Virology of the hepatitis A epidemic in Italy. Vox Sang 67(suppl 4):2–7, 1994.
153. Hutin YJ, Pool V, Cramer EH, et al. A multistate, foodborne outbreak of hepatitis A. N Engl J Med 340:595–602, 1999.
154. O'Grady J. Management of acute and fulminant hepatitis A. Vaccine 10(suppl 1):S21–S23, 1992.
155. Tibbs CJ, Williams R. Liver transplantation for acute and chronic viral hepatitis. J Viral Hepat 2:65–72, 1995.
156. Van Thiel DH. When should a decision to proceed with transplantation actually be made in cases of fulminant or subfulminant hepatic failure: at admission to hospital or when a donor organ is made available? J Hepatol 17:1–2, 1993.
157. Fagan E, Yousef G, Brahm J, et al. Persistence of hepatitis A virus in fulminant hepatitis and after liver transplantation. J Med Virol 30:131–136, 1990.
158. Tassopoulos NC, Papaevangelou GJ, Ticehurst JR, et al. Fecal excretion of Greek strains of hepatitis A virus in patients with hepatitis A and in experimentally infected chimpanzees. J Infect Dis 154:231–237, 1986.
159. Skinhoj P, Mathiesen LR, Kryger P. Fecal excretion of hepatitis A virus in patients with symptomatic hepatitis A infection. Ann Intern Med 106:221–226, 1987.
160. Rosenblum LS, Villarino ME, Nainan OV, et al. Hepatitis A outbreak in a neonatal intensive care unit: risk factors for transmission and evidence of prolonged viral excretion among preterm infants. J Infect Dis 164:476–482, 1991.
161. Krugman S, Ward R, Giles WP. The natural history of infectous hepatitis. Am J Med 32:717–728, 1962.
162. Lemon SM. The natural history of hepatitis A: the potential for transmission by transfusion of blood or blood products. Vox Sang 67(suppl 4):19–23, 1994.
163. Bell BP, Shapiro CN, Alter MJ, et al. The diverse patterns of hepatitis A epidemiology in the United States—implications for vaccination strategies. J Infect Dis 178:1579–1584, 1998.

164. Staes CJ, Schlenker TL, Risk I, et al. Sources of infection among persons with acute hepatitis A and no identified risk factors during a sustained community-wide outbreak. Pediatrics 106:E54, 2000.
165. Smith PF, Grabau JC, Werzberger A, et al. The role of young children in a community-wide outbreak of hepatitis A. Epidemiol Infect 118:243–252, 1997.
166. Armstrong GL, Bell BP. Hepatitis A virus infections in the United States: model-based estimates and implications for childhood immunization. Pediatrics 109:839–845, 2002.
167. McCaustland KA, Bond WW, Bradley DW, et al. Survival of hepatitis A virus in feces after drying and storage for 1 month. J Clin Microbiol 16:957–958, 1982.
168. Carl M, Francis DP, Maynard JE. Food-borne hepatitis A: recommendations for control. J Infect Dis 148:1133–1135, 1983.
169. Massoudi MS, Bell BP, Paredes V, et al. An outbreak of hepatitis A associated with an infected foodhandler. Public Health Rep 114:157–164, 1999.
170. Centers for Disease Control. Foodborne hepatitis A—Alaska, Florida, North Carolina, Washington. MMWR 39:228–232, 1990.
171. Desenclos JC, Klontz KC, Wilder MH, et al. A multistate outbreak of hepatitis A caused by the consumption of raw oysters. Am J Public Health 81:1268–1272, 1991.
172. Wang JY, Hu SL, Liu HY, et al. Risk factor analysis of an epidemic of hepatitis A in a factory in Shanghai. Int J Epidemiol 19:435–438, 1990.
173. Mele A, Stroffolini T, Palumbo F, et al. Incidence and risk factors for hepatitis A in Italy: public health indications from a 10-year surveillance. J Hepatol 26:743–747, 1997.
174. Germinario C, Lopalco PL, Chicanna M, et al. From hepatitis B to hepatitis A and B prevention: the Puglia (Italy) experience. Vaccine 18(suppl):S83–S85, 2000.
175. Hollinger FB, Khan NC, Oefinger PE, et al. Posttransfusion hepatitis type A. JAMA 250:2313–2317, 1983.
176. Soucie JM, Robertson BH, Bell BP, et al. Hepatitis A virus infections associated with clotting factor concentrate in the United States. Transfusion 38:573–579, 1998.
177. Mannucci PM, Gdovin S, Gringeri A, et al. Transmission of hepatitis A to patients with hemophilia by factor VIII concentrates treated with organic solvent and detergent to inactivate viruses. The Italian Collaborative Group. Ann Intern Med 120:1–7, 1994.
178. Benjamin RJ. Nucleic acid testing: update and applications. Semin Hematol 38:11–16, 2001.
179. Leikin E, Lysikiewicz A, Garry D, et al. Intrauterine transmission of hepatitis A virus. Obstet Gynecol 88:690–691, 1996.
180. McDuffie RS Jr, Bader T. Fetal meconium peritonitis after maternal hepatitis A. Am J Obstet Gynecol 180:1031–1032, 1999.
181. Tong MJ, Thursby M, Rakela J, et al. Studies on the maternal-infant transmission of the viruses which cause acute hepatitis. Gastroenterology 80:999–1004, 1981.
182. Watson JC, Fleming DW, Borella AJ, et al. Vertical transmission of hepatitis A resulting in an outbreak in a neonatal intensive care unit. J Infect Dis 167:567–571, 1993.
183. Coursaget P, Lebouleux D, Gharbi Y, et al. Etiology of acute sporadic hepatitis in adults in Senegal and Tunisia. Scand J Infect Dis 27:9–11, 1995.
184. Tsega E, Mengesha B, Hansson BG, et al. Hepatitis A, B, and delta infection in Ethiopia: a serologic survey with demographic data. Am J Epidemiol 123:344–351, 1986.
185. Bowden FJ, Currie BJ, Miller NC, et al. Should aboriginals in the "top end" of the Northern Territory be vaccinated against hepatitis A? Med J Aust 161:372–373, 1994.
186. Cianciara J. Hepatitis A shifting epidemiology in Poland and Eastern Europe. Vaccine 18(suppl):S68–S70, 2000.
187. Green MS, Block C, Slater PE. Rise in the incidence of viral hepatitis in Israel despite improved socioeconomic conditions. Rev Infect Dis 11:464–469, 1989.
188. Halliday ML, Kang LY, Zhou TK, et al. An epidemic of hepatitis A attributable to the ingestion of raw clams in Shanghai, China. J Infect Dis 164:852–859, 1991.
189. Gdalevich M, Grotto I, Mandel Y, et al. Hepatitis A antibody prevalence among young adults in Israel—the decline continues. Epidemiol Infect 121:477–479, 1998.
190. Innis BL, Snitbhan R, Hoke CH, et al. The declining transmission of hepatitis A in Thailand. J Infect Dis 163:989–995, 1991.
191. Kunasol P, Cooksley G, Chan VF, et al. Hepatitis A virus: declining seroprevalence in children and adolescents in Southeast Asia. Southeast Asian J Trop Med Public Health 29:255–262, 1998.
192. Lagos R, Potin M, Munoz A, et al. Serum antibodies against hepatitis A virus among subjects of middle and low socioeconomic levels in urban area of Santiago, Chile. Rev Med Chil 127:429–436, 1999.
193. Pinho JR, Sumita LM, Moreira RC, et al. Duality of patterns in hepatitis A epidemiology: a study involving two socioeconomically distinct populations in Campinas, Sao Paulo State, Brazil. Rev Inst Med Trop Sao Paulo 40:105–106, 1998.
194. Poovorawan Y, Vimolkej T, Chongsrisawat V, et al. The declining pattern of seroepidemiology of hepatitis A virus infection among adolescents in Bangkok, Thailand. Southeast Asian J Trop Med Public Health 28:154–157, 1997.
195. Das K, Jain A, Gupta S, et al. The changing epidemiological pattern of hepatitis A in an urban population of India: emergence of a trend similar to the European countries. Eur J Epidemiol 16:507–510, 2000.
196. Tapia-Conyer R, Santos JI, Cavalcanti AM, et al. Hepatitis A in Latin America: a changing epidemiologic pattern. Am J Trop Med Hyg 61:825–829, 1999.
197. Tufenkeji H. Hepatitis A shifting epidemiology in the Middle East and Africa. Vaccine 18(suppl 1):S65–S67, 2000.
198. Wang LY, Cheng YW, Chou SJ, et al. Secular trend and geographical variation in hepatitis A infection and hepatitis B carrier rate among adolescents in Taiwan: an island-wide survey. J Med Virol 39:1–5, 1993.
199. Ciocca M. Clinical course and consequences of hepatitis A infection. Vaccine 18(suppl 1):S71–S74, 2000.
200. Shah U, Habib Z, Kleinman RE. Liver failure attributable to hepatitis A virus infection in a developing country. Pediatrics 105:436–438, 2000.
201. Gil A, Gonzalez A, Dal Re R, et al. Prevalence of antibodies against varicella zoster, herpes simplex (types 1 and 2), hepatitis B and hepatitis A viruses among Spanish adolescents. J Infect 36:53–56, 1998.
202. Shapiro CN, Coleman PJ, McQuillan GM, et al. Epidemiology of hepatitis A: seroepidemiology and risk groups in the USA. Vaccine 10(suppl 1):S59–S62, 1992.
203. Prodinger WM, Larcher C, Solder BM, et al. Hepatitis A in Western Austria—the epidemiological situation before the introduction of active immunisation. Infection 22:53–55, 1994.
204. Termorshuizen F, Dorigo-Zetsma JW, de Melker HE, et al. The prevalence of antibodies to hepatitis A virus and its determinants in The Netherlands: a population-based survey. Epidemiol Infect 124:459–466, 2000.
205. Bottiger M, Christenson B, Grillner L. Hepatitis A immunity in the Swedish population: a study of the prevalence of markers in the Swedish population. Scand J Infect Dis 29:99–102, 1997.
206. Centers for Disease Control and Prevention. Summary of notifiable diseases, United States, 1997. MMWR 46:ii-87, 1998.
207. Centers for Disease Control and Prevention. Hepatitis Surveillance Report No. 57. Atlanta, Centers for Disease Control and Prevention, 2000.
208. Centers for Disease Control and Prevention. Prevention of hepatitis A through active or passive immunization: recommendations of the Advisory Committee on Immunization Practices (ACIP). MMWR 45(RR-15):1–30, 1996.
209. Cotter SM, Sansom S, Lee B, et al. Outbreak of hepatitis A among men who have sex with men: implications for hepatitis A vaccination. J Infect Dis. In press.
210. Friedman MS, Blake PA, Koehler JE, et al. Factors influencing a communitywide campaign to administer hepatitis A vaccine to men who have sex with men. Am J Public Health 90:1942–1946, 2000.
211. Harkess J, Gildon B, Istre GR. Outbreaks of hepatitis A among illicit drug users, Oklahoma, 1984–87. Am J Public Health 79:463–466, 1989.
212. Hutin YJ, Bell BP, Marshall KL, et al. Identifying target groups for a potential vaccination program during a hepatitis A communitywide outbreak. Am J Public Health 89:918–921, 1999.
213. Shaw FE Jr, Sudman JH, Smith SM, et al. A community-wide epidemic of hepatitis A in Ohio. Am J Epidemiol 123:1057–1065, 1986.

214. Craig AS, Sockwell DC, Schaffner W, et al. Use of hepatitis A vaccine in a community-wide outbreak of hepatitis A. Clin Infect Dis 27:531–535, 1998.
215. Averhoff F, Shapiro CN, Bell BP, et al. Control of hepatitis A through routine vaccination of children. JAMA 286:2968–2973, 2001.
216. Venczel LV, Desai MM, Vertz PD, et al. The role of child care in a community-wide outbreak of hepatitis A. Pediatrics 108:E78, 2001.
217. Shapiro CN, Hadler SC. Hepatitis A and hepatitis B virus infections in day-care settings. Pediatr Ann 20:435–441, 1991.
218. Jackson LA, Stewart LK, Solomon SL, et al. Risk of infection with hepatitis A, B or C, cytomegalovirus, varicella or measles among child care providers. Pediatr Infect Dis J 15:584–589, 1996.
219. Desenclos JC, MacLafferty L. Communitywide outbreak of hepatitis A linked to children in day care centers and with increased transmission in young adult men in Florida 1988–1989. J Epidemiol Community Health 47:269–273, 1993.
220. Hadler SC, Erben JJ, Matthews D, et al. Effect of immunoglobulin on hepatitis A in day-care centers. JAMA 249:48–53, 1983.
221. Szmuness W, Purcell RH, Dienstag JL, et al. Antibody to hepatitis A antigen in institutionalized mentally retarded patients. JAMA 237:1702–1705, 1977.
222. Shaw DD, Whiteman DC, Merritt AD, et al. Hepatitis A outbreaks among illicit drug users and their contacts in Queensland, 1997. Med J Aust 170:584–587, 1999.
223. O'Donovan D, Cooke RP, Joce R, et al. An outbreak of hepatitis A amongst injecting drug users. Epidemiol Infect 127:469–473, 2001.
224. Hutin YJ, Sabin KM, Hutwagner LC, et al. Multiple modes of hepatitis A virus transmission among methamphetamine users. Am J Epidemiol 152:186–192, 2000.
225. Ivie K, Spruill C, Bell BP. Prevalence of hepatitis A virus infection among illicit drug users, 1993–1994. Antiviral Ther 5(suppl 1):A.7, 2000.
226. Villano SA, Nelson KE, Vlahov D, et al. Hepatitis A among homosexual men and injection drug users: more evidence for vaccination. Clin Infect Dis 25:726–728, 1997.
227. Stokes ML, Ferson MJ, Young LC. Outbreak of hepatitis A among homosexual men in Sydney. Am J Public Health 87:2039–2041, 1997.
228. Henning KJ, Bell E, Braun J, et al. A community-wide outbreak of hepatitis A: risk factors for infection among homosexual and bisexual men. Am J Med 99:132–136, 1995.
229. Centers for Disease Control. Hepatitis A among homosexual men: United States, Canada, and Australia. MMWR 41:161–164, 1992.
230. Katz MH, Hsu L, Wong E, et al. Seroprevalence of and risk factors for hepatitis A infection among young homosexual and bisexual men. J Infect Dis 175:1225–1229, 1997.
231. Mah MW, Royce RA, Rathouz PJ, et al. Prevalence of hepatitis A antibodies in hemophiliacs: preliminary results from the Southeastern Delta Hepatitis Study. Vox Sang 67(suppl 1):21–22, 1994.
232. Mannucci PM, Santagostino E, Di Bona E, et al. The outbreak of hepatitis A in Italian patients with hemophilia: facts and fancies. Vox Sang 67(suppl 1):31–35, 1994.
233. Klein BS, Michaels JA, Rytel MW, et al. Nosocomial hepatitis A: a multinursery outbreak in Wisconsin. JAMA 252:2716–2721, 1984.
234. Noble RC, Kane MA, Reeves SA, et al. Posttransfusion hepatitis A in a neonatal intensive care unit. JAMA 252:2711–2715, 1984.
235. Weisfuse IB, Graham DJ, Will M, et al. An outbreak of hepatitis A among cancer patients treated with interleukin-2 and lymphokine-activated killer cells. J Infect Dis 161:647–652, 1990.
236. Goodman RA. Nosocomial hepatitis A. Ann Intern Med 103:452–454, 1985.
237. Papaevangelou GJ, Roumeliotou-Karayannis AJ, Contoyannis PC. The risk of nosocomial hepatitis A and B virus infections from patients under care without isolation precaution. J Med Virol 7:143–148, 1981.
238. Gibas A, Blewett DR, Schoenfeld DA, et al. Prevalence and incidence of viral hepatitis in health workers in the prehepatitis B vaccination era. Am J Epidemiol 136:603–610, 1992.
239. Steffen R, Rickenbach M, Wilhelm U, et al. Health problems after travel to developing countries. J Infect Dis 156:84–91, 1987.
240. Steffen R. Risk of hepatitis A in travellers. Vaccine 10(suppl 1): S69–S72, 1992.
241. Mele A, Sagliocca L, Palumbo F, et al. Travel-associated hepatitis A: effect of place of residence and country visited. J Public Health Med 13:256–259, 1991.
242. Steffen R, Kane MA, Shapiro CN, et al. Epidemiology and prevention of hepatitis A in travelers. JAMA 272:885–889, 1994.
243. Steffen R. Hepatitis A in travelers: the European experience. J Infect Dis 171(suppl 1):S24–S28, 1995.
244. Lange WR, Frame JD. High incidence of viral hepatitis among American missionaries in Africa. Am J Trop Med Hyg 43:527–533, 1990.
245. Christenson B. Epidemiological aspects of acute viral hepatitis A in Swedish travellers to endemic areas. Scand J Infect Dis 17:5–10, 1985.
246. Dalton CB, Haddix A, Hoffman RE, et al. The cost of a food-borne outbreak of hepatitis A in Denver, Colo. Arch Intern Med 156:1013–1016, 1996.
247. Lowry PW, Levine R, Stroup DF, et al. Hepatitis A outbreak on a floating restaurant in Florida, 1986. Am J Epidemiol 129:155–164, 1989.
248. Latham RH, Schable CA. Foodborne hepatitis A at a family reunion use of IgM-specific hepatitis a serologic testing. Am J Epidemiol 115:640-645, 1982.
249. Mishu B, Hadler SC, Boaz VA, et al. Foodborne hepatitis A: evidence that microwaving reduces risk? J Infect Dis 162:655–658, 1990.
250. Parkin WE, Marzinsky P, Griffin MR. Foodborne hepatitis A associated with cheeseburgers. J Med Soc N J 80:612–615, 1983.
251. Weltman AC, Bennett NM, Ackman DA, et al. An outbreak of hepatitis A associated with a bakery, New York, 1994: the 1968 "West Branch, Michigan" outbreak repeated. Epidemiol Infect 117:333–341, 1996.
252. Dentinger CM, Bower WA, Nainan OV, et al. An outbreak of hepatitis A associated with green onions. J Infect Dis 183:1273–1276, 2001.
253. Rosenblum LS, Mirkin IR, Allen DT, et al. A multifocal outbreak of hepatitis A traced to commercially distributed lettuce. Am J Public Health 80:1075–1079, 1990.
254. Niu MT, Polish LB, Robertson BH, et al. Multistate outbreak of hepatitis A associated with frozen strawberries. J Infect Dis 166:518–524, 1992.
255. Reid TM, Robinson HG. Frozen raspberries and hepatitis A. Epidemiol Infect 98:109–112, 1987.
256. Bloch AB, Stramer SL, Smith JD, et al. Recovery of hepatitis A virus from a water supply responsible for a common source outbreak of hepatitis A. Am J Public Health 80:428–430, 1990.
257. De Serres G, Cromeans TL, Levesque B, et al. Molecular confirmation of hepatitis A virus from well water: epidemiology and public health implications. J Infect Dis 179:37–43, 1999.
258. Bergeisen GH, Hinds MW, Skaggs JW. A waterborne outbreak of hepatitis A in Meade County, Kentucky. Am J Public Health 75:161–164, 1985.
259. Lerman Y, Chodik G, Aloni H, et al. Occupations at increased risk of hepatitis A: a 2-year nationwide historical prospective cohort. Am J Epidemiol 150:312–320, 1999.
260. Glas C, Hotz P, Steffen R. Hepatitis A in workers exposed to sewage: a systematic review. Occup Environ Med 58:762–768, 2001.
261. Poole CJ, Shakespeare AT. Should sewage workers and carers for people with learning disabilities be vaccinated against hepatitis A. BMJ 306:1102, 1993.
262. Trout D, Mueller C, Venczel L, et al. Evaluation of occupational transmission of hepatitis A virus among wastewater workers. J Occup Environ Med 42:83–87, 2000.
263. Weldon M, VanEgdom MJ, Hendricks KA, et al. Prevalence of antibody to hepatitis A virus in drinking water workers and wastewater workers in Texas from 1996 to 1997. J Occup Environ Med 42:821–826, 2000.
264. Venczel L, Brown S, Frumkin H, et al. Prevalence of hepatitis A virus infection among sewage workers in Georgia. American J. Industrial Med. In press.
265. Weiland O, Niklasson B, Berg R, et al. Clinical and subclinical hepatitis A occurring after immunoglobulin prophylaxis among Swedish UN soldiers in Sinai. Scand J Gastroenterol 16:967–972, 1981.
266. Pierce PF, Cappello M, Bernard KW. Subclinical infection with hepatitis A in Peace Corps volunteers following immune globulin prophylaxis. Am J Trop Med Hyg 42:465–469, 1990.

267. Kluge I. Gamma-globulin in the prevention of viral hepatitis: a study of the effect of medium-size doses. Acta Med Scand 174:469–477, 1963.

268. Mosley JW, Reisler DM, Brachott D, et al. Comparison of two lots of immune serum globulin for prophylaxis of infectious hepatitis. Am J Epidemiol 87:539–550, 1968.

269. Stokes J, Neefe JR. The prevention and attenuation of infectious hepatitis by gamma globulin. JAMA 127:144–145, 1945.

270. Stokes N. The prevention and attenuation of infectious hepatitis by gamma globulin. JAMA 127:144–145, 1945.

271. Aach RD, Elsea WR, Lyerly J, Henderson DA. Efficacy of varied doses of gamma globulin during an epidemic of infectious hepatitis, Hoonah, Alaska, 1961. Am J Pub Heath 53:1623–1629,1963.

272. Fowinkle EW, Guthrie N. Comparison of two doses of gamma globulin in the prevention of infectious hepatitis. Public Health Rep 79:634–637, 1964.

273. Cohn E, Oncley J, Strong LE. Chemical, clinical, and immunological studies on the products of human plasma fractionation: the characterization of the protein fractions of human plasma. J Clin Invest 23:417–432, 1944.

274. Lerman Y, Shohat T, Ashkenazi S, et al. Efficacy of different doses of immune serum globulin in the prevention of hepatitis A: a three-year prospective study. Clin Infect Dis 17:411–414, 1993.

275. Van Doorslaer E, Tormans G, van Damme P, et al. Cost effectiveness of alternative hepatitis A immunisation strategies. Pharmacoeconomics 8:5–8, 1995.

276. Fenn P, McGuire A, Gray A. An economic evaluation of vaccination against hepatitis A for frequent travelers. J Infect 36:17–22, 1998.

277. Ellis EF, Henney CS. Adverse reactions following administration of human gamma globulin. J Allergy 43:45–54, 1969.

278. Peetermans J. Production, quality control and characterization of an inactivated hepatitis A vaccine. Vaccine 10(suppl 1):S99–S101, 1992.

279. Armstrong ME, Giesa PA, Davide JP, et al. Development of the formalin-inactivated hepatitis A vaccine, VAQTA from the live attenuated virus strain CR326F. J Hepatol 18(suppl 2):S20–S26, 1993.

280. Karron RA, Daemer R, Ticehurst J, et al. Studies of prototype live hepatitis A virus vaccines in primate models. J Infect Dis 157:338–345, 1988.

281. Sjogren MH, Purcell RH, McKee K, et al. Clinical and laboratory observations following oral or intramuscular administration of a live attenuated hepatitis A vaccine candidate. Vaccine 10(suppl 1):S135–S137, 1992.

282. Midthun K, Ellerbeck E, Gershman K, et al. Safety and immunogenicity of a live attenuated hepatitis A virus vaccine in seronegative volunteers. J Infect Dis 163:735–739, 1991.

283. Cho MW, Ehrenfeld E. Rapid completion of the replication cycle of hepatitis A virus subsequent to reversal of guanidine inhibition. Virology 180:770–780, 1991.

284. Mao JS, Dong DX, Zhang HY, et al. Primary study of attenuated live hepatitis A vaccine (H2 strain) in humans. J Infect Dis 159: 621–624, 1989.

285. Cohen JI, Ticehurst JR, Feinstone SM, et al. Hepatitis A virus cDNA and its RNA transcripts are infectious in cell culture. J Virol 61:3035–3039, 1987.

286. Emerson SU, Huang YK, McRill C, et al. Molecular basis of virulence and growth of hepatitis A virus in cell culture. Vaccine 10(suppl 1):S36–S39, 1992.

287. Emerson SU, Huang YK, Purcell RH. 2B and 2C mutations are essential but mutations throughout the genome of HAV contribute to adaptation to cell culture. Virology 194:475–480, 1993.

288. Vidor E, Fritzell B, Plotkin S. Clinical development of a new inactivated hepatitis A vaccine. Infection 24:447–458, 1996.

289. Gluck R, Mischler R, Brantschen S, et al. Immunopotentiating reconstituted influenza virus virosome vaccine delivery system for immunization against hepatitis A. J Clin Invest 90:2491–2495, 1992.

290. Gust ID, Lehmann NI, Crowe S, et al. The origin of the HM175 strain of hepatitis A virus. J Infect Dis 151:365–367, 1985.

291. Flehmig B, Vallbracht A, Wurster G. Hepatitis A virus in cell culture. III. Propagation of hepatitis A virus in human embryo kidney cells and human embryo fibroblast strains. Med Microbiol Immunol (Berl) 170:83–89, 1981.

292. Heinricy U, Stierhof YD, Pfisterer M, et al. Properties of a hepatitis A virus candidate vaccine strain. J Gen Virol 68(pt 9):2487–2493, 1987.

293. Flehmig B, Heinricy U, Pfisterer M. Prospects for a hepatitis A virus vaccine. Prog Med Virol 37:56–71, 1990.

294. Flehmig B, Mauler RF, Noll G, et al. Progress in the development of an attenuated, live hepatitis A vaccine. In Zuckerman AJ (ed). Viral Hepatitis and Liver Disease. New York, Alan R. Liss, 1988, pp 87–90.

295. Ambrosch F, Wiedermann G, Jonas S, et al. Immunogenicity and protectivity of a new liposomal hepatitis A vaccine. Vaccine 15:1209–1213, 1997.

296. Ambrosch F, Wiedermann G, Jonas S, Althaus B, Finkel B, Glück R, Herzog C. Immunogenicity and protectivity of a new liposomal hepatitis A vaccine. Vaccine 15:1209–1213, 1997.

297. Dagan R, Greenberg D, Goldenbertg-Gehtman P, et al. Safety and immunogenicity of a new formulation of an inactivated hepatitis A vaccine. Vaccine 17:1919–1925, 1999.

298. López EL, Del Carmen Xifró M, Torrado LE, et al. Safety and immunogenicity of a pediatric formulation of inactivated hepatitis A vaccine in Argentinean children. Pediatr Infect Dis J 20:48–52, 2001.

299. Centers for Disease Control and Prevention. Notice to readers: FDA approval for a combined hepatitis A and B vaccine. MMWR 50:806–807, 2001.

300. Diaz-Mitoma F, Law B, Parsons J. A combined vaccine against hepatitis A and B in children and adolescents. Pediatr Infect Dis J 18:109–114, 1999.

301. Product Information: Avaxim® Aventis.

302. Product Information: Epaxal® Berna Biotech AG, 2002.

303. Product Information: TWINRIX Hepatitis A Inactivated and Hepatitis B (Recombinant) Vaccine. Philadelphia, GlaxoSmithKline, 2002.

304. Czeschinski PA, Binding N, Witting U. Hepatitis A and hepatitis B vaccinations: immunogenicity of combined vaccine and of simultaneously or separately applied single vaccines. Vaccine 18:1074–1080, 2000.

305. Van Herck K, van Damme P, Collard F, et al. Two-dose combined vaccination against hepatitis A and B in healthy subjects aged 11–18 years. Scand J Gastroenterol 12:1236–1240, 1999.

306. Connor BA, Phair J, Sack D, et al. Randomized double-blind study in healthy adults to assess the boosting effect of VAQTA or HAVRIX after a single dose of HAVRIX. Clin Infect Dis 34:396–401, 2001.

307. Bryan JP, Henry CH, Hoffman AG, et al. Randomized, cross-over controlled comparison of two inactivated hepatitis A vaccines. Vaccine 19:743–750, 2000.

308. Landry P, Tremblay S, Darioli R. Inactivated hepatitis A vaccine booster dose given ≥ 24 months after the primary dose. Vaccine 19:399–402, 2001.

309. Tilzey AJ, Palmer SJ, Barrow S, et al. Effect of hepatitis A vaccination schedules on immune response. Vaccine 10(suppl):S121–S123, 1992.

310. Tong MJ, Co RL, Bellak C. Hepatitis A vaccination. West J Med 158:602–605, 1993.

311. Product Information: Havrix®Hepatitis A Vaccine, Inactivated. Philadelphia, GlaxoSmithKline, 2002.

312. Product Information: VAQTA® Hepatitis A Vaccine, Inactivated. West Point, PA, Merck & Co., Inc, 2002.

313. Wiedermann G, Ambrosch F. Immunogenicity of an inactivated hepatitis A vaccine after exposure at 37 degrees C for 1 week. Vaccine 12:401–402, 1994.

314. Shouval D, Ashur Y, Adler R, et al. Single and booster dose responses to an inactivated hepatitis A virus vaccine: comparison with immune serum globulin prophylaxis. Vaccine 11(suppl 1):S9–S14, 1993.

315. van Damme P, Mathei C, Thoelen S, et al. Single dose inactivated hepatitis A vaccine: rationale and clinical assessment of the safety and immunogenicity. J Med Virol 44:435–441, 1994.

316. Hoke CH Jr, Binn LN, Egan JE, et al. Hepatitis A in the US Army: epidemiology and vaccine development. Vaccine 10(suppl 1):S75–S79, 1992.

317. Fujiyama S, Odoh K, Kuramoto I, et al. Current seroepidemiological status of hepatitis A with a comparison of antibody titers after infection and vaccination. J Hepatol 21:641–645, 1994.

318. Clemens R, Safary A, Hepburn A, et al. Clinical experience with an inactivated hepatitis A vaccine. J Infect Dis 171(suppl 1):S44–S49, 1995.

319. Balcarek KB, Bagley MR, Pass RF, et al. Safety and immunogenicity of an inactivated hepatitis A vaccine in preschool children. J Infect Dis 171(suppl 1):S70–S72, 1995.

320. Horng YC, Chang MH, Lee CY, et al. Safety and immunogenicity of hepatitis A vaccine in healthy children. Pediatr Infect Dis J 12:359–362, 1993.

321. McMahon BJ, Williams J, Bulkow L, et al. Immunogenicity of an inactivated hepatitis A vaccine in Alaska Native children and Native and non-Native adults. J Infect Dis 171:676–679, 1995.

322. Nalin DR. VAQTA, hepatitis A vaccine, purified, inactivated. Drugs Future 20:24–29, 1995.

323. Loutan L, Bouvier P, Althaus B, Glück R. Inactivated virosome hepatitis A vaccine. Lancet 343:322–324, 1994.

324. Holzer BR, Hatz C, Schmidt-Sissolak D, Glück R, Althaus B, Egger M. Immunogenicity and adverse effects of inactivated virosome versus alum-adsorbed hepatitis A vaccine: a randomized controlled trial. Vaccine 14:982–986, 1996.

325. Sjogren MH, Hoke CH, Binn LN, et al. Immunogenicity of an inactivated hepatitis A vaccine. Ann Intern Med 114:470–471, 1991.

326. Piazza M, Safary A, Vegnente A, et al. Safety and immunogenicity of hepatitis A vaccine in infants: a candidate for inclusion in the childhood vaccination programme. Vaccine 17:585–588, 1999.

327. Shapiro CN, Letson GW, Kuehn D. Effect of maternal antibody on immunogenicity of hepatitis A vaccine in infants [abstr H61]. In Abstracts of the 35th Annual Interscience Conference on Antimicrobial Agents and Chemotherapy, San Francisco, September 17–20, 1995.

328. Troisi CL, Hollinger FB, Krause DS, et al. Immunization of seronegative infants with hepatitis A vaccine (HAVRIX; SKB): a comparative study of two dosing schedules. Vaccine 15:1613–1617, 1997.

329. Dagan R, Amir J, Mijalovsky A, et al. Immunization against hepatitis A in the first year of life: priming despite the presence of maternal antibody. Pediatr Infect Dis J 19:1045–1052, 2000.

330. Lieberman JM, Marcy M, Partridge S, Ward JI. Evaluation of hepatitis A vaccine in infants: effect of maternal antibodies on the antibody response [abstr 76]. In Abstracts of the 36th Annual Meeting of the Infectious Diseases Society of America, Denver. Alexandria, VA, Infectious Diseases Society of America, 1998, p 38.

331. Fiore A, Shapiro CN, Sabin KM, et al. Persistence of protective antibody concentrations and response to a booster dose among children given hepatitis A vaccine during infancy: effect of maternal antibody status. Ped Infect Dis J. In press.

332. Franzen C, Frosner G. Placental transfer of hepatitis A antibody. N Engl J Med 304:427, 1981.

333. Linder N, Karetnyi Y, Gidony Y, et al. Decline of hepatitis A antibodies during the first 7 months of life in full-term and preterm infants. Infection 27:128–131, 1999.

334. Lieberman JM, Chang S, Partridge S, et al. Kinetics of maternal hepatitis A antibody decay in infants: implications for vaccine use. Pediatr Infect Dis J 21:347–348, 2002.

335. Neilsen GA, Bodsworth NJ, Watts N. Response to hepatitis A vaccination in human immunodeficiency virus-infected and -uninfected homosexual men. J Infect Dis 176:1064–1067, 1997.

336. Hess G, Clemens R, Bienzle U, et al. Immunogenicity and safety of an inactivated hepatitis A vaccine in anti-HIV positive and negative homosexual men. J Med Virol 46:40–42, 1995.

337. Keeffe EB, Iwarson S, McMahon BJ. Safety and immunogenicity of hepatitis A vaccine in patients with chronic liver disease. Hepatology 27:881–886, 1998.

338. Lee S-D, Chan CY, Yu MY. Safety and immunogenicity of inactivated hepatitis A vaccine in patients with chronic liver disease. J Med Virol 52:215–218, 1997.

339. Briem H, Safary A. Immunogenicity and safety in adults of hepatitis A virus vaccine administered as a single dose with a booster 6 months later. J Med Virol 44:443–445, 1994.

340. Reuman PD, Kubilis P, Hurni W, et al. The effect of age and weight on the response to formalin inactivated, alum-adjuvanted hepatitis A vaccine in healthy adults. Vaccine 15:1157–1161, 1997.

341. Lemon SM, Binn LN. Serum neutralizing antibody response to hepatitis A virus. J Infect Dis 148:1033–1039, 1983.

342. Shouval D, Ashur Y, Adler R, et al. Safety, tolerability, and immunogenicity of an inactivated hepatitis A vaccine: effects of single and booster injections, and comparison to administration of immune globulin. J Hepatol 18(suppl 2):S32–S37, 1993.

343. Lemon SM, Murphy PC, Provost PJ, et al. Immunoprecipitation and virus neutralization assays demonstrate qualitative differences between protective antibody responses to inactivated hepatitis A

vaccine and passive immunization with immune globulin. J Infect Dis 176:9–19, 1997.

344. Green MS, Cohen D, Lerman Y, et al. Depression of the immune response to an inactivated hepatitis A vaccine administered concomitantly with immune globulin. J Infect Dis 168:740–743, 1993.

345. Purcell RH, D'Hondt E, Bradbury R, et al. Inactivated hepatitis A vaccine: active and passive immunoprophylaxis in chimpanzees. Vaccine 10(suppl 1):S148–S151, 1992.

346. Centers for Disease Control and Prevention. Hepatitis A vaccination programs in communities with high rates of hepatitis A. MMWR 46:600–603, 1997.

347. McMahon BJ, Beller M, Williams J, et al. A program to control an outbreak of hepatitis A in Alaska by using an inactivated hepatitis A vaccine. Arch Pediatr Adolesc Med 150:733–739, 1996.

348. Werzberger A, Kuter B, Nalin D. Six years' follow-up after hepatitis A vaccination [letter]. N Engl J Med 338:1160, 1998.

349. Werzberger A, Mensch B, Kuter B, et al. A controlled trial of a formalin-inactivated hepatitis A vaccine in healthy children. N Engl J Med 327:453–457, 1992.

350. Shaw FE Jr, Shapiro CN, Welty TK, et al. Hepatitis transmission among the Sioux Indians of South Dakota. Am J Public Health 80:1091–1094, 1990.

351. Dentinger CM, Heinrich NL, Bell BP, et al. A prevalence study of hepatitis A virus infection in a migrant community: is hepatitis A vaccine indicated? J Pediatr 138:705–709, 2001.

352. Fan PC, Chang MH, Lee PI, et al. Follow-up immunogenicity of an inactivated hepatitis A virus vaccine in healthy children: results after 5 years. Vaccine 16:232–235, 1998.

353. Van Herck K, van Damme P. Inactivated hepatitis A vaccine-induced antibodies: follow-up and estimates of long-term persistence. J Med Virol 63:1–7, 2001.

354. Wiedermann G, Kundi M, Ambrosch F. Estimated persistence of anti-HAV antibodies after single dose and booster hepatitis A vaccination (0–6 schedule). Acta Trop 69:121–125, 1998.

355. Bouvier PA, Bock J, Loutan L, Farinelli T, Glueck R, Herzog C. Long-term immunogenicity of an inactivated virosome hepatitis A vaccine. J Med Virol 68:489–493, 2002.

355a Werzberger A, Mensch B, Nalin DR, et al. Effectiveness of hepatitis A in a former friendly affected community: 9 years' follow up after the Monroe field trial of VAQTA®. Vaccine 20:1699–1702,2002.

356. Robertson BH, D'Hondt EH, Spelbring J, et al. Effect of postexposure vaccination in a chimpanzee model of hepatitis A virus infection. J Med Virol 43:249–251, 1994.

357. Sagliocca L, Amoroso P, Stroffolini T, et al. Efficacy of hepatitis A vaccine in prevention of secondary hepatitis A infection: a randomised trial. Lancet 353:1136–1139, 1999.

358. Bell BP, Margolis HS. Efficacy of hepatitis A vaccine in prevention of secondary hepatitis A infection [letter]. Lancet 354:341, 1999.

359. American Academy of Pediatrics. Hepatitis A. In Pickering LK (ed). Red Book: Report of the Committee on Infectious Diseases (25th ed). Elk Grove Village, IL, American Academy of Pediatrics, 2000, pp 280–289.

360. Andre FE, D'Hondt E, Delem A, et al. Clinical assessment of the safety and efficacy of an inactivated hepatitis A vaccine: rationale and summary of findings. Vaccine 10(suppl 1):S160–S168, 1992.

361. Black S, Shinefield H, Su L, et al. Post-marketing safety evaluation of inactivated hepatitis A vaccine (VAQTA, Merck) in 9740 children and adults [abstr]. In Program and abstracts of the 38th Interscience Conference on Antimicrobial Agents and Chemotherapy. Washington, DC, ASM Press, 1998.

362. Niu MT, Salive M, Krueger C, et al. Two-year review of hepatitis A vaccine safety: data from the Vaccine Adverse Event Reporting System (VAERS). Clin Infect Dis 26:1475–1476, 1998.

363. Stark K, Günther M, Newhaus R, et al. Immunogenicity and safety of hepatitis A vaccine in liver and renal transplant recipients. J Infect Dis 180:2014–2017, 1999.

364. Bryan JP, Nelson M. Testing for antibody to hepatitis A to decrease the cost of hepatitis A prophylaxis with immune globulin or hepatitis A vaccines. Arch Intern Med 154:663–668, 1994.

365. Bonanni P, Colombai R, Franchi G, et al. Experience of hepatitis A vaccination during an outbreak in a nursery school of Tuscany, Italy. Epidemiol Infect 121:377–380, 1998.

366. Thorburn KM, Bohorques R, Stepak P, et al. Immunization strategies to control a community-wide hepatitis A epidemic. Epidemiol Infect 127:461–467, 2001.

367. Meltzer MI, Shapiro CN, Mast EE, et al. The economics of vaccinating restaurant workers against hepatitis A. Vaccine 19: 2138–2145, 2001.

368. Zanetti A, Pregliasco F, Andreassi A, et al. Does immunoglobulin interfere with the immunogenicity to Pasteur Merieux inactivated hepatitis A vaccine? J Hepatol 26:25–30, 1997.

369. Wagner G, Lavanchy D, Darioli R, et al. Simultaneous active and passive immunization against hepatitis A studied in a population of travellers. Vaccine 11:1027–1032, 1993.

370. Leentvaar-Kuijpers A, Coutinho RA, Brulein V, et al. Simultaneous passive and active immunization against hepatitis A. Vaccine 10(suppl 1):S138–S141, 1992.

371. Walter EB, Hornick RB, Poland GA. Concurrent administration of inactivated hepatitis A vaccine with immune globulin in healthy adults. Vaccine 17:1468–1473, 1999.

372. Ambrosch F, Andre FE, Delem A, et al. Simultaneous vaccination against hepatitis A and B: results of a controlled study. Vaccine 10(suppl 1):S142–S145, 1992.

373. Gil A, Gonzalez A, Dal Re R, et al. Interference assessment of yellow fever vaccine with the immune response to a single-dose inactivated hepatitis A vaccine (1440 EL.U.): a controlled study in adults. Vaccine 14:1028–1030, 1996.

374. Bienzle U, Bock HL, Kruppenbacher JP, et al. Immunogenicity of an inactivated hepatitis A vaccine administered according to two different schedules and the interference of other "travellers" vaccines with the immune response. Vaccine 14:501–505, 1996.

375. Jong EC, Valley J, Altman J, Taddeo C, Kuter B. Seroconversion rates when hepatitis A vaccine (VAQTA) is administered together with travelers' vaccines, typhoid fever vaccine and yellow fever vaccine [abstr]. Am J Trop Med Hyg 59(suppl 3):79, 1998.

376. Bouvier PA, Althaus B, Glueck R, Chippaux A, Loutan L. Tolerance and immunogenicity of the simultaneous administration of virosome hepatitis A and yellow fever vaccines. J Travel Med 6:228–233, 1999.

377. Emini EA, Hughes JV, Perlow DS, et al. Induction of hepatitis A virus-neutralizing antibody by a virus-specific synthetic peptide. J Virol 55:836–839, 1985.

378. Stapleton JT, Raina V, Winokur PL, et al. Antigenic and immunogenic properties of recombinant hepatitis A virus 14S and 70S subviral particles. J Virol 67:1080–1085, 1993.

379. Winokur PL, McLinden JH, Stapleton JT. The hepatitis A virus polyprotein expressed by a recombinant vaccinia virus undergoes proteolytic processing and assembly into viruslike particles. J Virol 65:5029–5036, 1991.

380. Rosen E, Stapleton JT, McLinden J. Synthesis of immunogenic hepatitis A virus particles by recombinant baculoviruses. Vaccine 11:706–712, 1993.

381. Bulkow LR, Wainwright RB, McMahon BJ, et al. Secular trends in hepatitis A virus infection among Alaska Natives. J Infect Dis 168:1017–1020, 1993.

382. Leach CT, Koo FC, Hilsenbeck SG, et al. The epidemiology of viral hepatitis in children in South Texas: increased prevalence of hepatitis A along the Texas–Mexico border. J Infect Dis 180:509–513, 1999.

383. Bialek S, Thoroughman D, Bell BP. Trends in hepatitis A incidence among American Indians, 1990–1999. Antiviral Ther 5(suppl 1):11, 2000.

384. Samandari T, Wasley A, Bell BP. Evaluating the impact of hepatitis A vaccination in the United States, 1990–2001. In Proceedings of the 51st annual Epidemic Intelligence Service (EIS) conference. Atlanta, Centers for Disease Control and Prevention, 2002.

385. Centers for Disease Control and Prevention. Summary of notifiable diseases, United States, 2000. MMWR 49:1–102, 2002.

386. Berge JJ, Drennan DD, Jacobs RJ, et al. The cost of hepatitis A infections in American adolescents and adults in 1997. Hepatology 31:469–473, 2000.

387. Jacobs RJ, Margolis HS, Coleman PJ. The cost-effectiveness of adolescent hepatitis A vaccination in states with the highest disease rates. Arch Pediatr Adolesc Med 154:763–770, 2000.

388. Meyerhoff AS, Jacobs RJ, Margolis HS, et al. Cost effectiveness of childhood hepatitis A vaccination in the USA. Antiviral Ther 5(suppl 1):10, 2000.

389. Goodman RA, Foster KL, Trowbridge FL, et al. Global disease elimination and eradication as public health strategies. Proceedings of a conference held in Atlanta, Georgia, USA, 23–25 February, 1998. Bull World Health Organ 76:1–162, 1998.

Chapter 16

Hepatitis B Vaccine

ERIC MAST • FRANK MAHONEY • MARK KANE • HAROLD MARGOLIS

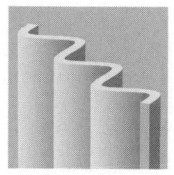

Viral hepatitis is a disease that has been recognized as a clinical entity since antiquity; however, the diversity of viruses causing hepatitis has only recently been recognized. Of the five viruses that are known to cause hepatitis in humans, hepatitis B virus (HBV) is responsible for the majority of the worldwide hepatitis disease burden. During the past 40 years, enormous progress has been made in the modern understanding of the etiology, natural history, epidemiology, and public health control of hepatitis B. Affordable vaccines and effective control strategies are now being deployed to control hepatitis B on a global basis; more than 160 countries use hepatitis B vaccine in their national immunization programs, and exciting new global initiatives have been implemented that allow the poorest countries in the world to afford this vaccine. In 10 to 15 years, chronic HBV infection in children should be essentially eliminated, and in 30 to 40 years there will be few victims of liver cancer and cirrhosis caused by HBV.

The first evidence that a form of hepatitis was transmitted by direct inoculation of blood or blood products was discovered when an outbreak of hepatitis occurred after a smallpox immunization campaign among shipyard workers in Bremen, Germany, in 1883.[1] In this outbreak, jaundice developed in 15% of 1289 shipyard workers several weeks to 8 months after receiving smallpox vaccine that had been prepared from human lymph, whereas several hundred unvaccinated workers did not become ill. Further evidence of a parenterally transmitted form of viral hepatitis was documented early in the 20th century, when numerous outbreaks of jaundice among patients attending venereal disease and diabetic clinics were associated with reuse of syringes and needles without sterilization.[2–8]

Blood products were confirmed as a source of hepatitis transmission through investigations of outbreaks of jaundice that occurred after administration of yellow fever vaccine,[9,10] administration of measles and mumps convalescent plasma,[11–13] and transfusion of whole blood.[14] The viral etiology of hepatitis outbreaks was first established during the 1940s through experimental transmission to human volunteers.[15–20] These studies provided evidence of two distinct forms of viral hepatitis based mainly on epidemiologic observations, including the incubation period and the route of infection. "Infectious hepatitis" was found to be transmitted by the fecal–oral route, had an incubation period of 2 to 6 weeks, and was primarily a disease of younger children. In contrast, "parenteral" or "serum hepatitis" was found to be transmitted by percutaneous exposure to blood products, had a longer incubation period of 2 to 6 months, and occurred more often in adults. The terms *hepatitis* A for "infectious hepatitis" and *hepatitis* B for "parenteral" or "serum hepatitis" were first introduced by MacCallum in 1947,[21] and later adopted by various expert committees to replace the multitude of terms for viral hepatitis.[22]

The largest recorded outbreak of hepatitis B was in 1942 during World War II, when 28,585 American soldiers inoculated with yellow fever vaccine developed jaundice and 62 of them died.[9] This outbreak was linked to a specific lot of vaccine that contained human serum. A follow-up study in the 1980s demonstrated that 97% of recipients of the serum-containing vaccine had serologic evidence of HBV infection, compared with 13% of people who received yellow fever vaccine that did not contain human serum, thus confirming that HBV was the cause of this outbreak.[23]

A series of transmission studies among human volunteers, including cross-challenge studies, conducted in the 1960s and 1970s by Krugman and collaborators at the Willowbrook Institute, ultimately confirmed the existence of two distinct forms of hepatitis.[24–26] These studies showed that the MS-1 strain of hepatitis (i.e., hepatitis A virus [HAV]) was transmitted by the fecal–oral route and had an incubation period of 30 to 38 days. In contrast, the MS-2 strain of hepatitis (i.e., HBV) had an incubation period of 41 to 108 days and was transmitted by percutaneous exposure. These studies also confirmed the existence of homologous immunity after infection with HAV or HBV.

The discovery of the etiologic agent for hepatitis B is among the remarkable scientific achievements of the 20th century. In 1965, Blumberg and colleagues described an isoprecipitin that was present in the serum of Australian aborigines, termed Australia antigen.[27] This antigen was found to have a variable distribution in healthy populations in different geographic areas of the world, with a low prevalence (<1%) in populations of North America and Europe and a high prevalence (6% to 25%) in the tropics and Southeast Asia. In addition, the antigen was found to occur more commonly among patients who had received multiple transfusions and blood products. The Australia antigen subsequently was shown to be related to HBV infection[28] and was ultimately shown to be the surface protein of HBV.

Within a decade after the discovery of Australia antigen, HBV was visualized by electron microscopy as 42-nm viral particles (Dane particles) that reacted with antisera to Australia antigen,[29] and immunoassays for the detection of antigens and antibodies associated with HBV infection were developed.[27,29,30] The development of sensitive and specific tests to detect HBV infection allowed investigators to define the natural history of HBV infection and to develop strategies to prevent transmission, including the screening of blood for hepatitis B surface antigen (HBsAg) to prevent transfusion-associated hepatitis B. In addition, units of blood that tested positive for antibody to HBsAg (anti-HBs) were used for the preparation of hepatitis B immune globulin (HBIG), which was shown to be effective in preventing or modifying the course of HBV infection.[31]

In 1970, in the course of studies on the natural history of HBV infection at Willowbrook, Krugman and colleagues boiled a serum preparation of the MS-2 strain of hepatitis for 1 minute to determine the effect of heat on infectivity of the virus.[32] The 1-minute boil destroyed the infectivity of the preparation, but the heat-inactivated material was subsequently shown to be immunogenic and partially protective when volunteers were challenged with the MS-2 strain after receiving the boiled preparation.[33] The realization that HBsAg could serve as an immunogen for the production of anti-HBs, and that this antibody was protective against HBV infection, led to development of prototype hepatitis B vaccines.[34,35] Beginning in the early 1980s, plasma-derived hepatitis B vaccines were manufactured and licensed in a number of countries. Subsequently, the development of recombinant DNA technology enabled the expression of large quantities of HBsAg in yeast and mammalian cells, which led to the production and licensing of recombinant hepatitis B vaccines.[36,37]

Epidemiologic studies conducted during the 1970s and 1980s demonstrated an association of chronic HBV infection with chronic liver disease, including hepatocellular carcinoma (HCC) and cirrhosis.[38,39] HBV-associated chronic liver disease was found to be among the leading causes of deaths in adults worldwide, particularly in countries with a high prevalence of chronic HBV infection.[40–42] The recognition of hepatitis B as a major global cause of morbidity and mortality led to a worldwide effort to reduce transmission of HBV and HBV-related chronic liver disease through routine infant vaccination.

Background

Clinical Description

Infection with HBV causes a broad spectrum of liver disease, including subclinical infection, acute self-limited hepatitis, and fulminant hepatitis.[43] Persons infected with HBV also may develop chronic infection, which can lead to chronic liver disease, and death from cirrhosis or HCC. The age at which HBV infection is acquired is the main factor determining clinical expression of disease and outcome of infection. Fewer than 10% of children under 5 years of age

who become infected have initial clinical signs or symptoms of disease (i.e., acute hepatitis B) compared with 30% to 50% of older children and adults.[44] The risk of developing chronic HBV infection varies inversely with age: approximately 80% to 90% of infants infected during the first year of life, 30% to 60% of children infected between 1 and 4 years of age, and 5% or less of adults develop chronic infection (Fig 16–1).[45,46] Persons with chronic diseases such as renal failure, human immunodeficiency virus (HIV) infection, and diabetes are at increased risk of developing chronic infection, presumably as a result of enhanced viral replication and ineffective immune clearance.[46–48]

Acute Hepatitis B

The clinical manifestations of acute hepatitis B are indistinguishable from other causes of viral hepatitis, and serologic testing is needed to make a definitive diagnosis. The incubation period is usually 3 to 4 months, with a range of 6 weeks to 6 months. The prodromal phase of disease is quite variable, and is characterized by insidious onset of constitutional symptoms that may include malaise, anorexia, nausea, occasional vomiting, low-grade fever, myalgias, and easy fatigability. In 5% to 10% of patients, a serum sickness–like syndrome may develop during the prodromal phase that is characterized by arthralgias or arthritis, rash, and angioedema. Other extrahepatic manifestations that have rarely been reported in association with acute HBV infection include polyarteritis nodosa, membranous glomerulonephritis,[49] Gianotti-Crosti syndrome,[50,51] and aplastic anemia.[52] In patients with icteric hepatitis, jaundice usually develops within 1 to 2 weeks after onset of illness; dark urine and clay-colored stools may appear 1 to 5 days before onset of clinical jaundice. During the icteric phase, constitutional prodromal symptoms usually diminish, and right upper quadrant pain may develop as the liver becomes enlarged and tender. In 10% to 30% of patients with acute hepatitis B, myalgias and arthralgias have been described without jaundice or other clinical signs of hepatitis; in one third of these patients, a maculopapular rash

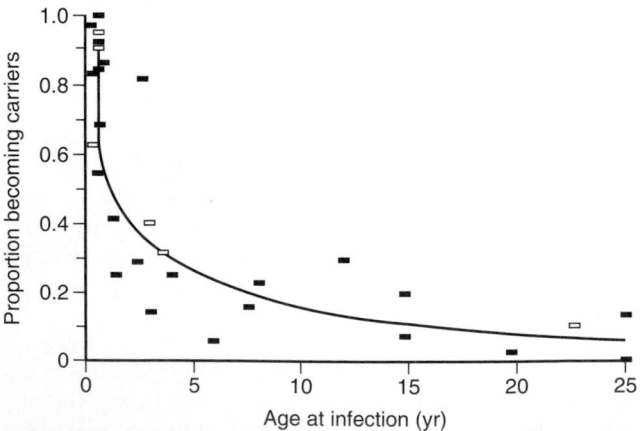

FIGURE 16–1 ▪ Studies evaluating the risk of chronic hepatitis B virus infection by age of infection. *Filled squares* represent data from developing countries; *open squares* represent data from developed countries. (From Edmunds WJ, Medley GF, Nokes DJ, et al. The influence of age on the development of the hepatitis B carrier state. Proc R Soc Lond B Biol Sci 253:197–201, 1993, with permission.)

appears with joint symptoms.[53] Clinical signs and symptoms of acute hepatitis B usually resolve within 1 to 3 months.

The severity of illness associated with acute hepatitis B usually does not require hospitalization. Approximately 30% of reported cases in the United States are hospitalized.[54] Higher rates of hospitalization may occur in other countries because of established patterns of medical care rather than disease severity. Fulminant liver failure occurs in approximately 0.5% to 1% of infected adults, but rarely in infected infants and children.[55,56] Higher rates of fulminant hepatitis may occur in association with HBV–hepatitis delta virus co-infection.[57] Patients with fulminant hepatitis usually present with features of hepatic encephalopathy, including disturbances in sleep patterns, asterixis, mental confusion, disorientation, somnolence, and coma. The case-fatality rate in patients who develop fulminant hepatitis is about 60% to 70%, unless liver transplantation can be performed.[58]

Chronic HBV Infection

Most of the disease burden associated with HBV infection occurs among persons with chronic infection. Persons who have persistence of HBsAg in serum for at least 6 months are classified as having chronic infection.[59] The natural history of chronic HBV infection is determined by the interaction between virus replication and host immune response. Additional factors that can contribute to progression include gender, alcohol consumption, and co-infection with other hepatotropic viruses. Chronic HBV infection is typically characterized by three phases in persons who acquire infection perinatally, and two phases in persons who acquire infection as older children and adults (Fig. 16–2). Perinatally acquired infections usually have a period of active viral replication without active liver disease,[60] which is followed by a replicative phase with active liver disease, and a later phase with low or absent viral replication and remission of active liver disease.[61] For persons who acquire infection as older children and adults, only the latter two phases generally occur.

The initial phase of perinatally acquired infections is characterized by high levels of virus replication, which is correlated with hepatitis B e antigen (HBeAg) positivity, and high levels of HBV DNA in serum. However, these patients usually have no evidence of active liver disease, with normal alanine aminotransferase (ALT) levels, no signs or symptoms of hepatitis, and minimal necroinflammatory activity on liver biopsy.[60,62] The absence of liver disease despite high levels of viral replication is believed to be due to immune tolerance. The initial phase of infection usually lasts 10 to 30 years. During this time, rates of spontaneous clearance of HBeAg from serum are less than 1% per year.[60,62,63] This low rate of HBeAg clearance accounts for the high prevalence of HBeAg among women of childbearing age in areas of the world where there are high rates of perinatal HBV transmission.

The second phase of perinatally acquired chronic infection and the first phase of chronic infection in older children and adults are characterized by high levels of virus replication with active liver disease (see Fig. 16–2). These patients are usually HBeAg positive, with high levels of HBV DNA in serum. Evidence of active liver disease includes elevated ALT levels and necroinflammatory

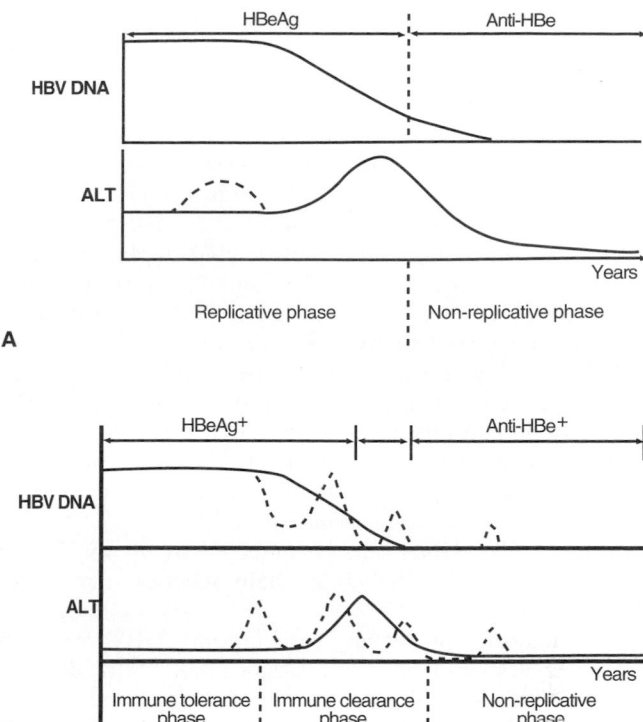

FIGURE 16–2 ■ Natural history of chronic hepatitis B virus infection. *A*, Adult-acquired infection. *B*, Perinatally acquired infection. *Solid* and *dashed lines* represent typical patterns of alanine aminotransferase (ALT) levels and hepatitis B virus DNA (HBV DNA) titers in patients with chronic HBV infection over time. (From Chan HL, Ghany MG, Lok ASF. Hepatitis B. *In* Schiff ER, Sorrell MF, Maddrey WC [eds]. Schiff's Diseases of the Liver [8th ed], Vol. 1. Philadelphia, Lippincott Williams & Wilkins, 1999, p 768, with permission.)

activity on liver biopsy. During this phase, fibrosis of the liver develops, which can lead to cirrhosis, an irreversible form of liver injury. Transition from this phase of chronic infection to the next phase occurs with clearance of HBV DNA and HBeAg from serum. The rate of spontaneous clearance of HBeAg is approximately 10% to 20% per year both in patients with perinatally acquired infections and in patients who acquire infection at older ages.[63–66] Most patients are asymptomatic during this phase, but conversion to HBeAg negativity may be accompanied by symptomatic exacerbations, with increased ALT levels.[64,65,67] Hepatic decompensation may occur in about 2% of patients during these exacerbations, which can rarely lead to death from hepatic failure.[68] In some patients with suboptimal immune response and abortive immune clearance, repeated exacerbations may occur, with intermittent clearance of HBV DNA from serum and transient loss of HBeAg.[69,70] Repeated episodes of necroinflammation may increase the risk of developing severe chronic liver disease. Ultimately, the outcome of chronic infection depends primarily on the severity of liver disease at the time HBeAg seroconversion occurs and HBV replication is arrested.

The last phase of chronic HBV infection (i.e., the third phase of perinatally acquired infection and the second phase of chronic infection acquired at older ages) is characterized by low or absent levels of virus replication and remission of active liver disease (see Fig. 16–2). These patients are typically HBeAg negative, are antibody to HBeAg (anti-HBe) positive, and have low or undetectable levels of HBV DNA in serum. Most of the patients who clear HBeAg have normal ALT levels and resolution of necroinflammation on liver biopsy, indicating resolution of active liver disease.[61,64,71,72] However, a small percentage continue to have moderate levels of HBV replication, elevated ALT levels, and chronic inflammation on liver biopsy despite HBeAg seroconversion.[71,73] These patients also can have residual liver disease, and can be misdiagnosed as having chronic liver disease of unknown etiology if they are HBsAg negative.[74,75] Patients who clear HBeAg generally remain HBsAg positive for long periods of time, even in the absence of detectable HBV DNA. The annual rate of HBsAg clearance among patients with chronic HBV infection is approximately 0.5% to 2%.[66,72,76,77] However, HBV DNA can be detected in up to 50% of these patients by polymerase chain reaction even after clearance of HBsAg.[78]

The majority of persons with chronic HBV infection remain healthy and die of unrelated causes.[79,80] In addition, persons with severe chronic liver disease are often asymptomatic until late in the course of their disease.[81] However, findings of long-term clinical follow-up studies indicate that chronic HBV infection is an important cause of morbidity and mortality worldwide. For example, in Taiwan, about 25% of persons who become chronically infected during childhood and 15% of those who become chronically infected at older ages die of HCC or cirrhosis.[38,82]

In one population-based study, the incidence of decompensated cirrhosis among persons with chronic HBV infection was 0.5 per 1000 person-years.[72] In studies of persons with chronic infection referred to clinical centers, the incidence of cirrhosis is as high as 2% to 3% per year.[83,84] Risk factors for the development of cirrhosis in persons with chronic infection include older age, HBeAg positivity, heavy use of alcohol (>40 g/day), and increased ALT levels.[83–85]

Persons with chronic HBV infection are also at high risk of developing HCC, which is the seventh most frequent human cancer worldwide.[40,42] In areas of high HBV endemicity, such as sub-Saharan Africa, China, and Southeast Asia, HCC is usually one of the top three fatal cancers in males.[41] Globally, it is estimated that approximately 60% of HCC occurs in persons with chronic HBV infection. Most cases occur in males, with an average male:female ratio of cases of 3.7:1. The reason for this male predominance is unknown. In a Taiwanese study, rates of HCC were approximately 100 times higher among men who were HBsAg positive (495 per 100,000 per year) than among those who were HBsAg negative (5 per 100,000 per year).[39,86] Other risk factors for HCC in persons with chronic HBV infection include older age, family history of HCC, presence of cirrhosis, and co-infection with hepatitis C virus (HCV).[39,72,87,88] Although HCC is more common in persons with cirrhosis, approximately 30% to 50% of HBV-associated HCC cases occur in persons who do not have cirrhosis.[72] Clearance of HBsAg may decrease the risk of HCC[75]; however, HCC can occur in persons who develop chronic HBV infection and then clear HBsAg.[72,76,89]

Virology

Hepatitis B virus is a 42-nm, double-shelled DNA virus of the Hepadnaviridae family that replicates in the liver and causes hepatic dysfunction.[90] The outer lipoprotein envelope contains HBsAg, which is produced in excess amounts and also circulates in the blood as 22-nm spherical and tubular particles (Fig. 16–3). The inner nucleocapsid is a 27-nm icosahedral structure consisting of 180 copies of the HBV core protein or hepatitis B core antigen (HBcAg), and surrounds a single molecule of partially double-stranded DNA and a DNA-dependent DNA polymerase (Fig. 16–4).

The HBV genome is a small, circular, partially double-stranded DNA molecule (complete minus strand and partial plus strand) that is approximately 3200 nucleotides in length (Fig. 16–5). The virus efficiently uses its genetic information to encode four groups of proteins and their regulatory elements by shifting the reading frames over the same genetic material.[91] The Pre-S/S gene has three separate open reading frames (ORFs) that encode three forms of HBsAg: the large, middle, and small structural proteins of the virus envelope. The C gene has two ORFs (C, pre-C). The C ORF encodes HBcAg, and the pre-C/C ORF encodes the *e* protein, which is processed to produce soluble HBeAg. The X gene encodes the X protein, a small transcriptional transactivator that influences the transcription of HBV genes by regulating the activity of transcriptional promoters.[92] The P gene encodes a large polymerase protein that functions as both a reverse transcriptase for synthesis of the negative DNA strand from genomic RNA

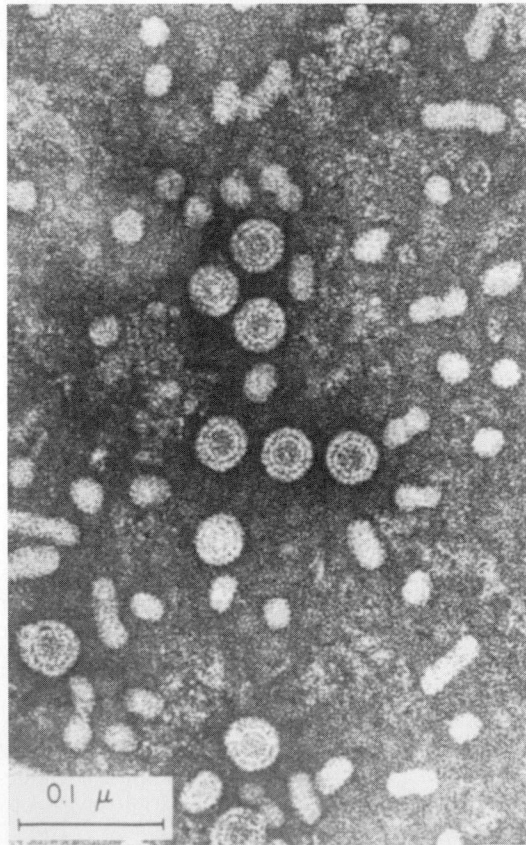

0.1 μ

FIGURE 16–3 ■ Electron micrograph of hepatitis B virus. Note Dane particles (43 nm) as well as spherical and tubular hepatitis B surface antigen particles (22 nm in diameter).

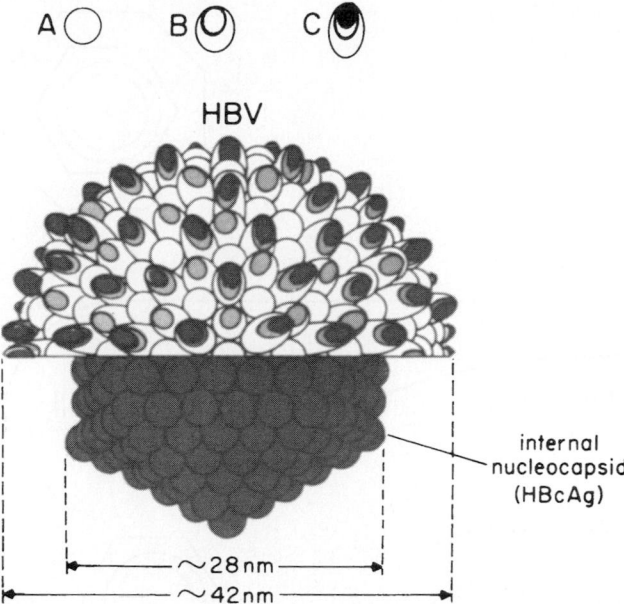

FIGURE 16–4 ▪ Schematic diagram of hepadnavirus particles. Individual subunits containing S protein only (*A*), S protein plus pre-S1 (*B*), and S protein plus pre-S1 and pre-S2 (*C*) are shown at the top of the figure. S proteins correspond to the white areas, pre-S2 to the gray areas, and pre-S1 to the black areas. The virus particles contain an internal nucleocapsid shown in the bottom split-open section. (From Neurath AR, Thanavala Y. Hepadnaviruses. *In* von Regenmortel MHV, Neurath AR [eds]. Immunochemistry of Virus, II. The Basis for Serodiagnosis and Vaccines. New York, Elsevier Science, 1990, pp 403–458, with permission.)

and an endogenous DNA polymerase for synthesis of the positive DNA strand using the negative strand as a template.

The HBV envelope contains a mixture of small, medium, and large HBsAg proteins in both glycosylated and nonglycosylated forms. The small HBsAg is expressed in the largest quantities and is coded for by the S gene alone. The middle HBsAg is coded for by the S gene and the pre-S2 region, and the large HBsAg is coded for by the S gene and both the pre-S1 and pre-S2 regions. Pre-S1 and pre-S2 proteins also are expressed individually in small quantities; these proteins appear to play an important role in the attachment of HBV to hepatocytes,[93–96] and they contain a number of T- and B-cell epitopes.[97] The role of the S protein in virus attachment has not been conclusively demonstrated; however, this protein contains the major site for binding of neutralizing antibody, designated the *a* determinant. Two other major determinants of the S protein also have been described; one has either *d* or *y* specificity, and the other has *w* or *r*. All combinations of these determinants have been found, resulting in four subtypes: adw, adr, ayw, and ayr. Antibodies to the *a* determinant confer protection in adults to all of these serotypes, whereas antibodies to the subtype determinants do not.[98] No apparent differences in infectivity or virulence of HBV have been attributed to HBsAg subtypes. However, these subtypes have a distinct geographic distribution worldwide and have been used in epidemiologic studies to identify patterns of virus transmission.[99] The most common subtype among per-

sons with chronic HBV infection in the United States is adw.[100]

Both the nucleocapsid protein (HBcAg) and the *e* protein are translated from the C gene. HBcAg is essential for viral packaging and is an integral part of the nucleocapsid. It is not detectable in serum by conventional techniques; however, it can be detected in liver tissue in patients with acute or chronic HBV infection. The *e* protein is processed by the endoplasmic reticulum, where it is cleaved and HBeAg (the precore fragment) is secreted. HBeAg is a soluble protein that is not a part of virus particles, but it can be detected in the serum of patients with acute hepatitis B and in persons with chronic HBV infection who have high virus titers. HBeAg also is expressed on the surface of hepatocytes[101] and may be an important target for the immune defense mechanisms leading to the destruction of hepatocytes.[102]

HBV replication begins with attachment of the virus to the cell surface and penetration, which likely occurs by direct membrane fusion (Fig. 16–6).[96,103] After uncoating in the cytoplasm, the nucleocapsid is transported to the nucleus. However, it is unclear whether the nucleocapsid enters the nucleus or disassembles in the cytoplasm and delivers the DNA to the nucleus at the nuclear pore. Once in the nucleus, the single-stranded gap in the viral genome is repaired and covalently closed circular DNA (cccDNA) is formed, which is completely double stranded. In contrast to classical retroviruses such as HIV, integration of

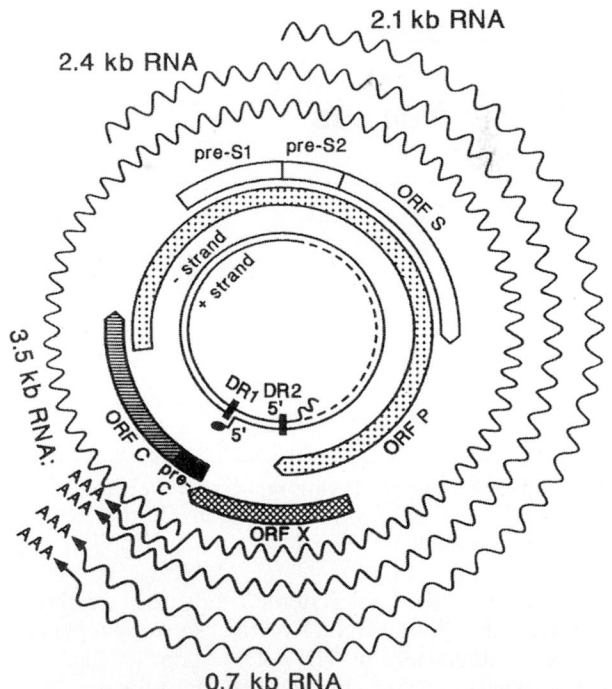

FIGURE 16–5 ▪ Hepatitis B virus coding organization. *Inner circle* represents virion DNA, with *dashes* signifying the single-stranded genomic region. *Boxes* denote viral coding regions, with *arrows* indicating direction of translation. Outermost *wavy lines* depict the viral RNAs identified in infected cells, with *arrows* indicating direction of transcription. (From Ganem D. Hepadnaviridae and their replication. *In* Fields BN, Knipe DM, Howley PM, et al [eds]. Fields Virology [3rd ed], Vol. 2. Philadelphia, Lippincott–Raven, 1996, p 2706, with permission.)

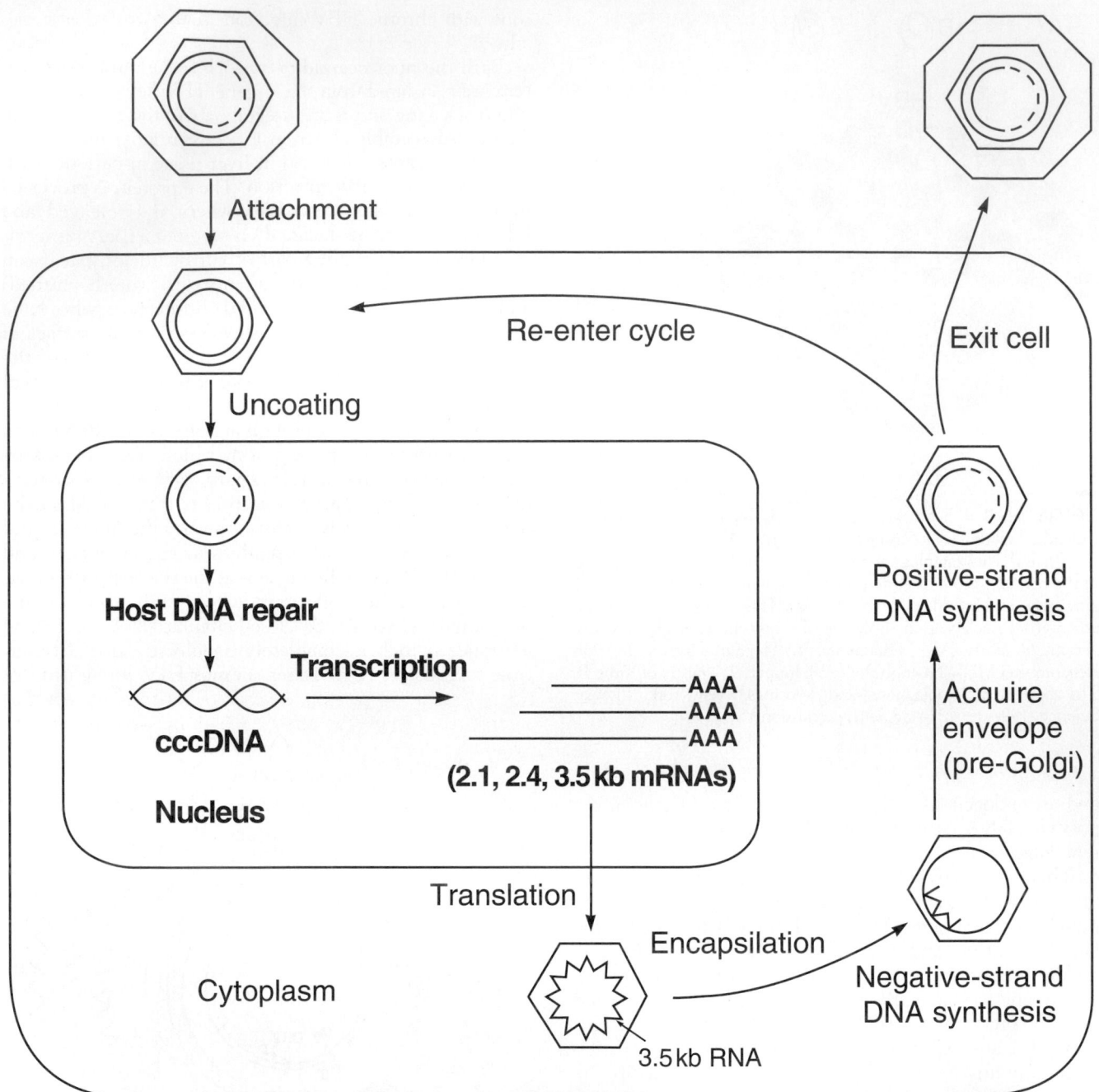

Attachment

Re-enter cycle   **Exit cell**

Uncoating

Positive-strand DNA synthesis

Host DNA repair

Transcription   ——————AAA
——————AAA
——————AAA

Acquire envelope (pre-Golgi)

cccDNA

(2.1, 2.4, 3.5 kb mRNAs)

Nucleus

Translation

Encapsilation

Cytoplasm   **Negative-strand DNA synthesis**

3.5 kb RNA

FIGURE 16–6 ■ Hepatitis B virus replication cycle (see text for details). cccDNA, covalently closed circular DNA. (From Butel JS, Lee TH, Slagle BL. Is the DNA repair system involved in hepatitis B virus-mediated hepatocellular carcinogenesis? Trends Microbiol 4:119, 1996, with permission.)

HBV DNA into the host genome is not necessary for viral messenger RNA (mRNA) synthesis or replication. However, integration of HBV DNA does occur during chronic infection, which may be important for the development of HCC. The cccDNA acts as the template for production of four mRNAs, each of which is expressed from its own promoter.[103] A 0.7-kb mRNA transcript encodes for the X protein; a 2.1-kb mRNA transcript encodes for pre-S2 and HBsAg proteins; a 2.4-kb mRNA transcript encodes for pre-S1, pre-S2, and S proteins; and a 3.5-kb mRNA encodes for HBcAg, HBeAg, and polymerase. These mRNA transcripts are transported into the cytoplasm,

where translation yields the viral envelope, core, precore, and X proteins and the viral DNA polymerase. The 3.5-kb mRNA is also a pregenomic RNA that serves as a template for HBV DNA synthesis. Viral packaging occurs in the cytoplasm, where the RNA pregenome is encapsulated by newly synthesized HBcAg, and the polymerase synthesizes negative-stranded DNA by reverse transcription. The RNA pregenome is then degraded by RnaseH, an enzyme that resides on the polymerase.[104] After the negative strand is synthesized, the polymerase starts to synthesize the positive DNA strand.[105] However, the process is not completed, resulting in replicative intermediates consisting of full-length minus-strand DNA plus variable-length (20% to 80%) positive-stranded DNA. Nucleocapsid particles containing these replicative intermediates bud from the pre-Golgi membranes, where they acquire HBsAg/pre-S protein-containing envelopes. Virus particles may then either exit the cell or be reimported into the nucleus and initiate another round of replication in the same cell.

HBV Mutants

Hepatitis B virus has a higher frequency of mutations than other DNA viruses because the virus replicates via an RNA intermediate, using a reverse transcriptase that appears to lack a proofreading function.[106] Mutations have been identified in all four HBV genes, and have been most fully characterized in the pre-C/C gene, the polymerase gene, and the preS/S gene.[106,107]

PRE-C/C GENE MUTANTS

The most common mutation in the precore/core region is a glycine-to-arginine point mutation at position 1896 that results in a translational stop codon (TAG); this codon stops expression of the e protein, which is processed to produce HBeAg.[108,109] Loss of HBeAg expression also has occurred with mutations in the core promotor region.[110] These mutations have been associated with fulminant hepatitis and with severe chronic liver disease.[111,112] However, fulminant hepatitis frequently occurs in the absence of the pre-C/C mutation,[113-115] and self-limited acute hepatitis has been reported in patients with this mutation.[116] Thus the role of pre-C/C mutations in increasing the severity of hepatitis is unclear, and other factors such as multiple pre-C/C mutations may be required to increase HBV virulence.[106]

POLYMERASE GENE MUTANTS

Mutations of the polymerase gene have been associated with resistance to treatment with nucleoside analogues[117-119] and with viral persistence.[120] The most common of these mutations occur at codon 528 (the template binding site of the polymerase) and at codon 552 of the YMDD motif (the catalytic site of the polymerase). Polymerase mutations have been demonstrated to emerge in up to one third of patients after treatment with nucleoside analogues, including lamivudine and famciclovir. These mutations significantly decrease the efficacy of treatment.[121] However, the majority of patients who develop these variants continue to benefit from treatment for at least 1 year, possibly because of decreased replication of mutant viruses.[121,122]

S GENE MUTANTS

Mutations in the S gene can lead to conformational changes in the a determinant, which is located between amino acids 124 and 147 of HBsAg, and has a double-loop structure projecting from the surface of the virus; the second loop (amino acids 139 to 147) is the major target for neutralizing anti-HBs (Fig. 16–7). S gene mutants most commonly result in amino acid changes at positions 143 to 145, but also have been found across the entire a determinant region. Concern has been expressed that these variants may allow replication of HBV in the presence of vaccine-induced anti-HBs or anti-HBs contained in HBIG (immunization escape mutants).[123] In addition, these mutants may not be detected by some commercially available HBsAg assays based on antibodies to the wild-type virus (diagnostic escape mutants).[124-127]

HBV infection with S mutant viruses has been reported to occur in the presence of protective levels of anti-HBs in infants born to HBV-infected mothers who received prophylaxis with HBIG and/or hepatitis B vaccine,[128-135] in children who responded to vaccination,[136] and in liver transplant recipients who received HBIG for prophylaxis of relapse of HBV infection.[137-139] However, in a population-based study of infants born to HBsAg- and HBeAg-positive mothers, 91% of 94 infants with immunization failures either were infected with wild-type virus or had mixed infections of wild-type and mutant viruses, and a similar frequency of mutant viruses was found in mothers who transmitted and those who did not transmit.[133,140] These findings suggest that S mutants were not associated with a failure of postexposure prophylaxis to prevent perinatal HBV transmission. In addition, pre-exposure vaccination of chimpanzees with currently licensed vaccines (not containing pre-S epitopes) conferred protection following intravenous challenge with the 145-HBV mutant.[141,142] Thus, there is no evidence at present that S variants have spread in immunized populations or that these mutants pose a threat to hepatitis B immunization programs.[143] Further studies and enhanced surveillance to detect the emergence of these variants are a high priority in monitoring the effectiveness of current immunization strategies.

Pathogenesis

HBsAg has been detected in organ tissues other than the liver, but there is little evidence to indicate primary replication in sites other than hepatocytes. Most available experimental evidence suggests that HBV is not directly cytopathic and that liver damage is produced by the cellular immune response to viral proteins in infected hepatocytes.[144] Extrahepatic manifestations that can appear during the prodromal phase of acute hepatitis B (e.g., arthritis, urticaria) and in patients with chronic infection (e.g., vasculitis, glomerulonephritis) appear to be mediated by immune complex formation.[53] Development of HCC in persons with chronic infection is apparently induced either directly by activating cellular oncogenes or inactivating tumor suppressor genes, or indirectly through chronic liver injury, inflammation, and the promotional effect of hepatocyte regeneration.[145]

Neonatal immune tolerance to viral antigens appears to play an important role in viral persistence in infants infected at birth, but the basis for poor T-cell response and the establishment of chronic infection in adults is not well understood. Patients with acute hepatitis B who resolve their infection have a vigorous T-cell response against multiple viral antigens, including the viral core, surface, and polymerase proteins. However, persons who develop chronic infection have a very weak or undetectable cellular immune response, suggesting that a less efficient T-cell response may permit persistence of HBV.

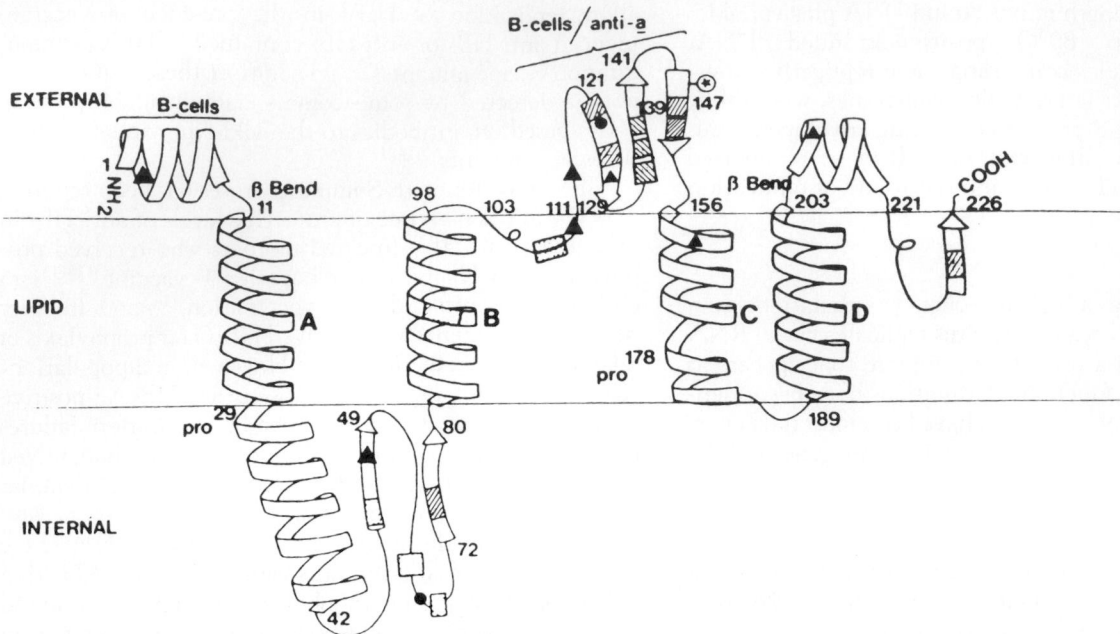

FIGURE 16–7 ▪ Secondary structure of hepatitis B virus s antigen in the lipid envelope as predicted by computer modeling. The *shaded areas* indicate the locations of sequence variations for *w/r* (▲) and *d/y* (●) subtypes. (From Howard C, Smith Stinh HJ, Brown SE, Steward MW. Towards the development of a synthetic hepatitis B vaccine. *In* Zuckerman A [ed]. Viral Hepatitis and Liver Disease: Proceedings of the International Symposium on Viral Hepatitis and Liver Disease, held at the Barbicon Centre, London, May 26–28, 1987. New York, Alan R. Liss, 1988, with permission.)

Diagnosis

Serologic tests are commercially available for a variety of antigens and antibodies associated with HBV infection, including HBsAg, anti-HBs, total (immunoglobulin [Ig] G and IgM) antibody to HBcAg (anti-HBc), IgM anti-HBc, HBeAg, and anti-HBe. In addition, hybridization assays and gene amplification techniques (e.g., polymerase chain reaction) are available to detect HBV DNA.

The clinical symptoms of acute hepatitis B are indistinguishable from those of other forms of viral hepatitis; thus definitive diagnosis requires serologic testing for HBV infection (Table 16–1). HBsAg, IgM anti-HBc, total anti-HBc, and HBeAg all can be detected in the serum as early as 1 to 2 months after exposure to HBV (Fig. 16–8). However, IgM anti-HBc is the only reliable marker of acute infection because the other three markers also can be

detected in persons with chronic HBV infection. IgM anti-HBc generally becomes undetectable within 6 to 9 months after the development of acute infection. In persons who recover following acute infection, HBsAg and HBeAg are usually cleared within 6 months following illness onset[44]; anti-HBs and anti-HBe develop during the convalescent phase (see Fig. 16–8). Anti-HBs is a protective antibody that neutralizes the virus. The presence of anti-HBs following acute infection indicates recovery and immunity from reinfection. Anti-HBs also can be detected in persons who have received hepatitis B vaccine and transiently in persons who have received HBIG.

In persons who develop chronic HBV infection, HBsAg and total anti-HBc remain persistently detectable, generally for life (Fig. 16–9). HBeAg and HBV DNA are variably present in chronically infected persons; the presence of

TABLE 16–1 ▪ Interpretations of Available Serologic Test Results for Hepatitis B Virus Infection

HBsAg	IgM Anti-HBc	Total Anti-HBc	Anti-HBs	Interpretation
+	–	–	–	Early HBV infection before antibody to hepatitis B core antigen (anti-HBc) is detectable
+	+	+	–	Early HBV infection. Onset is within 4–6 mo because IgM anti-HBc is detectable.
–	+	+	+ or –	Recent HBV infection (within 4–6 mo) with resolution (i.e., HBsAg is no longer detectable). Anti-HBs is usually detectable within several weeks after loss of HBsAg.
+	–	+	–	Probable chronic HBV infection. Onset was at least 4–6 mo ago because IgM anti-HBc is no longer detectable and HBsAg is present.
–	–	+	+	Past HBV infection, recovered

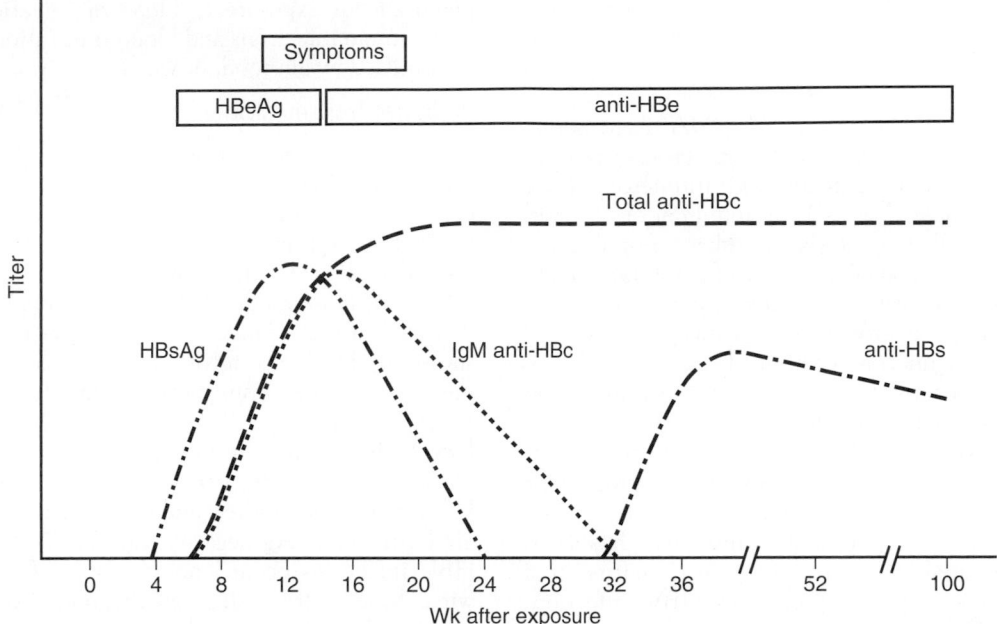

FIGURE 16–8 ■ Titer of hepatitis B surface antigen (HBsAg), antibody to hepatitis B core antigen (anti-HBc), immunoglobulin M (IgM) anti-HBc, and antibody to HBsAg (anti-HBs) in patients with acute hepatitis B with recovery.

HBeAg and/or HBV DNA in serum correlates with higher titers of HBV and greater infectivity.

Treatment

No specific treatment is recommended for persons with acute hepatitis B; supportive care is the mainstay of therapy. The goal of treatment for patients with chronic HBV infection is to stop progression of liver injury by suppressing or eliminating viral replication.[146–149] The endpoints used to assess response to treatment include normalization of ALT levels (biochemical response), sustained clearance of mark-

ers of active HBV replication (HBeAg and/or HBV DNA; virologic response), histologic improvement on liver biopsy (histologic response), and sustained clearance of HBsAg (complete response). Numerous treatments have been investigated for patients with chronic HBV infection, including interferon-alfa, nucleoside analogues, and immune modulators (e.g., cytokines, therapeutic vaccines). Two of these, interferon-alfa and lamivudine, have been approved by the U.S. Food and Drug Administration.

In 1976, the findings of two studies, one with leukocyte interferon and one with interferon-β, suggested that interferon can affect the serologic profile of people with chronic

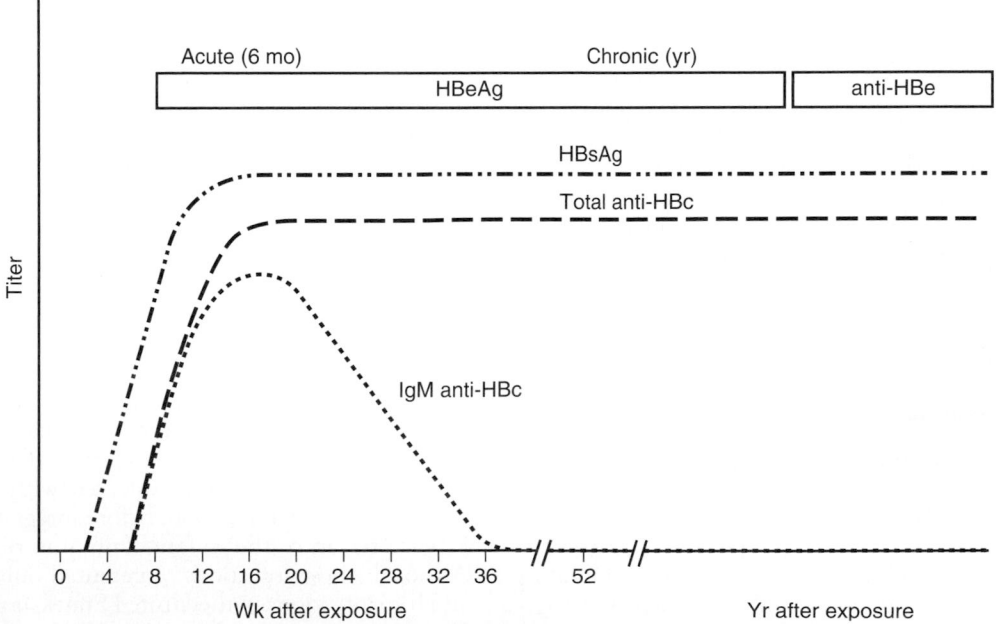

FIGURE 16–9 ■ Titer of HBsAg, anti-HBc, and IgM anti-HBc during progression to chronic hepatitis B virus infection. (See legend for Figure 16–8 for abbreviations.)

HBV infection.[150,151] Follow-up studies revealed that the most promising agent was interferon-alfa. However, the efficacy of interferon-alfa is limited to a small percentage of highly selected patients. In a meta-analysis of 15 clinical trials, clearance of HBeAg and HBV DNA from serum occurred in 33% and 37% of patients with HBeAg-positive chronic hepatitis B who were treated with interferon-alfa for 4 to 6 months, compared with 12% and 17% of controls, respectively.[152] In follow-up studies, virologic response has been found to be durable in 80% to 90% of patients after 4 to 8 years, and sustained virologic response usually was accompanied by histologic improvement on liver biopsy.[153-155] However, it remains unclear whether clearance of HBeAg and HBV DNA occurs more commonly with interferon treatment than it would eventually occur spontaneously over the natural course of disease.[147] In addition, data on the long-term clinical benefits of interferon treatment on progression to cirrhosis, HCC, and death are limited.

The nucleoside analogue lamivudine also has been extensively evaluated in clinical trials for treatment of patients with HBeAg-positive chronic HBV infection. Lamivudine is well tolerated after oral administration, with few if any side effects.[156-159] Short-term 12- or 24-week courses of lamivudine result in rapid declines in HBV DNA levels and improvements in ALT levels; however, pretreatment levels of HBV DNA rapidly return after discontinuation of treatment.[156] Studies of longer term treatment for 52 weeks have demonstrated sustained virologic response in 16% to 18% of patients compared with 4% to 6% of untreated controls, and histologic improvement on liver biopsy in 49% to 56% of treated patients compared to 23% to 25% of controls.[157-159] However, limited data are available on the durability of virologic response following lamivudine treatment, and the effect of treatment on long-term morbidity and mortality. The efficacy of interferon-alfa and lamivudine administered together appears to provide little, if any, added benefit compared to monotherapy with lamivudine or interferon-alfa alone.[159,160]

Studies evaluating administration of therapeutic hepatitis B vaccines in combination with interferon-alfa have suggested a possible benefit for treatment of chronic HBV infection.[161-163] In addition, a placebo-controlled trial in transgenic mice demonstrated that high-dose hepatitis B vaccine is effective in the treatment of chronic HBV infection.[164] However, no controlled trials of therapeutic vaccines for treatment of chronic HBV infection in humans have been reported in the medical literature.

Epidemiology

Routes of Transmission

Hepatitis B virus is transmitted by either percutaneous or mucous membrane contact with infected blood or other body fluids. The virus is found in highest concentrations in blood and serous exudates (as high as 10^8 to 10^9 virions/mL); 1- to 2-log lower concentrations are found in various body secretions, including saliva, semen, and vaginal fluid.[165] The primary routes of transmission are perinatal, early childhood exposure, sexual contact, and percutaneous exposure to blood or infectious body fluids (e.g., unsafe injections and blood transfusions). HBV is not transmitted by air, food, or water.

Perinatal Transmission

Perinatal transmission from infected mothers to their newborn infants is a major source of HBV infections in many countries.[166-172] Perinatal transmission occurs at the time of birth; in utero transmission is relatively rare, accounting for less than 2% of infections transmitted from mother to infant in most studies.[168,170-172] Although HBV can be detected in breast milk, there is no evidence that HBV is transmitted by breast-feeding.[173] The risk of perinatal transmission is higher from mothers with high titers of HBV DNA, which generally correlate with the presence of HBeAg in serum. The likelihood of an infant developing chronic HBV infection is 70% to 90% for those born to HBeAg-positive mothers and less than 10% from those who are born to HBeAg-negative mothers.[166,174] Most perinatal HBV infections occur among infants of pregnant women with chronic HBV infection. Pregnant women with acute hepatitis B in the first and second trimester rarely transmit HBV to the fetus or neonate.[175,176] However, the risk of transmission from pregnant women who acquire infection during the third trimester is approximately 60%.[176] In the United States, the race-adjusted prevalence of HBsAg among pregnant women is about 0.6%, and the prevalence of HBeAg among HBsAg-positive pregnant women is approximately 35% among women of Asian descent and 20% among other racial groups.[177,178] By applying race- and ethnicity-adjusted HBsAg prevalence estimates to U.S. natality data, approximately 22,000 infants are born to HBV-infected pregnant women each year; without immunoprophylaxis, approximately 6000 of these infants would develop chronic HBV infection.[179]

Early Childhood Transmission

Early childhood HBV transmission accounts for a high proportion of HBV infections worldwide.[180-195] Most early childhood transmission occurs in households of persons with chronic infection, but transmission also has been recognized in child day care centers and in schools.[196-201] The most probable mechanisms of early childhood transmission involve inapparent percutaneous or permucosal contact with infectious body fluids such as exudates from dermatologic lesions, breaks in the skin, or mucous membranes with blood or serous secretions.[165] HBV also may spread because of contact with saliva through bites or other breaks in the skin, as a consequence of the premastication of food, and through contact with virus from inanimate objects such as shared towels or toothbrushes or reuse of needles.[183,202-206] HBV remains infectious for at least 7 days outside the body and can be found in titers of 10^2 to 10^3 virions/mL on objects, even in the absence of visible blood.[195,207,208]

In the United States, an estimated 16,000 children less than 10 years of age were infected with HBV annually, beyond the postnatal period, before integration of hepatitis B vaccine into the infant immunization schedule.[209] Although these infections represented only 5% to 10% of all HBV infections in the United States, it is estimated that 18% of persons with chronic HBV infection acquired their infection postnatally during early childhood before implementation of perinatal hepatitis B immunization programs and routine infant hepatitis B immunization[210] (Fig. 16–10). In some populations, childhood transmission was more important than perinatal transmission as a cause of chronic HBV infection before hepatitis B immunization was widely implemented. For example, in studies conducted among U.S.-born children of Southeast Asian refugees during the 1980s, approximately 60% of chronic infections in young children were among children born to HBsAg-negative mothers.[191,193]

Sexual Transmission

HBV is efficiently transmitted by sexual contact, which can account for a high proportion of new HBV infections among adolescents and adults in countries with low and intermediate endemicity of chronic HBV infection.[211] It is estimated that sexual transmission accounts for about 50% of new infections among adults in the United States.[212] In countries where HBV infection is highly endemic, sexual transmission generally does not account for a high percentage of new cases because most persons are already infected during childhood.

The most common risk factors for sexual transmission among heterosexuals include multiple sexual partners (>1 partner in a 6-month period), history of a sexually transmitted disease (STD), or sex with a known infected person. Serologic evidence of HBV infection has ranged from 10% to 40% among adults at STD clinics.[211,213] Men who have sex with men are also at high risk of HBV transmission. Serosurveys conducted in the United States of young adult men who have sex with men indicate that 10% to 25% have serologic evidence of HBV infection and less than 10% have been vaccinated.[214] By comparison, approximately 5% of the general population has serologic evidence of HBV infection.[215]

Percutaneous Exposures (Such as Unsafe Injections)

Unsafe injections and other unsafe percutaneous or permucosal procedures conducted in medically related or other settings are a major source of blood-borne pathogen (HBV, HCV, HIV) transmission in many developing countries.[216–218] The risk of HBV infection from needle-stick exposures to HBsAg-positive blood is approximately 30% to 60% from inoculation with HBeAg-positive blood and 10% to 30% from HBeAg-negative blood.[219–221] By comparison, the risks of HCV and HIV transmission from percutaneous exposures are approximately 2% and 0.2%, respectively.[222,223] In addition to needle-stick exposures, blood transfusion is a major source of HBV transmission in countries where the blood supply is not screened for HBsAg.[224] Worldwide, unsafe injection practices may cause as many as 8 to 16 million HBV infections each year.[218] The primary nonmedical source of percutaneous exposures is injection of illicit drugs, which is a common mode of HBV transmission in many countries. For example, injection drug use accounts for approximately 15% of new HBV infections in the United States.[212]

Geographic Patterns of Transmission

The frequency and patterns of HBV transmission vary markedly in different parts of the world. Approximately 45% of the world's population live in areas where the prevalence of chronic HBV infection is high (i.e., ≥8% of the population is HBsAg positive); 43% live in areas where the prevalence is moderate (i.e., 2% to 7% of the population is HBsAg positive); and 12% live in areas of low endemicity (i.e., <2% of the population is HBsAg positive) (Fig. 16–11).

There are at least seven genotypes of the virus, which differ in geographic distribution.

In areas of high endemicity, the lifetime risk of HBV infection is more than 60% and most infections are acquired from perinatal and early childhood exposures, when the risk of developing chronic infection is greatest. In these areas, acute hepatitis B is rarely detected because most infections in early childhood are asymptomatic. However, rates of chronic liver disease and liver cancer are very high. Areas of high endemicity include most of Asia (except Japan and India), most of the Middle East, the Amazon basin, most Pacific Island groups, and Africa. In addition, some populations in low-endemicity areas have a high prevalence of infection, including Australian aborigines, New Zealand Maoris, and Alaskan Native Americans.

In areas of intermediate endemicity, the lifetime risk of HBV infection is 20% to 60% and infections occur in all age groups. Acute hepatitis B is common because many infections occur in adolescents and adults. However, high rates of chronic HBV infection are maintained primarily because of infections occurring in infants and children.

In areas of low endemicity, the lifetime risk of HBV infection is less than 20%. For example, the prevalence of chronic HBV infection in the United States is approximately 0.35%, and approximately 5% of the general population has serologic evidence of HBV infection.[215] Most HBV infections in areas of low endemicity occur in adults in relatively well-defined risk groups,[212] but a high proportion of chronic infections may occur as a consequence of perinatal and early childhood exposures. In the United States, more than one third of chronic HBV infections were acquired perinatally or in early childhood before perinatal

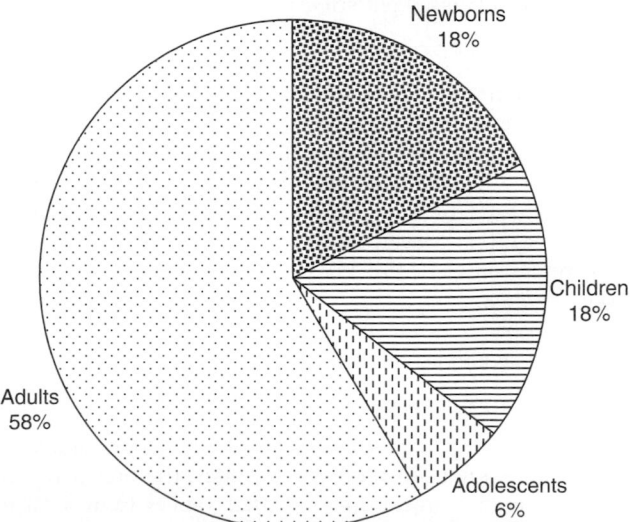

FIGURE 16–10 ■ Estimated age at infection of persons with chronic HBV Infection before implementation of hepatitis B immunization, United States. (Data from Margolis HS, Coleman PJ, Brown RE, et al. Prevention of hepatitis B virus transmission by immunization: an analysis of current recommendations. JAMA 274:1201–1208, 1995.)

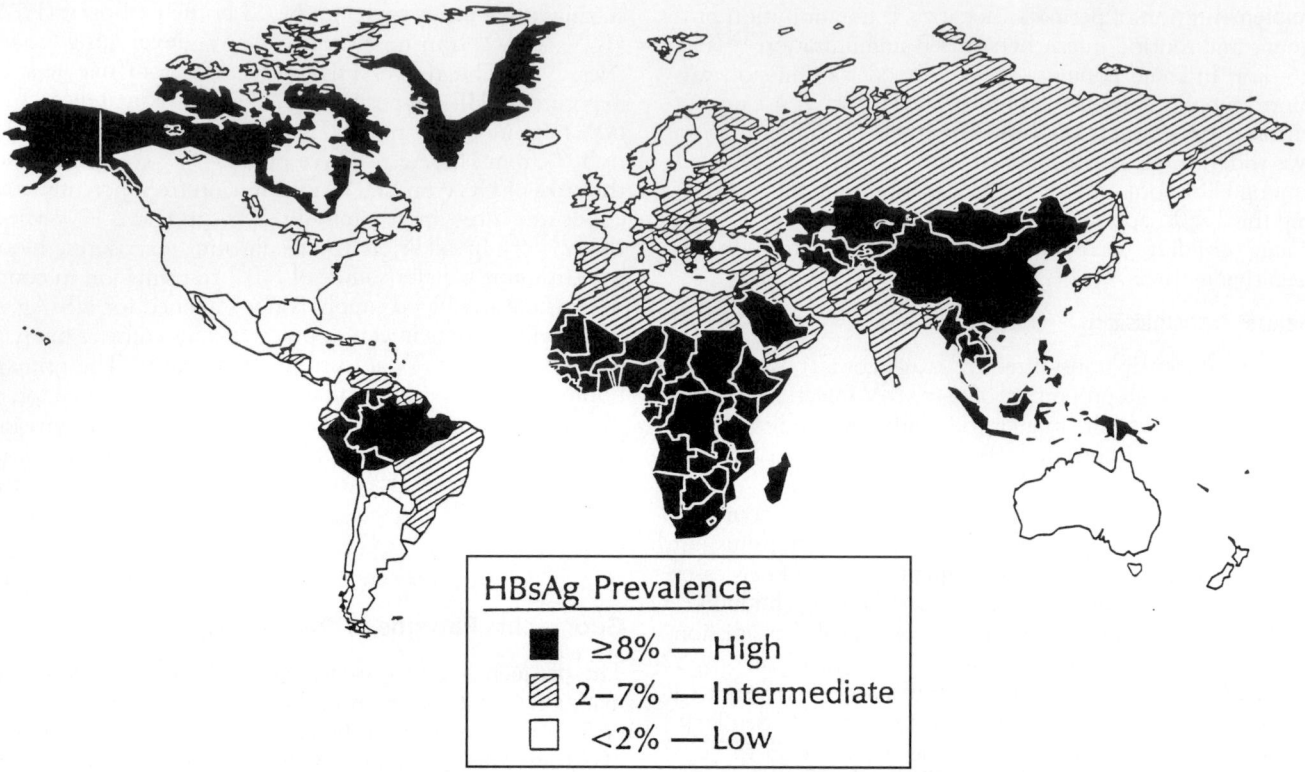

FIGURE 16-11 ■ Geographic distribution of chronic hepatitis B virus infection.

hepatitis B prevention programs and routine infant hepatitis B vaccination were implemented.[210]

The contribution of perinatal HBV transmission to the overall hepatitis B disease burden varies substantially in different geographic regions. In east and southeast Asian countries and the Pacific Islands, 35% to 50% of HBsAg-positive women are also HBeAg positive.[183,225–228] In these countries, approximately 3% to 5% of all infants may develop chronic HBV infection at birth and as many as 30% to 50% of all chronic infections among children result from perinatal transmission. In areas of high endemicity where the prevalence of HBeAg among pregnant women is low (i.e., Africa, South America, and the Middle East), perinatal HBV transmission contributes less to the pool of children with chronic infection than does postnatal early childhood transmission.[182,229–232] In general, less than 10% to 20% of all chronic infections among children in these areas result from perinatal exposures.

U.S. Risk Groups

Contacts of Persons with Chronic HBV Infection

In the United States, the prevalence of HBV infection among household and sexual contacts of persons with chronic HBV infection ranges from 25% to 50%.[233,234] The highest risk of infection is among sexual contacts. Among young children living in a household with an HBsAg-positive person, infection rates average 1% to 2% per year during the first decade of life.[186,191,193]

Hemodialysis Patients

Numerous studies documented a high risk of HBV infection among hemodialysis patients in the United States before initiation of strict infection control practices and hepatitis B vaccination.[235] Since these control measures were initiated, rates of HBV infection observed among patients undergoing hemodialysis have declined by over 95%.[236] However, the continued risk of infection among this population is evident from repeated outbreaks of HBV infection among unvaccinated patients.[237]

Incarcerated Persons

The prevalence of HBV infection among incarcerated adults in the United States ranges from 20% to 40% for both prison and jail inmates, and 1% to 2% have evidence of chronic infection.[238–241] The high prevalence of infection observed among adults primarily reflects infections acquired prior to incarceration. However, studies have demonstrated a 1% to 2% annual incidence of HBV infection in prison populations.[242,243] Among persons with acute hepatitis B, about 2% appear to have acquired their infection while incarcerated and 15% have a history of prior incarceration.[212]

Injection Drug Users

Direct parenteral exposure is the most efficient mode of HBV transmission. In the United States, the prevalence of infection among injection drug users ranges from 30% to 90%, and the risk of infection increases with number of years of drug use. It is estimated that greater than 80% of injection drug users are infected after 5 years of injecting.[244,245]

Persons with Occupational Exposure

In studies conducted in the United States during the 1970s and 1980s, the prevalence of HBV infection among health care workers was 10% to 30%.[246-251] Infection was associated with frequency of blood contact, needle-stick exposures, direct patient contact, and years of employment and was observed among a number of occupational categories, including physicians, nurses, laboratory technicians, and emergency medical technicians. However, the incidence of new infections has declined substantially in the United States with the widespread vaccination of heath care workers and implementation of standard precautions in health care settings, and is now less than that of the general population.[252]

Other groups with potential occupational risk of HBV infection include public safety workers with high-frequency exposure to blood.[253-255] However, the prevalence of HBV infection in groups such as police officers, firefighters, and corrections officers generally does not differ from the general population when adjusted for race and age.[253] Nonoccupational risk factors, such as a history of multiple sexual partners and STDs, are associated with HBV infection in these groups.[253] An increased risk of HBV infection resulting from occupational exposures has not been documented in persons infrequently exposed to blood or body fluids, such as ward clerks, dietary workers, maintenance workers, housekeeping personnel, lifeguards, schoolteachers, and persons employed in child day care settings.

Recipients of Clotting Factors for Bleeding Disorders

Prior to routine use of clotting factor concentrates manufactured by processes to inactivate viruses, most patients with hemophilia were at high risk of infections with blood-borne viruses, including HBV, HCV, HIV, and hepatitis delta virus.[256] Since 1987, clotting factor concentrates licensed in the United States have been manufactured by processes known to render HBV inactive.

Developmentally Disabled Persons

Very high rates of HBV infection were documented among residents in institutions for developmentally disabled persons before hepatitis B vaccine was used in these facilities.[257,258] In the United States, the risk of HBV infection in these institutions has declined substantially over the past three decades. However, because HBsAg-positive clients remain in institutions, it should be presumed that these persons can transmit HBV to other persons, especially if the disabled person behaves aggressively or has special medical problems (e.g., exudative dermatitis, open skin lesions) that increase the risk of exposure to blood or serous secretions.[259]

Travelers to HBV-Endemic Regions

Short-term travelers to areas where HBV infection is of high or intermediate endemicity (see Fig. 16–11) generally are not at risk of infection except when exposed to blood in medical, health care, or disaster relief activities; receiving medical care that involves parenteral exposures; or engaging in sexual or drug use activity.[260] However, persons working in these areas for 6 months or longer have infection rates of 2% to 5% per year.[261]

Passive Immunization

The discovery that passively acquired anti-HBs can protect individuals from acute hepatitis B and chronic HBV infection if given soon after exposure led to the development of HBIG, a specific immune globulin containing high titers of anti-HBs. In early studies, standard immune globulin also was shown to be effective for postexposure prophylaxis of HBV infection.[262] However, current blood donor screening practices exclude most persons who are anti-HBs positive, and immune globulin is no longer used for postexposure prophylaxis. HBIG was used for pre- and postexposure prophylaxis before hepatitis B vaccines became available, but currently is recommended only for postexposure prophylaxis (often in combination with hepatitis B vaccine) in the following settings: (1) perinatal exposure for an infant born to an HBsAg-positive mother, (2) percutaneous or mucous membrane exposure to HBsAg-positive blood, and (3) sexual exposure to an HBsAg-positive person. HBIG is also used to reduce the risk of recurrent HBV infection after liver transplantation.[263]

HBIG is prepared by the Cohn Oncly fractionation procedure from serum containing high titers of anti-HBs. The human plasma from which HBIG is prepared is screened for HBsAg and for antibodies to HIV and HCV. The process used to prepare HBIG inactivates and eliminates HIV from the final product.[264,265] Since 1996, all HBIG products available in the United States have been determined to be negative for HCV RNA by polymerase chain reaction, and since 1999 all of these products have been manufactured by methods that inactivate HCV and other viruses. HBIG should be stored at 2° to 8°C and should not be frozen.

HBIG is approximately 75% effective in preventing clinical hepatitis B or the development of chronic infection, if used shortly after exposure to the virus.[266-268] However, protection afforded by HBIG lasts only several months, leaving the recipient susceptible to HBV infection after antibody titers decline. In addition, it is expensive and is usually not affordable in the developing world.

One of the major uses of HBIG is as an adjunct to hepatitis B vaccine in preventing perinatal HBV transmission. Untreated, 70% to 90% of infants born to HBeAg-positive mothers become infected at birth and develop chronic HBV infection.[169,269] A regimen of three doses of HBIG, if started within 48 hours of birth, is approximately 75% effective in preventing chronic infection in infants.[167,270] However, children continuing to live in a household with an infected mother often become infected after the first year of life,[183] so HBIG administration alone is not sufficient for long-term protection of children born to HBV-infected mothers. With the development of hepatitis B vaccines, it was shown that immunoprophylaxis with both HBIG and hepatitis B vaccine could increase the efficacy of preventing perinatal HBV transmission to 85% to 95% and provide long-term protection.[169,177] More recent studies have shown that vaccine alone, when started at birth and at appropriate doses, provides protection similar to HBIG plus vaccine.[271]

HBIG is also indicated for postexposure prophylaxis after needle stick or other percutaneous injuries in susceptible individuals exposed to infectious body fluids from HBsAg-positive source patients. The efficacy of HBIG alone in preventing acute clinical hepatitis B in needle-stick recipients was demonstrated in two large, multicenter trials.[268,272] These trials demonstrated that, when untreated, approximately 30% of exposed people developed clinical disease after needle-stick exposure and that HBIG was approximately 75% effective in preventing clinical disease. With the availability of hepatitis B vaccine, postexposure prophylaxis protocols were developed that account for the vaccination and serologic status of the exposed person. These protocols recommend administration of HBIG to nonvaccinated individuals and to vaccine nonresponders.

The efficacy of HBIG in preventing clinical hepatitis B or chronic HBV infection following sexual exposure to an acutely infected partner is approximately 75% if given within 7 days of exposure.[273] Current recommendations for postexposure prophylaxis following sexual exposure to an infected person include the use of HBIG and hepatitis B vaccine.

Route of Administration and Dosage

The standard dose of HBIG for postexposure prophylaxis of infants born to HBsAg-positive mothers is 0.5 mL. In all other situations the dose is 0.06 mL/kg. For infants, HBIG should be administered intramuscularly in the anterolateral thigh using a 7/8- to 1-inch needle and can be given simultaneously with hepatitis B vaccine but at a separate site. For older children, adolescents and adults, an appropriate muscle mass (i.e., deltoid, gluteal) should be chosen in which to deliver the larger volumes of HBIG using a needle length appropriate for the person's age and size.[274] If the gluteal muscle is used, the central region of the buttock should be avoided; only the upper outer quadrant should be used, and the needle should be directed anteriorly to minimize possibility of injury to the sciatic nerve.[274]

Active Immunization

Development of Vaccines

Safe and effective hepatitis B vaccines have been commercially available since 1982. The first available vaccines were produced by harvesting HBsAg from the plasma of people with chronic infection. Subsequently, several vaccine manufacturers used recombinant DNA technology to express HBsAg in other organisms, which led to the development of recombinant DNA vaccines.[275–277] Recombinant DNA technology offered the potential to produce unlimited supplies of vaccine. Over the past decade, prices of recombinant DNA vaccines have declined considerably, and current United Nations International Children's Emergency Fund (UNICEF) contract prices for plasma-derived and recombinant DNA vaccines are essentially equivalent.[278] Both types of hepatitis B vaccine have been licensed and used in the United States. Plasma-derived vaccines are no longer produced by manufacturers in North America or western Europe, but are produced by manufacturers in Asia, and are used in many immunization programs worldwide (Table 16–2).

TABLE 16–2 ■ Hepatitis B Vaccines Available Internationally*

Manufacturer	Brand Name[†]	Country	Type[‡]
Berna Biotech	Hepavax-Gene	Switzerland	Recombinant DNA (mammalian cell)
Bhavat Biotech	Revac-B	India	Recombinant DNA (yeast)
Celltech Chiroscience	Hepagene	United Kingdom	Recombinant DNA (mammalian cell)
Center for Genetic Engineering and Biotechnology	Enivac-HB	Cuba	Recombinant DNA (yeast)
Chiel Jedang	Hepaccine-B	South Korea	Plasma-derived
Korea Green Cross	Hepavax-Gene	South Korea	Recombinant DNA (yeast)
LG Chemical	Euvax B	South Korea	Recombinant DNA (yeast)
Merck Sharp & Dohme	Recombivax HB	United States	Recombinant DNA (yeast)
	Comvax	United States	Combined Hib and recombinant DNA (yeast)
Pasteur Mérieux Connaught	Genhevac B	France	Recombinant DNA (mammalian cell)
Shantha Biotechnics	Shanevac-B	India	Recombinant DNA (yeast)
GlaxoSmithKline	Engerix-B	Belgium	Recombinant DNA (yeast)
	Infanrix-HB	Belgium	Combined DTaP and recombinant DNA (yeast)
	Infanrix HeXa	Belgium	Combined DTaP-IPV-Hib and recombinant DNA (yeast)
	Tritanrix-HB	Belgium	Combined DTwP and recombinant DNA (yeast)
	Tritanrix-HB-Hib	Belgium	Combined DTwP-Hib and recombinant DNA (yeast)
	Twinrix	Belgium	Combined hepatitis A and recombinant DNA (yeast)

*Numerous providers who sell only in country of production are not listed. Presence on this list does not imply endorsement of these products by the World Health Organization.

[†]Brand names may vary in different countries.

[‡]DTaP, diphtheria and tetanus toxoids and acellular pertussis; DTwP, diphtheria and tetanus toxoids and whole-cell pertussis; Hib, *Haemophilus influenzae* type B; IPV, inactivated poliovirus vaccine.

Hepatitis B vaccines are formulated to contain 3 to 40 μg of HBsAg protein per milliliter and have an aluminum phosphate or aluminum hydroxide adjuvant. Since 1999, hepatitis B vaccines available in the United States for use in infants and children have not contained thimerosal as a preservative because of concern about possible neurodevelopmental effects of mercury.[279] However, there is no evidence of any harmful effects of the small amounts of thimerosal in hepatitis B vaccine, and the risk, if any, is only theoretical.[280] Thimerosal continues to be used as a preservative in hepatitis B vaccines available in many countries, and is particularly important to prevent bacterial contamination when multidose vials are used.

Plasma-Derived Vaccines

Plasma-derived vaccines are prepared by harvesting the 22-nm particles of HBsAg from plasma of persons with chronic HBV infection.[275] The particles are highly purified, and any residual infectious particles are inactivated by various combinations of urea, pepsin, formaldehyde, and heat. Concerns about the safety of plasma-derived vaccine regarding transmission of blood-borne pathogens, including HIV, have proved to be unfounded.[281]

Recombinant DNA Vaccines

Most licensed recombinant DNA hepatitis B vaccines consist of a 226-amino-acid S gene product (HBsAg protein).[275] The yeast-produced vaccines, which are the most widely used, are obtained by inserting the S gene into a plasmid downstream of three genes from *Saccharomyces cerevisiae* that serve to promote production of HBsAg. A master seed of the transformed yeast is then made, from which working seeds are derived. Each time a lot of vaccine is needed, yeast from the working seed serves to start the fermentation in large vessels. The HBsAg is then purified to eliminate yeast components by various physical separation techniques, including chromatography and filtration. The expressed HBsAg polypeptide self-assembles into immunogenic spherical particles closely resembling the natural 22-nm particles found in the serum of persons with chronic HBV infection. The *a* determinant that is responsible for the most important immune response is exposed on the surface of the artificial HBsAg particle, as it is on the natural particle. The artificial particles differ from natural particles only in the glycosylation of HBsAg.

Combination Vaccines

Several vaccine manufacturers have produced combination vaccines containing a hepatitis B vaccine (HepB) component. These combination vaccines include diphtheria and tetanus toxoids and whole-cell pertussis (DTwP)–HepB vaccine; DTwP–*Haemophilus influenzae* type b conjugate (Hib)–HepB vaccine; diphtheria and tetanus toxoids and acellular pertussis (DTaP)–HepB vaccine; DTaP-Hib–inactivated poliovirus vaccine (IPV)–HepB vaccine; DtaP-IPV-HepB vaccine; Hib-HepB vaccine; and hepatitis A (HepA)–HepB vaccine. For each of these combination vaccines, the manufacturer has shown that the components remain sufficiently immunogenic to elicit protective levels of anti-HBs.[282–284] However, providers should not attempt to make extemporaneous mixtures of vaccine in the same syringe at point of

use because the results are unpredictable unless verified by the manufacturer and national control authorities. In the United States, Hib-HepB vaccine, and DtaP-IPV-HepB vaccine are licensed for use in children and HepA-HepB vaccine is licensed for use in adults. The diphtheria-tetanus-pertussis (DTP)–containing hepatitis B combination vaccines from one manufacturer are licensed in Europe and are used in immunization programs in many developing countries. Several other producers in a number of countries have DTP-containing hepatitis B combination vaccines under development.

Dosage and Route of Administration

The quantity of HBsAg protein per dose that induces a protective immune response in infants and children varies with the manufacturer, ranging from 1.5 to 10 μg, because of differences in hepatitis B vaccine production processes. In general, the vaccine dose for infants and adolescents is 50% lower than that required for adults. There is no international standard of vaccine potency expressed in micrograms of HBsAg protein, and the relative efficacy of different vaccines cannot be assessed on the basis of differences in HBsAg content. Vaccine produced by each manufacturer has been evaluated in clinical trials to determine the age-specific dose that achieves the maximum seroprotection rate. Persons who respond to hepatitis B vaccine with titers of anti-HBs of 10 milli–International Units (mIU)/mL or greater are protected against acute hepatitis B and chronic infection. The standard pediatric volume of administration is 0.5 mL. With lower volumes, the possibility exists of administering an inadequate dose to produce the required immune response using standard hubbed syringes. The types and formulations of hepatitis B vaccines can be interchanged. Vaccines of different types and from different manufacturers can be used for each dose that a child receives.[285] The recommended dose for hepatitis B vaccines licensed in the United States varies by product and the recipient's age (Table 16–3).

Hepatitis B vaccine should be given by intramuscular injection in the anterolateral aspect of the thigh of infants and children less than 24 months of age, and in the deltoid muscle of older children, adolescents, and adults. Administration in the buttock is not recommended because this route of administration has been associated with decreased protective antibody levels in some studies, probably because of inadvertent subcutaneous injection or injection into deep fat tissue.[286] In addition, there may be a risk of injury to the sciatic nerve if the vaccine is administered in the buttock. For infants and children, the vaccine should be administered using a 5/8- to 1-inch needle. A 1- to 1½-inch needle should be used for adolescents and adults to ensure delivery of vaccine into muscle tissue. If hepatitis B vaccine is administered on the same day as another injectable vaccine, it is preferable to give the two vaccines in different limbs. If more than one injection has to be given in the same limb, the thigh is the preferred site of injection because of the greater muscle mass, and the injection sites should be 1 to 2 inches apart so that any local reactions are unlikely to overlap.[274]

Although low doses of hepatitis B vaccine administered intradermally have been shown to reduce costs of vaccinating

TABLE 16–3 ■ Recommended Doses of Hepatitis B Vaccines Licensed in the United States[a]

Group	Comvax® Dose (μg)[b]	Engerix-B® Dose (μg)	Pediarix™ Dose (μg)[c]	Recombivax HB® Dose (μg)	Twinrix® Dose (μg)[d]
Infants[e], children and adolescents (<20 yrs)	5[f]	10	10[g]	5[h]	—
Adults (≥20 yrs)	—	20	—	10	20[i]
Hemodialysis patients and other immunocompromised persons	—	40	—	40	—

[a]Comvax and Recombivax HB are manufactured by Merck Sharp & Dohme; Engerix-B, Pediarix, and Twinrix are manufactured by GlaxoSmithKline.
[b]In addition to hepatitis B surface antigen, Comvax contains 7.5 μg *Haemophilus influenzae* type b polyribosylribitol phosphate and 125 μg *Neisseria menigitidis* outer membrane protein complex.
[c]In addition to hepatitis B surface antigen, Pediarix also contains 25 Lf units of diphtheria toxoid, 10 Lf units of tetanus toxoid, 3 pertussis antigens (25 μg of inactivated pertussis antigen, 25 μg of filamentous hemagglutinin, and 8 μg of peractin), 40 D-antigen units (DU) of type 1 poliovirus, 8 DU of type 2 poliovirus, and 32 DU of type 3 poliovirus.
[d]In addition to hepatitis B surface antigen, Twinrix contains 720 ELISA Units of inactivated hepatitis A vaccine.
[e]All infants, including those born to HBsAg-positive mothers, HBsAg-negative mothers, and mothers with unknown HBsAg status.
[f]Comvax should not be administered before 6 weeks of age. Comvax is licensed to use in infants and children aged 6 weeks to 15 months.
[g]Pediarix should not be administered before 6 weeks of age. Pediarix is licensed to use in infants and children aged 6 weeks to 6 years.
[h]A two-dose schedule of 10 μg of Recombivax HB is also licensed for adolescents 11–15 years of age.
[i]Twinrix is recommended for persons 18 years of age or greater who are at increased risk of both hepatitis B virus and hepatitis A virus infections.

adults,[287] this route of administration is not recommended because seroconversion rates among adults and children have been inconsistent and generally lower compared with three standard doses administered intramuscularly.[288] In addition, there are few data on the long-term protection afforded by this route of administration.

No clinically significant increase in adverse reactions or interference in antibody responses has been observed when hepatitis B vaccine has been given simultaneously, but at a different site, with other childhood or adult vaccines.[274,282,283,289–296] Thus hepatitis B vaccine can be given at the same time as other vaccines (e.g., DTP, oral poliovirus vaccine [OPV], IPV, HepA, Hib, measles, bacille Calmette-Guérin [BCG], and yellow fever vaccine). Hepatitis B vaccine also can be given at any time before or after a different inactivated or live vaccine because inactivated vaccines such as hepatitis B vaccine generally do not interfere with the immune response to other inactivated or live vaccines.[274]

Combination vaccines that include hepatitis B vaccine must not be used to give the birth dose of hepatitis B vaccine because DTP and Hib vaccines should not be administered at birth. Only monovalent hepatitis B vaccine should be used for the birth dose. Either monovalent hepatitis B vaccine or combination vaccines may be used for later doses in the hepatitis B vaccine schedule. Combination vaccines can be given whenever all the antigens in the vaccines are indicated.[297]

Available immunogenicity data from "off-schedule" vaccination suggest that, if the series is interrupted after the first dose, the second dose should be given as soon as possible and the second and third doses should be separated by an interval of at least 2 months; if only the third dose is delayed, it should be administered as soon as possible.[298–301] In any age group, when the vaccination schedule is interrupted it is not necessary to restart the vaccine series.

It is possible that people may have detectable HBsAg in serum if tested within a short time after vaccination (e.g., up to 18 days) because the vaccine contains HBsAg.[302–305]

Stability of Vaccine

The recommended storage temperature for hepatitis B vaccine is between 2° and 8°C. The vaccine is generally stable for at least 4 years from the date of manufacture if stored in this temperature range. However, there may be considerable variations in stability between hepatitis B vaccines from different manufacturers. Therefore, the package insert should be consulted in order to know the manufacturer's recommended shelf-life for each specific vaccine.

Most hepatitis B vaccines are relatively heat stable and have only a small loss of potency when stored between 20° and 26°C for up to 1 year, at 37°C for 2 to 6 months, and at 45°C for 1 week.[306,307] No significant differences were found in seroconversion rates and levels of protective antibody between infants who received a first dose that had been stored in the cold chain and those who received a first dose stored for up to a month at tropical temperatures.[308] The excellent heat stability of hepatitis B vaccine may allow the vaccine to be given at birth to prevent perinatal HBV transmission during home deliveries where refrigeration is not available. In demonstration projects, use of hepatitis B vaccine in prefilled single-use injection devices (e.g., Uniject™) outside the cold chain has been reported to simplify logistics, minimize vaccine wastage, and facilitate the speed and efficiency of immunization at birth during home visits.[308,309] The use of such devices outside the cold chain could greatly enhance hepatitis B vaccine delivery in outreach services.

Hepatitis B vaccine and combination vaccines that contain hepatitis B vaccine must not be frozen. The freezing of hepatitis B vaccine causes the HBsAg protein to dissociate from the alum adjuvant and thus to lose its immunogenicity/potency.[310,311] The freezing point of hepatitis B vaccine is about −0.5°C.[312]

Results of Vaccination

Vaccine Immunogenicity and Schedules

Historically, the standard three-dose hepatitis B vaccine series has consisted of two priming doses given 1 month apart and a third dose given 6 months after the third dose. In addition, multiple other schedules have been used successfully. Increasing the interval between the first and second dose of hepatitis B vaccine has little effect on immunogenicity or final antibody titer. Longer intervals between the last two doses result in higher final antibody levels.[312,313] A course of three doses of hepatitis B vaccine induces protective levels of anti-HBs in over 95% of healthy infants, children, and adolescents, and in more than 90% of healthy adults younger than 40 years.[314–316] After age 40 years, immunogenicity drops below 90%, and, by age 60 years, only 65% to 75% of vaccinees develop protective anti-HBs titers. Host factors in addition to age that contribute to decreased vaccine response include smoking, obesity, HIV infection, genetic factors, and the presence of a chronic disease.[286,317–325]

No differences in seroprotection exist between U.S.-licensed vaccines following the third vaccine dose, although some differences exist prior to complete vaccination.[326] Early differences in immunogenicity after one or two doses have little if any practical significance because there is little chance that HBV infection would occur prior to completion of the recommended vaccination schedule.

Infants and Children

A variety of hepatitis B vaccine schedules have been shown to induce levels of seroprotection of greater than 95% in infants, including doses administered at birth, 1, and 6 months of age; 2, 4, and 6 months of age; and 6, 10, and 14 weeks of age.[314,327–330] Programmatically, it is usually easiest if the three doses of hepatitis B vaccine are given at the same time as the three doses of other childhood vaccines (e.g., DTP vaccine, Hib vaccine) and these schedules will accommodate use of DTP- and Hib-containing combination vaccines. A hepatitis B vaccine schedule administered with DTP or Hib vaccines will prevent infections acquired during childhood, as well as infections acquired later in life. However, these schedules will not prevent perinatal HBV infections because they do not include a birth dose. Because of this, concerns have been expressed that increased use of combination vaccines may jeopardize perinatal hepatitis B prevention programs.[331] In order to prevent perinatal HBV transmission in settings where combination vaccines are used, a four-dose hepatitis B vaccination schedule may be needed, with the first dose administered at birth.

Certain premature infants with low birth weights (i.e., <2000 g) may have decreased seroconversion rates after administration of hepatitis B vaccine at birth.[332] However, by 1 month chronologic age, all premature infants, regardless of initial birth weight or gestational age, are as likely to respond adequately as older and larger infants, although this conclusion has been disputed.[333–335a]

For infant vaccination in the United States, the first dose of hepatitis B vaccine is recommended soon after birth and before hospital discharge (Table 16–4). The first dose also may be given by 2 months of age if the infant's mother has been appropriately tested for HBsAg and is verified to be HBsAg negative. The second dose is recommended at least 4 weeks after the first dose, except for Hib- and DTP-containing combination vaccines, which cannot be given before 6 weeks of age. The third dose is recommended at least 16 weeks after the first dose and at least 8 weeks after the second dose. The last dose in the series (third or fourth dose) is not recommended before 6 months of age. Infants born to HBsAg-negative mothers should complete the hepatitis B vaccine series by 18 months of age. Infants born to HBsAg-positive mothers and to mothers with unknown HBsAg status should complete the series by 6 months of age.

The World Health Organization (WHO) recommends multiple options for adding hepatitis B vaccine to existing infant immunization schedules that do not require additional visits for immunization[336] (Table 16–5). Schedules should optimize the percentage of children completing the hepatitis B vaccine series, which can be achieved with earlier administration of vaccines.[337] The WHO-recommended minimum interval between dose 1 and dose 2 is 4 weeks, and the minimum interval between dose 2 and dose 3 is 4 weeks. Schedules with these minimum intervals (e.g., 6, 10, and 14 weeks) have been demonstrated to have seroconversion rates similar to schedules with longer intervals, albeit with lower final anti-HBs titers. WHO minimum recommended intervals for infant hepatitis vaccination are shorter than those recommended in the United States. Although there are limited data regarding long-term protection for schedules with shorter intervals, alternative schedules often are not feasible. In addition, concerns about long-term protection are of little practical significance in high-endemicity countries where most HBV infections are acquired in childhood.

Adolescents

Hepatitis B vaccine schedules that have been demonstrated to induce seroprotection rates of greater than 95% in adolescents include doses administered at 0, 1, and 6 months; 0, 2, and 4 months; and 0, 12, and 24 months.[299,338–341] In addition, for adolescents 11 to 15 years of age, the adult dose (10 μg) of Recombivax HB® is licensed in the United States for administration on a 0- and 4- to 6-month schedule.[342] This two-dose schedule produced anti-HBs titers equivalent to those obtained with the pediatric dose (5 μg) administered on a three-dose schedule.[343] However, limited data are available regarding long-term protection with two-dose hepatitis B vaccine schedules.[343]

Adults

Three intramuscular doses of hepatitis B vaccine induce a protective antibody response in approximately 30% to 55% of healthy adults less than 40 years of age after the first dose, 75% after the second dose, and greater than 90% after the third dose.[36,37] However, the risk of failure to seroconvert increases by a relative risk of 1.76 in adults over 40 years of age.[343a] Because an increased risk for HBV infection is the indication for hepatitis B vaccination, and relatively high rates of seroprotection are achieved after each dose,

TABLE 16-4 ■ Recommended Schedule of Hepatitis B Vaccination for Different Age Groups, United States

Age Group	Dose	Schedule	Comments
Infants (<1 yr)		See separate schedules below for infants born to mothers who are HBsAg negative, HBsAg positive, and of unknown HBsAg status	• Only monovalent hepatitis B vaccine should be used for the birth dose. • Monovalent vaccine or combination vaccines containing hepatitis B vaccine may be used to complete the vaccine series; 4 doses of vaccine may be administered if the first dose is given at birth. • The second dose should be given at least 4 weeks after the first dose, except for combination vaccines, which should not be administered before 6 wk of age. The third dose should be given at least 16 wk after the first dose and at least 8 wk after the second dose. The last dose in the vaccination series (third or fourth dose) should not be administered before 6 mo of age
HBsAg-negative mother	1 2 3	Birth before hospital discharge (preferred) 1–4 mo 6–18 mo	• The first dose can also be given at age 1–2 mo, but only if the infant's mother is verified to be HBsAg negative. • For premature infants who weigh less than 2000 g at birth, the first dose of the hepatitis B vaccine series should be delayed until 1 month of chronologic age. Premature infants discharged from the hospital before 1 month chronologic age may be given hepatitis B vaccine at discharge if they are medically stable and showing consistent weight gain.
HBsAg-positive mother	1 2 3	Birth with HBIG (within 12 hr) 1–2 mo 6 mo	• HBIG (0.5 mL) and hepatitis B vaccine should be administered at separate sites • Postvaccination testing for HBsAg and antibody to HBsAg should be done at 9–15 mo of age. • For premature infants who weigh less than 2000 g at birth, the initial vaccine dose should not be counted toward completion of the hepatitis B vaccine series, and 3 additional doses of hepatitis B vaccine should be administered beginning when the infant is 1 mo of age.
Mother with unknown HBsAg status	1 2 3	Birth (within 12 hr) 1–2 mo 6 mo (6–18 mo if mother verified to be HBsAg negative)	• Mother should be tested for HBsAg; if the HBsAg test is positive, the infant should receive HBIG (0.5 mL) as soon as possible (no later than age 1 wk). • For premature infants who weigh less than 2000 g at birth, the initial vaccine dose should not be counted toward completion of the hepatitis B vaccine series, and 3 additional doses of hepatitis B vaccine should be administered beginning when the infant is 1 mo of age.
1–19 yr	1 2 3	All children and adolescents who have not been previously immunized against hepatitis B should begin the series during any visit. At least 4 wk after dose 1 At least 8 wk after dose 2 and at least 16 wk after dose 1	• The adult dose of Recombivax has been licensed for administration to adolescents 11–15 yr of age on a 2-dose schedule at 0 and 4–6 mo. If the adolescent is older than 15 yr of age when scheduled to receive the second dose, he or she should be switched to a 3-dose series, and the pediatric formulation should be used for doses 2 and 3.
≥20 yr	1 2 3	Adults with risk factors for HBV infection can begin the series at any visit At least 4 wk after dose 1 At least 8 wk after dose 2 and at least 16 wk after dose 1	• Twinrix (combined hepatitis A and hepatitis B vaccine) should be administered on a 0-, 1-, and 6-mo schedule.

TABLE 16–5 ■ Recommended Options for Adding Hepatitis B Vaccine to Childhood Immunization Schedules, World Health Organization

Age	Visit	Other Antigens	Hepatitis B Vaccine Options		
			No Birth Dose I	With Birth Dose	
				II	III
Birth	0	BCG (OPV0)[*]		HepB—birth[†]	HepB—birth[†]
6 wk	1	OPV1, DTP1	HepB1[‡]	HepB2[†]	DPT-HepB1[§]
10 wk	2	OPV2, DTP2	HepB2[‡]		DTP-HepB2[§]
14 wk	3	OPV3, DTP3	HepB3[‡]	HepB3[†]	DTP-HepB3[§]
9–12 mo	4	Measles			

[*]Only given in countries where polio is highly endemic.
[†]Monovalent vaccine.
[‡]Monovalent or combination vaccine.
[§]Combination vaccine.

vaccination should be initiated even if completion of the three-dose series cannot be assured.

Retrospective studies have suggested a difference in age-specific immunogenicity between the two vaccines licensed in the United States (Engerix-B® and Recombivax HB) when given to adults.[321,323] However, a prospective study found no differences in immunogenicity for people younger than 55 years.[320] For people older than 55 years, the likelihood of nonresponse was approximately two times greater among people receiving Recombivax HB compared with people receiving Engerix-B. However, this difference in immunogenicity would result in only a marginal difference in disease prevention and does not warrant the preferential use of one vaccine.

Hemodialysis Patients

Among adult hemodialysis patients, protective titers of anti-HBs developed in a median of 64% (range, 34% to 88%) and 86% (range, 40% to 98%) of those who received a three-dose and four-dose hepatitis B vaccine series, respectively.[235] Some studies have demonstrated higher seroprotection rates in patients with chronic renal failure before they become dialysis dependent, particularly patients with mild or moderate renal failure.[344]

Immunocompromised Persons

Immunocompromised persons (e.g., HIV positive, taking immunosuppressive drugs) have a suboptimal response to standard doses of hepatitis B vaccine.[317,345–348] Larger vaccine doses may be required to induce protective antibody titers in these persons, although few data are available on the response to higher doses.[349]

Induction of HBsAG Positivity

Vaccination has been found to be associated with transient presence of HBsAg in the serum.[349a]

Efficacy

Pre-Exposure Vaccine Efficacy

The efficacy of pre-exposure hepatitis B vaccination has been demonstrated in randomized, double-blind, placebo-controlled clinical trials involving several high-risk groups, including homosexual men, health care workers, hemodialysis staff members, and hemodialysis patients.[311,350–353] These studies demonstrated an overall efficacy of 80% to 100% (Table 16–6) and virtually complete protection among persons who developed anti-HBs titers of 10 mIU/mL or greater.

Postexposure Vaccine Efficacy

Among infants born to HBeAg-positive mothers, postexposure immunoprophylaxis with either plasma-derived or recombinant vaccines and HBIG is 80% to 100% effective

TABLE 16–6 ■ Randomized Clinical Studies of Pre-Exposure Hepatitis B Vaccine Efficacy

Group	Vaccine[*]	Dose (μg)	Schedule (mo)	No. of Subjects	Attack Rate[†]		Efficacy %
					Vaccinated	Unvaccinated	
Men who have sex with men[351]	MSD-P	20	0, 1, 6	1402	2.3	12.6	82
Men who have sex with men[350]	MSD-P	40	0, 1, 6	1083	3.5	27.1	87
Men who have sex with men[460]	CLN-P	3	0, 1, 2	800	5.0	24.0	80
Health care workers[458–460]	MSD-P	20	0, 1, 6	865	0.5	6.0	92
Health care workers[352]	Pasteur-P	5	0, 1, 2	354	0	8.0	100
Hemodialysis patients[459]	Pasteur-P	5	0, 1, 2	95	2.6	27.7	91
Hemodialysis patients[381]	MSD-P	40	0, 1, 6	1311	1.0	0.7	0[‡]
Hemodialysis patients[460]	CLN	3	0, 1, 2, 5	388	1.6	12.0	86

[*]CLN, Central Laboratory of the Netherlands Red Cross Blood Transfusion Service; MSD, Merck, Sharp & Dohme; P, plasma-derived vaccine.
[†]Attack rate (per 100 person-years) of hepatitis B virus infection defined as clinical hepatitis B and/or HBsAg positive greater than 3 months after starting vaccination series.
[‡]Although efficacy was not demonstrated in this study, no infections occurred among persons who developed and maintained protective levels of antibody to hepatitis B surface antigen.

in preventing chronic HBV infection (Table 16–7).[170–172,354–360] Several studies also have demonstrated a high efficacy of recombinant vaccine alone in preventing perinatal HBV transmission, including reports in which the administration of HBIG provided no additional protection (see Table 16–7). These findings indicate that the use of HBIG to prevent perinatal HBV transmission is not necessary, particularly in countries where pregnant women are not screened for HBsAg and hepatitis B vaccine is routinely given to all infants at birth. However, plasma-derived vaccines and lower doses of recombinant vaccine alone appear to be less effective in preventing perinatal HBV transmission when compared with vaccine and HBIG.[271,360,361] In most postexposure prophylaxis studies, hepatitis B vaccine has been administered to infants within 12 to 24 hours of birth. The efficacy of vaccine in preventing perinatal transmission declines the longer the first dose of vaccine is given after birth.[362]

Correlates of Protection

In vaccine efficacy studies, virtually complete protection has been achieved among people who developed anti-HBs titers of 10 mIU/mL or greater following vaccination.[311,350,351,353] However, cases of clinical hepatitis B and rarely of chronic HBV infection were observed among people with anti-HBs titers of less than 10 mIU/mL. Thus an anti-HBs response of 10 mIU/mL or greater as measured by commercial radioimmunoassay or enzyme immunoassay is considered to be the lower limit of adequate response to vaccine.[353,363]

Long-Term Protection and Booster Doses

Among infants and children who respond to a primary three-dose vaccination series, 15% to 50% lose detectable levels of anti-HBs within 5 to 15 years after vaccination (Table 16–8).[364–370] Among adult vaccinees, anti-HBs levels decline to less than 10 mIU/mL in 7% to 50% within 5 years after vaccination and in 30% to 60% within 9 to 11 years after vaccination (see Table 16–8).[371–375] In general, anti-HBs titers decline rapidly in the first 12 months after the third dose and then decline more gradually over time. However, no clinical cases of hepatitis B have been observed in follow-up studies among immune-competent vaccinated populations, and only rare chronic infections have been documented (see Table 16–8). Most breakthrough infections have been observed among vaccinated infants, whereas no chronic infections have been observed among adults who responded to vaccination. Thus hepatitis B vaccination provides long-term protection against clinical disease and chronic infection despite loss of detectable anti-HBs over time.

In studies conducted in immune-competent vaccinated populations where there is continued exposure to persons with chronic HBV infection, breakthrough infections detected by the presence of anti-HBc have been documented in a small percentage of persons (see Table 16–8).[366,368,376–380] However, these asymptomatic infections are unlikely to be a source of transmission to others and are not associated with development of chronic liver disease or HCC. Among immune-compromised persons such as hemodialysis patients, vaccine-induced protection (i.e., immune memory) appears

TABLE 16–7 ■ Studies of the Efficacy of Hepatitis B Vaccines in Neonates Born to Hepatitis B e Antigen–Positive Mothers

Study	HBIG at Birth	Vaccine*	Dose (µg)	Schedule (Age in mo)	No. of Subjects	HBsAg Positive (%)	Efficacy (%)†
Beasley et al.[354]	Yes	MSD-P	20	0, 1, 6	159	2.0–8.6	88–97
Lee et al.[172]	Yes	GSK-R	20	0, 1, 2, 12	54	7.4	89
	Yes	GSK-R	10	0, 1, 2, 12	56	1.8	97
	Yes	GSK-R	20	0, 1, 6	60	3.3	95
Lee et al.[461–465]	Yes	GSK-R	10	0, 1, 6	55	7	90
Lo et al.[356]	Yes	Pasteur	5	0, 1, 2, 12	72	8.1–11.4	84–88
Pongpipat et al.[357]	Yes	MSD-R	5	0, 1, 6	20	10.0	86
Poovorawan et al.[462]	Yes	GSK-R	10	0, 1, 2, 12	65	1.5	98
	Yes	GSK-R	10	0, 1, 6	60	0	100
Stevens et al.[361]	Yes	MSD-P	20	0, 1, 6	158	13.9	80
	Yes	MSD-P	10	0, 1, 6	152	10.9	84
	Yes	MSD-R	5	0, 1, 6	351	5.4	92
Wong et al.[168]	Yes	DRC-P	3	0, 1, 2, 6	124	9.2–14.4	79–87
Assateerawatt et al.[360]	No	MSD-R	2.5	0, 1, 2, 6	24	29	59
Beasley et al.[354]	No	MSD-P	20	0, 1, 6	40	22.5	68
Lo et al.[356]	No	Pasteur	5	0, 1, 2, 12	36	19.4	74
Milne et al.[463]	No	MSD-R	5	0, 1, 2	82	14.6	79
Moulia-Pelat et al.[464]	No	Pasteur-R	20	Mixed	16	6.2	91
Poovorawan et al.[360]	No	GSK-R	10	0, 1, 2, 12	59	3.4	95
	No	GSK-R	10	0, 1, 6	59	3.4	95
Tin[465]	No	MSD-P	20	0, 1, 2, 6	113	17.7	75
	No	MSD-P	10	0, 1, 6	58	12.1	83
	No	MSD-R	5	0, 1, 6	60	5	93
Wong et al.[168]	No	DRC-P	3	0, 1, 2, 6	64	24.3	65

*DRC, Dutch Red Cross; MSD, Merck, Sharpe & Dohme; P, plasma-derived; R, recombinant DNA; SKB, GlaxoSmithKline.
†Immunization efficacy calculation assumes 70% infection rate without postexposure prophylaxis.

to persist only as long as anti-HBs levels remain above 10 mIU/mL.[384] In these patients, annual anti-HBs testing is recommended and booster doses are required to maintain anti-HBs levels above 10 mIU/mL.[382]

The proposed mechanism for continued protection against clinically significant HBV infection, despite declining antibody titers, is an anamnestic immune response after HBV exposure.[383,384] An anamnestic response to a booster dose of vaccine has been demonstrated in greater than 95% of persons who responded to a primary vaccination series as infants, children, or adults and who lost detectable anti-HBs after 5 to 13 years.[385-396] A booster study in health care workers immunized 3–13 years previously showed uniform response to a single booster dose, suggesting that they would be protected if exposed to infection.[396a] These findings indicate that the immune system would be able to respond rapidly to HBV exposure. The long incubation period of HBV infection (6 weeks to 6 months), coupled with excellent anamnestic antibody response to low levels of HBsAg among previously immunized people, appears to limit breakthrough infections to those that do not produce detectable viremia, symptomatic disease, or chronic infection.

At present, vaccine advisory groups in the United States and in Europe do not recommend routine booster doses of hepatitis B vaccine or periodic serologic testing to monitor anti-HBs titers for immune-competent persons who have responded to vaccination.[382,397] Ongoing studies should provide information on the need for booster doses during the third decade after vaccination.

Prevention of Hepatocellular Carcinoma

In studies conducted in Taiwan, rates of HCC among cohorts of children born after routine infant immunization was started in the mid-1980s declined by greater than 50% (Fig. 16–12).[398,399] By comparison, rates of HCC in older age groups, and rates of other childhood cancers, remained stable or increased during this time period. These studies provide assurance that routine infant hepatitis B immunization is a well-conceived public health strategy that will benefit generations to come.

Side Effects

Hepatitis B vaccines have been shown to be safe when given to infants, children, adolescents, and adults. Globally, more than 1 billion hepatitis B vaccine doses have been administered, and in the United States more than 40 million infants and children and more than 30 million adults and adolescents have been vaccinated.

TABLE 16–8 ▪ Long-Term Protection from Hepatitis B Virus Infection Among Persons Who Responded to a Primary Vaccination Series

Group and Location	Persons Tested	Follow-up (yr)	Anti-HBs Loss (%)	HBV Infections	
				All, No. (%)	Chronic, No. (%)
INFANTS OF HBsAg/HBeAg-POSITIVE MOTHERS					
China[366]	74	9	49	7(9)	0(0)
China[377]	50	5	17	NA	1(2)
Taiwan[378]	199	6	3	0(0)	0(0)
Taiwan[466]	805	10	15	113(14)	3(0.4)
Taiwan[380]	165	5	17	11(7)	0(0)
Taiwan[364]	118	10	33	14(12)	0(0)
Thailand[462]	177	8	10	20(11)	0(0)
United States[361]	315	4–11	12	30(9)	0(0)
INFANTS AND YOUNG CHILDREN					
China[467-468]	318	12	20	2(0.7)	0(0)
Italy[307]	280	5	97	0(0)	0(0)
United States[372]	600	10	17	4(0.7)	0(0)
Venezuela[314]	280	6	29	6(2.1)	0(0)
The Gambia[136]	~700	7	25	(2.7)	0(0)
Samoa (unpublished data, CDC)	70	5	50	0(0)	0(0)
ADOLESCENTS AND ADULTS					
Germany—health care workers[468]	72	5	30	0(0)	0(0)
United States—men who have sex with men[361]	127	11	61	26(20)	0(0)
United States—men who have sex with men[371]	634	7–9	54	48(8)	0(0)
United States—Alaskan Natives[372]	272	10	38	6(2)	0(0)
France—health care workers[374]	143	5	7	4(3)	0(0)
New Zealand—adolescents[390]	173	5.5	7	0(0)	0(0)
Singapore—military personnel[373]	190	6	45	4(2)	0(0)
Singapore—medical and dental students[373]	100	5	19	1(6)	0(0)

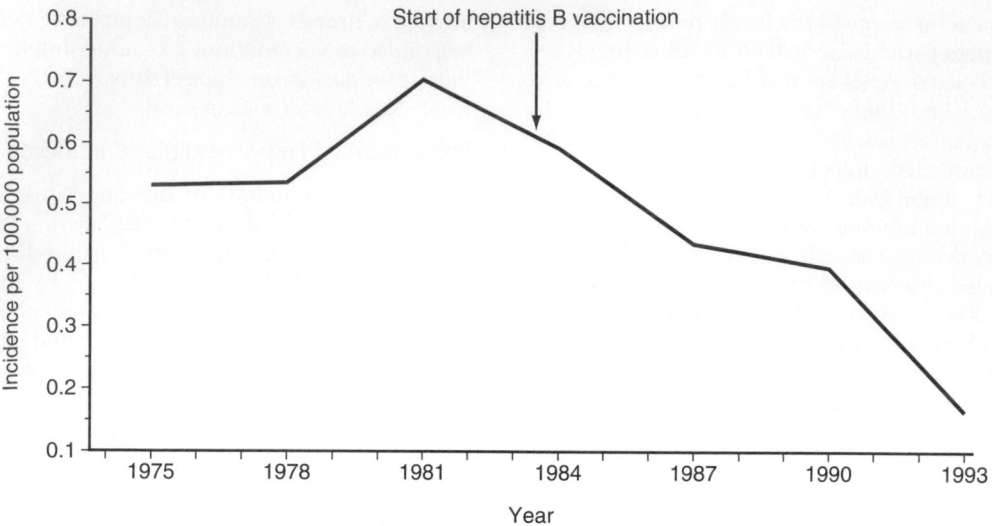

FIGURE 16–12 ■ Liver cancer death rates among children in Taiwan, 1975 to 1993. (Adapted from Lee CL, Ko YC. Hepatitis B vaccination and hepatocellular carcinoma in Taiwan. Pediatrics 99:351–353, 1997.)

Vaccine Reactogenicity

Local reactions to hepatitis B vaccine are generally mild and transient, lasting less than 24 hours. Pain at the injection site (3% to 29%) and temperature greater than 37.7°C (1% to 6%) are the most frequently reported side effects among adults and children receiving vaccine.[36,37,400] In placebo-controlled studies among adults, these side effects were reported no more frequently among persons receiving hepatitis B vaccine than among persons receiving placebo.[350,351] Among children receiving both hepatitis B vaccine and DTP vaccine, these mild side effects have been observed no more frequently than among children receiving DTP vaccine alone.[401] Although fever occasionally may occur after hepatitis B vaccination, administration of the vaccine soon after birth has not been associated with an increase in the number of febrile episodes or sepsis evaluations.[402]

Adverse Events

Numerous studies indicate that hepatitis B vaccines have an excellent safety profile. No serious adverse events were observed after hepatitis B vaccination in prelicensure clinical trials involving more than 200,000 recipients, including more than 50 studies of plasma-derived vaccines and studies of at least 12 separate recombinant vaccines.[403] In addition, evaluations of large-scale infant hepatitis B immunization programs in Alaska, Taiwan, New Zealand, and the United States have observed no association between vaccination and the occurrence of severe adverse events, including seizures, Guillain-Barré syndrome (GBS), or anaphylaxis.[403–407] Reports of serious adverse events after hepatitis B vaccination are exceedingly rare. However, reporting of an adverse event in temporal relationship with receipt of any vaccine, including hepatitis B vaccine, does not differentiate between a true causal association and a coincidental temporal relationship.

The most extensive review of possible serious adverse events after hepatitis B vaccination was conducted by the U.S. Institute of Medicine in 1993.[403] In this review, anaphylaxis was the only serious adverse event that met criteria for causality. For other serious adverse events that have been

rarely reported following hepatitis B vaccine, including GBS, demyelinating diseases of the central nervous system, arthritis, and sudden infant death syndrome, there was insufficient evidence to accept or reject a causal association.[408] Evaluating whether there is a causal relationship between these reported adverse events and hepatitis B vaccination is methodologically and logistically formidable because they are rare, and they occur in the absence of hepatitis B vaccination. In addition, most reported serious adverse events following hepatitis B vaccination have occurred in adults, and the peak incidence of these events in the absence of vaccination is in older age groups. Surveillance for vaccine-associated adverse events continues to be an important part of all immunization programs. Any presumed or confirmed risk of adverse events caused by hepatitis B vaccination must be balanced with the expected risk of HBV-related liver disease.

Early postlicensure surveillance of adverse events showed a possible association between GBS and receipt of the first vaccine dose of plasma-derived hepatitis B vaccine in adults in the United States.[409] In an analysis of GBS cases reported to the U.S. Centers for Disease Control and Prevention (CDC), the U.S. Food and Drug Administration, and vaccine manufacturers, among an estimated 2.5 million adults who received one or more doses of recombinant hepatitis B vaccine from 1986 to 1990, the rate of GBS did not exceed the background rate of this disease (unpublished data, CDC). In both of these studies, population-based rates for GBS derived from active surveillance studies were compared with rates derived from passive reporting of GBS, and cases reported after receipt of vaccine were not excluded even if other factors could have contributed to the disease. A study among more than 40,000 Alaskan Native children and adults given the same plasma-derived vaccine in which there was active surveillance for GBS cases also found no association between hepatitis B vaccination and GBS.[407]

A variety of chronic illnesses have been reported following hepatitis B vaccination, including demyelinating disorders (e.g., multiple sclerosis, optic neuritis, transverse myelitis),[410–412] chronic fatigue syndrome,[413] type 1 diabetes,[414] rheumatoid arthritis,[415,416] and autoimmune disorders.[417] In the mid-1990s, case-control studies conducted in

France found a possible association of recombinant hepatits B vaccine with multiple sclerosis that was not statistically significant.[418–420] These inconclusive findings led to a highly publicized decision by French health authorities to suspend school-based immunization of adolescents.[421] However, other studies have found no evidence of a causal association between hepatitis B immunization and the onset of multiple sclerosis, including a large case-control study among nurses,[422] a case-control study among members of three large U.S. managed care organizations,[423] and a study of the incidence of multiple sclerosis in adolescents before and after a hepatitis B vaccination program was begun.[424] A case-crossover study also showed no association between hepatitis B vaccination (and other vaccines) and short-term relapse in patients with multiple sclerosis.[425] In addition, expert panel reviews have concluded that available data do not demonstrate a causal association between hepatitis B vaccination and demyelinating diseases.[426,427] However, a report involving two episodes of leukoencephalitis in the same patient after hepatitis B vaccine has been published.[427a]

Controlled data on other chronic diseases that have been reported following hepatitis B immunization are limited. In one case-control study, no association was found between the receipt or timing of hepatitis B vaccine and the onset of diabetes mellitus in children.[428] Expert panel reviews have concluded that available data do not demonstrate a causal association between childhood vaccines, including hepatitis B vaccine, and type 1 diabetes.[429,430] Studies have also found no association of hepatitis B vaccination with an increased risk of asthma,[431] or wheezing lower respiratory disease.[432]

Case reports of anaphylaxis following hepatitis B vaccination have been recorded in the medical literature,[433] and a low rate of anaphylaxis has been observed in vaccine recipients based on reports to the Vaccine Adverse Events Reporting System (VAERS) in the United States, with an estimated incidence of 1 case in 600,000 vaccine doses distributed.[405] One anaphylactic reaction occurred in 43,358 adolescents vaccinated with recombinant vaccine in British Columbia, and no cases were observed among 166,757 children vaccinated with plasma-derived vaccine in New Zealand.[403] Although none of the persons who developed anaphylaxis died, anaphylaxis can be fatal, and hepatitis B vaccine may cause a life-threatening hypersensitivity reaction in certain individuals; therefore, further vaccination is contraindicated in persons with a history of anaphylaxis after a previous dose of hepatitis B vaccine.

Reports have been received by VAERS of alopecia in children and adults after administration of plasma-derived and recombinant hepatitis B vaccine, and some persons experienced hair loss following vaccination on more than one occasion.[434] Hair loss was temporary for more than two thirds of persons with follow-up information. Although a population-based epidemiologic study found no statistical association between alopecia and receipt of hepatitis B vaccine,[435] reported episodes of alopecia following rechallenge with hepatitis B vaccine suggest that vaccination may rarely trigger this event.

Rarely, infant deaths have been reported following hepatitis B vaccination[436]; however, available evidence indicates that hepatitis B vaccine is not causally associated with infant deaths. In a large case-control study conducted in New Zealand, no evidence was found that vaccination with hepatitis B vaccine or other vaccines increased the risk of sudden infant death syndrome (SIDS).[437] Another case-control study conducted in the United States found no evidence that newborn hepatitis B vaccination is associated with an increase in the number of febrile episodes, sepsis evaluations, or allergic or neurologic events.[438] Moreover, analyses of reports to VAERS have not found an increased frequency of reported adverse events, including SIDS, since implementation of routine infant hepatitis B vaccination in the United States.[436] Infant death rates, including rates of SIDS, have declined substantially in the United States during the 1990s, while infant hepatitis B vaccination coverage increased from less than 1% to greater than 90%.[436,439]

Contraindications to Vaccination

Hepatitis B vaccination is contraindicated for people with a history of allergic reactions to any vaccine component. In addition, people with a history of serious adverse events after receipt of hepatitis B vaccine should not receive additional doses. There is a theoretical contraindication to vaccination in people with allergy to *S. cerevisiae* (baker's yeast); however, there is little evidence documenting adverse reactions after vaccination of people with a history of yeast allergy. On the basis of limited data, there is no apparent risk of adverse events to developing fetuses when hepatitis B vaccine is administered to pregnant women.[440] In addition, the vaccine contains noninfectious HBsAg particles and should cause no risk to the fetus, and HBV infection affecting a pregnant woman may result in severe disease for the mother and chronic infection for the newborn. Therefore, neither pregnancy nor lactation should be a contraindication to vaccination of women at risk for infection.

Indications

Most of the serious consequences of HBV infection (i.e., liver cancer and cirrhosis) occur among persons with chronic HBV infection, and chronically infected persons serve as the main reservoir for the transmission of new infections. Thus the principal goal of hepatitis B immunization strategies is to reduce the prevalence of chronic HBV infections. A secondary goal is to prevent acute hepatitis B. Comprehensive hepatitis B immunization strategies prevent chronic HBV infections acquired in all age groups, and include the following components: routine infant vaccination, prevention of perinatal HBV transmission, and catch-up vaccination of persons not vaccinated as infants. The relative importance of each of these components varies depending on the epidemiology of HBV transmission in a particular country, including the proportion of chronic infections that are acquired in each age group. In addition to population-based immunization strategies, postexposure hepatitis B immunization is recommended for persons who have percutaneous and mucosal exposures to blood, for sexual contacts of persons with acute hepatitis B, and for household contacts with persons with acute hepatitis B if they have had a blood exposure to the index patient (i.e., sharing toothbrushes or razors). However, providing postexposure prophylaxis to these groups is expected to have little impact on the overall hepatitis B disease burden.

Routine Infant Vaccination

Routine infant immunization as an integral part of the childhood immunization schedule is a high priority in all countries because HBV transmission can be markedly reduced and potentially eliminated by attaining high hepatitis B vaccine coverage among successive cohorts of infants.[441] Even in countries with a low prevalence of chronic infection (see Fig. 16–11), a disproportionate number of persons with chronic HBV acquire their infection in early childhood when the risk of chronic infection is highest, emphasizing the importance of routine infant immunization as the key strategy. Many of these childhood infections occur among infants born to HBsAg-negative mothers, and would not be prevented by programs that screen pregnant women for HBsAg and provide immunoprophylaxis to infants born to HBsAg-positive mothers.[191,193] Long-term protection following infant vaccination is expected to last for decades and ultimately protect against infections acquired in all age groups.[383]

Prevention of Perinatal HBV Transmission

Postexposure immunization beginning at birth, with either hepatitis B vaccine alone or with hepatitis B vaccine and HBIG, is highly effective in preventing perinatal HBV transmission. Two different strategies can be used to prevent perinatal HBV transmission: (1) start the hepatitis B vaccine series for all infants at birth with a dose of vaccine that will prevent perinatal HBV transmission, or (2) screen all pregnant women for HBsAg and provide immunization at birth to infants of HBV-infected mothers. Use of a birth dose for all infants should be considered even in countries where pregnant women are screened for HBsAg in order to (1) safeguard against maternal hepatitis B testing errors and test reporting failures, (2) protect neonates discharged to households in which persons with chronic HBV infection other than the mother may reside, and (3) enhance the completion of the childhood immunization series.[442]

Catch-Up Vaccination

The implementation of routine infant immunization eventually will produce broad population-based immunity to HBV infection and prevent HBV transmission among all age groups. However, there may be a substantial disease burden from chronic infections acquired by older children, adolescents, and adults in countries with intermediate and low HBV endemicity. In these countries, vaccinating infants alone may not substantially lower the incidence of the disease for decades, and catch-up strategies targeted to unvaccinated persons in older age groups may be needed to hasten the development of population-based immunity and to more rapidly decrease the incidence of acute hepatitis B. Possible target groups for catch-up immunization include age-specific cohorts (e.g., routine immunization of young adolescents) and persons with risk factors for acquiring HBV infection.

In countries where chronic HBV infection is highly endemic, most infections are acquired among young children. In these countries, routine vaccination of infants rapidly reduces the transmission of HBV, and catch-up vaccination of older children is not usually required. It is particularly important that catch-up vaccination for older age groups in these countries should not hinder efforts to achieve a high level of completion of the vaccination series among infants and to prevent perinatal transmission with administration of a birth dose of hepatitis B vaccine.

U.S. Recommendations

In the United States, HBV transmission occurs in all age groups, and a comprehensive strategy is needed to provide widespread immunity and to effectively prevent HBV-related chronic liver disease. Beginning in the late 1980s, the Advisory Committee on Immunization Practices (ACIP) of the U.S. Public Health Service developed a comprehensive strategy to eliminate HBV transmission in the United States.[382,443] This strategy includes routine infant vaccination, screening of all pregnant women for HBsAg and provision of postexposure immunoprophylaxis beginning at birth to infants of HBsAg-positive mothers, catch-up vaccination of previously unvaccinated children and adolescents, and vaccination of adults in high-risk groups. Recommendations to vaccinate all infants were initially the subject of considerable debate among primary care providers in the United States, many of whom considered patients in their practice to be at low risk for acquiring HBV infection.[444] Providers also expressed concerns about the cost-effectiveness of infant vaccination and long-term protection after hepatitis B vaccination of infants, and routine adolescent vaccination was proposed as a more effective primary immunization strategy.[445] However, cost-effectiveness analysis has demonstrated that routine infant immunization is the most effective strategy to prevent HBV transmission in the United States because of the additional benefit in preventing early childhood transmission with infant immunization.[210] Despite the initial concerns of care providers, hepatitis B vaccination coverage of infants increased rapidly and reached levels as high as those observed for other childhood vaccines.[446] In 2000, more than 90% of children between 2 and 3 years of age had received three doses of hepatitis B vaccine.[447]

Recommendations by the ACIP for hepatitis B immunization in the United States are summarized below.

ROUTINE INFANT VACCINATION

1. Hepatitis B vaccination is recommended for all infants and should be completed by 18 months of age.
2. All infants should receive the first dose of hepatitis B vaccine soon after birth and before hospital discharge; the first dose also may be given by age 2 months, but only if the infant's mother is verified to be HBsAg negative.
3. Only monovalent hepatitis B vaccine can be used for the birth dose. Either monovalent hepatitis B vaccine or a combination vaccine containing hepatitis B vaccine may be used to complete the series; four doses of vaccine may be administered if the first dose is given at birth.
4. The second dose should be given at least 4 weeks after the first dose (except for Hib- and DTP-containing combination vaccines, which cannot be administered before age 6 weeks). The third dose should be given at least 16 weeks after the first dose and at least 8 weeks after the second dose. The last dose in the vaccination series (third or fourth dose) should not be administered before age 6 months.

PREVENTION OF PERINATAL HBV INFECTION

1. All pregnant women should be routinely tested for HBsAg during an early prenatal visit in *each* pregnancy. Testing should be repeated in late pregnancy for HBsAg-negative women at high risk of HBV infection (e.g., injection drug users, persons with intercurrent STDs, persons with multiple sexual partners) or who have had clinical hepatitis.

2. Infants born to HBsAg-positive mothers should receive monovalent hepatitis B vaccine (see Table 16–3) and HBIG (0.5 mL) within 12 hours of birth, administered at different sites. These infants should be provided case management in order to ensure (1) timely completion of the hepatitis B vaccination series, and (2) postvaccination testing for anti-HBs and HBsAg following the completion of the vaccine series at 9 to 15 months of age. Postvaccination testing is important to determine the success of immunoprophylaxis and to identify HBV-infected infants who require further medical management. Testing at 9 to 15 months of age minimizes the likelihood of detecting passively transferred anti-HBs from HBIG and maximizes the likelihood of detecting late HBsAg-positive infections. Infants who are anti-HBs positive and HBsAg negative are protected and do not need further medical management. Infants found to be anti-HBs and HBsAg negative should be revaccinated. Infants found to be HBsAg positive should be referred for medical management. All infants born to HBsAg-positive mothers can be breast-fed.

3. Women admitted for delivery without prenatal HBsAg testing should have blood drawn for testing. While test results are pending, the infant should receive hepatitis B vaccine within 12 hours of birth.

   a. If the mother is later found to be *HBsAg positive*, her infant should receive HBIG as soon as possible, but not after 7 days following birth. These infants should be tracked with active case management to ensure that the vaccination series is completed and postvaccination testing is done (see item 2 above).

   b. If the mother is found to be *HBsAg negative* or is never tested for HBsAg, her infant should complete the hepatitis B vaccine series as part of the routine vaccination schedule (see Table 16–4).

ROUTINE VACCINATION OF CHILDREN AND ADOLESCENTS

1. Hepatitis B vaccination is recommended for all children and adolescents (18 years of age and younger).

2. To ensure comprehensive vaccination coverage of adolescents, it is recommended that providers offer hepatitis vaccine to all adolescents at 11 to 12 years of age.

TABLE 16–9 ▪ Groups at Increased Risk for HBV Infection for Whom Hepatitis B Vaccination Is Recommended, United States

Group	Comments
Persons at increased risk of sexually transmitted HBV infection	Includes persons with more than one sex partner in the previous 6 mo, persons diagnosed with a recently acquired sexually transmitted disease
Men who have sex with men	
Injection drug users	
Household contacts and sexual partners of HBsAg-positive people	All household contacts, including infants, children, adolescents, and adults
People at occupational risk of infection through exposure to blood or blood-contaminated body fluid	Includes health care workers; public safety workers; trainees in health care fields in schools of medicine, dentistry, nursing, laboratory technology, and other allied health professions
Clients and staff of institutions for developmentally disabled persons	
Hemodialysis patients and patients with early renal failure before they require hemodialysis	The need for booster doses of vaccine in this group should be assessed by annual antibody testing and a booster dose given when antibody to hepatitis B surface antigen levels fall below 10 MIU/mL.
Patients who receive clotting-factor concentrates	Vaccine should be offered as soon as their specific clotting disorder is identified.
Adoptees and immigrants from countries where chronic HBV infection is of high or intermediate endemicity (see Fig. 16–11)	These individuals should be tested for HBsAg; if they are found to be HBsAg positive, all family members should be vaccinated.
International travelers	Includes persons who will be in areas where chronic HBV infection is of high or intermediate endemicity (see Fig. 16–11) for >6 mo, or who will be in these areas for any time period and have close contact with the local population, contact with blood (e.g., in a medical setting), or sexual contact with residents
Inmates of correctional facilities	Persons in juvenile and adult facilities, including jails, should be vaccinated.

TABLE 16–10 ■ Settings Where Hepatitis B Vaccine Should Be Routinely Offered, United States

Setting	Group Hepatitis B Vaccine Should Be Offered to
Sexuality transmitted disease clinics	All clients
HIV/AIDS testing and counseling programs	All clients
Correctional facilities (e.g., prisons, jails, juvenile detention)	All inmates; all staff with a risk of of percutaneous or permucosal exposures to blood or body fluids
Clinics for treatment of persons with HIV infection	All clients
Drug use prevention, treatment, and harm reduction clinics and programs (including needle-exchange programs)	All clients
Institutions for developmentally disabled persons	All clients and staff
Nonresidential day care programs for developmentally disabled persons (e.g., schools, sheltered workshops)	Staff should be vaccinated in settings attended by developmentally disabled persons known to be HBsAg positive. Classmates/attendees should be vaccinated if an HBsAg-positive client behaves aggressively or has special medical problems.
Health care facilities	All staff with a risk of percutaneous or permucosal exposures to blood or body fluids
Dialysis settings	All clients and staff

AIDS, acquired immunodeficiency syndrome.

VACCINATION OF ADOLESCENTS AND ADULTS IN HIGH-RISK GROUPS AND SETTINGS

1. Persons with risk factors for HBV infection should be vaccinated using the age-appropriate vaccine dose and schedule if not previously vaccinated as an infant, young child, or adolescent (Table 16–9).
2. Hepatitis B vaccination should be routinely offered to persons in high-risk settings (Table 16–10).

Immunization of Special Populations

ALASKAN NATIVES, PACIFIC ISLANDERS, AND FIRST-GENERATION IMMIGRANT POPULATIONS

In populations known to previously or currently have high rates of childhood HBV infection (i.e., Alaskan Natives, Pacific Islanders, and infants in immigrant or refugee families from countries in which HBV is of intermediate or high endemicity) (see Fig. 16–11), special efforts should be made to (1) ensure that hepatitis B vaccination is started at birth and completed for all infants by 12 months of age, and (2) ensure high vaccination coverage rates among children and adolescents who were not previously vaccinated at birth.

FAMILY MEMBERS OF INTERNATIONAL ADOPTEES

International adoptees and children who have immigrated from countries with intermediate and high endemicity of HBV infection (see Fig. 16–11) should be tested for HBsAg, and children determined to be HBsAg-positive should be monitored for the development of liver disease. Household members of HBsAg-positive children should be vaccinated. A child whose records indicate receipt of three or more doses of vaccine can be considered protected, and additional doses are not needed if at least one dose has been administered at 6 months of age or greater. Children who received their last hepatitis B vaccine dose at age less than 6 months should receive an additional dose at age 6 months or greater. Those who have received fewer than three doses should complete the series at the recommended intervals and ages (see Table 16–4).

PREMATURE INFANTS

Premature infants born to HBsAg-positive mothers must receive immunoprophylaxis with hepatitis B vaccine and hepatitis B immunoglobulin (HBIG) within 12 hours after birth. If these infants weigh less than 2,000 grams at birth, the initial vaccine dose should not be counted towards completion of the hepatitis B vaccine series, and three additional doses of hepatitis B vaccine should be administered, beginning when the infant is age 1 month.

For preterm infants born to mothers not tested for HbsAg during pregnancy, the maternal HBsAg status should be determined as soon as possible after delivery, and the infant should receive hepatitis B vaccine within 12 hours after birth. If these infants weigh less than 2,000 grams at birth, HBIG (0.5 mL) should also be given if the mother's HBsAg test result is not available within the initial 12 hours of birth, because of the potentially reduced immunogenicity of vaccine in these infants. In addition, the initial vaccine dose should not be counted toward the completion of the hepatitis B vaccine series, and three additional doses of hepatitis B vaccine should be administered, beginning when the infant is age 1 month.

If the infant's mother is assured to be HBsAg negative, premature infants with a birth weight of less than 2,000 grams can receive the first dose of the hepatitis B vaccine series at chronological age 1 month. Premature infants discharged from the hospital before chronological age 1 month also may be administered hepatitis B vaccine at discharge, if they are medically stable and have gained weight consistently.

POPULATIONS IN WHICH SCREENING OF PREGNANT WOMEN IS NOT FEASIBLE

In populations in which it is not feasible to screen pregnant women for HBsAg, *all* infants should receive their first dose of hepatitis B vaccine within 12 hours of birth, and should complete the hepatitis B vaccination series as part of the routine vaccination schedule, with the last dose administered no later than 12 months of age. Use of HBIG is not indicated in these populations.

Postexposure Prophylaxis

PERCUTANEOUS OR PERMUCOSAL EXPOSURES

After a percutaneous (needle stick, laceration, bite) or permucosal (ocular, mucous membrane) exposure to blood that contains or might contain HBV, the following should be done[448]:

1. Obtain a blood sample from the person who was the source of the exposure to determine his or her HBsAg status.
2. Review the vaccination and anti-HBs response status of the exposed person.

Prophylaxis for exposed people is dependent on the HBsAg status of the source patient and the immunization status of the exposed person (Table 16–11).

SEXUAL PARTNERS OF PEOPLE WITH ACUTE HEPATITIS B VIRUS INFECTION

All susceptible sexual partners of people with acute HBV infection should receive a single dose of HBIG (0.06 mL/kg) and should begin the hepatitis B vaccine series if prophylaxis can be started within 14 days of the last sexual contact.

HOUSEHOLD CONTACTS OF PEOPLE WITH ACUTE HEPATITIS B

An unvaccinated infant whose mother or primary caregiver has acute hepatitis B should receive HBIG (0.5 mL) and vaccination should be begun. For infants who have begun the hepatitis B vaccine series, no additional treatment is needed, and vaccination should be completed on schedule. Prophylaxis for other household contacts of people with acute HBV infection is not indicated unless a blood exposure to the index patient is identified (e.g., sharing toothbrushes or razors). Such exposures should be treated similarly to sexual exposures. If the index patient becomes chronically infected with HBV, all household contacts should be vaccinated.

Public Health Considerations

Worldwide, the prevention of chronic HBV infection has become a high priority as the consequences of acute and chronic HBV infection have been recognized to be a major public health problem. Approximately 30% of the world's population (i.e., about 2 billion people) have serologic evidence of infection with HBV.[449] Of these, 350 million have chronic HBV infection, about 500,000 to 750,000 of whom die each year from chronic liver disease. HBV is the leading cause of chronic hepatitis, cirrhosis, and HCC worldwide, and is second only to tobacco as a known human carcinogen.[226]

The acute and chronic outcomes of HBV infection also cause substantial morbidity and mortality in the United States. In the two decades prior to the introduction of routine infant hepatitis B immunization in the United States in 1991, approximately 200,000 to 300,000 persons were infected with HBV annually, and the average lifetime risk of

TABLE 16–11 ■ **Recommendations for Postexposure Immunoprophylaxis Following Percutaneous or Permucosal Exposure to Hepatitis B Virus, United States**

Vaccination and Antibody Response Status of Exposed Person	Treatment When Source Is:		
	HBsAg positive	HBsAg negative	Not tested or status unknown
Unvaccinated	HBIG* (1 dose), initiate HepB vaccination series	Initiate HepB vaccination series	Initiate HepB vaccination series
Previously vaccinated			
Known responder[†]	No treatment	No treatment	No treatment
Known nonresponder, no revaccination	HBIG (1 dose) and initiate revaccination[‡]	No treatment, consider revaccination[‡] for future protection	If known high-risk source, treat as if source is HBsAg positive
Known nonresponder to initial and revaccination series	HBIG × 2—second dose one month after first	No treatment	If known high-risk source, treat as if source is HBsAg positive
Antibody response unknown	Test exposed person for anti-HBs[§] 1. If adequate, no treatment 2. If inadequate, HBIG × 1 and initiate revaccination,[‡] evaluate antibody response at 6 mo[∥]	No testing, no treatment	Test exposed person for anti-HBs[§] 1. If adequate, no treatment 2. If inadequate, initiate revaccination,[‡] evaluate antibody response at 2–6 mo

*Hepatitis B immune globulin dose 0.06 mL/kg administered intramuscularly.
[†]Responder to hepatitis B vaccine is a person with antibody to hepatitis B surface antigen (anti-HBs) titer 10 mIU/mL or greater.
[‡]Revaccination with three-dose series.
[§]Adequate response is anti-HBs titer 10 mIU/mL or greater; inadequate response is less than 10 mIU/mL.
[∥]Testing before 6 months may detect passively acquired anti-HBs from HBIG.

HBV infection was approximately 5%.[450,451] In addition, approximately 1.25 million persons remain chronically infected and about 4000 to 5000 people die each year from HBV-related liver disease.[452] Approximately 300 of these deaths are due to fulminant hepatitis, 3000 to 4000 to cirrhosis, and 600 to 1000 to primary HCC.[179] Annually, HBV-related liver disease is estimated to produce medical and work-loss costs of at least $700 million. Cost–benefit analysis has shown that perinatal hepatitis B prevention and routine infant hepatitis B immunization can save $1 in medical and work-loss costs for each $1 spent on immunization.[210]

Since 1992, the WHO has called for all countries to add hepatitis B vaccine into their national childhood immunization services,[453,454] and substantial progress has been made in implementing this recommendation. In 2000, more than 100 countries adopted routine childhood hepatitis B vaccination, an increase from 20 countries in 1990. In addition, estimated infant hepatitis B vaccination coverage globally increased from less than 1% to greater than 30% from 1990 to 2000 (unpublished data, WHO/UNICEF). However, many low-income countries in sub-Saharan Africa and the Indian subcontinent did not introduce the vaccine during this period. The high cost of hepatitis B vaccine compared to other childhood vaccines included in the Expanded Programme on Immunization has historically been one of the main obstacles to its introduction in many of these countries.

In order to address inequities in the availability of hepatitis B vaccine in developing countries, the Global Alliance for Vaccines and Immunization (GAVI) and the Vaccine Fund began in 2000 to provide technical and financial support to introduce hepatitis B vaccine into national immunization services in 71 of the world's poorest countries. In addition, the cost of hepatitis B vaccine decreased dramatically during the 1990s from $3 to $6 per dose to $0.25 to $0.50 per dose (unpublished data, UNICEF). These factors have catalyzed a dramatic increase in the number of economically disadvantaged countries that have introduced routine infant hepatitis B vaccination. Since GAVI efforts began, more than 40 countries have introduced hepatitis B vaccine, and by 2003 more than 160 countries worldwide will have introduced the vaccine (Fig. 16–13). Special GAVI hepatitis B vaccination programs also have been started in China, India, and Indonesia, which represent approximately one third of the global birth cohort. In China, all newborns are expected to be eligible to receive hepatitis B vaccine free of charge within 5 years as part of the national immunization program. Presently, parents are required to pay for the vaccine. In India, 45 demonstration projects have been designed to transition the country into full integration of hepatitis B vaccination into the national immunization program during the next 5 years. In Indonesia, all newborns are expected to be eligible to get a birth dose of hepatitis B vaccine (usually at home) with Uniject™.

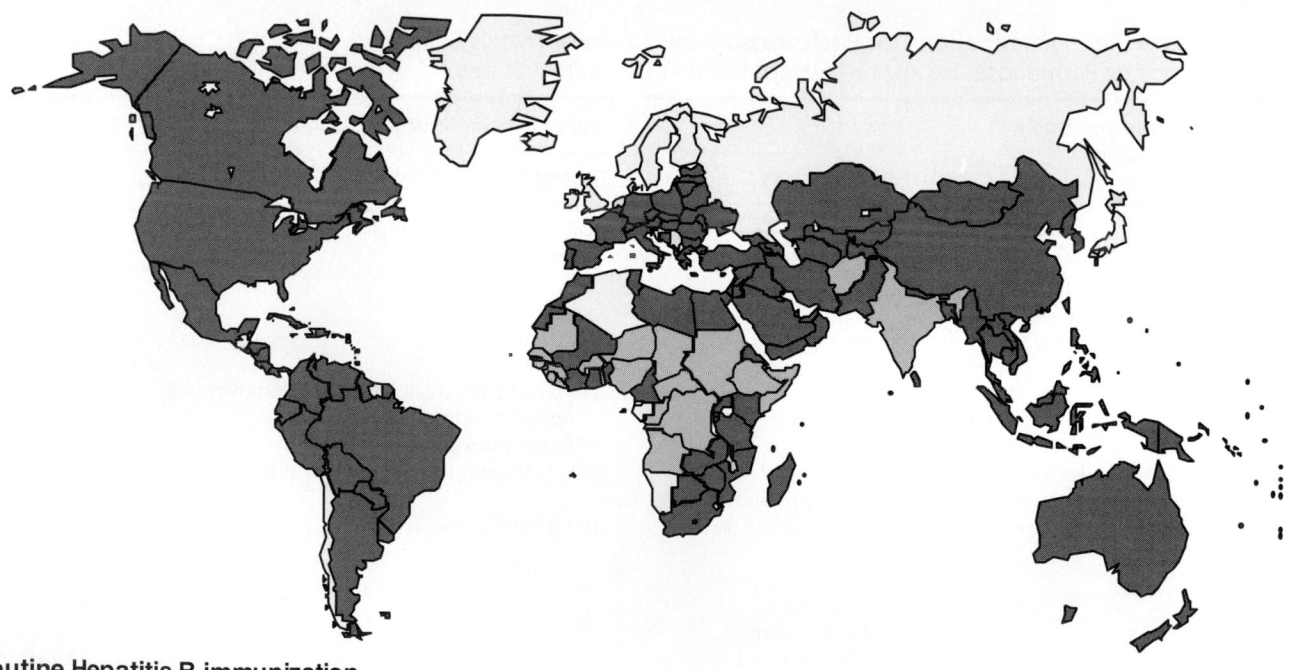

Routine Hepatitis B immunization

■ **Yes (N=165)** Includes countries with funding from The Vaccine Fund and plans to introduce vaccine in 2003

■ **No, eligible for The Vaccine Fund (N = 23)**

■ **No, not eligible for The Vaccine Fund (N = 26)**

FIGURE 16–13 ■ Countries using hepatitis B vaccine in their national childhood immunization schedule, 2003. (NOTE: The boundaries shown on this map do not imply the expression of any opinion whatsoever on the part of the World Health Organization concerning the legal status of any country, territory, city, or area or of its authorities, or concerning the delimitation of its frontiers or boundaries. Dotted lines on maps represent approximate border lines for which there may not yet be full agreement.) (Data from Expanded Programme on Immunization, World Health Organization.)

In addition to routine infant vaccination, the WHO recommends considering administration of a dose at birth to prevent perinatal HBV transmission. The priority for preventing perinatal HBV transmission in a particular country needs to take into account the relative contribution of perinatal transmission to the overall hepatitis B disease burden and the feasibility of delivering the first dose of hepatitis B vaccine at birth. In general, it is most feasible to deliver the vaccine at birth to infants who are born in health facilities. The WHO recommends that, in countries where a high proportion of chronic HBV infections is acquired perinatally (e.g., east and southeast Asia, Pacific Islands), a birth dose should be given to infants who are delivered in hospitals when hepatitis B vaccine is introduced into national immunization programs. Efforts also should be made in these countries to give hepatitis B vaccine as soon as possible after birth to infants delivered at home. In countries where a low proportion of chronic HBV infections is acquired perinatally (e.g., Africa), administration of a birth dose may be considered after evaluating the relative contribution of perinatal HBV infections to the overall disease burden, and the feasibility and cost-effectiveness of providing a birth dose.

In countries where a birth dose of hepatitis B vaccine is used to prevent perinatal HBV transmission, effective strategies have to be designed and implemented in order to deliver the vaccine. Hepatitis B vaccine can be administered at the same time as other vaccines that may be given close to the time of birth, including BCG and OPV. However, in order to prevent perinatal transmission, hepatitis B vaccine must be given as close as possible to the time of delivery, preferably within 24 hours. The design of strategies for administering the birth dose therefore must consider the roles of both obstetric staff (e.g., obstetricians, midwives, and birth attendants) and immunization service providers. In many developing countries, a high proportion of infants are born at home, which presents additional challenges to delivering hepatitis B vaccine at birth. Some of the prerequisites for providing hepatitis B vaccine for infants delivered at home may include motivated health staff, receptive communities, timely notification of births, adequate transport allowances, attention to cold chain issues, availability of single-dose vials of hepatitis B vaccine (e.g., Uniject™), and ensuring that injections can be safely administered. Home visits with serologic follow up may be necessary in disadvantaged populations to insure complete vaccination.[454a]

The effectiveness of routine infant hepatitis B immunization in significantly reducing or eliminating the prevalence of chronic HBV infection has been demonstrated in a variety of countries and settings. In general, studies conducted in high-HBV-endemicity areas have demonstrated declines in the prevalence of chronic HBV among children to less than 2% after introduction of the vaccine (Table 16–12). The greatest impact has been achieved in countries that have achieved high vaccine coverage among infants, and where a birth dose of vaccine was administered. In Alaska, where high vaccine coverage among infants has been achieved and all infants receive a birth dose of vaccine, HBV transmission among children has been eliminated.[441] The experience in Taiwan is particularly impressive. Universal vaccination decreased the prevalence of HBsAg carriage in children younger than 15 years of age from 9.8% in 1984 to 0.7% in 1999.[479] Careful studies have shown that exposed vaccinated children resist chronic hepatis B infection.[480] Similar results have been achieved in Gambia[481] and South Africa.[482] In South Africa, despite universal vaccination, escape variants of S antigen have not appeared.[483] The same conclusion was reached in Italy.[484] Many long-term hepatitis B immunization programs have demonstrated a greater than expected benefit in terms of disease reduction when compared with levels of vaccination coverage. A possible reason for this finding is that the pool of individuals who are highly infectious to others is greatly reduced by preventing chronic infections in children. Not only are new infections in children more likely to become chronic, but chronically infected children are likely to be HBeAg positive and highly infectious to others. Thus, by preventing infections in children, the number of HBeAg-positive persons declines rapidly over time because of the inherent clearance of HBeAg in older persons.

TABLE 16–12 ■ Studies Evaluating the Effectiveness of Routine Infant Hepatitis B Immunization in Reducing the Prevalence of Chronic HBV Infection in Children

Study and Site	No. Tested*	Follow-Up (yr)	Vaccine Coverage (%)	% with Chronic Infection Before	After
Alaska[441]	268	1–10	96	16	0.0
Rural China[469]	10,399	1–9	NA	14.6	1.6
FSM[†470]	364	3–4	82	NA[‡]	1.1
FSM[†470]	544	2	37	12	2.9
The Gambia[471]	675	9	100	10	0.6
Indonesia[472]	2519	4	>90	6.2	1.9
Saipan[464]	200	3–4	94	9	0.5
Samoa[473]	435	7–8	87	7	0.5
Saudi Arabia[474]	4791	1–8	85	6.7	0.3
Shanghai, China[469]	3193	1–9	NA	8.8	0.5
Taiwan[475]	424	7–10	73	10	1.1
Taiwan[476]	1337	7	90	9.7	0.7
Taiwan[477]	1500	6	92	10.5	1.7
Thailand[478]	3373	0–5	90	5.4	0.8

*Number of subjects tested in follow-up serosurveys after implementation of program.
†Federated States of Micronesia.
‡Not available.

Unlike the situation with other vaccine-preventable diseases, monitoring the efficacy of hepatitis B prevention programs is not based solely on surveillance of acute disease. In particular, because most infections in children are asymptomatic, acute disease surveillance will not reliably measure the initial impact of routine infant vaccination. However, trends in acute hepatitis B disease incidence can be used to evaluate the effectiveness of programs directed at adolescents and adults, who are more likely to have symptomatic infections after HBV exposure.[212,252,455] Because most of the HBV-associated morbidity and mortality is related to chronic infection, demonstrating a reduction in the prevalence of chronic infection in children is the major early indicator of program success. The serious adverse outcomes that are related to the acquisition of chronic HBV infection occur several decades after exposure; thus much of the benefit of infant immunization in prevention of cirrhosis and liver cancer will not be realized for decades after a program is started.

In 1993, the International Task Force for Disease Elimination proposed the elimination of chronic HBV infection as an achievable public health strategy.[456] Commitment of public health resources to eliminate HBV transmission will require recognition of the importance of this disease, persistent efforts to ensure that populations are protected, and patience to realize the goals of disease reduction, but the goal is achievable.[485]

REFERENCES

1. Lurman A. Eine icterus Epidemic. Berl Klin Woschenschr 22:20–23, 1885.
2. Ruge H. Die Zusammenhönge zwischen Syphilis, Salvarsan und der Sog: Katarrhalischen Gelbsucht auf Grund von 2500 der Marine von 1919–1929 beobachteten Föllen. Dermatol Wochenschr 94:278–286, 1932.
3. Sofer LJ. Postarsphenamine jaundice. Am J Syph 21:309–338, 1937.
4. MacCallum FO. Jaundice in syphilitics. Br J Vener Dis 19:63, 1943.
5. Murray DH. Acriflavine, its use by intravenous injection, in treatment of gonorrhea. J R Army Med Corps 54:19–27, 1930.
6. Flaum A, Malmros H, Persson E. Eine nosocomiale Ikterus Epidemic. Acta Med Scand 16(suppl):544–553, 1926.
7. Sherwood PM. Outbreak of syringe-transmitted hepatitis with jaundice in hospital diabetic patients. Ann Intern Med 33:380–396, 1950.
8. Droller H. An outbreak of hepatitis in a diabetic clinic. Br Med J 1:623–625, 1945.
9. Anonymous. Jaundice following yellow fever vaccination. JAMA 119:110, 1942.
10. Findlay GM, MacCallum FO. Note on acute hepatitis and yellow fever immunization. Trans R Soc Trop Med Hyg 51:297–308, 1937.
11. Beeson PB, Chesney G, McFarlan AM. Hepatitis following injection of mumps convalescent plasma. 1. Use of plasma in the mumps epidemic. Lancet 1:814–815, 1944.
12. McFarlan AM, Chesney G. Hepatitis following injection of mumps convalescent plasma. II. Epidemiology of the hepatitis. Lancet 1:816–817, 1944.
13. Propert SA. Hepatitis after prophylactic serum. Br Med J 2:677–678, 1938.
14. Beeson PB. Jaundice occurring one to four months after transfusion of blood or plasma: report of seven cases. JAMA 121:1332–1334, 1943.
15. Neefe JR, Gellis SS, Stokes J. Homologous serum hepatitis and infectious (epidemic) hepatitis: studies in volunteers bearing on immunological and other characteristics of etiologic agents. Am J Med Sci 1:3–22, 1946.
16. MacCallum FO, Bauer DJ. Homologous serum jaundice: transmission experiments with human volunteers. Lancet 1:622–627, 1944.
17. Voegt H. Zur Aetiologie der Hepatitis Epidemica. Munchen Med Wochenschr 89:76–79, 1942.
18. Cameron JDS. Infective hepatitis. Q J Med 12:139–155, 1943.
19. Medical Research Council. Infective Hepatitis: Studies in East Anglia during the Period 1943–1947 (Special Report Series, No 273). London, His Majesty's Stationery Office, 1937, 1951.
20. Havens WP. The etiology of infectious hepatitis. JAMA 134:653–655, 1947.
21. MacCallum FO. Homologous serum hepatitis. Lancet 2:691–692, 1947.
22. Zuckerman AJ. The history of viral hepatitis from antiquity to the present. In Deinhardt F, Deinhardt J (eds). Viral Hepatitis: Laboratory and Clinical Science. New York, Marcel Dekker, 1983, pp 3–32.
23. Seefe LB, Beebe GW, Hoofnagle JH, et al. A serologic follow-up of the 1942 epidemic of post-vaccination hepatitis in the United States Army. N Engl J Med 316:965–970, 1987.
24. Krugman S, Giles JP, Hammond J. Infectious hepatitis: evidence for 2 distinctive clinical, epidemiological and immunological types of infection. JAMA 200:365–373, 1967.
25. Krugman S, Giles JP. Viral hepatitis, type B (MS-2 strain): further observations on natural history and prevention. N Engl J Med 288:755–760, 1973.
26. Giles JP, McCollum RW, Berndtson LW, Krugman S. Viral hepatitis: relationship of Australia-SH antigen to the Willowbrook MS-2 strain. N Engl J Med 281:119–122, 1969.
27. Blumberg BS, Alter HJ, Visnich S. A "new" antigen in leukemia sera. JAMA 191:541–546, 1967.
28. Prince AM. An antigen detected in the blood of patients during the incubation period of serum hepatitis. Proc Natl Acad Sci U S A 60:814–821, 1968.
29. Dane DS, Cameroon CH, Briggs M. Virus-like particles in the serum of patients with Australia-antigen–associated hepatitis. Lancet 1:695–698, 1970.
30. Blumberg BS. A serum antigen (Australia antigen) in Down's syndrome, leukemia, and hepatitis. Ann Intern Med 66:924–931, 1967.
31. Krugman S, Giles JP, Hammond J. Viral hepatitis type B: prevention with specific hepatitis B immune serum globulin. JAMA 218:1665–1670, 1971.
32. Krugman S, Giles JP, Hammond JP. Viral hepatitis: effect of heat on the infectivity and antigenicity of the MS-1 and MS-2 strains. J Infect Dis 122:432–436, 1970.
33. Krugman S, Giles JP, Hammond J. Viral hepatitis type B MS-2 strain: studies on active immunization. JAMA 217:41–45, 1971.
34. Hilleman MR, Buynak EB, Roehm RR, et al. Purified and inactivated human hepatitis B vaccine: a progress report. Am J Med Sci 270:401–404, 1975.
35. Purcell RH, Gerin JL. Hepatitis B subunit vaccine: a preliminary report of safety and efficacy in chimpanzees. Am J Med Sci 270:395–399, 1975.
36. Zajac BA, West DJ, McAleer WJ, Scolnick EM. Overview of clinical studies with hepatitis B vaccine made by recombinant DNA. J Infect 13(suppl A):39–45, 1986.
37. Andre FE. Summary of safety and efficacy data on a yeast-derived hepatitis B vaccine. Am J Med 87(suppl 3A):14S–20S, 1989.
38. Beasley RP, Hwang L-Y. Overview on the epidemiology of hepatocellular carcinoma. In Hollinger FB, Lemon SM, Margolis HS (eds). Viral Hepatitis and Liver Disease. Proceedings of the 1990 International Symposium on Viral Hepatitis and Liver Disease: Contemporary Issues and Future Prospects. Baltimore, Williams & Wilkins, 1991, pp 532–535.
39. Beasley RP. Hepatitis B virus: the major etiology of hepatocellular carcinoma. Cancer 61:1942–1956, 1988.
40. International Agency for Research on Cancer. Hepatitis Viruses (IARC Monographs on the Evaluation of Carcinogenic Risks to Humans, Vol 59). Lyon, France, International Agency for Research on Cancer, 1994.
41. Parkin DM (ed). Cancer Occurrence in Developing Countries (Scientific Publication No 75). Lyon, France, International Agency for Research on Cancer, 1986.
42. Schafer DF, Sorrell MF. Hepatocellular carcinoma. Lancet 353:1253–1257, 1999.
43. Wright TL, Lau JY. Clinical aspects of hepatitis B virus infection. Lancet 342:1340–1344, 1993.
44. McMahon BJ, Alward WL, Hall DB, et al. Acute hepatitis B virus infection: relation of age to the clinical expression of disease and subsequent development of the carrier state. J Infect Dis 151:599–603, 1985.
45. Edmunds WJ, Medley GF, Nokes DJ, et al. The influence of age on the development of the hepatitis B carrier state. Proc R Soc Lond B Biol Sci 253:197–201, 1993.
46. Hyams KC. Risk of chronicity following acute hepatitis B virus infection: a review. Clin Infect Dis 20:992–1000, 1995.
47. Hadler SC, Judson FN, O'Malley PM, et al. Outcome of hepatitis B virus infection in homosexual men and its relation to prior human immunodeficiency virus infection. J Infect Dis 163:454–459, 1991.

48. Polish LB, Shapiro CN, Bauer F, et al. Nosocomial transmission of hepatitis B virus associated with the use of a spring-loaded fingerstick device. N Engl J Med 326:721–725, 1992.

49. Gilbert RD, Wiggelinkhuizen J. The clinical course of hepatitis B virus-associated nephropathy. Pediatr Nephrol 8:11–14, 1994.

50. Gianotti F. Papular acrodermatitis of childhood: an Australia antigen disease. Arch Dis Child 48:794–799, 1973.

51. Caputo R, Gelmetti C, Ermacora E, et al. Gianotti-Crosti syndrome: a retrospective analysis of 308 cases. J Am Acad Dermatol 26:207–210, 1992.

52. McSweeny PA, Carter JM, Green GJ, Romeril KR. Partial aplastic anemia associated with hepatitis B viral infection. Am J Med 85:255–256, 1988.

53. Dienstag JL. Immunogenesis of extrahepatic manifestations of hepatitis. Springer Semin Immunopathol 3:461–472, 1982.

54. Hepatitis Surveillance Report No 57. Atlanta, Centers for Disease Control and Prevention, 2000.

55. Pappas SC. Fulminant viral hepatitis. Gastroenterol Clin North Am 24:161–173, 1995.

56. Hoofnagle JH, Carithers RL, Shapiro C, Ascher N. Fulminant hepatic failure: summary of a workshop. Hepatology 21:240–252, 1995.

57. Smedile A, Farci P, Verme G, et al. Influence of delta infection on severity of hepatitis B. Lancet 2:945, 1982.

58. Bernuau J, Gordeau A, Poynard T, et al. Multivariate analysis of prognostic factors in fulminant hepatitis. Hepatology 6:648–651, 1986.

59. Hoofnagle JH. Chronic hepatitis B. N Engl J Med 323:337–339, 1990.

60. Lok ASF, Lai CL. A longitudinal follow-up of asymptomatic hepatitis B surface antigen-positive Chinese children. Hepatology 5:1130–1133, 1988.

61. Hoofnagle JH, Dusheiko GM, Seeff LB, et al. Seroconversion from hepatitis B e antigen to antibody in chronic type B hepatitis. Ann Intern Med 94:744–748, 1981.

62. Chang MH, Hwang LY, Hsu HC, et al. Prospective study of asymptomatic HBsAg carrier children infected in the perinatal period: clinical and liver histologic studies. Hepatology 8:374–377, 1988.

63. Liaw YF, Chu CM, Huang MJ, et al. Determinants for hepatitis B e antigen clearance in chronic type B hepatitis. Liver 4:301–306, 1984.

64. Lok AS, Lai CL, Wu PC, et al. Spontaneous hepatitis B e antigen to antibody seroconversion and reversion in Chinese patients with chronic hepatitis B virus infection. Gastroenterology 92:1839–1843, 1987.

65. Liaw YF, Chu CM, Su IJ, et al. Clinical and histological events preceding hepatitis B e antigen seroconversion in chronic type B hepatitis. Gastroenterology 89:732–735, 1985.

66. Alward WLM, McMahon BJ, Hall DB, et al. The long-term serological course of asymptomatic hepatitis B virus carriers and the development of primary hepatocellular carcinoma. J Infect Dis 151:604–609, 1985.

67. Bortolotti F, Cadrobbi P, Crivellaro C, et al. Long-term outcome of chronic type B hepatitis patients who acquire hepatitis B infection in childhood. Gastroenterology 99:805–810, 1990.

68. Sheen IS, Liaw YF, Tai DI, Chu CM. Hepatic decompensation associated with hepatitis B e antigen clearance in chronic type B hepatitis. Gastroenterology 89:732–735, 1985.

69. Liaw YF, Tai DI, Chu CM, et al. Acute exacerbation in chronic type B hepatitis: comparison between HBeAg and antibody-positive patients. Hepatology 7:20–23, 1987.

70. Lok ASF, Lai CL. Acute exacerbations in Chinese patients with chronic hepatitis B virus (HBV) infection: incidence, predisposing factors, and etiology. J Hepatol 10:29–34, 1990.

71. Fattovich G, Rugge M, Brollo L, et al. Clinical, virologic and histologic outcome following seroconversion from HBsAg to anti-HBe in chronic hepatitis type B. Hepatology, 6:167–172, 1986.

72. McMahon BJ, Holck P, Bulkow L, Snowball MM. Serologic and clinical outcomes of 1536 Alaska Natives chronically infected with hepatitis B virus. Ann Intern Med 135:759–768, 2001.

73. Lok AS, Hadziyannis SJ, Weller IV, et al. Contribution of low level HBV replication to continuing inflammatory activity in patients with anti-HBe positive chronic hepatitis B virus infection. Gut 25:1283–1287, 1984.

74. Brechot C, Degos F, Lugassy C, et al. Hepatitis B virus DNA in patients with chronic liver disease and negative tests for hepatitis B surface antigen. N Engl J Med 312:270–276, 1985.

75. Chung HT, Lai CL, Lok ASF. Pathogenic role of hepatitis B virus in hepatitis B surface antigen–negative decompensated cirrhosis. Hepatology 22:25–29, 1995.

76. Liaw YF, Sheen IS, Chen TJ, et al. Incidence, determinants and significance of delayed clearance of serum HBsAg in chronic hepatitis B virus infection: a prospective study. Hepatology 13:627–631, 1991.

77. Adachi J, Kaneko S, Matsushita E, et al. Clearance of HBsAg in seven patients with chronic hepatitis. Hepatology 16:1334–1337, 1992.

78. Gandhi MJ, Yang GG, McMahon BJ, Vyas GN. Hepatitis B virions isolated with antibodies to the pre-S1 domain reveal occult viremia by PCR in Alaska Native HBV carriers who have seroconverted. Transfusion 40:910–916, 2000.

79. Hoofnagle JH, Shafritz DA, Popper H. Chronic type B hepatitis and the "healthy" HBsAg carrier state. Hepatology 7:758–763, 1987.

80. McMahon BJ, Alberts SR, Wainwright RB, et al. Hepatitis B-related sequelae: prospective study in 1400 hepatitis B surface antigen-positive Alaska native carriers. Arch Intern Med 150:1051–1054, 1990.

81. Hoofnagle JH, Seef LB. Natural history of chronic type B hepatitis. Prog Liver Dis 7:469–479, 1982.

82. Hsieh CC, Tzonou A, Zavitsanos X, et al. Age at first establishment of chronic hepatitis B virus infection and hepatocellular carcinoma risk: a birth order study. Am J Epidemiol 136:1115–1121, 1992.

83. Yu MW, Hsu FC, Sheen IS, et al. Prospective study of hepatocellular carcinoma and liver cirrhosis in asymptomatic chronic hepatitis B virus carriers. Am J Epidemiol 145:1039–1047, 1997.

84. Liaw YF, Tai DI, Chu CM, Chen TJ. The development of cirrhosis in patients with chronic type B hepatitis: a prospective study. Hepatology 8:493–496, 1988.

85. Chevillotte G, Durbec JP, Gerolami A, et al. Interaction between hepatitis B virus and alcohol in liver cirrhosis: an epidemiologic study. Gastroenterology 85:141–145, 1983.

86. Beasley RP, Huang L-Y, Lin C, Chien C. Hepatocellular carcinoma and HBV: a prospective study of 22,707 men in Taiwan. Lancet 2:1129–1133, 1981.

87. McMahon BJ. Hepatocellular carcinoma and viral hepatitis. In Wilson RA (ed). Viral Hepatitis. New York, Marcel Dekker, 1997, pp 315–330.

88. Fattovich G, Giustina G, Schalm SW, et al. Occurrence of hepatocellular carcinoma and decompensation in western European patients with cirrhosis type B. The EUROHEP Study Group on Hepatitis B Virus and Cirrhosis. Hepatology 21:77–82, 1995.

89. Huo TI, Wu JC, Lee PC, et al. Sero-clearance of hepatitis B surface antigen in chronic carriers does not necessarily imply a good prognosis. Hepatology 28:231–236, 1998.

90. Seeger C, Mason WS. Hepatitis B virus biology. Microbiol Mol Biol Rev 64:51–68, 2000.

91. Tiollais P, Charnay P, Vyas GN. Biology of hepatitis B virus. Science 213:406–411, 1981.

92. Rossner MT. Review: Hepatitis B virus X gene product: a promiscuous transcriptional activator. J Med Virol 36:101–117, 1992.

93. Gerlich WH, Bruss V. Functions of hepatitis B virus proteins and molecular targets for protective immunity. In Ellis RW (ed). Hepatitis B Vaccines in Clinical Practice. New York, Marcel Dekker, 1993, pp 41–82.

94. Neurath AR, Kent SB, Strick N, Parker K. Identification and chemical synthesis of a host cell receptor binding site on hepatitis B virus. Cell 46:429–436, 1986.

95. Pontisso P, Petit MA, Bankowski MJ, Peeples ME. Human liver plasma membranes contain receptors for the hepatitis B virus pre-S1 region and, via polymerized human serum albumin, for the pre-S2 region. J Virol 63:1981–1988, 1989.

96. Gerlich WH, Lu X, Heerman KH. Studies on the attachment and penetration of hepatitis B virus. J Hepatol 17(suppl):S10–S14, 1993.

97. Koziel MJ. Immunology of viral hepatitis. Am J Med 100:98–109, 1996.

98. Prince AM, Ikram H, Hopp TP. Hepatitis B virus vaccine: identification of HBsAg/a and HBsAg/d but not HBsAg/y subtype antigenic determinants on a synthetic immunogenic peptide. Proc Natl Acad Sci U S A 79:579–582, 1982.

99. Courouce-Pauty AM, Plancon A, Soulier JP. Distribution of HBsAg subtypes in the world. Vox Sang 44:197–211, 1983.

100. Dodd RY, Holland PV, Ni LY, et al. Hepatitis B antigen: regional variation in incidence and subtype ratio in the American Red Cross donor population. Am J Epidemiol 97:111–115, 1973.
101. Mushahwar IK, McGrath LC, Drnec J, Overby LR. Radioimmunoassay for the detection of hepatitis B e antigen and its antibody: results of a clinical evaluation. Am J Clin Pathol 76:692–697, 1981.
102. Guidotti LG, Ishikawa T, Hobbs MV, et al. Intracellular inactivation of the hepatitis B virus by cytotoxic T lymphocytes. Immunity 4:25–36, 1996.
103. Lau JYN, Wright TL. Molecular virology and pathogenesis of hepatitis B. Lancet 342:1335–1340, 1993.
104. Chang LJ, Hirsch RC, Ganem D, Varmus HE. Effects of insertional and point mutations on the functions of the duck hepatitis B virus polymerase. J. Virol. 64:5553–5558, 1990.
105. Seeger C, Ganem D, Varmus HE. Biochemical and genetic evidence for the hepatitis B virus replication strategy. Science 232:477–484, 1986.
106. Hunt CM, McGill JM, Allen MI, Condreay LD. Clinical relevance of hepatitis B virus mutations. Hepatology 31:1037–1044, 2000.
107. François G, Kew M, Van Damme P, et al. Mutant hepatitis B viruses: a matter of academic interest only or a problem with far-reaching implications? Vaccine 19:3799–3815, 2001.
108. Carman WF, Jacyna MR, Hadziyannis S, et al. Mutation preventing formation of hepatitis B e antigen in patients with chronic hepatitis B infection. Lancet 2:588–591, 1989.
109. Scaglioni PP, Melegari M, Wands JR. Biologic properties of hepatitis B viral genomes with mutations in the precore promoter and precore open reading frame. Virology 233:374–381, 1997.
110. Laskus T, Rakela J, Nowicki MJ, Persing DH. Hepatitis B core promotor sequence analysis in fulminant and chronic hepatitis B. Gastroenterology 109:1618–1623, 1995.
111. Liang TJ, Hasegawa K, Rimon N, et al. A hepatitis B virus mutant associated with an episode of fulminant hepatitis. N Engl J Med 324:1705–1709, 1991.
112. Omata M, Ehata T, Kokosuka O, et al. Mutations in the precore region of hepatitis B virus DNA in patients with fulminant and severe hepatitis. N Engl J Med 324:1699–1704, 1991.
113. Hsu HY, Chang MH, Lee CY, et al. Precore mutant of hepatitis B virus in childhood fulminant hepatitis B: an infrequent association. J Infect Dis 171:776–781, 1995.
114. Liang TJ, Hasegawa K, Munoz SJ, et al. Hepatitis B virus precore mutation and fulminant hepatitis in the United States: a polymerase chain reaction-based assay for the detection of specific mutation. J Clin Invest 93:550–555, 1994.
115. Laskus T, Persing DH, Nowicku MJ, et al. Nucleotide sequence analysis of the precore region in patients with fulminant hepatitis B in the United States. Gastroenterology 105:1173–1178, 1993.
116. Hasegawa K, Huang J, Rogers SA, et al. Enhanced replication of a hepatitis B virus mutant associated with an epidemic of fulminant hepatitis. J Virol 68:1651–1659, 1994.
117. Ling R, Mutimer D, Ahmed M, et al. Selection of mutations in the hepatitis B virus polymerase during therapy of transplant recipients with lamivudine. Hepatology 24:711–713, 1996.
118. Tipples GA, Ma MM, Fischer KP, et al. Mutation in HBV RNA-dependent polymerase confers resistance to lamivudine in vivo. Hepatology 24:714–717, 1996.
119. Chayama K, Suzuki Y, Kobayashi M, et al. Emergence and takeover of YMDD motif mutant hepatitis B virus during long-term lamivudine therapy and re-takeover by wild type after cessation of therapy. Hepatology 27:1711–1716, 1998.
120. Blum HE, Galum E, Liang TJ, et al. Naturally occurring missense mutation in the polymerase gene terminating hepatitis B virus replication. J Virol 65:1836–1842, 1991.
121. Allen MI, Deslauriers M, Andrews CW, et al. Identification and characterization of mutations in hepatitis B virus resistant to lamivudine. Lamivudine Clinical Investigation Group. Hepatology 27:1670–1677, 1998.
122. Atkins M, Hunt CM, Brown N, et al. Clinical significance of YMDD mutant hepatitis B virus (HBV) in a large cohort of lamivudine-treated hepatitis B patients. Hepatology 28:398A, 1998.
123. Zuckerman AJ. Effect of hepatitis B virus mutants on efficacy of vaccination. Lancet 355:1382–1384, 2000.
124. Carman WF, Korula J, Wallace L, et al. Fulminant reactivation of hepatitis B due to envelope protein mutant of HBV that escaped detection by monoclonal HBsAg ELISA. Lancet 345:1406–1407, 1995.
125. Jongerius J, Wester M, Cuypers H, et al. New hepatitis B virus mutant form in a blood donor that is undetectable in several hepatitis B surface antigen screening assays. Transfusion 38:56–59, 1998.
126. Coleman PF, Chen YCJ, Mushahwar IK. Immunoassay detection of hepatitis B surface antigen mutants. J Med Virol 59:19–24, 1999.
127. Mimms L. Hepatitis B virus escape mutants: "pushing the envelope" of chronic hepatitis B virus infection. Hepatology 21:884–887, 1995.
128. Zanetti AR, Tanzi E, Manzillo G, et al. Hepatitis B variants in Europe. Lancet 2:1132–1133, 1988.
129. Carman WF, Zanetti AR, Karayiannis P, et al. Vaccine-induced escape mutant of hepatitis B virus. Lancet 336:325–329, 1990.
130. Harrison TJ, Hopes EA, Oon CJ, et al. Independent emergence of a vaccine-induced escape mutant of hepatitis B virus. J Hepatol 13(suppl):S105–S107, 1991.
131. Zuckerman AJ, Harrison TJ, Oon CJ. Mutation in S region of hepatitis B virus. Lancet 343:737–738, 1994.
132. Howard CR. The structure of hepatitis B envelope and molecular variants of hepatitis B virus. J Viral Hepat 2:165–170, 1995.
133. Nainan OV, Stevens CE, Taylor PE, Margolis HS. Hepatitis B virus (HBV) antibody resistant mutants among mothers and infants with chronic HBV infection. In Rizetto M, Purcell RH, Gerin JL, Verme G (eds). Viral Hepatitis and Liver Disease: Proceedings of the IXth Triennial Symposium on Viral Hepatitis and Liver Disease, Rome, 21–21 April 1996. Turin, Edzioni Minerva Medica, 1997, pp 132–134.
134. Hsu HY, Chang MH, Ni YH, et al. Surface gene mutants of hepatitis B virus in infants who develop acute or chronic hepatitis infections despite immunoprophylaxis. Hepatology 26:786–791, 1997.
135. Ngui SL, Andrews NJ, Underhill GS, et al. Failed perinatal immunoprophylaxis for hepatitis B: characteristics of maternal hepatitis B virus as risk factors. Clin Infect Dis 27:100–106, 1998.
136. Fortuin M, Karthigesu V, Allison L, et al. Breakthrough infections and identification of a viral variant in Gambian children immunized with hepatitis B vaccine. J Infect Dis 169:1374–1376, 1994.
137. McMahon G, Erlich PH, Moustapha ZA, et al. Genetic alterations in the gene encoding the major HBsAg: DNA and immunological analysis of recurrent HBsAg derived from monoclonal antibody–treated liver transplant patients. Hepatology 15:757–766, 1992.
138. Ghany MG, Ayola B, Villamil FG, et al. Hepatitis B virus S mutants in liver transplant recipients who were reinfected despite hepatitis B immune globulin prophylaxis. Hepatology 27:213–222, 1998.
139. Terrault N, Zhou S, McCory RW, et al. Incidence and clinical consequences of surface and polymerase gene mutations in liver transplant recipients on hepatitis B immune globulin. Hepatology 28:555–561, 1998.
140. Nainan OV, Khristova ML, Byun K-S, et al. Frequency and significance of hepatitis B virus antibody resistant mutants [abstract]. Antiviral Ther 5:29–30, 2000.
141. Purcell RH. Hepatitis B virus mutations and efficacy of vaccination. Lancet 356:769, 2000.
142. Ogata N, Cote PJ, Zanetti AR, et al. Licensed recombinant hepatitis B vaccines protect chimpanzees against infection with the prototype surface gene mutant of hepatitis B virus. Hepatology 30:779–786, 1999.
143. Mele A, Tancredi F, Romano L, et al. Effectiveness of hepatitis B vaccination in babies born to hepatitis B surface antigen-positive mothers in Italy. J Infect Dis 184:905–908, 2001.
144. Chisari F, Ferrari C. Hepatitis B virus immunopathogenesis. Annu Rev Immunol 13:29–60, 1995.
145. Di Bisceglie AM. Hepatocellular carcinoma. Ann Intern Med 108:390–401, 1988.
146. Malik AH, Lee WM. Chronic hepatitis B virus infection: treatment strategies for the next millennium. Ann Intern Med 132:723–731, 2000.
147. Lok AS, Heathcote EJ, Hoofnagle JH. Management of hepatitis B: 2000—summary of a workshop. Gastroenterology 120:1828–1853, 2001.
148. Lok ASF, McMahon BJ. Chronic hepatitis B: AASLD Practice Guidelines. Hepatology 34:1225–1241, 2001.
149. Hoofnagle JH, Di Bisceglie AM. The treatment of chronic viral hepatitis. N Engl J Med 336:347–356, 1997.

150. Greenberg HB, Pollard RB, Lutwick LI, et al. Effect of human leukocyte interferon on hepatitis B virus infection in patients with chronic active hepatitis. N Engl J Med 295:517–522, 1976.

151. Desmyter J, De Groote J, Desmet VJ, et al. Administration of human fibroblast interferon in chronic hepatitis B infection. Lancet 2:645–647, 1976.

152. Wong DKH, Cheung AM, O'Rourke K, et al. Effect of alpha-interferon treatment in patients with B e antigen-positive chronic hepatitis B: a meta-analysis. Ann Intern Med 119:312–323, 1993.

153. Lin SM, Sheen IS, Chien RN, et al. Long-term beneficial effect of interferon therapy in patients with chronic hepatitis B virus infection. Hepatology 29:971–975, 1999.

154. Lau DT, Everhart J, Kleiner DE, et al. Long-term follow-up of patients with chronic hepatitis B treated with interferon alfa. Gastroenterology 113:1660–1667, 1997.

155. Korenman J, Baker B, Wagonner J, et al. Long-term remission of chronic hepatitis B after alpha-interferon therapy. Ann Intern Med 114:629–634, 1991.

156. Dienstag JL, Perrillo RP, Schiff ER, et al. A preliminary trial of lamivudine for chronic hepatitis B infection. N Engl J Med 333:1657–1661, 1995.

157. Dienstag JL, Schiff ER, Wright TL, et al. Lamivudine as initial treatment of chronic hepatitis B in the United States. N Engl J Med 341:1256–1263, 1999.

158. Lai CL, Chien RN, Leung NW, et al. A one-year trial of lamivudine for chronic hepatitis B. Asia Lamivudine Study Group. N Engl J Med 339:61–68, 1998.

159. Schalm SW, Healthcote J, Cianciara J, et al. Lamivudine and alpha interferon treatment of patients with chronic hepatitis B infection: a randomized trial. Gut 46:562–568, 2000.

160. Schiff ER, Karayalcin S, Grimm I, et al. A placebo-controlled study of lamivudine and interferon alfa-2b in patients with chronic hepatitis B who previously failed interferon therapy. Hepatology 28:388A, 1998.

161. Pol S, Driss F, Michel ML, et al. Specific vaccine therapy in chronic hepatitis B infection. Lancet 344:342, 1994.

162. Wen YM, Wu XH, Hu DC, et al. Hepatitis B vaccine and anti-HBs complex as approach for vaccine therapy. Lancet 345:1575–1576, 1995.

163. McDermott AB, Madrigal JA, Sabin CA, et al. The influence of host factors and immunogenetics on lymphocyte responses to Hepagene vaccination. Vaccine 17:1329–1337, 1999.

164. Akbar SMF, Kajino K, Tanimoto K, et al. Placebo-controlled trial of vaccination with hepatitis B surface antigen in hepatitis B virus transgenic mice. J Hepatol 26:131–137, 1997.

165. Margolis HS, Alter MJ, Hadler SC. Viral hepatitis. In Viral Infections of Humans: Epidemiology and Control (4th ed). New York, Plenum Publishing Corporation, 1997, pp 363–418.

166. Okada K, Kamiyama I, Inomata M, et al. e antigen and anti-e in the serum of asymptomatic carrier mothers as indicators of positive and negative transmission of hepatitis B virus to their infants. N Engl J Med 294:746–749, 1976.

167. Beasley RP, Hwang LY, Stevens CE, et al. Efficacy of hepatitis B immune globulin for prevention of perinatal transmission of the hepatitis B virus carrier state: final report of a randomized double-blind, placebo-controlled trial. Hepatology 3:135–141, 1983.

168. Wong VCW, Ip HMP, Reesink HW, et al. Prevention of the HBsAg carrier state in newborn infants of mothers who are chronic carriers of HBsAg and HBeAg by administration of hepatitis-B vaccine and hepatitis-B immunoglobulin: double-blind randomised placebo-controlled study. Lancet 1:921–926, 1984.

169. Xu ZY, Liu CB, Francis DP, et al. Prevention of perinatal acquisition of hepatitis B virus carriage using vaccine: preliminary report of a randomized, double-blind, placebo-controlled, and comparative trial. Pediatrics 76:713–718, 1985.

170. Stevens CE, Taylor PE, Tong MJ, et al. Yeast-recombinant hepatitis B vaccine: efficacy with hepatitis B immune globulin in prevention of perinatal hepatitis B virus transmission. JAMA 257:2612–2616, 1987.

171. Poovorawan Y, Sanpavat S, Pongpunlert W, et al. Protective efficacy of a recombinant DNA hepatitis B vaccine in neonates of HBe antigen-positive mothers. JAMA 261:3278–3281, 1989.

172. Lee CY, Huang LM, Chang MH, et al. The protective efficacy of recombinant hepatitis B vaccine in newborn infants of hepatitis B e antigen-positive-hepatitis B surface antigen carrier mothers. Pediatr Infect Dis J 10:299–303, 1991.

173. Beasley RP, Stevens CE, Shiao IS, Meng HC. Evidence against breast-feeding as a mechanism for vertical transmission of hepatitis B. Lancet 2:740–741, 1975.

174. Beasley RP, Trepo C, Stevens CE, Szmuness W. The e antigen and vertical transmission of hepatitis B surface antigen. Am J Epidemiol 105:94–98, 1977.

175. Tong MJ, Thursby M, Rakela J, et al. Studies of the maternal–infant transmission of the viruses which cause acute hepatitis. Gastroenterology 80:999–1004, 1981.

176. Schweitzer IL, Dunn AEG, Peters RL, Spears RL. Viral hepatitis type B in neonates and infants. Am J Med 55:762–763, 1973.

177. Stevens CE, Toy PT, Tong MJ, et al. Perinatal hepatitis B virus transmission in the United States: prevention by passive-active immunization. JAMA 253:1740–1745, 1985.

178. Friedman SM, De Silva LP, Fox HE, Bernard G. Hepatitis B screening in a New York City obstetrics service. Am J Public Health 78:308–310, 1988.

179. Margolis HS, Alter MJ, Hadler SC. Hepatitis B: evolving epidemiology and implications for control. Semin Liver Dis 11:84–92, 1991.

180. Barrett DH, Burks JM, McMahon B, et al. Epidemiology of hepatitis B in two Alaska communities. Am J Epidemiol 105:118–122, 1977.

181. Leichtner AM, Leclair J, Goldmann DA, et al. Horizontal nonparenteral spread of hepatitis B among children. Ann Intern Med 94:346–349, 1981.

182. Whittle H, Inskip H, Bradley AK, et al. The pattern of childhood hepatitis B infection in two Gambian villages. J Infect Dis 161:1112–1115, 1990.

183. Beasley RP, Hwang LY. Postnatal infectivity of hepatitis B surface antigen-carrier mothers. J Infect Dis 147:185–190, 1983.

184. Kashiwagi S, Hayashi J, Ikematsu H, et al. Transmission of hepatitis B virus among siblings. Am J Epidemiol 120:617–625, 1984.

185. Marinier E, Barrois V, Larouze B, et al. Lack of perinatal transmission of hepatitis B virus infection in Senegal, West Africa. J Pediatr 106:843–849, 1985.

186. Franks AL, Berg CJ, Kane MA, et al. Hepatitis B infection among children born in the United States to southeast Asian refugees. N Engl J Med 321:1301–1305, 1989.

187. Davis LG, Weber DJ, Lemon SM. Horizontal transmission of hepatitis B virus. Lancet 1:889–893, 1989.

188. Botha JF, Ritchie MJ, Dusheiko GM, et al. Hepatitis B virus carrier state in black children in Ovamboland: role of perinatal and horizontal infection. Lancet 1:1210–1212, 1984.

189. Ko YC, Li SC, Yen YY, et al. Horizontal transmission of hepatitis B virus from siblings and intramuscular injection among preschool children in a familial cohort. Am J Epidemiol 133:1015–1023, 1991.

190. Craxi A, Tine F, Vinci M, et al. Transmission of hepatitis B and hepatitis delta viruses in the households of chronic hepatitis B surface antigen carriers: a regression analysis of indicators of risk. Am J Epidemiol 134:641–650, 1991.

191. Hurie MB, Mast EE, Davis JP. Horizontal transmission of hepatitis B virus infection to United States-born children of Hmong refugees. Pediatrics 89:269–273, 1992.

192. Pon EW, Ren H, Margolis H, et al. Hepatitis B virus infection in Honolulu students. Pediatrics 92:574–578, 1993.

193. Mahoney FJ, Lawrence M, Scott K, et al. Continuing risk for hepatitis B virus transmission among children born in the United States to southeast Asian children in Louisiana. Pediatrics 95:1113–1116, 1995.

194. Van Damme P, Cramm M, Van der Auwera JC, et al. Horizontal transmission of hepatitis B virus. Lancet 345:27–29, 1995.

195. Martinson FE, Weigle KA, Royce RA, et al. Risk factors for horizontal transmission of hepatitis B virus in a rural district in Ghana. Am J Epidemiol 147:478–487, 1998.

196. Hayashi J, Kashiwagi S, Nomura H, et al. Hepatitis B transmission in nursery schools. Am J Epidemiol 125:492–498, 1987.

197. Nigro G, Taliane G. Nursery-acquired asymptomatic B hepatitis. Lancet 1:1451–1452, 1989.

198. Shapiro CN, McCaig LF, Gensheimer KF, et al. Hepatitis B virus transmission between children in day care. Pediatr Infect Dis J 8:870–875, 1989.

199. Breuer B, Friedeman SM, Millner ES, et al. Transmission of hepatitis B virus to classroom contacts of mentally retarded carriers. JAMA 254:3190–3195, 1985.

200. David E, McIntosh G, Bek MD, et al. Molecular evidence of transmission of hepatitis B in a day-care centre. Lancet 347:118–119, 1996.

201. Oleske J, Minnefor A, Cooper R Jr, et al. Transmission of hepatitis B in a classroom setting. J Pediatr 97:770–772, 1980.

202. Villarejos VM, Visona KA, Guteirrez A, Rodriguez A. Role of saliva, urine and feces in the transmission of type B hepatitis. N Engl J Med 291:1375–1378, 1974.

203. Cancio-Bello TP, de Medina M, Shorey J, et al. An institutional outbreak of hepatitis B related to a human biting carrier. J Infect Dis 146:652–656, 1982.

204. Scott RM, Snitbhan R, Bancroft WH, et al. Experimental transmission of hepatitis B virus by semen and saliva. J Infect Dis 142:67–71, 1980.

205. Ward R, Borchert P, Wright A, et al. Hepatitis B antigen in saliva and mouth washings. Lancet 2:726–727, 1972.

206. Williams I, Smith MG, Sinha D, et al. Hepatitis B virus transmission in an elementary school setting. JAMA 278:2167–2169, 1997.

207. Bond WW, Favero MS, Peterson NJ, et al. Survival of hepatitis B virus after drying and storage for one week. Lancet 1:550–551, 1981.

208. Petersen NJ, Barrett DH, Bond WH, et al. HBsAg in saliva, impetiginous lesions and the environment in two remote Alaskan villages. Appl Environ Microbiol 32:572–574, 1976.

209. Armstrong GL, Mast EE, Wojczynski M, Margolis HS. Childhood hepatitis B virus infections in the United States before hepatitis B immunization. Pediatrics 108:1123–1128, 2001.

210. Margolis HS, Coleman PJ, Brown RE, et al. Prevention of hepatitis B virus transmission by immunization: an economic analysis of current recommendations. JAMA 274:1201–1208, 1995.

211. Alter MJ, Margolis HS. The emergence of hepatitis B as a sexually transmitted disease. Med Clin North Am 74:1529–1541, 1990.

212. Goldstein ST, Alter MJ, Williams IT, et al. Incidence and risk factors for acute hepatitis B in the United States, 1982–1998: implications for vaccination programs. J Infect Dis 185:713–719, 2002.

213. Thomas D, Cannon RO, Shapiro CN, et al. Hepatitis C, hepatitis B, and human immunodeficiency virus infections among non-intravenous drug-using patients attending clinics for sexually transmitted diseases. J Infect Dis 169:990–995, 1994.

214. MacKellar DA, Valleroy LA, Secura GM, et al. Two decades after vaccine license: hepatitis B immunization and infection among young men who have sex with men. Am J Public Health 91:965–971, 2001.

215. McQuillan GM, Townsend TR, Fields HA, et al. Seroepidemiology of hepatitis B virus in the United States, 1976 to 1980. Am J Med 87(suppl):5S–10S, 1989.

216. Kane A, Lloyd J, Zaffran M, et al. Transmission of hepatitis B, hepatitis C and human immunodeficiency viruses through unsafe injections in the developing world: model-based regional estimates. Bull World Health Organ 77:801–807, 1999.

217. Hutin YJF, Chen RT. Injection safety: a global challenge. Bull World Health Organ 77:787–788, 1999.

218. Hutin Y, Stilwell B, Hauri AM, Margolis H. Transmission of bloodborne pathogens through unsafe injections and proposed approach for the Safe Injection Global Network. In Margolis HS, Alter MJ, Liang TJ, Dienstag JL (eds). Viral Hepatitis and Liver Disease. London, International Medical Press, 2002, pp 219–227.

219. Anonymous. Relation of e antigen to infectivity of HBsAg-positive inoculations among medical personnel. Lancet 2:492–494, 1976.

220. Seeff LB, Wright EC, Zimmerman HJ, et al. Type B hepatitis after needlestick exposure: prevention with hepatitis B immune globulin. Final report of the Veterans Administration Cooperative Study. Ann Intern Med 88:285–293, 1978.

221. Grady GF, Lee VA, Prince AM, et al. Hepatitis B immune globulin for accidental exposures among medical personnel: final report of a multicenter controlled trial. J Infect Dis 138:625–638, 1978.

222. Gerberding JL. Management of occupational exposures to bloodborne viruses. N Engl J Med 332:444–451, 1995.

223. Centers for Disease Control and Prevention. Recommendations for prevention and control of hepatitis C virus (HCV) infection and HCV-related chronic disease. MMWR 47(RR-19):1–39, 1998.

224. World Health Organization. Global Database on Blood Safety: Summary Report 1998–1999. Available at www.who.int/bct/Main_areas_of_work/BTS/GDBS/GDBS_Report.pdf

225. Hu MD, Schenzle D, Dienhart F, Scheid R. Epidemiology of hepatitis A and B in Shanghai area: prevalence of serum markers. Am J Epidemiol 120:404–413, 1984.

226. Maynard JE, Kane MA, Alter MJ, Hadler SC. Control of hepatitis B by immunization: global perspectives. In Vyas GN, Dienstag JL, Hoofnagle JH (eds). Viral Hepatitis and Liver Disease. New York, Grune & Stratton, 1984, pp 967–969.

227. Lingao AL, Domingo EO, West S, et al. Seroepidemiology of hepatitis B in the Philippines. Am J Epidemiol 123:473–480, 1986.

228. Lee SD, Lo KJ, Wu JC, et al. Prevention of maternal–infant hepatitis B transmission by immunization: the role of serum hepatitis B virus DNA. Hepatology 6:369–373, 1986.

229. Toukan AU, Sharaiha ZK, Abu-El-Rub OA, et al. The epidemiology of hepatitis B virus among family members in the Middle East. Am J Epidemiol 132:220–232, 1990.

230. Bensebath G, Halder SC, Pereira Soares MC, et al. Epidemiologic and serologic studies of acute viral hepatitis in Brazil's Amazon Basin. Bull Pan Am Health Organ 21:16–27, 1987.

231. Hyams KC, Osman NM, Khaled EM, et al. Maternal–infant transmission of hepatitis B in Egypt. J Med Virol 24:191–197, 1988.

232. Toukan A. Strategy for control of hepatitis B virus infection in the Middle East and North Africa. Vaccine 8(suppl):117–121, 1990.

233. Bernier RH, Sampliner R, Gerety R, et al. Hepatitis B infection in households of chronic carriers of hepatitis B surface antigen. Am J Epidemiol 116:199–211, 1982.

234. Irwin GR, Allen AM, Bancroft WH, et al. Hepatitis B antigen and antibody: occurrence in families of asymptomatic HBsAg carriers. JAMA 227:1012–1013, 1974.

235. Centers for Disease Control and Prevention. Recommendations for preventing transmission of infections among chronic hemodialysis patients. MMWR 50(RR-5):1–43, 2001.

236. Alter MJ, Favero MS, Maynard JE. Impact of infection control strategies on the incidence of dialysis-associated hepatitis in the United States. J Infect Dis 153:1149–1151, 1986.

237. Centers for Disease Control and Prevention. Outbreaks of hepatitis B virus infection among hemodialysis patients—California, Nebraska, and Texas, 1994. MMWR 45:285–289, 1996.

238. Anda RF, Perlman SB, D'Alessio DJ, et al. Hepatitis B in Wisconsin male prisoners: considerations for serologic screening and vaccination. Am J Public Health 75:1182–1185, 1985.

239. Koplan JP, Wlaker JA, Bryan JA, Berquist KR. Prevalence of hepatitis B surface antigen and antibody at a state prison in Kansas. J Infect Dis 137:505–506, 1978.

240. Decker MD, Vaughn WK, Brodie JS, et al. Seroepidemiology of hepatitis B in Tennessee prisoners. J Infect Dis 150:450–459, 1984.

241. Tucker RM, Gaffey MJ, Fisch MJ, et al. Seroepidemiology of hepatitis D (delta agent) and hepatitis B among Virginia State prisoners. Clin Ther 9:622–628, 1987.

242. Hull HF, Lyons LH, Mann JM, et al. Incidence of hepatitis B in the penitentiary of New Mexico. Am J Public Health 75:1213–1214, 1985.

243. Decker MD, Vaughn WK, Brodie JS, et al. The incidence of hepatitis B in Tennessee prisoners. J Infect Dis 152:214–217, 1985.

244. Levine OS, Vlahov D, Koehler J, et al. Seroepidemiology of hepatitis B virus in a population of injecting drug users: association with drug injection patterns. Am J Epidemiol 142:331–341, 1995.

245. Levine OS, Vlahov D, Nelson KE. Epidemiology of hepatitis B virus infections among injecting drug users: seroprevalence, risk factors, and viral interactions. Epidemiol Rev 16:418–436, 1994.

246. Segal HE, Llewellyn CH, Irwin G, et al. Hepatitis B antigen and antibody in the U.S. Army: prevalence in health care personnel. Am J Public Health 66:667–671, 1976.

247. Pattison CP, Maynard JE, Berquist DR, Webster HM. Epidemiology of hepatitis B in hospital personnel. Am J Epidemiol 101:59–64, 1975.

248. Dienstag JL, Ryan DM. Occupational exposure to hepatitis B virus in hospital personnel: infection or immunization? Am J Epidemiol 115:26–39, 1982.

249. Smith JL, Maynard JE, Berquist KR, et al. Comparative risk of hepatitis B among physicians and dentists. J Infect Dis 133:705–706, 1978.

250. Hadler SC, Doto IL, Maynard JE, et al. Occupational risk of hepatitis B infection in hospital workers. Infect Control 6:24–31, 1985.

251. Hollinger FB, Grander JW, Nickel FR, Suarez M. Hepatitis B prevalence within a dental student population. J Am Dental Assoc 94:521–527, 1977.

252. Mahoney F, Stewart K, Hu H, Alter MJ. Progress towards the elimination of hepatitis B virus transmission among health care workers in the United States. Arch Intern Med 97:2601–2605, 1997.

253. Woodruff BA, Moyer LA, O'Rourke KM, Margolis HS. Blood exposure and the risk of hepatitis B virus infection in firefighters. J Occup Med 35:1048–1054, 1993.

254. Werman HA, Gwinn R. Seroprevalence of hepatitis B and C among rural emergency medical care personnel. Am J Emerg Med 15:248–251, 1997.

255. Spitters C, Zenilman J, Yeargain J, Pardoe K. Prevalence of antibodies to hepatitis B and C among fire department personnel prior to implementation of a hepatitis B vaccination program. J Occup Environ Med 37:663–664, 1995.

256. Centers for Disease Control. Public Health Service inter-agency guidelines for screening donors of blood, plasma, organs, tissues, and semen for evidence of hepatitis B and hepatitis C. MMWR 40(RR-4):1–17, 1991.

257. Chaudhary RK, Perry E, Cleary TE. Prevalence of hepatitis B infection among residents of an institution for the mentally retarded. Am J Epidemiol 105:123–126, 1977.

258. Vellinga A, Van Damme P, Meheus A. Hepatitis B and C in institutions for individuals with intellectual disability. J Intellect Disabil Res 4:445–453, 1999.

259. Shapiro CN, Hadler SC. Hepatitis A and hepatitis B virus infections in day-care settings. Pediatr Ann 20:435–441, 1991.

260. Steffen R. Risks of hepatitis B for travelers. Vaccine 8(suppl):S31–S32, 1990.

261. Lange WR, Frame JD. High incidence of viral hepatitis among American missionaries in Africa. Am J Trop Med Hyg 43:527–533, 1990.

262. Maynard JE. Passive immunization against hepatitis B: a review of recent studies and comment on current aspects of control. Am J Epidemiol 107:77–86, 1978.

263. Terrault NA, Zhou S, Combs C, et al. Prophylaxis in liver transplant recipients using a fixed dosing schedule of hepatitis B immune globulin. Hepatology 24:1327–1333, 1996.

264. Centers for Disease Control. Safety of therapeutic immune globulin preparations with respect to transmission for human T-lymphotrophic virus type III/lymphadenopathy-associated virus infection. MMWR 35:231–233, 1986.

265. Wells MA, Wittek AE, Epstein JS, et al. Inactivation and partition of human T-cell lymphotrophic virus, type III, during ethanol fractionation of plasma. Transfusion 26:210–213, 1986.

266. Seefe LB, Zimmerman HJ, Wright EL, et al. A randomized controlled double-blind trial of the efficacy of immune serum globulin for the prevention of posttransfusion hepatitis: a Veterans Administration Cooperative Study. Gastroenterology 72:111–121, 1977.

267. Palmovic D, Crnjakovic-Palmovic J. Prevention of hepatitis B virus infection in health care workers after accidental exposure: a comparison of two prophylactic schedules. Infection 21:42–45, 1993.

268. Grady GF, Lee VA, Prince AM, et al. Hepatitis B immune globulin for accidental exposures among medical personnel: final report of a multicenter controlled trial. J Infect Dis 138:625–638, 1978.

269. Stevens CE, Neurath RA, Beasley RP, Szmuness W. HBeAg and anti-HBe detection with radioimmunoassay: correlation with vertical transmission of hepatitis B virus in Taiwan. J Med Virol 3:237–241, 1979.

270. Dosik H, Jhaveri R. Prevention of neonatal hepatitis B infection by high-dose hepatitis B immune globulin. N Engl J Med 298:602–603, 1978.

271. Andre FJ, Zuckerman AJ. Review: protective efficacy of hepatitis B vaccines in neonates. J Med Virol 44:144–151, 1994.

272. Anonymous. Type B hepatitis after needle-stick exposure: prevention with hepatitis B immune globulin. Final report of the Veterans Administration Cooperative Study. Ann Intern Med 88:285–293, 1978.

273. Redeker AG, Mosley JW, Gocke DJ, et al. Hepatitis B immune globulin as a prophylactic measure for spouses exposed to acute type B hepatitis. N Engl J Med 293:1055–1059, 1975.

274. Centers for Disease Control and Prevention. General recommendations on immunization: recommendations of the Advisory Committee on Immunization Practices and the American Academy of Family Physicians. MMWR 51(RR-2):1–34, 2002.

275. Sitrin RD, Wampler DE, Ellis RW. Survey of licensed hepatitis B vaccines and their production processes. In Ellis RW (ed). Hepatitis B Vaccines in Clinical Practice. New York, Marcel Dekker, 1993, pp 83–101.

276. Emini EA, Ellis RW, Miller WJ, et al. Production and immunologic analysis of recombinant hepatitis B vaccine. J Infect 13(suppl A):3–9, 1986.

277. Stephenne J. Development and production aspects of a recombinant yeast-derived hepatitis B vaccine. Vaccine 8(suppl):S69–S73, 1990.

278. Global Alliance for Vaccines and Immunization and The Global Fund for Children's Vaccines. Vaccine & Immunization Products Guideline for Countries Eligible for Support from the Global Fund for Children's Vaccines. Geneva, Supply Division, UNICEF, 2001.

279. Centers for Disease Control and Prevention. Thimerosal in vaccines: a joint statement of the American Academy of Pediatrics and the Public Health Service. MMWR 48:563–565, 1999.

280. Stratton K, Gable A, McCormick MC (eds). *Immunization Safety Review. Thimerosal-containing vaccines and neurodevelopmental disorders.* Washington, DC, National Academy Press, 2001, pp 1–17.

281. Francis DP, Feorina PM, McDougal JS, et al. The safety of hepatitis B vaccine: inactivation of the AIDS virus during routine vaccine manufacture. JAMA 256:869–872, 1986.

282. Diez-Delgado J, Dal-Re R, Llorente M, et al. Hepatitis B component does not interfere with the immune response to diphtheria, tetanus, and whole-cell *Bordetella pertussis* components of a quadrivalent (DPTw-HB) vaccine: a controlled trial in healthy infants. Vaccine 15:1418–1422, 1997.

283. Bruguera M, Bayas JM, Vilella A, et al. Immunogenicity and reactogenicity of a combined hepatitis A and B vaccine in young adults. Vaccine 15:1407–1411, 1996.

284. West D, Hesley T, Jonas L, et al. Safety and immunogenicity of a bivalent *Haemophilus influenzae* type b/hepatitis B vaccine in healthy infants. Pediatr Infect Dis J 16:593–599, 1997.

285. Seto D, West DJ, Gilliam R, et al. Antibody responses of healthy neonates to two mixed regimens of hepatitis B vaccine. Pediatr Infect Dis J 18:840–841, 1999.

286. Shaw FE, Guess HA, Roets JM, et al. Effect of anatomic injection site, age, and smoking on the immune response to hepatitis B vaccination. Vaccine 7:425–430, 1989.

287. Redfield RR, Innis BL, Scott RM, et al. Clinical evaluation of low-dose intradermally administered hepatitis B virus vaccine. JAMA 254:3203–3206, 1985.

288. Bryan JP, Sjogren MH, Perine PL, Legters LJ. Low-dose intradermal and intramuscular vaccination against hepatitis B. Clin Infect Dis 14:697–707, 1992.

289. Coursaget P, Relyveld E, Brizaard A, et al. Simultaneous injection of hepatitis B vaccine with BCG and killed poliovirus vaccine. Vaccine 10:319–321, 1992.

290. Coursaget P, Yvonnet B, Telyveld EH, et al. Simultaneous administration of diphtheria-tetanus-pertussis-polio and hepatitis B vaccines in a simplified immunization program: immune response to diphtheria toxoid, tetanus toxoid, pertussis, and hepatitis B surface antigen. Infect Immun 51:784–787, 1986.

291. Aristegui J, Muniz J, Perez Legorburu A, et al. Newborn universal immunization against hepatitis B: immunogenicity and reactogenicity of simultaneous administration of diphtheria/tetanus/pertussis (DPT) and oral polio vaccines with hepatitis B vaccine at 0, 2, and 6 months of age. Vaccine 13:973–977, 1995.

292. Giammanco G, Li Volti S, Mauro L, et al. Immune response to simultaneous administration of a recombinant DNA hepatitis B vaccine and multiple compulsory vaccines in infancy. Vaccine 9:747–750, 1991.

293. Barone P, Mauro L, Leonardi S, et al. Simultaneous administration of HB recombinant vaccine with diphtheria and tetanus toxoid and oral polio vaccines: a pilot study. Acta Paediatr Jpn 33:455–458, 1991.

294. Coursaget P, Fritzell B, Blondeau C, et al. Simultaneous injection of plasma-derived or recombinant hepatitis B vaccines with yellow fever and killed polio vaccines. Vaccine 13:109–111, 1995.

295. Yvonnet B, Coursaget P, Deubel V, et al. Simultaneous administration of hepatitis B and yellow fever vaccines. Dev Biol Stand 65:205–207, 1986.

296. King GE, Hadler SC. Simultaneous administration of childhood vaccines: an important public health policy that is safe and efficacious. Pediatr Infect Dis J 13:394–407, 1994.

297. Advisory Committee on Immunization Practices. Combination vaccines for childhood immunization: recommendations of the Advisory Committee on Immunization Practices (ACIP), the American Academy of Pediatrics (AAP), and the American Academy of Family Physicians (AAFP). MMWR 48(RR-5):1–15, 1999.

298. Duval B, Deceuninck G. Seroprotection rates after late doses of hepatitis B vaccine. Pediatrics 109:350–351, 2002.

299. Halsey NA, Moulton LH, O'Donovan JC, et al. Hepatitis B vaccine administered to children and adolescents at yearly intervals. Pediatrics 103:1243–1247, 1999.

300. Mangione R, Stroffolini T, Tosti ME, et al. Delayed third hepatitis B vaccine dose and immune response. Lancet 345:1111–1112, 1995.

301. Keyserling HL, West DJ, Hesley TM, et al. Antibody responses of healthy infants to a recombinant hepatitis B vaccine administered at two, four, and twelve or fifteen months of age. J Pediatr 125:67–69, 1994.

302. Bernstein SR, Krieger P, Puppala BL, Costello M. Incidence and duration of hepatitis B surface antigenemia after neonatal hepatitis B immunization. J Pediatr 125:621–622, 1994.

303. Koksal N, Altinkaya N, Perk Y. Transient hepatitis B surface antigenemia after neonatal hepatitis B immunization. Acta Paediatr 85:1501–1502, 1996.

304. Kloster B, Kramer R, Eastlund T, et al. Hepatitis B surface antigenemia in blood donors following vaccination. Transfusion 35:475–477, 1995.

305. Lunn ER, Hoggarth BJ, Cook WJ. Prolonged hepatitis B surface antigenemia after vaccination. Pediatrics 105:E81, 2000.

306. Melnick JL. Thermostability of poliovirus, measles, and hepatitis B vaccines. Vaccine Res 4:1–11, 1995.

307. Van Damme P, Cramm M, Safary A, et al. Heat stability of a recombinant DNA hepatitis B vaccine. Vaccine 10:366–367, 1992.

308. Otto BF, Suarnawa IM, Stewart T, et al. At-birth immunization against hepatitis B using a novel pre-filled immunization device stored outside the cold chain. Vaccine 18:498–502, 2000.

309. Sutanto A, Suarnawa IM, Nelson CM, et al. Home delivery of hepatitis B vaccine to newborns in Indonesia: outreach immunization with a pre-filled, single-use injection device. Bull World Health Organ 77:119–126, 1999.

310. McLean AA, Shaw R Jr. Hepatitis B virus vaccine. Ann Intern Med 97:451, 1982.

311. Hadler SC, Francis DP, Maynard JE, et al. Long-term immunogenicity and efficacy of hepatitis B vaccine in homosexual men. N Engl J Med 315:209–214, 1986.

312. Galazka A, Milstein J, Zaffran M. Thermostability of vaccines (WHO/GPV/98.07). Geneva, World Health Organization, 1998. Available at *www.who.int/vaccines-documents/DocsPDF/www9661.pdf*

313. Middleman AB, Kozinetz CA, Robertson LM, et al. The effect of late doses on the achievement of seroprotection and antibody titer levels with hepatitis B immunization among adolescents. Pediatrics 107:1065–1069, 2001.

314. Hadler SC, Margolis HS. Hepatitis B immunization: vaccine types, efficacy, and indications for immunization. Curr Clin Top Infect Dis 12:282–308, 1992.

315. Hessel L, West DJ. Antibody responses to recombinant hepatitis B vaccines. Vaccine 20:2164–2165, 2002.

316. Andre FE. Overview of a 5-year clinical experience with a yeast-derived hepatitis B vaccine. Vaccine 8(suppl):S74–S78, 1990.

317. Collier AC, Corey L, Murphy VL, Handsfield HH. Antibody to human immunodeficiency virus (HIV) and suboptimal response to hepatitis B vaccine. Ann Intern Med 109:101–105, 1988.

318. Weber DJ, Rutala WA, Samsa GP, et al. Obesity as a predictor of poor antibody response to hepatitis B plasma vaccine. JAMA 254:3187–3189, 1985.

319. Clements ML, Miskovsky E, Davidson M, et al. Effect of age on the immunogenicity of yeast recombinant hepatitis B vaccines containing surface antigen (S) or PresS2 + S antigens. J Infect Dis 170:510–516, 1994.

320. Averhoff F, Mahoney FJ, Coleman P, et al. Risk factors for lack of response to hepatitis B vaccines: a randomized trial comparing the immunogenicity of recombinant hepatitis B vaccines in an adult population. Am J Prev Med 15:1–8, 1998.

321. Wood RC, MacDonald KL, White KE, et al. Risk factors for lack of detectable antibody following hepatitis B vaccination of Minnesota health care workers. JAMA 270:2935–2972, 1993.

322. Treadwell TL, Keeffe EB, Lake J, et al. Immunogenicity of two recombinant hepatitis B vaccines in older individuals. Am J Med 95:584–588, 1993.

323. Roome AJ, Walsh SJ, Cartter ML, et al. Hepatitis B vaccine responsiveness in Connecticut public safety personnel. JAMA 270:2931–2934, 1993.

324. Winter AP, Follett EAC, McIntyre J, et al. Influence of smoking on immunological responses to hepatitis B vaccine. Vaccine 12:771–772, 1994.

325. Alper CA, Kruskall MS, Marcus-Bagley D, et al. Genetic prediction of nonresponse to hepatitis B vaccine. N Engl J Med 321:708–712, 1989.

326. West DJ. Clinical experience with hepatitis B vaccines. Am J Infect Control 17:172–180, 1989.

327. Courseget P, Kane M. Overview of clinical studies in developing countries. In Ellis RW (ed). Hepatitis B Vaccines in Clinical Practice. New York, Marcel Dekker, 1993, pp 209–228.

328. Greenberg DP, Vadheim CM, Wong VK, et al. Comparative safety and immunogenicity of two recombinant hepatitis B vaccines given to infants at two, four, and six months of age. Pediatr Infect Dis J 15:590–596, 1996.

329. Da Villa G, Pelliccia MG, Peluso F, et al. Anti-HBs responses in children vaccinated with different schedules of either plasma-derived or HBV DNA recombinant vaccine. Res Virol 148:109–114, 1997.

330. Goldfarb J, Baley J, Medendorp SV, et al. Comparative study of the immunogenicity and safety of two dosing schedules of Engerix-B hepatitis B vaccine in neonates. Pediatr Infect Dis J 13:18–22, 1994.

331. Cooper A, Yusuf H, Rodewald L, et al. Attitudes, practices, and preferences of pediatricians regarding initiation of hepatitis B immunization at birth. Pediatrics 108:E98, 2001.

332. Lau YL, Tam AY, Ng KW, et al. Response of preterm infants to hepatitis B vaccine. J Pediatr 121:962–965, 1992.

333. Patel DM, Butler J, Feldman S, et al. Immunogenicity of hepatitis B vaccine in healthy very-low-birth-weight infants. J Pediatr 131:641–643, 1997.

334. Kim SC, Chung EK, Hodinka RL, et al. Immunogenicity of hepatitis B vaccine in preterm infants. Pediatrics 99:534–536, 1997.

335. Losonsky GA, Wasserman S, Stephens I, et al. Hepatitis B vaccination of premature infants: a reassessment of current recommendations for delayed immunization. Pediatrics 103(2):E14, 1999.

335a. Freitas da Motta M, Mussi-Pinhata MM, Jorge SM, et al. Immunogenicity of hepatits B vaccine in preterm and full term infants vaccinated within the first week of life. Vaccine 20:1557–1562, 2002.

336. Expanded Programme on Immunization. Introduction of Hepatitis B Vaccine into Childhood Immunization Services: Management Guidelines, Including Information for Health Workers and Parents (WHO/V&B/01.31). Geneva, World Health Organization, 2001. Available at *www.who.int/vaccines-documents/DocsPDF01/www613.pdf*

337. Yusuf HR, Daniels D, Smith P, et al. Association between administration of hepatitis B vaccine at birth and completion of the hepatitis B and 4:3:1:3 vaccine series. JAMA 284:978–983, 2000.

338. Jilg W, Schmidt M, Deinhardt F. Vaccination against hepatitis B: comparison of three different vaccination schedules. J Infect Dis 160:766–769, 1989.

339. Cassidy WM, Watson B, Ioli VA, et al. A randomized trial of alternative two- and three-dose hepatitis B vaccination regimens in adolescents: antibody responses, safety, and immunologic memory. Pediatrics 107:626–631, 2001.

340. Schiff GM, Sherwood JR, Zeldis JB, Krause DS. Comparative study of the immunogenicity and safety of two doses of recombinant hepatitis B vaccine in healthy adolescents. J Adolesc Health 16:12–17, 1995.

341. Milne A, Moyes CD, Allwood GK, et al. Antibody responses to recombinant, yeast-derived hepatitis B vaccine in teenage New Zealand children. N Z Med J 101:676–679, 1988.

342. Centers for Disease Control and Prevention. Alternate two-dose hepatitis B vaccination schedule for adolescents aged 11–15 years. MMWR 49:261, 2000.

343. Marsano LS, West DJ, Chan I, et al. A two-dose hepatitis B vaccine regimen: proof of priming and memory responses in young adults. Vaccine 16:624–629, 1998.

343a. Fisman DN, Agrawal D, Leder K. The effect of age on immunologic response to recombinant hepatitis B vaccine: a meta-analysis. Clin Infect Dis 35:1368–1375, 2002.

344. Fraser GM, Ochana N, Fenyves D, et al. Increasing serum creatinine and age reduce the response to hepatitis B vaccine in renal failure patients. J Hepatol 21:450–454, 1994.

345. Bruguera M, Cremades M, Slainas R, et al. Impaired response to recombinant hepatitis B vaccine in HIV-infected persons. J Clin Gastroenterol 14:27–30, 1992.

346. Zuccotti GV, Riva E, Flumine P, et al. Hepatitis B vaccination of infants of mothers infected with human immunodeficiency virus. J Pediatr 125:70–72, 1994.

347. Zuin G, Principi N, Tornaghi R, et al. Impaired response to hepatitis B vaccine in HIV infected children. Vaccine 10:857–860, 1992.

348. Diamant EP, Schechter C, Hodes DS, Peters VB. Immunogenicity of hepatitis B vaccine in human immunodeficiency virus-infected children. Pediatr Infect Dis J 12:877–878, 1993.

349. Polychronopoulou-Androulakaki S, Panagiotou JP, Kostaridou S, et al. Immune response of immunocompromised children with malig-

nancies to a recombinant hepatitis B vaccine. Pediatr Hematol Oncol 13:425–431, 1996.

349a. Lunn ER, Hoggarth BJ, Cook WJ. Prolonged hepatitis B surface antigenemia after vaccination. J Pediatr 105:E81, 2000.

350. Szmuness W, Stevens CE, Harley EJ, et al. Hepatitis B vaccine: demonstration of efficacy in a controlled trial in a high-risk population in the U.S. N Engl J Med 303:833–841, 1980.

351. Francis DP, Hadler SC, Thompson SE, et al. Prevention of hepatitis B with vaccine: report from the Centers for Disease Control Multi-Center Efficacy Trial Among Homosexual Men. Ann Intern Med 97:362–366, 1982.

352. Crosnier J, Jungers P, Courouce AM, et al. Randomised placebo-controlled trial of hepatitis B surface antigen vaccine in French haemodialysis units: I. Medical staff. Lancet 1:455–459, 1981.

353. Jack AD, Hall AJ, Maine N, et al. What level of hepatitis B antibody is protective? J Infect Dis 179:489–492, 1999.

354. Beasley RP, Hwang LY, Lee GC, et al. Prevention of perinatally transmitted hepatitis B virus with hepatitis B immune globulin and hepatitis B vaccine. Lancet 2:1099–1102, 1983.

355. Ip HMH, Lelie PN, Wong VCW, et al. Prevention of hepatitis B virus carrier state in infants according to maternal serum levels of HBV DNA. Lancet 1:406–409, 1989.

356. Lo K-W, Tsai Y-T, Lee S-D, et al. Immunoprophylaxis of infection with hepatitis B virus in infants born to hepatitis B surface antigen–positive carrier mothers. J Infect Dis 152:817–822, 1985.

357. Pongpipat D, Suvatte V, Assateerawats A. Hepatitis B immunization in high-risk neonates born from HBsAg-positive mothers: comparison between plasma derived and recombinant DNA vaccine. Asian Pac J Allergy Immunol 7:37–40, 1989.

358. Del Canho R, Grosheide PM, Mazel JA, et al. Ten-year neonatal hepatitis B vaccination program, the Netherlands, 1982–1992: protective efficacy and long-term immunogenicity. Vaccine 15:1624–1630, 1997.

359. Poovorawan Y, Sanpavat S, Pongpunlert W, et al. Long term efficacy of hepatitis B vaccine in infants born to hepatitis B e antigen positive mothers. Pediatr Infect Dis J 11:816–821, 1992.

360. Assateerawatt A, Tanphaichitr VS, Suvatte V, In-ngarm L. Immunogenicity and protective efficacy of low-dose recombinant DNA hepatitis B vaccine in normal and high-risk neonates. Asian Pac J Allergy Immunol 9:89–93, 1991.

361. Stevens CE, Toy PT, Taylor PE, et al. Prospects for control of hepatitis B virus infection: implications of childhood vaccination and long-term protection. Pediatrics 90(suppl):170–173, 1992.

362. Marion SA, Tomm Pastore M, Pi DW, Mathias RG. Long-term follow-up of hepatitis B vaccine in infants of carrier mothers. Am J Epidemiol 140:734–746, 1994.

363. Centers for Disease Control and Prevention. Sensitivity of the test for antibody to hepatitis B surface antigen—United States. MMWR 42:707–710, 1993.

364. Huang LM, Chiang BL, Lee CY, et al. Long-term response to hepatitis B vaccination and response to booster in children born to mothers with hepatitis B e antigen. Hepatology 29:954–959, 1999.

365. Resti M, Azzari C, Mannelli F, et al. Ten-year follow-up study of neonatal hepatitis B immunization: are booster injections indicated? Vaccine 15:1338–1340, 1997.

366. Ding L, Zhang M, Wang Y, et al. A 9-year follow-up study of the immunogenicity and long-term efficacy of plasma-derived hepatitis B vaccine in high-risk Chinese neonates. Clin Infect Dis 17:475–479, 1993.

367. Liao SS, Li RC, Li H, et al. Long-term efficacy of plasma-derived hepatitis B vaccine: a 15-year follow-up study among Chinese children. Vaccine 17:2661–2666, 1999.

368. Coursaget P, Leboulleux D, Soumare M, et al. Twelve-year follow-up study of hepatitis B immunization of Senegalese infants. J Hepatol 21:250–254, 1994.

369. Viviani S, Jack A, Hall AJ, et al. Hepatitis B vaccination in infancy in The Gambia: protection against carriage at 9 years of age. Vaccine 17:2946–2950, 1999.

370. Mintai Z, Kezhou L, Lieming D, Smego RA Jr. Duration and efficacy of immune response to hepatitis B vaccine in high-risk Chinese adolescents. Clin Infect Dis 16:165–167, 1993.

371. Hadler SC, Coleman PJ, O'Malley P, et al. Evaluation of long-term protection by hepatitis B vaccine for seven to nine years in homosexual men. In Hollinger FB, Lemon SM, Margolis HS (eds). Viral Hepatitis and Liver Disease. Proceedings of the 1990 International Symposium on Viral Hepatitis and Liver Disease: Contemporary

372. Wainwright RB, Bulkow LR, Parkinson AJ, et al. Protection provided by hepatitis B vaccine in a Yupik Eskimo population—results of a 10-year study. J Infect Dis 175:674–677, 1997.

373. Goh KT, Oon CJ, Heng BH, Lim GK. Long-term immunogenicity and efficacy of a reduced dose of plasma-based hepatitis B vaccine in young adults. Bull World Health Organ 73:523–527, 1995.

374. Courouce AM, Loplanche A, Benhamou E, Jungers P. Long-term efficacy of hepatitis B vaccination in healthy adults. In Zuckermann AJ (ed). Viral Hepatitis and Liver Disease: Proceedings of the International Symposium on Viral Hepatitis and Liver Disease, held at the Barbicon Centre, London, May 26–28, 1987. New York, Alan R Liss, 1988, pp 1002–1005.

375. Gibas A, Watkins E, Hinkle C, Dienstag JL. Long-term persistence of protective antibody after hepatitis B vaccination of healthy adults. In Zuckermann AJ (ed). Viral Hepatitis and Liver Disease: Proceedings of the International Symposium on Viral Hepatitis and Liver Disease, held at the Barbicon Centre, London, May 26–28, 1987. New York, Alan R Liss, 1988, pp 998–1001.

376. Xia G, Liu C, Yan T, et al. Prevalence of hepatitis B virus markers in children vaccinated by hepatitis B vaccine in five hepatitis B vaccine experimental areas of China. Chin J Exp Clin Virol 9:17–23, 1995.

377. Xu ZY, Duan SC, Margolis H. Long-term efficacy of postexposure immunization of infants for prevention of hepatitis B virus infection. United States–People's Republic of China Study Group on Hepatitis B. J Infect Dis 171:54–60, 1995.

378. Lo KJ, Lee SD, Tsai YT, et al. Long term immunogenicity and efficacy of hepatitis B vaccine in infants born to HBeAg-positive HBsAg-carrier mothers. Hepatology 8:1647–1650, 1988.

379. Hwang LY, Lee CY, Beasley RP. Five-year follow-up of HBV vaccination with plasma derived vaccine in neonates: evaluation of immunogenicity and efficacy against perinatal transmission. In Hollinger FB, Lemon SM, Margolis HS (eds). Viral Hepatitis and Liver Disease. Proceedings of the 1990 International Symposium on Viral Hepatitis and Liver Disease: Contemporary Issues and Future Prospects. Baltimore, Williams & Wilkins, 1991, pp 759–761.

380. Lee PI, Lee CY, Huang LM, Chang MH. Long-term efficacy of recombinant hepatitis B vaccine and risk of natural infection in infants born to mothers with hepatitis B e antigen. J Pediatr 126:716–721, 1995.

381. Stevens CE, Alter HJ, Taylor PE, et al for the Dialysis Vaccine Study Trial Group. Hepatitis B vaccine in patients receiving hemodialysis: immunogenicity and efficacy. N Engl J Med 311:496–501, 1984.

382. Centers for Disease Control. Hepatitis B virus: a comprehensive strategy for eliminating transmission in the United States through universal childhood vaccination. MMWR 40(RR-13):1–25, 1991.

383. Banatvala J, Van Damme P, Oehen S. Lifelong protection against hepatitis B: the role of vaccine immunogenicity in immune memory. Vaccine 19:877–885, 2000.

384. West DJ, Calandra GB. Vaccine-induced memory for hepatitis B surface antigen: implications for policy on booster vaccination. Vaccine 14:1019–1027, 1996.

385. Van Hattum J, Maikoe T, Poel J, De Gast GC. In vitro anti-HBs production by individual B cells of responders to hepatitis B vaccine who subsequently lost antibody. In Hollinger FB, Lemon SB, Margolis HS (eds). Viral Hepatitis and Liver Disease. Proceedings of the 1990 International Symposium on Viral Hepatitis and Liver Disease: Contemporary Issues and Future Prospects. Baltimore, Williams & Wilkins, 1991, pp 774–776.

386. Horowitz MM, Ershler WB, McKinney WP, Battiola RJ. Duration of immunity after hepatitis B vaccination: efficacy of low-dose booster vaccine. Ann Intern Med 108:185–189, 1988.

387. Da Villa G, Peluso F, Picciotto L, et al. Persistence of anti-HBs in children vaccinated against viral hepatitis B in the first year of life: follow-up at 5 and 10 years. Vaccine 14:1503–1505,1996

388. Resti M, Di Francesco G, Azzari C, et al. Anti-HBs and immunological memory to HBV vaccine: implication for booster timing. Vaccine 11:1079, 1993.

389. Milne A, Hopkirk N, Moyes CD. Hepatitis B vaccination in children: persistence of immunity at 9 years. J Med Virol 44:113–114, 1994.

390. Milne A, Waldon J. Recombinant DNA hepatitis B vaccination in teenagers: effect of a booster at 5½ years. J Infect Dis 166:942, 1992.

391. Milne A, Krugman S, Waldon JA, et al. Hepatitis B vaccination in children: five-year booster study. N Z Med J 105:336–338, 1992.

392. Davidson M, Krugman S. Recombinant yeast hepatitis B vaccine compared with plasma-derived vaccine: immunogenicity and effect of a booster dose. J Infect 13(suppl A):31–38, 1986.

393. Chan CY, Lee SD, Tsai YT, Lo KJ. Booster response to recombinant yeast-derived hepatitis B vaccine in vaccinees whose anti-HBs responses were initially elicited by a plasma-derived vaccine. Vaccine 9:765–767, 1991.

394. Trivello R, Chiaramonte M, Ngatchu T, et al. Persistence of anti-HBs antibodies in health care personnel vaccinated with plasma-derived hepatitis B vaccine and response to recombinant DNA HB booster vaccine. Vaccine 13:139–141, 1995.

395. Williams IT, Goldstein ST, Tufa J, et al. Long-term antibody response to hepatitis B vaccination beginning at birth and to subsequent booster vaccination. Pediatr Infect Dis J 22:157–163, 2003.

396. Watson B, West DJ, Chilkatowsky A, et al. Persistence of immunologic memory for 13 years in recipients of a recombinant hepatitis B vaccine. Vaccine 19:3164–3168, 2001.

396a. Williams JL, Christensen CJ, McMahon BJ, et al. Evaluation of the response to a booster dose of hepatitis B vaccine in previously immunized healthcare workers. Vaccine 19:4081–4085, 2001.

397. European Consensus Group on Hepatitis B Immunity. Are booster immunisations needed for lifelong hepatitis B immunity? Lancet 355:561–565, 2000.

398. Lee C-L, Ko Y-C. Hepatitis B vaccination and hepatocellular carcinoma in Taiwan. Pediatrics 99:351–353, 1997.

399. Chang MH, Chen CJ, Lai MS, et al. Universal hepatitis B vaccination in Taiwan and the incidence of hepatocellular carcinoma in children. Taiwan Childhood Hepatoma Study Group. N Engl J Med 336:1855–1859, 1997.

400. McLean AA, Hilleman MR, McAleer WJ, Buynak EB. Summary of worldwide experience with HB-Vax® (B,MSD). J Infect 7(suppl): 95–104, 1983.

401. Greenberg DP. Pediatric experience with recombinant hepatitis B vaccines and relevant safety and immunogenicity studies. Pediatr Infect Dis J 12:438–445, 1993.

402. Lewis E, Shinefield HR, Woodruff BA, et al for The Vaccine Safety Datalink Workgroup. Safety of neonatal hepatitis B vaccine administration. Pediatr Infect Dis J 20:1049–1054, 2001.

403. Institute of Medicine Vaccine Safety Committee. Stratton KR, Howe CJ, Johnston RB Jr (eds). Adverse events associated with childhood vaccines: evidence bearing on causality. Hepatitis B vaccines. Washington, DC, National Academy Press, pp 211–235, 1994.

404. Niu MT, Davis DM, Ellenberg S. Recombinant hepatitis B vaccination of neonates and infants: emerging safety data from the Vaccine Adverse Event Reporting System. Pediatr Infect Dis J 15:771–776, 1996.

405. Centers for Disease Control and Prevention. Update: vaccine side effects, adverse reactions and precautions. Recommendations of the Advisory Committee on Immunization Practices. MMWR 45(RR-12):1–35, 1996.

406. Chen D-S. Control of hepatitis B in Asia: mass immunization program in Taiwan. In Hollinger FB, Lemon SM, Margolis HS (eds). Viral Hepatitis and Liver Disease. Proceedings of the 1990 International Symposium on Viral Hepatitis and Liver Disease: Contemporary Issues and Future Prospects. Baltimore, Williams & Wilkins, 1991, pp 716–719.

407. McMahon BJ, Helminiak C, Wainwright RB, et al. Frequency of adverse reactions to hepatitis B vaccine in 43,618 persons. Am J Med 92:254–256, 1992.

408. Grotto I, Mandel Y, Ephrost M, et al. Major adverse reactions to yeast-derived hepatitis B vaccines: a review. Vaccine 16:329–334, 1998.

409. Shaw FE, Graham DJ, Guess HA, et al. Postmarketing surveillance for neurologic adverse events reported after hepatitis B vaccination. Am J Epidemiol 127:337–352, 1988.

410. Nadler JP. Multiple sclerosis and hepatitis B vaccination. Clin Infect Dis 17:928–929, 1993.

411. Herroelen L, de Keyser J, Ebinger G. Central nervous system demyelination after immunisation with recombinant hepatitis B vaccine. Lancet 338:1174–1175, 1991.

412. Trevisani F, Gattinara GC, Caraceni P, et al. Transverse myelitis following hepatitis B vaccination. J Hepatology 19:317–318, 1993.

413. Anonymous. Alleged link between hepatitis B vaccine and chronic fatigue syndrome. Can Dis Wkly Rep 17:215–216, 1991.

414. Classen JB. Childhood immunizations and diabetes mellitus. N Z Med J 109:195, 1996.

415. Maillefert JF, Sibilia J, Toussirot E, et al. Rheumatic disorders developed after hepatitis B vaccination. Rheumatology 38:978–983, 1999.

416. Pope JE, Stevens A, Howson W, Bell DA. The development of rheumatoid arthritis after recombinant hepatitis B vaccination. J Rheumatol 25:1687–1693, 1998.

417. Tudela P, Marti S, Bonal J. Systemic lupus erythematosus and vaccination against hepatitis B. Nephron 62:236, 1992.

418. Touze E, Gout O, Verdier-Taillefer MH, Lyon-Caen O, Alperovitch A. The first episode of central nervous system demyelinization and hepatitis B vaccination. Rev Neurol 156:242–246, 2000.

419. Touze E, Fourier A, Rue-Fenouche C, et al. Hepatitis B vaccination and first central nervous system demyelinating event: a case-control study. Neuroepidemiology 21:180–186, 2002.

420. Sturkenboom M, Abenhaim L, Wolfson C, et al. Vaccinations, demyelination, and multiple sclerosis study. Pharmacoepidemiol Drug Saf 8:S170–S171, 1999.

421. Balinska MA. L'affaire hepatite B en France. Esprit 276:34–48, 2001.

422. Ascherio A, Zhang SM, Hernan MA, et al. Hepatitis B vaccination and the risk of multiple sclerosis. N Engl J Med 344:327–332, 2001.

423. Verstraeten T, DeStefano F, Jackson L, et al. Risk of demyelinating disease after hepatitis B vaccination—West Coast, United States, 1995–1999 [abstract]. In Abstracts of the 50th Annual Epidemic Intelligence Service Conference, Atlanta, 2001.

424. Sadovnick AD, Scheifele DW. School-based hepatitis B vaccination programme and adolescent multiple sclerosis. Lancet 355:549–550, 2000.

425. Confavreux C, Suissa S, Saddier P, et al for the Vaccines in Multiple Sclerosis Study Group. Vaccinations and the risk of relapse in multiple sclerosis. N Engl J Med 344:319–326, 2001.

426. Halsey NA, Duclos P, VanDamme P, et al for the Viral Hepatitis Prevention Board. Hepatitis B vaccine and central nervous system demyelinating diseases. Pediatr Infect Dis J 18:23–24, 1999.

427. Institute of Medicine Immunization Safety Review Committee. Hepatitis B vaccine and demyelinating disorders. In Stratton K, Almario D, McCormick MC (eds). Immunization Safety Review: Multiple Immunizations and Immune Dysfunction. 2002. Washington, DC, National Academy Press, 2002.

427a. Konstantinou D, Paschalis C, Maraziotis T, et al. Two episodes of leukoencephalitis associated with recombinant hepatitis B vaccination in a single patient. Clin Infect Dis 33:1772–1773, 2001.

428. DeStefano F, Mullooly JP, Okoro CA, et al. Childhood vaccinations, vaccination timing, and risk of type 1 diabetes mellitus. Pediatrics 108:E112, 2001.

429. Institute for Vaccine Safety Diabetes Workshop Panel. Childhood immunization and type I diabetes: summary of an Institute for Vaccine Safety workshop. Pediatr Infect Dis J 18:217–222, 1999.

430. Stratton K, Wilson CB, McCormick MC (eds). Immunization Safety Review: Multiple Immunizations and Immune Dysfunction. Washington, DC, National Academy Press, 2002.

431. DeStefano F, Gu D, Kramarz P, et al. Childhood vaccinations and risk of asthma. Ped Infect Dis J 21:498–504, 2002.

432. Mullooly JP, Pearson J, Drew L, et al. Wheezing lower respiratory disease and vaccinations of full-term infants. Pharmacoepidemiol Drug Saf 11:21–30, 2002.

433. Lear JT, English JS. Anaphylaxis after hepatitis B vaccination. Lancet 345:1249, 1995.

434. Wise RP, Kiminyo KP, Salive ME. Hair loss after routine immunizations. JAMA 278:1176–1178, 1997.

435. Schwalbe JA, Ray P, Black SB, et al. Risk of alopecia after hepatitis B vaccination (poster), 38th Annual Interscience Conference on Antimicrobial Agents and Chemotherapy, September 24–27, San Diego, 1998.

436. Niu MT, Salive ME, Ellenberg SS. Neonatal deaths after hepatitis B vaccine: the Vaccine Adverse Event Reporting System, 1991–1998. Arch Pediatr Adolesc Med 153:1279–1282, 1999.

437. Mitchell EA, Stewart AW, Clements M. Immunisation and the sudden infant death syndrome. New Zealand Cot Death Study Group. Arch Dis Child 73:498–501, 1995.

438. Lewis E, Shinefield HR, Woodruff BA, et al. Safety of neonatal hepatitis B vaccine administration. Pediatr Infect Dis J 20:1049–1054, 2001.

439. Silvers LE, Ellenberg SS, Wise RP, et al. The epidemiology of fatalities reported to the Vaccine Adverse Event Reporting System, 1990–1997. Pharmacoepidemiol Drug Safety 10:279–285, 2001.

440. Levy M, Koren G. Hepatitis B vaccine in pregnancy: maternal and fetal safety. Am J Perinatol 8:227–232, 1991.

441. Harpaz R, Shapiro CN, Havron D, et al. Elimination of new chronic hepatitis B virus infections: results of the Alaska immunization program. J Infect Dis 181:413–418, 2000.

442. American Academy of Pediatrics. Recommended Childhood Immunization Schedule—United States, 2002. Pediatrics 109:162, 2002.

443. Centers for Disease Control and Prevention. Achievements in public health: hepatitis B vaccination—United States, 1982–2002. MMWR 51:549–552, 563, 2002.

444. Freed GL, Bordley WC, Clark SJ, Konrad TR. Reactions of pediatricians to a new CDC recommendation for universal immunization of infants with hepatitis B vaccine. Pediatrics 91:699–702, 1993.

445. Ganiats TR. Hepatitis B vaccination: are we jumping on the bandwagon too early? J Fam Pract 36:147–149, 1993.

446. Yusuf H, Daniels D, Mast EE, Coronado V. Hepatitis B vaccination coverage among United States children. Pediatr Infect Dis J 20(suppl):S30–S33, 2001.

447. Centers for Disease Control and Prevention. National, state, and urban area vaccination coverage levels among children aged 19–35 months—United States, 2000. MMWR 50:637–641, 2001.

448. Centers for Disease Control and Prevention. Updated U.S. Public Health Service guidelines for the management of occupational exposures to HBV, HCV, and HIV, and recommendations for postexposure prophylaxis. MMWR 50(RR-11):1–52, 2001.

449. Kane MA. Global status of hepatitis B immunization. Lancet 348:696, 1996.

450. McQuillan GM, Coleman PJ, Kruszon-Moran D, et al. Prevalence of hepatitis B virus infection in the United States: the National Health and Nutrition Examination Surveys, 1976 through 1994. Am J Public Health 89:14–18, 1999.

451. Coleman PJ, McQuillan GM, Moyer LA, et al. Incidence of hepatitis B virus infection in the United States, 1976–1994: estimates from the National Health and Nutrition Examination Surveys. J Infect Dis 178:954–959, 1998.

452. Mahoney F, Smith N, Alter MJ, Margolis H. Progress towards the elimination of hepatitis B virus transmission in the United States. Viral Hepatitis Rev 3:105–119, 1997.

453. World Health Organization. Expanded Programme on Immunization global advisory group. Wkly Epidemiol Rec 3:11–16, 1992.

454. Van Damme P, Kane M, Meheus A. Integration of hepatitis B vaccination into national immunisation programmes. BMJ 314:1033–1036, 1997.

454a. Euler GL, Copeland JR, Rangel MC, et al. Antibody response to postexposure prophylaxis in infants born to hepatitis B surface antigen-positive women. Pediatr Infect Dis J 22:123–129, 2003.

455. McMahon BJ, Rhoades ER, Heyward WL, et al. A comprehensive program to reduce the incidence of hepatitis B virus infection and its sequelae in Alaskan Natives. Lancet 2:1134–1136, 1987.

456. Centers for Disease Control and Prevention. Recommendations of the International Task Force for Disease Eradication. MMWR 42(RR-16):1–38, 1993.

457. Coutinho RA, Lelie N, Albrecht-Van Lent P, et al. Efficacy of a heat-inactivated hepatitis B vaccine in male homosexuals: outcome of a placebo-controlled double-blind trial. Br Med J 286:1305–1308, 1983.

458. Szmuness W, Stevens CE, Harley EJ, et al. Hepatitis B vaccine in medical staff of hemodialysis units: efficacy and subtype cross-protection. N Engl J Med 307:1481–1486, 1982.

459. Crosnier J, Jungers P, Courouce AM, et al. Randomized placebo-controlled trial of hepatitis B surface antigen vaccine in French haemodialyisis units: II. Haemodialysis patients. Lancet 1:797–800, 1981.

460. Desmyter J, Colaert J, De Groote G, et al. Efficacy of heat-inactivated hepatitis B vaccine in haemodialysis patients and staff: double-blind, placebo-controlled trial. Lancet 2:1323–1328, 1983.

461. Lee CY, Lee PI, Huang LM, et al. A simplified schedule to integrate the hepatitis B vaccine into an expanded program of immunization in endemic countries. J Pediatr 130:981–986, 1997.

462. Poovorawan Y, Sanpavat S, Chumdermpadetsuk S, Safary A. Long-term hepatitis B vaccine in infants born to hepatitis B e antigen positive mothers. Arch Dis Child 77:F47–F51, 1997.

463. Milne A, West DJ, Chinh DV, et al. Field evaluation of the efficacy and immunogenicity of recombinant hepatitis B vaccine without HBIG in newborn Vietnamese infants. J Med Virol 67:327–333, 2002.

464. Moulia-Pelat JP, Spiegel A, Martin PMV, et al. A 5-year immunization field trial against hepatitis B using a Chinese hamster ovary cell recombinant vaccine in French Polynesian newborns: results at 3 years. Vaccine 12:499–502, 1994.

465. Tin KM. Studies on the efficacy of hepatitis B vaccine in preventing perinatal HBV transmission in Burma. Presented at the Symposium on Control of Hepatitis B in Infants and Children in High-Risk Areas of the World, Whakatane, New Zealand, November 12–14, 1987.

466. Wu JS, Hwang LY, Goodman KJ, Beasley RP. Hepatitis B vaccination in high-risk infants: 10-year follow-up. J Infect Dis 179:1319–1325, 1999.

467. Yuen MF, Lim WL, Cheng CC, et al. Twelve-year follow-up of a prospective randomized trial of hepatitis B recombinant DNA yeast vaccine versus plasma-derived vaccine without booster doses in children. Hepatology 29:924–927, 1999.

468. Jilg W, Schmidt M, Deinhardt F. Persistence of specific antibodies after hepatitis B vaccination. J Hepatol 6:201–207, 1988.

469. Xu ZY, Cao CB, Liu SS, et al. Control of hepatitis B in China. In Rizzetto M, Purcell RH, Gerin JL, Verme G (eds). Viral Hepatitis and Liver Disease: Proceedings of the IXth Triennial Symposium on Viral Hepatitis and Liver Disease, Rome, 21–25 April 1996. Turin, Edizioni Minerva Medica, 1997, pp 689–690.

470. Mahoney FJ, Woodruff B, Auerbach S, et al. Progress on the elimination of hepatitis B virus transmission in Micronesia and American Samoa. Pac Health Dialog 3:140–146, 1996.

471. Viviani S, Jack A, Hall AJ, et al. Hepatitis B vaccination in infancy in The Gambia: protection against carriage at 9 years of age. Vaccine 17:2946–2950, 1999.

472. Ruff TA, Gertig DM, Otto BF, et al. Lombock hepatitis B model immunization project: toward universal infant hepatitis B immunization in Indonesia. J Infect Dis 171:290–296, 1995.

473. Mahoney F, Woodruff BA, Erben JJ, et al. Evaluation of a hepatitis B vaccination program on the prevalence of chronic HBV infection. J Infect Dis 167:203–207, 1993.

474. Al-Faleh FZ, Al-Jeffri M, Ramia S, et al. Seroepidemiology of hepatitis B virus infection in Saudi children 8 years after a mass hepatitis B vaccination programme. J Infect 38:167–170, 1999.

475. Chen HL, Chang MH, Ni YH, et al. Seroepidemiology of hepatitis B virus infection in children: ten years of mass vaccination in Taiwan. JAMA 276:906–908, 1996.

476. Shih HH, Chang MH, Hsu HY, et al. Long-term immune response of universal hepatitis B vaccination in infancy: a community-based study in Taiwan. Pediatr Infect Dis J 18:427–432, 1999.

477. Hsu HM, Lu CF, Lee SC, et al. Seroepidemiologic survey for hepatitis B virus infection in Taiwan: the effect of hepatitis B mass vaccination. J Infect Dis 179:367–370, 1999.

478. Chunsuttiwat S, Biggs BA, Maynard J, et al. Integration of hepatitis B vaccination into the Expanded Programme on Immunization in Chonburi and Chiangmai provinces, Thailand. Vaccine 15:769–774, 1997.

479. Lin Y-C, Chang M-H, Ni Y-H, et al. Long-term immunogenicity and efficacy of universal hepitis B virus vaccination in Taiwan. J Infect Dis 187:134–138, 2003.

480. Ni Y-H, Chang M-H, Huang L-M, et al. Hepatitis B virus infection in children and adolescents in a hyperendemic area: 15 years after mass hepatitis B vaccination. Ann Intern Med 135:796–800, 2001.

481. Whittle H, Jaffar S, Wansbrough M, et al. Observational study of vaccine efficacy 14 years after trial of hepatitis B vaccination in Gambian children. BMJ Sep 14;325 (7364):569, 2002.

482. Tsebe KV, Burnett RJ, Hlungwani NP, et al. The first five years of universal hepatitis B vaccination in South African: evidence for elimination of HBsAg carriage in under 5-year-olds. Vaccine 19:3919–3926, 2001.

483. Hino K, Katch Y, Vardas E. The effect of introduction of universal childhood hepatitis B immunization in South Africa on the prevalence of serologically negative hepatitis B virus infection and the selection of immune escape variants. Vaccine 19:3912–3918, 2001.

484. Mele A, Tancredi F, Romano L, et al. Effectiveness of hepatitis B vaccination in babies born to hepatitis B surface antigen-positive mothers in Italy. J Infect Dis 184:905–908, 2001.

485. Kao J-H, Chen D-S. Global control of hepatitis B virus infection. Lancet Inf Dis 2:395–403, 2002.

Chapter 17

Inactivated Influenza Vaccines

KEIJI FUKUDA • ROLAND A. LEVANDOWSKI •

CAROLYN B. BRIDGES • NANCY J. COX

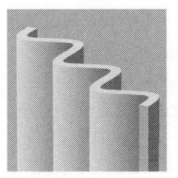

Epidemics and pandemics of respiratory disease, consistent with influenza, have been recorded since the 16th century.[1,2] During the 19th century, influenza was attributed to *Haemophilus influenzae* (Pfeiffer's bacillus), which had been isolated from patients with influenza and pneumonia.[3] Early efforts to vaccinate against influenza used extracts of *H. influenzae* as the immunizing material. However, isolation of the influenza A virus in 1933[4] rapidly led to the identification of influenza viruses as the cause of previous epidemics and pandemics of respiratory disease and to the development, testing, and first use of influenza vaccines in the 1930s and 1940s.[5-8]

During seasonal epidemics, large numbers of influenza infections can occur in all age groups. In most individuals, influenza is a self-limited illness, but serious secondary complications develop in many of those infected. The resulting illnesses, often requiring ambulatory medical care or hospitalization, substantially contribute to lost work and school time, overwhelmed hospitals and regional medical care systems,[9] and increases in "excess" hospitalizations and deaths.[10-15] Few other infectious diseases have adversely affected the health and economies of global populations as consistently and extensively as influenza.

The capacity of influenza A and B viruses to undergo gradual antigenic change in their two surface antigens, hemagglutinin (HA) and neuraminidase (NA), complicates vaccination against the disease. This type of antigenic change, which is known as antigenic drift, results from the accumulation of point mutations in the RNA genes encoding HA and NA and leads to the emergence of new variant strains. As the antibody prevalence to older variants increases in the population, the circulation of the older, previously dominant variants is suppressed, allowing new antigenic variants to become predominant. When the antibody prevalence to the new variant increases within a population, yet another antigenic variant emerges and the cycle is repeated. This ongoing process of antigenic drift ensures a constantly renewed pool of susceptible hosts and the repetitive occurrence of epidemics. Drift also necessitates annual changes in influenza vaccine strains and annual administration of vaccine.

On occasion, "antigenic shift" occurs when an influenza A virus with an HA or an HA–NA combination that has not recently infected humans is transmitted and causes disease. When such viruses are sufficiently transmissible among people, the result can be the rapid global spread of infection and disease. Such pandemics can be associated with rates of illness and death that are higher than usual. The effect of some pandemics, such as the infamous "Spanish flu" pandemic of 1918, has been catastrophic.[16]

The annual administration of influenza vaccine, especially to persons known to be at elevated risk for developing serious complications as a result of this infection, is the focus of current efforts to reduce the impact of this disease. Although the quality, availability, and use of inactivated influenza vaccine have increased substantially, influenza vaccine is underutilized in most countries, and influenza remains an uncontrolled infectious disease.

Background

Clinical Description

Symptoms do not result in approximately 30% to 50% of influenza infections[17-21]; however, asymptomatically infected persons can be infectious and transmit influenza to others. Although most symptomatic influenza infections are self-limited, acute febrile influenza illnesses can range in severity from mild to debilitating and, in some instances, become exacerbated by a variety of secondary complications.

Primary Influenza Illness

Primary influenza illness is characterized by the abrupt start of fever, sore throat, headache, myalgia, chills, anorexia, and extreme fatigue.[22] Fever usually ranges between 38°C and 40°C, but may be higher, and usually lasts for 3 to 5 days. Cough is usually unproductive of sputum, but a runny or

---

*Efficacy versus effectiveness: Efficacy is often measured using randomized placebo-controlled trials (RCTs). Properly conducted RCTs help to eliminate selection biases between intervention and nonintervention groups to isolate more precisely the effect of the intervention. The term *effectiveness* often is used to describe benefits seen from an intervention applied to a nonrandomized study population. Selection bias is often a concern in such studies. The difference between efficacy and effectiveness estimates can be significant.

All material in this chapter is in the public domain, with the exception of any borrowed figures or tables.

stuffy nose is common. Substernal tenderness, photophobia, abdominal pain, and diarrhea occur less frequently. Illness typically improves within a week, but cough and malaise may persist for several days to a few weeks longer. A minority of patients may experience fatigue for months.[23] In neonates, the primary manifestation may be unexplained fever. In children, fevers are often higher than in adults and sometimes lead to febrile seizures. Vomiting, abdominal pain, diarrhea, and other complications such as myositis, croup (tracheobronchitis), and otitis media also occur more frequently in children. In the elderly, fever may be absent and the presenting signs may include anorexia, lassitude, or confusion.

Complications of Influenza

The risk of developing serious complications from influenza infection is elevated in persons at both age extremes as well as in those with certain underlying conditions.[24] The most common serious complications of influenza include exacerbation of underlying chronic pulmonary and cardiopulmonary diseases, such as chronic obstructive pulmonary disease, asthma, and congestive heart failure, as well as development of bacterial pneumonia usually associated with Streptococcus pneumoniae, Staphylococcus aureus, and Haemophilus influenzae. Primary viral pneumonia occurs infrequently but often is fatal. In the pandemics of 1918 to 1919 and 1957 to 1958, some cases of viral pneumonia were associated with underlying cardiac valvular disease (frequently mitral stenosis from rheumatic heart disease) and pregnancy.[25,26] Pneumonias with both viral and bacterial features have been described.[26] Other complications involving the respiratory tract include bacterial sinusitis, bronchitis, croup, and otitis media.[27–30]

It is not certain if influenza is associated with Reye's syndrome. Reye's syndrome associated with influenza has been reported primarily in children with influenza B virus infection, but it has also been observed in children with influenza A infections.[31,32] The incidence of Reye's syndrome has decreased dramatically in the United States after warnings were issued in the 1980s regarding the use of aspirin to treat children.

Myocarditis and pericarditis were reported in association with influenza during the 1918 to 1919 pandemic, but since then have been documented infrequently. Minor electrocardiographic changes have been reported in patients with underlying heart disease and influenza. Myositis with rhabdomyolysis and myoglobinuria has been reported but is uncommon.[33,34] Toxic shock syndrome associated with secondary staphylococcal infection after acute influenza also has been reported.[35]

A number of central nervous system (CNS) complications, including encephalopathy, encephalitis, transverse myelitis, and Guillain-Barré syndrome (GBS), have been reported, but whether they are caused by influenza remains unclear. Recent reports, predominantly from Japan, suggest that children in some settings or populations can develop a frequently fatal or chronically debilitating encephalopathy in association with influenza infection.[36,37]

Virology

Taxonomy and Nomenclature

Influenza viruses, together with Thogoto-like viruses, form the family Orthomyxoviridae.[38] Influenza viruses are further divided into three genera, Influenzavirus A, Influenzavirus B, and Influenzavirus C virus, based on antigenic differences in two major structural proteins, the nucleoprotein (NP) and the matrix protein (M). Influenza A viruses are further classified into subtypes according to the properties of their major membrane glycoproteins, HA and NA. Fifteen HA subtypes and nine NA subtypes have been identified among influenza A viruses. The nomenclature of influenza viruses includes the type of isolate, the geographic location where it was isolated, the year of isolation, a laboratory identification number, and, for influenza A viruses, the subtype of the HA and NA (e.g., A/Panama/2007/99 [H_3N_2]).

Natural Hosts

Influenza A viruses naturally infect humans, causing epidemics and pandemics of respiratory disease. Virus isolation data indicate that influenza A viruses of the H_1N_1, H_1N_2, and H_3N_2 subtypes are currently circulating among humans, while H_2N_2 viruses circulated among humans in the mid-1900s. However, influenza A viruses of all 15 HA subtypes and all 9 NA subtypes have been isolated from wild aquatic birds, which serve as a natural reservoir and a source of novel genes for pandemic influenza viruses. Influenza A viruses also infect poultry, pigs, horses, and occasionally sea mammals. Interspecies transmission of influenza A viruses has been well documented and can result in severe illness, as amply demonstrated by the 1997 transmission of an influenza A (H_5N_1) virus from poultry to humans.[39–43] Although influenza B virus infection of seals in the Netherlands has been documented,[44] influenza B viruses appear to naturally infect primarily only humans and cause epidemics every few years. Influenza C viruses appear to infect only humans and pigs and usually cause sporadic cases or localized outbreaks of less severe upper respiratory tract infection in children and young adults.

Virus Structure

Influenza viruses are enveloped and contain segmented RNA-negative sense genomes (Fig. 17–1). Segmentation of the viral RNA allows exchange of genes (i.e., genetic reassortment) among influenza viruses of the same type (see below). The segmented RNA genome is associated with nucleoprotein and three viral polymerase proteins (PB1, PB2, and PA) within helical nucleocapsids that are surrounded by the virus envelope derived from the host cell membrane. The spherical, often pleomorphic, 80- to 120-nm virus particles have a surface layer of spike-like projections, 10 to 14 nm long, consisting of HA and NA proteins. HA is the major antigen against which the host's protective antibody response is directed and is responsible for attachment of influenza viruses to oligosaccharide-containing terminal sialic acids on the cell surface during early stages of infection. NA is less abundant on the viral surface and facilitates release of mature virus from infected cells. Antibody to NA is believed to restrict virus spread and reduce severity of the influenza infection.

The influenza A virus envelope also contains matrix (M1) and transmembrane (M2) proteins. M1 protein is located inside the viral membrane and is thought to add rigidity to the lipid bilayer, whereas M2 protein functions as a pH-activated ion channel[45] (see Adamantanes below).

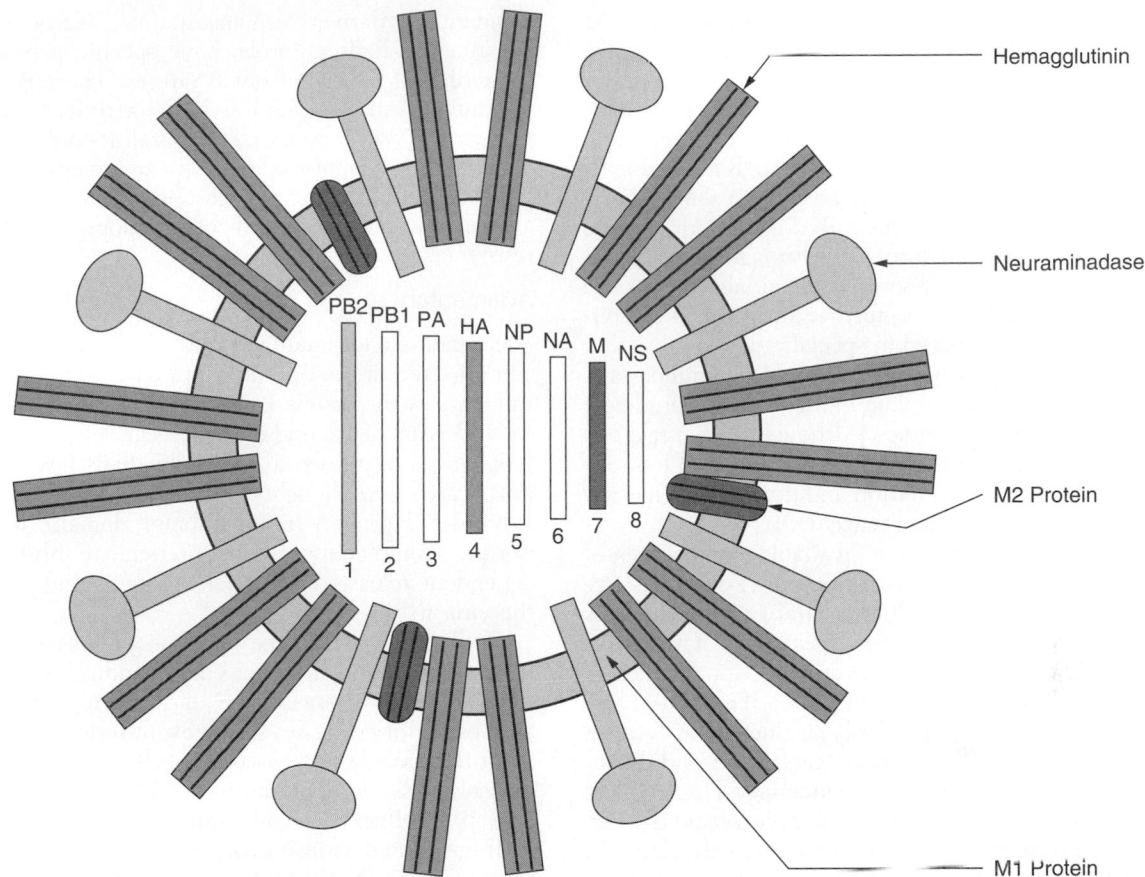

FIGURE 17–1 ■ Schematic representation of the influenza A virus. (Based on Lamb RA, Horvath CM: Diversity of coding strategies in influenza viruses. Trends Genet 7:261–266, 1991.)

Pathogenesis as It Relates to Prevention

Influenza viruses are spread by virus-laden aerosols produced by the coughing or sneezing of infectious individuals. The degree to which transmission occurs by airborne versus large droplets is uncertain. Transmission of virus by direct contact with infected respiratory secretions can also occur.

The incubation period for influenza is commonly 2 days but ranges from 1 to 4 days.[46] Virus can be isolated from the nasopharynx of adults for up to 5 days after illness. Children may shed virus for up to 2 weeks, while severely immunocompromised persons can shed virus for months.[47] The pathogenesis of influenza virus replication and its relationship to the clinical manifestations and complications of influenza are not well elucidated. However, studies conducted during the Asian influenza pandemic of 1957 to 1958 determined that infection and viral replication occurred primarily in the columnar epithelial cells of the respiratory tract,[48,49] but that viral replication can occur throughout the respiratory tract. After infection, ciliated columnar cells become vacuolated, lose cilia, and become necrotic. Regeneration of epithelium takes approximately 3 to 4 weeks, during which pulmonary abnormalities can persist. Although constitutional manifestations are pronounced in influenza, viremia has been reported rarely.[50,51]

Diagnosis

Infections by other pathogens, including respiratory syncytial virus (RSV), adenovirus, parainfluenza virus, rhinovirus, *Mycoplasma pneumoniae*, *Chlamydia pneumoniae*, and *Legionella pneumophila*, can result in individual illnesses similar to influenza. Nonetheless, certain epidemiologic features of influenza outbreaks and epidemics can greatly aid in the clinical diagnosis of influenza. For example, community-wide or institutional outbreaks of febrile respiratory illness cases during winter and spring months are characteristic of influenza, although RSV also can exhibit a similar epidemiologic pattern. In most instances, individual cases of influenza are difficult to identify reliably by clinical examination and routine laboratory findings alone, and the appropriate use of influenza diagnostic tests is helpful. Such tests include virus isolation (culture) and identification, direct detection of influenza virus in clinical specimens, point-of-care tests, molecular methods, and serologic tests.

Isolation of influenza viruses in cell culture or eggs followed by hemagglutination-inhibition (HI) testing to identify the virus has been considered the "gold standard" for influenza diagnosis for many years. Viral culture is very useful because the isolate can be typed, subtyped, and further characterized antigenically and genetically. However, the sensitivity of this technique depends on when in the course of illness the specimen is collected and its quality.[52] The specimen can be inoculated into embryonated hens' eggs or tissue culture systems, such as Madin-Darby canine kidney (MDCK), rhesus monkey kidney, or cynomolgus monkey kidney cell cultures and virus detected by hemagglutination, hemadsorption, or cytopathic effect. Results usually are not available for at least 3 days, although some laboratories use a rapid culture method that allows virus to be detected within 18 to 24 hours.[53] Although state health department laboratories and some hospital laboratories can type and subtype viral isolates, further antigenic characterization generally is conducted in specialized laboratories.

A variety of sensitive and specific radioimmunoassays, fluoroimmunoassays, and enzyme immunoassays can detect viral antigens in clinical samples. Although these assays can produce a result within a few hours, they are often less sensitive than standard virus isolation and they require specialized laboratory equipment and reagents.[52]

There are six commercially available "point-of-care" tests for rapid diagnosis of influenza. Five tests are immunoassays that detect influenza viral proteins and one test detects viral NA activity in specimens. Three tests detect influenza A and B viruses but do not distinguish between them (QuickVue Influenza Test, FLU OIA, and ZstatFlu). One test detects only influenza A viruses (Directigen Flu A), and two others can detect and distinguish between influenza A and B (Directigen Flu A+B and Binax NOW Flu A/B). In general, these diagnostic tests are useful for determining rapidly if influenza is the cause of outbreaks in institutions or other settings and for documenting circulation of influenza viruses in populations of patients. These tests have a sensitivity of 40% to 100% and a specificity of 52% to 100% according to the manufacturers. However, because point-of-care tests are often much less sensitive and specific than viral culture, collection of additional specimens for viral isolation is strongly recommended to confirm the rapid antigen test results.

Molecular methods now are being applied more widely to diagnose influenza virus infections and are likely to supplant virus culture as the "gold standard" for virus detection. Methods using reverse transcription of viral RNA followed by amplification with polymerase chain reaction are more rapid and sensitive than virus culture.[52] A new molecular approach uses DNA microarrays containing nucleic acid probes to type and subtype influenza viruses. A study by Li et al. demonstrated that a model microarray correctly identified influenza.[54]

Influenza virus infections also can be detected by measuring increases in influenza-specific antibody between acute and convalescent serum samples. Techniques for measuring antibody against influenza in sera include HI, virus neutralization, enzyme immunoassay, and complement fixation. In general, these tests are considered sensitive and may provide the only means for documenting influenza infection in situations where appropriate respiratory specimens are not available.

Treatment and Prevention with Antiviral Agents

Two classes of prescription medications, adamantanes and NA inhibitors, have been approved in the United States for use against influenza virus infections (Table 17–1). The adamantane derivatives, amantadine hydrochloride and rimantadine hydrochloride, have specific activity against influenza A viruses but not B viruses. The NA inhibitors, zanamivir and oseltamivir, have activity against both influenza A and B viruses. The four drugs differ by routes of administration, approved usage for treatment or chemoprophylaxis for different age groups, adverse events, costs, availability, and frequency of development of antiviral resistance.

Adamantanes

Amantadine and rimantadine are chemically related, orally administered drugs. Both are approved for the treatment of influenza A in persons 1 year of age and older and in persons 13 years of age and older, respectively, and for chemoprophylaxis of influenza A in individuals 1 year and older. Both drugs are thought to interfere with the influenza A virus M2 protein transmembrane domain, which functions as an ion channel. This interference inhibits the pH-dependent release of ribonucleoproteins and uncoating of the virus in cell culture assays.

Both drugs reduce the duration of illness by approximately 1 day and decrease viral shedding when administered within 48 hours of the start of symptoms. However, they have not been shown to prevent serious complications of influenza. When used for chemoprophylaxis, the adamantanes are approximately 70% to 90% effective in preventing illness caused by influenza A viruses.

It has been demonstrated, both in vitro and in vivo, that resistance to these drugs develops rapidly in influenza viruses, and that resistant viruses can transmit to contacts. Influenza A viruses resistant to one adamantane drug are also resistant to the other.

Amantadine and rimantadine are commonly used in the United States for chemoprophylaxis during institutional outbreaks of influenza A. When given as chemoprophylaxis to healthy adults and elderly nursing home residents in controlled studies, amantadine and rimantadine have been associated with gastrointestinal and CNS adverse effects, including lightheadedness, difficulty concentrating, nervousness, insomnia, and seizures in patients with pre-existing seizure disorders. Rimantadine has been associated with fewer CNS side effects than amantadine.

The usual therapeutic and prophylactic dosage of amantadine and rimantadine in adults less than 65 years is 100 mg orally twice a day (see Table 17–1). Doses should be reduced in children younger than 10 years and adults 65 years and older (especially those in nursing homes). Dosing of amantadine should be reduced in persons with renal insufficiency. Dosing of rimantadine should be reduced for severe hepatic or severe renal dysfunction. Treatment for influenza infection with the adamantanes should continue for 3 to 5 days or for 24 to 48 hours after disappearance of signs and symptoms. Duration of prophylaxis is variable, depending on the setting and the duration of influenza activity in the community or the institution.

Neuraminidase Inhibitors

The NA inhibitors, zanamivir and oseltamivir, are chemically related antiviral drugs active against both influenza A and B viruses. Zanamivir is an orally inhaled powdered drug that is approved for treatment of influenza in persons 7

TABLE 17–1 ■ Recommended Daily Dosage of Influenza Antiviral Medications for Treatment and Prophylaxis

Antiviral Agent[1]	Age Groups				
	1–6 yr	7–9 yr	10–12 yr	13–64 yr	≥65 yr
AMANTADINE[2]					
Treatment: influenza A	5 mg/kg/day up to 150 mg in two divided doses[3]	5 mg/kg/day up to 150 mg in two divided doses[3]	100 mg twice daily[4]	100 mg twice daily[4]	≤100 mg/day
Prophylaxis: influenza A	5 mg/kg/day up to 150 mg in two divided doses[3]	5 mg/kg/day up to 150 mg in two divided doses[3]	100 mg twice daily[4]	100 mg twice daily[4]	≤100 mg/day
RIMANTADINE[5]					
Treatment[6]: influenza A	NA[7]	NA	NA	100 mg twice daily[4,8]	100 mg/day[9]
Prophylaxis: influenza A	5 mg/kg/day up to 150 mg in two divided doses[3]	5 mg/kg/day up to 150 mg in two divided doses[3]	100 mg twice daily[4]	100 mg twice daily[4]	100 mg/day[9]
ZANAMIVIR[10,11]					
Treatment: influenza A and B	NA	10 mg twice daily	10 mg twice daily	10 mg twice daily	10 mg twice daily
OSELTAMIVIR					
Treatment[12]: influenza A and B	Dose varies by child's weight[13]	Dose varies by child's weight[13]	Dose varies by child's weight[13]	75 mg twice daily	75 mg twice daily
Prophylaxis: influenza A and B	NA	NA	NA	75 mg/day	75 mg/day

[1] Amantadine manufacturers include Endo Pharmaceuticals (Symmetrel®—tablet and syrup); Geneva Pharms Tech and Rosemont (Amantadine HCl—capsule); and Alpharma, Copley Pharmaceutical, HiTech Pharma, Mikart, Morton Grove, and Pharmaceutical Associates (Amantadine HCl—syrup). Rimantadine is manufactured by Forest Laboratories (Flumadine®—tablet and syrup) and Corepharma (Rimantadine HCl—tablet). Zanamivir is manufactured by GlaxoSmithKline (Relenza®—inhaled powder). Oseltamivir is manufactured by Hoffman-LaRoche, Inc. (Tamiflu®—tablet). (Information based on data published by the U.S. Food and Drug Administration at *www.fda.gov*, accessed January 29, 2002.)

[2] The drug package insert should be consulted for dosage recommendations for administering amantadine to persons with creatinine clearance of 50 mL/min/1.73m² or less.

[3] Note: 5 mg/kg of amantadine or rimantadine syrup = 1 tsp/22 lbs.

[4] Children 10 years of age and older who weigh less than 40 kg should be administered amantadine or rimantadine at a dosage of 5 mg/kg/day.

[5] A reduction in dosage to 100 mg/day of rimantadine is recommended for persons who have severe hepatic dysfunction or those with creatinine clearance of 10 mL/min or less. Other persons with less severe hepatic or renal dysfunction taking 100 mg/day of rimantadine should be observed closely, and the dosage should be reduced or the drug discontinued, if necessary.

[6] Only approved by the U.S. Food and Drug Administration (FDA) for treatment in adults.

[7] Not applicable.

[8] Rimantadine is approved by the FDA for treatment in adults. However, certain experts in the management of influenza consider it appropriate also for treatment in children.[275]

[9] Elderly nursing-home residents should be administered only 100 mg/day of rimantadine. A reduction in dosage to 100 mg/day should be considered for all persons 65 years of age and older if they experience possible side effects when taking 200 mg/day.

[10] Zanamivir administered via inhalation using a plastic device included in the package with the medication. Patients will benefit from instruction and demonstration of proper use of the device.

[11] Zanamivir is not approved for prophylaxis.

[12] A reduction in the dose of oseltamivir is recommended for persons with creatinine clearance less than 30 mL/min.

[13] The dose recommendation for children who weigh 15 kg or less is 30 mg twice a day; for children weighing more than 15 to 23 kg, the dose is 45 mg twice a day; for children weighing more than 23 to 40 kg, the dose is 60 mg twice a day; and for children weighing more than 40 kg, the dose is 75 mg twice a day.

years and older. Oseltamivir is an orally administered drug that is approved for treatment of influenza in persons older than 1 year and for chemoprophylaxis of influenza in persons 13 years and older (see Table 17–1). Both drugs block the active site of NA, common to both influenza A and influenza B viruses, which results in viral aggregation at the host cell surfaces and fewer viruses released from infected cells.

Similar to the adamantanes, the NA inhibitors decrease viral shedding and length of illness by approximately 1 day when treatment is initiated within 48 hours of illness. Both drugs can prevent symptoms of influenza infection in adults and adolescents, but it has not been established whether NA inhibitors can prevent serious complications of influenza, such as pneumonia, exacerbation of underlying chronic heart or lung conditions, or death.

Zanamivir and oseltamivir were approved in 1999, and, although few serious CNS adverse effects have been reported, postlicensure data are limited. Oseltamivir has been associated with nausea and vomiting during placebo-controlled treatment studies. Nausea, diarrhea, dizziness, headache, and cough have been reported during zanamivir treatment, but at frequencies similar to inhaled placebo. Zanamivir generally is not recommended for persons with underlying respiratory disease because of the risk of precipitating bronchospasm. Serious adverse respiratory events resulting from zanamivir use have been reported in persons with chronic pulmonary disease and in healthy adults.

NA inhibitor–resistant influenza viruses have been identified relatively infrequently compared to adamantane-resistant strains. In vitro studies indicate that cross-resistance may occur sometimes but not always between the NA inhibitor drugs. Resistance to NA inhibitor drugs does not affect susceptibility to adamantane drugs.

The recommended dosage of zanamivir is two inhalations (a total of 10 mg) twice daily about 12 hours apart for 5 days. The recommended dosage of oseltamivir for treatment in persons 13 years or older or in younger children who weigh more than 40 kg is 75 mg twice daily (see Table 17–1). Adjustments to dosing schedules for oseltamivi should be made based on age and renal function.

Epidemiology

Incidence and Prevalence

Epidemics and outbreaks of influenza occur in different seasonal patterns, depending on the region of the world. For countries in temperate climate zones (e.g., the United States), seasonal epidemics of influenza typically begin in the late fall to winter months and peak in mid- to late winter. Sporadic cases and institutional outbreaks can occur at any time of the year, including the summer months. Outbreaks associated with large groups of international travelers suggest that large outbreaks of influenza may begin to occur more frequently during unusual times of the year.[55-59] In tropical regions, seasonal patterns of influenza appear to be less pronounced, with epidemics interspersed with year-round isolation of influenza viruses. In some subtropical locations, such as Hong Kong, one or two smaller peaks of influenza activity have been noted to occur with regularity (*www.info.gov.hk/dh./diseases*). Within communities, epidemics or outbreaks typically last 6 to 8 weeks or longer.

The start, peak, duration, and size of individual seasons vary substantially from year to year. Nonetheless, influenza epidemics occurring during the interpandemic intervals are almost always smaller than those following the introduction of a new virus subtype (influenza pandemics). The size and impact of epidemics reflect the interplay of several factors, including the extent of the virus' antigenic variation, virulence, and transmissibility; the extent of immunity in the population; and the specific population groups that are affected.

Current Epidemiology as It Relates to Vaccination

Influenza B viruses have been documented to be in continuous circulation in the human populations since their first isolation in 1940, whereas influenza A (H_3N_2) viruses have been in circulation since their emergence in 1968. The influenza A (H_1N_1) viruses that re-emerged in

1977, after their disappearance in 1957, did not supplant the A (H_3N_2) subtype. The co-circulation of two subtypes of influenza A together with influenza B viruses since 1977 has complicated the epidemiology of influenza. During a given year, the predominant influenza viruses circulating may vary temporally and geographically within and among countries. It is noteworthy that the highest levels of influenza-associated mortality and hospitalization in the United States have occurred most often during seasons predominated by $A(H_3N_2)$ viruses.[10,13,60] Current influenza vaccine is trivalent and contains a representative virus from each circulating virus type and subtype.

Pandemics of Influenza

Although pandemics of influenza occur unpredictably and relatively infrequently, they are important because they result in the global circulation of a new influenza A virus and because they can lead to substantially increased morbidity and mortality in all age groups. Influenza pandemics are caused by the appearance and spread in humans of a new influenza A virus bearing either a novel HA or a novel HA and NA combination. Influenza viruses that have not circulated in humans in recent years are considered "novel" and arise through antigenic shift. Only influenza A viruses exhibit shift, which can occur in at least two ways.

In the first mechanism, the simultaneous infection of a host by influenza A viruses of two different subtypes allows corresponding viral genes to be exchanged (or reassort) between the infecting viruses. For example, infection of a pig simultaneously by both an avian influenza A virus and a human influenza A virus can allow genes from the virus normally in circulation among birds to reassort with genes of the influenza A viruses circulating among humans. The resulting "reassortment" of human and avian influenza genes could produce new influenza viruses containing many different combinations of genes. Some of the new progeny viruses will contain the HA or HA-NA genes from the avian influenza viruses. Pigs are thought to serve as "mixing vessels" for genetic reassortment among influenza A viruses because they are susceptible to infection by avian, swine, and human influenza A viruses. Avian species are considered to be the ultimate reservoir of influenza A viruses because viruses bearing all known HA subtypes circulate among wild birds. The viruses causing the 1957 and the 1968 pandemics showed evidence of genetic reassortment between avian and human influenza.

The second mechanism involves direct transmission of avian viruses to humans with subsequent adaptation to the new host. The direct infection of humans by an avian virus also was demonstrated in 1997 when 18 people in Hong Kong were hospitalized as a result of avian influenza A (H_5N_1) virus infections and six of these patients died. Previous to this outbreak, H_5N_1 viruses had been known to cause disease only in birds. Fortunately, the transmissibility of this avian H_5N_1 strain among humans was limited, and the likely immediate source of human infections, poultry in live markets and local farms in Hong Kong, was removed by their slaughter before the virus acquired greater transmissibility among humans.

Although pandemics are often associated with dramatic increases in mortality, the cumulative death toll from seasonal epidemic influenza in the United States since the 1968 pandemic exceeds the total U.S. influenza-related mortality for the 1918 pandemic, the most devastating pandemic of the 20th century. Between the spring of 1918 and the spring of 1919, three waves of "Spanish flu" caused by influenza A (H_1N_1) viruses swept around the world, leading to more than 550,000 deaths in the United States and more than 20 million deaths worldwide. For unknown reasons, influenza-related deaths in this pandemic occurred predominantly among people 20 to 40 years of age, a highly unusual pattern. Two subsequent pandemics, beginning in 1957 (the "Asian flu") and in 1968 ("Hong Kong flu"), were associated with the emergence of the influenza A (H_2N_2) virus and the influenza A (H_3N_2) virus, respectively. By contrast, the reappearance of influenza A (H_1N_1) virus in 1977 did not cause a true pandemic because illness largely was confined to people younger than 20 years of age. Based on these pandemics and earlier ones, and the continuing evolution of influenza A viruses, the occurrence of another pandemic is virtually certain.

Once a pandemic has begun, it will be too late to implement totally new activities that might be required to minimize its impact given the expected rapidity for pandemic viruses to spread worldwide. Therefore, planning and implementation of preparatory activities must start well in advance. Unlike most other health emergencies, influenza pandemics comprise several waves of infections and may last a year or two. Consequently, response efforts will require a sustained effort and close collaboration between public health and private sector groups.

During the current interpandemic phase, pandemic preparedness efforts must build on existing emergency response frameworks and focus on building routine influenza prevention and control activities. Such activities include increasing vaccine coverage of groups at high risk for complications from influenza, enhancing surveillance efforts, and pursuing research activities that will strengthen influenza pandemic responses.

Enhancing global surveillance for influenza is crucial because early warning of an impending pandemic might save hundreds of thousands of lives through more rapid national, regional, and international responses. Developing candidate pandemic influenza vaccine seeds now for influenza A subtypes that pose a pandemic threat could greatly speed up the process of making a pandemic vaccine available. Pilot experimental vaccine lots should be made with these seeds and tested in humans so the immune response can be better understood to a variety of HA and NA subtypes that pose a pandemic threat. Influenza pandemic plans also must address the probable shortage of vaccines and antivirals that are expected during the early pandemic stages. Investments in pandemic preparedness will have an immediate impact on the prevention and control of annual influenza epidemics.

Significance as a Public Health Problem

During influenza seasons, an estimated 10% to 20% of the U.S. population can develop influenza, but attack rates of 40% to 50% within institutions are not unusual. In communities, influenza cases often (but not exclusively) appear first among school-age children. Attack rates usually are the highest in this group and lowest among the elderly, whereas rates of serious disease are highest among the elderly, the very young, and those with certain underlying chronic conditions. Increases in the circulation of influenza viruses have been associated with elevations in acute respiratory illnesses, absenteeism in schools and the workplace, physician visits, hospitalizations, and deaths. The large numbers of medical care visits generated by influenza can overwhelm medical care systems, requiring hospitals and emergency services to divert patients.[9]

Attack Rates

Reported influenza infection attack rates vary considerably depending on the methods used to document infection, the season and predominating virus types and subtypes, the geographic location, the setting (e.g., community, institutions, households), and the age of the population studied. In general, virus isolation is considerably less sensitive than serology for documenting infection.

Among school-age children, rates of primary influenza illness exceed 30% in some years, whereas influenza infection rates among adults generally range from 1% to 15% during nonpandemic years.

Among community studies, one study of families in Seattle showed annual attack rates of 19% and 20%, respectively, for serologically confirmed influenza A and B infections between 1965 and 1969.[61] In the same study in 1978 to 1979, rates of influenza A (H_1N_1) infection soon after its re-emergence in 1977 were about 31%.[62] In Michigan, a community study of families during 1966 to 1971 found infection rates of 17% and 8% using serology for influenza A and B infections, respectively, but rates of only 1.4% and 1.5%, respectively, using virus isolation.[63] The attack rates by age group, based on serology for influenza A, were about 15% to 24% in children younger than 5 years, about 17% to 21% in children 5 to 19 years, and about 12% to 18% in persons older than 19 years. Rates were lower for influenza B infections. In Houston between 1976 and 1984, attack rates ranged from about 36% to 45% in children 5 years and younger, from about 40% to 48% in children 6 to 17 years, and from 21% to 23% in persons 18 years and older.

Attack rates among institutionalized populations can be much higher than those generally found in community studies. In military and boarding school populations, attack rates up to 87% and 90%, respectively, have been described. One review of outbreaks in nursing home populations estimated an average attack rate of 43%,[64] although higher rates have been described.[65] Influenza outbreaks also have been described in hospitals[66–69] and aboard cruise ships.[55,59]

Excess Hospitalization and Mortality

In population-based studies, influenza-related mortality is usually measured in terms of "excess" deaths. In this concept, developed by William Farr in the mid-19th century, increases in the number of deaths during an influenza epidemic beyond the expected number of deaths if there were no epidemic are attributed to influenza. In the United States during 1972 to 1992, the average annual toll of excess "all cause" deaths associated with influenza was about 20,000, with more than 40,000 deaths occurring during severe influenza seasons.[10] More recent analyses have estimated an average of about 36,000 annual deaths related to influenza during the 1990s, resulting in large part from aging of the U.S. population.[60] In the United States, the average annual number of hospitalizations associated with influenza has been estimated at 114,000 and as high as 200,000 during severe seasons.[13] The rates of influenza-associated hospitalization vary by age and risk group (Table 17–2).

Active Immunization

History of Vaccine Development and Current Vaccine

Efforts to develop influenza virus vaccines began soon after influenza A and B viruses were recognized as the etiologic agents of clinical influenza.[4,70–75] The first commercial vaccines were approved for use in the United States in 1945, based on efficacy studies performed in military recruits and college students using whole-virus inactivated influenza vaccines.[76,77] An influenza vaccine was of particular interest to the U.S. military during World War II, in part because of the devastation caused in both military and civilian populations by the 1918 to 1919 influenza pandemic during the late stages of World War I. The ability to grow large quantities of influenza viruses in eggs, elucidation of the physical properties of the viruses, and development of the principles of chemical inactivation made it possible to consider preparing thousands to millions of doses of vaccine.[78,79]

The processes used to make the current commercially available inactivated influenza virus vaccines share certain key features. All of the influenza viruses are replicated individually in substrates of animal origin and are harvested in liquid form. The majority of influenza vaccine viruses are replicated in the allantoic cavities of embryonated hens' eggs, but vaccines for commercial use also are now being produced using mammalian cell lines (MDCK or Vero), which could alter the current dependence on eggs.[80–84] For preparation of the monovalent intermediate vaccines, the harvested influenza viruses are inactivated by controlled treatment using either formalin or β-propiolactone, and several purification steps reduce nonviral proteins and other materials introduced during the manufacturing process. The monovalent vaccines are combined to formulate the final trivalent bulk vaccines, which then are filled into containers.

Although whole-virus vaccines are still in use in some countries and are highly effective, most vaccines manufactured since the 1970s have been subvirion preparations. These vaccines retain the immunogenic properties of the viral proteins but are associated with greatly reduced reac-

TABLE 17–2 ■ Estimated Rates of Influenza-Associated Hospitalization by Age Group and Risk Group for Selected Studies*

Study Years	Population	Age Group	Hospitalizations/ 100,000 Persons with High-Risk Conditions	Hospitalizations/ 100,000 Persons Without High-Risk Conditions
1973–1993[254]	Tennessee	0–11 mo	1900	496–1038[‡]
1973–1993[256†]	Medicaid	1–2 yr	800	186
		3–4 yr	320	86
		5–14 yr	92	41
1992–1997[253§]	Two health maintenance organizations	0–23 mo		144–187
		2–4 yr		0–25
		5–17 yr		8–12
1968–1969, 1970–1971, 1972–1973[249‖]	Health maintenance organization	15–44 yr	56–110	23–25
		45–64 yr	392–635	13–23
		≥65 yr	399–518	—
1969–1995[13‖]	National hospital discharge data	<65 yr		20–42[¶**]
		≥65 yr		125–228[¶**]

*Rates were estimated primarily in years and populations with low vaccination rates. Hospitalization can be expected to decrease as vaccination rates increase. Vaccination can be expected to reduce influenza-related hospitalizations by 30% to 70% in elderly persons and likely by even higher percentages in younger age groups when vaccine and circulating influenza virus strains are antigenically similar.

†Outcomes were for acute cardiac or pulmonary conditions.

‡The low estimate is for infants ages 6 to 11 months, and the high estimate is for infants ages 0 to 5 months.

§Outcomes were for acute pulmonary conditions. Influenza-attributable hospitalization rates for children at high risk were not included in this study.

‖Outcomes were limited to hospitalizations in which pneumonia or influenza was either listed as the first condition on discharge records[13] or included anywhere in the list of discharge diagnoses.[249]

¶Persons at high risk and not a high risk of influenza-related complications are combined.

**The low estimate is the average during seasons in which influenza A (H$_1$N$_1$) or influenza B viruses predominated and the high estimate is the average during influenza A (H$_3$N$_2$)–predominant seasons.

togenicity.[85–89] Subvirion vaccines are prepared by using a solvent (such as ether or a detergent) to dissolve or disrupt the viral lipid envelope. Additional purification steps can be taken to reduce the amounts of viral proteins (predominantly influenza matrix protein and nucleoprotein), resulting in subunit or purified surface antigen vaccine.

It is possible to produce purified influenza virus HA and NA vaccines using recombinant DNA technology,[90–93] but no such vaccine is yet commercially available. Although the original inactivated whole-virus influenza vaccines were relatively crude preparations, the purity of influenza virus vaccines has steadily increased,[94] aided greatly by the introduction of centrifugation and chromatographic steps to reduce residual egg materials. Since the recognition that dissolution of the lipid envelope allowed retention of immunogenicity with reduction in reactogenicity, "splitting" influenza viruses to produce subvirion preparations has become routine. An intact viral membrane is essential for infectivity of enveloped viruses. Therefore, disruption of the viral envelope adds assurance of viral inactivation. Subvirion vaccines were first prepared using ethyl ether and polysorbate 80, but a variety of detergents, including deoxycholate, tri-N-butyl phosphate, Triton X-100, Triton N101, and cetyltrimethylammonium bromide, are now used for commercial vaccine preparation.

The development of "high-growth" influenza A viruses suited to maximal replication in eggs has helped increase vaccine production. Since the early 1970s, influenza virus A/Puerto Rico/8/34 (PR8), a strain very well adapted to replication in eggs, has been used to develop influenza A virus reassortants that combine the HA and NA from wild-type viruses with the high growth properties of the PR8 donor virus.[95,96] Influenza A virus reassortants derived from PR8 often are more uniformly spherical than wild-type viruses,[96] which may facilitate recovery of virus during the various process steps. Although the matrix gene (RNA segment 7) mainly is associated with the high growth properties of PR8, and reassortants produced with PR8 often have the full complement of internal genes from PR8,[95] the growth characteristics of reassortants vary because the HA and NA also affect the adaptation and replication capabilities of the viruses in growth substrates. The effect of HA and NA on replication and the overall compatibility of genes from different influenza viruses probably also account for instances in which it is not possible to select high-growth reassortants using classic methods to reassort wild-type viruses with PR8. An area of continuing investigation is development of reliable high-growth donor strains of influenza B viruses suited to vaccine production.

Vaccine Constituents, Including Antibiotics and Preservatives

Hemagglutinin is the main immunogen in inactivated influenza vaccines, and its level (i.e., potency) is standardized by single radial immunodiffusion (SRID).[97–99] Although inactivated influenza vaccines contain NA, M, and NP in varying amounts depending on the process methods, their levels are not specifically quantified. Antibody to NA can add to the protective effect of vaccines, but the host response to NA is often limited in the presence of HA if, previously, the same or a closely related HA has elicited an immunologic response in the person vaccinated.[100] The immune responses to other viral proteins (e.g., M2)[101] are being investigated but their relative contributions to protection appear much less than the effects of antibodies directed against HAs. Therefore, HA content continues to be the primary concern in preparing inactivated vaccines.

The amount of HA, as measured by SRID, has been correlated with the immunogenicity of subvirion and whole-virion inactivated influenza virus vaccines.[86,87,102] Although chick cell agglutinating units may still be used to estimate vaccine potency (primarily for whole-virus vaccines), results need to be interpreted cautiously because chick cell agglutinating units may not correlate well with clinical immunogenicity, particularly for subvirion vaccines. To test commercially prepared influenza vaccines, most authorities favor SRID performed with influenza strain–specific antigens and antisera because other methods have correlated less well with immunogenicity.

Antibiotics are not added to inactivated influenza virus vaccines as active ingredients. Aminoglycoside antibiotics are used in some production schemes to reduce bacterial growth in eggs during processing steps, because eggs by their nature are not sterile. Antimicrobial agents associated with anaphylactic-type hypersensitivity responses, such as penicillin or other β-lactam antibiotics, however, are strongly discouraged for use at any phase of production. Antibiotics that are used in the production process are reduced to trace or undetectable amounts during purification of the viral proteins.

The agents used to disrupt the envelope of the virion are chosen based on both the acceptability for the process and suitability for human exposure. Each manufacturer uses only a specified agent or combination of agents. Minimal amounts of the detergents or solvents used for virus disruption may remain in the final vaccine preparation, but purification steps often reduce the amount to the limits of detection.

Thimerosal, a mercury-containing compound with broad, highly effective antimicrobial properties, is present in most inactivated influenza virus vaccines. Thimerosal is used to reduce bioburden (the total amount of bacteria and fungi) during production of influenza vaccines in eggs and/or as a preservative to prevent growth of bacteria and fungi in the final vaccine container, especially multidose containers. Although vaccines in single-dose containers theoretically can be formulated to contain no thimerosal or in amounts too low to have a preservative effect (such vaccines may be called "preservative free"), multidose containers are designed to be entered several times, which raises the possibility of entrainment and growth of bacteria or funguses. Thimerosal continues to be the preservative of choice for vaccine stored in multidose (or single-dose) containers, but additional preservatives such as phenoxyethanol are being evaluated to promote elimination of thimerosal as part of a continuing trend to limit the amount of mercury present in vaccines of all kinds.[103]

Either formalin or β-propiolactone is used in influenza vaccine to inactivate the viruses. If processed properly, β-propiolactone is chemically degraded, so that levels in the final vaccine product are below the limits of detection.[104] Although detectable quantities of formaldehyde persist in inactivated vaccines when formalin is used, the steps used for purification also reduce the amount of free formaldehyde, which, if it remains in high concentration, can reduce the potency of vaccines or interfere with SRID measurements of potency.[105-109]

Manufacture of Vaccine

The requirements of national authorities for influenza vaccines generally reflect the guidelines published by the World Health Organization (WHO),[110] but may include items that are specific to individual control authorities. Recommendations for the antigenic composition of influenza vaccines are made annually to ensure that current influenza vaccines are effective against recently circulating strains in both the northern and southern hemispheres.[111,112] As early as 1947, and within 2 years of the introduction of the first commercial vaccines, it was recognized that antigenic changes in the HAs of influenza viruses could reduce the effectiveness of vaccines.[113,114] As a result, the WHO global surveillance system was established in 1948. Laboratories from many countries participate and help determine whether significant changes have occurred in the antigenicity of the HAs of circulating influenza viruses. Surveillance has made it clear that antigenic changes occur not only by point mutations (antigenic drift), but also by way of antigenic shift (at irregular and unpredictable intervals). The WHO global influenza surveillance system has been expanded to improve the timely identification of antigenic changes necessary for updating vaccines.

Influenza vaccine viruses usually are isolates obtained through the WHO surveillance network. The WHO and various national authorities recommend use of certain strains based primarily on the antigenic characteristics of their HAs and NAs. Original isolates are passaged to develop reference strains that are distributed to manufacturers to develop seed viruses. Often the original wild-type strains grow relatively poorly in eggs, so considerable effort is expended examining several antigenically similar strains for several qualities needed to maximize virus yield during large-scale production, including their potential for development of high-growth reassortants, their growth characteristics, and their optimal incubation conditions (such as time and temperature). Because the available production time for trivalent influenza vaccine is limited by the need to distribute vaccine each fall, the total amount of vaccine that can be produced is limited by the least productive strain. In that context the influenza B virus component of trivalent influenza vaccines is becoming a limiting feature in expanding availability.

Currently, the strains used for manufacturing vaccines are isolated either in eggs or primary chick kidney cultures. This practice reflects the fact that embryonated hens' eggs have been the predominant "bioreactor" for replication of influenza viruses since the first inactivated vaccines were produced in the 1940s, but it also has been suggested that replication of influenza viruses in eggs provides a partial barrier to extraneous agents that might originate in the clinical source material.

The increasing interest in using mammalian cell substrates such as MDCK or Vero cells to replicate the viruses for production of inactivated influenza virus vaccine may promote changes in the way influenza viruses are isolated by surveillance laboratories for production use. Because most influenza surveillance laboratories are not prepared to handle tissue cultures in a way necessary to prevent introduction of extraneous agents, a concern is that the possible introduction and amplification of extraneous agents during subsequent passages could compromise the safety of vaccines. The interest in mammalian cell systems stems from concern that the availability of eggs could be reduced by an event requiring destruction of the egg-producing hens (e.g., an outbreak of avian influenza or Newcastle disease virus), and also from concern that the HAs of viruses grown in eggs may exhibit antigenic alterations, theoretically limiting vaccine effectiveness.[115-118] Therefore, strategies are being examined to implement direct isolation of influenza viruses in mammalian tissue culture to provide suitable starting seed viruses.

Regardless of the growth substrate used, the prevention of the introduction of extraneous agents is a concern. In relation to eggs, the main concern is the introduction of extraneous agents, such as avian leukosis virus, that originate in the flocks of chickens providing the eggs. In relation to mammalian tissue cultures, there are concerns that extraneous agents could be introduced from the original human host, from the tissue cultures used by the laboratory recovering the influenza virus, from the cell substrate used for manufacturing, or from one of the materials used to support the growth of the cell substrate.[119-122] For both eggs and mammalian tissue cultures, these concerns are reduced provided there is information to indicate that the process used to inactivate influenza viruses will inactivate other microorganisms effectively.

After replication of influenza viruses, a number of manufacturing steps are taken to increase the concentration of the active immunizing ingredients of the vaccines (mainly the viral HAs) and to reduce other (mainly nonviral) materials. For inactivated influenza virus vaccines produced using eggs or mammalian tissue cultures, removal and reduction of egg or tissue culture proteins occurs throughout the manufacturing process, beginning with concentration of virus by means of centrifugation through a sucrose gradient or passage of the virus-containing allantoic fluid over a chromatographic column. The resulting fluids may be additionally purified by dialysis or diafiltration, and the concentration of residual egg or cell proteins is reduced further during the final formulation when the HA concentration is adjusted to achieve final target levels.

Disruption of the lipid envelope permits further purification of the viral proteins and, in particular, the HAs and NAs. These proteins form rosette-like structures in which the hydrophilic heads of the proteins are on the exterior and the hydrophobic tail portions of the molecules are buried internally. The disruption process varies in efficiency, so that HA and NA still can be attached to lipid but in pieces smaller than the original virion. Dissolution of the viral envelope and removal of additional viral components results in vaccine products with reduced reactogenicity.[85-89,123,124]

Inactivated influenza virus vaccines are intended for parenteral administration, and must be sterile. Environmental bacteria and fungi colonize eggs, and the unintentional introduction of bacteria or fungi during manufacturing steps is also possible whether manufacturing is in eggs or mammalian tissue culture. Chemical inactivation steps are used to minimize the microbial load in the raw viral harvest from the growth substrate, and careful handling and use of component reagents and buffers also facilitate inactivated vaccine sterility. However, filtration steps ensure elimination of undesirable microbes. Generally, sterility can be achieved using filters with pore size sufficient (0.22 μ or less) to exclude small bacteria such as *Brevundimonas diminuta* (previously named *Pseudomonas diminuta*). Although the sterile filtration step does not eliminate endotoxins, which may have been formed previously by bacteria in the product, some of the purification steps can help to reduce endotoxin levels.[125] Because endotoxins contribute to febrile responses to injected vaccines, the limits for endotoxin levels on finished product are set well below clinically established thresholds for reactions.[126]

Producers

Each manufacturer has a somewhat different, proprietary process, but all of the processes result in vaccines standardized to ensure the immunogenicity of HA. Worldwide interest in the availability of inactivated influenza virus vaccine has increased as demand for vaccines has grown. As an example, annual inactivated influenza vaccine production for use in the United States increased from approximately 20 million doses in 1989 to more than 90 million doses in 2002. Significant commercial influenza vaccine production capability exists in Asia, Australia, Europe, and North America. However, there has been a steady consolidation of companies producing inactivated influenza virus vaccines, so that changes in names and contacts at pharmaceutical companies have been frequent. Information on influenza vaccine manufacturers can be obtained from the WHO web site (*www.who.int/emc/diseases/flu/manuf.html*).

Preparations Available, Including Combinations

Monovalent, bivalent, trivalent, quadrivalent, and even pentavalent influenza vaccines have been produced. Usually, the vaccines have included both influenza A and influenza B virus components. Monovalent vaccines have been used only in unusual circumstances, such as in 1986, when a supplemental A/Taiwan/21/86 vaccine was produced. Since 1978, most vaccines have been trivalent and have incorporated influenza A (H_1N_1) and A (H_3N_2) subtype viruses and an influenza B virus. During the 1990s, influenza B viruses diverged into two antigenically distinct lineages based on the HA.[127] This led to the use of a quadrivalent vaccine in at least one country.[128]

A number of adjuvants have been investigated for their potential to increase the immunogenicity of vaccines,[129-144] but only two have so far been licensed in Europe, one containing MF59 (an oil-in-water emulsion adjuvant) and the second using virosomes or immunopotentiating reconstituted influenza virosomes.[131,135] Most adjuvants have combined a lipid or fatty acid with a bacterial cell wall or bacterial protein, but other materials such as chitosan, polyinositol, aluminum, and cytokines also have been tried. Generally, adjuvants have modestly improved vaccine responses but often at the expense of increased reactogenicity, which has sometimes been strikingly severe.[138] For example, elderly recipients of an MF59-adjuvanted influenza vaccine developed geometric mean HI antibody titers that were 1.5 to 2 times higher against each of the three influenza vaccine components than those of recipients of standard subunit vaccine without adjuvant, and fourfold titer rises were also increased[135,145,146]; however, there were more local reactions and myalgia among recipients of vaccine containing MF59. For the virosome vaccine, influenza virus is inactivated, followed by extraction of the HA and NA proteins, which are then associated with lecithin to produce a conformation in which the influenza glycoproteins are exposed in a lipid particle. When compared with subunit vaccine in geriatric patients, the virosome vaccine elicited higher geometric mean antibody titers for two of the three virus components.[131,147] A small study in children with cystic fibrosis suggested that the virosome vaccine might be more immunogenic than subunit vaccine after one dose, but the differences were not striking.[144] No clinical efficacy studies have been done with either adjuvanted vaccine.

The components of influenza viruses themselves (including possibly the lipid envelope) play a role in producing reactions.[124] Because whole-virus preparations already include cellular lipids in the viral envelope, their increased immunogenicity in some studies may relate to an adjuvant effect of the lipid envelope. In parallel with the general adjuvant experience, the increased reactogenicity of whole-virus vaccines (e.g., febrile seizures in children) has restricted their use in some groups because of an unfavorable risk–benefit ratio.[88,89]

An adjuvant might permit conservation of antigen and increase the number of doses available for use in immunologically naïve adults, a potential benefit in a pandemic situation. Studies using experimental vaccines made with an influenza A (H_5N_3) virus from ducks both with and without MF-59 demonstrated that higher immune responses were obtained with the vaccine containing adjuvant.[141] However, some experiences suggest that responses of the immunologically naïve may not always be improved by incorporation of an adjuvant in influenza vaccines.[148]

Timeline for Influenza Vaccine Production

Production of influenza virus vaccines follows a similar schedule each year, reflecting the need to produce and administer vaccine before each influenza season (Fig. 17–2). The foundation for influenza vaccine production is the global influenza virus surveillance that continues throughout the year in both hemispheres. Starting in early winter (in either hemisphere), information from surveillance is used to inform manufacturers about trends in antigenic changes in influenza viruses, particularly trends that might signify the need to make changes in vaccine composition. As they are identified, strains showing antigenic changes are examined for their potential for use in manufacturing by regulatory authorities and by manufacturers, and high-growth influenza A reassortant viruses are produced.

Because several months are required for production of influenza virus vaccines, the time allotted for collecting and assessing surveillance data to ensure the best possible recommendations for vaccine composition must be balanced

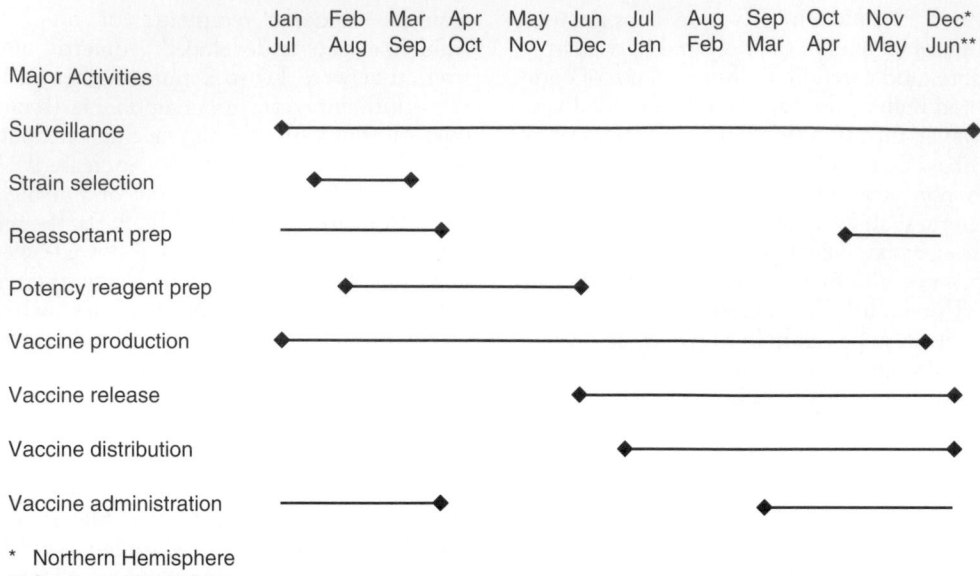

FIGURE 17–2 ■ Approximate influenza vaccine timetable.

against the time needed by manufacturers to produce all components of the vaccine. If recommendations are made too early, significant antigenic changes may be missed. However, if recommendations are made too late, the total vaccine output can be hampered. In addition to collecting and analyzing viral surveillance data, time is needed to allow experience to be gained in handling the vaccine candidate strains and to produce the reagents needed to standardize the new vaccine component viruses.

Manufacturing of monovalent vaccine components begins as early as possible and continues until sufficient material is available to produce the manufacturer's final targeted number of doses. The potency of monovalent vaccine components must be known before formulation of the trivalent vaccines can begin. Currently, the potency of monovalent components and trivalent vaccine is established using SRID.[97,99] This technique requires both an HA-specific antigen and an HA-specific antiserum. The antiserum is produced by immunizing animals with preparations of purified HA and takes at least 3 to 6 weeks.

Once the potency of all three components can be determined, formulation of the trivalent vaccine begins, followed by its filling into containers, labeling, packaging, and distribution. Despite increases in vaccine production and distribution of multimillions of doses, all manufacturing steps must be completed within 6 to 8 months because administration of vaccine typically begins and largely is completed during October to December in the northern hemisphere and during April to July in the southern hemisphere.

Dosage and Route

Inactivated influenza virus vaccines have been given by intramuscular, subcutaneous, intradermal, intranasal, and oral routes. The routes associated with the most reproducible immunogenicity and lowest reactogenicity have been the intramuscular and subcutaneous routes. Subcutaneous administration tends to be somewhat more reactogenic, and sometimes less immunogenic than the intramuscular route. Therefore, the intramuscular route is preferred in the United States. The intradermal route may require less antigen, but often results in more local reactogenicity than other routes.[149] The intranasal administration of inactivated influenza vaccine has not been studied as extensively as other routes of delivery. A commercially available nasally administered formulation was withdrawn recently because of its association with cranial nerve palsies.[150] The ability of oral administration to induce protective antibody responses has been studied, but generally very large doses or an adjuvant are required to promote mucosal and systemic immune responses.[151]

Current doses (based on the SRID content) recommended for inactivated influenza vaccines are 15 μg of each HA component per vaccine dose for persons 3 years of age and over and 7.5 μg of each HA per vaccine dose for children under 3 years of age. The inactivated influenza vaccine dosages are based on extensive clinical studies[86,87,89] undertaken when influenza A (H_1N_1) viruses reappeared and established themselves in human populations during the late 1970s. These studies demonstrated that children and adults who were unexposed to influenza through vaccine or natural infection required two doses of inactivated vaccine to achieve maximal antibody titers, whereas persons with some degree of pre-existing immunity needed only a single dose. The studies also established SRID as the preferred method for determining vaccine potency, because the HA content determined by SRID correlated well with antibody levels developing after whole-virus and subvirion vaccine preparations. The dose chosen balanced the desirability of inducing a maximum immune response in an individual (a higher dose increases the probability of achieving a maximum antibody titer) against the desirability of maximizing population coverage (a smaller dose will allow more individuals to be immunized, which might induce some degree of herd immunity) and the desirability of minimizing adverse reactions (a larger dose has a greater probability of causing immediate local and systemic reactions).

Vaccine Stability

Even though most influenza vaccine is used within 3 to 6 months after its production, the vaccine is expected to remain stable for a longer period. As part of good manufacturing practices and national regulatory requirements, vaccine manufacturers in the United States and elsewhere have ongoing programs to assess the stability of all vaccine products. Stability of a product results from careful attention to several factors, including the specific formulation of the product, the addition of stabilizing compounds (such as gelatin or polysorbate), the compatibility of the product with the intended container and closure and the preparative treatments needed to reduce adsorption or chemical interaction of the vaccine components with the container, and the vaccine's specific temperature limits. Stability assessment programs usually also examine sterility, pH, and the measurable content of preservatives and other chemical ingredients.

Experience indicates that inactivated influenza vaccines are sufficiently robust to maintain full potency above the minimum release specifications for more than 1 year, when stored at 4°C to 8°C. However, the potency of individual influenza virus vaccine components can decline at varying rates. For example, in 1996, the influenza A H_3N_2 component (but not the influenza A H_1N_1 or influenza B components) in the vaccine from one manufacturer lost potency faster than expected.[152] The possibility of unanticipated changes in potency highlights the need to monitor the stability of a product in which the key component, the viral HA, is frequently replaced.

Results of Vaccination

Immunogenicity of Vaccine

Measurement of Antibodies

Influenza vaccination induces antibodies against the major surface glycoproteins, HA and NA. While the HI and neutralization tests both measure levels of strain-specific antibodies, the HI test is most commonly used for measuring the antibody response to inactivated influenza vaccines because of its relative simplicity. In the HI test, antibodies present in an immune serum compete with red blood cells to bind the viral HA. Red blood cells from chickens or turkeys are used most often; however, guinea pig or human erythrocytes can be substituted in circumstances where avian red blood cells do not bind well to the influenza viruses in question. The HI assay can be complicated by nonspecific inhibitors of hemagglutination in human and animal serum. The inhibitors can be removed by pretreating serum with receptor-destroying enzyme from Vibrio cholerae or with periodate.

The neutralization test is a very sensitive and specific functional assay that measures antibody capable of preventing viral infectivity. However, classic neutralization methods based on plaque reduction or hemadsorption inhibition are labor intensive and require relatively large quantities of serum. More recently, neutralization-enzyme immunoassay tests have been used that are suitable for measuring neutralizing antibodies in small quantities of serum.[153,154] Titers of neutralizing antibody measured using this method correlate well with titers obtained by HI.[154]

Increasing the amount of influenza HA from 1 μg up to 6 to 10 μg of HA per vaccine dose generally results in increased levels of antibody to that strain. However, further increases in antigenic mass above 15 μg of HA per strain do not reproducibly elicit significantly higher antibody levels.[87] This type of "shallow" or flat dose-response effect over a wide range of antigen concentrations has been observed in both primed and unprimed individuals.[155–157] In elderly subjects, the serum antibody response to influenza vaccine is variable and generally lower than in younger subjects.[158]

Cellular Immune Responses

Cell-mediated immunity for influenza is frequently cross-reactive between different influenza virus subtypes, with T cells recognizing more conserved internal proteins, such as the M or NP proteins. The cytotoxic T-lymphocyte (CTL) responses in humans who have received inactivated influenza vaccines have not been studied extensively. In vaccinated healthy adults, increases in CTLs in peripheral blood have been short lived, returning to baseline levels within 6 months.[159,160]

Correlates of Protection

Neutralizing antibody directed against HA is the primary immune mediator of protection from influenza infection and illness. Currently, measurement of HI antibody titer in serum is the most useful correlate of protection. Elevated levels of serum anti-HA antibody are well correlated with resistance to influenza infection, whereas lower antibody levels are associated with increased risk of illness among persons exposed to influenza viruses.[161–164] Furthermore, challenge studies using live virus have shown that protection against influenza is also associated with local neutralizing antibody and secretory immunoglobulin A (IgA).[165,166] Although antibodies to NA do not efficiently neutralize influenza infection, they restrict virus release from infected cells, reduce the intensity of infection, and enhance recovery.[167,168]

Based on serologic studies of influenza using human serum, an HI titer of 32 to 40 is often referred to as the "protective titer." However, this terminology is misleading because this titer represents the level at which approximately 50% of individuals will be protected, and there is no titer value that can guarantee protection from infection.[162,169,170]

Herd Immunity

Influenza vaccination has been shown in certain settings, such as nursing homes and schools, to provide indirect benefits to those who remain unvaccinated,[171–173] a finding that is consistent with models of vaccine-induced herd immunity. Furthermore, it has been suggested that mass immunization might reduce the overall occurrence of influenza in the community, including in unvaccinated persons.[164,174] A more recent retrospective ecologic study suggested that mass immunization of schoolchildren in Japan had reduced excess mortality rates among older adults and that discontinuation of this vaccination program led to increases in excess mortality rates among elderly Japanese.[175] This study remains somewhat controversial because aging of the population and other variables were not controlled. In the United States, studies are underway to determine if vaccinating school-age children with trivalent live, attenuated influenza vaccine can reduce the spread of influenza in communities.

Efficacy and Effectiveness of Vaccine

Several factors affect the efficacy and effectiveness of influenza vaccine and their measurement. One major factor is the antigenic similarity between circulating strains and influenza vaccine strains. Improvements in global influenza virus surveillance have resulted in an increase in years with a good antigenic match between circulating and vaccine viruses. For example, in the United States from 1977–1978 through 1988–1989 and from 1990–1991 through 2001–2002, respectively, the vaccine and predominant circulating strains were well matched in 7 of 12 years (58%) and in 11 of 12 years (92%) (Centers for Disease Control and Prevention [CDC], unpublished data).

An important factor affecting the measurement of vaccine efficacy and effectiveness is the specificity of the outcome measure used in the study.[176] Some studies use highly specific outcomes, such as serologically confirmed influenza infection or culture-confirmed influenza, whereas others use clinically defined cases, such as influenza-like illness or influenza-related hospitalizations or deaths, which are unconfirmed by laboratory tests. More specific outcomes generally are associated with higher measurements of efficacy. For example, one study of the same healthy adult population in the same year showed a vaccine efficacy of 86% against serologically confirmed influenza illness, 34% against febrile respiratory illness, and 10% against upper respiratory infection.[177] When less specific outcomes are used, co-circulation of other pathogens causing similar clinical syndromes will reduce the calculated effectiveness. For example, if vaccine efficacy against influenza is 80%, but influenza is causing only half of the respiratory illnesses in a community, the calculated effectiveness against all respiratory illnesses will be 40%.

Influenza illness rates can also vary substantially from year to year, and, in years with low rates, the power of smaller studies to detect a difference in vaccine effectiveness may be compromised. Because of the year-to-year variability in illness rates and vaccine match, multiyear studies are preferred for estimating vaccine efficacy and effectiveness.

Despite these difficulties, some meta-analyses on influenza vaccine efficacy and effectiveness have been published.[161,163,178] Although the substantial differences in how vaccine efficacy and effectiveness are measured can make direct comparisons between studies and across years difficult, taken together, such studies can define an expected distribution of vaccine effectiveness over time.

Efficacy and Effectiveness Among Adults 65 Years and Older

Although a large number of influenza vaccine studies have been conducted among older populations (Table 17–3), only one randomized trial has been reported. This study, which included persons age 60 years or older without underlying health conditions, estimated that influenza vaccine

reduced symptomatic influenza by 58%,[128] but the study was not large enough to estimate vaccine effectiveness against influenza-related complications.

Nonrandomized studies among those age 65 and older either with or without chronic medical conditions have reported that vaccine reduces pneumonia and influenza hospitalization by 18% to 52% and death from all causes by 27% to 70%.[163,179–182] One meta-analysis estimated that influenza vaccine reduced influenza-like illness by 33% (95% confidence interval [CI]: 27% to 38%), hospitalization for pneumonia and influenza by 33% (27% to 38%), and mortality from all causes by 50% (46% to 56%) among community-dwelling elderly.[178] A second meta-analysis[163] included studies from both nursing home populations and noninstitutionalized groups of elderly. In the combined cohort studies, influenza vaccines were estimated to reduce respiratory illness by 56% (95% CI: 39% to 68%), pneumonia by 53% (35% to 66%), hospitalization by 50% (28% to 65%), and death by 68% (56% to 76%). In the same meta-analysis, the combined case-control studies estimated that vaccine reduced pneumonia and influenza hospitalization by 31% to 65% and death from any cause by 27% to 30%.[163]

Most influenza vaccination studies in the elderly have involved the retrospective analysis of large administrative databases, investigations of outbreaks, or case-control studies. One administrative database study covering three influenza seasons (1990 to 1993) estimated that vaccine reduced physician visits for pneumonia and influenza by 17%, pneumonia and influenza hospitalizations by 51%, and deaths from all causes during peak influenza weeks by 45%.[183] A two-year study (1996 to 1998) using data from health plan databases estimated that vaccine reduced pneumonia and influenza hospitalization by 18% to 24% and death by 35% to 61%.[182] The lower estimates occurred in years when the vaccine viruses were not well matched to the predominant circulating strains. Nonetheless, vaccine was estimated to substantially prevent influenza-related deaths even under these circumstances.

Several case-control studies have demonstrated the ability of influenza vaccine to prevent hospitalization. During the 1989 to 1990 influenza season in the United Kingdom, one study estimated that vaccine reduced influenza, pneumonia, bronchitis, and emphysema combined by 63%,[184] while a Spanish study estimated that vaccine reduced radiologically confirmed pneumonia by 79%.[185] In the United States, a 2-year study conducted in 1990 to 1992[186] estimated that vaccine reduced influenza-related hospitalization by 31% during an influenza A outbreak and by 32% during an influenza B outbreak. One study using 9 years of data from a health insurance plan estimated that vaccine reduced pneumonia and influenza hospitalization by 30% to 33% overall and by 51% to 83% in years when influenza A (H_3N_2) viruses predominated.[187] Another U.S. study during 1989 to 1990 estimated that the vaccine reduced pneumonia and influenza hospitalization by 45%.[188]

The effectiveness of vaccine against death has also been examined in case-control studies. A 1989 to 1990 U.K. study estimated that vaccine reduced influenza-related deaths by 75%,[189] while a Canadian study estimated that deaths during hospitalizations from any cause were reduced by 27% to 30%.[179]

TABLE 17–3 ■ Summary of Selected Vaccine Efficacy and Effectiveness Studies Conducted Among Elderly Persons

Reference	Population	Study Design	Year(s)	Outcome Measures and Vaccine Efficacy/Effectiveness Results	Comments
Govaert et al.[128] (1994)	≥60 yr, no high-risk medical conditions	RPCT	1991–92	Laboratory-confirmed influenza illness: VE 58%	65% of isolates antigenically well matched to vaccine strains
Gross et al.[163] (1995)	Institutionalized and noninstitutionalized elderly	Meta-analysis of 20 studies	NA	Respiratory illness: VE 56%; Hospitalization: VE 48%; Deaths: VE 68%	Included studies of years with and without drifted strains and nonepidemic years
Vu et al.[178] (2002)	≥65 yr, noninstitutionalized	Meta-analysis of 15 studies	NA	P&I hospitalization: VE 52%; All-cause deaths: VE 50%	Excluded studies with poor antigenic match between vaccine and circulating strains
Barker and Mullooly[249] (1980)	≥65 yr	Cohort study	1968–69, 1972–73	No VE in 1968–69; In 1972–73: P&I hospitalization: VE 72%; P&I hospitalization deaths: VE 87%	Antigenic shift occurred in 1968 with poor antigenic match
Fleming et al.[189] (1995)	≥55 yr	Cohort study	1989–90	All-cause deaths: VE 75%	Used administrative database
Nichol et al.[183] (1996)	≥65 yr	Cohort study	1990–93	P&I outpatient doctor visits: VE 17%; P&I hospitalization: VE 51%; All-cause deaths: VE 45%	Used administrative database
Nichol et al.[181] (1999)	≥65 yr with chronic lung disease	Cohort study	1993–96	P&I hospitalization: VE 52%; All-cause deaths: VE 70%	Used administrative database; A (H_3N_2) outbreaks and good antigenic matches in all 3 yr
Nordin et al.[182] (2001)	≥65 yr	Cohort study	1996–98	P&I hospitalization: VE 19%–24%; All-cause deaths: VE 35%–61%	Administrative database; lower VE estimates in 1997–98 with poor antigenic match
Mullooly et al.[187] (1994)	≥65 yr	Case-control	1980–89	P&I hospitalization: VE 30%–33% overall, range 15%–83%; P&I hospitalization deaths: not significant	VE 51%–83% when good antigenic match and A (H_3N_2) viruses predominated

Continued

TABLE 7–3 ■ Summary of Selected Vaccine Efficacy and Effectiveness Studies Conducted Among Elderly Persons—cont'd

Reference	Population	Study Design	Year(s)	Outcome Measures and Vaccine Efficacy/ Effectiveness Results	Comments
Fedson et al.[179] (1993)	≥45 yr, noninstitutionalized	Case-control	1982–83, 1985–86	P&I hospitalization: VE 32%–39% All-cause deaths: 27%–30%	72% study participants ≥65 years; administrative database
Ahmed et al.[184] (1997)	≥16 yr, 15% institutionalized	Case-control	1989–90	P&I, bronchitis, or emphysema hospitalization: VE 63%	84% study participants ≥65 yr
Foster et al.[188] (1992)	≥65 yr, noninstitutionalized	Case-control	1989–90	P&I hospitalization: VE 45%	
Ohmit and Monto[186] (1995)	≥65 yr	Case-control	1990–92	P&I hospitalization: VE 31%–32%	Influenza B predominated in year 1 and influenza A (H_3N_2) in year 2
Puig-Barbera et al.[185] (1997)	≥65 yr, noninstitutionalized	Case-control	1994–95	Radiologically confirmed pneumonia hospitalization: VE 79%	Controls were hospitalized for acute surgical abdomen or trauma

NA, nonapplicable; P&I, pneumonia and influenza; RPCT, randomized, placebo-controlled trial; VE, vaccine efficacy or effectiveness.

Vaccination of Nursing Home Populations

Vaccine effectiveness estimates in nursing home residents have varied widely, even during years when the vaccine and circulating virus strains were antigenically well matched.[190–194] For example, in years when the vaccine and circulating strains were well matched, studies have estimated that vaccine reduces influenza-like illness during nursing home outbreaks by zero to 80%, with most estimates approximating 40%.[190–196] Although the antibody response to influenza vaccination can be diminished in the frail elderly,[197–199] vaccination can prevent both hospitalization and death in this vulnerable population.[163,190,191,200–202] In this population, vaccine has been estimated to reduce hospitalizations and deaths by 47% to 90% and by 59% to 95%, respectively, with overall estimates of approximately 60% and 80%. Some studies suggest that vaccination rates of 80% or more of nursing home residents can induce herd immunity and decrease the risk of influenza outbreaks in nursing homes.[190,203] Vaccination of health care workers also can reduce morbidity and mortality in nursing home residents.[69,204,205]

Efficacy and Effectiveness in Adults Less Than 65 Years

In the 1940s, seminal studies conducted among U.S. military personnel established that vaccine could reduce influenza illness by 70% or more.[94] Several later studies were conducted among military personnel in different countries (Table 17–4). For example, a nonrandomized study of Finnish military personnel exposed to A/Sydney/5/97-like viruses found that vaccination reduced influenza illnesses by 57%.[206] An Israeli military study showed that vaccine reduced febrile respiratory illness by 42%.[207]

Additional studies have involved persons ages 18 to 64 years who were in the general population or were identified as workers (see Table 17–4). A 5-year placebo-controlled trial during 1985 to 1990[208] demonstrated that vaccine reduced culture-confirmed influenza by 70% to 79%.[208] Another 5-year placebo-controlled trial among 30- to 60-year-olds from 1983 to 1988 showed reductions of 47% to 73% against serologically or culture-confirmed influenza, including 1 year when the antigenic match between the vaccine and circulating strains was suboptimal.[209]

Two randomized, placebo-controlled studies have been conducted among healthy adult workers in the United States. One of them estimated that vaccination reduced upper respiratory illness by 25%, illness-related work absenteeism by 43%, and physician visits by 44%.[210] In the first year of the second study, the vaccine and circulating strains were not matched well. The estimated vaccine efficacy against serologically confirmed febrile respiratory illness was 50%, but there were no reductions in overall febrile respiratory illness, physician visits, or work absenteeism. In the second year of this study, vaccine was estimated to reduce laboratory-confirmed influenza illness by 86%, febrile respiratory illness by 34%, physician visits by 42%, and work absenteeism by 32%.[177]

Three randomized trials among health care workers have been reported.[20,21,211] A 1-year study during a year when the vaccine and circulating strains were antigenically dissimilar found no reductions of influenza-like illness or work absenteeism.[20] In a 3-year study, vaccine reduced serologically confirmed influenza by 88% to 89%,[21] febrile respiratory illness by 29%, and illness-related work absenteeism by 53%, but the findings were not statistically significant. Another 1-year study found no reduction in respiratory illnesses, although work absenteeism related to respiratory illness was reduced by 28%.[211]

Nonrandomized or quasi randomized studies among adult workers generally have found overall reductions in work absenteeism when the vaccine and circulating strains are well matched.[212–215] One meta-analysis of studies in healthy adults[161] estimated that, overall, inactivated influenza vaccine reduced laboratory-confirmed influenza by 68% and absenteeism from work by 0.4 days. However, some more recent studies were not included in the meta-analysis.[21,177,210,211] Overall, in years when the vaccine and circulating viruses are well matched, the vaccine can be expected to reduce laboratory-confirmed influenza by approximately 70% to 90%.

Vaccination in Groups with Chronic Medical Conditions

A limited number of influenza vaccine studies have been conducted in groups with underlying medical conditions. A study of diabetic persons estimated that influenza vaccine reduced influenza, pneumonia, or diabetes-related hospitalizations by 79% (95% CI: 19% to 95%) during two influenza seasons.[216] However, the control group had a significantly lower proportion of insulin-dependent diabetics, which could have inflated the vaccine effectiveness estimates. Another study used an administrative database to evaluate vaccine effectiveness against pneumonia and influenza hospitalization in persons 65 years and older with different medical conditions.[217] Vaccine effectiveness estimates were not statistically different among subgroups of elderly persons (healthy elderly; those with heart disease, lung disease, or diabetes; immune-compromised persons; or those with either dementia, stroke, vasculitis, or rheumatologic conditions). Estimates ranged from 43% to 56% when the vaccine and circulating viruses were antigenically well matched, and 21% to 42% when the match was not optimal. Another study among persons age 65 and older estimated that vaccine reduced pneumonia and influenza hospitalizations among those with heart or lung disease by 29%; those with either diabetes, renal or rheumatologic disease, stroke, or dementia by 32%; and those without a known underlying medical condition by 49%; deaths from any cause were reduced by 49%, 64%, and 55% in those groups, respectively, with overlapping confidence intervals.[180] A small randomized trial involving persons infected with human immunodeficiency virus estimated that vaccine reduced culture-confirmed influenza by 100%, but only 13% of the study population had a CD4+ count of less than 200 cells/mm^3, so the results may not be applicable to those with lower CD4+ counts.[218] Overall, vaccine efficacy and effectiveness estimates among persons with high-risk conditions are comparable to those among similar age groups of persons without high-risk conditions, although studies among severely immune-compromised persons are lacking.

Efficacy and Effectiveness in Children

Inactivated influenza vaccination studies among children are limited, and none has examined influenza hospitalization

TABLE 17—4 ■ Summary of Selected Vaccine Efficacy and Effectiveness Studies Conducted Among Adults Less Than 65 Years of Age

Reference	Population	Study Design	Year(s)	Outcome Measures and Vaccine Efficacy/Effectiveness Results	Comments
Demicheli et al.[161] (2000)	14–60 yr	Meta-analysis	NA	ILI decreased by 21%–37%, laboratory-confirmed influenza by 65%–72%, lost work days by 0.4 days/person	Included randomized and quasi-randomized studies published through 1997
Keitel et al.[209] (1997)	30–60 yr	RPCT	1983–88	VE against culture or serologically confirmed influenza: 47%–73%; VE against laboratory-confirmed influenza plus respiratory symptoms: 34%–60%	Poor vaccine antigenic match in one year
Weingarten et al.[20] (1988)	Health care workers	RPCT	1985–86	No significant decrease in ILI or work absenteeism	Poor antigenic match; no laboratory testing for influenza
Edwards et al.[208] (1994)	1–65 yr	RPCT	1986–90	VE against serologically confirmed influenza: 56%–79%; VE against serologically confirmed influenza plus ILI: 66%–94%	84% of participants > 16 yr; antigenically well matched in 2 of 4 yr efficacy data published
Kumpulainen and Makela[213] (1997)	18–62 yr	Randomized groups of workers	1990–91	VE against culture or serologically confirmed influenza: 100%	Low influenza attack rate of 0.8% among placebo group
Wilde et al.[21] (1999)	Health care workers <50 yr	RPCT	1992–95	VE against serologically confirmed influenza: 86%–100%; 53% reduction in work absenteeism: not statistically significant	Lack of absenteeism significance most likely result of small sample size of ~120 participants/year
Saxen and Virtanen[211] (1999)	Health care workers	RPCT	1996–97	10% nonsignificant reduction in respiratory illnesses; 28% reduction in total sick leave days	No laboratory testing done to confirm influenza illness
Nichol et al.[210] (1995)	18–64 yr, healthy	RPCT	1994–95	URI decreased by 25%, URI-related work absenteeism by 43%, URI-related physician visits by 44%	No laboratory testing done to confirm influenza illness

TABLE 17–4 ■ Summary of Selected Vaccine Efficacy and Effectiveness Studies Conducted Among Adults Less Than 65 Years of Age

Reference	Population	Study Design	Year(s)	Outcome Measures and Vaccine Efficacy/Effectiveness Results	Comments
Bridges et al.[177] (2000)	18–64 yr, healthy	RPCT	1997–99	*Year 1:* 50% VE against serologically confirmed febrile ILI not statistically significant, no reductions in ILI-related work absenteeism or doctors visits *Year 2:* VE 89% against serologically confirmed febrile ILI; 34%, 42%, and 32% reductions in all ILI and ILI-related physician visits and work absenteeism, respectively	Poor antigentic match in year 1
Leighton et al.[214] (1996)	Full-time workers	Retrospective cohort	1991–92	53% reduction in ILI of 4–14 days' duration and 50% reduction in ILI-related work absenteeism	Vaccinees self-selected; no laboratory confirmation of influenza infection
Campbell and Rumley[212] (1997)	Full-time workers	Prospective cohort	1992–93	59% reduction in proportion with ≥1 ILI 65% reduction in ILI-related lost workdays 15% reduction in proportion with ≥1 URI	Vaccinees self-selected; no laboratory confirmation of influenza infection
Grotto et al.[207] (1998)	Military	Prospective cohort	1995–96	VE 42% against febrile respiratory illness, 19% reduction in physician visits, and 11% reduction in use of any sick days	Some vaccinees self-selected and others vaccinated based on timing of entry into military; no influenza laboratory testing of study subjects
Pyhala et al.[206] (2001)	Military	Prospective cohort	1997–98	VE 57% against laboratory-confirmed influenza	Poor antigenic match

ILI, influenza-like illness; RPCT, randomized, placebo-controlled trial; URI, upper respiratory illness; VE, vaccine efficacy or effectiveness.

as an outcome (Table 17–5). In a randomized trial conducted over five influenza seasons in the United States among children 1 to 15 years, vaccine reduced influenza illness by 77% to 91%.[219] A 1-year study reported vaccine efficacies of 56% among healthy 3- to 6-year-olds and 100% among healthy 10- to 18-year-olds.[220] In Japan, efficacy studies, based on serologic confirmation of influenza infection, were carried out among children during 1982 to 1984.[172] For the 1983 influenza season, one or two subcutaneous doses of vaccine reduced illness by 76% among elementary schoolchildren and by 83% among junior and senior high schoolchildren.[172] In Russia, inactivated influenza vaccine was estimated to reduce respiratory illness by 24% in schoolchildren ages 7 to 10 years and by 30% in children 11 to 14 years in the 1989 to 1990 influenza season, and by 27% and 27% in the two groups, respectively, in the 1990 to 1991 season.[173] In Italy, a 1-year randomized trial of 344 children ages 1 to 6 years estimated that influenza-like illness was reduced by 67%.[221] In the United Kingdom, a study among adolescents at a boarding school during outbreaks in 1972 to 1973 and 1973 to 1974 estimated that vaccine reduced laboratory-confirmed influenza by 70%.[222–224] These studies by Hoskins et al.[223,224] concluded that annually vaccinated schoolchildren were just as likely to become ill with influenza over time as those who were not vaccinated, in spite of good protection after the first vaccination. This observation prompted some to question the wisdom of annual influenza vaccination. However, a careful reanalysis of data from the Hoskins studies[222] revealed that misclassification of the vaccination status of study subjects was responsible for the Hoskins findings; no negative effects of annual vaccination on protection were observed after the correct vaccination status was assigned to subjects.

Results are more varied in studies among very young children. In Japan, a study of 180 children ages 5 months to 7 years found that vaccine reduced influenza A cases by 66%, but no overall benefit was found among the small subset of children less than 2 years of age (n = 56).[225] In this study, children received subcutaneous primary and booster vaccinations rather than the intramuscular vaccinations recommended in the United States. In the United States, a randomized study of 127 children ages 24 to 60 months attending day care estimated that vaccine reduced serologically identified influenza infection by 45% (95% CI: 5% to 66%) for influenza A and B combined, influenza B by 45% (95% CI: −20% to +69%), influenza A (H_3N_2) by 31% (95% CI: −95% to +73%), and febrile influenza-like illness by 7% (95% CI: −30% to +23%).[226] In a 2-year randomized study among children 6 to 24 months of age, the vaccine was estimated to reduce respiratory illness by 66% in year 1 (n = 411) when influenza viruses circulated widely (attack rate of 20% in the unvaccinated). However, the vaccine was not efficacious in year 2 (n = 375), when influenza circulation was limited (attack rate of 3% in the unvaccinated).[227] Two studies found that vaccination decreased influenza-related otitis media by approximately 30%,[228,229] but a 2-year randomized study[227] reported vaccine did not reduce cases of otitis media, even when the vaccine reduced culture-confirmed influenza by 66%. However, the efficacy against laboratory-confirmed influenza-related otitis media was not reported. Overall, vaccine efficacy estimates in school-age children are similar to those found among healthy adults. Data for younger children are limited, but suggest that efficacy could be somewhat lower in the younger age groups.

Limited studies have been conducted among children with chronic medical conditions. In a nonrandomized study, vaccine reduced culture- or serologically confirmed influenza (against a drifted strain) by 22% to 54% in asthmatic children 2 to 6 years of age and by 60% to 78% in 7- to 14-year-olds.[230] A retrospective analysis using a computerized primary care database estimated that vaccine reduced medically attended visits for respiratory illness or otitis media among asthmatic children by 27% (95% CI: −7% to 51%) for those 0 to 12 years, by 55% (20% to 75%) for those less than 6 years, and by −5% (−81% to 39%) for those 6 to 12 years.[231] Overall, vaccine efficacy may be lower among high-risk children, particularly immune-suppressed children, compared with healthy adults or older healthy children.

Duration of Immunity and Protection

Inactivated vaccine induces a rapid systemic and local immune response in healthy young adults.[232] It has been shown that up to 90% of normal subjects develop serum HI titers of 1:40 or greater within 2 weeks of vaccination and that second doses provide little or no further increase in titers. Peak serum antibody levels develop within 4 to 6 weeks after vaccination,[233] and then antibody levels wane by as much as 50% within 6 months.[86]

Elderly subjects generally respond less well to influenza vaccines than young healthy adults, and those with chronic debilitating medical conditions generally respond less well than healthy subjects of similar age. Up to 50% of elderly vaccinees may fail to respond to inactivated influenza vaccine with a fourfold increase in HI antibodies.[234] In addition, antibody responses in the elderly may be somewhat delayed compared to those in younger individuals[235] and may return toward the baseline more rapidly than in young adults.[236]

The duration of protection from illness after influenza vaccination has been studied during several clinical trials. In 1968, a group of schoolchildren was vaccinated with the A/Hong Kong/68 vaccine and was observed over three successive influenza epidemics caused by the A/Hong Kong/68 virus. Three years after vaccination, the vaccine was still 67% effective in preventing influenza.[237] In randomized trials conducted among healthy college students, immunization with trivalent inactivated vaccine before the 1982 to 1983 epidemic provided 92% and 100% efficacy against influenza H_3N_2 and H_1N_1 infection-related illnesses, respectively, during the first year, and a 68% reduction against H_1N_1 infections during the second year without revaccination.[238] In a similar study of young adults in 1986 to 1987, vaccine reduced influenza A (H_1N_1) illness by 75% in the first year, H_3N_2 illness by 45% in the second year, and H_1N_1 illness by 61% during the third year after immunization.[213] Because elderly persons who have received repeated influenza vaccinations develop lower peak HI titers, and these antibody levels return to baseline faster than in young healthy adults receiving influenza vaccine for the first time, immunity is expected to be of shorter duration in this target group than in the young adults studied above.

TABLE 17–5 ■ Summary of Selected Vaccine Efficacy and Effectiveness Studies Conducted Among Children

Reference	Population	Study Design	Year(s)	Efficacy/Effectiveness	Comments
Clover et al.[220] (1991)	3–18 yr: n = 192	RPCT	1986–87	VE 56% 3–9 yr No lab-confirmed flu in 10–18 yr	Drifted strain
Neuzil et al.[219] (2001)	1–<3 yr: n = 102 3–<6 yr: n = 169 6–<11 yr: n = 302 11–<16 yr: n = 218	RPCT	1986–90	VE against culture-confirmed influenza, all ages: 77%–91% VE against serologically confirmed influenza: 1–<6 yr: 44%–49% 6–<11 yr: 74%–76% 11–<16 yr: 70%–81%	2 of 4 yr with drifted strains; all received single dose of vaccine
Rudenko et al.[173] (1993)	7–14 yr, schoolchildren: n = 8144	RPCT	1989–91	VE against respiratory illness: 24%–27% in 7–10 yr and 27%–30% in 11–14 yr	No laboratory confirmation of illness
Colombo et al.[221] (2001)	1–6 yr, healthy: n = 344	RCT	1995–96	VE against ILI of >72 hr duration: 67% No OM in vaccinated vs. 3 in unvaccinated (P = 0.07)	Randomized but no placebo used
Hurwitz et al.[226] (2000)	24–60 mo, day care attendees: n = 97	RPCT	1996–97	VE against serologically confirmed influenza: 45% VE against ILI: 7% (not significant)	Small sample size limits interpretation
Hoberman et al.[227] (2002)	6–24 mo, healthy: n = 786 person-yr	RPCT	1999–2001	VE against culture-confirmed influenza: 66% (CI: 34%–82%) in year 1 and –7% (–247%–67%) in year 2 No difference in OM	Low influenza illness rate in year 2
Monto et al.[164] (1970)	Nursery school age: n = 39 Elementary through high school age: n = 3682	Prospective cohort	1968–69	Overall, ~67% reduction in respiratory illness in vaccinated community among all ages	Vaccinated 86% of schoolchildren in one town and compared with unvaccinated community; herd immunity may have improved total VE

Continued

359

TABLE 7-5 ■ Summary of Selected Vaccine Efficacy and Effectiveness Studies Conducted Among Children—cont'd

Reference	Population	Study Design	Year(s)	Efficacy/Effectiveness	Comments
Hoskin et al.[223,224] (1973, 1979); Beyer et al.[222] (1998)	Schoolchildren: n = 797	Prospective cohort	1972–74	VE against serologic or culture-confirmed influenza: 70%	Self-selected vaccinees
Oya and Nerome[172] (1986)	Day care attendees: n = 501	Prospective cohort	1981–84	VE 51% against serologically confirmed influenza in 2 yr with good match and −3% in 1 yr with poor match	Parents self-selected vaccination for child
Heikkinen et al.[229] (1991)	1–3 yr, day care attendees: n = 374	Prospective cohort	1988–89	VE 83% against culture-confirmed influenza with OM and 30% reduction in all febrile OM	Vaccinated and unvaccinated children from different day care centers
Sugaya et al.[230] (1994)	2–14 yr, asthmatics: n = 1374	Prospective cohort	1992–93	VE against influenza H_3N_2: 54% in 2–6 yr and 78% in >6 yr VE against influenza B: 22% in 2–6 yr and 60% in >6 yr	Parents self-selected vaccination for children; drifted H_3N_2 strain
Clements et al.[228] (1995)	6–30 mo, day care attendees: n = 186	Prospective cohort	1993–94	31% reduction in OM	Mixture of some randomized, some self-selected vaccinees
Smith et al.[231] (2002)	0–12 yr, asthmatics: n = 349 year 1 n = 335 year 2	Retrospective cohort	1995–97	VE against acute respiratory disease: 55% (CI: 20%–75%) in <6 yr and −5% (−81%–39%) in ≥6 yr	Used administrative database; no laboratory confirmation
Maeda et al.[225] (2002)	Healthy children: <2 yr n = 13 2–7 yr n = 167	Prospective cohort	1999–2000	VE 66% against Directigen FLU-A–diagnosed influenza	Controls selected from hospital records; vaccine administered SQ with 2nd dose 2 wk after 1st

CI, 9_% confidence interval; ILI, influenza-like illness; OM, otitis media; RPCT, randomized, placebo-controlled trial; RCT, randomized, controlled trial; SQ, subcutaneous; VE, vaccine efficacy or effectiveness.

Although protection may persist for longer than a year after vaccination in young healthy adults, annual immunization with inactivated vaccine is recommended because one or more vaccine antigens usually are updated each year and because reductions in serum antibody levels have been well documented during the year after immunization. In particular, annual immunization of those 65 years of age and older close to the influenza season will help maximize antibody levels and protection in this important target group.

In contrast to the relatively short-lived antibody response to vaccination, serum antibody to HA can persist for decades after natural infection. During 1977 and 1978, influenza A (H_1N_1) viruses similar to those circulating in 1950 reappeared and spread throughout the world. Individuals born before 1950 were not affected, indicating that substantial immunity remained after almost 30 years. By contrast, disease occurred in individuals under 20 years of age, regardless of previous infection by influenza A (H_3N_2) viruses, showing that intersubtypic immunity in humans is weak.

Safety

Common Adverse Events

The most frequent adverse events associated with inactivated vaccines are local acute inflammatory reactions.[86,87,89] Pain, erythema, and induration, which generally are mild and rarely interfere with daily activities, occur at the site of vaccine administration in up to 65% of recipients. Local reactions rarely persist for longer than 24 to 48 hours. Although infection and bruising are possible, they occur no more often than with other injections.

The most common systemic reactions include fever, myalgia, arthralgia, and headache. These reactions occur much less frequently (generally less than 15%) than local reactions and tend to be seen most often in very young children and in others exposed to influenza virus vaccines or to one of the antigens in the vaccine for the first time.[85,88,102,123] In young children, whole-virus influenza vaccines and larger vaccine doses appear to produce more systemic reactions, including fever, than subvirion vaccines, and so subvirion inactivated vaccines are preferred for children.[88,89]

Rare Adverse Events (by Organ System)

The main concern identified in large-scale use of influenza virus vaccines has been GBS,[239] a rare neurologic syndrome characterized by ascending paralysis, paresthesia and dysesthesia, and oligoclonal antibodies in the cerebrospinal fluid (CSF) in the absence of CSF pleocytosis. GBS is a rare condition with an annual incidence of 10 to 20 cases per 1 million adult population,[240] and has been associated with many respiratory and gastrointestinal illnesses and, in particular, infection with *Campylobacter* species.[241] Although the etiology is not entirely understood, there is strong evidence that the induction of antibodies to glycolipids is central to the neuropathic changes. Most patients will make a complete or near-complete recovery, and plasmapheresis and administration of immune globulin appear to speed recovery.[242] However, paralysis of respiratory musculature requiring assisted ventilation can occur, and the case-fatality rate is approximately 6% and increases with age.[240,243]

During the 1976 swine influenza virus immunization campaign in the United States, which was held in anticipation of the spread of a swine influenza virus, an increased incidence of GBS cases occurred in vaccine recipients, halting the vaccination campaign.[239] The increase in GBS cases above the background rate was approximately 1 case for every 100,000 persons vaccinated with the swine influenza vaccine.[239]

Subsequent observational studies in the United States failed to identify a similar increase in GBS cases among recipients of inactivated vaccine between 1977 and 1991.[244,245] However, a study of the 1992 to 1994 influenza seasons estimated an increased incidence of approximately one GBS case per million recipients of inactivated influenza vaccine during the study years,[246] which is substantially less than the risk of developing severe complications from influenza infection. In the years since the 1976 swine influenza vaccine campaign, the question of whether GBS is associated with inactivated influenza vaccine has proven difficult to resolve by epidemiologic studies. Nonetheless, no experience similar to the 1976 vaccine campaign has since occurred, and the Advisory Committee on Immunization Practices (ACIP) has stated that "the potential benefits of influenza vaccination in preventing serious illness, hospitalization, and death greatly outweigh the possible risks for developing vaccine-associated GBS."[247] The CDC and the Food and Drug Administration jointly maintain the Vaccine Adverse Event Reporting System, a vaccine safety surveillance system for continuously monitoring for GBS and other adverse events potentially linked to influenza and other vaccines.

Indications for Vaccine

In the United States, the ACIP has the central role in establishing influenza vaccination policy. The ACIP, an advisory group to the CDC, is composed of voting and nonvoting liaison members who represent major medical organizations, the academic medical community, state and federal public health agencies, and vaccine manufacturers. The ACIP's recommendations for influenza vaccination are published annually in April or May in the *Morbidity and Mortality Weekly Report* in a document entitled "Prevention and Control of Influenza: Recommendations of the Advisory Committee on Immunization Practices."[248] Although the ACIP influenza vaccination recommendations can be considered permissive in tone because they indicate that vaccination is recommended for anyone (6 months or older) who wishes to avoid influenza, the primary goal of U.S. influenza vaccination policy since the early 1960s has been to foster influenza vaccination of persons at elevated risk for serious morbidity and death resulting from influenza. The current recommendations reflect this intent.[248]

The concern with certain groups at high risk for influenza-related complications stems from observations made at least as far back as the 1800s by William Farr, who noted that groups such as the elderly and persons with certain medical conditions were more likely to be adversely affected by influenza than others. Since then, numerous studies have confirmed that certain conditions, including chronic pulmonary or cardiac conditions, diabetes mellitus, an immunosuppressive state or condition,[180,216,217,249-251] and pregnancy,[252] increase the risk of hospitalization or death among individuals infected by influenza virus.

Current ACIP recommendations for the annual administration of influenza vaccine are summarized in Table 17–6. Broadly speaking, these recommendations state that the annual administration of influenza vaccine is indicated for

1. Persons at high risk for developing serious complications from influenza, including (a) all persons 65 years and older, (b) all persons 6 months of age and older with one or more of several medical conditions, and (c) persons living in certain institutional settings
2. All persons, especially health care workers and household members, who are in "close contact" with persons with high-risk conditions
3. Persons in other priority groups, such as those 50 to 64 years of age

Approximately 152 million people, including 75 million in the high-risk category and 77 million in the other targeted groups,[248] comprise the groups for whom influenza vaccination currently is recommended in the United States.

The reason for vaccinating persons "in close contact" with groups at "high risk" for developing serious complications from influenza is to reduce transmission of influenza virus infections from caregivers and other close contacts to these vulnerable persons. This approach has been supported by studies, conducted primarily in nursing home settings, suggesting that this strategy can reduce infections among nursing home residents.[54,69,204]

The recommendation to annually vaccinate all persons 50 years and older was made in 2000. This age group comprises approximately 43 million people, of whom 24% to 32% have one or more medical condition placing them at elevated risk for developing a serious complication from influenza.[248] Although the impact of influenza on this entire group has not been well demonstrated, the ACIP recommended vaccination of the entire group to increase the vaccination coverage of the persons with a high-risk condition in this age group and to derive other benefits, including decreased rates of illness and work absenteeism.

In 2002, the ACIP began *encouraging* vaccination of children 6 to 23 months in age and their close contacts. Although encouragement does not carry the full weight of a recommendation, it does signal the ACIP's recognition that healthy children in this age group are at elevated risk for hospitalization during periods when influenza viruses are in circulation[251,253-255] and the committee's intent to make a full recommendation once certain issues, such as those related to the feasibility of implementing such a recommendation, have been resolved.

In general, the recommended optimal timing in the United States for influenza vaccination is from October through November, a time period that balances the desirability of administering vaccine before significant influenza activity has started but not so far in advance that antibody titers in certain groups of vaccine recipients, particularly the elderly, begin to fall substantially before the influenza season begins. However, in 2000 and 2001, significant delays in the national distribution of influenza vaccine[256] led the ACIP to recommend that vaccination of high-risk groups and health care workers begin in October and that vaccination of others begin in November.[257,258] It is uncertain if staggered timing of vaccinations will continue to be recommended if the vaccine supply stabilizes. Regardless, it is clear that continuation of influenza vaccination activities through November and later is critical for substantially improving vaccination coverage and for fully utilizing vaccine supplies. In this regard, it is important to note that influenza seasons can begin early in the fall, but, in 21 of 25 consecutive influenza seasons between 1976 and 2001 in the United States, influenza activity peaked after December.

TABLE 17–6 ■ Groups Targeted by the U.S. Advisory Committee on Immunization Practices (ACIP) for Annual Vaccination

Groups at Elevated Risk of Influenza-Related Complications
Persons ≥65 yr
Residents of nursing homes and other chronic care facilities
Persons 6 mo–64 yr with certain medical conditions, including
    Chronic pulmonary disease, including asthma
    Chronic heart disease
    Chronic metabolic diseases, including diabetes
    Renal dysfunction
    Hemoglobinopathies
    Immunosuppression caused by medication or illness, such as HIV
Persons 6 mo–18 yr on long-term aspirin therapy
Pregnant women beyond 1st trimester during influenza season
Children 6–23 mo*
Persons Who Can Transmit Influenza to High-Risk Persons
Health care workers
Employees of nursing homes and other chronic care facilities or residences for persons in groups at high risk
Persons providing home care to high-risk groups
Household contacts of high-risk persons, including children <24 mo*
Persons Ages 50–64 Years

*The ACIP is encouraging vaccination of all children 6 to 23 months and the household members and out-of-home caregivers of children less than 24 months. A full recommendation may be forthcoming.

Contraindications and Precautions

Persons with previous allergic reactions to influenza vaccine should be medically evaluated to determine if further use of influenza vaccine is advisable. A distinction should be made between immunoglobulin E (IgE)–mediated hypersensitivity reactions, which are potentially life threatening, and non–IgE-mediated allergic reactions. Persons known to have an anaphylactic hypersensitivity to eggs or egg antigens or to influenza vaccine should not be vaccinated with an egg-replicated influenza vaccine until they are evaluated by a physician. True anaphylactic responses are rare, and, for suspected IgE-mediated reactions, desensitization may be considered if there is a strong indication for vaccine use.[259] In addition to egg antigens, it is possible (as with any vaccine) that other components may be sensitizing.

The risk–benefit ratio of vaccination needs to be assessed carefully for other types of allergic reactions. For example, allergic reactions to thimerosal are characterized by a delayed-type hypersensitivity that most often results in a local inflamed or indurated lesion similar to that seen with positive reactions to tuberculin skin tests used to document infection with tuberculosis.[260] Although the reaction may progress to vesiculation or ulceration, the reaction is not life threatening and can be managed with application of topical steroids. Current "preservative-free" influenza vaccines still contain trace amounts of thimerosal, but vaccines containing no thimerosal (which will contain an alternative preservative such as phenoxyethanol or no preservative) are being developed.

Vial stoppers or syringe plungers used for influenza vaccine can contain latex in the rubber composition, and concerns have been raised about reports of allergic reactions to latex rubber.[261] The contact surfaces of the rubber-containing parts are treated (usually with silicone) to reduce the possible introduction of latex rubber antigens into the vaccine. Nonetheless latex antigens might still enter influenza vaccine by way of repeated needle insertions through the stoppers of multidose containers, because a needle puncture could entrain small bits of the stopper. In recognition of these concerns, some manufacturers use alternate elastomeric products that do not contain latex, and others are making changes. The risk of exposure and sensitization to latex is exceedingly low, and this risk needs to be weighed against the potential benefit of vaccine. Information regarding the latex content of container components can be found in the package insert written specifically for each vaccine.

Influenza vaccine is recommended for women during their second or third trimester of pregnancy. Although vaccination during these periods is thought to be safe by many experts,[248] information on the administration of inactivated influenza vaccine during pregnancy is limited, and reproductive toxicologic studies generally have not been done in this group using inactivated influenza vaccines.[252,262-264]

Other Directions for Influenza Virus Vaccines

Inactivated influenza vaccines are highly safe and effective. Nonetheless, there is a strong interest in developing new and potentially improved influenza vaccines as well as expanding the availability of these vaccines.

Live, attenuated (cold-adapted) influenza vaccines are described in detail in Chapter 18 and are mentioned briefly here. These vaccines were developed to elicit an immune response, including production of secretory IgA antibodies in the mucosal tissues of the respiratory tract, that would be similar to the response developing after natural infection while minimizing the symptoms associated with viral replication. Live, attenuated influenza vaccines have been used extensively in countries of the former Soviet Union.

The use of mammalian cells to replicate influenza viruses for use in inactivated vaccine has received a great deal of attention in recent years and is anticipated to provide several advantages, including the potential availability of a product for use by those who are allergic to eggs or egg proteins. Antigenic selection often occurs when human influenza viruses are passaged in eggs but not when the same viruses are passaged solely in mammalian tissue culture. Therefore, it is also possible that human influenza viruses replicated only in mammalian tissue cultures will produce vaccines that are antigenically more similar to circulating viruses and increase vaccine effectiveness.[116,117]

Unlike other vaccines, influenza vaccine generally must be available for administration only 9 to 12 months after identification of a new vaccine virus, so that there is little time for investigating (and documenting) whether the seed virus is free of extraneous agents. The intense time pressure associated with the production and distribution of influenza vaccine, combined with the lack of field facilities that can maintain tissue cultures under conditions to prevent the introduction of extraneous agents, are currently obstacles to using tissue culture isolates in influenza vaccine production. Because antigenic changes occurring in eggs appear to be irreversible, influenza vaccines produced in tissue cultures using seed viruses originally recovered in eggs are not expected to improve vaccine effectiveness. An infrastructure capable of supporting use of influenza viruses passaged only in mammalian tissue cultures is required to realize the full theoretical benefits.

High-growth influenza virus reassortants play a central role in facilitating the production of large quantities of influenza vaccine. However, it has not always been possible to produce high-growth reassortants with the desired characteristics using classic reassorting procedures, because these procedures rely on co-infection of two different viruses followed by selection of viral clones with specific genotypic and phenotypic traits. Reverse genetics methods provide a powerful tool to improve the ability to produce reassortants with the desired properties.[265,266] Recent reverse genetic systems relying only on transfection of cells with all genes needed to make a complete virus are now available, so that influenza A and B reassortant viruses can be tailored specifically to growth substrates such as eggs and mammalian tissue cultures.

Other strategies for producing influenza vaccine have taken advantage of recent advances allowing rapid sequencing of influenza virus genes. For example, vectors containing influenza HA or NA genes have been used to infect tissue cultures in which the viral protein of interest (HA or NA) is produced in massive amount and can be purified for use as a vaccine. Clinical trials of purified HA or NA vaccines produced by using a baculovirus vector have demonstrated that such preparations can be standardized to produce immunogenic vaccines with reactogenicity profiles similar to or better than the profiles of vaccines produced by viral replication.[91-93] DNA vaccines, which are based on plasmids containing the relevant viral gene(s), also have been investigated. In animal models, DNA vaccines can stimulate both humoral and cellular immune mechanisms.[267] Although DNA vaccines could be relatively easy and inexpensive to produce and have been shown to have protective effects in animal models, progress has been slow on DNA vaccines for humans, in part because the immune response in humans has been relatively poor. It has been shown that specific CpG motifs in bacterial DNA have differential effects on the immune response, and work is proceeding to identify optimal motifs for immunogenic and protective effects in humans.[268-270]

Public Health Considerations

Vaccination Coverage Levels

Worldwide

The WHO recently issued a position paper encouraging influenza vaccine use in persons at increased risk for complications of influenza in all countries where epidemic surveillance is well established and where reduction of influenza and its complications are public health priorities.[271] Current recommendations for influenza vaccination vary among countries, with most recommending influenza vaccination for patients with cardiopulmonary disorders and somewhat fewer countries recommending vaccine for those with metabolic diseases and immunologic disorders and all persons above a certain age.[272] Although influenza vaccine use increased dramatically during the 1990s in a number of developed countries in Europe and the Americas,[272] vaccine distribution levels (i.e., the number of doses distributed per 1000 total resident population) among these countries have continued to vary by 5- to 10-fold or more during the past two decades. It appears that there are multiple factors that influence these differences; however, these factors remain poorly understood.[272] It is currently estimated that 250 million doses of trivalent inactivated influenza vaccine are produced worldwide.

United States

In the United States, influenza immunization rates have improved dramatically in recent years, especially among persons 65 years of age and older. Between 1989 and 1999, vaccination rates in this group rose from approximately 33% to 66%. In addition, vaccination rates among nursing home residents were estimated at about 83% in 1998.[248] In contrast, vaccination rates of high-risk persons less than 65 years old and of health care providers remain relatively low. For example, the overall vaccination rate for 18- to 64-year-olds with high-risk conditions was estimated at only 32% in 2000, and a study in four large health maintenance organizations found that only 9% to 10% of asthmatic children were vaccinated against influenza.[273] Furthermore, a 1998 study of health care workers found that only 37% were vaccinated.[248]

Prior to the 2000 to 2001 and 2001 to 2002 influenza seasons, delays in vaccine production and distribution by manufacturers occurred in the United States because of lower than anticipated yields and other manufacturing problems. Following these delays, two of the four manufacturers of influenza vaccine for the United States have withdrawn from the market during the past 3 years, heightening concerns about the supply of influenza vaccine and vaccine production delays in the future.

Disease Control Strategies

Current Strategies

In contrast to control efforts for some diseases, the primary goal of almost all current influenza vaccination programs is to reduce the number of serious complications, including deaths, resulting from influenza infections rather than to eliminate infections or disease. The development of this strategy reflects knowledge that influenza exerts a disproportionately severe impact on the elderly and those with chronic medical conditions, and the practical limitations of trying to vaccinate entire populations on an annual basis. The primary target groups of most vaccination recommendations are the elderly and others with chronic medical conditions.

Alternate Strategies

Two notable exceptions to this general tendency have been Japanese vaccination programs conducted between 1962 and 1987 that focused on immunizing children, and more recent efforts in Ottawa, Canada, to provide universal influenza vaccination to its population. Targeted vaccination of school-age children has been suggested recently in other countries because some studies indicated that vaccination of school-age children might provide the elderly and others in the community with protection against influenza through herd immunity (see *Herd Immunity* above).[164,175] However, no large prospective study has yet convincingly demonstrated that vaccinating school-age children will provide significant protection for other groups. Such a demonstration would be critical before considering such a recommendation because the risk of serious complications from influenza is generally low in healthy children in this age group. Some studies have suggested that vaccinating healthy adults against influenza might provide cost savings, but other studies have not shown this.[177,210,212,274]

Eradication or Elimination, If Feasible

Influenza cannot be considered an eradicable disease for several reasons. Most important, avian species are the natural host to all known influenza A viruses, while certain other animal species, particularly swine, also can support the circulation of some influenza A virus subtypes. Eradicating circulation of influenza A viruses among all animal species capable of hosting them is impossible. Furthermore, given the ability of influenza viruses to rapidly change their antigenicity, the need to update vaccines frequently is an insurmountable practical barrier to ever administering enough vaccine quickly enough to eliminate influenza virus circulation among human populations.

REFERENCES

1. Creighton C. A History of Epidemics in Britain, AD 1664–1666. New York, Cambridge University Press, 1891.
2. Thompson T. Annals of Influenza or Epidemic Catarrhal Fever in Great Britain from 1510 to 1837. London, Sydenham Society, 1852.
3. Pfeiffer RBM. Weitere Mitteilungen uber die Erreger der Influenza. Dtsch Med Wochenschr 18:465–467, 1892.
4. Smith W, Andrewes CH, Laidlaw PP. A virus obtained from influenza patients. Lancet 2:66–68, 1933.
5. Stokes J, Chenoweth A, Waltz A, et al. Results of immunization by means of active virus of human influenza. J Clin Invest 16:237–243, 1937.
6. A clinical evaluation of vaccination against influenza. JAMA 124:982–985, 1944.
7. Davenport FM. Current knowledge of influenza vaccine. JAMA 182:121–123, 1962.
8. Dowdle WR. Influenza immunoprophylaxis after 30 years' experience. In Nayak DP (ed). Genetic Variation Among Influenza Viruses. New York, Academic Press, 1981, pp 525–534.

9. Glaser CA, Gilliam S, Thompson WW, et al. Medical care capacity for influenza outbreaks, Los Angeles. Emerg Infect Dis 8:569–574, 2002.

10. Simonsen L, Clarke MJ, Williamson GD, et al. The impact of influenza epidemics on mortality: introducing a severity index. Am J Public Health 87:1944–1950, 1997.

11. Lui KJ, Kendal AP. Impact of influenza epidemics on mortality in the United States from October 1972 to May 1985. Am J Public Health 77:712–716, 1987.

12. Choi K, Thacker SB. Mortality during influenza epidemics in the United States, 1967–1978. Am J Public Health 72:1280–1283, 1982.

13. Simonsen L, Fukuda K, Schonberger LB, Cox NJ. The impact of influenza epidemics on hospitalizations. J Infect Dis 181:831–837, 2000.

14. Perrotta DM, Decker M, Glezen WP. Acute respiratory disease hospitalizations as a measure of impact of epidemic influenza. Am J Epidemiol 122:468–476, 1985.

15. Barker WH. Excess pneumonia and influenza associated hospitalization during influenza epidemics in the United States, 1970–1978. Am J Public Health 76:761–765, 1986.

16. Crosby A. America's Forgotten Pandemic: The Influenza of 1918. New York, Cambridge University Press, 1989.

17. Davis LE, Caldwell GG, Lynch RE, et al. Hong Kong influenza: the epidemiologic features of a high school family study analyzed and compared with a similar study during the 1957 Asian influenza epidemic. Am J Epidemiol 92:240–247, 1970.

18. Fox JP, Hall CE, Cooney MK, Foy HM. Influenzavirus infections in Seattle families, 1975–1979. I. Study design, methods and the occurrence of infections by time and age. Am J Epidemiol 116:212–227, 1982.

19. Elder AG, O'Donnell B, McCruden EA, et al. Incidence and recall of influenza in a cohort of Glasgow healthcare workers during the 1993–1994 epidemic: results of serum testing and questionnaire. BMJ 313:1241–1242, 1996.

20. Weingarten S, Staniloff H, Ault M, et al. Do hospital employees benefit from the influenza vaccine? A placebo-controlled clinical trial. J Gen Intern Med 3:32–37, 1988.

21. Wilde JA, McMillan JA, Serwint J, et al. Effectiveness of influenza vaccine in health care professionals: a randomized trial. JAMA 281:908–913, 1999.

22. Nicholson KG. Clinical features of influenza. Semin Respir Infect 7:26–37, 1992.

23. Imboden JB, Canter A, Cluff LE. Convalescence from influenza: a study of the psychological and clinical determinants. Arch Intern Med 108:115–121, 1961.

24. Noble GR. Epidemiological and clinical aspects of influenza. In Beare AS (ed). Basic and Applied Influenza Research. Boca Raton, FL, CRC Press, 1982, pp 11–50.

25. Stevens KM. The pathophysiology of influenzal pneumonia in 1918. Perspect Biol Med 25:115–125, 1981.

26. Louria DB, Blumenfeld HL, Ellis JT, et al. Studies on influenza in the pandemic of 1957–1958. II. Pulmonary complications of influenza. J Clin Invest 38:213–265, 1959.

27. Connolly AM, Salmon RL, Lervy B, Williams DH. What are the complications of influenza and can they be prevented? Experience from the 1989 epidemic of H_3N_2 influenza A in general practice. BMJ 306:1452–1454, 1993.

28. Heikkinen T, Thint M, Chonmaitree T. Prevalence of various respiratory viruses in the middle ear during acute otitis media. N Engl J Med 340:260–264, 1999.

29. Kim HW, Brandt CD, Arrobio JO, et al. Influenza A and B virus infection in infants and young children during the years 1957–1976. Am J Epidemiol 109:464–479, 1979.

30. Ruuskanen O, Arola M, Putto-Laurila A, et al. Acute otitis media and respiratory virus infections. Pediatr Infect Dis J 8:94–99, 1989.

31. Corey L, Rubin RJ, Hattwick MA, et al. A nationwide outbreak of Reye's syndrome: its epidemiologic relationship to influenza B. Am J Med 61:615–625, 1976.

32. Hurwitz ES, Nelson DB, Davis C, et al. National surveillance for Reye syndrome: a five-year review. Pediatrics 70:895–900, 1982.

33. Simon NM, Rovner RN, Berlin BS. Acute myoglobinuria associated with type A_2 (Hong Kong) influenza. JAMA 212:1704–1705, 1970.

34. Dietzman DE, Schaller JG, Ray CG, Reed ME. Acute myositis associated with influenza B infection. Pediatrics 57:255–258, 1976.

35. Sion ML, Hatzitolios AI, Toulis EN, et al. Toxic shock syndrome complicating influenza A infection: a two-case report with one case of bacteremia and endocarditis. Intensive Care Med 27:443, 2001.

36. Shinjoh M, Bamba M, Jozaki K, et al. Influenza A-associated encephalopathy with bilateral thalamic necrosis in Japan. Clin Infect Dis 31:611–613, 2000.

37. Togashi T, Matsuzono Y, Narita M. Epidemiology of influenza-associated encephalitis-encephalopathy in Hokkaido, the northernmost island of Japan. Pediatr Int 42:192–196, 2000.

38. Cox NJ, Fuller F, Kaverin N, et al. Orthomyxoviridae. In Regenmortal MHV et al. (eds). Virus Taxonomy: Classification and Nomenclature of Viruses. Seventh Report of the International Committee on Taxonomy of Viruses. San Diego, Academic Press, 2000, pp 585–597.

39. de Jong JC, Claas EC, Osterhaus AD, et al. A pandemic warning? Nature 389:554, 1997.

40. Subbarao K, Klimov A, Katz J, et al. Characterization of an avian influenza A (H_5N_1) virus isolated from a child with a fatal respiratory illness. Science 279:393–396, 1998.

41. Mounts AW, Kwong H, Izurieta HS, et al. Case-control study of risk factors for avian influenza A (H_5N_1) disease, Hong Kong, 1997. J Infect Dis 180:505–508, 1999.

42. Yuen KY, Chan PK, Peiris M, et al. Clinical features and rapid viral diagnosis of human disease associated with avian influenza A H_5N_1 virus. Lancet 351:467–471, 1998.

43. Centers for Disease Control and Prevention. Isolation of avian influenza A(H_5N_1) viruses from humans—Hong Kong, May–December 1997. MMWR 46:1204–1207, 1997.

44. Osterhaus AD, Rimmelzwaan GF, Martina BE, et al. Influenza B virus in seals. Science 288:1051–1053, 2000.

45. Cox NJ, Kawaoka Y. Orthomyxoviruses: influenza. In Topley WWC, Wilson GS, Parker MT, Collier LH (eds). Topley & Wilson's Principles of Bacteriology, Virology, and Immunity. London, Arnold, fourth edition, 1998, pp 385–433.

46. Treanor JJ. Influenza virus. In Mandell GL, Bennett JE, Dolin R (eds). Mandell, Douglas, & Bennett's Principles & Practice of Infectious Disease (5th ed). Philadelphia, Churchill Livingstone, 2000, pp 1823–1849.

47. Rocha E, Cox NJ, Black RA, et al. Antigenic and genetic variation in influenza A (H_1N_1) virus isolates recovered from a persistently infected immunodeficient child. J Virol 65:2340–2350, 1991.

48. Hers JF, Mulder J. Broad aspects of the pathology and pathogenesis of human influenza. Am Rev Resp Dis 83(pt 2):84–97, 1961.

49. Walsh JJ, Dietlein LF, Low FN, et al. Bronchotracheal response in human influenza. Arch Intern Med 108:376–388, 1961.

50. Kilbourne ED. Studies on influenza in pandemic of 1957. J Clin Invest 38:213–265, 1959.

51. Minuse E. An attempt to demonstrate viremia in cases of Asian influenza. J Lab Clin Med 59:1016–1019, 1962.

52. Cox NJ, Ziegler T. Influenza viruses. In Murray PR, Baron EJ (eds). Manual of Clinical Microbiology (8th ed). Washington, DC, ASM Press, pp. 1360–1367, 2003 [in press].

53. Ziegler T, Hall H, Sanchez-Fauquier A, et al. Type- and subtype-specific detection of influenza viruses in clinical specimens by rapid culture assay. J Clin Microbiol 33:318–321, 1995.

54. Li J, Chen S, Evans DH. Typing and subtyping influenza virus using DNA microarrays and multiplex reverse transcriptase PCR. J Clin Microbiol 39:696–704, 2001.

55. Miller JM, Tam TW, Maloney S, et al. Cruise ships: high-risk passengers and the global spread of new influenza viruses. Clin Infect Dis 31:433–438, 2000.

56. Centers for Disease Control and Prevention. Update: outbreak of influenza A infection—Alaska and the Yukon Territory, July–August 1998. MMWR 47:685–688, 1998.

57. Centers for Disease Control and Prevention. Update: outbreak of influenza A infection among travelers—Alaska and the Yukon Territory, May–June 1999. MMWR 48:545, 1999.

58. Influenza in travellers to Alaska, the Yukon Territory, and on west coast cruise ships, summer of 1999. Can Commun Dis Rep 25:137–139, 1999.

59. Uyeki T, Zane S, Bodnar U, et al. Large summertime influenza A outbreak among tourists in Alaska and the Yukon Territory. Clin Infect Dis 2003 [in press].

60. Thompson WW, Shay DK, Weintraub E, et al. Mortality associated with influenza and respiratory syncytial virus in the United States. JAMA 289:179–186, 2003.

61. Hall CE, Cooney MK, Fox JP. The Seattle virus watch. IV. Comparative epidemiologic observations of infections with influenza A and B viruses, 1965–1969, in families with young children. Am J Epidemiol 98:365–380, 1973.

62. Fox JP, Cooney MK, Hall CE, Foy HM. Influenzavirus infections in Seattle families, 1975–1979. II. Pattern of infection in invaded households and relation of age and prior antibody to occurrence of infection and related illness. Am J Epidemiol 116:228–242, 1982.

63. Monto AS, Kioumehr F. The Tecumseh Study of Respiratory Illness. IX. Occurrence of influenza in the community, 1966–1971. Am J Epidemiol 102:553–563, 1975.

64. Patriarca PA, Arden NH, Koplan JP, Goodman RA. Prevention and control of type A influenza infections in nursing homes: benefits and costs of four approaches using vaccination and amantadine. Ann Intern Med 107:732–740, 1987.

65. Arden N, Monto AS, Ohmit SE. Vaccine use and the risk of outbreaks in a sample of nursing homes during an influenza epidemic. Am J Public Health 85:399–401, 1995.

66. Cunney RJ, Bialachowski A, Thornley D, et al. An outbreak of influenza A in a neonatal intensive care unit. Infect Control Hosp Epidemiol 21:449–454, 2000.

67. Munoz FM, Campbell JR, Atmar RL, et al. Influenza A virus outbreak in a neonatal intensive care unit. Pediatr Infect Dis J 18:811–815, 1999.

68. Meibalane R, Sedmak GV, Sasidharan P, et al. Outbreak of influenza in a neonatal intensive care unit. J Pediatr 91:974–976, 1977.

69. Carman WF, Elder AG, Wallace LA, et al. Effects of influenza vaccination of health-care workers on mortality of elderly people in long-term care: a randomised controlled trial. Lancet 355:93–97, 2000.

70. Francis T. Transmission of influenza by a filterable virus. Science 80:457–459, 1934.

71. Francis T. A new type of virus from epidemic influenza. Science 92:405–408, 1940.

72. Lewis PA, Shope RE. Swine influenza. II. Hemophilic bacillus from the respiratory tract of infected swine. J Exp Med 54:361–371, 1931.

73. Magill TP. A virus from cases of influenza-like upper respiratory infection. Exp Biol Med 45:162–164, 1940.

74. Shope RE. Swine influenza. III. Filtration experiments and etiology. J Exp Med 54:373–385, 1931.

75. Shope RE. Swine influenza. I. Experimental transmission and pathology. J Exp Med 54:349–359, 1931.

76. Francis T, Salk JE, Brace WM. The protective effect of vaccination against epidemic influenza B. J Am Med Assoc 131:275–278, 1946.

77. Salk JE, Menke WJ, Francis T. A clinical, epidemiological and immunological evaluation of vaccination against epidemic influenza. Am J Hyg 42:57–93, 1945.

78. Francis T. Cultivation of human influenza virus in an artificial medium. Science 82:353–354, 1935.

79. Francis T. The development of the 1943 vaccination study of the Commission on Influenza. Am J Hyg 42:1–11, 1945.

80. Halperin SA, Smith B, Mabrouk T, et al. Safety and immunogenicity of a trivalent, inactivated, mammalian cell culture-derived influenza vaccine in healthy adults, seniors, and children. Vaccine 20:1240–1247, 2002.

81. Kistner O, Barrett PN, Mundt W, et al. A novel mammalian cell (Vero) derived influenza virus vaccine: development, characterization and industrial scale production. Wien Klin Wochenschr 111:207–214, 1999.

82. Palache AM, Brands R, van Scharrenburg GJ. Immunogenicity and reactogenicity of influenza subunit vaccines produced in MDCK cells or fertilized chicken eggs. J Infect Dis 176(suppl 1):S20–S23, 1997.

83. Palache AM, Scheepers HS, de Regt V, et al. Safety, reactogenicity and immunogenicity of Madin Darby Canine Kidney cell-derived inactivated influenza subunit vaccine: a meta-analysis of clinical studies. Dev Biol Stand 98:115–125, 1999.

84. Percheson PB, Trepanier P, Dugre R, Mabrouk T. A Phase I, randomized controlled clinical trial to study the reactogenicity and immunogenicity of a new split influenza vaccine derived from a non-tumorigenic cell line. Dev Biol Stand 98:127–132, 1999.

85. Cate TR, Couch RB, Kasel JA, Six HR. Clinical trials of monovalent influenza A/New Jersey/76 virus vaccines in adults: reactogenicity, antibody response, and antibody persistence. J Infect Dis 136(suppl):S450–S455, 1977.

86. Cate TR, Couch RB, Parker D, Baxter B. Reactogenicity, immunogenicity, and antibody persistence in adults given inactivated influenza virus vaccines—1978. Rev Infect Dis 5:737–747, 1983.

87. Quinnan GV, Schooley R, Dolin R, et al. Serologic responses and systemic reactions in adults after vaccination with monovalent A/USSR/77 and trivalent A/USSR/77, A/Texas/77, B/Hong Kong/72 influenza vaccines. Rev Infect Dis 5:748–757, 1983.

88. Wright PF, Thompson J, Vaughn WK, et al. Trials of influenza A/New Jersey/76 virus vaccine in normal children: an overview of age-related antigenicity and reactogenicity. J Infect Dis 136(suppl):S731–S741, 1977.

89. Wright PF, Cherry JD, Foy HM, et al. Antigenicity and reactogenicity of influenza A/USSR/77 virus vaccine in children—a multicentered evaluation of dosage and safety. Rev Infect Dis 5:758–764, 1983.

90. Johansson BE, Bucher DJ, Kilbourne ED. Purified influenza virus hemagglutinin and neuraminidase are equivalent in stimulation of antibody response but induce contrasting types of immunity to infection. J Virol 63:1239–1246, 1989.

91. Johansson BE, Price PM, Kilbourne ED. Immunogenicity of influenza A virus N2 neuraminidase produced in insect larvae by baculovirus recombinants. Vaccine 13:841–845, 1995.

92. Lakey DL, Treanor JJ, Betts RF, et al. Recombinant baculovirus influenza A hemagglutinin vaccines are well tolerated and immunogenic in healthy adults. J Infect Dis 174:838–841, 1996.

93. Powers DC, Smith GE, Anderson EL, et al. Influenza A virus vaccines containing purified recombinant H3 hemagglutinin are well tolerated and induce protective immune responses in healthy adults. J Infect Dis 171:1595–1599, 1995.

94. Williams MS, Wood JM. A brief history of inactivated influenza virus vaccines. In Hannoun C, Kendal AP, Klenk HD, Ruben FL (eds). Options for the Control of Influenza II. Proceedings of the International Conference on Options for the Control of Influenza, Courchevel, France, 1992. Amsterdam, Excerpta Medica, 1993, pp 169–171.

95. Baez M, Palese P, Kilbourne ED. Gene composition of high-yielding influenza vaccine strains obtained by recombination. J Infect Dis 141:362–365, 1980.

96. Kilbourne ED, Murphy JS. Genetic studies of influenza viruses. I. Viral morphology and growth capacity as exchangeable genetic traits: rapid in-ovo adaptation of early passage Asian strain isolates by combination with PR8. J Exp Med 111:387–406, 1960.

97. Williams MS, Mayner RE, Daniel NJ, et al. New developments in the measurement of the hemagglutinin content of influenza virus vaccines by single-radial-immunodiffusion. J Biol Stand 8:289–296, 1980.

98. Williams MS. Single-radial-immunodiffusion as an in vitro potency assay for human inactivated viral vaccines. Vet Microbiol 37:253–262, 1993.

99. Wood JM, Schild GC, Newman RW, Seagroatt V. An improved single-radial-immunodiffusion technique for the assay of influenza haemagglutinin antigen: application for potency determinations of inactivated whole virus and subunit vaccines. J Biol Stand 5:237–247, 1977.

100. Kilbourne ED, Cerini CP, Khan MW, et al. Immunologic response to the influenza virus neuraminidase is influenced by prior experience with the associated viral hemagglutinin. I. Studies in human vaccinees. J Immunol 138:3010–3013, 1987.

101. Frace AM, Klimov AI, Rowe T, et al. Modified M2 proteins produce heterotypic immunity against influenza A virus. Vaccine 17:2237–2244, 1999.

102. Ennis FA, Mayner RE, Barry DW, et al. Correlation of laboratory studies with clinical responses to A/New Jersey influenza vaccines. J Infect Dis 136(suppl):S397–S406, 1977.

103. Lowe I, Southern J. The antimicrobial activity of phenoxyethanol in vaccines. Lett Appl Microbiol 18:115–116, 1994.

104. LoGrippo GA. Investigations of the use of beta propiolactone in virus inactivation. Ann N Y Acad Sci 83:578–594, 1960.

105. Gard S. Theoretical considerations in the inactivation of viruses by chemical means. Ann N Y Acad Sci 83:638–648, 1960.

106. Ghandi SS. The effect of formaldehyde treatment of influenza virus on the assay of its haemagglutinin antigen content by the single-radial-immunodiffusion (SRD) technique. J Biol Stand 6:121–126, 1978.

107. Goldstein MA, Tauraso NM. Effect of formalin, beta-propiolactone, merthiolate, and ultraviolet light upon influenza virus infectivity chicken cell agglutination, hemagglutination, and antigenicity. Appl Microbiol 19:290–294, 1970.

108. Hoyle L. The chemical reactions of the haemagglutinins and neuraminidases of different strains of influenza viruses. I. Effect of reagents reacting with amino acids in the active centres. J Hyg (Lond) 67:289–299, 1969.

109. Reichert E, Majer M, Mauler R. Results of the single-radial-diffusion test with formaldehyde-treated influenza virus. Dev Biol Stand 39:187–191, 1977.

110. World Health Organization. Requirements for Influenza Vaccine (Inactivated): Revised at ECBS 1990. Geneva, World Health Organization, 1991.

111. World Health Organization. Recommended composition of influenza virus vaccines for use in the 2003 influenza season. Wkly Epidemiol Rec 77:344–348, 2002.

112. World Health Organization. Recommended composition of influenza virus vaccines for use in the 2002–2003 season. Wkly Epidemiol Rec 77:62–66, 2002.

113. Kilbourne ED, Smith C, Brett I, et al. The total influenza vaccine failure of 1947 revisited: major intrasubtypic antigenic change can explain failure of vaccine in a post-World War II epidemic. Proc Natl Acad Sci U S A 99:10748–10752, 2002.

114. Meyer HM Jr, Hopps HE, Parkman PD, Ennis FA. Review of existing vaccines for influenza. Am J Clin Pathol 70(1 suppl):146–152, 1978.

115. Katz JM, Webster RG. Efficacy of inactivated influenza A virus (H_3N_2) vaccines grown in mammalian cells or embryonated eggs. J Infect Dis 160:191–198, 1989.

116. Katz JM, Webster RG. Amino acid sequence identity between the HA1 of influenza A (H_3N_2) viruses grown in mammalian and primary chick kidney cells. J Gen Virol 73(pt 5):1159–1165, 1992.

117. Newman RW, Jennings R, Major DL, et al. Immune response of human volunteers and animals to vaccination with egg-grown influenza A (H_1N_1) virus is influenced by three amino acid substitutions in the haemagglutinin molecule. Vaccine 11:400–406, 1993.

118. Robertson JS, Nicolson C, Bootman JS, et al. Sequence analysis of the haemagglutinin (HA) of influenza A (H_1N_1) viruses present in clinical material and comparison with the HA of laboratory-derived virus. J Gen Virol 72(pt 11):2671–2677, 1991.

119. Garnick RL. Experience with viral contamination in cell culture. Dev Biol Stand 88:49–56, 1996.

120. Garnick RL. Raw materials as a source of contamination in large-scale cell culture. Dev Biol Stand 93:21–29, 1998.

121. Hay RJ. Operator-induced contamination in cell culture systems. Dev Biol Stand 75:193–204, 1991

122. Nettleton PF, Rweyemamu MM. The association of calf serum with the contamination of BHK21 clone 13 suspension cells by a parvovirus serologically related to the minute virus of mice (MVM). Arch Virol 64:359–374, 1980.

123. Barry DW, Mayner RE, Hochstein HD, et al. Comparative trial of influenza vaccines. II. Adverse reactions in children and adults. Am J Epidemiol 104:47–59, 1976.

124. Pickering JM, Smith H, Sweet C. Influenza virus pyrogenicity: central role of structural orientation of virion components and involvement of viral lipid and glycoproteins. J Gen Virol 73(pt 6):1345–1354, 1992.

125. Reichelderfer PS, Manischewitz JF, Wells MA, et al. Reduction of endotoxin levels in influenza virus vaccines by barium sulfate adsorption-elution. Appl Microbiol 30:333–334, 1975.

126. Hochstein HD, Fitzgerald EA, McMahon FG, Vargas R. Properties of US standard endotoxin (EC-5) in human male volunteers. J Endotoxin Res 1:52–66, 1994.

127. Rota PA, Hemphill ML, Whistler T, et al. Antigenic and genetic characterization of the haemagglutinins of recent cocirculating strains of influenza B virus. J Gen Virol 73(pt 10):2737–2742, 1992.

128. Govaert TM, Thijs CT, Masurel N, et al. The efficacy of influenza vaccination in elderly individuals: a randomized double-blind placebo-controlled trial. JAMA 272:1661–1665, 1994.

129. Arrington J, Braun RP, Dong L, et al. Plasmid vectors encoding cholera toxin or the heat-labile enterotoxin from Escherichia coli are strong adjuvants for DNA vaccines. J Virol 76:4536–4546, 2002.

130. Boyce TG, Hsu HH, Sannella EC, et al. Safety and immunogenicity of adjuvanted and unadjuvanted subunit influenza vaccines administered intranasally to healthy adults. Vaccine 19:217–226, 2000.

131. Conne P, Gauthey L, Vernet P, et al. Immunogenicity of trivalent subunit versus virosome-formulated influenza vaccines in geriatric patients. Vaccine 15:1675–1679, 1997.

132. Coombes AG, Major D, Wood JM, et al. Resorbable lamellar particles of polylactide as adjuvants for influenza virus vaccines. Biomaterials 19:1073–1081, 1998.

133. Coulter A, Wong TY, Drane D, et al. Studies on experimental adjuvanted influenza vaccines: comparison of immune stimulating complexes (ISCOMs) and oil-in-water vaccines. Vaccine 16:1243–1253, 1998.

134. Davenport FM, Hennessy AV, Askin FB. Lack of adjuvant effect of $AlPO_4$ on purified influenza virus hemagglutinins in man. J Immunol 100:1139–1140, 1968.

135. Gasparini R, Pozzi T, Montomoli E, et al. Increased immunogenicity of the MF59-adjuvanted influenza vaccine compared to a conventional subunit vaccine in elderly subjects. Eur J Epidemiol 17:135–140, 2001.

136. Hilbert AK, Fritzsche U, Kissel T. Biodegradable microspheres containing influenza A vaccine: immune response in mice. Vaccine 17:1065–1073, 1999.

137. Illum L, Jabbal-Gill I, Hinchcliffe M, et al. Chitosan as a novel nasal delivery system for vaccines. Adv Drug Deliv Rev 51:81–96, 2001.

138. Keitel W, Couch R, Bond N, et al. Pilot evaluation of influenza virus vaccine (IVV) combined with adjuvant. Vaccine 11:909–913, 1993.

139. Martin JT. Development of an adjuvant to enhance the immune response to influenza vaccine in the elderly. Biologicals 25:209–213, 1997.

140. Moldoveanu Z, Novak M, Huang WQ, et al. Oral immunization with influenza virus in biodegradable microspheres. J Infect Dis 167:84–90, 1993.

141. Nicholson KG, Colegate AE, Podda A, et al. Safety and antigenicity of non-adjuvanted and MF59-adjuvanted influenza A/Duck/Singapore/97 (H_5N_3) vaccine: a randomised trial of two potential vaccines against H_5N_1 influenza. Lancet 357:1937–1943, 2001.

142. Ramanathan RK, Potter DM, Belani CP, et al. Randomized trial of influenza vaccine with granulocyte-macrophage colony-stimulating factor or placebo in cancer patients. J Clin Oncol 20:4313–4318, 2002.

143. Rappuoli R, Pizza M, Douce G, Dougan G. Structure and mucosal adjuvanticity of cholera and Escherichia coli heat-labile enterotoxins. Immunol Today 20:493–500, 1999.

144. Schaad UB, Buhlmann U, Burger R, et al. Comparison of immunogenicity and safety of a virosome influenza vaccine with those of a subunit influenza vaccine in pediatric patients with cystic fibrosis. Antimicrob Agents Chemother 44:1163–1167, 2000.

145. De Donato S, Granoff D, Minutello M, et al. Safety and immunogenicity of MF59-adjuvanted influenza vaccine in the elderly. Vaccine 17:3094–3101, 1999.

146. Minutello M, Senatore F, Cecchinelli G, et al. Safety and immunogenicity of an inactivated subunit influenza virus vaccine combined with MF59 adjuvant emulsion in elderly subjects, immunized for three consecutive influenza seasons. Vaccine 17:99–104, 1999.

147. Gluck R, Mischler R, Finkel B, et al. Immunogenicity of new virosome influenza vaccine in elderly people. Lancet 344:160–163, 1994.

148. Hobson D, Lane CA, Beare AS, Chivers CP. Serologic studies on adult volunteers inoculated with oil-adjuvant Asian influenza vaccine. Br Med J 2:271–274, 1964.

149. Brown H, Kasel JA, Freeman DM, et al. The immunizing effect of influenza A/New Jersey/76 (Hsw_1N_1) virus vaccine administered intradermally and intramuscularly to adults. J Infect Dis 136(suppl):S466–S471, 1977.

150. Gluck R, Metcalfe IC. New technology platforms in the development of vaccines for the future. Vaccine 20(suppl 5):B10–B16, 2002.

151. Lazzell V, Waldman RH, Rose C, et al. Immunization against influenza in humans using an oral enteric-coated killed virus vaccine. J Biol Stand 12:315–321, 1984.

152. Poland GA. The role of sodium bisulfite in the 1996–1997 USA influenza vaccine recall. Vaccine 16:1865–1868, 1998.

153. Benne CA, Harmsen M, de Jong JC, Kraaijeveld CA. Neutralization enzyme immunoassay for influenza virus. J Clin Microbiol 32:987–990, 1994.

154. Okuno Y, Tanaka K, Baba K, et al. Rapid focus reduction neutralization test of influenza A and B viruses in microtiter system. J Clin Microbiol 28:1308–1313, 1990.

155. Mostow SR, Schoenbaum SC, Dowdle WR, et al. Studies on inactivated influenza vaccines. II. Effect of increasing dosage on antibody response and adverse reactions in man. Am J Epidemiol 92:248–256, 1970.

156. Palache AM, Beyer WE, Luchters G, et al. Influenza vaccines: the effect of vaccine dose on antibody response in primed populations during the ongoing interpandemic period: a review of the literature. Vaccine 11:892–908, 1993.

157. Nicholson KG, Tyrrell DA, Harrison P, et al. Clinical studies of monovalent inactivated whole virus and subunit A/USSR/77 (H_1N_1) vaccine: serological responses and clinical reactions. J Biol Stand 7:123–136, 1979.

158. Palache AM, Beyer WE, Sprenger MJ, et al. Antibody response after influenza immunization with various vaccine doses: a double-blind, placebo-controlled, multi-centre, dose-response study in elderly nursing-home residents and young volunteers. Vaccine 11:3–9, 1993.

159. Ennis FA, Rook AH, Qi YH, et al. HLA restricted virus-specific cytotoxic T-lymphocyte responses to live and inactivated influenza vaccines. Lancet 2:887–891, 1981.

160. Powers DC. Influenza A virus-specific cytotoxic T lymphocyte activity declines with advancing age. J Am Geriatr Soc 41:1–5, 1993.

161. Demicheli V, Jefferson T, Rivetti D, Deeks J. Prevention and early treatment of influenza in healthy adults. Vaccine 18:957–1030, 2000.

162. Dowdle WR, Coleman MT, Mostow SR, et al. Inactivated influenza vaccines. 2. Laboratory indices of protection. Postgrad Med J 49:159–163, 1973.

163. Gross PA, Hermogenes AW, Sacks HS, et al. The efficacy of influenza vaccine in elderly persons: a meta-analysis and review of the literature. Ann Intern Med 123:518–527, 1995.

164. Monto AS, Davenport FM, Napier JA, Francis T. Modification of an outbreak of influenza in Tecumseh, Michigan by vaccination of schoolchildren. J Infect Dis 122:16–25, 1970.

165. Clements ML, Betts RF, Tierney EL, Murphy BR. Comparison of inactivated and live influenza A virus vaccines. In Kendal AP, Patriarca PA (eds). Options for the Control of Influenza: Proceedings of a Viratek-UCLA Symposium, Keystone, Colorado, 1985. New York, Alan R Liss, 1986, pp 255–269.

166. Johnson PR, Feldman S, Thompson JM, et al. Immunity to influenza A virus infection in young children: a comparison of natural infection, live cold-adapted vaccine, and inactivated vaccine. J Infect Dis 154:121–127, 1986.

167. Kilbourne ED, Laver W, Schulman J, Webster R. Antiviral activity of antiserum specific for an influenza virus neuraminidase. J Virol 2:281–288, 1968.

168. Schulman J. Immunology of Influenza. In Edwin D. Kilbourne (ed.) The Influenza Viruses and Influenza. New York, Academic Press, 1975, pp 373–393.

169. Hobson D, Curry RL, Beare AS, Ward-Gardner A. The role of serum haemagglutination-inhibiting antibody in protection against challenge infection with influenza A_2 and B viruses. J Hyg (Lond) 70:767–777, 1972.

170. Davies JR, Grilli EA. Natural or vaccine-induced antibody as a predictor of immunity in the face of natural challenge with influenza viruses. Epidemiol Infect 102:325–333, 1989.

171. Patriarca PA, Weber JA, Parker RA, et al. Risk factors for outbreaks of influenza in nursing homes: a case-control study. Am J Epidemiol 124:114–119, 1986.

172. Oya A, Nerome K. Experiences with mass vaccination of young age groups with inactivated vaccines. In Kendal AP, Patriarca PA (eds). Options for the Control of Influenza: Proceedings of a Viratek-UCLA Symposium, Keystone, Colorado, 1985. New York, Alan R Liss, 1986, pp 183–192.

173. Rudenko LG, Slepushkin AN, Monto AS, et al. Efficacy of live attenuated and inactivated influenza vaccines in schoolchildren and their unvaccinated contacts in Novgorod, Russia. J Infect Dis 168:881–887, 1993.

174. Warburton MF. Immunization against influenza. Med J Aust 1:546–547, 1972.

175. Reichert TA, Sugaya N, Fedson DS, et al. The Japanese experience with vaccinating schoolchildren against influenza. N Engl J Med 344:889–896, 2001.

176. Orenstein WA, Bernier RH, Hinman AR. Assessing vaccine efficacy in the field: further observations. Epidemiol Rev 10:212–241, 1988.

177. Bridges CB, Thompson WW, Meltzer MI, et al. Effectiveness and cost–benefit of influenza vaccination of healthy working adults: a randomized controlled trial. JAMA 284:1655–1663, 2000.

178. Vu T, Farish S, Jenkins M, Kelly H. A meta-analysis of effectiveness of influenza vaccine in persons aged 65 years and over living in the community. Vaccine 20:1831–1836, 2002.

179. Fedson DS, Wajda A, Nicol JP, et al. Clinical effectiveness of influenza vaccination in Manitoba. JAMA 270:1956–1961, 1993.

180. Nichol KL, Wouremna J, von Sternberg T. Benefits of influenza vaccination for low-, intermediate-, and high-risk senior citizens. Arch Intern Med 158:1769–1776, 1998.

181. Nichol KL, Baken L, Nelson A. Relation between influenza vaccination and outpatient visits, hospitalization, and mortality in elderly persons with chronic lung disease. Ann Intern Med 130:397–403, 1999.

182. Nordin J, Mullooly J, Poblete S, et al. Influenza vaccine effectiveness in preventing hospitalizations and deaths in persons 65 years or older in Minnesota, New York, and Oregon: data from 3 health plans. J Infect Dis 184:665–670, 2001.

183. Nichol KL, Margolis KL, Wouremna J, von Sternberg T. Effectiveness of influenza vaccine in the elderly. Gerontology 42:274–279, 1996.

184. Ahmed AH, Nicholson KG, Nguyen-van Tam JS, Pearson JC. Effectiveness of influenza vaccine in reducing hospital admissions during the 1989–1990 epidemic. Epidemiol Infect 118:27–33, 1997.

185. Puig-Barbera J, Marquez-Calderon S, Masoliver-Fores A, et al. Reduction in hospital admissions for pneumonia in non-institutionalised elderly people as a result of influenza vaccination: a case-control study in Spain. J Epidemiol Community Health 51:526–530, 1997.

186. Ohmit SE, Monto AS. Influenza vaccine effectiveness in preventing hospitalization among the elderly during influenza type A and type B seasons. Int J Epidemiol 24:1240–1248, 1995.

187. Mullooly JP, Bennett MD, Hornbrook MC, et al. Influenza vaccination programs for elderly persons: cost-effectiveness in a health maintenance organization. Ann Intern Med 121:947–952, 1994.

188. Foster DA, Talsma A, Furumoto-Dawson A, et al. Influenza vaccine effectiveness in preventing hospitalization for pneumonia in the elderly. Am J Epidemiol 136:296–307, 1992.

189. Fleming DM, Watson JM, Nicholas S, et al. Study of the effectiveness of influenza vaccination in the elderly in the epidemic of 1989–1990 using a general practice database. Epidemiol Infect 115:581–589, 1995.

190. Arden NH, Patriarca PA, Kendal AP. Experiences in the use and efficacy of inactivated influenza vaccine in nursing homes. In Kendal AP, Patriarca PA (eds). Options for the Control of Influenza. New York, Alan R Liss, 1986, pp 155–168.

191. Deguchi Y, Takasugi Y, Tatara K. Efficacy of influenza vaccine in the elderly in welfare nursing homes: reduction in risks of mortality and morbidity during an influenza A (H_3N_2) epidemic. J Med Microbiol 49:553–556, 2000.

192. Meiklejohn G, Hall H. Unusual outbreak of influenza A in a Wyoming nursing home. J Am Geriatr Soc 35:742–746, 1987.

193. Monto AS, Hornbuckle K, Ohmit SE. Influenza vaccine effectiveness among elderly nursing home residents: a cohort study. Am J Epidemiol 154:155–160, 2001.

194. Staynor K, Foster G, McArthur M, et al. Influenza A outbreak in a nursing home: the value of early diagnosis and the use of amantadine hydrochloride. Can J Infect Control 9:109–111, 1994.

195. Morens DM, Rash VM. Lessons from a nursing home outbreak of influenza A. Infect Control Hosp Epidemiol 16:275–280, 1995.

196. Ohmit SE, Arden NH, Monto AS. Effectiveness of inactivated influenza vaccine among nursing home residents during an influenza type A (H_3N_2) epidemic. J Am Geriatr Soc 47:165–171, 1999.

197. de Bruijn IA, Remarque EJ, Jol-van der Zijde CM, et al. Quality and quantity of the humoral immune response in healthy elderly and young subjects after annually repeated influenza vaccination. J Infect Dis 179:31–36, 1999.

198. Fagiolo U, Amadori A, Cozzi E, et al. Humoral and cellular immune response to influenza virus vaccination in aged humans. Aging (Milano) 5:451–458, 1993.

199. Huang YP, Gauthey L, Michel M, et al. The relationship between influenza vaccine-induced specific antibody responses and vaccine-induced nonspecific autoantibody responses in healthy older women. J Gerontol 47:M50–M55, 1992.

200. Gross PA, Quinnan GV, Rodstein M, et al. Association of influenza immunization with reduction in mortality in an elderly population: a prospective study. Arch Intern Med 148:562–565, 1988.

201. Patriarca PA, Weber J, Parker RA, et al. Efficacy of influenza vaccine in nursing homes: reduction in illness and complications during an influenza A (H_3N_2) epidemic. JAMA 253:1136–1139, 1985.

202. Saah AJ, Neufeld R, Rodstein M, et al. Influenza vaccine and pneumonia mortality in a nursing home population. Arch Intern Med 146:2353–2357, 1986.

203. Oshitani H, Saito R, Seki N, et al. Influenza vaccination levels and influenza-like illness in long-term-care facilities for elderly people in Niigata, Japan, during an influenza A (H_3N_2) epidemic. Infect Control Hosp Epidemiol 21:728–730, 2000.

204. Potter J, Stott DJ, Roberts MA, et al. Influenza vaccination of health care workers in long-term-care hospitals reduces the mortality of elderly patients. J Infect Dis 175:1–6, 1997.

205. Saito R, Suzuki H, Oshitani H, et al. The effectiveness of influenza vaccine against influenza A (H_3N_2) virus infections in nursing homes in Niigata, Japan, during the 1998–1999 and 1999–2000 seasons. Infect Control Hosp Epidemiol 23:82–86, 2002.

206. Pyhala R, Haanpaa M, Kleemola M, et al. Acceptable protective efficacy of influenza vaccination in young military conscripts under circumstances of incomplete antigenic and genetic match. Vaccine 19:3253–3260, 2001.

207. Grotto I, Mandel Y, Green MS, et al. Influenza vaccine efficacy in young, healthy adults. Clin Infect Dis 26:913–917, 1998.

208. Edwards KM, Dupont WD, Westrich MK, et al. A randomized controlled trial of cold-adapted and inactivated vaccines for the prevention of influenza A disease. J Infect Dis 169:68–76, 1994.

209. Keitel WA, Cate TR, Couch RB, et al. Efficacy of repeated annual immunization with inactivated influenza virus vaccines over a five-year period. Vaccine 15:1114–1122, 1997.

210. Nichol KL, Lind A, Margolis KL, et al. The effectiveness of vaccination against influenza in healthy, working adults. N Engl J Med 333:889–893, 1995.

211. Saxen H, Virtanen M. Randomized, placebo-controlled double blind study on the efficacy of influenza immunization on absenteeism of health care workers. Pediatr Infect Dis J 18:779–783, 1999.

212. Campbell DS, Rumley MH. Cost-effectiveness of the influenza vaccine in a healthy, working-age population. J Occup Environ Med 39:408–414, 1997.

213. Kumpulainen V, Makela M. Influenza vaccination among healthy employees: a cost–benefit analysis. Scand J Infect Dis 29:181–185, 1997.

214. Leighton L, Williams M, Aubery D, Parker SH. Sickness absence following a campaign of vaccination against influenza in the workplace. Occup Med (Lond) 46:146–150, 1996.

215. Smith JW, Pollard R. Vaccination against influenza: a five-year study in the Post Office. J Hyg (Lond) 83:157–170, 1979.

216. Colquhoun AJ, Nicholson KG, Botha JL, Raymond NT. Effectiveness of influenza vaccine in reducing hospital admissions in people with diabetes. Epidemiol Infect 119:335–341, 1997.

217. Hak E, Nordin J, Wei F, et al. Influence of high-risk medical conditions on the effectiveness of influenza vaccination among elderly members of 3 large managed-care organizations. Clin Infect Dis 35:370–377, 2002.

218. Tasker SA, Treanor JJ, Paxton WB, Wallace MR. Efficacy of influenza vaccination in HIV-infected persons: a randomized, double-blind, placebo-controlled trial. Ann Intern Med 131:430–433, 1999.

219. Neuzil KM, Dupont WD, Wright PF, Edwards KM. Efficacy of inactivated and cold-adapted vaccines against influenza A infection, 1985 to 1990: the pediatric experience. Pediatr Infect Dis J 20:733–740, 2001.

220. Clover RD, Crawford S, Glezen WP, et al. Comparison of heterotypic protection against influenza A/Taiwan/86 (H_1N_1) by attenuated and inactivated vaccines to A/Chile/83-like viruses. J Infect Dis 163:300–304, 1991.

221. Colombo C, Argiolas L, La Vecchia C, et al. Influenza vaccine in healthy preschool children. Rev Epidemiol Sante Publique 49:157–162, 2001.

222. Beyer WE, de Bruijn IA, Palache AM, et al. The plea against annual influenza vaccination? "The Hoskins' Paradox" revisited. Vaccine 16:1929–1932, 1998.

223. Hoskins TW, Davies JR, Allchin A, et al. Controlled trial of inactivated influenza vaccine containing the A-Hong Kong strain during an outbreak of influenza due to the A-England-42-72 strain. Lancet 2:116–120, 1973.

224. Hoskins TW, Davies JR, Smith AJ, et al. Assessment of inactivated influenza-A vaccine after three outbreaks of influenza A at Christ's Hospital. Lancet 1:33–35, 1979.

225. Maeda T, Shintani Y, Miyamoto H, et al. Prophylactic effect of inactivated influenza vaccine on young children. Pediatr Int 44:43–46, 2002.

226. Hurwitz ES, Haber M, Chang A, et al. Studies of the 1996–1997 inactivated influenza vaccine among children attending day care: immunologic response, protection against infection, and clinical effectiveness. J Infect Dis 182:1218–1221, 2000.

227. Hoberman A, Greenberg DP, Paradise JI. Efficacy of inactivated influenza vaccine in preventing acute otitis media (AOM) in children. Presented at the Pediatric Academic Societies' annual meeting, 2002.

228. Clements DA, Langdon L, Bland C, Walter E. Influenza A vaccine decreases the incidence of otitis media in 6 to 30-month-old children in day care. Arch Pediatr Adolesc Med 149:1113–1117, 1995.

229. Heikkinen T, Ruuskanen O, Waris M, et al. Influenza vaccination in the prevention of acute otitis media in children. Am J Dis Child 145:445–448, 1991.

230. Sugaya N, Nerome K, Ishida M, et al. Efficacy of inactivated vaccine in preventing antigenically drifted influenza type A and well-matched type B. JAMA 272:1122–1126, 1994.

231. Smits AJ, Hak E, Stalman WA, et al. Clinical effectiveness of conventional influenza vaccination in asthmatic children. Epidemiol Infect 128:205–211, 2002.

232. Brokstad KA, Cox RJ, Olofsson J, et al. Parenteral influenza vaccination induces a rapid systemic and local immune response. J Infect Dis 171:198–203, 1995.

233. Gross PA, Russo C, Dran S, et al. Time to earliest peak serum antibody response to influenza vaccine in the elderly. Clin Diagn Lab Immunol 4:491–492, 1997.

234. Couch RB, Cate TR. Managing influenza in older patients. Geriatrics 38:61–64, 1983.

235. Strassburg MA, Greenland S, Sorvillo FJ, et al. Influenza in the elderly: report of an outbreak and a review of vaccine effectiveness reports. Vaccine 4:38–44, 1986.

236. Arroyo JC, Postic B, Brown A, et al. Influenza A/Philippines/2/82 outbreak in a nursing home: limitations of influenza vaccination in the aged. Am J Infect Control 12:329–334, 1984.

237. Foy HM, Cooney MK, McMahan R. A Hong Kong influenza immunity three years after immunization. JAMA 226:758–761, 1973.

238. Couch RB, Keitel WA, Cate TR, et al. Prevention of influenza virus infections by current inactivated influenza virus vaccines. In Brown LE, Hampson AW, Webster RG (eds). Options for the Control of Influenza III: Proceedings of the International Conference on Options for the Control of Influenza, Cairns, Australia, 1995. Amsterdam, Excerpta Medica, 1996, pp 97–106.

239. Schonberger LB, Bregman DJ, Sullivan-Bolyai JZ, et al. Guillain-Barré syndrome following vaccination in the National Influenza Immunization Program, United States, 1976–1977. Am J Epidemiol 110:105–123, 1979.

240. Ropper AH. The Guillain-Barré syndrome. N Engl J Med 326:1130–1136, 1992.

241. Willison HJ, Yuki N. Peripheral neuropathies and anti-glycolipid antibodies. Brain 125(pt 12):2591–2625, 2002.

242. Green DM. Advances in the management of Guillain-Barré syndrome. Curr Neurol Neurosci Rep 2:541–548, 2002.

243. Prevots DR, Sutter RW. Assessment of Guillain-Barré syndrome mortality and morbidity in the United States: implications for acute flaccid paralysis surveillance. J Infect Dis 175(suppl 1):S151–S155, 1997.

244. Kaplan JE, Katona P, Hurwitz ES, Schonberger LB. Guillain-Barré syndrome in the United States, 1979–1980 and 1980–1981: lack of an association with influenza vaccination. JAMA 248:698–700, 1982.

245. Hurwitz ES, Schonberger LB, Nelson DB, Holman RC. Guillain-Barré syndrome and the 1978–1979 influenza vaccine. N Engl J Med 304:1557–1561, 1981.

246. Lasky T, Terracciano GJ, Magder L, et al. The Guillain-Barré syndrome and the 1992–1993 and 1993–1994 influenza vaccines. N Engl J Med 339:1797–1802, 1998.

247. Centers for Disease Control and Prevention. Prevention and control of influenza: recommendations of the Advisory Committee on Immunization Practices (ACIP). MMWR 51(RR-3):12–13, 2002.

248. Bridges CB, Fukuda K, Uyeki TM, et al. Prevention and control of influenza: recommendations of the Advisory Committee on Immunization Practices (ACIP). MMWR 51(RR-3):1–31, 2002.

249. Barker WH, Mullooly JP. Impact of epidemic type A influenza in a defined adult population. Am J Epidemiol 112:798–811, 1980.

250. Neuzil KM, Wright PF, Mitchel EF, Griffin MR. The burden of influenza illness in children with asthma and other chronic medical conditions. J Pediatr 137:856–864, 2000.

251. Glezen WP, Decker M, Perrotta DM. Survey of underlying conditions of persons hospitalized with acute respiratory disease during influenza epidemics in Houston, 1978–1981. Am Rev Respir Dis 136:550–555, 1987.

252. Neuzil KM, Reed GW, Mitchel EF, et al. Impact of influenza on acute cardiopulmonary hospitalizations in pregnant women. Am J Epidemiol 148:1094–1102, 1998.

253. Izurieta HS, Thompson WW, Kramarz P, et al. Influenza and the rates of hospitalization for respiratory disease among infants and young children. N Engl J Med 342:232–239, 2000.

254. Neuzil KM, Mellen BG, Wright PF, et al. The effect of influenza on hospitalizations, outpatient visits, and courses of antibiotics in children. N Engl J Med 342:225–231, 2000.

255. Chiu SS, Lau YL, Chan KH, et al. Influenza-related hospitalizations among children in Hong Kong. N Engl J Med 347:2097–2103, 2002.

256. Fukuda K, O'Mara D, Singleton JA. How the delayed distribution of influenza vaccine created shortages in 2000 and 2001. P&T 27:235–242, 2002.

257. Centers for Disease Control and Prevention. Delayed supply of influenza vaccine and adjunct ACIP influenza vaccine recommendations for the 2000–2001 influenza season: Advisory Committee on Immunization Practices. MMWR 49:619–622, 2000.

258. Centers for Disease Control and Prevention. Delayed influenza vaccine availability for 2001–2002 season and supplemental recommendations of the Advisory Committee on Immunization Practices. MMWR 50:582–585, 2001.

259. Murphy KR, Strunk RC. Safe administration of influenza vaccine in asthmatic children hypersensitive to egg proteins. J Pediatr 106:931–933, 1985.

260. Audicana MT, Munoz D, del Pozo MD, et al. Allergic contact dermatitis from mercury antiseptics and derivatives: study protocol of tolerance to intramuscular injections of thimerosal. Am J Contact Dermat 13:3–9, 2002.

261. Sussman GL, Beezhold DH, Kurup VP. Allergens and natural rubber proteins. J Allergy Clin Immunol 110(2 suppl):S33–S39, 2002.

262. Freeman DW, Barno A. Deaths from Asian influenza associated with pregnancy. Am J Obstet Gynecol 78:1172–1175, 1959.

263. Harris JW. Influenza occurring in pregnant women: a statistical study of thirteen hundred and fifty cases. JAMA 72:978–980, 1919.

264. Widelock D, Csizmas L, Klein S. Influenza, pregnancy, and fetal outcome. Public Health Rep 78:1–11, 1963.

265. Hoffmann E, Krauss S, Perez D, et al. Eight-plasmid system for rapid generation of influenza virus vaccines. Vaccine 20:3165–3170, 2002.

266. Hoffmann E, Mahmood K, Yang CF, et al. Rescue of influenza B virus from eight plasmids. Proc Natl Acad Sci U S A 99:11411–11416, 2002.

267. Ulmer JB. Influenza DNA vaccines. Vaccine 20(suppl 2):S74–S76, 2002.

268. Gursel M, Verthelyi D, Gursel I, et al. Differential and competitive activation of human immune cells by distinct classes of CpG oligodeoxynucleotide. J Leukoc Biol 71:813–820, 2002.

269. Moldoveanu Z, Love-Homan L, Huang WQ, Krieg AM. CpG DNA, a novel immune enhancer for systemic and mucosal immunization with influenza virus. Vaccine 16:1216–1224, 1998.

270. Verthelyi D, Kenney RT, Seder RA, et al. CpG oligodeoxynucleotides as vaccine adjuvants in primates. J Immunol 168:1659–1663, 2002.

271. World Health Organization. Influenza vaccines. Wkly Epidemiol Rec 77:230–240, 2002.

272. Fedson DS. National immunization policies and vaccine distribution. In Nicholson KG, Webster RG, Hay AJ (eds). Textbook of Influenza. Oxford, Blackwell Science, 1998, pp 445–453.

273. Kramarz P, DeStefano F, Gargiullo PM, et al. Influenza vaccination in children with asthma in health maintenance organizations. Vaccine Safety Datalink Team. Vaccine 18:2288–2294, 2000.

274. Riddiough MA, Sisk JE, Bell JC. Influenza vaccination. JAMA 249:3189–3195, 1983.

275. Pickering LK (ed). 2000 Red Book: Report of the Committee on Infectious Diseases (25th ed). Elk Grove Village, IL, American Academy of Pediatrics, 2000.

Chapter 18

Influenza Vaccine—Live

ROBERT B. BELSHE • HUSEIN F. MAASSAB •
PAUL M. MENDELMAN

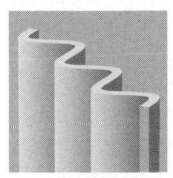

History

The human influenza viruses are members of the family Orthomyxoviridae and comprise three serologically distinct types: A, B, and C. Influenza A and B are the most significant pathogens in terms of morbidity and mortality and therefore are best studied. For example, the influenza A pandemic of 1918 to 1919 caused the deaths of an estimated 20 million people. Analysis of the extensive contemporary observations of that episode and efforts to explain it have been a dominant concern of students of respiratory disease and epidemiology ever since.[1] Modern knowledge of the causal agents of human influenza began in 1933 with the isolation in ferrets of a virus from patients with influenza.[2] In this study, it also was noted that sera of the convalescent patients contained neutralizing antibodies to the virus. The isolation of human virus was duplicated in 1934.[3] In 1940, a second etiologic type, type B influenza virus, was identified during the epidemic at that time and retrospectively associated with earlier episodes.[4,5] Both types A and B influenza have since been recognized in widespread outbreaks; however, only type A viruses have been associated with pandemics. Recent data support that the cause of the 1918 pandemic was a type A H_1N_1 virus.[6]

In view of the multiple types and subtypes and their relative independence in distribution, specific causation of waves and recurrences noted in descriptions of past epidemics and pandemics is uncertain. However, one point is clear: Effective prophylaxis is unquestionably desirable in view of the recurrent and enormously widespread disease caused by influenza viruses.

The conclusion that vaccine development for the control of influenza is desirable is based on observations that recovery from infection is accompanied by antibody development that confers resistance to reinfection and that circulating antibody levels similar to those observed in convalescent patients can be obtained by vaccination and presumably reflect an accompanying immunity. The use of trivalent inactivated influenza virus vaccine (TIV) in humans has been the subject of numerous studies, with an emphasis on providing an effective vaccine with minimal reactogenicity to all age groups. The results in field prophylaxis studies have been inconsistent, owing partly to transient protection related to the decline of vaccine-related homologous antibody and to constant changes in the two surface antigens of the virus. The use of vaccine for control of influenza has been shown to be effective when applied yearly to selected segments of the general population. The primary strategy for partial containment of influenza has been to concentrate efforts on prevention by vaccination of persons known to be at high risk. However, the variable efficacy of the killed vaccine, duration of effect, adverse reactions on parenteral administration, and failure to induce local or cellular immunity have stimulated research for alternative vaccination methods. An approach to immunization using live, attenuated virus has obvious merit, and the design and testing of vaccines attenuated by various methods that may be administered by an easy, natural route (e.g., nasal spray) are now being pursued. It is the purpose of this chapter to review the research that may lead to the licensing of an acceptable live, attenuated influenza virus vaccine of types A and B for use in humans.

Background

Why the Disease Is Important

Influenza is the most common cause of lower respiratory tract infections. It was estimated that, if one included all age groups, approximately 48 million cases of influenza occur in the United States each winter. However, this number varies depending on the susceptibility of the population to the virus and the infectiousness of the virus during an outbreak. Of the 48 million persons with influenza annually, approximately 3.9 million are hospitalized and 36,000

Contributors to this chapter in prior editions were Louise Herlocher, Marty Bryant, Michael Shaw, Carol Heilman, John LaMontagne, and Dan DeBorde.

die.[7] During major influenza epidemics in the United States, more than 40,000 influenza-associated deaths have occurred. In recent decades, more than 90% of the deaths attributed to influenza occurred among persons 65 years or older.[8] Influenza type A infection occurs most frequently and is responsible for the greatest amount of morbidity and mortality. Although influenza B has not caused a pandemic, it is responsible for regional epidemics that are less severe than influenza A epidemics.

Epidemic influenza tends to superimpose its profile on the existing pattern of respiratory disease, regardless of season. Influenza incidence rates vary with the nature of the epidemic virus strains and the population affected. Rates calculated from surveillance of individuals with upper respiratory illness suggest that influenza is responsible for roughly 10% to 20% of all respiratory illnesses per epidemic year,[9,10] with rates for influenza A being somewhat higher than those for influenza B. Nevertheless, an illness rate of 83% was observed in one epidemic season during an influenza B outbreak in an isolated Alaskan village.[11] Using the National Health Survey analysis of 101 million medically attended respiratory illnesses for 1977 to 1978, it has been estimated that 20 million cases could be attributed to influenza.[12] Most studies have found infection rates in preschool- and school-age children to be much higher than in adults, particularly during influenza B epidemics.[9,10,13,14] Consequently, families with school-age or younger children suffer disproportionately from influenza[12,13] as the result of frequent primary introduction from family members younger than 20 years of age.[13,15] These findings are consistent with the concepts that influenza is most likely to infect individuals with the least prior immunity and that children are a common source of influenza in the community.

Clinical Description

Influenza viruses are spread from person to person primarily through the coughing and sneezing of infected persons. The incubation period for influenza is 1 to 4 days, with an average of 2 days.[16] Adults and children typically are infectious from the day before symptoms begin until approximately 5 days after illness onset. Children can be infectious for a longer period, and very young children can shed virus for up to 6 days before their illness onset. Severely immunocompromised persons can shed virus for weeks.

Uncomplicated influenza illness is characterized by the abrupt onset of constitutional and respiratory signs and symptoms (e.g., fever, myalgia, headache, severe malaise, nonproductive cough, sore throat, and rhinitis). Respiratory illness caused by influenza is difficult to distinguish from illness caused by other respiratory pathogens on the basis of symptoms alone. Reported sensitivities and specificities of clinical definitions for influenza-like illness that include fever and cough have ranged from 63% to 78% and 55% to 71%, respectively, compared with viral culture. Sensitivity and predictive value of clinical definitions can vary, depending on the degree of co-circulation of other respiratory pathogens and the level of influenza activity.

Influenza illness typically resolves after a limited number of days for the majority of persons, although cough and malaise can persist for more than 2 weeks. Among certain persons, influenza can exacerbate underlying medical conditions (e.g., pulmonary or cardiac disease), lead to secondary bacterial pneumonia or primary influenza viral pneumonia, or occur as part of a co-infection with other viral or bacterial pathogens. Influenza infection also has been associated with encephalopathy, transverse myelitis, Reye's syndrome, myositis, myocarditis, and pericarditis.

Virology

Because of the complexity of the subject, it is beyond the scope of this chapter to address all aspects of influenza virology. Therefore, this section presents a simple review emphasizing those areas relevant to live virus vaccines. For a comprehensive review of the biology of influenza viruses, the reader is directed to another text.[17]

Orthomyxoviruses have segmented, single-stranded, negative-sense RNA genomes. Because they lack the proof-reading enzymes that maintain the fidelity of DNA replication, influenza viruses are subject to high rates of mutation during replication of their single-stranded RNA genome[18,19] and to high-frequency gene reassortment during mixed infections because of their segmented genome.[20,21] Because of these factors, influenza viruses undergo continual genetic changes that may affect their growth in vitro and in vivo, their pathogenicity in humans and animals, and the epidemiology of the resultant disease.[19] New antigenic changes, occurring by one or both of these mechanisms, allow the virus to overcome existing immunity in previously infected hosts.

Plaquing systems developed for influenza virus[22] and later modified by the addition of trypsin in the overlay medium[23] have allowed the determination of reassortment, reversion, and reactivation rates. Plaquing provided a cloning system for influenza virus, enabling the isolation of temperature-sensitive (ts) mutants.[24,25] These conditional lethal mutants, most of which varied from the parent by only a single mutational step, were used to map the influenza genome and dissect the viral replication cycle.[26] Biophysical analyses such as polyacrylamide gel electrophoresis were used to identify the genes having these mutations.[27,28] Similar analyses were performed using reassortants made between strains of influenza viruses showing clear differences in the electrophoretic mobility of their RNA genome segments.[29–33] The ability to clone specific mutants, organize them into complementation groups, and then correlate these groupings with phenotype and the RNA segment containing the mutation has allowed researchers to map the influenza virus genome, assigning each RNA segment to the encoded proteins and functions[34] (Table 18–1).

More recent investigations have examined influenza virus using a variety of molecular biology techniques: monoclonal antibodies,[35–38] cloning of isolated genes and expression of the encoded proteins,[39] sequence analyses of cloned gene segments or direct sequencing of the virion RNA[40,41] or sequencing using polymerase chain reaction techniques, and transfection of specifically modified genes.[42–46]

The mechanisms of antigenic drift and shift have been examined,[46] and the structure and function of the surface hemagglutinin (HA) and neuraminidase (NA) molecules and their antigenic and reactive sites have been eluci-

TABLE 18–1 ■ Products of Influenza A and B Virus Genes

RNA	Gene Products	Functions
1	PB2	Viral polymerase component involved in synthesis of capped messenger RNAs (mRNAs) and endonuclease, which cleaves host cell mRNA
2	PB1	Viral polymerase component with RNA transcription and replication activities
	PB-1 F2*	Viral protein generated from an alternate reading frame, triggers cell apoptosis
3	PA	Viral polymerase component involved in RNA replication
4	HA	Virion surface attachment and fusion glycoprotein, major antigenic determinant
5	NP	Major nucleocapsid structural component and type-specific antigen
6	NA	Virion surface glycoprotein with receptor-destroying enzyme activity, major antigenic determinant
	NB	Glycoprotein membrane ion channel found only in type B
7	M1	Membrane matrix protein and type-specific antigen
	M2	Nonglycosylated membrane ion channel, found only in type A
8	NS1	Nonstructural protein—unique post-transcriptional regulator that inhibits the nuclear transport of poly(A)–containing mRNAs and inhibits pre-mRNA splicing by binding to a specific region of U6 small nuclear RNA
	NS2	Cellular and virion protein of unknown function

*Recently described by Chen et al.[34]

dated.[46–49] Genes other than HA and NA also have been shown to change by the mechanisms similar to those responsible for antigenic shift and drift,[46] and sequence data have been compiled, allowing viral evolution and the rate of change of individual genes to be determined.[46,50–52]

Methods of Attenuation

The segmented and single-stranded RNA genome of influenza virus has a direct and immediate impact on its antigenicity, epidemiology, and hence the manner in which this virus may be controlled. Influenza A viruses exhibit both antigenic drift[53] and antigenic shift,[46] whereas influenza B viruses show only antigenic drift.[54] Antigenic drift is caused by the individual mutational changes in nucleotide sequence that occur because of the infidelity inherent in the replication of RNA genomes, with advantageous mutations becoming "fixed" in genomes of the replicating population. Although not subject to antigenic mediation, other genes also undergo this same mutational drift.[54] The rate of drift can vary among genes and viral types.[49,55–57] Antigenic shift, however, requires complete replacement of one or both of the surface glycoprotein genes. The accepted explanation is that these new genes are acquired through reassortment between human and animal influenza A viruses.[49] Burnet and Bull[58] suggested that attenuated live influenza virus suitable for vaccines might be produced by egg passage of the virus because of its inherent genetic instability. Thus, early on, investigators took advantage of the high mutation rate by passing the virus in nonhuman hosts, generating host-range (hr) mutant viruses for use as live virus vaccine candidates. Vaccines made by this method have not been shown to be reliably attenuated[59] and could result in disease. Attempts to further attenuate hr viruses in the presence of heated guinea pig serum produced a vaccine strain that was clinically safe in adults[60,61] but caused fever in children.[62] Thus hr viruses have been abandoned as potential vaccine candidates.

The high rate of genetic reassortment in orthomyxoviruses can be employed to quickly generate vaccine strains containing the genes for the surface antigens (HA and NA) of newly emergent wild-type (wt) viruses, while retaining other genes from attenuated strains.[63] Attenuated master strains must be shown to not cause significant illness in humans and to pass the property on to reassortants through the donation of genes other than the HA and NA genes.

Attenuated master strains have been made by several methods. They can be separated into three main classes: hr, ts, and cold-adapted (ca) mutants. Those master strains that have been used to generate live influenza reassortant vaccines for trials in humans are listed in Table 18–2.[61,64–95]

Although hr mutants were abandoned as vaccine candidates, they have been used as master attenuated strains in reassortant vaccines. Live reassortant vaccines made using A/Puerto Rico/8/34 (H_1N_1) (PR8) as the attenuating master strain have proved unsatisfactory because the six nonsurface antigen genes of PR8 did not reliably confer attenuation in combination with some wt surface genes. There was no simple means of determining which reassortants were attenuated and which were not.[64] Similar problems were noted

TABLE 18–2 ■ Influenza A Master Strains Used in the Preparation of Live Reassortant Virus Vaccines

Master Strain	Currently in Use	References
hr Mutants		
A/Puerto Rico/8/34 (H_1N_1)	No	61,64–72
A/Okuda/57/ (H_2N_2)	No	73
A/Mallard/6750/78 (H_2N_2)	No	73–77
A/Mallard/Alberta/88/76 (H_3N_8)	No	74–76, 78–81
ts Mutants		
ts 1[E]	No	82
ts1A2	No	67
ca Mutants		
A/Ann Arbor/6/60 (H_2N_2)	Yes	68, 83–85
B/Ann Arbor/1/66	Yes	86–91
A/Leningrad/134/17/57	Yes	88, 92–95
A/Leningrad/134/47/57	Yes	89, 91

with the A/Okuda/57 (H_2N_2) virus, which had had 280 passages in eggs and had been used in Japan.[65]

Ts master strains were generated by reassortment between A/Hong Kong/68 (H_3N_2) wt virus and ts mutants of A/Great Lakes/389/65 (H_2N_2) virus that had been grown in the presence of 5-fluorouracil.[66,67,69,82] Although several were shown to be attenuated in adults and children, some ts mutants reverted to virulence after passage in humans. Ts mutants have been abandoned because of this genetic instability.[96]

Cold adaptation has become the major means of generating live virus vaccines in master attenuated viruses.[97] Several methods have been used for cold-adapting influenza A virus. A/Ann Arbor/6/60 (H_2N_2) (A/AA/6/60) virus has been grown at successively lowered temperatures in primary chick kidney cells until a virus has been derived that grows as well at 25°C as it does at 33°C. All three polymerase genes have been shown to contribute to the attenuated phenotype of the ca A/AA/6/60 master strain.[98] The A/AA/6/60 virus derived in this manner has been shown to be both ca and ts. Ca implies that the virus will grow well at a reduced temperature (25°C) compared to permissive temperature (33°C), and ts implies that the vaccine virus replication is reduced by at least 2 logs of the median tissue culture infective dose ($TCID_{50}$) at the higher temperature 39°C. In addition, owing to the serial passages in primary chick kidney (PCK) cells and embryonated eggs, the master strain may well contain hr mutations. Although few sequence differences have been found between the ca A/AA/6/60 virus and its wt progenitor,[83] sequencing evidence has been found for changes in all eight genes of the attenuated ca A/AA/6/60 virus from its virulent wt counterpart.[24] Recently, Lu et al.[98a] used reverse genetics to identify the four major attenuating loci of the ca A/AA/6/60 ca strain. They are at base positions 1195 and 1766 of the PB1 gene, 821 of the PB2 gene, and 146 of the NP gene. There have been numerous human trials with reassortants made using ca A/AA/6/60 virus, and, in all cases, attenuation, antigenicity, and genetic stability have remained unaltered and consistent.[86] Similar procedures have been used for influenza B viruses,[87] and vaccine lines using ca B/Ann Arbor/1/66 (B/AA/1/66) virus as a master strain are being produced and evaluated.[88,89] The PA gene has been shown to be a major determinant of attenuation for the ca B/AA/1/66 vaccine strain.[99]

A ca master strain has also been used in Russia. Unlike the aforementioned ca A/AA/6/60 virus, the Russian master strain, A/Leningrad/134/57 virus, was produced by multiple passages primarily at 25° or 26°C and not by a gradual lowering of incubation temperatures. The original ca master strain A/Leningrad/134/17/57[92,100,101] was passaged an additional 30 times in embryonated eggs at 25°C to generate a new ca master strain, A/Leningrad/134/47/57 virus.[93] Reassortants made between this latter ca master strain and wt A/Leningrad/322/79 (H_1N_1) or A/Bangkok/1/79 (H_3N_2) virus were shown to be attenuated and immunogenic in children.[94] The A/Leningrad/134/47/57 master strain has been shown to contain changes in at least one of the polymerase genes as well as in the HA, NA, nucleocapsid protein (NP), and matrix (M) genes.[102] A/Aichi/2/68 virus has been adapted to growth at 25°C in a manner similar to that used for the Russian master strain, but with fewer passages.[97] This virus has been tested in both ferrets and human volunteers and is also immunogenic and attenuated.[103–105]

New techniques, such as recombinant DNA cloning and the transfection of in vitro mutagenized gene segments, are providing new possibilities for the production of live virus vaccines. Deletions also may be generated through site-specific mutagenesis in recombinant complimentary DNA (cDNA) clones. The ability to introduce RNA transcripts of specifically mutagenized cDNA clones into the influenza viruses as stable parts of the genome has opened new areas of research into vaccine development.[43,44] In addition, new techniques allow the rescue of virus via introduction of DNA plasmids into cells; in this case, no RNA transcripts are transfected. It is now possible to conceive of influenza vaccines genetically engineered for specific purposes.[106]

Pathogenesis as It Relates to Prevention

The pathology of influenza virus has been reviewed extensively.[107–110] The virus contacts the mucous lining of the respiratory tract and then attaches to ciliated columnar epithelial cells after release from the mucous layer.[110,111] The viral NA is probably involved in its release from mucous receptors and the liquefaction of the mucous layer. The ciliated columnar epithelial cell is most likely the major site of infection.[111] Bronchitis and tracheitis are common,[112] and there may be some lung involvement.[113] Otitis media is common in children. Viremia has been reported only sporadically[114,115] amidst numerous negative reports.[116–118] Influenza B demonstrates pathology similar to that of type A and is common in children.

Cleavage of the HA precursor protein into HA1 and HA2 proteins by post-translational processing is necessary for the glycoprotein to become membrane fusion competent.[119,120] Neuraminidase activity is often complementary to HA receptor specificity, allowing the two to act in concert.[121]

Influenza in humans is usually restricted to infection primarily of the trachea and upper respiratory tract, although, during severe pandemic periods, lung lesions may be present.[122] The amount of virus produced probably determines the extent and severity of symptoms.[96,123]

The most precise diagnosis of influenza is obtained by viral isolation in embryonated eggs or in cell cultures of nasopharyngeal or tracheal aspirates, or by using reverse transcriptase–polymerase chain reaction. Serologic diagnosis can be made by demonstrating fourfold rises in hemagglutinin-inhibiting (HAI) or complement-fixing antibodies.

The pattern of influenza infection is generally one of high morbidity and low mortality, although outbreaks also are reflected in excess mortality from subsequent pneumonia and hence an increase of total mortality. An epidemic may be defined by both serology and virus isolation to determine the dates of incidence and prevalence[12] and the impact of health on families and communities.[9,124]

By using excess mortality and morbidity resulting from influenza as an index, Collins[125] compiled an impressive record of influenza-associated mortality extending from 1887 through 1956. Over the period analyzed, the intervals between outbreaks and the sites affected varied greatly: After a decade of relative quiescence, the pandemic of 1889 to 1890 erupted violently and unexpectedly. The death toll between 1891 and 1892 was even greater, and high, sharp peaks of excess mortality recurred through 1908. Afterward, the disease was apparently much less virulent until the catastrophic pandemic of 1918 to 1920, in which over 20 million lives were lost worldwide. Subsequently, moderate to severe outbreaks have been amply documented.[123,126] Improved surveillance of influenza has been used as an accurate indicator and a valuable predictor of epidemic activity.[127]

Immunity Induced by Natural Infection

Naturally acquired immunity to influenza is mediated by serum antibodies and by antibodies present at the mucosal surface of the respiratory tract. In addition to serum and mucosal antibodies, natural infection with influenza also stimulates influenza-specific T cells that are thought to play a role in recovery. Other innate immune responses also may contribute to resistance to influenza infection, such as production of interferon or other antiviral factors by macrophages. Thus it appears that multiple mechanisms have evolved in humans to provide resistance to influenza.[128]

Immunity following natural infection provides long-lived protection against homologous influenza virus infection and disease in the absence of antigenic shift or drift. This effect was illustrated during the 1977 influenza season when H_1N_1 re-emerged after a 20-year absence. Epidemiologic surveys revealed that, compared to individuals born *after* 1955, individuals born *before* 1955 had a lower influenza attack rate in 1977. This is presumed to be due to prior exposure to nearly identical H_1N_1 strains in the 1950s. Immunity acquired by natural infection also can provide protection against influenza strains that have undergone antigenic drift. In British boarding school studies, protection provided by natural infection was compared with protection achieved by vaccination with inactivated influenza vaccine. The authors concluded that natural immunity afforded heterotypic protection against drifted strains that circulated 18 months later, whereas inactivated influenza vaccine did not.[129,130] These studies demonstrated that, although both natural infection and vaccination with inactivated vaccine stimulate serum HAI antibodies and provide protection against homologous wild-type influenza strains, the protection associated with natural infection is longer lived and broader than that induced by inactivated vaccine. Importantly, the fact that the differences in protection could not be accounted for by differences in serum HAI titers demonstrates that multiple immune mechanisms induced by natural infection confer resistance to influenza.

Immunity as It Relates to Vaccine Prevention

In order to prove that the influenza vaccines are effective, it is necessary to vaccinate a population prior to an influenza epidemic and compare the infection rates in vaccinated subjects with a group given a placebo. Case definitions of influenza vary according to study and may include culture-positive infection,[131,132] further fourfold antibody increase during the influenza epidemic, or clinical observations of influenza-like illnesses.[133] Specific point estimates of vaccine efficacy may be obtained by using culture-positive identification of cases, which eliminates clinical syndromes caused by other intercurrent viral infections. Efficacy field trials with culture-positive endpoints are optimally conducted in young children.[131,132] This population suffers a high attack rate of influenza, and, when young children are infected with influenza, they shed high quantities of wild-type virus for several days. This makes culture methodology a sensitive and specific case-finding method. Adult efficacy trials more commonly are conducted using clinical endpoints such as febrile respiratory illness.[133] Influenza is the most common cause of febrile respiratory illness in adults, and using cultures to identify influenza infection is problematic because adults may shed virus in low quantity and for brief duration. Use of fourfold antibody rise paired sera obtained pre- and postepidemic is also often used in adult studies, with case definition being any subject with a further fourfold antibody rise in response to the epidemic virus. However, the vaccine-induced serum antibodies interfere with detection of further fourfold increases. Subjects with vaccine-induced antibody may not produce sufficient antibody during the subsequent natural infection to result in a detectable, fourfold antibody increase. Therefore, this definition has inherent bias, unlike either the clinical endpoint for adult studies described above or the virus isolation endpoint for the pediatric efficacy trials as noted above.

Vaccine effectiveness and vaccine efficacy may be confused. In this chapter we refer to vaccine efficacy (*ve*) as the specific reduction in attack rates of laboratory-confirmed influenza (culture-positive cases), and *ve* is represented mathematically as

$$ve = (1 - Rv/Rp) \times 100\%$$

where Rv = attack rate in vaccinees and Rp = attack rate in placebo recipients. Vaccine effectiveness refers to the reduction in clinical events that may be expected to be associated with influenza, but could also be caused by other agents. Reduction of fever during the influenza season in all vaccinees compared to all placebo recipients, regardless of the culture result, is an example of vaccine effectiveness.[131–134]

History and Development of Cold-Adapted Intranasal Live, Attenuated Vaccine

The *ca* and *ts* A/AA/6/60 virus was derived in PCK cells from a virus originally isolated from an ill child and that was shown to produce clinical symptoms in ferrets. This virus was adapted to growth at 25°C, and a clone was selected by seven serial plaque-to-plaque purifications. This clone met the following criteria: high and equivalent virus yield in PCK cells and eggs at 33°C and 25°C, retention of *ca* and *ts* (reduction in replication titer at 39°C) markers in tissue culture, and attenuated behavior in ferrets. The *ca* B/AA/1/66 master strain was developed in the same manner, although it took fewer intermediate passages to achieve the final *ca* variant for type B virus than for type A.[87] The *wt* B/AA/1/66 influenza virus was restricted for growth at 36°C at the time of isolation, and therefore the *ts* phenotype is defined by a reduction in replication titer at 37°C compared with the achievable titer at 25°/33°C.[87]

Strategy and Advantages of the *ca* Reassortant Vaccines

Cold adaptation was found to be a reliable and efficient procedure for the derivation of live, attenuated influenza virus vaccines for humans. In addition, the process of genetic reassortment with the transfer of the six internal genes from a stable attenuated *ca* master donor strain of type A (A/AA/6/60) or type B (B/AA/1/66) to the new prevailing wild-type epidemic strain has yielded consistently attenuated cold-reassortant vaccines with the desired 6:2 gene profile for human use. These live *ca* reassortant vaccines for types A and B influenza viruses, developed at the University of Michigan, have been shown to have the proper level of attenuation and immunogenicity, and low or absent transmissibility combined with proven genetic stability, and are produced in acceptable tissue culture substrates or specific pathogen-free chicken eggs.[97]

Figure 18–1 presents the classical co-infection of the master donor viruses with wild-type influenza to develop a 6:2 reassortant vaccine strain.

Characteristics of CAIV-T

Influenza Virus Vaccine, Trivalent, types A and B, Live Cold-Adapted (CAIV-T) consists of approximately 10^7 $TCID_{50}$/dose of each influenza A/H_1N_1, influenza A/H_3N_2, and influenza B vaccine strain. The exact strains are updated each year to antigenically match the antigens recommended by national health authorities. CAIV-T is sprayed into the nose using a simple syringe-like device

that delivers a 0.25-mL volume of a large-particle aerosol into each nostril for a total volume of 0.5 mL (Fig. 18–2). To vaccinate children requires minimal cooperation to allow spraying the vaccine intranasally. The device is easy to use, and the vaccine is readily accepted and preferable to many over a parenteral injection by needle and syringe. The vaccine is produced in specific pathogen-free embryonated hen's eggs, contains egg allantoic fluid and sucrose-phosphate-glutamate stabilizer, and should not be given to persons with egg allergy. CAIV-T is free of preservatives.

Results of Vaccination

Immunogenicity of CAIV-T

Immunogenicity in Children

Following a single vaccination with CAIV-T of 10^4, 10^5, 10^6, or 10^7 $TCID_{50}$, serum HAI data indicated that increasing dosages of CAIV-T resulted in a higher percentage of children who seroconverted or developed a fourfold rise in HAI antibody titer following vaccination.[135] The dose-response effect was most apparent in seronegative subjects; 31%, 71%, and 91% of seronegative children seroconverted to H_3N_2 after 10^4, 10^5, or 10^6 $TCID_{50}$ of CAIV-T, respectively. Among seronegative children, a single dosage of 10^6 or 10^7 $TCID_{50}$ elicited 91% (40 of 44) seroconversion to the H_3N_2 strain, and 86% of vaccine recipients (38 of 44) developed a serum HAI titer of 1:32 or greater (data on file, MedImmune Vaccines, Inc.). Forty-eight percent of seronegative children (26 of 54) seroconverted to the B strain after doses of 10^6 or 10^7, and 19% (10 of 54) developed a serum HAI titer greater than 1:32 after a single dose of vaccine. Based on serum HAI results as the immunologic marker, the H_1N_1 strain was less immunogenic than the other strains after a single dose. This phenomenon may be due to viral competition or interference from the H_3N_2 and B viruses. Nevertheless, this phenomenon was observed only after the first dose in young children and is easily overcome with use of a second dose. Administration of two doses of CAIV-T separated by 60 ± 14 days induced fourfold or greater HAI titers in 96%, 96%, and 62% of children against H_3N_2, B, and H_1N_1, respectively.[131] Two doses of CAIV-T given a mean of 35 days apart (range, 28 to 60 days) containing the type A/Shenzhen H_1N_1 strain elicited a fourfold or greater rise in serum HAI response in 87% of seronegative children.[136] In this regard, it is much like using two doses of TIV as the primary vaccine in young children to develop an optimal antibody response, followed by a single annual revaccination in subsequent years.

Immunogenicity in Adults

A single-dose regimen in adults is supported by epidemiologic data indicating that the majority of adults are likely to be immunologically primed to influenza strains that have circulated in recent years and therefore should require only a single dose of vaccine to stimulate a protective immune response to current drift strains. The immunogenicity and efficacy results obtained in adults support that one dose of CAIV-T in adults conferred a high level of protection against laboratory-documented influenza illness due to

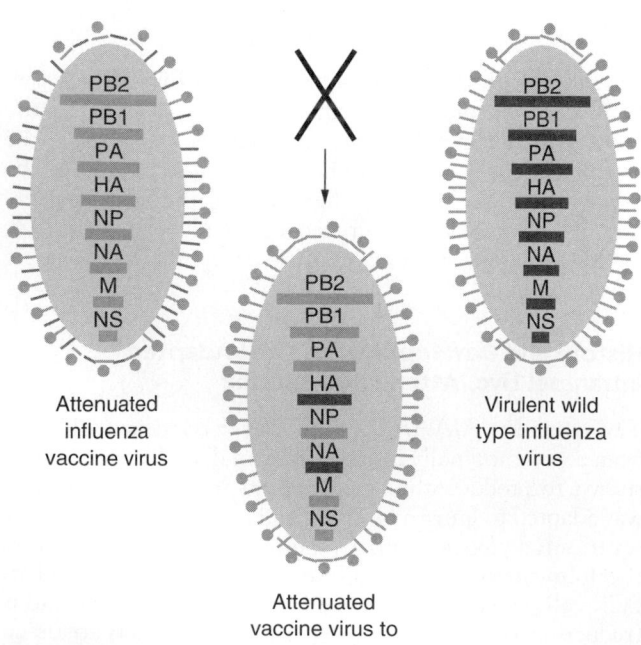

Attenuated influenza vaccine virus

Attenuated vaccine virus to new virus type

Virulent wild type influenza virus

FIGURE 18–1 ■ Diagram illustrating the process of genetic reassortment to generate vaccine strains. The cold-adapted master strain (*upper left*) is mated in tissue culture with a wild-type virus (*upper right*). Reassortant virus with the desired combination of attenuating genes (six "internal" genes) and contemporary HA and NA genes is selected for use in the vaccine. HA and NA genes are updated annually to exactly match those in the inactivated vaccine.

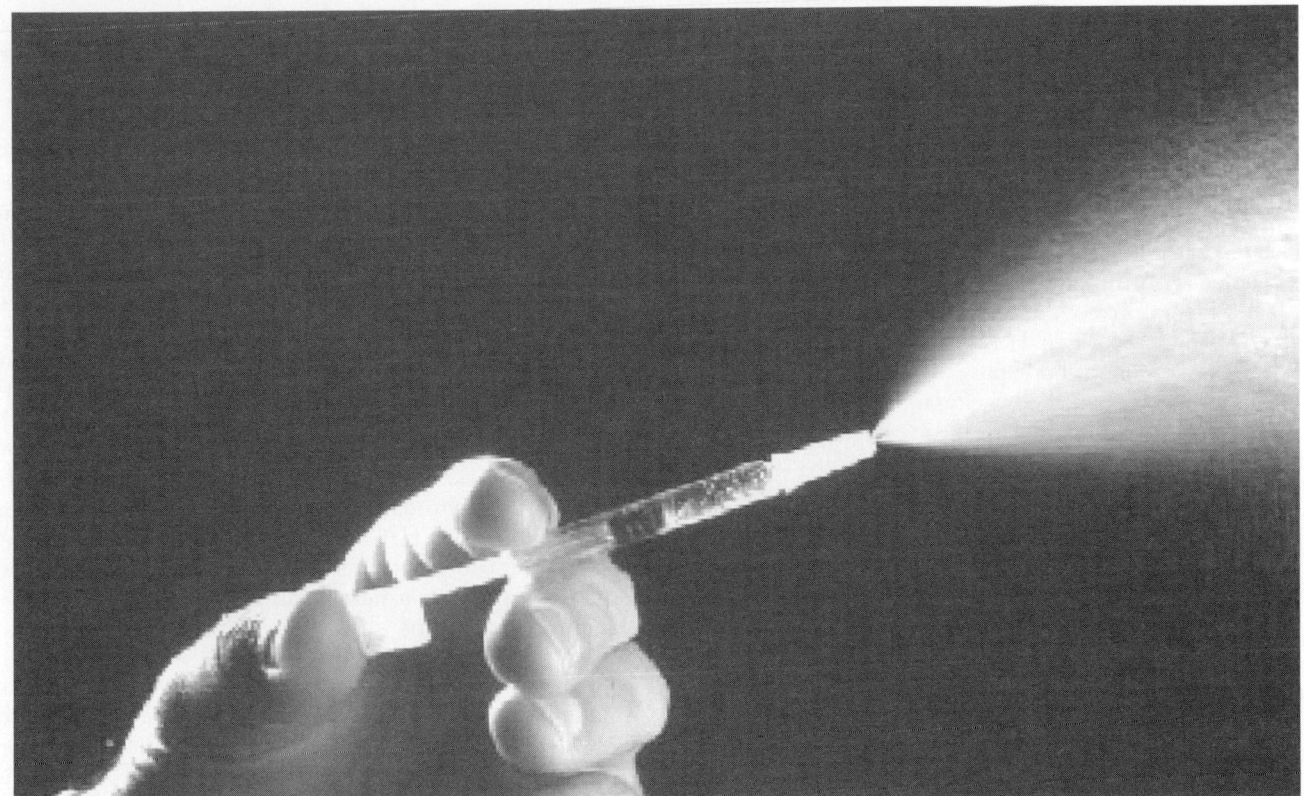

FIGURE 18–2 ■ Transilluminated illustration of large-particle aerosol generated for intranasal administration. The tip of the applicator is inserted into the anterior nares and the plunger depressed to administer the live, attenuated vaccine to a nostril. Removing the flange on the plunger allows a second spray to be administered into the other nostril.

wild-type H_1N_1, H_3N_2, or B strains, even though only a modest proportion of subjects developed a serum HAI titer of 1:32 or greater following vaccination.[137] These results suggested that a serum HAI titer of 1:32 or greater is not a strong correlate of protection for adults following immunization with CAIV-T. The results support that other important immunologic contributors to protection following immunization with CAIV-T, such as nasal immunoglobulin A (IgA) antibodies, could provide protection in the absence of a robust serum HAI response.[138,139] The mechanism(s) whereby vaccination with CAIV-T provides protection against influenza appear to mimic that of natural infection and to differ from that of TIV. TIV is believed to induce little secretory IgA and is not expected to stimulate $CD8^+$ cytotoxic T cells; this assertion is supported by previous studies in which adults immunized with either monovalent cold-adapted influenza virus vaccine (CAIV) or TIV were protected from challenge, although they had developed different serum HAI antibody and nasal IgA response profiles following vaccination.[140]

Correlates of Immune Protection Induced by CAIV-T

Many studies have characterized the immune response to cold-adapted influenza vaccines derived from the Maassab cold-adapted master strains that are used to produce CAIV-T. Because CAIV-T is a live, attenuated vaccine that is administered by the natural intranasal route of infection, the resulting immune response is expected to elicit the multiple immune mechanisms induced by natural infection with wild-type influenza viruses. Previous clinical studies have documented that influenza-specific IgA nasal antibodies, serum antibodies, T-cell responses, and interferon are produced in response to intranasal immunization with CAIV.[140,141]

Challenge studies with vaccine strains in children[139] or wild-type influenza in adults have elucidated some correlates of protection. Both serum and nasal wash antibodies in children and adults induced following immunization with CAIV-T are associated with protection from infection.[139] A high rate of serum HAI responses following immunization with CAIV-T predicts a high rate of protection against influenza in children.[131,132,134,139] Other important contributors to immunity, such as serum neutralizing antibodies, nasal IgA antibodies, or cytotoxic T cells, may provide protection.[139,142]

In order to evaluate the efficacy against H_1N_1 and also to obtain potential correlates of immune protection, children vaccinated previously with CAIV-T participated in a challenge study using H_1N_1 monovalent vaccine as the challenge virus. The endpoint was shedding of vaccine virus; despite the 5- to 8-month interval between vaccination and challenge, vaccine provided high efficacy (83%; 95% confidence interval, 60% to 93%) against shedding of type A/H_1N_1 challenge virus. Both serum antibody and nasal wash antibody were measured before H_1N_1 challenge, and there were significant differences in serum HAI antibody and nasal wash IgA antibody between the prior vaccinated children and the prior placebo subjects prior to challenge. Previously vaccinated subjects had significantly higher nasal wash and serum antibody titers. The presence of any serum antibody or nasal wash IgA significantly correlated with protection from viral shedding.[139]

Most studies of correlates of immune protection against influenza have focused on serum HAI antibody.[143–146] The results of these studies generally agree in that serum HAI is correlated with protection, but protective levels of antibody have varied with the prevalent virus subtype, specific assay used, and laboratory conducting the assay. Most of the studies were conducted when H_3N_2 viruses were present, and protective levels of antibody have varied from 1:20 to 1:80, with higher levels of antibody being more protective against H_3N_2.[138,142–146] The few studies on the correlates of immune protection against influenza A/H_1N_1 or influenza B have found that low levels of serum HAI antibody are correlated with protection against these viruses. In adults, a 1:10 HAI antibody titer correlated with protection against influenza B in one study[144] and 1:20 in another,[146] but the 1:20 HAI antibody titer did not protect children.[146] Another study found that a 1:64 HAI titer against B was protective in adults the following year.[145] Protection against H_1N_1 virus infection was given by a 1:20 HAI antibody titer in children, and any antibody titer protected adults.[146] A 1:32 HAI antibody titer is commonly said to be protective.[144] The multiple studies of serum HAI antibody indicate that clearly HAI antibody level does correlate with protection, but significant room for discussion is present on the absolute amount needed to confer protection. The above data suggest that H_3N_2 levels may need to be higher than HAI antibody to H_1N_1 or B; also the presence of nasal IgA with or without serum HAI antibody confounds analysis of correlates of protection. Clements et al. compared the correlates of immune protection induced by live, attenuated intranasal vaccine with inactivated parenteral vaccine after experimental challenge with wild-type influenza in adults.[147] A series of studies in which healthy adult volunteers were vaccinated with either inactivated or intranasal live, attenuated vaccines, followed by challenge with wild-type H_1N_1 or H_3N_2 viruses, revealed that serum HAI antibody titer correlated with protection against viral replication after inactivated vaccine (mean HAI titer, 6.4 log_2) but not live vaccine (mean HAI titer, 1.6 log_2); in contrast, live vaccine induced nasal IgA antibody (mean nasal wash IgA anti-HA titer, 6.9 log_2), which correlated with protection.[147]

Interference Between Strains

Interference between strains of closely related viruses during vaccination is a well-recognized phenomenon. Oral polio vaccine is the classical example cited because type 2 tends to overgrow types 1 or 3 after dose 1; multiple doses are given to overcome this interference. Multiple doses of oral rotavirus vaccine also have been given to ensure more solid immunity. Although the multivalent viral vaccine for measles, mumps, and rubella (M-M-R®) is immunogenic after a single dose, two doses are recommended to provide optimal protection. Interference between type A influenza H_1N_1 and H_3N_2 was previously identified.[148] A two-dose strategy as the primary regimen for influenza vaccination in young children optimizes a seroprotective response and

successfully overcomes interference if it occurs.[131,136] Subsequent annual revaccination requires only a single dose.

Heterotypic Antibody Data

One of the potential advantages of a live influenza vaccine is that it might be expected to stimulate broader immunity against antigenic drift strains, as demonstrated in young children. The basis for this expectation is that a live, replicating vaccine virus would present to the immune system a complete complement of influenza virus antigens in their native configurations. As a result, neutralizing antibodies would be produced to both surface proteins, HA and NA, and stimulate secretory antibodies in the respiratory tract as well as serum antibodies. In addition, highly conserved antigens such as M and NP may be presented in an immunologic context appropriate for stimulation of cross-reactive cytotoxic T cells and antibodies. Immune responses to native HA and NA antigens as well as internal proteins probably account for the observation that natural infection with a new strain induces some protection against drift strains that arise during the subsequent influenza seasons.

At least four field efficacy trials have demonstrated that immunization with CAIV can protect against antigenically drifted influenza strains, in addition to providing protection against homologous influenza strains.[132,133,140,149] In the more recent pivotal efficacy field trial of CAIV-T in children, the drifted variant A/Sydney/ (a H_3N_2 virus) caused the majority of disease in year 2 of the study.[132] CAIV-T contained A/Wuhan as its H_3N_2 antigen; Wuhan and Sydney were significantly different antigenically as determined by ferret antisera. CAIV-T was 86% efficacious at preventing culture-confirmed influenza from A/Sydney. In that same year an effectiveness study of CAIV-T in adults demonstrated significant reduction in work lost among vaccinated adults versus placebo recipients.[133]

The weight of evidence is that both natural infection[132] and immunization with CAIV[132,133,140,149] can provide protection against drifted strains. This remains an advantage of a live influenza vaccine because drift strains might arise unexpectedly in some seasons. To address the issue of whether CAIV-T stimulated immunity that was cross-reactive with antigenic drift strains, serum specimens obtained during the 1996 to 1997 pivotal efficacy trial were tested in the laboratory in HAI assays against a variety of H_3N_2 drift strains isolated during influenza seasons immediately preceding or following the 1996 to 1997 efficacy trial. Antigenic characterization performed with strain-specific ferret antiserum by the Centers for Disease Control and Prevention indicated that the strains included in the analysis were antigenic variants representative of the spectrum of H_3N_2 strains circulating during recent influenza seasons. The A/Sydney/5/97 (H_3N_2) strain was of particular interest because it was the predominant H_3N_2 strain circulating during the 1997 to 1998 influenza season and had undergone significant antigenic drift from the H_3N_2 vaccine strain A/Wuhan/359/95. Results of the analysis (Fig. 18–3) indicated that children vaccinated with CAIV-T developed serum HAI antibodies that cross-reacted with H_3N_2 strains that circulated either before or after the Wuhan strain. Specifically, following two doses of CAIV-T,

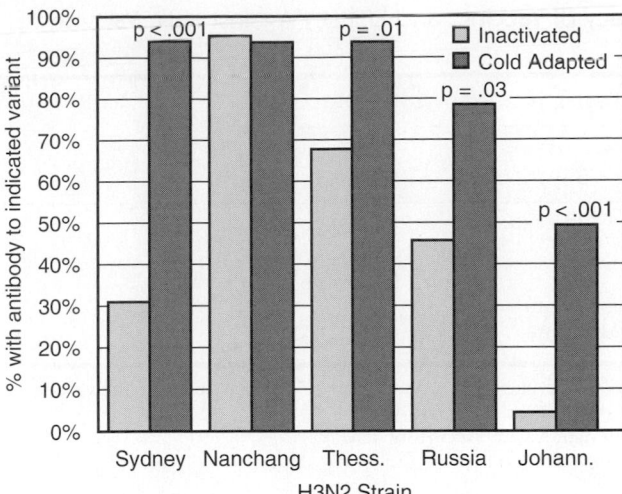

FIGURE 18–3 ■ Percentage of children given two doses of live, attenuated influenza vaccine (*dark bars*) or two doses of inactivated influenza vaccine (*light bars*) with HAI antibody postvaccine to the indicated variant of H_3N_2. Vaccines contained Nanchang antigen (inactivated vaccine) or Nanchang-like antigen (live vaccine containing A/Wuhan/359/95). P values indicate significant differences. The children given inactivated vaccines were younger than the children given live, attenuated vaccine. H_3N_2 virus antigens: Sydney, A/Sydney/5/97; Nanchang, A/Nanchang/933/95; Thess., A/Thessalonika 1/95; Russia, A/Russia/1319/95; Johann., A/Johannesburg/33/94. (Data from Belshe RB, Gruber WC. Prevention of otis media in children with live attenuated influenza vaccine given intranasally. Pediatr Infect Dis J 19(suppl):S66–S71, 2002.)

more than 90% of seronegative children seroconverted to the A/Thessalonika/1/95, A/Nanchang/933/95, A/Wuhan/359/95, and A/Sydney/5/97 strains, and approximately 80% and 50% seroconverted to the A/Russia/1319/95 and A/Johannesburg/33/94 strains, respectively, which were closely related viruses (Fig. 18–3). In addition, CAIV-T also can induce cross-reactive HAI antibody against antigenically drifted H_1N_1 and B viruses in seronegative children.[150] These results support the conclusion that CAIV-T stimulated a cross-reactive antibody response in children, and might be expected to provide a high level of protection against antigenic drift strains in an influenza season in which there was a similar suboptimal match between the vaccine strain and the epidemic strain.

Duration of Immunity Induced by CAIV-T

Longer term persistence of immunity may emerge as a characteristic of the host response induced by both CAIV vaccine and natural infection with longer follow-up of vaccine recipients.[132,134,139,151] Serum HAI antibodies and nasal IgA antibodies persist following immunization of children with CAIV-T, and this persistent immunity may provide protection against antigenic drift strains.[132,152,153] Nevertheless, the strains represented in CAIV-T need to be updated annually to provide optimal protection against newly emerging strains. Additional studies would need to be done to further understand the public health benefits of this vaccine in regard to duration of immunity.

TABLE 18–3 ■ Summary of a Wild-Type Influenza Challenge Efficacy Study in Adults After Live Attenuated (CAIV-T) or Inactivated (TIV) Vaccine

Vaccine	Number Vaccinated and Challenged	Number with Infection and Illness (%)	Efficacy*
CAIV-T	29	2(7)	85%
TIV	32	4(13)	71%
Placebo	31	14(45)	—

*Results of challenge with virulent H_1N_1, H_3N_2, and B viruses are combined.[137]
Strains in the CAIV-T were antigenically matched to TIV and were A/Shangdong/9/93 (H_3N_2), A/Texas/36/91 (H_1N_1)–like, and B/Panama/45/90 cold-adapted reassortant virus. TIV was the formulation used in 1994/95 (Fluvirin; Evans Medeva). Challenge wild-type viruses were homologous A/Shangdong/9/93 (H_3N_2), A/Texas/36/91 (H_1N_1), and B/Panama 45/90.

Efficacy/Effectiveness of CAIV-T

Adults

The results of a wild-type challenge study following a single vaccination with CAIV-T or inactivated vaccine (TIV) in adults is shown in Table 18–3. Placebo subjects had significantly more infection and illness than either vaccine group. CAIV-T had 85% efficacy and TIV had 71% efficacy against infection and illness after experimental challenge with H_1, H_3, or B viruses.[137]

A summary of key effectiveness results following a single dose of CAIV-T or placebo in healthy working adults is shown in Table 18–4. Vaccine significantly reduced the number of severe febrile illnesses and days of febrile upper respiratory tract illnesses among healthy, working adults.

TABLE 18–4 ■ Effectiveness of CAIV-T* in Healthy, Working Adults (Ages 18 to 64) During Influenza A/Sydney Outbreak of 1997 to 1998

Outcome	Reduction (95% CI) in Indicated Outcome in Vaccinated vs. Placebo Recipients
Number of severe febrile illnesses	19% (7%–29%)
Days of FURI	25% (14%–35%)
Days of missed work for FURI	28% (16%–39%)
Days of antibiotic use for FURI	45% (35%–54%)
Days of health care provider visits for FURI	41% (30%–50%)

*CAIV-T composition consisted of viruses antigenically equivalent to TIV for the 1997 to 1998 influenza season. These included A/Shenzhen/227/95 (H_1N_1), A/Wuhan/359/95 (H_3N_2) (a Nanchang-like virus), and, a B/Harbin/7/94-like virus.
CI, confidence interval; FURI, febrile upper respiratory illness.
Data from Nichol KL, Mendelman PM, Mallon KP, et al for the Live Attenuated Influenza Virus Vaccine in Healthy Adults Trial Groups. Effectiveness of live, attenuated intranasal influenza virus vaccine in healthy, working adults: a randomized controlled trial. JAMA 282:137–145, 1999.

TABLE 18–5 ■ Occurrence of Influenza in Years 1 and 2, Efficacy of Vaccine, and Efficacy Against H_1N_1 Vaccine Virus Challenge

Epidemic Virus	Year 1		
	Vaccine* (N = 1070)	Placebo (N = 532)	Efficacy, (95% CI)
A/Wuhan/359/95-like (H_3N_2)	7	63	95 (88–97)
A/Sydney/5/97-like (H_3N_2)	—	—	—
B	7	37	91 (79–96)
H_1N_1	0	0	
Any type	14	94 (100)‡	93 (87–96)

*The composition of vaccine in year 1 was A/Texas/36/91-like (H_1N_1), A/Wuhan/359/95-like (H_3N_2), and B/Harbin/7/94-like. In year 2 the vaccine composition for H_3N_2 and B was the same as year 1 and the H_1N_1 component was A/Shenzhen/227/95-like.
†The challenge virus was A/Shenzhen/227/95-like (H_1N_1) cold-adapted reassortant monovalent vaccine, titer $10^{7.0}$.
‡Six children had two illnesses, one caused by influenza A and one caused by influenza B.
CI, confidence interval.
Data from Belshe et al.[131, 132]

Vaccine also led to lower rates of work absenteeism, health care provider visits, and the use of prescription antibiotics and nonprescription medications. These benefits were observed during a season in which the predominant circulating influenza virus strain, A/Sydney/5/97 (H_3N_2), was not well matched to the A/Wuhan/359/95 strain contained in the vaccine.[133]

Children

CAIV-T was highly efficacious in the pivotal randomized controlled trial in children 15 to 71 months of age (mean 42 ± 16.6 months) conducted over two influenza seasons (Table 18–5 and Fig. 18–4). In year 1, children received either one dose or two doses of CAIV-T or placebo given 60 ± 14 days apart, and, in year 2, children received a single revaccination according to the original randomization. In year 1 of the study, there was 95% efficacy against H_3N_2 (Wuhan- or Nanchang-like viruses) and 91% efficacy against B. In year 2, the epidemic consisted largely of a variant not contained in the vaccine, influenza A/Sydney. In year 2, the epidemic of A/Sydney/5/97-like viruses caused 66 of 71 cases, with the remaining cases associated with A/Wuhan/359/95-like viruses (4 cases) or influenza B (1 case). Vaccine was 100% efficacious in year 2 against strains included in the vaccine and 86% efficacious against the variant, A/Sydney/5/97. Overall, during the 2 years of study, vaccine was 92% efficacious at preventing culture-confirmed influenza (see Fig. 18–4).

Influenza-associated otitis media was significantly reduced in each year of the study. In year 1, there was only one case of influenza-associated otitis media in the vaccine group, but there were 20 cases of otitis media among the placebo recipients associated with culture-positive

influenza (vaccine efficacy = 98%). In year 2, only two cases of otitis media were associated with influenza in the vaccine group, but 17 occurred in the placebo recipients (vaccine efficacy = 94%). Cases of lower respiratory disease associated with culture-positive influenza also were significantly reduced in the vaccine group; only 1 case occurred in the 2 years in the vaccine group, but there were 11 cases in the 2 years in the placebo recipients (vaccine efficacy = 95% against influenza culture-positive lower respiratory disease).

Several measures of vaccine effectiveness were assessed as indicators of benefit from annual vaccination (Table 18–6). In both study years there was a significant reduction in all febrile illness (regardless of result of viral cultures). In year 1, a significant reduction in febrile otitis media and reduction in associated antibiotic use was observed in the vaccine group. Similarly, vaccinated children also visited health care workers significantly less often.

Safety of CAIV-T

CAIV-T has been evaluated in at least 20 clinical trials in which more than 20,000 subjects received more than 28,000 doses of vaccine, including more than 15,000 healthy children 1 to 17 years of age and more than 3700 healthy adults 18 to 64 years of age. In randomized, placebo-controlled trials, over 8100 healthy children and over 3200 healthy adults received CAIV-T and over 3900 healthy children and over 1600 healthy adults received placebo. Among the placebo-controlled trials, the incidence of adverse reactions that may be complications of influenza (such as pneumonia, bronchitis, bronchiolitis, stomatitis, and central nervous system events) was similar

Year 2			H₁N₁ Vaccine Virus Challenge†		
Placebo (N = 917)	Efficacy (N = 441)	Vaccine (%)	Placebo (N = 144)	Efficacy, (N = 78)	(95% CI)
0	4	100 (54–100)			
15	51	86 (77–93)			
0	1	100 (84–100)	—	—	—
0	0		6	19	83 (60–93)
15	56	87 (78–93)	—	—	—

in CAIV-T and placebo groups (data on file, MedImmune Vaccines, Inc.). CAIV has been well-tolerated in clinical trials with 19 different 6:2 reassortant vaccine virus strains (7 H₁N₁, 9 H₃N₂, and 3 type B) conducted prior to those by MedImmune Vaccines and with at least 14 different 6:2 reassortants (4 H₁N₁, 5 H₃N₂, and 5 type B) in studies conducted by MedImmune Vaccines.

No serious adverse events were associated with vaccination in children in the 2-year efficacy trial.[131,132] Transient, minor symptoms of respiratory illness were present after dose 1 of year 1 (Table 18–7), when more vaccinated children, relative to placebo children, exhibited mild upper respiratory symptoms (rhinorrhea or nasal congestion on days 2, 3, 8, and 9 postvaccine), low-grade fever (on day 2 postvaccine), or decreased activity (on day 2 postvaccine).[131,132] After revaccination, no significant differences in rhinorrhea, fever, or decreased activity were present.[132,154]

Significant additional safety data were reported from a large, randomized, double-blind, placebo-controlled trial that evaluated medically attended events in the 42 days following vaccination in more than 9000 healthy children 1 to 17 years of age randomized 2:1 vaccine to placebo and concluded that CAIV-T appeared to be well tolerated.[155,156] These data are particularly helpful in regard to medically attended lower respiratory events; pneumonia, bronchiolitis, bronchitis, and croup were not significantly increased in vaccine recipients compared to placebo recipients. Asthma events were modestly increased in children 12 to 59 months of age but were not temporally clustered during the 42-day follow-up period.

In adults, CAIV-T is associated with minor upper respiratory symptoms, runny nose, and/or sore throat in approximately 10% of subjects. These symptoms are generally well tolerated.[133]

CAIV-T in High-Risk Populations

The safety and tolerability of CAIV-T in 48 children and adolescents 9 to 17 years of age with moderate to severe asthma has been evaluated.[157] Asthma stability following vaccination, measured by the percent change from baseline in forced expiratory volume at 1 second, change from baseline in peak expiratory flow rates, asthma symptom scores, nighttime awakening scores, and daily use of rescue medication, was similar in both CAIV-T and placebo groups. Mild exacerbations of asthma occurred in 2 of 24 CAIV-T recipients and 0 of 24 placebo recipients.

The safety and tolerability of CAIV-T when co-administered with TIV in 200 high-risk adults has been evaluated. Participants greater than or equal to 65 years of age with at least one additional risk factor for influenza morbidity received TIV co-administered with either CAIV-T or placebo. The safety and tolerability of CAIV-T plus TIV following vaccination was similar to that of placebo plus TIV with the exception of a higher incidence of sore throat (15% vs. 2%).[158]

The rationale for this combined approach to potentially offer improved efficacy over TIV alone in the elderly was initially shown by Treanor et al.[159] Subsequently, this approach did not provide statistically significant improved efficacy in adults with chronic obstructive pulmonary disease.[160]

CAIV-T has been administered to small numbers of adults and children with asymptomatic or mildly symptomatic human immunodeficiency virus infection.[161,162] These studies were conducted to assess safety in the event that CAIV-T was inadvertently given to immunosuppressed persons rather than to support use of CAIV-T in these populations. No untoward events or prolonged viral shedding resulted.

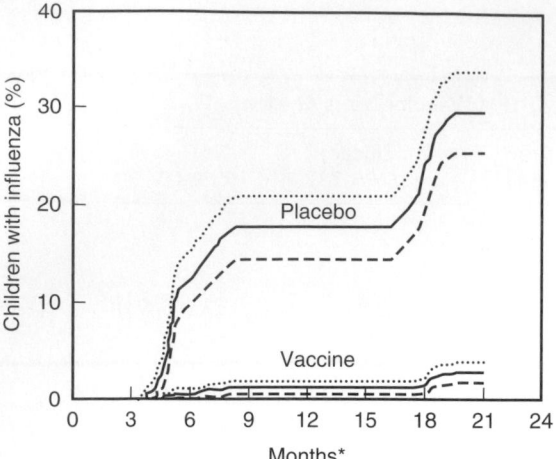

FIGURE 18–4 ■ Efficacy of live, attenuated influenza vaccine (FluMist) in a 2-year pediatric efficacy trial is indicated by differences in Kaplan Meier plot of the percentage of children developing culture-confirmed influenza in placebo or vaccine groups. Dashed lines represent 95% confidence interval. *Months from the start of the study. The composition of vaccine in year 1 was A/Texas/36/91-like (H_1N_1), A/Wuhan/395/95-like (H_3N_2), and B/Harbin/7/94-like. In year 2, the vaccine composition for H_3N_2 and B was the same as year 1 and the H_1N_1 component was A/Shenzhen/227/95-like. (Belshe RB, Gruber WC, Mendelman PM, et al. Efficacy of vaccination with live attenuated, cold-adapted, trivalent, intranasal influenza virus vaccine against a variant (A/Sydney) not contained in the vaccine. J Pediatr 136:168–175, 2000).

TABLE 18–6 ■ Effectiveness of Live, Attenuated Influenza Vaccine in Children in 1996 to 1997 (Year 1) and 1997 to 1998 (Year 2)

Effectiveness Measure*	% Reduction in Indicated Effectiveness Measure, Vaccine Group vs. Placebo Group	
	Year 1	Year 2
Febrile illness	21[†]	19[†]
OM	9	8
Febrile OM	33[†]	16
Febrile illness with Abx	29[†]	13
Febrile OM with Abx	33[†]	18
Days of missed day care	11	18[†]
Days of parent missing work	18	6
Visits to doctor	13[†]	8

*Effectiveness refers to all illnesses reported, regardless of culture result (not limited to the subset of influenza culture-positive cases). Vaccine antigens were the same as in Table 18–5.
[†]$P < 0.05$.
Abx, antibiotics; OM, otitis media.
Data from Belshe RB, Gruber WC. Prevention of otitis media in children with live attenuated influenza vaccine given intranasally. Pediatr Infect Dis J 19(suppl): S66–S71, 2000.

Genetic Stability of CAIV-T During Replication in Humans

Clinical studies of 6:2 CAIV strains demonstrated genetic stability of the vaccine during replication in humans. Vaccine virus isolates recovered from susceptible adults and seronegative children retain the vaccine phenotypes, indicating that reversion to virulence did not occur during replication of CAIV in humans.[163] It is likely that the observed stable attenuation is due to attenuating genetic sequences contained in multiple genes of CAIV vaccine strains.

To avoid contributing novel H and N genes to the environment, CAIV-T would not be used for vaccination against novel pandemic viruses until the virus was already widespread.

Transmission of CAIV-T

CAIV-T strains replicate in the nasopharynx of the recipient and are shed in the respiratory secretions. Data in the published literature failed to detect transmission of vaccine viruses derived from the passaged cold-adapted master donor viruses in multiple age groups and settings.[164–173] In an evaluation of direct transmissibility in a day care setting in children 8 to 36 months of age, 80% of the 98 FluMist recipients shed one or more vaccine strains, with a mean shedding duration of 7.6 days. One transmission event was observed among the 99 placebo recipients that was confirmed by phenotype and genotype analysis. The safety pro-

file for this child following transmission was similar to that of the other children in the study who received vaccine or placebo, and the child was not ill and did not experience a serious adverse event.[174]

Indications for Use of CAIV-T to Prevent Influenza

On June 17, 2003, CAIV-T was approved for use by the Food and Drug Administration as a vaccine to prevent influenza. The Advisory Committee on Immunization Practices developed draft guidelines for use of CAIV-T. CAIV-T is an important new option for active intranasal immunization to prevent disease caused by influenza A and B viruses in healthy children, adolescents, and healthy adults 5–49 years of age. Children 5–8 years of age should receive two doses 60 ± 14 days apart the first year of influenza vaccination; individuals 9–49 years of age should receive a single dose annually prior to exposure to influenza. In contrast to inactivated influenza vaccine which has been used largely in populations at high risk for death or other complications of influenza, CAIV-T is specifically indicated to prevent influenza in persons without underlying high risk conditions. CAIV-T and TIV are compared and contrasted in Table 18–7 (adapted from the ACIP draft guidelines)

The age range 5 to 49 years was selected for initial clinical use in healthy persons due to safety considerations for children less than 5 years of age. Provisional data in this age group raised concerns that CAIV-T might trigger or exacerbate reactive airway disease.[157] Although several lines of evidence do not support a causal link, further studies are

TABLE 18–7 ■ Comparison of CAIV-T with TIV

	CAIV-T	TIV
Route of Administration	Intranasal spray	Intramuscular injection
Type of vaccine	Live virus	Killed virus
Number of included virus strains	3 (2 influenza A, 1 influenza B)	3 (2 influenza A, 1 influenza B)
Vaccine virus strains updated	Annually	Annually
Frequency of administration	Annual	Annual
Can be administered to children and adults at high risk* from complications due to influenza	No	Yes
Can be administered to family members or close contacts of immunosuppressed persons	TIV is preferred	Yes[†]
Can be simultaneously administered with other vaccines	Yes[§]	Yes[‡]
If not simultaneously administered, can be administered within 4 weeks of another live vaccine	Prudent to space 4 weeks	Yes
If not simultaneously administered, can be administered within 4 weeks of an inactivated vaccine	Yes	Yes

*Populations at high risk from complications of influenza infection include persons aged ≥ 65 years; residents of nursing homes and other chronic-care facilities that house persons with chronic medical conditions; adults and children with chronic disorders of the pulmonary or cardiovascular systems; adults and children with chronic metabolic diseases (including diabetes mellitus), renal dysfunction, hemoglobinopathies, or immunosuppression; children and adolescents receiving long-term aspirin therapy (at risk for developing Reye syndrome after wild-type influenza infection); and women who will be in the second or third trimester of pregnancy during influenza season.
[†]Immunosuppressed persons include, but are not limited to those with human immunodeficiency virus (HIV), malignancy, or those receiving immuno-suppressive therapies.
[‡]TIV coadministration has been evaluated systematically only in adults with pneumococcal polysaccharide vaccine.
[§]No data exist regarding effect on efficacy.

needed. In addition, there were limited effectiveness data in persons 50–64 years old, a population universally recommended to receive trivalent inactivated vaccine.[133] The effectiveness trial in healthy working adults was specifically designed to examine the clinical benefits of CAIV-T in persons 18–64 years old but only 641 of 4561 adults (14%) were 50–64 years of age. Post hoc analysis among persons age 50–64 years revealed no statistically significant reductions in illness measures (proportion, episodes or days of illness) between vaccinees and placebo recipients, but there were significant reductions in illness associated missed work days and illness associated visits to their healthcare provider. While CAIV-T appeared to reduce more severe disease in older healthy adults, more data are needed before vaccine can be indicated for 50–64 year olds.

Contraindications to Use of CAIV-T

Persons Who Should Not Be Vaccinated with CAIV-T

The following populations should not be vaccinated with CAIV-T
- Persons aged < 5 years
- Persons aged ≥ 50 years*
- Persons with asthma, reactive airways disease or other chronic disorders of the pulmonary or cardiovascular systems; persons with other underlying medical conditions, including metabolic diseases such as diabetes, renal dysfunction, and hemoglobinopathies; or persons with known or suspected immune deficiency diseases or receiving immunosuppressive therapies*

- Children or adolescents receiving aspirin or other salicylates (because of the association of Reye syndrome with wild-type influenza infection)*
- Persons with a history of Guillain-Barré syndrome
- Pregnant women*
- Persons with a history of hypersensitivity, especially anaphylaxis, to any of the components of LAIV or to eggs

Close Contacts of Those at High Risk for Complication from Influenza

Close contacts of persons at high risk for complications from influenza should receive influenza vaccine to reduce transmission of wild type influenza viruses to contacts.
- There are no data assessing the risk of transmission of CAIV-T from vaccine recipients to immunosuppressed contacts; transmission in day care settings occurred with very low frequency and transmission to adults is considered highly unlikely. In the absence of direct data, use of TIV is preferred for vaccinating household members, healthcare workers, and others who have close contact with immunosuppressed individuals because of the theoretical risk that a live attenuated vaccine virus could be transmitted to the immunosuppressed individual and cause disease.
- For vaccination of healthy persons aged 5–49 years in close contact with all other immunocompetent high risk groups (i.e., persons with heart disease, lung disease, or diabetes), there is no preference between TIV and CAIV-T.

*These persons should receive TIV.

Administration of LAIV and Influenza Antiviral Use

It is unknown whether administering influenza antiviral medications affects the safety or efficacy of LAIV; LAIV should not be administered until 48 hours following cessation of influenza antiviral therapy, and influenza antiviral medications should not be administered for two weeks following receipt of LAIV.

Timing of CAIV-T Administration

The optimal time to vaccinate is usually in October and November. Children aged 5–8 years receiving LAIV for the first time should begin in October or earlier because those persons need a second dose 6–10 weeks after the initial dose. It is unknown whether concurrent administration of CAIV-T with other vaccines affects the safety or efficacy of either LAIV or the simultaneously administered vaccine. In the absence of specific data indicating interference, it is prudent to follow the ACIP General Recommendations on Immunization. Inactivated vaccines do not interfere with the immune response to other inactivated vaccines or to live vaccines. An inactivated vaccine can be administered either simultaneously or at any time before or after LAIV. A live vaccine not administered on the same day should be administered ≥ 4 weeks apart when possible.

Conclusions

CAIV-T has the potential to significantly contribute to the control of influenza and influenza-associated illnesses, including febrile otitis media and lower respiratory disease. CAIV-T has significant advantages in convenience of administration. The high efficacy of CAIV-T and efficacy in children against a significantly drifted strain of H_3N_2 (A/Sydney), a strain not contained in the vaccine, are compelling reasons to use the vaccine in children. Effectiveness in adults also was demonstrated using the same vaccine strain against this drifted H_3N_2 virus.

REFERENCES

1. Thomson D, Thomson R. Influenza with special reference to the complications and sequelae, bacteriology of influenzae pneumonia, pathology, epidemiological data, prevention and treatment. Ann Pickett-Thomson Research Lab 10:641–677, 1934.
2. Smith W, Andrewes CH, Laidlaw PO. A virus obtained from influenza patients. Lancet 2:66–68, 1933.
3. Francis T Jr. Transmission of influenza by a filterable virus. Science 80:457–459, 1934.
4. Francis T Jr. A new type of virus from epidemic influenza. Science 92:405–408, 1940.
5. Magill TP. A virus from cases of influenza-like upper respiratory infection. Proc Soc Exp Biol Med 45:73–164, 1940.
6. Taubenberger JK, Reid AH, Krafft AE, et al. Initial genetic characterization of the 1918 "Spanish" influenza virus. Science 275:1793–1796, 1997.
7. Thompson WW, Shay DK, Weintraub E, et al. Mortality associated with influenza and respiratory syncytial virus in the United States. JAMA 289:179–186, 2003.
8. Centers for Disease Control and Prevention. Prevention and control of influenza: recommendations of the Advisory Committee on Immunization Practices (ACIP). MMWR 45:1–24, 1996.
9. Monto AS, Kioumehr F. The Tecumseh Study of Respiratory Illness. IX. Occurrence of influenza in the community, 1966–1971. Am J Epidemiol 102:553–563, 1975.
10. Philip RN, Bell JA, Bean MO, et al. Epidemiologic studies on influenza in familial and general population groups, 1951–1956. II. Characteristics of occurrence. Am J Hyg 73:123–137, 1961.
11. Clark PS, Feltz ET, List-Young B, et al. An influenza B epidemic within a remote Alaskan community. JAMA 214:507–517, 1970.
12. Glezen WP. Serious morbidity and mortality associated with influenza epidemics. Epidemiol Rev 4:25–44, 1982.
13. Fox JP, Hall CE, Cooney MK, Foy HM. Influenza virus infection in Seattle families, 1975–1979. I. Study design, methods and the occurrence of infections by time and age. Am J Epidemiol 116:212–227, 1982.
14. Foy HM, Cooney MK, Allan I. Longitudinal studies of types A and B influenza among Seattle school children and families, 1969–1974. J Infect Dis 134:362–369, 1976.
15. Frank AL, Taber LH, Glezen PW, et al. Influenza B virus infections in the community and the family: the epidemics of 1976–1977 and 1979–1980 in Houston, Texas. Am J Epidemiol 118:313–325, 1983.
16. Centers for Disease Control and Prevention. Prevention and control of influenza: recommendations of the Advisory Committee on Immunization Practices (ACIP). MMWR 51:1–31, 2002.
17. Kilbourne ED. Influenza. New York, Plenum Publishing, 1987.
18. Portner A, Webster RG, Bean WH. Similar frequencies of antigenic variation in Sendai vesicular stomatitis and influenza A viruses. Virology 104:235–238, 1980.
19. Holland J, Spindler K, Horodyski F, et al. Rapid evolution of RNA genomes. Science 215:1577–1585, 1982.
20. Burnet FM, Lind PE. Recombination of characters between two influenza virus strains. Aust J Sci 12:109–110, 1949.
21. Hirst GK, Gotlieb T. The experimental production of combination forms of virus. II. A study of serial passage in the allantoic sac of agents that combine the antigens of two distinct influenza A strains. J Exp Med 98:53–70, 1953.
22. Simpson RW, Hirst GK. Genetic recombination among influenza viruses. I. Cross reactivation of plaque-forming capacity as a method for selecting recombinants from the progeny of crosses between influenza A strains. Virology 15:436–451, 1961.
23. Appleyard G, Maber HB. Plaque formation by influenza viruses in the presence of trypsin. J Gen Virol 25:351–357, 1974.
24. Simpson RW, Hirst GK. Temperature-sensitive mutants of influenza A virus: isolation of mutants and preliminary observations on genetic recombination and complementation. Virology 35:41–49, 1968.
25. Sugiura A, Tobita K, Kilbourne ED. Isolation and preliminary characterization of temperature-sensitive mutants of influenza virus. J Virol 10:639–647, 1972.
26. Mahy BWJ. Mutants of influenza virus. In Palese P, Kingsbury DW (eds). Genetics of Influenza Viruses. Vienna, Springer-Verlag, 1983, pp 194–254.
27. Almond JW, McGeoch D, Barry RD. Method for assigning temperature-sensitive mutations of influenza viruses to individual segments of the genome. Virology 81:62–73, 1977.
28. Almond JW, McGeoch D, Barry RD. Temperature-sensitive mutants of fowl plaque virus: isolation and genetic characterization. Virology 92:416–427, 1979.
29. Palese P, Ritchey MB, Schulman JL. P1 and P3 proteins of influenza virus are required for complementary RNA synthesis. J Virol 21:1187–1195, 1977.
30. Palese P, Schulman JL. Mapping of the influenza virus genome: identification of the hemagglutinin and the neuraminidase genes. Proc Natl Acad Sci U S A 73:2142–2146, 1976.
31. Schulman JL, Palese P. Selection and identification of influenza virus recombinants of defined genetic composition. J Virol 20:248–254, 1976.
32. Ritchey MB, Palese P, Schulman JL. Mapping of the influenza virus genome. III. Identification of genes coding for nucleoprotein, membrane protein, and nonstructural protein. J Virol 20:307–313, 1976.
33. Ritchey MB, Palese P, Schulman JL. Differences in protein patterns of influenza A viruses. Virology 76:122–128, 1977.
34. Chen W, Calvo PA, Malide D, et al. A novel influenza A virus mitochondrial protein that induces cell death. Nat Med 7:1306–1312, 2001.

35. Palese P, Ritchey MB, Schulman JL. Mapping of the influenza virus genome. II. Identification of the P1, P2 and P3 genes. Virology 76:114–121, 1977.

36. Laver WG, Air GM, Dopheide TA, Ward CW. Amino acid sequence changes in the hemagglutinin of A/Hong Kong (H3N2) influenza virus during the period 1968–77. Nature 283:454–457, 1980.

37. Van Wyke KL, Hinshaw VS, Bean WJ Jr, Webster RG. Antigenic variation of influenza A virus nucleoprotein detected with monoclonal antibodies. J Virol 35:24–30, 1980.

38. Webster RG, Kendal AP, Gerhard W. Analysis of antigenic drift in recently isolated influenza A (H1N1) viruses using monoclonal antibody preparations. Virology 96:258–264, 1979.

39. Webster RG, Hinshaw VS, Berton MT, et al. Antigenic drift in influenza viruses and association of biological activity with the topography of the hemagglutinin molecule. In Nayak DP, Fox CF (eds). Genetic Variation Among Influenza Viruses: ICN-UCLA Symposia on Molecular and Cellular Biology, Vol. 21. New York, Academic Press, 1981, pp 243–251.

40. Gething M-J, Sambrook J. Expression of cloned influenza virus genes. In Palese P, Kingsbury DW (eds). Genetics of Influenza Viruses. Vienna, Springer-Verlag, 1983, pp 169–191.

41. Lamb RA. The influenza virus RNA segments and their encoded proteins. In Palese P, Kingsbury DW (eds). Genetics of Influenza Viruses. Vienna, Springer-Verlag, 1983, pp 26–59.

42. Air GM, Compans RW. Influenza B and influenza C viruses. In Palese P, Kingsbury DW (eds). Genetics of Influenza Viruses. Vienna, Springer-Verlag, 1983, pp 280–304.

43. Enami M, Luytjes W, Krystal M, Palese P. Introduction of site-specific mutations into the genome of influenza virus. Proc Natl Acad Sci U S A 87:3802–3805, 1990.

44. Enami M, Palese P. High-efficiency formation of influenza virus transfectants. J Virol 65:2711–2713, 1991.

45. Luo G, Luytjes W, Enami M, Palese P. The polyadenylation signal of influenza virus mRNA involves a stretch of uridines followed by the RNA duplex of the panhandle structure. J Virol 65:2861–2867, 1991.

46. Webster RG, Bean WJ, Gorman OT, et al. Evolution and ecology of influenza A viruses. Microbiol Rev 56:152–179, 1992.

47. Wiley DC, Wilson IA, Skehel JJ. Structural identification of the antibody-binding sites of Hong Kong influenza hemagglutinin and their involvement in antigenic variation. Nature 238:373–378, 1981.

48. Wilson IA, Skehel JJ, Wiley DC. Structure of the hemagglutinin membrane glycoprotein of influenza virus at 3A resolution. Nature 289:366–373, 1981.

49. Webster RG, Laver WC, Air GM. Antigenic variation among type A influenza viruses. In Palese P, Kingsbury DW (eds). Genetics of Influenza Viruses. Vienna, Springer-Verlag, 1983, pp 309–322.

50. Colman PM. Neuraminidase: enzyme and antigen. In Krug RM (ed). The Influenza Viruses. New York, Plenum Press, 1991, pp 175–210.

51. Young JF, Desselberger U, Palese P. Evolution of human influenza A viruses in nature: sequential mutations in the genomes of new H1N1 isolates. Cell 18:73–83, 1979.

52. Krystal M, Young JF, Palese P, et al. Sequential mutations in the hemagglutinins of influenza B virus isolates: definition of antigenic domains. Proc Natl Acad Sci U S A 80:4527–4531, 1983.

53. Burnet FM. Principles of Animal Virology. New York, Academic Press, 1955.

54. Webster RG, Laver WG, Air GM, Schild GC. Molecular mechanisms of variation in influenza viruses. Nature 296:115–121, 1982.

55. Both GW, Sleigh MJ. Complete nucleotide sequence of the hemagglutinin gene from a human influenza virus of the Hong Kong subtype. Nucl Acids Res 8:2561–2757, 1980.

56. Krystal M, Buonagurio D, Young JF, Palese P. Sequential mutations in the NS genes of influenza virus field strains. J Virol 45:547–554, 1983.

57. Palese P, Young JF. Molecular epidemiology of influenza virus. In Palese P, Kingsbury DW (eds). Genetics of Influenza Viruses. Vienna, Springer-Verlag, 1983, pp 321–336.

58. Burnet FM, Bull DR. Changes in influenza virus associated with adaptation to passage in chick embryos. Aust J Exp Biol Med Sci 21:55–69, 1943.

59. Beare AS, Bynoe ML, Tyrrell DAJ. Investigation into the attenuation of influenza viruses by serial passage. Br Med J 4:482, 1968.

60. Minor TE, Dick EC, Dick RC, Inhorn SL. Attenuated influenza A vaccine (Alice) in an adult population: vaccine-related illness,

61. serum and nasal antibody production and intrafamily transmission. J Clin Microbiol 2:403, 1975.

61. Zaky DA, Douglas RG Jr, Betts RF, et al. Safety and efficacy of "Alice" influenza virus vaccine in normal healthy adults. J Infect Dis 133:669–675, 1976.

62. Hall CB, Douglas RG, Fralonardo SA. Live attenuated influenza virus vaccine trial in children. Pediatrics 56:991–998, 1975.

63. Mackenzie JS. Virulence of temperature-sensitive mutants of influenza virus. Br Med J 3:757–758, 1969.

64. Florent G. Gene constellation of live influenza A vaccines. Arch Virol 64:171–173, 1980.

65. Hay AJ, Bellamy AR, Abraham G, et al. Procedures for characterization of the genetic material of candidate vaccine strains. Dev Biol Stand 39:15–24, 1977.

66. Murphy BR, Tolpin MD, Massicot JG, et al. Escape of a highly defective influenza A virus mutant from its temperature-sensitive phenotype by extragenic suppression and other types of mutation. Ann N Y Acad Sci 354:172–182, 1980.

67. Murphy BR, Chanock RM. Genetic approaches to the prevention of influenza A virus infection. In Nayak DP (ed). Genetic Variation Among Influenza Viruses. New York, Academic Press, 1981, pp 601–616.

68. Wright PF, Okabe N, McKee KT Jr, et al. Cold-adapted recombinant influenza A virus vaccines in seronegative young children. J Infect Dis 146:71–79, 1982.

69. Tolpin MD, Clements ML, Levine MM, et al. Evaluation of a phenotypic revertant of the A/Alaska/77/ts-1A1 reassortant virus in hamsters and in seronegative adult volunteers: further evidence that the temperature-sensitive phenotype is responsible for attenuation of ts-1A2 reassortant viruses. Infect Immunol 36:645–650, 1982.

70. Kilbourne ED. Future influenza vaccines and the use of genetic recombinants. Bull World Health Organ 41:643–645, 1969.

71. Beare AS, Hall TS. Recombinant influenza-A viruses as live vaccines for man. Lancet 2:1271–1273, 1971.

72. Beare AS, Schild GC, Craig JW. Trials in man with live recombinants made from A/PR/8/34 (H1N1) and wild H3N2 influenza viruses. Lancet 2:729–732, 1975.

73. McCahon D, Beare AS, Stealey VM. The production of live attenuated influenza A strains by recombination with A/Okuda/57. Postgrad Med J 52:389–394, 1976.

74. Beare AS. Research into the immunization of humans against influenza by means of living viruses. In Beare AS (ed). Basic and Applied Influenza Research. Boca Raton, FL, CRC Press, 1982, pp 110–115.

75. Steinhoff MC, Halsey NA, Wilson MW, et al. Comparison of live-attenuated cold-adapted and avian-human influenza A/Bethesda/85-H3N2 reassortant virus vaccines in infants and children. J Infect Dis 162:394–401, 1990.

76. Murphy BR, Sly DL, Tierney EL, et al. Influenza A reassortant virus derived from avian and human influenza A viruses is attenuated and immunogenic in monkeys. Science 218:1330–1332, 1982.

77. Steinhoff MC, Halsey NA, Fries LF, et al. The A/Mallard/6750/78 avian/human, but not the A/Ann Arbor/6/60 cold-adapted, influenza A/Kawasaki/86 (H1N1) reassortant virus vaccine retains partial virulence for infants and children. J Infect Dis 163:1023–1028, 1991.

78. Murphy BR, Clements ML, Tierney EL, et al. Dose response of influenza A/Washington/897/80 (H3N2) avian-human reassortant virus in adult volunteers. J Infect Dis 152:225–229, 1985.

79. Murphy BR, Hinshaw VS, Sly DL, et al. Virulence of avian influenza A viruses for squirrel monkeys. Infect Immunol 37:1119–1126, 1982.

80. Snyder MH, Clements ML, Betts RF, et al. Evaluation of live avian-human reassortant influenza A H3N2 and H1N1 virus vaccines in seronegative volunteers. J Clin Microbiol 23:852–857, 1986.

81. Snyder MH, Clements ML, Herrington D, et al. Comparison of avian-human influenza A virus reassortants derived from different avian influenza virus donors: studies in squirrel monkeys, chimpanzees, and adult volunteers. J Clin Microbiol 24:467–469, 1986.

82. Kim HW, Arrobio JO, Brandt CD, et al. Temperature-sensitive mutants of influenza A virus: response of children to the influenza A/Hong Kong/68 ts-1 (E) (H3N2) candidate vaccine viruses and significance to neuraminidase antigen. Pediatr Res 10:238–242, 1976.

83. Herlocher ML, Maassab HF, Webster RG. Molecular and biological changes in the cold-adapted "master strain" A/AA/6/60 (H2N2) virus. Proc Natl Acad Sci U S A 90:6032–6036, 1993.

84. Herlocher ML, Clavo AC, Maassab HF. Sequence comparisons of A/AA/6/60 influenza viruses: mutations which may contribute to attenuation. Virus Res 42:11–25, 1996.

85. Maassab HF. Adaptation and growth characteristics of influenza virus at 25°C. Nature 213:612–614, 1967.

86. Maassab HF, Monto AS, DeBorde DC, et al. Development of cold recombinants of influenza virus as live virus vaccines. In Nayak D, Fox CF (eds). Genetic Variation Among Influenza Viruses. New York, Academic Press, 1981, pp 617–637.

87. Maassab HF. Development of variants of influenza virus. In Barry RD, Mahy BWJ (eds). The Biology of Large RNA Viruses. New York, Academic Press, 1970, pp 542–546.

88. Davenport FM, Hennessy AV, Maassab HF, et al. Pilot studies on recombinant cold-adapted live type A and B influenza virus vaccines. J Infect Dis 136:17–25, 1977.

89. Monto AS, Miller FD, Maassab HF. Evaluation of an attenuated, cold-recombinant influenza B virus vaccine. J Infect Dis 145:57–64, 1982.

90. LaMontagne JR, Wright PF, Clements ML, et al. Prospects for live, attenuated influenza vaccines using reassortants derived from the A/Ann Arbor/6/60 (H2N2) cold-adapted (ca) donor virus. In Laver WG (ed). The Origin of Pandemic Influenza Viruses. Amsterdam, Elsevier Science, 1983, pp 243–257.

91. Alexandrova GI, Smorodintsev AA. Obtaining of an additionally attenuated vaccinating cryophilic influenza strain. Rev Roum Inframicrobiol 2:179–189, 1965.

92. Ghendon YZ, Klimov AI, Alexandrova GI, Polezhaev FI. Analysis of genome composition and reactogenicity of recombinants of cold-adapted and virulent virus strains. J Gen Virol 53:215–224, 1981.

93. Ghendon YZ, Polezhaev FI, Lisovskaya KV, et al. Recombinant cold-adapted attenuated influenza A vaccines for use in children: molecular genetic analysis of the cold-adapted donor and recombinants. Infect Immunol 44:730–733, 1984.

94. Alexandrova GI, Polezhaev FI, Budilovsky GN, et al. Recombinant cold-adapted attenuated influenza A vaccines for use in children: reactogenicity and antigenic activity of cold-adapted recombinants and analysis of isolates from the vaccines. Infect Immunol 44:734–739, 1983.

95. Campbell D, Sweet C, Hay AJ, et al. Genetic composition and virulence of influenza virus: differences in facets of virulence between two pairs of recombinants with RNA segments of the same parental origin. J Gen Virol 58:387–398, 1982.

96. Chanock RM, Murphy BR, Kai C-J, et al. Prospects for stabilization of attenuation. In Stuart-Harris CH, Potter CW (eds). The Molecular Virology and Epidemiology of Influenza. New York, Academic Press, 1984, pp 115–120.

97. Maassab HF, DeBorde DC. Development and characterization of cold-adapted viruses for use as live virus vaccines. Vaccine 3:355–369, 1985.

98. Snyder MH, Betts RF, DeBorde D, et al. Four viral genes independently contribute to attenuation of live influenza A/Ann Arbor/6/60 (H2N2) cold-adapted reassortant virus vaccines. J Virol 62:488–495, 1988.

98a. Lu B, Zhou H, Kemble G, et al. Genetic basis of temperature-sensitive and attenuated phenotypes of FluMist vaccine strains derived from cold-adapted A/AA/6/60 influenza virus. [abstr. W43-4]. In Abstracts of American Societies for virology annual meeting, Davis, CA, July 12–16, 2002.

99. Donabedian AM, DeBorde DC, Cook S, et al. A mutation in the PA protein gene of cold-adapted B/Ann Arbor/1/66 influenza virus associated with reversion of temperature sensitivity and attenuated virulence. Virology 163:444–451, 1988.

100. Alexandrova GI, Garmashova LM, Golubev DB, et al. Experience in selection of safe thermosensitive recombinants of influenza virus [in Russian]. Vopr Virusol 4:342–346, 1979.

101. Kendal AP, Maassab HF, Alexandrova GI, Ghendon YZ. Development of cold-adapted recombinant live, attenuated influenza A vaccines in the U.S.A. and U.S.S.R. Antiviral Res 1:339–365, 1981.

102. Cox NJ, Kendal AP, Shilov AA, et al. Comparative studies on A/Leningrad/134/57 wild-type and 47-times passaged cold-adapted mutant influenza viruses: oligonucleotide mapping and RNA-RNA hybridization studies. J Gen Virol 66:1694–1704, 1985.

103. Maassab HF. Biologic and immunologic characteristics of cold-adapted influenza virus. J Immunol 102:728–732, 1969.

104. Beare AS, Maassab HF, Tyrrell DAJ, et al. A comparative study of attenuated influenza viruses. Bull World Health Organ 44:593, 1971.

105. Davenport FM, Hennessy AV, Minuse E, et al. Pilot studies on mono and bivalent live attenuated influenza virus vaccines. Proc Symp Live Influenza Vaccine, Yugoslav Acad Sci Arts, Zagreb 6/7:105–113, 1971.

106. Hoffman E, Neumann G, Kawaoka Y, et al. A DNA transfection system for generation of influenza A virus from eight plasmids. Proc Natl Acad Sci U S A 97:6108–6113, 2000.

107. Douglas GR. Influenza in man. In Kilbourne ED (ed). The Influenza Viruses and Influenza. New York, Academic Press, 1975, pp 395–447.

108. Stuart-Harris CH. Influenza and Other Virus Infections of the Respiratory Tract. Baltimore, Williams & Wilkins, 1965.

109. Stuart-Harris CH. Influenza—the human disease. In Stuart-Harris CW, Schild GC (eds). Influenza, the Viruses and the Disease. Littleton, MA, Publishing Sciences Group, 1976.

110. Klenk H-D, Rott R. The molecular biology of influenza virus pathogenicity. Adv Virus Res 34:247–281, 1988.

111. Tateno I, Suzuki S, Nakamura S, Kawamura A Jr. Rapid diagnosis of influenza by means of fluorescent antibody technic. I. Some basic information. Jpn J Exp Med 35:383, 1965.

112. Mulder J, Hers JF. Influenza. Groningen, Netherlands, Wolters-Noordhoff, 1972.

113. Smith H, Sweet C. Pathogenesis of influenza virus infection in ferrets, a model for human influenza. In Stuart-Harris CH, Potter CW (eds). The Molecular Virology and Epidemiology of Influenza. New York, Academic Press, 1984, pp 122–125.

114. Stanley ED, Jackson GG. Viraemia in Asian influenza. Trans Assoc Am Physicians 79:376, 1966.

115. Naficy K. Human influenza infection with proved viremia. N Engl J Med 269:964, 1963.

116. Minuse E, Willis PW III, Davenport FM, Francis T Jr. An attempt to demonstrate viremia in cases of Asian influenza. J Lab Clin Med 59:1016, 1962.

117. Morris JA, Kasel JA, Saglam M, et al. Immunity to influenza as related to antibody levels. N Engl J Med 274:527, 1966.

118. Khakpour M, Saidi A, Naficy K. Proved viraemia in Asian influenza (Hong Kong variant) during incubation period. Br Med J 4:208, 1969.

119. Lazarowitz SG, Choppin PW. Enhancement of infectivity of influenza A and B viruses by proteolytic cleavage of the hemagglutinin polypeptide. Virology 68:440–454, 1975.

120. Klenk H-D, Rott R, Orlich M, Biodorn J. Activation of influenza A viruses by trypsin treatment. Virology 68:426–439, 1975.

121. Baum LG, Paulson JC. The N2 neuraminidase of human influenza virus has acquired a specificity complementary to the hemagglutinin receptor specificity. Virology 180:10–15, 1991.

122. Shaw MW, Arden NH, Maassab HF. New aspects of influenza viruses. Clin Microbiol Rev 5:74–92, 1992.

123. Francis T, Jr, Maassab HF. Influenza viruses. In Horsfall FL Jr, Tarur I (eds). Viral and Rickettsial Infections of Man. Philadelphia, JB Lippincott, 1965, pp 689–740.

124. Glezen WP, Six HR, Frank AL, et al. Impact of epidemics upon communities and families. In Kendal AP, Patriarca PA (eds). Options for the Control of Influenza: Proceedings of a Viratek–UCLA Symposium. New York, Alan R Liss, 1986, pp 63–75.

125. Collins SD. Influenza in the United States, 1887–1956 (Public Health Monographs No 48). Bethesda, MD, U.S. Public Health Service, 1957.

126. Centers for Disease Control. Prevention and control of influenza: recommendation of the Advisory Committee on Immunization Practices (ACIP). MMWR 46(RR-9):1–25, 1977.

127. Choi K, Thacker SB. Improved accuracy and specificity of forecasting deaths attributed to pneumonia and influenza. J Infect Dis 144:606–608, 1981.

128. Hay AJ, Belshe RB, Anderson EL, et al. Influenza viruses. In Belshe RB (ed). Textbook of Human Virology. St. Louis, Mosby–Year Book, 1991, pp 307–341.

129. Hoskins TW, Davies JR, Smith AJ, et al. Assessment of inactivated influenza-A vaccine after three outbreaks of influenza A at Christ's Hospital. Lancet 1:33–35, 1979.

130. Davies JR, Grilli EA. Natural or vaccine-induced antibody as a predictor of immunity in the face of natural challenge with influenza viruses. Epidemiol Infect 102:325–333, 1989. [published erratum appears in Epidemiol Infect 103:217, 1989]

131. Belshe RB, Mendelman PM, Treanor J, et al. The efficacy of live attenuated, cold-adapted, trivalent, intranasal influenzavirus vaccine in children. N Engl J Med 338:1405–1412, 1998.

132. Belshe RB, Gruber WC, Mendelman PM, et al. Efficacy of vaccination with live attenuated, cold-adapted, trivalent, intranasal influenza virus vaccine against a variant (A/Sydney) not contained in the vaccine. J Pediatr 136:168–175, 2000.

133. Nichol KL, Mendelman PM, Mallon KP, et al for the Live Attenuated Influenza Virus Vaccine in Healthy Adults Trial Group. Effectiveness of live, attenuated intranasal influenza virus vaccine in healthy, working adults: a randomized controlled trial. JAMA 282:137–145, 1999.

134. Belshe RB, Gruber WC. Prevention of otitis media in children with live attenuated influenza vaccine given intranasally. Pediatr Infect Dis J 19(suppl):S66–S71, 2002.

135. King JC, Lagos R, Bernstein DL, et al. Safety and immunogenicity of low and high doses of trivalent live cold-adapted influenza vaccine administered intranasally as drops or spray to healthy children. J Infect Dis 177:1394–1397, 1998.

136. Zangwill KM, Droge J, Mendelman P, et al. Prospective, randomized, placebo controlled evaluation of the safety and immunogenicity of three lots of intranasal trivalent, influenza vaccine among young children. Pediatr Infect Dis J 20:740–746, 2001.

137. Treanor JJ, Kotloff K, Betts RF, et al Evaluation of trivalent, live, cold-adapted (CAIV-T) and inactivated (TIV) influenza vaccines in prevention of virus infection and illness following challenge of adults with wild-type influenza A (H1N1), A (H3N2), and B viruses. Vaccine 18:899–906, 1999.

138. Clements ML, Betts RF, Tierney EL, Murphy BR. Serum and nasal wash antibodies associated with resistance to experimental challenge with influenza A wild-type virus. J Clin Microbiol 24:157–160, 1986.

139. Belshe RB, Gruber WC, Mendelman PM, et al. Correlates of immune protection induced by live, attenuated, cold-adapted, trivalent intranasal influenza virus vaccine. J Infect Dis 181:1133–1137, 2000.

140. Clover RD, Crawford S, Glezen WP, et al. Comparison of heterotypic protection against influenza A/Taiwan/86 (H1N1) by attenuated and inactivated vaccines to A/Chile/83-like viruses. J Infect Dis 163:300–304, 1991.

141. Murphy BR, Clements ML. The systemic and mucosal immune response of humans to influenza A virus [review]. Curr Top Microbiol Immunol 146:107–116, 1989.

142. Gorse GJ, Belshe RB. Enhancement of anti-influenza A virus cytotoxicity following influenza A virus vaccination in older, chronically ill adults. J Clin Microbiol 28:2539–2550, 1990.

143. Potter CW. Determinants of immunity to influenza infection in man. Br Med Bull 335:69–75, 1979.

144. National Institutes of Health. Specific immunity in influenza B: summary of Influenza Workshop III. J Infect Dis 127:220–236, 1973.

145. Fox JP, Cooney MK, Hall CE, Hjordis MF. Influenza virus infections in Seattle families, 1975–1979. II. Pattern of infection in invaded households and relation of age and prior antibody to occurrence of infection and related illness. Am J Epidemiol 116:228–242, 1982.

146. Hjordis MF, Cooney MK, McMahan R, et al. Single-dose monovalent A₂/Hong Kong influenza vaccine efficacy 14 months after immunization. JAMA 217:1067–1071, 1971.

147. Clements ML, Betts RF, Tierney EL, Murphy BR. Resistance of adults to challenge with influenza A wild-type virus after receiving live or inactivated virus vaccine. J Clin Microbiol 23:73–76, 1986.

148. Gruber WC, Belshe RB, King JC, et al for the National Institute of Allergy and Infectious Diseases Vaccine and Treatment Evaluation Program and the Wyeth-Ayerst *ca* Influenza Vaccine Investigators Group. Evaluation of live attenuated influenza vaccines in children 6–18 months of age: safety, immunogenicity, and efficacy. J Infect Dis 173:1313–1319, 1996.

149. Edwards KM, Dupont WD, Westrich MK, et al. A randomized controlled trial of cold-adapted and inactivated vaccines for the prevention of influenza A disease. J Infect Dis 169:68–76, 1994.

150. Nolan T, Lee MS, Zangwill KM, et al. Safety and immunogenicity of a live-attenuated vaccine blended and filled at two manufacturing facilities. Vaccine 21:1224–1231, 2003.

151. Bernstein DI, Treanor J, Yan L, et al. Effect of four yearly vaccinations with cold-adapted, trivalent, intranasal influenza virus vaccines (CAIV-T) on antibody response to vaccine virus [abstr 1640]. In Abstracts of the Pediatric Academic Societies annual meeting, Baltimore, May 4–7, 2002.

152. Bernstein DI, Yan L, Treanor J, et al. Effect of yearly vaccinations with live, attenuated, cold adapted, trivalent, intranasal influenza vaccines on antibody responses in children. Pediatr. Infect. Dis. J. 22:28–34, 2003.

153. Piedra PA, Glezen WP, Mbawuike I, et al. Studies on reactogenicity and immunogenicity of attenuated bivalent cold recombinant influenza type A (CRA) and inactivated trivalent influenza virus (TI) vaccine in infants and young children. Vaccine 11:718–724, 1993.

154. Piedra PA, Yan L, Kotloff K, et al. Safety of the trivalent, cold-adapted influenza vaccine in preschool-aged children. Pediatrics 110:662–672, 2002.

155. Black S, Shinefield H, Hansen J, et al. Large scale safety study of FluMist in 9,689 children 1–17 years of age [abstract]. In Abstracts of the Third International Pediatric Infectious Disease Conference, Monterey, CA, 2001.

156. Black S, Shinefield H, Hansen J, et al. Large scale safety study of FluMist in 9,689 children 1–17 years of age [abstract]. In Abstracts of the Fifth Annual Conference on Vaccine Research, Baltimore, 2002.

157. Redding G, Walker RE, Hessel C, et al. Safety and tolerability of cold-adapted influenza virus vaccine in children and adolescents with asthma. Pediatr Infect Dis J 21:44–48, 2002.

158. Jackson LA, Holmes SJ, Mendelman PM, et al. Safety of a trivalent live attenuated intranasal influenza vaccine, FluMist, administered in addition to parenteral trivalent inactivated influenza vaccine to seniors with chronic medical conditions. Vaccine 17:1905–1909, 1999.

159. Treanor JJ, Mattison HR, Dumyati G, et al. Protective efficacy of combined live intranasal and inactivated influenza A virus vaccines in the elderly. Ann Intern Med 117:625–633, 1992.

160. Gorse G, O'Connor T, Young S, et al. Efficacy of live, cold-adapted, and inactivated influenza virus vaccines in older adults with chronic obstructive pulmonary disease (COPD): A VA Cooperative Study. Vaccine 21:2142–2153, 2003.

161. King JC Jr, Treanor J, Fast PF, et al. Comparison of the safety, vaccine virus shedding, and immunogenicity of influenza virus vaccine, trivalent, types A and B, live cold-adapted, administered to human immunodeficiency virus (HIV)-infected and non-HIV-infected adults. J Infect Dis 181:725–728, 2000.

162. King JC Jr, Fast PE, Zangwill KM, et al for the HIV Influenza Study Group. Safety, vaccine virus shedding and immunogenicity of trivalent, cold-adapted, live attenuated influenza vaccine administered to human immunodeficiency virus-infected and noninfected children. Pediatr Infect Dis J 10:1124–1131, 2001.

163. Cha T-A, Kao K, Zhao J, et al. Genotypic stability of cold-adapted influenza virus vaccine in an efficacy clinical trial. J Clin Microbiol 38:839–845, 2000.

164. Belshe RB, Van Voris LP. Cold-recombinant influenza A/California/10/78 (H1N1) virus vaccine (CR-37) in seronegative children: infectivity and efficacy against investigational challenge. J Infect Dis 149:735–740, 1984.

165. Clements ML, Snyder MH, Sears SD, et al. Evaluation of the infectivity, immunogenicity, and efficacy of live cold-adapted influenza B/Ann Arbor/1/86 reassortant virus vaccine in adult volunteers. J Infect Dis 161:869–877, 1990.

166. Couch RB, Quarles JM, Cate TR, et al. Clinical trials with live cold-reassortant influenza virus vaccines. In Kendal AP Patriarca PA, ed. Options for the Control of Influenza. New York, Alan R Liss, 1986, pp 223–241.

167. Davenport FM, Hennessy AV, Minuse E, et al. Pilot studies on mono and bivalent live attenuated influenza virus vaccines. In Proceedings of the Symposium on Live Influenza Vaccine 1971, pp 105–113.

168. Davenport FM, Hennessy AV, Maassab HF, et al. Pilot studies on recombinant cold-adapted live type A and B influenza virus vaccines. J Infect Dis 136:17–25, 1977.

169. Moritz AJ, Kunz C, Hofman H, et al. Studies with a cold-recombinant A/Victoria/3/75 (H3N2) virus. II. Evaluation in adult volunteers. J Infect Dis 142:857–860, 1980.

170. Reeve P, Gerendas B, Moritz A, et al. Studies in man with cold-recombinant influenza virus (H1N1) live vaccines. J Med Virol 6:75–83, 1980.

171. Van Voorthuizen F, Jens D, Saes F. Characterization and clinical evaluation of live influenza A vaccine prepared from a recombinant of the A/USSR/92/77 (H1N1) and the cold-adapted A/Ann Arbor/6/60 (H2N2) strains. Antiviral Res 1:107–122, 1981.

172. Wright PF, Okabe N, McKee KT Jr, et al. Cold-adapted recombinant influenza A virus vaccines in seronegative young children. J Infect Dis 146:71–79, 1982.
173. Wright PF, Johnson PR, Karzon DT. Clinical experience with live, attenuated vaccines in children. *In* Kendal AP, Patriarca PA (eds). Options for the Control of Influenza. New York, Alan R Liss, 1986, pp 243–253.
174. Vesikari T, Karvonen A, Korhonen T, et al. A randomized, double-blind, placebo-controlled trial of the safety, transmissibility and phenotypic stability of a live, attenuated, cold-adapted influenza virus vaccine (CAIV-T) in children attending day care [abstr G-450]. In Abstracts of the 41st Interscience Conference on Antimicrobial Agents and Chemotherapy, Chicago, December 16–19, 2001.

Chapter 19

Measles Vaccine

PETER M. STREBEL[*] • MARK J. PAPANIA • NEAL A. HALSEY

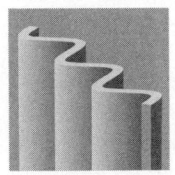 The written history of measles is classically traced to the writings of the Persian physician Rhazes, also known as Abu Becr, who lived during the 10th century.[1-4] However, the disease was apparently recognized as early as the seventh century by such ancients as the Hebrew physician Al Yehudi.[2,3] Rhazes referred to measles as *hasbah*, which means "eruption" in Arabic.[2,3] *Rubeola* and *morbilli* are descriptive Latin words first used in the Middle Ages. The latter is a diminutive of *morbus*, meaning "disease," which was reserved to refer to the bubonic plague; *morbilli* referred to a minor disease. "Measles" is probably derived from *mesels*, the anglicized form of *misellus*, which in turn is a diminutive of the Latin word *miser*, meaning miserable and referring to the sufferer of various eruptions or sores. The presence of nonspecific leprous sores was incorrectly identified with the disease called *morbilli* in Latin. Thus, *mesels* came to be equated with the disease and not the sufferer of ill-defined skin lesions.[4]

Rhazes appears to have been the first to make the distinction between measles and smallpox.[3,4] He considered measles to be a severe disease, "more to be dreaded than smallpox."[3] Although Rhazes did distinguish between the two diseases, he and others still probably considered them to be closely related.[4] Furthermore, although he was aware of the seasonal nature of measles, he did not think the disease was infectious.[3]

As noted by Wilson,[4] the distinction between measles and smallpox was becoming clearer by the beginning of the 17th century, when annual bills of mortality in London in 1629 listed the two diseases separately. Thomas Sydenham clearly described the clinical characteristics of measles during this period and believed the disease to be infectious.[3-5] It was, however, Francis Home, a Scottish physician who worked in Edinburgh in the mid-18th century, who truly recognized the infectious nature of the illness in his attempts to prevent it.[6] In 1758, he used an approach similar to variolation, the scarification technique used to induce mild smallpox before jennerian vaccination. The absence of vesicular or pustular lesions, such as those seen in smallpox and from which the variolation material was obtained, presented a challenge to Home. Lacking the knowledge that viremia precedes the rash of measles, he inoculated 12 children with material from the blood of a measles patient taken at the peak of the fever and onset of the rash. Ten of them developed a rash that was typical of the disease, preceded by symptoms of upper respiratory infection. This technique came to be known as morbillization but was never widely adopted.

Understanding of the epidemiology of measles was greatly enhanced by the classic investigation of a measles epidemic on the Faroe Islands in 1846 by the young Danish physician Peter Panum.[7] He not only confirmed that measles was contagious but also defined the 14-day interval between exposure and appearance of exanthem, recognized the higher mortality at the extremes of age, and observed that infection provided lifelong immunity.

In 1911, using infected material from acute cases, Goldberger and Anderson[8] transmitted human measles infection to monkeys, clearly demonstrating the existence of an infectious agent or substance responsible for measles. This finding antedated the technology to isolate and culture the measles virus. In 1954, Enders and Peebles[9] successfully isolated the measles virus in human and monkey kidney tissue cultures. Adaptation of the virus to chicken embryos[10] and cultivation in chicken embryo tissue culture[11] paved the road to vaccine development and licensure in 1963.[12-22]

Widespread vaccination of children in this country[23-28] and others[29-42] has had a dramatic effect on the incidence of measles and its associated complications. Reductions in morbidity and mortality have been so great that global eradication has been proposed[43-45] and judged feasible.[46,47] This would be a fitting end to a disease once confused with smallpox, the first infectious disease eradicated from the world.

Background

Clinical Description

Usual Clinical Course

The first symptoms of measles occur after a 10- to 12-day incubation period that follows airborne or droplet exposure. If infection occurs after parenteral exposure, the incubation

[*]Prior versions of this chapter were authored by Stephen Preblud, Samuel Katz, Lauri Markowitz, and Stephen Redd. Substantial sections of this chapter were taken from their previous work.

period is shortened by 2 to 4 days.[3,12,48–50] Immunosuppressed persons may have a prolonged incubation period.[51] The prodromal stage is heralded by the onset of fever, malaise, conjunctivitis, coryza, and tracheobronchitis (manifesting as cough) and lasts 2 to 4 days. This symptom complex is similar to that seen with any upper respiratory infection. The temperature rises during the ensuing 4 days and may reach as high as 40.6°C (105°F). Koplik's spots, the enanthema believed to be pathognomonic of measles, appear on the buccal mucosa 1 to 2 days before the onset of rash and may be noted for an additional 1 to 2 days after rash onset.[52] The rash is an erythematous maculopapular eruption that usually appears 14 days after exposure and spreads from the head (face, forehead, hairline, ears, and upper neck) over the trunk to the extremities during a 3- to 4-day period. The exanthem is usually most confluent on the face and upper body and initially blanches on pressure. During the next 3 to 4 days, the rash fades in the order of its appearance and assumes a nonblanching brownish appearance.

Virus can be isolated from both the nasopharynx and blood during the latter part of the incubation period and during the early stages of rash development.[9,53] Although virus has been isolated from the urine as late as 4 to 7 days after rash onset,[54] viremia generally clears 2 to 3 days after rash onset in parallel with the appearance of antibody.[55] Individuals with measles are generally considered to be infectious 2 to 4 days before through 4 days after rash onset.

Measles virus infection causes simultaneous activation and suppression of the immune system.[56–60] Measurement of cytokines released during measles suggests activation of CD8+ T cells, which are important for viral clearance, and type 2 CD4+ T cells, which provide optimal antibody production. Measles virus infection leads to a decrease of CD4+ lymphocyte counts that begins before the onset of rash and lasts for up to 1 month.[61] A study of measles patients in The Gambia found marked suppression of the production of interleukin-12, a known regulator of cellular immunity, and suggests a mechanism for the immune suppression associated with measles infection.[60] Recovery from infection is associated with the production of serum and secretory antibodies[55,62–70] as well as the establishment of cellular immunity.[58,59,71–77] Although subclinical infection with boosting of antibody may occur with subsequent exposure,[63,65] immunity after natural infection is believed to be lifelong.[7,78]

Complications

The complications associated with measles infection have been the subject of much description and review.[2,48,50,79–100] In industrialized countries, the most commonly cited complications associated with measles infection are otitis media (7% to 9%), pneumonia (1% to 6%), diarrhea (8%), postinfectious encephalitis (1 per 1000 to 2000 cases of measles), subacute sclerosing panencephalitis (SSPE) (1 per 100,000 cases), and death (1.0 to 3.0 per 1000 cases). Complications are likely to be present if the fever has not lysed within 1 to 2 days of rash onset. The risk of serious complications and death is increased in children less than 5 years and adults greater than 20 years of age.[2,3,90,91,95,98] Pneumonia, which is responsible for approximately 60% of deaths, is more common in young patients whereas acute encephalitis occurs more frequently in adults.[90,98] Pneumonia may occur as a primary viral pneumonia

(Hecht's pneumonia) or as a bacterial superinfection, most commonly with staphylococcus, pneumococcus, or typable (encapsulated) *Haemophilus influenzae*. Other described complications include thrombocytopenia, laryngotracheobronchitis, stomatitis, hepatitis, appendicitis and ileocolitis, pericarditis and myocarditis, glomerulonephritis, hypocalcemia, and Stevens-Johnson syndrome.[48,50] Although it has long been assumed that measles infection exacerbates or activates tuberculosis,[101] it is no longer certain that this is the case.[102]

Measles infection runs a devastating course in children in developing countries, where the mortality rates can be as high as 2% to 15%.[3,48,50,103–117] Pneumonia is the most common severe complication from measles and is associated with the greatest number of measles-associated deaths.[118,119] The rash is intense and often hemorrhagic (black measles), and it resolves after marked desquamation. Inflammation of the mucosa leads to stomatitis and diarrhea. Diarrhea is a frequent cause of death because it may persist long after the acute insult and further aggravate a pre-existing malnourished state.[99,120,121] Mediastinal and subcutaneous emphysema, keratitis, corneal ulceration, and gangrene of the extremities are not uncommon. The combination of vitamin A deficiency and keratitis results in a high incidence of blindness.[122–124] Secondary bacterial infections, often with staphylococci, produce pustules, furuncles, pneumonia, osteomyelitis, and other pyogenic complications.

SSPE is a rare degenerative central nervous system (CNS) disease caused by a persistent infection with a defective measles virus.[125–129] The agent has been noted in affected brain tissue by use of antigen detection assays, electron microscopy, polymerase chain reaction (PCR), and in situ RNA hybridization (and has been cultured by co-cultivation techniques). Signs and symptoms of mental and motor deterioration begin an average of 7 years after measles infection, which frequently has occurred before the age of 2 years. Patients have progressive personality changes, develop myoclonic seizures and motor disability, lapse into a coma, and die. The average age at onset is 9 years. Males outnumber females 2:1 to 4:1.[92,93,97,130] Patients with SSPE have high titers of measles-specific antibodies in their sera and cerebrospinal fluid. Measles viruses that have been isolated from affected brain tissue have mutations that prevent normal replication and budding from the host membrane; such mutations can occur in M, H, or F genes of the virus.[126,131] SSPE occurs as a complication of measles infection with a frequency of about 1 per 100,000 measles cases.

A team of investigators in the United Kingdom has suggested that infection with measles virus or measles vaccine virus results in a persistent infection of the gastrointestinal tract leading to Crohn's disease or ulcerative colitis later in life.[132–134] They hypothesized further that the etiology of inflammatory bowel disease is multifactorial and may involve infection with measles virus at a very young age, intense exposure, concurrent infections with other viruses, and a special genetic predisposition.[135] These investigators have gone on to study a subset of children with developmental disorder and ileocolonic lymphonodular hyperplasia and report finding evidence of measles virus in biopsies from the terminal ileum of these children using reverse transcriptase–polymerase chain reaction (RT-PCR) techniques.[136] The findings of this group of investigators have led to speculation that combined vaccination with measles-mumps-rubella (MMR) vaccine may be responsible not only for some forms of inflammatory bowel disease but also the increasing incidence of childhood autism. Other researchers, however, have been unable to replicate earlier laboratory findings using similar as well as more sensitive and specific methods.[137,138] Subsequent well-conducted epidemiologic studies have not found an association between measles vaccination and development of inflammatory bowel disease[139–141] or autism.[141,142] In summary, the available laboratory and epidemiologic evidence does not support hypotheses that measles or measles-containing vaccines might contribute to or induce inflammatory bowel disease or autism[143] (see *Adverse Events* below).

Measles has been proposed to be a causal factor for several other diseases. Studies from different laboratories have revealed conflicting evidence for persistence of measles virus in affected tissues from patients with otosclerosis[144] and Paget's disease.[145] Current evidence is inconclusive regarding a possible role of measles infections in the pathogenesis of multiple sclerosis.[146]

Infection during pregnancy is associated with an increased risk of miscarriage and prematurity,[147,148] although there is no convincing evidence that maternal infection with measles is associated with congenital malformations.[149,150] Clinical illness in the newborn after intrauterine exposure follows a shortened incubation period and may vary from mild to severe.[150,151]

Clinical Variants

The typical course of measles described in the preceding section can be modified by the presence of antibody.[2,3,48,50] This situation usually arises in the infant with residual maternal transplacental antibody or in the individual given immune globulin (IG) after exposure in an attempt to abort or attenuate disease.[65,152–155] Although some individuals have subclinical infection,[156] most will have a mild abbreviated illness that confers lasting immunity.[155,157] A second clinical measles infection may occur, however, if immunity is incomplete.[2,50,158] Typical or modified measles illness also may rarely follow reinfection after either natural infection[159,160] or vaccination.[160–169] Schaffner and colleagues[159] reported a case of typical albeit mild measles in a 16-year-old girl who reportedly had measles 8 years previously. She had a hemagglutination-inhibition (HI) antibody titer of 1:200 on the second day of rash and titers of 1:1600 and 1:320 at 23 days and 6 months after rash onset, respectively. The rapidity of antibody appearance, the high titer achieved, and the absence of immunoglobulin (Ig) M antibody in all of the specimens suggested a secondary immune response. Although reports examining immunity after infection rely on antibody determination, immunity relies heavily on T-lymphocyte memory and function.

Measles infection in the immunocompromised host can be prolonged, severe, and frequently fatal.[170–175] Infection in these persons may occur in the absence of rash.[170,173,174,176] The severity of illness is believed to be due primarily to impaired cell-mediated immunity.[177–180] Two especially severe complications are an acute progressive encephalitis (measles inclusion body encephalitis)[96,181,182] and a characteristic giant cell pneumonia (Hecht's pneumonia).[170–172,183]

Measles has been found to be more severe in persons with human immunodeficiency virus (HIV) infection. In the United States, the case-fatality rate has been reported to be as high as 50% in HIV-infected children.[184]

An atypical variant of measles occurred in some recipients of killed measles vaccine who were subsequently exposed to wild-type virus.[48,50,158,160,185–197] Patients with atypical measles lacked antibody to the measles virus fusion (F) protein[125,197,198] and had exaggerated cellular responses to measles antigen.[73,199] Exposure resulted in an unbalanced response between cellular and humoral immunity with production of extremely high levels of measles-specific circulating antibody.[50,73,74,186,197] Studies in monkeys have shown that this illness is caused by antigen-antibody immune complexes.[200] After an incubation period of 1 to 2 weeks, a prodrome consisting of high fever, headache, abdominal pain, myalgia, and cough ensued. In the next 2 to 3 days, an unusual rash erupted on the extremities and spread centripetally. Whereas the exanthem could be erythematous and maculopapular, it was frequently petechial or vesicular and accompanied by edema, and was occasionally pruritic. Hepatocellular enzymes were sometimes strikingly elevated. The illness was frequently mistaken for Rocky Mountain spotted fever and had to be differentiated from meningococcemia, Henoch-Schönlein purpura, and drug eruptions.[48,50,201] A nodular pneumonitis with pleural effusion was common.[194,202] In spite of the potential for serious illness, there was only one report of a possible atypical measles–related fatality.[203] This syndrome also has been reported rarely after receipt of live measles vaccine exclusively.[204,205] Individuals with atypical measles are believed to be noncontagious.[50,186,187] On the basis of humoral and cellular immunity studies, they also are thought to be protected from subsequent illness after exposure to measles.[73,74,197] The syndrome probably can be prevented by appropriate immunization with live vaccine.[73,74,206,207]

Virology

The measles virus is a spherical, nonsegmented, single-stranded, negative-sense RNA virus with a diameter of 120 to 250 nm.[125,198,208] It is a member of the genus *Morbillivirus* in the family Paramyxoviridae and is closely related to the canine distemper, rinderpest, and *peste-des-petits-ruminants* viruses and a phocine distemper virus of seals.[209,210] There are six structural proteins. Three are complexed with the RNA and form the nucleocapsid: the phosphoprotein (P), the large protein (L), and the nucleoprotein (N). Three are complexed with the envelope: F protein, hemagglutinin protein (H), and matrix protein (M).[198] The F and H envelope proteins are glycosylated; the innermost of the three envelope proteins, the M protein, is not. The F and H proteins are responsible for fusion of virus and host cell membranes, allowing viral penetration and hemolysis. Virions enter the cell by binding to the human cellular receptor CD46,[211] fusing with the membrane, and releasing the nucleocapsid into the cytoplasm. Viral replication takes about 24 hours. After synthesis of viral proteins and RNA, infectious viral particles bud from the cell membrane. Human signaling lymphocyte activation molecules (SLAMs; also known as CD150) have recently been identified as additional cellular receptors for measles virus. Human SLAM is a membrane glycoprotein expressed on cells of the immune system and seems to mediate lymphocyte activation and control cytokine production.[212]

The entire 15,894-nucleotide-long genome of the prototype Edmonston strain of measles as well as the genomes of the Edmonston-derived vaccines[213–215] and several wild-type strains[216,217] have been sequenced. Although measles virus is considered a monotypic virus, sequence analysis of the N, H, P, and M genes has shown that there are multiple, distinct lineages of wild-type viruses.[218–225] This sequence variability has made it possible to use molecular techniques to help monitor the transmission pathways of measles virus.[226] Molecular epidemiologic data, when analyzed in conjunction with standard epidemiologic information, can confirm or suggest the source of outbreaks and, over time, can provide a measurement of the effectiveness of vaccination control programs and monitor elimination.[224] For example, genetic analysis of wild-type viruses isolated in the United States from 1988 to 2000 helped to document the interruption of endemic transmission in the United States.[227] Comparison of genetic sequences from wild-type strains isolated in the United States with those isolated elsewhere in the world has suggested international importations of measles virus as sources of outbreaks.[226] To facilitate the expansion of virologic surveillance activities, the World Health Organization (WHO) has recommended a standard nomenclature and analysis protocol.[228] The WHO currently recognizes 20 genotypes and one proposed genotype (Fig. 19–1) of measles virus based on phylogenetic analysis of the N gene and has established a set of reference

sequences.[229,230] The WHO is attempting to build a global database to describe that pattern of endemic genotypes in each part of the world. The biologic significance of differences in the genetic sequence of wild-type strains is not known; the immune response generated through vaccination protects against all strains.

Measles virus is difficult to culture from clinical specimens and is best isolated in the marmoset lymphocyte cell line B95a,[231] although primary human fetal or infant kidney or primary monkey kidney cells also may be used.[125] However, after initial passage in the laboratory, many other primary and continuous cell lines of both human and nonhuman origin are permissive (e.g., human amnion, human embryonic lung, human carcinoma [HeLa, Hep-2, and KB], and chick embryo).[125,232,233]

Measles virus is inactivated rapidly in the presence of sunlight, heat, and extremes of pH.[125] It can, however, be safely stored for long periods at −70°C (−94°F).

In cell cultures, the virus causes two distinct cytopathic effects.[20,125,234,235] The first is formation of multinucleated syncytia (giant cells) containing numerous nuclei of fused cells. This corresponds to the predominant pathologic process observed in infected tissues, including skin and Koplik's spots.[236] When observed in lymphoid tissue, the giant cells are referred to as Warthin-Finkeldey cells; otherwise they are known as epithelial giant cells.[125] Both intracytoplasmic and intranuclear inclusions are characteristic. Whereas this cytopathic effect is characteristic of wild-type virus isolates, the cytopathic effects of passaged virus may additionally include spindle cell transformation. This difference in cytopathic effects as well as other factors, such as ability to grow in chick embryo fibroblasts, plaque morphology, interferon production, and optimal growth temperature, help differentiate wild-type virus from attenuated vaccine virus strains.[125,237–239]

Pathogenesis as It Relates to Prevention

The sequence of events between exposure to measles virus and subsequent primary acute illness in the normal host has been extensively studied, described, and reviewed[48,50,79–81]; it is based on information from both monkeys and humans. First there is localized infection of the respiratory epithelium of the nasopharynx, and possibly of the conjunctivae,[240] with spread to regional lymphatics. Further events then occur in a manner similar to those observed in the Fenner ectromelia–mouse experimental model.[241] Specifically, 2 to 3 days after exposure, there is a primary viremia with further replication of virus at the site of inoculation as well as in regional and distant reticuloendothelial tissue. Then, 5 to 7 days after exposure, there is an intense secondary viremia of 4 to 7 days' duration that leads to infection of and further replication in the skin, conjunctivae, respiratory tract, and other distant organs.[242] The amount of virus in blood and infected tissues peaks 11 to 14 days after exposure and then falls rapidly during the next 2 to 3 days. The characteristic rash is probably a manifestation of a hypersensitivity reaction and may not be seen in persons with suppression of the cell-mediated immune system.

The pathogenesis of measles infection indicates that prevention through immunization could be accomplished by

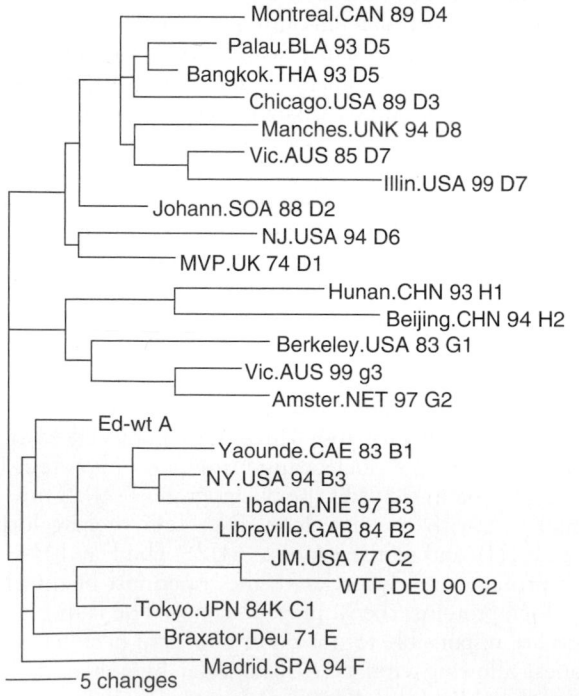

FIGURE 19–1 ■ Genetic relationship of the nucleoprotein gene from measles viruses. The World Health Organization currently recognizes 20 genotypes (A, B1, B2, B3, C1, C2, D1, D2, D3, D4, D5, D6, D7, D8, E, F, G1, G2, H1, and H2) and one proposed genotype (g3). The figure shows the names of reference strains followed by the genotype designation. The horizontal scale is proportional to genetic relatedness.

inhibiting replication at and dissemination from the nasopharynx or by inhibiting the viremia that occurs during the incubation period. The first approach requires the presence of local secretory IgA antibody or transudated IgG[243]; the second approach requires circulating antibody, either actively or passively acquired, to neutralize the virus. Although infection can be prevented solely after administration of antibody,[152–155] induction of cellular immunity would also seem to be desirable.[3,239] Children with primary agammaglobulinemia do not have more severe measles infections than do children with normal immune systems, and both develop long-lasting immunity after infection.[178,179] These observations indicate that the cell-mediated immune system alone is adequate to prevent measles.

On re-exposure, it is uncertain whether prevention of the primary viremia is necessary or even feasible, but it is obvious that the secondary viremia should be prevented. In fact, an initial limited replication and the circulation of a small amount of viral antigen may be necessary to restimulate the immune system and to elicit an anamnestic antibody response.

Diagnosis

Measles should be suspected in children who present with an acute erythematous rash and fever, preceded by a 2- to 4-day prodrome of cough, coryza, conjunctivitis, and photophobia. Recent experience suggests that clinical measles may be difficult to distinguish from other causes of febrile rash illness, particularly in areas where the incidence of measles has been low. Clinical features that support the diagnosis of measles include the following: the presence of Koplik's spots, the characteristic 2 to 4 days of intensifying prodromal symptoms, the progression of the rash from the head to the trunk and out to the extremities, and the lysis of fever shortly after the appearance of the rash. Health care providers working in measles-endemic areas may be more familiar with these clinical findings than are health care providers working in areas with a low incidence of measles. A clinical case definition for epidemiologic purposes is the presence of rash lasting 3 or more days; a temperature of 38.4°C (101°F) or higher, if it is measured; and cough, conjunctivitis, or coryza.[207] Its use for clinical diagnosis is limited, particularly because of the criterion requiring at least 3 days of rash before the diagnosis is made. In some parts of the world, a less specific clinical definition not requiring 3 days' duration of rash is being used for epidemiologic purposes. Laboratory tests are necessary to confirm the diagnosis, especially when measles is rare. Other illnesses, such as rubella, dengue, parvovirus B19, human herpesvirus type 6, and measles vaccine reactions, can meet these clinical definitions.[244–246] In the United States, it is recommended that clinicians obtain a blood or other suitable specimen for laboratory confirmation from all patients suspected of having measles, unless the patient is part of an already documented measles outbreak.

Although virus isolation, direct cytologic examination of clinical material, or demonstration of virus antigen can be used to diagnose measles,[53,54,247–252] detection of measles-specific IgM antibody is the most commonly used method. An increase in measles antibodies between acute and convalescent serum specimens is also diagnostic but requires the collection of two blood specimens. RT-PCR can be used to identify measles virus RNA in urine, blood, and nasopharyngeal mucus.[253–255] Because measles is an RNA virus, RNA must be reverse transcribed to DNA before PCR analysis, resulting in a much reduced sensitivity for diagnosing measles compared with diagnosing DNA viruses.[256]

In primary acute infection, detectable antibodies generally appear in the serum within the first few days of rash onset, peak within about 4 weeks, and subsequently decline somewhat but persist for life[48,50,62–65,257–259] (Fig. 19–2). Both IgG and IgM antibodies are initially produced.[260–263] However, IgG antibodies are detectable long after infection, whereas IgM antibodies are rarely detected after 6 to 8 weeks. Serum and secretory IgA antibodies are also produced.[68–70,264,265] Re-exposure usually induces a characteristic anamnestic response with a rapid boosting of IgG antibody; IgM may not be detected after re-exposure with use of some currently available serologic assays.[65,166,261,262] If IgM is detected after re-exposure, it will be at a lower ratio to IgG than the IgM-to-IgG ratio in a previously unexposed person.[266]

The tests for complement fixation (CF), HI, and neutralization (Nt) have been the assays historically employed to detect fourfold rises in measles IgG antibody between acute and convalescent sera.[125] However, the CF test has been shown to be less sensitive,[63–65,78,267] and the HI and Nt tests have undergone technical modifications over time.[268] The plaque reduction neutralization (PRN) test has remained the "gold standard" to which other more rapid and simpler methods are compared, but, because it is time and personnel intensive, it is generally limited to specialized reference laboratories and research work.[268] Fluorescence tests are available,[269] as are enzyme immunoassays (EIAs), also referred to as enzyme-linked immunosorbent assays (ELISAs).[270–276] Currently EIA tests for measles IgG are the most widely used because they are generally sensitive and convenient. Good correlation has been shown between HI and Nt antibody in many studies,[277] as well as between EIA and other serologic methods for the diagnosis of acute measles.[271,272,278] The EIA for measles IgG is based on

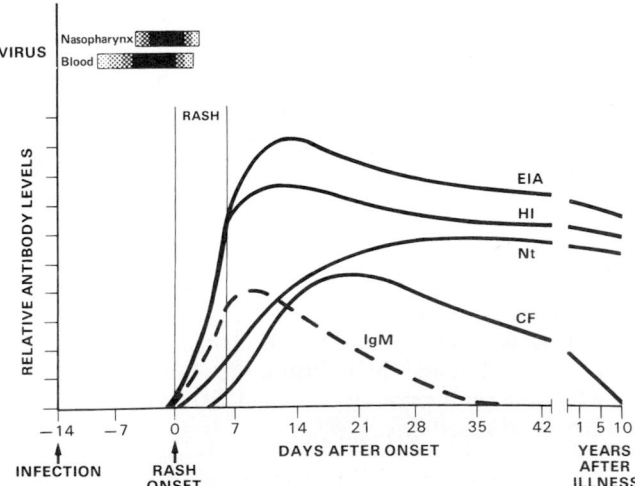

FIGURE 19–2 ■ Schematic of immune response in acute measles infection. EIA, enzyme immunoassay; HI, hemagglutination; Nt, neutralization; CF, complement fixation; IgM, immunoglobulin M.

significant changes in optical density values and cannot be translated directly to antibody concentrations or titers.

Currently, the recommended laboratory method for the confirmation of clinically diagnosed measles is a serum-based IgM EIA collected at the time the patient first presents for medical care.[279] A single specimen is adequate to detect the presence of IgM antibody.[265,275,276] A number of commercial kits using an indirect EIA method (with removal of the patient's IgG antibody before testing for IgM) or an antibody capture EIA technique (without removal of IgG) are now available and have been shown to have similar sensitivity (83% to 92%) and specificity (87% to 100%).[280] However, if measles prevalence is low (e.g., 1%), a modest reduction in the specificity of the assay from 99% to 95% will decrease the positive predictive value of the assay from 48% to 15% (i.e., only 15% of IgM-positive clinical cases will be true measles). Patients with parvovirus B19 or rubella infections may have false-positive reactions (rate of about 4%) when tested with measles IgM EIAs.[244,281]

Correct interpretation of serologic data depends on proper timing of specimens with regard to rash onset. This is especially important in interpreting negative IgM results. For example, in one study, the sensitivity of an antibody capture IgM assay was approximately 80% within the first 72 hours after rash onset and rose to 100% between 3 and 14 days after rash onset.[282] Sensitivity of the assay within the first 3 days of rash onset is thought to be similar for other commercially available kits. If the validity of the initial measles IgM test is in doubt, a second convalescent specimen should be taken and tested for both IgG and IgM. In some cases, interpretation may be difficult and requires precise information regarding dates of rash onset, prior measles vaccination, and specimen collection.

Two new approaches provide alternatives to venipuncture for collection of diagnostic specimens: oral fluid and blood spots on filter paper. In the United Kingdom, a radioimmunoassay has been developed to detect IgM antibodies in saliva or oral secretions.[283] The test was 92% sensitive and 98% specific compared with serum tests to detect IgM and is routinely used to diagnose measles. Use of oral fluid samples has appeal because the technique is noninvasive, can be used for rubella testing, and does not require processing in the field, and it may be possible to detect not only measles IgM but the measles virus genome for molecular characterization. Disadvantages are that commercial assays are not yet available to test the specimens and a confirmatory serum specimen or second oral fluid specimen may be required in some cases.[284] Although still considered an invasive technique, fingerstick as a method for sample collection may be more acceptable to parents than phlebotomy.[256] Blood spots collected onto filter paper do not require processing in the field, or a cold chain for transport to the laboratory, and can be used to test for measles and rubella as well as for molecular characterization of the measles virus genome. In addition, the eluted serum can be tested using commercially available EIAs without loss of sensitivity or specificity.[285–287]

Treatment

A number of preparations, such as interferon,[288,289] thymic humoral factor,[290] thymostimulin,[291] levamisole,[292] rib-

avirin,[293] and IG,[152] have been used to treat measles. None of these is commonly used to treat uncomplicated measles, although limited studies with ribavirin have shown reduced duration of illness.[293] Ribavirin and interferon may be effective in treating severe measles in immunocompromised persons.[294]

High doses of vitamin A have been shown to decrease mortality and morbidity in young children hospitalized with measles in developing countries.[295–297] The WHO currently recommends vitamin A for children with acute measles.[298] Treatment with vitamin A is once daily for 2 days at 200,000 IU for children ages 12 months or older, 100,000 IU for infants 6–11 months of age, and 50,000 IU for infants less than 6 months of age. In the United States as well as in developing countries, children with measles have been found to have low levels of serum retinol, and those with more severe illness have lower levels.[299–301] The American Academy of Pediatrics (AAP) recommends a single dose of vitamin A for hospitalized children ages 6 months to 2 years with measles, 200,000 IU for children ages 12 to 23 months, and 100,000 IU for those ages 6 to 11 months.[206] In addition, vitamin A therapy should be administered to children with measles who are immunosuppressed, who have clinical evidence of vitamin A deficiency, or who have recently immigrated from areas with a high mortality rate from measles.[206]

Antibiotics, in the absence of pneumonia, sepsis, or other signs of a secondary bacterial complication, are not recommended.[302]

Various chemotherapeutic agents have also been used in patients with SSPE in an attempt to treat or at least alter the clinical course of the disease.[128,303–306] Of these, inosiplex (Isoprinosine) and interferon have been the most extensively studied[304–308]; despite anecdotal evidence of their effectiveness, controlled trials are lacking.

Epidemiology

General Epidemiology

In the absence of an immunization program, measles is a ubiquitous, highly contagious, seasonal disease affecting nearly every person in a given population by adolescence.[2,3,309–311] An important exception is island populations, which can remain free of infection for variable periods and then, after reintroduction of the virus, experience epidemic disease that involves all age groups not affected by the last wave of infection.[3,7,78,83,87,310] Thus, whereas peak transmission usually occurs among young children, outbreaks in isolated communities involve many older individuals. This is exemplified by Panum's description of measles on the Faroe Islands, in which the disease affected individuals of all ages who were not affected by the last epidemic that had occurred 65 years previously.[7]

Measles is transmitted primarily from person to person by large respiratory droplets but also can be spread by the airborne route as aerosolized droplet nuclei.[2,3,312–315] The period of maximal contagion occurs during the prodrome.[8,48,50,88] Secondary attack rates in susceptible household (and institutional) contacts are high and can be on the order of 90% or greater.[49,63,257,316–318] Because virus is excreted before and after the appearance of rash, the onset of exanthem in secondary household cases occurs an average of 14 to 15 days (range of 7 to 18 days) after that in the index case.[317] Almost all primary infections (except those modified by maternal antibody or parenteral IG) are thought to be clinically overt.[2,3] Asymptomatic transmission from exposed immune persons has not been demonstrated.[319,320] Although susceptible monkeys may contract measles, there is no significant animal reservoir.[3,48,125]

Before the introduction of vaccines in most developed countries, school-age children had the highest risk of infection and accounted for the largest proportion of cases.[2,3,309] However, in dense urban areas, transmission among preschoolers took on greater importance.[309,321] Although serious complications did occur, they were relatively rare compared with the situation in developing countries. In the United States before the introduction of vaccine in 1963, major epidemics occurred approximately every 2 to 3 years.[2,3,322–324] Each year, disease peaked in late winter and early spring. The highest occurrence of disease was in children 5 to 9 years of age, who accounted for more than 50% of reported cases (Table 19–1). More than 95% of cases had occurred by age 15 years.[2,3,309] The highest risk of death was in children younger than 1 year and in adults.[2,90,91]

The measles virus is so contagious that it can be expected to circulate wherever a relatively large number of susceptibles congregate, even in the face of a low population susceptibility rate.[3] This explains the outbreaks that were typical among military recruits before the institution of routine measles vaccination.[325] Outbreaks among high-school and college students, most of whom have been vaccinated, demonstrate the virus's capability to seek out the small number of remaining susceptibles.[325–329]

Before widespread vaccination, in many developing countries, the average age at infection was much lower than that observed in developed countries.[3,103–109] In some areas of Africa, more than 50% of 2-year-old and 100% of 4-year-old children may be expected to have had measles. Poor nutrition and rapid loss of maternal antibody may explain why a greater proportion of these infants are susceptible at an earlier age than are those in developed areas,[277,330–334] and infection, in turn, results from the early age at which infants are exposed to the community at large.[103] This is in contrast to developed countries, where infants are usually homebound until they enter day care or school. Although young age at infection contributes to the high risk of serious complications and death, malnutrition,

especially vitamin A deficiency, also may be an important factor leading to the marked severity of measles in the developing world because of defects in cellular (and possibly humoral) immunity.[110,335] However, there is some evidence that crowding, which leads to an increased dose of virus, may be a more significant determinant of the severity of infection than is protein-calorie malnutrition.[336–338]

Significance as a Public Health Problem

Although remarkable control of measles has been achieved in some areas of the world,[40,339] in 2000, measles was still the leading cause of vaccine-preventable deaths in children and the fifth leading cause of all deaths among children less than 5 years of age.[340] Measles is also responsible for much diarrhea, respiratory disease, and blindness in the developing world.[114,119,120] In 2000, approximately 1.07 million measles-associated deaths were prevented because of the impact of vaccination programs. The Global Burden of Disease 2000 Study estimated that measles resulted in 777,000 deaths worldwide in 2000, of which 452,000 (58%) deaths were in the African Region of the WHO.[340]

In the United States in the prevaccine era, approximately 500,000 cases of measles were reported each year, but, in reality, an entire birth cohort of approximately 4 million persons was infected annually.[27] Associated with these cases were an estimated 500 deaths; 150,000 cases with respiratory complications; 100,000 cases of otitis media; 48,000 hospitalizations; 7000 seizure episodes; and 4000 cases of encephalitis, which left up to one quarter of patients permanently brain damaged or deaf.[27] On the basis of a 1985 dollar value, the annual cost was in excess of $670 million.[341] Using a 1992 dollar value, the annual estimated costs of measles in 1994 in the absence of vaccination would have been $2.2 billion in direct costs and $1.6 billion in indirect costs.[342]

Passive Immunization

Human IG provides sufficient measles antibodies to prevent or modify the disease when given within 6 days of exposure to measles.[152–155] Unfortunately, the immunity conferred by IG is only temporary (approximately 3 to 4 weeks, assuming that neither modified nor typical disease occurs).[153,343] However, there are certain situations in which immediate and relatively reliable prophylaxis against measles is

TABLE 19–1 ■ Age Distribution and Mean Annual Incidence of Reported Measles Cases by Age Group

Age (yr)	1960–1964*		1981–1988†		1989–1991†		1993–1996†		1997–2001†	
	Total (%)	Cases/ 100,000	Total (%)	Cases/ 100,000	Total (%)	Cases/ 100,000	Total (%)	Cases/ 100,000	Total (%)	Cases/ 100,000
0–4	37.2	766.0	31.9	4.9	43.6	43.7	29.1	0.84	35.5	0.10
5–9	52.8	1236.9	11.7	1.8	10.4	10.4	9.9	0.28	6.4	0.17
10–14	6.5	169.1	19.7	3.3	9.2	9.8	12.9	0.36	7.0	0.19
≥15	3.4	10.0	35.6	0.6	36.9	3.5	48.1	0.12	51.1	0.13

*Data represent prevaccine years and are from four reporting areas: New York City, District of Columbia, Illinois, and Massachusetts.
†Data from the entire United States.

desirable. These situations include household exposure to measles in children younger than 1 year, pregnant women, immunocompromised patients, and other persons with a contraindication to the receipt of live vaccine.

In the 1940s, Janeway demonstrated that administration of IG in a dose of 0.18 to 0.22 mL/kg within 6 days following intimate exposure prevented measles in about three of four individuals, with mild measles occurring in the fourth.[153] Presumably IG donors in 1945 had high measles antibody titers resulting from measles disease. Currently, large proportions of many populations have vaccine-induced measles immunity, which results in lower measles antibody titers. A study in Japan demonstrated a relationship between the measles antibody titer measured in the IG lot given and the level of protection from measles in persons exposed to measles. The study subjects received 0.33 mL/kg of IG intramuscularly at 3.3 days (± 1.1 days) after exposure. Measles attack rates were 45% (9 of 20) among those who received IG with 16 to 33 IU/mL of measles antibody compared to 0% (0 of 13) among those who received IG with 40 to 45 IU/mL.[344] In the United States, the Food and Drug Administration (FDA) requires that IG preparations contain a measles neutralizing antibody level that demonstrates adequate potency when compared with the FDA reference standard IG.[345]

Current U.S. recommendations suggest intramuscular immune globulin (IMIG) for susceptible household contacts for whom vaccine either is contraindicated or was not given with 3 days of initial exposure. Prophylaxis with IG is especially important for household contacts at increased risk for complications from measles (i.e., infants less than 12 months of age, pregnant women, or immunocompromised persons). The recommended dose of IMIG is 0.25 mL/kg within 6 days of initial exposure. The dose should be increased to 0.50 mL/kg for immunocompromised persons. The maximum dose in all cases is 15 mL.[206,207] Infants younger than 5 to 6 months of age usually have partial or complete immunity to measles as a result of passive maternal antibody. However, infants whose mothers develop measles are not protected by maternal antibody and should receive IMIG. IMIG is not indicated for household contacts who have received at least one dose of measles vaccine at 12 months of age or older unless they are immunocompromised. Persons who receive IMIG and do not develop clinical measles should receive measles vaccine 5 to 6 months later (depending on the dose administered), as long as the patient is at least 12 months of age and there are no contraindications to vaccination.[207,346]

All persons with HIV infection (and children of unknown infection status born to HIV-infected women) who are exposed to wild-type measles should receive IMIG (0.5 mL/kg, maximum dose 15 mL), regardless of their immunization status.[347] An exception is the patient receiving intravenous immune globulin (IVIG) therapy of at least 100 mg/kg within 3 weeks prior to exposure.[207] IVIG is commonly used in immunocompromised patients with primary immunodeficiency, HIV infection, or B-cell chronic lymphocytic leukemia. Although IVIG is not licensed for measles prophylaxis in exposed patients, IVIG preparations meet the same minimum standard for measles antibody titers as do IMIG preparations.[346] Taking into account the relative protein concentrations, an IVIG dose of 82.5 mg/kg would have roughly the same amount of measles antibody as the recommended 0.5 mL/kg of IMIG for immunocompromised patients.[346] Therefore, the IVIG doses commonly used (100 to 400 mg/kg) for immunocompromised patients should be sufficient to prevent measles.

Active Immunization

Vaccine Strains

Origin and Development

After the isolation and propagation of measles virus in tissue culture by Enders and Peebles[9] in 1954, vaccine development, testing, and licensure quickly followed.[12–22] The Edmonston strain, named after the youth from whom the virus was isolated, was used for many of the vaccines developed worldwide[348–365] (Fig. 19–3). To make the now-famous Edmonston B vaccine, Enders and colleagues[13,20,239] further passaged the Edmonston strain at 35°C to 36°C (95°F to 96.8°F) 24 times in primary kidney cells and 28 times in primary human amnion cells, adapted it to chicken embryos (6 passages), and then passaged it in chicken embryo cells. This attenuated Edmonston B vaccine was licensed in the United States in March 1963 along with another Edmonston B virus strain that had been adapted to primary dog kidney cells.[366–368] Although the administration of the Edmonston B vaccine was associated with a high rate of fever (temperature of 39.4°C [103°F] or higher; 20% to 40%) and rash (approximately 50%), the recipients remained remarkably well. However, simultaneous administration of a small dose of IG (eventually set at 0.02 mL/kg) reduced the occurrence of high fever and rash by approximately 50%[257,351,354,355,366,367,369–374] (Fig. 19–4). Approximately 18.9 million doses of Edmonston B vaccine were administered in the United States between 1963 and 1975 (Table 19–2 and Fig. 19–5).

Killed Vaccine

A formalin-inactivated, alum-precipitated vaccine derived from the Edmonston strain was also licensed in the United States in 1963 and used until 1967 (see Table 19–2). This vaccine was also used in some provinces in Canada. Usually, three doses of killed vaccine or two doses of killed and one dose of live vaccine were administered at monthly intervals with few side effects.[65,257,351,354,375–382] Use of killed vaccine was eventually not recommended when it became apparent that this vaccine produced short-lived immunity and placed many recipients at risk for atypical measles infection.[383] It has been estimated that between 600,000 and 900,000 persons in the United States received the 1.8 million doses of killed measles vaccine that were administered[384] (see Table 19–2 and Fig. 19–5).

Further Attenuated Live Vaccines

Many further attenuated vaccines have been developed and are in active use worldwide (Table 19–3; see Fig. 19–3). Most were derived from the Edmonston strain. These further attenuated vaccines differ in the viral isolate of origin, the number and temperature of cell culture passages, the type of cell culture used for the passage and production, and

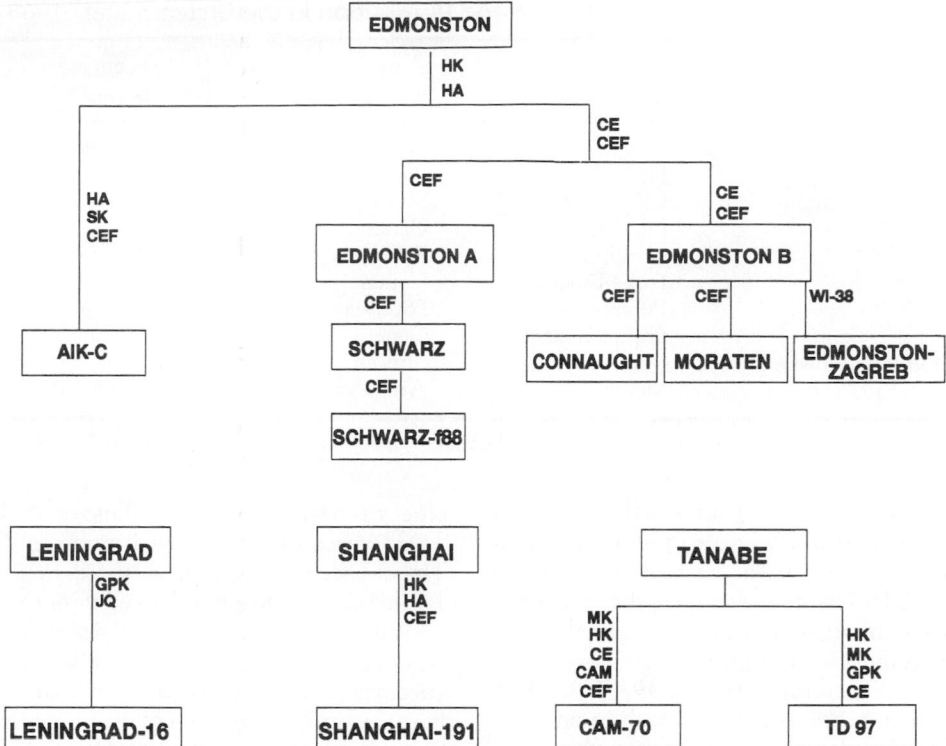

FIGURE 19–3 ■ Attenuation history of selected measles vaccine strains. Cell cultures in which strains were passed during attenuation: CAM, chick chorioallantoic membrane; CE, chick embryo intra-amniotic cavity; CEF, chick embryo fibroblast; GPK, guinea pig kidney; HA, human amnion; HK, human kidney; JQ, Japanese quail; MK, monkey kidney; SK, sheep kidney; WI-38, human diploid cell line.

whether plaquings were performed during the passages.[13,20,357,361,362,365,385] Although differences in plaque size,[357,386] subgenomic particles,[387] temperature sensitivity,[388] and pathogenicity in severe combined immune-deficient mice containing human thymic tissue implants[389] have been described among the further attenuated vaccine strains, their significance is uncertain.

Nucleotide sequence analysis of the F, H, N, and M genes showed no more than 0.6% variability among vaccine strains derived from the Edmonston strain.[223] Mori et al.[388] sequenced the entire genome of the AIK-C vaccine and found only 56 nucleotide differences, from a total of 15,894 bases, compared with the Edmonston sequence. More divergent sequences were found in the non–Edmonston-derived vaccines, CAM-70 and S-191, confirming the independent origin of these vaccines. However, all the vaccine strains, whether derived from Edmonston or from other wild-type viruses, are members of the same genotype, genotype A.[223,230]

Studies have identified nucleotide sequence substitutions in the H gene that appear to mediate some of the biologic characteristics of the Moraten strain of vaccine.[390] Comparison of the noncoding regions of a low-passage Edmonston wild-type strain and five Edmonston vaccine viruses found 21 nucleotide positions at which the wild type and one or more of the vaccine types differed. Five nucleotide substitutions were conserved in all of the vaccine strains. Comparison of protein-encoding nucleotide sequences of the N, P, M, F, H, and L genes of these vaccine strains with Edmonston wild-type virus identified amino acid substitutions in each of the genes; however, the overall level of heterogeneity did not exceed 0.3%.[214,215] The role

that these sequence differences in both the coding and non-coding regions of the genome play in attenuation of measles viruses remains to be evaluated using recently developed reverse genetics systems.[391]

Two further attenuated live measles vaccines derived from the Edmonston strain were licensed in the United States, the Schwarz strain in 1965 and the Moraten strain in 1968 (see Table 19–2 and Fig. 19–3). The Schwarz vaccine was derived from Edmonston virus passaged an addi-

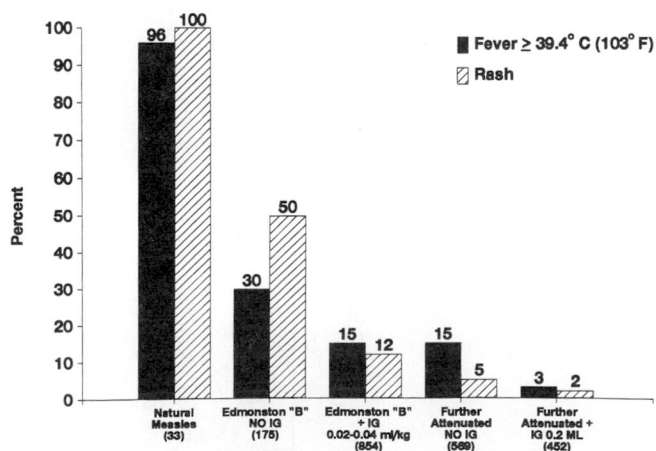

FIGURE 19–4 ■ Incidence of fever and rash after natural measles infection and vaccination. Number of susceptibles is included in parentheses; IG, immune globulin. (Adapted from Krugman S, Giles JP, Jacobs AM, Friedman H. Studies with a further attenuated live measles-virus vaccine. Pediatrics 31:919–928, 1963.)

TABLE 19–2 ■ History of Measles Vaccine Manufacture and Distribution in the United States, 1963 to 2001

Vaccine	Strain	Manufacturer	Brand	Years in Use	Doses Distributed
Inactivated	—	Lilly	Generic	1963–1967	1.8 million
		Pfizer	Pfizer Vax, Measles-K		
Live, attenuated	Edmonston B	Lederle	M-Vac	1963–1975	18.9 million
		Lilly	Generic		
		Merck	Rubeovax		
		Parke Davis	Generic		
		Pfizer	Pfizer-vax, Measles-L		
		Philips Roxane	Generic		
Live, further attenuated	Schwarz	Pitman Moore–Dow	Lirugen	1965–1976	>255 million
	Moraten	Merck	Attenuvax	1968 to 2001	

Adapted from Hayden GF. Measles vaccine failure: a survey of causes and means of prevention. Clin Pediatr 18:155–167, 1979.

tional 85 times at 32°C (89.6°F) in chicken embryo cells.[392-395] The Moraten strain was also passaged at this lower temperature, but only an additional 40 times.[396] Compared with the Edmonston B vaccine, the frequency and severity of side effects attributed to these and other further attenuated vaccines were significantly lower[257,351,356,392-397] (see Fig. 19–4). A temperature of 39.4°C (103°F) or higher occurred in only 5% to 15% and rash in only 3% to 5% of vaccinees. Simultaneous administration of specially titered IG in a low dose (0.02, 0.1, or 0.2 mL/kg) further reduced the incidence of high fever and rash to approximately 3% each[257] (see Fig. 19–4). These doses of IG did not interfere with seroconversion, but the peak geometric mean antibody titer was lower than that observed without IG administration. The further attenuated vaccines were intended for use without IG.[398]

The Moraten vaccine (Attenuvax, Merck) is now the only measles vaccine used in the United States; the Schwarz vaccine is the predominant product in many other nations.[360] Several different further attenuated measles vaccines, including AIK-C, Schwarz F88, CAM-70, and TD97, have been developed and are being used in Japan.[361,362,365,385] The vaccine developed by Smorodintsev (Leningrad-16) was introduced in Russia in 1967 and was the principal vaccine virus strain in eastern Europe.[358] The CAM-70 and TD97 vaccines were derived from the Tanabe strain.[365,385] These vaccines, as well as those in use in China since 1965,[363] are the few not derived from the Edmonston virus.

Whereas most measles vaccines were attenuated and are produced in chick embryo fibroblasts, a few currently used vaccines were attenuated in human diploid cells. The Edmonston-Zagreb vaccine, used extensively in Yugoslavia since 1969, was derived from the Edmonston strain and underwent additional passage in WI-38 cells.[357] This vaccine is now produced by several other manufacturers (see Table 19–3). Other vaccine strains have been adapted to MRC-5 and R-17 human diploid cells in Iran[359,364] and in China.[363]

Dosage and Route of Administration

According to current regulations in the United States, measles vaccine must contain at least 1000 median tissue culture infective doses ($TCID_{50}$) at the end of the expiration date of the vaccine.[399] This amount is administered in a 0.5-mL dose. The minimum dose required to immunize a seronegative child has been found to be as low as 20 $TCID_{50}$ in some studies but higher in others.[400-403] The dose in the

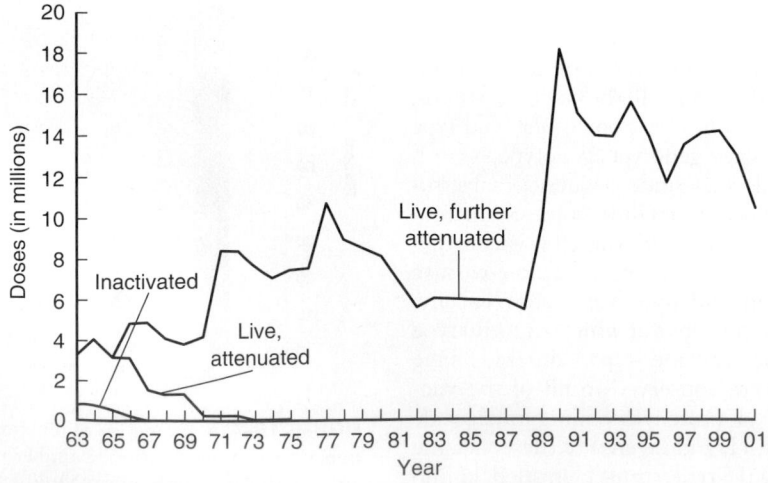

FIGURE 19–5 ■ Doses of measles virus vaccine distributed, by vaccine type, United States, 1963 to 2001. Live, attenuated is the Edmonston B strain; live, further attenuated is the Schwarz and Moraten strains combined.

TABLE 19–3 ■ Measles Vaccine Manufacturers and Vaccine Strains Produced

Manufacturer	Vaccine Strain
Merck (United States)	Moraten
RIVM (Netherlands)	Moraten
Aventis Pasteur (Canada)	Connaught
National Institute of Health (Pakistan)	Connaught
Glaxo-Smith-Kline (Belgium)	Schwarz
Aventis-Pasteur (France)	Schwarz
Chiron (Italy)	Schwarz
Sevapharma (Czech Republic)	Schwarz
Cantacuzino Institute (Romania)	Schwarz
Takeda Chemical Industries, Ltd (Japan)	Schwarz F88
Berna Biotech (Switzerland)	Edmonston-Zagreb
Serum Institute of India	Edmonston-Zagreb
Institute of Immunology (Croatia)	Edmonston-Zagreb
Birmex (Mexico)	Edmonston-Zagreb*
Research Foundation for Microbial Diseases (Japan)	CAM-70
BioManguinhos (Brazil)	CAM-70
Perum BioFarma (Indonesia)	CAM-70
The Kitasato Institute (Japan)	AIK-C
The Razi State Serum Institute (Iran)	AIK-HDC†/ Schwarz (a composite)
Chiba-Serum (Japan)	TD97
VECTOR (Russia)	Leningrad-16
National Vaccine and Serum Institute (China)	Shanghai-191
Lanzhou Institute of Biological Products (China)	Shanghai-191
Shanghai Institute of Biological Products (China)	Shanghai 191

*Not in production (as of September 2002).
†AIK-C vaccine produced on human diploid cells.

commercial product is designed to compensate for some of the virus deterioration that may result either from improper storage or reconstitution or from exposure to light or heat before injection.

The recommended route of administration is subcutaneous injection. Although there are only limited data on the intramuscular route, it appears to be as effective as subcutaneous vaccination.[404] Studies with the Edmonston B and further attenuated vaccines have examined the effectiveness of other routes of administration, such as intranasal and conjunctival inoculation.[12,16,49,243,366,367,405–407] Most of the results were not favorable. In contrast, aerosol administration, which was evaluated during the early 1960s and 1970s in Japan, the former Soviet Union, and the United States, showed promising results.[407] During the 1980s, studies were undertaken to determine whether aerosol administration of measles vaccine could overcome maternal antibody and immunize younger infants.[407–412] Many of these studies have found the Edmonston-Zagreb vaccine strain to be more immunogenic than the Schwarz strain when it is administered by aerosol.[413] However, whereas some investigators reported high seroconversion rates after administration by this route in young infants,[408–410,412] others found it inferior to subcutaneous administration.[411]

More recently, aerosol administration of measles vaccine in South Africa[414] and of combined measles and rubella vaccines in Mexico[415] resulted in boosting of antibody responses among schoolchildren. These studies have led to enthusiasm about the possible use of aerosol administration as a less invasive alternative to needle-and-syringe administration during mass vaccination campaigns, especially among schoolchildren. However, data on the primary immune response following aerosol vaccination as well as safety among naïve preschool-age children are limited. The challenge remains to demonstrate immunization safety with this new approach and license an aerosol device together with an existing measles vaccine strain. The WHO has formed a Product Development Group to test and bring to licensure such a product before 2009.[416]

Combination with Rubella and Mumps Vaccines

In the United States, vaccination against measles is most often accomplished with combined live vaccines that also contain attenuated rubella and mumps vaccine viruses. Such combined vaccines were licensed in the United States in 1971. They contain at least 1000 $TCID_{50}$ of the measles Moraten strain, at least 5000 $TCID_{50}$ of the mumps Jeryl Lynn strain, and at least 1000 $TCID_{50}$ of the RA27/3 strain of rubella vaccine virus. The RA27/3 strain of rubella virus replaced the HPV-77:DE-5 strain as the rubella component in 1979. Currently, the only licensed MMR vaccine is produced by Merck & Company (M-M-R II). Measles vaccine is also available in a measles-rubella formulation (M-R-VAX II; Merck). More combination products have been developed as other countries began vaccinating children against rubella or mumps along with measles.[32–35,38,417,418] For example, GlaxoSmithKline produces a vaccine that contains Schwarz measles vaccine, RIT 4385 mumps vaccine strain (derived from the Jeryl Lynn strain), and the RA27/3 strain of rubella vaccine. GlaxoSmithKline also produces a combined vaccine that contains the Schwarz measles vaccine, the Urabe mumps vaccine, and the RA27/3 rubella vaccine. Aventis-Pasteur produces a combined formulation with Schwarz measles vaccine, Urabe mumps vaccine, and RA27/3 rubella vaccine. In Japan, several formulations of combined vaccines are available, including one containing the AIK-C measles virus, the Hoshino mumps virus, and the Takahashi rubella virus strains.[419] Two other combined vaccines are also licensed, one containing the CAM-70 measles strain and one the Schwarz F88 strain. The MMR vaccine containing the Urabe mumps strain is no longer being produced in Japan. A triple vaccine with the Edmonston-Zagreb strain of measles vaccine is being produced by the Institute of Immunology, Zagreb,[420] Berna Biotec (formerly Swiss Serum Institute),[421] and the Serum Institute of India (Leningrad-Zagreb mumps strain and RA27/3 rubella strain).

Safety and immunogenicity data indicate that combining the measles antigen with rubella and mumps antigens is both safe and effective.[417–438]

Production and Constitution of Vaccine

Preparation methods for the Merck vaccine provide generally applicable information regarding the production and constitution of measles vaccines.[439] Although there are minor differences in dose, antibiotic content, and other details among manufacturers, there are no reports of significant differences in side effects or vaccine efficacy.

The vaccine virus is cultured in primary chick embryo cells. After an initial cell growth phase, the cultures are inoculated with the further attenuated Moraten strain of measles virus. After several days' incubation at 32°C (89.6°F), the cells are washed to remove fetal bovine serum and the medium is replaced with one containing 50 μg/mL of neomycin, sucrose, buffered salts, amino acids, and human albumin. Fluids containing virus can be removed from the cultures for a period of time as the cells are maintained at the same temperature. These fluids are frozen until determinations of the virus titer have been performed on retained aliquots. Harvested virus fluids having sufficient virus potency and satisfactorily passing tests are thawed, pooled, sampled for safety testing, clarified, dispensed, and refrozen.

When bulk vaccine has passed all quality control tests, portions of the vaccine are thawed, dispensed into vials, and lyophilized. At the time of use, the vaccine is reconstituted with fluid (sterile distilled water) provided by the manufacturer. A preservative-containing reconstitution fluid is not recommended for general use because it may inactivate the vaccine. Each vaccine dose contains approximately 25 μg of neomycin. Sorbitol and hydrolyzed gelatin are added as stabilizers. When reconstituted with the provided diluent, the vaccine is clear and yellow in color.

In 1996, the existence of reverse transcriptase in several vaccines that were grown in chick embryo fibroblast tissue culture was reported, including measles vaccine,[440] by use of a new and highly sensitive technique to detect the reverse transcriptase activity. With use of similar assays, other laboratories have confirmed the existence of the reverse transcriptase activity.[441] In subsequent studies, evidence was found that this reverse transcriptase activity is associated with the endogenous avian retrovirus EAV-0[442] and endogenous avian leukosis viruses ALV-E.[443] Extensive efforts to identify a transmissible virus have failed to link the reverse transcriptase activity with a transmissible virus. A study of 206 recipients of combined MMR vaccine found no evidence of infection with either avian leukosis virus or endogenous avian retrovirus.[444] These findings and the fact that transmission of retroviruses across disparate species may be restricted,[445] indicate no apparent risk to vaccine recipients.

Stability of Vaccine

Measles vaccine is extremely stable between −70°C (−94°F) and −20°C (−4°F).[405,446] Although measles vaccine is affected adversely by higher temperatures, the introduction of more heat-stable vaccines in 1979 has led to increased stability under normal working conditions, which is especially important in the developing world.[447] In the United States, manufacturers must demonstrate that a minimum titer of 1000 TCID$_{50}$ is maintained at the end of the dating period when the vaccine is stored at 2°C to 8°C. The WHO has a requirement that lyophilized measles vaccine, after exposure to 37°C for at least 1 week, cannot lose more than 1 log$_{10}$ and must maintain a titer of at least 1000 TCID$_{50}$.[448]

For the currently available vaccine in the United States, when it is stored at 2°C to 8°C (35.6°F to 46.4°F), a mini-

mum titer of 1000 TCID$_{50}$ can be maintained in unreconstituted vaccine for 2 years or more. This potency can be maintained for 8 months at room temperature and 4 weeks at 37°C (98.6°F). Reconstituted vaccine loses 50% of its potency in 1 hour at 20°C to 25°C (68°F to 77°F) and almost all its potency when it is held at 37°C (98.6°F) for 1 hour. Vaccine is also sensitive to sunlight; however, colored glass vials further minimize loss of potency. Notwithstanding its improved thermostability, the vaccine still needs to be handled with care according to the recommendations of the manufacturer.

As stated in the package insert, Merck recommends that its product be shipped at a temperature of 10°C (50°F) or less and stored, before reconstitution, at 2°C to 8°C (35.6°F to 46.4°F) and protected from sunlight. After reconstitution, the product should be kept in a dark place at 2°C to 8°C (35.6°F to 46.4°F) and used within 8 hours.

Results of Vaccination

The Immune Response

The immune response after successful vaccination is similar in almost all respects to that noted after natural infection. Although the interval between vaccination and an immune response is a few days shorter than that observed after natural infection,[12,52] immunization induces both humoral[22,65,68,70,257] and cellular[74-76] immunity and the production of interferon.[449-451]

Laboratory evidence of immunity is most conveniently documented by use of antibody assays because tests for cell-mediated immunity are not standardized. However, even with antibody assays, results of studies on vaccine-induced immunity may vary depending on the sensitivity of the antibody assay used.[63-65,78,267-273,452-460] Although the presence of antibodies detected by HI, ELISA, or CF correlates with immunity, Nt antibodies are probably most important in clinical protection.[2,3,63,78,277]

IgG, IgM, and IgA antibodies can be detected in both serum and nasal secretions.[68,70,261,263,461] IgM antibody can be detected in the serum between 2 and 6 weeks (peak at 3 weeks) after vaccination and disappears soon thereafter.[261,263,462] Although only small amounts of IgA have been detected in serum, IgA is the predominant antibody found in nasal secretions.[68,70] Although detectable serum IgA and IgM antibodies are transient, IgG antibodies generally persist for many years. The antibody titers elicited by vaccination do decline over time (as do those induced by natural infection) and may become undetectable.[65,258,259,437,453,463-468] Vaccine-induced antibody titers are typically lower than those induced by natural infection. Vaccine-induced immunity is subject to boosting on challenge, by either vaccine or wild-type virus; likewise, similar boosting can be observed after natural infection.[63,65,258,259,394,461,465,466] Thus, as discussed in more detail later, immunization usually provides immunity as solid as that induced by natural infection.

Although many investigators have described the initial antibody response elicited by live measles vaccination, the studies by Krugman and colleagues[65,156,257-259] serve as an excellent example. Depending on the antibody assay used (CF, HI, or Nt), antibodies first appear between 12 (HI and

Nt) and 15 (CF) days and peak 21 to 28 days after vaccination. Although antibodies were detected in 95% or more of susceptible vaccinees, regardless of the vaccine strain, the CF geometric mean titer did vary by strain of vaccine (Table 19–4). The geometric mean titer for children 1 month after receipt of Edmonston B vaccine alone, Edmonston B vaccine plus IG, Schwarz vaccine, and Schwarz vaccine with IG were 1:208,[156] 1:96, 1:56, and 1:24 to 1:32, respectively.[257] The titer observed in 33 children 1 month after natural infection was 1:128.[257] Hilleman and colleagues[396] also noted a difference in the geometric mean titer by vaccine strain using the HI assay (Table 19–5). Although 98% or more of vaccinees seroconverted, the HI geometric mean antibody titer associated with the Edmonston B vaccine was 1:25, whereas that noted after vaccination with either the Schwarz or Moraten further attenuated strains was 1:16. Despite these differences in geometric mean antibody titer, receipt of these vaccines was associated with a markedly reduced risk of infection that did not decrease over time.[65,258,259]

Measles-specific cell-mediated immunity after live, attenuated vaccine has seldom been studied because of the lack of a simple in vitro assay. With the importance that cell-mediated immunity plays in natural infection,[58,177–180] it would seem that successful vaccination would stimulate such immunity. In studies that have been conducted, cell-mediated immune responses after live, attenuated vaccine appear to be similar to but less pronounced than those after natural infection.[177–180,469] For example, Gallagher and co-workers[76] reported that a positive lymphocyte stimulation index was noted in 9 of 9 subjects with natural immunity and in 10 of 16 vaccinees. More recently, Pabst and colleagues[470] found good correlation between antibody titers and lymphoproliferative responses in 124 children receiving their first dose of MMR. However, a study of the immune response to measles vaccination at 9 months of age among 55 Peruvian children found that 93% developed a humoral response and only 23% had lymphoproliferative responses.[471] Gans and co-workers[472] studied the ability of infants ages 6, 9, or 12 months to respond to measles vaccine and found that, unlike humoral responses, T-cell responses can be established despite the presence of passive antibodies. Ward and co-workers[473] studied revaccinated children and found good lymphoproliferative responses after revaccination, even

among those whose antibody titers dropped to low levels. It appears that both wild-type virus and vaccine infection result in a biphasic immune response, beginning with transient production of interleukin-2 and interferon-γ followed by more sustained production of interleukin-4. First, CD8+ T cells are activated, which are important for viral clearance. Later, beginning about the time of rash onset, CD4+ T cells are activated and are involved in antibody production.[58] These responses by the cell-mediated immune system correspond to an initial T-helper (Th) 1-type response with a shift to a Th2-type response.

Vaccination suppresses cell-mediated immune function (as does natural infection).[101,469,474–478] This manifests in vitro as suppression of lymphocyte stimulation or in vivo as suppression of cutaneous delayed hypersensitivity to various antigens. Fireman and colleagues[475] noted suppressed cellular immune function up to 4 weeks after administration of live vaccine. Suppression did not occur after receipt of killed vaccine. A study of Bangladeshi infants found that delayed-type hypersensitivity reactions to *Candida* antigen were significantly reduced at 6 weeks postvaccination.[479] Data suggest that this suppression is due to down-regulation of interleukin-12, which is needed for cell-mediated immunity.[480] Although there was concern initially that this temporary suppression of cellular immunity might be harmful, for example, in patients with unrecognized tuberculosis,[102] it is now clear that there is no such risk.[481,482]

One would assume that the presence of a rash after parenteral injection of vaccine would be associated with viremia. The generalized stimulation of T and B lymphocytes after vaccination also suggests viremia. Few studies documented viremia after vaccination. Early studies with the canine cell vaccine isolated vaccine virus from blood,[366–368] and, more recently, van Binnendijk and colleagues[483] have isolated Schwarz strain vaccine virus from monkeys 7 to 9 days after vaccination. There are no reports of isolation of vaccine virus from blood in normal humans.[12–14,19,49] Although Mitus and associates[170] did isolate vaccine virus from the throat and conjunctivae of a susceptible leukemic patient who died of giant cell pneumonia after administration of Edmonston B vaccine, they failed to isolate virus from the blood. The apparent difficulty of isolating vaccine virus may reflect the low level of viremia after vaccination.

TABLE 19–4 ▪ Antibody Response 21 to 28 Days After Measles Vaccination With or Without Immune Globulin[*]

Vaccination Regimen	Total Number	Seroconversion (%)	GMT[†]
Edmonston B Vaccine			
Alone	171	96	—
	27	—	1 : 208
Immune globulin, 0.02 mL/kg	185	99	1 : 96
Further Attenuated Vaccine[‡]			
Alone	121	99	1 : 56
Immune globulin, 0.1 mL total	89	95	1 : 32
Immune globulin, 0.2 mL total	452	98	1 : 32
Immune globulin, 0.02 mL/kg	193	95	1 : 24

[*]Neutralizing titer of 1:400/0.1 mL.
[†]Complement fixation assay geometric mean antibody titer.
[‡]Schwarz strain.
Adapted from Krugman S, Giles JP, Jacobs AM, Friedman H. Studies with live attenuated measles-virus vaccine. Am J Dis Child 103:353–363, 1962; and Krugman S, Giles JP, Jacobs AM, Friedman H. Studies with a further attenuated live measles-virus vaccine. Pediatrics 31:919–928, 1963.

TABLE 19–5 ■ Antibody Response 28 Days After Attenuated and Further Attenuated Measles Vaccine

Vaccine	Total Number	Seroconversion (%)	GMT
Edmonston B[†]	258	99	1 : 25
Schwarz[‡]	250	98	1 : 16
Moraten[‡]	273	98	1 : 16

[*]Hemagglutination-inhibition assay.
[†]Attenuated vaccine.
[‡]Further attenuated vaccine.
GMT, geometric mean antibody titer.
Adapted from Hilleman MR, Buynak EB, Weibel RE, et al. Development and evaluation of the Moraten measles virus vaccine. JAMA 206:587–590, 1968.

Because wild-type virus is so highly transmissible, both virologic and clinical studies with susceptible contacts were conducted in early vaccine investigations.[12,14–19,49,366,368] These studies showed no evidence of virus excretion by vaccinees. Measles vaccine virus was isolated from a throat swab taken from a 3-year-old boy who presented with fever only 12 days after vaccination with MMR vaccine.[484] This case report suggests that subcutaneous vaccination with live, attenuated measles virus can result in respiratory excretion of the vaccine virus. Person-to-person transmission of vaccine virus has never been documented.

Response to Revaccination

The immune response after revaccination depends on the results of the initial vaccination. Persons who had no response to initial vaccination typically generate a primary immune response to revaccination, with a significant rise in antibody titer and the production of IgM antibody. After revaccination of an individual with some level of immunity, a fourfold or greater rise in antibody may appear sooner than that seen after initial vaccination, but there are no signs of clinical infection.[65,258,259,261,263,459,460,467,485] IgG antibodies are first detected within 5 to 6 days and peak around 12 days. IgM antibodies are not produced. As is the case with immunity after natural infection, these are the characteristics of an anamnestic immune response.[260,262] Such a boost is more likely to occur in the presence of a low or undetectable pre-existing antibody titer, whereas persons with a high level of circulating antibody may not boost.[65,258,259,453,465–467,486] Krugman and co-workers[65] reported that, after revaccination, a significant increase in HI titer occurred in only 1 of 6 children with HI titers of 1:16 or 1:32 but in 25 of 36 children with titers of 1:8 or less. Similar findings were noted in vaccinees exposed to wild-type virus.

Boosting of antibody titers appears to be transient, with several investigators finding decay of antibody levels to the pre-revaccination level within months to years.[472,487–489] In one study, antibody titers against measles in children with low levels of antibody before revaccination decayed during a 6-month period after revaccination; however, cellular immunity, measured in a lymphocyte proliferation assay, appeared to persist.[473]

The booster phenomenon is not unique to vaccine-induced immunity. It can also be observed after exposure to measles or after vaccination in persons who have had measles, but it occurs less frequently because antibody titers after natural infection are usually higher than those after

vaccination.[63,65] Stokes and colleagues[63] reported that, on re-exposure to wild-type virus, 6 of 12 naturally immune persons with pre-exposure Nt titers ranging from 1:2 to 1:8 experienced a boost in titer. However, such boosts were not seen in any of 22 individuals with titers between 1:16 and 1:128. These data indicate that subclinical reinfection may occur after both natural infection and successful vaccination.

Studies of the response to revaccination[472,484,490–492] have shown that a high proportion of vaccinated persons who lack detectable antibody to measles will respond to the second dose. Among persons initially vaccinated after 12 months of age, at least 90% will respond.

Effectiveness of Protection

Measures of Protection

An individual's risk of measles is the product of his or her susceptibility to measles and risk of exposure to measles virus. Measles vaccine provides both *personal immunity* to prevent disease when exposed to measles virus and *population immunity* through decreased intensity of transmission as the proportion of immune persons in a population increases. The population immunity effect decreases the risk of measles among immunized as well as unimmunized persons.

The most direct method of measuring the personal immunity effect of measles vaccine would be to challenge vaccinees and controls with wild-type measles virus and document the clinical outcome. Such studies are not done in humans because of the harmful effects of exposure to measles virus. In studies in animals challenged with wild-type measles virus, vaccinated animals have significant decreases in clinical symptoms and measles virus replication compared to unvaccinated animals.[493] These studies are performed to evaluate the response to new vaccines in terms of clinical protection, reduced viral load, and development of serologic and cellular immunity.[483,494,495]

Because tests of cell-mediated immunity to measles are less widely available, antibody titers are most often used as evidence of protection from measles (i.e., as a *correlate of protection*). Despite the fact that any detectable level of measles antibody has been interpreted as evidence of protection after vaccination, the development of more sensitive antibody tests[268] has raised concerns that low levels of antibody[459] may not be protective. A school blood drive before a measles outbreak permitted correlation of pre-exposure measles antibody titers using the PRN test with the level of clinical protection.[496] Eight of nine students with low but detectable levels of measles antibody (PRN titer ≤120) developed typical measles, compared with none of 71 with pre-exposure PRN titers of greater than 120. Seven of 11 students with pre-exposure PRN titers of 216 to 874 had a fourfold or greater rise in antibody titer compared with none of 7 with a pre-exposure PRN titer of 1052 or greater, indicating that high titers were associated with protection against both infection and disease. Although it is likely that many persons with low antibody titers will not develop disease after exposure, available data suggest that these low levels of antibody may not be fully protective.

Protection also can be evaluated by examining the immune response of vaccinees challenged with vaccine virus through revaccination.[162,259,467,483,487,497,498] Such challenges most often result in an anamnestic immune response (see *Response to Revaccination* above).

The most commonly used method to quantify the protective effect of measles vaccine is to identify individuals with similar likelihood of exposure to measles virus and compare the attack rate of disease in unvaccinated and vaccinated persons. The decrease in attack rate among vaccinated compared to unvaccinated individuals is called *vaccine effectiveness* or *vaccine efficacy*.[499,500] (Refer to Chapter 56 for a more detailed discussion of this topic, including formulas and methods for calculating vaccine effectiveness.) In outbreak settings in which a high proportion of the population is vaccinated, the proportion of cases that are vaccinated will also be high, and it may appear erroneously that the vaccine effectiveness is low.[501,502] However, approximately 50% of cases can be expected to be vaccinated with vaccine efficacy and vaccine coverage each 90%.[499] This proportion increases to 60% with a 95% coverage rate. The majority of available data indicate vaccine effectiveness in the United States of 90% to 95% or greater,[503] consistent with seroconversion data.

Reduction in the occurrence of measles after the introduction of vaccine is a common measure of vaccine-induced protection at the population level. Both Krugman and colleagues[257] and Baba and co-workers[504] noted virtual elimination of measles from a population of institutionalized children after vaccination became routine, despite high levels of infection in the surrounding community. Similarly, nationwide surveillance in many countries with high levels of immunization has documented a significant reduction in reported measles cases following vaccine licensure.[23–42] For more examples of the impact of measles vaccination on measles incidence, see *Experiences with Measles Control and Elimination in Various Countries* later in this chapter.

Monitoring the reproductive rate, or *R* value, is another method of assessing the impact of vaccination on a population. The basic reproductive rate (R_0) is the average number of cases that would be expected to spread from a single case of measles in a completely susceptible population. Measles is a highly infectious disease, and R_0 has been estimated as 12.5 to 18.[505] The effective reproductive rate (R) incorporates the level of immunity in a population with the factors that determine R_0. In a completely susceptible population, $R = R_0$. In other populations, the difference between R and R_0 is the effect of population immunity. When R is greater than 1, the number of cases increases from one generation to the next and an epidemic begins. As the spread of disease increases immunity in the population,

R falls below 1, the number of cases decreases from one generation to the next, and the epidemic ends. To achieve interruption of endemic transmission of measles, it is necessary to achieve a level of population immunity that maintains *R* less than 1 (see Chapter 56). In the United States, assessment of the reproductive rates through surveillance data documented *R* less than 1 for the period from 1992 to 1999.[506] Recent analysis of vaccination programs in Western Europe found that four of eight countries had vaccine coverage sufficiently high to eventually eliminate measles.[507]

Host Factors Affecting Protection

The quality and durability of measles vaccine–induced immunity is dependent on a number of factors that relate both to the vaccine and to the host.[258,508] In considering factors affecting protection, it is important to distinguish between primary vaccine failure—that is, a failure to seroconvert after vaccination—and secondary vaccine failure—that is, loss of protection after demonstrated seroconversion.

MATERNAL ANTIBODY AND AGE AT VACCINATION

A number of host factors may be responsible for primary vaccine failure. The most important and well described is maternal antibody. Passively acquired measles antibodies may neutralize vaccine virus before a complete immune response develops. The most common sources of these antibodies are maternal transfer, IG, and other blood products. The presence of maternally derived transplacental antibody is particularly important in evaluating the immunogenicity of live measles vaccine in early childhood.[277,509]

As noted by Orenstein and colleagues,[509] recommendations for the age at vaccination must balance two factors: (1) the earliest age at which high rates of seroconversion can be obtained and (2) the age group with the greatest risk of severe infection. A balance must be met that optimizes vaccine-induced protection while minimizing the risk of morbidity and mortality that would occur by delaying vaccination.[277,332] The age at vaccination that achieves this balance is lower in developing countries than in developed nations because of the increased risk of measles exposure and because of earlier loss of maternally derived antibody. The reasons for the variation in duration of passive protection from maternal antibody include differences in (1) levels of measles antibody in mothers, (2) efficiency of transport of IgG across the placenta, and (3) rate of loss of passively acquired antibody by the infant.[277,510]

Early in the clinical investigations of live measles virus vaccine, it was recognized that maternal antibody interfered with seroconversion by in vivo neutralization of vaccine virus before adequate replication had occurred.[508] On the basis of data available at the time, it appeared that maternal antibody rarely persisted beyond 7 months of age and that an adequate immune response could be achieved if vaccination was limited to infants 9 months of age and older.[63,65,455,457,511] Whereas only 60% to 70% of infants younger than 9 months seroconverted, 95% or more of older infants produced antibodies.[22,509] Accordingly, when vaccine was licensed in 1963, the recommended age for routine vaccination was 9 months.[512]

In the first few years after licensure, it became apparent, however, that maternal antibodies actually persisted in many infants until 11 months of age.[65,454,455,458] On the basis of these data, vaccination before 1 year would be expected to be associated with a high risk of primary vaccine failure and subsequent infection in exposed vaccinees.[158,162, 457,513–516] Thus, in 1965, the recommended age for vaccination was raised to 12 months.[398] The importance of this change is illustrated by Krugman's data showing that only 86% of 123 infants 9 months of age seroconverted after administration of Edmonston B vaccine and IG, compared with 97% of 899 children vaccinated at 12 months of age or older.[517]

In 1965, it was also recommended that children vaccinated before 1 year of age be revaccinated because a large proportion of these children were susceptible and were expected to respond well to revaccination. A number of studies confirmed these findings,[467,513,514,518] but there are also some data indicating that early vaccination may alter the immune response after revaccination. Wilkins and Wehrle[457] first raised concerns by reporting that 19 (51.4%) of 37 children who did not respond when they were initially vaccinated at 6 to 10 months of age did not have detectable HI antibodies 8 months after revaccination. All 37 did, however, have detectable Nt antibody. Similarly, Linnemann and colleagues[519] reported that 29 (40.3%) of 72 children vaccinated before 10 months of age were HI negative at a mean of 4.8 years after revaccination. In contrast, Lampe and colleagues[498] did not find any difference in seroconversion rates in children vaccinated once at 15 months of age or later compared with children revaccinated after first being vaccinated before 1 year of age. Using an EIA assay, Murphy and colleagues[520] observed high seroprevalence rates at a mean of 6 months after vaccination in 302 children revaccinated after early vaccination and in 300 vaccinated once at 15 months of age or older (98% for both groups). However, they did observe that the titers in the revaccinated group were lower than those in the children vaccinated once. These findings were confirmed by McGraw.[404]

One of the most complete descriptions of an altered immune response is provided by Stetler and colleagues.[460] These authors reported that children revaccinated after an initial vaccination before 1 year had no difficulty seroconverting; post-revaccination HI antibody was detected in 116 (95.9%) of 121 children lacking HI antibody before revaccination. Eight months later, HI antibodies were undetectable in 58 (47.9%), but, after retesting with a cytopathic effect neutralization (CPEN) test, only 5 (4.2%) of 120 sera were negative. Successful priming in some of the early vaccinees was also suggested by the finding that IgM was detected in the sera of only 22.2% of 63 revaccinated children lacking HI, EIA, and CPEN antibody, compared with 74.0% of 50 random control vaccinees. These findings were similar to those noted by Black and co-workers.[497]

Although there may be some alteration of the immune response, the most reliable indicator of the actual effectiveness of revaccination of these children is the evaluation of their risk of infection. Although revaccination may not be 100% effective, available data indicate that revaccination is efficacious.[514,518] Shasby and colleagues[513] reported that, in an outbreak, the attack rate in 73 children vaccinated once before 12 months of age was 35.6%, whereas the attack rate in 55 children revaccinated after 12 months of age was only

1.8%. Davis and co-workers[518] noted that none of 80 students revaccinated after their first vaccination before 12 months of age became infected during an outbreak. For comparison, the attack rate in children vaccinated twice at 12 months of age or older was 1.4% (2 of 138), that in children vaccinated once at 12 months of age or older was 1.8% (21 of 1191), and that in unvaccinated children was 57.1% (4 of 7). Hutchins and colleagues reported a vaccine effectiveness of 99.5% for children vaccinated with a first dose at age 6 to 11 months and a second dose after age 12 months.[521] Thus the available data indicate that revaccination of children first vaccinated before 1 year of age will result in good vaccine-induced protection, although it may be associated with an altered immune response, manifested as a lower antibody titer. This conclusion is especially important because vaccination of children as young as 6 months, with subsequent revaccination, is recommended in certain outbreak situations.[206,207]

The recommended age at vaccination was again changed in 1976 from 12 months to 15 months because newer data indicated that children vaccinated at 15 months of age and older were even more likely to make and maintain antibodies and were less likely to be infected in outbreak situations than those children vaccinated earlier.[509] Although some studies provide contrary results, examination of data on seroconversion rates and prevalence of antibodies after vaccination indicates that, in general, 79% to 89% of children vaccinated at 12 months of age have detectable antibodies, compared with 87% to 99% of those vaccinated at 15 months or later.[454–456,458,509,513,522–524] Similarly, a number of studies measuring the risk of measles in vaccinated and unvaccinated children indicated that measles occurred in children vaccinated at 12 months of age approximately 1.5 to 5.0 times more frequently than in those vaccinated later than 12 months.[509,513,516,525–528]

Data on measles antibody titers in umbilical cord blood and in infants suggested that infants whose mothers have vaccine-induced immunity may be receiving less maternal antibody than infants whose mothers had natural measles.[470,524,529–531] Many mothers born in the vaccine era have antibodies induced by vaccination, which typically results in lower titers than does measles disease. Also, an increased proportion of mothers born since the introduction of measles vaccine may not have any measles antibodies because they have not had measles or been vaccinated. In 1998, over 87% of women giving birth in the United States were born after 1963, the year measles vaccine was licensed.[532] In a national serologic survey, Hutchins and colleagues noted a 19% seronegativity rate among women born between 1967 and 1976.[533]

Infants whose mothers were born in the vaccine era are susceptible to disease at a younger age and are more likely to respond to vaccination at an early age. In a 1992 cohort study in the United States, Papania and co-workers documented a greater than 2.5 relative risk of measles among infants whose mothers were born in the vaccine era compared to infants whose mothers were born before 1963.[534] Higher rates of seroconversion at 12 months also have been found in children born to women with vaccine-induced immunity (SC Redd, GE King, J Nordin, et al., Centers for Disease Control and Prevention [CDC], unpublished data, 1994).[529,531] Based on these findings, in 1994, the age of vaccination in the United States was changed again to be between 12 and 15 months.[207]

Factors that alter the efficiency of transport of IgG across the placenta also can affect the amount of antibody infants receive. Maternal measles antibody is transferred across the placenta from mother to infant via an active transport system, which results in a higher antibody titer in the infant than the mother. Because the majority of the maternal measles antibody transfer occurs late in the third trimester, infants born prematurely often have low antibody titers.[535] Several diseases that affect the mother, most importantly malaria and HIV infection, have been shown to decrease the placental transfer of maternal measles antibody and result in lower infant titers.[536,537]

Because infants in developing countries may lose maternal measles antibody at an early age and may be exposed to measles virus at an early age as a result of intense transmission, the WHO recommendations indicate that 9 months is the most appropriate age for delivery of the first dose of measles vaccine in most developing countries.[538] In addition to receiving less maternal antibody, and becoming susceptible to measles at an earlier age, infants of HIV-infected mothers may be less likely to respond to vaccination at an older age if they become HIV infected. Therefore, the WHO recommends that infants of HIV-infected mothers should routinely be vaccinated against measles at 6 months of age, with a follow-up dose given after 9 months of age.[539]

Two studies of the immunogenicity of measles vaccine found that, even in the absence of detectable maternal measles antibody, infants age 6 months had lower seroconversion rates and lower geometric mean antibody titers compared with older infants or toddlers. These findings suggest age-related maturation during the first year of life in the humoral immune response to measles vaccine unrelated to passively transferred maternal antibody.[540,541]

INTERCURRENT ILLNESS AND MALNUTRITION

There is a theoretical concern that interferon produced by an intercurrent infection may interfere with successful vaccination.[466,542] Studies addressing this question, which have been conducted in developing and in developed countries, have produced discordant results. Two studies in developing countries found no differences in seroconversion rates in ill and well children after receipt of measles vaccine.[333,543] However, a small study in the United States found that 80% of children with rhinorrhea seroconverted, compared with 98% of well children.[544] Subsequent studies conducted in the United States and Canada have found equivalent seroconversion rates among children with upper respiratory infections or mild illness and well children.[545-547] In a study of 128 mildly ill and 258 well children given MMR, seroconversion to measles was 97% in well children compared with 99% in those with mild illnesses, mostly upper respiratory tract infection[547]; no differences were observed in seroconversion to mumps or rubella. A study conducted in Wisconsin found no association of vaccine failure and vaccination during the high-risk season for respiratory infections.[548] One study conducted in Thailand found lower geometric mean antibody titers for children vaccinated at 9 months of age among those who experienced an upper respiratory

tract infection in the 2 weeks after vaccination.[549] However, vaccination of mildly ill children and vaccination during the upper respiratory infection season appear to outweigh the theoretical risk of lower seroconversion rates.[550] Several studies have found seroconversion rates in malnourished children similar to those in children who are well nourished.[332,551,552]

IMMUNOSUPPRESSION AND HIV INFECTION

Measles vaccination is not recommended for most immunocompromised patients, and as a result few data are available on the immune response in such patients. However, the increasing number of children with HIV infection, the high risk of severe measles in these children, and few demonstrated side effects to measles vaccine have resulted in recommendations for vaccination. Studies in the United States have found that HIV-infected children have poor responses to vaccination, lose antibody more quickly after vaccination, and respond poorly to revaccination.[173,546,553-555] Retrospective studies have found that only 12% of 24[173] and 59% of 37[554] vaccinated children with HIV infection had detectable measles antibody. Seroconversion rates in prospective studies range from 33% of 39 children to 60% of 25 children.[184,553] In the Democratic Republic of Congo (formerly Zaire), seroconversion rates after vaccination at 9 months were 77% in asymptomatic HIV-infected children and 36% in symptomatic HIV-infected children (36%).[556] In two other studies in Africa, seroconversion rates after vaccination at 6 months were greater than 75% in HIV-infected children.[557,558] A study in Thailand found that, by age 9 months, 100% of 30 infants of HIV-infected mothers had lost their maternally acquired antibodies and that, by 12 weeks postvaccination, HIV-positive infants had lower seroconversion and median antibody levels when compared with HIV-negative infants.[559] HIV-infected children may respond better when they are vaccinated at earlier ages, before they become severely immunocompromised.[560] This point is illustrated by a case report of an HIV-infected boy with evidence of moderate immunosuppression who developed fever, diarrhea, and rash following vaccination with MMR vaccine at age 14 months.[561] Serum collected 13 days after vaccination was measles IgM positive, IgG negative, and measles PCR positive, with genomic sequencing indicating vaccine strain. Follow-up serum showed good IgG seroconversion.

Adults who were vaccinated in childhood before becoming infected with HIV appear to retain protective levels of measles antibody. High seroprevalence of measles antibody in HIV-infected adults in the United States has been documented,[562] and antibody levels are maintained, even as immunosuppression progresses.

VITAMIN A SUPPLEMENTATION

Investigators in Indonesia found a lower rate of seroconversion among children vaccinated at 6 months of age who received supplementary vitamin A compared with children not receiving such a supplement.[563] Subsequent studies conducted in Guinea-Bissau, India, and West Java found similar rates of seroconversion among 9-month-old children receiving and not receiving vitamin A supplements.[564-566] Among malnourished children in the Indian study, the postvaccination geometric mean antibody titer was significantly higher in the group receiving vitamin A compared with the placebo group.[565] A large multicenter clinical trial confirmed the safety of vitamin A supplementation administered with routine immunizations at 6, 10, and 14 weeks of age and at 9 months with measles immunization.[567] The balance of evidence supports the WHO recommendation that, in vitamin A–deficient countries, infants should receive a vitamin A supplement at the time of measles immunization.[568]

OTHER HOST FACTORS

Even after receipt of potent vaccine, approximately 2% to 5% of vaccinees will fail to respond for unknown reasons.[22,65,257] Studies of genetic factors have found associations with particular human lymphocyte antigen (HLA) types and nonresponse (HLA-B8, -B13, -B44, and -C5) or hyper-response (HLA-B7 and -B51) to measles vaccination.[569,570] The same investigators also found an association between homozygosity for class I and class II HLA alleles and poor response to measles vaccination.[571] Together these genetic factors appear to account for the majority of nonresponders.

Although there may be some exceptions in the very young,[404,457,460,497] revaccination has been found in both epidemiologic and serologic studies to induce the same high rate of immune response that follows initial vaccination.[459,467,490–492,513,514,519]

Vaccine Factors Affecting Protection

VACCINE ANTIGEN AND STRAIN

Although most further attenuated measles vaccines have been found to be equally immunogenic in older children,[396,408] differences in the ability of vaccine strains to immunize young infants have been reported.[409,411,572–576] High measles morbidity and mortality among infants younger than the recommended age for vaccination (9 months) in developing countries[577,578] has stimulated research on strategies for immunization of younger infants. Sabin and associates in the early 1980s investigated aerosol administration of two measles vaccines, the Edmonston-Zagreb and Schwarz strains.[408,409] Their finding of higher seroconversion rates after Edmonston-Zagreb than after Schwarz vaccine focused attention on this vaccine strain. Several subsequent studies found that the Edmonston-Zagreb strain was more immunogenic than the Schwarz vaccine in this age group. The AIK-C strain of measles vaccine also has been found to be highly immunogenic in young infants and, in some studies, more immunogenic than either Schwarz or Edmonston-Zagreb vaccines.[579–581] The reasons for these differences are not known.

VACCINE DOSE

Small doses of vaccine can effectively immunize older infants and children; however, the dose of vaccine administered has been shown to be important in immunizing young infants.[572,573,575] Increasing the Edmonston-Zagreb vaccine dose from 10,000 to 40,000 plaque-forming units (PFU) in The Gambia resulted in an increase in response rate from 73% to 100% in 4- to 6-month-old infants.[577] In Mexico, serologic response to vaccination of 6-month-olds increased for both Schwarz (66% to 91%) and Edmonston-Zagreb

(92% to 98%) vaccines, with a 100-fold increase in dose[573]; the effect was greater for Schwarz than for Edmonston-Zagreb vaccine. Because of these data and interest in a vaccination strategy for children younger than 1 year in developing countries, in 1990 the WHO recommended that a higher dose (initially defined as >100,000 PFU and later changed to >50,000 PFU) Edmonston-Zagreb vaccine be administered at 6 months of age in areas where measles mortality in young infants was a major health problem.[582,583] However, problems with vaccine availability resulted in little use of the vaccine on a large scale. Questions have been raised regarding the safety of high-dose measles vaccine, with a higher mortality rate in girls in several developing countries who received high-titer vaccines at 5 to 6 months of age compared with those who received standard-titer vaccines at 9 to 10 months.[584,585] Increased mortality rates after vaccination with a high-titer vaccine were not observed in developed countries or in countries with an infant mortality rate below 100 per 1000 births.[586] High-titer measles vaccines are not currently recommended.[587]

VACCINE HANDLING

Primary vaccine failures with live vaccine have stemmed from improper handling. Loss of potency of live vaccines can result from poor shipping or storage practices.[588,589] Although administration of impotent vaccine had previously been implicated in outbreaks of measles in vaccinated persons, the likelihood of this occurring now has been greatly reduced by the addition in 1979 of the new stabilizers discussed previously.[402,446]

Persistence of Immunity

The majority of data suggest that a dose of live vaccine properly administered to an appropriate host that results in seroconversion will afford lifelong protection to nearly all vaccinees.[590] The duration of vaccine-induced immunity has been documented by studying the persistence of measurable antibody, the clinical characteristics and serologic response of measles cases in vaccinated persons, the effects of vaccine challenge, and the attack rate in vaccinees as a function of the time since vaccination.

Although vaccine-induced antibody titers are lower than those achieved after natural infection, this difference does not appear to be biologically significant. Serologic studies limited to children vaccinated at 12 months of age or older indicate that, although antibody titers do decline over time, detectable antibodies are present in most vaccinees.[65,258,259,437,452,453,456,459,461,463–465,591] Because titers can fall to levels undetectable with some assays, the test used is important in the assessment of immune status. Furthermore, many individuals lacking detectable antibody manifest a secondary immune response on revaccination or exposure to wild-type virus, indicating persistence of some level of immunity.[266]

Krugman[65,258,259] followed the serologic status of a population of institutionalized children for 16 years. The HI geometric mean antibody titer in 70 individuals who received further attenuated vaccine was 1:333 at 1 month but, in the absence of exposure, had fallen to 1:6 after 16 years[259] (Fig. 19–6). Thirteen percent had a HI titer of 1:4, 10% had a titer of 1:2, and 13% had no detectable antibody. In con-

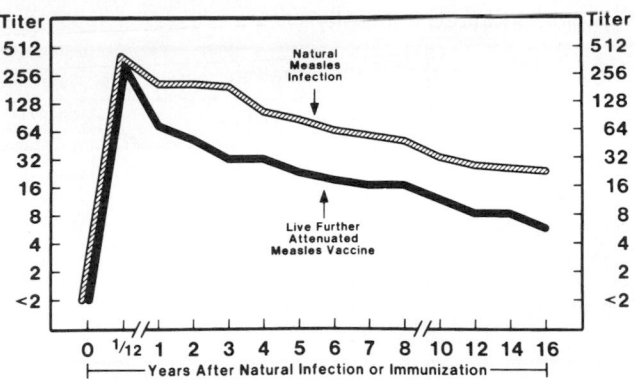

FIGURE 19–6 ■ Measles geometric mean hemagglutination-inhibition antibody titers after natural infection and immunization with live, further attenuated vaccine. (Courtesy of S. Krugman.)

trast, whereas 47 naturally infected children had a comparable 1-month HI geometric mean antibody titer of 1:410, 16 years after disease the geometric mean titer was 1:22 (see Fig. 19–6). Only 4% had a HI titer of 1:2, and none had undetectable antibodies. Sixteen sera with HI titers ranging from below 1:2 to 1:4, obtained from persons vaccinated 6 to 15 years earlier, were retested with the more sensitive PRN assay[268]; the PRN titers ranged from 1:4 to 1:46.[259] Typical booster responses after revaccination of some of the HI-negative individuals were also found.

Dine and associates followed up adults vaccinated in a vaccine trial in the 1970s. The 56 participants, who were all seropositive by HI tests after vaccination, all had detectable measles antibody by PRN at least 26 years after vaccination.[592] PRN titers greater than 1:120 were found in 92% of the subjects, and the strongest predictor of lower titers was lower HI titers in the original study. None of the subjects had been revaccinated in the interim period, or had had measles or known exposure to measles. Fewer than five cases were reported annually from Cincinnati, the study setting, over the 12 years before the follow-up study began. Therefore, boosting of antibody titers from exposure to wild-type measles virus was unlikely to play a major role in sustaining antibody titers in most of the study subjects.

Seroprevalence studies also provide useful information about duration of immunity, but, because information on seroconversion is lacking, one cannot be sure whether persons are seronegative because of primary or secondary vaccine failure. In addition, sensitivity of the assay procedure is important. These variables account for some discrepancies in reported findings. For example, Bass and co-workers[453] reported that HI antibodies were detectable in 73% of 40 children more than 8 years after vaccination; however, 98% had Nt antibody. Orenstein and colleagues[437] reported that the seroprevalence among 1871 high-school students (10th, 11th, and 12th graders), 98.1% of whom had been vaccinated at 14 months of age or older and who had no history of measles, was 86.9% by an HI assay. However, 98.8% were positive with both the HI assay and the same PRN assay used in the Krugman study.[268] Orenstein and colleagues[459] further documented the specificity of the PRN assay by vaccinating HI-negative children. IgM was detected in 14 of 16 students with a PRN titer below 1:4 but in only 1 of 68 who were PRN positive.

Although live virus vaccine–induced immunity is accepted as durable, there have been case reports of measles in persons who had a previously documented seroconversion after vaccination, which indicates that secondary vaccine failure can occur.[165,167,593] Also, there have been reports of measles, or modified measles, occurring in vaccinees who had laboratory evidence of infection, although IgM was not detected, which suggests a secondary immune response.[160–164,166] A secondary immune response indicates a pre-existing level of immunity, although such reports are limited by the sensitivity of the assays used to detect IgM antibody. These studies also suggest that the clinical reinfection can be mild and may be more likely to occur in persons vaccinated at younger than 12 months. One study that provides data on the risk of clinical reinfection after vaccination was conducted in Canada; 5% (9 of 175) of persons who initially seroconverted after receipt of measles vaccine developed measles within 10 years of vaccination.[165] In this study, persons who developed measles had lower postvaccination titers than those who did not.

In epidemiologic studies of persons vaccinated with live measles vaccine at 12 months of age or older, some studies have shown that people with increased time since vaccination have slight increases in attack rates compared to those more recently vaccinated; however, none has yet documented a significant increase[513,514,516,518,526,594–596] (Table 19–6). During outbreaks, observed attack rates in persons vaccinated 15 years or more before infection have been on the order of 5% or less, and calculated vaccine efficacies have generally been 90% to 95% or greater. These results are consistent with the expected frequency of primary vaccine failure that occurs in everyday practice. Data from the United Kingdom, the United States, and other countries[328,590,591,597,598] have not found increases in vaccine failures with time since vaccination. With overall incidence of measles in the United States at record low levels and no evidence of increasing incidence among previously vaccinated persons, waning immunity does not appear to constitute a problem. Although secondary vaccine failures have been documented, taken collectively, the serologic and epidemiologic data during the past 35 years indicate that vaccine provides long-term immunity.

Combined Vaccines and Simultaneous Vaccination

Live measles vaccine has been administered successfully in combination or in conjunction with a variety of immunizing agents, such as yellow fever vaccine, poliovirus vaccine, diphtheria and tetanus toxoids and whole-cell pertussis vaccine (DTP), meningococcal vaccine, hepatitis B vaccine, and smallpox vaccine.[426,429,433,599–608] There is one report of interference with the measles antibody response after simultaneous administration of meningococcal A and C vaccine,[604] although a different team of investigators did not find interference with simultaneous administration of measles vaccine and meningococcal A vaccine.[603]

Measles vaccine is most commonly administered today along with rubella and mumps vaccines as a combined vaccine (MMR) as part of routine childhood immunization programs.[206,207] Use of MMR vaccine instead of single-antigen measles vaccine increases the benefit/cost ratio of the measles vaccination program in the United States from

TABLE 19–6 ■ Epidemiologic Studies of Duration of Measles Vaccine–Induced Immunity

Study	Attack Rate (%) by Years Since Vaccination*			
	0–4	5–9	>10	≥15
Shasby et al.[513†]	9.4 (3/32)[‡]	6.9 (7/101)	5.4 (8/52)	—
Nkowane et al.[514§]	0 (0/18)	1.1 (1/21)	1.4 (10/158)	—
Davis et al.[518]	1.1 (2/187)	1.7 (11/661)	2.6 (8/308)	0 (0/35)
Marks et al.[516‖]	4.0/1000	4.2/1000	5.4/1000	11.7/1000
Hutchins et al.[594]	0 (0/33)	0 (0/143)	2.2 (12/549)	3.1 (6/192)
Robertson et al.[787]	0 (0/2)	1.4 (1/74)	3.4 (10/292)	0 (0/3)
Guris et al.[596]	11.8 (2/17)	0 (0/7)		18.2 (2/11)

*Single vaccination at 15 months of age or older except for Shasby, Nkowane, and Davis (12 months of age or older).
†Years since vaccination: 5 to 8 and 9 or more.
‡Number ill/total number.
§Projected from a 25% random sample.
‖Cases per 1000 person-weeks at 0 to 3 (2 of 499), 4 to 6 (6 of 1420), 7 to 9 (5 of 929), and 10 to 12 (4 of 343) years since vaccination.
Adapted from Markowitz LE, Preblud SR, Fine PE, et al. Duration of live measles vaccine–induced immunity. Pediatr Infect Dis J 9:101–109, 1990.

17.2:1 to 21.3:1.[342] Measles vaccine is also frequently administered to susceptible adults, either as MMR or combined with only rubella vaccine.

Studies consistently show that combinations of these three antigens, regardless of the virus strain, elicit the same high rates of seroconversion seen with each component individually and that there is no increased risk of reactions in persons susceptible to all three antigens[418–436,438] (Tables 19–7 and 19–8). Furthermore, vaccination of persons already immune to one or more of the antigens, from either previous vaccination or infection, is not associated with any increased risk of vaccine-associated adverse events.[605,609–612] Although there are reports of directly mixing measles vaccine with DTP,[613] this should not be done routinely. Rather, the vaccines should be administered in separate syringes and at separate sites.[614]

Immunization against varicella along with measles, rubella, and mumps, either as two vaccines (varicella and MMR) or as a quadrivalent vaccine (MMRV), has been studied.[615,616] Seroconversion rates have been reported to be 95% or greater to all antigens, although titers against varicella were lower among persons receiving the quadrivalent vaccine.

Postexposure Prophylaxis

Routine measles vaccination before natural exposure provides the best protection against measles. However, persons without measles immunity who are exposed can receive some protection through measles vaccination or IG administration after exposure.

Use of Vaccine

Exposure to measles is not a contraindication to measles immunization. Available data suggest that live virus measles vaccine, if given within 72 hours of measles exposure, will provide protection in some cases.[379,482,617,618] Also, the vaccine should induce protection against subsequent measles exposures should the initial exposure fail to result in protection. Therefore, vaccine is the intervention of choice for persons older than 12 months of age who are exposed to measles in most settings (e.g., day care facilities, schools, colleges, health care facilities), unless contraindicated (see *Precautions and Contraindications* below). Infants 6 to 11 months of age may receive measles vaccine instead of IG if the initial exposure is detected within 72 hours. Infants vaccinated before age 12 months must be revaccinated on or

TABLE 19–7 ■ Antibody Response After Administration of Measles Vaccine Alone and in Combination with Mumps and Rubella Vaccines

Vaccine	Total Number	Measles		Mumps		Rubella	
	%	%	GMT*	%	GMT†	%	GMT*
Measles[‡]	23	100	82	—	—	—	—
Measles,[‡] mumps,[§] rubella (RA27/3)	91	96	89	90	31	100	301
Measles,[‡] mumps,[§] rubella (HPV-77:DE-5)	85	99	77	89	15	99	144

*Hemagglutination-inhibition assay geometric mean antibody titer.
†Indirect immunofluorescent assay geometric mean antibody titer.
‡Moraten strain.
§Jeryl Lynn strain.
Adapted from Lerman SJ, Bollinger M, Brunken JM. Clinical and serologic evaluation of measles, mumps, and rubella (HPV-77:DE5 and RA27/3) virus vaccines, singly and in combination. Pediatrics 68:18–22, 1981.

TABLE 19–8 ■ Proportion of Children with Fever and Rash After Administration of Measles
Vaccine Alone and in Combination with Mumps and Rubella Vaccines[*]

Vaccine	Total Number	Fever (%) (≥39.4°C)	Rash (%)
Measles[†]	43	5	12
Measles,[†] mumps,[‡] rubella (RA27/3)	141	11	20
Measles,[†] mumps,[‡] rubella (HPV-77:DE-5)	142	8	17
Placebo	42	0	9

[*]During the 6 weeks after vaccination.
[†]Moraten strain.
[‡]Jeryl Lynn strain.
Adapted from Lerman SJ, Bollinger M, Brunken JM. Clinical and serologic evaluation of measles, mumps and rubella (HPV-77:DE5 and RA27/3) virus
    vaccines, singly and in combination. Pediatrics 68:18–22, 1981.

after the first birthday with two doses of MMR vaccine separated by at least 28 days (see *Indications* below).

Use of Immune Globulin

Because measles is infectious during the prodrome and often is not diagnosed until the rash onset, many exposed persons are not identified until more than 72 hours after initial exposure. This is typically the situation for household contacts. IG can be given to prevent or modify measles in a susceptible person within 6 days of exposure.[152–155] However, any immunity conferred is temporary unless modified or typical measles occurs.[153,343] IG should not be used to control measles outbreaks.

Administration of IG within 6 days of initial exposure is indicated for susceptible contacts of measles patients for whom measles vaccination is not indicated. This includes those for whom risk of complications is increased (i.e., infants ≤12 months of age, pregnant women, or immunocompromised persons), those for whom the vaccine is contraindicated (see *Precautions and Contraindications* below), and those who are not vaccinated within 72 hours of initial exposure. IG prophylaxis is not indicated for exposed persons who have received at least one dose of measles vaccine on or after the first birthday, unless they are immunocompromised. All immunocompromised patients (including anyone with HIV infection and children of unknown infection status born to HIV-infected women) who are exposed to wild-type measles should receive IG prophylaxis, regardless of their immunization status. An exception is the patient receiving IVIG at regular intervals whose last dose was received within 3 weeks of exposure (see *Passive Immunization* above).[206,207]

Most infants less than 6 months of age are immune because of passively acquired maternal antibodies. However, if measles is diagnosed in a mother, unvaccinated children of all ages in the household who lack other evidence of measles immunity should receive IG or vaccine. All persons who receive IG should subsequently receive MMR vaccine after the appropriate interval unless it is otherwise contraindicated.

Adverse Effects

Adverse reactions after receipt of live, further attenuated measles vaccines (alone and in combination) are generally mild. With the exception of hypersensitivity reactions, adverse reactions are limited to susceptible vaccinees and

occur primarily during the 6 to 12 days after vaccination when the peak in replication of the live virus occurs.[257,351–356,392–395,418,419,422,425–433,435,605,614,619–628]

Fever of 39.4°C or higher (≥103°F) occurs in approximately 5% to 15% of vaccinees between the 7th and 12th day after vaccination and lasts approximately 1 to 2 days. In a study of twins, when one twin received MMR vaccine while the other received placebo, increased rates of fever occurred almost exclusively 9 or 10 days after vaccination.[418]

Rash occurs in approximately 5% of recipients beginning 7 to 10 days after vaccination and lasting for 1 to 3 days. Determining the etiology of a rash illness following measles vaccination can be difficult because other infections, such as human herpesvirus type 6 and human papillomavirus type 19, can often occur early in life and can be confused with a vaccine reaction.[245]

When the vaccine is administered to an individual already incubating natural disease, it is not usually possible to determine if fever and rash are caused by the vaccine or if the child has a modified case of measles unless wild-type virus is isolated from urine or the respiratory tract. The frequency of fever, rash, and other side effects after second doses of measles-containing vaccines is lower than after the first because most children are already immune from the initial vaccination, thus preventing significant viral replication.[620] One study found a slightly higher rate of adverse effects after a second dose of MMR when that dose was given to 10- to 12-year-olds compared with 4- to 6-year-olds.[627] This difference was most likely due to a higher rate of susceptibility among 10- to 12-year-olds and the recognized increase rate of arthralgia caused by rubella vaccine in older children. Adverse events resulting in medical visits within 1 month after vaccination of 10- to 12-year-olds were still rare (attributable risk 1.7/1000) and consisted mainly of rashes and joint pain.

Measles vaccine is associated with a mild decrease in platelet counts within a few days after the vaccine is given, and rare cases of idiopathic thrombocytopenic purpura (ITP) have been associated with measles-containing vaccines.[629,630] In the United Kingdom, an increased risk of ITP was documented following measles vaccination at a rate of one case in every 22,300 doses, with most cases occurring in the 6 weeks following immunization. Therefore, advisory committees recommend caution when administering measles-containing vaccines to children with thrombocytopenia or a past history of ITP.[206,207]

Immediate hypersensitivity reactions, including hives and anaphylaxis, occur rarely.[631] The rate of anaphylaxis is less than one case in every 1 million doses administered. Measles vaccine is produced in chick embryo tissue culture, and for many years there were concerns about administering these vaccines to children with egg allergy. However, several studies using sensitive methods have demonstrated that there is no evidence of egg protein in measles vaccine, and many children with immediate hypersensitivity reactions to measles-containing vaccines have reacted to the gelatin stabilizer.[631-633] Children with immediate hypersensitivity to eggs can be safely immunized with measles vaccines, and no special precautions are necessary.[632]

Febrile seizures are the most commonly reported neurologic adverse event following measles vaccination.[239,621,625-628] Fever from any source lowers the threshold for seizures, and a febrile seizure is not a sign of CNS infection or disease. Febrile seizures occur primarily in the second and third year of life and are not associated with long-term sequelae. The risk of febrile seizures is increased approximately threefold in the 8 to 14 days after receipt of MMR.[628] The rates of fever and febrile seizures following measles vaccines are much lower than the rates following measles disease. There has been no increased risk of adverse events observed in children who received measles vaccine combined with rubella and mumps vaccines (MMR) as compared with measles vaccine administered alone.[628]

Postinfectious encephalitis is a recognized complication of measles, but there is uncertainty as to whether or not encephalitis is caused by further attenuated measles vaccines in normal hosts. In children who have died during the rash phase of measles, measles virus has been found in brain tissue, but measles virus rarely has been found anywhere in the CNS with postinfectious encephalitis, which is thought to be due to an altered immune response to myelin proteins.[207,634] Encephalitis has been reported after measles immunization at a rate of approximately one case per 1 million vaccine recipients.[635] This rate is lower than the background rate of encephalitis of unknown etiology in unvaccinated children in the general population. There is temporal clustering of reports in the 5 to 15 days after immunization when other adverse effects from the vaccine occur. There has been one report of a vaccine isolate recovered from the cerebrospinal fluid of a normal individual who received Edmonston B strain vaccine.[636] There have been no cases of vaccine-strain virus causing encephalitis in persons with intact immune systems confirmed by neuropathologic studies. Nine cases of encephalitis following measles-containing vaccines were reported in the United States during 1979 to 1986, when 22.7 million doses of measles antigen–containing vaccine were distributed, for a rate of 1 per 2.5 million doses (0.4 per 1 million doses).[612] This rate is lower than that noted for severe neurologic disorders of unknown etiology in unimmunized children of the same age range, suggesting a possible chance temporal association.[637] In the United Kingdom, the National Childhood Encephalopathy Study found an increased rate of encephalopathy or prolonged or complicated convulsions within 7 to 14 days after measles vaccination, but none of the children had any serious permanent sequelae.[638,639] Some experts believe that the vaccine can cause encephalitis; if this is true, the rate is at least 1000 times less than the rate after natural infection. The Institute of Medicine concluded in 1994 that there was inadequate evidence to accept or reject a causal relation between measles vaccine and encephalitis or encephalopathy.[630]

There are case reports, but no evidence of increased risk or causal associations, of several other disorders following measles vaccines, including Reye's syndrome, oculomotor palsy, optic neuritis, retinopathy, hearing loss, cerebellar ataxia, arthralgia, arthritis, and soft tissue reactions.[239,612,640-649] There is no increased risk of Guillain-Barré syndrome following measles vaccine.[650,651] In a cohort study of 167,240 children, no significant association between timing of the receipt of measles vaccine and asthma was found.[652]

SSPE is caused by persistence of measles virus in the CNS through as-yet undefined mechanisms. SSPE develops in approximately 8.5 per 1 million children who have measles. No specific immune deficiency has been identified in children with SSPE to explain the failure of the immune system to eliminate the virus. There has been concern that measles vaccine virus could also cause a persistent CNS infection because some patients with SSPE who have received vaccine had no history of disease.[92,97,130] However, when investigated carefully, most of these individuals have histories of measles-like illnesses and/or known exposures to measles followed by administration of passive IG.[630,653] Genetic sequencing of viruses obtained from the brains of patients with SSPE to date, including patients with no history of having had measles, has revealed only viruses of wild-type origin.[654,655] Case-control studies and the marked decline of SSPE in parallel with the decline in measles following the introduction and widespread use of measles vaccine demonstrate that the vaccine protects against SSPE (Fig. 19–7). It is not known if measles virus persists in immunologically normal individuals who do not develop SSPE. Measles virus genomic RNA was detected frequently in persons who had been immunized or exposed to measles more than 2 months before testing in one study, and one group of investigators found evidence for persistence of measles virus nucleocapsid in a variety of tissues many years after measles.[656,657] An HIV-infected intravenous drug user developed progressive measles retinitis and subsequent progressive CNS disease diagnosed as SSPE at 30 years of age.[658] His illness resembled measles encephalitis in immunocompromised individuals. He had a history of measles at 2 years of age, and HIV infection most likely occurred in later life secondary to intravenous drug abuse or sexual contact.

Measles encephalitis in immunosuppressed children, including children with HIV infection or leukemia, is sometimes referred to as subacute or inclusion body measles encephalitis and is caused by progressive measles virus infection.[659,660] Onset is usually 5 weeks to 6 months after acute measles, and virus has been identified in brain tissue and cerebrospinal fluid specimens. Virus isolated from brain tissue specimens from several patients have been shown to be wild-type measles virus.[655,659] One patient with an undefined immune disorder who developed this disorder at 21 months of age was found to have measles vaccine virus in brain tissue.[661]

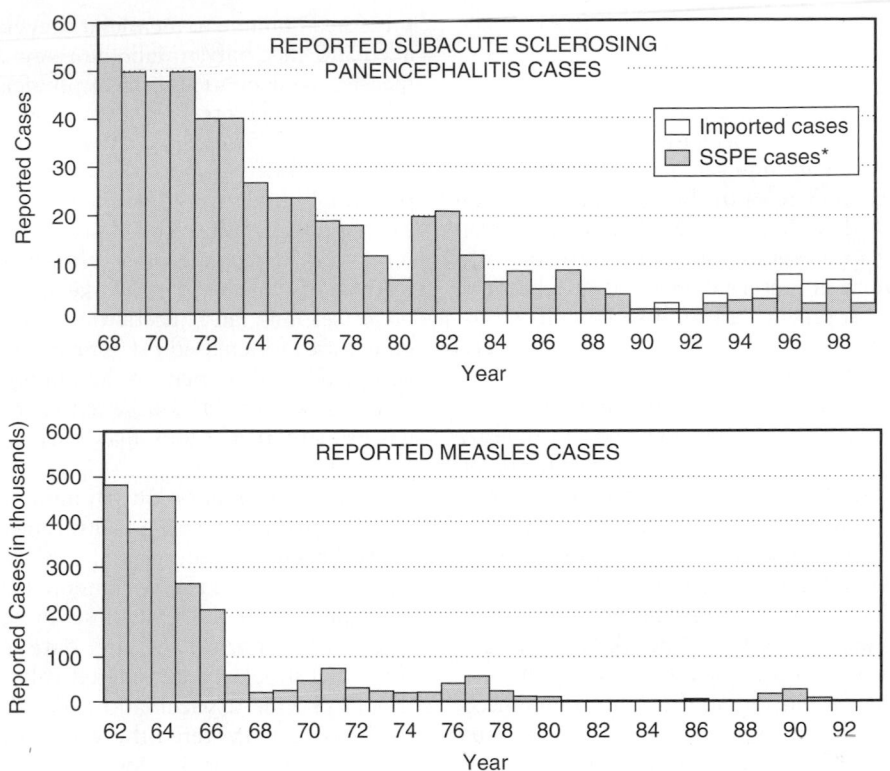

FIGURE 19–7 ■ Reported measles cases, 1962 to 1993, and subacute sclerosing panencephalitis (SSPE) cases, 1968 to 1999, United States. SSPE data are provisional. Distinction between imported and nonimported SSPE cases was not determined before 1990. (SSPE data courtesy of P. Dyken and S. Cunningham.)

In persons with severe immune suppression, there is an increased risk of progressive measles vaccine virus replication and severe complications, including fatal pneumonia.[662,663] HIV infection has not been associated with increased risks of adverse events in the few weeks following measles vaccination[664,665] (see Chapter 11 for additional information on immunization of HIV-infected persons). Only one well-documented instance of a severe complication following measles vaccine in an HIV-infected person has been documented. Measles vaccine virus was identified in the lung of a 20-year-old man who died of progressive pneumonitis that was recognized about 9 months after receiving a second dose of measles vaccine.[663,666] One HIV-infected child who had received MMR vaccine at 15 months of age was found to have characteristic inclusion bodies on brain biopsy at 18 months of age, but no specific testing was performed to determine the source or identity of the virus.[659] Also, a 19-year-old HIV-infected man with hemophilia had paramyxovirus nucleocapsids in intranuclear inclusion bodies, and there was evidence of measles antigen on immunohistochemical staining, but the virus was not sequenced.[660] He had received measles vaccine at 10 years of age, and there was no history of measles exposure in the year preceding the biopsy. The age at which he acquired HIV infection and possible subsequent exposures to measles were not reported. The WHO recommends measles vaccine for all children regardless of possible HIV infection because of the high risk of serious complications from measles in HIV-infected persons.[665] Advisory committees in the United States, where the risk of measles exposure is low, recommend withholding measles vaccine

from persons with severe immunosuppression (CD4 cells <15%).[667]

The possibility that measles virus persists in selected tissues following measles has been proposed by investigators who found evidence for measles antigen or genomic material in human tissues including brain, lung, intestine, and bone years after measles disease.[657] The investigators proposed that these viruses contribute to or cause inflammatory diseases in these organs, including Paget's disease,[145,668,669] otosclerosis,[144] and inflammatory bowel disease.[670] However, other investigators have found no evidence for measles viruses or measles genomic material in tissues from affected or normal patients.[671] One group of investigators promoted the hypothesis that measles vaccine given in combination with mumps and rubella vaccines (MMR) predisposed genetically susceptible children to develop inflammatory bowel disease and autism.[670,672,673] In-depth reviews conducted by the Institute of Medicine[143] concluded that the evidence favors rejection of the MMR-autism hypothesis, and an expert review by the AAP[671] concluded that the evidence does not support either of these hypotheses. Advisory committees in many countries recommend the use of MMR to protect against these three diseases.[206,207,674,675]

Revaccination of persons who had received killed measles vaccine in the 1960s who have not been rendered immune from revaccination or exposure to measles sometimes results in enhanced swelling and other reactions.[73,74,186,187,622–624] Nevertheless, these persons should be vaccinated in order to protect them against atypical measles and the associated increased risk of complications following exposure to wild-type measles.[207]

Indications

General

The goal of measles vaccination programs is to protect people from the severe consequences of measles infection by providing lifelong individual immunity to vaccinees and by reducing susceptibility to measles in the population to prevent transmission of this disease. The major source of measles susceptibility in a population is the birth of children, who will all lose their maternal antibody and become susceptible in the first or second year of life. The most critical task of any vaccination program is the timely delivery of the first dose of measles vaccine to young children. The timing of the first dose must balance the proportion of infants who have lost maternal antibody and are able to respond to vaccination at a given age against the risk of measles infection before that age.[509] Therefore, recommendations for measles vaccination vary by country.

The WHO recommends that, for most developing countries, measles vaccine be administered at 9 months of age because of the high level of measles morbidity and mortality that occur in the first year of life.[538] In 2000, the WHO recommended that countries provide a second opportunity for measles vaccination, to vaccinate those not immunized at the recommended age and to provide a second opportunity to those who did not respond to the first dose.[298] In the WHO region of the Americas, most countries have reduced the incidence of measles through mass campaigns and increased the recommended age for the first dose of measles vaccine to 12 months to maximize the proportion of infants who respond to the first dose.[676]

Many developed and some developing countries now have schedules for two doses. In developed countries, the first dose is usually recommended early in the second year of life; the age for the second dose varies.[31-34,207,677] The following section provides detailed recommendations of measles vaccination for the United States.

General Immunization Guidelines

MMR is the vaccine of choice when protection against any of these three diseases is required on or after the first birthday, unless any of its component vaccines is contraindicated.[206,207] Use of combined MMR vaccine for both measles doses and all other indications should provide an additional safeguard against primary vaccine failures and facilitate elimination of rubella and congenital rubella syndrome and continued reduction of mumps incidence. Data also indicate that the favorable benefit/cost ratio for routine measles, rubella, and mumps vaccination is even greater when the vaccines are administered as combined MMR vaccine.[341,342]

Measles or MMR vaccine may be administered simultaneously with other vaccines to persons at the recommended age to receive these vaccines. Neither theoretical considerations nor practical experience indicate that the simultaneous administration at separate anatomic sites of measles vaccine or MMR and other live or inactivated vaccines will produce a diminished immune response or increase the incidence of adverse events among vaccinated persons.[207]

Specific criteria for documentation of measles immunity have been established to identify the appropriate level of immunization for different groups. People can generally be presumed immune to measles if they have documentation of adequate vaccination, laboratory evidence of immunity to measles, or documentation of physician-diagnosed measles or were born before 1957 (few people in the United States born before 1957 escaped natural infection). In general, one dose of MMR is considered adequate vaccination for preschool children and adults who are not at high risk of exposure to measles. Two doses of MMR are indicated for schoolchildren, students at post–high school educational institutions, health care workers, people in measles outbreak settings, and international travelers because these groups are at increased risk for exposure to measles. Criteria accepted as evidence of immunity for the purpose of meeting school or college entry requirements or other government regulations may vary among state and local jurisdictions.[206,207]

Proper documentation of immunization is critical to assuring that every individual receives the appropriate vaccines. Vaccination status and date of administration of all vaccinations should be documented in the patient's permanent medical record. Only doses of vaccine for which written documentation of the date of administration is presented should be considered valid. Health care workers should provide a vaccination record for a patient only if they have administered the vaccine or have seen a record that documents vaccination.[206,207]

Because of reduced efficacy of measles vaccine when it is administered to young children, doses of measles vaccine administered to children younger than 12 months are not considered valid doses. Children vaccinated at ages younger than 12 months should be revaccinated at 12 to 15 months of age (provided at least 28 days have elapsed) to be considered to have received a single dose of measles vaccine.[206,207]

Routine Vaccination Schedule

PRESCHOOL CHILDREN

All children should receive the first dose of measles-containing vaccine at 12 to 15 months of age (Table 19–9). Children living in high-risk areas should be vaccinated at 12 months of age. A second dose may be given as early as 28 days after the first dose (e.g., during an outbreak or for international travel), based on the principle that live virus vaccines not administered at the same time should be separated by at least 1 month.[206,207]

SCHOOLCHILDREN

The second dose of MMR vaccine is recommended when children are age 4 to 6 years (i.e., before a child enters kindergarten or first grade). This recommended timing for the second dose of MMR vaccine has been adopted jointly by the Advisory Committee on Immunization Practices (ACIP), the AAP, and the American Academy of Family Physicians (AAFP).[206,207] Evidence now indicates that (1) the major benefit of administering the second dose is a reduction in the proportion of persons who remain susceptible because of primary vaccine failure, (2) waning immunity is not a major cause of vaccine failure and has little influence on measles transmission, and (3) revaccination of children who have low levels of measles antibody produces only a transient rise in antibody levels.[165,472,488]

TABLE 19–9 ▪ **Recommendations for Measles Vaccination in the United States**

Routine childhood schedule	
Most areas	Two doses* First dose: 12–15 mo Second dose: 4–6 yr
High-risk areas†	Two doses* First dose: 12 mo Second dose: 4–6 yr
Colleges and other post–high school educational institutions	Documentation of receipt of two doses of measles vaccine on or after the first birthday‡ or other evidence of measles immunity§
Persons working in health care facilities	Documentation of receipt of two doses of measles vaccine on or after the first birthday‡ or other evidence of measles immunity§

*Both doses should preferably be given as a combined measles-mumps-rubella vaccine (MMR). The American Academy of Pediatrics and the Advisory Committee on Immunization Practices recommend the second dose at 4 to 6 years of age.
†A county with more than five cases among preschool-age children during each of the last 5 years; a county with a recent outbreak among unvaccinated preschool-age children; or a county with a large inner-city urban population. These recommendations may be applied to an entire county or identified risk areas within a county.
‡No less than 1 month apart. If there is no documentation of any dose of vaccine, vaccine should be given at the time of entry or employment and no less than 1 month later.
§Prior physician-diagnosed measles disease, laboratory evidence of measles immunity, or birth before 1957.

As part of comprehensive health services for all adolescents, the ACIP, AAP, and AAFP recommend a health maintenance visit at age 11 to 12 years. This visit should serve as an opportunity to evaluate vaccination status and administer MMR vaccine to all persons who have not received two doses at the recommended ages.[206,207] Children who do not have documentation of adequate vaccination against measles or other acceptable evidence of immunity should be admitted to school only after administration of the first dose of MMR vaccine. If required, the second MMR dose should be administered as soon as possible, but no sooner than 28 days after the first dose. As of the 2001 to 2002 school year, 82% of children in schools in the United States are in grades that have been covered by state immunization requirements for two doses of measles vaccine. The estimated two-dose coverage rate in children in grades covered by state requirements is 97% to 98%.[678]

Vaccination of High-Risk Groups

COLLEGES AND OTHER POST–HIGH SCHOOL EDUCATIONAL INSTITUTIONS

Risks for transmission of measles at post–high school educational institutions can be high because these institutions may bring together large concentrations of persons who may be susceptible to measles.[679] College entry requirements for measles immunity substantially reduce the risk for measles outbreaks on college campuses where they are implemented and enforced.[680] Therefore, colleges, universities, technical and vocational schools, and other institutions for post–high school education should require that all undergraduate and graduate students have received two doses of MMR vaccine or have other acceptable evidence of immunity before enrollment. Students without documentation of any measles immunization or immunity should receive a dose on entry, followed by a second dose 4 weeks later.[206,207]

OUTBREAK SETTINGS

During outbreaks in schools and other institutions, all students, and personnel born in 1957 or later, should have doc-

umentation of two doses of measles-containing vaccine on or after the first birthday.[206,207] All persons who do not have such documentation or other evidence of immunity should be revaccinated or excluded from the school until at least 2 weeks after the onset of rash in the last case of measles. Persons receiving their second dose, as well as unimmunized persons receiving their first dose as part of the outbreak control program, may be readmitted immediately to school. In outbreaks where there is increased risk of exposure for infants younger than 1 year, vaccination with monovalent measles vaccine is recommended for infants as young as 6 months. If monovalent vaccine is not available, MMR may be given. Children who are vaccinated before their first birthday should be revaccinated when they are 12 months of age (provided at least 28 days have elapsed since the first dose given before age 12 months) and again at school entry. During outbreaks, IG should be administered to immunocompromised persons, susceptible pregnant women, and unvaccinated children younger than 12 months who are exposed to measles. However, IG should not be used to control outbreaks. Likewise, serologic screening before vaccination generally is not recommended during an outbreak because waiting for results on, contacting, and then vaccinating persons identified as susceptible can impede the rapid vaccination needed to curb the outbreak.

Every suspected measles case should be reported immediately to the local health department, and every effort must be made to verify that the illness is measles, especially if this may be the first case in the community. Subsequent prevention of the spread of measles depends on prompt immunization of persons at risk of exposure or already exposed who cannot readily provide documentation of measles immunity, including the date of immunization.[206,207]

If an outbreak occurs in a health care setting, all employees who were born in 1957 or later who cannot provide documentation that they have received two doses of measles vaccine on or after their first birthday or other evidence of immunity to measles should receive a dose of measles vaccine. Because some health care personnel who have acquired measles in health care facilities were born before 1957, immunization of older employees who may have occupational exposure to measles also should be considered. Susceptible personnel who have been exposed should be relieved from direct patient contact from the 5th to the 21st day after exposure, regardless of whether they received vaccine or IG after the exposure. Personnel who become ill should be relieved from patient contact until 4 days after rash develops.[206,207]

HEALTH CARE WORKERS

People who work in health care facilities are at greater risk for acquiring measles than the general population. During 1985 to 1989, physicians had an eightfold increased risk and nurses a twofold increased risk compared with non–health care workers of the same age.[681] In the 120 measles outbreaks occurring during 1993 through 2001, health care facilities were the most commonly reported settings, with 24 outbreaks reported.[682] Because persons working in medical settings have been infected with and have transmitted measles to patients and co-workers, the ACIP and AAP have recommended that persons born in or after 1957 working in health care facilities be required to provide evidence of two MMR vaccinations, documentation of physician-diagnosed measles, or laboratory evidence of measles immunity. Health care workers who need a second dose of measles-containing vaccine should be revaccinated 1 month (at least 28 days) after their first dose. In addition, because measles has occurred in persons born before 1957, health care facilities also may consider requiring MMR vaccination for health care workers born before 1957 who do not have a history of measles or documentation of immunity to measles.[206,207]

Because any health care worker who is not immune to measles can contract and transmit this disease, all health care facilities should ensure that those who work in their facilities are immune to measles. Serologic screening need not be done before vaccinating for measles and rubella unless the medical facility considers it cost-effective.[683,684] Serologic testing is appropriate only if persons who are identified as susceptible are subsequently vaccinated in a timely manner. Serologic screening ordinarily is not necessary for persons who have documentation of appropriate vaccination or other acceptable evidence of immunity.[206,207]

INTERNATIONAL TRAVELERS

Measles is endemic in many countries. Protection against measles is especially important for persons planning foreign travel. Before their departure from the United States, children 12 months of age or older should have received two doses of MMR vaccine separated by at least 28 days, with the first dose administered on or after the first birthday. Children ages 6 to 11 months should receive a dose of monovalent measles vaccine before departure. If monovalent measles vaccine is not available, MMR may be used. For infants vaccinated before 12 months of age, revaccination should be at 12 to 15 months of age (12 months of age for those remaining in areas of endemic or epidemic measles). The second revaccination should be administered at least 28 days later.[206,207]

Because the risk of complications from measles is increased in adults, it is also important to protect susceptible adults. Most persons born in the United States before 1957 are likely to be immune. However, for persons born after 1956 who travel abroad, two doses of measles vaccine should be administered separated by at least 28 days, unless there is documentation of receipt of two doses, other evidence of immunity, or a contraindication.[206,207]

PERSONS INFECTED WITH HUMAN IMMUNODEFICIENCY VIRUS

HIV-infected persons are at increased risk for severe complications if infected with measles.[176,184] Among HIV-infected persons who did not have evidence of severe immunosuppression, no serious or unusual adverse events have been reported after measles vaccination.[184,685] Therefore, MMR vaccination is recommended for all asymptomatic HIV-infected persons who do not have evidence of severe immunosuppression and for whom measles vaccination would otherwise be indicated. MMR vaccination also should be considered for all symptomatic HIV-infected persons who do not have evidence of severe immunosuppression.[686] Testing asymptomatic persons for HIV infection is not necessary before administering MMR or other measles-containing vaccines.[206,207]

Because the immunologic response to live and killed-antigen vaccines may decrease as HIV disease progresses, vaccination early in the course of HIV infection may be more likely to induce an immune response.[560] Therefore, HIV-infected infants without severe immunosuppression should routinely receive MMR vaccine as soon as possible on reaching the first birthday (i.e., at age 12 months).[687] Consideration should be given to administering the second dose of MMR vaccine as soon as 28 days (i.e., 1 month) after the first dose rather than waiting until the child is ready to enter kindergarten or first grade. In addition, if at risk for exposure to measles, HIV-infected infants who are not severely immunocompromised should be administered single-antigen measles vaccine or MMR vaccine at age 6 to 11 months. These children should receive another dose, administered as MMR vaccine, as soon as possible on reaching the first birthday, provided at least 1 month has elapsed since the administration of the previous dose of measles-containing vaccine. An additional dose of MMR vaccine can be administered as early as 1 month after the second dose. Newly diagnosed HIV-infected adults and children age 12 months or older without acceptable evidence of measles immunity should receive MMR vaccine as soon as possible after diagnosis, unless they have evidence of severe immunosuppression.

CLOSE CONTACTS OF IMMUNOSUPPRESSED PATIENTS

To minimize the risk of exposure to measles among patients with immunosuppression, including HIV infection, all family and other close contacts of these patients should be vaccinated with two doses of MMR vaccine, unless they are immunosuppressed, have other contraindications, or have other acceptable evidence of measles immunity.

PATIENTS TREATED WITH CHEMOTHERAPY, ORGAN TRANSPLANT, OR BONE MARROW TRANSPLANT

When cancer chemotherapy or immunosuppressive treatment is being considered, measles vaccination ideally should precede the initiation of chemotherapy or immunosuppression by at least 2 weeks.[687] Measles vaccination is contraindicated during the period of immunosuppression. Patients exposed to measles or at high risk of exposure while immunosuppressed should be given IG regardless of previous immunization status (see *Postexposure Prophylaxis* above). For patients who have received hematopoietic stem cell transplants, MMR or its component vaccines should be given 24 months after transplantation if the recipient is presumed to be immunocompetent.[688-691] Persons with leukemia in remission who were not immune to measles when diagnosed with leukemia may receive measles-containing vaccine. At least 3 months should elapse after termination of chemotherapy before administration of the first dose of measles vaccine.[207]

REVACCINATION OF PERSONS VACCINATED ACCORDING TO EARLIER RECOMMENDATIONS

Anyone vaccinated at any age with killed vaccine alone or killed vaccine followed by live vaccine within a 3-month period, and anyone vaccinated between 1963 and 1967 with a vaccine of unknown type, should be revaccinated to ensure protection and to prevent atypical measles illness. Revaccinating persons who received an unknown type of vaccine is recommended because Edmonston B, inactivated, and further attenuated live vaccines all were in use during this interval (see Fig. 19-5). As noted previously, vaccination of an immune individual is not associated with any increased risk of adverse events. However, revaccination of recipients of killed vaccine may be associated with local reactions of pain, swelling, erythema, and regional lymphadenopathy lasting 1 to 2 days.[73,74,186,187,622-624] These reactions have been reported to occur in 4% to 55% of vaccinees. More severe reactions have been noted, but only rarely.[74] Whereas revaccination has not been proved to totally eliminate the risk for atypical measles,[193] available data suggest that the risk is reduced considerably.[73,74,197] Thus the risk of these reactions is outweighed by the risk associated with atypical measles.[207]

A dose of further attenuated live vaccine with IG administered simultaneously should not be considered adequate vaccination. This recommendation is based on the theoretical consideration that passively derived antibody might interfere with seroconversion. Whereas low doses of IG do not appear to interfere with seroconversion,[257] there is no information available about the dose used in general practice shortly after the introduction of further attenuated vaccines in the United States. Furthermore, at least one study has suggested that there is an increased rate of seronegativity when further attenuated vaccine was administered with IG.[513] Finally, and perhaps most important, revaccination is indicated if there is any uncertainty about the vaccination record.[528]

Precautions and Contraindications

In general, measles vaccination is contraindicated for patients with acute severe illness, immunosuppression, pregnancy, or a personal history of an anaphylactic reaction to measles-containing vaccines. For the rare patient with a personal history of an anaphylactic reaction to gelatin or neomycin, measles vaccine should be administered with extreme caution and in consultation with an immunologist. Following administration of IG or other blood products, vaccination should be delayed for the recommended interval, unless the patient is exposed to measles or at high risk of exposure.[207] Clinical judgment must be used in deciding whether to vaccinate a patient with a history of thrombocytopenia. Mild illness, personal or family history of seizures, steroid therapy that is not immunosuppressive, and allergic reactions to eggs, chicken, feathers, or penicillin are not contraindications to measles vaccination. Persons with contraindications to measles vaccination should receive IG if they are exposed to measles or at high risk of exposure. Unfortunately, this only provides protection for a short time (see *Passive Immunization* above). To reduce the risk of exposure to measles in persons for whom the vaccine is contraindicated, their household contacts should be immune to measles or be vaccinated (unless contraindicated). To prevent nosocomial exposure to measles in patients with contraindications, all health care workers should be immune to measles or be vaccinated (unless contraindicated) (see *Indications* above).

Severe Illness

Measles-containing vaccines should not be administered to patients with acute severe illnesses, including those with significant fever or evolving neurologic conditions. To avoid confusing the evolution of the illness with possible complications resulting from measles vaccine, vaccination should be deferred until the acute severe illness is resolved.

Withholding vaccination for false contraindications is a major cause of late vaccination and low vaccine coverage. Measles vaccination should not be deferred in the presence of mild conditions such as mild upper respiratory infections, otitis media, or diarrhea.[550] Multiple large studies, in the United States and in other countries, have documented that children with mild illness have similar serologic responses to measles vaccination compared to well children. These studies also showed that the ill children had no increased risk of adverse events following vaccination compared to well children.[207,543,545,547]

Tuberculosis

Because of a theoretical concern that measles vaccination might exacerbate tuberculosis, patients with untreated active tuberculosis should begin antituberculosis therapy before measles vaccination. This theoretical concern is based on the reputed role of measles disease as an aggravating factor in tuberculosis and the similar suppression of delayed hypersensitivity for up to 4 to 6 weeks seen following both measles disease and measles vaccination.[474,476] However, a 1976 review of studies examining the effect of measles disease on tuberculosis patients showed that none of the studies provided conclusive evidence that measles disease has a deleterious effect on tuberculosis.[102] In several small studies in the 1960s, measles vaccine did not exacerbate tuberculosis in children receiving antituberculosis therapy.[481,482,692] However, there are no data available on the effect of measles vaccine on patients with untreated tuberculosis.

Tuberculin skin testing is not a prerequisite for measles immunization. In patients for whom tuberculin skin testing is indicated, such testing can be undertaken at the same time that vaccine is administered. If skin testing is not done at that time, it is advisable to wait 4 to 6 weeks after vaccination before administering a tuberculosis skin test.[206,207]

Immunosuppression

Live virus measles vaccine should not be administered to persons who are immunosuppressed because of medication (e.g., high-dose steroids, alkylating agents, and antimetabolites), other therapy such as radiation, or underlying illness (e.g., congenital immunodeficiency, leukemia, lymphoma, generalized malignant disease) (see *Indications* above). Although patients with severe immunosuppression related to HIV infection should not receive measles vaccine, HIV-infected individuals who are not severely immunosuppressed may be vaccinated. Immunosuppressed patients who are exposed to measles or at risk of exposure should receive IG regardless of their history of measles disease, vaccination, or serology, because they are at high risk of complications and death from measles (see *Passive Immunization* above). Replication of live vaccine virus may be augmented and prolonged in patients who are immunocompromised, and adverse events following vaccination, including death, are more common in immunosuppressed patients[659,693] (see *Adverse Effects* above).

Systemic corticosteroid treatment can result in immunosuppression. Because the minimum dose and duration of steroid therapy necessary to induce immunosuppression are not well defined, clinical judgment must be used to assess whether a patient on steroid therapy is immunosuppressed. Most experts would consider a steroid dose equivalent to or greater than a prednisone dose of 2 mg/kg of body weight per day (or a total of 20 mg/day) administered daily or on alternate days for 14 days or more to be sufficiently immunosuppressive to contraindicate measles vaccination.[207] Patients receiving immunosuppressive doses of steroids should not receive measles vaccine until 1 month after the end of steroid therapy. Vaccination is not contraindicated in persons receiving topical, localized (e.g., intra-articular, bursal, or tendon injection), or low- to moderate-dose steroids, or physiologic steroid replacement. Patients who receive high-dose steroids for less than 14 days generally can be vaccinated immediately after cessation of steroid therapy. Measles vaccine is contraindicated in any patient on any dose of steroids with clinical or laboratory evidence of immunosuppression or an underlying disease that is immunosuppressive.[207,687]

MMR and other measles-containing vaccines are not recommended for HIV-infected persons in the United States with evidence of severe immunosuppression because of the risk of adverse events, the impaired immune response to MMR vaccination, and the current low risk of exposure to measles in the United States.[206,207,667] Severe immunosuppression is defined as (1) a CD4+ count of less than 200 cells/mm³ for persons 6 years of age and older, a CD4+ count of less than 500 cells/mms³ for children 1 to 5 years old, and a CD4+ count of less than 750 cells/mm³ for children younger than 12 months of age; or (2) CD4+ cells less than 15% of total lymphocytes for children younger than 13 years.[686] One case of fatal vaccine-associated pneumonitis has been documented in a severely immunocompromised patient with HIV infection[661,664] (see *Adverse Events* above). Because of continued high incidence of measles in many countries and the severity of measles in HIV-infected individuals, the WHO recommends measles vaccine for all children regardless of HIV infection status.[663] Available

data suggest that persons with HIV infection who are not severely immunosuppressed may be vaccinated safely.[184,557,558,667] Because measles has been documented to be severe in HIV-infected persons in both the United States and developing countries,[694] measles vaccine is recommended routinely for asymptomatic HIV-infected children and adults without evidence of measles immunity and should be considered for those with symptomatic HIV infections who are not severely immunosuppressed. Asymptomatic patients at risk for HIV infection do not need to be screened for HIV before vaccination[206,207,667] (see *Indications* above).

Pregnancy

On theoretical grounds, live virus vaccines, including measles vaccine, should not be administered to a pregnant woman. However, in contrast to rubella and mumps vaccines, measles vaccine virus has not been shown to cross the placenta and infect the fetus. Susceptible women of childbearing age may be vaccinated after asking them if they are pregnant (excluding them if they are) and explaining the theoretical risks.

Allergies

Severe immediate hypersensitivity reactions (urticaria, angioneurotic edema, wheezing, hypotension, and shock) are very rare serious complications following measles vaccination. From 1991 to 2000, the U.S. Vaccine Adverse Event Reporting System received reports of events that were classified as probable or possible anaphylaxis at an average of two reports per 1 million doses of MMR distributed.[695] No anaphylaxis deaths have been reported in association with measles vaccination, but anaphylaxis can be life threatening. Persons with a history of anaphylaxis following measles-containing vaccines should not receive further doses but should be tested to document immune status. However, most patients with anaphylactic reactions following measles vaccination do not have clinically evident risk factors for anaphylaxis. Adequate treatment for hypersensitivity reactions, including epinephrine injection, should be available for immediate use whenever measles vaccines are administered, along with staff trained in treatment of anaphylactic reactions.[206]

Measles vaccines typically contain hydrolyzed gelatin as a stabilizer. Allergic reaction to gelatin has been recognized as a major cause of anaphylaxis after MMR vaccination.[696–699] Persons with previous systemic allergic reactions to gelatin should be vaccinated with extreme caution and in consultation with an immunologist.[207] Vaccine skin testing may be useful in these patients, but there is no protocol available. Patients with severe immediate hypersensitivity reactions have been shown to have high levels of antigelatin IgE and IgG and increased gelatin-specific T-cell responses.[667,696,697] In a study in Japan, 24 of 26 children who had allergic reactions to vaccines had antigelatin IgE. Only two of the children had allergic reactions to gelatin (in food) prior to vaccination.[698] In contrast, substantially fewer children (6 of 22) with severe allergic reactions to MMR in the United States had antigelatin IgE, and none had a reported history of allergic reactions to gelatin in food.[695] Measles vaccines contain trace amounts of the antibiotic neomycin. Allergic reactions to topical or systemic neomycin are rare and typically consist of delayed or cell-mediated immune responses such as contact dermatitis. The rare patients with systemic allergic reactions to either topical or systemic administration of neomycin should be vaccinated with extreme caution and in consultation with an immunologist.[206] Measles vaccines do not contain other antibiotics, such as penicillin; therefore penicillin allergy is not a contraindication to vaccination.

Measles (and mumps) vaccines are grown in chick embryo fibroblast cultures. Fasano and colleagues measured 37 pg/dose of ovalbumin cross-reacting protein in the MMR vaccine currently licensed in the United States.[700] Because some children with egg allergy have had anaphylactic reactions to measles vaccines,[701] previous recommendations included an algorithm of vaccine skin testing and desensitization for children who have had anaphylactic reactions after egg ingestion.[702] However, in some studies more than 1200 children with severe allergic reactions to eggs have been vaccinated safely.[703,704] Vaccine skin testing and desensitization are no longer recommended for persons with severe egg allergies.[206] These persons may be vaccinated using the same precautions (treatment for anaphylaxis immediately available) as for persons without severe egg allergy. Also, persons with less severe allergic reactions to eggs, or allergy to chicken or feathers, may be vaccinated as usual.[206,207]

Administration of Immune Globulin and Other Blood Products

Because passively derived antibody may interfere with vaccine seroconversion, vaccination should be deferred for 3 to 11 months after receipt of IG and other blood products, depending on the dose of the blood product received.[206,207,705] In addition, vaccination should precede receipt of IG by at least 2 weeks whenever possible. However, unvaccinated persons may not be fully protected during the entire time interval suggested following blood product administration. Therefore, additional doses of IG or measles vaccination may be necessary if the patient is exposed to measles or at high risk of exposure to measles. If measles vaccination is given before the recommended interval has elapsed, the dose should be repeated (at least 1 month after the measles vaccination and after the recommended interval from the time of blood product administration has elapsed).

Thrombocytopenia

Oski and Naiman reported significant depression of platelet counts without clinical symptoms following vaccination with Edmonston B vaccine, including one infant who had thrombocytopenia repeatedly after three doses. Previous immunity to measles did not prevent depression of the platelet count.[629] ITP has been associated with measles-containing vaccines currently in use.[630] The increased risk of ITP following MMR vaccination is estimated at three to four cases for every 100,000 doses.[706–708] There are no reports in which ITP solely associated with measles vaccines has resulted in death.

It is difficult to assess the risk of recurrence of ITP associated with measles vaccines given to people who have had previous ITP. At least two cases of recurrent MMR-associated ITP have been reported in patients with ITP associated with a previous MMR dose,[709,710] and one case of

MMR-associated exacerbation of chronic ITP was reported in a 19-year-old female whose onset of chronic ITP was associated with rubella vaccination in the second year of life.[711] In a study including 21 children with ITP before their first dose of MMR, Miller and co-workers reported that none had a recurrence of ITP following vaccination.[706] However, there has been no study of the risk of an additional dose of MMR in patients who developed ITP following a previous dose. Therefore, advisory committees recommend caution when administering measles-containing vaccines to children with thrombocytopenia or a past history of ITP, especially when the prior episode of ITP was associated with measles vaccination.[206,207] Serologic assessment of immunity may be useful in assessing the risk and benefits of immunization in such patients.

Family or Personal History of Seizures

Measles vaccination, like other causes of fever, may cause febrile seizures in young children. The 5% to 7% of children who have either a personal or family history of seizures may have an increased risk of febrile seizures following measles vaccination.[712] Febrile seizures following vaccination do not increase the risk of epilepsy or other neurologic disorders. The benefits of administering measles vaccine to children with personal or family history of seizures substantially outweigh the risks, and these children should be vaccinated following the standard recommendations. Their parents should be advised of the benefits for the vaccination and the minimal increased risk of febrile seizures. Because the fever induced by measles vaccine occurs between 6 and 12 days after vaccination and seizures may occur with the onset of fever, it is difficult to use antipyretics to prevent febrile seizures after measles vaccination. Patients taking anticonvulsants should continue this medication after measles immunization.[206,207]

Future Vaccines

Although measles vaccines are highly effective, the need to delay immunization until passively acquired maternal antibodies have declined has been an impediment to the global control and eradication of measles.[713] Research is being conducted to develop new vaccines that might effectively immunize children at younger ages or be administered by routes that allow easy delivery during mass campaigns. Advances have been made in the development of subunit and vectored measles vaccines that could avoid the problems experienced with the previously used formalin-inactivated measles vaccine and may be immunogenic in young infants in the presence of maternal antibody.[714]

Oral vaccination using an enteric-coated live, attenuated measles vaccine was not successful in monkeys.[715] However, oral administration of a measles peptide incorporated into a vesicle induced a cell-mediated immune response to measles.[716] DNA vaccines boosted by plant-derived measles virus hemagglutinin have been shown to induce neutralizing antibodies,[717,718] and orally administered adenovirus modified to express measles nucleocapsid antigen induced both measles antibody and cytotoxic T-cell responses.[719] Aerosol administration of live, attenuated vaccines has been successful, and, if delivery devices can be made practical, this approach could be feasible, especially in large-scale campaigns.[413,720] Mucosal administration of a vesicular stomatitis virus expressing measles hemagglutinin was effective and overcame the inhibitory effect of maternal antibodies in a cotton rat model.[721]

Public Health Considerations

Epidemiologic Results of Vaccination

Measles is one of the most contagious diseases of humans and is a classic communicable disease of childhood. The goal of measles vaccination is to prevent illness and death caused by measles directly among vaccinated persons and indirectly among unvaccinated persons as a result of decreased transmission.[3,722] In the absence of vaccination, measles occurs in epidemic cycles. The magnitude and frequency of the epidemics depends on the population size, contact rates between individuals, and the rate at which new susceptible individuals are added to the population through births or migration.[723,724] In England and Wales in the 1940s, epidemics occurred every second year, starting in the large cities of London, Manchester, and Liverpool and spreading outward to towns and rural villages.[40,725] In the large population centers, chains of transmission were sustained during the periods between epidemics and these *cities were the reservoirs of measles*. In towns and villages, transmission died out after an epidemic and had to be reintroduced for each subsequent epidemic. Epidemic cycles of measles also can be described in terms of the effective reproduction number, *R*, defined as the average number of secondary cases produced by a typical case in a population (see Chapter 56).[726,727] When *R* is less than 1, the average case gives rise to less than one case and the number of cases occurring subsequently begins to decrease.

Introduction of measles vaccination leads to a reduction in the size of epidemics and an increase in the interval between measles epidemics.[722] The widened interepidemic interval has been referred to as the "honeymoon period."[728,729] Vaccination of successive cohorts of young children results in a decrease in incidence among vaccinated cohorts, an overall decline in measles incidence in all age groups (because of dampened transmission), and, when outbreaks occur, an increase in the proportion of cases among older children.[328,729,730] Susceptibility to measles among older cohorts occurs most often because these individuals missed natural disease as young children and either missed getting vaccinated (program failure), or failed to respond to vaccination (primary vaccine failure). Waning of vaccine-induced immunity (secondary vaccine failure) has been found to occur in 0% to 5% of vaccinees but does not appear to play a major role in reducing overall population immunity to measles.[165,590,598]

As vaccination coverage increases among successive birth cohorts, measles transmission decreases, reducing the risk of measles even among unvaccinated individuals. At some vaccine-induced immunity level lower than 100%, measles virus transmission is interrupted.[731–733] Mathematical models have estimated the *herd immunity threshold* for measles in the United States at 93% to 95%.[734] If this level of population immunity is maintained by a vaccina-

tion program, endemic transmission of measles will die out and measles elimination is achieved. *Elimination* does not result in zero measles cases because importations of measles from endemic areas continue to occur. However, spread from these importations is short lived and will end without intervention. Documenting the elimination of measles is challenging. De Serres and associates have proposed using the proportion of cases imported and the distribution of outbreak sizes to monitor elimination.[735] These surveillance parameters can be used to estimate *R*, which must be maintained at less than 1 to achieve elimination. *Global eradication* of measles will occur when the last chain of transmission of measles virus is interrupted and can be defined as the simultaneous achievement of measles elimination in every country.

In industrialized countries, a single dose of measles vaccine administered in the second year of life induces immunity in about 95% of vaccinees.[503] With a primary vaccine failure rate of 5%, 100% of the population would have to be vaccinated to reach a 95% immunity level with a single-dose strategy. Approximately 95% of persons who fail to respond to the first dose respond to a *second dose*,[490] and with high vaccine coverage the herd immunity target can be reached if two doses are administered.

In developing countries, high morbidity and mortality resulting from measles among infants led to a recommendation to vaccinate infants at 9 months of age, a time when maternal antibody may interfere with seroconversion.[736] Studies have found the median seroconversion rate with vaccination at age 9 months to be 85% (range, 70% to 98%).[737] This leaves three times more infants susceptible (15% of vaccinees) than does a rate of 95%. After a single dose with 90% coverage and 85% seroconversion, 77% of the population would be immune. To improve immunity, some have considered providing a second dose, usually through routine health services at an older age, when seroconversion is 95%. However, this could raise immunity levels, given 90% coverage with both doses, to only 90%, leaving 10% susceptible. Alternatively, if vaccination were provided outside the health services, such that many children never vaccinated could receive a first dose while previously vaccinated children receive a second dose, the resulting population immunity level would be much higher. This is known as a *second opportunity strategy*. For example, if the second opportunity reached 90% coverage of prior first-dose recipients and previously unvaccinated children, population immunity would increase to greater than 95%. In countries with poor access to preventive services, the second opportunity for measles vaccination is most often provided through nationwide supplementary immunization activities, or mass campaigns because these are more effective at reaching children who have never been vaccinated.

Experiences with Measles Control and Elimination in Various Countries

Industrialized Countries

Experience in industrialized countries has shown that a single dose of measles vaccine, widely administered, can reduce measles transmission, but a two-dose strategy is necessary for elimination of indigenous transmission.[738–744]

Many countries introduced measles vaccine as a single-dose schedule and then added a second opportunity for vaccination because of the persistence of outbreaks despite high single-dose coverage (Table 19–10). Industrialized countries have found that the costs of patient care and outbreak control outweigh the cost of a second opportunity for immunization.[745] Some countries (e.g., Canada, United Kingdom, Australia, and New Zealand) have adopted a two-dose schedule and have conducted a one-time, nationwide vaccination campaign to reduce susceptibility among school-age children. Other countries (e.g., the United States, Finland, and Sweden) have relied on a two-dose schedule alone.

In the *United States*, the distribution and use of more than 255 million doses of live measles vaccine between the year of licensure (1963) and the end of 2000 (see Fig. 19–5) has been associated with a marked reduction in measles (Fig. 19–8) and its associated complications and an estimated savings of billions of dollars.[27,342] Whereas approximately 4 million cases occurred annually in prevaccine years, on average 400,000 to 500,000 cases were reported. In 1999, 2000, and 2001, only 100, 100, and 108 cases, respectively, were reported, a reduction of more than 99.9% compared with the years preceding vaccine licensure.[28] The reported occurrence of SSPE also has declined greatly (see Fig. 19–7) and was virtually eliminated in the late 1980s and early 1990s. A small number of cases have been reported each year during the late 1990s as a result of the resurgence of measles during 1989 to 1991. Approximately half of the recent SSPE cases result from measles acquired outside the United States (P. Dyken, personal communication, 2002).

The United States has embarked on three elimination efforts (see Fig. 19–8).[23,24,732,746,747] The first, in 1966, was based on a single-dose strategy with vaccination at 12 months of age (see Table 19–10). The second, announced in 1978, had three components: (1) a high level of population immunity through vaccination with a single dose of measles vaccine, (2) disease surveillance, and (3) prompt response to outbreaks.[23,24] To reach high coverage, vaccination requirements for school entry were enacted and enforced in every state. These requirements, which mandated not only measles vaccination but also other childhood vaccinations, have become the major legacy of this elimination initiative. Although sustained interruption of transmission of measles was not achieved, measles was eliminated from most of the country; 54% of counties in the United States were measles free for the entire decade from 1980 to 1989, and only 17 (0.5%) counties reported measles every year during that period.[747] During this interval, outbreaks continued to occur in schools among school-age persons with histories of vaccination and among unvaccinated preschool-age children.[326,514,518,528,594,748] In 1989, the United States introduced a routine second dose of measles vaccine at 4 to 6 years or 11 to 12 years to address the problem of school outbreaks (see Table 19–10).

After relatively low incidence during the 1980s, a 3-year epidemic of measles began in 1989 and resulted in over 55,000 cases and 123 deaths.[749,750] The average annual incidence during 1989 to 1991 was 7.4 per 100,000 population, compared with an average incidence for 1981 to 1988 of 1.8 per 100,000. Incidence was increased in all age groups; however, the greatest increases were in children younger than 1 year and 1 to 4 years, resulting in almost half of all cases occurring in children younger than 5 years (see Table 19–1). This epidemic was due to low measles vaccination levels among preschool-age children, particularly in inner cities,[751-754] and was part of a hemisphere-wide measles epidemic.[755]

In 1993, the third elimination initiative was launched based on increasing preschool immunization levels to greater than 90% and vaccination of all schoolchildren with a sec-

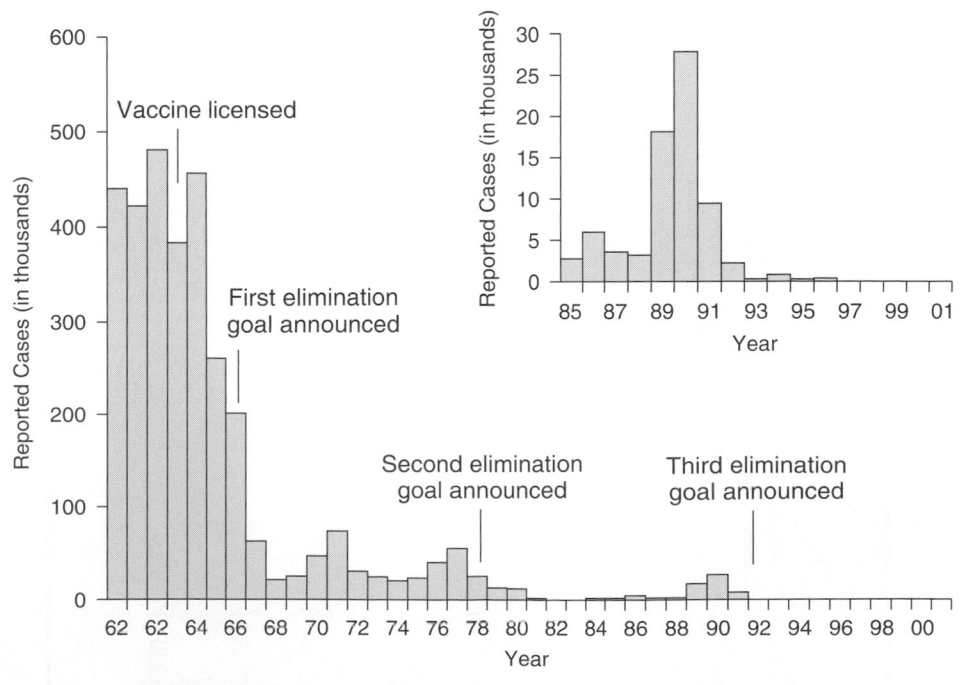

FIGURE 19–8 ■ Reported measles cases, United States, 1960 to 2001.

TABLE 19–10 ■ Evolution of Measles Vaccination Policy in Selected Countries and the Expanded Programme on Immunisation (EPI), 1963 to 2001

Country	First Opportunity		Second Opportunity			
	First Dose in Schedule		Second Dose in Schedule		Supplementary Campaign	
	Year	Recommended Age	Year	Recommended Age	Year	Age Range
United States	1963	9 mo				
	1965	12 mo				
	1976	15 mo	1989	4–6 or 11–12 yr		
	1994	12–15 mo				
Canada	1963	9 mo				
	1968	12 mo	1999	4–6 yr		
United Kingdom	1968	12–23 mo				
	1988	13–15 mo	1996	18 mo or 4–6 yr	1996	5–16 yr
Brazil	1973	8 mo				
	1976	7 mo	1996	Before school entry	1994	5–16 yr
	1982	9 mo				
			1992	12–15 mo	1992	9 mo–14 yr
					1995	1–3 yr
					1997	6 mo–4 yr
					2000	1–4 yr
China	1965	8–12 mo	1986	7 yr		
WHO EPI Program	1983	9 mo				
	1989	6 mo	2001	(either routine second dose or periodic supplementary campaigns)		
	1991	9 mo				

ond dose. To implement these vaccination strategies, between 11 and 16 million doses of measles vaccine were distributed annually between 1994 and 2001 (see Fig. 19–5). Since 1997, the annual incidence has been less than one case per 1 million population, and the majority of cases are internationally imported or linked to imported cases.[28] During the resurgence, a single genotype (D3) was isolated from at least eight different sites. In contrast, since 1993, multiple genotypes have been isolated and all are known to circulate in other countries.[226,227] In March 2000, the CDC convened a panel of experts to review the pattern of measles transmission in the United States. Each participant concluded that measles was no longer an endemic disease in the United States. During 1999 through 2001, 21 of 33 outbreaks (64%) have been either epidemiologically or virologically linked to an importation, and the distribution of outbreak sizes is consistent with an absence of endemic measles transmission (Table 19–11). The achievement of measles elimination in the United States is the result of three major factors: (1) 90% or greater vaccination coverage with the first dose among preschool-age children, (2) administration of a second dose to more than 80% of all school-age children, and (3) reduction in measles importations from Latin America as a result

of aggressive control measures recommended by the Pan American Health Organization (PAHO).[28]

Canada began a measles immunization program in 1963 (see Table 19–10). Despite achieving coverage in excess of 95% with a single dose of measles vaccine throughout the 1980s, measles outbreaks continued to occur.[743,744] In 1995, 2362 measles cases were reported in Canada (i.e., more than one third of the total in the Western Hemisphere). School outbreaks among children who had received a single dose of measles-containing vaccine accounted for most cases. Mathematical modeling predicted a sizable measles epidemic, and cost-benefit analyses showed that a national vaccination campaign to prevent the predicted epidemic would save $2.50 for every dollar spent.[745,756] On the basis of these analyses, 11 of the 12 provinces of Canada undertook mass vaccination campaigns targeting school-age children using measles-rubella vaccine in the spring of 1996. A coverage level of more than 90% was achieved. In addition, a second dose was added to the routine schedule at age 18 months or 4 to 6 years (see Table 19–10). From 1997 through 2001, Canada has interrupted endemic measles transmission as evidenced by the occurrence of only a few small outbreaks, many linked to importation.[757] Occasional

TABLE 19–11 ■ Measles Outbreaks in the United States by Location, Epidemiologic Linkage to Importation, and Virus Genotype, 1999, 2000, and 2001

Year	State	County	Number of Cases	Epidemiologic Link	Virus Genotype
1999	OR/WA	3 counties	13	Unknown	—
	CA	Santa Cruz	6	India	D4
	CA	2 counties	4	India	—
	CA	2 counties	3	Unknown	—
	VA	Prince William	3	Vietnam	—
	WA	2 counties	3	Italy	D8
	MA	2 counties	4	Unknown	—
	TX	2 counties	3	England	D8
	VA	Bedford	15	Unknown	D4
	AR	St. Francis	4	Unknown	—
	MI	Oakland	6	England	D6
2000	NYC	2 counties	8	England	D6
	UT	Summit	3	Japan	—
	CA/WA/CO	4 counties	4	Las Vegas, NV	—
	CA	Santa Cruz	3	Germany	—
	NY	3 counties	9	Unknown	—
	NV/CA	2 counties	4	Unknown	—
	CA	Los Angeles	5	Unknown	G2
	IL	2 counties	3	Unknown	—
	VT/NH	3 counties	6	Ethiopia	D4
	CA	San Mateo	3	Philippines	D3
2001	WA*	King	4	Korea	H1
	WA*	King	7	Unknown	H1
	MA	2 counties	3	Pakistan	D4
	MD/PA	2 counties	4	Philippines	D3
	9 States	12 counties	14†	China	—
	CA	2 counties	5	Japan	—
	PA	Bedford	3	Philippines	—
	NYC	Manhattan	4	Japan	D5
	CA	San Diego	4	Germany	—
	CA*	San Francisco	3	England	D7
	CA*	San Francisco	6	Unknown	D7

*Epidemiologically distinct clusters.
†Includes 13 adoptees from an orphanage and 1 contact case.

larger outbreaks have occurred among communities with a religious objection to vaccination.

In 1968, the *United Kingdom* introduced measles vaccine for children between the ages of 1 and 2 years, but throughout the 1970s and early 1980s coverage remained below 80%. In 1988, combined MMR vaccine was introduced in place of measles vaccine at age 13 to 15 months (see Table 19–10) and coverage improved to over 90%. In November 1994, all children ages 5 to 16 years in England and Wales were offered combined measles-rubella vaccine, regardless of prior vaccination history, in an attempt to prevent a predicted epidemic of measles. During the campaign, 6.2 million doses were administered for a reported coverage of 92%.[740,741,758] Between 1995 and 2000, among 594 confirmed measles cases, 212 (36%) were sporadic and 382 (64%) were associated with 51 clusters. Forty-eight sporadic cases (23%) and 18 of 51 clusters (35%) were associated with an importation of infection from overseas. A wide variety of measles virus genotypes were identified over this period. The pattern of sporadic cases and small clusters associated with importations is consistent with elimination of sustained indigenous measles transmission.[758] However, unfounded concerns about vaccine safety have led to a decline in MMR coverage and an outbreak of measles in South London during the first quarter of 2002 that resulted in 90 confirmed cases.[759]

Excellent control of measles has been achieved in other industrialized countries. In 1982, *Finland* initiated a measles elimination program based on a two-dose vaccination strategy. Efforts to improve vaccination coverage included mass media, a registry system to track defaulters, and an intensive outreach program.[35] By 1993, coverage was above 95% for both doses and measles virus circulation was interrupted.[739] Measles elimination has been maintained in Finland as a result of consistently high two-dose vaccination coverage.[760] *Sweden* has reported similar success with a two-dose schedule.[33] However, in other Western European countries (e.g., Italy,[761] Germany,[762] France[763]), measles remains endemic, in part because of the perception that vaccination may be more risky than the disease itself. However, from April 1999 to February 2000, 2961 cases of measles were reported in *the Netherlands* among members of a religious group opposed to vaccination. Three patients died and 68 were hospitalized as a result of complications.[764,765]

The *European Region* of WHO, which includes the countries of the Former Soviet Union, has established a goal for the regional elimination of measles by 2007.[765] In addition to the United Kingdom, Finland, and Sweden, a number of European countries are close to, or have already achieved, elimination (e.g., Hungary, Poland, the Netherlands, Slovenia).[766] Successful catch-up vaccination campaigns using combined measles-rubella vaccine have been conducted in Romania (in 1998),[767] Albania (in 2000),[768] and Kyrgyzstan (in 2001),[769] and these countries have used this opportunity to introduce programs to prevent congenital rubella syndrome.

Less Industrialized Countries

Beginning in the late 1970s, the *Expanded Programme on Immunisation* (EPI) has played a major role in the development of immunization programs in less industrialized countries. Measles vaccination coverage in these countries rose from 18% in 1981 to 76% in 1990, and an estimated 1.7 million measles deaths were prevented in 1995 alone.[770] During the 1990s, donor support for the EPI decreased substantially and measles vaccination coverage levels plateaued or decreased, with the estimated annual number of measles deaths stabilizing at about 1 million.[339]

Worldwide in 2000, measles was estimated to cause 777,000 deaths (i.e., 1.4% of 55.7 million total deaths).[340] Among children less than 5 years of age, measles was the fifth leading cause of death, accounting for 5.4% of the 10.9 million total deaths in this age group. The vast majority of *measles deaths* (>95%) occur in less industrialized countries because of lower measles vaccination coverage (i.e., underdeveloped routine health services and lack of a second opportunity for measles vaccination) and a higher casefatality ratio in these countries. The higher risk of death from measles in less industrialized countries compared to industrialized countries has been associated with a younger median age of cases, increased intensity of exposure, increased likelihood of secondary infections, and malnutrition, especially vitamin A deficiency. Poverty, crowded living conditions, and large family size are the underlying socioeconomic factors contributing to this epidemiologic pattern.[736]

During the late 1980s and early 1990s in less industrialized countries, two different approaches were developed to address the problem of severe measles in children younger than 9 months, the age for vaccination recommended by the WHO (see Table 19–10). First, *high titer measles vaccines* (e.g., Edmonston-Zagreb measles vaccine) were developed to overcome interference by maternal measles antibody when administered at 4 to 6 months of age.[582] Although high-titer vaccines were more immunogenic than standardtiter vaccines, they were unexpectedly associated with delayed excess mortality among females, and these vaccines are no longer recommended.[587] The second approach, developed by the PAHO,[676] was based on the observation that older siblings were often the source of measles infection for infants. The concept of a one-time nationwide mass vaccination campaign for children ages 9 months to 14 years regardless of prior disease or vaccination history was pioneered in Cuba in 1987.[771] The objective of this socalled *catch-up campaign* was to interrupt measles virus transmission by rapidly reducing susceptibility among older children and thereby prevent transmission to infants less than 9 months of age. This approach proved highly effective and has been developed further into the PAHO strategy for measles elimination.

THE PAHO STRATEGY

In 1994, ministers of health of countries of North and South America established the goal of eliminating measles from the Western Hemisphere by the end of 2000. To accomplish this goal, the PAHO developed a strategy with three essential vaccination components: (1) catch-up—a one-time mass vaccination covering all children ages 1 to 14 years regardless of prior disease or vaccination status; (2) keep-up—achievement of 90% or greater immunization coverage in each successive birth cohort; and (3) followup—subsequent mass campaigns conducted every 3 to 5 years covering all children ages 1 to 5 years irrespective of prior disease or vaccination history.[676] After the catch-up campaigns, some countries have increased the measles vaccination age to 12 months to maximize vaccine efficacy. In addition to the vaccination strategy, case-based surveillance with laboratory confirmation of suspected measles cases has been established in all countries of the Americas.[772]

In *Brazil*, the National Immunization Program was created in 1973 and routine measles vaccination was recommended at 8 months of age.[773] National measles control was intensified in 1980 to 1981 with campaigns focused in areas of low coverage. The minimum recommended age for measles vaccination was changed to 7 months in 1976 and then to 9 months in 1982. In 1992, with the adoption of a measles elimination goal by 2000, a second dose was recommended at age 12 to 15 months (see Table 19–10). Based on the success of statewide mass vaccination campaigns in Parana and Sao Paulo in 1987, Brazil conducted a nationwide "catch-up" campaign in 1992 during which 48 million doses of measles vaccine were administered to children ages 9 months to 14 years. In 1995, the first national "follow-up" campaign for children ages 1 to 3 years was conducted; the state of Sao Paulo did not participate in this campaign.

In 1997, after a 4-year period of good control, Brazil experienced a major resurgence of measles with a total of 53,335 cases and 61 deaths.[773] Transmission was concentrated in the metropolitan area of Sao Paulo State but subsequently spread to involve all states. The highest age-specific incidence rates were among children less than 1 year of age (1577 per 100,000), young adults ages 20 to 29 years (539 per 100,000), and children ages 1 to 4 years (205 per 100,000). This age distribution was similar throughout Brazil, with 55% of cases occurring among adults ages 20 to 29 years, a cohort born between 1968 and 1977, when the vaccination program was being initiated. Characterization of measles viruses during the outbreak in 1997 identified the D6 genotype. This same genotype was identified in subsequent measles outbreaks in Argentina and Uruguay in 1998 and Chile, Bolivia, and the Dominican Republic during 1999 to 2001.[774]

The resurgence of measles in Brazil in 1997 led to a nationwide follow-up campaign in 1997 for children ages 6 months to 4 years. A third follow-up campaign was conducted in 2000 for children ages 1 to 4 years. After two follow-up campaigns, measles transmission appears to have been interrupted in Brazil—of 8358 suspected measles cases reported in 2000, only 36 cases (0.4%) were confirmed. The last recorded measles outbreak was in February 2000, with 15 cases.[773]

Implementation of the PAHO strategy in the *Western Hemisphere* has resulted in a greater than 99% decline in reported measles cases from a high of almost 250,000 cases in 1990 to 537 cases in 2001, the lowest annual total ever (Fig. 19–9).[772] The pattern of measles importations into the United States confirms the success of the PAHO strategy.[775] In 1990, at the height of the regionwide resurgence in measles, 242 of 300 importations of measles were from Latin America; in contrast, of 53 importations in 2001, none was from Latin America (CDC, unpublished data). During 2001, measles outbreaks in Haiti and the Dominican Republic were brought under control, ending known transmission of the D6 measles virus genotype in the Western Hemisphere. In the first 6 months of 2002, Venezuela and Colombia were the only countries in the Western Hemisphere experiencing large outbreaks affecting predominantly preschool-age children and young adults.[776]

The success of the PAHO strategy has led to expansion of its use outside the Western Hemisphere. In *Africa*, where an estimated 452,000 measles deaths occurred in 2000, the PAHO strategy has been adopted in an effort to reduce measles mortality. Between 1996 and 1999, seven Southern African countries (South Africa, Namibia, Zimbabwe, Swaziland, Malawi, Botswana, and Lesotho) conducted catch-up vaccination campaigns and introduced case-based measles surveillance.[42] Reported measles deaths in these

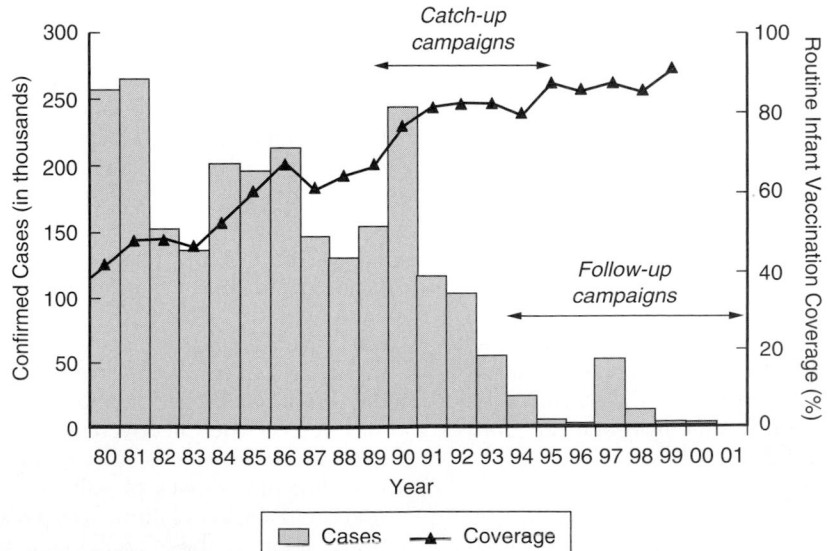

FIGURE 19–9 ■ Reported measles cases, Latin America and the Caribbean, 1980 to 2001. (Data courtesy of the Special Programme on Vaccines and Immunizations, Pan American Health Organization.)

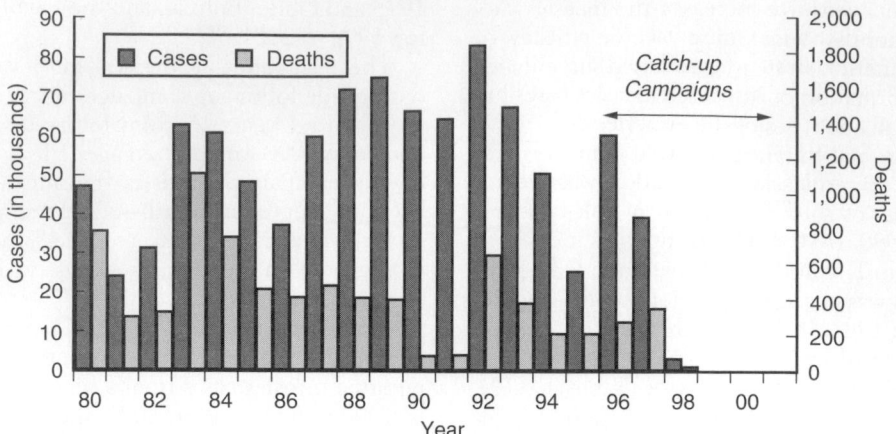

FIGURE 19–10 ■ Reported measles cases and reported measles deaths, seven southern African countries, 1980 to 2001. (Data courtesy of R. Biellik.)

countries decreased from 350 in 1996 to zero in 2000 and 2001 (Fig. 19–10).

MORTALITY REDUCTION STRATEGIES

In February 2001, at a meeting hosted by the American Red Cross, a new partnership was formed to advocate for reduction of measles mortality in Africa. In the first year of the *measles partnership*, supplementary measles vaccination campaigns were conducted in eight countries (Benin, Burkina Faso, Cameroon, Ghana, Mali, Tanzania, Togo, and Uganda) vaccinating 21 million children, and these campaigns are predicted to prevent an estimated 47,000 measles deaths over the next 3 years.[777]

The impact of measles vaccination on overall childhood mortality in developing countries was questioned by one study that reported *replacement mortality* (i.e., later death from other causes).[113] However, several subsequent studies have documented that measles vaccination increases overall child survival.[778–781] In Bangladesh, investigators found that the overall mortality rate in measles-vaccinated children was 45% lower than in unvaccinated children and that this difference persisted for several years after vaccination.[778]

In 2001, the WHO and the United Nations International Children's Emergency Fund (UNICEF) published a *strategic plan for global measles control* during 2001 to 2005.[298] Its goals are to reduce measles mortality by 50% by 2005 and to achieve and maintain interruption of indigenous measles transmission in large geographic areas with established elimination goals (viz., the Americas, European, and Eastern Mediterranean regions of the WHO). The plan recommends a second opportunity for measles immunization for all children and endorses mass vaccination campaigns, if well planned and implemented, as an effective method for delivering measles vaccine. In effect, this plan has made two opportunities for measles immunization the standard of care in all countries regardless of development status or routine vaccination coverage (see Table 19–10).

Measles Eradication

The feasibility of measles eradication has been debated for many years.[43,45–47,782–784] Hopkins and colleagues have pro-

posed global measles eradication and pointed out both the similarities and differences between measles and smallpox.[43] Measles will be substantially more difficult to eradicate than smallpox because of its higher contagiousness, younger median age at infection, and older age at which vaccine is effective.

In 1996, the WHO, PAHO, and CDC convened a meeting to review progress in global measles control and the elimination effort in the Western Hemisphere.[46] The consultative group concluded that eradication was feasible using currently available vaccines and that a strategy based on periodic mass campaigns and strengthening of immunization services will be needed in most developing countries. Recognizing the need to first complete polio eradication, the WHO-UNICEF strategic plan for measles, issued in 2001, postpones discussion about establishing a target date for global measles eradication to 2005.[298] The threat of bioterrorism has made the prospect of stopping measles vaccination after global eradication unlikely. However, it may be possible to drop one dose, and this, together with the lives saved and the treatment and outbreak control costs averted, may still make global measles eradication a cost-effective public health goal.[47]

Available evidence indicates measles meets the criteria for a disease that can be eradicated: (1) there is no animal or environmental reservoir and humans are critical to maintaining transmission; (2) accurate diagnostic tests are available; (3) measles vaccine and existing vaccination strategies are effective and safe; and (4) measles transmission has been interrupted in a large geographic area (e.g., nationwide) for a prolonged period of time.[47] Major challenges to global measles eradication will include: (1) increasing urbanization and population density that will require very high vaccination coverage; (2) war and civil unrest; (3) the frequency of international travel and forced migrations that facilitate importations of measles; and (4) the HIV epidemic, which may reduce the effectiveness of measles vaccination and increase the transmissibility of measles.[694] Other potential impediments are lack of political will, risk of unsafe injections, and the possibility of transmission among adults.

To address these challenges, research is ongoing to improve diagnostic tests for measles using filter paper blood spots[286,287] and oral fluid[284] and to develop alternative routes for administration of existing measles vaccines (e.g., aerosol vaccination[413-415]), needle-free jet injectors to reduce the risk of unsafe injections, and new candidate vaccines that could be administered in the presence of maternal antibodies ("stealth vaccines").[416,785] In addition, disease surveillance and program monitoring are being strengthened to learn from recent field experience with measles mortality reduction and regional elimination activities. These efforts provide optimism that, in the future, the goal of global measles eradication may be achieved.

REFERENCES

1. Abu Becr M. A Discourse on the Smallpox and Measles [Mead R, English trans]. London, J Brindley, 1748.
2. Babbott FL Jr, Gordon JE. Modern measles. Am J Med Sci 228:334–361, 1954.
3. Black FL. Measles. *In* Evans AS (ed). Viral Infections of Humans: Epidemiology and Control (3rd ed). New York, Plenum Publishing, 1989, pp 451–465.
4. Wilson GS. Measles as a universal disease. Am J Dis Child 103:219–223, 1962.
5. Sydenham T. The Works of Thomas Sydenham. Vol. 2. London, Sydenham Society, 1922, pp 250–251.
6. Enders JF. Francis Home and his experimental approach to medicine. Bull Hist Med 38:101–112, 1964.
7. Panum PL. Observation made during the epidemic of measles on the Faroe Islands in the year 1846. Med Classics 3:839–886, 1939.
8. Goldberger J, Anderson JF. An experimental demonstration of the presence of the virus of measles in the mixed buccal and nasal secretions. J Am Med Assoc 57:476–478, 1911.
9. Enders JF, Peebles TC. Propagation in tissue cultures of cytopathogenic agents from patients with measles. Proc Soc Exp Biol Med 86:277–286, 1954.
10. Milovanovic MV, Enders JF, Mitus A. Cultivation of measles virus in human amnion cells and developing chick embryo. Proc Soc Exp Biol Med 95:120–127, 1957.
11. Katz SL, Milovanovic MV, Enders JF. Propagation of measles virus in cultures of chick embryo cells. Proc Soc Exp Biol Med 97:23–29, 1958.
12. Katz SL, Enders JF. Immunization of children with a live attenuated measles virus. Am J Dis Child 98:605–607, 1959.
13. Enders JF, Katz SL, Milovanovic MV, Holloway A. Studies on an attenuated measles-virus vaccine. I. Development and preparation of the vaccine: techniques for assay of effects of vaccination. N Engl J Med 263:153–159, 1960.
14. Katz SL, Enders JF, Holloway A. Studies on an attenuated measles-virus vaccine. II. Clinical, virologic and immunologic effects of vaccine in institutionalized children. N Engl J Med 263:159–161, 1960.
15. Kempe CH, Ott EW, St. Vincent L, Maesel JC. Studies on an attenuated measles-virus vaccine. III. Clinical and antigenic effects of vaccine in institutionalized children. N Engl J Med 263:162–165, 1960.
16. Black FL, Sheridan SR. Studies on an attenuated measles-virus vaccine. IV. Administration of vaccine by several routes. N Engl J Med 263:165–169, 1960.
17. Lepow ML, Gray N, Robbins FC. Studies on an attenuated measles-virus vaccine. V. Clinical, antigenic and prophylactic effects of vaccine in institutionalized and home-dwelling children. N Engl J Med 263:170–173, 1960.
18. Krugman SL, Giles JP, Jacobs AM. Studies on an attenuated measles-virus vaccine. VI. Clinical, antigenic and prophylactic effects of vaccine in institutionalized children. N Engl J Med 263:174–177, 1960.
19. Katz SL, Kempe HC, Black FL, et al. Studies on an attenuated measles-virus vaccine. VIII. General summary and evaluation of the results of vaccination. N Engl J Med 263:180–184, 1960.
20. Enders JF. Measles virus: historical review, isolation and behavior in various systems. Am J Dis Child 103:282–287, 1962.
21. Enders JF, Katz SL, Holloway A. Development of attenuated measles-virus vaccines: a summary of recent investigation. Am J Dis Child 103:335–340, 1962.
22. Seminar on the Epidemiology and Prevention of Measles and Rubella. Arch Virusforsch 16:1–551, 1965.
23. Centers for Disease Control. Goal to eliminate measles from the United States. MMWR 41:391, 1978.
24. Hinman AR, Brandling-Bennett AD, Nieberg PI. The opportunity and obligation to eliminate measles from the United States. JAMA 242:1157–1162, 1979.
25. Hinman AR, Orenstein WA, Bloch AB, et al. Impact of measles in the United States. Rev Infect Dis 5:439–444, 1983.
26. Markowitz LE, Preblud SR, Orenstein WA, et al. Patterns of transmission in measles outbreaks in the United States, 1985–1986. N Engl J Med 320:75–81, 1989.
27. Bloch AB, Orenstein WA, Stetler HC, et al. Health impact of measles vaccination in the United States. Pediatrics 76:524–532, 1985.
28. Centers for Disease Control and Prevention. Measles—United States, 2000. MMWR 51:120–123, 2002.
29. White FMM. Policy for measles elimination in Canada and program implications. Rev Infect Dis 5:577–582, 1983.
30. Ikic DM. Edmonston-Zagreb strain of measles vaccine: epidemiologic evaluation in Yugoslavia. Rev Infect Dis 5:558–563, 1983.
31. Sejda J. Control of measles in Czechoslovakia (CSSR). Rev Infect Dis 5:564–567, 1983.
32. Rabo E, Taranger J. Scandinavian model for eliminating measles, mumps, and rubella. Br Med J (Clin Res Ed) 289:1402–1404, 1984.
33. Bottiger M, Christenson B, Romanus V, et al. Swedish experience of two-dose vaccination programme aiming at eliminating measles, mumps, and rubella. Br Med J (Clin Res Ed) 295:1264–1267, 1987.
34. Peltola H, Kurki T, Virtanen M, et al. Rapid effect on endemic measles, mumps, and rubella of nationwide vaccination programme in Finland. Lancet 1:137–139, 1986.
35. Paunio M, Virtanen M, Peltola H, et al. Increase of vaccination coverage by mass media and individual approach: intensified measles, mumps, and rubella prevention program in Finland. Am J Epidemiol 133:1152–1160, 1991.
36. Yihao Z, Wannian S. Introduction to the control of measles by vaccination in the People's Republic of China. Rev Infect Dis 5:568–573, 1983.
37. Wang L, Zeng G, Lee L, et al. Progress in accelerated measles control in the People's Republic of China: 1991–2000. J Infect Dis, 187 (Suppl 1):S252–S257, 2003.
38. van Druten JAM, de Boo T, Plantinga AD. Measles, mumps, and rubella control by vaccination. Dev Biol Stand 65:53–63, 1986.
39. Henderson RH, Keja J, Hayden G, et al. Immunizing the children of the world: progress and prospects. Bull World Health Organ 66:535–543, 1988.
40. Cliff A, Haggett P, Smallman-Raynor M. Measles: An Historical Geography of a Major Human Viral Disease. Cambridge, MA, Blackwell Scientific Publications, 1993.
41. Hersh BS, Tambina G, Nogueira C, et al. Review of regional measles surveillance data in the Americas, 1996–1999. Lancet 355:1943–1948, 2000.
42. Biellik R, Madema S, Taole A, et al. First 5 years of measles elimination in southern Africa: 1996–2000. Lancet 359:1564–1568, 2002.
43. Hopkins DR, Hinman AR, Koplan JP, Lane JM. The case for global measles eradication. Lancet 1:1396–1398, 1982.
44. Hinman AR, Bart KJ, Hopkins DR. Costs of not eradicating measles. Am J Public Health 75:713–715, 1985.
45. de Quadros CA. Global eradication of poliomyelitis and measles: another quiet revolution. Ann Intern Med 127:156–158, 1997.
46. Centers for Disease Control and Prevention. Measles eradication: recommendations from a meeting cosponsored by the World Health Organization, the Pan American Health Organization, and CDC. MMWR 46(RR-11):1–20, 1997.
47. Orenstein WA, Strebel PM, Papania M, et al. Measles eradication: is it in our future? Am J Public Health 90:1521–1525, 2000.
48. Robbins FC. Measles: clinical features. Pathogenesis, pathology, and complications. Am J Dis Child 103:266–273, 1962.
49. Katz SL, Enders JF, Holloway A. Use of Edmonston attenuated measles strain: a summary of three years' experience. Am J Dis Child 103:340–344, 1962.
50. Kempe CH, Fulginiti VA. The pathogenesis of measles virus infection. Arch Ges Virusforsch 16:103–128, 1965.
51. Case Records of the Massachusetts General Hospital: Weekly Clinicopathological Exercises. Case 34-1988. Progressive pulmonary consolidations in a 10-year-old boy with Evans' syndrome. N Engl J Med 319:495–509, 1988.

52. Koplik H. The diagnosis of the invasion of measles from a study of the exanthema as it appears on the buccal mucous membrane. Arch Pediatr 13:918–922, 1896.

53. Gresser I, Chany C. Isolation of measles virus from the washed leukocyte fraction of blood. Proc Soc Exp Biol Med 113:695–698, 1963.

54. Gresser I, Katz SL. Isolation of measles virus from urine. N Engl J Med 263:452–454, 1960.

55. Ruckle G, Rogers KD. Studies with measles virus. II. Isolation of virus and immunologic studies in persons who have had natural disease. J Immunol 78:341–355, 1957.

56. Griffin DE, Ward BJ, Jauregui E, et al. Immune activation in measles. N Engl J Med 320:1667–1672, 1989.

57. McChesney MB, Oldstone BA. Virus-induced immunosuppression: infections with measles virus and human immunodeficiency virus. Adv Immunol 45:335–380, 1989.

58. Griffin DE. Immune responses during measles virus infection. Curr Top Microbiol Immunol 191:117–134, 1995.

59. Moss WJ, Polack FP. Immune responses to measles and measles vaccine: challenges for measles control. Viral Immunol 14:297–309, 2001.

60. Atabani SF, Byrnes AA, Jaye A, et al. Natural measles causes prolonged suppression of interleukin-12 production. J Infect Dis 184:1–9, 2001.

61. Okada H, Kobune F, Sato TA, et al. Extensive lymphopenia due to apoptosis of uninfected lymphocytes in acute measles patients. Arch Virol 145:905–920, 2000.

62. Bech V. Studies on the development of complement fixing antibodies in measles patients: observations during a measles epidemic in Greenland. J Immunol 83:267–275, 1959.

63. Stokes J Jr, Reilly CM, Buynak EB, Hilleman MR. Immunologic studies of measles. Am J Hyg 74:293–303, 1961.

64. Enders-Ruckle G. Methods of determining immunity, duration, and character of immunity resulting from measles. Arch Ges Virusforsch 16:182–207, 1965.

65. Krugman S, Giles JP, Friedman H, Stone S. Studies on immunity to measles. J Pediatr 66:471–488, 1965.

66. Norrby E, Gollmar Y. Appearance and persistence of antibodies against different virus components of regular measles infections. Infect Immun 6:240–247, 1972.

67. Kibler R, ter Meulen V. Antibody-mediated cytotoxicity after measles virus infection. J Immunol 114:93–98, 1975.

68. Bellanti JA, Sanga RL, Klutinis B, et al. Antibody responses in serum and nasal secretions of children immunized with inactivated and attenuated measles-virus vaccines. N Engl J Med 280:628–633, 1969.

69. Polna I, Aleksandrowicz J, Krawczynski K, et al. Measles antibodies in nasal secretions and sera of children with measles. Acta Virol 21:331–337, 1977.

70. Friedman M, Hadari I, Goldstein V, Sarov I. Virus-specific secretory IgA antibodies as a means of rapid diagnosis of measles and mumps infection. Isr J Med Sci 19:881–884, 1983.

71. Ruckdeschel JC, Graziano KD, Mardiney MR Jr. Additional evidence that the cell-associated system is the primary host defense against measles (rubeola). Cell Immunol 17:11–18, 1975.

72. Graziano KD, Ruckdeschel JC, Mardiney MR Jr. Cell-associated immunity to measles (rubeola): the demonstration of in vitro lymphocyte tritiated thymidine incorporation in response to measles complement fixation antigen. Cell Immunol 15:347–359, 1975.

73. Krause PJ, Cherry JD, Naiditch MJ, et al. Revaccination of previous recipients of killed measles vaccine: clinical and immunologic studies. J Pediatr 93:565–571, 1978.

74. Krause PJ, Cherry JD, Carney JM, et al. Measles-specific lymphocyte reactivity and serum antibody in subjects with different measles histories. Am J Dis Child 134:567–571, 1980.

75. Whittle HC, Werblinska J. Cellular cytotoxicity to measles virus during natural measles infection. Clin Exp Immunol 42:136–143, 1980.

76. Gallagher MR, Welliver R, Yamanaka T, et al. Cell-mediated immune responsiveness to measles: its occurrence as a result of naturally acquired or vaccine-induced infection and in infants of immune mothers. Am J Dis Child 135:48–51, 1981.

77. Sissons JGP, Colby SD, Harrison WO, Oldstone MBA. Cytotoxic lymphocytes generated in vivo with acute measles virus infection. Clin Immunol Immunopathol 34:60–68, 1985.

78. Black FL, Rosen L. Patterns of measles antibodies in residents of Tahiti and their stability in the absence of re-exposure. J Immunol 88:725–731, 1962.

79. Krugman S, Katz SL, Gershon AA, et al. Measles. In Krugman S (ed). Infectious Diseases of Children (8th ed). St. Louis, CV Mosby, 1985, pp 152–166.

80. Cherry JD. Measles. In Feigen RD, Cherry JD (eds). Textbook of Pediatric Infectious Diseases (2nd ed). Philadelphia, WB Saunders, 1987, pp 1607–1628.

81. Hilleman MR. Current overview of the pathogenesis and prophylaxis of measles with focus on practical implications. Vaccine 20:651–665, 2002.

82. Appelbaum E, Dolgopol VB, Dolgin J. Measles encephalitis. Am J Dis Child 77:25–48, 1949.

83. Christensen PE, Schmidt H, Bang HO, et al. An epidemic of measles in southern Greenland, 1951. Measles in virgin soil. II. The epidemic proper. Acta Med Scand 144:430–449, 1953.

84. Peart AFW, Nagler FP. Measles in the Canadian Arctic, 1952. Can J Public Health 45:146–156, 1954.

85. Miller HG, Stanton JB, Gibbons JL. Para-infectious encephalomyelitis and related syndromes: a critical review of the neurologic complications of certain specific fevers. Q J Med 25:247–505, 1956.

86. Miller DL. Frequency of complication of measles, 1963: report on a national inquiry by the Public Health Laboratory Service in collaboration with the Society of Medical Officers of Health. Br Med J 2:75–78, 1964.

87. Bech V. The measles epidemic in Greenland in 1962. Arch Ges Virusforsch 16:53–56, 1965.

88. Littauer J, Sorensen K. The measles epidemic at Umanak in Greenland in 1962. Dan Med J 12:43–50, 1965.

89. McLean DM, Best JM, Smith PA, et al. Viral infections of Toronto children during 1965. II. Measles encephalitis and other complications. Can Med Assoc J 94:906–910, 1966.

90. Barkin RM. Measles mortality: a retrospective look at the vaccine era. Am J Epidemiol 102:341–349, 1975.

91. Barkin RM. Measles mortality: analysis of the primary cause of death. JAMA 129:307–309, 1975.

92. Modlin JF, Jabbour JT, Witte JJ, Halsey NA. Epidemiologic studies of measles, measles vaccine, and subacute sclerosing panencephalitis. Pediatrics 59:505–512, 1977.

93. Modlin JF, Halsey NA, Eddins DL, et al. Epidemiology of subacute sclerosing panencephalitis. J Pediatr 94:231–236, 1979.

94. Becroft DMO, Osborne DRS. The lungs in fatal measles infection in childhood: pathological, radiological and immunological correlations. Histopathology 4:401–412, 1980.

95. Englehandt SF, Halsey NA, Eddins DL, Hinman AR. Measles mortality in the United States 1971–1975. Am J Public Health 70:1166–1169, 1980.

96. Johnson RT, Griffin DE, Hirsch RL, et al. Measles encephalomyelitis—clinical and immunologic studies. N Engl J Med 310:137–141, 1984.

97. Centers for Disease Control. Subacute sclerosing panencephalitis surveillance—United States. MMWR 31:585–588, 1982.

98. Atkinson WL, Markowitz LE. Measles and measles vaccine. Semin Pediatr Infect Dis 2:100–107, 1991.

99. Greenberg BL, Sack RB, Salazar-Lindo, et al. Measles associated diarrhea in hospitalized children in Lima, Peru: pathogenic agents and impact on growth. J Infect Dis 164:495–502, 1991.

100. Perry RT, Halsey NA. The clinical significance of measles. J Infect Dis 2003 [in press].

101. von Pirquet CE. Das Verhalten der kutanen Tuberkulinreaktion wahrend der Masern. Dtsch Med Wochenschr 34:1297–1300, 1908.

102. Flick JA. Does measles really predispose to tuberculosis? Am Rev Respir Dis 114:257–265, 1976.

103. Morley D, Woodland M, Martin WJ. Measles in Nigerian children: a study of the disease in West Africa, and its manifestations in England and other countries during difficult epochs. J Hyg (Camb) 61:115–134, 1963.

104. Morley D. Severe measles in the tropics. Br Med J 1:297–300, 363–365, 1969.

105. Scheifele DW, Forbes CE. The biology of measles in African children. East Afr Med J 50:169–173, 1973.

106. Assaad F. Measles: summary of worldwide impact. Rev Infect Dis 5:452–459, 1983.

107. Borgono JM. Current impact of measles in Latin America. Rev Infect Dis 5:417–421, 1983.

108. Hull HF, Williams PJ, Oldfield F. Measles mortality and vaccine efficacy in rural West Africa. Lancet 1:972–975, 1983.

109. Loening UE, Coovadia HM. Age specific occurrence rates of measles in urban, periurban, and rural environments and implication for time of vaccination. Lancet 2:324–326, 1983.

110. Nieberg P, Dibley MJ. Risk factors for fatal measles infections. Int J Epidemiol 15:309–311, 1986.

111. Porter JDH, Gastellu-Etchegorry M, Navarre I, et al. Measles outbreaks in the Mozambican refugee camps in Malawi: the continued need for an effective vaccine. Int J Epidemiol 19:1072–1077, 1989.

112. Narain JP, Khare S, Rana SRS, Banerjee KB. Epidemic measles in an isolated unvaccinated population, India. Int J Epidemiol 18:952–958, 1989.

113. The Kasongo Project Team. Influence of measles vaccination on survival pattern of 7–35-month-old children in Kasongo, Zaire. Lancet 1:764–767, 1981.

114. Foster SO, McFarland DA, John MA. Health sector priorities review, measles. In Jamison DT, Mosley WH (eds). Evolving Health Sector Priorities in Developing Countries. Washington, DC, The World Bank, 1993, pp 161–183.

115. Singh J, Sharma RS, Verghese T. Measles mortality in India: a review of community-based studies. J Commun Dis 26:203–214, 1994.

116. Mgone JM, Mgone CS, Duke T, et al. Control measures and the outcome of the measles epidemic of 1999 in the Eastern Highlands Province. P N G Med J 43:91–97, 2000.

117. Singh J, Kumar A, Rai RN, et al. Widespread outbreaks of measles in rural Uttar Pradesh, India, 1996: high-risk areas and groups. Indian Pediatr 36:249–256, 1999.

118. Hussey GD, Clements CJ. Clinical problems in measles case management. Ann Trop Paediatr 16:307–317, 1996.

119. Markowitz LE, Neiburg P. The burden of acute respiratory infection due to measles in developing countries and the potential impact of measles vaccine. Rev Infect Dis 13(suppl 6):S555–S561, 1991.

120. Koster F, Curlin G, Aziz KMA, Haque A. Synergistic impact of measles and diarrhoea in nutrition and mortality in Bangladesh. Bull World Health Organ 59:901–908, 1981.

121. Sarker SA, Wahed MA, Rahaman MM, et al. Persistent protein losing enteropathy in post measles diarrhea. Arch Dis Child 61:739–743, 1986.

122. Expanded Programme on Immunisation, Programme for the Prevention of Blindness Nutrition. Joint WHO/UNICEF statement on vitamin A for measles. Wkly Epidemiol Rec 62:133–134, 1987.

123. Gilbert CE, Wood M, Waddel K, Foster A. Causes of childhood blindness in east Africa: results in 491 pupils attending 17 schools for the blind in Malawi, Kenya, and Uganda. Ophthalmic Epidemiol 2:77–84, 1995.

124. Foster A, Sommer A. Corneal ulceration, measles, and childhood blindness in Tanzania. Br J Ophthalmol 71:331–343, 1987.

125. Gershon AA, Krugman S. Measles virus. In Lennette EH, Schmidt NJ (eds). Diagnostic Procedures for Viral, Rickettsial, and Chlamydial Infections (5th ed). Washington, DC, American Public Health Association, 1979, pp 665–693.

126. Sever JL. Persistent measles infection of the central nervous system: subacute sclerosing panencephalitis. Rev Infect Dis 5:467–473, 1983.

127. Sakaguchi M, Yoshikawa Y, Yamanouchi K, et al. Characteristics of fresh isolates of wild measles virus. Jpn J Exp Med 56:61–67, 1986.

128. Gascon GG. Subacute sclerosing panencephalitis. Semin Pediatr Neurol 3:260–269, 1996.

129. Dyken PR. Neuroprogressive disease of post-infectious origin: a review of a resurging subacute sclerosing panencephalitis (SSPE). Ment Retard Dev Disabil Res Rev 7:217–225, 2001.

130. Halsey NA, Modlin JF, Jabbour JT, et al. Risk factors in subacute sclerosing panencephalitis: a case control study. Am J Epidemiol 3:415–420, 1980.

131. Billeter MA, Cattaneo R, Spielhofer P, et al. Generation and properties of measles virus mutations typically associated with subacute sclerosing panencephalitis. Ann N Y Acad Sci 724:367–377, 1994.

132. Ebkom A, Wakefield AJ, Zack M, Adami HO. Perinatal measles infection and subsequent Crohn's disease. Lancet 344:508–510, 1994.

133. Wakefield AJ, Ekbom A, Dhillon AP, et al. Crohn's disease: pathogenesis and persistent measles virus infection. Gastroenterology 108:991–996, 1995.

134. Thompson NP, Montgomery SM, Pounder RE, Wakefield AJ. Is measles vaccination a risk factor for inflammatory bowel disease? Lancet 345:1071–1074, 1995.

135. Wakefield AJ, Montgomery SM. Measles virus a risk factor for inflammatory bowel disease: an unusually tolerant approach. Am J Gastroenterol 95:1389–1392, 2000.

136. Uhlmann V, Martin CM, Sheils O, et al. Potential viral pathogenic mechanism for new variant inflammatory bowel disease. Mol Pathol 55:84–90, 2002.

137. Iizuka M, Nakagomi O, Chiba M, et al. Absence of measles virus in Crohn's disease [letter]. Lancet 345:199, 1995.

138. Afzal MA, Armitage E, Ghosh S, et al. Further evidence of the absence of measles virus genome sequence in full thickness intestinal specimens from patients with Crohn's disease. J Med Virol 62:377–382, 2000.

139. Feeney M, Clegg A, Winwood P, Snook J. A case-control study of measles vaccination and inflammatory bowel disease. Lancet 350:764–766, 1997.

140. Davis RL, Kramarz P, Bohlke K, et al. Measles-mumps-rubella and other measles-containing vaccines do not increase the risk for inflammatory bowel disease. Arch Pediatr Adolesc Med 155:354–359, 2001.

141. Taylor B, Miller E, Lingam R, et al. Measles, mumps, rubella vaccination and bowel problems or developmental regression in children with autism: population study. BMJ 324:393–396, 2002.

142. Madsen KM, Hviid A, Vestergaard M, et al. A population-based study of measles, mumps, and rubella vaccination and autism. N Engl J Med 347:1477–1482, 2002.

143. Straton K, Gable A, Shetty P, McCormick M, for the Institute of Medicine. Immunization Safety Review: Measles-Mumps-Rubella Vaccine and Autism. Washington, DC, National Academy Press, 2001.

144. Niedermeyer HP, Arnold W, Neubert WJ, Sedlmeier R. Persistent measles virus infection as a possible cause of otosclerosis: state of the art. Ear Nose Throat J 79:552–554, 556, 558 passim, 2000.

145. Reddy SV, Menaa C, Singer FR, et al. Measles virus nucleocapsid transcript expression is not restricted to the osteoclast lineage in patients with Paget's disease of bone. Exp Hematol 27:1528–1532, 1999.

146. Ohara Y. Multiple sclerosis and measles virus. Jpn J Infect Dis 52:198–200, 1999.

147. Atmar RL, Englund JA, Hammill H. Complications of measles in pregnancy. Clin Infect Dis 14:217–226, 1992.

148. Eberhart-Phillips JE, Frederick PD, Baron RC, Mascola L. Measles in pregnancy: a descriptive study of 58 cases. Obstet Gynecol 82:797–801, 1993.

149. Siegel M. Congenital malformations following chickenpox, measles, mumps, and hepatitis: results of a cohort study. JAMA 226:1521–1524, 1973.

150. Jesperson CS, Littover J, Saglid V. Measles as a cause of fetal defects: a retrospective study of ten measles epidemics in Greenland. Acta Paediatr Scand 66:367–376, 1977.

151. Siegel M, Fuerst HT, Peress NS. Comparative fetal mortality in maternal virus diseases: a prospective study on rubella, measles, mumps, chicken pox, and hepatitis. N Engl J Med 274:768–771, 1966.

152. Stokes J Jr, Maris EP, Gellis SS. Chemical, clinical, and immunologic studies on the products of human plasma fractionation. XI. The use of concentrated normal human serum gamma globulin (human immune serum globulin) in the prevention and attenuation of measles. J Clin Invest 23:531–540, 1944.

153. Janeway CA. Use of concentrated human serum γ-globulin in the prevention and attenuation of measles. Bull N Y Acad Med 21:202–222, 1945.

154. Brody JA, Bridenbraugh E. Prophylactic g-globulin and live measles vaccine in an island epidemic of measles. Lancet 2:811–813, 1964.

155. Perkins FT. Passive prophylaxis of measles. Arch Ges Virusforsch 16:210–217, 1965.

156. Krugman S, Giles JP, Jacobs AM, Friedman H. Studies with live attenuated measles-virus vaccine. Am J Dis Child 103:353–363, 1962.

157. Karlitz S, Markham FS. Immunity after modified measles. Am J Dis Child 103:682–687, 1962.

158. Linnemann CC Jr. Measles vaccine: immunity, reinfection, and revaccination. Am J Epidemiol 97:365–371, 1973.

159. Schaffner W, Schluederberg AES, Byrne EB. Clinical epidemiology of sporadic measles in a highly immunized population. N Engl J Med 279:783–789, 1968.

160. Cherry JD, Feigen RD, Lobes JA Jr, et al. Urban measles in the vaccine era: a clinical, epidemiologic, and serologic study. J Pediatr 81:217–230, 1972.

161. Linnemann CC, Hegg ME, Rotte TC, et al. Measles IgM response during reinfection of previously vaccinated children. J Pediatr 82:798–801, 1973.

162. Schluederberg A, Lamm SH, Landrigan PJ, Black FL. Measles immunity in children vaccinated before one year of age. Am J Epidemiol 97:402–409, 1973.

163. Smith FR, Curran AS, Raciti A, Black FL. Reported measles in persons immunologically primed by prior vaccination. J Pediatr 101:391–393, 1982.

164. Nagy G, Kosa S, Takatsy S, Koller M. The use of IgM tests for analysis of the causes of measles vaccine failures: experience gained in an epidemic in Hungary in 1980 and 1981. J Med Virol 13:93–103, 1984.

165. Mathias R, Meekison J, Arcand T, et al. The role of secondary vaccine failures in measles outbreaks. Am J Public Health 79:475–478, 1989.

166. Edmonson MB, Addiss DG, McPherson JT, et al. Mild measles and secondary vaccine failure during sustained outbreak in a highly vaccinated population. JAMA 263:2467–2471, 1990.

167. Reyes MA, Franky De Borrero M, Roa J, et al. Measles vaccine failure after documented seroconversion. Pediatr Infect Dis J 6:848–851, 1987.

168. Dai B, Chen ZH, Liu QC, et al. Duration of immunity following immunization with live measles vaccine: 15 years of observation in Zhejiang Province, China. Bull World Health Organ 69:415–423, 1991.

169. Ishiwada N, Addae MM, Tetteh JK, et al. Vaccine-modified measles in previously immunized children in Accra, Ghana: clinical, virological and serological parameters. Trop Med Int Health 6:694–698, 2001.

170. Mitus A, Enders JF, Craig JM, Holloway A. Persistence of measles virus and depression of antibody formation in patients with giant cell pneumonia after measles. N Engl J Med 261:882–889, 1959.

171. Mitus A, Enders JF, Edsall G, Holloway A. Measles in children with malignancy: problems and prevention. Arch Ges Virusforsch 16:331–337, 1965.

172. Siegel MM, Walter TK, Ablin AR. Measles pneumonia in childhood leukemia. Pediatrics 60:38–40, 1977.

173. Krasinski K, Borkowsky W. Measles and measles immunity in children infected with human immunodeficiency virus. JAMA 261:2512–2516, 1989.

174. Gray MM, Hann IM, Glass S, et al. Mortality and morbidity caused by measles in children with malignant disease attending four major treatment centres: a retrospective review. Br Med J (Clin Res Ed) 295:19–22, 1987.

175. Kaplan LJ, Daum RS, Smaron M, McCarthy CA. Severe measles in immunocompromised patients. JAMA 267:1237–1241, 1992.

176. Markowitz LE, Chandler FW, Roldan EO, et al. Fatal measles pneumonia without rash in a child with AIDS. J Infect Dis 158:480–483, 1988.

177. Nahmias AJ, Griffith D, Salsbury C, Yoshida K. Thymic aplasia and lymphopenia, plasma cells and normal immunoglobulins: relation to measles virus infection. JAMA 201:729–734, 1967.

178. Good RA, Zak SJ. Disturbances in gamma globulin synthesis as "experiments of nature." Pediatrics 18:109–149, 1956.

179. Burnet FM. Measles as an index of immunological function. Lancet 2:610–613, 1968.

180. Coovadia HM, Brain P, Hallett AF, et al. Immunoparesis and outcome in measles. Lancet 1:619–621, 1977.

181. Aicardi J, Goutiere SF, Arsenio-Nunes ML, Lebon P. Acute measles encephalitis in children with immunosuppression. Pediatrics 59:232–239, 1977.

182. Roos RP, Graves MC, Wollmann RL, et al. Immunologic and virologic studies of measles inclusion body encephalitis: the relationship to subacute sclerosing panencephalitis. Neurology 31:1263–1270, 1981.

183. Enders JF, McCarthy K, Mitus A, Cheatham WJ. Isolation of measles virus at autopsy in cases of giant-cell pneumonia without rash. N Engl J Med 261:875–881, 1959.

184. Palumbo P, Hoyt L, Demasio K, et al. Population-based study of measles and measles immunization in human immunodeficiency virus–infected children. Pediatr Infect Dis J 11:1008–1014, 1992.

185. Rauh LW, Schmidt R. Measles immunization with killed virus vaccine: serum antibody titers and experience with exposure to measles epidemic. Am J Dis Child 109:232–237, 1965.

186. Fulginiti VA, Eller JJ, Downie AW, Kempe CH. Altered reactivity to measles virus: atypical measles in children previously immunized with inactivated measles virus vaccines. JAMA 202:1075–1080, 1967.

187. Nader PR, Horowitz MS, Rousseau J. Atypical exanthem following exposure to natural measles: eleven cases in children previously inoculated with killed vaccine. J Pediatr 72:22–28, 1968.

188. Gokiert JG, Beamish WE. Altered reactivity to measles virus in previously vaccinated children. Can Med Assoc J 103:724–727, 1970.

189. Buser F, Montagnon B. Severe illness in children exposed to natural measles after prior vaccination against the disease. Scand J Infect Dis 2:157–160, 1970.

190. O'Neil AE. The measles epidemic in Calgary 1969–1970: the protective effect of vaccination for the individual and the community. Can Med Assoc J 105:819–825, 1971.

191. Welliver RC, Cherry JD, Holtzman AE. Typical, modified, and atypical measles: an emerging problem in the adolescent and adult. Arch Intern Med 137:39–41, 1977.

192. Weiner LB, Corwin RM, Nieberg PI, Feldman HA. A measles outbreak among adolescents. J Pediatr 90:17–20, 1977.

193. Chatterji M, Mankad V. Failure of attenuated viral vaccine in prevention of atypical measles. JAMA 238:2635, 1977.

194. Hall WW, Breese Hall C. Atypical measles in adolescents: evaluation of clinical and pulmonary function. Ann Intern Med 90:882–886, 1979.

195. Martin DB, Weiner LB, Nieberg PI, Blair DC. Atypical measles in adolescents and young adults. Ann Intern Med 90:877–881, 1979.

196. Fulginiti VA, Helfer RE. Atypical measles in adolescent siblings 16 years after killed measles virus vaccine. JAMA 244:804–806, 1980.

197. Annuziato D, Kaplan MH, Hull WW, et al. Atypical measles syndrome: pathologic and serologic findings. Pediatrics 70:203–209, 1982.

198. Norrby E. Measles. In Fields BN (ed). Virology. New York, Raven Press, 1985, pp 1305–1321.

199. Lennon RG, Isacson P, Rosales T, et al. Skin tests with measles and poliomyelitis vaccines in recipients of inactivated measles virus vaccine. JAMA 200:275–280, 1967.

200. Polack FP, Auwerter PG, Lee SH, et al. Production of atypical measles in rhesus macaques: evidence for disease mediated by immune complex formation and eosinophils in the presence of fusion-inhibiting antibody. Nat Med 5:629–634, 1999.

201. Brooks JB, McDade JE, Alley CC. Rapid differentiation of Rocky Mountain spotted fever from chickenpox, measles, and enterovirus infections and bacterial meningitis by frequency-pulsed electron capture gas-liquid chromatography analysis of sera. J Clin Microbiol 14:165–172, 1981.

202. Laptook A, Wind A, Nussbaum M, Shenker IR. Pulmonary lesions in atypical measles. Pediatrics 62:42–46, 1978.

203. Centers for Disease Control. Death from measles, possibly atypical—Michigan. MMWR 28:298–299, 1979.

204. Cherry JD, Feigen RD, Lobes LA, Shakelford PG. Atypical measles in children previously immunized with attenuated measles virus vaccines. Pediatrics 50:712–717, 1972.

205. St. Geme JW Jr, Bush BM, George BL. Exaggerated natural measles following attenuated virus immunization: a refraction–toxic shock syndrome [letter]. Pediatrics 67:942, 1981.

206. American Academy of Pediatrics. Measles. In Pickering LK (ed). 2000 Red Book: Report of the Committee on Infectious Diseases (25th ed). Elk Grove Village, IL, American Academy of Pediatrics, 2000, pp 385–396.

207. Centers for Disease Control and Prevention. Recommendations of the Advisory Committee on Immunization Practices (ACIP): measles, mumps, and rubella—vaccine use and strategies for elimination of measles, rubella, and congenital rubella syndrome and control of mumps. MMWR 47(RR-8):1–57, 1998.

208. Waterson AP. Measles virus. Arch Ges Virusforsch 16:57–80, 1965.

209. Bostock CJ, Barrett T, Crowther JR. Characterization of the European seal morbillivirus. Vet Microbiol 23:351–360, 1990.

210. Imagawa DT. Relationships among measles, canine distemper, and rinderpest viruses. Prog Med Virol 10:160–193, 1968.

211. Naniche D, Varior-Krishnan G, Cervoni F, et al. Human membrane cofactor protein (CD46) acts as a cellular receptor for measles virus. J Virol 67:6025–6032, 1993.

212. Tatsuo H, Yanagi Y. The morbillivirus receptor SLAM (CD150). Microbiol Immunol 46:135–142, 2002.

213. Crowley JC, Dowling PC, Menonna J, et al. Sequence variability and function of measles virus 3' and 5' ends and intercistronic regions. Virology 164:498–506, 1988.

214. Parks CL, Lerch RA, Walpita P, et al. Analysis of the noncoding regions of measles virus strains in the Edmonston vaccine lineage. Pearl River, NY, Department of Viral Vaccine Research, Wyeth-Lederle Vaccines, J Virol 75(2):921–933, 2001.

215. Parks CL, Lerch RA, Walpita P, et al. Comparison of predicted amino acid sequences of measles virus strains in the Edmonston vaccine lineage. Pearl River, New York Department of Viral Vaccine Research, Wyeth-Lederle Vaccines, J Virol 75(2):910–920, 2001.

216. Takeda M, Kato A, Kobune F, et al. Measles virus attenuation associated with transcriptional impediment and a few amino acid changes in the polymerase and accessory proteins. J Virol 72:8690–8696, 1998.

217. Takeuchi K, Miyajima N, Kobune F, Tashiro M. Comparative nucleotide sequence analyses of the entire genomes of B95a cell-isolated and Vero cell-isolated measles viruses from the same patient. Virus Genes 20:253–257, 2000.

218. Giraudon P, Jacquier MF, Wild TF. Antigenic analysis of African measles virus field isolates: identification and localization of one conserved and two variable epitope sites on the NP protein. Virus Res 10:137–152, 1988.

219. Baczko D, Brinckmann U, Padowitz I, et al. Nucleotide sequence of the genes encoding the matrix protein of two wild-type measles virus strains. J Gen Virol 72:2279–2282, 1991.

220. Taylor MJ, Godfrey E, Baczko K, et al. Identification of several different lineages of measles virus. J Gen Virol 72:83–88, 1991.

221. Rota JS, Hummel KB, Rota PA, Bellini WJ. Genetic variability of the glycoprotein genes of current wildtype measles isolates. J Virol 188:135–142, 1992.

222. Rota PA, Bloom AE, Vanchiere JA, Bellini WJ. Evolution of the nucleoprotein and matrix genes of wild-type strains of measles virus isolated from recent epidemics. Virology 198:724–730, 1994.

223. Rota JS, Wang ZD, Rota PA, Bellini WJ. Comparison of sequences of the H, F, and N coding genes of measles virus vaccine strains. Virus Res 31:317–330, 1994.

224. Mulders MN, Truong AT, Muller CP. Monitoring of measles elimination using molecular epidemiology. Vaccine 19:2245–2249, 2001.

225. Rota JR, Bellini WJ, Rota PA. Measles. In Thompson RCA (ed). Molecular Epidemiology of Infectious Diseases. London, Kluwer Academic & Lippincott–Raven Publishers, 2000, pp 168–180.

226. Rota J, Heath JL, Rota PA, et al. Molecular epidemiology of measles virus: identification of pathways of transmission and implications for measles elimination. J Infect Dis 173:32–37, 1996.

227. Rota JS, Rota PA, Redd SB, et al. Genetic analysis of measles viruses isolated in the United States, 1995–1996. J Infect Dis 177:204–208, 1998.

228. World Health Organization. Standardization of the nomenclature for describing the genetic characteristics of wild-type measles viruses. Wkly Epidemiol Rec 73:265–272, 1998.

229. World Health Organization. Nomenclature for describing the genetic characteristics of wild-type measles viruses (update). Wkly Epidemiol Rec 76:241–247, 2001.

230. World Health Organization. Nomenclature for describing the genetic characteristics of wild-type measles viruses (update)—Part II. Wkly Epidemiol Rec 76:249–251, 2001.

231. Kobune F, Sakata H, Sugiura A. Marmoset lymphoblastoid cells as a sensitive host for isolation of measles virus. J Virol 64:700–705, 1990.

232. Matumoto M. Multiplication of measles virus in cell cultures. Bacteriol Rev 30:152–176, 1966.

233. Forthal DN, Blanding J, Aarnaes S, et al. Comparison of different methods and cell lines for isolating measles virus. J Clin Microbiol 31:695–697, 1993.

234. Enders JF, Katz SL, Grogran E. Markers for Edmonston measles virus. Am J Dis Child 103:473–474, 1962.

235. McCarthy K. Measles in laboratory hosts and tissue culture systems. Am J Dis Child 103:314–319, 1962.

236. Suringa DWR, Bank LJ, Ackerman AB. Role of measles virus in skin lesions and Koplik's spots. N Engl J Med 283:1139–1142, 1970.

237. Buynak EB, Peck JM, Creamer AA, et al. Differentiation of virulent from avirulent measles strains. Am J Dis Child 103:460–473, 1962.

238. DeMaeyer E, Enders JF. Growth characteristics, interferon production and plaque formation with different lines of Edmonston measles virus. Arch Ges Virusforsch 16:151–160, 1965.

239. Katz SL. Immunization with live attenuated measles virus vaccines: five years' experience. Arch Virusforsch 16:222–230, 1965.

240. Papp K. Experiences prouvant que la voie d'infection de la rougeole est la contamination de la muqueuse conjunctival. Rev Immunol Ther Antimicrob 20:27–36, 1956.

241. Fenner F. The pathogenesis of the acute exanthems. Lancet 2:915–920, 1948.

242. Moench TR, Griffin DE, Obriecht CR, et al. Acute measles in patients with and without neurological involvement: distribution of measles virus antigen and RNA. J Infect Dis 158:433–442, 1988.

243. Ogra PL, Fishaut M, Gallagher MR. Viral vaccination via mucosal routes. Rev Infect Dis 2:352–369, 1980.

244. Thomas HI, Barret E, Hesketh LM, et al. Simultaneous IgM reactivity by EIA against more than one virus in measles, parvovirus B19, rubella infection. J Clin Virol 14:107–118, 1999.

245. Oliveira MI, Curti SP, Figueiredo CA, et al. Rash after measles vaccination: laboratory analysis of cases reported in Sao Paulo, Brazil. Rev Saude Publica 36:155–159, 2002.

246. Ramsay M, Reacher M, O'Flynn C, et al. Causes of morbilliform rash in a highly immunized English population. Arch Dis Child 87:202–206, 2002.

247. Llanes-Rodas R, Liu C. Rapid diagnosis of measles from urinary sediments stained with fluorescent antibody. N Engl J Med 275:515–523, 1966.

248. Lightwood R, Nolan R, Franco M, White AJS. Epithelial giant cells in measles as an aid in diagnosis. J Pediatr 77:59–64, 1970.

249. Fulton RE, Middleton PJ. Immunofluorescence in diagnosis of measles infection in children. J Pediatr 86:17–22, 1975.

250. Olding-Stenkvist E, Bjorvatn B. Rapid detection of measles virus in skin rashes by immunofluorescence. J Infect Dis 134:463–469, 1976.

251. Nommensen FE, Dekkers NWHM. Detection of measles antigen in conjunctival epithelial lesions staining by Lissamine green during measles virus infection. J Med Virol 7:157–162, 1981.

252. Boyd JF. A fourteen year study to identify measles antigen in urine specimens by fluorescent-antibody methods. J Infect 6:163–170, 1983.

253. Jin L, Richards A, Brown DW. Development of a dual target–PCR for detection and characterization of measles virus in clinical specimens. Mol Cell Probes 10:191–200, 1996.

254. Rota PA, Khan AS, Durigon E, et al. Detection of measles virus RNA in urine specimens from vaccine recipients. J Clin Microbiol 33:2485–2488, 1995.

255. Riddell MA, Chibo D, Kelly HA, et al. Investigation of optimal specimen type and sampling time for detection of measles virus RNA during a measles epidemic. J Clin Microbiol 39:375–376, 2001.

256. Wassilak SGF, Bernier RH, Herrmann KL, et al. Measles seroconfirmation using dried capillary blood specimens in filter paper. Pediatr Infect Dis 3:117–121, 1984.

257. Krugman S, Giles JP, Jacobs AM, Friedman H. Studies with a further attenuated live measles-virus vaccine. Pediatrics 31:919–928, 1963.

258. Krugman S. Present status of measles and rubella immunization in the United States: a medical progress report. J Pediatr 90:1–12, 1977.

259. Krugman S. Further-attenuated measles vaccine: characteristics and use. Rev Infect Dis 5:477–481, 1983.

260. Schluederberg A. Immune globulins in human viral infections. Nature 205:1232–1233, 1965.

261. Heffner RR Jr, Schluederberg A. Specificity of the primary and secondary antibody responses to myxoviruses. J Immunol 98:668–672, 1967.

262. Polna I, Aleksandrowicz J, Roszkowska K. Localization of measles antibody and inhibitor activity in fractions of human sera at different stages of the disease, and sera of animals immunized with measles virus. I. Dynamics of increase in measles antibody activity and its localization in children sera after natural infection. Acta Microbiol Pol A 5:131–138, 1973.

263. Aleksandrowicz J, Polna I, Sadowski W. II. Primary and secondary immunological response of experimental animals to attenuated and nonattenuated measles virus. Acta Microbiol Pol A 5:139–145, 1973.

264. Friedman MG, Philip M, Dagan R. Virus-specific IgA in serum, saliva, and tears of children with measles. Clin Exp Immunol 75:58–64, 1989.

265. Erdman DD, Anderson LJ, Adams DR, et al. Evaluation of mono-clonal antibody–based capture enzyme immunoassays for detection of specific antibodies to measles virus. J Clin Microbiol 29:1466–1471, 1991.

266. Erdman DD, Heath JL, Watson JC, et al. Immunoglobulin M anti-body response to measles virus following primary and secondary vac-cination and natural virus infection. J Med Virol 41:44–48, 1993.

267. Cutchins EC. A comparison of the hemagglutination-inhibition, neutralization and complement fixation tests in the assay of antibody to measles. J Immunol 88:788–795, 1962.

268. Albrecht P, Herrmann K, Burns GR. Role of virus strain in conven-tional and enhanced measles plaque neutralization test. J Virol Methods 3:251–260, 1981.

269. Roesing TG, Meeker J, Garfinkle B, et al. Determination of antibody to measles virus by a fluoroimmunoassay (FIAX). J Biol Stand 9:401–407, 1981.

270. Forghani B, Schmidt NJ. Antigen requirements, sensitivity, and specificity of enzyme immunoassays for measles and rubella viral anti-bodies. J Clin Microbiol 9:657–664, 1979.

271. Kleiman MB, Blackburn CKL, Zimmerman SE, French ML. Comparison of enzyme-linked immunosorbent assay for acute measles with hemagglutination inhibition, complement fixation, and fluorescent-antibody methods. J Clin Microbiol 14:147–152, 1981.

272. Neumann PW, Weber JM, Jessamine AG, O'Shaughnessy MV. Comparison of measles antihemolysin test, enzyme-linked immunosorbent assay, and hemagglutination inhibition test with neutralization test for determination of immune status. J Clin Microbiol 22:296–298, 1985.

273. Weigle KA, Murphy MD, Brunell PA. Enzyme-linked immunosor-bent assay for evaluation of immunity to measles virus. J Clin Microbiol 19:376–379, 1984.

274. Hummel KB, Erdman DD, Heath J, Bellini WJ. Baculovirus expres-sion of the nucleoprotein gene of measles virus and the utility of the recombinant protein in diagnostic enzyme immunoassays. J Clin Microbiol 30:2874–2880, 1992.

275. Rossier E, Miller H, McCulloch B, et al. Comparison of immunoflu-orescence and enzyme immunoassay for detection of measles-specific immunoglobulin M antibody. J Clin Microbiol 29:1069–1071, 1991.

276. Mayo DR, Brennan T, Cormier DP, et al. Evaluation of a commercial measles virus immunoglobulin M enzyme immunoassay. J Clin Microbiol 29:2865–2867, 1991.

277. Black FL. Measles active and passive immunity in a worldwide per-spective. Prog Med Virol 36:1–33, 1989.

278. Ratnam S, Gadag V, West R, et al. Comparison of commercial enzyme immunoassay kits with plaque reduction neutralization test for detection of measles virus antibody. J Clin Microbiol 33:811–815, 1995.

279. Bellini WJ, Helfand RF. Current challenges in the laboratory diagno-sis of measles infections. J Infect Dis 187(Suppl 1): S283–S290, 2003.

280. Ratnam S, Tipples G, Head C, et al. Performance of indirect immunoglobulin M (IgM) serology tests and IgM capture assays for laboratory diagnosis of measles. J Clin Microbiol 38:99–104, 2000.

281. Jenkerson SA, Beller M, Middaugh JP, Erdman DD. False positive rubeola IgM tests. N Engl J Med 332:1103–1104, 1995.

282. Helfand RF, Heath JL, Anderson LJ, et al. Diagnosis of measles with an IgM capture EIA: the optimal timing of specimen collection after rash onset. J Infect Dis 175:195–199, 1997.

283. Brown DW, Ramsay ME, Richards AF, Miller E. Salivary diagnosis of measles: a study of notified cases in the United Kingdom, 1991–1993. BMJ 308:1015–1017, 1994.

284. Ramsay M, Brugha R, Brown D. Surveillance of measles in England and Wales: implications of a national saliva testing programme. Bull World Health Organ 75:515–521, 1997.

285. Condorelli F, Scalia G, Stivala A, et al. Detection of immunoglobu-lin G to measles virus, rubella virus, and mumps virus in serum sam-ples and in microquantities of whole blood dried on filter paper. J Virol Methods 49:25–36, 1994.

286. Helfand RF, Keyserling HL, Williams I, et al. Comparative detection of measles and rubella IgM and IgG derived from filter paper blood and serum samples. J Med Virol 65:751–757, 2001.

287. De Swart RL, Nur Y, Abdallah A, et al. Combination of reverse tran-scriptase PCR analysis and immunoglobulin M detection on filter paper blood samples allows diagnosis and epidemiological studies of measles. J Clin Microbiol 39:270–273, 2001.

288. Olding-Stenkvist E, Forsgren M, Henley D, et al. Measles encephalopathy during immunosuppression: failure of treatment. Scand J Infect Dis 14:1–4, 1982.

289. Simpson R, Eden OB. Possible interferon response in a child with measles encephalitis during immunosuppression. Scand J Infect Dis 16:315–319, 1984.

290. Beatty DW, Handzel ZT, Pecht M, et al. A controlled trial of treat-ment of acquired immunodeficiency in severe measles with thymic humoral factor. Clin Exp Immunol 56:479–485, 1984.

291. Tovo PA, Pugliese A, Palomba E, et al. Thymostimulin therapy in patients with measles meningoencephalitis. Thymus 8:91–94, 1986.

292. Wesley AG, Coovadia HM, Kiepiela P. Levamisole therapy in children at risk from severe measles. Ann Trop Paediatr 2:23–29, 1982.

293. Banks G, Fernandez H. Clinical use of ribavirin in measles: a sum-marized review. In Smith RA, Knight V, Smith JAD (eds). Clinical Applications of Ribavirin. New York, Academic Press, 1984, pp 203–209.

294. Ross LA, Kim KS, Mason WH, Gomperts E. Successful treatment of disseminated measles in a patient with acquired immunodeficiency syndrome: consideration of antiviral and passive immunotherapy. Am J Med 88:313–314, 1990.

295. Hussey GD, Klein M. A randomized, controlled trial of vitamin A in children with severe measles. N Engl J Med 323:160–164, 1990.

296. Barclay AJG, Foster A, Sommer A. Vitamin A supplements and mor-tality related to measles: a randomized clinical trial. Br Med J (Clin Res Ed) 294:294–296, 1987.

297. D'Souza RM, D'Souza R. Vitamin A for preventing secondary infec-tions in children with measles—a systematic review. J Trop Paediatr 48:72–77, 2002.

298. World Health Organization and United Nations Children's Fund. Measles Mortality Reduction and Regional Elimination: Strategic Plan, 2001–2005 (WHO/V&B/01.13). Geneva, World Health Organization, 2001.

299. Butler JC, Havens PL, Sowell AL, et al. Measles severity and serum retinol (vitamin A) concentration among children in the United States. Pediatrics 91:1176–1181, 1993.

300. Frieden TR, Sowell AL, Henning KJ, et al. Vitamin A levels and severity of measles: New York City. Am J Dis Child 146:182–186, 1992.

301. Arrieta AC, Zaleska M, Stutman HR, Marks MI. Vitamin A levels in children with measles in Long Beach, California. J Pediatr 121:75–78, 1992.

302. Shann F. Meta-analysis of trials of prophylactic antibiotics for chil-dren with measles: inadequate evidence. BMJ 314:334–336, 1997.

303. Freeman JM. Treatment for subacute sclerosing panencephalitis with 5-bromo-2-deoxyuridine and Pyran copolymer. Neurology 18(pt 2):176–192, 1968.

304. Steiner I, Wirguin I, Morag A, Abramsky O. Intraventricular alpha interferon for subacute sclerosing panencephalitis. J Child Neurol 4:20–23, 1989.

305. Gascon GG, Yamani S, Cafege A. Treatment of subacute sclerosing panencephalitis with alpha interferon. Ann Neurol 30:227–228, 1991.

306. DuRant RH, Dyken PR, Swift AV. The influence of inosiplex treat-ment on the neurological disability of patients with subacute scleros-ing panencephalitis. J Pediatr 101:288–293, 1982.

307. Anlar B, Yalaz K, Kose G, Saygi S. Beta-interferon plus inosiplex in the treatment of subacute sclerosing panencephalitis. J Child Neurol 13:557–559, 1998.

308. Yazaki M, Yamazaki M, Urasawa N, et al. Successful treatment with alpha-interferon of a patient with chronic measles infection of the brain and parkinsonism. Eur Neurol 44:184–186, 2000.

309. Langmuir AD. Medical importance of measles. Am J Dis Child 103:224–226, 1962.

310. Black FL. Measles antibody prevalence in diverse populations. Am J Dis Child 103:242–249, 1962.

311. Preblud SR, Gross F, Halsey NA, et al. Assessment of susceptibility to measles and rubella. JAMA 247:1134–1137, 1982.

312. deJong JG. The survival of measles virus in air, in relation to the epi-demiology of measles. Arch Ges Virusforsch 16:97–102, 1965.

313. Riley RC, Murphy G, Riley RL. Airborne spread of measles in a sub-urban elementary school. Am J Epidemiol 107:421–432, 1978.

314. Bloch AB, Orenstein WA, Ewing WM, et al. Measles outbreak in a pediatric practice: airborne transmission in an office setting. Pediatrics 75:676–683, 1985.
315. Ehresmann KR, Hedberg CW, Grimm MB, et al. An outbreak of measles at an international sporting event with airborne transmission in a domed stadium. J Infect Dis 171:679–683, 1995.
316. Top FH. Measles in Detroit, 1935. I. Factors influencing the secondary attack rate among susceptibles at risk. Am J Public Health 28:935–943, 1938.
317. Hope-Simpson RE. Infectiousness of communicable diseases in the household. Lancet 2:549–554, 1952.
318. Sutter RW, Markowitz LE, Bennetch JM, et al. Measles among the Amish: a comparative study of measles severity in primary and secondary cases in households. J Infect Dis 163:12–16, 1991.
319. Brandling-Bennett AD, Landrigan PJ, Baker EL. Failure of vaccinated children to transmit measles. JAMA 224:616–618, 1973.
320. Lievano F, Papania M, Helfand R, et al. Lack of evidence of measles virus shedding in people with inapparent measles infections. J Infect Dis Suppl 2003 [in press].
321. The National Vaccine Advisory Committee. The measles epidemic: the problems, barriers, and recommendations. JAMA 266:1547–1552, 1991.
322. Hedrich AW. The corrected average attack rate from measles among city children. Am J Hyg 11:576–600, 1930.
323. London WP, Yorke JA. Recurrent outbreaks of measles, chickenpox, and mumps. I. Seasonal variation in contact rates. Am J Epidemiol 98:453–468, 1973.
324. Yorke JA, London WP. Recurrent outbreaks of measles, chickenpox, and mumps. II. Systematic differences in contact rates and stochastic effects. Am J Epidemiol 98:469–482, 1973.
325. Crawford GE, Gremillion DH. Epidemic measles and rubella in Air Force recruits: impact of immunization. J Infect Dis 144:403–410, 1981.
326. Chen RT, Goldbaum GM, Wassilak SGF, et al. An explosive point-source outbreak in a highly vaccinated population. Am J Epidemiol 129:173–182, 1989.
327. Centers for Disease Control and Prevention. Measles outbreak among school-aged children—Juneau, Alaska, 1996. MMWR 45:777–780, 1996.
328. Hennessy KA, Ion-Nedelcu N, Craciun M, et al. Measles epidemic in Romania, 1996–1998: assessment of vaccine effectiveness by case-control and cohort studies. Am J Epidemiol 150:1250–1257, 1999.
329. Lambert SB, Morgan ML, Riddel MA, et al. Measles outbreak in young adults in Victoria, 1999. Med J Aust 173:467–471, 2000.
330. Collaborative study by Ministry of Health of Kenya and World Health Organization: measles immunity in the first year after birth and the optimum age for vaccination in Kenyan children. Bull World Health Organ 55:21–31, 1977.
331. Ministries of Health of Brazil, Chile, Costa Rica, and Ecuador and the Pan American Health Organization. Seroconversion rates and measles antibody titers induced by measles vaccination in Latin American children 6 to 12 months of age. Rev Infect Dis 5:596–605, 1983.
332. Halsey NA. The optimal age for administering measles vaccine in developing countries. In Halsey NA, de Quadros CA (eds). Recent Advances in Immunization: A Bibliographic Review (publication no 451). Washington, DC, Pan American Health Organization, 1983, pp 4–17.
333. Halsey NA, Boulos R, Mode F, et al. Responses to measles vaccine in Haitian infants 6 to 12 months old: influence of maternal antibodies, malnutrition, and concurrent illnesses. N Engl J Med 313:544–549, 1985.
334. Black FL, Berman LL, Borgono JM, et al. Geographic variation in infant loss of maternal measles antibody and in prevalence of rubella antibody. Am J Epidemiol 124:442–452, 1986.
335. Whittle HC, Mee J, Werblinska J, et al. Immunity to measles in malnourished children. Clin Exp Immunol 42:144–151, 1980.
336. Aaby P, Bukh J, Hoff G, et al. High measles mortality in infancy related to intensity of exposure. J Pediatr 109:40–44, 1986.
337. Morley DC, Aaby P. Managing measles: size of infecting dose may be important [letter]. BMJ 314:1692, 1997.
338. Paunio M, Peltola H, Valle M, et al. Explosive school-based measles outbreak: intense exposure may have resulted in high risk, even among revaccinees. Am J Epidemiol 148:1103–1110, 1998.
339. Centers for Disease Control and Prevention. Progress toward global measles control and regional elimination, 1990–1997. MMWR 47:1049–1054, 1998.
340. Murray CJL, Lopez AD, Mathers CD, Stein C. The Global Burden of Disease 2000 Project: Aims, Methods, and Data Sources (Global Programme for Evidence for Health Policy—Discussion Paper No 36). Geneva, World Health Organization, 2001. Available at www3.who.int/whosis/burden/papers/Discussion%20Paper%2036%20Revised.doc
341. White CC, Koplan JP, Orenstein WA. Benefits, risks, and costs of immunization for measles, mumps, and rubella. Am J Public Health 75:739–744, 1985.
342. Hatziandreu EJ, Brown RE, Halpern MT. A Cost Benefit Analysis of Measles-Mumps-Rubella Vaccine: Final Report. Arlington, VA, Battelle, 1994, pp 1–66.
343. Stiehm ER. Standard and special human immune serum globulins as therapeutic agents. Pediatrics 63:301–319, 1979.
344. Endo A, Izumi H, Miyashita M, et al. Current efficacy of postexposure prophylaxis against measles with immunoglobulin. J Pediatric 138:926–928, 2001.
345. Department of Health and Human Services, Food and Drug Administration. Revision of requirements applicable to albumin (human), plasma protein fraction (human), and immune globulin (human) (21 CFR Part 640 [Docket No. 98N-0608]). Fed Reg 64:26282–26287, 1999.
346. Siber GR, Werner BG, Halsey NA, et al. Interference of immune globulin with measles and rubella immunization. J Pediatr 122:204–211, 1993.
347. American Academy of Pediatrics, Committee on Infectious Diseases and Committee on Pediatric AIDS. Measles immunization in HIV-infected children. Pediatrics 103:1057–1060, 1999.
348. Okuno Y, Takahashi M, Toyoshima K, et al. Studies on the prophylaxis of measles with attenuated living virus. III. Inoculation tests in man and monkey with chick embryo passage measles virus. Biken J 3:115–122, 1960.
349. Katz SL, Morley DC, Krugman S. Attenuated measles vaccine in Nigerian children. Am J Dis Child 103:402–405, 1962.
350. Smorodinstev AA, Boychuk LM, Shikina ES, et al. Further experiences with live measles vaccines in U.S.S.R. Am J Dis Child 103:384–386, 1962.
351. Report of a WHO Scientific Group: measles vaccine. World Health Organ Tech Rep Ser 263:5–37, 1963.
352. Medical Research Council. Vaccination against measles: a study of clinical reactions and serological response of young children. Br Med J 1:817–823, 1965.
353. Medical Research Council. Vaccination against measles: a clinical trial of live measles vaccine given alone and live vaccine preceded by killed vaccine. Br Med J 1:441–446, 1966.
354. Bolotovskij VM, Nefedova LA, Gelikman BG, et al. Comparative studies of measles vaccine in a controlled trial in the USSR. Bull World Health Organ 34:859–864, 1966.
355. Cockburn WC, Pecenka J, Sundaresan T. WHO supported comparative studies of attenuated live measles vaccines. Bull World Health Organ 34:223–231, 1966.
356. Swartz T, Klingberg W, Nishmi M, et al. A comparative study of four live measles vaccines in Israel. Bull World Health Organ 39:285–292, 1968.
357. Ikic D, Juzasic M, Beck M, et al. Attenuation and characterization of Edmonston-Zagreb measles virus. Ann Immunol Hung 16:175–181, 1972.
358. Peradze TV, Smorodintsev AA. Epidemiology and specific prophylaxis of measles. Rev Infect Dis 5:487–490, 1983.
359. Mirchamsy H. Measles immunization in Iran. Rev Infect Dis 5:491–494, 1983.
360. Clements CJ, Milstein JB, Grabowsky M, Gibson J. Research into Alternative Measles Vaccines in the 1990s (EPI/Gen/88.11 Rev 1). Geneva, World Health Organization, 1988.
361. Hirayama M. Measles vaccine used in Japan. Rev Infect Dis 5:495–503, 1983.
362. Makino S. Development and characteristics of live AIK-C measles virus vaccine: a brief report. Rev Infect Dis 5:504–505, 1983.
363. Jianzhi X, Zhihui C. Measles vaccine in the People's Republic of China. Rev Infect Dis 5:506–510, 1983.

364. Mirchamsy H, Bahrami S, Shafyi A, et al. The isolation and characterization of a human diploid cell strain and its use in production of measles vaccine. J Biol Stand 14:75–79, 1986.

365. Okuno Y, Ueda S, Kurimura T, et al. Studies on further attenuated live measles vaccine. VII. Development and evaluation of CAM-70 measles virus vaccine. Biken J 14:253–258, 1971.

366. McCrumb FR, Kress S, Saunders E, et al. Studies with live attenuated measles-virus vaccine. I. Clinical and immunologic responses in institutionalized children. Am J Dis Child 101:689–700, 1961.

367. Kress S, Schluederberg AE, Hornick RB, et al. Studies with live attenuated measles-virus vaccine. II. Clinical and immunologic response of children in an open community. Am J Dis Child 101:701–707, 1961.

368. Hornick RB, Schluederberg AE, McCrumb FR Jr. Vaccination with live attenuated measles virus. Am J Dis Child 103:344–347, 1962.

369. Stokes J Jr, Hilleman MR, Weibel RE, et al. Efficacy of live attenuated measles-virus vaccine given with human immune globulin. N Engl J Med 265:507–513, 1961.

370. Weibel R, Halenda R, Stokes J Jr, et al. Administration of Enders' live measles virus vaccine with immune globulin. JAMA 180:1086–1094, 1962.

371. Morley D, Katz SL, Krugman S. The clinical reaction of Nigerian children to measles vaccine with and without gamma globulin. J Hyg (Camb) 61:135–141, 1963.

372. Benson PF, Butler NR, Goeffe AP, et al. Vaccination of infants with living attenuated measles vaccine (Edmonston strain) with and without gamma-globulin. Br Med J 2:851–853, 1964.

373. Weibel RE, Stokes J Jr, Halenda R, et al. Durable immunity two years after administration of Enders' live measles-virus vaccine with immune globulin. N Engl J Med 270:172–175, 1964.

374. Warren RJ, Nader PR, Levine RH. Measles immune globulin: proposed standard dose given with live attenuated measles virus vaccine. JAMA 203:186–188, 1968.

375. Warren J, Gallian MJ. Concentrated inactivated measles-virus vaccine: preparation and antigenic potency. Am J Dis Child 103:418–423, 1962.

376. Feldman HA. Protective value of inactivated measles vaccine. Am J Dis Child 103:423–424, 1962.

377. Karzon DT, Winkelstein W Jr, Jenss R, et al. Field trial of inactivated measles vaccine. Am J Dis Child 103:425–426, 1962.

378. Karlitz S, Berliner BC, Orange M, et al. Inactivated measles virus vaccine: subsequent challenge with attenuated live virus vaccine. JAMA 184:673–679, 1963.

379. Fulginiti VA, Kempe CH. Measles exposure among vaccine recipients. Am J Dis Child 106:450–461, 1963.

380. Krugman S, Stone S, Hu R, Friedman H. Measles immunization incorporated in the routine schedule for infants: efficacy of a combined inactivated-live vaccination regimen. Pediatrics 34:795–797, 1964.

381. Karzon DT, Rush D, Winkelstein W. Immunization with inactivated measles virus vaccine: effect of booster dose and response to natural challenge. Pediatrics 36:40–50, 1965.

382. Guinee VF, Henderson DA, Casey HL, et al. Cooperative measles vaccine field trial. I. Clinical efficacy. II. Serologic studies. Pediatrics 37:649–665, 1966.

383. Centers for Disease Control. Recommendations of the Public Health Service Advisory Committee on Immunization Practice: measles vaccines. MMWR 16:269–271, 1967.

384. Orenstein WA, Halsey NA, Hayden GF, et al. Current status of measles in the United States, 1973–1977. J Infect Dis 137:847–853, 1978.

385. Suzuki K, Morita M, Katoh M, et al. Development and evaluation of the TD97 measles virus vaccine. J Med Virol 32:194–901, 1990.

386. Mann GF, Allison LMC, Copeland JA, et al. A simplified plaque assay system for measles virus. J Biol Stand 8:219–225, 1980.

387. Bellocq C, Roux L. Wide occurrence of measles virus subgenomic RNAs in attenuated live-virus vaccines. Biologicals 18:337–343, 1990.

388. Mori T, Sasaki K, Hashimoto H, Makino S. Molecular cloning and complete sequence of genomic RNA of the AIK-C strain of attenuated measles virus. Virus Genes 7:67–81, 1993.

389. Valsamakis A, Kaneshima H, Griffin DE. Strains of measles vaccine and their ability to replicate in and damage human thymus. J Infect Dis 183:498–502, 2001.

390. Lecouturier V, Fayolle J, Caballero M, et al. Identification of two amino acids in the hemagglutinin glycoprotein of measles virus (MV) that govern hemadsorption, HeLa cell fusion, and CD46 downregulation: phenotypic markers that differentiate vaccine and wild-type MV strains. J Virol 70:4200–4204, 1996.

391. Radecke F, Spielhofer P, Schneider H, et al. Rescue of measles viruses from cloned DNA. EMBO J 14:5773–5784, 1995.

392. Andelman SL, Schwarz A, Andelman MB, Zackler J. Experimental vaccination against measles: clinical evaluation of a highly attenuated live measles vaccine. JAMA 184:721–723, 1963.

393. Schwarz AJ. Immunization against measles: development and evaluation of a highly attenuated live measles vaccine. Ann Paediatr 202:241–252, 1964.

394. Schwarz AJF, Anderson JT. Immunization with a further attenuated live measles vaccine. Arch Virusforsch 16:273–278, 1965.

395. Schwarz AJF, Anderson JT, Ramos-Alvarez M, et al. Extensive clinical evaluations of a highly attenuated live measles vaccine. JAMA 199:84–88, 1967.

396. Hilleman MR, Buynak EB, Weibel RE, et al. Development and evaluation of the Moraten measles virus vaccine. JAMA 206:587–590, 1968.

397. Krugman S, Constantinidis P, Medovy H, Giles JP. Comparison of two further attenuated live measles-virus vaccines. Am J Dis Child 117:137–138, 1969.

398. Centers for Disease Control. Recommendations of the Public Health Service Advisory Committee on Immunization Practice. MMWR 14:64–67, 1965.

399. Potency test. 21 C.F.R. § 630.34.

400. Sassani A, Mirchamsy H, Shafyi A, et al. Excessive attenuation of measles virus as a possible cause of failure in measles immunization. Ann Inst Pasteur Virol 138:491–501, 1987.

401. Makino S, Sasaki K, Nakayama T, et al. A new combined trivalent live measles (AIK-C strain), mumps (Hoshino strain) and rubella (Takahashi strain) vaccine. Am J Dis Child 144:905–910, 1990.

402. McAleer WJ, Markus HZ, McLeam AA, et al. The stability on storage at various temperatures of the live measles, mumps, and rubella virus vaccines in a new stabilizer. J Biol Stand 8:281–287, 1980.

403. Wallace RB, Landrigan PJ, Smith A, et al. Trial of a reduced dose of measles vaccine in Nigerian children. Bull World Health Organ 53:361–364, 1976.

404. McGraw TT. Reimmunization following early immunization with measles vaccine: a prospective study. Pediatrics 77:45–48, 1986.

405. Lee GC-Y. Intranasal vaccination with attenuated measles virus. Proc Soc Exp Biol Med 112:656–658, 1963.

406. Kok PW, Kenya PR, Ensering H. Measles immunization with further attenuated heat-stable measles vaccine using five different methods of administration. Trans R Soc Trop Med Hyg 77:171–176, 1983.

407. Sabin AB. Immunization against measles by aerosol. Rev Infect Dis 5:514–523, 1983.

408. Sabin AB, Arechiga AF, Fernandez de Castro J, et al. Successful immunization of infants with and without maternal antibody by aerosolized measles vaccine. I. Different results with undiluted human diploid cell and chick embryo fibroblast vaccines. JAMA 240:2651–2652, 1983.

409. Sabin AB, Arechiga AF, Fernandez de Castro J, et al. Successful immunization of infants with and without maternal antibody by aerosolized measles vaccine. II. Vaccine comparisons and evidence for multiple antibody response. JAMA 251:2363–2371, 1984.

410. Whittle HC, Rowland MG, Mann GF, et al. Immunization of 4–6-month-old Gambian infants with Edmonston-Zagreb measles vaccine. Lancet 2:834–837, 1984.

411. Khanum S, Garelick H, Uddin N, et al. Comparison of Edmonston-Zagreb and Schwarz strains of measles vaccine given by aerosol or subcutaneous injection. Lancet 1:150–153, 1987.

412. Ekunwe EO. Immunization by inhalation of aerosolized measles vaccine. Ann Trop Pediatr 10:145–149, 1990.

413. Cutts FT, Clements CJ, Bennett JV. Alternative routes of measles immunization: a review. Biologicals 25:323–338, 1997.

414. Dilraj A, Cutts F, de Castro J, et al. Response to different measles vaccines strains given by aerosol and subcutaneous routes to school-children: a randomized trial. Lancet 355:798–803, 2000.

415. Sepulveda-Amor J, Valdespino-Gomez JL, Garcia-Garcia Mde L, et al. A randomized trial demonstrating successful boosting responses following simultaneous aerosols of measles and rubella (MR) vaccines in school age children. Vaccine 20:2790–2795, 2002.

416. World Health Organization, Department of Vaccines and Biologicals. Report of a meeting on Research Related to Measles Control and Elimination (V&B/01.13). Geneva, World Health Organization, 2001.

417. Walker D, Carter H, Jones IG. Measles, mumps, and rubella: the need for a change in immunization policy. Br Med J (Clin Res Ed) 292:1501–1502, 1986.

418. Peltola H, Heinonen OP. Frequency of true adverse reactions to measles-mumps-rubella vaccine: a double-blind placebo-controlled trial in twins. Lancet 1:939–942, 1986.

419. Isozaki M, Kuno-Sakai H, Hoshi N, et al. Effects and side effects of a new trivalent combined measles-mumps-rubella (MMR) vaccine. Tokai J Exp Clin Med 7:547–550, 1982.

420. Beck M, Smerdel S, Dedic I, et al. Immune response to Edmonston-Zagreb measles virus strain in monovalent and combined MMR vaccine. Dev Biol Stand 65:95–100, 1986.

421. Just M, Berger R, Glueck R, Wegmann A. Evaluation of a combined vaccine against measles-mumps-rubella produced on human diploid cells. Dev Biol Stand 65:25–27, 1986.

422. Buynak EB, Weibel RE, Whitman JE Jr, et al. Combined live measles-mumps-rubella virus vaccines: findings in clinical-laboratory studies. JAMA 207:2259–2262, 1969.

423. Smorodintsev AA, Nasibov MN, Jakovleva NV. Experience with live rubella virus vaccine combined with live vaccines against measles and mumps. Bull World Health Organ 42:283–289, 1970.

424. Krugman S, Muriel G, Fontana VJ. Combined live measles, mumps, rubella vaccine: immunological response. Am J Dis Child 121:380–381, 1971.

425. Stokes J Jr, Weibel RE, Vallarejos VM, et al. Trivalent combined measles-mumps-rubella vaccine: findings in clinical-laboratory studies. JAMA 218:57–61, 1971.

426. Karchmer AW, Friedman JP, Casey HL, et al. Simultaneous administration of live virus vaccines: measles, mumps, poliomyelitis, and smallpox. Am J Dis Child 121:382–388, 1971.

427. Landrigan PJ, Murphy KB, Meyer HM Jr, et al. Combined measles-rubella vaccines: virus dose and serologic response. Am J Dis Child 125:65–67, 1973.

428. Schwarz AJF, Jackson JE, Ehrenkranz NJ, et al. Clinical evaluation of a new measles-mumps-rubella trivalent vaccine. Am J Dis Child 129:1408–1412, 1975.

429. Krugman RD, Witte JJ, Parkman PD, et al. Combined administration of measles, mumps, rubella, and trivalent poliovirus vaccines. Public Health Rep 92:220–222, 1977.

430. Weibel RE, Carlson AJ Jr, Villarejos VM, et al. Clinical and laboratory studies of combined live measles, mumps, and rubella vaccines using the RA 27/3 rubella virus (40979). Proc Soc Exp Biol Med 165:323–326, 1980.

431. Lerman SJ, Bollinger M, Brunken JM. Clinical and serologic evaluation of measles, mumps and rubella (HPV-77:DE5 and RA 27/3) virus vaccines, singly and in combination. Pediatrics 68:18–22, 1981.

432. Sugiura A, Ohtawara M, Hayami M, et al. Field trial of trivalent measles-rubella-mumps vaccine in Japan. J Infect Dis 146:709, 1982.

433. Parkman PD, Hopps HE, Albrecht P, Meyer HM Jr. Simultaneous administration of vaccines. In Halsey NA, de Quadros CA (eds). Recent Advances in Immunization: A Bibliographic Review (publication no 451). Washington, DC, Pan American Health Organization, 1983, pp 65–80.

434. Brunell PA, Weigle K, Murphy MD. Antibody response following measles-mumps-rubella vaccine under conditions of customary use. JAMA 250:1409–1412, 1983.

435. Vesikari T, Ala-Laurila E-L, Heikkinen A, et al. Clinical trial of a new trivalent measles-mumps-rubella vaccine in young children. Am J Dis Child 138:843–847, 1984.

436. Wegmann A, Gluck R, Just M, et al. Comparative study and evaluation of further attenuated, live measles vaccines alone and in combination with mumps and rubella vaccines. Dev Biol Stand 65:69–74, 1986.

437. Orenstein WA, Herrmann KL, Albrecht P, et al. Immunity against measles and rubella in Massachusetts school children. Dev Biol Stand 65:75–83, 1986.

438. Andre FE, Peetermans J. Effect of simultaneous administration of live measles vaccine on the "take rate" of live mumps vaccine. Dev Biol Stand 65:101–107, 1986.

439. Elliott AY. Manufacture and testing of measles, mumps and rubella vaccine. In Proceedings of the 19th Immunization Conference, Boston, May 21–24, 1984, pp 79–86.

440. Böni J, Stadler J, Reigel F, Schüpbach J. Detection of reverse transcriptase activity in live attenuated virus vaccines. Clin Diagn Virol 5:43–53, 1996.

441. Mahy BWJ, Hadler SC. Editorial. Clin Diagn Virol 5:1–2, 1996.

442. Weissmahr RN, Schüpbach J, Böni J. Reverse transcriptase activity in chicken embryo fibroblast culture supernatants is associated with particles containing endogenous avian retrovirus EAV-0 RNA. J Virol 71:3005–3012, 1997.

443. Johnson JA, Heneine W. Characterization of endogenous avian leucosis viruses in chicken embryonic fibroblast substrates used in production of measles and mumps vaccines. J Virol 75:3605–3612, 2001.

444. Hussain AI, Shanmugam V, Switzer WM, et al. Lack of evidence of endogenous avian leucosis virus and endogenous avian retrovirus transmission to measles, mumps, and rubella vaccine recipients. Emerg Infect Dis 7:66–72, 2001.

445. Waters TD, Anderson PS, Beebe GW, Miller RW. Yellow fever vaccination, avian leukosis virus, and cancer risk in man. Science 177:76–77, 1972.

446. Peetermans J, Colinet G, Stephenne J, Bouillet A. Stability of freeze-dried and reconstituted measles vaccines. Dev Biol Stand 41:259–264, 1978.

447. Heyman DL, Smith EL, Nakano JH, et al. Further field testing of the more heat-stable measles vaccines in Cameroon. Br Med J (Clin Res Ed) 285:531–533, 1982.

448. WHO Expert Committee on Biological Standardization. Requirements for measles, mumps, and rubella vaccines and combined vaccines (live). World Health Organ Tech Rep Ser 840, annex 3, pp. 100–201, 1994.

449. Petralli JK, Merigan TC, Wilbur JC. Action of endogenous interferon against vaccinia infection in children. Lancet 2:401–405, 1965.

450. Trubina LM, Yakovenko ZF, Itkis SN, Zakharchenko EM. Interferon formation induced by various viruses in cultures of leukocytes from children vaccinated against measles. Acta Virol 16:446, 1972.

451. Nakayama T, Urano T, Osano M, et al. Long-term regulation of interferon production by lymphocytes from children inoculated with live measles virus vaccine. J Infect Dis 158:1386–1390, 1988.

452. Kalis JM, Quie PG, Balfour HH Jr. Measles (rubeola) susceptibility among elementary schoolchildren. Am J Epidemiol 101:527–531, 1975.

453. Bass JW, Halstead SB, Fischer GW, et al. Booster vaccination with further live attenuated measles vaccine. JAMA 235:31–34, 1976.

454. Albrecht P, Ennis FA, Saltzman EJ, Krugman S. Persistence of maternal antibody in infants beyond 12 months: mechanism of measles vaccine failure. J Pediatr 91:715–718, 1977.

455. Krugman RD, Rosenberg R, McIntosh K, et al. Further attenuated live measles vaccine: the need for revised recommendations. J Pediatr 91:766–767, 1977.

456. Balfour HH, Amren DD. Rubella, measles, and mumps antibodies following vaccination of children: a potential rubella problem. Am J Dis Child 132:573–577, 1978.

457. Wilkins J, Wehrle PF. Additional evidence against measles vaccine administration to infants less than 12 months of age: altered immune response following active/passive immunization. J Pediatr 94:865–869, 1979.

458. Sato H, Albrecht P, Reynolds DW, et al. Transfer of measles, mumps, and rubella antibodies from mother to infant: its effect on measles, mumps, and rubella immunization. Am J Dis Child 133:1240–1243, 1979.

459. Orenstein WA, Albrecht P, Herrman KL, et al. Evaluation of low levels of measles antibody: the plaque neutralization test as a measure of prior exposure to measles virus. J Infect Dis 155:146–149, 1986.

460. Stetler HC, Orenstein WA, Bernier RH, et al. Impact of revaccinating children who initially received measles vaccine before 10 months of age. Pediatrics 77:471–476, 1986.

461. Pedersen IR, Mordhorst CH, Ewald T, von Magnus H. Long-term antibody response after measles vaccination in an isolated arctic society in Greenland. Vaccine 4:173–178, 1986.

462. Helfand RF, Kebede S, Gary HE, et al. Timing of development of measles-specific immunoglobulin M and G after primary measles vaccination. Clin Diagn Lab Immunol 6:178–180, 1999.

463. Brown P, Gajdusek C, Tasi T. Persistence of measles antibody in the absence of circulating natural virus five years after immunization of an isolated virgin population with Edmonston B vaccine. Am J Epidemiol 90:514–518, 1969.

464. Weibel RE, Buynak EB, McLean AA, et al. Persistence of antibody in human subjects 7 to 10 years following administration of combined live attenuated measles, mumps, and rubella virus vaccines (40967). Proc Soc Exp Biol Med 165:260–263, 1980.

465. Isomura S, Morishima T, Nishikawa K, et al. A long-term follow-up study on the efficacy of further attenuated live measles vaccine, Biken CAM vaccine. Biken J 29:19–26, 1986.

466. Linnemann CC, Dine MS, Bloom JE, Schiff GM. Measles antibody in previously vaccinated children: the need for revaccination. Am J Dis Child 124:53–57, 1972.

467. Arbeter AM, Arthur JH, Blakeman GJ, McIntosh K. Measles immunity: reimmunization of children who previously received live measles vaccine and gamma globulin. J Pediatr 81:737–741, 1972.

468. Mossong J, O'Callaghan CJ, Ratnam S. Modelling antibody response to measles vaccine and subsequent waning of immunity in a low exposure population. Vaccine 19:523–529, 2000.

469. Ward BJ, Griffin DE. Changes in cytokine production after measles virus vaccination: predominant production of IL-4 suggests induction of a Th2 response. Clin Immunol Immunopathol 67:171–177, 1993.

470. Pabst HF, Spady DW, Marusyk RG, et al. Reduced measles immunity in infants in a well vaccinated population. Pediatr Infect Dis J 11:525–529, 1992.

471. Bautista-Lopez NL, Vaisberg A, Kanashiro R, et al. Immune response to measles vaccine in Peruvian children. Bull World Health Organ 79:1038–1046, 2001.

472. Gans H, Yasukawa L, Rinki M, et al. Immune responses to measles and mumps vaccination of infants at 6, 9, and 12 months. J Infect Dis 184:817–826, 2001.

473. Ward BJ, Boulianne N, Ratnam S, et al. Cellular immunity in measles vaccine failure: demonstration of measles antigen–specific lymphoproliferative responses despite limited serum antibody production after revaccination. J Infect Dis 172:1591–1595, 1995.

474. Starr S, Berkowitz S. Effects of measles, gamma-globulin modified measles and vaccine measles on the tuberculin test. N Engl J Med 270:386–391, 1964.

475. Fireman P, Friday G, Kumate J. Effect of measles vaccine on immunologic responsiveness. Pediatrics 43:264–272, 1969.

476. Zweiman B, Pappagianis D, Maibach H, Hildreth EA. Effect of measles immunization on tuberculin hypersensitivity and in vitro lymphocyte reactivity. Int Arch Allergy 40:834–841, 1971.

477. Arneborn P, Biberfeld G. T-lymphocyte subpopulations in relation to immunosuppression in measles and varicella. Infect Immun 39:29–37, 1983.

478. Griffin DE, Moench TR, Johnson RT, et al. Peripheral blood mononuclear cells during natural measles virus infection: cell surface phenotypes and evidence for activation. Clin Immunol Immunopathol 40:305–312, 1986.

479. Schnorr JJ, Cutts FT, Wheeler JG, et al. Immune modulation after measles vaccination of 6–9-months-old Bangladeshi infants. Vaccine 19:1503–1510, 2001.

480. Karp CL, Wysocka M, Wahl LM, et al. Mechanism of suppression of cell-mediated immunity by measles virus. Science 273:228–231, 1996.

481. Kempe CH. Measles vaccine in children with asthma and tuberculosis. Am J Dis Child 103:409, 1962.

482. Berkovich S, Starr S. Use of live-measles-virus vaccine to abort an expected outbreak of measles within a closed population. N Engl J Med 269:75–77, 1963.

483. van Binnendijk RS, Poelen MC, van Amerongen G, et al. Protective immunity in macaques vaccinated with live attenuated, recombinant, and subunit measles vaccines in the presence of passively acquired antibodies. J Infect Dis 175:524–532, 1997.

484. Morfin F, Beguin A, Lina B, Thouvenot D. Detection of measles vaccine in the throat of a vaccinated child. Vaccine 20:1541–1543, 2002.

485. Wittler RR, Veit BC, Mcintyre S, Schydlower M. Measles revaccination response in a school-age population. Pediatrics 88:1024–1030, 1991.

486. Christenson B, Bottiger M. Measles antibody: comparison of long-term vaccination titres, early vaccination titres and naturally acquired immunity to and booster effects on the measles virus. Vaccine 12:129–133, 1994.

487. Deseda-Tous J, Cherry JD, Spencer MJ, et al. Measles revaccination: persistence and degree of antibody titer by type of immune response. Am J Dis Child 132:287–290, 1978.

488. Markowitz LE, Albrecht P, Orenstein WA, et al. Persistence of measles antibody after revaccination. J Infect Dis 166:205–208, 1992.

489. Bartoloni A, Cutts FT, Guglielmetti P, et al. Response to measles revaccination among Bolivian school-aged children. Trans R Soc Trop Med Hyg 91:716–718, 1997.

490. Watson JC, Pearson JA, Markowitz LE, et al. An evaluation of measles revaccination among school-entry-aged children. Pediatrics 97:613–618, 1996.

491. Poland GA, Jacobson RM, Thampy AM, et al. Measles reimmunization in children seronegative after initial immunization. JAMA 277:1156–1158, 1997.

492. Cote TR, Sivertson D, Horan JM, et al. Evaluation of a two-dose measles, mumps, and rubella vaccination schedule in a cohort of college athletes. Public Health Rep 108:431–435, 1993.

493. Zhu YD, Heath J, Collins J, et al. Experimental measles. II. Infection and immunity in the rhesus macaque. Virology 233:85–92, 1997.

494. Wyde PR, Stittelaar KJ, Osterhaus AD, et al. Use of cotton rats for preclinical evaluation of measles vaccines. Vaccine 19:42–53, 2000.

495. Zhu Y, Rota P, Wyatt L, et al. Evaluation of recombinant vaccinia virus measles vaccines in infant rhesus macaques with preexisting measles antibody. Virology 276:202–213, 2000.

496. Chen RT, Markowitz LE, Albrecht P, et al. Measles antibody: reevaluation of protective titers. J Infect Dis 162:1036–1042, 1990.

497. Black FL, Berman LL, Libel M, et al. Inadequate immunity to measles in children vaccinated at an early age: effect of revaccination. Bull World Health Organ 62:315–319, 1984.

498. Lampe RM, Weir MR, Scott RMC, Weeks JL. Measles reimmunization in children immunized before 1 year of age. Am J Dis Child 139:33–35, 1985.

499. Orenstein WA, Bernier RH, Dondero TJ, et al. Field evaluation of vaccine efficacy. Bull World Health Organ 63:1055–1068, 1985.

500. Marks JS, Hayden GF, Orenstein WA. Methodologic issues in the evaluation of vaccine effectiveness: measles vaccine at 12 vs. 15 months. Am J Epidemiol 116:510–523, 1982.

501. Wyll SA, Witte JJ. Measles in previously vaccinated children: an epidemiological study. JAMA 216:1306–1310, 1971.

502. Landrigan PJ. Epidemic measles in a divided city. JAMA 221:567–570, 1972.

503. King GE, Markowitz LE, Patriarca PA, Dales LG. Clinical efficacy of measles vaccine during the 1990 measles epidemic. Pediatr Infect Dis J 10:883–887, 1991.

504. Baba R, Yabuuchi H, Takahashi M, et al. Seroepidemiologic behavior of varicella zoster virus infection in a semiclosed community after introduction of VZV vaccine. J Pediatr 105:712–716, 1984.

505. Anderson RM, May RM. Directly transmitted infectious diseases: control by vaccination. Science 215:1053–1060, 1982.

506. De Serres G, Gay NJ, Farrington CP. Epidemiology of transmissible diseases after elimination. Am J Epidemiol 151:1039–1048, 2000.

507. Wallinga J, Levy-Bruhl D, Gay NJ, Wachmann CH. Estimation of measles reproduction ratios and prospects for elimination of measles by vaccination in some Western European countries. Epidemiol Infect 127:281–295, 2001.

508. Hayden GF. Measles vaccine failure: a survey of causes and means of prevention. Clin Pediatr 18:1555–1567, 1979.

509. Orenstein WA, Markowitz L, Preblud SR, et al. Appropriate age for measles vaccination in the United States. Dev Biol Stand 65:13–21, 1986.

510. Caceras VM, Strebel PM, Sutter RW. Factors determining prevalence of maternal antibody to measles virus throughout infancy: a review. Clin Infect Dis 31:110–119, 2000.

511. Reilly CM, Stokes J Jr, Buynak EB, et al. Living attenuated measles-virus vaccine in early infancy: studies of the role of passive antibody in immunization. N Engl J Med 265:165–169, 1961.

512. American Academy of Pediatrics. Report of the Committee on the Control of Infectious Diseases. Evanston, IL, American Academy of Pediatrics, 1964, p 8.

513. Shasby DM, Shope TC, Downs H, et al. Epidemic measles in a highly vaccinated population. N Engl J Med 296:585–589, 1977.

514. Nkowane BM, Bart SW, Orenstein WA, Baltier M. Measles outbreak in a vaccinated school population: epidemiology, chains of transmission and the role of vaccine failures. Am J Public Health 77:434–438, 1987.

515. Reynolds DW, Start A. Immunity to measles in children vaccinated before and after one year of age. Am J Dis Child 124:848–849, 1972.

516. Marks JS, Halpin TJ, Orenstein WA. Measles vaccine efficacy in children previously vaccinated at 12 months of age. Pediatrics 62:955–960, 1978.

517. Krugman S. Present status of measles and rubella immunization in the United States: a medical progress report. J Pediatr 78:1–16, 1971.

518. Davis RM, Whitman ED, Orenstein WA, et al. A persistent outbreak of measles despite appropriate prevention and control measures. Am J Epidemiol 126:438–449, 1987.

519. Linnemann CC Jr, Dine MS, Rosella GA, Askey MT. Measles immunity after revaccination: results in children vaccinated before 10 months of age. Pediatrics 69:332–335, 1982.

520. Murphy MD, Brunell PA, Lievens AW, Schehab ZM. Effect of early immunization on antibody response to reimmunization with measles vaccine as demonstrated by enzyme-linked immunosorbent assay (ELISA). Pediatrics 74:90–93, 1984.

521. Hutchins SS, Dezayas A, Le Blond K, et al. Evaluation of an early two-dose measles vaccination schedule. Am J Epidemiol 154:1064–1071, 2001.

522. Yeager AS, Davis JH, Ross LA, Harvey B. Measles immunization: successes and failures. JAMA 237:347–351, 1977.

523. Wilkins J, Wehrle PF. Evidence for reinstatement of infants 12 to 14 months of age into routine measles immunization programs. Am J Dis Child 132:164–166, 1978.

524. Yeager AS, Harvey B, Crosson FJ Jr, et al. Need for measles revaccination in adolescents: correlation with birth date prior to 1972. J Pediatr 102:191–195, 1983.

525. Judelsohn RG, Fleissner ML, O'Mara DJ. School-based measles outbreaks: correlation of age at immunization with risk of disease. Am J Public Health 70:1162–1165, 1980.

526. Faust HS, Thompson FE. Age at and time since vaccination during a measles outbreak in a rural community. Am J Dis Child 137:977–980, 1983.

527. Shelton JD, Jacobson JE, Orenstein WA, et al. Measles vaccine efficacy: influence of age at vaccination vs duration of time since vaccination. Pediatrics 62:961–964, 1978.

528. Hull HF, Montes JD, Hays PC, Lucero RL. Risk factors for measles vaccine failure among immunized students. Pediatrics 76:518–523, 1985.

529. Maldonado YA, Lawrence EC, DeHovitz R, et al. Early loss of passive measles antibody in infants of mothers with vaccine-induced immunity. Pediatrics 96:447–450, 1995.

530. Kacica MA, Venezia RA, Miller J, et al. Measles antibodies in women and infants in the vaccine era. J Med Virol 45:227–229, 1995.

531. Markowitz LE, Albrecht P, Rhodes P, et al. Changing levels of measles antibody titers in women and children in the United States: impact on response to revaccination. Pediatrics 97:53–58, 1996.

532. Ventura SJ, Martin JA, Curtin SC, et al. Births: final data for 1998. Natl Vital Stat Rep 48:1–100, 2000. Available at *www.cdc.gov/nchs/data/nvsr/nvsr48/nvs48_03.pdf*

533. Hutchins SS, Redd SC, Schrag S, et al. National serologic survey of measles immunity among persons 6 years of age and older, 1988–1994. Medscape Gen Med 3(1), 2001. Available at *www.medscape.com/viewarticle/408098*

534. Papania MJ, Baughman AL, Lee S, et al. Increased susceptibility to measles in infants in the United States. Pediatrics 104:E59, 1999. Available at *www.pediatrics.org/cgi/content/full/104/5/e59*

535. Ozbek S, Vural M, Tastan Y, et al. Passive immunity of premature infants against measles during early infancy. Acta Paediatr 88:1254–1257, 1999.

536. Okoko BJ, Wesuperuma LH, Ota MO, et al. Influence of placental malaria and maternal hypergammaglobulinemia on materno-foetal transfer of measles and tetanus antibodies in a rural west African population. J Health Popul Nutr 19:59–65, 2001.

537. de Moraes-Pinto MI, Verhoff F, Chimsuku L, et al. Placental antibody transfer: influence of maternal HIV infection and placental malaria. Arch Dis Child Fetal Neonatal Ed 79:F202–F205, 1998.

538. World Health Organization, Global Programme for Vaccines and Immunization, Expanded Programme on Immunisation. Immunization Policy (WHOGPV/GEN/95.02 Rev. 1). Geneva, World Health Organization, 1996.

539. World Health Organization, Vaccines, Immunization and Biologicals. EPI Vaccines in HIV-Infected Individuals. Geneva, World Health Organization, 2001. Available at *www.who.int/vaccines-diseases/diseases/HIV.shtml*

540. Kumar ML, Johnson CE, Chui LW, et al. Immune response to measles vaccine in 6-month-old infants of measles seronegative mothers. Vaccine 16:2047–2051, 1998.

541. Gans HA, Arvin AM, Galinus J, et al. Deficiency of the humoral immune response to measles vaccine in infants immunized at 6 months. JAMA 280:527–532, 1998.

542. Wheelock EF, Larke RPB, Caroline NL. Interference in human viral infections: present status and prospects for the future. Prog Med Virol 10:286–347, 1968.

543. Ndikuyeze A, Munoz A, Stewart J, et al. Immunogenicity and safety of measles vaccine in ill African children. Int J Epidemiol 17:448–455, 1988.

544. Krober MS, Stracener CE, Bass JW. Decreased measles antibody response after measles-mumps-rubella vaccine in infants with colds. JAMA 265:2095–2096, 1991.

545. Dennehy PH, Saracen CL, Peter G. Seroconversion rates to combined measles-mumps-rubella-varicella (MMRV) vaccine of children with upper respiratory tract infection. Pediatrics 94:514–516, 1994.

546. Ratman S, West R, Gadag V. Measles and rubella antibody response after measles-mumps-rubella vaccination in children with afebrile upper respiratory tract infection. J Pediatr 127:432–434, 1995.

547. King GE, Markowitz LE, Heath J, et al. Antibody response to measles-mumps-rubella vaccine of children with mild illness at the time of vaccination. JAMA 275:704–707, 1996.

548. Edmonson MB, Davis JP, Hopfensperger DJ, et al. Measles vaccination during the respiratory virus season and risk of vaccine failure. Pediatrics 98:905–910, 1996.

549. Simasathien S, Migasena S, Bellini W, et al. Measles vaccination of Thai infants by intranasal and subcutaneous routes: possible interference from respiratory infections. Vaccine 15:329–334, 1997.

550. Peter G. Measles immunization: recommendations, challenges, and more information. JAMA 265:2111–2112, 1991.

551. McMurray DN, Loomis AS, Cassazza LJ, Rey H. Influence of moderate malnutrition on morbidity and antibody response following vaccination with live, further attenuated measles virus vaccine. Bull Pan Am Health Organ 13:52–57, 1979.

552. Ifekwunigwe AE, Grasset N, Glass R, Foster S. Immune response to measles and smallpox vaccinations in malnourished children. Am J Clin Nutr 33:621–624, 1980.

553. Rudy BJ, Rutstein RM, Pinto-Martin JP. Responses to measles immunization in children infected with human immunodeficiency virus. J Pediatr 25:72–74, 1994.

554. al-Attar I, Reisman J, Muehlmann M, McIntosh K. Decline of measles antibody titers after immunization in human immunodeficiency virus infected children. Pediatr Infect Dis J 14:149–151, 1995.

555. Hilgartner MW, Maeder MA, Mahoney EM, et al. Response to measles, mumps, and rubella revaccination among HIV-positive and HIV-negative children and adolescents with hemophilia. Am J Hematology 66:92–98, 2001.

556. Oxtoby MJ, Ryder R, Mvula M, et al. Patterns of immunity to measles among African children infected with human immunodeficiency virus [abstract]. In Proceedings of the 38th Epidemic Intelligence Service Conference, Atlanta, April 3–7, 1989.

557. Lepage P, Dabis F, Msellati P, et al. Safety and immunogenicity of high-dose Edmonston-Zagreb measles vaccine in children with HIV-1 infection. Am J Dis Child 146:550–555, 1992.

558. Cutts FT, Mandala K, St. Louis M, et al. Immunogenicity of high-titer Edmonston-Zagreb measles vaccine in human immunodeficiency virus–infected children in Kinshasa, Zaire. J Infect Dis 167:1418–1421, 1993.

559. Thaithumyanon P, Punnahitananda S, Thisyakorn U, et al. Immune responses to measles immunization and the impact on HIV-infected children. Southeast Asian J Trop Med Public Health 31:658–662, 2000.

560. Arpadi SM, Markowitz LE, Baughman AL, et al. Measles antibody in vaccinated human immunodeficiency virus type 1–infected children. Pediatrics 97:653–657, 1996.

561. Goon P, Cohen B, Jin L, et al. MMR vaccine in HIV-infected children—potential hazard? Vaccine 19:3816–3819, 2001.

562. Zolopa AB, Kemper CA, Shiboski S, et al. Progressive immunodeficiency due to infection with human immunodeficiency virus does not lead to waning immunity to measles in a cohort of homosexual men. Clin Infect Dis 18:636–638, 1994.

563. Semba RD, Munasir 7, Beeler J, et al. Reduced seroconversion to measles in infants given vitamin A with measles vaccination. Lancet 345:1330–1332, 1995.

564. Benn CS, Aaby P, Baleá C, et al. Randomised trial of effect of vitamin A supplementation on antibody response to measles vaccine in Guinea-Bissau, west Africa. Lancet 350:101–105, 1997.

565. Bahl R, Kumar R, Bhandari N, et al. Vitamin A administered with measles vaccine to nine-month-old infants does not reduce vaccine immunogenicity. J Nutr 129:1569–1573, 1999.

566. Semba RD, Akib A, Beeler J, et al. Effect of vitamin A supplementation on measles vaccination in nine-month-old infants. Public Health 111:245–247, 1997.

567. Randomized trial to assess benefits and safety of vitamin A supplementation linked to immunization in early infancy. WHO/CHD Immunization-Linked Vitamin A Supplementation Study Group. Lancet 352:1257–1263, 1998.

568. Ross DA, Cutts FT. Vindication of policy of vitamin A with measles vaccination. Lancet 350:81–82, 1997.

569. Hayney MS, Poland GA, Jacobson RM, et al. The influence of the HLA-DRB1*13 allele on measles vaccine response. J Invest Med 44:261–263, 1996.

570. Poland GA, Jacobson RM, Schaid D, et al. The association between HLA class I alleles and measles vaccine-induced antibody response: evidence for a significant association. Vaccine 16:1869–1871, 1998.

571. St. Sauver JL, Ovsyannikova IG, Jacobson RM, et al. Associations between human leucocyte antigen homozygosity and antibody levels to measles vaccine. J Infect Dis 185:1545–1559, 2002.

572. Whittle HC, Mann G, Eccles M, et al. Effects of dose and strain of vaccine on success of measles vaccination in infants aged 4–5 months. Lancet 1:963–966, 1988.

573. Markowitz LE, Sepulveda J, Diaz-Ortega JL, et al. Immunization of six-month old infants with different doses of Edmonston-Zagreb and Schwarz measles vaccines. N Engl J Med 322:580–587, 1990.

574. Tidjani O, Grunitsky B, Guerin N, et al. Serological effects of Edmonston-Zagreb, Schwarz and AIK-C measles vaccine strains given at ages 4–5 or 8–10 months. Lancet 2:1357–1360, 1989.

575. Kiepiela P, Coovadia HM, Loening WEK, et al. Lack of efficacy of the live standard potency Edmonston-Zagreb live, attenuated measles vaccine in African infants. Bull World Health Organ 69:221–227, 1991.

576. Job JS, Halsey NA, Boulos R, et al. Successful immunization of infants at 6 months of age with high dose Edmonston-Zagreb measles vaccine. Pediatr Infect Dis J 10:303–311, 1991.

577. Dabis F, Sow A, Waldman R, et al. The epidemiology of measles in a partially vaccinated African city: implications for immunization programmes. Am J Epidemiol 127:171–178, 1988.

578. Kambarami RA, Nathoo KJ, Nkrumah FK, Pirie DJ. Measles epidemic in Harare, Zimbabwe, despite high measles immunization coverage rates. Bull World Health Organ 69:213–219, 1991.

579. Tsai HY, Huang LM, Shih YT, et al. Immunogenicity and safety of standard-titer AIK-C measles vaccine in nine-month-old infants. Viral Immunol 12:343–348, 1999.

580. Nkrumah FK, Osei-Kwasi M, Dunyo SK, et al. Comparison of AIK-C measles vaccine in infants at 6 months with Schwarz vaccine at 9 months: a randomized controlled trial in Ghana. Bull World Health Organ 76:353–359, 1998.

581. Pabst HF, Spady DW, Carson MM, et al. Cell-mediated and antibody immune responses to AIK-C and Connaught monovalent measles vaccine given to 6-month-old infants. Vaccine 17:1910–1918, 1999.

582. Expanded Programme on Immunization. Measles immunization before 9 months of age. Wkly Epidemiol Rec 2:8, 1990.

583. Expanded Programme on Immunization. Safety and efficacy of high titre measles vaccine at 6 months of age. Wkly Epidemiol Rec 66:249–251, 1991.

584. Garenne M, Leroy O, Beau FP, Sene I. Child mortality after high titer measles vaccines: prospective study in Senegal. Lancet 338:903–907, 1991.

585. Aaby P, Samb B, Simondon F, et al. Divergent mortality for male and female recipients of low-titre and high-titre measles vaccines in rural Senegal. Am J Epidemiol 138:756–765, 1993.

586. Libman MD, Ibrahim SA, Omer MI, et al. No evidence for short- or long-term morbidity after increased titer measles vaccination in Sudan. Pediatr Infect Dis J 21:112–119, 2002.

587. Expanded Programme on Immunization. Safety of high-titre measles vaccines. Wkly Epidemiol Rec 67:357–361, 1992.

588. Krugman RD, Meyer BC, Parkman PD, et al. Impotency of vaccines as a result of improper handling in clinical practice. J Pediatr 85:512–514, 1972.

589. Lerman SJ, Gold E. Measles in children previously vaccinated against measles. JAMA 216:1311–1314, 1971.

590. Markowitz LE, Preblud SR, Fine PE, et al. Duration of live measles vaccine–induced immunity. Pediatr Infect Dis J 9:101–109, 1990.

591. Miller C. Live measles vaccine: a 21-year follow-up. Br Med J (Clin Res Ed) 295:22–24, 1987.

592. Dine MS, Hutchins SS, Thomas A, et al. Persistence of vaccine-induced antibody to measles 26–33 years after vaccination. J Infect Dis [in press].

593. Hirose M, Hidaka Y, Miyazaki C, et al. Five cases of measles secondary vaccine failure with confirmed seroconversion after live measles vaccination. Scand J Infect Dis 29:187–190, 1997.

594. Hutchins SS, Markowitz LE, Mead P, et al. School-based measles outbreak: the effect of a selective revaccination policy and risk factors for vaccine failure. Am J Epidemiol 132:157–168, 1990.

595. O'Neil AE. The measles epidemic in Calgary, 1974–1975: the duration of protection conferred by the vaccine. Can J Public Health 69:325–333, 1978.

596. Guris D, McCready J, Watson JC, et al. Measles vaccine effectiveness and duration of vaccine-induced immunity in the absence of boosting from exposure to measles virus. Pediatr Infect Dis J 15:1082–1086, 1996.

597. Ramsay ME, Moffatt D, O'Connor M. Measles vaccine: a 27-year follow-up. Epidemiol Infect 112:409–412, 1994.

598. Anders JF, Jacobson RM, Poland GA, et al. Secondary failure rates of measles vaccines: a meta-analysis of published studies. Pediatr Infect Dis J 15:62–66, 1996.

599. Meyer HM Jr. Field experience with combined live measles, smallpox, and yellow fever vaccines. Arch Ges Virusforsch 16:366–374, 1965.

600. Sherman RM, Hendrickse RG, Montifiore D. Simultaneous administration of live measles virus vaccine and smallpox vaccine. Br Med J 2:672–676, 1967.

601. Weibel RE, Stokes J Jr, Buynak EB, et al. Clinical laboratory experiences with a more attenuated Enders measles virus vaccine (Moraten) combined with smallpox vaccine. Pediatrics 43:567–572, 1969.

602. Ruben FL, Smith EA, Foster SO, et al. Simultaneous administration of smallpox, measles, yellow fever, and diphtheria-pertussis-tetanus antigens to Nigerian children. Bull World Health Organ 48:175–181, 1973.

603. Lapeyssonnie L, Omer IA, Nicolas A, Roumiantzeff M. A study of the serological response of Sudanese children to three associated immunizations (measles, tetanus, meningococcal A meningitis). Med Trop (Mars) 39:71–79, 1979.

604. Ajjan N, Fayet MT, Biron G, et al. Combination of attenuated measles vaccine (Schwarz) with meningococcus A and A + C vaccine. Dev Biol Stand 41:209–216, 1978.

605. Deforest A, Long SS, Lischner HW, et al. Simultaneous administration of measles-mumps-rubella vaccine with booster doses of diphtheria-tetanus-pertussis and oral poliovirus vaccines. Pediatrics 81:237–246, 1988.

606. Huang L, Lee C, Hsu C, et al. Effect of monovalent measles and trivalent measles-mumps-rubella vaccines at various ages and concurrent administration with hepatitis B vaccine. Pediatr Infect Dis J 9:461–465, 1990.

607. Lhuillier M, Mazzariol MJ, Zadi S, et al. Study of combined vaccination against yellow fever and measles in infants from six to nine months. J Biol Stand 17:9–15, 1989.

608. Adu FD, Omotade OO, Oyedele OI, et al. Field trial of combined yellow fever and measles vaccines among children in Nigeria. East Afr Med J 73:579–582, 1996.

609. Centers for Disease Control. Recommendations of the Immunization Practices Advisory Committee (ACIP): new recommended schedule for active immunization of normal infants and children. MMWR 35:577–579, 1986.

610. King GE, Hadler SC. Simultaneous administration of childhood vaccines: an important public health policy that is safe and efficacious. Pediatr Infect Dis J 13:394–407, 1994.

611. Giammanco G, Li Volti S, Salemi I, et al. Immune response to simultaneous administration of a combined measles, mumps, and rubella vaccine with booster doses of diphtheria-tetanus and poliovirus vaccine. Eur J Epidemiol 9:199–202, 1993.

612. Centers for Disease Control. Adverse Events Following Immunization Surveillance Report No. 3, 1985–1986. Atlanta, Centers for Disease Control, 1989.

613. John TJ, Selvakumar R, Balrai V, Simoes EAF. Antibody response to measles vaccine with DTPP [letter]. Am J Dis Child 141:14, 1987.

614. Chen RT, Haber P, Mullen JR. Surveillance of the safety of simultaneous administration of vaccines. The Centers for Disease Control and Prevention experience. Ann N Y Acad Sci 754:309–320, 1995.

615. Englund JA, Swarez CS, Kelly J, et al. Placebo-controlled trial of varicella vaccine given with or after measles-mumps-rubella vaccine. J Pediatr 114:37–44, 1989.

616. Watson BM, Laufer DS, Kuter BJ, et al. Safety and immunogenicity of a combined live attenuated measles, mumps, rubella and varicella vaccine (MMRIIV) in healthy children. J Infect Dis 173:731–734, 1996.

617. Fulginiti V. Simultaneous measles exposure and immunization. Arch Ges Virusforsch 16:300–304, 1965.

618. Ruuskanen O, Salmi TT, Halonen P. Measles vaccination after exposure to natural measles. J Pediatr 93:43–46, 1978.

619. Byrne EB, Rosenstein BJ, Jaworski AA, Jaworski RA. A statewide mass measles immunization program. JAMA 199:619–623, 1967.

620. Chen RT, Moses JM, Markowitz LE, Orenstein WA. Adverse events following measles-mumps-rubella and measles vaccinations in college students. Vaccine 9:297–299, 1991.

621. Griffin MR, Ray WA, Mortimer EA, et al. Risk of seizures after measles-mumps-rubella immunization. Pediatrics 88:881–885, 1991.

622. Scott TFM, Bonanno DE. Reactions to live-measles-virus vaccine in children previously vaccinated with killed-virus vaccine. N Engl J Med 277:248–250, 1967.

623. Harris RW, Isacson P, Karzon DT. Vaccine-induced hypersensitivity: reactions to live measles and mumps vaccine in prior recipients of inactivated measles vaccine. J Pediatr 74:552–563, 1969.

624. Stetler HC, Gens RD, Seastrom GR. Severe local reactions to live measles virus vaccine following an immunization program. Am J Public Health 73:899–900, 1983.

625. Landrigan PJ, Witte JJ. Neurologic disorders following live measles-virus vaccination. JAMA 223:1459–1462, 1973.

626. Abe T, Nonaka C, Hiraiwa M, et al. Acute and delayed neurologic reaction to inoculation with attenuated live measles virus. Brain Dev 7:421–423, 1985.

627. Davis RL, Marcuse E, Black S, et al. MMR2 immunization at 4 to 5 years and 10 to 12 years of age: a comparison of adverse clinical events after immunization in the Vaccine Safety Datalink (VSD) project. Pediatrics 100:767–771, 1997.

628. Barlow WE, Davis RL, Glasser JW, et al. The risk of seizures after receipt of whole-cell pertussis or measles, mumps, and rubella vaccine. N Engl J Med 345:656–661, 2001.

629. Oski FA, Naiman JL. Effect of live measles vaccine on the platelet count. N Engl J Med 275:352–356, 1966.

630. Institute of Medicine. Measles and mumps vaccine. In Adverse Events Associated With Childhood Vaccines: Evidence Bearing on Causality. Washington, DC, National Academy Press, 1994, p 130.

631. Carapetis JR, Curtis N, Royle J. MMR immunisation: true anaphylaxis to MMR vaccine is extremely rare. BMJ 323:869, 2001.

632. James JM, Burks AW, Roberson PK, Sampson HA. Safe administration of the measles vaccine to children allergic to eggs. N Engl J Med 332:1262–1266, 1995.

633. Bruno G, Grandolfo M, Lucenti P, et al. Measles vaccine in egg allergic children: poor immunogenicity of the Edmonston-Zagreb strain. Pediatr Allergy Immunol 8:17–20, 1997.

634. Johnson RT. Inflammatory and demyelinating diseases. In Viral Infections of the Nervous System (2nd ed). Philadelphia, Lippincott–Raven, 1998, pp 227–264.

635. Duclos P, Ward BJ. Measles vaccines: a review of adverse events. Drug Safety 6:435–454, 1998.

636. Forman ML, Cherry JD. Isolation of measles virus from the cerebrospinal fluid of a child with encephalitis following measles vaccination [abstract 13]. In Proceedings of the 77th Annual Meeting of the American Pediatric Society, April 26–29, 1967.

637. Bloch AB, Orenstein WA, Wassilak SG, et al. Epidemiology of measles and its complications. In Gruenberg EM, Lewis C, Goldston SE (eds). Vaccinating Against Brain Syndromes: The Campaign Against Measles and Rubella (Monographs in Epidemiology and Biostatistics, Vol. 9). New York, Oxford University Press, 1986, pp 5–20.

638. Committee on Safety of Medicines and the Joint Committee on Vaccination and Immunization. Whooping Cough. London, Her Majesty's Stationery Office, 1981, pp 79–169.

639. Miller D, Wadsworth J, Diamond J, Ross E. Measles vaccination and neurological events. Lancet 349:730–731, 1997.

640. Morens DM, Halsey NA, Schoenberger LB, Baublis JV. Reye syndrome associated with vaccination with live virus vaccines: an exploration of possible etiologic relationships. Clin Pediatr 18:42–44, 1979.

641. Chan CC, Sogg RL, Steinman L. Isolated oculomotor palsy after measles immunization. Am J Ophthalmol 89:446–448, 1980.

642. Karzarian EL, Gager WE. Optic neuritis complicating measles, mumps, and rubella vaccination. Am J Ophthalmol 86:544–547, 1978.

643. Marshall GS, Wright PF, Fenichel GM, Karzon DT. Diffuse retinopathy following measles, mumps, and rubella vaccination. Pediatrics 76:989–991, 1985.

644. Brodsky L, Stanievich J. Sensorineural hearing loss following live measles virus vaccination. Int J Pediatr Otorhinolaryngol 10:159–163, 1985.

645. Trump RC, White TR. Cerebellar ataxia presumed due to live, attenuated measles virus vaccine. JAMA 199:165–166, 1967.

646. Glenn MP, McKendrick DW. Varicella bullosa associated with measles vaccine. Br J Dermatol 83:595–596, 1970.

647. Shoss RG, Rayhanzadeh S. Toxic epidermal necrolysis following measles vaccination. Arch Dermatol 110:766–770, 1974.

648. Buntain WL, Missall SR. Local subcutaneous atrophy following measles, mumps, and rubella vaccination [letter]. Am J Dis Child 130:335, 1976.

649. Buck BE, Yang LC, Caleb MH, et al. Measles virus panniculitis subsequent to vaccine administration. J Pediatr 101:366–373, 1982.

650. da Silveira CM, Salisbury DM, de Quadros CA. Measles vaccination and Guillain-Barré syndrome. Lancet 349:14–16, 1997.

651. Patja A, Paunio M, Kinnunen E, et al. Risk of Guillain-Barré syndrome after measles-mumps-rubella vaccination. J Pediatr 138:250–254, 2001.

652. DeStefano F, Gu D, Kramarz P, et al. Childhood vaccinations and risk of asthma. Pediatr Infect Dis J 21:498–504, 2002.

653. Halsey NA, Modlin JF, Jabbour JT. Subacute sclerosing panencephalitis (SSPE): an epidemiologic review. In Stevens JG, Todaro GJ, Fox CF (eds). Persistent Viruses. New York, Academic Press, 1978, pp 101–114.

654. Miki K, Komase K, Mgone CS, et al. Molecular analysis of measles virus genome derived from SSPE and acute measles patients in Papua, New Guinea. J Med Virol 68:105–112, 2002.

655. Jin L, Beard S, Hunjan R, et al. Characterization of measles virus strains causing SSPE: a study of 11 cases. J Neurovirol 8:335–344, 2002.

656. Sonoda S, Nakayama T. Detection of measles virus genome in lymphocytes from asymptomatic healthy children. J Med Virol 65:381–387, 2001.

657. Katayama Y, Kohso K, Nishimura A, et al. Detection of measles virus mRNA from autopsied human tissues. J Clin Microbiol 36:299–301, 1998.

658. Park DW, Boldt HC, Massicotte SJ, et al. Subacute sclerosing panencephalitis manifesting as viral retinitis: clinical and histopathologic findings. Am J Ophthalmol 123:533–542, 1997.

659. Koppel BS, Poon TP, Khandji A, et al. Subacute sclerosing panencephalitis and acquired immunodeficiency syndrome: role of electroencephalography and magnetic resonance imaging. J Neuroimaging 6:122–125, 1996.

660. Budka H, Urbanits S, Liberski PP, et al. Subacute measles virus encephalitis: a new and fatal opportunistic infection in a patient with AIDS. Neurology 46:586–587, 1996.

661. Bitnun A, Shannon P, Durward A, et al. Measles inclusion body encephalitis caused by the vaccine strain of measles virus. Clin Infect Dis 29:855–861, 1999.

662. Monafo WJ, Haslam DB, Roberts RL, et al. Disseminated measles infection after vaccination in a child with a congenital immunodeficiency. J Pediatr 124:273–276, 1994.

663. Centers for Disease Control and Prevention. Measles pneumonitis following measles-mumps-rubella vaccination of a patient with HIV infection. MMWR 45:603–606, 1996.

664. Moss WJ, Monze M, Ryon JJ, et al. Prospective study of measles in hospitalized, human immunodeficiency virus (HIV)-infected and HIV-uninfected children in Zambia. Clin Infect Dis 35:189–196, 2002.

665. Moss WJ, CJ Clements, Halsey NA. Immunization of children at risk for infection with the human immunodeficiency virus. Bull World Health Organ 81:61–70, 2003.

666. Angel JB, Walpita P, Lerch RA, et al. Vaccine-associated measles pneumonitis in an adult with AIDS. Ann Intern Med 129:104–106, 1998.

667. American Academy of Pediatrics, Committee on Infectious Diseases and Committee on Pediatric AIDS. Measles immunization in HIV-infected children. Pediatrics 103(5 pt 1):1057–1060, 1999.

668. Singer FR. Update on the viral etiology of Paget's disease of bone. J Bone Miner Res 14:29–33, 1999.

669. Kurihara N, Reddy SV, Menaa C, et al. Osteoclasts expressing the measles virus nucleocapsid gene display a pagetic phenotype. J Clin Invest 105:607–614, 2000.

670. Wakefield AJ, Murch SH, Anthony A. Ileal-lymphoid-nodular hyperplasia, non-specific colitis, and pervasive developmental disorder in children. Lancet 351:637–641, 1998.

671. Halsey NA, Hyman SL. Measles-mumps-rubella vaccine and autistic spectrum disorder: report from the New Challenges in Childhood Immunizations Conference convened in Oak Brook, IL, June 12–13, 2000. Pediatrics 107:E84, 2001.

672. Wakefield AJ, Montgomery SM. Measles, mumps, rubella vaccine: through a glass, darkly. Adverse Drug React 19:1–19, 2000.

673. Wakefield AJ, Anthony A, Murch SH. Enterocolitis in children with developmental disorders. Am J Gastroenterol 95:2285–2295, 2000.

674. Glismann S, Ronne T, Schmidt JE. The EUVAC-NET survey: national measles surveillance systems in the EU, Switzerland, Norway, and Iceland. Eurosurveill Monthly 6:105–110, 2001.

675. Measles, rubella, and congenital rubella syndrome—United States and Mexico, 1997–1999. MMWR 49:1048–1050, 1059, 2000.

676. de Quadros CA, Olivé JM, Hersh BS, et al. Measles elimination in the Americas: evolving strategies. JAMA 275:224–229, 1996.

677. Rosenthal SR, Clements CJ. Two-dose measles vaccination schedules. Bull World Health Organ 71:421–428, 1993.

678. Kolasa M, Klemperer-Johnson S, Papania M. Second dose measles immunization requirements for school children—progress toward implementation for all school children in all states. J Infect Dis Suppl 2003 [in press].

679. Hersh BS, Markowitz LE, Hoffman RE, et al. A measles outbreak at a college with a prematriculation immunization requirement. Am J Public Health 81:360–364, 1991.

680. Baughman AL, Williams WW, Atkinson WL, et al. The impact of college pre-matriculation requirements on risk for measles outbreaks. JAMA 255:1127–1132, 1994.

681. Atkinson WL, Markowitz LE, Adams NC, Seastrom GR. Transmission of measles in medical settings, 1985–1989. Am J Med 91(suppl 3B):320S–324S, 1991.

682. Yip F, Redd S, Papania M. Patterns of measles outbreaks, United States, 1993–2000. J Infect Dis Suppl 2003 [in press].

683. Subbarao EK, Amin S, Kumar ML. Prevaccination serologic screening for measles in health care workers. J Infect Dis 163:876–878, 1991.

684. Grabowsky M, Markowitz L. Serologic screening, mass immunization and implications for immunization programs. J Infect Dis 164:1237–1238, 1991.

685. McLaughlin M, Thomas P, Onorato I, et al. Live viral vaccines in human immunodeficiency virus infected children: a retrospective survey. Pediatrics 82:229–233, 1988.

686. Centers for Disease Control and Prevention. 1994 Revised classification system for human immunodeficiency virus infection in children less than 13 years of age. Official authorized addenda: Human immunodeficiency virus infection codes and official guidelines for coding and reporting ICD-9-CM. MMWR 43(RR-12):1–19, 1994.

687. Centers for Disease Control and Prevention. Recommendations of the Advisory Committee on Immunization Practices (ACIP): use of vaccines and immune globulins in persons with altered immunocompetence. MMWR 42(RR-4):1–18, 1993.

688. Henning KJ, White MH, Sepkowitz KA, Armstrong D. A national survey of immunization practices following allogenic bone marrow transplantation. JAMA 277:1148–1151, 1997.

689. Ljungman P, Fridell E, Lonnqvist B, et al. Efficacy and safety of vaccination of marrow transplant recipients with a live attenuated measles, mumps, and rubella vaccine. J Infect Dis 159:610–615, 1989.

690. Ljungman P, Lewensohn-Fuchs I, Hammarstrom V, et al. Long-term immunity to measles, mumps, and rubella after allogeneic bone marrow transplantation. Blood 84:657–663, 1994.

691. Centers for Disease Control and Prevention. General recommendations on immunization: recommendations of the Advisory Committee on Immunization Practices and the American Academy of Family Physicians. MMWR 51(RR-2):23, 2002.

692. Starr S, Berkovich S. The effect of measles, gamma globulin modified measles, and attenuated measles vaccine on the course of treated tuberculosis in children. Pediatrics 35:97–102, 1965.

693. Bellini WJ, Rota JS, Greer PW, Zaki SR. Measles vaccination death in a child with severe combined immunodeficiency: report of a case [abstract]. Presented at the Annual Meeting of Laboratory Investigation, 1992.

694. Moss WJ, Cutts F, Griffin DE. Implications of the human immunodeficiency virus epidemic for control and eradication of measles. Clin Infect Dis 29:106–112, 1999.

695. Pool V, Braun MM, Celso JM, et al. Prevalence of anti-IgE antibodies in persons with anaphylaxis following measles-mumps-rubella vaccination in the United States. Pediatrics 110:E71, 2002.

696. Kelso JM, Jones RT, Yunginger JW. Anaphylaxis to measles, mumps, and rubella vaccine mediated by IgE to gelatin. J Allergy Clin Immunol 91:867–872, 1993.

697. Sakaguchi M, Ogura H, Inouye S. IgE antibody to gelatin in children with immediate-type reactions to measles and mumps vaccines. J Allergy Clin Immunol 96:563–565, 1995.

698. Sakaguchi M, Nakayama T, Inouye S. Food allergy to gelatin in children with systemic immediate-type reactions, including anaphylaxis, to vaccines. J Allergy Clin Immunol 98:1058–1061, 1996.

699. Patja A, Makinen-Kiljunen S, Davidkin I, et al. Allergic reactions to measles-mumps-rubella vaccination. Pediatrics 107:E27, 2001. Available at www.pediatrics.org/cgi/content/full/107/2/e27

700. Fasano MB, Wood RA, Cooke SK, Sampson HA. Egg hypersensitivity and adverse reactions to measles, mumps, and rubella vaccine. J Pediatr 120:878–881, 1992.

701. Herman JJ, Radin R, Schneiderman R. Allergic reactions to measles (rubeola) vaccine in patients hypersensitive to egg protein. J Pediatr 102:196–199, 1983.

702. American Academy of Pediatrics. Active immunization. In Peter G (ed). 1988 Red Book: Report of the Committee on Infectious Diseases (21st ed). Elk Grove Village, IL, American Academy of Pediatrics, 1998, pp 5–28.

703. Kemp A, Van Asperen P, Mukhi A. Measles immunization in children with clinical reactions to egg protein. Am J Dis Child 144:33–35, 1990.

704. James JM, Burks AW, Roberson PK, Sampson HA. Safe administration of the measles vaccine to children allergic to eggs. N Engl J Med 332:1262–1266, 1995.

705. Siber GR, Werner BG, Halsey NA, et al. Interference of immune globulin with measles and rubella immunization. J Pediatr 122:204–211, 1993.

706. Miller E, Waight P, Farrington CP, et al. Idiopathic thrombocytopenic purpura and MMR vaccine. Arch Dis Child 84:227–229, 2001.

707. Nieminen U, Peltola H, Syrjälä MT, et al. Acute thrombocytopenic purpura following measles, mumps, and rubella vaccination: a report on 23 patients. Acta Pediatr 82:267–270, 1993.

708. Böttiger M, Christenson B, Romanus V, et al. Swedish experience of two-dose vaccination programme aiming at eliminating measles, mumps, and rubella. BMJ 295:1264–1267, 1993.

709. Vlacha V, Forman EN, Miron D, et al. Recurrent thrombocytopenic purpura after repeated measles-mumps-rubella vaccination. Pediatrics 97:738–739, 1996.

710. Beeler J, Varricchio F, Wise R. Thrombocytopenia after immunization with measles vaccines: review of the Vaccine Adverse Event Reporting System (1990 to 1994). Pediatr Infect Dis J 15:88–90, 1996.

711. Drachtman RA, Murphy S, Ettinger LJ. Exacerbation of chronic idiopathic thrombocytopenic purpura following measles-mumps-rubella immunization. Arch Pediatr Adolesc Med 148:326–327, 1994.

712. Centers for Disease Control. Adverse Events Following Immunization (Surveillance report no. 3, 1985–1986). Atlanta: Centers for Disease Control, 1989.

713. Polack FP, Hoffman SJ, Moss WJ, Griffin DE. Altered synthesis of interleukin-12 and type 1 and type 2 cytokines in rhesus macaques during measles and atypical measles. J Infect Dis 185:13–19, 2002.

714. Osterhaus AD, de Vries P, van Binnendijk RS. Measles vaccines: novel generations and new strategies. J Infect Dis 170(suppl 1):S42–S55, 1994.

715. Stittelaar KJ, de Swart RL, Vos HW, et al. Enteric administration of a live attenuated measles vaccine does not induce protective immunity in a macaque model. Vaccine 20:2906–2912, 2002.

716. Conacher M, Alexander J, Brewer JM. Oral immunisation with peptide and protein antigens by formulation in lipid vesicles incorporating bile salts (bilosomes). Vaccine 19:2965–2974, 2001.

717. Huang Z, Dry I, Webster D, et al. Plant-derived measles virus hemagglutinin protein induces neutralizing antibodies in mice. Vaccine 19:2163–2171, 2001.

718. Webster DE, Cooney ML, Huang Z, et al. Successful boosting of a DNA measles immunization with an oral plant-derived measles virus vaccine. J Virol 76:7910–7912, 2002.

719. Sharpe S, Fooks A, Lee J, et al. Single oral immunization with replication deficient recombinant adenovirus elicits long-lived transgene-specific cellular and humoral immune responses. Virology 293:210–216, 2002.

720. Sepulveda-Amor J, Valdespino-Gomez JL, Garcia-Garcia M de L, et al. A randomized trial demonstrating successful boosting responses following simultaneous aerosols of measles and rubella (MR) vaccines in school age children. Vaccine 20:2790–2795, 2002.

721. Niewiesk S. Studying experimental measles virus vaccines in the presence of maternal antibodies in the cotton rat model (*Sigmodon hispidus*). Vaccine 19:2250–2253, 2001.

722. Cutts FT, Markowitz LE. Successes and failures in measles control. J Infect Dis 170(suppl 1):S32–S41, 1994.

723. Bartlett MS. Measles periodicity and community size. J R Stat Soc 120:48–70, 1957.

724. Black FL. Measles endemicity in insular populations: community size and its evolutionary implication. J Theor Biol 11:207–211, 1966.

725. Grenfell BT, Bjornstad ON, Kappey J. Travelling waves of measles and spatial hierarchies in measles epidemics. Nature 414:716–723, 2001.

726. Anderson RM, May RM. Vaccination and herd immunity to infectious diseases. Nature 318:323–329, 1985.

727. Nokes DJ, Williams JR, Butler AR. Towards eradication of measles virus: global progress and strategy evaluation. Vet Microbiol 44:333–350, 1995.

728. Mclean AR, Anderson RM. Measles in developing countries. Part II. The predicted impact of mass immunization. Epidemiol Infect 100:419–442, 1988.

729. Chen RT, Weierbach R, Bisoffi Z, et al. A "post-honeymoon period" measles outbreak in Muyinga sector, Burundi. Int J Epidemiol 23:185–193, 1994.

730. Agocs MM, Markowitz LE, Straub I, Dômôk I. The 1988–1989 measles epidemic in Hungary: assessment of vaccine failure. Int J Epidemiol 21:1007–1013, 1992.

731. Thacker SB, Millar DJ. Mathematical modeling and attempts to eliminate measles: a tribute to the late professor George Macdonald. Am J Epidemiol 133:517–525, 1991.

732. Conrad JL, Wallace R, Witte JJ. The epidemiologic rationale for the failure to eradicate measles in the United States. Am J Public Health 61:2304–2310, 1971.

733. Fine PEM. Herd immunity: history, theory, practice. Epidemiol Rev 15:265–302, 1993.

734. Hethcote HW. Measles and rubella in the United States. Am J Epidemiol 117:2–13, 1983.

735. De Serres G, Gay NJ, Farrington CP. Epidemiology of transmissible diseases after elimination. Am J Epidemiol 151:1039–1048, 2000.

736. Cutts FT, Henderson RH, Clements CJ, et al. Principles of measles control. Bull World Health Organ 69:1–7, 1991.

737. Cutts FT, Grabowsky M, Markowitz LE. The effect of dose and strain of live attenuated measles vaccines on serological responses in young infants. Biologicals 23:95–106, 1995.

738. Centers for Disease Control and Prevention. Measles—United States, 1996 and the interruption of indigenous transmission. MMWR 46:242–246, 1997.

739. Peltola H, Heinonen OP, Valle M, et al. The elimination of indigenous measles, mumps, and rubella from Finland by a 12-year, two-dose vaccination program. N Engl J Med 331:1397–1402, 1994.

740. Ramsay ME, Gay NJ, Miller E, et al. The epidemiology of measles in England and Wales: rationale for the 1994 national vaccination campaign. Commun Dis Rep CDR Rev 4:R141–R146, 1994.

741. Babad HR, Nokes DJ, Gay NJ, et al. Predicting the impact of measles vaccination in England and Wales—model validation and analysis of policy options. Epidemiol Infect 114:319–344, 1995.

742. Gay N, Ramsay M, Cohen B, et al. The epidemiology of measles in England and Wales since the 1994 vaccination campaign. Commun Dis Rep CDR Rev 7:R17–R21, 1997.

743. Duclos P, Paulsen E. Measles elimination in Canada. Can J Public Health 86:370, 1995.

744. Duclos P, Redd SC, Varughese P, Hersh BS. Measles in adults in Canada and the United States: implications for measles elimination and eradication. Int J Epidemiology 28:141–146, 1999.

745. Pelletier L, Chung P, Duclos P, et al. A benefit-cost analysis of two-dose measles immunization in Canada. Vaccine 9:989–996, 1998.

746. Sencer DJ, Dull HB, Langmuir AD. Epidemiologic basis for eradication of measles in 1967. Public Health Rep 82:253–256, 1967.

747. Hersh BS, Markowitz LE, Maes EF, et al. The geography of measles in the United States, 1980–1989. JAMA 267:1936–1941, 1992.

748. Gustafson TL, Lievens AW, Brunell PA, et al. Measles outbreak in a fully immunized secondary school population. N Engl J Med 316:771–774, 1987.

749. Atkinson WL, Orenstein WA, Krugman S. The resurgence of measles in the United States, 1989–1990. Annu Rev Med 43:451–463, 1992.

750. Gindler JS, Atkinson WL, Markowitz LE, Hutchins SS. The epidemiology of measles in the United States in 1989 and 1990. Pediatr Infect Dis J 11:841–846, 1992.

751. National Vaccine Advisory Committee. The measles epidemic: the problems, barriers, and recommendations. JAMA 266:1547–1552, 1991.

752. Centers for Disease Control and Prevention. Measles vaccination levels among selected groups of preschool-aged children—United States. MMWR 40:36–39, 1990.

753. Centers for Disease Control and Prevention. Vaccination coverage of 2-year-old children—United States, 1991–1992. MMWR 42:985–988, 1993.

754. Zell ER, Dietz V, Stevenson J, et al. Low vaccination levels of US preschool and school-age children: retrospective assessments of vaccination coverage, 1991–1992. JAMA 271:833–839, 1994.

755. Measles in Canada, 1989. Can Dis Wkly Rep 16:213–218, 1990.

756. Gay NJ, Pelletier L, Duclos P. Modelling the incidence of measles in Canada: an assessment of the options for vaccination policy. Vaccine 16:794–801, 1998.

757. King A, Varughese P, De Serres G, et al. The epic of measles in Canada: from endemic to epidemic to elimination. J Infect Dis Suppl [in press].

758. Ramsay ME, Li J, White J, et al. The elimination of indigenous measles transmission in England and Wales. J Infect Dis 187(Suppl 1): S198–S207, 2003.

759. Public Health Laboratory Services. London measles outbreak. CDR Wkly 12:1–2, 2002.

760. Peltola H, Davidkin I, Paunio M, et al. Mumps and rubella eliminated from Finland. JAMA 284:2643–2647, 2000.

761. Surveillance report: epidemic measles in the Campania region of Italy leads to 13 cases of encephalitis and 3 deaths. Eurosurveill Wkly 6(27), 2002. Available at *www.eurosurveillance.org/ew/ 2002/020704.asp*

762. Hillebrand W, Siedler A, Tischer A, et al. Progress towards measles elimination in Germany. J Infect Dis 187 (Suppl 1): S208–S216, 2003.

763. Bonmarin I, Levy-Bruhl D. Measles in France: the epidemiological impact of suboptimal immunisation coverage. Eurosurveill Monthly 7:55–60, 2002. Available at *www.eurosurveillance.org/em/ v07n04/0704-221.asp*

764. Centers for Disease Control and Prevention. Measles outbreak—Netherlands, April 1999–January 2000. MMWR 49:299–303, 2000.

765. van den Hof S, Meffre CM, Conyn van Spaendonck MA, et al. Measles outbreak in a community with very low vaccine coverage, the Netherlands. Emerg Infect Dis 7(3 suppl):593–597, 2001.

766. Spika JS, Wassilak S, Pebody R, et al. Measles and rubella in the World Health Organization European Region: diversity creates challenges. J Infect Dis 187 (Suppl 1): S191–S197, 2003.

767. Ion-Nedelcu N, Craciun D, Pitigoi D, et al. Measles elimination: a mass immunization campaign in Romania. Am J Public Health 91:1042–1045, 2001.

768. Bino S, Kakarriqi E, Xibinaku M, et al. Measles-rubella mass immunization campaign in Albania, 2000. J Infect Dis 187 (Suppl 1): S235–S240, 2003.

769. Dayan GH, Zimmerman L, Shtcinke L, et al. Investigation of a rubella outbreak in Kyrgyzstan 2001: implications for an integrated approach to measles elimination and prevention of congenital rubella syndrome. J Infect Dis 187 (Suppl 1): S223–S229, 2003.

770. Cutts FT, Olive J-M. Vaccination programs in developing countries. *In* Plotkin SA, Orenstein WA (eds). Vaccines (3rd ed). Philadelphia, WB Saunders, 1999, pp 1047–1073.
771. Molinert HT, Rodriguez R, Galindo M. Principales Aspectos del Programa Nacional de Immunizacion de la Republica de Cuba. Havana, Cuba, Ministry of Health, 1993.
772. World Health Organization. Progress towards interrupting indigenous measles transmission, WHO Region of the Americas. Wkly Epidemiol Rec 77:21–24, 2002.
773. Prevots DR, Parise MS, Segatto TCV, et al. Interruption of measles transmission in Brazil, 2000. J Infect Dis 187 (Suppl 1): S111–S120, 2003.
774. Rota PA, Bellini WJ. Update on global distribution of wild-type measles viruses. J Infect Dis 187 (Suppl 1): S270–S276, 2003.
775. Vitek CR, Redd SC, Redd SB, Hadler SC. Trends in importation of measles to the United States, 1986–1994. JAMA 277:1952–1956, 1997.
776. Centers for Disease Control and Prevention. Outbreak of measles—Venezuela and Colombia. MMWR 51:757–760, 2002.
777. Grabowsky M, Strebel P, Gay A, et al. Measles elimination in southern Africa [letter]. Lancet 360:716, 2002.
778. Clemens JD, Stanton B, Chakraborty J, et al. Measles vaccination and childhood mortality in rural Bangladesh. Am J Epidemiol 128:1330 1339, 1988.
779. Holt EA, Boulos R, Halsey NA, et al. Childhood survival in Haiti: protective effect of measles vaccination. Pediatrics 85:188–194, 1990.
780. Koenig MA, Khan MA, Wojtyniak B, et al. Impact of measles vaccination on childhood mortality in rural Bangladesh. Bull World Health Organ 68:441–447, 1990.
781. Aaby P, Pedersen IR, Knudsen K, et al. Child mortality related to seroconversion or lack of seroconversion after measles vaccination. Pediatr Infect Dis J 8:197–200, 1989.
782. Cutts FT, Henao-Restrepo A-M, Olive J-M. Measles elimination: progress and challenges. Vaccine 17:S47–S52, 1999.
783. Cutts FT, Steinglass R. Should measles be eradicated? BMJ 316:765–767, 1998.
784. Olive J-M, Aylward BR, Melgaard B. Disease eradication as a public health strategy: is measles next? World Health Stat Q 50:185–187, 1997.
785. The Bill and Melinda Gates Foundation. Measles: Closing the Window of Vulnerability for Children. 2002. Available at *www.gatesfoundation.org/storygallery/measles.htm*
786. Robertson SE, Markowitz LE, Berry DA, et al. A million dollar measles outbreak: epidemiology, risk factors and a selective re-vaccination strategy. Public Health Rep 107:24–31, 1992.

Chapter 20

Mumps Vaccine

STANLEY A. PLOTKIN

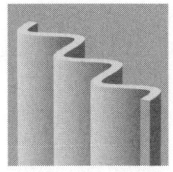Hippocrates was the first to describe the clinical picture of mumps in the fifth century BC. His description of an illness characterized by swelling about one or both ears and, in some instances, painful swelling of one or both testes is reported in Book 1 of his *Book of Epidemics*. In 1790, the Royal Society of Edinburgh published a paper by Hamilton titled "An Account of a Distemper by the Common People of England Vulgarly Called the Mumps."[1] Hamilton reported for the first time that some patients with mumps had evidence of involvement of the central nervous system. He also emphasized the importance of orchitis as a manifestation of the disease in adult males. The origin of the word *mumps* is obscure but may be related to the old English verb, which means "grimace, grin, or mumble."

Although mumps generally is viewed as an acute communicable disease of childhood, it gained notoriety as an illness that substantially affected armies during times of mobilization. Gordon drew attention to this phenomenon in a series of two reviews of the epidemiology of mumps written during the 1940s.[2,3] He noted that mumps was the leading cause of days lost from active duty in the U.S. Army in France during World War I. The average annual rate of hospitalization resulting from mumps during World War I was 55.8 per 1000 (a total of 230,356 cases), which was exceeded only by the rates for influenza and gonorrhea.[4,5] In 1940, the Surgeon General of the United States stated that, next to the venereal diseases, mumps was the most disabling of the acute infections among recruits.[6] Mumps continues to occur in military settings even in the vaccine era. In the 1980s, mumps was reported frequently among Soviet military recruits,[7] and outbreaks occurred among U.S. military personnel stationed in Korea in 1986[8] and on board a ship in the western Pacific in 1992.[9]

In 1934, in a landmark study, Johnson and Goodpasture identified the etiologic agent of mumps as a virus.[10] They obtained saliva from patients with epidemic parotitis and produced nonsuppurative parotitis in monkeys by inoculating the filtered, bacteria-free infectious material into Stensen's duct. The Koch postulates were fulfilled when filtrate from affected monkey parotid glands caused parotitis in uninfected monkeys and children.[11] Cultivation of the mumps virus in the developing chick embryo was first achieved by Habel[12] and Enders[13] in 1945. Propagation of the mumps virus in chick embryo and tissue culture made it possible to develop inactivated and live virus vaccines. An experimental inactivated vaccine developed in 1946[14] was tested in humans in 1951.[15] The first live, attenuated mumps virus vaccines were developed during the 1960s in the former Soviet Union[16] and the United States.[17]

These live vaccines have been adopted into public health practice in most developed countries as part of a triple vaccine with measles and rubella. Where systematically applied, they have exerted good control over the disease, although perhaps not as successfully as the other two components. Safety problems also have impinged on the use of mumps vaccines.

Background

Clinical Description

The major manifestations of mumps are listed in Table 20–1. The classical symptom of mumps is parotitis, which may be unilateral or, more commonly, bilateral and develops an average of 16 to 18 days after exposure.[18] Parotitis may be preceded by several days of nonspecific symptoms, including fever, headache, malaise, myalgias, and anorexia. Data from longitudinal studies have suggested that 15% to 20% of mumps virus infections produce typical acute parotitis; as many as 40% to 50% of infections in some studies have been associated with nonspecific or primarily respiratory symptoms.[19,20] Particularly in children younger than 5 years, mumps commonly may appear as lower respiratory disease.[21] Inapparent infection may be more common in adults than in children,[22] and parotitis may occur more commonly in children ages 2 to 9 years than in other children.[20] Serious complications of mumps virus infection can occur without evidence of parotitis. Fever usually lasts 1 to 6 days, but enlargement of the parotid gland may persist 10 days or longer. An average of 7 days is lost from work or school.[9,19,23,24]

Some complications of mumps are known to occur at higher rates in adults than in children.[19,25] Orchitis occurs in

---

Contributors to this chapter in previous editions were Steve Cochi, Melinda Wharton, and Robert Weibel.

TABLE 20–1 ■ Major Manifestations of Mumps

Manifestation	Frequency (%)
Glandular	
Parotitis	60–70
Submandibular and/or sublingual adenitis	10
Epididymo-orchitis	25 (postpubertal men)
Oophoritis	5 (postpubertal women)
Pancreatitis	4
Neurologic	
Asymptomatic pleocytosis of CSF	50
Aseptic meningitis	1–10
Encephalitis	0.02–0.3
Deafness (usually transient)	4
Other	
Mild renal function abnormalities	30–60
Electrocardiogram abnormalities	5–15

From Galazka AM, Robertson SE, Kraigher A. Mumps and mumps vaccine: a global review. Bull World Health Organ, 77:4, 1999, with permission.

as many as 37% of postpubertal men who develop mumps.[7,22,26] The virus can be recovered from the testis,[27] and the pathology may involve both Leydig and germ cells, leading to decreased testosterone production as well as loss of reproductive function.[28] Although orchitis can be bilateral in as many as 30% of men with mumps orchitis, sterility is thought to occur only rarely.[27,28] Nevertheless, oligospermia and hypofertility occur in 13% of men with bilateral mumps orchitis, and interferon-γ has been used to attempt prevention of this complication.[28] An increased risk of testicular cancer has been reported after mumps orchitis.[29–31]

Mastitis has been reported in as many as 31% of female patients older than 15 years who have mumps,[22] and pelvic pain thought to represent oophoritis also has been observed. An association with subsequent infertility has been suggested but remains unconfirmed.[32] An increase in fetal death has been observed among women who develop mumps during the first trimester of pregnancy.[33]

No overall increased incidence of congenital malformations resulting from maternal mumps infection during pregnancy has been demonstrated,[34] although mumps virus has been shown to cross the placenta and infect the fetus.[35] Endocardial fibroelastosis has long been suspected to be a complication of intrauterine or postnatal mumps infection, based on serologic data and positive reactions to mumps skin test antigen.[36] Ni and colleagues reported detecting the mumps virus genome by the polymerase chain reaction (PCR) in cardiac muscle from 21 of 29 (72%) patients with endocardial fibroelastosis.[37] Endocardial fibroelastosis has become less common, perhaps because of the widespread use of mumps vaccine, and mumps does not appear to be a cause of other myopathies.[38–40]

Virus has been isolated at birth from infants born to women with mumps.[41] Mumps is generally considered a benign infection among neonates,[42] but severe disease may occur.[41,43–45]

Pancreatitis, usually mild, may be present in 4% of cases.[19] Although an association with diabetes mellitus has been suggested,[46–49] it remains unproved.

Central nervous system involvement is reported in 4% to 6% of clinical cases in both population-based studies and large outbreaks.[19,26,50,51] Adults are at more risk for mumps meningoencephalitis than are children.[19,25] Typically, the illness is mild, appearing as aseptic meningitis that is clinically indistinguishable from other forms of aseptic meningitis,[52] and most patients recover fully. However, other more serious clinical presentations include encephalitis and rarely cerebellar ataxia,[53,54] with the possibility of permanent sequelae, including paralysis, seizures, cranial nerve palsies, aqueductal stenosis, hydrocephalus, and death.[53,55–59] As many as half of patients with mumps meningoencephalitis have no evidence of parotid gland involvement.[52,60] Typical abnormalities of the cerebrospinal fluid in people with mumps virus infection of the central nervous system include mononuclear pleocytosis, elevated protein levels, and normal or low glucose levels. Subclinical involvement of the central nervous system appears to be common, and cerebrospinal fluid pleocytosis is common in people with clinically uncomplicated mumps virus infection.[61] Chronic encephalitis has been reported rarely.[62–64]

Mumps is a major cause of sensorineural deafness among children. Deafness may be sudden in onset, bilateral, and permanent.[65–67] Mumps virus has been isolated from perilymph.[68]

Nephritis is not uncommon but is generally not clinically significant.[69] The pathogenesis of nephritis is uncertain; it may be due to either direct viral infection of the kidney or immune complex glomerulonephritis. Although a limited number of pathologic specimens have been examined, there is evidence to suggest that immune complex deposition may play a role in some cases.[70] Autoimmune hemolytic anemia associated with mumps also has been reported.[71]

Mumps arthropathy is a rare complication that reportedly is most common in young adults and more common in men than in women. The arthropathy may be manifested as arthralgias, polyarticular migratory arthritis, or monoarticular arthritis of the knee, hip, or ankle and may have a protracted course.[72,73] The pathogenesis of mumps arthritis is unknown. Although mumps virus has not been isolated from affected joints, mumps virus can replicate in explants of human joint tissue.[74,75]

Electrocardiographic abnormalities are sometimes detected in people with mumps virus infection between days 5 and 10 of illness,[76] but clinically apparent myocarditis is rare. The myocarditis is usually self-limited, but fatal cases have been reported.[77,78] Conduction abnormalities, including complete heart block, may occur.[79]

Virology

Mumps virus is a member of the genus *Rubulavirus* in the family Paramyxoviridae, which also includes Newcastle disease virus; human parainfluenza virus types 2, 4a, and 4b; and simian virus 5. It is an enveloped, negative-strand RNA virus consisting of 15,384 nucleotides encoding seven genes.[80] Two surface glycoproteins, the hemagglutinin-neuraminidase (HN) protein and the fusion (F) protein, are responsible for viral adsorption and fusion of the virion membrane with the host cell membrane, respectively, but both are required for cell-to-cell fusion. The ability to fuse cells is directly related to the neurovirulence of mumps strains.[81] Antibodies to the HN protein neutralize the infectivity of mumps virus.

The five other structural proteins that have been characterized are located within the virion and are not thought to be important targets of a protective immune response. The nucleocapsid (NP) protein confers helical symmetry on the RNA complex. RNA transcriptase activity has been ascribed to both the phospho-(or polymerase) (P) protein and the large (L) protein. The membrane-associated, or matrix (M), protein is thought to play an important role in the assembly of viral proteins and in the budding of virions from the cell surface. Sequencing of the mumps virus genome revealed an additional open reading frame that could encode a small hydrophobic (SH) protein,[82] which has the characteristics of an integral membrane protein[83] of unknown function. Two nonstructural proteins, V and I, are encoded by the P gene and are synthesized as a result of co-transcriptional editing of messenger RNA.[84,85] The V protein is thought to play a role in regulating replication of the genome.

The genomic organization of the virus from 3' to 5' ends is NP-P-M-F-SH-HN-L.[86] The most variable part of the mumps virus genome is in the SH gene. Several different methods have been described for differentiating wild-type and vaccine strains of mumps virus. Strains have been differentiated by amplification and sequencing of segments of the F gene,[87,88] the HN gene,[89] and the SH gene.[90,91] Yamada and associates sequenced a 223-nucleotide segment of the P gene from several vaccine strains and wild-type strains and from isolates obtained from patients who developed meningitis or parotitis after vaccination.[92] They found unique nucleotide changes for the Urabe, Hoshino, Miyahara, and Torii vaccine strains, and the postvaccination isolates were identical to the corresponding vaccine strain. They also noted a specific nucleotide change in the Urabe vaccine strain that resulted in the loss of one restriction endonuclease cleavage site. Thus the Urabe strain could be distinguished from other strains by restriction endonuclease digestion of PCR-amplified P gene segments.[92]

Nucleotide sequence analysis of different segments of the mumps virus genome has allowed mumps vaccine strains and circulating wild-type strains to be grouped on the basis of similarity. Although relationships among mumps virus strains have been inferred from nucleotide sequence analyses of the P,[93] F,[87] and HN[94] genes, the SH gene sequence has been studied the most extensively.[95–100] On the basis of sequence variation in the SH gene, eight genotypes have been identified.[101,102,102a] Group A includes the Jeryl Lynn vaccine strain and the Kilham, Enders, Urabe, and SBL-1 strains. Group B included the Urabe wild-type and vaccine strains and other isolates from Japan. Group C included isolates from the United Kingdom. Sequence analysis of the SH gene has demonstrated similarity between the two strains that constitute the Jeryl Lynn vaccine.[95] Strains isolated during outbreaks in Switzerland from 1992 to 1993 were later demonstrated to be closely related to isolates from the United Kingdom.[97,98]

Although there seems to be no strict geographic localization of genotypes, data from Britain suggest that, in the vaccine era, unlike the homogeneity seen before, mumps strains of varying genotypes are being imported. The sequence of a contemporary genotype G strain differs from a genotype B strain by 71 amino acids (1.5%).[102] Several genotypes of mumps virus are currently co-circulating in Japan.[103]

Varying degrees of homology of amino acid sequences have been demonstrated to analogous proteins in related paramyxoviruses. There is moderate homology between the F protein of mumps virus and that of other paramyxoviruses,[104,105] and similarities also exist between the mumps virus HN protein and that of other paramyxoviruses.[106,107] These similarities account for the serologic cross-reactions that are observed among paramyxoviruses.[108–110] Likewise, homology has been demonstrated for the L,[80] M,[111,112] NP,[113] and P[114] protein sequences of mumps virus and those of other paramyxoviruses.

Before monoclonal antibodies were available, no antigenic differences among mumps viruses had been demonstrated.[115,116] However, by using monoclonal antibodies to distinguish among structural proteins of the mumps virus, researchers have demonstrated a variety of antigenic differences.[94,117,118] Strain-specific differences in neutralizing activity have been identified,[94] and symptomatic mumps virus reinfections have been reported.[119]

Several mumps vaccines have been found to contain more than one strain of mumps virus. The Jeryl Lynn vaccine has been demonstrated to contain two distinct but related viruses in an approximate 1:5 ratio.[95] The Urabe Am9 vaccine from two manufacturers has been demonstrated to contain two viruses in a 1:3 ratio.[120] The Leningrad-3 mumps vaccine also has been reported to contain more than one strain of virus.[121,122]

Although extensive sequencing data are now available for multiple strains of wild-type mumps virus and vaccine strains, the molecular basis of attenuation is not understood. Differences in the neuroinvasiveness of various strains of mumps virus have been demonstrated in a neonatal hamster model.[123] In a 1993 mumps outbreak in Japan, a high incidence of aseptic meningitis was noted. Subsequent analysis of strains from the outbreak revealed that some circulating strains had lost a restriction endonuclease cleavage site in the P gene, a change previously reported to be specific for the Urabe strain.[92,124] However, sequencing of one of these strains demonstrated other changes that allowed it to be distinguished from the Urabe vaccine strain.[125] Additional sequencing data may lead to a better understanding of the relationship between these findings and the high rate of aseptic meningitis observed in this outbreak. Brown and colleagues reported that the two virus variants in Urabe vaccine differ in neurovirulence.[120] Sequencing demonstrated a single nucleotide change resulting in an amino acid change at position 335 in the HN glycoprotein, from glutamine to lysine. However, other mumps virus strains (including vaccine strains) also have lysine at that position.[94] There is evidence based on neutralization studies with monoclonal antibodies that amino acid 335 occupies an important domain, but other amino acid changes have been observed in the variant as well.[126]

Pathogenesis as It Relates to Prevention

Mumps can be understood as a respiratory infection that is frequently accompanied by viremia, which leads commonly to organ involvement, particularly of the salivary glands. Mumps virus can be recovered from the saliva approximately 7 days before the onset of symptoms, and it persists for several days thereafter.[127] Infection of the kidneys, whether accompanied by clinical nephritis or not, is accompanied by viruria that lasts 10 to 14 days; most patients with mumps show viruria.[13] Because mumps virus is present in the saliva and urine for long periods, infection is probably transmitted by large droplets that infect the upper respiratory tract. Approximately one third of infected individuals do not manifest salivary gland or other involvement. Because mumps virus has been isolated from patients with undifferentiated respiratory disease, one can infer that many infections do not go beyond the respiratory tract.[21].

Viremia is likely to occur late in the incubation period, which in terms of the interval until parotitis is 12 to 25 days, 16 to 18 days being the usual.[18,128] In view of the protective effect on the infant exerted by maternal mumps antibodies (see subsequent discussion), it is probable that the viremia is cell free.

Viremia leads to the involvement of many different glandular and other tissues. Parotitis or other salivary gland involvement is certainly the most common, occurring in two thirds of infections. The second most common is meningitis, which may occur in the absence of parotitis. The incidence of central nervous system involvement is difficult to judge. If lumbar punctures are performed routinely, as many as half of the infections show inflammation of the meninges.[19,129] If the diagnosis is based only on clinical evidence of meningitis, only 0.5% to 15.0% of cases are considered to involve the central nervous system.[130]

In a newborn hamster model of mumps encephalitis, both the HN and F glycoproteins appear to be important in pathogenesis.[131] Wolinsky and colleagues found that monoclonal antibodies to the HN glycoprotein—but not the F glycoprotein—of mumps virus protected newborn hamsters from fatal experimental mumps encephalitis.[132] A monoclonal antibody to F was found by Löve and colleagues to protect newborn hamsters from developing necrotizing mumps encephalitis, but large amounts of viral antigen were present in tissue.[133] The monkey neurovirulence test does not correlate well with neurovirulence in humans, although the test has been improved and is used to qualify seed virus and lots of attenuated vaccine strains.[134–136] Data suggest that the monkey test could be replaced by a neurovirulence test in neonatal rats inoculated intracranially.[137]

In any case, virus isolation from the cerebrospinal fluid confirms that meningitis is a complication of viremia, which also explains mumps nephritis, orchitis, oophoritis, pancreatitis, mastitis, thyroiditis, arthritis, and endolymph infections that lead to deafness. Mumps virus has been recovered from the testis during mumps orchitis.[27]

Viremia during infection in a pregnant woman explains reports of the isolation of mumps virus from the placenta[138] and the fetus.[35]

The point at which the mumps virus is most susceptible to immune attack is therefore the period of viremia, when antibodies can prevent viral spread. However, it is possible that local antibodies induced by mumps live virus vaccine also act to prevent respiratory infection by the virus. Cellular immunity probably plays a role in protection, because administration of immune globulin has been gener-ally ineffective in preventing mumps after exposure.[139] Nevertheless, the considerable although transient efficacy of an inactivated mumps virus vaccine suggests that antibodies are the most important means of protection.[140]

Although antigenic differences among mumps strains appear to be minor, symptomatic reinfection has been reported.[119] Reinfections may be common, usually resulting in asymptomatic rises in antibody but occasionally accompanied by mild illness.

Diagnosis

The diagnosis of mumps is usually made clinically, based on the presence of parotitis. Although parotitis can result from infection with other viruses, such as coxsackieviruses, parainfluenza viruses,[141] and Epstein-Barr virus, these agents do not produce parotitis on an epidemic scale. In the absence of high levels of mumps vaccination, most cases of parotitis that are clinically suspected to be mumps are caused by infection with the mumps virus[131]; nonetheless, before the introduction of mumps vaccination in Alberta, one third of sporadic cases reported by participating family practitioners from 1980 to 1982 could not be confirmed serologically as mumps.[19] The inadequacy of clinical diagnosis is even more apparent when disease incidence is low; and thus, as disease incidence declines, laboratory confirmation becomes increasingly important.[142–145] Brunell and colleagues evaluated 20 children with parotitis who had received mumps vaccine 3 to 39 months previously.[146] The diagnosis of mumps could be confirmed in only 8 children, and serologic studies and virus isolation failed to identify any infectious cause in the other 12 children. Only 32 of 252 suspected cases reported to the Texas Department of Health in the first 11 months of 1995 could be confirmed, based on documentation of mumps immunoglobulin M (IgM) antibody testing or epidemiologic linkage to a laboratory-confirmed case.[147] In England and Wales, only 3% of 1333 reported clinically diagnosed cases that were tested for salivary mumps IgM antibody were confirmed as mumps.[144]

Mumps virus may be readily isolated from swabs of the opening of Stensen's duct, saliva, urine, or cerebrospinal fluid during the first 5 days of illness. Primary rhesus monkey kidney or HeLa cells are ordinarily used for virus isolation, but the marmoset lymphoblastoid cell line B95a appears to be equally sensitive.[148]

Direct detection of mumps virus in clinical specimens (oropharyngeal swabs or cerebrospinal fluid) by reverse transcription–PCR (RT-PCR) has been reported.[88] Cusi and colleagues evaluated the use of RT-PCR to detect mumps virus in clinical specimens from children with suspected mumps in Siena, Italy, during the period 1993 to 1995.[88] RT-PCR was more sensitive than mumps IgM enzyme-linked immunosorbent assay (ELISA), detecting evidence of mumps infection in 22 of 27 oropharyngeal swabs from children with parotitis, compared with 18 of 27 positive tests for mumps IgM antibody by ELISA. Afzal and colleagues used RT-PCR in evaluation of clinical specimens from patients during the 1996 outbreak in Portugal.[149] In this series, mumps virus was detected more frequently from saliva than from throat swabs by RT-PCR.

Interestingly, Poggio et al.[150] reported that 96% of patients with clinically diagnosed mumps meningitis had a positive

RT-PCR in the spinal fluid, although virus was isolated in only 39%. No data are available on PCR results in patients without clinical central nervous system involvement.

Historically, serologic assays, including complement fixation, neutralization, and hemagglutination inhibition, have been employed for the diagnosis of mumps. Paired sera are required for these assays, and the acute serum should be obtained as early as possible in the course of illness. Cross-reactions with other paramyxoviruses may occur. Demonstration of neutralizing antibodies is extremely laborious, and both complement fixation and hemagglutination-inhibition assays are relatively insensitive. The hemolysis-in-gel assay is simple enough to perform to make it feasible for serologic screening.[151] However, both false-positive and false-negative results may occur.[152]

At present, ELISAs for mumps immunoglobulin G (IgG) and IgM antibody are widely available commercially. The use of IgM antibody assays allows for the diagnosis of mumps from the analysis of a single acute serum sample, and cross-reactions with other paramyxoviruses do not occur.[108,109] Compared with the complement fixation, hemagglutination-inhibition, and hemolysis-in-gel tests, the IgM ELISA is more sensitive.[153] IgM antibodies are detectable within the first few days of illness, reach a maximum level about a week after the onset of symptoms, and remain elevated for several weeks or months.[153,154] Comparison of antibody levels in serum and cerebrospinal fluid may provide support for local synthesis of antibody in the central nervous system.[155,156] Maximum antibody titers in cerebrospinal fluid occur 1 to 2 weeks after the onset of meningeal symptoms.

Researchers have described a capture radioimmunoassay for mumps IgM antibody in saliva.[157,158] The method is highly sensitive compared with serology 1 to 4 weeks after onset, but data are more limited during the first week after onset, and after the fourth week. Based on the measured declines in IgM antibody in saliva in a small number of cases, the test appears to have limited usefulness after 5 to 6 weeks.

Indirect fluorescent antibody assays for mumps IgM antibody testing are offered by some laboratories. False-positive test results for mumps IgM antibody by this technique have been reported.[159]

Immunity to mumps may be documented by the presence of neutralizing antibodies or by the detection of IgG antibodies by ELISA. In several studies of vaccinated people, seroconversion was demonstrated by ELISA even in the absence of demonstrable neutralizing antibody.[152,160–162] The reason for this finding may be related to antibody directed primarily against the F protein or simply to strain specificity of neutralization.[161] With the addition of complement, neutralizing antibodies may be detectable.[163] The mumps skin test is not reliable and should not be used for identification of susceptible individuals.[164]

Correlates of Immunity

Unfortunately, there is poor correlation between neutralizing, hemagglutination-inhibiting and ELISA antibodies, which makes determination of immunity dependent on the method.[165] This problem has created difficulty in evaluating the immunogenicity of attenuated viruses (see below).

Although humoral immunity is undoubtedly key in the prevention of viremia, and cellular immune responses are known to develop after vaccination, no definite correlate with protection is known. Nojd et al.[166] have described a case of reinfection that suggests that neutralizing antibodies are strain specific. If this is the case, techniques that measure antibodies against all viral components should correlate better with immunity.

Epidemiology

In the years before the introduction of mumps vaccine in the United States, mumps was most commonly reported among young school-age children, with more than half the reported cases of mumps among children 5 to 9 years of age.[167,168] Preschool-age children also may have played an important role in the epidemiology of mumps. The longitudinal Seattle Virus Watch Study (1965 to 1969) found that infants and preschool-age children (many of whom did not develop typical parotitis) accounted for the majority of probable primary infections in households.[20]

Data on the incidence of mumps in the U.S. military in the 20th century suggest that there have been significant shifts in morbidity from adults to children associated with increasing urbanization. During World War I, when mumps was a major cause of days lost from active duty among U.S. troops, cases occurred predominantly among men from rural backgrounds.[169] During World War II, outbreaks still occurred among military recruits, but reported rates were less than one tenth of those documented during World War I. Large outbreaks tended to occur only among groups of soldiers from rural areas.[26] Serosurveys of military recruits in 1962 demonstrated little difference in rates of susceptibility to mumps among men from urban, town, and rural backgrounds.[170] A serosurvey of U.S. Army recruits in 1989 found no differences among recruits from urban, suburban, small town, and rural backgrounds, but people from the western United States were more likely to be seronegative than others (relative risk 1.31; 95% confidence interval, 0.94 to 1.82). Black non-Hispanic recruits were significantly more likely to be seropositive than recruits from other racial or ethnic backgrounds.[171]

Serosurveys from around the world have demonstrated that, in the absence of mumps vaccination, there is substantial variation in the average age at infection with mumps virus. A seroepidemiologic study in St. Lucia demonstrated that 70% of children are seropositive for mumps at 4 years of age,[172] whereas studies from the Netherlands,[173] Singapore,[174] Turkey,[175] and Scotland[176] demonstrated that most children 4 years of age and younger remained susceptible. In the Netherlands, peak acquisition occurred between ages 4 and 6 years; more than 90% of people age 14 years had mumps-neutralizing antibodies, as did 95% of adults ages 18 to 65 years.[173] Before the initiation of routine mumps vaccination of children in 1988, the average age at infection in the United Kingdom was reported to be 6 to 7 years.[177] Evidence from England indicates that there has been some decrease in the average age at infection, perhaps because of increased contacts among preschool-age children.[178,179] Before the introduction of mass vaccination in Spain, two thirds of 3- to 5-year-old children and more

TABLE 20–2 ■ Average Annual Reported Mumps Incidence in Several Countries in the World Health Organization European Region Before and After Introduction of Mumps Vaccine and in Two Countries with No Mumps Vaccination.

Country	Prevaccine		Postvaccine		
	Years	Average Annual Incidence (per 100,000)	Years	Average Annual Incidence (per 100,000)	% Reduction
TWO-DOSE SCHEDULE					
Denmark	1977–1979	726	1993–1995	1	>99
Finland	1977–1979	226	1993–1995	<1	>99
Norway	1977–1979	371	1993–1995	11	97
Slovenia	1977–1979	410	1993–1995	4	>99
Sweden	1977–1979	435	1993–1995	<1	>99
ONE-DOSE SCHEDULE					
America	1983–1985	280	1993–1995	16	94
Croatia	1983–1985	101	1993–1995	12	88
England and Wales	1983–1985	40	1993–1995	5	88
Israel	1983–1985	102	1993–1995	10	90
Latvia	1983–1985	141	1993–1995	3	98
NO MUMPS VACCINE					
Poland	1983–1985	415	1993–1995	361	—
Romania	1983–1985	242	1993–1995	217	—

From Galazka AM, Robertson SE, Kraigher A. Mumps and mumps vaccine: a global review. Bull World Health Organization 77:5, 1999, with permission.

than half of 6- to 7-year-old children were susceptible to mumps. The trend within each age group, however, was toward decreased susceptibility with more siblings and years in school.[180]

Galazka et al.[181] reviewed the prevaccine epidemiology of mumps. Annual incidences in various countries are shown in Table 20–2. An incidence of 300 per 100,000 population was about average, but perhaps 90% of cases remained unreported. The incidence in one developing country, Oman, was in the average range, while in Thailand mumps encephalitis seemed to be uncommon.[182] In most studies seropositivity is high by adolescence, indicating high infection rates in school-age children.

Hope-Simpson demonstrated in household contact studies that mumps is less infectious than measles or varicella.[18] Secondary attack rates among susceptible household contacts younger than 15 years were 75.6% for measles, 61.0% for varicella, and 31.1% for mumps. Some of the observed differences were undoubtedly due to a higher rate of subclinical infection with mumps, but the higher average age at infection observed for mumps also supports the less efficient transmission of mumps virus.[183]

Most epidemiologic reports suggest an interepidemic period for mumps of approximately 3 years.[177,179] In temperate zones, mumps exhibits seasonality, with peak incidence occurring during the winter and spring and a

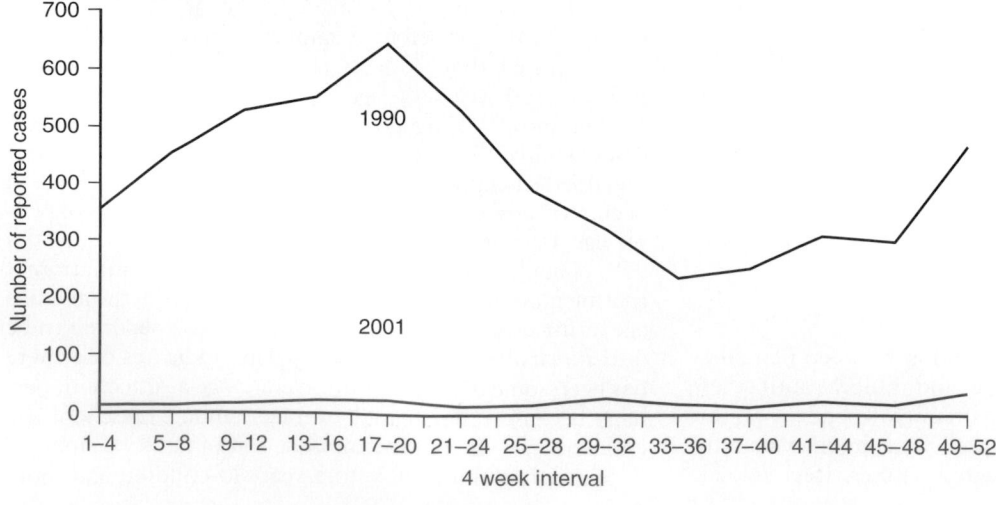

FIGURE 20–1 ■ Reported mumps cases, by 4-week interval, in the United States, 1990 and 2001. (From National Notifiable Diseases Surveillance System, Centers for Disease Control and Prevention, Atlanta, GA, 2002.)

nadir in the summer.[178] This seasonal pattern was seen in the United States until the mid-1990s but is no longer apparent (Fig. 20–1). Seasonality of mumps has not been noted in tropical areas.

Passive Immunization

Immune globulin has not been demonstrated to be effective for postexposure prophylaxis against mumps or for the prevention of complications.[139,184] Likewise, mumps immune globulin has not been proven to be effective and is no longer available in the United States.[130,139] In a study that resulted from an outbreak of mumps in Alaska, administration of mumps immune globulin to susceptible people did not appear to decrease attack rates or prevent clinical complications.[50] However, maternal antibody is transferred across the placenta and appears to protect infants from developing mumps during the first year of life.[128,185]

Active Immunization

Vaccine Strains

Origin and Development

Soon after the initial isolation of mumps virus, attempts were made to develop vaccines based on formalin-inactivated virus.[14,15] Although these vaccines were somewhat effective, the duration of immunity was short, and their use was abandoned in the United States in the 1950s.[186,187]

More than 10 mumps vaccine strains, listed in Table 20–3, are in use throughout the world. Strains have been adapted to the embryonated egg,[188] chick embryo fibroblast cell culture,[188–192] human diploid cell culture,[193,194] quail embryo fibroblast cell culture,[195] and primary guinea pig kidney cell culture.[196]

Description of Vaccines and Producers: Vaccine Dosage, Route of Administration, and Composition

The live virus mumps vaccine produced in the United States by Merck & Company is derived from the Jeryl Lynn strain of mumps virus isolated from the throat of Jeryl Lynn Hilleman and attenuated by passage in embryonated hen's eggs and chick embryo cell culture.[189] The vaccine is available both as monovalent mumps vaccine and in combination with measles and rubella vaccines (MMR).

In its monovalent form, mumps vaccine is supplied as a lyophilized powder containing 20,000 times the median tissue culture infective dose ($TCID_{50}$) of virus, which is reconstituted with sterile, preservative-free water. Sorbitol and hydrolyzed gelatin are used as stabilizers, and 25 µg of neomycin is present in each dose of vaccine. The volume of 0.5 mL is injected subcutaneously above the deltoid area. The vaccine should be kept at 2° to 8°C and should not be exposed to light.

GlaxoSmithKline selected a specific clone of the Jeryl Lynn strain (JL-1) and passaged it an unstated number of times in chick embryo fibroblasts to obtain a strain called RIT 4385. This further passaged strain appears to have the same properties as Jeryl Lynn.

The Urabe Am9 strain was developed by the Biken Institute in Japan from an isolate obtained from the saliva of a mumps patient. The vaccine was produced in Europe by GlaxoSmithKline, Chiron, and Aventis Pasteur. Reports of vaccine-associated meningitis (see subsequent discussion) led to the withdrawal of Urabe-containing vaccines from several countries, but it is still produced by Aventis Pasteur and Chiron. Each dose contains 5000 $TCID_{50}$ of lyophilized virus and is administered subcutaneously after rehydration with sterile water in a volume of 0.5 mL. The Rubini mumps vaccine virus was derived from a mumps isolate obtained from the urine of a child named Carlo Rubini in Switzerland in 1974.[94,193] Subsequent nucleotide sequence analysis has demonstrated that the strain is closely related to a wild-type strain isolated in Germany from 1987 to 1992[90] as well as to the tissue culture–adapted Enders strain.[94]

Most of the other strains listed in Table 20–3 have had limited usage, often being sold in one country only.[191] The exception is the Leningrad-Zagreb strain, which is purchased by the United Nations International Children's Emergency Fund as part of a triple MMR

TABLE 20–3 ■ Mumps Vaccine Strains Currently in Use

Strain	Manufacturer	Cell Substrate[†]	Main Area of Distribution
Jeryl Lynn	Merck	CEF	Worldwide
RIT 4385[*]	GlaxoSmithKline	CEF	Worldwide
Urabe	Aventis Pasteur	CEF	Worldwide
	Biken	CEF	Japan
Hoshino	Kitasato Institute	CEF	Japan
Rubini	Swiss Serum Institute	HDCS	Europe
Leningrad-3	Bacterial Medicine Institute, Moscow	CEF	Russia
Leningrad-Zagreb	Institute of Immunology of Zagreb	CEF	Yugoslavia
	Serum Institute of India	CEF	Worldwide
Miyahara	Chem-Sero Therapeutic Research Institute	CEF	Japan
Torii	Takeda Chemicals	CEF	Japan
NK M-46	Chiba	CEF	Japan
S-12	Razi State Serum & Vaccine Institute	HDCS	Iran

[*]Derived from the Jeryl Lynn strain.
[†]CEF, chick embryo fibroblast; HDCS, human diploid cell strain.

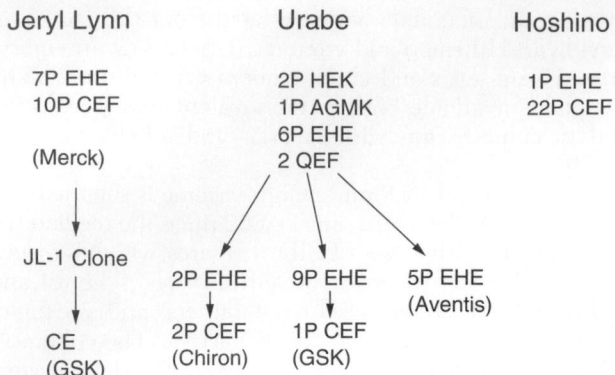

FIGURE 20–2 ▪ Derivation of some attenuated mumps strains. GSK, GlaxoSmithKline.

vaccine. Figure 20–2 gives the history of passage during the attenuation of some of the strains listed in Table 20–3 that have gained prominence.

At least three of the major vaccine strains have been shown to be composed of mixed virus populations. The Jeryl Lynn strain has two distinct viruses, both probably originating from U.S. wild-type isolates and maintained in passage.[95] The Urabe vaccine strain from two manufacturers also has been demonstrated to contain two distinct strains, one of which may be more neurovirulent than the other.[120] The Leningrad-3 strain used in the former Soviet Union is a mixture of large-plaque and small-plaque variants.[121] The significance of these findings is not entirely clear, but studies of the Urabe strain variants suggest that different populations may have different biologic characteristics. As shown in Figure 20–2, the Urabe strain was passaged differently by different manufacturers, and it is therefore not surprising that sequencing revealed numerous mutants in the products.[197]

The route of administration for mumps vaccine is intramuscular or subcutaneous. However, Cusi et al.[198] have reported that several strains could induce neutralizing antibodies in mice after intranasal administration.

Stability of Vaccine

A study of the stability of the Jeryl Lynn strain of vaccine showed that the lyophilized vaccine could be stored for at least 3 years at –20°C without significant loss of infectivity.[199] A loss of infectivity of 0.5 log $TCID_{50}$ is seen after storage at 4°C after 1 year, at room temperature after 2 months, and at 37°C after 1 week. When reconstituted to a liquid state, the mumps vaccine remains stable at 4°C for about 8 hours.[200]

Combinations Including Mumps Vaccine

Mumps vaccine is available as monovalent vaccine or as part of combined formulations with measles and rubella vaccines (MMR). The administration of MMR vaccine results in immune responses similar to those produced by the administration of individual measles, mumps, and rubella vaccines at different sites or at different times. MMR combinations are manufactured by Merck, using Moraten (further attenuated Edmonston) measles, RA

27/3 rubella, and Jeryl Lynn mumps strains; by GlaxoSmithKline using Schwarz measles, RA 27/3 rubella, and RIT 4385 mumps strains; by Aventis Pasteur using Schwarz measles, RA 27/3 rubella, and Urabe mumps strains; by Berna using the Edmonston-Zagreb measles, RA 27/3 rubella, and Rubini mumps strains; and by the Serum Institute of India using Edmonston-Zagreb measles, RA 27/3 rubella, and Leningrad-Zagreb (L-Zagreb) mumps strains. Combination products including measles, mumps, rubella, and varicella vaccines are currently under development (see Chapter 29).

Results of Vaccination

Immune Responses

In one of the first prelicensure immunogenicity studies of the Jeryl Lynn strain, conducted in Philadelphia in 1965, the seroconversion rate in children who tested initially as seronegative for mumps neutralization antibody was 98.1% (355 of 362 children).[17,201] Similar results have been reported from other studies.[202–205] The total prelicensure experience in U.S. children showed that 96.9% of 6283 initially seronegative children developed neutralizing antibody after vaccination.[201] One study after licensure suggested that, in some recipients of mumps vaccine, the immune response may not be completed by 4 weeks after immunization; seroconversion rates were 86.6% at 4 weeks and 93.3% at 5 weeks after immunization.[206]

In studies of monovalent Urabe vaccine, 94% of recipients seroconverted.[207] In Germany, a total of 94.4% of previously seronegative children developed neutralizing antibody after administration of vaccine from any of four lots of Urabe vaccine. The antibody response was demonstrated to persist for at least 32 months after vaccination.[207] Researchers in Finland compared the immunogenicity of the Urabe vaccine with that of the Jeryl Lynn vaccine in children 14 to 20 months of age. According to the results of the hemolysis-in-gel and neutralization assays, 55 of 58 (94.8%) of the recipients of the Urabe vaccine experienced seroconversion, as did 58 of 60 children (96.7%) who received the Jeryl Lynn vaccine.[208]

Ninety-three percent of children receiving monovalent Hoshino strain vaccine seroconverted.[209] In another study, 122 previously seronegative children received the Hoshino vaccine, and 95% developed neutralizing antibody to mumps.[191] In a study of preschool-age children attending day care, 712 of 775 (92%) who received the Leningrad-3 mumps vaccine seroconverted based on the hemagglutination-inhibition assay.[210]

In early field trials of the L-Zagreb vaccine conducted in preschool-age children, 88% to 94% of children in various districts were demonstrated to have developed mumps antibodies as documented by hemagglutination inhibition. Later trials of the L-Zagreb strain combined with measles and rubella vaccines demonstrated seroconversion rates as high as 98%.[188]

The level of mumps-neutralizing antibody in children 6 to 8 weeks after vaccination is substantially lower than the level after natural mumps. In the Philadelphia prelicensure study, mean neutralization antibody titers were 1:9 after vaccination and 1:6 after natural disease.[17]

The immunogenicity of mumps vaccine has been evaluated as a component of triple MMR vaccines. The Jeryl Lynn strain gave between 90% conversion (geometric mean antibody titer, 31) and 98% conversion in two studies.[211,212] The Urabe and Jeryl Lynn strains were compared in several studies as part of two different trivalent vaccines.[213-216] In Finland, seroconversion rates of 96% to 98% based on hemagglutination-inhibition assays were demonstrated for MMR preparations containing Urabe or Jeryl Lynn strains in children 14 to 24 months of age.[215] A comparison of Urabe and Jeryl Lynn vaccines administered with measles vaccine in Austria suggested that the Urabe vaccine produced higher antibody responses as determined by ELISA.[216] In the United Kingdom, 88% of 13- to 15-month-old recipients of Urabe-containing MMR were demonstrated to develop neutralizing antibody.[217] Table 20–4 presents results of four studies comparing seroconversion after Jeryl Lynn or Urabe administered as part of MMR.[215,216,218] Urabe appeared to be more immunogenic than Jeryl Lynn.

The RIT 4385 derivative of Jeryl Lynn was compared directly with Jeryl Lynn in a study of two MMR vaccines. Table 20–5 shows that the two vaccines were similar in immunogenicity, both at day 60 and at 1 year following vaccination.[219] Results at 18 months were also comparable.[220]

The immunogenicity of the Rubini mumps vaccine given as MMR has been evaluated in several clinical studies. Among children 15 to 24 months of age, 95% of recipients of Rubini mumps vaccine and 100% of recipients of Jeryl Lynn vaccine seroconverted, based on immunofluorescence.[221] In a study comparing the immunogenicity of Jeryl Lynn, Urabe, and Rubini vaccines given as MMR among children 15 to 24 months of age, all children who received vaccines containing Jeryl Lynn or Urabe as the mumps component seroconverted as measured by immunofluorescence. In contrast, the seroconversion rate after use of Rubini vaccine varied among the four lots tested and was as low as 71% for one lot.[222] Another comparative study[105] showed equal seroconversion with the use of Jeryl Lynn and Rubini vaccines when measured by

the indirect immunofluorescence test but not by ELISA. An extensive serologic study of specimens obtained in clinical trials of three different MMR vaccines showed high seroconversion for the measles and rubella components (>95%), but a difference between Jeryl Lynn and Urabe (>95%) and Rubini (38%) in ELISA tests, but not in immunofluorescence and neutralization tests.[223] Nevertheless, poor effectiveness of Rubini vaccine has been reported (see later).

Equivalent rates of seroconversion after the administration of monovalent and trivalent vaccines have been demonstrated for the Hoshino vaccine.[191] Similarly, studies with the L-Zagreb vaccine have demonstrated similar rates of seroconversion (approximately 90%) when vaccine is administered to 12- to 14-month-old children as single-antigen mumps vaccine or combined with measles and rubella vaccines.[188,224]

The Leningrad 3 strain gave similar seroconversion.[195]

Factors Influencing Seroconversion

Mild illnesses do not affect seroconversion to mumps vaccine. King and colleagues studied serologic responses to MMR in children receiving routine vaccination, who fre-

TABLE 20–4 ■ Comparative Immunogenicity of Urabe (U) and Jeryl Lynn (JL) Strains

Study	Antibody Test*	% Seroconversion	
		U	JL
Christenson et al.[213]	Neut.	60/64 (94%)	66/64 (91%)
	HIG	66/77 (86%)	66/80 (63%)
Vesikari et al.[214]	Neut.	76/91 (84%)	38/57 (67%)
	HIG	67/85 (79%)	44/61 (72%)
Vesikari et al.[215]	EHI	90/93 (97%)	49/51 (96%)
Popow-Kraupp et al.[216]	EIA	190/196 (97%)	171/190 (90%)
Overall		84%–97%	63%–96%

*EHI, enhanced hemagglutination; EIA: ELISA; HIG: hemolysis-in-gel; Neut., neutralization.

TABLE 20–5 ■ Seroconversion (SC) and Geometric Mean Antibody Titer (GMT) in 9 to 24-Month-Old Children Given One of Two MMR Vaccines

Antibodies	Vaccine	42–60 Days		One Year*	
		%SC†	GMT	%SC‡	GMT
Measles	Moraten (Merck)	96.9	3270	100	3190
	Schwarz (GSK)	98.7	2958	100	3058
Mumps	Jeryl Lynn (Merck)	96.9	1526	87.0	1049
	RIT-4385 (GSK)	95.5	1400	88.4	1010
Rubella	RA 27/3 (Merck)	99.5	79.3	100	75.6
	RA 27/3 (GSK)	99.5	72.5	100	76.5

*Seroconversion only.
†N = approximately 1050 for GlaxoSmithKline (GSK), 380 for Merck.
‡N = approximately 140 in both groups.
From Usonis V, Bakasenas V, Denis M. Neutralization activity and persistence of antibodies induced in response to vaccination with a novel mumps strain, RIT 4385. Infection 29:159–162, 2001, with permission.

quently have mild illness afterward.[225] Seroconversion to the Jeryl Lynn mumps valence was not influenced by the illnesses, and the children exhibited an overall seroconversion rate of 83% as determined by ELISA.

Age at the time of vaccination does affect seroconversion. A small study examined the immune responses to the Jeryl Lynn strain among seronegative infants without a documented exposure to mumps virus.[200] The seroprevalence of prevaccination mumps antibody varied by age from 50% (4 of 8) in infants ages 3 to 5 months to 9% (2 of 23) in those ages 6 to 8 months to 10% (2 of 21) in those ages 9 to 11 months. Seroconversion rates among the initially seronegative children also varied among these age groups and were 50%, 95%, and 95%, respectively. A larger study of mumps antibodies showed a seroprevalence of 93%, 80%, 33%, 12%, and 4% at 0 to 0.5, 0.5 to 3, 3 to 6, 6 to 9 and 9 to 12 months, respectively.[226] Wagenvoort and associates demonstrated that most infants born to mothers with naturally acquired mumps antibody became seronegative by 4 months of age.[173] Seroconversion after Jeryl Lynn vaccination reached 70% at age 6 months and more than 90% at 9 or 12 months, but in the lowest age group an additional 20% of infants showed a T-cell proliferation response, suggesting that they had been immunized despite the absent serologic response.[227]

The response to Urabe strain mumps vaccine given as MMR has been evaluated among children younger than 12 months. In a study in India, children 9, 12, and 15 months of age were vaccinated, and their seroresponses as measured by hemagglutination-inhibition assay were reduced from 92% when the vaccine was given at 1 year of age to 75% when vaccine was given at 9 months of age.[228] In contrast, in Brazil, 99% of children seroconverted after vaccination at 9 months of age as measured by neutralization, and 100% seroconverted after vaccination at 15 months of age[229]; similar results were reported from South Africa.[230]

Whether or not immune globulin interferes with the immune response to mumps vaccine has not been well studied. Among 23 children 2 to 13 years of age who were initially seronegative to mumps, co-administration of mumps vaccine and 0.1 to 0.2 mL of immune globulin per pound resulted in 100% seroconversion and no difference in the levels of postvaccination mumps antibody titers compared with those of 11 control children who had received vaccine only.[200]

MMR is now often recommended for older children, and seroconversion rates of mumps-susceptible children vaccinated at 18 months or 12 years of age were compared in Sweden. Whereas 93% of the toddlers converted, only 80% of the 12-year-olds did so.[218]

Seroconversion rates among adults are generally slightly lower than those for children. A prelicensure immunogenicity study demonstrated neutralizing antibody responses after vaccination of 19 of 20 (95%) initially seronegative adults.[231] The total prelicensure experience in adults vaccinated with the Jeryl Lynn strain showed an overall seroconversion rate of 92.6% among 163 initially susceptible adults (132 men and 31 women).[205]

Mumps vaccine administered after exposure to mumps does not provide clinical protection or alter the severity of the disease.[204] However, evidence from an observational study suggests that mass vaccination during a mumps outbreak may help terminate the outbreak.[232]

Persistence of Antibodies

Serologic studies have shown that neutralizing antibody titers of 1:2 or higher persisted for at least 12 years after vaccination in a follow-up study of children involved in a clinical efficacy trial.[233–236] Weibel[236] has summarized data on antibody persistence from this longitudinal study, which demonstrate that, with the passage of time, antibody levels after vaccination remain consistently lower than those after clinical mumps (Table 20–6). In the final report of the mumps data from this longitudinal study,[233] the mumps-neutralizing antibody titers of 22 vaccinated children, all of whom had remained free of clinical mumps disease during the 12 years of follow-up, were compared with those of 24 unvaccinated control children from the original 20-month trial who had developed natural mumps. Antibody measurements had been taken on the two groups of children at intervals of 3 to 4 years, 7 to 8 years, and 11 to 12 years after vaccination and mumps disease, respectively.

Although the initial level of neutralizing antibody reached after vaccination was generally less than that after natural disease, the geometric mean titers after vaccination decreased by 27% in nearly 12 years, whereas those following natural mumps fell 80% during approximately the same time period. Thus the mean titers after vaccination (mean 9.1) and natural mumps (mean 11.5) were comparable. There was evidence during the follow-up period, however, that suggested asymptomatic boosting of antibody levels as a result of subclinical natural reinfection, particularly among the vaccinees.[234]

Miller and colleagues followed children given Jeryl Lynn or Urabe vaccine 4 years previously at 12 to 18 months of age.[237] Seronegativity by neutralization assay had developed in 19% of the Jeryl Lynn recipients and 15% of Urabe recipients, a difference that was statistically significant. Among seropositive children, however, geometric mean antibody titers were higher among Jeryl Lynn recipients than among

TABLE 20–6 ■ Persistence of Mumps-Neutralizing Antibody in Seropositive Children After Clinical Mumps or Vaccination with Jeryl Lynn Strain of Mumps Vaccine

	Mumps-Neutralizing Antibody Geometric Mean Titers	
Time	Vaccine (34 Children)	Clinical Mumps (36 Children)
1 mo	10.1	62.8
1 yr	12.8	27.6
2 yr	11.9	42.1
4 yr	11.8	34.5
7 yr	10.3	18.6
9.5 yr	12.5	24.4

From Weibel RE. Mumps vaccine. In Plotkin SA, Mortimer EA (eds). Vaccines (2nd ed). Philadelphia, WB Saunders, 1988, p 231, with permission.

recipients of Urabe vaccine.[237] Canadian children who had received MMR vaccines containing Jeryl Lynn or Urabe strains at 12 to 24 months of age were later evaluated at 6 to 7 years of age. As measured by ELISA, 15% of Jeryl Lynn recipients and 7% of Urabe recipients were seronegative at 6 to 7 years of age.[238] Finnish workers provided data on children vaccinated with Jeryl Lynn vaccine at 14 to 18 months of age and again at 6 years of age. Seroconversion was 86% after the first dose, 76% at 6 years of age, 95% after booster, and 86% 9 years later.[239] A follow-up done in Sweden 10 years after vaccination of toddlers with Jeryl Lynn showed persistent antibodies in 73%.[240]

A follow up study of infants vaccinated with the RIT 4385 clone of Jeryl Lynn showed 95% neutralization positives at 18 months after vaccination.[240a]

Immunocompromised Persons

Data are limited on the immunogenicity of mumps vaccine among immunocompromised people. A study in pediatric patients who had received bone marrow transplants revealed that MMR vaccination 2 or more years after transplantation resulted in an increase in seropositivity from 31% to 87%.[241] Among 20 bone marrow transplant patients ages 1 to 29 years who were vaccinated with MMR vaccine 2 to 3 years after transplantation, 11 were seronegative before vaccination and 7 of the 11 seronegative patients seroconverted.[242] In a small study of children with end-stage renal disease undergoing maintenance hemodialysis, only 5 of 10 children seroconverted after receiving mumps vaccine as MMR.[243]

Protective Efficacy in Controlled Clinical Trials

Before the licensure of the Jeryl Lynn strain of mumps vaccine in the United States, two different clinical trials demonstrated that a single dose of live, attenuated mumps vaccine was 95% to 96% effective in preventing mumps disease in people who were followed for as many as 20 months after vaccination.[201,204,244] The first clinical trial was conducted in Philadelphia from 1965 to 1967 among selected children and their siblings attending nursery school or kindergarten (Table 20–7).[201,244] The children initially were screened serologically, and those lacking mumps antibody were randomized to the vaccinated and control groups (although complete randomization of the siblings was not achieved). Both groups were followed for a total of 20 months for the acquisition of a laboratory-confirmed case of clinical mumps or the documented exposure to a laboratory-confirmed case in a classroom or household setting. Laboratory confirmation was defined as the isolation of mumps virus from mouth or throat specimens or the indication of a fourfold or greater increase in mumps antibody titer by hemagglutination-inhibition or neutralization antibody assays. Of the 867 children enrolled, 398 children (174 vaccinees and 224 control subjects) had a documented exposure to mumps during the 20-month follow-up period. Five cases of mumps occurred in the vaccinated group, compared with 133 cases among the control children. The overall protective efficacy of the vaccine was 95% (95% confidence interval, 88% to 98%), and the point estimates of efficacy varied from 92% to 96% by subgroups of exposed individuals (families vs. classrooms) and by interval from vaccination to exposure (0 to 10 months vs. 11 to 20 months).

The second clinical trial was a double-blind, placebo-controlled study conducted from 1966 to 1967 of first- and second-grade children attending 44 schools in Forsyth County, North Carolina (Table 20–8).[204] Every tenth study child in each school received the placebo vaccine, and no study participants were excluded based on mumps antibody status. After sera were drawn from a sample of children for mumps antibody testing by neutralization, all vaccinations were given during a 2-day period at the onset of the trial, and the children were followed for 6 months. Initial susceptibility to mumps did not differ significantly between the two study groups in the sample of children tested. During the follow-up period from 30 to 180 days after vaccination, there were 5 cases of mumps among the 2965 children who received mumps vaccine, compared with 13 cases among the 316 control children, giving a vaccine efficacy of 96% (95% confidence interval, 88% to 99%).

Smorodintsev and co-workers reported a small clinical trial of the Leningrad-3 strain among children 3 1/2 to 6 years of age.[16] Two (2.3%) of the 85 vaccinated children developed mumps disease, compared with 42 (38.8%) of the

TABLE 20–7 ■ Protective Efficacy of Jeryl Lynn Strain of Mumps Vaccine Among Initially Susceptible Children, by Months Since Vaccination, Philadelphia, 1965 to 1967

Interval Between Vaccination and Mumps Exposure (mo)	Study Group	Vaccinated Group			Unvaccinated Group			Vaccine Efficacy (%)
		No. of Cases	No. at Risk	Attack Rate (%)	No. of Cases	No. at Risk	Attack Rate (%)	
0–10	Household	2*	29	6.9	50	59	84.7	91.7
	Classroom	2*	114	1.8	49	113	43.4	95.9
11–20	Household	1†	14	7.1	22	24	91.7	92.3
	Classroom	1†	28	3.6	24	40	60.0	94.1
Total period	All children‡	5	174	2.9	133	224	59.4	95.2

*Three of these children showed postvaccination neutralizing antibody titers of 1:1; one failed to respond.
†This child, who was in both household and classroom groups, failed to respond serologically to vaccination.
‡Among vaccinated children, 11 counted twice, one of whom contracted mumps; among control children, 12 counted twice, and mumps developed in all 12.
From Hilleman MR, Weibel RE, Buynak EB, et al. Live, attenuated mumps-virus vaccine. 4. Protective efficacy as measured in a field evaluation. N Engl J Med 276:252–258, 1967, with permission from *The New England Journal of Medicine.*

TABLE 20–8 ■ Protective Efficacy of Jeryl Lynn Strain of Mumps Vaccine Among Primary School Children,* North Carolina, 1966 to 1967

Study Group	No. of Cases	No. at Risk	Attack Rate (%)	Vaccine Efficacy (%)	95% Confidence Interval† (%)
Vaccines	5	2965	0.17	96	88–99
Control subjects	13	329	3.95		

*Children were enrolled without serologic screening to exclude those who were already immune.
†By the Fisher exact text, two-tailed.

children in the control group, giving a vaccine efficacy of 94% (95% confidence interval, 76% to 98%). Subsequent studies of efficacy gave protection rates from 91% to 99%, but it was not clear whether the unvaccinated controls were chosen at random.[245]

Effectiveness in Field Use and Duration of Immunity

Effectiveness of the Jeryl Lynn strain of mumps vaccine in the United States under conditions of routine use has been consistently lower in outbreak-based studies (i.e., 78% to 91%) than in the original efficacy trials (i.e., 95% to 96%) (Table 20–9)[24,232,246–252] Although low vaccine effectiveness may be the result of true low efficacy, the methods used in postlicensure field evaluations of vaccine effectiveness have limited our ability to draw firm conclusions about the reasons for the lower estimates for vaccine efficacy compared with the results in controlled clinical trials. Kim-Farley and colleagues have demonstrated that errors such as inaccurate case definition, incomplete surveillance with limited case

TABLE 20–9 ■ Published Clinical Studies of Mumps Vaccine Efficacy and Effectiveness

Study Population	Vaccine Strain*	Year	Vaccine Efficacy (%)	95% Confidence Interval (%)
PROSPECTIVE CLINICAL TRIALS				
Philadelphia	J	1965–1967	95	88–98
North Carolina	J	1966–1967	96	88–99
Russia	L-3	1970	91–99†	?
OUTBREAK STUDIES				
			Effectiveness (%)	
New York	J	1973	79	53–91
Yugoslavia	L-Z	1974	97–100	?
Canada	J	1977	75	49–87
Ohio	J	1981	81	71–88
Ohio	J	1982	85	39–94
New Jersey	J	1983	91	77–93
Tennessee	J	1986	78	64–87
Spain	J/U	1987	86	65–95
Kansas	J	1988–1989	83	57–94
Spain	J/U	1990	75	53–86
Switzerland	J	1993–1996	61	0–85
	U	1993–1996	73	42–88
	R	1993–1996	6	–45 to 40
Switzerland	J	1994	65	11–86
	U	1994	76	36–91
	R	1994	12	–102 to 62
France	U	1995	76	66–83
Belgium	J/U	1995–1996	67	50–79
United Kingdom	J	1996	68	24–86
Italy	J/U	1996	1.0‡	Ref.
	R	1996	2.4‡	1.4–4.4
Spain	J	1997	1.0‡	Ref.
	R	1997	6.5‡	3.6–11.8
Canada	J	1997	80	29–96
Switzerland	J	1998	78	64–82
	U	1998	87	76–94
	R	1998	–4	–218 to 15

*J, Jeryl Lynn; L-3, Leningrad 3; L-Z, Leningrad-Zagreb; R, reference group; R, Rubini; U, Urabe.
‡Relative risk of mumps.
†Uncertain as to randomization.

ascertainment, and inaccurate determination of vaccination status all are factors that potentially contribute to falsely low estimates of vaccine efficacy in observational studies.[248]

The occurrence of serologically or virologically confirmed mumps cases in vaccinated people is also predictable, as with any vaccine of less than 100% efficacy. This problem becomes more prominent as vaccination coverage increases. Although the overall rate of susceptibility decreases, the proportion of previously vaccinated people increases among the remaining susceptibles, and hence cases occur among vaccinated people even when vaccine efficacy is high.[253] Incomplete case ascertainment with selectively better identification of vaccinated than unvaccinated cases may result in low vaccine efficacy estimates. Factors that can confound the analyses include prior mumps disease and subclinical infection occurring before the outbreak and unequal levels of exposure of vaccinees and non-vaccinees to mumps virus during the outbreak. Inaccuracies in determining mumps vaccination status from parent histories or school records also may result in misleadingly low estimates of efficacy.[232,248,249,253]

Despite these methodologic limitations, the outbreak-based studies taken together suggest that mumps vaccine effectiveness is lower than the estimates derived from the controlled efficacy trials with relatively short follow-up periods. Although earlier studies had not identified the waning of vaccine-induced immunity as an important factor,[232,250] several more recent outbreaks in highly vaccinated populations have raised the possibility of waning immunity.[24,254,255] Two outbreaks occurred in U.S. high schools in which more than 95% of students were vaccinated. In a Tennessee school, serologic data suggested that most of the mumps cases resulted from primary failure of the first dose to produce seroconversion; however, students vaccinated more than 3 years earlier had higher attack rates than those vaccinated more recently, suggesting that waning immunity also may have contributed to the outbreak.[254] In a Texas outbreak, 18% of students developed mumps despite prior vaccination. However, there was no evidence for an increase in attack rate with increased time since vaccination.[255] A school outbreak in Quebec also included many vaccinated children.[256] However, in an outbreak in Vancouver secondary to a "rave," young vaccinated adults showed 80% protection.[257] Thus it remains uncertain whether failure to seroconvert after a first vaccination or waning immunity is the major risk factor for mumps among vaccinated people.

The efficacy of the Urabe strain was studied in an outbreak that occurred in a French community. The focus of the epidemic was a primary school in which the calculated efficacy was 76%.[258] Analysis of reported mumps cases in Switzerland and Singapore, supplemented by serologic data, suggest that the Rubini strain has little or no efficacy.[259,260] That stark conclusion was supported by a study conducted in five primary schools in Geneva, in which secondary attack rates were calculated in children exposed in school according to the vaccine they had received. The protective efficacy of Jeryl Lynn vaccine was 65%, that of Urabe vaccine 76%, and that of the Rubini vaccine only 12%.[261] The same group performed a study of efficacy in family contacts, and found efficacies of 62%, 73%, and 6% respectively for

Jeryl Lynn, Urabe, and Rubini.[262] Another study conducted in Eastern Switzerland concluded an efficacy of 78% for Jeryl Lynn, 87% for Urabe, and −4% for Rubini.[263] An efficacy analysis performed in Southern Italy found an odds ratio for vaccine failure of 2.4 for Rubini compared to Jeryl Lynn or Urabe. Interestingly the odds ratio increased with age of the vaccinee.[264] In Seville, Spain, a comparison of Rubini and Jeryl Lynn strains indicated a relative risk of 6.5 for the former strain.[265] The decreased ELISA antibody response to the Rubini strain has been mentioned above.

An outbreak in a well-vaccinated lower school in Belgium was analyzed by Vandermeulen et al.,[266] who found that prior vaccination was 67% effective against clinical mumps. Time from vaccination did not appear to influence seropositivity or effectiveness.

An outbreak has been described in a Japanese primary school in which some of the students had been vaccinated with two Japanese attenuated strains: the Urabe strain (given as MMR) and the Torii strain.[241] Calculations from the reported data suggest a protection level of 61%. The Leningrad-3 strain was reported to have a vaccine effectiveness of 96.4% when given to children attending 19 day care centers in a program to control an outbreak of mumps.[210]

Although the relative contributions of primary vaccine failure and secondary vaccine failure (i.e., waning immunity) remain uncertain, it seems reasonable to assume that a second dose of MMR vaccine given at school entry for the prevention of measles would result in a further decrease in the proportion of children susceptible to mumps on entering school. In one study, U.S. children who had previously received Jeryl Lynn vaccine given as MMR were evaluated before receiving a second dose of MMR at either 4 to 6 or 11 to 13 years of age. As determined by ELISA, 97% of 4- to 6-year-old children and 100% of 11- to 13-year-old children were seropositive for mumps antigen, and 100% of both age groups were seropositive after revaccination.[267]

In the United States, the Advisory Committee on Immunization Practices and the American Academy of Pediatrics have recommended since 1989 that all children receive two doses of measles vaccine.[268] Because measles vaccine is generally given to children in the United States as MMR vaccine, the effect of implementation of this recommendation has been that most children receive two doses of mumps vaccine. Although there is limited information on the effectiveness of a second dose of mumps vaccine, a two-dose schedule of MMR vaccine should protect most people who do not respond to initial vaccination. Since this recommendation has been implemented in the United States, reported cases of mumps have decreased dramatically.

Risk Factors for Vaccine Failure

Epidemiologic studies of mumps outbreaks have examined potential risk factors for mumps vaccine failure by comparing the characteristics of vaccinated cases and vaccinated control subjects. Several studies demonstrated that use of the measles vaccine before 15 months of age was associated with vaccine failure during the 1980s, when most mothers had immunity resulting from prior infection with mumps rather than vaccination.[269] In contrast, mumps vaccination at 12 to 14 months of age has not been associated with mumps vaccine failure.[24,232,250,254,255,270] One study conducted in 9-month-old children showed a decreased rate of seroconversion.[228] Two studies have shown a trend toward a lower attack rate among children who have received two doses of mumps vaccine as opposed to those who have received one dose, but in both instances the findings did not reach statistical significance.[24,255] The type of mumps vaccine preparation (i.e., monovalent vs. MMR) has not been found to affect the risk of vaccine failure.[232,250,254,255,270] Studies have not shown clear evidence of increased risk with increasing number of years since vaccination (i.e., waning immunity), but such studies have been hampered by an inability to measure the independent effect of this potential risk factor. Reinfection likely resulted in boosting of immunity in vaccinees when mumps incidence was high. With near-elimination of mumps in several countries that have achieved high levels of vaccination coverage with two doses of MMR, boosting probably no longer plays a role in maintaining immunity. Further surveillance for mumps in highly vaccinated populations will be required to determine the importance (if any) of boosting in maintaining mumps immunity.

A provocative case report of a patient with chronic mumps parotitis suggested that reinfection with a different mumps genotype is possible because the neutralizing response is genotype specific.[271] If this is the case, it would provide a possible mechanism for vaccine failures, and could explain the failure of the Rubini strain.

Transmission of Vaccine Virus

In the Philadelphia prelicensure immunogenicity study, none of the 365 children who were classroom or household contacts of the vaccinated children developed mumps vaccine virus infection.[17] This conclusion was based on an analysis of paired serum specimens that documented the absence of contact transmission of the virus. Other studies have shown that recipients of the Jeryl Lynn strain of mumps virus vaccine do not spread this virus to susceptible contacts and that the vaccine virus cannot be isolated from blood, urine, or saliva.[138,203] However, the RNA genome of the vaccine viruses has been isolated from children given the Japanese Miyahara and Hoshino strains.[272] Yamauchi and colleagues isolated mumps virus from placental tissues of two of three seronegative women who were administered the vaccine 7 to 10 days before planned abortions.[138] One study demonstrated transmission of the Urabe strain to a sibling from a child who developed parotitis after vaccination.[273]

Possibility of Herd Immunity

Mathematical models of the potential impact of mass vaccination on the incidence of mumps disease predict that an 85% to 90% level of vaccination coverage by 2 years of age would be required to eliminate the transmission of the mumps virus in western Europe or the United States.[177] High levels of vaccine coverage with two doses of MMR in Sweden and Finland have resulted in dramatic reductions in disease incidence (see later). By 1996, 91% of 19- to 35-month-old children in the United States had received at least one dose of measles-containing vaccine (almost all of

which was administered as MMR), and many children had received two doses of MMR. The number of mumps cases was at an all-time low, with only 751 cases reported.[274,275]

Simultaneous Administration with Other Vaccines

Simultaneous administration of mumps vaccine as MMR with diphtheria and tetanus toxoids and whole-cell pertussis vaccine, with diphtheria and tetanus toxoids and acellular pertussis vaccine, or with oral poliovirus vaccine, *Haemophilus influenzae* type b conjugate vaccine, or hepatitis B vaccine does not impair antibody responses or increase rates of serious adverse events.[271,276–279] Simultaneous administration of varicella vaccine either in combination with separate measles, mumps, and rubella vaccines or with MMR vaccine but in separate sites has been shown to be safe and immunogenic.[280–283]

Adverse Events

The most common adverse reactions to mumps vaccination are parotitis and low-grade fever. Vaccine-associated parotitis occurs most commonly 10 to 14 days after vaccination.[284] Rash, pruritus, and purpura have been reported after mumps vaccination but are uncommon and usually mild and transient. In one study of Jeryl Lynn and Urabe strains, parotid and/or submaxillary swelling was noted in 1.6% of children who received Jeryl Lynn vaccine and in 1% to 2% of children who received Urabe vaccine.[216] In a large study of Urabe vaccine, there was a 0.7% incidence of parotitis.[285] The Hoshino strain vaccine virus has been isolated from vaccine recipients who developed parotitis 14 to 24 days after vaccination.[286]

Three strains of mumps vaccine, Jeryl Lynn, Urabe, and Edmonston-Zagred, were compared in Brazil.[286a] Parotid enlargement following vaccination occurred respectively in 0.5%, 1.3%, and 3.1% of vaccinees, compared with 0.2% of controls.

Assessing complications after mumps vaccination is made more difficult by the fact that most mumps vaccine is given in combination with measles and rubella vaccines. Based on biologic plausibility, however, orchitis,[287] arthritis,[209,288] sensorineural deafness,[289,290] and acute myositis[291] may rarely follow vaccination. The role of mumps vaccine in reports of diffuse retinopathy,[292] gait disturbances,[293] and thrombocytopenic purpura[294–296] after MMR vaccination is difficult to evaluate. Moreover, strain identification is essential when a complication occurs after mumps vaccination because it may be due to coincidental wild-type virus infection.[297]

Despite the use of chicken embryo as the substrate for mumps vaccine, few serious allergic reactions are attributable to egg protein. Allergy to gelatin included in the vaccine is more frequently associated with acute reactions.[298] The chicken embryo cell substrate of mumps vaccines does contain endogenous avian leukosis virus and other endogenous avian viruses,[299] but there is no evidence for acquisition of these viruses by vaccinees.[300]

A search for mumps virus replication in children with symptomatic human immunodeficiency virus (HIV) infection gave negative results.[301] Mumps virus could not be found in the intestines of patients with inflammatory bowel disease.[302]

Encephalitis within 30 days after mumps vaccination does not occur more frequently than the background rate of central nervous system dysfunction in the normal population; only 0.4 case of encephalitis has been reported in the United States per million doses of live virus mumps vaccine distributed.[130] Febrile seizures following mumps vaccination have been rarely reported.[303] A large study in Finland found no increase in the background incidence of Guillain-Barré syndrome, which was about 1 in 500,000 toddlers.[298]

Aseptic Meningitis

As noted previously, one of the most frequent complications of natural mumps infection is meningitis.[22,50] Mumps strains used as attenuated vaccines have lost most of their potential for viremia, and therefore for meningitis as a complication of viremia, but this potential has not been lost entirely. The reported rate of aseptic meningitis that occurs after vaccination ranges widely, from approximately 1 in 800,000 for the Jeryl Lynn strain[304] to as high as 1 in 1000 for the Leningrad-3 strain.[305] The incubation period of the illness has generally been between 2 and 3 weeks after vaccination, and the clinical symptoms and signs, including lymphocytic pleocytosis in the cerebrospinal fluid, have been similar to those of the natural disease.[306]

Of course, coincidental meningitis after vaccination may occur as a result of other viruses and even wild-type mumps virus,[90] and confirmation of the causative role of vaccine virus requires definitive identification of the mumps virus isolate as the vaccine strain (see earlier discussion under *Virology*). However, because viruses similar or identical in sequence to the vaccine virus previously administered have been isolated from people with postvaccination meningitis,[87,89,92] there is no doubt that some vaccine strains can cause meningitis.

Data bearing on meningitis after vaccination are available from many countries, including the United States, the United Kingdom, Canada, Germany, Japan, France, and Brazil. In the United States, meningitis after vaccination with the Jeryl Lynn strain has been a rare event that is perhaps coincidental with vaccination, occurring after only 1 in 1.8 million doses administered, according to passive surveillance.[307] In a large cohort of children 12 to 23 months of age for whom vaccination and hospitalization records were available, for every 100,000 doses administered, one child was hospitalized for aseptic meningitis within 30 days of receiving MMR. In a nested case-control study, receipt of MMR within 8 to 14, 14, or 30 days was not demonstrated to be a risk factor for hospitalization for aseptic meningitis, but the number of cases was very small; odds ratios were 1.00 (95% confidence interval, 0.1 to 9.2), 0.50 (0.1 to 4.5), and 0.84 (0.2 to 3.5), respectively.[308] In Germany, the Jeryl Lynn strain was associated with a meningitis rate of 1 in 1 million doses,[284] and isolation of a Jeryl Lynn–like strain was reported from one patient who developed aseptic meningitis after vaccination.[309] Post-licensure surveillance in Germany over two years, during which approximately 600,000 doses of Jeryl Lynn and 500,000 doses of its derivative RIT-4385 were given, both as part of triple vaccines, failed to detect any cases of associated aseptic meningitis.[309a]

Reported rates of postvaccine meningitis for strains used in Japan have been 1 in 120,000, 30,000, 20,000, and 5000 for the Hoshino, Torii, Miyahara, and Chiba strains, respectively (S. Makino, personal communication, 1998), but these rates are based on passive surveillance.

The Urabe strain has been linked with aseptic meningitis wherever adverse reactions have been studied. In Japan, the rate of meningitis after vaccination with the Urabe strain was reported to be as high as 1 in 2000 doses, and the rate of meningitis with Urabe strain isolated from cerebrospinal fluid was 1 in 9000.[310,311] In one prefecture, the rate of proven Urabe meningitis was 1 in 900.[311] A prospective study of meningitis after vaccination with Urabe-containing MMR produced by four different Japanese manufacturers revealed no cases after administration of one of the vaccines but similar incidence after administration of any of three others.[312] Retrospective data collected by the Ministry of Health also suggested variation between one case in 933 vaccinations to one case in 18,686 vaccinations. A follow-up study further confused the picture. Urabe vaccine manufactured by Biken gave an incidence of 25 per 10,000 doses administered in one formulation but 0 per 10,000 doses in another formulation. The rates for Urabe vaccines made by Takeda and Kitasato were 14 and 7.4 per 10,000 doses administered, respectively.[313]

A retrospective study conducted in Korea could not differentiate between the effects of Urabe and Hoshino strains, as both were used. However, the conclusion was that the rate of aseptc meningitis following one or the other of those strains was 1 in 10,500 doses.[313a]

In Canada, the observed rate of meningitis after vaccination with Urabe strain was calculated to be 1 in 62,000 doses of the vaccine manufactured by GlaxoSmithKline.[314] In Europe, Urabe strain mumps vaccines manufactured by GlaxoSmithKline and Aventis Pasteur were extensively used. Estimates by the capture-recapture method[315] and by retrospective passive surveillance[316] of the rate of meningitis in France after administration of the Urabe strain produced by Aventis Pasteur elicited a rate of one case of meningitis per 28,400 vaccinations; for GlaxoSmithKline, the estimated rate was one case per 120,000 vaccinations.

In the United Kingdom, a cluster of cases in the Nottingham area prompted an investigation that disclosed that the incidence of vaccine-associated mumps meningitis after vaccination with the Urabe strain was higher than had been previously thought.[317] By linking virology laboratory and hospital discharge records with vaccination histories, 1 case of postvaccination meningitis was found per 3800 doses of MMR administered in the Nottingham health district. During this period, 80% of the MMR used in the district contained the Urabe strain, and all cases of meningitis identified followed inoculation with vaccines that contained the Urabe strain.[318] Data for the entire United Kingdom, based on Public Health Laboratory Service surveillance, suggested a rate of one aseptic meningitis case in 11,000 doses among the 85% of the children who received Urabe-containing vaccine, compared with no cases after vaccination among the 15% of children who received Jeryl Lynn–containing vaccine.[319] Convulsions occurred 15 to 35 days after vaccination with Urabe strain vaccine in 1 of 2600 doses.[320] In Salvador, Brazil, an epidemic of meningitis followed a mass vaccination campaign with MMR containing Urabe. A case-control analysis showed a relative risk of 14.3 within 3 weeks of vaccination, with an attributable risk of 1 in 14,000 doses.[321] The relationship of vaccination with Urabe to aseptic meningitis cases in Italian military recruits was confirmed by sequencing isolates from

TABLE 20–10 ■ Rates of Aseptic Meningitis After Vaccination with Urabe Strains of Various Manufacturers

Manufacturer	Country	Reference	Rates (Doses for 1 Case)
AvP, GSK	UK (Nottingham)	317	11,000
Takeda	Japan	311	862
Kitasato	Japan	313	3125
All Japanese	Japan	310, 313	933–18,686
Aventis Pasteur	France	316	28,400
GlaxoSmithKline	France	315	121,951
Aventis Pasteur	Saudi Arabia	373	2,439,000
GlaxoSmithKline	Brazil	321	14,000
GlaxoSmithKline	Canada	314	62,000

cerebrospinal fluid.[372] As a result of these findings, vaccines containing the Urabe strain were withdrawn from use in several countries. Table 20–10 summarizes the various incidence rates reported for aseptic meningitis after Urabe, and illustrates their wide range.

Brown and co-workers demonstrated that the strain isolated from cases of aseptic meningitis was one of two variants present in the Urabe vaccine.[120] The meningitis-associated variant had a mutation from guanine to adenine at base 1081, which resulted in a glutamine-to-lysine change in amino acid 335 of the HN protein. Further analysis showed that the adenine mutants could be either temperature sensitive or not, and that it was non–temperature-sensitive mutants that were recovered from meningitis cases.[323] However, this conclusion has been disputed, and it may be that other mutations are more important to attenuation.[324] Moreover, it appears that, because of different passage histories, all strains labeled Urabe are not the same, a conclusion supported by sequence data.[324]

The L-Zagreb strain caused an outbreak of mumps parotitis, meningitis, and orchitis after a mass vaccination campaign in Surinam.[325] In Brazil, the same strain elicited a large number of meningitis cases, and it was estimated that there was one case for each 6–20,000 doses of vaccine.[326] Another study from Brazil estimated an incidence of 1 meningitis per 3390 doses of L-Zagreb.[326a]

Fortunately, sequelae to postvaccine meningitis have been rare or absent. Unpublished follow-up data from France, Canada, and the United Kingdom have not revealed sequelae clearly attributable to the illness, although possible sequelae have been noted in about 3% to 5% of cases.

In conclusion, it appears that many attenuated mumps vaccine strains cause aseptic meningitis, although the rates of this complication vary according to the vaccine strain, the manufacturer, the index of clinical suspicion, and the intensity of surveillance. For Urabe strain vaccine, the variation lies between 1 per 1000 and 1 per 20,000 vaccinations. However, in evaluating the importance of this complication, one has to consider the incidence of meningitis that would occur in natural mumps (variously reported as between 1% and 50%, but a conservative estimate would be 1 in 400 cases).[327] and the possible differences in efficacy between strains. The data summarized in Table 20–10 sug-

gest that Urabe gives higher rates of protection than Jeryl Lynn. Nokes and Anderson have argued that, if the Urabe strain is more efficacious than the Jeryl Lynn strain, the risk-benefit ratio would be in favor of the former strain when vaccination coverage is low and mumps virus continues to circulate in the population.[328] Assuming a rate of Urabe-associated meningitis of 1 in 11,000 and an incidence of mumps greater than 1% per year, vaccination is better than not vaccinating. The choice between Jeryl Lynn and Urabe should depend on weighing the relatively higher efficacy of the latter, the higher price of the former, and the cost of caring for vaccine reactions to the latter. Different countries have made different judgments regarding the use of Jeryl Lynn or Urabe strain vaccines for the prevention of mumps,[329,329a] and the WHO considers all strains beside Rubini to be acceptable.[329b]

Indications for Vaccination

In the United States, the Advisory Committee on Immunization Practices has recommended two doses of MMR vaccine for all children and certain high-risk groups of adolescents and adults. The first dose of MMR vaccine should be administered to all children at age 12 to 15 months, and the second dose administered routinely at age 4 to 6 years. Certain adults who may be at increased risk for exposure to and transmission of mumps should receive special consideration for vaccination. These people include international travelers, people attending colleges and other higher educational institutions, and people who work at health care facilities.[330]

In general, people can be considered immune to mumps who (1) have documentation of vaccination with live mumps virus vaccine on or after their first birthday, (2) have laboratory evidence of mumps immunity, (3) have documentation of physician-diagnosed mumps, or (4) were born before 1957. People born before 1957 in the United States are likely to have been infected naturally between 1957 and 1977 and may be presumed immune even if they have not had clinically recognizable mumps disease. However, birth before 1957 does not guarantee mumps immunity. Therefore, during mumps outbreaks, vaccination with MMR should be considered for people born before 1957 who may be exposed to mumps and who may be susceptible. Laboratory testing for mumps susceptibility before vaccination is not necessary.[330] There is no increased risk of adverse reactions to vaccination of people who are already immune.

Precautions and Contraindications

Because mumps vaccine produced in chick embryo cell culture contains small quantities of ovalbumin, there have been concerns about the risk for serious allergic reactions in people with egg allergy. However, studies have demonstrated that the risk for serious allergic reactions such as anaphylaxis after the administration of mumps vaccine in people allergic to eggs is extremely low and that skin testing with vaccine is not predictive of allergic reaction to vaccination.[331–335] Therefore, skin testing is not required before administering mumps vaccine to these individuals. Similarly, the administration of gradually increasing doses of vaccine is not required.[330]

Data suggest that most anaphylactic reactions to mumps-containing vaccines are associated with hypersensitivity not to egg antigens but to other components of the vaccines. MMR and its component vaccines contain hydrolyzed gelatin as a stabilizer. There are several case reports of people with an anaphylactic sensitivity to gelatin, who had anaphylactic reactions after receiving MMR vaccine.[336-338] Therefore, extreme caution should be exercised when administering MMR or its component vaccines to people who have a history of an anaphylactic reaction to gelatin or gelatin-containing products. Skin testing for sensitivity to gelatin could be considered, but no specific protocols for this purpose have been published.[330] Likewise, people who have a history of anaphylactic reactions to neomycin should not receive the vaccine; a history of contact dermatitis to neomycin is not a contraindication to vaccination. Mumps vaccine does not contain penicillin.

Mumps vaccine should be given at least 2 weeks before the administration of immune globulin or deferred until 3 months after such administration, because passively acquired antibody can interfere with response to the vaccine.

The live virus mumps vaccine should not be given to pregnant women because of the theoretical risk of fetal damage; there is no evidence, however, that the vaccine can cause congenital malformations in humans. Vaccinated women should avoid pregnancy for 1 month after vaccination.

People with severe febrile illnesses should in general not be vaccinated until they have recovered. Vaccination should not be postponed because of minor illness.

Live virus mumps vaccine should not be given to people with acquired immunodeficiency or suppressed immunity (e.g., leukemia, lymphoma, generalized malignancy, or therapy with corticosteroids, alkylating drugs, antimetabolites,

or radiation). An exception is children infected with HIV. MMR vaccination is recommended for all asymptomatic HIV-infected people who do not have evidence of severe immunosuppression and for whom measles vaccination would otherwise be indicated. MMR vaccination also should be considered for all asymptomatic HIV-infected people who do not have evidence of severe immunosuppression. Because the immunologic response to vaccines may decrease as HIV disease progresses, HIV-infected infants without severe immunosuppression should routinely receive MMR at age 12 months. Consideration should be given to administering the second dose of MMR vaccine as soon as 1 month after the first dose.[330] Patients with leukemia in remission who have not received chemotherapy in at least 3 months may receive live virus mumps vaccine, as may people who have received short-term (i.e., less than 2 weeks' duration) steroid therapy.[330]

Public Health Considerations

Epidemiologic Effects of Vaccination—United States

Live, attenuated mumps vaccine was licensed in the United States in 1967. Since that time, the incidence of mumps in this country has decreased dramatically. However, outbreaks of mumps in the 1980s raised new questions about vaccine efficacy and the duration of immunity (see under *Effectiveness in Field Use and Duration of Immunity*).

Following the licensure of the live virus mumps vaccine in 1967, reported cases of mumps decreased from more than 185,000 in 1967 to 2982 by 1985, a decrease of more than

MUMPS. Reported cases per 100,000 population by year — United States, 1975–2000

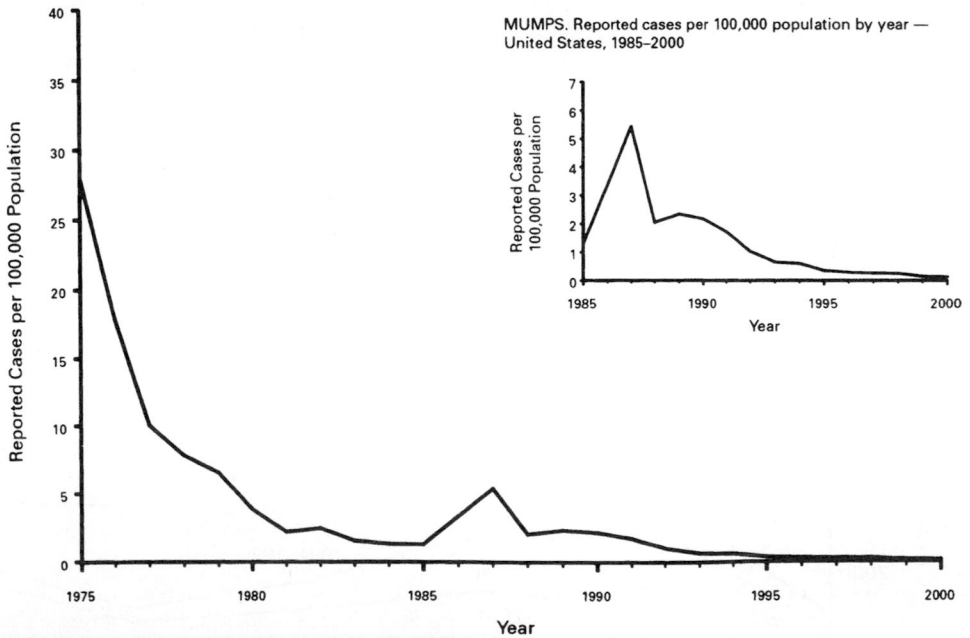

MUMPS. Reported cases per 100,000 population by year — United States, 1985–2000

Because of the recommendation of two doses of measles-mumps-rubella (MMR) vaccine and its high coverage rate in the United States, mumps is at record low levels. During the 1990s, mumps cases declined substantially from 5,292 reported cases in 1990 to 338 reported cases in 2000, meeting the *Healthy People 2000* objective of <500 cases per year.

Note: A mumps vaccine was first licensed in December 1967.

FIGURE 20–3 ■ Reported cases of mumps per 100,000 population by year in the United States, 1985 to 2000. Because of the recommendation of two doses of measles-mumps-rubella (MMR) vaccine and its high coverage rate in the United States, mumps is at record low levels. During the 1990s, mumps declined substantially from 5292 reported cases in 1990 to 338 reported cases in 2000, meeting the *Healthy People 2000* objective of less than 500 cases per year. (*Note:* Mumps vaccine was first licensed in December 1967.) (From Mumps: Reported cases per 100,000 population by year—United States, 1985–2000. MMWR 49:52, 2002.)

98% (Fig. 20–3). In 1986 and 1987, however, a relative resurgence of mumps occurred, with 7790 cases reported in 1986 and 12,848 in 1987. Outbreaks were reported in high schools,[232] in colleges,[24,339] and in the workplace among young adults.[340]

That resurgence was the result of incomplete vaccination coverage of adolescents and young adults in the years after the introduction of the live virus vaccine. Since 1989, reported cases of mumps have again decreased: In 2000, only 338 mumps cases were reported in the United States, an all-time low. Reductions have been most dramatic among those 5 to 19 years of age (Fig. 20–4). This pattern reflects an increasing implementation of school immunization requirements for two doses of MMR vaccine as well as improved specificity in the reporting of mumps in some states.[147]

During the prevaccine era, mumps was classically a disease of children 5 to 9 years of age. From 1986 to 1991, however, the highest age-specific incidence shifted to children 10 to 14 years of age.[341-343] From the beginning of the vaccine era, the average age of people with mumps infection gradually increased, resulting in an increasing proportion of cases reported among people 15 years and older. From 1967 to 1971, only 8% of reported cases were among this age group, compared with more than one third from 1987 to 1992 (Fig. 20–5).[342,343] This shift in reported cases of mumps from school-age children to adolescents and young adults was an expected result of the implementation of immunization programs, which historically were directed at preschool-age children and led to widespread interruption of mumps virus transmission; a similar shift was previously observed for measles and rubella.

Several lines of evidence suggest that the increase in reported mumps was primarily the result of failure to vaccinate susceptible people and only secondarily the result of vaccine failures.[344] National immunization policy in the United States historically was slow to endorse mumps vaccine as a routine immunization of childhood. Thus a decade elapsed between licensure of the vaccine in 1967 and the recommendation at the end of 1977 that it be given routinely to all children. The sluggish pattern of distribution of mumps vaccine during this decade confirmed that the vaccine only gradually came into widespread use. However, during the decade after licensure of mumps vaccine, the incidence of reported mumps declined markedly. Presumably, this decline was a result of the incremental uptake of sufficient mumps vaccine in the U.S. population to interrupt substantially the transmission of the mumps virus. Data from secondary attack rate studies and mathematical models show that clinical mumps is substantially less communicable than measles, leading to reductions in the transmission of mumps at immunization levels that would have only a minimal impact on measles transmission.[18,345] Consequently, a cohort of children born between about 1967 and 1977 (i.e., people between 10 and 20 years of age in 1987) grew up when the chance of exposure to wild mumps virus for a preschool-age or young school-age child was markedly declining while the opportunity to receive mumps vaccine was uncertain. The greater mobility of older children and adolescents increased the potential for contact among susceptible people in these age groups, which led to mumps outbreaks when mumps disease was introduced into these populations.

At the same time, there was a gradual movement toward the routine use of mumps vaccine in children born since 1977. Although the increasing use of MMR vaccine and the enactment of mumps immunization school laws by states led to higher levels of mumps immunization in U.S. children, the timing of these events varied among state immunization programs and the many private providers of vaccine. The gradual implementation of these changes likely resulted in isolated pockets of susceptible, unvaccinated children.

Immunization policy influenced not only the age groups affected but also the areas where outbreaks have occurred. During the relative resurgence of mumps that began in 1986, large outbreaks generally were confined to states that did not have comprehensive (i.e., kindergarten through grade 12) requirements for mumps vaccination for school attendance. In 1986, the reported incidence of mumps in 15 states without any requirement for mumps vaccination was 14-fold higher than that observed in states that had a com-

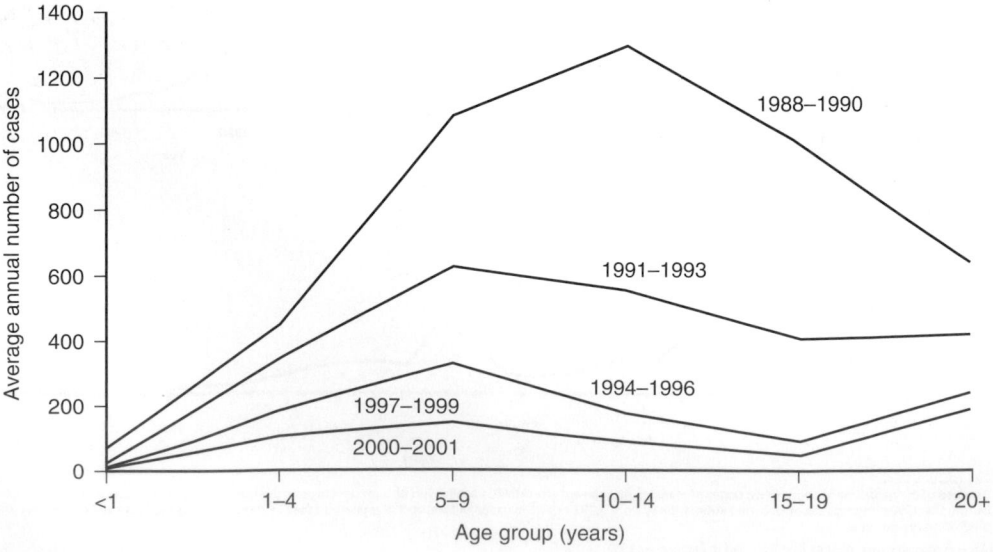

FIGURE 20–4 ■ Average annual number of reported cases by age group and by 3-year period, 1988 to 2001. (From National Notifiable Diseases Surveillance System, Centers for Disease Control and Prevention, Atlanta, GA, 2002.)

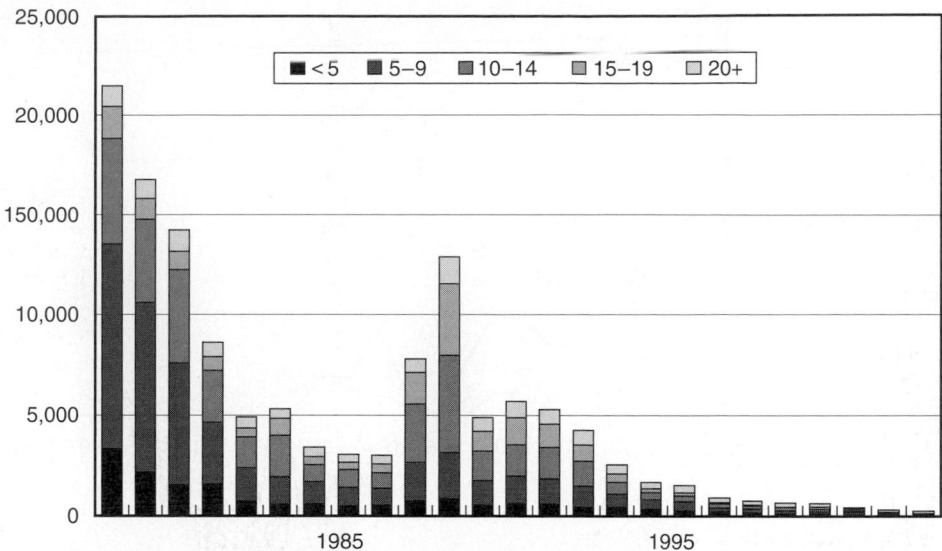

FIGURE 20–5 ▪ Reported cases of mumps by age group, United States, 1977 to 2001. In each year, the age distribution of cases of known age has been applied to the cases of unknown age. (From National Notifiable Diseases Surveillance System, Centers for Disease Control and Prevention, Atlanta, GA, 2002.)

prehensive requirement. The incidence in states with requirements that affected only some students (e.g., a requirement that applied only to children first entering school) was more than twice as high as that observed in states with comprehensive laws.[344] More recent data demonstrate that, as mumps incidence has decreased nationally, differences in incidences between states with and without comprehensive school vaccination laws have been less striking (Fig. 20–6).[343]

School laws regarding mumps vaccination have consistently been shown to be effective in decreasing the incidence of mumps.[25,247,344] The occurrence of a cluster of outbreaks of mumps on university campuses from 1986 to 1987 underscored the need for prematriculation immunization requirements that include inoculation with mumps vaccine.[23] The dramatic reduction in reported cases of mumps in the United States since 1991 reflects increasing implementation of school immunization laws requiring two doses of MMR. In 1998, the Advisory Committee on Immunization Practices recommended that all states take immediate steps to implement the two-dose MMR schedule so that, by the year 2001, all children in kindergarten through grade 12 will have received two doses of MMR.[330] This protocol should result in further decreases in mumps

among school-age children. However, with disease now at an all-time record low in the United States, national surveillance data will be inadequate for documenting further decreases without improved case investigation and increased use of laboratory testing for confirmation of mumps.

From 1975 to 1984, there was approximately 1 death from mumps per 5000 reported cases and 1 case of mumps encephalitis per 500 reported cases (Fig. 20–7). Since 1984, these proportions have been more variable owing to smaller numbers of reported events, and, since 1995, mumps encephalitis has not been a reportable disease in the United States.[346] Because of under-reporting of both mumps and mumps encephalitis, these figures probably overestimate the risk of mortality and underestimate the rate of mumps encephalitis. Indeed, before the introduction of mumps vaccination, mumps was the most commonly diagnosed cause of encephalitis in childhood; introduction of routine vaccination has resulted in the virtual elimination of mumps encephalitis in some areas.[347,348]

Previous cost-benefit analyses have shown that $7 to $14 are saved for every dollar spent on a program of vaccination with either mumps or MMR vaccine.[349,350] A more recent analysis found cost-benefit ratios of 6.1 (direct costs only)

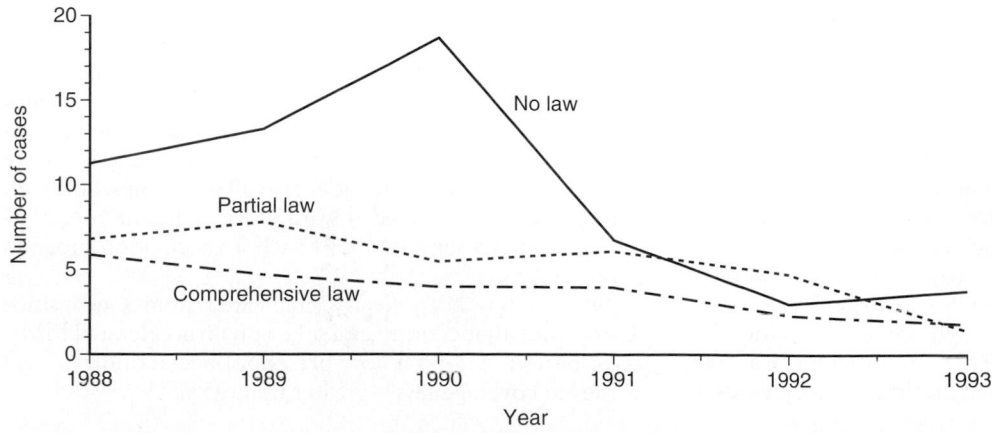

FIGURE 20–6 ▪ Reported incidence of mumps for people 5 to 19 years of age by type of state immunization requirement, United States, 1988 to 1993. (From van Loon FPL, Holmes SJ, Sirotkin BI, et al. Mumps surveillance—United States, 1988–1993. Mor Mortal Wkly Rep CDC Surveill Summ 44:1–14, 1995.)

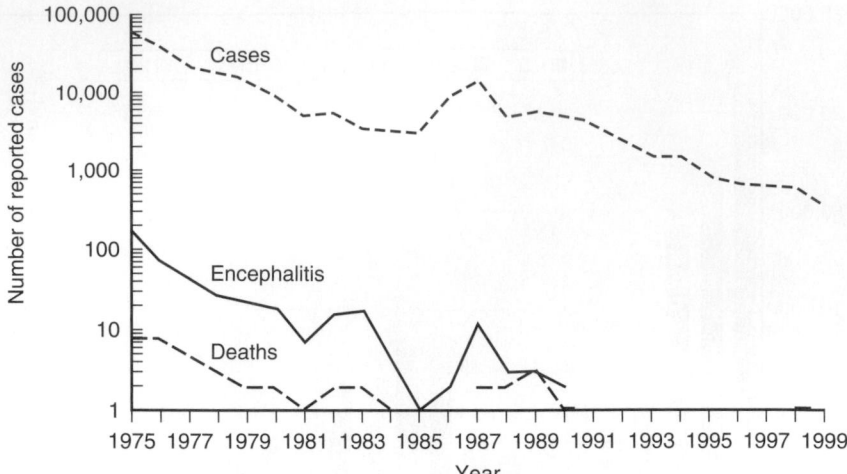

FIGURE 20–7 ■ Reported cases of mumps and mumps encephalitis and deaths from mumps, United States, 1975 to 1995. There were no deaths due to mumps from 1985 to 1986 and from 1992 to 1995; mortality data for 1996 are not yet available. No cases of mumps encephalitis were reported in 1991 and 1993; beginning in 1995, mumps encephalitis was no longer nationally notifiable.

and 13.0 (direct and indirect costs) for use of monovalent mumps vaccine and 16.3 (direct costs only) and 21.3 (direct and indirect costs) for MMR vaccine (Centers for Disease Control and Prevention, unpublished data).

Epidemiologic Effects of Vaccination—Countries Other Than the United States

Compulsory immunization with mumps vaccine was introduced in Croatia in 1976, and a greater than 90% reduction in morbidity was reported by 1978.[188]

In Finland, a two-dose schedule of vaccination with MMR was introduced in November 1982, with a first dose being given at 14 to 18 months of age and the second at 6 years of age. During the first 2 ½ years of the vaccination program, 81% of targeted children had been vaccinated, with a resulting 87% decrease in the incidence of mumps.[351] By 1986, more than 95% of eligible children had been vaccinated.[352] In 1989, Koskiniemi and Vaheri reported that no cases of mumps encephalitis had been seen at Helsinki Children's Hospital, the pediatric referral hospital for southern Finland, since the introduction of the vaccination program.[347]

By 1994, Peltola and colleagues noted that there were fewer than 30 cases of laboratory-confirmed mumps reported each year and that these were probably imported.[353] The incidence of new cases of type 1 (insulin-dependent) diabetes, which had been rising in Finland, has leveled off since 1990 and has been accompanied by a decrease in mumps antibodies in diabetic children, although a causal relationship has not been established.[354] By 1997, indigenous mumps disappeared from Finland, with only the rare imported cases remaining (Fig. 20–8).[355] The success of the Finnish program, achieved by the routine two-dose schedule of MMR vaccination, serves as a model for other countries that wish to eradicate measles, rubella, and mumps.[356]

In Sweden, a two-dose vaccination schedule with MMR at 18 months and 12 years of age was introduced in 1982, with approximately 90% coverage for each of the two doses. Before the second dose, according to one study, 27% of prior vaccinees had lost mumps antibodies, but the booster seroconverted all but 7%.[240] Although mumps vaccine was licensed in Sweden in the 1970s, the vaccine was not widely used until 1982. Subsequently, dramatic decreases in

reported morbidity for all three diseases were observed.[357] Serologic screening demonstrated an increase in the proportion of unvaccinated 12-year-old children who tested seronegative to mumps virus, from 13% in 1985 to 39% in 1989. This trend suggests a decrease in naturally acquired immunity after the introduction of widespread vaccination, thus providing another reason for a two-dose schedule.[358]

Routine vaccination with MMR at 12 to 15 months of age was introduced in England and Wales in 1988. Preschool-age children also were offered MMR in a 3-year catch-up program, and, in some districts, catch-up vaccination was extended to children up to 10 years of age. Vaccination coverage reached 91% of 24-month-old children by 1996.[359] The impact of vaccination on disease incidence was prompt, as reflected in notified cases, which decreased 79% from 1989 to 1990.[360] Based on reports from sentinel surveillance, the annual incidence decreased from 160 per 100,000 population in 1989 to 17 per 100,000 in 1995, with the most dramatic decrease occurring among children 0 to 14 years of age. Since November 1994, salivary mumps IgM antibody testing has been offered for confirmation of clinically diagnosed mumps, and 46% of 2868 notified cases have been tested. Mumps IgM antibody was detected in only 40 (3%) of these specimens, one of which was obtained from a person who had been recently vaccinated. Serologic surveillance demonstrated an increase in seronegativity among people 9 to 20 years of age, reflecting a decreased circulation of mumps virus. With the introduction of a routine second dose of MMR at 4 years of age, further reductions in incidence of mumps are expected.[144]

In January 1989, Israel incorporated mumps and rubella vaccine with measles vaccine into the routine immunization schedule at 15 months of age. The incidence of mumps dropped from 11.6 to 0.6 per 10,000 between the prevaccine era and 1991.[361] By 1998, mumps incidence was only 0.3 per 100,000, with a reduction in all age groups, although the age peak had shifted toward older children.[362] A cost-benefit analysis suggested that such a vaccination program was cost saving.[363]

Mumps has been nearly eradicated from Cuba since 1988, when that country embarked on an accelerated MMR vaccination program of preschool-age children and achieved coverage levels greater than 95%.[364]

Year	Immunization Program Recipients/*Vaccine*	No. of Mumps Cases
1960		14656
1961		7990
1962		10395
1963		11405
1964		13543
1965		14734
1966		18233
1967		20325
1968		11881
1969		11780
1970	Military Recruits / *Inactivated Vaccine**	20794
1971		22980
1972		7895
1973		6729
1974		7162
1975		8949
1976		8790
1977		5076
1978		4462
1979		22324
1980		12026
1981		2992
1982		2182
1983		1468
1984		514
1985		414
1986		555
1987		77
1988		122
1989	*Jeryl Lynn Strain*† / National Immunization Program Children at 14 to 18 mo and 6 y / *Jeryl Lynn Strain*†	44
1990		19
1991		9
1992		13
1993		15
1994		18
1995		6
1996		2
1997		0 (2)‡
1998		0 (1)§
1999		0 (1)‖

FIGURE 20–8 ■ Indigenous mumps in Finland from 1960 to 1999. *Unshaded area* indicates number of cases through 1986 based on reported cases; *shaded area* indicates number of cases after 1986 based on serologic confirmation. *Inactivated mumps vaccine was used for recruits of the defense forces in 1960 to 1986. †Component of measles-mumps-rubella vaccine. ‡Two cases of mumps imported from Russia. §One case imported from Estonia. One case imported from Africa. (Redrawn from Peltola H, Davidkin I, Paunio M, et al. Mumps and rubella eliminated from Finland. JAMA 284:2643–2647, 2000.)

A contrasting experience has been reported from Switzerland. The Jeryl Lynn strain mumps vaccine (given as MMR) first became available in Switzerland in 1971, and MMR vaccine including the Urabe strain was introduced in 1983. Routine vaccination of children at 15 to 24 months of age was recommended by Swiss public health authorities in 1985. MMR containing the Rubini mumps vaccine became available in 1986 and subsequently accounted for more than half the doses of MMR vaccine used in the country. Reports from a sentinel network of physicians demonstrated an increase in reported cases of mumps beginning in

1991. Increases in mumps cases were seen among all age groups but were most striking among children 5 to 9 years of age. Based on information from the sentinel network and manufacturer-specific coverage estimates, the effectiveness of the Rubini vaccine among children 1 to 19 years of age from 1991 to 1993 was estimated at 13% to 73%, compared with 69% to 92% for the Jeryl Lynn and Urabe vaccines.[365] However, subsequent studies described above showed very low efficacy for the Rubini strain. By 1993 to 1994, 59% of reported cases were noted to occur in children previously vaccinated, compared with only 9% from 1986 to 1987.[366] A 1991 to 1992 seroprevalence survey suggested that mumps immunity in young children was lagging behind that for measles and rubella, perhaps reflecting the relatively poor immunogenicity of the Rubini strain vaccine.[367]

In Portugal, routine vaccination with MMR at 15 months of age was begun in 1987. In 1990, a second dose of MMR was recommended at 11 to 13 years of age. Reported cases of mumps decreased from 2197 in 1987 to 627 in 1993. In 1994, however, reported cases increased to 1445 and continued to increase from 1995 to 1996. The outbreak accelerated dramatically in early 1996; during the first 8 months of that year, 7620 cases were reported. Although incidence increased among all age groups, rates were highest among children 1 to 4 years of age. This finding was unexpected because reported MMR vaccination coverage among children 12 to 23 months of age had exceeded 90% since 1991. Three different mumps vaccines—Urabe, Rubini, and Jeryl Lynn strains—were initially available in Portugal as MMR. Following recognition of aseptic meningitis after vaccination with Urabe mumps vaccine, the sale of Urabe-containing vaccine was suspended in Portugal in October 1992, and subsequently only Rubini-containing MMR was used.[368] Substitution of Rubini for Urabe vaccine was followed by a mumps epidemic.[368]

Disease Control Strategies and Possible Eradication

The experience with aseptic meningitis after vaccination with several strains of mumps vaccine creates a dilemma. On the one hand, these reactions underscore the importance of careful postlicensure monitoring of safety to detect other uncommon events that may be causally related to vaccination and the incidence of aseptic meningitis with any new mumps vaccines. On the other hand, the trade-off between efficacy of vaccination and adverse reactions must be carefully evaluated. The selection of a vaccine strain must be decided by the balance between adverse reactions and the complications of wild-type mumps that are prevented.

A second critical issue for further study concerns the extent and duration of protection conferred by a single dose of mumps vaccine. Widespread use of the live virus mumps vaccine since its licensure in 1967 has resulted in a marked decrease in the incidence of mumps in the United States. However, the outbreaks reported from 1986 to 1991 illustrate both the potential for continued epidemics in susceptible unvaccinated populations and the importance of vaccine failure. The question of whether vaccine failure is due to low seroconversion or to waning immunity remains unresolved.

A two-dose MMR vaccination schedule was adopted in Sweden[369] and Finland[347] in 1982 with the aim of eradicating measles, mumps, and rubella within a decade. Likewise, the two-dose schedule in the United States has reduced reported cases of mumps to a record low. These programs have had a marked impact on the incidence of all three diseases, suggesting that the goal of eradication may be feasible if high immunization coverage levels with two doses of MMR can be achieved. However, an effect on mumps incidence may not be seen when only part of the childhood population is vaccinated, as noticed in the Piedmont region of Italy.[370]

In 1991, the International Task Force for Disease Eradication concluded that mumps is potentially eradicable through the use of MMR vaccine but that more data are needed to document the impact of mumps and the use of the vaccine in developing countries.[371] With national and regional measles and rubella elimination efforts now underway in the Americas and Europe,[372] programs may be established that could lead to elimination and ultimately eradication of mumps if MMR vaccine is used. In the absence of such an effort, it remains to be seen whether the benefits of mumps vaccination are of sufficient value globally to incorporate mumps vaccine into the routine childhood vaccination schedule of the Expanded Programme on Immunisation of the World Health Organization.

REFERENCES

1. Hamilton R. An account of a distemper by the common people of England vulgarly called the mumps. London Med J 11:190–211, 1790.
2. Gordon JE. The epidemiology of mumps. Am J Med Sci 200:412–428, 1940.
3. Gordon JE. Ten years in the epidemiology of mumps. Am J Med Sci 218:338–359, 1949.
4. Stokes J. Mumps. In Historical Unit, U.S. Army Medical Service (ed). Preventive Medicine in World War II. Vol. IV. Communicable Diseases Transmitted Chiefly Through Respiratory and Alimentary Tracts. Washington, DC, U.S. Army Medical Service, 1958, pp 135–140.
5. Feldman HA. Mumps. In Evans AS (ed). Viral Infections of Humans: Epidemiology and Control (3rd ed). New York, Plenum Medical Books, 1990, pp 471–491.
6. Parran T. Health and medical preparedness. JAMA 115:49–51, 1940.
7. Postovit VA. Epidemic parotitis in adults. Voen Med Zh 3:38–41, 1983.
8. Arday DR, Kanjarpane DD, Kelley PW. Mumps in the US Army 1980–1986: should recruits be immunized? Am J Public Health 79:471–474, 1989.
9. Kuhlman JC. Mumps outbreak aboard the USS Reuben James. Mil Med 159:255–257, 1994.
10. Johnson CD, Goodpasture EW. An investigation of the etiology of mumps. J Exp Med 59:1–19, 1934.
11. Johnson CD, Goodpasture EW. The etiology of mumps. Am J Hyg 21:46–57, 2002.
12. Habel K. Cultivation of mumps virus in the developing chick embryo and its application to studies of immunity to mumps in man. Public Health Rep 60:201–212, 2002.
13. Enders JF. Mumps: Techniques of laboratory diagnosis, tests for susceptibility, and experiments on specific prophylaxis. J Pediatr 29:129–142, 1946.
14. Habel K. Preparation of mumps vaccine and immunization of monkeys against experimental mumps infection. Public Health Rep 61:1655–1664, 1946.
15. Habel K. Vaccination of human beings against mumps: vaccine administered at the start of an epidemic. I. Incidence and severity of mumps in vaccinated and control groups. Am J Hyg 54:295–311, 1951.
16. Smorodintsev AA, Luzianina TY, Mikutskaya BA. Data on the efficiency of live mumps vaccine from chick embryo cell cultures. Acta Virol 9:240–247, 1965.
17. Weibel RE, Stokes J Jr, Buynak EB, et al. Live attenuated mumps-virus vaccine. 3. Clinical and serologic aspects in a field evaluation. N Engl J Med 276:245–251, 1967.
18. Hope-Simpson RE. Infectiousness of communicable diseases in the household (measles, chickenpox, and mumps). Lancet 2:549–554, 1952.
19. Falk WA, Buchan K, Dow M, et al. The epidemiology of mumps in southern Alberta 1980–1982. Am J Epidemiol 130:736–749, 1989.
20. Cooney MK, Fox JP, Hall CE. The Seattle Virus Watch. VI. Observations of infections with and illness due to parainfluenza, mumps and respiratory syncytial viruses and Mycoplasma pneumoniae. Am J Epidemiol 101:532–551, 1975.
21. Foy HM, Cooney MK, Hall CE. Isolation of mumps virus from children with acute lower respiratory tract disease. Am J Epidemiol 94:467–472, 1971.
22. Philip RN, Reinhard KR, Lackman DB. Observation on a mumps epidemic in a virgin population. Am J Hyg 69:91–111, 1959.
23. Centers for Disease Control. Mumps outbreaks on university campuses—Illinois, Wisconsin, South Dakota. MMWR 36:496–498, 503–505, 1987.
24. Hersh BS, Fine PE, Kent WK, et al. Mumps outbreak in a highly vaccinated population. J Pediatr 119:187–193, 1991.
25. U.S. Department of Health. Mumps, Surveillance, January 1997—December 1982. Atlanta, U.S. Department of Health and Human Services, 1984.
26. McGuinnes AC, Gall EA. Mumps at army camps in 1943. War Med 5:95–104, 1944.
27. Bjorvatn B. Mumps virus recovered from testicles by fine-needle aspiration biopsy in cases of mumps orchitis. Scand J Infect Dis 5:3–5, 1973.
28. Dejucq N, Jegou B. Viruses in the mammalian male genital tract and their effects on the reproductive system. Microbiol Mol Biol Rev 65:208–231, 2001.
29. Beard CM, Benson RC Jr, Kelalis PP, et al. The incidence and outcome of mumps orchitis in Rochester, Minnesota, 1935 to 1974. Mayo Clin Proc 52:3–7, 1977.
30. Swerdlow AJ, Huttly SR, Smith PG. Testicular cancer and antecedent diseases. Br J Cancer 55:97–103, 1987.
31. Brown LM, Pottern LM, Hoover RN. Testicular cancer in young men: the search for causes of the epidemic increase in the United States. J Epidemiol Community Health 41:349–354, 1987.
32. Prinz W, Taubert HD. Mumps in pubescent females and its effect on later reproductive function. Gynaecologia 167:23–27, 1968.
33. Siegel MS, Fuerst HT, Peress NS. Comparative fetal mortality in maternal virus diseases: a prospective study on rubella, measles, mumps, chicken pox, and hepatitis. N Engl J Med 274:768–771, 1966.
34. Siegel MS. Congenital malformations following chickenpox, measles, mumps and hepatitis: results of a cohort study. JAMA 226:1521–1524, 1973.
35. Kurtz JB, Tomlinson AH, Pearson J. Mumps virus isolated from a fetus. Br Med J (Clin Res Ed) 284:471, 1982.
36. Noren GR, Adams P, Anderson RC. Positive skin test reactivity to mumps virus antigen in endocardial fibroelastosis. J Pediatr 62:604–606, 1963.
37. Ni J, Bowles NE, Kim YH, et al. Viral infection of the myocardium in endocardial fibroelastosis: molecular evidence for the role of mumps virus as an etiologic agent. Circulation 95:133–139, 1997.
38. Leff RL, Love LA, Miller FW, et al. Viruses in idiopathic inflammatory myopathies: absence of candidate viral genomes in muscle. Lancet 339:1192–1195, 1992.
39. Nishino H, Engel AG, Rima BK. Inclusion body myositis: the mumps virus hypothesis. Ann Neurol 25:260–264, 1989.
40. Fox SA, Ward BK, Robbins PD, et al. Inclusion body myositis: investigation of the mumps virus hypothesis by polymerase chain reaction. Muscle Nerve 19:23–28, 1996.
41. Jones JF, Ray CG, Fulginiti VA. Perinatal mumps infection. J Pediatr 96:912–914, 1980.
42. Sterner G, Grandien M. Mumps in pregnancy at term. Scand J Infect Dis Suppl 71:36–38, 1990.
43. Groenendaal F, Rothbarth PH, van den Anker JN, Spritzer R. Congenital mumps pneumonia: a rare cause of neonatal respiratory distress. Acta Paediatr Scand 79:1252–1254, 1990.

44. Lacour M, Maherzi M, Vienny H, Suter S. Thrombocytopenia in a case of neonatal mumps infection: evidence for further clinical presentations. Eur J Pediatr 152:739–741, 1993.

45. Reman O, Freymuth F, Laloum D, Bonte JF. Neonatal respiratory distress due to mumps. Arch Dis Child 61:80–81, 1986.

46. Dacou-Voutetakis C, Constantinidis M, Moschos A, et al. Diabetes mellitus following mumps: insulin reserve. Am J Dis Child 127:890–891, 1974.

47. Sultz HA, Hart BA, Zielezny M, Schlesinger ER. Is mumps virus an etiologic factor in juvenile diabetes mellitus? J Pediatr 86:654–656, 1975.

48. Otten A, Helmke K, Stief T, et al. Mumps, mumps vaccination, islet cell antibodies and the first manifestation of diabetes mellitus type I. Behring Inst Mitt 75:83–88, 1984.

49. Hyöty H, Leinikki P, Reunanen A, et al. Mumps infections in the etiology of type 1 (insulin-dependent) diabetes. Diabetes Res 9:111–116, 1988.

50. Reed D, Brown G, Merrick R, et al. A mumps epidemic on St. George Island, Alaska. JAMA 199:113–117, 1967.

51. Russell RR, Donald JC. The neurological complications of mumps. Br Med J 2:27–30, 1967.

52. Levitt LP, Rich TA, Kinde SW, et al. Central nervous system mumps: a review of 64 cases. Neurology 20:829–834, 1970.

53. Miller HG, Stanton JB, Gibbons JL. Para-infectious encephalomyelitis and related syndromes. Q J Med 25:427–505, 1956.

54. Cohen HA, Ashkenazi A, Nussinovitch M, et al. Mumps-associated acute cerebellar ataxia. Am J Dis Child 146:930–931, 1992.

55. Timmons GD, Johnson KP. Aqueductal stenosis and hydrocephalus after mumps encephalitis. N Engl J Med 283:1505–1507, 1970.

56. Bray PF. Mumps—a cause of hydrocephalus? Pediatrics 49:446–449, 1972.

57. Lahat E, Aladjem M, Schiffer J, Starinsky R. Hydrocephalus due to bilateral obstruction of the foramen of Monro: a "possible" late complication of mumps encephalitis. Clin Neurol Neurosurg 95:151–154, 1993.

58. Oldfelt V. Sequelae of mumps-meningoencephalitis. Acta Med Scand 134:405–414, 1949.

59. Oran B, Çeri A, Yilmaz H, et al. Hydrocephalus in mumps meningoencephalitis: case report. Pediatr Infect Dis J 14:724–725, 1995.

60. Azimi PH, Cramblett HG, Haynes RE. Mumps meningoencephalitis in children. JAMA 207:509–512, 1969.

61. Bang HO, Bang J. Involvement of the central nervous system in mumps. Acta Med Scand 113:487–505, 1943.

62. Julkunen I, Lehtokoski-Lehtiniemi E, Koskiniemi M, Vaheri A. Elevated mumps antibody titers in the cerebrospinal fluid suggesting chronic mumps virus infection in the central nervous system. Pediatr Infect Dis 4:99, 1985.

63. Ito M, Go T, Okuno T, Mikawa H. Chronic mumps virus encephalitis. Pediatr Neurol 7:467–470, 1991.

64. Julkunen I, Koskiniemi M, Lehtokoski-Lehtiniemi E, et al. Chronic mumps virus encephalitis: mumps antibody levels in cerebrospinal fluid. J Neuroimmunol 8:167–175, 1985.

65. Hall R, Richards H. Hearing loss due to mumps. Arch Dis Child 62:189–191, 1987.

66. Vuori M, Lahikainen EA, Peltonen T. Perceptive deafness in connection with mumps: a study of 298 servicemen suffering with mumps. Acta Otolaryngol 55:213–236, 1987.

67. Okamoto M, Shitara T, Nakagawa M, et al. Sudden deafness accompanied by asymptomatic mumps. Acta Otolaryngol Suppl 514:45–48, 1994.

68. Westmore GA, Pickard BH, Stern H. Isolation of mumps virus from the inner ear after sudden deafness. Br Med J 1:14–15, 1979.

69. Utz JP, Houk VN, Alling DW. Clinical and laboratory studies of mumps. IV. Viruria and abnormal renal function. N Engl J Med 270:1283–1286, 1964.

70. Lin CY, Chen WP, Chiang H. Mumps associated with nephritis. Child Nephrol Urol 10:68–71, 1990.

71. Ozen S, Damarguc I, Besbas N, et al. A case of mumps associated with acute hemolytic crisis resulting in hemoglobinuria and acute renal failure. J Med 25:255–259, 1994.

72. Gordon SC, Lauter CB. Mumps arthritis: a review of the literature. Rev Infect Dis 6:338–344, 1984.

73. Harel L, Amir J, Reish O, et al. Mumps arthritis in children. Pediatr Infect Dis J 9:928–929, 1990.

74. Huppertz HI, Chantler JK. Restricted mumps virus infection of cells derived from normal human joint tissue. J Gen Virol 72 (pt 2):339–347, 1991.

75. Huppertz HI, Niki NP, Chantler JK. Susceptibility of normal human joint tissue to viruses. J Rheumatol 18:699–704, 1991.

76. Rosenberg DH. Electrocardiographic changes in epidemic parotitis (mumps). Proc Soc Exp Biol Med 58:9–11, 1945.

77. Roberts WC, Fox SM III. Mumps of the heart: clinical and pathologic features. Circulation 32:342–345, 1965.

78. Chaudary S, Jaski BE. Fulminant mumps myocarditis. Ann Intern Med 110:569–570, 1989.

79. Arita M, Ueno Y, Masuyama Y. Complete heart block in mumps myocarditis. Br Heart J 46:342–344, 1981.

80. Okazaki K, Tanabayashi K, Takeuchi K, et al. Molecular cloning and sequence analysis of the mumps virus gene encoding the L protein and the trailer sequence. Virology 188:926–930, 1992.

81. Tecle T, Johansson B, Yun Z, Orvell C. Antigenic and genetic characterization of the fusion (F) protein of mumps virus strains. Arch Virol 145:1199–1210, 2000.

82. Elango N, Varsanyi TM, Kövamees J, Norrby E. Molecular cloning and characterization of six genes, determination of gene order and intergenic sequences and leader sequence of mumps virus. J Gen Virol 69(pt 11):2893–2900, 1988.

83. Takeuchi K, Tanabayashi K, Hishiyama M, Yamada A. The mumps virus SH protein is a membrane protein and not essential for virus growth. Virology 225:156–162, 1996.

84. Elliott GD, Yeo RP, Afzal MA, et al. Strain-variable editing during transcription of the P gene of mumps virus may lead to the generation of non-structural proteins NS1 (V) and NS2. J Gen Virol 71(pt 7):1555–1560, 1990.

85. Paterson RG, Lamb RA. RNA editing by G-nucleotide insertion in mumps virus P-gene mRNA transcripts. J Virol 64:4137–4145, 1990.

86. Clarke DK, Sidhu MS, Johnson JE, Udem SA. Rescue of mumps virus from cDNA. J Virol 74:4831–4838, 2000.

87. Forsey T, Mawn JA, Yates PJ, et al. Differentiation of vaccine and wild mumps viruses using the polymerase chain reaction and dideoxynucleotide sequencing. J Gen Virol 71(pt 4):987–990, 1990.

88. Cusi MG, Bianchi S, Valassina M, et al. Rapid detection and typing of circulating mumps virus by reverse transcription/polymerase chain reaction. Res Virol 147:227–232, 1996.

89. Brown EG, Furesz J, Dimock K, et al. Nucleotide sequence analysis of Urabe mumps vaccine strain that caused meningitis in vaccine recipients. Vaccine 9:840–842, 1991.

90. Künkel U, Driesel G, Henning U, et al. Differentiation of vaccine and wild mumps viruses by polymerase chain reaction and nucleotide sequencing of the SH gene: brief report. J Med Virol 45:121–126, 1995.

91. Turner PC, Forsey T, Minor PD. Comparison of the nucleotide sequence of the SH gene and flanking regions of mumps vaccine virus (Urabe strain) grown on different substrates and isolated from vaccinees. J Gen Virol 72(pt 2):435–437, 1991.

92. Yamada A, Takeuchi K, Tanabayashi K, et al. Differentiation of the mumps vaccine strains from the wild viruses by the nucleotide sequences of the P gene. Vaccine 8:553–557, 1990.

93. Yamada A, Takeuchi K, Tanabayashi K, et al. Sequence variation of the P gene among mumps virus strains. Virology 172:374–376, 1989.

94. Yates PJ, Afzal MA, Minor PD. Antigenic and genetic variation of the HN protein of mumps virus strains. J Gen Virol 77(pt 10):2491–2497, 1996.

95. Afzal MA, Pickford AR, Forsey T, et al. The Jeryl Lynn vaccine strain of mumps virus is a mixture of two distinct isolates. J Gen Virol 74(pt 5):917–920, 1993.

96. Yeo RP, Afzal MA, Forsey T, Rima BK. Identification of a new mumps virus lineage by nucleotide sequence analysis of the SH gene of ten different strains. Arch Virol 128:371–377, 1993.

97. Künkel U, Schreier E, Siegl G, Schultze D. Molecular characterization of mumps virus strains circulating during an epidemic in eastern Switzerland 1992/93. Arch Virol 136:433–438, 1994.

98. Ströhle A, Bernasconi C, Germann D. A new mumps virus lineage found in the 1995 mumps outbreak in western Switzerland identified by nucleotide sequence analysis of the SH gene. Arch Virol 141:733–741, 1996.

99. Afzal MA, Buchanan J, Heath AB, Minor PD. Clustering of mumps virus isolates by SH gene sequence only partially reflects geographical origin. Arch Virol 142:227–238, 1997.

100. Örvell C, Kalantari M, Johansson B. Characterization of five conserved genotypes of the mumps virus small hydrophobic (SH) protein gene. J Gen Virol 78(pt 1):91–95, 1997.

101. Jin L, Beard S, Brown DW. Genetic heterogeneity of mumps virus in the United Kingdom: identification of two new genotypes. J Infect Dis 180:829–833, 1999.
102. Jin L, Beard S, Hale A, et al. The genomic sequence of a contemporary wild-type mumps virus strain. Virus Res 70:75–83, 2000.
102a. Amexis G, Rubin S, Chatterjee N, et al. Identification of a new genotype H wild-type mumps virus strain and its molecular relatedness to other virulent and attenuated strains. J Med Virol 70:284–286, 2003.
103. Takahashi M, Nakayama T, Kashiwagi Y, et al. Single genotype of measles virus is dominant whereas several genotypes of mumps virus are co-circulating. J Med Virol 62:278–285, 2000.
104. Waxham MN, Server AC, Goodman HM, Wolinsky JS. Cloning and sequencing of the mumps virus fusion protein gene. Virology 159:381–388, 1987.
105. Schwarzer S, Reibel S, Lang AB, et al. Safety and characterization of the immune response engendered by two combined measles, mumps and rubella vaccines. Vaccine 16:298–304, 1998.
106. Waxham MN, Aronowski J, Server AC, et al. Sequence determination of the mumps virus HN gene. Virology 164:318–325, 1988.
107. Kövamees J, Norrby E, Elango N. Complete nucleotide sequence of the hemagglutinin-neuraminidase (HN) mRNA of mumps virus and comparison of paramyxovirus HN proteins. Virus Res 12:87–96, 1989.
108. Ukkonen P, Väisänen O, Penttinen K. Enzyme-linked immunosorbent assay for mumps and parainfluenza type 1 immunoglobulin G and immunoglobulin M antibodies. J Clin Microbiol 11:319–323, 1980.
109. Meurman O, Hänninen P, Krishna RV, Ziegler T. Determination of IgG- and IgM-class antibodies to mumps virus by solid-phase enzyme immunoassay. J Virol Methods 4(4-5):249–256, 1982.
110. Örvell C, Rydbeck R, Löve A. Immunological relationships between mumps virus and parainfluenza viruses studied with monoclonal antibodies. J Gen Virol 67(pt 9):1929–1939, 1986.
111. Elango N. Complete nucleotide sequence of the matrix protein mRNA of mumps virus. Virology 168:426–428, 1989.
112. Elliott GD, Afzal MA, Martin SJ, Rima BK. Nucleotide sequence of the matrix, fusion and putative SH protein genes of mumps virus and their deduced amino acid sequences. Virus Res 12:61–75, 1989.
113. Elango N, Varsanyi TM, Kövamees J, Norrby E. The mumps virus fusion protein mRNA sequence and homology among the paramyxoviridae proteins. J Gen Virol 70(pt 4):801–807, 1989.
114. Elango N, Kövamees J, Norrby E. Sequence analysis of the mumps virus mRNA encoding the P protein. Virology 169:62–67, 1989.
115. Beveridge WIB, Lind PE. Virus haemagglutination and serological relations. Aust J Exp Biol 24:127–132, 1946.
116. Leprat R, Aymard M. Selective inactivation of hemagglutinin and neuraminidase on mumps virus. Arch Virol 61:273–281, 1979.
117. Server AC, Merz DC, Waxham MN, Wolinsky JS. Differentiation of mumps virus strains with monoclonal antibody to the HN glycoprotein. Infect Immun 35:179–186, 1982.
118. Örvell C. The reactions of monoclonal antibodies with structural proteins of mumps virus. J Immunol 132:2622–2629, 1984.
119. Gut JP, Lablache C, Behr S, Kirn A. Symptomatic mumps virus reinfections. J Med Virol 45:17–23, 1995.
120. Brown EG, Dimock K, Wright KE. The Urabe AM9 mumps vaccine is a mixture of viruses differing at amino acid 335 of the hemagglutinin-neuraminidase gene with one form associated with disease. J Infect Dis 174:619–622, 1996.
121. Boriskin YS, Yamada A, Kaptsova TI, et al. Genetic evidence for variant selection in the course of dilute passaging of mumps vaccine virus. Res Virol 143:279–283, 1992.
122. Boriskin YS, Kaptsova TI, Booth JC. Mumps virus variants in heterogeneous mumps vaccine. Lancet 341:318–319, 1993.
123. McCarthy M, Jubelt B, Fay DB, Johnson RT. Comparative studies of five strains of mumps virus in vitro and in neonatal hamsters: evaluation of growth, cytopathogenicity, and neurovirulence. J Med Virol 5:1–15, 1980.
124. Forsey T, Bentley ML, Minor PD, Begg N. Mumps vaccines and meningitis. Lancet 340:980, 1992.
125. Saito H, Takahashi Y, Harata S, et al. Isolation and characterization of mumps virus strains in a mumps outbreak with a high incidence of aseptic meningitis. Microbiol Immunol 40:271–275, 1996.
126. Afzal MA, Yates PJ, Minor PD. Nucleotide sequence at position 1081 of the hemagglutinin-neuraminidase gene in the mumps Urabe vaccine strain. J Infect Dis 177:265–266, 1998.
127. Ennis FA, Jackson D. Isolation of virus during the incubation period of mumps infection. J Pediatr 72:536–537, 1968.
128. Meyer MB. An epidemiologic study of mumps: its spread in schools and families. Am J Hyg 75:259–281, 1962.
129. Brown JW, Kirkland HB, Hein GE. Central nervous system involvement during mumps. Am J Med Sci 215:434–441, 1948.
130. Centers for Disease Control. Mumps prevention. MMWR 38:397–400, 1989.
131. Merz DC, Wolinsky JS. Biochemical features of mumps virus neuraminidases and their relationship with pathogenicity. Virology 114:218–227, 1981.
132. Wolinsky JS, Waxham MN, Server AC. Protective effects of glycoprotein-specific monoclonal antibodies on the course of experimental mumps virus meningoencephalitis. J Virol 53:727–734, 1985.
133. Löve A, Rydbeck R, Utter G, et al. Monoclonal antibodies against the fusion protein are protective in necrotizing mumps meningoencephalitis. J Virol 58:220–222, 1986.
134. Rubin SA, Snoy PJ, Wright KE, et al. The mumps virus neurovirulence safety test in Rhesus monkeys: a comparison of mumps virus strains. J Infect Dis 180:521–525, 1999.
135. Afzal MA, Marsden SA, Hull RM, et al. Evaluation of the neurovirulence test for mumps vaccines. Biologicals 27:43–49, 1999.
136. Furesz J. Safety of live mumps virus vaccines. J Med Virol 67:299–300, 2002.
137. Rubin SA, Pletnikov M, Taffs R, et al. Evaluation of a neonatal rat model for prediction of mumps virus neurovirulence in humans. J Virol 74:5382–5384, 2000.
138. Yamauchi T, Wilson C, St. Geme JW Jr. Transmission of live, attenuated mumps virus to the human placenta. N Engl J Med 290:710–712, 1974.
139. Utz JP. Viruria in man, an update. Prog Med Virol 17:77–90, 1974.
140. Meyer MB, Stifler WC, Joseph JM. Evaluation of mumps vaccine given after exposure to mumps, with special reference to the exposed adult. Pediatrics 37:304–315, 1966.
141. Meurman O, Vainionpää R, Rossi T, Hänninen P. Viral etiology of parotitis. Scand J Infect Dis 15:145–148, 1983.
142. Gaulin C, DeSerres G. Need for a specific definition of mumps in a highly immunized population. Can Commun Dis Rep 23:14–16, 1997.
143. Centers for Disease Control and Prevention. Manual for the Surveillance of Vaccine-Preventable Diseases. Atlanta, Centers for Disease Control and Prevention, 1997.
144. Gay N, Miller E, Hesketh L, et al. Mumps surveillance in England and Wales supports introduction of two-dose vaccination schedule. Commun Dis Rep CDR Rev 7:R21–R26, 1997.
145. Lennette EH, Jensen FW, Guenther RW, et al. Serologic responses to para-influenza viruses in patients with mumps virus infection. J Lab Clin Med 61:780–788, 1963.
146. Brunell PA, Brickman A, Steinberg S, Allen E. Parotitis in children who had previously received mumps vaccine. Pediatrics 50:441–444, 1972.
147. Pelosi JW, Besselink LC. Reducing mumps morbidity in Texas [abstract]. In Abstracts of the 30th National Immunization Conference, Washington, DC, April 9–12, 1996.
148. Knowles WA, Cohen BJ. Efficient isolation of mumps virus from a community outbreak using the marmoset lymphoblastoid cell line B95a. J Virol Methods 96(1):93–96, 2001.
149. Afzal MA, Buchanan J, Dias JA, et al. RT-PCR based diagnosis and molecular characterisation of mumps viruses derived from clinical specimens collected during the 1996 mumps outbreak in Portugal. J Med Virol 52:349–353, 1997.
150. Poggio GP, Rodriguez C, Cisterna D, et al. Nested PCR for rapid detection of mumps virus in cerebrospinal fluid from patients with neurological diseases. J Clin Microbiol 38:274–278, 2000.
151. Grillner L, Blomberg J. Hemolysis-in-gel and neutralization tests for determination of antibodies to mumps virus. J Clin Microbiol 4:11–15, 1976.
152. Christenson B, Böttiger M. Methods for screening the naturally acquired and vaccine-induced immunity to the mumps virus. Biologicals 18:213–219, 1990.
153. Ukkonen P, Granström ML, Penttinen K. Mumps-specific immunoglobulin M and G antibodies in natural mumps infection as measured by enzyme-linked immunosorbent assay. J Med Virol 8:131–142, 1981.
154. Benito RJ, Larrad L, Lasierra MP, et al. Persistence of specific IgM antibodies after natural mumps infection. J Infect Dis 155:156–157, 1987.

155. Ukkonen P, Granström ML, Räsänen J, et al. Local production of mumps IgG and IgM antibodies in the cerebrospinal fluid of meningitis patients. J Med Virol 8:257–265, 1981.

156. Vandvik B, Nilsen RE, Vartdal F, Norrby E. Mumps meningitis: specific and non-specific antibody responses in the central nervous system. Acta Neurol Scand 65:468–487, 1982.

157. Ramsay ME, Brown DW, Eastcott HR, Begg NT. Saliva antibody testing and vaccination in a mumps outbreak. CDR (Lond Engl Rev) 1:R96–R98, 1991.

158. Perry KR, Brown DW, Parry JV, et al. Detection of measles, mumps, and rubella antibodies in saliva using antibody capture radioimmunoassay. J Med Virol 40:235–240, 1993.

159. Schluter WW, Reef SE, Dykewicz CA, Jennings CE. Pseudo-outbreak of mumps—Illinois, 1995 [abstr 338]. In Abstracts of the 30th National Immunization Conference, Washington, DC, April 9–12, 1996.

160. Leinikki PO, Shekarchi I, Tzan N, et al. Evaluation of enzyme-linked immunosorbent assay (ELISA) for mumps virus antibodies. Proc Soc Exp Biol Med 160:363–367, 1979.

161. Sakata H, Hishiyama M, Sugiura A. Enzyme-linked immunosorbent assay compared with neutralization tests for evaluation of live mumps vaccines. J Clin Microbiol 19:21–25, 1984.

162. Fedová D, Bruckova M, Plesnik V, et al. Detection of postvaccination mumps virus antibody by neutralization test, enzyme-linked immunosorbent assay and sensitive hemagglutination inhibition test. J Hyg Epidemiol Microbiol Immunol 31:409–422, 1987.

163. Hishiyama M, Tsurudome M, Ito Y, et al. Complement-mediated neutralization test for determination of mumps vaccine-induced antibody. Vaccine 6:423–427, 1988.

164. Brickman A, Brunell PA. Susceptibility of medical students to mumps: comparison of serum neutralizing antibody and skin test. Pediatrics 48:447–450, 1971.

165. Pipkin PA, Afzal MA, Heath AB, Minor PD. Assay of humoral immunity to mumps virus. J Virol Methods 79(2):219–225, 1999.

166. Nojd J, Tecle T, Samuelsson A, Örvell C. Mumps virus neutralizing antibodies do not protect against reinfection with a heterologous mumps virus genotype. Vaccine 19:1727–1731, 2001.

167. Collins SD. Age incidence of the common communicable diseases of children. Public Health Rep 44:763–826, 1929.

168. Mumps Surveillance. Report No 1. Atlanta, U.S. Department of Health, Education and Welfare, 1968.

169. Brooks H. Epidemic parotitis as a military disease. Med Clin North Am 2:493–505, 1918.

170. Black FL. A nationwide serum survey of United States military recruits, 1962. III. Measles and mumps antibodies. Am J Hyg 80:304–307, 1964.

171. Kelley PW, Petruccelli BP, Stehr-Green P, et al. The susceptibility of young adult Americans to vaccine-preventable infections: a national serosurvey of US Army recruits. JAMA 266:2724–2729, 1991.

172. Cox MJ, Anderson RM, Bundy DA, et al. Seroepidemiological study of the transmission of the mumps virus in St. Lucia, West Indies. Epidemiol Infect 102:147–160, 1989.

173. Wagenvoort JH, Harmsen M, Boutahar-Trouw BJ, et al. Epidemiology of mumps in the Netherlands. J Hyg (Lond) 85:313–326, 1980.

174. Seroepidemiology of measles, mumps, and rubella. Wkly Epidemiol Rec 67:231–233, 1992.

175. Aksit S, Egemen A, Ozacar T, Kurugol Z. Mumps seroprevalence in an unvaccinated population in Izmir, Turkey. Acta Paediatr 89:370–371, 2000.

176. Narayan KM, Moffat MA. Measles, mumps, rubella antibody surveillance: pilot study in Grampian, Scotland. Health Bull (Edinb) 50:47–53, 1992.

177. Anderson RM, Crombie JA, Grenfell BT. The epidemiology of mumps in the UK: a preliminary study of virus transmission, herd immunity and the potential impact of immunization. Epidemiol Infect 99:65–84, 1987.

178. Galbraith NS, Young SE, Pusey JJ, et al. Mumps surveillance in England and Wales 1962–1981. Lancet 1:91–94, 1984.

179. Nokes DJ, Wright J, Morgan-Capner P, Anderson RM. Serological study of the epidemiology of mumps virus infection in northwest England. Epidemiol Infect 105:175–195, 1990.

180. Arroyo M, Alia JM, Mateos ML, et al. Natural immunity to measles, rubella and mumps among Spanish children in the pre-vaccination era. Int J Epidemiol 15:95–100, 1986.

181. Galazka AM, Robertson SE, Kraigher A. Mumps and mumps vaccine: a global review. Bull World Health Organ 77:3–14, 1999.

182. Chokephaibulkit K, Kankirawatana P, Apintanapong S, et al. Viral etiologies of encephalitis in Thai children. Pediatr Infect Dis J 20:216–218, 2001.

183. Anderson RM, May RM. Vaccination and herd immunity to infectious diseases. Nature 318:323–329, 1985.

184. Gellis SS, McGuinnes AC, Peters M. A study on the prevention of mumps orchitis by gamma globulin. Am J Med Sci 210:661–664, 1945.

185. Hodes D, Brunell PA. Mumps antibody: placental transfer and disappearance during the first year of life. Pediatrics 45:99–101, 1970.

186. Hilleman MR. The development of live attenuated mumps virus vaccine in historic perspective and its role in the evolution of combined measles-mumps-rubella. In Plotkin SA, Fantini B (eds). Vaccinia, Vaccination, Vaccinology: Jenner, Pasteur, and Their Successors. Paris, Elsevier, 1996, pp 283–292.

187. Hilleman MR. Past, present, and future of measles, mumps, and rubella virus vaccines. Pediatrics 90(1 pt 2):149–153, 1992.

188. Beck M, Welsz-Malecek R, Mesko-Prejac M, et al. Mumps vaccine L-Zagreb, prepared in chick fibroblasts. I. Production and field trials. J Biol Stand 17:85–90, 1989.

189. Buynak EB, Hilleman MR. Live attenuated mumps virus vaccine. 1. Vaccine development. Proc Soc Exp Biol Med 123:768–775, 1966.

190. Sasaki K, Higashihara M, Inoue K, et al. Studies on the development of a live attenuated mumps virus vaccine. I. Attenuation of the Hoshino "wild" strain of mumps virus. Kitasato Arch Exp Med 49:43–52, 1976.

191. Makino S, Sasaki K, Nakayama T, et al. A new combined trivalent live measles (AIK-C strain), mumps (Hoshino strain), and rubella (Takahashi strain) vaccine: findings in clinical and laboratory studies. Am J Dis Child 144:905–910, 1990.

192. Yamanishi K, Takahashi M, Ueda S, et al. Studies on live mumps virus vaccine. V. Development of a new mumps vaccine "AM 9" by plaque cloning. Biken J 16:161–166, 1973.

193. Glück R, Hoskins JM, Wegmann A, et al. Rubini, a new live attenuated mumps vaccine virus strain for human diploid cells. Dev Biol Stand 65:29–35, 1986.

194. Sassani A, Mirchamsy H, Shafyi A, et al. Development of a new live attenuated mumps virus vaccine in human diploid cells. Biologicals 19:203–211, 1991.

195. Smorodintsev AA, Kiyachko NS, Nasibov NM, Schickina ES. Experience with live mumps virus vaccine in the USSR. In Proceedings of the First International Conference of Vaccines Against Viral and Rickettsial Diseases of Man. Washington, DC, Pan-American Health Organization, 1967.

196. Odisseev H, Gacheva N. Vaccinoprophylaxis of mumps using mumps vaccine, strain Sofia 6, in Bulgaria. Vaccine 12:1251–1254, 1994.

197. Amexis G, Colau B, Fineschi N, et al. Sequence comparison among various Urabe strains. Virology 300:171–179, 2000.

198. Cusi MG, Correale P, Valassina M, et al. Comparative study of the immune response in mice immunized with four live attenuated strains of mumps virus by intranasal or intramuscular route. Arch Virol 146:1241–1248, 2001.

199. McAleer WJ, Markus HZ, McLean AA, et al. Stability on storage at various temperatures of live measles, mumps and rubella virus vaccines in new stabilizer. J Biol Stand 8:281–287, 1980.

200. Buynak EB, Hilleman MR, Leagus MB, et al. Jeryl Lynn strain live attenuated mumps virus vaccine: influence of age, virus dose, lot, and gamma-globulin administration on response. JAMA 203:9–13, 1968.

201. Hilleman MR, Buynak EB, Weibel RE, Stokes J Jr. Live, attenuated rubella-virus vaccine. N Engl J Med 279:300–303, 1968.

202. Roth A. Immunization with live attenuated mumps virus vaccine in Honolulu: a field trial. Am J Dis Child 115:459–460, 1968.

203. Stokes J Jr, Weibel RE, Buynak EB, Hilleman MR. Live attenuated mumps virus vaccine. II. Early clinical studies. Pediatrics 39:363–371, 1967.

204. Sugg WC, Finger JA, Levine RH, Pagano JS. Field evaluation of live virus mumps vaccine. J Pediatr 72:461–466, 1968.

205. Young ML, Dickstein B, Weibel RE, et al. Experiences with Jeryl Lynn strain live attenuated mumps virus vaccine in a pediatric outpatient clinic. Pediatrics 40:798–803, 1967.

206. Brunell PA, Brickman A, Steinberg S. Evaluation of a live attenuated mumps vaccine (Jeryl Lynn): with observations on the optimal time for testing serologic response. Am J Dis Child 118:435–440, 1969.

207. Ehrengut W, Georges AM, André FE. The reactogenicity and immunogenicity of the Urabe Am9 live mumps vaccine and persistence of vaccine induced antibodies in healthy young children. J Biol Stand 11:105–113, 1983.

208. Vesikari T, André FE, Simoen E, et al. Evaluation in young children of the Urabe Am9 strain of live attenuated mumps vaccine in comparison with the Jeryl Lynn strain. Acta Paediatr Scand 72:37–40, 1983.

209. Nakayama T, Urano T, Osano M, et al. Evaluation of live trivalent vaccine of measles AIK-C strain, mumps Hoshino strain and rubella Takahashi strain, by virus-specific interferon-gamma production and antibody response. Microbiol Immunol 34:497–508, 1990.

210. Garaseferian MG, Bolotovskii VM, Shatrova LP, Titova NS. Prevention of mumps in preschool institutions using a live mumps vaccine made from strain L-3 [in Russian]. Zh Mikrobiol Epidemiol Immunobiol 4:39–42, 1988.

211. Lerman SJ, Bollinger M, Brunken JM. Clinical and serologic evaluation of measles, mumps, and rubella (HPV-77:DE-5 and RA 27/3) virus vaccines, singly and in combination. Pediatrics 68:18–22, 1981.

212. Brunell PA, Weigle K, Murphy MD, et al. Antibody response following measles-mumps-rubella vaccine under conditions of customary use. JAMA 250:1409–1412, 1983.

213. Christenson B, Heller L, Böttiger M. The immunizing effect and reactogenicity of two live attenuated mumps virus vaccines in Swedish schoolchildren. J Biol Stand 11:323–331, 1983.

214. Vesikari T, André FE, Simoen E, et al. Comparison of the Urabe Am 9-Schwarz and Jeryl Lynn-Moraten combinations of mumps-measles vaccines in young children. Acta Paediatr Scand 72:41–46, 1983.

215. Vesikari T, Ala-Laurila EL, Heikkinen A, et al. Clinical trial of a new trivalent measles-mumps-rubella vaccine in young children. Am J Dis Child 138:843–847, 1984.

216. Popow-Kraupp T, Kundi M, Ambrosch F, et al. A controlled trial for evaluating two live attenuated mumps-measles vaccines (Urabe Am 9-Schwarz and Jeryl Lynn-Moraten) in young children. J Med Virol 18:69–79, 1986.

217. Edees S, Pullan CR, Hull D. A randomised single blind trial of a combined mumps measles rubella vaccine to evaluate serological response and reactions in the UK population. Public Health 105:91–97, 1991.

218. Christenson B, Böttiger M. Vaccination against measles, mumps and rubella (MMR): a comparison between the antibody responses at the ages of 18 months and 12 years and between different methods of antibody titration. J Biol Stand 13:167–172, 1985.

219. Usonis V, Bakasenas V, Kaufhold A, et al. Reactogenicity and immunogenicity of a new live attenuated combined measles, mumps and rubella vaccine in healthy children. Pediatr Infect Dis J 18:42–48, 1999.

220. Usonis V, Bakasenas V, Denis M. Neutralization activity and persistence of antibodies induced in response to vaccination with a novel mumps strain, RIT 4385. Infection 29:159–162, 2001.

221. Just M, Berger R, Glück R, Wegmann A. Evaluation of a combined vaccine against measles-mumps-rubella produced on human diploid cells. Dev Biol Stand 65:25–27, 1986.

222. Berger R, Just M, Glück R. Interference between strains in live virus vaccines, I. Combined vaccination with measles, mumps and rubella vaccine. J Biol Stand 16:269–273, 1988.

223. Tischer A, Gerike E. Immune response after primary and re-vaccination with different combined vaccines against measles, mumps, rubella. Vaccine 18:1382–1392, 2000.

224. Bhargava I, Chhaparwal BC, Phadke MA, et al. Immunogenicity and reactogenicity of indigenously produced MMR vaccine. Indian Pediatr 32:983–988, 1995.

225. King GE, Markowitz LE, Heath J, et al. Antibody response to measles-mumps-rubella vaccine of children with mild illness at the time of vaccination. JAMA 275:704–707, 1996.

226. Nicoara C, Zach K, Trachsel D, et al. Decay of passively acquired maternal antibodies against measles, mumps, and rubella viruses. Clin Diagn Lab Immunol 6:868–871, 1999.

227. Gans H, Yasukawa L, Rinki M, et al. Immune responses to measles and mumps vaccination of infants at 6, 9, and 12 months. J Infect Dis 184:817–826, 2001.

228. Singh R, John TJ, Cherian T, Raghupathy P. Immune response to measles, mumps and rubella vaccine at 9, 12, and 15 months of age. Indian J Med Res 100:155–159, 1994.

229. Forleo-Neto E, Carvalho ES, Fuentes IC, et al. Seroconversion of a trivalent measles, mumps, and rubella vaccine in children aged 9 and 15 months. Vaccine 15:1898–1901, 1997.

230. Schoub BD, Johnson S, McAnerney JM, et al. Measles, mumps and rubella immunization at nine months in a developing country. Pediatr Infect Dis J 9:263–267, 1990.

231. Davidson WL, Buynak EB, Leagus MB, et al. Vaccination of adults with live attenuated mumps virus vaccine. JAMA 201:995–998, 1967.

232. Wharton M, Cochi SL, Hutcheson RH, et al. A large outbreak of mumps in the postvaccine era. J Infect Dis 158:1253–1260, 1988.

233. Weibel RE, Buynak EB, McLean AA, Hilleman MR. Follow-up surveillance for antibody in human subjects following live attenuated measles, mumps, and rubella virus vaccines. Proc Soc Exp Biol Med 162:328–332, 1979.

234. Weibel RE, Buynak EB, McLean AA, Hilleman MR. Persistence of antibody after administration of monovalent and combined live attenuated measles, mumps, and rubella virus vaccines. Pediatrics 61:5–11, 1978.

235. Weibel RE, Buynak EB, McLean AA, et al. Persistence of antibody in human subjects for 7 to 10 years following administration of combined live attenuated measles, mumps, and rubella virus vaccines. Proc Soc Exp Biol Med 165:260–263, 1980.

236. Weibel RE. Mumps vaccine. In Plotkin SA, Mortimer EA (eds). Vaccines (2nd ed). Philadelphia, WB Saunders, 1988, p 231.

237. Miller E, Hill A, Morgan-Capner P, et al. Antibodies to measles, mumps and rubella in UK children 4 years after vaccination with different MMR vaccines. Vaccine 13:799–802, 1995.

238. Boulianne N, De Serres G, Ratnam S, et al. Measles, mumps, and rubella antibodies in children 5–6 years after immunization: effect of vaccine type and age at vaccination. Vaccine 13:1611–1616, 1995.

239. Davidkin I, Valle M, Julkunen I. Persistence of anti-mumps virus antibodies after a two-dose MMR vaccination: a nine-year follow-up. Vaccine 13:1617–1622, 1995.

240. Broliden K, Abreu ER, Arneborn M, Böttiger M. Immunity to mumps before and after MMR vaccination at 12 years of age in the first generation offered the two-dose immunization programme. Vaccine 16:323–327, 1998.

240a. Usonis V, Bakasenas V, Denis M. Neutralization activity and persistence of antibodies induced in response to vaccination with a novel mumps strain, RIT 4385. Infection 29:159–162, 2001.

241. King SM, Saunders EF, Petric M, Gold R. Response to measles, mumps and rubella vaccine in paediatric bone marrow transplant recipients. Bone Marrow Transplant 17:633–636, 1996.

242. Ljungman P, Fridell E, Lönnqvist B, et al. Efficacy and safety of vaccination of marrow transplant recipients with a live attenuated measles, mumps, and rubella vaccine. J Infect Dis 159:610–615, 1989.

243. Schulman SL, Deforest A, Kaiser BA, et al. Response to measles-mumps-rubella vaccine in children on dialysis. Pediatr Nephrol 6:187–189, 1992.

244. Hilleman MR, Weibel RE, Buynak EB, et al. Live attenuated mumps-virus vaccine. IV. Protective efficacy as measured in a field evaluation. N Engl J Med 276:252–258, 1967.

245. Smorodintsev AA, Nasibov MN, Jakovleva NV. Experience with live rubella virus vaccine combined with live vaccines against measles and mumps. Bull World Health Organ 42:283–289, 1970.

246. Centers for Disease Control. Mumps in an elementary school—New York. MMWR 22:185–186, 1973.

247. Chaiken BP, Williams NM, Preblud SR, et al. The effect of a school entry law on mumps activity in a school district. JAMA 257:2455–2458, 1987.

248. Kim-Farley R, Bart S, Stetler H, et al. Clinical mumps vaccine efficacy. Am J Epidemiol 121:593–597, 1985.

249. Lewis JE, Chernesky MA, Rawls ML, Rawls WE. Epidemic of mumps in a partially immune population. Can Med Assoc J 121:751–754, 1979.

250. Sullivan KM, Halpin TJ, Marks JS, Kim-Farley R. Effectiveness of mumps vaccine in a school outbreak. Am J Dis Child 139:909–912, 1985.

251. Pena AA, Pitarch SM, Adsuara LS. Epidemia de paratiditis en una población escolar y eficacia de la vacunación antiparotiditis. Med Clin (Barc) 93:607–610, 1989.

252. Guimbao J, Moreno MP, Gutiérrez V, et al. La parotiditis en época posvacunal: patrón epidemiolólgico y efectividad vacunal en un brote epidémico. Med Clin (Barc) 99:281–285, 1992.

253. Orenstein WA, Bernier RH, Dondero TJ, et al. Field evaluation of vaccine efficacy. Bull World Health Organ 63:1055–1068, 1985.

254. Briss PA, Fehrs LJ, Parker RA, et al. Sustained transmission of mumps in a highly vaccinated population: assessment of primary

vaccine failure and waning vaccine-induced immunity. J Infect Dis 169:77–82, 1994.

255. Cheek JE, Baron R, Atlas H, et al. Mumps outbreak in a highly vaccinated school population: evidence for large-scale vaccination failure. Arch Pediatr Adolesc Med 149:774–778, 1995.

256. Savard C, Godin C. Outbreak of mumps, Montreal, October 1998 to March 1999—with a particular focus on a school. Can Commun Dis Rep 26:69–71, 2000.

257. Buxton J, Craig C, Daly P, et al. An outbreak of mumps among young adults in Vancouver, British Columbia, associated with "rave" parties. Can J Public Health 90:160–163, 1999.

258. Baron S, Lorente C. Investigation d'une Épidémie d'Orcillons dans la Commune de Millau (Aveyron), Janvier-Août 1995. Paris, Réseau National de Santé Publique Français, 1995, pp 1–22.

259. Germann D, Ströhle A, Eggenberger K, et al. An outbreak of mumps in a population partially vaccinated with the Rubini strain. Scand J Infect Dis 28:235–238, 1996.

260. Goh KT. Resurgence of mumps in Singapore caused by the Rubini mumps virus vaccine strain. Lancet 354:1355–1356, 1999.

261. Toscani L, Batou M, Bouvier P, Schlaepfer A. [Comparison of the efficacy of various strains of mumps vaccine: a school survey.] Soz Praventivmed 41:341–347, 1996.

262. Chamot E, Toscani L, Egger P, et al. [Estimation of the efficacy of three strains of mumps vaccines during an epidemic of mumps in the Geneva canton (Switzerland).] Rev Epidemiol Sante Publique 46:100–107, 1998.

263. Schlegel M, Osterwalder JJ, Galeazzi RL, Vernazza PL. Comparative efficacy of three mumps vaccines during disease outbreak in Eastern Switzerland: cohort study. BMJ 319:352, 1999.

264. Field evaluation of the clinical effectiveness of vaccines against pertussis, measles, rubella and mumps. The Benevento and Compobasso Pediatricians Network for the Control of Vaccine-Preventable Diseases. Vaccine 16:818–822, 1998.

265. Mora JL, Lopez TM, Camacho JC. Efectividad communitaria de las vacunas frente a la paratiditis infecciosa estudio de casos. Rev Esp Salud Publica 73:455–464, 1999.

266. Vandermeulen C, Hoppenbrouwers K, Roelants M, et al. Investigation of a mumps epidemic among an adequately immunized maternal and primary school population [abstract]. In Abstracts of the Congress of the European Society of Pediatric Infectious Diseases (ESPID), Istanbul, March, 2001.

267. Johnson CE, Kumar ML, Whitwell JK, et al. Antibody persistence after primary measles-mumps-rubella vaccine and response to a second dose given at four to six vs. eleven to thirteen years. Pediatr Infect Dis J 15:687–692, 1996.

268. Centers for Disease Control. Measles prevention. MMWR 38(suppl 9):1–18, 1989.

269. Orenstein WA, Markowitz L, Preblud SR, et al. Appropriate age for measles vaccination in the United States. Dev Biol Stand 65:13–21, 1986.

270. Centers for Disease Control. Efficacy of mumps vaccine—Ohio. MMWR 32:391–398, 1983.

271. Nojd J, Tecle T, Sameulsson A, et al. Mumps virus neutralizing antibodies do not protect against reinfection with a heterologous mumps virus genotype. Vaccine 19:1727–1731, 2001.

272. Nagai T, Nakayama T. Mumps vaccine virus genome is present in throat swabs obtained from uncomplicated healthy recipients. Vaccine 19:1353–1355, 2001.

273. Sawada H, Yano S, Oka Y, Togashi T. Transmission of Urabe mumps vaccine between siblings. Lancet 342:371, 1993.

274. Centers for Disease Control and Prevention. Status report on the Childhood Immunization Initiative: national, state, and urban area vaccination coverage levels among children aged 19–35 months—United States, 1996. MMWR 46:657–664, 1997.

275. Centers for Disease Control and Prevention. Status report on the Childhood Immunization Initiative: reported cases of selected vaccine-preventable diseases—United States, 1996. MMWR 46: 665–671, 1997.

276. Rothstein EP, Bernstein H, Glode M, et al. Simultaneous administration of an acellular pertussis-DT vaccine (ADTP) with MMR and OPV vaccines [abstract]. In Program and Abstracts of the 32nd Interscience Conference on Antimicrobial Agents and Chemotherapy, Anaheim, CA, October 11–14, 1992.

277. Dashefsky B, Wald E, Guerra N, Byers C. Safety, tolerability, and immunogenicity of concurrent administration of Haemophilus influenzae type b conjugate vaccine (meningococcal protein conjugate)

with either measles-mumps-rubella vaccine or diphtheria-tetanus-pertussis and oral poliovirus vaccines in 14- to 23-month-old infants. Pediatrics 85(4 pt 2):682–689, 1990.

278. Huang LM, Lee CY, Hsu CY, et al. Effect of monovalent measles and trivalent measles-mumps-rubella vaccines at various ages and concurrent administration with hepatitis B vaccine. Pediatr Infect Dis J 9:461–465, 1990.

279. King GE, Hadler SC. Simultaneous administration of childhood vaccines: an important public health policy that is safe and efficacious. Pediatr Infect Dis J 13:394–407, 1994.

280. Arbeter AM, Baker L, Starr SE, et al. Combination measles, mumps, rubella and varicella vaccine. Pediatrics 78(4 pt 2):742–747, 1986.

281. Arbeter AM, Baker L, Starr SE, Plotkin SA. The combination measles, mumps, rubella and varicella vaccine in healthy children. Dev Biol Stand 65:89–93, 1986.

282. Englund JA, Suarez CS, Kelly J, et al. Placebo-controlled trial of varicella vaccine given with or after measles-mumps-rubella vaccine. J Pediatr 114:37–44, 1989.

283. Just M, Berger R, Gluck R, Wegmann A. Evaluation of a combined vaccine against measles-mumps-rubella produced on human diploid cells. Dev Biol Stand 65:25–27, 1986.

284. Fescharek R, Quast U, Maass G, et al. Measles-mumps vaccination in the FRG: an empirical analysis after 14 years of use. II. Tolerability and analysis of spontaneously reported side effects. Vaccine 8:446–456, 1990.

285. Miller C, Miller E, Rowe K, et al. Surveillance of symptoms following MMR vaccine in children. Practitioner 233:69–73, 1989.

286. Nakayama T, Oka S, Komase K, et al. The relationship between the mumps vaccine strain and parotitis after vaccination. J Infect Dis 165:186–187, 1992.

286a.Dos Santo BA, Ranieri TS, Bercini M, et al. An evaluation of the adverse reaction potential of three measles-mumps-rubella combination vaccines. Pan Am J Public Health 12(4):240–246, 2002.

287. Kuczyk MA, Denil J, Thon WF, et al. Orchitis following mumps vaccination in an adult. Urol Int 53:179–180, 1994.

288. Nussinovitch M, Harel L, Varsano I. Arthritis after mumps and measles vaccination. Arch Dis Child 72:348–349, 1995.

289. Stewart BJ, Prabhu PU. Reports of sensorineural deafness after measles, mumps, and rubella immunisation. Arch Dis Child 69:153–154, 1993.

290. Nabe-Nielsen J, Walter B. Unilateral total deafness as a complication of the measles-mumps-rubella vaccination. Scand Audiol Suppl 30:69–70, 1988.

291. Rose C, Viget N, Copin MC, et al. Severe and transient acute myositis after mumps vaccination (Imovax-Oreillons) [in French]. Therapie 51:87, 1996.

292. Marshall GS, Wright PF, Fenichel GM, Karzon DT. Diffuse retinopathy following measles, mumps, and rubella vaccination. Pediatrics 76:989–991, 1985.

293. Plesner AM. Gait disturbances after measles, mumps, and rubella vaccine [letter]. Lancet 345:316, 1995.

294. Drachtman RA, Murphy S, Ettinger LJ. Exacerbation of chronic idiopathic thrombocytopenic purpura following measles-mumps-rubella immunization. Arch Pediatr Adolesc Med 148:326–327, 1994.

295. Jonville-Béra AP, Autret E, Galy-Eyraud C, Hessel L. Thrombocytopenic purpura after measles, mumps and rubella vaccination: a retrospective survey by the French Regional Pharmacovigilance Centres and Pasteur-Mèrieux Sérums et Vaccins. Pediatr Infect Dis J 15:44–48, 1996.

296. Nieminen U, Peltola H, Syrjälä MT, et al. Acute thrombocytopenic purpura following measles, mumps and rubella vaccination: a report on 23 patients. Acta Paediatr 82:267–270, 1993.

297. Cohen BJ, Jin L, Brown DW, Kitson M. Infection with wild-type mumps virus in army recruits temporally associated with MMR vaccine. Epidemiol Infect 123:251–255, 1999.

298. Patja A, Makinen-Kiljunen S, Davidkin I, et al. Allergic reactions to measles-mumps-rubella vaccination. Pediatrics 107:E27, 2001.

299. Johnson JA, Heneine W. Characterization of endogenous avian leukosis viruses in chicken embryonic fibroblast substrates used in production of measles and mumps vaccines. J Virol 75:3605–3612, 2001.

300. Hussain AI, Shanmugam V, Switzer WM, et al. Lack of evidence of endogenous avian leukosis virus and endogenous avian retrovirus transmission to measles, mumps, and rubella vaccine recipients. Emerg Infect Dis 7:66–72, 2001.

301. Frenkel LM, Nielsen K, Garakian A, Cherry JD. A search for persistent measles, mumps, and rubella vaccine virus in children with human immunodeficiency virus type 1 infection. Arch Pediatr Adolesc Med 148:57–60, 1994.

302. Iizuka M, Saito H, Yukawa M, et al. No evidence of persistent mumps virus infection in inflammatory bowel disease. Gut 48:637–641, 2001.

303. Griffin MR, Ray WA, Mortimer EA, et al. Risk of seizures after measles-mumps-rubella immunization. Pediatrics 88:881–885, 1991.

304. Nalin DR. Mumps vaccine complications: which strain? Lancet 2:1396, 1989.

305. Cizman M, Mozetic M, Radescek-Rakar R, et al. Aseptic meningitis after vaccination against measles and mumps. Pediatr Infect Dis J 8:302–308, 1989.

306. McDonald JC, Moore DL, Quennec P. Clinical and epidemiologic features of mumps meningoencephalitis and possible vaccine-related disease. Pediatr Infect Dis J 8:751–755, 1989.

307. Nalin DR. Evaluating mumps vaccines. Lancet 339:305, 1992.

308. Black S, Shinefield H, Ray P, et al. Risk of hospitalization because of aseptic meningitis after measles-mumps-rubella vaccination in one-to two-year-old children: an analysis of the Vaccine Safety Datalink (VSD) Project. Pediatr Infect Dis J 16:500–503, 1997.

309. Ehrengut W, Zastrow K. Complications after preventive mumps vaccination in West Germany (including multiple preventive vaccinations). Monatsschr Kinderheilkd 137:398–402, 1989.

309a.Schlipkoter U, Muhlberger N, von Kries R, Weil J. Surveillance of measles-mumps-rubella vaccine-associated asept meningitis in Germany. Infection 30:351–355, 2003.

310. Sugiura A, Yamada A. Aseptic meningitis as a complication of mumps vaccination. Pediatr Infect Dis J 10:209–213, 1991.

311. Fujinaga T, Motegi Y, Tamura H, Kuroume T. A prefecture-wide survey of mumps meningitis associated with measles, mumps and rubella vaccine. Pediatr Infect Dis J 10:204–209, 1991.

312. Ueda K, Miyazaki C, Hidaka Y, et al. Aseptic meningitis caused by measles-mumps-rubella vaccine in Japan. Lancet 346:701–702, 1995.

313. Kimura M, Kuno-Sakai H, Yamazaki S, et al. Adverse events associated with MMR vaccines in Japan. Acta Paediatr Jpn 38:205–211, 1996.

313a.Ki M, Park T, Yi SG, et al. Risk analysis of aseptic meningitis after measles-mumps-rubella vaccination in Korean children by using a case-crossover design. Am J Epidemiol 157:158–165, 2003.

314. Furesz J, Contreras G. Vaccine-related mumps meningitis—Canada. Can Dis Wkly Rep 16:253–254, 1990.

315. Rebiere I, Galy-Eyraud C. Estimation of the risk of aseptic meningitis associated with mumps vaccination, France, 1991–1993. Int J Epidemiol 24:1223–1227, 1995.

316. Jonville-Béra AP. Aseptic meningitis following mumps vaccine: a retrospective survey by the French Regional Pharmacovigilance Centres and by Pasteur-Mèrieux Sérums & Vaccins. Pharmacoepidemiol Drug Safety 5:33–37, 1996.

317. Balraj V, Miller E. Complications of mumps vaccines. Rev Med Virol 5:219–227, 1995.

318. Colville A, Pugh S. Mumps meningitis and measles, mumps, and rubella vaccine. Lancet 340:786, 1992.

319. Miller E, Goldacre M, Pugh S, et al. Risk of aseptic meningitis after measles, mumps, and rubella vaccine in UK children. Lancet 341:979–982, 1993.

320. Farrington P, Pugh S, Colville A, et al. A new method for active surveillance of adverse events from diphtheria/tetanus/pertussis and measles/mumps/rubella vaccines. Lancet 345:567–569, 1995.

321. Dourado I, Cunha S, Teixeira MG, et al. Outbreak of aseptic meningitis associated with mass vaccination with a Urabe-containing measles-mumps-rubella vaccine: implications for immunization programs. Am J Epidemiol 151:524–530, 2000.

322. Lista F, Faggioni G, Peragallo MS, et al. Molecular analysis of early postvaccine mumps-like disease in Italian military recruits. JAMA 287:1114–1115, 2002.

323. Wright KE, Dimock K, Brown EG. Biological characteristics of genetic variants of Urabe AM9 mumps vaccine virus. Virus Res 67:49–57, 2000.

324. Amexis G, Fineschi N, Chumakov K. Correlation of genetic variability with safety of mumps vaccine Urabe AM9 strain. Virology 287:234–241, 2001.

325. Bakker WJ, Mathias RG. Mumps caused by an inadequately attenuated measles, mumps and rubella vaccine. Can J Infect Dis 12:144–148, 2001.

326. da Cunha SS, Rodrigues LC, Barreto ML, Dourado I. Outbreak of aseptic meningitis and mumps after mass vaccination with MMR vaccine using the Leningrad-Zagreb mumps strain. Vaccine 20:1106–1112, 2002.

326a.da Silveira CM, Kmetzsch CI, Mohrdieck R, et al. The risk of aseptic meningitis associated with the Leningrad-Zagreb mumps vaccine strain following mass vaccination with measles-mumps-rubella vaccine, Rio Grande do Sul, Brazil, 1999. Int J Epidemiol 31:978–982, 2002.

327. Mumps Surveillance. Report No 2. Atlanta, U.S. Department of Health, Education and Welfare, 1972.

328. Nokes DJ, Anderson RM. Vaccine safety versus vaccine efficacy in mass immunisation programmes. Lancet 338:1309–1312, 1991.

329. Peltola H. Mumps vaccination and meningitis. Lancet 341:994–995, 1993.

329a.Fullerman KE, Reef SE. Commentary: Ongoing debate over the safety of the different mumps vaccine strains impacs mumps disease control. Intern J of Epidem 31:983–984, 2002.

329b.WHO position paper: Mumps virus vaccines. Weekly Epidem Rocord 45(9):346–355, 2001.

330. Advisory Committee on Immunization Practices. Measles, mumps, and rubella—vaccine use and strategies for measles, rubella, and congenital rubella syndrome elimination and mumps control. MMWR 47(RR-8): 1–57, 1998.

331. Fasano MB, Wood RA, Cooke SK, Sampson HA. Egg hypersensitivity and adverse reactions to measles, mumps, and rubella vaccine. J Pediatr 120:878–881, 1992.

332. Kemp A, Van Asperen P, Mukhi A. Measles immunization in children with clinical reactions to egg protein. Am J Dis Child 144:33–35, 1990.

333. James JM, Burks AW, Roberson PK, Sampson HA. Safe administration of the measles vaccine to children allergic to eggs. N Engl J Med 332:1262–1266, 1995.

334. Lavi S, Zimmerman B, Koren G, Gold R. Administration of measles, mumps, and rubella virus vaccine (live) to egg-allergic children. Crit Care Nurse 10(4):80–82, 1990.

335. Beck SA, Williams LW, Shirrell MA, Burks AW. Egg hypersensitivity and measles-mumps-rubella vaccine administration. Pediatrics 88:913–917, 1991.

336. Kelso JM, Jones RT, Yuninger JW. Anaphylaxis to measles, mumps, and rubella vaccine mediated by IgE to gelatin. J Allergy Clin Immunol 91:867–872, 1993.

337. Sakaguchi M, Ogura H, Inouye S. IgE antibody to gelatin in children with immediate-type reactions to measles and mumps vaccines. J Allergy Clin Immunol 96:563–565, 1995.

338. Sakaguchi M, Nakayama T, Inouye S. Food allergy to gelatin in children with systemic immediate-type reactions, including anaphylaxis, to vaccines. J Allergy Clin Immunol 98(6 pt 1):1058–1061, 1996.

339. Sosin DM, Cochi SL, Gunn RA, et al. Changing epidemiology of mumps and its impact on university campuses. Pediatrics 84:779–784, 1989.

340. Kaplan KM, Marder DC, Cochi SL, Preblud SR. Mumps in the workplace: further evidence of the changing epidemiology of a childhood vaccine-preventable disease. JAMA 260:1434–1438, 1988.

341. Summary of notifiable diseases, United States, 1986. MMWR 35:1–57, 1986.

342. Summary of notifiable diseases, United States, 1987. MMWR 36:1–59, 1988.

343. van Loon FP, Holmes SJ, Sirotkin BI, et al. Mumps surveillance—United States, 1988–1993. Mor Mortal Wkly Rep CDC Surveill Summ 44:1–14, 1995.

344. Cochi SL, Preblud SR, Orenstein WA. Perspectives on the relative resurgence of mumps in the United States. Am J Dis Child 142:499–507, 1988.

345. Anderson RM, May RM. Directly transmitted infections diseases: control by vaccination. Science 215:1053–1060, 1982.

346. Summary of notifiable diseases, United States 1994. MMWR 43:1–80, 1994.

347. Koskiniemi M, Vaheri A. Effect of measles, mumps, rubella vaccination on pattern of encephalitis in children. Lancet 1:31–34, 1989.

348. Rantala H, Uhari M. Occurrence of childhood encephalitis: a population-based study. Pediatr Infect Dis J 8:426–430, 1989.

349. Koplan JP, Preblud SR. A benefit-cost analysis of mumps vaccine. Am J Dis Child 136:362–364, 1982.

350. White CC, Koplan JP, Orenstein WA. Benefits, risks and costs of immunization for measles, mumps and rubella. Am J Public Health 75:739–744, 1985.

351. Peltola H, Karanko V, Kurki T, et al. Rapid effect on endemic measles, mumps, and rubella of nationwide vaccination programme in Finland. Lancet 1:137–139, 1986.

352. Paunio M, Virtanen M, Peltola H, et al. Increase of vaccination coverage by mass media and individual approach: intensified measles, mumps, and rubella prevention program in Finland. Am J Epidemiol 133:1152–1160, 1991.

353. Peltola H, Heinonen OP, Valle M, et al. The elimination of indigenous measles, mumps, and rubella from Finland by a 12-year, two-dose vaccination program. N Engl J Med 331:1397–1402, 1994.

354. Hyöty H, Hiltunen M, Reunanen A, et al. Decline of mumps antibodies in type 1 (insulin-dependent) diabetic children and a plateau in the rising incidence of type 1 diabetes after introduction of the mumps-measles-rubella vaccine in Finland. Childhood Diabetes in Finland Study Group. Diabetologia 36:1303–1308, 1993.

355. Peltola H, Davidkin I, Paunio M, et al. Mumps and rubella eliminated from Finland. JAMA 284:2643–2647, 2000.

356. Heisler MB, Richmond JB. Lessons from Finland's successful immunization program. N Engl J Med 331:1446–1447, 1994.

357. Böttiger M, Christenson B, Romanus V, et al. Swedish experience of two-dose vaccination programme aiming at eliminating measles, mumps, and rubella. Br Med J (Clin Res Ed) 295:1264–1267, 1987.

358. Christenson B, Böttiger M. Changes of the immunological patterns against measles, mumps and rubella: a vaccination programme studied 3 to 7 years after the introduction of a two-dose schedule. Vaccine 9:326–329, 1991.

359. Vaccination coverage statistics for children up to two years of age in the United Kingdom. Commun Dis Rep CDR Wkly 6:262, 1996.

360. Jones AG, White JM, Begg NT. The impact of MMR vaccine on mumps infection in England and Wales. CDR (Lond Engl Rev) 1:R93–R96, 1991.

361. Slater PE, Roitman M, Costin C. Mumps incidence in Israel—impact of MMR vaccine. Public Health Rev 18:88–93, 1990.

362. Slater PE, Anis E, Leventhal A. The control of mumps in Israel. Eur J Epidemiol 15:765–767, 1999.

363. Berger SA, Ginsberg GM, Slater PE. Cost-benefit analysis of routine mumps and rubella vaccination for Israeli infants. Isr J Med Sci 26:74–80, 1990.

364. Krugman S, de Quadros C. Eradication of Measles, Rubella and Routine Mumps in Cuba: Report of a Technical Advisory Group. Washington, DC, Pan-American Health Organization, 1989.

365. Zimmermann H, Matter HC, Kiener T. [Mumps epidemiology in Switzerland: results from the Sentinella surveillance system 1986–1993. Sentinella Work Group.] Soz Praventivmed 40:80–92, 1995.

366. Matter HC, Cloetta J, Zimmermann H. Measles, mumps, and rubella: monitoring in Switzerland through a sentinel network, 1986–94. Sentinella Arbeitsgemeinschaft. J Epidemiol Community Health 49(suppl 1):4–8, 1995.

367. Matter L, Germann D, Bally F, Schopfer K. Age-stratified seroprevalence of measles, mumps and rubella (MMR) virus infections in Switzerland after the introduction of MMR mass vaccination. Eur J Epidemiol 13:61–66, 1997.

368. Dias JA, Cordeiro M, Afzal MA, et al. Mumps epidemic in Portugal despite high vaccine coverage—preliminary report. Eurosurveillance 1:25–28, 1996.

369. Fahlgren K. Two doses of MMR vaccine—sufficient to eradicate measles, mumps and rubella? Scand J Soc Med 16:129–135, 1988.

370. Zotti C, Ossola O, Barberis R, et al. Mumps: a current epidemiologic pattern as a necessary background for the choice of a vaccination strategy. Eur J Epidemiol 15:659–663, 1999.

371. Recommendations of the International Task Force for Disease Eradication. MMWR 42(RR-16):1–38, 1993.

372. Measles eradication: recommendations from a meeting cosponsored by the World Health Organization, the Pan American Health Organization, and CDC. MMWR 46(RR-11):1–20, 1997.

373. Al-Mazrou Y, Tumsah S, Khali M, et al. Safety evaluation of MMR vaccine during a primary school campaign in Saudi Arabia. J Trop Pediatr 48:354–358, 2002.

Chapter 21

Pertussis Vaccine

KATHRYN M. EDWARDS • MICHAEL D. DECKER

History

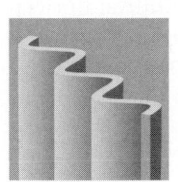

Pertussis (whooping cough) is a bacterial respiratory infection caused by *Bordetella pertussis*, a gram-negative bacillus. Its major manifestation is a protracted cough illness that lasts many weeks. The disease is most severe in infants and young children, many of whom suffer the intense paroxysmal coughing that terminates in an inspiratory "whoop."

The first known description of an outbreak of pertussis is that of Guillaume De Baillou, who described an epidemic that occurred in Paris in the summer of 1578.[1] The epidemic primarily affected infants and young children and resulted in high mortality. Apparently the disease had been known previously in France, because De Baillou referred to its common name of *quinte*, which he hypothesized might have reflected the characteristic sound of the cough or the 5-hour periodicity of the paroxysms.

A disease known in Britain from the early 16th century as *chyne-cough* probably was pertussis, and the terms *whooping cough* and *chincough* appeared in the London Bills of Mortality in 1701.[2] The causative organism was grown by Jules Bordet and Octave Gengou in 1906, and the first crude vaccines appeared soon thereafter.[3]

Importance

Prior to widespread use of whole-cell pertussis vaccine, there were as many as 270,000 cases of pertussis reported each year in the United States (indeed, the true case count likely approximated the annual birth cohort), with 10,000 deaths.[4] The occurrence of pertussis declined markedly after the introduction of whole-cell vaccine, to a nadir of 1010 cases reported in 1976.[5] The occurrence of pertussis has since progressively increased, with 7867 cases reported for 2000, the highest total since 1964.[6] The increase in pertussis in the United States has been greatest among older children and adults, probably reflecting waning vaccine-induced immunity. Because pertussis often goes undiagnosed in adolescents and adults, it is likely that the actual number of cases greatly exceeds the number reported. Recent reports also indicate that pertussis incidence continues to increase in infants too young to have received three doses of pertussis-containing vaccine.[6]

Worldwide, pertussis remains an important killer of children. The World Health Organization (WHO) estimates that 45 million cases occur worldwide annually, with 400,000 deaths.[7,8]

Background

Clinical Description

Infants and Young Children

The incubation period of pertussis averages 9 or 10 days (range, 6 to 20 days). The onset is insidious, and symptoms are indistinguishable from those of a minor upper respiratory infection. Fever is usually minimal throughout the course of infection. Cough, initially intermittent, progresses within 1 or 2 weeks to become paroxysmal. The paroxysms increase in both frequency and severity and then gradually subside, rarely lasting longer than 2 to 6 weeks. In the absence of immunization, most children experience the full-blown disease; however, some children appear to develop either clinical immunity or serologic evidence of prior infection without a history of clinical pertussis, suggesting that mild atypical cases occur.[9,10]

It is during the paroxysmal stage, when the cough is most severe, that the characteristic whoop occurs. The whoop is caused by forced inspiration through a narrowed glottis immediately after a paroxysm of a dozen or more rapid, short coughs without intervening inspiration. The paroxysms apparently result from difficulty in expelling thick mucus from the tracheobronchial tree. During a paroxysm, cyanosis may occur and vomiting may ensue. The clinical picture of a young infant in a severe paroxysm is distressing indeed. After the episode, the child is often exhausted; unfortunately, several paroxysms may occur successively within a few minutes. Between paroxysms, the child may be playful and appear quite normal. Paroxysms may be induced by eating, laughing, crying, and a variety of other stimuli and are usually worse at night.

Recovery is gradual. The paroxysms become less frequent and milder, and the whoop disappears. Nonparoxysmal cough may persist for many weeks. During the convalescent phase, intercurrent respiratory infections may trigger a recurrence of the paroxysmal cough.

COMPLICATIONS AND SEQUELAE

Complications were observed in 5.8% of patients with confirmed pertussis infection in one German series.[10] Children less than 6 months of age were noted to have complications more frequently than older children (23.8% and 5.1%, respectively). Minor complications of pertussis include subconjunctival hemorrhages and epistaxis secondary to the paroxysms. Edema of the face may occur. An ulcer of the lingual frenulum is frequently seen, owing to protrusion of the tongue during paroxysms. Suppurative otitis media frequently occurs (caused by the usual bacteria, such as *Streptococcus pneumoniae* or *Haemophilus influenzae*, not *B. pertussis*).

Major complications, which are sometimes fatal, are of three types: pulmonary, encephalitic, and nutritional. Of these, pulmonary complications are the most frequent.[10] The vast majority of full-blown pertussis cases likely exhibit some degree of atelectasis or bronchopneumonia. Pathologically, the pneumonia is both interstitial and alveolar, and the usual exudate is primarily mononuclear.[11] Pneumonic involvement may be sufficiently severe to compromise respiratory function and cause death. Indeed, 54% of the deaths associated with pertussis are attributed to pneumonia. However, in children who survive pneumonia, permanent lung damage usually does not occur.[12]

Acute encephalopathy associated with pertussis, generally occurring during the paroxysmal stage, has been recognized for many years. There may be a wide variety of manifestations, the most common of which are convulsions and altered consciousness. Only limited data on the incidence of encephalopathy are available; estimates from population-based studies have ranged from 8 to 80 per 100,000 cases.[13,14] More recently, of those cases reported to the Centers for Disease Control and Prevention (CDC) between 1997 and 2000, 26 (0.9 per 100,000) were complicated by encephalopathy.[6,15] Approximately one third of children with pertussis encephalopathy succumb to the acute illness, one third survive with permanent brain damage, and one third recover without obvious neurologic sequelae (D. Annunziato, personal communication, 1985).[16]

Nutritional deficiencies resulting from repeated vomiting can also be problematic. Inability to maintain adequate caloric intake in previously malnourished children who develop pertussis is a particularly severe problem in developing countries.

Adolescents and Adults

It is becoming clear that pertussis plays an important role in the etiology of cough illness in older children and adults, particularly among populations with high rates of childhood immunization with whole-cell pertussis vaccine (see below under *Epidemiology*). Recent U.S. data demonstrate that the pertussis incidence rates among adolescents and adults have increased 62% and 60%, respectively.[6] Furthermore, older children and adults have been demonstrated to be a reservoir for pertussis infection and serve as a source of spread to young children.[17] In a study from Canada, the clinical characteristics of pertussis in 88 adults with laboratory-confirmed disease were reported.[18] The largest proportion of the cases (40%) was seen in individuals 20 to 39 years of age. Pertussis accounted for 33% of the prolonged cough in participants 12 to 19 years old, 19% in those 20 to 39 years, 19% in those 40 to 59 years

old, and 16% in those over 60 years old. Females comprised 71% of the reported cases. Nearly 60% of the subjects reported prior pertussis vaccination, with less than 10% having prior natural infection. Subjects with confirmed pertussis had a median of 56 days of cough and 43 days with violent cough. Vomiting was seen in 46% of the subjects, night cough in 84%, and apnea for 30 seconds after cough in 14%. Adults had higher rates of complications than adolescents, including pneumonia.[18a]

German household contact studies have provided another comprehensive description of the signs and symptoms of adult pertussis.[19,20] In contrast to adults in the United States, of 79 German adults with symptomatic pertussis, 34% had been diagnosed with pertussis as children; 72 (91%) had cough with their present illness, 63 (80%) had cough lasting longer than 21 days, and 1 had had a cough for 8 months.[20] Prolonged paroxysmal cough was experienced by 50 patients (63%), cough resulting in sleep disturbance was reported in 41 (52%), cough followed by vomiting occurred in 33 (42%), and whoops occurred in 6 (8%). The adults usually expectorated "a glassy, viscous mucus." Malaise was reported in 24 patients and arthralgia in 12. Eleven patients reported attacks involving flushing and sweating. These episodes lasted 1 to 2 minutes, occurred several times a day, and continued for 2 to 8 weeks.

Family studies of children with culture-confirmed pertussis disease and seroprevalence studies have both shown that asymptomatic infections are common in older children and adults.[21–23] Frequently, these asymptomatic adults have been implicated in the spread of infection to susceptible children. For example, in one study, 4 children with confirmed pertussis infection and their 18 family members were evaluated with culture and serology for *B. pertussis*. The attack rate for pertussis infection in contacts was 83%, but two thirds of the cases in immunized contacts were subclinical. All infected family contacts had diagnostically elevated serologic tests for pertussis at the time the index case was diagnosed. However, culture identified only 20% of infected contacts. Symptomatic infection was characterized by a higher pertussis toxin (PT) antibody response and asymptomatic infection by a higher filamentous hemagglutinin (FHA) antibody response. These data suggest that, after pertussis immunization, immunity to disease is greater than is protection from infection.[23]

COMPLICATIONS AND SEQUELAE

Complications of pertussis were seen in 18 (23%) of the 79 adult patients in the German study.[20] These included otitis media (four patients), pneumonia (two patients), urinary incontinence (three patients), rib fracture (one patient), and severe weight loss (one patient). Other known complications of pertussis in adults include cough syncope, in which a prolonged coughing attack is followed by unconsciousness; seizures; loss of concentration; and loss of memory.[24–26]

Bacteriology

Overview

The causative agent of pertussis is *B. pertussis*, a small, gram-negative, pleomorphic bacillus. Although the organism was identified before the turn of the century in stained preparations of respiratory secretions from children with pertussis and from pathology specimens,[27] the organism was not recovered in culture until 1906 by Bordet and Gengou.[3] The culture medium originally employed, now called Bordet-Gengou medium, is still used in many clinical laboratories, although more complex synthetic media have been devised and are employed in some laboratories to grow this relatively fastidious organism.

Two closely related organisms in the genus *Bordetella* are *B. parapertussis* and *B. bronchiseptica*. The former is responsible for a pertussis-like syndrome in humans, which usually is less severe than pertussis. The latter produces respiratory illnesses in domestic animals.[27] Because the DNA structure of these two organisms is essentially identical to that of *B. pertussis*, it may be that the three organisms are actually subspecies of the same bacterium.[28] Of all the *Bordetella* species, only *B. pertussis* synthesizes PT. Although the chromosomes of *B. parapertussis* and *B. bronchiseptica* contain the PT loci, they are transcriptionally silent because of defective promotors.[29] In their virulent phase, these three organisms all produce nearly identical virulence factors.[30] Indeed, some have suggested that the curious absence of descriptions of pertussis before the 16th century may represent the adaptation of an animal organism to humans as recently as five centuries ago.[28] However, others see evidence of pertussis in the ancient folklore of southern India and Malabar.[2]

Although many of the biologic activities of *B. pertussis* have been recognized for some time, attempts to determine the components responsible for these various activities were unsuccessful for many years. However, newer techniques have facilitated the identification of several components that apparently contribute to disease manifestations and immunity. This increased understanding of the organism's biology has led to an enhanced understanding of the pathogenesis of the disease and has spurred development of purified component (acellular) vaccines.

Bordetella pertussis has a marked tropism for and attaches strongly to ciliated respiratory tract epithelial cells.[31,32] The bacteria may be internalized by epithelial cells but do not penetrate submucosal cells or invade the blood stream. However, toxins produced by the organism can enter the blood stream and produce systemic effects. *Bordetella pertussis* antigens that have been incorporated in acellular vaccines, as well as other known components of the pertussis organism, are listed in Table 21–1.

Key Components

PERTUSSIS TOXIN

PT, previously termed lymphocytosis-promoting factor, is a major contributor to the pathogenesis of pertussis and is generally believed to play an important role in the induction of clinical immunity. PT is an oligomeric structure composed of five different subunits, S1 through S5 (Fig. 21–1). Structurally it belongs to the A-B class of bacterial toxins. The S1 component (A protomer) catalyzes the ADP ribosylation of GTP-binding regulatory proteins involved in signal transduction in the eukaryotic cell. The A protomer is largely responsible for the recognized bio-

TABLE 21–1 ■ Key Components of the Bordetella Pertussis Organism

Component	Biological Activity
Pertussis toxin	A secreted exotoxin that induces lymphocytosis, sensitivity to histamine, pancreatic islet cell activation, and immune enhancement.
Filamentous hemagglutinin	Involved in attachment to ciliated respiratory epithelium.
Fimbriae	Involved in attachment to ciliated respiratory epithelium.
Pertactin	An outer membrane protein that promotes adhesion to ciliated respiratory epithelium.
BrkA	An outer membrane protein that mediates adherence and resists complement.
Adenylate cyclase	Inhibits phagocytic function.
Endotoxin	Contributes to fever and local reactions in animals and, probably, in humans.
Tracheal cytotoxin	Causes ciliary stasis and cytopathic effects on tracheal mucosa.
Dermonecrotic or heat-labile toxin	Causes dermal necrosis and vasoconstriction in animals.

logic activities of PT, including promotion of lymphocytosis, stimulation of islet cells,[33] sensitization to histamines, clustering of Chinese hamster ovary cells, and adjuvant properties. The B oligomer is a ring-shaped structure that consists of one copy each of subunits S2, S3, and S5 and two copies of S4. S5 serves to link the two dimers, S2-S4 and S3-S4.[34] The primary function of the B oligomer is to facilitate the attachment of PT to the ciliated cells of the respiratory tract.[35,36] However, the B oligomer does have some enzymatic activities, including hemagglutination and T-cell mitogenicity. The entire PT molecule is required for the majority of the enzymatic activities of the A protomer (the A protomer does not function in the absence of the B oligomer).[33,37] PTs produced by different agglutinogen-type strains of *B. pertussis* appear to have a single biologic and serologic identity.[38] PT is not produced by *B. parapertussis* or *B. bronchiseptica*; although these organisms contain genes that encode for biologically active forms of PT, the relevant promoters are inactive and toxin is not produced.[39]

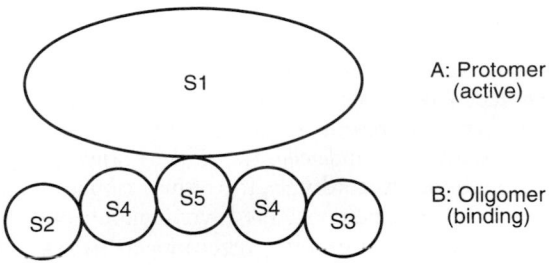

FIGURE 21–1 ■ Diagrammatic representation of the pertussis toxin (see text).

PT appears to play two major roles in the pathogenesis of pertussis, although the precise mechanisms are not entirely clear. First, it facilitates the attachment of *B. pertussis* to ciliated respiratory cells. Second, it appears to be of major importance in cell toxicity. PT is a strong immunogen. Antibodies to PT are associated with clinical immunity to pertussis, and many researchers believe these antibodies to be the most important (some, the sole) mediators of clinical protection.[40] In the laboratory, antibodies to PT protect mice that undergo intracerebral challenge with live *B. pertussis* (the mouse protection test). These antibodies are similarly protective of mice after aerosol challenge.[33,41] Studies employing intracerebral or aerosol challenge of mice that have been actively immunized with subunits of PT or passively immunized with monoclonal antibodies to various PT subunits have suggested that the entire molecule is required for optimum protection.[33,36,37,42] PT is chemically or genetically inactivated (toxoided) for incorporation into acellular pertussis vaccines. Interestingly, however, intravenous injection of substantial quantities of active PT into adult human volunteers caused no adverse effects.[43]

FILAMENTOUS HEMAGGLUTININ

FHA, a large, hairpin-shaped molecule, is synthesized as a 367-kDa precursor that is modified at both ends and cleaved to form the mature 220-kDa protein. In vitro studies suggest that the molecule has four separate binding domains that facilitate binding to monocytes and macrophages, ciliated respiratory epithelial cells, and nonciliated epithelial cells.[30] Data suggest that FHA may also have an immunomodulatory function. The interaction of FHA with receptors on macrophages suppresses the proinflammatory cytokine interleukin-12 via an interleukin-10–dependent mechanism and results in persistence of the organism by curbing the protective Th1 response.[44] Another study demonstrates that FHA stimulates proinflammatory and proapoptotic responses in human monocytes and respiratory epithelial cells.[45] Mutant organisms deficient in FHA adhere poorly in vitro.[31,46,47] Mice immunized with FHA are protected against lethal respiratory challenge with pertussis but not against intracerebral challenge.[41,48] FHA is a strong immunogen, and serum antibodies to FHA are found after natural infection and after immunization with vaccines containing this protein. The results of one epidemiologic study in Finland suggested that antibodies to FHA in immunized schoolchildren correlated with protection against pertussis disease (correlates of protection are discussed more fully in a subsequent section).[49]

FIMBRIAE AND AGGLUTININS

Bordetella organisms express filamentous, polymeric, protein cell surface structures called fimbriae. More than a dozen agglutinogens are present on the cell envelope of the three species of the genus *Bordetella*; two of the known agglutinogens are fimbriae. Accordingly, the terms *fimbriae* and *agglutinogens* should not be considered synonymous, and should not be used interchangeably. Agglutinogen patterns differ among the three species. As many as eight are found in *B. pertussis*, six of which are unique to that species, but only agglutinogens 1, 2, and 3 are considered to be of importance in disease pathogenesis and immunity. Antibodies to these agglutinogens have been useful in seroepidemiologic studies.

In vivo studies have shown that fimbriae-negative strains of *B. pertussis* are defective in their ability to multiply in the nasopharynx and trachea of mice.[50] *Bordetella bronchiseptica* strains devoid of fimbriae but unaltered in expression of FHA and other putative adhesins are unable to colonize animal trachea.[51] Serum antibodies to the fimbriae are found almost universally after natural disease or after immunization with vaccines containing these proteins.

Evidence is conflicting regarding the role of antibodies to these agglutinogens in clinical immunity. The major evidence for such a role is that the efficacy of whole-cell pertussis vaccines appears to be compromised in the absence of a "match" between the agglutinogens in the vaccine and those of prevalent *B. pertussis* strains. There is some in vitro evidence of shifts in serotypes of *B. pertussis* on serial culture.[52] There is also evidence that a change in serotype occurs during the course of clinical pertussis in some instances.[53] Seroepidemiologic data from the United Kingdom indicate that, between 1941 and 1953, the circulating strains of *B. pertussis* contained agglutinogens 1, 2, and 3. By 1968, however, 75% of isolated strains contained only agglutinogens 1 and 3.[54] There is suggestive evidence (but no proof) that this change resulted from the use of vaccines that contained relatively little agglutinogen 3.[53,55,56] The one product that contained considerable agglutinogen 3 was far more effective than the others in preventing pertussis during this time. Subsequent manufacturing changes that incorporated more agglutinogen 3 resulted in higher efficacy.[53] It is, of course, possible that serotype differences are markers for some other antigenic differences in strains of *B. pertussis*; however, the biologic activities of PT from different serotypes of *B. pertussis* do not appear to differ.[38] Because of the evidence that the agglutinogens play some role in the induction of clinical immunity to pertussis, the WHO has recommended that whole-cell pertussis vaccines contain agglutinogens 1, 2, and 3.[57]

PERTACTIN

Pertactin (PRN), originally known as the 69-kDa protein, is a surface-associated protein that is exported to the outer membrane, where it undergoes proteolytic cleavage.[58] Somewhat similar proteins are produced by *B. parapertussis* and *B. bronchiseptica*.[59] PRN participates in attachment through its Arg-Gly-Asp (RGD) motif to facilitate eukaryotic cell binding[59–61] and invasion.[62]

PRN is highly immunogenic. Antibodies to PRN are found after natural disease or immunization with vaccines containing this protein.[63,64] Mice that have been protected passively with antibodies to PRN are highly resistant to an otherwise fatal aerosol challenge with virulent *B. pertussis*.[65] However, in the intracerebral mouse protection test, mice that have been actively immunized with PRN are protected only when also immunized with FHA.[59]

Studies from the Netherlands have shown that genetic variation in PRN (and PT) molecules exists, with a shift over time in the circulating strains toward variants not represented in the pertussis vaccine(s) used in the community.[66] Subsequent mouse-model studies have shown that the Dutch whole-cell pertussis vaccine is less effective against some PRN variants than others. In contrast, a study from France indicates that, despite lyophilization, multiple Aventis Pasteur whole-cell vaccine lots stored since 1984 had conserved genomes and still expressed the major toxins and adhesins.[67] Studies from the same investigators confirmed that the vaccine lots were highly immunogenic in mice.[68] Additional studies are needed from other geographic areas using different whole-cell vaccines to determine whether selection pressure may have contributed to variation in the PRN molecule, leading to less effective vaccines.[69,70] It is not known whether such variation might be seen with acellular vaccines; the presence of high concentrations of multiple antigens may decrease the likelihood of changes occurring in the PRN molecule, although this will need to be evaluated over time. Thus far, the available clinical[71,72] and experimental[73,74] data do not show reduced effectiveness of current diphtheria and tetanus toxoids and acellular pertussis (DTaP) vaccines against variant strains.

ADENYLATE CYCLASE

Adenylate cyclase, present in all virulent strains of B. pertussis, is synthesized as a protoxin monomer that is cleaved into an active molecule, which allows it to enter a variety of eukaryotic cells. Once inside the cell, it is activated by calmodulin and catalyzes the production of large quantities of cyclic AMP. Purified adenylate cyclase inhibits chemotaxis, chemiluminescence, and superoxide anion generation by monocytes and neutrophils in vitro, and in vivo augments production within the phagocyte of cyclic AMP from ATP, resulting in an excessive accumulation of cyclic AMP and paralysis of the various phagocytic functions.[30,75] In vivo studies have shown that, compared to wild-type organisms, mutants in adenylate cyclase are defective in their ability to cause lethal infection. These findings suggest that adenylate cyclase serves as an anti-inflammatory and antiphagocytic factor during infection. In the mouse model of aerosol infection, PT and adenylate cyclase appear to be the two most important virulence factors.[76] Adenylate cyclase is immunogenic[77]; in the mouse models of intracerebral and aerosol challenge, prior active immunization with adenylate cyclase was shown to be similar in protective efficacy to whole-cell vaccine.[78] In addition, it has been shown that adenylate cyclase antibodies interfere with the multiplication of organisms in these models.[78]

TRACHEAL CYTOTOXIN

Of the virulence factors produced by Bordetella organisms, only tracheal cytotoxin induces paralysis and destruction of respiratory ciliated epithelium, the hallmark of the disease. Tracheal cytotoxin is a fragment released from the peptidoglycan of the B. pertussis cell wall.[79–81] Its activities were studied in vitro in tracheal organ and cell cultures and found to induce mitochondrial bloating, disruption of the tight junctions, extrusion of the ciliated epithelial cells, and little or no damage to the nonciliated cells.[30] There is also evidence to suggest that the cytopathology is due to tracheal cytotoxin's increasing production of nitric oxide that then diffuses into the neighboring ciliated cells, causing cell death.

HEAT-LABILE TOXIN

Heat-labile toxin, so called because it is inactivated at 56°C, is also known as the dermonecrotic or mouse-lethal toxin because of its effects in experimental animals.[82] It is produced by all virulent Bordetella species. Located intracellularly, it can be recovered by disruption of B. pertussis cells. The mechanism of production of cutaneous lesions after injection of the toxin in animals appears to be vasoconstriction.[83] The toxin is lethal to mice when injected intravenously. The role, if any, of heat-labile toxin in the pathogenesis of pertussis is unknown. No consistent effects on cells have been recognized in vitro. It is a weak immunogen, antibodies to it are nonprotective in animal challenge tests, and its absence does not diminish the lethality of experimental pertussis infection in mice.[76]

BrkA

BrkA (Bordetella resistance to killing genetic locus, frame A), another outer membrane protein of B. pertussis similar in structure to PRN, protects the bacterium against classical-pathway complement-mediated killing.[84] It has been shown that antibodies to BrkA augment killing of B. pertussis.[85] Although increased susceptibility to complement during acute bacterial growth would seem to mark the organism for elimination, antibody is needed for classical complement activation. Antibody after a primary infection takes some time to develop, and rapid multiplication might arise before killing could occur. In contrast to the primary infection, if antibody has already been stimulated by natural disease or vaccine, a secondary response can be generated rapidly and killing might occur. This may explain why pertussis tends to be a milder disease after vaccination.[86]

ENDOTOXIN

The endotoxin or lipopolysaccharide of B. pertussis exhibits many of the in vivo activities of endotoxins produced by other gram-negative organisms, but its role in the disease process or in recovery is unclear.[87] Organisms with incomplete endotoxin production have shown decreased colonization of the respiratory tract in the mouse model.[88] The endotoxin content of whole-cell vaccines may have contributed to the immediate adverse systemic and local reactions to those vaccines.[89]

Pathogenesis

Current knowledge of the components of B. pertussis and their actions permits construction of a reasonable hypothesis regarding the pathogenesis of whooping cough in humans.[30,90,91] Transmission occurs when airborne bacteria from symptomatic patients reach the ciliated respiratory epithelium of a susceptible host. Bordetella pertussis overcomes the mucosal immune defenses of the upper respiratory tract and causes disease in healthy individuals. The organisms attach strongly to the ciliated cells through several adhesins. Although PT and FHA are important attachment proteins, fimbrial proteins, PRN, and BrkA participate in this process as well.[32,46,58,91,92] The bacteria do not invade beyond the epithelial layers of the respiratory tract, but PT enters the bloodstream and exerts its biologic effects on systemic sites. PT, adenylate cyclase, and BrkA have marked effects on host immune function.[32,75,84,93] Adenylate cyclase induces production of high levels of cyclic AMP, disrupting the functions of several cell types of the immune system; PT inhibits chemotaxis of phagocytic cells into the site of inflammation; and BrkA protects the bacteria against classical complement attack.[84] Tracheal cytotoxin and heat-labile toxin are likely involved in the damage to the tracheobronchial epithelium that is so characteristic of the disease.[80-82]

Although this sequence may explain the respiratory manifestations of pertussis, the pathogenesis of the encephalopathy that can complicate clinical disease remains unclear.[94] Suggested pathogenic mechanisms have included anoxia secondary to severe paroxysms, metabolic disturbances, hypoglycemia, or minute intracranial hemorrhages[94]; a direct toxic effect on the brain seems unlikely, given the fact that intravenous injection of substantial quantities of active PT into adult human volunteers caused no adverse effects.[43]

Diagnosis

The etiologic agent responsible for an infectious disease is generally determined by culture of the organism, detection of antigens or nucleic acids produced by the organism, or measurement of the immune response to the organism. Even when using all these criteria, the confirmation of B. pertussis infection is still one of the most difficult diagnostic challenges facing the clinician, particularly in adolescents and adults. Pertussis organisms can be detected in the nasopharynx of patients with pertussis only early in the illness, when the symptoms are similar to those of the common cold. By the time severe cough appears, the organism typically has decreased in number or disappeared from the nasopharynx, making culture or antigen detection extremely difficult.

Bacteriologic Diagnosis

CULTURE

Culture of B. pertussis from the nasopharynx of symptomatic patients is compelling evidence of the disease and remains the "gold standard" for laboratory diagnosis of pertussis.[95,96] The optimum likelihood of isolating the organism is achieved by immediate inoculation of a nasopharyngeal aspirate specimen onto fresh media early in the illness in a laboratory experienced with handling B. pertussis. At best, these conditions are difficult to meet, but, even under optimum circumstances, the organism is frequently not recovered because of its fastidious nature and its disappearance early in the disease process.[97] Cultures obtained after 21 days of cough are significantly less likely to yield organisms.[98-101] Because the human nasopharynx is colonized with many respiratory bacteria, the use of selective media containing antibiotics such as cloxacillin and cephalexin may increase the yield of positive pertussis cultures by suppressing normal flora and allowing Bordetella to grow.[99] Two media are specialized for pertussis cultures: Bordet-Gengou medium, containing defibrinated horse blood and cloxacillin; and Regan-Lowe medium, containing charcoal agar, defibrinated horse blood, and cephalexin. Although Granstrom and colleagues have shown that the two media detect comparable numbers of positive cultures in symptomatic unimmunized children with pertussis,[102] others have reported better yield with Regan-Lowe medium.[99] Direct plating of the specimen at the bedside or clinic has also been shown to increase the yield of positive cultures, whereas prior therapy with erythromycin or sulfamethoxazole reduces the likelihood of positive cultures. Data from pertussis vaccine efficacy studies suggest that immunized individuals with pertussis have lower rates of positive cultures than unimmunized control subjects and that isolation rates are negatively correlated with increasing age,[103] which further complicates the diagnosis of pertussis in partially or fully immunized children or adults.

In preparation for the Swedish efficacy trials of the acellular vaccines, investigators evaluated the parameters associated with optimal culture yields.[96] They concluded that the method of collection of the specimens was important, with nasopharyngeal aspirates yielding better samples than nasopharyngeal swabs. When swabs were used, Dacron was better than calcium alginate, which was shown to inhibit polymerase chain reaction (PCR) assays, and better than cotton, which was shown to be toxic to bacteria. The aspirate was obtained by placing an infant feeding tube through the nose into the posterior pharynx. Material was aspirated, and the tube was removed and then flushed with 1 mL of normal saline. Although direct plating of the aspirate was optimal, if that was not possible, Regan-Lowe transport medium was used, incubated, and plated at 72 hours after inoculation. This enrichment process increased the number of positive cultures by 7% to 14%.[101] These investigators preferred Regan-Lowe medium to Bordet-Gengou and incubated the plates for at least 7 days. However, in spite of these refinements that increased the sensitivity of culture, the senior investigator in this group concluded that "Although the culture is the 'gold standard' for the diagnosis of pertussis, its position should be reconsidered, as the diagnostic sensitivity is insufficient even when technical conditions are optimal."[96]

ANTIGEN DETECTION: DIRECT FLUORESCENT ANTIBODY TEST AND POLYMERASE CHAIN REACTION

Antigen detection tests offer the important advantage that organisms do not have to be viable for detection and therefore can be detected later in the disease and in the presence of antibiotics.

The first such test, the direct fluorescent antibody (DFA) test, can achieve a specificity of up to 99.6% but a sensitivity of only 61% (compared with culture) in experienced laboratories.[96,99,100,104] When properly performed, the DFA test can provide a useful addition to culture and serology, particularly for the confirmation of clinically suspected cases. However, as with any test of less than perfect specificity, the positive predictive value of the test can be quite low when the true prevalence of disease is low in the tested population. The replacement of polyclonal with monoclonal DFA reagents has been reported to enhance the assay performance and may be used in some situations.[105] More recently, PCR assays have been developed for the identification of unique gene sequences of B. pertussis in respiratory secretions.[99,106-111] Although bacteria can no longer be cultured after 5 days of therapy, the PCR can remain positive for an additional week.[112] Although still rather labor intensive and demanding of scrupulous technique to avoid cross-contamination, this rapid, highly sensitive and specific diagnostic method is steadily becoming more widely available. Improved techniques, such as immunomagnetic and solid-phase detection methods, offer the promise that a single organism might be detected with this improved technology.

Two types of clinical samples have been tested in PCR assays: nasopharyngeal aspirates and nasopharyngeal swab specimens. During the investigation of pertussis epidemics, most studies have demonstrated that the PCR assay is more sensitive than culture in the diagnosis of pertussis and that nasopharyngeal swabs provide adequate samples for analysis. Several PCR assays have been developed, the majority of which target one of four chromosomal regions of the organism for PCR amplification: (1) the PT promoter region, (2) repeated insertion sequences, (3) a region upstream from the porin gene, and (4) the adenylate cyclase toxin gene. Some have suggested that assays with repeated insertion sequences as the target are more sensitive with a low number of amplification cycles, but there also is an increased risk for cross-reaction with other species. A comparative trial examined the nationwide use of a PCR assay in Finland and Switzerland from nearly 4000 clinical samples and found that the sensitivity of the PT promoter–based PCR was higher than that of the insertion sequence–based PCR.[113] In these studies, the PCR remained positive longer than culture and offered results more rapidly. Bordetella pertussis cultures typically take 3 to 7 days to become positive, whereas PCR can be completed in 1 to 2 days.[113]

The various acellular pertussis vaccine efficacy trials conducted in the 1990s (see below) have provided information about the sensitivity and specificity of various PCR methods. In the Erlangen trial, 392 symptomatic subjects had nasopharyngeal samples for PCR compared with culture and serology. PCR and culture were positive in 22% and 6% of the samples, respectively. When serologic criteria were the gold standard, the sensitivity of the PCR was 61% and the specificity was 88%.[114] In another study conducted in Germany, 7153 samples were taken from symptomatic children. Bordetella pertussis was identified by culture in 3% and by PCR in 7.6%, a 2.6-fold increase.[115] Studies by Swedish investigators have shown that rates of PCR positivity increased from 87.5% to 95% when aspirates were treated with cation-exchange resins. Overall, PCR increased the yield of positive samples by 38.6%.[96]

Increasing reports of the successful use of PCR in clinical laboratories and of the development of "real-time" methods for the diagnosis of pertussis infections are encouraging and suggest that the diagnosis of pertussis infections may become easier for the clinician in the years ahead.[95,116–120]

Serologic Diagnosis

Serologic tests for antibodies to various components of the B. pertussis organism have been used extensively in the research environment for the diagnosis of pertussis in children and, particularly, in adults.[96,99,114,121–123] Serologic testing avoids the lack of sensitivity and other known limitations of culture methods and has improved our understanding of the clinical spectrum of pertussis, particularly by demonstrating asymptomatic, mild, or atypical infections in partially immune individuals.[23,124–126] Serologic studies have been used to examine the natural history of pertussis in unimmunized populations by determining the prevalence of antibodies at various ages,[127,128] and they have been shown to be useful in monitoring the incidence of pertussis during regional outbreaks.[129] Serologic studies have been of considerable value in monitoring clinical outcomes in trials of newer pertussis vaccines, because partially immune individuals may incur pertussis infection but display few or no symptoms.[103] Finally, serologic studies have enabled an understanding of the role of pertussis in the etiology of cough illness in adolescents and adults.[130]

Tests used to measure serum antibodies to B. pertussis include complement fixation, agglutination tests, toxin neutralization, and enzyme-linked immunosorbent assays (ELISAs).[99] Of these tests, ELISA methods are used most frequently because they are the easiest to perform and standardize and they can detect specific immunoglobulin isotype responses. Another advantage of the ELISA method is that serum antibodies against specific antigens of B. pertussis can be readily measured; for example, antibodies to PT and FHA are among those commonly assayed. Considerable effort has been expended to develop a standardized ELISA method that can be used in the evaluation of vaccine candidates and in the diagnosis of pertussis disease.[131–133] Methods of quantitation of antibody have also been refined.[134] Standardization has been important for the evaluation of vaccine candidates, but has not resulted in the widespread availability of serologic tests for the diagnosis of pertussis in most clinical laboratories. The diagnosis of a case of pertussis based on serology is dependent on the definition used. The most conclusive serologic evidence of an infection is the demonstration of a significant rise in specific antibodies as a consequence of the infection. Serologic definitions of many infectious diseases are made by fourfold titer rises between the pre- and the postimmunization samples. However, pertussis presents a considerable problem in this regard, because the frequently subtle early course of the disease does not excite suspicion of the diagnosis for several weeks. By this time, a substantial rise in serum antibodies has already occurred, thus compromising the likelihood of a significant increase between the acute and convalescent serum specimens. Indeed, the delay in clinical suspicion and thus in obtaining the acute specimen may result in higher antibody levels in the acute than in the convalescent specimen; it has been demonstrated that fourfold decreases in antibody between the acute and convalescent specimens can also be associated with culture-confirmed pertussis.[123]

An approach that avoids this problem of specimen timing has been taken in studies of people with respiratory illnesses who are suspected of having pertussis.[124–127] In these studies, the range of antibody levels is determined in a comparable control population of people who are not suspected to have pertussis. The distribution of antibody levels in single specimens from the population under investigation is determined and compared with that of the normal population. Those subjects whose antibody levels, singly or in various combinations, exceed the mean of the control population by a selected factor (typically, 2 or 3 standard deviations) are assumed to have experienced recent infection.[127,135–138] An example of the effect of case definition on the number of subjects diagnosed with pertussis and on the estimates of pertussis disease prevalence is shown in Table 21–2. In this study, Senzilet et al. enrolled patients 12 years of age or older with persistent cough of 1 to 8 weeks' duration from nine health units in eight Canadian provinces. Only two cases were diagnosed with positive culture, and three additional cases were detected with PCR. When serologic measures were used, only seven had a fourfold rise in titer between the acute and convalescent samples. However, 36 persons had a single antibody titer that exceeded the 99.9th percentile for controls, and 84 had single antibody titers that exceeded 3 standard deviations from that of the control subjects. As shown in Table 21–2, the calculated prevalence of pertussis disease in this population is highly dependent on the serologic definition.[18]

A somewhat different problem is presented by the use of serologic testing to detect pertussis in field trials of pertussis vaccine. As mentioned above, the laboratory routine used and the criteria applied for serologic case confirmation in vaccine efficacy trials have a direct influence on the identification of cases, which consequently may also affect the estimation of vaccine efficacy. Some differences in the application of serologic confirmation criteria among the clinical studies of acellular pertussis vaccines include the level of increase in titer required and the use of single-specimen diagnostics. Additionally, the availability of pre-exposure serum specimen collections increases the sensitivity of serologic confirmation. In the 1992 to 1995 Stockholm trial, a regimen was introduced to collect serum samples systematically; using acute- and convalescent-phase sera from the cough episodes, the proportion of all cases that was serologically confirmed was 25%. When pre-exposure sera also were available, the proportion was 35%; the change in sensitivity was differential by vaccine group and thus had some effect on the calculation of vaccine efficacy. Therefore, given the different application of serologic methods among the various efficacy studies, direct comparisons of efficacy rates between these studies should be made with caution.[139] Another concern with serologic diagnosis is that, although it may be appropriate for nonimmunized control subjects, detection of antibody increases may be compromised in those who were recently immunized, because immunization itself leads to increases in antibody titer. In this situation, the evaluation of antibodies against

an antigen of B. pertussis that was not included in the vaccine can be useful, if such an antigen exists.

Treatment and Prevention with Antibiotics

All patients with suspected pertussis should receive erythromycin therapy. However, treatment can ameliorate symptoms only if it is begun early in the catarrhal phase. Once the individual has developed paroxysmal cough, antibiotic therapy has little effect on the course of disease.[140] Treatment is still beneficial, however, because antibiotics hasten clearance of the organism and limit spread to other susceptible contacts.[4,141,142]

Erythromycin, especially the estolate form, has been considered the most active drug against pertussis.[141,142] The dosage of erythromycin is 40 to 50 mg/kg/day, with a maximum of 2 g/day, given every 6 hours. Because bacterial relapses have been reported with shorter courses of therapy, it has traditionally been recommended that treatment continue for 14 days. A trial comparing therapy with erythromycin estolate for 7 days (74 patients) and 14 days (94 patients) found overall failure rates of 2.70% and 1.06%, respectively.[140] Although these rates did not differ significantly and both failure rates are quite low, the point estimates nonetheless indicate a more than twofold higher failure rate with 7-day therapy. Another study has suggested that the required duration of therapy is related to the age of the patient, with very young patients requiring longer therapy than older patients.[143] If macrolides are not tolerated, trimethoprim-sulfamethoxazole (8 mg of trimethoprim/kg/day in two divided doses) has been recommended, although few data exist to confirm its efficacy.[144]

The newer macrolides azithromycin and clarithromycin have good penetration into relevant tissues, are effective in vitro, and offer reduced adverse effects and a simplified dosing regimen. A small study conducted in Japan compared once-daily azithromycin for 5 days (8 patients) with twice-daily clarithromycin for 7 days (9 patients), with matched historical control subjects given erythromycin for 14 days.[145] Eradication rates after azithromycin and clarithromycin were both 100%, compared with 13 of 16 and 16 of 18 among the respective matched controls; no bacterial relapses were detected. In a third study, 37 children ages 2 to 18 months with culture-confirmed pertussis were randomized to receive either 3 or 5 days of azithromycin. Two

TABLE 21–2 ▪ Adolescents and Adults with Prolonged Cough Illness (7–56 Days) Who Met Various Case Definitions for Laboratory Confirmation or Evidence of Pertussis*

Case definition	Criteria	No. positive/ no. tested	Prevalence, % (95% CI)	Mean age, years (range)
1	Culture positive for Bordetella pertussis	2/440	0.5 (0.1–1.8)	18.4 (12.6–24.1)
2	PCR positive for B. pertussis	3/314	1.0 (0.2–3.0)	24.0 (12.6–37.8)
3	Fourfold increase in antibody titer	7/393	1.8 (0.8–3.8)	28.1 (12.3–70.6)
4	Antibody titer >99.99 percentile for control values	36/440	8.3 (5.9–11.2)	36.6 (14.1–69.4)
5	Antibody titer >3 SDs greater than GMT for control subjects	84/440	19.1 (15.6–23.0)	39.0 (12.3–87.7)

*Includes all subjects with at least one biologic specimen.
CI, confidence interval; GMT, geometric mean titer; PCR, polymerase chain reaction; SD, standard deviation
Adapted from Senzilet LD, Halperin SA, Spika JS, et al. Pertussis is a frequent cause of prolonged cough illness in adults and adolescents. Clin Infect Dis 32:1691–1697, 2001.

patients who received 3 days of therapy remained pertussis culture positive at 7 days but were culture negative at 14 days. Patients who received the 5 days of therapy were culture negative at both the 7- and 14-day cultures. Although these studies are supportive for the use of abbreviated courses of azithromycin, further evaluation is needed.

The ability of antibiotics to prevent pertussis in contacts was re-evaluated in a randomized, placebo-controlled trial of erythromycin estolate chemoprophylaxis for household contacts of children with culture-positive B. pertussis infection.[146] Based on random allocation, either erythromycin or placebo was used for 10 days in 135 households with 310 contacts. There were no differences between the two groups in the development of respiratory symptoms compatible with a case definition of pertussis. There were 19 households with secondary culture-positive cases of pertussis, 4 in the erythromycin-treated group and 15 in the placebo group (eradication efficacy 67.5% [range 7.6 to 88.7]), but adverse events associated with medication were noted in 34% of the antibiotic-treated and in 16% of the placebo-treated contacts. The authors concluded that "erythromycin prevented culture positive pertussis in household contacts but did not prevent clinical disease." Additional randomized studies of new agents in similar settings are needed.

Another problem associated with the use of erythromycin chemoprophylaxis in infants has been the association with increased rates of pyloric stenosis.[147,148] These findings suggest caution in defining the groups at risk for pertussis, particularly in young infants, and careful observation for signs of obstruction.

One final concern with the use of erythromycin for chemoprophylaxis of pertussis is the increasing prevalence of antibiotic resistance. Erythromycin resistance was first recognized in Arizona in 1994.[149] Since then, additional erythromycin-resistant isolates have been reported.[150,151] Screening of isolates from around the United States suggests that the rates of erythromycin resistance remain very low, but reports of a novel resistance phenotype that appears only after a 7-day incubation period suggest that clinicians should remain alert to potential treatment failures.[152]

In summary, a 14-day course of erythromycin is recommended for antibiotic prophylaxis of household and other close contacts, regardless of vaccination status, and for health care workers with a high risk of, or known, exposure to pertussis.[153–155] Prophylaxis reduces, but does not eliminate, the risk of pertussis.[156,157] Prophylaxis within a household is substantially more effective if given before the appearance of the first secondary case.[157] Cases and inadequately vaccinated contacts younger than 7 years of age should be excluded from school, day care, and similar settings until they have received at least 5 days of prophylaxis or therapy.[153]

Epidemiology

Overview

Pertussis is an endemic disease with epidemic peaks occurring every 2 to 5 (typically, 3 to 4) years.[158–161] Widespread pertussis vaccination of children and the consequent reduction in the incidence of disease do not appear to have altered these intervals,[158,162,163] suggesting that ongoing endemic circulation of the organism in the community continues.[164,165] There is no consistent seasonal pattern. Some studies have reported a summertime peak; others have failed to demonstrate seasonal peaks or have indicated that peaks are more apt to occur during the winter months.[163,166,167] From 1980 to 1989, the peak incidence in the United States occurred during the early summer in the warmer states and between June and October in the northern states.[159] During 1990 to 1996, cases occurred in all seasons, with seasonality varying by age group.[160] In some reports morbidity and mortality rates have been higher in females than in males.[159] There is no evidence that females are more susceptible to infection than males; furthermore, before the development of pertussis vaccine, it was expected that every child would have whooping cough sooner or later. It is therefore likely that the disease is more severe in female patients, which results in more ready recognition and higher mortality than in male patients. One explanation for this phenomenon is that, for the first 6 months of life, male infants have considerably higher levels of testosterone than do female infants, which perhaps results in a larger laryngeal airway and thus less likelihood of obstruction (J. Germak, personal communication, 1986).[168] Another explanation might be that the sexes differ in their immune responses to pertussis infection, but no data exist to confirm this theory.

Pertussis is acquired through direct transmission from close respiratory contact. Transmission by the indirect route from airborne droplet nuclei or organisms on fomites or in dust occurs extremely rarely, if ever. Whooping cough is highly contagious: as many as 90% of susceptible household contacts acquire the disease. Rates of transmission in school settings range from 50% to 80%.[169]

Pertussis may occur at any age. Infants are susceptible to pertussis within the first few weeks or months of life, when mortality from whooping cough is highest. For many years, it was assumed that one attack of pertussis provided lifelong immunity. Before widespread vaccination, this belief was reflected by the age distribution of pertussis: approximately 20% of all whooping cough cases occurred in infants younger than 1 year, and nearly 60% occurred among children ages 1 to 4 years.[166] Anecdotal information indicated that second attacks of pertussis did occur in the prevaccine era, such as in older persons exposed to grandchildren with the disease, although these instances were rarely described and incompletely documented.[170] More recent data from Germany suggest that second attacks of pertussis may not be uncommon. Geometric mean titers of agglutinins and antibody to PT, FHA, fimbrial proteins, and PRN were two- to threefold higher in sera from American students than in sera from German recruits. In contrast, the geometric mean immunoglobulin A (IgA) values and the percentage of subjects with detectable IgA antibodies to the four antigens were similar in the two populations. The authors proposed that, because IgA antibody results mainly from infection and not from immunization, B. pertussis infections are common among both American and German young adults, despite the marked difference in rates of clinical pertussis in the two countries.[171] A chronic carrier state has not been demonstrated,[172] but evidence for such a state may be compromised by the insensitivity of culture methods.[173]

Incidence of Pertussis in the United States

Disease caused by *B. pertussis* was once a major cause of morbidity and mortality among infants and children. From the 1920s (when pertussis was first a reportable disease) until the early 1940s, there were 115,000 to 270,000 cases of pertussis reported each year, with 5000 to 10,000 deaths. These figures represented approximately 150 cases and 6 deaths per 100,000 population.[4] As pertussis vaccine came to be used commonly in infants and children, the incidence of pertussis markedly decreased (Fig. 21–2).[159] By the 1970s, the annual incidence of reported disease had been reduced by 99%, and the lowest annual number of cases of pertussis—1010—was reported in 1976. Reported cases began to increase in the 1980s: From 1980 to 1989, 27,826 cases of pertussis were reported to the CDC, for a crude incidence of 1.2 cases per 100,000 population. The U.S. pertussis case-fatality rate during the 1980s was estimated to be 0.6%.[159] Cyclical peaks in pertussis incidence were noted in 1983, 1986, 1990, 1993, 1996, and 2002, with each peak surpassing the last.[6] The highest number of cases since 1964 (7796 cases) was reported in 2000 (7867 cases). From 1997 to 2000, a total of 28,187 cases of pertussis were reported. The largest number was seen in individuals 10 to 19 years of age (8273), with the next highest number of cases noted in infants less than 6 months of age (7203). Average annual incidence rates were highest among infants less than 1 year old (55.5 cases per 100,000 population) and lower in chil-dren ages 1 to 4 years (5.5), children ages 5 to 9 years (3.6), persons ages 10 to 19 years (5.5), and persons over 20 years of age (0.8). The proportion who were hospitalized or had complications was highest in the infants less than 6 months and decreased with increasing age. In infants less than 6 months, 63% were hospitalized, 12% had radiologically confirmed pneumonia, and 1% had seizures. Fifty-six of the total 62 deaths seen with pertussis from 1997 to 2000 occurred in children less than 6 months of age.

Several large pertussis outbreaks have been reported in recent years.[106,129,174–177] In the 1993 outbreak in Chicago, the median age of patients was 8 months, with most children having received fewer than three vaccine doses.[174] In contrast, during the Cincinnati outbreak, the median age was 17 months, and most of the children had received at least three doses of vaccine.[175] A statewide outbreak of pertussis in 1996 in Vermont, a highly vaccinated population, affected primarily school-age children and adults.[177] Multiple outbreaks of disease have also been reported from Canada.[106,129] Many researchers have speculated about the reasons for this increase in pertussis disease. Some have noted that the two commercial whole-cell vaccines used prior to conversion to acellular pertussis vaccine in the United States produced substantially different antibody responses, with one generating little antibody to PT and the other little antibody to FHA. These individuals have suggested that the increase in pertussis disease in the early 1990s was the result of vaccines that were less immunogenic than previously believed.[178,179] Evidence for this

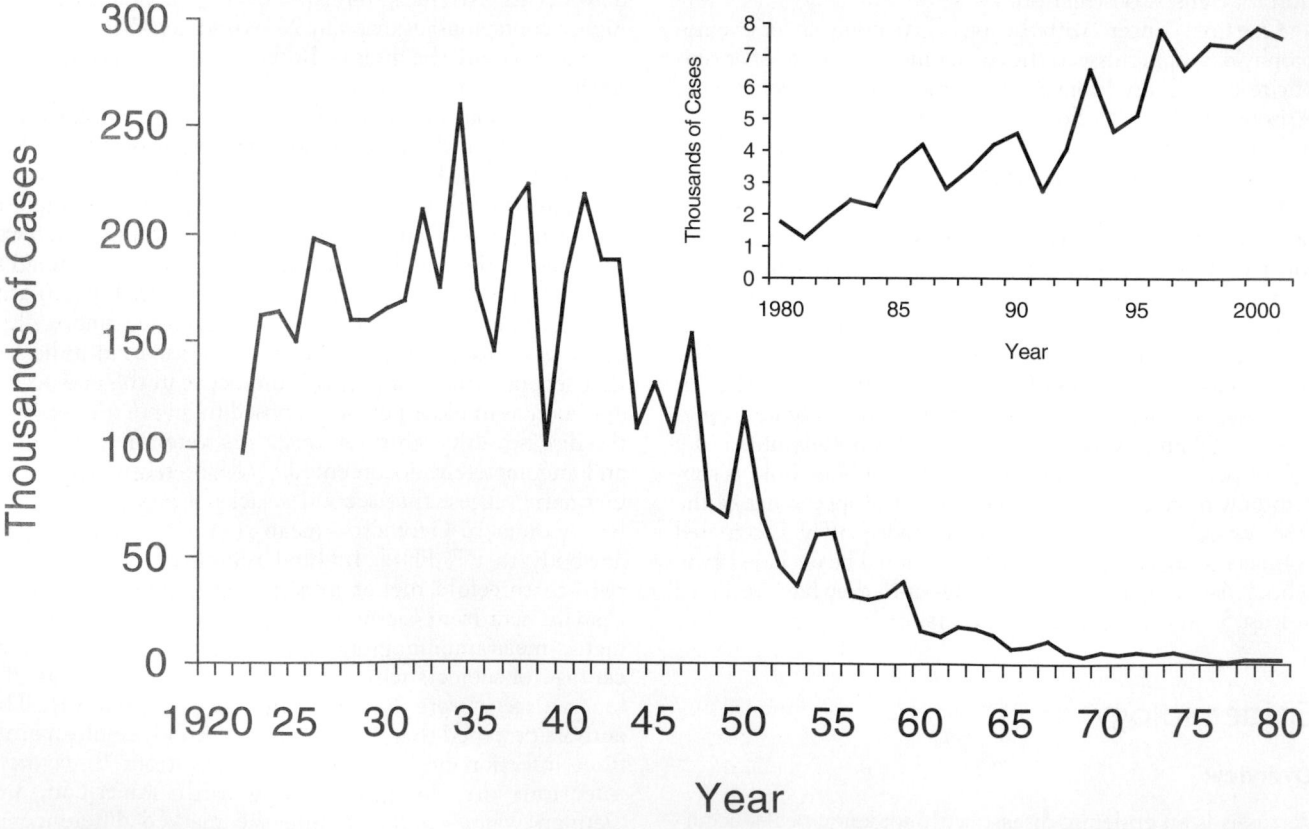

FIGURE 21–2 ■ Number of reported pertussis cases, by year, in the United States from 1922 to 2001. Data for 1922–1996 from W. Orenstein, personal communication, Centers for Disease Control and Prevention; data for subsequent years from "Provisional cases of selected notifiable dieases preventable by vaccination [52nd week]", as published annually in Morbidity and Mortality Weekly Report (see also http://www.cdc.gov).

concern was provided by the pertussis vaccine efficacy trials conducted in Europe in the early 1990s, which found adequate efficacy after three doses for one U.S. whole-cell vaccine[180] but quite low efficacy for the other.[181,182] Most cases of pertussis among recipients of the latter vaccine occurred after the age at which a fourth dose of vaccine is recommended in the United States.[181,182] These results are completely consistent with U.S. surveillance data from 1992 to 1994 that found an overall whole-cell pertussis vaccine efficacy of 64% after three doses and of 82% after four or more doses.[15]

In 1996, acellular pertussis vaccines were licensed and introduced for routine immunization of children. Since licensure of these vaccines, pertussis incidence has continued to increase in infants too young to receive three doses of pertussis-containing vaccine and in adolescents and adults. Prevention efforts have been directed at maintaining high vaccination coverage rates and managing pertussis cases and outbreaks. The effectiveness of pertussis vaccine among children ages 7 to 18 months of age who had received at least three doses of vaccine was estimated by the CDC to be 88% (95% confidence interval [CI], 79% to 93%) during 1998 to 1999, a period in which approximately 66% of children less than 18 months of age had received DTaP and 33% had received diphtheria and tetanus toxoids and (whole-cell) pertussis (DTP) vaccine.[6]

During the 1990s in the United States, an average of fewer than 10 deaths from pertussis was recorded annually. The remarkable decline in mortality from the disease since the 1950s is clearly attributable to widespread use of whole-cell vaccine.[183] Nonetheless, as noted, pertussis appears to be increasing in the United States, particularly among adolescents and adults, and continues to pose a substantial burden.

More recently, in countries such as the United States in which pertussis vaccination is common, the age distribution of pertussis has changed markedly. Before the advent of widespread vaccination,[166] 41% of cases providing age data occurred in infants younger than 1 year.[184] Of cases reported during 1990 to 1993, 44% occurred among children younger than 1 year of age, 22% among children ages 1 to 4 years, 10% among children ages 5 to 9 years, and 24% among individuals 10 years and older.[15] During 1994 to 1996, these proportions were 34% in children younger than 1 year and 16% in children 1 to 4 years of age. The proportion of cases occurring in 5- to 9-year-old children rose to 12%, and the greatest increase was observed in persons 10 to 19 years of age, where the percentage doubled.[160] Data from 1997 to 2000 indicate further increases in incidence rates among adolescents and adults (62% and 60%, respectively).[6] Rates also increased 11% among infants, decreased 8% among children ages 1 to 4 years, and remained constant among 5- to 9-year-old children. As always, such changes could represent changes in reporting, true changes in disease rates, or both.

Although pertussis in adolescents has been increasing recently, outbreaks in this age group have been reported for some time. In 1965, Lambert reported an outbreak in Michigan, in which the highest attack rates were seen in individuals older than 10 years, and concluded that "the direct relationship of increased pertussis incidence in vaccinated people to increased interval since the last injection of pertussis-containing vaccine was the most significant study finding."[170] During an outbreak in an immunized popula-

tion in Finland, the attack rate (per 100,000) of laboratory-confirmed pertussis was 317 in children younger than 4 years, 1838 in children 4 to 6 years of age, and 2535 in children 7 to 15 years of age.[185] In a Wisconsin outbreak, adolescents were at a higher risk than any other age group for the acquisition of pertussis.[186] Reports of pertussis outbreaks in middle-school and high-school populations are not uncommon, and statewide surveillance in Massachusetts has shown that the incidence of confirmed pertussis in people 11 to 19 years of age has increased remarkably.[135,159,187] From 1989 to 1998, the incidence of pertussis in adolescents and adults in Massachusetts increased to 71 and 5 per 100,000, respectively, compared to 5 and 0.8 per 100,000 respectively nationally. By 1998, 92% of pertussis cases reported in Massachusetts were in adolescents and adults, compared to only 47% nationally. The availability of a specific serologic test and active public health surveillance in the state might explain many of the differences in rates. Adolescents and adults with pertussis diagnosed in Massachusetts had clinically significant disease: over 80% of the cases had paroxysmal cough, over 40% had cough associated with vomiting, and nearly 50% had cough duration greater than 1 month.[136]

However, in many adolescent and adult infections, symptoms are mild or even absent, and cases are recognized only because of the presence of an outbreak. Serologic studies during outbreaks have demonstrated the occurrence of frequent asymptomatic infections or illnesses, indistinguishable from mild viral upper respiratory disorders, among previously vaccinated people or among those with a past history of pertussis.[23,124–126] How contagious these infections are is unknown, but it is clear that infected adults have been responsible for the transmission of disease to young infants and children.[17,23] In the Chicago outbreak, for example, young mothers were an important source of pertussis for their infants.[174]

Pertussis has also become recognized as an important cause of chronic cough. Of 218 Australian adults referred for investigation of chronic cough, 56 (26%) had pertussis IgA antibody levels more than 3 standard deviations higher than normal.[188] Similarly, Mink and colleagues found that 26% of students presenting to a university student health service with cough of at least 6 days' duration had serologic evidence of pertussis.[125] During the 1993 pertussis epidemic in Chicago, 10 (26%) of 38 adults presenting to a clinic with unexplained cough had serologic evidence of pertussis.[174] Of adults presenting to an emergency department with cough persisting 2 weeks or longer, 21% had serologic evidence of pertussis.[189] Of adult patients in a large California health care plan who were referred for chronic cough, 12.4% had evidence of recent pertussis,[190] representing an incidence of 176 per 100,000 person-years—a rate greater than the annual incidence of reported pertussis (157 per 100,000) in the United States in the prevaccine era. Two studies, one from Canada and another from the United States, sought to determine the prevalence of pertussis in adolescents and adults with cough illness. In the Canadian study, as described earlier, nearly 20% of 442 adolescents and adults with cough illness lasting greater than 7 days were diagnosed with laboratory confirmed or suspected pertussis. The greatest number of cases of pertussis were confirmed in participants 20 to 39 years of age, but the highest proportion of cough illness resulting from pertussis was seen in adolescents 12 to 19 years of age.[18,130] In the U.S. study, members of a managed care organization with cough were followed prospectively to estimate the incidence of pertussis. Of 212 patients 10 to 49 years of age enrolled over a 2-year period, at least one positive laboratory test result for pertussis was found in 13% of the subjects. On the basis of these data, the incidence of pertussis was estimated to be 507 cases per 100,000 person-years.[137] These reports have also shown clearly that chronic cough may be the sole manifestation of pertussis among adolescents and adults and that adults with pertussis cannot be differentiated on clinical grounds from other adult patients with cough.[189]

Further insight into the epidemiology of pertussis in a highly vaccinated population comes from a serosurvey of 600 normal healthy individuals ages 1 to 65 years (Fig. 21–3).[127] The results demonstrated not only the expected peak in PT and FHA titers in the 4- to 6-year-old group, reflecting the administration of booster doses of pertussis vaccine, but also a second, larger peak in the 13- to 17-year-old group, suggesting that natural exposure to pertussis is frequent during the adolescent years.

In part, the increase in recognized cases of pertussis in older individuals may represent enhanced suspicion and recognition, improved reporting of adult pertussis, or better diagnostic methods. However, the most important factor has probably been waning vaccine-induced immunity, coupled with the infrequency of pertussis in well-immunized populations and thus fewer opportunities for the reinforcement of immunity by casual exposure. Immunity after vaccination was previously thought to be of shorter duration than that after natural disease, but this concept has been challenged by the frequent diagnosis of pertussis in German adults who had experienced previous natural infection.[19,20,171] It is also possible that vaccine-induced immunity is less vigorous or that it provides more protection against disease manifestations than against infection.[23] Whatever the reasons, the increased recognition of pertussis in older individuals has stimulated interest in booster immunization of adolescents and adults. International pertussis experts have advocated such immunization.[191]

Significance of Pertussis as a Global Public Health Problem

In the developing world, the situation is very different and is reminiscent of that existing in the United States earlier in the century. Data collected by the Expanded Programme

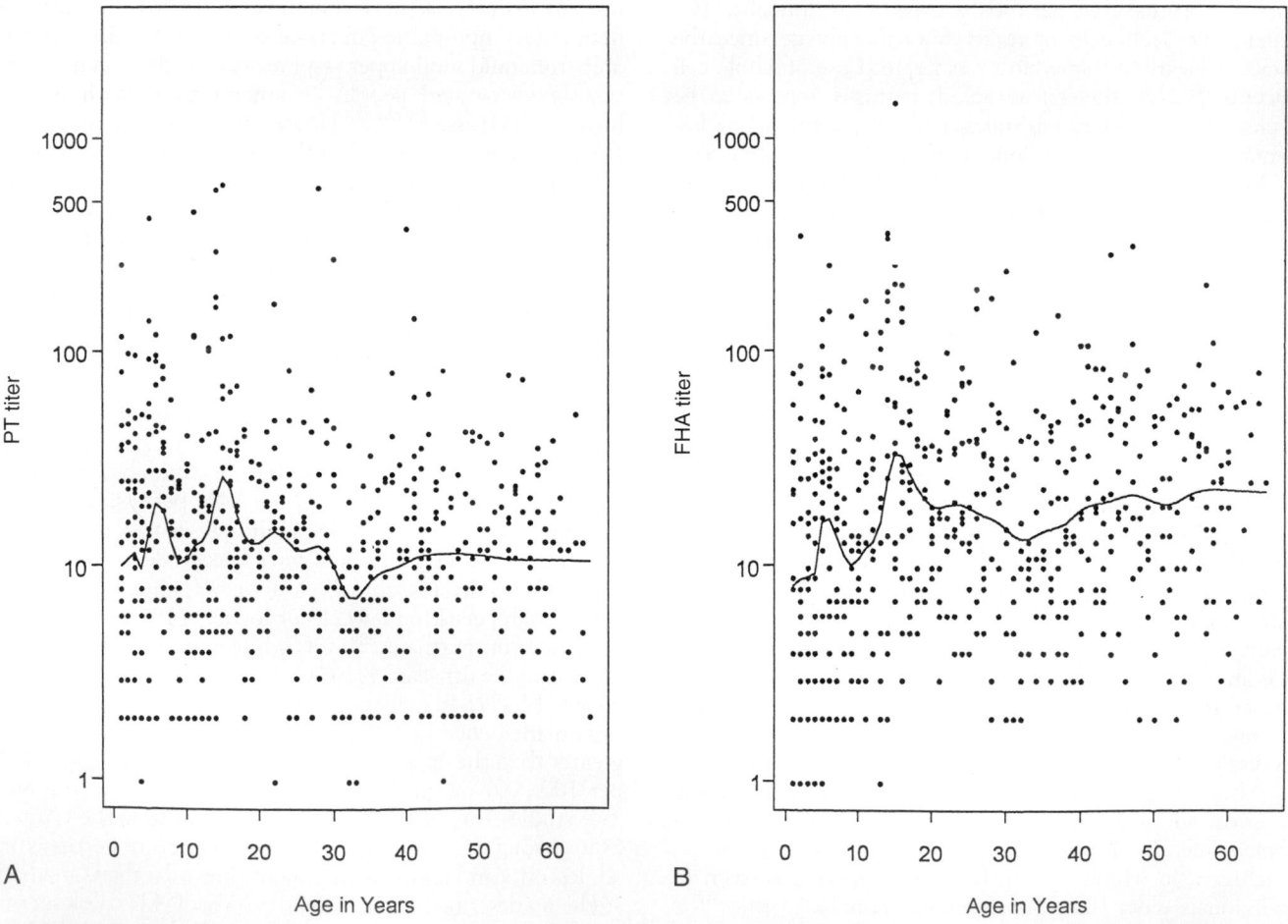

FIGURE 21–3 ■ Serologic responses (as measured by enzyme-linked immunosorbent assay) to pertussis toxin (PT; A) and filamentous hemagglutinin (FHA; B) of 600 normal healthy individuals ages 1 to 65 years. *Solid lines* show geometric mean titers by age; each dot represents one subject. (Adapted from Cattaneo LA, Reed G, Haase DH, et al. The seroepidemiology of *Bordetella pertussis* infections: a study of persons aged 1–65 years. J Infect Dis 173:1256–1259, 1996.)

on Immunization (EPI) of the WHO in 1992 indicated that 850,000 of the approximately 110 million children born annually in the developing world a decade earlier succumbed to pertussis before their fifth birthdays. Obviously, complicating factors such as low birth weight, malnutrition, and other infections, particularly intestinal and respiratory, contribute to mortality from pertussis in these population groups. A WHO estimate illustrates both the success of the EPI and the substantial work yet to be done. In 1994, 40 million pertussis infections resulted in 5 million episodes of pneumonia, 360,000 deaths (a nearly 60% reduction), and 50,000 patients with long-term neurologic complications (including permanent brain damage).[7]

Passive Immunization

Transplacental

Antibodies to PT and FHA readily cross the placenta and are found in infant sera in concentrations comparable to those in maternal sera. The half-life of transplacental antibodies is about 6 weeks, with disappearance by 4 months of age.[192] Transplacental antibodies appear to offer little or no clinical protection, because infants of mothers who are presumed to be immune to pertussis, whether because of immunization or disease, are susceptible on exposure. From 1990 to 1996, children younger than 1 year of age accounted for the highest proportion of pertussis cases, but their proportion has decreased over time. During the period from 1990 to 1993, 44% of the cases were reported in children younger than 1 year. From 1994 to 1996, 34% of the cases were seen in children less than 1 year. When the intervals were further divided, 82% of the children less than 1 year of age with reported pertussis from 1990 to 1996 were actually less than 6 months of age, too young for three primary pertussis vaccine doses. Thirty-five percent of these children were less than 2 months of age, too young to have received any doses of vaccine and yet, evidently, not protected by maternal antibody.[160]

Therapeutic

Before the widespread use of pertussis vaccine and the availability of antibiotics, passive immunization using whole serum was employed in an effort to prevent the spread of disease to exposed susceptible people and to modify the course of the illness in those who had already acquired whooping cough.[193] Most of the studies of preventive efficacy in exposed individuals were not controlled; a few studies that did include control subjects suggested that as many as 40% of recipients were protected.[11,40,193]

The subsequent development of methods for purification of serum immune globulins led to the commercial production of pertussis hyperimmune globulin, composed largely of immunoglobulin G (IgG).[194] Although this preparation was widely used for prophylaxis and treatment, controlled studies indicated that it had no effect, and production was discontinued.[195,196]

More recently, new preparations of pertussis immune globulin have been produced and evaluated in animal models and humans. Sato and Sato demonstrated that both monoclonal and polyclonal antibodies to PT improved survival of suckling mice after aerosol challenge with live pertussis organisms.[41] The ability to generate high-titer immune globulin by immunizing adults with less reactogenic acellular pertussis vaccines led to a reassessment of the use of immune globulin as therapy for pertussis. In 1991, Granstrom and colleagues conducted a double-blind, randomized, placebo-controlled trial of a pertussis immune globulin prepared from adults immunized with an acellular pertussis vaccine containing either PT or PT plus FHA.[197] A significant reduction in the duration of whoops was demonstrated in the recipients of the pertussis immune globulin compared with placebo recipients (8.7 vs. 20.6 days; $P = 0.0041$). A pertussis immune globulin has been prepared by the Massachusetts Biologic Laboratories using serum from adults immunized with monovalent pertussis toxoid vaccine. This product has been evaluated in the mouse aerosol model of pertussis and in Phase I trials in infants.[198] Preliminary studies demonstrated clinical improvement, but larger, more definitive trials have not been completed.

Active Immunization

History

The isolation and propagation of B. pertussis on artificial media in 1906 led to the development of vaccine for the prevention of whooping cough, a disease that at the turn of the century killed more than 5 of every 1000 children born in the United States. Initial steps to develop a vaccine were empirical, given the lack of understanding of the biology of the organism and its relationship to the pathogenesis of the disease. An improved understanding of the different phases of the organism led to refinement in the methods of vaccine production and resulted in a whole-cell vaccine prepared in a standardized and reproducible fashion. During the 1980s and 1990s, knowledge of the components of the pertussis organism and their biologic roles expanded and led to the development of the acellular pertussis vaccines.

Whole-cell pertussis vaccines were first licensed in the United States in 1914 and became available combined with diphtheria and tetanus toxoids (DTP) in 1948. They were recommended and widely used for routine vaccination of children in the United States. Because of state laws mandating vaccination for school entry, almost all U.S. children are vaccinated.

In 1996, less reactogenic acellular pertussis vaccines were licensed and recommended for routine use among infants. DTP vaccine use in the United States has declined precipitously and has been replaced by the acellular DTaP vaccines.[5]

Development of Whole-Cell Vaccines

Whole-cell pertussis vaccines are suspensions of killed B. pertussis organisms. One of the first clinical trials of a whole-cell vaccine conducted during an epidemic of pertussis in the Faroe Islands provided evidence of efficacy.[199] In the 1930s, steps taken to improve vaccines included increasing the number of bacteria in the vaccine; using standardized culture media; inactivating the organisms by "gentler" methods; and using fresh, rapidly growing Phase 1 organisms.[27,40]

TABLE 21–3 ■ Key Characteristics of Selected Acellular Pertussis Vaccines*

Manufacturer or Distributor	Vaccine†	Evaluated in MAPT	Micrograms of Pertussis Antigen per Dose				Diphtheria Toxoid‡	Tetanus Toxoid‡
			PT	FHA	PRN	FIM		
Aventis Pasteur (Canada)§	Tripacel; DAPTACEL	Yes	10	5	3	5	15	5
Aventis Pasteur (Canada)§	HCPDT	No	20	20	3	5	15	5
Aventis Pasteur (France)	Triavax; Triaxim	Yes	25	25	—	—	15	5
Aventis Pasteur (USA)	Tripedia	Yes	23.4	23.4	—	—	6.7	5
Baxter Laboratories	Certiva	No	40	—	—	—	15	6
Chiron Vaccines	Acelluvax	Yes	5	2.5	2.5	—	25	10
GlaxoSmithKline	Infanrix	Yes	25	25	8	—	25	10
Japan National Institutes of Health	JNIH-6‖	No	23.4	23.4	—	—	—	—
Japan National Institutes of Health	JNIH-7	No	37.7	—	—	—	—	—
SmithKline Beecham Biologicals	SKB-2	Yes	25	25	—	—	25	10
Wyeth Pharmaceuticals¶	ACEL-IMUNE	Yes	3.5	35	2	0.8	9	5

*Compositions may differ in various markets; local suppliers should be consulted as necessary.
†Trade names (in italics; most common trade names, if multiple names exist) except as follows: HCPDT is the "hybrid" formulation of Tripacel evaluated in the 1993 Stockholm trial (otherwise, used only in combinations); JNIH-6 and JNIH-7 were the acellular vaccines used in the 1986 Swedish trial; SKB-2 was an experimental two-component DTaP evaluated in the 1992 Stockholm trial.
‡Measured in Limit of Flocculation units per dose.
§FIM (agglutinogen) component is a mixture of FIM-2 and FIM-3. In MAPT, PT was 10 μg; FHA, 5 μg.
‖A Biken vaccine, similar to Tripedia.
¶Contains approximately 40 μg (but not more than 60 μg) of pertussis antigen proteins, consisting of approximately 86% FHA, approximately 8% PT, approximately 4% PRN, and approximately 2% FIM-2.
FHA, filamentous hemagglutinin; FIM, fimbrial proteins; MAPT, Multicenter Acellular Pertussis Trial; PRN, pertactin; PT, pertussis toxin.

A major stumbling block in the development and assessment of pertussis vaccines was the lack of a suitable means other than clinical trials for assessing the immunizing capability of a vaccine. After World War II, the mouse protection test was designed and it reproducibly measured vaccine potency. In this test, mice were immunized with pertussis vaccine and then challenged by intracerebral inoculation of living B. pertussis organisms.[200] Although several antigens of B. pertussis affected the results of the mouse protection test, and it was not clear that the mouse-protective and human-protective antigens were identical, the results of the mouse protection test were shown to correlate well with protective efficacy in humans and allowed vaccine to be reliably standardized.[201,202] Whole-cell pertussis vaccines have been produced in the United States by methods that vary somewhat among manufacturers.[27] The organisms have been grown in liquid or solid media, and have been inactivated by several methods (usually by formalin). In the United States, pertussis vaccine is almost always administered to children in combination with diphtheria and tetanus toxoids (DT). This combination is adsorbed onto an aluminum salt, which results in greater immunogenicity and less reactivity.

TABLE 21–4 ■ Additional Characteristics of Selected Acellular Pertussis Vaccines*

Manufacturer or Distributor	Vaccine†	How Toxoided
Aventis Pasteur (Canada)	Tripacel; DAPTACEL	Glutaraldehyde
Aventis Pasteur (Canada)	HCPDT	Glutaraldehyde
Aventis Pasteur (France)	Triavax; Triaxim	Glutaraldehyde
Aventis Pasteur (USA)	Tripedia	Formaldehyde
Baxter Laboratories	Certiva	H_2O_2
Chiron Vaccines	Tricelluvax¶	Genetic
GlaxoSmithKline	Infanrix	Formaldehyde**
Japan National Institutes of Health	JNIH-6	Formaldehyde
Japan National Institutes of Health	JNIH-7	Formaldehyde
SmithKline Beecham Biologicals	SKB-2	Formaldehyde
Wyeth Pharmaceuticals	ACEL-IMUNE	Formaldehyde

*Compositions may differ in various markets; local suppliers should be consulted as necessary. Aluminum content is per dose.
†Trade names (in italics; most common trade name, if multiple names exist) except as follows: HCPDT is the "hybrid" formulation of Tripacel evaluated in the 1993 Stockholm trial (otherwise, used only in combinations); JNIH-6 and JNIH-7 were the acellular vaccines used in the 1986 Swedish trial; SKB-2 was an experimental two-component DTaP evaluated in the 1992 Stockholm trial.
‡As aluminum phosphate.

Development of Acellular Vaccines

The common occurrence of minor but burdensome adverse reactions, the rare occurrence of more severe adverse reactions, and public anxiety over allegations of possible devastating complications following immunization with whole-cell vaccine stimulated the search for effective, less reactogenic pertussis vaccines. Research under the leadership of Margaret Pittman, Charles Manclark, and others led to an improved understanding of the biology of B. pertussis and to the isolation of components of the organism important in disease pathogenesis and induction of clinical immunity. This fundamental knowledge contributed to the production in Japan, by Sato and colleagues, of the first purified component (acellular) vaccines. The initial vaccines consisted predominantly of FHA, along with smaller amounts of inactivated PT and, in some cases, fimbrial proteins and PRN, and are known as Takeda-type vaccines. They soon were followed by additional acellular vaccines containing equal quantities of PT and FHA (termed Biken-type vaccines). Criteria for the licensure of the acellular vaccines in Japan included low toxicity in the mouse, documentation of mouse potency, diminished systemic and local reactivity in children, and antibody production in children similar to or exceeding that of the whole-cell vaccine. Demonstration of clinical protection by field trials was not required, although household-contact studies and pertussis surveillance after implementation of the acellular vaccines gave clear evidence of effectiveness. Since 1981, acellular pertussis vaccines have been used exclusively in Japan and have been very effective.[203–207] Reported pertussis currently is at an all-time low in Japan.[208]

The encouraging results in Japan stimulated efforts in other industrialized nations to evaluate further the Japanese acellular vaccines and to develop other acellular vaccines. Nearly two dozen acellular pertussis vaccines were developed, many were evaluated in immunogenicity and reactogenicity trials, and the efficacy and safety of a number were evaluated in field trials. We focus here on those products that have been licensed and are in use internationally.

These vaccines vary from one another with respect to their source, number of components, quantity of each component, method of purification, method of toxin inactivation, incorporated adjuvants, and excipients (Tables 21–3 and 21–4).[209] Unfortunately, identifying the optimum formulation for an acellular vaccine has proven difficult, because no simple method exists to determine the protective capability of a pertussis vaccine. The results of the mouse intracerebral protection test correlate reasonably well with the clinical protection afforded by whole-cell vaccine, but the test does not predict the efficacy of acellular pertussis vaccines.[210] Guiso and colleagues have found that the results of intranasal challenge in a murine model correlated with efficacy of selected acellular pertussis vaccines,[211] suggesting the possible utility of such tests in preclinical evaluation of candidate vaccines. Although human immunologic correlates of protection have been avidly sought, these efforts have met with only partial success, as described later in this chapter.

Acellular pertussis vaccines have entirely replaced whole-cell pertussis products in the United States, Canada, Australia, some Asian, and many European markets (Table 21–5).

Vaccine Producers

The vaccine industry has undergone dramatic consolidation over the past 20 years; both long-established companies and new biotechnology start-ups have been acquired or merged. These changes render nomenclature problematic. For vaccines currently marketed, we will use the name of the current manufacturer, even when describing studies conducted by a predecessor company. For products not presently marketed, we will use the name of the company that produced them, even if that company now is owned by or operates under a successor name. To further assist the reader, Table 21–6 lists the current major vaccine manufacturers along with the names of predecessor, component, or acquired companies.

Aluminum (mg)	Diluent	Preservative	Trace Constituents
0.33[‡]	PBS	Phenoxyethanol	Glutaraldehyde, PS
0.33[‡]	PBS	Phenoxyethanol	Glutaraldehyde, PS
0.30[§]	n/a	Thimerosal	n/a
0.17[‖]	PBS	None	Formaldehyde, gelatin, PS
0.50[§]	PBS	Thimerosal	none
1.0[§]	n/a	Thimerosal	n/a
0.625[§**]	Saline	Phenoxyethanol	Formaldehyde, PS
0.08	PBS	Thimerosal	Formaldehyde
0.075	PBS	Thimerosal	Formaldehyde
0.50[§]	Saline	Phenoxyethanol	Formaldehyde, PS
0.23[††]	PBS	Thimerosal	Formaldehyde, gelatin, PS

[§]As aluminum hydroxide.
[‖]As aluminum potassium sulfate.
[¶]Pertussis components are formaldehyde-stabilized. Aluminum content was 0.35 mg in MAPT.
[**]PT component detoxified with both formaldehyde and glutaraldehyde. In MAPT, aluminum content was 0.50 mg.
[††]A mixture of aluminum hydroxide and aluminum phosphate.
MAPT, Multicenter Acellular Pertussis Trial; n/a, information not available; PBS, phosphate-buffered saline; PS, polysorbate 80.

Available Whole-Cell Pertussis Vaccine Preparations

Despite availability of acellular vaccines, whole-cell vaccines remain the most widely used globally. Whole-cell vaccines are produced locally in many regions of the world, are generally efficacious, and are inexpensive to produce. Each country has to evaluate, based on its own circumstances, the costs, relative efficacy, and rate of adverse reactions to both whole-cell and acellular vaccines in designing its pertussis immunization strategy.

There are far too many whole-cell vaccines produced globally to permit a complete listing here. Internationally distributed vaccines include those produced by Aventis Pasteur, GlaxoSmithKline, Evans Vaccines, and Chiron Behring GmbH & Co. Some whole-cell vaccines are available in combination with conjugate *Haemophilus influenzae* type b (Hib) vaccine, enhanced inactivated poliovirus vaccine (IPV), or hepatitis B virus (HBV) vaccine (see Chapter 29).

Available Acellular Pertussis Vaccine Preparations

Constituents and Stability, Storage and Handling, Dosage and Route

Details of the composition and other key characteristics of selected acellular pertussis vaccines are listed below and are shown in Tables 21–3 and 21–4. Unless otherwise noted, all vaccines listed should be stored refrigerated at 2° to 8°C (36° to 46°F; do not freeze). The standard dose of pertussis vaccine is 0.5 mL given intramuscularly in the anterolateral thigh or, if necessary, the deltoid. It is inappropriate to give a partial dose in the hope of reducing adverse effects.

Preparations Licensed in the United States

The vaccines discussed in this section are licensed in the United States as of spring 2002. They may also be licensed, or under application for licensure, in other jurisdictions. In those jurisdictions, their compositions and trade names may vary from those provided here; local suppliers should be consulted as necessary.

Because the intracerebral mouse protection test does not provide a valid measure of the protective capability of the acellular pertussis vaccines, the potency of individual lots of these vaccines produced for the U.S. marketplace is evaluated by measurement of the antibody response to PT (plus FHA, PRN, and fimbrial proteins, as applicable) in immunized mice, using an ELISA.

WYETH-LEDERLE VACCINES AND PEDIATRICS (ACEL-IMUNE)

The Lederle-Takeda DTaP, marketed as ACEL-IMUNE, was licensed in the United States on December 17, 1991, for use as the fourth and fifth (booster) doses in the pertussis series following a primary series of whole-cell vaccine. A reformulation of the Lederle-Takeda vaccine was licensed

for use in the infant primary series on December 30, 1996, and subsequently received licensure for the fourth and fifth doses as well. ACEL-IMUNE was produced by Wyeth-Lederle Vaccines and Pediatrics and combined the acellular pertussis vaccine manufactured by Takeda Chemical Industries, Ltd. (Osaka, Japan), with diphtheria and tetanus toxoids manufactured by Wyeth-Lederle Laboratories (Pearl River, NY). The acellular pertussis vaccine component contained approximately 3.5 µg PT, 35 µg FHA, 2 µg PRN, and 0.8 µg FIM-2. All components were detoxified with formaldehyde. Early in 2001, Wyeth-Lederle ceased manufacture and distribution of this vaccine.

AVENTIS PASTEUR, UNITED STATES (TRIPEDIA)

The Aventis Pasteur–Biken DTaP, marketed as Tripedia, was licensed August 21, 1992, for use as the fourth and fifth (booster) doses in the pertussis series following a primary series of whole-cell vaccine. Tripedia was licensed for use in the infant primary series on July 31, 1996, and was subsequently licensed for the fourth and fifth doses after a primary series of the vaccine. Tripedia is produced by Aventis Pasteur (United States) and combines the acellular pertussis vaccine manufactured by Biken and Tanabe Corporation (Osaka, Japan) with diphtheria and tetanus toxoids manufactured by Aventis Pasteur. The acellular pertussis vaccine component contains approximately 23.4 µg PT and 23.4 µg FHA. The vaccine is supplied in preservative-free single-dose vials and in 7.5-mL multidose vials containing thimerosal as a preservative. The acellular pertussis component also is marketed as a stand-alone product in Germany.

For toddlers, Tripedia may be used to reconstitute Aventis Pasteur's conjugate Hib vaccine, ActHIB, so that the fourth dose of DTaP and the booster dose of conjugate Hib vaccine (representing either the third or the fourth Hib dose, depending on the choice of prior Hib vaccine) may be given via a single injection. The two vaccines are marketed together for this purpose under the trade name TriHIBit (see Chapters 14 and 29).

GLAXOSMITHKLINE (INFANRIX)

On January 29, 1997, the Food and Drug Administration (FDA) licensed a three-component acellular pertussis vaccine distributed by GlaxoSmithKline Pharmaceuticals for use in infants and children. The GlaxoSmithKline DTaP, marketed as Infanrix, consists of acellular pertussis components manufactured by GlaxoSmithKline Biologicals (Rixensart, Belgium) plus diphtheria and tetanus toxoids manufactured by Chiron Behring GmbH & Co (Marburg, Germany). The acellular pertussis vaccine component contains not less than 25 µg PT, 25 µg FHA, and 8 µg PRN. The vaccine is supplied as a turbid white suspension in packages of 10 single-dose thimerosal-free vials or prefilled syringes. The vaccine currently is not licensed in the United States for the fifth dose in children who have received any prior doses of DTaP. Infanrix is marketed in many countries, often in combination with other components such as IPV, Hib vaccine, or HBV vaccine.

TABLE 21-5 ■ Pertussis Immunization Schedules Recommended by Selected National Authorities, as of July 2002*†

Country	Primary Vaccination Schedule	Pediatric Boosters	Adolescent-Adult Boosters
GLOBAL: MOST COUNTRIES IN AFRICA, THE MIDDLE EAST, AND ASIA (EXCEPT AS SHOWN OTHERWISE HEREIN)			
EPI Programs	6, 10, 14 wk: DTP	18 mo to 4 yr: DTP	
NORTH AMERICA			
Canada	2, 4, 6 mo: DTaP-IPV-Hib	18 mo: DTaP-IPV-HIB; 4-6 yr: DTaP-IPV	14-16 yr: Tdap (or Td)
United States	2, 4, 6 mo: DTaP	15-18 mo and 4-6 yr: DTaP	
Mexico	2, 4, 6 mo: DTP-Hib-HB	2 and 4 yr: DTP	
EUROPE			
Austria	2, 3, 4 mo: DTaP-IPV-Hib-HB	13-18 mo: DTaP-IPV-Hib-HB; 7 yr: Tdap-IPV	14-15 yr: Tdap-IPV
Belgium	2, 3, 4 mo: DTaP-Hib-IPV	13-18 mo: DTaP-Hib-IPV; 5 yr: Tdap-IPV or Td-IPV	
Czech Republic	3, 4, 5 mo: DTP	18 mo and 5 yr: DTP	
Denmark	3, 5, 12 mo: DTaP-IPV-Hib		
Finland	3, 4, 5 mo: DTP	20-24 mo: DTP	
France	2, 3, 4 mo: DTP	16 mo: DTP	
Germany	2, 3, 4 mo: DTaP-IPV-Hib-Hb	11 mo: DTaP-IPV-Hib-Hb	9-17 yr: Tdap
Greece	Approx 2, 4, 6 mo: DTaP or DTP	18 mo and 4-5 yr: DTP or DTaP	
Hungary	3, 4, 5 mo: DTP	3 yr and 6 yr: DTP	
Iceland	3, 5, 12 mo: DTaP-IPV	5 yr: DTaP	
Ireland	2, 4, 6 mo: DTaP-IPV-Hib	4-5 yr: DTaP-IPV	
Israel	2, 4, 6 mo: DTP	12 mo: DTP	
Italy	2, 4, 10 mo: DTaP	4-5 yr: DTaP	
Luxembourg	2, 3, 4 mo: DTaP-IPV-Hib	11 mo: DTaP-IPV-Hib	
The Netherlands	2, 3, 4 mo: DTP-IPV	11 mo: DTP-IPV; 4 yr: DTaP-IPV	
Norway	3, 5, 12 mo: DTaP		
Poland	2, 3-4, 5 mo: DTP	18 mo: DTP	
Portugal	2, 4, 6 mo: DTP	15 mo and 5 yr: DTP	
Russia	3, 4, 5 mo: DTP	18 mo: DTP	
Slovakia	2, 3, 9 mo: DTP	24 mo: DTP	
Spain	2, 4, 6 mo: DTP or DTaP	18 mo and 6 yr: DTP or DTaP	
Sweden	3, 5, 12 mo: DTaP		
Switzerland	2, 4, 6 mo: DTaP-IPV-Hib	15 mo: DTaP-IPV-Hib; 4 yr: DTaP	
United Kingdom	2, 3, 4 mo: DTP-Hib	3-5 yr: DTaP	
CENTRAL AND SOUTH AMERICA (MOST COUNTRIES NOT SHOWN FOLLOW A SCHEDULE SIMILAR TO ONE OF THE FOLLOWING)			
Argentina	2, 4, 6 mo: DTP-Hib	18 mo: DTP-Hib; 4-5 yr: DTP	
Brazil	2, 4, 6 mo: DTP	15 mo: DTP	
Chile	2, 4, 6 mo: DTP	18 mo and 4 yr: DTP	
El Salvador	2, 3, 4 mo: DTP	15 mo and 4-5 yr: DTP	
French Guiana	2, 3, 4 mo: DTP	1 and 5 yr: DTP	10 yr: DTP
Peru	2, 3, 4 mo: DTP		
Trinidad/Tobago	3, 4.5, 6 mo: DTP	18 mo and 4-5 yr: DTP	
Uruguay	2, 4, 6 mo: DTP-Hib	12 mo: DTP-Hib	
ASIA (MOST COUNTRIES NOT SHOWN GENERALLY FOLLOW THE EPI SCHEDULE)			
Australia	2, 4, 6 mo: DTaP or DTaP-HB	18 mo and 4 yr: DTaP	
China	3, 4, 5 mo: DTP	18-24 mo: DTP	
Indonesia	2-11 mo: 3 doses DTP		
Japan	3-12 mo: 3 doses DTaP	12-18 mo: DTaP	
Republic of Korea	2, 4, 6 mo: DTaP		
Malaysia	3, 4, 5 mo: DTP	18 mo: DTP	
New Zealand	6 wk, 3mo, 5 mo: DTaP	15 mo: DTaP	
Taiwan	2, 4, 6 mo: DTP	18 mo: DTP	
Thailand	2, 4, 6 mo: DTP	18-30 mo and 4-6 yr: DTP	

*Complied from multiple sources. In many countries, products based on whole-cell pertussis vaccine are used in the national or public programs (shown in the above table), whereas products based on acellular vaccines often are used in private practice. In such countries, recommended schedules for private practice typically are based on U.S. or Western European schedules.

†As of August 2002, the WHO maintained an interactive resource that displayed demographic data, incidence of vaccine-preventable diseases, and recent (but not necessarily current) immunization schedules by selected country, at *www-nt.who.int/vaccines/globalsummary/Immunization/CountryProfileSelect.cfm*.

TABLE 21–6 ■ Current Major Vaccine Manufacturers and Their Merged, Acquired, or Component Companies

Name as of July 2002	Former, Merged, Acquired, or Component Companies or Names
Aventis Pasteur	Connaught Laboratories; Pasteur Mérieux; Pasteur Mérieux Connaught
Baxter Laboratories	Acambis (20% ownership); AMVAX; North American Vaccine
Berna Biotech	Berna; Swiss Serum Institute (SSI); Rhein Biotech; Korean Green Cross
Chiron Vaccines	Behring; Biocine; Sclavo
GlaxoSmithKline	Glaxo; Glaxo Wellcome; SmithKline Beecham; Wellcome; SmithKline–RIT; RIT (Recherche et Industrie Thérapeutiques)
Merck & Co	
Powderject Vaccines	Evans Vaccines; Medeva Vaccines; SBL Vaccines
Wyeth Pharmaceuticals	American Home Products; Lederle Laboratories; Praxis; Wyeth-Ayerst Laboratories; Wyeth Lederle; Wyeth Vaccines

BAXTER PHARMACEUTICALS (CERTIVA)

Certiva was licensed for use in infants and children on July 29, 1998. It is a monovalent pertussis vaccine (the pertussis component consists solely of 40 µg inactivated PT). The vaccine was developed by the National Institute of Child Health and Human Development (NICHD) and is unique in that the pertussis component is detoxified with hydrogen peroxide. Certiva was manufactured by North American Vaccine (AMVAX) prior to their purchase by Baxter. The vaccine currently is not being marketed in the United States, but continues to be produced in bulk for inclusion in the Danish DTaP-IPV combination vaccine.

AVENTIS PASTEUR, CANADA (TRIPACEL, DAPTACEL, TRIACEL, MONOCEL)

Aventis Pasteur Ltd (Willowdale, Ontario, Canada) produces a multicomponent acellular pertussis vaccine that is marketed in most countries as Tripacel (Tables 21–3 and 21–4) but in the United States as DAPTACEL and in Latin America as Triacel or Monocel. The acellular pertussis vaccine component contains approximately 10 µg PT, 5 µg FHA, 3 µg PRN, and 5 µg of combined FIM-2 and FIM-3. A formulation (known as the "hybrid" version) that differs by increasing the PT and FHA concentrations to 20 µg each is used in the production of combination vaccines (e.g., combined with IPV as Quadracel, or combined with IPV and Hib as Pediacel; see Chapter 29 for further details, including additional combinations). Because these vaccines contain PT, FHA, PRN, and both FIM-2 and FIM-3, they are commonly referred to as five-component vaccines. Daptacel is supplied in packages of one or five thimerosal-free single-dose vials.

Preparations Licensed Only in Countries Other than the United States

As of spring 2002, several acellular pertussis vaccines have been licensed in other countries but have not (as yet) been licensed in the United States. The characteristics and trade names of these vaccines may vary in some jurisdictions from those given here; local suppliers should be consulted as necessary.

AVENTIS PASTEUR, FRANCE (TRIAVAX IN EUROPE, TRIAXIM ELSEWHERE)

This two-component DTaP vaccine was developed by Aventis Pasteur (Lyon, France) and is marketed in Europe as Triavax and outside Europe as Triaxim. The acellular pertussis vaccine component contains approximately 25 µg PT and 25 µg FHA. The vaccine is available combined with Hib as Tetravac or combined with Hib and IPV as Pentavac.

AVENTIS PASTEUR, CANADA (ADACEL, COVAXIS; ALSO AVAILABLE COMBINED WITH IPV AS REPEVAX)

Aventis Pasteur Ltd (Willowdale, Ontario, Canada) produces an adolescent-adult formulation of their five-component acellular pertussis vaccine that differs from Tripacel (see Table 21–3) by containing reduced quantities of PT (2.5 µg) and FHA (5 µg). Combined with adult diphtheria and tetanus toxoids (Td) (2 Lf D and 5 Lf T) , this adult-formulation acellular pertussis vaccine and tetanus and diphtheria toxoids (Tdap) vaccine is marketed in Canada as Adacel and in Europe as Covaxis. A fully liquid combination of Adacel plus IPV is marketed in Europe as Repevax (see Chapter 29).

CHIRON VACCINES (ACELLUVAX, TRIACELLUVAX, ACELLUVAX DTP)

Triacelluvax is a three-component acellular pertussis vaccine manufactured by Chiron Vaccines SpA (Siena, Italy; previously Biocine Sclavo). Triacelluvax contains 5 µg PT, 2.5 µg FHA, and 2.5 µg PRN. The vaccine is unique in that the pertussis toxoid component consists of a recombinant PT that is genetically detoxified using molecular techniques to alter two amino acids for the S1 subunit of B. pertussis toxin,[212] resulting in the lack of PT enzymatic activity. A number of prelicensure clinical trials were conducted in U.S. children, but in 1999 Chiron withdrew its FDA license application. On October 15, 2001, the European marketing authorization for Triacelluvax was voluntarily withdrawn. Combined with diphtheria and tetanus toxoids, the vaccine continues to be marketed as Triacelluvax in Italy and Acelluvax DTP elsewhere.

GLAXOSMITHKLINE (BOOSTRIX)

GlaxoSmithKline produces an adolescent-adult formulation of their three-component acellular pertussis vaccine that differs from Infanrix (see Table 21–3) by containing reduced quantities of PT (8 µg), FHA (8 µg), and PRN (2.5 µg), combined with diphtheria (2.5 Lf) and tetanus (5 Lf) toxoids manufactured by Chiron Behring GmbH & Co (Marburg, Germany). This Tdap vaccine is licensed in Australia, Europe, and elsewhere.

Preparations Not Submitted for Licensure

Several additional acellular pertussis vaccines were developed during the 1980s and 1990s but have not been licensed anywhere and are not known to be undergoing further development. Interested readers are referred to the prior edition of this text[213] for further details.

Vaccine Schedule Deviations

A failure to adhere to the recommended schedule, causing a delay between doses, should not interfere with the final immunity achieved by any of the pertussis vaccines. There is no need to start the series over again, regardless of the time between doses. Partial doses should not be given; there is no evidence that doing so reduces the frequency of serious adverse events, and there is the risk that efficacy might be impaired.

Interchangeability of Vaccines

Few data are available demonstrating the effects of a change during the scheduled immunization series from one brand of DTaP to another. Recommendations of the Advisory Committee on Immunization Practices (ACIP) and the American Academy of Pediatrics Committee on Infectious Diseases (Red Book Committee) therefore have indicated a preference to use the same brand of DTaP vaccine for all doses of the vaccination series for a given child. However, the recommendations also state that, if the vaccine provider does not know, or does not have available, the brand of DTaP previously administered to a child, any of the licensed DTaP vaccines may be used to complete the vaccination series. Moreover, the one published study evaluating a change from one DTaP (Tripedia) to another (Infanrix) during the primary series found no adverse effect on safety or immunogenicity.[214] As a practical matter, free interchange of the various acellular pertussis vaccines has become commonplace, fueled by periodic changes in public distribution systems, the vagaries of patient migration and shifting provider purchases, and intermittent shortages of one vaccine or another.

Simultaneous Administration with Other Vaccines

DTP and DTaP are routinely administered concomitantly with polio vaccine (oral or injectable), conjugate Hib vaccine, conjugate pneumococcal vaccine, HBV vaccine, measles-mumps-rubella vaccine, and varicella vaccine, as appropriate to the age and previous vaccination status of the child, using separate syringes for injections at separate sites. Most studies have found that the adverse reactions after multiple simultaneous vaccinations are only slightly greater than would be expected from the most reactogenic vaccine alone. Further reductions in adverse reactions can often be obtained by using vaccines that combine various of these entities (see Chapter 29), thereby reducing the number of injections given. Although reduced immunogenicity to the pertussis antigens has occasionally been seen when given in combination or association with one or more of the other vaccines, no data exist to suggest that concomitant administration of any of these other vaccines decreases the efficacy of pertussis vaccine.[215,216] Because whole-cell pertussis vaccine has adjuvant properties, replacement of the whole-cell component with acellular vaccine has resulted in reports of diminution of the immune responses to some of the simultaneously administered vaccines (see Chapter 29), without evidence of impairment of efficacy.

Results of Vaccination: Whole-Cell Pertussis Vaccines

Overview

Although some observers have challenged whole-cell pertussis vaccine as being ineffective, dangerous, or superfluous,[217,218] most authorities agree that the widespread use of the vaccine has had enormous benefits.[183,219,220] Observations that have led to this conclusion include the results of clinical trials; the rapid decline in morbidity and mortality from pertussis concomitant with the implementation of vaccine programs; the recurrence of disease in countries in which immunization has been discontinued, rates of acceptance have declined markedly, or vaccines have become ineffective; the inverse correlation of the pertussis attack rate with the proportion of immunized children in communities in which pertussis becomes epidemic; and the lower attack rates in previously immunized children than in unimmunized children under both endemic and epidemic conditions.

Immune Responses to Whole-Cell Vaccines

Many of the world's children are immunized with whole-cell pertussis vaccines produced locally. Few data exist that compare the safety, immunogenicity, and efficacy of individual whole-cell products produced in various countries. Most authorities had presumed that all whole-cell vaccines were very similar and that one was as immunogenic and effective as another. However, when significant differences in immune responses were noted with whole-cell pertussis products produced by different manufacturers in the United States and Canada, it became apparent that all whole-cell vaccines were not the same.[178,221,222] The

European acellular pertussis vaccine efficacy trials, using whole-cell vaccines produced in several different countries, demonstrated substantial differences in efficacy among the various products. Thus it appears possible that some of the whole-cell pertussis vaccines produced in various countries in the world and administered to infants and children might be less effective than others. The impact of these differences on the global burden of pertussis disease is unknown.

Another concern with whole-cell pertussis vaccines is the negative impact of high maternal antibody levels on infant immune responses. It has been demonstrated that the magnitude of the primary antibody response to whole-cell vaccine in infants depends on the preimmunization (transplacental) levels of antibody to PT, with higher circulating levels of maternally derived antibody being associated with significantly lower levels of postimmunization antibody.[192] In contrast, PT antibody responses to an acellular vaccine containing 12.5 µg each of PT and FHA were superior to those of the whole-cell vaccine and were not affected by prevaccination antibody levels.[192] Studies in developing countries have not evaluated the impact of maternal antibody on immune responses to locally produced whole-cell vaccines in young children.

Controlled Clinical Trials of Whole-Cell Vaccines

It is well documented by controlled clinical trials that pertussis vaccine provides protection against clinical whooping cough after exposure in the majority of immunized people. The first convincing evidence was provided by studies in the Faroe Islands during two epidemics.[199] These studies showed that pertussis vaccine not only protected against disease but also ameliorated the severity of disease in immunized individuals who contracted the illness. Although studies with early vaccines produced inconsistent results,[11,183,220,223] clinical trials subsequent to standardization of the vaccines by the mouse protection test[219] demonstrated clear-cut, consistent efficacy.[219,224,225]

In more recent years, a number of field trials of acellular pertussis vaccines (see below under *Efficacy Trials, 1992 to 1997*) have incorporated whole-cell pertussis vaccines as controls and have provided some of the best data ever obtained about the efficacy of the conventional whole-cell vaccines. As mentioned previously, these studies suggest that whole-cell vaccines vary substantially in efficacy. (The following estimates reflect efficacy after three doses and, to the extent possible, consistent case definitions; however, none of these studies was fully blinded and randomized, and these estimates may be generous.) The Mainz[226] and Munich[227] studies produced efficacy estimates of 98% and 96%, respectively, for the German-produced Behringwerke vaccine; the U.S.-made Wyeth-Lederle whole-cell vaccine was reported to be 83% efficacious in the Erlangen trial[180,228]; and the Senegal trial reported the French-made Aventis Pasteur whole-cell vaccine to be 96% efficacious.[229] In each of these trials, the whole-cell vaccine was more efficacious than the acellular product.

In marked contrast, the U.S.-made Connaught whole-cell vaccine had very low rates of efficacy after three doses: 48% in Sweden and 36% in Italy.[181,182] Vaccine efficacy of the Connaught whole-cell vaccine was nearly 74% for the first 6 months after the third dose of vaccine but declined rapidly after that time.[181]

A British national survey of reported whooping cough from 1989 to 1990 determined that the efficacy of the Wellcome whole-cell vaccine, administered at 3, 5, and 10 months of age, was 87% and 93% during epidemic and nonepidemic periods, respectively.[230] Efficacy declined with age but remained high until the age of 8 years. A repeat survey was conducted in 1994 to determine whether efficacy had been altered by the change to an accelerated schedule of immunization at 2, 3, and 4 months of age (with no subsequent booster). Efficacy was not altered and was 94% overall for those subjects between 6 months and 5 years of age.[231] This accelerated schedule was also associated with a reduced rate of adverse reactions compared with the prior schedule.[232]

Other Evidence of Effectiveness of Whole-Cell Vaccines

Secular Changes in Morbidity and Mortality

There is no question that the widespread use of whole-cell pertussis vaccine in developed countries has been associated with a remarkable decline in reported pertussis.[162,163,183,233] However, it is also clear that mortality rates from pertussis were declining in at least some of these countries even before the advent of the vaccine.[162,183,219,234,235] The latter reductions likely reflect a decrease in case-fatality rates as a result of such factors as improved social and economic conditions, better nutrition, and declines in concomitant infections that may have enhanced pertussis mortality.

Effects of the Withdrawal of Pertussis Immunization

Strong evidence of the benefits of pertussis vaccine was provided by unintended experiments that occurred in three developed countries when vaccine use was curtailed or abandoned. Japan initiated widespread immunization against pertussis in 1950, and over the ensuing years the numbers of reported cases and the numbers of deaths declined remarkably (Fig. 21–4).[163,236] However, beginning in 1975, adverse events temporally associated with administration of whole-cell pertussis vaccine to young children led to a near-boycott of the vaccine and epidemic pertussis recurred. Hundreds of children died of pertussis during this period.[163] A similar experience occurred in England and Wales, in the context of negative publicity surrounding adverse events associated with vaccine. Rates of vaccine acceptance fell from approximately 75% to nearly 25% during the mid-1970s, major epidemics of pertussis ensued, and numerous children died.[162,237] In Sweden, the administration of pertussis vaccine was suspended in 1979 when pertussis outbreaks occurred despite high vaccination coverage, suggesting poor efficacy of the vaccine then in use. The incidence of whooping cough then increased more than fourfold from 1980 to 1985, with several major outbreaks in subsequent years.[238,239] With the advent of routine pertussis immunization using acellular vaccines, pertussis rates in Sweden have now declined markedly.[240] A review of French experience over a period of 30 years showed persistent high efficacy of whole-cell vaccine.[241]

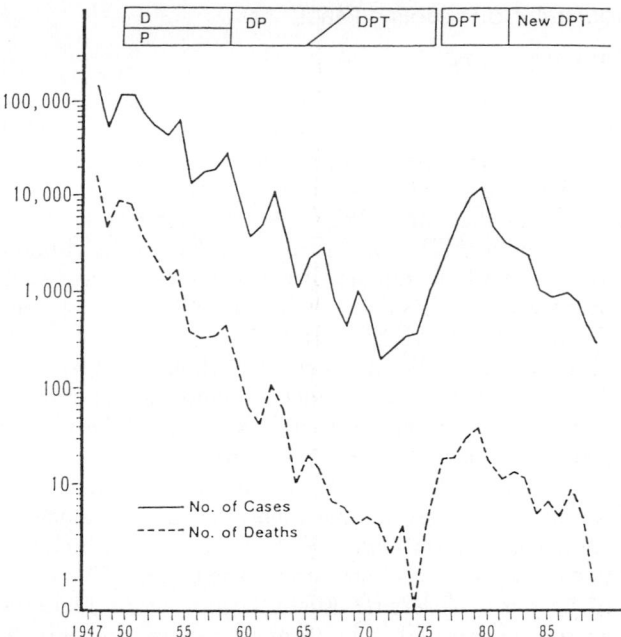

FIGURE 21–4 ■ Number of reported pertussis cases and deaths, by year, in Japan from 1947 to 1990. "New DPT" refers to the Biken- and Takeda-type acellular vaccines (see text). (From Kimura M. Japanese clinical experiences with acellular pertussis vaccines. Dev Biol Stand 73:5–9, 1991, with permission.)

Pertussis Rates in Vaccinated and Unvaccinated Communities

Further evidence of the efficacy of whole-cell pertussis vaccine is provided by the observation that the reported incidence of pertussis disease varies inversely with vaccine acceptance rates. A study in England and Wales found that communities with low pertussis vaccine acceptance rates (<30%) had a 59% higher reported incidence of pertussis among children than did areas with high (>50%) acceptance rates; areas with intermediate acceptance rates had intermediate pertussis rates.[242] These findings were not explained by differences among the communities such as crowding and social class; indeed, after adjustment for these two social indicators, the inverse correlation with immunization status was, if anything, stronger. In the United States, where infant immunization for pertussis has been routine since the late 1940s or early 1950s, national surveillance demonstrated a greater than 95% reduction in pertussis; surveillance data from 1992 to 1994 found an overall whole-cell pertussis vaccine efficacy of 64% after three doses and of 82% after four or more doses.[15]

Pertussis Attack Rates in Immunized and Unimmunized Children During Outbreaks

Additional evidence for the efficacy of whole-cell pertussis vaccine is provided by community outbreaks of pertussis in which the attack rates of the disease in immunized children were compared with the rates in those who were incompletely or never immunized.[162,243,244] Although the methods of ascertainment and analysis vary, most studies indicate that the efficacy of three or more doses of pertussis vaccine in protecting children against clinical disease during outbreaks is 80% to 90%, with incomplete immunization offering partial protection.[243] In children who contracted pertussis in spite of immunization, the disease was milder and complications were far less frequent, despite the fact that younger infants and children are more likely to have received inadequate or no immunization.[245,246]

Herd Immunity After Immunization

In view of the fact that whole-cell pertussis vaccine is not 100% effective, it could be considered curious that morbidity and mortality from clinical pertussis have been negligible in countries with widespread immunization programs. This is a particularly interesting finding because surveillance statistics and studies demonstrating pertussis to be a common cause of protracted cough illness in adolescents and adults suggest that B. pertussis remains ubiquitous in these countries.[125,127,135,188–190] Attempts to model mathematically the decline in pertussis incidence attributable to widespread immunization with vaccines of 85% efficacy have underestimated the rates of decline of the disease.[247] Although other factors, such as social and economic changes, likely play a role, the most probable explanation is herd immunity, a complex phenomenon that varies among different infectious diseases and is difficult to measure with precision[248] (see Chapter 56). Herd immunity undoubtedly explains the cycles of outbreaks of pertussis every 3 or 4 years; after an outbreak, several years are required for the proportion of susceptible individuals to increase to a level that facilitates a new wave of rapid spread within a population. Finally, recent studies describing higher rates of pertussis disease in immunized children living in communities with large numbers of unimmunized children provide additional evidence for the role of herd immunity.[249]

Duration of Immunity After Whole-Cell Vaccines

A number of studies have evaluated the duration of protection after immunization with whole-cell vaccine. Those that provide the longest period of evaluation indicate that protection declines by 50% over a period of 6 to 12 years.[250–252] These data are consistent with the incidence and serosurvey data cited previously that suggest an increase in rates of pertussis among 13- to 17-year-olds, representing an interval of 7 to 12 years since last vaccination.[127] It is likely that the duration of protection is influenced by the vaccine used, the number of doses given, the vaccination schedule, and the level of circulating B. pertussis capable of stimulating an amnestic response in previously immunized individuals.

Adverse Events with Whole-Cell Vaccines

Overview

Despite their clear benefits in reducing the substantial mortality and morbidity of pertussis, the whole-cell vaccines have long been recognized as our least satisfactory vaccines with respect to adverse reactions. They commonly cause reactions that are minor but burdensome, occasionally cause reactions that are transient but frightening, and uncommonly cause more serious, generally self-limited, adverse effects. For some time, there was substantial suspicion that whole-cell vaccines might be causally related to devastating outcomes such as encephalopathy or sudden infant death syndrome (SIDS), but several careful epidemiologic studies have largely dispelled these concerns.

Untoward events after pertussis immunization began to be of increasing concern to the public and to physicians in the early 1970s, particularly in countries where widespread vaccination had eliminated most disease. Vaccine-associated adverse events loomed large in the eyes of young parents and physicians who had never witnessed the morbidity and mortality of whooping cough. Widespread publicity about the alleged dangers of pertussis vaccine, coupled with declining disease rates in some countries and doubts about vaccine efficacy in others, resulted in near-abandonment of pertussis vaccine in several countries. Consequently, pertussis disease recurred.[162,163,238] In the United States, strong school-entry immunization laws enabled vaccination rates to be maintained despite widespread publicity about these concerns. Extensive litigation over alleged personal injuries caused by the vaccine cost millions of dollars and contributed to the cessation of pertussis vaccine production by several manufacturers.

Establishing or disproving cause and effect, particularly for events of major consequence, proved difficult. Although the original allegations of causation were largely anecdotal and based on the fallacious assumption that *subsequences* and *consequences* were synonymous, they raised great concern and stimulated the search for an improved vaccine. The relationships between whole-cell pertussis vaccine and fatal or disabling events were difficult to evaluate because of the rarity of such events; because vaccine was administered to infants at an age when disorders such as encephalopathy, infantile spasms, neurologic conditions, and SIDS were most likely to occur; because these disorders can arise from other causes; and because an absolute negative can never be proved. Earlier estimates of the rates of adverse events were not optimal because of lack of consideration of background rates, ill-defined criteria, and uncertainty of denominators. However, in the 1980s, more rigorous epidemiologic or interventional studies greatly improved the understanding of the incidence and spectrum of adverse events after whole-cell pertussis vaccine. Many of these studies, particularly those related to serious untoward events, were evaluated by a special committee of the Institute of Medicine (IOM) of the U.S. National Academy of Sciences.[141-143] Although these evaluations were reassuring to health care providers and parents alike, it was the development of less reactogenic acellular pertussis vaccines and their replacement of the whole-cell products that put an end to the long debate in developed countries over adverse events associated with whole-cell vaccines. Whole-cell pertussis vaccines remain widely used in the United Kingdom, France, and developing countries, where concerns regarding adverse events do not seem to be important local issues.

In light of the continuing move toward acellular vaccines, we restrict the discussion of adverse events associated with whole-cell vaccines to a summary of the key studies and conclusions. Readers interested in a more thorough review of these data are referred to the second edition of this text.[253]

Nonfatal, Nondisabling Reactions

COMMON REACTIONS

Minor local reactions, consisting of redness, swelling, and pain at the site of injection, occur in about half of DTP recipients. Reactions occur five times more frequently after DTP than DT.[254] Similarly, minor systemic reactions such as fever, irritability, and drowsiness are significantly more common after DTP than DT.[254] About half of the children who receive whole-cell pertussis vaccine experience some minor fever, with less than 1% having an elevation in temperature to 40.5°C (105°F).[254,255]

Participants in the Multicenter Acellular Pertussis Trial (MAPT; see below) experienced somnolence at rates of 62% for whole-cell recipients and 43% for acellular vaccine recipients,[255] suggesting that the somnolence was, at least in part, an effect of the DTP vaccine. Some children are reported to have an unusual high-pitched cry. Somewhat more remarkable is a period of excessive crying, which may last several hours or longer after an injection. This incessant, inconsolable crying usually begins within 12 hours. Persistent crying of 1 hour or more occurred in both the DTP and DT groups in the Cody et al. study but was at least four times more common after DTP. Among those with persistent crying, the cry was described as high-pitched or unusual in 3.5% of the children.[254] This reaction appears to be a unique response to inoculation with DTP.

These common reactions vary somewhat in frequency and severity among lots[256] and manufacturers.[220] The vaccine schedule followed also may affect the incidence and severity of adverse reactions. In 1990, the schedule for DTP vaccination in the United Kingdom was changed from 3, 5, and 10 months of age to 2, 3, and 4 months of age. The new schedule has been associated with a substantial reduction in postvaccination fever and redness of the injection site.[232] With the accelerated vaccination schedule in the United Kingdom, reaction rates for the whole-cell vaccine did not differ significantly from those of several acellular vaccines.[232]

Reaction rates also vary with the number of prior DTP injections. In the Cody et al. study, local reactions increased in frequency with successive doses, including the preschool booster.[254] The incidence of fever also increased with successive doses through the 18-month booster, but was lower with the preschool booster. Conversely, persistent, inconsolable crying occurred most frequently with the initial dose and less often thereafter. In the MAPT, the incidence and severity of fever increased substantially with successive primary doses of the reference whole-cell vaccine.[255,257] Redness increased modestly; the frequency of pain, fussiness, anorexia, vomiting, and the use of antipyretics did not materially increase or decrease with successive doses; and drowsiness decreased.[255] In general, children who have experienced local or systemic reactions after pertussis vaccine have an enhanced likelihood of experiencing the same reaction with a subsequent dose.[258]

UNCOMMON REACTIONS

DTP is associated with febrile seizures (0.06% in the Cody et al. trial), and seizures occur at increased rates after DTP in children with personal or family histories of convulsions.[254, 259-265] However, simple convulsions, although distressing, are considered to be benign.[259,266] There is no evidence to support the concern that seizures after the receipt of DTP might induce epilepsy in some children.[267]

Another worrisome but uncommon reaction to DTP is that of a strange shock-like state, termed a *hypotonic-hyporesponsive episode* (HHE), that usually has its onset within 12 hours of inoculation and may last for several hours but always resolves.[268] Neither death nor adverse sequelae have been observed after these episodes. The Cody et al. study detected nine HHEs, for an incidence of 0.06%.[254] The mechanism of this phenomenon is unknown. HHE has been seen with other vaccines, including acellular pertussis products, as described later.

Serious Reactions Allegedly Caused by Whole-Cell Pertussis Vaccine

ENCEPHALOPATHY

The most serious reaction that has been attributed to whole-cell pertussis vaccine is acute encephalopathy, the first anecdotal report of which was made in 1933.[199] The National Childhood Encephalopathy Study, conducted in Great Britain from 1976 to 1979, examined whether the frequency of vaccination in children with encephalopathy was greater than expected. It compared children ages 2 months to 3 years admitted to a hospital for serious acute neurologic disease with a control group of normal children. Based on 11 subjects who appeared to have residua 18 months later, it was estimated that acute encephalopathy with permanent brain damage occurred at the widely quoted rate of 1 per 310,000 doses, with a 95% CI of 1 in 54,000 to 5,310,000 doses. However, subsequent investigations cast doubt on most of these 11 diagnoses.[269-271] A 10-year follow-up evaluation was conducted of all the children included in the original study and their age-matched control subjects. More than 80% of these individuals were traced. The prevalence rates for death or other sequelae were similar regardless of whether or not the onset of acute neurologic illness was temporally associated with DTP vaccination. The investigators concluded that whole-cell pertussis immunization "may on rare occasions be associated with the development of severe acute neurologic illness that can have serious sequelae."[272]

The results of the National Childhood Encephalopathy Study have been subjected to extensive analysis, reanalysis, challenge, and debate,[271-277] none of which has overturned the investigators' initial cautious interpretation that the data suggested but did not prove a causal relationship between pertussis vaccine and permanent neurologic damage. Several U.S. studies also failed to show a relation between vaccine and acute encephalopathy leading to brain damage.[260-262] In 1994, the IOM concluded that the "balance of evidence is consistent with a causal relation between DTP and chronic nervous system dysfunction in children whose serious acute neurologic illness occurred within 7 days of DTP vaccination."[278] However, the IOM was not able to determine whether the pertussis vaccine increased the number of children with chronic neurologic illness or was simply a precipitating event in children who would have nonetheless developed chronic neurologic dysfunction as a result of underlying brain or metabolic abnormalities.

INFANTILE SPASMS

Infantile spasms, which occur in about 40 per 100,000 infants,[279] have been reported in temporal association with pertussis vaccination.[280] Because infantile spasms typically present between 2 and 8 months of age, it is obvious that an association is occasionally seen by chance alone. Four studies have demonstrated no foundation for concern that DTP causes infantile spasms.[270,281-283]

SUDDEN INFANT DEATH SYNDROME

Because SIDS occurs most often in the first 6 months of life,[284] it is to be expected by chance alone that some instances would be observed within a day or two of receipt of DTP. Several early reports suggested clustering of SIDS cases within a few days after the administration of DTP,[285-289] but subsequent studies found no evidence of a causal relationship between SIDS and receipt of DTP.[290-297] The IOM panel, after a careful review of all studies, also concluded that no causal relationship existed.[298-300]

OTHER SERIOUS CONDITIONS

The IOM panel examined the evidence concerning an association between DTP and a variety of syndromes; their conclusions are summarized in Table 21–7.[298-300]

TABLE 21–7 ■ **Institute of Medicine Conclusions Regarding Causation of Serious Adverse Events by DTP**

Event	Conclusion
Evidence indicates causation	Anaphylaxis Prolonged or inconsolable crying Febrile seizures
Evidence consistent with causation	Acute encephalopathy Hypotonic-hyporesponsive episodes
Evidence does not indicate causation	Afebrile seizures Hypsarrhythmia Infantile spasms Reye's syndrome Sudden infant death syndrome
Insufficient evidence to draw a conclusion	Aseptic meningitis Chronic neurologic damage Epilepsy Erythema multiforme or other rashes Guillain-Barré syndrome Hemolytic anemia Juvenile diabetes Learning or attention disorders Peripheral mononeuropathy Thrombocytopenia
No evidence available either way	Autism

Data from Howson CP, Howe CJ, Fineberg HV (eds). Adverse effects of pertussis and rubella vaccines: a report of the Committee to Review the Adverse Consequences of Pertussis and Rubella Vaccines. Washington, DC: National Academy Press, 1991; Howson CP, Fineberg HV. Adverse events following pertussis and rubella vaccines: summary of a report of the Institute of Medicine. JAMA 267:392–396, 1992; and Howson CP, Fineberg HV. The ricochet of magic bullets: summary of the Institute of Medicine report, Adverse effects of pertussis and rubella vaccines. Pediatrics 89:318–324, 1992.

U.S. National Childhood Vaccine Injury Act

Increasing litigation over alleged vaccine injuries and withdrawal from the marketplace of vaccines by several DTP manufacturers prompted the U.S. Congress in 1986 to pass the National Childhood Vaccine Injury Act, which provides compensation for certain untoward events that occur within specified time periods after vaccination. In 1995, program rules were revised in light of the report of the IOM committee.[298-300] The replacement of whole-cell with acellular pertussis vaccines has markedly reduced the rates of adverse reactions temporally associated with vaccine,[301] resulting in a corresponding decline in vaccine injury claims.[302]

Results of Vaccination: Acellular Pertussis Vaccines

Immune Responses to Acellular Vaccines

Humoral Immunity

Numerous immunogenicity and reactogenicity studies have been published, each evaluating one of the various acellular pertussis vaccines. Making comparisons across such studies, however, is an uncertain process, given the variations in study design, study populations, and serologic assays. To provide such comparisons and facilitate selection of candidate vaccines for anticipated efficacy trials, the National Institute of Allergy and Infectious Diseases (NIAID) sponsored the MAPT in six of its Vaccine Treatment and Evaluation Units from 1991 to 1992. Thirteen acellular and two whole-cell vaccines were evaluated in the MAPT, including all but one of the acellular vaccines subsequently evaluated in efficacy trials. Although this last vaccine was not made available for the MAPT, it was evaluated thereafter at one of the Vaccine Treatment and Evaluation Units using the MAPT protocol, procedures, and data forms; sera were evaluated in one of the MAPT reference laboratories. Immunogenicity and reactogenicity results from that study are presented here, along with the MAPT results, to provide the most complete available comparison of these vaccines.

Healthy infants enrolled in the MAPT were randomized to receive one of the study vaccines (see Table 21-3) at 2, 4, and 6 months of age. Whole-cell vaccines made by Lederle Laboratories (the reference or control vaccine) and the Massachusetts Public Health Biologic Laboratories also were evaluated. Sera were obtained before the first immunization and 1 month after the third immunization. Serologic assays included ELISA antibody to PT, FHA, PRN, and fimbrial proteins; Chinese hamster ovary cell and agglutination assays; and assays of diphtheria and tetanus antitoxin.[209]

Each vaccine produced significant increases in antibodies directed against its included antigens, which most often equaled or exceeded those produced by the reference whole-cell vaccine (Table 21-8).[209] Nonetheless, postimmunization antibody levels differed substantially among the acellular vaccines. For PRN and fimbrial proteins, and to some extent for FHA, antibody levels tended to correlate with the quantity of antigen included in the vaccine. For

TABLE 21-8 ■ Antibody Levels One Month Following Third Dose of Vaccine: Results from the Multicenter Acellular Pertussis Trial and a Follow-up Trial*

Manufacturer or Distributor	Vaccine[†]	Geometric Mean Antibody Level (95% CI) Following Immunization at 2, 4, and 6 Mo			
		PT	FHA	PRN	FIM
Aventis Pasteur (Canada)	*Tripacel*	36 (32–41)	37 (32–42)	114 (93–139)	240 (204–282)
Aventis Pasteur (Canada)	CLL-3F$_2$	38 (33–44)	36 (31–41)	3.4 (3.1–3.6)	230 (183–290)
Aventis Pasteur (France)	*Triavax*	68 (60–76)	143 (126–161)	3.3 (3.1–3.6)	1.9 (1.6–2.1)
Aventis Pasteur (USA)	*Tripedia*	127 (111–144)	84 (73–95)	3.5 (3.2–3.9)	2.0 (1.7–2.3)
Baxter Laboratories	*Certiva*	54 (41–71)	1.1 (1.0–1.2)	n/a	n/a
Biocine Sclavo	BSc-1	180 (163–200)	1.2 (1.1–1.4)	3.4 (3.1–3.7)	1.8 (1.7–2.0)
Chiron Vaccines	*Acelluvax*	99 (87–113)	21 (18–25)	65 (53–79)	1.9 (1.7–2.1)
GlaxoSmithKline	*Infanrix*	54 (46–64)	103 (88–120)	185 (148–231)	1.9 (1.7–2.2)
Massachusetts Public Health Biologic Labs	SSVI-1	99 (87–111)	1.2 (1.1–1.3)	3.4 (3.1–3.6)	2.1 (1.8–2.4)
Michigan Department of Public Health	Mich-2	66 (59–75)	237 (213–265)	3.2 (3.0–3.4)	2.0 (1.8–2.3)
SmithKline Beecham Biologicals	SKB-2	104 (94–116)	110 (99–122)	3.3 (3.1–3.5)	1.9 (1.7–2.1)
Speywood (Porton) Pharmaceuticals	Por-3F$_2$	29 (25–33)	20 (17–23)	3.0 (3.0–3.1)	361 (303–430)
Wyeth Lederle Vaccines and Pediatrics	LPB-3P	39 (32–48)	144 (127–163)	128 (109–150)	19 (13–27)
Wyeth Pharmaceuticals	*ACEL-IMUNE*	14 (12–17)	49 (45–54)	54 (47–62)	51 (41–63)
Wyeth Lederle Vaccines and Pediatrics	Whole-cell	67 (54–83)	3.0 (2.7–3.4)	63 (54–74)	191 (161–227)

*Results for Certiva are from a separate study conducted at a MAPT study center after completion of the MAPT, using the MAPT protocol, procedures, and data forms; sera were assayed at one of the MAPT reference laboratories.

†For those vaccines without known trade names, designation reflects source and composition of vaccine.[209] For branded products (in italics), note that the licensed vaccine's formulation may differ from that of the vaccine evaluated in MAPT.

CI, confidence interval; FHA, filamentous hemagglutinin; FIM, fimbrial proteins; MAPT, Multicenter Acellular Pertussis Trial; n/a, not available; PRN, pertactin; PT, pertussis toxin.

Adapted from Edwards KM, Meade BD, Decker MD, et al. Comparison of 13 acellular pertussis vaccines: overview and serologic response. Pediatrics 96:548–557, 1995.

PT, postimmunization antibody levels did not correlate well with the quantity of antigen in the vaccine, suggesting that manufacturing techniques were important in determining the immunogenicity of the particular PT component of each vaccine. No acellular vaccine was most or least immunogenic with respect to all included antigens.

Cell-Mediated Immunity

Animal studies,[303-306] persistent pertussis infection in human immunodeficiency virus–infected patients,[307,308] and clinical trials demonstrating protection against pertussis in the face of persistence of cell-mediated immunity (CMI) and waning antibody levels have suggested an important role for CMI in the host defense against pertussis. Mills and colleagues showed that the rate of B. pertussis clearance following respiratory challenge of immunized mice correlated with vaccine efficacy in children.[309] Using mice with targeted disruptions of the interferon-γ (IFN-γ) receptor, interleukin-4, or immunoglobulin heavy-chain genes, they demonstrated an absolute requirement for antibody in bacterial clearance and a critical role for IFN-γ in immunity generated by previous infection or immunization with the whole-cell pertussis vaccine.[309] Passive immunization experiments suggested that protection early after immunization with acellular pertussis vaccines was mediated by antibody against multiple protective antigens. In contrast, more complete protection conferred by previous infection or immunization with the whole-cell pertussis vaccines reflected the induction of Th1 cells. These findings suggested that the mechanism of immunity against B. pertussis involved both humoral and cellular immune responses directed against several protective antigens.

As part of the comprehensive evaluation of acellular vaccines in adults and children, investigators characterized pertussis-specific CMI after the administration of acellular pertussis vaccine. Initial studies in adults[310-314] and subsequent studies in infants[315] and toddlers[316,317] demonstrated that acellular pertussis vaccine induced specific T-cell responses to the antigens included in the vaccine, which increased progressively with time after vaccination.[313] Interleukin-2 and IFN-γ were induced preferentially, and Th1 cells were involved in the immune responses.[323] It was also learned that CMI responses persisted with time, while

antibody levels waned, as shown in Table 21-9. A small cohort of children had CMI responses evaluated on multiple occasions during the Italian acellular pertussis vaccine efficacy trial. A marked decline in anti-PT IgG levels was noted and was inversely correlated with substantial increases in the proportion and magnitude of CMI responses to the same antigen more than 42 months after vaccination.[317-319] Further support for the role of CMI in disease prevention was provided by an investigation of a pertussis outbreak in a Finnish school; students with persistent CMI responses were protected from disease, whereas no correlation was found between protection and antibody levels.[320]

Studies of CMI in recipients of acellular pertussis vaccines, in those infected with wild-type B. pertussis, and in individuals suffering adverse reactions to acellular vaccines should continue. An improved understanding of the full range of immune responses to both vaccination and disease is sorely needed.

Immune Correlates of Protection

The establishment of an immune correlate of protection is important for all vaccines, but is particularly needed for acellular pertussis vaccines given that the old "gold standard," the mouse protection test, does not appear to predict vaccine potency adequately. Immune correlates of protection typically are established in randomized, placebo-controlled efficacy trials in which the attainment of a particular postvaccination level of immunity is correlated with prevention of disease. Early studies from the United Kingdom had suggested that measurable agglutinin titers in serum after whole-cell vaccination correlated with protection against pertussis disease.[202,224,321] One of the stated goals of the 1986–1987 Swedish efficacy trial evaluating the one- or two-component Japanese-made acellular vaccines was to establish serologic correlates of protection. However, much to everyone's dismay, postvaccination antibody levels of PT and FHA did not correlate with clinical protection. A number of possible explanations were proposed for this disappointing result[322]: postimmunization antibody levels may have poorly predicted antibody levels at the time of exposure, reflecting the lack of data on the kinetics of antibody decline after immunization; antibody assays may have

TABLE 21–9 ■ Antibody and Cell-Mediated Immune Responses to Pertussis Toxin in a Cohort of Children 48 Months Old or Less Who Were Followed Longitudinally After Acellular Vaccine

Age (mo)	Months After Vaccine	Immunoglobulin Responses		CMI Proliferative Responses	
		Seroresponders/Total*	GMT (95%CI)	CMI Responders/Total†	Mean SI‡
2		1/19	1.3 (0.9–1.8)	0/19	1.2 (0.3–3)
7	1	19/19	103 (103–104)	4/19	2.7 (0.3–12.8)
20	14	8/19	6.4 (5.7–7.1)	8/19	6.7 (0.5–26.3)
48	42	1/19	2.0 (1.5–2.6)	17/19	31.5 (1–203)

*Seroresponse is defined as a serum antibody titer greater than four times the minimal detection limit.
†A CMI response is defined as an SI greater than 4.
‡Stimulation index (SI) is the ratio of counts per minute for stimulated versus unstimulated lymphocytes.
CMI, cell-mediated immunity; GMT, geometric mean antibody titer.
Adapted from Cassone A, Mastrantonio P, Ausiello CM. Are only antibody levels involved in the protection against pertussis in acellular pertussis vaccine recipients? JID 182:1575–1576, 2000.

measured the wrong epitopes; or perhaps protection was conferred not by humoral antibody but instead by CMI or mucosal immunity.

In several of the acellular pertussis vaccine efficacy trials conducted in Europe in the mid-1990s, efforts were made to determine immune correlates of protection. A nested household study was conducted as part of the 1992 Stockholm efficacy trial, which included a DT (placebo) arm, a U.S. whole-cell DTP vaccine, a two-component acellular vaccine, and a five-component acellular vaccine. Serum samples obtained at 1 and 2.5 years of age and within 4 months prior to exposure, or acute serum samples obtained at least 6 months after the third dose, were used as pre-exposure serum samples for 209 household-exposed children.[323] The results of this study indicated that vaccine efficacy against typical pertussis after household exposure to *B. pertussis* was 75% for the five-component acellular vaccine, 42% for the two-component vaccine, and 29% for the licensed U.S. whole-cell vaccine when compared to the DT placebo. Logistic regression analyses demonstrated statistically significant correlations between clinical protection and the presence in pre-exposure sera of IgG antibodies against pertactin, FIM-2/3, and pertussis toxin. The authors concluded that multicomponent pertussis vaccines of proven high efficacy used in the Swedish efficacy trials induced higher antibody levels against PRN and FIM-2/3 than did the less efficacious vaccines evaluated in the same trials, and that anti-PRN, anti–FIM-2/3, and anti-PT may be used as surrogate markers of protection against pertussis for multicomponent acellular and whole-cell vaccines.

A different U.S.-licensed DTP vaccine, a four-component acellular vaccine, and an open control group were compared in a randomized, controlled trial conducted in Erlangen, Germany.[180,324] Sera were collected from vaccinees after the third and fourth doses of vaccine and at comparable time periods in DT vaccine recipients. In addition, sera were collected from a random sample of subjects in each vaccine group at approximately 3-month intervals to construct antibody kinetics curves. This allowed estimation of the specific levels of antibody to PT, FHA, PRN, and FIM-2 at the time of exposure in the household setting. The imputed geometric mean antibody titers to PT, PRN, and FIM-2 at the time of household exposure to pertussis infection were higher ($P < 0.07$ or lower) in noncases compared with cases. A multivariate classification tree analysis found that only PRN and PT were significantly associated with protection. Subjects with an imputed PRN value of 7 EU/mL or less had a 67% chance of infection, regardless of the PT value. No subjects with a PRN value of 7 EU/mL or greater and a PT value of 66 EU/mL or greater were cases, but, if the PRN value was 7 EU/mL or greater and the PT value was 66 EU/mL or less, the predicted probability of being a case was 31%. Logistic regression analysis also found that high versus low PRN values were associated with prevention of illness following household exposure. In the presence of antibody to PRN, PT, and FIM-2, the additional presence of antibody to FHA did not contribute to protection.

The similarities in the findings in these two studies are noteworthy, but it must be remembered that no efficacious one- or two-component acellular pertussis vaccines were evaluated in those studies; the results may inform us well as

to the correlates of protection for the specific vaccines evaluated, while failing to elucidate correlates that are generalizable to all acellular pertussis vaccines. As Hewlett and Halperin stated in their editorial accompanying the publication of these data, "Over interpretation of these data is a significant risk and must be assiduously avoided." They cautioned that a vaccine containing PT alone was shown to be efficacious in the Göteborg trial and that the presence of PRN and fimbrial proteins therefore is not essential to protection afforded by acellular vaccines.[325]

Controlled Clinical Trials of Acellular Vaccines

Results are available from nine large efficacy trials of acellular pertussis vaccine that were initiated between 1985 and 1993 in Europe or Africa. The efficacy trials differed by many characteristics: type of study, study population, prevalence of pertussis and other diseases in the community, number of immunizations, timing of immunizations, choice of comparison or control vaccines, methods of surveillance, case definitions, and details of the laboratory support used to evaluate fulfillment of the case definition. These differences confound interpretation of the trials and prevent a simple, direct comparison of their primary efficacy results.

In evaluating these efficacy trials, we have several independent goals: to determine whether the candidate vaccine performs well enough to warrant licensure, to position correctly the evaluated vaccine within the spectrum of available vaccines, to draw inferences concerning the influence on efficacy of various vaccine characteristics, and to draw inferences concerning the effect on vaccine evaluation of various study design characteristics. Various deviations from the ideal study design (Table 21–10) are likely to affect these goals differentially; that is, a study that poses difficulties in accomplishing one goal may nonetheless be useful for accomplishing other goals.

The objectives of pertussis vaccination also play a role in evaluating measurements of efficacy. If the societal goal is focused on the prevention of severe disease, then a study's inability to detect mild illness (or determine efficacy against that endpoint) may not be important. However, if the goal is to prevent pertussis infection, then mild illnesses must be detected, even though such illnesses may be more difficult to ascertain than classical whooping cough. To the extent that vaccines modify but do not prevent illness, the case definition chosen could have a major impact on interpretation of the efficacy, and hence the benefits, of the vaccine.

Although frustration with the limitations of these trials has led to calls for "definitive studies" that would resolve remaining questions,[327] it is doubtful that any sponsor, public or private, would find the enormous expense of such a study to be both in their interest and of sufficient priority to compete successfully for funds. Thus these trials will likely remain our only sources of efficacy data, and we must make use of them as best we can.

1986 Swedish Efficacy Trial

The first large-scale efficacy trial of acellular vaccine was conducted in 1986 in Sweden, where routine pertussis immunization had been discontinued in 1979 and pertussis had since become endemic.[238] The randomized, dou-

TABLE 21–10 ■ Characteristics of the Ideal Pertussis Efficacy Trial

Characteristic	Comment
Prospective	Avoids recall and other biases.
Randomized	Minimizes risk of unbalanced allocation of confounders.
Fully blinded	Minimizes risk of selection, response, detection, diagnostic, and other biases. Using an unblinded, unimmunized control group is very likely to bias efficacy estimates upward, because parents who know their coughing children are unprotected are more likely to suspect pertussis and seek care.
Employs a commonly used immunization schedule.	Permits comparison of results to largest possible number of other studies.
Uses a whole-cell control group (ideally, one used in other efficacy trials).	Provides direct comparison with presumed gold standard; improves ability to link results of one study to another.
Also uses a placebo control group, if ethically permissible.	Allows calculation of absolute efficacy, which is the most useful result. Relative risk (RR), which is the only measure available without a placebo group, can be very misleading. For example, if DTaP #1 and DTP #1 have efficacies of 80% and 90%, then RR = 2. If DTaP #2 and DTP #2 have efficacies of 92% and 98%, then RR = 4. Thus, DTaP #2, which is better than #1, looks worse.
Conducts active surveillance for pertussis and obtains diagnostic specimens in accord with a protocol designed to detect mild as well as severe disease.	Minimizes detection bias; improves efficiency, power. Especially in cohort studies, poor surveillance biases toward the null hypothesis (i.e., hides differences between vaccines). In addition, obtaining diagnostic specimens only in more severe cases can bias efficacy estimates upward.[326]
Employs the WHO criteria (at least 21 days of paroxysmal cough plus bacteriologic, serologic, or epidemiologic confirmation) as the primary case definition.	Permits comparison of results to largest possible number of other studies.
Obtains specimens for culture from all suspected cases.	Cornerstone of bacteriologic confirmation. Improves specificity, compared to clinical criteria alone.
Obtains specimens for antigen detection from all suspected cases.	May be positive after culture turns negative; improves sensitivity, compared to culture alone.
Obtains specimens for serology (acute and convalescent) from all suspected cases.	Improves sensitivity and reduces diagnostic bias, compared to bacteriologic confirmation alone (culture is less likely to be positive in immunized than unimmunized cases).
Uses serologic definitions appropriate to the vaccines being evaluated (e.g., looks for rises to antigens not included in the vaccine itself).	Immunized subjects who acquire pertussis are less likely than unimmunized subjects to manifest a diagnostic rise in an antibody that has already risen substantially in response to vaccine.
Close contacts of pertussis cases evaluated for pertussis infection.	Permits epidemiologic confirmation of clinical cases, thereby improving sensitivity and reducing impact of diagnostic biases of culture and serology.
If booster given, analyzes separately time at risk before and after booster.	Necessary for valid comparison to results of other studies.
Provides alternate analyses that differ in case definition or diagnostic tools employed.	Permits evaluation of: vaccine's ability to protect against mild disease; effect of variations in case definition; contribution of various confirmatory criteria.

ble-blind, placebo-controlled trial (Table 21–11) evaluated a Biken vaccine containing 23.4 μg each of PT and FHA (denoted JNIH-6; see Tables 21–3 and 21–4),[332] a monocomponent vaccine prepared for the purposes of this study and containing 37.7 μg of PT (denoted JNIH-7),[332] and vaccine diluent given as a placebo.[103] There was no whole-cell control group. A two-dose schedule was used; infants were enrolled and immunized at 5 to 11 months of age, with the second dose given 8 to 12 weeks later.

Antibody responses to PT were dose dependent, being higher in the children who received the monovalent vaccine; FHA antibody rose only in the bivalent vaccine group. Efficacy for both vaccines was less than anticipated (Tables 21–12 and 21–13); for culture-confirmed cough of any duration, efficacy was 69% for the two-component vaccine and 54% for the monocomponent vaccine.[103]

During the surveillance period, four vaccinees (one JNIH-7 and three JNIH-6 recipients) died of bacterial infections.[339] Review of hospitalizations for infection found no differences among the three study groups. Analyses of immunoglobulins from prevaccination and postvaccination sera showed no abnormalities, nor did leukocyte counts obtained in a subsample of subjects 2 to 4 months after the second dose.

In January 1989, the Swedish National Bacteriology Laboratory withdrew the acellular vaccine licensure application, citing both the impression that efficacy was lower than that of whole-cell vaccines and the possible association with deaths resulting from serious bacterial infections. The laboratory called for studies that would directly compare acellular and whole-cell vaccines.[340]

In light of these safety concerns and of animal data suggesting that PT might enhance the susceptibility of animals

TABLE 21–11 ■ Overview of Nine Acellular Pertussis Vaccine Efficacy Trials

Location, Year Begun	Study Groups and Vaccines Evaluated			Ages of Vaccination	Duration†	Surveillance		Comments on Study Design
	Acellular*	Whole-Cell	Placebo			Active	Passive	
RANDOMIZED, FULLY BLINDED, CONTROLLED COMPARATIVE STUDIES								
Stockholm, 1986[328]	JNIH-6 JNIH-7	None	Diluent	5–11 mo, then 8–12 wk later	15 mo‡	Telephone q. mo	Parents instructed to report	Lack of whole-cell control hampered interpretation. Schedule (2 doses, relatively late in infancy) makes comparisons to other trials difficult. Later analyses revealed differential sensitivity of culture and of serology in vaccine vs. placebo groups.
Stockholm, 1992[181]	SKB-2 Tripacel§	Connaught‖	DT	2, 4, 6 mo	23.3 mo 23.8 mo	Telephone q. 6–8 wk	Parents instructed to report	Stockholm 1992 and Italy are the benchmark studies: prospective, fully randomized, and blinded, with both whole-cell and placebo (DT) control groups. Each study evaluated 2 candidate acellular vaccines head to head, using the same immunization schedules and nearly identical case definitions and diagnostic procedures.
Italy, 1992[182]	Infanrix Acelluvax	Connaught‖	DT	2, 4, 6 mo	17 mo	Telephone q. mo	Parents instructed to report	
Stockholm, 1993[329]	SKB-2 Acelluvax HCPDT§	Wellcome	None	88% at 3, 5, 12 mo; 12% at 2, 4, 6 mo	7.2 mo 21.5 mo 21.5 mo	Clinic visits at 5, 12, 18 mo	Daily check of culture reports	No placebo control group, thus no absolute efficacy estimates, hampering comparisons to other studies. Formulation of Connaught Canada 5-component vaccine changed since Stockholm 1992, further hampering comparisons; however, Acelluvax arm presumably comparable to Italy.
RANDOMIZED, FULLY BLINDED, CONTROLLED STUDIES								
Göteborg (Sweden), 1991[330]	Certiva	None	DT	3, 5, 12 mo	17.5 mo	Telephone q. mo	Parents instructed to report	Vaccination schedule and lack of whole-cell control group hamper comparisons to other studies.

Study	Trade name	Manufacturer	Control	Doses	Mean duration	Active surveillance	Passive surveillance	Comments
Senegal, 1990[229]	*Triavax*	Pasteur Mérieux	DT	2, 4, 6 mo	21 mo	Field worker visit q. wk	None	Prospective, double-blind, randomized for relative risk of DTaP vs. DTP. Absolute efficacy based on case-contact study using nonrandomized DT/no vaccine group that was unblinded to parents and, probably, to field workers performing initial case detection. Investigating physicians said to be blinded.
Erlangen (Germany), 1991[180]	*ACEL-IMUNE*	Lederle[‖]	DT	3, 5, 7, 17 mo	25.6 mo	Telephone q. 2 wk	Parents instructed to report to PMD	Prospective, double-blind, randomized for relative risk of DTaP vs. DTP. Absolute efficacy based on comparison to a nonrandomized DT group that was unblinded to parents and, occasionally, to investigators.
Mainz (Germany), 1992[226]	*Infanrix*	Behringwerke or SmithKline Beecham	DT	3, 4, 5 mo	23 mo	None	Physician report of contact by parent	Household contact study. Vaccine assignment not randomized; parents and physicians responsible for initial case detection not blinded. Central case investigators were said to be blinded.
Munich, 1993[227,331]	*Tripedia*	Behringwerke	DT	3, 5, 7 mo	n/a	None	Physician report of contact by parent	Nonrandomized (vaccine chosen by parents), unblinded (parents and investigators knew vaccine status) case-control study.

*Descriptive name given for those without trade name (trade names in italics). See Tables 21–3 and 21–4 for further details.

[†]Mean duration of surveillance. Subjects were eligible for inclusion as cases from time of last dose (Stockholm 1992, Stockholm 1993), from 28 to 30 days after last dose (Stockholm 1986, Italy, Göteborg, Senegal, Mainz), or from 14 days after last dose (Erlangen) of DTaP.

[‡]Passive unblinded surveillance, augmented with inquiries mailed to parents every 6 months and follow-up of positive cultures reported to the National Bacteriology Laboratory, continued for an additional 3 years.

[§]*Tripacel* and HCPDT are similar, except that *Tripacel* contains 10 μg PT and 5 μg FHA, as compared to 20 μg of each in HCPDT.

[‖]U.S.-licensed whole-cell vaccine.

HCPDT, hybrid component pertussis-diphtheria-tetanus vaccine; n/a, not available or not applicable; PMD, private physician.

TABLE 21–12 ■ Results of Nine Acellular Pertussis Vaccine Efficacy Trials, Based on Case Definition Most Similar to That of the WHO Definition*

Study	Case Definition†	Vaccine‡ (# Components)	Efficacy (95% CI)			Comment
			Cases	Absolute %	Relative Risk	
RANDOMIZED, FULLY BLINDED, CONTROLLED, COMPARATIVE STUDIES						
Stockholm 1986[328]	≥21 days cough + ≥9 coughing spasms on at least 1 day + positive culture	JNIH-6 (2)	10	81 (61–90)		Differential sensitivity of culture, lack of serologic or epi-link criteria may bias estimates upward.
Stockholm 1992[181]	≥21 days paroxysmal cough, plus either: positive culture, confirmed by SA or PCR; 2-fold PT or FHA IgG rise; or epi link to culture-positive case	JNIH-7 (1)	12	75 (53–87)		
		SKB-2 (2)	159	59 (51–66)	0.83 (0.66–1.1) vs. DTP	Because of unusually low DTP efficacy, relative risks difficult to compare to other studies.
		Tripacel§ (4)	59	85 (81–89)	0.29 (0.21–0.40) vs. DTP	
		Connaught DTP	148	48 (37–58)		
Italy 1992[182]	≥21 days paroxysmal cough, plus either: positive culture, confirmed by SA or PCR; 4-fold CHO or 2-fold PT or FHA IgG or IgA rise; no epi-link criterion	Infanrix (3)	37	84 (76–89)	0.25 (0.17–0.36) vs. DTP	Because of unusually low DTP efficacy, relative risks difficult to compare to other studies.
		Acelluvax (3)	36	84 (76–90)	0.25 (0.17–0.36) vs. DTP	
		Connaught DTP	141	36 (14–52)		
Stockholm 1993[329]	≥21 days paroxysmal cough plus positive culture (no information on confirmation); no serologic or epi-link criteria	HCPDT§ (4)	13		0.85 (0.41–1.79) vs. DTP	Comparison is to the Wellcome DTP used in this study (see Table 21–11).
		Acelluvax (3)	21		1.38 (0.71–2.69) vs. DTP	Acelluvax, unchanged from Italy, provides a link to the Italy study (and thus to Stockholm 1992).
		SKB-2 (2)	99		2.3 (1.5–3.5) vs. DTP‖	
		HCPDT§ (4)	38		0.62 (0.31–1.2) vs. Acelluvax‖	
		SKB-2 (2)	99		2.0 (1.4–2.8) vs. Acelluvax‖	
RANDOMIZED, FULLY BLINDED, CONTROLLED STUDIES						
Göteborg 1991[330]	≥21 days paroxysmal cough plus either: positive culture confirmed by SA, PCR; 3-fold PT or FHA IgG rise; epi link	Certiva (1)	72	71 (63–78)		Lack of FHA in vaccine enhanced sensitivity of serologic criteria, improving accuracy of estimate.

Location/Year	Case definition	Vaccine		Efficacy % (CI)	Relative	Comments
Senegal 1990[229]	≥21 days paroxysmal cough plus either: positive culture confirmed by DIF; 2-fold PT or FHA IgG rise; epi link	Triavax (2)	24	74 (51–86)	2.42 (1.4–4.3) vs. DTP	Few cases, thus broad CIs. Open DT group may bias absolute efficacy estimates upward.
Erlangen 1991[180]	≥21 days cough with paroxysms, whoop, or vomiting, plus confirmation[¶]	PMC-Fr DTP	7	92 (81–97)		Open DT group, incomplete case ascertainment may bias absolute efficacy estimates upward.
		ACEL-IMUNE (4)	≤45	78 (60–88)	1.5 (0.7–3.4) vs. DTP[228]	
		Lederle DTP	≤18	93 (83–97)		
Mainz 1992[226]	21 days paroxysmal cough plus either: positive culture confirmed by DIF or SA; 2-fold PT or FHA IgG or IgA rise	Infanrix (3)	7	89 (77–95)	4.7 (0.6–37.3) vs. DTP	Few cases, thus broad CIs. Note how misleading relative risk is if DTP result is close to 100%.
		Behring, SKB DTP	1	98 (83–100)		
Munich 1993[227,331]	21 days paroxysmal cough plus either: positive culture confirmed by SA; epi link; no serologic criteria	Tripedia (2)	4	93 (63–99)**	2.0 (n/a) vs. DTP	Few cases, thus broad CIs. Lack of serologic criteria, blinding, or randomization may bias efficacy estimates upward.
		Behring DTP	1	96 (71–100)		

*Results shown are for complete primary infant immunization series (three doses, except Stockholm 1986, two doses); effects of any booster dose are not included. Some results obtained by recalculation from data provided in the referenced source; such results may represent crude, rather than adjusted, efficacies. Blank cells: not applicable or no data. WHO case definition: 21 or more days of paroxysmal cough, plus bacteriologic, serologic, or epidemiologic confirmation that cough is due to B. pertussis.

†Unless otherwise noted: All cultures were nasopharyngeal; FHA rises were considered diagnostic only if culture (and PCR, if done) were negative for B. parapertussis, "epi link" means documented contact with a culture-confirmed (PCR-confirmed, for Senegal) case within 28 days before or after illness onset in the subject (for Erlangen or Munich, no time limit was specified). Criteria shown are for the case definition most similar to that of the WHO; different criteria may have been used for alternative case definitions.

‡Descriptive name given for those without trade name (trade names in italics). Letters before hyphen indicate source; characters after hyphen indicate number and type of components. All single-component vaccines contain PT; all two-component vaccines contain PT and FHA; three-component vaccines contain PT and FHA plus either PRN or FIM; four-component vaccines contain PT, FHA, PRN, and FIM. See Tables 21–3 and 21–4 for further details.

§Tripacel and HCPDT are similar, except that Tripacel contains 10 μg PT and 5 μg FHA, as compared to 20 μg of each in HCPDT.

‖For time from first dose to soon after the third dose, when SKB-2 recipients were unblinded and boosted with another vaccine.

¶Confirmation criteria: Positive culture (confirmed by PCR in last year of study); "significant" PT IgG or IgA result; or household contact to a culture-confirmed case. "Significant" serologic result defined as a ratio of convalescent to acute antibody level that exceeded the 95th, 99th, or 99.9th percentile of a distribution of similar ratios determined among randomly selected subjects at roughly the same time post-immunization. Selection of the percentile limit was determined by how many, and which, antibody ratios were elevated. Efficacy rates reflect adjustment for single adult households and households in which all siblings were unimmunized. Other published efficacy estimates[180] may have used FHA, PRN, or FIM IgG or IgA values or fourfold AGG rises as well, and may not have reflected such adjustment.

**Differs from efficacy reported in FDA-approved patient package insert, which is based on the primary case definition (≥21 days of any cough) rather than the WHO definition. AGG, agglutination; CHO, Chinese hamster ovary cell assay; CI, confidence interval; DIF, direct immunofluorescence; FHA, filamentous hemagglutinin; FIM, fimbrial proteins; HCPDT, hybrid component pertussis-diphtheria-tetanus vaccine; IgA, immunoglobulin A; IgG, immunoglobulin G; n/a, not available or not applicable; PCR, polymerase chain reaction; PMC-Fr, Pasteur Mérieux Connaught–France; PRN, pertactin; PT, pertussis toxin; SA, slide agglutination; SKB, SmithKline Beecham.

to bacterial infection,[341] several studies were conducted that demonstrated, if anything, a decreased risk of severe invasive bacterial disease after DTP immunization[342–344] and no increased risk of minor infections.[343] Data from Japan indicated that there was no enhanced risk from the acellular vaccines.[345] Thus it appears that the four deaths were chance events, with no causal relationship to vaccination.

SUBSEQUENT FOLLOW-UP AND ANALYSES

Later evaluations of various case definitions and confirmatory criteria showed that the two-component and monocomponent vaccines were 81% and 75% effective, respectively, in preventing culture-confirmed disease with at least 21 days of coughing spasms.[333] Estimates of efficacy were profoundly influenced by case definition, ranging (using the monocomponent vaccine as an example) from 5% efficacy in preventing spasmodic cough lasting 1 day or longer to 100% efficacy in preventing culture-confirmed pertussis with spasmodic cough lasting 28 days or longer, with whoops on at least 1 day.[333]

It was also found that prior receipt of pertussis vaccine reduced the likelihood of finding positive pertussis cultures or significant antibody rises in patients with cough.[295] Thus pertussis infection could be confirmed more readily in placebo recipients than in vaccinees, which would tend to bias efficacy estimates upward.

Although the initial results from the 1986 Swedish trial had suggested that the efficacies of the monocomponent and two-component vaccines did not differ, long-term follow-up showed the two-component vaccine to be significantly more efficacious (Fig. 21–5).[239] Following unblinding of the study after 15 months of active observation, passive surveillance continued for 3 additional years, during which vaccine efficacy ranged from 77% to 92% for the bivalent vaccine and from 65% to 82% for the monovalent vaccine, depending on the case definition (see Table 21–13).[239] Clinical immunity after immunization with acellular pertussis vaccine was maintained for at least 4 years.[239]

The monocomponent vaccine, with 50% more PT, appeared to be more effective than the two-component vaccine in preventing the most severe manifestations of disease. Its efficacy exceeded that of the two-component vaccine for every case definition involving whoops (see Table 21–13), a difference that was statistically significant for 28 or more days of cough with whoops.[333] On the other hand, the two-component vaccine appeared to be more effective in preventing mild or moderate disease (e.g., shorter durations of cough or cough without whoops).[239,333,346] Thus efficacy was influenced by both the choice of antigens and the quantity of antigen included.

The initial efficacy results[103] gave the impression that these acellular vaccines were substantially less efficacious than whole-cell vaccine.[103,239,328] As a result, Japan remained the only country in which they were licensed. However, results of later studies suggest that efficacy would have been higher had a standard three-dose schedule been used. Most important, inclusion of a whole-cell control group might have led to markedly different conclusions regarding the relative efficacy of these vaccines.

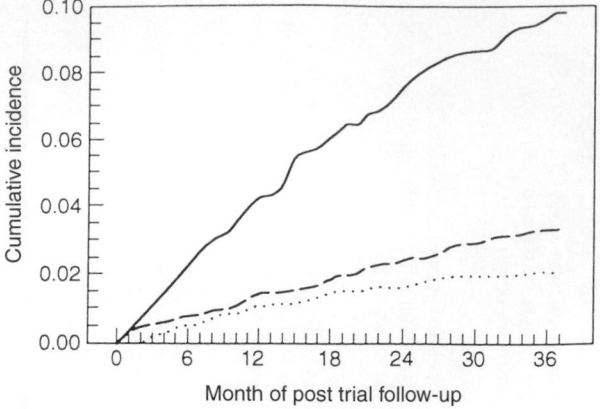

FIGURE 21–5 ■ Cumulative incidence curves for culture-confirmed pertussis during unblinded post-trial follow-up, in the placebo group (*solid line*), in the monocomponent (JNIH-7) vaccine group (*dashed line*), and in the two-component (JNIH-6) vaccine group (*dotted line*). Unblinded follow-up started August 27, 1987, and ended September 9, 1990. (From Storsaeter J, Olin P. Relative efficacy of two acellular pertussis vaccines during three years of passive surveillance. Vaccine 10:142–144, 1992, with permission.)

World Health Organization Case Definition of Pertussis

In response to the demonstration in the 1986 Swedish trial of the strong influence of pertussis case definition on estimates of vaccine efficacy, and in expectation of the efficacy trials that would be conducted to evaluate the new vaccines being developed, the WHO convened a group of pertussis experts in January 1991 to develop a consensus pertussis case definition for use in clinical trials. The resulting WHO case definition requires the presence of paroxysmal cough for at least 21 days plus confirmation that the cough illness actually is due to pertussis. This confirmation can be based on laboratory results (e.g., a positive culture for *B. pertussis* or a significant rise in a specific antibody, such as IgG or IgA against PT, FHA, or FIM-2 or -3) or on an epidemiologic link (e.g., a household contact with a laboratory-confirmed case within 28 days before or after the onset of illness in the subject).[347] The consensus statement recognized that future laboratory developments might add to the tools available for bacteriologic or serologic confirmation (e.g., DFA, PCR, assay of antibody to PRN).

Although the WHO case definition has played an essential role in improving comparability of subsequent field trials, its limitations should be recognized. First, it improves but does not eliminate the problem of differential sensitivity of the case definition with respect to detecting pertussis in the various arms of a comparative trial. The yield of cultures is lower in immunized than in unimmunized pertussis patients and varies inversely with the efficacy of the vaccine.[181,334,337,346,348] Thus a cough illness that is really pertussis is more likely to be confirmed by culture in the unvaccinated group than in the vaccinated group. This disparity leads to a disproportionate discarding of true pertussis cases in the vaccinated group, which can result in falsely elevated estimates of vaccine efficacy. Similarly, the differences between a less effective and a more effective vaccine are likely to be exaggerated because more cases will be

TABLE 21–13 ■ Results of Nine Acellular Pertussis Vaccine Efficacy Trials for Various Case Definitions or Surveillance Periods*

Study	Vaccine(s)†	Case Definition‡	Efficacies (95% CI)	
			Absolute, %	Relative Risk (vs. DTP)
RANDOMIZED, FULLY BLINDED, CONTROLLED, COMPARATIVE STUDIES				
Stockholm (1986)	JNIH-6, JNIH-7	≥1 day of any cough + positive culture[103]	69 (47–82), 54 (26–72)	
		Same; but including cases from date of first dose[103]	65 (44–78), 53 (28–69)	
		Same; but for first 60 days after first dose only[328]	41 (0–79), 42 (0–79)	
		≥1 day cough with spasms (defined in Table 21–12)[333]	16 (3–27), 5 (–10, 17)	
		≥1 day cough with spasms + ≥1 day whoops[333]	39 (16–56), 51 (30–65)	
		≥1 day cough with spasms + culture[333]	75 (54–86), 60 (33–76)	
		≥1 day cough with spasms + whoops + culture[33≡]	85 (67–94), 89 (72–96)	
		≥21 days cough with spasms[333]	41 (23–55), 27 (6–43)	
		≥21 days cough with spasms + whoops[333]	60 (37–75), 62 (39–76)	
		≥21 days cough with spasms + culture[333]	**81 (61–90), 75 (53–87)**	
		≥21 days cough with spasms + whoops + culture[333]	84 (63–93), 90 (73–97)	
		3 additional years of passive surveillance: positive culture[239]	77 (65–85), 65 (50–75)	
		3 additional years: ≥30 days cough + positive culture[239]	92 (84–96), 79 (67–87)	
		3 additional years: ≥9 cough spasms/day + positive culture[239]	89 (76–97), 82 (67–90)	
Stockholm (1992)	SKB-2, Tripacel	≥21 days paroxysmal cough, confirmed as in Table 21–12[181]	59 (51–66), 85 (81–89)	0.83 (0.66–1.1), 0.29 (0.21–0.40)
		Same; but including cases from date of first dose[181]	59 (51–66), 84 (80–88)	0.83 (0.66–1.1), 0.30 (0.22–0.42)
		≥1 day any cough, confirmed as in Table 21–12[18≡]	42 (33–51), 78 (73–82)	
		≥21 days any cough, confirmed as in Table 21–12[334]	54 (46–62), 81 (76–85)	
Italy	*Infanrix, Acelluvax*	≥21 days paroxysmal cough + positive culture[182]	85 (n/a), 87 (n/a)	
		≥21 days paroxysmal cough, confirmed as in Table 21–12[182]	84 (76–89), 84 (76–90)	0.25 (0.17–0.36), 0.25 (0.17–0.36)
		Same; but including cases from date of first dose[182]	82 (73–87), 84 (76–89)	0.28 (0.20–0.39), 0.25 (0.17–0.36)
		Same; but from 30 days after 1st dose to 29 days after 3rd[182]	19 (0–84), 83 (0–98)	0.49 (0.17–1.44), 0.10 (0.01–0.79)
		≥7 days any cough, confirmation as above[182]	71 (60–78), 71 (61–79)	0.38 (0.30–0.49), 0.38 (0.29–0.48)
		≥21 days any cough, confirmation as above[182]	79 (70–85), 77 (68–84)	0.29 (0.21–0.39), 0.31 (0.24–0.42)
Stockholm (1993)	HCPTD, *Acelluvax*	Positive culture, with or without (±) cough[329]		1.40 (0.78–2.52), 2.55 (1.50–4.33)
		≥21 days paroxysmal cough + positive culture[325]		**0.85 (0.41–1.79), 1.38 (0.71–2.69)**
		Positive culture, ± cough; from date of first dose[325]		1.25 (0.90–1.75), 1.84 (1.36–2.51)
		≥21 d paroxysmal cough + positive culture; from first dose[329]		1.25 (0.82–1.89), 1.65 (1.12–2.45)
		Same; but from date of first dose to date of second dose[335]		1.49 (0.80–2.77), 1.42 (0.76–2.65)
		Same; but from date of second dose to date of third dose[329]		1.42 (0.54–3.74), 3.14 (1.34–7.34)
RANDOMIZED, FULLY BLINDED, CONTROLLED STUDIES				
Göteborg	*Certiva*	≥7 days any cough, confirmed as in Table 21–12[330]	54 (43–63)	
		≥7 days any cough, confirmed by Göteborg criteria[330]	62 (51–70)	
		≥21 days any cough, confirmed as in Table 21–12[330]	63 (52–71)	
		≥21 days any cough, confirmed by Göteborg criteria[330]	69 (60–77)	
		≥21 days paroxysmal cough, confirmed by Göteborg criteria[330]	77 (69–83)	

Table continued on following page

TABLE 21–13 ■ Results of Nine Acellular Pertussis Vaccine Efficacy Trials for Various Case Definitions or Surveillance Periods*—cont'd

Study	Vaccine(s)†	Case Definition‡	Efficacies (95% CI)	
			Absolute, %	Relative Risk (vs. DTP)
Senegal	Triavax	Same; from 30 days after 2nd dose to 29 days after 3rd[336]	39 (0–66)	
		≥21 days paroxysmal cough, confirmed as in Table 21–12[330]	71 (63–78)	
		Same; from first dose to 29 days after second dose[330]	≤16 (0–≤64)	
		Same; from 30 days after 2nd dose to 29 days after 3rd[330]	55 (12–78)	
		Same; from 18.5 to 24.5 months after third dose[337]	77 (65–85)	

OTHER STUDIES

Study	Vaccine(s)†	Case Definition‡	Absolute, %	Relative Risk (vs. DTP)
Senegal	Triavax	≥21 days any cough, confirmed as in Table 21–12[229]	31 (7–49)	1.54 (1.23–1.94)
		As above, plus epi-link cases confirmed by PCR[229]	53 (23–71)	1.87 (1.38–2.52)
		≥8 days paroxysmal cough, confirmed as in Table 21–12[338]		3.26 (2.08–5.10)
		≥21 days paroxysmal cough, confirmed as in Table 21–12[229]	74 (51–86)	2.42 (1.35–4.34)
		As above, plus epi-link cases confirmed by PCR[229]	85 (66–93)	2.80 (1.36–5.74)
Erlangen	ACEL-IMUNE	≥7 days any cough, confirmed as in Table 21–12[180]	62 (38–77)§	3.1 (n/a)
		≥21 days paroxysmal cough, confirmed as in Table 21–12[180]	78 (60–88)	
Mainz	Infanrix	≥1 day paroxysmal cough[226]	64 (51–73)	1.5 (0.7–3.4)
		≥7 days paroxysmal cough, confirmed as in Table 21–12[226]	81 (68–89)	
		≥21 days paroxysmal cough, with or without confirmation[226]	83 (71–90)	
Munich	Tripedia	≥21 days paroxysmal cough, confirmed as in Table 21–12[226]	89 (77–95)	4.7 (0.6–37.3) vs DTP
		≥21 days any cough, confirmed as in Table 21–12[227]	80 (63–89)‖	4.0 (n/a) vs DTP
		≥21 days paroxysmal cough, confirmed as in Table 21–12[227]	93 (63–99)	2.0 (n/a) vs DTP

*Results shown are for complete primary infant immunization series (three doses, except Stockholm 1986, two doses); effects of any booster dose are not included. Some results obtained by recalculation from data provided in the referenced source; such results may represent crude, rather than adjusted, efficacies. Lower confidence limits less than zero are shown as zero. Blank cells: not applicable or no data. WHO case definition: 21 or more days of paroxysmal cough, plus bacteriologic, serologic, or epidemiologic confirmation that cough is due to *B. pertussis*. See Tables 21–7 and 21–8 for additional details, including confirmation methods used by each study.

†Descriptive name given for those without trade name (trade names in italics). See Tables 21–3 and 21–4 for further details.

‡Definition most similar to that of the WHO (≥21 days paroxysmal cough, confirmed as pertussis by culture, serology, or epidemiologic link to a culture-confirmed case) is shown in boldface; see Table 21–12 for details. Göteborg criteria: positive culture; or IgG against both PT and FHA 6000 or greater in a single convalescent specimen; or two major criteria; or one major and one minor criterion. Major criteria: threefold rise in PT or FHA IgG; household contact with confirmed pertussis. Minor criteria: threefold change in PT or FHA IgA or IgM; positive PCR. Unless otherwise specified, subjects were eligible for inclusion as cases from time of last dose (Stockholm 1992, Stockholm 1993), from 28 to 30 days after last dose (Stockholm 1986, Italy, Göteborg, Senegal, Mainz), or from 14 days after last dose (Erlangen) of DTaP (see Table 21–11 for vaccination schedule).

§Not adjusted for single-adult households and households in which all siblings were unimmunized (see Table 21–12).

‖This result, which is based on the primary case definition rather than the WHO definition, is the one reported in the FDA-approved patient package insert.

CI, confidence interval; FHA, filamentous hemagglutinin; FIM, fimbrial proteins; HCPDT, hybrid component pertussis-diphtheria-tetanus vaccine; IgG, immunoglobulin G; n/a, data not available; PCR, polymerase chain reaction; PRN, pertactin; PT, pertussis toxin; SKB, SmithKline Beecham.

confirmed by culture in the group that received the less effective vaccine. Those subjects who have already had a substantial increase in the level of a pertussis antibody, as a result of the receipt of a highly immunogenic vaccine, will be less likely to show a fourfold (or other diagnostic) rise in the level of that antibody after infection than those subjects who did not receive a vaccine containing that antigen (or a vaccine substantially less immunogenic with respect to that antigen).[337,346] When comparing two vaccines, one of which stimulates the antibody being tested for and one of which does not, there will be a diagnostic bias favoring the vaccine that stimulates the antibody. If both vaccines contain the antigen in question, the bias will favor the more immunogenic vaccine.

Second, setting the clinical cutoff at "paroxysmal cough of 21 days or more" has been shown to result in the removal from efficacy calculations of a substantial number of laboratory-confirmed pertussis cases.[239,333,349] Because these mild cases are more common in vaccinees than in control subjects, it might be argued that the effect is to inflate efficacy estimates, reducing the ability to discriminate among vaccines. However, if one's intent is to measure the vaccine's efficacy in preventing classical whooping cough, and mild disease is of lesser interest, then this quality is not a defect.

Third, the case definition permits the use of a variety of serologic assays for confirmation as well as the future use of additional serologic assays or other bacteriologic techniques to detect B. pertussis organisms. Although commendable, this flexibility means that studies that differ in the laboratory tools employed for case confirmation, and thus in the sensitivity and specificity of case confirmation, nonetheless may characterize themselves as using the WHO case definition. Thus, as always, the burden is on the reader to consider carefully the methods employed in each trial.

Efficacy Trials, 1992 to 1997

After the 1986 Swedish clinical trial, worldwide efforts to develop additional acellular pertussis vaccines continued, culminating in eight additional efficacy trials initiated between 1990 and 1993 (see Table 21–11). Four of the trials were randomized, prospective, and fully blinded; of these, three incorporated a whole-cell control arm and evaluated several candidate acellular vaccines head to head. The four remaining trials each evaluated only a single vaccine, using a variety of study designs; all made use of placebo (DT or no vaccine) groups that were neither randomized nor fully blinded.

Key characteristics of all nine efficacy studies are summarized in Tables 21–12 and 21–13. For each trial, Table 21–12 presents results for the case definition that we consider most similar to the WHO standard case definition, and Table 21–13 presents selected results reflecting a variety of alternative case definitions or surveillance intervals. For studies not incorporating a placebo control group (e.g., DT), only relative risks (usually calculated relative to a DTP vaccine used in the same trial) are available. However, relative risks must be interpreted with great caution, and can be directly compared across trials only if the reference (e.g., DTP) vaccines are identical. Unfortunately, no two studies conducted without placebo control groups incorporated a common DTP vaccine, and thus relative risks can be compared meaningfully only within the studies that evaluated multiple acellular vaccines.

SWEDEN AND ITALY, 1992 TO 1993

Of the 13 acellular vaccines evaluated in the MAPT, four were selected, based on evaluations of their safety, immunogenicity, and purity, for evaluation in two NIAID-funded efficacy trials conducted in Sweden and Italy.[181,182] These two NIAID-sponsored studies were of rigorous design and serve as the benchmarks against which others must be compared. The studies were prospective, double blinded, and randomized and incorporated both placebo (DT) and whole-cell control arms. The two studies used closely coordinated protocols, serologic assays, and case definitions (however, the Italian case definition did not include epidemiologically linked cases, and pre-exposure sera were not collected routinely in Italy as they were in Sweden). Infants were immunized at 2, 4, and 6 months of age, and no booster was given. Each study compared two candidate acellular vaccines head to head. The control whole-cell vaccine used in both was produced by Connaught Laboratories (Swiftwater, PA) and was licensed for use in the United States.

During the main follow-up period of the Swedish study (hereafter referred to as Stockholm 1992), 737 cases of pertussis were diagnosed that met the primary case definition. Efficacy was 59% for the SmithKline Beecham bivalent vaccine (SKB-2), 85% for the Aventis Pasteur five-component vaccine (Tripacel), and 48% for the Connaught whole-cell vaccine (see Table 21–12).[181] The efficacy of the five-component vaccine was sustained during the 2 years of follow-up, whereas the efficacy of the whole-cell vaccine declined substantially.

The performance of the two-component vaccine was much lower than had been anticipated. (JNIH-6, a similar vaccine, was 81% effective in the 1986 trial, using the most similar case definition.) It was noted that the SmithKline Beecham two-component vaccine produced significantly less antibody to PT in Sweden than it had in the MAPT,[350] prompting both the investigators[181] and other reviewers[350] to speculate that the vaccine's performance in Stockholm 1992 may, in part, have reflected characteristics unique to the batch of vaccine used in that trial.

The five-component vaccine was 78% effective against laboratory-confirmed pertussis with at least 1 day of cough, suggesting substantial protection against mild or atypical pertussis. In contrast, for this case definition the two-component and Connaught whole-cell vaccines were 42% and 41% effective, respectively.[181]

During the main follow-up period of the Italian trial, 288 cases of pertussis met the primary case definition. The GlaxoSmithKline (Infanrix) and Chiron Vaccines (Triacelluvax) three-component acellular vaccines were both 84% effective; efficacy for the Connaught whole-cell vaccine was 36%.[182] Since completion of the main follow-up period, unblinded surveillance of the study cohort has continued. During the first 9 months of extended follow-up, efficacy of the two vaccines differed significantly: 36 cases were detected among recipients of the GlaxoSmithKline vaccine, as compared with 18 among recipients of the Chiron vaccine (efficacies of 78% and 89%, respectively).[351] However, a more complete analysis that incorporated results through April 1997 found no material differences in long-term efficacy. For the GlaxoSmithKline and Chiron vaccines, respectively, efficacies by year of observation were: 1994, 82.7% and 82.1%; 1995, 81.5% and 85.9%; and 1996, 87.6% and 87.7%.[352] Additional follow-up through 6 years of age has demonstrated continued high efficacy of these vaccines.[353]

The similarity in efficacy of the three multicomponent vaccines is noteworthy, particularly given their substantially different compositions (see Tables 21–3 and 21–4). Triacelluvax has only one fifth the PT, one tenth the FHA, and one third the PRN content of Infanrix (but the PT is genetically inactivated, rather than being a toxoided natural protein). The Canadian five-component vaccine, Tripacel, had far less than half the PT, FHA, and PRN of Infanrix but contained FIM-2 and FIM-3. These facts strongly suggest that the efficacy of an acellular pertussis vaccine is influenced by both the choice of components and the particular characteristics of those components.

SWEDEN, 1993 TO 1996

After completion of the immunization phase of Stockholm 1992 (but before completion of the surveillance phase), the Swedish investigators launched another NIAID-supported prospective, randomized, double-blind trial (henceforth referred to as Stockholm 1993) that compared four vaccines: (1) the two-component SmithKline Beecham vaccine evaluated in Stockholm 1992; (2) a five-component Aventis Pasteur Canada vaccine (HCPDT) similar to the one evaluated in Stockholm 1992 (Tripacel) but reformulated to contain more PT and FHA; (3) the three-component Chiron acellular vaccine (Triacelluvax) evaluated in Italy; and (4) a different whole-cell vaccine, the Medeva Wellcome whole-cell vaccine (now produced by Evans Medical) used in the United Kingdom.[329] Because of the safety and efficacy of acellular pertussis vaccine demonstrated in Stockholm 1992, Stockholm 1993 did not incorporate a placebo group. Conducted in 22 of 25 Swedish counties, the trial randomized 82,892 children to be immunized at 3, 5, and 12 months of age (the Swedish schedule for DT). Surveillance was predominantly passive; detected rates of pertussis were markedly lower than in Stockholm 1992. Surveillance was terminated early for the group receiving the two-component SmithKline Beecham vaccine, and the subjects were immunized with the Canadian five-component acellular vaccine when results from the Stockholm 1992 study showed the two-component vaccine to be of substantially lower efficacy than the others.

The relative performances of the evaluated vaccines are shown in Tables 21–12 and 21–13 (the absence of a placebo control group precludes calculation of absolute vaccine efficacies.) Relative risks of culture-confirmed *B. pertussis* infection with at least 21 days of paroxysmal cough were 0.85 and 1.38 for the five-component and three-component vaccines, respectively, as compared with whole-cell vaccine. The relative risk of pertussis occurring between administration of the second dose (5 months of age) and third dose (12 months of age) of vaccine was 1.42 for the five-component vaccine, 3.13 for the three-component vaccine, and 7.81 for the two-component vaccine (as compared with whole-cell vaccine). Efficacy of the two-

component vaccine differed significantly from that of the other three.

The Stockholm 1993 study provides important new data, but several factors complicate the direct comparison of its results to those of other trials. As noted, there was no placebo control group, precluding calculations of absolute efficacy. The Wellcome whole-cell vaccine was not used in any other efficacy trial. The five-component Aventis Pasteur Canada vaccine evaluated was the "hybrid" formulation developed for use in combination vaccines, containing twice the PT and four times the FHA as in the "classical" formulation. The SmithKline Beecham two-component vaccine was used in Stockholm 1992, but surveillance of this group was terminated early in the second Stockholm study. Thus the Chiron three-component vaccine represents the only link to the prior trials.

Based on the Stockholm 1992 and Italy 1992 trials (see Table 21–12), Infanrix, Triacelluvax, and the classical (CLL-4F$_2$) formulation of Tripacel appear to be of equal efficacy. In Stockholm 1993, however, the relative risk of typical pertussis with the reformulated (hybrid or HCPDT) version of Tripacel was 0.62 (95% CI, 0.28 to 1.29) compared to Triacelluvax. For combined mild and severe pertussis, the hybrid five-component vaccine was equal to the whole-cell vaccine but significantly better than Triacelluvax.[326] Taken together, these observations suggest to us that the hybrid formulation of Tripacel is more efficacious than the classical formulation, and accordingly, that increasing the amount of PT and FHA in a vaccine can increase its efficacy. Of note, serologic studies performed on small subsets of subjects in the 1992[334] and 1993[336] Stockholm trials found significantly higher FHA responses with the hybrid formulation used in 1993 compared with the classical formulation used in 1992. There were no differences in antibody responses to the SmithKline Beecham bivalent vaccine lots used in the 1992 and 1993 trials.

GÖTEBORG, SWEDEN

A randomized, double-blind, placebo-controlled trial sponsored by the NICHD was conducted in Göteborg, Sweden, from September 1991 to July 1994. This trial evaluated the monocomponent (PT toxoid only) acellular vaccine (Certiva) developed by the NICHD and manufactured at that time by North American Vaccine.[330] Children were immunized with DTaP or DT at 3, 5, and 12 months of age; there was no whole-cell control group.

During the period from 30 days after the third (12-month) vaccination to the end of the study, 72 DTaP and 240 DT recipients met the WHO case definition, for an efficacy of 71%. Other case definitions produced efficacy estimates ranging from 54% to 77%, depending on the stringency of the definition. A nested analysis of subjects with household exposure to pertussis found 66% efficacy after two doses and 75% efficacy after three doses.[354] During an additional 6 months of surveillance after unblinding of the study (representing a period averaging 18.5 to 24.5 months after the third injection), efficacy was 77% for the full cohort and 76% in a nested household-contact study.[337]

Because this vaccine included only PT toxoid, serologic rises of antibodies to FHA were an unbiased indicator of possible pertussis. Thus pertussis could be identified more readily among vaccine recipients than if the vaccine had contained FHA. Other vaccines to which this vaccine is compared may have benefited from a lower case ascertainment rate in the vaccine groups, biasing their efficacy estimates upward.

The only other efficacy trial that immunized subjects at 3, 5, and 12 months of age was Stockholm 1993. However, comparing results with that study cannot readily be done; the two studies evaluated no acellular vaccines in common, and there was no DT arm in Stockholm 1993 or whole-cell arm in Göteborg.

Follow-up for 2 years following immunization showed no diminution in protection among the DTaP group, as compared to the DT group.[337] Subsequent mass immunization in the Göteborg area using the PT toxoid vaccine has resulted in significant decreases in *B. pertussis* isolates and hospitalizations in all age groups.[355]

MUNICH, GERMANY

An unblinded, nonrandomized case-control study sponsored by Aventis Pasteur was conducted in 63 German pediatric practices from February 1993 to May 1995.[227] A cohort of children was enrolled prospectively to receive, according to parental choice, either the Aventis Pasteur–Biken two-component DTaP (Tripedia), the Behringwerke DTP, a DT vaccine, or no vaccine at approximately 3, 5, and 7 months of age.

All infants 2 to 24 months of age who presented to a participating pediatrician with cough for 7 days or more, or with suspected exposure to pertussis, had nasopharyngeal specimens obtained for culture (whether the children were part of the above cohort or not). There were 11,237 such children, including 3245 who were part of the prospective cohort. Children whose cultures were positive and whose cough persisted for 21 days or more were each matched with four control patients from the same practice who were born within 30 days of the subject. Pertinent clinical, demographic, and immunization data were entered into a conditional logistic regression analysis to calculate the relative odds of pertussis while controlling for confounding factors.

Eighty-seven subjects met the case definition of 21 or more days of paroxysmal cough plus either positive culture or household contact with a laboratory-confirmed case. These individuals were matched to 344 control subjects. Eighty-one of the case subjects and 186 of the control subjects had received no pertussis vaccine; 4 and 55, respectively, had received three doses of DTaP; and 1 and 61, respectively, had received three doses of DTP. Adjusted estimates of efficacy were 96% for the DTP and 93% for the DTaP.[227]

This study raises issues that may be applicable to any study that is not completely blinded and randomized. Although these efficacy estimates reflect adjustment for risk factors that differed between cases and controls, such as the number of siblings in day care, it is not possible to adjust for, or even confirm the existence or magnitude of, any bias that might have arisen because the study was not blinded or randomized. The analysis rested on comparing the proportions of vaccinated patients in two groups: those patients who were brought in because of possible pertussis, and control subjects who were selected in a systematic manner. If unvaccinated children were more likely than vaccinated children to be brought to the pediatrician with suspicious

cough, they would be over-represented in the case (but not control) groups, biasing upward the estimates of efficacy for DTaP and DTP.

Could this bias have happened? Parents knew what vaccine their child received; those whose child received no pertussis vaccine might have been more likely to seek care when their child had a cough illness. (Conversely, parents who selected a pertussis-containing vaccine may have been more health conscious and more likely to seek medical attention than other parents. Lack of blinding can bias in either direction.) It is reassuring that 76% of cultures in the prospective cohort were from infants receiving DTaP, and infants receiving DTaP comprised 75% of the cohort, suggesting that any bias was negligible.

Even if the parents did not differ in their response to cough illness, we know that vaccinated children who develop pertussis have a milder illness. Such children are less likely to have been brought to the pediatrician and are thus less likely to have been included in the case group. Because the case definition did not allow for serologic confirmation of possible cases, confirmation depended on obtaining a positive culture, thus increasing the risk of diagnostic bias (as described after the 1986 Swedish trial).

These factors, coupled with the small number of cases detected, led us to interpret the point estimates of efficacy from the Munich trial with caution. Some reassurance, however, is derived from the fact that the Munich and Mainz studies generated similar estimates of efficacy for the referent whole-cell vaccine that was common to both.

The Munich investigators continued to follow the study cohort through the end of 2001. During the period from 2 years through 6 years (1997 to 2001) following the fourth dose of pertussis vaccine (given at 15 to 24 months of age), the crude overall efficacy against typical pertussis (defined as 21 or more days of paroxysmal cough) was 93% (95% CI, 79% to 98%) for those receiving Tripedia and 96% (95% CI, 76% to 99%) for those receiving the Behring whole-cell vaccine; adjusted for various confounders, the respective efficacies were 96% (85% to 99%) and 97% (81% to 99.6%). Protection was materially lower among those not receiving four doses: crude and adjusted efficacies for those receiving three or fewer doses of Tripedia were 82% (7% to 96%) and 83% (− 5% to 97%), respectively. Adjusted efficacy against milder pertussis (defined as 7 or more days of any cough) was 71% (45% to 84%) for those receiving four doses of Tripedia and 80% (40% to 93%) for those receiving four doses of Behring whole-cell vaccine. (Note that long-term follow-up results from the various efficacy trials should not be compared directly to the results obtained in the original trials, given the substantial differences in surveillance methods and sensitivities.)

ERLANGEN, GERMANY

A prospective, randomized, double-blind clinical trial conducted from May 1991 to December 1994 in Erlangen, Germany, compared two U.S.-licensed vaccines produced by study sponsor Wyeth-Lederle: the Lederle-Takeda four-component DTaP (ACEL- IMUNE) and the U.S. DTP that served as the control vaccine in the MAPT.[180,228] Participants were immunized at approximately 3, 5, 7, and 17 months of age. Infants whose parents declined pertussis immunization received a German DT vaccine at approximately 3, 5, and 17 months of age and served as the control group for estimates of absolute efficacy.

Based on a case definition of 21 or more days of cough with paroxysms, whoop, or post-tussive vomiting plus either positive culture, positive serology, or household contact with a culture-proven case, efficacies after three doses of vaccine were 78% for DTaP and 93% for DTP.[180] (The abstract of this trial's published report cites an efficacy of 83% for the DTaP, but that figure reflects the benefit of a fourth, booster dose of vaccine and thus is not comparable to the data presented for any other trial.) As reported in the FDA-approved labeling for ACEL-IMUNE, the relative risk of pertussis was 1.5 for DTaP compared with DTP.[228] A household-contact study nested within the overall trial found efficacy rates similar to those reported from the cohort study.[356]

Although this study also used an unblinded, nonrandomized placebo control group for estimates of absolute efficacy, the potential for ascertainment bias may have been reduced by the use of active surveillance (telephone calls every 2 weeks) to detect possible cases. In a follow-up analysis that has implications for all of the efficacy studies, the local physicians who served as study investigators were stratified into three groups based on the proportion of their patients who underwent investigation for pertussis.[357] For subjects attended by physicians who sought pertussis diligently, efficacy of the DTaP in preventing laboratory-confirmed pertussis with 7 or more days of cough was only 40%, whereas efficacy was 78% and 75% in the physician groups of moderate and low diligence, respectively. These results are not surprising, in that the less diligent physicians detected only the more obvious (i.e., more severe) cases, and it has long been known that the efficacy of pertussis vaccine appears higher when one uses case definitions that focus on more severe disease. Nonetheless, this analysis has illuminated the extent to which fairly subtle differences in diagnostic diligence can alter estimates of efficacy, and it alerts us to another factor that might confound efforts to compare the results of different studies.

The Lederle-Takeda is a four-component vaccine, but it predominantly consists of FHA (86%; about 35 μg), with very little PT, fimbrial proteins, or PRN, as reflected by both its formulation (see Table 21–3) and its immunogenicity (see Table 21–8). It appears to be of somewhat lower efficacy than the three-component vaccines evaluated in Italy (although the 95% CIs do overlap). If so, this represents further evidence that the quantity of the individual components can be as important as the number of components in determining the efficacy of the vaccine.

Following unblinding of the study, physicians and parents of approximately one third of study participants agreed to respond to semiannual questionnaires regarding cough illness and pertussis among study participants. Surveillance from 1995 through 2000 showed no diminution in pertussis protection in either the DTaP or the DTP group, as compared to the DT group.[358]

NIAKHAR, SENEGAL

A prospective, randomized, double-blind study conducted in Senegal from 1990 to 1994 compared a two-component DTaP produced by study sponsor Aventis Pasteur (Triavax)

with that company's European DTP in children immunized at 2, 4, and 6 months of age.[229] Estimates of absolute efficacy were derived from a nested case-contact study that compared rates of pertussis (after exposure to an index case) among study subjects and nonstudy children (who thus had received either DT or no vaccine) living in the same villages and housing compounds. Thus the study design was analogous to that of a household-contact study.

Surveillance detected 197 DTaP and 123 DTP recipients who met the primary case definition of confirmed pertussis (see Table 21–12) with cough for 21 or more days, yielding a relative risk of pertussis 1.54 times higher in the DTaP than the DTP group. Requiring the cough to be paroxysmal (the WHO definition) reduced the case counts to 41 and 16, respectively, for a relative risk with DTaP of 2.42 compared with DTP.

When cases were stratified by age, the relative risk of meeting the primary case definition was 1.16 for children younger than 18 months versus 1.76 for older children, suggesting that protection waned more quickly among DTaP than DTP recipients.

The case-contact study included 197 DTaP recipients, 190 DTP recipients, and 17 unvaccinated children exposed to pertussis, of whom 24, 7, and 8, respectively, met the WHO case definition; the absolute efficacy estimates were 74% for DTaP and 92% for DTP. Owing to the small number of cases, confidence limits for these estimates are wide (95% CIs, 51% to 86% and 81% to 97% for DTaP and DTP, respectively). In addition, although field surveillance workers and physician evaluators were blinded to the vaccination status of the randomized children, it is obvious that parents knew whether their children had been vaccinated, a situation that may have increased case detection among unimmunized children. For both reasons, the relative rates are likely to be more reliable than the absolute efficacy estimates.

Initial reports from the investigators cited efficacies of 85% to 86% for DTaP and 95% to 96% for DTP,[359] and some early reviews echo those figures.[360,361] However, these higher efficacies are based on a requirement that epidemiologically linked cases be confirmed by PCR, a case definition more strict than that of the WHO.

Compared with whole-cell vaccine, relative risks of WHO-defined pertussis were 0.85 and 1.38 in Stockholm 1993 for the five-component Aventis Pasteur and three-component Chiron vaccines, respectively, as compared with 2.42 for the two-component DTaP evaluated in Senegal. Unless the Aventis Pasteur whole-cell vaccine used in the Senegal trial is substantially more effective than the Wellcome whole-cell vaccine used in the Stockholm 1993 trial, it would appear that this two-component acellular vaccine is less efficacious than the three- and five-component vaccines evaluated in Sweden and Italy. (The data do not permit a direct comparison with the two-component vaccine evaluated in Sweden.)

MAINZ, GERMANY

A prospective household-contact study was conducted from October 1992 to September 1994 in six areas of Germany, in which 22,505 children had been immunized with study sponsor GlaxoSmithKline's three-component acellular pertussis vaccine (Infanrix) in a prior safety and immunogenicity trial. Other children in these regions were unimmunized against pertussis or had been immunized with the Behringwerke whole-cell vaccine at 3, 4, and 5 months of age, in accord with the standard German schedule. Passive surveillance for pertussis identified households that contained both an index case of pertussis and at least one contact age 6 to 47 months who could be evaluated. Prospective surveillance of the 360 eligible contacts identified 104 secondary cases of pertussis (defined as 21 or more days of spasmodic cough plus either culture or serologic confirmation of *B. pertussis* infection): 96 of the 173 unvaccinated children, 7 of the 112 DTaP recipients, and 1 of the 75 DTP recipients. The corresponding estimates of vaccine efficacy were 89% for the DTaP and 98% for the Behringwerke DTP.[226]

The use of a household-contact study design largely eliminated the potential for ascertainment bias that would otherwise arise from the fact that study groups were not blinded or randomized, because family members were intensely surveyed by blinded field supervisors for pertussis in households with an index case. However, the authors noted that the efficacy of the Behringwerke whole-cell vaccine may have been overestimated owing to more frequent erythromycin use among contacts who had received the whole-cell vaccine.[226] The simplest explanation for the higher efficacy estimate for Infanrix in this study (89%) than in the more rigorous, prospective Italian trial (84%) is that the small number of cases in this study reduced the precision of the estimate, as reflected by the wide confidence limits (95% CI, 77% to 95%).

Conclusions from the Efficacy Trials

Although the efficacy trials and other studies have greatly enriched our understanding of pertussis vaccines, they have left many important questions unresolved. Despite attempts to standardize key variables, no two studies are perfectly comparable. No study has evaluated a multicomponent vaccine directly against versions of itself that contain alternate components or different quantities of each component, and there is no reasonable expectation of such a study. Although the comparative merits of the various acellular vaccines will remain a subject of debate, decisions must nonetheless be made. The following comments reflect our opinion of the relevant data, as presented in the text and tables elsewhere in this chapter.

DIFFERENCES AMONG ACELLULAR VACCINES

The fact that numerous DTaP vaccines are licensed, and are treated evenhandedly by government purchasers or distributors, does not mean they are equivalent to each other. They differ in source, number of components, amount of each component, and method of manufacture, resulting in differences in efficacy and in the frequency of adverse effects.

COMPARATIVE EFFICACY OF ACELLULAR VERSUS WHOLE-CELL VACCINES

Acellular and whole-cell vaccines overlap in their ranges of efficacies. If we could match all the vaccines head to head in a prospective, blinded, randomized trial, we would probably find that whole-cell efficacies range from 85% to 95%, with one or two much lower. We would probably find that acellular efficacies range from 75% to 90%, with one or two

much lower. Vaccine efficacy is not the sole determinant of the effectiveness of an immunization program; factors such as the comprehensiveness of coverage and the immunization schedule (especially the timing and number of boosters) are of greater importance in determining program effectiveness. For example, pediatric pertussis was well controlled in the United States using one whole-cell vaccine of moderate efficacy and another whose efficacy (without a booster dose) was startlingly low (see Table 21–12).

Acellular vaccines may be preferable for booster immunization. A case-control study performed in Canada showed that a single booster of acellular vaccine given to children either at 18 months or at 5–6 years, substantially decreased the risk of pertussis compared with children who received a booster of whole cell vaccine.[361a]

COMPARATIVE EFFICACY OF THE VARIOUS ACELLULAR VACCINES

It is virtually certain that there are real differences in efficacy among the acellular vaccines. However, vaccine efficacy is only one—and probably not the most important—factor in determining the effectiveness of a vaccine program, and it is only one of the qualities that should be considered in choosing a vaccine. Of the evaluated acellular pertussis vaccines, all except SKB-2 appear to have demonstrated sufficient efficacy in the prevention of whooping cough (and all are sufficiently safe) to warrant their licensure. Licensed vaccines are generally considered equally acceptable; in the United States, for example, recommending bodies (such as the ACIP or the Red Book Committee) have expressed no preference for one licensed acellular vaccine over another. Thus one should not accord undue importance to the following ranking.

When we consider the results of the efficacy studies as well as the confidence the design of each study permits us to have in its results, we conclude that the three- and five-component vaccines evaluated in Stockholm 1992, Stockholm 1993, and Italy (Triacelluvax, Infanrix, and the two formulations [classical and hybrid] of Tripacel) are probably the most efficacious. The vaccines evaluated in Munich and Senegal (Tripedia and Triavax) may be in an intermediate tier, with the remaining vaccines somewhat less efficacious. Owing to study design limitations, however, we cannot exclude the possibility that the middle and lower tiers are equivalent (or even that the middle and upper tiers are equivalent), let alone try to place those vaccines in order.

Note that we have categorized the Biken and Takeda vaccines as middle or lower tier; however, these are the acellular vaccines used in Japan, where national surveillance statistics have shown them to control pertussis exceedingly well (at least as well as whole-cell vaccine; see Fig. 21–4). Note also that widespread use of Certiva in the Göteborg area since mid-1995 has been associated with the near-eradication of pertussis disease. Either we have incorrectly categorized these vaccines, or "middle or lower tier" is more than good enough (we believe the latter to be the case).

There is good evidence from Japan that acellular vaccines can induce substantial herd immunity. During a period when only children 2 years or older were being immunized, pertussis rates fell dramatically not only in that group but also among all younger age groups. The experience in Göteborg, Sweden, in household studies and after implementation in 1995 of mass vaccination with Certiva provides further evidence of herd immunity. Whether the acellular vaccines differ in their ability to decrease spread of pertussis, independent of any differences in efficacy, is unclear.

DETERMINANTS OF EFFICACY

The number of components, the quantity of each component, and the methods of producing the components (particularly the PT) all influence the efficacy of an acellular vaccine; no one of these factors is determinative irrespective of the others. For example, a vaccine with few components might be more effective than another vaccine that has more components but has them in lesser quantity or of lesser immunogenicity.

Everyone seems to agree that PT is the essential component; most seem to think that adding other components is helpful. The three vaccines previously mentioned as appearing to be the most effective all contain PRN. However, that does not prove that PRN is more important than FHA or fimbrial proteins; no study has made the necessary comparisons (e.g., PT/FHA plus fimbrial proteins versus the same PT/FHA plus PRN). Moreover, as noted previously, the available studies attempting to define correlates of protection are limited by the fact that their data derive from vaccination with only certain vaccines; even if they correctly identify correlates for those vaccines, they can offer no insight into the correlates of protection with other vaccines.

ONSET OF PROTECTION AND EFFECT OF VACCINE SCHEDULE

It appears that some protection (perhaps 15% to 20%) accrues with the first dose, and substantially more with the second dose (see Tables 21–13 and 21–14). A reanalysis of data in the Technical Report of the Stockholm 1993 trial indicates that the incidence of pertussis was markedly lower after the second dose than after the first dose, and was reduced somewhat further by the third dose (Table 21–14).[335] These data also illustrate that patterns of protection vary by dose; the whole-cell vaccine offered relatively greater protection with a single dose, lower incremental benefit with the next dose, and a more rapid decline in protection with time following the third dose. It is also apparent that acellular vaccines differ, sometimes markedly, in the degree of protection afforded by the initial doses. However, for most of the efficacy studies, the data necessary for a proper analysis of this question have not been published.

In general, three doses appear to be necessary for acceptable protection, and, for most of the vaccines and schedules, a booster dose at around 15 months of age will provide substantial additional benefit. There is probably little difference between schedules that immunize at ages 2, 4, and 6 months; 3, 5, and 7 months; or even 2, 3, and 4 months. Immunizing at 3, 5, and 12 months of age gives a little less protection in the second half-year of life and better protection thereafter, as one would intuitively expect.

COMPARATIVE RATES OF ADVERSE REACTIONS

Common adverse events (e.g., fever, pain, irritability) and uncommon adverse events (e.g., seizures, shock-like episodes) both appear to be reduced by about two thirds with acellular as compared to whole-cell vaccine. Of course, using acellular vaccine will not reduce the risk of events such as SIDS that are not caused by pertussis vaccine. Among the acellular vaccines, the MAPT study allows us to directly compare rates of common adverse reactions. As shown in Table 21–15, no one vaccine is the most or least reactogenic across all reactions, but there are some trends. Of the seven vaccines presently licensed in one or more countries, the fewest reactions are seen with Triacelluvax and Certiva and ACEL-IMUNE (perhaps because of its low content of antigens other than FHA). Vaccines more reactogenic than average for all DTaPs evaluated in the MAPT include Infanrix and Tripacel, two of the highest efficacy vaccines, as well as Triavax. The seventh vaccine, Tripedia, had average reactogenicity. With respect to the less common, more severe adverse effects, one presumes that the acellular vaccines must differ from one another at least somewhat, but the safety data from the efficacy trials (Table 21–16) cannot be compared across studies. Once again, we must caution the reader against according too much importance to these rankings, even if he or she agrees with them. The reduction in reactogenicity of every acellular vaccine, compared with whole-cell vaccine, is far greater than any differences among the acellular vaccines.

CHOICE OF VACCINE

For those providers free to choose among vaccines, we recommend consideration of five factors (some may not apply in every situation): efficacy, rate of adverse effects, cost, convenience (e.g., how is the vaccine supplied?), and service (e.g., reliability of supply, provision of educational materials, etc.). Choices can then be made based on the relative weights assigned to each of those factors.

TABLE 21–14 ■ Incidence of Pertussis (per Million Days at Risk) by Dose, Stockholm 1992 Efficacy Trial*

Interval	SKB-2	Acelluvax	HCPDT	Evans-Medeva WCV
Primary Analyses (follow-up from study start until October 1996)				
Dose 1 to dose 3	n/a	8.1	6.7	4.4
Dose 3 to study end (approx 21 mo)	n/a	1.8	1.1	1.3
Secondary Analyses (follow-up from study start until 28 July 1995, when SKB-2 group was reimmunized with HCPDT)				
Dose 1 to dose 2	19.6	16.0	16.9	11.3
Dose 2 to dose 3	14.3	5.8	2.6	1.8
Dose 3 to early termination (approx 7 mo)	4.2	1.3	1.0	0.5

*Data derived from Tables 12.1.1, 12.1.3, 12.2.1, 12.2.3, and 12.2.4 in Olin T, Gustafsson L, Rasmussen F et al. Efficacy Trial of Acellular Pertussis Vaccines: Technical Report Trial II, with Preplanned Analysis of Efficacy, Immunogenicity and Safety. Stockholm, Swedish Institute for Infectious Disease Control, 1997.

TABLE 21–15 ■ Adverse Reaction Results from the Multicenter Acellular Pertussis Trial and a Follow-up Trial*

Manufacturer or Distributor	Vaccine†	Fever, °F 100.1–101	>101.1	Redness, mm 1–20	>20	Swelling, mm 1–20	>20	Pain‡	Fussiness§	Drowsiness	Anorexia	Vomiting	Crude Overall Average|	# of Values Exceeding MAPT DTAP Average¶
Aventis Pasteur (Canada)	Tripacel	29.2%	3.6%	32.8%	3.6%	21.9%	4.4%	5.1%	18.2%	42.3%	19.0%	12.4%	17.5%	6
Aventis Pasteur (Canada)	3-component	22.4%	3.2%	44.0%	2.4%	22.4%	8.0%	12.0%	21.6%	45.6%	27.2%	21.6%	20.9%	8
Aventis Pasteur (France)	Triavax	24.1%	4.6%	42.9%	4.5%	28.6%	5.3%	8.3%	12.0%	42.1%	20.3%	7.5%	18.2%	7
Aventis Pasteur (USA)	Tripedia	19.3%	5.2%	27.4%	5.2%	16.3%	3.7%	9.6%	19.3%	41.5%	22.2%	7.4%	16.1%	5
Baxter Laboratories	Certiva	20.0%	2.5%	20.0%	2.5%	7.5%	2.5%	7.5%	22.5%	30.0%	20.0%	2.5%	12.5%	2
Biocine Sclavo	1-component	18.6%	3.6%	28.3%	5.3%	24.8%	3.5%	3.6%	20.4%	52.2%	25.7%	17.7%	18.5%	6
Chiron Vaccines	Triacelluvax	19.0%	1.6%	29.4%	1.6%	17.5%	2.4%	1.6%	16.7%	41.3%	19.0%	9.5%	14.5%	0
GlaxoSmithKline	Infanrix	28.3%	3.3%	35.0%	4.2%	24.2%	5.8%	10.8%	15.0%	46.7%	19.2%	12.5%	18.6%	7
Massachusetts Public Health Biologic Labs	1-component	21.2%	4.1%	36.3%	1.4%	21.9%	6.2%	8.2%	16.4%	48.6%	22.6%	14.4%	18.3%	8
Michigan Department of Public Health	2-component	22.1%	2.2%	30.1%	5.9%	19.1%	3.7%	13.2%	16.2%	46.3%	23.5%	14.0%	17.8%	5
SmithKline Beecham Biologicals	2-component	18.8%	3.1%	31.3%	2.1%	23.4%	4.2%	6.2%	17.2%	37.0%	17.7%	10.9%	15.6%	2
Speywood (Porton) Pharmaceuticals	3-component	17.6%	5.0%	36.1%	2.5%	21.0%	4.2%	4.2%	24.4%	45.4%	18.5%	10.9%	17.3%	5
Wyeth Lederle Vaccines and Pediatrics	3-component	16.0%	5.9%	15.1%	2.5%	10.9%	0.8%	5.9%	12.6%	29.4%	22.7%	12.6%	12.2%	2
Wyeth Pharmaceuticals	ACEL-IMUNE	16.6%	3.2%	23.5%	2.8%	12.4%	3.2%	3.7%	14.3%	40.6%	24.9%	13.4%	14.4%	2
Average for all DTaPs in MAPT	—	20.8%	3.7%	31.4%	3.3%	20.1%	4.2%	6.9%	17.1%	42.7%	21.7%	12.6%	16.8%	5
Wyeth Lederle Vaccines and Pediatrics	whole-cell	44.5%	15.9%	56.3%	16.4%	38.5%	22.4%	40.2%	41.5%	62.0%	35.0%	13.7%	—	—

Abbreviations: CI, confidence interval; FHA, filamentous hemagglutinin; FIM, fimbrial proteins; MAPT, Multicenter Acellular Pertussis Trial; PRN, pertactin; PT, pertussis toxin

*Results for Certiva are from a separate study conducted at an MAPT study center after completion of the MAPT, using the MAPT protocol, procedures, and data forms.

†Number of pertussis components, for those vaccines without known trade names. For branded products, note that the licensed vaccine's formulation may differ from that of the vaccine evaluated in MAPT. See Table 21–3 and its footnotes for details.

‡Moderate (cried or protested to touch) or severe (cried when leg moved).

§Moderate (prolonged crying and refused to play) or severe (persistent crying and could not be comforted).

|An unweighted average of the 11 specific rates shown to the left of this value. Has the effect of giving more weight to less serious reactions, but provides a crude overall comparison that may be useful.

¶Of the 11 specific rates, the number for which this vaccine's reaction rate exceeded the average for all DTaPs evaluated in the MAPT (see the next-to-last row of the table). Treats small differences and large differences as though they were the same, but provides a crude overall comparison that may be useful.

Adapted with permission from Decker MD, Edwards KM, Steinhoff MC, Rennels MB, Pichichero ME, Englund JA, Anderson EL, Deloria MA, Reed GF. Comparison of 13 acellular pertussis vaccines: adverse reactions. Pediatrics 1995;96:557–566.

511

Other Evidence of Effectiveness of Acellular Vaccines

Both the whole-cell and acellular pertussis vaccines have been highly effective in controlling pertussis in Japan. From 1948 to 1975, pertussis was well controlled by a program that initiated immunization at the age of 3 months (see Fig. 21–4).[205] In response to concerns regarding adverse reactions, in 1975 the age of immunization was raised to 24 months, effectively suspending immunization for 2 years. During this period, reported pertussis cases in Japan rose dramatically, with more than 40,000 cases and nearly 200 deaths for the 8 years from 1976 to 1983.[163,205] By 1980, vaccine acceptance rates were again above 70%, and pertussis cases began to decline.[205] In 1981, whole-cell vaccine was replaced by the new acellular vaccines, and the decline in cases and deaths continued[205]; by 1988, reported pertussis cases were approximately 400, with 5 deaths.[362]

It was hoped that a program that vaccinated children beginning at 2 years of age would prevent transmission of disease to younger children,[205] and national surveillance data indeed revealed that pertussis rates declined sixfold to ninefold among unimmunized children younger than 2 years.[363] Unfortunately, even with this decline, 1984 pertussis rates still remained sixfold higher among these unimmunized children than they had been in 1974, prior to the suspension of whole-cell immunization. For children 3 years and older, however, the incidence of pertussis was essentially the same in 1984 as it had been in 1974.[205] Consequently, the national immunization policy was changed once again, and beginning in 1989, it was recommended that pertussis immunization commence at age 3 months.

A later study provided data showing that the incidence of pertussis among children 2 years and younger continued to decline between 1987 and 1989.[207] Thus it would appear that use of the acellular pertussis vaccines among older children was capable of protecting younger, unimmunized children but that the full effect did not appear until vaccination had continued long enough, and widely enough, to substantially reduce overall pertussis rates.

Household-contact studies in Japan found that the efficacy of the acellular vaccines ranged from 78% to 94%.[205, 206, 364–367] Studies of the Lederle-Takeda[209,255,362,368–375] and Aventis Pasteur–Biken[209,255,376–378] vaccines found that their immunogenicities were comparable to those of whole-cell vaccine and were similar in Japanese and U.S. infants. In addition, these vaccines caused fewer adverse reactions than the whole-cell vaccine. These data justified licensure of these vaccines in the United States for the fourth and fifth doses, prior to completion of the efficacy trials.[332,379]

An active, nationwide, hospital-based surveillance system in Germany (where acellular vaccines have predominated since their introduction) has demonstrated an age-adjusted effectiveness of completed primary vaccination of 99.8% (95% CI, 98.9% to 100%) for prevention of hospitalization as a result of pertussis.[380] Even a single dose gave 68% effectiveness.

Efficacy of Acellular Vaccines Against Mild Disease

Persons with mild disease may play an important role in the spread of pertussis, and vaccines may differ in their effectiveness against mild disease. If so, those vaccines that are more effective against mild disease may be more effective at interrupting the transmission of pertussis, resulting in a greater herd immunity effect.

It has been suggested that vaccines containing attachment proteins (e.g., FHA, PRN, and perhaps fimbrial proteins) may have a relative advantage in preventing mild disease and may therefore better curtail the spread of pertussis. Figure 21–6 shows the efficacy of various vaccines in preventing culture-confirmed pertussis associated with cough of selected durations. The slope of each line reflects the change in efficacy from mild to severe disease (a horizontal line means that efficacies are the same for mild and severe disease). None of the lines is perfectly horizontal; every vaccine was more efficacious against severe than against mild illness (see also Table 21–13). The acellular vaccine with the lowest overall efficacy (the SmithKline Beecham–GlaxoSmithKline two-component acellular vaccine [SKB-2]) has a line that is noticeably steeper than most, and the line for the Aventis Pasteur Canada five-component vaccine (Tripacel) appears more horizontal than most. Many lines have surprisingly similar slopes, despite representing quite dissimilar vaccines (e.g., slopes are virtually identical for the monocomponent vaccine Certiva and the three-component vaccine Infanrix). Thus it does not appear that the number of components in the vaccine necessarily affects efficacy against mild disease separately from efficacy against severe disease.

Duration of Immunity After Acellular Vaccines

The available data from follow-up of various efficacy trial cohorts, covering periods ranging from 2 to 6 years, show no diminution in protection from pertussis for the evaluated acellular pertussis vaccines, with the single exception of the experimental two-component GSK DTaP evaluated in Sweden.

Long-term follow-up of subjects in the 1986 Swedish efficacy trial did not demonstrate any decline in efficacy of the JNIH-6 or JNIH-7 vaccines through the end of the fourth year after immunization (although it did make clear the higher efficacy of the JNIH-6 vaccine).[239] In the Stockholm 1992 trial, efficacy of the Aventis Pasteur five-component vaccine was sustained above 80% during 2 years of follow-up, whereas that of the control whole-cell vaccine declined sharply.[181] During 6 years of extended follow-up in the Italian trial, efficacies of both the Chiron and the GlaxoSmithKline three-component vaccines were fully maintained.[182,352] Follow-up of subjects given Certiva in the Göteborg trial showed that protection remained unchanged for at least 2 years after the third dose. Follow-up of the Erlangen cohort for 6 years showed no diminution in protection for the Lederle-Takeda DTaP or the Lederle DTP. Five-year follow-up results for the Aventis Pasteur–Biken vaccine used in the Munich cohort are expected in mid-2002.

A British study of children immunized at ages 3, 5, and 9 months with acellular or Wellcome whole-cell vaccine found significantly better PT antibody persistence at age 4 to 5 years among recipients of the Aventis Pasteur two-component acellular vaccine compared with the whole-cell or Lederle-Takeda vaccines.[232] In contrast, the efficacy trial

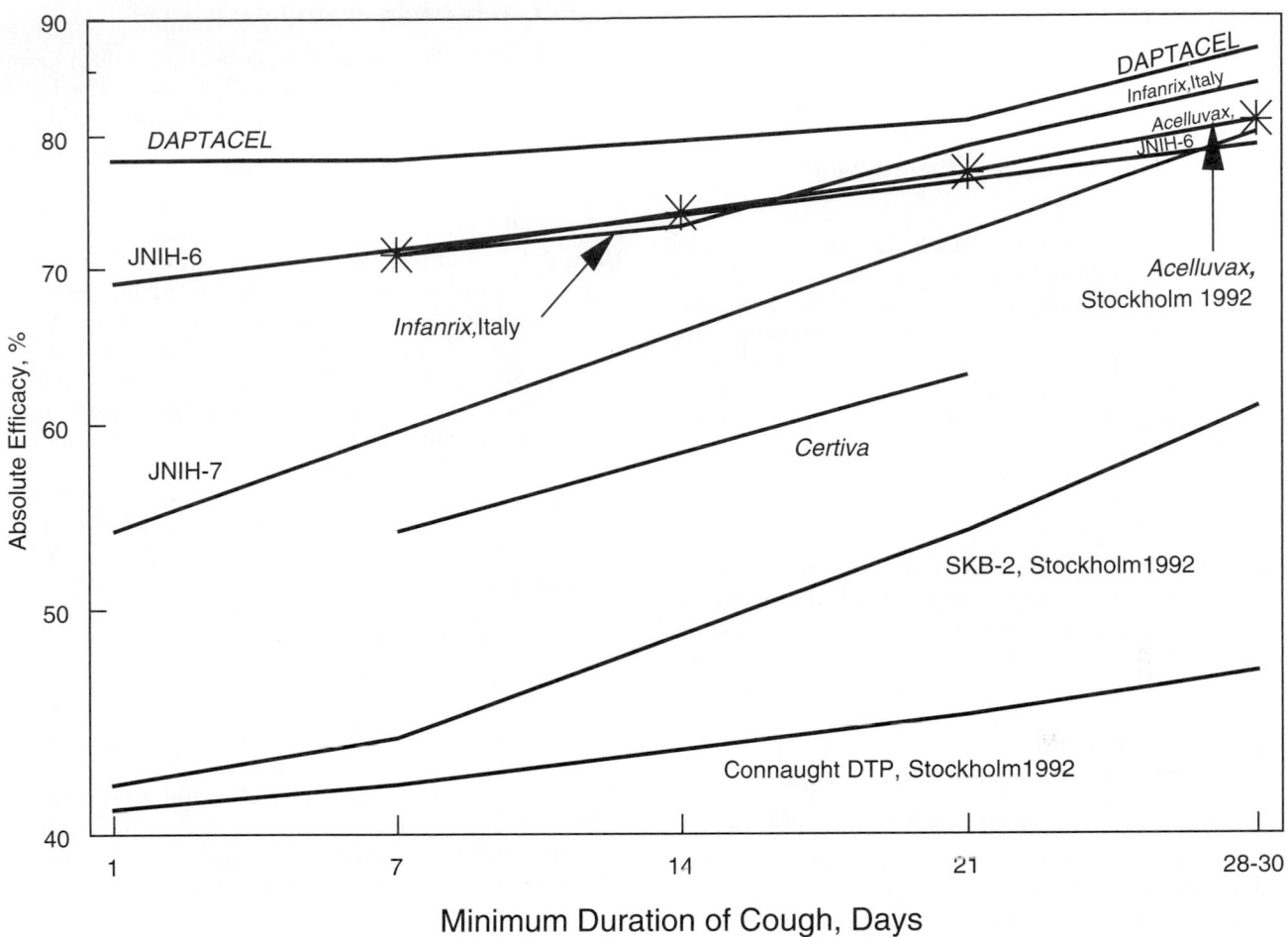

FIGURE 21–6 ■ Efficacy of pertussis vaccines evaluated in prospective, randomized trials (names defined in Table 21–3) for preventing various durations of any cough associated with culture-confirmed pertussis. A slope of zero (horizontal line) would indicate equal protection for mild and severe disease; steeper slopes reflect lesser protection for mild than severe disease. Because estimates were obtained in separate studies, only the slopes, and not the actual values, should be compared.

in Senegal found that the protective efficacy of the same Aventis Pasteur vaccine, given at ages 2, 4, and 6 months, declined after 18 months of age as compared with the Aventis Pasteur whole-cell vaccine.[229]

The duration of immunity will likely depend on the vaccine used, the schedule followed, and the number of doses administered. Although further long-term data are needed, the available results strongly suggest improved duration of immunity with most licensed acellular vaccines, as compared to whole-cell vaccine.

An outbreak of pertussis in an American elementary school revealed an efficacy of 80% for all vaccines with no evidence for waning of immunity.[380a]

Guiso and colleagues analyzed B. pertussis strains isolated in Japan before and after the introduction of acellular vaccines and found no evidence for antigenic divergence induced by vaccination.[380b]

Adverse Events with Acellular Vaccines

Numerous safety and immunogenicity studies of the acellular vaccines have been conducted in infants and children[376,381–386] and have invariably found the acellular

vaccines to be associated with lower rates of adverse reactions than whole-cell vaccine. Although most trials have not compared one acellular vaccine with another to detect differences in the rates of adverse reactions, the MAPT evaluated 13 acellular and 2 whole-cell vaccines and thus offers the best comparison of common reactions with these vaccines.[255] The various efficacy trials maintained surveillance for severe adverse events among much larger numbers of infants and thus supplement the MAPT data by providing more precise estimates of rates for these less common events.

Common Adverse Events: Comparative Rates

The MAPT included all acellular vaccines studied in the efficacy trials except one, a monovalent PT vaccine similar to Certiva, produced by North American Vaccine. Fortunately, this vaccine was evaluated using the MAPT protocol in a subsequent trial at one of the MAPT study sites, which allows it to be directly compared with the other vaccines (see Table 21–15).

Among the acellular vaccines, there were significant differences with respect to redness, swelling, pain, and vomiting but not fussiness, drowsiness, anorexia, or antipyretic use.[255] No acellular vaccine was consistently the most or least reactogenic. Compared with the reference whole-cell vaccine, all the acellular vaccines were associated with significantly lower rates and severity of every reaction except vomiting.

Common and Severe Adverse Events: Data from the Efficacy Trials

Adverse reaction data from the efficacy trials, organized by vaccine, are summarized here and in Table 21–16. Definitions and methods may have differed from study to study, and thus caution should be used in comparing rates between trials. Note also that Table 21–16 presents reaction rates per dose of vaccine, whereas the rates presented in the following paragraphs are per subject (these two approaches will produce different rates unless every child with a reaction has the same reaction with every dose).

ACEL-IMUNE (LEDERLE-TAKEDA)

In the Erlangen trial, minor local and systemic reactions and antipyretic use occurred at nearly identical rates among DTaP and DT recipients but were significantly more common after DTP.[387] Persistent inconsolable crying was experienced by 3.3% of recipients of DTP and 0.7% of recipients of DTaP or DT; convulsions within 72 hours of vaccination occurred in 4, 1, and 0 recipients, respectively.[388] One case of HHE occurred, in a DTP recipient.

TRIACELLUVAX (CHIRON) AND INFANRIX (GLAXOSMITHKLINE)

In the Italian trial, adverse events were significantly more common among recipients of DTP than DTaP or DT. Temperature of 40.5°C or greater was seen in 6.8% of recipients of DTP, 0.8% of recipients of Infanrix, 1.1% of recipients of Triacelluvax, and 1.3% of recipients of DT; crying 3 or more hours in 11.5%, 1.9%, 1.3%, and 0%, respectively; and HHE in 1.7%, 0.2%, 0%, and 1.3%, respectively.[389] Seizures within 48 hours of vaccination occurred in one Infanrix recipient and in three DTP recipients.[182] The Stockholm 1993 trial also found significantly fewer of these adverse reactions with Triacelluvax than whole-cell vaccine.[329]

CERTIVA (BAXTER PHARMACEUTICALS)

Of 1724 children given Certiva in the Göteborg trial, there were no episodes of persistent crying, HHE, afebrile seizures, or withdrawal from the study because of an adverse reaction.[330] Two acellular vaccine recipients (0.1%) developed febrile convulsions within 48 hours after vaccination. Invasive bacterial infections occurred at a lower rate among Certiva than DT recipients.

TRIAVAX (AVENTIS PASTEUR, FRANCE)

In the Senegal efficacy study, Triavax and Aventis Pasteur's French whole-cell vaccine were each given to approximately 2200 children. Persistent crying was significantly more common among whole-cell recipients (eight vs. zero episodes). Two subjects in each group experienced febrile seizures within 48 hours of vaccine administration. No episodes of HHE or anaphylactic reactions were seen. In the pilot study preceding this trial, fever, crying, and local reactions were significantly more common with whole-cell than acellular vaccine.[390]

TRIPACEL (AVENTIS PASTEUR LTD, CANADA)

Of the 2552 children given the classical (CLL-4F$_2$) formulation of Tripacel in Stockholm 1992, 1 (0.04%) had HHE and another was withdrawn as a result of pronounced local reactions.[181] There were seven episodes of convulsions, but none occurred within 48 hours of vaccination, making a causal association unlikely. Of 17,686 children given the hybrid (HCPDT) formulation of Tripacel in Stockholm 1993, 0.04% had fever of 40°C or greater and 0.02% had convulsions within 48 hours of vaccine administration.[329] Minor local and systemic reactions were significantly less common with HCPDT than with whole-cell vaccine. The investigators made a special effort to detect HHE in Stockholm 1993, and thus higher HHE rates were recorded for vaccines evaluated in that study than for the same, or similar, vaccines evaluated in other studies. HHE rates were, for Tripacel, 0.47 per 1000 in Stockholm 1993 (hybrid formulation) versus 0.13 per 1000 in Stockholm 1992 (classical formulation); and for Triacelluvax, 0.26 per 1000 in Stockholm 1993 versus 0.07 per 1000 in Italy 1992.

TRIPEDIA (AVENTIS PASTEUR, USA)

Of 12,514 children given Tripedia in the Munich trial, 2.2% experienced the following adverse events related to vaccination: fever, 0.9%; local reactions, 0.4%; unusual crying, 0.3%; irritability, 0.3%; somnolence, 0.2%; crying more than 3 hours, 0.04%; HHE, 0.02%; and febrile seizure, 0.01%.[227] Ten children given Tripedia had culture-confirmed invasive bacterial disease, but the rate of disease was not significantly higher than that seen in the control group.

Severe Adverse Events: National Surveillance Data

The claims paid by the Japanese Vaccine Compensation System provide a comparison of severe neurologic reactions and deaths with whole-cell versus acellular vaccine and with immunization beginning at 3 months versus 2 years.[205,207,391] As shown in Table 21–17, changing the age of administration of whole-cell vaccine from 3 months to 2 years was associated with a dramatic reduction in compensable adverse neurologic events and deaths; a further reduction occurred with the change from whole-cell to acellular vaccine. The data strongly suggest that this low rate of serious adverse events was maintained after the initiation in 1989 of immunization with acellular vaccine at the age of 3 months. Severe neurologic events and deaths both were reduced more than eightfold during 13 years of acellular vaccine use, as compared with the preceding 11 years of whole-cell vaccine use (see Table 21–17).

The Alberta, Canada, public health system provided all immunizations and conducted uniform surveillance for postimmunization adverse events during the years preceding and following the transition in Canada from whole-cell to acellular pertussis vaccines. Prior to July 1, 1997, a pentavalent DTP-IPV-Hib combination vaccine was used in the province; beginning July 1, a DTaP-IPV-Hib combination was used (this combination, Pentacel, is based on the HCPDT version of Tripacel that was studied in Stockholm 1993). The switch to the acellular combination was associated with an 89% reduction in fever greater than 40°C, an 82% reduction in unusual cry, and a 74% reduction in HHE.[392] These results were confirmed by Scheifele et al.,

TABLE 21–16 ■ Incidence (per 1000 Doses) of Major Adverse Reactions Following Primary Immunization: Data from Efficacy Trials, 1992–1997*

Product	Trial	Vaccine	Doses	High Fever[†]	HHE	Persistent Crying[‡]	Seizures[§]
ACEL-IMUNE	Erlangen[180]	DTaP	16,644	0.06	0	2.0[‡]	0.06
		DTP	16,424	0.19	0.06	8.8[‡]	0.18
Tripedia	Munich[227]	DTaP	41,615	n/a[†]	0.05	0.12	0.02
Infanrix	Italy[182]	DTaP	13,761	0.36	0	0.44	0.07
		DTP	13,520	2.4	0.67	4.0	0.22
		DT	4,540	0.44	0.44	0	0
Acelluvax	Italy[182]	DTaP	13,713	0.29	0.07	0.66	0
		DTP	13,520	2.4	0.67	4.0	0.22
		DT	4,540	0.44	0.44	0	0
	Stockholm 1993[329]	DTaP	61,219	0.24	0.26	n/a	0.03
		DTP	60,792	0.61	0.56	n/a	0.21
Certiva	Göteborg[330]	DTaP	5,124	2.6	0	0[‡]	0.4
		DT	5,130	1.9	0	0[‡]	0
Tripacel	Stockholm 1992[181,334]	DTaP	7,699	0.26	0.13	0.9	0
		DTP	6,143	4.4	0.81	4.8	0.16
		DT	7,667	0.39	0	0.52	0.26
HCPDT	Stockholm 1993[329]	DTaP	61,220	0.11	0.47	n/a	0.06
		DTP	60,792	0.61	0.55	n/a	0.21
Triavax	Senegal[229]	DTaP	6,881	n/a	0	0	0.29
		DTP	6,595	n/a	0	1.2	0.39

*Note that duration of surveillance or definitions of adverse reactions may have varied from trial to trial. Thus, comparisons within trials are more valid than comparisons across trials. Trade names in italics.
[†]Fever 40°C or higher, except: 40.5°C or higher for Erlangen; for Munich, rate of "fever" was 2.8 per 1000 but "fever" was not defined.
[‡]Crying persisting 3 hours or longer, except that duration not specified for Erlangen and Göteborg.
[§]Within 48 hours of vaccination.
HCPDT, hybrid component pertussis-diphtheria-tetanus vaccine; n/a, data not available.

who evaluated emergency room visits and hospitalizations at tertiary-care pediatric centers across Canada and found an 86% decline in febrile seizures and a 75% decline in HHE coincident with the transition from whole-cell to acellular-based combination vaccines in Canada.[393]

Similar data, albeit less dramatic, are available from the U.S. Vaccine Adverse Event Reporting System (VAERS), maintained by the CDC and the FDA.[394] From 1991 to 1993, rates of reported adverse events after the fourth and fifth doses in the pertussis immunization series were significantly lower for DTaP than DTP. These events included fever (1.9 vs. 7.5 events per 100,000 vaccinations), seizures (0.5 vs. 1.7), and hospitalization (0.2 vs. 0.9), for a total of 2.9 versus 9.8 cases per 100,000 vaccinations, respec-

tively.[395] There were three reports of encephalopathy after DTP, but none after DTaP. A follow-up report in 1990, covering the period between January 1, 1995 (when whole-cell vaccine was in exclusive use), and June 30, 1998 (when acellular vaccine was in predominant use), revealed steadily declining annual numbers of VAERS reports involving immunization against pertussis, from 2071 in 1995 to 491 in the first half of 1998.[396]

Results of Booster Doses Given to Children Previously Primed with Acellular Vaccine

A continuation study of the MAPT evaluated the safety and immunogenicity of a fourth dose of acellular vaccine given at 15 to 20 months to children who had been primed with

TABLE 21–17 ■ Japanese Vaccine Injury Compensation System Claims, 1970–1993

Reporting Period	Vaccines in Use	Doses (millions)	Vaccination Age, 1st dose	Number of Claims		Claims per 10⁶ Doses	
				Neurologic Events[*]	Total Deaths[†]	Neurologic Events[‡]	Total Deaths[‡]
Jan 1970–Jan 1975	Whole cell		3 mo	86	37		
Feb 1975–Aug 1981	Whole cell		2 yr	23	3		
Sep 1981–Dec 1984	Acellular		2 yr	11	2		
1970–1980, overall	Whole cell	44.9	3 mo, 1970–75; 2 yr, 1975–1980			18.5	7.4
1981–1993, overall	Acellular	62.6	2 yr, 1981–1988; 3 mo thereafter			2.4	0.9

[*]Claims approved for neurologic illnesses within 7 days after DTP immunization. Data from Kimura M, Kuno-Sakai H. Current epidemiology of pertussis in Japan. Pediatr Infect Dis J 9:705–709, 1990.
[†]Number of deaths included among claims paid. Data from Noble GR, Bernier RH, Esber EC et al. Acellular and whole-cell pertussis vaccine in Japan: Report of a visit by U.S. scientists. JAMA 257:1351–1356, 1987.
[‡]Rate per 10 million doses of cases applied to the compensation system. Data from Kuno-Sakai H, Kimura M. Epidemiology of pertussis and use of acellular pertussis vaccines in Japan. Dev Biol Stand 89:331–332, 1997.

either acellular or whole-cell vaccine at 2, 4, and 6 months of age.[397] For children who received four consecutive doses of an acellular vaccine, fever and injection site redness, swelling, and pain were seen more frequently with the fourth dose than with the primary series. Of children given a booster with acellular vaccine, those who had been primed with acellular vaccine had local redness and swelling significantly more frequently than did those who had been primed with whole-cell vaccine. However, children who had received four consecutive doses of whole-cell vaccine had significantly higher rates of irritability, redness, swelling, and pain after the booster than did either of the groups that were given a fourth dose of acellular vaccine. None of 1293 evaluated children experienced seizures, HHEs, or fever greater than 105°F. Also of note, several cases of entire limb swelling were observed after administration of the fourth dose of acellular vaccine to children previously primed with DTaP.

A report from Germany of entire limb swelling occurring after the fourth dose of one three-component DTaP had appeared in 1997. Among children from whom adverse reactions were specifically solicited, the rate of entire thigh swelling was 2.4%, whereas it was reported to occur in only 0.5% of those not specifically followed for reactions.[398] With this report in mind, Rennels et al. evaluated the cases of entire limb swelling after the fourth dose of acellular pertussis vaccine in MAPT.[399] Although extensive swelling reactions had not been anticipated in MAPT and had not been prospectively studied, parents in MAPT had been provided with diary cards that contained a section for them to report other reactions of concern. Parents of 20 (2%) of the 1015 children who had received the same DTaP vaccine throughout the primary and booster series described swelling of the entire thigh after the fourth dose. In contrast, none of the 246 children primed with DTP and boosted with DTaP were reported to have entire thigh swelling. Differences in rates between the whole-cell and acellular-primed groups were significant ($P = 0.02$). An interesting observation was that 40% of these children with whole-limb swelling were judged by their parents to have experienced no pain and 40% were judged not to have erythema, in spite of the extensive swelling reactions. The only significant association between rates of entire thigh swelling following dose 4 and the composition of the associated vaccine was with the quantity of diphtheria toxoid ($P = 0.02$). Antibody levels to pertussis toxoid, diphtheria toxoid, and tetanus toxoid were evaluated for subjects with extensive swelling and three controls per case in an attempt to determine whether the swelling might be due to an Arthus reaction. No difference was noted in the comparative distribution of pre- and postvaccination antibody titers between cases and controls, but sample sizes were small. In contrast, a large study of children given a fifth dose of Tripedia found that higher prevaccination antibody titers were associated with a higher frequency of large local reactions.[400] Thus, there is some evidence that high IgG antibody levels prebooster might play a role in the large limb swelling and may be related to excessive antigen content.

Children enrolled in MAPT were also studied after the fifth dose of DTaP.[401] Given the 5-year interval between initial enrollment and the fifth dose, many children were not located for enrollment in the study. None of 121 children given five doses of the same DTaP, versus 4 (2.7%) of 146

children receiving a mixed DTaP series, were reported to have experienced swelling of the whole upper arm following the fifth dose ($P = 0.13$). For children with swelling after the fifth dose, the onset of swelling was noted by parents on days 1 and 2 postvaccination and generally resolved by day 4, with no sequelae.

Rennels and colleagues reanalyzed data from the fourth-dose and fifth-dose MAPT studies and found no consistent relation between the quantity of aluminum in various DTaP vaccines and their rates of extensive swelling.[402] Further review of the literature regarding extensive swelling reactions reveals other sporadic reports in early studies of acellular pertussis vaccines in Japan[403] and Sweden.[404] The proposed explanation at that time was that immunizations had been given by the deep subcutaneous and not the intramuscular route. This observation was supported by the report that shorter needle length was associated with increased local reactions.[405] However, in the MAPT studies, the extensive swelling was seen with 9 of the 12 DTaP vaccines (containing from one to five pertussis antigens), which were given intramuscularly by experienced vaccine study nurses.[399] The pathophysiology of the large local reactions seen after booster injections of DTaP vaccine probably is multifactorial and may represent a cumulative increased response to several component antigens. Both whole-cell pertussis vaccine and tetanus toxoid have been documented to cause large local reactions. Previous studies have shown an association between severe local reactions and immunoglobulin E antibody levels to the toxoid vaccines, which are enhanced by aluminum absorption.[406-408] CMI may play a role in sensitization of certain individuals to repeated doses of toxoid vaccines, a possibility that needs further assessment.[316,409] In addition, there are data indicating that children with large erythematous reactions after DTaP vaccines more commonly react to skin test patches containing DT or acellular pertussis antigens.[410]

Summary of Adverse Events

Almost every study has found minor local and systemic adverse reactions to be less common with acellular than whole-cell vaccine. Although HHEs and seizures are seen after acellular vaccine, they occur less frequently than with whole-cell vaccine.

Rates of rare adverse effects cannot be determined reliably even with large efficacy trials, and they require postmarketing surveillance for their determination. Of course, adverse events temporally but not causally associated with vaccination will continue to occur at their background rates regardless of the vaccine used. Among children primed and boosted with acellular vaccine, reaction rates increase successively with each booster dose but remain lower than seen among children primed and boosted with whole-cell vaccine.

Vaccination of Adolescents and Adults

Numerous acellular pertussis vaccines have been evaluated in adults.[411-417] All appear highly immunogenic, with few adverse reactions. As noted previously, Tdap vaccines have been licensed in various jurisdictions (but not yet in the

United States) for immunization of adolescents and adults under the brand names Adacel, Boostrix, Covaxis, and (combined with IPV) Repevax.

Several groups of experts[191,418] have encouraged development and use of acellular pertussis vaccines for adolescents and adults. The International Consensus Group on Pertussis Immunisation[191] and the Global Pertussis Initiative[418] both have recommended universal adolescent booster vaccination combined with targeted immunization of those adults most likely to have contact with babies, including parents and other close family members, health care workers, and day care workers; universal immunization of young adults; and routine use of Tdap rather than Td for all adult booster immunizations. Some experts have identified a need for stand-alone acellular pertussis vaccines for adolescents and adults, to supplement the available Tdap vaccines and permit pertussis vaccination when boosting with Td would be inappropriate (e.g., if recently done).

Tdap is not yet licensed in the United States, and there are no relevant ACIP recommendations. In Canada, where Adacel has been licensed for several years, the National Advisory Committee on Immunization has recently recommended that Tdap should be used to replace the adolescent booster of Td, and that unimmunized children older than 6 and immigrants of uncertain immunization status should receive two doses of Tdap with a 4-week interval, followed by a third dose at 12 months after the first.[419] Similarly, the Austrian Standing Commission on Immunization's 2002 Immunization Plan notes the increasing incidence of pertussis in adolescents and adults and calls for routine use of Tdap (Tdap-IPV, when available) at 7 years, 14 to 15 years, and every 10 years thereafter.[420]

An additional strategy that has been discussed is the use of Tdap, rather than DTaP, at the 4- to 6-year booster, to reduce the adverse reactions associated with the current approach. In that regard, it is of interest that the European licensing authority has just modified the marketing authorization of Boostrix to include children age 4 and above; presumably, similar approval will be sought for other markets and other Tdap vaccines (e.g., Adacel).

Adverse Reactions in Adolescents and Adults

In a Swedish study of the Biken vaccine in adults, local reactions were common (85%) but described by most subjects as insignificant. One of 20 placebo recipients and 2 of 47 vaccine recipients reported substantial discomfort.[421] In the vaccine group, two distinct patterns of local swelling and redness were noted: an early-onset reaction at 2 to 3 days and a late-onset reaction at 7 to 14 days. Fever of 38°C or greater was seen in one placebo and two vaccine recipients. A study of the Aventis Pasteur two-component acellular vaccine noted fever of 37.8°C or greater in 9 of 164 adults.[414] Local redness or swelling was present in one third of subjects, with a maximum diameter of 8 cm. Early and late reactions were seen. In another trial, redness was noted at the injection site in 4 of 76 volunteers given a monovalent PT vaccine similar to Certiva; no fever or late local reactions were seen.[415] In a Tennessee study that randomized 120 adults to receive standard Td or full-, half-, or quarter-strength Lederle-Takeda acellular vaccine combined with Td, local and systemic adverse reactions were rare and

did not differ significantly among the study groups.[413] A series of studies in adolescents and adults of the Chiron Biocine three-component acellular pertussis vaccine demonstrated no serious adverse reactions; rates of minor reactions generally did not differ between the vaccine and placebo groups.[412]

A National Institutes of Health (NIH)–sponsored multicenter trial evaluated the immunogenicity and reactogenicity in adults of varying strengths of five acellular pertussis vaccines (variants of Certiva, Triacelluvax, Infanrix, ACEL-IMUNE, and a PT-FHA vaccine supplied by the Massachusetts Public Health Biologic Laboratories).[411,417] All vaccine dose strengths were well tolerated, although dose-related increases in the rates of injection-site symptoms and the duration of injection-site discomfort were seen in some subjects. Late-onset or biphasic reactions, generally minor, were also noted in this study. The frequency of these late reactions seemed to be greater for the higher strength doses and for vaccines with more antigens.

Immunogenicity in Adolescents and Adults

All the studies just mentioned demonstrated excellent immunogenicity of the acellular vaccines in adults, even with doses substantially lower than the standard pediatric dose. In the Tennessee study of the Lederle-Takeda vaccine, antibody responses to PT, FHA, fimbrial proteins, and PRN, even at the lowest dose, exceeded those seen in infants after complete primary immunization with the same vaccine.[413] No interference was noted with diphtheria or tetanus antibody responses in any of the groups. Similar findings were reported with the same vaccine when studied in German adults.[416] In the NIH dose-ranging study, dose-related increases in serum antibody levels against known vaccine antigens were seen in all vaccine groups.[411,417] For several vaccines, significant antibody responses were seen against antigens not known to be present in the vaccines, suggesting that the vaccines contained those antigens in trace quantities and were stimulating an anamnestic response in these adults, who had been immunized in childhood with whole-cell vaccine.

Efficacy in Adolescents and Adults

An NIH-sponsored study, the APERT trial, evaluated the efficacy of an acellular pertussis vaccine in adolescents and adults.[422] This prospective trial, conducted at eight centers across the United States, randomized 2781 healthy subjects ages 15 to 65 years to receive either an acellular pertussis vaccine (Boostrix minus the Td components) or hepatitis A vaccine. For 2 years, subjects were actively followed for pertussis illness with phone calls every 2 weeks (a total of more than 58,000 person-months of surveillance). Serum specimens were obtained at routine intervals; for any cough illness lasting 5 days or longer, serum specimens and nasopharyngeal aspirates for culture and PCR were obtained.

The acellular pertussis vaccine was well tolerated, with fewer than 5% of subjects reporting minor local or systemic adverse reactions. The study and control groups did not differ in the rate of severe adverse events, none of which were considered vaccine related. Local reactions were detected more commonly in females than males.

Cough illnesses lasting 5 or more days were reasonably common (more than one per every 2 person-years) and were seen equally in both study groups. There were 4 well-documented pertussis infections per 1000 patient-years of follow-up; the incidence was highest in subjects 15 to 30 years of age and in those with cough illnesses of longest duration. A variety of case definitions were evaluated based on the strength of the laboratory evidence (positive culture, PCR, or rise in pertussis-specific antibodies in paired acute-convalescent specimens). There was a significantly lower incidence of pertussis in acellular pertussis vaccinees than controls; the point estimate of vaccine efficacy was 92% (95% CI, 32% to 99%). The rate of pertussis seen in the APERT trial is quite consistent with rates identified in other studies of adult pertussis (see *Epidemiology*, above) and suggests that there are between 1 and 1.5 million pertussis illnesses per year in the United States among adolescents and adults.

Many authorities have thought that licensure of acellular pertussis vaccine for adult use was warranted even without specific efficacy data, based on immunogenicity and safety data in adults coupled with efficacy and other data from studies conducted in children. Certainly, now that efficacy of an adult-formulation acellular vaccine has been demonstrated, routine use of these vaccines to boost immunity in adolescents and adults should be considered. Health care workers, child care workers, and adolescents and adults in households containing children (particularly newborns) are among the likely high-priority target groups for immunization.[423]

Use of Vaccine in Outbreaks—Adolescents and Adults

The reduced adverse reaction profile of acellular vaccines has already stimulated use, or recommendations for use, of pediatric formulations among health care workers during hospital-based or community outbreaks.[424,425] Pending licensure of acellular pertussis vaccines for adult use, the available data suggest that booster immunization of previously immunized health care workers, using one third to one half of the standard pediatric dose of a licensed acellular pertussis vaccine, is safe and immunogenic. Availability of adult formulations will facilitate such use and likely will lead to relevant recommendations.

Although DTaP was used in the cited outbreaks, if monocomponent acellular pertussis vaccine were available, its use would be preferred to avoid possible Arthus reactions among people who recently received a booster with Td. The efficacy of such immunization is as yet unproved; pertussis attack rates already were declining in both outbreaks when vaccination was implemented. Clearly, however, vaccination is most likely to be beneficial if it is begun as early as possible in the epidemic. During an outbreak, such booster immunization may also be appropriate for other adolescents and adults at high risk of complications from acute pertussis, but data are lacking.

Indications for Vaccine

With licensure of the combination DTaP vaccine for primary vaccination of infants, recommendations for the use of pertussis vaccine in the United States have been modified extensively. Both the ACIP and the Red Book Committee have recommended that the acellular vaccine be preferred for all doses in the vaccination schedule, although DTP remains an acceptable alternative for any of the five doses (albeit no longer commercially available).

Immunization of Infants and Children

In the United States, unless specifically contraindicated (see later), every infant should receive pertussis vaccine at ages 2, 4, and 6 months and 12 to 18 months; a booster is indicated at 4 to 6 years of age. The timing of infant vaccination is determined by birth age, without regard to prematurity.[144,426] Children whose vaccination series has been interrupted need not have prior doses repeated but should have their series resumed at the earliest opportunity.

At present, no formulation of DTaP combined with Hib vaccine is licensed in the United States for primary immunization of infants; one such formulation (TriHIBit) is approved for the fourth (booster) dose of the DTaP series (the third or fourth dose of the Hib series, depending on the prior Hib vaccine[s] used). Combination vaccines containing DTaP, IPV, and either Hib or HBV are likely to become available in the United States for use in infants, and many such combinations already are licensed elsewhere (see Chapter 29).

Immunization of Adolescents and Adults

With the development of acellular vaccines that are safe and immunogenic for use in adults (see earlier in this chapter), discussions are ongoing about whether pertussis vaccines should be given routinely to adolescents and adults or only to certain high-risk populations.

Use of Vaccine in Outbreaks—Children

Immunization initiated after a pertussis exposure does not protect from that exposure; in an outbreak, however, exposure opportunities are ongoing and the existence of an outbreak should reinvigorate efforts to properly immunize those children who have not completed a full vaccination schedule. An accelerated infant vaccination schedule (e.g., 4, 8, and 12 weeks of age) may be indicated.[153] There is no evidence that supplemental doses of pertussis vaccine are required during an outbreak for the protection of normal children who have received pertussis immunization in accord with the recommended schedule. Supplemental immunization of children who have immunologic or cardiopulmonary compromise may be considered if the benefits of vaccination are believed to outweigh the risks of adverse reactions.

Precautions and Contraindications

Normal Infants and Children

Older recommendations regarding contraindications and precautions reflected concerns that are not supported by more recent data. At present, there are but two true contraindications to the use of pertussis vaccine: anaphylaxis or encephalopathy following prior administration of a vaccine containing a pertussis component.[144,426]

An anaphylactic reaction occurring immediately after administration of DTaP or whole-cell DTP is a contraindication to further vaccination with separate diphtheria, tetanus, or pertussis (acellular or whole-cell) components, absent proof as to which of these three components was responsible. Given the importance of tetanus vaccination, referral to an allergist for tetanus toxoid desensitization may be indicated. Acute encephalopathy occurring within 7 days after administration of DTP or DTaP, not attributable to another identifiable cause, is a contraindication to further pertussis immunization. DT vaccine should be administered for the remaining doses in the vaccination schedule, although it may be appropriate to delay vaccination until the patient's neurologic status clears.[144,426]

The following are now considered precautions, not contraindications, to pertussis vaccine: temperature 40.5°C (105°F) or greater within 48 hours of pertussis vaccination, not due to another identified cause; collapse or shock-like state (HHE) within 48 hours; persistent, inconsolable crying lasting 3 or more hours, occurring within 48 hours after vaccination; and convulsions occurring within 3 days, with or without fever. Decisions regarding the further administration of pertussis vaccine should be guided by an individualized evaluation of benefits and risks.[144,426] Those risks are likely to be substantially lower if acellular, rather than whole-cell, pertussis vaccine is used.

A family history of seizures, of adverse reactions to vaccine, or of allergy to vaccine is not a contraindication to the receipt of DTP or DTaP. Administration of pertussis vaccine should be deferred briefly for children with moderate or severe acute illnesses, with or without fever; they may be vaccinated as soon as they recover. Children who are immunocompromised or are receiving immunosuppressive therapy may be vaccinated with DTP or DTaP. If immunosuppressive therapy will be discontinued soon, deferral of vaccination until 1 month after therapy may permit better immune responses.

Children with Neurologic Disorders

As is discussed above under *Adverse Events with Whole-Cell Vaccines*, pertussis vaccine may precipitate febrile convulsions and may unmask neurologic disorders that would soon have become evident anyway, but it does not appear to cause or worsen chronic neurologic disorders. Because children with neurologic impairments are as needful—indeed, perhaps more needful—of protection from pertussis disease as are normal children, any decision to decline pertussis vaccination should reflect a careful consideration of risks and benefits, particularly in light of the increasing incidence of pertussis.[144,426] It may be appropriate to delay pertussis vaccination of infants with neurologic disorders until their status is clarified, but again careful consideration is required. The highest risk of pertussis is in the first 6 months of life, whereas the risk of febrile convulsions is higher thereafter; both factors therefore argue for adherence to the standard schedule.

Children with prior convulsions should probably have pertussis vaccine deferred until the cause of the convulsions is assessed and any necessary treatment is established. Febrile seizures unrelated to pertussis vaccine are not a contraindication to further vaccination, nor is a family history of seizures.[426] Administration of acetaminophen at a dose of 15 mg/kg should also be considered at the time of vaccination and every 4 hours for the ensuing 24 hours.[426]

False Contraindications

A number of situations have been considered incorrectly to be contraindications, and deferral of pertussis vaccination on these bases is inappropriate: redness, swelling, or pain at the injection site; temperature less than 40.5°C (105°F); mild acute illness, even involving diarrhea or low-grade fever; current antibiotic therapy; recent exposure to an infectious disease; prematurity; personal or family history of allergies; and family history of SIDS, convulsions, or adverse event after pertussis vaccination.[426] Prior pertussis infection is not a contraindication to vaccination; although a previously infected child may not require vaccination for immunity, proceeding with vaccination obviates the risk that the prior illness was not in fact pertussis.

Public Health Considerations

Disease Control Strategies

There is but one disease control strategy for pertussis: vaccination. But with which vaccine? Numerous whole-cell and acellular pertussis vaccines have been evaluated in efficacy trials. Which should be licensed, and which should be recommended for use?

In the United States, the answers are relatively simple, inasmuch as the efficacy trials demonstrated superior efficacy and fewer adverse effects for acellular pertussis vaccines than for a whole-cell vaccine widely used in the United States.[179] Numerous acellular vaccines have now been licensed in the United States; absent relevant head-to-head trials, the efficacies of the licensed acellular vaccines appear to be sufficiently similar that all are recommended equally over whole-cell vaccine by the advisory bodies. Purchase prices of the whole-cell and acellular vaccines differed little, and all the licensed products are made available to the states by the Federal Vaccines for Children program (see Chapter 53). Given the long-standing public concern regarding the adverse effects of whole-cell vaccine, it is not surprising that this vaccine disappeared relatively quickly from the U.S. market.

Other countries will have to apply their own relative weights when evaluating the comparative cost, efficacy, and adverse effects of the acellular and whole-cell vaccines.[427] Many countries may decide that their present whole-cell vaccine offers unsurpassed efficacy at low cost; if the vaccine is well accepted by the public, no change would be indicated.

Among the acellular vaccines, there will likely be trade-offs between efficacy and cost. Countries electing to use acellular vaccine are likely to choose among those that they perceive as the most efficacious. However, because the effectiveness of a pertussis immunization program depends not only on the efficacy of the vaccine but also on the coverage achieved by the program, countries with comprehensive programs that wish to use an acellular vaccine might elect to use a vaccine that is somewhat less efficacious but materially less expensive. For all countries, the effectiveness of the immunization program is more important than the effectiveness of the pertussis vaccine, given the excellent performance of all licensed vaccines. With the increasing availability of combination vaccines, these decisions are likely to become even more complex (see Chapter 29).

Eradication or Elimination

Humans are the only reservoir for pertussis, and chronic carriage is not known to occur. In principle, then, pertussis can be eradicated. Acellular vaccines, as discussed previously, appear suitable for use among all age groups, but it remains to be seen whether their widespread use can interrupt transmission of pertussis within a region. Global eradication, although perhaps possible, clearly must be many years away.

REFERENCES

1. Holmes WH. Bacillary and Rickettsial Infections. New York, Macmillan, 1940, pp 395–398.
2. Hardy A. Whooping cough. In Kiple KF (ed). The Cambridge World History of Human Disease. New York, Cambridge University Press, 1993, pp 1094–1096.
3. Bordet J, Gengou O. Le microbe de la coqueluche. Ann Inst Pasteur 20:731–741, 1906.
4. Cherry JD, Brunell PA, Golden GS, et al. Report of the task force on pertussis and pertussis immunization—1988. Pediatrics 81(suppl): 933–984, 1988.
5. Pertussis vaccination: Use of acellular pertussis vaccines among infants and young children. Recommendations of the Advisory Committee on Immunization Practices (ACIP). MMWR 46(RR-7):1–25, 1997.
6. Pertussis—United States, 1997–2000. MMWR 51:73–76, 2002.
7. Global Programme on Vaccines. State of the World's Vaccines and Immunization. Geneva, World Health Organization; and New York, UNICEF, 1996.
8. Pertussis Reported Cases (interactive online data table). Geneva, World Health Organization, accessed August 8, 2002. Available at *www.nt.who.int/vaccines/globalsummarry/timeseries/TSincidencePer.htm*
9. Zackrisson G, Taranger J, Trollfors B. History of whooping cough in nonvaccinated Swedish children, related to serum antibodies to pertussis toxin and filamentous hemagglutinin. J Pediatr 116:190–194, 1990.
10. Heininger U, Klich K, Stehr K, et al. Clinical findings in *Bordetella pertussis* infections: results of a prospective multicenter surveillance study. Pediatrics 100:E10, 1997.
11. Lapin LH. Whooping Cough. Springfield, IL, Charles C Thomas, 1943.
12. Johnston ID, Bland JM, Ingram D, et al. Effect of whooping cough in infancy on subsequent lung functions and bronchial reactivity. Am Rev Respir Dis 134:270–275, 1986.
13. Department of Health and Social Security, Committee on Safety of Medicines and Joint Committee on Vaccination and Immunisation. Whooping Cough. London, Her Majesty's Stationery Office, 1981, pp 1–184.
14. Litvak AM, Gibel H, Rosenthal SE, et al. Cerebral complications in pertussis. J Pediatr 32:357–379, 1948.
15. Pertussis—United States, January 1992–June 1995. MMWR 44:525–529, 1995.
16. Miller DL, Ross EM, Alderslade R, et al. Pertussis immunisation and serious acute neurological illness in children. Br Med J (Clin Res Ed) 282:1595–1599, 1981.

17. Nelson JD. The changing epidemiology of pertussis in young infants: the role of adults as reservoirs of infection. Am J Dis Child 132:371–373, 1978.
18. Senzilet LD, Halperin SA, Spika JS, et al. Pertussis is a frequent cause of prolonged cough illness in adults and adolescents. Clin Infect Dis 32:1691–1697, 2001.
18a. DeSerres G, Shadmani R, Duval B, et al. Morbidity of pertussis in adolescents and adults. J Infect Dis 182:174–179, 2000.
19. Schmitt-Grohe S, Cherry JD, Heininger U, et al. Pertussis in German adults. Clin Infect Dis 21:860–866, 1995.
20. Postels-Multani S, Schmitt HJ, Wirsing von Konig CH, et al. Symptoms and complications of pertussis in adults. Infection 23:139–142, 1995.
21. Long SS, Lischner HW, Deforest A, et al. Serologic evidence of subclinical pertussis in immunized children. Pediatr Infect Dis J 9:700–705, 1990.
22. Cromer BA, Goydos J, Hackell J, et al. Unrecognized pertussis infection in adolescents. Am J Dis Child 147:575–577, 1993.
23. Long SS, Welkon CJ, Clark JL. Widespread silent transmission of pertussis in families: antibody correlates of infection and symptomatology. J Infect Dis 161:480–486, 1990.
24. Jenkins P, Clarke SW. Cough syncope: a complication of adult whooping cough. Br J Dis Chest 75:311–313, 1981.
25. Halperin SA, Marrie TJ. Pertussis encephalopathy in an adult: case report and review. Rev Infect Dis 13:1043–1047, 1991.
26. MacLean DW. Adults with pertussis. J R Coll Gen Pract 32:298–300, 1982.
27. Manclark CR, Cowell JL. Pertussis. In Germanier R (ed). Bacterial Vaccines. New York, Academic Press, 1984, pp 69–106.
28. Kloos WE, Mohapatra N, Dobrogosz WJ, et al. Deoxyribonucleotide sequence relationships among *Bordetella* species. Int J Syst Bacteriol 31:173–176, 1981.
29. Arico B, Rappuoli R. *Bordetella parapertussis* and *Bordetella bronchiseptica* contain transcriptionally silent pertussis toxin genes. J Bacteriol 169:2847–2853, 1987.
30. Mattoo S, Foreman-Wykert AK, Cotter PA, et al. Mechanisms of *Bordetella* pathogenesis. Front Biosci 6:E168–E186, 2001.
31. Tuomanen E. *Bordetella pertussis* adhesins. In Wardlaw AC, Parton R (eds). Pathogenesis and Immunity in Pertussis. Chichester, John Wiley & Sons Ltd, 1988, pp 75–94.
32. Weiss A. Mucosal immune defenses and the response of *Bordetella pertussis*. ASM News 63:22–28, 1997.
33. Sato H, Sato Y. Relationship between structure and biological and protective activities of pertussis toxin. Dev Biol Stand 73:121–132, 1991.
34. Farizo KM, Huang T, Burns DL. Importance of holotoxin assembly in PT-mediated secretion of pertussis toxin from *Bordetella pertussis*. Infect Immun 68:4049–4054, 2000.
35. Tamura M, Nogimori K, Murai S, et al. Subunit structure of islet-activating protein, pertussis toxin, in conformity with the A-B model. Biochemistry 21:5516–5522, 1982.
36. Halperin SA, Issekutz TB, Kasina A. Modulation of *Bordetella pertussis* infection with monoclonal antibodies to pertussis toxin. J Infect Dis 163:355–361, 1991.
37. Nencioni L, Pizza MG, Volpini G, et al. Properties of the B oligomer of pertussis toxin. Infect Immun 59:4732–4734, 1991.
38. Watanabe M. Biological activities of pertussigen from *Bordetella pertussis* of various agglutinogen types. Microbiol Immunol 28:509–515, 1984.
39. Hausman SZ, Cherry JD, Heininger U, et al. Analysis of proteins encoded by the ptx and ptl genes of *Bordetella bronchiseptica* and *Bordetella parapertussis*. Infect Immun 64:4020–4026, 1996.
40. Pittman M. The concept of pertussis as a toxin-mediated disease. Pediatr Infect Dis J 3:467–486, 1984.
41. Sato H, Sato Y. *Bordetella pertussis* infection in mice: correlation of specific antibodies against two antigens, pertussis toxin, and filamentous hemagglutinin with mouse protectivity in an intracerebral or aerosol challenge system. Infect Immun 46:415–421, 1984.
42. Arciniega JL, Shahin RD, Burnette WN, et al. Contribution of the B oligomer to the protective activity of genetically attenuated pertussis toxin. Infect Immun 59:3407–3410, 1991.
43. Griffith AH. Permanent brain damage and pertussis vaccination: is the end of the saga in sight? Vaccine 7:199–210, 1989.
44. McGuirk P, McCann C, Mills KH. Pathogen-specific T regulatory 1 cells induced in the respiratory tract by a bacterial molecule that stimulates interleukin 10 production by dendritic cells: a novel strategy for

evasion of protective T helper type 1 responses by *Bordetella pertussis*. J Exp Med 195:221–231, 2002.

45. Abramson T, Kedem H, Relman DA. Pro-inflammatory and pro-apoptotic activities associated with *Bordetella pertussis* filamentous hemagglutinin. Infect Immun 69:2650–2658, 2001.

46. Tuomanen E, Weiss A, Rich R, et al. Filamentous hemagglutinin and pertussis toxin promote adherence of *Bordetella pertussis* to cilia. Dev Biol Stand 61:197–204, 1985.

47. Tuomanen E, Weiss A. Characterization of two adhesions of *Bordetella pertussis* for human ciliated respiratory-epithelial cells. J Infect Dis 152:118–125, 1985.

48. Oda M, Cowell JL, Burstyn DG, Manclark CR. Protective activities of the filamentous hemagglutinin and the lymphocytosis-promoting factor of *Bordetella pertussis* in mice. J Infect Dis 150:823–833, 1984.

49. He Q, Viljanen MK, Olander RM, et al. Antibodies to filamentous hemagglutinin of *Bordetella pertussis* and protection against whooping cough in schoolchildren. J Infect Dis 170:705–708, 1994.

50. Geuijen CA, Willems RJ, Bongaerts M, et al. Role of the *Bordetella pertussis* minor fimbrial subunit, FimD, in colonization of the mouse respiratory tract. Infect Immun 65:4222–4228, 1997.

51. Cotter PA, Yuk MH, Mattoo S, et al. Filamentous hemagglutinin of *Bordetella bronchiseptica* is required for efficient establishment of tracheal colonization. Infect Immun 66:5921–5929, 1998.

52. Stanbridge TN, Preston NW. Variation of serotype in strains of *Bordetella pertussis*. J Hyg (Camb) 73:305–310, 1974.

53. Preston NW, Stanbridge TN. Efficacy of pertussis vaccines: a brighter horizon. Br Med J 3:448–451, 1972.

54. Bronne-Shanbury C, Miller D, Standfast AF. The serotypes of *Bordetella pertussis* isolated in Great Britain between 1941 and 1968 and a comparison with the serotypes observed in other countries over this period. J Hyg (Camb) 76:265–275, 1976.

55. Efficacy of whooping-cough vaccines used in the United Kingdom before 1968. Br Med J 1:259–262, 1973.

56. Preston NW. Prevalent serotypes of *Bordetella pertussis* in non-vaccinated communities. J Hyg (Camb) 77:85–91, 1976.

57. WHO Expert Committee on Biological Standardization. Requirements for Diphtheria, Pertussis, Tetanus and Combined Vaccines (WHO Technical Report Series 800, 40th report). Geneva, World Health Organization, 1990, pp 87–179.

58. Brennan MJ, Li ZM, Cowell JL, et al. Identification of a 69-kilodalton nonfimbrial protein as an agglutinogen of *Bordetella pertussis*. Infect Immun 56:3189–3195, 1988.

59. Novotny P, Chubb AP, Cownley K, et al. Biologic and protective properties of the 69-kDa outer membrane protein of *Bordetella pertussis*: a novel formation for an acellular pertussis vaccine. J Infect Dis 164:114–122, 1991.

60. Leininger E, Kenimer JG, Brennan MJ. Surface proteins of *Bordetella pertussis*: role in adherence. *In* Manclark CR (ed). Proceedings of the Sixth International Symposium on Pertussis (DHHS Publication No. [FDA] 90–1164). Bethesda, MD, U.S. Public Health Service, 1990, pp 100–104.

61. Emsley P, McDermott G, Charles IG, et al. Crystallographic characterization of pertactin, a membrane-associated protein from *Bordetella pertussis*. J Mol Biol 235:772–773, 1994.

62. Ewanowich CA, Leininger E, Kenimer JG, et al. Mechanisms of *Bordetella pertussis* invasion of HeLa 229 cells. *In* Manclark CR (ed). Proceedings of the Sixth International Symposium on Pertussis (DHHS Publication No. [FDA] 90–1164). Bethesda, MD, U.S. Public Health Service, 1990, pp 106–113.

63. Thomas MG, Redhead K, Lambert HP. Human serum antibody responses to *Bordetella pertussis* infection and pertussis vaccination. J Infect Dis 159:211–218, 1989.

64. Trollfors B, Zackrisson G, Taranger J, et al. Serum antibodies against a 69-kilodalton outer-membrane protein, pertactin, from *Bordetella pertussis* in nonvaccinated children with and without a history of clinical pertussis. J Pediatr 120:924–926, 1992.

65. Shahin RD, Brennan MJ, Li ZM, et al. Characterization of the protective capacity and immunogenicity of the 69-kD outer membrane protein of *Bordetella pertussis*. J Exp Med 171:63–73, 1990.

66. Mooi FR, van Oirschot H, Heuvelman K, et al. Polymorphism in the *Bordetella pertussis* virulence factor P.69/pertactin and pertussis toxin in The Netherlands: temporal trends and evidence for vaccine-driven evolution. Infect Immun 66:670–675, 1998.

67. Njamkepo E, Rimlinger F, Thiberge S, et al. Thirty-five years' experience with the whole-cell pertussis vaccine in France: vaccine strains analysis and immunogenicity. Vaccine 20:1290–1294, 2002.

68. Weber C, Boursaux-Eude C, Coralie G, et al. Polymorphism of *Bordetella pertussis* isolates circulating for the last 10 years in France, where a single effective whole-cell vaccine has been used for more than 30 years. J Clin Microbiol 39:4396–4403, 2001.

69. King AJ, Berbers G, van Oirschot HF, et al. Role of the polymorphic region 1 of the *Bordetella pertussis* protein pertactin in immunity. Microbiology 147(pt 11):2885–2895, 2001.

70. Mooi FR, van Loo IH, King AJ. Adaptation of *Bordetella pertussis* to vaccination: a cause for its reemergence? Emerg Infect Dis 7(3 suppl):526–528, 2001.

71. Mastrantonio P, Spigaglia P, van Oirschot H, et al. Antigenic variants in *Bordetella pertussis* strains isolated from vaccinated and unvaccinated children. Microbiology 145:2069–2075, 1999.

72. Mastrantonio P, Cerquetti M, Cardines R, et al. Immunogenicity issues in the quality control of the new acellular pertussis vaccines. Biologicals 27:119–121, 1999.

73. Poolman J. Efficacy of Infanrix in promoting lung clearance of *B. pertussis* strains expressing pertactin antigenic variants in a mouse respiratory model [abstr 234]. *In* Abstracts of the 39th Interscience Conference on Antimicrobial Agents and Chemotherapy, September 1999, p 356.

74. Boursaux-Eude C, Thiberge S, Carletti G, et al. Intranasal murine model of *Bordetella pertussis* infection, II: sequence variation and protection induced by a tricomponent acellular vaccine. Vaccine 17:2651–2660, 1999.

75. Hewlett EL, Gordon VM. Adenylate cyclase toxin of *Bordetella pertussis*. *In* Wardlaw AC, Parton R (eds). Pathogenesis and Immunity in Pertussis. New York, John Wiley & Sons, 1988, pp 193–209.

76. Weiss AA, Goodwin M St. M, Allison N. Investigation of the role of *Bordetella pertussis* virulence factors in disease. *In* Manclark CR (ed). Proceedings of the Sixth International Symposium on Pertussis (DHHS Publication No. [FDA] 90–1164). Bethesda, MD, U.S. Public Health Service, 1990, pp 202–205.

77. Arciniega JL, Hewlett EL, Johnson FD, et al. Human serologic response to envelope-associated proteins and adenylate cyclase toxin of *Bordetella pertussis*. J Infect Dis 163:135–142, 1991.

78. Guiso N, Szatanik M, Rocancourt M. *Bordetella pertussis* adenylate cyclase: a protective antigen against lethality and bacterial colonization in murine respiratory and intracerebral models. *In* Manclark CR (ed). Proceedings of the Sixth International Symposium on Pertussis (DHHS Publication No. [FDA] 90–1164). Bethesda, MD, U.S. Public Health Service, 1990, pp 207–231.

79. Cookson BT, Cho HL, Herwaldt LA, et al. Biological activities and chemical composition of purified tracheal cytotoxin of *Bordetella pertussis*. Infect Immun 57:2223–2229, 1989.

80. Goldman WE. Tracheal cytotoxin of *Bordetella pertussis*. *In* Wardlaw AC, Parton R (eds). Pathogenesis and Immunity in Pertussis. New York, John Wiley & Sons, 1988, pp 231–246.

81. Goldman WE, Collier JL, Cookson BL, et al. Tracheal cytotoxin of *Bordetella pertussis*: biosynthesis, structure, and specificity. *In* Manclark CR (ed). Proceedings of the Sixth International Symposium on Pertussis (DHHS Publication No. [FDA] 90–1164). Bethesda, MD, U.S. Public Health Service, 1990, pp 5–10.

82. Nakase Y, Endoh M. Heat-labile toxin of *Bordetella pertussis*. *In* Wardlaw AC, Parton R (eds). Pathogenesis and Immunity in Pertussis. New York, John Wiley & Sons, 1988, pp 211–229.

83. Endoh M, Nagai M, Burns DL, et al. Effects of exogenous agents on the action of *Bordetella parapertussis* in heat-labile toxin on guinea pig skin. Infect Immun 58:1456–1460, 1990.

84. Fernandez RC, Weiss AA. Cloning and sequencing of a *Bordetella pertussis* serum resistance locus. Infect Immun 62:4727–4738, 1994.

85. Oliver DC, Fernandez RC. Antibodies to BrkA augment killing of *Bordetella pertussis*. Vaccine 20:235–241, 2001.

86. Barnes MG, Weiss AA. Growth phase influences complement resistance of *Bordetella pertussis*. Infect Immun 70:403–406, 2002.

87. Chaby R, Caroff M. Lipopolysaccharides of *Bordetella pertussis* endotoxin. *In* Wardlaw AC, Parton R (eds). Pathogenesis and Immunity in Pertussis. Chichester, John Wiley & Sons Ltd, 1988, pp 247–271.

88. Harvill ET, Preston A, Cotter PA, et al. Multiple roles for *Bordetella* lipopolysaccharide molecules during respiratory tract infection. Infect Immun 68:6720–6728, 2000.

89. Baraff LJ, Manclark CR, Cherry JD, et al. Analyses of adverse reactions to diphtheria and tetanus toxoids and pertussis vaccine by vaccine lot, endotoxin content, pertussis vaccine potency and percentage of mouse weight gain. Pediatr Infect Dis J 8:502–507, 1989.

90. Weiss AA, Hewlett EL. Virulence factors of *Bordetella pertussis*. Annu Rev Microbiol 40:661–686, 1986.

91. Hewlett EL. Pertussis: current concepts of pathogenesis and prevention. Pediatr Infect Dis J 16(4 suppl):S78–S84, 1997.

92. Zhang JM, Cowell JL, Steven AC, et al. Purification of serotype 2 fimbriae of *Bordetella pertussis* and their identification as a mouse protective antigen. Dev Biol Stand 61:173–185, 1985.

93. Confer DL, Eaton JW. Phagocyte impotence caused by an invasive bacterial adenylate cyclase. Science 217:948–950, 1982.

94. Olson LC. Pertussis. Medicine 54:427–469, 1975.

95. Muller FM, Hoppe JE, Wirsing von Konig CH. Laboratory diagnosis of pertussis: state of the art in 1997. J Clin Microbiol 35:2435–2443, 1997.

96. Hallander HO. Microbiological and serological diagnosis of pertussis. Clin Infect Dis 28(suppl 2):S99–S106, 1999.

97. Broome CV, Fraser DW, English WJ II. Pertussis—diagnostic methods and surveillance. *In* Manclark CR, Hill JC (eds). International Symposium on Pertussis. Bethesda, MD, U.S. Public Health Service, 1979, pp 19–22.

98. Strebel PM, Cochi SL, Farizo KM, et al. Pertussis in Missouri: evaluation of nasopharyngeal culture, direct fluorescent antibody testing, and clinical case definitions in the diagnosis of pertussis. Clin Infect Dis 16:276–285, 1993.

99. Onorato IM, Wassilak SGF. Laboratory diagnosis of pertussis: the state of the art. Pediatr Infect Dis J 6:145–151, 1987.

100. Halperin SA, Bortolussi R, Wort AJ. Evaluation of culture, immuno-fluorescence, and serology for the diagnosis of pertussis. J Clin Microbiol 27:752–757, 1989.

101. Hallander HO, Reizenstein E, Renemar B, et al. Comparison of nasopharyngeal aspirates with swabs for culture of *Bordetella pertussis*. J Clin Microbiol 31:50–52, 1993.

102. Granstrom G, Wretlind B, Granstrom M. Diagnostic value of clinical and bacteriological findings in pertussis. J Infect 22:17–26, 1991.

103. Placebo-controlled trial of two acellular pertussis vaccines in Sweden—protective efficacy and adverse events. Ad Hoc Group for the Study of Pertussis Vaccines. Lancet 1:955–960, 1988.

104. Donaldson P, Whitaker JA. Diagnosis of pertussis by fluorescent antibody staining of nasopharyngeal smears. Am J Dis Child 99:423–427, 1960.

105. Stadel AJ. Use of monoclonal fluorescent antibodies for the detection of *B. pertussis* and *B. parapertussis*. Am Clin Lab 19:14, 2000.

106. Ewanowich CA, Chui LW-L, Paranchych MG, et al. Major outbreak of pertussis in northern Alberta, Canada: analysis of discrepant direct fluorescent-antibody and culture results by using polymerase chain reaction methodology. J Clin Microbiol 31:1715–1725, 1993.

107. He Q, Mertsola J, Soini H, et al. Sensitive and specific polymerase chain reaction assays for detection of *Bordetella pertussis* in nasopharyngeal specimens. J Pediatr 124:421–426, 1994.

108. Schlapfer G, Cherry JD, Heininger U, et al. Polymerase chain reaction identification of *Bordetella pertussis* infections in vaccinees and family members in a pertussis vaccine efficacy trial in Germany. Pediatr Infect Dis J 14:209–214, 1995.

109. Olcen P, Backman A, Johansson B, et al. Amplification of DNA by the polymerase chain reaction for the efficient diagnosis of pertussis. Scand J Infect Dis 24:339–345, 1992.

110. Reizenstein E, Lofdahl S, Granstrom M, et al. Evaluation of an improved DNA probe for diagnosis of pertussis. Diagn Microbiol Infect Dis 15:569–573, 1992.

111. Glare EM, Paton JC, Premier RR, et al. Analysis of a repetitive DNA sequence from *Bordetella pertussis* and its application to the diagnosis of pertussis using the polymerase chain reaction. J Clin Microbiol 28:1982–1987, 1990.

112. Edelman K, Nikkari S, Ruuskanen O, et al. Detection of *Bordetella pertussis* by polymerase chain reaction and culture in the nasopharynx of erythromycin-treated infants with pertussis. Pediatr Infect Dis J 15:54–57, 1996.

113. He Q, Schmidt-Schlapfer G, Just M, et al. Impact of polymerase chain reaction on clinical pertussis research: Finnish and Swiss experiences. J Infect Dis 174:1288–1295, 1996.

114. Heininger U, Schmidt-Schlapfer G, Cherry JD, et al. Clinical validation of a polymerase chain reaction assay for the diagnosis of per-

115. Schmidt-Schlapfer G, Liese JG, Porter F, et al. Polymerase chain reaction (PCR) compared with conventional identification in culture for detection of *Bordetella pertussis* in 7153 children. Clin Microbiol Infect 3:462–467, 1997.

116. Sloan LM, Hopkins MK, Mitchell PS, et al. Multiplex LightCycler PCR assay for detection and differentiation of *Bordetella pertussis* and *Bordetella parapertussis* in nasopharyngeal specimens. J Clin Microbiol 40:96–100, 2002.

117. Kosters K, Riffelmann M, Wirsing von Konig CH. Evaluation of a real-time PCR assay for detection of *Bordetella pertussis* and *B. parapertussis* in clinical samples. J Med Microbiol 50:436–440, 2001.

118. Reischl U, Lehn N, Sanden GN, et al. Real-time PCR assay targeting IS481 of *Bordetella pertussis* and molecular basis for detecting *Bordetella holmesii*. J Clin Microbiol 39:1963–1966, 2001.

119. Tilley PA, Kanchana MV, Knight I, et al. Detection of *Bordetella pertussis* in a clinical laboratory by culture, polymerase chain reaction, and direct fluorescent antibody staining: accuracy and cost. Diagn Microbiol Infect Dis 37:17–23, 2000.

120. Loeffelholz MJ, Thompson CJ, Long KS, et al. Comparison of PCR, culture, and direct fluorescent-antibody testing for detection of *Bordetella pertussis*. J Clin Microbiol 37:2872–2876, 1999.

121. Meade BD, Mink CM, Manclark CR. Serodiagnosis of pertussis. *In* Manclark CR (ed). Proceedings of the Sixth International Symposium on Pertussis (DHHS Publication No. [FDA] 90–1164). Bethesda, MD, U.S. Public Health Service, 1990, pp 322–329.

122. Wirsing von Konig CH, Gounis D, Laukamp S, et al. Evaluation of a single-sample serological technique for diagnosing pertussis in unvaccinated children. Eur J Clin Microbiol Infect Dis 18:341–345, 1999.

123. Simondon F, Iteman I, Preziosi MP, et al. Evaluation of an immunoglobulin G enzyme-linked immunosorbent assay for pertussis toxin and filamentous hemagglutinin in diagnosis of pertussis in Senegal. Clin Diagn Lab Immunol 5:130–134, 1998.

124. Steketee RW, Burstyn DG, Wassilak SG, et al. A comparison of laboratory and clinical methods for diagnosing pertussis in an outbreak in a facility for the developmentally disabled. J Infect Dis 157:441–449, 1988.

125. Mink CM, Cherry JD, Christenson P, et al. A search for *Bordetella pertussis* infection in university students. Clin Infect Dis 14:464–471, 1992.

126. Addiss DG, Davis JP, Meade BD, et al. A pertussis outbreak in a Wisconsin nursing home. J Infect Dis 164:704–710, 1991.

127. Cattaneo LA, Reed GW, Haase DH, et al. The seroepidemiology of *Bordetella pertussis* infections: a study of persons age 1–65 years. J Infect Dis 173:1256–1259, 1996.

128. Giammanco A, Chiarini A, Stroffolini T, et al. Seroepidemiology of pertussis in Italy. Rev Infect Dis 13:1216–1220, 1991.

129. Halperin SA, Bortolussi R, MacLean D, et al. Persistence of pertussis in an immunized population: results of the Nova Scotia Enhanced Pertussis Surveillance Program. J Pediatr 115:686–693, 1989.

130. Edwards KM. Is pertussis a frequent cause of cough in adolescents and adults? Should routine pertussis immunization be recommended? Clin Infect Dis 32:1698–1699, 2001.

131. Meade BD, Deforest A, Edwards KM, et al. Description and evaluation of serologic assays used in a multicenter trial of acellular pertussis vaccines. Pediatrics 96(3 pt 2):570–575, 1995.

132. Lynn F, Reed GF, Meade BD. A comparison of enzyme immunoassays used to measure serum antibodies to components of *Bordetella pertussis*. Dev Biol Stand 89:197–204, 1997.

133. Lynn F, Reed GF, Meade BD. Collaborative study for the evaluation of enzyme-linked immunosorbent assays used to measure human antibodies to *Bordetella pertussis* antigens. Clin Diagn Lab Immunol 3:689–700, 1996.

134. Reizenstein E, Hallander HO, Blackwelder WC, et al. Comparison of five calculation modes for antibody ELISA procedures using pertussis serology as a model. J Immunol Methods 183:279–290, 1995.

135. Marchant CD, Loughlin AM, Lett SM, et al. Pertussis in Massachusetts, 1981–1991: incidence, serologic diagnosis, and vaccine effectiveness. J Infect Dis 169:1297–1305, 1994.

136. Yih WK, Lett SM, des Vignes FN, et al. The increasing incidence of pertussis in Massachusetts adolescents and adults, 1989–1998. J Infect Dis 182:1409–1416, 2000.

137. Strebel P, Nordin J, Edwards K, et al. Population-based incidence of pertussis among adolescents and adults, Minnesota, 1995–1996. J Infect Dis 183:1353–1359, 2001.

138. de Melker HE, Versteegh FG, Conyn-Van Spaendonck MA, et al. Specificity and sensitivity of high levels of immunoglobulin G antibodies against pertussis toxin in a single serum sample for diagnosis of infection with *Bordetella pertussis*. J Clin Microbiol 38:800–806, 2000.

139. Hallander HO. Diagnostic pertussis serology in the recent clinical efficacy studies of acellular vaccines. Dev Biol Stand 89:205–212, 1997.

140. Halperin SA, Bortolussi R, Langley JM, et al. Seven days of erythromycin estolate is as effective as fourteen days for the treatment of *Bordetella pertussis* infections. Pediatrics 100:65–71, 1997.

141. Bass JW, Klenk EL, Kotheimer JB, et al. Antimicrobial treatment of pertussis. J Pediatr 75:768–781, 1969.

142. Hewlett EL. *Bordetella* species. *In* Mandell GL, Bennett JE, Dolin R (eds). Mandell, Douglas and Bennett's Principles and Practice of Infectious Diseases (4th ed). New York, Churchill Livingstone, 1995, pp 2078–2083.

143. Kawai H, Aoyama T, Goto A, et al. Evaluation of pertussis treatment with erythromycin ethylsuccinate and stearate according to age. Kansenshogaku Zasshi 68:1324–1329, 1994.

144. Peter G, Hall CB, Halsey NA, et al. (eds). Red Book 1997: Report of the Committee on Infectious Diseases (24th ed). Elk Grove Village, IL, American Academy of Pediatrics, 1997.

145. Aoyama T, Sunakawa K, Iwata S, et al. Efficacy of short-term treatment of pertussis with clarithromycin and azithromycin. J Pediatr 129:761–764, 1996.

146. Halperin SA, Bortolussi R, Langley JM, et al. A randomized, placebo-controlled trial of erythromycin estolate chemoprophylaxis for household contacts of children with culture-positive *Bordetella pertussis* infection. Pediatrics 104:E42, 1999.

147. Centers for Disease Control and Prevention. Hypertrophic pyloric stenosis in infants following pertussis prophylaxis with erythromycin—Knoxville, Tennessee, 1999. JAMA 283:471–472, 2000.

148. Honein MA, Paulozzi LJ, Himelright IM, et al. Infantile hypertrophic pyloric stenosis after pertussis prophylaxis with erythromycin: a case review and cohort study. Lancet 354:2101–2105, 1999.

149. Centers for Disease Control and Prevention. Erythromycin-resistant *Bordetella pertussis*—Yuma County, Arizona, May–October 1994. JAMA 273:13–14, 1995.

150. Gordon KA, Fusco J, Biedenbach DJ, et al. Antimicrobial susceptibility testing of clinical isolates of *Bordetella pertussis* from northern California: report from the SENTRY Antimicrobial Surveillance Program. Antimicrob Agents Chemother 45:3599–3600, 2001.

151. Korgenski EK, Daly JA. Surveillance and detection of erythromycin resistance in *Bordetella pertussis* isolates recovered from a pediatric population in the Intermountain West region of the United States. J Clin Microbiol 35:2989–2991, 1997.

152. Bartkus J, Juni BA, Ehresman K, et al. Proposed mechanism of erythromycin resistance in *Bordetella pertussis* [abstr C1–1817]. In Abstracts of the 41st Interscience Conference on Antimicrobial Agents and Chemotherapy, Chicago, IL, December 16–19, 2001, p 102.

153. Pertussis. *In* Benenson AS (ed). Control of Communicable Disease Manual (16th ed). Washington, DC, American Public Health Association, 1995.

154. Weber DJ, Rutala WA. Management of healthcare workers exposed to pertussis. Infect Control Hosp Epidemiol 15:411–415, 1994.

155. Decker MD, Schaffner W. Nosocomial diseases of health care workers spread by the airborne or contact route (other than tuberculosis). *In* Mayhall CG (ed). Hospital Epidemiology and Infection Control. Baltimore, Williams & Wilkins, 1996, pp 871–872.

156. Wirsing von Konig CH, Schmitt HJ, Bogaerts H, et al. Factors influencing the analysis of secondary prevention of pertussis. Dev Biol Stand 89:175–179, 1997.

157. De Serres G, Boulianne N, Duval B. Field effectiveness of erythromycin prophylaxis to prevent pertussis within families. Pediatr Infect Dis J 14:969–975, 1995.

158. Fine PE, Clarkson JA. The recurrence of whooping cough: possible implications for assessment of vaccine efficacy. Lancet 1:666–669, 1982.

159. Farizo KM, Cochi SL, Zell ER, et al. Epidemiological features of pertussis in the United States, 1980–1989. Clin Infect Dis 14:708–719, 1992.

160. Guris D, Strebel PM, Bardenheier B, et al. Changing epidemiology of pertussis in the United States: increasing reported incidence among adolescents and adults, 1990–1996. Clin Infect Dis 28:1230–1237, 1999.

161. Centers for Disease Control and Prevention. Pertussis—United States, 1997–2000. JAMA 287:977–979, 2002.

162. Cherry JD. The epidemiology of pertussis and pertussis vaccine in the United Kingdom and the United States: a comparative study. Curr Probl Pediatr 14:1–78, 1984.

163. Kanai K. Japan's experience in pertussis epidemiology and vaccination in the past thirty years. Jpn J Med Sci Biol 33:107–143, 1980.

164. Cherry JD, Baraff LJ, Hewlett E. The past, present, and future of pertussis: the role of adults in epidemiology and future control. West J Med 150:319–328, 1989.

165. Cherry JD. Pertussis in adults. Ann Intern Med 128:64–66, 1998.

166. Luttinger P. The epidemiology of pertussis. Am J Dis Child 12:290–315, 1916.

167. Friedlander A. Whooping cough. *In* Abt IA (ed). Pediatrics. Vol. 11. Philadelphia, WB Saunders, 1925, pp 128–147.

168. Forest MG, Cathiard AM, Bertrand JA. Evidence of testicular activity in early infancy. J Clin Endocrinol Metab 37:148–151, 1973.

169. Clark AC, Bradford WL, Berry GP. An epidemiological study of an outbreak of pertussis in a public school. Am J Public Health 36:1156–1162, 1946.

170. Lambert HS. Epidemiology of a small pertussis outbreak in Kent County, Michigan. Public Health Rep 80:365–369, 1965.

171. Cherry JD, Beer T, Chartrand SA, et al. Comparison of values of antibody to *Bordetella pertussis* antigens in young German and American men. Clin Infect Dis 20:1271–1274, 1995.

172. Linnemann CC Jr, Bass JW, Smith MH. The carrier state in pertussis. Am J Epidemiol 88:422–427, 1968.

173. Lambert HP. The carrier state: *Bordetella pertussis*. J Antimicrob Chemother 18(suppl A):13–16, 1986.

174. Rosenthal S, Strebel P, Cassiday P, et al. Pertussis infection among adults during the 1993 outbreak in Chicago. J Infect Dis 171:1650–1652, 1995.

175. Christie CD, Marx ML, Marchant CD, et al. The 1993 epidemic of pertussis in Cincinnati: resurgence of disease in a highly immunized population of children. N Engl J Med 331:16–21, 1994.

176. Resurgence of pertussis—United States, 1993. MMWR 42:952–953, 959–960, 1993.

177. Pertussis outbreak—Vermont, 1996. MMWR 46:822–826, 1997.

178. Edwards KM, Decker MD, Halsey NA, et al. Differences in antibody response to whole-cell pertussis vaccines. Pediatrics 88:1019–1023, 1991.

179. Edwards KM, Decker MD. Acellular pertussis vaccines for infants. N Engl J Med 334:391–392, 1996.

180. Stehr K, Cherry JD, Heininger U, et al. A comparative efficacy trial in Germany in infants who received either the Lederle/Takeda acellular pertussis component DTP (DTaP) vaccine, the Lederle whole-cell component DTP vaccine, or DT vaccine. Pediatrics 101:1–11, 1998.

181. Gustafsson L, Hallander HO, Olin P, et al. A controlled trial of a two-component acellular, a five-component acellular, and a whole-cell pertussis vaccine. N Engl J Med 334:349–355, 1996.

182. Greco D, Salmaso S, Mastrantonio P, et al. A controlled trial of two acellular vaccines and one whole-cell vaccine against pertussis. Progetto Pertosse Working Group. N Engl J Med 334:341–348, 1996.

183. Mortimer EA Jr, Jones PK. An evaluation of pertussis vaccine. Rev Infect Dis 1:927–934, 1979.

184. Pertussis surveillance—United States 1989–1991. MMWR Morb Mortal Wkly Rep 41(SS-8):11–19, 1992.

185. He Q, Viljanen MK, Nikkari S, et al. Outcomes of *Bordetella pertussis* infection in different age groups of an immunized population. J Infect Dis 170:873–877, 1994.

186. Biellik RJ, Patriarca PA, Mullen JR, et al. Risk factors for community- and household-acquired pertussis during a large-scale outbreak in central Wisconsin. J Infect Dis 157:1134–1141, 1988.

187. Mink CA, Sirota NM, Nugent S. Outbreak of pertussis in a fully immunized adolescent and adult population. Arch Pediatr Adolesc Med 148:153–157, 1994.

188. Robertson PW, Goldberg H, Jarvie BH, et al. *Bordetella pertussis* infection: a cause of persistent cough in adults. Med J Aust 146:522–525, 1987.

189. Wright SW, Edwards KM, Decker MD, et al. Pertussis infection in adults with persistent cough. JAMA 273:1044–1046, 1995.

190. Nennig ME, Shinefield HR, Edwards KM, et al. Prevalence and incidence of adult pertussis in an urban population. JAMA 275:1672–1674, 1996.

191. Campins-Marti M, Cheng HK, Forsyth K, et al. Recommendations are needed for adolescent and adult pertussis immunisation: rationale and strategies for consideration. Vaccine 20:641–646, 2001.

192. Van Savage J, Decker MD, Edwards KM, et al. Natural history of pertussis antibody in the infant and effect on vaccine response. J Infect Dis 161:487–492, 1990.

193. Bradford WL. Use of convalescent blood in whooping cough. Am J Dis Child 50:918–928, 1935.

194. Department of Health and Human Services, Food and Drug Administration. Biological products; bacterial vaccines and toxoids; implementation of efficacy review; proposed rule. Fed Register 50:51002–51117, 1985.

195. Balagtas RC, Nelson KE, Levin S, et al. Treatment of pertussis with pertussis immune globulin. J Pediatr 79:203–208, 1971.

196. Morris D, McDonald JC. Failure of hyperimmune gamma globulin to prevent whooping cough. Arch Dis Child 32:236–239, 1957.

197. Granstrom M, Olinder-Nielsen AM, Holmblad P, et al. Specific immunoglobulin for treatment of whooping cough. Lancet 338:1230–1233, 1991.

198. Bruss JB, Malley R, Halperin S, et al. Treatment of severe pertussis: a study of the safety and pharmacology of intravenous pertussis immunoglobulin. Pediatr Infect Dis J 18:505–511, 1999.

199. Madsen T. Vaccination against whooping cough. JAMA 101:187–188, 1933.

200. Kendrick PL, Eldering G, Dixon MK, et al. Mouse protection tests in the study of pertussis vaccine: a comparative series using intracerebral route for challenge. Am J Public Health 37:803–810, 1947.

201. Eldering G. Symposium on pertussis immunization, in honor of Dr. Pearl L. Kendrick in her eightieth year: historical notes on pertussis immunization. Health Lab Sci 8:200–205, 1971.

202. Medical Research Council. Vaccination against whooping cough: relation between protection tests in children and results of laboratory tests. Br Med J 2:454–462, 1956.

203. Sato Y, Kimura M, Fukumi H. Development of a pertussis component vaccine in Japan. Lancet 1:122–126, 1984.

204. Kimura M, Hikino N. Results with a new DTP vaccine in Japan. Dev Biol Stand 61:545–561, 1985.

205. Noble GR, Bernier RH, Esber EC, et al. Acellular and whole-cell pertussis vaccine in Japan: report of a visit by U.S. scientists. JAMA 257:1351–1356, 1987.

206. Aoyama T, Murase Y, Gonda T, et al. Type-specific efficacy of acellular pertussis vaccine. Am J Dis Child 142:40–42, 1988.

207. Kimura M, Kuno-Sakai H. Current epidemiology of pertussis in Japan. Pediatr Infect Dis J 9:705–709, 1990.

208. Kimura M. Japanese clinical experiences with acellular pertussis vaccines. Dev Biol Stand 73:5–9, 1991.

209. Edwards KM, Meade BD, Decker MD, et al. Comparison of 13 acellular pertussis vaccines: overview and serologic response. Pediatrics 96(3 pt 2):548–557, 1995.

210. Robinson A, Funnell SG. Potency testing of acellular pertussis vaccines. Vaccine 10:139–141, 1992.

211. Guiso N, Capiau C, Carletti G, et al. Intranasal murine model of Bordetella pertussis infection. I. Prediction of protection in human infants by acellular vaccines. Vaccine 17:2366–2376, 1999.

212. Pizza M, Covacci A, Bartoloni A, et al. Mutants of pertussis toxin suitable for vaccine development. Science 246:497–500, 1989.

213. Edwards KM, Decker MD, Mortimer EA Jr. Pertussis vaccine. In Plotkin S, Mortimer EA, Orenstein WA, eds. Vaccines (3rd ed). Philadelphia, WB Saunders, 1999, pp 293–344.

214. Greenberg DP, Pickering LK, Senders SD, et al. Interchangeability of 2 diphtheria-tetanus-acellular pertussis vaccines in infancy. Pediatrics 109:666–672, 2002.

215. Edwards KM, Decker MD. Combination vaccines consisting of acellular pertussis vaccines. Pediatr Infect Dis J 16(4 suppl):S97–S102, 1997.

216. Gold R, Scheifele D, Barreto L, et al. Safety and immunogenicity of Haemophilus influenzae vaccine (tetanus toxoid conjugate) administered concurrently or combined with diphtheria and tetanus toxoids, pertussis vaccine and inactivated poliomyelitis vaccine to healthy infants at two, four and six months of age. Pediatr Infect Dis J 13:348–355, 1994.

217. Hinman AR, Koplan JP. Pertussis and pertussis vaccine: reanalysis of benefits, risks and costs. JAMA 251:3109–3113, 1984.

218. Miller DL, Alderslade R, Ross EM. Whooping cough and whooping cough vaccine: the risks and benefits debate. Epidemiol Rev 4:1–24, 1982.

219. Kendrick P, Eldering G. Progress report on pertussis immunization. Am J Public Health 26:8–12, 1936.

220. Sauer LW. Whooping cough: new phases of the work of immunization and prophylaxis. JAMA 112:305–308, 1939.

221. Baker JD, Halperin SA, Edwards K, et al. Antibody response to Bordetella pertussis antigens after immunization with American and Canadian whole-cell vaccines. J Pediatr 121:523–527, 1992.

222. Steinhoff MC, Reed GF, Decker MD, et al. A randomized comparison of reactogenicity and immunogenicity of two whole-cell pertussis vaccines. Pediatrics 96(3 pt 2):567–570, 1995.

223. Doull JA, Shibley GS, McClelland JS. Active immunization against whooping cough: interim report of the Cleveland experience. Am J Public Health 26:1097–1105, 1936.

224. Sako W. Studies on pertussis immunization. J Pediatr 30:29–40, 1947.

225. Medical Research Council. Vaccination against whooping-cough: the final report to the Immunization Committee of the Medical Research Council and to the medical officers of health for Battersea and Wandsworth, Bradford, Liverpool and Newcastle. Br Med J 1:994–1000, 1959.

226. Schmitt H-J, von Konig CH, Neiss A, et al. Efficacy of acellular pertussis vaccine in early childhood after household exposure. JAMA 275:37–41, 1996.

227. Liese JG, Meschievitz CK, Harzer E, et al. Efficacy of a two-component acellular pertussis vaccine in infants. Pediatr Infect Dis J 16:1038–1044, 1997.

228. Lederle Laboratories. ACEL-IMUNE® product labeling. In Physician's Desk Reference. Montvale, NJ, Medical Economics Company, 1997.

229. Simondon F, Preziosi MP, Yam A, et al. A randomized double-blind trial comparing a two-component acellular to a whole-cell pertussis vaccine in Senegal. Vaccine 15:1606–1612, 1997.

230. Ramsay ME, Farrington CP, Miller E. Age-specific efficacy of pertussis vaccine during epidemic and non-epidemic periods. Epidemiol Infect 111:41–48, 1993.

231. White JM, Fairley CK, Owen D, et al. The effect of an accelerated immunization schedule on pertussis in England and Wales. Commun Dis Rep CDR Rev 6:R86–R91, 1996.

232. Miller E, Ashworth LA, Redhead K, et al. Effect of schedule on reactogenicity and antibody persistence of acellular and whole-cell pertussis vaccines: value of laboratory tests as predictors of clinical performance. Vaccine 15:51–60, 1997.

233. Lautrop H, Mikkelson OS. The effect of prophylactic whooping-cough vaccination: an attempt at an evaluation based on experiences in Denmark. Ugeskr Laeger 131:735–741, 1969.

234. Sutter RW, Cochi SL. Pertussis hospitalizations and mortality in the United States, 1985–1988: evaluation of the completeness of national reporting. JAMA 267:386–391, 1992.

235. Dauer CC. Reported whooping cough morbidity and mortality in the United States. Public Health Rep 58:661–676, 1943.

236. Kimura M, Kuno-Sakai H. Immunization system in Japan: its history and present situation. Acta Paediatr Jpn 30:109–126, 1988.

237. Stuart-Harris CH. Experiences of pertussis in the United Kingdom. In Manclark CR, Hill JC (eds). International Symposium on Pertussis. Bethesda, MD, U.S. Public Health Service, 1979, pp 256–261.

238. Romanus V, Jonsell R, Bergquist SO. Pertussis in Sweden after the cessation of general immunization in 1979. Pediatr Infect Dis J 6:364–371, 1987.

239. Storsaeter J, Olin P. Relative efficacy of two acellular pertussis vaccines during three years of passive surveillance. Vaccine 10:142–144, 1992.

240. Taranger J, Trollfors B, Bergfors E, et al. Immunologic and epidemiologic experience of vaccination with a monocompetent pertussis toxoid vaccine. Pediatrics 108:E115, 2001.

241. Baron S, Njamkepo E, Grimprel E, et al. Epidemiology of pertussis in French hospitals in 1993 and 1994: 30 years of routine use of vaccination. Pediatr Infect Dis J 17:412–418, 1998.

242. Pollard R. Relation between vaccination and notification rates for whooping cough in England and Wales. Lancet 1:1180–1182, 1980.

243. Onorato IM, Wassilak SG, Meade B. Efficacy of whole-cell pertussis vaccine in preschool children in the United States. JAMA 267:2745–2749, 1992.

244. Khetsuriani N, Bisgard K, Prevots DR, et al. Pertussis outbreak in an elementary school with high vaccination coverage. Pediatr Infect Dis J 20:1108–1112, 2001.

245. Vesselinova-Jenkins CK, Newcombe RG, Gray OP, et al. The effects of immunisation upon the natural history of pertussis: a family study in the Cardiff area. J Epidemiol Community Health 32:194–199, 1978.

246. Grob PR, Crowder MJ, Robbins JF. Effect of vaccination on severity and dissemination of whooping cough. Br Med J (Clin Res Ed) 282:1925–1928, 1981.

247. Cvjetanovic B, Grab B, Uemura K. Diphtheria and whooping cough: diseases affecting a particular age group. Bull World Health Organ 56(suppl 1):103–133, 1978.

248. Fox JP, Elveback L, Scott W, et al. Herd immunity: basic concept and relevance to public health immunization practices. Am J Epidemiol 94:179–189, 1971.

249. Feikin DR, Lezotte DC, Hamman RF, et al. Individual and community risks of measles and pertussis associated with personal exemptions to immunizations. JAMA 284:3145–3150, 2000.

250. Jenkinson D. Duration of effectiveness of pertussis vaccine: evidence from a 10-year community study. Br Med J (Clin Res Ed) 296: 612–614, 1988.

251. Fine PE, Clarkson JA. Reflections on the efficacy of pertussis vaccines. Rev Infect Dis 9:866–883, 1987.

252. Weiss ES, Kendrick PL. The effectiveness of pertussis vaccine: an application of Sargent and Merrell's method of measurement. Am J Hyg 38:306–309, 1943.

253. Mortimer E. Pertussis. In Plotkin S, Mortimer E (eds): Vaccines (2nd ed). Philadelphia, WB Saunders, 1994.

254. Cody CL, Baraff LJ, Cherry JD, et al. Nature and rates of adverse reactions associated with DTP and DT immunizations in infants and children. Pediatrics 68:650–660, 1981.

255. Decker MD, Edwards KM, Steinhoff MC, et al. Comparison of 13 acellular pertussis vaccines: adverse reactions. Pediatrics 96(3 pt 2):557–566, 1995.

256. Baraff LJ, Cody CL, Cherry JD. DTP-associated reactions: an analysis by injection site, manufacturer, prior reactions, and dose. Pediatrics 73:31–36, 1984.

257. Pichichero ME, Christy C, Decker MD, et al. Defining the key parameters for comparing reactions among acellular and whole-cell pertussis vaccines. Pediatrics 96(3 pt 2):588–592, 1995.

258. Deloria MA, Blackwelder WC, Decker MD, et al. Association of reactions after consecutive acellular or whole-cell pertussis vaccine immunizations. Pediatrics 96(3 pt 2):592–594, 1995.

259. Hirtz DG, Nelson KB, Ellenberg JH. Seizures following childhood immunizations. J Pediatr 102:14–18, 1983.

260. Walker AM, Jick H, Perera DR, et al. Neurologic events following diphtheria-tetanus-pertussis immunization. Pediatrics 81:345–349, 1988.

261. Griffin MR, Ray WA, Mortimer EA, et al. Risk of seizures and encephalopathy after immunization with the diphtheria-tetanus-pertussis vaccine. JAMA 263:1641–1645, 1990.

262. Gale JL, Thapa PB, Bobo JK, et al. Acute neurological illness and DTP: report of a case-control study in Washington and Oregon. In Manclark CR (ed). Sixth International Symposium on Pertussis Abstracts (DHHS Publication No. [FDA] 90–1162). Bethesda, MD, U.S. Public Health Service, 1990.

263. Stetler HC, Orenstein WA, Bart KJ, et al. History of convulsions and use of pertussis vaccine. J Pediatr 107:175–179, 1985.

264. Bellman MH, Ross EM. Pertussis immunization and fits. In Ross E, Reynolds E (eds). Paediatric Perspectives on Epilepsy. New York, John Wiley & Sons, 1985.

265. Livengood JR, Mullen JR, White JW, et al. Family history of convulsions and use of pertussis vaccine. J Pediatr 115:527–531, 1989.

266. Ellenberg JH, Hirtz DG, Nelson KB. Do seizures in children cause intellectual deterioration? N Engl J Med 314:1085–1088, 1986.

267. Shields WD, Nielsen C, Buch D, et al. Relationship of pertussis immunization to the onset of neurologic disorders: a retrospective epidemiologic study. J Pediatr 113:801–805, 1988.

268. Braun MM, Terracciano G, Salive ME, et al. Report of a US Public Health Service workshop on hypotonic-hyporesponsive episode (HHE) after pertussis immunization. Pediatrics 102:E52, 1998.

269. Miller DC, Wadsworth MJ, Ross EM. Pertussis vaccine and severe acute neurological illnesses: response to a recent review by members of the NCES team. Vaccine 7:487–489, 1989.

270. Bellman MH, Ross EM, Miller DL. Infantile spasms and pertussis immunisation. Lancet 1:1031–1034, 1983.

271. Safety of pertussis vaccine [letter]. Lancet 335:655–656, 1990.

272. Miller D, Madge N, Diamond J, et al. Pertussis immunisation and serious acute neurological illnesses in children. BMJ 307:1171–1176, 1993.

273. Griffith AH. Pertussis vaccines and permanent brain damage [letter]. Vaccine 7:489–490, 1989.

274. Bowie C. Viewpoint: lessons from the pertussis vaccine court trial. Lancet 335:397–399, 1990.

275. Stephenson JB. A neurologist looks at neurological disease temporally related to DTP immunization. Tokai J Exp Clin Med 13(suppl):157–164, 1988.

276. Leviton A. Neurologic sequelae of pertussis immunization—1989. J Child Neurol 4:311–314, 1989.

277. MacRae KD. Epidemiology, encephalopathy, and pertussis vaccine. In FEMS—Symposium Pertussis: Proceedings of the Conference Organized by the Society for Microbiology and Epidemiology of the GDR, Berlin, April 20–22, 1988, pp 302–311.

278. Stratton KR, Howe CJ, Johnston RB Jr (eds). DPT Vaccine and Chronic Nervous System Dysfunction: A New Analysis. Division of Health Promotion and Disease Prevention, Institute of Medicine. Washington, DC, National Academy Press, 1994.

279. Riikonen R, Donner M. Incidence and aetiology of infantile spasms from 1960 to 1976: a population study in Finland. Dev Med Child Neurol 21:333–343, 1979.

280. Millichap JG. Etiology and treatment of infantile spasms: current concepts, including the role of DPT immunization. Acta Paediatr Jpn 29:54–60, 1987.

281. Melchior JC. Infantile spasms and early immunization against whooping cough: Danish survey from 1970 to 1975. Arch Dis Child 52:134–137, 1977.

282. Fukuyama Y, Tomori N, Sugitate M. Critical evaluation of the role of immunization as an etiological factor of infantile spasms. Neuropaediatrie 8:224–237, 1977.

283. Lombroso CT. A prospective study of infantile spasms: clinical and therapeutic correlations. Epilepsia 24:135–158, 1983.

284. Guyer B, Martin JA, MacDorman MF, et al. Annual summary of vital statistics 1996. Pediatrics 100:905–918, 1997.

285. Bernier RH, Frank JA Jr, Dondero TJ Jr, et al. Diphtheria-tetanus toxoids-pertussis vaccination and sudden infant deaths in Tennessee. J Pediatr 101:419–421, 1982.

286. Baraff LJ, Ablon WJ, Weiss RC. Possible temporal association between diphtheria-tetanus toxoid-pertussis vaccination and sudden infant death syndrome. Pediatr Infect Dis 2:7–11, 1983.

287. Torch WC. Diphtheria-pertussis-tetanus (DPT) immunization: a potential cause of the sudden infant death syndrome (SIDS). J Pediatr 101:169–170, 1982.

288. Torch WC. Characteristics of diphtheria-pertussis-tetanus (DPT) postvaccinal deaths and DPT-caused sudden infant death syndrome (SIDS): a review. Neurology 36(suppl 1):148, 1986.

289. Nickerson BG, Robison BK. How many sudden infant death syndrome victims were recently immunized? Western Soc Pediatr Res Clin Res 33:121A, 1985.

290. Taylor EM, Emergy JL. Immunization and cot deaths. Lancet 2:721, 1982.

291. Hoffman HS, Hunter JC, Damus K, et al. Diphtheria-tetanus-pertussis immunization and sudden infant death: results of the National Institute of Child Health and Human Development Cooperative Epidemiological Study of Sudden Infant Death Syndrome Risk Factors. Pediatrics 79:698–711, 1987.

292. Bouvier-Colle MH, Flahaut A, Messiah A, et al. Sudden infant death and immunization: an extensive epidemiological approach to the problem in France—winter 1986. Int J Epidemiol 18:121–126, 1989.

293. Griffin MR, Ray WA, Livengood JR, et al. Risk of sudden infant death syndrome (SIDS) after immunization with the diphtheria-tetanus-pertussis vaccine. N Engl J Med 319:618–623, 1988.

294. Geraghty KC. Presentation to the Immunization Practices Advisory Committee, Centers for Disease Control, Atlanta, GA, October 25, 1985.

295. Walker AM, Jick H, Perera DR, et al. Diphtheria-tetanus-pertussis immunization and sudden infant death syndrome. Am J Public Health 77:945–951, 1987.

296. Solberg LK. DTP immunization, visit to child health center and sudden infant death syndrome (SIDS). Report to the Oslo Health Council, Norway, 1985, 131 pp.

297. Wennergren G, Milerad J, Lagercrantz H, et al. The epidemiology of sudden infant death syndrome and attacks of lifelessness in Sweden. Acta Paediatr Scand 76:898–906, 1987.

298. Howson CP, Howe CJ, Fineberg HV (eds). Adverse Effects of Pertussis and Rubella Vaccines: Report of the Committee to Review the Adverse Consequences of Pertussis and Rubella Vaccines, Institute of Medicine. Washington, DC, National Academy Press, 1991.

299. Howson CP, Fineberg HV. Adverse events following pertussis and rubella vaccines: summary of a report of the Institute of Medicine. JAMA 267:392–396, 1992.
300. Howson CP, Fineberg HV. The ricochet of magic bullets: summary of the Institute of Medicine report, Adverse Effects of Pertussis and Rubella Vaccines. Pediatrics 89:318–324, 1992.
301. Skowronski DM, De Serres G, MacDonald D, et al. The changing age and seasonal profile of pertussis in Canada. J Infect Dis 185:1448–1453, 2002.
302. Ridgway D. Disputed claims for pertussis vaccine injuries under the National Vaccine Injury Compensation Program. J Invest Med 46:168–174, 1998.
303. Mills KH, Barnard A, Watkins J, et al. Cell-mediated immunity to Bordetella pertussis: role of Th1 cells in bacterial clearance in a murine respiratory infection model. Infect Immun 61:399–410, 1993.
304. Petersen JW, Andersen P, Ibsen PH, et al. Proliferative responses to purified and fractionated Bordetella pertussis antigens in mice immunized with whole-cell pertussis vaccine. Vaccine 11:463–472, 1993.
305. Petersen JW, Ibsen PH, Haslov K, Heron I. Proliferative responses and gamma interferon and tumor necrosis factor production by lymphocytes isolated from tracheobronchial lymph nodes and spleens of mice aerosol infected with Bordetella pertussis. Infect Immun 60:4563–4570, 1992.
306. Redhead K, Watkins J, Barnard A, et al. Effective immunization against Bordetella pertussis respiratory infection in mice is dependent on induction of cell-mediated immunity. Infect Immun 61:3190–3198, 1993.
307. Adamson PC, Wu TC, Meade BD, et al. Pertussis in a previously immunized child with human immunodeficiency virus infection. J Pediatr 115:589–592, 1989.
308. Bromberg K, Tannis G, Steiner P. Detection of Bordetella pertussis associated with the alveolar macrophages of children with immunodeficiency virus infection. Infect Immun 59:4715–4719, 1991.
309. Mills KH, Ryan M, Ryan E, Mahon BP. A murine model in which protection correlates with pertussis vaccine efficacy in children reveals complementary roles for humoral and cell-mediated immunity in protection against Bordetella pertussis. Infect Immun 66:594–602, 1998.
310. De Magistris MT, Romano M, Nuti S, et al. Dissecting human T cell responses against Bordetella species. J Exp Med 168:1351–1362, 1988.
311. Gearing AJ, Bird CR, Redhead K, et al. Human cellular immune responses to Bordetella pertussis infection. FEMS Microbiol Immunol 1:205–211, 1989.
312. Peppoloni S, Nencioni L, Di Tommaso A, et al. Lymphokine secretion and cytotoxic activity of human CD4+ T cell clones against Bordetella pertussis. Infect Immun 59:3768–3773, 1991.
313. Petersen JW, Ibsen PH, Bentzon MW, et al. The cell-mediated and humoral immune response to vaccination with acellular and whole-cell pertussis vaccine in adult humans. FEMS Microbiol Immunol 3:279–287, 1991.
314. Podda A, Nencioni L, De Magistris MT, et al. Metabolic, humoral, and cellular responses in adult volunteers immunized with the genetically inactivated pertussis toxin mutant PT-9K/129G. J Exp Med 172:861–868, 1990.
315. Zepp F, Knuf M, Habermehl P, et al. Pertussis-specific cell-mediated immunity in infants after vaccination with a tricomponent acellular pertussis vaccine. Infect Immun 64:4078–4084, 1996.
316. Ausiello CM, Lande R, Urbani F, et al. Cell-mediated immunity and antibody responses to Bordetella pertussis antigens in children with a history of pertussis infection and in recipients of an acellular pertussis vaccine. J Infect Dis 181:1985–1995, 2000.
317. Ausiello CM, Lande R, Urbani F, et al. Cell-mediated immune responses in four-year-old children after primary immunization with acellular pertussis vaccines. Infect Immun 67:4064–4071, 1999.
318. Cassone A, Ausiello CM, Urbani F, et al. Cell-mediated and antibody responses to Bordetella pertussis antigens in children vaccinated with acellular or whole-cell pertussis vaccines. The Progetto Pertosse-CMI Working Group. Arch Pediatr Adolesc Med 151:283–289, 1997.
319. Cassone A, Mastrantonio P, Ausiello CM. Are only antibody levels involved in the protection against pertussis in acellular pertussis vaccine recipients? J Infect Dis 182:1575–1577, 2000.
320. Tran Minh NN, He Q, Edelman K, et al. Cell-mediated immune responses to antigens of Bordetella pertussis and protection against pertussis in school children. Pediatr Infect Dis J 18:366–370, 1999.
321. Miller JJ, Silverberg RJ, Saito TM. An agglutinative reaction for Haemophilus pertussis, II: its relation to clinical immunity. J Pediatr 22:644–651, 1943.
322. Olin P, Hallander HO, Gustafsson L, et al. How to make sense of pertussis immunogenicity data. Clin Infect Dis 33(suppl 4):S288–S291, 2001.
323. Storsaeter J, Hallander HO, Gustafsson L, et al. Levels of antipertussis related to protection after household exposure to Bordetella pertussis. Vaccine 16:1907–1916, 1998.
324. Cherry JD, Gornbein J, Heininger U, et al. A search for serologic correlates of immunity to Bordetella pertussis cough illnesses. Vaccine 16:1901–1906, 1998.
325. Hewlett EL, Halperin SA. Serological correlates of immunity to Bordetella pertussis. Vaccine 16:1899–1900, 1998.
326. Plotkin SA, Cadoz M. Acellular vaccine efficacy trials. Pediatr Infect Dis J 16:913–914, 1997.
327. Poland GA. Still more questions on pertussis vaccines. Lancet 350:1564–1565, 1997.
328. Olin P, Storsaeter J. Vaccine efficacy. In A Clinical Trial of Acellular Pertussis Vaccines in Sweden: Technical Report. Stockholm, National Bacteriological Laboratory, 1988, pp 1–28.
329. Olin P, Rasmussen F, Gustafsson L, et al. Randomised controlled trial of two-component, three-component, and five-component acellular pertussis vaccines compared with whole-cell pertussis vaccine. Ad Hoc Group for the Study of Pertussis Vaccines. Lancet 350:1569–1577, 1997.
330. Trollfors B, Taranger J, Lagergård T, et al. A placebo-controlled trial of a pertussis-toxoid vaccine. N Engl J Med 333:1045–1050, 1995.
331. Pasteur Mérieux Connaught. Tripedia® product labeling. In Physician's Desk Reference. Montvale, NJ, Medical Economics Company, 1997, pp 908–911.
332. Pertussis vaccination: acellular pertussis vaccine for reinforcing and booster use—supplementary ACIP statement. Recommendations of the Immunization Practices Advisory Committee (ACIP). MMWR 41(RR-1):1–10, 1992.
333. Blackwelder WC, Storsaeter J, Olin P, et al. Acellular pertussis vaccines: efficacy and evaluation of clinical case definitions. Am J Dis Child 145:1285–1289, 1991.
334. Gustafsson L, Hallander HO, Olin P, et al. Efficacy Trial of Acellular Pertussis Vaccines: Technical Report, Trial I, with Results of Preplanned Analysis of Safety, Efficacy and Immunogenicity. Stockholm, Swedish Institute for Infectious Disease Control, 1995.
335. Olin P, Gustafsson L, Rasmussen F, et al. Efficacy Trial of Acellular Pertussis Vaccines: Technical Report Trial II, with Results of Preplanned Analysis of Efficacy, Immunogenicity and Safety. Stockholm, Swedish Institute for Infectious Disease Control, 1997.
336. Taranger J, Trollfors B, Lagergård T. Clinical Trials of a Monocomponent Pertussis Toxoid Vaccine (NICHD Ptxd)—A Technical Report. Göteborg, Sweden, Göteborg University, 1995.
337. Taranger J, Trollfors B, Lagergård T, et al. Unchanged efficacy of a pertussis toxoid vaccine throughout the two years after the third vaccination of infants. Pediatr Infect Dis J 16:180–184, 1997.
338. Knudsen KM. Statistical Report on Vaccine Efficacy, Senegal Pertussis Study. Report 3 (May 13, 1996). Copenhagen, Denmark, Statens Seruminstitut, 1996.
339. Storsaeter J, Olin P, Renemar B, et al. Mortality and morbidity from invasive bacterial infections during a clinical trial of acellular pertussis vaccines in Sweden. Pediatr Infect Dis J 7:637–645, 1988.
340. License application for pertussis vaccine withdrawn in Sweden. Lancet 1:114, 1989.
341. Samore MH, Siber GR. Effect of pertussis toxin on susceptibility of infant rats to Haemophilus influenzae type b. J Infect Dis 165:945–948, 1992.
342. Black SB, Cherry JD, Shinefield HR, et al. Apparent decreased risk of invasive bacterial disease after heterologous childhood immunization. Am J Dis Child 145:746–749, 1991.
343. Davidson M, Letson GW, Ward JI, et al. DTP immunization and susceptibility to infectious diseases: is there a relationship? Am J Dis Child 145:750–754, 1991.
344. Joffe LS, Glode MP, Gutierrez MK, et al. Diphtheria-tetanus toxoids-pertussis vaccination does not increase the risk of pertussis hospitalization with an infectious illness. Pediatr Infect Dis J 11:730–735, 1992.
345. Kimura M, Kuno-Sakai H. Acellular pertussis vaccines and fatal infections [letter]. Lancet 1:881–882, 1988.

346. Storsaeter J, Hallander H, Farrington CP, et al. Secondary analyses of the efficacy of two acellular pertussis vaccines evaluated in a Swedish Phase III trial. Vaccine 8:457–461, 1990.

347. WHO Meeting on Case Definition of Pertussis: Geneva, January 10–11, 1991 (General document MIM/EPI/PERT/91.01 [1245]). Geneva, World Health Organization, 1991, pp 4–5.

348. Hallander HO, Storsaeter J, Mollby R. Evaluation of serology and nasopharyngeal cultures for diagnosis of pertussis in a vaccine efficacy trial. J Infect Dis 163:1046–1054, 1991.

349. Heininger U, Cherry JD, Eckhardt T, et al. Clinical and laboratory diagnosis of pertussis in the regions of a large vaccine efficacy trial in Germany. Pediatr Infect Dis J 12:504–509, 1993.

350. Edwards KM, Decker MD. Comparison of serologic results in the NIAID Multicenter Acellular Pertussis Trial with recent efficacy trials. Dev Biol Stand 89:265–273, 1997.

351. Greco D, Salmaso S, Mastrantonio P, et al. A difference in relative efficacy of two DTaP vaccines in continued blinded observation of children following a clinical trial [abstract 1021]. Pediatr Res 39:173A, 1996.

352. Salmaso S, Anemona A, Mastrantonio P, et al. Long-term efficacy of pertussis vaccines in Italy. PROPER Study Working Group. Dev Biol Stand 95:189–194, 1998.

353. Salmaso S, Mastrantonio P, Tozzi AE, et al. Sustained efficacy during the first 6 years of life of 3-component acellular pertussis vaccines administered in infancy: the Italian experience. Pediatrics 108:E81, 2001.

354. Trollfors B, Taranger J, Lagergård T, et al. Efficacy of a monocomponent pertussis toxoid vaccine after household exposure to pertussis. J Pediatr 130:532–536, 1997.

355. Taranger J, Trollfors B, Bergfors E, et al. Mass vaccination of children with pertussis toxoid—decreased incidence in both vaccinated and nonvaccinated persons. Clin Infect Dis 33:1004–1010, 2001.

356. Heininger U, Cherry JD, Stehr K, et al. Comparative efficacy of the Lederle/Takeda acellular pertussis component DTP (DTaP) vaccine and Lederle whole-cell component DTP vaccine in German children after household exposure. Pertussis Vaccine Study Group. Pediatrics 102:546–553, 1998.

357. Cherry JD, Heininger U, Stehr K, et al. The effect of investigator compliance (observer bias) on calculated efficacy in a pertussis vaccine trial. Pediatrics 102(4 pt 1):909–912, 1998.

358. Lugauer S, Heininger U, Cherry JD, et al. Long-term clinical effectiveness of an acellular pertussis component vaccine and a whole cell pertussis component vaccine. Eur J Pediatr 161:142–146, 2002.

359. Simondon F. Senegal pertussis trial. Dev Biol Stand 89:63–66, 1997.

360. Plotkin SA, Cadoz M. The acellular pertussis vaccine trials: an interpretation. Pediatr Infect Dis J 16:508–517, 1997.

361. Cherry JD. Comparative efficacy of acellular pertussis vaccines: an analysis of recent trials. Pediatr Infect Dis J 16(4 suppl):S90–S96, 1997.

361a. De Serres G, Shadmani R, Boulianne N, et al. Effectiveness of a single dose of acellular pertussis vaccine to prevent pertussis in children primed with pertussis whole cell vaccine. Vaccine 19:3004–3008, 2001.

362. Kimura M, Kuno-Sakai H. Pertussis vaccines in Japan. Acta Paediatr Jpn 30:143–153, 1988.

363. Kimura M, Kuno-Sakai H. Epidemiology of pertussis in Japan. Tokai J Exp Clin Med 13(suppl):1–7, 1988.

364. Sato Y, Sato H. Further characterization of Japanese acellular pertussis vaccine prepared in 1988 by 6 Japanese manufacturers. Tokai J Exp Clin Med 13(suppl):79–88, 1988.

365. Ginnaga A, Morokuma K, Aihara K, et al. Characterization and clinical study on the acellular pertussis vaccine produced by a combination of column purified pertussis toxin and filamentous hemagglutinin. Tokai J Exp Clin Med 13(suppl):59–69, 1988.

366. Kimura M, Kuno-Sakai H. Developments in pertussis immunisation in Japan. Lancet 336:30–32, 1990.

367. Pittman M. History of the development of pertussis vaccine. Dev Biol Stand 73:13–29, 1991.

368. Aoyama T, Murase Y, Kato M, et al. Efficacy and immunogenicity of acellular pertussis vaccine by manufacturer and patient age. Am J Dis Child 143:655–659, 1989.

369. Isomura S, Suzuki S, Sato Y. Clinical efficacy of the Japanese acellular pertussis vaccine after intrafamilial exposure to pertussis patients. Dev Biol Stand 61:531–537, 1985.

370. Mortimer EA Jr, Kimura M, Cherry JD, et al. Protective efficacy of the Takeda acellular pertussis vaccine combined with diphtheria and tetanus toxoids following household exposure of Japanese children. Am J Dis Child 144:899–904, 1990.

371. Cherry JD, Mortimer EA, Hackell JG, et al. Clinical trials in the United States and Japan with the Lederle-Takeda and Takeda acellular pertussis-diphtheria-tetanus (APDT) vaccines. The Multicenter APDT Vaccine Study Group. Dev Biol Stand 73:51–58, 1991.

372. Kuno-Sakai H, Kimura M, Ozaki K, et al. Japanese clinical trials with Takeda acellular pertussis vaccine. Tokai J Exp Clin Med 13(suppl):15–19, 1988.

373. Morgan CM, Blumberg DA, Cherry JD, et al. Comparison of acellular and whole-cell pertussis-component DTP vaccines: a multicenter double-blind study in 4- to 6-year-old children. Am J Dis Child 144:41–45, 1990.

374. Glode M, Joffe L, Reisinger K, et al. Safety and immunogenicity of acellular pertussis vaccine combined with diphtheria and tetanus toxoids in 17- to 24-month-old children. Pediatr Infect Dis J 11:530–535, 1992.

375. Blumberg D, Mink CM, Cherry JD, et al. Comparison of an acellular pertussis-component diphtheria-tetanus-pertussis (DTP) vaccine with a whole-cell pertussis-component DTP vaccine in 17- to 24-month-old children, with measurement of 69-kilodalton outer membrane protein antibody. J Pediatr 117(1 pt 1):46–51, 1990.

376. Blumberg DA, Mink CM, Cherry JD, et al. Comparison of acellular and whole-cell pertussis-component diphtheria-tetanus-pertussis vaccines in infants. The APDT Vaccine Study Group. J Pediatr 119:194–204, 1991.

377. Watson B, Cawein A, McKee BL, et al. Safety and immunogenicity of acellular pertussis vaccine, combined with diphtheria and tetanus as the Japanese commercial Takeda vaccine, compared with the Takeda acellular pertussis component combined with Lederle's diphtheria and tetanus toxoids in two-, four- and six-month-old infants. Pediatr Infect Dis J 11:930–935, 1992.

378. Kamiya H, Nii R, Matsuda T, et al. Immunogenicity and reactogenicity of Takeda acellular pertussis-component diphtheria-tetanus-pertussis vaccine in 2- and 3-month-old children in Japan. Am J Dis Child 146:1141–1147, 1992.

379. Pertussis vaccination: Acellular pertussis vaccine for the fourth and fifth doses of the DTP series: update to supplementary ACIP statement. Recommendations of the Advisory Committee on Immunization Practices (ACIP). MMWR 41(RR-15):1–5, 1992.

380. Juretzko P, Von Kries R, Hermann M, et al. Effectiveness of acellular pertussis vaccine assessed by hospital-based active surveillance in Germany. Clin Infect Dis 35:162–167, 2002.

380a. Khetsuriani N, Bisgard K, Prevots R, et al. Pertussis outbreak in an elementary school with high vaccination coverage. Pediatr Infect Dis J 20: 1108–1112, 2001.

380b. Guiso N, Boursaux-Eude C, Weber C, et al. Analysis of *Bordatella pertussis* isolates collected in Japan before and after introduction of acellular pertussis vaccines. Vaccine 19: 3248–3252, 2001.

381. Edwards KM, Karzon DT. Pertussis vaccines. Pediatr Clin North Am 37:549–566, 1990.

382. Lewis K, Cherry JD, Holroyd J, et al. A double-blind study comparing an acellular pertussis-component DTP vaccine with a whole-cell pertussis-component DTP vaccine in 18-month-old children. Am J Dis Child 140:872–876, 1986.

383. Edwards KM, Lawrence E, Wright PF. Diphtheria, tetanus, and pertussis vaccine: a comparison of the immune response and adverse reactions to conventional and acellular pertussis components. Am J Dis Child 140:867–871, 1986.

384. Edwards KM, Bradley RB, Decker MD, et al. Evaluation of a new highly purified pertussis vaccine in infants and children. J Infect Dis 160:832–837, 1989.

385. Pichichero ME, Badgett JT, Rodgers GC Jr, et al. Acellular pertussis vaccine: immunogenicity and safety of an acellular pertussis vs. a whole cell pertussis vaccine combined with diphtheria and tetanus toxoids as a booster in 18- and 24-month old children. Pediatr Infect Dis J 6:352–363, 1987.

386. Anderson EL, Belshe RB, Bartram J. Differences in reactogenicity and antigenicity of acellular and standard pertussis vaccines combined with diphtheria and tetanus in infants. J Infect Dis 157:731–737, 1988.

387. Schmitt-Grohe S, Stehr K, Cherry JD, et al. Minor adverse events in a comparative efficacy trial in Germany in infants receiving either the Lederle/Takeda acellular pertussis component DTP (DTaP) vaccine, the Lederle whole-cell component DTP (DTP) or DT vaccine. The Pertussis Vaccine Study Group. Dev Biol Stand 89:113–118, 1997.

388. Uberall MA, Stehr K, Cherry JD, et al. Severe adverse events in a comparative efficacy trial in Germany in infants receiving either the Lederle/Takeda acellular pertussis component DTP (DTaP) vaccine, the Lederle whole-cell component DTP (DTP) or DT vaccine. The Pertussis Vaccine Study Group. Dev Biol Stand 89:83–89, 1997.

389. Ciofi degli Atti ML, Olin P. Severe adverse events in the Italian and Stockholm I pertussis vaccine clinical trials. Dev Biol Stand 89:77–81, 1997.

390. Simondon F, Yam A, Gagnepain JY, et al. Comparative safety and immunogenicity of an acellular versus whole-cell pertussis component of diphtheria-tetanus-pertussis vaccines in Senegalese infants. Eur J Clin Microbiol Infect Dis 15:927–932, 1996.

391. Kuno-Sakai H, Kimura M. Epidemiology of pertussis and use of acellular pertussis vaccines in Japan. Dev Biol Stand 89:331–332, 1997.

392. McDermott C, Grimsrud K, Waters J. Acellular pertussis vaccine and whole cell pertussis vaccine: a comparison of reported selected adverse events [abstr P41]. In Abstracts of the Third Canadian National Conference on Immunization, Calgary (Alberta) Canada, December 1998.

393. Scheifele D, Halperin S, Pless R, et al. Marked reduction in febrile seizures and hypotonic-hyporesponsive episodes with acellular pertussis-based vaccines: results of Canada-wide surveillance [abstr 31]. Paper presented at the 37th Annual Meeting of the Infectious Diseases Society of America, Philadelphia, PA, November 1999.

394. Chen RT, Rastogi SC, Mullen JR, et al. The Vaccine Adverse Event Reporting System (VAERS). Vaccine 12:542–550, 1994.

395. Rosenthal S, Chen R, Hadler S. The safety of acellular pertussis vaccine vs whole-cell pertussis vaccine: a postmarketing assessment. Arch Pediatr Adolesc Med 150:457–460, 1996.

396. Braun MM, Mootrey GT, Salive ME, et al. Infant immunization with acellular pertussis vaccines in the United States: assessment of the first two years' data from the Vaccine Adverse Event Reporting System (VAERS). Pediatrics 106:E51, 2000.

397. Pichichero ME, Deloria MA, Rennels MB, et al. A safety and immunogenicity comparison of 12 acellular pertussis vaccines and one whole-cell pertussis vaccine given as a fourth dose in 15 to 20 month old children. Pediatrics 100:772–788, 1997.

398. Schmitt HJ, Beutel K, Schuind A, et al. Reactogenicity and immunogenicity of a booster dose of a combined diphtheria, tetanus, and tricomponent acellular pertussis vaccine at fourteen to twenty-eight months of age. J Pediatr 130:616–623, 1997.

399. Rennels MB, Deloria MA, Pichichero ME, et al. Extensive swelling after booster doses of acellular pertussis-tetanus-diphtheria vaccines. Pediatrics 105:E12, 2000.

400. Liese JG, Stojanov S, Zink TH, et al. Safety and immunogenicity of Biken acellular pertussis vaccine in combination with diphtheria and tetanus toxoid as a fifth dose at four to six years of age. Munich Vaccine Study Group. Pediatr Infect Dis J 20:981–988, 2001.

401. Pichichero ME, Edwards KM, Anderson EL, et al. Safety and immunogenicity of six acellular pertussis vaccines and one whole-cell pertussis vaccine given as a fifth dose in 4- to 6-year-old children. Pediatrics 105:E11, 2000.

402. Rennels MB, Deloria MA, Pichichero ME, et al. Lack of consistent relationship between quantity of aluminum in diphtheria-tetanus-acellular pertussis vaccines and rates of extensive swelling. Vaccine 20(suppl 20):S44–S47, 2002.

403. Isomura S. Efficacy and safety of acellular pertussis vaccine in Aichi Prefecture, Japan. Pediatr Infect Dis J 7:258–262, 1988.

404. Blennow M, Granström M. Adverse reactions and serologic response to a booster dose of acellular vaccine in children immunized with acellular or whole-cell vaccine as infants. Pediatrics 84:62–67, 1989.

405. Diggle L, Deeks J. Effect of needle length on incidence of local reactions to routine immunisation in infants aged 4 months: randomised controlled trial. BMJ 321:931–1033, 2000.

406. Nagel J, Svec D, Waters T, et al. IgE synthesis in man. I. Development of specific IgE antibodies after immunization with tetanus-diphtheria (Td) toxoids. J Immunol 118:334–341, 1977.

407. Mark A, Björkstén B, Granström M. Immunoglobulin E responses to diphtheria and tetanus toxoids after booster with aluminum-adsorbed and fluid DT-vaccines. Vaccine 13:669–673, 1995.

408. Hedenskog S, Björkstén B, Blennow M, et al. Immunoglobulin E response to pertussis toxin in whooping cough and after immunization with a whole-cell and an acellular pertussis vaccine. Int Arch Allergy Appl Immunol 89:156–161, 1989.

409. Ausiello CM, Urbani F, la Sala A, et al. Vaccine- and antigen-dependent type 1 and type 2 cytokine induction after primary vaccination of infants with whole-cell or acellular pertussis vaccines. Infect Immun 65:2168–2174, 1997.

410. Scheifele DW, Halperin SA, Ferguson AC. Assessment of injection site reactions to an acellular pertussis-based use of skin tests with vaccine antigens. Vaccine 19:4720–4726, 2001.

411. Keitel WA, Muenz LR, Decker MD, et al. A randomized clinical trial of acellular pertussis vaccines in healthy adults: dose-response comparisons of 5 vaccines and implications for booster immunization. J Infect Dis 180:397–403, 1999.

412. Decker MD, Cates KL, Maida A, et al. Safety and immunogenicity in adults and adolescents of Biocine acellular pertussis (aP) vaccine [abstr 123.002]. In Abstracts of the 7th International Congress for Infectious Diseases, Hong Kong, June 1996.

413. Edwards KM, Decker MD, Graham BS, et al. Adult immunization with acellular pertussis vaccine. JAMA 269:53–56, 1993.

414. Cadoz M, Arminjon F, Quentin-Millet MJ, et al. Safety and immunogenicity of Mérieux acellular pertussis in adult volunteers. In Transcript of the Workshop on Acellular Pertussis Vaccines. Washington, DC, U.S. Department of Health and Human Services, 1986, pp 131–134.

415. Sekura RD, Zhang YL, Robertson R, et al. Clinical, metabolic and antibody responses of adult volunteers to an investigational vaccine composed of pertussis toxin inactivated by hydrogen peroxide. J Pediatr 113:806–813, 1988.

416. Stehr K, Lugauer S, Heninger U, et al. Immunogenicity and reactogenicity of Lederle/Takeda acellular pertussis vaccine in 185 German adults. Pediatr Res 37:189A, 1995.

417. Keitel W. Adult pertussis study results using five acellular vaccines. Acellular pertussis vaccine trials: results and impact on US public health. Paper presented at the National Institutes of Health Pertussis Conference, Washington, DC, June 3–5, 1996.

418. Forsyth K, Tan T, Wirsing von Konig C-H, et al. Evaluation of the pertussis evidence base and immunization strategies to improve disease control: interim findings of the Global Pertussis Initiative [abstract]. Paper presented at 7th International Symposium on Pertussis, Cambridge, England, September 2002.

419. National Advisory Committee on Immunization. Canada Immunization Guide (6th ed). Ottawa (Ontario), Canada, Population and Public Health Branch, Health Canada, 2002.

420. Obersten Sanitätsrates (Impfausschuss). Impfplan 2002 Österreich: Empfehlungen des Obersten Sanitätsrates (Impfausschuss), Stand 2002, accessed July 14, 2002. Available at www.reisemed.at/Impfplan%202000.html

421. Granstrom M, Thoren M, Belnnow M, et al. Acellular pertussis vaccine in adults: adverse reactions and immune response. Eur J Clin Microbiol 6:18–21, 1987.

422. Ward J. Acellular pertussis vaccines in adolescents and adults [abstr 1291]. In Abstracts of the 41st Interscience Conference on Antimicrobial Agents and Chemotherapy, Chicago, IL, December 16–19, 2001, p 520.

423. Wright SW, Edwards KM, Decker MD, et al. Pertussis seroprevalence in emergency department staff. Ann Emerg Med 24:413–417, 1994.

424. Shefer A, Dales L, Nelson M, et al. Use and safety of acellular pertussis vaccine among adult hospital staff during an outbreak of pertussis. J Infect Dis 171:1053–1056, 1995.

425. Christie CD, Garrison KM, Kiely L, et al. A trial of acellular pertussis vaccine in hospital workers during the Cincinnati pertussis epidemic of 1993. Clin Infect Dis 33:997–1003, 2001.

426. Diphtheria, tetanus and pertussis: recommendations for vaccine use and other preventive measures. Recommendations of the Immunization Practices Advisory Committee (ACIP). MMWR 40(RR-10):1–28, 1991.

427. Decker MD, Edwards KM. Acellular pertussis vaccines: the authors reply. N Engl J Med 334:1547–1548, 1996.

Chapter 22

Pneumococcal Polysaccharide Vaccine

DAVID S. FEDSON • DANIEL M. MUSHER

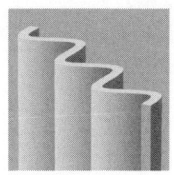

The modern development of pneumococcal polysaccharide vaccine exemplifies the full cycle of scientific discovery regarding the pathogenesis, treatment, and eventual prevention of a major infectious disease. At each stage, new knowledge has brought forth questions not only about the basic biology of pneumococcal infections and the immune response to pneumococcal vaccination, but also about the epidemiologic importance of pneumococcal infections and the benefits that might be realized if pneumococcal vaccine were widely used.

In recent years, several reviews have added to classical older works[1-4] providing comprehensive summaries of all aspects of pneumococcal infections[5-14] and pneumococcal vaccine.[15-19] For more than 100 years, the study of *Streptococcus pneumoniae* and pneumococcal infections has occupied a central position in the development of a scientific basis for the control of infectious diseases.[3,20,21] The organism was first isolated and grown in the laboratory almost simultaneously by Sternberg and Pasteur in 1881 (Table 22–1). During the next decade, the pneumococcus was shown to be the chief cause of lobar pneumonia. By the early 20th century, the importance of humoral immunity had been recognized, in large measure as a result of studies of *S. pneumoniae*, and there was the beginning of an understanding of the potential protective effects of antiserum and vaccines.

The first large-scale clinical trial of a crude whole-cell pneumococcal vaccine was conducted in 1911, at a time when the importance of type-specific immunity was not understood. During the next two decades, the experimental foundation was laid for understanding the importance of antibody to pneumococcal capsular polysaccharide and for developing an effective polyvalent, type-specific pneumococcal polysaccharide vaccine. The first clinical trial of a tetravalent vaccine was reported at the close of World War II. Two hexavalent vaccines were marketed in 1946, only to be withdrawn within a few years. Physicians had little interest in a vaccine to prevent a disease they could now treat successfully with penicillin.

It remained for Austrian and Gold to demonstrate, in the early 1960s, that pneumococcal infections were still lethal in spite of appropriate antimicrobial therapy.[22] Led by Austrian, efforts to develop a modern pneumococcal capsular polysaccharide vaccine were undertaken once again. Within a decade, the efficacy of pneumococcal polysaccharide vaccine was conclusively demonstrated in clinical trials conducted among gold miners in South Africa.[23,24] This was soon followed by licensure of a 14-valent capsular polysaccharide vaccine in the United States in 1977 and a 23-valent polysaccharide vaccine in 1983.

In the meantime, the poor immunogenicity of pneumococcal polysaccharide vaccine in children less than 2 years of age led to the development of second-generation vaccines in which capsular polysaccharides were conjugated to one of several different proteins.[25] This effort culminated in a clinical trial that demonstrated the remarkable efficacy of a 7-valent pneumococcal conjugate vaccine in young children.[26] In recent years, several pneumococcal virulence factors have been shown to induce protection against experimental pneumococcal infections, leading to preliminary studies demonstrating the immunogenicity of a pneumococcal protein-based vaccine (pneumococcal surface protein A [PspA]) in humans.[27] Finally, in 2001, the complete genome sequence of a virulent isolate of *S. pneumoniae* was published,[28] raising the possibility that other protective antigens might soon be discovered.

In previous editions of this book, all pneumococcal vaccines were covered in a single chapter. In this edition, pneumococcal conjugate vaccines and newer protein-based vaccines are discussed in a separate chapter (see Chapter 23). Because pneumococcal conjugate vaccines have been developed primarily for children, many aspects of childhood pneumococcal disease also are discussed in the same chapter. This chapter focuses more on adult pneumococcal disease and its prevention with pneumococcal polysaccharide vaccine.

Background

Clinical Pneumococcal Infections

The major clinical syndromes caused by *S. pneumoniae* are widely recognized and discussed in all standard medical

TABLE 22-1 ■ Historical Milestones in the Study of Pneumococcal Disease and Pneumococcal Vaccines

1881	Pasteur, Sternberg—Pneumococus first isolated and grown in vitro
1880s	Pneumococcus shown to be a major cause of lobar pneumonia
1884	Gram's stain developed
1891	Klemperer, Klemperer—Protective effect of antiserum demonstrated
1897	Bezancon, Griffin—Distinct pneumococcal serotypes demonstrated
1902	Neufeld—Capsular swelling (quellung) with specific antiserum shown
1904	Neufeld, Rimpau—Opsonization by immune serum demonstrated
1910	Neufeld, Handel—Type-specific immunity discovered
1911	Wright—Clinical trials of whole-cell pneumococcal vaccine conducted in South Africa
1913	Lister—Type-specific antibodies develop after infection or injection of heat-killed organisms
1917–27	Avery, Dochez, Heidelberger, Goebel—Capsular antigens shown to be complex polysaccharides that are antigenic and determine serologic reactivity
1928	Griffith—Capsular transformation demonstrated
1930	Francis, Tillett—Purified capsular polysaccharides shown to be immunogenic in humans
1931	Dubos, Avery—Capsular polysaccharide determines pneumococcal virulence
1931	Finland, Sutliff—Serum therapy for lobar pneumonia shown to be effective
1938	Felton—Clinical protection against type-specific disease shown in persons injected with purified capsular polysaccharides
	Ekwurzel—Clinical trial of capsular polysaccharides shown to reduce incidence of pneumonia and its mortality
1941	Abraham, Chain and co-workers—Penicillin successful in treating gram-positive infections
1944	Avery, MacLeod, McCarty—Capsular transformation by DNA demonstrates that DNA is the bearer of genetic information
1945	MacLeod, Heidelberger and co-workers—Successful clinical trial of tetravalent pneumococcal vaccine conducted in military recruits
1946–48	Hexavalent pneumococcal vaccines introduced but soon withdrawn
1964	Austrian, Gold—Pneumococcal infections shown to be a continuing problem in patients treated with antibiotics
1967	Hansman, Bullen—Penicillin-resistant pneumococcus reported
1968	Pneumococcal polysaccharide vaccine development begun
1976	Austrian, Smit—Efficacy of pneumococcal polysaccharide vaccine demonstrated in healthy adults in South Africa
1977	14-valent pneumococcal polysaccharide vaccine licensed
1983	23-valent pneumococcal polysaccharide vaccine licensed
1980s	Pneumococcal conjugate vaccine development begun
1990s	Pneumococcal protein vaccine development begun
2000	Black, Shinefield—Efficacy of pneumococcal conjugate vaccine demonstrated in infants in Northern California
2000	Briles, Nabors and co-workers—Immunogenicity of pneumococcal protein (PspA) vaccine demonstrated in healthy adults
2001	Tettelin and co-workers—Complete genome sequence of S. pneumoniae published

textbooks.[14] Infections of the middle ear (otitis media), sinuses, tracheobronchial tree, and lung are the result of direct spread of the organism from the nasopharynx. Invasive pneumococcal disease is defined by the detection of S. pneumoniae in the bloodstream or when the organisms have spread hematogenously to the central nervous system (meningitis), heart valves (endocarditis), and, rarely, other sites such as joints or the peritoneal cavity. Primary (occult) bacteremia usually affects children but also can be diagnosed, less commonly, in adults. The organism also may spread directly to adjacent sites; from the lung to the pleural space (pleuritis), from the nasopharynx to the central nervous system through a defect in the dura (cerebrospinal fluid [CSF] leak), or from the female genital tract to the peritoneum. Pneumococcal infections occur throughout the year, although the number of cases is usually higher during winter months when there are outbreaks of viral diseases and an increase in air pollution.

Bacteriology of *Streptococcus pneumoniae*

The microorganism initially observed by Sternberg and Pasteur was called Pneumococcus by Fraenkel in 1886.[3] It was renamed *Diplococcus pneumoniae* in 1920 because of its distinctive morphology. Its name was changed to *Streptococcus pneumoniae* in 1974 because of its many similarities to other streptococci. Historically, the demonstration in 1944 by Avery, MacLeod, and McCarty that DNA is the active substance responsible for the genetic transformation from rough (nonencapsulated) to smooth (encapsulated) cells is one of the cornerstones of modern molecular biology.[29-31] Other biologic markers, such as type specificity and antibiotic resistance, are also genetically transferable.

Pneumococci are relatively fastidious, facultative anaerobic organisms that grow in short chains in broth culture and appear as gram-positive diplococci when examined microscopically. *Streptococcus pneumoniae* serotypes 3 and 37 grow as large mucoid colonies, but other serotypes produce smooth colonies that are not obviously mucoid. Hydrogen peroxide is one of the end products of bacterial metabolism. Because pneumococci lack catalase or peroxidase, adding red blood cells to the growth medium inactivates hydrogen peroxide and enhances their viability. Under aerobic conditions, colonies of S. pneumoniae alter hemoglobulin, producing a greenish discoloration of the surrounding blood-containing medium that has been called incorrectly *alpha* hemolysis. A similar discoloration can be seen around colonies grown on chocolate agar. The sensitivity of pneumococci but not most other streptococci to growth inhibition by ethylhydrocupreine (Optochin) has been widely used for laboratory identification. Some pneumococcal isolates, however, are resistant to Optochin,[32] and solubility of the colony in bile is usually regarded as definitive for routine diagnostic purposes.

Cell wall (C-) polysaccharide is unique to *S. pneumoniae* and is present in all isolates (Fig. 22–1).[14,33,34] It consists of teichoic acid that is covalently linked to a peptidoglycan backbone on the outer surface of the cell wall. Peptidoglycan plays a major role in stimulating the inflammatory response associated with pneumococcal infections.[5,35] C-polysaccharide is responsible for serologic cross-reactivity between *S. pneumoniae* and other streptococci. It reacts with a specific β-globulin in human serum (C-reactive protein) in the early stages of the inflammatory response and activates the alternative complement pathway. Antibody to C-polysaccharide appears early in life and can be found in virtually all children and adults, but it does not protect against pneumococcal infection.[36]

The capsular polysaccharide on the cell surface is one of the primary factors responsible for the virulence of *S. pneumoniae* in the normal host.[14,33,34] Invasiveness depends more on the composition than on the amount of capsular polysaccharide produced; for example, types 3 and 37 are both heavily encapsulated, but type 3 is highly invasive whereas type 37 seldom causes disease.[37] Invasiveness also depends on spontaneous phase variation. Transparent strains are adapted to the nasopharynx (they have less capsule, more surface choline and cell wall–associated teichoic acid, and more of certain adhesins). In order to survive better in the bloodstream they become opaque (they have more capsule, less choline, and more of certain protective antigens).[38–40] The genetic control of phase variation is not understood. Unlike peptidoglycan, capsular polysaccharide does not induce an inflammatory response in the host. Instead it

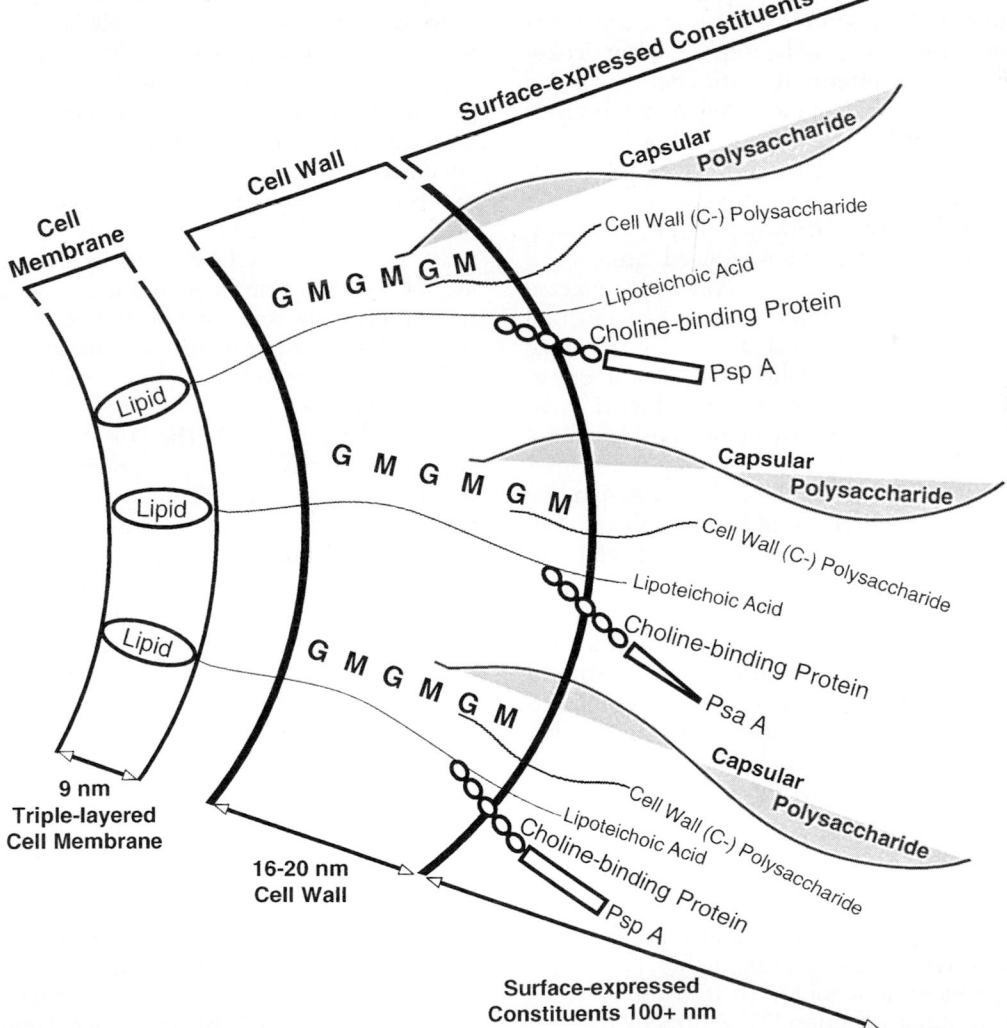

FIGURE 22–1 ■ A representation of the cell membrane, cell wall, and capsule of *Streptococcus pneumoniae*. Within the cell wall, M is *N*-acetylmuramic acid and G is *N*-acetyl-D-glucosamine. The stem peptides and the cross-linked pentaglycine bridges that extend from the long M-G-M-G chains are not shown. Cell wall (C-) polysaccharide consists of teichoic acid with peptidoglycan and phosphorylcholine (not shown). F antigen is the lipid/teichoic acid moiety in the cell membrane that extends into the cell wall. (From Musher DM. *Streptococcus pneumoniae*. In Mandell GL, Bennett JE, Dolin R (eds). Principles and Practice of Infections Diseases (5th ed). New York, Churchill Livingstone, 2001, p 2130, with permission.)

inhibits phagocytosis, presumably by preventing polymor-phonuclear leukocytes from recognizing antibodies to cell wall constituents or complement adherent to the bacterial cell wall.[41] In addition, capsular polysaccharide interferes with intracellular killing of phagocytized pneumococci by activating a mechanism that is not dependent on immune globulin or complement.[42] Although opaque phenotypes have greater virulence, transparent phenotypes have greater competence for genetic transformation.[40]

Several other virulence factors have been identified in S. pneumoniae (see Fig. 22–1).[5,6,14,33,43–46] Pneumolysin is a non–surface-exposed, thiol-activated cytoplasmic toxin that can damage a wide range of cells. It binds to cholesterol in the host cell membrane and, in a two-stage process, leads to pore formation and the osmotic lysis of the cell.[47–49] Pneumolysin is toxic to ciliated epithelial cells, slowing cil-iary beating and reducing mucus clearance. It disrupts the tight junctions of alveolar epithelial cells, damaging the alveolar-capillary barrier and leading to edema and hemor-rhage.[50,51] In the brain, it is toxic to the ciliated ependymal cells that line the ventricles and cerebral aqueducts.[52] Pneumolysin inhibits the respiratory burst and suppresses the antimicrobial activities of polymorphonuclear leuko-cytes and macrophages by interfering with chemotaxis and the production of lymphokines, including tumor necrosis factor-α (TNF-α) and interleukin (IL)-1.[47,48] It also inhibits the proliferative response of lymphocytes to mitogens, induces nitric acid formation in macrophages, and activates the classical complement pathway. A pneumolysin-negative mutant of S. pneumoniae has reduced virulence in experimental infections in mice.[53,54] Antibody directed against pneumolysin protects mice against experimental infection, and patients hospitalized with nonbacteremic pneumococcal pneumonia have higher levels of antibody to pneumolysin that do those with bacteremic disease.[55] An inactivated pneumolysin is currently being considered as a possible vaccine.[47,56]

Autolysin (lytA) is one of a family of choline-binding proteins that are noncovalently bound to the phosphoryl-choline of teichoic acid on the pneumococcal cell sur-face.[57,58] LytA degrades the peptidoglycan backbone of S. pneumoniae. It was thought to release pneumolysin and several components of the pneumococcal cell wall known to be inflammatory,[5,44] but recent research has questioned its essential role in the release of pneumolysin.[59] Mutations in the lytA gene render pneumococci avirulent,[60,61] but antibodies to lytA alone are not protective, indicating that lytA facilitates the activity of other virulence factors.

Pneumococcal surface protein A (PspA) is an antigeni-cally variable choline-binding protein that can be found on the surface of every pneumococcus.[62,63] It prevents C3-mediated binding of host cell complement, thus reducing complement-mediated phagocytosis and clearance.[64] PspA binds lactoferrin, interfering with immune function in the host and perhaps securing a source of iron for bacterial metabolism at the site of infection.[65,66] Antibody to PspA partially protects mice against pneumococcal chal-lenge,[67,68] and PspA is actively being studied as a possi-ble vaccine.[27] In a study of patients hospitalized with pneumococcal pneumonia, however, antibody levels to PspA were similar in those with and without bacteremic disease.[55]

Pneumococcal surface antigen A (PsaA) is not an adhesin as was originally thought.[44,69] It appears to function in a transporter system that brings Mn^{2+} and Zn^{2+} into the bacterial cytoplasm.[44] It also appears necessary for adher-ence and the ability of S. pneumoniae to colonize mucosal surfaces. Antibody to PsaA appears after pneumococcal col-onization or infection, and the presence of this antibody reduces colonization in experimental animals.[70]

Choline-binding protein A (CbpA, also known as PspC or SpsA) is another member of the family of choline-bind-ing proteins and was the first adhesin to be described in S. pneumoniae.[44] CbpA creates a bridge between the choline moieties of teichoic or lipoteichoic acid in the pneumococ-cal cell wall and glycoconjugates on the surface of host cells. Its activity is evident only with cytokine-activated cells that express receptors (e.g., platelet activating factor [PAF] receptor) that bind to phosphocholine of the pneumococ-cal cell wall. It has also been shown to bind to the secretory component of IgA, to C3, and to factor H, which regulates complement.[43,71,72]

Hyaluronate lyase (hyaluronidase) is one of a group of enzymes that break down extracellular matrix, and thus it functions as a "spreading factor."[44] It is directly involved in host invasion[73] and interacts with several receptor-binding proteins on host cell surfaces. Immunoglobulin A (IgA) protease cleaves serum and secretory IgA1 and may help pneumococci evade host defenses at the mucosal surface, but its precise role in pathogenesis is uncertain.[74] Two neu-raminidases, NanA and NanB, cleave N-acetylneuraminic acid, exposing host cell surface molecules that pneumococci use for adherence and colonization.[75] Several other puta-tive virulence factors have been described.[76,77] It is likely that analysis of the genome of S. pneumoniae will identify additional virulence factors and suggest some as candidate vaccine antigens.[43,78,79]

Since the early 1980s, the Danish system for classifying S. pneumoniae has been used worldwide. Differences in the chemical structures of pneumococcal capsular polysaccha-rides provide the basis for classifying them into serotypes. Currently, 90 different serotypes have been described.[80,81] Some serogroups include several serotypes that are serolog-ically related. Thus, for example, in serogroup 7 the original type 7 was called 7F (for "first") and related serotypes iden-tified later were named 7A, 7B, and so forth.

Only a limited number of serotypes account for most pneumococcal disease in humans. Lower numbered serotypes are generally responsible for causing invasive dis-ease, but shifts in the prevalence of individual serotypes within geographic areas or populations occur over time.[82] For example, type 1 used to be a prominent cause of pneu-mococcal disease in the United States but now causes no more than 1% to 2% of cases, whereas type 3 remains a fre-quently isolated serotype from patients with invasive dis-ease. The reasons for these shifts are unknown, but the ability to colonize, antibiotic susceptibility, and socioeco-nomic factors are probably important. Fundamental differ-ences in the epidemiology of individual serogroups have been demonstrated among different age groups in different regions during the same time period.[83,84]

Each serotype can be identified by its chemical structure and its reaction with type-specific antisera. The most widely used method for serotyping is the quellung test.[81] When bacteria in suspension are mixed with homologous antiserum and methylene blue, a distinct capsular precipitin reaction can be observed microscopically. Simple macroscopic agglutination by specific antisera also can be used. Serotyping of *S. pneumoniae* is usually accomplished using antisera provided by the Statens Serum Institut in Copenhagen, Denmark. The antisera are available commercially as (1) Omniserum, which reacts with all 90 serotypes; (2) 14 pooled sera, each of which reacts with 7 to 12 types; and (3) 46 sera, each specific for a single serotype or serogroup. A special set of 12 pooled sera (A through F, H, and P through T) are available commercially as Pneumotest. They cover 23 different vaccine-related serotypes and 25 other cross-reacting serotypes. Used in checkerboard fashion, they can serotype 90% or more of all invasive pneumococcal isolates.[85] In addition, several monovalent antisera have been prepared to selected serogroups, but they generally do not distinguish between individual serotypes within a serogroup.[86]

Coagglutination[87] and latex agglutination[88] tests also have been developed for serotyping, with results that are equivalent to those obtained with the quellung test.[89] The simplicity and low cost of the coagglutination test has allowed it to be used in epidemiologic studies in developing countries. More elaborate molecular typing methods employ pulsed-field gel electrophoresis (PFGE)[90] or polymerase chain reaction (PCR)[91] techniques. The most advanced method uses multilocus enzyme electrophoresis as the basis for multilocus sequence typing (MLST).[92,93] This has become the basis for describing the molecular epidemiology of *S. pneumoniae*. Usually there is good agreement between serotypes determined by the quellung test and genotypes determined by MLST, but exceptions can occur as a result of capsular switching. When this happens, a single serotype may be shown to have several distantly related MLST genotypes.[93]

Pathogenesis and Host Defense as They Relate to Prevention

Many nonimmunologic and immunologic factors act together to defend the host against pneumococcal infection.[14] Nonimmunologic factors include normal function of the gag and cough reflexes and intact clearance mechanisms in the bronchial tree. Immunologic factors include a sufficient number of normally functioning phagocytic cells and sufficient concentrations of antibody and complement. A deficiency of one or more of these factors can be implicated in most cases of pneumococcal infection.

Suppression of the gag or cough reflex can be induced by alcohol, opiates, or aging. Inflammatory damage to clearance mechanisms in the respiratory tract follows long-term exposure to cigarette smoke or other air pollutants. Cigarette smoking alone accounts for 51% of the attributable risk of invasive pneumococcal disease in nonelderly adults.[94] Crowding in day care centers, prisons, or homeless shelters increases the risk of exposure to both antecedent viral respiratory infections and *S. pneumoniae*. Alcohol ingestion, renal or hepatic insufficiency, glucocorticoid treatment, and diabetes mellitus adversely affect the migration of and/or bacterial killing by polymorphonuclear leukocytes. Splenectomized individuals lose the benefit of

blood clearance mechanisms that function in the absence of anticapsular antibody and are at risk of overwhelming infection. Antibody production is deficient in human immunodeficiency virus (HIV) infection, myeloma, and lymphoma, and may be altogether absent in congenital or acquired hypogammaglobulinemia. The extremes of age are associated with the highest incidence of pneumococcal infection. The susceptibility of infants and young children primarily reflects the initial exposure of an immature immune system to new pathogens. In contrast, the susceptibility of elderly persons is multifactorial and nonimmunologic factors predominate, with chronic cardiopulmonary and other diseases and poor nutrition being among the most important.

A clearer understanding has emerged of the relationships between the various constituents of *S. pneumoniae* and the molecular events that characterize pneumococcal infections.[5,6,9,11] Successful nasopharyngeal colonization occurs with organisms that exhibit transparent, not opaque, colonial morphology.[38,39] The process of phase variation serves to modify cell surface proteins and cell wall structure, exposing CbpA. CbpA appears to function as an adhesin[95] that binds to the polymeric immunoglobulin receptor plgR expressed by human nasopharyngeal epithelial cells.[96]

Once aspirated into the lung, transparent phase variants attach themselves to specific glycoconjugates on type II pneumocytes.[11,97] Adherence occurs in a two-stage process: an initial, rapid phase stimulated by a thrombin-dependent mechanism and a later, more prolonged phase stimulated by the cytokines TNF-α and IL-1. Adherence also involves an interaction between CbpA and the complement component C3 that is expressed on the epithelial cell surface.[98] The cells are then activated, leading to up-regulation of their expression of platelet activating factor (PAF) receptor.[97,99] Choline on teichoic acid serves as a direct ligand with the PAF receptor. Intracellular invasion of activated epithelial cells involves internalization of the pneumococcus into a vacuole in a PAF receptor–dependent process, followed by translocation across the cell and recycling of the PAF receptors.[9,11] The intense inflammatory response to pulmonary infection is mediated by cell wall components, not capsular polysaccharide, and the two most potent are phosphorylcholine-containing C-polysaccharide and teichoic acid. Mixtures of cell wall components and pneumolysin[100] can recreate the characteristic pathologic findings that accompany pneumococcal pneumonia, including the intense edema, complement activation, deposition of fibrin, and hemorrhage (red hepatization). These inflammatory changes are mediated by several cytokines[7] and probably nitric oxide.[101] Left unchecked, the process inevitably leads to bacteremia (opaque phase variants) and death. It can be reversed when leukocytes are recruited to the site of infection. Leukocytes accumulate through a two-step process, one dependent on adhesin molecules (integrin CD18) and the other on a non–CD18-dependent process. Cell wall components, PAF, and C5a contribute to their influx (gray hepatization). Pneumococci are opsonized by serotype-specific immunoglobulins (immunoglobulin G [IgG] and polymeric IgA) and complement and are then bound to the surface of alveolar macrophages, engulfed, and killed in a process classically known as surface phagocytosis.[11,102,103]

In pneumococcal meningitis, organisms can invade either directly from the nasopharynx or through the blood stream.[6,104,105] Transparent, not opaque, phenotypes cross the blood-brain barrier through PAF receptor–mediated endocytosis.[106] Once this is accomplished, pneumococci encounter minimal host resistance because of low CSF levels of immunoglobulins and complement-mediated humoral defense mechanisms. Pneumococcal cell wall components stimulate the release of several proinflammatory cytokines (e.g., TNF-α, IL-1, IL-6), leading to cerebral edema, increased intracranial pressure, impaired autoregulation of cerebral blood flow, ischemic necrosis, and neuronal loss. Matrix metalloproteinases contribute to the breakdown of the blood-brain barrier and to the ingress of leukocytes.[104] Direct neurotoxicity and damage to microvascular endothelial cells is mediated by pneumolysin,[107] nitric acid, and several reactive oxygen species.[104,108] Neuronal damage, commonly affecting the dentate gyrus of the hippocampus, occurs as a result of the release of an apoptosis-inducing factor from mitochondria.[109,110]

The molecular events that occur during pneumococcal infection help explain several of the clinical features of disease. The classical crisis of pneumococcal pneumonia followed by the lysis of fever was commonly seen with antiserum treatment and later with antibiotic treatment. It can now be understood as the consequence of the sudden release of inflammatory cell wall components. Once bacterial replication and lysis are controlled, the inflammatory process abates and fever declines. In overwhelming infection, however, antibiotic treatment can release massive amounts of cell wall components that exacerbate the inflammatory response and lead to death. Until treatments are developed that down-regulate or interrupt this process, the host's ability to respond effectively to vaccination by producing antibody to capsular polysaccharide and perhaps other virulence factors will remain the single best mechanism of protection against pneumococcal disease.

The antibody responses to pneumococcal capsular polysaccharides in very young children are poor,[111] largely because of delayed maturation of specific subsets of B cells.[112] Antibody responses of adults, however, can vary considerably and are subject to genetic factors that are inherited in a co-dominant pattern.[113] Those who possess the G2m(23) allele, an antigenic marker on the heavy chain of the IgG2 idiotype, may have higher antibody levels to some serotype capsular polysaccharides than those who lack this gene. Interactions between Gm and Km allotypes, which are responsible for the γ- and κ-type light chains, are also well known.[114] In addition, differences in the antibody responses between individuals appear to reflect different expression of VH3 genes.[115] Antibody responses within individuals also appear to be governed by a small number of VH genes[116,117] and the antibodies produced are derived from a small number of clones of memory B cells.[117,118]

An important genetic determinant of susceptibility to pneumococcal infection is Fcγ receptor (FcγR) polymorphism. This receptor is found on the surface of polymorphonuclear leukocytes and ligates with the Fc region of IgG2.[119] Leukocytes that are homozygous for the recessive allotype (FcγRIIa-R131) have a reduced ability to phagocytize pneumococci that have been opsonized by type-specific antibody. Patients who are homozygous for this allotype more often experience bacteremia when they have pneumococcal pneumonia than do those who are not.[120] Similar receptor activity has been described for IgA-initiated leukocyte function.[121] It is not known whether genetic factors are responsible for difference in the intrinsic ability of IgG anti–capsular polysaccharide antibodies to opsonize pneumococci in patients with bacteremic compared with non-bacteremic pneumococcal pneumonia.[122] Other proposed genetically related risk factors for invasive pneumococcal disease await confirmation.[123-125]

IgG antibodies to pneumococcal capsular polysaccharides can activate and fix complement through the classical pathway, promoting opsonization and phagocytosis. The Fc receptor of attached immunoglobulin and the presence of complement play critical roles in mediating the protective effect of type-specific antibody. The third component of complement (C3) is the site of convergence of the classical and alternative complement pathways and the source of the opsonically active fragments C3b and iC3b.[72,98] Polymorphonuclear leukocytes possess receptors for each of these fragments, and phagocytosis is initiated through their interaction. In the absence of antibody, complement can be activated via the alternative pathway by peptidoglycan, although capsular polysaccharides may contribute to this reaction. Complement components are not fixed to the bacterial surface, but generate C5a, thereby causing inflammation. This process does not lead to successful opsonization, because Fc components are found at the cell wall and are not recognized by phagocytic cells.

Attempts to explain differences in the virulence of pneumococcal serotypes according to differences in their abilities to fix complement by the alternative pathway have provided inconsistent results.[126] Individual serotypes differ in the amount and site of covalently bound C3b and iC3b. Highly immunogenic and virulent serotypes such as serotype 3 do not inhibit C3b deposition; instead, they alter its proteolytic degradation to fragments, some of which do not function as ligands for phagocytic cell receptors.[127] Some of these fragments (e.g., C3d) appear to interact with receptors on B cells to promote antibody synthesis. Thus complement seems to play a role in regulating antibody production.

The spleen is of critical importance in host defense against pneumococcal bacteremia. In the absence of opsonizing antibody, virulent organisms are cleared from the bloodstream during their slow passage through the sinusoids of Billroth. The spleen also may be involved in regulating the antibody response to capsular polysaccharides.[128] This seems to depend on the structure of the polysaccharide. For example, following splenectomy in mice, other antibody-producing tissues compensate by synthesizing antibodies to some capsular polysaccharides (e.g., serotype 3) but not to others (e.g., serotype 14). This important difference may be due to the tendency of neutral polysaccharides such as serotype 14 to localize to the marginal zone of the spleen, whereas highly acidic polysaccharides such as serotype 3 localize to the red pulp. Pneumococcal capsular polysaccharides that are bound to C3d preferentially localize to the marginal zone and can be found at the surface of CD21+ B cells, the C3d receptors, leading to a rapid immune response.[129] Immaturity of the marginal zone may help explain why infants fail to make antibodies to serotype 14 polysaccharides but respond well to serotype 3.

Diagnosis of Pneumococcal Infections

Pneumococcal infections are diagnosed with certainty when the organism is cultured from blood or a normally sterile extrapulmonary site (e.g., cerebrospinal, pleural, or synovial fluid). Blood cultures that eventually grow *S. pneumoniae* are usually positive within 12 to 14 hours,[130] and commercially available tests for identifying laboratory isolates are reliable.[131] Positive cultures of specimens obtained by transthoracic needle aspiration can often increase the diagnostic yield.[132] Yet if cultures from normally sterile sites are negative, establishing a reliable diagnosis of pneumococcal infection becomes problematic.

The issue of whether microscopic examination or culture of sputum can be used to diagnose nonbacteremic pneumococcal pneumonia has been discussed extensively.[14,133–137] The diagnosis can seldom be questioned when criteria used to interpret a Gram-stained sputum specimen are stringent: 25 or more polymorphonuclear leukocytes and 1 to 2 squamous epithelial cells per low-power field and 5 or more elongated Gram-positive cocci for each white blood cell under oil immersion.[8,135] Sometimes, more liberal criteria are used.[138] Several studies have reaffirmed the value of microscopic examination of a Gram-stained sputum specimen in providing useful information about the cause of community-acquired pneumonia and in guiding the initial choice of antimicrobial therapy.[8,133,138] Unfortunately, many patients with pneumonia, especially those who are elderly, are unable to provide adequate sputum specimens. In one series, only 210 (35%) of 513 hospitalized patients were able to produce a sputum specimen that could be meaningfully interpreted.[138] Moreover, the quality of processing of sputum specimens for Gram's stain and culture by anyone other than trained laboratory staff is variable and often imprecise.[137,139] In the hands of well-trained laboratory staff, however, interpretations of the Gram's stain are usually reliable.[140] The accuracy and utility of the examination can be greatly improved by excluding poor specimens and those obtained from patients previously treated with antibiotics. Nonetheless, it is often difficult for clinicians to interpret individual laboratory reports, and this uncertainty confounds the interpretation of many case series reported in the literature.[135]

Considerable attention has been given to improving the accuracy of diagnosing pneumococcal infections by detecting pneumococcal antigen in sputum, blood, CSF, and urine specimens.[141–145] Most of these newer techniques have not added substantially to the diagnostic utility of classical bacteriologic methods alone. Enzyme immunoassay and enzyme-linked immunosorbent assay (ELISA) tests for C-polysaccharide in sputum have been shown to have good positive predictive values,[146,147] but the results of these and other antigen detection tests are often difficult to interpret because of cross-reactions with the antigens of *viridans* streptococci.[148] The tests may sometimes increase the proportion of patients who are diagnosed as having pneumococcal pneumonia, especially those who have been treated previously with antibiotics and have negative sputum cultures. They may also increase the diagnostic yield of bronchoalveolar lavage[149] and transthoracic needle[150,151] and pleural fluid[152] aspirates.

Latex agglutination has been useful for detecting urinary excretion of type-specific pneumococcal capsular polysaccharides. In one study of 285 patients who had community-acquired pneumonia, the test increased diagnostic yield 2.2-fold.[153] Among 203 patients in this study who were culture negative, the specificity of positive urinary antigen tests was not confounded by nasopharyngeal carriage of *S. pneumoniae*. In 1999, a rapid immunochromatographic test for urinary C-polysaccharide (Binax NOW) became commercially available. In an early study of fewer than 100 patients with community-acquired pneumonia, the test was positive in 82% of those with bacteremic pneumococcal disease and 44% to 78% of those with presumptive pneumococcal pneumonia.[154] Only 6% of those with no microbial diagnosis had a positive test, although many such patients were thought to have pneumococcal infections. No patients without pneumonia were included in this study. In a larger study of 420 pneumonia patients, 120 (30%) had a positive rapid urinary antigen test, including 80% of those with pneumococcal bacteremia and 52% of those with positive sputum cultures.[153] Positive tests for urinary antigen also were obtained in 46 culture-negative pneumonia patients, some of whom may have had pneumococcal pneumonia.[154] The test may not be very specific, however, because it can be positive in persons who have only been colonized with *S. pneumoniae*. Moreover, healthy children who live in settings where nasopharyngeal colonization rates are high often have positive rapid urinary antigen tests.[155,156] These findings suggest that the rapid immunochromatographic test cannot be relied on to diagnose pneumococcal pneumonia.

Pneumococcal antigen also has been sought in the CSF of patients with meningitis.[145,157] Investigators in developing countries have been enthusiastic about these tests because reliable bacteriologic cultures are often unavailable, but antigen tests add little to what can be learned from a properly prepared CSF Gram's stain and culture.[158] In developed countries, nonselective overuse of CSF antigen tests[159] and technical factors such as changes in CSF pH[160] reduce their usefulness. Similarly, the rapid immunochromatographic test for urinary C-polysaccharide has not been shown to be useful for diagnosing cases of pneumococcal meningitis.[161–163]

Diagnostic tests also have been developed that are based on detecting antibodies to pneumolysin in circulating immune complexes.[164–166] In the largest experience to date, Finnish investigators have used this technique to diagnose children with lower respiratory tract infections. In one study, each of three antibody tests was insensitive by itself.[167] In a large study of 350 Filipino children with acute lower respiratory tract infections, tests for immune complexes to capsular polysaccharide and C-polysaccharide were positive in only a few patients.[168] Results in adults indicate that IgG antibodies to pneumolysin in immune complexes cannot be relied on for diagnosing pneumococcal pneumonia.[169,170] Moreover, the serologic methods present formidable technical problems that appear to outweigh their utility.[171]

A promising approach to diagnosing pneumococcal pneumonia has used an ELISA assay to detect increases in antibodies to PsaA.[172] The test had high sensitivity and specificity when patients with pneumococcal pneumonia diagnosed by sterile site culture or urinary antigen detection were compared with controls. Because the test could be used regardless of whether patients had received antibiotic treatment, the diagnostic yield was substantially increased. As yet, there is no information on anti-PsaA antibody responses to nasopharyngeal colonization.

The newest approach to diagnosing pneumococcal infections has been to use PCR techniques.[173] Primers derived from the genes for pneumolysin,[174-178] autolysin (*lytA*),[179,180] and penicillin-binding protein 2B[181,182] have been used in clinical studies. Almost all culture-proven cases of invasive pneumococcal disease also have been identified by PCR.[175,178,179,182-186] PCR testing of specimens obtained by transthoracic needle aspiration has increased the proportion of definitive diagnoses in patients with pneumococcal pneumonia.[151] Similarly promising results have been obtained in PCR studies of CSF specimens taken from patients with meningitis.[183,184,187] Almost all sputum specimens from patients with culture-proven pneumococcal pneumonia[188] and specimens of middle-ear fluid from children with pneumococcal otitis media[189-191] are PCR positive. In one study of sputum specimens, the positive and negative predictive values of the PCR test were 100% and 95%, respectively.[188] Nonetheless, when patients with pneumococcal infections were studied with a full range of diagnostic tests (urinary antigen, serology, and PCR), statistical agreement among the individual tests was poor.[174,192] Moreover, whether a person with a positive PCR assay truly has pneumococcal disease cannot be determined by PCR assay alone. In settings where nasopharyngeal colonization rates are high, PCR assays are often positive in the absence of clinical respiratory disease.[175] In settings where colonization is infrequent, the test is seldom positive, but study populations have been small.[174] PCR assays are still expensive and labor intensive, and they have yet to be modified for routine use. If this could be done, PCR might become most useful in a universal assay designed to detect common pathogens responsible for acute meningitis.[173,193,194]

In spite of considerable efforts to develop and evaluate non–culture-based methods for diagnosing pneumococcal infections, results thus far have been disappointing. Some assays have problems with sensitivity and others with specificity. A non–culture-based test with markedly improved diagnostic sensitivity and specificity remains elusive.

Treatment and Antibiotic Resistance

In many patients with pneumococcal pneumonia, the causative organism is not known at the time treatment is begun.[14] As a result, treatment generally includes antibiotics that are effective against *S. pneumoniae* and other potential pathogens. Unfortunately, the increasing resistance of pneumococci to penicillin and other commonly used antimicrobial agents has made treatment decisions more difficult.

In the late 1960s, isolates of *S. pneumoniae* emerged in Papua New Guinea[195] that were moderately resistant to penicillin at a minimal inhibitory concentration (MIC) of 0.1 or greater to 1.0 μg/mL. A decade later, isolates with greater penicillin resistance and/or resistance to several other antibiotics were reported.[196] Since then, antibiotic-resistant pneumococci have been isolated from patients

with increasing frequency throughout the world. Excellent reviews have been published on the molecular mechanisms underlying antibiotic resistance[197-199] and the laboratory diagnosis,[200] epidemiology,[200-205] and management[206-209] of infections caused by resistant pneumococci.

Isolates of *S. pneumoniae* are considered intermediately resistant to penicillin if the MIC is between 0.1 and 1 μg/mL. High-level resistance is present if the MIC is 2 μg/mL or greater. Some laboratories still screen pneumococcal isolates for penicillin resistance using oxacillin-containing disks, whereas others go directly to microbroth dilution or the E-test.[14,200] Once resistant strains have been identified, other techniques can be used to define their molecular determinants, including multilocus enzyme analysis and PFGE of the macrorestriction pattern of chromosomal DNA.[210-213] Amplified fragments of DNA can be further analyzed by restriction fragment end-labeling, ribotyping, and BOX fingerprinting.

Enzymes that are essential for replication of *S. pneumoniae* have an affinity for penicillin and are called penicillin-binding proteins (PBPs). Resistance to penicillin and other β-lactam antibiotics is due to alterations in one or more PBPs (1a, 1b, 2x, 2a, 2b, and 3) that reduce their affinity for the antibiotic.[197,199,214] In highly resistant strains, up to five PBPs can be affected. The modified genes encoding each of these PBPs have acquired new DNA sequences from heterologous DNA donors, many of which appear to be *viridans* streptococci. Because these changes occur as independent events, the resultant PBP patterns exhibit a wide degree of variation, and each resistant isolate, with its "mosaic" of altered PBP genes, represents a distinct clone. This mosaic of penicillin-resistant PBP genes can spread "horizontally" to other pneumococcal strains. Individual penicillin-resistant strains characterized by unique PBP patterns also can share other characteristics such as resistance to other antibiotics and rates of autolysis. Clonal expansion allows resistant strains to become established in populations and to spread to distant geographic sites.[205]

Once penicillin resistance is acquired, the level of resistance can increase by point mutation. External pressure from antibiotic overuse and the unique resistance-selecting capacity of different β-lactam antibiotics may account for some of these changes. Resistance to some β-lactam antibiotics, including third-generation cephalosporins, can be acquired more rapidly than penicillin resistance, most likely because no more than two genetic determinants are involved. Penicillin-resistant pneumococci also can acquire new and different capsular serotypes, again through genetic transformation.[215-217]

Acquired resistance to other antimicrobial agents is not due to changes in PBPs, but to other factors.[197,198] The mechanisms and clinical significance of resistance to macrolides,[198,218,219] fluroquinolones[198,220,221] and tetracyclines, chloramphenicol, and other antibiotics[197,198] are reviewed elsewhere.

Bactericidal antibiotics act by inhibiting cell wall biosyntheses, but cell death requires the activation of the autolysin (*lytA*). Certain strains of *S. pneumoniae* have been identified, however, that stop growing in the presence of an antibiotic but do not die. Growth resumes once treatment stops. Vancomyin tolerance has been described in a few clinical isolates of *S. pneumoniae*.[222,223] A mutation in the

VncS gene, part of a two-component signal transduction system that regulates cell death, appears to be responsible.

In the United States, an increasing proportion of invasive isolates of S. pneumoniae are resistant to penicillin and other antibiotics.[201,224-226] In one study, more than 75% of recent penicillin-resistant isolates were included in the 12 most prevalent PFGE types.[227] Multidrug resistance was identified in virtually all of the isolates of 9 of these 12 clones, and 5 were closely related to clones circulating in other parts of the world. Thus the growth in antibiotic resistance of S. pneumoniae has been due largely to increased circulation of a few multidrug-resistant clones. Serotypes included in 23-valent pneumococcal vaccine accounted for 88% of these isolates.[201]

In other parts of the world, antibiotic resistance also has continued to increase.[200,202,203,225,228-231] Variations in resistance also have been observed according to season and age group as well as serotype.[232] Higher rates of penicillin resistance have been associated with higher rates of β-lactam consumption,[233-235] and similar relationships have been observed for the macrolides[234,235] and fluoroquinolones.[236,237] These findings appear to contradict other evidence that increasing resistance is due to widespread circulation of a limited number of multidrug-resistant clones. Mathematical models have helped to reconcile these different observations.[205,234,235,238-240]

The treatment of pneumococcal infections caused by antibiotic-resistant strains has been widely discussed.[14,206-209,225,241-244] In adults with community-acquired pneumococcal pneumonia, there is probably no difference in the response to treatment of most cases caused by strains that are resistant to penicillins and cephalosporins compared with those that are sensitive.[241,245-248] However, in one retrospective study of patients with bacteremic pneumococcal pneumonia who died 4 or more days after treatment had begun, those infected with strains with high-level resistance to penicillin or cefuroxime had a three- and sevenfold increased risk of death, respectively (Table 22-2).[249] Fortunately, they accounted for a very small proportion of all study patients.

Several expert groups have published guidelines for the management of adults with community-acquired pneumonia.[242,250-252] The Centers for Disease Control and Prevention (CDC) guidelines assume clinicians already know the identity and antibiotic sensitivity of the infecting organism.[242] Recognizing that this information is seldom available, the Infectious Diseases Society of America[250] and the Canadian Infectious Disease Society[251] recommend that outpatients with pneumonia be treated with one of several agents that will be effective against S. pneumoniae and other organisms that might be involved. Treatment of inpatient pneumococcal pneumonia usually requires intravenous penicillin or ceftriaxone in all but those with very high-level resistance. Quinolones are becoming more commonly used, but vancomycin should be reserved for patients who are allergic to β-lactams. For pneumococcal meningitis, higher doses of penicillin or ceftriaxone usually suffice for those infected with penicillin-sensitive strains.

Children treated for pneumococcal bacteremia and/or pneumonia have similar outcomes, regardless of the antibiotic sensitivity of the infecting organism, although there are occasional exceptions.[253,254] Children with meningitis caused by resistant S. pneumoniae, however, present a more serious therapeutic challenge. Even high doses of penicillin and other β-lactam antibiotics may not adequately penetrate into the CSF, and treatment failures occur.[255,256] Because the causative organisms also may be resistant to other antibiotics, combination therapy with ceftriaxone and vancomycin has become common in the initial treatment of childhood meningitis.[256]

Infection with antibiotic-resistant pneumococci in children less than 2 years of age has added to the urgency of developing more effective pneumococcal vaccines for this age group. Yet resistant strains account for an increasing proportion of pneumococcal infections in older individuals, and the overall burden of disease caused by these strains is probably greater in older persons than it is in young children. Concern about antibiotic resistance is clearly an important factor underlying renewed interest in pneumococcal polysaccharide vaccine.

TABLE 22-2 ■ Mortality from Bacteremic Pneumococcal Pneumonia, 1995–1997: Effects of Antibiotic Resistance, Age, and Underlying Conditions

Risk Factor	Number of Patients	Characteristic	Adjusted Odds Ratio*	% of All Patients
Penicillin resistance, death ≥ 4 days	1151	MIC < 0.12 μg/mL	—	88
		MIC ≥ 4.0 μg/mL	7.1[†]	1.7
Cefotaxime resistance, death ≥ 4 days	1134	MIC < 1.0 μg/mL	—	96
		MIC ≥ 2.0 μg/mL	5.9[†]	1.4
Age	2376	<17 yr	—	7
		18–64 yr	5.1	50
		65–74 yr	5.8	16
		≥75 yr	12.0	27
Underlying condition(s)	2376	Absent	—	38
		Present	2.8	62

*Compared with the reference groups, all odds ratios were statistically significant (95% confidence intervals excluded 1.0).
[†]Odds ratios were adjusted for age, race, location, and underlying conditions.
MIC, minimal inhibitory concentration.
Adapted from Feikin DR, Schuchat A, Kolczak M, et al. Mortality from invasive pneumococcal pneumonia in the era of antibiotic resistance, 1995–1997. Am J Public Health 90:223–229, 2000.

Epidemiology of Pneumococcal Infections

The Carrier State

Virtually all pneumococcal infections occur in persons who are asymptomatic nasopharyngeal carriers of S. pneumoniae. Thus it is not surprising that the greater incidence of pneumococcal infections in young children compared with adults is paralleled by higher carrier rates. Studies conducted in the 1970s showed carrier rates of 38% to 60% in preschool children, 29% to 35% in primary school children, and 9% to 25% in middle school students.[257] Carrier rates were lower among adults: 18% to 29% in those with children at home, but only 6% in those without children at home. In a study of 300 elderly residents of a long-term care institution, 6% were nasopharyngeal carriers.[258]

After the disappearance of maternal antibodies, infants 5 to 6 months of age or older generally lack antibodies to pneumococcal capsular polysaccharides. Once nasopharyngeal colonization occurs, either alone or in association with an infection such as otitis media,[259,260] they acquire type-specific antibodies.[261–263] Season of the year and concomitant viral upper respiratory tract infection can affect the acquisition of carriage. Close contact with others, either in or outside the household, is essential. A good example of this is a household study that was conducted in Finland, where families are small and day care uncommon.[264] During a 2-year period, 34 (37%) of 92 families had more than one carrier, and in 85% of this group the same serotype was shared by two or more individuals. In day care centers, rates of colonization are very high[265–268]; antibiotic-resistant strains predominate, often because of recent antibiotic treatment[14,265,268–271]; and the clonal spread of a few strains is common.[265–267,272–274]

Most adults also lack antibodies to most pneumococcal serotypes, but specific antibodies appear after colonization.[275] In an outbreak of pneumococcal pneumonia among military recruits that was due to serotype 1, serum antibody was detected in only 4% of unexposed controls but was found in 28% of the asymptomatic contacts of those who were infected. In a second pneumonia outbreak caused by serotypes 7F and 8, 36% of colonized subjects initially had antibody to one or both serotypes, and an additional 31%

developed such antibody in the ensuing month in the absence of recognized local or systemic disease.

The relationship between the acquisition of nasopharyngeal carriage of individual serotypes and their likelihood to cause invasive disease is not well understood.[276] Some serotypes (e.g., types 6, 14, 19, and 23) are acquired frequently and carried for extended periods, whereas others (e.g., types 3 and 12) are acquired infrequently and are rapidly eliminated. A longitudinal study of the acquisition and duration of nasopharyngeal carriage among children in Papua New Guinea showed that serotypes regarded as more immunogenic (e.g., types 3, 7, and 9) were less frequently acquired than were less immunogenic (e.g., types 6, 19, and 23) serotypes, and they were also carried for shorter periods of time.[276] No relationship was found, however, between the immunogenicity of the individual serotypes and their invasiveness.

Pneumococcal Infections in Adults

Pneumonia is the most frequently recognized pneumococcal infection of adults. Studies conducted during the preantibiotic era showed that about 20% of cases were associated with positive blood cultures.[1] Bacteremic pneumococcal pneumonia is by far the most common form of invasive pneumococcal disease, accounting for approximately 90% or more of all cases (Fig. 22–2). Pneumococcal meningitis, with or without accompanying bacteremia, is the next most common form of invasive disease, while other types of invasive disease occur infrequently. Acute bacterial sinusitis caused by S. pneumoniae may be common, but it is rarely diagnosed with certainty.

The terms pneumococcal pneumonia and pneumococcal bacteremia (or invasive pneumococcal disease) are often used in ways that suggest the two conditions are mutually exclusive. This is not so; there is considerable overlap between the two.[277] Recognizing this overlap is essential for understanding the epidemiology of pneumococcal infections in adults and for interpreting studies of the efficacy of pneumococcal vaccine and the effectiveness of vaccination.

Pneumococcal Pneumonia

Streptococcus pneumoniae is the major bacterial cause of adult community-acquired pneumonia requiring hospital

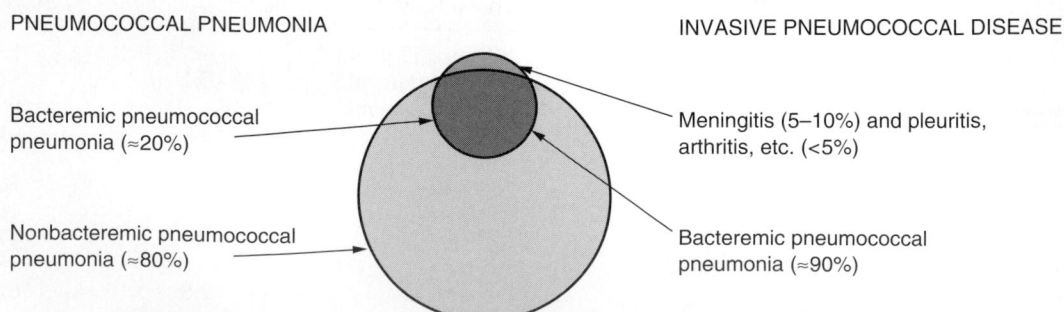

FIGURE 22–2 ▪ The overlap between pneumococcal pneumonia (large circle) and invasive pneumococcal disease (small circle). Bacteremic pneumococcal pneumonia accounts for approximately 20% of all cases of pneumococcal pneumonia that are hospitalized. Among patients with pneumococcal pneumonia who are managed as outpatients, the proportion with bacteremic disease is not well known. (Adapted from Fedson DS. Pneumococcal vaccination for older adults—the first 20 years. Drugs Aging 15(suppl 1):21–30, 1999.)

admission. Several excellent reviews of community-acquired pneumonia[278-282] and pneumococcal pneumonia[8,10,283-285] have been published. Clinical research on pneumonia in the United States has often focused on defining prognostic factors that can be used as criteria for intensive care unit admission or for outpatient rather than inpatient treatment.[286,287] Yet, in the United States and more so in other countries, considerable attention also has been given to accurately determining the annual incidence of community-acquired pneumonia and the proportion of all pneumonia cases caused by S. pneumoniae.

A comprehensive study of all cases of community-acquired pneumonia was conducted in Finland in the early 1980s.[288] The overall incidence (both outpatient and inpatient) was 11.6 cases per 1000 persons per year. Men had higher incidence and mortality rates than women. Among all cases, 31% were 60 years of age or older, and the incidence in this group was 20 cases per 1000. Among elderly patients, 67% were admitted to the hospital and the case-fatality rate was 11%. Surprisingly, 54% of elderly patients were free of major underlying medical conditions that are associated with an increased risk for pneumonia. In younger adults 15 to 59 years in age, the incidence was 6 cases per 1000 and the case-fatality rate 0.6%.

In the United States, a study conducted in Franklin County, Ohio, reported that, in 1991, rates of hospitalization for community-acquired pneumonia were 2.8 and 10.1 per 1000 persons ages 45 to 64 years and 65 years or older, respectively.[289] Rates were higher in blacks than in whites, and overall mortality was 4.6% and 12.5% in persons less than 65 years and 65 years of age or greater, respectively. More recently, a national study of hospitalization for community-acquired pneumonia in persons 65 years of age or older reported an incidence of 18.3 per 1000 and a case-fatality rate of 10.6%.[290] The nationwide costs of treating these patients were estimated to be $4.4 billion, 6.3% of all expenditures on hospital care for the elderly. Almost 50% of these costs were incurred in intensive care units. In the United Kingdom, similar hospital care costs for community-acquired pneumonia have been reported.[291]

The clinical and laboratory features and the prognoses for cases of community-acquired pneumonia caused by different microorganisms show considerable overlap, and consequently the causative agent cannot be reliably predicted in more than half of cases.[292] Previous reviews of community-acquired pneumonia indicated that approximately 30% to 50% of all cases requiring hospitalization were caused by S. pneumoniae.[293,294] In almost all studies, S. pneumoniae ranked first among all known causes. Several prospective studies of community-acquired pneumonia have been reported since the earlier reviews that provide further insight into the incidence of pneumococcal pneumonia (Table 22–3).[151,287,289,295-325] In almost all reports, a definitive diagnosis of pneumococcal pneumonia was based on positive blood cultures or, in a few instances, cultures of pleural fluid or transthoracic needle aspirates. In many studies, however, blood cultures were not obtained in many patients. Even in studies in which almost all patients were cultured, a substantial proportion had been treated with antibiotics before blood cultures were obtained, making it unlikely the cultures would be positive. Nonetheless, in spite of these limitations, in 10 studies in which blood cultures were obtained in more than two thirds of patients (and in which 14% to 39% of all pneumonia patients had been treated with antibiotics before hospitalization), blood cultures were positive for S. pneumoniae in 4.6% to 8.0% of patients.[287,289,295,296,299,303,305,312,319,324a,325] In two additional studies, cultures of transthoracic needle aspirates or urinary antigen detection also were used in large proportions of study subjects, many of whom had previously received antibiotics.[302,305] Definitive pneumococcal pneumonia was diagnosed in 12% and 15% of all pneumonia patients, respectively.

These findings have a direct bearing on determining the proportion of all community-acquired pneumonias that are caused by S. pneumoniae. Earlier studies indicated that approximately 20% of all cases of pneumococcal pneumonia were accompanied by bacteremia.[1,326] If these findings are accepted, at least 25% to 30% of all pneumonias can be assumed to be due to S. pneumoniae. Given the underdiagnosis of pneumococcal bacteremia in all pneumonia studies, it is reasonable to conclude that pneumococcal pneumonia still accounts for at least 30% to 50% of all cases of community-acquired pneumonia admitted to the hospital. It follows that, if the incidence of community-acquired pneumonia in elderly persons in the United States in 1997 was 18.3 cases per 1000, the incidence of pneumococcal pneumonia was probably 5.5 to 9.2 cases per 1000 elderly persons, and the annual cost of hospital care for pneumococcal pneumonia alone was on the order of $1.3 to $2.2 billion.[290]

In the absence of more precise methods for diagnosing cases of nonbacteremic pneumococcal pneumonia, better estimates of the overall incidence of pneumococcal pneumonia could be obtained if more attention were paid to accurately documenting the proportion of all pneumonia patients who have pneumococcal bacteremia. This will require studies in which blood cultures are obtained from all patients and the investigators know which patients who were cultured were previously treated with antibiotics (Table 22–4). To date, no published report on community-acquired pneumonia has included this information.

S. pneumoniae is an underappreciated cause of nosocomial pneumonia on hospitals wards and pneumonia in intensive care units (see Table 22–3).[327-329] Patients are usually elderly and often immunocompromised, and outbreaks are sometimes due to antibiotic-resistant organisms.[327,330] Pneumonia occurs with much greater frequency among residents of nursing homes and long-term care institutions than it does in those who live in the community, often accounting for 10% to 15% of all pneumonia hospitalizations.[331-333] S. pneumoniae is the organism most frequently responsible, antibiotic resistance is frequent, and case-fatality rates can be very high.[332,334-337] S. pneumoniae also is the most common bacterial cause of nonsevere community-acquired pneumonia that does not require hospital admission (see Table 22–3).[315,319,324] Focal outbreaks of pneumococcal pneumonia can occur in any setting where there is severe crowding and poor ventilation.[338]

The generally accepted mortality rate for community-acquired pneumonia is 5% to 10% in persons of all ages and 10% to 30% in persons 65 years of age or older (see Table 22–3). Reported mortality rates for pneumococcal bacteremia range from 5% to 36% in all adults and from 18% to 51% in the elderly (see below). Most of these patients die

TABLE 22–3 ■ Adult Community-Acquired Pneumococcal Pneumonia

Country, Location	Year(s) of Study	Total No. of Cases	Mean/ Median Age (yr)	Site of Care			Diagnostic	
				Out-patient (%)	Hospital (%)	(% ICU)	Blood Culture (%)	Previous Antibiotics (%)
United States								
Ohio	1991	2776	—§	—	100	(—)	76	20
Seattle	1994–96	522	~45	0	100	(18)	82	14
US, Canada								
3 cities	1991–94	1343	—	41	59	(13)	71	—
France								
Amiens	1991–95	53	56	0	100	(0)	—	43
Clermont-Fd	1998–99	215	67	0	100	(6)	83	37
Spain								
Balearas	1992–94	91	51	74	26	(—)	—	21
Lleida	1993–94	109	51	0	100	(—)	100	43
Barcelona	1994–96	392	54	13	87	(10)	98	25
Girona	1995	198	55	—	—	(—)	93	—
La Coruña	18 months	366	60	0	100	(7)	100	19
Barcelona	1995–97	533	64	0	100	(8)	97	27
Barcelona	1996–97	395	68	0	100	(16)	66	16
Barcelona	1993–95	241	53	39	61	(9)	67	—
Italy								
Rimini	1991–94	210	27	—	—	(—)	57	26
25 centers	1994–96	613	56	10	90	(1)	33	24
United Kingdom								
Nottingham	1998–99	267	65	0	100	(6)	84	39
Finland								
Kuopio	1981–82	304	49	56	44	(—)	3	—
8 countries								
124 centers	1990–92	808	~54	—	—	(—)	—	2
N. Zealand								
Christchurch	1999–00	474¶	64	0	100	(3)	94	27
Japan								
Kurashiki	1994–97	326	65	10	90	(—)	86	38
Kawasaki	1998–00	84	> 65	0	100	(—)	—	39
Malaysia								
K. Lumpur	1997–99	127	55	0	100	(—)	—	21
Penang	1999–00	98	56	0	100	(—)	—	8
Argentina								
Buenos Aires	1997–98	346	64	25	75	(11)	100	34
Slovenia								
Ljubljana	1996–97	211	57	0	100	(—)	92	28
Kenya								
Kilifi	1994–96	281	~30	0	100	(—)	100	54
14 countries	1998–99	383	56	0	100	(—)	100	0
United States								
Buffalo	1996–99	104	82	0	100	(100)	89	23
France								
Tourcoing	1987–95	505¶	63	0	100	(100)	~100	15
Spain								
Barcelona	1996–98	89	65	0	100	(100)	~100	17
N. Zealand								
Wellington	1997–98	32	59	0	100	(100)	100	25
Canada								
Halifax	1991–94	149	41	95	5	(0)	2	44
Switzerland								
Neuchatel	4 yr	170	43	92	—	(0)	~100	5
Spain								
Lleida	1997–99	247	50	100	0	(0)	96	34

*"Enhanced" diagnostic studies included one or more of the following: transthoracic needle aspiration (TNA), protected brush bronchoalveolar lavage, sputum antigen, urinary antigen, serum antigen, serum antibody, or serum polymerase chain reaction studies specific for S. pneumoniae.
†Isolation of S. pneumoniae from blood, pleural fluid, or TNA.
‡Includes diagnoses based on sputum culture ± Gram's stain and "positive enhanced studies."
§Indicates no information provided in the report.
¶Retrospective study. All other reports were prospective studies.

| Studies | | Cases of Pneumococcal Pneumonia | | | | | Unknown Cause | | |
"Enhanced" Studies*	CAP Case Fatality Rate (%)‖	Definitive†	Presumptive‡	Total No.	Total (%)	Rank	No.	(%)	Ref.
No	9	154	197	351	(13)	2	1545	(56)	289
No	5	29	25	54	(10)	1	229	(44)	295
No	11	63	59	122	(9)	1	942	(70)	287,297
Yes	—	4	9	13	(25)	1	21	(40)	298
No	7	17	1	18	(8)	1	160	(74)	296
Yes	—	3	6	9	(10)	2	43	(47)	300
Yes	—	27	0	27	(25)	1	19	(17)	151
Yes	7	68	26	94	(24)	1	164	(42)	302
Yes	3	—	—	36	(18)	1	119	(60)	304
Yes	7	17	9	26	(7)	2	267	(73)	299
Yes	10	82	53	135	(25)	1	250	(47)	305
Yes	5	30	35	65	(16)	1	213	(54)	303
Yes	5	6	21	27	(11)	1	128	(53)	301
—	2	13	25	38	(18)	1	95	(45)	306
Yes	2	4	32	36	(6)	1	429	(70)	307
Yes	15	9	120	129	(48)	1	68	(25)	309
Yes	6	0	125	125	(41)‖	1	121	(40)	310
Yes	4	46	122	168	(21)	1	489	(60)	311
No	4	22	45	67	(14)	1	277	(58)	312
Yes	6	7	68	75	(23)	1	127	(39)	308
No	9	—	—	11	(13)	1	44	(52)	314
No	10	4	3	7	(6)	2	74	(58)	313
Yes	9	1	2	3	(3)	5	56	(57)	320
No	18	10	25	35	(10)	1	199	(58)	317
No	8	12	0	12	(6)	1	—	—	325
Yes	10	74	55	129	(46)	1	101	(36)	322
No	1	24	84	108	(28)	1	78	(46)	324a
Yes	55	≥6	≤6	12	(12)	2	49	(47)	318
Yes	28	40	97	137	(27)	1	196	(39)	316
Yes	26	≥13	≤8	21	(24)	1	42	(47)	323
Yes	31	3	3	3	(19)	1	19	(60)	321
No	0	—	1	1	(1)	—	72	(48)	315
Yes	1	6	28	34	(20)	1	78	(46)	319
Yes	—	≥11	58	69	(28)	1	85	(34)	324

‖ Indicates community–acquired pneumonia.

TABLE 22-4 ■ Obtaining Blood Cultures Before Antibiotic Treatment in Patients Hospitalized with Community-Acquired Pneumonia

Blood Culture Obtained (%)	Previous Antibiotic Treatment (%)		
	Yes	No	Total
Yes	13	35	48
No	23	29	52
Total	36	64	100

The study of 119 patients was conducted in the Tameside General Hospital, United Kingdom, 1993 to 1994. Only 35% of pneumonia patients were cultured before antibiotic treatment was begun. (P. McDonald, unpublished observations.)

within the first week of illness. The overall mortality rate for pneumococcal pneumonia, however, is not known with accuracy, largely because the diagnosis of nonbacteremic cases remains elusive. Yet nonbacteremic pneumococcal pneumonia is a serious disease; when defined by stringent criteria (including no previous antibiotic treatment), it has a 30-day mortality of 13%, a rate two thirds that of bacteremic cases.[8]

Invasive Pneumococcal Disease

Invasive pneumococcal disease is any infection in which *S. pneumoniae* is isolated from the blood or another normally sterile site.[14] Among all bacteremic infections in hospitalized patients, *S. pneumoniae* accounts for 4% to 12% of cases,[339–343] and, among all patients hospitalized with community-acquired pneumonia, approximately 5% to 10% will have pneumococcal bacteremia (see Table 22–3). In adults, invasive disease is more common in winter than in summer months and its occurrence is highly correlated with virus infections, lower temperatures, and air pollution.[344] It is also more common in men than in women and in persons with lower incomes and less education. Infection with antibiotic-resistant organisms, however, is more likely to occur in persons with higher incomes.[345]

Most hospital-based reports of invasive pneumococcal disease include all cases of pneumococcal bacteremia,[346–358] although some reports focus on bacteremic pneumococcal pneumonia[246,249,359–364] or pneumococcal meningitis.[365–368] Among all cases of pneumococcal bacteremia, anywhere from 70% to 98% are associated with pneumococcal pneumonia[343,346,348–351,353,357,362,368a] (although the usual rate is ~90%) and 5% to 10% with pneumococcal meningitis (see Fig. 22–2).[8,349,353,355,357,368a,369] Other clinical syndromes such as endocarditis,[370,370a,371] arthritis,[372,373] and intra-abdominal infection[374,375] are far less common. More than 90 unusual and infrequent manifestations of pneumococcal infection have been described.[376] Postsplenectomy patients account for only 1% to 2% of bacteremic patients,[77,348,349,353,355] and nosocomial infection for approximately 5% to 10% of cases,[343,346–348,351,360] in most series. Recurrent pneumococcal bacteremia caused by the same or a different serotype is usually a sign of underlying immunocompromise[377–380] or complement deficiency.[381] HIV infection has been noted in 20% to 30% or more of bacteremic patients in reports from institutions that see large numbers of such patients.[246,353,363,368a] Surprisingly, 7% to 16% of

adults with pneumococcal bacteremia have had no identified source of infection.[346,348,350,353,357] In addition, approximately 20% to 30% of patients have had no identifiable underlying high-risk medical condition,[350,353] although in many of them the conditions were probably overlooked. In one study, every patient had one or more of the conditions known to be associated with pneumococcal pneumonia.[8]

Mortality rates in case series of invasive disease or pneumococcal bacteremia have ranged widely: 5% to 36% in all adults [8,22,246,249,341,343,346–349,352,353,356,359,362–364] and 18% to 51% in persons greater than or equal to 65 years of age or greater than or equal to 70 years of age.[249,346,348–351,353,357,368a] The low mortality rates reported from Stockholm and Halifax[355,359] were unusual and may have been due to the unequal circulation of certain clones or serotypes in different communities.[245] In most case series, mortality rates have generally been 12% to 25%. In pneumococcal meningitis, case-fatality rates of 20% to 40% have been the rule.[355,365–368,382,383] In case series that have reported the serotypes of isolates, 90% or more have been vaccine-type organisms.[8,349,353,365]

Reports of laboratory-based surveillance of defined populations provide a better indication than case series of the burden of invasive pneumococcal disease. In the United States during the 1980s, the annual incidence of pneumococcal bacteremia or invasive pneumococcal disease in adults was reported to be 9 to 19 cases per 100,000 persons (Table 22–5).[384–387] In persons 65 years of age or older, the incidence was 22 to 57 cases per 100,000 persons. Subsequent studies from Franklin County, Ohio,[388] Atlanta, Georgia,[389] and Dallas, Texas[390] reported rates of 19 to 30 cases per 100,000 adults of all ages and 80 to 85 cases per 100,000 elderly persons. Lower rates were reported from several other sites.[391–395,397] In 1998, the Acute Bacterial Core (ABC) Surveillance study estimated a national incidence of 23 cases per 100,000 in all persons and 60 cases per 100,000 in elderly persons.[396] No association was found between the proportion of multidrug-resistant invasive isolates and the incidence of invasive disease in adults.[396a]

Several reports have provided estimates of the incidence of invasive pneumococcal disease in Canada,[228,398] nine countries in western Europe,[339,357,399–414] Israel,[415] Australia,[416–418] and New Zealand[369] (see Table 22–5). In several countries, invasive disease rates have been similar to the higher rates observed in many areas in the United States. In other countries, the rates have been much lower.

Substantial geographic variations have been reported in rates of invasive pneumococcal disease between different areas of the United States[396] and between different countries in western Europe and elsewhere (see Table 22–5). Because approximately 90% of patients with invasive pneumococcal disease have bacteremic pneumococcal pneumonia, variation in the frequency with which blood cultures are obtained in pneumonia patients probably explains most of these differences. In Finland in the 1980s, for example, blood cultures were obtained in very few patients with community-acquired pneumonia[310] and reported rates for invasive disease were low.[412] In contrast, in Franklin County, Ohio, a few years later, 76% of all patients hospitalized with pneumonia were cultured[289] and rates for pneumococcal bacteremia were high.[388] Furthermore, large variations in rates of invasive disease have been observed between different regions of the same country in the same year (Fig. 22–3) (Å. Örtqvist, personal communication, 2002).[401,419] Some of the differences between regions in these countries might reflect differences in population density, but it is unlikely that variations this large have been due solely to the epidemiologic behavior of S. pneumoniae. Moreover, even in regions where blood cultures have been obtained in most pneumonia patients, cultures are unlikely to have been positive in patients who had already been treated with antibiotics. In a revealing study conducted in Manchester, England; Stockholm, Sweden; Barcelona, Spain; and Huntington, WV, 67% of pneumonia patients in Manchester had a blood culture but 42% had previously received antibiotics.[355] In Stockholm, only 21% of patients

TABLE 22–5 ▪ Incidence of Invasive Pneumococcal Disease in Developed Countries

Country, Location	Year(s)	Number of Cases	Annual Incidence per 100,000 People		Mortality (%)		Serogroup/ Serotype Coverage by 23-Valent Vaccine (%)	Reference
			All Ages	Older Than 65 Years	All Ages	Older Than 65 Years		
United States								
Hawaii	1986–87	220*	9†	22	16	35	—‡	384
Oklahoma City, OK	1990	144	17	42	15	—	86	385
Charleston, SC	1986–87	110*	19	53	18	44	—	386
Monroe County, NY	1985–89	671*	19	57	15	29	—	387
Southern California	1992–95	814	13	32	8	16	—	391
Franklin County, OH	1991–93	419*	19§	83	19	26	92	388
Atlanta, GA	1994	712	30	85	—	—	—	389
Dallas County, TX	1995	432	22	80	16	30	—	390
Huntington, WV	1993–97	—	—	45‖	—	16 (≥50)	—	392
San Francisco, CA	1994–96	500	34	48	12	24	—	397
Baltimore, MD								
White	1995–96	615	18	—	—	—	—	393
Black		766	59	—	—	—	—	
Rhode Island	1998–99	413	21	—	10	—	—	394
Alaska, non-native	1991–98	672	16	—	—	—	92	395
ABC surveillance	1998	—	23	60	—	—	86 (≥65 yr)	396
Canada								
Toronto	1995	470	15	63	19	28	94	398
Quebec	1996–98	3650	17	—	7	11	90	228
United Kingdom								
England & Wales	1993–95	11,028	7	24		—	97	399
England & Wales	1995–97	10,535	7	21	—	—	—	400
Oxford	1995–97	1288	10	36	—	—	—	400
South & West England	1995	668	10	45 (≥75)	—	—	—	401
Aberdeen	1993–95	104	10	—	24	43	94	402
France								
National	1996	4991	9	31	—	—	—	403
Puy de Dôme	1994–98	214	7	18	25	28	—	404
Netherlands								
6 sites	1992	—	8	24	—	—	—	405
	1996	—	15	63	—	—	—	405
	1998	—	9	39	—	—	—	405
Utrecht	1993–95	177*	10	—	24	31	—	406
Belgium								
Flemish Brabant	1995–97	—	—	36	—	—	—	407
Denmark								
National	1992	821	16	—	—	—	~90	408
	1996	1410	27	—	—	—	—	414
	1999	877	17	64	—	—	—	409, 414
Sweden								
Stockholm County	1993–95	—	—	34	—	12	—	407
National	1995	—	15	41	—	—	—	410
Lünd	1996	64*	15	—	—	33	96	339
Göteborg	1981–95	904	10	27 (≥60)	15	19	—	411
Norway								
National	1996	885	21	62	—	—	90	419
Finland								
3 areas	1983–92	1045	9§	27	—	—	95	412

Continued

TABLE 22–5 ■ Incidence of Invasive Pneumococcal Disease in Developed Countries—cont'd

Country, Location	Year(s)	Number of Cases	Annual Incidence per 100,000 People		Mortality (%)		Serogroup/ Serotype Coverage by 23-Valent Vaccine (%)	Reference
			All Ages	Older Than 65 Years	All Ages	Older Than 65 Years		
Spain								
Valencia	1995	274	—	57	—	—	—	407
Barcelona	1988–99	321	10	32	18	24	—	413
Israel								
National	1994–96	603*	15§	55	28	36	94	415
Australia								
Victoria	1995–98	~1200	8	25	12	23	91	416
New South Wales	1997–99	1270	14	—	20 (≥15)	28	~90	417
Northern Territory, nonindigenous	1994–98	425	15	63	10	—	90	418
New Zealand								
Auckland	1998–00	96*	9	—	18	—	>90	369

*Pneumococcal bacteremia only.
†Reported rates have been rounded to the nearest whole number.
‡Indicates no data available.
§Persons older than 16 to 18 years.
‖Bacteremic pneumococcal pneumonia.

had received antibiotics, but only 38% were cultured. In both Barcelona and Huntington, 72% of patients were cultured, but in Barcelona 36% of patients had been given antibiotics before cultures were obtained, whereas in Huntington only 16% had been previously treated. Higher rates for positive blood cultures have been reported in patients who have not previously been given antibiotics compared with those who have.[298,303,309,312,388] Thus previous antibiotic treatment has a direct bearing on ascertaining the true incidence of invasive disease. If reports on disease incidence were accompanied by information on the proportion of pneumonia patients who had blood cultures before antibiotics were given (see Table 22–4), interpreting reported rates for disease incidence would be less difficult. It is reasonable to conclude that all reported rates of invasive disease are underestimates. Given the information in Table 22–5, the true rates of invasive disease are probably at least

approximately 15 to 20 cases per 100,000 people of all ages and approximately 50 per 100,000 in those 65 years of age and older.[13]

Several investigators believe that increasing rates of invasive pneumococcal disease observed in Sweden,[339,411,420–422] Norway,[419] Finland,[423] Denmark,[424] the Netherlands,[405] and the United Kingdom[425] during the 1990s represented a true increase in disease occurrence rather than improved case ascertainment. It is clear that increasing disease rates were not due to changes in the age or sex of patients, the emergence of antimicrobial resistance among S. pneumoniae, or changes in the use of pneumococcal vaccine. It is also likely that more accurate blood culturing techniques could not have accounted for more than a small proportion of the increase. In Sweden, investigators have argued that the increase was due to a sevenfold increase in the number of serotype 14 isolates.[422] In the United Kingdom, Finland,

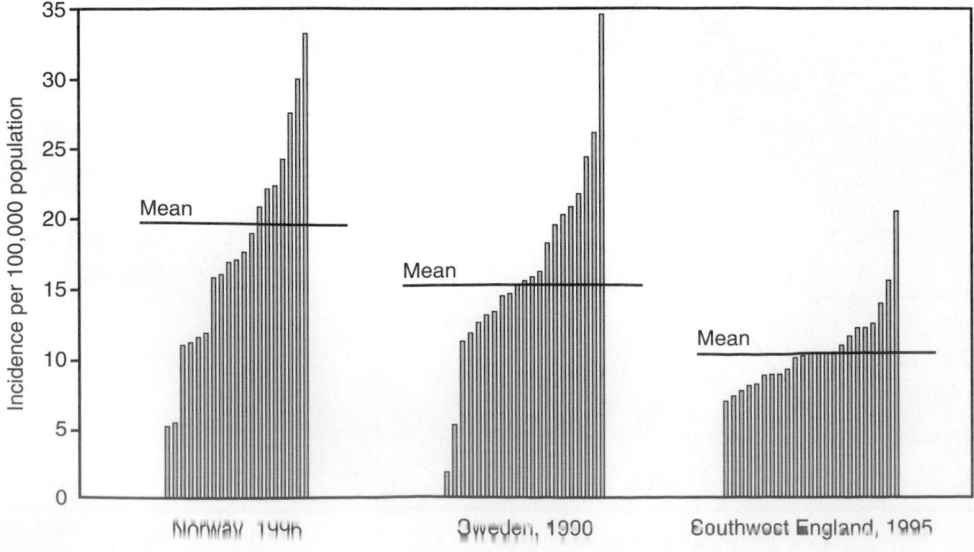

FIGURE 22–3 ■ Geographic variations in the incidence of invasive pneumococcal disease in counties in Norway and Sweden and in districts in southwest England. The mean values are for the region (southwest England) or the two countries as a whole (Norway and Sweden). (Data from Smith et al.,[405] Hasseltvedt et al.,[424] and Å Örtqvist, personal communication, 2002.)

and Denmark, however, the incidence of serotype 14 disease was much lower and did not increase during this period.[401,412,424] Also, it is well known that, as rates of pneumococcal disease caused by some serotypes increase, those caused by other serotypes decline.[82,426,427] Swedish investigators have argued that increased rates of invasive disease cannot be ascribed to higher numbers of blood cultures.[339,420,421] Yet, in North Jutland County in Denmark, a fourfold increase in the rate of pneumococcal bacteremia between 1981 and 1996 was highly correlated with the annual number of blood cultures taken.[428] Similar findings were reported for laboratory districts in England in 1995.[401] Moreover, in Sweden and Denmark, the increases in invasive disease have affected older people but not children and have been seen for pneumococcal bacteremia but not pneumococcal meningitis.[408,410,411] It is difficult to see how such large and selective increases in disease occurrence could have been caused by changes in the microorganism or the immunologic status of the populations. Changes in human behavior seem a more likely explanation.

A more interesting change in the epidemiology of invasive pneumococcal disease is the decrease in its incidence in several western European countries since 1996 (see Table 22–5). None of these countries adopted widespread pneumococcal vaccination after 1996, and the use of influenza vaccine also did not change.[429] Thus far, no satisfactory explanation for this change has been forthcoming.

Several studies in the United States document substantially higher rates of invasive pneumococcal disease in blacks than in whites and Hispanics.[386–390,393,396,397] These findings apply to both elderly persons and younger adults, regardless of HIV status. Even higher rates of invasive disease have been reported among the White Mountain Apaches in Arizona,[430] the Alaskan Native population,[395,431] and aboriginal populations in Australia.[418,432,433] In these groups, rates for invasive disease have been 156, 62, and 120 to 297 cases per 100,000 persons of all ages, respectively.

The data on mortality from invasive pneumococcal disease obtained in population-based studies confirm those reported in case series; rates range from 7% to 28% in persons of all ages and from 11% to 44% in the elderly (see Table 22–5). Mortality estimates for entire populations, however, can be problematic. In the United States, for example, an earlier population-based estimate of 40,000 deaths from pneumococcal pneumonia (nonbacteremic as well as bacteremic) each year[434] was recently lowered to 7000 to 12,500.[249] This newer estimate, however, is based on an underlying case fatality rate of only 12%, and this rate is lower than those reported in many case series.

As in reports of case series, virtually all population-based laboratory studies of invasive disease that include serogroup/serotype data show that approximately 90% of the isolates belong to the serogroups or serotypes included in 23-valent pneumococcal vaccine (see Table 22–5).[228,435]

Pneumococcal Infections in Children

In developed countries, virtually every child becomes a nasopharyngeal carrier of S. pneumoniae during the first year of life.[14] Many go on to develop one or more episodes of otitis media associated with pneumococcal infection. A smaller number develop more serious pneumococcal infections: pneumococcal bacteremia without an identified focus of infection, pneumococcal pneumonia, and, far less commonly, pneumococcal meningitis.

Pneumococcal conjugate vaccines have been developed primarily for use in children. For this reason, the epidemiology of pneumococcal infections in children is discussed in Chapter 23.

Pneumococcal Infections in Developing Countries

Most studies of the epidemiology of pneumococcal infections in developing countries focus on children less than 5 years of age. The World Health Organization (WHO) estimates that 1.6 to 2.2 million children die of acute respiratory infections (ARIs) each year, almost all in developing countries.[436] Most of these deaths are concentrated in the first year of life, especially in the first 3 months.[436–438] The bacterial causes of childhood ARI mortality are not well defined, and there is considerable variation in the findings from different study sites. Nonetheless, in most studies the leading cause is S. pneumoniae.[437,438] It is also the leading cause of nonepidemic childhood meningitis in Africa and other regions of the developing world.[439] Recent studies of childhood pneumococcal infections in developing countries have been designed to guide policy decisions for vaccine development and implementation.[437,440,441] A more complete discussion of these issues can be found in Chapter 23.

In contrast to children, the epidemiology of adult pneumococcal infections is not well known.[13] Population-based studies of invasive pneumococcal disease, pneumococcal pneumonia, and pneumococcal meningitis have been reported from very few developing countries, and much of what is known of their epidemiology is based on indirect estimates derived from other sources. In addition, it is difficult to generalize from a study conducted in one country to studies conducted in other countries at different stages of economic development and/or urbanization. In spite of these limitations, the evidence suggests that S. pneumoniae causes appreciable morbidity and mortality among adults.

Few prospective studies of adult community-acquired pneumonia have been reported from developing countries (see Table 22–3),[313,317,320,322,442] but at least two provide useful information. In a hospital-based study of 343 patients conducted in Buenos Aires (Argentina is considered to be a rapidly developing country), blood cultures were obtained in all patients.[317] Definite or presumptive pneumococcal pneumonia was documented in only 35 (10%) (see Table 22–3). However, no bacterial etiology was found in 58% of patients, perhaps in part because 34% of all patients had previously been treated with antibiotics. All 113 patients managed as outpatients survived, but 50 (22%) of the 230 who were hospitalized died. A more comprehensive hospital-based study was reported from Kenya, a less well-developed country.[322] Paired blood cultures were obtained in all 281 patients and transthoracic aspirates were cultured in 259 (92%). In addition, pneumococcal antigen (10 serotypes) was sought in 248 (88%) pretreatment urine specimens using a latex tube agglutination test. Overall, pneumococcal pneumonia was diagnosed in 129 (46%) of all patients; 57% of diagnoses were made by culture and 43% by antigen detection alone. The true proportion with pneumococcal pneumonia was probably higher because

54% of the patients had previously taken antibiotics. Earlier studies from hospitals in sub-Saharan Africa estimated that 38% to 58% of all adult pneumonias were due to *S. pneumoniae*.[13] Given difficult laboratory conditions, previous antibiotic treatment, and the frequent failure to undertake any diagnostic studies, it is likely that *S. pneumoniae* accounts for an even higher proportion of adult community-acquired pneumonias in developing countries.

Several hospital-based studies have sought to determine the bacterial etiology of febrile illness in patients who were thought to have bloodstream infections.[443-448] Most blood cultures have been negative, often because of previous antibiotic treatment, but pneumococcal bacteremia has been relatively common, especially in dry seasons. Moreover, in a study of 502 patients with febrile illness thought to be bacterial meningitis, pneumococcal infection was confirmed in 88 (17%) and was the probable cause of many of the 68 additional cases of probable bacterial meningitis.[449] In a South African teaching hospital, *S. pneumoniae* accounted for 70% of all cases of bacterial meningitis.[450]

There have been only two reports of the incidence of invasive pneumococcal disease among adults in a developing country, both from Soweto in South Africa.[451,452] The more recent report, based on 254 cases, estimated the incidence of pneumococcal bacteremia in persons 25 to 44, 45 to 64, and 65 or more years of age to be 45, 42, and 50 per 100,000, respectively.[452] These rates probably represent only a small portion of the burden of invasive pneumococcal disease in the community. The earlier report, based on only 66 cases, estimated the incidence of invasive disease in HIV-positive and HIV-negative patients ages 18 to 40 years to be 197 and 24 per 100,000 persons, respectively.[451] By comparison, in San Francisco the incidence of invasive disease in HIV-positive and HIV-negative African-Americans ages 18 to 64 years was 2385 and 60 per 100,000, respectively.[397] The different rates in the two communities provide some measure of the under-reporting of invasive disease in Soweto.

The remarkable effect of HIV infection on the incidence of invasive pneumococcal disease in sub-Saharan Africa was shown most clearly in a clinical trial of 23-valent pneumococcal vaccine in HIV-infected younger adults in Uganda.[453] In the placebo group, the invasive disease incidence was 17 per 1000 patient-years (1700 per 100,000). An earlier study of HIV-positive sex workers in Kenya reported an incidence of invasive disease of 42.5 per 1000 patient-years (1 in 24), and for recurrent disease it was 264 cases per 1000 patient-years (1 in 4).[454]

A major reason for underestimating the incidence of adult invasive pneumococcal disease in developing countries is the failure to obtain blood cultures from patients with pneumonia. In reports from India[455] and Uruguay,[456] the numbers of adults with bacteremic pneumococcal pneumonia and pneumococcal meningitis were similar, whereas in developed countries pneumonia patients usually outnumber those with meningitis by a factor of 8 to 10 or more (see Fig. 22–2). This suggests that the incidence of pneumococcal meningitis might be used to give a crude estimate of the overall incidence of invasive disease. For example, in Niger the incidence of pneumococcal meningitis was almost 8 per 100,000 in persons 40 years and older.[457] This rate was 10 times that observed in the United States,[383] and it suggests that the incidence of invasive disease was easily 100 per 100,000 in this age group and probably much higher.

A "surrogate" estimate of the incidence of invasive pneumococcal disease in developing countries has been obtained from community-based studies of indigenous populations living in Arizona,[430] Alaska,[395,431] and western, central, and northern Australia.[418,432,433] These populations have had rates of invasive disease well above those of neighboring nonindigenous populations. For persons 20 to 59 and 60 or 65 years of age or greater, annual rates of 53 to 178 and 46 to 222 per 100,000, respectively, have been reported. The findings from disadvantaged populations in these two countries provide probably the best indication of the invasive disease experience of adults who live under similar socioeconomic conditions in many less developed countries.

The serogroup/serotype distribution of invasive disease isolates obtained from adults in developing countries is similar to what is found in developed countries. In a weighted analysis of reports from many developing countries, 80% to 90% or more of all isolates were included in 23-valent pneumococcal vaccine.[458] Although antibiotic resistance is increasing in developing countries, in most it is less severe than it is in developed countries.

Because microbiologically defined outcomes in population-based studies are imprecise, investigators have come to favor "vaccine probe" studies.[13,441,459] In these studies, the burden of disease is defined by the difference in disease rates between vaccinated and control groups. One such study was carried out in adults in Papua New Guinea in the 1970s, well before the concept of a vaccine probe study had been suggested.[460] Over a 3-year period, the difference in all-cause mortality rates between the placebo group and a group that received 14-valent pneumococcal vaccine was 1.9 per 1000 population per year, a result suggesting that vaccine-type pneumococcal disease accounted for 21% of all deaths in the study population. A WHO report on priorities for pneumococcal vaccine development has called for several studies of the burden of adult pneumococcal disease to be undertaken in developing countries.[461] The report suggested that a vaccine probe trial of pneumococcal conjugate or a conjugate/polysaccharide combination could be used to define the vaccine-preventable disease burden in adults. Although not mentioned in the WHO report, a vaccine probe study using only the polysaccharide vaccine also could be considered. The polysaccharide vaccine would not induce herd immunity, but it would provide a direct measure of the burden of vaccine-type pneumococcal disease in the community.

Passive Immunization

In the preantibiotic era, type-specific antisera prepared in animals were used successfully to treat patients with pneumococcal infections.[462-464] Human immune globulin has been used for both prophylaxis and treatment of experimental pneumococcal infections.[465,466] Increasing antimicrobial resistance, the poor response to active immunization of immunocompromised patients, and technological progress in producing safer, more specific human immunoglobulins[462] have led to renewed interest in passive immunization for preventing pneumococcal infections.

Intravenous immune globulin (IVIG) preparations commercially available in the United States contain varying amounts of antibody to pneumococcal capsular polysaccharides.[467,468] Each is safe to administer and has not been shown to transmit hepatitis B or HIV infections. IVIG should not be given to patients with selective IgA deficiency because approximately 40% of these patients produce antibodies to IgA that have been implicated in IVIG-associated anaphylactic reactions.[469] The low levels of anti–capsular polysaccharide antibodies present in commercially available IVIG preparations require that relatively high doses be given, usually 400 mg/kg every 28 days.

Monthly infusions of IVIG significantly reduced the occurrence of pneumococcal infections in adults with lymphoma[469] and myeloma.[470] When IVIG has been given to children with HIV infections, however, it has not been effective in those with low CD4+ counts and has had no effect on overall mortality.[471] In addition, its annual cost for a 70-kg adult is more than $45,000.[469] Its cost-effectiveness for HIV-infected and other immunocompromised patients has not been established.[472]

Active Immunization

Pneumococcal Polysaccharide Vaccine

The first pneumococcal polysaccharide vaccines marketed in the United States were two hexavalent preparations. They were licensed in the late 1940s but were soon withdrawn. The first 14-valent vaccine was licensed in the United States in 1977. Each 0.5-mL dose contained 50 µg of each purified capsular polysaccharide. The amount of each antigen was reduced to 25 µg per 0.5 mL dose for the 23-valent vaccine that was introduced in 1983.[473]

Current pneumococcal vaccines contain capsular polysaccharides of serotypes 1, 2, 3, 4, 5, 6B, 7F, 8, 9N, 9V, 10A, 11A, 12F, 14, 15B, 17F, 18C, 19A, 19F, 20, 22F, 23F, and 33F.[474] The polysaccharides are dissolved in isotonic saline, and either phenol (0.25%) or thimerosal (0.01%) is added as a preservative. The vaccines contain no adjuvants. They should be stored at 2° to 8°C, and should not be frozen; under these conditions, they are stable for 24 months. Techniques that simultaneously measure the consistency of molecular size and the antigenicity of individual polysaccharides over time have helped to ensure uniformity between different lots of vaccine.[475] In the United States, two vaccines have been marketed: Pneumovax® 23 by Merck & Company and Pnu-Imune® 23 by Wyeth Lederle. In November 2002, Wyeth Lederle stopped producing Pnu-Imune 23. In Canada, Pneumo® 23 (Aventis Pasteur) and Pneumovax®23 are available. These two vaccines are marketed in countries in western Europe and in other regions of the world.

The serotypes included in 23-valent pneumococcal vaccine were chosen on the basis of the relative distribution of the individual serotypes that cause invasive pneumococcal infections. These serotypes have accounted for approximately 90% or more of the types responsible for invasive pneumococcal infections in developed and developing countries (see Table 22–5). The choice of a specific serotype, however, reflects more than the frequency with which it causes invasive disease.[473] Most serotypes within serogroups (e.g., 7F, 10A, 11A, 22F, and 33F) were chosen solely because of their epidemiologic occurrence, but serotypes 9N and 9V and 19F and 19A were included because heterologous antibody responses to the individual capsular polysaccharides are poor. The polysaccharides of types 15B and 15C are nearly identical and their antibodies are highly cross-reactive; hence only serotype 15B was included. Serotypes 6A and 6B are frequent causes of invasive disease, and antibodies to the two serotypes are highly cross-reactive. Type 6B was included instead of 6A because it is a more stable antigen. Type 5 was included because it is a frequent cause of infection in Africa and other developing regions.

Vaccine Administration

Pneumococcal polysaccharide vaccine should be administered as a single 0.5-mL dose, preferably intramuscularly rather than subcutaneously.[474] It should not be administered intradermally because this can cause severe local reactions. The vaccine can be administered simultaneously with influenza and other vaccines, including those used for routine childhood immunization. When given with influenza vaccine, but at a separate site, there is no decrease in the pneumococcal and influenza antibody responses.[476] Malaria prophylaxis with chloroquine and proguanil does not affect antibody responses to pneumococcal vaccination.[477]

Adverse Reactions and Contraindications

There are no contraindications to administering pneumococcal polysaccharide vaccine other than a severe reaction to a previous dose of the vaccine.

Local side effects such as erythema, induration, and pain appear in approximately 30% to 50% of all recipients of pneumococcal vaccine. These reactions last 1 to 3 days and are well tolerated.[474,478] They are more prominent in young and middle-aged adults, but their severity diminishes with advancing age, such that older persons usually have little or no local discomfort. When intramuscular and subcutaneous injections are compared, local soreness lasts longer after the former, but erythema is more common after the latter. In general, local and systemic adverse reactions are more likely to occur in persons with higher concentrations of antibodies to pneumococcal polysaccharides.[479] These reactions probably reflect Arthus-like phenomena. More severe systemic reactions are infrequent, and severe febrile reactions (>103°F) are decidedly rare.[478]

Healthy children tolerate pneumococcal vaccination well,[480,481] and no serious local reactions have been reported following vaccination and revaccination of infants.[482] Although there is an association between pre-existing antibody levels and local or systemic reactions in adults, no such correlation has been observed in children,[483] perhaps because they generally have lower antibody levels.

There is one report of an anaphylactic reaction following administration of 23-valent pneumococcal polysaccharide vaccine to a 2-year-old nonatopic boy who had small bowel and liver disease and was awaiting transplantation.[484] Bronchospasm and cutaneous and laryngeal edema developed immediately following vaccination, but resolved with appropriate treatment. A diagnostic evaluation demonstrated immunoglobulin E (IgE) antibodies specific for pneumococcal polysaccharides, suggesting that previous nasopharyngeal carriage or occult infection with *S. pneumoniae* induced IgE-dependent sensitization. Another report describes a 67-year-old woman who developed lymphadenopathy, hyperglobulinemia, and minimal change nephrotic syndrome 1 week after receiving pneumococcal vaccine.[485] After a prolonged and severe illness, she recovered with intensive steroid treatment.

Local reactions and fever but not other systemic reactions are more frequent in children who are given *Haemophilus influenzae* type b and meningococcal vaccines at the same time as pneumococcal vaccine.[486] The antibody responses to each vaccine are not compromised by giving them simultaneously.

Pneumococcal vaccination of HIV-infected individuals may be followed by a transient increase in viral load,[487] but the same increase has been observed following vaccination with other inactivated vaccines (e.g., influenza, tetanus toxoid)[488] and it is not thought to be of any clinical significance. A few patients with immunologic disorders have had more serious reactions following pneumococcal vaccination, but these events are likely to have been chance occurrences that were not causally related. Neurologic disorders such as Guillain-Barré syndrome have not been reported.

When pneumococcal vaccine is given simultaneously with influenza vaccine, there is no increase in the rate of systemic reactions compared with influenza vaccine alone and little or no increase in the rate of local reactions, although two injections are given.[476,489]

Results of Vaccination

Methods of Assessing Antibody Response

Until the late 1980s, antibody responses to pneumococcal vaccine were measured by radioimmunoassay (RIA).[490] The RIA technique was sensitive and reproducible, but it had several disadvantages, including expense, the need to use radiolabeled type-specific polysaccharides, and the inability to distinguish between different antibody classes. In addition, the antibodies measured by RIA were not specific for capsular polysaccharides. This was due to the use of test antigens that contained both capsular and C-polysaccharides.[491-496] Thus RIA measured both protective anticapsular and nonprotective anti–C-polysaccharide antibodies.

Once this methodologic problem became apparent, several unexplained features of earlier reports could be understood. First, many persons tested by RIA appeared to have antibody to nearly every serotype of *S. pneumoniae*. This was a surprising finding because infections caused by some of these serotypes were exceedingly uncommon. Second, because there were measurable levels of antibody before vaccination, antibody responses following vaccination had to be reported as fold increases, and it was difficult to determine which levels might be associated with protection.

Third, there was a poor correlation between RIA antibody levels and measures of opsonophagocytosis in vitro[497,498] and protection in vivo. This could now be explained because RIA did not accurately measure the anti–capsular polysaccharide antibodies responsible for these activities.

Several ELISA[491-493,499] and other enzyme immunoassays[500,501] have been developed for measuring antibodies to pneumococcal polysaccharides. These assays are simple and inexpensive and do not require radiolabeled reagents. They can also distinguish between immunoglobulin M (IgM), IgG, and IgA antibodies. Because antigens used in ELISA assays often contain C-polysaccharides,[494,502] an adsorption step is required to remove antibody to C-polysaccharide from sera that are to be tested. Unencapsulated mutants of *S. pneumoniae* have been created for this purpose.[503] A commercial C-polysaccharide preparation is supplied by the Statens Serum Institute in Copenhagen. After C-polysaccharide has been removed from test sera, residual cross-reactivity may still be present.[504-506] This is probably due to nonspecific antibodies that bind to novel epitopes that contaminate commercial preparations of capsular polysaccharides. Differences in specificity have been found for different lots of individual serotypes from the same and different manufacturers,[506] calling into question the accuracy of some ELISA antibody measurements. A heterologous type 22F pneumococcal polysaccharide can be used to adsorb out antibodies to these common epitopes.[507] Doing so improves the correlation between IgG levels determined by ELISA and in vitro measures of functional activity. These and other measures have been used to establish quality standards for ELISA testing among many laboratories.[508,509]

ELISA measurements of anti–capsular polysaccharide antibodies after C-polysaccharide adsorption show that, before vaccination, most normal individuals lack antibodies to most pneumococcal serotypes.[510] Following vaccination, antibodies develop to most vaccine serotypes. Both IgM and IgG antibodies can be detected within 5 to 8 days of vaccination. IgG antibody levels, however, may not reach their peak until 70 to 100 days following vaccination.[112] A short-lived secretory IgA response also occurs.[511] IgM antibody levels decline rapidly and are no longer detectable after a few months, whereas IgG antibody levels usually persist, albeit at reduced levels, for 5 or more years.

Unfortunately, ELISA cannot distinguish between functional and nonfunctional antibodies. The antibodies that develop after pneumococcal vaccination facilitate opsonization, activate complement, promote bacterial phagocytosis by polymorphonuclear leukocytes and alveolar macrophages, and protect experimental animals against pneumococcal infection.[512] Measurements of antibody avidity often provide a better correlation than ELISA antibody levels, with more direct measures of antibody protection.[117,513-515] In some adults, however, high levels of avidity before vaccination may make it difficult to detect increases in functional activity after vaccination.[516]

One way to measure functional activity is the classical opsonophagocytic killing assay 1, but the test is laborious and not often used. Several flow-cytometric opsonophagocytic assays (OPAs) have been developed to measure functional activity.[514,517-519] Some of these complement-dependent assays use cultured HL-60 cells as effector cells rather than harvested leukocytes.[514,518,519] Using leukocytes from healthy donors may be more efficient, but HL-60 cells can be standardized for large-scale studies[520] and allow 50 or more specimens to be processed each day.[517,519] Correlations between ELISA antibody levels and OPA activity vary, depending on the serotype and the OPA method that is used. Better correlations are observed for serotypes 6B and 23F than for 19F.[521] ELISA antibody levels that do not correlate well with OPA activity may reflect the need for complement in the assay, the inability to distinguish between bacteria that are adherent to the surface of the phagocyte and those that have been internalized and killed, and discordant FcγR allotypes for the test sera and effector phagocytes.[119,522,523] A double-fluorescent method that distinguishes between adherent and internalized particles and matches donor and effector cell FcγR allotypes enhances the sensitivity of the assay.[523,524] Other methods also have been developed to improve the efficiency of OPA assays.[525,526]

Another way to measure functional activity is to administer graded doses of antibody to animals such as mice and then challenge them with varying doses of S. pneumoniae. Experiments using postvaccination sera from healthy young adults have demonstrated a close correlation between the level of antibody and the degree of protection.[502] With older subjects, especially those that have diseases that affect immunity, antibody is not as protective.[514] A major limitation of these in vivo studies is that only a few S. pneumoniae serotypes (e.g., types 1, 2, 3, 4, 5, and 8) reliably cause disease in mice. Serotypes 6A and 6B cause disease in newborn mice, but other serotypes of great epidemiologic interest, such as 14, 19, and 23F, produce no experimental illness. Several additional serotypes cause illness after aerosol inoculation of infant rats, but this is a difficult model to work with.[527]

There is no consensus on what constitutes a minimally protective level of human antibody for each pneumococcal serotype. One study suggested that levels of about 0.05 µg/mL were protective against serotypes 1, 3, and 4,[502] whereas another suggested that protective levels against infection caused by six different serotypes varied from less than 0.05 to greater than 0.4 µg/mL, depending on serotype.[528] Sera used in these studies were obtained 6 to 8

weeks after vaccination, and perhaps sera obtained several years later would have been more protective at equivalent levels of ELISA-measured antibody. In another study of pulmonary infection caused by 10 different pneumococcal serotypes, infant rats were passively immunized with a bacterial polysaccharide immune globulin preparation (BPIG-8).[527] With the exception of serotype 14, serum antibody levels ranging from 0.10 to 1.15 µg/mL significantly reduced morbidity and mortality; serotype 14 infection required 2.32 µg/mL. No attempt was made to correlate in vivo protection with in vitro OPA activity.

Thus a given level of IgG antibody as measured by ELISA does not necessarily indicate a predictable degree of protection against pneumococcal infection. This is further illustrated by the results of laboratory studies shown in Table 22–6.[514] In two elderly individuals, similar levels of IgG antibodies measured by ELISA were associated with very different levels of functional activity.

Pneumococcal polysaccharides are T-cell–independent antigens. Thus it is not surprising that little is known about cell-mediated immune responses following vaccination. The number of interferon-γ–secreting cells (a T-helper [Th]-1 marker) tends to increase following vaccination, but there are no changes in IL-4 and IL-5 (Th-2 markers).[529] Vaccination is also followed by a transient decline in the immune responses to protein antigens. The clinical relevance of these changes is not known.

Immunogenicity in Normal Adults

In early comparative studies conducted in healthy adults, antibody levels measured by RIA were similar following vaccination with 25 or 50 µg of each pneumococcal capsular polysaccharide.[473] Similar comparisons have not been made using ELISA methods.

Healthy adults develop good antibody responses after vaccination with 23-valent pneumococcal vaccine. In one study, the IgG responses to 10 representative serotypes were evaluated in 72 subjects.[530] Among 720 possible responses, 86% were positive. The capacity of these individuals to generate antibody responses to individual serotypes was not randomly distributed among study subjects: 53% had IgG responses to all 10 polysaccharides, whereas 11% responded

TABLE 22–6 ■ Immunoglobulin G (IgG) Antibody Levels and Functional Measures of Protection Against Pneumococcal Infection in Two Elderly Adults*

		Functional Measures of Protection		
Patient Age (yr)	ELISA IgG (µg/mL)	Antibody Avidity NaSCN[†]	Opsonic Titer (50% Killing)	% of Mice Surviving After Challenge
90	2.7	1.67	8142	100
74	2.4	0.013	4	0

*Four doses of serotype-specific antibody (6, 18, 50, and 150 ng) were administered to groups of mice infected intraperitoneally with 100 times the median infective dose of S. pneumoniae serotype 4.
†Molar concentration of sodium thiocyanate (NaSCN) necessary to yield an 85% reduction in enzyme-linked immunosorbent assay (ELISA) IgG optical density.
Adapted from Table 3 in Romero-Steiner S, Musher DM, Cetron MS, et al. Reduction in functional antibody activity against *Streptococcus pneumoniae* in vaccinated elderly individuals highly correlates with decreased IgG antibody avidity. Clin Infect Dis 29:281–288, 1999.

to 5 or fewer polysaccharides. Those with a larger number of antibody responses also had higher mean IgG levels than did those who responded to fewer antigens.

Among IgG subclasses, IgG2 antibodies have shown the greatest increase following pneumococcal vaccination.[500,531] Small amounts of IgG1 antibody have been detected in some persons, and barely measurable levels of IgG3 or IgG4 antibody have been found in a few.[530] The failure of some healthy adults to make IgG antibodies is not associated with abnormal levels of serum IgG, IgM, or IgA; a failure to switch from IgM to IgG; or a global defect in the production of IgG2. Interestingly, patients who have recovered from community-acquired pneumonia may have lower levels of IgG subclass antibody compared with normal controls. Nonetheless, they respond as well as controls to pneumococcal vaccine.[532]

Pneumococcal vaccination also induces IgM and IgA antibody responses. The brisk polymeric serum IgA2 subclass antibody response often seen may reflect previous contact with pneumococcal antigens at mucosal surfaces.[533] The IgA response to vaccination persists much longer than the IgA response to pneumococcal infection.

Some healthy adults respond vigorously to all or nearly all of the polysaccharides in pneumococcal vaccine, whereas others respond to fewer antigens and with lower levels of IgG antibody. Genes that govern the Gm and Km allotypes of IgG are thought to influence antibody responses to the pneumococcal capsular polysaccharides.[114] In general, persons who have the G2m(23) allotype (an antigenic marker on the heavy chain of the IgG2 idiotype) or who lack the Km (1) allotype have increased antibody responses. Studies in twins have provided useful insights into the genetic regulation of antibody responses to pneumococcal vaccination. In spite of a closer correlation in mean IgG and IgG2 antibody levels after vaccination in monozygotic compared with dizygotic twins,[534,535] differences have still been found within pairs of monozygotic twins.[536] The differences may be due to individual variability in V-region genes that determine the final specificity of B cells.

Not surprisingly, human leukocyte antigen (HLA) type has no effect on antibody responses following pneumococcal vaccination. Polysaccharide antigens interact directly with surface receptors of B cells to stimulate the generation of a clone of antibody-producing cells, whereas protein antigens are broken down into relatively small sequences of amino acids for surface presentation, a process that requires major histocompatibility class participation.[537]

Immunogenicity in Normal Children

Mean IgG levels for individual polysaccharides in 2-month-old infants are higher than those found in older infants, reflecting transplacental transfer of maternal IgG1 antibodies.[538,539] Subsequent nasopharyngeal colonization and infection induce variable antibody responses to capsular polysaccharides, depending on the age of the child and the capsular serotype.[539,540]

After receiving one dose of pneumococcal polysaccharide vaccine, infants develop good antibody responses to types 3, 4, 8, and 9N; intermediate responses to types 1, 2, 7F, 18C, 19F, and 25; and poor responses to types 12, 14,

23F, and 6A and 6B.[483,538,541,542] All immunoglobulin classes are included in these responses, although among IgG subclasses, IgG2 and IgG4 predominate.[543] A second dose of vaccine does not, as a rule, lead to higher antibody levels. Several studies of the relative immunogenicity of different serotypes have been reported.[481,538,540] In Papua New Guinea, for example, good antibody responses were seen to types 2, 3, 5, 7F, and 23F, and poor responses to types 6B and 19F.[540,544] In The Gambia, pneumococcal vaccine was given to groups of children starting either at 2 or 9 months of age.[538] Modest IgG responses were seen to types 1, 3, and 5 in children of both age groups. Children vaccinated at 9 months were the only ones to develop antibodies to types 19F and 23F, and few children in either group responded to type 6A. IgA antibody responses were similar to those seen for IgG, although levels were generally lower. Antibody responses to vaccination in children more than 2 years of age are generally good.[481]

The mucosal immune response may help to protect children from acute and recurrent pneumococcal otitis media. Secretory IgA antibodies frequently are detected in nasopharyngeal secretions of children with otitis media.[545,546] During the acute phase of otitis media, a considerable amount of specific anti–capsular polysaccharide antibody, both IgA and IgG, is transferred from serum into the middle ear cavity.[547] In these children, pneumococcal vaccine elicits an antibody response in middle-ear fluid as well as in the serum.

Because capsular polysaccharides induce antibodies primarily by T-cell–independent mechanisms, most are poor immunogens in children whose immune systems are still under development.[548] Although highly immunogenic serotypes such as type 3 can induce antibodies in infants as young as 3 months of age, antibody responses to most other pneumococcal capsular polysaccharides are generally poor in children less than 2 years of age, and pneumococcal polysaccharide vaccine is not recommended for these children.[474]

Immunogenicity in Persons with High-Risk Conditions

Immunocompetent Persons

THE ELDERLY

Most healthy older adults respond well to pneumococcal polysaccharide vaccine. When measured by ELISA, antibody levels,[549–553] antibody avidity,[550,553] and 5-year antibody persistence[554] in older persons are generally similar to what is observed in younger individuals. In one study of 350 elderly subjects, antibody levels to certain serotypes before and after vaccination were higher in elderly men than in women. Unlike antibody levels in women, those in men showed little decline with increasing age.[555] Most studies, however, suggest that antibody levels decline substantially after vaccination. In one study of 15 persons, the decline in antibody levels was such that, after 5 years, 60% were considered candidates for revaccination.[554] In another report, geometric mean antibody levels to serotypes 4, 6B, 9V, 19F, and 23F declined to prevaccination levels 3 years after vaccination.[556] The most important factor predicting sustained antibody levels was the magnitude of the initial antibody response to vaccination.

Approximately 20% of elderly men appear to be poor responders to most of the 23 capsular polysaccharides in pneumococcal vaccine (Fig. 22–4).[552] (The antibody responses of elderly women to all 23 polysaccharide antigens have not been studied.) A similar proportion of men also appear to be unable to generate good functional antibody responses.[550] Not all of these individuals have low levels of IgG or IgG2.[557] These observations appear to be clinically relevant: Sera taken from persons who have had an episode of bacteremic or nonbacteremic pneumococcal pneumonia fail to opsonize the infecting serotype in in vitro assays and also fail to protect mice against challenge infection in passive transfer experiments.[122] Moreover, persons with a history of bacteremic pneumococcal infections have lower antibody responses to subsequent pneumococcal vaccination than do persons without such a history.[557] Attempts to improve the antibody responses of older adults by coadministration of IL-12 as an adjuvant have been unsuccessful.[558]

CHRONIC CARDIOVASCULAR AND PULMONARY DISEASES

Antibody responses to pneumococcal vaccine in older patients with chronic cardiovascular diseases are usually similar to those of older persons who are healthy and those of younger persons.[559] Heart failure patients often have multiple immune system abnormalities, yet they respond normally to pneumococcal vaccine.[560] Asthmatic patients treated with alternate-day corticosteroids (10 to 35 mg) have antibody levels before and after vaccination that are similar to those of age-matched normal controls.[561] One study of patients with chronic obstructive pulmonary disease (COPD), however, showed that they developed significantly lower antibody levels and responded to fewer serotypes when compared with controls.[559] Adults with α_1-antitrypsin deficiency and recurrent pulmonary infections generally respond well to pneumococcal vaccine, although the responses in those with bronchiectasis tend to be lower.[562] In adults with IgA deficiency, recurrent pulmonary

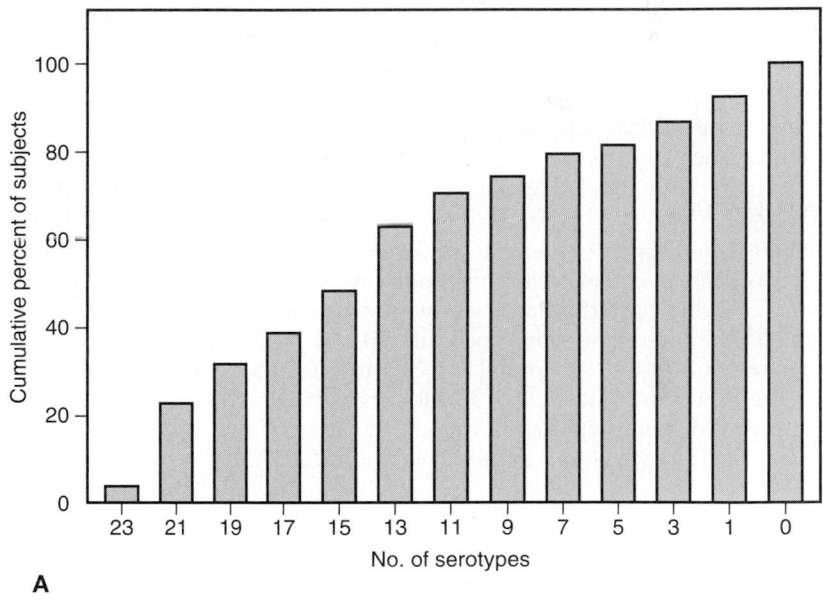

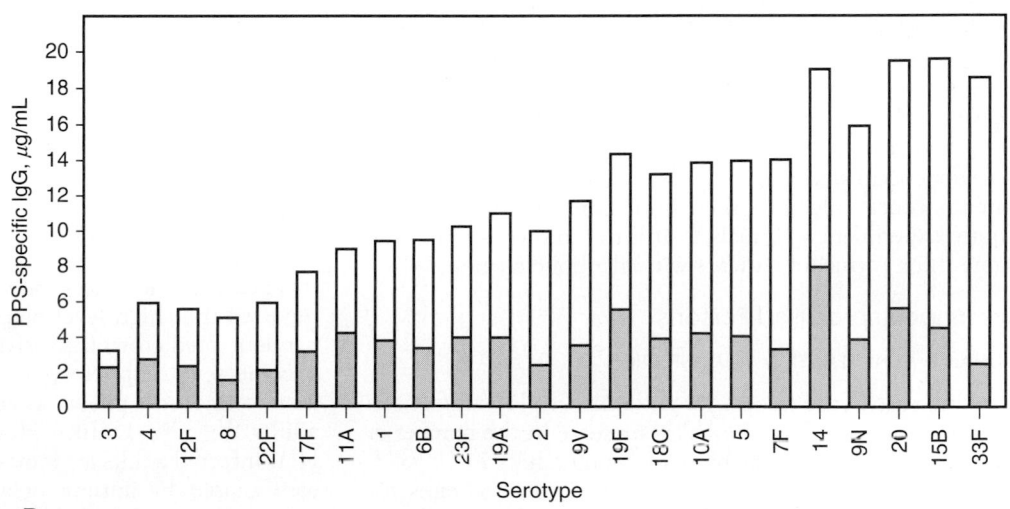

FIGURE 22–4 ■ Cumulative two-fold antibody increases (*A*) and geometric mean immunoglobulin G antibody increases (*B*) for 23 individual vaccine serotypes following pneumococcal polysaccharide vaccination of 53 elderly men. (Redrawn from Rubins JB, Alter M, Loch J, Janoff EN. Determination of antibody responses of elderly adults to all 23 capsular polysaccharides after pneumococcal vaccination. Infect Immun 67: 5979–5984, 1999.)

infections affect only those who also have low levels of IgG2 and IgG4.

Children who experience recurrent episodes of sinopulmonary infection often have low or nondetectable levels of anti-pneumococcal antibodies.[563–569] One study compared antibody levels to 12 different serotypes in 66 affected children 2 to 5 years of age with those in 28 age-matched controls.[569] Antibody levels in those with recurrent infections were generally lower both before and after vaccination compared with controls. In other studies of children with recurrent sinopulmonary infections and normal serum IgG levels, 4% to 14% failed to mount any antibody response to pneumococcal vaccine[565–568] and 40% to 50% failed to generate an IgG2 antibody response,[567] in spite of often normal IgG2 levels.[566] Similar findings have been demonstrated in otitis-prone children.[570] The nature of these apparent defects in anti-pneumococcal antibody production is not known; many children with low IgG2 levels do not experience recurrent sinopulmonary infections.

Some children with ataxia-telangiectasia and atopic eczema experience frequent sinopulmonary infections and respond poorly to pneumococcal vaccine.[571,572] Not surprisingly, most children in whom a humoral immunodeficiency is already evident also respond poorly to pneumococcal vaccine.[565,567] Age appears to be an important factor for children who have normal IgG concentrations but experience recurrent infections; antibody responses are better in those who are older.

DIABETES MELLITUS

Diabetes mellitus is a frequent underlying condition in patients with pneumococcal bacteremia, although one or more comorbid conditions are usually present. Early studies using RIA showed that adults and children with type 1 diabetes respond as well as normal subjects to pneumococcal vaccine. A more recent study of 30 patients with either type 1 or type 2 diabetes reported normal antibody responses to pneumococcal vaccination as measured by ELISA.[573]

CHRONIC ALCOHOLISM AND CIRRHOSIS

Patients with chronic alcoholism and cirrhosis usually have adequate antibody responses to pneumococcal vaccine,[574, 575] although occasional differences between patients and control subjects have been observed for some serotypes.[574] In one study, antibody levels before vaccination were higher in alcoholic subjects than in controls.[575] One month after vaccination, IgG, IgM, and IgA antibodies in alcoholic subjects were significantly increased over baseline levels, but by 6 months they had declined to levels lower than those in controls. Pneumococcal vaccination induces less protection against pneumococcal infection in cirrhotic compared with noncirrhotic experimental animals.[576] It is not known whether the same thing is true for patients with alcoholic cirrhosis.

Immunocompromised Persons

HUMAN IMMUNODEFICIENCY VIRUS INFECTION

The increase in the number of patients with HIV infections has brought with it a remarkable increase in the number of pneumococcal infections both in young adults[353, 361, 577–582] and in children.[583–585] Nasopharyngeal carriage rates for S. pneumoniae are similar in HIV-positive and HIV-negative individuals.[586–588] Carriage may persist for long periods, however, increasing the likelihood that the organism will develop antimicrobial resistance. This occurs frequently in persons receiving prophylaxis with trimethoprim-sulfamethoxazole.

Population-based studies in the 1980s and early 1990s showed that hospital admissions for community-acquired pneumonia rose rapidly in persons between 25 and 50 to 60 years in age, largely as a result of HIV infection.[589] In a large multicenter study in the United States, the hospitalization rate for bacterial pneumonia was 5.5 per 1000 person-years.[306,579] Community-acquired pneumonia often was seen as the first manifestation of HIV infection.[578,590,591]

Streptococcus pneumoniae has been the leading cause of bacterial pneumonia in HIV-infected adults in developed countries.[306,579,592–594] Together with nontyphoidal salmonellae, S. pneumoniae also has been the leading nonmycobacterial cause of pneumonia in developing countries.[595] In San Francisco in the early 1990s, the rate for pneumococcal bacteremia in patients with acquired immunodeficiency syndrome (AIDS) was 1 case per 100 patient-years, a rate greater than 100 times that reported in the same age group in the pre-AIDS era.[596] In several centers, HIV-infected individuals accounted for 40% or more of all cases of invasive pneumococcal disease in adults up to 55 years in age.[353,577,580] One report even suggested that surveillance for invasive pneumococcal disease in younger adults was useful in estimating the size of the HIV-infected population.[597] With the introduction of highly active antiretroviral therapy (HAART), the morbidity and mortality of pneumococcal infections among adults in the United States has declined dramatically.[598,599] For example, during the period from 1994 to 1997, the rate of invasive pneumococcal disease in HIV-infected younger adults in San Francisco declined more than 2.5-fold.[397] Similar declines no doubt have occurred in other countries where HAART regimens have been introduced.

The clinical features and risk factors associated with pneumococcal pneumonia and invasive pneumococcal disease in HIV-infected adults[306,578,600–605] and children[583,584] are generally similar to those seen in persons without HIV infection. HIV-infected pneumonia patients are more often bacteremic than are those without HIV infection.[442,578,606] Mortality rates in the two groups are generally similar,[353,397,451,594,601,606] although two studies suggest that death rates in HIV-infected patients may be higher.[361,580] A few patients may present with manifestations of disease not commonly seen since the preantibiotic era.[600] After one episode of pneumococcal disease, HIV-infected individuals are at greatly increased risk of a second episode.[353,606] Antibiotic-resistant S. pneumoniae do not usually present difficult management problems, and rates of colonization,[577] invasive disease,[353] and death[607] do not appear to be increased. Nonetheless, one study of HIV-infected adults reported that high-level penicillin resistance was an independent predictor of invasive disease mortality.[608] Finally, vaccine serogroup/serotype organisms account for 90% or more of invasive pneumococcal infections in HIV-infected adults.[353,451,580] Unlike HIV-negative adults, however, HIV-infected adults are more likely to develop invasive disease caused by antimicrobial-resistant serotypes that are commonly found in children.[451,601,609,610]

Several studies have reported the antibody responses of HIV-infected adults[611–619] and children[620–622] to pneumococcal capsular polysaccharides. Because of polyclonal B-cell activation, many unvaccinated HIV-infected adults have higher total IgG levels than non–HIV-infected controls, but antibody levels to capsular polysaccharides are reduced both before[614,618,623] and after[606,612,616–628] vaccination. Antibody responses to pneumococcal vaccine tend to be lower in those with lower CD4+ counts,[611,624] but in several reports antibody responses have been similar regardless of CD4+ count.[612,613] Responses are also similar in those with and without a history of previous pneumococcal disease.[618] Studies of functional antibody responses following pneumococcal vaccination are limited, but opsonophagocytic activity appears to be reduced compared with activity in non–HIV-infected controls.[616,618] In addition, IgM and IgA antibody responses to vaccination are frequently suboptimal.[613,614] One small study suggested that the poor antibody response to pneumococcal vaccination in HIV-infected individuals could be due to aberrant VH3 gene expression.[115]

In HIV-infected children, antibody responses to pneumococcal vaccination range from poor to near normal.[620–622] Children born of HIV-infected mothers also have low levels of maternally transferred anti-pneumococcal antibodies.[625]

Following vaccination of adults with HIV infection, antibody levels to most serotypes decline more rapidly than they do in healthy controls, and after 1 to 3 years usually return to prevaccination levels.[615,617,624]

A few investigators have reported on the combined use of pneumococcal conjugate and polysaccharide vaccines in HIV-infected adults. Antibody responses to the conjugate vaccine alone were generally reduced compared with those in healthy controls,[626,627] but they were similar to[626,627] or better than[628] those seen in HIV-infected adults who had been given one dose of polysaccharide vaccine. In the last study, the conjugate vaccine also elicited a better opsonophagocytic response than did the polysaccharide vaccine, perhaps because sera were tested after adsorbing out non–serotype-specific antibodies with heterologous serotype 22F polysaccharide.[628] A second dose of conjugate vaccine had little effect on antibody levels observed after the first dose of conjugate vaccine.[626,628] In contrast, in one study a dose of polysaccharide vaccine boosted antibody levels in persons with CD4+ cell counts of 200 or more /μL,[626] but in another it had little effect.[628] To date, there have been no reports on the duration of antibody responses (ELISA or functional) in HIV-infected adults given both conjugate and polysaccharide vaccines compared with the duration in those given only the polysaccharide vaccine.

An early study showed that HIV-infected adults who were treated with zidovudine had better antibody responses following pneumococcal vaccination than did comparable individuals who were not being treated.[629] Vaccination with pneumococcal[487] and other[488] vaccines can be followed by a transient increase in plasma HIV viral load in adults[487,628,630] and children.[631,632] There is no indication, however, that this has any effect on the overall course of HIV disease. There have been no published reports on the antibody responses to pneumococcal vaccination of HIV-infected patients who are being treated with HAART regimens, are in clinical remission, and have low or undetectable plasma HIV levels. Vaccination, however, appears to have no appreciable effect on plasma viral load in these individuals.[633]

The increased risk of pneumococcal infections in persons with HIV infection is largely due to deficiencies in the amount or functional capacity of antibodies to pneumococcal capsular polysaccharides. Decreased levels of antibodies to other important determinants of pneumococcal virulence may also be important.[634] Antibody responses to pneumococcal polysaccharide vaccine are better in the early stage of infection when patients are asymptomatic and CD4+ counts are high, indicating that, once the diagnosis of HIV infection is made, pneumococcal vaccine should be given without delay.

SPLENECTOMY

Children and adults are at greatly increased risk of bacterial infection following splenectomy.[635] Overwhelming postsplenectomy infection (OPSI) is more common in persons with immunologic or hematologic disorders than it is in those who have undergone splenectomy for trauma. In one study from Australia, the overall incidence of OPSI was approximately 4 cases per 1000 patient-years, a 12.6-fold increase in risk compared with the general population.[636] Another report estimated an incidence of 3.3 cases per 1000 patient-years for patients with Hodgkin's disease, 1.7 for those with idiopathic thrombocytopenia, 0.7 for those with hereditary spherocytosis, and 0.3 for those following trauma.[637] Approximately half of all episodes of OPSI occur more than 5 years after splenectomy,[638] and case-fatality rates are 50% or higher.[635,638] S. pneumoniae is the most common cause of OPSI, accounting for 30% to 60% or more of all cases.[635,638,639] In one study from Norway, the rate for pneumococcal bacteremia in postsplenectomy patients was 2.7 cases per 1000 patient-years, a rate greater than 25 times that for the general population.[640]

Antibody responses to pneumococcal vaccine in postsplenectomy patients vary, largely because some patients are immunocompromised and others are not. Following splenectomy for trauma, IgG antibody responses measured by ELISA are similar to those in normal controls.[641,642] Opsonophagocytic antibody levels, however, are lower in those vaccinated 1 or 7 days compared with those vaccinated 14 days after splenectomy.[641] Whether it is better to postpone pneumococcal vaccination for at least 2 weeks following splenectomy is not entirely clear. A large study from Denmark, where 91% of postsplenectomy patients had been vaccinated, suggested this would be worthwhile.[643] Unfortunately, the analysis did not control for underlying conditions in the study subjects.

Previous splenectomy may be the strongest single indication for vaccination with pneumococcal polysaccharide vaccine.[474,644] This includes children 2 years of age or older who have previously received pneumococcal conjugate vaccine.[645] Most physicians know that postsplenectomy patients are at increased risk for pneumococcal infections,[646] but patients themselves are usually unaware of their risk or have difficulty remembering what preventive measures they should take.[647,648] Organized programs for identifying postsplenectomy patients have been successful in vaccinating most of them,[643,647] but, in the absence of such programs, vaccination rates are low.[638] Periodic measurement of antibody levels after vaccination has been recommended but is seldom done except for research purposes.[643] Postsplenectomy patients remain at increased risk indefinitely, and for this reason revaccination after 5 years or earlier is generally recommended.[642,643] Long-term antimicrobial prophylaxis also has been recommended, but compliance is difficult, and it is usually more practical to instruct vaccinated patients to begin self-treatment with an oral antimicrobial agent at the first sign of febrile illness.[638] This sound advice is seldom followed, and increasing antibiotic resistance may make such treatment less effective. Nonetheless, a comprehensive strategy to prevent OPSI that includes vaccination can be highly effective; in one county in Denmark where 60% of postsplenectomy patients had been vaccinated, only 1 of 38 bacteremias that were observed in these patients over a 10-year period was due to S. pneumoniae.[649]

SICKLE CELL DISEASE

Children with homozygous sickle cell disease (hemoglobin SS) are at greatly increased risk of pneumococcal infections compared with normal children[650]; they may be 600 times more likely to develop pneumococcal meningitis and are more likely to experience fulminant pneumococcal sepsis. The most significant period of risk begins approximately 4 months after birth and continues until at least 4 to 5 years of age. In the Cooperative Study of Sickle Cell Disease, infants with homozygous (SS) and heterozygous (SC) disease were followed for a mean of 1.2 years.[651] Those with SS disease who were 6 to 12 months of age had an incidence of 9.9 episodes of pneumococcal bacteremia per 100 person-years, while those who were 3 years of age had a rate of 4.7 cases per 100 person-years. Infection rates for children with SC disease (32% of all subjects) were only slightly lower. Many of the infections were due to antibiotic-resistant organisms. Among all children enrolled in this study, the mortality rate from pneumococcal bacteremia was 15%, a rate similar to what has been reported in smaller case series.[652,653]

The most important pathophysiologic defect that predisposes sickle cell patients to pneumococcal infection is functional asplenia. Reduced serum opsonic activity caused by defects in the classical and alternative complement pathways may be present, often in association with deficiencies in type-specific antibody.[654,655] Susceptibility to pneumococcal infection is not due to genotypic variation in the binding of IgG2 and altered clearance of encapsulated organisms.[656]

Children with sickle cell disease who are 2 years of age or older may respond initially to pneumococcal polysaccharide vaccine, but their responses are usually short lived.[657] Revaccination at 5 years of age is followed by poor serotype-specific antibody responses in most, and, in those who respond, almost half show a twofold or greater decline in antibody levels 10 to 15 months later. Older children and young adults may respond better than younger children to primary vaccination and revaccination.[658,659] Prevaccination sera from these subjects may show little opsonophagocytic activity, but increased activity usually can be found following vaccination.[659]

In the past, penicillin prophylaxis in young children with sickle cell disease reduced the overall rate of nasopharyngeal colonization with S. pneumoniae,[660] but it also increased the risk that colonizing organisms would be antibiotic resistant.[661,662] Prophylaxis also reduced their risk of pneumococcal bacteremia, whether or not they had received pneumococcal vaccine.[660] Discontinuing penicillin prophylaxis at 5 years of age was not followed by an increased rate of bacteremic disease. The management of children with sickle cell disease has improved dramatically over the past two decades.[663] Hospitalization and death from pneumococcal infection have been largely eliminated by meticulous adherence to penicillin prophylaxis during the first 5 years of life. It is unclear whether pneumococcal vaccination has contributed significantly to the improved outcome of these children. Nonetheless, given the steady increase in antibiotic-resistant S. pneumoniae, it is uncertain for how long penicillin prophylaxis will be beneficial. Pneumococcal conjugate vaccine will be important for the control of pneumococcal infections in children with sickle cell disease. In those 2 years of age or older, however, 23-valent polysaccharide vaccine will continue to be indicated and recommended.[645]

HEMATOLOGIC NEOPLASMS

Patients with chronic lymphocytic leukemia, Hodgkin's disease, and multiple myeloma are at increased risk for severe pneumococcal infections.[664,665] In one report, the annual incidence of invasive pneumococcal disease in these patients was 2.6%.[664] Several factors influence their antibody responses to pneumococcal vaccine, including the stage of disease, whether or not a splenectomy has been performed, the extent of previous radiation therapy or chemotherapy, and the time between completion of treatment and vaccination.[665]

Few patients with chronic lymphocytic leukemia respond to pneumococcal vaccine, even when they are not receiving chemotherapy.[666–668] Those who do respond have less advanced disease and higher levels of IgG, IgG2, and IgG4.[668] Children with acute leukemia who are on maintenance chemotherapy have poor antibody responses, but the levels achieved in some may be protective.[669] In contrast, those who have been in remission for 2 or more years respond well to pneumococcal vaccination.[670]

Patients with Hodgkin's disease respond to vaccination as well as normal persons if they are vaccinated before treatment begins.[671,672] In patients with non-Hodgkin's lymphoma, antibody levels before vaccination tend to be lower than those of normal subjects or patients with Hodgkin's disease.[671–673] Once treatment begins, antibody responses to vaccination are reduced. In some patients, antibody levels fall below what they were before vaccination, and in others the response is delayed for several months. After completion of treatment, antibody levels may not return to pretreatment levels, and patients seldom respond to revaccination.[673] These findings indicate that they should be vaccinated as soon as possible after the diagnosis is established, before treatment begins.

Patients with multiple myeloma have low antibody levels before vaccination. After vaccination, antibody responses are poor, although a few patients respond to a few serotypes.[470,674] The capacity to respond does not correlate with the severity of the disease or the timing of chemotherapy, and antibody levels are seldom sustained. Prophylactic

IVIG (0.4 g/kg body weight monthly) given to stable multiple myeloma patients can provide significant protection against pneumonia and septicemia,[470] in spite of the rapid decline in antibody levels.

OTHER NEOPLASMS

Antibody responses of patients with nonhematologic neoplasms to pneumococcal vaccine have received little attention. In one small study, antibody levels after vaccinating patients with solid tumors were similar to those in healthy vaccinated controls.[675] Mild to moderate immunosuppressive treatment had minimal effect on their responses.

RENAL DISEASES

Children with nephrotic syndrome are at increased risk for serious pneumococcal infections, as are renal transplant and hemodialysis patients.[676] Patients with chronic renal disease, those on hemodialysis, and those who have received renal transplants[677] usually have good antibody responses to a first dose of pneumococcal vaccine, although levels may be lower than the levels seen in normal subjects.[678] Over the next 2 years, antibody levels decline markedly. Revaccination leads to modest increases in antibody levels, but they seldom reach those seen initially.[679] Children with nephrotic syndrome[680] and other chronic renal diseases[681] usually respond adequately to vaccination. Except in those with minimal change nephrotic syndrome or a history of relapse, however, antibody levels rapidly decline.[680] Revaccination 1 year later leads to good antibody responses in about half of renal disease patients, but levels decline rapidly over the next few months.[681]

BONE MARROW, CARDIAC, AND LIVER TRANSPLANTATIONS

Recipients of allogeneic bone marrow transplants are at increased risk of pneumococcal infections. Infection does not usually occur during the first 6 months after transplantation, probably because antibiotics are given to prevent *Pneumocystis carinii* pneumonia. Patients who develop pneumococcal infections have decreased IgG, IgG subclass, IgM, and type-specific antibodies and diminished serum opsonic activity.[682-684] Pneumococcal vaccination of matched sibling donors before transplantation does not increase antibody levels in transplant recipients.[684] If vaccine is given 6 months after transplantation or during corticosteroid treatment of graft-versus-host disease, antibody responses, especially IgG2 antibodies, are limited.[684-687] If vaccination is delayed until 12 months following transplantation or if two doses are given at 12 and 24 months, antibody responses are still poor.[688] Antibody levels do not return to pretransplantation levels until 1 to 2 years after transplantation. The slow return of IgG2 levels to normal and the poor response to pneumococcal vaccination is similar to the pattern of immunologic maturation of young children.[685,687] Prevention of pneumococcal infection during this interval depends on other measures such as antimicrobial prophylaxis.

In contrast to recipients of allogeneic bone marrow transplants, some patients who receive autologous transplants have normal levels of IgG2 antibodies to pneumococcal capsular polysaccharides and maintain these levels for at least 1 year after transplantation.[686] Nonetheless, most adults[689] and children[690] who are vaccinated 12 or more months after autologous transplantation have reduced antibody levels both before and after vaccination. For adults, this is true regardless of whether the stem cells are derived from peripheral blood or bone marrow.[689] In western Europe, most bone marrow transplant centers rely on antimicrobial prophylaxis to prevent pneumococcal infections.[691] Only 25% of centers that perform both types of transplants, and only 12% of those performing only autologous transplants administer pneumococcal vaccine to their patients.

Persons who receive cardiac and liver transplants are also at increased risk of pneumococcal infections.[692,693] One study of 31 cardiac and liver transplant patients who were given pneumococcal vaccine 4 to 85 months after transplantation showed that antibody responses to six of nine vaccine serotypes tested were similar to those of healthy controls.[694] However, two reports of older adults vaccinated 5 or more years after cardiac transplantation showed geometric mean antibody levels that were significantly reduced when compared with those of healthy, age-matched controls.[695] In patients who receive liver transplants, antibody levels fall below prevaccination levels 3 months later, probably as a result of immunosuppressive therapy. Although pneumococcal vaccine is not very immunogenic in these patients, it is well tolerated.[694]

Children with cardiac transplants are at increased risk of invasive pneumococcal disease.[696] When transplanted early in life, they respond poorly to pneumococcal vaccine compared with those who are transplanted when they are older. In younger children, azathioprine has an irreversible cytotoxic effect on B cells, whereas cyclosporine interrupts cytokine gene expression.[697] Defects in isotype switching from IgM to IgG also may contribute to the failure of these children to respond to vaccination.[698]

OTHER DISORDERS

Patients with systemic lupus erythematosus,[699-701] rheumatoid arthritis,[700] Felty's syndrome,[702] and celiac sprue[703] are at increased risk for pneumococcal infections, mainly because they have functional asplenia. Earlier studies of patients with systemic lupus erythematosus showed that antibody responses to pneumococcal vaccine were either normal or somewhat lower than those seen in normal subjects. Responses were not correlated with drug therapy, renal function, immunoglobulin levels, or disease activity. In a more recent study, pneumococcal vaccination of patients with systemic lupus erythematosus and rheumatoid arthritis did not increase disease activity, and antibody responses were good in some but not all patients.[700] Patients with celiac sprue respond normally to pneumococcal vaccine.[703]

Inherited deficiencies of the complement system are known to predispose to pneumococcal infections. One report of four patients with C3 deficiency noted that three were almost totally deficient in antibodies to pneumococcal capsular polysaccharides.[704] Only a few individuals with other types of complement deficiency had such defects. Whether C3-deficient patients respond normally to pneumococcal vaccine is not known.

Older persons with low serum vitamin B_{12} levels may have antibody responses to pneumococcal vaccination that are significantly lower than those of age-matched normal controls.[705] No clinical or epidemiologic data suggest that they are at increased risk of pneumococcal infection.

Vaccination in Pregnancy

The safety of pneumococcal vaccination in early pregnancy has not been determined.[474] There is no reason to expect that vaccination in the first trimester should have any adverse effect on fetal development, although it is preferable to vaccinate high-risk women before rather than during pregnancy. Vaccination during the third trimester, however, is well tolerated.[706–709]

Vaccinating women of child-bearing age before they become pregnant does not appear to result in increased levels of pneumococcal-specific antibodies at the time of later delivery, nor do their newborn infants have higher antibody levels than those of infants born of unvaccinated women.[710] Vaccinating women during the third trimester of pregnancy, however, could provide valuable protection against pneumococcal infections in their newborns infants.[708,709,711]

In developed countries, pneumococcal colonization of the female genital tract and maternal pneumococcal sepsis are very uncommon.[712–714] Pneumococcal bacteremia in newborns is rare, but case-fatality rates approach 50%.[712,714–717] The annual incidence of maternal pneumococcal bacteremia is approximately 4 cases per 100,000 persons,[718] and in neonates it is 4 to 6 cases per 100,000.[718,719] Rarely, concomitant infections of mother and infant with the same serotype organism have been observed.[714,720] In infants less than 6 months of age, S. pneumoniae is a common cause of bacterial sepsis and meningitis,[711] and otitis media is extremely common. Higher cord blood levels of antibodies to serotypes 3, 14, and 19F are associated with fewer episodes of otitis media during this period, and protection is better correlated with serum IgG1 than with IgG2 levels.[721,722]

Maternal immunization with pneumococcal vaccine is safe for newborn infants. Six clinical trials that were conducted in developing countries showed it had no effect on perinatal mortality, stillbirths, or prematurity.[723] A higher number of early neonatal deaths occurred in infants born to vaccinated mothers, but these deaths were considered unlikely to have been related to maternal immunization. Moreover, in developing countries, maternal antibody levels following vaccination in late pregnancy were higher than they were in women living in developed countries.[707,708]

Active transplacental transfer of pneumococcal IgG antibodies is well documented.[724–727] Even in infants born of unvaccinated mothers, serum IgG1 antibody levels may be slightly higher than maternal levels,[727] although this is not true for preterm and low-birth-weight infants.[727,728] When pregnant women are vaccinated in the third trimester, type-specific IgG antibody levels in cord blood are usually higher than levels in infants whose mothers have not been vaccinated.[706,707] However, serotype-specific cord blood IgG antibody levels show wide variation when compared with maternal levels. For example, in Papua New Guinea, infants born of women vaccinated during the third trimester had good antibody levels to serotypes 5, 14, and 23F, but poor antibody levels to serotype 7F.[709] In addition, several studies have shown that the half life of these anti-

bodies is little more than 1 month, and by 3 months antibody levels in children born of vaccinated and unvaccinated mothers are often similar.[706–709] Nonetheless, during the first 2 to 3 months of life, antibody levels to important serotypes such as 6B, 14, and 19F are often higher in infants born of vaccinated compared with unvaccinated mothers. Moreover, these infants have higher levels of opsonophagocytic antibodies to several pneumococcal serotypes.[708]

Maternal vaccination during the third trimester has been suggested as a way to confer protection on breast-fed newborns. In the postpartum period, unvaccinated women usually have measurable levels of breast milk antibodies to some pneumococcal serotypes that can be detected for as long as 5 months after delivery.[707] However, breast milk antibody levels are often low and not well correlated with rates of nasopharyngeal colonization or otitis media in breast-fed infants.[729] Nonetheless, a case-control study from Brazil suggested that infants who were breast-fed had a much lower risk of hospitalization for pneumonia than did those who were not.[730] In vaccinated women, levels of breast milk IgA antibodies to several serotypes are higher than they are in breast milk from unvaccinated mothers and may persist for at least 7 months.[708] These IgA antibodies may be important because half are IgA2 antibodies that are resistant to the protease activity of bacterial flora in the upper respiratory tract.[711]

Maternal immunization with pneumococcal polysaccharide vaccine does not affect the antibody responses of older infants who are given polysaccharide vaccine at 8 to 9 months in age; these infants respond as well as those born of unvaccinated mothers.[709]

Maternal immunization with pneumococcal polysaccharide vaccine is likely to be a clinically effective and perhaps also a cost-effective way to prevent serious pneumococcal infections in infants during the first 6 months of life. Clinical trials should be undertaken to confirm this, especially in developing countries.[723]

Revaccination

In the 1980s, revaccination with 14-valent pneumococcal vaccine was not recommended.[731–733] Unwillingness to recommend revaccination was based on a few small studies that reported frequent local Arthus-like reactions and systemic reactions when revaccination occurred within 1 to 2 years of primary vaccination. In later studies, however, revaccination of adults with 14-valent[734] or 23-valent[735–737] vaccine (especially 4 or more years after the initial dose) was associated with rates of local and systemic adverse reactions that were no more frequent or severe than what had been seen following primary vaccination. None of these earlier studies, however, directly compared adverse reactions following revaccination with those following primary vaccination.

A more recent comparative study has shown that revaccination is well tolerated.[738] Among 1514 subjects ages 50 to 74 years, 901 received 23-valent vaccine for the first time and 513 were revaccinated, in all cases 5 or more years following initial vaccination. Local and systemic adverse reactions in the two groups are summarized in Table 22–7. Revaccinated subjects experienced sizable local adverse reactions more frequently than primary vaccinees (11% vs.

TABLE 22–7 ■ Adverse Reactions Following Primary Vaccination or Revaccination with Pneumococcal Polysaccharide Vaccine*

Adverse Reactions	Days 0–2			Days 3–6		
	Primary (%)	Revaccination (%)	P value	Primary (%)	Revaccination (%)	P value
Local[†]						
Any tenderness at injection site	51	69	<.001	10	15	0.02
Severe arm soreness	2	5	0.01	1	0	—
Cannot raise arm above head	3	10	<.001	1	1	—
Cannot raise arm above shoulder	1	5	<.001	0	0	—
Systemic[‡]						
Myalgia	9	10	—	7	7	—
Temp ≥ 37.5°C	8	10	—	7	7	—
Temp ≥ 38.6°C	0.4	1	—	0.2	1	—

*Primary vaccination = 901 subjects; revaccination = 513 subjects.
[†]Very few local adverse reactions persisted more than 6 days, and after 6 days there were no significant differences ($P > 0.05$) between the two groups.
[‡]Other systemic adverse reactions evaluated were nausea, headache, arthralgia, and fatigue. For all systemic reactions there were no significant differences between the two groups.
Adapted from Jackson LA, Benson P, Sneller VP, et al. Safety of revaccination with pneumococcal polysaccharide vaccine. JAMA 281:243–248, 1999.

3%), but limitations in arm movement were modest and lasted only a few days. Local reactions tended to occur more frequently among those with higher levels of serum antibody before revaccination, a finding similar to what has been observed following primary vaccination.[479] Rates for systemic adverse reactions were similar in the two groups. In another study of revaccination in older adults, reactions serious enough to require hospitalization were not observed.[739]

After adults are revaccinated, increases in antibody levels to most serotypes are somewhat lower than those observed after primary vaccination.[510,735,738,740] In addition, no anamnestic response is seen. Thus a second dose of vaccine should not be considered a booster dose.

Revaccination is most strongly recommended for persons with surgical or functional asplenia. After primary vaccination, 50% or more of these patients experience a decline in antibody to prevaccination levels after 5 to 10 years.[740,741] Revaccination is well tolerated.[658,741,742] In patients with chronic renal disease, antibody levels following primary vaccination decline rapidly, especially in those who have had splenectomies.[679] Revaccination of these patients after only 2 years is also well tolerated.

In persons with HIV infection who were initially vaccinated within 1 year of HIV seroconversion and were revaccinated 5 or more years later, antibody responses were lower and less frequent than those in recently HIV-seroconverted patients after their first dose of vaccine.[743] The results are difficult to interpret, however, because the study was small and different antiretroviral treatments were used in the two study groups. Revaccination of HIV-infected individuals who have failed to respond to their initial dose of vaccine has no effect.[615]

Little is known about the long-term antibody persistence following pneumococcal revaccination. In one study of children and adolescents with sickle cell disease, antibody levels measured 3 to 7 years after revaccination were substantially lower than levels observed shortly after revaccination.[658] Except for postsplenectomy patients,[740] the clinical effectiveness of revaccination is unknown.

Pneumococcal Vaccine Efficacy and Vaccination Effectiveness

Definitions

The words *efficacy* and *effectiveness* are often used interchangeably, but they actually have different meanings.[744] For vaccine efficacy, the question asked is, "Does the vaccine work?" A prospective clinical trial is the most widely accepted method for evaluating whether a vaccine "works." The trial evaluates the vaccine's efficacy as a biologic product under conditions that optimize the chance of obtaining a positive result with the least amount of effort and expense. In contrast, effectiveness deals with a different question: "Does vaccination help people?" In other words, what benefits can be expected when an efficacious vaccine is used in routine clinical practice? Vaccination effectiveness is usually evaluated in a retrospective, observational study.

Pneumococcal polysaccharide vaccine is not a single vaccine; it is 23 individual vaccines. Consequently, any statement about its efficacy (or effectiveness) must be understood to indicate the aggregate efficacy of its 23 capsular polysaccharide antigens. Most monovalent vaccines have efficacies of 90% or greater. This level of protection is unlikely to be achieved with a 23-valent vaccine, as can be shown by the following example. Consider a person who lacks protective antibody to three pneumococcal serotypes and who therefore is at risk of infection resulting from any one of them. Assume the efficacy of each serotype capsular polysaccharide is 90%. Consider also that, if this person is vaccinated but later develops an infection resulting from one of these three serotypes, the vaccine as a whole is considered to lack protective efficacy. In this example, the aggregate efficacy of the vaccine can be calculated as a compound probability ($.9 \times .9 \times .9$) and will never be greater than 73%. In principle, the aggregate efficacy of pneumococcal vaccine could be calculated precisely by multiplying the point estimates of efficacy for all 23 polysaccharide antigens, adjusting for the relative frequency of infection caused by each individual capsular type. In practical terms, this would be extremely difficult to do and it has never been done. Nonetheless, the concept of aggregate efficacy or effectiveness is of fundamental importance for understanding the benefits that should be expected from pneumococcal polysaccharide vaccine. Unfortunately, this concept is often misunderstood, unappreciated, or simply not recognized.

The Carrier State

Studies conducted during outbreaks of pneumococcal disease in military camps during World War II showed a 50% reduction in nasopharyngeal carriage of S. pneumoniae in subjects given an experimental pneumococcal vaccine.[745] Later, long-term studies in nonoutbreak settings compared patterns of pneumococcal carriage before and after vaccination with 14-valent vaccine.[263,746–748] None showed a significant reduction in carrier rates among vaccinees or a shift among carriers in the distribution of vaccine-type and non–vaccine-type organisms. Because 14-valent vaccine did not appreciably affect nasopharyngeal carriage of pneumococci, similar studies with 23-valent vaccine have not been undertaken in normal subjects.

Vaccine Efficacy and Vaccination Effectiveness in Children

Several randomized controlled trials in the 1980s assessed the efficacy of 14-valent pneumococcal polysaccharide vaccine in preventing otitis media. In Australia, a study of 1158 healthy children showed no consistent differences between vaccinees and controls in the mean number of episodes of otitis media per child nor in rates for a variety of clinical signs and symptoms, restricted activity, physician visits, and hospital admissions.[749] These findings were observed in children 2 years of age or older as well as in those who were younger. Other studies in otitis-prone children younger than 2 years of age gave mixed results.[750–752] Considered together, these studies have been interpreted as showing the limited efficacy of pneumococcal vaccine in preventing otitis media in young children.

In contrast to its equivocal protection against otitis media, pneumococcal polysaccharide vaccine was shown to reduce mortality from acute lower respiratory tract infections that commonly affect children in developing countries.[748,753,754] In a study of more than 7000 children in Papua New Guinea, half of whom were immunized between 6 months and 5 years of age, pneumococcal vaccination reduced mortality by 59% in children of all ages (P = 0.008; 95% confidence interval [CI], 19% to 79%), and by 50% in children vaccinated at 2 years of age or younger (P = 0.043; 95% CI, 1% to 75%). However, vaccination was only marginally protective against moderate to severe disease and did not protect against mild illness.[754] More recently, investigators using an indirect cohort method showed that pneumococcal vaccination of children 2 to 5 years of age was 62% effective (95% CI, 35% to 78%) in preventing invasive pneumococcal disease due to vaccine serotypes.[755] Vaccination effectiveness was lower in children with sickle cell disease, perhaps as a result of concomitant antimicrobial prophylaxis.

Vaccine Efficacy and Vaccination Effectiveness in Adults

In the 1940s, clinical trials established the efficacy of experimental trivalent and tetravalent pneumococcal polysac-charide vaccines in preventing pneumococcal pneumonia and bacteremia in military recruits.[745] In the same decade, clinical trials of 2- and 3-valent polysaccharide vaccines conducted among residents of a long-term care facility also showed reductions in the occurrence of vaccine-type pneumococcal bacteremia and pneumococcal pneumonia.[756] Reductions also were seen, however, in non–vaccine-type illness.

Evidence of the efficacy of modern pneumococcal vaccines emerged in the early 1970s from prospective randomized controlled trials conducted among novice gold miners in South Africa.[23,24] These young men experienced very high rates of pneumococcal disease, ensuring that clinical trials with several thousand subjects would yield definitive results. In one of these studies, the efficacy of a 13-valent pneumococcal vaccine was shown to be 82% against vaccine-type pneumococcal bacteremia, 78.5% against vaccine-type bacteremia and pneumonia combined, and approximately 53% against clinical pneumonia confirmed by chest radiograph, irrespective of microbial cause.[24] In addition to providing unequivocal evidence of vaccine efficacy, the trials also showed that a reduction in vaccine-type disease was not accompanied by replacement disease caused by non–vaccine-type S. pneumoniae or other microorganisms. Another clinical trial of 14-valent vaccine was carried out in Papua New Guinea.[460] Among 5273 adults, pneumococcal vaccine reduced the occurrence of definite pneumococcal pneumonia (blood and/or lung aspirate culture positive) by 90% (2 vs. 14 cases; P < 0.005) and clinically and radiologically diagnosed pneumonia by 25% (36 vs. 48 cases; P > 0.05). Among all 11,950 adults studied, pneumonia mortality was reduced by 44% (23 vs. 41 cases; P < 0.05) and total mortality was reduced by 22% (130 vs. 179 cases; P < 0.05).

Pneumococcal vaccine was first licensed in the United States on the basis of the results of the efficacy trials conducted in South Africa. However, the vaccine was intended for use primarily in elderly and high-risk adults. Because there were no data from efficacy trials in older persons, a number of postlicensure clinical trials were undertaken. Ten separate prospective clinical trials were conducted in these groups.[757–765] One randomized controlled trial also was undertaken in HIV-infected adults in Uganda.[453] The results of these 11 trials have been discussed in several reviews,[18,277,766–770] and they have been the subject of five published meta-analyses.[771–775] The primary focus in almost all of these studies has been to determine the efficacy of pneumococcal vaccine in preventing pneumococcal pneumonia. The overall conclusion of the investigators has been that pneumococcal vaccine is not protective. Others who have considered the evidence regard these studies as inconclusive.

The investigators who conducted the clinical trials in older individuals encountered numerous methodologic problems. Three of the trials were small immunogenicity and safety studies and cannot be regarded as serious efforts to evaluate vaccine efficacy in preventing clinical disease.[760–762] In the late 1970s, Austrian conducted two clinical trials, one among residents of a long-term care institution and the other among enrollees of a managed care organization in California.[757] Approximately one third of the subjects in each trial were 65 years of age or older.

Neither study showed that pneumococcal vaccine was protective. In France, an open, randomized clinical trial was conducted among 1686 residents of 48 long-term care institutions.[758] The investigators concluded that 14-valent pneumococcal vaccine significantly reduced the occurrence of all pneumonias, yet their randomization process generated study groups of surprisingly uneven size (933 vs. 749), clinical follow-up by the more than 80 study physicians was highly variable, and approximately one third of subjects enrolled in the two study groups either died or were lost to follow-up. In the Veterans Administration Cooperative Study, investigators were unable to demonstrate the efficacy of 14-valent vaccine in preventing pneumococcal pneumonia.[759] There were important differences in the two study groups, however: significantly more vaccinated subjects had previous histories of pneumococcal pneumonia and significantly more died of all causes during the follow-up period. Moreover, almost half of all diagnosed outcomes were pneumococcal bronchitis, a condition for which no investigator has suggested pneumococcal vaccine offers protection.

Three clinical trials were reported from Finland[763,765] and Sweden[764] in the late 1990s. One of the Finnish studies evaluated 14-valent vaccine during the period from 1982 to 1985.[763] Investigators found that vaccine prevented pneumococcal pneumonia only in elderly persons with underlying medical risk conditions (vaccine efficacy = 59%; 95% CI, 6% to 82%), but not in all elderly persons studied (vaccine efficacy = 15%; 95% CI, –43% to 50%). Vaccine also was not protective when all episodes of pneumonia were considered. A larger and more recent Finnish trial randomized subjects by year of birth.[765] Investigators found that 23-valent vaccine did not reduce the occurrence of pneumococcal pneumonia or all pneumonia. The clinical trial of 23-valent vaccine in Sweden was conducted among persons who had been hospitalized previously for pneumonia.[764] Like the two Finnish studies, it too failed to show that vaccination prevented pneumococcal pneumonia. In each of these three clinical trials, most cases of pneumococcal pneumonia were diagnosed by demonstrating antibody to pneumolysin in circulating immune complexes. This method is known to give false-positive diagnoses.[169,170]

Six clinical trials included pneumococcal bacteremia as a study outcome.[758–761,764,765] Two showed fewer cases of bacteremic disease in vaccinated compared with control subjects,[764,765] but none showed that vaccine provided a statistically significant degree of protection.

The prospective clinical trials have been criticized for many reasons, but one criticism that applies to all of them is that their sample sizes were too small. This issue was recently examined quantitatively.[776] The analysis was based on the proposition that it is possible to determine whether a clinical trial was large enough by using the rate of outcome events observed in the control group during the trial period to calculate retrospectively the number of trial subjects (i.e., person-years of observation) that would have been needed to rule out a false-negative result.[777] In this analysis, only two conditions—pneumococcal bacteremia and all pneumonia—were considered valid study outcomes because of the uncertainties about the diagnosis of individual cases of pneumococcal pneumonia and other trial endpoints.[776] Calculations assumed vaccine efficacies of 50% and 70% for pneumococcal bacteremia (all serotypes) and

15% and 25% for all pneumonia. (If 30% or 50% of all pneumonias are due to pneumococcal infections and if vaccine efficacy is 50%, vaccine efficacy in preventing all pneumonia will be 15% or 25%.) The results of this analysis are summarized in Table 22–8. They show that, for each trial, the number of person-years of observation in the vaccine and control groups was far smaller than the number needed to rule out a false-negative result for reasonable levels of vaccine efficacy. The findings provide convincing evidence that, given their sample sizes, the prospective clinical trials were destined to be inconclusive.

When the results of several clinical trials are inconclusive, investigators often perform a meta-analysis. By pooling the results of the individual trials, they hope to assemble a study population that is large enough to give a definitive result. Nonetheless, a meta-analysis, like a clinical trial, cannot avoid the requirement for an adequate sample size. The retrospective sample size approach described above also was used to analyze the results of five published meta-analyses that have evaluated pneumococcal polysaccharide vaccine. Results in Table 22–8 show that for preventing pneumococcal bacteremia, none of the five meta-analyses was able to rule out false-negative results for vaccine efficacies of of 50% and 70%. In addition, for preventing all pneumonia, none could rule out a false-negative result for a vaccine efficacy of 15%.

The five published meta-analyses differed from each other in many ways. No two studies assembled the same groups of clinical trials for analysis. Each meta-analysis contained miscounts of the numbers of subjects and/or the numbers of episodes of outcome events in some of the trials that were analyzed. A substantial proportion of pneumonia episodes in the clinical trials affected persons living in institutions, not the community. In four of the meta-analyses,[771,772,774,775] only two thirds of study subjects could be considered to represent immunocompetent community-dwelling elderly and high-risk adults, yet approximately 95% of elderly persons targeted for pneumococcal vaccination live in the community. The remaining meta-analysis[773] excluded several trials that should have been analyzed, but included the trial of untreated HIV-infected younger adults in Uganda that should have been excluded. For all meta-analyses, there was no way to determine what proportion of pneumonia episodes were managed as outpatients; although 30% to 50% of cases of adult community-acquired pneumonia that require hospitalization are probably caused by S. pneumoniae, the proportion of outpatient pneumonia cases that are pneumococcal in origin is not known. None of the five meta-analyses evaluated the adequacy of the sample sizes for the individual trials or for the meta-analysis. For these and other reasons,[776] the meta-analyses do not provide firm evidence that pneumococcal vaccine fails to prevent pneumococcal pneumonia (in other words, cases of nonbacteremic as well as bacteremic disease) in populations of community-dwelling elderly and high-risk adults for whom the vaccine is primarily intended.

One randomized controlled trial of 23-valent vaccine was conducted in untreated HIV-infected adults in Uganda.[453] Investigators found that vaccine did not prevent cases of invasive pneumococcal disease and that cases of all-cause pneumonia were actually more frequent in vaccinated

TABLE 22-8 ■ Retrospective Calculation of Sample Sizes Required to Rule Out False-Negative Results in Prospective Clinical Trials and Meta-Analyses of Pneumococcal Vaccine in Elderly and High-Risk Adults*

Principal Investigator (Reference)	Unadjusted RR†		Person-Years of Observation in Both Vaccine and Control Groups					
			Pneumococcal Bacteremia			All Pneumonia		
	Pneumococcal Bacteremia	All Pneumonia	Approximate No. During the Clinical Trial	Retrospective Sample Size Requirement		Approximate No. During the Clinical Trial	Retrospective Sample Size Requirement	
				VE = 50%	VE = 70%		VE = 15%	VE = 25%
Clinical Trials								
Austrian-1[757]	—‡	1.30§	—	—	—	2913	13,400	4700
Austrian-2[757]	—	.98	—	—	—	34,462	118,000	28,000
Gaillat[758]	nd	.20¶	3372	147,300	70,000	3372	58,000	25,000
Simberkoff[759]	2.01	1.39	6656	340,000	157,300	6656	87,400	37,600
Koivula[763]	—	1.13	7944	—	—	7944	54,600	30,000
Örtqvist[764]	.21	1.18	1666	17,200	8200	1666	18,100	6800
Honkanen[765]	.37	1.16	64,000	638,000	295,000	38,037	175,700	75,550
Meta-Analyses								
Fine[771]	1.23	.73	10,650	170,000	76,600	10,603	102,700	44,400
Hutchison[772]	1.22	—	10,377	170,000	78,600	—	—	—
Moore[773]	.51	1.01	2009	17,200	8200	16,841	56,200	13,400
Cornu[774]	.35	1.02	11,741	72,800	32,100	23,826	47,000	20,200
Watson[775]	.46	1.00	43,697	176,000	79,400	95,625	118,000	28,000

*The table excludes three smaller clinical trials of Klastersky et al.,[760] Leech et al.,[761] and Davis et al.,[762] and the trial of French et al.[453] that was conducted in HIV-1–infected patients in Uganda. Retrospective calculations of the sample size requirements for these four trials indicated that each trial was not large enough to rule out false negative results for the vaccine efficacies (VEs) shown in the table.

†Unadjusted relative risk (RR). The 95% confidence intervals (95% CI) of the RRs were not statistically significant unless otherwise indicated.

‡Not studied.

§95% CI = 1.13 to 1.48.

||Not done because there was no case of pneumococcal bacteremia in the vaccine group.

¶95% CI = 0.09 to 0.46.

subjects than in controls (adjusted first-event analysis, hazard ratio = 2.02; 95% CI, 1.19 to 3.45). This finding suggested to the investigators that pneumococcal vaccine was harmful. Yet the hazard ratio describing the difference between vaccine and control subjects was lower for invasive disease, a specific outcome, than it was for all pneumonia, a less specific outcome.[778] In addition, all-cause mortality rates were the same (28%) in the two study groups over the 18-month study period.

A large-scale community vaccination program was reported from Stockholm County.[779] In the fall of 1998, all persons 65 years of age or older were offered influenza and pneumococcal vaccines and approximately 40% accepted one or both. During the first 6 months of follow-up, vaccinated individuals had 29% fewer hospital admissions for all-cause pneumonia (95% CI, 24% to 34%) and 52% fewer admissions for invasive pneumococcal disease (95% CI, 1% to 77%). The investigators, however, did not report results for pneumococcal vaccine alone, nor did they adjust for differences in the distribution of risk factors between vaccinated and unvaccinated subjects. In the absence of risk adjustment, it is difficult to know whether pneumococcal vaccine contributed to the apparent protection seen in vaccinated individuals.

Because randomized controlled trials of pneumococcal vaccine in older high-risk adults are difficult to conduct, investigators have turned to observational studies to evaluate the clinical effectiveness of pneumococcal vaccination.[780,781] Six case-control studies have been reported (Table 22–9).[782–787] In each, pneumococcal bacteremia, not pneumococcal pneumonia, was the outcome evaluated. The Philadelphia[784] and Charlottesville[786] studies showed vaccination effectiveness rates of 70% and 81%, respectively.

Vaccination effectiveness rates in the New Haven[782] and Connecticut[785] studies were lower. The Oxford study has been reported only as an abstract, and full details are awaited.[787] Failure to demonstrate clinical effectiveness in the Denver study[783] was likely due to incomplete ascertainment of the vaccination status of study subjects and possible bias in the selection of controls.[767]

The most convincing case-control study was reported from Connecticut.[785] In this study the aggregate effectiveness of pneumococcal vaccination in preventing pneumococcal bacteremia caused by vaccine and vaccine-related serotype organisms was 56%, and it was 47% effective in preventing all pneumococcal bacteremias, regardless of serotype (see Table 22–9). In a subset of 175 immunocompromised patients, clinical effectiveness against vaccine and vaccine-related serotype infection was only 21% (95% CI, −55% to 60%). However, in the remaining 808 immunocompetent patients (82% of all patients studied), vaccination was 61% protective (95% CI, 47% to 72%). The effectiveness of vaccination declined with increasing patient age and time since vaccination. Nonetheless, in immunocompetent patients ages 65 to 74 years, vaccination effectiveness over a 5-year period was 71% (95% CI, 30% to 88%), and for those 75 to 84 years of age its effectiveness over 3 years was 67% (95% CI, 20% to 87%). Not surprisingly, vaccination was not effective in preventing pneumococcal bacteremia caused by non–vaccine-type organisms (see Table 22–9).

The effectiveness of pneumococcal vaccination also has been assessed using an indirect cohort method.[788,789] The method assumes that, if pneumococcal vaccination is effective, fewer illnesses caused by vaccine-type organisms will occur in vaccinated compared with unvaccinated persons,

TABLE 22–9 ▪ Clinical Effectiveness of Pneumococcal Vaccination in Preventing Invasive Pneumococcal Disease in Observational Studies Conducted in Older Adults*

Type of Infection	Location	Number of Cases/Controls	Vaccination Effectiveness		Reference
			%	95% CI	
All serotypes	Oxford	247/247	32	−26 to 63	787
	Connecticut	1054/1054	47	30 to 59	785
	Seattle	—†	44	7 to 67	792
	Toronto	—‡	63	13 to 85	789
	New Haven	90/90	67	13 to 87	782
	Philadelphia	122/244	70	37 to 86	784
	Charlottesville	85/152	81	34 to 94	786
Vaccine type ± VT-related	Denver	—§	−21	−221 to 55	783
	Connecticut	983/983	56	42 to 67	785
	CDC	—‖	57	45 to 66	788
Non VT ± VT-related	Connecticut	170/170	−73	−263 to 18	785

*The results of a case-control study conducted in Alaska were reported in a letter (Davidson M, Parkinson AJ, Bulkow LR, et al. Epidemiology of invasive pneumococcal disease—reply. J Infect Dis 171:1065–1066, 1995) and were cited in the third edition of this chapter. The full results of this study have never been published, however, and they have been deleted from the table in this edition.
†Retrospective cohort study of 47,365 subjects 65 years or older in age followed for 3 years. The Cox proportional hazard model controlled for age, sex, smoking, immunosuppression, other high-risk conditions, nursing home residency, outpatient visits and hospital admission in the previous year, and receipt of influenza vaccine. Pneumococcal vaccination was a time-dependent variable. Vaccination effectiveness in immunocompetent persons was 54% (95% CI, 13% to 76%).
‡Indirect cohort study based on surveillance of a population of 3.1 million persons in 1995. Vaccination effectiveness in immunocompetent persons was 89% (95% CI, 59% to 97%).
§Indirect cohort study that evaluated 26 vaccinated and 63 unvaccinated subjects.
‖Indirect cohort study that evaluated 515 vaccinated and 2322 unvaccinated subjects.
CI, confidence interval; VT, vaccine-type pneumococcal infection; CDC, Centers for Disease Control and Prevention.

whereas infections caused by non–vaccine-type organisms will occur with equal frequency in both groups. Using 14 years of data from a nationwide surveillance program, CDC investigators showed that pneumococcal vaccine was 57% effective in preventing bacteremic disease caused by vaccine-type organisms (see Table 22–9).[788] Moreover, vaccination was effective in preventing bacteremia in persons with diabetes mellitus (vaccination effectiveness = 84%; 95% CI, 50% to 95%), coronary vascular disease (vaccination effectiveness = 73%; 95% CI, 23% to 90%), congestive heart failure (vaccination effectiveness = 69%; 95% CI, 17% to 88%), and chronic pulmonary disease (vaccination effectiveness = 65%; 95% CI, 14% to 95%). In all immunocompetent persons 65 years of age or older, it was 75% protective (95% CI, 57% to 85%). The Connecticut investigators also validated the indirect cohort method using data from their case-control study.[785] In immunocompetent adults, the 62% effectiveness (95% CI, 24% to 81%) determined by the indirect cohort method was virtually the same as the 61% effectiveness shown in the case-control study.

Two observational studies have used a retrospective cohort approach to analyze the large administrative data sets of managed care organizations.[790–792] The Seattle study showed that pneumococcal vaccination was 43% effective in preventing pneumococcal bacteremia (all serotypes in all study subjects), but it did not reduce hospital admissions for pneumonia (see Table 22–9).[792] The Minneapolis study focused on patients with COPD and showed that, during the influenza season, pneumococcal vaccination helped to reduce hospitalizations for all pneumonia and reduce all-cause mortality.[790] Protection afforded by pneumococcal vaccination was in addition to that of influenza vaccination and continued during the noninfluenza season.

Observational studies also have shown that pneumococcal vaccination benefits adults with HIV infection. CDC investigators reported findings from a case-control study of invasive pneumococcal disease.[605] After adjusting for race, smoking, close contact with children, and CD4+ cell count, they found that pneumococcal vaccination was 76% effective in white subjects (95% CI, 35% to 91%) but not effective in blacks (vaccination effectiveness = 24%; 95% CI, −50% to 61%). There was no ready explanation for the racial difference observed. Three additional case-control studies[604,793,794] and two retrospective cohort studies[795,796] also showed that pneumococcal vaccination was 60% to 70% protective in HIV-infected individuals with higher CD4+ cell counts. None of these studies showed that giving pneumococcal vaccine to HIV-infected patients was harmful. In a preliminary report of case-control study, pneumococcal vaccination was 21% effective in preventing invasive disease in Navaho adults, a result that was not statistically significant.[794a]

Many observers have been reluctant to accept the results of observational studies on the effectiveness of pneumococcal vaccination. It is important, however, to recognize that there is neither a theoretical nor an empirical justification for regarding observational studies as inferior to randomized controlled trials simply because, in the absence of an experimental design, they cannot account for unrecognized differences between cases and controls.[277,776,797] Observational studies that are well conducted give results that are comparable to and no more variable than those of prospective clinical trials. The results of both types of studies, if properly conducted, should be regarded as complementary. The findings from well-conducted observational studies convincingly show that pneumococcal vaccination is effective in preventing invasive pneumococcal disease in immunocompetent older adults, many of whom have high-risk conditions. In spite of this evidence, many observers, basing their conclusions solely on the results of prospective clinical trials, still believe that pneumococcal vaccine lacks efficacy in older individuals.[766,771,773–775,798–801a] Yet the prospective clinical trials and their meta-analyses have had numerous methodologic problems, including study populations that were too small. Furthermore, the failure to demonstrate that pneumococcal vaccination prevents nonbacteremic as well as bacteremic pneumococcal pneumonia does not diminish the public health importance of using pneumococcal vaccine to prevent bacteremic or invasive pneumococcal disease.[802,802a]

Cost-Effectiveness of Pneumococcal Vaccination

When 14-valent pneumococcal polysaccharide vaccine was first licensed, the U.S. Congress Office of Technology Assessment (OTA) evaluated its cost-effectiveness in preventing pneumococcal pneumonia in elderly persons.[803] When 23-valent pneumococcal vaccine became available, the OTA re-evaluated its earlier study.[804] The results compared very favorably with the cost-effectiveness of other preventive, screening, and treatment interventions for elderly persons.[804,805] Other investigators also examined the cost-effectiveness of pneumococcal vaccination for preventing pneumococcal pneumonia in the United States,[806] the Netherlands,[807,808] Belgium,[809] and Spain.[810,811] Each study demonstrated that vaccinating elderly persons would be similarly cost-effective.

Acceptance of the earlier findings on cost-effectiveness was limited by uncertainty about the efficacy of pneumococcal vaccine in preventing pneumococcal pneumonia.[766,771,773–775,798–800,812] For this reason, it was suggested that the cost-effectiveness of vaccination to prevent pneumococcal bacteremia alone should be evaluated.[802] One such study was reported for the United States,[813,814] another for five countries in western Europe,[407] and a third for France.[815] In each study, investigators used the most recent data on the incidence of invasive pneumococcal disease in the elderly[13,387] and the best available evidence on the clinical effectiveness of vaccination.[785] The analyses showed that pneumococcal vaccination of elderly persons to prevent pneumococcal bacteremia alone would be cost-saving in the United States and very cost-effective in western Europe (Table 22–10).

In the United States, the cost-effectiveness of pneumococcal vaccination is comparable to or considerably better than that of a large number of medical and surgical interventions widely used in the care of older adults.[804,816] Vaccination has been found to be cost-effective when vaccine is given in nontraditional settings[817,818] or administered to active-duty military personnel.[819] A Canadian study has shown that it would be cost-effective for HIV-infected individuals.[820] Importantly, a study in western Europe has shown that the cost-effectiveness of vaccinating older adults is greatly improved if, in addition to preventing cases of bacteremic pneumococcal pneumonia, vaccination prevents only a small portion (10% to 20%) of all cases of nonbacteremic pneumococcal pneumonia.[821]

TABLE 22–10 ■ Cost-Effectiveness of Pneumococcal Vaccination to Prevent Invasive Pneumococcal Disease

Country	Cost-Effectiveness Ratio (US $)*
United States[†]	Cost saving
Belgium[‡]	6530
Scotland[‡]	6370
France[‡]	4395
Spain[‡]	4310
Sweden[‡]	3860

*Cost to gain one quality-adjusted life-year in the population. Costs in European currency units were converted to dollars; 1.18 ecus = US $1.00, January 1995.

[†]From Sisk et al.[813] Disease incidence was assumed to be 57 cases per 100,000 persons 65 years of age or older and the case-fatality rate was assumed to be 29%.

[‡]From Ament et al.[407] Disease incidence was assumed to be 50 cases per 100,000 persons 65 years of age or older and the case-fatality rate was assumed to be 30%.

Vaccine Failure

Not everyone who receives pneumococcal polysaccharide vaccine will be protected against serious pneumococcal infection; the 23-valent vaccine does not cover approximately 10% of the serotypes responsible for invasive disease, and persons at greatest risk are usually those with the poorest antibody responses to vaccination. Published reports of vaccine failure have focused on postsplenectomy patients[822] and those with immunocompromise,[873] HIV infection,[616,824] or alcoholism.[825,826] In some persons with vaccine failure, infections have been caused by serotypes that are relatively weak vaccine antigens (e.g., types 6B, 19F, and 23F). Even among fully immunocompetent individuals, some are unable to mount antibody responses to more than a few individual serotypes.[552] In those who do respond, antibody levels may decline so that protection present 1 year after vaccination is no longer present after 5 years. In the absence of information about what antibody levels ensure protection against infection by individual serotypes, it is difficult to draw meaningful conclusions about relationships between serologic responses to vaccination and vaccine failure.

Public Health Considerations

Immunization Policies and Vaccine Use

Recommendations and Reimbursement for Pneumococcal Polysaccharide Vaccination

THE UNITED STATES

The Advisory Committee on Immunization Practices (ACIP) strongly recommends vaccination for all persons 65 years of age or older and for those between 2 and 65 years of age who are at increased risk for serious pneumococcal infection (Table 22–11).[474] Persons with functional or anatomic asplenia (e.g., sickle cell disease and postsplenectomy patients) should be informed that fulminant pneumococcal disease has a high mortality rate and should be vaccinated. When possible, pneumococcal vaccine should be given 2 weeks before elective splenectomy. Vaccination does not ensure complete protection, so any unexplained febrile illness requires prompt medical evaluation and treatment if pneumococcal bacteremia is suspected. It is prudent for asplenic individuals to carry a 12- to 24-hour supply of an oral antibiotic active against S. pneumoniae and to begin self-treatment if prompt access to medical care is unavailable.

TABLE 22–11 ■ Recommendations for Pneumococcal Polysaccharide Vaccination and Revaccination in the United States, 1997

Vaccination*	Revaccination
IMMUNOCOMPETENT PERSONS ≥2 YR OF AGE	
≥65 yr of age	Once if vaccinated before 65 yr of age and vaccine was given more than 5 yr previously
≤65 yr with	
Functional or anatomic asplenia	Once after 5 yr if >10 yr of age; if ≤10 yr, consider revaccination after 3 yr
Chronic cardiovascular or pulmonary disease, diabetes mellitus, alcoholism and chronic liver disease, cerebrospinal fluid leaks, and persons living in special environments or social settings (e.g., Alaskan Natives, American Indians)	Not routinely recommended
IMMUNOCOMPROMISED PERSONS ≥2 YR OF AGE	
HIV infection, congenital immunodeficiency, leukemia, lymphoma, Hodgkin's disease, multiple myeloma, generalized malignancy, immunosuppressive or corticosteriod therapy, chronic renal failure, and organ or bone marrow transplantation	Once after 5 yr
Nephrotic syndrome	If ≤10 yr of age, consider revaccination after 3 yr

*If previous vaccination status is unknown, pneumococcal vaccine should be given.

Adapted from Centers for Disease Control and Prevention. Prevention of pneumococcal disease: recommendations of the Advisory Committee on Immunization Practices (ACIP). MMWR 46(RR-8): 1–24, 1997.

The ACIP recommends that adults should review their vaccination status at 50 years of age to determine whether they have one or more high-risk conditions[474]; among those 50 to 64 years of age, at least 36% will have cardiovascular conditions and 12% will have pulmonary conditions that are indications for pneumococcal vaccination.[827] Persons living in nursing homes and chronic care facilities and those who live in homeless shelters should be vaccinated because outbreaks of pneumococcal disease have occurred in these settings.[335,828–830] Pneumococcal vaccine is not recommended for children in day care or for those with recurrent upper respiratory tract disease, otitis media, and sinusitis.

Pneumococcal vaccination is recommended for immunocompromised persons because of their increased risk of disease.[474] Vaccination is safe and its cost is low, but many of these patients are likely to derive little if any benefit. Persons with HIV infection should be vaccinated as soon as the diagnosis is confirmed. Persons who are being considered for immunosuppressive therapy should be vaccinated at least 2 weeks before treatment begins or, if this is not possible, 3 months after treatment stops because the antibody response to vaccination during or shortly after chemotherapy or radiation therapy is poor.

In the United States, routine revaccination with 23-valent pneumococcal vaccine is not recommended (see Table 22–11).[481] It is contraindicated for anyone who has experienced a severe reaction to a first dose of pneumococcal vaccine. Revaccination once is recommended for persons 65 years of age or older who were vaccinated more than 5 years before reaching the age of 65. It is also recommended for those with functional or anatomic asplenia and those who are immunocompromised. Revaccination after 3 years should be considered for children 10 years of age or younger with asplenia or conditions associated with a rapid decline in antibody levels. The clinical effectiveness of revaccination and the need for additional doses are unknown; thus a second revaccination is not recommended. Although many persons have received three or more doses of pneumococcal vaccine, there is no information on the safety of repeated revaccination.

Reimbursement for the cost of pneumococcal vaccine and its administration is provided by the federal government to all persons enrolled in the Medicare program, most of whom are 65 years of age or older.[474] Reimbursement for younger persons with high-risk conditions is sometimes provided by managed care organizations and private health insurance.

OTHER DEVELOPED COUNTRIES

Current (2002) recommendations for pneumococcal vaccination vary among developed countries. Many countries did not register the 23-valent vaccine or issue national recommendations until the 1990s (Table 22–12).[831] Not all developed countries have national recommendations, but, among those that do, all include persons with functional or anatomic asplenia and almost all include those with chronic cardiopulmonary diseases, diabetes mellitus, and conditions associated with immunocompromise.[831] Several countries that recommend vaccinating certain high-risk individuals, however, do not recommend vaccinating elderly persons above a certain age. In the United Kingdom,

France, Switzerland, Portugal, Finland, and The Netherlands. National recommendations are not issued in Italy and Spain; instead, they are the responsibility of regional governments. Thus far, only a few regions in Italy and a few autonomous communities in Spain have recommended vaccinating all elderly persons. Unlike the United States, several other countries (Belgium, France, and Germany) recommend routine revaccination every 3 to 5 years for all persons covered by their national recommendations (D. S. Fedson, unpublished observations).[832]

A substantial number of countries do not provide reimbursement for pneumococcal vaccination by national or social health insurance (see Table 22–12). In some countries, partial reimbursement is provided or full reimbursement or free vaccine is available in a few communities. Most persons in these countries who wish to be vaccinated must pay for it themselves.

Use of Pneumococcal Polysaccharide Vaccine

THE UNITED STATES

As many as 50 million persons in the United States are candidates for pneumococcal vaccination, including more than 33 million who are 65 years of age or older. During the 14-year period from 1978 through 1991, approximately 23 million doses of pneumococcal vaccine were distributed nationwide.[293] During the 5-year period from 1992 through 1996, an additional 23 million doses were distributed,[831] and approximately 28 million doses were distributed from 1997 through 2000 (R. A. Strikas, personal communication, 2001). Data from the CDC's Behavioral Risk Factor Surveillance Study showed that, in 1997, 46% of persons 65 years of age or older had been vaccinated with pneumococcal vaccine.[434,833] Vaccination rates were higher in whites (47%) than in Hispanics (34%) or African-Americans (30%). Among elderly urban-dwelling Native Americans, coverage was only 21%,[834] and in persons with diabetes mellitus it was only 33%.[835] Vaccination rates tended to be higher in persons with more education, a recent physician visit, and self-reported health problems.[434,836] Substantial geographic variation in vaccination coverage was reported among the 50 states (range, 32% to 59%), and regional surveys showed coverage rates in the same range.[837,838] Variations of greater magnitude have been reported among individual physician practices.[839]

Surveys of pneumococcal vaccine coverage in the United States are reliable and, if anything, tend to underestimate coverage levels: The sensitivity of self-reported vaccination is .90 and the specificity is .64.[840] Among elderly persons who have not been vaccinated, the most important reason is not knowing about the vaccine.[841] This is largely due to the failure of physicians to recommend vaccination. In the late 1980s, a CDC study showed that, regardless of whether elderly persons had positive or negative attitudes toward pneumococcal vaccination, the recommendation of a health care provider determined whether an individual was vaccinated: If vaccination was not recommended, only 5% to 7% were immunized, whereas, if it was recommended, 63% to 84% were immunized.[842] Similar findings were reported a decade later.[837,843] Cost was rarely a reason for not being vaccinated.[841]

TABLE 22–12 ■ Pneumococcal Vaccination in 22 Developed Countries: Relationship Between Vaccine Registration, Recommendations, Reimbursement, Disease Incidence, Health Economic Studies, and Vaccine Distribution

Country	Year 23-Valent Vaccine Registered*	Age-Based Vaccination Recommendation for Elderly Adults*	Public Reimbursement Available*	Reported Annual Incidence of Invasive Pneumococcal Disease per 100,000 Elderly Adults[†]	Health Economic Studies Published Before Vaccine Was Introduced[‡]	Cumulative No. of Doses Distributed per 10,000 Population, 1996–2000[§]
Belgium	1995	Yes	—[‖]	36	Yes	661
United Kingdom	1989	—[¶]	Yes	36	—**	597
Iceland	—[††]	Yes	—	64	—	541
Norway	1996	Yes	—	62	—	528
Sweden	1984	Yes	—	41	—	476
Germany	1984	Yes	Yes	—	—	439
Ireland	1985	Yes	(Yes)[‡‡]	—	—	357
Austria	1995	Yes	—	—	—	344
Spain	—	(Yes)	(Yes)	57	Yes	300
Denmark	1996	Yes	—	64	—	237
France	1983	—	Yes	31	—	171
Greece	1998	Yes	Yes	—	—	124
Switzerland	1983	Yes	—	—	—	121
Luxembourg	1995	Yes	—	—	—	121
Italy	1992	(Yes)	(Yes)	—	—	83
Portugal	—	—	—	—	—	58
Finland	1984	Yes	—	27	Yes	36
Netherlands	1984	—	—	63	Yes	19
United States	1983	Yes	Yes	60	Yes	1300
Canada	1983	Yes	Yes	63	—	1169
Australia	1996	Yes	(Yes)	25	—	906
New Zealand	1984	Yes	—	—	—	50

*Data from D. S. Fedson (ref. 831 and unpublished observations).
[†]See Table 22–5.
[‡]D. S. Fedson, unpublished observations.
[§]See Figure 22–5.
[‖]No reimbursement for vaccination of recommended groups by national or social health insurance.
[¶]No age-based vaccination recommendation for elderly adults.
**No health economic studies published.
[††]Vaccine registration is not required in Iceland.
[‡‡]Parentheses indicate age-based recommendation or public reimbursement applies to some but not all regions or individuals in the country.

Most physicians in the United States recognize which patients are at risk for pneumococcal infection and understand the benefits of pneumococcal vaccination.[836] Little is known, however, about the vaccination practices of office-based physicians who are responsible for giving most vaccinations. Some still have doubts about the efficacy of the vaccine and the groups for whom it is recommended, but more often they overlook vaccination because they are focused on other, more immediate problems. In outpatient settings, substantial improvements in vaccination rates have followed the introduction of educational programs and reminder/recall systems for patients and of interventions that remind physicians to vaccinate.[844–849] Improvements in coverage also have been reported for community-based delivery programs,[850–852] and vaccination in such nontraditional settings is safe and well accepted.[853] In almost every instance, higher coverage rates have been achieved with administrative and organizational changes in the way vaccination is offered.[854,855] Nurses, pharmacists, and other health care providers have contributed to these efforts,[844,856]

and standing orders for vaccine delivery by nonphysicians have been especially important. [838,844,855] In many instances, pneumococcal vaccination has been incorporated into yearly programs for influenza vaccination without causing any falloff in the delivery of influenza vaccine.[857]

One often overlooked setting for pneumococcal vaccination is the hospital.[858] Previous hospital care is a useful marker for identifying high-risk individuals: Approximately two thirds of patients hospitalized with pneumococcal bacteremia or pneumonia (all causes) have been discharged from a hospital at least once within the previous 5 years.[858,859] Unfortunately, most efforts to vaccinate them before hospital discharge have met with mixed results, but systems-oriented approaches that include standing orders have been the most effective (Table 22–13).[858,860–862] Vaccination programs also have been reported from hospital emergency departments[863,864] and long-term care institutions.[865,866] Greater attention is now being given to hospital-based pneumococcal vaccination by hospital administrators and quality assurance programs.[867,868]

TABLE 22–13 ■ Effectiveness of Pneumococcal Vaccination Programs for Patients Discharged from the Hospital

Study (Reference)	Year	Intervention	Vaccination Rate (%)	
			Control	Intervention
Metersky[861]	2001	Clinical pathway chart prompt	1	1
Overhage	1996	Computer reminder, house staff	2	2
Klein	1983	Chart reminder	2	10
Klein	1983	Chart reminder + poster	2	20
Vondracek	1998	Chart reminder	0	24
Landis	1996	Standing order, nurse	4	32
Dexter[860]	2001	Computer reminder	1	36
Shelvin[862]	2002	Chart reminder	5	38
Clancy	1992	Computer reminder	4	50
Bloom	1988	Pamphlet + nurse + volunteer	0	75
Klein	1986	Standing order, nurse	0	78

All studies except those with specific references were reviewed by D.S. Fedson et al.[858]

Several population-based programs to improve pneumococcal vaccine delivery have been organized by large health care organizations[869] and by state[870] and local[871] public health departments. One noteworthy program targeted a remote population of high-risk Alaskan Natives, increasing vaccination rates from 30% to 84% within 3 years.[872] The National Coalition for Adult Immunization continues to sponsor National Adult Immunization Awareness Week each October to emphasize the importance of vaccinating adults against pneumococcal disease.[873]

Several initiatives have been undertaken at the federal level to increase pneumococcal vaccination coverage. In the early 1980s, the Surgeon General established the goal of vaccinating 60% of the elderly by 1990. The same goal was set for the year 2000,[874] and a goal of 90% has been set for the year 2010.[836] In 1993, the federal government authorized Medicare reimbursement for influenza vaccine and established a separate billing code for providing reimbursement for the administration of (not just the cost of) pneumococcal vaccine. This improved the overall level of physician reimbursement for pneumococcal vaccination. In 1994, the National Vaccine Advisory Committee report on adult immunization recommended several initiatives to improve pneumococcal vaccination,[875] many of which have been incorporated into federal programs. These efforts are reflected in the cumulative annual level of pneumococcal vaccine distribution seen in the United States during the period from 1996 to 2000 (Fig. 22–5). This level exceeded that in all other developed countries.

OTHER DEVELOPED COUNTRIES

Figure 22–5 shows the cumulative distribution of pneumococcal vaccine in 22 developed countries during the periods from 1991 to 1995 and from 1996 to 2000. Before 1991, no country other than the United States used appreciable amounts of vaccine. Since then, Canada has greatly increased it vaccine use. As in the United States, pneumococcal vaccine was registered in Canada in the late 1970s and recommendations for its use by the National Advisory Committee on Immunization have always been similar to those issued by the ACIP.[876] What was missing, however, were decisions by provincial health departments to pur-

chase pneumococcal vaccine and distribute it free of charge to practitioners. (Provincial health departments purchase 90% or more of the doses of influenza vaccine used in Canada, and since the 1980s the level of influenza vaccine use throughout Canada has been similar to that in the United States.[876]) In 1996, health officials in the province of Ontario decided to purchase enough pneumococcal vaccine to vaccinate all persons 65 years of age or older over a 3-year period.[877] As a result of this decision and a public awareness and professional education program, Ontario accounted for 91% of all pneumococcal vaccine used in Canada in 1996. Over the next four years, publicly funded programs for pneumococcal vaccination were adopted by all of Canada's 13 provinces and territories.[878] Eight programs covered all elderly persons, asplenic individuals, persons with other high-risk conditions, and residents of long-term care facilities. The other five programs covered three of the four high-risk groups. In addition, special programs targeted inner city areas with high rates of homelessness, substance abuse, and HIV infection.[889] Although coverage rates for elderly persons have not been reported, a national cross-sectional survey in 1999 showed that 71% of residents of long-term care facilities had received pneumococcal vaccine.[880]

The use of pneumococcal vaccine in Australia increased dramatically in the late 1990s (see Fig. 22–5). Initial recommendations by the National Health and Medical Research Council were similar to those in North America. However, pneumococcal vaccine was the only vaccine on the standard schedule that was not funded by federal grants to the states.[881] In 1998, the state of Victoria began a program of offering free pneumococcal vaccine to people over the age of 65 years. During the 2-year period from 1997 to 1998, an estimated 42% of the elderly in the state were vaccinated. Pneumococcal vaccine also has been provided free of charge to Aboriginal and Torres Strait Islander adults ages 50 years and older.[882] In 2000, vaccination was recommended for indigenous persons 15 years of age or older in the Northern Territories and 2 years of age or older in central Australia.[418] Vaccination in far north Queensland has been associated with a noticeable decline in the incidence of invasive pneumococcal disease among indigenous adults.[883] Some observers have recommended that the age

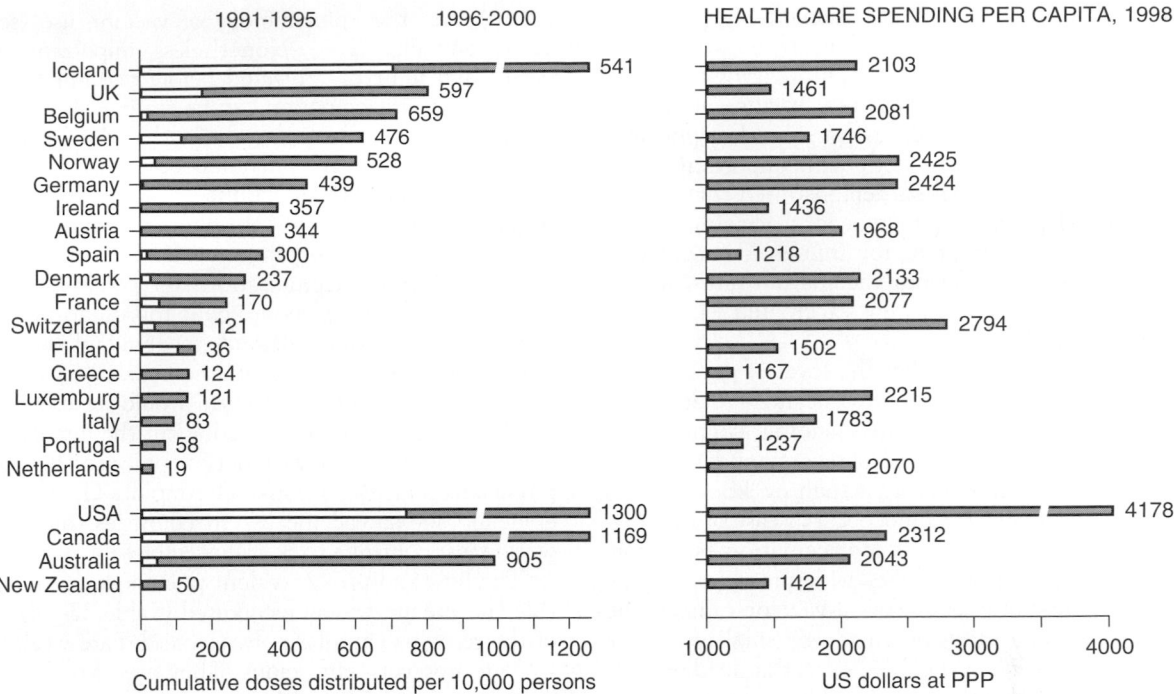

FIGURE 22–5 ■ Pneumococcal vaccination in 22 developed countries, 1991 to 2000 (D. S. Fedson, unpublished observations). The figure shows the cumulative number of doses of pneumococcal vaccine distributed per 10,000 total population during two 5-year periods from 1991 to 1995 (open bars) and from 1996 to 2000 (closed bars and numbers). Also shown is health care spending per capita in each country for the year 1998. These data were obtained from the Office of Economic Cooperation and Development and have been adjusted for purchasing power parity (PPP).

limit for vaccination should be lowered to 25 years for all indigenous groups and to 60 years for other adults.[884]

The greatest disparities in the use of pneumococcal vaccine between countries have occurred in western Europe (see Fig. 22–5). In 1988, the WHO's Regional Office for Europe convened a technical advisory group to consider the status of pneumococcal vaccination.[885] The advisory group's main conclusion was to recommend vaccinating all elderly persons and persons of any age who are at increased risk of pneumococcal infection. Iceland began to use pneumococcal vaccine in 1991, but other countries did not begin to respond to the WHO recommendation until the mid-1990s.[831] Belgium became the leading western European country in using pneumococcal vaccine during the 5-year period from 1996 to 2000 (see Fig. 22–5). To a great extent this was due to the work of a group of experts who formulated the Belgian Consensus on Pneumococcal Vaccine.[886,887] The group took the lead in establishing national recommendations, launching programs for public awareness and professional education, and evaluating the effectiveness of vaccine delivery. During the first 2 years of the program, approximately 20% of the target population was vaccinated.[888]

In the United Kingdom, recommendations to vaccinate high-risk (but not all elderly) persons in the United Kingdom began to be implemented in 1994. Several reports described various aspects of vaccination programs run by general practitioners, focusing on the need to educate patients and to structure programs for offering them vaccine.[889–896] A survey of Scottish nursing homes documented low rates of pneumococcal vaccination (11%), highlighting the need for a national recommendation to vaccinate nursing home residents.[897] In Ireland, a recommendation to

vaccinate all elderly people came into effect only in 2000. A survey of two general practices showed that 82% of elderly patients who received a written invitation to be vaccinated accepted the vaccine.[898]

Other countries in western Europe also demonstrated success with pneumococcal vaccination. In the Nordic countries, Sweden,[410,899,900] Norway,[901] and, to a lesser extent, Denmark[902] began vaccinating in the mid-1990s and maintained a steady if unremarkable level of use each year (see Fig. 22–5). Finland, however, used very little vaccine. Vaccine use remained modest in Switzerland, and one report found that only 6% of elderly and high-risk patients seen in primary care had been vaccinated.[903] Vaccine use was somewhat better in Austria. In 1998, Germany adopted a recommendation to vaccinate all persons above 60 years of age,[904] and over the next 2 years this was followed by a remarkable increase in vaccine use, more so in states that had previously been part of East Germany (D. S. Fedson, unpublished observations). In Italy, several smaller regions began to vaccinate elderly adults starting in 1998, although the national level of vaccine use remained low. In Spain, comprehensive programs for vaccinating persons over 65 years of age were begun in Catalonia in 1999[905] and in Galicia in 2000. In both autonomous communities, vaccination rates quickly approached 60% (D. S. Fedson, unpublished observations). Greece recommends vaccinating all elderly persons and has begun using vaccine. Portugal has no recommendation and vaccine use is low.

The Netherlands is the country in western Europe in which pneumococcal vaccine use is lowest (see Fig. 22–5). In contrast, the Netherlands leads all countries in western Europe in the use of influenza vaccine.[429,906] Pneumococcal vaccination is recommended only for persons with functional or anatomic asplenia. Remarkably, however, Dutch health officials recommend that, in the event of an influenza pandemic, when supplies of influenza vaccine are likely to be insufficient, pneumococcal vaccine should be used because it offers protection against secondary pneumococcal infections.[907] A recent study with important implications for Dutch policy makers demonstrated that, in the setting of general practice, pneumococcal vaccine can be added to an existing program for influenza vaccination without compromising influenza vaccination rates. In this study, 75% of elderly patients were vaccinated with pneumococcal vaccine.[908]

Figure 22–5 shows clearly that the level of pneumococcal vaccine use in a developed country bears no relationship to its per capita level of health care spending. Higher levels of vaccine use depend more on broad recommendations and some form of public reimbursement than on knowledge of reported rates of invasive pneumococcal disease or information about the cost-effectiveness of vaccination (see Table 22–12). More than anything else, widespread geographic variations in the use of pneumococcal vaccine indicate the importance of specific decisions made by small groups of public health officials. It is their decisions that lead to comprehensive recommendations and public reimbursement. This is an important lesson for health officials in other countries to keep in mind when they begin to consider issues of public policy for pneumococcal vaccination.[909]

Considerations for the Future

Since pneumococcal polysaccharide vaccine was first licensed in 1977, much has been learned about the burden of pneumococcal disease (see Tables 22–3 and 22–5), the clinical effectiveness of pneumococcal vaccination (see Table 22–9), the value of vaccination to society (see Table

22–10), and the epidemiology of vaccine use (see Table 22–12 and Fig. 22–5). Nonetheless, important questions persist and must be answered before the full potential of pneumococcal vaccination can be realized. In many developed countries, reliable population-based estimates of the occurrence of invasive pneumococcal disease still are not available and need to be obtained. Additional retrospective studies are needed to assess the effectiveness of pneumococcal vaccination not only in preventing invasive disease but also in reducing hospitalizations for community-acquired pneumonia. Knowing more about the duration of protection after vaccination will guide recommendations for periodic revaccination. Additional comparative studies of the cost-effectiveness of vaccination would be useful. Finally, much more needs to be learned about the microepidemiology of pneumococcal vaccination practices by individual physicians and institutions. The rapidly changing macroepidemiology of vaccine use in countries throughout the world must continue to be followed closely.

The limitations of 23-valent pneumococcal polysaccharide vaccine are widely recognized (Table 22–14).[910] Some of the serotype capsular polysaccharides are weak antigens and are not very efficacious. They are also the serotypes most often associated with antibiotic resistance. Moreover, antibody levels and clinical protection decline within a few years of vaccination. Revaccination does not elicit a booster antibody response. Yet, in spite of these limitations, pneumococcal vaccination of older and high-risk adults is clearly worthwhile.

The potential benefits of pneumococcal polysaccharide vaccine for children and adults who live in developing countries have been ignored, in spite of the findings from clinical trials conducted in Papua New Guinea in the 1970s.[460,753] Maternal immunization is currently being considered because it might prevent pneumococcal infections

TABLE 22–14 ■ Limitations of Pneumococcal Polysaccharide Vaccine in Older Adults

Serotype*	Antimicrobial Resistance†	Antibody Persistence (yr)‡	Vaccination Effectiveness§	
			%	95% CI
1	—‖	—	77	50 to 90
3	—	—	42	5 to 65
4	—	4.5	76	6 to 58
5	—	—	—	—
6B	Yes	3.0	46	−4 to 72
7	—	—	53	8 to 76
9V	Yes	5.0	52	12 to 74
14	Yes	7.7	62	44 to 75
18C	—	—	36	−20 to 66
19F	Yes	3.8	27	−50 to 65
23F	Yes	4.7	15	−24 to 41

*Eleven serotypes considered for future pneumococcal conjugate vaccines.
†Data from Butler and Cetron.[204]
‡Data from Sankilampi et al.[556] The investigators calculated the time intervals required for postvaccination serum antibody levels to decline to prevaccination levels following administration of one dose of 23-valent pneumococcal polysaccharide vaccine. Sixty-two subjects who were 65 to 88 years of age were evaluated.
§Data from Butler et al.[788] Serotype-specific effectiveness against invasive pneumococcal disease was determined for older adults whose mean age was greater than 50 years. CI indicates confidence interval.
‖No data or not mentioned.
Adapted from Fedson DS. Pneumococcal conjugate vaccination for adults: why it's important for children. Pediatr Infect Dis J 19:183–186, 2000.

in very young infants, and there has been a renewed call for a clinical trial of polysaccharide vaccine in children 8 to 9 months of age.[911,912] Yet in developing countries, mortality from respiratory tract infections, although greatest in young children, extends across the life span and greatly exceeds that seen in developed countries.[913] Children in developing countries who survive to adulthood continue to have high mortality rates throughout their adult years.[914] Many deaths are undoubtedly due to pneumococcal infections. It is possible that pneumococcal polysaccharide vaccine could benefit adults as well as children in developing countries, but the research needed to support vaccination programs has not been done.

There is a good possibility that pneumococcal conjugate[910] and/or protein-based[27] vaccines could have a major impact on pneumococcal disease in adults as well as children in both developing and developed countries. Eventually, however, investigators will have to address the question of whether these newer vaccines will be used as replacement or as supplemental vaccines. If they are to replace the existing polysaccharide vaccine, it will be extremely difficult to obtain evidence of their clinical efficacy because placebo-controlled clinical trials probably will not be permitted, except perhaps in a few developing countries. However, if these newer vaccines are intended to supplement the existing polysaccharide vaccine, large clinical trials may not be necessary. A conjugate vaccine for adults (an 11-valent vaccine would be preferable because of its broader serotype coverage) could be licensed if it were shown that a conjugate prime/polysaccharide boost schedule is just as safe and more immunogenic than polysaccharide vaccine alone.[910] The schedule works in children,[25] but the results of studies in adults have been mixed and in general are regarded as disappointing.[628,910,915] Whether such a schedule would provide adults with more long-lasting protection against infection caused by the conjugate vaccine serotypes is not yet known. A protein-based vaccine also might be licensed as a supplemental vaccine if there were experimental evidence to justify a combined schedule, if it were safe, and if it did not compromise the immunogenicity of the polysaccharide vaccine. In either case, 23-valent pneumococcal polysaccharide vaccine would still be used. The clinical effectiveness of either of the two combined regimens could then be evaluated in observational studies, much as a postlicensure study of the effectiveness of 7-valent pneumococcal conjugate vaccination of infants[916] confirmed the efficacy of the vaccine demonstrated earlier in a randomized controlled trial.[26]

In the 25 years since pneumococcal polysaccharide vaccine first became commercially available, it still is misunderstood, undervalued, and underused.[917] Yet it is difficult to imagine that it will be completely replaced by one of the newer vaccines in the foreseeable future. By itself, the polysaccharide vaccine provides important benefits that justify its wider use. Used in combination with newer vaccines to immunize persons of all ages, it could bring enormous improvements in public health worldwide.

Acknowledgment

The authors thank Astutie Michel, Cecile Silarakis, and Marie-Christine Auger for assistance in preparing the manuscript.

REFERENCES

1. Heffron R. Pneumonia with Special Reference to Pneumococcus Lobar Pneumonia. (A Commonwealth Fund book.) Cambridge, MA, Harvard University Press, 1979.
2. White B. The Biology of Pneumococcus: The Bacteriologic, Biochemical and Immunological Characters and Activities of *Diplococcus pneumoniae*. (A Commonwealth Fund book.) Cambridge, MA, Harvard University Press, 1979.
3. Austrian R. Pneumococcus: the first one hundred years. Rev Infect Dis 3:183–189, 1981.
4. Austrian R. Maxwell Finland Lecture. Random gleanings from a life with the pneumococcus. J Infect Dis 131:474–484, 1975.
5. Tuomanen E. Molecular and cellular biology of pneumococcal infection. Curr Opin Microbiol 2:35–39, 1999.
6. Gillespie SH, Balakrishnan I. Pathogenesis of pneumococcal infection. J Med Microbiol 49:1057–1067, 2000.
7. Dallaire F, Ouellet N, Bergeron Y, et al. Microbiological and inflammatory factors associated with the development of pneumococcal pneumonia. J Infect Dis 184:292–300, 2001.
8. Musher DM, Alexandraki I, Graviss EA, et al. Bacteremic and non-bacteremic pneumococcal pneumonia: a prospective study. Medicine (Baltimore) 79:210–221, 2000.
9. Ring A, Tuomanen E. Host cell invasion by *Streptococcus pneumoniae*. Subcell Biochem 33:125–135, 2000.
10. Light RB. Pulmonary pathophysiology of pneumococcal pneumonia. Semin Respir Infect 14:218–226, 1999.
11. Novak R, Tuomanen E. Pathogenesis of pneumococcal pneumonia. Semin Respir Infect 14:209–217, 1999.
12. Catterall JR. *Streptococcus pneumoniae*. Thorax 54:929–937, 1999.
13. Fedson DS, Scott JAG. The burden of pneumococcal disease among adults in developed and developing countries: what is and is not known. Vaccine 17(suppl 1):S11–S18, 1999.
14. Musher DM. *Streptococcus pneumoniae*. In Mandell GL, Bennett JE, Dolin R (eds). Principles and Practice of Infections Diseases (5th ed). New York, Churchill Livingstone, 2001, pp 2128–2147.
15. Poland GA. The prevention of pneumococcal disease by vaccines: promises and challenges. Infect Dis Clin North Am 15:97–122, 2001.
16. Whitney CG, Schaffner W, Butler JC. Rethinking recommendations for use of pneumococcal vaccines in adults. Clin Infect Dis 33:662–675, 2001.
17. Örtqvist Ä. Pneumococcal vaccination: current and future issues. Eur Respir J 18:184–195, 2001.
18. Fedson DS. The clinical effectiveness of pneumococcal vaccination: a brief review. Vaccine 17(suppl 1):S85–S90, 1999.
19. Butler JC, Shapiro ED, Carlone GM. Pneumococcal vaccines: history, current status, and future directions. Am J Med 107(suppl 1A):69S–76S, 1999.
20. Austrian R, Oswald T. Avery: the Wizard of York Avenue. Am J Med 107(suppl 1A):7S–11S, 1999.
21. Krause RM. Paul Ehrlich and O.T. Avery: pathfinders in the search for immunity. Vaccine 17(suppl 3):S64–S67, 1999.
22. Austrian R, Gold J. Pneumococcal bacteremia with especial reference to bacteremic pneumococcal pneumonia. Ann Intern Med 60:759–776, 1964.
23. Smit P, Oberholzer D, Hayden-Smith S, et al. Protective efficacy of pneumococcal polysaccharide vaccines. JAMA 238:2613–2616, 1977.
24. Austrian R, Douglas RM, Schiffman G, et al. Prevention of pneumococcal pneumonia by vaccination. Trans Assoc Am Physicians 89:184–194, 1976.
25. Eskola J, Anttila M. Pneumococcal conjugate vaccines. Pediatr Infect Dis J 18:543–551, 1999.
26. Black S, Shinefield H, Fireman B, et al. Efficacy, safety and immunogenicity of heptavalent pneumococcal conjugate vaccine in children. Northern California Kaiser Permanente Vaccine Study Center Group. Pediatr Infect Dis J 19:187–195, 2000.
27. Nabors GS, Braun PA, Herrmann DJ, et al. Immunization of healthy adults with a single recombinant pneumococcal surface protein A (PspA) variant stimulates broadly cross-reactive antibodies to heterologous PspA molecules. Vaccine 18:1743–1754, 2000.
28. Tettelin H, Nelson KE, Paulsen IT, et al. Complete genome sequence of a virulent isolate of *Streptococcus pneumoniae*. Science 293:498–506, 2001.
29. Avery OT, MacLeod CM, McCarty M. Studies on the chemical nature of the substance inducing transformation of pneumococcal types: induction of transformation by a desoxyribonucleic acid

fraction isolated from pneumococcus type III [republication of a 1944 paper]. Mol Med 1:344–365, 1995.

30. Lederberg J. The transformation of genetics by DNA: an anniversary celebration of Avery, MacLeod and McCarty (1944). Genetics 136:423–426, 1994.

31. McCarty M. A retrospective look: how we identified the pneumococcal transforming substance as DNA. J Exp Med 179:385–394, 1994.

32. Pikis A, Campos JM, Rodriguez WJ, Kaith JM. Optochin resistance in Strptococcus pneumoniae: mechanism, significance, and clinical implications. J Infect Dis 184:582–590, 2001.

33. Watson DA, Musher DM, Verhoef J. Pneumococcal virulence factors and host immune responses to them. Eur J Clin Microbiol Infect Dis 14:479–490, 1995.

34. Cundell D, Masure HR, Tuomanen EI. The molecular basis of pneumococcal infection: a hypothesis. Clin Infect Dis 21(suppl):S204–S212, 1995.

35. Tuomanen E, Tomasz A, Heugstler B, Zak O. The relative role of bacterial cell wall and capsule in the induction of inflammation in pneumococcal meningitis. J Infect Dis 151:535–540, 1985.

36. Musher DM, Watson DA, Baughn RE. Does naturally acquired IgG antibody to cell wall polysaccharide protect human subjects against pneumococcal infection? J Infect Dis 161:736–740, 1990.

37. Bruyn GA, Zegers BJ, van Furth R. Mechanisms of host defense against infection with Streptococcus pneumoniae. Clin Infect Dis 14:251–262, 1992.

38. Weiser JN, Markiewicz Z, Tuomanen EI, Wani JH. Relationship between phase variation in colony morphology, intrastrain variation in cell wall physiology, and nasopharyngeal colonization by Streptococcus pneumoniae. Infect Immun 64:2240–2245, 1996.

39. Kim JO, Weiser JN. Association of intrastrain phase variation in quantity of capsular polysaccharide and teichoic acid with the virulence of Streptococcus pneumoniae. J Infect Dis 177:368–377, 1998.

40. Weiser JN, Kapoor M. Effect of intrastrain variation in the amount of capsular polysaccharide on genetic transformation of Streptococcus pneumoniae: implications for virulence studies of encapsulated strains. Infect Immun 67:3690–3692, 1999.

41. Kim JO, Romero-Steiner S, Sorensen UB, et al. Relationship between cell surface carbohydrates and intrastrain variation on opsonophagocytosis of Streptococcus pneumoniae. Infect Immun 67:2327–2333, 1999.

42. Schweinle JE. Pneumococcal intracellular killing is abolished by polysaccharide despite serum complement activity. Infect Immun 54:876–881, 1986.

43. Hollingshead SK, Briles DE. Streptococcus pneumoniae: new tools for an old pathogen. Curr Opin Microbiol 4:71–77, 2001.

44. Jedrzejas MJ. Pneumococcal virulence factors: structure and function. Microbiol Mol Biol Rev 65:187–207, 2001.

45. Rieux V. Virulence factors of Streptococcus pneumoniae [in French]. Med Mal Infect 32(suppl 1):1–12, 2002.

46. Gray BM. Pneumococcal microbiology and immunity. Pediatr Ann 31:233–240, 2002.

47. Paton JC. The contribution of pneumolysin to the pathogenicity of Streptococcus pneumoniae. Trends Microbiol 4:103–106, 1996.

48. Rubins JB, Janoff EN. Pneumolysin: a multifunctional pneumococcal virulence factor. J Lab Clin Med 131:21–27, 1998.

49. Cockeran R, Anderson R, Feldman C. The role of pneumolysin in the pathogenesis of Streptococcus pneumoniae infection. Curr Opin Infect Dis 15:235–239, 2002.

50. Rayner CF, Jackson AD, Rutman A, et al. Interaction of pneumolysin-sufficient and -deficient isogenic variants of Streptococcus pneumoniae with human respiratory mucosa. Infect Immun 63:442–447, 1995.

51. Rubins JB, Charboneau D, Paton JC, et al. Dual function of pneumolysin in the early pathogenesis of murine pneumococcal pneumonia. J Clin Invest 95:142–150, 1995.

52. Hirst RA, Sikand KS, Rutman A, et al. Relative roles of pneumolysin and hydrogen peroxide from Streptococcus pneumoniae in inhibition of ependymal ciliary beat frequency. Infect Immun 68:1557–1562, 2000.

53. Benton KA, Everson MP, Briles DE. A pneumolysin-negative mutant of Streptococcus pneumoniae causes chronic bacteremia rather than acute sepsis in mice. Infect Immun 63:448–455, 1995.

54. Berry AM, Alexander JE, Mitchell TJ, et al. Effect of defined point mutations in the pneumolysin gene on the virulence of Streptococcus pneumoniae. Infect Immun 63:1969–1974, 1995.

55. Musher DM, Phan HM, Baughn RE. Protection against bacteremic pneumococcal infection by antibody to pneumolysin. J Infect Dis 183:827–830, 2001.

56. Alexander JE, Lock RA, Peeters CC, et al. Immunization of mice with pneumolysin toxoid confers a significant degree of protection against at least nine serotypes of Streptococcus pneumoniae. Infect Immun 62:5683–5688, 1994.

57. Swiatlo E, Champlin FR, Holman SC, et al. Contribution of choline-binding proteins to cell surface properties of Streptococcus pneumoniae. Infect Immun 70:412–415, 2002.

58. Gosink KK, Mann ER, Guglielmo C, et al. Role of novel choline binding proteins in virulence of Streptococcus pneumoniae. Infect Immun 68:5690–5695, 2000.

59. Balachandran P, Hollingshead SK, Paton JC, Briles DE. The autolytic enzyme LytA of Streptococcus pneumoniae is not responsible for releasing pneumolysin J Bacteriol 183:3108–3116, 2001.

60. Berry AM, Lock RA, Hansman D, Paton JC. Contribution of autolysin to virulence of Streptococcus pneumoniae. Infect Immun 57:2324–2330, 1989.

61. Berry AM, Paton JC. Additive attenuation of virulence of Streptococcus pneumoniae by mutation of the genes encoding pneumolysin and other putative pneumococcal virulence proteins. Infect Immun 68:133–140, 2000.

62. Briles DE, Tart RC, Swialto E, et al. Pneumococcal diversity: consideration for new vaccine strategies with emphasis on pneumococcal surface protein A (PspA). Clin Microbiol Rev 11:645–657, 1998.

63. Hollingshead SK, Becker R, Briles DE. Diversity of PspA: mosaic genes and evidence for past recombination in Streptococcus pneumoniae. Infect Immun 68:5889–5900, 2000.

64. Tu AH, Fulgham RL, McCrory MA, et al. Pneumococcal surface protein A inhibits complement activation by Streptococcus pneumoniae. Infect Immun 67:4720–4724, 1999.

65. Hakansson A, Roche H, Mirza S, et al. Characterization of binding of human lactoferrin to pneumococcal surface protein A. Infect Immun 69:3372–3381, 2001.

66. Hammerschmidt S, Bethe G, Remane PH, Chhatwal GS. Identification of pneumococcal surface protein A as a lactoferrin-binding protein of Streptococcus pneumoniae. Infect Immun 67:1683–1687, 1999.

67. McDaniel LS, Sheffield JS, Delucchi P, Briles DE. PspA, a surface protein of Streptococcus pneumoniae, is capable of eliciting protection against pneumococci of more than one capsular type. Infect Immun 59:222–228, 1991.

68. Briles DE, King JD, Gray MA, et al. PspA, a protection-eliciting pneumococcal protein: immunogenicity of isolated native PspA in mice. Vaccine 14:858–867, 1996.

69. Berry AM, Paton JC. Sequence heterogeneity of PsaA, a 37-kilodalton putative adhesin essential for virulence of Streptococcus pneumoniae. Infect Immun 64:5255–5262, 1996.

70. Johnson SE, Dykes JK, Jue DL, et al. Inhibition of pneumococcal carriage in mice by subcutaneous immunization with peptides from the common surface protein pneumococcal surface adhesin A. J Infect Dis 185:489–496, 2002.

71. Janulczyk R, Iannelli F, Sjoholm AG, et al. Hic, a novel surface protein of Streptococcus pneumoniae that interferes with complement function. J Biol Chem 275:37257–37263, 2000.

72. Hostetter MK. Opsonic and nonopsonic interactions of C3 with Streptococcus pneumoniae. Microb Drug Resist 5:85–89, 1999.

73. Berry AM, Lock RA, Thomas SM, et al. Cloning and nucleotide sequence of the Streptococcus pneumoniae hyaluronidase gene and purification of the enzyme from recombinant Escherichia coli. Infect Immun 62:1101–1108, 1994.

74. Lomholt H. Evidence of recombination and an antigenically diverse immunoglobulin A1 protease among strains of Streptococcus pneumoniae. Infect Immun 63:4238–4243, 1995.

75. Tong HH, Blue LE, James MA, DeMaria TF. Evaluation of the virulence of a Streptococcus pneumoniae neuraminidase-deficient mutant in nasopharyngeal colonization and development of otitis media in the chinchilla model. Infect Immun 68:921–924, 2000.

76. Bethe G, Nau R, Wellmer A, et al. The cell wall-associated serine protease PrtA: a highly conserved virulence factor of Streptococcus pneumoniae. FEMS Microbiol Lett 205:99–104, 2001.

77. Holmes AR, McNab R, Millsap KW, et al. The pavA gene of Streptococcus pneumoniae encodes a fibronectin-binding protein that is essential for virulence. Mol Microbiol 41:1395–1408, 2001.

78. Polissi A, Pontiggia A, Feger G, et al. Large-scale identification of virulence genes from Streptococcus pneumoniae. Infect Immun 66:5620–5629, 1998.

79. Paton JC, Giammarinaro P. Genome-based analysis of pneumococcal virulence factors: the quest for novel vaccine antigens and drug targets. Trends Microbiol 9:515–518, 2001.

80. Henrichsen J. Six newly recognized types of *Streptococcus pneumoniae*. J Clin Microbiol 33:2759–2762, 1995.

81. Henrichsen J. Typing of *Streptococcus pneumoniae*: past, present, and future. Am J Med 107(suppl 1A):50S–54S, 1999.

82. Feikin DR, Klugman KP. Historical changes in pneumococcal serogroup distribution: implications for the era of pneumococcal conjugate vaccines. Clin Infect Dis 35:547–555, 2002.

83. Scott JAG, Hall AJ, Dagan R, et al. Serogroup-specific epidemiology of *Streptococcus pneumoniae*: associations with age, sex, and geography in 7,000 episodes of invasive disease. Clin Infect Dis 22:973–981, 1996.

84. Inostroza J, Vinet AM, Retamal G, et al. Influence of patient age on *Streptococcus pneumoniae* serotypes causing invasive disease. Clin Diagn Lab Immunol 8:556–559, 2001.

85. Sorensen UB. Typing of pneumococci by using 12 pooled antisera. J Clin Microbiol 31:2097–2100, 1993.

86. Henrichsen J, Robbins JB. Production of monovalent antisera by induction of immunological tolerance for capsular typing of *Streptococcus pneumoniae*. FEMS Microbiol Lett 73:89–93, 1992.

87. Lalitha MK, Thomas K, Kumar RS, Steinhoff MC. Serotyping of *Streptococcus pneumoniae* by coagglutination with 12 pooled antisera. J Clin Microbiol 37:263–265, 1999.

88. Park MK, Briles DE, Nahm MH. A latex bead-based flow cytometric immunoassay capable of simultaneous typing of multiple pneumococcal serotypes (Multibead assay). Clin Diagn Lab Immunol 7:486–489, 2000.

89. Lalitha MK, Pai R, John TJ, et al. Serotyping of *Streptococcus pneumoniae* by agglutination assays: a cost-effective technique for developing countries. Bull World Health Organ 74:387–390, 1996.

90. Lefevre JC, Faucon G, Sicard AM, Gasc AM. DNA fingerprinting of *Streptococcus pneumoniae* strains by pulsed-field gel electrophoresis. J Clin Microbiol 31:2724–2728, 1993.

91. van Belkum A, Sluijuter M, de Groot R, et al. Novel BOX repeat PCR assay for high-resolution typing of *Streptococcus pneumoniae* strains. J Clin Microbiol 34:1176–1179, 1996.

92. Enright MC, Spratt BG. A multilocus sequence typing scheme for *Streptococcus pneumoniae*: identification of clones associated with serious invasive disease. Microbiology 144(pt 11):3049–3060, 1998.

93. Enright MC, Spratt BG. Multilocus sequence typing. Trends Microbiol 7:482–487, 1999.

94. Nuorti JP, Butler JC, Farley MM, et al. Cigarette smoking and invasive pneumococcal disease. Active Bacterial Core Surveillance Team. N Engl J Med 342:681–689, 2000.

95. Rosenow C, Ryan P, Weiser JN, et al. Contribution of novel choline-binding proteins to adherence, colonization and immunogenicity of *Streptococcus pneumoniae*. Mol Microbiol 25:819–829, 1997.

96. Zhang JR, Mostov KE, Lamm ME, et al. The polymeric immunoglobulin receptor translocates pneumococci across human nasopharyngeal epithelial cells. Cell 102:827–837, 2000.

97. Tuomanen EI, Masure HR. Molecular and cellular biology of pneumococcal infection. Microb Drug Resist 3:297–308, 1997.

98. Smith BL, Hostetter MK. C3 as substrate for adhesion of *Streptococcus pneumoniae*. J Infect Dis 182:497–508, 2000.

99. Cundell DR, Gerard NP, Gerard C, et al. *Streptococcus pneumoniae* anchor to activated human cells by the receptor for platelet-activating factor. Nature 377:435–438, 1995.

100. Cockeran R, Theron AJ, Steel HC, et al. Proinflammatory interactions of pneumolysin with human neutrophils. J Infect Dis 183:604–611, 2001.

101. Orman KL, Shenep JL, English BK. Pneumococci stimulate the production of the inducible nitric oxide synthase and nitric oxide by murine macrophages. J Infect Dis 178:1649–1657, 1998.

102. Gordon SB, Irving GR, Lawson RA, et al. Intracellular trafficking and killing of *Streptococcus pneumoniae* by human alveolar macrophages are influenced by opsonins. Infect Immun 68:2286–2293, 2000.

103. Janoff EN, Fasching C, Orenstein JM, et al. Killing of *Streptococcus pneumoniae* by capsular polysaccharide-specific polymeric IgA, complement, and phagocytes. J Clin Invest 104:1139–1147, 1999.

104. Nathan BR, Scheld WM. New advances in the pathogenesis and pathophysiology of bacterial meningitis. Curr Infect Dis Rep 2:332–336, 2000.

105. Meli DN, Christen S, Leib SL, Tauber MG. Current concepts in the pathogenesis of meningitis caused by *Streptococcus pneumoniae*. Curr Opin Infect Dis 15:253–257, 2002.

106. Ring A, Weiser JN, Tuomanen EI. Pneumococcal trafficking across the blood-brain barrier: molecular analysis of a novel bidirectional pathway. J Clin Invest 102:347–360, 1998.

107. Zysk G, Schneider-Wald BK, Hwang JH, et al. Pneumolysin is the main inducer of cytotoxicity to brain microvascular endothelial cells caused by *Streptococcus pneumoniae*. Infect Immun 69:845–852, 2001.

108. Braun JS, Sublett JE, Freyer D, et al. Pneumococcal pneumolysin and H(2)O(2) mediate brain cell apoptosis during meningitis. J Clin Invest 109:19–27, 2002.

109. Braun JS, Novak R, Murray PJ, et al. Apoptosis-inducing factor mediates microglial and neuronal apoptosis caused by pneumococcus. J Infect Dis 184:1300–1309, 2001.

110. Nau R, Soto A, Bruck W. Apoptosis of neurons in the dentate gyrus in humans suffering from bacterial meningitis. J Neuropathol Exp Neurol 58:265–274, 1999.

111. Soininen A, Lahdenkari M, Kilpi T, et al. Antibody response to pneumococcal capsular polysaccharides in children with acute otitis media. Pediatr Infect Dis J 21:186–192, 2002.

112. Goldblatt D. Immunisation and the maturation of infant immune responses. Dev Biol Stand 95:125–132, 1998.

113. Musher DM, Watson DA, Baughn RE. Genetic control of the immunologic response to pneumococcal capsular polysaccharides. Vaccine 19:623–627, 2000.

114. Pandey JP. Immunoglobulin GM and KM allotypes and vaccine immunity. Vaccine 19:613–617, 2000.

115. Chang Q, Abadi J, Alpert P, Pirofski L. A pneumococcal capsular polysaccharide vaccine induces a repertoire shift with increased VH3 expression in peripheral B cells from human immunodeficiency virus (HIV)-uninfected but not HIV-infected persons. J Infect Dis 181:1313–1321, 2000.

116. Sun Y, Park MK, Kim J, et al. Repertoire of human antibodies against the polysaccharide capsule of *Streptococcus pneumoniae* serotype 6B. Infect Immun 67:1172–1179, 1999.

117. Baxendale HE, Davis Z, White HN, et al. Immunogenetic analysis of the immune response to pneumococcal polysaccharide. Eur J Immunol 30:1214–1223, 2000.

118. Lucas AH, Moulton KD, Tang VR, Reason DC. Combinatorial library cloning of human antibodies to *Streptococcus pneumoniae* capsular polysaccharides: variable region primary structures and evidence for somatic mutation of Fab fragments specific for capsular serotypes 6B, 14, and 23F. Infect Immun 69:853–864, 2001.

119. Jansen WT, Breukels MA, Snippe H, et al. Fcgamma receptor polymorphisms determine the magnitude of in vitro phagocytosis of *Streptococcus pneumoniae* mediated by pneumococcal conjugate sera. J Infect Dis 180:888–891, 1999.

120. Yee AM, Phan HM, Zuniga R, et al. Association between FcgammaRIIa-R131 allotype and bacteremic pneumococcal pneumonia. Clin Infect Dis 30:25–28, 2000.

121. van der Pol W, Vidarsson G, Vile HA, et al. Pneumococcal capsular polysaccharide-specific IgA triggers efficient neutrophil effector functions via FcalphaRI (CD89). J Infect Dis 182:1139–1145, 2000.

122. Musher DM, Phan HM, Watson DA, Baughn RE. Antibody to capsular polysaccharide of *Streptococcus pneumoniae* at the time of hospital admission for pneumococcal pneumonia. J Infect Dis 182:158–167, 2000.

123. Roy S, Knox K, Segal S, et al. MBL genotype and risk of invasive pneumococcal disease: a case control study. Lancet 359:1569–1573, 2002.

124. Kronborg G, Weis N, Madsen HO, et al. Variant mannose-binding lectin alleles are not associated with susceptibility to or outcome of invasive pneumococcal infection in randomly included patients. J Infect Dis 185:1517–1520, 2002.

125. Roy S, Hill AV, Knox K, et al. Association of common genetic variant with susceptibility to invasive pneumococcal disease. BMJ 324:1369, 2002.

126. Hostetter MK. Serotypic variations among virulent pneumococci in deposition and degradation of covalently bound C3b: implications for phagocytosis and antibody production. J Infect Dis 153:682–693, 1986.

127. Angel CS, Ruzek M, Hostetter MK. Degradation of C3 by *Streptococcus pneumoniae*. J Infect Dis 170:600–608, 1994.

128. Cohn DA, Schiffman G. Immunoregulatory role of the spleen in antibody responses to pneumococcal polysaccharide antigens. Infect Immun 55:1375–1380, 1987.

129. Peset Llopis MJ, Harms G, Hardonk MJ, Timens W. Human immune response to pneumococcal polysaccharides: complement-mediated localization preferentially on CD21-positive splenic marginal zone B cells and follicular dendritic cells. J Allergy Clin Immunol 97:1015–1024, 1996.

130. Neuman MI, Harper MB. Time to positivity of blood cultures for children with Streptococcus pneumoniae bacteremia. Clin Infect Dis 33:1324–1328, 2001.

131. Kellogg JA, Bankert DA, Elder CJ, Gibbs JL, Smith MC. Identification of Streptococcus pneumoniae revisited. J Clin Microbiol 39:3373–3375, 2001.

132. Scott JA, Hall AJ. The value and complications of percutaneous transthoracic lung aspiration for the etiologic diagnosis of community-acquired pneumonia. Chest 116:1716–1732, 1999.

133. Gleckman R, DeVita J, Hibert D, et al. Sputum Gram stain assessment in community-acquired bacteremic pneumonia. J Clin Microbiol 26:846–849, 1988.

134. Perlino CA. Laboratory diagnosis of pneumonia due to Streptococcus pneumoniae. J Infect Dis 150:139–144, 1984.

135. Musher DM. Gram stain and culture of sputum to diagnose bacterial pneumonia [letter]. J Infect Dis 152:1096, 1985.

136. Heineman HS, Chawla JK, Lopton WM. Misinformation from sputum cultures without microscopic examination. J Clin Microbiol 6:518–527, 1977.

137. Reed WW, Byrd GS, Gates RH, et al. Sputum Gram's stain in community-acquired pneumococcal pneumonia—a meta-analysis. West J Med 165:197–204, 1996.

138. Roson B, Carratala J, Verdaguer R, et al. Prospective study of the usefulness of sputum Gram stain in the initial approach to community-acquired pneumonia requiring hospitalization. Clin Infect Dis 31:869–874, 2000.

139. Fine MJ, Orloff JJ, Rihs JD, et al. Evaluation of housestaff physicians' preparation and interpretation of sputum Gram stains for community-acquired pneumonia. J Gen Intern Med 6:189–198, 1991.

140. Parry CM, White RR, Ridgeway ER, et al. The reproducibility of sputum gram film interpretation. J Infect 41:55–60, 2000.

141. Gillespie SH, Smith MD, Dickens A, et al. Detection of C-polysaccharide in serum of patients with Streptococcus pneumoniae bacteraemia. J Clin Pathol 48:803–806, 1995.

142. Jesudason MV, Sridharan G, Arulselvan K, et al. C substance–specific latex agglutination for early and rapid detection of Streptococcus pneumoniae in blood cultures. Indian J Med Res 102:258–260, 1995.

143. Boersma WG, Lowenberg A, Holloway Y, et al. Pneumococcal antigen persistence in sputum from patients with community-acquired pneumonia. Chest 102:422–427, 1992.

144. Salih MA, Ahmed AA, Sid Ahmed H, Olcen P. An ELISA assay for the rapid diagnosis of acute bacterial meningitis. Ann Trop Paediatr 15:273–278, 1995.

145. Camargos PA, Almeida MS, Cardoso I, et al. Latex particle agglutination test in the diagnosis of Haemophilus influenzae type B, Streptococcus pneumoniae and Neisseria meningitidis A and C meningitis in infants and children. J Clin Epidemiol 48:1245–1250, 1995.

146. Gillespie SH, Smith MD, Dickens A, et al. Diagnosis of Streptococcus pneumoniae pneumonia by quantitative enzyme-linked immunosorbent assay of C-polysaccharide antigen. J Clin Pathol 47:749–751, 1994.

147. Parkinson AJ, Rabiego ME, Sepulveda C, et al. Quantitation of pneumococcal C polysaccharide in sputum samples from patients with presumptive pneumococcal pneumonia by enzyme immunoassay. J Clin Microbiol 30:318–322, 1992.

148. Boersma WG, Lowenberg A, Holloway Y, et al. The role of antigen detection in pneumococcal carriers: a comparison between cultures and capsular antigen detection in upper respiratory tract secretions. Scand J Infect Dis 25:51–56, 1993.

149. Jimenez P, Meneses M, Saldias F, Velasquez M. Pneumococcal antigen detection in bronchoalveolar lavage fluid from patients with pneumonia. Thorax 49:872–874, 1994.

150. Bella F, Tort J, Morera MA, et al. Value of bacterial antigen detection in the diagnostic yield of transthoracic needle aspiration in severe community acquired pneumonia. Thorax 48:1227–1229, 1993.

151. Ruiz-Gonzalez A, Falguera M, Nogues A, Rubio-Caballero M. Is Streptococcus pneumoniae the leading cause of pneumonia of unknown etiology? A microbiologic study of lung aspirates in consecutive patients with community-acquired pneumonia. Am J Med 106:385–390, 1999.

152. Boersma WG, Lowenberg A, Holloway Y, et al. Rapid detection of pneumococcal antigen in pleural fluid of patients with community acquired pneumonia. Thorax 48:160–162, 1993.

153. Scott JA, Hannington A, Marsh K, Hall AJ. Diagnosis of pneumococcal pneumonia in epidemiological studies: evaluation in Kenyan adults of a serotype-specific urine latex agglutination assay. Clin Infect Dis 28:764–769, 1999.

154. Dominguez J, Gali N, Blanco S, et al. Detection of Streptococcus pneumoniae antigen by a rapid immunochromatographic assay in urine samples. Chest 119:243–249, 2001.

155. Dowell SF, Garman RL, Liu G, et al. Evaluation of Binax NOW, an assay for the detection of pneumococcal antigen in urine samples, performed among pediatric patients. Clin Infect Dis 32:824–825, 2001.

156. Adegbola RA, Obaro SK, Biney E, Greenwood BM. Evaluation of Binax NOW Streptococcus pneumoniae urinary antigen test in children in a community with a high carriage rate of pneumococcus. Pediatr Infect Dis J 20:718–719, 2001.

157. Finlay FO, Witherow H, Rudd PT. Latex agglutination testing in bacterial meningitis. Arch Dis Child 73:160–161, 1995.

158. Dunbar SA, Eason RA, Musher DM, Clarridge JE 3rd. Microscopic examination and broth culture of cerebrospinal fluid in diagnosis of meningitis. J Clin Microbiol 36:1617–1620, 1998.

159. Perkins MD, Mirrett S, Reller LB. Rapid bacterial antigen detection is not clinically useful. J Clin Microbiol 33:1486–1491, 1995.

160. Cunniffe JG, Whitby Strevens S, Wilcox MH. Effect of pH changes in cerebrospinal fluid specimens on bacterial survival and antigen test results. J Clin Pathol 49:249–253, 1996.

161. Tarafdar K, Rao S, Recco RA, Zaman MM. Lack of sensitivity of the latex agglutination test to detect bacterial antigen in the cerebrospinal fluid of patients with culture-negative meningitis. Clin Infect Dis 33:406–408, 2001.

162. Alonso-Tarres C, Cortes-Lletget C, Casanova T, Domenech A. False-positive pneumococcal antigen test in meningitis diagnosis. Lancet 358:1273–1274, 2001.

163. Marcos MA, Martinez E, Almela M, et al. New rapid antigen test for diagnosis of pneumococcal meningitis. Lancet 357:1499–1500, 2001.

164. Korppi M, Heiskanen-Kosma T, Leinonen M, Halonen P. Antigen and antibody assays in the aetiological diagnosis of respiratory infection in children. Acta Paediatr 82:137–141, 1993.

165. Nohynek H, Eskola J, Laine E, et al. The causes of hospital-treated acute lower respiratory tract infection in children. Am J Dis Child 145:618–622, 1991.

166. Leinonen M, Syrjala H, Jalonen E, et al. Demonstration of pneumolysin antibodies in dissociated immune complexes—a new method for etiological diagnosis of pneumococcal pneumonia. Serodiagn Immunother Infect Dis 4:451–458, 1990.

167. Korppi M, Koskela M, Jalonen E, Leinonen M. Serologically indicated pneumococcal respiratory infection in children. Scand J Infect Dis 24:437–443, 1992.

168. Lankinen KS, Ruutu P, Nohynek H, et al. Pneumococcal pneumonia diagnosis by demonstration of pneumolysin antibodies in precipitated immune complexes: a study in 350 Philippine children with acute lower respiratory infection. Scand J Infect Dis 31:155–161, 1999.

169. Musher DM, Mediwala R, Phan HM, et al. Nonspecificity of assaying for IgG antibody to pneumolysin in circulating immune complexes as a means to diagnose pneumococcal pneumonia. Clin Infect Dis 32:534–538, 2001.

170. Scott JA, Hall AJ, Leinonen M. Validation of immune-complex enzyme immunoassays for diagnosis of pneumococcal pneumonia among adults in Kenya. Clin Diagn Lab Immunol 7:64–67, 2000.

171. Leinonen M, Makela PH. Diagnosis of pneumococcal pneumonia. Clin Infect Dis 33:1440–1441, 2001.

172. Scott JAG, Obiero J, Hall AJ, Marsh K. Validation of immunoglobulin G enzyme-linked immunosorbent assay for antibodies to pneumococcal surface adhesin A in the diagnosis of pneumococcal pneumonia among adults in Kenya. J Infect Dis 186:220–226, 2002.

173. Gillespie SH. The role of the molecular laboratory in the investigation of Streptococcus pneumoniae infections. Semin Respir Infect 14:269–275, 1999.

174. Toikka P, Nikkari S, Ruuskanen O, et al. Pneumolysin PCR-based diagnosis of invasive pneumococcal infection in children. J Clin Microbiol 37:633–637, 1999.

175. Dagan R, Shriker O, Hazan I, et al. Prospective study to determine clinical relevance of detection of pneumococcal DNA in sera of children by PCR. J Clin Microbiol 36:669–673, 1998.

176. Dominguez J, Gali N, Matas L, et al. PCR detection of *Streptococcus pneumoniae* DNA in serum samples for pneumococcal pneumonia diagnosis. Clin Microbiol Infect 7:164–166, 2001.

177. Lorente ML, Falguera M, Nogues A, et al. Diagnosis of pneumococcal pneumonia by polymerase chain reaction (PCR) in whole blood: a prospective clinical study. Thorax 55:133–137, 2000.

178. Menendez R, Cordoba J, de La Cuadra P, et al. Value of the polymerase chain reaction assay in noninvasive respiratory samples for diagnosis of community-acquired pneumonia. Am J Respir Crit Care Med 159:1868–1873, 1999.

179. Hassanking M, Baldeh I, Secka O, et al. Detection of *Streptococcus pneumoniae* DNA in blood cultures by PCR. J Clin Microbiol 32:1721–1724, 1994.

180. McAvin JC, Reilly PA, Roudabush RM, et al. Sensitive and specific method for rapid identification of *Streptococcus pneumoniae* using real-time fluorescence PCR. J Clin Microbiol 39:3446–3451, 2001.

181. Zhang Y, Isaacman DJ, Wadowsky RM, et al. Detection of *Streptococcus pneumoniae* in whole blood by PCR. J Clin Microbiol 33:596–601, 1995.

182. du Plessis M, Smith AM, Klugman KP. Rapid detection of penicillin-resistant *Streptococcus pneumoniae* in cerebrospinal fluid by a semi-nested-PCR strategy. J Clin Microbiol 36:453–457, 1998.

183. Hall LM, Duke B, Urwin G. An approach to the identification of the pathogens of bacterial meningitis by the polymerase chain reaction. Eur J Clin Microbiol Infect Dis 14:1090–1094, 1995.

184. Olcen P, Lantz PG, Backman A, Radstrom P. Rapid diagnosis of bacterial meningitis by a seminested-PCR strategy. Scand J Infect Dis 27:537–539, 1995.

185. Salo P, Örtqvist A, Leinonen M. Diagnosis of bacteremic pneumococcal pneumonia by amplification of pneumolysin gene fragment in serum. J Infect Dis 171:479–482, 1995.

186. Friedland LR, Menon AG, Reising SF, et al. Development of a polymerase chain reaction assay to detect the presence of *Streptococcus pneumoniae* DNA. Diagn Microbiol Infect Dis 20:187–193, 1994.

187. Isaacman DJ, Zhang Y, Rydquist White J, et al. Identification of a patient with *Streptococcus pneumoniae* bacteremia and meningitis by the polymerase chain reaction (PCR). Mol Cell Probes 9:157–160, 1995.

188. Gillespie SH, Ullman C, Smith MD, Emery V. Detection of *Streptococcus pneumoniae* in sputum samples by PCR. J Clin Microbiol 32:1308–1311, 1994.

189. Post JC, Preston RA, Aul JJ, et al. Molecular analysis of bacterial pathogens in otitis media with effusion. JAMA 273:1598–1604, 1995.

190. Jero J, Virolainen A, Salo P, et al. PCR assay for detecting *Streptococcus pneumoniae* in the middle ear of children with otitis media with effusion. Acta Otolaryngol (Stockh) 116:288–292, 1996.

191. Virolainen A, Salo P, Jero J, et al. Comparison of PCR assay with bacterial culture for detecting *Streptococcus pneumoniae* in middle-ear fluid of children with acute otitis media. J Clin Microbiol 32:2667–2670, 1994.

192. Michelow IC, Lozano J, Olsen K, et al. Diagnosis of *Streptococcus pneumoniae* lower respiratory infection in hospitalized children by culture, polymerase chain reaction, serological testing, and urinary antigen detection. Clin Infect Dis 34:E1–E11, 2002.

193. Lu JJ, Perng CL, Lee SY, Wan CC. Use of PCR with universal primers and restriction endonuclease digestions for detection and identification of common bacterial pathogens in cerebrospinal fluid. J Clin Microbiol 38:2076–2080, 2000.

194. Balganesh M, Lalitha MK, Nathaniel R. Rapid diagnosis of acute pyogenic meningitis by a combined PCR dot-blot assay. Mol Cell Probes 14:61–69, 2000.

195. Hansman D, Bullen MM. A resistant pneumococcus. Lancet 2:264–265, 1967.

196. Jacobs MR, Koornhof HJ, Robins-Browne RM, et al. Emergence of multiply resistant pneumococci. N Engl J Med 299:735–740, 1978.

197. Charpentier E, Tuomanen E. Mechanisms of antibiotic resistance and tolerance in *Streptococcus pneumoniae*. Microbes Infect 2:1855–1864, 2000.

198. Widdowson CA, Klugman KP. Molecular mechanisms of resistance to commonly used non-betalactam drugs in *Streptococcus pneumoniae*. Semin Respir Infect 14:255–268, 1999.

199. Tomasz A. New faces of an old pathogen: emergence and spread of multidrug-resistant *Streptococcus pneumoniae*. Am J Med 107(suppl 1A):55S–62S, 1999.

200. Forward KR. The epidemiology of penicillin resistance in *Streptococcus pneumoniae*. Semin Respir Infect 14:243–254, 1999.

201. Whitney CG, Farley MM, Hadler J, et al. Increasing prevalence of multidrug-resistant *Streptococcus pneumoniae* in the United States. N Engl J Med 343:1917–1924, 2000.

202. Collignon PJ, Turnidge JD. Antibiotic resistance in *Streptococcus pneumoniae*. Med J Aust 173(suppl):S58–S64, 2000.

203. Blondeau JM, Tillotson GS. Antimicrobial susceptibility patterns of respiratory pathogens—a global perspective. Semin Respir Infect 15:195–207, 2000.

204. Butler JC, Cetron MS. Pneumococcal drug resistance: the new "special enemy of old age." Clin Infect Dis 28:730–735, 1999.

205. Levin BR, Lipsitch M, Perrot V, et al. The population genetics of antibiotic resistance. Clin Infect Dis 24(suppl 1):S9–S16, 1997.

206. Kaplan SL, Mason EO Jr. Management of infections due to antibiotic-resistant *Streptococcus pneumoniae*. Clin Microbiol Rev 11:628–644, 1998.

207. Campbell GD Jr, Silberman R. Drug-resistant *Streptococcus pneumoniae*. Clin Infect Dis 26:1188–1195, 1998.

208. Schrag SJ, Beall B, Dowell SF. Limiting the spread of resistant pneumococci: biological and epidemiologic evidence for the effectiveness of alternative interventions. Clin Microbiol Rev 13:588–601, 2000.

209. Harwell JI, Brown RB. The drug-resistant pneumococcus: clinical relevance, therapy, and prevention. Chest 117:530–541, 2000.

210. Dunne WM Jr, Kehl KS, Holland-Staley CA, et al. Comparison of results generated by serotyping, pulsed-field restriction analysis, ribotyping, and repetitive-sequence PCR used to characterize penicillin-resistant pneumococci from the United States. J Clin Microbiol 39:1791–1795, 2001.

211. Vilhelmsson SE, Tomasz A, Kristinsson KG. Molecular evolution in a multidrug-resistant lineage of *Streptococcus pneumoniae*: emergence of strains belonging to the serotype 6B Icelandic clone that lost antibiotic resistance traits. J Clin Microbiol 38:1375–1381, 2000.

212. Zhou J, Enright MC, Spratt BG. Identification of the major Spanish clones of penicillin-resistant pneumococci via the Internet using multilocus sequence typing. J Clin Microbiol 38:977–986, 2000.

213. McGee L, McDougal L, Zhou J, et al. Nomenclature of major antimicrobial-resistant clones of *Streptococcus pneumoniae* defined by the Pneumococcal Molecular Epidemiology Network. J Clin Microbiol 39:2565–2571, 2001.

214. Hakenbeck R. Beta-lactam-resistant *Streptococcus pneumoniae*: epidemiology and evolutionary mechanism. Chemotherapy 45:83–94, 1999.

215. Doern GV, Brueggemann AB, Blocker M, et al. Clonal relationships among high-level penicillin-resistant *Streptococcus pneumoniae* in the United States. Clin Infect Dis 27:757–761, 1998.

216. Nesin M, Ramirez M, Tomasz A. Capsular transformation of a multidrug-resistant *Streptococcus pneumoniae* in vivo. J Infect Dis 177:707–713, 1998.

217. Gherardi G, Whitney CG, Facklam RR, Beall B. Major related sets of antibiotic-resistant pneumococci in the United States as determined by pulsed-field gel electrophoresis and pbp1a-pbp2b-pbp2x-dhf restriction profiles. J Infect Dis 181:216–229, 2000.

218. Gay K, Stephens DS. Structure and dissemination of a chromosomal insertion element encoding macrolide efflux in *Streptococcus pneumoniae*. J Infect Dis 184:56–65, 2001.

219. Shortridge VD, Doern GV, Brueggemann AB, et al. Prevalence of macrolide resistance mechanisms in *Streptococcus pneumoniae* isolates from a multicenter antibiotic resistance surveillance study conducted in the United States in 1994–1995. Clin Infect Dis 29:1186–1188, 1999.

220. Janoir C, Podglajen I, Kitzis MD, et al. In vitro exchange of fluoroquinolone resistance determinants between *Streptococcus pneumoniae* and *viridans* streptococci and genomic organization of the parE-parC region in *S. mitis*. J Infect Dis 180:555–558, 1999.

221. Ho PL, Que TL, Tsang DN, et al. Emergence of fluoroquinolone resistance among multiply resistant strains of *Streptococcus pneumoniae* in Hong Kong. Antimicrob Agents Chemother 43:1310–1313, 1999.

222. McCullers JA, English BK, Novak R. Isolation and characterization of vancomycin-tolerant *Streptococcus pneumoniae* from the cerebrospinal fluid of a patient who developed recrudescent meningitis. J Infect Dis 181:369–373, 2000.

223. Novak R, Henriques B, Charpentier E, et al. Emergence of vancomycin tolerance in *Streptococcus pneumoniae*. Nature 399:590–593, 1999.

224. Butler JC, Hofmann J, Cetron MS, et al. The continued emergence of drug-resistant *Streptococcus pneumoniae* in the United States: an update from the Centers for Disease Control and Prevention's Pneumococcal Sentinel Surveillance System. J Infect Dis 174:986–993, 1996.

225. Appelbaum PC. Resistance among *Streptococcus pneumoniae*: implications for drug selection. Clin Infect Dis 34:1613–1620, 2002.

226. Centers for Disease Control and Prevention. Resistance of *Streptococcus pneumoniae* to fluoroquinolones—United States, 1995–1999. MMWR 50:800–804, 2001.

227. Richter SS, Heilmann KP, Coffman SL, et al. The molecular epidemiology of penicillin-resistant *Streptococcus pneumoniae* in the United States, 1994–2000. Clin Infect Dis 34:330–339, 2002.

228. Jette LP, Delage G, Ringuette L, et al. Surveillance of invasive *Streptococcus pneumoniae* infection in the province of Quebec, Canada, from 1996 to 1998: serotype distribution, antimicrobial susceptibility, and clinical characteristics. J Clin Microbiol 39:733–737, 2001.

229. Hoban DJ, Doern GV, Fluit AC, et al. Worldwide prevalence of antimicrobial resistance in *Streptococcus pneumoniae*, *Haemophilus influenzae*, and *Moraxella catarrhalis* in the SENTRY Antimicrobial Surveillance Program, 1997–1999. Clin Infect Dis 32(suppl 2): S81–S93, 2001.

230. Lee NY, Song JH, Kim S, et al. Carriage of antibiotic-resistant pneumococci among Asian children: a multinational surveillance by the Asian Network for Surveillance of Resistant Pathogens (ANSORP). Clin Infect Dis 32:1463–1469, 2001.

231. Felmingham D, Gruneberg RN. The Alexander Project 1996–1997: latest susceptibility data from this international study of bacterial pathogens from community-acquired lower respiratory tract infections. J Antimicrob Chemother 45:191–203, 2000.

232. Marco F, Bouza E, Garcia-de-Lomas J, Aguilar L. *Streptococcus pneumoniae* in community-acquired respiratory tract infections in Spain: the impact of serotype and geographical, seasonal and clinical factors on its susceptibility to the most commonly prescribed antibiotics. J Antimicrob Chemother 46:557–564, 2000.

233. Clavo-Sanchez AJ, Giron-Gonzalez JA, Lopez-Prieto D, et al. Multivariate analysis of risk factors for infection due to penicillin-resistant and multidrug-resistant *Streptococcus pneumoniae*: a multicenter study. Clin Infect Dis 24:1052–1059, 1997.

234. Garcia-Rey C, Aguilar L, Baquero F, et al. Importance of local variations in antibiotic consumption and geographical differences of erythromycin and penicillin resistance in *Streptococcus pneumoniae*. J Clin Microbiol 40:159–164, 2002.

235. Bronzwaer SLAM, Cars O, Buchholz U, et al. A European study on the relationship between antimicrobial use and antimicrobial resistance. Emerg Infect Dis 8:278–282, 2002.

236. Ho PL, Tse WS, Tsang KW, et al. Risk factors for acquisition of levofloxacin-resistant *Streptococcus pneumoniae*: a case-control study. Clin Infect Dis 32:701–707, 2001.

237. Davidson R, Cavalcanti R, Brunton JL, et al. Resistance to levofloxacin and failure of treatment of pneumococcal pneumonia. N Engl J Med 346:747–750, 2002.

238. Lipsitch M. Measuring and interpreting associations between antibiotic use and penicillin resistance in *Streptococcus pneumoniae*. Clin Infect Dis 32:1044–1054, 2001.

239. Austin DJ, Kristinsson KG, Anderson RM. The relationship between the volume of antimicrobial consumption in human communities and the frequency of resistance. Proc Natl Acad Sci U S A 96:1152–1156, 1999.

240. Pihlajamaki M, Kotilainen P, Kaurila T, et al. Macrolide-resistant *Streptococcus pneumoniae* and use of antimicrobial agents. Clin Infect Dis 33:483–488, 2001.

241. Musher DM, Bartlett JG, Doern GV. A fresh look at the definition of susceptibility of *Streptococcus pneumoniae* to beta-lactam antibiotics. Arch Intern Med 161:2538–2544, 2001.

242. Heffelfinger JD, Dowell SF, Jorgensen JH, et al. Management of community-acquired pneumonia in the era of pneumococcal resistance: a report from the Drug-Resistant *Streptococcus pneumoniae* Therapeutic Working Group. Arch Intern Med 160:1399–1408, 2000.

243. File TM Jr. Appropriate use of antimicrobials for drug-resistant pneumonia: focus on the significance of beta-lactam-resistant *Streptococcus pneumoniae*. Clin Infect Dis 34(suppl 1):S17–S26, 2002.

244. Lynch JP III, Martinez FJ. Clinical relevance of macrolide-resistant *Streptococcus pneumoniae* for community-acquired pneumonia. Clin Infect Dis 34(suppl 1):S27–S34, 2002.

245. Henriques B, Kalin M, Örtqvist Å, et al. Molecular epidemiology of *Streptococcus pneumoniae* causing invasive disease in 5 countries. J Infect Dis 182:833–839, 2000.

246. Metlay JP, Hofmann J, Cetron MS, et al. Impact of penicillin susceptibility on medical outcomes for adult patients with bacteremic pneumococcal pneumonia. Clin Infect Dis 30:520–528, 2000.

247. Ewig S, Ruiz M, Torres A, et al. Pneumonia acquired in the community through drug-resistant *Streptococcus pneumoniae*. Am J Respir Crit Care Med 159:1835–1842, 1999.

248. Jehl F, Bedos JP, Poirier R, et al. Nationwide survey on community-acquired pneumococcal pneumonia necessitating hospitalization [in French]. Med Mal Infect 32:267–283, 2002.

249. Feikin DR, Schuchat A, Kolczak M, et al. Mortality from invasive pneumococcal pneumonia in the era of antibiotic resistance, 1995–1997. Am J Public Health 90:223–229, 2000.

250. Bartlett JG, Dowell SF, Mandell LA, et al. Practice guidelines for the management of community-acquired pneumonia in adults. Infectious Diseases Society of America. Clin Infect Dis 31:347–382, 2000.

251. Mandell LA, Marrie TJ, Grossman RF, et al. Canadian guidelines for the initial management of community-acquired pneumonia: an evidence-based update by the Canadian Infectious Diseases Society and the Canadian Thoracic Society. The Canadian Community-Acquired Pneumonia Working Group. Clin Infect Dis 31:383–421, 2000.

252. Huchon G, Woodhead M. European Study on Community-acquired Pneumonia (ESOCAP) Committee. Guidelines for management of adult community acquired lower respiratory tract infections. Eur Resp J 11:986–991, 1998.

253. Buckingham SC, Brown SP, Joaquin VH. Breakthrough bacteremia and meningitis during treatment with cephalosporins parenterally for pneumococcal pneumonia. J Pediatr 132:174–176, 1998.

254. Dowell SF, Smith T, Leversedge K, Snitzer J. Failure of treatment of pneumonia associated with highly resistant pneumococci in a child. Clin Infect Dis 29:462–463, 1999.

255. Friedland IR, McCracken GH. Drug therapy—management of infections caused by antibiotic-resistant *Streptococcus pneumoniae*. N Engl J Med 331:377–382, 1994.

256. Bradley JS, Scheld WM. The challenge of penicillin-resistant *Streptococcus pneumoniae* meningitis: current antibiotic therapy in the 1990s. Clin Infect Dis 25(24 suppl 2):213–221, 1997.

257. Hendley JO, Sande MA, Stewart PM, Gwaltney JM Jr. Spread of *Streptococcus pneumoniae* in families. I. Carriage rates and distribution of types. J Infect Dis 132:55–61, 1975.

258. Raz R, Soboh S, Much A, et al. Pneumococcal carriage in geriatric institute residents. Infect Dis Clin Pract 8:291–293, 1999.

259. Syrjanen RK, Kilpi TM, Kaijalainen TH, et al. Nasopharyngeal carriage of *Streptococcus pneumoniae* in Finnish children younger than 2 years old. J Infect Dis 184:451–459, 2001.

260. Soininen A, Pursiainen H, Kilpi T, Käyhty H. Natural development of antibodies to pneumococcal capsular polysaccharides depends on the serotype: association with pneumococcal carriage and acute otitis media in young children. J Infect Dis 184:569–576, 2001.

261. Hansman D, Morris S. Pneumococcal carriage amongst children in Adelaide, South Australia. Epidemiol Infect 101:411–417, 1988.

262. Gray BM, Dillon HC Jr. Epidemiological studies of *Streptococcus pneumoniae* in infants: antibody to types 3, 6, 14, and 23 in the first two years of life. J Infect Dis 158:948–955, 1988.

263. Douglas RM, Hansman D, Miles HB, Paton JC. Pneumococcal carriage and type-specific antibody: failure of a 14-valent vaccine to reduce carriage in healthy children. Am J Dis Child 140:1183–1185, 1986.

264. Leino T, Auranen K, Jokinen J, et al. Pneumococcal carriage in children during their first two years: important role of family exposure. Pediatr Infect Dis J 20:1022–1027, 2001.

265. Nilsson P, Laurell MH. Carriage of penicillin-resistant *Streptococcus pneumoniae* by children in day-care centers during an intervention program in Malmo, Sweden. Pediatr Infect Dis J 20:1144–1149, 2001.

266. Sa-Leao R, Tomasz A, Sanches IS, et al. Carriage of internationally spread clones of *Streptococcus pneumoniae* with unusual drug resistance patterns in children attending day care centers in Lisbon, Portugal. J Infect Dis 182:1153–1160, 2000.

267. Raymond J, Le Thomas I, Moulin F, et al. Sequential colonization by *Streptococcus pneumoniae* of healthy children living in an orphanage. J Infect Dis 181:1983–1988, 2000.

268. Kellner JD, Ford-Jones EL. *Streptococcus pneumoniae* carriage in children attending 59 Canadian child care centers. Toronto Child Care Centre Study Group. Arch Pediatr Adolesc Med 153:495–502, 1999.

269. Gunnarsson O, Ekdahl K. Previous respiratory tract infections and antibiotic consumption in children with long- and short-term carriage of penicillin-resistant *Streptococcus pneumoniae*. Epidemiol Infect 121:523–528, 1998.

270. Dagan R, Leibovitz E, Greenberg D, et al. Dynamics of pneumococcal nasopharyngeal colonization during the first days of antibiotic treatment in pediatric patients. Pediatr Infect Dis J 17:880–885, 1998.

271. Skull S, Shelby-James T, Morris P, et al. *Streptococcus pneumoniae* antibiotic resistance in Northern Territory children in day care. J Paediatr Child Health 35:466–471, 1999.

272. Robinson DA, Edwards KM, Waites KB, et al. Clones of *Streptococcus pneumoniae* isolated from nasopharyngeal carriage and invasive disease in young children in central Tennessee. J Infect Dis 183:1501–1507, 2001.

273. Samore MH, Magill MK, Alder SC, et al. High rates of multiple antibiotic resistance in *Streptococcus pneumoniae* from healthy children living in isolated rural communities: association with cephalosporin use and intrafamilial transmission. Pediatrics 108:856–865, 2001.

274. Bogaert D, Engelen MN, Timmers-Reker AJ, et al. Pneumococcal carriage in children in the Netherlands: a molecular epidemiological study. J Clin Microbiol 39:3316–3320, 2001.

275. Musher DM, Groover JE, Reichler MR, et al. Emergence of antibody to capsular polysaccharides of *Streptococcus pneumoniae* during outbreaks of pneumonia: association with nasopharyngeal colonization. Clin Infect Dis 24:441–446, 1997.

276. Smith T, Lehmann D, Montgomery J, et al. Acquisition and invasiveness of different serotypes of *Streptococcus pneumoniae* in young children. Epidemiol Infect 111:27–39, 1993.

277. Fedson DS. Pneumococcal vaccination for older adults—the first 20 years. Drugs Aging 15(suppl 1):21–30, 1999.

278. Feldman C. Pneumonia in the elderly. Clin Chest Med 20:563–573, 1999.

279. Torres A, El Ebiary M, Riquelme R, et al. Community-acquired pneumonia in the elderly. Semin Respir Infect 14:173–183, 1999.

280. Macfarlane J. Lower respiratory tract infection and pneumonia in the community. Semin Respir Infect 14:151–162, 1999.

281. Ewig S. Community-acquired pneumonia: definition, epidemiology, and outcome. Semin Respir Infect 14:94–102, 1999.

282. Finch R. Community-acquired pneumonia: the evolving challenge. Clin Microbiol Infect 7(suppl 3):30–38, 2001.

283. Pallares R. Treatment of pneumococcal pneumonia. Semin Respir Infect 14:276–284, 1999.

284. Marrie TJ. Pneumococcal pneumonia: epidemiology and clinical features. Semin Respir Infect 14:227–236, 1999.

285. Klugman KP, Feldman C. *Streptococcus pneumoniae* respiratory tract infections. Curr Opin Infect Dis 14:173–179, 2001.

286. Fine MJ, Auble TE, Yealy DM, et al. A prediction rule to identify low-risk patients with community-acquired pneumonia. N Engl J Med 336:243–250, 1997.

287. Fine MJ, Stone RA, Singer DE, et al. Processes and outcomes of care for patients with community-acquired pneumonia: results from the Pneumonia Patient Outcomes Research Team (PORT) cohort study. Arch Intern Med 159:970–980, 1999.

288. Jokinen C, Heiskanen L, Juvonen H, et al. Incidence of community-acquired pneumonia in the population of four municipalities in eastern Finland. Am J Epidemiol 137:977-988, 1993.

289. Marston BJ, Plouffe JF, File TM Jr, et al. Incidence of community-acquired pneumonia requiring hospitalization. Arch Intern Med 157:1709–1718, 1997.

290. Kaplan V, Angus DC, Griffin MF, et al. Hospitalized community-acquired pneumonia in the elderly: age- and sex-related patterns of care and outcome in the United States. Am J Respir Crit Care Med 165:766–772, 2002.

291. Guest JF, Morris A. Community-acquired pneumonia: the annual cost to the National Health Service in the UK. Eur Respir J 10:1530–1534, 1997.

292. Farr BM, Kaiser DL, Harrison BD, Connolly CK. Prediction of microbial aetiology at admission to hospital for pneumonia from the presenting clinical features. British Thoracic Society Pneumonia Research Subcommittee. Thorax 44:1031–1035, 1989.

293. Fedson DS, Musher DM. Pneumococcal vaccine. *In* Plotkin SA, Mortimer EA Jr (eds). Vaccines (2nd ed). Philadelphia, WB Saunders, 1994, pp 517–564.

294. Fedson DS, Musher DM, Eskola J. Pneumococcal vaccine. *In* Plotkin SA, Orenstein WA (eds). Vaccines (3rd ed). Philadelphia, WB Saunders, 1999, pp 553–607.

295. Park DR, Sherbin VL, Goodman MS, et al. The etiology of community-acquired pneumonia at an urban public hospital: influence of human immunodeficiency virus infection and initial severity of illness. J Infect Dis 184:268–277, 2001.

296. Laurichesse H, Sotto A, Bonnet E, et al. Pre- and in-hospital management of community-acquired pneumonia in southern France, 1998–1999. Eur J Clin Microbiol Infect Dis 20:770–778, 2001.

297. Brandenburg JA, Marrie TJ, Coley CM, et al. Clinical presentation, processes and outcomes of care for patients with pneumococcal pneumonia. J Gen Intern Med 15:638–646, 2000.

298. Glerant JC, Hellmuth D, Schmit JL, et al. Utility of blood cultures in community-acquired pneumonia requiring hospitalization: influence of antibiotic treatment before admission. Respir Med 93:208–212, 1999.

299. Juega J, Montero Martinez C, Pedreira JD, et al. Community acquired pneumonia requiring admission to hospital: etiology and follow-up of 366 cases [in Spanish]. An Med Interna 15:421–426, 1998.

300. Santos de Unamuno C, Llorente San Martin MA, Carandell Jager E, et al. Site of care provision, etiology and treatment of community-acquired pneumonia in Palma de Mallorca [in Spanish]. Med Clin (Barc) 110:290–294, 1998.

301. Almirall J, Bolibar I, Vidal J, et al. Epidemiology of community-acquired pneumonia in adults: a population-based study. Eur Respir J 15:757–763, 2000.

302. Sopena N, Sabria M, Pedro-Botet ML, et al. Prospective study of community-acquired pneumonia of bacterial etiology in adults. Eur J Clin Microbiol Infect Dis 18:852–858, 1999.

303. Ruiz M, Ewig S, Marcos MA, et al. Etiology of community-acquired pneumonia: impact of age, comorbidity, and severity. Am J Respir Crit Care Med 160:397–405, 1999.

304. Castro-Guardiola A, Armengou A, Garcia D, et al. Prospective study of 198 community acquired pneumonias in a general hospital [in Spanish]. Enferm Infecc Microbiol Clin 17:213–218, 1999.

305. Roson B, Carratala J, Dorca J, et al. Etiology, reasons for hospitalization, risk classes, and outcomes of community-acquired pneumonia in patients hospitalized on the basis of conventional admission criteria. Clin Infect Dis 33:158–165, 2001.

306. Boschini A, Smacchia C, Di Fine M, et al. Community-acquired pneumonia in a cohort of former injection drug users with and without human immunodeficiency virus infection: incidence, etiologies, and clinical aspects. Clin Infect Dis 23:107–113, 1996.

307. Logroscino CD, Penza O, Locicero S, et al. Community-acquired pneumonia in adults: a multicentric observational AIPO study. Monaldi Arch Chest Dis 54:11–17, 1999.

308. Ishida T, Hashimoto T, Arita M, et al. Etiology of community-acquired pneumonia in hospitalized patients: a 3-year prospective study in Japan. Chest 114:1588–1593, 1998.

309. Lim WS, Macfarlane JT, Boswell TC, et al. Study of community acquired pneumonia aetiology (SCAPA) in adults admitted to hospital: implications for management guidelines. Thorax 56:296–301, 2001.

310. Jokinen C, Heiskanen L, Juvonen H, et al. Microbial etiology of community-acquired pneumonia in the adult population of 4 municipalities in eastern Finland. Clin Infect Dis 32:1141–1154, 2001.

311. Lode H, Garau J, Grassi C, et al. Treatment of community-acquired pneumonia: a randomized comparison of sparfloxacin, amoxycillin-clavulanic acid and erythromycin. Eur Respir J 8:1999–2007, 1995.

312. Laing R, Slater W, Coles C, et al. Community-acquired pneumonia in Christchurch and Waikato 1999–2000: microbiology and epidemiology. N Z Med J 114:488–492, 2001.

313. Liam CK, Lim KH, Wong CM. Community-acquired pneumonia in patients requiring hospitalization. Respirology 6:259–264, 2001.

314. Kobashi Y, Okimoto N, Matsushima T, Soejima R. Clinical analysis of community-acquired pneumonia in the elderly. Intern Med 40:703–707, 2001.

315. Marrie TJ, Peeling RW, Fine MJ, et al. Ambulatory patients with community-acquired pneumonia: the frequency of atypical agents and clinical course. Am J Med 101:508–515, 1996.

316. Georges H, Leroy O, Vandenbussche C, et al. Epidemiological features and prognosis of severe community-acquired pneumococcal pneumonia. Intensive Care Med 25:198–206, 1999.

317. Luna CM, Famiglietti A, Absi R, et al. Community-acquired pneumonia: etiology, epidemiology, and outcome at a teaching hospital in Argentina. Chest 118:1344–1354, 2000.
318. El Solh AA, Sikka P, Ramadan F, Davies J. Etiology of severe pneumonia in the very elderly. Am J Respir Crit Care Med 163(3 pt 1):645–651, 2001.
319. Bochud PY, Moser F, Erard P, et al. Community-acquired pneumonia: a prospective outpatient study. Medicine (Baltimore) 80:75–87, 2001.
320. Hooi LN, Looi I, Ng AJ. A study on community acquired pneumonia in adults requiring hospital admission in Penang. Med J Malaysia 56:275–284, 2001.
321. Gowardman J, Trent L. Severe community acquired pneumonia: a one-year analysis in a tertiary referral intensive care unit. N Z Med J 113:161–164, 2000.
322. Scott JA, Hall AJ, Muyodi C, et al. Aetiology, outcome, and risk factors for mortality among adults with acute pneumonia in Kenya. Lancet 355:1225–1230, 2000.
323. Ruiz M, Ewig S, Torres A, et al. Severe community-acquired pneumonia: risk factors and follow-up epidemiology. Am J Respir Crit Care Med 160:923–929, 1999.
324. Falguera M, Sacristan O, Nogues A, et al. Nonsevere community-acquired pneumonia: correlation between cause and severity or comorbidity. Arch Intern Med 161:1866–1872, 2001.
324a. Ortiz-Ruiz G, Caballero-Lopez J, Friedland IR, et al. A study evaluating the efficacy, safety, and tolerability of Ertapenem versus Ceftriaxone for the treatment of community-acquired pneumonia in adults. Clin Infect Dis 34:1076–1083, 2002.
325. Socan M, Marinic-Fiser N, Kraigher A, et al. Microbial aetiology of community-acquired pneumonia in hospitalised patients. Eur J Clin Microbiol Infect Dis 18:777–782, 1999.
326. Ostergaard L, Andersen PL. Etiology of community-acquired pneumonia: evaluation by transtracheal aspiration, blood culture, or serology. Chest 104:1400–1407, 1993.
327. Paradisi F, Corti G, Cinelli R. *Streptococcus pneumoniae* as an agent of nosocomial infection: treatment in the era of penicillin-resistant strains. Clin Microbiol Infect 7(suppl 4):34–42, 2001.
328. Rubins JB, Cheung S, Carson P, et al. Identification of clinical risk factors for nosocomial pneumococcal bacteremia. Clin Infect Dis 29:178–183, 1999.
329. Canet JJ, Juan N, Xercavins M, et al. Hospital-acquired pneumococcal bacteremia. Clin Infect Dis 35:697–702, 2002.
330. Weiss K, Restieri C, Gauthier R, et al. A nosocomial outbreak of fluoroquinolone-resistant *Streptococcus pneumoniae*. Clin Infect Dis 33:517–522, 2001.
331. Muder RR. Pneumonia in residents of long-term care facilities: epidemiology, etiology, management, and prevention. Am J Med 105:319–330, 1998.
332. Lim WS, Macfarlane JT. A prospective comparison of nursing home acquired pneumonia with community acquired pneumonia. Eur Respir J 18:362–368, 2001.
333. Gleason PP, Meehan TP, Fine JM, et al. Associations between initial antimicrobial therapy and medical outcomes for hospitalized elderly patients with pneumonia. Arch Intern Med 159:2562–2572, 1999.
334. McNeeley DF, Lyons J, Conte S, et al. A cluster of drug-resistant *Streptococcus pneumoniae* among nursing home patients [letter]. Infect Control Hosp Epidemiol 19:476–477, 1998.
335. Nuorti JP, Butler JC, Crutcher JM, et al. An outbreak of multidrug-resistant pneumococcal pneumonia and bacteremia among unvaccinated nursing home residents. N Engl J Med 338:1861–1868, 1998.
336. Gleich S, Morad Y, Echague R, et al. *Streptococcus pneumoniae* serotype 4 outbreak in a home for the aged: report and review of recent outbreaks. Infect Control Hosp Epidemiol 21:711–717, 2000.
337. Centers for Disease Control and Prevention. Outbreak of pneumococcal pneumonia among unvaccinated residents of a nursing home—New Jersey, April 2001. MMWR 50:707–710, 2001.
338. Hoge CW, Reichler MR, Dominguez EA, et al. An epidemic of pneumococcal disease in an overcrowded, inadequately ventilated jail. N Engl J Med 331:643–648, 1994.
339. Ekdahl K, Martensson A, Kamme C. Bacteraemic pneumococcal infections in Southern Sweden 1981–1996: trends in incidence, mortality, age-distribution, serogroups and penicillin-resistance. Scand J Infect Dis 30:257–262, 1998.
340. Goldstein FW, Acar JF. Antimicrobial resistance among lower respiratory tract isolates of *Streptococcus pneumoniae*: results of a 1992–1993 western Europe and USA collaborative surveillance study. The Alexander Project Collaborative Group. J Antimicrob Chemother 38(suppl A):71–84, 1996.
341. Schonheyder HC. Two thousand seven hundred and thirty nine episodes of bacteremia in the county of Northern Jutland 1996–1998: presentation of a regional clinical database [in Danish]. Ugeskr Laeger 162:2886–2891, 2000.
342. Gosbell IB, Newton PJ, Sullivan EA. Survey of blood cultures from five community hospitals in southwestern Sydney, Australia, 1993–1994. Aust N Z J Med 29:684–692, 1999.
343. Javaloyas M, Garcia-Somoza D, Gudiol F. Epidemiology and prognosis of bacteremia: a 10-year study in a community hospital. Scand J Infect Dis 34:436–441, 2002.
344. Kim PE, Musher DM, Glezen WP, et al. Association of invasive pneumococcal disease with season, atmospheric conditions, air pollution, and the isolation of respiratory viruses. Clin Infect Dis 22:100–106, 1996.
345. Chen FM, Breiman RF, Farley M, et al. Geocoding and linking data from population-based surveillance and the US Census to evaluate the impact of median household income on the epidemiology of invasive *Streptococcus pneumoniae* infections. Am J Epidemiol 148:1212–1218, 1998.
346. Afessa B, Greaves WL, Frederick WR. Pneumococcal bacteremia in adults: a 14-year experience in an inner-city university hospital. Clin Infect Dis 21:345–351, 1995.
347. Gomez J, Banos V, Gomez JR, et al. Clinical significance of pneumococcal bacteraemias in a general hospital: a prospective study 1989–1993. J Antimicrob Chemother 36:1021–1030, 1995.
348. Laaveri T, Nikoskelainen J, Meurman O, et al. Bacteraemic pneumococcal disease in a teaching hospital in Finland. Scand J Infect Dis 28:41–46, 1996.
349. Mirzanejad Y, Roman S, Talbot J, et al. Pneumococcal bacteremia in two tertiary care hospitals in Winnipeg, Canada. Chest 109:173–178, 1996.
350. Holm A, Berild D, Ringertz S, Hoiby EA. Incidence and characteristics of invasive pneumococcal infections 1993–1996 in Aker University Hospital, Oslo [abstract]. *In* Abstracts of the 37th Interscience Conference on Antimicrobial Agents and Chemotherapy, Toronto, September 28–October 1, 1997, p 343.
351. Farinas-Alvarez C, Farinas MC, Garcia-Palomo JD, et al. Prognostic factors for pneumococcal bacteremia in a university hospital. Eur J Clin Microbiol Infect Dis 19:733–741, 2000.
352. Mufson MA, Kruss DM, Wasil RE, Metzger WI. Capsular types and outcome of bacteremic pneumococcal disease in the antibiotic era. Arch Intern Med 134:505–510, 1974.
353. Frankel RE, Virata M, Hardalo C, et al. Invasive pneumococcal disease: clinical features, serotypes, and antimicrobial resistance patterns in cases involving patients with and without human immunodeficiency virus infection. Clin Infect Dis 23:577–584, 1996.
354. Crowe M, Ispahani P, Humphreys H, et al. Bacteraemia in the adult intensive care unit of a teaching hospital in Nottingham, UK, 1985–1996. Eur J Clin Microbiol Infect Dis 17:377–384, 1998.
355. Kalin M, Örtqvist Å, Almela M, et al. Prospective study of prognostic factors in community-acquired bacteremic pneumococcal disease in 5 countries. J Infect Dis 182:840–847, 2000.
356. Balakrishnan I, Crook P, Morris R, Gillespie SH. Early predictors of mortality in pneumococcal bacteraemia. J Infect 40:256–261, 2000.
357. Vaqueiro SM, Sampere VM, Font CB, et al. Pneumococcal bacteremia in patients aged over 65 years: a study of 161 cases [in Spanish]. Med Clin (Barc) 117:241–245, 2001.
358. Huebner RE, Wasas AD, Klugman KP. Trends in antimicrobial resistance and serotype distribution of blood and cerebrospinal fluid isolates of *Streptococcus pneumoniae* in South Africa, 1991–1998. Int J Infect Dis 4:214–218, 2000.
359. Örtqvist Å, Kalin M, Julander I, Mufson MA. Deaths in bacteremic pneumococcal pneumonia: a comparison of two populations—Huntington, WVa, and Stockholm, Sweden. Chest 103:710–716, 1993.
360. Marfin AA, Sporrer J, Moore PS, Siefkin AD. Risk factors for adverse outcome in persons with pneumococcal pneumonia. Chest 107:457–462, 1995.

361. Pesola GR, Charles A. Pneumococcal bacteremia with pneumonia: mortality in acquired immunodeficiency syndrome. Chest 101:150–155, 1992.

362. Waterer GW, Jennings SG, Wunderink RG. The impact of blood cultures on antibiotic therapy in pneumococcal pneumonia. Chest 116:1278–1281, 1999.

363. Moroney JF, Fiore AE, Harrison LH, et al. Clinical outcomes of bacteremic pneumococcal pneumonia in the era of antibiotic resistance. Clin Infect Dis 33:797–805, 2001.

364. Waterer GW, Somes GW, Wunderink RG. Monotherapy may be suboptimal for severe bacteremic pneumococcal pneumonia. Arch Intern Med 161:1837–1842, 2001.

365. Urwin G, Yuan MF, Hall LM, et al. Pneumococcal meningitis in the North East Thames Region UK: epidemiology and molecular analysis of isolates. Epidemiol Infect 117:95–102, 1996.

366. Fiore AE, Moroney JF, Farley MM, et al. Clinical outcomes of meningitis caused by Streptococcus pneumoniae in the era of antibiotic resistance. Clin Infect Dis 30:71–77, 2000.

367. Stanek RJ, Mufson MA. A 20-year epidemiological study of pneumococcal meningitis. Clin Infect Dis 28:1265–1272, 1999.

368. Auburtin M, Porcher R, Bruneel F, et al. Pneumococcal meningitis in the intensive care unit: prognostic factors of clinical outcome in a series of 80 cases. Am J Respir Crit Care Med 165:713–717, 2002.

368a. Torres JM, Cardenas O, Vasquez A, Schlossberg D. Streptococcus pneumoniae bacteremia in a community hospital. Chest 113:387–390, 1998.

369. Drinkovic D, Wong CG, Taylor SL, et al. Pneumococcal bacteraemia and opportunities for prevention. N Z Med J 114:326–328, 2001.

370. Lindberg J, Fangel S. Recurrent endocarditis caused by Streptococcus pneumoniae. Scand J Infect Dis 31:409–410, 1999.

370a. Aronin SI, Mukherjee SK, West JC, Cooney EL. Review of pneumococcal endocarditis in adults in the penicillin era. Clin Infect Dis 26:165–171, 1998.

371. Lefort A, Mainardi JL, Selton-Suty C, et al. Streptococcus pneumoniae endocarditis in adults: a multicenter study in France in the era of penicillin resistance (1991–1998). The Pneumococcal Endocarditis Study Group. Medicine (Baltimore) 79:327–337, 2000.

372. Ispahani P, Weston VC, Turner DPJ, Donald FE. Septic arthritis due to Streptococcus pneumoniae in Nottingham, United Kingdom, 1985–1998. Clin Infect Dis 29:1450–1454, 1999.

373. James PA, Thomas MG. Streptococcus pneumoniae septic arthritis in adults. Scand J Infect Dis 32:491–494, 2000.

374. Dugi DD III, Musher DM, Clarridge JE III, Kimbrough R. Intraabdominal infection due to Streptococcus pneumoniae. Medicine (Baltimore) 80:236–244, 2001.

375. Capdevila O, Pallares R, Grau I, et al. Pneumococcal peritonitis in adult patients: report of 64 cases with special reference to emergence of antibiotic resistance. Arch Intern Med 161:1742–1748, 2001.

376. Taylor SN, Sanders CV. Unusual manifestations of invasive pneumococcal infection. Am J Med 107(suppl 1A):12S–27S, 1999.

377. Rodriguez-Creixems M, Munoz P, Miranda E, et al. Recurrent pneumococcal bacteremia: a warning of immunodeficiency. Arch Intern Med 156:1429–1434, 1996.

378. Turett GS, Blum S, Telzak EE. Recurrent pneumococcal bacteremia—risk factors and outcomes. Arch Intern Med 161:2141–2144, 2001.

379. Coccia MR, Facklam RR, Saravolatz LD, Manzor O. Recurrent pneumococcal bacteremia: 34 episodes in 15 patients. Clin Infect Dis 26:982–985, 1998.

380. McEllistrem MC, Mendelsohn AB, Pass MA, et al. Recurrent invasive pneumococcal disease in individuals with human immunodeficiency virus infection. J Infect Dis 185:1364–1368, 2002.

381. Ekdahl K, Truedsson L, Sjoholm AG, Braconier JH. Complement analysis in adult patients with a history of bacteremic pneumococcal infections or recurrent pneumonia. Scand J Infect Dis 27:111–117, 1995.

382. Hussein AS, Shafran SD. Acute bacterial meningitis in adults: a 12-year review. Medicine (Baltimore) 79:360–368, 2000.

383. Schuchat A, Robinson K, Wenger JD, et al. Bacterial meningitis in the United States in 1995. N Engl J Med 337:970–976, 1997.

384. Campbell JF, Donohue MA, Mochizuki RB, et al. Pneumococcal bacteremia in Hawaii: initial findings of a pneumococcal disease prevention project. Hawaii Med J 48:513–514, 1989.

385. Haglund LA, Istre GR, Pickett DA, et al. Invasive pneumococcal disease in central Oklahoma: emergence of high-level penicillin resistance and multiple antibiotic resistance. Pneumococcus Study Group. J Infect Dis 168:1532–1536, 1993.

386. Breiman RF, Spika JS, Navarro VJ, et al. Pneumococcal bacteremia in Charleston County, South Carolina: a decade later. Arch Intern Med 150:1401–1405, 1990.

387. Bennett NM, Buffington J, LaForce FM. Pneumococcal bacteremia in Monroe County, New York. Am J Public Health 82:1513–1516, 1992.

388. Plouffe JF, Breiman RF, Facklam RR. Bacteremia with Streptococcus pneumoniae: implications for therapy and prevention. Franklin County Pneumonia Study Group. JAMA 275:194–198, 1996.

389. Hofmann J, Cetron MS, Farley MM, et al. The prevalence of drug-resistant Streptococcus pneumoniae in Atlanta. N Engl J Med 333:481–486, 1995.

390. Pastor P, Medley F, Murphy TV. Invasive pneumococcal disease in Dallas County, Texas: results from population-based surveillance in 1995. Clin Infect Dis 26:590–595, 1998.

391. Zangwill KM, Vadheim CM, Vannier AM, et al. Epidemiology of invasive pneumococcal disease in southern California: implications for the design and conduct of a pneumococcal conjugate vaccine efficacy trial. J Infect Dis 174:752–759, 1996.

392. Mufson MA, Stanek RJ. Bacteremic pneumococcal pneumonia in one American city: a 20-year longitudinal study, 1978–1997. Am J Med 107(suppl 1A):34S–43S, 1999.

393. Harrison LH, Dwyer DM, Billmann L, et al. Invasive pneumococcal infection in Baltimore, MD: implications for immunization policy. Arch Intern Med 160:89–94, 2000.

394. Cooper TA, Bandy U. Invasive disease attributed to Streptococcus pneumoniae, 1998–1999. Med Health R I 84(1):24–25, 2001.

395. Rudolph KM, Parkinson AJ, Reasonover AL, et al. Serotype distribution and antimicrobial resistance patterns of invasive isolates of Streptococcus pneumoniae: Alaska, 1991–1998. J Infect Dis 182:490–496, 2000.

396. Robinson KA, Baughman W, Rothrock G, et al. Epidemiology of invasive Streptococcus pneumoniae infections in the United States, 1995–1998: opportunities for prevention in the conjugate vaccine era. JAMA 285:1729–1735, 2001.

396a. Morita JY, Zell ER, Danila R, et al. Association between antimicrobial resistance among pneumococcal isolates and burden of invasive pneumococcal disease in the community. Clin Infect Dis 35:420–427, 2002.

397. Nuorti JP, Butler JC, Gelling L, et al. Epidemiologic relation between HIV and invasive pneumococcal disease in San Francisco County, California. Ann Intern Med 132:182–190, 2000.

398. McGeer A, Landry L, Goldenberg E, Green K. Population-based surveillance for invasive pneumococcal infections in Toronto, Canada: implications for prevention [abstract]. In Abstract of the 36th Interscience Conference on Antimicrobial Agents and Chemotherapy, New Orleans, September 15–18, 1996, p 251.

399. Laurichesse H, Grimaud O, Waight P, et al. Pneumococcal bacteraemia and meningitis in England and Wales, 1993 to 1995. Commun Dis Public Health 1:22–27, 1998.

400. Sleeman K, Knox K, George R, et al. Invasive pneumococcal disease in England and Wales: vaccination implications. J Infect Dis 183:239–246, 2001.

401. Smith MD, Stuart J, Andrews NJ, et al. Invasive pneumococcal infection in South and West England. Epidemiol Infect 120:117–123, 1998.

402. McKenzie H, Reid N, Dijkhuizen RS. Clinical and microbiological epidemiology of Streptococcus pneumoniae bacteraemia. J Med Microbiol 49:361–366, 2000.

403. The National Laboratory Surveillance Network (EPIBAC). Surveillance of Bacterial Meningitis and Bacteraemia of Selected Bacteria. Saint-Maurice, Réseau National de Santé Publique, 1997.

404. Laurichesse H, Romaszko JP, Nguyen LT, et al. Clinical characteristics and outcome of patients with invasive pneumococcal disease, Puy-de-Dome, France, 1994–1998. Eur J Clin Microbiol Infect Dis 20:299–308, 2001.

405. de Neeling AJ, van Pelt W, Hol C, et al. Temporary increase in incidence of invasive infection due to Streptococcus pneumoniae in the Netherlands. Clin Infect Dis 29:1579–1580, 1999.

406. van Ampting JMA, Bonter KP, Diepersloot RJA, et al. Pneumococcal bacteraemia: incidence, outcome and predisposing factors. Eur J Intern Med 9:145–150, 1998.

407. Ament A, Baltussen R, Duru G, et al. Cost-effectiveness of pneumococcal vaccination of older people: a study in 5 western European countries. Clin Infect Dis 31:444–450, 2000.

408. Konradsen HB. *Streptococcus pneumoniae.* Epi-News 18, 1998.
409. Konradsen HB. *Streptococcus pneumoniae.* Epi-News 14, 2000.
410. Örtqvist Å. Pneumococcal disease in Sweden: experiences and current situation. Am J Med 107(suppl 1A):44S–49S, 1999.
411. Dahl MS, Trollfors B, Claesson BA, et al. Invasive pneumococcal infections in southwestern Sweden: a second follow-up period of 15 years. Scand J Infect Dis 33:667–672, 2001.
412. Sankilampi U, Herva E, Haikala R, et al. Epidemiology of invasive *Streptococcus pneumoniae* infections in adults in Finland. Epidemiol Infect 118:7–15, 1997.
413. Dominguez A, Salleras L, Cardenosa N, et al. The epidemiology of invasive *Streptococcus pneumoniae* disease in Catalonia (Spain): a hospital-based study. Vaccine 20:2989–2994, 2002.
414. Konradsen HB, Kaltoft MS. Invasive pneumococcal infections in Denmark from 1995 to 1999: epidemiology, serotypes, and resistance. Clin Diagn Lab Immunol 9:358–365, 2002.
415. Raz R, Elhanan G, Shimoni Z. Pneumococcal bacteremia in hospitalized Israeli adults: epidemiology and resistance to penicillin. Clin Infect Dis 24:1164-1168, 1997.
416. Hogg GG, Strachan JE, Lester RA. Invasive pneumococcal disease in the population of Victoria. Med J Aust 173(suppl):S32–S35, 2000.
417. McIntyre PB, Gilmour RE, Gilbert GL, et al. Epidemiology of invasive pneumococcal disease in urban New South Wales, 1997–1999. Med J Aust 173(suppl):S22–S26, 2000.
418. Krause VL, Reid SJ, Merianos A. Invasive pneumococcal disease in the Northern Territory of Australia, 1994–1998. Med J Aust 173(suppl):S27–S31, 2000.
419. Hasseltvedt V, Hoiby EA, Iversen BG, Nokelby H. Systemisk pneumokokksydom 1996. MSIS-Rapport 25:8, 1997.
420. Hedlund J, Svenson SB, Kalin M, et al. Incidence, capsular types, and antibiotic susceptibility of invasive *Streptococcus pneumoniae* in Sweden. Clin Infect Dis 21:948–953, 1995.
421. Giesecke J, Fredlund H. Increase in pneumococcal bacteraemia in Sweden [letter]. Lancet 349:699–700, 1997.
422. Kallenius G, Hedlund J, Swenson SB, et al. Pneumococcal bacteraemia in Sweden [letter]. Lancet 349:1910, 1997.
423. Baer M, Vuento R, Vesikari T. Increase in bacteraemic pneumococcal infections in children [letter]. Lancet 345:661, 1995.
424. Nielsen SV, Henrichsen J. Incidence of invasive pneumococcal disease and distribution of capsular types of pneumococci in Denmark, 1989–1994. Epidemiol Infect 117:411–416, 1996.
425. Aszkenasy OM, George RC, Begg NT. Pneumococcal bacteraemia and meningitis in England and Wales 1982 to 1992. Commun Dis Rep CDR Wkly 5:R45–R50, 1995.
426. Henrichsen J. The pneumococcal typing system and pneumococcal surveillance. J Infect 1(suppl 2):31–37, 1979.
427. Geslin P, Fremaux A, Sissia G, Spicq C. *Streptococcus pneumoniae:* serotypes, invasive and antibiotic resistant strains. Current situation in France [in French]. Presse Med 27(suppl 1):21–27, 1998.
428. Schonheyder HC, Sorensen HT. Reasons for increase in pneumococcal bacteraemia [letter]. Lancet 349:1554, 1997.
429. Van Essen GA, Palache AM, Forleo E, Fedson DS. Influenza vaccination in 2000: vaccination recommendations and vaccine use in 50 developed and rapidly developing countries. Vaccine 21:1780–1785, 2003.
430. Cortese MM, Wolff M, Almeido-Hill J, et al. High incidence rates of invasive pneumococcal disease in the White Mountain Apache population. Arch Intern Med 152:2277–2282, 1992.
431. Davidson M, Parkinson AJ, Bulkow LR, et al. The epidemiology of invasive pneumococcal disease in Alaska, 1986–1990—ethnic differences and opportunities for prevention. J Infect Dis 170:368–376, 1994.
432. Torzillo PJ, Hanna JN, Morey F, et al. Invasive pneumococcal disease in Central Australia. Med J Aust 162:182–186, 1995.
433. Mak DB, Plant AJ, Rushworth RL. Where the data are deficient: a field evaluation of the effectiveness of pneumococcal vaccination in remote Australia. Aust J Rural Health 9(1):38–46, 2001.
434. Centers for Disease Control and Prevention. Influenza and pneumococcal vaccination levels among adults aged > or =65 years—United States, 1997. MMWR 47:797–802, 1998.
435. Flamaing J, Verhaegen J, Peetermans WE. *Streptococcus pneumoniae* bacteraemia in Belgium: differential characteristics in children and the elderly population and implications for vaccine use. J Antimicrob Chemother 50:43–50, 2002.
436. Williams BG, Gouws E, Boschi-Pinto C, et al. Estimates of worldwide distribution of child deaths from acute respiratory infections. Lancet Infect Dis 2:25–32, 2002.
437. Mulholland K. Magnitude of the problem of childhood pneumonia. Lancet 354:590–592, 1999.
438. Bacterial etiology of serious infections in young infants in developing countries: results of a multicenter study. The WHO Young Infants Study Group. Pediatr Infect Dis J 18(10 suppl):S17–S22, 1999.
439. Peltola H. Burden of meningitis and other severe bacterial infections of children in Africa: implications for prevention. Clin Infect Dis 32:64–75, 2001.
440. Kertesz DA, di Fabio JL, de Cunto Brandileone MC, et al. Invasive *Streptococcus pneumoniae* infection in Latin American children: results of the Pan American Health Organization Surveillance Study. Clin Infect Dis 26:1355–1361, 1998.
441. Mulholland K, Levine O, Nohynek H, Greenwood BM. Evaluation of vaccines for the prevention of pneumonia in children in developing countries. Epidemiol Rev 21:43–55, 1999.
442. Koulla-Shiro S, Kuaban C, Belec L. Acute community-acquired bacterial pneumonia in human immunodeficiency virus (HIV) infected and non-HIV-infected adult patients in Cameroon: aetiology and outcome. Tuber Lung Dis 77:47–51, 1996.
443. Archibald LK, McDonald LC, Nwanyanwu O, et al. A hospital-based prevalence survey of bloodstream infections in febrile patients in Malawi: implications for diagnosis and therapy. J Infect Dis 181:1414–1420, 2000.
444. Bell M, Archibald LK, Nwanyanwu O, et al. Seasonal variation in the etiology of bloodstream infections in a febrile inpatient population in a developing country. Int J Infect Dis 5:63–69, 2001.
445. Gordon MA, Walsh AL, Chaponda M, et al. Bacteraemia and mortality among adult medical admissions in Malawi—predominance of non-typhi salmonellae and *Streptococcus pneumoniae.* J Infect 42:44–49, 2001.
446. Ssali FN, Kamya MR, Wabwire Mangen F, et al. A prospective study of community-acquired bloodstream infections among febrile adults admitted to Mulago Hospital in Kampala, Uganda. J Acquir Immune Defic Syndr Hum Retrovirol 19:484–489, 1998.
447. Dougle ML, Hendriks ER, Sanders EJ, Dorigo Zetsma JW. Laboratory investigations in the diagnosis of septicaemia and malaria. East Afr Med J 74:353–356, 1997.
448. Arthur G, Nduba VN, Kariuki SM, et al. Trends in bloodstream infections among human immunodeficiency virus-infected adults admitted to a hospital in Nairobi, Kenya, during the last decade. Clin Infect Dis 33:248–256, 2001.
449. Gordon SB, Walsh AL, Chaponda M, et al. Bacterial meningitis in Malawian adults: pneumococcal disease is common, severe, and seasonal. Clin Infect Dis 31:53–57, 2000.
450. Schutte CM, Van der Meyden CH, Magazi DS. The impact of HIV on meningitis as seen at a South African academic hospital (1994 to 1998). Infection 28:3–7, 2000.
451. Jones N, Huebner R, Khoosal M, et al. The impact of HIV on *Streptococcus pneumoniae* bacteraemia in a South African population. AIDS 12:2177–2184, 1998.
452. Karstaedt AS, Khoosal M, Crewe-Brown HH. Pneumococcal bacteremia in adults in Soweto, South Africa, during the course of a decade. Clin Infect Dis 33:610–614, 2001.
453. French N, Nakiyingi J, Carpenter LM, et al. 23-Valent pneumococcal polysaccharide vaccine in HIV-1-infected Ugandan adults: double-blind, randomised and placebo controlled trial. Lancet 355:2106–2111, 2000.
454. Gilks CF, Ojoo SA, Ojoo JC, et al. Invasive pneumococcal disease in a cohort of predominantly HIV-1 infected female sex-workers in Nairobi, Kenya. Lancet 347:718–723, 1996.
455. Prospective multicentre hospital surveillance of *Streptococcus pneumoniae* disease in India. Invasive Bacterial Infection Surveillance (IBIS) Group, International Clinical Epidemiology Network (INCLEN). Lancet 353:1216–1221, 1999.
456. Hortal M, Camou T, Palacio R, et al. Ten-year review of invasive pneumococcal diseases in children and adults from Uruguay: clinical spectrum, serotypes, and antimicrobial resistance. Int J Infect Dis 4:91–95, 2000.
457. Campagne G, Schuchat A, Djibo S, et al. Epidemiology of bacterial meningitis in Niamey, Niger, 1981–1996. Bull World Health Organ 77:499–508, 1999.
458. Hausdorff WP, Bryant J, Paradiso PR, Siber GR. Which pneumococcal serogroups cause the most invasive disease: implications for conjugate vaccine formulation and use, part I. Clin Infect Dis 30:100–121, 2000.

459. Clemens J, Brenner R, Rao M, et al. Evaluating new vaccines for developing countries: efficacy or effectiveness? JAMA 275:390–397, 1996.

460. Riley ID, Tarr PI, Andrews M, et al. Immunisation with a polyvalent pneumococcal vaccine: reduction of adult respiratory mortality in a New Guinea Highlands community. Lancet 1:1338–1341, 1977.

461. Department of Vaccines and Biologicals. Report of a meeting on priorities for pneumococcal and *Haemophilus influenzae* type b (Hib) vaccine development and introduction. Bull World Health Organ 1999.

462. Casadevall A, Scharff MD. Serum therapy revisited: animal models of infection and development of passive antibody therapy. Antimicrob Agents Chemother 38:1695–1702, 1994.

463. Keller MA, Stiehm ER. Passive immunity in prevention and treatment of infectious diseases. Clin Microbiol Rev 13:602–614, 2000.

464. Skerrett SJ. Antibody treatment of lower respiratory tract infections. Semin Respir Infect 16:67–75, 2001.

465. Chudwin DS. Prophylaxis and treatment of pneumococcal bacteremia by Immune Globulin Intravenous in a mouse model. Clin Immunol Immunopathol 50:62–71, 1989.

466. Shurin PA, Giebink GS, Wegman DL, et al. Prevention of pneumococcal otitis media in chinchillas with human bacterial polysaccharide immune globulin. J Clin Microbiol 26:755–759, 1988.

467. Hamill RJ, Musher DM, Groover JE, et al. IgG antibody reactive with five serotypes of *Streptococcus pneumoniae* in commercial intravenous immunoglobulin preparations. J Infect Dis 166:38–42, 1992.

468. Weisman LE, Cruess DF, Fischer GW. Opsonic activity of commercially available standard intravenous immunoglobulin preparations. Pediatr Infect Dis J 13:1122–1125, 1994.

469. Buckley RH, Schift RI. The use of intravenous immune globulin in immunodeficiency diseases. N Engl J Med 325:110–117, 1991.

470. Chapel HM, Lee M, Hargreaves R, et al. Randomised trial of intravenous immunoglobulin as prophylaxis against infection in plateau-phase multiple myeloma. The UK Group for Immunoglobulin Replacement Therapy in Multiple Myeloma. Lancet 343:1059–1063, 1994.

471. Intravenous immune globulin for the prevention of bacterial infections in children with symptomatic human immunodeficiency virus infection. N Engl J Med 325:73–80, 1991.

472. Weeks JC, Tierney MR, Weinstein MC. Cost effectiveness of prophylactic immune globulin in chronic lymphocytic leukemia. N Engl J Med 325:81–86, 1991.

473. Robbins JB, Austrian R, Lee CJ, et al. Considerations for formulating the second-generation pneumococcal capsular polysaccharide vaccine with emphasis on the cross-reactive types within groups. J Infect Dis 148:1136–1159, 1983.

474. Centers for Disease Control and Prevention. Prevention of pneumococcal disease: recommendations of the Advisory Committee on Immunization Practices (ACIP). MMWR 46(RR-8):1–24, 1997.

475. Sweeney JA, Sumner JS, Hennessey JP Jr. Simultaneous evaluation of molecular size and antigenic stability of PNEUMOVAX 23, a multivalent pneumococcal polysaccharide vaccine. Dev Biol (Basel) 103:11–26, 2000.

476. Fletcher TJ, Tunnicliffe WS, Hammond K. Simultaneous immunisation with influenza vaccine and pneumococcal polysaccharide vaccine in patients with chronic respiratory disease. BMJ 314:1663–1665, 1997.

477. Gyhrs A, Pedersen BK, Bygbjerg I, et al. The effect of prophylaxis with chloroquine and proguanil on delayed-type hypersensitivity and antibody production following vaccination with diphtheria, tetanus, polio, and pneumococcal vaccines. Am J Trop Med Hyg 45:613–618, 1991.

478. Nichol KL, MacDonald RM, Hauge M. Side effects associated with pneumococcal vaccination. Am J Infect Control 25:223–228, 1997.

479. Sankilampi U, Honkanen PO, Pyhala R, Leinonen M. Associations of prevaccination antibody levels with adverse reactions to pneumococcal and influenza vaccines administered simultaneously in the elderly. Vaccine 15:1133–1137, 1997.

480. Sell SH, Wright PF, Vaughn WK. Clinical studies of pneumococcal vaccines in infants. I. Reactogenicity and immunogenicity of two polyvalent polysaccharide vaccines. Rev Infect Dis 3(suppl):S97–S107, 1981.

481. Lee HJ, Kang JH, Henrichsen J, et al. Immunogenicity and safety of a 23-valent pneumococcal polysaccharide vaccine in healthy children and in children at increased risk of pneumococcal infection. Vaccine 13:1533–1538, 1995.

482. Borgono JM, Mclean AA, Vella PP. Vaccination and revaccination with polyvalent pneumococcal polysaccharide vaccines in adults and infants. Proc Soc Exp Biol Med 157:148–154, 1978.

483. Koskela M, Leinonen M, Haiva VM. First and second dose antibody responses to pneumococcal polysaccharide vaccine in infants. Pediatr Infect Dis J 5:45–50, 1986.

484. Ponvert C, Ardelean-Jaby D, Colin-Gorski AM, et al. Anaphylaxis to the 23-valent pneumococcal vaccine in child: a case-control study based on immediate responses in skin tests and specific IgE determination. Vaccine 19:4588–4591, 2001.

485. Kikuchi Y, Imakiire T, Hyodo T, et al. Minimal change nephrotic syndrome, lymphadenopathy and hyperimmunoglobulinemia after immunization with a pneumococcal vaccine. Clin Nephrol 58:68–72, 2002.

486. Eskola J, Käyhty H, Takala A, et al. Reactogenicity and immunogenicity of combined vaccines for bacteraemic diseases caused by *Haemophilus influenzae* type b, meningococci and pneumococci in 24-month-old children. Vaccine 8:107–110, 1990.

487. Brichacek B, Swindells S, Janoff EN, et al. Increased plasma human immunodeficiency virus type 1 burden following antigenic challenge with pneumococcal vaccine. J Infect Dis 174:1191–1199, 1996.

488. Stanley SK, Ostrowski MA, Justement JS, et al. Effect of immunization with a common recall antigen on viral expression in patients infected with human immunodeficiency virus type I. N Engl J Med 334:1222–1230, 1996.

489. Honkanen PO, Keistinen T, Kivela SL. Reactions following administration of influenza vaccine alone or with pneumococcal vaccine to the elderly. Arch Intern Med 156:205–208, 1996.

490. Schiffman G, Douglas RM, Bonner MJ, et al. A radioimmunoassay for immunologic phenomena in pneumococcal disease and for the antibody response to pneumococcal vaccines. I. Method for the radioimmunoassay of anticapsular antibodies and comparison with other techniques. J Immunol Meth 33:133–144, 1980.

491. Koskela M. Serum antibodies to pneumococcal C polysaccharide in children: response to acute pneumococcal otitis media or to vaccination. Pediatr Infect Dis J 6:519–526, 1987.

492. Siber GR, Priehs C, Madore DV. Standardization of antibody assays for measuring the response to pneumococcal infection and immunization. Pediatr Infect Dis J 8(1 suppl):S84–S91, 1989.

493. Musher DM, Luchi MJ, Watson DA, et al. Pneumococcal polysaccharide vaccine in young adults and older bronchitics: determination of IgG responses by ELISA and the effect of adsorption of serum with non-type-specific cell wall polysaccharide. J Infect Dis 161:728–735, 1990.

494. Goldblatt D, Levinsky RJ, Turner MW. Role of cell wall polysaccharide in the assessment of IgG antibodies to the capsular polysaccharides of *Streptococcus pneumoniae* in childhood. J Infect Dis 166:632–634, 1992.

495. Goldblatt D, Jadresic LP, Levinsky RJ, Turner MW. Antibody responses to pneumococcal capsular polysaccharide: what is being measured? Immunodeficiency 4(1-4):47–50, 1993.

496. Sorensen UB. Pneumococcal polysaccharide antigens: capsules and C-polysaccharide. An immunochemical study. Dan Med Bull 42:47–53, 1995.

497. Musher DM, Chapman AJ, Goree A, et al. Natural and vaccine-related immunity to *Streptococcus pneumoniae*. J Infect Dis 154:245–256, 1986.

498. Fine DP, Kirk JL, Schiffman G, et al. Analysis of humoral and phagocytic defenses against *Streptococcus pneumoniae* serotypes 1 and 3. J Lab Clin Med 112:487–497, 1988.

499. Nieuwhof WN, Hodgen AN. An enzyme-linked immunosorbent assay suitable for the routine estimation of specific immunoglobulin G responses to polyvalent pneumococcal polysaccharide vaccine in humans. J Immunol Methods 84:197–202, 1985.

500. Shyamala GN, Roberton DM, Hosking CS. Human-isotype-specific enzyme immunoassay for antibodies to pneumococcal polysaccharides. J Clin Microbiol 26:1575–1579, 1988.

501. Verheul AF, Versteeg AA, Westerdaal NA, et al. Measurement of the humoral immune response against *Streptococcus pneumoniae* type 14-derived antigens by an ELISA and ELISPOT assay based on biotin-avidin technology. J Immunol Methods 126:79–87, 1990.

502. Musher DM, Johnson B Jr, Watson DA. Quantitative relationship between anticapsular antibody measured by enzyme-linked immunosorbent assay or radioimmunoassay and protection of mice against challenge with *Streptococcus pneumoniae* serotype 4. Infect Immun 58:3871–3876, 1990.

503. Watson DA, Musher DM. Interruption of capsule production in *Streptococcus pneumoniae* serotype 3 by insertion of transposon Tn916. Infect Immun 58:3135–3138, 1990.

504. Concepcion N, Frasch CE. Evaluation of previously assigned antibody concentrations in pneumococcal polysaccharide reference serum 89SF by the method of cross-standardization. Clin Diagn Lab Immunol 5:199–204, 1998.

505. Yu X, Sun Y, Frasch C, et al. Pneumococcal capsular polysaccharide preparations may contain non-C-polysaccharide contaminants that are immunogenic. Clin Diagn Lab Immunol 6:519–524, 1999.

506. Soininen A, van den Dobbelsteen G, Oomen L, Käyhty H. Are the enzyme immunoassays for antibodies to pneumococcal capsular polysaccharides serotype specific? Clin Diagn Lab Immunol 7:468–476, 2000.

507. Concepcion NF, Frasch CE. Pneumococcal type 22f polysaccharide absorption improves the specificity of a pneumococcal-polysaccharide enzyme-linked immunosorbent assay. Clin Diagn Lab Immunol 8:266–272, 2001.

508. Plikaytis BD, Goldblatt D, Frasch CE, et al. An analytical model applied to a multicenter pneumococcal enzyme-linked immunosorbent assay study. J Clin Microbiol 38:2043–2050, 2000.

509. Quataert S, Martin D, Anderson P, et al. A multi-laboratory evaluation of an enzyme-linked immunoassay quantitating human antibodies to *Streptococcus pneumoniae* polysaccharides. Immunol Invest 30:191–207, 2001.

510. Musher DM, Groover JE, Rowland JM, et al. Antibody to capsular polysaccharides of *Streptococcus pneumoniae*: prevalence, persistence, and response to revaccination. Clin Infect Dis 17:66–73, 1993.

511. Nieminen T, Käyhty H, Virolainen A, Eskola J. Circulating antibody secreting cell response to parenteral pneumococcal vaccines as an indicator of a salivary IgA antibody response. Vaccine 16:313–319, 1998.

512. Vioarsson G, Jonsdottir I, Jonsson S, Valdimarsson H. Opsonization and antibodies to capsular and cell wall polysaccharides of *Streptococcus pneumoniae*. J Infect Dis 170:592–599, 1994.

513. Usinger WR, Lucas AH. Avidity as a determinant of the protective efficacy of human antibodies to pneumococcal capsular polysaccharides. Infect Immun 67:2366–2370, 1999.

514. Romero-Steiner S, Musher DM, Cetron MS, et al. Reduction in functional antibody activity against *Streptococcus pneumoniae* in vaccinated elderly individuals highly correlates with decreased IgG antibody avidity. Clin Infect Dis 29:281–288, 1999.

515. Sun Y, Hwang Y, Nahm MH. Avidity, potency, and cross-reactivity of monoclonal antibodies to pneumococcal capsular polysaccharide serotype 6B. Infect Immun 69:336–344, 2001.

516. Anttila M, Voutilainen M, Jantti V, et al. Contribution of serotype-specific IgG concentration, IgG subclasses and relative antibody avidity to opsonophagocytic activity against *Streptococcus pneumoniae*. Clin Exp Immunol 118:402–407, 1999.

517. Jansen WT, Gootjes J, Zelle M, et al. Use of highly encapsulated *Streptococcus pneumoniae* strains in a flow-cytometric assay for assessment of the phagocytic capacity of serotype-specific antibodies. Clin Diagn Lab Immunol 5:703–710, 1998.

518. Romero-Steiner S, Libutti D, Pais LB, et al. Standardization of an opsonophagocytic assay for the measurement of functional antibody activity against *Streptococcus pneumoniae* using differentiated HL-60 cells. Clin Diagn Lab Immunol 4:415–422, 1997.

519. Martinez JE, Romero-Steiner S, Pilishvili T, et al. A flow cytometric opsonophagocytic assay for measurement of functional antibodies elicited after vaccination with the 23-valent pneumococcal polysaccharide vaccine. Clin Diagn Lab Immunol 6:581–586, 1999.

520. Guy B, Testart C, Gimenez S, et al. Comparison of polymorphonuclear cells from healthy donors and differentiated HL-60 cells as phagocytes in an opsonophagocytic assay using antigen-coated fluorescent beads. Clin Diagn Lab Immunol 7:314–317, 2000.

521. Jansen WT, Vakevainen-Anttila M, Käyhty H, et al. Comparison of a classical phagocytosis assay and a flow cytometry assay for assessment of the phagocytic capacity of sera from adults vaccinated with a pneumococcal conjugate vaccine. Clin Diagn Lab Immunol 8:245–250, 2001.

522. Vakevainen M, Jansen W, Saeland E, et al. Are the opsonophagocytic activities of antibodies in infant sera measured by different pneumococcal phagocytosis assays comparable? Clin Diagn Lab Immunol 8:363–369, 2001.

523. Rodriguez ME, van der Pol WL, Sanders LA, van de Winkel JG. Crucial role of FcgammaRIIa (CD32) in assessment of functional anti-*Streptococcus pneumoniae* antibody activity in human sera. J Infect Dis 179:423–433, 1999.

524. Rodriguez ME, van der Pol WL, van de Winkel JG. Flow cytometry-based phagocytosis assay for sensitive detection of opsonic activity of pneumococcal capsular polysaccharide antibodies in human sera. J Immunol Methods 252:33–44, 2001.

525. Nahm MH, Briles DE, Yu X. Development of a multi-specificity opsonophagocytic killing assay. Vaccine 18:2768–2771, 2000.

526. Lin JS, Park MK, Nahm MH. Chromogenic assay measuring opsonophagocytic killing capacities of antipneumococcal antisera. Clin Diagn Lab Immunol 8:528–533, 2001.

527. Stack AM, Malley R, Thompson CM, et al. Minimum protective serum concentrations of pneumococcal anti-capsular antibodies in infant rats. J Infect Dis 177:986–990, 1998.

528. Johnson SE, Rubin L, Romero-Steiner S, et al. Correlation of opsonophagocytosis and passive protection assays using human anti-capsular antibodies in an infant mouse model of bacteremia for *Streptococcus pneumoniae*. J Infect Dis 180:133–140, 1999.

529. Wuorimaa T, Käyhty H, Eskola J, et al. Activation of cell-mediated immunity following immunization with pneumococcal conjugate or polysaccharide vaccine. Scand J Immunol 53:422–428, 2001.

530. Musher DM, Groover JE, Watson DA, Pandey JP. Genetic regulation of the capacity to make immunoglobulin G to pneumococcal capsular polysaccharides. J Invest Med 45:57–68, 1997.

531. Bardardottir E, Jonsson S, Jonsdottir I, et al. IgG subclass response and opsonization of *Streptococcus pneumoniae* after vaccination of healthy adults. J Infect Dis 162:482–488, 1990.

532. Herer B, Labrousse F, Mordelet-Dambrine M, et al. Selective IgG subclass deficiencies and antibody responses to pneumococcal capsular polysaccharide antigen in adult community-acquired pneumonia. Am Rev Respir Dis 142:854–857, 1990.

533. Johnson S, Opstad NL, Douglas JM Jr, Janoff EN. Prolonged and preferential production of polymeric immunoglobulin A in response to *Streptococcus pneumoniae* capsular polysaccharides. Infect Immun 64:4339–4344, 1996.

534. Konradsen HB, Henrichsen J, Wachmann H, Holm N. The influence of genetic factors on the immune response as judged by pneumococcal vaccination of mono- and dizygotic Caucasian twins. Clin Exp Immunol 92:532–536, 1993.

535. Konradsen HB, Oxelius VA, Hahn Zoric M, Hanson LA. The importance of G1m and 2 allotypes for the IgG2 antibody levels and avidity against pneumococcal polysaccharide type 1 within mono- and dizygotic twin-pairs. Scand J Immunol 40:251–256, 1994.

536. Konradsen HB, Hahn Zoric M, Nagao AT, Hanson LA. Differences within mono- and dizygotic twin-pairs in spectrotypes and clones of IgG2 antibodies to pneumococcal polysaccharide type 1 and C-polysaccharide after vaccination. Scand J Immunol 40:423–428, 1994.

537. Kantor AB, Leonore AH. Origin of murine B cells lineages. Annu Rev Immunol 11:501–538, 1993.

538. Temple K, Greenwood B, Inskip H, et al. Antibody response to pneumococcal capsular polysaccharide vaccine in African children. Pediatr Infect Dis J 10:386–390, 1991.

539. Brussow H, Baensch M, Sidoti J. Seroprevalence of immunoglobulin M (IgM) and IgG antibodies to polysaccharides of *Streptococcus pneumoniae* in different age groups of Ecuadorian and German children. J Clin Microbiol 30:2765–2771, 1992.

540. Witt CS, Pomat W, Lehmann D, Alpers MP. Antibodies to pneumococcal polysaccharides in pneumonia and response to pneumococcal vaccination in young children in Papua New Guinea. Clin Exp Immunol 83:219–224, 1991.

541. Douglas RM, Paton JC, Duncan SJ. Antibody response to pneumococcal vaccination in children younger than five years of age. J Infect Dis 148:131–137, 1983.

542. Leinonen M, Sakkinen A, Kalliokoski R. Antibody response to 14-valent pneumococcal capsular polysaccharide vaccine in pre-school age children. Pediatr Infect Dis J 5:39–44, 1986.

543. Lim PL, Lau YL. Occurrence of IgG subclass antibodies to ovalbumin, avidin, and pneumococcal polysaccharide in children. Int Arch Allergy Immunol 104:137–143, 1994.

544. Pomat WS, Lehmann D, Sanders RC, et al. Immunoglobulin G antibody responses to polyvalent pneumococcal vaccine in children in the highlands of Papua New Guinea. Infect Immun 62:1848–1853, 1994.

545. Virolainen A, Vero J, Käyhty H, et al. Nasopharyngeal antibodies to pneumococcal capsular polysaccharides in children with acute otitis media. J Infect Dis 172:1115–1118, 1995.

546. Virolainen A, Jero J, Käyhty H, et al. Nasopharyngeal antibodies to pneumococcal pneumolysin in children with acute otitis media. Clin Diagn Lab Immunol 2:704–707, 1995.

547. Virolainen A, Jero J, Käyhty H. Antibodies to pneumolysin and pneumococcal capsular polysaccharides in middle ear fluid of children with acute otitis media. Acta Otolaryngol 115:796–803, 1995.

548. Rijkers GT, Sanders EAM, Breukels MA, Zegers BJM. Responsiveness of infants to capsular polysaccharides: implications for vaccine development. Rev Med Microbiol 7:3–12, 1996.

549. Musher DM, Groover JE, Graviss EA, Baughn RE. The lack of association between aging and postvaccination levels of IgG antibody to capsular polysaccharides of *Streptococcus pneumoniae*. Clin Infect Dis 22:165–167, 1996.

550. Rubins JB, Puri AK, Loch J, et al. Magnitude, duration, quality, and function of pneumococcal vaccine responses in elderly adults. J Infect Dis 178:431–440, 1998.

551. Lottenbach KR, Mink CM, Barenkamp SJ, et al. Age-associated differences in immunoglobulin G1 (IgG1) and IgG2 subclass antibodies to pneumococcal polysaccharides following vaccination. Infect Immun 67:4935–4938, 1999.

552. Rubins JB, Alter M, Loch J, Janoff EN. Determination of antibody responses of elderly adults to all 23 capsular polysaccharides after pneumococcal vaccination. Infect Immun 67:5979–5984, 1999.

553. Carson PJ, Nichol KL, O'Brien J, et al. Immune function and vaccine responses in healthy advanced elderly patients. Arch Intern Med 160:2017–2024, 2000.

554. Konradsen HB. Quantity and avidity of pneumococcal antibodies before and up to five years after pneumococcal vaccination of elderly persons. Clin Infect Dis 21:616–620, 1995.

555. Sankilampi U, Honkanen PO, Bloigu A, et al. Antibody response to pneumococcal capsular polysaccharide vaccine in the elderly. J Infect Dis 173:387–393, 1996.

556. Sankilampi U, Honkanen PO, Bloigu A, Leinonen M. Persistence of antibodies to pneumococcal capsular polysaccharide vaccine in the elderly. J Infect Dis 176:1100–1104, 1997.

557. Ekdahl K, Braconier JH, Svanborg C. Impaired antibody response to pneumococcal capsular polysaccharides and phosphorylcholine in adult patients with a history of bacteremic pneumococcal infection. Clin Infect Dis 25:654–660, 1997.

558. Hedlund J, Langer B, Konradsen HB, Örtqvist Å. Negligible adjuvant effect for antibody responses and frequent adverse events associated with IL-12 treatment in humans vaccinated with pneumococcal polysaccharide. Vaccine 20:164–169, 2001.

559. Bruyn GA, Hiemstra PS, Matze-van der Lans A, van Furth R. Pneumococcal anticapsular antibodies in patients with chronic cardiovascular and obstructive lung disease in the Netherlands. J Infect Dis 162:1192–1194, 1990.

560. Doing A, Griffin D, Jacobson JA, et al. B-cell function in chronic heart failure: antibody response to pneumococcal vaccine. J Card Fail 7:318–321, 2001.

561. Lahood N, Emerson SS, Kumar P, Sorensen RU. Antibody levels and response to pneumococcal vaccine in steroid-dependent asthma. Ann Allergy 70:289–294, 1993.

562. Miravitelles M, de Gracia J, Rodrigo MJ, et al. Specific antibody response against the 23-valent pneumococcal vaccine in patients with alpha(1)-antitrypsin deficiency with and without bronchiectasis. Chest 116:946–952, 1999.

563. Shapiro GG, Virant FS, Furukawa CT, et al. Immunologic defects in patients with refractory sinusitis. Pediatrics 87:311–316, 1991.

564. Zora JA, Silk HJ, Tinkelman DG. Evaluation of postimmunization pneumococcal titers in children with recurrent infections and normal levels of immunoglobulin. Ann Allergy 70:283–288, 1993.

565. Sanders LA, Rijkers GT, Kuis W, et al. Defective antipneumococcal polysaccharide antibody response in children with recurrent respiratory tract infections. J Allergy Clin Immunol 91(1 pt 1):110–119, 1993.

566. Epstein MM, Gruskay F. Selective deficiency in pneumococcal antibody response in children with recurrent infections. Ann Allergy Asthma Immunol 75:125–131, 1995.

567. Sanders LA, Rijkers GT, Tenbergen Meekes AM, et al. Immunoglobulin isotype-specific antibody responses to pneumococcal polysaccharide vaccine in patients with recurrent bacterial respiratory tract infections. Pediatr Res 37:812–819, 1995.

568. Hidalgo H, Moore C, Leiva LE, Sorensen RU. Preimmunization and postimmunization pneumococcal antibody titers in children with recurrent infections. Ann Allergy Asthma Immunol 76:341–346, 1996.

569. Silk H, Zora J, Goldstein J, et al. Response to pneumococcal immunization in children with and without recurrent infections. J Asthma 35:101–112, 1998.

570. Dhooge IJ, van Kempen MJP, Sanders LAM, Rijkers GT. Deficient IgA and IgG2 anti-pneumococcal antibody levels and response to vaccination in otitis prone children. Int J Pediatr Otorhinolaryngol 64:133–141, 2002.

571. Sanal O, Ersoy F, Yel L, et al. Impaired IgG antibody production to pneumococcal polysaccharides in patients with ataxia-telangiectasia. J Clin Immunol 19:326–334, 1999.

572. Arkwright PD, Patel L, Moran A, et al. Atopic eczema is associated with delayed maturation of the antibody response to pneumococcal vaccine. Clin Exp Immunol 122:16–19, 2000.

573. Eibl N, Spatz M, Fischer GF, et al. Impaired primary immune response in type-1 diabetes: results from a controlled vaccination study. Clin Immunol 103:249–259, 2002.

574. McMahon BJ, Parkinson AJ, Bulkow L, et al. Immunogenicity of the 23-valent pneumococcal polysaccharide vaccine in Alaska Native chronic alcoholics compared with nonalcoholic Native and non-Native controls. Am J Med 95:589–594, 1993.

575. McCashland TM, Preheim LC, Gentry MJ. Pneumococcal vaccine response in cirrhosis and liver transplantation. J Infect Dis 181:757–760, 2000.

576. Preheim LC, Mellencamp MA, Snitily MU, Gentry MJ. Effect of cirrhosis on the production and efficacy of pneumococcal capsular antibody in a rat model. Am Rev Respir Dis 146:1054–1058, 1992.

577. Janoff EN, O Brien J, Thompson P, et al. *Streptococcus pneumoniae* colonization, bacteremia, and immune response among persons with human immunodeficiency virus infection. J Infect Dis 167:49–56, 1993.

578. Garcia-Leoni ME, Moreno S, Rodeno P. Pneumococcal pneumonia in adult hospitalized patients infected with the human immunodeficiency virus. Arch Intern Med 152:1808–1812, 1992.

579. Hirschtick RE, Glassroth J, Jordan MC, et al. Bacterial pneumonia in persons infected with the human immunodeficiency virus: pulmonary complications of HIV infection study group. N Engl J Med 333:845–851, 1995.

580. Hibbs JR, Douglas RM Jr, Judson FN, et al. Prevalence of human immunodeficiency virus infection, mortality rate, and serogroup distribution among patients with pneumococcal bacteremia at Denver General Hospital, 1984–1994. Clin Infect Dis 25:195–199, 1997.

581. Schneider RF, Rosen MJ. Pneumococcal infections in HIV-infected adults. Semin Respir Infect 14:237–242, 1999.

582. Janoff EN, Breiman RF, Daley CL, Hopewell PC. Pneumococcal disease during HIV infection: epidemiologic, clinical, and immunologic perspectives. Ann Intern Med 117:314–324, 1992.

583. Gesner M, Desiderio D, Kim M, et al. *Streptococcus pneumoniae* in human immunodeficiency virus type 1-infected children. Pediatr Infect Dis J 13:697–703, 1994.

584. Farley JJ, King JC, Nair P, et al. Invasive pneumococcal disease among infected and uninfected children of mothers with human immunodeficiency virus infection. J Pediatr 124:853–858, 1994.

585. Mao C, Harper M, McIntosh K, et al. Invasive pneumococcal infections in human immunodeficiency virus-infected children. J Infect Dis 173:870–876, 1996.

586. Rusen IA, Fraser-Roberts L. Nasopharyngeal pneumococcal colonization among Kenyan children: antibiotic resistance, strain types and associations with human immunodeficiency virus type 1 infection. Pediatr Infect Dis J 16:656–662, 1997.

587. Falguera M, Perez-Mur J, Galindo C, Garcia M. Prevalence and outcome of pneumococcal carrier human immunodeficiency virus-infected patients [letter]. J Infect Dis 168:511, 1993.

588. Rodriguez-Barradas MC, Tharapel RA, Groover JE, et al. Colonization by *Streptococcus pneumoniae* among human immunodeficiency virus-infected adults: prevalence of antibiotic resistance, impact of immunization, and characterization by polymerase chain reaction with BOX primers of isolates from persistent *S. pneumoniae* carriers. J Infect Dis 175:590–597, 1997.

589. Drucker E, Webber MP, McMaster P, Vermund SH. Increasing rate of pneumonia hospitalizations in the Bronx: a sentinel indicator for human immunodeficiency virus. Int J Epidemiol 18:926–933, 1989.

590. Selwyn PA, Feingold AR, Hartel D, et al. Increased risk of bacterial pneumonia in HIV-infected intravenous drug users without AIDS. AIDS 2:267–272, 1988.

591. Manos GE, van Deutekom H, Peerbooms PG, et al. Community-acquired pneumonia in drug abusers in Amsterdam [letter]. Lancet 336:939–940, 1990.

592. Miller RF, Foley NM, Kessel D, Jeffrey AA. Community acquired lobar pneumonia in patients with HIV infection and AIDS. Thorax 49:367–368, 1994.

593. Mundy LM, Auwaerter PG, Oldach D, et al. Community-acquired pneumonia: impact of immune status. Am J Respir Crit Care Med 152(4 pt 1):1309–1315, 1995.

594. Afessa B, Green B. Bacterial pneumonia in hospitalized patients with HIV infection: the Pulmonary Complications, ICU Support, and Prognostic Factors of Hospitalized Patients with HIV (PIP) Study. Chest 117:1017–1022, 2000.

595. Hart CA, Beeching NJ, Duerden BI, et al. Infections in AIDS. J Med Microbiol 49:947–967, 2000.

596. Redd SC, Rutherford GW 3rd, Sande MA, et al. The role of human immunodeficiency virus infection in pneumococcal bacteremia in San Francisco residents. J Infect Dis 162:1012–1017, 1990.

597. Schuchat A, Broome CV, Hightower A, et al. Use of surveillance for invasive pneumococcal disease to estimate the size of the immunosuppressed HIV-infected population. JAMA 265:3275–3279, 1991.

598. McNaghten AD, Hanson DL, Jones JL, et al. Effects of antiretroviral therapy and opportunistic illness primary chemoprophylaxis on survival after AIDS diagnosis. Adult/Adolescent Spectrum of Disease Group. AIDS 13:1687–1695, 1999.

599. Palella FJ Jr, Delaney KM, Moorman AC, et al. Declining morbidity and mortality among patients with advanced human immunodeficiency virus infection. HIV Outpatient Study Investigators. N Engl J Med 338:853–860, 1998.

600. Rodriguez Barradas MC, Musher DM, Hamill RJ, et al. Unusual manifestations of pneumococcal infection in human immunodeficiency virus-infected individuals: the past revisited. Clin Infect Dis 14:192–199, 1992.

601. Feldman C, Glatthaar M, Morar R, et al. Bacteremic pneumococcal pneumonia in HIV-seropositive and HIV-seronegative adults. Chest 116:107–114, 1999.

602. Osmond DH, Chin DP, Glassroth J, et al. Impact of bacterial pneumonia and Pneumocystis carinii pneumonia on human immunodeficiency virus disease progression. Pulmonary Complications of HIV Study Group. Clin Infect Dis 29:536–543, 1999.

603. Baril L, Astagneau P, Nguyen J, et al. Pyogenic bacterial pneumonia in human immunodeficiency virus-infected inpatients: a clinical, radiological, microbiological, and epidemiological study [see comments]. Clin Infect Dis 26:964–971, 1998.

604. Navin TR, Rimland D, Lennox JL, et al. Risk factors for community-acquired pneumonia among persons infected with human immunodeficiency virus. J Infect Dis 181:158–164, 2000.

605. Breiman RF, Keller DW, Phelan MA, et al. Evaluation of effectiveness of the 23-valent pneumococcal capsular polysaccharide vaccine for HIV-infected patients. Arch Intern Med 160:2633–2638, 2000.

606. Falco V, Fernandez de Sevilla T, Alegre J, et al. Bacterial pneumonia in HIV-infected patients: a prospective study of 68 episodes. Eur Respir J 7:235–239, 1994.

607. Meynard JL, Barbut F, Blum L, et al. Risk factors for isolation of Streptococcus pneumoniae with decreased susceptibility to penicillin G from patients infected with human immunodeficiency virus. Clin Infect Dis 22:437–440, 1996.

608. Turett GS, Blum S, Fazal BA, et al. Penicillin resistance and other predictors of mortality in pneumococcal bacteremia in a population with high human immunodeficiency virus seroprevalence. Clin Infect Dis 29:321–327, 1999.

609. Crewe Brown HH, Karstaedt AS, Saunders GL, et al. Streptococcus pneumoniae blood culture isolates from patients with and without human immunodeficiency virus infection: alterations in penicillin susceptibilities and in serogroups or serotypes. Clin Infect Dis 25:1165–1172, 1997.

610. Nuorti JP, Butler JC, Gelling L, et al. Epidemiologic relation between HIV and invasive pneumococcal disease in San Francisco County, California. Ann Intern Med 132:182–190, 2000.

611. Rodriguez-Barradas MC, Musher DM, Lahart C. Antibody to capsular polysaccharides of Streptococcus pneumoniae after vaccination of human immunodeficiency virus-infected subjects with 23-valent pneumococcal vaccine. J Infect Dis 165:533–536, 1992.

612. Weiss PJ, Wallace MR, Oldfield EC 3rd, et al. Response of recent human immunodeficiency virus seroconverters to the pneumococcal polysaccharide vaccine and Haemophilus influenzae type b conjugate vaccine. J Infect Dis 171:1217–1222, 1995.

613. Mascartlemone F, Gerard M, Libin M, et al. Differential effect of human immunodeficiency virus infection on the IgA and IgG antibody responses to pneumococcal vaccine. J Infect Dis 172:1253–1260, 1995.

614. Carson PJ, Schut RL, Simpson ML, et al. Antibody class and subclass responses to pneumococcal polysaccharides following immunization of human immunodeficiency virus-infected patients. J Infect Dis 172:340–345, 1995.

615. Rodriguez-Barradas MC, Groover JE, Lacke CE, et al. IgG antibody to pneumococcal capsular polysaccharide in human immunodeficiency virus-infected subjects: persistence of antibody in responders, revaccination in nonresponders, and relationship of immunoglobulin allotype to response. J Infect Dis 173:1347–1353, 1996.

616. French N, Gilks CF, Mujugira A, et al. Pneumococcal vaccination in HIV-1-infected adults in Uganda: humoral response and two vaccine failures. AIDS 12:1683–1689, 1998.

617. Nielsen H, Kvinesdal B, Benfield TL, et al. Rapid loss of specific antibodies after pneumococcal vaccination in patients with human immunodeficiency virus-1 infection. Scand J Infect Dis 30:597–601, 1998.

618. Janoff EN, Fasching C, Ojoo JC, et al. Responsiveness of human immunodeficiency virus type 1-infected Kenyan women with or without prior pneumococcal disease to pneumococcal vaccine. J Infect Dis 175:975–978, 1997.

619. Moore D, Nelson M, Henderson D. Pneumococcal vaccination and HIV infection. Int J STD AIDS 9:1–7, 1998.

620. Arpadi SM, Back S, O Brien J, Janoff EN. Antibodies to pneumococcal capsular polysaccharides in children with human immunodeficiency virus infection given polyvalent pneumococcal vaccine. J Pediatr 125:77–79, 1994.

621. Peters VB, Diamant EP, Hodes DS, Cimino CO. Impaired immunity to pneumococcal polysaccharide antigens in children with human immunodeficiency virus infection immunized with pneumococcal vaccine. Pediatr Infect Dis J 13:933–934, 1994.

622. Gibb D, Spoulou V, Giacomelli A, et al. Antibody responses to Haemophilus influenzae type b and Streptococcus pneumoniae vaccines in children with human immunodeficiency virus infection. Pediatr Infect Dis J 14:129–135, 1995.

623. Talesnik E, Vial PA, Labarca J, et al. Time course of antibody response to tetanus toxoid and pneumococcal capsular polysaccharides in patients infected with HIV. J Acquir Immune Defic Syndr Hum Retrovirol 19:471–477, 1998.

624. Kroon FP, van Dissel JT, Ravensbergen E, et al. Antibodies against pneumococcal polysaccharides after vaccination in HIV-infected individuals: 5-year follow-up of antibody concentrations. Vaccine 18:524–530, 1999.

625. de Moraes Pinto MI, Almeida AC, Kenj G, et al. Placental transfer and maternally acquired neonatal IgG immunity in human immunodeficiency virus infection. J Infect Dis 173:1077–1084, 1996.

626. Kroon FP, van Dissel JT, Ravensbergen E, et al. Enhanced antibody response to pneumococcal polysaccharide vaccine after prior immunization with conjugate pneumococcal vaccine in HIV-infected adults. Vaccine 19:886–894, 2000.

627. Ahmed F, Steinhoff MC, Rodriguez-Barradas MC, et al. Effect of human immunodeficiency virus type 1 infection on the antibody response to a glycoprotein conjugate pneumococcal vaccine: results from a randomized trial. J Infect Dis 173:83–90, 1996.

628. Feikin DR, Elie CM, Goetz MB, et al. Randomized trial of the quantitative and functional antibody responses to a 7-valent pneumococcal conjugate vaccine and/or 23-valent polysaccharide vaccine among HIV-infected adults. Vaccine 20:545–553, 2001.

629. Glaser JB, Volpe S, Aguirre A, et al. Zidovudine improves response to pneumococcal vaccine among persons with AIDS and AIDS-related complex. J Infect Dis 164:761–764, 1991.

630. Farber CM, Barath AA, Dieye T. The effects of immunization in human immunodeficiency virus type 1 infection [letter]. N Engl J Med 335:817, 1996.

631. Keller M, Deveikis A, Cutillar-Garcia M, et al. Pneumococcal and influenza immunization and human immunodeficiency virus load in children. Pediatr Infect Dis J 19:613–618, 2000.

632. Vigano A, Bricalli D, Trabattoni D, et al. Immunization with both T cell-dependent and T cell-independent vaccines augments HIV viral load secondarily to stimulation of tumor necrosis factor alpha. AIDS Res Hum Retroviruses 14:727–734, 1998.

633. Negredo E, Domingo P, Sambeat MA, et al. Effect of pneumococcal vaccine on plasma HIV-1 RNA of stable patients undergoing effective highly active antiretroviral therapy. Eur J Clin Microbiol Infect Dis 20:287–288, 2001.

634. Amdahl BM, Rubins JB, Daley CL, et al. Impaired natural immunity to pneumolysin during human immunodeficiency virus infection in the United States and Africa. Am J Respir Crit Care Med 152(6 pt 1):2000–2004, 1995.

635. Bisharat N, Omari H, Lavi I, Raz R. Risk of infection and death among post-splenectomy patients. J Infect 43:182–186, 2001.

636. Cullingford GL, Watkins DN, Watts AD, Mallon DF. Severe late postsplenectomy infection. Br J Surg 78:716–721, 1991.

637. Styrt BA. Risks of infection and protective strategies for the asplenic patient. Infect Dis Clin Pract 5:94–100, 1996.

638. Waghorn DJ. Overwhelming infection in asplenic patients: current best practice preventive measures are not being followed. J Clin Pathol 54:214–218, 2001.

639. Schutze GE, Mason EO Jr, Barson WJ, et al. Invasive pneumococcal infections in children with asplenia. Pediatr Infect Dis J 21:278–282, 2002.

640. Aavitsland P, Froholm LO, Hoiby EA, Lystad A. Risk of pneumococcal disease in individuals without a spleen [letter]. Lancet 344:1504, 1994.

641. Shatz DV, Schinsky MF, Pais LB, et al. Immune responses of splenectomized trauma patients to the 23-valent pneumococcal polysaccharide vaccine at 1 versus 7 versus 14 days after splenectomy. J Trauma 44:760–765; discussion 765–766, 1998.

642. Molrine DC, Siber GR, Samra Y, et al. Normal IgG and impaired IgM responses to polysaccharide vaccines in asplenic patients. J Infect Dis 179:513–517, 1999.

643. Konradsen HB, Rasmussen C, Ejstrud P, Hansen JB. Antibody levels against Streptococcus pneumoniae and Haemophilus influenzae type b in a population of splenectomized individuals with varying vaccination status. Epidemiol Infect 119:167–174, 1997.

644. Anonymous. Guidelines for the prevention and treatment of infection in patients with an absent or dysfunctional spleen. Working Party of the British Committee for Standards in Haematology Clinical Task Force. BMJ 312:430–434, 1996.

645. Overturf GD. Technical report: prevention of pneumococcal infections, including the use of pneumococcal conjugate and polysaccharide vaccines and antibiotic prophylaxis. American Academy of Pediatrics Committee on Infectious Diseases. Pediatrics 106(2 pt 1):367–376, 2000.

646. Palejwala AA, Hong LY, King D. Managing patients with an absent or dysfunctional spleen: under half of doctors know that antibiotic prophylaxis should be life long. BMJ 312:1360, 1996.

647. Sarangi J, Coleby M, Trivella M, Reilly S. Prevention of postsplenectomy sepsis: a population-based approach. J Public Health Med 19:208–212, 1997.

648. Hegarty PK, Tan B, O'Sullivan R, et al. Prevention of postsplenectomy sepsis: how much do patients know? Hematol J 1:357–359, 2000.

649. Ejstrud P, Kristensen B, Hansen JB, et al. Risk and patterns of bacteraemia after splenectomy: a population-based study. Scand J Infect Dis 32:521–525, 2000.

650. Knight-Madden J, Serjeant GR. Invasive pneumococcal disease in homozygous sickle cell disease: Jamaican experience 1973–1997. J Pediatr 138:65–70, 2001.

651. Gill FM, Sleeper LA, Weiner SJ, et al. Clinical events in the first decade in a cohort of infants with sickle cell disease. Cooperative Study of Sickle Cell Disease. Blood 86:776–783, 1995.

652. Chesney PJ, Wilimas JA, Presbury G, et al. Penicillin- and cephalosporin-resistant strains of Streptococcus pneumoniae causing sepsis and meningitis in children with sickle cell disease. J Pediatr 127:526–532, 1995.

653. Wang WC, Wong WY, Rogers ZR, et al. Antibiotic-resistant pneumococcal infection in children with sickle cell disease in the United States. J Pediatr Hematol Oncol 18:140–144, 1996.

654. Bjornson AB, Lobel JS. Direct evidence that decreased opsonization of Streptococcus pneumoniae via the alternative complement pathway in sickle cell disease is related to antibody deficiency. J Clin Invest 79:388–398, 1987.

655. Rautonen N, Martin NL, Rautonen J, et al. Low number of antibody producing cells in patients with sickle cell anemia. Immunol Lett 34:207–211, 1992.

656. Norris CF, Surrey S, Bunin GR, et al. Relationship between Fc receptor IIA polymorphism and infection in children with sickle cell disease. J Pediatr 128:813–819, 1996.

657. Bjornson AB, Falletta JM, Verter JI, et al. Serotype-specific immunoglobulin G antibody responses to pneumococcal polysaccharide vaccine in children with sickle cell anemia: effects of continued penicillin prophylaxis. J Pediatr 129:828–835, 1996.

658. Rao SP, Rajkumar K, Schiffman G, et al. Anti-pneumococcal antibody levels three to seven years after first booster immunization in children with sickle cell disease, and after a second booster. J Pediatr 127:590–592, 1995.

659. Vernacchio L, Romero-Steiner S, Martinez JE, et al. Comparison of an opsonophagocytic assay and IgG ELISA to assess responses to pneumococcal polysaccharide and pneumococcal conjugate vaccines in children and young adults with sickle cell disease. J Infect Dis 181:1162–1166, 2000.

660. Gaston MH, Verter JI, Woods G, et al. Prophylaxis with oral penicillin in children with sickle cell anemia: a randomized trial. N Engl J Med 314:1593–1599, 1986.

661. Steele RW, Warrier R, Unkel PJ, et al. Colonization with antibiotic-resistant Streptococcus pneumoniae in children with sickle cell disease. J Pediatr 128:531–535, 1996.

662. Norris CF, Mahannah SR, Smith-Whitley K, et al. Pneumococcal colonization in children with sickle cell disease. J Pediatr 129:821–827, 1996.

663. Pearson HA. Prevention of pneumococcal disease in sickle cell anemia [editorial]. J Pediatr 129:788–789, 1996.

664. Gowda R, Razvi FM, Summerfield GP. Risk of pneumococcal septicaemia in patients with chronic lymphoproliferative malignancies. BMJ 311:26–27, 1995.

665. Griffiths H, Lea J, Bunch C, et al. Predictors of infection in chronic lymphocytic leukaemia (CLL). Clin Exp Immunol 89:374–377, 1992.

666. Mellemgaard A, Brown P, Heron I. Ranitidine improves the vaccination response in patients with chronic lymphocytic leukemia—a randomized, controlled study. Immunol Infect Dis 3:109–111, 1993.

667. Sinisalo M, Aittoniemi J, Oivanen P, et al. Response to vaccination against different types of antigens in patients with chronic lymphocytic leukaemia. Br J Haematol 114:107–110, 2001.

668. Hartkamp A, Mulder AH, Rijkers GT, et al. Antibody responses to pneumococcal and haemophilus vaccinations in patients with B-cell chronic lymphocytic leukaemia. Vaccine 19:1671–1677, 2001.

669. Rautonen J, Siimes MA, Lundstrom U, et al. Vaccination of children during treatment for leukemia. Acta Paediatr Scand 75:579–585, 1986.

670. Smith S, Schiffman G, Karayalcin G, Bonagura V. Immunodeficiency in long-term survivors of acute lymphoblastic leukemia treated with Berlin-Frankfurt-Munster therapy. J Pediatr 127:68–75, 1995.

671. Grimfors G, Bjorkholm M, Hammarstrom L, et al. Type-specific antipneumococcal antibody subclass response to vaccination after splenectomy with special reference to lymphoma patients. Eur J Haematol 43:404–410, 1989.

672. Grimfors G, Soderqvist M, Holm G, et al. A longitudinal study of class and subclass antibody response to pneumococcal vaccination in splenectomized individuals with special reference to patients with Hodgkin's disease. Eur J Haematol 45:101–108, 1990.

673. Petrasch S, Kuhnemund O, Reinacher A, et al. Antibody responses of splenectomized patients with non-Hodgkin's lymphoma to immunization with polyvalent pneumococcal vaccines. Clin Diagn Lab Immunol 4:635–638, 1997.

674. Robertson JD, Nagesh K, Jowitt SN, et al. Immunogenicity of vaccination against influenza, Streptococcus pneumoniae and Haemophilus influenzae type B in patients with multiple myeloma. Br J Cancer 82:1261–1265, 2000.

675. Nordoy T, Aaberge IS, Husebekk A, et al. Cancer patients undergoing chemotherapy show adequate serological response to vaccinations against influenza virus and *Streptococcus pneumoniae*. Med Oncol 19:71–78, 2002.

676. Pesanti EL. Immunologic defects and vaccination in patients with chronic renal failure. Infect Dis Clin North Am 15:813–832, 2001.

677. Kazancioglu R, Sever MS, Yuksel-Onel D, et al. Immunization of renal transplant recipients with pneumococcal polysaccharide vaccine. Clin Transplant 14:61–65, 2000.

678. Rytel MW, Dailey MP, Schiffman G, et al. Pneumococcal vaccine immunization of patients with renal impairment. Proc Soc Exp Biol Med 182:468–473, 1986.

679. Linnemann CC, First R, Schiffman G. Revaccination of renal transplant and hemodialysis patients with pneumococcal vaccine. Arch Intern Med 146:1554–1556, 1986.

680. Spika JS, Halsey NA, Le CT, et al. Decline of vaccine-induced antipneumococcal antibody in children with nephrotic syndrome. Am J Kidney Dis 7:466–470, 1986.

681. Fuchshuber A, Kuhnemund O, Keuth B, et al. Pneumococcal vaccine in children and young adults with chronic renal disease. Nephrol Dial Transplant 11:468–473, 1996.

682. Giebink GS, Warkentin PI, Ramsay NK, Kersey JH. Titers of antibody to pneumococci in allogeneic bone marrow transplant recipients before and after vaccination with pneumococcal vaccine. J Infect Dis 154:590–596, 1986.

683. Sheridan JF, Tutschka PJ, Sedmak DD, Copelan EA. Immunoglobulin G subclass deficiency and pneumococcal infection after allogeneic bone marrow transplantation. Blood 75:1583–1586, 1990.

684. Lortan JE, Vellodi A, Jurges ES, Hugh Jones K. Class- and subclass-specific pneumococcal antibody levels and response to immunization after bone marrow transplantation. Clin Exp Immunol 88:512–519, 1992.

685. Ambrosino DM. Impaired polysaccharide responses in immunodeficient patients: relevance to bone marrow transplant patients. Bone Marrow Transplant 7(suppl 3):48–51, 1991.

686. Hammarstrom V, Pauksen K, Azinge J, et al. Pneumococcal immunity and response to immunization with pneumococcal vaccine in bone marrow transplant patients: the influence of graft versus host reaction. Support Care Cancer 1:195–199, 1993.

687. Avanzini MA, Carra AM, Maccario R, et al. Antibody response to pneumococcal vaccine in children receiving bone marrow transplantation. J Clin Immunol 15:137–144, 1995.

688. Guinan EC, Molrine DC, Antin JH, et al. Polysaccharide conjugate vaccine responses in bone marrow transplant patients. Transplantation 57:677–684, 1994.

689. Gandhi MK, Egner W, Sizer L, et al. Antibody responses to vaccinations given within the first two years after transplant are similar between autologous peripheral blood stem cell and bone marrow transplant recipients. Bone Marrow Transplant 28:775–781, 2001.

690. Spoulou V, Victoratos P, Ioannidis JP, Grafakos S. Kinetics of antibody concentration and avidity for the assessment of immune response to pneumococcal vaccine among children with bone marrow transplants. J Infect Dis 182:965–969, 2000.

691. Ljungman P, Cordonnier C, de Bock R, et al. Immunisations after bone marrow transplantation: results of a European survey and recommendations from the Infectious Diseases Working Party of the European Group for Blood and Marrow Transplantation. Bone Marrow Transplant 15:455–460, 1995.

692. Amber IJ, Gilbert EM, Schiffman G, Jacobson JA. Increased risk of pneumococcal infections in cardiac transplant recipients. Transplantation 49:122–125, 1990.

693. Barkholt LB, Ericson BG, Tollemar J. Infections in human liver recipients: different patterns early and late after transplantation. Transplant Int 6:77–84, 1993.

694. Dengler TJ, Strnad N, Zimmermann R, et al. Pneumococcal vaccination after heart and liver transplantation: immune responses in immunosuppressed patients and in healthy controls. German. Dtsch Med Wochenschr 121:1519–1525, 1996.

695. Blumberg EA, Brozena SC, Stutman P, et al. Immunogenicity of pneumococcal vaccine in heart transplant recipients. Clin Infect Dis 32:307–310, 2001.

696. Stovall SH, Ainley KA, Mason EO Jr, et al. Invasive pneumococcal infections in pediatric cardiac transplant patients. Pediatr Infect Dis J 20:946–950, 2001.

697. Gennery AR, Barge D, Spickett GP, Cant AJ. Lymphocyte subset populations in children with polysaccharide antibody deficiency following cardiac transplantation. J Clin Immunol 21:37–42, 2001.

698. Gennery AR, Cant AJ, Baldwin CI, Calvert JE. Characterization of the impaired antipneumococcal polysaccharide antibody production in immunosuppressed pediatric patients following cardiac transplantation. J Clin Immunol 21:43–50, 2001.

699. Liote F, Angle J, Gilmore N, Osterland CK. Asplenism and systemic lupus erythematosus. Clin Rheumatol 14:220–223, 1995.

700. Elkayam O, Paran D, Caspi D, et al. Immunogenicity and safety of pneumococcal vaccination in patients with rheumatoid arthritis or systemic lupus erythematosus. Clin Infect Dis 34:147–153, 2002.

701. Uthman I, Soucy JP, Nicolet V, Senecal JL. Autosplenectomy in systemic lupus erythematosus. J Rheumatol 23:1806–1810, 1996.

702. Brzeski M, Smart L, Baird D, et al. Pneumococcal septic arthritis after splenectomy in Felty's syndrome. Ann Rheum Dis 50:724–726, 1991.

703. McKinley M, Leibowitz S, Bronzo R, et al. Appropriate response to pneumococcal vaccine in celiac sprue. J Clin Gastroenterol 20:113–116, 1995.

704. Hazlewood MA, Kumararatne DS, Webster AD, et al. An association between homozygous C3 deficiency and low levels of antipneumococcal capsular polysaccharide antibodies. Clin Exp Immunol 87:404–409, 1992.

705. Fata FT, Herzlich BC, Schiffman G, Ast AL. Impaired antibody responses to pneumococcal polysaccharide in elderly patients with low serum vitamin B$_{12}$ levels. Ann Intern Med 124:299–304, 1996.

706. O'Dempsey TJ, McArdle T, Ceesay SJ, et al. Immunization with a pneumococcal capsular polysaccharide vaccine during pregnancy. Vaccine 14:963–970, 1996.

707. Shahid NS, Steinhoff MC, Hoque SS, et al. Serum, breast milk, and infant antibody after maternal immunisation with pneumococcal vaccine. Lancet 346:1252–1257, 1995.

708. Munoz FM, Englund JA, Cheesman CC, et al. Maternal immunization with pneumococcal polysaccharide vaccine in the third trimester of gestation. Vaccine 20:826–837, 2002.

709. Lehmann D, Pomat WS, Combs B, et al. Maternal immunization with pneumococcal polysaccharide vaccine in the highlands of Papua New Guinea. Vaccine 20:1837–1845, 2002.

710. Santosham M, Englund JA, McInnes P, et al. Safety and antibody persistence following *Haemophilus influenzae* type b conjugate or pneumococcal polysaccharide vaccines given before pregnancy in women of childbearing age and their infants. Pediatr Infect Dis J 20:931–940, 2001.

711. Glezen WP. Maternal vaccines. Prim Care 28:791–806, 2001.

712. Westh H, Skibsted L, Korner B. *Streptococcus pneumoniae* infections of the female genital tract and in the newborn child. Rev Infect Dis 12:416–422, 1990.

713. Singh J, Dick J, Santosham M. Colonization of the female urogenital tract with *Streptococcus pneumoniae* and implications for neonatal disease. Pediatr Infect Dis J 19:260–262, 2000.

714. Gomez M, Alter S, Kumar ML, et al. Neonatal *Streptococcus pneumoniae* infection: case reports and review of the literature. Pediatr Infect Dis J 18:1014–1018, 1999.

715. Johnsson H, Bergstrom S, Ewald U, Schwan A. Neonatal septicemia caused by pneumococci. Acta Obstet Gynecol Scand 71:6–11, 1992.

716. Primhak RA, Tanner MS, Spencer RC. Pneumococcal infection in the newborn. Arch Dis Child 69:317–318, 1993.

717. Simpson JM, Patel JS, Ispahani P. *Streptococcus pneumoniae* invasive disease in the neonatal period: an increasing problem? Eur J Pediatr 154:563–566, 1995.

718. Kaplan M, Rudensky B, Beck A. Perinatal infections with *Streptococcus pneumoniae*. Am J Perinatol 10:1–4, 1993.

719. Johnsson H, Ewald U. The incidence of neonatal pneumococcal septicemia in Sweden 1991–1992: the result of a national survey. Ups J Med Sci 99:161–165, 1994.

720. Hughes BR, Mercer JL, Gosbel LB. Neonatal pneumococcal sepsis in association with fatal maternal pneumococcal sepsis. Aust N Z J Obstet Gynaecol 41:457–458, 2001.

721. Lockhart NJ, Daly KA, Lindgren BR, et al. Low cord blood type 14 pneumococcal IgG1 but not IgG2 antibody predicts early infant otitis media. J Infect Dis 181:1979–1982, 2000.

722. Becken ET, Daly KA, Lindgren BR, et al. Low cord blood pneumococcal antibody concentrations predict more episodes of otitis media. Arch Otolaryngol Head Neck Surg 127:517–522, 2001.

723. WHO meeting on maternal and neonatal pneumococcal immunization. Wkly Epidemiol Rec 73:187–188, 1998.

724. Chudwin DS, Wara DW, Schiffman G, et al. Maternal-fetal transfer of pneumococcal capsular polysaccharide antibodies. Am J Dis Child 139:378–380, 1985.

725. Lee CJ, Takaoka Y, Saito T. Maternal immunization and the immune response of neonates to pneumococcal polysaccharides. Rev Infect Dis 9:494–510, 1987.

726. Anderson P, Porcelli S, Pichichero M. Natural maternal and cord serum antibodies to pneumococcal serotypes 6A, 14, 19F, and 23F polysaccharides. Pediatr Infect Dis J 11:677–679, 1992.

727. Carvalho B, Carneiro Sampaio MM, Sole D, et al. Transplacental transmission of serotype-specific pneumococcal antibodies in a Brazilian population. Clin Diagn Lab Immunol 6:50–54, 1999.

728. Okoko BJ, Wesumperuma LH, Hart AC. Materno-foetal transfer of H. influenzae and pneumococcal antibodies is influenced by prematurity and low birth weight: implications for conjugate vaccine trials. Vaccine 20:647–650, 2001.

729. Rosen IAV, Hakansson A, Aniansson G, et al. Antibodies to pneumococcal polysaccharides in human milk: lack of relationship to colonization and acute otitis media. Pediatr Infect Dis J 15:498–507, 1996.

730. Cesar JA, Victora CG, Barros FC, et al. Impact of breast feeding on admission for pneumonia during postneonatal period in Brazil: nested case-control study. BMJ 318:1316–1320, 1999.

731. Centers for Disease Control. Pneumococcal polysaccharide vaccine. MMWR 38:64–68, 1989.

732. Mufson MA. Antibody response of pneumococcal vaccine: need for booster dosing? Int J Antimicrob Agents 14:107–112, 2000.

733. Nichol KL. Revaccination of high-risk adults with pneumococcal polysaccharide vaccine [editorial]. JAMA 281:280–281, 1999.

734. Mufson MA, Krause HE, Schiffman G, Hughey DF. Pneumococcal antibody levels one decade after immunization of healthy adults. Am J Med Sci 293:279–284, 1987.

735. Mufson MA, Hughey DF, Turner CE, Schiffman G. Revaccination with pneumococcal vaccine of elderly persons 6 years after primary vaccination. Vaccine 9:403–407, 1991.

736. Rodriguez R, Dyer PD. Safety of pneumococcal revaccination. J Gen Intern Med 10:511–512, 1995.

737. Davidson M, Bulkow LR, Grabman J, et al. Immunogenicity of pneumococcal revaccination in patients with chronic disease. Arch Intern Med 154:2209–2214, 1994.

738. Jackson LA, Benson P, Sneller VP, et al. Safety of revaccination with pneumococcal polysaccharide vaccine. JAMA 281:243–248, 1999.

739. Snow R, Babish JD, McBean AM. Is there any connection between a second pneumonia shot and hospitalization among Medicare beneficiaries? Public Health Rep 110:720–725, 1995.

740. Konradsen HB, Henrichsen J. The need for revaccination 10 years after primary pneumococcal vaccination in splenectomized adults [letter]. Scand J Infect Dis 23:397, 1991.

741. Konradsen HB, Pedersen FK, Henrichsen J. Pneumococcal revaccination of splenectomized children. Pediatr Infect Dis J 9:258–263, 1990.

742. Rutherford EJ, Livengood J, Higginbotham M, et al. Efficacy and safety of pneumococcal revaccination after splenectomy for trauma. J Trauma 39:448–452, 1995.

743. Tasker SA, Wallace MR, Rubins JB, et al. Reimmunization with 23-valent pneumococcal vaccine for patients infected with human immunodeficiency virus type 1: clinical, immunologic, and virologic responses. Clin Infect Dis 34:813–821, 2002.

744. Fedson DS. Measuring protection: efficacy versus effectiveness. Dev Biol Stand 95:195–201, 1998.

745. MacLeod M, Hodges RG, Heidelberger M, Bernhard WG. Prevention of pneumococcal pneumonia by immunization with specific capsular polysaccharides. J Exp Med 82:445–465, 1945.

746. Herva E, Luotonen J, Timonen M. The effect of polyvalent pneumococcal polysaccharide vaccine on nasopharyngeal and nasal carriage of Streptococcus pneumoniae. Scand J Infect Dis 12:97–100, 1980.

747. Rosen C, Christensen P, Hovelius B, Prellner K. A longitudinal study of the nasopharyngeal carriage of pneumococci as related to pneumococcal vaccination in children attending day-care centres. Acta Otolaryngol (Stockh) 98:524–532, 1984.

748. Riley ID, Lehmann D, Alpers MP. Pneumococcal vaccine trials in Papua New Guinea: relationships between epidemiology of pneumococcal infection and efficacy of vaccine. Rev Infect Dis 13(suppl 6):S535–S541, 1991.

749. Douglas RM, Miles HB. Vaccination against Streptococcus pneumoniae in childhood: lack of demonstrable benefit in young Australian children. J Infect Dis 149:861–869, 1984.

750. Karma P, Pukander J, Sipila M. Prevention of otitis media in children by pneumococcal vaccination. Am J Otolaryngol 6:173–184, 1985.

751. Teele DW, Klein JO. Use of pneumococcal vaccine for prevention of recurrent acute otitis media in infants in Boston. Rev Infect Dis 3(suppl):S113–S118, 1981.

752. Howie VM, Ploussard J, Sloyer JL, Hill JC. Use of pneumococcal polysaccharide vaccine in preventing otitis media in infants: different results between racial groups. Pediatrics 73:79–81, 1984.

753. Riley ID, Lehmann D, Alpers MP, et al. Pneumococcal vaccine prevents death from acute lower-respiratory-tract infections in Papua New Guinean children. Lancet 2:877–881, 1986.

754. Lehmann D, Marshall TF, Riley ID, Alpers MP. Effect of pneumococcal vaccine on morbidity from acute lower respiratory tract infections in Papua New Guinean children. Ann Trop Paediatr 11:247–257, 1991.

755. Fiore AE, Levine OS, Elliott JA, et al. Effectiveness of pneumococcal polysaccharide vaccine for preschool-age children with chronic disease. Emerg Infect Dis 5:828–831, 1999.

756. Kaufman P. Pneumonia in old age: active immunization against pneumonia with pneumococcal polysaccharide—results of a six year study. Arch Intern Med 79:518–531, 1947.

757. Austrian R. Surveillance of pneumococcal infection for field trials of polyvalent pneumococcal vaccines. (NIH Publication DAB-VPD-12-84, Contract No IA13257). Bethesda, MD, National Institutes of Health, 1980.

758. Gaillat J, Zmirou D, Mallaret MR, et al. Clinical trial of an antipneumococcal vaccine in elderly subjects living in institutions [in French]. Rev Epidemiol Sante Publ 33:437–444, 1985.

759. Simberkoff MS, Cross AP, Al-Ibrahim M, et al. Efficacy of pneumococcal vaccine in high-risk patients: results of a Veterans Administration Cooperative Study. N Engl J Med 315:1318–1327, 1986.

760. Klastersky J, Mommen P, Cantraine F, Safary A. Placebo controlled pneumococcal immunization in patients with bronchogenic carcinoma. Eur J Cancer Clin Oncol 22:807–813, 1986.

761. Leech J, Gervais A, Ruben F. Efficacy of pneumococcal vaccine in severe chronic obstructive pulmonary disease. CMAJ 136:361–365, 1987.

762. Davis AL, Aranda CP, Schiffman G, Christianson LC. Pneumococcal infection and immunologic response to pneumococcal vaccine in chronic obstructive pulmonary disease: a pilot study. Chest 92:204–212, 1987.

763. Koivula I, Stén M, Leinonen M, Mäkelä PH. Clinical efficacy of pneumococcal vaccine in the elderly: a randomized, single-blind population-based trial. Am J Med 103:281–290, 1997.

764. Örtqvist Å, Hedlund J, Burman LA, et al. Randomized trial of 23-valent pneumococcal capsular polysaccharide vaccine in the prevention of pneumonia in middle-aged and elderly people. Lancet 351:399–403, 1998.

765. Honkanen PO, Keistinen T, Miettinen L, et al. Incremental effectiveness of pneumococcal vaccine on simultaneously administered influenza vaccine in preventing pneumonia and pneumococcal pneumonia among persons aged 65 years or older. Vaccine 17:2493–2500, 1999.

766. Hirschmann JV, Lipsky BA. The pneumococcal vaccine after 15 years of use. Arch Intern Med 154:373–377, 1994.

767. Fedson DS, Shapiro ED, LaForce FM, et al. Pneumococcal vaccine after 15 years of use: another view. Arch Intern Med 154:2531–2535, 1994.

768. Nguyen-van-Tam JS, Neal KR. Clinical effectiveness, policies, and practices for influenza and pneumococcal vaccines. Semin Respir Infect 14:184–195, 1999.

769. Lehmann D. Efficacy and effectiveness of pneumococcal polysaccharide vaccines and their use in industrialised countries. Med J Aust 173(suppl):S41–S44, 2000.

770. Rubins JB, Janoff EN. Pneumococcal disease in the elderly: what is preventing vaccine efficacy? Drugs Aging 18:305–311, 2001.

771. Fine MJ, Smith MA, Carson CA, et al. Efficacy of pneumococcal vaccination in adults: a meta-analysis of randomized controlled trials. Arch Intern Med 154:2666–2677, 1994.

772. Hutchison BG, Oxman AD, Shannon HS, et al. Clinical effectiveness of pneumococcal vaccine: meta-analysis [see comments]. Can Fam Physician 45:2381–2393, 1999.

773. Moore RA, Wiffen PJ, Lipsky BA. Are the pneumococcal polysaccharide vaccines effective? Meta-analysis of the prospective trials. BMC Fam Pract 1(1):1, 2000.

774. Cornu C, Yzebe D, Leophonte P, et al. Efficacy of pneumococcal polysaccharide vaccine in immunocompetent adults: a meta-analysis of randomized trials. Vaccine 19:4780–4790, 2001.

775. Watson L, Wilson BJ, Waugh N. Pneumococcal polysaccharide vaccine: a systematic review of clinical effectiveness in adults. Vaccine 20:2166–2173, 2002.

776. Fedson DS, Liss C. Precise answers to the wrong question: prospective clinical trials and the meta-analyses of pneumococcal vaccine in elderly and high-risk adults. Vaccine [in press] 2003.

777. Detsky AS, Sackett DL. When was a "negative" clinical trial big enough? How many patients you needed depends on what you found. Arch Intern Med 145:709–712, 1985.

778. Fedson DS, Watson M. Pneumococcal vaccine and HIV-1 infection. Lancet 356:1272–1273, 2000.

779. Christenson B, Lundbergh P, Hedlund J, Örtqvist Å. Effects of a large-scale intervention with influenza and 23-valent pneumococcal vaccines in adults aged 65 years or older: a prospective study. Lancet 357:1008–1011, 2001.

780. Clemens JD, Shapiro ED. Resolving the pneumococcal vaccine controversy: are there alternatives to randomized clinical trials? Rev Infect Dis 6:589–600, 1984.

781. Rodrigues LC, Smith PG. Use of the case-control approach in vaccine evaluation: efficacy and adverse effects. Epidemiol Rev 21:56–72, 1999.

782. Shapiro ED, Clemens JD. A controlled evaluation of the protective efficacy of pneumococcal vaccine for patients at high risk of serious pneumococcal infections. Ann Intern Med 101:325–330, 1984.

783. Forrester HL, Jahnigen DW, LaForce FM. Inefficacy of pneumococcal vaccine in a high-risk population. Am J Med 83:425–430, 1987.

784. Sims RV, Steinmann WC, McConville JH, et al. The clinical effectiveness of pneumococcal vaccine in the elderly. Ann Intern Med 108:653–657, 1988.

785. Shapiro ED, Berg AT, Austrian R, et al. The protective efficacy of polyvalent pneumococcal polysaccharide vaccine. N Engl J Med 325:1453–1460, 1991.

786. Farr BM, Johnston BL, Cobb DK, et al. Preventing pneumococcal bacteremia in patients at risk: results of a matched case-control study. Arch Intern Med 155:2336–2340, 1995.

787. Knox K, Moore H, Griffiths D, et al. Efficacy of pneumococcal vaccination in adults in the Oxford Region, UK [abstract]. In Abstracts of the 3rd International Symposium on Pneumococci and Pneumococcal Diseases, Anchorage, May 5–8, 2002, pp 91–92.

788. Butler JC, Breiman RF, Campbell JF, et al. Pneumococcal polysaccharide vaccine efficacy: an evaluation of current recommendations. JAMA 270:1826–1831, 1993.

789. Green K, Landry L, Goldenberg E, et al. Effectiveness of a pneumococcal vaccination program in preventing invasive pneumococcal disease [abstract]. In Abstracts of the 39th Interscience Conference on Antimicrobial Agents and Chemotherapy, San Francisco, September 26–29, 1999, p 673.

790. Nichol KL, Baken L, Wuorenma J, Nelson A. The health and economic benefits associated with pneumococcal vaccination of elderly persons with chronic lung disease. Arch Intern Med 159:2437–2442, 1999.

791. Nichol KL. The additive benefits of influenza and pneumococcal vaccinations during influenza seasons among elderly persons with chronic lung disease. Vaccine 17(suppl 1):S91–S93, 1999.

792. Jackson LA, Neuzil LA, Yu O et al. Effectiveness of pneumococcal polysaccharide vaccine in older adults. N Eng J Med 348:1747–1755, 2003.

793. Gebo KA, Moore RD, Keruly JC, Chaisson RE. Risk factors for pneumococcal disease in human immunodeficiency virus-infected patients. J Infect Dis 173:857–862, 1996.

794. Guerrero M, Kruger S, Saitoh A, et al. Pneumonia in HIV-infected patients: a case-control survey of factors involved in risk and prevention. AIDS 13:1971–1975, 1999.

794a. Benin A, O' Brien K, Watt J, et al. Effectivness of 23-valent pneumococcal vaccine against invasive pneumococcal disease in Navaho adults [abstract]. In Abstracts of the 39th Annual Meeting of the Infectious Diseases Society of America, San Francisco, October 25–28, abstract 351, 2001.

795. Dworkin MS, Ward JW, Hanson DL, et al. Pneumococcal disease among human immunodeficiency virus-infected persons: incidence, risk factors, and impact of vaccination. Clin Infect Dis 32:794–800, 2001.

796. Rodriguez-Barradas MC, Petersen N. Do HIV-infected persons have an increased risk of pneumococcal disease following immunization with pneumococcal polysaccharide vaccine (PV)? [abstract]. In Abstracts of the 39th Annual Meeting of the Infectious Diseases Society of America, San Francisco, October 25–28, 2001, p 1148.

797. Abel U, Koch A. The role of randomization in clinical studies: myths and beliefs. J Clin Epidemiol 52:487–497, 1999.

798. Simberkoff MS. Pneumococcal vaccine in the prevention of community-acquired pneumonia: a skeptical view of cost-effectiveness. Semin Respir Infect 8:294–299, 1993.

799. Hak E, van Essen GA, Grobbee DE, Verheij ThJM. Effectiveness of pneumococcal vaccine [letter]. Lancet 351:1283, 1998.

800. Moller K, Kronborg G, Dirksen A. Is polysaccharide pneumococcal vaccine effective in adults [in Danish]? Ugeskr Laeger 163:6112–6117, 2001.

801. Jefferson T, Demicheli V. Polysaccharide pneumococcal vaccines. BMJ 325:292–293, 2002.

801a. Mangtani P, Cutts F, Hall AJ. Efficacy of polysaccharide pneumococcal vaccine in adults in more developed countries: the state of the evidence. Lancet Infect Dis 3:71–78, 2003.

802. Fedson DS. Pneumococcal vaccination in the prevention of community-acquired pneumonia: an optimistic view of cost-effectiveness. Semin Respir Infect 8:285–293, 1993.

802a. Fedson DS. Efficacy of polysaccharide pneumococcal vaccine in adults in more developed countries: another view of the evidence. Lancet Infect Dis 3:271–272, 2003.

803. Willems JS, Sanders CR, Riddiough MA, Bell JC. Cost effectiveness of vaccination against pneumococcal pneumonia. N Engl J Med 303:553–559, 1980.

804. Fedson DS. Influenza and pneumococcal vaccination of the elderly: newer vaccines and prospects for clinical benefits at the margin. Prev Med 23:751–755, 1994.

805. Tengs TO, Adams ME, Pliskin JS, et al. Five-hundred life-saving interventions and their cost-effectiveness. Risk Anal 15:369–390, 1995.

806. Gable CB, Botteman M, Savage G, Joy K. The cost effectiveness of pneumococcal vaccination strategies. Pharmacoeconomics 12(2 pt 1):161–174, 1997.

807. Baltussen RMPM, Ament AJHA, Leidl RM, van Furth R. Cost-effectiveness of vaccination against pneumococcal pneumonia in the Netherlands. Eur J Public Health 7:153–161, 1997.

808. Postma MJ, Heijnen MLA, Jager JC. Cost-effectiveness analysis of pneumococcal vaccination for elderly individuals in the Netherlands. Pharmacoeconomics 19:215–222, 2001.

809. De Graeve D, Lombaert G, Goossens H. Cost-effectiveness analysis of pneumococcal vaccination of adults and elderly persons in Belgium. Pharmacoeconomics 17:591–601, 2000.

810. Plans Rubio P, Garrido Morales P, Salleras Sanmarti L. The cost-effectiveness of pneumococcal vaccination in Catalonia [in Spanish]. Rev Esp Salud Publica 69:409–417, 1995.

811. Jimenez FJ, Guallar P. Cost-effectiveness analysis of pneumococcal vaccination in the elderly Spanish population. Br J Med Econ 10:193–202, 1996.

812. Beutels P, Postma MJ. Economic evaluations of adult pneumococcal vaccination strategies. Expert Rev Pharmacoeconomics Outcomes Res 1:47–58, 2001.

813. Sisk JE, Moskowitz AJ, Whang W, et al. Cost-effectiveness of vaccination against pneumococcal bacteremia among elderly people. JAMA 278:1333–1339, 1997.

814. Whang W, Sisk JE, Heitjan DF, Moskowitz AJ. Probabilistic sensitivity analysis in cost-effectiveness: an application from a study of vaccination against pneumococcal bacteremia in the elderly. Int J Technol Assess Health Care 15:563–572, 1999.

815. Amazian K, Nicoloyannis N, Colin C, et al. Cost effectiveness analysis of pneumococcal vaccination of older people in France [in French]. Med Mal Infect 32:405–417, 2002.

816. Chapman RH, Stone PW, Sandberg EA, et al. A comprehensive league table of cost-utility ratios and a sub-table of "panel-worthy" studies. Med Decis Making 20:451–467, 2000.

817. Mukamel DB, Taffet GH, Bennett NM. Cost utility of public clinics to increase pneumococcal vaccines in the elderly. Am J Prev Med 21:29–34, 2001.

818. Weaver M, Krieger J, Castorina J, et al. Cost-effectiveness of combined outreach for the pneumococcal and influenza vaccines. Arch Intern Med 161:111–129, 2001.

819. Vold PP, Owens DK. Cost-effectiveness of the pneumococcal vaccine in the United States Navy and Marine Corps. Clin Infect Dis 30:157–164, 2000.

820. Marra CA, Patrick DM, Marra F. A cost-effectiveness analysis of pneumococcal vaccination in street-involved, HIV-infected patients. Can J Public Health 91:334–339, 2000.

821. Ament A, Fedson DS, Christie P. Pneumococcal vaccination and pneumonia: even a low level of clinical effectiveness is highly cost-effective. Clin Infect Dis 33:2078–2079, 2001.

822. Klinge J, Hammersen G, Scharf J, et al. Overwhelming postsplenectomy infection with vaccine-type *Streptococcus pneumoniae* in a 12-year-old girl despite vaccination and antibiotic prophylaxis. Infection 25:368–371, 1997.

823. Rege K, Mehta J, Treleaven J, et al. Fatal pneumococcal infections following allogeneic bone marrow transplant. Bone Marrow Transplant 14:903–906, 1994.

824. Begemann M, Policar M. Pneumococcal vaccine failure in an HIV-infected patient with fatal pneumococcal sepsis and HCV-related cirrhosis. Mt Sinai J Med 68:396–399, 2001.

825. McMahon BJ, Parkinson AJ, Rudolph K, et al. Sepsis due to *Streptococcus pneumoniae* in a patient with alcoholism who received pneumococcal vaccine. Clin Infect Dis 28:1162–1163, 1999.

826. Hanna JN, Wenck DJ, Murphy DN. Three fatal pneumococcal polysaccharide vaccine failures. Med J Aust 173:305–307, 2000.

827. Centers for Disease Control and Prevention. Assessing adult vaccination status at age 50 years. MMWR 44:561–563, 1995.

828. Centers for Disease Control and Prevention. Outbreaks of pneumococcal pneumonia among unvaccinated residents of chronic-care facilities—Massachusetts, October 1995, Oklahoma, February, 1996, and Maryland, May-June 1996. MMWR 46(3):60–62, 1997.

829. Quick RE, Hoge CW, Hamilton DJ, et al. Underutilization of pneumococcal vaccine in nursing home in Washington State: report of a serotype-specific outbreak and a survey. Am J Med 94:149–152, 1993.

830. Musher DM. Pneumococcal outbreaks in nursing homes [editorial; comment]. N Engl J Med 338:1915–1916, 1998.

831. Fedson DS. Pneumococcal vaccination in the United States and 20 other developed countries, 1981–1996. Clin Infect Dis 26:1117–1123, 1998.

832. Ständige Impfkommission. Impfempfehlungen der Ständigen Impfkommission (STIKO) am Robert-Koch-Institut. Epidemiol Bull 28:203–218, 2001.

833. Singleton JA, Greby SM, Wooten KG, et al. Influenza, pneumococcal, and tetanus toxoid vaccination of adults—United States, 1993–7. MMWR 49(SS-9):39–62, 2000.

834. Buchwald D, Sheffield J, Furman R, et al. Influenza and pneumococcal vaccination among Native American elders in a primary care practice. Arch Intern Med 160:1443–1448, 2000.

835. Centers for Disease Control and Prevention. Influenza and pneumococcal vaccination rates among persons with diabetes mellitus—United States, 1997. MMWR 48(42):961–967, 1999.

836. Mieczkowski TA, Wilson SA. Adult pneumococcal vaccination: a review of physician and patient barriers. Vaccine 20:1383–1392, 2002.

837. Nichol KL, MacDonald R, Hauge M. Factors associated with influenza and pneumococcal vaccination behavior among high-risk adults. J Gen Intern Med 11:673–677, 1996.

838. Petersen RL, Saag K, Wallace RB, Doebbeling BN. Influenza and pneumococcal vaccine receipt in older persons with chronic disease: a population-based study. Med Care 37:502–509, 1999.

839. Solberg LI, Kottke TE, Brekke ML. Variation in clinical preventive services. Eff Clin Pract 4:121–126, 2001.

840. MacDonald R, Baken L, Nelson A, Nichol KL. Validation of self-report of influenza and pneumococcal vaccination status in elderly outpatients. Am J Prev Med 16:173–177, 1999.

841. Centers for Disease Control and Prevention. Reasons reported by Medicare beneficiaries for not receiving influenza and pneumococcal vaccinations—United States, 1996. MMWR 48:886–890, 1999.

842. Centers for Disease Control. Adult immunization: knowledge, attitudes and practices—Dekalb and Fulton Counties, Georgia, 1988. MMWR 37:657–661, 1988.

843. Ehresmann KR, Ramesh A, Como-Sabetti K, et al. Factors associated with self-reported pneumococcal immunization among adults 65 years of age or older in the Minneapolis–St. Paul metropolitan area. Prev Med 32:409–415, 2001.

844. Rhew DC, Glassman PA, Goetz MB. Improving pneumococcal vaccine rates: nurse protocols versus clinical reminders. J Gen Intern Med 14:351–356, 1999.

845. Herman CJ, Speroff T, Cebul RD. Improving compliance with immunization in the older adult: results of a randomized cohort study. J Am Geriatr Soc 42:1154–1159, 1994.

846. Latessa RA, Cummings DM, Lilley SH, Morrissey SL. Changing practices in the use of pneumococcal vaccine. Fam Med 32:196–200, 2000.

847. Kleschen MZ, Holbrook J, Rothbaum AK, et al. Improving the pneumococcal immunization rate for patients with diabetes in a managed care population: a simple intervention with a rapid effect. Jt Comm J Qual Improv 26:538–546, 2000.

848. Jacobson TA, Thomas DM, Morton FJ, et al. Use of a low-literacy patient education tool to enhance pneumococcal vaccination rates: a randomized controlled trial. JAMA 282:646–650, 1999.

849. Redfield JR, Wang TW. Improving pneumococcal vaccination rates: a three-step approach. Fam Med 32:338–341, 2000.

850. Shenson D, Quinley J, DiMartino D, et al. Pneumococcal immunizations at flu clinics: the impact of community-wide outreach. J Community Health 26:191–201, 2001.

851. Stancliff S, Salomon N, Perlman DC, Russell PC. Provision of influenza and pneumococcal vaccines to injection drug users at a syringe exchange. J Subst Abuse Treat 18:263–265, 2000.

852. Krieger JW, Castorina JS, Walls ML, et al. Increasing influenza and pneumococcal immunization rates: a randomized controlled study of a senior center-based intervention. Am J Prev Med 18:123–131, 2000.

853. D'heilly S, Bauman WL, Nichol KL. Safety and acceptability of pneumococcal vaccinations administered in nontraditional settings. Am J Infect Control 30:261–268, 2002.

854. Gyorkos TW, Tannenbaum TN, Abrahamowicz M, et al. Evaluation of the effectiveness of immunization delivery methods. Can J Public Health 85(suppl 1):S14–S30, 1994.

855. Shefer A, Briss P, Rodewald L, et al. Improving immunization coverage rates: an evidence-based review of the literature. Epidemiol Rev 21:96–142, 1999.

856. Grabenstein JD, Guess HA, Hartzema AG, et al. Effect of vaccination by community pharmacists among adult prescription recipients. Med Care 39:340–348, 2001.

857. Terrell-Perica SM, Effler PV, Houck PM, et al. The effect of a combined influenza/pneumococcal immunization reminder letter. Am J Prev Med 21:256–260, 2001.

858. Fedson DS, Houck P, Bratzler D. Hospital-based influenza and pneumococcal vaccination: Sutton's Law applied to prevention. Infect Control Hosp Epidemiol 21:692–699, 2000.

859. Fedson DS, Harward MP, Reid RA, Kaiser DL. Hospital-based pneumococcal immunization: epidemiologic rationale from the Shenandoah study. JAMA 264:1117–1122, 1990.

860. Dexter PR, Perkins S, Overhage JM, et al. A computerized reminder system to increase the use of preventive care for hospitalized patients. N Engl J Med 345:965–970, 2001.

861. Metersky ML, Fine JM, Tu GS, et al. Lack of effect of a pneumonia clinical pathway on hospital-based pneumococcal vaccination rates. Am J Med 110:141–143, 2001.

862. Shevlin JD, Summers-Bean C, Thomas D, et al. A systematic approach for increasing pneumococcal vaccination rates at an inner-city public hospital. Am J Prev Med 22:92–97, 2002.

863. Slobodkin D, Kitlas J, Zielske P. Opportunities not missed—systematic influenza and pneumococcal immunization in a public inner-city emergency department. Vaccine 16:1795–1802, 1998.

864. Stack SJ, Martin DR, Plouffe JF. An emergency department-based pneumococcal vaccination program could save money and lives. Ann Emerg Med 33:299–303, 1999.

865. Nichol KL, Grimm MB, Peterson DC. Immunizations in long-term care facilities: policies and practice. J Am Geriatr Soc 44:349–355, 1996.

866. Stevenson KB, McMahon JW, Harris J, et al. Increasing pneumococcal vaccination rates among residents of long-term care facilities: provider-based improvement strategies implemented by peer-review organizations in four western states. Infect Control Hosp Epidemiol 21:705–710, 2000.

867. Providers debate pros and cons of pneumonia vaccination at discharge. Clin Resource Manag 2(2):29–31, 18, 2001.

868. Hospital public health: protocol for immunizing inpatients. Hosp Case Manag 9(10):151–153, 2001.

869. Centers for Disease Control and Prevention. Increasing pneumococcal vaccination rates among patients of a National Health-Care Alliance—United States, 1993. MMWR 44(40):741–744, 1995.

870. Campbell JF, Donohue MA, Nevin-Woods C, et al. The Hawaii pneumococcal disease initiative. Am J Public Health 83:1175–1176, 1993.

871. Centers for Disease Control. Comprehensive delivery of adult vaccination—Minnesota, 1986–1992. MMWR 42(39):768–770, 1993.

872. Davidson M, Chamblee C, Campbell HG, et al. Pneumococcal vaccination in a remote population of high-risk Alaska Natives. Public Health Rep 108:439–446, 1993.

873. Centers for Disease Control and Prevention. Pneumococcal and influenza vaccination levels among adults aged > or = 65 years—United States, 1993. MMWR 45(40):853–859, 1996.

874. Fedson DS. Clinical practice and public policy for influenza and pneumococcal vaccination of the elderly. Clin Geriatr Med 8:183–199, 1992.

875. Fedson DS. Adult immunization: summary of the National Vaccine Advisory Committee report. JAMA 272:1133–1137, 1994.

876. Fedson DS. Influenza and pneumococcal vaccination in Canada and the United States, 1980–1993: what can the two countries learn from each other? Clin Infect Dis 20:1371–1376, 1995.

877. McGeer A, Green K, Laudry L, et al. Assessing the potential impact of vaccination programs on invasive pneumococcal disease: data from population-based surveillance. Can J Infect Dis 10(suppl A):24A–26A, 1999.

878. Squires SG, Pelletier L. Publicly-funded influenza and pneumococcal immunization programs in Canada: a progress report. Can Commun Dis Rep 26:141–148, 2000.

879. Buxton J, Weatherill S, Hockin J, Daly P. Influenza and pneumococcal immunization "blitz" in an inner city area: downtown eastside of Vancouver, British Columbia. Can Commun Dis Rep 26:117–122, 2000.

880. Stevenson CG, McArthur MA, Naus M, et al. Prevention of influenza and pneumococcal pneumonia in Canadian long-term care facilities: how are we doing? CMAJ 164:1413–1419, 2001.

881. Andrews RM, Lester RA. Improving pneumococcal vaccination coverage among older people in Victoria. Med J Aust 173(suppl):S45–S47, 2000.

882. Forrest JM, McIntyre PB, Burgess MA. Pneumococcal disease in Australia. Commun Dis Intell 24:89–92, 2000.

883. Hanna JN, Young DM, Brookes DL, et al. The initial coverage and impact of the pneumococcal and influenza vaccination program for at-risk indigenous adults in Far North Queensland. Aust N Z J Public Health 25:543–546, 2001.

884. Are current recommendations for pneumococcal vaccination appropriate for Western Australia? The Vaccine Impact Surveillance Network—Invasive Pneumococcal Study Group. Med J Aust 173(suppl):S36–S40, 2000.

885. Fedson D, Henrichsen J, Makela PH, Austrian R. Immunization of elderly people with polyvalent pneumococcal vaccine. Infection 17:437–441, 1989.

886. Peetermans WE, Bachez P, Peleman R, et al. Belgian consensus on pneumococcal vaccine. Acta Clin Belg 51:350–356, 1996.

887. Peleman RA, Peetermans WE, Van Laethem Y, et al. Prevention of pneumococcal disease: an update on the Belgian Consensus Report. Acta Clin Belg 54:321–327, 1999.

888. Peetermans WE, Lacante P. Pneumococcal vaccination by general practitioners: an evaluation of current practice. Vaccine 18:612–617, 1999.

889. McDonald P, Friedman E, Banks A, et al. Pneumococcal vaccine campaign based in general practice. BMJ 314:1094–1098, 1997.

890. Siriwardena AN. Targeting pneumococcal vaccination to high-risk groups: a feasibility study in one general practice. Postgrad Med J 75:208–212, 1999.

891. Turner DP, Finch G. Pneumococcal vaccine uptake in medical patients discharged from a district hospital. Commun Dis Public Health 2:291–292, 1999.

892. Kyaw MH, Nguyen-van-Tam JS, Pearson JC. Family doctor advice is the main determinant of pneumococcal vaccine uptake. J Epidemiol Community Health 53:589–590, 1999.

893. Findlay PF, Gibbons YM, Primrose WR, et al. Influenza and pneumococcal vaccination: patient perceptions. Postgrad Med J 76:215–217, 2000.

894. Wahid ST, Nag S, Bilous RW, et al. Audit of influenza and pneumococcal vaccination uptake in diabetic patients attending secondary care in the Northern Region. Diabet Med 18:599–603, 2001.

895. Cummins A, Millership S. Local review of the provision of prophylaxis and advice to patients without functioning spleens. Commun Dis Public Health 4:144–145, 2001.

896. Kyaw MH, Bramley JC, Chalmers J, et al. Pneumococcal vaccination: opinion of general practitioners and hospital doctors in Scotland, 1999–2000. Commun Dis Public Health 4:42–48, 2001.

897. Kyaw MH, Wayne B, Holmes EM, et al. Influenza and pneumococcal vaccination in Scottish nursing homes: coverage, policies and reasons for receipt and non-receipt of vaccine. Vaccine 20:2516–2522, 2002.

898. Bedford D, Igoe G, White M, et al. The acceptability of pneumococcal vaccine to older persons in Ireland. Ir Med J 93:48–49, 2000.

899. Örtqvist Å, Hedlund J, Kalin M. The elderly should be vaccinated against pneumococci [in Swedish]. Lakartidningen 96:1305–1308, 1999.

900. Örtqvist Å, Jonsson B, Baltussen R, Ament A. Vaccination of the elderly against pneumococcal disease is cost-efficient: mass vaccination of all aged 65 and over is recommended [in Swedish]. Lakartidningen 97:5120–5125, 2000.

901. Flo RW, Solberg CO. Pneumococcal vaccine [in Norwegian]. Tidsskr Nor Laegeforen 118:3799–3802, 1998.

902. Konradsen HB. Pneumococcal vaccine is clinically effective [in Danish]. Ugeskr Laeger 163(48):6771–6774, 2001.

903. Bovier PA, Chamot E, Bouvier GM, Loutan L. Importance of patients' perceptions and general practitioners' recommendations in understanding missed opportunities for immunisations in Swiss adults. Vaccine 19:4760–4767, 2001.

904. Hulsse C, Littmann M, Fiedler K, et al. Epidemiologic and serologic studies of pneumococcal infections with reference to the new STIKO recommendations [in German]. Gesundheitswesen 61:393–397, 1999.

905. Salleras L, Urbiztondo L, Parron I. A pneumococcal vaccination program for the elderly in Catalonia [in Spanish]. Vacunas 1:91–94, 2000.

906. Ambrosch F, Fedson DS. Influenza vaccination in 29 countries: an update to 1997. Pharmacoeconomics 16(suppl 1):47–54, 1999.

907. Health Council of the Netherlands. Vaccination Policies in Case of an Influenza Pandemic (Publication no 2000/01). The Hague, Health Council of the Netherlands, 2000.

908. Opstelten W, Hak E, Verheij TJ, van Essen GA. Introducing a pneumococcal vaccine to an existing influenza immunization program: vaccination rates and predictors of noncompliance. Am J Med 111:474–479, 2001.

909. Pneumococcal vaccines: WHO position paper. Wkly Epidemiol Rec 74:177–183, 1999.

910. Fedson DS. Pneumococcal conjugate vaccination for adults: why it's important for children. Pediatr Infect Dis J 19:183–186, 2000.

911. Shann F. Pneumococcal vaccine: time for another controlled trial. Lancet 351:1600–1601, 1998.

912. Shann F. Bacterial pneumonia: commoner than perceived. Lancet 357:2070–2072, 2001.

913. Murray CJL, Lopez AD. Mortality by cause for eight regions of the world: global burden of disease study. Lancet 349:1269–1276, 1997.

914. Kitange HM, Machibya H, Black J. Outlook for survivors of childhood in sub-Saharan Africa: adult mortality in Tanzania. BMJ 312:216–220, 1996.

915. Chan CY, Molrine DC, George S, et al. Pneumococcal conjugate vaccine primes for antibody responses to polysaccharide pneumococcal vaccine after treatment of Hodgkin's disease. J Infect Dis 173:256–258, 1996.

916. Black SB, Shinefield HR, Hansen J, et al. Postlicensure evaluation of the effectiveness of seven valent pneumococcal conjugate vaccine. Pediatr Infect Dis J 20:1105–1107, 2001.

917. An undervalued vaccine for adults. Lancet 354:2011, 1999.

Chapter 23

Pneumococcal Conjugate Vaccines*

JUHANI ESKOLA • STEVEN BLACK • HENRY SHINEFIELD

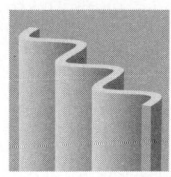

Although the safety and efficacy profiles of the 23-valent pneumococcal polysaccharide vaccine are well documented and recognized, in common with other capsular-type polysaccharides it has limitations such as weak antigenicity, an apparent decline in the level of clinical protection within a few years of vaccination, and no booster antibody response on revaccination. Moreover, the vaccine is insufficiently immunogenic in infants and children, whose immune systems are still developing.[1-5] Impaired responses to the polysaccharide vaccine also are seen in certain groups of people with increased risk of pneumococcal infections, such as people with human immunodeficiency virus (HIV) infection,[6-10] patients with hematologic neoplasms,[11-14] and bone marrow transplant recipients.[15-17] The ability of the polysaccharide vaccine to reduce mucosal carriage of pneumococci is limited,[18,19] and therefore it does not provide any significant protection against mucosal pneumococcal infections[3,20-22] or against spread of resistant pneumococcal strains. In spite of these limitations, health authorities recommend wider use of the polysaccharide vaccine, especially among the elderly and some groups of people at increased risk of pneumococcal infections.[23,24]

The need for safe and more immunogenic vaccines for prevention of pneumococcal infections in both infants and young children as well as among the high-risk patient groups is, however, evident. Recent estimates of children dying from acute respiratory infections largely caused by pneumococci range up to 1.9 million per year.[25,26] A vaccine that was efficacious during the first months of life could prevent a substantial proportion of these fatalities. Rapidly increasing antibiotic resistance of pneumococci[27-31] further emphasizes the need for development of effective prophylactic means to prevent the spread of pneumococcal infections.

Polysaccharide-protein conjugates,[32-34] pneumococcal proteins,[35] nucleic acids as vaccines,[36,37] use of live vectors as delivery agents,[36] and stronger adjuvantation of current antigens[38-40] offer promising avenues for wider coverage and increased efficacy compared with the current polysaccharide vaccine. In addition to traditional intramuscular administration of the antigens, mucosal administration of polysaccharide-based or protein vaccines has been evaluated.[41-44] Conjugate vaccines are the most advanced of these new approaches; one polysaccharide-protein conjugate vaccine is already licensed and widely used, and a few others are at different stages of development. The development of protein antigens as vaccines is still at an early stage and other approaches merely at the drawing board.

Goebel and Avery showed in 1929 that the immunogenicity of weakly immunogenic carbohydrate antigens could be improved if they were coupled covalently to an immunogenic carrier protein.[45,46] After the principle was discovered and published, it took half a century before the first *Haemophilus influenzae* type b (Hib),[47-49] meningococcal,[50-52] and pneumococcal[33,53-56] conjugate vaccines arrived at the clinical testing phase. Examples of these three first conjugates have now been licensed and are becoming part of routine vaccination programs in various countries. During the last few years, research has continued to be active, and several other candidate polysaccharide-protein conjugate vaccines, including streptococcal,[57,58] typhoid,[59,60] and staphylococcal,[61-64] are in clinical development.

To manufacture pneumococcal conjugate vaccines, purified capsular polysaccharides are taken from the most

---

*We will use the following abbreviations for pneumococcal vaccines throughout the chapter:

- PncPS (pneumococcal polysaccharide vaccine; various manufacturers)
- PncD (pneumococcal conjugate vaccine using diphtheria toxoid as a carrier; manufactured by Aventis Pasteur)
- PncT (pneumococcal conjugate vaccine using tetanus protein as a carrier; manufactured by Aventis Pasteur)
- PncDT (pneumococcal conjugate using diphtheria and tetanus as carrier proteins; manufactured by Aventis Pasteur)
- PncCRM (pneumococcal conjugate using CRM$_{197}$ protein as a carrier; manufactured by Wyeth)
- PncOMPC (pneumococcal conjugate using meningococcal outer membrane protein complex as a carrier; manufactured by Merck)
- PncH (pneumococcal conjugate using *Haemophilus influenzae* protein D as a carrier; manufactured by GlaxoSmithKline)

prevalent serotypes of pneumococci (1, 3, 4, 5, 6B, 7F, 9V, 14, 18C, 19F, and 23F).[v1] Each of these saccharides is coupled individually to a carrier protein. The carrier proteins used in Hib conjugate vaccines all have been applied to develop pneumococcal conjugate vaccines: tetanus and diphtheria toxoids,[48,49,54,65] a nontoxic mutant of diphtheria toxin (CRM$_{197}$ protein),[47,66] and the outer membrane protein complex (OMPC) of *Neisseria meningitidis* group B.[67,68] Another pneumococcal conjugate already tested in humans uses Hib protein D as a carrier.[69,70] The final vaccines are mixtures of 7 to 11 saccharide-protein conjugates, eventually adjuvanted with aluminum salts.

Pathogenesis

The only natural reservoir of *Streptococcus pneumoniae* is the human nasopharynx, from which it can be transmitted through respiratory droplets to other individuals. In most cases, pneumococcus is carried in the upper respiratory mucosa without apparent symptoms, and disease occurs in only a small proportion of persons. From the nasopharynx, pneumococci may spread locally into the paranasal sinuses to cause sinusitis, into the middle ear cavity to cause otitis media, or, by inhalation into the lungs to cause pneumonia. In addition, pneumococcus may cause systemic infections with considerable mortality, including bacteremia or meningitis or, in rare cases, infections in remote foci such as joints, bones, and soft tissues.

Capsular polysaccharide is the most important virulence factor of *S. pneumoniae*. It protects pneumococci from phagocytosis by physically shielding the inner structures of the bacterium from antibodies and complement, separating bound opsonins from receptors on phagocytes, and serving as a barrier to the deposition of the complement. Pneumococci that lack the capsule are normally avirulent,[71] while antibodies to the capsular polysaccharides are protective.[72-74] The virulence depends on the chemical composition and molecular size of the capsular polysaccharide.[75,76] Different serotypes of pneumococci have been suggested to vary in virulence depending on their abilities to activate the alternative pathway of the complement,[77] to deposit and degrade the complement components on the capsule,[78] and to resist phagocytosis,[79] and in their ability to induce antibodies.[80]

Epidemiology

Pneumococcal Infections in Children

In the United States, *S. pneumoniae* causes approximately 17,000 cases of invasive disease per year in children less than 5 years old, resulting in 700 cases of meningitis and 200 deaths.[81] The annual incidence of invasive pneumococcal diseases is 165 cases per 100,000 population in children less than 12 months of age, and 203 per 100,000 in children 12 to 23 months, with the peak incidence occurring among children 6 to 11 months (235 per 100,000).[81] The incidence then declines between 2 and 4 years of age to 35.2 per 100,000, reaching its lowest levels in older children, 5 to 17 years of age (3.9 per 100,000).[82] A similar distribution of incidence by age is seen in Canada.[83]

Bacteremia without focus is more common in young children than in the general population,[81,84-86] and comprises 60% to 70% of invasive pneumococcal disease encountered in this age group.[81,87,88] Pneumonia and meningitis are the next most common, but meningitis remains the diagnosis with the highest case fatality rate.[84,85] Since the introduction of the Hib vaccine, *S. pneumoniae* has become the leading cause of bacterial meningitis and occult bacteremia in the United States.[81,89] As children grow older, the proportions of pneumococcal infections classified as meningitis and bacteremia without focus decline, and the proportion of pneumonia increases.[87]

The burden of pneumococcal disease is greatest for those populations in which the PncPS vaccine is least immunogenic: children less than 2 years of age; the elderly; immunocompromised individuals, including those infected with HIV, with functional or anatomic asplenia, or with malignancies; and individuals with chronic cardiovascular, pulmonary, or liver diseases.[90-92] In Europe and in the United States, as in developing countries, children less than 2 years of age comprise the population that is most vulnerable to pneumococcal infections. In one study, 64% of all invasive infections, and 74% where there was no underlying illness, occurred in children 2 years of age or less, although mortality rates are lower in this age group than in older children and adults.[87] There is evidence that this level of risk is increased further by spending time in crowded or communal settings such as day care centers.[88,93]

Children from minority groups suffer disproportionately: Although the overall incidence of invasive pneumococcal disease in children less than 2 years of age is 167 cases per 100,000 person-years in the United States, black children of the same age have an incidence of 400, Alaskan Native children have an incidence of 624, and Native American children less than 2 years of age have an overwhelming incidence of 2396 cases per 100,000 (Table 23–1).[94]

Boys are more likely than girls to contract pneumococcal infections,[95,96] and there are often seasonal peaks in incidence,[97,98] with infection most likely in the winter months. Recent influenza infection in children may be a risk factor for severe pneumococcal pneumonia.[99] In addition to attendance at day care, recent ear infections, recent antibiotic use, and a lack of breast-feeding are associated with increased incidence of invasive pneumococcal diseases in children.[88] These risk factors may not be independent, because children in day care are less likely to breast-feed, and those with recent ear infections are also likely to have had recent antibiotic use. The association of invasive pneumococcal diseases with recent ear infections may indicate that the middle ear is an important route of *S. pneumoniae* invasion.[88]

In Europe as in the United States, the highest levels of infection are in children of 2 years of age or less (and are highest in the second 6 months of life), declining steadily thereafter into the teenage years.[85,86] However, the incidence of pneumococcal infections is generally reported to be much lower in Europe than in the United States.[100] For example, in England and Wales, the annual incidence of invasive pneumococcal diseases in infants between 6 and 11 months is 35.8 per 100,000,[101] compared with 235 per 100,000 in the United States. In Finland, the annual incidence of invasive pneumococcal diseases is 45.3 per 100,000 among those less than 2 years of age.[86] This

TABLE 23–1 ■ Incidence of Invasive Pneumococcal Disease in Children in the United States, by Age and Ethnic Group

Age (yr)	Incidence per 100,000 Person-Years			
	All Races	Blacks	Alaskan Natives	Native American (Navajo or Apache)
<2	167	400	624	2396
2–4	36	116*	98†	227†
5–9	6	9	23	54
10–19	3	5	5	35

* Age 2 to 3 years.
† Age 2 to 5 years.
Adapted from Preventing pneumococcal disease among infants and young children: recommendations of the Advisory Committee on Immunization Practices. MMWR 49(RR-9):1–35, 2000.

difference in incidence is somewhat surprising given that these regions are similar in socioeconomic status and access to health care. Hausdorff et al. hypothesized that this difference is largely due to a difference in blood culturing practices.[102] In Europe, most pediatric blood cultures are performed on samples obtained from hospitalized children and are likely to show serious disease, whereas blood cultures are less likely to be obtained from young children with unexplained fevers.[103,104] In the United States, however, blood cultures are often obtained from outpatient populations with more frequent but less severe bacteremias.[102]

In developing countries, S. pneumoniae is estimated to result in up to 1.9 million deaths in children 2 years of age or younger, surpassing the number of deaths caused by any other infectious disease.[25,26,105] However, the true burden of disease is difficult to quantify in countries where disease surveillance systems and diagnostic facilities are lacking, and most children with pneumococcal infections are diagnosed only if hospitalized.[94,106]

In developing countries, children with pneumococcal meningitis have a younger mean age than those in industrialized countries and neonatal infections are not uncommon.[106] Conservative estimates put the incidence of pneumococcal disease in The Gambia at 500 per 100,000 in children in their first year of life, and 250 per 100,000 in those younger than 5 years of age.[106] Studies from Latin America[97,107] confirm that children less than 2 years of age are at particular risk for invasive pneumococcal diseases, and that a significant risk is present in infants less than 6 months of age. Pneumonia and meningitis are the first and second most frequent presentations, respectively, and are more common in males than in females.

In Southern India, more than 80% of infants are nasopharyngeal carriers of S. pneumoniae by 6 months of age[108] and more than 50% have been colonized by the age of 2 months. This is considerably younger than in the United States, where children, on average, acquire their first strain at 6 months of age.[108] The risk of carriage at 2 months of age is increased in infants born to uneducated mothers, those exposed to 20 or more cigarettes a day, and, interestingly, those who received colostrum at birth. Maternal night blindness is also associated with early colonization in this region with high rates of vitamin A deficiency.

Echoing what is seen in native populations in North America, indigenous people in Australia have much higher rates of pneumococcal disease than do non-native populations. Indigenous children less than 2 years of age have an incidence of invasive pneumococcal diseases of 2053 cases per 100,000 person-years,[109] whereas nonindigenous children have rates intermediate between those of Europe and the United States.[110] Minority populations in Israel also have a higher incidence of pneumococcal infections, although the difference is not as pronounced as in Australia and the United States.[98] This difference appears to be socioeconomically based, because minority groups in Israel are not a single ethnic population but as a group have higher birthrates, more crowded living conditions, less education, and lower socioeconomic status than the majority Jewish population.[98,111]

Pneumococcal Infections in Immunocompromised Individuals

A compromised immune system, whether caused by HIV infection, malignancy, or asplenia, is a major risk factor for pneumococcal disease. Infection with S. pneumoniae occurs over 100 times more frequently in HIV-infected individuals than among the general population,[112–114] Recurrent bacterial sepsis can be the first indicator of acquired immunodeficiency syndrome in pediatric patients,[6] and otitis media has been reported to be three times more frequent in HIV-infected children than in uninfected children.[6,115] In the United States, rates of invasive pneumococcal diseases for HIV-infected children less than 5 years of age are 2.8 times those of HIV-negative children of the same age; the rate is 12.6 times higher for HIV-infected children less than 3 years of age.[81]

In South Africa, the incidence of pneumococcal bacteremia is increased 36.9-fold in HIV-infected children, compared with HIV-negative individuals.[116] Between 1997 and 1999, 5% of all children born in Soweto, South Africa, were infected with HIV.[94] In addition, many of these children have other predisposing conditions, including malnutrition and tuberculosis.[94,117] The rates of pneumococcal bacteremia doubled between 1987 and 1997 as the rates of HIV infection rose.[117] Overall, the disease spectrum is similar in HIV-positive and HIV-negative populations, except that pneumonia is more common in HIV-infected children.

Individuals with sickle cell disease and other hemoglobinopathies resulting in functional asplenia are also at increased risk for serious infections with *S. pneumoniae*.[118-120] Although in the general population most cases of bacteremia occur in children less than 2 years of age, bacteremia occurs more often in older children who also have HIV infection or sickle cell disease,[121] and pneumococcal infection accounts for as many as 25% of deaths from sickle cell disease.[122] Without immunization, the rate of invasive pneumococcal disease in children with sickle cell disease is 30 to 100 times greater than that of healthy children and is greatest in children less than 2 years of age. Even with vaccination with the PncPS vaccine, invasive pneumococcal disease among children with sickle cell disease who are less than 5 years of age is still 10-fold more frequent than in children without sickle cell disease.[122]

Children with nephrotic syndrome also are susceptible to pneumococcal disease, with the majority of infections occurring within the first 2 years after presentation. *Streptococcus pneumoniae* is responsible for 50% to 60% of sepsis and peritonitis in children with nephrotic syndrome, which accounts for a large portion of infective episodes in this population.[123] Patients who have received a bone marrow transplant are also more vulnerable to pneumococcal disease than the general public,[124] in part because they often have impaired opsonization function and lose protection from previous immunizations because of T-cell and B-cell depletion.[125] Patients with Hodgkin's disease have an increased risk of pneumococcal infection, a risk that can persist long after the underlying condition has been successfully treated.[126]

Serotype Distribution

Development of the Hib conjugate vaccine was simplified by the need to protect only against a single serotype. In contrast, 40 serogroups comprising 90 serotypes have been described for *S. pneumoniae*. Among this large number of serotypes, a relatively small number account for most of the invasive disease in young children around the globe, with fewer than 10 serogroups accounting for most invasive pneumococcal disease within each region.[100] However, the distribution of disease-causing serotypes varies between regions (Table 23–2), and by age and disease within regions.

The PncPS vaccine is made by combining purified polysaccharides from 23 pneumococcal serotypes. Because of the more technically difficult process of manufacturing conjugate vaccines, it is impractical to combine so many valencies into one vaccine. To date, conjugate vaccines containing the saccharides of 7, 9, and 11 serotypes have

been proposed or created; the first to be licensed was a 7-valent vaccine (PncCRM), representing the serotypes 4, 6B, 9V, 14, 18C, 19F, and 23F. All the current vaccine candidates have been designed based on knowledge about the relative importance of the disease-causing serotypes. Although comprehensive information about serotypes is not available for many parts of the world,[100] it is important to determine which serogroups or types cause disease in a variety of populations in order to design the most effective vaccines for regional or global use.

Worldwide, serogroups 14, 6, and 19 represent the most frequent sterile-site isolates from sick children regardless of country. In a meta-analysis of 19 studies conducted in 16 countries, Sniadack et al.[127] found the most common serogroups to be (in descending order) 14, 6, 19, 18, 9, 23, 7, 4, 1, and 15 for developed countries and 6, 14, 8, 5, 1, 19, 9, 23, 18, 14, and 7 for developing countries. Based on this information, the authors suggested a vaccine against 1, 5, 6B, 7F, 9V, 14, 18C, 19F, and 23F as the optimal 9-valent vaccine for global use. Although serotype 4 is included in the licensed PncCRM vaccine, in this study it was not found to be one of the seven most common serotypes in developed or developing countries.

Hausdorff and colleagues published a pair of reports describing the global distribution of serogroups, based on an analysis of 72 previously published studies.[100,128] The first examined which serogroups cause most invasive disease worldwide. In most regions, 50% of invasive pneumococcal disease is caused by two or three serotypes in young children, and by four to five serotypes in older children and adults. For young children, serogroups 6 and 14 are first or second in each region except Asia, and 19 is among the fourth most common (except in Latin America, where it is fifth). For older children and adults, no single serogroup is particularly common. Serogroups in the 7-valent vaccine are responsible for almost 90% of invasive pneumococcal diseases in young children in the United States and Canada and for 60% or more in all other regions except Asia (43%) (see Table 23–2). The nonvaccine serotypes 6A and 19A account for a substantial portion of disease within their serogroups,[100] but within-serogroup cross-reactivity may allow the 7-valent vaccine to provide protection against these serotypes, particularly 6A.[129] Serogroups 1 and 5 contribute much more to invasive pneumococcal diseases in young children in Europe than in the United States, Canada, or Oceania.[100] A 9-valent vaccine that includes serotypes 1 and 5 in addition to the serotypes covered in the 7-valent vaccine also would markedly increase disease coverage in older children

TABLE 23–2 ■ Most Prevalent Serotypes in Invasive Diseases in Young Children by Geographic Location and Vaccine Coverage

Geographic Area	7 Most Common Serogroups, in Descending Order	% Vaccine Coverage
United States and Canada	14, 6, 19, 18, 23, 9, 4	88.7
Oceania	14, 6, 19, 18, 23, 9, 4	77.6
Europe	14, 6, 19, 8, 23, 9, 1	74.4
Africa	6, 14, 1, 19, 23, 5, 15	67.3
Latin America	14, 6, 5, 1, 19, 23, 18	63.4
Asia	1, 19, 6, 5, 14, 7, 23	43.1

From Hausdorff WP, Bryant J, Paradiso PR, et al. Which pneumococcal serogroups cause the most invasive disease: implications for conjugate vaccine formulation and use, part I. Clin Infect Dis 30:100–121, 2000, with permission.

and adults in all regions. Serotypes not included in the 11-valent vaccine (which contains 3 and 7F in addition to the serotypes found in the 9-valent vaccine) cause a substantial proportion of disease in the older age groups.

In their second report, Hausdorff and colleagues[128] correlated serotype with the form of disease. Serogroups 1 and 14 were found to be isolated more often from blood, and serogroups 6, 10, and 23 from cerebrospinal fluid (CSF). In young children, serotypes 3, 19, and 23 were isolated more often from middle-ear fluid.[128] Although some serotypes were associated more closely with one disease state than another, none of the most prominent serotypes was found exclusively in one clinical site, and all seem to have the potential to invade each of the normally sterile sites and to cause disease from those sites.[128] Whether the same is true for the more minor serotypes remains unclear.

Within a single region and age group, the number of serogroups responsible for a given percentage of blood isolates does not appear to be substantially different from the number of serogroups responsible for the same percentage of CSF or middle-ear fluid (MEF) isolates.[128] There is, however, a difference in serogroup diversity as a function of age: The diversity of serogroups in blood or CSF is lower for young children than for older children and adults. Therefore, fewer serogroups are responsible for the majority of bacteremic disease and meningitis in young children than in older children and adults. The serogroups that are covered by the conjugate vaccines were isolated slightly less frequently from CSF than from blood or middle-ear fluid; still, serogroups represented in the 9-valent vaccine comprised approximately 75% of pneumococcal isolates from the CSF of young children in Europe, the United States, and Canada.[128]

Among preschool children, serotype 14 is the most prevalent,[84,87,130] and serotypes 14, 6B, and 19F account for more than 50% of invasive pneumococcal infections.[130] The distribution of serotypes varies somewhat by clinical site of isolation: 6B is isolated more often from CSF than from blood and causes more meningitis than 14,[121] whereas 9V is isolated less often from CSF than from blood. Serotypes 3, 19A, and 23F are isolated more often from MEF than from blood, and 4, 9V, 14, and 18C less often.[130] Serotype 14 is most frequently associated with cellulitis, and is also frequently associated with pneumonia.[87]

In the United States, the proportion of invasive disease caused by serotypes covered by the currently licensed 7-valent vaccine is more than 80%,[82,84,121,130,131] and is potentially somewhat higher because of cross-reactivity between serotypes within a serogroup. The coverage is better for young children than for older children.[130] The proportion of isolates of the nonvaccine serogroups 1 and 3 increases with age, as does the vaccine serogroup 23, so that vaccine coverage is 94% in children 2 years of age or younger, but drops to 82% in children 2 to 5 years of age.[87] In children less than 17 years of age, vaccine serogroups account for 94.1% of CSF isolates,[121] and coverage is also very high (98%) for occult bacteremia in children less than 2 years of age.[89]

Because the 7-valent conjugate vaccine was designed around the serotypes that are predominant in the United States, and serotype distribution varies considerably across geographic regions, coverage by the vaccine can also vary in different countries. For example, the 7-valent vaccine, which gives greater than 80% coverage against invasive disease in

the United States, would give only 52% coverage in Germany.[85] This coverage would rise to 62% with a 9-valent vaccine and to 71% with an 11-valent vaccine. Similar rates would be predicted from a study of nasopharyngeal carriage in the Netherlands,[132] but coverage would be slightly higher in Scotland.[133] In Finland, serogroups 14, 6, and 19 were found to be the most prevalent, in that order, together accounting for 54% of invasive pneumococcal infections. Serotype 14 was more prevalent in children 2 years of age or younger, being replaced by serogroup 18 in older children. The serogroups 14, 6, 19, 7, 18, and 23 comprised 78% of all invasive infections; five of these six are included in the 7-valent vaccine.[86] In Denmark, the 10 leading serotypes, responsible for 82% of invasive pneumococcal diseases in children less than 6 years of age, were 1, 4, 6A, 6B, 7F, 9V, 14, 18C, 19F, and 23F.[134] Serotypes 1, 3, 5, and 7F were more common in newborns and children more than 2 years of age, whereas 6B and 14 were more common in children between 6 months and 2 years of age. In contrast to the data from Finland,[86] in Denmark serotype 18C was more common in children less than 1 year of age than in older children.[134] Consistent with other studies, the proportion of isolates with serotypes 1 and 14 was significantly higher in blood than CSF, but serotype 6B was found more often in CSF isolates.[134] In Denmark, the 7-valent vaccine would provide better coverage in children less than 2 years of age (65.9%) than in children between 2 and 6 years of age (47.7%).[134] Unlike many other European and even other Scandinavian countries, serogroup 7, which is not included in the 7-valent vaccine, is prominent in Sweden, particularly in cases of bacteremia.[104]

A sampling of individual studies from around the world gives the flavor of the serotype diversity that is seen in pneumococcal disease. In a small study in Turkey,[135] the coverage of a proposed 9-valent vaccine for developing countries (see below)[127] would provide 90% coverage for Turkish children less than 2 years of age, but only 43% coverage for older children. The serotype distributions in Santiago, Chile,[107] and Uruguay[97] were similar to each other. In Uruguay, the seven most common serotypes accounted for 80% of the invasive isolates, although 21 serotypes were identified overall. In South Indian infants, the serogroup distribution of nasopharyngeal colonization changed over the first 6 months of life. Although serotypes 6, 14, 15, 19, and 23 persisted in the top seven over the 6 months, their relative frequency changed. Furthermore, serotype 10 became less frequent after 2 months of age, and serotype 33 appeared in the top four at 6 months.[108] In Israeli children, serotype 14 was associated primarily with bacteremia without focus, and an ethnic difference was found for serotype 1, which was more prevalent among non-Jews than among Jews.[98]

Six serotypes (14, 6B, 23F, 19F, 9V, and 6A) accounted for 90% of the isolates that were resistant to at least three classes of drugs. Serotypes included in the now-licensed 7-valent vaccine, PncCRM, comprised 78% of all penicillin-resistant strains and 81% of those isolated from children less than 5 years of age. If the vaccine provides cross-protection against serotypes 6A and 19A, an additional 15% of penicillin-resistant infections would be covered, a total coverage of 96% in children less than 5 years of age. However, recombination is frequent among pneumococcal strains and can lead to serotype changes among resistant bacteria, creating resistance among serotypes that were previously susceptible.[136]

Resistance is caused in part by the abundant overuse of antibiotics, and limiting antibiotic use can reduce the prevalence of resistant organisms, as has been shown in Iceland.[137] However, given that the most prevalent serotypes included in the vaccine are also the most likely to be resistant, vaccination has taken on a new importance. The conjugate vaccine will be potentially most useful in young children, who not only are underserved by the current polysaccharide vaccine, but who also provide the largest pool of resistant bacteria.

As discussed earlier, a much lower incidence of invasive pneumococcal diseases has been reported in Europe than in the United States, which can be attributed in part to a difference in blood culture practices.[102] The reported serotype distribution also could be skewed by this sampling bias if some serotypes are more likely to cause severe disease requiring hospitalization, because these virulent serotypes would have a higher apparent prevalence in regions that perform blood cultures only on hospitalized patients. In fact, although the most common serotypes (14, 6, 19, 18, 23, 9, and 4) have a much higher incidence in the United States than in Europe, the low incidence of disease caused by serogroups 7, 1, and 5 is similar in both regions.[102] This pattern might indicate that serogroups 7, 1, and 5 cause severe rather than mild disease in both regions. As an example, serotype 1 causes 5% of invasive pneumococcal diseases in western Europe and only 0.5% of invasive pneumococcal diseases in the United States, yet the rate of serotype 1 disease is about 0.9 per 100,000 person-years in each region.[102] This supports the idea that certain serogroups are intrinsically highly virulent[102] and could account for the high prevalence of serotypes 1 and 5 in the developing world, where, as in Europe, blood cultures rarely are performed on an outpatient basis.

Active Immunization

The reader is referred to Chapter 22 for information on pneumococcal polysaccharide vaccines.

T-cell Dependent Immune Response and Conjugate Vaccines

Native polysaccharides belong among the T-cell–independent (TI) types of antigens,[138,139] whereas polysaccharide-protein conjugates are T-cell–dependent (TD) antigens.[32,140] TI antigens—polysaccharides, polypeptides, and polynucleotides—are believed to activate only mature B cells; therefore, there is as a rule no response to polysaccharides in early infancy. A response to TI antigen shows limited memory induction, affinity maturation, or isotype switch.[141–143]

The immune response to the polysaccharide-protein conjugate starts in nonlymphoid tissue when dendritic cells capture the conjugate molecules (Fig. 23–1).[144–146] During the migration to local secondary lymph tissues,[147] dendritic cells process the carrier protein intracellularly into peptides,[148] to be presented later in context with major histocompatibility complex (MHC) class II molecules to antigen-specific T cells.[145,149–151] Recently, it has been suggested that even in TI immunity T-cell help is involved, although in a different form than in the classic TD immunity, and that antibody

responses to pneumococcal capsular polysaccharides require another type of T-cell help. According to this hypothesis, an MHC class I–like molecule, CD1, presents polysaccharide antigens to CD8+ type T helper (Th) cells.[152]

Epitopes of each capsular polysaccharide antigen bind to specific membrane-bound antibodies that are expressed on the surfaces of B lymphocytes and dendritic cells.[153] The serotype of pneumococcal polysaccharide can alter the peptide specificities of T-cell responses.[150] This interaction triggers receptor-mediated endocytosis, a process that involves the invagination of the antigen-antibody binding complex by a patch of the surrounding cell membrane. The internalized vesicle fuses with endosomes, and their acidic microenvironment facilitates enzyme-mediated catabolism of the conjugated vaccine. After molecular processing, peptidic epitopes of carrier protein associate with MHC class II proteins, which then are targeted to the external membrane surface of the antigen-presenting cells. The expression of foreign peptide epitopes by MHC class II proteins is a molecular signal to CD4+ Th precursor cells that the antigen-presenting cell has encountered a pathogen.[154]

An array of cytokine-mediated events then is initiated involving complex interactions between different subsets of T cells. Interleukin-2 secretion by Th precursor cells induces a clone of activated T cells (Th0), which in turn secrete interleukin-4.[154] Interleukin-4 secretion by Th0 clones gives rise to subsets 1 and 2 of Th lymphocytes (Th1 and Th2), the latter secreting interleukin-4, -5 and -6.[155] Th2 secretion of cytokines stimulates the differentiation and proliferation of B cells into plasma and memory B-cell progenitors of the same specificity that produce antibodies against the original pneumococcal polysaccharide antigens.

T-cell help in response to polysaccharide-protein conjugates is limited in a primary immune response.[156] Specialized antigen-presenting cells are required for the T-cell priming, because naive B cells may fail to activate naive T cells.[157] After priming, polysaccharide-specific B cells are able to function as antigen-presenting cells for mature T cells. They detect and internalize conjugates by receptor-mediated endocytosis and present the carrier peptides in MHC class II molecules on their surfaces (see Fig. 23–1).[158] This is followed by direct contact between T and B cells.[159] The cognate stimulatory interaction results in B cell activation and proliferation in germinal centers.[146,158,160,161] The activated B cells differentiate into antibody-secreting plasma cells or memory cells.[162] The carrier protein of PncOMPC vaccine acts both as carrier and adjuvant and thereby enhances even stronger TD-responses in infants.[162a]

The initial encounter with an antigen activates a large number of B cells with a wide variety of affinities.[144,156] During B-cell proliferation in germinal centers, the genes encoding variable regions of antibodies undergo somatic hypermutations.[163] The continued selection of high-affinity B-cell clones in the presence of diminishing antigen concentration leads to maturation of affinity.[164,165] The competition for free antigen drives affinity maturation in the early stage, but, after the disappearance of free antigen, follicular dendritic cells control the process.[160,166] B cells with high affinity to antigens adhering to follicular dendritic cell surfaces survive, and B cells with low affinity are destroyed by apoptosis.[166,167]

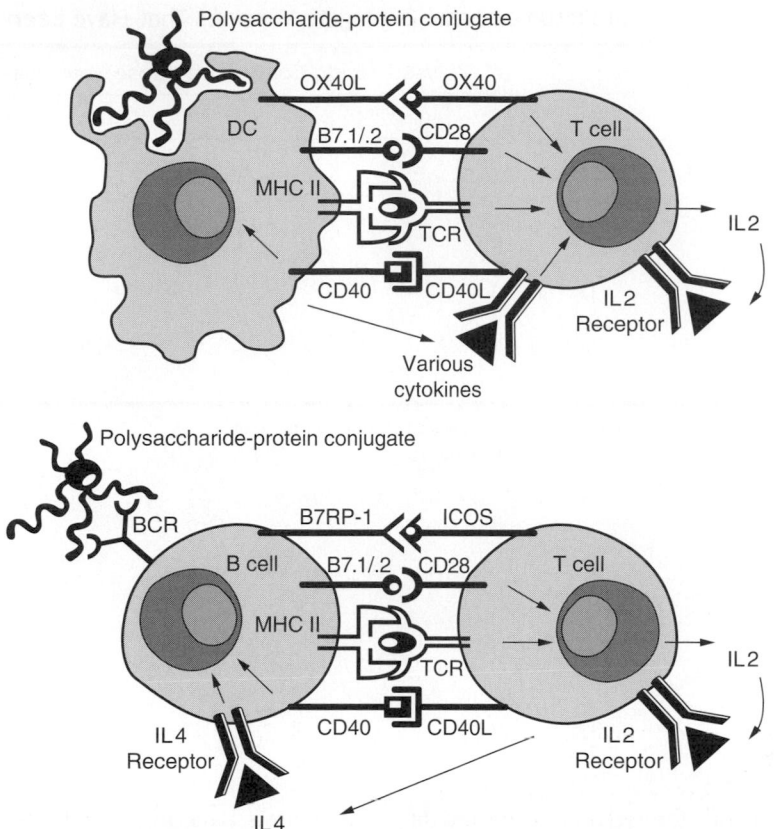

FIGURE 23–1 ■ Priming of naive T cells requires an interaction between dendritic cells (DC) and carrier protein–specific T cells. This interaction necessitates antigenic stimulation via the major histocompatibility complex class II–T-cell receptor (MHC II–TCR) pathway and co-stimulatory support via subsequent CD40-CD40L and B7-CD28 pathways. Various cytokines, including interleukin (IL)-12, interferon-α (IFNα), and IL-18, promote Th1 development, and IL-4 promotes Th2 development. After priming, T cells interact with B cells. The pneumococcal polysaccharide–specific B cells internalize the conjugate and present carrier protein peptides in the context of MHC II molecules to T cells. The activation of B cells necessitates MHC II–TCR signaling and co-stimulatory support via CD40-CD40L, B7-CD28, and B7RP-1–ICOS pathways. Eventually, cytokines including IL-4 and IL-5 induce B-cell proliferation and generation of germinal centers. The activated B cells differentiate into antibody-secreting plasma cells and memory B cells.[146,158] BCR, B-cell receptor. KOS = inducible co-stimulator. (Figure taken from Guttormsen HK, Sharpe AH, Chandraker AK, et al. Cognate stimulatory B-cell–T-cell interactions are critical for T-cell help recruited by glycoconjugate vaccines. Infect Immun 67:6375–6384, 1999. Adapted by Tomi Wuorimaa, KTL, Finland.)

Antibody-secreting cells appear rapidly in bone marrow after primary immunization. However, these cells secreting low-avidity antibodies soon die, within 2 weeks.[168] Fresh plasma cells with increased avidity arrive from germinal centers and replace the early cells in bone marrow, reaching a plateau within 6 to 7 weeks.[162] Eventually, as the amount of antigen diminishes in germinal centers, high-affinity antibody-antigen complexes are formed near the surfaces of dendritic cells. High-affinity B cells interact simultaneously with antibodies and the antigen within the complex via Fcγ and B-cell receptors. Cross-linking of Fcγ II and B-cell receptors impedes B-cell proliferation and further formation of plasma cells,[169] but promotes formation of memory B cells.[162]

Attention has been increasingly focused on the role of conjugate vaccine–induced immunologic memory in conferring protection against invasive infections caused by encapsulated bacteria.[170,171] Memory is based on the increased number of mature antigen-specific T and B cells that enable rapid immune responses, with high concentration of high-avidity antibodies, to subsequent antigen exposure. Development of memory is dependent on activation of carrier protein–specific T cells and is mediated by long-

living polysaccharide-specific memory B cells expressing antibodies with high avidity.[158,172,173] Although the longevity of memory T cells seems to require the presence of the antigen,[174] persistence of memory B cells appears to be independent of exposure to the antigen.[175]

Vaccines

Over the past 15 years, several manufacturers have developed pneumococcal conjugate vaccines through different approaches. These vaccines differ in the included serotypes, the carrier proteins, and their conjugation chemistry (Table 23–3).

The number of pneumococcal serotypes included in current vaccine candidates in clinical development range from 7 to 11. Serotypes 4, 6B, 9V, 14, 18C, 19F, and 23F are common to all vaccines. The Wyeth 9-valent candidate vaccine includes serotypes 1 and 5 in addition to the previous seven, while GlaxoSmithKline and Aventis Pasteur[†] have included serotypes 1, 3, 5, and 7 in their 11-valent vaccines.

[†]Aventis Pasteur decided in 2002 to stop development of the 11-valent PncDT vaccine.

TABLE 23–3 ■ Chemical Composition of Pneumococcal Conjugate Vaccines That Have Been Tested in Clinical Trials

Manufacturer	Product Name	Polysaccharide Content (mg/dose) per Serotype							
		1	3	4	5	6B	7F	9V	14
Wyeth	Prevnar	—	—	2	—	4	—	2	2
	—	2	—	2	2	4	—	2	2
GlaxoSmithKline	—	1	1	1	1	1	1	1	1
Aventis Pasteur	—	1*	3	1*	1*	10	1*	1*	3
Merck	—	—	—	1	—	3–3.5	—	1.5	1

*Polysaccharide conjugated to tetanus protein; other serotypes conjugated to diphtheria toxoid.
ADH, adipic acid dihydrazide; OMPC, outer membrane protein complex.

The amount of polysaccharide for each conjugate also differs between the vaccines, ranging from 1 to 10 μg per serotype. In general, pneumococcal conjugates contain less polysaccharide per serotype than the licensed Hib conjugate vaccines. This most likely reflects both the desire to reduce the total amounts of carrier protein and polysaccharide in the vaccine and a perceived greater immunogenicity for pneumococcal serotypes compared with Hib. Although it would be preferable to include a larger number of different polysaccharides in a conjugate vaccine, technically this becomes challenging. In addition, incremental benefits in coverage from increasing the number of serotypes remain low after the standard 11 serotypes have been included. Moreover, the total amount of carrier protein in the final vaccine may need to be limited because too much carrier protein can impair the antibody response to the polysaccharide antigen.[176–179]

Several different carriers have been used, four being the same proteins used in Hib conjugates. Wyeth continues using CRM_{197}, a nontoxic mutant of diphtheria toxin, in their pneumococcal vaccine.[47,66] The Aventis Pasteur vaccine candidate has two different carriers: pneumococcal polysaccharides from serotypes 3, 6B, 14, and 18C are conjugated to diphtheria toxoid and those from serotypes 1, 4, 5, 7F, 9V, 19F, and 23F to tetanus protein.[48,49,54] Merck uses OMPC, modified from N. meningitidis,[67,68,180] as in their Hib conjugate. GlaxoSmithKline has decided to conjugate pneumococcal polysaccharides to the H. influenzae protein D.[69,70] Other potential carrier proteins that have been tested in animal studies include bovine serum albumin, human immunoglobulin G (IgG), complement C3d, keyhole limpet hemocyanin, flagellar protein of Salmonella, pertussis toxoid, and pneumolysin toxoid.[181–184] Conjugates between the carrier and hapten parts have been made using a variety of procedures.[56,185] Vaccine man-

ufacturers have in general adapted their Hib conjugation technology to covalently link the carrier and hapten parts together.[56,185] The basic procedure used by Wyeth[186] first activates the polysaccharide by reaction with periodate. The carrier protein is then coupled directly to the polysaccharide through reductive amination. Aventis Pasteur covalently links each polysaccharide to either tetanus protein or diphtheria toxoid using adipic acid dihydrazide linker methodology.[48,187] Polysaccharides are activated and derivatized with adipic acid dihydrazide and cyanoborohydride. The activated, derivatized polysaccharides are coupled to the carrier protein with a carbodiimide. In this manner, the carrier is cross-linked at multiple points, forming a lattice structure. Merck uses a bigeneric linker to couple polysaccharides to carrier protein.[180,186] The polysaccharides are derivatized to introduce amino groups, which are subsequently converted to bromoacetyl groups. In parallel, the OMPC is derivatized to introduce thio groups. The thiolated protein is coupled to the bromacetylated polysaccharide, forming the conjugate. The conjugation chemistry for GlaxoSmithKline's candidate vaccine has not yet been published. Aluminum adjuvants are used in two pneumococcal conjugate vaccines. Wyeth uses aluminum phosphate[53] while Merck uses aluminum hydroxyphosphate.[180]

The only currently licensed pneumococcal conjugate vaccine, Prevnar™, is manufactured by Wyeth as a liquid preparation. Each 0.5-mL dose is formulated to contain 2 μg of each saccharide for serotypes 4, 9V, 14, 18C, 19F, and 23F, and 4 μg of serotype 6B per dose (16 μg total saccharide); approximately 20 μg of CRM_{197} carrier protein; and 0.125 mg of aluminum per 0.5-mL dose as aluminum phosphate adjuvant. After shaking, the vaccine is a homogeneous, white suspension.

18C	19F	23F	Chemistry	Carrier(s)	Adjuvant
2	2	2	Direct coupling through reductive amination	CRM_{197}	Aluminum phosphate
2	2	2			
1	1	1	?	*H. influenzae* protein D	—
3	1*	1*	Covalently coupled using ADH	Diphtheria toxoid, tetanus protein	—
1	2–2.5	1	Bigeneric linker OMPC	*N. meningitidis*	Aluminum hydroxy-phosphate

Results of Vaccination

Immunogenicity of the Vaccine

Measurement of Immunity

Antibodies against capsular polysaccharides are protective against diseases caused by encapsulated bacteria. In pneumococcal infections, this is indirectly demonstrated by the increased incidence of serious infections in groups with lower antibody concentrations (e.g., infants, patients with hypo- or agammaglobulinemia, and patients recovering from bone marrow transplantation).[6-17] Direct evidence of the protective effect of anti-capsular antibodies comes from studies where passively administered antibodies have provided protection from otitis media or invasive pneumococcal disease.[72,74] Vaccines that induce antibodies to pneumococcal capsular polysaccharides are protective against invasive pneumococcal infections.[2]

Immune responses to pneumococcal vaccines have been evaluated by radioimmunoassay (RIA) and enzyme immunoassay (EIA), both of which measure the binding of antibodies to pneumococcal polysaccharide antigens.[188,189] Very recently, a new fluorescent assay has been described for measuring antibodies.[189a] Although it looks promising, its real value remains to be seen in the years to come. In addition to anti-polysaccharide antibody concentrations as such, assays that measure the functional activity of antibodies in vitro are widely used. These include analysis of high-avidity antibodies or an opsonophagocytosis assay (OPA). Validation of EIA methods for measuring concentrations of serotype-specific antibodies to pneumococci has advanced,[190] and validation of OPAs is ongoing.

RADIOIMMUNOASSAY AND ENZYME IMMUNOASSAY

Radioimmunoassay used to be the method of choice for measuring the amount of antibodies to pneumococci.[189] However, it has features that limit its use. Preparation of radiolabeled antigens in a consistent manner is difficult, and RIA cannot be used to determine antibody isotypes because it measures not only IgG but also immunoglobulin A (IgA) and immunoglobulin M (IgM) antibodies. In contrast, EIA is a sensitive, convenient, and rapid method to perform even for a large number of samples. Concentrations of IgA, IgM, and IgG isotypes and of total immunoglobulin,[169] as well as of IgG subclasses,[191] can be determined using a reference serum.

Interpretation of the early RIA results is problematic because a significant proportion of antibodies thought to be type-specific are directed toward pneumococcal C polysaccharide[192] that are neither opsonic nor protective. Therefore, their inhibition from serum samples by neutralization is needed in the conduct of both RIA as well as EIA.[193] Another problem is that adult human sera also seem to contain other polyreactive antibodies that recognize pneumococcal polysaccharides of different serotypes in EIA.[194-196] These antibodies, present in sera of individuals who have naturally acquired antibodies but less so in sera of those immunized with pneumococcal vaccines, most probably are directed to contaminants in the pneumococcal polysaccharide preparations that are used as antigens in the assays or directed to polyreactive epitopes present in the polysaccharide antigens. Their removal by inhibition of antibody binding by soluble polysaccharides of an irrelevant serotype (e.g., by using a polysaccharide of serotype 22F) improves the specificity.[194]

Substantial progress has been made in the past 4 years in the standardization of the pneumococcal polysaccharide

EIA antibody assay. The Food and Drug Administration (FDA) has made available a reference serum from pooled human sera (89SF), and concentrations of several IgG anti-pneumococcal polysaccharide antibodies in this serum have been reported. All major pneumococcal reference laboratories are now using this reference to control for interlaboratory variation. Plikaytis et al. analyzed the degree of agreement among 12 laboratories quantifying an identical series of serum specimens using a consensus IgG EIA developed for this study.[190]

Specific antibody-secreting cells (ASCs) to pneumococcal polysaccharide and to carrier proteins can be detected with an enzyme-linked immunospot assay (ELISPOT) in various lymphatic tissues or in the peripheral blood. Because the B cells are continuously circulating through the lymphatics and blood back to the peripheral tissues, cells committed to mucosal sites also are present in the peripheral blood for a limited period of time, before homing to different exocrine tissues. The appearance of these antigen-specific ASCs thus can be measured in peripheral blood after an antigen challenge, and the magnitude of this response is thought to reflect the immune response on mucosal membranes.[197–202]

AVIDITY

Antibody avidity describes the strength with which an antibody binds to a complex antigen. Several methods based on RIA[203] or EIA[204–211] have been described for determining relative antibody avidity to different types of antigens. In EIA techniques, the binding of antibody to the coated antigen may be prevented by competitive inhibition using decreasing concentrations of free antigen[205,208] or by eluting the antibody from the antigen by a dissociating agent, such as thiocyanate,[206–208,211] urea,[209] or diethylamine.[205,207,208] (Thiocyanate anion and urea interfere with the antibody-antigen binding primarily through disrupting the hydrophobic bonds;[208] diethylamine is a protein denaturing agent.) Because the elution assays are based on dissociation of the antibody-antigen complexes of low avidity, they allow ranking of the antibodies by their avidity. Experience with Hib conjugate vaccines suggest that measurement of antibody avidity may prove useful in assessing the induction of memory, and that avidity assays could be used to distinguish between those individuals who are primed for memory and those who are not.[212,213]

OPSONOPHAGOC YTIC ACTIVITY

Because opsonin-dependent phagocytosis is the primary defense mechanism against S. pneumoniae, a variety of techniques to measure the OPA of antibodies to pneumococci have been developed.[214–220] These include radioisotopic, flow cytometric, microscopic, and viability (or killing) assays. Most are performed using human polymorphonuclear leukocytes as the effector cells, but some assays have been adapted to utilize culturable phagocytes (differentiated HL-60 cells).[217,218] Although several methods have been described, no standard assay is available.

Generally, the results obtained by the various techniques correlate well, although serotype-specific differences were found.[221]

The correlation between the IgG antibody concentration and OPA results is relatively strong in immune sera,[218,219,221] but is weaker at low antibody concentrations.[221–225] The correlation is especially poor in unimmunized children. In general, the correlation between antibody concentration and OPA seems to be good in infants[226] who have been immunized with conjugate vaccines[220,227] but lower in adults.[195,225,226] The reason for this, as already mentioned, is that the serum samples from adults contain antibodies that are detected by standard EIA but are not functionally active.[195,225,228]

Because antibody OPA more closely resembles the mechanism of immunity than antibody binding to a solid polysaccharide antigen, in animal models it provides better correlation with protection than the concentration of IgG antibodies as measured by EIA.[224,229] Therefore, it has been recommended as the primary assay to evaluate the functional activity of pneumococcal conjugate vaccine immune response.

Antibody Response

INFANTS AND YOUNG CHILDREN

Infants are the main target group for pneumococcal conjugate vaccines. Most clinical trials therefore have focused on safety and immunogenicity of candidate vaccines in infants. The youngest children have received the conjugate vaccine according to the Expanded Programme on Immunization schedule, at the age of 6, 10, and 14 weeks. The schedule that has been studied most extensively is a three-dose primary immunization series either at 2, 3, and 4 months or at 2, 4, and 6 months of age, followed eventually by a booster dose during the second year of life.

Only a few studies have been published in which different schedules, different numbers of vaccine doses, or different dosages of antigens have been compared directly. It appears, however, that three doses may be needed for optimal immune response to PncOMPC[230] and PncCRM[231] vaccines in early infancy. Dose-response evaluation results have been published from tetravalent PncT and PncD vaccines (1, 3, or 10 μg of each polysaccharide). For PncT vaccine, no dose dependency was seen after the primary immunization, whereas the booster response was highest in the group primed with the lowest dose of the conjugate vaccine.[232] In contrast, with PncD vaccine, the highest dose induced the strongest response after primary immunization, but the booster response was greatest in the group primed with the lowest dose.[233]

To demonstrate the general tendencies of the responses in the immunogenicity studies, data from various vaccines are compiled in Table 23–4. Immune responses to the licensed 7-valent PncCRM vaccine (Prevnar) are presented in more detail in Figure 23–2 and in Table 23–5. In young children and infants who do not respond at all to the pneu-

TABLE 23–4 ■ Antibody Geometric Mean Concentrations (µg/mL) 1 Month After Dose 3 of Various Pneumococcal Conjugate Vaccines*

Site	N	Simultaneous Pertussis Vaccine	Vaccination Schedule (mo)	Pneumococcal Serotype											Reference
				1	3	4	5	6B	7F	9V	14	18C	19F	23F	
AVENTIS PASTEUR (PncDT)															
Israel	90	acP	2, 4, 6	0.52	1.84	1.49	1.34	0.65	1.43	0.49	1.00	0.77	2.17	0.34	369
Finland	51	wcP	2, 4, 6	2.46	1.45	3.22	2.10	0.68	2.22	1.41	1.93	0.90	3.98	1.20	369–371
Israel	65	wcP	2, 4, 6	4.16	2.60	5.26	2.20	1.29	3.61	1.85	2.01	1.17	6.55	1.78	369–371
Finland	38	wcP	2, 4, 6	1.55	1.26	3.86	1.98	0.97	4.37	2.03	1.01	0.81	5.60	1.23	369, 370, 372–376
Israel	57	wcP	2, 4, 6	1.65	1.55	3.14	1.84	1.05	4.11	1.54	1.82	0.76	4.88	1.44	369, 370, 372–376
Iceland	65	wcP	3, 4, 6	2.67	3.98	4.17	1.86	0.81	3.96	1.95	2.71	1.87	6.2	1.32	373, 377–380
Chile	65	wcP	2, 4, 6	4.28	2.58	9.41	4.56	1.79	6.66	3.67	3.34	1.36	11.4	2.95	381
WYETH (PncCRM)															
NCKP	156	wcP	2, 4, 6			1.3		1.22		1.01	3.72	1.44	1.95	2.54	245, 247
NCKP	75	acP	2, 4, 6			1.37		2.14		1.23	5.04	1.88	1.52	1.21	247
U.S.	90	wcP	2, 4, 6			1.36		1.37		0.98	3.48	1.24	3.45	1.8	309
NCKP	88	wcP	2, 4, 6			1.46		4.7		1.99	4.6	2.16	1.39	1.88	240
NCKP	32	acP	2, 4, 6			1.47		2.18		1.52	5.05	2.24	1.54	1.48	240
U.S.	159	acP	2, 4, 6			2.03		2.97		1.18	4.64	1.96	1.91	1.71	240
Germany	83	acP	2, 4, 6			3.5		2.5		2.3	4.7	2.6	4.1	1.9	382
South Africa	250	wcP	6, 10, 14 wk	5.30		4.02	6.18	5.87		3.24	3.61	4.78	2.99	2.73	383
South Africa	122–135	wcP	6, 10, 14 wk	5.82		4.22	7.31	5.60		3.62	3.76	5.68	2.91	2.95	241
The Gambia	91–97	wcP	2, 3, 4	6.94		4.90	5.84	4.93		4.07	4.45	4.89	2.91	2.85	308
Finland	57	wcP	2, 4, 6			1.7		2.0		2.5	6.3	3.6	3.3	2.5	300
MERCK (PncOMPC)															
Apache & Navajo	34	wcP	2, 4, 6			1.80		0.19		1.15	2.03	0.90	0.87	0.14	384
Alaskan Native	30	wcP	2, 4, 6			1.97		0.36		2.57	1.52	1.39	1.17	0.72	384
U.S.	32	wcP	2, 4, 6			2.59		0.47		2.77	2.97	1.31	1.32	0.43	384
GLAXOSMITHKLINE (PncH)															
Costa Rica	30	?	3, 4, 5	2.8	2.3	2.8	3.2	1.44	2.5	3.3	6.52	2.0	4.15	1.69	385
Philippines	150	wcP	6, 10, 14 wk					1.2			3.5		4.2	1.5	386

*Note that the studies have been conducted in different populations, at different time periods, and the antibody assays have been performed in different laboratories; results from separate studies are therefore not directly comparable.

acP, acellular pertussis; NCKP, Northern California Kaiser Permanente medical centers; wcP, whole-cell pertuss s.

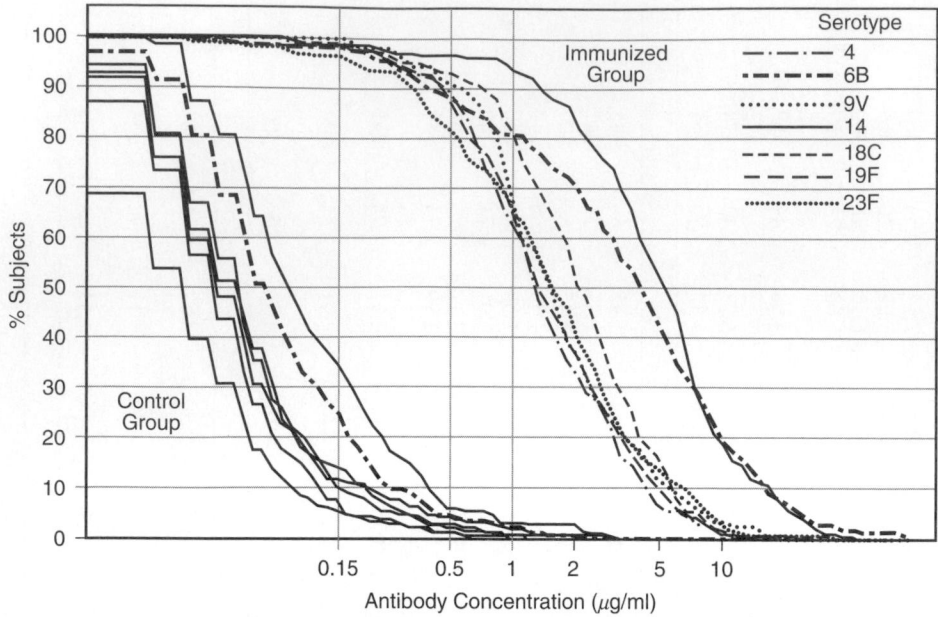

FIGURE 23–2 ■ Reverse cumulative distribution curves of post–dose 3 antibody concentrations when PncCRM vaccine was given concurrent with diphtheria and tetanus toxoids and pertussis (DTP) or diphtheria and tetanus toxoids and acellular pertussis (DTaP) vaccines.[245,247]

mococcal serotypes most frequently causing infections in children (i.e., 6B and 23F), a clear response can be seen when the same serotype polysaccharides are administered in the conjugate vaccines. Generally, 5- to 10-fold rises in geometric mean concentrations (GMCs) of anti-capsular antibodies usually can be demonstrated when postimmunization concentrations are compared with the preimmunization concentrations. Antibody concentrations at 7 months of age, 1 month after the third dose, range from 0.49 to 9.41 µg/mL depending on the serotype and vaccine (see Table 23–4). For some serotypes (14, 18C, and 19F) even one dose in early infancy may be enough to induce antibody production in some infants, whereas for other serotypes (6B and 23F) three doses are needed. Because the same pattern of response is common to conjugates with different carrier proteins, it is plausible that the type of response—strong or weak—is an inherent property of the polysaccharide itself.

Antibody concentrations achieved after the initial series of three doses usually are sustained only for a few months and decline thereafter to close to preimmunization levels. However, a dose of the pneumococcal vaccine, either polysaccharide or conjugate, administered during the second year of life to children primed with any of the conjugates generally induces an approximately 10-fold increase in antibody concentrations. This response has three features typical of an anamnestic response. First, there is a large, rapid response of both IgG1 and IgG2 antibodies. The increase in GMC is much stronger than that seen if the same vaccines were given at the same age without priming.[232-238] The rapidity of the response was shown by an increase in GMCs of anti-capsular antibodies in samples taken 7 to 10 days after immunization at 24 months of age, provided children had received primary doses with the conjugate.[236,238] Second, there is a shift of IgG subclass distribution after the booster dose as compared to the

TABLE 23–5 ■ Geometric Mean Concentrations (µg/mL) of Pneumococcal Antibodies Following the Third and Fourth Doses of PncCRM or Control Vaccine When Administered Concurrently with DTP-HbOC or DTaP and HbOC in the Kaiser Permanente Efficacy Study

Serotype	After Dose 3 (DTP-HbOC)		After Dose 3 (DTaP and HbOC)		After Dose 4 (DTP-HbOC)	
	PncCRM*	Control	PncCRM*	Control	PncCRM*	Control
	(N = 88)	(N = 92)	(N = 32)	(N = 32)	(N = 68)	(N = 61)
4	1.46 (1.19, 1.78)	0.03	1.47 (1.08, 2.02)	0.02	2.38 (1.88, 3.03)	0.04
6B	4.70 (3.59, 6.14)	0.08	2.18 (1.20, 3.96)	0.06	14.45 (11.17, 18.69)	0.17
9V	1.99 (1.64, 2.42)	0.05	1.52 (1.04, 2.22)	0.04	3.51 (2.75, 4.48)	0.06
14	4.60 (3.70, 5.74)	0.05	5.05 (3.32, 7.70)	0.04	6.52 (5.18, 8.21)	0.06
18C	2.16 (1.73, 2.69)	0.04	2.24 (1.65, 3.02)	0.04	3.43 (2.70, 4.37)	0.07
19F	1.39 (1.16, 1.68)	0.09	1.54 (1.09, 2.17)	0.10	2.07 (1.66, 2.57)	0.18
23F	1.85 (1.46, 2.34)	0.05	1.48 (0.97, 2.25)	0.05	3.82 (2.85, 5.11)	0.09

*Geometric mean concentration (95% confidence interval).

DTP-HbOC, diphtheria and tetanus toxoids and pertussis–*H. influenzae* type b oligosaccharide conjugate; DTaP, diphtheria and tetanus toxoids and acellular pertussis.

Data from Shinefield HR, Black S, Ray P, et al. Safety and immunogenicity of heptavalent pneumococcal CRM197 conjugate vaccine in infants and toddlers. Pediatr Infect Dis J 18:757–763, 1999; and Black S, Shinefield H, Fireman B, et al. Efficacy, safety and immunogenicity of heptavalent pneumococcal conjugate vaccine in children. Northern California Kaiser Permanente Vaccine Study Center Group. Pediatr Infect Dis J 19:187–195, 2000.

response to the primary immunization. The serotype-specific pneumococcal IgG antibody response is virtually restricted to the IgG1 subclass after primary immunization, but secondary immunization elicits antibodies of both IgG1 and IgG2 subclasses.[226,234]

The third feature of a memory response is the maturation of antibody avidity.[212] The avidity of antibodies was increased in children given a conjugate booster but not a polysaccharide vaccine booster.[204,239] This suggests that the response to a pneumococcal conjugate was a TD response, but the TI pneumococcal polysaccharide vaccine only triggered the existing memory B cells.[232]

CONCURRENT ADMINISTRATION WITH OTHER VACCINES

During the licensure process of a new vaccine, the manufacturer has to demonstrate that the antibody responses to other routinely administered childhood vaccines are not adversely affected. This has been shown with Prevnar in studies where it was administered simultaneously with diphtheria and tetanus toxoids and pertussis–*H. influenzae* type b oligosaccharide conjugate (DTP-HbOC) or diphtheria and tetanus toxoids and acellular pertussis (DTaP) and HbOC, oral or inactivated poliovirus, hepatitis B, measles-mumps-rubella, and varicella vaccines.[240] In general, the results demonstrate that the pneumococcal conjugate vaccine is compatible with other recommended childhood vaccines when administered concurrently (Table 23–6). Inconsistent differences in response to pertussis antigens after primary immunizations and some suppression of Hib response after booster dose were observed, but these were considered to have no clinical significance and did not prevent licensure of the vaccine.

The response to HbOC (the Hib conjugate vaccine with the same CRM_{197} carrier as in the PncCRM vaccine) and diphtheria toxoid is higher when PncCRM is administered concurrently with HbOC and DTP than when it is administered without concurrent PncCRM.[241,242] The increase in anti–Hib polysaccharide antibody concentrations is depen-

dent on the amount of PncCRM.[242] For the PncT vaccine, the opposite seems to be true: The response to polyribosylribitol phosphate conjugated with tetanus toxoid (Hib conjugate with tetanus protein carrier) and tetanus toxoid is lower among recipients of concurrent PncT than in those who did not receive PncT.[179] Furthermore, the effect seems to be dose-dependent: the higher the PncT dose, the lower the anti-Hib and antitetanus responses.[243,244]

There is only a limited amount of published data on how concurrent vaccinations with other childhood vaccines influence the response to pneumococcal conjugates, and the clinical relevance of these findings—if any—is not clear. When Shinefield et al. gave the primary series of PncCRM with or without hepatitis B vaccine, there was no significant effect on the anti–pneumococcal polysaccharide concentrations measured after the third dose.[245] In the same study, PncCRM booster was administered either with or without concurrent HbOC-DTaP vaccine. The responses to pneumococcal polysaccharides—as well as to Hib, diphtheria, and pertussis—tended to be lower in the group that had received HbOC-DTaP concurrently with the PncCRM vaccine.[245] In the study of Choo et al., PncCRM was given mixed or as a separate injection with HbOC simultaneously with diphtheria and tetanus toxoids and whole-cell pertussis (DTwP). The mean fold rises after the primary immunizations in the group receiving the vaccines separately tended to be higher than in the group receiving the PncCRM-HbOC vaccine mixture. In both groups, anamnestic responses were noted after the booster dose.[246]

OLDER CHILDREN AND ADULTS

To determine an appropriate schedule of the PncCRM vaccine for children 7 months of age or older at the time of the first immunization, 483 children in four studies received PncCRM at various schedules (Table 23–7). GMCs for most serotypes among older infants and children were

TABLE 23–6 ■ Antibody Responses Following Concurrent Administration of Prevnar with Other Vaccines

	Primary Series				Booster Dose			
	GMC[†]		% Responders[‡]		GMC[†]		% Responders[‡]	
Antigen*	Prevnar	Control[§]	Prevnar	Control[§]	Prevnar	Control[§]	Prevnar	Control[§]
Hib	6.2	4.4	99.5, 88.3	97.0, 88.1	22.7	47.9	100, 97.9	100,100
Diphtheria	0.9	0.8	100	97.0	2.0	3.2	100	100
Tetanus	3.5	4.1	100	100	14.4	18.8	100	100
Pertussis antigens								
PT	19.1	17.8	74.0	69.7	68.6	121.2	68.1	73.1
FHA	43.8	46.7	66.4	69.7	29.0	48.2	68.1	84.6
Pertactin	40.1	50.9	65.6	77.3	84.4	83.0	83.0	96.2
Fimbriae 2	3.3	4.2	44.7	62.5	5.2	3.8	63.8	50.0
Hepatitis B	—	—	99.4	96.2				
IPV type 1	—	—	89.0	93.6				
IPV type 2	—	—	94.2	93.6				
IPV type 3	—	—	83.8	80.8				

*HiB vaccine was HibTITER®, DTaP vaccine was ACEL-IMUNE®.
[†]Geometric mean concentration: Hib, µg/mL; diphtheria and tetanus toxoids, IU/mL; pertussis antigens, units/mL.
[‡]Positive response Hib, ≥0.15 µg/mL or greater; diphtheria and tetanus, 0.1 IU/mL or greater; pertussis antigens four-fold rise; IPV, 1:10 or higher; hepatitis B, 10 mIU/mL or greater.
[§]Concurrent vaccines only.
FHA, filamentous hemagglutinin; Hib, *H. influenzae* type b; IPV, inactivated poliovirus vaccine; PT, pertussis toxin.
Data from package insert (see Table 23-7).

comparable to immune responses of infants who received three doses of conjugate in the Kaiser Permanente efficacy study.[247] Based on these data, the recommendation is to use PncCRM at 2, 4, 6, and 12 to 15 months of age. For children 12 to 23 months of age, two doses are recommended at least 2 months apart, and for those above the age of 24 months through 9 years of age, one dose is sufficient.

To date there is no evidence that conjugate vaccines are more immunogenic than the PncPS vaccine in older adults, although only a few studies have addressed the issue. A 5-valent PncCRM vaccine (6B, 14, 18C, 19F, and 23F) elicited a larger response to serotype 6B than a polysaccharide vaccine in young adults, but did not increase the immunity to serotype 14.[248] In another study using the same vaccines, antibody responses for 6B, 18C, and 23F were higher with conjugate than the polysaccharide vaccine, but not for 14 and 19F.[183] When measured as functional activity, the conjugate was clearly superior to the PncPS vaccine, the increase in OPA titers to 6B being 3-fold after the PncPS vaccine but 59-fold after the conjugate vaccine.[249]

It is also controversial whether revaccination further enhances immune responses in adults. Although immunization with PncPS after previous immunization with conjugate vaccine can induce a modest increase in antibody concentration, the increase is only additive and not consistent with a priming effect.[248] The potential reasons for rather low responses may include that the dose of the polysaccharide or the interval after the primary vaccination was not optimal. Because adults have natural antibodies to pneumococcal polysaccharides and to the carrier protein, the initial vaccination with the conjugate vaccine already represents a booster vaccination.[249a]

IMMUNOCOMPROMISED INDIVIDUALS

Three small studies have been conducted to test the idea that children with recurrent infections have impairment in their responses to pneumococci, and that conjugate vaccine can enhance their protection. In 17 children who responded poorly to polysaccharide vaccine, there was a modest increase in their antibody concentrations in response to PncCRM vaccine.[250] In general, children with recurrent episodes of otitis media may have deficient IgG2 antibody responses to polysaccharide antigens, but, after conjugate priming, a group

of five such children responded to polysaccharide immunization with a brisk IgG2 antibody response.[159] A third study compared immune responses to polysaccharide and conjugate vaccines in otitis-free and otitis-prone children. Postimmunization GMCs were significantly higher for children receiving conjugate than for those receiving polysaccharide vaccine; the difference was primarily due to a better response to conjugate in the otitis-prone group.[95]

Both 5- and 7-valent PncCRM conjugate vaccines have been tested in HIV-positive individuals. Five-valent PncCRM conjugate vaccine elicited significantly higher antibody concentrations than did polysaccharide vaccine for serotypes 6B, 18C, and 23F in HIV-negative individuals, and both vaccines elicited similar GMCs in HIV-infected persons.[183] Although the responses after the first two vaccinations are rather modest in children with advanced HIV, the third dose overcame any difference.[251] Antibody concentrations after the primary series were higher than those seen previously in a similar population with the polysaccharide vaccine.[251] In HIV-positive children between the ages of 2 and 9 years, there was a trend toward higher antibody GMCs for serotypes 6B, 14, 18C, and 23F following 5-valent PncCRM conjugate vaccine as compared to the PncPS vaccine.[252] Because no consistent evidence of boosting was seen in response to the polysaccharide vaccine, more than one dose of conjugate vaccine may be needed to prime for immunologic memory in children with HIV infection. HIV-positive adults with a CD4 cell count of less than 200/μL had only a modest response to vaccination with a 4-valent PncOMPC vaccine as well as to a second dose 1 month later.[253] In contrast, HIV-positive individuals with a CD4 cell count of 200/μL or greater had a significant increase in antibodies, which was further strengthened through a PncPS booster.[253] In another study in a similar patient population, conjugate priming seemed to be clearly beneficial as compared with the PncPS vaccine.[253a]

In infants with sickle cell disease, a three-dose primary series of 7-valent PncCRM vaccine, given at 2, 4, and 6 months, or a single dose given at 12 months induced significant increases in serum antibody concentration for all serotypes.[122] In children 2 years of age or older with sickle cell disease, two doses of 7-valent conjugate vaccine, given 8 weeks apart, followed by a polysaccharide booster 8 weeks

TABLE 23-7 ■ Geometric Mean Concentration (GMC; μg/mL) of Pneumococcal Antibodies Following Immunization of Children from 7 Months Through 9 Years of Age with PncCRM

Age Group	No. of Doses	Number of Children	GMC per Serotype						
			4	6B	9V	14	18C	19F	23F
7–11 mo	3	22	2.34	3.66	2.11	9.33	2.31	1.60	2.50
		39	3.60	4.63	2.04	5.48	1.98	2.15	1.93
12–17 mo	2	82–84	3.91	4.67	1.94	6.92	2.25	3.78	3.29
		33	7.02	4.25	3.26	6.31	3.60	3.29	2.92
18–23 mo	2	52–54	3.36	4.92	1.80	6.69	2.65	3.17	2.71
		45	6.85	3.71	3.86	6.48	3.42	3.86	2.75
24–35 mo	1	53	5.34	2.90	3.43	1.88	3.03	4.07	1.56
36–59 mo	1	52	6.27	6.40	4.62	5.95	4.08	6.37	2.95
5–9 yr	1	101	6.92	20.84	7.49	19.32	6.72	12.51	11.57

From Prevnar™; Pneumococcal 7-Valent Conjugate Vaccine (Diphtheria CRM$_{197}$ Protein) [package insert]. Pearl River, NY, Lederle Laboratories, 2000

later resulted in higher GMCs than polysaccharide vaccine alone.[118] Functional activity of antibodies, as measured by OPA, was higher in the group of sickle cell patients receiving two doses of conjugate and one dose of polysaccharide than in a group receiving the polysaccharide alone.[118]

The immune response of patients with treated Hodgkin's disease to PncOMPC vaccine has been tested in two studies. Although the response to a single dose of 7-valent vaccine PncOMPC is lower than to a polysaccharide vaccine,[126] one dose of conjugate is able to induce immunologic priming even in this patient group.[254] There is currently no direct evidence that a pneumococcal conjugate vaccine would be beneficial in bone marrow transplant patients, but experience with Hib conjugates suggest that this might be expected.[15,17,124]

MUCOSAL IMMUNE RESPONSE

Parenterally administered pneumococcal vaccines, both polysaccharides and conjugates, are able to induce mucosal antibody responses. Serotype-specific salivary antibodies are found rarely after the primary immunizations (IgG in 0% to 3% and IgA in 3% to 33% of children, depending on the serotype), but more frequently (IgG in 4% to 60% and IgA in 12% to 80%) after the booster either with the conjugate or with polysaccharide vaccine.[235] Similar results have been reported with the PncT and PncD vaccines.[255] The question about induction of mucosal memory is still open. Even though only the IgA mean concentrations for serotype 14 in saliva were higher in vaccinees than in the nonvaccinated control group in a United Kingdom study, there was a significant increase to mucosal antibodies after the booster dose of polysaccharide at 13 months, leading the authors to suggest that conjugate had primed children for memory responses.[256] However, another study found no clear differences in salivary antibody responses between children primed with conjugate and those who received their first pneumococcal vaccine during the second year of life.[255] The IgG detected in saliva is suggested to be derived from serum, with high serum IgG concentrations potentially leading to leakage of the antibodies into mucosal secretions. Serum and salivary IgG concentrations indeed correlate strongly, in accordance with this concept.

A high number of IgA ASCs detected with ELISPOT is considered to be an indicator of the mucosal IgA response after parenteral pneumococcal vaccination. The ASC response to parenteral protein vaccines is generally dominated by IgG-producing cells,[201,257] whereas that to polysaccharide antigens is dominated by IgA-producing cells.[202,258,259] The IgA:IgG ratio of the ASC response to a polysaccharide that is conjugated to a protein carrier is altered towards a pattern typical of TD antigen.[198,259] For the PncPS vaccine, the response is dominated by the IgA ASCs,[200] but after the conjugate the IgG ASC responses are higher.[199,260] The ASC responses to the PncT and PncD vaccines in toddlers were lower than those seen in adults after administration with conjugate vaccine, but comparable to those in adults after PncPS vaccine. In toddlers, the ASC response was clearly dominated by IgA-secreting cells.[200]

ANTIBODY SUBCLASSES, AVIDITY, AND OPSONOPHAGOCYTIC ACTIVITY

The IgG antibody response in infants is mainly of the subclass IgG1. After the booster in the second year of life, IgG2 also starts to appear, and the response in adults to both pneumococcal polysaccharide and conjugate vaccines is mainly of the IgG2 subclass.[219,226,234,236,261,262] The response to protein antigens is different; it consists mainly of the IgG1 subclass, both in adults and in children. In adults, some differences have been found in the IgG1:IgG2 ratio after vaccination with pneumococcal polysaccharide versus conjugate vaccines or between different conjugate vaccines.[219,226,262,263] However, the relevance of these findings for estimating the T-cell dependence of the response in infants to the same vaccines and the functional activity of antibodies remains to be elucidated.

Notable increases in OPA are induced by pneumococcal polysaccharide and conjugate vaccines (Table 23–8). In adults the increases were 59-fold in the conjugate vaccine groups versus 2.6-fold in the polysaccharide vaccine group. Infants immunized with a conjugate vaccine demonstrate increased opsonic activities comparable with those of adults immunized with polysaccharide vaccine.

The avidity of the antibodies seems to differ after different conjugates, at least when serotype 6B antibodies were studied. PncT and PncCRM induce high avidity, which increases from postprimary samples taken at 7 months to prebooster samples at 14 months, and boosting with conjugate but not with the polysaccharide vaccine further increases the avidity.[204] This may be because the conjugate booster promotes affinity maturation by the TD mechanisms or because the amount of the antigen in the polysaccharide vaccine is high enough to induce both low- and

TABLE 23–8 ■ Geometric Mean Concentrations (GMC; μg/mL), Mean Avidities, and Opsonophagocytic Activity (OPA) of Antibodies to Pneumococcal Serotype 6B

	Adults*		Children†		
	Pre	Post	7 mo	15 mo	16 mo
GMC	1.35	9.93	1.72	0.60	17.4
Avidity index	53.4	60.3	337.6	55.1	61.9
OPA	13.9	461.8	37.2	6.20	892.4

*Values for pre- and postvaccination sera.
†Values obtained after primary immunization series (7 months), before booster (15 months), and after booster (16 months).
From Anttila M, Voutilainen M, Jantti V, et al: Contribution of serotype-specific IgG concentration, IgG subclasses and relative antibody avidity to opsonophagocytic activity against *Streptococcus pneumoniae*. Clin Exp Immunol 118:402–407, 1999, with permission.

high-avidity B cell clones to produce antibodies, whereas only clones with high avidity are induced by the lower concentrations of PS in the conjugate vaccines. A study performed recently with an 11-valent vaccine prepared by Aventis Pasteur demonstrated increasing avidity for most serotypes after primary vaccination, and higher avidity after the booster. Most of the antibodies produced were of the IgG1 subclass.[263a]

When the contribution of total IgG concentration, IgG2:IgG1 ratio, and relative antibody avidity to OPA was evaluated, only the total antibody level had a significant positive correlation with opsonophagocytosis.[226] Although no direct contribution of avidity to opsonophagocytic activity has been found, a negative correlation between the concentration needed for killing and avidity suggests that fewer antibodies of high rather than of low avidity are required for killing of bacteria. The negative effect of IgG2:IgG1 ratio on OPA seen in adults suggests that IgG1 may act more efficiently as an opsonin than does IgG2.[226] It remains to be determined from the efficacy trial data which of the above-mentioned analyses (total antibody concentration, OPA, avidity, subclass distribution), either alone or in any of the potential combinations, is the most reliable laboratory surrogate for protection.

Variables Influencing Immunogenicity of Conjugate Vaccines

Several factors affect the magnitude of the antibody response. In addition to the composition of the vaccine, these include the number of vaccine doses, the vaccination schedule, and possible interference with simultaneously administered vaccines. Clear-cut differences exist in the antibody responses to different capsular-type polysaccharides in the conjugate vaccines. Polysaccharide-based PncCRM vaccines (bi-, penta-, or heptavalent) have been shown to be immunogenic in infants, whereas the antibody responses to the corresponding oligosaccharide formulations have remained relatively modest.[234,242,264,265] Inclusion of additional serotypes does not seem to significantly affect the immunogenicity of each individual conjugated polysaccharide.[266] Serotypes 6B and 23F appear to be poor immunogens in spite of conjugation, whereas serotype 19F induces a relatively high antibody concentration. Serotypes such as 3 and 18C are usually satisfactory immunogens even after the first dose. A significant increase in anti-6B IgG can be seen only after the third dose. For serotype 4, there is already a marked response after the first dose, and a further increase after the second dose, but not after the third dose. Serotype 19F induces an antibody response after the second dose, and the third dose does not increase the mean antibody concentrations.

The immunogenicity of conjugates is dependent on chemical characteristics, polysaccharide:protein ratio, and length of the carbohydrate molecules.[56,150,267,268] In pneumococcal conjugates, polysaccharides seem to be more immunogenic than oligosaccharides.[234,242,269] Other variables influencing immunogenicity include inherent properties of carrier proteins, the nature of chemical linkage[270] sites of carbohydrate attachment to protein carriers,[140,270] conformational changes in epitopes after conjugation,[56] availability of antigenic structural components,[150,242] presence of free polysaccharides or carrier proteins in the vaccine,[178,244] and the carbohydrate:protein ratio.[271]

The optimal carrier may be different for each serotype. Thus far, direct comparisons have been made only between diphtheria and tetanus carriers. Polysaccharides from serotypes 3, 9V, and 14 evoke a better response in infants when conjugated to diphtheria toxoid, and polysaccharides from serotype 4 evoke a better response when conjugated to tetanus protein.[272,273] No carrier-specific differences in immunogenicity have been shown for serotypes 6B, 18C, 19F, and 23F. Furthermore, different vaccines seem to have different capacities to induce a mucosal immune response: Whereas diphtheria toxoid conjugates induce a better mucosal response, tetanus conjugates seem more efficient in inducing systemic responses.[198]

Immunity to carrier proteins is beneficial for the improved immunogenicity of conjugate vaccines. Early priming with carrier proteins enhances the immune response to polysaccharides in subsequent immunizations with conjugates.[244,274–276] Although this T-cell immunity against carrier proteins is essential for responses to polysaccharides, B-cell immunity to carrier protein may become detrimental on induction of anti-carrier antibodies.[277] In a situation where polysaccharide- and protein-specific B cells compete to capture conjugates, high amounts of antibodies to carrier proteins may result in a suppressed immune response to polysaccharides.[178,179,244,274,278] This argues for minimizing the amount of antigen and implementing mixed carrier vaccines.

Correlates of Protection

To avoid the expensive and time-consuming efficacy trials for new pneumococcal vaccines, it would be extremely valuable to be able to predict the vaccine efficacy on the basis of serologic studies. In addition to huge resource needs, efficacy trials with new conjugates also are becoming difficult from an ethical viewpoint when a conjugate vaccine is already available for the population. Different means used to predict protective efficacy include concentration of serum IgG antibodies, distribution of IgG1/IgG2 subclasses,[191] IgG avidity,[212,243] IgG OPA,[218,220,225] and animal models for pneumococcal infections.[279,280]

Determination of serologic correlates or surrogates of protection against pneumococcal diseases has proved complicated. First, even if the level of specific antibody were considered an adequate surrogate,[281] it may vary between serotypes and the disease in question. Second, the quantitative assessment of immune response alone may be insufficient, and measurement of the qualitative characteristics of antibodies also should be included in the analyses.[282] Finally, induction of immunologic memory has to be taken into consideration,[170,171,212,213,282,283] because, even after a low antibody response, immunologic memory can be induced.

Traditionally, methods for assessing the association between the immunogenicity and the disease have relied on comparisons of aggregate measures such as vaccine efficacy and GMC of antibodies. The relationship at the aggregate level does not, however, necessarily represent the underlying individual-level relationship. Correlates of protection can be sought in populations by comparing cross-sectional information on antibody concentrations and estimates of protection in the same group of subjects as well as on the individual level by investigating longitudinal follow-up data on children who contract pneumococcal infection in spite of vaccination.

ANIMAL MODELS

In addition to in vitro assays, many laboratories have developed animal models to study the immunogenicity and efficacy of pneumococcal conjugate vaccines using mice, rats, chinchillas, or infant monkeys.[41,180,266,284-288] In the immunogenicity studies, animals are actively immunized with the experimental vaccine and then bled before and after vaccination, to obtain sera for in vitro analyses.[180,285,287,288] The protection models are usually based on active immunization. The animals are subsequently challenged with the infecting bacteria.[42,266,279,286] The route of the challenge varies depending on the required outcome (carriage, acute otitis media [AOM], bacteremia, pneumonia). Adult and infant mice as well as rats have been used in these models to determine the protective capacity of human anti–pneumococcal polysaccharide antibodies against colonization, different types of pneumococcal infections (bacteremia, meningitis), or death.[224,229,289-295]

SEROLOGIC CORRELATES

In February 2001, a workshop sponsored by the Center for Biologics Evaluation and Research and the National Institute of Allergy and Infectious Diseases was convened to discuss correlates of immunity for pneumococcal conjugate vaccines. National control authorities expect information on both the seven serotypes in the current vaccine as well as the new ones. The current view seems to be that noninferiority immunogenicity trials comparing a vaccine with the licensed one should be sufficient for inferring efficacy against invasive pneumococcal disease. The main conclusions from this workshop are summarized in Table 23–9.

Experience from the Hib conjugate vaccines licensure is of interest in this regard. The FDA approved three Hib conjugates for licensure. The first two were licensed in 1990 based on clinical efficacy data. The third Hib conjugate vaccine was licensed without a direct efficacy demonstration. However, the manufacturer was able to demonstrate comparative immunogenicity with the licensed vaccines, good persistence of antibodies, induction of the immunologic memory, and the functional activity of the antibodies.

The data from both the Kaiser Permanente invasive infection efficacy trial and the Finnish AOM efficacy trial have been analyzed. Based on the data from the Kaiser Permanente efficacy trial,[30] Siber et al. proposed using one threshold level of 0.20 μg/ml for all serotypes.[23] The arguments for their proposal were

1. An antibody level of 0.20 μg/mL or greater corresponds to the threshold of opsonic antibody of 1/8, and this threshold appears to predict the age-specific disease rates.
2. This threshold is consistent with data from passive immunization studies, and appears to discriminate between conjugate vaccinees and controls in immunogenicity studies.
3. Infants with antibody levels of 0.20 μg/mL or greater after conjugate vaccine show evidence for priming for the capsular polysaccharide, and antibody response after dose 3 correlates with the magnitude of the booster response.

Analysis of data from the Finnish AOM trials,[227] however, showed no correlation between the post–dose 3 antibody GMC and efficacy against AOM. This was true for both the PncOMPC and PncCRM vaccines. Preliminary results suggest that association between the antibody concentration and the risk of AOM differs between the pneumococcal serotypes.[227] The Finnish group used generalized linear modeling to study the association between the antibody concentrations to serotypes 6B, 19F, and 23F and the risk of AOM caused by the homologous serotypes in the 5 months following immunizations. Association was most clear-cut for serotype 23F, and poorest for serotype 19F. Even low concentrations (GMC 0.5 μg/mL) predicted vaccine efficacy of 50% for 6B, while a GMC of 2 μg/mL was required for the same efficacy for 23F. For 19F, results suggested that, in order to achieve protective efficacy, much higher concentrations (GMC >10 μg/mL) might be required. Thus these results indicate a very different behavior of serotypes, discouraging the setting of a unique serologic correlate of protection for all serotypes. Therefore, the Finnish group suggested that GMC may not be an appropriate measure to predict protection against otitis. Even if it were to be used, serotype-specific criteria need to be established.[227]

Finding reliable predictors for protection may prove to be even more complicated. Experience with Hib conjugate vaccines has taught us that antibody levels cited as correlates long-term of protection and developed following the study of polysaccharide vaccines or passive immunization studies failed to accurately predict the subsequent success of Hib conjugates.[171] This failure was likely due to the fact that conjugate vaccines not only induce antibodies, but also prime the immune system for later, protective memory

TABLE 23–9 ■ Conclusions from February 2001 Meeting on Correlates of Immunity to Pneumococcal Conjugate Vaccines

1. Antibody concentration is important for short-term protection, and induction of memory will be important for long-term protection.
2. Animal data support opsonophagocytic assay as the functional assay that could be used as surrogate of protection, although antibody avidity may contribute to protection.
3. Both geometric mean concentration of antibodies and percent responders are important parameters in comparison of vaccines.
4. One should focus on a "threshold" level, for percent responders, rather than on a "protective" level.
5. Direct comparisons of vaccines in randomized trials will reduce the effects of assay variability.

responses. It may be, therefore, that pneumococcal antibody levels alone do not adequately predict protection from infection. If induction of memory or quality of antibodies is important for the protection, antibody concentrations referred to above may set the bar too high. Furthermore, different levels of antibodies, or indeed memory, may be required to prevent invasive rather than mucosal pneumococcal infections.[213] It may also be that, for prevention of mucosal infection, local immunity may be needed, or that only local immunity is sufficient.

Efficacy and Effectiveness of the Vaccine

Invasive Disease

In a double-blind study conducted at 23 Northern California Kaiser Permanente (NCKP) medical centers, 37,868 infants were randomized to receive either the pneumococcal conjugate vaccine or a meningococcus group C conjugate vaccine as a control.[247] Study vaccine was given at 2, 4, 6, and 12 to 15 months of age, along with other routine childhood vaccines. Children with sickle cell disease, known immunodeficiency, any serious chronic or progressive disease, a history or seizures, or a history of pneumococcal or meningococcal disease were excluded from the study.

The primary outcome measure was the incidence of invasive pneumococcal disease caused by vaccine serotypes. Secondary outcome measures included the incidence of otitis media and pneumonia, which are addressed later in this section. To be included in the main efficacy analysis, invasive disease must have been caused by a vaccine serotype, occurred more than 14 days after the third dose of the vaccine, and occurred in a subject vaccinated according to protocol. Children less than 16 months old were considered to be fully vaccinated if they had received three or more doses of vaccine; children 16 months old or older were considered to be fully vaccinated after receipt of a fourth dose. In addition to the per-protocol analysis, an intent-to-treat (ITT) analysis was performed that included all invasive disease caused by any pneumococcal serotype occurring after randomization regardless of vaccination status.

In the per-protocol analysis, 40 cases of invasive pneumococcal diseases were seen in the study population (Table 23–10). Of these, 39 were in the control group. This represents a vaccine efficacy of 97% (95% confidence interval [CI]: 82% to 100%; P < 0.0001). The one vaccine failure was a child who had received four doses of

vaccine, yet developed bacteremic pneumonia caused by serotype 19F.

In the ITT analysis, there were 52 cases of vaccine-serotype invasive pneumococcal diseases, three of which were in vaccinated children, representing a vaccine efficacy of 94%. The three failures included the one described above, a case of 19F disease in a child who developed leukemia after vaccination and was receiving immunosuppressive chemotherapy, and a partially vaccinated child who developed a 6B infection 317 days after a single dose of vaccine. Point estimates of serotype-specific efficacy were able to be determined for four vaccine serotypes, and ranged from 85% for serotype 19F to 100% for serotypes 14, 18C, and 23F.

There was no evidence of an increased risk of disease caused by nonvaccine serotypes. Nine cases of invasive pneumococcal diseases caused by nonserotype pneumococci occurred during the study, six in the control group and three in vaccinated children. Only one case was caused by a potentially cross-reactive serotype in a vaccinated child. Overall, in an ITT analysis including disease caused by both vaccine and nonvaccine serotypes, an 89.1% reduction was seen in the burden of invasive pneumococcal diseases in children who had received at least one dose of conjugate vaccine.

Efficacy of the 7-valent conjugate vaccine also was analyzed separately for the low-birth-weight and preterm infants who had been included in the NCKP study.[296] Although the study protocol required that patients be vaccinated at outpatient clinics, healthy low-birth-weight and preterm infants were eligible for this evaluation once they were discharged from the hospital. No difference in mean age of administration of vaccine resulted for low-birth-weight and preterm infants compared with normal-birth-weight and full-term infants. For low-birth-weight infants who received the control vaccine, the relative risk of invasive pneumococcal diseases was 2.6 compared with normal-birth-weight infants, and for preterm infants the relative risk was 1.6 compared with full-term infants. However, no low-birth- weight or preterm recipient of pneumococcal vaccine contracted an invasive pneumococcal disease, as compared with six low-birth-weight infants and nine preterm controls who received the meningococcal vaccine; the pneumococcal vaccine was therefore 100% efficacious for both groups.

A postlicensure follow-up study was conducted after the vaccine was approved for use in infants in February 2000. In April 2000, the vaccine was introduced into the general

TABLE 23–10 ■ Invasive Disease Efficacy Results as of April 20, 1999, in Kaiser Permanente Efficacy Trial

	Number of Episodes		Vaccine Efficacy %	
	PncOMPC	Control Group	Point Estimate	95% CI
Per-protocol fully vaccinated	39	1	97.4	82.7–99.9
Intent to treat	49	3	93.9	79.6–98.5
Partially vaccinated only	7	1	85.7	0–100
All cases	55	6	89.1	73.7–95.8

CI, confidence interval.
Data from Black S, Shinefield H, Fireman B, et al. Efficacy, safety and immunogenicity of heptavalent pneumococcal conjugate vaccine in children. Pediatr Infect Dis J 19:187–195, 2000, with permission.

Kaiser Permanente population and began to be used routinely. Between April 2000 and March 2001, of the more than 200,000 children in the Kaiser Permanente system less than 5 years of age, 44,946 children received 152,041 doses of the conjugate vaccine. Age-specific disease incidence during the year following vaccine licensure was compared with age-specific disease within the Kaiser Permanente population during the 5 years before vaccine licensure (Table 23–11). In children less than 1 year of age, an 87% reduction was seen in invasive pneumococcal diseases caused by vaccine serotypes. In children less than 2 years of age, the reduction was 58%, and in children less than 5 years of age, the reduction was 62%. There was no corresponding increase in disease caused by nonvaccine serotypes. In fact, the magnitude of the reduction in disease was substantially greater than both the percentage of children who had received at least one dose of the vaccine and the percentage of fully vaccinated children, suggesting the vaccine may provide some degree of herd immunity.

Preliminary results have been published from another invasive infection efficacy trial.[297] This community-randomized, controlled efficacy trial of PncCRM[298] was conducted between April 1997 and October 2000 among Navajo and White Mountain Apache children, who have some of the highest rates of invasive pneumococcal disease in the world. Meningococcal vaccine was used as a control. A per-protocol analysis was performed of the 5792 children under 2 years old who were enrolled in the primary efficacy portion of the study. Eight cases of vaccine-serotype invasive disease occurred in the control group, as compared to two in the PncCRM group, yielding an efficacy of 76.8% (95% CI: 9.4% to 95.1%).[297] In an ITT analysis, 14 cases of vaccine-serotype disease occurred in the control group, as compared to 2 cases in the PncCRM group, for an efficacy of 86.4% (95% CI: 40.3% to 96.9%).[297] These efficacy estimates demonstrate that, even in the context of the intense bacterial transmission that occurs in this high-risk population, the vaccine is highly efficacious.

Pneumonia

The data from the NCKP trial also were analyzed for the efficacy of the conjugate vaccine in the prevention of pneumonia.[299] Cases of pneumonia were identified by the presence in the NCKP database of a diagnosis of pneumonia by the treating physician in the outpatient, emergency room, or hospital setting in which the patient was seen. Diagnoses of "bronchopneumonia" and "viral pneumonia" also were included. Per-protocol analyses began 14 days after the completion of the primary series of vaccinations, whereas ITT analyses began at randomization.

The cases of pneumonia were divided into four categories, which also represent the four outcome measures of the study: (1) all cases; (2) those in which a chest radiograph was obtained; (3) those in which a chest radiograph showed only perihilar findings; and (4) those in which a chest radiograph was positive for infiltrates beyond the perihilar area, or for consolidation or empyema ("positive film"). An a priori hypothesis was that positive films were more likely to be indicative of pneumococcal infection than negative or perihilar films.

In the control group, the incidence of a first episode of pneumonia was 45.8 per 1000 person-years. Of these cases, a radiograph was obtained in 28.9 per 1000 person-years, a radiograph with perihilar findings in 3.4, and a positive film in 10.1. The conjugate vaccine significantly reduced the number of episodes of pneumonia in which there was a positive film, to 8.3 per 1000 person-years, for an estimated efficacy of 17.7% (95% CI: 4.8 to 28.9; $P = 0.01$). When stratified by age, the vaccine had a significant effect for children less than 12 or less than 24 months of age with positive films. The vaccine also significantly reduced all clinical pneumonia for children less than 24 months of age. This shows the efficacy of the vaccine against pneumonia in children less than 2 years of age, and supports the initial hypothesis that positive films are more likely to be indicative of pneumococcal disease than films with other findings. The effect of race and ethnicity on the risk of pneumonia was examined in the subset of control subjects for whom information about race or ethnicity was available. Asians, blacks, and Hispanics all were found to be at a greater risk of pneumonia than whites. Asians and Hispanics also were more likely to have a positive film than whites. However, there was no evidence that the vaccine was more or less effective in these groups.

Acute Otitis Media

Streptococcus pneumoniae is the most commonly reported bacterial cause of AOM. Statistics from the United States

TABLE 23–11 ▪ Postlicensure Efficacy of the 7-Valent PncCRM Vaccine Against Vaccine Serotypes in the Year Following Licensure Versus Disease Incidence Prior to Licensure in the Kaiser Permanente Population

| | Incidence per 100,000 Person-Years | | % Partially or Fully Vaccinated (April 2000–March 2001) | | |
| | April 1996–March 2000 (95% CI) | April 2000– March 2001 | Partially | Fully | % Reduction in |
Age (yr)					Invasive Disease
<1	73.75 (51.52–98.15)	9.35	57.8	16.2	87.3
<2	91.31 (81.67–113.80)	38.22	52.6	14.1	58.1
<5	47.58 (42.21–59.59)	17.89	34.3	13.6	62.4

CI, confidence interval.
From Black SB, Shinefield H, Fireman B, et al. Efficacy against pneumonia of heptavalent conjugate pneumococcal vaccine (Wyeth Lederle) in 37,868 infants and children: expanded data analysis including duration of protection. *In* Abstracts of the 3rd International Symposium on Pneumococci and Pneumococcal Diseases, Anchorage, May 5–8, 2002.

suggest that there are about 20 million office visits annually as a result of AOM, and costs caused by otitis are estimated to be between $2 and $3.8 million US per year.[299a,299b] The proportion of pneumococcus as an etiologic agent recovered from MEF has varied from 18% to 55% in published materials. By choosing 7 to 11 common serotypes, one could cover 71% to 95% of pneumococcal otitis. Thus a vaccine providing full protection against all serotypes would prevent in theory 12% to 52% of all cases of AOM. The reality seems, however, to be ruder.

The Finnish Otitis Media Vaccine Trial was a prospective, randomized, double-blind study conducted from 1995 to 1999, designed to evaluate the efficacy of the PncCRM and PncOMPC 7-valent pneumococcal vaccines against AOM in Finnish infants and children between the ages of 2 months and 24 months.[300,301] Both vaccines contained pneumococcal serotypes 4, 6B, 9V, 14, 18C, 19F, and 23F, and were used in parallel and compared with the same control vaccine (hepatitis B).

A total of 2497 children were enrolled at the age of 2 months and randomized to receive either the PncCRM (n = 831) or PncOMPC (n = 835) vaccine or a control vaccine (n = 831) at 2, 4, 6, and 12 months of age, and were followed up to 24 months of age. Whenever AOM was diagnosed, myringotomy was performed and MEF aspirated for identification of bacteria. During the follow-up from 6.5 to 24 months of age, the overall incidence of AOM was 1.16 episodes per person-year in the PncCRM group, 1.25 in the PncOMPC group, and 1.24 in the control group. Of the AOM episodes attributed to vaccine serotypes, 107 occurred in the PncCRM-vaccinated children and 110 in the PncOMPC-vaccinated children. In the control group, there were 250 such episodes. Based on these figures, the efficacy of the PncCRM vaccine against serotype-specific AOM was 57% (95% CI: 44% to 67%), and that of the PncOMPC vaccine 56% (95% CI: 44% to 66%). The serotype-specific efficacies ranged from 25% to 84% (Table 23–12). AOM episodes caused by serotypes potentially cross-reactive with the vaccine serotypes were reduced by 51% in the PncCRM. The rate of AOM episodes caused by all other serotypes was 3390 higher among the recipients of both the PncCRM than in the control group. This finding suggests that pneumococcal conjugate vaccines that reduce carriage of vaccine serotypes may leave open an ecologic niche easily filled by serotypes not included in the vaccine.

In the NCKP efficacy trial,[247] the investigators were able to look at the impact of vaccinations on other clinical entities than invasive infections by using the computerized database of their health maintenance organization. Vaccine recipients had 9% fewer visits resulting from otitis media, had 7% fewer new episodes of AOM, were 20% less likely to require tympanostomy tubes, and were 23% less likely to have recurrent otitis during the period from after the first dose of vaccine to the end of the 3-year trial.

Pneumococcal Carriage

Three Israeli studies have established that conjugate vaccines are effective in reducing nasopharyngeal carriage of vaccine serotypes.[302–304] In the first, open study,[302] one and two doses of a 7-valent PncOMPC vaccine were compared with a single dose of PncPS vaccine in children 12, 15, or 18 months of age. One month after a single dose of vaccine, no change was seen from prevaccination levels in PncOMPC vaccine and PncPS vaccine groups, nor was there any difference between the groups in carriage of vaccine serotypes. By contrast, the group receiving two doses of PncOMPC had a significant reduction in carriage 3 months after the first dose of vaccine (just before receiving a second dose), and carriage was reduced further after the second dose. One year after the initial vaccination, there was still no difference in carriage in the group that had received PncPS vaccine, but the two conjugate vaccine groups had significantly lower rates of vaccine serotype carriage. However, carriage of nonvaccine serotypes increased from 15% to 20% prior to immunization to 32% to 39% one year later.

The second study was a double-blind, placebo-controlled study in infants.[303] PncD and PncT conjugate vaccines were used. Each infant was immunized with conjugate vaccine at 2, 4, and 6 months of age, followed by a PncPS vaccine booster at 12 months. Carriage was low at 2 months but increased with age. For vaccine serotypes, however, there was no overall increase in carriage over time in vaccinated infants, whereas carriage increased from less than 10% to approximately 30% in the placebo group.

Most recently, the Israeli group conducted a study in toddlers attending day care centers to test the efficacy of a 9-valent PncCRM on nasopharyngeal carriage of *S. pneumoniae* in general, and antibiotic-resistant *S. pneumoniae* in particular.[304] In this study, 264 toddlers ages 12 to 35 months were enrolled in eight day care centers in Beer-Shiva, Israel. They received either PncCRM or meningococcal C conjugate vaccine in a randomized, double-blind fashion. Subjects ages 12 to 17 months received two doses 2 to 3 months apart, and all others received a single dose. The children were followed every month during the first year after the completion of vaccination, and every 2 to 3 months for the second year. At each visit, a nasopharyngeal culture was obtained, along with a history of any disease or antibiotic use. For all age groups, the rate of carriage was lower among subjects who had received PcnCRM than among controls, with the greatest effect (68%) in the 15- to 23-month age group. Single-serotype reductions were seen for four serotypes, with 6B having the maximal reduction. Even if vaccine-type pneumococci were acquired, the density of carriage often was lower in vaccinated children.[305] In addition, carriage of serotype 6A was reduced, although the vaccine contained only the 6B antigen. Carriage of nonvaccine serotypes, with the exception of 6A, increased in vaccinated children in all age groups, as compared to controls.[305] The reduction in the carriage of antibiotic-resistant *S. pneumoniae* was most prominent in the age group that had the most disease and antibiotic use, 15 to 35 months.

TABLE 23–12 ■ Episodes of Acute Otitis Media (AOM) from Various Causes and Estimates of Protective Efficacy of PncOMPC and PncCRM Vaccines During Per-Protocol Follow-Up of the Finnish Otitis Media Efficacy Trial

| | Number of Episodes | | | Vaccine Efficacy (%) | | | |
| | | | | PncOMPC | | PncCRM | |
Cause of AOM	PncOMPC Group	Control Group	PncCRM Group	Point Estimate	95% CI	Point Estimate	95% CI
VACCINE SEROTYPES							
All 7 combined	110	250	107	56	44 to 66	57	44 to 67
4	1	4	2	75	−122 to 97	49	−176 to 91
6B	12	56	9	79	58 to 89	84	62 to 93
9V	2	11	5	82	12 to 96	54	−48 to 86
14	11	26	8	58	10 to 80	69	20 to 88
18C	8	17	7	53	−28 to 83	58	−4 to 83
19F	37	58	43	37	1 to 59	25	−14 to 51
23F	40	82	33	52	28 to 68	59	35 to 75
CROSS-REACTIVE SEROTYPES							
All combined		84	41			51	27 to 67
6A		45	19			57	24 to 76
9N		8	2			75	−24 to 95
18B		1	2			−103	−213 to 82
19A		26	17			34	−26 to 65
23A		4	1			75	−151 to 97
OTHER PNEUMOCOCCAL SEROTYPES							
All combined		95	125			−33	−80 to 1
3		13	13				
10		5	32				
11		24	24				
15		23	5				
22		7	7				
33		0	6				
35		10	14				
38		3	7				
Rough		2	6				
Other		11	11				
OTHER CAUSES							
Any type of S. pneumoniae	314	414	271	25	11 to 37	34	21 to 45
Haemophilus influenzae		287	315			−11	−34 to 8
Moraxella catarrhalis		381	379			−1	−19 to 15
Any confirmed by presence of middle ear fluid	1279	1267	1177	0	−12 to 10	7	−5 to 17
Any	1364	1345	1251	−1	−12 to 10	6	−4 to 16

CI, confidence interval.

Data from Eskola J, Kilpi T, Palmu A et al. Efficacy of a pneumococcal conjugate vaccine against acute otitis media. N Engl J Med 344: 403–409, 2001, and Kilpi T, Palmu A, Leinomen M, et al. Efficacy of a Seven-Valent penumococcal conjugate vaccine (PncOMPC) against Serotyp-specific acute otitis media (AOM) caused by streptococcus pneumoniae (Pnc). In Abstracts of the 40th ICAAC, Toronto, September, 2002.

The efficacy of a 9-valent PncCRM vaccine against nasopharyngeal carriage was evaluated in a placebo-controlled study of South African infants.[241] The infants were vaccinated at 6, 10, and 14 weeks of age, because nasopharyngeal carriage occurs at a very young age in South Africa. Overall carriage rates increased with age for both groups, rising from 26% and 30% at 6 weeks in controls and vaccinees, respectively, to 61% and 54% at 9 months. The minimum length of carriage was estimated to be 1.4 months. At 9 months, carriage rates of vaccine serotypes were lower in vaccinees (18%) than in controls (36%), but carriage of nonvaccine serotypes was higher in vaccinees (36%) than in controls (25%). As was also seen in the Israeli studies, carriage was not reduced 1 month after vaccination, suggesting that the vaccine does not eliminate strains already present in the nasopharynx. Although nonvaccine serotypes were found to have increased following vaccination, it is unclear whether these were in fact acquired after vaccination, or whether these serotypes were subdominant clones that were not detected in culture in the presence of the more common vaccine-type pneumococci.

TABLE 23–13 ■ Percent of children with Adverse Reactions in Recipients of the PncCRM Conjugate and Control (Hepatis B) Vaccines Within 3 Days After Immunization in the Finnish Otitis Media Efficacy Trial

Reaction	Dose 1 (at 2 mo)*			Dose 2 (at 4 mo)*		
	PncCRM (N = 831)	Control Vaccine (N = 831)	P Value	PncCRM (N = 827)	Control Vaccine (N = 829)	P Value
Pain (any)	3	2	0.091	4	2	0.020
Redness						
Any	14	9	0.004	16	13	0.060
>2.5 cm	0	0.1	1	0.2	0.4	0.993
Swelling						
Any	6	2	<0.001	5	3	0.162
>2.5 cm	1.1	0.2	0.07	1.0	0.4	0.221
Fever (temperature >39.0°C)	0.4	0.2	1	1.0	0.5	0.380
Crying (more than usual)	42	37	0.029	42	33	<0.001

Data from Eskola J, Kilpi T, Palmu A, et al. Efficacy of a pneumococcal conjugate vaccine against acute otitis media. N Engl J Med 344:403–409, 2001.
*Concomitant vaccine: DTwP-Hib
†Concomitant vaccine: Inactivated Polio Vaccine

Herd Immunity

The ability of pneumococcal conjugate vaccines to reduce nasopharyngeal carriage of the vaccine serotypes[302,303] potentially extends the benefits beyond those children who are vaccinated. Dagan et al. have shown that the younger siblings of children attending day care are at increased risk of carriage, but vaccination of children in day care also reduces the nasopharyngeal carriage in their younger siblings.[29]

Postlicensure evaluation of the efficacy of the PncCRM vaccine[306] found that the reduction in disease was greater than the percentage of children who had been vaccinated. Disease incidence prelicensure in vaccinated and unvaccinated infants less than 1 year, less than 2 years, and less than 5 years of age fell from between 40 and 110 cases per 100,000 person-years to less than 1 case per 100,000 person-years. In the age group 5 to 19 years, the incidence fell from 2.6 cases to 2.1 cases per 100,000 person-years; in those 20 to 39 years of age from 5.7 to 2.4; in those 40 to 59 years from 10.2 to 8.7; and in those 60 years of age and older the incidence fell from 35.4 to 30.3 cases per 100,000 person-years. The reduction for all ages greater than 5 years was between 9.3% and 11.4%, with the greatest reduction at 58% in 20- to 39-year olds.

Safety

Children Less Than Two Years of Age

The safety of pneumococcal conjugate vaccines has been most extensively examined in children less than 2 years of age. Local reactions, including swelling, redness, and indura-

tion, are not uncommon[246,247,296,307,308] but are generally mild and self-limiting (Table 23–13).

Local reactions have been reported to occur both more frequently[247,300,308] and less frequently[242,245,246,300,308,309] following conjugate vaccination than following concurrent vaccinations given into a different limb (e.g., DTP), or vaccinations used as a control (e.g., meningococcal conjugate vaccine or inactivated polio vaccine). Some studies reported no differences.[241,269] Fever (temperature ≥38°C) is more frequent in infants receiving pneumococcal conjugate vaccine than in controls.[242,247,296,300] Fever greater than or equal to 39°C also has been reported to be more common in conjugate vaccine recipients in some studies,[247,300] but only after either the second[90] or third[300] dose within the primary series.

Generalized systemic symptoms, such as irritability, drowsiness, and crying more than usual, sometimes have been seen in conjugate vaccine recipients,[246] but these symptoms have been mild. Other events that could possibly be attributed to conjugate vaccine include urticaria, rash, excessive crying, hypotonic-hyporesponsive episodes, and transient granulocytopenia.[245,300,309]

In the NCKP efficacy trial,[247] multiple methods were used to assess the safety of the 7-valent PncCRM vaccine. In addition to obtaining information about local and systemic reactions by telephone interview 48 to 72 hours and 14 days after each dose, the frequency of uncommon events requiring medical attention after vaccination was evaluated through the use of comprehensive hospitalization and emergency room utilization databases. The incidence of these events was followed for 30 days after vaccination for events in hospitalized children and for 60 days for events seen in

	DXose 3 (at 6 mo)*			Dose 4 (at 12 mo)†		
	PncCRM (N = 822)	Control Vaccine (N = 824)	P Value	PncCRM (N = 813)	Control Vaccine (N = 815)	P Value
	5	3	0.023	8	2	<0.001
	20	16	0.025	15	14	0.601
	0.4	0.1	0.622	0.9	0.1	0.075
	5	4	0.155	6	6	0.827
	0.5	0.4	0.996	1.3	0.4	0.094
	2.0	0.5	0.013	1.6	1.7	0.966
	40	31	<0.001	28	19	<0.001

the emergency department. Adverse events that were severe, unexpected, or possibly had been caused by the study vaccine were followed up through chart review, parent contact, or both. Of 92 diagnostic categories, significant differences were seen for only two: febrile seizures and elective admissions. Febrile seizures requiring hospitalization were more common in recipients of PncCRM than controls, but only in those patients who had received DTwP at the same time; there was no difference in rate of seizure between recipients of PncCRM and control vaccine who had received a concomitant DTaP vaccine. There was no clustering of febrile seizures within the 3-day period following vaccine administration, and the rates of seizure in this study were below the historical rates of seizure seen following DTwP vaccination.[81] Rates of sudden infant death syndrome also were similar to or lower than those expected from historical data. Elective admissions, including ventilatory ear tube placement, occurred more frequently in the control group.[247] In an analysis of selected categories of outpatient clinic visits, there were no significant differences between PncCRM recipients and controls in any category except overall seizures, which occurred more frequently in controls; no seizure subcategory was different between the two groups, and there was no temporal clustering of the seizures relative to vaccination.

A preliminary analysis of safety has been conducted following the widespread use of Prevnar in the community since it has been licensed.[30] Patients were used as their own controls by separating adverse events into those that occurred 0 to 2 days, 0 to 7 days, 0 to 14 days, and 0 to 30 days postvaccination, and comparing the rates of adverse events during these periods with those that occurred 31 to 60 days postvaccination (and therefore were unlikely to be caused by vaccine). Febrile illness, all seizure events, allergic reactions, asthma, croup, breath-holding, and gastroenteritis were the specific events chosen for analysis. The rates of other conditions, such as asthma, neutropenia, and death, also were compared with their rates in historical controls. The only within-subject reaction that significantly increased following PncCRM vaccination was febrile illness. The relative risk of febrile illness seen in the emergency department was 2.61 in the 2 days following the first dose of the primary series and 1.94 in the 2 days following any dose of the primary series. Within 30 days of dose three, there was also an increased risk of a febrile illness diagnosed in an outpatient clinic compared with the period before the vaccination. Compared with historical controls, infants receiving PncCRM were less likely to receive a diagnosis of asthma; no significant differences were seen in the rates of other diseases.

Older Children and Adults

As with children less than 2 years of age, pain at the injection site is the most common adverse reaction in older children, occurring in 20% to 56% of patients.[252,310] Swelling is the next most commonly reported local reaction,[310] but there were no significant differences between those receiving conjugate vaccines and those receiving control vaccinations. Fever was seen more frequently in children receiving PncPS vaccine than conjugate vaccines, but temperature greater than 38°C was rare in any group.[95,267,310] Vaccination by a strictly deep intramuscular route appeared to prevent prominent local reactions.[311] Reactogenicity did not increase with repeated doses.[310,312]

Special Groups

A study is currently underway to examine whether vaccination of a pregnant woman with a 9-valent PncCRM vaccine affects the response of the infant to the regular immunization schedule with 7-valent vaccine, and to compare the adverse events in the mothers following vaccination with 9-valent pneumococcal conjugate vaccine versus control.[313] This study design also will allow the investigators to evaluate the natural decline of transplacental antibodies for the two serotypes included in the 9-valent but not the 7-valent vaccine (serotypes 1 and 5). To date, 57 women have been vaccinated and 46 babies have been born. No significant adverse events have occurred that were thought to be related to the vaccine.

King et al.[251] compared a three-dose vaccine series of 5-valent PncCRM vaccine in HIV-positive and HIV-negative children, all greater than 2 years of age. Saline was used in HIV-negative children as a control. Only minor adverse reactions were observed. The reactogenicity of PncCRM was not different between children with and without sickle cell disease[118,122]; however, those who had a three-dose primary series had slightly stronger reactions to a PncPS booster than those who had a single dose at 12 months. Low-birth-weight infants had higher rates of extensive redness and swelling (greater than 3 cm) than normal-birth-weight infants following the third dose in the primary series, and low-birth-weight infants receiving PncCRM had higher rates of hives compared with those receiving control vaccine, but not compared with normal-birth-weight infants.[296] Preterm infants had swelling greater than 2.4 cm more often than full-term infants. Preterm infants receiving PncCRM had stronger reactions than those receiving control meningococcal vaccine[296]: fever greater than 38°C, swelling, tenderness at injection site, irritability, loss of appetite, vomiting, diarrhea, and hives all occurred more frequently than in preterm infants receiving control vaccine. However, these reactions were not severe enough to preclude the use of PncCRM in preterm infants.

Indications for Vaccine

Three organizations in the United States, the Advisory Committee on Immunization Practices (ACIP), the American Academy of Pediatrics (AAP), and the American Academy of Family Physicians , have made recommendations regarding the use of and appropriate schedule for vaccination with the licensed PncCRM, based on available clinical data on efficacy, immunogenicity, and safety.[247,296,307]

Based on large-scale efficacy trials, the three organizations recommend routine PncCRM vaccination of all infants, and catch-up vaccination of children younger than 24 months (Table 23–14). The first dose should be given at 2 months of age, although it can be given as early as 6 weeks. For infants receiving the first dose before 6 months, the three primary doses should be given 6 to 8 weeks apart (at approximately 2, 4, and 6 months of age), and one booster dose should be given between the ages of 12 and 15 months.

All children less than 24 months of age who did not receive PncCRM before 6 months of age should be given catch-up doses. If the first dose is given between the ages of 7 and 11 months, two doses should be given 6 to 8 weeks apart, with a booster dose at 12 to 15 months of age. If the first dose is given between 12 and 23 months of age, two doses should be given 6 to 8 weeks apart, with no booster dose. If no dose has been given before 24 months, a single dose should be given at that time. Premature infants should be given the vaccine at the appropriate chronologic age along with other routine vaccinations, regardless of calculated gestational age.

There is currently insufficient evidence to suggest whether the conjugate vaccine will be superior to the PncPS vaccine in healthy children over 5 years old. The ACIP therefore declines to recommend the replacement of the PS vaccine with PncCRM in older children and adults, although the use of PncCRM is not contraindicated. An advantage of the conjugate vaccine is that it initiates immunologic memory and produces an enhanced immune

TABLE 23–14 ■ Recommended Vaccination Schedule

PRIMARY SERIES AND "CATCH UP" IMMUNIZATION		
Age at First Dose (mo)	**Primary Series**	**Booster Dose**
2–6	3 doses 6–8 wk apart	1 dose at 12–15 mo of age
7–11	2 doses 6–8 wk apart	1 dose at 12–15 mo of age
12–23	2 doses 6–8 wk apart	None
≥24	1 dose	None
CHILDREN AT HIGH RISK		
Age (mo)	**No. Previous Doses**	**Recommended**
≤23	None	Conjugate, 4 doses
24–59	Conjugate, 4 doses	PS, 1 dose
	Conjugate, 1–3 doses	PS, 1 dose
	PS, 1 dose	Conjugate, 2 doses
	None	Conjugate, 2 doses; PS 1 dose

PS, polysaccharide.
From Preventing pneumococcal disease among infants and young children: recommendations of the Advisory Committee on Immunization Practices. MMWR 49(RR-9):1–35, 2000.

response in children 2 to 5 years of age. However, the wider serotype coverage of the PncPS vaccine might be more appropriate in children older than 5 years, in whom the serotypes covered by the conjugate vaccine are responsible for a smaller proportion of pneumococcal disease. In addition, the PncPS vaccine is less expensive. The AAP considers immunization with a single dose of either vaccine to be acceptable; if both vaccines are used, their administration should be separated by 6 to 8 weeks.

The currently available data are inadequate to recommend universal vaccination with PncCRM for children older than 24 months who are at moderate risk: children 24 to 35 months of age; children of Alaskan Native, Native American, or African-American descent; and children who attend day care centers at least 4 hours per week with two or more unrelated children.[314] However, vaccination with PncCRM should be considered on an elective basis for all children ages 24 to 59 months, with priority given to children who are at moderate risk.[81] Priority for vaccination also should be considered for children at social or economic disadvantage, who live in crowded or substandard housing, are homeless, experience chronic exposure to tobacco smoke, or have a history of recurrent otitis media.[314]

Catch-up vaccination is recommended for children 24 to 59 months of age who are at high risk for invasive pneumococcal diseases. At high risk are children with sickle cell disease or other types of asplenia, HIV infection, primary immunodeficiency, chronic cardiac or pulmonary disease, cerebrospinal fluid leaks, diabetes mellitus, and immunocompromising conditions such as malignancies, chronic renal failure or nephrotic syndrome, immunosuppressive chemotherapy, and solid organ transplant.

The ACIP and AAP recommend that a dose of PncPS be given to high-risk children older than 24 months at least 2 months after their last dose of PncCRM. For those children who did not receive PncCRM before 24 months of age (including those who received a dose of PncPS), two doses of PncCRM should be given, 2 months apart, followed by a dose of PncPS at least 2 months after the second dose of PncCRM. For children with sickle cell disease or who are immunocompromised, but not for children with chronic illness, revaccination with PncPS after 5 years is recommended. Scheduled vaccinations should be given at least 2 weeks before an elective splenectomy is performed for any reason or before immune-compromising therapy. In addition to vaccination, antibiotic prophylaxis is recommended for children with sickle cell disease or functional or anatomic asplenia.

The pneumococcal conjugate vaccine may be given concurrently with other recommended vaccines. However, separate syringes should be used for each vaccination, and injections should be made at separate sites even if given on the same extremity. Each 0.5-mL dose of PncCRM should be injected intramuscularly.

Future Vaccines

In spite of their good safety record and demonstrated high efficacy against invasive infections, there are several questions related to pneumococcal conjugate vaccines. The main issue is the potential for replacement disease with nonvaccine serotypes that may attenuate the overall benefit seen from reduction in disease caused by vaccine serotypes. There are also challenges related to the complexity of manufacture of conjugate vaccines. Therefore, there is increasing interest in protein vaccines.

The development of an effective protein-based vaccine depends on a thorough understanding of the roles of the various putative virulence proteins in pathogenesis. Several pneumococcal proteins, including pneumococcal surface protein A (PspA), pneumococcal surface adhesin A (PsaA), and pneumolysin (Ply) are considered essential for bacterial virulence.[279,315] Following the availability of the pneumococcal genome sequence in 1997, additional members of the choline-binding protein family[316-318] and other pneumococcal surface proteins[319,320] have been identified, and their role in pneumococcal pathogenesis and potential as pneumococcal vaccines—either as such or as carrier proteins for pneumococcal conjugates—is being examined.

In animals, PspA,[321-326] PsaA,[327-330] and Ply[331-333] have been shown to be immunogenic and protective against pneumococcal challenge. Limited data on the development of antibodies to these pneumococcal proteins in humans, especially in children, are also available.[334-340] Lower concentrations of antibodies to PsaA in children with pneumococcal AOM as compared with those with nonpneumococcal AOM,[341] to PsaA in children with pneumococcal carriage compared to noncarriers,[337] and to PspA in children with pneumococcal invasive infection as compared to children with nonpneumococcal invasive infection[335] have been demonstrated. Increases in anti-PsaA and anti-Ply titres are seen in adults with pneumococcal pneumonia, the increase being more evident in those with bacteremic pneumonia. However, anti-PspA levels showed a twofold increase in only 15% of Finnish children with invasive pneumococcal diseases.

PspA is a surface protein present in all clinically relevant strains of S. pneumoniae.[342] Although PspAs from different pneumococcal strains are serologically variable, some elicit antibodies that are cross-reactive with PspAs from unrelated strains. Active immunization of mice with PspA or with truncated PspA generates antibodies that protect against subsequent challenge with several strains of pneumococci.[323,343,344] Moreover, orally administered PspA given with the mucosal adjuvant cholera toxin induces significant levels of serum IgG and IgA antibodies and protects mice against challenge infection.[22] A Phase I clinical trial demonstrated that the PspA vaccine, a recombinant family 1 PspA protein, is safe and elicits human antibodies that can protect mice from challenge with pneumococci expressing either family 1 or family 2 PspAs.[326,345,346] Immune responses in the vaccinated individuals were cross-reactive to distantly related PspA proteins, and these antibodies persisted at high levels at least 6 months after vaccination.[347] In addition, the titre of antibody elicited in human serum was more than 1000 times higher than the titre required to protect mice from fatal infection.[347]

PsaA is a membrane-associated, cell surface–exposed lipoprotein that is common to all serotypes of pneumococcus.

It functions in the transport of Mn^{++} and Zn^{++}, and appears to be important for pneumococcal virulence.[348] PsaA is immunogenic and protective in mice.[344] It has been cloned, sequenced and expressed. Antibodies to PsaA reduce but do not eliminate adherence to epithelial cells. Thus there may be other adhesion molecules that play a role in adhesion of pneumococci to epithelial cells. It is not known whether this would result in some form of replacement phenomenon. This will obviously need to be monitored closely in clinical trials.

Pneumolysin is a cytolytic toxin produced by all pneumococci, regardless of serotype.[349] Genetically engineered Ply-negative mutants of pneumococci have significantly reduced virulence for mice.[324] Mice injected with inactivated Ply or recombinant Ply toxoid exhibit enhanced survival when challenged with different pneumococcal serotypes.[331,349] PdB is a mutant form of Ply that has only 0.1% of the hemolytic toxic activity of Ply but seems to retain full complement activation activity. Immunization with PdB protects mice against lung inflammation caused by Ply and against pneumonia following challenge. It also protects against intraperitoneal challenge, but not for all tested strains.

Development of a pneumococcal vaccine containing PspA, PsaA, Ply, and/or other proteins could result in a broad-spectrum TD vaccine that protects against a wide variety of strains and elicits immunologic memory.[345] Because it seems likely that different virulence factors of S. pneumoniae function at different stages of the pneumococcal infection, it is possible that immunization with a combination of these antigens will provide supplementary protection.[350,351]

Public Health Considerations

Serotype Replacement

At best, the conjugate vaccine can only protect against a limited number of the 90 pneumococcal serotypes. In theory, reduction in the carriage of vaccine serotypes may pave the way for nonvaccine serotypes to increase in prevalence.[352,353] Both mathematical modeling and animal challenge data suggest that serotype replacement may occur after conjugate vaccination.[354–357]

In clinical studies, the results have been conflicting. Some studies,[91,241,300,302] but not all,[122,303,306] have found an increase in nonvaccine serotypes accompanying the decrease in vaccine serotypes in nasopharyngeal culture samples following vaccination. Some of these discrepancies could be explained by small sample sizes and short follow-up periods. To us, it would seem logical that pneumococcal conjugates would be able to affect acquisition of carriage, in a way similar to that which takes place with Hib conjugate vaccines.[358–362] The more important question is whether serotype replacement leads to changes in the incidence or clinical picture of clinical infections. In efficacy trials, mucosal infections seem to behave differently than invasive disease. In the Finnish otitis media efficacy trial, although there was a reduction of 57% in episodes caused by serotypes in the 7-valent PncCRM vaccine and a 51% reduction in episodes caused by cross-reactive serotypes, there was an increase of 33% in episodes caused by other pneumococcal serotypes and an 11% increase in those caused by H. influenzae (see Table 23–12).[300] No similar increase has occurred in the incidence of invasive pneumococcal infections in the follow-up of the Kaiser Permanente efficacy trial.[306] In theory, these differences may be explained by different pathogenesis of mucosal versus invasive infections. It is, however, also possible that the follow-up time is not yet sufficient to know the extent of the replacement phenomenon in invasive infections.

One needs to distinguish between serotype unmasking and serotype replacement.[241,354,356] In most cases, nasopharyngeal carriage is determined by serotyping a single colony after a sample is cultured. This method almost always identifies the most abundant serotype present in the nasopharynx, but may overlook other serotypes that are also present but in lower abundance. If these minority pneumococci are of nonvaccine serotype, they are obviously more likely to be detected following vaccination, when the presence of vaccine serotypes is reduced. The current view is, however, that the shift in the relative frequencies of pneumococcal serotypes in carriage and otitis media studies is real, and is an indication of replacement—and not due only to increased sensitivity of the diagnostics or unmasking.

Among the 90 serogroups, a relatively small number account for most of the invasive disease in young children around the globe. In each region, 10 or fewer serogroups account for most invasive pneumococcal diseases, with those represented in the 9-valent vaccine accounting for two thirds or more in each region.[100] This is consistent with the hypothesis that vaccine serotypes as a group have a higher level of intrinsic virulence relative to other serotypes. If nonvaccine serotypes are newly detected because of unmasking rather than replacement, it seems likely that they are not virulent and will not contribute to disease. However, there may be interactions between serotypes that affect the frequency of colonization or that result in nonvaccine serotypes being kept in check by competition with vaccine serotypes.[352,357] If this is true, then nonvaccine serotypes may or may not prove to be virulent when this competition is removed.[356]

The serotypes included in pneumococcal conjugate vaccines are those that are currently most resistant to antibiotics. These serotypes are often less immunogenic in children than other serotypes, so that they are carried longer and have greater exposure to antibiotics.[363] If replacement serotypes are more immunogenic, they will be carried for a shorter period of time, and consequently will have less chance to become antibiotic resistant. Although the vaccine covers most of the strains that are now resistant to antibiotics, pneumococci readily switch their capsule genes[136] and subsequently their serotype. If serotype switch occurs in the nasopharynx where nonvaccine serotypes are already present, the resistant pneumococci are likely to adopt these nonvaccine serotypes. Because the capsule is a major determinant of virulence, the new strains may remain less invasive,[241] and therefore they may not cause disease that requires antibiotic treatment. However, some studies suggest a complicated relationship between capsular type and other genes responsible for virulence, so that existing associations between capsular type and virulence may change in response to vaccine-induced selective pressure.[356]

It will be important not to become complacent with the widespread use of the conjugate vaccines. Careful monitoring will be required to determine whether serotype replacement is occurring in carriage and in disease.[81,81a]

Economic Evaluations

Vaccine cost-effectiveness is dependent on many factors, including the incidence of disease, the efficacy of the vaccine, the sequelae of disease, and the cost per dose of the vaccine. Any of these factors may change over time as prices change, as more is learned about vaccine efficacy, or when standards of medical care improve. Any determination of cost-effectiveness therefore will be limited by the time- and place-specific variables that were used for the analysis. In addition, there are significant nonmedical costs associated with pneumococcal disease, most notably the cost of work time lost by parents caring for ill children.[364,365]

Lieu et al. analyzed the potential cost-effectiveness of the PncCRM vaccine[364] using data from the NCKP randomized trial[247] as well as the opinions of a panel of experts. The analysis was based on a comparison of "vaccination" with "no vaccination," assuming the use of four doses for routine vaccination of healthy infants and one dose for catch-up vaccination of children older than 2 years. In addition, the conservative assumption was made that a vaccinated infant would experience reductions in pneumococcal diseases only until his or her fifth birthday, and that vaccine efficacy against invasive disease would decrease from 100% in children less than 2 years old to 93% in children 2 to 5 years old. High-risk infants were excluded from this analysis. The cost-effectiveness of PncCRM from the perspectives of both society (medical and nonmedical costs) and health care payers (medical costs only) were calculated. From the societal perspective, vaccination of healthy infants would result in savings if the vaccine cost $46 or less per dose. From the health care payer perspective, net savings would occur if the vaccine cost $18 or less per dose. It is unclear at this point whether these costs per dose can be achieved. As of 2001, the private sector cost for PncCRM was $58.75 and the public sector cost was $45.99.[366] At these prices, a full series of PncCRM is much more expensive in the United States than two other new vaccines, against varicella and hepatitis A, and in most developing countries a single dose of PncCRM would substantially exceed the total cost of administering the nine antigens currently in use during the first month of life.

Future Use

Many areas remain to be examined with regard to the use of pneumococcal conjugate vaccines. To date, the efficacy of the conjugates has been examined only in young children, and it is still unclear to what extent they are efficacious in other risk groups. The licensed PncCRM was designed to protect against the serotypes most prevalent in infants in the United States. Infections in other target groups may have a different spectrum of serotypes.

Important questions to be answered in the very near future include how high a level of protection pneumococcal conjugates can afford to other risk groups, namely to HIV-infected and various other immunocompromised patient populations. Another area to be investigated urgently is the extent of protection conjugate vaccines to provide to the elderly, especially whether the vaccines are able to protect against pneumonia. If protection is sufficient, manufacturers, regulatory agencies, and public health authorities need to define the optimal composition of the vaccine and recommend how the vaccine should be used in an efficient way.

Very young infants also remain at high risk. There are two ways to extend the protection into the very first months of life: either start immunization immediately after birth or provide passive protection to the infant through maternal immunization. Although immunization of pregnant women with PncPS does provide elevated antibody levels to the infant for 14 to 22 weeks after birth,[367] at which time the primary series of vaccination would be nearly complete, it is not known whether this interferes with the vaccinations normally given during the first 6 months of life. Studies in animals have suggested that prenatal vaccination can protect against otitis media and invasive pneumococcal diseases in neonates,[368] and studies are underway in humans to determine the safety and immunogenicity of such a procedure.[313]

As additional efficacy trials of pneumococcal conjugate vaccines will be expensive and perhaps ethically questionable, licensure of additional combinations of conjugated polysaccharides will depend on agreement with regard to serological correlates of immunity. Unfortunately, variation between serotypes, quality of antibody, genetic background of the population, and the influence of simultaneously administered vaccines all make extraction of correlates difficult.[369]

Other topics that are either currently under investigation or where research is necessary include the optimal vaccination schedule, the use of a pneumococcal conjugate vaccine combined with other routine vaccinations in order to reduce the number of injections, and the duration of protection afforded by the vaccine.[81]

REFERENCES

1. Rijkers GT, Sanders EAM, Breukels MA, et al. Responsiveness of infants to capsular polysaccharides: implications for vaccine development. Rev Med Microbiol 7:3–12, 1996.
2. Fedson DS, Musher DM, Eskola J. Pneumococcal vaccine. In Plotkin SA, Orenstein WA (eds). Vaccines (4th ed.). Philadelphia, WB Saunders, 2003.
3. Mäkelä PH, Sibakov M, Herva E, et al. Pneumococcal vaccine and otitis media. Lancet 2:547–551, 1980.
4. Douglas RM, Paton JC, Duncan SJ, et al. Antibody response to pneumococcal vaccination in children younger than five years of age. J Infect Dis 148:131–137, 1983.
5. Leinonen M, Sakkinen A, Kalliokoski R, et al. Antibody response to 14-valent pneumococcal capsular polysaccharide vaccine in preschool age children. Pediatr Infect Dis 5:39–44, 1986.
6. Gibb D, Spoulou V, Giacomelli A, et al. Antibody responses to Haemophilus influenzae type b and Streptococcus pneumoniae vaccines in children with human immunodeficiency virus infection. Pediatr Infect Dis J 14:129–135, 1995.
7. Carson PJ, Schut RL, Simpson ML, et al. Antibody class and subclass responses to pneumococcal polysaccharides following immunization of human immunodeficiency virus-infected patients. J Infect Dis 172:340–345, 1995.

8. Rodriguez-Barradas MC, Groover JE, Lacke CE, et al. IgG antibody to pneumococcal capsular polysaccharide in human immunodeficiency virus-infected subjects: persistence of antibody in responders, revaccination in nonresponders, and relationship of immunoglobulin allotype to response. J Infect Dis 173:1347–1353, 1996.

9. Arpadi SM, Back S, O'Brien J, et al. Antibodies to pneumococcal capsular polysaccharides in children with human immunodeficiency virus infection given polyvalent pneumococcal vaccine. J Pediatr 125:77–79, 1994.

10. Peters VB, Diamant EP, Hodes DS, et al. Impaired immunity to pneumococcal polysaccharide antigens in children with human immunodeficiency virus infection immunized with pneumococcal vaccine. Pediatr Infect Dis J 13:933–934, 1994.

11. Mellemgaard A. Ranitidine improves the vaccination response in patients with chronic lymphocytic leukemia—a randomized, controlled study. Immunol Infect Dis 3:109–111, 1993.

12. Rautonen J, Siimes MA, Lundström U, et al. Vaccination of children during treatment for leukemia. Acta Paediatr Scand 75:579–585, 1986.

13. Grimfors G, Soderqvist M, Holm G, et al. A longitudinal study of class and subclass antibody response to pneumococcal vaccination in splenectomized individuals with special reference to patients with Hodgkin's disease. Eur J Haematol 45:101–108, 1990.

14. Grimfors G, Bjørkholm M, Hammarström L, et al. Type-specific antipneumococcal antibody subclass response to vaccination after splenectomy with special reference to lymphoma patients. Eur J Haematol 43:404–410, 1989.

15. Parkkali T, Kayhty H, Ruutu T, et al. A comparison of early and late vaccination with Haemophilus influenzae type b conjugate and pneumococcal polysaccharide vaccines after allogeneic BMT. Bone Marrow Transplant 18:961–967, 1996.

16. Parkkali T, Väkeväinen M, Käyhty H, et al. Opsonophagocytic activity against Streptococcus pneumoniae type 19F in allogeneic BMT recipients before and after vaccination with pneumococcal polysaccharide vaccine. Bone Marrow Transplant 27:207–211, 2001.

17. Parkkali T, Käyhty H, Anttila M, et al. IgG subclasses and avidity of antibodies to polysaccharide antigens in allogeneic BMT recipients after vaccination with pneumococcal polysaccharide and Haemophilus influenzae type b conjugate vaccines. Bone Marrow Transplant 24:671–678, 1999.

18. MacLeod CM, Hodges RG, Heidelberger M, et al. Prevention of pneumococcal pneumonia by immunization with specific capsular polysaccharides. J Exp Med 82:445–465, 1945.

19. van den Dobbelsteen GP, van Rees EP. Mucosal immune responses to pneumococcal polysaccharides: implications for vaccination. Trends Microbiol 3:155–159, 1995.

20. Mäkelä PH, Karma P. Pneumococcal vaccine in otitis media. Lancet 1:152–153, 1981.

21. Fedson DS. Pneumococcal vaccination for older adults: the first 20 years. Drugs Aging 15:21–30, 1999.

22. Fedson DS. Pneumococcal vaccination: four issues for western Europe. Biologicals 25:215–219, 1997.

23. Siber G. WHO meeting: definition and evaluation of immune correlates of protection against pneumococcal infection in children that can serve as the basis for licensure of future pneumococcal conjugate vaccines. In Abstracts of the 3rd International Symposium on Pneumococci and Pneumococcal Diseases, Anchorage, May 5–8, 2002.

24. Herman CJ, Speroff T, Cebul RD. Improving compliance with immunization in the older adult: results of a randomized cohort study. J Am Geriatr Soc 42:1154–1159, 1994.

25. Mulholland K. Magnitude of the problem of childhood pneumonia. Lancet 354:590–592, 1999.

26. Williams BG, Gouws E, Boschi-Pinto C, et al. Estimates of world-wide distribution of child deaths from acute respiratory infections. Lancet Infect Dis 2:25–32, 2002.

27. Jacobs MR. Antibiotic-resistant Streptococcus pneumoniae in acute otitis media: overview and update. Pediatr Infect Dis J 17:947–952, 1998.

28. Butler JC, Hoffmann J, Cetron M. The continued emergence of drug-resistant Streptococcus pneumoniae in the United States: an update from the Centers for Disease Control and Prevention's Pneumococcal Sentinel Surveillance System. J Infect Dis 174:986–993, 1996.

29. Dagan R, Melamed R, Muallem M, et al. Nasopharyngeal colonization in southern Israel with antibiotic-resistant pneumococci during the first 2 years of life: relation to serotypes likely to be included in pneumococcal conjugate vaccines. J Infect Dis 174:1352–1355, 1996.

30. Black SB, Shinefield H, Fireman B, et al. Efficacy against pneumonia of heptavalent conjugate pneumococcal vaccine (Wyeth Lederle) in 37,868 infants and children: expanded data analysis including duration of protection. In Abstracts of the 3rd International Symposium on Pneumococci and Pneumococcal Diseases, Anchorage, May 5–8, 2002.

31. Resistance of Streptococcus pneumoniae to fluoroquinolones—United States, 1995–1999. MMWR 50:800–804, 2001.

32. Robbins JB, Schneerson R. Polysaccharide-protein conjugates: a new generation of vaccines. J Infect Dis 161:821–832, 1990.

33. Siber GR. Pneumococcal disease: prospects for a new generation of vaccines. Science 265:1385–1387, 1994.

34. Eskola J, Anttila M. Pneumococcal conjugate vaccines. Pediatr Infect Dis J 18:543–551, 1999.

35. Briles DE, Hollingshead SK, Nabors GS, et al. The potential for using protein vaccines to protect against otitis media caused by Streptococcus pneumoniae. Vaccine 19(suppl):S87–S95, 2000.

36. Lesinski GB, Smithson SL, Srivastava N, et al. A DNA vaccine encoding a peptide mimic of Streptococcus pneumoniae serotype 4 capsular polysaccharide induces specific anti-carbohydrate antibodies in Balb/c mice. Vaccine 19:1717–1726, 2001.

37. Nayak AR, Tinge SA, Tart RC, et al. A live recombinant avirulent oral Salmonella vaccine expressing pneumococcal surface protein A induces protective responses against Streptococcus pneumoniae. Infect Immun 66:3744–3751, 1998.

38. Buchanan RM, Briles DE, Arulanandam BP, et al. IL-12-mediated increases in protection elicited by pneumococcal and meningococcal conjugate vaccines. Vaccine 19:2020–2028, 2001.

39. Chu RS, McCool T, Greenspan NS, et al. CpG oligodeoxynucleotides act as adjuvants for pneumococcal polysaccharide-protein conjugate vaccines and enhance antipolysaccharide immunoglobulin G2a (IgG2a) and IgG3 antibodies. Infect Immun 68:1450–1456, 2000.

40. Dullforce P, Sutton DC, Heath AW. Enhancement of T cell-independent immune responses in vivo by CD40 antibodies. Nat Med 4:88–91, 1998.

41. Jakobsen H, Saeland E, Gizurarson S, et al. Intranasal immunization with pneumococcal polysaccharide conjugate vaccines protects mice against invasive pneumococcal infections. Infect Immun 67:4128–4133, 1999.

42. Jakobsen H, Schulz D, Pizza M, et al. Intranasal immunization with pneumococcal polysaccharide conjugate vaccines with nontoxic mutants of Escherichia coli heat-labile enterotoxins as adjuvants protects mice against invasive pneumococcal infections. Infect Immun 67:5892–5897, 1999.

43. Arulanandam BP, Lynch JM, Briles DE, et al. Intranasal vaccination with pneumococcal surface protein A and interleukin-12 augments antibody-mediated opsonization and protective immunity against Streptococcus pneumoniae infection. Infect Immun 69:6718–6724, 2001.

44. Cho NH, Seong SY, Chun KH, et al. Novel mucosal immunization with polysaccharide-protein conjugates entrapped in alginate microspheres. J Control Release 53:215–224, 1998.

45. Avery OT, Goebel WF. Chemo-immunological studies on conjugated carbohydrate-proteins. II. Immunological specificity of synthetic sugar-protein antigen. J Exp Med 50:533–550, 1929.

46. Goebel WF, Avery OT. Chemo-immunological studies on conjugated and carbohydrate-proteins. I. The synthesis of ρ-aminophenol β-glucoside, ρ-aminophenol β-lactoside, and their coupling with serum globulin. J Exp Med 50:521–531, 1929.

47. Anderson P. Antibody responses to Haemophilus influenzae type b and diphtheria toxin induced by conjugates of oligosaccharides of the type b capsule with the nontoxic protein CRM197. Infect Immun 39:233–238, 1983.

48. Schneerson R, Barrera O, Sutton A, et al. Preparation, characterization, and immunogenicity of Haemophilus influenzae type b polysaccharide-protein conjugates. J Exp Med 152:361–376, 1980.

49. Gordon LK. Characterization of a hapten-carrier conjugate vaccine: H. influenzae–diphtheria conjugate vaccine. In Chanok RM, Lerner RL (eds). Modern Approaches to Vaccines. Cold Spring Harbor, NY, Cold Spring Harbor Laboratory, 1984, pp 393–396.

50. Jodar L, Feavers IM, Salisbury D, et al. Development of vaccines against meningococcal disease. Lancet 359:1499–1508, 2002.

51. Lakshman R, Finn A. Meningococcal serogroup C conjugate vaccine. Expert Opin Biol Ther 2:87–96, 2002.

52. Richmond P, Borrow R, Findlow J, et al. Evaluation of de-O-acetylated meningococcal C polysaccharide-tetanus toxoid conjugate vaccine in infancy: reactogenicity, immunogenicity, immunologic

priming, and bactericidal activity against O-acetylated and de-O-acetylated serogroup C strains. Infect Immun 69:2378–2382, 2001.

53. Katkocin DM. Characterization of multivalent pneumococcal conjugate vaccines. Dev Biol 103:113–119, 2000.

54. Chu C, Schneerson R, Robbins JB, et al. Further studies on the immunogenicity of *Haemophilus influenzae* type b and pneumococcal type 6A polysaccharide-protein conjugates. Infect Immun 40:245–256, 1983.

55. Moreau M, Schulz D. Polysaccharide-based vaccines for the prevention of pneumococcal infections. J Carbohydrate Chemistry 19:419–434, 2000.

56. Eby R. Pneumococcal conjugate vaccines. Pharm Biotechnol 6:695–718, 1995.

57. Brigtsen AK, Kasper DL, Baker CJ, et al. Induction of cross-reactive antibodies by immunization of healthy adults with types Ia and Ib group B streptococcal polysaccharide-tetanus toxoid conjugate vaccines. J Infect Dis 185:1277–1284, 2002.

58. Guttormsen HK, Baker CJ, Nahm MH, et al. Type III group B streptococcal polysaccharide induces antibodies that cross-react with *Streptococcus pneumoniae* type 14. Infect Immun 70:1724–1738, 2002.

59. Lin FY, Ho VA, Khiem HB, et al. The efficacy of a *Salmonella typhi* Vi conjugate vaccine in two-to-five-year-old children. N Engl J Med 344:1263–1269, 2001.

60. Szu SC, Taylor DN, Trofa AC, et al. Laboratory and preliminary clinical characterization of Vi capsular polysaccharide-protein conjugate vaccines. Infect Immun 62:4440–4444, 1994.

61. Fattom A, Li X, Cho YH, et al. Effect of conjugation methodology, carrier protein, and adjuvants on the immune response to *Staphylococcus aureus* capsular polysaccharides. Vaccine 13:1288–1293, 1995.

62. Shinefield H, Black S, Fattom A, et al. Use of a *Staphylococcus aureus* conjugate vaccine in patients receiving hemodialysis. N Engl J Med 346:491–496, 2002.

63. Fattom AI, Sarwar J, Basham L, et al. Antigenic determinants of *Staphylococcus aureus* type 5 and type 8 capsular polysaccharide vaccines. Infect Immun 66:4588–4592, 1998.

64. Fattom AI, Sarwar J, Ortiz A, et al. A *Staphylococcus aureus* capsular polysaccharide (CP) vaccine and CP-specific antibodies protect mice against bacterial challenge. Infect Immun 64:1659–1665, 1996.

65. Fritzell B, Plotkin S. Efficacy and safety of a *Haemophilus influenzae* type b capsular polysaccharide-tetanus protein conjugate vaccine. J Pediatr 121:355–362, 1992.

66. Flanagan MP, Michael JG. Oral immunization with a *Streptococcal pneumoniae* polysaccharide conjugate vaccine in enterocoated microparticles induces serum antibodies against type specific polysaccharides. Vaccine 17:72–81, 1999.

67. Black S, Shinefield H, Ray P. Efficacy of heptavalent conjugate pneumococcal vaccine (Wyeth Lederle) in 37,000 infants and children: results of the Northern California Kaiser Permanente efficacy trial. *In* Abstracts of the 38th Interscience Conference on Antimicrobial Agents and Chemotherapy, San Diego, CA, September 24–27, 1998.

68. Vella PP, Ellis RW. Immunogenicity of *Haemophilus influenzae* type b conjugate vaccines in infant rhesus monkeys. Pediatr Res 29:10–13, 1991.

69. Janson H, Heden LO, Grubb A, et al. Protein D, an immunoglobulin D-binding protein of *Haemophilus influenzae*: cloning, nucleotide sequence, and expression in *Escherichia coli*. Infect Immun 59:119–125, 1991.

70. Akkoyunlu M, Melhus A, Capiau C, et al. The acylated form of protein D of *Haemophilus influenzae* is more immunogenic than the nonacylated form and elicits an adjuvant effect when it is used as a carrier conjugated to polyribosyl ribitol phosphate. Infect Immun 65:5010–5016, 1997.

71. Watson DA, Musher DM. Interruption of capsule production in *Streptococcus pneumoniae* serotype 3 by insertion of transposon Tn916. Infect Immun 58:3135–3138, 1990.

72. Shurin PA, Rehmus JM, Johnson CE, et al. Bacterial polysaccharide immune globulin for prophylaxis of acute otitis media in high-risk children. J Pediatr 123:801–810, 1993.

73. Bruyn GA, Zegers BJ, Van Furth R. Mechanisms of host defense against infection with *Streptococcus pneumoniae*. Clin Infect Dis 14:251–262, 1992.

74. Siber GR, Thompson C, Reid GR, et al. Evaluation of bacterial polysaccharide immune globulin for the treatment or prevention of *Haemophilus influenzae* type b and pneumococcal disease. J Infect Dis 165(suppl):S129–S133, 1992.

75. CJ, Banks SD, Li JP. Virulence, immunity, and vaccine related to *Streptococcus pneumoniae*. Crit Rev Microbiol 18:89–114, 1991.

76. Knecht JC, Schiffman G, Austrian R. Some biological properties of *Pneumococcus* type 37 and the chemistry of its capsular polysaccharide. J Exp Med 132:475–487, 1970.

77. Fine DP. Pneumococcal type-associated variability in alternate complement pathway activation. Infect Immun 12:772–778, 1975.

78. Hostetter MK. Serotypic variations among virulent pneumococci in deposition and degradation of covalently bound C3b: implications for phagocytosis and antibody production. J Infect Dis 153:682–693, 1986.

79. Brown EJ, Joiner KA, Cole RM, et al. Localization of complement component 3 on *Streptococcus pneumoniae*: anti-capsular antibody causes complement deposition on the pneumococcal capsule. Infect Immun 39:403–409, 1983.

80. van Dam JE, Fleer A, Snippe H. Immunogenicity and immunochemistry of *Streptococcus pneumoniae* capsular polysaccharides. Antonie Van Leeuwenhoek Int J Gen Mol Microbiol 58:1–47, 1990.

81. Preventing pneumococcal disease among infants and young children: recommendations of the Advisory Committee on Immunization Practices (ACIP). MMWR 49(RR-9):1–35, 2000.

81a. Pelton SI, Klein JO. The future of pneumococcal conjugate vaccines for prevention of pneumococcal diseases in infants and children. Pediatrics 110:805–814, 2002.

82. Robinson KA, Baughman W, Rothrock G, et al. Epidemiology of invasive *Streptococcus pneumoniae* infections in the United States, 1995–1998—opportunities for prevention in the conjugate vaccine era. JAMA 285:1729–1735, 2001.

83. Bjornson G, Scheifele D, Binder F, et al. Population-based incidence rate of invasive pneumococcal infection in children: Vancouver, 1994–1998. Can Commun Dis Rep 26:149–151, 2000.

84. Scheifele D, Halperin S, Pelletier L, et al. Invasive pneumococcal infections in Canadian children, 1991–1998: implications for new vaccination strategies. Canadian Paediatric Society/Laboratory Centre for Disease Control Immunization Monitoring Program, Active (IMPACT). Clin Infect Dis 31:58–64, 2000.

85. von Kries R, Siedler A, Schmitt HJ, et al. Proportion of invasive pneumococcal infections in German children preventable by pneumococcal conjugate vaccines. Clin Infect Dis 31:482–487, 2000.

86. Eskola J, Takala AK, Kela E, et al. Epidemiology of invasive pneumococcal infections in children in Finland. JAMA 268:3323–3327, 1992.

87. Kaplan SL, Mason EO Jr, Wald E, et al. Six year multicenter surveillance of invasive pneumococcal infections in children. Pediatr Infect Dis J 21:141–147, 2002.

88. Levine OS, Farley M, Harrison LH, et al. Risk factors for invasive pneumococcal disease in children: a population-based case-control study in North America. Pediatrics 103:E28, 1999.

89. Alpern ER, Alessandrini EA, McGowan KL, et al. Serotype prevalence of occult pneumococcal bacteremia. Pediatrics 108:E23, 2001.

90. Leophonte P, Neukirch F. Anti-pneumococci vaccination: role and indications in the prevention of community acquired infections of the lower respiratory tract [in French]. Med Mal Infect 31:181–194, 2001.

91. Obaro SK, Adegbola RA, Banya WA, et al. Carriage of pneumococci after pneumococcal vaccination. Lancet 348:271–272, 1996.

92. Black S, Shinefield H, Fireman B, et al. Efficacy, safety, and immunogenicity of heptavalent pneumococcal conjugate vaccine in children. Am J Managed Care 6(suppl):S536–S549, 2001.

93. Klein DL. Pneumococcal disease and the role of conjugate vaccines. Microb Drug Resist 5:147–157, 1999.

94. Madhi SA, Petersen K, Madhi A, et al. Impact of human immunodeficiency virus type 1 on the disease spectrum of *Streptococcus pneumoniae* in South African children. Pediatr Infect Dis J 19:1141–1147, 2000.

95. Barnett ED, Pelton SI, Cabral HJ, et al. Immune response to pneumococcal conjugate and polysaccharide vaccines in otitis-prone and otitis-free children. Clin Infect Dis 29:191–192, 1999.

96. Kolberg J, Hoiby EA, Ase A, et al. *Streptococcus pneumoniae* heat shock protein 70 does not induce human antibody responses during infection. FEMS Immunol Med Microbiol 29:289–294, 2000.

97. Hortal M, Algorta G, Bianchi I, et al. Capsular type distribution and susceptibility to antibiotics of *Streptococcus pneumoniae* clinical strains isolated from Uruguayan children with systemic infections. Pneumococcus Study Group. Microb Drug Resist 3:159–163, 1997.

98. Dagan R, Engelhard D, Piccard E, et al. Epidemiology of invasive childhood pneumococcal infections in Israel. The Israeli Pediatric Bacteremia and Meningitis Group. JAMA 268:3328–3332, 1992.

99. O'Brien KL, Walters MI, Sellman J, et al. Severe pneumococcal pneumonia in previously healthy children: the role of preceding influenza infection. Clin Infect Dis 30:784–789, 2000.

100. Hausdorff WP, Bryant J, Paradiso PR, et al. Which pneumococcal serogroups cause the most invasive disease? Implications for conjugate vaccine formulation and use, part I. Clin Infect Dis 30:100–121, 2000.

101. Miller E, Waight P, Efstratiou A, et al. Epidemiology of invasive and other pneumococcal disease in children in England and Wales 1996–1998. Acta Paediatr Suppl 89:11–16, 2000.

102. Hausdorff WP, Siber G, Paradiso PR. Geographical differences in invasive pneumococcal disease rates and serotype frequency in young children. Lancet 357:950–952, 2001.

103. Ziebold C, von Kries R, Siedler A, et al. Epidemiology of pneumococcal disease in children in Germany. Acta Paediatr Suppl 89:17–21, 2000.

104. Eriksson M, Henriques B, Ekdahl K. Epidemiology of pneumococcal infections in Swedish children. Acta Paediatr Suppl 89:35–39, 2000.

105. Poland GA. The burden of pneumococcal disease: the role of conjugate vaccines. Vaccine 17:1674–1679, 1999.

106. Obaro SK. Prospects for pneumococcal vaccination in African children. Acta Trop 75:141–153, 2000.

107. Levine MM, Lagos R, Levine OS, et al. Epidemiology of invasive pneumococcal infections in infants and young children in metropolitan Santiago, Chile, a newly industrializing country. Pediatr Infect Dis J 17:287–293, 1998.

108. Coles CL, Kanungo R, Rahmathullah L, et al. Pneumococcal nasopharyngeal colonization in young South Indian infants. Pediatr Infect Dis J 20:289–295, 2001.

109. Krause VL, Reid SJ, Merianos A. Invasive pneumococcal disease in the Northern Territory of Australia, 1994–1998. Med J Aust 173(suppl):S27–S31, 2000.

110. McIntyre PB, Nolan TM. Conjugate pneumococcal vaccines for non-indigenous children in Australia. Med J Aust 173(suppl): S54–S57, 2000.

111. Fraser D, Givon-Lavi N, Bilenko N, et al. A decade (1989–1998) of pediatric invasive pneumococcal disease in 2 populations residing in 1 geographic location: implications for vaccine choice. Clin Infect Dis 33:421–427, 2001.

112. Jain A, Jain S, Gant V. Should patients positive for HIV infection receive pneumococcal vaccine? Br Med J 310:1060–1062, 1995.

113. Dworkin MS, Ward JW, Hanson DL, et al. Pneumococcal disease among human immunodeficiency virus-infected persons: incidence, risk factors, and impact of vaccination. Clin Infect Dis 32:794–800, 2001.

114. Poland GA. The prevention of pneumococcal disease by vaccines: promises and challenges. Infect Dis Clin North Am 15:97–122, 2001.

115. Barnett ED, Klein JO, Pelton SI, et al. Otitis media in children born to human immunodeficiency virus-infected mothers. Pediatr Infect Dis J 11:360–364, 1992.

116. Jones N, Huebner R, Khoosal M, et al. The impact of HIV on Streptococcus pneumoniae bacteraemia in a South African population. AIDS 12:2177–2184, 1998.

117. Karstaedt AS, Khoosal M, Crewe-Brown HH. Pneumococcal bacteremia during a decade in children in Soweto, South Africa. Pediatr Infect Dis J 19:454–457, 2000.

118. Vernacchio L, Neufeld EJ, MacDonald K, et al. Combined schedule of 7-valent pneumococcal conjugate vaccine followed by 23-valent pneumococcal vaccine in children and young adults with sickle cell disease. J Pediatr 133:275–278, 1998.

119. Gill FM, Sleeper LA, Weiner SJ, et al. Clinical events in the first decade in a cohort of infants with sickle cell disease. Cooperative Study of Sickle Cell Disease. Blood 86:776–783, 1995.

120. Zarkowsky HS, Gallagher D, Gill FM, et al. Bacteremia in sickle hemoglobinopathies. J Pediatr 109:579–585, 1986.

121. Babl FE, Pelton SI, Theodore S, et al. Constancy of distribution of serogroups of invasive pneumococcal isolates among children: experience during 4 decades. Clin Infect Dis 32:1155–1161, 2001.

122. O'Brien KL, Swift AJ, Winkelstein JA, et al. Safety and immunogenicity of heptavalent pneumococcal vaccine conjugated to CRM(197) among infants with sickle cell disease. Pneumococcal Conjugate Vaccine Study Group. Pediatrics 106:965–972, 2000.

123. McIntyre P, Craig JC. Prevention of serious bacterial infection in children with nephrotic syndrome. J Pediatr Child Health 34:314–317, 1998.

124. Guinan EC, Molrine DC, Antin JH, et al. Polysaccharide conjugate vaccine responses in bone marrow transplant patients. Transplantation 57:677–684, 1994.

125. Schutze GE, Mason EO Jr, Wald ER, et al. Pneumococcal infections in children after transplantation. Clin Infect Dis 33:16–21, 2001.

126. Molrine DC, George S, Tarbell N, et al. Antibody responses to polysaccharide and polysaccharide-conjugate vaccines after treatment of Hodgkin disease. Ann Intern Med 123:828–834, 1995.

127. Sniadack DH, Schwartz B, Lipman H, et al. Potential interventions for the prevention of childhood pneumonia: geographic and temporal differences in serotype and serogroup distribution of sterile site pneumococcal isolates from children—implications for vaccine strategies. Pediatr Infect Dis J 14:503–510, 1995.

128. Hausdorff WP, Bryant J, Kloek C, et al. The contribution of specific pneumococcal serogroups to different disease manifestations: implications for conjugate vaccine formulation and use, part II. Clin Infect Dis 30:122–140, 2000.

129. Giebink GS, Meier JD, Liebeler CL, et al. Immunogenicity and efficacy of Streptococcus pneumoniae polysaccharide-protein conjugate vaccines against homologous and heterologous serotypes in the chinchilla otitis media model. J Infect Dis 173:119–127, 1996.

130. Butler JC, Breiman RF, Lipman HB, et al. Serotype distribution of Streptococcus pneumoniae infections among preschool children in the United States, 1978–1994: implications for development of a conjugate vaccine. J Infect Dis 171:885–889, 1995.

131. Butler JC, Breiman RF, Campbell JF, et al. Pneumococcal polysaccharide vaccine efficacy: an evaluation of current recommendations. JAMA 270:1826–1831, 1993.

132. Bogaert D, Engelen MN, Timmers-Reker AJ, et al. Pneumococcal carriage in children in the Netherlands: a molecular epidemiological study. J Clin Microbiol 39:3316–3320, 2001.

133. Kyaw MH, Clarke S, Edwards GF, et al. Serotypes/groups distribution and antimicrobial resistance of invasive pneumococcal isolates: implications for vaccine strategies. Epidemiol Infect 125:561–572, 2000.

134. Kaltoft MS, Zeuthen N, Konradsen HB. Epidemiology of invasive pneumococcal infections in children aged 0–6 years in Denmark: a 19-year nationwide surveillance study. Acta Paediatr Suppl 89:3–10, 2000.

135. Kanra G, Erdem G, Ceyhan M, et al. Serotypes and antibacterial susceptibility of pneumococci isolated from children with infections in Ankara in relation to proposed pneumococcal vaccine coverage. Acta Pediatr Jpn 40:437–440, 1998.

136. Coffey TJ, Enright MC, Daniels M, et al. Recombinational exchanges at the capsular polysaccharide biosynthetic locus lead to frequent serotype changes among natural isolates of Streptococcus pneumoniae. Mol Microbiol 27:73–83, 1998.

137. Harwell JI, Brown RB. The drug-resistant pneumococcus: clinical relevance, therapy, and prevention. Chest 117:530–541, 2000.

138. Harding CV, Roof RW, Allen PM, et al. Effects of pH and polysaccharides on peptide binding to class II major histocompatibility complex molecules. Proc Natl Acad Sci U S A 88:2740–2744, 1991.

139. Ishioka GY, Lamont AG, Thomson D, et al. MHC interaction and T cell recognition of carbohydrates and glycopeptides. J Immunol 148:2446–2451, 1992.

140. Stein KE. Thymus-independent and thymus-dependent responses to polysaccharide antigens. J Infect Dis 165(suppl):S49–S52, 1992.

141. Baker PJ, Amsbaugh DF, Stashak PW, et al. Regulation of the antibody response to pneumococcal polysaccharide by thymus-derived cells. Rev Infect Dis 3:332–341, 1981.

142. Mosier DE, Zaldivar NM, Goldings E, et al. Formation of antibody in the newborn mouse: study of T-cell-independent antibody response. J Infect Dis 136(suppl):S14–S19, 1977.

143. Pabst HF, Kreth HW. Ontogeny of the immune response as a basis of childhood disease. J Pediatr 97:519–534, 1980.

144. Delves PJ, Roitt IM. The immune system: first of two parts. N Engl J Med 343:37–49, 2000.

145. Delves PJ, Roitt IM. The immune system: second of two parts. N Engl J Med 343:108–117, 2000.

146. Schwartz RH. Immunology: it takes more than two to tango. Nature 409:31–32, 2001.

147. Lanzavecchia A, Sallusto F. Dynamics of T lymphocyte responses: intermediates, effectors, and memory cells. Science 290:92–97, 2000.

148. Klein J, Sato A. The HLA system: first of two parts. N Engl J Med 343:702–709, 2000.

149. Hwang Y, Nahm MH, Briles DE, et al. Acquired, but not innate, immune responses to Streptococcus pneumoniae are compromised by neutralization of CD40L. Infect Immun 68:511–517, 2000.

150. McCool TL, Harding CV, Greenspan NS, et al. B- and T-cell immune responses to pneumococcal conjugate vaccines: divergence between carrier- and polysaccharide-specific immunogenicity. Infect Immun 67:4862–4869, 1999.

151. Turley SJ, Inaba K, Garrett WS, et al. Transport of peptide-MHC class II complexes in developing dendritic cells. Science 288:522–527, 2000.

152. Lee MC, Kobzik L, De Sousa AO, et al. Antibody responses to pneumococcal capsular polysaccharides require CD1 mediated antigen presentation to CD8+ helper T cells. In Abstracts of the 3rd International Symposium on Pneumococci and Pneumococcal Diseases, Anchorage, May 5–8, 2002.

153. Banchereau J, Steinman RM. Dendritic cells and the control of immunity. Nature 392:245–252, 1998.

154. Abbas AK, Murphy KM, Sher A. Functional diversity of helper T lymphocytes. Nature 383:787–793, 1996.

155. Ada G. Vaccines and vaccination. N Engl J Med 345:1042–1053, 2001.

156. MacLennan IC, Liu YJ, Johnson GD. Maturation and dispersal of B-cell clones during T cell-dependent antibody responses. Immunol Rev 126:143–161, 1992.

157. Ronchese F, Hausmann B. B lymphocytes in vivo fail to prime naive T cells but can stimulate antigen-experienced T lymphocytes. J Exp Med 177:679–690, 1993.

158. Guttormsen HK, Sharpe AH, Chandraker AK, et al. Cognate stimulatory B-cell–T-cell interactions are critical for T-cell help recruited by glycoconjugate vaccines. Infect Immun 67:6375–6384, 1999.

159. Breukels MA, Rijkers GT, Voorhorst-Ogink MM, et al. Pneumococcal conjugate vaccine primes for polysaccharide-inducible IgG2 antibody response in children with recurrent otitis media acuta. J Infect Dis 179:1152–1156, 1999.

160. Berek C. The development of B cells and the B-cell repertoire in the microenvironment of the germinal center. Immunol Rev 126:5–19, 1992.

161. Wu ZQ, Khan AQ, Shen Y, et al. B7 requirements for primary and secondary protein- and polysaccharide-specific Ig isotype responses to Streptococcus pneumoniae. J Immunol 165:6840–6848, 2000.

162. Tarlinton DM, Smith KG. Dissecting affinity maturation: a model explaining selection of antibody-forming cells and memory B cells in the germinal centre. Immunol Today 21:436–441, 2000.

162a. Pérez-Melgosa M, Ochs HD, Linsley PS, et al. Carrier-mediated enhancement of logmate T cell help: the basis for enhanced immunogenicity of meningococcal outer membrane protein polysaccharide conjugate vaccine. Eur J Imm 31:2373–2378, 2001.

163. Hougs L, Juul L, Ditzel HJ, et al. The first dose of a Haemophilus influenzae type b conjugate vaccine reactivates memory B cells: evidence for extensive clonal selection, intraclonal affinity maturation, and multiple isotype switches to IgA2. J Immunol 162:224–237, 1999.

164. Berek C, Ziegner M. The maturation of the immune response. Immunol Today 14:400–404, 1993.

165. Smith KG, Light A, Nossal GJ, et al. The extent of affinity maturation differs between the memory and antibody-forming cell compartments in the primary immune response. EMBO J 16:2996–3006, 1997.

166. Nossal GJ. The molecular and cellular basis of affinity maturation in the antibody response. Cell 68:1–2, 1992.

167. Choe J, Li L, Zhang X, et al. Distinct role of follicular dendritic cells and T cells in the proliferation, differentiation, and apoptosis of a centroblast cell line, L3055. J Immunol 164:56–63, 2000.

168. Smith KG, Hewitson TD, Nossal GJ, et al. The phenotype and fate of the antibody-forming cells of the splenic foci. Eur J Immunol 26:444–448, 1996.

169. Pearse RN, Kawabe T, Bolland S, et al. SHIP recruitment attenuates Fc gamma RIIB-induced B cell apoptosis. Immunity 10:753–760, 1999.

170. Lucas AH, Granoff DM. Imperfect memory and the development of Haemophilus influenzae type B disease. Pediatr Infect Dis J 20:235–239, 2001.

171. Eskola J, Ward J, Dagan R, et al. Combined vaccination of Haemophilus influenzae type b conjugate and diphtheria-tetanus-pertussis containing acellular pertussis. Lancet 354:2063–2068, 1999.

172. Goldblatt D. Immunisation and the maturation of infant immune responses. Dev Biol Stand 95:125–132, 1998.

173. Guttormsen HK, Wetzler LM, Finberg RW, et al. Immunologic memory induced by a glycoconjugate vaccine in a murine adoptive lymphocyte transfer model. Infect Immun 66:2026–2032, 1998.

174. van Essen D, Dullforce P, Brocker T, et al. Cellular interactions involved in Th cell memory. J Immunol 165:3640–3646, 2000.

175. Maruyama M, Lam KP, Rajewsky K. Memory B-cell persistence is independent of persisting immunizing antigen. Nature 407:636–642, 2000.

176. Herzenberg LA, Tokuhisa T. Epitope-specific regulation. I. Carrier-specific induction of suppression for IgG anti-hapten antibody responses. J Exp Med 155:1730–1740, 1982.

177. Renjifo X, Wolf S, Pastoret PP, et al. Carrier-induced, hapten-specific suppression: a problem of antigen presentation? J Immunol 161:702–706, 1998.

178. Fattom A, Cho YH, Chu C, et al. Epitopic overload at the site of injection may result in suppression of the immune response to combined capsular polysaccharide conjugate vaccines. Vaccine 17:126–133, 1999.

179. Dagan R, Eskola J, Leclerc C, et al. Reduced response to multiple vaccines sharing common protein epitopes that are administered simultaneously to infants. Infect Immun 66:2093–2098, 1998.

180. Vella PP, Marburg S, Staub JM, et al. Immunogenicity of conjugate vaccines consisting of pneumococcal capsular polysaccharide types 6B, 14, 19F, and 23F and a meningococcal outer membrane protein complex. Infect Immun 60:4977–4983, 1992.

181. Kuo J, Douglas M, Ree HK, et al. Characterization of a recombinant pneumolysin and its use as a protein carrier for pneumococcal type 18C conjugate vaccines. Infect Immun 63:2706–2713, 1995.

182. Test ST, Mitsuyoshi J, Connolly CC, et al. Increased immunogenicity and induction of class switching by conjugation of complement C3d to pneumococcal serotype 14 capsular polysaccharide. Infect Immun 69:3031–3040, 2001.

183. Ahmed F, Steinhoff MC, Rodriguez-Barradas MC, et al. Effect of human immunodeficiency virus type 1 infection on the antibody response to a glycoprotein conjugate pneumococcal vaccine: results from a randomized trial. J Infect Dis 173:83–90, 1996.

184. Powers DC, Anderson EL, Lottenbach K, et al. Reactogenicity and immunogenicity of a protein-conjugated pneumococcal oligosaccharide vaccine in older adults. J Infect Dis 173:1014–1018, 1996.

185. Lindberg AA. Glycoprotein conjugate vaccines. Vaccine 17(suppl):S28–S36, 1999.

186. Eby R. Modern approaches to new vaccines including prevention of AIDS. In Plotkin SA, Orenstein WA (eds). Vaccines (2nd ed). Philadelphia, WB Saunders, 1994, pp 119–124.

187. Schneerson R, Robbins JB, Parke JC Jr, et al. Quantitative and qualitative analyses of serum antibodies elicited in adults by Haemophilus influenzae type b and pneumococcus type 6A capsular polysaccharide-tetanus toxoid conjugates. Infect Immun 52:519–528, 1986.

188. Quataert SA, Kirch CS, Wiedl LJ, et al. Assignment of weight-based antibody units to a human antipneumococcal standard reference serum, lot 89-S. Clin Diagn Lab Immunol 2:590–597, 1995.

189. Schiffman G, Douglas RM, Bonner MJ, et al. A radioimmunoassay for immunologic phenomena in pneumococcal disease and for the antibody response to pneumococcal vaccines. I. Method for the radioimmunoassay of anticapsular antibodies and comparison with other techniques. J Immunol Methods 33:133–144, 1980.

189a. Pickering JW, Martins TB, Greer RW, et al. A multiplexed fluorescent microsphere immunoassay for antibodies to pneumococcal capsular polysaccharides. Am J Clin Pathol 117:589–596, 2002[DG4].

190. Plikaytis BD, Goldblatt D, Frasch CE, et al. An analytical model applied to a multicenter pneumococcal enzyme-linked immunosorbent assay study. J Clin Microbiol 38:2043–2050, 2000.

191. Soininen A, Seppälä I, Wuorimaa T, et al. Assignment of immunoglobulin G1 and G2 concentrations to pneumococcal capsular polysaccharides 3, 6B, 14, 19F, and 23F in pneumococcal reference serum 89-SF. Clin Diagn Lab Immunol 5:561–566, 1998.

192. Siber GR, Priehs C, Madore DV. Standardization of antibody assays for measuring the response to pneumococcal infection and immunization. Pediatr Infect Dis J 8(suppl):S84–S91, 1989.

193. Koskela M. Serum antibodies to pneumococcal C polysaccharide in children: response to acute pneumococcal otitis media or to vaccination. Pediatr Infect Dis J 6:519–526, 1987.

194. Concepcion NF, Frasch CE. Pneumococcal type 22F polysaccharide absorption improves the specificity of a pneumococcal-polysaccha-

ride enzyme-linked immunosorbent assay. Clin Diagn Lab Immunol 8:266–272, 2001.

195. Coughlin RT, White AC, Anderson CA, et al. Characterization of pneumococcal specific antibodies in healthy unvaccinated adults. Vaccine 16:1761–1767, 1998.

196. Yu X, Sun Y, Frasch C, et al. Pneumococcal capsular polysaccharide preparations may contain non-C-polysaccharide contaminants that are immunogenic. Clin Diagn Lab Immunol 6:519–524, 1999.

197. Gowans JL, Knight EJ. The route of re-circulation of lymphocytes in the rat. Proc R Soc (Ser B) 159:257–282, 1964.

198. Nieminen T, Eskola J, Käyhty H. Pneumococcal conjugate vaccination in adults: circulating antibody secreting cell response and humoral antibody responses in saliva and in serum. Vaccine 16:630–636, 1998.

199. Lue C, Prince SJ, Fattom A, et al. Antibody- secreting peripheral blood lymphocytes induced by immunization with a conjugate consisting of Streptococcus pneumoniae type 12F polysaccharide and diphtheria toxoid. Infect Immun 58:2547–2554, 1990.

200. Nieminen T, Käyhty H, Virolainen A, et al. Circulating antibody secreting cell response to parenteral pneumococcal vaccines as an indicator of a salivary IgA antibody response. Vaccine 16:313–319, 1998.

201. Lue C, van den Wall Bake AW, Prince SJ, et al. Intraperitoneal immunization of human subjects with tetanus toxoid induces specific antibody-secreting cells in the peritoneal cavity and in the circulation, but fails to elicit a secretory IgA response. Clin Exp Immunol 96:356–363, 1994.

202. Heilmann C, Pedersen FK. Quantitation of blood lymphocytes secreting antibodies to pneumococcal polysaccharides after in vivo antigenic stimulation. Scand J Immunol 23:189–194, 1986.

203. Griswold WR, Lucas AH, Bastian JF, et al. Functional affinity of antibody to the Haemophilus influenzae type b polysaccharide. J Infect Dis 159:1083–1087, 1989.

204. Anttila M, Eskola J, Åhman H, et al. Avidity of IgG for Streptococcus pneumoniae type 6B and 23F polysaccharides in infants primed with pneumococcal conjugates and boosted with polysaccharide or conjugate vaccines. J Infect Dis 177:1614–1621, 1998.

205. Devey ME, Bleasdale K, Lee S, et al. Determination of the functional affinity of IgG1 and IgG4 antibodies to tetanus toxoid by isotype-specific solid-phase assays. J Immunol Methods 106:119–125, 1988.

206. Feldman RG, Hamel ME, Breukels MA, et al. Solid-phase antigen density and avidity of antibodies detected in anti-group B streptococcal type III IgG enzyme immunoassays. J Immunol Methods 170:37–45, 1994.

207. Goldblatt D, van Etten L, van Milligen FJ, et al. The role of pH in modified ELISA procedures used for the estimation of functional antibody affinity. J Immunol Methods 166:281–285, 1993.

208. Goldblatt D. Simple solid phase assays for avidity. In Turner MW, Johnston AP (eds). Immunochemistry: A Practical Approach, 2nd ed. Oxford IRL Press at Oxford University Press 1997, pp 31–51.

209. Hedman K, Lappalainen M, Seppälä I, et al. Recent primary toxoplasma infection indicated by a low avidity of specific IgG. J Infect Dis 159:736–740, 1989.

210. Macdonald RA, Hosking CS, Jones CL. The measurement of relative antibody affinity by ELISA using thiocyanate elution. J Immunol Methods 106:191–194, 1988.

211. Pullen GR, Fitzgerald MG, Hosking CS. Antibody avidity determination by ELISA using thiocyanate elution. J Immunol Methods 86:83–87, 1986.

212. Goldblatt D, Vaz AR, Miller E. Antibody avidity as a surrogate marker of successful priming by Haemophilus influenzae type b conjugate vaccines following infant immunization. J Infect Dis 177:1112–1115, 1998.

213. Goldblatt D. Correlates of protection: role of memory. In Abstracts of the 3rd International Symposium on Pneumococci and Pneumococcal Diseases, Anchorage, May 5–8, 2002.

214. Esposito AL, Clark CA, Poirier WJ. An assessment of the factors contributing to the killing of type 3 Streptococcus pneumoniae by human polymorphonuclear leukocytes in vitro. APMIS 98:111–121, 1990.

215. Jansen WT, Gootjes J, Zelle M, et al. Use of highly encapsulated Streptococcus pneumoniae strains in a flow-cytometric assay for assessment of the phagocytic capacity of serotype-specific antibodies. Clin Diagn Lab Immunol 5:703–710, 1998.

216. Lortan JE, Kaniuk AS, Monteil MA. Relationship of in vitro phagocytosis of serotype 14 Streptococcus pneumoniae to specific class and

217. Martinez JE, Romero-Steiner S, Pilishvili T, et al. A flow cytometric opsonophagocytic assay for measurement of functional antibodies elicited after vaccination with the 23-valent pneumococcal polysaccharide vaccine. Clin Diagn Lab Immunol 6:581–586, 1999.

218. Romero-Steiner S, Libutti D, Pais LB, et al. Standardization of an opsonophagocytic assay for the measurement of functional antibody activity against Streptococcus pneumoniae using differentiated HL-60 cells. Clin Diagn Lab Immunol 4:415–422, 1997.

219. Vidarsson G, Sigurdardottir ST, Gudnason T, et al. Isotypes and opsonophagocytosis of pneumococcus type 6B antibodies elicited in infants and adults by an experimental pneumococcus type 6B-tetanus toxoid vaccine. Infect Immun 66:2866–2870, 1998.

220. Vidarsson G, Jonsdottir I, Jonsson S, et al. Opsonization and antibodies to capsular and cell wall polysaccharides of Streptococcus pneumoniae. J Infect Dis 170:592–599, 1994.

221. Väkeväinen M, Jansen W, Saeland E, et al. Are the opsonophagocytic activities of antibodies in infant sera measured by different pneumococcal phagocytosis assays comparable? Clin Diagn Lab Immunol 8:363–369, 2001.

222. Anttila M, Soininen A, Nieminen T, et al. Contribution of serotype specific IgG concentration, subclass ratio, and relative avidity to opsonophagocytic activity against Streptococcus pneumoniae. In Abstracts of the Pneumococcal Vaccines for the World 1998 Conference, Washington, DC, October 12–14, 1998.

223. Bardardottir E, Jonsson S, Jonsdottir I, et al. IgG subclass response and opsonization of Streptococcus pneumoniae after vaccination of healthy adults. J Infect Dis 162:482–488, 1990.

224. Johnson SE, Rubin L, Romero-Steiner S, et al. Correlation of opsonophagocytosis and passive protection assays using human anticapsular antibodies in an infant mouse model of bacteremia for Streptococcus pneumoniae. J Infect Dis 180:133–140, 1999.

225. Nahm MH, Olander JV, Magyarlaki M. Identification of cross-reactive antibodies with low opsonophagocytic activity for Streptococcus pneumoniae. J Infect Dis 176:698–703, 1997.

226. Anttila M, Voutilainen M, Jäntti V, et al. Contribution of serotype-specific IgG concentration, IgG subclasses and relative antibody avidity to opsonophagocytic activity against Streptococcus pneumoniae. Clin Exp Immunol 118:402–407, 1999.

227. Jokinen J, Åhman H, Kilpi T, et al. The concentration of anti-pneumococcal antibodies as a serological correlate of protection— a case study of acute otitis media. In Abstracts of the 3rd International Symposium on Pneumococci and Pneumococcal Diseases, Anchorage, May 5–8, 2002.

228. Soininen A, van den Dobbelsteen G, Oomen L, et al. Are the enzyme immunoassays for antibodies to pneumococcal capsular polysaccharides serotype specific? Clin Diagn Lab Immunol 7:468–476, 2000.

229. Saeland E, Vidarsson G, Jonsdottir I. Pneumococcal pneumonia and bacteremia model in mice for the analysis of protective antibodies. Microb Pathog 29:81–91, 2000.

230. Käyhty H, Åhman H, Rönnberg PR, et al. Pneumococcal polysaccharide-meningococcal outer membrane protein complex conjugate vaccine is immunogenic in infants and children. J Infect Dis 172:1273–1278, 1995.

231. Leach A, Ceesay SJ, Banya WA, et al. Pilot trial of a pentavalent pneumococcal polysaccharide/protein conjugate vaccine in Gambian infants. Pediatr Infect Dis J 15:333–339, 1996.

232. Åhman H, Käyhty H, Vuorela A, et al. Dose dependency of antibody response in infants and children to pneumococcal polysaccharides conjugated to tetanus toxoid. Vaccine 17:2726–2732, 1999.

233. Åhman H, Käyhty H, Lehtonen H, et al. Streptococcus pneumoniae capsular polysaccharide-diphtheria toxoid conjugate vaccine is immunogenic in early infancy and able to induce immunologic memory. Pediatr Infect Dis J 17:211–216, 1998.

234. O'Brien KL, Steinhoff MC, Edwards K, et al. Immunologic priming of young children by pneumococcal glycoprotein conjugate, but not polysaccharide, vaccines. Pediatr Infect Dis J 15:425–430, 1996.

235. Nurkka A, Åhman H, Korkeila M, et al. Serum and salivary anticapsular antibodies in infants and children immunized with the heptavalent pneumococcal conjugate vaccine. Pediatr Infect Dis J 20:25–33, 2001.

236. Obaro SK, Huo Z, Banya WA, et al. A glycoprotein pneumococcal conjugate vaccine primes for antibody responses to a pneumococcal polysaccharide vaccine in Gambian children. Pediatr Infect Dis J 16:1135–1140, 1997.

IgG subclass antibody levels in healthy adults. Clin Exp Immunol 91:54–57, 1993.

237. Dagan R, Melamed R, Zamir O, et al. Safety and immunogenicity of tetravalent pneumococcal vaccines containing 6B, 14, 19F, and 23F polysaccharides conjugated to either tetanus toxoid or diphtheria toxoid in young infants and their boosterability by native polysaccharide antigens. Pediatr Infect Dis J 16:1053–1059, 1997.

238. Anderson EL, Kennedy DJ, Geldmacher KM, et al. Immunogenicity of heptavalent pneumococcal conjugate vaccine in infants. J Pediatr 128:649–653, 1996.

239. Anttila M, Eskola J, Åhman H, et al. Differences in the avidity of antibodies evoked by four different pneumococcal conjugate vaccines in early childhood. Vaccine 17:1970–1977, 1999.

240. Prevnar™: Pneumococcal 7-valent Conjugate Vaccine (Diphtheria CRM$_{197}$ Protein) [package insert]. Pearl River, NY, Lederle Laboratories, 2000.

241. Mbelle N, Huebner RE, Wasas AD, et al. Immunogenicity and impact on nasopharyngeal carriage of a nonavalent pneumococcal conjugate vaccine. J Infect Dis 180:1171–1176, 1999.

242. Daum RS, Hogerman D, Rennels MB, et al. Infant immunization with pneumococcal CRM197 vaccines: effect of saccharide size on immunogenicity and interactions with simultaneously administered vaccines. J Infect Dis 176:445–455, 1997.

243. Herzenberg LA, Tokuhisa T, Herzenberg LA. Carrier-priming leads to hapten-specific suppression. Nature 285:664–667, 1980.

244. Insel RA. Potential alterations in immunogenicity by combining or simultaneously administering vaccine components. Ann N Y Acad Sci 754:35–47, 1995.

245. Shinefield HR, Black S, Ray P, et al. Safety and immunogenicity of heptavalent pneumococcal CRM197 conjugate vaccine in infants and toddlers. Pediatr Infect Dis J 18:757–763, 1999.

246. Choo S, Seymour L, Morris R, et al. Immunogenicity and reactogenicity of a pneumococcal conjugate vaccine administered combined with a Haemophilus influenzae type B conjugate vaccine in United Kingdom infants. Pediatr Infect Dis J 19:854–862, 2000.

247. Black S, Shinefield H, Fireman B, et al. Efficacy, safety and immunogenicity of heptavalent pneumococcal conjugate vaccine in children. Northern California Kaiser Permanente Vaccine Study Center Group. Pediatr Infect Dis J 19:187–195, 2000.

248. Shelly MA, Jacoby H, Riley GJ, et al. Comparison of pneumococcal polysaccharide and CRM197-conjugated pneumococcal oligosaccharide vaccines in young and elderly adults. Infect Immun 65:242–247, 1997.

249. Eskola J. Immunogenicity of pneumococcal conjugate vaccines. Pediatr Infect Dis J 19:388–393, 2000.

249a. Baxendale HE, Davis Z, White HN, et al. Immunogenetic analysis of the immune response to pneumococcal polysaccharide. Eur J Immunol 30:1214–1223, 2000.

250. Sorensen RU, Leiva LE, Giangrosso PA, et al. Response to a heptavalent conjugate Streptococcus pneumoniae vaccine in children with recurrent infections who are unresponsive to the polysaccharide vaccine. Pediatr Infect Dis J 17:685–691, 1998.

251. King JCJ, Vink PE, Farley JJ, et al. Safety and immunogenicity of three doses of a five-valent pneumococcal conjugate vaccine in children younger than two years with and without human immunodeficiency virus infection. Pediatrics 99:575–580, 1997.

252. King JCJ, Vink PE, Farley JJ, et al. Comparison of the safety and immunogenicity of a pneumococcal conjugate with a licensed polysaccharide vaccine in human immunodeficiency virus and non-human immunodeficiency virus-infected children. Pediatr Infect Dis J 15:192–196, 1996.

253. Kroon FP, Van Dissel JT, Ravensbergen E, et al. Enhanced antibody response to pneumococcal polysaccharide vaccine after prior immunization with conjugate pneumococcal vaccine in HIV-infected adults. Vaccine 19:886–894, 2001.

253a. Feikin DR, Elic CM, Goetz MB, et al. Randomized trial of the quantitative and functional antibody responses to a 7-valent pneumococcal conjugate vaccine and/or 23-valent polysaccharide vaccine among HIV infected adults. Vaccine 20:545–553, 2001.

254. Chan CY, Molrine DC, George S, et al. Pneumococcal conjugate vaccine primes for antibody responses to polysaccharide pneumococcal vaccine after treatment of Hodgkin's disease. J Infect Dis 173:256–258, 1996.

255. Korkeila M, Lehtonen H, Åhman H, et al. Salivary anti-capsular antibodies in infants and children immunised with Streptococcus pneumoniae capsular polysaccharides conjugated to diphtheria or tetanus toxoid. Vaccine 18:1218–1226, 2000.

256. Choo S, Zhang Q, Seymour L, et al. Primary and booster salivary antibody responses to a 7-valent pneumococcal conjugate vaccine in infants. J Infect Dis 182:1260–1263, 2000.

257. Trollmo C, Sollerman C, Carlsten H, et al. The gut as an inductive site for synovial and extra-articular immune responses in rheumatoid arthritis. Ann Rheum Dis 53:377–382, 1994.

258. Lue C, Tarkowski A, Mestecky J. Systemic immunization with pneumococcal polysaccharide vaccine induces a predominant IgA2 response of peripheral blood lymphocytes and increases of both serum and secretory anti-pneumococcal antibodies. J Immunol 140:3793–3800, 1988.

259. Tarkowski A, Lue C, Moldoveanu Z, et al. Immunization of humans with polysaccharide vaccines induces systemic, predominantly polymeric IgA2-subclass antibody responses. J Immunol 144:3770–3778, 1990.

260. Santosham M, Englund JA. Safety and antibody persistence following Haemophilus influenzae type b conjugate or pneumococcal polysaccharide vaccines given before pregnancy in women of childbearing age and their infants. Pediatr Infect Dis J 20:931–940, 2001.

261. Wuorimaa T, Käyhty H, Leroy O, et al. Tolerability and immunogenicity of an 11-valent pneumococcal conjugate vaccine in adults. Vaccine 19:1863–1869, 2001.

262. Soininen A, Seppälä I, Nieminen T, et al. IgG subclass distribution of antibodies after vaccination of adults with pneumococcal conjugate vaccines. Vaccine 17:1889–1897, 1999.

263. Rappuoli R. Conjugates and reverse vaccinology to eliminate bacterial meningitis. Vaccine 19:2319–2322, 2001.

263a. Wuorimaa T, Dagan R, Väkevainen M, et al. Avidity and subclasses of IgG after immunization of infants with an 11-valent pneumococcal conjugate vaccine with or without aluminum adjuvant. J Infect Dis 184:1211–1215, 2001.

264. Anttila M, Eskola J, Käyhty H. Opsonic activity and concentration of antibodies to Streptococcus pneumoniae type 6B polysaccharide. In Abstracts of the 35th Annual Meeting of the Infectious Diseases Society of America, San Francisco, CA, September 17–20, 1997.

265. Lu CH, Lee CJ, Kind P. Immune responses of young mice to pneumococcal type 9V polysaccharide-tetanus toxoid conjugate. Infect Immun 62:2754–2760, 1994.

266. Giebink GS, Koskela M, Vella PP, et al. Pneumococcal capsular polysaccharide-meningococcal outer membrane protein complex conjugate vaccines: immunogenicity and efficacy in experimental pneumococcal otitis media. J Infect Dis 167:347–355, 1993.

267. Pichichero ME, Porcelli S, Treanor J, et al. Serum antibody responses of weanling mice and two-year-old children to pneumococcal-type 6A-protein conjugate vaccines of differing saccharide chain lengths. Vaccine 16:83–91, 1998.

268. Laferriere CA, Sood RK, de Muys JM, et al. Streptococcus pneumoniae type 14 polysaccharide-conjugate vaccines: length stabilization of opsonophagocytic conformational polysaccharide epitopes. Infect Immun 66:2441–2446, 1998.

269. Steinhoff MC, Edwards K, Keyserling H, et al. A randomized comparison of three bivalent Streptococcus pneumoniae glycoprotein conjugate vaccines in young children: effect of polysaccharide size and linkage characteristics. Pediatr Infect Dis J 13:368–372, 1994.

270. Stein KE. Glycoconjugate vaccines: what next? Int J Technol Assess Health Care 10:167–176, 1994.

271. Mawas F, Feavers IM, Corbel MJ. Serotype of Streptococcus pneumoniae capsular polysaccharide can modify the Th1/Th2 cytokine profile and IgG subclass response to pneumococcal-CRM(197) conjugate vaccines in a murine model. Vaccine 19:1159–1166, 2000.

272. Nurkka A, Åhman H, Yaich M, et al. Serum and salivary anti-capsular antibodies in infants and children vaccinated with octavalent pneumococcal conjugate vaccines, PncD and PncT. Vaccine 20:194–201, 2001.

273. Åhman H, Käyhty H, Tamminen P, et al. Pentavalent pneumococcal oligosaccharide conjugate vaccine PncCRM is well-tolerated and able to induce an antibody response in infants. Pediatr Infect Dis J 15:134–139, 1996.

274. Peeters CC, Tenbergen-Meekes AM, Poolman JT, et al. Effect of carrier priming on immunogenicity of saccharide-protein conjugate vaccines. Infect Immun 59:3504–3510, 1991.

275. Granoff DM, Holmes SJ, Belshe RB, et al. Effect of carrier protein priming on antibody responses to Haemophilus influenzae type b conjugate vaccines in infants. JAMA 272:1116–1121, 1994.

276. Kurikka S. Priming with diphtheria-tetanus-pertussis vaccine enhances the response to the *Haemophilus influenzae* type b tetanus conjugate vaccine in infancy. Vaccine 14:1239–1242, 1996.

277. Barington T, Skettrup M, Juul L, et al. Non-epitope-specific suppression of the antibody response to *Haemophilus influenzae* type b conjugate vaccines by preimmunization with vaccine components. Infect Immun 61:432–438, 1993.

278. Barington T, Juul L, Gyhrs A, et al. Heavy-chain isotype patterns of human antibody-secreting cells induced by *Haemophilus influenzae* type b conjugate vaccines in relation to age and preimmunity. Infect Immun 62:3066–3074, 1994.

279. De Velasco EA, Dekker BAT, Verheul AFM, et al. Anti-polysaccharide immunoglobulin isotype levels and opsonic activity of antisera: relationships with protection against *Streptococcus pneumoniae* infection in mice. J Infect Dis 172:562–565, 1995.

280. Romero-Steiner S, Musher DM, Cetron MS, et al. Reduction in functional antibody activity against *Streptococcus pneumoniae* in vaccinated elderly individuals highly correlates with decreased IgG antibody avidity. Clin Infect Dis 29:281–288, 1999.

281. Robbins JB, Schneerson R, Szu SC. Perspective: Hypothesis: serum IgG antibody is sufficient to confer protection against infectious diseases by inactivating the inoculum. J Infect Dis 171:1387–1398, 1995.

282. Granoff DM, Lucas AH. Laboratory correlates of protection against *Haemophilus influenzae* type b disease: importance of assessment of antibody avidity and immunologic memory. Ann N Y Acad Sci 754:278–288, 1995.

283. Goldblatt D, Richmond P, Millard E, et al. The induction of immunologic memory after vaccination with *Haemophilus influenzae* type b conjugate and acellular pertussis-containing diphtheria, tetanus, and pertussis vaccine combination. J Infect Dis 180:538–541, 1999.

284. van der Ven LT, van den Dobbelsteen GP, Nagarajah B, et al. A new rat model of otitis media caused by *Streptococcus pneumoniae*: conditions and application in immunization protocols. Infect Immun 67:6098–6103, 1999.

285. Rodriguez ME, van den Dobbelsteen GP, Oomen LA, et al. Immunogenicity of *Streptococcus pneumoniae* type 6B and 14 polysaccharide-tetanus toxoid conjugates and the effect of uncoupled polysaccharide on the antigen-specific immune response. Vaccine 16:1941–1949, 1998.

286. Lee CJ, Lock RA, Andrew PW, et al. Protection of infant mice from challenge with *Streptococcus pneumoniae* type 19F by immunization with a type 19F polysaccharide–pneumolysoid conjugate. Vaccine 12:875–878, 1994.

287. Peeters CC, Tenbergen-Meekes AM, Poolman JT, et al. Immunogenicity of a *Streptococcus pneumoniae* type 4 polysaccharide–protein conjugate vaccine is decreased by admixture of high doses of free saccharide. Vaccine 10:833–840, 1992.

288. Paton JC, Lock RA, Lee CJ, et al. Purification and immunogenicity of genetically obtained pneumolysin toxoids and their conjugation to *Streptococcus pneumoniae* type 19F polysaccharide. Infect Immun 59:2297–2304, 1991.

289. Musher DM, Johnson B Jr, Watson DA. Quantitative relationship between anticapsular antibody measured by enzyme-linked immunosorbent assay or radioimmunoassay and protection of mice against challenge with *Streptococcus pneumoniae* serotype 4. Infect Immun 58:3871–3876, 1990.

290. Stack AM, Malley R, Thompson CM, et al. Minimum protective serum concentrations of pneumococcal anti-capsular antibodies in infant rats. J Infect Dis 177:986–990, 1998.

291. Saeland E, Jakobsen H, Ingolfsdottir G, et al. Serum samples from infants vaccinated with a pneumococcal conjugate vaccine, PncT, protect mice against invasive infection caused by *Streptococcus pneumoniae* serotypes 6A and 6B. J Infect Dis 183:253–260, 2001.

292. Madore DV, Strong N, Eby R. Use of animal testing for evaluating glycoconjugate vaccine immunogenicity. Dev Biol Stand 101:49–56, 1999.

293. Giebink GS. The pathogenesis of pneumococcal otitis media in chinchillas and the efficacy of vaccination in prophylaxis. Rev Infect Dis 3:342–353, 1981.

294. Malley R, Stack AM, Ferretti ML, et al. Anticapsular polysaccharide antibodies and nasopharyngeal colonization with *Streptococcus pneumoniae* in infant rats. J Infect Dis 178:878–882, 1998.

295. Kadioglu A, Gingles NA, Grattan K, et al. Host cellular immune response to pneumococcal lung infection in mice. Infect Immun 00.432 501, 2000.

296. Shinefield H, Black S, Ray P, et al. Efficacy, immunogenicity and safety of heptavalent pneumococcal conjugate vaccine in low birth weight and preterm infants. Pediatr Infect Dis J 21:182–186, 2002.

297. O'Brien KL, Moulton L, Reid RR, et al. Invasive disease efficacy of a 7-valent pneumococcal conjugate vaccine among Navajo and White Mountain Apache (N/WMA) children. *In* Abstracts of the 19th Meeting of the European Society for Paediatric Infectious Diseases, Istanbul, March 26–28, 2001.

298. Moulton LH, O'Brien KL, Kohberger R, et al. Design of a group-randomized *Streptococcus pneumoniae* vaccine trial. Control Clin Trials 22:438–452, 2001.

299. Black S, Shinefield H, Ling S, et al. Effectiveness of heptavalent pneumococcal conjugate vaccine in children younger than five years of age for prevention of pneumonia. Pediatr Infect Dis J 21:810–815, 2002.

299a. Berman. Otitis media in children. NEJM 332:1560–1565, 1995.

299b. Freid VM, Makuc DM, Rooks RN. Ambulatory health care visits by children: principal diagnosis and place of visits. Vital and Health Statistics. 13(137):1–23. Washington, DC, 1998.

300. Eskola J, Kilpi T, Palmu A, et al. Efficacy of a pneumococcal conjugate vaccine against acute otitis media. N Engl J Med 344:403–409, 2001.

301. Kilpi T, Palmu A, Leinomen M, et al. Efficacy of a seven-valent pneumococcal conjugate vaccine (PncOMPC) against serotype-specific acute otitis media (AOM) caused by streptococcus pneumaniae (Pnc). *In* Abstracts of the 40th ICAAC, Toronto, September, 2002.

302. Dagan R, Melamed R, Muallem M, et al. Reduction of nasopharyngeal carriage of pneumococci during the second year of life by a heptavalent conjugate pneumococcal vaccine. J Infect Dis 174:1271–1278, 1996.

303. Dagan R, Muallem M, Melamed R, et al. Reduction of pneumococcal nasopharyngeal carriage in early infancy after immunization with tetravalent pneumococcal vaccines conjugated to either tetanus toxoid or diphtheria toxoid. Pediatr Infect Dis J 16:1060–1064, 1997.

304. Dagan R, Givon-Lavi N, Zamir O, et al. Reduction of nasopharyngeal carriage of *Streptococcus pneumoniae* after administration of a 9-valent pneumococcal conjugate vaccine to toddlers attending day care centers. J Infect Dis 185:927–936, 2002.

305. Fraser D, Dagan R, Givon-Lavi N, et al. Density of nasopharyngeal colonization of vaccine-type and non-vaccine type pneumococci after administration of 9-valent CRM_{197} conjugate pneumococcal vaccine. *In* Abstracts of the 2nd International Symposium on Pneumococci and Pneumococcal Disease, Sun City, March 19–23, 2000.

306. Black SB, Shinefield HR, Hansen J, et al. Postlicensure evaluation of the effectiveness of seven valent pneumococcal conjugate vaccine. Pediatr Infect Dis J 20:1105–1107, 2001.

307. Blum MD, Dagan R, Mendelman PM, et al. A comparison of multiple regimens of pneumococcal polysaccharide-meningococcal outer membrane protein complex conjugate vaccine and pneumococcal polysaccharide vaccine in toddlers. Vaccine 18:2359–2367, 2000.

308. Obaro SK, Adegbola RA, Chang I, et al. Safety and immunogenicity of a nonavalent pneumococcal vaccine conjugated to CRM_{197} administered simultaneously but in a separate syringe with diphtheria, tetanus and pertussis vaccines in Gambian infants. Pediatr Infect Dis J 19:463–469, 2000.

309. Rennels MB, Edwards KM, Keyserling HL, et al. Safety and immunogenicity of heptavalent pneumococcal vaccine conjugated to CRM_{197} in United States infants. Pediatrics 101:604–611, 1998.

310. Zielen S, Buhring I, Strnad N, et al. Immunogenicity and tolerance of a 7-valent pneumococcal conjugate vaccine in nonresponders to the 23-valent pneumococcal vaccine. Infect Immun 68:1435–1440, 2000.

311. Wuorimaa T, Dagan R, Eskola J, et al. Tolerability and immunogenicity of an eleven-valent pneumococcal conjugate vaccine in healthy toddlers. Pediatr Infect Dis J 20:272–277, 2001.

312. Pichichero ME, Shelly MA, Treanor JJ. Evaluation of a pentavalent conjugated pneumococcal vaccine in toddlers. Pediatr Infect Dis J 16:72–74, 1997.

313. Giebink GS, Daly KA, Le CT, et al. Pneumococcal (Pnc) conjugate vaccine (PCV) as maternal and infant immunogens. *In* Abstracts of the 3rd International Symposium on Pneumococci and Pneumococcal Diseases, Anchorage, May 5–8, 2002.

314. American Academy of Pediatrics, Committee on Infectious Diseases. Policy statement: recommendations for the prevention of pneumococcal infections, including the use of pneumococcal conju-

gate vaccine (Prevnar), pneumococcal polysaccharide vaccine, and antibiotic prophylaxis. Pediatrics 106:362–366, 2000.

315. Watson DA, Musher DM, Verhoef J. Pneumococcal virulence factors and host immune responses to them. Eur J Clin Microbiol Infect Dis 14:479–490, 1995.

316. Gosink KK, Mann ER, Guglielmo C, et al. Role of novel choline binding proteins in virulence of *Streptococcus pneumoniae*. Infect Immun 68:5690–5695, 2000.

317. Overweg K, Kerr A, Sluijter M, et al. The putative proteinase maturation protein A of *Streptococcus pneumoniae* is a conserved surface protein with potential to elicit protective immune responses. Infect Immun 68:4180–4188, 2000.

318. Hollingshead SK, Briles DE. *Streptococcus pneumoniae*: new tools for an old pathogen. Curr Opin Microbiol 4:71–77, 2001.

319. Wizemann TM, Heinrichs JH, Adamou JE, et al. Use of a whole genome approach to identify vaccine molecules affording protection against *Streptococcus pneumoniae* infection. Infect Immun 69:1593–1598, 2001.

320. Adamou JE, Heinrichs JH, Erwin AL, et al. Identification and characterization of a novel family of pneumococcal proteins that are protective against sepsis. Infect Immun 69:949–958, 2001.

321. Briles DE, Creech TR, Swiatlo E, et al. Pneumococcal diversity: considerations for new vaccine strategies with emphasis on pneumococcal surface protein A (PspA). Clin Microbiol Rev 11:645–657, 1998.

322. Briles DE, Tart RC, Wu HY, et al. Systemic and mucosal protective immunity to pneumococcal surface protein A. Ann N Y Acad Sci 797:118–126, 1996.

323. McDaniel LS, Sheffield JS, Delucchi P, et al. PspA, a surface protein of *Streptococcus pneumoniae*, is capable of eliciting protection against pneumococci of more than one capsular type. Infect Immun 59:222–228, 1991.

324. Tart RC, McDaniel LS, Ralph BA, et al. Truncated *Streptococcus pneumoniae* PspA molecules elicit cross-protective immunity against pneumococcal challenge in mice. J Infect Dis 173:380–386, 1996.

325. Crain MJ, Waltman WD, Turner JS, et al. Pneumococcal surface protein A (PspA) is serologically highly variable and is expressed by all clinically important capsular serotypes of *Streptococcus pneumoniae*. Infect Immun 58:3293–3299, 1990.

326. Wu HY, Nahm MH, Guo Y, et al. Intranasal immunization of mice with PspA (pneumococcal surface protein A) can prevent intranasal carriage, pulmonary infection, and sepsis with *Streptococcus pneumoniae*. J Infect Dis 175:839–846, 1997.

327. Srivastava N, Zeiler JL, Smithson SL, et al. Selection of an immunogenic and protective epitope of the PsaA protein of *Streptococcus pneumoniae* using a phage display library. Hybridoma 19:23–31, 2000.

328. Talkington DF, Brown BG, Tharpe JA, et al. Protection of mice against fatal pneumococcal challenge by immunization with pneumococcal surface adhesin A (PsaA). Microb Pathog 21:17–22, 1996.

329. Briles DE, Ades E, Paton JC, et al. Intranasal immunization of mice with a mixture of the pneumococcal proteins PsaA and PspA is highly protective against nasopharyngeal carriage of *Streptococcus pneumoniae*. Infect Immun 68:796–800, 2000.

330. De BK, Sampson JS, Ades EW, et al. Baculovirus expression, purification and evaluation of recombinant pneumococcal surface adhesin A of *Streptococcus pneumoniae*. Pathobiology 67:115–122, 1999.

331. Alexander JE, Lock RA, Peeters CC, et al. Immunization of mice with pneumolysin toxoid confers a significant degree of protection against at least nine serotypes of *Streptococcus pneumoniae*. Infect Immun 62:5683–5688, 1994.

332. Paton JC, Lock RA, Hansman DJ. Effect of immunization with pneumolysin on survival time of mice challenged with *Streptococcus pneumoniae*. Infect Immun 40:548–552, 1983.

333. Lock RA, Hansman D, Paton JC. Comparative efficacy of autolysin and pneumolysin as immunogens protecting mice against infection by *Streptococcus pneumoniae*. Microb Pathog 12:137–143, 1992.

334. Simell B, Korkeila M, Pursiainen H, et al. Pneumococcal carriage and otitis media induce salivary antibodies to pneumococcal surface adhesin A, pneumolysin, and pneumococcal surface protein A in children. J Infect Dis 183:887–896, 2001.

335. Virolainen A, Russell W, Crain MJ, et al. Human antibodies to pneumococcal surface protein A in health and disease. Pediatr Infect Dis J 19:134–138, 2000.

336. Virolainen A, Jero J, Käyhty H, et al. Antibodies to pneumolysin and pneumococcal capsular polysaccharides in middle ear fluid of children with acute otitis media. Acta Otolaryngol 115:796–803, 2001.

337. Obaro SK, Adegbola RA, Tharpe JA, et al. Pneumococcal surface adhesin A antibody concentration in serum and nasopharyngeal carriage of *Streptococcus pneumoniae* in young African infants. Vaccine 19:411–412, 2000.

338. Virolainen A, Jero J, Chattopadhyay P, et al. Comparison of serum antibodies to pneumolysin with those to pneumococcal capsular polysaccharides in children with acute otitis media. Pediatr Infect Dis J 15:128–133, 1996.

339. Lindell E, Quiambo B, Mikkola E, et al. Serum antibodies to pneumococcal surface adhesin A (PsaA), pneumolysin (Ply) and pnemococcal surface protein A (PspA), in Filipino pregnant women and their offspring. *In* Abstracts of the 41st Interscience Conference on Antimicrobial Agents and Chemotherapy, Chicago, September 22–25, 2001.

340. Käyhty H, Mikkola E, Quiambo B, et al. Serum antibodies to pneumococcal (Pnc) surface adhesin A (PsaA) in Filipino pregnant women and their offspring. *In* Abstracts of the 2nd World Congress of Pediatric Infectious Diseases, Manila, November 2–6, 1999.

341. Rapola S, Kilpi T, Lahdenkari M, et al. Antibody response to the pneumococcal proteins pneumococcal surface adhesin A and pneumolysin in children with acute otitis media. Pediatr Infect Dis J 20:482–487, 2001.

342. Yamamoto M, McDaniel LS, Kawabata K, et al. Oral immunization with PspA elicits protective humoral immunity against *Streptococcus pneumoniae* infection. Infect Immun 65:640–644, 1997.

343. Briles DE, King JD, Gray MA, et al. PspA, a protection-eliciting pneumococcal protein: immunogenicity of isolated native PspA in mice. Vaccine 14:858–867, 1996.

344. Berry AM, Paton JC. Sequence heterogeneity of PsaA, a 37-kilodalton putative adhesin essential for virulence of *Streptococcus pneumoniae*. Infect Immun 64:5255–5262, 1996.

345. Brooks-Walter A, Hollingshead S, Briles D. PspA and its sister molecule, PspC, both show potential eliciting wide-spread immunity to pneumococcal infection. *In* Abstracts of the 2nd International Symposium on Pneumococci and Pneumococcal Disease, Sun City, March 19–23, 2000.

346. Hollingshead S, Nabors GS, Braun P, et al. Vaccines based on pneumococcal proteins. *In* Abstracts of the 2nd International Symposium on Pneumococci and Pneumococcal Disease, Sun City, March 19–23, 2000.

347. Nabors GS, Braun PA, Herrmann DJ, et al. Immunization of healthy adults with a single recombinant pneumococcal surface protein A (PspA) variant stimulates broadly cross-reactive antibodies to heterologous PspA molecules. Vaccine 18:1743–1754, 2000.

348. Wischnack LL, Jacobson RM, Poland GA, et al. The surprisingly high acceptability of low-efficacy vaccines for otitis media: a survey of parents using hypothetical scenarios. Pediatrics 95:350–354, 1995.

349. Paton JC, Andrew PW, Boulnois GJ, et al. Molecular analysis of the pathogenicity of *Streptococcus pneumoniae*: the role of pneumococcal proteins. Annu Rev Microbiol 47:89–115, 1993.

350. Briles DE, Hollingshead S, Brooks-Walter A, et al. The potential to use PspA and other pneumococcal proteins to elicit protection against pneumococcal infection. Vaccine 18:1707–1711, 2000.

351. Ogunniyi AD, Folland RL, Briles DE, et al. Immunization of mice with combinations of pneumococcal virulence proteins elicits enhanced protection against challenge with *Streptococcus pneumoniae*. Infect Immun 68:3028–3033, 2000.

352. Spratt BG, Greenwood BM. Prevention of pneumococcal disease by vaccination: does serotype replacement matter? Lancet 356:1210–1211, 2000.

353. Moxon ER. Natural history and pathogenesis as they affect clinical trials. Dev Biol Stand 95:61–67, 1998.

354. Lipsitch M. Interpreting results from trials of pneumococcal conjugate vaccines: a statistical test for detecting vaccine-induced increases in carriage of nonvaccine serotypes. Am J Epidemiol 154:85–92, 2001.

355. Lipsitch M, Dykes JK, Johnson SE, et al. Competition among *Streptococcus pneumoniae* for intranasal colonization in a mouse model. Vaccine 18:2895–2901, 2000.

356. Lipsitch M. Bacterial vaccines and serotype replacement: lessons from *Haemophilus influenzae* and prospects for *Streptococcus pneumoniae*. Emerg Infect Dis 5:336–345, 1999.

357. Lipsitch M. Vaccination against colonizing bacteria with multiple serotypes. Proc Natl Acad Sci U S A 94:6571–6576, 1997.

358. Takala AK, Eskola J, Leinonen M, et al. Reduction of oropharyngeal carriage of *Haemophilus influenzae* type b (Hib) in children immunized with an Hib conjugate vaccine. J Infect Dis 164:982–986, 1991.

359. Takala AK, Santosham M, Almeido-Hill J, et al. Vaccination with *Haemophilus influenzae* type b meningococcal protein conjugate vaccine reduces oropharyngeal carriage of *Haemophilus influenzae* type b among American Indian children. Pediatr Infect Dis J 12:593–599, 1993.

360. Mohle-Boetani JC, Ajello G, Breneman E, et al. Carriage of *Haemophilus influenzae* type b in children after widespread vaccination with conjugate *Haemophilus influenzae* type b vaccines. Pediatr Infect Dis J 12:589–593, 1993.

361. Barbour ML, Booy R, Crook DW, et al. *Haemophilus influenzae* type b carriage and immunity four years after receiving the *Haemophilus influenzae* oligosaccharide-CRM$_{197}$ (HbOC) conjugate vaccine. Pediatr Infect Dis J 12:478–484, 1993.

362. Adegbola RA, Mulholland EK, Secka O, et al. Vaccination with a *Haemophilus influenzae* type b conjugate vaccine reduces oropharyngeal carriage of *H. influenzae* type b among Gambian children. J Infect Dis 177:1758–1761, 1998.

363. Dagan R, Fraser D. Conjugate pneumococcal vaccine and antibiotic-resistant *Streptococcus pneumoniae*: herd immunity and reduction of otitis morbidity. Pediatr Infect Dis J 19(suppl):S79–S87, 2000.

364. Lieu TA, Ray GT, Black SB, et al. Projected cost-effectiveness of pneumococcal conjugate vaccination of healthy infants and young children. JAMA 283:1460–1468, 2000.

365. Capra AM, Lieu TA, Black SB, et al. Costs of otitis media in a managed care population. Pediatr Infect Dis J 19:354–355, 2000.

366. Jacobs RJ, Meyerhoff AS. Comparative cost effectiveness of varicella, hepatitis A, and pneumococcal conjugate vaccines. Prev Med 33:639–645, 2001.

367. Shahid NS, Steinhoff MC, Hoque SS, et al. Serum, breast milk, and infant antibody after maternal immunisation with pneumococcal vaccine. Lancet 346:1252–1257, 1995.

368. Hajek DM, Quartey M, Giebink GS. Maternal pneumococcal conjugate immunization protects infant chinchillas in the pneumococcal otitis media model. Acta Otolaryngol 122:262–269, 2002.

369. Kayhty H, Ahman H. Bridging phase 2 and phase 3 pneumococcal immunologic data for future combination vaccines. Clin Inf Dis 33(Suppl 4):S292–S298, 2001.

Chapter 24

Poliovirus Vaccine—Inactivated

STANLEY A. PLOTKIN • EMMANUEL VIDOR*

Historical Introduction

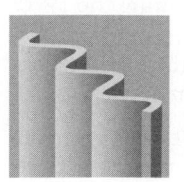

Not since the introduction of rabies vaccine by Louis Pasteur was public interest in vaccines stirred as much as by the development and testing of inactivated poliovirus vaccine (IPV), and not since Einstein did a scientist receive the public adulation accorded to Jonas Salk, the vaccine's inventor. Contributing to this phenomenon were the rise of poliomyelitis as an epidemic disease, its notoriety with the public (augmented by the paralysis suffered by President Franklin Roosevelt), the publicity diffused by the March of Dimes Foundation in its efforts to raise money for research, and the involvement of hundreds of thousands of U.S. children in the field trial that demonstrated the efficacy of IPV.

The efficacy trial was organized by Dr. Thomas Francis of the University of Michigan and sponsored by the National Foundation for Infantile Paralysis. It was a hallmark in vaccine science and the prototype for many later efficacy trials.[1] Francis insisted on a double-blind protocol, with only partial success. Of 217 study areas in 44 states, only 90 followed a placebo-controlled protocol, but they involved 419,000 vaccinees and 330,000 placebo recipients. Unblinded observations were also made on more than 1,000,000 children, 232,000 of whom were vaccinated. The trial began in April 1954, and the successful results were announced on April 12, 1955.[2] Licensure followed rapidly, with broad vaccination of American children.

Nevertheless, in the early 1960s, IPV was eclipsed by oral poliovirus vaccine (OPV), except in some northern European countries. More recent changes in public health conditions, the accelerating disappearance of poliomyelitis as an epidemic disease, and both sporadic and epidemic cases of paralysis caused by the attenuated OPV have restored interest in IPV. An increasing number of countries have adopted its use, and more are likely to do so.

The disease itself is ancient. A famous Egyptian stele dating from 1580 to 1350 BC shows a man with flaccid paralysis of a leg. However, presumably owing to almost universal infection under the protection of maternal antibodies, only sporadic cases were described (perhaps

including that of Sir Walter Scott) until the 19th century. Early in that century, small outbreaks were noted, usually among infants living in rural areas. In 1870, Jean-Martin Charcot described the pathologic lesions in the gray matter of the spinal cord, and in 1890 Oscar Medin described a major outbreak in Sweden, where epidemics subsequently continued to occur. Epidemics were reported in the United States at the end of the century, and in 1916 thousands of children were paralyzed during an epidemic in the northeastern United States. Fortunately, in 1908 Karl Landsteiner and Eric Popper isolated the virus of poliomyelitis in monkeys, and scientific study of the agent began.[3]

The key scientific discoveries that led to IPV were as follows:

1. Definition of the three serotypes of poliovirus by David Bodian and colleagues[4]
2. Determination that polio viremia precedes paralysis[5]
3. Confirmation that neutralizing antibodies protect against disease[6]
4. Demonstration by John Enders and colleagues that the virus could be grown in cell culture[7]

These discoveries permitted Salk, fresh from his success in developing an inactivated influenza vaccine and also experienced in working with poliovirus, to start efforts at vaccine development. Large quantities of virus were grown in roller tubes of monkey testicular and kidney cells, and the kinetics of inactivation by formalin were studied. Salk concluded that if aggregates of virus were removed by filtration, poliovirus could be inactivated at a constant first-order rate, permitting complete killing if the process was of sufficient duration. Pools of trivalent vaccine were prepared at Connaught Laboratories in Toronto for use in a field trial of efficacy, which was conducted by Thomas Francis and his associates in 1954. The trial decisively demonstrated that IPV was protective, and in 1955 IPV was licensed in the United States.[8]

Years later, two major developments improved the quality of IPV. The first was the invention by Anton Van Wezel in Holland of techniques to select the best sources of

---

*Contributing to this chapter in prior editions were Jonas Salk, Jacques Drucker, Denis Malvy, and Andrew Murdin.

monkey kidney cells, to grow the cells to high density on microbeads, and concentrate the virus produced.[9] The second development was the adaptation of the Vero continuous African green monkey kidney cell line to the production of poliovirus by Bernard Montagnon at the Institut Mérieux (now Aventis Pasteur) of Lyon, France.[10] The result of these improvements was the enhanced-potency IPV, which is the subject of this chapter.

Licensure of IPV was the first result of the cell culture revolution that permitted the development of many other vaccines. At the time of licensure, more than 20,000 cases of polio were reported annually in the United States. Polio was a worldwide disease with an incidence in the tropics that was as great as that in the developed world but was unrecognized owing to the concentration of cases in infants younger than 2 years.[11-12] The description of poliomyelitis as a disease, in addition to its virology, pathogenesis, and epidemiology, is covered in Chapter 25.

Passive Immunization

A field trial using human γ-globulin verified the importance of viremia in the pathogenesis of the disease poliomyelitis and proved the concept that antibodies were protective. This field experience, conducted in 1952 by Hammon and colleagues,[6] involved more than 54,000 children, half of whom received γ-globulin and half of whom received injections of gelatin. From the second to the eighth week after injection, paralytic poliomyelitis was reduced about 80%. Unfortunately, despite the large dose used in the study (0.3 mL/kg), the protection proved temporary (8 weeks), rendering γ-globulin administration impractical as a public health strategy except in household contacts.

Maternally produced antibodies transmitted via the placenta are also protective, but their half-life is only 21 days. By 6 months of age few unvaccinated infants are protected.[13]

Active Immunization

Prior Approaches to Inactivated Poliovirus Vaccines

Before the work of Salk, two disastrous attempts were made in the 1930s to inactivate poliovirus in monkey spinal cord for the purposes of vaccination. Formalin was used by Brodie and Park,[14] whereas Kolmer[15] used ricinoleate. Both attempts failed because of inadequate inactivation and probably also inadequate immunogenicity. The occurrence of polio cases probably caused by the vaccines terminated their development, and instilled a sense of caution.

Description of Inactivated Poliovirus Vaccine

IPV is a mixture of the three polioviruses made by harvesting cell culture supernatants and submitting them to inactivation by formalin. The first version of IPV was produced in primary rhesus monkey kidney cell culture, with all the problems of finding healthy monkeys and of excluding simian viruses that might be latent or replicating actively in cultured cells. The poliovirus strains used by Salk and still used by most manufacturers are Mahoney (Salk type 1; Brunenders is used in Sweden and Denmark); MEF1 (Salk type 2); and Saukett (Salk type 3). The final vaccine mixture is adjusted to achieve the right concentration of antigens (see below). Attempts have been made recently to produce IPV from the three Sabin strains. This appears to be possible; however, the immunogenicity of the Sabin type 2 virus is much reduced compared with the MEF1, and the antigenicity of the Sabin type 3 strain is reduced compared with Saukett.[16]

Although the results of the field trial of efficacy were dramatically positive (described under *Efficacy of Inactivated Poliovirus Vaccine* below), the Cutter incident (described under *Adverse Events* below) led to a change in manufacturing processes that lowered the immunogenicity of the vaccine.[17] The occurrence of paralytic polio in vaccinated children during the early 1960s weakened confidence in IPV.[18] However, several technical advances during the 1970s permitted the development of an enhanced-potency IPV that, although based on principles similar to those of the first-generation vaccine, differs in three important aspects:

1. The cell substrate on which the virulent seed viruses are inoculated is either secondary or tertiary subcultures of kidneys from pathogen-free monkeys, human diploid cell strains, or the Vero African green monkey kidney cell line, rather than primary cultures from newly captured monkeys.
2. To increase density, cells are grown on microbeads in large fermenters.
3. The virus harvest is concentrated before inactivation to increase the final antigen content.

The production of enhanced-potency IPV in Vero cells is outlined in Figure 24–1.[19-21] The substrate cell culture is expanded by cell division of the working cell bank (at about passage 137) adapted to grow on microcarrier beads (Fig. 24–2) in large vessels until a density of about 1.5×10^{12} cells (corresponding to about passage 142) is reached in each 1000-L fermenter (Fig. 24–3). Growth medium is then removed, the cells are washed, and one of the three types of poliovirus is inoculated. By 72 to 96 hours of incubation at 37°C, the cells have been lysed by viral replication, and the supernatant fluids are collected. After clarification through a 0.2-μm filter, the virus is concentrated 500-fold by ultrafiltration. To remove cellular proteins and DNA, the concentrated virus is passed through column chromatography to yield 15 L of purified material. At this point, there is less than 10 pg of DNA in the material, a level considered to pose no hazard to recipients.[22]

The concentrated, purified virus is inactivated by the addition of formalin to a final concentration of 1:4000, followed by incubation at 37°C for 12 days. By 4 days viral inactivation should be almost complete, as confirmed by sampling for residual live virus. During inactivation of the virus, it is important to avoid viral clumping and to maintain a neutral pH. An extra filtration is included during inactivation to remove viral clumps.[23]

The final monovalent material is subjected to tests for residual infectivity, which of course must be negative. The three monovalent lots are then mixed to form the trivalent enhanced-potency IPV. Concentrations of the three vaccine types are adjusted by determination of the poliovirus D antigen (which is expressed only on intact poliovirus

Expansion of cell culture seeds by passage on microbeads to reach density of 10^{12} cells per 1000-L fermenter

↓

Inoculation of seed virus (types 1, 2, or 3)

↓

Incubation at 37°C for 3 to 4 days

↓

Harvest 1000 L supernatant

↓

Filter for clarification

↓

Concentrate to 2 L by ultrafiltration

↓

Purify by column chromatography to volume of 15 L

↓

Filter for sterility

↓

Dilution in medium 199 and new filtration

↓

Inactivate with 1/4000 formalin for 6 days at 37°C

↓

Filter again for elimination of clumps

↓

On days 9 and 12, sample for control*

↓

Combine with other serotypes for trivalent vaccine; adjust antigen concentration*

FIGURE 24–1 ■ Production of enhanced-potency inactivated poliovirus vaccine. *Sampling of an equivalent of at least 1500 human doses for control of effective inactivation.

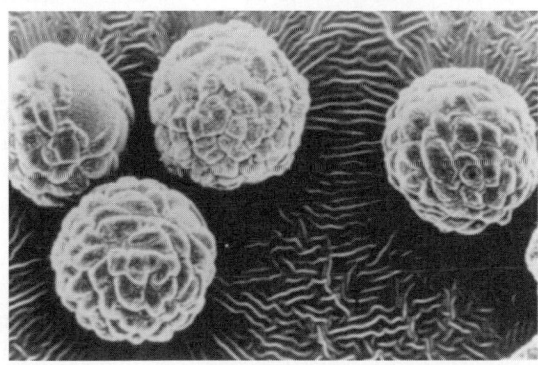

FIGURE 24–2 ■ Kidney cells from monkeys (Vero) growing on microcarrier beads in cultivation. (Courtesy of Dr. B. Montagnon, Institut Mérieux, Lyon.)

particles) using gel diffusion or enzyme-linked immunosorbent assays. The final formula in D units is 40 of type 1, 8 of type 2, and 32 of type 3. The original IPV used in the United States had contained 20 units of type 1, 2 units of type 2, and 4 units of type 3.

Formalin inactivation does modify some of the epitopes of the virus, particularly the antigenic site 1 of viral types 2 and 3.[24] Although this modification has little effect on the overall neutralizing antibody response, it does alter the specificity of that response, which may have some epidemiologic effect (see section on Finland under *Public Health Considerations* below).

Producers

Table 24–1 lists the manufacturers of enhanced-potency IPV, which are principally based in Europe. The enhanced-

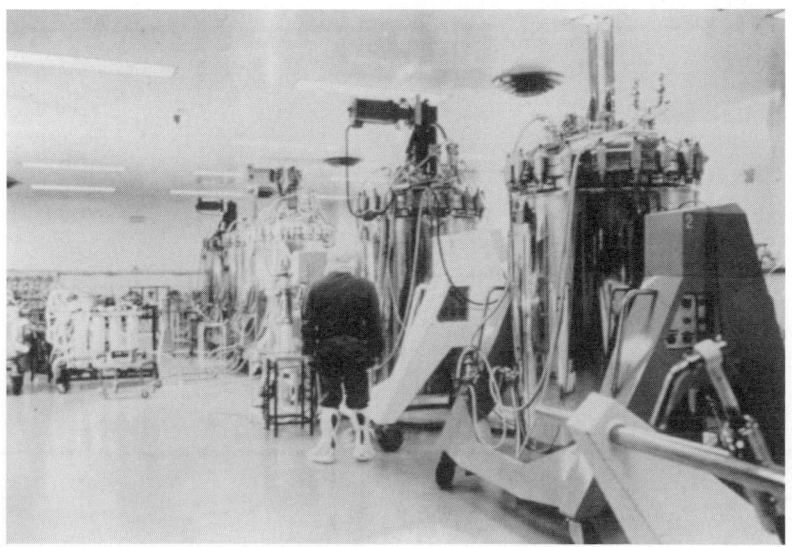

FIGURE 24–3 ■ Tanks of 1000-L capacity in which cells are grown for virus cultivation. (Courtesy of Dr. B. Montagnon, Institut Mérieux, Lyon.)

TABLE 24–1 ■ Manufacturers of IPV

Manufacturer	Where Made	Cell Substrate
Aventis Pasteur*	France, Canada	Vero, MRC-5
Chiron-Behring	Italy	Vero
GlaxoSmithKline*	Belgium	Vero
National Biological Laboratory (S.B.L.)	Sweden	Vero
Rijks Institute	The Netherlands	Vero
Statens Seruminstitut	Denmark	Rhesus monkey kidney†

*Current U.S. manufacturers.
†Recently switched to Vero.

potency IPV predominantly used in the United States is produced in Vero cells by Aventis Pasteur. The only other cell substrate in use for IPV production is human diploid cell strains. Because all IPV now in use is of enhanced potency, the chapter hereafter uses the designation IPV to refer to enhanced-potency IPV vaccines. Current production capacity is estimated at about 80 million doses per year, although expansion of capacity is underway.

Dosage and Route

Salk established that the immune response to polio vaccine was directly related to the dose of viral antigen (Table 24–2).[25] Recommended dosage for IPV given as a primary vaccination in adults is three doses (0.5 mL/dose). The first two doses can be given 1 or preferably 2 months apart, with the third dose given 6 to 12 months later. If there is urgency, the third dose can be given earlier, but the immune response will not be as good. IPV may be inoculated either subcutaneously or intramuscularly; however, when given in combination with other antigens such as diphtheria, tetanus, and pertussis (DTP) or hepatitis B, the vaccine should be administered by the intramuscular route only.

When IPV is used for primary vaccination of infants, the schedule is two or three doses during the first 6 months of life, followed by a booster during the second year of life and another booster before school entry. Two doses are sufficient as priming for the booster in the second year, but, when IPV is included in combination vaccines with DTP, convenience may dictate using three doses. In any case, the first two doses should be followed by a third dose at least 6 months later.[26] In the United States, infants immunized with IPV alone receive doses at ages 2 months, 4 months, 6 to 18 months, and 4 to 6 years. In France, the first three doses are given earlier at 2, 3, and 4 months of age, whereas in Scandinavia the schedule is spread out, with only two doses before 1 year of age. The schedules used in various countries are shown in Table 24–3. The issue of additional boosters after the preschool dose is considered later (see under *Duration of Immunity* below).

Few data are available on the primary immunization of seronegative adults. However, indications are that three doses should be given on a schedule of 0, 1, and 6 months. Adults who are already seropositive need only one booster dose to develop high titers (Aventis Pasteur, unpublished data).

Available Preparations

Three IPVs are currently licensed in the United States: produced in France, Canada, and Belgium. The French and Belgian vaccines are produced in Vero cell culture, whereas

TABLE 24–2 ■ Comparative Estimation of Type 1 Immune Status: Detectable Serum Antibody Versus Secondary-type Responsiveness

No. of Subjects*	Primary Dose†	% of Group with Detectable Antibody (≥1:4)		% of Group with Secondary-type Antibody Response (≥1:32)‡ 2 Weeks After Booster Doses§
		2 Weeks After One Dose	1 Year After Two Doses	
33	None	—	—	6
24	2	100	92	100
21	1	100	85	100
26	1/2	96	60	96
27	1/4	93	73	100
30	1/8	87	45	93
26	1/16	77	35	96

*In the group evaluated 2 weeks after booster dose.
†Milliliters of reference vaccine A given in each of two doses 2 weeks apart.
‡Antibody titer of 1:32 arbitrarily chosen as criterion for hyperreactive secondary-type antibody response.
§One milliliter of vaccine J.
From Salk J, Salk D. Vaccination against poliomyelitis. *In* Voller A, Friedman H (eds). New Trends and Developments in Vaccines. Lancashire, England, MTP Press, 1978, pp 117–154, with permission.

TABLE 24-3 ■ Administration Schedules of IPV

Vaccines	Schedules
Children	
United States	2 mo, 4 mo, 6–18 mo, 4–6 yr
	2 mo, 4 mo, 6 mo, 12–18 mo*
Canada	2 mo, 4 mo, 6 mo, 12–18 mo, 4–6 yr
France	2 mo, 3 mo, 4 mo, 12–18 mo, 6 yr,
	11 yr, 16 yr
Sweden	3 mo, 5 mo, 12 mo, 6 yr
Netherlands	3 mo, 4 mo, 5 mo, 12 mo, 4 yr, 9 yr
Adults in all countries	0, 1–2, and 6–12 mo

*Permissible with combination vaccines, and may be recommended for IPV alone in the future.

the Canadian vaccine is produced in MRC-5 human diploid cell culture.

In the United States IPV is available in its monovalent form, and very recently in a combination with diphtheria, tetanus, acellular pertussis and hepatitis B vaccines. However, in Canada, Europe, and elsewhere, IPV is administered in combination with diphtheria, tetanus, and acellular pertussis (DTaP) and *Haemophilus influenzae* type b (Hib). Hexavalent combinations that also contain hepatitis B vaccine are now available in Europe and the rest of the world excluding North America. A combination of whole-cell DTP and IPV is also available. These combinations are produced principally by Aventis Pasteur and GlaxoSmithKline.

Worldwide, the market for vaccines containing IPV is dominated by those two large companies, but other smaller manufacturers are likely to expand their production (see Table 24–1). Table 24–7 and Figure 24–6 (see *Combination Vaccines Containing Inactivated Poliovirus Vaccine* below) present data obtained with IPV produced in MRC-5 cells in the course of studies of combination vaccines. After three doses at 2, 4, and 6 months of age, excellent responses were seen, which were markedly augmented after a booster dose at 18 months. Additional data on the MRC-5–produced IPV are provided in Table 24–8 (see *Combination Vaccines Containing Inactivated Poliovirus Vaccine* below), which also contains information on IPV produced in primary monkey kidney cells.

Vaccine Constituents Other Than Immunizing Antigens

With regard to the vaccines produced in Vero cell culture, streptomycin, neomycin, and polymyxin B are used during the manufacturing process to control bacterial contamination but are largely eliminated during production. Test results for these antibiotics in the final product are negative, but trace amounts (<200 ng of streptomycin, <5 ng of neomycin, and <25 ng of polymyxin B) may still be present. Preservation is conferred by residual formalin (0.02%) and 2-phenoxyethanol (0.5%), which are sufficient to maintain sterility. Thimerosal has never been used to preserve polio vaccines because it destroys the polio antigens.

The MRC-5–produced vaccine contains trace amounts of streptomycin and neomycin as well as formalin (27 ppm), 2-phenoxyethanol (0.5%), human albumin (0.5%), and Tween 80 (20 ppm).

Stability

In contrast to OPV, IPV is relatively heat stable. The vaccine is stable for 4 years at 4°C and for 1 month at 25°C. At 37°C, there is significant loss of potency of the type 1 component after 1 to 2 days, and of types 2 and 3 after 2 weeks.[27] Freezing diminishes the in vitro potency of IPV and should be avoided.[28]

Results of Vaccination

Immune Responses

Although it is possible to measure serum antibodies to poliovirus by a variety of methods, neutralizing antibodies are considered to correlate with protection, and only these are considered here.

IPV is a classical killed antigen vaccine. Immune responses depend on the concentration of antigens, the number of doses, the interval between doses, and the suppressive response of antibodies already present. Either two or three doses have been administered during the first year of life. When two doses were given, it was usually at 2 and 4 months of age. Data collected from 30 studies of IPV-containing vaccines involving more than 4500 subjects are summarized in Table 24–4. Seroresponse ranged from 89% to 100% for poliovirus type 1, from 92% to 100% for poliovirus type 2, and from 70% to 100% for poliovirus type 3. Table 24–4 also summarizes responses after three doses. Responses after three doses are clearly better than after two, particularly when the schedule is 2-4-6 months. However, schedules of 3-4-5 and 2-3-4 months also give good responses, though lower than after 2-4-6. After two or three doses in the first year, antibody levels fall subsequently, although the vaccinees usually retain a positive titer and a

TABLE 24-4 ■ Summary of Immunogenicity of IPV after Two or Three Doses in the First Year of Life

	One Month After Last Vaccination							
	Type 1		Type 2		Type 3		Study	Approximate
Schedule	Seropositives	GMT	Seropositives	GMT	Seropositives	GMT	Groups	No. Subjects
2-4 mo	89–100%	17–355	92–100%	17–709	70–100%	50–1200	30	4500
2-4, 12-18 mo	94–100%	495–2629	98–100%	1518–6637	97–100%	1256–4332	10	2000
2-4-6 mo	96–100%	143–2459	96–100%	78–2597	95–100%	187–3010	48	6000
3-4-5 mo	85–100%	110–475	98–100%	92–944	86–100%	89–1244	8	500
2-3-4 mo	93–100%	143–595	89–100%	91–561	95–100%	221–1493	18	2200
6-10-14 wk	66–99%	49–535	63–99%	68–571	91–100%	90–731	8	840

GMT, geometric mean antibody titer.

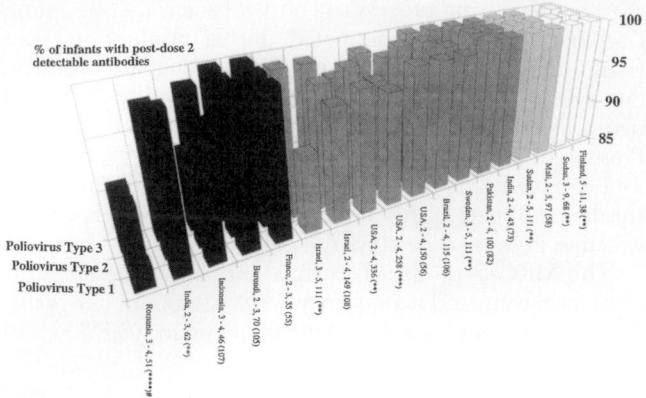

FIGURE 24–4 ■ Immunogenicity of Vero cell–produced vaccines containing enhanced-potency inactivated poliovirus vaccine administered in two doses during the first year of life. The country, age at vaccination, and number of infants enrolled at the beginning of the study are shown; reference numbers in parentheses refer to the original publication. (From Vidor E, Meschievitz C, Plotkin S. Fifteen years of experience with Vero-produced enhanced potency inactivated poliovirus vaccine. Pediatr Infect Dis J 16:312–322, 1997, with permission.)

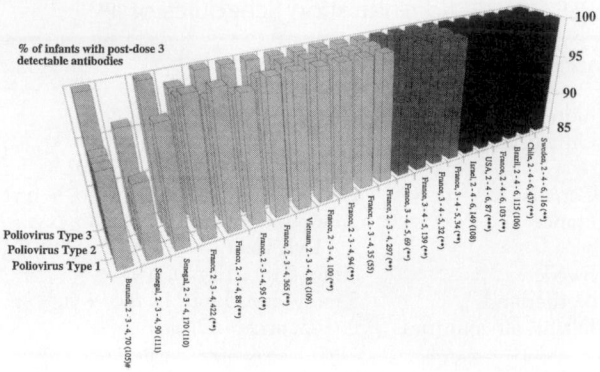

FIGURE 24–5 ■ Immunogenicity of Vero cell–produced vaccines containing enhanced-potency inactivated poliovirus vaccine administered in three doses during the first year of life. The country, age at vaccination, and number of infants enrolled at the beginning of the study are shown; reference numbers in parentheses refer to the original publication. (From Vidor E, Meschievitz C, Plotkin S. Fifteen years of experience with Vero-produced enhanced potency inactivated poliovirus vaccine. Pediatr Infect Dis J 16:312–322, 1997, with permission.)

third or fourth injection in the second year of life gives a marked anamnestic response.

Figure 24–4 and Table 24–5 present data on the neutralizing antibody responses after two or three doses of Vero cell–produced IPV.[29-34] The studies represented in Figure 24–4 were conducted in a wide range of geographic locations, including tropical countries, with a range of schedules starting at 2 to 5 months of age. More than 85% of infants responded to all three serotypes, and in many cases the percent seroconversion was close to 100. Five more recent studies conducted in the United States are presented in Table 24–5, along with titer values and percent seropositivity. In the U.S. studies, nearly all infants were already seropositive after the second dose, although their titers were generally below 1:100. The data in Figure 24–4 also show that, in terms of immunogenicity, an interval of 2 months between the first two doses is preferable to an interval of 1 month, as is the case for other vaccine antigens in infants.

Figure 24–5 presents the findings of 22 studies in which titers were measured after three doses of IPV. Virtually all infants are seropositive to the three polioviruses. The U.S. data in Table 24–5 confirm this point and show that the geometric mean titers after three doses are well over 1:100. In the U.S. trials, the third dose of IPV was given either at 6 months of age or in the second year of life. In the former case, titers were between 1:100 and 1:1000, whereas, when the third dose was administered after a longer interval, titers rose to more than 1:1000.

Effect of Maternal Antibodies and Neonatal Vaccination

Many studies have documented that high levels of maternally transmitted poliovirus antibodies do diminish the height of antibody response to a full IPV schedule.[35-43] This effect can be corrected by giving three doses of IPV during the first year of life, or by giving a booster late in the first year of life or during the second year of life.

Swartz and colleagues[44] showed that a single dose of IPV at birth primed infants to a uniform response to a second dose given at age 6 months. Israeli infants who were immunized at birth with IPV concomitant with hepatitis B vaccine showed higher mean antibody levels for polio types 2 and 3 at 1 and 3 months of age than infants who received IPV at 2 months of age, but the difference disappeared at 7 months of age after both groups had received one additional dose of IPV and two doses of OPV.[39] However, Hovi et al.[45] did show priming for higher titers in Pakistani infants whose three OPV doses at 8, 12, and 16 weeks of age were supplemented by a birth dose of IPV. Thus IPV at birth appears to prime the immune system, but this strategy has not been tried in public health practice.

Combination Vaccines Containing Inactivated Poliovirus Vaccine

IPV has been combined with DTP, DTaP, hepatitis B, and Hib vaccines without major effect on its immunogenicity,[28,46-49] and those combinations are now widely used in countries outside the United States (Table 24–6). Table 24–7 gives the results of vaccination with three different combinations produced by different manufacturers[50-53] (see also Chapter 21).

Table 24–8 and Figure 24–6 present data obtained with IPV produced in MRC-5 cells in the course of studies of combination vaccines. After three doses at 2, 4, and 6 months of age, excellent responses were seen, which were markedly augmented after a booster dose at 18 months. Additional data on the MRC-5–produced IPV are provided in Table 24–9, which also contains information on IPV produced in primary monkey kidney cells.

Inactivated Poliovirus Vaccine in the Expanded Program on Immunization Schedule

To achieve rapid immunization in developing countries with high rates of endemic infections, vaccines are given on a 6-10-14–week schedule, which is clearly not optimal for immune response, due to the short interval between doses

TABLE 24–5 ■ U.S. Studies with the Vero Cell–Produced IPV Given Alone or in Mixed IPV/OPV Sequential Schedules

Investigators and Reference	No.*	Vaccine Administered at Given Age				% of Neutralizing Antibody to Indicated Strain ≥1/8 (Geometric Mean Titer)											
		2 Months	4 Months	6 Months	Booster 12–18 Months	After Second Dose			After Third Dose†			Before Booster			After Booster‡		
						Type 1	Type 2	Type 3	Type 1	Type 2	Type 3	Type 1	Type 2	Type 3	Type 1	Type 2	Type 3
Faden et al.[29]	116	IPV	IPV	IPV	IPV	96 (184)	100 (631)	96 (634)				90 (61)	96 (135)	92 (102)	96 (1954)	100 (5835)	100 (5187)
	34	IPV	IPV	IPV	OPV	100 (283)	100 (481)	100 (1132)				100 (128)	100 (334)	93 (151)	100 (3044)	100 (10,693)	100 (2347)
	94	IPV	IPV	IPV	IPV	97 (44)	96 (105)	95 (83)				92 (22)	65 (42)	87 (23)	100 (2070)	100 (3419)	100 (1968)
Blatter and Starr[34]	68	IPV	IPV	IPV	IPV	98 (88)	100 (256)	98 (162)				100 (41)	100 (71)	93 (35)	100 (2029)	100 (4388)	100 (2580)
	75	IPV	IPV	IPV	OPV	94 (28)	98 (91)	96 (63)				85 (18)	96 (47)	81 (20)	100 (1568)	100 (7199)	96 (297)
	99	IPV	IPV	IPV	OPV	99 (90)	99 (120)	95 (126)				98 (47)	96 (61)	88 (29)	100 (1765)	100 (7516)	99 (709)
Halsey et al.[33]	87	IPV	IPV	IPV	OPV	97 (74)	98 (82)	100 (110)	100 (463)	100 (652)	100 (605)	100 (72)	100 (98)	100 (91)	100 (2141)	100 (7169)	100 (1824)
McBean et al.[30]	331	IPV	IPV		IPV	99	99	99							99	100	100
	332	IPV	IPV		IPV	99	100	100							100	100	100
Modlin et al.[31]	101	IPV	IPV		IPV	97	92	78							100	100	100

*Number of enrolled subjects at beginning of study.

†In infancy.

‡Booster is third or fourth dose, depending on the schedule.

IPV, inactivated poliovirus vaccine; OPV, live oral poliovirus vaccine.

631

TABLE 24–6 ▪ IPV-Containing Combinations for Infants

Manufacturer	Other Valences in Combination	Trade Name	Where Licensed*
Aventis Pasteur	DTP	Tetracoq	EU, LA, AA
	DTP/Hib	Pentacoq	EU, LA, AA
	DTaP	Tetravac	EU, LA, AA
	DTaP5	Quadracel	CA, LA, AA
	DTaP/Hib	Pentavac	EU, LA, AA
	DTaP5/Hib	Pentacel	CA, LA, AA
	DTaP/Hib/HBV	Hexavac	EU, AA
GlaxoSmithKline	DT	DT-Polio	EU
	DTaP	Infanrix IPV	CA, EU, LA, AA
	DTaP/Hib	Infanrix IPV Hib	EU, LA, AA
	DTaP/HBV	Infanrix PeNta†	EU, AA, US
	DTaP/HBV/Hib	Infanrix Hexa	EU, LA, AA
Statens Serum Inst. (Baxter)	DTaP	Certib-IPV	EU
	DTaP/Hib	DiTeKi Pol/Act-Hib	EU

*AA, Asia and Africa; CA, Canada; EU, Europe; LA, Latin America; US, United States.
†Called Pediarix in the U.S.
DTaP, diphtheria, tetanus, and acellular pertussis vaccine; DTP, diphtheria, tetanus, and whole-cell pertussis vaccine; HBV, hepatitis B vaccine; Hib, *Haemophilus influenzae* type b vaccine.

TABLE 24–7 ▪ Post–Primary Series Geometric Mean Antibody Titer (GMT) and Percentages of Subjects with Poliovirus Neutralizing Antibodies (NA) After Primary Series Performed with Quadrivalent, Pentavalent, and Hexavalent Combination IPV-Containing Vaccines

Country, Date (Reference) Schedule	Poliovirus Antibodies* Post–Dose 3					
	Type 1		Type 2		Type 3	
France, 1996–1997 (52) 2-4-6 months of age	7 MONTHS OF AGE					
N	334 (1)	333 (2)	334 (1)	333 (2)	334 (1)	333 (2)
GMT	470	343	505	315	846	707
% with NA ≥ 1:5	100%	100%	100%	100%	100%	100%
Moldavia, 1998 (53) 6-10-14 weeks of age	18 WEEKS OF AGE					
N	144 (3)	150 (4)	144 (3)	150 (4)	144 (3)	150 (4)
GMT	170	535	97.9	154	544.1	731
% with NA ≥ 1:8	99.3%	98.7%	97.2%	98.0%	100%	98.7%
Sweden, 1999 (51) 3-5 months of age	6 MONTHS OF AGE					
N	178 (5)	178 (6)	178 (5)	178 (6)	178 (5)	178 (6)
GMT	621	774	1097	1190	499	668
% with NA ≥ 1:4	99.5%	100%	100%	100%	99.5%	100%
USA, 2001 (188) 2-4-6 months of age	7 MONTHS OF AGE					
N	86–91 (7)		86–91 (7)		86–91 (7)	
GMT	415		514		1729	
% with NA ≥ 18:	100%		99%		100%	

*Vaccines used (manufacturer):
1: DTaP/IPV/HBV/PRP-T fully liquid vaccine (Aventis Pasteur/Merck)
2: DTaP/IPV vaccine (Aventis Pasteur) reconstituting lyophilized PRP-T vaccine (Aventis Pasteur)
3: DTaP/HBV/IPV vaccine (GlaxoSmithKline)
4: DTP/IPV vaccine (Aventis Pasteur) reconstituting lyophilized PRP-T vaccine (Aventis Pasteur)
5: DTaP/IPV vaccine (Statens Serum Institute/North American Vaccine Inc.) reconstituting lyophilized PRP-T vaccine (Aventis Pasteur)
6: DTaP/IPV vaccine (Statens Serum Institute/North American Vaccine Inc.)
7: DTaP/IPV/HBV vaccine (GlaxoSmithKline)
DTaP, diphtheria, tetanus, and acellular pertussis vaccine; DTP, diphtheria, tetanus, and whole-cell pertussis vaccine; HBV, hepatitis B vaccine; IPV, inactivated poliovirus vaccine; PRP-T, *Haemophilus* b conjugate vaccine.

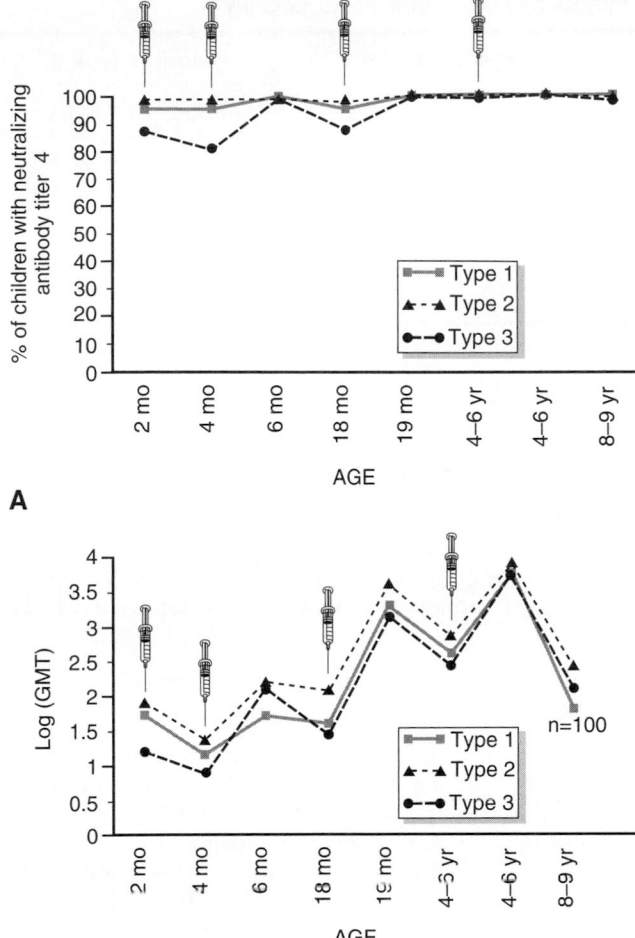

A

B

FIGURE 24–6 ■ Eight- to 9-year follow-up study of poliovirus-neutralizing antibodies in children immunized with MRC-5–produced inactivated polio vaccine. Vaccinees received a two-dose primary series at 2 and 4 months of age and booster vaccinations at 18 months and 4 to 6 years of age (indicated by the syringe symbol). A, Percentage of children with a neutralizing antibody titer of 4 or greater. B, Natural logarithm of the geometric mean antibody titer (GMT). The number of sera (n) tested at each time is shown. (Reprinted from Murdin A, Barreto L, Plotkin S. Inactivated poliovirus vaccine: past and present experience. Vaccine 14:735–746, 1996, with permission from Elsevier Science.)

and the higher levels of maternal antibodies at early ages. In a study sponsored by the World Health Organization (WHO),[54] three doses of IPV were given to infants in Oman and Thailand. Whereas 90% to 96% of the Omani infants responded to the three serotypes, the Thai infants showed seroconversion rates of only 67% and 65% to types 1 and 2, respectively. The low responses in Thailand were attributed to high maternal antibody titers (as shown in Fig. 24–7), the onset of vaccination at 6 weeks of age, and an interval of 1 rather than 2 months between doses.[42,55] The results of eight studies in which IPV was given by the Expanded Programme on Immunisation (EPI) schedule are given in Table 24–10.[40,41,53,56–59] Taken overall, the data support the utility of IPV even with an early schedule, although the results are less satisfactory than with more extended schedules. In evaluating these results, the rela-

tively low "take rate" of OPV in routine immunization of infants in tropical countries should be taken into account. The persistence of poliovirus antibodies after the EPI schedule and the effect of boosters have not yet been documented.

Immunogenicity of Sequential Schedule of Inactivated and Oral Poliovirus Vaccines

For several years, the United States used a schedule of mixed IPV/OPV vaccination, in which two doses of IPV were administered at 2 and 4 months of age, followed by two doses of OPV administered at 6 to 18 months of age and again at school entry. Table 24–5 provides data on the excellent immunogenicity of this schedule. Israel and Denmark also use a mixed schedule, with successful induction of immune responses and protection. The Israeli experience is large because of concern regarding circulation of live virus. Two schedules have been used: IPV at 2, 4, 6, and 12 months of age, with OPV at 7 and 13 months of age; or IPV at 2, 4, and 12 months plus OPV at 4, 6, and 12 months.[60] A study in the United Kingdom showed the advantages of a mixed schedule in terms of immunogenicity.[61]

A particular use of mixed schedules was undertaken in Romania because of an unusually high rate of vaccine-associated paralytic poliomyelitis (VAPP) owing to concurrent intramuscular injections.[62] Infants in one province of Romania received IPV at 2, 3, and 4 months of age, together with OPV at 4 and 9 months of age.[63] The schedule was well tolerated and highly immunogenic. No cases of polio occurred subsequently in this region, but too few children were involved to draw conclusions about the prevention of VAPP.

The WHO study mentioned previously[54] compared four doses of OPV, three doses of IPV, and a mixed schedule consisting of four doses of OPV and three doses of IPV. The

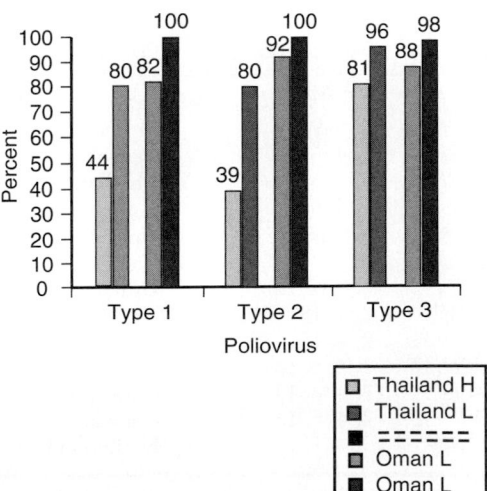

FIGURE 24–7 ■ Seroconversion to poliovirus types 1, 2, and 3 after three IPV doses (24 weeks), by maternal antibody (H ≥ 64, L < 64), in Thailand and Oman. (WHO Collaborative Study Group on Oral and Inactivated Poliovirus Vaccines. J Infect Dis 175(suppl 1):S215–S227, 1997, with permission.)

TABLE 24–8 ■ Poliovirus Neutralizing Antibody Responses in Infants to MRC-5 Cell–Produced IPV*

Time of Administration (mo)	Type of Vaccine	No. of Subjects	Poliovirus Type 1		Poliovirus Type 2		Poliovirus Type 3	
			% Antibody ≥4[†]	GMT[‡]	% Antibody ≥4	GMT	% Antibody ≥4	GMT
7	Combined	211	100	252	99.5	222	100	919
	Separate	211	100	282	99.5	209	100	1024
18	Combined	188	94	47	88	34.2	98	109
	Separate	188	95	44	90	35.7	98	121
19	Combined	189	100	4961	100.0	4289	100	5180
	Separate	187	100	4686	100.0	4907	100	4572

*Vaccine given at 7, 18, and 19 months of age after a three-dose primary series at 2, 4, and 6 months of age and a booster at 18 months of age with DPT/IPV and PRP-T given combined or simultaneously at separate sites.
[†]Percentage of children with a poliovirus-neutralizing antibody titer of ≥4.
[‡]Geometric mean titer of poliovirus-neutralizing antibodies.
DPT, diphtheria, pertussis, and tetanus; IPV, inactivated poliovirus vaccine; GMT, geometric mean titer; PRP-T, *Haemophilus* b conjugate vaccine.
From Murdin A, Barreto L, Plotkin S. Inactivated poliovirus vaccine: past and present experience. Vaccine 14:735–746, 1996, with permission.

vaccines were administered to infants in Oman, The Gambia, and Thailand. Seroconversion rates and geometric mean titers were highest in the mixed OPV/IPV group. In addition, when children of the three groups were challenged with another dose of OPV, virus excretion was as low in the mixed vaccine group as in the OPV group, confirming the presence of mucosal immunity.

Another mixed schedule was tested in the Ivory Coast, with the objective of correcting deficiencies in response to OPV in tropical settings.[64] A single dose of IPV or OPV was given after three doses of OPV. Of those 9-month-old children who remained seronegative after the third dose of OPV, 81%, 100%, and 67% seroconverted to types 1, 2,

and 3 polio, respectively, after the IPV booster. The corresponding percentages for an OPV booster were 14, 27, and 5.

Immunogenicity in the Immunocompromised Patient

Because IPV is indicated for immunocompromised people even in countries that recommend OPV, the immunogenicity of IPV in these patients is an important issue.

Prematurity does not appear to reduce the response to IPV when the vaccine is given at the usual postnatal age[65,66] unless the infants are chronically ill.[67] However, vaccination of full-term infants at birth results in lower immune

TABLE 24–9 ■ Neutralization Antibody Responses to Non–Vero Cell–Produced IPVs*

IPV Used[†]	Age at Vaccination (mo)	Country	No. of Subjects[‡]	% Positive for Neutralizing Antibodies to Indicated Strain								
				After Second Dose			After Third Dose			Before Fourth Dose		
				Type 1	Type 2	Type 3	Type 1	Type 2	Type 3	Type 1	Type 2	Type 3
PMKC 40/8/32	1.5, 10 or 2.5, 5, 11	India	114	97	88	97						
PMKC 40/8/32	3, 8–9, 14	Burkina Faso	179	94	99	78						
PMKC 40/8/32	2, 4, 6	Kenya	84	94	88	97	100	98	100			
PMKC 40/8/32	2, 4, 6	Thailand	94	100	99	97	100	100	100			
MRC-5 40/8/32	2, 4, 6	Canada	120	90	99	97	99	100	100			
MRC-5 40/8/32	2.4, 15	United States	279	92	94	74	81	92	53	99	100	100
PMKC 40/4/16	2, 3.5, 10	Israel	115	100	97	100	97	95	96	100	100	100
MRC-5 40/8/32	2.4, 18	United States	377	99	100	99	98	99	99	100	100	100
PMKC 40/4/16	2, 4, 18	United States	371	99	99	99	99	99	98	99	100	100
MRC-5 40/8/32	2, 4, 18	Canada	329	99	99	99	98	95	97	87	99	100
MRC-5 40/8/32	2, 4, 6, 18	Canada	443	94	97	96	99	99	99	100	100	100
MRC-5 40/8/32	2, 4, 6, 18	Canada	211	NA	NA	NA	NA	100	99	100	94	88
MRC-5 40/8/32	2, 4, 6, 18	Canada	211	NA	NA	NA	100	99	100	95	90	98
PMKC 40/4/8	3, 4, 5, 18	Netherlands	118	NA	NA	NA	97	95	94	100	99	96

*Two or three doses of IPV were administered during the first year of life, with or without a booster dose during the second year of life.
[†]Cell substrate and poliovirus D antigen formulation of the used vaccine.
[‡]Number of subjects enrolled at beginning of study.
IPV, inactivated poliovirus vaccine; MRC-5, Medical Research Council strain 5 of human diploid fibroblasts; NA, data not available or analysis not performed; PMKC, primary monkey kidney culture.
From Vidor E, Meschiewitz C, Plotkin S. Fifteen years of experience with Vero-produced enhanced potency inactivated poliovirus vaccine. Pediatr Infect Dis J 16:312–322, 1997, with permission.

TABLE 24–10 ■ Geometric Mean Antibody Titer (GMT) and Percentages of Subjects with Poliovirus Neutralizing Antibodies (NA) after IPV Vaccines Given at 6, 10, and 14 Weeks of Age

Country, Date (Reference)*	Pre–Dose 1			Post–Dose 3		
	Type 1	Type 2	Type 3	Type 1	Type 2	Type 3
India, 1989 (56)	6 wk; N = 106–107			18 wk; N = 49–54		
GMT	38.9	53.0	16.2	239	204	309
% with NA ≥ 1:5	_____NA_____			_____NA_____		
Oman, 1990–1992 (40, 41)	24 wk; N = 161–169					
GMT	NA			447	571	251
% with NA ≥ 1:8				88%	92%	91%
Gambia, 1990–1991 (40)				24 wk; N = 87–105		
GMT	NA			79	144	241
% with NA ≥ 1:8				81%	82%	98%
Thailand, 1991–1992 (40)				24 wk; N = 92–134		
GMT	NA			49	68	136
% with NA ≥ 1:8				66%	63%	92%
India, 1995–1996 (57)				18 wk; N = 39 (1)		
GMT	NA			120	125	90
% with NA ≥ 1:4				90%	80%	98%
Moldavia, 1998 (53)				18 wk		
N	NA			144(2) 150(3)	144(2) 150(3) 144(2)	150(3)
GMT				170 535	98 154 544	731
% with NA ≥ 1:8				99.3% 98.7%	97.2% 98.0% 100%	98.7%
South Africa, 1998 (58)	6 wk; N = 119 (2)			18 wk; N = 119 (2)		
GMT	20.3	23.1	16.0	116	93	166
% with NA ≥ 1:8	63.1%	73.0%	46.7%	99.2%	99.2%	99.2%
Philippines, 1999 (59)	6 wk; N = 65 (4)			18 wk; N = 65 (4)		
GMT	34.5	36.4	13.5	863	768	901
% with NA ≥ 1:8	81.5%	81.5%	76.9%	100%	100%	100%

*Vaccines used:

India 1989: DTP/IPV (Tetracoq®, Aventis Pasteur)

Oman/Gambia/Thailand 1990–1992: DTP/IPV (Tetracoq®, Aventis Pasteur)

India 1995–1996: IPV (Imovax polio®, Aventis Pasteur)

Moldavia 1998: DTaP/HBV/IPV (GlaxoSmithKline) and PRP-T (GlaxoSmithKline) versus DTP/IPV/PRP-T Pentacoq®, Aventis Pasteur) and HBV (Engerix-B®, GlaxoSmithKline)

South Africa 1998: DTP/IPV/PRP-T (Pentacoq®, Aventis Pasteur)

Philippines 1999: DTaP/IPV/PRP-T (Pediacel®, Aventis Pasteur)

†Method of vaccination:

1: Intradermal administration of 0.1 mL of IPV concomitantly with DTP at a separate site.

2: Vaccination with DTP/IPV reconstituting lyophilized PRP-T vaccine.

3: Vaccination with DTaP/HBV/IPV vaccine.

4: Vaccination with DTaP/IPV/PRP-T fully liquid vaccine.

DTaP, diphtheria, tetanus, and acellular pertussis vaccine; DTP, diphtheria, tetanus, and whole-cell pertussis vaccine; HBV, hepatitis B vaccine; IPV, inactivated poliovirus vaccine; PRP-T, *Haemophilus* b conjugate vaccine.

responses than does vaccination later in life, presumably because maternal antibody levels are higher in newborns.[66,68]

Children infected with human immunodeficiency virus (HIV) who were given two doses of IPV in early infancy responded reasonably well, probably because their immune systems were largely intact.[69] In hemophilic adults, however, HIV seropositivity had a negative effect on titer levels after IPV, although all adults responded to some degree.[70] Chronic renal dialysis patients also seroconverted in 90% or more of cases.[71] In patients who had undergone a bone marrow transplantation and were reimmunized after transplantation, vaccination was usually successful in inducing antibodies, although at least two and often three doses were needed.[72,73]

Secretory Immunoglobulin A Responses and Local Immunity

In general, the secretory immunoglobulin A (IgA) response to IPV is not as high as is the response to OPV. Many of the data come from the laboratory of Ogra, who found that about 90% of IPV recipients showed poliovirus-specific secretory IgA, compared with 100% of OPV recipients.[48,74–76] Moreover, titers were on average three to four times higher in the OPV vaccinees than in the IPV recipients. Local and systemic antibody responses after three doses of IPV, OPV, or a mixed schedule are shown in Table 24–11.[48] One study conducted in another laboratory showed equal secretory IgA levels in pharyngeal and stool samples of prior IPV and OPV vaccinees, suggesting that the titers equalize after a time.[77]

Significant secretory IgA responses to IPV were shown in the breast milk of Pakistani mothers. Both premature and full-term infants developed nasopharyngeal IgA anti-polio antibody after immunization in about 90% of cases.[78] Hovi[36] has studied IgA production in the intestine of IPV vaccinees, but found little IgA until the vaccinees had been challenged with OPV. A correlation was found between the detection of intestinal IgA and diminution of virus excretion.

Effect of Inactivated Poliovirus Vaccine on Poliovirus Excretion

Early in the history of IPV, it was shown that IPV vaccinees could excrete poliovirus after challenge,[79–82] which was considered an important disadvantage in relation to OPV. Time has shown that the difference is not between black and white but between two shades of gray. Studies in monkeys demonstrated that pharyngeal excretion of poliovirus was inhibited in IPV vaccinees.[83–85] Marine and colleagues followed families exposed to a natural type 1 outbreak and found that pharyngeal infection was prevented by low levels of neutralizing antibodies, whereas higher levels reduced intestinal infection (Table 24–12).[86] In a more recent study by Onorato and colleagues, children who had received three doses of IPV or OPV were challenged with two different doses of type 1 OPV.[77] The results (summarized in Table 24–13) reveal that, whereas few subjects in either group excreted virus from the pharynx, intestinal infection occurred in both groups but was lower in the OPV group. The persistence of local immunity has not been well studied, but there is evidence that resistance to reinfection wanes and that protection ultimately depends on the level of serum antibodies.[87,88] Two challenge studies have been accomplished using type 3. In one, 93% of IPV-vaccinated infants excreted type 3 after challenge with 300,000 median tissue culture infective doses ($TCID_{50}$), but there was no control group.[89] However, in the other study, a challenge with 600,000 $TCID_{50}$ induced only 5% to 10% excretion in infants who received either OPV alone or mixed IPV and OPV.[90] In the Finnish study, the median length of

poliovirus excretion in IPV vaccinees was 35 to 42 days, and the peak virus titers were $10^{5.6}$ $TCID_{50}$ per gram.[36] The issue of gastrointestinal immunity after IPV is discussed in more detail elsewhere.[28,87]

Studies have examined the effect of IPV on the mutation of OPV strains in the intestinal tract.[91–93] This phenomenon, referred to as *reversion to virulence*, is a regular feature of the replication of attenuated strains, whereby the mutations in those strains responsible for attenuation in humans revert to the virulent genotype. Although the suggestion has been made that prior IPV immunization potentiates that reversion,[94,95] a relatively large study failed to show a significant difference in the mutation of excreted virus between the IPV and OPV groups.[96]

Efficacy of Inactivated Poliovirus Vaccine

The efficacy of IPV in its original version was proved beyond a doubt in the original field trial conducted by Thomas Francis.[97] In that trial, approximately 400,000 children randomly received vaccine or placebo, and another 200,000 were vaccinated and observed together with unvaccinated children. There were 71 cases of paralytic polio in vaccinees versus 445 in control subjects. In the placebo-controlled part of the study, 70 cases occurred in the placebo arm versus 11 in the vaccinated arm.[97] The calculated efficacy of the vaccine was 80% to 90% against paralytic polio and 60% to 70% against all forms of polio.

The efficacy of IPV was later confirmed in several settings. Melnick and colleagues calculated an efficacy of 96%

TABLE 24–12 ■ Percent Excretion of Wild Poliovirus Type 1 in Children According to Level of Vaccine-Induced Serum Neutralizing Antibody

Antibody titer	% Excretion at Given Time After Infection			
	1–2 Weeks		3–4 Weeks,	5–6 Weeks,
	P	S	S	S
<8	75	93	82	60
8–64	38	97	81	54
>64	25	88	59	28

P, pharynx sample; S, stool sample.
Data from Vidor et al.[28] and Marine et al.[86]

TABLE 24–11 ■ Levels of Serum Neutralizing or Nasopharyngeal Immunoglobulin A Antibodies in Children After Three Doses of IPV, OPV, or a Combined Schedule

	OPV-OPV-OPV			IPV-IPV-IPV			IPV-IPV-OPV		
	Type 1	Type 2	Type 3	Type 1	Type 2	Type 3	Type 1	Type 2	Type 3
Serum neutralizing antibodies									
% Positive	100	100	100	96	100	100	100	100	100
GMT	1470	3578	1522	1954	5835	5187	3044	10,693	2348
Nasopharyngeal secretory immunoglobulin A antibodies									
% Positive	100	100	100	89	91	89	75	81	81
GMT	69	97	128	24	25	31	19	22	23

GMT, geometric mean titer; IPV, inactivated poliovirus vaccine; OPV, oral poliovirus vaccine.
From Faden H, Modlin J, Thoms M, et al. Comparative evaluation of immunization with live attenuated and enhanced-potency inactivated trivalent poliovirus vaccines in childhood: systemic and local immune responses. J Infect Dis 162;1291–1297, 1990, with permission.

TABLE 24–13 ■ Isolation of Poliovirus from Stool or Pharynx of Prior Recipients of IPV or OPV After Challenge with Type 1 OPV

Challenge Dose	No. of Pharyngeal Isolations (%)		No. of Stool Isolations (%)	
	IPV	OPV	IPV	OPV
High (5,000,000 TCID$_{50}$)	1/45 (2)	3/45 (7)	37/45 (82)	14/45 (31)
Low (500 TCID$_{50}$)	0/48 (0)	0/34 (0)	22/48 (46)	6/34 (18)
Total	1/93 (1)	3/79 (4)	59/93 (63)	20/79 (25)

IPV, inactivated poliovirus vaccine; OPV, oral poliovirus vaccine; TCID$_{50}$, median tissue culture infective dose.
From Onorato I, Modlin J, McBean A, et al. Mucosal immunity induced by enhanced-potency inactivated and oral polio vaccines. J Infect Dis 163:1–6, 1991, with permission.

through two polio seasons in Houston.[98] In Senegal, two doses of DTP/IPV were given in the Kolda area, which subsequently suffered an epidemic of type 1 polio. According to case-control analysis, the efficacy of one dose was 36% and of two doses was 89% (95% confidence limits, 62% to 97%).[99–101] In another study conducted in the North Arcot region of India, John compared OPV in one district with IPV vaccination in two other districts.[102] Vaccination coverage with three doses rose to 85% to 90% in the OPV districts and 75% to 80% in the IPV districts. Case-control analysis revealed an efficacy of 92% for IPV and 66% for OPV. During the introduction of IPV into Canada, efficacy of the vaccine was calculated at more than 90%.[103]

Herd Immunity

Perhaps the best evidence for a herd immunity effect of IPV is the experience in the United States. IPV was introduced into routine use in 1955 and was replaced by OPV in 1962. A sharp drop in the numbers of cases of paralytic and nonparalytic polio is evident during the years 1955 to 1962 (Fig. 24–8). The apparent reduction in the total number of cases observed exceeded the expectation based on the percentage of children vaccinated (Fig. 24–9). More specific regional data were also published that suggested a greater than expected reduction in polio cases.[104] An important point to consider is that studies conducted in families, in which contact is intimate, may show less blockage of transmission than community-based studies. The fecal-oral route may be more important to transmission in families, whereas contact with pharyngeal secretions may be more important to community spread.

The second example of herd immunity is furnished by the example of the Netherlands. Vaccination is refused by a particular religious community of 200,000 individuals who are well dispersed throughout this country, although IPV is routinely administered to the rest of the population. Two outbreaks of polio have occurred in this religious group, one caused by type 1 virus in 1978 (110 cases) and the second by type 3 virus in 1992 (71 cases). Despite the wide circulation of virus in the sect members, there was only a single case of polio in other Dutch people. Approximately 400,000 unvaccinated individuals not belonging to the sect also remained unaffected.[105–110] The virulent viruses were passed to religious groups in North America in both

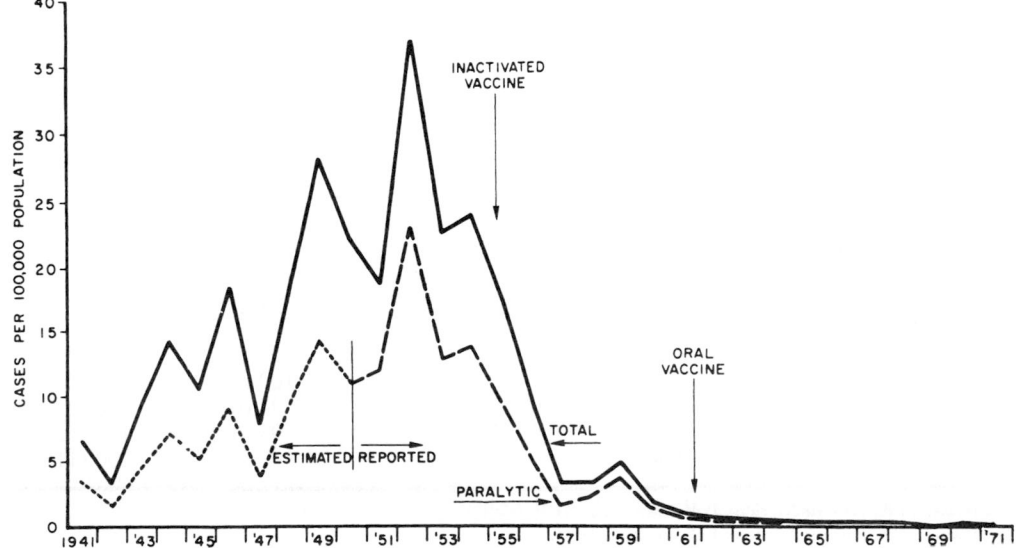

FIGURE 24–8 ■ Incidence of polio in the United States. The oral poliovirus vaccine was introduced from 1961 to 1962. The *dashed line* indicates the incidence of paralytic polio only; the *solid line* measures the incidence of both paralytic and nonparalytic polio. (From Centers for Disease Control. Immunization Against Disease—1972. Atlanta, Centers for Disease Control, 1973.)

schedule is a single dose at 2, 4, and 6 to 18 months, followed by a booster at 4 to 6 years. OPV is no longer available to physicians, and is dispensed by the CDC from a stockpile only in emergencies, which would essentially be an outbreak of wild poliovirus. In Canada and a number of other countries, principally in Europe, IPV is also the routine vaccine against polio.[139]

Children

For children who need rapid vaccination because they are traveling to a zone of endemic polio, or for those who have not been vaccinated previously, the recommended schedule is two doses 1 month apart followed by a booster 6 months later (or, if pressed for time, at least 1 month later).

Adults, Including Travelers[138]

Routine vaccination of adults is not recommended in the United States, but it is recommended in many European countries. If adults need primary polio vaccination, they should always receive IPV, because VAPP after OPV appears to be more common after the age of 18 years. Combinations of adult diphtheria and tetanus toxoids plus IPV have been developed in Europe and in Canada.[140] In principle, vaccination of previously unvaccinated adults, to protect them from VAPP, is recommended when they are in contact with children excreting OPV. At this time in the United States this would apply only to parents whose children are being vaccinated overseas.

Those adults traveling to polio epidemic or polio-endemic areas should receive IPV as a booster before their first trip. Laboratory personnel working with wild polioviruses should have previously completed vaccination. Health care workers should also be vaccinated because they may come into contact with wild poliovirus or reverted attenuated viruses being excreted by vaccinees.

IPV is universally recommended for patients with congenital or acquired immunodeficiency, including HIV infection, in view of the VAPP risk in those patients after OPV.[141] Those receiving systemic steroid therapy or chemotherapy are included in this indication. In developing countries, OPV is recommended for asymptomatic HIV-seropositive people because the risk of polio is considered larger than the risk of VAPP. In those countries where OPV is routinely used, family contacts of immunosuppressed people should receive IPV instead of OPV.

Contraindications to Inactivated Poliovirus Vaccine[137,138]

Formal contraindications to IPV consist of previous severe reaction to IPV or to streptomycin, neomycin, or polymyxin B. Neither pregnancy nor breast-feeding is a contraindication.

Simultaneous Use with Other Vaccines

No significant interference effects have been described when IPV was used in association with DTP, Hib, or hepatitis B vaccines. The largest experiences with IPV combinations have been with DTP/IPV and DTP/IPV/Hib in France, Canada, and elsewhere (see Chapter 29).[28,96,116] In combination vaccines, IPV is compatible with DTP, DTaP, Hib, and hepatitis B, although generalization is difficult owing to the many combinations and the rapidly changing picture of the availability of these vaccines. Spontaneous mixtures should not be made by the physician because IPV is destroyed by certain substances, such as thimerosal, which is used as a preservative in some other vaccines. Bypass syringes have been used to prevent inactivation of IPV by DTP before injection.

Public Health Considerations

Results of Vaccination with Inactivated Poliovirus Vaccine

Experience with IPV in national programs has been longest in Europe and in Canada. Some countries have used IPV exclusively, and some as part of a mixed schedule with OPV, as reviewed by Murdin and colleagues[96] and Plotkin.[139] Table 24–15 lists the countries using IPV for routine pediatric vaccination as of this writing, either exclusively or as part of a sequential scheme with OPV.

Sweden

Sweden has used IPV since 1957. In 1989, enhanced-potency IPV replaced the original vaccine. Indigenous circulation of wild poliovirus was stopped by 1962,[142] although a subsequent case occurred in an unvaccinated religious sect without spread to the larger population.[143] Data showing the persistence of antibodies in Swedish children despite the absence of circulating virus were discussed earlier under *Duration of Immunity*.

Finland

IPV has been used in Finland for many years, starting with first-generation vaccine and changing to enhanced-potency IPV in 1985. The only outbreak of polio since the introduction of vaccine involved 10 cases in 1984 under the following circumstances[144,145]:

1. The type 3 component of the first-generation IPV being used in Finland was of low potency, with the minority of vaccinees responding with antibodies.[146]
2. Vaccination coverage had slipped to 80%.

TABLE 24–15 ■ Countries Where IPV Is Recommended by Health Authorities or by Medical Associations, 2002[†]

Andorra	Ireland
Austria	Israel*
Belgium	Italy*
Belarus*	Latvia*
Canada	Lithuania*
Croatia*	Luxembourg
Denmark	Netherlands
Egypt*	New Zealand
Finland	Norway
France	Poland*
Germany	Sweden
Hungary*	Ukraine*
Iceland	USA

*Sequential schedule.
[†]Australia and the United Kingdom are likely to be added in the near future.

3. A type 3 wild virus was introduced, probably from Turkey, that was genetically distinct from the Saukett virus in the vaccine.[105] The mutation in the wild type 3 virus had occurred at neutralization antigenic site 1. This site is present on inactivated polioviruses and is one of the sites that induce neutralizing antibodies. However, the three other sites present on the virus were destroyed by inactivation, and thus protection depended on the presence of antibody to site 1. Because the circulating virus had mutated at this site, it escaped neutralization.[146]

4. A trypsin-treated vaccine was developed in an attempt to correct the specificity of the type 3 response,[146a] but tests showed that it did not improve the immunogenicity.[89]

5. OPV was brought in to stop the outbreak, after which the Finns returned to the use of IPV, but in the form of the enhanced-potency vaccine also used in Sweden. The new IPV did induce antibodies neutralizing to the Finnish mutant virus. No spread of polio to Sweden occurred during the epidemic.[142]

Denmark

Denmark chose a mixed schedule in 1968. Starting in1970, Danish children received IPV at 5, 6, and 15 months of age, followed by OPV at 2, 3, and 4 years of age. Single polio cases were diagnosed in 1969, 1976, 1980, and 1986, the last two being imported. No wild virus has been identified in sewage samples since 1968. Not surprisingly, seroimmunity has been virtually 100% at all age levels of the Danish population.[96,159] No VAPP has occurred among 1.5 million Danes who have received two or more doses of IPV. Recently Denmark changed to an all-IPV schedule.

The Netherlands

Enhanced-potency IPV was developed in the Netherlands in the late 1970s and reached its current form by 1982.[147] Polio has been prevented ever since in the general population, who receive a combined DTP/IPV or more recently DTaP/IPV vaccine. In 2001, a survey of immunity in the general Dutch population revealed seropositivity rates of 97%, 93%, and 90%, respectively for polioviruses types 1, 2, and 3.[148] As recounted earlier, however, two outbreaks have occurred in Protestant sects refusing vaccination, without spread to others (see under *Herd Immunity*).

Iceland

Polio disappeared from Iceland in 1960 after the introduction of IPV vaccination in 1956.[142]

Norway

Norway started vaccination with IPV in the late 1950s but switched to OPV in 1965. After that switch, there were six cases of VAPP, of which five were in unvaccinated people and the sixth in an individual given IPV 10 years earlier (L. Flagstrud and H. Nokleby, personal communication, 1996). Because most of the susceptible population had received IPV previously but nevertheless VAPP was concentrated in the remaining unvaccinated population, it appears that VAPP had been almost completely prevented by prior IPV vaccination. Norway switched back to IPV in 1979, and since then the only reported poliomyelitis has been imported from abroad.[142]

France

France is perhaps the best example of a sizable country exposed to immigration from polio-endemic areas in Africa that has kept the disease at bay with IPV vaccination only. France started vaccination with an IPV in 1956, but in 1965 OPV became the recommended vaccine. Both OPV and IPV were in use until 1983, when the Vero cell–produced IPV received official recommendation. Doses are recommended at ages 2, 3, 4, and 15 to 18 months; 5 to 6 years; and 11 years. VAPP occurred sporadically during the use of OPV but ceased to be seen after 1986.[149–151] The last wild polio case was reported in 1989, and attempts to find virus in sewage have not been successful since 1988.[149–152] The occurrence of polio in France from 1977 to 1992 is shown in Figure 24–10.[149]

Germany

A switch from OPV to IPV was made in 1998 in Germany, because in the last decade there were 15 cases of VAPP but

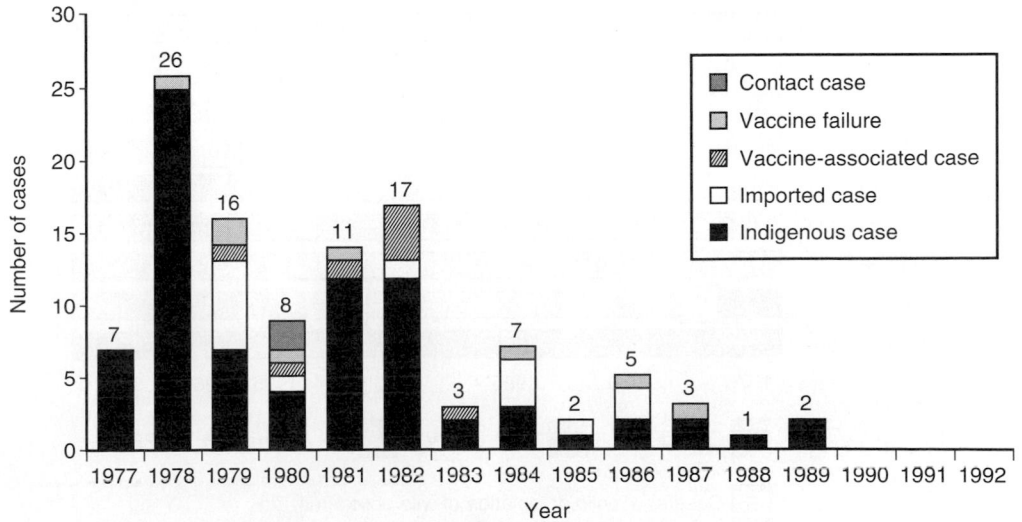

FIGURE 24–10 ■ Sources of poliomyelitis in France, 1977 to 1992.

only 2 caused by imported wild viruses. Doses are recommended at 2, 4, and 11 to 14 months of age, with a booster in adolescence. However, because combination vaccines are in general use, most infants receive IPV doses at 2, 3, 4, and 11 to 14 months of age.

Canada

Canadian provinces have used IPV, OPV, or a mixed schedule since the inception of vaccination in 1955. At present, nearly all provinces are using IPV, and the experience has been particularly large in Ontario, Canada's most populous province. Since 1988, the IPV vaccine has been produced in human diploid cells. The last indigenous case of polio occurred in 1988, related to importation of the virus. Introductions of poliovirus from the Netherlands in 1979 and 1992 and from the Indian subcontinent in 1996 failed to result in spread to the general population.[28,103,153]

Figure 24–11 shows the close relationship between OPV use in individual provinces and VAPP. All of the provinces have now switched to IPV alone. Also shown in Figure 24–11 are the most recent introductions of wild poliovirus into Canada from overseas. Ontario, the largest province with the largest immigrant population, has had the most introductions, but provinces using OPV have also had wild poliovirus introduced. In every case, the wild virus was confined to unvaccinated immigrant groups or unvaccinated religious cults, while the general population was unscathed.

Israel

Israel has used both polio vaccines in an attempt to solve their particular epidemiologic situation, in which two communities that live close together have different hygienic conditions and levels of vaccination coverage. After brief experience with IPV, Israel started routine OPV vaccination in 1960. Vaccination coverage reached high levels among both Jewish and Arab children. Nevertheless, sporadic poliomyelitis continued among Jews, and small epidemics continued to occur in the West Bank and Gaza.[154–158]

In view of the failure of OPV to control polio, in 1978 the Israelis introduced a combined schedule: OPV was administered at 1, 2 ½, 4, 5 ½, and 12 months of age, and IPV (as DTP/IPV) was given at 2 ½ and 4 months of age. For a time in the 1980s, there were no cases in Israel proper and only sporadic cases in the Palestinian areas.[154,156] All was more or less well until 1988, when an epidemic of 15 cases of type 1 polio occurred in Israel,[157,158] localized in one of two districts that had adopted IPV vaccination of infants. Although the analysis of this epidemic is controversial, it is clear that antibody responses to OPV were suboptimal, resulting in a low level of resistance among Israeli young adults. Conversely, the wild virus may have circulated among infants immunized with IPV only, allowing spread to their parents.[158]

The response to the epidemic included mass vaccination with OPV and the institution of three doses of DTP/IPV in the routine vaccination scheme, together with four doses of OPV. Since 1988, no cases of polio have been reported in Israel or its territories, despite an outbreak in neighboring Jordan from 1991 to 1992 that caused wild virus circulation in Gaza.[157]

Other European Countries

As of this writing, only Greece, Portugal, Spain, and the United Kingdom use OPV. All the rest use all-IPV schedules, except for Italy, which uses a sequential schedule. In addition, as the use of five- and six-component combination vaccines containing IPV becomes more general, the remaining countries are likely to switch.

United States

Early use of first-generation IPV in the United States was discussed previously (see under *Herd Immunity*). Despite incomplete application of the vaccine, polio incidence fell 95% between the introduction of the vaccine in 1955 and its abandonment in 1961 (see Fig. 24–8). The remaining cases, however, many of them in IPV vaccinees, sapped

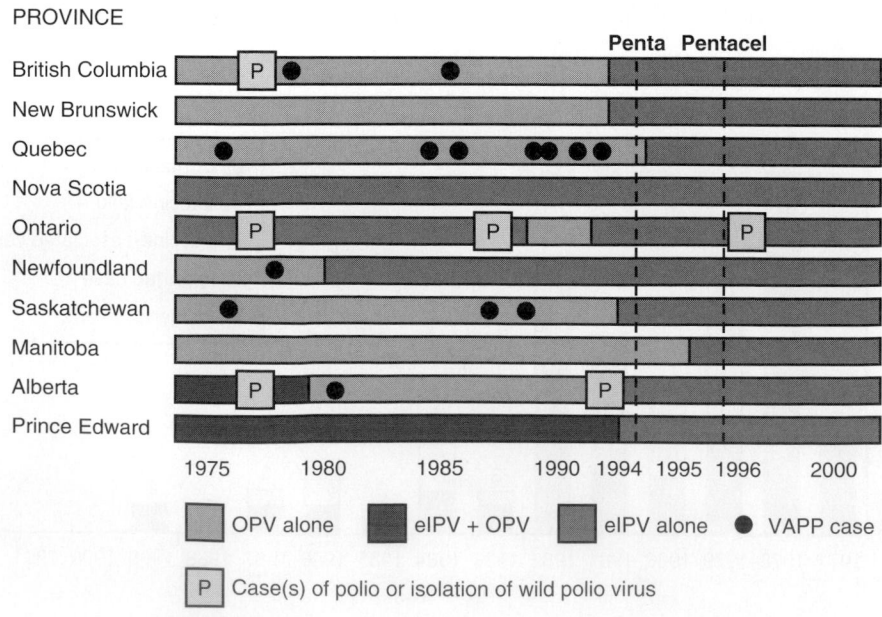

FIGURE 24–11 ■ Canadian polio experience, 1975 to 2001.

confidence in the vaccine and caused its replacement by OPV.[96,139]

The last cases of paralytic poliomyelitis in the United States occurred in 1979 among unvaccinated Amish children in Pennsylvania, Missouri, Iowa, and Wisconsin. The evolution in polio vaccine policy in the United States is summarized in Table 24–16. Opinion gradually shifted away from OPV and toward IPV, but with the preference for a combination vaccine. Although a combination containing IPV has not yet been licensed, IPV was reintroduced into routine use in the United States in its enhanced-potency form in 1997 as part of a sequential schedule consisting of two doses of IPV at 2 and 4 months of age, followed by two doses of OPV at 18 months and 4 to 6 years of age.[32] VAPP cases immediately decreased to three in 1997 and one in 1998. All of these cases occurred in children whose physicians had elected to start immunization with OPV rather than the recommended IPV. Three years later, in 2000, the United States chose four doses of IPV as the accepted regimen.[137,138,160]

The primary reason for the reintroduction of IPV in the United States was the perception that polio is vanishing from the world, whereas paralysis associated with OPV was exacting a yearly toll of 8 to 10 cases.[139,141,161,162] Before the switch occurred, concern was expressed that the use of monovalent IPV might decrease immunization rates because of the necessity of additional injections. However, the opposite has been the case, and immunization rates were unaffected by the change to partial and then complete IPV schedules.[163–166]

Australia and New Zealand

New Zealand is now using a combination of DTaP and IPV, whereas Australia has decided to switch from OPV to IPV

TABLE 24–16 ■ Steps in U.S. Decisions Regarding Polio Vaccination

1955	IPV licensed
1961	Polio outbreak shows partial effectiveness of IPV; epidemiologic data show that IPV does not completely prevent poliovirus circulation
1963	OPV licensed, replaces IPV as recommended vaccine
1964	Surgeon General's committee concludes that 57 cases of VAPP occurred between 1961 and 1964 (reversion to virulence first recognized in 1955)
1970s	Van Wezel and Cohen at RIVM improve immunogenicity of IPV
1977	IOM report recommends OPV for children, IPV for adults
1978	Mérieux makes IPV in Vero cells, monkeys no longer needed
1988	IOM report recommends staying with OPV until IPV combination available, or 90% coverage reached
1995	IOM workshop recommends moving toward IPV
1995	ACIP recommends IPV/OPV sequential schedule
1997	Sequential schedule adopted
1999	ACIP recommends sequential schedule or all IPV; OPV not recommended
2000	All IPV recommended

ACIP, Advisory Committee on Immunization Practices; IOM, Institute of Medicine; IPV, inactivated poliovirus vaccine; OPV, oral poliovirus vaccine; RIVM, Rijksinstituut Voor Volksgezondheid en Milien; VAPP, vaccine-associated paralytic poliomyelitis.

as soon as a combination vaccine is licensed, based on a cost analysis showing that the introduction of IPV in a combination vaccine costing $10 or less would be cost-effective.[167]

Developing Countries

Although not routinely recommended in developing countries, IPV has been studied in those areas (Aventis Pasteur, unpublished data).[28,54,55,100,168] The viewpoint of the WHO and other authorities is that only OPV should be used as the principal tool for eradicating polio in developing countries.[169] However, John and his colleagues, working in Southern India, have shown that IPV can be highly effective in preventing polio without the problems of OPV (VAPP and the need for repeated administration to obtain uniform seroconversion).[170] Arguments for using IPV in developing countries are explored below under *Role of Inactivated Poliovirus Vaccine in Polio Eradication.*

Recommendations for the Use of Inactivated Poliovirus Vaccine

IPV is the polio vaccine of choice for immunosuppressed individuals and in most circumstances is the vaccine of choice for adults. Since the 1960s, the controversy that has consumed much ink is the choice of IPV or OPV for routine vaccination in infancy. Table 24–17 summarizes the advantages and disadvantages of IPV, OPV, or mixed IPV/OPV schedules.[139] In essence, the arguments for IPV are safety, predictable immunogenicity, and the possibility of its inclusion in combination vaccines. The arguments for OPV are induction of mucosal immunity, ease of administration to large populations, and low cost. The argument for a mixed schedule is to fuse the immunogenicity advantages of each vaccine, with less risk of VAPP.

VAPP, which is discussed in detail in Chapter 25, is an inescapable phenomenon that has been consistently observed after OPV.[32,136,171,172] In our view, the following circumstances should lead to the choice of IPV for routine vaccination of infants at the beginning of the 21st century in a particular country:

1. Absence of paralytic polio and the likelihood that wild polioviruses are not circulating. This criterion applies to countries where eradication of polio has been certified, even if importation is possible through carriage by immigrants. As stated previously, the WHO still recommends OPV in this circumstance.
2. High prior vaccine coverage with either IPV or OPV, equivalent to 80% or better of infants and children, so that introduction of wild virus is unlikely to result in spread.
3. Ability of the medical system or of individual families to afford the higher costs of IPV, although the cost issue may be exaggerated. Reduced wastage and lower need for a "cold chain" compensate to some degree for the difference in price, and the cost differential between IPV and OPV varies from country to country. In the United States, for example, because of liability tax and other factors, the difference in price is not so evident. In developing countries, while the relative cost of IPV versus OPV is high, the absolute price of IPV is lower because of the system of

TABLE 24-17 ■ Advantages and Disadvantages of all-OPV, all-IPV, or Mixed Vaccination Schedules

Feature	All OPV	All IPV	IPV/OPV
VAPP	1 case per 790,000 first vaccinations	No cases	Estimated 50–75% reduction in VAPP cases
Safety (other than VAPP)	Excellent	Excellent	Excellent
Systemic immunity	Good	Good	Good
Mucosal immunity	Excellent	Slight to moderate in intestine Marked in pharynx Overall less than OPV	Excellent
Efficacy	Excellent	Excellent	Excellent
Transmission to contacts and secondary vaccination	Yes	No	Some
Extra injections	No	Yes if monovalent No if part of combination vaccine	Same as for all IPV
Reduced compliance	No	Possible if monovalent vaccine	Possible if monovalent vaccine
Availability of combinations	None	Yes	Yes
Cost	Low	Higher, though price difference depends on volume, use of combinations	Intermediate

two-tiered pricing. The costs of National Vaccination Days with OPV, in which large populations are mobilized, must also be taken into account.

The criteria for a mixed schedule are the same, but with the addition of a public health policy factor: the desire to prevent polio by all possible means, taking advantage of both vaccines but also maximizing safety.[173,174] Although this point refers to schedules beginning with IPV and ending with OPV, in view of the sometimes low rates of seroconversion after the primary vaccination, IPV might be considered in a single booster dose for children living in tropical areas who have been previously vaccinated with OPV.[64]

Role of Inactivated Poliovirus Vaccine in Polio Eradication

Wild polioviruses have been eradicated from the Western Hemisphere, Europe, and the Western Pacific. The principal weapon in the eradication campaign has been OPV, given in national campaigns, although the same goal was achieved in many European countries using IPV. OPV campaigns are also having a marked impact on the incidence of polio in traditionally endemic areas, such as the Indian subcontinent and Africa.[175] At some point, there will be no clinical evidence of paralytic polio caused by wild virus in the world, and thus questions will arise concerning how to verify eradication and what to do about vaccination. The role of IPV in facilitating eradication and its verification is much disputed, ranging from no role at all[169,176] to complete substitution of IPV for OPV.[177]

Various strategies for the "endgame" have been suggested. One strategy would be to stop all vaccination and simply observe for wild virus circulation and cases of poliovirus-induced paralysis. A second strategy would be to continue OPV vaccination while attempting to detect circulating wild poliovirus. The difficulty here would be in detecting the wild virus in a sea of excreted attenuated viruses, some mutated toward virulence and some recombinants with other polioviruses.[178,179] VAPP would continue to occur, so paralysis caused by poliovirus would not be truly eradicated. Moreover, reports of immunosuppressed individ-

uals who excrete poliovirus for long periods of time[180] raise the specter of reintroduction of the virus. Even more concern has been generated by the recent realization that virulent revertants of Sabin strains, as a result of recombination with other enteroviruses,[181,182] have themselves become epidemic in Egypt, Haiti, the Dominican Republic, and the Philippines. These strains now pose a danger for poorly vaccinated populations, and would be a greater danger if all countries had stopped vaccination.

A third strategy could be proposed, consisting of a gradual switch from OPV to combined pediatric vaccines containing IPV (e.g., DTP/Hib/hepatitis B/IPV) as wild poliovirus disappears from more and more countries. Vaccination with IPV would facilitate the search for polioviruses in the environment, because screening would not be obscured by OPV vaccine strains and yet protection against polio would be maintained. Such a strategy may be all the more valuable because it has been calculated that, even after a 5-year period without polio cases, there is still a 0.1% to 1.0% probability of silent transmission.[183]

It is evident that developed countries are already using or will soon switch to IPV, principally to avoid sporadic or epidemic VAPP associated with OPV. Some of the more affluent developing countries will also avail themselves of IPV. In view of the possible use of poliovirus as a biologic warfare weapon, many countries will continue to use IPV even if eradication of wild virus is achieved.[184] Developing countries may also be loath to risk resurgence of polio if OPV immunization is stopped, as a result of uncertainties concerning persistent circulation of wild or revertant vaccine viruses in normal and immunosuppressed individuals.[185,186]

The principal arguments offered against conversion from OPV to IPV in developing countries are cost and shortage of vaccine supply. To some extent these problems are related because large production volumes reduce cost. However, the more cogent response to cost is that IPV should not be used as a monovalent vaccine with the attendant expenses of separate administration, but rather as part of a combination vaccine, such as the one mentioned above. Combinations containing IPV based on acellular pertussis vaccines are also available. If there were a demand,

and bearing in mind the oft-stated desire to bring new vaccines to the EPI schedule, the cost of IPV would be negligible as part of DTP- or DTaP-based combinations.

Vaccine supply is a problem, in that there are currently only two major manufacturers of IPV, and their joint capacity would not permit vaccination of every child in the world. If all industrialized countries used IPV, about 40 million doses would be needed, about half of current production capacity, leaving insufficient vaccine for developing countries. Of course, this problem is somewhat circular in that the manufacturers have not received the call to increase their capacity. An annual production of between 200 and 300 million doses of IPV is probably feasible in the immediate future. However, to reduce the need for a larger supply, the use of IPV in developing countries could be targeted to countries or regions of countries where the hidden presence of wild polio is most feared (a so-called *cordon sanitaire*), so that recrudescence of the virus could be recognized by isolation from excreta, rather than by outbreaks of paralysis.

Although OPV vaccination must be continued in countries where wild virus still circulates, countries with high vaccination coverage and absent wild virus should consider switching to sequential IPV/OPV schedules or to IPV alone.

Conclusion

More than 40 years after its invention, IPV is renascent, owing to improvements in its manufacture and its outstanding safety record. In the immediate future, this vaccine is certain to have more widespread use, as the world moves toward the eradication of poliovirus with the use of two potent vaccines that can be synergistic for public health programs in terms of safety, immunogenicity, and other attributes.[187]

REFERENCES

1. Monto AS. Francis field trial of inactivated poliomyelitis vaccine: background and lessons for today. Epidemiol Rev 21:7–23, 1999.
2. Lambert SM, Markel H. Making history: Thomas Francis Jr, MD, and the 1954 Salk Poliomyelitis Vaccine Field Trial. Arch Pediatr Adolesc Med 154:512–517, 2000.
3. Gear J. The history of the Poliomyelitis Research Foundation. Rivonia, South Africa, Poliomyelitis Research Foundation, 1996, pp 4–13.
4. Bodian D, Morgan I, Howe H. Differentiation of types of poliomyelitis viruses: the grouping of fourteen strains into three basic immunologic types. Am J Hyg 49:234–245, 1949.
5. Horstman DM, McCollum R, Mascola A. Viremia in human poliomyelitis. J Exp Med 99:355–369, 1954.
6. Hammon W, Coriell LL, Wehrle PF, Stokes J Jr. Evaluation of Red Cross gamma globulin as a prophylactic agent for poliomyelitis. J Am Med Assoc 151:1272–1285, 1953.
7. Enders J, Weller T, Robbins F. Cultivation of the Lansing strain of poliomyelitis virus in cultures of various human embryonic tissues. Science 109:85–87, 1949.
8. Beale J. The development of IPV. *In* Plotkin S, Fantini B (eds). Vaccinia, Vaccination, Vaccinology: Jenner, Pasteur and Their Successors. Paris, Elsevier, 1996, pp 85–87.
9. van Wezel AL. Growth of cell-strains and primary cells on microcarriers in homogeneous culture. Nature 216:64–65, 1967.
10. Montagnon B. Polio and rabies vaccines produced in continuous cell lines: a reality for Vero cell line. Dev Biol Stand 70:27–47, 1988.
11. Paul JR, Melnick PJ, Barnett V, Goldblum N. A survey of neutralizing antibodies to poliomyelitis in Cairo, Egypt. Am J Hyg 55:402–413, 1952.
12. Lebrun A, Cerf J, Gelfand H, Fantini B. Vaccination with the CHAT strain of type I attenuated poliomyelitis virus in Leopoldville, Belgian Congo. I. Description of the city, its history of poliomyelitis, and the plan of vaccination campaign. Bull World Health Organ 22:203–213, 1960.
13. Plotkin S, Koprowski H, Stokes J Jr. Clinical trials in infants of orally administered attenuated poliomyelitis viruses. Pediatrics 23:1041–1062, 1960.
14. Brodie M, Park W. Active immunization against poliomyelitis. Am J Public Health 26:119–125, 1936.
15. Kolmer J. Vaccination against acute anterior poliomyelitis. Am J Public Health 26:126–135, 1936.
16. Kersten G, Hazendonk T, Beuvery C. Antigenic and immunogenic properties of inactivated polio vaccine made from Sabin strains. Vaccine 17:2059–2066, 1999.
17. Murray R. Standardization licensing and availability of live polio virus vaccine. JAMA 175:843–846, 1961.
18. Berkovich S, Pickering J, Kibrick S. Paralytic poliomyelitis in Massachusetts. N Engl J Med 264:1325–1329, 1959.
19. Montagnon BJ, Fanget B, Vincent-Falquet JC. Industrial-scale production of inactivated poliovirus vaccine prepared by culture of Vero cells on microcarrier. Rev Infect Dis 6(suppl 2):S341–S344, 1984.
20. Duchene M, Peetermans J, D'Hont E, et al. Production of poliovirus vaccines: past, present, and future. Viral Immunol 3:243–272, 1990.
21. Montagnon BJ, Vincent-Falquet JC, Saluzzo JF. Experience with Vero cells at Pasteur Merieux Connaught. Dev Biol Stand 98:137–140, 1999.
22. Horaud F. Viral vaccines and residual cellular DNA. Biologicals 23:225–228, 1995.
23. Melnick JL. Virus inactivation: lessons from the past. Dev Biol Stand 75:29–36, 1990.
24. Ferguson M, Wood DJ, Minor PD. Antigenic structure of poliovirus in inactivated vaccines. J Gen Virol 74:685–690, 1993.
25. Salk J. One-dose immunization against paralytic poliomyelitis using a noninfectious vaccine. Rev Infect Dis 6(suppl 2):S444–S450, 1984.
26. Mellander L, Bottiger M, Hanson LA, et al. Avidity and titers of the antibody response to two inactivated poliovirus vaccines with different antigen content. Acta Paediatr 82:552–556, 1993.
27. Sawyer LA, McInnis J, Patel A, et al. Deleterious effect of thimerosal on the potency of inactivated poliovirus vaccine. Vaccine 12:851–856, 1994.
28. Vidor E, Caudrelier P, Plotkin SA. The place of DTP/eIPV vaccine in routine paediatric vaccination. Rev Med Virol 4:261–277, 1994.
29. Faden H, Modlin JF, Thoms ML, et al. Comparative evaluation of immunization with live attenuated and enhanced-potency inactivated trivalent poliovirus vaccines in childhood: systemic and local immune responses. J Infect Dis 162:1291–1297, 1990.
30. McBean AM, Thoms ML, Albrecht P, et al, for the Field Staff and Coordinating Committee. Serologic response to oral polio vaccine and enhanced-potency inactivated polio vaccines. Am J Epidemiol 128:615–628, 1988.
31. Modlin JF, Halsey NA, Thoms ML, et al. Humoral and mucosal immunity in infants induced by three sequential inactivated poliovirus vaccine-live attenuated oral poliovirus vaccine immunization schedules. Baltimore Area Polio Vaccine Study Group. J Infect Dis 175(suppl 1):S228–S234, 1997.
32. Advisory Committee on Immunization Practices. Poliomyelitis prevention in the United States: introduction of a sequential vaccination schedule of inactivated poliovirus vaccine-live attenuated poliovirus vaccine immunization schedules. MMWR 46(RR-3):1–25, 1997.
33. Halsey NA, Blatter M, Bader G. Safety and immunogenicity of a combination DPT/IPV vaccine administered to infants in a dual-chamber syringe: final report. Swiftwater, PA, Connaught Laboratories, 1994.
34. Blatter M, Starr S. Safety and immunogenicity of a combination DPT/eIPV vaccine administered to infants in a dual-chamber syringe, in 2-month-old infants. Swiftwater, PA, Connaught Laboratories, 1994.
35. Sormunen H, Stenvik M, Eskola J, Hovi T. Age- and dose-interval-dependent antibody responses to inactivated poliovirus vaccine. J Med Virol 63:305–310, 2001.

36. Hovi T. Inactivated poliovirus vaccine and the final stages of poliovirus eradication. Vaccine 19:2268–2272, 2001.

37. Singh J, Ravi RN, Dutta AK, et al. Immunogenicity of enhanced potency inactivated polio vaccine. Indian Pediatr 29:1353–1356, 1992.

38. Kok PW, Leeuwenburg J, Tukei P, et al. Serological and virological assessment of oral and inactivated poliovirus vaccines in a rural population in Kenya. Bull World Health Organ 70:93–103, 1992.

39. Linder N, Handsher R, German B, et al. Controlled trial of immune response of preterm infants to recombinant hepatitis B and inactivated poliovirus vaccines administered simultaneously shortly after birth. Arch Dis Child Fetal Neonatal Ed 83(1):F24–F27, 2000.

40. Combined immunization of infants with oral and inactivated poliovirus vaccines: results of a randomized trial in The Gambia, Oman, and Thailand. WHO Collaborative Study Group on Oral and Inactivated Poliovirus Vaccines. Bull World Health Organ 74:253–268, 1996.

41. Sutter RW, Suleiman AJ, Malankar PG, et al. Sequential use of inactivated poliovirus vaccine followed by oral poliovirus vaccine in Oman. J Infect Dis 175(suppl 1):S235–S240, 1997.

42. Simoes EA, Padmini B, Steinhoff MC, et al. Antibody response of infants to two doses of inactivated poliovirus vaccine of enhanced potency. Am J Dis Child 139:977–980, 1985.

43. Simoes EA, John TJ. The antibody response of seronegative infants to inactivated poliovirus vaccine of enhanced potency. J Biol Stand 14:127–131, 1986.

44. Swartz TA, Handsher R, Stoeckel P, et al. Immunologic memory induced at birth by immunization with inactivated polio vaccine in a reduced schedule. Eur J Epidemiol 5:143–145, 1989.

45. Hovi T, Stenvik M, Agboatwalla M. Effect of administering oral and inactivated polio vaccines immediately after birth. Eur J Clin Microbiol Infect Dis 18:526–528, 1999.

46. Baker JD, Halperin SA, Edwards K, et al. Antibody response to Bordetella pertussis antigens after immunization with American and Canadian whole-cell vaccines. J Pediatr 121:523–527, 1992.

47. Halperin SA, Langley JM, Eastwood BJ. Effect of inactivated poliovirus vaccine on the antibody response to Bordetella pertussis antigens when combined with diphtheria-pertussis-tetanus vaccine. Clin Infect Dis 22:59–62, 1996.

48. Halperin SA, Eastwood BJ, Langley JM. Immune responses to pertussis vaccines concurrently administered with viral vaccines. Ann N Y Acad Sci 754:89–96, 1995.

49. Kurikka S, Kayhty H, Saarinen L, et al. Comparison of five different vaccination schedules with Haemophilus influenzae type b-tetanus toxoid conjugate vaccine. J Pediatr 128:524–530, 1996.

50. Mallet E. Aventis Pasteur study E2119: data on file. Swiftwater, PA, Aventis Pasteur, 2002.

51. Knutsson N, Trollfors B, Taranger J, et al. Immunogenicity and reactogenicity of diphtheria, tetanus and pertussis toxoids combined with inactivated polio vaccine, when administered concomitantly with or as a diluent for a Hib conjugate vaccine. Vaccine 19:4396–4403, 2001.

52. Mallet E, Fabre P, Pines E, et al. Immunogenicity and safety of a new liquid hexavalent combined vaccine compared with separate administration of reference licensed vaccines in infants. Pediatr Infect Dis J 19:1119–1127, 2000.

53. Gylca R, Gylca V, Benes O, et al. A new DTPa-HBV-IPV vaccine co-administered with Hib, compared to a commercially available DTPw-IPV/Hib vaccine co-administered with HBV, given at 6, 10 and 14 weeks following HBV at birth. Vaccine 19:825–833, 2000.

54. Combined immunization of infants with oral and inactivated poliovirus vaccines: results of a randomized trial in The Gambia, Oman, and Thailand. WHO Collaborative Study Group on Oral and Inactivated Poliovirus Vaccines. J Infect Dis 175(suppl 1):S215–S227, 1997.

55. Krishnan R, Jadhav M, John TJ. Efficacy of inactivated poliovirus vaccine in India. Bull World Health Organ 61:689–692, 1983.

56. Desai AM. Aventis Pasteur study MAS01489: data on file. Swiftwater, PA, Aventis Pasteur, 1989.

57. Nirmal S, Cherian T, Samuel BU, et al. Immune response of infants to fractional doses of intradermally administered inactivated poliovirus vaccine. Vaccine 16:928–931, 1998.

58. Hussey G, Malan H, Hughes J, et al. Aventis Pasteur study HIT40: data on file. Swiftwater, PA, Aventis Pasteur, 1998.

59. Capeding MR. Aventis Pasteur study EUV07199/HE9810: data on file. Swiftwater, PA, Aventis Pasteur, 1999.

60. Eskola J, Dagan R. Aventis Pasteur study PNF06: data on file. Swiftwater, PA, Aventis Pasteur, 1997.

61. Ramsay ME, Begg NT, Gandhi J, Brown D. Antibody response and viral excretion after live polio vaccine or a combined schedule of live and inactivated polio vaccines. Pediatr Infect Dis J 13:1117–1121, 1994.

62. Strebel P, Ion-Nedelcu N, Baughman AL, et al. Intramuscular injections within 30 days of immunization with oral poliovirus vaccine—a risk factor for vaccine-associated paralytic poliomyelitis. N Engl J Med 332:500–506, 1995.

63. Ion-Nedelcu N, Strebel P, Toma F, et al. Sequential and combined use of inactivated and oral poliovirus vaccines: Dolj District, Romania, 1992–1994. J Infect Dis 175(suppl):S241–S246, 1997.

64. Morinière BJ, van Loon FP, Rhodes PH, et al. Immunogenicity of a supplemental dose of oral versus inactivated poliovirus vaccine [see comments]. Lancet 341:1545–1550, 1993.

65. Adenyi-Jones SCA, Faden H, Ferdon MB, et al. Systemic and local immune responses to enhanced-potency inactivated poliovirus vaccine in premature and term infants. J Pediatr 120:686–689, 1992.

66. Linder N, Yaron M, Handsher R, et al. Early immunization with inactivated poliovirus vaccine in premature infants. J Pediatr 127:128–130, 1995.

67. O'Shea TM, Dillard RG, Gillis DC, et al. Low rate of response to enhanced inactivated polio vaccine in preterm infants with chronic illness. Clin Res Reg Aff 10(1):49–57, 1993.

68. Weckx LY, Schmidt BJ, Herrmann AA, et al. Early immunization of neonates with trivalent oral poliovirus vaccine. Bull World Health Organ 70:85–91, 1992.

69. Barbi M, Bardare M, Luraschi C, et al. Antibody response to inactivated polio vaccine (E-IPV) in children born to HIV positive mothers. Eur J Epidemiol 8:211–216, 1992.

70. Varon D, Handsher R, Dardik R, et al. Response of hemophilic patients to poliovirus vaccination: correlation with HIV serology and with immunological parameters. J Med Virol 40:91–95, 1993.

71. Sipila R, Hortling L, Hovi T. Good seroresponse to enhanced-potency inactivated poliovirus vaccine in patients on chronic dialysis. Nephrol Dial Transplant 5:352–355, 1990.

72. Engelhard D, Handsher R, Naparstek E, et al. Immune response to polio vaccination in bone marrow transplant recipients. Bone Marrow Transplant 8:295–300, 1991.

73. Ljungman P, Duraj V, Magnius L. Response to immunization against polio after allogeneic marrow transplantation. Bone Marrow Transplant 7:89–93, 1991.

74. Ogra PL, Karzon D, Righthand F, et al. Immunoglobulin response in serum and secretions after immunization with live and inactivated poliovaccine and natural infection. N Engl J Med 279:893–900, 1968.

75. Zhaori G, Sun M, Faden HS, Ogra PL. Nasopharyngeal secretory antibody response to poliovirus type 3 virion proteins exhibits different specificities after immunization with live or inactivated poliovirus vaccines. J Infect Dis 159:1018–1024, 1989.

76. Faden H, Duffy L. Effect of concurrent viral infection on systemic and local antibody responses to live attenuated and enhanced-potency inactivated poliovirus vaccines. Am J Dis Child 146:1320–1323, 1992.

77. Onorato IM, Modlin JF, McBean AM, et al. Mucosal immunity induced by enhanced-potency inactivated and oral polio vaccines. J Infect Dis 163:1–6, 1991.

78. Hanson LA, Carlsson B, Jalil F, et al. Different secretory IgA antibody responses after immunization with inactivated and live poliovirus vaccines. Rev Infect Dis 6(suppl 2):S356–S360, 1984.

79. Fox JP, Gelfand HM, LeBlanc DR, et al. The influence of natural and artificially induced immunity on alimentary infections with poliovirus. Am J Public Health 48:1181–1192, 1958.

80. Horstman DM, Paul JR, Melnick JL, Deutsch JV. Infection induced by oral administration of attenuated poliovirus to persons possessing homotypic antibody. J Exp Med 105:159–177, 1957.

81. David D, Lipson M, Carver D, et al. The degree and duration of poliomyelitis virus excretion among vaccinated household contacts of clinical cases of poliomyelitis. Pediatrics 22:33–40, 1958.

82. Gelfand HM, LeBlanc DR, Potash L, Fox JP. Studies on the development of natural immunity to poliomyelitis in Louisiana. IV. Natural infections with polioviruses following immunization with a formalin-inactivated vaccine. Am J Hyg 70:312–327, 1959.

83. Howe HA, O'Leary W, Bender W, et al. Day-by-day response of vaccinated chimpanzees to poliomyelitis infection. Am J Public Health 47:871–875, 1956.

84. Craig DE, Brown GC. The relationship between poliomyelitis antibody and virus excretion from the pharynx and anus of orally infected monkeys. Am J Hyg 69:1–12, 1959.

85. Selvakumar R, John TJ. Intestinal immunity induced by inactivated poliovirus vaccine. Vaccine 5:141, 1987.

86. Marine WM, Chin TDY, Gravelle CR. Limitation of fecal and pharyngeal poliovirus excretion in Salk-vaccinated children. Am J Hyg 76:173–195, 1962.

87. Ghendon Y, Robertson SE. Interrupting the transmission of wild polioviruses with vaccines: immunological considerations. Bull World Health Organ 72:973–983, 1994.

88. Nishio O, Ishihara Y, Sakae K, et al. The trend of acquired immunity with live poliovirus vaccine and the effect of revaccination: follow-up of vaccinees for ten years. J Biol Stand 12:1–10, 1984.

89. Piirainen L, Stenvik M, Roivainen M, et al. Randomised, controlled trial with the trypsin-modified inactivated poliovirus vaccine: assessment of intestinal immunity with live challenge virus. 17:1084–1090, 1999.

90. Parent du Chatelet I, Merchant A, Fisher-Hoch S, et al. Serological response and poliovirus excretion following different combined oral and inactivated poliovirus vaccines immunization schedules. Vaccine 2002 [in press].

91. Minor PD. The molecular biology of poliovaccines. J Gen Virol 73:3065–3077, 1992.

92. Macadam AJ, Arnold C, Howlett J, et al. Reversion of the attenuated and temperature-sensitive phenotypes of the Sabin type 3 strain of poliovirus in vaccinees. Virology 172:408–414, 1989.

93. Chumakov KM, Powers LB, Noonan KE, et al. Correlation between amount of virus with altered nucleotide sequence and the monkey test for acceptability of oral poliovirus vaccine. Proc Natl Acad Sci U S A 88:199–203, 1991.

94. Abraham R, Minor P, Dunn G, et al. Shedding of virulent poliovirus revertants during immunization with oral poliovirus vaccine after prior immunization with inactivated polio vaccine. J Infect Dis 168:1105–1109, 1993.

95. Ogra PL, Faden HS, Abraham R, et al. Effect of prior immunity on the shedding of virulent revertant virus in feces after oral immunization with live attenuated poliovirus vaccines. J Infect Dis 164:191–194, 1991.

96. Murdin AD, Barreto L, Plotkin SA. Inactivated poliovirus vaccine: past and present experience. Vaccine 14:735–746, 1996.

97. Francis T, Korns R, Voight R, et al. An evaluation of the 1954 poliomyelitis vaccine trials. Ann Arbor, University of Michigan, 1955.

98. Melnick JL, Benyeh-Melnick M, Peña R, Yow M. Effectiveness of Salk vaccine: analysis of virologically confirmed cases of paralytic and nonparalytic poliomyelitis. JAMA 175:1159–1162, 1961.

99. Stoeckel P, Schlumberger M, Parent G, et al. Use of killed poliovirus vaccine in a routine immunization program in West Africa. Rev Infect Dis 6(suppl 2):S463–S466, 1984.

100. Robertson SE, Traverso HP, Drucker J, et al. Clinical efficacy of a new enhanced-potency, inactivated poliovirus vaccine. Lancet 1:897–899, 1988.

101. Centers for Disease Control. Paralytic poliomyelitis—Senegal, 1986–1987: update on the N-IPV efficacy study. MMWR 37:257–259, 1988.

102. John T. Poliovirus vaccine and poliomyelitis control in India [abstract]. Abstracts of the World Conference on Poliomyelitis and Measles, New Delhi, 1992.

103. Varughese PV, Carter AO, Acres SE, Furesz J. Eradication of indigenous poliomyelitis in Canada: impact of immunization strategies. Can J Public Health 80:363–368, 1989.

104. Chin TD. Immunity induced by inactivated poliovirus vaccine and excretion of virus. Rev Infect Dis 6(suppl 2):S369–S370, 1984.

105. Hofman B. Poliomyelitis in The Netherlands before and after vaccination with inactivated poliovaccine. J Hyg 65:547–557, 1967.

106. van Wijngaarden JK, van Loon AM. The polio epidemic in The Netherlands, 1992–1993. Public Health Rev 21(1-2):107–116, 1993.

107. Bijkerk H. Poliomyelitis in The Netherlands. Dev Biol Stand 47:233–240, 1981.

108. Bijkerk H. Poliomyelitis epidemic in The Netherlands. Dev Biol Stand 43:195–206, 1979.

109. Oostvogel PM, van Wijngaarden JK, van der Avoort HG, et al. Poliomyelitis outbreak in an unvaccinated community in The Netherlands, 1992–93. Lancet 344:665–670, 1994.

110. Schaap GJP, Bijkerk H, Coutinho RA, et al. The spread of wild poliovirus in the well-vaccinated Netherlands in connection with the 1978 epidemic. Prog Med Virol 29:124–140, 1984.

111. Centers for Disease Control. Epidemiological notes and reports: follow-up on poliomyelitis—United States, Canada, Netherlands, 1979. MMWR 28:345, 1979.

112. Centers for Disease Control and Prevention. Lack of evidence for wild poliovirus circulation—United States, 1993. MMWR 43:957–959, 1995.

113. Rumke HC. Vaccination against polio: inactivated polio vaccine used in The Netherlands and Burkina Faso. Trop Geogr Med 45(5):202–205, 1993.

114. Oostvogel PM, Rumke HC, Conyn-Van Spaendonck MA, et al. Poliovirus circulation among schoolchildren during the early phase of the 1992–1993 poliomyelitis outbreak in The Netherlands. J Infect Dis 184:1451–1455, 2001.

115. Faden H, Duffy L, Sun M, Shuff C. Long-term immunity to poliovirus in children immunized with live attenuated and enhanced-potency inactivated trivalent poliovirus vaccines. J Infect Dis 168:452–454, 1993.

116. Vidor E, Meschievitz C, Plotkin SA. Fifteen years of experience with Vero-produced enhanced potency inactivated poliovirus vaccine. Pediatr Infect Dis J 16:312–322, 1997.

117. Bottiger M. Polio immunity to killed vaccine: an 18-year follow-up. Vaccine 8:443–445, 1990.

118. Swartz TA, Roumiantzeff M, Peyron L, et al. Use of a combined DTP-polio vaccine in a reduced schedule. Dev Biol Stand 65:159–166, 1986.

119. Salk J, Drucker J, Malvy D. Noninfectious poliovirus vaccine. In Plotkin S, Mortimer E Jr (eds). Vaccines (2nd ed). Philadelphia, WB Saunders, 1994, pp 205–227.

120. Taranger J, Trollfors B, Knutsson N, et al. Vaccination of infants with a four-dose and a three-dose vaccination schedule. Vaccine 18:884–891, 1999.

121. Carlsson RM, Claesson BA, Fagerlund E, et al. Antibody persistence in 5 year old children who received a pentavalent vaccine in infancy. Pediatr Infect Dis J 21: 535–541, 2002.

122. Langue J, Thebault C, Boisnard F, Blondeau C. Antibody persistence against diphtheria, tetanus, pertussis, poliomyelitis and *Haemophilus influenzae* type B (Hib) in 5–6 years old children. Paper presented at the 19th annual meeting of the European Society for Paediatric Infectious Diseases, Istanbul, Turkey, 2001.

123. Salk J. Persistence of immunity after administration of formalin-treated poliovirus vaccine. Lancet 2:715–723, 1960.

124. Salk J. Are booster doses of poliovirus vaccine necessary? Vaccine 8:419–420, 1990.

125. Salk D, van Wezel ALSJ. Induction of long-term immunity to paralytic poliomyelitis by use of non-infectious vaccine. Lancet 2:1317–1321, 1984.

126. Product Information: IPOL: Poliovirus Vaccine Inactivated. Swiftwater, PA, Aventis Pasteur, Inc, 1997.

127. Wattigney WA, Mootrey GT, Braun MM, Chen RT. Surveillance for poliovirus vaccine adverse events, 1991 to 1998: impact of a sequential vaccination schedule of inactivated poliovirus vaccine followed by oral poliovirus vaccine. Pediatrics 107(5):E83, 2001.

128. Reinert P, Boucher J, Pines E, et al. Primary and booster immunization with DTaP-IPV vaccine administered either in combination or in association with a *Haemophilus influenzae* type b vaccine (Act-HIB): a large scale safety study. Paper presented at the 15th Annual Meeting of the European Society for Pediatric Infectious Diseases, Paris, 1997.

129. Nathanson N, Langmuir AD. The Cutter incident: poliomyelitis following formaldehyde-inactivated poliovirus vaccination in the United States during the spring of 1955. III. Comparison of the clinical character of vaccinated and contact cases occurring after use of high rate lots of Cutter vaccine. Am J Hyg 78:61–81, 1963.

130. Nathanson N, Langmuir AD. The Cutter incident: poliomyelitis following formaldehyde-inactivated poliovirus vaccination in the United States during the spring of 1955. I. Background. Am J Hyg 78:16–28, 1963.

131. Nathanson N, Langmuir AD. The Cutter incident: poliomyelitis following formaldehyde-inactivated poliovirus vaccination in the United States during the spring of 1955. II. Relationship of poliomyelitis to Cutter vaccine. Am J Hyg 78:29–60, 1963.

132. Plotkin SA. Inactivated polio vaccine for the United States: a missed vaccination opportunity. Pediatr Infect Dis J 14:835–839, 1995.

133. Butel JS, Lednicky JA. Cell and molecular biology of simian virus 40: implications for human infections and disease. J Natl Cancer Inst 91:119–134, 1999.

134. Vilchez RA, Madden CR, Kozinetz CA, et al. Association between simian virus 40 and non-Hodgkin's lymphoma. Lancet 359:817–823, 2002.

135. Shivapurkar N, Harada K, Reddy J, et al. Presence of simian virus 40 DNA sequences in human lymphomas. Lancet 359:851–852, 2002.

136. Schattner A, Ben Chetrit E, Schmilovitz H. Poliovaccines and the course of systemic lupus erythematosus—a retrospective study of 73 patients. Vaccine 10:98–100, 1992.

137. Poliovirus infections. In Peter G, Hall C, Halsey N, et al (eds). Red Book Report of the Committee on Infectious Diseases (24th ed). Elk Grove Village, IL, American Academy of Pediatrics, 1997, pp 424–433.

138. Prevots DR, Burr RK, Sutter RW, Murphy TV. Poliomyelitis prevention in the United States. MMWR 49:1–22, 2000.

139. Plotkin SA. Developed countries should use inactivated polio vaccine for the prevention of poliomyelitis. Rev Med Virol 7:75–81, 1997.

140. Laroche P, Barrand M, Wood SC, et al. The immunogenicity and safety of a new combined diphtheria, tetanus and poliomyelitis booster vaccine (Td-eIPV). Infection 27:49–56, 1999.

141. Sutter RW, Prevots DR. Vaccine-associated paralytic poliomyelitis among immunodeficient persons. Infect Med June:438, 1994.

142. Bottiger M. The elimination of polio in the Scandinavian countries. Public Health Rev 21:27–33, 1993.

143. Bottiger M, Mellin P, Romanus V, et al. Epidemiological events surrounding a paralytic case of poliomyelitis in Sweden. Bull World Health Organ 57:99–103, 1979.

144. Hovi T, Cantell K, Huovilainen A, et al. Outbreak of paralytic poliomyelitis in Finland: widespread circulation of antigenically altered poliovirus type 3 in a vaccinated population. Lancet 1:1427–1432, 1986.

145. Lapinleimu K. Elimination of poliomyelitis in Finland. Rev Infect Dis 6(suppl 2):S457–S460, 1984.

146. Magrath DI, Evans DM, Ferguson M, et al. Antigenic and molecular properties of type 3 poliovirus responsible for an outbreak of poliomyelitis in a vaccinated population. J Gen Virol 67(pt 5):899–905, 1986.

146a. Piirainen L, Roivainen M, Litmanen L, et al. Immunogenicity of a pilot activated poliovirus vaccine with trypsin-treated type 3-component. Vaccine 15: 237–243, 1997.

147. van Wezel AL, van Steenis G, van deer Marel P, Osterhaus AD. Inactivated poliovirus vaccine: current production methods and new developments. Rev Infect Dis 6(suppl 2):S335–S340, 1984.

148. Conyn-Van Spaendonck MA, de Melker HE, Abbink F, et al. Immunity to poliomyelitis in The Netherlands. Am J Epidemiol 153:207–214, 2001.

149. Malvy DJ, Drucker J. Elimination of poliomyelitis in France: epidemiology and vaccine status. Public Health Rev 21:41–49, 1993.

150. Roure C, Rebiere I, Aymard M, et al. Surveillance de la poliomyelite en France. Bull Epidemiol Hebd 15:59–61, 1993.

151. Guerin N, Bregere P, Caudrelier P, Raynaud O. Neutralising antibody response to oral poliovirus vaccine after primary immunisation with inactivated poliovirus vaccine. Eur J Clin Microbiol Infect Dis 17:815–816, 1998.

152. Drucker J. Poliomyelitis in France: epidemiology and vaccination status. Pediatr Infect Dis J 10:967–969, 1991.

153. Ministry of Health Ontario. Wild-type poliovirus isolated in Hamilton. Public Health Epidemiol Rep 7:51–52, 1996.

154. Tulchinsky T, Abed Y, Shaheen S, et al. A ten-year experience in control of poliomyelitis through a combination of live and killed vaccines in two developing countries. Am J Public Health 79:1648–1652, 1989.

155. Lasch EE, Abed Y, Abdulla K, et al. Successful results of a program combining live and inactivated poliovirus vaccines to control poliomyelitis in Gaza. Rev Infect Dis 6(suppl 2):S467–S470, 1984.

156. Swartz TA, Ben Porath E, Kanaaneh H, et al. Comparison of inactivated poliovirus vaccine and oral poliovirus vaccine programs in Israel. Rev Infect Dis 6(suppl 2):S556–S561, 1984.

157. Tulchinsky T. Combined OPV and IPV program in control of poliomyelitis in two endemic areas—a potential tool in the struggle to eradicate poliomyelitis. Public Health Rev 21:153–156, 1997.

158. Slater PE, Orenstein WA, Morag A, et al. Poliomyelitis outbreak in Israel in 1988: a report with two commentaries. Lancet 335:1192–1195, 1990.

159. von Magnus H, Petersen I. Vaccination with inactivated poliovirus vaccine and oral poliovirus vaccine in Denmark. Rev Infect Dis 6(suppl 2):S471–S474, 1984.

160. Poliovirus Infections. In Pickering LK (ed). Red Book Report of the Committee on Infectious Diseases (25th ed). Elk Grove Village, IL, American Academy of Pediatrics, 2000, pp 467–470.

161. Strebel PM, Sutter RW, Cochi SL, et al. Epidemiology of poliomyelitis in the United States one decade after the last reported case of indigenous wild virus-associated disease. Clin Infect Dis 14:568–579, 1992.

162. Yogev R, Edwards KM. Polio vaccination schedules in the United States: the rationale for change. Semin Pediatr Infect Dis 10:249–257, 1999.

163. Kolasa MS, Desai SN, Bisgard KM, et al. Impact of the sequential poliovirus immunization schedule: a demonstration project. Am J Prev Med 18:140–145, 2000.

164. Lakhiani CN, Vivier PM, Alario AJ, et al. Analysis of the transition from oral polio vaccine to inactivated polio vaccine for primary immunization in a hospital-based primary care practice. Pediatr Infect Dis J 19:575–576, 2000.

165. Davis RL, Lieu TA, Mell LK, et al. Impact of the change in polio vaccination schedule on immunization coverage rates: a study in two large health maintenance organizations. Pediatrics 107:671–676, 2001.

166. Lieu TA, Davis RL, Capra AM, et al. Variation in clinician recommendations for multiple injections during adoption of inactivated polio vaccine. Pediatrics 107(4):E49, 2001.

167. Tucker AW, Isaacs D, Burgess M. Cost-effectiveness analysis of changing from live oral poliovirus vaccine to inactivated poliovirus vaccine in Australia. Aust N Z J Public Health 25:411–416, 2001.

168. John TJ. Immunisation against polioviruses in developing countries. Rev Med Virol 3:149–160, 1993.

169. Hull HF, Aylward RB. Ending polio immunization [see comments]. Science 277:780, 1997.

170. John TJ. Anomalous observations on IPV and OPV vaccination. Dev Biol (Basel) 105:197–208, 2001.

171. Estevrs K. Safety of oral poliomyelitis vaccine: results of a WHO enquiry. Bull World Health Organ 66:739–746, 1988.

172. Andrus JK, Strebel PM, de Quadros CA, Olive JM. Risk of vaccine-associated paralytic poliomyelitis in Latin America, 1989–91. Bull World Health Organ 73:33–40, 1995.

173. McBean AM, Modlin JF. Rationale for the sequential use of inactivated poliovirus vaccine and live attenuated poliovirus vaccine for routine poliomyelitis immunization in the United States. Pediatr Infect Dis J 6:881–887, 1987.

174. Faden H. Poliovirus vaccination: a trilogy. J Infect Dis 168:25–28, 1993.

175. Hull HF, Birmingham ME, Melgaard B, Lee JW. Progress toward global polio eradication. J Infect Dis 175(suppl 1):S4–S9, 1997.

176. Henderson DA. Countering the posteradication threat of smallpox and polio. Clin Infect Dis 34:79–83, 2002.

177. John TJ. The final stages of the global eradication of polio. N Engl J Med 343:806–807, 2000.

178. Georgescu MM, Delpeyroux F, Tardy-Panit M, et al. High diversity of poliovirus strains isolated from the central nervous system from patients with vaccine-associated paralytic poliomyelitis. J Virol 68:8089–8101, 1994.

179. Dove AW, Racaniello VR. The polio eradication effort: should vaccine eradication be next? [see comments]. Science 277:779–780, 1997.

180. Prolonged poliovirus excretion in an immunodeficient person with vaccine-associated paralytic poliomyelitis. MMWR 46(28):641–643, 1997.

181. Guillot S, Caro V, Cuervo N, et al. Natural genetic exchanges between vaccine and wild poliovirus strains in humans. J Virol 74:8434–8443, 2000.

182. Kew O, Morris-Glasgow V, Landaverde M, et al. Outbreak of poliomyelitis in Hispaniola associated with circulating type 1 vaccine-derived poliovirus. Science 296:356–359, 2002.

183. Eichner M, Dietz K. Eradication of poliomyelitis: when can one be sure that polio virus transmission has been terminated? Am J Epidemiol 143:816–822, 1996.

184. Racaniello VR. It is too early to stop polio vaccination. Bull World Health Organ 78:359–360, 2000.

185. Schoub BD. The risks of stopping vaccination: perspectives from the developing world. Bull World Health Organ 78:360–361, 2000.

186. Fine PE. Gaps in our knowledge about transmission of vaccine-derived polioviruses. Bull World Health Organ 78:358–359, 2000.

187. Plotkin SA. An end to Manicheism. Public Health Rev 21:135–138, 1993.

188. Yeh SH, Ward JI, Partridge S, et al. Safety and immunogenicity of a pentavalent diphtheria, tetanus, pertussis, hepatitis B and polio combination vaccine in infants. Pediatr Infect Dis J 20(10): 973–980, 2001.

Chapter 25

Poliovirus Vaccine—Live

ROLAND W. SUTTER • OLEN M. KEW • STEPHEN L. COCHI

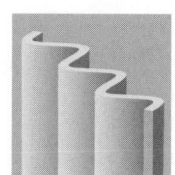

HISTORY

The written history of poliomyelitis can be traced to the first description of the disease as a separate clinical entity by Michael Underwood in 1789, more than 200 years ago.[1] Since then, many important scientific discoveries and public health milestones have been associated with poliomyelitis. Undoubtedly, the most consequential of these were the development of effective poliovirus vaccines,[2] which paved the way for the implementation of control programs, and a resolution by the World Health Assembly that established the goal of global eradication of poliomyelitis by the year 2000.[3] Although the 2000 eradication target was not achieved, the polio eradication initiative is operational in all polio-endemic countries (including those affected by conflict) and is approaching its final stage, with interruption of the last chains of poliovirus transmission expected in the next 12 to 24 months, and the world could be certified as free of wild poliovirus as early as 3 years after detection of the last circulating virus.

Although the written history of poliomyelitis is relatively succinct, an Egyptian stele from the 18th dynasty (1580 to 1350 BC) depicts a "crippled young man, apparently a priest, with a withered and shortened right leg, and with his foot held in a typical equinus position characteristic of flaccid paralysis."[4] This inscription demonstrates that poliomyelitis probably has affected humankind since ancient times. Underwood[1] introduced the term *debility of the lower extremities* in 1789; other researchers suggested a series of alternative terms, including *Lähmungszustände der unteren Extremitäten* in 1840,[5] *morning paralysis* in 1843,[6] *paralysie essentielle chez les enfants* in 1851,[7] *paralysie atrophiques graisseues de l'enfance* in 1855,[8] *spinale Kinderlähmung* in 1860,[9] *tephromyelitis anterior acuta parenchymatose* in 1872,[10] and *poliomyelitis anterior acuta* in 1874.[11] The last term is based on anatomic location of lesions within the spinal cord—which was discovered in the early 1870s—and constructed from the Greek words *polios* (i.e., gray) and *myelos* (i.e., marrow, the gray matter of the spinal cord) with the ending -*itis* to imply inflammation. Although the terms *Heine-Medin disease* in 1907,[12] *infantile paralysis*, and *polio* were proposed subsequently, poliomyelitis prevailed and became the standard designation for the disease.

In the late 19th century and early 20th century, a change in the epidemiology of poliomyelitis from a predominantly endemic to an epidemic form was observed in Sweden and Norway,[12–14] heralding similar changes in other industrialized countries. Our understanding of these changes in the epidemiology was greatly aided by groundbreaking investigations of the three largest poliomyelitis outbreaks of the time: (1) 132 cases in Rutland County, Vermont, in 1894 by Charles Caverly,[15] (2) 1031 cases in Sweden in 1905 by Ivar Wickman,[12,14] and (3) more than 9000 cases in New York in 1916.[16] Wickman was the first to recognize that abortive cases might equal or outnumber cases with paralytic manifestations and that these cases may be significant in the propagation of the infection.[14] These outbreaks were due to an accumulation of a sufficient number of susceptible children to sustain epidemic transmission of poliovirus, presumably because improvements in hygiene and sanitation had delayed poliovirus exposure from infancy to later in life.

Landsteiner and Popper[17] reported in 1908 that a "filtrable agent" (i.e., virus) was the cause of poliomyelitis on the basis of microscopic examination of spinal cords from two monkeys that had been injected intraperitoneally with a suspension of ground-up cord from a fatal human case. Burnet and Macnamara[18] determined in 1931 that more than one strain of virus could cause poliomyelitis and that immunity to one strain did not confer immunity to another strain. These investigators based their findings on cross-immunity and serologic tests and, most importantly, showed that three monkeys that had recovered from one strain (and should have been immune) developed paralytic disease after injection of another strain. This report had profound implications, although not immediately appreciated at the time, both in terms of redefining the epidemiology of the disease and with respect to directing the subsequent development of vaccines. In 1948, an effort was launched to determine the number of distinct poliovirus strains. This effort was coordinated by the Committee on Typing of the National Foundation for Infantile Paralysis, which reported in 1951 that three and only three types of poliovirus, designated types I, II, and III, were the cause of poliomyelitis.[19] Enders, Weller, and Robbins[20] demonstrated in 1949 that poliovirus could be grown in non-nervous, human embryonic tissue, work that was later honored with the Nobel Prize. Thus the determination of the number of poliovirus strains, the ability for large-scale growth of the virus, and the finding that circulating antibody had a protective effect against poliomyelitis[21-26] all were essential preconditions for the development of effective poliovirus vaccines.

Two different approaches for vaccine development pursued at the time were successful: inactivation of poliovirus by formalin pioneered by Dr. Jonas Salk, licensed as inactivated poliovirus vaccine (IPV) in 1955 after one of the largest controlled field trials ever conducted[2]; and the attenuation of the three serotypes of poliovirus by Dr. Albert Sabin, licensed in 1961 as monovalent oral poliovirus vaccine (OPV) and in 1963 as trivalent OPV.[27] The widespread use of IPV and OPV rapidly controlled poliomyelitis.

The construction of the Drinker respirator (i.e., "iron lung") beginning in 1928 and its widespread use in the 1930s and 1940s rapidly decreased the case-fatality ratio of bulbar forms of poliomyelitis.[28] Epidemic poliomyelitis in the early part of the 20th century was associated with a high case-fatality rate (27.1% during the New York epidemic of 1916).[16,29,30] Further improvements in hygiene and sanitation delayed the median age of poliovirus infection from younger than 5 years in the 1910s to 5 to 9 years in the 1940s[31,32] and allowed the accumulation of large numbers of people susceptible to poliomyelitis. Epidemics of ever-increasing magnitude began to occur in the United States and Europe until the mid- to late 1950s when vaccines became available. Because increasing age appeared to be the primary risk factor for bulbar paralysis—the basis for the "central dogma" of the epidemiology of poliomyelitis[33]—an increasing proportion of cases required respiratory support, and whole wards of iron lungs were devoted to caring for poliomyelitis victims in the 1940s and 1950s.

Poliomyelitis is intimately linked with some of the greatest triumphs in medicine, including scientific breakthroughs, public health achievements, and advancements in social justice. The concept of social justice, the indiscriminate benefit of scientific discoveries or access to care and rehabilitation, was pioneered by the National Foundation for Infantile Paralysis, which raised funds through annual March of Dimes campaigns that covered treatment and rehabilitation costs of poliomyelitis victims.[34] The Vaccines for Children Act (1993) ensures that poliovirus vaccines are available for poor children in the United States. Ultimately, the successful conclusion of the poliomyelitis eradication initiative will benefit all children equally, whether rich or poor, whether white or black, and whether living in industrialized or developing countries.

The history of poliomyelitis has been reviewed in detail by Paul[4] and in Chapter 2 of this edition of *Vaccines*.

Why Is the Disease Important?

Poliomyelitis was the leading cause of permanent disability in the prevaccine era.[31] Besides the considerable disease burden, poliomyelitis was much feared in the prevaccine era because it could strike anybody, no means existed of pro-

tecting oneself or one's children, and, unlike the situation with other diseases such as measles, from which most children either recover or die rapidly, society was reminded every day of the devastating effects of this crippling disease.

Disease control programs using poliovirus vaccines have prevented and continue to prevent millions of children from becoming paralyzed. In 1988, when the global eradication target was adopted, the World Health Organization (WHO) estimated that approximately 350,000 cases of paralytic poliomyelitis were occurring annually,[35] despite availability of effective vaccines over the prior three decades. Poliomyelitis has gained renewed attention in recent years because the feasibility of its eradication has been demonstrated[35,36] and because of the visibility of the ongoing global effort to eradicate poliovirus.[37-39]

Background

Clinical Description

Poliomyelitis is an acute infection caused by any of three serotypes of poliovirus that replicate initially in the gastrointestinal tract and rarely in the motor neurons of the anterior horn cells in the spinal cord, where replication of virus results in cell destruction and flaccid paralysis of the muscles the cells innervate (i.e., spinal poliomyelitis). On occasion, brain stem cells innervating respiratory muscles can be affected, resulting in difficulties in breathing (i.e., bulbar paralysis). In addition to the acute paralysis, late manifestations with exacerbation of weakness or new paralysis (i.e., postpolio syndrome) can be observed in a significant proportion of patients decades after the acute paralytic episode.

Poliovirus exposure in a person susceptible to poliomyelitis results in one of the following consequences: (1) inapparent infection without symptoms, (2) minor illness, (3) nonparalytic poliomyelitis (aseptic meningitis), or (4) paralytic poliomyelitis.[31,40-42] Inapparent infection without symptoms is the most frequent outcome (72%) after poliovirus exposure in susceptible people.[43] Minor illness is the most frequent form (24%) of the disease, characterized by transient illness associated with a few days of fever, malaise, drowsiness, headache, nausea, vomiting, constipation, or sore throat, in various combinations.[43] Nonparalytic poliomyelitis (aseptic meningitis) is a relatively rare outcome (4%) of poliovirus infection. It begins usually as a minor illness characterized by fever, sore throat, vomiting, and malaise. One to 2 days later, signs of meningeal irritation become apparent, including stiffness of the neck or back; vomiting; severe headache; and pain in the limbs, back, and neck.[40] This form of the disease lasts 2 to 10 days, and recovery is usually rapid and complete. In a small proportion of these cases, the disease advances to transient mild muscle weakness or paralysis.

Paralytic poliomyelitis is a rare outcome (usually <1%) of poliovirus infections among susceptible people. Its clinical course is characterized by a minor illness of several days and a symptom-free period of 1 to 3 days, followed by rapid onset of flaccid paralysis with fever and progression to the maximum extent of paralysis within a few days. This characteristic clinical course of a minor illness followed by the major illness with paralysis has been related to the two humps of the dromedary.[44] In actuality, this is a misnomer, because the dromedary is a one-humped camel. Among adolescent and adult cases of poliomyelitis, the minor illness is often absent, and these groups also appear to experience more severe pain in the affected extremities. After temperature returns to normal, there is usually no further progression of paralysis. If paralysis of an extremity is not complete, it is more pronounced proximally. Paralysis is usually asymmetric, associated with diminished or complete loss of deep tendon reflexes and an intact sensory system. Paralytic manifestations in extremities begin proximally and progress to involve distal muscle groups (i.e., descending paralysis). Depending on the anatomic location of motor neuron damage in the spinal cord or in the brain stem, spinal, mixed spinal–bulbar, or bulbar paralysis involving primarily respiratory muscles may be observed. The anterior horn cells (and brain stem cells), just like other nerve cells of the central nervous system (CNS), cannot be regenerated or replaced, and paralysis is permanent. Nevertheless, because of compensation of other, still functioning muscles, partial or total recovery can be achieved, usually within the first 6 months after onset of disease. Detailed clinical descriptions may be found in a number of reviews and books.[45–48]

Postpolio syndrome, a term invented in the early 1980s, refers to a disease entity that encompasses the late manifestations of acute paralytic poliomyelitis.[49] Aside from previously published case reports and case series, the first systematic investigation of postpolio syndrome was published in 1984.[50] After an interval of 15 to 40 years, many people (25% to 40%) who contracted paralytic poliomyelitis in their childhood may experience muscle pain and exacerbation of existing weakness or may develop new weakness or paralysis. Factors that enhance the risk of postpolio syndrome include (1) increasing length of time since acute poliovirus infection, (2) presence of permanent residual impairment after recovery from the acute illness, and (3) female gender. The exact cause of these late effects is currently unknown, although it is not a consequence of persistent infection. The pathogenesis of postpolio syndrome is thought to involve late attrition of oversized motor units that developed during the recovery process of paralytic poliomyelitis.[49] Postpolio syndrome has been described in people infected during the era of wild-type poliovirus circulation. An excellent summary of the current scientific knowledge of postpolio syndrome has been published.[51]

Virology

Polioviruses are part of the *Enterovirus* genus and belong to the family Picornaviridae (Italian: *pico*, implying small, and

RNA, the nucleic acid component).[52] Polioviruses are small (27 to 30 nm in diameter), nonenveloped viruses with capsids of icosahedral symmetry enclosing a single-stranded, positive-sense RNA genome about 7500 nucleotides long. Polioviruses share most of their biochemical and biophysiologic properties with the other enteroviruses. They are stable at acid pH (3.0 to 5.0) for 1 to 3 hours and resistant to inactivation by many common detergents and disinfectants, including soaps, nonionic detergents, and lipid solvents such as ethanol, ether, and chloroform. Polioviruses are rapidly inactivated by treatment with 0.3% formaldehyde or 0.5 ppm free residual chlorine, by desiccation, or by exposure to ultraviolet light. Infectivity is stable for weeks at 4°C and for days at 30°C. Polioviruses are readily inactivated at 55°C, but $MgCl_2$ stabilizes infectivity.[53]

There are three antigenic types (serotypes 1, 2, and 3)[19,54–57] (Table 25–1), which, apart from their antigenic differences, are otherwise very similar. The complete genomic sequences have been determined for representatives of each serotype,[58] including those of the three Sabin OPV strains. Only the sequences encoding the capsid proteins are unique to polioviruses, because the flanking sequences are frequently exchanged by recombination with closely related enteroviruses during circulation in nature.[59,60] The poliovirion consists of 60 copies each of four capsid proteins (VP1 through VP4) that form a highly structured capsid shell.[61] The three major proteins (VP1, VP2, VP3) share a similar basic architecture, and were probably derived from a common ancestral protein. The smallest protein, VP4, internalized in the native virion, is formed by the cleavage of the precursor VP0 (VP4 + VP2) during the final maturation of the virion. The external surface of the poliovirion is decorated by peptide loops extending from VP1, VP2, and VP3, which form the neutralizing antigenic sites.[61,62] Four neutralizing antigenic sites have been identified by patterns of reactivity with neutralizing monoclonal antibodies, and the assignments have been confirmed by high-resolution x-ray crystallography.[62] Sites 2, 3, and 4 are discontinuous and formed from loops contributed by different capsid proteins. The major type-specific differences in the sequences of the capsid polypeptides primarily reside on the most surface-accessible peptide loops, which represent less than 4% of the total capsid protein. Amino acid sequences of the underlying framework of the capsid are highly conserved across poliovirus serotypes.[58] Although the neutralizing antigenic sites vary within each serotype, the range of variability is constrained, such that all polioviruses within a serotype can be neutralized by type-specific antisera.

TABLE 25–1 ■ Polioviruses

Poliovirus Serotype	Prototype* Strain Designation	Geographic Origin	Illness in Person Yielding Virus	Investigators
1	Brunhilde	Maryland	Paralytic poliomyelitis[†]	Bodian et al.[55]
2	Lansing	Michigan	Fatal paralytic poliomyelitis[‡]	Armstrong[54]
3	Leon	California	Fatal paralytic poliomyelitis[‡]	Kessel and Pait[56]

*Prototype strains for serotypes.
†Virus recovered from feces.
‡Virus recovered from spinal cord.

Polioviruses attach to and enter cells via a specific poliovirus receptor (PVR, or CD155) on the cytoplasmic membrane, a glycoprotein of the immunoglobulin superfamily whose host function is unknown.[63] The terminal residues of the receptor specifically interact with sequences forming a canyon-like channel on the virion surface. Each poliovirion has 60 receptor-binding sites.[64,65] The PVR is expressed on the surface of human and simian cells supporting poliovirus infection, but is absent on cells from nonprimates, rendering them resistant to infection. The human PVR gene has been cloned.[63] On introduction into resistant cells, the human gene converts them into susceptible cells.[66] The gene for the human PVR has been introduced into a germ line of mice.[67,68] The resulting transgenic animals become susceptible to polioviruses, demonstrating that the primary block to infection of normal mice by such strains is at the level of cell entry.[67] Transgenic mice expressing the human PVR gene become paralyzed on intraspinal or intracerebral inoculation with wild-type poliovirus but do not develop disease on inoculation with attenuated Sabin strains.[67] Such transgenic mice have proven useful for neurovirulence testing of OPV lots, for study of field isolates, and for detailed studies of poliovirus pathogenesis. Because of concerns that transgenic mice infected with poliovirus may escape the laboratories, breed with nontransgenic mice, and potentially establish a nonhuman reservoir of poliovirus transmission, specific guidelines have been issued to address this theoretical risk.[69]

Polioviruses are among the simplest viruses in terms of genetic organization and replication cycle.[52] However, they grow very rapidly, yielding up to 10,000 infectious particles per cell in a growth cycle of 4 to 5 hours. After attachment and entry, the genomic RNA is uncoated and translated under the control of the "internal ribosomal entry site" (IRES) to produce a single polypeptide, the polyprotein. The polyprotein is cleaved after translation into the virus-specific proteins, which include the capsid proteins, two virus-specific proteases controlling proteolytic processing, and an RNA-dependent RNA polymerase catalyzing the synthesis of RNA molecules of negative and positive polarity. The negative-polarity RNA serves as a template for synthesis of positive-polarity messenger and genomic RNA. Host protein synthesis is rapidly inhibited by the cleavage of a cellular protein required for initiation of translation of host messenger RNA but not for the initiation of translation from the poliovirus IRES. Infected cells are rapidly converted into factories for poliovirus synthesis, show cytopathic effects after several hours, and release virus through cell lysis and death. Once virion assembly has started, production of capsid protein and replication of RNA are closely linked, and integration of viral RNA into the virion follows within several minutes. Morphogenesis appears to involve the combination of viral RNA with a shell of viral proteins (VP0, VP1, VP3), during which the VP0 procapsid protein is cleaved to yield VP2 and VP4.

Pathogenesis as It Relates to Prevention

The pathogenesis of poliovirus infection indicates that prevention through immunization can be accomplished by inhibiting replication at and dissemination from the gastrointestinal tract, by inhibiting the viremia that follows, or by doing both. After the individual is exposed to poliovirus by way of the oral cavity, the virus attaches and enters specific cells that express the PVR.[63] The virus replicates locally at the sites of virus implantation (e.g., tonsils, intestinal M cells, and Peyer's patches of the ileum) or at the lymph nodes that drain these tissues. The first approach requires the presence of local secretory immunoglobulin (Ig) A antibody. The second approach—because spread occurs primarily by way of the bloodstream to other susceptible tissues (i.e., other lymph nodes, brown fat, and the CNS) or by way of retrograde axonal transport to the CNS—requires the presence of neutralizing antibody.

The host range of poliovirus and tissue tropism is determined by the expression of the PVR, which belongs to the immunoglobulin superfamily.[63] Tissue tropism refers to the ability of poliovirus to replicate in specific cells.[70] Early studies on poliovirus pathogenesis were conducted in primates, but the development of PVR transgenic mice has led to a renaissance in pathogenesis studies.[71,72] Most of the earlier observations with primates[45,46,48] have been confirmed in the PVR transgenic mouse model,[72] and new tools have been used to investigate important unresolved questions about poliovirus pathogenesis. For example, in situ hybridization with nucleic acid probes of the PVR in transgenic mice suggested a limited expression of the PVR to the CNS, thymus, lung, kidney, and adrenal glands and more recently in monocytes (mononuclear phagocytes).[73] Replication of poliovirus in motor neurons results in cell destruction and paralysis. The chief limitation of the mouse model is the low level of expression of the PVR in mouse intestinal tissue, resulting in very inefficient replication of virus at the primary site of natural infection.[72]

Poliovirus may be found in the blood of patients with the abortive form ("minor illness"), and it can be detected several days before onset of clinical signs of CNS involvement in patients who develop nonparalytic or paralytic poliomyelitis.[24,74] The virus is regularly present in the throat and in the stools before the onset of illness. In individuals who have either clinical or subclinical infection, virus is excreted in the feces for several weeks[43] and in saliva for 1 to 2 weeks. The mean duration of wild poliovirus type 1 excretion in fecal specimens is 24 days (median, 20 to 29 days), with a range of 1 to 114 days.[43]

For further details of pathogenesis and pathology, see Bodian,[45] Bodian and Horstmann,[46] Sabin,[48] and Racaniello and Ren.[72]

Diagnosis

Paralytic poliomyelitis caused by imported wild-type poliovirus or by vaccine-related poliovirus has become a rare disease in the United States and other industrialized countries. Therefore, physicians may not be familiar with the disease or consider the diagnosis of poliomyelitis until other more frequent causes of acute flaccid paralysis (AFP) have been ruled out. The diagnosis of paralytic poliomyelitis is dependent on (1) clinical course, (2) virologic testing, (3) special studies, and (4) residual neurologic deficit 60 days after onset of symptoms. For surveillance purposes, any case with physician-diagnosed suspected poliomyelitis is investigated in the United States, and a case is confirmed if a panel of independent experts determines that the case definition* for paralytic poliomyelitis has been met. The WHO is using a sensitive case definition: any case of AFP in a person less than 15 years of age, or a case in a person of any age from which poliomyelitis is suspected. This definition attempts to capture all cases of paralysis that might be caused by poliovirus, including those erroneously diagnosed as other clinical syndromes such as Guillain-Barré syndrome. This sensitive screening definition is balanced by a specific case classification system (i.e., virologic case classification scheme) that relies on isolation of poliovirus from stool specimens to confirm cases of AFP as poliomyelitis. As countries improve the quality and timeliness of AFP surveillance, the virologic case classification has now replaced the clinical case classification scheme in almost all endemic and recently endemic countries (see *Disease Control Strategies* below).

Clinical Course

The clinical course (see *Clinical Description* above) is helpful in ruling in or ruling out paralytic poliomyelitis. Several studies in the developing world have attempted to assess the sensitivity and specificity of different clinical case definitions for paralytic poliomyelitis and compared these with the "gold standard" of virologically confirmed poliomyelitis based on poliovirus isolation from stool specimens. These studies reported similar findings.[75-77] The largest study reported a sensitivity of 64% and a specificity of 82% for a case definition that included age younger than 6 years, fever at onset, and rapid progress to maximum extent of paralysis (≤4 days).[75] The addition of a specific pattern of paralysis (proximal, unilateral, or absence of paralysis in all four extremities) increased the specificity with varying degrees of loss in sensitivity. The case definitions and case classification schemes have been reviewed.[78] Data from India suggest that residual paralysis 60 days after onset of paralysis is the strongest predictor for confirmed poliomyelitis (i.e., isolating wild-type poliovirus in stool samples during the initial examination). These findings highlight the importance of a 60-day follow-up examination to assess whether areas with wild-type poliovirus circulation may have been missed.

Virologic Testing

Because AFP has many etiologies, including Guillain-Barré syndrome, transverse myelitis, and infection with nonpolio enteroviruses (see *Differential Diagnosis* below), laboratory confirmation is critical to establishing the diagnosis of poliomyelitis. The basic approach is to attempt to isolate poliovirus from the stools of patients with AFP, and to characterize any poliovirus isolates to determine whether they are vaccine-related or wild-type. Detailed descriptions of standard laboratory principles and procedures for investigation of enterovirus infections are available,[79] and standard typing antisera for identifying enteroviral isolates are available through the WHO.[80] The WHO has published a manual for the virologic investigation of poliomyelitis cases that includes protocols for the isolation of poliovirus.[81] This manual has become the standard guide for the isolation and characterization of polioviruses for laboratories in the WHO's Global Laboratory Network for Poliomyelitis Eradication[82] and is widely used in other diagnostic laboratories.[83]

Two cell lines are recommended for the isolation of polioviruses in stool specimens: (1) RD cells, derived from human rhabdomyosarcoma, and (2) L20B cells, derived from the mouse L cell line and genetically altered to express the human PVR.[66] RD cells have the advantage of being very sensitive to poliovirus infection and yielding high poliovirus titers in culture. RD cells will support the replication of other human enteroviruses, but not Coxsackie B viruses. L20B cells will support the replication of polioviruses, but, like their parenteral mouse L cells, are resistant to infection by most nonpolio enteroviruses. Thus L20B cells are used for the selective cultivation of polioviruses. HEp-2C (Cincinnati) cells, derived from a human epidermoid sarcoma, had been used by Global Laboratory Network laboratories for poliovirus isolation. However, because the use of HEp-2C cells did not increase the sensitivity for poliovirus detection above that obtained with the combined use of RD and L20B cells, routine use of HEp-2C cells in the Network was discontinued. HEp-2C cells are useful for the study of nonpolio enteroviruses because they can support the replication of many different enterovirus serotypes, including Coxsackie B viruses.

Poliovirus may be recovered from stool, throat swabs, or cerebrospinal fluid taken soon after the onset of illness and from stool specimens collected over longer periods of time (usually up to 8 weeks after the start of infection).[84] Poliovirus isolation rates from cerebrospinal fluid are generally low; however, when virus is found, a causal relationship between a poliovirus serotype and paralytic disease is strongly suggested. The WHO recommends that two stool samples be collected at least 24 hours apart to confirm the diagnosis, because excretion of virus can be intermittent and the sensitivity of isolation is less than 100%.† Wild-type poliovirus has been found in stool samples of 63% to 93% of patients during the first 2 weeks of illness, in 35% to 75% during the third and fourth weeks, and in less than 50% during the fifth and sixth weeks.[84] The duration of viral shedding is reduced among children who were previously vaccinated, had pre-existing homologous antibody, or had a previous intestinal infection with homologous poliovirus.[84]

Clinical specimens are processed to produce a virus suspension largely free of bacteria and other debris, to which antibiotics are added to inhibit the growth of residual bacteria, and the suspension is inoculated onto cell cultures. Cells are monitored daily for cytopathic effects, which appear typically within 3 to 6 days of incubation. Poliovirus isolates are identified by serotype in neutralization tests using pools of specific antiserum. Polioviruses also can be identified by the polymerase chain reaction (PCR) using group-specific[85] and serotype-specific[86] primer sets. Intratypic differentiation

---

*"A patient must have had paralysis clinically and epidemiologically compatible with poliomyelitis and, at 60 days after onset of symptoms, had residual neurologic deficit, had died, or had no information available on neurologic residua."[495] This case definition was formerly known as the Best Available Paralytic Poliomyelitis Case Count (BAPPCC).

†Extensive evaluations of the Global Laboratory Network in the Americas have demonstrated that, with a well-functioning transport system for specimens and high-quality laboratories that pass proficiency tests, one stool sample is adequate. This is the only region in which there is a recommendation that one stool specimen be collected from AFP cases.

(ITD) of poliovirus isolates (testing whether they are vaccine-related or wild-type) is performed throughout the Global Laboratory Network using one antigenic and one molecular method.[82] The standard antigenic ITD method uses an enzyme-linked immunosorbent assay system with preparations of highly specific cross-adsorbed antisera.[87,88] The molecular ITD methods use genotype-specific nucleic acid probes,[89,90] genotype-specific PCR primers,[91–93] or PCR coupled to analyses of restriction fragment length polymorphism.[94] Some Network laboratories use panels of neutralizing monoclonal antibodies for preliminary ITD testing.[87]

The purpose of ITD is to screen out polioviruses that are closely related (>99% VP1 sequence identity) to the Sabin OPV strains, and are unlikely to be of current epidemiologic importance. The remaining poliovirus isolates are either wild-type polioviruses or atypical vaccine-derived polioviruses (VDPVs) (see *Vaccine-Derived Polioviruses* below). Since the beginning of 2001, Network laboratories routinely sequence the complete VP1 region of any wild-type poliovirus isolated from an AFP case. Analysis of the full approximately 900-nucleotide VP1 region, performed to obtain the degree of phylogenetic resolution necessary to distinguish among wild-type poliovirus isolates, has permitted reconstruction of individual chains of transmission from sequence data.[95] The use of genomic sequencing has given rise to a new discipline that combines the tools and concepts of classical epidemiology with those of microbiology, biochemistry, genetics, and evolutionary biology (see *Molecular Epidemiology of Poliovirus* below).[96]

Serologic testing may be helpful in establishing the diagnosis but often does not contribute and sometimes may cause confusion because (1) antibody rises have already occurred by the time the first specimen has been collected, (2) antibody may be present to one or more serotypes because of previous or recent vaccination, and (3) heterotypic responses may be observed to one serotype after exposure to another serotype. There are no reliable means of distinguishing antibody induced by vaccine-related or wild-type poliovirus. Standard protocols for neutralization assays to determine levels of antibody to poliovirus are available.[81,97,98] Paired serum specimens are required to demonstrate a fourfold or greater rise in antibody titer between acute and convalescent sera. The first serum specimen should be collected as soon as possible after onset of paralytic manifestations, and the second specimen should be collected 2 to 3 weeks later. Neutralizing antibodies appear early and are usually already detectable at the time of onset of paralysis. However, if the first specimen is taken early enough, a rise in titer may be demonstrated during the course of the disease. In a study from Louisiana, specimens were collected as soon as possible after hospital admission from poliomyelitis patients and about 6 weeks later; in 36% of patients, a fourfold rise in poliovirus antibody titer could be demonstrated; in 61%, reciprocal titers were above 320 and did not change; and in 3%, reciprocal titers were below 320 and remained unchanged.[99]

Neutralizing assays continue to be the gold standard method for the detection of type-specific antibody in sera.[22] Neutralization antibody induced by a single serotype may not be completely serotype specific. In practical terms, this seldom constitutes a problem because the heterotypic response results in low levels of neutralizing antibody

Because of the limitations described, serology may be more important in excluding (e.g., no detectable antibody) the diagnosis of poliomyelitis than in confirming it. However, intrathecal immune responses can be measured and offer the advantage of attributing a causal relationship between a poliovirus serotype and paralytic disease.[100] Other assays have been proposed but are used infrequently, including indirect immunofluorescence,[101] paper-radioactive virus method,[102] enzyme-linked immunosorbent assay,[103] and microindirect hemagglutination and hemagglutination-inhibition.[104]

Special Studies

Nerve conduction and electromyography studies can point to the anatomic location of the paralysis[105]—destruction of anterior horn cells in the spinal cord versus a demyelinating process in the peripheral nerves—helping to exclude the most frequent cause of AFP, Guillain-Barré syndrome. Magnetic resonance imaging has been used infrequently, but, in at least one patient with poliomyelitis, magnetic resonance imaging has highlighted the anterior column of the spinal cord.[106] Analysis of spinal fluid may be helpful in ruling out other causes. In paralytic poliomyelitis, the cerebrospinal fluid contains an increased number of leukocytes—usually 10 to 200/mL, and seldom more than 500/mL.[107,108] At the onset of signs of CNS involvement, the ratio of polymorphonuclear cells to lymphocytes is high, but within a few days the ratio is reversed. The total white blood cell count slowly subsides to normal levels. The protein content of the cerebrospinal fluid initially is elevated only slightly (average, about 46 mg/100 mL [range, 15 to 165 mg/100 mL] in nonparalytic cases and 68 mg/100 mL [range, 25 to 250 mg/100 mL] among paralytic cases), but it rises gradually in paralytic cases until the third week, generally returning to normal by the sixth week.[107] Glucose levels are usually within the normal range. In fatal cases, spinal cord and brain stem tissue samples should be examined for the typical lesions caused by viral replication and destruction of the motor neuron cells.

Residual Neurologic Deficit

The clinical case definition for paralytic poliomyelitis requires a residual neurologic deficit at 60 days after onset of paralysis. Such a neurologic deficit may be apparent as complete flaccid paralysis of one or more extremities or partial paralysis or weakness of muscles or muscle groups. In the latter instance, because of functional recovery (intact muscles may compensate for muscles that are not innervated), it may be more difficult to establish a neurologic deficit. The most severe cases of poliomyelitis in terms of complications and fatal outcomes occur in people with underlying immunodeficiency disorders.

Differential Diagnosis

The differential diagnoses of AFP have been reviewed.[109] The list of underlying causes of AFP is extensive (Table 25–2). The causes can be classified according to the pathophysiologic mechanisms and anatomic sites of the etiologic factors. For example, poliovirus damages primarily the anterior horn cells of the spinal cord. This damage leads secondarily to paralysis of extremity muscles (Fig. 25–1). The distinguishing features of poliomyelitis, Guillain-Barré syn-

TABLE 25–2 ■ Causes and Differential Diagnosis of Acute Flaccid Paralysis

Infectious	
Viral	
Enteroviruses	Poliomyelitis, Coxsackie A (A7, A9; A4, A5, A10), Coxsackie B (B1–B5), echoviruses (6, 9; 1–4, 7, 11, 14, 16–18, 30), enterovirus 70, enterovirus 71
Other viruses	Myxoviruses (mumps virus), toga and arboviruses, Epstein-Barr virus; human immuno-deficiency virus (HIV), Japanese B encephalitis virus, West Nile virus
Bacterial	*Campylobacter jejuni* (leading cause of Guillain-Barré syndrome)
Metabolic—transient and periodic paralyses	
Hypokalemic	Familial, Sjögren's syndrome, hyperthyroidism, gossypol induced (toxic phenolic pigment in cottonseed), association with barium poisoning, association with hyperaldosteronism
Normo- or hyperkalemic	Familial, adynamia episodica hereditaria of Gamstorp
Hypophosphatemia	
Drug induced	
Heroin	
Antibiotics	Aminoglycosides, polymyxin B, tetracyclines
Organic	
Volatile hydrocarbons	Hexane, methyl butyl ketone, carbon disulfide
Trecresyl phosphate	Jamaican ginger tonic; contaminant of cooking oil, mustard oil, or flour
Other	Cantharidin, diethyltoluamide (DEET), dithiobiuret (rat poison), triethyldodecyl-ammonium bromide (mouse poison)
Toxins	
Bacterial	Botulinum, diphtheria, tetanus (cephalic form), *moraxella*
Fungal—mycotoxins	*Penicillium citrea-viridae*, *Penicillium islandicum*, *Penicillium citrinum*
Insect	Tick paralysis; spider venom; cockroach, beetle; wasp venom; *Lepidoptera* larvae
Parasite/protozoa/dinoflagellates	Paralytic shellfish poisoning—saxitoxin, ichthyotoxism (sardines)
Reptiles—snake venom	Cobra, Australian elapid, krait, mamba, Sea snake
Plants and plant toxin	*Gloriosa superba* (daisy) [root], *Lathyrus* species (sweet pea), *Aconitum* (monkshood), hemlock (parsley), *Karwinskia humboldtiana*/coyotillo (buckthorn) [berries], *Calliopsis* species (daisy), *Cassia* (bean), *Cycas* (evergreen), [seeds], *Gelsemium* [blossoms], *Heliotropium* (bush tea shrub), *Melochia* species [stems], *Oenanthe* species (parsnips)
Metals	Organic tin compounds, lead
Pesticides	EPN, trichlorfon (Dipterex), dichlorvos (DDVP), DEF, isofenphos (Oftanol), leptophos (Phosvel)
Inherited/congenital/acquired	Werdnig-Hoffmann disease, Wohlfart-Kugelberg-Welander disease, porphyric polyneuropathy
Unknown/multiple causes	Guillain-Barré syndrome, China paralytic syndrome, Bell's palsy, transverse myelitis
Asthma	Polio-like Hopkins' syndrome

drome, transverse myelitis, and traumatic neuritis (neuritis secondary to the trauma of injections) are contained in Table 25–3.

In general, in the absence of wild-type virus–induced poliomyelitis, Guillain-Barré syndrome accounts for 50% or more of the cases of AFP in industrialized countries such as the United Kingdom and Australia as well as in developing countries in Latin America.[110-112] At times, nonpolio enteroviruses have been associated with cases of polio-like paralytic disease, but this has been uncommon. Coxsackievirus A7 has been associated with outbreaks of paralytic disease,[113,114] and enterovirus 71 has been involved in several outbreaks of CNS disease, including polio-like paralysis, with some fatal cases.[115] Two motor neuron diseases in childhood are Werdnig-Hoffmann disease, a rapidly progressing, often fatal disorder of early childhood, and Wohlfart-Kugelberg-Welander disease, a more benign disorder with a generally later onset.[116] Electromyographic findings are useful in establishing the diagnosis of these disorders.[117] China paralytic syndrome, a distinct disease entity that appears different from Guillain-Barré syndrome and poliomyelitis, has been described among children and adults in northern China.[118] Early symptoms of this disease include leg weakness and resistance to neck flexion. The weakness ascends rapidly, affects symmetrically the arms and respiratory muscles, and progresses to a maximum extent of weakness within 6 days on average. Electromyography indicates denervation potentials in weak muscles and suggests that this entity may be a reversible distal motor nerve terminal or anterior horn lesion. Tick bite paralysis occurs infrequently and is manifested by flaccid ascending paralysis that usually resolves rapidly after tick removal. Botulism toxins can also cause descending paralysis—characterized by symmetric impairment of cranial nerves, followed by a descending pattern of weakness or paralysis of the extremities and trunk.[119] A relatively frequent complication among approximately 10% to 15% of diphtheria patients is paralysis of the soft palate and peripheral nerves resulting from diphtheria toxin[120]; tetanus toxin can cause a flaccid paralysis of the muscles innervated by the affected cranial nerves (i.e., cephalic tetanus).[121] Case reports have linked AFP and West Nile virus infection (a flavivirus) among elderly adults in Mississippi and Louisiana, suggesting that West Nile virus may damage the anterior horn cells of the spinal cord to cause paralytic disease.[122-124]

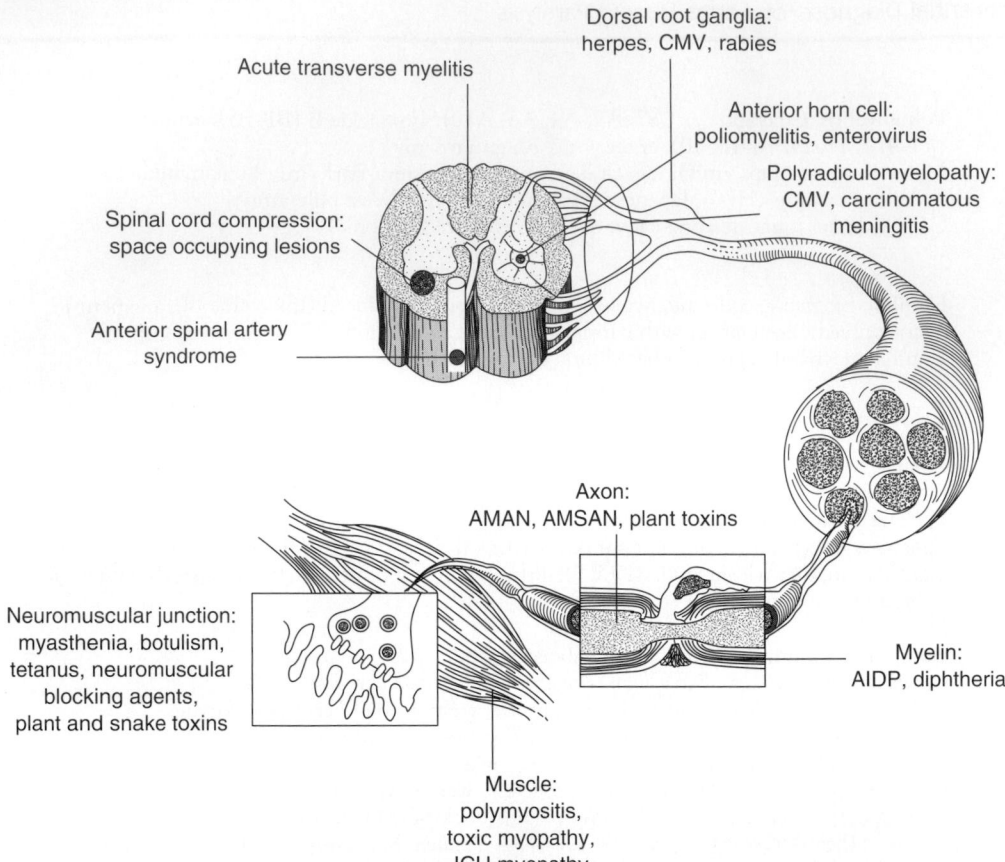

FIGURE 25–1 ▪ Pathophysiologic mechanisms and anatomic sites of etiologic factors for acute flaccid paralysis. AIDP, acute inflammatory demyelinating polyneuropathy; AMAN, acute motor axonal neuropathy; AMSAN, acute motor-sensory axonal neuropathy; CMV, cytomegalovirus; ICU, intensive care. (Redrawn from Marx et al.[109] and Ho et al.[494] Adapted and reprinted with permission from the *Annual Review of Neuroscience,* volume 21 © 1998 by Annual Reviews www.annualreviews.org.

The following signs and symptoms help in distinguishing poliomyelitis from other causes of AFP: (1) fever is present at onset; (2) there is rapid progression to maximum paralysis; (3) paralysis is usually asymmetric; and (4) paralysis is more pronounced proximally than distally (i.e., descending paralysis). However, as poliomyelitis becomes an increasingly rare disease, unusual clinical presentations, such as symmetric paralysis of the lower extremities (many cases caused by intramuscular injections, which increase the risk of paralytic manifestations in the extremity that, in the absence of intramuscular injections, would not have become paralyzed)[125] or mild paralysis or weakness in partially immune children, may be seen.

Epidemiology

General Epidemiology

Poliomyelitis is a ubiquitous, highly contagious, seasonal viral disease (more pronounced in moderate-climate countries) caused by three serotypes of poliovirus (types 1, 2, and 3) that infect nearly every person in a given population in the absence of vaccination.[31] Paralytic manifestations are a rare outcome (less than 1%) of poliovirus infections. Important exceptions are island or isolated populations (e.g., Eskimo), which can remain unaffected by the virus for varying periods and, after reintroduction, can experience outbreaks of poliomyelitis that affect all age groups that were not affected by the previous wave of infection.[126]

Poliovirus type 1 appears to be the most neurovirulent of the three serotypes.[127] Most epidemic and endemic cases of poliomyelitis are caused by poliovirus type 1, followed by type 3 and type 2. Peak transmission occurs among infants and young children (tropical areas) and school-aged children (temperate zones). However, outbreaks in isolated communities can give rise to paralytic cases in many older individuals.[31,126]

Poliomyelitis is transmitted by person-to-person spread through fecal–oral and oral–oral routes or, less frequently, by a common vehicle (e.g., water, milk).[128,129] People remain most infectious immediately before and 1 to 2 weeks after onset of paralytic disease, although poliovirus replicates for substantially longer periods and is excreted for 3 to 6 weeks in feces and approximately 2 weeks in saliva.[43] Thus the period of communicability may be 4 to 8 weeks. Secondary infection rates of susceptible household or institutional contacts, probably mediated by fecal–oral spread, are high, more than 90%.[43] The incubation period between infection and first symptoms (minor illness) is 3 to 6 days and from infection to onset of paralytic disease usually 7 to 21 days, with a range of 3 to 35 days.[130] Most exposures to polioviruses result in inapparent infections.[31,40,41] On the basis of serologic surveys in the prevaccine era[131,132] and lameness surveys in developing countries, it appears that, in the absence of a control program with vaccines, approximately 1 in 200 children (0.5%) will develop paralytic disease after exposure to polioviruses.[133]

Until recently, excretion of poliovirus was thought to be limited to 4 to 6 weeks among immune-competent

TABLE 25–3 ■ Distinguishing Features of Four Common Diagnoses of Acute Flaccid Paralysis

Feature	Poliomyelitis	Guillain-Barré Syndrome	Traumatic Neuritis (After Injection)	Transverse Myelitis
Development of paralysis	24–48-hr onset to full paralysis	From hours to 10 days	From hours to 4 days	From hours to 4 days
Fever at onset	High, always present at onset of flaccid paralysis, gone when progression of paralysis stops	Not common	Commonly present before, during, and after flaccid paralysis	Rarely present
Flaccid paralysis	Acute, usually asymmetric, principally proximal	Generally acute, symmetric, and distal	Asymmetric, acute, and affecting only one limb	Acute, lower limbs, symmetric
Progression of paralysis	"Descending"	"Ascending"		
Muscle tone	Reduced or absent in affected limb	Global hypotonia	Reduced or absent in affected limb	Hypotonia in affected limbs
Deep tendon reflexes	Decreased or absent	Globally absent	Decreased or absent	Absent in lower limbs early, hyperreflexia late
Sensation	Severe myalgia, backache, no sensory changes	Cramps, tingling, hypoanesthesia of palms and soles	Pain in gluteus, hypothermia	Anesthesia of lower limbs with sensory level
Cranial nerve involvement	Only when bulbar involvement is present	Often present, affecting nerves VII, IX, X, XI, XII	Absent	Absent
Respiratory insufficiency	Only when bulbar involvement is present	In severe cases, enhanced by bacterial pneumonia	Absent	Sometimes
Autonomic signs and symptoms	Rare	Frequent blood pressure alterations, sweating, blushing, and body temperature fluctuations	Hypothermia in affected limb	Present
Cerebrospinal fluid	Inflammatory	Albumin-cytologic dissociation	Normal	Normal or mild in cells
Bladder dysfunction	Rare	Transient	Never	Present
Nerve conduction velocity: third week	Abnormal: anterior horn cell disease (normal during first 2 wk)	Abnormal: slowed conduction, decreased motor amplitudes	Abnormal: axonal damage	Normal or abnormal, no diagnostic value
Electromyography at 3 wk	Abnormal	Normal	Normal	Normal
Sequelae at 3 mo and up to a year	Severe, asymmetric atrophy, skeletal deformities developing later	Symmetric atrophy of distal muscles	Moderate atrophy, only in affected limbs	Flaccid diplegia atrophy after years

Adapted from Global Program for Vaccines and Immunization. Field Guide for Supplementary Activities Aimed at Achieving Polio Eradication. Geneva, World Health Organization, 1996.

individuals and less than 3 years among immune-deficient persons. In 1997, a case report suggested that an immune-deficient patient with common variable immunodeficiency disorder (CVID) who acquired vaccine-associated paralytic poliomyelitis (VAPP) in 1981 may have excreted VDPV for approximately 7 years prior to onset of paralysis.[134,135] Subsequent investigations have revealed that as many as 15 patients with either CVID, agammaglobulinemia, or severe combined immunodeficiency disorder (SCID) have excreted poliovirus for periods of approximately 12 months or longer, and rarely for more than 10 years, based on epidemiologic data and molecular sequencing information[136] (see *Molecular Epidemiology of Poliovirus* below) and WHO unpublished data (Table 25–4).[134,135,137–145] Many of these long-term carriers stopped excreting poliovirus sponta-

neously. As of 2002, 3 of the 15 long-term carriers are known to continue to excrete polioviruses. None of the viruses examined from these carriers showed recombination with other nonpolio enteroviruses. The absence of recombination may suggest that the poliovirus had replicated in a single individual rather than through person-to-person transmission in the community (see *Vaccine-Derived Poliovirus* below).[134–143]

Between 1976 and 1995, 48 outbreaks involving approximately 17,000 cases of paralytic poliomyelitis were reported in the literature.[146] These outbreaks involved primarily unvaccinated or inadequately vaccinated subgroups and were caused predominantly by poliovirus type 1 (74%). On the basis of this review, cases in developing countries occurred mostly among children younger than 2 years,

TABLE 25–4 ■ Summary of Individuals Excreting Poliovirus for Approximately 12 Months or Longer, 1962 to 2001

Reference	Country	Year*	Age†	Sex	Immuno-deficiency Disorders
MacCallum[137]	UK	1962	3	M	Hypogamma
MacCallum,[137] Martin et al.[138]	UK	1962	20	F	
Hara et al.,[139] Abo et al.[140]	Japan	1977	3	M	
Kew et al.[134,135]	USA	1981	17	M	CVID
CDC	USA	1986	11	F	CVID
Misbah et al.[141]	UK	1987	34	M	CVID
Bellmunt et al.[142]	Germany	1990	7	M	CVID
CDC	USA	1990	1.3	F	SCID
Maclennan et al.[143]	UK	1995	25	M	CVID
CDC	USA	1995	0.3	F	SCID
Unpublished	Iran	1995	1.5	F	Ab deficiency
Unpublished	Argentina	1998	3	M	Agamma
Unpublished	Germany	2000	24	F	Ab deficiency
Buttinelli et al.[144]	Italy	2000	1.75	F	Agamma
Certification report[145]	Taiwan	2001	8	M	Ab deficiency

*Year of onset of paralysis or year first sample collected for nonparalytic cases.
†Age (in years) at onset of paralysis or at first sample collection for nonparalytic cases.
‡Interval from last dose of oral poliovirus vaccine to last poliovirus isolate.
Ab, antibody; Agamma, agammaglobulinemia; CDC, Centers for Disease Control and Prevention; CVID, common variable immunodeficiency disorder; Hypogamma, hypogammaglobulinemia; SCID; severe combined immunodeficiency disorder; NA, not available; XLA, X-linked agammaglobulinemia.

whereas cases in industrialized countries tended to occur in older people who had remained susceptible to poliomyelitis.

Besides age and being unvaccinated or inadequately vaccinated, several factors have been shown to increase the risk of acquiring paralytic manifestations, including intramuscular injections with diphtheria and tetanus toxoids and pertussis vaccine (DTP)[147,148] or antibiotics,[149,150] strenuous exercise,[151–153] injury such as fractures, and pregnancy.[154] *Provocation poliomyelitis* describes the enhanced risk of paralytic manifestations that follows injection in the 30 days preceding paralysis onset. Bodian and Nathanson demonstrated 40 years ago that retrograde axonal transport is responsible for the poliovirus invasion of the CNS in provocation poliomyelitis.[155] More recently, Gromeier and Wimmer suggested that the temporary expression of the human PVR on peripheral neurons during the repair process of injured nerves may enhance poliovirus access into peripheral neurons.[71,156] Retrograde transport in the axon via the fast system appears to shorten further the period from initial access of the poliovirus to the peripheral neuron to the virus reaching the motor neuron cells of the CNS.[157] This limits the time during which the immune system could develop an effective response. *Aggravation poliomyelitis* describes the elevated risk of paralytic disease that follows strenuous exercise shortly (preceding 24 to 48 hours) before paralysis onset.

Removal of tonsils and adenoids predisposes to bulbar poliomyelitis.[158] Clinical observations on this fact were reported in the early part of the 20th century.[158,159] Rhesus monkeys, when inoculated with poliovirus in the tonsillopharyngeal region developed poliomyelitis with greater frequency than when they were inoculated by other routes.[4] Later, von Magnus and Melnick[160] demonstrated that, if cynomolgus monkeys were given poliovirus by the oral route, their susceptibility was greatly enhanced in animals that had had their tonsils recently removed. Ogra and Karzon[161,162] studied 40 children before and after removal of tonsils and adenoids. The children ranged from 3 to 11 years of age and had been immunized with live, attenuated poliovirus vaccine 6 months to 6 years previously. Before tonsillectomy, IgA poliovirus antibody was present in appreciable titers in the nasopharynx of all children, but no IgM or IgG antibody was detectable. Significantly, however, after tonsillectomy, the pre-existing IgA poliovirus antibody level in the nasopharynx sharply declined in all children studied. Mean antibody titers decreased threefold to fourfold. Thus removal of tonsils may eliminate a valuable source of immunocompetent tissue particularly important in conferring resistance to poliovirus.

Lower socioeconomic status has been shown to be a risk for paralytic poliomyelitis in developing countries,[163] probably because children belonging to the lower socioeconomic group experience more intense exposure to poliovirus (i.e., a higher virus inoculum, which has been shown in experimental studies to be a risk factor for paralytic disease[29]). In addition, these children are also at higher risk for primary vaccine failure after OPV because of more frequent concurrent enterovirus infections.[163–166]

In a study of twins, concordance with regard to paralytic poliomyelitis was found in 36% of monozygous pairs compared with 6% of dizygous pairs.[167] The authors concluded that the data were consistent with "the theory that susceptibility may

Paralysis Present	Poliovirus Serotype	%VP1 Maximum Divergence from Sabin Parent Strain	Recombination with Other Nonpolio Enteroviruses	Interval‡
No	1	NA	NA	32 mo
No	3	2.3	No	21 mo
Yes	2	NA	NA	2 yr
Yes	1	10.0	No	7.5 yr
No	2	10.8	No	9.6 yr
No	2	4.1	No	>1 yr
Yes	1	8.3	No	~8.5 yr
Yes	2	1.8	No	9 mo
No	2	12.9	No	> 10 yr
Yes	2	2.2	No	3.7 yr
Yes	2	2.0	No	Unvaccinated
Yes	1	2.0	No	Unvaccinated
Yes	1	3.5	NA	2 yr
Yes	2	0.9	No	9 mo
Yes	1	3.4	NA	2.5 yr

be conditioned by the homozygous state of a recessive gene."[167] A human leukocyte antigen (HLA) complex study suggested that HLA-encoded genetic factors control resistance to the paralytic form of poliomyelitis.[168] Data on genetic susceptibility to poliomyelitis were reviewed by Wyatt,[169] who proposed that multiple-linked genes determine whether an infection with poliovirus results in paralytic disease.

The case-fatality rate is variable and depends primarily on the age groups affected. The highest case-fatality rates have been reported from epidemic cases in the early 20th century[16,29,30] and among adolescents and young adults, but are commonly between 5% and 10%.[29,31] Even in the 1990s, the case-fatality rate can be high, as occurred in a large outbreak of poliomyelitis in Albania in 1996, which reported a case-fatality rate of 10%.[170] More recently, an outbreak of poliomyelitis occurred on the Cape Verde Islands in 2000. Of the 33 reported cases, 7 died, for a case-fatality ratio (CFR) of 21%. The CFR was 0%, 20%, and 57% among cases ages less than 5 years, 5 to 14 years, and 15 years or older, respectively.[171]

Apes, such as chimpanzees, gorillas, and orangutans, are susceptible to poliovirus and can experience paralytic disease after poliovirus infection; outbreaks of poliomyelitis have been reported both in captivity and in the wild.[172–174] It is unlikely that they play any role in the sustained transmission of this virus,[175] because of the limited size of the ape populations. Most monkeys cannot be infected by oral administration of poliovirus and would not be expected to participate in the chain of transmission. In short, there is no significant animal reservoir for poliovirus.[175]

Results from mathematical modeling suggest that the force of poliovirus infection, measured primarily by the average age at infection among populations in the prevaccine era, is substantially higher in developing countries compared with industrialized countries. For example, the basic reproductive number (a measure of infectivity) of wild-type poliovirus is between 3 and 5 in the United States, which means that, on average, an infected individual introduced into a fully susceptible population would transmit the poliovirus to three to five other individuals in contact with the infected individual. In contrast, the average infected person in a developing tropical setting would be expected to have transmitted the infection to 10 to 12 contacts.[176,177] As population immunity increases, and many of the contacts of an infected person are no longer susceptible, the number of transmissions decreases. When the reproductive rate is less than 1 because of high population immunity, transmission ceases. The herd immunity threshold is the level of immunity in the population (e.g., in the "herd") at which an infected person, on average, would transmit the infection to less than one susceptible contact.

Whereas poliomyelitis outbreaks in industrialized countries can be prevented with overall population immunity levels of approximately 66% to 80%, outbreaks in developing countries with poor sanitation and hygiene could still occur with immunity levels as high as 94% to 97% (Fig. 25-2). These findings may be helpful in explaining why there was no spread to the general population after the outbreaks in the Netherlands, Canada, and the United States[178,179] and why widespread transmission among well-vaccinated populations occurred in many outbreaks in developing countries.[180,181]

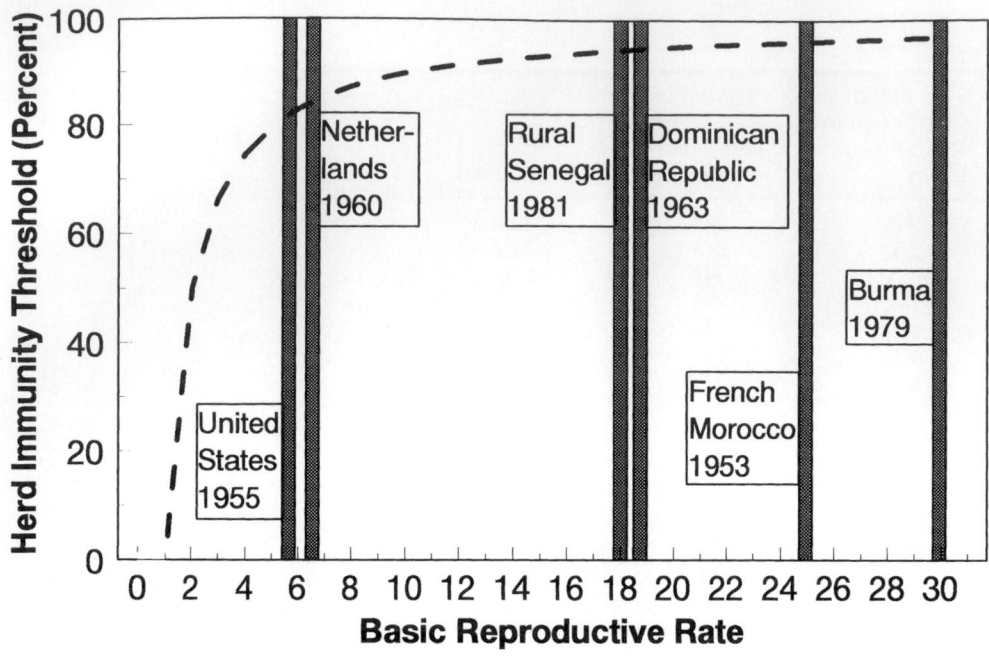

FIGURE 25–2 ▪ Herd immunity threshold levels for selected industrialized and developing countries, based on basic reproductive rate, or R_0. Threshold values for herd immunity were calculated using $1 - (1/R_0)$, where R_0 is $1 +$ (life expectancy/average age at infection with poliovirus). Herd immunity threshold values are shown by the *dashed line*. The *solid bars* are the basic reproductive rate in a given population. (From Patriarca PA, Sutter RW, Oostvogel PM. Outbreaks of paralytic poliomyelitis, 1976–1995. J Infect Dis 175[suppl 1]:S165–S172, 1997, with permission.)

Epidemiologic Patterns and Incidence of Poliomyelitis

The epidemiology of poliomyelitis changed substantially during the last century. Three epidemiologic patterns have been observed: (1) *endemic*, (2) *epidemic* (prevaccine), and (3) *vaccine era*. Polioviruses probably circulated in an uninterrupted *endemic* fashion for many centuries, infecting new cohorts of susceptible infants continuously, almost all early in life, when maternally derived antibody transferred from mother to the newborn still provided some protection.

A change from endemic transmission to periodic *epidemics* was first observed in some temperate-climate countries (e.g., Norway, Sweden, the United States) late in the 19th century and at the beginning of the 20th century.[12–15] The delay in median age of poliovirus exposure permitted the accumulation of sufficient children susceptible to poliomyelitis to permit periodic outbreaks. In the United States, the median age of poliovirus infection increased from younger than 5 years at the beginning of the century to 5 to 9 years in the 1940s, before poliovirus vaccine licensure.[31] In contrast, approximately 80% of the cases were in children younger than 5 years during the large epidemic in New York in 1916.[16] The generally accepted explanation, supported by numerous studies, is that, in a temperate-zone climate with increased economic development and correspondingly improved resources for community sanitation and household hygiene, exposure to polioviruses was postponed to later in life. Epidemic transmission became the primary epidemiologic pattern in temperate climate countries, such as the industrialized countries in Europe and North America, until poliomyelitis was brought under control after introduction of effective vaccines (Fig. 25–3).

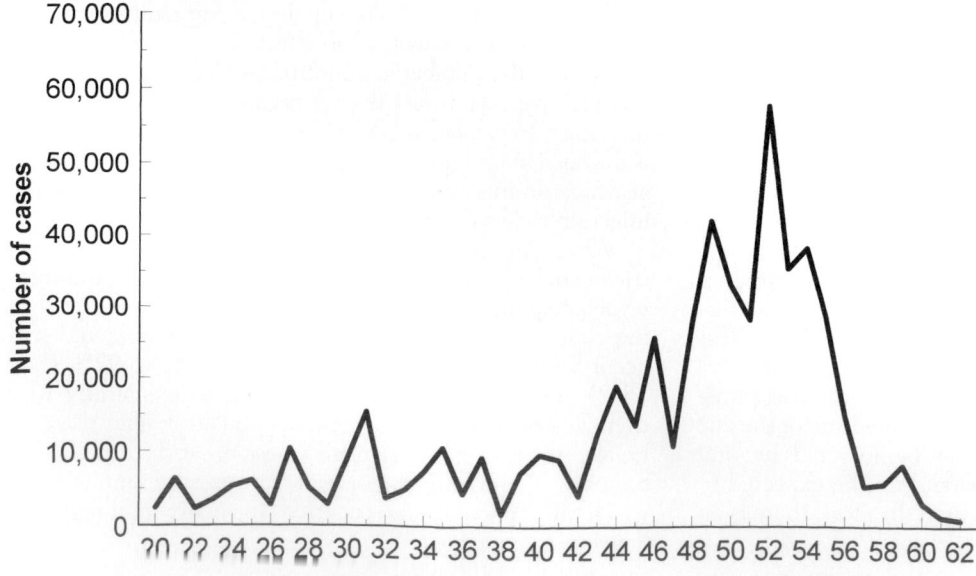

FIGURE 25–3 ▪ Reported cases of poliomyelitis, United States, 1920 to 1962. (Centers for Disease Control and Prevention)

In developing countries, particularly tropical areas, an endemic epidemiologic pattern predominated until recently. Poliovirus exposure occurred early in life. Although earlier theories suggested that paralytic poliomyelitis was not a health burden in tropical countries because of early exposure of infants to virus at a time when levels of maternally derived antibodies protected them from paralytic disease, more recent studies have disproved these theories. The history and scientific evidence for this misconception—that poliomyelitis was not a significant public health problem in developing countries—has been reviewed in detail in the corresponding chapter of the second edition of *Vaccines*.[182] In the last three decades, a series of lameness surveys were conducted in many developing countries that reported between 5 and 10 lameness cases per 1000 children in the age group studied,[133] suggesting that approximately 1 in 100 to 1 in 200 children acquire paralytic disease attributable to poliovirus. The WHO estimates that, in the absence of vaccination, there would be 600,000 cases of paralytic disease annually, the great majority of which would occur in children from developing countries. With improving vaccination coverage, a shift from an endemic to an epidemic pattern of poliovirus transmission has been observed in some developing countries that experienced large epidemics.[146,181,183-185]

The *vaccine era* began in the United States and in many European countries, Canada, Australia, New Zealand, and Japan after introduction of IPV in 1955.[2] The incidence of paralytic poliomyelitis decreased rapidly from 18,308 reported cases in the United States in 1954, the year immediately preceding IPV licensure, to 2499 cases in 1957, a decline of 86% only 3 years after the availability and widespread use of IPV. The relative upswing in reported cases in 1959 (6289 cases), with many cases having a history of receiving several prior doses of IPV, raised concerns regarding the clinical efficacy of IPV in preventing paralytic disease, although the concerns were probably unfounded.[186] Nevertheless, continued and accelerated IPV use decreased the incidence of paralytic poliomyelitis to nearly record low levels (2525 cases) in the United States by 1960. Widespread use of IPV in other countries was followed by substantial decreases in the incidence of poliomyelitis and, in some European countries, including Finland, the Netherlands, and Sweden, resulted in the apparent elimination of indigenous wild-type poliovirus transmission.[187,188]

The OPV era started in the United States with licensure of monovalent OPV in 1961, followed by licensure of trivalent OPV in 1963.[27] Although live, attenuated oral poliovirus vaccine was developed in the United States, the first large-scale production, as well as the large field trials that proved the safety and efficacy of the vaccine, took place in the former Soviet Union. A mass immunization program was initiated in the Soviet Union in 1959 and completed in 1960, covering 77.5 million people or 36.7% of the entire population. The immunization campaign was followed by a sharp decrease in the incidence of poliomyelitis: from 10.6 per 100,000 population in 1958 to 0.43 per 100,000 population in 1963. Between 1964 and 1979, the incidence had remained at a level of 0.01 to 0.1 per 100,000 population.[189] Similar declines in the incidence of poliomyelitis were observed in other European countries, Australia, New Zealand, Canada, and the United States after the introduction of OPV. In the United States, monovalent OPV was administered initially in mass vaccination campaigns in 1962—called Sabin Oral Saturdays/Sundays (SOS)—followed by a routine vaccination program that administered vaccine to infants year-round.[27,190,191] The impact of administering OPV to a population that already had high immunity levels generated by previous natural infection or vaccination with IPV was impressive. Substantial reductions in the reported number of poliomyelitis cases were observed from 988 cases in 1961 to 61 cases in 1965. In 1973, only seven cases of poliomyelitis were reported. Epidemic poliomyelitis also was brought under control, with the last outbreak in the general population occurring in Texas along the United States–Mexico border in 1970, followed by small outbreaks occurring in 1972 and 1979 among religious groups whose members object to vaccination.[179] The last indigenously acquired case of poliomyelitis due to wild-type poliovirus was detected in 1979. Between 1985 and 2000, aside from three imported cases of poliomyelitis (the most recent was reported in 1993), all cases have been vaccine associated.[192] Rarely has a serious disease been controlled as rapidly and dramatically as has poliomyelitis in the United States and other industrialized countries of the world.

The history of controlling poliomyelitis in many developing, particularly tropical countries has been more recent. There is a notable exception: Cuba appears to have interrupted wild-type poliovirus after two rounds of mass vaccination campaigns in 1962.[193] In many other developing countries, however, national vaccination programs were not operational until the late 1970s and early 1980s, and global OPV coverage with three doses among children age 1 year only reached 80% by 1990.[194] Wherever moderately high levels of OPV coverage were achieved, the incidence of poliomyelitis decreased by more than would be expected,[195] but endemic transmission of polioviruses continued, and cases of poliomyelitis continued to be reported. In addition to achieving high routine coverage with three doses of OPV, control of poliomyelitis required additional supplemental doses of OPV that were incorporated into the routine vaccination schedule in some countries; other countries needed to administer supplemental doses of OPV in mass campaigns. For example, in Brazil, control of poliomyelitis could not be accomplished until mass vaccination campaigns were initiated in 1980 (Fig. 25–4). The impact of these mass campaigns on poliomyelitis incidence was dramatic; the number of reported cases decreased from 1290 in 1980 to 122 in 1981, a decrease of more than 90%.[196]

Significance as a Public Health Problem

In the absence of effective control programs with poliovirus vaccine, approximately 1 of every 200 children (see *General Epidemiology* above) develops paralysis after exposure to polioviruses,[133] followed in most instances by permanent disability; 5% to 10% of patients with paralytic disease have a fatal outcome.[29,31] Thus, with a worldwide birth cohort of approximately 131 million in 2002, approximately 600,000 people would be expected to acquire paralytic poliomyelitis resulting in permanent disability each year, and between 30,000 and 60,000 of the cases would result in poliomyelitis-associated deaths. In the United

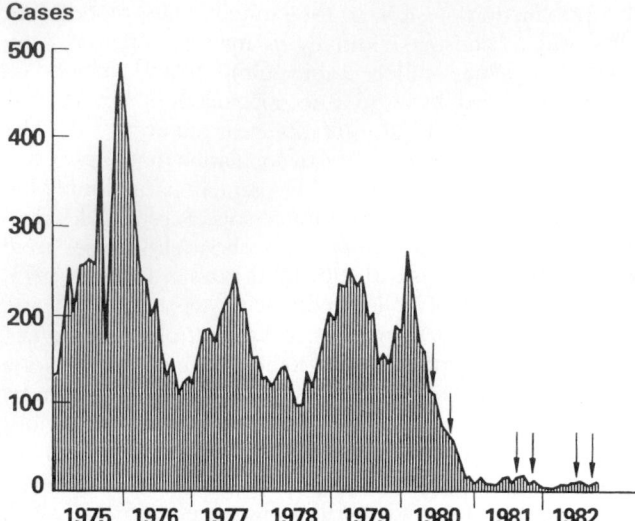

Cases

FIGURE 25–4 ▪ Cases of poliomyelitis by 4-week periods in Brazil, 1975 to 1982. *Arrows* indicate national immunization days. (From Risi JB. The control of poliomyelitis in Brazil. Rev Infect Dis 6[suppl 2]:S400–S403, 1984, with permission.)

States, a report estimated that, in the absence of a control program, more than $3 billion ($926 million in direct costs and $2.1 billion in indirect costs) would be required each year to cover the treatment and other related costs of patients with poliomyelitis.[197] In addition to the acute manifestations of poliomyelitis, patients may experience postpolio syndrome decades after the acute episode; postpolio syndrome is associated with new muscle pain, exacerbation of existing muscle weakness, or the development of new weakness or paralysis[49] that may require additional therapy, rehabilitation, and respiratory support.

In spite of the availability of two highly effective vaccines, poliomyelitis still exerts a significant public health impact in the world. In the United States in the prevaccine era, the peak incidence year of poliomyelitis was in 1952, when 57,879 cases of poliomyelitis were reported (including 21,269 cases of paralytic disease).[198] After the availability and widespread use of poliovirus vaccines beginning in 1955, poliomyelitis was rapidly controlled in industrialized countries and in other areas where vaccines were used effectively. Globally, the Expanded Programme on Immunization, a program of the WHO established in 1974, provided leadership to national programs in virtually all developing countries to improve vaccination coverage. Coverage levels reached 80% with three doses of OPV among children 1 year of age for the first time in 1990,[194] resulting in substantial decreases in the global morbidity and mortality burden of poliomyelitis. Despite this success, the WHO estimated that approximately 350,000 cases of paralytic poliomyelitis associated with permanent disability occurred in 1988, the year the global polio eradication target was adopted.[35] Because of rapid progress toward polio eradication, the worldwide reported incidence of poliomyelitis was only 494 cases in 2001[37] (and the number of cases associated with wild-type poliovirus isolation was 480). As of 25 February 2003, a total of 1915 virologically confirmed poliomyelitis cases had been reviewed by the World Health

Organization for 2002. The increase in cases was due to better reporting completion (Nigeria) and epidemic spread in India. The reporting completeness improved concurrently[37,199]; thus it is unlikely that many cases of poliomyelitis remained undetected in 2001 (and even more unlikely that significant areas of poliovirus circulation were missed).

Paralytic poliomyelitis continues to be a serious, albeit declining, threat to children in polio-endemic countries and occasionally to people residing in industrialized countries that have primarily achieved good control of poliomyelitis for many years.[200,201] Even in countries with well-vaccinated populations that have eliminated indigenous wild-type poliovirus circulation for decades, gaps in population immunity may persist, particularly in groups objecting to vaccination (e.g., religious groups such as the Amish in the United States, and the Netherlands Reformatory Church in the Netherlands and related groups in Canada) or groups that are not reached effectively by national vaccination programs (e.g., Roma, previously referred to as "gypsies").[178,202–204] In the United States, the last two outbreaks of poliomyelitis occurred in 1972 and 1979 among members of religious groups objecting to vaccination.[179] The 1979 outbreak was an extension of an outbreak affecting first the Netherlands in 1978 and then Canada.[178,203] An outbreak of poliomyelitis affecting the same religious group in the Netherlands also occurred in 1992 to 1993.[201] On the basis of genomic sequence,[93,94] the poliovirus type 1 strain causing the epidemic in the Netherlands in 1978 had its origin in Turkey. The recent outbreak was due to poliovirus type 3, which was most likely imported from the Indian subcontinent.[205] In Spain, the last cases of poliomyelitis in 1980 to 1981 were detected among Roma children.[202] In both outbreaks in Bulgaria in 1990 to 1991 and in 2000,[206,207] as well as in the Romanian outbreak in 1991 to 1992,[208] Roma children either were exclusively affected or constituted a substantial proportion of poliomyelitis cases. Although no cases of paralytic poliomyelitis were detected in the outbreaks in the United States (1979), Canada (1978), and the Netherlands (1978 and 1992 to 1993) beyond the affected unvaccinated or inadequately vaccinated subpopulations, wild-type poliovirus exposure of people in the general population and the establishment of subsequent endemic and epidemic transmission remain a concern.

Molecular Epidemiology of Poliovirus

The application of molecular tools, such as genomic sequencing of poliovirus, has added a new dimension and resolution power to our understanding of the epidemiology of poliomyelitis.[96,209] Because the poliovirus genome evolves rapidly (1% to 2% nucleotide substitutions per site per year) (Fig. 25–5), links between poliomyelitis cases can now be determined and importations from the remaining poliovirus reservoirs can be established. These molecular methods offer an additional tool to monitor the progress of the global polio eradication initiative and suggest that lineages of poliovirus genotypes (differing by less than 15% in their nucleotide sequences) disappear sequentially through intensive immunization efforts.[96,210] The experience in the Americas suggests that, if a genotype is not detected for a

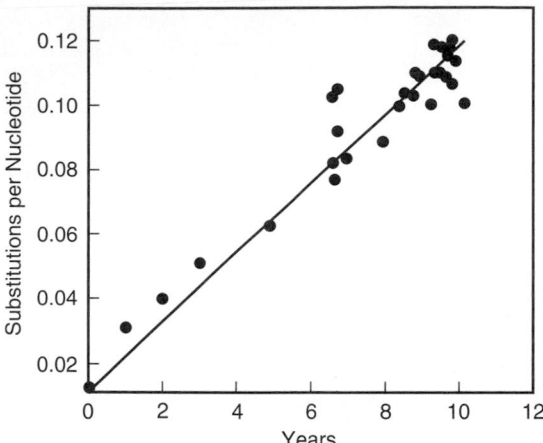

FIGURE 25–5 ■ Rate of fixation of nucleotide substitutions in the VP1 gene (906 nucleotides) over a 10-year period (1981 to 1991) for wild poliovirus type 1 (NWSA genotype, from the northern Andean region of South America).

year or more despite adequate surveillance, it probably has become extinct.[211] These methods have established the existence of numerous poliovirus genotypes endemic to different regions of the world,[96] the former Soviet Union,[91] Europe, the Middle East, and the Indian subcontinent[212] and demonstrated that poliovirus type 2 is usually the first serotype to be eliminated,[213] that poliovirus type 3 appears to circulate more locally than other serotypes, and that poliovirus type 1 appears to be most commonly associated with importations from neighboring countries and with intercontinental or global spread of the virus.[210,211,214] Genomic sequencing of polioviruses suggested that the viruses responsible for the epidemic in the Netherlands in 1992 to 1993 (type 3) and Albania in 1996 (type 1), as well as that in Bulgaria and Georgia in 2001 (type 1),[214] were probably imported from reservoirs in the Indian subcontinent.[212] These molecular methods have shown that, in some instances, different genotypes of poliovirus can circulate concomitantly and cause poliomyelitis cases in a geographically limited area.[184,211]

Most of the genotypes found in 1988 appear now to be extinct (Fig. 25–6). The remaining wild-type poliovirus reservoirs are localized to areas with pockets of low OPV coverage and where demographic and environmental conditions favor poliovirus circulation. During the peak months of poliovirus circulation (summer through fall in many areas), virus spreads from the reservoir communities (where poliovirus circulation is sustained throughout the year) to adjacent nonreservoir indicator communities (where the density of nonimmune susceptible children can support some poliovirus circulation during the peak transmission season). Within a country or region, it is important to identify and target reservoir communities for intensified mass vaccination campaigns (see *Disease Control Strategies* below). Molecular epidemiologic methods also have been used to characterize unusual VDPVs isolated from immunodeficient patients or from outbreaks associated with the circulation of OPV-derived virus (see *Vaccine-Derived Polioviruses* below).

Molecular epidemiologic methods are routinely used to help identify reservoir communities.[37] This has led to a

refinement in the concept of *virus importation*, which in previous usage referred to virus transmission across political boundaries. Although many importations over long distances have been documented,[96] reservoir communities and their associated indicator communities frequently overlap international borders,[215] underscoring the importance of regional synchronization of national immunization days. Even more important are the patterns of importation from reservoir communities to indicator communities within a country. Effective intervention in the reservoir communities, especially during the low transmission season, prevents the subsequent spread to indicator communities.

Molecular epidemiologic methods have opened a new avenue for detecting gaps in polio surveillance. In areas with good surveillance, poliovirus isolates representing frequent sampling of a single chain of transmission are typically closely related (usually >99.5 VP1 sequence identity among the closest relatives). These closely related viruses are represented on phylogenetic trees as short-branch connections between sequences.[59,95] Long-branch connections between isolate sequences indicate missing information. If the virus is imported, the missing information may be recovered from the sequence relationships among viruses from the source reservoir.[96] However, in other circumstances, no closely related viruses can be found, and the recent virologic history of the isolate lineage is indeterminate. For example, gaps in surveillance in southern Egypt were inferred from the sequence data, because indigenous type 3 isolates in 1999 appeared as "orphan lineages" on phylogenetic trees, and the closest relatives were isolated nearly 3 years earlier.[216]

A serious challenge to the integrity of poliovirus surveillance data is the occurrence of poliovirus contamination of cultures. Very high workloads in poliovirus laboratories increase the risk of contamination. Fortunately, sequence analysis usually can distinguish contaminants from true clinical isolates. Contaminants are easily recognized when they are standard wild-type reference strains, such as Mahoney, MEF1, or Saukett (Sabin strain contaminants are of little current programmatic importance), but are more difficult to recognize when they are the wild-type polioviruses indigenous to a country or community. However, when wild-type polioviruses isolated at different times and locations have identical VP1 sequences, contamination is suspected, because such sequence identities are inconsistent with the rapid rate of evolution of the poliovirus genomes.[217] If the surveillance question is crucial, the sequencing window may be expanded to increase confidence in the observed genetic relationships. At the advanced stages of polio eradication, laboratory contamination could have severe programmatic consequences if unrecognized, prompting the diversion of resources into unnecessary immunization campaigns mobilizing large populations and costing millions of dollars, as well as potentially delaying certification of a WHO region as polio-free (see *Certification of Polio Eradication* below).

Passive Immunization

Therapeutic use of convalescent serum for poliomyelitis was first recommended as early as 1915.[218] Several trials using convalescent serum, administered by a single intrathecal

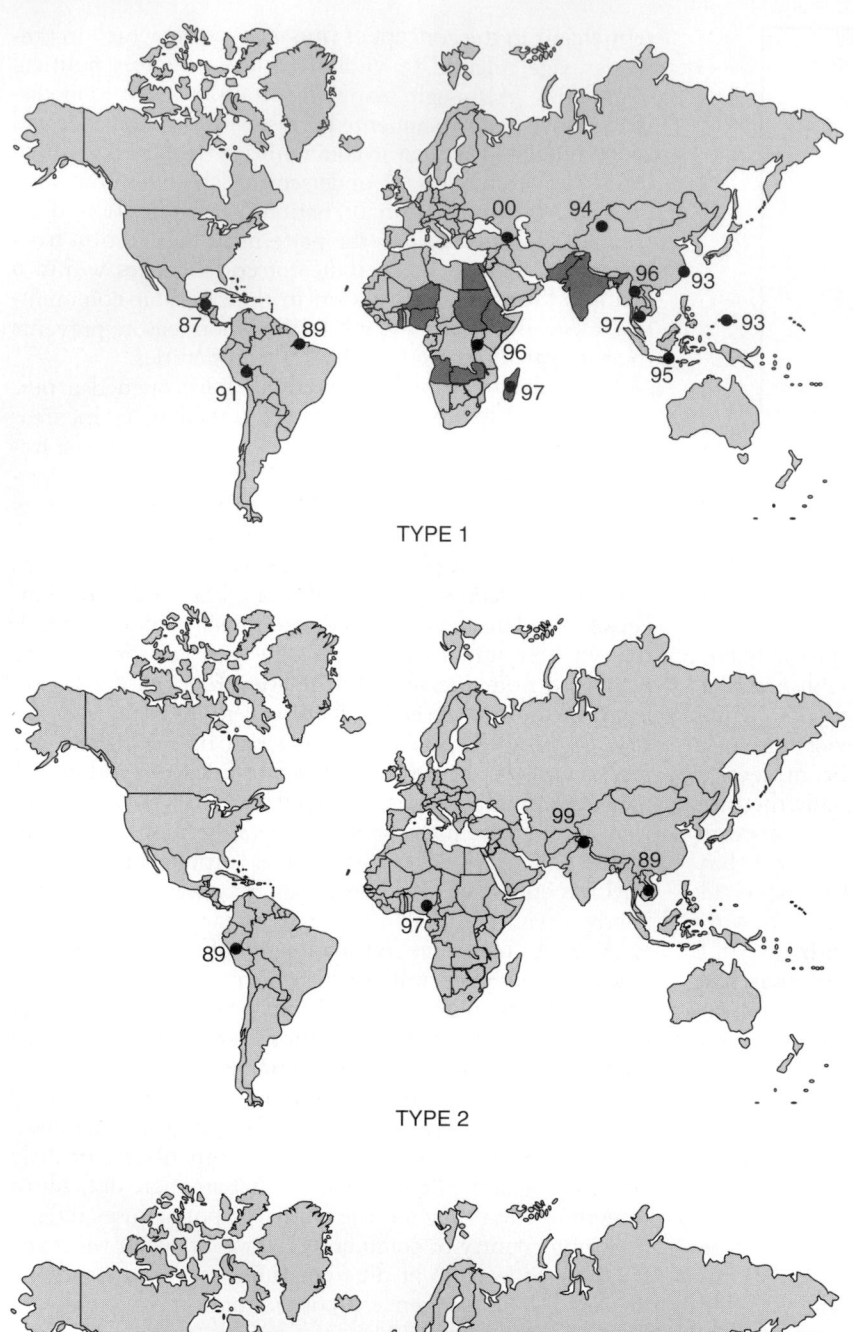

TYPE 1

TYPE 2

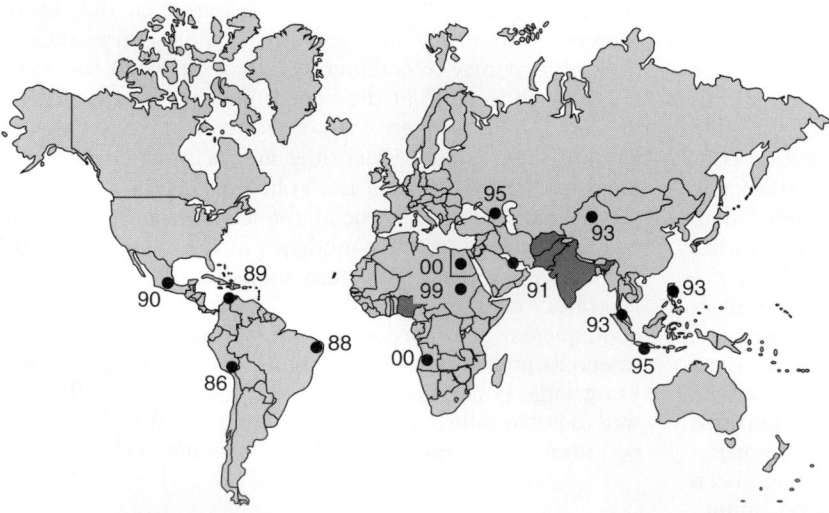

TYPE 3

FIGURE 25–6 ■ Progressive eradication of poliovirus genotypes,* 1986 to 2000. Darker shaded countries represent those from which wild-type polioviruses were isolated in 2001 as a result of either ongoing endemic transmission or virus importation. The numbers next to the black circles represent the year a poliovirus genotype was last detected. Since 1986, 11 genotypes of poliovirus type 1 have disappeared; 4 genotypes continue to circulate. Between 1989 and 1999, all four known genotypes of poliovirus type 2 have disappeared. Since 1986, 13 genotypes of poliovirus type 3 have been eliminated; 3 genotypes continue to circulate. (Redrawn from Kew OM, Pallansch MA. The mechanism of polio eradication. *In* Semler BL, Wimmer E [eds], Molecular Biology of Picornaviruses. Washington, DC, ASM Press, 2002, pp 481–491.)

*Note: A genotype shares less than 85% nucleotide sequence homology with another genotype of the same serotype.

injection, intraspinally, intravenously, or subcutaneously, reported conflicting results.[219] However, convalescent serum use was advocated by some until a well-controlled trial during a poliomyelitis outbreak in 1931 provided no statistical evidence that the therapy was of value.[220]

Administration of antibody was pursued again in the late 1940s and early 1950s as a means of preventing poliomyelitis by passive immunization. It had been demonstrated previously that low levels of circulating neutralizing antibody were protective against the paralytic manifestations of poliomyelitis both in experimental animal models and in humans.[220] In addition, infants in the first few months of life rarely acquired paralytic poliomyelitis, presumably because maternally derived type-specific poliovirus antibodies provided some protection. However, this protective effect is relatively short lived. Maternally derived antibody declines with a half-life of approximately 28 days and can rarely be detected in infants older than 6 months.[221]

A large field trial funded by the National Foundation for Infantile Paralysis demonstrated in 1952 that immune globulin (i.e., gamma globulin) was effective in preventing paralytic disease if it was administered before the presumed exposure to poliovirus, but that the protective effect was relatively short lived, about 5 to 8 weeks.[222] In this study, a single dose of 0.14 mL/kg body weight was administered intramuscularly.[222] However, evaluation of large-scale use of gamma globulin in 1953 by the National Advisory Committee for the Evaluation of Gamma Globulin in the Prophylaxis of Poliomyelitis concluded that "its preventive effect in community prophylaxis during 1953 has not been demonstrated. Also, no modification of the severity of paralysis was shown. Nevertheless, the committee cannot say that the use of gamma globulin by mass inoculation produced no effect."[223] Although these conclusions were modified somewhat by Hammon et al.—who pointed out that this evaluation had serious, perhaps fatal flaws, including (1) the gamma globulin was given far too late to be expected to have much or any effect and (2) this was not a controlled experiment with appropriate controls[222]—the committee report nevertheless dampened enthusiasm for this approach. In addition, in view of the progress toward the subsequent development of effective poliovirus vaccines that induced active immunity, presumably for life, gamma globulin as a tool to prevent poliomyelitis was not further pursued.

Passive immunity to poliomyelitis (and other diseases) among immunodeficient people, particularly those with agammaglobulinemia or hypogammaglobulinemia, is achieved through substitution therapy, namely, the regular administration (monthly) of intravenous immune globulin to those individuals. Monthly doses of 100 to 400 mg/kg body weight given intravenously are used.[224] Intramuscular immune globulin also may be used, but appears less effective. Immune globulin, whether it is formulated to be administered intramuscularly or intravenously, must pass the requirements of the Food and Drug Administration in the United States, which include minimum titers for antibody to polioviruses. In addition, immune globulin or hyperimmune sera may be used to eliminate chronic enterovirus infections,[225] including chronic infections with poliovirus,[226] and the oral route of administration sometimes has been used.[225]

Active Immunity

Early Approaches

Research on inducing active immunity in monkeys by administering ground-up spinal cord and observing whether the animals succumbed to poliomyelitis began as early as 1910.[227] Inactivation of poliovirus by formalin was first reported in 1911.[228] Brodie and Goldblum[229,230] first used subinfective doses of live poliovirus and later mixed live poliovirus with hyperimmune serum before using phenol and formalin as inactivating substances. After further small-scale experiments to optimize formalin inactivation and administration of the inactivated vaccine to small numbers of rhesus monkeys, adult volunteers, and children, the vaccine was administered to approximately 3000 children.[231,232] However, this approach was controversial and not pursued further because of concerns about the efficacy and safety of this vaccine. Kolmer in 1935 pioneered the use of attenuated live poliovirus that had been passaged continually in monkeys and prepared a suspension of monkey spinal cord in 1% sodium ricinoleate. The vaccine was administered to approximately 10,000 children, at least 10 of whom acquired paralytic poliomyelitis shortly after vaccination, for a rate of approximately 1 case per 1000 children vaccinated.[233,234] In short, both approaches—inactivation by formalin and attenuation of live poliovirus—that were successfully used later by Salk and Sabin had been employed during these trials. In retrospect, it is clear that, without knowledge of the number of poliovirus serotypes, these early vaccine development efforts were doomed to failure.

Advances in tissue culture growth of poliovirus in the late 1940s[20] renewed interest in poliovirus vaccines, and some of the first reports on attenuation of wild-type poliovirus for vaccine purposes were published in the early 1950s.[235-238] Essentially, attenuated strains were developed by several passages of virus at high concentration in cell cultures of rodent CNS tissue or non–nervous system tissue from monkeys, followed by selection of attenuated variants at limiting dilutions or from single plaques.

Description of Vaccine: How Strains Were Developed

The history of early developments of oral vaccines can be reviewed in detail in reports of meetings published between 1958 and 1961[239-242] and in the corresponding chapter of the second edition of Vaccines.[182] As with most major scientific achievements, crucial contributions came from a number of different investigative teams.[27,243-245] Hilary Koprowski and colleagues[235] reported the successful immunization of humans against poliomyelitis with a live poliovirus vaccine as early as 1950. Although these attenuated strains were not selected for licensing, this work meant that, by 1960, when not only his strains but also several other candidate vaccines were well into their testing and field trial use, a 10-year record of evidence was available on patterns of response in humans who had received the type 2 strain in 1950.[246]

Continued development and testing of candidate strains were conducted in three institutions: the Children's Hospital Research Foundation, Cincinnati (A. B. Sabin);

Lederle Laboratories, Wayne, NJ (V. J. Cabasso et al.); and the Wistar Institute, Philadelphia (H. Koprowski et al.).[241,242] The work with attenuated polioviruses was advanced toward practical usefulness, particularly by Sabin, who meticulously studied a number of progeny of single virus particles for neurotropism in monkeys and finally selected three for small experimental trials in humans.[247] Much of the early efforts in the development of candidate strains were devoted to (1) maintaining high degrees of infectivity in cell culture and the human intestinal tract, (2) inducing detectable levels of neutralizing antibody in a high proportion of susceptible (seronegative) recipients, (3) displaying low neurovirulence in monkeys, (4) demonstrating a lack of association with paralytic disease in humans, and (5) maintaining genetic stability after replication in the human host.[180] The efforts of a number of investigators to develop and test suitable attenuated poliovirus strains came to fruition during 1955 to 1959, and large-scale field trials were held in many countries under a variety of conditions. Many of these trials in humans involved the sequential administration of monovalent formulations of poliovirus types 1, 2, and 3. A number of investigators around the world participated in studies in which these candidate strains were fed to millions of people. At the two conferences held by the Pan American Health Organization (1959 and 1960), these investigators joined in assessing the results.[241,242]

The field trials[241,242] and subsequent studies focused not only on the human populations fed candidate virus but also on the virus populations recovered from stool samples of vaccinees. Because the attenuated polioviruses are living organisms that must multiply to immunize, it was essential to know as much as possible about the progeny viruses let loose in nature—agents that still retain their property of infecting humans. All poliovirus strains, regardless of how highly attenuated, retain the property of multiplying and destroying cells in the monkey spinal cord. The degree to which this property is retained, however, varies over an enormous range as one progresses from the virulent strains to the highly attenuated ones suitable for vaccine use. The laboratory techniques are such that different degrees of neurotropism, even among attenuated strains, can be detected.

In 1958, a detailed comparison of candidate strains was conducted.[248,249] The attenuated strains that had been developed at the Yale Poliomyelitis Study Unit had already been shown to have too high a degree of reversion in chimpanzees and were dropped from consideration.[237,250] At Baylor College of Medicine in Houston, extensive comparison was made of the Sabin strains and the Lederle-Cox strains for neurovirulence in hundreds of monkeys inoculated by the intracerebral and intraspinal routes.[248–251] At the Division of Biologics Standards of the National Institutes of Health, Murray and colleagues[252] compared three sets of candidate strains as follows: Lederle-Cox, Sabin, and Koprowski-Wistar. In spite of the fact that the studies had been done in two different laboratories and with some variations in methodology, the overall findings were essentially in agreement. It was clear that the Lederle and Wistar strains were more neurotropic for monkeys than the Sabin strains. Because the results favored the Sabin strains, these strains are the ones that have been licensed, manufactured and used almost universally since then.

TABLE 25–5 ■ Poliovirus Type 1, Sabin Strain, Passage History

Year	Manipulation	Designation
1941	*Francis and Mack:* Isolation of Mahoney strain	Mahoney strain
	Salk: 14 MKTC and 2 monkey testicular cell passages	
1953	*Li and Schaeffer:* 11 MKTC passages	LS strain
	Additional tissue culture passages in monkey kidney and skin	LS-a / LS-b / LS-c
1954	*Sabin:* 5 passages in cynomolgus MKTC (3 terminal dilutions) 3 single-plaque passages	
	Selection by neurovirulence testing	LS-c, 2ab
1956	*Sabin:* 2 passages in cynomolgus MKTC	LS-c, 2ab/KP$_2$ = SO
1956	*MSD:* 1 passage in rhesus MKTC	LS-c, 2ab/KP$_3$ SO + 1 = SOM

MKTC, monkey kidney tissue culture; MSD, Merck Sharp & Dohme.
Data from WHO Consultative Group on Poliomyelitis Vaccines, 1985.

The passage histories of the three Sabin vaccine seeds now in use are shown in Tables 25–5 through 25–8.[253] For example, the type 1 strain was derived from the Mahoney strain, initially isolated by Francis and Mack in 1941. Salk made additional monkey kidney and monkey testicular passages. In 1953, Li and Schaeffer made 11 monkey kidney tissue culture passages, yielding the partially attenuated LS strain, and additional passages in monkey kidney and skin to yield the further attenuated strain LS-c. Then Sabin, in 1954, carried the LS-c strain through terminal dilutions and single-plaque passages, carefully selecting by neurovirulence testing, and finally obtaining strain LS-c, 2ab. Two further passes, in cynomolgus kidney, yielded LS-c, 2ab/KP$_2$, designated SO (Sabin original). Dr. Bettylee Hampil at Merck Sharp & Dohme made one additional passage in rhesus

TABLE 25–6 ■ Poliovirus Type 2, Sabin Strain, Passage History

Year	Manipulation	Designation
—	*Fox and Gelfand:* P 712 strain isolated	P 712
1954	*Sabin:* 4 passages (3 terminal dilutions) in cynomolgus MKTC	
	3 serial passages of plaque isolates	
	Selection by neurovirulence testing	
	Fed to chimpanzees	P 712, Ch
	3 single-plaque passages	P 712, Ch, 2ab
1956	*Sabin:* 2 passages in cynomolgus MKTC	P 712, Ch, 2ab/KP$_2$ = SO
1956	*MSD:* 1 passage in rhesus MKTC	P 712, Ch, 2ab/KP$_3$ SO + 1 = SOM

MKTC, monkey kidney tissue culture; MSD, Merck Sharp & Dohme.
Data from WHO Consultative Group on Poliomyelitis Vaccines, 1985.

TABLE 25–7 ■ Poliovirus Type 3, Sabin Strain, Passage History

Year	Manipulation	Designation
1937	*Kessel and Stimpert:* Leon strain isolated 20 intracerebral passages in rhesus monkeys	Leon strain
1952	*Melnick:* 8 passages in rhesus testicular tissue culture	
1953	*Sabin:* 3 passages in cynomolgus MKTC 30 rapid passages at low dilution in cynomolgus MKTC 3 terminal dilution passages 1 low-dilution pass 9 plaques isolated, single-plaques passed 3 times Selection by neurovirulence testing	Leon 12a,b
1956	*Sabin:* 3 passages in cynomolgus MKTC	Leon 12a,b/KP$_3$ = SO
1956	*MSD:* 1 passage in rhesus MKTC	Leon 12a,b/KP$_4$ SO + 1 = SOM

MKTC, monkey kidney tissue culture; MSD, Merck Sharp & Dohme.
Data from WHO Consultative Group on Poliomyelitis Vaccines, 1985.

monkey kidney tissue culture to derive LS-c, 2ab/KP$_3$, designated SO + 1 or SOM. The current vaccine is SO + 4, four tissue culture passages beyond the SO. A maximum of five passages are permitted, after which earlier (grandmother) seeds must be thawed and used to prepare new mother seeds. Because of inherent difficulties in maintaining the genetic stability of the Sabin type 3 seed stock, manufacturers have turned to an RNA-derived passage and clone of the strain, labeled SOR. This seed has yielded a vaccine of greater consistency and stability than the original Sabin seed. Adequate grandmother seeds are available through the WHO Consultative Group to last for centuries.

The genetic basis for the attenuation of the Sabin OPV strains has been intensively investigated. Two basic approaches have been taken: (1) sequence comparisons between the Sabin strains and their neurovirulent wild-type parents (types 1 and 3) or neurovirulent revertants (types 2 and 3) obtained from patients with VAPP; and (2) investi-

TABLE 25–8 ■ Poliovirus Type 3, Sabin Strain, RNA-Derived, Passage History

Year	Manipulation	Designation
1959	*Pfizer:* 1 passage of SOM in cercopithecoid MKTC with SV40 antiserum	SO + 2 = 127-B-111
1962	*Pfizer:* RNA extraction and plaque cloning, selection by rct40° marker test 2 plaque purifications	SO + 3 = 457-111 SO + 5 = SOR
1978	Seed stocks acquired by Institute Mérieux and distributed to others when Pfizer ceased operations	

MKTC, monkey kidney tissue culture; SV40, simian virus 40.
Data from WHO Consultative Group on Poliomyelitis Vaccines, 1985.

gation of the contribution of specific nucleotide substitutions to attenuation using infectious complementary DNA (cDNA) clones (see also *Genetic Stability of Vaccine Seed Strains* below). The 57 nucleotide substitutions distinguishing the Sabin 1 strain from its neurovirulent parent, Mahoney/USA41, are scattered throughout the genome.[254] Six mapped to the 5′-untranslated region (UTR), 49 mapped to the coding region (21 of which encoded amino acid substitutions), and 2 mapped to the 3′-UTR. Infectious cDNA constructs containing different combinations of Sabin 1 and Mahoney/USA41 sequences were tested for neurovirulence in monkeys or transgenic mice, for temperature sensitivity, and for other phenotypic properties distinguishing Sabin 1 from Mahoney/USA41.[254,256] The single most important determinant for attenuation in Sabin 1 was the A→G substitution at position 480 (abbreviated as A480G) in the 5′-UTR.[257] Four other determinants mapped to the capsid region (one in VP4, one in VP3, and two in VP1), and a weak determinant of attenuation and temperature sensitivity mapped to the RNA polymerase encoded by the 3D gene (Fig. 25–7).[255,256,258] Only two nucleotide substitutions (G481A in the 5′-UTR, and C2909U encoding a threonine→isoleucine substitution at position 143 of VP1) appear to be responsible for the attenuated phenotype of Sabin 2.[259,260] The total number of sequence differences between P712/USA54 and Sabin 2 is uncertain. However, because P712/USA54 has inherently low neurovirulence,[261] identification of critical attenuating sites in Sabin 2 involved determination of the effects of introduction of sequences derived from a neurovirulent revertant of Sabin 2 (obtained from a case of VAPP) into infectious cDNA constructs derived from Sabin 2.[259,260] Of the 10 nucleotide substitutions distinguishing Leon/USA37 and Sabin 3, only three substitutions (C472U in the 5′-UTR, C2034U encoding a serine→phenylalanine substitution at position 91 of VP3, and U2493C encoding an isoleucine→threonine substitution at position 6 of VP1) appear to be the main determinants of attenuation.[262–264]

As with Sabin 1,[257] the most important determinants of attenuation in Sabin 2 and 3 map to the 5′-UTR,[257,260,264] and appear to reduce the efficiency of initiation of translation of the poliovirus RNA template.[265,266] The other substitutions are thought to contribute to the stability of the attenuated phenotype. The high stability of the attenuated phenotype of Sabin 1 is attributed to the larger number of attenuating substitutions and their relative contributions to the phenotype. Quantitative determination of the contributions of each substitution is complicated by several factors: (1) the role of minor determinants of attenuation is difficult to measure, (2) some substitutions have pleiotropic effects on phenotype, (3) some Sabin strain phenotypes require a combination of substitutions, (4) second-site mutations can suppress the attenuated phenotype in various ways, and (5) the outcome of experimental neurovirulence tests may vary with the choice of experimental animals (monkeys vs. transgenic mice) or the route of injection (intraspinal vs. intracerebral). Examples of substitutions with pleiotropic effects are (1) the serine→phenylalanine substitution at position 91 of VP3, which confers both attenuation and temperature sensitivity to Sabin 3[267]; and (2) the tyrosine→histidine substitution at position 73 of the 3D polymerase of Sabin 1, which is an important

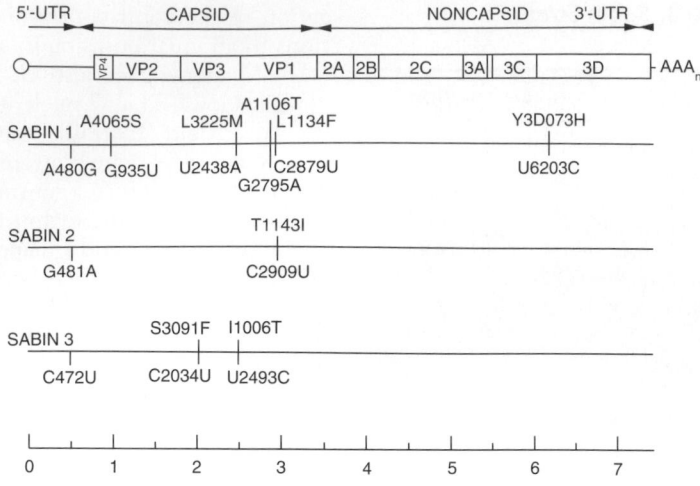

FIGURE 25–7 ■ Location of principal attenuating nucleotide (*lower bars*) and amino acid (*upper bars*) substitutions in each of the three Sabin OPV strains. Abbreviations of nucleotide residues: A, adenine; C, cytosine; G, guanine; U, uracil. Abbreviations for amino acid residues: A, alanine; C, cysteine; F, phenylalanine; H, histidine; I, isoleucine; L, leucine; M, methionine; S, serine; T, threonine; Y, tyrosine. Substitutions are shown as nonattenuated parent–position–Sabin strain; nucleotide positions are numbered consecutively from residue 1 of the RNA genome; and amino acid positions are indicated by the abbreviated name for viral protein (4, VP4; 2, VP2; 3, VP3; 1, VP1; 3D, 3D-polymerase) and numbered consecutively from residue 1 of each protein. For example, a guanine (Mahoney)→uracil (Sabin 1) substitution at RNA position 935 (G935U) encodes an alanine (Mahoney)→serine (Sabin 1) replacement at residue 65 of VP4 (A4065S). The Y3D073H substitution in Sabin 1 and the S3091F substitution in Sabin 3 are important determinants of temperature sensitivity. (Constructed from findings reported by Bouchard et al.,[254] Ren et al.,[259] Macadam et al.,[261] Tatem et al.,[262] and Westrop et al.[263])

determinant of temperature sensitivity[255,258] and a minor contributor to attenuation.[258] The relationship between poliovirus neurovirulence in experimental animals (where virus is introduced directly into the CNS) and pathogenicity for humans (where virus is introduced by ingestion) cannot be measured in controlled experiments, and remains ambiguous. Clearly the Sabin OPV strains are several orders of magnitude less pathogenic than wild-type polioviruses, as indicated by the very low incidence of VAPP[192] compared with the high incidence of paralytic poliomyelitis in areas where wild-type polioviruses are circulating.

The attenuating substitutions of the Sabin strains are sometimes described as mutations impairing the specific determinants of poliovirus neurovirulence. However, attenuation is a specific phenotype of each Sabin strain. Poliovirus neurovirulence, by contrast, is a much more complex property. Expression of a neurovirulent phenotype requires the efficient function of numerous steps in the natural life cycle of the virus and, thus, the efficient expression of several viral genes.[52,268] Impairment in the expression of any of these poliovirus genes can reduce replicative fitness and confer a more attenuated phenotype.[268] However, such mutants may not be suitable candidates for live virus vaccines. The Sabin strains contain specific genetic defects that are not found among the highly diverse population of circulating wild-type polioviruses. These exceptional defects are unstable to replication in the human intestine, and variants with higher replicative fitness are regularly selected. Other combinations of substitutions can produce highly attenuated polioviruses potentially suitable for vaccine use.[269] However, the attenuating substitutions of the Sabin strains were shown to confer highly favorable biologic properties, making these strains the best available candidates for licensure as viral poliovirus vaccines.

How Trivalent Vaccine Was Developed

Viral replication in the gastrointestinal tract and seroconversion were usually demonstrated in 80% to 100% of seronegative recipients with a single dose of monovalent vaccines at dosage levels of 10^5 median tissue culture infective doses ($TCID_{50}$).[270–274] However, when doses of 10^5 $TCID_{50}$ of each poliovirus serotype were mixed and administered as trivalent preparations, the replication and antibody production were consistently lower for some types compared with the sequential administration of monovalent vaccines.[275–281] This effect could be modified somewhat by increasing the doses of each type ($\geq 10^7$ $TCID_{50}$).[282,283] In addition, these studies showed that trivalent OPV of similar potency for each serotype was associated with a predominance of poliovirus type 2 excretion, and significantly higher type 2 antibody titers, than for poliovirus types 1 and 3. These early trials did not evaluate the impact of increasing the quantity of one serotype or reducing the quantity of another on seroconversion to all three serotypes because the interference effect of type 2 often could be overcome by administering three or more doses of the trivalent vaccine.

In 1961, a large study in Canada tested a "balanced" formulation of trivalent OPV (10^6 $TCID_{50}$ for Sabin type 1, 10^5 $TCID_{50}$ for Sabin type 2, and $10^{5.5}$ $TCID_{50}$ for Sabin type 3).[284] A single dose of this balanced (10:1:3) vaccine was administered to nearly 24,000 people, including 106 previously seronegative subjects, 103 (97%) of whom seroconverted to all three serotypes. Although one could conclude from this study that a single dose of OPV may be sufficiently immunogenic for a routine program, only triple-seronegative infants were included in this analysis of the Canadian trial, so the results represent the best possible scenario for inducing optimal levels of seroconversion because the infants lacked maternally derived antibody that can interfere with seroconversion. On the basis of these findings and an unpublished study from Guam, the balanced formulation of OPV was licensed in Canada in 1962 and in the United States in 1963.

Dosage and Route

According to current regulations in the United States, trivalent live, attenuated oral poliovirus vaccine (OPV) must contain at least $10^{5.5}$ TCID$_{50}$ for poliovirus type 1, $10^{4.5}$ TCID$_{50}$ for type 2, and $10^{5.2}$ TCID$_{50}$ for type 3.[285,286] However, the U.S. manufacturer routinely exceeds these minimum requirements, and an evaluation by a WHO reference laboratory found potency levels of $10^{6.5}$, $10^{5.4}$, and $10^{6.3}$ TCID$_{50}$ per dose of types 1, 2, and 3, respectively (WHO unpublished data). The WHO requires the following minimum TCID$_{50}$ values for each vaccine poliovirus serotype: $10^{5.9} \pm 0.5$ TCID$_{50}$ for type 1, $10^{5.0} \pm 0.5$ TCID$_{50}$ for type 2, and $10^{5.7} \pm 0.5$ TCID$_{50}$ for type 3. However, because of evidence from an evaluation in Brazil that poliovirus type 3 immunogenicity is not satisfactory with $10^{5.5}$ (300,000) TCID$_{50}$, particularly in tropical countries,[287] the WHO's Global Advisory Group recommended in 1990 that the type 3 component of OPV should be increased to $10^{5.8}$ (600,000) TCID$_{50}$.[235] OPV purchased by the United Nations International Children's Emergency Fund (UNICEF) beginning with the 1992 to 1993 tender period complied with this recommendation.

The recommended route of administration of OPV is the oral route, by releasing the vaccine volume (0.5 mL) contained in single-dose droppers into the oral cavity[289] for vaccine manufactured in the United States (prior to 2000, when OPV production was discontinued), or by providing two drops (~0.1 mL) of OPV contained in multidose vials produced by many non-U.S. manufacturers.[290] Although in the early 1960s some manufacturers put OPV into dragees, at present only OPV produced in China is in dragee form; before administration, the dragee must be ground up and mixed with water.

Producers

At least 12 manufacturers around the world are producing OPV[‡] using the Sabin vaccine seeds (now under the control of the WHO) (Table 25–9). This includes producers in Belgium, China, France, Indonesia, Iran, Italy, Japan, Mexico, Russia, Vietnam, and Yugoslavia. In addition, manufacturers in Egypt, Pakistan, Brazil, India, and Korea are filling and finishing bulk OPV produced by one of the primary manufacturers.

Most of these manufacturers use seed strains of types 1 and 2 no more than two passages away from the WHO master seed (SO + 1, i.e., Sabin original plus one passage). There is more variation in the type 3 seed used; most manufacturers are now using the Pfizer RNA-derived seed (SOR + 1). The type 3 seed used by China, the CHUNG-3 strain,

---

[‡]In the past, several U.S. companies produced OPV: Merck Sharp & Dohme, Wyeth, Pfizer, Lederle, and Wyeth-Lederle Vaccines and Pediatrics. Currently, no manufacturer produces OPV in the United States.

TABLE 25–9 ■ Manufacturers of Oral Poliovirus Vaccine (2002)[*]

Manufacturer[†]	City	Country
Aventis Pasteur	Lyon	France
Beijing Institute of Biological Products	Beijing	China
BioFarma	Bandung	Indonesia
Birmex (Instituto Nacional de Virologia)	Mexico City	Mexico
Chiron Vaccines	Siena	Italy
Chumakov Institute (Institute of Poliomyelitis and Viral Encephalitides)	Moscow	Russia
GlaxoSmithKline	Rixensart	Belgium
Poliomyelitis Research Center (POLIOVAC)	Hanoi	Viet Nam
Japan Poliomyelitis Research Institute	Tokyo	Japan
Kunming Institute of Medical Sciences	Kunming	China
Razi Institute (Vaccine and Serum Institute)	Hessarak	Iran
Institute of Immunology and Virology (TORLAK)	Belgrade	Yugoslavia

[*]Since 1997, three manufacturers (Chiron Behringwerke, Marburg, Germany; Evans Medical Ltd., Medeva-Speke, Liverpool, United Kingdom; and Wyeth-Lederle Vaccines and Pediatrics, Pearl River, NY) have discontinued production of OPV.

[†]In addition, manufacturers in Egypt, India, Brazil, Korea, and Pakistan produce OPV from imported bulk.

has been shown by oligonucleotide mapping to be similar to Sabin type 3. Vero cells and human diploid cells are employed by at least one manufacturer each for growing their vaccine viruses; the others continue to employ primary monkey kidney cells. It is recommended that the cells for cultivation be taken from monkeys bred in captivity. Like the cell cultures used, the monkey colony should be shown to be free of extraneous viruses and other pathogens.

Preparations Available (Including Combinations)

Although monovalent OPV formulations of the three poliovirus serotypes were used widely in the early 1960s, they were replaced by trivalent OPV starting in 1963 in the United States and other countries. Exceptions include Hungary, which used all three types of monovalent OPV sequentially until the early 1990s,[291] and South Africa, which routinely used monovalent type 1 OPV in its routine immunization program until the early 1990s.[292] Monovalent OPV formulations, although licensed and used extensively in many countries in the early 1960s, are not licensed anymore. The absence of licensed products precludes their use in routine vaccination programs. However, their use is being discussed as the product of choice for a stockpile of vaccine available for potential outbreak control during the posteradication era.[274] Therefore, trivalent OPV is the only preparation available, either in single-, 10-, 20-, or 50-dose vials. No combination products with OPV as one of the components have been licensed.

Constituents (Including Antibiotics and Preservatives)

The growth medium for the cells consists of Eagle's basal medium, the components of which include Earle's balanced salt solution, amino acids, antibiotics, and calf serum. After the cells have grown out, the medium is removed and replaced with fresh medium that contains the inoculating virus but no calf serum. The final vaccine is diluted with a modified cell culture maintenance medium that usually contains stabilizer. Each dose of vaccine may contain trace amounts of penicillin, neomycin, polymyxin, and strepto-mycin (see *Contraindications and Precautions* below) as well as $MgCl_2$ as a stabilizer. The vaccine contains phenol red as an indicator of pH.

Vaccine Stability

Before any vaccine lot can be released, it must be tested and meet the requirements of the national control authorities. If the vaccine is purchased by UNICEF, it also must meet the WHO requirements for manufacture, safety, and potency. Because OPV is a live viral vaccine, it is unstable unless it is stored at low temperatures (frozen). Thermostability requirements were defined by the WHO as OPV that loses less than 0.5 log_{10} of titer of each of the three vaccine strains after exposure to 37°C for 2 days.[293] In addition, current regulations require that, for maintenance of potency, the vaccine must be stored and shipped frozen and that, after thawing, it must be held in the refrigerator at no more than 10°C for a period not to exceed 30 days, after which time it must be discarded.

In the early 1960s, it was found that the infectivity of the enteroviruses could be preserved even when they were heated at 50°C if molar $MgCl_2$ was added,[294] a property that is still used in their identification and characterization. This discovery was applied rapidly to live vaccines[56] not only in the laboratory[295] but also in the field, where stabilized vaccines were used effectively to halt type 1 and type 3 outbreaks.[296] In laboratory studies with OPV containing $MgCl_2$ as a stabilizer,[297] the vaccine showed so little loss in virus titer after long-term storage at −20°C that the predicted half-life was calculated as 92 years. It also was noted that vaccine stabilized with $MgCl_2$ suffered no significant loss of potency after as many as nine cycles of alternate warm and cold conditions. Both sucrose and sorbitol have been used as stabilizers, but they have been less effective, particularly at high temperatures.[289] One manufacturer has introduced concentrated phosphate buffer–lactalbumin hydrolysate as a stabilizer; it works well at 4°C, but more data are needed to learn how effective it would be in the field at higher temperatures. It has recently been shown that D_2O (deuterium oxide) with $MgCl_2$ improves the thermal stability[298]; however, no OPV vaccines in use today contain D_2O.

Individual vaccine vial monitors (VVMs) were introduced in 1996 for all OPV procured by UNICEF.[299] VVMs respond to heat exposure with a change in color. The potential benefits of VVMs include (1) ability to keep opened vials without having to discard partially used vials at the end of the day, (2) decrease of at least 30% in vaccine wastage rates, (3) flexibility to take the vaccine beyond the cold chain to reach remote locations, and, most important,

(4) reassurance for the vaccinator at peripheral vaccination sites that the vaccine is potent.[299]

Regulatory Requirements for OPV Licensure

National control or regulatory agencies, such as the Food and Drug Administration in the United States or the National Institute for Biological Standards and Control in the United Kingdom, provide guidance to manufacturers for the production and licensing of OPV.[285] In addition, the WHO provides regulations that manufacturers must follow to be eligible to sell vaccine through the UNICEF tender. The WHO regulations contain three sections: (1) manufacturing requirements, (2) national control requirements, and (3) requirements for Poliomyelitis Vaccine (Oral) prepared in primary cultures of monkey kidney cells. In addition, a summary protocol for Poliomyelitis Vaccine (Oral) production is provided in Appendix 7 of that document.[293]

The WHO recommends that all candidate vaccine strains be evaluated in large-scale field trials before licensure because of the possibility that neurovirulence testing in monkeys may not always predict the actual behavior of vaccine strains (i.e., reversion to neurovirulence and potential for epidemic spread) in humans under field conditions.[300] USOL-D bac, a new poliovirus type 3 vaccine strain, was developed by the Institute of Sera and Vaccines in Prague, Czechoslovakia, in 1962.[301] Virus isolated in stool after administration of Sabin type 3 possessed a higher degree of neurovirulence than the corresponding mutants of USOL-D bac. In addition, this vaccine strain had passed all neurovirulence tests as determined in monkeys and appeared to be safer than the Sabin type 3 strain. In 1968, an extensive outbreak of poliomyelitis caused by poliovirus type 3 occurred in Poland 4 months after a small vaccine trial with Sabin type 3 and USOL-D bac vaccine strains had been carried out.[302] Subsequent molecular investigations indicated that USOL-D bac had been responsible for the epidemic.[303–305] This experience in humans indicates that monkey neurovirulence testing alone is insufficient to ensure vaccine safety. This conclusion is supported by data from the United States. Neurovirulence information, based on monkey neurovirulence tests, from more than 80 individual vaccine lots of Sabin type 3 virus produced between 1964 and 1983 was reviewed.[306] The authors of this study concluded that "type 3 OPV is, if anything, less neurovirulent than is type 1 OPV. However, in field use type 3 OPV has been associated with vaccine-related poliomyelitis more frequently than has type 1 OPV."[306] The molecular mechanisms for poliovirus attenuation and experiences with neurovirulence testing during the last 40 years were reviewed in a meeting in 1991.[307]

Genetic Stability of Vaccine Seed Strains

Live virus vaccines for RNA viruses present special challenges for development, manufacture, and administration because the mutation rates of RNA genomes are many orders of magnitude higher than those of DNA genomes.[268,308,309] The underlying cause of this high mutability is that the viral RNA polymerases (replicases) lack the proofreading mechanisms associated with DNA polymerases of DNA viruses and cellular organisms.[309] The absence of proofreading mechanisms in viral RNA replicases limits the size of RNA virus genomes (the largest is ~32,000 nucleotides in length) because the likelihood of incorporation of deleterious mutations increases with genome length. RNA virus populations exist as "quasi species," that is, as a heterogeneous collection of sequence variants distributed about an average "master" sequence.[310] Quasi species are capable of rapid evolution under challenging environmental conditions because variants with higher genetic fitness for the new conditions may be pre-existent in the populations.

The above considerations are of particular relevance to OPV. OPV preparations have been shown to be quasi species, with revertant variants of the critical attenuating 5'-UTR mutations representing approximately 0.1% of the population.[311] The biologic pressures applied in the selection for the attenuated OPV strains[261] are partially reversed when the strains are propagated at large scale for OPV production. The stringent growth and postproduction testing requirements for OPV are designed to limit the enrichment for variants with increased neurovirulence and to assure a product of uniform high safety. Several key measures were implemented to limit the enrichment for variants: (1) use of cell substrates favoring maintenance of the attenuated variants, (2) limitation of the number of production passages from the original OPV seed strains, (3) reselection from the OPV seed stocks of clones with low neurovirulence, and (4) incubation of OPV production cultures at temperatures (~34°C) favoring the maintenance of the temperature-sensitive phenotypes of the OPV strains.

The advent of recombinant DNA technology has opened a new avenue for the development of OPV seed stocks of enhanced genetic uniformity. Building on the finding of Racaniello and Baltimore[312] that infectious cDNA clones of poliovirus can be maintained as plasmids in the bacterium *Escherichia coli*, Nomoto and colleges[313,313a] developed infectious cDNA clones for each of the Sabin OPV strains. The poliovirus sequences contained within the recombinant plasmids are well defined and are genetically stable, because the DNA polymerases replicating the plasmid sequences have high-fidelity proofreading mechanisms. Moreover, the recombinant plasmid sequences can be readily confirmed by DNA sequencing. Thus OPV seed strain sequences can be maintained indefinitely in recombinant DNA plasmids. RNA transcripts produced in vitro from recombinant DNA plasmids are not genetically homogeneous, because the bacterial RNA polymerase catalyzing the transcription does not have proofreading mechanisms. However, unlike when OPV strains are propagated in cell culture, there is no biologic selection during the transcription process for variant genomes with reduced attenuation. Thus the RNA used to transfect cultured cells is more homogeneous, and the OPV seed stocks produced from the transfections of cultured cells have uniform biologic properties that are indistinguishable from those of the most stable OPV strains.[314]

Results of Vaccination

Viral Excretion and Immune Response

OPV administration, similar to natural exposure to polioviruses, initiates a complex process that eventually results in both humoral (systemic) and mucosal (local) immunity. The kinetics of this immune response have been reviewed in detail by Ogra and Karzon.[162] Production of IgM antibody predominates initially, can be detected as early as 1 to 3 days after infection, and disappears after 2 to 3 months. IgG antibody increases during this same period, eventually constitutes the predominant class of persistent antibody, and may last for life.[315] The development of both serum and secretory antibody responses to OPV compared with IPV is shown in Figure 25–8.[162] The broader response of nasal and duodenal IgA associated with OPV administration is apparent. The humoral immune response is not completely serotype specific,[127,316] and some degree of cross-protection (heterotypic cross-reaction) has been observed. Pre-existing antibody to poliovirus type 2 may modify the risk of paralytic poliomyelitis after exposure to poliovirus type 1.[317] The significance of cell-mediated immunity to poliovirus exposure remains to be shown,[318] although cytotoxic T-cell responses may contribute to the inflammation and cell necrosis that characterize poliovirus infections of the CNS.

Viremia has been demonstrated commonly after ingestion of type 2 OPV. Free virus is present in serum between days 2 and 5 after vaccination, and virus, bound to antibody, can be detected for an additional few days.[319,320] Bound virus in serum is detected by acid treatment, which inactivates the antibody and liberates active virus.

The majority of infants (70% to 90%) susceptible to poliomyelitis excrete poliovirus after administration of OPV. A study conducted during the winter of 1960 in Houston reported that 72%, 88%, and 75% of infants 0 to 6 months of age excreted homologous poliovirus types 1, 2, and 3, respectively, after vaccination with monovalent poliovirus vaccines[321] (Fig. 25–9). The same study showed that familial and extrafamilial contacts of vaccinated children get exposed secondarily to excreted poliovirus and in turn also excrete poliovirus in feces. The highest proportion of type 2 monovalent OPV–vaccinated infants excreted

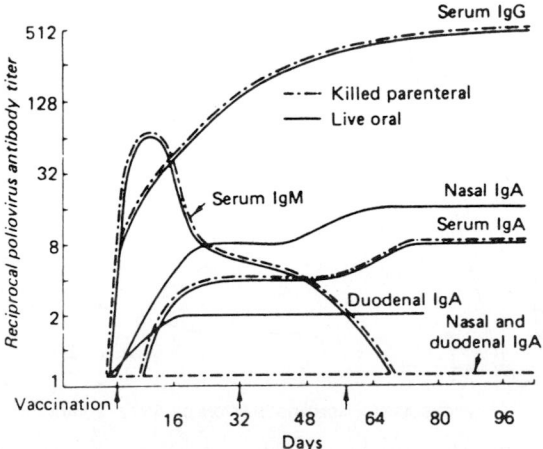

FIGURE 25–8 ▪ Serum and secretory antibody responses to orally administered, live, attenuated poliovirus vaccine (OPV) and to intramuscularly administered inactivated poliovirus vaccine (IPV). (From Ogra PL, Fishaut M, Gallagher MR. Viral vaccination via the mucosal routes. Rev Infect Dis 2:352–369, 1980, with permission.)

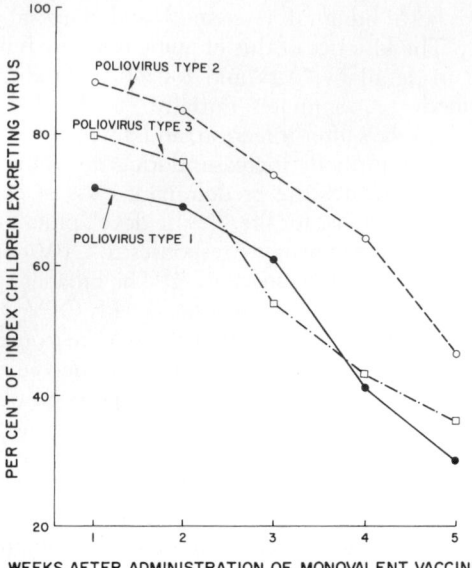

FIGURE 25–9 ■ Weekly excretion rates of homotypic virus by index children after administration of monovalent poliovaccines. (From Benyesh-Melnick M, Melnick JL, Rawls WE, et al. Studies on the immunogenicity, communicability, and genetic stability of oral poliovaccine administered during the winter. Am J Epidemiol 86:112–136, 1967, with permission.)

homologous virus in the first week after vaccination, the highest proportion of familial contacts excreted virus during the second week, and the highest proportion of nonfamilial contacts excreted virus during the fourth week (Fig. 25–10).

In industrialized countries, after complete primary vaccination with three doses of OPV, 95% or more of recipients seroconvert and develop long-lasting immunity to all three poliovirus serotypes. In a trial in the United States, 39% of vaccinees seroconverted to poliovirus type 1, 84% to

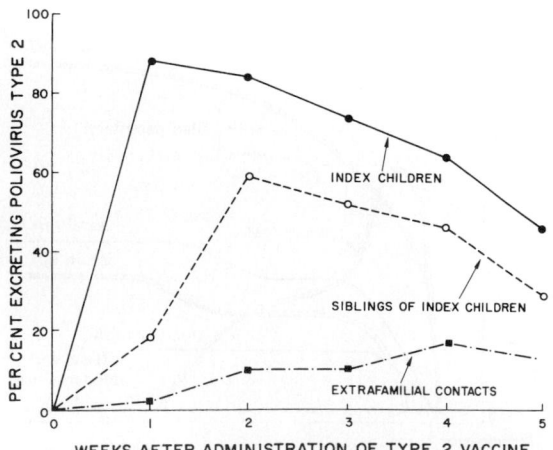

FIGURE 25–10 ■ Weekly excretion rates of homotypic virus following administration of type 2 monovalent vaccine, for index children, their siblings younger than 5 years, and extrafamilial contacts. (From Benyesh-Melnick M, Melnick JL, Rawls WE, et al. Studies on the immunogenicity, communicability, and genetic stability of oral poliovaccine administered during the winter. Am J Epidemiol 86:112–136, 1967, with permission.)

poliovirus type 2, and 71% to poliovirus type 3 after a single dose of OPV.[322] After receipt of two doses of OPV, seroprevalence was 92% to poliovirus type 1, 100% to poliovirus type 2, and 96% to poliovirus type 3; and after three doses of OPV, 97% had antibodies to poliovirus type 1, 100% to poliovirus type 2, and 100% to poliovirus type 3.[322] This study used a formulation of at least $10^{5.5}$, $10^{4.5}$, and $10^{5.2}$ $TCID_{50}$ of types 1, 2, and 3, respectively, of trivalent OPV vaccine produced in the United States and confirmed earlier studies conducted between 1959 and 1962, which administered OPV to infants and children who were initially seronegative. These earlier studies reported that, after two doses, the proportion of recipients seroconverting was 90% to 93% for type 1, 99% to 100% for type 2, and 76% to 98% for type 3; after a third dose, all converted to types 1 and 2, and 87% to 100% seroconverted to type 3.[102,221,240–242]

However, OPV appears to be considerably less immunogenic in developing countries. A comprehensive review of the immunogenicity of OPV in developing countries reported that a weighted average of only 73% (range, 36% to 99%), 90% (range, 77% to 100%), and 70% (range, 40% to 99%) of children participating in these studies have detectable antibody to poliovirus types 1, 2, and 3, respectively, after three OPV doses[180] (Table 25–10). Results of controlled trials conducted after the review[180] have confirmed the lower immunogenicity of OPV, particularly to poliovirus type 3, in developing countries.[323–325] A number of hypotheses attempt to explain the differences in OPV performance between industrialized and developing countries. These include interference from concurrent infections with other enteroviruses or diarrhea, both of which are more prevalent in developing countries.[323–326] In addition, there may be nonspecific factors not yet known; and colostrum contains secretory IgA, which can influence seroconversion.[327–329] Children with higher levels of maternal antibody have lower seroconversion rates. Maternally derived antibodies are higher in newborns in developing countries compared with newborns in the industrialized world[322,323]; and OPV is administered at an earlier age (birth, 6, 10, and 14 weeks), an age when the influence of maternally derived antibody on seroconversion is more distinct.[180] Increasing the potency of OPV can correct some of these limitations of the currently formulated OPV[325,330]; this also can be achieved by administering additional doses of OPV in the routine program or through mass campaigns.[78]

Mucosal immunity is measured primarily by resistance to poliovirus replication and excretion in the pharynx and intestine after challenge with monovalent or trivalent OPV.[241,242] After challenge, lower titers of virus are excreted for significantly shorter periods among vaccinees compared with unvaccinated children[331] (Table 25–11). Secretory IgA can be measured directly in stool, saliva, and breast milk to assess the degree of mucosal immunity. These methods are difficult to perform, require tedious standardization, and are rarely used. Mucosal immunity may exist even when levels of serum antibody are negligible,[243,332] although the degree of mucosal immunity appears most closely correlated with the titer of homologous humoral antibody[333]: the lower the titer, the more likely excretion of challenge virus can be demonstrated. One study reported that mucosal immunity may be strain specific, and mucosal immunity induced by one vaccine poliovirus strain may not induce mucosal

TABLE 25–10 ■ Seroconversion/Seroprevalence After Receipt of Three Doses of Oral Poliovirus Vaccine (OPV) in the Developing World

Country	Percentage with Neutralizing Antibody to Indicated Serotype			Age at First OPV Dose (mo)	Interval Between Doses (mo)	No. Studied	Lowest Dilution Tested*	Vaccine Formulation†
	Type 1	Type 2	Type 3					
Thailand	69	95	69	3	1.5	92	1:4	2:2:2
Thailand	90	100	100	3	1.5	82	1:4	5:1:2
Mexico	75	93	59	6	1	75	NA	3:3:3
India	61	77	40	3	1	74	1:10	4:4:4
South Africa	85	96	90	2	1.5	956	1:10	4:2:2
Iran	77	77	60	2	1	354	1:10	5:1:3
Iran	91	92	77	2	1	595	1:10	5:1:3
South Africa	86	96	75	0	1.5	176	1:8	6:2:3
China	99	98	99	0	3	100	1:4	10:1:3
Sri Lanka	97	98	98	3	2	65	1:8	10:1:3
Israel	95	98	93	2	1.5	121	1:10	10:1:3
Kenya	92	98	90	2	2	45	1:8	10:1:3
Brazil	91	98	94	2	2	75	1:5	10:1:3
South Africa	87	95	90	3	1	77	1:10	10:1:3
India	86	84	62	3	1.5	158	1:4	10:1:3
Mali	82	90	76	2	2	118	1:8	10:1:3
The Gambia	81	95	56	2	1	182	1:10	10:1:3
Brazil	80	95	56	2	>2	161	1:8	10:1:3
India	73	87	63	0	1	139	1:8	10:1:3
India	72	88	79	1.5	1	86	1:8	10:1:3
Sri Lanka	69	91	78	2	2	68	1:4	10:1:3
India	66	95	72	1.5	1	61	1:8	10:1:3
Kenya	63	92	60	6	2	65	1:8	10:1:3
India	63	75	68	2	1	71	1:10	10:1:3
India	58	92	83	3	1	78	1:10	10:1:3
Brazil	55	71	65	3	1.5	30	1:8	10:1:3
Nigeria	48	92	52	2	1.5	56	1:8	10:1:3
India	47	75	59	3	1.5	50	1:16	10:1:3
Kenya	44	77	60	6	2	31	1:8	10:1:3
India	40	75	51	2	2	87	1:8	10:1:3
Ghana	36	73	61	3	6	75	1:8	10:1:3
Morocco	89	95	74	2	1	122	1:10	20:2:13

*Lowest antibody dilution tested.
†The ratio of potencies of type 1 to type 2 to type 3.
Adapted from Patriarca PA, Wright PF, John TF. Factors affecting the immunogenicity of oral poliovirus vaccine in developing countries: review. Rev Infect Dis 13:926–939, 1991.

immunity against another strain.[334] Intestinal mucosal immunity induced by IPV is less effective against infection than that induced by OPV, as measured by the proportion of vaccinees excreting virus or the duration of excretion. However, the clinical importance of these differences in reducing wild-type virus spread in highly immunized populations in industrialized countries is not clear because (1) IPV appears to reduce shedding compared with no vaccine, and (2) pharyngeal spread may be important in industrialized countries, and IPV induces pharyngeal immunity.[335,336] IPV and OPV induce equivalent pharyngeal mucosal immunity based on studies in industrialized countries that rely on

TABLE 25–11 ■ Intestinal Immunity in Vaccinated (OPV or IPV) and Naturally Immune and Susceptible Children

Study Group	Proportion Excreting	Mean Duration of Excretion (days)	Mean Titer of Virus Excreted (log TCID$_{50}$)	Excretion Index (million)*	Reduction in Viral Excretion (%)
Susceptible control subjects	0.80	20.4	5.15	2.305	Reference
IPV vaccinated	0.74	12.3	4.11	0.1173	95
OPV vaccinated	0.37	4.6	2.18	0.00026	99
Naturally immune	0.37	5.4	2.03	0.00022	99

*Excretion index: proportion of children excreting challenge type 1 virus × mean duration of excretion days × titer of virus excreted.
Constructed from data in Fine and Carneiro,[177] Global Programme for Vaccines and Immunization,[489] and Ghedon and Sanakoyeva.[490]

vaccine virus challenge to assess mucosal immunity.[337] In contrast, in developing countries with poor hygiene and great potential for fecal–oral spread of enteric viruses, the clear increase in mucosal (intestinal) immunity induced by OPV over IPV would appear to offer a major advantage to OPV in reducing the circulation of polioviruses. Secretory IgA has an important role in defense against poliovirus infections,[162,337,338] and all available evidence indicates that the immune response after vaccination with OPV is similar to that after infection with wild-type poliovirus.

Few studies have provided data on the persistence of mucosal immunity. No data are currently available from developing countries regarding the duration of mucosal immunity for polioviruses. Several studies have assessed resistance to oral challenge by vaccine viruses years after the initial administration of OPV. One study reported that children were completely resistant to intestinal infection 10 years after vaccination, unless prechallenge serum antibodies were 1:8 or lower.[333] Another study reported similar findings on the relationship of humoral antibody and resistance to excretion.[339] No data are available on the long-term persistence of secretory IgA for polioviruses. However, looking at the mucosal immunity induced by another enterovirus, echovirus type 6, might provide some insights. A study assessing the falloff in secretory IgA titer to echovirus type 6 in the pharynx and intestine reported no declines during a 4-year follow-up period,[340] although the possibility of boosting with echovirus 6 or other enteroviruses in the follow-up period cannot be excluded.

When poliovirus is ingested, the virus has contact with proteolytic enzymes such as trypsin, which may alter viral antigens.[338] Secretory and humoral antibody responses after OPV include those against the new antigens associated with trypsin-cleaved virus. Such antigens are not accessible in IPV, and consequently the immune response after IPV is more limited.[341]

Evidence of OPV Effectiveness

A large body of empirical and scientific evidence has accumulated since the late 1950s that demonstrates the effectiveness of OPV in preventing paralytic disease. OPV use was pioneered in the former Soviet Union,[342–344] and the approaches developed in the Soviet Union led to rapid control or elimination of poliomyelitis in many countries. The most prominent example of the effectiveness of OPV is the success of the global polio eradication program,[37] including the Western Hemisphere, and the WHO's Western Pacific and European Regions, which were certified free of wild-type poliovirus by Regional Certification Commissions in 1994, 2000, and 2002, respectively.[345–347] OPV has curtailed epidemics and has greatly reduced the incidence of poliomyelitis, often eliminating the pattern of expected seasonal increase in poliomyelitis cases.[46,191,195,296,344,348–356] Two vaccine effectiveness studies have been conducted in recent years.[181,356] The study in Oman estimated that the effectiveness of three doses of OPV in preventing paralytic disease was approximately 90%.[181] Much of the earlier evidence of both small and large trials is contained in meeting reports.[241,242]

The ability of OPV to infect contacts of vaccine recipients (i.e., "contact spread") and "indirectly vaccinate" these contacts against poliomyelitis is considered by many to be another advantage of OPV compared with IPV. OPV

vaccine virus spread has been demonstrated by prospective virologic studies and by serologic studies in both industrialized and developing countries.[321,324,358–361] Serologic surveys have shown that the proportion of people who possess antibodies is considerably greater than would be expected either by vaccination or by the circulation of wild-type polioviruses. After OPV introduction in Yaoundé, Cameroon, the incidence of paralytic poliomyelitis decreased by 85%, although only 35% of children 12 to 13 months of age received three doses of OPV.[195] Among infants who received IPV in Oman, the seroconversion rates were significantly higher among those whose study period coincided with a mass OPV campaign that was conducted elsewhere in the country[324] (Fig. 25–11). A serologic survey among unvaccinated inner-city children in the United States also demonstrated that a substantial proportion of these children are exposed secondarily to vaccine viruses[360] (Fig. 25–12). In a study conducted in the United Kingdom, infants received a dose of IPV at 2 months of age. In the ensuing 1-month period and before any OPV was administered, 11% of infants excreted poliovirus type 1 and 4% excreted poliovirus type 2 in stool specimens.[361] These data indicate that vaccine virus spreads easily from OPV recipients to contacts both in industrialized and in developing countries.

Duration of Immunity

Because attenuated viruses contained in OPV are live viruses that induce the same types of antibody as wild-type poliovirus does, and because wild-type virus infection is believed to induce lifelong immunity, it has been reasoned by analogy that immunity induced by OPV is also lifelong. In an isolated Eskimo population, antibodies induced by wild-type poliovirus were shown to have persisted for at least 40 years in the absence of any further exposure during the intervening period.[315] The best evidence of the persistence of vaccine-induced immunity is the absence of disease in adolescents and adults who had been vaccinated previously with OPV and the persistence of type-specific antibody assessed in population-based surveys.[362,363] However, interpretation of these data is difficult because of potential repeated exposures to shed virus. In prospective studies in which the same vaccinees were observed for several years, antibodies to types 1 and 2 were found in more than 90% of children and to type 3 in 83% to 95%.[27,364–369] Data from population-based studies of antibody seroprevalence conducted among Army recruits in the United States in 1989 (>95% to poliovirus types 1 and 2, and >85% to poliovirus type 3)[363] and among school-age children in Massachusetts in 1981 (>99% to poliovirus type 1, >99% to poliovirus type 2, and >99% to poliovirus type 3)[362] and in The Gambia (88.1% to poliovirus type 1 and 89.3% to poliovirus type 3 among 3- to 4-year-old children)[370] have demonstrated that poliovirus antibodies induced by OPV persist for many years.

Adverse Events

Vaccine-Associated Paralytic Poliomyelitis

In the early 1990s, the Institute of Medicine reviewed adverse events associated with childhood vaccines, including poliovirus vaccines.[371] The major adverse event associ-

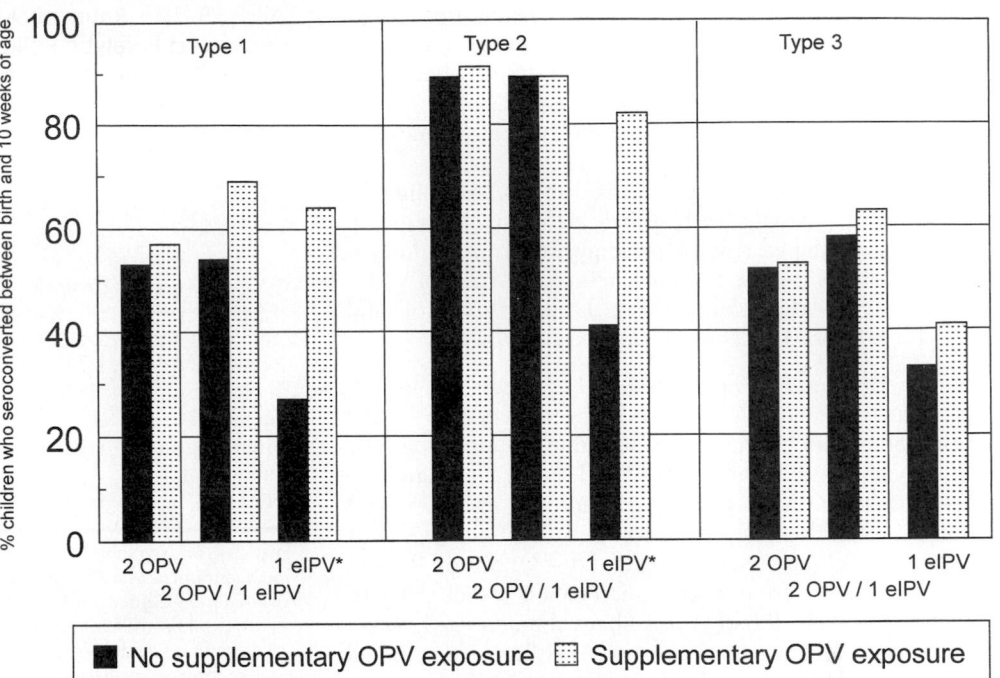

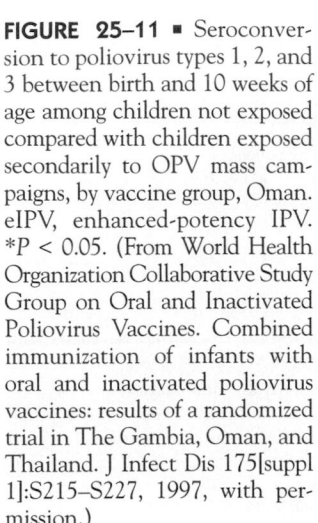

FIGURE 25–11 ▪ Seroconversion to poliovirus types 1, 2, and 3 between birth and 10 weeks of age among children not exposed compared with children exposed secondarily to OPV mass campaigns, by vaccine group, Oman. eIPV, enhanced-potency IPV. *P < 0.05. (From World Health Organization Collaborative Study Group on Oral and Inactivated Poliovirus Vaccines. Combined immunization of infants with oral and inactivated poliovirus vaccines: results of a randomized trial in The Gambia, Oman, and Thailand. J Infect Dis 175[suppl 1]:S215–S227, 1997, with permission.)

ated with OPV is VAPP. Shortly after licensure and widespread use of monovalent OPV, cases with paralytic manifestations followed vaccination with monovalent type 3 vaccines. These cases were considered clinically consistent with poliomyelitis and were supported by laboratory findings that did not exclude a possible causal relationship to the administration of oral vaccine. This report by the Surgeon General describes the earliest cases of VAPP.[372]

In 1969, the WHO coordinated a collaborative study to obtain data on the potential risks associated with OPV use. The findings of the first 5- and 10-year follow-up studies were published.[373,374] During the 5-year period from 1980 to 1984, 395 cases of acute persisting spinal paralysis were reported from 13 countries with a total population of 547

million.[375] The risk of VAPP (in either recipients or contacts of recipients) was less than 0.3 cases per million doses of OPV distributed (or less than 1 case per 3.3 million doses), and the average annual incidence of VAPP was 0.14 per 1 million people (range, 0.0 to 0.33), excluding Romania. Romania reported an average annual incidence of 2.7 per 1 million people. Although some have challenged the existence of VAPP,[27,376,377] believing that the cases of paralysis have different etiologic factors, the following evidence supports vaccine viruses as causative:

1. Clinical syndromes are typical of poliomyelitis.
2. Vaccine virus is frequently isolated from cases.
3. History of exposure to vaccine is often obtained.

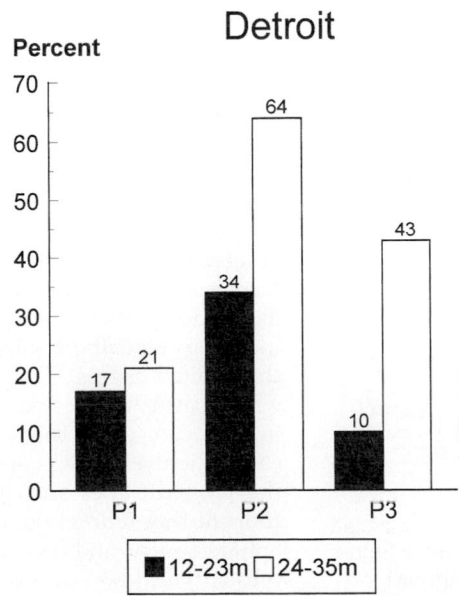

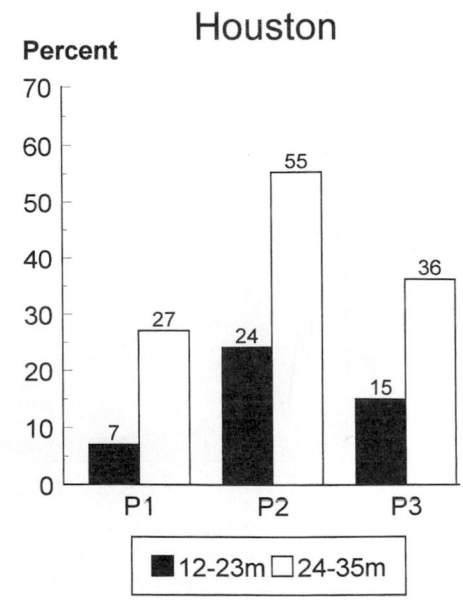

FIGURE 25–12 ▪ Poliovirus antibody seroprevalence among unvaccinated inner-city preschool children, by age groups, Detroit and Houston, 1990 to 1991. P1, poliovirus type 1; P2, poliovirus type 2; P3, poliovirus type 3; 12-23m, 12 to 23 months of age; 24-35m, 24 to 35 months of age. (Constructed from data in Chen RT, Hausinger S, Dajani AS, et al. Seroprevalence of antibody against polivirus in inner-city preschool children: implications for vaccination policy in the United States. JAMA 275:1639–1645,1996.

4. Both recipient and contact cases cluster after receipt of the first dose of OPV (one would expect virtually equal numbers of cases after each dose if there were other etiologic agents causing the illnesses).

5. Shed viruses have been shown to have mutated toward neurovirulence.

6. The incidence of VAPP is highest in immunodeficient people with B-cell deficiencies, a group also at higher risk of poliomyelitis from wild-type poliovirus.[378] The completeness of reporting of VAPP cases to the Centers for Disease Control and Prevention (CDC) was estimated to be 81%.[379]

Between 1980 and 1994, a total of 125 cases (94% of all reported cases) classified as VAPP were reported in the United States, including 49 (39%) among immunologically normal vaccine recipients, 46 (37%) among immunologically normal contacts of vaccine recipients, and 30 (24%) among immunologically compromised OPV recipients or contacts of OPV recipients[379] (Fig. 25–13). Six of 46 contact VAPP cases were not epidemiologically associated with vaccine; however, all had virus isolates characterized as vaccine related. Most contact cases were either unvaccinated or inadequately vaccinated. Therefore, if contacts had been concomitantly vaccinated and immunized, the risk of contact cases would have been smaller or nonexistent.

For the period 1980 to 1994, the risk of VAPP in the United States was estimated as 1 case per 2.4 million doses of OPV distributed; for children receiving the first doses of OPV, the risk was estimated as 1 case per 750,000 children vaccinated[380] (Table 25–12). The risk of VAPP is highest after the first dose of OPV. Recipients of a first dose and their contacts had a 6.8-fold higher risk of VAPP than did recipients of subsequent doses and their contacts. People with immunodeficiency disorders are at highest risk for VAPP. The risk of VAPP among immunocompromised people is elevated to more than 3200 times the risk of immunocompetent people.[381] Almost all cases occurred in people with congenital or acquired immunodeficiency. Immunedeficient people with VAPP primarily had abnormalities affecting the B-cell system (humoral immunity), with agammaglobulinemia or hypogammaglobulinemia most frequently associated with VAPP.[381] With the exception of one VAPP case with immunodeficiency disorder, in all other cases, the precipitating event for the diagnosis of immuno-

TABLE 25–12 ■ Ratio of Number of Cases of Vaccine-Associated Paralytic Poliomyelitis to Number of Doses of Oral Poliovirus Vaccine Distributed, United States, 1980 to 1994

| Case Category | Ratio of Number of Cases per Million Doses of OPV Distributed | | | Relative Risk* |
	Overall	First Dose	Subsequent Doses	
Recipient	1:6.2	1:1.4	1:27.2	19.4
Contact	1:7.6	1:2.2	1:17.5	8.0
Community acquired	1:50.5	NA	NA	NA
Immunologically abnormal	1:10.1	1:5.8	1:12.9	2.2
Total†	1:2.4	1:0.75	1:5.1	6.8

*First dose ratio to subsequent dose ratio. NA, Not available.
†Includes normal as well as immunologically abnormal cases.
Adapted from Centers for Disease Control and Prevention. Poliomyelitis prevention in the United States: introduction of a sequential vaccination schedule of inactivated poliovirus vaccine followed by oral poliovirus vaccine. Recommendations of the Advisory Committee on Immunization Practices. MMWR 46(RR-3): 1–25, 1997.

deficiency was the onset of paralytic disease. Poliovirus type 3 is the virus most frequently isolated from immunocompetent people with VAPP. In contrast, poliovirus type 2 is the most common virus detected in immunodeficient cases with VAPP. Poliovirus type 1 is rarely isolated from cases with VAPP.[192]

Romania and Hungary have consistently reported higher rates of VAPP than other countries with well-developed surveillance systems. Until recently, both Romania and Hungary used trivalent OPV and monovalent OPV, respectively, solely in campaigns.[208,291] The high risk of VAPP in Hungary was associated primarily with the administration of monovalent type 3 OPV.[291] The high risk of VAPP in Romania can be attributed to provocation poliomyelitis (i.e., multiple intramuscular injections in the 30 days before paralytic manifestations).[382] VAPP cases in Romania had received, on average, 16.8 intramuscular injections, primarily for antibiotics, in the 30 days before onset of paralysis. Analysis of VAPP cases in the United States between 1980 and 1993 suggested that cases with a history of intramuscular injections received an average of only 1.5 intramuscular injections in the 45 days before onset of paralysis; no clustering of injections during the 45-day period was observed.[383] In contrast, in Romania, most injections were received in the periods from 0 to 7 days and from 8 to 14 days before onset. It appears unlikely that intramuscular injections contribute substantially to the VAPP burden in the United States. The risk of VAPP in the Americas, where Latin America administered large quantities of OPV in mass campaigns (national immunization days) to eradicate poliomyelitis, was similar to the VAPP risk reported in the United States and other countries.[384] An analysis in India further refined the risk estimates for one large developing country, and demonstrated that the risk of VAPP is substantially lower in this country despite large quantities of

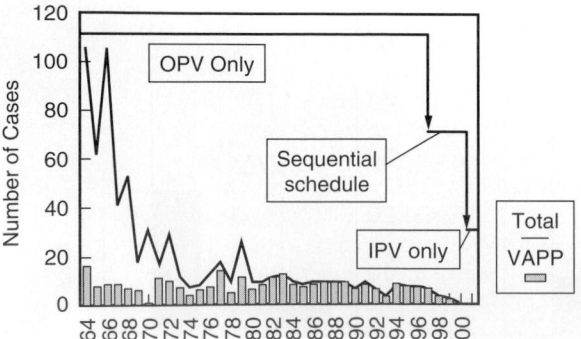

FIGURE 25–13 ■ Total reported paralytic poliomyelitis cases and vaccine-associated paralytic poliomyelitis (VAPP), United States, 1961 to 2000 (Centers for Disease Control and Prevention).

OPV administered in mass vaccination campaigns and through routine immunization programs (more than 700 million doses of OPV in 1999 alone). The risk among first-dose recipients was estimated as 1 case per 2.8 million children (compared with a first-dose recipient risk of 1 case per 1.4 million children in the United States). The lower risk estimates in India may be explained in part because (1) both the proportion with and the titers of maternally derived antibody are high among newborns because wild-type poliovirus circulated widely until recently and may have led to frequent virus exposure and boosting of titers in the general population; (2) a birth dose of OPV is recommended for institutional births (thus inducing immunity when the newborn is still under protection against poliomyelitis from maternally derived antibody); and (3) the routine vaccination schedule calls for OPV doses at 6, 10, and 14 weeks of age (again immunity is induced at earlier ages than in industrialized countries). Thus high levels of maternal antibody, and OPV vaccination at an age when maternal antibody would be expected to protect against VAPP, appear to be the main reasons why the observed risk of VAPP in India (and probably in other countries under similar circumstances) appears to be lower than that in industrialized countries.[385]

A recent evaluation of the global burden of vaccine-associated paralytic poliomyelitis (VAPP) by the WHO estimated that between 250–500 cases occur each year.[386]

Immunodeficient children are subject to infection, frequently fatal, by a wide variety of normally benign or avirulent agents. Nonpolio enteroviruses may cause serious or fatal illnesses in immunocompromised people.[387,388] A prominent feature of such infections is the patient's inability to eradicate the virus from the CNS; some patients continue to yield virus from cerebrospinal fluid for up to 3 years.[389] As of 2002, a total of 15 persons with immunodeficiency disorders have been shown to excrete poliovirus for periods of approximately 12 months or longer (see *General Epidemiology* above) since the early 1960s. Two cases in this series deserve attention. A patient with VAPP in the United States may have excreted virus for approximately 7 years prior to onset of paralytic disease in 1981,[134,135] and a person from the United Kingdom who does not have paralytic disease has excreted poliovirus for more than 10 years (as of 2002).[136] In immunodeficient individuals, poliovirus infection, either by a wild-type virus or by a vaccine strain, may develop in an atypical manner, with an incubation period longer than 28 days, a high mortality rate after a long chronic illness, and unusual lesions in the CNS.[22,226,381,390]

Vaccine-Derived Polioviruses

In principle, all clinical and environmental poliovirus isolates that are related to the OPV strains are VDPVs. However, derivatives of the Sabin OPV strains have been classified into two broad categories: (1) "OPV-like" isolates that have close sequence relationships (>99% VP1 sequence identity) to the original OPV strains; and (2) VDPV isolates that have sequence properties (≤99% VP1 sequence identity from the parental Sabin strains) indicative of prolonged replication of the vaccine virus. VDPV isolates, in turn, have been subdivided into two groups, reflective of the differing conditions that lead to their appearance: (1) immunodeficient VDPVs (iVDPVs),

isolated from immunodeficient patients who become chronically infected after exposure to OPV; and (2) circulating VDPVs (cVDPVs) that arise in communities with inadequate OPV coverage. VDPVs are of particular interest because of their implications for current and future strategies for global polio eradication.[136,177,391]

The large majority of vaccine-related isolates are OPV-like. Capsid sequences of OPV-like isolates (usually surveyed by VP1 sequencing) closely match those of the parental Sabin strains. Because poliovirus genomes evolve rapidly (approximately 1% per year), the extent of VP1 sequence divergence can be used to approximate duration of a poliovirus infection.[135,138,142] However, the confidence intervals for these time estimates are wide because of the stochastic nature of mutation and because some VP1 sites in the Sabin strains are subject to negative selection during replication of OPV in the human intestine.[392] Confidence intervals narrow when the sequencing window is extended to include the complete capsid region or the complete genome. The number of VP1 nucleotide substitutions expected from the poliovirus molecular clock to accumulate during infection of an immunologically normal primary vaccine recipient (assuming a maximum duration of infection of ~8 weeks) is zero to three. Selected reversion may add one or two additional VP1 substitutions during a normal infection. Thus the 1% (equivalent to approximately nine nucleotide substitutions in VP1) demarcation between OPV-like isolates and VDPVs should include virtually all OPV-like isolates. Some VDPVs could be included among isolates with 0.5% and 1% divergence from the OPV strains. However, such isolates are relatively rare, and, when found, the epidemiologic data are reviewed for evidence of conditions favoring appearance of VDPVs.

Many OPV-like isolates have recombinant genomes.[142,393-395] The large majority of OPV-like recombinants were generated by heterotypic genetic exchange among Sabin strains. OPV-like isolates with non-Sabin strain sequences are rare.[395] The abundance of vaccine-related recombinants results from the trivalent formulation of OPV and the likelihood that some recombinants have higher fitness for replication in the human intestine than the original OPV strains. Crossovers are most frequently found in the noncapsid region, less frequently in the 5′-UTR, and least frequently in the 3′-terminal sequences of the capsid region.[396] Vaccine-related recombinants are more often associated with types 3 and 2 than with type 1.[393-395,397] Because capsid and noncapsid sequences co-evolve, the extent of VP1 sequence identity to the corresponding Sabin OPV strain is generally reflective of the evolutionary history of the overall genome.

It seems likely that many OPV-like isolates have recovered the capacity for higher neurovirulence and possibly increased transmissibility. The small number of substitutions controlling neurovirulence in experimental animals were found to have reverted among many OPV-like isolates, especially among isolates of types 2 and 3.[392,398-400] Because the critical and unstable attenuating mutations in the 5′-UTRs of the Sabin strains also affect fitness for virus replication in the human intestine,[399] it appears possible that revertants at these sites would have a higher fitness for person-to-person spread. However, spread is normally limited by high OPV coverage.

It has long been recognized that immunodeficient patients with defects in antibody production (especially those with CVID or X-linked agammaglobulinemia) could become chronically infected when exposed to OPV.[381] Unambiguous demonstration that vaccine-related poliovirus isolates from immunodeficient patients had unusual sequence properties awaited the application of molecular tools, such as oligonucleotide fingerprinting[401] and genomic sequencing,[135,138,142] to poliovirus diagnostics. As expected, the extent of sequence divergence is related to the duration of the chronic infection. Not all isolates from immunodeficient patients would be classified as iVDPVs. Some isolates are specimens taken early in the chronic infection and no subsequent specimens were taken. In other situations, either the chronic infections had resolved spontaneously or the patient died from complications of the immunodeficiency (including fatal poliomyelitis). However, some iVDPV isolates are highly divergent (~90% VP1 sequence identity to the parental OPV strain), suggesting that the chronic poliovirus infections had persisted for 10 years or more.[136,402] Chronic iVDPV infections are independent events,[192,381] and the isolates obtained from such infection trace separate pathways of divergence from the original OPV strains.[135,138] Many of the iVDPV isolates are recombinant, but, as with most OPV-like isolates, the recombinant sequences of all known iVDPV isolates have been derived from the Sabin strains. This pattern of recombination has permitted the recognition of iVDPV isolates from their sequence properties. The underlying reason for this pattern of recombination may be that chronically infected immunodeficient patients are generally resistant to superinfection by other enteroviruses.

Chronic infection of immunodeficient patients with VDPVs is problematic because such infections cannot be prevented by high OPV coverage. So far, all reports of persistent iVDPV infections have been from countries with high to intermediate levels of development, where the rates of OPV coverage are high and where the survival times of immunodeficient patients may be extended by their access to appropriate clinical management. The survival rates for hypogammaglobulinemic patients are probably very low in developing countries at highest risk for poliovirus spread. The population of chronic iVDPV excreters is declining in developed countries because some patients have died, some have cleared their infections, and no new iVDPV infections have been found in countries that have shifted to IPV. Although there is no evidence of spread of iVDPVs from immunodeficient patients to the wider community,[136,192] the potential for such spread may be limited by high vaccine coverage in the communities where immunodeficient patients have extended survival times.

The cVDPVs have been recognized more recently. Polio outbreaks associated with cVDPVs have been recognized in four different parts of the world (Table 25–13). In Egypt, type 2 cVDPV was isolated from 30 polio patients during the years 1988 to 1993.[403] The rate and pattern of VP1 divergence from the Sabin type 2 OPV strain suggested that all lineages were derived from a single OPV infection that occurred around 1983. Phylogenetic analysis showed that the cVDPVs circulated widely in Egypt along several independent chains of transmission, and established independent foci of endemicity in separate communities. cVDPV circulation ceased when OPV coverage rates increased. In Hispaniola (Haiti and the Dominican Republic), an outbreak of 21 confirmed cases (including two fatal cases) in 2000 to 2001 was associated with type 1 cVDPV.[59] A more limited outbreak, associated with an independent-lineage type 1 cVDPV, occurred in the Philippines in 2001.[404] A fourth outbreak, involving two separate type 2 cVDPV lineages, was detected in Madagascar in 2002.[405] The cVDPVs have recovered the essential properties of wild-type polioviruses: (1) the capacity to cause paralytic disease in humans, and (2) the capacity for continuous person-to-person transmission. The common risk factors for cVDPV circulation were major gaps in OPV coverage, providing large numbers of susceptibles for virus circulation; environmental conditions favoring poliovirus spread; and the prior eradication of the corresponding serotype of indigenous wild-type poliovirus.

All outbreak-associated cVDPV isolates described thus far have been recombinants with related enteroviruses.[59,403,406] However, this observation does not imply that recombination is essential to the phenotypic reversion of the Sabin strains, because the main determinants of attenuation of all three Sabin strains map to the 5′-UTR and capsid region sites[254,268,392,402] and most of the crossovers in cVDPV isolates map to the noncapsid region. The high frequency of back-

TABLE 25–13 ▪ Outbreaks of Circulating Vaccine-Derived Poliovirus, 1988 to 2002

Country	Year	No. cVDPV Cases	Serotype	% nt Divergence	Virus Recombined with Nonpolio Enterovirus	Immunization Coverage with Three Doses of OPV	Duration of Circulation
Egypt[403]	1988–1993	30*	2	4% to 7%	Yes	Reported high	6–11 yr
Haiti[59]	2000–2001	8	1	2.6%	Yes	<30% nationwide	~2 yr
Dominican Republic[59]	2000–2001	13	1	1.9%	Yes	<30% in most affected areas	>6 mo
Philippines[404]	2001	3	1	~2%	Yes	OPV shortage over past 2 yr	~2 yr
Madagascar[405]	2001, 2002	5†	2	1%, 2.5%	Yes	<50% nationwide	1 yr, 2.5 yr

*Cited paper specifies 32 cases; however, further investigations removed two of these because of identical genomic nucleotide sequences.
†Two separate clusters of infections, one with a single case in 2001 and another with four cases in 2002, respectively.
nt, nucleotide.

mutation of the attenuating 5′-UTR sites during replication of OPV in the human intestine[397,399,400] suggests that back-mutations would usually precede recombination. Recombination within the capsid region is infrequent,[407] and none of the cVDPV isolates characterized so far show evidence of any such recombination.[59,405,406] The observed successive recombination events involving the noncapsid region[59] and the 5′-UTR sequences may not be associated with any progressive increase in replicative fitness. Rather, recombination with other enteroviruses is likely to be a random process that occurs during mixed infection, the probability of which increases with the total number of people infected. Thus the combination in a vaccine-related isolate of significant divergence of capsid nucleotide sequences (>1% from the parental OPV strains) and recombination with other enteroviruses is a likely indicator of VDPV circulation. VP1 sequence divergence of greater than 1% in a cVDPV isolate would suggest that circulation had occurred for at least a year, raising the possibility that immunization activities during the preceding year had failed to stop VDPV circulation.

The cVDPV outbreaks in developing countries challenge the assumption that poliovirus endemicity can be restored only by reintroduction of wild-type poliovirus, underscore the urgency of reaching the goal of global polio eradication as quickly as possible, and have important implications for the endgame strategy of polio eradication (see *Stopping Polio Vaccination After Eradication Has Been Achieved* below). The immediate priority is to eliminate the remaining pockets of wild-type poliovirus endemicity in South Asia and sub-Saharan Africa.[37] At the same time, it is essential to maintain high levels of vaccination coverage against polioviruses in all countries, both to prevent the spread of imported wild-type polioviruses and to suppress the emergence of cVDPVs. Areas at highest risk for emergence of cVDPVs are those where vaccination coverage rates have declined, the competing wild-type polioviruses have been eliminated, and epidemiologic conditions had previously favored wild-type poliovirus transmission. In response to the recent cVDPV outbreaks, the WHO has recommended the reinstatement of mass immunization campaigns to close the immunity gap in areas where coverage through routine immunization has been insufficient to prevent widening susceptibility to polio.[408] The frequency of the mass campaigns shall be determined by the rate of accumulation of susceptibles in the population and the basic reproduction number for poliovirus in the highest risk populations in each area.[146,177] No additional measures have been recommended for the remaining polio-endemic countries, because activities currently planned for elimination of the last pockets of types 1 and 3 poliovirus circulation would also effectively prevent dissemination of cVDPVs.

Simian Virus 40

During the early years of OPV production, some cell cultures were contaminated with simian virus 40 (SV40), a virus that causes cancer in rodents.[409] Although concerns were raised about the carcinogenic potential of the SV40 in vaccinees and their offspring, long-term follow-up studies do not support such an association.[410,411] A meeting convened at the National Institutes of Health in 1997 re-examined the available evidence and concluded that "no measurable increase in neoplastic diseases has occurred in

humans exposed to SV40 contaminated polio vaccines."[412] Subsequently, a report evaluated the cancer risks of birth cohorts potentially exposed to SV40 and concluded that these cohorts did not experience a significantly increased risk for the cancer outcomes studied.[413] Nevertheless, the question of whether SV40 exposure can increase cancer risk continues to be debated, and additional research is needed to accept or reject this association.[414,415] A review by the Immunization Safety Committee (under the auspices of the Institute of Medicine) concluded in 2002 that, because the epidemiologic studies were sufficiently flawed, the evidence was inadequate to conclude whether or not SV40-contaminated polio vaccine caused cancer.[416] Cell lines currently used for OPV production come from monkeys raised in colonies free of SV40 or from well-characterized continuous cell lines (Vero cells). In addition, OPV must be screened for known viruses; thus, SV40 is not present in current lots of OPV vaccine.

Guillain-Barré Syndrome

A review by the Institute of Medicine in 1992 suggested that "the evidence favors acceptance of a causal relationship between OPV and Guillain-Barré syndrome."[371] This conclusion was based primarily on data from Finland, where an OPV mass campaign was conducted to control an outbreak of poliomyelitis and 27 patients developed Guillain-Barré syndrome within 10 weeks after initiation of the campaign.[417,418] However, after the Institute of Medicine review was completed, the Finnish data were reanalyzed and an observational study was completed in the United States.[419,420] The observational study in the United States showed that rates of Guillain-Barré syndrome after OPV were similar to rates that would have been expected in the absence of vaccination. The reanalysis in Finland suggested that the increase in Guillain-Barré syndrome risk began before the mass vaccination campaign had been initiated, and noted that an influenza epidemic occurred concurrently with the mass campaign. Thus the available data do not support a causal relationship between OPV and Guillain-Barré syndrome.

Contraindications and Precautions

Contraindications for OPV administration differ somewhat depending on whether the vaccine recipient resides in the industrialized or the developing world (Table 25–14). The risk-benefit ratio of OPV versus no vaccine among children residing in countries with endemic poliomyelitis or recent endemic poliomyelitis favors OPV administration in almost all circumstances. Because of the availability of IPV in a number of industrialized countries and because the need for mucosal (intestinal) immunity is not as great, industrialized countries may have more contraindications than developing countries. In general, OPV is contraindicated in people with known immunodeficiency disorders and those receiving cancer chemotherapy. Age older than 18 years and pregnancy were precautions in the United States, and OPV doses should be repeated in children who vomit within 30 minutes of OPV receipt. In developing countries, OPV doses administered to children with diarrhea also should be repeated. More details on contraindications and precautions are discussed below.

TABLE 25–14 ■ Contraindications and Precautions for Use of Oral Poliovirus Vaccine in the United Kingdom, the United States, and Developing Countries

Type		U.K.[420]	U.S.[379,419]	Developing Country (WHO)
Contraindications	Known or suspected immunodeficiency disorder or immunocompromised	Yes	Yes	Yes*
	Family member known to have or suspected of having immunodeficiency disorder or being immunocompromised	Yes	Yes	NA
	HIV infection	No†	Yes	No‡
	Age ≥ 18 yr	No	Yes (use IPV)	NA
	Allergic reaction to previous doses of OPV or one of its components	No	Yes	NA
Precautions	Pregnancy	Yes	Yes§	NA
	Diarrhea	Yes (postpone)	No	Yes (repeat doses)

*If immunodeficiency is known.
†For HIV-positive symptomatic individuals, IPV may be used instead of OPV at the discretion of the clinician.
‡Yes, if clinical disease.
§If immediate protection against poliomyelitis is necessary, IPV or OPV can be used.
HIV, human immunodeficiency virus; IPV, inactivated poliovirus vaccine; NA, not applicable; OPV, oral poliovirus vaccine.

Altered Immune States

In industrialized countries, people with known or suspected immunodeficiency disorders, such as SCID, CVID, agammaglobulinemia, and hypogammaglobulinemia, should not receive OPV.[380,381,421,422] Similarly, in people with altered immune states resulting from diseases such as leukemia, lymphoma, or generalized malignant disease or with immune systems compromised by therapy with corticosteroids, alkylating drugs, antimetabolites, or radiation, OPV is contraindicated. Because of the potential for vaccine spread, OPV should not be given to a child who is a member of a family in which there are immunocompromised people. Also, where there has been a family member with immunodeficiency in the past, OPV should not be given to another child unless that child is known to be immunocompetent.

Human Immunodeficiency Virus Infection

In many industrialized countries, OPV in people infected with human immunodeficiency virus (HIV) is considered either a precaution or a contraindication. OPV also should not be used for immunizing household contacts of patients with the immunodeficiency disorder; instead, IPV is recommended.

In developing countries, the HIV status of infants is often not known, and IPV is not available as an alternative vaccine. In these settings, OPV is administered early in life (i.e., 6, 10, and 14 weeks of age) on the basis of WHO recommendations; this is at an age when HIV infection would not be expected to have caused immunodeficiency. Several studies showed that OPV induces antibody to polioviruses in a similar proportion of HIV-infected infants compared with the response in non–HIV-infected infants.[423,424] HIV infection does not appear to be a risk factor for paralytic poliomyelitis caused by wild-type poliovirus[425] or for VAPP. There are only two case reports in the literature, one from Romania and one from Zimbabwe, that link HIV infection and VAPP.[426,427]

Previous Allergic Reaction

OPV may contain trace amounts of penicillin, neomycin, polymyxin, and streptomycin, and a previous allergic reaction to OPV or a similar reaction to these antibiotics constitutes a contraindication to further OPV receipt.[380,422]

Adult Use

The recommendations for use of OPV among unvaccinated adults 18 years of age and older in industrialized countries is not uniform. In the United States, these adults should not receive OPV, because of concerns about a slightly elevated risk of VAPP in adults.[372] In the United Kingdom, no such restrictions are recommended.[422] Nevertheless, adults in the United States at risk may receive OPV if they had been primed by OPV previously.[380]

Pregnancy

In most industrialized countries, pregnancy is either a contraindication or a precaution to OPV receipt.[422] Two evaluations have found no link between adverse outcomes and administration of OPV to pregnant women.[428,429] Nevertheless, most immunization authorities recommend that immunization during pregnancy generally should be avoided for reasons of theoretical risk. However, if immediate protection against poliomyelitis is needed, IPV or OPV can be used.[380,421]

Diarrhea

In the United Kingdom, vomiting or diarrhea are criteria for exclusion for OPV administration.[422] In developing countries, OPV may be given to a child with diarrhea; however, because of the lower immunogenicity of OPV in these countries, the dose should not be counted as a valid dose toward completing the routine schedule and should be repeated 4 weeks later.[323,324,380,421,430]

Simultaneous Administration with Other Vaccines

In industrialized countries as well as in developing countries, OPV is usually administered with other vaccines, including (where appropriate) bacille Calmette-Guérin, DTP, hepatitis B, measles, *Haemophilus influenzae* type b, and other vaccines used routinely,[380,430] because no interference between these vaccines and OPV has been observed.

Sequential and Combined Schedules

With the progress reported toward polio eradication, many industrialized countries are reviewing and revising their routine vaccination schedules from using OPV exclusively to either a sequential schedule of IPV followed by OPV, or using IPV exclusively for the prevention of poliomyelitis. For example, the United States shifted from an exclusive OPV schedule to a preferred sequential schedule of two doses of IPV followed by two doses of OPV in 1997, and to an IPV-only schedule in 2000.[431,432] Many countries in Europe and elsewhere are examining the advantages and disadvantages of sequential vaccination schedules for adoption into national vaccination policies. Sequential schedules offer the following scientific and programmatic advantages:

1. The schedule should reduce the number of VAPP cases among recipients by 95% and to some degree among contacts because the mucosal immunity induced by two doses of IPV should reduce spread of vaccine virus.
2. Continued use of OPV will induce effective intestinal immunity,[433] thereby enhancing community resistance to transmission of imported wild-type poliovirus.
3. There is opportunity for spread of vaccine virus, thus immunizing people missed by routine immunization (this becomes less important as immunization coverage reaches high levels).
4. The number of injections in the second year of life is reduced from what would be required with use of an IPV-only schedule, making compliance with the overall schedule easier.
5. The schedule will lead to stocking of both poliovirus vaccines by health care providers, facilitating choice by both parents and providers.

As of 2002, sequential schedules of IPV followed by OPV have been recommended in six industrialized countries and two reporting entities, including Bermuda, Belarus, Croatia, Latvia, Lithuania, Hungary, Israel, and the West Bank and Gaza.[434] The immunogenicity of sequential schedules depends on the vaccines used, the age at administration, the number of doses, and the interval between doses. In addition to the results of the immunogenicity studies, there is a growing body of evidence suggesting the effectiveness of this approach in controlling poliomyelitis.[435]

In the United States, a small trial first demonstrated the immunogenicity of two sequential schedules of IPV and OPV in inducing antibody.[436] Subsequently, a series of studies were conducted in the United States to assess the immunogenicity of sequential schedules of IPV followed by OPV. In general, these studies showed that a series of at least three doses of either vaccine—IPV or OPV or with sequential or combined use—was necessary to induce antibody to all three poliovirus serotypes in more than 90% of vaccinees.[437–439]

To assess the effectiveness of three sequential schedules in inducing mucosal immunity in the United States, vaccinees received a dose of OPV at age 18 months (3 months

after the last dose of poliovirus vaccine), and stool specimens were obtained before challenge (day 0) and 3, 7, and 21 days thereafter. One dose of OPV after IPV reduced shedding of poliovirus types 2 and 3 (after challenge with OPV) but did not decrease poliovirus type 1 shedding. Two doses of OPV after IPV decreased shedding of poliovirus type 1 and further decreased shedding of poliovirus type 3. The study, conducted by The Johns Hopkins University, demonstrated that at least two doses of OPV were needed to induce mucosal immunity sufficient to significantly decrease the proportion of vaccinees excreting poliovirus.[433] The proportion of study subjects who had received prior IPV and excreted type 1 (18%) was much lower than expected based on other challenge studies with OPV. The reasons for this discrepancy are not known, because other challenge studies of IPV vaccinees with trivalent OPV led to 80% shedding of poliovirus type 1[440] and with monovalent OPV led to 70% excretion.[338] We believe the most likely explanation is that the study duration (16 months) may have allowed participants (including those receiving only IPV) to be exposed to vaccine virus excreted from other OPV-vaccinated infants, masking differences that may have existed shortly after the completion of the primary series.

No combined schedules of IPV and OPV have been evaluated in the United States, except for one study arm, which was part of a larger study of sequential schedules, that used one dose of OPV and IPV simultaneously at 4 months of age (IPV at 2 months, IPV/OPV at 4 months, OPV at 6 and 15 months).[433] In this trial, two doses of IPV and three doses of OPV resulted in seroprevalence levels of 99% to 100% against poliovirus types 1, 2, and 3 compared with 99% to 100% after three doses of IPV and 96% to 100% after three doses of OPV.

In developing countries, the major issue is how to improve the immunogenicity of OPV. In these settings, schedules using OPV followed by IPV were evaluated. These studies demonstrated that IPV after a primary series of OPV can correct the low immunogenicity of OPV alone that was commonly reported from tropical developing countries. In the Ivory Coast, schedules that added a dose of IPV administered simultaneously with measles vaccine, after a course of three doses of OPV administered by the routine program, resulted in a significantly higher proportion of children with antibodies against poliovirus types 1 and 3 compared with a control group that received an additional dose of OPV. Administration of a dose of IPV increased seroprevalence from 85% to 97% for poliovirus type 1 and from 76% to 92% for poliovirus type 3.[441] The experiences in the Gaza Strip are of particular interest. In this area, a new combined and sequential schedule of OPV and IPV (monovalent type 1 OPV during the first month, simultaneous administration of OPV and IPV at 2 to 3 and 3 to 4 months, and OPV at 5 to 6 and 12 to 14 months) reduced the incidence of poliomyelitis during the first 3 years after the change in vaccination schedule from an annual incidence of 10 per 100,000 population to 2.2 per 100,000 population.[435,442,443] In Israel, after the outbreak in 1988,[444] a sequential schedule of IPV and OPV has been adopted for routine use.[445]

In the developing world, however, a large randomized trial in The Gambia, Oman, and Thailand compared the immunogenicity of (1) a combined schedule of four doses of OPV administered at birth, 6, 10, and 14 weeks and IPV administered simultaneously with OPV at 6, 10, and 14 weeks; (2) four doses of OPV administered at birth, 6, 10, and 14 weeks; and (3) three doses of IPV administered at 6, 10, and 14 weeks. The combined schedule with seven doses of poliovirus vaccines performed significantly better (95% to 99% for poliovirus type 1, 99% to 100% for poliovirus type 2, and 97% to 100% for poliovirus type 3) compared with four doses of OPV or three doses of IPV[324] (Table 25–15). In addition, the combined schedule was not affected by socioeconomic status or level of maternal antibody, in contrast to the comparison groups that received OPV or IPV, respectively. This study demonstrated that a combined schedule could correct the lower immunogenicity of OPV in developing countries, but additional doses of vaccine are required.[180] Mucosal immunity induced by the combined schedule in the IPV/OPV group was similar to that of the OPV group and significantly better than that of the IPV group.[324]

One study reported no benefit of one dose of OPV after three doses of IPV in terms of type 3 seroprevalence and geometric mean antibody titer (GMT)[446]; however, a larger study in Oman demonstrated that additional doses of OPV significantly increased seroprevalence and GMT to polioviruses types 1 and 3.[447] This study confirmed earlier observations about the incremental benefit of adding additional doses of OPV in terms of seroconversion and GMT.[78,180,330,447]

Limited data are available on the persistence of poliovirus antibody induced by combined or sequential schedules of poliovirus vaccines. A single study in the United States evaluated the persistence of antibody 4 years after a primary series of sequential schedules.[448] Antibody persistence was excellent, but titers decreased by 10- to 100-fold during the first 2 years of follow-up, and thereafter the titers remained relatively stable.

Results of Controlled Trials of Protection Against Disease

There are no data from controlled trials of sequential schedules that were used as the outcome measure of the prevention of paralytic disease. Because detectable antibody to polioviruses provides an excellent correlate for protection, results of controlled trials are redundant and would be unethical to conduct.[22]

Potential Adverse Reactions with Sequential Schedules

Genetic sequencing studies suggest that reversion of Sabin strains to potentially more neurovirulent phenotypes occurs commonly after OPV administration.[396–398,400,449–454] Two relatively small studies[455,456] indicated that the use of a sequential schedule may not reduce the frequency of such mutations. However, one larger study suggests that the use of a dose of IPV before two or more doses of OPV may reduce the amount of type 3 virus shed, the most common cause of VAPP, but probably will not influence the shedding of type 1 or type 2 viruses or the extent of reversion.[457]

Recommendations for Vaccine Use

Two major objectives of vaccination, protection at the youngest possible age and minimum rates of attrition (i.e., dropout) between OPV doses, govern the development of routine vaccination schedules in industrialized and developing countries. In each of these settings, an optimal balance must be found between these objectives.[78]

Industrialized Countries

Most industrialized countries, including many western European countries, have recommended schedules in the past that relied exclusively on OPV for the prevention of poliomyelitis. More recently, encouraged by progress of the global polio eradication initiative and by the desire to reduce or eliminate the burden of VAPP, many of these industrialized countries are re-evaluating their vaccination policy options. As of 2002, a total of 22 countries and reporting entities with a combined birth cohort of 6.8 million rely exclusively on IPV (i.e., Andorra, Austria, Belgium, Canada, Denmark, Finland, France, Germany, Guam, Iceland, Ireland, Italy, Luxembourg, the Netherlands, New Zealand,

TABLE 25–15 ■ Proportion Seropositive for Neutralizing Antibody to Poliovirus Types 1, 2, and 3 in Infants Immunized with OPV Alone, IPV Alone, or OPV and IPV Simultaneously, The Gambia, Oman, and Thailand

Age and Type of Vaccines Administered					Proportion Seropositive (%)		
Birth	6 wk	10 wk	14 wk	Serotype	The Gambia (N = 118)	Oman (N = 183)	Thailand (N = 145)
OPV	OPV	OPV	OPV	1	88	90	98
				2	97	98	100
				3	72	73	100
	IPV	IPV	IPV	1	81	88	66
				2	82	92	63
				3	98	91	92
OPV	OPV/IPV	OPV/IPV	OPV/IPV	1	97	95	99
				2	100	99	100
				3	99	97	100

Constructed from data in WHO Collaborative Study Group on Oral and Inactivated Poliovirus Vaccines. Combined immunization of infants with oral and inactivated poliovirus vaccines: results of a randomized trial in The Gambia, Oman, and Thailand. J Infect Dis 175(suppl 1):S215–S227, 1997.

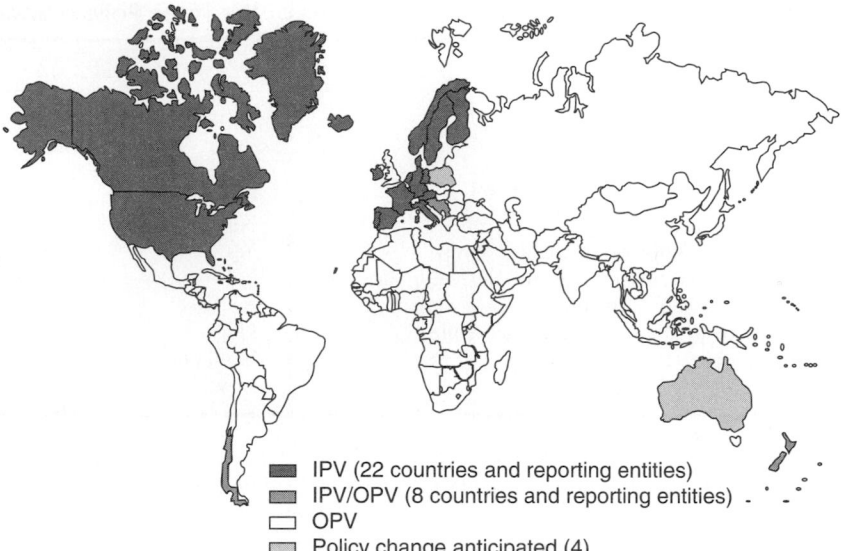

FIGURE 25–14 ■ Countries using IPV only, a sequential schedule of IPV followed by OPV, or OPV only in their national routine immunization program as vaccine of choice for the prevention of poliomyelitis.

the Northern Mariana Islands, Norway, Monaco, San Marino, Sweden, Switzerland, and the United States), whereas 6 countries and 2 reporting entities with a combined birth cohort of 0.5 million use sequential schedules of both IPV and OPV (i.e., Bermuda, Belarus, Croatia, Latvia, Lithuania, Hungary, Israel, and the West Bank and Gaza). Australia, Japan, Poland, and Slovenia, with a combined birth cohort of 1.8 million, are planning to change current national polio vaccination policy, which relies on OPV, to IPV either in a sequential schedule or an IPV-only schedule (Figure 25–14). The rest of the world, with a combined birth cohort of 122.7 million, is using OPV. The major differences in the recommended schedules between industrialized and developing countries include (1) age at first dose, (2) vaccines used for each dose, and (3) interval between doses. The recommendations for poliomyelitis prevention in the United States were revised most recently in 2000.[432] A schedule relying only on IPV is now recommended by the CDC and the American Academy of Pediatrics for primary poliovirus vaccination of children in the United States. The schedule calls for three doses of IPV administered at 2 and at 4 months and between 6 and 18 months. A preschool booster dose of IPV is recommended after age 4 years. In contrast, the United Kingdom continues to rely exclusively on OPV given at 2, 3, and 4 months of age[422] (Table 25–16). The minimum recommended interval between doses of OPV for routine vaccination varies; in the United States, 6 to 8 weeks are recommended. For the United Kingdom, intervals between OPV doses of 4 weeks are preferred.[422] The major advantages and disadvantages of

the three poliovirus vaccination schedules are shown in Table 25–17.

Routine immunization for adults residing in the continental United States and many other industrialized countries is not believed to be necessary because of the small risk of exposure to wild-type poliovirus.[380,421,422] However, adults who are at increased risk because of contact with a patient infected with wild-type poliovirus or who are working with polioviruses and those who are planning travel to an epidemic or endemic area should be immunized. Parents and other household members who do not have definite evidence of having been completely immunized should receive IPV at the time the child is vaccinated.[380,421]

Developing Countries

The WHO-recommended schedule that calls for the administration of four doses of OPV at birth, 6, 10, and 14 weeks of age should be used for polio-endemic or recently polio-endemic countries. This is particularly important in areas in which frequent importation or endemic circulation of wild-type polioviruses takes place and in which a majority of infants are exposed to all three poliovirus types early in life.[146,180,435,442] For these areas, the primary immunization schedules not only should begin early, with the first dose being given to newborns, but also—and most important—should be completed as early as possible. Many countries also recommend a dose of OPV in the second year of life, usually at age 18 months given simultaneously with DTP.

This four-dose WHO-recommended schedule is supported by data from China,[458] where a schedule that included a birth

TABLE 25–16 ■ Current Poliovirus Vaccination Schedules in the United States and the United Kingdom, 2002

Country	Vaccine	Schedule			
		Month/Year of Age of Vaccine Administration			
United States	IPV	2 mo	4 mo	6–18 mo	4–6 yr
United Kingdom	OPV	2 mo	3 mo	4 mo	School entry

TABLE 25–17 ▪ Advantages and Disadvantages of the Three Poliovirus Vaccination Schedules

Attribute	OPV Only	IPV Only	IPV/OPV Sequential
VAPP	1 case/700,000 OPV recipients*	None	50% to 75% reduction from OPV-only schedule
Other serious adverse events	None known	None known	None known
Systemic immunity	High	High	High
Mucosal immunity	High	Lower	High
Secondary transmission of vaccine virus	Yes	No	Some
Emergence of circulating vaccine-derived poliovirus	Yes	No	Probably reduced
Extra injections or visits needed	No	Yes	Yes
Compliance with immunization schedule	High	Possibly reduced	Possibly reduced
Future combination vaccines	Unlikely	Likely	Likely (IPV)
Current cost	Low	Higher	Intermediate

*First-dose recipient risk.
Adapted from Centers for Disease Control and Prevention. Poliomyelitis prevention in the United States: introduction of a sequential vaccination schedule of inactivated poliovirus vaccine followed by oral poliovirus vaccine. Recommendations of the Advisory Committee on Immunization Practices. MMWR 46(RR-3):1–25, 1997.

dose of OPV performed considerably better than a schedule without a birth dose, particularly for type 3 (97% vs. 74% seroprevalence). These recommendations have been further supported and extended by a review of the available literature on the efficacy of early immunization with DTP and OPV.[165,459–461]

Public Health Considerations

Epidemiologic Results of Vaccination

Surveillance data since 1980 suggest that continuing transmission of indigenous wild-type poliovirus has been interrupted in the United States, during a period when the country relied on OPV for immunization.[192,378] As part of the certification of the Western Hemisphere as polio free, all countries in the Americas, including the United States, were certified free of indigenous wild-type poliovirus in 1994 by an International Commission convened by the Pan American Health Organization on the basis of a detailed review of available data by national committees.[345] Data on poliomyelitis incidence during 1988 to 2001 by WHO region, a period during which the polio eradication initiative has been implemented in all WHO regions, can be found in Figure 25–15. Progress has been impressive. In 1988, 125 countries were polio-endemic; by the end of 2001, only 10 countries in South Asia and Africa were considered polio-endemic (i.e., demonstration of indigenous virus transmission; importation with limited transmission in time and space does not constitute re-establishment of endemicity). Cases of poliomyelitis decreased more than 99% from an estimated 350,000 in 1988 to 494 in 2001. Wild poliovirus type 2 was last detected in October 1999 in Uttar Pradesh, India.[37] These achievements occurred under conditions of increasing surveillance sensitivity. Wild poliovirus type 3 was detected in five countries in 2001 (Afghanistan, India, Nigeria, Pakistan, and Somalia). Wild poliovirus type 1 was detected in the same 5 countries, as well as in 10 additional countries: Algeria (importation), Angola, Bulgaria (importation), Ethiopia, Egypt, Georgia (importation), Mauritania (virus of unknown origin presumed to be an importation), Niger, Sudan, and Zambia

(importation). Between 1988 and 2001, the polio eradication initiative prevented more than 4 million children from the crippling consequences of poliomyelitis, and averted more than 1 million deaths, some as a result of poliomyelitis prevention and most because vitamin A supplements are administered to the same target children in many polio-endemic countries during national and subnational immunization campaigns.[462,463]

Disease Control Strategies

In 1988, the World Health Assembly, the governing body of the WHO, resolved to eradicate polio globally by the year 2000.[3] The global resolution followed the 1990 regional elimination goal established in 1985 by the countries of the Western Hemisphere. The last case of poliomyelitis associated with wild-type poliovirus isolation in the Americas was reported from Peru in 1991, and the entire hemisphere was certified free of indigenous wild-type poliovirus by an International Certification Commission in 1994.[345]

The following strategies to achieve polio eradication, developed in the Western Hemisphere, were adopted by the WHO for worldwide implementation in all polio-endemic countries[35]:

1. Achieving and maintaining high routine coverage in infants younger than 1 year with at least three doses of oral poliovirus vaccine (OPV3)
2. Administering supplemental doses of OPV to all young children (usually those younger than 5 years) during national immunization days to rapidly interrupt poliovirus transmission
3. Conducting "mopping-up" vaccination campaigns—localized campaigns targeting high-risk areas where poliovirus transmission is most likely to persist at low levels
4. Developing sensitive systems of epidemiologic and laboratory surveillance, including establishing surveillance of cases of AFP[§]

§A confirmed case of polio is defined as AFP and at least one of the following: (1) laboratory-confirmed wild-type poliovirus infection, (2) residual paralysis at 60 days, (3) death, or (4) no follow-up investigation at 60 days.

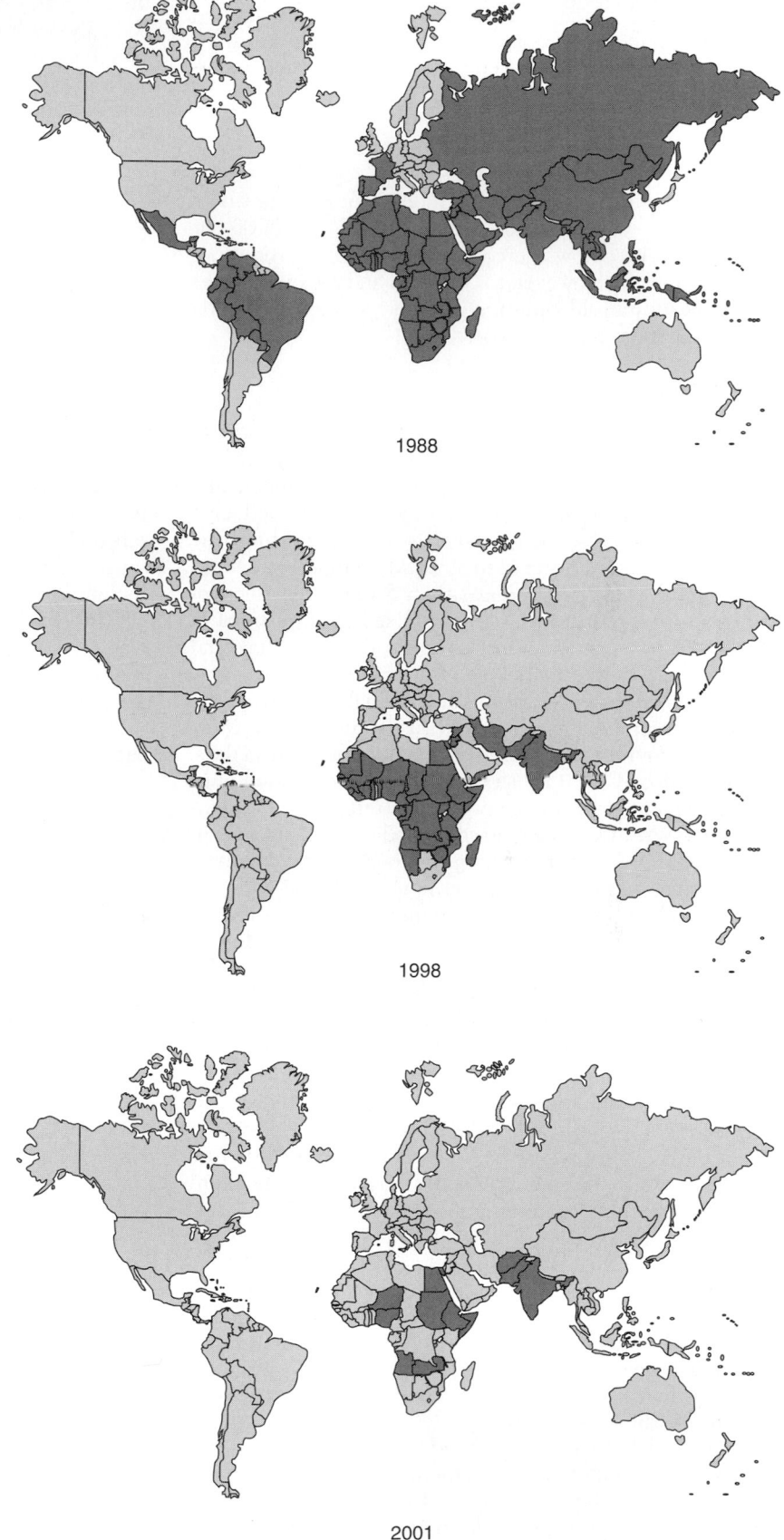

1988

1998

2001

FIGURE 25–15 ▪ Countries that isolated wild-type poliovirus in 1988, 1998, and 2001. Darker shaded countries isolated wild-type poliovirus as a result of ongoing endemic transmission or importation; the remaining countries did not isolate wild-type poliovirus. (Redrawn from Kew OM, Pallansch MA. The mechanism of polio eradication. *In* Semler BL, Wimmer E [eds], Molecular Biology of Picornaviruses. Washington, DC, ASM Press, 2002, pp 481–491.)

Routine Immunization

Control of poliomyelitis and the global eradication initiative are greatly aided by well-functioning routine immunization programs that deliver potent OPV to a high proportion of infants in the first year of life. Global coverage with three doses of OPV among infants younger than 1 year was 82% in 2000. All WHO regions reported a coverage of more than 80% except for the African Region, where coverage improved from 40% in 1988 to 55% in 2000 but continues to be below the coverage achieved in the other WHO regions.[194] However, these global and regional figures may mask substantial variation in coverage reported among and within individual countries.

National Immunization Days

Mass campaigns with OPV—administered during national immunization days—are the only proven strategy to reduce widespread transmission of wild-type poliovirus in endemic countries.[464,465] National immunization days are conducted twice annually for a short period (1 to 3 days) in which one dose of OPV is administered to all children in the target age group, usually children younger than 5 years, regardless of prior vaccination history. A second dose is administered in the same way after an interval of 4 to 6 weeks. National immunization days usually take place during the low transmission season when conditions are optimal to interrupt the few remaining chains of poliovirus transmission. Most countries provide OPV during national immunization days, relying primarily on fixed sites, including vaccination clinics supplemented by a large number of temporary vaccination sites. With the acceleration of eradication activities in 1999, many of the remaining polio-endemic countries began using a strategy relying on house-to-house administration of OPV during national immunization days.

National immunization days are necessary in developing countries to rapidly increase immunity levels in the population to achieve and surpass herd immunity threshold levels for poliomyelitis and, hence, rapidly interrupt the transmission of poliovirus. OPV administered in campaigns also appears to be more immunogenic compared with OPV administered in the routine program,[466,467] probably because (1) national immunization days are conducted during the low poliovirus transmission season because this is the period when the fewest chains of poliovirus transmission are maintained, (2) national immunization days are conducted during the low transmission season for other enteroviruses that may interfere with poliovirus seroconversion,[468] (3) the cold chain can be better maintained for these short campaigns, and (4) massive use of OPV probably also results in intensive secondary spread of shed virus.[324] Children residing in polio-endemic countries using national immunization days may receive 13 to 14 doses of OPV by the time they reach their fifth birthday.[78,330] These OPV doses are administered both by the routine program (three or four doses) and through national immunization days (two doses annually during the first 5 years of life). These additional doses of OPV, administered during national immunization days, should correct the lower immunogenicity of OPV commonly observed in tropical areas.

All endemic and most recently endemic countries continued to conduct supplementary immunization activities

during 2001. An estimated 575 million children younger than 5 years (more than 80% of all children younger than 5 years) in 94 countries received nearly 2 billion doses of OPV during 300 rounds of national immunization days, sub–national immunization days, or mopping-up activities. All countries used well supervised house-to-house vaccination in part or all of the target area for supplementary immunization activities to further increase the quality and reach the highest possible coverage among children less than 5 years of age. Coordinated national immunization days have been conducted in Western Africa since 2000, and in Central Africa since 2001.[37] The national immunization days in India—vaccinating as many as 145 million children in a single round—represent the largest mass campaigns ever conducted.

"Mopping-Up" Campaigns

To eliminate the last potential or known reservoirs of wild-type poliovirus circulation, "mopping-up" vaccination campaigns are conducted. These mopping-up campaigns usually target children younger than 5 years with two doses of OPV separated by an interval of 4 to 6 weeks. These campaigns include house-to-house administration of OPV to reach any children who may have been missed by national immunization days. Mopping up is a critical component to achieve interruption of the final chains of poliovirus transmission in all polio-endemic countries. Risk areas (often targeting more than 1 million children younger than 5 years to have the optimal impact), usually defined at county or district levels, to be included in mopping up include those with recent circulation of wild-type poliovirus (usually within the last 3 years), low vaccination coverage, suboptimal surveillance, large migrant or refugee populations, and common borders with known poliovirus-endemic areas.

These supplemental immunization activities have been successful in decreasing the number of reported poliomyelitis cases globally from 35,251 (estimated to be approximately 350,000 cases) in 1988 (when the polio eradication target was adopted) to 494 in 2001, a decrease of more than 99%[37] (Fig. 25–16). Figure 25–17 displays the remaining AFP cases associated with wild-type poliovirus isolation during a 12-month period from mid-2001 to mid-2002. A detailed review

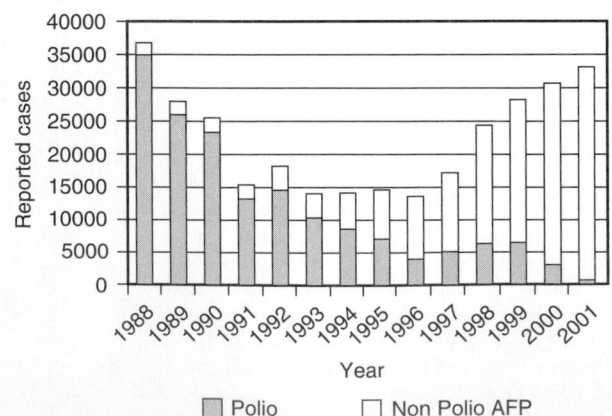

FIGURE 25-16 ■ Total reported acute flaccid paralysis (AFP) cases and confirmed poliomyelitis cases, 1988 to 2001 (World Health Organization).

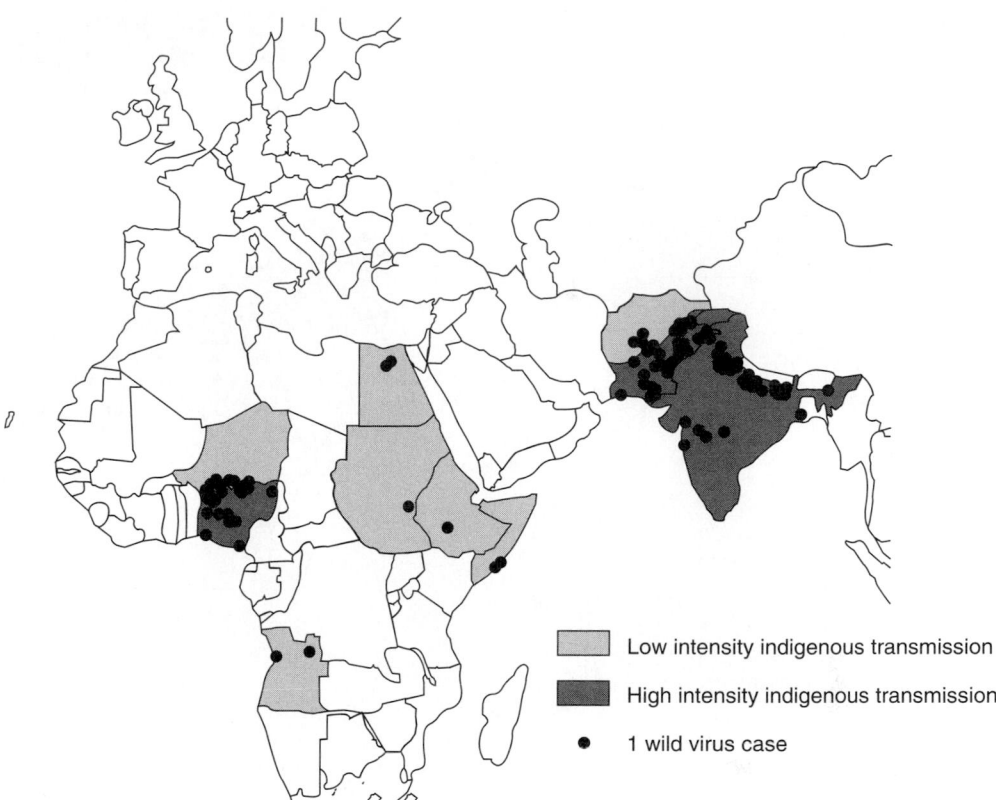

FIGURE 25–17 ■ Acute flaccid paralysis cases associated with wild-type poliovirus isolation, and countries considered at high or low poliovirus transmission intensity, mid-2001 to mid-2002 (World Health Organization).

☐ Low intensity indigenous transmission

■ High intensity indigenous transmission

● 1 wild virus case

of the current status of the polio eradication initiative was published in 1997[469] with annual progress reports, the most recent in 2002.[37]

Surveillance

Surveillance for cases of AFP and for wild-type poliovirus is critical for guiding programmatic activities as well as for contributing to the eventual certification of polio-free status. Systems for AFP surveillance have been established in all polio-endemic or recently endemic countries. Surveillance relies on two complementary and mutually reinforcing components: 1) AFP case investigations, and 2) virologic studies of polioviruses obtained from clinical specimens. The major reason for using a symptom (e.g., AFP) rather than a diagnosis (e.g., poliomyelitis) is to ensure that the sensitivity of the surveillance system can be maximized; all possible cases of poliomyelitis, including those with atypical presentations, will be included in the surveillance system. In addition, AFP surveillance helps to monitor the quality of surveillance even in the absence of cases of poliomyelitis. In the last stages of the eradication program, no cases of poliomyelitis (except for rare cases of VAPP) would be expected to be detected. Thus it would be impossible to determine whether the absence of poliomyelitis cases represents "true" absence or deficiencies in surveillance. On the basis of the experience in the Americas, in each population a rate of 1 case of nonpolio AFP per 100,000 population younger than 15 years would be expected annually, and achievement of such a rate would indicate adequate surveillance, defined as the ability of the surveillance system to detect wild-type poliovirus circula-

tion resulting from indigenous transmission or virus importation, should it occur. A global network of 145 formally accredited laboratories has been established to process all stool specimens collected from AFP cases worldwide for virologic investigations (Fig. 25–18). The formal annual accreditation process relies on six criteria (Table 25–18). Standard methods and reagents are used to isolate virus in tissue cultures and perform intratypic differentiation as wild-type, Sabin-derived (<1% genomic sequencing divergence from Sabin parent strains), or vaccine-derived (>1% genomic sequencing divergence from Sabin parent strains) poliovirus. All wild-type poliovirus strains and all VDPVs are sequenced in specialized network laboratories to guide programmatic action. Based on additional virologic and epidemiologic data, VDPVs can further be classified as circulating (cVDPV) or associated with prolonged replication in an immunodeficient individual (iVDPV) (see *Vaccine-Derived Polioviruses* above).

All six regions of the WHO have achieved a rate of slightly more than 1 nonpolio AFP case per 100,000 population younger than 15 years of age. Table 25–19 contains the AFP rates for the different WHO regions in 2001.[37] Five WHO regions also have surpassed the second most important quality indicator for adequate surveillance (i.e., the proportion of AFP cases from which two stool samples had been collected within 14 days of paralysis onset). This indicator reached 84% in 2001 globally; it also increased rapidly in the WHO's African Region from 50% in 2000 to 71% in 2001.[37] A comprehensive list of performance indicators used to monitor the quality of AFP surveillance can be found in Table 25–20.

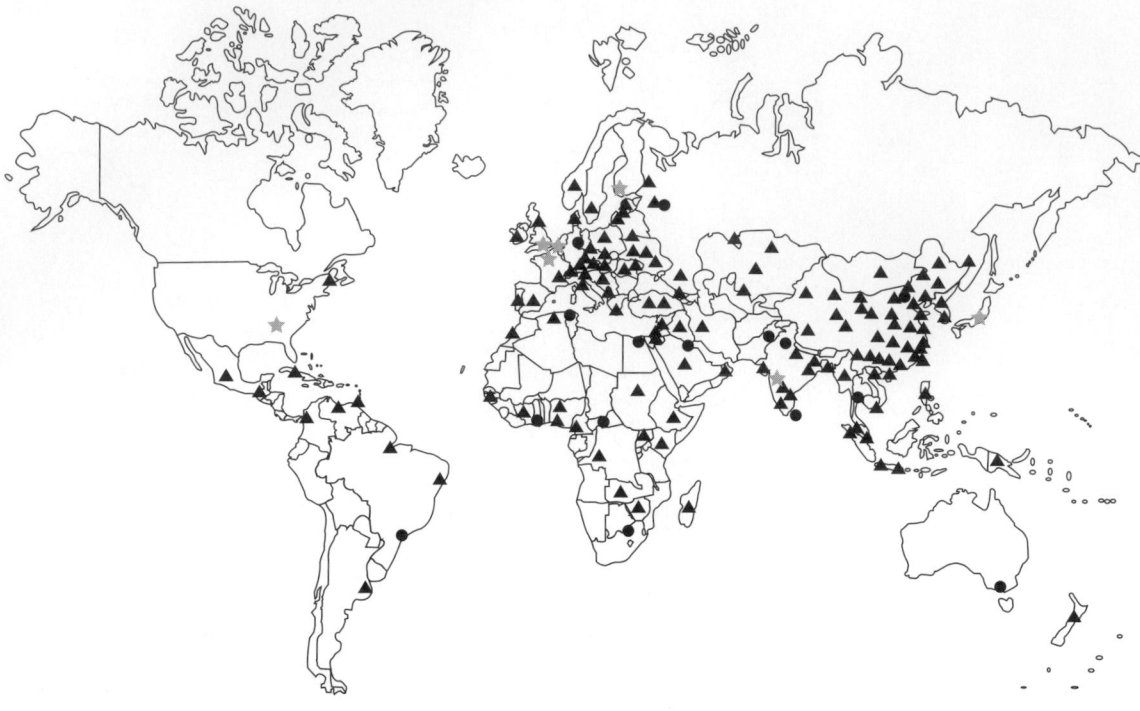

★ Specialized Reference Laboratory
● Regional Reference Laboratory
▲ National/Sub-national Laboratory

FIGURE 25–18 ■ Laboratories participating in the Global Laboratory Network for Poliomyelitis Eradication, by tier (national, regional, and specialized laboratory), 2002.

Stopping Polio Vaccination After Eradication Has Been Achieved

The goal of any eradication program is to make the need for the preventive intervention unnecessary (i.e., discontinuation of vaccination against poliomyelitis).[470,471] Successful certification of global poliomyelitis eradication will enable consideration of stopping of poliovirus vaccination, thereby

TABLE 25–18 ■ **Standards Used for the Annual Accreditation of Laboratories Participating in the World Health Organization Global Laboratory Network for Poliomyelitis Eradication**

Standard	Indicator
Results of processing of stool samples reported within 28 days after arrival in laboratory	≥80%
Minimal number of specimens processed	≥150
Accuracy of poliovirus typing (compared with typing performed at Regional Network Laboratory)	≥90%
Poliovirus isolates forwarded to Regional Network Laboratory within 7 days (after serotyping results) for intratypic differentiation as wild-type or vaccine-derived poliovirus	≥80%
Internal quality control procedures implemented	≥ Quarterly
Results on most recent quality assurance panels	≥80%
Score on on-site review	≥80%

preventing the occurrence of VAPP, eliminating the possibility that cVDPV will emerge to reseed the population with a wild phenotype of a VDPV genotype, and obtaining the substantial economic savings from no longer having to vaccinate each successive birth cohort with OPV. A number of issues need to be resolved before vaccination can be stopped, including assurance that (1) wild-type poliovirus transmission has been interrupted (i.e., global certification); (2) laboratory stocks of poliovirus-containing or potentially infectious materials have been contained, so that these will not serve as a reservoir to reseed a susceptible population; (3) the vaccine viruses will not continue to circulate (and potentially emerge into cVDPV) after vaccination is stopped; (4) long-term shedders of VDPVs will not reseed the population; and (5) a stockpile of polio vaccine is in place to respond to any detection of poliovirus, should it occur. Some of the critical issues that need to be addressed for these five areas of work are summarized in Table 25–21.

A stockpile of polio vaccine is necessary if a decision is made to change the current vaccination recommendations to either (1) use IPV globally or in selected areas, (2) discontinue OPV use completely in all countries, or (3) develop and introduce a new vaccine. Many of the basic stockpile issues, such as the size, the vaccine (monovalent OPV, trivalent OPV, or IPV) and the composition (filled vaccine vials, bulk, or a combination), how many storage sites, and release protocols (e.g., who retains the authority to release vaccine), are currently under discussion.[472] In

TABLE 25–19 ■ Confirmed Poliomyelitis Cases and Acute Flaccid Paralysis Surveillance Indicators, by World Health Organization Region, 2000 to 2001[*]

Region	AFP Cases Reported		Nonpolio AFP Rate		Total Confirmed (Clinical + Virus)		Virus Confirmed Cases	
	2000	2001	2000	2001	2000	2001	2000	2001
Africa	5936	8442	1.5	3.0	1863	69	160	69
Americas	2076	2197	1.2	1.1	12[†]	10[†]	0	0
Eastern Mediterranean	3253	3865	1.4	1.9	505	140	287	140
Europe	1645	1764	1.1	1.2	0	3[‡]	0	3
South-East Asia	10,758	10,615	1.8	1.8	591	268	272	268
Western Pacific	6894	6529	1.5	1.4	0	3[‡]	0	0
Total	30,562	33,512	1.6	1.6	2971	494	719	480

[*]Data available from the WHO as of June 18, 2002.
[†]Circulating vaccine-derived poliovirus (cVDPV).
[‡]Imported poliovirus.

addition, a world switching to IPV for maintaining polio immunity after certification of eradication may require a relatively much smaller stockpile to control subsequent polio outbreaks, should they occur, compared to a world in which no vaccine is produced. Furthermore, a stockpile may have to grow with an increasing number of susceptible infants born into a world without polio vaccination. Because such a stockpile would be used primarily for outbreak control should any poliovirus be introduced again into a population (because of unintentional or deliberate release), the immunogenicity and the kinetics of the immune response become critical decision determinants. Monovalent (i.e., type-specific) OPVs might be the most appropriate stockpile vaccines,[274] because (1) immuno-

TABLE 25–20 ■ Indicators of Acute Flaccid Paralysis (AFP) Disease Surveillance and Laboratory Performance

Indicator	Target
Nonpolio AFP rate in children <15 yr	≥1/100,000
Completeness of monthly reporting	≥90%
Timeliness of monthly reporting	≥80%
Reported AFP cases investigated ≤48 hr after report	≥80%
Reported AFP cases with 2 stool specimens collected ≤14 days since onset	≥80%
Reported AFP cases with a follow-up examination at least 60 days after paralysis onset to verify the presence or absence of residual paralysis	≥80%
Specimens arriving at national laboratory within <3 days of being sent	≥80%
Specimens arriving at laboratory in good condition[*]	>80%
Specimens with a turnaround time of ≤28 days between receipt and reporting of results	≥80%
Stool specimens from which nonpolio enterovirus was isolated	≥10%

[*]Good condition means that, on arrival, (1) there is ice or frozen icepacks or a temperature indicator (showing <8°C) in the container, (2) the specimen volume is adequate (>5 g), (3) there is no evidence of leakage or desiccation, and (4) appropriate documentation (laboratory request/reporting form) is completed.

genicity per dose is substantially higher compared to trivalent OPV or IPV (one dose of monovalent OPV may provide an immune response to the one serotype that is equivalent to three doses of trivalent OPV); (2) monovalent OPVs are faster in inducing a type-specific immune response (one would not have to wait for administration of several doses); and (3) their use would be directed against a specific serotype of poliovirus, without introducing unnecessary serotypes ("fighting fire with fire"). However, because monovalent OPVs are not licensed anymore, it is not known whether regulatory authorities would be willing to relicense these products. Development of a noninfectious vaccine that would induce humoral immunity comparable to IPV and mucosal immunity comparable to OPV (without serious adverse effects) might reduce the size of a stockpile, although the prospects of development for such a vaccine are not good.[473]

Certification of Polio Eradication

A process that started with the constitution of an International Commission for the Certification of Polio Eradication in the WHO Region of the Americas in 1990 (which certified the entire Western Hemisphere free of polio in 1994[345]) is being replicated in each of six WHO regions, guided by the Global Certification Commission.[474] The Commission in the Americas defined four criteria on the basis of which possible poliovirus eradication could be assessed: (1) the absence of virologically confirmed cases for a period of 3 years in the presence of adequate surveillance; (2) the absence of detected wild-type poliovirus in tests of stools from healthy children (e.g., from the contacts of cases of AFP being investigated) and, when indicated, from waste water; (3) evaluation by a national certification committee convened for that purpose in the country, eventually reporting to the regional commission; and (4) establishment of appropriate measures to deal with wild-type poliovirus importations.

In recently polio-endemic countries, the certification process will rely primarily on data from AFP surveillance; in countries that have been free of poliovirus for many years (and that have not implemented AFP surveillance), the process will evaluate data from all relevant sources (i.e., VAPP surveillance, virologic surveillance, environmental

TABLE 25–21 ▪ Major Issues for the Formulation of Postcertification Polio Vaccination Policies

Category	Issues
Certification	Is the global certification process sufficiently robust to reliably document the absence of wild-type poliovirus?
	Given the emergence of and outbreaks caused by cVDPVs, should the certification process address these viruses?
	Ultimately, because all live polioviruses have the potential to circulate and acquire the characteristics of wild-type polioviruses, should the certification process address all live polioviruses (and, if OPV is discontinued, require that all live polioviruses be adequately contained)?
Containment	Will high levels of IPV coverage prevent the emergence of cVDPVs or eliminate cVDPVs should they circulate?
	What level of IPV coverage will be required, especially in a low-hygiene tropical setting, to prevent the circulation of VDPVs?
	Will routine vaccination with IPV in countries manufacturing IPV from wild-type polioviruses be necessary?
	Will routine vaccination with IPV be implemented or continued in industrialized countries, and for what periods?
Circulation in population	What vaccination strategy will be most effective in preventing polioviruses from after OPV is discontinued (will mass campaigns be required to boost "population immunity")?
	What will be the potential contribution of IPV (can IPV decrease or eliminate the risk of circulation of cVDPVs in a transition period to no OPV use [i.e., should IPV be added to the routine vaccination program before OPV discontinuation])?
	What is the risk period for the emergence of cVDPVs (and can the risk be further minimized, and the risk period further shortened) depending on the vaccination strategy selected?
Chronic shedders	Will chronic carriers of poliovirus be a risk for reseeding populations with poliovirus?
	When will this risk be greatest: shortly after stopping polio vaccination or 10–20 yr in the future, when many cohorts of newborns are added to the pool of the poliovirus-susceptible population?
	What can and should be done to eliminate or decrease this risk (e.g., enhance identification and treatment of long-term poliovirus carriers)?
	Will HIV-infected (or severely immune-compromised acquired immunodeficiency syndrome) constitute a potential reservoir for poliovirus?
Stockpile	How do different postcertification vaccination options affect vaccine stockpile decisions?
	Given the need for a stockpile, what is the appropriate size (how many doses), vaccine (monovalent OPV, trivalent OPV, IPV, or new vaccine), and composition (what proportion of vaccine is in bulk, what proportion is filled into vials for immediate use) of a stockpile?
	Will the stockpile size need to grow over time to correspond to an increasing population susceptible to poliovirus?
	What decision-making process needs to be in place for release of stockpile vaccine?
	Where will the stockpile vaccine be stored (single or multiple storage sites, industrialized or developing countries)?
	What arrangements need to be made to ensure continued manufacturing capacity of OPV (in the event OPV use will be discontinued globally), or restart OPV production, if necessary?
	If live poliovirus vaccines will be used to control outbreak in the post–stopping OPV era, what will be necessary to ensure that these outbreak vaccines will not reseed a population (and the world) with poliovirus (what is the risk of "fighting fire with fire")?
Vaccination policy	Is a coordinated approach to discontinue polio vaccination globally feasible?
	How much OPV will be needed after recommendations for discontinuation of routine OPV use have been made?
	What risk (in terms of establishing vaccine virus transmission) will areas that continue OPV use pose to areas that have discontinued OPV use?
	Should IPV be used either in a transition period from OPV use to stopping all vaccination or for the foreseeable future in routine vaccination programs?

surveillance [e.g., Finland], adverse events reporting systems). It is not clear what role environmental surveillance will have in the certification process of recently polio-endemic countries. Ongoing evaluations in Egypt and India have highlighted the strength of this form of surveillance in (1) confirming wild-type poliovirus circulation in areas of Egypt where AFP surveillance has not detected cases, and (2) demonstrating frequent episodes of importation of wild-type poliovirus into Mumbai from an endemic state in Northern India.

In addition to the Americas, the process of certification has been concluded in the Western Pacific Region (a region that includes China, the world's most populated country) in 2000[345] and the European Region in 2002.[347] The experience with certification in these three regions has demonstrated that the criteria applied are sound, and no wild-type poliovirus previously indigenous to these regions has ever re-emerged from a certified region as of mid-2002.

The Global Commission for the Certification of Polio Eradication is responsible for certifying the world as free of wild-type polioviruses. It also started discussions in 2001[475] of the implications of the outbreaks of cVDPVs in Haiti and the Dominican Republic[59] for the global certification process, but postponed a decision as to whether or not to extend their mandate and include cVDPVs as part of the process. Since then, the outbreak in the Philippines in 2001,[404] the outbreak under investigation in Madagascar in 2001 to 2002,[405] and the retrospective investigation of a cVDPV outbreak in Egypt during 1988 to 1993[403] have highlighted further the importance of this issue.

Laboratory Containment of Poliovirus

In 1997, the second meeting of the global certification commission added the requirement to effectively contain any laboratory stock of wild-type poliovirus as a condition for eventual global certification.[476] In contrast to the smallpox eradication program, in which the virus was restricted to a selected group of laboratories, poliovirus is used in many laboratories conducting serology, research, or vaccine production. Many laboratories store potentially infectious materials that may contain polioviruses. These specimens could have been collected for studies unrelated to poliomyelitis, including studies of other enteric pathogens from countries during periods when wild-type polioviruses were still circulating either in an endemic or epidemic manner. In addition, the manufacturing process for IPV relies on wild-type polioviruses. Thus polioviruses, either vaccine derived or wild type, may be found in many laboratories and freezers, known or unknown to the laboratory personnel.[477,478]

The containment guidelines attempt to minimize the risk of inadvertent transmission from the laboratory to the community[477] through emphasis on (1) identification and documentation of infectious and potentially infectious materials in laboratories through a detailed national inventory; (2) destruction of these materials (or storage in repositories with appropriate biosafety levels); and (3) enhancement of containment in manufacturing sites for IPV (because the viral concentration required for vaccine production needs to be very high, these sites may be at highest risk for inadvertent transmission). Past experiences with laboratory workers exposed to wild-type poliovirus demonstrate that containment is more than a theoretical consideration.[479] Furthermore, implementation of effective containment requires validation of the process. A recent investigation of potentially infectious materials from South Asia collected more than 20 years ago and stored at the CDC found 6 wild-type polioviruses in 265 stool samples.[480] The containment process has been linked deliberately to the process of regional certification of polio eradication, and substantial progress toward containment had to be demonstrated to the Regional Certification Commissions in the Western Pacific and European Regions before regional certification was declared.

Vaccine-Derived Poliovirus Circulation in the Population

Once wild-type poliovirus transmission has been interrupted, Sabin-derived and vaccine-derived polioviruses (see *Vaccine-Derived Polioviruses* above) will be the only viruses replicating in the gastrointestinal tracts of vaccinees and possibly circulating in their contacts. However, our under-

standing of the risks that these viruses pose to re-establishment of circulation is limited. Answers to a number of questions would greatly improve our current knowledge:

1. Will vaccine-derived viruses continue to circulate and cause VAPP if vaccination is stopped?[177]
2. What are the risk factors for VDPVs to mutate toward greater neurovirulence, acquire the transmission characteristics of wild-type poliovirus, and cause outbreaks of cVDPV?
3. What is the frequency of (and risk factors for) long-term carriers of VDPVs among immunodeficient people to potentially reseed the population at large?

Although no formal global burden of VAPP has been published, it is likely that more than 250 cases would be occurring each year globally if current OPV vaccination policies are maintained. This global disability burden would have to be born by communities using OPV in the absence of naturally occurring poliomyelitis. The likelihood of establishing ongoing circulation of VDPV in a population has been studied in Cuba. Cuba administers OPV twice a year (usually in February and April) in mass campaigns (no OPV is available during the rest of the year). A series of studies among infants and young children (i.e., serology, stool surveys) and in the environment demonstrated that the virus persisted in this country for only 8 to 12 weeks following a campaign.[481–483] Because Cuba has better sanitation, hygiene, and nutrition and a smaller average family size than most developing countries, these studies need to be replicated in other tropical countries where conditions favor poliovirus transmission (i.e., low population immunity, high contact rates, and low hygiene and sanitation).

Long-Term Carriers of Poliovirus

Billions of doses of OPV have been administered during 40 years of worldwide use. During these more than three decades of OPV use, there have been 15 documented instances of human carriage of vaccine virus for approximately 12 months or longer.[136,390] All identified carriers reside in industrialized countries or middle-income countries (Argentina, Taiwan), where the quality of the health systems allows both diagnosis and therapeutic intervention (e.g., the use of intravenous immune globulin is credited with substantial decreases in opportunistic infections among immune-deficient patients) that permit longer survival of these patients. The only exception is Iran, where a child with antibody deficiency died in 1995 from whom extensively drifted VDPVs were isolated. It remains unclear whether these rare carriers have the potential to reseed the population at large once poliovirus has been eradicated and new cohorts of infants susceptible to poliomyelitis are added each year to the population. It is currently unknown whether immune-deficient infants born in developing countries survive sufficiently long to pose a threat to reseeding the population with poliovirus.

Many industrialized countries (including the United States) have discontinued OPV, use IPV instead (often as a combination vaccine), and may continue IPV vaccination after a global recommendation for OPV discontinuation has been made because they may consider themselves at increased risk for (1) intentional release of poliovirus through acts of bioterrorism or biologic warfare, (2) unintentional escape of poliovirus through containment failures, or (3) reseeding of poliovirus from long-term carriers. The potential biologic weapons threats and potential biologic terrorism agents have been assessed, but poliovirus was not included in either assessment, presumably because the current high population immunity against polioviruses precludes their use.[484,485] Nevertheless, should vaccination against polioviruses be stopped, cohorts susceptible to poliomyelitis will accumulate rapidly, and the risk assessment would likely change.[177] More recently, the full-length poliovirus cDNA has been synthesized by assembling oligonucleotides of plus and minus strand polarity. The synthetic poliovirus cDNA was transcribed by RNA polymerase into viral RNA that translated and replicated in a cell-free extract, resulting in de novo synthesis of infectious poliovirus,[486] demonstrating that, even if poliovirus has become extinct, laboratories could create fully infectious polioviruses again.

A series of studies has been carried out or are in progress in industrialized countries (i.e., the United States and the United Kingdom) and in developing countries (i.e., Brazil, Ethiopia, Guatemala, Kenya, Haiti, the Ivory Coast, and Pakistan) to assess what proportion of immunodeficient people with or without VAPP excrete poliovirus chronically and to characterize the findings by type of immunodeficiency disorder. In general, these studies have demonstrated that the risk of chronic poliovirus excretion is low (even among immune-deficient patients), estimated to be between 0.1% and 1% (Neal Halsey, Johns Hopkins University, personal communication, 1999). Cases of VAPP among immunodeficient patients represent a group that appears to be at high risk for chronic poliovirus excretion. In many instances, these cases are identified both as immune deficient and as long-term poliovirus excreters during the diagnostic work-up after onset of paralytic manifestations.

In developing countries, children with HIV infection have been evaluated for persistence of poliovirus excretion. Several small unpublished studies, evaluating approximately 200 HIV-infected children, have not identified a single HIV-infected child with prolonged poliovirus excretion. Additional studies are planned to extend these small studies and to evaluate HIV-infected adults, a group that is much larger than HIV-infected children, and correlate poliovirus excretion with markers for immunodeficiency. Although selected IgA-deficient persons excrete virus for periods of up to 6 months,[487] none has been shown to excrete virus for longer periods. Therefore, it is unlikely that this group poses a threat, although the number of IgA-deficient subjects evaluated at the end of 2001 is small. All identified long-term poliovirus carriers have been diagnosed with agammaglobulinemia, CVID, or SCID. Mathematical modeling and a detailed review of the available scientific data are necessary to further define parameters that may be important for the development of a strategy to stop poliovirus vaccination.

Vaccination Options for the Posteradication Era

Several WHO consultative meetings have been convened during the past 4 years to review available evidence, identify key scientific questions, and guide the WHO toward the development of a postcertification immunization policy, if necessary, for the prevention of poliomyelitis.[171,100] The

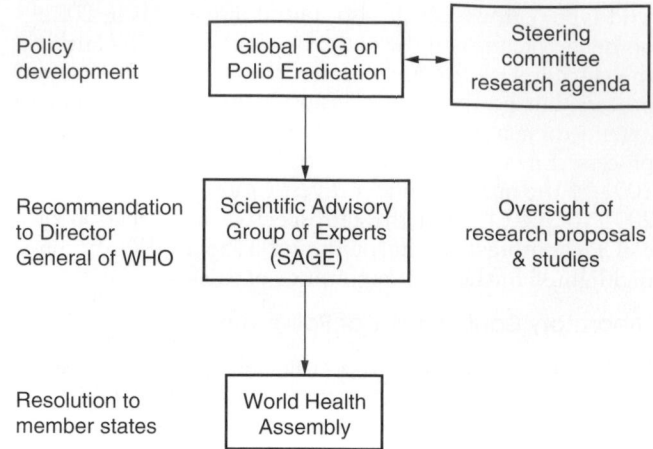

FIGURE 25–19 ■ Decision-making tree for posteradication polio vaccination policy.

WHO has put in place a structure for decision making (Fig. 25–19) that places at its center the Technical Consultative Group (TCG) on the Global Eradication of Poliomyelitis, which would receive data and information emanating from the research guided by the WHO Steering Committee on Stopping Vaccination. In turn, the TCG will report to the Scientific Advisory Group of Experts (the WHO's principal advisory group on immunization). Ultimately, a decision of this magnitude (i.e., whether to stop or continue poliovirus vaccination) will be made by the World Health Assembly, the WHO's governing body representing the 191 member states of the organization. In principle, the process can be reduced to two major decisions: (1) whether or not to stop OPV after certification of eradication, and (2) whether IPV is needed or not for an interim period worldwide after OPV has been discontinued. The rationale and options for a postcertification vaccination policy have been outlined by the TCG.[474] Although some experts argue that polio vaccination may need to be continued indefinitely, the TCG has concluded, based on the rationale cited previously (see *Stopping Polio Vaccination after Eradication Has Been Achieved* above), that there are compelling reasons to stop vaccination, provided it is safe to do so.[391,489–491]

Options for discontinuing OPV in the postcertification era have been described,[136,488] and include (1) discontinuing OPV after a mass campaign with OPV to maximize population immunity and minimize the risk of VDPV emergence and circulation, (2) switching to vaccination with IPV, and (3) developing new vaccines for the postcertification era that will not cause VAPP and ideally also would not be transmissible.[136,391,488] The TCG has outlined some of the most important considerations for each of these options,[488] which are modified slightly here:

1. Coordinated discontinuation of OPV worldwide after polio eradication has been certified by the Global Certification Commission. Under this scenario, mass vaccination campaigns with OPV (to maximize population immunity) would be followed by coordinated OPV discontinuation. The major advantage of this option would be the cessation of OPV at a time when the population immunity is likely to be at the highest levels, levels that will not be achieved again for many

years, if ever, once vaccination is discontinued. The major disadvantage is the potential risk of circulating VDPV emergence for an indefinable risk window (probably not exceeding 3–5 years). Countries would have the option of continuing vaccinating with IPV.[488]

2. Increase the use of IPV, including in the developing world. The major advantage of this scenario would be that populations would have at least some level of protection against polio, including circulating vaccine-derived poliovirus, for the foreseeable future. This would reduce the likelihood and magnitude of polio outbreaks should virus be introduced and may decrease consideration of polio as a bioterrorism agent. A major disadvantage would be low population immunity if coverage levels are not high and the low seroconversion rates for IPV when given at the usual immunization contact ages in developing countries.[323,324] In addition, the increased costs of IPV may prove prohibitive in the absence of the disease. Because some countries may elect to continue using IPV as part of the routine vaccination program, it would be desirable to have an IPV that does not require wild poliovirus for production since this raises the potential of accidental release as has been documented previously.[473]

3. Developing new live vaccines for the post-eradication period, vaccines that would not cause VAPP and are not transmissible.[473] This option appears to be a formidable task, and one that may not be feasible based on current scientific knowledge and regulatory concerns. The costs involved in developing, testing and seeking regulatory approval for a new vaccine would be enormous. Since OPV causes VAPP on the order of 1 case per million first doses administered, any field trial testing a new vaccine would need to be very large. The molecular basis of transmissibility is unknown thus hampering efforts at the rational design of less transmissible strains. In addition, it is not known for how long a new vaccine would be used, further reducing the financial incentives to manufacturers to develop, test and produce such a product.[492] Some experts believe that such a vaccine would only be needed for a relatively short period (until absence of any kind of poliovirus [i.e., wild, vaccine-derived] has been proven and containment validated). For these reasons, it appears unlikely that a new vaccine could be available during the expected time frame of the polio eradication initiative or even ever in the post-eradication era unless substantial public sector investments were made.

The first option described above currently appears to be the most attractive in terms of programmatic feasibility and costs, although substantial uncertainties remain. After global eradication of poliovirus has been achieved, many countries will be ready and indeed anxious to stop vaccinating against a disease that no longer exists. Individual decisions by countries to stop OPV could however place populations that no longer benefit from vaccination at risk for imported circulating VDPV from countries that elect to continue using

that vaccine, as well as spread of wild viruses from laboratories that did not adequately contain their viruses. For this reason, stopping OPV requires a coordinated approach. However, it would be premature to endorse any strategy until the risk of circulating VDVP reintroduction and various costs are better understood. Thus, OPV will be required in the global immunization program for the foreseeable future."

Conclusion

Poliomyelitis has affected humankind since ancient times. It appeared as an epidemic disease in industrialized countries in the 19th century and the beginning of the 20th century. Development and widespread use of poliovirus vaccines have effectively controlled poliomyelitis in industrialized countries. The global poliomyelitis eradication initiative, adopted in 1988, has led to dramatic decreases in the incidence of poliomyelitis in developing countries. Although some issues remain in regard to defining a strategy to stop vaccination after poliomyelitis eradication has been achieved, it appears likely that the eradication target will be accomplished, thus relegating this once much-feared crippling disease to one that future generations will know only by history.[39]

REFERENCES

1. Underwood M. A Treatise of Children with General Directions for Management of Infants from Birth (2nd ed). London, Matthews, 1789.
2. Poliomyelitis Vaccine Evaluation Center. Evaluation of the 1954 Field Trial of Poliomyelitis Vaccine. Ann Arbor, MI, Edwards Brothers, 1957.
3. World Health Assembly. Global Eradication of Poliomyelitis by the Year 2000. Geneva, World Health Organization, 1988.
4. Paul JR. A History of Poliomyelitis. New Haven, CT, Yale University Press, 1971.
5. Heine J. Beobachtungen über Lähmungszustände der unteren Extremitäten und deren Behandlung. Stuttgart, Köhler, 1840.
6. West C. On some forms of paralysis incidental to infancy and childhood. London Med Gaz 32:829–836, 1843.
7. Rilliet F. De la paralysie essentielle chez les enfants. Gaz Med Paris 6:681–704, 1851.
8. de Boulogne D. De l'Electrisation Localisée et de son Application a la Physiologie, a la Pathologie et a la Thérapeutique. Paris, Baillières, 1855.
9. von Heine J. Spinale Kinderlähmung. Stuttgart, Cotta, 1860.
10. Charcot JM. Groupe des myopathies de cause spinal: paralysie infantile. Rev Phot Hop 4:1–36, 1872.
11. Frey A. Ein Fall von subakuter Lähmung Erwachsener, wahrscheinlich Poliomyelitis. Berl Klin Wochenschr 11:549–566, 1874.
12. Wickman I. Beiträge zur Kentniss der Heine-Medinschen Krankheit (Poliomyelitis acuta und verwandte Erkrankungen). Berlin, Karger, 1907.
13. Leegaard C. Die akute Poliomyelitis in Norwegen. Dtsch Z Nervenheilk 53:145–262, 1890.
14. Wickman I. Studien über Poliomyelitis acuta: Zugleich ein Beiträge zur Kentniss der Myelitis acuta. Arb Path Inst Univ Helsingfors. Vol. 1. Berlin, Karger, 1905.
15. Caverly CS. Preliminary report of an epidemic of paralytic disease, occurring in Vermont, in the summer of 1894. Yale Med J i:1–5, 1894–1895.
16. Lavinder CH, Freeman AW, Frost WH. Epidemiologic studies of poliomyelitis in New York City and the northeastern United States during the year 1916. Public Health Bull (Wash) 91, 1918.
17. Landsteiner K, Popper E. Mikroskopische Präparate von einem menschlichen und zwei Affenrückenmarken. Wien Klin Wochenschr 21:1830, 1908.

18. Burnet FM, Macnamara J. Immunological differences between strains of poliomyelitis virus. Br J Exp Pathol 12:57–61, 1931.

19. Committee on Typing of the National Foundation for Infantile Paralysis. Immunologic classification of poliomyelitis viruses: a cooperative program for the typing of one hundred strains. Am J Hyg 54:191–274, 1951.

20. Enders JF, Weller TH, Robbins FC. Cultivation of the Lansing strain of poliomyelitis virus in cultures of various human embryonic tissue. Science 109:85–87, 1949.

21. Hammon WM, Coriell LI, Stokes J. Evaluation of Red Cross gamma globulin as a prophylactic agent for poliomyelitis. I. Plan of controlled field tests and results of 1951 pilot study in Utah. J Am Med Assoc 150:739–749, 1952.

22. Sutter RW, Pallansch MA, Sawyer LA, et al. Defining surrogate serologic tests with respect to predicting protective vaccine efficacy: poliovirus vaccination. Ann N Y Acad Sci 754:289–299, 1995.

23. Brown GC, Rabson AS, Schieble JH. The effect of gamma globulin on subclinical infection in familial associates of poliomyelitis cases: II. Serological studies and virus isolations from pharyngeal secretions. J Immunol 74:71–80, 1955.

24. Horstmann DM, McCollum RW, Mascola AD. Viremia in human poliomyelitis. J Exp Med 99:355–369, 1954.

25. McKay HW, Fodor AR, Kokko UP. Viremia following administration of live poliovirus vaccines. Am J Public Health 53:274–285, 1963.

26. Nathanson N, Bodian D. Experimental poliomyelitis following intramuscular virus injection. III. The effect of passive antibody on paralysis and viremia. Bull Johns Hopkins Hosp 111:198–220, 1962.

27. Sabin AB. Oral poliovirus vaccine: history of its development and use and current challenge to eliminate poliomyelitis from the world. J Infect Dis 151:420–436, 1985.

28. Drinker P, Shaw LA. Apparatus for prolonged administration of artificial respiration: I. A design for adults and children. J Clin Invest 7:229–247, 1929.

29. Sabin AB. Paralytic consequences of poliomyelitis infection in different parts of the world and in different population groups. Am J Public Health 41:1215–1230, 1951.

30. Greenberg M, Siegel M, Magee MC. Poliomyelitis in New York City, 1949. N Y State Med J 50:1119–1123, 1950.

31. Sabin AB. Epidemiologic patterns of poliomyelitis in different parts of the world. In Poliomyelitis. Papers and Discussions Presented at the First International Poliomyelitis Conference. Philadelphia, JB Lippincott, 1949, pp 3–33.

32. Das AN. A Study of the Trend of the Age Selection of Poliomyelitis in the United States Since 1910. Baltimore, Johns Hopkins University, 1932.

33. Olin G. The epidemiologic pattern of poliomyelitis in Sweden from 1905 to 1950. In Poliomyelitis: Papers and Discussions Presented at the Second International Poliomyelitis Conference. Philadelphia, JB Lippincott, 1951, pp 367–375.

34. Paul JR. The National Foundation for Infantile Paralysis. In A History of Poliomyelitis. New Haven, CT, Yale University Press, 1971, pp 308–323.

35. Hull HF, Ward NA, Hull BP, et al. Paralytic poliomyelitis: seasoned strategies, disappearing disease. Lancet 343:1331–1337, 1994.

36. de Quadros CA, Hersh BS, Olive JM, et al. Eradication of wild poliovirus from the Americas: acute flaccid paralysis surveillance, 1988–1995. J Infect Dis 175(suppl 1):S37–S42, 1997.

37. World Health Organization. Progress towards the global eradication of poliomyelitis, 2001. Wkly Epidemiol Rec 77:98–107, 2002.

38. de Quadros CA. Global eradication of poliomyelitis and measles: another quiet revolution. Ann Intern Med 127:156–158, 1997.

39. Foege WH. A world without polio: "Future generations will know by history only . . . ." JAMA 270:1859–1860, 1993.

40. Horstmann DM. Clinical aspects of acute poliomyelitis. Am J Med 6:592–605, 1949.

41. Horstmann DM. Poliomyelitis: severity and type of disease in different age groups. Ann N Y Acad Sci 61:956–967, 1955.

42. Paul JR. Clinical epidemiology of poliomyelitis. Medicine (Baltimore) 20:495–520, 1941.

43. Gelfand HM, LeBlanc DR, Fox JP, Conwell DP. Studies on the development of natural immunity to poliomyelitis in Louisiana. II. Description and analysis of episodes of infection observed in study households. Am J Hyg 65:367–385, 1957.

44. Draper G. Acute Poliomyelitis. Philadelphia, Blakiston's, 1917.

45. Bodian D. Poliomyelitis: pathogenesis and histopathology. In Rivers TM, Horsfall FL (eds). Viral and Rickettsial Infections of Man. Philadelphia, JB Lippincott, 1959, pp 479–498.

46. Bodian D, Horstmann DM. Polioviruses. In Horsfall FL, Tamm I (eds). Viral and Rickettsial Infections of Man (4th ed). Philadelphia, JB Lippincott, 1965, pp 430–473.

47. Morens DM, Pallansch MA, Moore M. Polioviruses and other enteroviruses. In Belshe RB (ed). Textbook of Human Virology (2nd ed). St. Louis, Mosby, 1991, pp 427–497.

48. Sabin AB. Poliomyelitis. In Braude AI, Davis CE, Fierer J (eds). International Textbook of Medicine. Vol. II. Infectious Diseases and Medical Microbiology (2nd ed). Philadelphia, WB Saunders, 1986, pp 1147–1161.

49. Ramlow J, Alexander M, LaPorte R, et al. Epidemiology of postpolio syndrome. Am J Epidemiol 136:769–786, 1992.

50. Dalakas MC, Sever JL, Madden DL, et al. Late post-poliomyelitis muscular atrophy: clinical, virological and immunological studies. Rev Infect Dis 6(suppl 2):S562–S567, 1984.

51. Dalakas MC, Bartfeld H, Kurland LT. The postpolio syndrome: advances in the pathogenesis and treatment. Ann N Y Acad Sci 753:1–412, 1995.

52. Racaniello VR. Picornaviridae: the viruses and their replication. In Knipe DM, Howley PM, Griffin DE, et al (eds). Fields Virology. Philadelphia, Lippincott Williams & Wilkins, 2001, pp 685–722.

53. Melnick JL, Ashkenazi A, Midulla VC, et al. Immunogenic potency of MgCl$_2$-stabilized oral poliovaccine. JAMA 185:406–408, 1963.

54. Armstrong C. The experimental transmission of poliomyelitis to the Eastern cotton rat, Sigmodon hispidus hispidus. Public Health Rep 54:1719–1721, 1939.

55. Bodian D, Morgan IM, Howe HA. Differentiation of types of poliomyelitis viruses. III. The grouping of fourteen strains into three basic immunologic types. Am J Hyg 49:234–245, 1949.

56. Kessel JF, Pait CF. Differentiation of three groups of poliomyelitis virus. Proc Soc Exp Biol Med 70:315–316, 1949.

57. Murdin AD, Lu HH, Murray MG, Wimmer E. Poliovirus antigenic hybrids simultaneously expressing antigenic determinants from all three serotypes. J Gen Virol 73:607–611, 1992.

58. Toyoda H, Kohara MM, Kataoka Y, et al. Complete nucleotide sequences of all three poliovirus serotype genomes: implication for genetic relationship, gene function and antigenic determinants. J Mol Biol 174:561–585, 1984.

59. Kew OM, Morris-Glasgow V, Landaverde M, et al. Outbreak of poliomyelitis in Hispaniola associated with circulating type 1 vaccine-derived poliovirus. Science 296:356–359, 2002.

60. Liu HM, Zheng DP, Zhang LB, et al. Rapid divergence of wild type 1 poliovirus into separate lineages by recombination and mutation [abstr W34-6]. In Abstracts of the annual meeting of the American Society for Virology, Ft. Collins, CO, 2000, p 114.

61. Hogle JM, Chow M, Filman DJ. Three-dimensional structure of poliovirus at 2.9 A resolution. Science 229:1358–1365, 1985.

62. Minor PD. Antigenic structure of picornaviruses. Curr Top Microbiol Immunol 161:121–154, 1990.

63. Mendelsohn CL, Wimmer E, Racaniello VR. Cellular receptor for poliovirus: molecular cloning, nucleotide sequence, and expression of a new member of the immunoglobulin superfamily. Cell 56:855–865, 1989.

64. Belnap DM, McDermott BM, Filman DJ, et al. Three-dimensional structure of poliovirus receptor bound to poliovirus. Proc Natl Acad Sci U S A 97:73–78, 2000.

65. He YN, Bowman VD, Mueller S, et al. Interaction of the poliovirus receptor with poliovirus. Proc Natl Acad Sci U S A 97:79–84, 2000.

66. Pipkin PA, Wood DJ, Racaniello VR, Minor PD. Characterization of L cells expressing the human poliovirus receptor for the specific detection of polioviruses in vitro. J Virol Methods 41:333–340, 1993.

67. Ren R, Constantini F, Gorgacz EJ, et al. Transgenic mice expressing a human poliovirus receptor: a new model for poliomyelitis. Cell 63:353–362, 1990.

68. Koike S, Taya C, Kurata T, et al. Transgenic mice susceptible to poliovirus. Proc Natl Acad Sci U S A 88:951–955, 1991.

69. World Health Organization. Maintenance and distribution of transgenic mice susceptible to human viruses: memorandum from a WHO meeting. Bull World Health Organ 71:497–502, 1993.

70. Freistadt MS, Stoltz DA, Eberle KE. Role of poliovirus receptors in the spread of infection. Ann N Y Acad Sci 753:37–47, 1995.

71. Gromeier M, Wimmer E. Mechanisms of injury-provoked poliomyelitis. J Virol 72:5056–5060, 1998.

72. Racaniello VR, Ren R. Poliovirus biology and pathogenesis. Curr Top Microbiol Immunol 206:305–325, 1996.

73. Freistadt MS, Fleit HB, Wimmer E. Poliovirus receptor on human blood cells: a possible extraneural site of poliovirus replication. Virology 195:798–803, 1993.

74. Bodian D, Paffenbarger RS. Poliomyelitis infection in households: frequency of viremia and specific antibody response. Am J Hyg 60:83–98, 1954.

75. Andrus JK, de Quadros CA, Olive JM, et al. Screening of cases of acute flaccid paralysis for poliomyelitis eradication: Ways to improve specificity. Bull World Health Organ 70:591–596, 1992.

76. Dietz V, Lezana M, Garcia Sancho C, Montesano R. Predictors of poliomyelitis case confirmation at initial clinical evaluation: implications for poliomyelitis eradication in the Americas. Int J Epidemiol 21:800–806, 1992.

77. Biellik RJ, Bueno H, Olive JM, de Quadros C. Poliomyelitis case confirmation: characteristics for use by national eradication programmes. Bull World Health Organ 70:79–84, 1992.

78. Patriarca PA, Linkins RW, Sutter RW, Orenstein WA. Optimal schedule for the administration of oral poliovirus vaccine. In Kurstak E (ed). Measles and Poliomyelitis: Vaccine, Immunization, and Control. Wien, Springer-Verlag, 1993, pp 303–313.

79. Melnick JL. Enteroviruses: polioviruses, coxsackieviruses, echoviruses, and newer enteroviruses. In Fields BN, Knipe DM, Chanock RM, et al (eds). Fields Virology (2nd ed). New York, Raven Press, 1990, pp 549–605.

80. Melnick JL, Mordhorst CH, Pervikov Y. Worldwide use of LBM combination pools for typing enteroviruses. Bull World Health Organ 67:327–332, 1989.

81. Expanded Programme on Immunization and Division of Communicable Diseases. Manual for the Virological Investigation of Poliomyelitis. Geneva, World Health Organization, 1990.

82. Centers for Disease Control and Prevention. Developing and expanding contributions of the Global Laboratory Network for Poliomyelitis Eradication, 1997–1999. MMWR 49:156–160, 2000.

83. Centers for Disease Control and Prevention. Status of the Global Laboratory Network for Poliomyelitis Eradication. MMWR 46:692–694, 1997.

84. Alexander JP, Gary HE, Pallansch MA. Duration of poliovirus excretion and its implications for acute flaccid paralysis surveillance: a review of the literature. J Infect Dis 175(suppl 1):S176–S182, 1997.

85. Kilpatrick DR, Nottay B, Yang CF, et al. Group-specific identification of polioviruses by PCR primers containing mixed-base or deoxyinosine residues at positions of codon degeneracy. J Clin Microbiol 34:2990–2996, 1996.

86. Kilpatrick DR, Nottay B, Yang CF, et al. Serotype-specific identification of polioviruses by PCR primers containing mixed-base or deoxyinosine residues at positions of codon degeneracy. J Clin Microbiol 36:352–357, 1998.

87. van der Avoort HGAM, Hull BP, Hovi T, et al. Comparative study of five methods for intratypic differentiation of polioviruses. J Clin Microbiol 33:2562–2566, 1995.

88. van Wezel AL, Hazendonk AG. Intratypic differentiation of poliomyelitis virus strains by strain-specific antisera. Intervirology 11:2–8, 1979.

89. De L, Nottay BK, Yang CF, et al. Identification of vaccine-related polioviruses by hybridization with specific RNA probes. J Clin Microbiol 33:562–571, 1995.

90. De L, Yang CF, da Silva E, et al. Genotype-specific RNA probes for the direct identification of wild polioviruses by blot hybridization. J Clin Microbiol 35:2834–2840, 1997.

91. Lipskaya GY, Chervonskaya EA, Belova GI, et al. Geographic genotypes (geotypes) of poliovirus case isolates from the former Soviet Union: relatedness to other known poliovirus genotypes. J Gen Virol 76:1687–1699, 1995.

92. Yang CF, De L, Holloway BP, et al. Detection and identification of vaccine-related polioviruses by the polymerase chain reaction. Virus Res 20:159–179, 1991.

93. Yang CF, De L, Yang SJ, et al. Genotype-specific in vitro amplification of sequences of the wild type 3 polioviruses from Mexico and Guatemala. Virus Res 24:277–296, 1992.

94. Balanant JS, Guillot S, Candrea A, et al. The natural genomic variability of poliovirus analyzed by a restriction fragment polymorphism assay. Virology 184:645–654, 1991.

95. Shulman LM, Handsher R, Yang SJ, et al. Resolution of the pathways of poliovirus type 1 transmission during an outbreak. J Clin Microbiol 38:945–952, 2000.

96. Kew OM, Mulders MN, Lipskaya GY, et al. Molecular epidemiology of polioviruses. Semin Virol 6:401–414, 1995.

97. Albrecht P, Enterline JC, Boone EJ, Klutch MJ. Poliovirus and polioantibody assay in Hep-2 and Vero cell cultures. J Biol Stand 11:91–97, 1983.

98. Expanded Programme on Immunization. Report of a WHO Consultation on Polio Neutralization Antibody Assays, Nashville, TN, 5–6 December 1991. Geneva, World Health Organization, 1990.

99. Bhatt PN, Brooks M, Fox JP. Extent of infection with poliomyelitis virus in household associates of clinical cases as determined serologically and by virus isolation using tissue culture methods. Am J Hyg 61:287–301, 1955.

100. Rovainen M, Agboatwalla M, Stenvik M, et al. Intrathecal immune response and virus-specific immunoglobulin M antibodies in laboratory diagnosis of acute poliomyelitis. J Clin Microbiol 31:2427–2432, 1993.

101. Pettit C, Minnich LL, Shehab ZM, Ray GC. Comparison between indirect immunofluorescence and microneutralization for detection of antibodies to polioviruses. J Clin Microbiol 25:1325–1326, 1987.

102. Hodes HL, Berger R, Ainbender E, et al. Study of viral antibodies by the paper-reactive virus method. Pediatrics 37:7–18, 1966.

103. Hagenaars AM, van Delft RW, Nagel J, et al. A modified ELISA technique for the titration of antibodies to polio virus as an alternative to a virus neutralization test. J Virol Methods 6:233–239, 1983.

104. Esposito JJ. Detection of poliovirus antigens and antibodies: microindirect haemagglutination and haemagglutination inhibition tests for poliovirus types I, II, and III. Microbios 16:29–36, 1976.

105. Wiechers D. Electrophysiology of acute polio revisited: utilizing newer EMG techniques in vaccine-associated disease. Ann N Y Acad Sci 753:111–119, 1995.

106. Malzberg MS, Rogg JM, Tate CA, et al. Poliomyelitis hyperintensity of the anterior horn cells on MR images of the spinal cord. AJR Am J Roentgenol 161:863–865, 1993.

107. Bernstein HGG, Clark JMP, Tunbridge RE. Acute anterior poliomyelitis among service personnel in Malta: account of epidemic. Br Med J 1:763–767, 1945.

108. Fraser FR. A study of the cerebrospinal fluid in acute poliomyelitis. J Exp Med 18:242–251, 1913.

109. Marx A, Glass J, Sutter RW. Differential diagnoses of acute flaccid paralysis and its role in poliomyelitis surveillance. Epidemiol Rev 22:298–316, 2000.

110. Salisbury DM, Ramsay ME, White JM, Brown DW. Polio eradication: surveillance implications for the United Kingdom. J Infect Dis 175(suppl 1):S156–S159, 1997.

111. Olive JM, Castillo C, Castro RG, de Quadros CA. Epidemiologic study of Guillain-Barré syndrome in children <15 years of age in Latin America. J Infect Dis 175(suppl 1):S160–S164, 1997.

112. Herceg A, Kennett M, Antony J, Longbottom H. Acute flaccid paralysis surveillance in Australia: the first year. Commun Dis Intell 20:403–405, 1996.

113. Grist NR, Bell EG. Enteroviral etiology of the paralytic poliomyelitis syndrome. Arch Environ Health 21:382–387, 1970.

114. Voroshilova MK, Chumakov MP. Poliomyelitis-like properties of AB-IV-Coxsackie A7 group of viruses. Prog Med Virol 2:106–170, 1959.

115. Melnick JL. Enterovirus type 71 infections: a varied clinical pattern sometimes mimicking paralytic poliomyelitis. Rev Infect Dis 6(suppl 2):S387–S390, 1984.

116. Dyken P, Krawiecki N. Neurodegenerative diseases in infancy and childhood. Ann Neurol 13:351–364, 1983.

117. Daube JR. Electrophysiologic studies in the diagnosis and prognosis of motor neuron diseases. Neurol Clin 3:473–493, 1985.

118. McKhann GM, Cornbluth DR, Ho T, et al. Clinical and electrophysiological aspects of acute paralytic diseases of children and young adults in northern China. Lancet 338:593–597, 1991.

119. Weber JT, Hatheway CL, St. Louis ME. Botulism. In Hoeprich PD, Colin Jordan M, Ronald AR (eds). Infectious Diseases: A Treatise of the Infectious Process (5th ed). Philadelphia, JB Lippincott, 1994, pp 1185–1194.

120. Hoeprich PD. Diphtheria. *In* Hoeprich PD, Colin Jordan M, Ronald AR (eds). Infectious Diseases: A Treatise of the Infectious Process (5th ed). Philadelphia, JB Lippincott, 1994, pp 373–380.

121. Sutter RW, Orenstein WA, Wassilak SG. Tetanus. *In* Hoeprich PD, Colin Jordan M, Ronald AR (eds). Infectious Diseases: A Treatise of the Infectious Process (5th ed). Philadelphia, JB Lippincott, 1994, pp 1175–1185.

122. Leis A, Stokic D, Plok K, et al. Acute flaccid paralysis syndrome associated with West Nile virus infection—Mississippi and Louisiana, July–August 2002. MMWR 51:825–828, 2002.

123. Leis AA, Stokic DS, Plok JL, et al. A polio-like syndrome from West Nile virus infection. N Engl J Med 347:1280–1281, 2002.

124. Glass JD, Samuels O, Rich MM. Poliomyelitis due to West Nile Virus. N Engl J Med 347:1281–1282, 2002.

125. Wyatt HV. Poliomyelitis and infantile paralysis: changes in host and virus. Hist Phil Life Sci 15:357–396, 1993.

126. Paul JR, Riordan JT, Melnick JL. Antibodies to three different antigenic types of poliomyelitis virus in sera of North Alaskan Eskimos. Am J Hyg 54:275–285, 1951.

127. Salk J. Requirements for persisting immunity to poliomyelitis. Trans Assoc Am Physicians 69:105–114, 1956.

128. Aycock WL. A milk-borne epidemic of poliomyelitis. Am J Hyg 7:791–803, 1927.

129. Bancroft PM, Engelhard WE, Evans C. Poliomyelitis in Huskerville (Lincoln) Nebraska: studies indicating a relationship between clinically severe infection and proximate fecal pollution of water. JAMA 164:836–847, 1957.

130. Horstmann DM, Paul JR. The incubation period in human poliomyelitis and its implications. J Am Med Assoc 135:11–14, 1947.

131. Melnick JL, Ledinko N. Development of neutralizing antibodies against the three types of poliomyelitis virus during an epidemic period: the ratio of inapparent infection to clinical poliomyelitis. Am J Hyg 58:207–222, 1953.

132. Penttinen K, Patiala R, Bremer D. The paralytic/infected ratio in a susceptible population during a polio type 1 epidemic. Ann Med Exp Fenn 39:195–202, 1961.

133. Bernier RH. Some observations on poliomyelitis lameness surveys. Rev Infect Dis 6(suppl 2):S371–S375, 1984.

134. Centers for Disease Control and Prevention. Prolonged poliovirus excretion in an immunodeficient person with vaccine-associated paralytic poliomyelitis. MMWR 46:641–643, 1997.

135. Kew OM, Sutter RW, Nottay BK, et al. Prolonged replication of a type 1 vaccine-derived poliovirus in an immunodeficient patient. J Clin Microbiol 36:2893–2899, 1998.

136. Wood D, Sutter RW, Dowdle W. Stopping vaccination following poliomyelitis eradication: issues and challenges. Bull World Health Organ 78:847–857, 2000.

137. MacCallum FO. The Role of Humoral Antibodies in Protection Against and Recovery from Bacterial and Virus Infections in Hypogammaglobulinemia (Medical Research Council Special Report Series, 310). London, Medical Research Council, 1971, pp 72–85.

138. Martin J, Dunn G, Hull R, et al. Evaluation of the Sabin strain of type 3 poliovirus in an immunodeficient patient during the entire 637-day period of excretion. J Virol 74:3001–3010, 2000.

139. Hara M, Saito Y, Komatsu T, et al. Antigenic analysis of poliovirus isolated from a child with agammaglobulinemia. Microbiol Immunol 25:905–913, 1981.

140. Abo W, Chiba S, Yamanaka T, et al. Paralytic poliomyelitis in a child with agammaglobulinemia. Eur J Pediatr 132:11–16, 1979.

141. Misbah SA, Lawrence PA, Kurtz JB, Chapel HM. Prolonged faecal excretion of poliovirus in a nurse with common variable hypogammaglobulinemia. Postgraduate Med J 67:301–303, 1991.

142. Bellmunt A, May G, Zell R, et al. Evolution of a poliovirus type 1 during 5.5 years of prolonged enteral replication in an immunodeficient patient. Virology 36:178–184, 1999.

143. Maclennan CA, Dunn G, Wood P, et al. Chronic infection with vaccine-derived neurovirulent poliovirus in a common variable immunodeficiency and implications for world health. J Allergy Clin Immunol 107(suppl):S304–S305, 2001.

144. Buttinelli G, Donati V, Fiore S, et al. Nucleotide variation in Sabin type 2 poliovirus from an immunodeficient patient with poliomyelitis. J Gen Virol, 2003 [in press].

145. Taiwan Polio Eradication Certification Committee. National Documentation for Maintenance of Poliomyelitis Eradication in Taiwan for the Period July 2000–December 2001. Taipei, Taiwan Polio Eradication Certification Committee, April 2000.

146. Patriarca PA, Sutter RW, Oostvogel PM. Outbreaks of poliomyelitis, 1976–1995. J Infect Dis 175(suppl 1):S165–S172, 1997.

147. Bradford Hill AB, Knowelden J. Inoculation and poliomyelitis: a statistical investigation in England and Wales in 1949. Br Med J 2:1–6, 1950.

148. Sutter RW, Patriarca PA, Suleiman AJM, et al. Attributable risk of DTP (diphtheria-tetanus toxoids and pertussis vaccine) injection in provoking paralytic poliomyelitis during a large outbreak in Oman. J Infect Dis 165:444–449, 1992.

149. Lambert SM. A yaws campaign and an epidemic of poliomyelitis in Western Samoa. J Trop Med Hyg 39:41–46, 1936.

150. Korns RF, Albrecht RM, Locke FB. The association of parenteral injections with poliomyelitis. Am J Public Health 42:153–169, 1952.

151. Trueta J, Hodes R. Provoking and localising factors in poliomyelitis: an experimental study. Lancet 1:998–1001, 1954.

152. Horstmann DM. Acute poliomyelitis: relation of physical activity at the time of onset to the course of the disease. J Am Med Assoc 142:236–241, 1950.

153. Talmey M. Predisposing factors in infantile paralysis. N Y Med J 104:202–204, 1916.

154. Aycock WL. Frequency of poliomyelitis in pregnancy. N Engl J Med 225:405–408, 1941.

155. Nathanson N, Bodian D. Experimental poliomyelitis following intramuscular virus injection. I. The effect of neural block on a neurotropic and a pantropic strain. II. Viremia and the effect of antibody. Bull Johns Hopkins Hosp 108:308–333, 1961.

156. Gromeier M, Solcki D, Patel DD, Wimmer E. Expression of the human poliovirus receptor/CD155 gene during development of the central nervous system: implications for the pathogenesis of poliomyelitis. Virology 74:7381–7390, 2000.

157. Ohka S, Yang WX, Terada E, et al. Retrograde transport of intact poliovirus through the axon via the fast transport system. Virology 250:67–75, 1998.

158. Aycock WL. Tonsillectomy and poliomyelitis. I. Epidemiological considerations. Medicine (Baltimore) 21:65–94, 1942.

159. Sabin AB. Experimental poliomyelitis by the tonsillopharyngeal route with special reference to the influence of tonsillectomy on the development of bulbar paralysis. J Am Med Assoc 111:605–610, 1938.

160. von Magnus H, Melnick JL. Tonsillectomy in experimental poliomyelitis. Am J Hyg 48:113–125, 1948.

161. Ogra PL. Effect of tonsillectomy and adenoidectomy on nasopharyngeal antibody response to poliovirus. N Engl J Med 284:59–64, 1971.

162. Ogra PL, Karzon DT. Formation and function of poliovirus antibody in different tissues. Prog Med Virol 13:156–193, 1971.

163. Bernkopf H, Medalie J, Yekutiel M. Antibodies to poliomyelitis virus and socioeconomic factors influencing their frequency in children in Israel. Am J Trop Med 1957:697–703, 1957.

164. Pal SR, Banerjee G, Aikat BK. Serological investigation on endemicity of poliomyelitis in Calcutta and in a neighboring rural area. Indian J Med Res 54:507–511, 1966.

165. Sutter RW, Patriarca PA, Suleiman AJM, et al. Paralytic poliomyelitis in Oman: association between regional differences in attack rate and variations in antibody responses to oral poliovirus vaccine. Int J Epidemiol 22:936–944, 1993.

166. Swartz TA, Skalska P, Gerichter CG, Cockburn WC. Routine administration of oral polio vaccine in a subtropical area: factors possibly affecting sero-conversion. J Hyg (Camb) 70:719–726, 1972.

167. Herndon CN, Jennings RG. A twin-family study of susceptibility to poliomyelitis. Am J Hum Genet 3:17–46, 1951.

168. van Eden W, Persijn GG, Bijerk H, et al. Differential resistance to paralytic poliomyelitis controlled by histocompatibility leukocyte antigens. J Infect Dis 147:422–426, 1983.

169. Wyatt HV. Is poliomyelitis a genetically-determined disease? I. A genetic model. Med Hypotheses 1:35–42, 1975.

170. Prevots DR, Ciofi M, Sallabanda A, et al. Outbreak of paralytic poliomyelitis in Albania, 1996: high attack rate among adults and apparent interruption of transmission following nationwide mass vaccination. Clin Infect Dis 26:419–425, 1998.

171. Centers for Disease Control and Prevention. Outbreak of poliomyelitis—Cape Verde, 2000. MMWR 49:1070, 2000.

172. Allmond W, Froeschle JE, Gilloud NB. Paralytic poliomyelitis in large laboratory primates. Am J Epidemiol 85:229–239, 1967.

173. Goodall J. The Chimpanzees of Gombe. Boston, Belknap Press of Harvard University, 1986, pp 92–94.

174. Ruch TC. Diseases of Laboratory Primates. London, WB Saunders, 1967, pp 408–410.

175. Dowdle WR, Birmingham ME. The biologic principles of poliovirus eradication. J Infect Dis 175(suppl 1):S286–S292, 1997.

176. Fine PEM. Herd immunity: history, theory, practice. Epidemiol Rev 15:265–302, 1993.

177. Fine PEM, Carneiro IAM. Transmissibility and persistence of oral polio vaccine viruses: implications for the global poliomyelitis initiative. Am J Epidemiol 150:1001–1021, 1999.

178. Furesz J, Armstrong RE, Contreras G. Viral and epidemiological links between poliomyelitis outbreaks in unprotected communities in Canada and the Netherlands [letter]. Lancet 2:1248, 1978.

179. Schonberger LR, Kaplan J, Kim-Farley R, et al. Control of paralytic poliomyelitis in the United States. Rev Infect Dis 6(suppl 2):S424–S426, 1984.

180. Patriarca PA, Wright PF, John TJ. Factors affecting the immunogenicity of oral poliovirus vaccine in developing countries: review. Rev Infect Dis 13:926–939, 1991.

181. Sutter RW, Patriarca PA, Brogan S, et al. Outbreak of paralytic poliomyelitis in Oman: evidence for widespread transmission among fully vaccinated children. Lancet 338:715–720, 1991.

182. Melnick JL. Live attenuated poliovirus vaccines. In Plotkin SA, Mortimer EA (eds). Vaccines (2nd ed). Philadelphia, WB Saunders, 1994, pp 155–204.

183. Otten MW, Deming MS, Jaiteh KO, et al. Epidemic poliomyelitis in The Gambia following the control of poliomyelitis as an endemic disease. I. Descriptive findings. Am J Epidemiol 135:381–392, 1992.

184. Afif H, Sutter RW, Kew OM, et al. Outbreak of poliomyelitis in Gizan, Saudi Arabia: cocirculation of wild type 1 polioviruses from three separate origins. J Infect Dis 175(suppl 1):S71–S75, 1997.

185. Reichler MR, Abbas A, Kharabsheh S, et al. Outbreak of paralytic poliomyelitis in a highly immunized population in Jordan. J Infect Dis 175(suppl 1):S62–S70, 1997.

186. Melnick JL, Benyesh-Melnik M, Pena R, Yow M. Effectiveness of Salk vaccine: analysis of virologically confirmed cases of paralytic and nonparalytic poliomyelitis. JAMA 175:1159–1162, 1961.

187. Bottiger M. Long-term immunity following vaccination with killed poliovirus vaccine in Sweden, a country with no circulating poliovirus. Rev Infect Dis 6(suppl 2):S548–S551, 1984.

188. Lapinleimu K. Elimination of poliomyelitis in Finland. Rev Infect Dis 6(suppl 2):S456–S460, 1984.

189. Grachev VP. Long-term use of oral poliovirus vaccine from Sabin strains in the Soviet Union. Rev Infect Dis 6(suppl 2):S321–S322, 1984.

190. Nathanson N. Epidemiologic aspects of poliomyelitis eradication. Rev Infect Dis 6(suppl 2):S308–S312, 1984.

191. Sabin AB. Oral poliovirus vaccine—recent results and recommendations for optimum use. R Soc Health J 82:51–59, 1962.

192. Strebel PM, Sutter RW, Cochi SL, et al. Epidemiology of poliomyelitis in the United States one decade after the last reported case of indigenous wild virus–associated disease. Clin Infect Dis 14:568–579, 1992.

193. Cruz RR. Cuba: mass polio vaccination program. Rev Infect Dis 6(suppl 2):S408–S412, 1984.

194. Expanded Programme on Immunization. EPI Information System: Global Summary, August 1997. Geneva, World Health Organization, 1997.

195. Heymann DL, Murphy K, Brigaud M, et al. Oral poliovirus vaccine in tropical Africa: greater impact on incidence of paralytic disease than expected from coverage surveys and seroconversion rates. Bull World Health Organ 65:495–501, 1987.

196. Risi JB. The control of poliomyelitis in Brazil. Rev Infect Dis 6(suppl 2):S400–S403, 1984.

197. Hatziandreu EJ, Palmer CS, Halpern MT, Brown RE. A Cost Benefit Analysis of OPV: Final Report. Arlington, VA, Battelle, 1994.

198. Centers for Disease Control. Summary of notifiable diseases, United States, 1990. MMWR 39:1–61, 1991.

199. World Health Organization. Poliomyelitis in 1980. Parts 1 and 2. Wkly Epidemiol Rec 56:329–332, 337–341, 1981.

200. Kubli D, Steffen R, Schar M. Importation of poliomyelitis in industrialised nations between 1975 and 1984: evaluation and conclusions for vaccination recommendations. Br Med J (Clin Res Ed) 295:169–171, 1987.

201. Oostvogel PM, van Wijngaarden JK, van der Avoort HGAM, et al. Poliomyelitis in an unvaccinated community in the Netherlands, 1992–1993. Lancet 344:665–670, 1994.

202. Bernal A, Garcia-Saiz A, Liacer A, et al. Poliomyelitis in Spain, 1982–1984: virologic and epidemiologic studies. Am J Epidemiol 126:69–76, 1987.

203. Centers for Disease Control. Poliomyelitis—Pennsylvania, Maryland. MMWR 28:49–50, 1979.

204. Aylward RB, Porta D, Fiore L, et al. Unimmunized gypsy populations and implications for the eradication of poliomyelitis in Europe. J Infect Dis 175(suppl 1):S86–S88, 1997.

205. Mulders NM, van Loon AM, van der Avoort HGAM, et al. Molecular characterization of a wild poliovirus type 3 epidemic in the Netherlands (1992 and 1993). J Clin Microbiol 33:3252–3256, 1995.

206. World Health Organization. Poliomyelitis outbreak, Bulgaria. Wkly Epidemiol Rec 67:336–337, 1992.

207. Centers for Disease Control and Prevention. Imported poliovirus causing poliomyelitis—Bulgaria, 2001. MMWR 50:1033–1035, 2001.

208. Strebel PM, Aubert-Cambiescu A, Ion-Nedelcu N, et al. Paralytic poliomyelitis in Romania, 1984–1992: evidence for a high risk of vaccine-associated disease and reintroduction of wild-virus infection. Am J Epidemiol 140:1111–1124, 1994.

209. Kew OM, Nathanson N. Molecular epidemiology of viruses. Semin Virol 6:357–358, 1995.

210. Rico-Hesse R, Pallansch MA, Nottay BK, Kew OM. Geographic distribution of wild poliovirus type 1 genotypes. Virology 160:311–322, 1987.

211. Kew OM, Nottay BK, Rico-Hesse R, Pallansch M. Molecular epidemiology of wild poliovirus transmission. In Kurstak E, Marusyk RG, Murphy FA, van Regenmortel MHV (eds). Applied Virology Research. Vol 2. Virus Variability, Epidemiology and Control. New York, Plenum Publishing, 1990, pp 199–221.

212. Mulders MN, Lipskaya GY, van der Avoort HGAM, et al. Molecular epidemiology of wild poliovirus type in Europe, the Middle East, and the Indian subcontinent. J Infect Dis 171:1399–1405, 1995.

213. Centers for Disease Control and Prevention. Apparent global interruption of wild poliovirus type 2 transmission. MMWR 50:222–224, 2001.

214. Kew OM, Pallansch MA. The mechanism of polio eradication. In Semler BL, Wimmer E (eds), Molecular Biology of Picornaviruses. Washington, DC, ASM Press, 2002, pp 481–491.

215. Yoshida H, Li J, Yoneyama T, et al. Two major strains of type 1 wild poliovirus circulating in Indochina. J Infect Dis 175:1233–1237, 1997.

216. Centers for Disease Control and Prevention. Progress toward poliomyelitis eradication—Egypt, 2001. MMWR 51:305–307, 2002.

217. Pinheiro FP, Kew OM, Hatch MH, da Silveira CM. Eradication of wild poliovirus from the Americas: wild poliovirus surveillance—laboratory issues. J Infect Dis 175(suppl 1):S43–S49, 1997.

218. Netter A. Serotherapie de la poliomyélite. Nos résultats chez 30 malades: indications, techniques, incidents possibles. Bull Acad Med Paris 74:403–423, 1915.

219. Paul JR. Convalescent serum therapy. In A History of Poliomyelitis. New Haven, CT, Yale University Press, 1971, pp 190–199.

220. Flexner S, Lewis PA. Experimental poliomyelitis in monkeys: active immunization and passive protection. JAMA 54:1780–1782, 1910.

221. Gelfand HM, Fox JP, LeBlanc DR, Elveback L. Studies on the development of natural immunity to poliomyelitis in Louisiana: V. Passive transfer of polio antibody from mother to fetus, and natural decline and disappearance of antibody in the infant. J Immunol 85:46–55, 1960.

222. Hammon WM, Coriell LL, Wehrle PF. Evaluation of Red Cross gamma globulin as a prophylactic agent for poliomyelitis. IV. Final report of results based on clinical diagnosis. JAMA 151:1272–1285, 1953.

223. National Advisory Committee for the Evaluation of Gamma Globulin in the Prophylaxis of Poliomyelitis. An Evaluation of the Efficacy of Gamma Globulin in the Prophylaxis of Paralytic Poliomyelitis as Used in the United States 1953 (Publication No 358). Washington, DC, U.S. Public Health Service, 1954.

224. Department of Drugs. Drug Evaluations: Annual 1991. Milwaukee, American Medical Association, 1991.

225. O'Neal KM, Pallansch MA, Winkelstein JA, et al. Chronic group A coxsackievirus infection in agammaglobulinemia: demonstration of genomic variation of serotypically identical isolates persistently excreted by the same patient. J Infect Dis 157:183–186, 1988.

226. Davis LE, Bodian D, Price D, et al. Chronic progressive poliomyelitis secondary to vaccination of an immunodeficient child. N Engl J Med 297:214–245, 1977.

227. Flexner S, Lewis PA. Experimental poliomyelitis in monkeys: seventh and eighth notes. J Am Med Assoc 54:1789, 1910.

228. Romer PH. Die epidemische Kinderlähmung (Heine-Medinsche Krankheit). Berlin, Springer, 1911.

229. Brodie M, Goldblum A. Active immunization against poliomyelitis in monkeys. J Exp Med 53:885–893, 1931.

230. Brodie M. Active immunization against poliomyelitis. J Exp Med 56:493–505, 1932.

231. Brodie M, Park WH. Active immunization against poliomyelitis. N Y State J Med 35:815–818, 1935.

232. Brodie M, Park WH. Active immunization against poliomyelitis. JAMA 105:1089–1093, 1935.

233. Kolmer JA. Susceptibility and immunity in relation to vaccination in acute anterior poliomyelitis. JAMA 105:1956–1963, 1935.

234. Leake JP. Poliomyelitis following vaccination against this disease. JAMA 105:2152, 1936.

235. Koprowski H, Jervis GA, Norton TW. Immune responses in human volunteers upon oral administration of a rodent-adapted strain of poliomyelitis virus. Am J Hyg 55:108–126, 1952.

236. Li CP, Schaeffer M, Nelson DB. Experimentally produced variants of poliomyelitis virus combining in vivo and in vitro techniques. Ann N Y Acad Sci 61:902–910, 1955.

237. Melnick JL. Variation in poliomyelitis virus on serial passage through tissue culture. Cold Spring Harb Symp Quant Biol 18:178–179, 1953.

238. Sabin AB, Hennessen WA, Winsser J. Studies on variants of poliomyelitis virus. I. Experimental segregation and properties of avirulent variants of three immunologic types. J Exp Med 99:551–576, 1954.

239. Poliomyelitis: Papers and Discussions Presented at the 4th International Poliomyelitis Conference. Philadelphia, JB Lippincott, 1958.

240. Poliomyelitis: Papers and Discussions Presented at the 5th International Poliomyelitis Conference. Philadelphia, JB Lippincott, 1961.

241. Pan American Health Organization. Proceedings of the Second International Conference on Live Poliovirus Vaccines. Washington, DC, Pan American Health Organization, 1960.

242. Pan American Sanitary Bureau. Proceedings of the First International Conference on Live Poliovirus Vaccines. Washington, DC, Pan American Sanitary Bureau, 1959.

243. Sabin AB. Present position of immunization against poliomyelitis with live virus vaccines. Br Med J 1:663–680, 1959.

244. Koprowski H. Live poliomyelitis virus vaccines. JAMA 178: 1151–1155, 1961.

245. Paul JR. Status of vaccination against poliomyelitis, with particular reference to oral vaccination. N Engl J Med 264:651–658, 1961.

246. Koprowski H. The 10th anniversary of the development of live poliovirus vaccine. In Proceedings of the Second International Conference on Live Poliovirus Vaccines. Washington, DC, Pan American Health Organization, 1960.

247. Sabin AB. Properties and behaviour of orally administered attenuated poliovirus vaccine. JAMA 164:1216–1223, 1957.

248. Melnick JL. Problems associated with the use of live poliovirus vaccine. Am J Public Health 50:1013–1031, 1960.

249. Melnick JL. Tests for safety of live poliovirus vaccine. Acad Med N J Bull 6:146–167, 1960.

250. Melnick JL, Benyesh-Melnick M, Brennan JC. Studies on live poliovirus vaccine: its neurotropic activity in monkeys and its increased neurovirulence after multiplication in vaccinated children. JAMA 171:1165–1172, 1959.

251. Melnick JL. Attenuation of poliomyelitis viruses on passage through tissue culture. Fed Proc 13:505, 1954.

252. Murray R, Kirschstein R, van Hoosier G, Baron S. Comparative virulence for rhesus monkeys of poliovirus strains used for oral administration. In Proceedings of the First International Conference on Live Poliovirus Vaccines. Washington, DC, Pan American Sanitary Bureau, 1959, pp 39–64.

253. Westrop GD, Wareham KA, Evans DMA, et al. Genetic basis of attenuation of the Sabin type 3 oral poliovirus vaccine. J Virol 63:1338–1344, 1989.

254. Nomoto A, Omata T, Toyoda H, et al. Complete nucleotide sequence of the attenuated poliovirus Sabin 1 genome. Proc Natl Acad Sci U S A 79:5793–5797, 1982.

255. Bouchard MJ, Lam DH, Racaniello VR. Determinants of attenuation and temperature sensitivity in type 1 poliovirus Sabin strain. J Virol 69:4972–4978, 1995.

256. Omata T, Kohara M, Kuge S, et al. Genetic analysis of the attenuation phenotype of poliovirus type 1. J Virol 58:348–358, 1986.

257. Kawamura N, Kohara M, Abe S, et al. Determinants in the 5′ noncoding region of poliovirus Sabin 1 RNA that influence the attenuating phenotype. J Virol 63:1302–1309, 1989.

258. Tardy-Panit M, Blondel B, Martin A, et al. A mutation in the RNA polymerase of the poliovirus type 1 contributes to attenuation in mice. J Virol 67:4630–4638.

259. Macadam AJ, Pollard SR, Ferguson G, et al. Genetic basis of attenuation of the Sabin type 2 vaccine strain of poliovirus in primates. Virology 192:18–26, 1993.

260. Ren R, Moss EG, Racaniello VR. Identification of two determinants that attenuate vaccine-related type 2 poliovirus. J Virol 65:1377–1382, 1991.

261. Sabin AB, Boulger LR. History of Sabin attenuated poliovirus oral live vaccine strains. J Biol Stand 1:115–118, 1973.

262. Macadam AJ, Arnold C, Howlett J, et al. Reversion of the attenuated and temperature-sensitive phenotypes of the Sabin type 3 strain poliovirus in vaccinees. Virology 172:408–414, 1989.

263. Tatem J, Weeks-Levy C, Georgiu A, et al. A mutation present in the amino terminus of Sabin 3 poliovirus VP1 protein is attenuating. J Virol 66:3194–3197, 1992.

264. Westrop GD, Wareham KA, Evans DMA, et al. Genetic basis of attenuation of the Sabin type 3 oral poliovirus vaccine. J Virol 63:1338–1344, 1989.

265. Muzychenko AR, Lipskaya GY, Maslova SV, et al. Coupled mutations in the 5′-untranslated region of the Sabin poliovirus strains during in vivo passage: structural and functional implications. Virus Res 21:111–122, 1991.

266. Svitkin YV, Pestova T, Maslova SV, Agol VI. Point mutations modify the response of poliovirus RNA to a translation initiation factor: a comparison of neurovirulent and attenuated strains. Virology 166:394–404, 1988.

267. Macadam A, Ferguson G, Arnold C, Minor PD. An assembly defect as a result of an attenuating mutation in the capsid proteins of the poliovirus type 3 vaccine strain. J Virol 65:5225–5231, 1991.

268. Wimmer E, Hellen CU, Cao X. Genetics of poliovirus. Annu Rev Genet 27:353–436, 1993.

269. Martin J, Minor PD. Characterization of CHAT and Cox type 1 live-attenuated poliovirus vaccine strains. J Virol 76:5339–5349.

270. Horwitz A, Martins da Silva M, Bica AN. Large-scale field studies with live attenuated polioviruses in the Americas. In Proceedings of the Fifth International Poliomyelitis Conference. Philadelphia, JB Lippincott, 1961, pp 221–227.

271. Cox HR, Cabasso VJ, Markham FS, et al. Immunologic response to trivalent oral poliomyelitis vaccine. In Proceedings of the First International Conference on Live Poliovirus Vaccines. Washington, DC, Pan American Sanitary Bureau, 1959, pp 229–248.

272. Voroshilova MK. Influence of dose and schedule of oral immunization of people with live poliovirus vaccine on antibody response. In Proceedings of the Fifth International Poliomyelitis Conference. Philadelphia, JB Lippincott, 1961, pp 296–303.

273. Verlinde JD, Wilterdink JB. A small-scale trial on vaccination and revaccination with live attenuated polioviruses in the Netherlands. In Proceedings of the First International Conference on Live Poliovirus Vaccines. Washington, DC, Pan American Sanitary Bureau, 1959, pp 355–366.

274. Caceres VM, Sutter RW. Sabin monovalent oral polio vaccines: review of past experiences and their potential use after polio eradication. Clin Infect Dis 33:531–541, 2001.

275. Embil J, Gervais L, Hernandez Miyares C, Cardelle G. Use of attenuated live poliovirus vaccine in Cuban children. In Proceedings of the Second International Conference on Live Poliovirus Vaccines. Washington, DC, Pan American Health Organization, 1960, pp 365–370.

276. Kimball AC, Barr RN, Bauer H, et al. Minnesota studies with oral poliomyelitis vaccine: community spread of orally administered attenuated poliovirus vaccine strains. In Proceedings of the Second

International Conference on Live Poliovirus Vaccines. Washington, DC, Pan American Health Organization, 1960, pp 161–173.

277. Krugman S, Warren J, Eiger MS, et al. Immunization of new-born infants with live attenuated poliovirus vaccine. *In* Proceedings of the Second International Conference on Live Poliovirus Vaccines. Washington, DC, Pan American Health Organization, 1960, pp 315–321.

278. Paul JR, Horstmann DM, Riordan JT, et al. The capacity of live attenuated polioviruses to cause human infection and to spread within families. *In* Proceedings of the Second International Conference on Live Poliovirus Vaccines. Washington, DC, Pan American Health Organization, 1960, pp 174–184.

279. Tomlinson AJH, Davies J. Trial of live attenuated poliovirus vaccine: a report to the Public Health Laboratory Service from the Poliomyelitis Vaccines Committee of the Medical Research Council. Br Med J 2:1037–1044, 1961.

280. Voroshilova MK, Zhevandrova VI, Tolskaya EA, et al. Virologic and serologic investigations of children immunized with trivalent live vaccine from A. B. Sabin's strains. *In* Proceedings of the Second International Conference on Live Poliovirus Vaccines. Washington, DC, Pan American Health Organization, 1960, pp 240–265.

281. Zhdanov VM, Chumakov MP, Smorodintsev AA. Large-scale practical trials and use of live poliovirus vaccine in the USSR. *In* Proceedings of the Second International Conference on Live Poliovirus Vaccines. Washington, DC, Pan American Health Organization, 1960, pp 576–588.

282. Ramos Alvarez M, Gomez Santos F, Rivera LR, Mayes O. Viral and serological studies in children immunized with live poliovirus vaccine—preliminary report of a large trial conducted in Mexico. *In* Proceedings of the First International Conference on Live Poliovirus Vaccines. Washington, DC, Pan American Sanitary Bureau, 1959, pp 483–494.

283. Ramos Alvarez M, Bustamante ME, Alvarez Alba R. Use of Sabin's live poliovirus vaccine in Mexico: results of a large-scale trial. *In* Proceedings of the Second International Conference on Live Poliovirus Vaccines. Washington, DC, Pan American Health Organization, 1960, pp 386–409.

284. Robertson HE, Acker MS, Dillenberg HO, et al. Community-wide use of a "balanced" trivalent oral poliovirus vaccine (Sabin): a report of the 1961 trial at Prince Albert, Saskatchewan. Can J Public Health 53:179–191, 1962.

285. Food and Drug Administration. Additional standards for viral vaccines; poliovirus vaccine live oral; final rule (21 CFR Part 630). Fed Reg 56:21418–21438, 1991.

286. Public Health Service. Public Health Service Regulations: Biological Products. Title 42, Part 73. Washington, DC, U.S. Department of Health, Education and Welfare, 1967.

287. Patriarca PA, Laender F, Palmeira G, et al. Randomised trial of alternative formulations of oral poliovaccine in Brazil. Lancet 1:429–433, 1988.

288. World Health Organization. Report of the 13th Global Advisory Group Meeting, Cairo, 14–18 October 1990. Geneva, World Health Organization, 1991.

289. Lederle Laboratories. Poliovirus Vaccine Live Oral Trivalent [package insert]. Pearl River, NY, Lederle Laboratories, 1993.

290. Global Programme for Vaccines and Immunization. International List of Availability of Vaccines and Sera. Geneva, World Health Organization, 1995.

291. Domok I. Experiences associated with the use of live poliovirus vaccine in Hungary, 1959–1982. Rev Infect Dis 6(suppl 2):S413–S418, 1984.

292. Schoub BD, Johnson S, McAnererney J, et al. Monovalent neonatal polio immunization—a strategy for the developing world. J Infect Dis 157:836–839, 1988.

293. World Health Organization. Requirements for Poliomyelitis Vaccine (Oral). Requirements for Biological Substances No. 7 (Revised 1989). Geneva, World Health Organization, 1990.

294. Wallis C, Melnick JL. Stabilization of poliovirus by cations. Tex Rep Biol Med 19:683–700, 1961.

295. Petersen I, von Magnus H. Polio neutralization tests with MgCl$_2$-stabilized virus. Acta Pathol Microbiol Scand 61:652–653, 1964.

296. Yofe J, Goldblum N, Eylan E, Melnick JL. An outbreak of poliomyelitis in Israel in 1961 and the use of attenuated type 1 vaccine in its control. Am J Hyg 76:225–238, 1962.

297. Mirchamsy H, Shafyi A, Mahinpour M, Nazari P. Stabilizing effect of magnesium chloride and sucrose on Sabin live polio vaccine. Dev Biol Stand 41:255–257, 1978.

298. Milstien JB, Lemon SM, Wright PF. Development of a more thermostable poliovirus vaccine. J Infect Dis 175(suppl 1):S247–S253, 1997.

299. Expanded Programme on Immunization. The Vaccine Vial Monitor. Geneva, World Health Organization, 1994.

300. Ghendon Y. WHO recommendations on potential use of a new poliomyelitis vaccine. Dev Biol Stand 78:133–139, 1993.

301. Vonka V, Janda Z, Simon J, et al. A new type 3 attenuated poliovirus for possible use in oral poliovirus vaccine. Prog Med Virol 9:204–255, 1967.

302. Melnick JL, Berencsi G, Biberi-Moroeanu S, et al. WHO collaborative studies on poliovirus type 3 strains isolated during the 1968 poliomyelitis epidemic in Poland. Bull World Health Organ 47:287–294, 1972.

303. Kew OM, Nottay BK. Molecular epidemiology of polioviruses. Rev Infect Dis 6(suppl 2):S499–S504, 1984.

304. Kew OM, De L, Yang CF, et al. The role of virologic surveillance in the global initiative to eradicate poliomyelitis. *In* Kurstak E (ed). Control of Virus Diseases. New York, Marcel Dekker, 1993, pp 215–246.

305. Martin J, Ferguson GL, Wood DJ, Minor PD. The vaccine origin of the 1968 epidemic of the type 3 poliomyelitis in Poland. Virology 278:42–49, 2000.

306. Nathanson N, Horn SD. Neurovirulence tests of type 3 poliovirus vaccine manufactured by Lederle Laboratories, 1964–1988. Vaccine 10:469–474, 1992.

307. Brown F, Lewis BP (eds). Poliovirus attenuation: molecular mechanisms and practical aspects. Dev Biol Stand 78:1–187, 1993.

308. de la Torre JC, Giacchetti C, Semler BL, Holland JJ. High frequency of single-base transitions and extreme frequency of precise multiple-base reverse mutations in poliovirus. Proc Natl Acad Sci U S A 89:2531–2535, 1992.

309. Drake JW. Rates of spontaneous mutations among RNA viruses. Proc Natl Acad Sci U S A 90:4171–4175, 1993.

310. Domingo E, Holland JJ. RNA virus mutations and fitness for survival. Annu Rev Microbiol 51:151–178, 1997.

311. Chumakov KM, Norwood LP, Parker ML, et al. RNA sequence variants in live poliovirus vaccine and their relation to neurovirulence. J Virol 66:966–970, 1992.

312. Racaniello VR, Baltimore D. Cloned poliovirus complementary DNA is infectious in mammalian cells. Science 214:915–919, 1981.

313. Kohara M, Abe S, Kuge S, et al. An infectious cDNA clone of the poliovirus Sabin strain could be used as a stable repository and inoculum for the oral live vaccine. Virology 151:21–30, 1986.

313a. Kawamura N, Kohara M, Abe S, et al. Determinants in the 5' noncoding region of poliovirus Sabin 1 RNA that influence the attenuating phenotype. J Virol 63:1302–1309, 1989.

314. Kohara M, Omata T, Kameda T, et al. In vitro phenotypic markers of a poliovirus recombinant constructed from infectious cDNA clones of the neurovirulent Mahoney strain and the attenuated Sabin 1 strain. J Virol 53:786–792, 1985.

315. Paul JR, Riordan JT, Melnick JL. Antibodies to three different antigenic types of poliomyelitis virus in sera from North American Eskimos. Am J Hyg 54:275–285, 1951.

316. Sabin AB. Transitory appearance of type 2 neutralizing antibody in patients infected with type 1 poliomyelitis virus. J Exp Med 96:99–106, 1956.

317. Hammon WM, Ludwig EH. Possible protective effect of previous type 2 infection against paralytic poliomyelitis due to type 1 virus. Am J Hyg 66:274–280, 1957.

318. Bogger-Goren S, Baba K, Hurly P, et al. Antibody response to varicella-zoster virus after natural and vaccine-induced infection. J Infect Dis 146:260–265, 1982.

319. Horstmann DM, Opton EM, Klemperer R, et al. Viremia in infants vaccinated with oral poliovirus vaccine (Sabin). Am J Hyg 79:47–63, 1964.

320. Melnick JL, Proctor RO, Ocampo AR, et al. Free and bound virus in serum after administration of oral poliovirus vaccine. Am J Epidemiol 84:329–342, 1966.

321. Benyesh-Melnick M, Melnick JL, Rawls WE, et al. Studies on the immunogenicity, communicability and genetic stability of oral poliovaccine administered during the winter. Am J Epidemiol 86:112–136, 1967.

322. McBean AM, Thoms ML, Albrecht P, et al. Serologic response to oral polio vaccine and enhanced-potency inactivated polio vaccines. Am J Epidemiol 128:615–628, 1988.
323. WHO Collaborative Study Group on Oral and Inactivated Poliovirus Vaccines. Response to an Infant Immunization Schedule Combining Oral and Inactivated Poliovirus Vaccines: Compared With Either Vaccine Alone. Results of a Randomized Trial in The Gambia, Oman, and Thailand. Final Report. Geneva, World Health Organization, 1995.
324. WHO Collaborative Study Group on Oral and Inactivated Poliovirus Vaccines. Combined immunization of infants with oral and inactivated poliovirus vaccines: results of a randomized trial in The Gambia, Oman, and Thailand. J Infect Dis 175(suppl 1):S215–S227, 1997.
325. World Health Organization Collaborative Study Group on Oral Poliovirus Vaccine. Factors affecting the immunogenicity of oral poliovirus vaccine: a prospective evaluation in Brazil and The Gambia. J Infect Dis 171:1097–1106, 1995.
326. Posey DL, Linkins RW, Oliveria MJ, et al. The effect of diarrhea on oral poliovirus vaccine failure in Brazil. J Infect Dis 175(suppl 1):S258–S263, 1997.
327. Zaman S, Carlsson B, Morikawa A, et al. Poliovirus antibody titres, relative affinity, and neutralizing capacity in maternal milk. Arch Dis Child 68:198–201, 1993.
328. Ogra SS, Weintraub DI, Ogra PL. Immunologic aspects of human colostrum and milk: interaction with the intestinal immunity of the neonate. Adv Exp Med Biol 107:95–107, 1978.
329. Palmer EL, Gary GW, Black R, Martin ML. Antiviral activity of colostrum and serum immunoglobulins A and G. J Med Virol 5:123–129, 1980.
330. Patriarca PA, Linkins RW, Sutter RW. Poliovirus vaccine formulations. In Kurstak E (ed). Measles and Poliomyelitis: Vaccine, Immunization, and Control. Wien, Springer-Verlag, 1993, pp 265–277.
331. Sutter RW, Patriarca PA. Inactivated and live, attenuated poliovirus vaccines: mucosal immunity. In Kurstak E (ed). Measles and Poliomyelitis: Vaccines, Immunization and Control. Wien, Springer-Verlag, 1993, pp 279–294.
332. Smorodintsev AA, Davidenkova EF, Drobyshevskaya AI, et al. Results of a study of the reactogenic and immunogenic properties of live antipoliomyelitis vaccine. Bull World Health Organ 20:1053–1074, 1959.
333. Nishio O, Ishihara Y, Sakae K, et al. The trend of acquired immunity with live poliovirus vaccine and the effect of revaccination: follow-up of vaccinees for ten years. J Biol Stand 12:1–10, 1984.
334. Janda Z, Adam E, Vonka V. Properties of a new type 3 attenuated poliovirus. VI. Alimentary tract resistance in children fed previously with type 3 Sabin vaccine to reinfection with homologous and heterologous type 3 attenuated poliovirus. Arch Virusforsch 20:87–98, 1967.
335. Soloviev VD. Problems connected with live polio vaccine. In Proceedings of the Fifth International Poliomyelitis Conference. Philadelphia, JB Lippincott, 1961, pp 403–410.
336. Rossen RD, Kasel JA, Couch RB. The secretory immune system: its relation to respiratory viral infections. Prog Med Virol 13:194–238, 1971.
337. Onorato IM, Modlin JF, McBean AM, et al. Mucosal immunity induced by enhanced-potency inactivated and oral polio vaccines. J Infect Dis 163:1–6, 1991.
338. Ogra PL, Fishaut M, Gallagher MR. Viral vaccination via the mucosal routes. Rev Infect Dis 2:352–369, 1980.
339. Smith JWG, Lee JA, Fletcher WB, et al. The response of oral polio-vaccine in persons aged 16–18 years. J Hyg (Camb) 76:235–247, 1976.
340. Ogra PL. Distribution of echovirus antibody in serum, nasopharynx, rectum and spinal fluid after natural infection with echovirus type 6. Infect Immun 2:150–155, 1970.
341. Rovainen M, Hovi T. Cleavage of VP1 and modification of antigenic site 1 of type 2 polioviruses by intestinal trypsin. J Virol 62:3536–3539, 1988.
342. Agol VI, Drozdov SG. Russian contribution to OPV. Biologicals 21:321–325, 1993.
343. Sabin AB. Role of my cooperation with Soviet scientists in the elimination of polio. Perspect Biol Med 31:57–64, 1987.
344. Chumakov MP, Voroshilova MK, Drozdov SG, et al. Some results of the work on mass immunization in the Soviet Union with live

345. Centers for Disease Control and Prevention. Certification of poliomyelitis eradication—the Americas, 1994. MMWR 43:720–722, 1994.
346. Centers for Disease Control and Prevention. Certification of poliomyelitis eradication—Western Pacific Region, October 2000. MMWR 50:1–3, 2001.
347. World Health Organization. Certification of poliomyelitis eradication, European region, June 2002. Wkly Epidemiol Rec 77:221–223, 2002.
348. Hale JH, Doraisingham M, Kanagaratnam K, et al. Large-scale use of Sabin type 2 attenuated poliovirus vaccine in Singapore during a type 1 poliomyelitis epidemic. Br Med J 1:1537–1549, 1959.
349. Knowelden J, Hale JH, Gardner PS, Lee JH. Measurement of the protective effect of attenuated poliovirus vaccine. Br Med J 1:1418–1420, 1961.
350. Fox JP, Gelfand HM, LeBlanc DR, Rowan DF. The influence of natural and artificially induced immunity on alimentary infections with polioviruses. Am J Public Health 48:1181–1192, 1958.
351. Koprowski H, Norton TW, Jervis GA, et al. Clinical investigations of attenuated strains of poliomyelitis virus: use as a method of immunization of children with living virus. JAMA 160:954–966, 1956.
352. Paul JR, Horstmann DM, Niederman JC. Immunity in poliomyelitis infection: observations in experimental epidemiology. In Najjar VA (ed). Immunity and Virus Infection. New York, John Wiley & Sons, 1959, pp 233–245.
353. Skovranek V, Zacek K. Oral poliovirus vaccine (Sabin) in Czechoslovakia: effectiveness of nationwide use in 1960. JAMA 176:524–526, 1961.
354. Plotkin SA, Koprowski H. Epidemiological studies on the safety and efficacy of vaccination with the CHAT strain of attenuated poliovirus in Leopoldville, Belgian Congo. In Proceedings of the First International Conference on Live Poliovirus Vaccines. Washington, DC, Pan American Sanitary Bureau, 1959, pp 419–436.
355. Rangelova SM. Control of poliomyelitis in Bulgaria: experiences of two decades. Prog Med Virol 31:183–211, 1984.
356. Dong DX. Immunization with oral poliovirus vaccine in China. Prog Med Virol 31:168–182, 1984.
357. Deming MS, Jaiteh KO, Otten MW, et al. Epidemic poliomyelitis in The Gambia following the control of poliomyelitis as an endemic disease. II. Clinical efficacy of trivalent oral polio vaccine. Am J Epidemiol 135:393–408, 1992.
358. Horstmann DM, Emmons J, Gimpel L, et al. Enterovirus surveillance following a community-wide oral poliovirus vaccination program: a seven-year study. Am J Epidemiol 97:173–186, 1973.
359. Sabin AB, Ramos-Alvarez M, Alvarez-Amezquita J, et al. Live, orally given poliovirus vaccine—effect of rapid mass immunization on population under conditions of massive enteric infections with other viruses. JAMA 173:1521–1526, 1960.
360. Chen RT, Hausinger S, Dajani AS, et al. Seroprevalence of antibody against poliovirus in inner-city preschool children: implications for vaccination policy in the United States. JAMA 275:1639–1645, 1996.
361. Ramsay ME, Begg NT, Ghandi J, Brown D. Antibody response and viral excretion after live polio vaccine or a combined schedule of live and inactivated polio vaccines. Pediatr Infect Dis J 13:1117–1121, 1994.
362. Orenstein WA, Wassilak SGF, DeForest A, et al. Seroprevalence of poliovirus antibodies among Massachusetts schoolchildren [abstr 512]. In Abstracts of the 28th Interscience Conference on Antimicrobial Agents and Chemotherapy, New Orleans, September 28–October 1, 1988, p 198.
363. Kelley PW, Petruccelli BP, Stehr-Green P, et al. The susceptibility of young adult Americans to vaccine-preventable infections: a national serosurvey of US army recruits. JAMA 266:2724–2729, 1991.
364. WHO Consultative Group. Evidence on the safety and efficacy of live poliomyelitis vaccines currently in use, with special reference to type 3 poliovirus. Bull World Health Organ 40:925–945, 1969.
365. Oberhofer TR, Brown GC, Monto AS. Seroimmunity to poliomyelitis in an American community. Am J Epidemiol 101:333–339, 1975.
366. Horstmann DM. Maxwell Finland lecture: Viral vaccines and their ways. Rev Infect Dis 1:502–516, 1979.
367. Cabasso VJ, Nozell H, Rueggsegger JM, Cox HR. Poliovirus antibody three years after oral trivalent vaccine (Sabin strains). J Pediatr 68:199–203, 1966.

poliovirus vaccine prepared from Sabin strains. Bull World Health Organ 25:79–91, 1961.

368. Krugman RD, Hardy GE, Sellers C, et al. Antibody persistence after primary immunization with trivalent oral poliovirus vaccine. Pediatrics 60:80–82, 1977.

369. Rousseau WE, Noble GR, Tegtmeier GE, et al. Persistence of poliovirus neutralizing antibodies eight years after immunization with live attenuated virus vaccine. N Engl J Med 289:1357–1359, 1973.

370. Fortuin M, Maine N, Mendy M, et al. Measles, polio and tetanus toxoid antibody levels in Gambian children aged 3 to 4 years following routine vaccination. Trans R Soc Trop Med Hyg 89:326–329, 1995.

371. Stratton KR, Howe CJ, Johnston RB. Adverse Events Associated with Childhood Vaccines: Evidence Bearing on Causality. Washington, DC, National Academy Press, 1994.

372. Terry L. The Association of Cases of Poliomyelitis with the Use of Type 3 Oral Poliomyelitis Vaccines. Washington, DC, U.S. Department of Health, Education and Welfare, 1962.

373. WHO Collaborative Study Group. The relationship between persisting spinal paralysis and poliomyelitis vaccine—results of a ten-year enquiry. Bull World Health Organ 60:231–242, 1982.

374. WHO Collaborative Study Group. The relationship between acute and persisting spinal paralysis and poliomyelitis vaccine (oral): results of a WHO enquiry. Bull World Health Organ 53:319–331, 1976.

375. Esteves K. Safety of oral poliomyelitis vaccine: results of a WHO enquiry. Bull World Health Organ 66:739–746, 1988.

376. Sabin AB. Commentary on report on oral poliomyelitis vaccine. JAMA 190:52–55, 1964.

377. Sabin AB. Paralytic poliomyelitis: old dogmas and new perspectives. Rev Infect Dis 3:543–564, 1981.

378. Wyatt HV. Poliomyelitis in hypogammaglobulinemics. J Infect Dis 128:802–806, 1973.

379. Prevots DR, Sutter RW, Strebel PM, et al. Completeness of reporting for paralytic poliomyelitis, United States, 1980 through 1991. Arch Pediatr Adolesc Med 148:479–485, 1994.

380. Centers for Disease Control and Prevention. Poliomyelitis prevention in the United States: introduction of a sequential vaccination schedule of inactivated poliovirus vaccine followed by oral poliovirus vaccine. Recommendations of the Advisory Committee on Immunization Practices. MMWR 46 (RR-3):1–25, 1997.

381. Sutter RW, Prevots DR. Vaccine-associated paralytic poliomyelitis among immunodeficient persons. Infect Med 11:426, 429–430, 435–438, 1994.

382. Strebel PM, Ion-Nedelcu N, Baughman AL, et al. Intramuscular injections within 30 days of immunization with oral poliovirus vaccine—a risk factor for vaccine-associated paralytic poliomyelitis. N Engl J Med 332:500–506, 1995.

383. Izurieta HS, Sutter RW, Baughman AL, et al. Vaccine-associated paralytic poliomyelitis in the United States: no evidence of elevated risk after simultaneous intramuscular injections with vaccine. Pediatr Infect Dis J 14:840–846, 1995.

384. Andrus JK, Strebel PM, de Quadros CA, Olive JM. Risk of vaccine-associated paralytic poliomyelitis in Latin America, 1989–91. Bull World Health Organ 73:33–40, 1995.

385. Kohler KA, Banerjee K, Hlady WG, et al. Vaccine-associated paralytic poliomyelitis in India during 1999: decreased risk despite massive use of oral polio vaccine. Bull World Health Organ 80:210–216, 2002.

386. Vaccines and Biologicals. Report of the interim meeting of the technical consultative group (TCG) on the global eradication of poliomyelitis, Geneva, November 9–11, 2002. World Health Organization, Geneva, 2003.

387. Wilfert CM, Buckley RH, Mohanakumar T, et al. Persistent and fatal central-nervous-system echovirus infections in patients with agammaglobulinemia. N Engl J Med 296:1485–1489, 1977.

388. Ziegler JB, Penny R. Fatal echo 30 virus infection and amyloidosis in X-linked hypogammaglobulinemia. Clin Immunol Immunopathol 3:347–352, 1975.

389. Hodes DS, Espinoza DV. Temperature sensitivity of isolates of echovirus type 11 causing chronic meningoencephalitis in an agammaglobulinemic patient. J Infect Dis 144:377, 1981.

390. Gorson KC, Ropper AH. Nonpoliovirus poliomyelitis simulating Guillain-Barré syndrome. Arch Neurol 58:1460–1464, 2001.

391. Technical Consultative Group to the World Health Organization on the Global Eradication of Poliomyelitis. "Endgame" issues for the global polio eradication initiative. Clin Infect Dis 34:72–77, 2002.

392. Macadam AJ, Pollard SR, Ferguson G, et al. Genetic basis of attenuation of the Sabin type 2 vaccine strain of poliovirus in primates. Virology 192:18–26, 1993.

393. Agol VI. Recombination and other genomic rearrangements in picornaviruses. Semin Virol 8:77–84, 1997.

394. Cuervo NS, Guillot S, Romanenkova N, et al. Genomic features of intratypic recombinant Sabin poliovirus strains excreted by primary vaccinees. J Virol 75:5740–5751, 2001.

395. Georgescu MM, Delpeyroux F, Crainic R. Tripartite genome organization of a natural type 2 vaccine/nonvaccine recombinant poliovirus. J Gen Virol 76:2343–2348, 1995.

396. Martin JE, Samoilovich E, Dunn G, et al. Isolation of an intertypic poliovirus capsid recombinant from a child with vaccine-associated paralytic poliomyelitis. J Virol 76:10921–10928, 2002.

397. Cammack NJ, Philipps A, Dunn G, et al. Intertypic genomic rearrangements of poliovirus strains in vaccinees. Virology 167:507–514, 1989.

398. Macadam AJ, Arnold C, Howlett J, et al. Reversion of the attenuated and temperature-sensitive phenotypes of the Sabin type 3 strain of poliovirus in vaccinees. Virology 172:408–414, 1989.

399. Minor PD, Dunn G. The effect of sequences in the 5′ non-coding region on the replication of polioviruses in the human gut. J Gen Virol 69:1091–1096, 1988.

400. Yoshida H, Horie H, Matsuura K, et al. Prevalence of vaccine-derived poliovirus in the environment. J Gen Virol 83:1107–1110, 2002.

401. Yoneyama T, Hagiwar A, Hara M, Shimojo H. Alteration in oligonucleotide fingerprint patterns of the viral genome in poliovirus type 2 isolated from paralytic patients. Infect Immun 37:46–53, 1982.

402. Kawamura N, Kohara M, Abe S, et al. Determinants in the 5′ non-coding region of poliovirus Sabin 1 RNA influence the attenuating phenotype. J Virol 63:1302–1309, 1989.

403. Centers for Disease Control and Prevention. Circulation of a type 2 vaccine-derived poliovirus—Egypt, 1982–1993. MMWR 50:41–42, 51, 2001.

404. Centers for Disease Control and Prevention. Acute flaccid paralysis associated with circulating vaccine-derived poliovirus—Philippines. MMWR 50:874–875, 2001.

405. World Health Organization. Paralytic poliomyelitis in Madagascar, 2002. Wkly Epidemiol Rec 77:241–242, 2002.

406. Thorley B, Paladin F, Shimizu H. Paper presented at the XIIth International Congress of Virology, Paris, 27 July–1 August 2002.

407. Liu HM, Zheng DP, Zhang LB, et al. Molecular evolution of a type 1 wild-vaccine poliovirus recombinant during widespread circulation in China. J Virol 74:11153–11161, 2000.

408. Vaccines and Biological Division. Seventh Meeting of the Technical Consultative Group (TCG) on the Global Eradication of Poliomyelitis, 9–11 April, 2002 (WHO/V&B/02.12). Geneva, World Health Organization, 2002.

409. Eddy BE, Borman GS, Berkeley WH, Young RD. Tumors induced in hamsters by injection of rhesus monkey kidney cell extracts. Proc Soc Exp Biol Med 107:191–197, 1961.

410. Mortimer EA, Lepow ML, Gold E, et al. Long-term follow up of persons inadvertently inoculated with SV40 as neonates. N Engl J Med 305:1517–1518, 1981.

411. Shah K, Nathanson N. Human exposure to SV40: review and comment. Am J Epidemiol 103:1–12, 1976.

412. Lewis AM, Egan W. Meeting report. Workshop on simian virus 40 (SV40): a possible human polyomavirus. Biologicals 25:355–358, 1997.

413. Strickler HD, Rosenberg PS, Devesa SS, et al. Contamination of poliovirus vaccines with simian virus 40 (1955–1963) and subsequent cancer rates. JAMA 279:292–295, 1998.

414. Butel JS, Lednicky JA. Cell and molecular biology of simian virus 40: implications for human infections and disease. J Natl Cancer Institute 91:119–134, 1999.

415. Butel JS. Simian virus 40, poliovirus vaccines, and human cancer: research progress versus media and public interest. Bull World Health Organ 78:195–197, 2000.

416. Stratton K, Almario DA, McCormick MC (eds). Immunization Safety Review: SV40 Contamination of Polio Vaccine and Cancer. Washington, DC, National Academy Press, 2002.

417. Uhari M, Rantala M, Niemela M. Cluster of childhood Guillain-Barré cases after an oral polio vaccine campaign. Lancet 2:440–441, 1989.

418. Kinnunen E, Farkkila M, Hovi T, et al. Incidence of Guillain-Barré syndrome during a nationwide oral poliovirus campaign. Neurology 39:1034–1036, 1989.

419. Rantala H, Cherry JD, Shields WD, Uhari M. Epidemiology of Guillain-Barré syndrome in children: relationship of oral polio vaccine administration to occurrence. J Pediatr 124:220–223, 1994.

420. Kinnunen E, Junttila O, Haukka J, Hovi T. Nationwide oral poliovirus vaccination campaign and the incidence of Guillain-Barré syndrome. Am J Epidemiol 147:69–73, 1998.

421. American Academy of Pediatrics. Poliovirus infections. In Peter G (ed). 1997 Red Book: Report of the Committee on Infectious Diseases. Elk Grove Village, IL, American Academy of Pediatrics, 1997, pp 424–433.

422. Salisbury DM, Begg NT (eds). Immunisation against Infectious Disease. 1996 Edition. Department of Health, Welsh Office, Scottish Office Home and Health Department, DHHS (Northern Ireland). London, Her Majesty's Stationery Office, 1996.

423. Onorato IM, Strebel PM, Sutter RW. Immunizations, vaccine-preventable diseases, and HIV infection. In Wormser GP (ed). AIDS and Other Manifestations of HIV Infection (3rd ed). Philadelphia, Lippincott–Raven, 1998, pp 745–758.

424. Ryder RW, Oxtoby MJ, Mvula M, et al. Safety and immunogenicity of bacille Calmette-Guérin, diphtheria-tetanus-pertussis, and oral polio vaccines in newborn children in Zaire infected with human immunodeficiency virus type 1. J Pediatr 122:697–702, 1993.

425. Vernon A, Okwo B, Lubamba N, Miaka MB. Paralytic poliomyelitis and HIV infection in Kinshasa, Zaire. In Proceedings of the Sixth International Conference on AIDS, San Francisco, CA, June 20–24, 1990.

426. Ion-Nedelcu N, Dobrescu A, Strebel PM, Sutter RW. Vaccine-associated paralytic poliomyelitis and HIV infection [letter]. Lancet 343:51–52, 1994.

427. Chitsike I, van Furth R. Paralytic poliomyelitis associated with live oral poliomyelitis vaccine in child with HIV infection in Zimbabwe: case report. BMJ 318:841–843, 1999.

428. Harjulehto-Mervaala T, Aro T, Hiilesmaa VK, et al. Oral polio vaccination during pregnancy: no increase in the occurrence of malformations. Am J Epidemiol 138:407–414, 1993.

429. Harjulehto-Mervaala T, Aro T, Hiilesmaa VK, et al. Oral polio vaccination during pregnancy: lack of impact on fetal development and perinatal outcome. Clin Infect Dis 18:414–420, 1994.

430. Myaux JA, Unicomb L, Besser RE, et al. Effect of diarrhea on the humoral response to oral polio vaccination. Pediatr Infect Dis J 15:204–209, 1996.

431. American Academy of Pediatrics. 1997 Red Book: Report of the Committee on Infectious Diseases. Elk Grove Village, IL, American Academy of Pediatrics, 1997.

432. Centers for Disease Control and Prevention. Poliomyelitis prevention in the United States: updated recommendations of the Advisory Committee on Immunization Practices (ACIP). MMWR 49(RR-5):1–22, 2000.

433. Modlin JF, Halsey NA, Thoms ML, et al. Humoral and mucosal immunity in infants induced by three sequential inactivated poliovirus vaccine–live attenuated oral poliovirus vaccine immunization schedules. J Infect Dis 175(suppl 1):S228–S234, 1997.

434. Vaccines and Biologicals. WHO vaccine-preventable diseases: monitoring system. 2002 Global Summary. World Health Organization, Geneva, 2002.

435. Lasch EE, Abed Y, Marcus O, et al. Combined live and inactivated poliovirus vaccine to control poliomyelitis in a developing country—five years after. Dev Biol Stand 65:137–143, 1985.

436. Faden H, Modlin JF, Thoms ML, et al. Comparative evaluation of immunization with live attenuated and enhanced-potency poliovirus vaccines in childhood: systemic and local immune response. J Infect Dis 162:1291–1297, 1990.

437. Blatter MM, Starr S. Safety and Immunogenicity of a Combination DTP/eIPV Vaccine Presented in a Dual Chamber Syringe, in 2-Month-Old Infants. Swiftwater, PA, Connaught Laboratories, 1993.

438. Halsey NA, Blatter MM, Bader G. Safety and Immunogenicity of a Combination DTP/IPV Vaccine Administered to Infants in a Dual Chamber Syringe. Swiftwater, PA, Connaught Laboratories, 1994.

439. Halsey N, Blatter M, Bader G, et al. Inactivated poliovirus vaccine alone or sequential inactivated and oral poliovirus vaccine in two-, four-, and six-month-old infants with combination Haemophilus influenzae type b/hepatitis B vaccine. Pediatr Infect Dis J 16:675–679, 1997.

440. Ion-Nedelcu N, Strebel PM, Toma F, et al. Sequential use of inactivated and oral poliovirus vaccines: Dolj district, Romania, 1992–1994. J Infect Dis 175(suppl 1):S241–S246, 1997.

441. Moriniere BJ, van Loon FPL, Rhodes PH, et al. Immunogenicity of a supplemental dose of oral versus inactivated poliovirus vaccine. Lancet 341:1545–1550, 1993.

442. Tulchinsky T, Abed Y, Handsher R, et al. Successful control of poliomyelitis by a combined OPV/IPV polio vaccine program in the West Bank and Gaza, 1978–1993. Isr J Med Sci 30:489–494, 1994.

443. Goldblum N, Gerichter CB, Tulchinsky TH, Melnick JL. Poliomyelitis control in Israel, the West Bank and Gaza Strip: changing strategies with the goal of eradication in an endemic area. Bull World Health Organ 72:783–796, 1994.

444. Slater PE, Orenstein WA, Morag A, et al. Poliomyelitis outbreak in Israel in 1988: a report with two commentaries. Lancet 335:1192–1198, 1990.

445. Swartz TA, Handsher R. Israel in the elimination phase of poliomyelitis—achievements and remaining problems. Public Health Rev 21:99–106, 1993–1994.

446. Hanlon P, Hanlon L, Marsh V, et al. Serological comparisons of approaches to polio vaccination in The Gambia. Lancet 1:800–801, 1987.

447. Sutter RW, Suleiman AJM, Malankar PG, et al. Sequential use of inactivated poliovirus vaccine followed by oral poliovirus vaccine in Oman. J Infect Dis 175(suppl 1):S235–S240, 1997.

448. Faden H, Duffy L, Sun M, Shuff C. Long-term immunity to poliovirus in children immunized with live attenuated and enhanced-potency inactivated trivalent poliovirus vaccines. J Infect Dis 168:452–454, 1993.

449. Kew OM, Nottay BK, Hatch MH, et al. Multiple genetic changes can occur in the oral poliovaccines upon replication in humans. J Gen Virol 56(pt 2):337–347, 1981.

450. Cann AJ, Stanway G, Hughes PJ, et al. Reversion to virulence of the live attenuated Sabin type 3 oral poliovirus vaccine. Nucleic Acids Res 12:7787–7792, 1984.

451. Pollard SR, Dunn G, Cammack N, et al. Nucleotide sequence of a neurovirulent variant of the type 2 oral poliovirus vaccine. J Virol 63:4949–4951, 1989.

452. Evans DMA, Dunn G, Minor PD, et al. Increased neurovirulence associated with a single nucleotide change in a noncoding region of Sabin type 3 poliovaccine genome. Nature 314:548–550, 1985.

453. Dunn G, Begg NT, Cammack N, Minor PD. Virus excretion and mutation by infants following primary vaccination with live oral poliovaccine from two sources. J Med Virol 32:92–95, 1990.

454. Tatem JM, Weeks-Levy C, Mento SJ, et al. Oral poliovirus vaccine in the United States: molecular characterization of Sabin type 3 after replication in the gut of vaccinees. J Med Virol 35:101–109, 1991.

455. Ogra PL, Faden HS, Abraham R, et al. Effect of prior immunity on the shedding of virulent revertant virus in feces after oral immunization with live attenuated poliovirus vaccines. J Infect Dis 161:191–194, 1991.

456. Abraham R, Minor P, Dunn G, et al. Shedding of virulent poliovirus revertants during immunization with oral poliovirus vaccine after prior immunization with inactivated polio vaccine. J Infect Dis 168:1105–1109, 1993.

457. Murdin AD, Barreto L, Plotkin S. Inactivated poliovirus vaccine: past and present experience. Vaccine 14:735–746, 1996.

458. De-Xiang D, Xi-Min H, Wan-Jun L, et al. Immunisation of neonates with trivalent oral poliomyelitis vaccine (Sabin). Bull World Health Organ 64:853–860, 1986.

459. Halsey N, Galazka A. The efficacy of DTP and oral poliomyelitis immunization schedules initiated from birth to 12 weeks of age. Bull World Health Organ 63:1151–1169, 1985.

460. Galazka AM, Lauer BA, Henderson RH, Keja J. Indications and contraindications for vaccines used in the Expanded Programme on Immunization. Bull World Health Organ 62:357–366, 1984.

461. Weckx LY, Schmidt BJ, Hermann AA, et al. Early immunization of neonates with trivalent oral poliovirus vaccine. Bull World Health Organ 70:85–91, 1992.

462. Goodman T, Dalmiya N, de Benoist B, Schultink W. Polio as a platform: using national immunization days to deliver vitamin A supplements. Bull World Health Organ 78:305–314, 2000.

463. Ching P, Birmingham M, Goodman T, et al. The childhood mortality impact of integrating vitamin A supplements with immunization campaigns. Am J Public Health 90:1526–1529, 2000.

464. Birmingham ME, Aylward RB, Cochi SL, Hull HF. National Immunization Days: state of the art. J Infect Dis 175(suppl 1):S183–S188, 1997.

465. Expanded Programme on Immunization. Field Guide for Supplementary Activities Aimed at Achieving Polio Eradication. Geneva, World Health Organization, 1997.

466. Reichler MR, Kharabsheh S, Rhodes P, et al. Increased immunogenicity of oral poliovirus vaccine administered in mass vaccination campaigns compared with the routine vaccination program in Jordan. J Infect Dis 175(suppl 1):S198–S204, 1997.

467. Richardson G, Linkins RW, Eames M, et al. Immunogenicity of oral poliovirus vaccine administered in mass campaigns versus routine immunization programs. Bull World Health Organ 73:769–777, 1995.

468. Deming MS, Linkins RW, Jaiteh KO, Hull HF. The clinical efficacy of trivalent oral polio vaccine in The Gambia by season of vaccine administration. J Infect Dis 175(suppl 1):S254–S257, 1997.

469. Cochi SL, Hull HF, Sutter RW, et al. Global poliomyelitis eradication initiative: status report. J Infect Dis 175(suppl 1):1–292, 1997.

470. Dowdle WR, Hopkins DR (eds). The Eradication of Infectious Diseases: Report of the Dahlem Workshop on the Eradication of Infectious Diseases. Chichester, John Wiley & Sons, 1998.

471. Goodman RA, Foster KL, Throwbridge FL, Figueroa JP. Global disease elimination and eradication as public health strategies: proceedings of a conference held in Atlanta, Georgia, USA, 23–25 February 1998. Bull World Health Organ 76(suppl):S1–S162, 1998.

472. Fine PEM, Sutter RW, Orenstein WA. Stopping a polio outbreak in the post-eradication era. *In* Brown F (ed), Progress in Polio Eradication: Vaccine Strategies for the End Game. Development in Biology. Karger, Basel 105:129–147, 2001.

473. Department of Vaccines and Biologicals. New Polio Vaccines for the Post-Eradication Era, Geneva, 19–20 January 2000 (WHO/V&B/00.20). Geneva, World Health Organization, 2000.

474. Expanded Programme on Immunization. Report of the First Meeting of the Global Commission for the Certification of Poliomyelitis (WHO/EPI/GEN/95.6). Geneva, World Health Organization, 1995.

475. Department of Vaccines and Biologicals. Certification of Eradication of Poliomyelitis: Report of the Sixth Meeting of the Global Commission for the Certification of the Eradication of Poliomyelitis, Washington, DC, 28–29 March 2001 (WHO/V&B/01.15). Geneva, World Health Organization, 2001.

476. Global Programme for Vaccines and Immunization. Report of the Second Meeting of the Global Commission for the Certification of the Eradication of Poliomyelitis, Geneva, 1 May 1997 (WHO/EPI/GEN 98.03). Geneva, World Health Organization, 1998.

477. Department of Vaccines and Biologicals. WHO Global Action Plan for Laboratory Containment of Wild Polioviruses (WHO/V&B/99.32). Geneva, World Health Organization, 1999.

478. Centers for Disease Control and Prevention. Global progress toward laboratory containment of wild polioviruses, June 2001. MMWR 50:620–623, 2001.

479. Mulders MN, Reimerink JHJ, Koopmans MPG, van Loon AM, van der Avoort HGAM. Genetic analysis of wild poliovirus importations into the Netherlands (1979–1995). J Infect Dis 176:617–624, 1997.

480. Pallansch M, Staples M. Wild poliovirus found in stored potential infectious materials. Polio Lab Network Q Update 8:1–2, 2002.

481. Mas Lago P. Eradication of poliomyelitis in Cuba: a historical perspective. Bull World Health Organ 77:681–687, 1999.

482. Mas Lago P, Caceres VM, Galindo MA, et al. Persistence of vaccine-derived poliovirus following a mass vaccination campaign in Cuba: implications for stopping polio vaccination after global eradication. Int J Epidemiol 30:1029–1034, 2001.

483. Plotkin SA. Commentary: Cuba libre of poliovirus. Int J Epidemiol 30:1034, 2001.

484. Kortepeter MG, Parker GW. Potential biological weapons threats. Emerg Infect Dis 5:523–527, 1999.

485. Rotz LD, Khan AS, Lillibridge SR, et al. Public health assessment of potential biological terrorism agents. Emerg Infect Dis 8:225–230, 2002.

486. Cello J, Paul AV, Wimmer E. Chemical synthesis of poliovirus cDNA: generation of infectious virus in the absence of natural template. Science 297:1016–1018, 2002.

487. Savilahti E, Klemola T, Carlsson B, et al. Inadequacy of mucosal IgM antibodies in selective IgA deficiency: excretion of attenuated polio viruses is prolonged. J Clin Immunol 8:89–94, 1988.

488. Expanded Programme on Immunization. Report of the Meeting on the Scientific Basis for Stopping Polio Immunization, Geneva, 23–25 March 1998 (WHO/EPI/GEN/98.12). Geneva, World Health Organization, 1998.

489. Dove AW, Racaniello VR. The polio eradication effort: should vaccine eradication be next? Science 277:779–780, 1997.

490. Hull HF, Aylward RB. Ending polio immunization. Science 277:780, 1997.

491. Henderson DA. Countering the posteradication threat of smallpox and polio. Clin Infect Dis 34:79–83, 2002.

492. Global Programme for Vaccines and Immunization. Vaccine Research and Development: Report of the Technical Review Group Meeting, 9–10 June 1997. Achievements and Plan of Action, July 1997–June 1998. Geneva, World Health Organization, 1997.

493. Ghendon YUZ, Sanakoyeva II. Comparison of the resistance of the intestinal tract to poliomyelitis vaccine (Sabin strains) in persons after naturally and experimentally acquired immunity. Acta Virol 5:265–273, 1961.

494. Ho TW, McKhann GM, Griffin JW. Human autoimmune neuropathies. Annu Rev Neurosci 21:187–226, 1998.

495. Sutter RW, Brink EW, Cochi SL, et al. A new epidemiologic and laboratory classification system for paralytic poliomyelitis cases. Am J Public Health 79:495–498, 1989.

Chapter 26

Rubella Vaccine

STANLEY A. PLOTKIN • SUSAN REEF

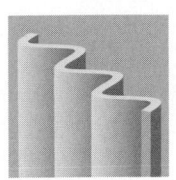

Rubella

just
a dead comma of flesh where
the ear should hang, a poxed hole
mottled in bone, and she holds you, as you
shiver
curled against the muffled songs we sing as
we pass by
in our doctor's clothes and then leave you alone
again, to redefine
the white surgery waiting-room with glazed dum-dum eyes,
not even warming
the living gel of your pulped brain.

MICHAEL O'REILLY. FALLING ON DEAF EARS.
PERSPECT BIOL MED 39:204, 1992.

Discovered in the late 18th century, becoming prominent in 1941, and controlled in developed countries during the last 30 years, rubella is an interesting case history in relation to vaccine development and application. Although rubella is ordinarily a mild exanthematous viral infection in children and young adults, it assumes greater importance in pregnant women, from whom the causative virus is often transmitted to their fetuses, with disastrous effects.

The first researchers to distinguish the disease from other exanthemas were German physicians, hence, the common English language eponym *German measles*.[1] In 1841, a British physician reported an outbreak in a boys' school in India and coined the term *rubella*, a Latin diminutive meaning "little red."[2] For the next hundred years, rubella received scant attention, but in 1941, Norman McAlister Gregg,[3] an Australian ophthalmologist, published a report relating congenital cataracts to maternal rubella. Gregg noticed an unusual number of infants with cataracts, and he was curious enough to investigate. It is said that a crucial clue was a conversation he overheard in his waiting room between two mothers who were discussing the rubella they both had sustained in pregnancy during the Australian outbreak of 1940.[4] After several years of inattention and skepticism, Gregg's original observation was followed by reports of Australian,[5] Swedish,[6] American,[7] and British[8] epidemiologists and teratologists confirming the role of rubella in congenital cataracts and also noting the simultaneous

association of heart disease and deafness in the infants. Thus the characteristic congenital rubella triad was established.

The next 20 years were spent in trying to isolate the causative agent and in obtaining statistics on the risk of fetal abnormality after maternal rubella. Various estimates of the risk of fetal disease were made, ranging from high to low. The disparity in estimates stemmed from the absence of a definitive diagnostic test and consequent misdiagnosis of rubella in the mother. In late 1962, a breakthrough came in the form of the first isolations of rubella virus by Weller and Neva[9] in Boston and by Parkman, Beuscher, and Artenstein[10] in Washington, DC. The former group detected the presence of rubella virus by cytopathic effect in human amnion cells, whereas the latter group developed a technique dependent on interference with the growth of enteroviruses in African green monkey kidney (AGMK) cell culture. The AGMK technique soon became the standard method for virus isolation.

Meanwhile, a pandemic of rubella started in Europe in the 1962 to 1963 season, with spread to the United States and pandemic disease in 1964 to 1965. As a result, from 1964 to 1966, thousands of pregnancies were affected by rubella, leaving behind a wake of medically induced abortions and abnormal infants.[11,12] The pandemic led to the recognition of an expanded congenital rubella syndrome (CRS), which added hepatitis, splenomegaly, thrombocytopenia, encephalitis, mental retardation, and numerous other anomalies to the already described deafness, cataracts, and heart disease.[1,2,13] The pandemic also made it obvious that a vaccine was needed, and many groups set to work.

Between 1965 and 1967, several attenuated rubella strains were developed and reached clinical trials.[14–16] In 1969 and 1970, rubella vaccine entered into commercial use in Europe and North America. Since the late 1970s, vaccination has had a major impact on the epidemiology of rubella and CRS.

Background

Clinical Description

Acquired Rubella

Rubella is spread by aerosols, and primary implantation and replication occurs in the nasopharynx. The incubation period of rubella is 14 to 21 days, with most patients developing a rash 14 to 17 days after exposure.[17] During the first week after exposure, there are no symptoms. In the second week, lymphadenopathy may be noted, particularly occipital and postauricular, and virus cultures reveal rubella virus in the nasopharynx. Later in the second week, virus appears in the blood. At about this time, there may be a prodromal illness consisting of low-grade fever (<39.0°C), malaise, and mild conjunctivitis. If not already present, the aforementioned lymphadenopathy is likely to develop.

At the end of the incubation period, a maculopapular erythematous rash appears on the face and neck. The rash may be difficult to detect, particularly on pigmented skin, and is more prominent after hot showers or baths. During a course of 1 to 3 days, the rash spreads downward and begins to fade. Pharyngeal virus excretion is particularly important up to 4 days after rash onset, and virus excretion in the pharynx and urine may continue for another 1 to 2 weeks, but viremia ends with the onset of the rash.[18] The evolution of acquired rubella is illustrated in Figure 26–1.

Although acquired rubella is thought of as a benign disease, arthralgia and arthritis commonly are observed in adults, and chronic arthritis has been reported after rubella infection.[19,20] Other less common complications are thrombocytopenia[21] and encephalitis, which may be fatal.[22,23] Encephalitis occurs in approximately 1 in 6000 cases and is of the postinfectious type, although the limited available pathologic data show little evidence of demyelination.[24] In a Japanese outbreak, the incidence of encephalitis was 1 in 1600 cases of rubella.[25] In addition, there is a rare late syndrome of progressive rubella panencephalitis.[26,27] Guillain-Barré syndrome after rubella has also been reported.[28] Antibodies to rubella and measles structural proteins are elevated in autoimmune chronic active hepatitis, but whether this is related to viral persistence is unknown.[29]

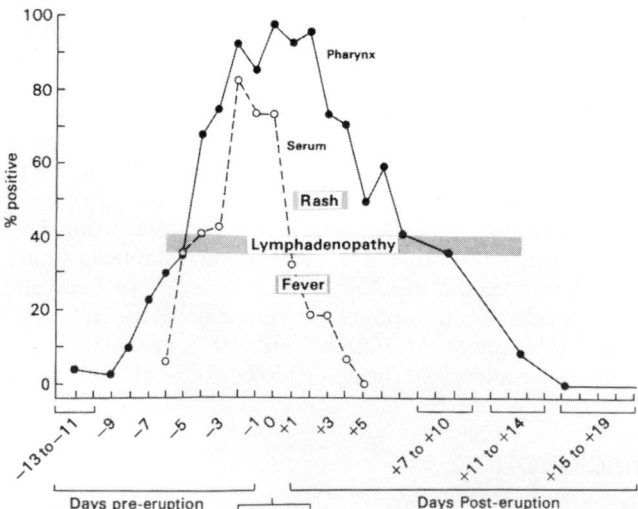

FIGURE 26–1 ■ The sequence of events in acquired rubella infections, showing the relationship between onset of rash and other clinical symptoms and recovery of rubella virus from diagnostic specimens.

TABLE 26–1 ■ Prominent Clinical Findings in Congenital Rubella Syndrome

Cataracts	Intrauterine growth retardation
Retinitis	Metaphyseal rarefactions
Microphthalmia	
Glaucoma	Hepatosplenomegaly
	Thrombocytopenic purpura
Cochlear deafness	
Central auditory imperception	Interstitial pneumonitis
Patent ductus arteriosus	Diabetes
Peripheral pulmonic artery	Hypothyroidism
stenosis	
Encephalitis	
Microcephaly	
Mental retardation	
Autism	

Modified from Cooper LZ, Preblud SR, Alford CA. Rubella. *In* Remington JS, Klein JO (eds). Infectious Diseases of the Fetus and Newborn Infant (4th ed). Philadelphia, WB Saunders, 1995, p 288.

Congenital Rubella

Rubella is the archetypical fetal infectious pathogen (see *Pathogenesis as It Relates to Prevention* below). Because all organs of the fetus are affected, it is not surprising that CRS comprises a lengthy list of abnormalities, both teratologic, resulting from interference with organogenesis, and inflammatory, involving organs such as the liver and spleen[30] (Table 26–1).

The time of infection during gestation is important in relation to the fetal outcome; early infection tends to result in serious ocular or cardiac disease, whereas infection late in the first half of pregnancy is likely to result in deafness. However, the relationship between gestational age and abnormality can be overemphasized because fetal infection, once established, spreads to all organs, and damage may be cumulative. Table 26–2 demonstrates that organ specificity is only generally related to the stage of gestational infection with rubella virus. The most common congenital defects are sensorineural deafness, cataracts, pigmentary retinopathy,

TABLE 26–2 ■ Age of Gestation at Time of Rubella in Relation to Abnormalities Observed

	Month of Gestation Measured from Last Menstrual Period				
	0*	1	2	3	4
Birth weight <2500 g	0/1[†]	9/21	9/21	10/18	0/2
<38 weeks' gestation	0/1	5/21	2/21	4/18	0/2
Growth retardation	0/1	7/21	5/20	7/17	0/2
Ocular defects	0/1	14/21	9/21	9/18	0/2
Cardiac defects	0/1	17/21	13/21	6/18	0/2
Deafness	0/1	8/18	10/18	11/17	2/2
Mental retardation	1/1	7/20	7/20	8/16	0/2
Microcephaly	1/1	3/18	2/19	4/17	0/2

*Before conception.

†Ratio of number of patients with condition to total number for whom information is available.

From Plotkin SA, Cochran W, Lindquist J, et al. Congenital rubella syndrome in late infancy. JAMA 200:435–441, 1967, with permission. Copyright 1967, American Medical Association.

and patent ductus arteriosus, but a myriad of other defects occur, including glaucoma, peripheral pulmonic stenosis, endocrinopathies including diabetes, hyperimmunoglobulinemia M,[31] microcephaly, and mental retardation. Ocular defects are particularly varied, including abnormalities of the cornea, the lens, and the retina.[32] A recent analysis of prospective studies for distribution of clinical manifestations of CRS is summarized in Table 26–3.[33]

Various estimates have been made of the incidence of fetal abnormalities after internal infection.[7,34–39] Most prospective studies of the incidence of fetal rubella have accepted clinical diagnosis of rubella in the mother for case inclusion. If only virologically confirmed maternal rubella is considered, the rate of transmission to the fetus during the first trimester of pregnancy is about 80%.[35,40–42] The two most reliable studies, one from United States data[36] and the other from United Kingdom data,[35] are tabulated in Table 26–4. The first 12 weeks of pregnancy are clearly the most dangerous time for rubella infection in the mother. The incidence of fetal disease declines during the next 4 weeks, and in the 16th to the 20th weeks only deafness has been reported as a complication. Preconceptional rubella rarely results in fetal infection, but rashes that occur within 12 days of the last menstrual period carry proven risk.[43,44] In an Irish epidemic, 71% of fetuses infected early in pregnancy were affected.[45] In contrast, some Japanese workers[46] have claimed that rubella virus is less teratogenic in their country, but these claims have not been supported.[25]

Damage caused by congenital rubella infection does not stop at birth. Hearing may worsen, glaucoma may become apparent, and even late cataracts are possible. Retinal detachments and esophageal problems are common later in life.[47] Interestingly, autism is a feature of some late-onset neurologic disease in CRS patients. In addition, a variety of syndromes thought to be autoimmune, including diabetes

TABLE 26–4 ■ Fetal Abnormality Induced by Confirmed Rubella at Various Stages of Pregnancy

Stage of Pregnancy (wk)	United Kingdom Study (% Defective)*	United States Study (% Defective)†
≤4		70
5–8		40
≤10	90	
11–12	33	
9–12		25
13–14	11	
15–16	24	
13–16		40
≥17	0	8

*Data from Miller E, Cradock-Watson JE, Pollock TM. Consequences of confirmed maternal rubella at successive stages of pregnancy. Lancet 2:781–784, 1982.
†Data from South MA, Sever JL. Teratogen update: the congenital rubella syndrome. Teratology 31:297–307, 1985.

mellitus and thyroiditis, each occur in about 6% of CRS survivors.[47,48]

Virology

The agent of rubella is a cubical, medium-sized (60 to 70 nm), lipid-enveloped virus with an RNA genome belonging to the togavirus family and the genus *Rubivirus*. Although the other togaviruses are arthropod borne, there is no evidence for such transmission of rubella. Frey[49] has reviewed the virology of rubella. Apart from the complex lipid envelope derived from the host cell, rubella virus is composed of three proteins, two embedded in the envelope in the form of spikes (E1 and E2) and one (C) composing the capsid. E1 is a glycoprotein with neutralizing and hemagglutinating

TABLE 26–3 ■ Frequencies of Selected Defects in Infants with Congenital Rubella Syndrome: Comparison of Data from Prospective Studies and Data Presented in a Standard Pediatric Infectious Disease Textbook

Clinical Manifestation	No. of Studies	Study Subjects*	Previously Reported Subjects (%)†
Hearing impairment	10	68/113 (60)	80–90
Heart defect	9	45/100 (45)	—
Patent ductus arteriosus	3	9/45 (20)	30
Peripheral pulmonic stenosis	3	6/49 (12)	25‡
Microcephaly	3	13/49 (27)	Rare
Cataracts	3	16/65 (25)	35
Low birth weight (<2500 g)	2	5/22 (23)	50–85
Hepatosplenomegaly	6	13/67 (19)	10–20
Purpura	5	11/65 (17)	5–10
Mental retardation	2	2/15 (13)	10–20
Meningoencephalitis	3	5/49 (10)	10–20
Radiolucent bone	3	3/43 (7)	10–20
Retinopathy	3	2/44 (5)	35

*Number of infants with congenital rubella syndrome/number of study subjects (percentage in parentheses).
†Frequencies presented in textbook data.
‡Includes pulmonary arterial hypoplasia, supravalvular stenosis, valvular stenosis, and peripheral branch stenosis.
From Reef SE, Plotkin S, Cordero JF, et al. Preparing for elimination of congenital rubella syndrome (CRS): summary of a workshop on CRS elimination in the United States. Clin Infect Dis 31:85–95, 2000, with permission.

epitopes, while the function of the E2 glycoprotein is unclear.[50] The three proteins, which have molecular masses of 60,000 kDa (E1), 42,000 to 47,000 kDa (E2), and 30,000 kDa (C), are derived from a polypeptide of 110 kDa that is translated from a 245-kDa messenger RNA.[51–53]

The RNA genome of rubella virus contains about 10,000 nucleotides and is infectious,[54,55] and complementary DNA copies facilitate study of its transcripts.[56] The replication strategy of rubella virus is similar to that of the alpha viruses in that both full-length and subgenomic RNAs are produced, and it is from the subgenomic RNA that viral structural proteins are translated. Three other proteins are produced by the virus in infected cells but are not incorporated into the virion.[57]

There is only one serotype of rubella virus, and analyses of sequence variation among occidental isolates show high conservation of amino acid structure (0% to 3.3% differences), with less conservation of isolates from Asia (up to 7%).[58,59] An international collaborative group[60] confirmed that isolates from North America, Europe, and Japan were closely related to each other and form genotype I, whereas genotype II comprises some strains from China, Korea, and India.[61] The genetic differences between genotypes do not appear to translate into antigenic differences, despite amino acid changes of 3% to 6% in viral proteins.[62] No significant antigenic drift has occurred in recent years, and isolates from vaccinees showed little variation from vaccine strains.

Rubella virus grows in many different primary, semicontinuous, and continuous cells of mammalian origin. In human amnion cells, it produces a subtle cytopathic effect. More pronounced cytopathic effects, sufficient to allow plaque formation, are produced in continuous cell lines, such as rabbit kidney (RK13) and baby hamster kidney (BHK-21).[18] Even in those cell lines, fresh isolates frequently are not highly cytopathogenic and require adaptation by serial passage. High passage generates defective-interfering RNA and particles.[63] The virus also can be grown in monolayers of RK13 or BHK-21 cell lines, in which plaque morphology varies by virus strain.

Virus isolation is generally performed in primary AGMK cell culture, in which virus growth is detected by "challenging" the cultures with a cytopathogenic agent such as echovirus 11. If rubella virus has infected the cultures, the action of echovirus 11 is blocked; the presence of rubella virus is inferred by this interference. Confirmation is performed by another technique, such as neutralization or fluorescence with specific antirubella serum.[64]

Pathogenesis as It Relates to Prevention

The pathogenesis of acquired rubella infection provides two points at which immune intervention could have an effect. The first point is in the nasopharynx, where the virus first replicates and from which it spreads to local lymph nodes. Secretory immunoglobulin (Ig) A antibody in the nasopharynx, induced by prior disease or vaccination, can block mucosal replication. The second point begins about a week into the incubation period, at which time the viremia can be blocked by the presence of antibody, either passively or actively acquired.

During viremia in a pregnant woman, the virus may infect the placenta. Placental replication appears to precede fetal infections, leading to entrance of virus into the fetal circulation, from which it infects fetal organs.[65] In vitro experiments show that human embryonic cells of many different lineages are susceptible to the virus and develop chronic infection.[66] The same phenomenon occurs in vivo, except that only a few cells are infected at any one time.[67] If the infected cells are stimulated to divide, either artificially in vitro or in the course of embryologic development in vivo, there is an inhibition of mitosis[66,68] that may be mediated in part by a soluble protein inhibitor[69] or by the induction of apoptosis.[70a,70–72] Organogenesis is thus disrupted. In a few organs, including the lens, cochlea, and brain, the damage caused by the virus is more cytopathic.[73] Destruction of endothelial cells leads to vasculitis and ischemia. Cytologic studies show that the cell skeleton and mitochondria both are damaged by rubella virus replication.[74] In summary, the action of rubella virus on the fetus is mediated by a combination of intracellular pathology, inhibition of cellular replication, and apoptosis.[74,75]

Diagnosis

Methods for the diagnosis of acquired and congenital rubella are summarized in Table 26–5. Clinical diagnosis of acquired infection is so inaccurate as to be useless without laboratory support. Isolation of virus can be accomplished from the blood and nasopharynx during the prodromal period and from the nasopharynx for as long as 2 weeks after eruption, although the likelihood of virus recovery is

TABLE 26–5 ■ Laboratory Diagnosis of Acquired and Congenital Rubella

Test	Specimen	When Positive	
		Acquired Rubella	Congenital Rubella
Virus isolation	Throat, urine, blood	First week of illness	At birth, declining thereafter
RT-PCR	Amniotic fluid, placenta	NA	Throughout pregnancy
IgM antibody	Serum	2 mo postillness	At birth and first year of life
IgG antibody rise	Sera	Fourfold increase between acute and convalescent	NA
Low IgG antibody avidity	Serum	2 mo postillness	At birth and years later
IgG antibody persistence	Serum	NA	Beyond 6 mo of age, until exposure to infection or vaccination

IgG, immunoglobulin G; IgM, immunoglobulin M; NA, not applicable; RT-PCR, reverse transcriptase–polymerase chain reaction.

sharply reduced by 4 days after the rash. AGMK cells or the RK13 cell line are generally used for virus isolation. Owing to the slow growth of the virus in tissue culture, virus isolation is often bypassed in favor of serologic diagnosis.

The initial serologic diagnosis was feasible because rubella virus hemagglutinates red blood cells, particularly of avian origin.[76] This viral hemagglutinin is used as an antigen for measurement of antibodies by hemagglutination-inhibition (HI) testing. Because HI tests are labor intensive, other serologic examinations that are amenable to mass testing have come into use, such as latex agglutination, indirect hemagglutination, enzyme-linked immunosorbent assay (ELISA), and fluorescence inhibition.[42,77] Any of these methods may be used to detect seropositivity to rubella. Detection of antibodies in saliva or urine could simplify testing in developing countries, but commercial kits are not available.[78–81]

Serologic diagnosis depends on the demonstration of a fourfold rise in titer between acute and convalescent specimens or a demonstration of IgM antibody in the acute specimen.[77] The standard serologic test was the HI test, but other tests that are easier to perform and are more sensitive have come into use, including latex agglutination, hemolysis in gel, and ELISA. For IgM testing, ELISA is the predominant assay in use, and results may be positive for up to 6 weeks after the acute infection. Newer methods for detection of IgM antibodies are more accurate.[82]

Susceptibility has been defined as an HI antibody titer of less than 1:8, a hemolysis in gel result of less than 10 IU, or an optical density by ELISA below the limit set by the manufacturer. Titers at the borderline level are difficult to evaluate, but the consensus is that, although in the majority of cases they reflect immunity, vaccination is the safest response.[83]

Assays for antibody avidity and for responses to specific proteins or peptides have come into use for diagnosis of recent infection.[84] Low-avidity antibodies indicate recent infection, with maturation to high avidity by about 2 months postexanthem. Pustowoit and Liebert[85] studied various serologic modalities and found that low levels of antibody to the major neutralizing epitope on the E1 protein, poor response to the E2 protein, and low IgG avidity for rubella virus were highly predictive of recent infection in both mother and infant.

In contrast to the situation with acquired infection, the recognition of the combination of cataracts, heart disease, and deafness provides a clinical means of diagnosis of CRS that is reasonably accurate.[86] However, laboratory confirmation is always desirable both because isolated abnormalities may occur and for public health reasons.

Congenital rubella infection can be diagnosed in the infant by the detection of virus, viral genome, IgM antibodies, low-avidity IgG antibodies, or antibodies persisting beyond the predicted decay of passively transmitted maternal antibodies. Virus often can be isolated from tissues obtained at biopsy or autopsy or during surgical procedures such as cataract extraction,[87] but more often nasopharyngeal swabs, urine specimens, or cerebrospinal fluid serve as the sources. Almost always one or more of these sources are positive for virus at birth, gradually becoming negative during the first year of life.[88] In severe cases, virus excretion may persist for several years.[89]

The polymerase chain reaction (PCR) has been adapted to the detection of rubella RNA by reverse transcription and amplification.[90] The method appears to be sensitive and specific[91,92] and is particularly useful for prenatal detection of rubella infection of the fetus.[93] A negative PCR performed on fetal material is good evidence against intrauterine rubella.[44]

IgM antibodies are present in the infant for as long as a year after birth, and low-avidity IgG antibodies may persist for longer periods. Persistence of IgG antibodies beyond 6 months of age can be detected in 95% of infants with CRS.[94] An infant with seropositive results for rubella after 6 months of age who has not received rubella vaccine is likely to have been congenitally infected. Moreover, sensitization to proliferation of lymphocytes after stimulation with rubella antigens is often negative in CRS infants, even when they are seropositive,[95] and this test may be used for diagnosis in children younger than 3 years.

Epidemiology

Acquired Infection

Rubella is a worldwide infection, as may be inferred from serologic surveys conducted in many different countries.[96,97] The factors that give rubella its epidemiologic characteristics are respiratory spread that is greater in crowded societies, different age at infection, and periodic disappearance from geographic areas, only to reappear in epidemic form when susceptibles accumulate. As is true of other diseases, some individual rubella patients excrete large amounts of virus in respiratory secretions and are highly infectious "spreaders."[98] The basic reproductive rate before vaccination was estimated to be 6 to 7 in developed countries and up to 12 in crowded developing countries.[99,100] In Europe there was wide variation in rubella force of infection between countries, with reproductive rates ranging from 3 to 8.[101] Much childhood infection is asymptomatic and therefore unrecognized. Day care centers also promote early infection with rubella. In island countries and in countries that are less crowded, the average age at rubella infection is older, and many children reach puberty still in a seronegative state.[102] Under these circumstances, introduction of the virus into places where young people congregate results in epidemic spread.[98] Thus schools, colleges, and military camps are all places where rubella is likely to become epidemic. Outbreaks at the stock exchange on Wall Street illustrate the potential effect of bringing seronegative individuals together in close quarters. In fact, rubella is highly efficient at infecting susceptible persons in certain epidemiologic situations.[103–105]

In the United States, the epidemiology of rubella before vaccination was both endemic and epidemic.[11] Rubella tended to occur each spring, primarily in schoolchildren 6 to 10 years of age but also in older individuals. Superimposed on this occurrence was a cycle of major epidemics at 7-year intervals (Fig. 26–2). Susceptibility in young adults varied from 10% to 20%, with the lower figure being found after an epidemic. Similarly, in Israel, approximately 9% of women were infected during a 1972 rubella outbreak[106]; however, even after the epidemic, a significant pool of susceptible individuals remained.

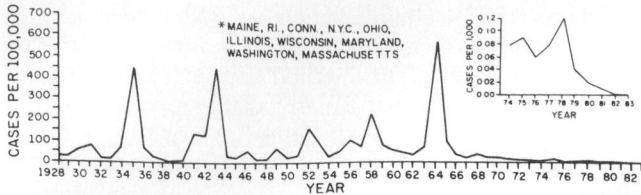

FIGURE 26–2 ■ Rubella incidence in 10 selected areas* of the United States, 1928 to 1983. (From Williams NM, Preblud SR. Rubella and congenital rubella surveillance, 1983. MMWR 33:1SS–10SS, 1984, with permission.)

The epidemiology of rubella in developing countries can be deduced from the seroprevalence of rubella antibodies. The large variation seen in seroprevalence suggests that rubella occurs in sporadic epidemics except where population density is high. In the metropolis of São Paulo, Brazil, nearly everyone is seropositive by 20 years of age,[107] whereas in rural Mexico, seropositivity varies from 29% to 76%.[108] Surveillance of rash disease in South America shows that rubella infection is ubiquitous. Cutts and colleagues[108a] reviewed rubella susceptibility data from 45 developing countries and found remarkable differences among them not correlated with geography. For example, Malaysia, Peru, and Nigeria were among the countries where more than 25% of women were found to be seronegative. Studies done in Lagos, Nigeria, and Izmir, Turkey, confirm the low seroprevalence in women of child-bearing age.[109,110]

Congenital Infection

Most information on the epidemiology of CRS is available from the United Kingdom and the United States. Table 26–6 presents the tally of fetal damage caused by rubella subsequent to the 1963 to 1964 outbreak.[12] A minimum of 30,000 infants were damaged by intrauterine rubella, for an incidence rate of 100 per 10,000 pregnancies. In Philadelphia, the rate was also as high as 1% of pregnancies.[111] After that outbreak, CRS rates fell to 4 to 8 per

TABLE 26–6 ■ **Estimated Morbidity Associated with the 1963 to 1964 Rubella Epidemic**

Clinical Events	Cases
Rubella cases	12,500,000
Arthritis-arthralgia	159,375
Encephalitis	2084
Deaths	
Excess neonatal deaths	2100
Other deaths	60
Total deaths	2160
Excess fetal wastage	6250
Congenital rubella syndrome	
Deaf children	8055
Deaf-blind children	3580
Mentally retarded children	1790
Other congenital rubella syndrome	6575
Total congenital rubella syndrome	20,000
Therapeutic abortions	5000

From National Communicable Disease Center. Rubella surveillance. Bethesda, MD, U.S. Department of Health, Education, and Welfare, 1969.

10,000 pregnancies until 1970, when the first vaccines were licensed. Since then, the rate has declined further to a vanishingly low incidence of less than 0.01 per 10,000 pregnancies.[112] Table 26–7 gives the current surveillance criteria for CRS in the United States.[33] The epidemiology of CRS in the United Kingdom has been similar to that in the United States, with rates of approximately 4.6 per 10,000 births in the prevaccine era.[113]

The epidemiology of CRS is really known only for a few countries of the world. Little information is available for the countries in South America, Africa, and most of Asia, although such data suggest that CRS is common even in the developing world.[114,115] For example, in India, 26% of 90 infants investigated for congenital malformations had serologic evidence of CRS.[116] Two other Indian studies[117,118] showed that 10–25% of children with nontraumatic cataracts and 15% of infants suspected of having congenital infection were rubella positive. Rubella was also frequently the cause of sensorineural hearing loss in Saudi Arabian children.[118] Retrospective analysis of a recent epidemic in Kumasi, Ghana, gave an incidence of 0.8 per 1000 live births.[119] A review of worldwide data concerning CRS revealed rates in developing countries varying between 0.6 and 2.2 per 1000 live births, similar to rates seen in developed countries before universal vaccination.[100]

A virulence factor has been postulated for rubella strains, and it has been argued from laboratory and clinical data that rubella virus is not teratogenic in Japan. Kono and colleagues[46] reported that Japanese strains had no effect on pregnant rabbits, whereas American strains were transmitted across the placenta from dams to fetal rabbits. In addition, they reported that on the main island of Honshu, no CRS was reported even though rubella outbreaks were evident.[120] However, after careful analysis of rubella on the southern Japanese island of Kyushu, Ueda and associates[121] showed that the rates of both rubella and CRS were high. They concluded that the apparently low rate of CRS on Honshu is due to a high seropositivity rate in adult women and a low clinical reporting rate of CRS.

CRS shows a predisposition to affect infants of young mothers, presumably because these women are more likely to enter pregnancy in a seronegative state. Women in contact with populations in which rubella outbreaks occur frequently, such as military recruits and school-age children, are more likely to be exposed. Military dependents and schoolteachers are thus at increased risk. Pregnant women with older children are also at greater risk.

Although rubella outbreaks may be explosive, they frequently do not exhaust all susceptible persons in large populations, and thus a history of having been exposed to a rubella outbreak does not necessarily indicate immunity to rubella. Even more important is the fact that 10% to 85% of infections in various outbreaks have been inapparent or at least have been without evidence of eruption.[104] Infection without rash in pregnancy can still lead to fetal disease, although the risk may be lower than that after symptomatic infection with rash.[122]

Significance as a Public Health Problem

The seriousness of congenital rubella as a public health problem can be gauged by the results of the last major

TABLE 26–7 ■ Clinical Description and Criteria for Congenital Rubella Syndrome (CRS) Case Definition for the United States

	1999 Revised Definition	Case Classification
Clinical case definition	Presence of defect(s) or laboratory data consistent with congenital rubella infection. Infants with CRS usually present with >1 sign or symptom consistent with congenital rubella infection. However, infants may present with a single defect. Hearing impairment is the most common single defect.	Confirmed if lab findings also positive.
Clinical description	An illness usually manifests in infancy, resulting from rubella infection in utero and characterized by signs or symptoms in the following categories: category A—cataracts/ congenital glaucoma, congenital heart disease (most commonly patent ductus arterious or peripheral pulmonary artery stenosis), hearing impairment, pigmentary retinopathy; category B—purpura, hepatosplenomegaly, jaundice, microcephaly, developmental delay, mental retardation, meningoencephalitis, radiolucent bone disease.	Probable if ≥2 findings. Possible if only one finding.
Laboratory criteria for diagnosis	Isolation of rubella virus or demonstration of rubella-specific IgM antibody or of infant rubella IgG antibody level that persists at a higher level and for a longer period than expected from passive transfer of maternal antibody (i.e., does not drop at the expected rate of a two-fold dilution per month); PCR positive for rubella virus.	Congenital rubella infection (CRI), if laboratory finding only.

IgG, immunoglobulin G; IgM, immunoglobulin M; PCR, polymerase chain reaction.
From Reef SE, Plotkin S, Cordero JF, et al. Preparing for elimination of congenital rubella syndrome (CRS): summary of a workshop on CRS elimination in the United States. Clin Infect Dis 31:89, 2000, with permission.

American epidemic in 1964 to 1965 (see Table 26–6). An estimated 12.5 million rubella cases occurred, including approximately 2000 cases of encephalitis. Over 30,000 pregnancies were affected by this epidemic. Of these pregnancies, about 5000 pregnant women chose to have surgical abortions, and about 6250 lost fetuses to spontaneous abortions. Another 2100 infants were stillborn or died soon after birth.[12] CRS occurred in 20,000 infants who survived pregnancy. Of these, 11,600 were deaf, 3580 blind, and about 1800 mentally retarded. The human misery imposed by such severe damage can well be imagined. The economic burden has been estimated to be $221,660 per child with CRS, and the total cost of the epidemic may have been $1.5 billion.[12]

Before the use of vaccine, rubella epidemics involved about 5% of the population, although only approximately 10% of these cases were reported to public health authorities.[123] In the years between epidemics, rates were about one tenth of the epidemic peaks, but CRS continued at a low endemic rate even in those years.

Analysis of the age distribution of acquired rubella in the prevaccine era showed 60% of cases in children younger than 10 years and 23% in those older than 15 years.[124] As discussed subsequently, application of vaccine in children did not reduce by much the incidence in adolescents and adults, and CRS continued to occur for some years after the introduction of vaccination.

Lest it be thought that rubella infection in pregnancy has lost its danger, a more recent outbreak among unvaccinated Amish people living in Pennsylvania serves as a corrective.[125] Young Amish women were 20% seronegative at the beginning of the outbreak, and infections in pregnancy were common. More than 8% of Amish infants gave laboratory evidence of infection, and more than 2% had CRS. Of infants born after first-trimester infection, 90% had confirmed or possible CRS. Aside from isolated religious or philosophical objectors, the contemporary main foci of acquired and congenital rubella in the United States are immigrants from Latin America, where vaccination has not been practiced.[126]

In the United Kingdom, CRS estimates before the use of vaccine were only about 200 to 300 cases per year, but that figure was from a passive ascertainment system.[113] In Australia, about one baby with CRS per 2000 births was recorded before vaccine.[127] During an outbreak of rubella in Israel, there were 1441 confirmed infections in pregnant women, most of whom had abortions.[128] Projection of the experience to the United States would be equivalent to 75,000 pregnancies complicated by rubella. In France, 16% of congenital cataract cases were attributable to CRS.[129] A follow-up study of an epidemic in Poland showed that 15% of pregnant women had been infected. The rate of CRS after first-, second-, and third-trimester infection was 78%, 33%, and 0%, respectively.[130] The picture of rubella in the developing world is complex.[100,131] Although a frequent seroepidemiologic finding has been a high rate of infection early in life,[105] there are many exceptions, including island populations,[132] several West African countries, the city of Calcutta, and Morocco.[133] Thus the pattern is that of a disease that comes in epidemic waves, and that may be absent from an area for some time.

Clusters of CRS have been reported in developing countries,[134,135] and there is little doubt that, wherever seronegative pregnant women are exposed to a rubella outbreak,

CRS cases will follow. A study conducted in Chennai, India, confirmed the presence of rubella virus in 10% of congenital cataract cases, with serologic evidence of infection in 25%.[136]

The most complete analysis of CRS in developing countries was performed by Cutts and Vynnycky.[137] They modeled the incidence of the disease in the many countries not using vaccination and derived an estimate of 110,000 annual cases of CRS throughout the world, although the confidence limits were wide, ranging from 14,000 to 308,000 cases. Their estimates are shown in Table 26–8, which suggests a mean incidence of about 1.7 CRS cases per 1000 live births.

Passive Immunization

Ordinary Immune Serum Globulin

Because most adults have had rubella, ordinary immune serum globulin (ISG) contains rubella antibody.[138] By the HI test, rubella antibody titers of about 1:16 are found in immune globulins.[139] Before the development of vaccine, ISG frequently was offered to pregnant women who had been exposed to rubella in the hope that it would prevent fetal infection. The results were equivocal, but, if large doses (20 to 30 mL) of material with high titer were given, frank symptoms and viremia could be prevented.[140–143] Experimental studies confirmed the efficacy of passive antibody in preventing clinical rubella,[144,145] but there were numerous failures of γ-globulin to prevent congenital fetal abnormality in actual practice.[142,145] In one study of CRS patients, 6% of mothers gave histories of receipt of γ-globulin after exposure.[94] Thus, whatever the real efficacy of ISG, it is unlikely to be complete.

The sole current indication for ISG is the exposure to rubella of a pregnant seronegative woman who will not accept abortion if infection is proved. If 1 week or less has elapsed since exposure and a serum specimen is taken first to confirm susceptibility, ISG in large amounts (20 mL) can be given intramuscularly. Convalescent specimens should be obtained 3 and 4 weeks later to search for IgM antibody

and a rise in IgG titer. The absence of a rash in the exposed woman does not mean that viremia and fetal infection have been prevented. The newer intravenous γ-globulins do not have high concentrations of rubella antibodies.[139]

Hyperimmune Rubella Globulin

To overcome the deficiencies of ISG, a hyperimmune globulin was prepared by Cutter Laboratories from the sera of normal individuals who had high rubella antibody titers. The titer of this preparation was 1:8000 by HI. A controlled clinical trial of the preparation was performed in volunteers who were inoculated first with live, unattenuated rubella virus and then given hyperimmune rubella globulin 24 to 96 hours later. With a challenge given intranasally, viremia was detected in 2 of 5 control subjects and in 1 of 10 subjects given γ-globulin. Pharyngeal excretion was similar in the two groups.[146] Although a previous experimental study with high-titered globulin had given better results,[144] the production of hyperimmune globulin was stopped, and it is not now commercially available.

Active Immunization

Nonliving Vaccines

Advances in molecular biology have allowed consideration of a subunit-inactivated vaccine against rubella. The genome of the virus has been sequenced, in particular the genetic code for the E1 protein,[147,148] which carries multiple neutralizing epitopes located between amino acids 214 and 285 of the 481 amino acids contained in the polypeptide.[149–151] T-cell epitopes also were defined on the E1 protein, although no single epitope was recognized by a majority of individuals.[152–156] The E1 protein has been produced in quantity in baculovirus vectors by truncating the C terminus to allow secretion.[157–160] So far, the immunogenicity of bioengineered E1 has been moderate,[159] but strong adjuvants have produced good responses in animals.[161] Synthetic peptides also have generated neutralizing antibodies,[162] and virus-like particles containing the

TABLE 26–8 ■ Estimated Incidence Rate of Congenital Rubella Syndrome (CRS) per 100,000 Live Births and Number of Cases of CRS by WHO Region, 1996

WHO Region	Mean Incidence Rate of CRS per 100,000 Live Births	No. of CRS Cases Mean	95% CI
Africa	104	22,471	6127–51,472
Americas			
Island	171		
Mainland	175		
Total		15,994	4552–35,950
Eastern Mediterranean	77	12,080	1008–30,950
South-East Asia	136	46,621	1016–168,910
Western Pacific	173	12,634	1545–21,396
Global total		109,800	14,248–308,438

CI, confidence interval; WHO, World Health Organization.
From Cutts FT, Vynnycky E. Modelling the incidence of congenital rubella syndrome in developing countries. Int J Epidemiol 28:1176–1184, 1999, with permission.

three main viral proteins have been produced from transfected cell lines, with retention of immunogenicity.[163,164] Other possible strategies for rubella vaccines include nucleic acid vaccine. Research findings show that DNA plasmids can induce immune responses. Pougatcheva et al.[165] raised neutralizing antibodies in mice by injecting complementary DNA coding for the envelope glycoproteins. Although it is doubtful that an inactivated vaccine could provide protection from infancy throughout the child-bearing period, such a vaccine might be useful for immunizing adult women.

Live Virus Vaccine

Vaccine Strains: Origin and Development[166]

Several vaccine strains were developed soon after the isolation of rubella virus in tissue culture. Three vaccines were licensed in the United States in 1969 to 1970 as follows: HPV-77 (duck embryo),[167] HPV-77 (dog kidney),[14] and Cendehill (rabbit kidney).[15] Soon thereafter, the RA27/3 human diploid fibroblast vaccine was licensed in Europe.[16] During the succeeding years, both HPV-77 (dog kidney) and Cendehill were withdrawn from American licensure. Finally, in 1979, RA27/3 was licensed in the United States, and HPV-77 (duck embryo) was withdrawn, leaving RA27/3 as the only American rubella vaccine. The RA27/3 strain is also the most widely used throughout the world with the exception of Japan[168] (Table 26–9). This strain was adopted because of its consistent immunogenicity, induction of resistance to reinfection, and low rate of side effects.[169] Accordingly, most of the information presented hereafter concerns the RA27/3 strain, with the addition of data on the other strains that can be extrapolated to the currently used vaccine.

RA27/3 was isolated from a fetus infected with rubella in early 1965.[166,170] Culture fluid from a tissue explant was passaged directly into WI-38 cells, and eight serial passages were made in WI-38 cultures incubated at 37°C. Additional passages then were done in cultures incubated at 30°C. After seven passages at 30°C, studies using human volunteers showed that the strain was attenuated. To reduce the pathogenicity even further, 10 additional passages were made.[171] The RA27/3 strain is produced as a vaccine strain between the 25th and 33rd passages in human diploid cells

(WI-38 or MRC-5).[169] The relatively rapid attenuation by passage may be attributable to the use of cold adaptation, whereas the retention of high immunogenicity may be attributable to the low number of passages required to attenuate.[172] The nucleotide sequence of the envelope genes of RA27/3 has been sequenced, revealing 31 amino acid changes in the vaccine compared with the sequence in the wild strain.[173] In comparison, only five changes were noted in the HPV-77 strain.[174]

Strain-specific nucleotide sequences have been demonstrated in the RA27/3 strain, permitting specific identification.[175] Although some antigenic variations have been discerned with rabbit antibodies against *Escherichia coli*–expressed proteins,[176] monoclonal antibody studies employing a panel of monoclonal antibodies showed no significant differences[177] (see *Virology* above).

The Japanese strains were isolated in AGMK cultures and then passaged in chick embryos, guinea pig kidney, swine kidney, rabbit testicle, or bovine kidney cells before production in quail embryo fibroblasts or rabbit kidney cells.[178] One Japanese vaccine strain, TO-336, has been sequenced before and after attenuation.[179] Nucleotide mutations were discovered at 21 sites, 13 in the genes for nonstructural proteins, five in the genes for structural proteins, and three in noncoding regions. Although these mutations gave rise to 10 amino acid changes, none could be associated with attenuation. Moreover, the mutations were different from those of two other attenuated strains (RA 27/3 and Cendehill).

Dosage and Route of Administration

The vaccine dose of RA27/3 is required to be at least 1000 plaque-forming units (PFU) of virus delivered subcutaneously. However, titration studies in humans showed that, in keeping with its being a live vaccine, even small subcutaneous doses (<3 PFU) of RA27/3 are immunogenic.[180] A peculiar attribute of RA27/3, not so far demonstrated with any other rubella vaccine strain, is its immunogenicity when administered intranasally.[181–187] Some studies suggested that intranasal administration might confer an advantage on the vaccinees in terms of quality of the immune response.[188] However, the subcutaneous administration of vaccine gave similar humoral antibody with only slightly less secretory antibody.[170,188] Moreover, the

TABLE 26–9 ■ Current Manufacturers of Rubella Vaccines

Manufacturer	Virus Strain	Cell Substrate
Merck (United States)	RA27/3	HDCS
SmithKline-RIT (Belgium)	RA27/3	HDCS
Berna (Switzerland)	RA27/3	HDCS
Aventis Pasteur (France)	RA27/3	HDCS
Sclavo (Italy)	RA27/3	HDCS
Institute of Immunology (Yugoslavia)	RA27/3	HDCS
Serum Institute of India	RA27/3	HDCS
Chemo-sero-therapeutic Research Institute (Japan)	Matsuba	Rabbit kidney
Chiba Serum Institute (Japan)	TCRB 19	Rabbit kidney
Kitasato Institute (Japan)	Takahashi	Rabbit kidney
Osaka University (Japan)	Matsuura	Quail embryo fibroblast
Takeda Chemical Industries (Japan)	TO-336	Rabbit kidney

HDCS, human diploid cell strain.
Modified from Perkins FT. Licensed vaccines. Rev Infect Dis 7:S73–S76, 1985.

intranasal dose of RA27/3 required for consistent immunization is high: 10,000 PFU.[183] Lower doses result in frequent failures,[189] particularly in children, possibly owing to the mechanics of administration. Nevertheless, under careful conditions, some workers have been able to achieve 95% seroconversion rates, only slightly inferior to those rates achieved with subcutaneous injection of RA27/3.[186] Mexican workers have attempted vaccination against both measles and rubella by a small-particle aerosol, and have achieved seroconversion rates indistinguishable from those obtained with subcutaneous inoculation.[190] Aerosol administration may have public health advantages, and is being explored further.

Combination with Measles and Mumps

In the United States and increasingly elsewhere, rubella vaccination is accomplished with a triple vaccine that also contains measles and mumps vaccine viruses (MMR). The American triple formulation (MMR II; Merck Sharp & Dohme) contains the Moraten attenuated measles virus (1000 median tissue culture infective doses [$TCID_{50}$]), the Jeryl Lynn mumps virus (5000 $TCID_{50}$), and the RA27/3 rubella virus (1000 $TCID_{50}$). Four formulations are available in Europe and elsewhere. Pluserix (GlaxoSmithKline) contains the Schwarz measles virus (1000 $TCID_{50}$), the Jeryl Lynn–like Mumps strain (20,000 $TCID_{50}$), and RA 27/3 rubella virus (1000 $TCID_{50}$). Trimovax (Aventis Pasteur) contains the Schwarz measles virus (1000 $TCID_{50}$), the Urabe mumps virus (20,000 $TCID_{50}$), and the RA27/3 rubella virus (1000 $TCID_{50}$). Morupar (Chiron) contains the same three viruses, but the mumps virus concentration is given as at least 5000 $TCID_{50}$. A fourth European formulation (Triviraten, Berna) contains Edmonston-Zagreb measles virus and Rubini mumps, but is no longer on the market. For those who prefer not to vaccinate against mumps, a measles and rubella combination is produced by Aventis Pasteur.

Another major manufacturer is the Serum Institute of India, which manufactures three different rubella-containing formulations: rubella-only vaccine (Wistar RA 27/3; 1000 $TCID_{50}$), measles-rubella (MR) (with the addition of EZ measles virus; 1000 $TCID_{50}$), and MMR (Trestivac, with the addition of L-Zagreb mumps strain; 5000 $TCID_{50}$).

Production and Constituents of Vaccine

RA27/3 is manufactured on a human diploid cell substrate, either WI-38 or MRC-5 fetal lung fibroblasts. Cell cultures inoculated with the seed virus are incubated at 30°C. After 4 to 7 days of initial incubation, there is sufficient virus in the supernatant medium to harvest. Fresh medium is added, and subsequent harvests can be made every 2 to 3 days for several weeks. Stabilizer is added to the harvest fluids, which are frozen for later safety testing and pooling before eventual lyophilization.[191,192] The final RA27/3 vaccine is essentially free of animal serum but does contain 0.4% human albumin, 25 to 50 µg/mL neomycin, and, in one case (Sclavo), 50 µg/mL of kanamycin. The lyophilization medium varies according to the manufacturer; however, it generally contains sucrose or sorbitol, glutamic acid and other amino acids, and buffering salts. When lyophilized, the vaccine is hypertonic. Reconstitution is accomplished

with sterile distilled water (0.5 to 1.0 mL) according to the manufacturer's directions, which restores the vaccine to a normal or slightly hypertonic state. The water added for reconstitution should not include a preservative because it would kill the live vaccine virus. All manufacturers provide water for reconstitution with the vaccine.

RA27/3 is produced in the United States, the United Kingdom, France, Belgium, Italy, Switzerland, Yugoslavia, and India by the manufacturers listed in Table 26–9. Despite minor differences in dose, antibiotic content, and other details among manufacturers, differences in vaccine efficacy or in the nature or severity of side effects have not been reported.

Stability of Vaccine

Rubella vaccine is highly stable in the frozen state at ~70°C or ~20°C. At 4°C, the viability of the virus and the potency of the vaccine also are maintained for at least 5 years. At room temperature, there is significant loss after 3 months; at 37°C, a 3-week period is sufficient to damage vaccine potency.[193] The vaccine should be stored at 2° to 8°C and protected from light. The virus is labile after reconstitution and should be used within 8 hours.

Results of Vaccination

Immune Responses

Vaccination induces antibodies of both IgM and IgG classes and cellular immune responses. The induction of secretory IgA responses depends on the type of immunization, as described below.

Most studies of immunogenicity have been done by measuring HI responses, although the neutralizing responses may be more important biologically. By the HI technique, 95% to 100% of RA27/3 vaccinees experience seroconversion by 21 to 28 days after vaccination, with geometric mean antibody titers ranging from 1:30 to 1:300, depending on the method of titration.[16,171,194,195] Some of the apparent failures, at least in young adults, may be explained by pre-existing low levels of antibody that neutralize the vaccine virus but are detectable only by sensitive tests.[196]

Several direct comparative immunogenicity studies have been done with different strains. A trial comparing the administration of the RA27/3 and Cendehill strains to Scottish schoolgirls resulted in a 98% seroconversion for the former and 90% for the latter.[197] In Sweden, Bottiger and Heller[198] found a 98% response after inoculation with RA27/3 and 96% after inoculation with Cendehill. In another Swedish trial, Grillner[199] tested neutralizing titers after vaccination, and 95% of RA27/3 vaccinees were seropositive compared with 56% of Cendehill vaccinees. Menser and colleagues[200] tested RA27/3 and Cendehill in Australian schoolgirls and adults; they found no differences in seroconversion but better boosting of seropositive individuals by RA27/3. Weibel and associates[201] conducted large comparative studies of RA27/3 and HPV-77, obtaining results that are summarized in Table 26–10. The Japanese TO-336 and the Chinese BRD-2 strains compared favorably with RA27/3 in parallel studies.[202,203]

RA27/3 elicits complement-fixing and precipitating antibody titers in nearly all vaccinees.[170] In a precipitin test system, RA27/3 was the only vaccine strain that evoked

TABLE 26–10 ▪ Comparison of Hemagglutination-Inhibiting (HI) Antibody Response Among Initially Seronegative Children and Adults Who Received RA27/3 or HPV-77 Duck Embryo Rubella Virus Vaccines

	Children			Adults		
Vaccine	Seroconverting/Total (N)	HI Titer Range	Mean	Seroconverting/Total (N)	HI Titer Range	Mean
RA27/3	153/153 (100%)	8–1024	153*	98/99 (99)	<8–512	84*
HPV-77:DE	152/156 (97%)	<8–512	81	85/94 (90)	<8–512	35

*Significantly greater than geometric mean antibody titer for HPV-77:DE group (P <0.001).
Modified from Weibel RE, Villarejos VM, Klein EB, et al. Clinical laboratory studies of live attenuated RA27/3 and HPV-77 DE rubella virus vaccines. Proc Soc Exp Biol Med 165:44–49, 1980. Copyright 1980, Society for Experimental Biology and Medicine.

antibodies to the iota internal antigen of rubella virus.[204] Vaccination induces antibodies predominantly binding the E1 protein as detected by immunoblot, but those antibodies mature in avidity less rapidly than after natural infection and do not reach the same level.[205]

The induction of neutralizing antibody is particularly significant and is seen regularly and promptly after the administration of RA27/3. Figure 26–3 and Table 26–11 present comparative data obtained in New Haven, Connecticut,[124] and in Sweden.[198] Immunoblot analysis confirmed the persistence of antibodies for at least 3 years to the E1 protein that bears neutralizing epitopes. Antibodies to the C protein also persisted, but antibodies to E2 disappeared in some cases.[206]

A crucial property of RA27/3 is its ability to induce secretory IgA antibody in the nasopharynx, which, as discussed subsequently, may prevent reinfection with wild virus. This property makes vaccination with RA27/3 similar to natural infection, which also induces local immunity. Although secretory IgA responses are higher after

intranasal vaccination, they also are induced by subcutaneous vaccination with RA27/3.[207,208] Whereas some workers believe that secretory antibodies are important in protection against rubella, Cradock-Watson and colleagues[209] published evidence that nasal antibodies were transient in appearance, and they doubted the ability of these antibodies to prevent reinfection.

Not surprisingly, vaccination, like disease, is followed by the early production of IgM-class antibodies. These antibodies reach a peak at 1 month after vaccination[209] and last approximately 1 month more.[210,211]

Cellular immune responses have been studied, although their significance is unclear. A proliferation of lymphoblasts in response to rubella antigen appears 2 weeks after vaccination, without suppression of tuberculin hypersensitivity.[212] Honeyman and co-workers[213] found sensitization of lymphocytes from Cendehill vaccinees to rubella antigen, which disappeared 1 year later. Relatively short-lived cellular responses also were seen in other studies.[214,215] Human leukocyte antigen–restricted T-cell cytotoxicity was shown to increase after immunization.[216] Morag and co-workers[217] showed that cytotoxic T-lymphocyte activity was high in tonsillar lymphocytes after intranasal vaccination (with RA27/3) but was low after subcutaneous vaccination (with HPV-77). Unfortunately, subcutaneous administration of RA27/3 was not evaluated.

Although early studies done with relatively insensitive detection systems suggested that rubella vaccines did not cause viremia, viremia has been documented between 7 and 11 days after inoculation.[218] However, the viremia is low and inconstant. Pharyngeal excretion of virus is more frequent, occurring from about 7 to 21 days after vaccina-

FIGURE 26–3 ▪ Comparison of neutralizing antibodies and hemagglutination-inhibiting (HI) antibodies in three groups of individuals: naturally infected children, children given HPV-77 duck embryo vaccine, and children given RA27/3 vaccine. (From Horstmann DM. Viral vaccines and their ways. Rev Infect Dis 1:502–516, 1979, with permission.)

TABLE 26–11 ▪ Neutralizing Antibody Response in 114 Rubella-Vaccinated Women Who Demonstrated Seroconversion with Hemagglutination-Inhibiting Antibodies

Vaccine	Before Vaccination*	After Vaccination	
		8 Wk	2 yr
Cendehill	1/45	24/43 (56%)	27/33 (82%)
HPV-77 duck	2/29	23/29 (79%)	16/17 (94%)
RA27/3	1/40	37/39 (95%)	20/20 (100%)

*Number positive/number tested.
From Grillner L. Neutralizing antibodies after rubella vaccination of newly delivered women: comparison between three vaccines. Scand J Infect Dis 7:169–172, 1975, with permission.

tion, in low titer of usually less than 10 PFU per swab. Excretion peaks on approximately the 11th day after vaccination; if properly tested, essentially all vaccinees will be shown to excrete virus from the nasopharynx.[219,220]

In view of the excretion of rubella virus by vaccinees, considerable effort has been made to detect the spread of vaccine virus to susceptible contacts. Initially, contact studies were focused on children in institutions and on families, and no evidence for spread of vaccine virus was found.[15,16,168] For example, none of 393 seronegative family members was infected by contact with RA27/3 vaccinees.[16] Veronelli[221] studied 347 familial contacts of HPV-77 vaccinees and also found no evidence of spread.

Subsequently, experience in studies of contact spread produced largely negative results, with the rare asymptomatic seroconversion that could not be explained fully.[222,223] Scott and Byrne[224] observed 121 seronegative pregnant women exposed to HPV-77 vaccines during a vaccination campaign in Rhode Island; only one experienced seroconversion. Fifteen seronegative husbands who had been exposed to wives vaccinated with Cendehill did not acquire infection.[225] Negative results were also obtained in 67 elementary school teachers exposed to vaccinated pupils.[226] Fleet and colleagues[227] performed a large population surveillance study in Nashville, Tennessee, in which 24,000 children were vaccinated. More than 11,000 pregnancies were assessed by virologic studies of newborns and abortuses and by serologic study of the mothers, without a demonstrated effect of vaccine virus.[227] A possible case of symptomatic reinfection by contact has been reported, but the evidence was unconvincing.[228] Low percentages of seroconversion among contacts were found in large studies of HPV-77 and Cendehill vaccinees.[229,230] The general lack of evidence for spread by vaccine virus may reflect the maintenance of attenuated markers by excreted virus, as demonstrated for RA27/3.[231]

Responses to rubella as part of MMR combinations are equal to those seen after rubella vaccination as a single antigen. Table 26–12 is taken from a study by Weibel and colleagues[201] that compared MMR formulated with RA27/3 to RA27/3 alone. The excellent responses in both groups of vaccinees have been confirmed by other investigators,[232,233] who also found RA27/3 to be superior to the earlier HPV-77 component.[232] Seroconversion to rubella vaccination with any of the other triple combinations (see above) is usually 97% to 98%.[234,235] Bivalent measles-rubella and mumps-rubella vaccines also produced rubella antibody levels that were equivalent to those of the monovalent vaccine.[232] A triple vaccine that contained Cendehill virus gave a 96% seroconversion rate to the rubella component.[236] Comparative studies between the Merck and GlaxoSmithKline triple combinations showed some statistical differences of doubtful clinical importance, but excellent seroconversion to rubella after both vaccines.[237,238]

In summary, rubella vaccine induces immune responses that are similar in quality but lesser in quantity than those after natural disease.[239] The live virus produces viremia and pharyngeal excretion, but both are of low magnitude and are noncommunicable. IgG and IgM antibody responses follow vaccination. Natural infection elicits nasal secretory antibody that may be useful in the prevention of reinfection, and RA27/3 vaccine also has the same property.

Protective Effects

The protective efficacy of rubella vaccination has been assessed (1) by observation of vaccinees and control subjects during natural epidemics and (2) by intranasal challenge of vaccinated volunteers with unattenuated or attenuated viruses.

During an institutional outbreak of rubella, Davis and colleagues[240] were able to evaluate the effect of natural rubella exposure on persons who had been vaccinated with HPV-77. Clinical rubella occurred in 22 of 33 unvaccinated seronegative individuals but in none of 22 vaccinees and 66 naturally immune individuals. Asymptomatic reinfection without viremia was noted in five vaccinees (23.0%) and in one naturally immune subject (1.5%). Grayston and associates[241] compared the effect of HPV-77 vaccine with placebo during an epidemic on Taiwan. Rubella incidence began to drop in the vaccinated group within 2 to 3 weeks, and vaccine efficacy was estimated at 94%. In a separate study undertaken during the same outbreak, RA27/3 vaccine gave a 97% protection rate. A group of children in day care was observed by Chang and colleagues[242] after some had been vaccinated with Cendehill. The vaccine afforded complete protection against disease, but 50% of the vaccinees were re-infected.

A dramatic example of protection by vaccine was reported from Japan.[243] An outbreak started in a school for apprentices at the Toyota automobile factory. RA27/3 vaccine was given randomly to a third of the boys. As shown in Figure 26–4, the epidemic continued for 7 weeks, but rubella ceased to occur in vaccinees 2 weeks after they were vaccinated.

TABLE 26–12 ■ Antibody Responses in Initially Seronegative Children Who Received Combined Measles (Moraten)–Mumps (Jeryl Lynn)–Rubella (RA27/3) or Monovalent RA27/3 Rubella Vaccine

	Antibody Responses Versus								
	Measles (HI) Conversion			Mumps (Neutralizing) Conversion			Rubella (HI) Conversion		
Vaccine	N/Total	%	Geometric Mean	N/Total	%	Geometric Mean	N/Total	%	Geometric Mean
Combined	64/68	94	57	65/68	96	8	68/68	100	136
Monovalent	—	—	—	—	—	—	67/67	100	159

HI, hemagglutination inhibition.
From Weibel RE, Carlson AJ, Villarejos VM, et al. Clinical and laboratory studies of combined live measles, mumps, and rubella vaccines using the RA27/3 rubella virus. Proc Soc Exp Biol Med 165:323–326, 1980, with permission.

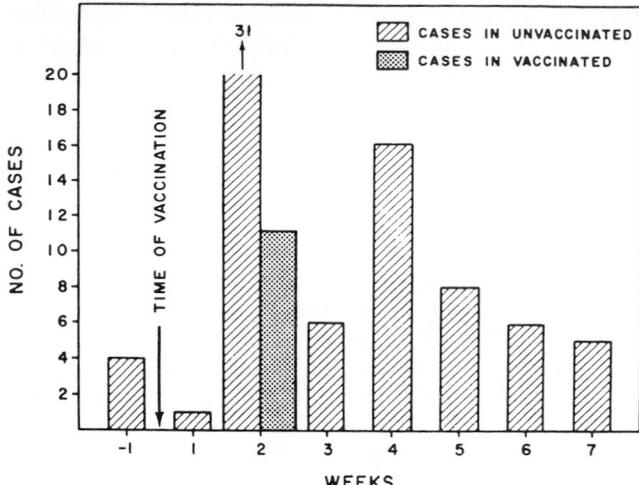

FIGURE 26–4 ■ Demonstration of protection against rubella during an epidemic in a boys' school at the Toyota car factory near Nagoya, Japan. Boys were selected at random to receive RA27/3 vaccine at the time indicated, and about one third received the vaccine. (From Furukawa T, Miyata T, Kondo K, et al. Rubella vaccination during an epidemic. JAMA 213:987–990, 1970, with permission. Copyright 1970, American Medical Association.)

An outbreak of rubella in a primary school in France during 1997 permitted a calculation of effectiveness, because only about 75% of children had been vaccinated. Effectiveness of RA 27/3 was 95% (85% to 99% confidence interval).[244] An effectiveness study done in Italian military recruits gave a figure of 94.5% for rubella vaccination.[245]

In Olmstead County, Minnesota, adolescent girls were vaccinated with Cendehill; unvaccinated boys were used as control subjects, which permitted a calculation of efficacy at 94% during a 1972 outbreak.[246] The introduction of rubella vaccination of recruits at Lackland Air Force Base resulted in a 95% reduction in rubella by 1979.[247] A more recent outbreak in Sanford, Maine, during 1980 to 1981 allowed an assessment of vaccine efficacy 8 years after vaccination; it was 90%.[248]

In Finland, five cases of rubella encephalitis were seen at Helsinki Children's Hospital during a 15-year period starting in the late 1960s, whereas none has been seen since the advent of MMR vaccination in 1982.[249]

Correlates of Immunity

The immune response that correlates best with protection is neutralizing antibodies.[250] However, on the one hand, even vaccinees with low levels of serum antibodies are protected,[251] while on the other hand, reinfection may take place in some individuals with measurable antibodies (see below). Moreover, closing off of viral excretion in CRS cases appears to correlate with the appearance of cellular immune responses. (J Best, personal communication, 2001.) Because measurement of neutralizing antibodies is not routinely available, 15 IU of antibodies measured by other methods may be considered as a correlate of protection.[252] However, infants with CRS have been born to mothers who have antibody levels of 15 IU or greater. Review of epidemiologic data in the United States has demonstrated pro-tection at 10 IU, so the cutoff for protection was set at 10 IU in the United States.[83]

Reinfection and Herd Immunity

Early in rubella vaccine studies, it became evident that, under conditions of exposure to wild virus, reinfection of persons vaccinated with HPV-77 and Cendehill could occur with a frequency of 50% or greater.[253–257] Herd immunity was shown to be ineffective when rubella broke out in a company of military recruits who were studied by Horstmann and co-workers.[258] Although most recruits had antibodies as a result of vaccination or prior infection at the start of the epidemic, 100% of the remaining susceptible individuals were infected. Moreover, 80% of the recruits vaccinated with HPV-77 were reinfected. The same conclusion was reached in another study of recruits, in which rubella singled out the susceptible individuals despite high levels of immunity in the group.[259]

Bermuda experienced a rubella outbreak in 1971. A vaccination campaign with Cendehill resulted in prompt termination of the epidemic, and vaccine efficacy was estimated to be 94%.[260] However, a rubella epidemic in Casper, Wyoming, in the same year showed that, although the vaccine (HPV-77) prevented rubella in immunized elementary school children, unimmunized adolescents and adults still suffered an attack rate that was 50% of that expected without vaccination.[261,262] Fogel and colleagues[253] used intranasal RA27/3 as a challenge to RA27/3, Cendehill, and HPV-77 vaccinees. Their results showed a higher rate of reinfection in the last two groups compared with that in RA27/3 vaccinees (Table 26–13). Among RA27/3 vaccinees, approximately 5% had low titers 6 to 16 years after vaccination.[263] A 9.8% incidence of asymptomatic reinfection was reported 5 years after vaccination.[264]

Harcourt and associates[254] concluded that reinfection is dependent on a number of immunologic factors, including but not restricted to the presence of nasopharyngeal IgA rubella antibody. When the RA27/3 virus itself was given intranasally as a challenge virus, O'Shea and co-workers[251] found that reinfection as determined by titer rises was infrequent in those who had significant titers (>15 IU) of rubella antibody from previous infection or vaccination but was frequent in vaccinees who had low titers (<15 IU). However, reinfection was not associated with lack of

TABLE 26–13 ■ **Reinfection* of Vaccinees After Virus Challenge**

Previous Vaccine Given	Total Vaccinees	Vaccinees Showing Reinfection	
		N	Percentage
Cendehill	27	18	66.7
HPV-77	30	14	45.7
RA27/3	28	2	7.1

*As revealed by a positive booster in at least one of four serologic tests.
From Fogel A, Gerichter CB, Barena B, et al. Response to experimental challenges in persons immunized with different rubella vaccines. J Pediatr 92:26–29, 1978, with permission.

TABLE 26–14 ■ Viremia and Virus Excretion in Volunteers After Subcutaneous or Intranasal Challenge with RA27/3 Rubella Virus Vaccine

Antibody Status Before Vaccination	No. of Vaccinees	Viremia	Virus Excretion
Seronegative	21	15	12 (6–14)*
Seropositive (>15 IU)	10	0	1 (7)
Low titer (≤15 IU)			
Natural infection	12	0	0
Previous vaccination			
RA27/3	7	0	0
Other strains	12	1 (12)	3 (6–9)

*Numbers in parentheses indicate days after vaccination on which findings were positive.
Adapted from O'Shea S, Best J, Banatvala JE. Viremia, virus excretion, and antibody responses after challenge to volunteers with low levels of antibody to rubella virus. J Infect Dis 148:639–647, 1983.

neutralizing antibodies, and viremia as part of the reinfection was rare (Table 26–14).

The significance of reinfection is hotly debated. In some studies, reinfection leads only to an IgG booster response, without IgM,[265] whereas in others the appearance of IgM antibody suggested significant viral replication.[266,267] Nevertheless, clinical rubella has been documented during reinfection of vaccinees[268] and naturally immune individuals.[269,270] Moreover, maternal reinfection during pregnancy has resulted in congenital rubella.[45,271–285] In a prospective study, Morgan-Capner and associates[286] found definite evidence of passage of virus from reinfected mothers to their fetuses in two of three cases in which exposure had occurred in the first trimester and fetal tissue was available. However, follow-up of seven live-born infants did not reveal CRS. O'Shea and colleagues[287] measured rubella immunity in reinfected women and reinfected seropositive volunteers undergoing a challenge with rubella virus. The presence or absence of neutralizing antibodies or cellular immunity did not correlate with the likelihood of reinfection. However, Matter and co-workers[252] suggested that reinfection may be more likely at low levels of antibody as measured by hemolysis in gel (10 to 15 IU), and Mitchell and colleagues[288] reported that reinfection was correlated with lack of prior antibodies to a peptide of the E1 protein.

It is not always easy to distinguish between primary and secondary responses in a person with prior low or undetectable antibodies who has been exposed to natural infection or been revaccinated. If that distinction is important for clinical care or research, detection of IgM antibodies or low-avidity IgG antibodies may be helpful.[252,266] The best conclusion at this time is that reinfection with fetal transmission of wild rubella virus is a fact, in the presence of both natural and vaccine-induced immunity, but that the risk is probably less than 5% in the first trimester of pregnancy compared with at least 80% in primary infection. The danger of reinfection is another reason for immunizing contacts of pregnant women.

Persistence of Immunity and Revaccination

Numerous data are available on persistence of antibody after vaccination. Liebhaber and colleagues[289] found antibodies in all 18 vaccinees 2 years after vaccination with

RA27/3. In response to a challenge with unattenuated rubella virus, 16 of the 18 vaccinees showed resistance to reinfection. Amazonian Indians given RA27/3 by Black and co-workers[290] had persistent antibodies in the absence of any possible re-exposure to the virus, although there was a twofold drop during 2.5 years. A 98% to 99% persistence of antibody was noted in schoolchildren 4 years after vaccination.[291] Zealley and Edmond[292] reported on a long-term study of Edinburgh schoolgirls, 97% of whom retained antibodies 6 to 7 years after vaccination with RA27/3. The longest observation periods after vaccination with RA27/3 thus far have been 12 to 17 years,[172] 15 years,[293] and 10 to 21 years.[294] In the latter study, 97% of subjects retained their positive antibody status. In one long-term study, 75 (96%) of 78 vaccinees retained measurable antibody[172] (Fig. 26–5). In a follow-up of Baltimore schoolchildren, there was a decline of less than fourfold in titer during a 15-year postvaccination period, and 97% remained seropositive.[295]

Miller and colleagues[296] studied 475 children 4 years after vaccination with MMR and found 97% to be positive for rubella antibodies. A Canadian study of a similar number of children tested 5 to 6 years after vaccination with MMR gave identical results.[297] Bottiger[298] observed 220 Swedish children given MMR at 18 months of age. At 12 years of age, 97% had rubella antibodies, although not at the same levels seen immediately after vaccination. A second dose given at 12 years of age raised the titer levels to those seen after primary vaccination. Christenson and Bottiger[299] also observed a cohort of almost 500 girls vaccinated at age 12 years. After 8 years, 96% were still seropositive, and 94% were still so at 16 years after vaccination, although the mean titers had dropped from 1:110 to 1:18 (Table 26–15).

Different results were reported by Johnson and co-workers,[300] who studied 95 children given MMR at 15 months of age. Children studied at age 4 to 6 years were 100% positive for rubella-neutralizing antibodies, but only 63% of children ages 11 to 13 years were positive. They suggested that immunity had waned. After a second dose of MMR, 100% of children became seropositive, with almost a threefold rise in the geometric mean titer of rubella antibodies. In Newfoundland, Ratnam and associates[301] found that 16.5% of children 8 to 17 years of age were seronegative after prior

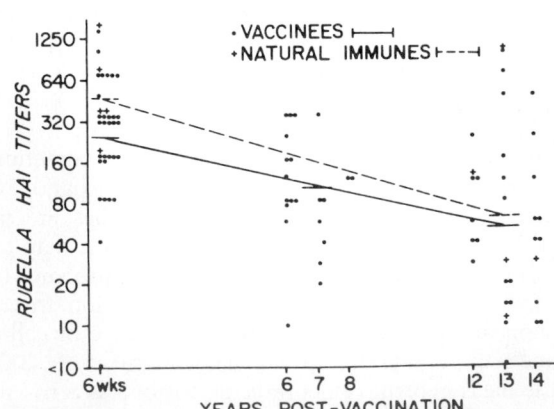

FIGURE 26–5 ■ Persistence of hemagglutination-inhibiting antibody (HAI) to rubella after natural infection or the administration of RA27/3 vaccine. (From Plotkin SA, Buser F. History of RA27/3 rubella vaccine. Rev Infect Dis 7[suppl]:S77–S78, 1985, with permission.)

TABLE 26–15 ■ Persistence of Rubella Antibodies
After Vaccination of Seronegative Schoolgirls

Time After Vaccination	N	% HI Titers ≥1:8	GMT (HI)
8 wk	486	100	110
2 yr	346	99	80
4 yr	136	99	53
8 yr	486	96	34
16 yr	190	94	18

HI, hemagglutination inhibition; GMT, geometric mean antibody titer.
Data from Christenson B, Bottinger M. Long-term follow-up study of
rubella antibodies in naturally immune and vaccinated young adults.
Vaccine 12:41–45, 1994.

vaccination at 1 year of age. Elsewhere in Canada, Mitchell et al.[302] found ELISA antibodies, "subprotective" neutralizing antibodies, and lymphocyte proliferation responses in 92%, 77%, and 74%, respectively, of adolescents 14 to 16 years after their first dose.

A Dutch seroprevalence study showed that, 9 years after the introduction of universal rubella vaccination of infants, more than 95% of vaccinees were still seropositive. Moreover, only 5% of reported rubella cases occurred in vaccinees.[303] In Finland, titrations were done in children followed over 15 years. Five to 7 years after a single dose, 98% to 100% of the children were still seropositive. They were given a booster dose, after which seroprevalence continued to be 100%. However, at 15 years after a first rubella vaccination and 9 years after a second dose, 30% of children had low titers. Children given a second dose at 11 to 13 years still had elevated titers.[304] Reports of persistence of antibody to Cendehill vaccine from Australia, Switzerland, the United States, and the United Kingdom gave, in order, 95% persistence at 5 years,[200] 96% at 15 years,[305] 98% at 10 years,[306] and 100% at 8 to 18 years[292,307] after vaccination.

Persistence of antibodies after vaccination with the HPV-77 vaccines used earlier has been variable. Whereas some reports were favorable,[294,307–309] other reports indicated that antibody was less persistent.[310,311] Follow-up of those vaccinated with Cendehill or HPV-77:DE 20 years previously in Hawaii showed persistent antibody in 92.8%.[312] A study in Milwaukee revealed 13% seronegativity 12 years after vaccination.[313] Best[314] summarized published studies of antibody persistence 9 to 21 years after vaccination and found a seronegativity rate of 1% for RA27/3 vaccinees, 2.7% for Cendehill vaccinees, and 7.3% for HPV-77 vaccinees.

An epidemic of rubella occurred during 1981 to 1982 among students at the University of California at Los Angeles. Strassburg and colleagues[315] performed a case-control study and found that prior immunization with unspecified rubella vaccines conferred 97% protection, even though some students had been immunized 10 years previously. Natural immunity to rubella lasts at least 26 years.[316]

One study reported good persistence of antibody 10 years after inoculation with the Japanese TO-336 virus.[317] Persistent antibody and protection also followed the use of the Matsuba strain.[318] A follow-up study of subjects given the Matsuura strain also showed good persistence of antibodies and T-cell activation.[319]

Rossier and associates[320] studied persistence of cellular immunity to rubella and found that, in contrast to naturally infected individuals, most HPV-77 vaccinees lacked cellular immunity 5 years after vaccination. A similar difference was noted between Cendehill vaccinees and naturally infected adults.[213] Mitchell and associates[302] found positive lymphoproliferative responses to rubella antigens in all of 39 adolescents who presumably had been vaccinated more than 10 years previously. In a small group of vaccinees followed 23 years after receipt of the Matsuba strain, 15% were negative by HI, but reimmunization nevertheless induced secondary responses.[321]

It thus appears that rubella seropositivity wanes after vaccination, but most vaccinees remain seropositive and the others may still be immune, judging from the absence of outbreaks in the United States. Reimmunization has been advocated by some of those who have studied the persistence of antibodies to HPV-77:DEV and Cendehill,[322,323] and subcutaneous RA27/3 could be given as a booster vaccine for those previously immunized.[324,325] However, ostensibly seronegative individuals usually show secondary immunologic responses after boosters, indicating that they had been immune.[326,327] A study of two doses of rubella vaccine (as part of MMR) showed persistent immunity in 95% of children 2–4 years after the first dose, with a boost in GMT from 41 IU to 72 IU after a second dose.[327a] The authors commented that within three years of the booster, antibodies fall to prior levels. In any case, the question has now been rendered in part moot by the adoption in many countries of a routine second dose of measles vaccine, usually as a triple vaccine containing rubella. Revaccination is a suggested strategy to augment rubella immunity before the age of reproduction. Individuals who fail to seroconvert after rubella vaccination should be given a single repeated dose. Failure to respond to the second dose may be evidence for tolerance to rubella virus antigens,[328] which is definitely seen in survivors of CRS.[329]

In summary, the need for a second dose of rubella vaccine is unproven. Although titers decrease with time, high rates of seropositivity are maintained. However, the routine indication for a second dose of a measles-containing vaccine, the general use of combination vaccines containing rubella for that purpose, the innocuity of a second dose of rubella vaccine, the success of two-dose national strategies in eliminating rubella, and the need to maintain protection during the years of child-bearing all argue for a two-dose schedule. However, the rare cases of rubella occurring in the United States are in unvaccinated persons, without signs of spread to the general population, suggesting that a second dose of rubella vaccine may be unneeded. Although a second dose of rubella vaccine would be preferable just before adolescence, measles control and convenience are better with a second dose at school entry.[330]

Combined and Associated Vaccines

As mentioned previously, when rubella vaccine is given to preschool-age children, it is almost always given in combination with measles and mumps vaccines as MMR vaccine. Excellent results have been reported for both RA27/3 and Cendehill as components of triple vaccines.[201,331] There is no contraindication to giving MMR even in the presence of immunity to one or two of its components, and American authorities prefer to use MMR exclusively in vaccination programs. Rubella or MMR vaccine can be given simultaneously (but separately) with diphtheria and tetanus toxoids and pertussis vaccine, *Haemophilus influenzae* vaccine, inactivated poliovirus vaccine, hepatitis B vaccine, oral poliovirus vaccine,[332] and varicella vaccine.[333]

Adverse Reactions

Common Side Effects

Vaccinees sometimes develop mild rubella, including rash, lymphadenopathy, fever, sore throat, and headache. The incidence of each of these side effects varies directly with age, being almost absent in infants but present in up to 50% of women. As stated previously, the severity of reactions is greatest in older women. Fortunately, the minor side effects are seldom severe enough to cause days to be lost from school or work.[198,200,334,335]

A double-blind study of vaccination with MMR in children gave a 1% incidence of arthropathy and little evidence of other reactions.[336] This study was conducted in twins, one of whom received vaccine and the other placebo. The results are given in Table 26–16, which shows that the differences in reactions between vaccinees and placebos were small. The twin study was repeated by the same Finnish workers in 6-year-old children receiving second doses of MMR. The only symptom appearing to be associated with vaccination was arthralgia.[337] Another controlled study revealed no significant differences in reactions of children receiving either MMR or measles vaccines.[338] Female children are more likely than males to have fever and rash after vaccination.[339]

Serious Reactions

In 1991, the Institute of Medicine of the National Academy of Sciences published a committee report on four possible adverse effects of rubella vaccine: acute arthritis, chronic arthritis, neuropathies, and thrombocytopenia.[340] The committee concluded that RA27/3 causes acute arthritis. With regard to chronic arthritis, the committee stated, "The evidence is consistent with a causal relation between the currently used rubella vaccine strain (RA27/3) and chronic arthritis in adult women, although the evidence is limited in scope and confined to reports from one institution." However, the committee found insufficient evidence to indicate a causal relationship between use of the vaccine and incidence of radiculoneuritis, other neuropathies, and thrombocytopenia. As discussed in the following sections, some of these conclusions remain controversial.

ARTHRITIS AND ARTHRALGIA

A review of adverse events in Canada gave a reaction rate for rubella vaccine of 28.7 per 100,000 doses distributed, of which 0.3 per 100,000 was arthritis or arthralgia.[341] Acute arthropathy is part of the disease caused by rubella virus, at least in adults, and is also the most important side effect of vaccination.[342] Although the HPV-77 strain is no longer in use, much information on joint reactions was obtained by studying reactions to vaccination with this strain. The HPV-77 dog kidney vaccine was particularly likely to cause reactions in joints, even in children.[343,344] At times, the reactions included neuropathies, such as the "catcher's crouch" syndrome.[343-348] The HPV-77 duck embryo vaccine produced reactions that were age related; for example, in one study, 0% of girls younger than 13 years, 2% of those 13 to 16 years old, 6% of those 17 to 19 years old, 25% of women 20 to 24 years old, and 50% of women older than 25 years developed reactions in the joints.[349,350] Symptoms could be prolonged.[351] In two different studies, Cendehill vaccine was reported to cause these reactions in 23% and 16% of women.[352,353] RA27/3 produced infrequent reactions in children,[354] but approximately 25% of adults had temporary joint symptoms.[334]

Polk and associates[355] performed a comparative trial of rubella vaccines in adult women. Some of their comparative data are represented in Table 26–17. In addition, they reviewed other reports and concluded that the incidence of transient

TABLE 26–16 ▪ Symptoms and Signs Caused by MMR Vaccination and Day of Peak Occurrence in Finnish Twin Study

Symptoms and Signs	Maximum Difference in Rate* (%)	95% CI	Peak Frequency (Days After Vaccination)
Local erythema (>2 cm)	0.8	0.1–1.4	2
Other local reaction	0.4	0–1.4	2
Mild fever (≤38.5°C rectal)	2.7	0–6.1	10
Moderate fever (38.6–39.5°C)	2.9	1.6–4.3	9
High fever (≥39.5°C)	1.4	0.7–2.1	10
Irritability	4.1	2.1–6.1	10
Drowsiness	2.5	1.4–3.6	11
Willingness to stay in bed	1.4	0.5–2.3	11
Generalized rash	1.6	0–3.0	11
Conjunctivitis	2.1	0.9–3.2	10
Arthropathy	0.8	0.2–1.3	7–9
Peripheral tremor	0.4	0–0.9	9
Cough and/or coryza	−1.5†	−4.6–1.6	9
Nausea and/or vomiting	−0.8†	−1.6–0	7–8
Diarrhoea	0.7	0–1.7	11

*Between MMR group and placebo group.
†More in placebo-injected children.
From Peltola H, Heinonen OP. Frequency of true adverse reactions to measles-mumps-rubella vaccine: a double-blind placebo-controlled trial in twins. Lancet 1:939–942, 1986, with permission.

TABLE 26–17 ■ Side Effects Among Seronegative Adult Female Vaccinees Receiving Measles-Mumps-Rubella (MMR) or Measles-Mumps-Rubella II (MMR II) and Among Seropositive Control Subjects

	MMR (HPV-77:DE-5)	MMR II (RA27/3)	Control Subjects
N			
Age (yr)	59	53	60
X̄ ± SD	29.29 ± 9.09	30.00 ± 9.81	30.70 ± 10.36
Median	26	27	27
Range	19–58	19–58	20–58
Any joint manifestation	17 (28.8%)	14 (26.4%)	2 (3.3%)
Arthritis only	9 (15.3%)	6 (11.3%)	0 (0)
Paresthesias	2	0	0
Fever	5	1	4
Rash	4	4	2
Days of work missed because of joint pains*	8 (4)	3 (1)	0

*Number of vaccinees who missed work in parentheses.
From Polk BF, Modlin JF, White JA, DeGirolami PC. A controlled comparison of joint reactions among women receiving one of two rubella vaccines. Am J Epidemiol 115:19–25, 1982, with permission.

arthralgia or arthritis was 35% to 63% with the use of HPV-77 (dog kidney), 27% to 33% with HPV-77 (duck embryo), 8% to 10% with Cendehill, and 13% to 15% with RA27/3. Although many different joints can be involved in the reaction to rubella vaccines, knees and fingers are the most common, whereas the hips are seldom involved. Conflicting evidence has been reported regarding the influence of the stage of the menstrual cycle on joint symptoms.[202,349,351]

The mechanism of joint inflammation appears to be direct infection of the synovial tissue by the virus, if one extrapolates from recoveries of the virus from joints of patients with arthritis after occurrence of natural rubella[356] and after inoculation with HPV-77 vaccine.[357] Laboratory studies suggesting that rubella RNA and rubella peptides might induce autoimmunity also have been published.[358,359] Women who possess class II human leukocyte antigen DR2 or DR5 have elevated risk of acute joint reactions after rubella vaccine.[360] Human joint tissue infected in vitro by Miki and Chantler[361] supported high-titer replication of wild viruses and of HPV-77 but 100- to 1000-fold less replication of RA27/3. The Cendehill strain grew hardly at all in joint tissue, and genetic mapping showed that the mutations giving restriction were mostly located in the 5′ noncoding region.[362] Although RA27/3 has not been recovered from joints, Tingle and associates[363] reported isolating vaccine virus from the peripheral blood mononuclear cells of two women who had prolonged arthritis after administration of the vaccine. Joint reactions were not associated with elevated IgG or prolonged IgM responses.[363] Bosma et al.[364] tested synovial fluids or biopsies from 79 patients with chronic inflammatory arthritis and detected rubella RNA in only two specimens, one from a patient who had rheumatoid arthritis and the other from an immunodeficient patient with arthritis caused by mycoplasma. They concluded that rubella was not etiologic for chronic arthritis, but might rarely persist within the joints.

Tingle and co-workers[365] reported a prospective study conducted in British Columbia of arthritis after RA27/3 vaccination or natural disease. The incidence of acute arthritis was 52% in the disease group and 14% in the vaccinees. Recurrent arthropathy developed in 30% of women who had the disease and 5% of women who had been vaccinated.

Symptoms were not associated with circulating immune complexes.[366] The occurrence of chronic viremia and the determination of an etiologic relationship between rubella vaccination and chronic arthritis await confirmation.

The Institute of Medicine committee suggested the need for prospective, double-blind, controlled trials of rubella vaccine in adult women, associated with attempts to isolate rubella virus, to resolve the controversy.[367] Six studies touching on this issue have since been reported. Phillips and colleagues[368] and subsequently Frenkel et al.[369] and Nielsen and co-workers[370] were unable to confirm the presence of viremia in vaccinees complaining of chronic arthritis. Rubella genomic RNA was not demonstrated by Zhang and associates[371] in blood and synovial fluid from cases of rheumatoid arthritis. Slater and colleagues[372] observed two cohorts of Israeli women, one of which had received rubella vaccine. Five to 10 years later, the incidence of arthritis in vaccinees and control subjects was 3.9% and 3.2%, respectively, an insignificant difference. At the Kaiser Permanente Northern California Health Maintenance Organization, Ray and colleagues[373] linked rubella vaccination records with cases of chronic arthritis and found no association between the two.

Finally, the British Columbia group performed a placebo-controlled prospective study of approximately 500 women, half of whom were vaccinated and observed for 1 year.[374] Their results are summarized in Table 26–18. Not surprisingly, acute arthralgia and arthritis were more common in vaccinees, although the excess attributable to vaccine was only 5%. In evaluating women with persistent arthropathy, they defined "Persistent arthropathy . . . as occurrence of arthralgia or arthritis at any time during the 12 months after vaccination in women who experienced acute arthropathy and for whom joint complaints could not be attributed to other causes." The frequency of chronic arthropathy was 15% in the placebo group and 22% in the vaccine arm. However, whereas 58 (72%) of 81 women in the vaccine group with acute arthropathy later developed chronic arthropathy, 41 (75%) of the 55 women in the placebo arm with acute arthropathy also developed chronic arthropathy. Thus chronic arthropathy

TABLE 26–18 ■ Frequencies of Acute and Chronic Reactions to Rubella Vaccine or Placebo in Adult Women

	Group (%)		
	Placebo (N = 275)	Vaccine (N = 268)	Odds Ratio (95% Confidence Interval)
ACUTE REACTIONS			
Sore throat	32	34	1.09 (0.75–1.59)
Cervical Lymphadenopathy	10	19	2.21 (1.31–3.76)
Rash	11	25	2.57 (1.58–4.21)
Myalgia	16	21	1.36 (0.88–2.10)
Paresthesias	7	7	1.09 (0.57–2.09)
Arthralgia	16	21	1.42 (0.92–2.19)
Arthritis	4	9	2.36 (1.13–4.92)
Arthralgia or arthritis	20	30	1.73 (1.17–2.57)
CHRONIC REACTIONS			
Myalgia	9	15	1.68 (0.99–2.84)
Paresthesias	4	5	1.12 (0.50–2.50)
Arthralgia or arthritis	15	22	1.58 (1.01–2.45)

Adapted from Tingle A, Mitchell L, Grace M, et al. Randomised double-blind placebo-controlled study on adverse effects of rubella immunisation in seronegative women. Lancet 349:1277–1281, 1996.

was associated with prior acute arthropathy but not with rubella vaccine. In addition, there was no description of the severity or frequency or duration of the symptoms of the women in either group. Moreover, by the authors' case definition, a woman who had an episode of acute arthralgia for 3 days and then one episode of arthralgia of any duration more than a month later would meet the chronic or persistent arthropathy case definition. Thus it is unclear what relationship these findings have to the chronic rubella arthropathy previously reported.

More recently, the British Columbia group retested the seronegative women in the original study with several additional tests for antibodies, and found that 21.7% were positive.[375] The group then revised its hypothesis, arguing that low, nonfunctional responses to prior rubella infection predisposed women to joint complaints when vaccinated. However, the original placebo group apparently was not retested, and the statistical significance of the new conclusions remains doubtful.

Thus, taking the evidence as a whole, one is left with the conclusion that, although chronic arthropathy caused by RA27/3 is plausible biologically, it is unconfirmed by virology or epidemiology, and is rare if it occurs at all. Nevertheless, on the basis of the Institute of Medicine report, the National Vaccine Injury Compensation Program has been accepting claims of chronic arthropathy resulting from rubella vaccination, and compensation has been awarded to 23 of 56 completed cases.[376]

Chiba and colleagues[377] reported a depression of rubella-specific cellular immune responses in children with arthritis. Circulating immune complexes containing rubella antigen were found in 11 of 33 vaccinees who developed arthralgia after vaccination but in only 3 of 19 who did not.[378]

NEUROLOGIC ADVERSE EVENTS

Although few neurologic events after vaccination with RA27/3 have been reported, it is useful to review this type of information for all vaccine strains.[379] Polyneuropathy is part of natural rubella and is among the most frequent of the unusual complications of rubella vaccination. Schaffner and associates,[380] who reviewed the problem in 1974, found 299 reports of polyneuropathy after vaccination. The cases they reviewed followed immunization with HPV-77:DEV, HPV-77:DK, and, less frequently, Cendehill vaccines. The symptoms began about 40 days after vaccination, appearing in the form of two syndromes, one consisting of paresthesias and pain in the arms and the other involving pain in the knee and preference for a crouching position. The second syndrome tended to recur. Carpal tunnel syndrome and Horner's syndrome also were seen. Children with polyneuropathy showed impairment of motor and sensory nerve conduction. Cusi et al.[381] studied a case of mild peripheral neuropathy in a young seronegative woman that began 4 weeks postvaccination. Antibodies to myelin basic protein were detected in the patient, and the authors induced anti–rubella binding antibodies in mice by immunization with a peptide derived from myelin that is homologous with a peptide in the rubella C protein. Attempts to demonstrate rubella virus or genome in the patient's white blood cells were negative.

Two cases of optic neuritis after vaccination for rubella have been reported, the vaccine being HPV-77 in one instance[382] and an unstated vaccine in the other.[383] Two cases of anterior uveitis after MMR vaccination were reported from Saudi Arabia.[384] Transverse myelitis has been reported on two occasions[385] and diffuse myelitis on three occasions after inoculation with RA27/3, Cendehill, and an unstated vaccine.[386,387] Four cases of transverse myelitis have been reported after vaccination with MMR containing RA27/3.[388] Facial paresthesias were reported after vaccination with RA27/3.[389] A case of disseminated encephalomyelitis was reported in Japan after vaccination with the Takahashi strain.[390] Two cases of Guillain-Barré syndrome have been noted after the use of HPV-77:DEV, but an etiologic association could not be confirmed.[385,391]

There are rare reports of Guillain-Barré syndrome after rubella vaccination in combined vaccines,[392] but an epidemiologic study in the United Kingdom after an MR vaccination campaign revealed rates of Guillain-Barré less than that expected by the background rate (1 per 100,000 children).[393] In addition, a large retrospective study of Guillain-Barré syndrome was conducted in Finland. No clustering of cases occurred after MMR vaccination, nor did subsequent MMR vaccination cause relapses in patients with the syndrome.[394] Another Finnish study showed no relationship of MMR vaccination to encephalitis, aseptic meningitis or autism.[394a] Chantler and associates[395] showed that rubella viruses grow in human astrocytes but poorly in oligodendrocytes, suggesting that demyelinating disease is not likely to be associated with rubella virus replication.

OTHER ADVERSE EVENTS

A case of "bone changes" after rubella vaccination was reported,[396] but the negative virus isolation, absence of IgM antibodies, and lack of detail make the association dubious.

One case of mild orchitis after the administration of rubella vaccine was reported.[397]

Thrombocytopenia has followed vaccination for rubella on several occasions[398,399] and has been reported frequently after the administration of triple vaccine.[400,401] A decrease in platelets may be seen in some asymptomatic vaccinees after vaccination, and symptomatic thrombocytopenia has been reported after natural rubella. A rate of 1 in 3000 is accepted for thrombocytopenia after wild rubella,[402] whereas rates 10 times lower have been reported after rubella vaccination.[400] It appears that either measles or rubella vaccines may be responsible for thrombocytopenia after MMR.[403] In addition, exacerbation of chronic thrombocytopenia has been reported after MMR,[404] as has recurrent thrombocytopenia after repeated administration.[405] A British study concluded that the risk of thrombocytopenia within 6 weeks of MMR vaccination was 1 in 22,300 doses, but only two thirds of cases were attributable to the vaccine, for a risk of 1 in 33,000 doses.[406] Revaccination is not recommended by the Advisory Committee on Immunization Practices for children who suffered thrombocytopenic purpura after MMR,[407] but the balance of risk and benefit should be weighed, particularly because the British study found no recurrences after MMR in children with prior thrombocytopenia.[408]

A Swedish study examined autoantibodies to pancreatic islet cells and to thyroid cells before and after MMR vaccination, and found no increase, making it unlikely that vaccination contributes to diabetes or thyroiditis.[409]

Rubella vaccines have been noted to depress nonspecific cellular immunity transiently,[410] including the tuberculin reaction, cell-mediated immunity to Candida, phytohemagglutinin responses, and delayed-type hypersensitivity to recall antigens; they also increase suppressor T cells.[411-413] Follow-up study of RA27/3 vaccinees has shown no increase in cancer incidence.[414]

Indications for Rubella Vaccine

The targets of rubella vaccination are listed in Table 26–19.

Infants

Rubella vaccine is given to preschool-aged children in the United States and many other developed countries in an effort to immunize them for the future and to protect their mothers through reduction of rubella virus circulation. In view of the lack of evidence of contagiousness of vaccinees, infants whose mothers are pregnant may be vaccinated.

Rubella vaccine is usually given at 12 to 15 months of age as part of the MMR vaccine. Children who miss the

TABLE 26–19 ■ Target Groups for Rubella Vaccination

Infants ≥12 mo
Older unvaccinated children and adolescents
College students
Childcare personnel
Health care workers
Military personnel
Adult women before pregnancy
Adult seronegative women postpartum
Adult men in contact with pregnant women
All of the above as part of a two-dose elimination strategy

vaccine at that time can receive it at any later age and in most states must receive it at the time of school entry. The age at first vaccination does not seem to be as critical for rubella as for measles vaccine. Passively transmitted maternal antibodies are present in only 5% of infants from 9 to 12 months and 2% from 12 to 15 months of age.[415] From 9 months of age on, vaccination is almost 100% successful,[234,416-421] but there is little need to prevent rubella in those younger than 1 year.[422] A study done in Brazil showed reliable seroconversion after rubella vaccine from about 6 months of age.[107] The presence of acute respiratory infection at the time of vaccination of infants 12 to 18 months of age was shown in three separate studies to have no influence on seroconversion.[423-425]

Adolescents

Vaccination is recommended for all adolescents, male and female, who have not been previously vaccinated. In addition, revaccination with rubella vaccine as part of MMR is recommended in many countries, either at entry to primary school or at 11 to 13 years. The justification for this practice lies mainly in the prevention of measles outbreaks caused by accumulation of susceptibles resulting from primary vaccine failure. However, it has been argued that revaccination also will boost waning immunity to rubella and mumps. Although the evidence for the need to revaccinate against rubella is slim, two-dose regimens are now standard in the United States and other countries (see *Persistence of Immunity and Revaccination* above and *Epidemiologic Results of Vaccination* below).

In the United Kingdom, public health policy formerly emphasized vaccination of 11- to 14-year-old girls, with the idea that a cohort of immune women could be created during a period of 10 to 20 years. The success of this policy is considered subsequently (see *Epidemiologic Results of Vaccination* below); in brief, its advantage was narrowing the target group to potential mothers, and its disadvantages were a high refusal rate and the lack of effect on the circulation of virus. However, Schiff and colleagues[426] succeeded in vaccinating 97% of the high-school girls in a rural town in Wisconsin, with excellent results. Immunization of adolescent girls has been done with and without the addition of contraception, depending on the known sexual activity in the particular population.[427,428]

Adults

The most directed vaccination program, in the sense of having the most immediate impact on CRS, is vaccination of women. The principal problem with this approach is the possibility of unsuspected pregnancy, although, as described subsequently (see *Pregnancy* below), the actual risk to the fetus may be nonexistent.

Identification of seronegative women cannot be done accurately on the basis of history because clinical diagnosis of prior rubella is unreliable.[429] Vaccination of women who give negative histories of prior vaccinations is advocated without confirmatory serologic testing.[422] A frequent practice has been to test women for immune status and then to vaccinate them while oral contraceptives or other forms of pregnancy precaution are taken.[430-433] Vaccination can be practiced as part of routine gynecologic care, premarital screening, and occupational health care or at other medical opportunities, as long as contraception can be ensured for 1 month. A frequently expressed concern is whether to vaccinate women with low positive titers, such as those with ELISA values just beyond the cutoff value, with hemolysis in gel values of 10 to 15 IU, or with HI titers of 1:8. Current evidence suggests that those women usually are immune but may be at higher risk of reinfection,[434] and thus one dose of vaccine should be offered (see *Reinfection and Herd Immunity* above). There is no evidence that vaccination of seropositive women is attended by increased risk of untoward reactions.

The use of rubella vaccine during the puerperium (postpartum vaccination) has been widely advocated.[352,435–441] Because 56% of CRS children in the United Kingdom were born to multiparae,[442] this practice should prevent a significant portion of CRS. Indeed, Edmond and Zealley[443] observed that CRS was prevented in Edinburgh by vaccination of girls and postpartum vaccination of women, with most of the failures occurring in women who had been screened but not vaccinated. However, pregnancy can occur even in the immediate postpartum period,[444] and contraceptive measures such as the use of depot progestogen have been advocated.[445] Administration of blood or blood products such as $Rh_0(D)$ immune globulin before vaccination requires postvaccination tests for seroconversion.

Although the postpartum genital tract is not susceptible to rubella vaccine virus,[446] vaccinated parturient women do excrete vaccine virus in their breast milk.[447] The vaccine virus then may be transmitted to their newborns, but they remain asymptomatic and do not develop tolerance to subsequent vaccination.[448–450] Thus breast-feeding is not a contraindication to vaccination.

Adult men not in high-risk groups are not generally targeted for vaccination, although they are also a reservoir of susceptibles and may serve as the source of infection of pregnant women.[451] An outbreak in Croatia showed that infection can propagate among men even if they do not live in a collectivity, despite routine vaccination of infants and women.[452]

Military Recruits and College Students

Vaccination is routinely practiced in the armed forces of the United States, with the consequence being the virtual eradication of rubella.[247] Rubella also was eradicated in the armed forces of Singapore several years after commencement of routine vaccination.[453] The consequences of failure to vaccinate were illustrated by an epidemic in British troops in Bosnia.[454] The French army, which until recently has not practiced routine rubella vaccination of its recruits, has had perennial epidemics.[455] In view of the congregation of large numbers of susceptible young adults in colleges and universities, routine vaccination with MMR at matriculation also is advocated.[422] In principle, these vaccinations will be second doses, but they are considered important to prevent outbreaks of measles and perhaps rubella on college campuses.

Hospital Employees

Outbreaks of rubella in hospitals,[456–459] with the resultant exposure of pregnant women, have led to the recommendation of compulsory rubella vaccination for both male and female hospital employees.[460] In one hospital outbreak,[461] those departments that had a compulsory vaccination policy escaped unscathed, whereas those departments that had

a voluntary vaccination policy suffered numerous cases, including infections of pregnant women. A comprehensive evaluation reconfirmed the recommendation for vaccination of hospital personnel.[462]

International Travelers

Unimmunized women of child-bearing age who travel overseas should be vaccinated to protect against the greater likelihood of exposure to the disease in countries that do not use rubella vaccine.

Contraindications

General Contraindications[422]

Rubella vaccine can be given to patients with minor respiratory illnesses, febrile or afebrile (see *Indications for Rubella Vaccine* above). Those with congenital immune deficiencies should never receive a live virus vaccine, although family members should be vaccinated to protect the patients against rubella, measles, and mumps. It also would be prudent to wait until systemic immunosuppressant drug therapy has been terminated for 3 months before vaccinating patients receiving such regimens. A 16-year-old boy with acute lymphoblastic leukemia who received RA27/3 rubella vaccine developed chronic infection of leukocytes and high antibody titers. Symptoms of arthritis required temporary interruption of immunosuppression, but fortunately the patient recovered spontaneously.[463] Short-term (less than 2 weeks) corticosteroid therapy is not a contraindication to the administration of rubella vaccine. Patients whose immunity had been ablated during bone marrow transplantation were given rubella vaccine as part of MMR 2 years later by Ljungman and associates.[464] They observed a 75% seroconversion to the rubella component with no safety problems. King and colleagues[465] performed a similar study and found 91% seroconversion.

Children with chronic renal disease who are on hemodialysis can be immunized successfully before transplantation.[466]

Persons who have had anaphylactic reactions to neomycin should not receive rubella vaccines containing that antibiotic.[467] Whereas monovalent RA27/3 vaccine is grown in human diploid cells, MMR does contain other viruses grown in avian tissue, but reactions in egg-sensitive individuals are very rare.

Concurrent IgG

Vaccination within 2 weeks before receipt of IgG or 3 months after receipt of IgG is inadvisable.[139,422] However, anti-$Rh_0(D)$ globulin did not interfere with vaccination of postpartum women.[441] Women who are vaccinated after receiving anti-$Rh_0(D)$ globulin should be tested 6 weeks later for rubella antibodies.

Human Immunodeficiency Virus Infection

Asymptomatic children who are infected with the human immunodeficiency virus (HIV) should receive rubella vaccine as part of MMR. Virologic study of 10 HIV-infected patients who received MMR failed to detect rubella virus.[468] MMR also should be considered for symptomatic children who are not severely immunosuppressed. Older children and adults who were rubella seropositive before becoming infected with HIV maintain high-avidity rubella antibodies and do not need revaccination.[469]

Pregnancy

Pregnancy remains a contraindication to rubella vaccination, and women are advised to take precautions against pregnancy for 1 month (28 days) after vaccination. On the basis of a case of wild virus transmission to a fetus conceived 7 weeks after vaccination,[469] a prior recommendation had been for a 3-month delay, but evidence for damage to the fetus by rubella vaccine strains is nonexistent.[470] Several summaries of the accumulated American, British, and German data have been published[471–473] (Table 26–20). Transplacental passage of vaccine virus is evidently a rare event, having occurred 4 times in 708 pregnancies complicated by RA27/3 vaccination. More important, there was no CRS case demonstrated in more than 1000 pregnancies during which rubella vaccines were given. Hoffman et al. reported the case of a woman vaccinated 3 weeks after conception who gave birth to an infant who excreted RA 27/3 virus until 8 months of age. Nevertheless, the infant was free of abnormalities.[474]

On the basis of data in Table 26–20, the theoretical maximum risk for CRS after the administration of vaccine is 1.3%, considerably lower than the risk with wild rubella virus or indeed the risk of non–CRS-induced congenital defects in pregnancy. If only the American women known to be seronegative who received RA27/3 are considered in the calculation, the theoretical risk to the fetus still does not rise above 2.1%. For these reasons, and because the observed risk has been zero, rubella vaccination during pregnancy is no longer considered an indication for abortion.[475,476]

Children with Congenital Rubella Syndrome

Children with CRS probably will not respond to parenteral rubella vaccine, even when they are seronegative.[477] They can be immunized with RA27/3 intranasally,[478] but there is no official recommendation to vaccinate these children.

Public Health Considerations

Epidemiologic Results of Vaccination

The goal of rubella vaccination programs is the prevention of the intrauterine infection that causes CRS. Since the licensure of the rubella vaccine in 1969, the global epidemiology of rubella and CRS has changed dramatically. In 2000, the World Health Organization (WHO) convened a meeting to review the worldwide status of CRS and its prevention.[479,480] This meeting was prompted by the availability of more data on the CRS disease burden in developing countries, an increase in the number of countries with national rubella immunization programs, and advances in laboratory diagnosis since the last international meeting on CRS and rubella in 1984. In 1996, only 78 countries/territories used rubella vaccine in their national immunization programs. As of April 2000, this number had increased to 111 (52%) of the world's 214 countries and territories. The proportion of countries using rubella vaccine varies markedly by WHO region: Africa, 2%; South-East Asia, 20%; Eastern Mediterranean, 50%; Western Pacific, 57%; Europe, 68%; and the Americas, 89%. Much of the recent increase occurred in the WHO regions of the Americas and the Western Pacific, where polio eradication has allowed national immunization programs to address new challenges.

Incorporation of rubella vaccine in the national immunization program also is related to a country's economic status. None of the 46 least developed countries has introduced rubella vaccine, compared with 50% (13/26) of countries with economies in transition (Eastern European countries and the newly independent states of the former Soviet Union); 60% (53/88) of developing countries; 74% (20/27) of territories, protectorates, or self-governing areas; and 93% (25/27) of developed countries.

United States

Rubella vaccine has had spectacular success in the United States, in terms of the number of people vaccinated and the declining numbers of rubella cases reported. Figure 26–2 shows that since the licensing of the vaccine in 1969, no major epidemic of rubella has occurred, despite the previously observed 6- to 9-year cycle.

These impressive results were obtained initially by the vaccination of children, with a dependence on herd immunity to protect pregnant women. However, assessment in 1977 to 1978 revealed that, although the program was having a major impact on rubella in children, rubella rates in those older than 15 years were not substantially different from prevaccination rates.[481] Specific experiences in institutional or citywide outbreaks showed that the concept of herd immunity had only limited validity, giving a protection of perhaps 50%.[261,482,483] Moreover, some doubted that children were the sole source of infection for their mothers.[484] Serologic surveys showed a persistence of 12% to 24% seronegativity in adolescent and adult populations. As a consequence, programs to expand vaccination of adolescents and adults were increased. Since then, the disease rate in age groups old enough to bear children has dropped markedly, as have the number of CRS cases (see Fig. 26–2). From an average of 106 cases a year during the 1970s, the number fell to 20 per year, and the prospect of elimination of CRS was discussed.[485,486] Subsequently, the incidence of rubella dropped to less than 1 per 100,000 population, and the incidence of CRS dropped to less than 0.1 per 100,000 births.[112] In fact, only seven cases of CRS were reported in 1983 in the United States, two in 1984, and two in 1985.[112,481,485–487]

In 1988, a nadir was reached in reported postnatal rubella, and only one case of CRS was registered in 1989. A large outbreak of rubella occurred in unimmunized immigrants to California and was followed by the expected cluster of CRS cases.[488] A serologic survey conducted between 1988 and 1994 showed 92% seropositivity in 6- to 11-year-old children, but only 85% in persons ages 20 to 29 years.[489] Nevertheless, the rubella vaccination program appears to be successful, and reported cases are now at record low levels (Fig. 26–6).

Since the mid-1990s, rubella has occurred mainly among foreign-born Hispanic adults who are unvaccinated or whose vaccination status is unknown, with very limited spread and circulation among the U.S. resident population.[490] From 1997 to 1999, 20 (83%) of 24 infants with CRS were born to Hispanic mothers, and 21 (91%) of the 23 infants were born to foreign-born mothers.[491] Mothers' countries of birth include mainly Mexico, Central

TABLE 26–20 ■ Summary of Data on Accidental Vaccination Before Pregnancy and During Early Pregnancy of Women in the United States and Germany

Study Location and Vaccine	Vaccinated Women (N)	Mother's Immune Status Before Vaccination		
		Susceptible	Immune	Unknown
Cendehill and HPV-77	538	149	25	364
RA27/3	683	272	32	379
Cendehill	340	130	61	149
RA27/3	25	16	4	5

CRS, congenital rubella syndrome.
Data from Centers for Disease Control and Prevention. Rubella prevention: recommendation of the Immunization Practices Advisory Committee. MMWR Rep 39(RR-15):1–18, 1990; Rubella vaccination during pregnancy—United States, 1971–1988. MMWR 38:289–293, 1989; and Enders G. Rubella antibody titers in vaccinated and nonvaccinated women and results of vaccination during pregnancy. Rev Infect Dis 7(suppl):S103–S107, 1985.

American countries, and countries of the Spanish-speaking Caribbean. Genomic sequencing suggests the strains circulating earlier have disappeared, while imported strains have featured in several recent outbreaks. Another more diffuse group of strains appears to be sporadic and indigenous[491] (Fig. 26–7).

In the debate over vaccine policy, cost-benefit analyses were made to assess the various strategies. For every dollar spent on childhood rubella vaccination in the United States, $7.70 was saved.[492] An analysis made in Israel also reached the same favorable conclusion.[493] However, Schoenbaum and colleagues[494] argued that vaccination of schoolgirls would be economically preferable to vaccination of infants.

Meanwhile, the growing resurgence of measles resulted in a recommendation for a routine second dose of measles vaccine, usually in the form of MMR.[495,496] Thus revaccination with rubella became standard, practiced at either entrance to primary school (4 to 6 years) or entrance to sec-

ondary school (11 to 12 years of age). Although there are theoretical arguments in favor of revaccinating older preadolescent children,[330] the United States is moving toward uniform revaccination at 4 to 6 years.

Europe

Every country in western Europe has introduced rubella vaccination into routine childhood vaccination as part of MMR. The Scandinavian countries and the Netherlands have adopted a policy of two doses of MMR, and the other countries give a second dose of rubella vaccine to adolescent girls.[497]

Pebody et al.[498] have studied the seroepidemiology of rubella in western Europe. They found high rates of seropositivity across age groups in Finland and the Netherlands; gaps in immunity in Denmark, England, France, and Germany; and high susceptibility in Italy, which had poor coverage rates. Modeling of the vaccine coverage and seroprevalence data showed that Italy and Germany are in danger of rubella outbreaks and CRS.[101,499] However, Italy recently had introduced routine MMR vaccination of infants (S Salmaso, personal communication, 2002).

UNITED KINGDOM

The policy of vaccinating schoolgirls was adopted by the British in 1970.[481,500] During subsequent years, the number of reported rubella cases decreased only slightly, although the reported cases of CRS decreased approximately 75%.[501] About 15% of schoolgirls did not accept the vaccine,[502,503] which explained why 88% of women reporting for assessment for rash disease had not been immunized.[61] Although serologic studies showed that vaccination had reduced seronegativity of young women,[61,504–506] many susceptible persons still remained.[506,507] A national program to promote vaccination was started, and acceptance of rubella vaccine among schoolgirls increased.[500]

After original hesitation, opinion in Britain changed to favor the inclusion of young children in rubella vaccination

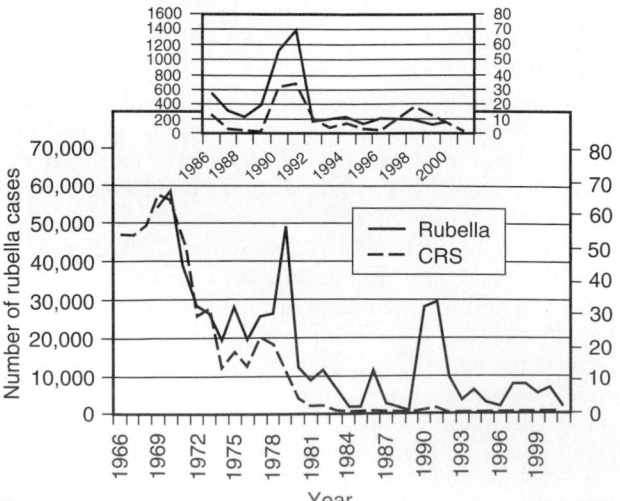

FIGURE 26–6 ■ Reported rubella and CRS cases, United States, 1966 to 2001.

Outcome for Live Births					
Total Live Born	Live Born to Susceptible Mothers	Asymptomatic Infection	CRS Defect	Products of Conception Positive When Tested for Rubella	Theoretical Risk of CRS Defect (%)
UNITED STATES					
290	94	8	0	17/85	0–3.8
562	226	3	0	1/35	0–1.6
GERMANY					
177	107	2	0	1/34	
17	12	0	0		

practice, as is now done in the United States.[508–511] Since October 1988, rubella vaccine as part of MMR has been recommended to all infants,[512] and in 1994, a large-scale vaccination campaign was conducted with MR combined vaccine. Congenital rubella and terminations of pregnancy for rubella have decreased markedly in England and Wales,[513] with only one CRS case reported in 1995.[514,515] In 1996, however, the United Kingdom experienced a resurgence of rubella, primarily in adult and adolescent males who were unvaccinated.[515] As might be predicted, cases of CRS followed the outbreak. Pregnant women immigrating into the United Kingdom from Asia and Africa are at increased risk for CRS.[515a] Additional outbreaks in universities have resulted from imported rubella in Greek students.[516] More recently, public concern relating to allegations of a relation between MMR vaccination and autism reduced rubella coverage, but the impact on CRS has not yet been manifest.

SCANDINAVIA

In 1982, Sweden adopted a two-stage vaccination scheme involving the use of MMR at two ages: 18 months and 12 years.[517] The rationale for this scheme was as follows[518]:

1. Vaccination at 18 months will reduce the incidence of rubella among schoolchildren and, ultimately, among child-bearing women when these same children reach maturity.
2. A more immediate effect on rubella in pregnancy is obtained by vaccinating young girls.
3. The second dose also reinforces immunity and replaces the boosters formerly provided by natural infection.

An acceptance rate of 88% was achieved among Swedish schoolgirls and an even higher rate among other children. Some problems with seroconversion for mumps and measles among the 12-year-old girls were reported, but rubella vaccine gave good results in both age groups.[519] Christenson and Bottiger[520] studied the rubella serology of 1343 suscep-

tible 12-year-olds in the Swedish program and found that 100% seroconverted after vaccination. Before 1974, a yearly average of 14 CRS cases were recorded in Sweden; there were 2 cases per year between 1975 and 1985, and there have been no cases since 1985.[521]

The Finns vaccinate with MMR at 14 to 18 months and at 6 years. The peak incidence has shifted to adults, whereas children appear to be protected.[522] The success of the MMR two-dose vaccination policy in Finland has been spectacular. Peltola and colleagues[523] summarized the results of the program that succeeded in eliminating indigenous cases of rubella, measles, and mumps. This program was supported by improved surveillance of disease and by ancillary studies demonstrating lack of significant reactions to vaccine and persistence of antibodies. Ukkonen[524] provided data on the disappearance of rubella and the state of rubella immunity in the Finnish population. As shown in Figure 26–8, the two-dose policy has erased seronegativity in adolescents and caused rubella to disappear. Since 1986, no case of CRS has been reported. The last indigenous rubella case occurred in 1996. In 1997 and 1998, one imported rubella case was reported each year with no secondary cases identified.[525]

FRANCE

Between 1982 and 1994, during which MMR was recommended for all 1-year-old French children, rubella infections in pregnancy dropped from 45 to 9 cases per 100,000 births.[526] Vaccine coverage is now over 90% in children less than 10 years of age, but considerably lower in adolescents.[527] French authorities have instituted a second dose of MMR at 6 years of age.[528]

OTHER EUROPEAN COUNTRIES

The Netherlands replaced selective vaccination of girls with mass vaccination of infants in 1987. Although the program has successfully prevented CRS, circulation of rubella virus persists, perhaps because some religious communities have low coverage.[529]

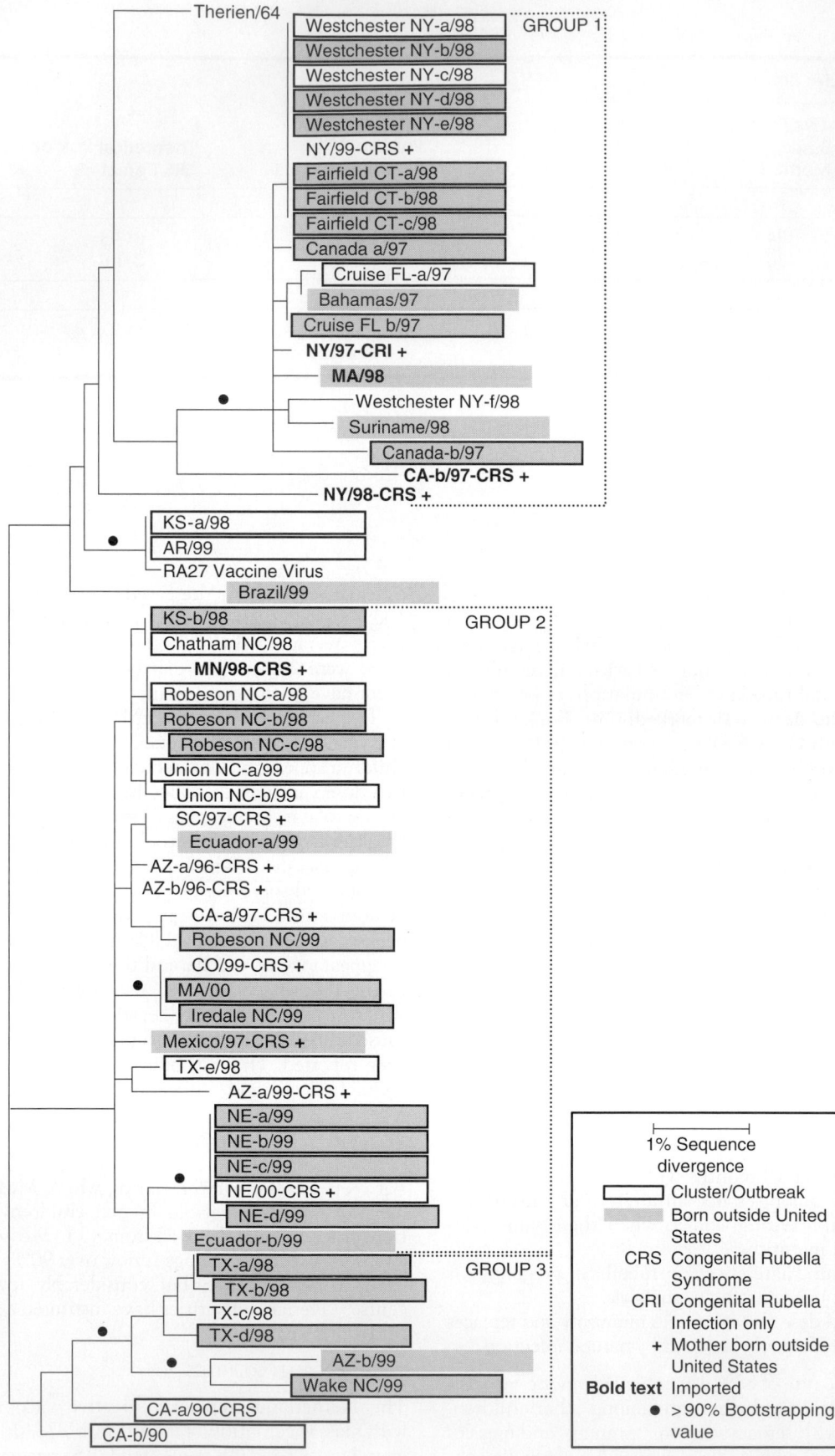

FIGURE 26–7 ■ Phylogenetic analysis of rubella isolates in the Americas during the 1990s. (Redrawn from Reef S, Frey TK, Theall K, et al. The changing epidemiology of rubella in the 1990s: on the verge of elimination and new challenges for control and prevention. JAMA 287:464-472, 2002.)

Coverage rates in Switzerland are also uncertain, and Matter and colleagues[530] reported the persistence of rubella and CRS cases.

Canada

The provinces of Canada adopted a policy either of mass vaccination of infants or of selective vaccination of preschool-age girls.[481,531] Total rubella incidence dropped in the provinces that adopted mass vaccination of infants but was not much changed in those adopting vaccination of preschool-age girls. However, reported CRS decreased throughout Canada. As of 1983, all provinces give vaccine to infants and also to 12-year-old girls who have not been immunized previously.[531]

Israel

Israel at first adopted the British policy of vaccination of schoolgirls. Subsequent observations showed that, whereas the youngest girls were being protected, epidemics could still infect large numbers of pregnant women. Accordingly, family health clinics, which most Israeli women attend, started to screen for rubella antibodies and to vaccinate seronegative women. Universal vaccination of children with MMR was started.[128] The problem of eliminating rubella in Israel has been exacerbated by the early emphasis

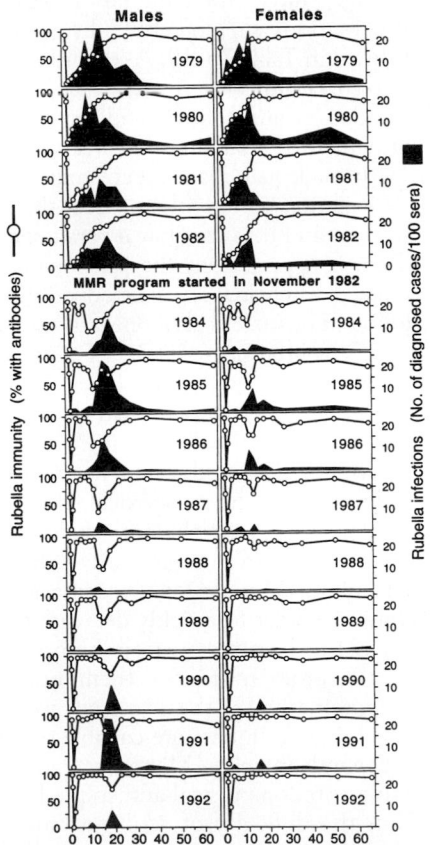

FIGURE 26–8 ■ Gradual increase in rubella immunity and disappearance of rubella infections as a consequence of measles, mumps, and rubella (MMR) vaccination. *Top,* Before the MMR program (1979 to 1982). *Bottom,* During the MMR program (1984 to 1992). (From Ukkonen P. Rubella immunity and morbidity: impact of different vaccination programs in Finland 1979–1992. Scand J Infect Dis 28:31–35, 1996, with permission.)

on vaccination of women only, by immigration of unvaccinated populations, and by the existence of religious communities that do not accept vaccination. Thus progress has been slow, and in 1992 five cases of CRS were reported.[532,533]

Australia

Australia also adopted the policy of vaccinating schoolgirls. By 1983, 12 years after the program had started, 96% of pregnant women were seropositive. MMR vaccination of children began in 1988 to 1989, followed by vaccination of adolescents of both sexes in 1994 to 1996. A second dose of MMR at age 4 to 5 years has been recommended.[534] Vaccine coverage is high, and 97% of children with documented rubella immunization are seropositive.[535] Cases of reported CRS have fallen from approximately 120 per year (prevaccine) to 20 per year, despite continued circulation of virus among children.[127] Vaccine efficacy is high,[536] and in Western Australia the CRS incidence is below 2 cases per 10,000 births.[537] In South Australia, CRS incidence has fallen from 6.5 per 100,000 births in 1965 to 1979 to 1.5 per 100,000 in 1980 to 1986.[538]

Latin America

The Technical Advisory Group of the Pan-American Health Organization has recommended routine rubella immunization throughout the Americas, after concluding that 20,000 infants with CRS are born each year to that region even in the absence of an epidemic.[539] Of 47 countries in the Americas, all will have instituted rubella vaccination by 2003 with the exception of Haiti and the Dominican Republic. Cuba has already eradicated rubella.[539a] The English-speaking Caribbean countries have added rubella to their measles vaccination campaigns and included rubella elimination in the goals of the program.[540]

Previously, a model immunization program for rubella had been conducted in Saõ Paulo, Brazil, by Massad and co-workers.[541,542] All children 1 to 10 years old were included in a mass campaign with MMR, accompanied by routine MMR vaccination of infants at 15 months of age. Immunity to rubella in the population jumped from 40% to 97%, and, more important, the number of CRS cases dropped from 29 confirmed and suspected in 1992 to none in 1994. However, immigration of new children into Saõ Paulo and the absence of a vaccination program for older individuals led to a subsequent increase in the overall incidence of rubella. Although the highest incidence in 1997 was still among children ages 1 to 9 years of age, by 1999 to 2000 the incidence in the older age groups (15 to 29 years) had risen from 7 to 13 per 100,000 and exceeded that of the younger age groups. Accordingly, a two-phase vaccination plan was developed to accelerate CRS prevention. In November 2001, a total population of 16,437,881 females in 13 states received MMR vaccine. Each state in Brazil established a target group based on the introduction date of the vaccine. In the first phase, vaccination coverage reached 93%. Women who were pregnant during the first phase would be vaccinated later. During the next phase, over 12 million women of child-bearing age were to be vaccinated in 11 states during June and July 2002.[540]

The strategy employed in the English-speaking Caribbean is a combination of routine MMR vaccination of infants combined with mass campaigns with MMR or MR in 5- to 39-year-old persons of both sexes.[543] This strategy appears to be having success.[544]

Costa Rica had introduced MMR vaccination for infants as early as 1986, but serologic studies showed that coverage was incomplete, particularly in young adults. In 1999, a large rubella outbreak occurred, with 84% of cases in persons more than 15 years old. A mass vaccination campaign was launched in 2001, aimed at all persons 15 to 39 years of age.[545]

Chile began MMR vaccination of infants in 1990 and booster vaccination of 6-year-old children in 1993. However, rubella outbreaks were observed in 1997 and 1998 involving adolescents and adults. The Chileans launched a mass vaccination program for women ages 10 to 29 years, excluding pregnant women. The latter are being vaccinated postpartum.[546]

Developing Countries

The facts concerning rubella and CRS described earlier under *Epidemiology* suggest that many developing countries have a significant incidence of CRS and could benefit from rubella vaccination. Robertson and colleagues[547] have reviewed the use of rubella vaccine in developing countries. They documented use of rubella vaccine in about 30% of nonindustrialized countries. In South Africa, the rubella component of an MMR vaccine elicited seroconversion in 94% of black African infants.[418] Although combined childhood and adult female vaccination was the strategy employed by the majority of countries, 40% did not do so, and Robertson et al. expressed concern that selective vaccination of infants might increase the risk of infection in pregnant women by reducing the now-prevalent exposure in childhood.[133] The picture described by Robertson and colleagues[547] is spotty: Cuba has succeeded in eliminating rubella, and most developing countries, notably Malaysia, Hong Kong, and the Middle Eastern states, are starting to vaccinate against rubella. However, in Korea, only vaccination of female infants has been practiced.[548] Large countries like China and India are not vaccinating all of their children against rubella, and most of Asia and Africa is virgin territory in that respect.

Hinman and colleagues[548a] have examined the cost-benefit ratios for rubella vaccination in developing countries. They found that the economic argument for rubella vaccination was as strong as for hepatitis B and Hib vaccination, certainly in Latin America and the Caribbean and probably in Asia and Africa, although more data are needed.

Strategies for Rubella Vaccination

Possible strategies for the control of rubella are many. In principal, assuming high coverage, routine vaccination of infants would eliminate CRS in 30 to 40 years; vaccination of adolescent girls would eliminate CRS in 10 to 20 years; and vaccination of all women of child-bearing age would eliminate CRS immediately. However, the first strategy is complicated by the fear of a paradoxical temporary increase in rubella susceptibility of pregnant women, the second strategy is impeded by the difficulty in vaccinating adolescents, and the last strategy is dogged by the contraindication to vaccination of pregnant women.

The choice of a strategy for vaccination for rubella should be based on local circumstances. Rubella vaccination of infants should be practiced if the two following conditions are fulfilled: (1) rubella is given as part of MMR or MR, and (2) vaccine acceptance rates are high. Schoolgirl vaccination is an alternative strategy only if high acceptance rates can be guaranteed. Vaccination of seronegative women is now feasible because of the availability of simple serologic methods and the evidence described previously that rubella vaccine is not teratogenic. Vaccination of this group has the advantage of a direct effect on the group at highest risk. Vaccination of infants is an excellent strategy, but only if a high immunization rate is achieved. Because 100% acceptance of vaccine is unlikely and one does not wish to wait for the eradication of CRS, some combination of the aforementioned strategies is necessary. Knox[549] and Anderson and May[550] have argued that, where vaccine acceptance rates are less than 84%, the adult vaccination policy is best; where acceptance rates are higher, the childhood vaccination policy is best.[551] The adoption of a two-dose strategy by many developed countries has been highly successful in eliminating pockets of susceptibility, and this policy is likely to be extended as part of efforts to maintain control of infectious diseases in adolescents and adults.

In the United States, a decision was made to eliminate rubella and CRS,[486] and the goal was for elimination by the year 2000.[552] The strategy for elimination was essentially childhood vaccinations supplemented by vaccination of women as outlined in Table 26–19. As described above, this policy has been successful.

Knox,[549] Anderson and May,[550] and Gay et al.[553] have shown by mathematical modeling that institution of infant vaccination with inadequate vaccine coverage will decrease rubella virus circulation sufficiently to affect the susceptibility of adult women and thus to allow a paradoxical increase in CRS. Indeed, it appears that the phenomenon actually occurred in Greece, where low-level introduction of MMR in infants was followed by increased seronegativity of Athenian women and a CRS outbreak in 1993.[554] Figure 26–9, based on the mathematical modeling of Nigel Gay ("Modeling the impact of strategy options," unpublished document, 2002), gives the relation between rubella vaccine coverage and the predicted incidence of CRS, and shows that 80% infant coverage is needed to prevent the paradoxical effect.

Thus, in order to prevent the introduction of rubella vaccination in a country from temporarily increasing CRS, two steps are possible: (1) to do rapid vaccination of all prepubertal children in order to quickly decrease rubella virus circulation, or (2) to do a mass vaccination of all postpubertal females in order to render them nonsusceptible. Obviously, a combination of the two steps would be best, but not all developing countries are capable of carrying out vaccination beyond infancy. Moreover, vaccination of adults inevitably entails more real and coincidental adverse reactions. Thus the difficulty of adult vaccination should not act as a barrier to moving forward with elimination of rubella.[480] Instead, measles elimination should be done with combined vaccines (MR or MMR) to take advantage of mass campaigns to deal with both diseases. Of course, there must be a commitment to continue universal routine use of the same vaccines in infancy. Although CRS will decline slowly with this strategy, it will eventually disappear, and to

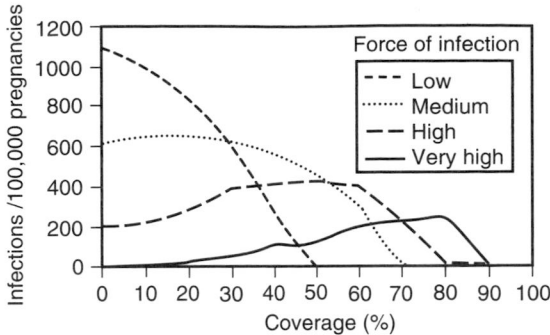

FIGURE 26–9 ■ Predicted long-term effect of infant vaccination. (Courtesy of Nigel Gay)

finish the job a country can avail itself of adult vaccination as soon as it is able.

Rubella virus and the congenital syndrome it causes are legitimate targets for eradication.[555] The virus is carried only by humans, the only chronically infected reservoir is babies with CRS, who do eventually stop excreting; the vaccine is highly effective; and combination vaccination with measles and/or mumps reduces the cost and avoids any additional expenses of administration.[556,557] The implementation of universal immunization throughout the world would mean the end of CRS within 100 years of its description.[558,559]

REFERENCES

1. Smith JL. Rothelin (epidemic roseola-German measles-hybrid measles, etc.). Arch Dermatol 1:1–13, 1875.
2. Veale H. History of an epidemic of röteln, with observation on its pathology. Edin Med J 12:404–414, 1866.
3. Gregg NM. Congenital cataract following German measles in the mother. Trans Ophthalmol Soc Aust 3:35–46, 1941.
4. Burgess MA. Gregg's rubella legacy 1941–1991. Med J Aust 155:355–357, 1991.
5. Pitt D, Keir EH. Results of rubella in pregnancy. Med J Aust 2:647–651, 1965.
6. Lundstrom R. Rubella during pregnancy: a follow-up study of children born after an epidemic of rubella in Sweden, 1951, with additional investigations on prophylaxis and treatment of maternal rubella. Acta Paediatr Scand 133(suppl):1–110, 1962.
7. Greenberg M, Pellitteri O, Barton J. Frequency of defects in infants whose mothers had rubella during pregnancy. JAMA 165:675–678, 1957.
8. Manson MM, Logan WPD, Loy RM. Rubella and other virus infections during pregnancy (Report on Public Health and Mechanical Subjects No 101). London, Her Royal Majesty's Stationery Office, 1960.
9. Weller TH, Neva FA. Propagation in tissue culture of cytopathic agents from patients with rubella-like illness. Proc Soc Exp Biol Med 111:215–225, 1962.
10. Parkman PD, Buescher EL, Artenstein MS. Recovery of rubella virus from army recruits. Proc Soc Exp Biol Med 111:225–230, 1962.
11. Witte JJ, Karchmer AW. Epidemiology of rubella. Am J Dis Child 118:107–112, 1969.
12. Rubella surveillance. Bethesda, MD, National Communicable Disease Center, 1969, p 1.
13. Plotkin SA, Oski FA, Hartnett EM, et al. Some recently recognized manifestations of the rubella syndrome. J Pediatr 67:182–191, 1965.
14. Meyer HM, Parkman PD, Hobbins TE, et al. Attenuated rubella viruses: laboratory and clinical characteristics. Am J Dis Child 118:155–169, 1969.
15. Prinzie A, Huygelen C, Gold J, et al. Experimental live attenuated rubella virus vaccine: clinical evaluation of Cendehill strain. Am J Dis Child 118:172–177, 1969.
16. Plotkin SA, Farquhar J, Katz M, Buser F. Attenuation of RA27/3 rubella virus in WI-38 human diploid cells. Am J Dis Child 118:178–185, 1969.
17. Heggie AD, Robbins FC. Natural rubella acquired after birth. Am J Dis Child 118:12–17, 1969.
18. Plotkin SA. Rubella viruses. In Lennette EH, Schmidt NJ (eds). Diagnostic Procedures for Viral and Rickettsial Infections (4th ed). Washington, DC, American Public Health Association, 1969, pp 364–413.
19. Kanto TG, Tanner M. Rubella arthritis and rheumatoid arthritis. Arthritis Rheum 5:378–383, 1962.
20. Fraser FRE, Cunningham A, Hayes K, et al. Rubella arthritis in adults: isolation of virus, cytology and other aspects of infection. Clin Exp Rheumatol 1:287–293, 1983.
21. Morse EE, Zinkham WH, Jackson DP. Thrombocytopenic purpura following rubella infection in children and adults. Arch Intern Med 117:573–579, 1966.
22. Sherman FE, Michaels RH, Kenny FM. Acute encephalopathy (encephalitis) complicating rubella: reports of cases with virologic studies, cortisol-production determinations and observations at autopsy. JAMA 192:675–681, 1965.
23. Pisternick D, Hopps J, Dannecker GE, et al. Fulminant verlaufende Rotelnenzephalitis mit latalem Ausgang. Monatsschr Kinderheilkd 145:105–108, 1997.
24. Katz M, Plotkin SA. Parainfectious encephalopathies associated with measles, mumps, chickenpox and German measles. In Goldensohn ES, Appel SH (eds). Scientific Approaches to Clinical Neurology. Vol. 1. Philadelphia, Lea & Febiger, 1977, pp 405–425.
25. Moriuchi H, Yamasaki S, Mori K, et al. A rubella epidemic in Sasebo, Japan in 1987, with various complications. Acta Paediatr Jpn 32:67–75, 1990.
26. Townsend JJ, Baringer JR, Wolinsky JS, et al. Progressive rubella panencephalitis: late onset after congenital rubella. N Engl J Med 292:990–993, 1975.
27. Weil ML, Itabashi H, Cremer NE, et al. Chronic progressive panencephalitis due to rubella virus simulating subacute sclerosing panencephalitis. N Engl J Med 292:994–998, 1975.
28. Yaginuma Y, Kawamura M, Ishikawa M. Landry-Guillain-Barre-Strohl syndrome in pregnancy. J Obstet Gynaecol Res 22:47–49, 1996.
29. Kalvenes MB, Kalland KH, Haukenes G. Radioimmunoprecipitation and immunoblot studies of antibodies to rubella virus in patients with chronic liver disease. Arch Virol 136:73–85, 1994.
30. Cooper L, Preblud SR, Alford CA. Rubella. In Remington JS, Klein JO (eds). Infectious Diseases of the Fetus and Newborn Infant (4th ed). Philadelphia, WB Saunders, 1995, pp 268–311.
31. Cosachow J, Frieri M. Hyper-IgM syndrome with congenital rubella. Pediatr Asthma Allergy Immunol 9(2):79–85, 1995.
32. O'Neill JF. The ocular manifestations of congenital infection: a study of the early effect and long-term outcome of maternally transmitted rubella and toxoplasmosis. Trans Am Ophthalmol Soc 96:813–879, 1998.
33. Reef SE, Plotkin S, Cordero JF, et al. Preparing for elimination of congenital rubella syndrome (CRS): summary of a workshop on CRS elimination in the United States. Clin Infect Dis 31:85–95, 2000.
34. Siegel M, Fuerst HT, Peress NS. Fetal mortality in maternal rubella: results of a prospective study from 1957 to 1964. Am J Obstet Gynecol 96:247–253, 1966.
35. Miller E, Cradock-Watson JE, Pollock TM. Consequences of confirmed maternal rubella at successive stages of pregnancy. Lancet 2:781–784, 1982.
36. South MA, Sever JL. Teratogen update: the congenital rubella syndrome. Teratology 31:297–307, 1985.
37. Ingalls TH. German measles and German measles in pregnancy. Am J Dis Child 93:555–558, 1957.
38. Grillner L, Forsgren M, Barr B, et al. Outcome of rubella during pregnancy with special reference to the 17th–24th weeks of gestation. Scand J Infect Dis 15:321–325, 1983.
39. Sheridan MD. Final report of a prospective study of children whose mothers had rubella in early pregnancy. Br Med J 2:536–539, 1964.
40. Rawls WE, Desmyter J, Melnick JL. Serologic diagnosis and fetal involvement in maternal rubella: criteria for abortion. JAMA 203:627–631, 1968.
41. Thompson KM, Tobin JO. Isolation of rubella virus from abortion material. Br Med J 1:264–266, 1970.
42. Cradock-Watson JE, Bourne MS, Vandervelde EM. IgG, IgA and IgM responses in acute rubella determined by the immunofluorescent technique. J Hyg (Lond) 70:473–485, 1972.

362. Lund KD, Chantler JK. Mapping of genetic determinants of rubella virus associated with growth in joint tissue. J Virol 74:796–804, 2000.

363. Tingle AJ, Kettyls GD, Ford DK. Studies on vaccine-induced rubella arthritis: serologic findings before and after immunization. Arthritis Rheum 22:400–402, 1979.

364. Bosma TJ, Etherington J, O'Shea S, et al. Rubella virus and chronic joint disease: is there an association? J Clin Microbiol 36:3524–3526, 1998.

365. Tingle AJ, Allen M, Petty RE, et al. Rubella-associated arthritis. I. Comparative study of joint manifestations associated with natural rubella infection and RA 27/3 rubella immunisation. Ann Rheum Dis 45:110–114, 1986.

366. Singh VK, Tingle AJ, Schulzer M. Rubella-associated arthritis. II. Relationship between circulating immune complex levels and joint manifestations. Ann Rheum Dis 45:115–119, 1986.

367. Howson CP, Katz M, Johnston RB Jr, Fineberg HV. Chronic arthritis after rubella vaccination. Clin Infect Dis 15:307–312, 1992.

368. Phillips P, Dougherty R, Mican J. Failure to isolate rubella virus (RV) from blood of adults after vaccination. Arthritis Rheum 32:113, 1989.

369. Frenkel L, Garakian A, Cherry JD. Rubella virus (RV): no evidence of persistent infection following immunization with RA27/3 or wild type infection [abstr]. In Abstracts of the 31st Interscience Conference on Antimicrobial Agents and Chemotherapy, Chicago, IL, 1991, p 1294.

370. Nielsen K, Garakian A, Frenkel LM, Cherry JD. The in vitro growth and serial passage of RA 27/3 rubella vaccine virus in cord blood mononuclear leukocytes from normal babies. Pediatr Res 37:623–625, 1995.

371. Zhang D, Nikkari S, Vainionpaa R, et al. Detection of rubella, mumps, and measles virus genomic RNA in cells from synovial fluid and peripheral blood in early rheumatoid arthritis. J Rheumatol 24:1260–1265, 1997.

372. Slater PE, Ben-Zvi T, Fogel A, et al. Absence of an association between rubella vaccination and arthritis in underimmune postpartum women. Vaccine 13:1529–1532, 1995.

373. Ray P, Black S, Shinefield H, et al. Risk of chronic arthropathy among women after rubella vaccination. Vaccine Safety Datalink Team [see comments]. JAMA 278:551–556, 1997.

374. Tingle AJ, Mitchell LA, Grace M, et al. Randomised double-blind placebo-controlled study on adverse effects of rubella immunisation in seronegative women. Lancet 349:1277–1281, 1997.

375. Mitchell LA, Tingle AJ, Grace M, et al. Rubella virus vaccine associated arthropathy in postpartum immunized women: influence of preimmunization serologic status on development of joint manifestations. J Rheumatol 27:418–423, 2000.

376. Weibel RE, Benor DE. Chronic arthropathy and musculoskeletal symptoms associated with rubella vaccines: a review of 124 claims submitted to the National Vaccine Injury Compensation Program. Arthritis Rheum 39:1529–1534, 1996. (published erratum appears in Arthritis Rheum 39:1930, 1996)

377. Chiba Y, Sadeghi E, Ogra PL. Abnormalities of cellular immune response in arthritis induced by rubella vaccination. J Immunol 117(5 pt 1):1684–1687, 1976.

378. Coyle PK, Wolinsky JS, Buimovici-Klein E, et al. Rubella-specific immune complexes after congenital infection and vaccination. Infect Immun 36:498–503, 1982.

379. Centers for Disease Control. Adverse Events Following Immunization (Report No 1, 1979–1982). Atlanta, Centers for Disease Control, 1984.

380. Schaffner W, Fleet WF, Kilroy AW, et al. Polyneuropathy following rubella immunization: a follow-up study and review of the problem. Am J Dis Child 127:684–688, 1974.

381. Cusi MG, Bianchi S, Santini L, et al. Peripheral neuropathy associated with anti-myelin basic protein antibodies in a woman vaccinated with rubella virus vaccine. J Neurovirol 5:209–214, 1999.

382. Kazarian EL, Gager WE. Optic neuritis complicating measles, mumps, and rubella vaccination. Am J Ophthalmol 86:544–547, 1978.

383. Kline LB, Margulies SL, Oh SJ. Optic neuritis and myelitis following rubella vaccination. Arch Neurol 39:443–444, 1982.

384. Islam SM, El Sheikh HF, Tabbara KF. Anterior uveitis following combined vaccination for measles, mumps and rubella (MMR): a report of two cases. Acta Ophthalmol Scand 78:590–592, 2000.

385. Centers for Disease Control. Rubella Surveillance No 2. Atlanta, Centers for Disease Control, 1970.

386. Holt S, Hudgins D, Krishnan KR, Critchley EM. Diffuse myelitis associated with rubella vaccination. Br Med J 2:1037–1038, 1976.

387. Behan PO. Diffuse myelitis associated with rubella vaccination. Br Med J 1:166, 1977.

388. Joyce KA, Rees J. Transverse myelitis after measles, mumps, and rubella vaccine. BMJ 311:422, 1995.

389. Morton-Kute L. Rubella vaccine and facial paresthesias. Ann Intern Med 102:563, 1985.

390. Tsuru T, Mizuguchi M, Ohkubo Y, et al. Acute disseminated encephalomyelitis after live rubella vaccination. Brain Dev 22:259–261, 2000.

391. Gunderman JR. Guillain-Barré syndrome: occurrence following combined mumps-rubella vaccine. Am J Dis Child 125:834–835, 1973.

392. Rees J, Hughes R. Guillain-Barré syndrome after measles, mumps, and rubella vaccine. Lancet 343:733, 1994.

393. Hughes R. Vaccines and Guillain-Barré syndrome. BMJ 312:1475–1476, 1996.

394. Patja A, Paunio M, Kinnunen E, et al. Risk of Guillain-Barré syndrome after measles-mumps-rubella vaccination. J Pediatr 138:250–254, 2001.

394a. Makela A, Nuorti JP, Peltola H. Neurologic disorders after measles-mumps-rubella vaccination. Pediatrics 110: 957–963, 2002.

395. Chantler JK, Smyrnis L, Tai G. Selective infection of astrocytes in human glial cell cultures by rubella virus. Lab Invest 72:334–340, 1995.

396. Peters ME, Horowitz S. Bone changes after rubella vaccination. AJR Am J Roentgenol 143:27–28, 1984.

397. Zeffer KB, Sauer MV. Orchitis after a rubella vaccination: a case report. J Reprod Med 33:80–81, 1988.

398. Sharma ON. Thrombocytopenia following measles-mumps-rubella vaccination in a one-year-old infant. Clin Pediatr (Phila) 12:315, 1973.

399. Neiderud J. Thrombocytopenic purpura after a combined vaccine against morbilli, parotitis and rubella. Acta Paediatr Scand 72:613–614, 1983.

400. Nieminen U, Peltola H, Syrjälä MT, et al. Acute thrombocytopenic purpura following measles, mumps and rubella vaccination: a report on 23 patients. Acta Paediatr 82:267–270, 1993.

401. Chang SK, Farrell DL, Dougan K, Kobayashi B. Acute idiopathic thrombocytopenic purpura following combined vaccination against measles, mumps, and rubella. J Am Board Fam Pract 9:53–55, 1996.

402. Bayer WL, Sherman FE, Michaels RH, et al. Purpura in congenital and acquired rubella. N Engl J Med 273:1362–1366, 1965.

403. Autret E, Jonville-Bera AP, Galy-Eyraud C, Hessel L. Thrombocytopenic purpura after isolated or combined vaccination against measles, mumps and rubella.. Thérapie 51:677–680, 1996.

404. Drachtman RA, Murphy S, Ettinger LJ. Exacerbation of chronic idiopathic thrombocytopenic purpura following measles-mumps-rubella immunization. Arch Pediatr Adolesc Med 148:326–327, 1994.

405. Vlacha V, Forman EN, Miron D, Peter G. Recurrent thrombocytopenic purpura after repeated measles-mumps-rubella vaccination. Pediatr Infect Dis J 97:738–739, 1996.

406. Miller E, Waight P, Farrington CP, et al. Idiopathic thrombocytopenic purpura and MMR vaccine. Arch Dis Child 84:227–229, 2001.

407. Advisory Committee on Immunization Practices (ACIP). Update: vaccine side effects, adverse reactions, contraindications, and precautions. MMWR 45(RR-12):1–35, 1996.

408. Pool V, Chen R, Rhodes P. Indications for measles-mumps-rubella vaccination in a child with prior thrombocytopenic purpura. Pediatr Infect Dis J 16:423–424, 1997.

409. Lindberg B, Ahlfors K, Carlsson A, et al. Previous exposure to measles, mumps, and rubella—but not vaccination during adolescence—correlates to the prevalence of pancreatic and thyroid autoantibodies. Pediatrics 104:E12, 1999

410. Midulla M, Businco L, Moschini L. Some effects of rubella vaccination of immunologic responsiveness. Acta Paediatr Scand 61:609–611, 1972.

411. Ganguly R, Cusumano CL, Waldman RH. Suppression of cell-mediated immunity after infection with attenuated rubella virus. Infect Immun 13:464–469, 1976.

412. Arneborn P, Biberfeld G, Wasserman J. Immunosuppression and alterations of T-lymphocyte subpopulations after rubella vaccination. Infect Immun 29:36–41, 1980.

413. Munyer TP, Mangi RJ, Dolan T, Kantor FS. Depressed lymphocyte function after measles-mumps-rubella vaccination. J Infect Dis 132:75–78, 1975.

414. Mellor JA, Langford DT, Zealley H, et al. A survey of cancer morbidity and mortality in vaccinees seven to 12 years after the administration of live vaccine propagated in human diploid cells. J Biol Stand 11:221–225, 1983.

415. Nicoara C, Zach K, Trachsel D, et al. Decay of passively acquired maternal antibodies against measles, mumps, and rubella viruses. Clin Diagn Lab Immunol 6:868–871, 1999.

416. Herrmann KL, Wende RD, Witte JJ. Rubella immunization with HPV-77 DE5 vaccine during infancy. Am J Dis Child 121:474–476, 1971.

417. Wilkins J, Wehrle PF. Further evaluation of the optimum age for rubella vaccine administration. Am J Dis Child 133:1237–1239, 1979.

418. Schoub BD, Johnson S, McAnerney JM, et al. Measles, mumps and rubella immunization at nine months in a developing country. Pediatr Infect Dis J 9:263–267, 1990.

419. Volti SL, Giammanco-Bilancia G, Grassi M, et al. Duration of the immune response to MMR vaccine in children of two age-different groups. Eur J Epidemiol 9:311–314, 1993.

420. Singh R, John TJ, Cherian T, Raghupathy P. Immune response to measles, mumps & rubella vaccine at 9, 12 & 15 months of age. Indian J Med Res 100:155–159, 1994.

421. Ratnam S, Chandra R, Gadag V. Maternal measles and rubella antibody levels and serologic response in infants immunized with MMR II vaccine at 12 months of age. J Infect Dis 168:1596–1598, 1993.

422. Rubella prevention. Recommendations of the Immunization Practices Advisory Committee (ACIP). MMWR 39(RR-15):1–18, 1990.

423. Dennehy PH, Saracen CL, Peter G. Seroconversion rates to combined measles-mumps-rubella-varicella vaccine of children with upper respiratory tract infection. Pediatrics 94:514–516, 1994.

424. Ratnam S, West R, Gadag V. Measles and rubella antibody response after measles-mumps-rubella vaccination in children with afebrile upper respiratory tract infection. J Pediatr 127:432–434, 1995.

425. Cilla G, Pena B, Marimon JM, Pérez-Trallero E. Serologic response to measles-mumps-rubella vaccine among children with upper respiratory tract infection. Vaccine 14:492–494, 1996.

426. Schiff GM, Linnemann CC Jr, Rotte T, Ashe HS. Rubella surveillance and immunization: susceptibility in nonurban adolescents. JAMA 226:554–556, 1973.

427. Rauh JL, Schiff GM, Johnson LB. Rubella surveillance and immunization among adolescent girls in Cincinnati. Am J Dis Child 124:71–75, 1972.

428. Mann JM, Montes JM, Hull HF, et al. Risk of pregnancy among adolescent schoolgirls participating in a measles mass immunization program. Am J Public Health 73:527–529, 1983.

429. Lerman SJ, Lerman LM, Nankervis GA, Gold E. Accuracy of rubella history. Ann Intern Med 74:97–98, 1971.

430. Tattersall JM, Freestone DS. Rubella vaccination in young women attending a family planning clinic. Practitioner 211:769–772, 1973.

431. Halstead E, Halstead SB, Jackson RS, et al. Rubella vaccination: fertility control in a large-scale vaccination program for postpubertal women. Am J Obstet Gynecol 121:1089–1094, 1975.

432. Gringras M, Reisler R, Caisley J, et al. Vaccination of rubella-susceptible women during oral contraceptive care in general practice. Br Med J 2:245–246, 1977.

433. Rowlands S, Bethel RG. Contraceptive cover for rubella vaccination. Practitioner 226:1155–1156, 1982.

434. Schiff GM, Young BC, Stefanovic GM, et al. Challenge with rubella virus after loss of detectable vaccine-induced antibody. Rev Infect Dis 7(suppl 1):S157–S163, 1985.

435. Kelly CS, Gibson JL, Williams CS, Leibovitz A. Postpartum rubella immunization: results with the HPV-77 strain. Obstet Gynecol 37:338–342, 1971.

436. Tobin JO. Rubella vaccination of postpartum women and of adolescents in the Northwest of England. Can J Public Health 62:634–667, 1971.

437. Beazley JM, Hurley R, Middlebrook C, Rumpus MF. Rubella vaccination in the puerperium. Br J Prev Soc Med 25:140–143, 1971.

438. Grillner L, Hedstrom CE, Bergstrom H, et al. Vaccination against rubella of newly delivered women. Scand J Infect Dis 5:237–241, 1973.

439. Cheldelin LV, Francis DP, Tilson H. Postpartum rubella vaccination: a survey of private physicians in Oregon. JAMA 225:158–159, 1973.

440. Griffiths PD, Baboonian C. Is post partum rubella vaccination worthwhile? J Clin Pathol 35:1340–1344, 1982.

441. Black NA, Parsons A, Kurtz JB, et al. Post-partum rubella immunisation: a controlled trial of two vaccines. Lancet 2:990–992, 1983.

442. Marshall WC, Peckham CS, Dudgeon JA, et al. Parity of women contracting rubella in pregnancy: implications with respect to rubella vaccination. Lancet 1:1231–1233, 1976.

443. Edmond E, Zealley H. The impact of a rubella prevention policy on the outcome of rubella in pregnancy. Br J Obstet Gynaecol 93:563–567, 1986.

444. Baldwin JA, Freestone DS. Risk of early post-partum pregnancy in context of post-partum vaccination against rubella. Lancet 2:366–367, 1971.

445. Sharp DS, Macdonald H. Use of medroxyprogesterone acetate as a contraceptive in conjunction with early postpartum rubella vaccination. Br Med J 4:443–446, 1973.

446. Bolognese RJ, Corson SL, Fuccillo DA, Traub R. The susceptibility of the postpartum and postabortal cervix and uterine cavity to infection with attenuated rubella virus. Am J Obstet Gynecol 125:525–527, 1976.

447. Buimovici-Klein E, Hite RL, Byrne T, Cooper LZ. Isolation of rubella virus in milk after postpartum immunization. J Pediatr 91:939–941, 1977.

448. Landes RD, Bass JW, Millunchick EW, Oetgen WJ. Neonatal rubella following postpartum maternal immunization. J Pediatr 97:465–467, 1980.

449. Losonsky GA, Fishaut JM, Strussenberg J, Ogra PL. Effect of immunization against rubella on lactation products. I. Development and characterization of specific immunologic reactivity in breast milk. J Infect Dis 145:654–660, 1982.

450. Losonsky GA, Fishaut JM, Strussenberg J, Ogra PL. Effect of immunization against rubella on lactation products. II. Maternal-neonatal interactions. J Infect Dis 145:661–666, 1982.

451. Perez-Trallero E, Cilla G, Urbieta M. Rubella immunisation of men: advantages of herd immunity. Lancet 348:413, 1996.

452. Bakasun V, Suzanic-Karnincic S. A rubella outbreak in the region of Rijeka, Croatia. Int J Epidemiol 24:453–456, 1995.

453. Lim MK, Fong YF, Soh CS. Rubella seroprevalence in the Singapore Armed Forces (SAF) and the changing need of the SAF rubella immunisation programme. Ann Acad Med Singapore 26(1):37–39, 1997.

454. Adams MS, Croft AM, Winfield DA, Richards PR. An outbreak of rubella in British troops in Bosnia. Epidemiol Infect 118:253–257, 1997.

455. Migliani R, Renaudat-Olivaud A, Barneche JP, et al. Epidémie de rubéole en 1996 dans un centre d'instruction militarie dans le centre de la France. Bull Epidémiol Hebd 28:124–125, 1996.

456. Weiss KE, Falvo CE, Buimovici-Klein E, et al. Evaluation of an employee health service as a setting for a rubella screening and immunization program. Am J Public Health 69:281–283, 1979.

457. Polk BF, White JA, DeGirolami PC, Modlin JF. An outbreak of rubella among hospital personnel. N Engl J Med 303:541–545, 1980.

458. Nosocomial rubella infection—North Dakota, Alabama, Ohio. MMWR Morb Mortal Wkly Rep 29:630–631, 1981.

459. Rubella in hospitals—California. MMWR 32:37–39, 1983.

460. Greaves WL, Orenstein WA, Stetler HC, et al. Prevention of rubella transmission in medical facilities. JAMA 248:861–864, 1982.

461. Heseltine PN, Ripper M, Wohlford P. Nosocomial rubella—consequences of an outbreak and efficacy of a mandatory immunization program. Infect Control 6:371–374, 1985.

462. Weber DJ, Rutala WA, Orenstein WA. Prevention of mumps, measles, and rubella among hospital personnel. J Pediatr 119:322–326, 1991.

463. Geiger R, Fink FM, Sölder B, et al. Persistent rubella infection after erroneous vaccination in an immunocompromised patient with acute lymphoblastic leukemia in remission. J Med Virol 47:442–444, 1995.

464. Ljungman P, Fridell E, Lonnqvist B, et al. Efficacy and safety of vaccination of marrow transplant recipients with a live attenuated measles, mumps, and rubella vaccine. J Infect Dis 159:610–615, 1989.

465. King SM, Saunders EF, Petric M, Gold R. Response to measles, mumps, and rubella vaccine in paediatric bone marrow transplant recipients. Bone Marrow Transplant 17:633–636, 1996.

466. Flynn JT, Frisch K, Kershaw DB, et al. Response to early measles-mumps-rubella vaccination in infants with chronic renal failure and/or receiving peritoneal dialysis. Adv Perit Dial 15:269–272, 1999.

467. Kwitten PL, Rosen S, Sweinberg SK. MMR vaccine and neomycin allergy. Pediatr Forum 147:128–129, 1993.
468. Frenkel LM, Nielsen K, Garakian A, Cherry JD. A search for persistent measles, mumps, and rubella vaccine virus in children with human immunodeficiency virus type 1 infection. Arch Pediatr Adolesc Med 148:57–60, 1994.
469. Fleet WF Jr, Benz EW Jr, Karzon DT, et al. Fetal consequences of maternal rubella immunization. JAMA 227:621–627, 1974.
470. Centers for Disease Control and Prevention. Revised ACIP recommendation for avoiding pregnancy after receiving a rubella-containing vaccine. MMWR 50:1117, 2001.
471. Rubella vaccination during pregnancy—United States, 1971–1983. MMWR Morb Mortal Wkly Rep 33:365–368, 373, 1984.
472. Bart SW, Stetler HC, Preblud SR, et al. Fetal risk associated with rubella vaccine: an update. Rev Infect Dis 7(suppl 1):S95–S102, 1985.
473. Enders G. Rubella antibody titers in vaccinated and nonvaccinated women and results of vaccination during pregnancy. Rev Infect Dis 7(suppl 1):S103–S107, 1985.
474. Hofmann J, Kortung M, Pustowoit B, et al. Persistent fetal rubella vaccine virus infection following inadvertent vaccination during early pregnancy. J Med Virol 61:155–158, 2000.
475. Rubella vaccination during pregnancy—United States, 1971–1986. MMWR 36:457–461, 1987.
476. Sheppard S, Smithells RW, Dickson A, Holzel H. Rubella vaccination and pregnancy: preliminary report of a national survey. Br Med J 292:727, 1986.
477. Cooper LZ, Florman AL, Ziring PR, Krugman S. Loss of rubella hemagglutination inhibition antibody in congenital rubella: failure of seronegative children with congenital rubella to respond to HPV-77 rubella vaccine. Am J Dis Child 122:397–403, 1971.
478. Ingalls TH, Plotkin SA, Philbrook FR, Thompson RF. Immunisation of schoolchildren with rubella (RA27-3) vaccine: intranasal and subcutaneous administration. Lancet 1:99–101, 1970.
479. World Health Organization. Rubella vaccines: WHO position paper. 75:161–172, 2000.
480. World Health Organization Weekly Epid. Record. Report of a meeting on preventing congenital rubella syndrome: immunization strategies, surveillance needs, Geneva, 12–14 January 2000 (WHO/V&B/00.10). Geneva, Department of Vaccines and Biologicals, World Health Organization, 2000, pp 101–177.
481. Preblud SR, Serdula MK, Frank JA Jr, et al. Rubella vaccination in the United States: a ten-year review. Epidemiol Rev 2:171–194, 1980.
482. Weinstein L, Chang TW. Rubella immunization. N Engl J Med 288:100–101, 1973.
483. Farquhar JD. Experience with rubella and rubella immunization in institutionalized children. J Pediatr 83:51–56, 1973.
484. Schoenbaum SC, Biano S, Mack T. Epidemiology of congenital rubella syndrome: the role of maternal parity. JAMA 233:151–155, 1975.
485. Cochi SL, Edmonds LE, Dyer K, et al. Congenital rubella syndrome in the United States, 1970–1985. Am J Epidemiol 129:349–361, 1989.
486. Bart KJ, Orenstein WA, Preblud SR, Hinman AR. Universal immunization to interrupt rubella. Rev Infect Dis 7(suppl 1):S177–S184, 1985.
487. Rubella and congenital rubella syndrome—United States, 1984–1985. MMWR 35:129–135, 1986.
488. Increase in rubella and congenital rubella syndrome—United States, 1988–1990. MMWR 40:93–99, 1991.
489. Dykewicz CA, Kruszon-Moran D, McQuillan GM, et al. Rubella seropositivity in the United States, 1988–1994. Clin Infect Dis 33:1279–1286, 2001.
490. Danovaro-Holliday MC, LeBaron CW, Allensworth C, et al. A large rubella outbreak with spread from the workplace to the community. JAMA 284:2733–2739, 2000.
491. Reef SE, Frey TK, Theall K, et al. The changing epidemiology of rubella in the 1990s: on the verge of elimination and new challenges for control and prevention. JAMA 287:464–472, 2002.
492. White CC, Koplan JP, Orenstein WA. Benefits, risks and costs of immunization for measles, mumps and rubella. Am J Public Health 75:739–744, 1985.
493. Berger SA, Ginsberg GM, Slater PE. Cost-benefit analysis of routine mumps and rubella vaccination for Israeli infants. Isr J Med Sci 26:74–80, 1990.
494. Schoenbaum SC, Hyde JN Jr, Crampton K. Benefit-cost analysis of rubella vaccination policy. N Engl J Med 294:306–310, 1976.
495. Centers for Disease Control. Measles prevention. MMWR 38:1–18, 1989.
496. American Academy of Pediatrics Committee on Infectious Diseases. Measles: reassessment of the current immunization policy. Pediatrics 84:1110–1113, 1989.
497. Galazka A. Rubella in Europe. Epidemiol Infect 107:43–54, 1991.
498. Pebody RG, Edmunds WJ, Conyn-van Spaendonck M, et al. The seroepidemiology of rubella in western Europe. Epidemiol Infect 125:347–357, 2000.
499. Edmunds WJ, van de Heijden OG, Eerola M, Gay NJ. Modelling rubella in Europe. Epidemiol Infect 125:617–634, 2000.
500. Dudgeon JA. Selective immunization: protection of the individual. Rev Infect Dis 7(suppl 1):S185–S190, 1985.
501. Smithells RW, Sheppard S, Marshall WC, Milton A. National Congenital Rubella Surveillance Programme 1971–81. Br Med J 285:1363, 1982.
502. Peckham CS, Marshall WC, Dudgeon JA. Rubella vaccination of schoolgirls: factors affecting vaccine uptake. Br Med J 1:760–761, 1977.
503. Noah ND, Fowle SE. Immunity to rubella in women of childbearing age in the United Kingdom. BMJ 297:1301–1304, 1988.
504. Freestone DS. Vaccination against rubella in Britain: benefits and risks. Dev Biol Stand 43:339–348, 1979.
505. Hambling MH. Changes in the distribution of rubella antibodies in women of childbearing age during the first eight years of a rubella vaccination programme. J Infect 2:341–346, 1980.
506. Clarke M, Seagroatt V, Schild GC, et al. Surveys of rubella antibodies in young adults and children. Lancet 1(8326 pt 1):667–669, 1983.
507. Gilmore D, Robinson ET, Gilmour WH, Urquhart GE. Effect of rubella vaccination programme in schools on rubella immunity in a general practice population. Br Med J 284:628–630, 1982.
508. Miller CL, Miller E, Sequeira PJ, et al. Effect of selective vaccination on rubella susceptibility and infection in pregnancy. Br Med J 291:1398–1401, 1985.
509. Anderson RM, Grenfell BT. Control of congenital rubella syndrome by mass vaccination. Lancet 2:827–828, 1985.
510. Anderson RM, Grenfell BT. Quantitative investigations of different vaccination policies for the control of congenital rubella syndrome (CRS) in the United Kingdom. J Hyg (Lond) 96:305–333, 1986.
511. Walker D, Carter H, Jones IG. Measles, mumps, and rubella: the need for a change in immunisation policy. Br Med J 292:1501–1502, 1986.
512. Hutchinson A. Rubella prevention—a new era? J R Coll Gen Pract 38:193–194, 1988.
513. Miller E. Rubella in the United Kingdom. Epidemiol Infect 107:31–42, 1991.
514. Miller E, Tookey P, Morgan-Capner P, et al. Rubella surveillance to June 1994: third joint report from the PHLS and the National Congenital Rubella Surveillance Programme. Commun Dis Rep CDR Rev 4:R146–R152, 1994
515. Miller E, Waight P, Gay N, et al. The epidemiology of rubella in England and Wales before and after the 1994 measles and rubella vaccination campaign: fourth joint report from the PHLS and the National Congenital Rubella Surveillance Programme. Commun Dis Rep CDR Rev 7:R26–R32, 1997
515a. Sheridan E, Aitken C, Jeffries D, et al. Congenital rubella syndrome: a risk in immigrant populations. Lancet 359:674–675, 2002.
516. Editor. Communicable Disease Report. Rubella in Students. CDR Wkly 9:113, 1999.
517. Christenson B, Bottiger M, Heller L. Mass vaccination programme aimed at eradicating measles, mumps, and rubella in Sweden: first experience. Br Med J 287:389–391, 1983.
518. Rabo E, Taranger J. Scandinavian model for eliminating measles, mumps, and rubella. Br Med J 289:1402–1404, 1984.
519. Bottiger M, Christenson B, Taranger J, Bergman M. Mass vaccination programme aimed at eradicating measles, mumps and rubella in Sweden: vaccination of schoolchildren. Vaccine 3:113–116, 1985.
520. Christenson B, Bottiger M. Changes of the immunological patterns against measles, mumps and rubella: a vaccination programme studied 3 to 7 years after the introduction of a two-dose schedule. Vaccine 9:326–329, 1991.
521. Bottiger M, Forsgren M. Twenty years' experience of rubella vaccination in Sweden: 10 years of selective vaccination (of 12-year-old girls and of women postpartum) and 13 years of a general two-dose vaccination. Vaccine 15:1538–1544, 1997.

522. Peltola H, Kurki T, Virtanen M, et al. Rapid effect on endemic measles, mumps, and rubella of nationwide vaccination programme in Finland. Lancet 1:137–139, 1986.

523. Peltola H, Heinonen OP, Valle M, et al. The elimination of indigenous measles, mumps, and rubella from Finland by a 12-year, two-dose vaccination program. N Engl J Med 331:1397–1402, 1994.

524. Ukkonen P. Rubella immunity and morbidity: impact of different vaccination programs in Finland 1979–1992. Scand J Infect Dis 28:31–35, 1996.

525. Peltola H, Davidkin I, Paunio M, et al. Mumps and rubella eliminated from Finland. JAMA 284:2643–2647, 2000.

526. Marret H, Golfier F, Di Maio M, et al. Rubella in pregnancy: management and prevention. Presse Med 28:2117–2122, 1999.

527. Antona D, Guerin N. Couverture vaccinale rougeole-rubéole-oreillons en France en 1998: première et deuxième doses. Bull Epidémiol Hebd 19:74–75, 1999.

528. Che D, Baron S, Levy-Bruhl D. Epidemiology of rubella in France, 20 years after the advent of vaccination. Rev Prat 50:1629–1631, 2000.

529. van der Heijden OG, Conyn-van Spaendonck MA, Plantinga AD, Kretzschmar ME. A model-based evaluation of the national immunization programme against rubella infection and congenital rubella syndrome in The Netherlands. Epidemiol Infect 121:653–671, 1998.

530. Matter L, Bally F, Germann D, Schopfer K. The incidence of rubella virus infections in Switzerland after the introduction of the MMR mass vaccination programme. Eur J Epidemiol 11:305–310, 1995.

531. Furesz J, Varughese P, Acres SE, Davies JW. Rubella immunization strategies in Canada. Rev Infect Dis 7(suppl 1):S191–S193, 1985.

532. Fogel A, Barnea BS, Aboudy Y, Mendelson E. Rubella in pregnancy in Israel: 15 years of follow-up and remaining problems. Isr J Med Sci 32:300–305, 1996.

533. Slater PE, Roitman M, Leventhal A, Anis E. Control of rubella in Israel: progress and challenge. Public Health Rev 24:183–192, 1996.

534. Coulter C, Wood R, Robson J. Rubella infection in pregnancy. Commun Dis Intell 23:93–96, 1999.

535. Causer J, Mira M, Karr M, et al. Serological survey of measles and rubella immunity in Sydney preschool children. J Paediatr Child Health 36:418–421, 2000.

536. Cheah D, Hall R, Mead C, Passaris I. The effectiveness of rubella vaccine. Med J Aust 158:434–435, 1993.

537. Condon RJ, Bower C. Rubella vaccination and congenital rubella syndrome in Western Australia. Med J Aust 158:379–382, 1993.

538. Cheffins T, Chan A, Keane RJ, et al. The impact of rubella immunisation on the incidence of rubella, congenital rubella syndrome and rubella-related terminations of pregnancy in South Australia. Br J Obstet Gynaecol 105:998–1004, 1998.

539. Pan-American Health Organization. SVI Technical Advisory Group meets. EPI Newsletter 19:371–374, 1997.

539a. Pan-American Health Organization. Accelerated rubella control and prevention of CRS evolving strategies. EPI Newsletter 24(5):2–3, 2002.

540. Pan-American Health Organization. Brazil accelerates control of rubella and prevention of congenital rubella syndrome. EPI Newsletter 24(2):1–3, 2002.

541. Massad E, Nascimento Burattini M, de Azevedo Neto RS, et al. A model-based design of a vaccination strategy against rubella in a non-immunized community of Sao Paulo state, Brazil. Epidemiol Infect 112:579–594, 1994.

542. Massad E, de Azevedo Neto RS, Burattini MN, et al. Assessing the efficacy of a mixed vaccination strategy against rubella in Sao Palo, Brazil. Int J Epidemiol 24:842–850, 1995.

543. Hinman AR, Hersh BS, de Quadros CA. Rational use of rubella vaccine for prevention of congenital rubella syndrome in the Americas. Rev Panam Salud Publica 4:156–160, 1998.

544. Irons B, Lewis MJ, Dahl-Regis M, et al. Strategies to eradicate rubella in the English-speaking Caribbean. Am J Public Health 90:1545–1549, 2000.

545. Centers for Disease Control and Prevention. Nationwide campaign for vaccination of adults against rubella and measles—Costa Rica, 2001. MMWR Morb Mortal Wkly Rep 50:976–979, 2001.

546. Pan-American Health Organization. Rubella campaign in Chile. EPI Newsletter 21:3–4, 1999.

547. Robertson SE, Cutts FT, Samuel R, Diaz-Ortega JL. Control of rubella and congenital rubella syndrome (CRS) in developing countries, Part 2: Vaccination against rubella. Bull World Health Organ 75:69–80, 1997.

548. Park KS, Kim HS. Seroprevalence of rubella antibodies and effects of vaccination among healthy university women students in Korea. Yonsei Med J 37:420–426, 1996.

548a. Hinman AR, Irons B, Lewis M, et al. Economic analyses of rubella and rubella vaccines: a global review. Bull WHO 80:264–270, 2002.

549. Knox EG. Epidemiology of prenatal infections: an extension of the congenital rubella model. Stat Med 2:1–12, 1983.

550. Anderson RM, May RM. Vaccination against rubella and measles: quantitative investigations of different policies. J Hyg (Lond) 90:259–325, 1983.

551. Forster J. Rubella vaccination. Eur J Pediatr 147:570–573, 1988.

552. Public Health Service. Healthy People 2000: National Health Promotion and Disease Prevention Objectives—Full Report with Commentary (publ no 91-50212). Washington, DC, U.S. Department of Health and Human Services, 1991.

553. Gay NJ, Valambia S, Galasko D, Miller E. Selective rubella vaccination programmes: a survey of districts in England & Wales. Rev Med Virol 4:261–277, 1994.

554. Panagiotopoulos T, Antoniadou I, Valassi-Adam E. Increase in congenital rubella occurrence after immunisation in Greece: retrospective survey and systematic review. Br Med J 319:1462–1467, 1999.

555. Fenner F. Candidate viral diseases for elimination or eradication. Bull World Health Organ 76(suppl 2):68–70, 1998.

556. Plotkin SA, Katz M, Cordero JF. The eradication of rubella. JAMA 281:561–562, 1999.

557. Plotkin SA. Rubella eradication. Vaccine 19:3311–3319, 2001.

558. Plotkin SA. Birth and death of congenital rubella syndrome. JAMA 251:2003–2004, 1984.

559. Orenstein WA, Bart KJ, Hinman AR, et al. The opportunity and obligation to eliminate rubella from the United States. JAMA 251:1988–1994, 1984.

Chapter 27

Tetanus Toxoid

STEVEN G. F. WASSILAK • MARTHA H. ROPER •
TRUDY V. MURPHY • WALTER A. ORENSTEIN

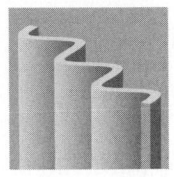 Tetanus is unique among diseases for which immunization is routinely recommended because it is not communicable. *Clostridium tetani*, the causative agent of tetanus, is widespread in the environment; many animals in addition to humans can harbor and excrete the organism and its spores. When spores of C. *tetani* are introduced into the anaerobic/hypoaerobic conditions found in devitalized tissue or punctures, they germinate to vegetative bacilli that elaborate toxin. The clinical presentation results from the actions of this toxin on the central nervous system (CNS). Many animal species besides humans are susceptible to the disease.

The clinical characteristics of tetanus were recognized as distinct early in human history because of the constancy and severity of the symptoms in animals and humans. Although the first medical description appears in the writings of Hippocrates, the etiology of tetanus was unknown until 1884. Carle and Rattone[1] demonstrated that, when the contents of a pustule from a fatal human case were injected into sciatic nerve in a rabbit model, the typical symptoms of tetanus resulted; the disease could subsequently be passed to other rabbits from infected nervous tissue. Inoculation of soil samples into animals also resulted in tetanus. Gram-positive bacilli often were noted in the exudate at the inoculation site but generally not in nervous tissue, leading Nicolaier[2] to hypothesize that a poison produced at the site of inoculation led to the nervous system symptoms. In 1886, spore-forming bacilli were observed in the exudate obtained from a human case.[3] In 1889, the spores of C. *tetani*, in contrast to the vegetative organisms, were shown to survive heating and to germinate under anaerobic conditions; injection of pure cultures reproducibly caused the disease in animals.[4] After identification and purification of the toxin in 1890, repeated inoculation of animals with minute quantities of toxin led to the production in survivors of antibodies that neutralized the effects of the toxin.[5] Preparations of antibodies derived from animal sera, particularly from horses, became the first means to prevent and treat tetanus. The culmination of these efforts was in the preparation of "anatoxin"—chemically inactivated toxin, now termed a *toxoid*—in 1924.[6] Toxoid induced active immunity against the disease before exposure.

The impetus to prevent tetanus through immunization originated from the striking and highly fatal disease in both industrialized and developing nations, predominantly associated with injuries to otherwise healthy persons, and particularly during military conflicts. In the developing world, the continuing health burden from tetanus is largely among neonates. Prevention of tetanus is now almost universally achievable by use of highly immunogenic and safe toxoid-containing vaccines. Tetanus also can be prevented or modified by use of exogenous antibody.

Background

Clinical Description

Although the incubation period for tetanus has been reported to vary from 1 day to several months following a wound, the majority of cases occur within 3 days to 3 weeks after inoculation of spores. In the United States during 1998 to 2000, the median interval between the injury and onset of tetanus was 7 days (range 0 to 112 days) for 89 nonneonatal cases with reported information. The time between injury and the onset of symptoms was 30 days or less for 94% of the cases, and 2 days or less for 12% of the cases.[7]

There is a direct relationship between the site of inoculation and the incubation period, with the longest intervals occurring after injuries farthest from the CNS; injuries of the head and trunk generally are associated with the shortest incubation periods.[8,9] As historically noted, the incubation period is inversely related to severity of illness,[10–16] and the incubation period has been considered one of the best prognostic indicators.[17,18] Incubation periods of 10 days or more tend to result in mild disease, whereas incubation periods within 7 days of injury tend to result in more severe disease.

Three clinical syndromes are associated with tetanus infection: (1) localized, (2) generalized, and (3) cephalic.[8] Localized tetanus, which is unusual in humans, consists of spasm of muscles in a confined area close to the site of the injury.[19,20] Painful contractions may persist for several weeks to months before gradually subsiding. Localized disease is thought to occur when transport of toxin produced at the site of the injury is restricted to the local nerves.[9] The symptoms can be produced experimentally by simultaneously injecting toxin into a muscle and antitoxin into blood to prevent hematogenous dissemination.[9] Although localized tetanus per se is generally mild, with death-to-case ratios of less than 1%, progression to generalized tetanus and more serious outcomes can occur.[19]

More than 80% of cases of tetanus are generalized. The most common initial sign is spasm of the muscles of mastication—trismus, or lockjaw—occurring in more than 50% of the cases.[8,21] Trismus associated with spasm of the facial muscles results in a characteristic facial expression—risus sardonicus—consisting of raised eyebrows, tight closure of the eyelids, wrinkling of the forehead, and extension of the corners of the mouth laterally. Trismus may be followed by spasm of other muscles in the neck, thorax and back, abdomen, and extremities. Sustained spasm of back muscles can give rise to opisthotonos. Generalized tonic tetanic seizure–like activity (termed tetanospasm), often triggered by mild external stimuli such as sudden noises, consists of sudden painful contraction of all muscle groups resulting in opisthotonos, adduction at the shoulders, flexion of the elbows and wrists, and extension of the legs. Frank convulsions can occur in severely affected patients. Spasm of the glottis can result in immediate death. Temperature elevations of 2°C to 4°C are often associated with severe spasms. Patients exhibit generalized hyperreflexia. Cognitive functions are not overtly affected.

Tetanus can be accompanied by severe autonomic nervous system abnormalities, particularly among the elderly and narcotic addicts, that consist of systemic arterial hypertension or hypotension, flushing, diaphoresis, tachycardia, and arrhythmias.[22–26] Tetanus also is associated with a variety of spasm-related complications, including fractures of the long bones and vertebrae, asphyxia from glottic obstruction, and traumatic glossitis. Toxin can induce urinary retention and dysphagia. Complications can result from chronic debility: pulmonary embolism, decubitus ulcers, pneumonia, catheter-associated infections, and contrac-

tures. Long-term consequences—including prolonged muscle fatigue, hyperostoses and osteoarthritis, and difficulties with speech, memory, and mental capacity—have been documented.[27–29]

Tetanus neonatorum, the most common presentation of the disease in developing countries, is a form of generalized tetanus occurring in newborn infants, most often as a result of an infected umbilical cord stump.[8] The illness typically begins 3 to 14 days after birth with poor sucking and excessive crying in an infant with normal ability to suck in the first 2 days of life.[8,30] This is followed by variable degrees of trismus, difficulty swallowing, opisthotonos, and other tetanic spasms.

The clinical course of generalized tetanus is highly variable. The disease frequently remains intense for 1 to 4 weeks and then gradually subsides. Death-to-case ratios for reported cases of generalized tetanus have varied from 25% to 70% overall, with fatality ratios in the past approaching 100% at the extremes of age.[15,16] With modern intensive care, mortality currently can be reduced to 10% to 20%.[18,31–37] In the United States during 1972 to 2000, reported death-to-case ratios have declined from approximately 50% to less than 20% overall, but ratios vary depending on age (Fig. 27–1) and immunization status.[7,38–40] A higher death-to-case ratio has been reported when tetanus results from intramuscular injection of quinine.[41]

Cephalic tetanus is a rare manifestation of the disease generally associated with lesions of the head or face, especially in the distribution of the facial nerve and the orbits.[8,30] It also has been associated with chronic otitis media.[42] On occasion, a portal of injury cannot be identified. The incubation period is usually 1 to 2 days. In contrast to generalized tetanus, which is associated with spasm, cephalic tetanus is manifested by atonic cranial nerve palsies involving nerves III, IV, VII, IX, X, and XII, singly or in combination. Nonetheless, trismus can be present. The disease may progress to generalized tetanus and has a similar prognosis.[8,43]

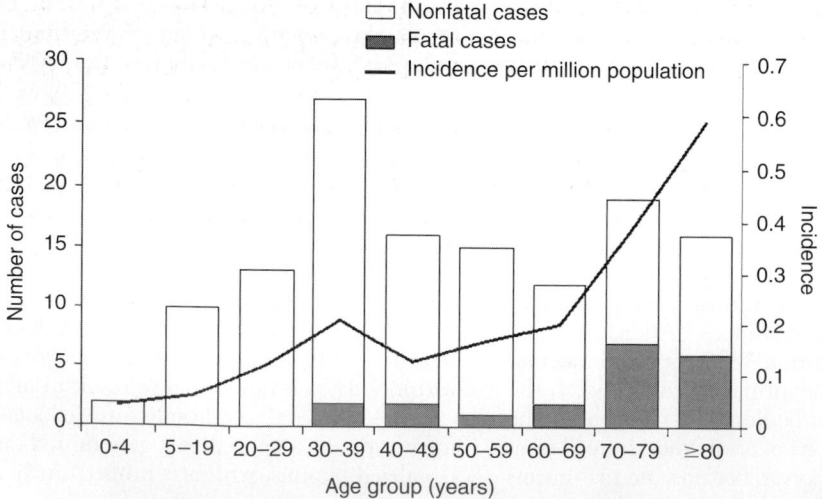

FIGURE 27–1 ■ The number of reported cases of tetanus, survival status of patients, and average annual incidence rates by age group in the United States, 1998 to 2000. (Based on data from the Centers for Disease Control and Prevention.)

Bacteriology

Clostridium tetani is a gram-positive, spore-forming, motile, anaerobic bacillus.[44-48] Typically measuring 0.3 to 0.5 μm in width and 2 to 2.5 μm in length, the vegetative form often develops long filament-like cells in culture. Flagellae are attached bilaterally on non–spore-forming bacteria. With sporulation, *C. tetani* takes on the more characteristic drumstick-like appearance. Spores usually form in the terminal position. *C. tetani* is considered a strict anaerobe that grows optimally at 33°C to 37°C; however, depending on the strain, growth can occur at 14°C to 43°C. *C. tetani* can be cultured in a variety of media used in growing anaerobes, such as thioglycolate, casein hydrolysate, and cooked meat. Growth is enhanced in media supplemented with reducing substances at a neutral to alkaline pH. On blood agar, the organism produces characteristic compact colonies extending in a meshwork of fine filaments. Growth is usually accompanied by the production of gas and is associated with a fetid odor.

Sporulation is dependent on a variety of factors that include pH, temperature, and media composition. Sporulation can be promoted at 37°C and in the presence of oleic acid, phosphates, 1% to 2% sodium chloride or protein, and magnesium.[44,45] Aging also promotes sporulation. In contrast, acidification, high (>41°C) or low (<25°C) temperatures, glucose, assorted saturated fatty acids, antibiotics, and potassium can inhibit spore formation. The germination of spores requires anaerobic conditions and is enhanced by the presence of lactic acid and chemicals toxic to cells.[47]

If not exposed to sunlight, the spores can persist in soil for months to years.[8,44,45] The spores are resistant to boiling and a variety of disinfectants. Inactivation of spores requires 15 to 24 hours in solutions of phenol (5%), formalin (3%), chloramine (1%), or hydrogen hyperoxidates (6%). Heating to 120°C for 15 to 20 minutes more easily destroys the spores. Use of aqueous iodine or 2% glutaraldehyde at pH 7.5 to 8.5 kills spores within 3 hours.

The most common source of environmental exposure to *C. tetani* bacilli and spores is the soil, where the organism is widely but variably distributed. It is difficult to compare studies of the distribution of the organism in nature because of differences in methodology.[48] A method of quantifying spores that was described in 1984 may provide a standardized method for future studies.[49] Most studies suggest that viable spores are more commonly present in soils with an alkaline pH and in nutrient-rich soils in warm, moist climates that could more easily support multiplication of the bacillus.[50,51] Within the contiguous United States, however, a limited study in 1975 found spores in 30% of the samples without any apparent geographic or chemical influence on the distribution.[52]

Soil is not the only reservoir of the organism. Animals, both herbivores and omnivores, can carry *C. tetani* bacilli and spores in their intestines and readily disseminate the organism in their feces. Fecal carriage has been reported in 10% to 20% of horses and 25% to 30% of dogs and guinea pigs; fecal specimens from several other species, including sheep, cattle, and small mammals, also were found to contain *C. tetani*.[53,54] Attempts to quantify the frequency of human intestinal colonization have produced varied results ranging from 0% to 40%.[47,55-61] Rural residents tend to have higher rates of intestinal carriage than city dwellers. *C. tetani* spores also have been detected in street dust[61,62] and the dust and air of surgical operating theaters.[61]

Pathogenesis

Clostridium tetani produces two exotoxins, tetanolysin and tetanospasmin.[8,46,47] Tetanolysin is an oxygen-sensitive hemolysin related to streptolysin and the θ-toxin of *Clostridium perfringens*. It may play a role in establishing infection at the site of inoculation but is not otherwise involved in pathogenesis of the disease.[63] Tetanospasmin, a neurotoxin and the cause of the manifestations of tetanus, is a highly toxic protein that accumulates intracellularly during the logarithmic phase of growth and is released into the medium on autolysis. The toxin has an approximate molecular weight of 150,000 and is synthesized as a single polypeptide prototoxin chain. When released in culture medium, the prototoxin is cleaved by proteases into light (toxic moiety) and heavy (binding) chains with molecular weights of 50,000 and 100,000, respectively, containing two disulfide bonds—one between chains and one internal to the heavy chain.[64-67] The C-terminal end of the heavy chain (fragment C) is the moiety that binds to gangliosides; although the heavy chain may mediate pore formation after binding, it is otherwise totally inactive.[68,69] The light chain is an endopeptidase that cleaves a membrane protein of synaptic vesicles.[70] Toxin production appears to be under the control of a plasmid.[71,72]

Tetanus toxin is one of the most potent known poisons on a weight basis. As little as 1 ng/kg may kill a mouse, and 0.3 ng/kg will kill a guinea pig.[73] The estimated minimum human lethal dose is less than 2.5 ng/kg. Various species have different levels of responsiveness to the toxin. For example, cats, dogs, and particularly birds and poikilotherms appear to be relatively resistant to its effects; guinea pigs, monkeys, sheep, goats, and particularly horses are sensitive to the toxin.[74] As reviewed by Smith,[53] the presence of pre-existing antitoxin does not generally account for the differences in animal susceptibility to tetanus toxin.

Infection usually begins with the inoculation of spores through the epithelium. Wounds accompanied by tissue injury and necrosis (with or without the presence of aerobic organisms) leading to anaerobic or hypoaerobic conditions are generally necessary for the spores to germinate and bacilli to replicate. Ionic calcium appears to increase local necrosis and increase the likelihood of *C. tetani* infection, and it may be a factor in soil contamination that particularly enhances germination.[75] The umbilical stump serves as a nontraumatic site where spore contamination can easily lead to germination and bacterial replication, but traditional surgeries or piercings also can be associated with neonatal tetanus.[36,76,77]

Transport of toxin from the injured site into the CNS is complex. Toxin injected under the skin appears to enter underlying muscle; infiltration of muscle with antitoxin before subcutaneous toxin injection can block the development of tetanus.[8] Once in the muscle, some toxin makes its way to the CNS directly by intra-axonal transport; the major portion is transported by the lymphatics to the bloodstream and then disseminated to a variety of tissues.[8,78]

Tetanus toxin does not cross the blood-brain barrier[78]; neuronal transport is the sole means of entry into the CNS.[8,79–82] The toxin can be demonstrated in motor end plates of muscle nerves. After it gains entry at neuromuscular junctions by binding to gangliosides,[69,83] toxin proceeds up the nerve by intra-axonal transport to the ventral horns of the spinal cord or motor nuclei of the cranial nerves.[84–86] The disease can progress clinically despite use of parenteral antitoxin. Neuronal binding of toxin is not reversible[87]; intracranial injection studies in animals suggest that recovery may depend on new functional connections, whereas spinal cord culture studies suggest that recovery depends on toxin degradation.[88,89]

Tetanospasmin can act at the peripheral motor end plates, the spinal cord, the brain, and the sympathetic nervous system.[8,22–26,90,91] The toxic moiety cleaves the synaptic vesicle membrane protein synaptobrevin and causes disinhibition of spinal cord reflex arcs by interfering with release of the neurotransmitters glycine and γ-aminobutyric acid (GABA) from presynaptic inhibitory fibers.[8,70,90–95] Once inhibition is blocked, excitatory reflexes multiply unchecked, causing the tetanic spasms or, at the cerebral level, convulsions. The clinical syndrome appears almost identical to strychnine poisoning, which acts by competitively binding to postsynaptic glycine receptors at the motor neurons.[96] Tetanospasmin also has been shown to interfere with release of a variety of other neurotransmitters, including acetylcholine in peripheral somatic and autonomic nerves.[97] More detailed information on the nature of the toxin and its effects can be found in reviews by Bizzini[65] and van Heyningen.[98]

Diagnosis

The diagnosis of tetanus is established primarily on clinical grounds and secondarily supported by epidemiologic setting. A history of a wound contaminated by soil or other material and the presence of a local skin infection are helpful in the diagnosis, although these criteria are not always present.[8] Bacteriologic investigations are frequently negative. Characteristic-appearing gram-positive bacilli, some with terminal or subterminal spores, occasionally may be seen in aspirates from the affected area; anaerobic cultures of tissues or aspirates are usually not positive.[33,99] Low or undetectable levels of circulating antitoxin at the time of onset of symptoms are compatible with the diagnosis; however, there are a number of case reports in which moderately high levels of antitoxin were noted at the time of presentation.[100–107] Changes in antitoxin levels in convalescence are not reliably seen.[108] Given the mild nature of some presentations, electromyography has been suggested to aid in the diagnosis,[109] and elicitation of trismus by posterior pharyngeal stimulation has been reported to help in clinical differentiation.[110]

The differential diagnosis depends on the clinical form of tetanus and the presenting symptoms. Cephalic tetanus may be confused with Bell's palsy and trigeminal neuritis. However, cephalic tetanus often is accompanied by other cranial nerve symptoms, including dysphagia, and signs of trismus and nuchal rigidity.[8,30] Trismus has a variety of causes, including caries, tonsillitis, peritonsillar abscess, temporomandibular joint dysfunction, parotitis, and CNS

disturbances other than tetanus. Rabies patients also can present with hyperreflexia; however, rabies is more likely to be associated with hallucinations, hydrophobia, mania, stupor, and a history of an animal bite, and is unlikely to be accompanied by trismus. In addition, seizures with rabies are usually clonic, whereas tetanospasms are prolonged and tonic. Encephalitis is rarely associated with trismus and is much more likely to be accompanied by disturbances of consciousness than is tetanus. Because of nuchal rigidity, bacterial meningitis could be confused with tetanus.

A variety of metabolic conditions and poisonings can resemble tetanus. Although muscle spasm may be seen with hypocalcemic tetany, it is not generally associated with trismus.[111] A determination of low serum calcium can confirm tetany. Strychnine poisoning can mimic generalized tetanus.[96] However, such poisoning is characterized by (1) rare association with persistent trismus, (2) greater muscle relaxation between spasms, (3) normal body temperature, and (4) presence of detectable strychnine in gastric contents or in urine. Phenothiazine toxicity may be associated with a variety of dystonias, including trismus. Detection of phenothiazines in the blood or amelioration by treatment with diphenhydramine confirms the diagnosis. Hysteria can mimic tetanus; however, hysterical patients usually relax during prolonged observation or when they are distracted and are more likely to display clonic rather than tonic spasms.[112]

Because of the unique presentation of neonatal tetanus, postmortem history (even taken by nonclinical personnel) can permit accurate classification of the illness as the cause of death with a high degree of probability, simply by determining the timing of symptoms and verifying that the child was normal after birth. The World Health Organization (WHO) defines neonatal tetanus as an illness occurring in a child who has the normal ability to suck and cry in the first 2 days of life, loses this ability between 3 and 28 days of life, and becomes rigid or has convulsions; or any neonate that has a hospital diagnosis of tetanus (see Chapter 55).

Treatment

At the time a patient presents with tetanus, toxin has entered the nervous system, is circulating in the lymphatics and bloodstream, and is continuing to be produced by C. tetani at the site of infection. The purpose of tetanus therapy is (1) to prevent additional circulating toxin from reaching the CNS, (2) to prevent further toxin production by eliminating the organism, and (3) to give supportive care for the duration of the illness. General principles for use of human tetanus immune globulin (TIG) and pharmacotherapy are outlined here. Detailed information on treatment can be obtained from review articles and chapters.[37,95,113–116]

TIG should be given at the time of diagnosis to neutralize circulating toxin before it reaches the nervous system.[8,116] The optimal dose of therapeutic TIG has not been established. When TIG became available in the 1960s, a dose range of 3000 to 6000 units given intramuscularly in a single administration was chosen based on calculations of the quantity of immunoglobulin necessary to achieve antibody levels in excess of those found to be minimally protective against the effects of tetanus toxin.[117] Despite the absence of evidence to support the choice of this dose range, 3000 to 6000 units of TIG was adopted as the standard for TIG therapy.[8] A retrospective analysis of tetanus cases reported in the United States from 1965 to 1971 subsequently suggested that a TIG dose of 500 units might be as effective as higher doses in reducing mortality.[118] Although some authorities continue to recommend 3000 to 6000 units of TIG,[37,119,120] others now recommend 500 units.[87,115,116] The results of an observational study involving 236 patients with severe tetanus admitted to two hospitals during 1981 to 2001 also suggested that the reduction in TIG dose from 3000 to 65000 units to 500 units midway through the study did not appear to adversely affect patient outcome. The study was not designed to compare the effects of the two TIG doses, and the substantial improvement in patient survival related to advances in overall management could have obscured modest negative effects produced by the reduction in TIG dose.[18]

Equine antitoxin can be given intravenously but is associated with serious allergic side effects such as anaphylaxis and serum sickness.[121–123] Following intramuscular TIG administration, peak serum levels of antitoxin are achieved by 48 to 72 hours, a theoretical disadvantage of TIG, which by product labeling cannot be given intravenously in the United States.[124] Regardless, no evidence to date suggests that intravenous equine antitoxin is more efficacious than intramuscularly administered human TIG, and therefore equine antitoxin is not recommended when TIG is available.[125] Intravenous immune globulin (IVIG) has been proposed as an alternative to TIG when TIG is unavailable or when intramuscular injections must be avoided.[120,124,126,127] Although the quantity of tetanus antitoxin in IVIG produced by different manufacturers varies, it appears that commercial IVIG preparations contain sufficient anti-tetanus antibody to achieve protective antibody levels when given in doses of 200 to 400 mg/kg.[124,127] IVIG is not licensed for this indication in the United States.

Use of intrathecal antitoxin for therapy is controversial.[128,129] Because systemically administered antibody does not cross the blood-brain barrier, intrathecal administration theoretically offers the possibility of neutralizing unbound toxin in the CNS. Two controlled trials and several uncontrolled studies reported decreased mortality with intrathecal administration of equine antitoxin or TIG.[128–133] Other studies, including randomized controlled trials, failed to show benefit in either adults or neonates.[134–137] Abrutyn and Berlin performed a meta-analysis of English-language reports of trials examining the utility of intrathecal antitoxin; they concluded that intrathecal equine or human immunoglobulin has no proven benefit in the treatment of tetanus, and that this route of administration should be used only in the context of well-designed controlled clinical trials.[129] Because it is unclear whether intrathecal TIG therapy affords any benefit, and because TIG available in the United States is not licensed for this indication, use of intrathecal TIG cannot be recommended.

All suspected tetanus patients should start or complete a primary series of vaccination with tetanus toxoid, or receive a booster dose, at the time of diagnosis. Tetanus itself may not induce immunity to tetanospasmin.[108] Relapsing or recurrent cases have been reported.[42,104,138–140] Patients with tetanus appear to respond to tetanus toxoid less vigorously than other individuals, but do nevertheless achieve protective levels of antitoxin.[141,142]

Continuing production of tetanus toxin should be prevented by appropriate antimicrobial therapy and surgical drainage or débridement. In the past, penicillin was the antibiotic of choice. Procaine penicillin, 1.2 million units daily, or aqueous crystalline penicillin G, 4 million units daily divided every 6 hours, was administered for 5 to 10 days to kill the vegetative form of the organism.[8] However, penicillin is a central GABA antagonist and may potentiate the effects of tetanus toxin.[115,116] A controlled trial from Indonesia found significantly improved prognosis with use of metronidazole compared with penicillin.[143] Whether this result was due to the meritorious effects of metronidazole, and/or the deleterious effects of penicillin, is unclear. Nonetheless, metronidazole, given as 500 mg every 6 hours either intravenously or orally, has become the accepted antibiotic of choice for tetanus antimicrobial therapy. Erythromycin, tetracycline, and clindamycin are acceptable alternatives.

Meticulous supportive care is critical to the management of patients with tetanus.[33,34,128] To minimize spasms, the patient should be kept in a quiet, dimly lit room equipped to avoid sudden environmental stimuli, including loud noises. Pharmacologic treatment of hypertonicity and spasms depends on the severity of disease. The objective is to control spasms and increased tone without impairing voluntary movement, consciousness, or spontaneous respiration, if possible. Because tetanospasmin blocks GABA release from inhibitory neurons in the CNS, the ideal therapeutic agent would reverse or counteract this blockade.[95,115,116] Experimental work with benzodiazepines such as diazepam demonstrated that the $GABA_A$ agonist action of these agents indirectly counteracts the effects of the toxin.[115,144,145] Intravenous diazepam is generally given in doses of 0.5 to 15 mg/kg/day.[99,146–149] Some clinicians use standard doses administered every 2 to 8 hours; others give doses at the time of spasms, using 5 to 10 mg as often as three times per hour or more.[8,34] Higher doses may be used if the lower doses fail; some adults require and tolerate doses of more than 600 mg in 24 hours. Lorazepam is also effective and may be preferred because of its longer duration of action.[115] Midazolam given as a continuous infusion also has been effective and has the advantage of being free of propylene glycol, a preservative present in parenteral diazepam and lorazepam preparations that can produce lactic acidosis.[113,115,116] Other muscle relaxants that have been used include dantrolene and intrathecal baclofen.[37,113,115,116,150] Propofol by continuous infusion has been used as an adjunct sedative to benzodiazepine therapy.[37,115,116,151] Magnesium sulfate, a presynaptic neuromuscular blocker, also has been used by some to control muscle spasms in generalized tetanus as well as manifestations of autonomic dysfunction (see below).[37,152,153]

Other drugs used to treat tetanus in the past include the short-acting barbiturates, particularly secobarbital sodium and pentobarbital.[8,99] In contrast to diazepam, barbiturates are more likely to result in respiratory depression and coma. Chlorpromazine has been used with and without barbiturate therapy.[8,114] Paraldehyde and meprobamate also were used to treat tetanus patients in the past.[8] None of these older agents is generally recommended.[115,116]

Some studies suggest that pyridoxine is a useful adjunct to the treatment of neonatal tetanus.[154,155] Although systemic corticosteroids were associated with improved outcome in two studies, the mechanism of steroid action in tetanus is unclear; their use should be considered experimental.[113,115,156,157]

If conservative therapy fails to control muscle spasms, or if the patient presents in extreme spasm, neuromuscular blockade with assisted ventilation is indicated. Vecuronium is now the agent of choice because it causes minimal autonomic instability; an alternative is atracurium.[37,95,115,116] Older agents can be used in their absence.[8,99] When neuromuscular blocking agents are used, sedation is still required to suppress consciousness and memory of the period of paralysis.[115,116]

Although effective in controlling spasms, the agents discussed above may not decrease sympathetic overactivity that can complicate the course of tetanus and increase the risk of fatal outcome. Autonomic dysfunction has been successfully treated with labetalol or morphine.[26,95,116,158–160] β-Blockers should not be given in isolation because their use can result in unopposed α-adrenergic activity leading to severe hypertension. Other agents used for managing autonomic dysfunction include continuous intravenous magnesium sulfate, clonidine, and fentanyl.[37,113,152,161,162] Spinal anesthesia given with catecholamine infusion has been reported useful in extreme instances of hemodynamic instability.[163,164]

Acute respiratory failure caused by thoracic, abdominal, diaphragmatic, or laryngeal spasm is a common early complication of generalized tetanus. Respiratory decompensation in tetanus can be precipitous; close observation of patients early in their course is essential. Assisted ventilation may be required for only a short period, even in cases requiring neuromuscular blockade. Tracheotomy is indicated if prolonged mechanical ventilation is likely, if endotracheal intubation exacerbates upper airway spasm, or if the patient is unable to cough or swallow.[8,33,165]

Moderate and severe tetanus often results in high metabolic demands and a protein-catabolic state. Attention to providing adequate nutritional support is important, starting from the time of hospital admission. Parenteral alimentation is sometimes required.[37,95,115,166,167] Other supportive measures include prophylaxis for thromboemboli, gastrointestinal hemorrhage, and pressure sores.

Epidemiology

Incidence and Descriptive Epidemiology of Non-Neonatal Tetanus

The epidemiology of tetanus reflects the degree to which effective immunization programs are implemented. In spite of the availability of a highly effective immunizing agent, tetanus continues to exert a substantial health burden in the world.[168,169] In 1984, estimates based on mortality surveys suggested that there were approximately 1 million annual deaths caused by neonatal tetanus alone.[170] At the same time, estimates based on reports from the developing world (excluding China) suggested that 310,000 to 700,000 non-neonatal tetanus cases and 122,000 to 300,000 deaths occurred annually. In contrast, an estimated 2000 tetanus cases and under 1000 resultant deaths occurred annually in the developed world during the same period.

Major declines in the incidence of reported cases of tetanus since the 1950s occurred in the Americas (particularly Cuba and North America), European countries, Japan, Australia and New Zealand, and the former USSR; tetanus is now considered rare in most developed countries.[34,35,39,40,51,169,171–174] The declines have been attributed to improved hygiene and childbirth practices, improved wound care, reduction in exposure to tetanus spores, and improved rates of active immunization over many birth cohorts.[51,168,172,173] The majority of European countries have a reported annual incidence below 0.01 per 100,000 population.[169] Those European countries with crude incidence rates higher than 0.01 are in southern, central, and eastern Europe and the Caucasus, where differences in soil exposure or bacterial concentration of C. tetani could play a role, but also where routine childhood immunization may not have been consistently implemented. In general, the current distribution of tetanus in developed nations reflects incomplete toxoid coverage, with the predominance of cases occurring in the elderly.[34,35,171–175]

In the United States, death certificate data from the early 1900s, and national reporting of cases starting in 1947, documented a relatively constant decline in the annual rate of deaths from tetanus. The decline may have accelerated with introduction of equine antitoxin for prophylaxis and treatment starting in the mid-1920s (Fig. 27–2).[176] In 1947, when national reporting began, the incidence of reported cases was 0.39 per 100,000. A decline in the incidence of reported cases continued at a rate that was more gradual than the rate of decline for deaths. The efficiency of the reporting of tetanus deaths in the United States was estimated at 40% in the 1980s, and it is likely that substantial under-reporting of deaths and cases is still occurring.[177] A resurgence in the 1990s of tetanus cases reported among illegal injecting drug users, a recognized risk group,[7,40,178–181] resulted in a leveling of the average annual incidence rates for cases among persons 20 to 39 years of age (Fig. 27–3). In 1998 to 2000, the overall average annual incidence of tetanus reported in the United States was 0.016 cases per 100,000 population (see Fig. 27–2).[7]

Tetanus generally follows a distinct seasonal trend with a midsummer or "wet" season peak, which may reflect soil and spore conditions as well as more frequent injuries during the warmer months.[14,51,182,183] The global distribution of tetanus generally focuses in areas with a moist, warm climate and fertile soil. The highest rates of tetanus remain in the developing world, particularly in countries near the equator.[168,169] Historically in the United States, although all states reported cases, tetanus was predominantly a disease of the Southeast.[14–16,176,182–184] In recent years, cases have routinely been reported from throughout the United States, and geographic and climatic distinctions in incidence have been less apparent.[7,38–40]

Aside from neonatal tetanus, the largest proportion of cases in developing countries is among male older children and young adults. Wherever immunization programs are in place, the rates of tetanus decline,[51] and the sex and age distributions shift to mirror the underimmunized population. In the 1950s, more than one third of the deaths from tetanus in the United States were among neonates and

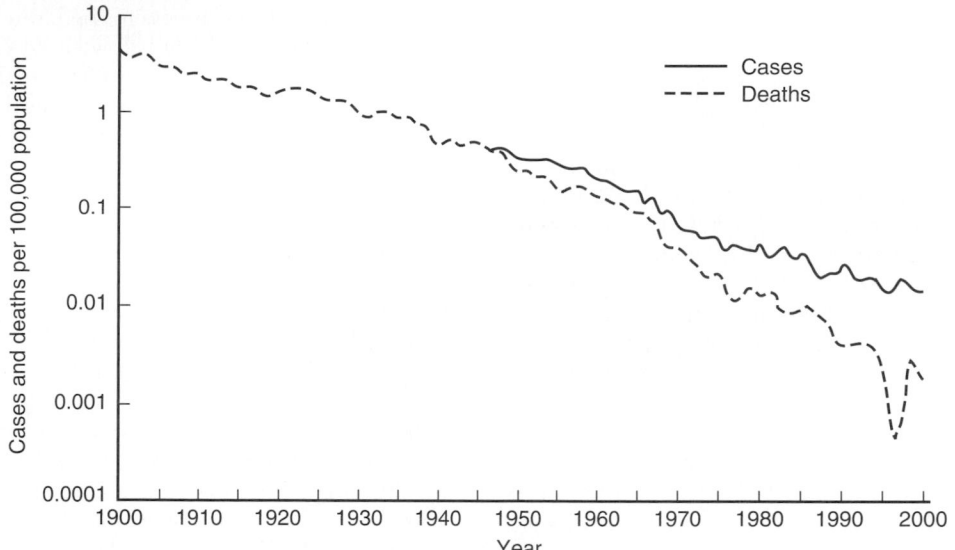

FIGURE 27–2 ■ Mortality and incidence rates of tetanus reported in the United States, 1900 to 2000. Note: Not all states reported deaths from tetanus until after 1932. The estimated rates shown here are based on the population of the reporting states. National reporting of cases began in 1947. (Based on data from the Centers for Disease Control and Prevention.)

infants less than 1 year old.[182,183] In contrast, from 1998 to 2000, no deaths from tetanus occurred among neonates or children, and three fourths of the deaths occurred among persons 60 years of age or older.[7]

In the 1950s, nonwhite individuals had an incidence of tetanus more than five times higher than that of whites.[182,183] Data from 1998 to 2000 indicate that this disparity no longer exists. In contrast, adult, non–U.S.-born immigrants, particularly Hispanics, may be at substantial increased risk for tetanus compared with the rest of the population. During 1998 to 2000, Hispanics had an average annual incidence of tetanus in the United States that was 2.7 times higher than that of non-Hispanics.[7] A national

survey conducted in 1988 to 1994 found a substantially lower prevalence of protective tetanus antibody among adult Mexican-Americans than among other groups.[185] In the late 1990s, large, inner-city emergency departments in Los Angeles and New York City also identified adult immigrants, predominantly from the Americas, to be at increased risk for tetanus, because of no vaccination or lapsed vaccination with toxoid.[186,187]

Since the early toxoid era, acute wounds have been the most common associated site of infection leading to tetanus, including relatively minor wounds and abrasions. In a small proportion of cases, no history of injury can be elicited.[7,14,184,188–190] Illegal injection drug use is known to

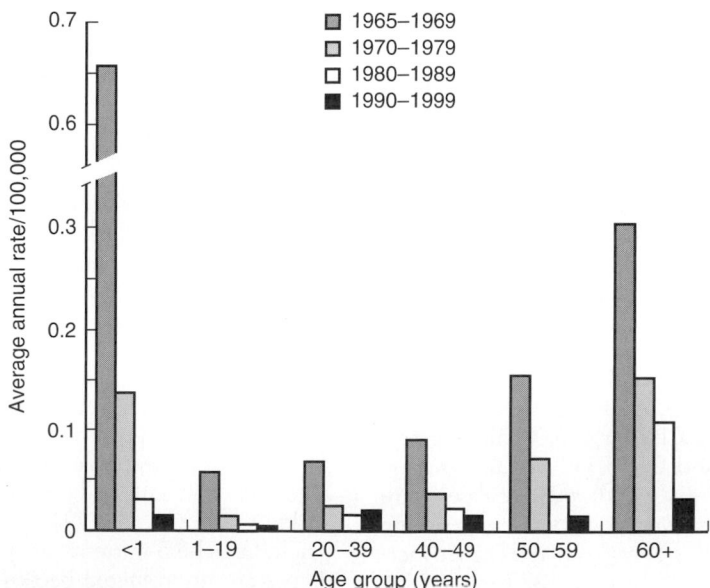

FIGURE 27–3 ■ Age group–specific incidence rates of tetanus for cases reported in the United States, 1965 to 1999. (Based on data from the Centers for Disease Control and Prevention.)

place individuals at increased risk for tetanus.[178,181,191] Operative procedures, particularly bowel surgery, have infrequently resulted in tetanus.[192,193] In recent years, tattoos and body piercing also have anecdotally been associated with tetanus.[7,40,194,195]

There has been debate over whether humans can develop circulating antitoxin against tetanus in the absence of vaccination or disease. In the era before active immunization and standardization of the neutralization test, humans colonized with *C. tetani* were not consistently found to have antibodies to toxin and other *C. tetani* antigens.[56,57] The majority of studies that purport to show natural immunity did not use toxin neutralization assays in mice, the accepted definitive method of testing that correlates with clinical protection (see *Assessment of Immune Responses* below). Studies using other generally acceptable assays (e.g., enzyme-linked immunosorbent assay [ELISA] and passive hemagglutination) showed that substantial proportions of some reportedly unimmunized populations in Brazil, China, Ethiopia, India, Italy, Israel, Spain, and the former USSR have detectable levels of antitoxin.[196–201] Specifically, up to 80% of people in India and up to 95% of people in a group of Ethiopian refugees had levels of antitoxin by these methods exceeding 0.01 IU/mL.[196,197,199] This information has led some to suggest that, at least in some areas of the developing world, asymptomatic colonization or infection with *C. tetani* may stimulate production of antitoxin. Such studies have been criticized because the absence of vaccination cannot be confirmed and because in vitro assays were used in most of the studies[53,202]; there may be substantial overestimation of protective immunity (see *Assessment of Immune Responses* below). This would not explain the findings in full, because some studies did include toxin neutralization assays. However, if seropositivity were indicative of immunity from natural exposure, the prevalence of seropositive individuals should increase with increasing age as a result of cumulative exposure; this does not appear to be the case, arguing against these levels being indicative of natural immunity.[196,199] Serosurveys in the United States have found 25% or more of reportedly unimmunized individuals to have circulating antitoxin, although negative immunization histories are perhaps more likely to be unreliable than in developing countries.[203–207] If natural immunity occurs in some unimmunized populations, it has no substantial importance in the control of tetanus.

The current epidemiology of tetanus in the United States outside of the neonatal period is here derived from detailed information of 129 cases reported from 1998 to 2000.[7] Of the 115 cases with the clinical presentation reported, 81% were generalized, 17% were localized, and 2% were cephalic. The average annual incidence was 0.016 cases per 100,000 population. Age and sex were reported for all 129 cases; the average annual incidence was 0.005 per 100,000 among persons less than 20 years of age, 0.016 per 100,000 among persons 20 to 59 years of age, and 0.035 per 100,000 among persons 60 years of age or older. Overall, 60% of cases were male. The gender distribution was age-dependent. Among persons 1 month to 59 years of age, males had a higher incidence of tetanus than females (0.018 vs. 0.007 per 100,000, respectively). Among persons 60 years of age or older, males had a lower incidence of tetanus than females (0.031 vs. 0.039 per 100,000, respectively).

Similarly, past serosurveys in the United States measured levels of tetanus antibody below those considered protective in 38% to 59% of men and 53% to 71% of women 60 years of age or older.[203–207] The seroprevalence of protective levels of antibody in younger individuals was substantially higher.[204–208] A national, population-based serosurvey of more than 18,000 people older than 5 years in the United States reaffirmed the heightened susceptibility in older age. The survey was conducted during 1988 to 1994; antibody levels were measured by ELISA, and were defined as protective if greater than 0.15 IU/mL (see *Assessment of Immune Responses* below). Overall, 72% of the population 6 years and older had protective levels, falling from more than 90% in children 6 to 11 years of age to 31% in people 70 years of age or older.[185,207] Among persons 40 years and older, the percentage with protective levels decreased more rapidly with age among women than among men. At age 70 years, only 45% of men and 21% of women had protective levels of antibody to tetanus.[185]

Acute trauma of diverse severity was reported for 73% of 129 current cases of non-neonatal tetanus (1998 to 2000).[7] The most frequently reported injuries were puncture wounds (50%), lacerations (33%), and abrasions (9%). Injuries incurred in outdoor settings accounted for 54% of wound-associated cases. Other wound-associated injuries included crush injuries, fractures, and other acute trauma accounting for 6% of cases, and a spider bite and recent tattoo accounting for 2% of cases. No surgical wounds were reported among current cases. Twenty-three percent of 129 cases were associated with chronic wounds and infections (e.g., skin ulcers, gangrene, abscesses), with diabetes, or with illegal injection drug use. Dental infections accounted for 2% of cases. Patients with diabetes made up 12% of cases. The estimated average annual incidence of tetanus among known diabetics (National Center for Health Statistics)[209] was 0.026 per 100,000 population for diabetic persons 20 to 59 years of age, and 0.070 per 100,000 population among diabetic persons 60 years of age and older. Patients with history of illegal injection drug use accounted for 15% of cases, and an increasing proportion of cases during the second half of the last decade.[38–40,210,211] Many of these patients had multiple subcutaneous abscesses from subcutaneous injection of drugs. Black tar heroin was the type of drug reported for 71% of 14 heroin users among current cases.

No known acute injury, chronic wound, or medical condition was reported for 3% of cases. Cases associated with minor or chronic wounds, and a variable proportion without recent history of a wound, have been described during many decades, as pointed out in the review article by Bytchenko.[51]

The immunization status was known for 38% (49) of the 129 current cases. Five non-neonatal pediatric cases were in children who had received no tetanus toxoid because their parents had philosophic or religious objection to vaccines. A review of 15 reported cases of tetanus in neonates (2) and children (13) from 1992 to 2000 in the United States (including the 5 current cases) found that 85% of the children were unprotected because of religious or philosophic objection to vaccination.[212]

Twenty (15%) of the 129 non-neonatal cases had received at least a primary series (i.e., three or more doses) of tetanus toxoid before onset of tetanus (Table 27–1). Of these cases, eight reported that the last dose of the primary series or booster dose of toxoid was received less than 10 years before the illness. Cases in previously immunized individuals generally exhibit a milder clinical course and lower case-fatality rate than those in unimmunized individuals.[213–215] Among 20 current cases who reported having had a primary series of tetanus toxoid, one death (6%) occurred in an injecting drug user whose last dose of tetanus toxoid was received more than 10 years before the onset of tetanus. All other deaths (19 cases; 20%) occurred among 94 cases with fewer than three doses of tetanus toxoid, or with unknown vaccination history.[7]

Of the 90 current patients with acute wounds and available medical history, only 33 (37%) sought medical care for the injury, and a tetanus toxoid–containing vaccine was given as prophylaxis in wound management to 20 (61%) of these. A review of previous cases reported in the 1980s and 1990s in the United States indicated that fewer than 60% of persons with injuries for which a tetanus and diphtheria toxoid vaccine was indicated received a dose during wound management.[216] Most current patients who sought medical care for the acute injury also were candidates for, but did not receive, TIG (see *Tetanus Prophylaxis in Wound Management* below).

Incidence and Descriptive Epidemiology of Neonatal Tetanus

Tetanus occurring within the first month of life results from *C. tetani* infection of a child born to a mother who did not possess sufficient circulating antitoxin to passively protect the infant by transplacental transfer. The epidemiology of tetanus neonatorum is distinct from that of tetanus outside the neonatal period. Neonatal tetanus symptoms occur 3 to 14 days after birth in approximately 90% of cases but can occur from 1 up to 28 days of age.[183,217–220] This predictable incubation period has led several cultures to apply time-related names to the condition, for example, "three-six disease" in China and "eight-day disease" in the Pacific Islands and other locations.[220,221] Cases often are associated with nonsterile conditions of childbirth, with delivery personnel untrained in sterile care of the umbilical cord and stump or not adequately washing their hands,[222–224] with traditional surgeries,[36,76,77] and particularly with births followed by unhygienic cultural rituals involving the umbilical stump—

such as application of herbs, clarified butter, or animal dung.[218,222,223,225–232] Unless their mothers have received two or more doses of tetanus toxoid, newborns are susceptible.[233] The magnitude of the occurrence of neonatal tetanus is particularly important given a death rate of more than 95% without specific therapy and 10% to 90% with therapy, depending on the intensity of supportive care.[36,217–220,225–228,234–237] Long-term residual effects on neurologic and growth status can be seen.[238,239]

The global burden of neonatal tetanus was long underestimated. The incidence of tetanus neonatorum in developing nations in the 1960s had been estimated to be approximately 0.1 per 1000 live births on the basis of reported disease.[51] Using hospital-based reporting, an estimate was made in 1981 of 600,000 neonatal tetanus deaths worldwide, corresponding to approximately 5 neonatal tetanus deaths per 1000 live births.[168] A better assessment of the occurrence of neonatal tetanus throughout the globe was only possible with the use of community-based, house-to-house surveys of neonatal deaths, which documented that the actual incidence of neonatal tetanus was more than 50 per 1000 live births in some areas.[217,220] In the early 1980s, by use of these surveys, an estimated 1.2 million deaths per year occurred as a result of tetanus neonatorum, corresponding to approximately 10 deaths per 1000 live births.[220] The full impact of neonatal tetanus had not previously been evident because the populations at highest risk live in rural areas with greater exposure to contaminated soil, higher risk peripartum conditions and practices, poor access to health care services, and unreliable birth and death registration. With better recognition of the global health burden of tetanus in neonates, a risk to mothers and pregnant women also has been appreciated. It has been estimated that up to 30,000 cases of maternal tetanus occurred each year in the early 1990s[240,241]; a review of the published reports of cases indicated that 27% occurred after abortion (surgical or spontaneous) and 67% occurred in the postpartum period.[241] Programmatically, efforts at prevention and elimination of neonatal tetanus are linked with prevention and elimination of maternal tetanus.

There is some indication that the risk of neonatal tetanus is lower at higher altitudes.[242] In many areas, there is a striking male predominance (2:1 or greater) of tetanus neonatorum as detected by surveillance or by population-based surveys; in other areas, this predominance is less striking or nonexistent.[172,183,189,220] In addition to possible

TABLE 27–1 ■ Immunization History for Non-Neonatal Cases of Tetanus Reported in the United States, 1998 to 2000

Immunization Status	Number of Cases (%)	Time Since Last Dose		
		<10 yr	≥10 yr	Unknown
0 doses	19 (14.7)	—	—	—
1 dose	10 (7.7)	2	8	—
2 doses	0 (0.0)	—	—	—
3 doses	2 (1.6)	2	0	0
≥4 doses	18 (14.0)	6	8	4
Unknown	80 (62.0)	6*	17*	57
Total	129 (100.0)	15	34	61

*Among the 80 cases for whom the total number of doses of toxoid was unknown, the interval from the last (or only) dose of tetanus toxoid was reported as less than 10 years for 6 cases and 10 years or greater for 17 cases.

gender differences in traditional practices, it has been noted that separation of the cord stump occurs later in boys[243] and that this may account in part for the tendency toward a male predominance.[244]

In the United States, neonatal tetanus deaths during the 20th century became progressively less common before tetanus toxoid was used widely in women, perhaps because of improvements in puerperal hygiene.[221] Because tetanus among infants (children <1 year of age) occurs almost exclusively in the neonatal period, tetanus in this age group can be used as a surrogate measure of neonatal disease. Deaths from tetanus among infants declined from 0.64 per 1000 live births in 1900 to 0.07 in 1930, and to 0.01 by the 1960s.[221] The overall decline in tetanus mortality reflects an increased prevalence of maternal immunity acquired through routine childhood tetanus toxoid vaccination beginning in the late 1940s, as well as more hygienic birth practices, including hospital delivery. Starting in 1961, the incidence of tetanus among infants was more closely monitored; trends in incidence paralleled those in mortality. From 1967 to 1968, a precipitous decrease occurred in the incidence of reported tetanus cases and deaths among infants. This decrease corresponded to a sharp decline in reported cases from Texas after a rigorous vaccination campaign among high-risk mothers. After 1968, the incidence of tetanus among infants continued to decline more gradually (see Fig. 27–3). Other developed nations have witnessed similar declines.[168] In Europe in the 1990s, neonatal tetanus cases occasionally were reported from southern, central, and eastern European and Caucasus countries. More recently, only Turkey has reported neonatal tetanus cases; the national reported incidence rate has fallen below 0.05 per 1000 live births and the estimated incidence is under 0.2 per 1000.[240,245]

Of the 31 cases of neonatal tetanus reported in the United States from 1972 to 2000, 27 (87%) were among infants born outside of a hospital. Nineteen of the cases (61%) occurred in Texas, which had only 6.5% of United States births during that period. Only six mothers (19%) had a history of having received tetanus toxoid, and only one mother was reported to have received more than one dose of toxoid. Twenty-one infants (75%) survived of the 28 with known outcome.

Since 1984, only three cases of neonatal tetanus have been reported in the United States: one each in 1989, 1995, and 1998.[246-248] The first case was an infant born at home under nonsterile conditions to an unvaccinated foreign-born mother who had received no prenatal care.[246] The second case was an infant born in a hospital following routine prenatal care. The mother also was foreign-born; she had received a single lifetime dose of tetanus toxoid, although she had delivered another child in the United States.[247] The third case was an infant whose U.S.-born mother chose not to receive toxoid because of philosophic objection to vaccination. The infant was delivered in a hospital by cesarean section; at home, the umbilical stump was treated with a nonsterile, commercial clay powder thought to accelerate healing.[212,248] These cases highlight the importance of obtaining vaccination histories from all pregnant women, particularly those who are foreign born, and of counseling women who decline vaccination about the risk of neonatal tetanus.

Passive Immunization and Correlation of Serum Antitoxin with Protection

Early researchers were able to prevent, modify, or treat tetanus in animal models using antitoxin prepared from large animals. The therapeutic doses required were much larger than the prophylactic ones.[53] Passive immunization with equine tetanus antitoxin for treatment and for prophylaxis after wounds became common practice in World War I, and there was some evidence of prophylactic efficacy.[10,47,249] However, equine antitoxin is associated with frequent adverse reactions, including anaphylaxis and serum sickness.[121-123,250] As a means of decreasing the antigenicity of equine antitoxin for human use, proteolytic treatment was introduced to obtain cleaved Fab fragments with preserved neutralizing activity.[251] Further steps to produce purified equine immunoglobulin G (IgG) antitoxin were developed, and a pasteurization step to reduce the risk of virus transmission has been tested.[252] Despite improvements in the quality of equine antitoxin, the passive immunity it confers is of limited duration. The half-life of refined equine antitoxin in humans is less than 2 weeks and may be considerably less in previously sensitized individuals.[252-254]

TIG was introduced in the early 1960s and was found to have a fairly constant half-life of 28 days in humans.[250,255] The frequency of local and systemic reactions associated with TIG is considerably lower than with equine antitoxin.[117,250] The greater safety and longer half-life of TIG has made it the preferred tetanus antitoxin for passive immunization. Even in the developing world, TIG is beginning to replace equine antitoxin as it becomes more widely available, although the high cost of TIG compared to equine antitoxin precludes its use in many countries.[114,256] TIG is produced by cold-ethanol fractionation of the plasma of hyperimmunized adults. This preparation has been shown not to pose a risk of hepatitis transmission. It is distributed in 1-mL vials with 250 IU/mL (see Appendix 2 of this text for a list of U.S. producers). Recommendations for the use of TIG in patients with tetanus-prone wounds or conditions are given in the section on *Tetanus Prophylaxis in Wound Management* below. Tetanus toxoid is always given with TIG to induce long-lasting immunity in those with past exposure to toxoid and to initiate active immunization in those without any prior exposure.[257-260]

Quantitation of the potency of antitoxin of animal or human origin has been standardized by comparison with an international standard antitoxin using fixed doses of toxin. The international antitoxin unit defined in 1928 represented half the potency of the unit defined by the U.S. National Institutes of Health (NIH). In 1950, the WHO reset the international standard unitage to agree with that of the NIH. Assay results before that time generally were reported in antitoxin units (or American units) per milliliter (AU/mL) using the NIH reference standard. Results using the current standard are reported as international units per milliliter (IU/mL). Prior to 1992, the only international reference antitoxin was of equine origin; the WHO Expert Committee on Biological Standardization established the first international standard for human anti-tetanus immunoglobulin in 1992.[261]

The minimum level of tetanus antitoxin needed to ensure protection against tetanus is generally accepted to be 0.01 IU/mL as measured by in vivo neutralization assay.[255,262–264] This level is based primarily on animal studies of the protective effects of active and passive immunization. A review by McComb in 1964 of data on the reduction of tetanus in horses following homologous passive immunization found an absence of clinical tetanus in horses following injection of 1500 IU of antitoxin after acute injury (approximately 2.5 IU/kg), corresponding to a serum antitoxin level of 0.01 IU/mL.[255] These results were in agreement with earlier work showing that guinea pigs with serum antitoxin levels of 0.01 IU/mL or higher did not succumb to challenge with inocula of fixed lethal doses of C. tetani spores.[265] Of interest, although none of the guinea pigs with antitoxin levels of 0.01 IU/mL or higher died, 13% developed mild, nonfatal tetanus; 7% with levels less than 0.01 IU/mL were completely protected. The only experimental studies in humans followed active immunization.

A number of articles describing cases of tetanus in neonates and adults with tetanus antitoxin levels of 0.01 IU/mL or higher challenge the assumption that an antitoxin level of 0.01 IU/mL is always protective.[100–107] Serum antitoxin levels detected at the time of presentation ranged from 0.15 to 25 IU/mL. The measurement of serum antitoxin levels in many of the reports was performed with in vitro methods that are known to overestimate the amount of neutralizing antibody present (see *Assessment of Immune Responses* below). In one study, the patient described had a level of 0.2 IU/mL by ELISA and a result of less than 0.01 IU/mL by neutralization assay.[104] Thus, in some of these cases, levels of biologically active anti-tetanus antibody may have been less than 0.01 IU/mL. However, a number of other patients described had levels well above 0.01 IU/mL by neutralization assay.[100,102,105,106] Some of these patients had deep necrotic wounds. It is possible that, when large quantities of toxin are produced, a serum concentration of anti-tetanus antibody of 0.01 IU/mL is insufficient to provide protection. Alternatively, the wounds in these patients may have been sufficiently sequestered from circulating antitoxin that toxin gained access to the nervous system before neutralization could occur. In addition, it is possible that, in previously vaccinated individuals, large doses of tetanus toxin could lead to an anamnestic response before anti-tetanus antibody testing was performed. Nonetheless, these case reports suggest that protection at a 0.01-IU/mL level of antitoxin is not absolute. Given the consistent results in animal studies, it is reasonable to conclude that antitoxin levels of 0.01 IU/mL by neutralization assay at the time of exposure are indicative of protection in most situations.

Active Immunization: Toxoid

Early Approaches

The purification of tetanus toxin led to efforts to inactivate it chemically without eliminating immunogenicity. Initially, researchers used iodine trichloride. An early human challenge study and seroconversion studies supported the applied use of tetanus toxoid for prophylaxis in humans. Later, formaldehyde emerged as the most convenient and efficient means of inactivation. In 1927, Ramon and Zoeller combined tetanus toxoid with diphtheria toxoid and demonstrated that there was no antigenic competition for immune responses; they also recognized neonatal tetanus as a disease to be prevented by immunization of pregnant women.[266] Tetanus toxoid became commercially available in the United States in 1938 but was not widely used until the military began routine prewound prophylactic inoculation in 1941.

Toxoid Description

Currently, a high-yielding strain of C. tetani is cultured in liquid medium in large-capacity fermenters (up to 1000 L) to produce commercial toxoid. The medium, modified by Latham from that of Mueller and Miller, consists of a tryptic digest of casein, free of Berna and Witte peptones and other allergenic substances.[45] In the United States, media containing human blood group–specific substances, such as beef heart infusion broth, are specifically avoided. Data suggest that tetanus toxin production can be enhanced by bubbling nitrogen through the liquid media.[267] Extracellular toxin is harvested by filtration, purified, and detoxified with 40% formaldehyde at 37°C. Some manufacturers detoxify the crude toxin before purification in order to enhance the safety of the production process for personnel.

In 1965, the WHO standardized the calibration of the potency of tetanus toxoid–containing vaccines and established the first international standard for Tetanus Toxoid, Adsorbed, shortly after the establishment of the first international standard for Tetanus Toxoid, Plain.[268] Comparison with a standard preparation using mouse bioassays allowed the establishment of international units (IU) of toxoid potency. However, the international standard assay has not been adopted in the United States for licensure and lot standardization of tetanus toxoid content because of inconsistencies in results obtained from mice assays, particularly relative to persistent (>6 months) serologic responses in humans.[269–271] The immune response in mice varies greatly depending on the mouse strain used.[270,271] In the United States, tetanus toxoid potency regulations require antitoxin induction of at least 2 IU/mL in the guinea pig potency test.[272] In 2000, the third international standard was established, replacing the second international standard of 1981.[273] The collaborative study to assess the suitability of the candidate preparation for the second international standard also confirmed previous observations that potency testing in guinea pigs yielded more consistent results than those in mice.[273]

In 1979, the WHO set potency standards for tetanus toxoid preparations. Until 1982, 30 IU was the unitage required per human dose; this was changed in 1982 to 40 IU (60 IU in preparations of diphtheria and tetanus toxoids and pertussis vaccine).[274] Some authors have used the results of the limits of flocculation (Lf) test as a surrogate measure of potency. Manufacturers of tetanus toxoid licensed in the United States indicate the quantity of toxoid in preparations by Lf content and the purity by Lf per milligram of protein nitrogen (pure toxoid has 3000 Lf/mg).[65] However, the Lf assay measures overall antigen content, which may not perfectly correlate with the level of antibody elicited. U.S. requirements for antigen content and potency for commercial tetanus toxoid products are discussed below in the section on *Dosage and Route*.

WHO standards apply as recommendations for commercial and governmental producers and also serve as a requirement for supply to United Nations (UN) agencies, including the WHO and the United Nations Children's Fund (UNICEF).

Producers

In the United States, several manufacturers distribute adsorbed tetanus toxoid (TT) singly or in combination with diphtheria toxoid (DT [for pediatric use], Td [adult formulation]), with or without acellular pertussis vaccine (DTaP), and with *Haemophilus influenzae* type b (Hib) conjugate vaccine (DTaP-Hib); in 2003, a DTaP vaccine in combination with hepatitis B and inactivated poliovirus vaccine was licensed* (see Appendix 2 of this text for all current U.S. producers). Fluid TT is produced by a single manufacturer and is only available in limited quantities. In Canada and many western European nations, inactivated poliomyelitis vaccine may be combined with diphtheria and tetanus toxoids and whole-cell pertussis (DTP), DT, or DTaP. Other combinations have been introduced outside the United States for use in childhood, including whole-cell DTP with hepatitis B (HepB) vaccine and DTaP combinations with HepB vaccine with or without Hib conjugate vaccines.

Producers who are eligible to supply TT-containing products to UN agencies and meet WHO requirements ("prequalified") as of March 2003 include Aventis Pasteur, Canada (DTP); Aventis Pasteur, France (DTP, DT, TT, and Td); Bio Farma, Indonesia (DTP, DT, and TT); Chiron Behring, Germany (DTP); Chiron Vaccines, Italy (DTP and DTP-Hib); CSL, Ltd., Australia (DTP, DT, and TT); GlaxoSmithKline, Belgium (DTP-HepB and DTP-HepB to be combined with Hib); and the Serum Institute of India (DTP, DT, TT, and Td). Although previously tetanus toxoid–containing products were widely made by local manufacturers, the volume of products so produced is decreasing. In response to problems evident with tetanus toxoid potency in many developing countries (see *Public Health Perspective* below),[275] in 1992 the World Health Assembly resolved to work toward the exclusive use of vaccines that meet WHO requirements.[276] In 1992, there were 63 producers of DTP/TT vaccines in 42 countries. Twenty-two developing countries with commercial or state producers of tetanus toxoid were evaluated in 1995 and products had serious impediments to meeting WHO standards[275]; as of August 2002, 9 no longer have manufacturers of these products and 11 have strengthened their regulatory authorities and standards (including two with producers of UN-prequalified vaccines).[†]

Dosage and Route

As with other inactivated vaccines and toxoids, the immunologic response to tetanus toxoid requires more than one dose to confer protection and persisting immunity. There is no need to repeat doses if scheduled doses are delayed. Even with long intervals between doses, the immune response to subsequent doses appears similar to or better than that with shorter intervals.[277,278]

In North America, the preparations available are given as 0.5-mL doses. The adsorbed toxoid is administered intramuscularly; the fluid TT preparation can be given subcutaneously. Either can be given by jet injector. The toxoid content of commercial products is assessed by flocculation with standard antitoxin and measured in Lf units. This measure of toxoid protein content does not necessarily correspond to immunogenicity as measured by potency in guinea pigs. Adsorbed products available in the United States have a content of 2 to 10 Lf/dose; the fluid TT contains 4 Lf. Potency is determined by animal bioassays: for the fluid preparation, immunized guinea pigs are tested for survival after a toxin challenge; for precipitated toxoid, a serum pool from immunized guinea pigs must exceed 2 IU/mL.

Available Preparations

DTaP and DT are combinations used in infants and children younger than 7 years. In the United States, one DTaP formulation is approved for combined administration in the same syringe with Hib conjugate vaccine for dose four of the five-dose DTaP series.

Universal use of DTP/DTaP in infancy and childhood is recommended unless there are contraindications to pertussis vaccine.[120,279,280] Td is used in persons 7 years of age and older because it contains less diphtheria toxoid (2 Lf or less) than the pediatric preparation (DT; more than 10 Lf). Single-antigen tetanus toxoid is also available in the United States for use in persons 7 years of age and older either as an adsorbed or fluid preparation, the latter in limited quantities. Td is preferred for tetanus prophylaxis in adults under all circumstances because most adults in need of tetanus toxoid are likely to be susceptible to diphtheria; Td is the recommended formulation for routine boosting of older children, adolescents, and adults. Clinically significant reactions are not substantially more frequent after receipt of Td than single-antigen tetanus toxoid. Although more than 70% of tetanus toxoid for adult use (Td or TT) distributed in the 1960s was single-antigen tetanus toxoid, only 9.5% of the 76 million doses of tetanus toxoid distributed for adult use in 1997 to 2001 was single-antigen tetanus toxoid.[281]

Many tetanus toxoid adsorbed preparations are available with various precipitating salt adjuvants. In the United States, aluminum hydroxide, aluminum potassium sulfate, or aluminum phosphate is used as the adjuvant. These adjuvants induce an adequate immune response after fewer doses of toxoid than with the fluid preparation.[282] The primary immunization schedule for fluid toxoids requires four doses, whereas the adsorbed toxoid requires three. In neonatal tetanus prevention trials, three doses of fluid toxoid for pregnant women were necessary to achieve protective levels of antitoxin, as opposed to two doses of adsorbed toxoid.[264] At constant levels of antigen content, geometric mean antibody responses may or may not be higher after adsorbed toxoid.[264,283] Because fluid and adsorbed preparations are essentially equivalent with regard to the frequency

---

*Centers for Disease Control and Prevention. Notice to readers: FDA licensure of diphtheria and tetanus toxoid and acellular pertussis adsorbed, hepatitis B (recombinant), and poliovirus vaccine combined (Pediarix) for use in infants. MMWR 52:203–204, 2003.
†WHO, unpublished data.

of adverse events following immunization, adsorbed toxoid is preferred because it confers protective levels of antitoxin for a longer time.[283,284] Response to either form of toxoid as a booster dose is equally brisk. In combined active-passive immunization, TIG does not substantially alter the response to adsorbed toxoid as it does with fluid toxoid.[255,260,285] In the United States, therefore, adsorbed products are recommended over fluid. The fluid TT preparation is only available on special request to the manufacturer. Td preparations are available only as adsorbed products. Outside the United States, a calcium phosphate–adsorbed product is also available.[286] Interest has focused on the theoretical but unproved possibility that calcium-adsorbed preparations may be associated with fewer reactions than the aluminum-adsorbed products.[287–289]

Constituents

According to WHO standards, the final product should contain 0.5% formaldehyde or less. In the United States, minimum requirements stipulate residual formaldehyde content of 0.02% or less. In adsorbed products, precipitating calcium or aluminum salt adjuvants are present. A single human dose must contain less than 1.25 mg of aluminum in the United States. Preparations outside the United States may contain larger amounts of aluminum. Multiple-dose preparations of DTaP, DT, Td, and tetanus toxoid products must contain an additive to prevent bacterial contaminant overgrowth. Historically the preservative used was thimerosal to a final concentration up to 0.1%, but more typically 0.01%. Recently, phenoxyethanol has been used as an alternative to thimerosal in preparations for children, usually with a final concentration of 0.01%. Concerns over exposure to mercury led the Food and Drug Administration to undertake a review of all medicinal products containing the metal, including vaccines. Currently, all routinely recommended vaccines for administration to infants in the United States, including DTaP are either thimerosal free or contain only trace amounts (<1 µg/dose). All single-dose preparations of DTaP in the United States have either no added preservative or phenoxyethanol, but may contain trace amounts of thimerosal from the manufacturing process. Other preparations (DT, Td, and tetanus toxoid) do still contain thimerosal. DTaP vaccines also may contain trace amounts of gelatin and polysorbate 80.

Stability

Preparations should be stored at 2°C to 8°C and generally have a 2- or 3-year expiration date. Use of this preparation in the developing world is not as dependent on the "cold chain" as are other immunobiologics. Higher ambient temperatures should be avoided, particularly for periods longer than 7 days; however, exposure to ambient temperature for weeks does not substantially reduce the potency of the toxoid except at temperatures of 45°C or greater.[290] Tetanus toxoid exposed to 60°C is destroyed in 3 to 5 hours. Freezing also can reduce potency, particularly when the toxoid is adsorbed.[8,291,292] Adsorbed tetanus toxoid, whether monovalent or combined, can appear granulated after freezing has induced changes in the adsorbent, but granulation is not a reliable way to determine if toxoid previously was frozen.

The effect of freezing on DT or DTP is variable. The effect of repeated freezing on adsorbed and fluid single-antigen tetanus toxoids has been shown to reduce mean antitoxin response.[293] The available data on temperature stability have been reviewed.[294,295]

Results of Active Immunization

Assessment of Immune Responses

Active immunization confers immunity to tetanus by stimulating production of serum antitoxin. Primary immunization with tetanus toxoid also induces cellular immune responses (T-helper type 1 [Th1] or type IV hypersensitivity) in 74% to 90% of recipients, which are not thought to be relevant to serologic protection per se but rather related to an anamnestic response.[296] Intradermal skin testing with tetanus toxoid has been used as a screen for anergy,[297–299] although false-positive reactions occur.[300]

The gold standard for assessing a serologic immune response to tetanus toxoid is the toxin neutralization test, which measures biologically active antitoxin in serum.[278,301,302] Neutralization tests are performed in mice injected with serial dilutions of test serum that have been preincubated with a lethal dose of tetanus toxin and standardized to a reference serum specimen. Toxin neutralization tests detect antitoxin titers as low as 0.001 IU/mL. These assays are believed to be most reliable because they assess actual neutralization in a living host. Because in vivo neutralization tests are time consuming and expensive, a variety of in vitro serologic tests have been developed. Among these are passive hemagglutination (PHA), ELISA, radioimmunoassays, immunofluorescent assays, latex agglutination, and a variety of methods using agar gel precipitation. The advantages and disadvantages of each technique have been reviewed.[202,303] In general, any of the in vitro techniques for tetanus antitoxin detection can be useful, provided that correlation with toxin neutralization has been confirmed. However, most in vitro assays have the important limitation that they do not discriminate between biologically active antibody and non-neutralizing antibody, leading to a lack of specificity that is most apparent at low antibody titers.[202] PHA and ELISA are currently the most commonly used in vitro techniques to determine tetanus antitoxin levels; the following discussion is limited to these two types of assays.

PHA techniques were the first widely used in vitro alternatives to neutralization assays.[303–309] Although results vary among PHA techniques, there is a good correlation with toxin neutralization at high and moderate titers of antibody. Consistency in testing among laboratories has been aided by the use of turkey erythrocytes in the assay.[303,307] However, PHA tests measure both IgG and immunoglobulin M (IgM), perhaps preferentially IgM.[309] Only IgG has biologically relevant neutralizing activity.[262,310] Thus antibodies detected at low titers by PHA, particularly those produced early in a primary immunization series, may not represent neutralizing antitoxin.[202]

Standard (indirect) ELISAs measure antibody binding to tetanus toxin or toxoid that has been passively adsorbed to wells in microtiter plates (solid-phase antigen). Studies comparing the results of standard ELISA to neutralization assays in mice have demonstrated good correlation between the two tests when ELISA titers are above 0.16 to 0.2 IU/mL; ELISA titers below that level significantly overestimate effective antibody concentrations.[202,311-317] Factors contributing to this lack of specificity include nonspecific antibody binding to contaminant proteins adhering to the surface of the test plate, detection of IgM in addition to IgG, and detection of antibody with little or no neutralization activity. Biologically inactive antibody can result from low avidity, asymmetric (monovalent) structure, and/or binding sites that recognize biologically unimportant epitopes, including those created on the toxin or toxoid molecules by the denaturing effects of solid-phase binding.[314,315,317,318]

Several modifications to the standard ELISA have been used to overcome the problem of detecting biologically inactive antibody. In competitive-antigen ELISA, soluble toxin or toxoid antigen is mixed with the test serum solution and the amount of antibody binding to soluble antigen is calculated. This assay produces results that correlate well with neutralization assays at titers as low as 0.004 IU/mL.[318,319] Another modification of ELISA that increases specificity at low antibody titers is toxin-binding inhibition. In this technique, a measured amount of toxin is preincubated with the serum specimen and subsequently exposed to antitoxin-coated plates to detect unbound toxin.[320-322] The most recent modification is the double-antigen ELISA, in which biotin-labeled toxin or toxoid is added to test serum that has been incubated in microtiter wells precoated with toxoid. In this assay, only antibody that is bound to both solid-phase antigen and the labeled soluble antigen is detected. The double-antigen method also shows good correlation with in vivo neutralization at antibody titers below 0.10 IU/mL.[323]

When reporting results of tetanus antitoxin tests, the assay method used should be stated, as well as the correlation with a neutralization assay, if known. Recent serosurveys to determine the prevalence of protective tetanus antitoxin in U.S. and Canadian populations have used standard ELISA to measure antitoxin levels. Protective immunity was defined as an antitoxin level greater than 0.15 IU/mL.[185,207,324] The use of this relatively high cutoff value underestimates the level of protection in the study populations because some individuals with lower antitoxin levels will be protected; however, use of a cutoff value below 0.16 IU/mL would clearly overestimate the level of protection. The use of a more specific modified ELISA technique as discussed above may permit more accurate determinations of protective immunity against tetanus in future serosurveys.

Effectiveness

Results of Controlled Studies of Protection Against Disease

A double-blind, randomized, controlled clinical trial in rural Colombia showed that two or three doses of tetanus toxoid administered to women of child-bearing age protected their babies against neonatal tetanus.[278,325] Control infants had a neonatal tetanus mortality rate of 78 per 1000 live births, whereas no neonatal tetanus cases occurred in the children of women who received at least two doses

A mean antitoxin level of 0.01 AU/mL in pregnant women has been associated with protection of infants from neonatal tetanus.[264]

Other Evidence of Effectiveness

Early data suggesting the efficacy of active immunization with tetanus toxoid come from Wolters and Dehmel,[326] who immunized themselves with toxoid and achieved serum levels of 0.007 to 0.01 AU/mL. This allowed them to resist challenge with "two or three fatal doses" of tetanus toxin, but the actual challenge dose is unknown.[326]

The reduction in neonatal tetanus where tetanus toxoid is used in pregnant women supports the preceding findings. Field assessment of the efficacy of two or more tetanus toxoid doses has been made in neonatal tetanus mortality surveys, reporting 70% to 100% effectiveness.[202,327-331] Formal assessments of the efficacy of tetanus toxoid against disease in ages outside the neonatal period have not been made because of the rarity of the disease. Nonetheless, the efficacy of a standard pre-exposure immunization regimen plus postwound booster doses was demonstrated in the application of tetanus toxoid use in the military: Only 12 cases of tetanus occurred among 2.73 million wounded U.S. Army personnel on all fronts in World War II (0.44 per 100,000) versus 70 of 520,000 wounded in World War I (13.4 per 100,000); only 4 of the 12 had completed primary immunization.[332] A similar experience occurred in British personnel.[249]

Based on the results of the initial studies in neonatal tetanus prevention and the effect that programs of prenatal immunization to prevent neonatal tetanus have had, as well as the correlation of immunogenicity with protection, routine use of toxoid has been assumed also to be highly effective.[264,278] As indicated in the next section, primary immunization of infants and children leads to antitoxin responses well above protective levels in virtually all recipients.

Indications for Use

Because of the success of active immunization in the military, wide C. tetani spore distribution, the high death-to-case ratio of tetanus, and frequent reactions with and incomplete efficacy of equine antitoxin,[333] routine inoculation in childhood was recommended in 1944 by the American Academy of Pediatrics (AAP). In the mid-1940s, tetanus toxoid was combined with diphtheria toxoid and pertussis vaccine (DTP), which permitted administration of all three antigens with a single injection. In 1951, the AAP recommended routine use of DTP in infancy, and generalized use by practitioners became more common. Since that time, advisory groups in the United States, including the Advisory Committee on Immunization Practices (ACIP), have recommended that all people receive three or more doses of tetanus toxoid in the appropriate combination based on age, followed by routine booster doses every 10 years.[120,280]

Administration to Infants and Children

The recommended schedule for routine tetanus immunization in the United States is given in Table 27-2.[120,279,280,334,335] The WHO-recommended schedule for

TABLE 27–2 ■ Recommendations for Primary Immunization with Tetanus Toxoid by Age at Beginning Immunization, United States[*]

Interval Before	Age Group and Vaccine			
	<1 Yr (DTaP[*] or DT[†,‡])	1–6 yrs		≥7 yr (Td[‖])
		DTaP[*]	DT[†,§]	
Dose 1	First visit	First visit	First visit	First visit
Dose 2	1–2 mo	1–2 mo	1–2 mo	1–2 mo
Dose 3	1–2 mo	1–2 mo	6–12 mo	6–12 mo
Dose 4	Approximately 1 yr[¶]	Approximately 1 yr[¶]	—	—

[*]DTaP is the pertussis vaccine preparation for all doses in the series in the United States. Whole-cell DTP is an acceptable alternative throughout the world.

[†]DT for those with contraindications to pertussis vaccine.

[‡]Boosters with DT or DTaP (dose 5) indicated at 4 to 6 years of age. Boosters with Td at 11 to 12 years of age and every 10 years thereafter. First visit generally at 2 months of age.

[§]Dose 4 of DT indicated at 4 to 6 years of age unless dose 3 administered at 4 years of age or older. In this instance, dose 4 is not needed. Boosters with Td indicated at 11 to 12 years of age and every 10 years thereafter.

[‖]Boosters with Td indicated at 11 to 12 years of age and every 10 years thereafter.

[¶]Dose 5 of DTaP (DTP) indicated at 4 to 6 years of age unless dose 4 administered at 4 years of age or older. In this instance, dose 5 is not needed. Boosters with Td indicated at 11 to 12 years of age and every 10 years thereafter.

DT, diphtheria and tetanus toxoids for pediatric use; DTaP, diphtheria and tetanus toxoids and acellular pertussis vaccine; DTP, diphtheria and tetanus toxoids and whole-cell pertussis vaccine; Td, tetanus and diphtheria toxoids for adult use.

the developing world of DTP at 6, 10, and 14 weeks of age also is being used in many countries in Europe and elsewhere and is discussed in more detail below.[336]

Tetanus toxoid is one of the most potent immunizing agents used routinely in children. Protective levels can be obtained with schedules starting in the newborn period.[272,336–341] Premature infants have immune responses at a given chronologic age comparable to those of term infants.[340,342]

In contrast to the immunologic response to diphtheria toxoid, which may be impeded in the presence of passively transferred maternal antitoxin, the immune response to tetanus toxoid has been considered to be minimally inhibited by maternal antitoxin.[338,339,343–345] Many of the studies examining inhibition of response to tetanus toxoid were performed at a time before most mothers were likely to be immune.[346] The majority of women of child-bearing age in the United States have previously been immunized and have received a booster dose in adolescence; increasing numbers of adult women in the developing world also have been previously immunized. Studies in the United States have shown that term infants have high geometric mean titers (GMTs) of circulating tetanus antitoxin at 2 months of age, before immunization, implying that most term infants currently have levels of antitoxin well above protective levels before beginning immunization.[347–349] Edwards and colleagues[349] evaluated 13 candidate acellular pertussis (DTaP) vaccines (with a U.S. schedule of doses at 2, 4, and 6 months of age) and compared the serologic responses with a whole-cell DTP vaccine licensed in the United States. Before the first dose at 2 months of age, GMTs varied from 1.115 to 7.43 IU/mL as measured by modified PHA. After the third dose at 6 months of age, all infants had levels of antibody of 0.01 IU/mL or higher, and GMTs ranged from 3.094 to 22.513 IU/mL. High preimmunization antitoxin titers do not inhibit the induction of active immunity, including in children of mothers vacci-

nated in pregnancy.[350,351] With an accelerated schedule (e.g., 2, 3, and 4 months), the tetanus toxoid response may be lower in infants with higher pre-existing maternal antitoxin.[352] However, infants are protected after immunization, and, by 6 months after completing an accelerated schedule, mean titers are still well above protective levels.[353]

During the first year of life, the older a child is at the time of receipt of the third dose of tetanus toxoid, the higher the level of antitoxin produced. Brown and co-workers[354] studied infants beginning immunization at 3 to 7 months of age with three doses of DTP inoculated at 1- or 2-month intervals. In general, regardless of interval, GMTs were higher in infants completing the schedule at older ages (21.2 to 29.1 AU/mL) versus younger ages (13.5 to 24.0 AU/mL). However, these differences are probably of no clinical significance: all infants, regardless of schedule, had antitoxin titers much higher than 0.01 AU/mL for at least 12 to 18 months after completing the initial three-dose series (the lowest was 0.125 AU/mL), and both groups had comparable GMTs (2.0–2.9 AU/mL vs. 1.2–2.0 AU/mL). Response to the booster dose was similar under all schedules tested, confirming that immunization against tetanus can begin at an early age with good results. More recent studies support the results of Brown and co-workers. In the United Kingdom, the routine schedule for DTP was changed in 1992 from three doses at 3, 4½ to 5, and 8½ to 11 months to 2, 3, and 4 months.[336,353] Children vaccinated with the accelerated schedule (completed at 4 months of age) had only about one sixth the GMT of tetanus antitoxin at approximately 8 weeks after the third dose, compared with children who completed immunization at the older age (0.522 vs. 3.43 IU/mL, as assessed by radioimmunoassay). By 1 year after the third dose, the differences had narrowed (0.197 IU/mL for the accelerated schedule vs. 0.341 IU/mL). No child with either schedule had levels less than 0.01 IU/mL.

Single doses of standard- or high-potency tetanus toxoids have induced protective levels in some studies.[283,288,355-357] However, in general, these levels do not greatly exceed 0.01 IU/mL, and long-term follow-up has been lacking. A minimum of two doses of standard-potency tetanus toxoids are considered necessary to reach protective levels of circulating antitoxin in infants during the first year of life.[272,358-362] Data collected in trials of DTP vaccines in the United States imply that three doses may be needed in infants before significant production of antitoxin takes place.[347-349]

Most primary immunization schedules used in the developed world consist of two or three doses in the first year of life followed by a reinforcing dose approximately 6 months to 1 year afterward.[120,279,280,334,363] When combined DTP is used, the schedule for tetanus immunization is often tied to the scheduling requirements of immunization with diphtheria toxoid and pertussis vaccines. Immunization against pertussis is generally recommended as three doses in the first year of life. The Expanded Programme on Immunisation (EPI) of the WHO, with its emphasis on protection in early infancy, recommends a total of three doses of DTP early in the first year, starting as early as 6 weeks of age, with a minimum of 4 weeks between doses.[364]

Intervals for the first two or three doses are generally 1 to 2 months, and there appears to be little reason to prefer one interval over another with regard to tetanus antitoxin production. Data from Brown and colleagues[354] indicated that, whereas infants vaccinated at 2-month intervals made higher levels of antitoxin than infants vaccinated at 1-month intervals, all groups of infants had similar GMTs at the time of reinforcing doses.

After two- or three-dose primary schedules during infancy, antibody levels tend to wane.[344,353,354,365-367] Although children who receive two or three doses of vaccine at 1- or 2-month intervals rarely have lost protective levels of antibody 1 year after the last dose, reinforcing doses at this time lead to high levels of antitoxin production and long-term immunity, generally exceeding 10 years.[284,344,347,348,350,352-354,362,366-370]

In children older than 1 year, two doses at intervals of 1 to 2 months appear to induce protective levels of antitoxin that persist at least 6 to 12 months.[365] A reinforcing dose at this time is associated with a marked booster response and persistent high levels of antitoxin. Therefore, most immunization schedules for children older than 1 year call for three doses: the first two separated by 1 to 2 months and the third dose 6 to 12 months after the second. However, when tetanus toxoid is combined with pertussis vaccine, which requires a minimum of three doses, a schedule similar to that for infants often is used, with three doses 1 to 2 months apart followed by a fourth dose 6 to 12 months later.

Administration to Adults

The immune response to tetanus toxoid appears to decrease with increasing age. In comparative studies, children generally will develop higher levels of antitoxin than adults.[371] Despite the decrease in immunogenicity, the majority of adult vaccinees achieve and maintain protective levels of antitoxin for many years.[277,284] Most schedules in use in the world today call for two doses 1 to 2 months apart followed by a third dose 6 to 12 months later.

After two doses 4 weeks or more apart, almost all adults produce antitoxin levels higher than 0.01 IU/mL.[371] GMTs vary according to type of vaccine and schedule but in general are below 1.0 IU/mL. In one large-scale field trial in New Guinea, titers persisted at protective levels for 40 months in as many as 78% of adult women given two doses of aluminum phosphate–adsorbed vaccine and for 54 months in 33%.[372] Other studies, particularly in older adults, have confirmed that persistence of protective levels of antitoxin without a reinforcing dose is short lived.[373,374]

A reinforcing dose 6 to 12 months after the first two doses is associated with production of high levels of antitoxin (>5 IU/mL) that have long-term duration.[371] Immune response in the elderly may be somewhat impaired. Only 77% of elderly subjects in one study had protective levels of antitoxin 8 years after a three-dose primary series.[373] Other workers also have indicated a weaker immune response in elderly individuals.[375-378] Nevertheless, in most adults, routine boosters every 10 years are sufficient to maintain immunity.[277,284,370,376]

Administration to Women of Child-Bearing Age for Prevention of Neonatal Tetanus

A minimum of two doses of tetanus toxoid at least 1 month apart with the last dose at least 2 weeks before the estimated date of delivery appears to provide protective levels of antibody for well above 80% of newborns.[202] Data do not support sufficient protection from neonatal tetanus when only one dose of standard potency is administered in pregnancy.[202,327] Efficacy above 80% and long-term protection are desired, so the WHO has adopted a schedule of five tetanus toxoid doses administered during a minimum of 2.6 years and preferably more than 10 years to induce sustained levels of circulating antitoxin in all vaccinated women for the duration of their reproductive years[379] (Table 27–3).

The EPI, established in 1974 to provide multiple vaccines to infants, also included the immunization of women in pregnancy to prevent tetanus neonatorum. In communities where routine immunization has been systematically implemented, many expectant mothers and women of child-bearing age will have a history of having completed childhood immunization and/or vaccination in adulthood. An immunization schedule for women of child-bearing age has been recommended that considers the woman's prior history of vaccination in infancy, childhood, adolescence, and later child-bearing years so that an excessive number of doses are not given—a maximum of six doses is administered from infancy through the reproductive years to prevent neonatal tetanus[202,379] (see Table 27–3).

Duration of Immunity and Booster Immunization

After each subsequent tetanus toxoid injection, antitoxin levels peak within 2 weeks, fall rapidly during 2 months, and then fall more gradually in the years following.[380] A constant log-linear decline in antitoxin level has been described.[284,369,370,381] Long-term protection has been reviewed by Simonsen.[382] These data generally support long-lasting persistence of protective antitoxin levels but with the need for booster doses after a primary series

TABLE 27–3 ■ Recommendations of the World Health Organization for Immunization of Women of Child-Bearing Age for Prevention of Neonatal Tetanus*

NOT PREVIOUSLY IMMUNIZED	
Dose No.*	When Given
TT (or Td) 1	First contact or as early in pregnancy as possible
TT (or Td) 2	At least 4 wk after dose 1
TT (or Td) 3	6–12 mo after dose 2 or during subsequent pregnancy
TT (or Td) 4	1–5 yr after dose 3 or during subsequent pregnancy
TT (or Td) 5	1–10 yr after dose 4 or during subsequent pregnancy; no further doses indicated

PREVIOUSLY IMMUNIZED			
		Recommended Immunizations*	
Age at Last Immunization	Previous Immunization	At Present (Contact/ Pregnancy)	Later (at Interval of at Least 1yr)
Infancy	3 doses of DTP	2 doses TT (or Td) (at least 4 wk apart)	1 dose of TT (or Td)
Childhood	4 doses of DTP	1 dose of TT (or Td)	1 dose of TT (or Td)
School age	3 doses of DTP	1 dose of TT (or Td)	1 dose of TT (or Td)
School age	4 doses of DTP + 1 dose of DT/Td	1 dose of TT (or Td)	None
Adolescence	4 doses of DTP + 1 dose of DT/Td at 4–6 yr + 1 dose of TT/Td at 14–16 yr of age	None	None

*The 1998 Strategic Advisory Group of Experts for the Vaccines and Biologics Department of the WHO recommended that programs replace TT by Td in a phased manner. For covering the gap in immunity against tetanus created by the respective strategies of primary immunization with three doses of DTP during infancy and TT to women of child-bearing age, and for boosting diphtheria immunity, Td should be administered to school-age children. In addition, TT can be replaced by Td for adult vaccination. (World Health Organization, the Children's Vaccine Initiative [CVI] and WHO's Global Programme for Vaccines and Immunization [GPV]. Recommendations from the Scientific Advisory Group of Experts [SAGE], Part I. Wkly Epidemiol Rec 73:281–284, 1998.)

DT, diphtheria and tetanus toxoids for pediatric use; DTP, diphtheria and tetanus toxoids and whole-cell pertussis vaccine, Td, tetanus and diphtheria toxoids for adult use; TT, tetanus toxoid.

Adapted from Galazka AM. The Immunologic Basis for Immunization: Tetanus (WHO/EPI/GEN/93. 13). Geneva, World Health Organization, 1993; and World Health Organization. Field Manual for Neonatal Tetanus Elimination (WHO/V&B/99.14). Geneva, World Health Organization, 1999.

throughout life. The best information on the long-term duration of protective levels of tetanus antitoxin comes from studies in Denmark, where there was consistent use of three doses of single-source, 12-Lf adsorbed tetanus toxoid from 1950 through 1960 and four doses of a 7-Lf toxoid since 1961 in a homogeneous population. These data indicate that, after a three-dose primary series consisting of two doses separated by 1 month, followed by a third dose 9 months to 1 year later, protective levels of antitoxin persist in 96% of recipients for 13 to 14 years and in 72% of recipients for more than 25 years.[368,381,382] A study in Sweden indicated that, after a series of three doses 4 to 6 weeks apart, protective levels of antibody were retained by more than 94% after 10 years.[383] Information from an American study showed persistence in 91% of recipients for 7 to 13 years after a three-dose primary series 1 month apart without a reinforcing dose.[384] In U.S. children who received four or more doses of tetanus toxoid, none was found to have an antitoxin level below 0.08 IU/mL in the 90 months of follow-up.[370] On the basis of this information and other studies with similar results, immunization advisory bodies in the United States have recommended that boosters for routine, pre-exposure prophylaxis are needed no more frequently than every 10 years.[120,280]

An acceptable immune response is achieved after booster doses of tetanus toxoid even when intervals of longer than 20 years have elapsed since the last dose, although the briskness and height of response, and duration of protective antitoxin levels, are somewhat dependent on the length of time since primary vaccination.[369,376,381,385-388] Because cases of tetanus are rarely seen in persons who received a primary series of vaccine and then received a booster dose of toxoid as part of wound prophylaxis, it appears that some delay in antitoxin response is not a substantial concern for the majority of persons with extended periods of time since their previous dose (see *Tetanus Prophylaxis in Wound Management* below). The duration of immunity induced by fluid toxoid is shorter lived than that induced by adsorbed toxoid, thus, booster immunization within 3 years has been recommended for those previously immunized with fluid toxoid, preferably with adsorbed tetanus toxoid.[389]

Historically, the policy of administering tetanus boosters every 10 years was based on the possibility that fluid tetanus toxoid was used in prior doses and that dose potencies of available preparations were highly variable.[260] The studies of duration of immunity in Scandinavia cited above in which adsorbed toxoid of constant antigen content and potency was used may not be representative of the situation elsewhere. For the Danish population, Simonsen et al.[381] proposed a school-age booster after primary immunization and subsequent routine boosters at least every 20 years. If applied to other populations with a more heterogeneous exposure to tetanus toxoid preparations, that recommendation might lead to a significant proportion of unprotected individuals.

The need for booster doses every 10 years has been questioned by some experts because few cases of tetanus, and even fewer associated deaths, are reported among people who received a primary series of three or more doses, regardless of whether they have received booster doses.[38-40,382,390-394] This low morbidity and mortality in vaccinated populations has occurred despite poor adherence to the recommendation for decennial boosters; only 50% of adults in the United States report having received a tetanus booster during the previous 10 years.[395] The proposed alternative is that, following a primary childhood series and adolescent booster, no further routine assessment of tetanus immunization status should occur until individuals reach the age of 50 years.[394,396] Tetanus toxoid prophylaxis in wound management would still be recommended. Gardner has argued that this alternative schedule is justified on the basis of excess adverse events attributed to tetanus toxoid use, and because this schedule could be more effectively monitored for compliance.[394] The frequencies of adverse events attributable to tetanus toxoid, in particular brachial plexus neuropathy, may have been overestimated (see *Adverse Events Following Immunization* below).[397]

The most important rationale for the current recommendation of decennial adult tetanus boosters in North America is to maintain serum antitoxin well above protective levels for nearly all members of the population. Although primary vaccination alone has an effect on disease severity, severe tetanus cases and deaths have been reported despite receipt of prior toxoid doses.[14,106,107,332,398] The consequences to population immunity of the lack of compliance with the decennial booster policy are evident in the results of the recent population-based tetanus antitoxin serosurvey in the United States: The proportion of the population with protective levels of antitoxin declines with increasing age, leaving 20% of those 40 to 49 years of age unprotected and 70% unprotected by the age of 70 years.[185] In addition, the elderly may not have as great or long-lasting a response to a single dose of toxoid as younger individuals; a single booster dose at 50 years of age may not provide adequate protection.[203,296,373,377] Because tetanus boosters are not always administered for wounds and other conditions associated with tetanus (see *Epidemiology* above), reliance on prophylaxis provided during wound care does not guarantee that those at high risk will be protected. A cost-effectiveness analysis comparing the decennial booster strategy with that of a single booster in later life was performed by Balestra and Littenberg.[393] They estimated that decennial boosting prevented four times as many cases as a single booster at 65 years of age. They also estimated that decennial boosters were substantially less cost-effective—$143,138 in 1993 dollars for every year of life saved with decennial booster versus $4527 with a single booster at age 65 years. However, the analysis did not take the costs of prophylactic tetanus boosters with wound care into account, thereby overestimating the difference in cost between the two strategies.

The final consideration underlying the recommendation to give adults decennial boosters specifically with Td is the fact that diphtheria antitoxin levels decline more rapidly than tetanus antitoxin levels, requiring booster doses every 10 years.[200,300] Given the greater health impact of decennial

boosters, the ACIP has continued to recommend them.[87,120,280]

Booster Immunization for Prevention of Maternal and Neonatal Tetanus

The WHO recommendation for tetanus immunization of women of child-bearing age in countries with and without well-established routine childhood vaccination is shown in Table 27–3.[379,400] These recommendations are intended to elicit high antitoxin titers during pregnancy in order to prevent neonatal tetanus. The schedule recommends boosting at each subsequent pregnancy unless five to six doses have been administered previously. Analyses of data collected in Bangladesh over 13 years from women vaccinated with one, two, or no doses of tetanus toxoid have shown a substantial reduction in overall neonatal mortality in the 4- to 14-day interval after birth for the offspring of vaccinated mothers.[401] The duration of immunity was up to 10 years for women who received two doses and up to 4 years after one dose. These data not only show the high efficacy of tetanus toxoid and long duration of immunity but also confirm the major contribution neonatal tetanus makes to overall mortality 4 to 14 days after birth.

Immunization in Immunodeficiency

Because tetanus toxoid–containing vaccines (DTP, DTaP, DT, Td, and TT) are inactivated, they are safe for use in immunocompromised individuals, including those with congenital immunodeficiencies, human immunodeficiency virus (HIV) infection, hematologic or other malignancies, stem cell transplants (SCTs) or organ transplants, and chronic renal failure (CRF).[402,403] Most of these conditions are associated with reduced responsiveness to tetanus toxoid vaccination or shorter duration of protection, although data defining abnormalities in tetanus immunity are incomplete for many conditions.[404-415] With the exception of modified guidelines to be used for SCT recipients and patients with CRF, the general schedule for primary and booster vaccination with tetanus toxoid–containing vaccine presented above under *Indications for Use* also are recommended for persons with known or suspected immunodeficiency.[402,403] Anti-tetanus antibody determinations may be indicated in immunocompromised individuals to assess responses to vaccination and duration of protection, and to guide the use of supplemental tetanus toxoid doses.

Adults and infants infected with HIV generally respond to tetanus toxoid vaccination with increases in serum antitoxin levels.[403,405,406,409,416] Adults who received primary vaccination before acquiring HIV infection develop protective levels of antitoxin following a booster dose of tetanus toxoid.[416] Antitoxin levels in HIV-infected subjects tend to be lower than in uninfected controls, particularly in those whose CD4+ cell counts are less than $300 \times 10^6/L$.[403,405,406] Although most infants with perinatally acquired HIV infection respond normally to tetanus toxoid–containing vaccines, serologic responses to vaccination decline as HIV disease progresses.[403,408,409,417] The duration of protective tetanus antitoxin levels in HIV-infected individuals is uncertain, although there is some evidence that protective antibody levels are shorter lived than in those who are uninfected.[403,407]

Vaccination recommendations for transplant patients differ for SCT recipients and solid organ recipients. Following SCT, patients are initially severely immunocompromised and require reconstitution of immunity against vaccine-preventable diseases once their acquired immune system has matured.[418] Three doses of DTaP or DT in children less than 7 years, or Td in children 7 years or older and adults, are recommended; the doses should be given at 12, 14, and 24 months after transplant.[411,418] There is evidence that vaccinating the stem cell donor 6 to 10 days before marrow harvest results in the transfer of both antibody-synthesizing B cells and antigen-specific T cells to the recipient, thereby conferring some protection during the first year following SCT, and augmenting the response to active immunization given during the second year.[411]

In contrast to SCT, information about tetanus immunity and responsiveness to tetanus toxoid following solid organ transplantation is sparse. Solid organ transplant patients require lifelong immunosuppression to prevent organ rejection and to preserve allograft function, and are therefore at increased risk for infections. Children who undergo successful renal or hepatic transplantation appear to retain normal responses to tetanus toxoid despite immunosuppressive therapy.[419,420] Adult renal transplant patients also retain responsiveness to tetanus toxoid, although the level of antitoxin produced is significantly lower than in healthy controls.[412] Vaccination strategies vary among transplant centers, and sufficient information is not currently available to mandate a change in the formal recommendations for vaccination in solid organ transplant recipients. Thus the standard schedule for primary and booster tetanus toxoid vaccination continues to be recommended for both child and adult solid organ transplant recipients.[411]

CRF is associated with immune deficits caused by uremia-induced alterations in cell-mediated immunity and IgG_1 production.[412,419,421] Studies of adults with CRF, including those receiving chronic dialysis, demonstrate a variety of defects in responsiveness to tetanus toxoid. The proportion of CRF patients with protective levels of tetanus antitoxin at baseline is lower than in healthy populations, as is the proportion of patients who seroconvert in response to tetanus toxoid.[412,413] Mean antitoxin levels produced by CRF patients who respond to toxoid are lower than those produced by healthy controls, and the duration of protective immunity in CRF patients is reduced.[412,414,415] More than one booster dose may be necessary to achieve protective antitoxin levels in adult patients with CRF, and boosters may be required more frequently than every 10 years to maintain protection. Monitoring antitoxin levels following vaccination and at periodic intervals thereafter is indicated in this population to direct individual vaccination strategies. In contrast to adults, children receiving hemodialysis for CRF have a normal initial response to vaccination with DTP, although the duration of protection has not been determined.[422] Most infants receiving peritoneal dialysis also have a normal response to routine DTP vaccination, maintaining protective levels for 24 months.[423]

Adverse Events Following Immunization

Whereas mild local reactions are relatively common after receipt of tetanus toxoid, more serious reactions, including neurologic and hypersensitivity reactions, are exceedingly rare. The rates and severity of adverse events in recipients of tetanus toxoid are influenced by the number of prior doses and level of pre-existing antitoxin, perhaps the amount of toxoid in the dose, the type and quantity of adjuvant, the route of injection, the presence of other antigens in the preparation, and perhaps the presence of organomercurials used as preservative.

The most common adverse event following injection of tetanus toxoid is a local reaction. Local reactions are reported in 0% to 95% of recipients, depending on the definition. Most studies suggest increasing rates of local reactions with an increasing number of doses.[371,424–426] Among recipients of a booster dose of adsorbed toxoid, 50% to 85% experience pain or tenderness at the injection site and 25% to 30% experience edema and erythema.[427–431] More severe local reactions characterized by marked swelling occur in fewer than 2% of vaccinees.[424,432]

Some investigators claim that increasing antigen content (Lf) increases local reactions, but there is no clear evidence of this.[424,425,433] However, higher levels of pre-existing antitoxin are associated with higher rates of local reactions and with reactions of greater severity.[389,424,425,427,428,433–436] Persons who have a rapid immunologic response (within 4 days), suggestive of priming by past doses, have higher rates of local reactions than persons whose immunologic response is slower.[425,433–436] Massive local reactions, such as swelling from elbow to shoulder, have occurred most often in persons with a history of multiple booster doses of toxoid. Typically, these reactions began within 2 to 8 hours after toxoid administration in the deltoid. Serum antitoxin levels in these persons ranged from 2 to 160 IU/mL, manyfold higher on average than levels in persons without reactions, or in those with systemic adverse events.[433,437–440] The pathogenesis of massive local reactions is not fully understood. Preformed antibody apparently forms complexes with the deposited toxoid to induce an inflammatory response (Arthus reaction, or type III hypersensitivity).[437,440] Other undefined host factors are involved because the range of antitoxin levels in individuals who exhibit this response is wide and includes levels seen in individuals without such a response. In persons with a history of massive local reactions after tetanus toxoid, boosting with lower than standard doses of tetanus toxoid (1 Lf) has been proposed by some researchers to lead to an adequate immune response without significant adverse events.[425,433,441] Antitoxin levels in such persons should be evaluated before booster doses are given to ascertain whether there is a need for additional doses. Most other severe local reactions can be prevented by avoiding unnecessary boosters of tetanus toxoid in wound management (see *Tetanus Prophylaxis in Wound Management* below).

There have been conflicting reports as to whether aluminum adjuvants increase the incidence of local reactions compared with fluid toxoids.[282,427,428,436,442] Aluminum adjuvant in adsorbed products theoretically can invoke local inflammatory responses more frequently than fluid toxoid because the presence of adjuvant can induce activation of complement and stimulate macrophages.[443] Differences in study results could be due to differences in the manufacturing process of adsorbed toxoids resulting in variable adsorption and adjuvant activity.[443] Alternatively, differences in the potency of the toxoid administered to the study groups may have varied (with or without equivalent Lf content), a problem found in all comparisons of adverse events after tetanus toxoid administration. Histologic evidence suggests that aluminum hydroxide crystals may remain at the injection site following intramuscular injection of aluminum hydroxide–adsorbed vaccines in some persons. The clinical implications of this finding, if any, are unclear.[444-446]

The frequency of local reactions is increased when toxoid is administered subcutaneously rather than intramuscularly.[424] This is particularly true for adsorbed toxoid[447]; aluminum adjuvant can cause sterile abscesses when given subcutaneously.[443] Use of jet injectors, which deposit some toxoid in the subcutaneous tissue, results in twofold higher rates of edema at the administration site than intramuscular injection by needle.[448]

In the United States, tetanus toxoid is given as a single antigen, or in combination with diphtheria toxoid, with or without pertussis antigens.[120,279,280,334] (Adverse effects of diphtheria toxoid– and pertussis-containing vaccines are addressed, respectively, in Chapters 13 and 21.) In some controlled trials, minor adverse events, such as swelling or pain, occurred more frequently after Td than after tetanus toxoid alone (TT).[426,429] The same lot of tetanus toxoid was not used in both the Td and TT preparations, limiting the conclusions that could be drawn from these trials. Other studies have not found a substantial difference in the rates of local reactions with Td compared with TT, or TT was associated with higher rates of local reactions than Td.[430,431,449] Increasing frequencies of large local reactions after use of DTaP vaccines recently have been observed; the pathogenesis of these reactions is not well understood.[450,451]

The preservative used in the U.S. preparations of tetanus toxoid has, until recently, been exclusively thimerosal. This mercury-containing compound has been linked to delayed-type hypersensitivity reactions in some individuals.[441,452] It is uncertain to what degree hypersensitivity to thimerosal influences local reactions when given intramuscularly. Reports have rarely linked reactions with an exaggerated delayed-type hypersensitivity response to tetanus toxoid itself.[437,453-455] No long-term effects of thimerosal use have been identified.[456] Concerns over exposure to mercury led the U.S. Food and Drug Administration to undertake a review of all medicinal products containing the metal, including vaccines. Similarly, the European Medicines Evaluation Agency's Committee for Proprietary Medicinal Products has requested vaccine manufacturers to submit manufacturing plans to eliminate organomercurials as preservatives in their products. In the United States, all routinely recommended vaccines administered to infants (including DTaP) are either thimerosal free or contain trace amounts (see *Constituents* above).[457-459]

Systemic reactions following tetanus toxoid inoculation are less common than local reactions. Fever can accompany a local response, particularly when there is a marked local reaction or antitoxin levels are high.[429,432,440] Uncommonly, persons with high antitoxin levels experience high fever and malaise without experiencing substantial local reactions, primarily after receiving booster doses of toxoid.[440] Booster doses of Td are associated with fever in 0.5% to 7% of recipients; temperatures above 39°C are rare.[426,429,432] Other sys-

temic symptoms such as headache or malaise are reported less frequently than fever.[425,426,432] Lymphadenopathy also can occur after toxoid inoculation.[428,437]

Peripheral neuropathy, particularly brachial plexus neuropathy, has been reported to occur hours to weeks after tetanus toxoid administration.[460-467] These reports and laboratory findings have been reviewed.[397,467,468] Although anecdotal, the reports are consistent with neuropathy as a manifestation of immune complex disease similar to that occurring after equine tetanus antitoxin.[469] The Vaccine Safety Committee of the U.S. Institute of Medicine concluded in 1994 that there is evidence to support a causal association between tetanus toxoid and brachial plexus neuropathy.[397] The evidence was considered inadequate to accept or reject a causal relationship of tetanus toxoid with mononeuropathy. On the basis of two published case series from the Mayo Clinic of brachial plexus neuropathy that included cases following tetanus toxoid exposure,[465,466] the Institute of Medicine committee estimated that 0.5 to 1 case of brachial neuropathy per 100,000 recipients was attributable to tetanus toxoid within 1 month of immunization.[397] Given that this estimate was based solely on open case series that include six toxoid-exposed patients with unknown total immunization histories,[465,466] the calculated attributable risk may have been overestimated for the contemporary general population.

There have been reports of at least 25 cases of Guillain-Barré syndrome (GBS) after tetanus toxoid.[397,460-463] One patient had relapsing GBS signs and symptoms after each of three injections of toxoid.[461] Although there may be a causal relationship between tetanus toxoid and GBS, the occurrence is rare. An estimate of the incidence of GBS following tetanus toxoid administration is 0.4 per million doses.[397] Population studies do not support a causal role for tetanus toxoids in GBS. A study of 700,000 children who received DTP found a frequency of GBS after immunization similar to expected background rates.[470] After administration of tetanus toxoids to an estimated 1.2 million children and adults, another study found a lower frequency of GBS after immunization than expected by chance alone.[471]

Other neurologic events, including seizures and acute encephalopathy, have been reported after tetanus toxoid or DT.[397,440,472,473] There are insufficient data to support a causal relationship with any of these other illnesses.[397] As is true with all immunizations, the occurrence of systemic symptoms soon after inoculation does not in itself indicate causation; the association may instead reflect an unrelated chance occurrence.

Tetanus toxoid occasionally induces an immunoglobulin E (IgE) response, particularly with aluminum salt–adsorbed toxoid.[287,474-476] True anaphylactic (type I hypersensitivity) reactions to purified tetanus toxoid are rare.[397,477-479] Before 1942 in the United States, contaminating peptones from the culture media and silk fibers from the filtering process were present in toxoid preparations. Two cases of anaphylaxis were reported after administration of 61,000 doses (0.003%) of these vaccines.[480-483] In a large series using Air Force recruits in the early 1960s, serious allergic reactions attributable to toxoid occurred in 0.001%.[484] Passive surveillance in the United States in 1991 to 1995 for serious allergic reactions including laryngospasm, bronchospasm, or anaphylaxis yielded a rate of 1.6 serious allergic reactions reported per million doses of publicly distributed Td.[‡]

Skin testing has been suggested as an aid to assessing the risk of anaphylaxis with tetanus toxoid administration in persons with a history of hypersensitivity reactions following tetanus vaccine. However, skin tests are of limited benefit and confer some risk themselves.[441,485] In a study of Air Force recruits with a history of an anaphylactic reaction after a prior tetanus toxoid dose, an intradermal skin test was negative in 94 of 95.[441] All recruits tolerated full-dose challenges of toxoid, suggesting lack of IgE-mediated hypersensitivity in the prior reaction. Positive skin test responses were found in study subjects who subsequently tolerated full-dose challenges.[441] However, in another study, anaphylaxis was reported in 3 of 200 persons undergoing skin testing who had a history of sensitivity. Similar reports of anaphylaxis have been made by others.[479,485] Thus undue weight should not be put on the results of the tests alone because of the lack of specificity,[486] and caution must be used if skin testing is performed.

When eliciting a history of allergic reactions to tetanus toxoid, attention should be paid to the details of the injection and the reaction. One potential problem with histories of reactions in older subjects is confusion between equine antitoxin and tetanus toxoids. An adverse reaction after a "tetanus shot" received before tetanus toxoid became widely available may suggest that equine antitoxin or another product was received. When the history is consistent with an immediate hypersensitivity reaction, testing for serum antitoxin level may be helpful to evaluate the actual need for a booster of toxoid. In the context of emergency wound care, such results are unlikely to be immediately available. In that case, skin testing before challenge could be attempted in a setting equipped to manage anaphylaxis (Table 27–4). If skin testing is not feasible, or deemed imprudent, TIG can be used for immediate tetanus prophylaxis, and decisions about the approach to booster administration can be deferred until the results of serum antitoxin testing are available.

Tetanus immunization in pregnancy has rarely been related to mild hemolytic disease of the newborn when the toxoid was produced with media containing human blood group–related antigens such as beef heart infusion.[487,488] Such substances are excluded from growth media used by U.S. manufacturers; therefore, this has not been a relevant issue in the United States and can be similarly avoided elsewhere if producers adhere to WHO standards.

Simultaneous Administration with Other Vaccines

Tetanus toxoid has been combined with diphtheria toxoid, pertussis vaccines (both whole cell and acellular), and Hib conjugate vaccines without compromising the immune response or substantially enhancing adverse events associated with the tetanus component (see *Available Preparations* above). Combination with whole-cell pertussis vaccines enhances the serologic response to diphtheria and tetanus toxoids because of the adjuvant properties of whole-cell vaccines.

With the use of Hib–polyribosylribitol phosphate (PRP) polysaccharide conjugate vaccine covalently linked to tetanus toxoid (PRP-T), theoretical concerns were raised as to whether tetanus toxoid in the conjugate vaccine could inhibit or enhance a response to tetanus toxoid. These concerns have not been shown to be clinically relevant. Initial antitoxin responses are slightly higher after simultaneous administration of DTP vaccines with PRP-T compared with DTP alone, but overall antitoxin levels are well above protective levels regardless of whether or not DTP is administered with PRP-T. Maternally acquired tetanus antitoxin does not interfere with the immune response to PRP-T.[489] PRP-T alone induces a tetanus antitoxin response that is substantial but lower than the response to tetanus toxoid,[490] thus PRP-T vaccines cannot substitute for tetanus toxoid. Use of simultaneous PRP-T with DTP does not appear to increase the frequency of common adverse events and does not appear to differ in this respect from other Hib conjugate vaccines.[491] DTP combined with PRP-T vaccine in the same syringe is equivalent in immunogenicity and safety to DTP with PRP-T vaccine administered separately.[492,493]

[‡]Centers for Disease Control and Prevention, unpublished data.

TABLE 27–4 ■ Protocol for Skin Testing for Acute Hypersensitivity and Challenge to Tetanus Toxoid[*]

Step	Preparation	Volume (mL)	Concentration	Route
1	TT, fluid	—	1:10	Skin prick
2	TT, fluid	0.02	1:100,000	ID
3	TT, fluid	0.02	1:10,000	ID
4	TT, fluid	0.02	1:1000	ID
5	TT, fluid	0.02	1:100	ID
6	Td, adsorbed	0.02	1:10	SC
7	Td, adsorbed	0.1	1:10	SC
8	Td, adsorbed	0.1	Full strength	SC
9	Td, adsorbed	0.4	Full strength	SC

[*]Wait 15 minutes between steps for observation of reaction.
ID, intradermal injection; SC, subcutaneous; Td, tetanus and diphtheria toxoids for adult use; TT, tetanus toxoid.
Modified from Jacobs RL, Lowe RS, Lanier BQ. Adverse reactions to tetanus toxoid. JAMA 247:40–42, 1982; Mansfield LE, Ting S, Rawls DO, Frederick R. Systemic reactions during cutaneous testing for tetanus toxoid hypersensitivity. Ann Allergy 57:135–137, 1986.

Contraindications and Precautions

A careful history of possible adverse events is necessary because some patients may have confused equine antitoxin with toxoid. Conditions recognized by the ACIP and the Committee on Infectious Diseases of the AAP as contraindications to the use of tetanus toxoid include a history of severe hypersensitivity or a neurologic event after a prior dose.[120,280] The evaluation should distinguish between a serious neurologic illness for which further doses are contraindicated and other syndromes, such as syncope, for which they are not. When toxoid is contraindicated, TIG should be given if immune status is unknown and a wound occurs that is not clean and minor. TIG is not necessary for clean and minor wounds. Delayed-type hypersensitivity to thimerosal is not a contraindication to products containing this preservative because it would be manifested as a subcutaneous/cutaneous reaction without systemic effects.

Although studies have failed to suggest that tetanus toxoid with or without diphtheria toxoid is teratogenic or has any other harmful effect when it is given in pregnancy,[494,495] in industrialized nations, when providers believe that the woman will return for visits later in pregnancy, it may be prudent to delay immunization to the second trimester to minimize any concern of a perceived relationship with any observed birth defect.[496]

Tetanus Prophylaxis in Wound Management

All individuals presenting for care of skin wounds or infections should be evaluated for tetanus prophylaxis. The lesion should be treated as medically indicated, including removal of foreign bodies, débridement of devitalized tissue, incision and drainage, and irrigation to prevent or eliminate an anaerobic environment and bacterial contamination.[497-500] The patient's history of tetanus toxoid immunization should be obtained, with attention to the number of prior doses as well as the interval since the last dose. In the 1950s, a booster dose of toxoid was recommended for every wound if more than 1 year had elapsed since the last dose. The association of Arthus-type reactions with frequently repeated tetanus boosters, and a better understanding of the kinetics of antibody responses following booster administration, led to a reappraisal of this practice.[284,366,370,384,439] Guidelines for the use of tetanus toxoid and TIG for tetanus prophylaxis in wound management based on the current recommendations of the ACIP are given in Table 27–5.[120,280,500]

Although any wound can give rise to tetanus, clean wounds are considered to have a low likelihood of tetanus spore contamination and of developing the anaerobic and acidic conditions that promote spore germination. For people with this category of wound, a tetanus toxoid booster is recommended if the patient has received fewer than three doses of adsorbed toxoid in the past, or if more than 10 years has passed since the previous toxoid dose. TIG administration is not necessary. With some exceptions, most individuals in the United States will have protective antitoxin levels before exposure (see *Epidemiology* above for groups more likely to be unprotected). Individuals with a history of three or more doses of toxoid but without detectable antitoxin develop detectable antibodies within 4 to 7 days following the receipt of a subsequent dose.[385,386,388,501,502] Experimental evidence suggests that protection begins before a rise in antitoxin level is detectable.[503]

Wounds contaminated with dirt, feces, or saliva; deep wounds and punctures; and wounds with devitalized tissue, such as burns, frostbite, gangrene, and crush injures, are considered more likely to develop *C. tetani* infection and toxin production. Abscesses, cellulitis, chronic ulcers, and other wounds in patients with diabetes mellitus or illicit injection drug use also should be considered "tetanus prone." Most patients who received fluid toxoid in the past, and, less commonly, those who received adsorbed toxoid, may have circulating antitoxin levels below 0.01 IU/mL after 5 years.[370,384,389] Therefore, the current recommendation for patients with tetanus-prone wounds is to receive a dose of toxoid if more than 5 years have elapsed since the last dose. In addition, patients who have received fewer than three prior toxoid doses, those whose vaccination histories are uncertain, and those with immunodeficiencies (see *Immunization in Immunodeficiency* above) should receive prophylactic TIG for such wounds (see below). When administered at a separate site, TIG does not interfere with the immune response to adsorbed tetanus toxoid.[255,260,285]

TABLE 27–5 ▪ Summary Guide to Tetanus Prophylaxis in Routine Wound Management, United States

History of Adsorbed Tetanus Toxoid (Doses)	Clean, Minor Wounds		All Other Wounds*	
	Td[†]	TIG	Td[†]	TIG
Unknown or <3	Yes	No	Yes	Yes
≥3[‡]	No[§]	No	No[¶]	No

*Including, but not limited to, wounds contaminated with dirt, feces, soil, saliva; puncture wounds; avulsions; and wounds resulting from missiles, crushing, burns, and frostbite.

[†]For children less than 7 years old, DTaP (DT, if pertussis vaccine is contraindicated) is preferred to tetanus toxoid alone. For persons 7 years of age and older, Td is preferred to tetanus toxoid alone. Diphtheria and tetanus toxoids and whole-cell pertussis vaccine (DTP) may be used instead of DTaP as indicated, or in other countries.

[‡]If only three doses of *fluid* toxoid have been received, then a fourth dose of toxoid, preferably an adsorbed toxoid, should be given.

[§]Yes, if more than 10 years since last dose.

[¶]Yes, if more than 5 years since last dose. (More frequent boosters are not needed and can accentuate side effects.)

From Centers for Disease Control and Prevention. Diphtheria, tetanus and pertussis: guidelines for vaccine prophylaxis and other preventive measures. Recommendations of the Immunization Practices Advisory Committee (ACIP). MMWR 40(RR-10):1–28, 1991.

The dose currently recommended by the ACIP and the AAP for prophylactic TIG is 250 IU given intramuscularly.[120,280] This dose will provide antitoxin levels above 0.01 IU/mL beginning 2 to 3 days after administration and lasting for at least 4 weeks in almost all individuals.[123,260,504–508] A concern that higher TIG doses are necessary to guarantee protection has led some authorities to recommend the range of 250 to 500 IU for wound prophylaxis.[116,500,509] The uncertainty about the optimal dose for prophylactic TIG stems from reports of tetanus in individuals with circulating levels of antitoxin greater than 0.01 IU/mL (see *Passive Immunization and Correlation of Serum Antitoxin with Protection* above), and the report of fatal tetanus despite prophylactic administration of 250 IU of TIG.[510] Doses of 400 to 500 IU may induce protective levels earlier than doses of 250 IU,[511] and produce serum antitoxin levels of up to 1.0 IU/mL.[123,250,512] Because patients who receive prophylactic TIG do so in the context of professional wound care, they are less likely to develop tetanus, or tetanus infection with high levels of toxin. Thus a TIG dose of 250 IU is appropriate in most circumstances; however, if wound care has been delayed or a wound appears to present a particularly high risk of tetanus, the higher dose of 500 IU may be considered.

Before TIG was widely available, antibiotics were used for tetanus prophylaxis in wound management as a substitute for or adjunct to equine antitoxin.[513] Smith and earlier researchers demonstrated the efficacy of prophylactic antibiotics in animal models[514]; however, efficacy superior or equal to that of antitoxin in the prevention of tetanus in humans was never proven.[515,516] Antimicrobials are not currently recommended for tetanus prophylaxis per se.[497,515] Instead, wounds should be observed for signs of infection and treatment should be initiated promptly if any infection occurs.

Reviews of tetanus cases reported in the United States from 1989 to 2000 demonstrated that many individuals who subsequently developed tetanus received less than the recommended prophylactic care when medical treatment was sought for wounds.[7,38–40,216] Two studies suggested that, when patients with wounds do seek care in the United States, 1% to 6% receive fewer prophylactic measures than recommended, and 12% to 17% receive Td, with or without TIG, when not indicated.[517,518] Confusion about optimal prophylactic measures has been described outside the United States as well.[519,520] Education of physicians regarding the recommendations for tetanus prophylaxis in wound management is needed to improve the level of appropriate prophylactic care.

Public Health Perspective

Disease Control Strategies

Elimination of environmental exposure to *C. tetani* is impossible. However, tetanus toxoid is one of the most effective and safest biologics available, thus the health burden of tetanus is almost completely preventable through routine immunization. Although there have been advances in the care of tetanus patients, tetanus remains a severe and lengthy disease with a significant case-fatality rate. The direct cost of care for tetanus patients in the United States can exceed $150,000.[521]

In the developed world, the lowest seroprevalence rates of antitoxin and the highest incidence rates of tetanus are in the oldest age groups. For further progress in preventing tetanus in the United States, efforts are needed to increase compliance with the ACIP recommendation for primary immunization and routine decennial Td booster doses in adults, particularly in the elderly.[396,496] Serosurveys of the prevalence of tetanus antitoxin show that susceptibility to tetanus increases with increasing age as a result of lack of adequate immunization[185,201,203–208,377,395,522–527]; the age distribution of tetanus cases in developed countries reflects this susceptibility. Although elderly individuals have a diminished response to antigenic stimulation in general, primary immunization and recommended booster doses of tetanus toxoid successfully confer protection against tetanus.[203,296,375–378,380–382,525,528]

Maternal and Neonatal Tetanus Elimination (MNTE)

Despite remarkable progress in preventing tetanus worldwide, a significant burden of the disease remains in the developing world, particularly in the neonatal period. According to WHO estimates, in 2000 there were 200,000 deaths caused by neonatal tetanus and 109,000 deaths caused by non-neonatal tetanus (see also *Epidemiology* above).[169] Efforts to decrease the incidence of tetanus in the developing world began in earnest when the EPI was launched by the WHO in 1974. Although the true burden of neonatal tetanus was grossly underestimated at that time, the WHO recommended neonatal tetanus prevention through training of traditional birth attendants to provide "clean" delivery services and administration of at least two doses of tetanus toxoid to pregnant women.[379] Following the discovery of the extent of tetanus occurring in the neonatal period in the 1980s,[220] but also recognizing progress in the application of WHO recommendations, the 1989 World Health Assembly announced a goal to eliminate neonatal tetanus worldwide by 1995.[529,530] By 1990, the estimated annual number of neonatal tetanus deaths had fallen from 1.2 million in 1980 (about 10 deaths per 1000 live births) to 408,000 (about 3.0 deaths per 1000 live births).[531,532] In 1993, neonatal tetanus elimination was defined as less than one case of neonatal tetanus for every 1000 live births per year in each administrative district.[533] The estimated 200,000 deaths caused by neonatal tetanus in 2000 represents about 1.5 tetanus deaths per 1000 live births overall.

Much of this recent progress reflects the use of the "high-risk" approach toward prevention of neonatal tetanus, initially pioneered in the Americas in the early 1990s. The high-risk approach uses supplemental immunization campaigns for women of child-bearing age, targeting high-risk areas identified by surveillance or other indicators.[240,400] In 1999, progress toward neonatal tetanus elimination was reassessed, and WHO, UNICEF, and the United Nations Population Fund (UNFPA) forged a stronger partnership. The partnership revised the global goal to include maternal tetanus elimination with neonatal tetanus elimination and the operational target to 2005.[240] As a result of enhanced immunization of women, the estimated number of deaths from maternal tetanus associated with puerperal infection and septic abortion has fallen from 30,000 per year in 1990 to 10,000 in 2000.[241,534] The partnership's strategic goal is to provide three properly spaced doses of tetanus toxoid to at least 80% of women of child-bearing age in high-risk areas, and to promote the traditional strategies of routine immunization of pregnant women, clean delivery practices, and effective neonatal tetanus surveillance.[240]

In 1980, global tetanus toxoid use of two or more doses in pregnant women was reported to be 4%; by 1990, coverage with two or more doses had increased to 57%, and to 64% in 1997.[532] Since the elimination goal was set, the reported coverage of pregnant women with two or more doses of tetanus toxoid ("TT2+") has not exceeded 50% in much of the developing world.[245] However, TT2+ coverage figures underestimate the true level of protection from tetanus for infants: Doses received during childhood, in prior pregnancies, in other health encounters, or in mass campaigns may have been ignored if undocumented.[533,535,536] By including maternal verbal histories of prior immunization, even if undocumented, the degree of underestimation in coverage is reduced but still present. The WHO currently recommends monitoring progress in programs for neonatal tetanus elimination by the use of the mother's cumulative immunization history to determine the proportion of children protected at birth.[400] Protection at birth (PAB) can be estimated during dedicated EPI cluster surveys or multiple-indicator cluster surveys (MICS). EPI surveys are designed to determine immunization coverage in children 12 to 23 months of age; PAB can be simultaneously estimated for a sample of children younger than 12 months by determining the lifetime history of toxoid doses and timing of last dose for their mothers at the time the children were born.[400,537] MICS are typically large enough to include a subsample of women with children younger than 12 months in addition to older children. Serosurveys in specialized studies have allowed an immunologic assessment of the true protection of mothers and infants.[319,536,538,539] A study in Burundi confirmed the correlation of serologic protection with the child's estimated PAB based on maternal recall of cumulative tetanus toxoid immunizations.[536] A study in the Central African Republic indicated the potential for underestimation of protection with this method as well; estimated PAB by maternal recall of tetanus toxoid status was 74%, whereas seroprevalance testing for antitoxin level of 0.01 IU/mL or higher by double-antigen ELISA estimated protection at 89%.[540]

The WHO also encourages routine monitoring of the cumulative tetanus immunization status of women when they bring their infants for the first dose of DTP[400,530]; inadequately immunized women who do not have contraindications should be immunized at that health encounter. Although monitoring in this way does not provide information on women who do not bring their children for DTP1, it is a more accurate assessment of the effectiveness of national, regional, or local programs aimed at maternal and neonatal tetanus elimination than monitoring of TT2+.[541]

The expansion of the MNTE target group beyond only pregnant women is an important step. The immunization of all women of child-bearing age can be more effective than limiting vaccination to pregnant women, and circumvents poor access to health services.[400,533,542] Many countries demonstrated substantial progress in controlling neonatal tetanus when they began immunizing all women of child-bearing age whenever possible, with booster inoculation offered during pregnancy[226,327,400,401,530,533,543–547]§ Data from Bangladesh have shown a substantial reduction in overall neonatal mortality in the 4- to 14-day interval after birth for up to 10 years for women who received two doses and up to 4 years after one dose.[401] In addition, vaccination of women of child-bearing age addresses tetanus following wounds and also following septic spontaneous or induced abortions among primiparae.[241,548] The 1998 Scientific Advisory Group of Experts to the WHO recommended that programs replace TT by Td in a phased manner.[549] For covering the gap in immunity against tetanus created by the respective strategies of primary immunization with three doses of DTP during infancy and TT to women of child-bearing age, and for boosting diphtheria immunity, Td should be administered to school-age children; however, immunization in schools is only an effective option where school enrollment and attendance rates are high. In addition, TT can be replaced by Td for adult vaccination. Immunization schedules have been developed to take the mother's entire prior immunization status, if known, into account (see Table 27–3).[202,379,400] After nearly 30 years of the EPI, most countries have a substantial proportion of women of child-bearing age with some prior exposure to tetanus toxoid. Global coverage of children with DTP has increased during the 1980s and has been estimated to exceed 70% since 1990.[245] A study of adolescent girls in Nigeria, Malawi, and Pakistan suggested that protective levels of antibody may be present in a high proportion even without booster/reinforcing doses after infant immunization.[550]

The high-risk approach focuses available public health resources on districts with a reported incidence of disease of more than 1.0 neonatal tetanus case per 1000 births or, if surveillance is limited, other indicators suggesting there is a substantial disease burden.[226,400,530,542–545,547] Once high-risk districts are identified, all women of child-bearing age are targeted for immunization through well-prepared, focal mass campaigns. The effectiveness of the campaigns is closely monitored, assuring 80% or greater coverage. Ideally, three rounds of immunization are performed, with appropriate spacing to provide effective and long-term protection. The WHO Region of the Americas (Pan American Health Organization) systematically targeted neonatal tetanus using the high-risk approach in 16 countries of the region.§ From 1992 to 1996, the proportion of districts with an incidence of 1.0 or higher per 1000 live births decreased from 2.5% to 1.0%. As of 2000, the only country in the Americas that has not reached elimination is Haiti.[534]

Since 1994, more than 30 countries have used the high-risk approach.[532] China immunized 23 million women of child-bearing age with campaigns in 320 of 560 identified high-risk districts in 1996, reducing overall neonatal tetanus mortality to less than 0.6 per 1000 live births nationally in 1997, from over 3 per 1000 in 1990.[532,543] Improved detection of neonatal tetanus cases after imple-

---

§da Silva and deQuadros, Pan American Health Organization, unpublished data. April, 1996.

menting the high-risk approach helps to focus intervention activities on areas and populations of greatest need.[331] Neonatal tetanus case investigations are performed to determine whether the case occurred as a result of the mother's failure to access the health care system or the failure of the health care system to provide toxoid during visits made by the mother (missed opportunities).[331,400,537]

The current WHO/UNICEF/UNFPA initiative continues to emphasize hygienic delivery practices in all three aspects: "clean" hands, "clean" delivery surface and perineum, and "clean" cord-cutting and care.[400] Although immunization per se is more effective than the presence of trained attendants in reducing tetanus mortality, training of birth attendants reduces overall neonatal mortality resulting from tetanus, other infections, and other causes.[226,325,551–553] Clean cord care is ensured by attendant training and provision of a water supply, soap, sterile ties/clamps, scissors/blades, gauze, and topical antimicrobials; disposable, prepackaged delivery kits are available. The estimated proportion of pregnant women who have access to "clean" deliveries has not increased greatly since 1989 and remains well below 50% globally. Each aspect of clean deliveries has been shown to be important; hand cleaning is particularly protective.[222,224,554] Three case-control studies have indicated that the use of topical antibiotics at the time of delivery and in postnatal care decreased the risk of neonatal tetanus by up to 80% above and beyond other protective measures; antiseptics were also protective, while dry cord care in itself did not appear to reduce risk.[554–556]

On the basis of these findings, a comprehensive approach using immunization of women of child-bearing age, attended birth, clean delivery practices, improved cord care, and topical antimicrobials can provide optimal protection against neonatal tetanus. Currently, more than 134 countries and areas (Fig. 27–4) have succeeded in reaching the WHO definition of elimination—less than 1 case per 1000 live births for all districts—including 33 countries considered "endemic" for neonatal tetanus in 1990.[532,534] Fifty-seven countries have not reached or validated elimination of neonatal tetanus as defined; 20 of these account for 90% of all estimated cases, and 9 of these 20 are in the African continent.[240,532,534]

A concern about the potency of tetanus toxoid–containing vaccines manufactured in the developing world arose in the 1990s. Immunization with two doses of tetanus toxoid, given 4 weeks or more apart, with the second at least 2 weeks before delivery, significantly reduces mortality resulting from neonatal tetanus and confers an appropriate immune response for several years.[325,350,372,401,557,558] Nonetheless, cases of neonatal tetanus have been reported in children of vaccinated women.[103,105,223,559–562] A study in Bangladesh in 1990 estimated the efficacy of two doses of tetanus toxoid to be below 50%; a small serosurvey of vaccinated women was consistent with these findings.[223] Subsequent testing at a WHO reference laboratory of samples from three consecutive toxoid lots produced in Bangladesh indicated no detectable potency. This prompted the WHO to review the quality control procedures in 22 countries that reported neonatal tetanus and had local manufacture of tetanus toxoid; only four of these countries had a functioning national control authority. Eighty lots of toxoid from 21 manufacturers in 14 of those countries were tested for potency; 15 of the 80 failed to meet WHO minimum potency standards.[275] Major efforts then were made to standardize the production of vaccines, and to initiate and strengthen the biologics control authorities in these 22 countries. These steps were successful: as of 2002, 9 countries no longer produce these products and use UN-prequalified vaccines exclusively; 11 others have strengthened their regulatory authorities and apply WHO standards, including 2 with manufacturers of UN-prequalified vaccines.[¶]

[¶]WHO, unpublished data.

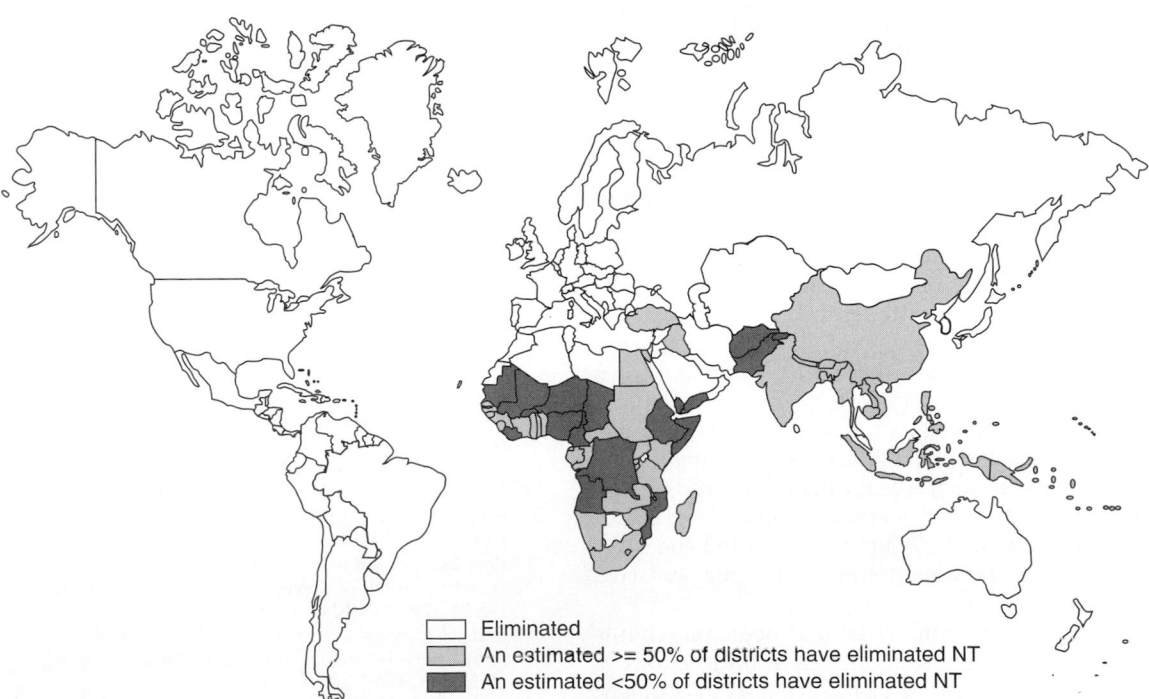

FIGURE 27–4 ■ Global neonatal tetanus elimination status, by country, 2000. Note: Elimination is defined as less than one case per 1000 live births in each district of the country. (Based on data from the World Health Organization.)

Other potential reasons for apparent tetanus toxoid failure include inaccurate or unverified histories of prior vaccination, use of inadequate immunization schedules with inappropriately short intervals between doses,[294] and poor toxoid handling, particularly repeated freezing.[8,291-294] Decreased transport of antitoxin across the placenta in some populations[563,564] or unusually high toxin challenges that overcome maternal antitoxin may play some role in a small proportion of apparent failures of toxoid to prevent neonatal tetanus. Dietz and colleagues[294] reviewed other factors that may affect the response to tetanus toxoid, including malarial infection, which can decrease the response; malarial chemoprophylaxis, which can enhance it; and malnutrition, which appears not to substantially affect induction of immunity. Case investigations and the use of other indicators are critical to determine whether the predominant cause of neonatal tetanus in a given area is vaccine failure or failure to vaccinate. Lack of adequate vaccination is a far greater cause of neonatal tetanus than is vaccine failure, particularly given the improved quality of toxoid products currently used.

A major impediment to program implementation in some countries has been the active distribution of misinformation about the purpose of vaccination campaigns. Allegations that tetanus toxoid is a covert contraceptive or sterilizing agent have circulated and disrupted the immunization of adolescents and women in Cambodia, Mexico, Nicaragua, the Philippines, and Tanzania.[565,566] Such allegations, which "travel" easily by Internet throughout the world, are based on the suspicions and fears of some organizations and leaders that the true aim of tetanus immunization is to reduce fertility. Because maternal and neonatal tetanus prevention campaigns specifically target only women of child-bearing age, local populations are particularly vulnerable to these rumors when there is already some level of distrust of government personnel. In areas where the fervor of public accusation has been extreme—leading to court injunctions or political posturing—the level of disruption has greatly affected women's and even children's immunization.[565-567] These accusations continue to circulate and must be combated with vigorous education campaigns involving credible community leaders in anticipation of problems.

Use of tetanus toxoid to prevent neonatal tetanus is highly cost effective. With routine toxoid administration costing approximately $1.14 (circa 1989 dollars), the median cost per death averted has been estimated to be $105 with routine administration and $115 with administration through campaigns. Reduction of tetanus following wounds and maternal tetanus (about 4 for every 100 cases of neonatal tetanus) were not included in these calculations. Assuming an estimated cost of treatment of $592, the combination of repeated campaigns and continuing immunization of pregnant women was estimated to produce the maximum number of cases averted compared to either approach alone, at a cost of $595 per case averted and a net savings ratio (ratio of treatment costs saved to cumulative 30-year costs) of 1.2.[568-572]

Once countries achieve maternal and neonatal tetanus elimination, ongoing support to health infrastructures is essential to maintain high TT2+ coverage in women, increase and maintain routine DTP immunization of children, and ensure the provision of appropriate booster doses. For all programs, enhanced neonatal tetanus surveillance and ongoing monitoring of immunization program quality indicators are necessary to identify areas of increased risk for maternal and neonatal disease.

To achieve maternal and neonatal tetanus elimination in the 57 countries not yet meeting the target criterion, additional resources, political commitment, and time for implementation of plans are required. Unfortunately, 17 countries where neonatal tetanus incidence remains high have substantial health infrastructure weaknesses, in part because of ongoing civil unrest or conflict and severely limited health budgets.[240,531] WHO/UNICEF/ UNFPA are seeking additional partners for the coming years to support the national programs in these 17 countries. Forty countries are approaching elimination: 22 countries have fewer than 10% of districts at continued high risk; 18 others with weaker infrastructures have less than 50% of districts with 1.0 case or more per 1000 live births.

REFERENCES

1. Carle A, Rattone G. Studio esperimentale sull'etiologia del tetano. G Accad Med Torrino 32:174, 1884.
2. Nicolaier A. Über infektiösen Tetanus. Dtsch Med Wochenschr 10:842–844, 1884.
3. Rosenbach AJF. Zur Ätiologie des Wundstarrkrampfes beim Menschen. Arch Klin Chir 34:306–317, 1886.
4. Kitasato S. Über den Tetanusbazillus. Z Hyg 7:225–234, 1889.
5. von Behring E, Kitasato S. Über das Zustandekommen der Diphtherie-Immunität bei Tieren. Dtsch Med Wochenschr 16:1113–1114, 1890.
6. Descombey P. L'anatoxine tetanique. Can R Soc Biol 91:239–241, 1924.
7. Pascual FB, McGinley E, Zanardi L, et al. Tetanus surveillance—United States, 1998–2000. MMWR (SS) [Accepted for publication].
8. Weinstein L. Tetanus. N Engl J Med 289:1293–1296, 1973.
9. Kryzhanovsky GN. Pathophysiology. In Veronesi R (ed). Tetanus: Important New Concepts. Amsterdam, Excerpta Medica, 1981, pp 109–182.
10. Bruce D. Tetanus. J Hyg (Camb) 19:1–32, 1920.
11. Garcia-Palmieri MR, Ramirez R. Generalized tetanus: analysis of 202 cases. Ann Intern Med 47:721–730, 1957.
12. Adams EB. The prognosis and prevention of tetanus. S Afr Med J 42:739–743, 1968.
13. Patel JC, Mehta BC, Modi KN. Prognosis in tetanus. In Patel JC (ed). Proceedings of the International Conference on Tetanus, 1963. Bombay, PH Ramans Printers, 1965, p 181.
14. LaForce FM, Young LS, Bennett JV. Tetanus in the United States (1965–1966). N Engl J Med 280:569–574, 1969.
15. Buchanan TM, Brooks GF, Martin S, Bennett JV. Tetanus in the United States, 1968 and 1969. J Infect Dis 122:564–567, 1970.
16. Blake PA, Feldman RA. Tetanus in the United States, 1970–1971. J Infect Dis 131:745–748, 1975.
17. Armitage P, Cliffard R. Prognosis in tetanus: use of data from therapeutic trials. J Infect Dis 138:1–8, 1978.
18. Brauner JS, Rios Vieira SR, Bleck TP. Changes in severe accidental tetanus mortality in the ICU during two decades in Brazil. Intensive Care Med 28:930–935, 2002.
19. Millard AH. Local tetanus. Lancet 2:844–846, 1954.
20. Roistacher K, Griffin JW. Local tetanus. Johns Hopkins Med J 149:84–88, 1981.
21. Pratt EL. Clinical tetanus: a study of fifty-six cases with special reference to methods of prevention and a plan for evaluating treatment. JAMA 129:1243–1247, 1945.
22. Kerr JH, Corbett JL, Prys-Roberts C, et al. Involvement of the sympathetic nervous system in tetanus: studies on 82 cases. Lancet 2:236–241, 1968.
23. Zacks SI, Shef MF. Tetanus toxin: fine structure, localization of binding sites in striated muscle. Science 159:643–644, 1968.

24. Kanarek DJ, Kaufman B, Zwi S. Severe sympathetic hyperactivity associated with tetanus. Arch Intern Med 132:602–604, 1973.

25. Hollow VM, Clarke GM. Autonomic manifestations of tetanus. Anaesth Intensive Care 3:142–147, 1975.

26. Buchanan N, Cane GW, DeAndrade M. Autonomic dysfunction in tetanus: the effects of a variety of therapeutic agents, with special reference to morphine. Intensive Care Med 5:65–68, 1979.

27. Luisto M. Outcome and neurological sequelae of patients after tetanus. Acta Neurol Scand 80:504–511, 1989.

28. Luisto M, Seppalainen AM. Electroencephalopathy in tetanus. Acta Neurol Scand 80:157–161, 1989.

29. Luisto M, Zitting A, Tallroth K. Hyperostosis and osteoarthritis in patients surviving after tetanus. Skeletal Radiol 23:31–35, 1994.

30. Veronesi R, Focaccia R. The clinical picture. In Veronesi R (ed). Tetanus: Important New Concepts. Amsterdam, Excerpta Medica, 1981, pp 459–463.

31. Trujillo MJ, Castillo A, Espana JV, et al. Tetanus in the adult: intensive care and management experience with 233 cases. Crit Care Med 8:419–423, 1980.

32. Garnier MJ. Tetanus in patients 3 years of age and up. Am J Surg 129:459–463, 1975.

33. Edmondson RS, Flowers MW. Intensive care in tetanus: management, complications and mortality in 100 cases. Br Med J 1:1401–1404, 1979.

34. Humbert G, Fillastre JP, Dordain M, et al. One hundred cases of tetanus. Scand J Infect Dis 4:129–131, 1972.

35. Peetermans WE, Schepens D. Tetanus—still a topic of present interest: a report of 27 cases from a Belgian referral hospital. J Intern Med 239:249–252, 1996.

36. Sow PS, Diop BM, Barry HL, et al. Tetanos et pratiques traditionnelles a Dakar (a propos de 141 cas). Dakar Med 38:55–59, 1993.

37. Cook TM, Protheroe RT, Handel JM. Tetanus: a review of the literature. Br J Anaesth 87:477–487, 2001.

38. Prevots R, Sutter RW, Strebel PM, et al. Tetanus surveillance—United States, 1989–1990. MMWR 41(SS-8):1–9, 1992.

39. Izurieta HS, Sutter RW, Strebel PM, et al. Tetanus surveillance—United States, 1991–1994. MMWR 46(SS-2):16–24, 1997.

40. Bardenheier B, Prevots DR, Khetsuriani N, Wharton M. Tetanus surveillance—United States, 1995–1997. MMWR 47 (SS-2):1–13, 1998.

41. Yen LM, Dao LM, Day NPJ, et al. Role of quinine in the high mortality of intramuscular injection tetanus. Lancet 344:786–787, 1994.

42. Oyelami OA, Aladekomo TA, Ononye FO. A 10-year retrospective evaluation of cases of postneonatal tetanus seen in a paediatric unit of a university teaching hospital in southwestern Nigeria (1985 to 1994). Cent Afr J Med 42:73–75, 1996.

43. Jagoda A, Riggio S, Burguieres T. Cephalic tetanus: a case report and review of the literature. Am J Emerg Med 6:128–130, 1988.

44. Bytchenko B. Microbiology of tetanus. In Veronesi R (ed). Tetanus: Important New Concepts. Amsterdam, Excerpta Medica, 1981, pp 28–39.

45. Bizzini B. Tetanus. In Germanier R (ed). Bacterial Vaccines. Orlando, FL, Academic Press, 1984, pp 38–68.

46. Hatheway CL, Johnson EA. Clostridium: the spore-bearing anaerobes. In Collier L, Balows A, Sussman M (eds). Topley & Wilson's Microbiology and Microbial Infections (9th ed). Vol. 2. London, Arnold, 1998, pp 731–782.

47. Tulloch WJ. Report of bacteriological investigation of tetanus carried out on behalf of the War Office Committee for the Study of Tetanus. J Hyg (Camb) 18:103–202, 1919.

48. Sanada I, Nishida S. Isolation of Clostridium tetani from soil. J Bacteriol 89:626–629, 1965.

49. Ebisawa I, Kurata M. A quantitative study of C. tetani in the earth. In Nistico G, Mastroeni P, Pitzurra M (eds). Proceedings of the Seventh International Conference on Tetanus, Copanello, Italy, September 10–15, 1984. Rome, Gangeni Publishing Company, 1985, pp 7–10.

50. Dubovsky J, Meyer K. The occurrence of C. tetani in soil and in vegetables. J Infect Dis 31:614–616, 1922.

51. Bytchenko B. Geographical distribution of tetanus in the world, 1951–1960. Bull World Health Organ 34:71–104, 1966.

52. Smith LD. The occurrence of Clostridium botulinum and Clostridium tetani in the soil of the United States. Health Lab Sci 15:74–80, 1978.

53. Smith JWG. Tetanus. In Wilson G, Miles A, Parker MT (eds). Topley and Wilson's Principles of Bacteriology, Virology and Immunity. Vol. 3. Baltimore, Williams & Wilkins, 1984, pp 345–368.

54. Kerrin JC. The distribution of C. tetani in the intestines of animals. Br J Pathol 10:370–373, 1929.

55. TenBroeck C, Bauer JH. The tetanus bacillus as an intestinal saprophyte in man. J Exp Med 36:261–271, 1922.

56. TenBroeck C, Bauer JH. Studies on the relation of tetanus bacilli in the digestive tract to tetanus antitoxin in the blood. J Exp Med 37:479–489, 1923.

57. Coleman GE, Meyer KF. Study of tetanus agglutinins and antitoxin in human serums. J Infect Dis 39:332–336, 1926.

58. Bauer JH, Meyer KF. Human intestinal carriers of tetanus spores in California. J Infect Dis 38:295–305, 1926.

59. Kerrin JC. The incidence of C. tetani in human feces. Br J Pathol 9:69–71, 1928.

60. Bandmann F. Zum Nachweis von Tetanusbacillen im Darm von Ulcus-und Carcinomträgern. Z Hyg 136:559–567, 1953.

61. Lowbury EJL, Lilly HA. Contamination of operating-theatre air with C tetani. Br Med J 2:1334–1336, 1958.

62. Gilles EC. The isolation of tetanus bacilli from street dust. JAMA 109:484–486, 1937.

63. Smith JWG. Tetanus and its prevention. Prog Drug Res 19:391–401, 1975.

64. Matsuda M, Yoneda M. Isolation and purification of two antigenically active, "complementary" polypeptide fragments of tetanus neurotoxin. Infect Immun 12:1147–1153, 1975.

65. Bizzini B. The chemistry of tetanus toxin as a basis for understanding its immunological and biological activities. In Nistico G, Mastroeni P, Pitzurra M (eds). Proceedings of the Seventh International Conference on Tetanus, Copanello, Italy, September 10–15, 1984. Rome, Gangeni Publishing Company, 1985, pp 11–28.

66. Robinson JP, Hash JH. A review of the molecular structure of tetanus toxin. Mol Cell Biochem 48:33–44, 1982.

67. Schiavo G, Papini E, Genna G, Montecucco C. An intact interchain disulfide bond is required for the neurotoxicity of tetanus toxin. Infect Immun 58:4136–4141, 1990.

68. Ahnert-Hilger G, Dauzenroth MW, Habermann E, et al. Chains and fragments of tetanus toxin, and their contribution to toxicity. J Physiol 84:229–236, 1990.

69. Parton RG, Critchley DR, Ockleford CD. Tetanus toxin binding to mouse spinal cord cells: an evaluation of the role of gangliosides in toxin internalization. Brain Res 475:118–127, 1988.

70. Pellizzari R, Rossetto O, Washbourne P, et al. In vitro biological activity and toxicity of tetanus and botulinum neurotoxins. Toxicol Lett 102:191–197, 1998.

71. Laird WJ, Aaronson W, Silver RP, et al. Plasmid-associated toxigenicity in Clostridium tetani. J Infect Dis 142:623, 1980.

72. Finn LW Jr, Silver RP, Habig HW, et al. The structural gene for tetanus neurotoxin is on a plasmid. Science 224:881–884, 1984.

73. Gill DM. Bacterial toxins: a table of lethal amount. Microbiol Rev 46:86–94, 1982.

74. Wright GP. The neurotoxins of Clostridium botulinum and Clostridium tetani. Pharmacol Rev 7:413–456, 1955.

75. Bulloch WE, Cramer W. On a new factor in the mechanism of bacterial infection. Proc R Soc B 90:513–528, 1919.

76. Eregie CO. Uvulectomy as an epidemiological factor in neonatal tetanus mortality: observations from a cluster survey. West Afr J Med 13:56–58, 1994.

77. Bennett J, Breen C, Traverso H, et al. Circumcision and neonatal tetanus: disclosure of risk and its reduction by topical antibiotics. Int J Epidemiol 28:263–266, 1999.

78. Abel JJ, Firor WM, Chalain W. Researches on tetanus. IX. Further evidence to show that tetanus toxin is not carried to central nervous system by way of the axis cylinders of motor nerves. Bull Johns Hopkins Hosp 63:373–403, 1938.

79. Friedemann U, Zuger B, Hollander A. Investigations on the pathogenesis of tetanus. J Immunol 36:473–488, 1939.

80. Bizzini B. Tetanus toxin. Microbiol Rev 43:224–240, 1979.

81. Green J, Erdmann JG, Wellhoner HH. Is there retrograde axonal transport of tetanus toxin in both alpha and beta fibres? Nature 265:370, 1977.

82. Schwab ME, Thoenen H. Selective binding, uptake and retrograde transport of tetanus toxin by nerve terminals in the rat iris. J Cell Biol 77:1–13, 1978.

83. Fedinec AA. Current studies on pathogenesis of tetanus. In Nistico G, Mastroeni P, Pitzurra M (eds). Proceedings of the Seventh International Conference on Tetanus, Copanello, Italy, September 10–15, 1984. Rome, Gangeni Publishing Company, 1985, pp 61–68.

84. Price DL, Griffin JW, Young A, et al. Tetanus toxin: direct evidence for retrograde axonal transport. Science 188:945–957, 1975.

85. Manning KA, Erichsen JT, Evinger C. Retrograde transneuronal transport properties of fragment C of tetanus toxin. Neuroscience 34:251–263, 1990.

86. Parton RG, Critchley DR, Ockleford CD. A study of the mechanism of internalisation of tetanus toxin by primary mouse spinal cord cultures. J Neurochem 49:1057–1068, 1987.

87. Sanford JP. Tetanus—forgotten but not gone [editorial]. N Engl J Med 332:812–813, 1995.

88. Habig WH, Nelson PG, Hardegree MC, et al. Tetanus toxin in dissociated spinal cord cultures: long-term characterization of form and action. J Neurochem 47:930–937, 1986.

89. Empson RM, Gutnick MJ, Jefferys JG, Amitai Y. Injection of tetanus toxin into the neocortex elicits persistent epileptiform activity but only transient impairment of GABA release. Neuroscience 57:235–239, 1993.

90. Brooks VB, Curtis DR, Eccles JC. Mode of action of tetanus toxin. Nature 175:120–121, 1955.

91. Brooks VB, Asanuma H. Action of tetanus toxin in the cerebral cortex. Science 137:674–676, 1962.

92. Bergey GK, Nelson PG, Bigalke H. Differential effects of tetanus toxin on inhibitory and excitatory synaptic transmission in mammalian spinal cord neurons in culture: a presynaptic locus of action for tetanus toxin. J Neurophysiol 57:121–131, 1987.

93. Schiavo G, Benfenati R, Poulain B, et al. Tetanus and botulism-B neurotoxins block neurotransmitter release by proteolytic cleavage of synaptobrevin. Nature 359:832–835, 1992.

94. Cornille F, Fournie-Zaluski MC, Roques BP, et al. Cooperative exosite-dependent cleavage of synaptobrevin by tetanus toxin light chain. J Biol Chem 272:3459–3464, 1997.

95. Bleck TP. Tetanus: pathophysiology, management, and prophylaxis. Dis Mon 37:545–603, 1991.

96. Boyd RE, Brennan PT, Denj J-F, et al. Strychnine poisoning. Am J Med 74:507–512, 1983.

97. Wellhoner JJ. Tetanus neurotoxin. Rev Physiol Biochem Pharmacol 93:1–68, 1982.

98. van Heyningen S. Tetanus toxin. Pharmacol Ther 11:141–157, 1980.

99. Alfery DD, Rauscher LA. Tetanus: a review. Crit Care Med 7:176–181, 1979.

100. Goulon M, Girard O, Grosbuis S, et al. Les anticorps antitetaniques. Nouv Presse Med 1:3049–3050, 1972.

101. Berger SA, Cherubin LE, Nelson S, et al. Tetanus despite preexisting antitetanus antibody. JAMA 240:769–770, 1978.

102. Passen EL, Andersen BR. Clinical tetanus despite a 'protective' level of toxin-neutralizing antibody. JAMA 255:1171–1173, 1986.

103. Maselle SY, Matre R, Mbise R, Hofstad T. Neonatal tetanus despite protective serum antitoxin concentration. FEMS Microbiol Immunol 3:171–175, 1991.

104. Crone NE, Reder AT. Severe tetanus in immunized patients with high anti-tetanus titers. Neurology 42:761–764, 1992.

105. de Moraes-Pinto MI. Neonatal tetanus despite immunization and protective antitoxin antibody. J Infect Dis 171:1076–1077, 1995.

106. Pryor T, Onarecker C, Coniglione T. Elevated antitoxin titers in a man with generalized tetanus. J Fam Pract 44:299–303, 1997.

107. Abrahamian FM, Pollack CV, LoVecchio F, et al. Fatal tetanus in a drug abuser with "protective" antitetanus antibodies. J Emerg Med 18:189–193, 2000.

108. Turner TB, Velasco-Joven EA, Prudovsky S. Studies on the prophylaxis and treatment of tetanus. II. Studies pertaining to treatment. Bull Johns Hopkins Hosp 102:71–84, 1958.

109. Steinegger T, Wiederkehr M, Ludin HP, Roth F. Elektromyogramm als diagnostische Hilfe beim Tetanus. Schweiz Med Wochenschr 126:379–385, 1996.

110. Apte NM, Karnad DR. Short Report: The spatula test: a simple bedside test to diagnose tetanus. Am J Trop Med Hyg 53:386–387, 1995.

111. Smith WD, Tobias MA. Tetany, tetanus or drug reaction? Br J Anaesth 48:703–705, 1976.

112. Barnes V, Ware MR. Tetanus, pseudotetanus, or conversion disorder: a diagnostic dilemma? South Med J 86:591–592, 1993.

113. Ernst ME, Klepser ME, Fouts M, Marangos MN. Tetanus: pathophysiology and management. Ann Pharmacother 31:1507–1513, 1997.

114. Farrar JJ, Yen LM, Cook T, et al. Tetanus. J Neurol Neurosurg Psychiatry 69:292–301, 2000.

115. Bleck TP, Brauner JS. Tetanus. In Scheld WM, Whitley RJ, Durack DT (eds). Infections of the Central Nervous System (2nd ed). Philadelphia, Lippincott–Raven, 1997, pp 629–653.

116. Bleck TP. Clostridium tetani (Tetanus). In Mandell GL, Bennet JE, Dolin R (eds). Principles and Practice of Infectious Diseases (5th ed). New York, Churchill Livingstone, 2000, pp 2537–2543.

117. Nation NS, Pierce NF, Adler SJ, et al. Tetanus: the use of human hyperimmune globulin in treatment. Calif Med 98:305–307, 1963.

118. Blake PA, Feldman RA, Buchanan TM, et al. Serologic therapy of tetanus in the United States, 1965–1971. JAMA 235:42–44, 1976.

119. Abrutyn E. Tetanus. In Braunwald E, Fauci AS, Kasper DL, et al. (eds). Harrison's Principles of Internal Medicine (15th ed). New York, McGraw-Hill, 2001, pp 918–920.

120. American Academy of Pediatrics. Tetanus (lockjaw). In Pickering LK (ed). 2000 Red Book: Report of the Committee on Infectious Diseases (25th ed). Elk Grove Village, IL, American Academy of Pediatrics, 2000, pp 563–570.

121. Moynihan NH. Serum-sickness and local reactions in tetanus prophylaxis. Lancet 2:264–266, 1955.

122. Merson MH, Hughs JM, Dowell VR, et al. Current trends in botulism in the United States. JAMA 229:1305–1308, 1974.

123. Rubenstein HM. Studies on human tetanus antitoxin. Am J Hyg 76:276–292, 1962.

124. Lee DC, Lederman HM. Anti-tetanus toxoid antibodies in intravenous gamma globulin: an alternative to tetanus immune globulin. J Infect Dis 166:642–645, 1992.

125. McCracken GH Jr, Dowell DL, Marschall FN. Double-blind trial of equine antitoxin and human immune globulin in tetanus neonatorum. Lancet 1:1146–1149, 1971.

126. Bleck TP. Intravenous immune globulin for passive tetanus prophylaxis. J Infect Dis 167:498–499, 1993.

127. Krause I, Wu R, Sherer Y, et al. In vitro antiviral and antibacterial activity of commercial intravenous immunoglobulin preparations—a potential role for adjuvant intravenous immunoglobulin therapy in infectious diseases. Transfusion Med 12:133–139, 2002.

128. Rey M, Diop-Mar I, Robert D. Treatment of tetanus. In Veronesi R (ed). Tetanus: Important New Concepts. Amsterdam, Excerpta Medica, 1981, pp 207–237.

129. Abrutyn E, Berlin JA. Intrathecal therapy in tetanus: a meta-analysis. JAMA 266:2262–2267, 1991.

130. Gupta PS, Kapoor R, Goyal S, et al. Intrathecal human tetanus immunoglobulin in early tetanus. Lancet 2:439–440, 1980.

131. Sun KO, Li PC, Yu YL, et al. Management of tetanus: a review of 18 cases. J R Soc Med 87:135–137, 1994.

132. Agarwal M, Thomas K, Peter JV, et al. A randomized double-blind sham-controlled study of intrathecal human anti-tetanus immunoglobulin in the management of tetanus. Nat Med J India 11:209–212, 1998.

133. Menon J, Mathews L. Intrathecal immunoglobulin in the treatment of tetanus. Indian Pediatr 39:654–657, 2002.

134. Vakil BJ, Armitage P. Therapeutic trial of intracisternal human tetanus immunoglobulin in clinical tetanus. Trans R Soc Trop Med Hyg 73:579–583, 1979.

135. Sedaghatian MR. Intrathecal serotherapy in neonatal tetanus: a controlled trial. Arch Dis Child 54:623–625, 1979.

136. Neequaye J, Nkrumah FR. Failure of intrathecal antitetanus serum to improve survival in neonatal tetanus. Arch Dis Child 58:276–278, 1983.

137. Beague RE, Lindo-Soriano I. Failure of intrathecal tetanus antitoxin in the treatment of tetanus neonatorum. J Infect Dis 164:419–420, 1991.

138. Spenney JG, Lamb RN, Cobbs CG. Recurrent tetanus. South Med J 64:859–862, 1971.

139. Bhatt AD, Dastur FD. Relapsing tetanus: a case report. J Postgrad Med 27:184–186, 1981.

140. Cain HD, Falco FG. Recurrent tetanus. Calif Med 97:31–33, 1962.

141. Naranyanan K, Gupta PS, Kumar N, Agarwal SK. Antitoxin response in tetanus. Indian J Med Res 74:482–485, 1981.

142. Yeni P, Carbon C, Tremolieres F, Gibert C. Serum levels of antibody to toxoid during immunization and after specific immunization of patients with tetanus. J Infect Dis 145:278, 1982.

143. Ahmadsyah I, Salim A. Treatment of tetanus: an open study to compare the efficacy of procaine penicillin and metronidazole. Br Med J (Clin Res Ed) 291:648–650, 1985.

144. Tallman JF, Gallager DW. The GABA-ergic system: a locus of benzodiazepine action. Annu Rev Neurosci 8:21–44, 1985.

145. Davidoff RA. Antispasticity drugs: mechanisms of action. Ann Neurol 17:107–116, 1985.

146. Joseph A, Pulimood BM. Use of diazepam in tetanus—a comparative study. Indian J Med Res 68:489–491, 1978.

147. Dasta JF, Brier KL, Kidwell GA, et al. Diazepam infusion in tetanus: correlation of drug levels with effect. South Med J 74:278–280, 1981.
148. Tekur U, Gupta A, Tayal G, et al. Blood concentrations of diazepam and its metabolites in children and neonates with tetanus. J Pediatr 102:145–147, 1983.
149. Vassa T, Yajnik VH, Joshi KR, et al. Comparative clinical trial of diazepam with other conventional drugs in tetanus. Postgrad Med J 50:755–758, 1974.
150. Checketts MR, White RJ. Avoidance of intermittent positive pressure ventilation in tetanus with dantrolene therapy. Anaesthesia 48:969–971, 1993.
151. Borgeat A, Popovic V, Schwander D. Efficiency of a continuous infusion of propofol in a patient with tetanus. Crit Care Med 19:295–297, 1991.
152. Attygalle D, Rodrigo N. Magnesium sulphate for control of spasms in severe tetanus: can we avoid sedation and artificial ventilation? Anaesthesia 52:956–962, 1997.
153. Attygalle D, Rodrigo N. Magnesium as first-line therapy in the management of tetanus: a prospective study of 40 patients. Anaesthesia 57:778–817, 2002.
154. Dianto, Mustadjab I. The influence of pyridoxin in the treatment of tetanus neonatorum. Paediatr Indones 31:165–169, 1991.
155. Caglar MK. Pyridoxine in the treatment of tetanus neonatorum. Paediatr Indones 29:233–236, 1989.
156. Paydas S, Akoglu TF, Akkiz H, et al. Mortality-lowering effect of systemic corticosteroid therapy in severe tetanus. Clin Ther 10:276–280, 1988.
157. Chandry ST, Peter JV, Joh L, et al. Betamethasone in tetanus patients: an evaluation of its effect on the mortality and morbidity. J Assoc Phys India 40:373–376, 1992.
158. Domenighetti GM, Savary G, Stricker H. Hyperadrenergic syndrome in severe tetanus: extreme rise in catecholamines responsive to labetalol. Br Med J (Clin Res Ed) 288:1483–1484, 1984.
159. Rie M, Wilson RS. Morphine therapy controls autonomic hyperactivity in tetanus. Ann Intern Med 88:653–654, 1978.
160. Wright DK, Lalloo UG, Nayiager S, Govender P. Autonomic nervous system dysfunction in severe tetanus: current perspectives. Crit Care Med 17:371–375, 1989.
161. Sutton DN, Tremlett MR, Woodcock TE, Nielsen MS. Management of autonomic dysfunction in severe tetanus: the use of magnesium sulfate and clonidine. Intensive Care Med 16:75–80, 1990.
162. Moughabghab AV, Prevost G, Socolovsky C. Fentanyl therapy controls autonomic hyperactivity in tetanus. Br J Clin Pract 50:477–478, 1996.
163. Southorn PA, Blaise GA. Treatment of tetanus-induced autonomic nervous system dysfunction with continuous epidural blockade. Crit Care Med 14:251–252, 1986.
164. Shibuya M, Sugimoto H, Sugimoto T, et al. The use of continuous spinal anesthesia in severe tetanus with autonomic disturbance. J Trauma 29:1423–1429, 1989.
165. Mukherjee DR. Tetanus and tracheostomy. Ann Otol Rhinol Laryngol 86:67–72, 1977.
166. O'Keefe SJD, Wesley A, Jialal I, Epstein S. The metabolic response and problems with nutritional support in acute tetanus. Metabolism 33:482–487, 1984.
167. Hiraide A, Katayama M, Sugimoto H, et al. Metabolic changes in patients severely affected by tetanus. Ann Surg 213:66–69, 1991.
168. Bytchenko BD, Causse G, Grab B, Kereselidze TS. Tetanus: recent trends of world distribution. In Mérieux C (ed). Proceedings of the Sixth International Conference on Tetanus, Lyon, France, December 3–5, 1981. Lyon, Collection Foundation Mérieux, 1981, pp 97–111.
169. World Health Organization. World Health Report 2001, Annex Table 2. Geneva, World Health Organization, 2001.
170. Galazka A, Cook R. Neonatal tetanus today and tomorrow. In Nistico G, Mastroeni P, Pitzurra M (eds). Proceedings of the Seventh International Conference on Tetanus, Copanello, Italy, September 10–15, 1984. Rome, Gangeni Publishing Company, 1985, pp 350–363.
171. Rey M, Tikhomirov E. Nonneonatal tetanus over the world. In Nistico G, Bizzini B, Bytchenko M, Triau R (eds). Proceedings of the Eighth International Conference on Tetanus, Leningrad, USSR, August 25–28, 1987. Rome, Pythagora Press, 1989, pp 506–518.
172. Luisto M. Epidemiology of tetanus in Finland from 1969 to 1985. Scand J Infect Dis 21.655–663, 1989.
173. Galazka A, Kardymowicz B. Tetanus incidence and immunity in Poland. Eur J Epidemiol 5:474–480, 1989.
174. Antona D. Le tetanos en France en 2000 et 2001. Bull Epidemiol Hebdomadaire 40:197–199, 2002.
175. Prospero E, Appignanesi R, D'Errico MM, Carle F. Epidemiology of tetanus in the Marches Region of Italy, 1992–1995. Bull World Health Organ 76:47–54, 1998.
176. Fraser DW. Tetanus in the United States, 1900–1969: analysis by cohorts. Am J Epidemiol 96:306–312, 1972.
177. Sutter RW, Cochi SL, Brink EW, Sirotkin BI. Assessment of vital statistics and surveillance data for monitoring tetanus mortality, 1979–1984. Am J Epidemiol 131:132–142, 1990.
178. Levinson AK, Marske RL, Shein MD. Tetanus in heroin addicts. JAMA 157:658–660, 1955.
179. Cherubin CE. Urban tetanus: the epidemiologic aspects of tetanus in narcotic addicts in New York City. Arch Environ Health 14:802–808, 1967.
180. Cherubin CE, Millian SJ, Palusci E, et al. Investigations in tetanus in narcotics addicts in New York City. Am J Epidemiol 88:215–223, 1968.
181. Cherubin CE. Epidemiology of tetanus in narcotic addicts. N Y State J Med 70:267–271, 1970.
182. Axnick NW, Alexander ER. Tetanus in the United States: a review of the problem. Am J Public Health 47:1493–1501, 1957.
183. Heath CW, Zusman J, Sherman IL. Tetanus in the United States, 1950–1960. Am J Public Health 54:769–779, 1964.
184. Moore RM, Singleton AO. Tetanus at the John Sealy Hospital. Surg Gynecol Obstet 69:146–154, 1939.
185. McQuillan GM, Kruszon-Moran D, Deforest A, et al. Serologic immunity to diphtheria and tetanus in the United States. Ann Intern Med 136:660–666, 2002.
186. Jacobs DH, Tovar JM, Hung OL, et al. Behavioral risk factor and preventive health care practice survey of immigrants in the emergency department. Academic Emergency Med 9:599–608, 2002.
187. Henderson SO, Mody T, Growth DE, et al. The presentation of tetanus in an emergency department. J Emerg Med 16:705–708, 1998.
188. Christensen NA, Thurber DL. Clinical experience with tetanus: 91 cases. Proc Mayo Clin 32:146–158, 1957.
189. Faust RA, Vickers OR, Cohn I. Tetanus: 2,449 cases in 68 years at Charity Hospital. J Trauma 16:704–712, 1976.
190. Bowen V, Johnson J, Boyle J, Snelling CF. Tetanus—a continuing problem in minor injuries. Can J Surg 31:7–9, 1988.
191. Sangalli M, Chierchini P, Aylward RB, Forastiere F. Tetanus: a rare but preventable cause of mortality among drug users and the elderly. Eur J Epidemiol 12:539–540, 1996.
192. Postoperative tetanus [editorial]. Lancet 2:964–965, 1984.
193. Federmann M, Kotzerke M. Postoperative tetanus. Dtsch Med Wochenschr 114:1833–1836, 1989.
194. O'Malley CD, Smith N, Braun R, Prevots DR. Tetanus associated with body piercing [letter]. Clin Infect Dis 27:1343–1344, 1998.
195. Dyce O, Bruno JR, Hong D, et al. Tongue piercing . . . the new "rusty nail"? Head Neck 22:728–732, 2000.
196. Ray SN, Ray K, over SS. Sero-survey of diphtheria and tetanus antitoxin. Indian J Med Res 68:901–904, 1978.
197. Dastur FD, Awatramani VP, Dixit SK. Response to single dose of tetanus vaccine in subjects with naturally acquired tetanus antitoxin. Lancet 2:219–222, 1981.
198. Veronesi R, Bizzini B, Focaccia R, et al. Naturally acquired antibodies to tetanus toxin in humans and animals from the Galapagos Islands. J Infect Dis 147:308–311, 1983.
199. Matzkin H, Regev S. Naturally acquired immunity to tetanus toxin in an isolated community. Infect Immun 48:267–268, 1985.
200. Veronesi R. Naturally acquired tetanus immunity: still a controversial theme? In Nistico G, Mastroeni P, Pitzurra M (eds). Proceedings of the Seventh International Conference on Tetanus, Copanello, Italy, September 10–15, 1984. Rome, Gangeni Publishing Company, 1985, pp 365–372.
201. Leshem Y, Herman J. Tetanus immunity in kibbutz women. Isr J Med Sci 25:127–130, 1989.
202. Galazka AM. The Immunologic Basis for Immunization: Tetanus (WHO/EPI/GEN/13.13). Geneva, World Health Organization, 1993.
203. Ruben FL, Nagel J, Fireman P. Antitoxin responses in the elderly to tetanus-diphtheria (Td) immunization. Am J Epidemiol 108:145–149, 1978.
204. Crossley K, Irvine P, Warren B, et al. Tetanus and diphtheria immunity in urban Minnesota adults. JAMA 242:2298–2300, 1979.

205. Weiss BP, Strassburg MA, Feeley JC. Tetanus and diphtheria immunity in an elderly population in Los Angeles County. Am J Public Health 73:802–804, 1983.
206. Stair TO, Lippe MA, Russell H, Feeley JC. Tetanus immunity in emergency department patients. Am J Emerg Med 7:563–566, 1989.
207. Gergen PJ, McQuillan GM, Kiely M, et al. A population-based serologic survey of immunity to tetanus in the United States. N Engl J Med 332:761–766, 1995.
208. Koblin BA, Townsend TR. Immunity to diphtheria and tetanus in inner-city women of childbearing age. Am J Public Health 79:1297–1298, 1989.
209. National Center for Health Statistics. National Health Interview Survey, 1998, 1999, and 2000. Available at www.cdc.gov/nchs/nhis.htm
210. Centers for Disease Control and Prevention. Tetanus among injecting drug users—California, 1997. MMWR 47:149–151, 1998.
211. Rezza G, Pizzuti R, De Campora E, et al. Tetanus and injection drug use: rediscovery of a neglected problem? Eur J Epidemiol 12:665–666, 1996.
212. Fair E, Murphy TV, Golaz A, et al. Philosophic objection to vaccination as a risk for tetanus among children younger than 15 years. Pediatrics 109:E2, 2002. (Available at www.pediatrics.org/cgi/content/full/109/1/e2)
213. Can modified tetanus occur? [editorial]. N Engl J Med 266:1117–1118, 1962.
214. McComb JA. Tetanus in a previously immunized person [letter]. N Engl J Med 273:452–453, 1965.
215. Luisto M, Iivananinen M. Tetanus in immunized children. Dev Med Child Neurol 35:351–355, 1993.
216. Centers for Disease Control and Prevention. Tetanus—Puerto Rico, 2002. MMWR 51:613–615, 2002.
217. Suleman O. Mortality from tetanus neonatorum in Punjab (Pakistan). Pakistan Pediatr J 6:152–183, 1982.
218. Marshall FN. Tetanus of the newborn: with special reference to experiences in Haiti, W. I. Adv Pediatr 15:65–110, 1968.
219. Adams JM, Kenny JD, Rudolph AJ. Modern management of tetanus neonatorum. Pediatrics 64:472–477, 1979.
220. Stanfield JP, Galazka A. Neonatal tetanus in the world today. Bull World Health Organ 62:647–669, 1984.
221. Hinman AR, Foster SO, Wassilak SGF. Neonatal tetanus: potential for elimination in the USA and the world. Pediatr Infect Dis 6:813–816, 1987.
222. Leroy O, Garenne M. Risk factors of neonatal tetanus in Senegal. Int J Epidemiol 20:521–526, 1991.
223. Hlady WG, Bennett JV, Samadi AR, et al. Neonatal tetanus in rural Bangladesh: risk factors and toxoid efficacy. Am J Public Health 82:1365–1369, 1992.
224. Quddus A, Luby S, Rahbar M, Pervaiz Y. Neonatal tetanus: mortality rate and risk factors in Loralai District, Pakistan. Int J Epidemiol 31:648–653, 2002.
225. Jagetiya P, Bhandari B. Analysis of tetanus neonatorum cases admitted in a hospital during 1976–1977. Indian J Public Health 23:103–105, 1979.
226. Hamid ED, Daulay AP, Lubis CP, et al. Tetanus neonatorum in babies delivered by traditional birth attendants in Medan, Indonesia. Paediatr Indones 25:167–174, 1985.
227. Cliff J. Neonatal tetanus in Maputo, Mozambique. Part I: Hospital incidence and childbirth practices. Cent Afr J Med 31:9–12, 1985.
228. Traverso HD, Bennett JV, Kahn AJ, et al. Ghee application to the umbilical cord: a risk factor for tetanus. Lancet 1:486–488, 1989.
229. Bennett J, Azhar, Rahim F, et al. Further observations on ghee as a risk factor for tetanus. Int J Epidemiol 24:643–647, 1995.
230. Bennett J, Schooley M, Traverso H, et al. Bundling, a newly identified risk factor for neonatal tetanus: implications for global control. Int J Epidemiol 25:879–884, 1996.
231. Roison AJ, Prazuch T, Tall F, et al. Risk factor for neonatal tetanus in west Burkina Faso: a case-control study. Eur J Epidemiol 12:535–537, 1996.
232. Bennett J, Ma C, Traverso H, et al. Neonatal tetanus associated with topical umbilical ghee: covert role of cow dung. Int J Epidemiol 28:1172–1175, 1999.
233. Baltazar JC, Sarol JN. Prenatal tetanus immunization and other practices associated with neonatal tetanus. Southeast Asian J Trop Med Public Health 26:137–138, 1994.
234. Salimpour R. Cause of death in tetanus neonatorum: study of 233 cases with 54 necropsies. Arch Dis Child 52:587–594, 1977.
235. Bhat GJ, Joshi MK, Kandoth PW. Neonatal tetanus: a clinical study of 100 cases. Indian Pediatr 16:159–166, 1979.
236. Gupta SM, Takkar VP, Verma AK. A retrospective study of tetanus neonatorum and comparative assessment of diazepam in its treatment. Indian Pediatr 16:343–346, 1979.
237. Paul SS, Utal DS, Gupta GS. Tetanus neonatorum. Indian Pediatr 21:683–687, 1984.
238. Teknetzi P, Manios S, Katsouyanopoulos V. Neonatal tetanus—long-term residual handicaps. Arch Dis Child 58:68–69, 1983.
239. Anlar B, Yalaz K, Dizmen R. Long-term prognosis after neonatal tetanus. Dev Med Child Neurol 31:76–80, 1989.
240. United Nations Children's Fund, World Health Organization, and United Nations Population Fund. Maternal and Neonatal Tetanus Elimination by 2005: Strategies for Achieving and Maintaining Elimination, November 2000 (WHO/V&B/02.09). Geneva, World Health Organization, 2002.
241. Farveau V, Mamdani M, Steinglass R, Koblinsky M. Maternal tetanus: magnitude, epidemiology and potential control measures. Int J Gynecol Obstet 40:3–12, 1993.
242. Ball K, Norboo T, Gupta U, et al. Is tetanus rare at high altitudes? [letter]. Trop Doct 24:78–80, 1994.
243. Oudesluys-Murphy AM, Eilers GA, de Groot CJ. The time of separation of the umbilical cord. Eur J Pediatr 146:387–389, 1987.
244. Oudesluys-Murphy AM. Umbilical cord care and neonatal tetanus [letter]. Lancet 1:843, 1989.
245. World Health Organization. WHO Vaccine-Preventable Diseases: Monitoring System 2001 Global Summary (WHO/V&B/02.20). Geneva, World Health Organization, 2002.
246. Kumar S, Malecki JM. A case of neonatal tetanus. South Med J 84:396–398, 1991.
247. Craig AS, Reed GW, Mohon RT, et al. Neonatal tetanus in the United States: a sentinel event in the foreign-born. Pediatr Infect Dis J 16:955–959, 1997.
248. Centers for Disease Control and Prevention. Neonatal tetanus—Montana, 1998. MMWR 47:928–930, 1998.
249. Boyd JSK. Tetanus in the African and European theatres of war 1939–1945. Lancet 1:113–119, 1946.
250. Rubbo SD, Suri JC. Passive immunization against tetanus with human immune globulin. Br Med J 2:79–81, 1962.
251. Pope CG. Development of knowledge of antitoxins. Br Med Bull 19:230–234, 1963.
252. Lang J, Kamga-Fotso L, Peyrieux JC, et al. Safety and immunogenicity of a new equine tetanus immunoglobulin associated with tetanus-diphtheria vaccine. Am J Trop Med Hyg 63:298–305, 2000.
253. Reisman RE, Rose NR, Witebsky E, Arbesman CE. Serum sickness: II. Demonstration and characteristics of antibodies. J Allergy 32:531–543, 1961.
254. Suri JC, Rubbo SD. Immunization against tetanus. J Hyg (Camb) 59:29–48, 1961.
255. McComb JA. The prophylactic dose of homologous tetanus antitoxin. N Engl J Med 270:175–178, 1964.
256. Wilde H, Thipkong P, Sitprija V, Chaiyabutr N. Heterologous antisera and antivenoms are essential biologicals: perspectives on a worldwide crisis. Ann Intern Med 125:233–236, 1996.
257. Smith JWG, Evans DG, Jones DA, et al. Simultaneous active and passive immunization against tetanus. Br Med J 1:237–238, 1963.
258. Eckmann L. Active and passive immunization. N Engl J Med 271:1087–1091, 1964.
259. Smith JWG. Simultaneous active and passive immunization of guinea pigs against tetanus. J Hyg (Camb) 62:379–388, 1964.
260. Levine L, McComb JA, Dwyer RC, Latham WC. Active-passive tetanus immunization. N Engl J Med 274:186–190, 1966.
261. Sesardic D, Wong MY, Gaines Das RE, Corbel MJ. The first international standard for Antitetanus Immunoglobulin, Human: pharmaceutical evaluation and international collaborative study. Biologicals 21:67–75, 1993.
262. Edsall G. Problems in the immunology and control of tetanus. Med J Aust 2:216–220, 1976.
263. Smith JWG. Diphtheria and tetanus toxoids. Br Med Bull 25:177–182, 1969.
264. MacLennan R, Schofield FD, Pittman M, et al. Immunization against neonatal tetanus in New Guinea: antitoxin response of pregnant women to adjuvant and plain toxoids. Bull World Health Organ 32:683–697, 1965.

265. Sneath PAT, Kerlake EG, Sruby F. Tetanus immunity: resistance of guinea pigs to lethal spore doses induced by active and passive immunization. Am J Hyg 25:464–476, 1937.

266. Ramon G, Zoeller C. L'anatoxine tetanique et l'immunisation active de l'homme vis-à-vis du tetanos. Ann Inst Pasteur 41:808–825, 1927.

267. De Luca MM, Basualdo JA, Bernagozzi JA, Abeiro HD. Nitrogen-gas bubbling during the cultivation of Clostridium tetani produces a higher yield of tetanus toxin for the preparation of its toxoid. Microbiol Immunol 41:161–163, 1997.

268. WHO Expert Committee on Biological Standardization. International Standards for Tetanus Vaccine (Adsorbed) (WHO/BS/66.839). Geneva, World Health Organization, 1965.

269. Pitman M, Kolb RW, Barile MF, et al. Immunization against neonatal tetanus in New Guinea: 5. Laboratory assayed potency of tetanus toxoids and relationship to human antitoxin response. Bull World Health Organ 43:469–478, 1970.

270. Hardegree MC, Pittman M, Maloney CJ. Influence of mouse strain on the assayed potency (unitage) of tetanus toxoid. Appl Microbiol 24:120–126, 1972.

271. Lyng J, Nyerges G. The second international standard for Tetanus Toxoid (Adsorbed). J Biol Stand 12:121–130, 1984.

272. Hardegree MC, Fornwald RE, Farber J, et al. Titration of tetanus toxoids in international units: relationship to antitoxin responses of rhesus monkeys. In Mérieux C (ed). Proceedings of the Sixth International Conference on Tetanus, Lyon, France, December 3–5, 1981. Lyon, Collection Foundation Mérieux, 1981, pp 409–424.

273. Sasardic D, Winsness R, Rigsby P, et al. Calibration of replacement international standard and European Pharmacopoeia Biological Reference preparation for Tetanus Toxoid, Adsorbed. Biologicals 30:49–68, 2002.

274. Manahilov R, Solomonova K. Evaluation of the quality of tetanus toxoid preparations. In Nistico G, Bizzini B, Bytchenko M, Triau R (eds). Eighth International Conference on Tetanus, Leningrad, USSR, August 25–28, 1987. Rome, Pythagora Press, 1989, pp 235–237.

275. Dietz V, Milstien JB, van Loon F, et al. Performance and potency of tetanus toxoid: implications for eliminating neonatal tetanus. Bull World Health Organ 74:619–628, 1996.

276. World Health Assembly. Resolution 45.17: Immunization and vaccine quality, 1992. In Handbook of Resolutions and Decisions of the World Health Assembly and the Executive Board (1985–1992), Vol. 3 (3rd ed). Geneva, World Health Organization, 1993. Available at policy.who.int/cgi-bin/om_isapi.dll?softpage=Policy42

277. McCarroll JR, Abrahams I, Skudder PA. Antibody response to tetanus toxoid 15 years after initial immunization. Am J Public Health 52:1669–1675, 1962.

278. Newell KW, LeBlank DR, Edsall G, et al. The serological assessment of a tetanus toxoid field trial. Bull World Health Organ 45:773–785, 1971.

279. Centers for Disease Control and Prevention. Pertussis vaccination: use of acellular pertussis vaccines among infants and young children. Recommendations of the Advisory Committee on Immunization Practices (ACIP). MMWR 46(RR-7):1–25, 1997.

280. Centers for Disease Control and Prevention. Diphtheria, tetanus and pertussis: guidelines for vaccine prophylaxis and other preventive measures. Recommendations of the Immunization Practices Advisory Committee (ACIP). MMWR 40(RR-10):1–28, 1991.

281. Zhou W, Pool V, Iskander JK, et al. Surveillance for safety after immunization: Vaccine Adverse Event Reporting System (VAERS)–United States, 1991–2001. MMWR 52(SS-1):1–24, 2002.

282. Jones FG, Moss JM. Studies on tetanus toxoid. I: The antitoxic titer of human subjects following immunization with tetanus toxoid and tetanus alum precipitated toxoid. J Immunol 30:115–125, 1936.

283. MacLennan R, Levine L, Newell KW, Edsall G. The early primary immune response to adsorbed tetanus toxoid in man: a study of the influence of antigen concentration, carrier concentration, and sequence of dosage on the rate, extent, and persistence of the immune response to one and to two doses of toxoid. Bull World Health Organ 49:615–626, 1973.

284. Gottlieb S, McLaughlin FX, Levine L, et al. Long-term immunity to tetanus: a statistical evaluation and its clinical implications. Am J Public Health 54:961–971, 1964.

285. Mahoney LJ, Aprile MA, Moloney PJ. Combined active-passive immunization against tetanus in man. Can Med Assoc J 96:1401–1404, 1967.

286. Relyveld E, Bengounia A, Huet M, Kreeftenberg JG. Antibody response of pregnant women to two different adsorbed tetanus toxoids. Vaccine 9:369–372, 1991.

287. Vassilev TL. Aluminum phosphate but not calcium phosphate stimulates the specific IgE response in guinea-pigs to tetanus toxoid. Allergy 33:155–159, 1978.

288. Kielmam AA, Vohra SR. Control of tetanus neonatorum in rural communities—immunization effects of high-dose calcium phosphate–adsorbed tetanus toxoid. Indian J Med Res 66:906–916, 1977.

289. Relyveld EH, Bizzini B, Gupta RK. Rational approaches to reduce adverse reactions in man to vaccines containing tetanus and diphtheria toxoids. Vaccine 16:1016–1023, 1998.

290. Kumar V, Sahai G, Kumar A. Studies on the stability of tetanus and pertussis components of DTP vaccine on exposure to different temperatures. Indian J Pathol Microbiol 23:50–54, 1982.

291. World Health Organization, Expanded Programme on Immunisation. The effects of freezing on the appearance, potency and toxicity of adsorbed and unadsorbed DPT vaccines. Wkly Epidemiol Rec 55:385–390, 1980.

292. World Health Organization, Expanded Programme on Immunisation. The effects of freezing on the appearance, potency and toxicity of adsorbed and unadsorbed DPT vaccines. Wkly Epidemiol Rec 55:396–398, 1980.

293. Menon PS, Sahai G, Joshi VB, et al. Field trial on frozen and thawed tetanus toxoid. Indian J Med Res 64:25–32, 1976.

294. Dietz V, Galazka A, van Loon F, Cochi S. Factors affecting the immunogenicity and potency of tetanus toxoid: implications for the elimination of neonatal and non-neonatal tetanus as public health problems. Bull World Health Organ 75:81–93, 1997.

295. Galazka A, Milstien J, Zaffran M. Thermostability of Vaccines (WHO/GPV/98.07). Geneva, World Health Organization, 1998.

296. Schatz D, Ellis T, Ottendorfer E, et al. Aging and the immune response to tetanus toxoid: diminished frequency and level of cellular immune reactivity to antigenic stimulation. Clin Diagn Lab Immunol 5:894–896, 1998.

297. Borut TC, Ank BJ, Gard SE, Stiehm ER. Tetanus toxoid skin test in children: correlation with in vitro lymphocyte stimulation and monocyte chemotaxis. J Pediatr 97:567–573, 1980.

298. Johnson C, Walls RS, Ruwoldt A. Delayed hypersensitivity to tetanus toxoid in man: in vivo and in vitro studies. Pathology 15:369–372, 1983.

299. Delafuente JC, Eisenberg JD, Hoelzer DR, Slavine RG. Tetanus toxoid as an antigen for delayed cutaneous hypersensitivity. JAMA 249:3209–3211, 1983.

300. Kaufman DB, deMendonca WC, Newton J. Diphtheria-tetanus skin testing. Am J Dis Child 134:479–483, 1980.

301. Barile MF, Hardegree MC, Pittman M. Immunization against neonatal tetanus in New Guinea. 3. The toxin-neutralization test and the response of guinea pigs to the toxoids as used in the immunization schedules in New Guinea. Bull World Health Organ 43:453–459, 1970.

302. Christiansen G. Quantification of tetanus antitoxin by toxin neutralization test in mice: a comparison between lethal and paralytic techniques. J Biol Stand 9:453–460, 1981.

303. Marconi P, Pitzurra M, Bistoni F. Passive hemagglutination as the reference method for evaluation of tetanus immunity. In Nistico G, Mastroeni P, Pitzurra M (eds). Proceedings of the Seventh International Conference on Tetanus, Copanello, Italy, September 10–15, 1984. Rome, Gangeni Publishing Company, 1985, pp 259–273.

304. Hardegree MC, Barile MF, Pittman M, et al. Immunization against neonatal tetanus in New Guinea. 4. Comparison of tetanus antitoxin titers obtained by haemagglutination and toxin neutralization in mice. Bull World Health Organ 43:461–468, 1970.

305. Winsnes R, Christiansen G. Quantification of tetanus antitoxin in human sera. II. Comparison of counter-immunoelectrophoresis and passive haemagglutination with toxin neutralisation in mice. Acta Pathol Microbiol Scand B 87:197–200, 1979.

306. Peel MM. Measurement of tetanus antitoxin I. Indirect haemagglutination. J Biol Stand 8:177–189, 1980.

307. Pitzurra LF, Bistoni M, Pitzurra L, et al. Comparison of passive haemagglutination with turkey erythrocyte assay, enzyme-linked immunosorbent assay and counter immunoelectrophoresis assay for serological evaluation of tetanus immunity. J Clin Microbiol 17:432–435, 1983.

308. Gupta RK, Maheshwari SC, Singh H. The titration of tetanus antitoxin. I. Factors affecting the sensitivity of the indirect haemagglutination test. J Biol Stand 12:11–17, 1984.

309. Gupta RK, Maheshwari SC, Singh H. The titration of tetanus anti-toxin. II. A comparative evaluation of the indirect haemagglutina-tion and toxin neutralization tests. J Biol Stand 12:137–143, 1984.

310. Ourth PP, MacDonald AB. Neutralization of tetanus toxin by human and rabbit immunoglobulin classes and subunits. Immunology 3:807–815, 1977.

311. Melville-Smith ME, Seagroatt VA, Watkins JT. A comparison of enzyme-linked immunosorbent assay (ELISA) with the toxin neu-tralization test in mice as a method for the estimation of tetanus anti-toxin in human sera. J Biol Stand 11:137–144, 1983.

312. Cox JC, Permier RR, Finger W, et al. A comparison of enzyme immunoassay and bioassay for the quantitative determination of anti-bodies to tetanus toxin. J Biol Stand 11:123–128, 1983.

313. Sedgwick AK, Ballow M, Sparks K, et al. Rapid quantitative micro-enzyme–linked immunosorbent assay for tetanus antibodies. J Clin Microbiol 18:104–109, 1983.

314. Hagenaars AM, van Delft RW, Nagel J. Comparison of ELISA and toxin neutralization for the determination of tetanus antibodies. J Immunoassay 5:1–11, 1984.

315. Simonsen O, Bentzon MW, Heron I. ELISA for the routine determina-tion of antitoxic immunity to tetanus. J Biol Stand 14:231–239, 1986.

316. Virella G, Hyman B. Quantitation of anti-tetanus and anti-diphthe-ria antibodies by enzymoimmunoassay: methodology and applica-tions. J Clin Lab Anal 5:43–48, 1991.

317. Dokmetjian J, Della Valle C, Lavigne V, et al. A possible explanation for the discrepancy between ELISA and neutralising antibodies to tetanus toxin. Vaccine 18:2698–2703, 2000.

318. Simonsen O, Schou C, Heron I. Modification of the ELISA for the estimation of tetanus antitoxin in human sera. J Biol Stand 15:143–157, 1987.

319. Vernacchio L, Madico G, Verastegui M, et al. Neonatal tetanus in Peru: risk assessment with modified enzyme-linked immunosorbent assay and toxoid skin test. Am J Public Health 83:1754–1756, 1993.

320. Hendriksen CFM, van der Gun JW, Kreeftenberg JG. The toxin-binding inhibition test as a reliable in vitro alternative to the toxin neutralization test in mice for the estimation of tetanus antitoxin in human sera. J Biol Stand 16:287–297, 1988.

321. Hendriksen CFM, van der Gun JW, Kreeftenberg JG. Combined esti-mation of tetanus and diphtheria antitoxin in human sera by the in vitro toxin-binding inhibition (ToBi) test. J Biol Stand 17:191–200, 1989.

322. Hong HA, Ke NT, Nhon TN, et al. Validation of the combined toxin-binding inhibition test for determination of neutralizing anti-bodies against tetanus and diphtheria toxins in a vaccine field study in Vietnam. Bull World Health Organ 74:275–282, 1996.

323. Kristiansen M, Aggerbeck H, Heron I. Improved ELISA for determi-nation of anti-diphtheria and/or anti-tetanus antitoxin antibodies in sera. APMIS 105:843–853, 1997.

324. Yuan L, Lau W, Thipphawong J, et al. Diphtheria and tetanus immu-nity among blood donors in Toronto. CMAJ 156:985–990, 1997.

325. Newell KW, Duenas Lehman A, LeBlanc DR, Garces Osorio N. The use of toxoid for the prevention of tetanus neonatorum: final report of a double-blind controlled field trial. Bull World Health Organ 35:863–871, 1966.

326. Wolters KL, Dehmel H. Abschliessende Untersuchungen über die Tetanusprophylaxe durch aktive Immunisierung. Z Hyg 124: 326–332, 1942.

327. Rahman M, Chen LC, Chakraborty J, et al. Use of tetanus toxoid for the prevention of neonatal tetanus. 1. Reduction of neonatal mortal-ity by immunization of non-pregnant and pregnant women in rural Bangladesh. Bull World Health Organ 60:261–267, 1982.

328. Kumar V, Kumar R, Mathur VN, et al. Neonatal tetanus mortality in a rural community of Haryana. Indian Pediatr 25:167–169, 1986.

329. Maru M, Geahun A, Hosana S. A house-to-house survey on neona-tal tetanus in urban and rural areas in the Gondar region, Ethiopia. Trop Geogr Med 40:233–236, 1986.

330. Expanded Programme on Immunization. Neonatal tetanus mortality surveys, Egypt. Wkly Epidemiol Rec 62:332–335, 1987.

331. Cardenas Ayala VM, Nunez Urquiza RM, Brogan DR, et al. Neonatal tetanus mortality in Veracruz, Mexico, 1989. Bull Pan Am Health Organ 29:116–128, 1995.

332. Long AP, Sartwell PE. Tetanus in the U.S. Army in World War II. Bull US Army Med Dept 7:371–385, 1947.

333. Press E. Desirability of the routine use of tetanus toxoid. N Engl J Med 239:50–56, 1948.

334. Centers for Disease Control and Prevention. General recommenda-tions on immunization: recommendations of the Advisory Committee on Immunization Practices (ACIP) and the American Academy of Family Physicians (AAFP). MMWR 51 (RR-2):1–36, 2002.

335. Adkins SB. Immunizations: current recommendations. Am Fam Physician 56:865–874, 1997.

336. Ramsay ME, Corbel MJ, Redhead K, et al. Persistence of antibody after accelerated immunisation with diphtheria/tetanus/pertussis vac-cine. BMJ 302:1489–1491, 1991.

337. Cooke JV, Holowach J, Atkins JE, et al. Antibody formation in early infancy against diphtheria and tetanus toxoids. J Pediatr 33:141–146, 1948.

338. Barrett CD, McLeon IW, Molner JG, et al. Multiple antigen immu-nization of infants against poliomyelitis, diphtheria, pertussis and tetanus: an evaluation of antibody responses of infants one day old to seven months of age at start of inoculations. Pediatrics 30:720–736, 1962.

339. Di Sant'Agnese PA. Combined immunization against diphtheria, tetanus, and pertussis in newborn infants. I. Production of antibodies in early infancy. Pediatrics 3:20–33, 1949.

340. Di Sant'Agnese PA. Combined immunization against diphtheria, tetanus, and pertussis in newborn infants. III. Relationship of age to antibody production. Pediatrics 3:333–344, 1949.

341. Di Sant'Agnese PA. Simultaneous immunization of newborn infants against diphtheria, tetanus, and pertussis: production of antibodies and duration of antibody levels in an Eastern Metropolitan area. Am J Public Health 40:674–680, 1950.

342. Bernbaum JC, Daft A, Anolik R, et al. Response of preterm infants to diphtheria-tetanus-pertussis immunizations. J Pediatr 107: 184–188, 1985.

343. Barr M, Glenny AT, Butler NR. Immunization of babies with diph-theria-tetanus-pertussis prophylactic. Br Med J 2:635–639, 1955.

344. Di Sant'Agnese PA. Combined immunization against diphtheria, tetanus, and pertussis in newborn infants II. Duration of antibody levels; antibody titers after booster dose; effect of passive immunity to diphtheria on active immunization with diphtheria toxoid. Pediatrics 13:181–194, 1949.

345. Peterson JC, Christie A. Immunization in the young infant: response to combined vaccines. VI. Tetanus. Am J Dis Child 81:518–529, 1951.

346. Halsey NA, Galazka A. The efficacy of DPT and oral poliomyelitis immunization schedules initiated from birth to 12 weeks of age. Bull World Health Organ 63:1151–1169, 1985.

347. Barkin RM, Samuelson JS, Gotlin LP. DTP reactions and serologic response with a reduced dose schedule. J Pediatr 105:189–194, 1984.

348. Barkin RM, Pichichero ME, Samuelson JS, et al. Pediatric diphthe-ria and tetanus toxoids vaccine: clinical and immunologic response when administered as the primary series. J Pediatr 106:779–781, 1985.

349. Edwards KM, Meade BD, Decker MD, et al. Comparison of 13 acel-lular pertussis vaccines: overview and serologic response. Pediatrics 96:548–557, 1995.

350. Kutukculer N, Kurugol Z, Egemen A, et al. The effect of immuniza-tion against tetanus during pregnancy for protective antibody titres and specific antibody responses of infants. J Trop Pediatr 42:308–309, 1996.

351. Habig WH, Tankersley DL. Tetanus. In Cryz SJ (ed). Vaccines and Immunotherapy. New York, Pergamon Press, 1991, pp 13–19.

352. Booy R, Aitken SJM, Taylor S, et al. Immunogenicity of combined diphtheria, tetanus, pertussis vaccine given at 2, 3, and 4 months ver-sus 3, 5, and 9 months of age. Lancet 339:505–510, 1992.

353. Ramsay MEB, Rao M, Begg NT, et al. Antibody response to acceler-ated immunisation with diphtheria, tetanus, pertussis vaccine. Lancet 342:203–205, 1993.

354. Brown GC, Volk VK, Gottshall RY, et al. Responses of infants to DTP-P vaccine used in nine injection schedules. Public Health Rep 79:585–602, 1964.

355. Breman JG, Wright GG, Levine L, et al. The primary serologic response to a single dose of adsorbed tetanus toxoid, high concentra-tion type. Bull World Health Organ 59:745–752, 1981.

356. Stanfield JP, Gall D, Bracken PM. Single-dose antinatal tetanus immunisation. Lancet 1:215–219, 1973.

357. Agarwal K, Pandit K, Kannan AT. Single-dose tetanus toxoid—a review of trials in India with special reference to control of tetanus neonatorum. Indian J Pediatr 81:283–285, 1984.

358. Dick G. Combined vaccines. Can J Public Health 57:435–446, 1966.
359. Someya S, Mizuhara H, Murata R, et al. Studies on the adequate composition of diphtheria and tetanus toxoids with reference to the amounts of toxoids and aluminum adjuvant. Jpn J Med Sci Biol 34:21–35, 1981.
360. Ruben FL, Smith EA, Foster SO, et al. Simultaneous administration of smallpox, measles, yellow fever, and diphtheria-pertussis-tetanus antigens to Nigerian children. Bull World Health Organ 48:175–181, 1973.
361. Miller JJ, Saito TM. Concurrent immunization against tetanus, diphtheria and pertussis: a comparison of fluid and alum-precipitated toxoids. J Pediatr 21:31–44, 1942.
362. Orenstein WA, Weisfeld JS, Halsey NA. Diphtheria and tetanus toxoids and pertussis vaccine, combined. In Recent Advances in Immunization: A Bibliographic Review (PAHO Scientific Publ No 451). Washington, DC, Pan American Health Organization, 1983, pp 30–51.
363. World Health Organization. Immunization Policies in Europe: Report on a WHO Meeting, Karlovy Vary, Czechoslovakia, December 10–12, 1984 (ICP/EPI 001 m01, 1430G, 1986 PS4). Geneva, World Health Organization, 1986.
364. Expanded Programme on Immunization. Global Advisory Group. Wkly Epidemiol Rec 60:13–16, 1985.
365. Volk VK. Safety and effectiveness of multiple antigen preparations in a group of free-living children. Am J Public Health 39:1299–1313, 1949.
366. Barrett CD, Timm EA, Molner JG, et al. Multiple antigen immunization of infants against poliomyelitis, diphtheria, pertussis and tetanus. II. Response of infants and young children to primary immunization and eighteen-month booster. Am J Public Health 49:644–655, 1959.
367. Pichichero ME, Barkin RM, Samuelson JS. Pediatric diphtheria and tetanus toxoids–adsorbed vaccine: immune response to the first booster following the diphtheria and tetanus toxoids primary series. Pediatr Infect Dis 5:428–430, 1986.
368. Scheibel I, Bentzon MW, Christensen PE, et al. Duration of immunity to diphtheria and tetanus after active immunization. Acta Pathol Microbiol Scand 67:380–392, 1966.
369. Simonsen O, Kjeldsen K, Heron I. Immunity against tetanus and effect of revaccination 25–30 years after primary vaccination. Lancet 2:1240–1242, 1984.
370. Peebles TC, Levine L, Eldred ML, et al. Tetanus-toxoid emergency boosters: a reappraisal. N Engl J Med 280:575–581, 1969.
371. Myers MG, Beckman CW, Vosdingh RA, et al. Primary immunization with tetanus and diphtheria toxoids: reaction rate and immunogenicity in older children and adults. JAMA 248:2478–2480, 1982.
372. Hardegree ML, Barile MF, Pittman M, et al. Immunization against neonatal tetanus in New Guinea. 2. Duration of primary antitoxin responses to adjuvant tetanus toxoids and comparison of booster responses to adjuvant and plain toxoids. Bull World Health Organ 43:439–451, 1970.
373. Ruben FL, Fireman P. Follow-up study: protective immunization in the elderly [letter]. Am J Public Health 73:1330, 1983.
374. Solomonova K, Vizev S. Secondary response to boostering by purified aluminum-hydroxide–adsorbed tetanus antitoxin in aging and in aged adults. Immunobiology 158:312–319, 1981.
375. Kishimoto S, Tomino S, Mitsuya H, et al. Age-related decline in the in vitro and in vivo syntheses of anti-tetanus toxoid antibody in humans. J Immunol 125:2347–2352, 1980.
376. Simonsen O, Block AV, Klærke A, et al. Immunity against tetanus and response to revaccination in surgical patients more that 50 years of age. Surg Gynecol Obstet 164:329–334, 1987.
377. Murphy SM, Hegarty DM, Feighery CS, et al. Tetanus immunity in elderly people. Age Ageing 24:99–102, 1995.
378. Masar I, Kamienicka L, Novakova I. Immune response of elderly to booster of tetanus. In Nistico G, Bizzini B, Bytchenko M, Triau R (eds). Proceedings of the Eighth International Conference on Tetanus, Leningrad, USSR, August 25–28, 1987. Rome, Pythagora Press, 1989, pp 251–253.
379. World Health Organization, Expanded Programme on Immunization. Prevention of Neonatal Tetanus Through Immunization (WHO/EPI/GEN/86/9). Geneva, World Health Organization, 1986.
380. Evans DG. Persistence of antitoxin in man following active immunisation. Lancet 2:316–317, 1943.
381. Simonsen O, Badsberg JH, Kjeldsen K, et al. The fall-off in serum concentration of tetanus antitoxin after primary and booster vaccination. Acta Pathol Microbiol Scand C 94:77–82, 1986.
382. Simonsen O. Vaccination against tetanus and diphtheria. Danish Med Bull 36:24–47, 1989.
383. Christenson B, Böttiger M. Immunity and immunization of children against tetanus in Sweden. Scand J Infect Dis 23:643–647, 1991.
384. Volk VK, Gottshall RY, Anderson HD, et al. Antigenic response to booster dose of diphtheria and tetanus toxoids, seven to thirteen years after primary inoculation of noninstitutionalized children. Public Health Rep 77:185–194, 1962.
385. Looney JM, Edsall G, Ipsen J, Chasen WH. Persistence of antitoxin levels after tetanus-toxoid inoculation in adults, and effect of a booster dose after various intervals. N Engl J Med 254:6–12, 1956.
386. Simonsen O, Klærke M, Jensen JEB, et al. Revaccination against tetanus 17 to 20 years after primary vaccination: kinetics of antibody response. J Trauma 27:1358–1361, 1987.
387. Simonsen O, Bentzon MW, Kjeldsen J, et al. Evaluation of vaccination requirements to secure continuous antitoxin immunity to tetanus. Vaccine 5:115–122, 1987.
388. Kaiser GC, King RD, Lempe RE, Ruster MH. Delayed recall of active tetanus immunization. JAMA 178:914–916, 1961.
389. White WG, Gall D, Barnes GM, et al. Duration of immunity after active immunisation against tetanus. Lancet 2:95–96, 1969.
390. Mathias RG, Schechter MT. Booster immunization for diphtheria and tetanus: no evidence for need in adults. Lancet 1:1089–1091, 1985.
391. Gardner P, LaForce FM. Protection against tetanus [letter]. N Engl J Med 333:599, 1995.
392. Bowie C. Tetanus toxoid for adults—too much of a good thing [editorial]. Lancet 348:1185–1186, 1996.
393. Balestra DJ, Littenberg B. Should adult tetanus immunization be given as a single vaccination at age 65? J Gen Intern Med 8:405–412, 1993.
394. Gardner P. Issues related to the decennial tetanus-diphtheria toxoid booster recommendations in adults. Infect Dis Clin North Am 15:143–153, 2001.
395. Singleton JA, Greby SM, Wooten KG, et al. Influenza, pneumococcal, and tetanus toxoid vaccination of adults—United States, 1993–1997. MMWR 49(SS-9):39–52, 2000.
396. Task Force on Immunization of the American College of Physicians. Guide for Adult Immunization (4th ed). Philadelphia, American College of Physicians, 1997.
397. Institute of Medicine Vaccine Safety Committee. Diphtheria and tetanus toxoids. Adverse events associated with childhood vaccines: evidence bearing on causality. In Stratton KR, Howe CJ, Johnston RB (eds). Research Strategies for Assessing Adverse Effects Associated with Vaccines. Washington, DC, National Academy Press, 1994, pp 67–117.
398. Murphy KJ. Fatal tetanus with brain-stem involvement and myocarditis in an ex-serviceman. Med J Aust 57:542–544, 1970.
399. Sutter RW, Hadler SC, McQuilllan G, Gergen PJ. Protection against tetanus [letter reply]. N Engl J Med 333:600, 1995.
400. World Health Organization. Field Manual for Neonatal Tetanus Elimination (WHO/V&B/99.14). Geneva, World Health Organization, 1999.
401. Koenig MA, Roy NC, McElrath T, et al. Duration of protective immunity conferred by maternal tetanus toxoid immunization: further evidence from Matlab, Bangladesh. Am J Public Health 88:903–907, 1998.
402. Centers for Disease Control. Use of vaccines and immune globulins in persons with altered immunocompetence: recommendations of the Advisory Committee on Immunization Practices (ACIP): MMWR 42(RR-4):1–18, 1993.
403. Moss WJ, Clements CJ, Halsey NA. Immunization of children at risk of infection with human immunodeficiency virus. Bull WHO 81:61–70, 2003.
404. Webster ADB, Latif AAA, Brenner MK, Bird D. Evaluation of test immunization in the assessment of antibody deficiency syndromes. Br Med J (Clin Res Ed) 288:1864–1866, 1984.
405. Kroon FP, Van Dissel JT, Labadie J, et al. Antibody response to diphtheria, tetanus, and poliomyelitis vaccines in relation to the number of CD4+ T lymphocytes in adults infected with human immunodeficiency virus. Clin Infect Dis 21:1197–1203, 1995.
406. Dieye TN, Sow PS, Simonart T, et al. Immunologic and virologic response after tetanus toxoid booster among HIV-1- and HIV-2-infected Senegalese individuals. Vaccine 20:905–913, 2002.

407. Talesnik E, Vial PA, Labarca J, et al. Time course of antibody response to tetanus toxoid and pneumococcal capsular polysaccharides in patients infected with HIV. J Acquir Immune Defic Syndr 19:471–477, 1998.

408. Von Reyn CF, Clements CJ, Mann JM. Human immunodeficiency virus infection and routine childhood immunisation. Lancet 1:669–672, 1987.

409. Ryder RW, Oxtoby MJ, Mvula M, et al. Safety and immunogenicity of bacille Calmette-Guerin, diphtheria-tetanus-pertussis, and oral polio vaccines in newborn children in Zaire infected with human immunodeficiency virus type 1. J Pediatr 122:697–702, 1993.

410. Hammarstrom V, Pauksen K, Svensson H, et al. Tetanus immunity in patients with hematological malignancies. Support Care Cancer 6:469–472, 1998.

411. Molrine DC, Hibberd PL. Vaccines for transplant recipients. Infect Dis Clin North Am 15:273–305, 2001.

412. Grindt M, Pietsch M, Kohler H. Tetanus immunization and its association to hepatitis B vaccination in patients with chronic renal failure. Am J Kid Dis 26:454–460, 1995.

413. Kruger S, Seyfarth M, Sack K, Kreft B. Defective immune response to tetanus toxoid in hemodialysis patients and its association with diphtheria vaccination. Vaccine 17:1145–1150, 1999.

414. Kruger S, Muller Steinhardt M, Kirchner H, Kreft B. A 5-year follow-up on antibody response after diphtheria and tetanus vaccination in hemodialysis patients. Am J Kid Dis 38:1264–1270, 2001.

415. Guerin A, Buisson Y, Nutini MT, et al. Response to vaccination against tetanus in chronic haemodialysed patients. Nephrol Dial Transplant 7:323–326, 1992.

416. Kurtzhals JAL, Kjeldsen K, Heron I, Skinhoj P. Immunity against diphtheria and tetanus in human immunodeficiency virus-infected Danish men born 1950–1959. APMIS 100:803–808, 1992.

417. World Health Organization. HIV infection and immunization. In Immunization Policy (WHOGPV/GEN/95.03 Rev.1). Geneva, World Health Organization, 1996, pp 36–39.

418. Centers for Disease Control and Prevention. Guidelines for preventing opportunistic infections among hematopoietic stem cell transplant recipients: recommendations of CDC, the Infectious Disease Society of America, and the American Society of Blood and Marrow Transplantation. MMWR 49(RR-10):1–125, 2000.

419. Balloni A, Assael BM, Ghio L, et al. Immunity to poliomyelitis, diphtheria and tetanus in pediatric patients before and after renal or liver transplantation. Vaccine 17:2507–2511, 1999.

420. Enke BU, Bokenkamp A, Offner G, et al. Response to diphtheria and tetanus booster vaccination in pediatric renal transplant recipients. Transplantation 64:237–241, 1997.

421. Beaman M, Michael J, MacLennan ICM, Adu D. T-cell-independent and T-cell-dependent antibody responses in patients with chronic renal failure. Nephrol Dial Transplant 4:216–221, 1989.

422. Kleinknecht C, Margolis A, Bonnissol C, et al. Serum antibodies before and after immunisation in haemodialysed children. Proc Eur Dial Transplant Assoc 14:209–214, 1977.

423. Neu AM, Warady BA, Furth SL, et al. Antibody levels to diphtheria, tetanus and rubella in infants vaccinated while on PD: a study of the Pediatric Peritoneal Dialysis Study Consortium. Adv Perit Dial 13:297–299, 1997.

424. Relihan M. Reactions to tetanus toxoid. J Irish Med Assoc 62:430–434, 1969.

425. White WG, Barnes GM, Barker E, et al. Reactions to tetanus toxoid. J Hyg (Camb) 71:283–297, 1973.

426. Williams JJ, Ellingson HV. Field trial of commercially prepared diphtheria-tetanus toxoid: immunization reactions among recruits. Unpublished report to the Armed Forces Epidemiologic Board, 1954.

427. Collier LH, Polakoff S, Mortimer J. Reactions and antibody responses to reinforcing doses of adsorbed and plain tetanus vaccines. Lancet 1:1364–1368, 1979.

428. Jones AE, Melville-Smith M, Watkins J, et al. Adverse reactions in adolescents to reinforcing doses of plain and adsorbed tetanus vaccines. Community Med 7:99–106, 1985.

429. Macko MB. Comparison of the morbidity of tetanus toxoid boosters with tetanus-diphtheria toxoid boosters. Ann Emerg Med 14:33–35, 1985.

430. Deacon SP, Langford DT, Shepard WM, Knight PA. A comparative clinical study of adsorbed tetanus vaccine and adult-type tetanus-diphtheria vaccine. J Hyg (Camb) 89:513–519, 1982.

431. Zurrer G, Steffen R. Side effects in tetanus vs. diphtheria tetanus vaccination in travellers [abstract WPO3.3]. In Proceedings of the First Conference on International Travel Medicine, Zurich, Switzerland, April 5–8, 1988.

432. Sisk CW, Lewis CE. Reactions to tetanus-diphtheria toxoid (adult). Arch Environ Health 11:34–36, 1965.

433. McComb JA, Levine L. Adult immunization. II. Dosage reduction as a solution to increasing reactions to tetanus toxoid. N Engl J Med 265:1152–1153, 1961.

434. Levine L, Ipsen J, McComb JA. Adult immunization: preparation and evaluation of combined fluid tetanus and diphtheria toxoids for adult use. Am J Hyg 73:20–35, 1961.

435. Ipsen J. Immunization of adults against diphtheria and tetanus. N Engl J Med 251:459–466, 1954.

436. Holden JM, Strang DU. Reactions to tetanus toxoid: comparison of fluid and adsorbed toxoids. N Z Med J 64:574–577, 1965.

437. Eisen AH, Cohen JJ, Rose B. Reaction to tetanus toxoid: report of a case with immunologic studies. N Engl J Med 269:1408–1411, 1963.

438. Schneider CH. Reactions to tetanus toxoid: a report of five cases. Med J Aust 1:303–305, 1964.

439. Edsall G, Elliot MW, Peebles TC, et al. Excessive use of tetanus toxoid boosters. JAMA 202:17–19, 1967.

440. Levine L, Edsall G. Tetanus toxoid: what determines reaction proneness? J Infect Dis 144:376, 1981.

441. Jacobs RL, Lowe RS, Lanier BQ. Adverse reactions to tetanus toxoid. JAMA 247:40–42, 1982.

442. Griffith AH. Clinical reactions to tetanus toxoid. In Eckmann L (ed). Principles of Tetanus. Bern, Hans Huber, 1967, p 299.

443. Edelman R. Vaccine adjuvants. Rev Infect Dis 2:370–383, 1980.

444. Gherardi RK, Coquet M, Cherin P, et al. Macrophagic myofasciitis lesions assess long-term persistence of vaccine-derived aluminum hydroxide in muscle. Brain 124:1821–1831, 2001.

445. World Health Organization. Vaccine safety: Vaccine Safety Advisory Committee [Macrophagic myofasciitis and aluminum-containing vaccines]. Wkly Epidemiol Rec 74:337–340, 1999.

446. World Health Organization. Corrigendum to No. 41, pp 338–339: vaccine safety. Wkly Epidemiol Rec 74:354, 1999.

447. Expanded Programme on Immunization. Reactions to tetanus toxoid. Wkly Epidemiol Rec 57:193–194, 1982.

448. Middaugh JP. Side effects of diphtheria-tetanus toxoid in adults. Am J Public Health 69:246–249, 1979.

449. Ullberg-Olsson K. Vaccinationsreaktioner efter injektion: av tetanustoxoid med och utan tillsats av difteritoxoid. Lakartidningen 76:2976, 1979.

450. Rennels MB, Deloria MA, Pichichero ME, et al. Extensive swelling after booster doses of acellular pertussis-tetanus-diphtheria vaccines. Pediatrics 105:E12, 2000.

451. Centers for Disease Control and Prevention. Use of diphtheria toxoid-tetanus toxoid-acellular pertussis vaccine as a five-dose series: supplemental recommendations of the Advisory Committee on Immunization Practices (ACIP). MMWR 49(RR-13):1–8, 2000.

452. Reisman RE. Delayed hypersensitivity to merthiolate preservative. J Allergy 43:245–248, 1969.

453. Gold H. Sensitization induced by tetanus toxoid, alum precipitated. J Lab Clin Med 27:26–36, 1941.

454. Church JA, Richards W. Recurrent abscess formation following DTP immunizations: association with hypersensitivity to tetanus toxoid. Pediatrics 75:899–900, 1985.

455. Osawa J, Kitamura K, Ikezawa Z, Nakejima H. A probable role for vaccines containing thimerosal in thimerosal hypersensitivity. Contact Dermatitis 24:178–182, 1991.

456. Institute of Medicine, Immunization Safety Review Committee, Stratton KR, Howe CJ, Johnston RB (eds). Thimerosal-Containing Vaccines and Neurodevelopmental Disorders. Washington, DC, National Academy Press, 2001.

457. Centers for Disease Control and Prevention. Thimerosal in vaccines: a joint statement of the American Academy of Pediatrics and the Public Health Service. MMWR 48:563–565, 1999.

458. World Health Organization. Thimersal as a vaccine preservative. Wkly Epidemiol Rec 75:12–16, 2000.

459. European Agency for the Evaluation of Medicinal Products. Public Statement on Thimersal Containing Medicinal Products, 8 July 1999 (EMEA/20962/99), London, European Agency for the Evaluation of Medicinal Products, 1999. Available at *www.emea.eu.int/ pdfs/human/press/pus/2096299EN.pdf*

460. Quast U, Hennessen W, Widmark RM. Mono- and polyneuritis after tetanus vaccination (1970–1977). Dev Biol Stand 43:25–32, 1979.

461. Pollard JD, Selby G. Relapsing neuropathy due to tetanus toxoid: report of a case. J Neurol Sci 37:113–125, 1978.

462. Holliday PL, Bauer RB. Polyradiculoneuritis secondary to immunization with tetanus and diphtheria toxoids. Arch Neurol 40:56–57, 1983.

463. Newton N, Janati A. Guillain-Barré syndrome after vaccination with purified tetanus toxoid. South Med J 80:1053–1054, 1987.

464. Kiwit JCW. Neuralgic amyotrophy after administration of tetanus toxoid [letter]. J Neurol Neurosurg Psychiatry 47:320, 1984.

465. Tsairis P, Dyck PJ, Mulder DW. Natural history of brachial plexus neuropathy: report on 99 patients. Arch Neurol 2:116–120, 1965.

466. Beghi E, Kurland LT, Mulder DW, Nicolosi A. Brachial plexus neuropathy in the population of Rochester, Minnesota, 1970–1981. Ann Neurol 18:320–323, 1985.

467. Dittman S. Tetanusschutzimpfung. Beitr Hyg Epidemiol 25:239–240, 1981.

468. Rutledge SL, Snead OC. Neurologic complications of immunizations. J Pediatr 109:917–923, 1986.

469. Garvey JL. Serum neuritis: 20 cases following use of antitetanic serum. Postgrad Med 13:210–213, 1953.

470. Rantala J, Cherry JD, Shields WD, et al. Epidemiology of Guillain-Barré syndrome in children: relationship of oral polio vaccine occurrence. J Pediatr 124:220–223, 1994.

471. Tuttle J, Chen RT, Rantala H, et al. The risk of Guillain-Barré syndrome after tetanus-toxoid-containing vaccines in adults and children in the United States. Am J Public Health 87:2045–2048, 1997.

472. Schlenska GK. Unusual neurologic complications following tetanus toxoid administration. J Neurol 215:299–302, 1977.

473. Schwarz G, Lanzer G, List WF. Acute midbrain syndrome as an adverse reaction to tetanus toxoid. Intensive Care Med 15:53–54, 1988.

474. Nagel J, Svec D, Waters T, Fireman P. IgE synthesis in man. I. Development of specific IgE antibodies after immunization with tetanus-diphtheria (Td) toxoids. J Immunol 118:334–341, 1977.

475. Matuhasi T, Ikegami H. Elevation of levels of IgE antibody to tetanus toxin in individuals vaccinated with diphtheria-pertussis-tetanus vaccine. J Infect Dis 146:290, 1982.

476. Cogne M, Ballet JJ, Schmitt C, Bizzini B. Total and IgE antibody levels following booster immunization with aluminum adsorbed and nonadsorbed tetanus toxoid in humans. Ann Allergy 54:148–151, 1985.

477. Zalogna GP, Chernow B. Life-threatening anaphylactic reactions to tetanus toxoid. Ann Allergy 49:107–108, 1982.

478. Ratliff DA, Burns-Cox CJ. Anaphylaxis to tetanus toxoid (unreviewed reports). Br Med J (Clin Res Ed) 288:114, 1983.

479. Engler RJM, Zalogna G. Anaphylaxis to tetanus toxoid: IgE mediated disease [abstract 422]. J Allergy Clin Immunol 75(pt 2):210, 1985.

480. Cooke RA, Hampton S, Sherman WB, Stull A. Allergy induced by immunization with tetanus toxoid. JAMA 114:1854–1858, 1940.

481. Whittingham HE. Anaphylaxis following administration of tetanus toxoid. Br Med J 1:292–293, 1940.

482. Parrish HJ, Oakley CL. Anaphylaxis after injection of tetanus toxoid: report of a case. Br Med J 1:294–295, 1940.

483. Miller HG, Stanton JB. Neurologic sequelae of prophylactic inoculation. Q J Med 23:1–27, 1954.

484. Smith RE, Wolnisty C. Allergic reactions to tetanus, diphtheria, influenza, and poliomyelitis immunization. Ann Allergy 20:809–813, 1962.

485. Mansfield LE, Ting S, Rawls DO, Frederick R. Systemic reactions during cutaneous testing for tetanus toxoid hypersensitivity. Ann Allergy 57:135–137, 1986.

486. Facktor MA, Bernstein RA, Fireman P. Hypersensitivity to tetanus toxoid. J Allergy Clin Immunol 52:1–12, 1973.

487. Gupte SC, Bhatia HM. Anti-A and anti-B titre response after tetanus toxoid injections in normal adults and pregnant women. Indian J Med Res 70:221–228, 1979.

488. Gupte SC, Bhatia HM. Increased incidence of haemolytic disease of the newborn caused by ABO-incompatibility when tetanus toxoid is given during pregnancy. Vox Sang 38:22–28, 1980.

489. Kurikka S, Olander RM, Eskola J, Kayhty H. Passively acquired anti-tetanus and anti-Haemophilus antibodies and the response to Haemophilus influenzae type b–tetanus toxoid conjugate vaccine in infancy. Pediatr Infect Dis J 15:530–535, 1996.

490. Carlsson RM, Claesson BA, Iwarson S, et al. Antibodies against Haemophilus influenzae type b and tetanus in infants after subcutaneous vaccination with PRP-T/diphtheria, or PRP-OMP/diphtheria-tetanus vaccines. Pediatr Infect Dis J 13:27–33, 1994.

491. Holmes SJ, Fritzell B, Guito KP, et al. Immunogenicity of Haemophilus influenzae type b polysaccharide–tetanus toxoid conjugate vaccine in infants. Am J Dis Child 147:832–836, 1993.

492. Avendano A, Ferreccio C, Lagos R, et al. Haemophilus influenzae type b polysaccharide–tetanus protein conjugate vaccine does not depress serologic responses to diphtheria, tetanus or pertussis antigens when coadministered in the same syringe with diphtheria-tetanus-pertussis vaccine at two, four and six months of age. Pediatr Infect Dis J 12:638–643, 1993.

493. Kaplan SL, Lauer BA, Ward MA, et al. Immunogenicity and safety of Haemophilus influenzae type b–tetanus protein conjugate vaccine alone or mixed with diphtheria-tetanus-pertussis vaccine in infants. J Pediatr 124:323–327, 1994.

494. da Silveira CM, Caceres VM, Dutra MG, et al. Safety of tetanus toxoid in pregnant women: a hospital-based case-control study of congenital anomalies. Bull World Health Organ 73:605–608, 1995.

495. Catindig N, Abad-Viola G, Magboo F. Tetanus toxoid and spontaneous abortions: is there epidemiological evidence of an association? [letter] Lancet 348:1098–1099, 1996.

496. Centers for Disease Control and Prevention. Update on adult immunization recommendations of the Advisory Committee on Immunization Practices (ACIP). MMWR 40(RR-12):1–52, 1991.

497. Smith JWG, Laurence DR, Evans DG. Prevention of tetanus in the wounded. Br Med J 3:453–455, 1975.

498. Percy AS, Kukora JS. The continuing problem of tetanus. Surg Gynecol Obstet 160:307–312, 1985.

499. Furste W. Four keys to 100 per cent success in tetanus prophylaxis. Am J Surg 128:616–623, 1974.

500. Committee on Trauma, American College of Surgeons. Prophylaxis against tetanus in wound management. Am Coll Surg Bull 69:22–23, 1984. Revised 1995. Available at www.facs.org/dept/trauma/publications/tetanus.pdf.

501. Banton HJ, Miller PA. An observation of antitoxin titers after booster doses of tetanus toxoid. N Engl J Med 240:13–14, 1949.

502. Trinca JC. Active immunization against tetanus: the need for a single all-purpose toxoid. Med J Aust 2:116–120, 1945.

503. Ipsen J. Changes in immunity and antitoxin level immediately after secondary stimulus with tetanus toxoid in rabbits. J Immunol 86:50–55, 1961.

504. McComb JA, Dwyer RC. Passive-active immunization with tetanus immune globulin. N Engl J Med 268:857–862, 1963.

505. Moloney PJ. Active-passive immunization against tetanus. In Eckmann L (ed). Principles of Tetanus. Bern, Hans Huber, 1967, pp 393–396.

506. Rubbo SD. New approaches to tetanus prophylaxis. Lancet 2:449–453, 1966.

507. Cohen H, Leussink AB. Passive-active immunization with human tetanus immunoglobulin and adsorbed toxoid. J Biol Stand 1:313–320, 1973.

508. Wahlbert T, Leibl H, Brauner A, et al. Tetanus antibody levels of female volunteers after injection with solvent/detergent-treated human tetanus immunoglobulin (Tetabulin S/D). Vox Sanguinis 80:159–161, 2001.

509. Lindsey D. Tetanus prophylaxis—do our guidelines assure protection? [editorial]. J Trauma 24:1063–1064, 1984.

510. Johnson DM. Fatal tetanus after prophylaxis with human tetanus immune globulin [letter]. JAMA 207:1519, 1969.

511. Pontecorvo M. The prophylactic dose of TIG. In Nistico G, Mastroeni P, Pitzurra M (eds). Proceedings of the Seventh International Conference on Tetanus, Copanello, Italy, September 10–15, 1984. Rome, Gangeni Publishing Company, 1985, pp 375–379.

512. Forrat R, Dumas R, Seiberling M, et al. Evaluation of the safety and pharmacokinetic profile of a new, pasteurized, human tetanus immunoglobulin administered as sham, postexposure prophylaxis of tetanus. Antimicrob Agents Chemother 42:298–305, 1998.

513. Smith JWG, MacIver AG. Studies in experimental tetanus infection. J Med Microbiol 2:385–393, 1969.

514. Smith JWG. Penicillin in prevention of tetanus. Br Med J 2:1293–1296, 1964.

515. Lucas AO, Willis AJP. Prevention of tetanus. Br Med J 2:1333–1336, 1965.

516. Lowbury EJL, Kidson A, Lilly HA, et al. Prophylaxis against tetanus in non-immune patients with wounds: the role of antibiotics and of human antitetanus globulin. J Hyg (Camb) 80:267–274, 1978.

517. Brand DA, Acampora D, Gottlieg L, et al. Adequacy of antitetanus prophylaxis in six hospital emergency rooms. N Engl J Med 309:636–640, 1983.

518. Giangrosso J, Smith RK. Misuse of tetanus immunoprophylaxis in wound care. Ann Emerg Med 14:573–579, 1985.

519. Ribero ML, Gastaldi G, Fara GM. Ongoing tetanus prophylaxis of injured patients in five hospital emergency rooms. Boll Ist Sieroter Milan 64:70–76, 1985.

520. Elkharrat D, Chammard AB, Raskine L, et al. Impact of guidelines to alter antitetanus prophylaxis practices and reduce costs in the Emergency Department. Am J Therapeutics 6:203–209, 1999.

521. Centers for Disease Control and Prevention. Tetanus—Kansas, 1993. MMWR 43:309–311, 1994.

522. Galazka A, Sporzynska Z. Immunity to tetanus and diphtheria in various age groups of the Polish population. Arch Immunol Ther Exp 27:715–726, 1979.

523. Matzkin H, Regev S, Kedem R, Nili E. A study of factors influencing tetanus immunity in Israeli male adults. J Infect 11:71–78, 1985.

524. Bouleaud J, Huet M. Contribution in the study of tetanus in France. In Nistico G, Mastroeni P, Pitzurra M (eds). Proceedings of the Seventh International Conference on Tetanus, Copanello, Italy, September 10–15, 1984. Rome, Gangeni Publishing Company, 1985, pp 495–497.

525. Gareau AB, Eby RJ, McLellan BA, Williams DR. Tetanus immunization status and immunologic response to a booster in an emergency department geriatric population. Ann Emerg Med 19:1377–1382, 1990.

526. Bottiger M, Gustavsson O, Svensson A. Immunity to tetanus, diphtheria and poliomyelitis in the adult population of Sweden in 1991. Int J Epidemiol 27:916–925, 1998.

527. de Melker HE, van den Hof S, Berbers GA, et al. A population-based study on tetanus antitoxin levels in the Netherlands. Vaccine 18:100–108, 1999.

528. Shohat T, Marva E, Sivan Y, et al. Immunologic response to a single dose of tetanus toxoid in older people. J Am Geriatr Soc 48:949–951, 2000.

529. World Health Assembly. Resolution 42.32: Expanded Programme on Immunization, 1989. In Handbook of Resolutions and Decisions of the World Health Assembly and the Executive Board (1985–1992). Vol. 3 (3rd ed). Geneva, World Health Organization, 1993. Available at policy.who.int/cgi-bin/om_isapi.dll?softpage=Policy42

530. Expanded Programme on Immunization. Global Advisory Group—Part I. Wkly Epidemiol Rec 65:5–11, 1990.

531. Expanded Programme on Immunization. Eliminating Neonatal Tetanus: How Near, How Far? (WHO/EPI/GEN/96.01). Geneva, World Health Organization, 1996..

532. World Health Organization. Progress towards the global elimination of neonatal tetanus, 1990–1998. Wkly Epidemiol Rec 74:73–80, 1999.

533. Expanded Programme on Immunization. Global Advisory Group—Part II. Wkly Epidemiol Rec 69:29–31, 34–35, 1994.

534. World Health Organization. Progress towards the global elimination of neonatal tetanus, 1999–2001. Wkly Epidemiol Rec [in press].

535. Aylward RB, Mansour E, Cummings F. Surveillance for neonatal tetanus in high-risk areas [letter]. Lancet 347:690–691, 1996.

536. Expanded Programme on Immunization. Estimating tetanus protection of women by serosurvey, Burundi. Wkly Epidemiol Rec 71:117–124, 1997.

537. Expanded Programme on Immunization. Training for Mid-Level Managers: EPI Coverage Survey (WHO/EPI/MLM/91.10). Geneva, World Health Organization, 1991.

538. Perez-Trallero E, Urbieta M, Diaz-de-Tuesta JL, et al. Anti-tetanus toxin titers in sera of the women who gave birth in 1985 and 1989 in Gipuzkoa (Basque Country, Spain). Eur J Epidemiol 11:231–234, 1995.

539. De Francisco A, Chakraborty J. Maternal recall of tetanus toxoid vaccination. Ann Trop Paediatr 16:49–54, 1996.

540. Deming MS, Roungou J-B, Kristiansen M, et al. Tetanus toxoid coverage as an indicator of serological protection against neonatal tetanus. Bull World Health Organ 80:696–703, 2002.

541. World Health Organization. Protection-at-birth (PAB) method, Tunisia. Wkly Epidemiol Rec 25:203–206, 2000.

542. Ekanem EE, Asindi AA, Antia-Obong OE. Factors influencing tetanus toxoid immunization among pregnant women in Cross Rivers State, Nigeria. Nigerian Med Pract 27:3–5, 1994.

543. Expanded Programme on Immunization. Reassessment of the neonatal tetanus problem, China. Wkly Epidemiol Rec 68:201–204, 1993.

544. Expanded Programme on Immunization. Elimination of neonatal tetanus, Thailand. Wkly Epidemiol Rec 68:337–341, 1993.

545. Expanded Programme on Immunization. Progress towards neonatal tetanus elimination, 1988–1994. Wkly Epidemiol Rec 71:33–36, 1996.

546. Bennett J, Seward J, Sakai S, Wang LD. Identifying areas at high-risk for neonatal tetanus [letter]. Lancet 346:1628–1629, 1995.

547. Aylward RB, Mansour E, Aly Oon ES, et al. The role of surveillance in "high risk" approach to the elimination of neonatal tetanus in Egypt. Int J Epidemiol 25:1286–1291, 1996.

548. Brabin L, Kemp J, Maxwell S, et al. Protecting adolescent girls against tetanus. Br Med J 311:73–74, 1995.

549. World Health Organization, The Children's Vaccine Initiative (CVI) and WHO's Global Programme for Vaccines and Immunization (GPV). Recommendations from the Scientific Advisory Group of Experts (SAGE), Part I. Wkly Epidemiol Rec 73:281–284, 1998.

550. Brabin L, Fazio-Tirrozzo G, Shahid S, et al. Tetanus antibody levels among adolescent girls in developing countries. Trans R Soc Trop Med Hyg 94:455–459, 2000.

551. Rahman S. The effect of traditional birth attendants and tetanus toxoid in reduction of neonatal mortality. J Trop Pediatr 28:163–165, 1982.

552. Berggren GG, Verly A, Garnier N, et al. Traditional midwives, tetanus immunization, and infant mortality in rural Haiti. Trop Doct 13:79–87, 1983.

553. Kessel E. Strategies for the control of neonatal tetanus. J Trop Pediatr 30:145–149, 1984.

554. Parashar UD, Bennett J, Boring JR, Hlady WG. Topical antimicrobials applied to the umbilical cord stump: a new intervention against neonatal tetanus. Int J Epidemiol 27:904–908, 1998.

555. Traverso H, Kamil S, Rahim H, et al. A reassessment of risk factors for neonatal tetanus. Bull World Health Organ 69:573–579, 1991.

556. Bennett J, Macia J, Traverso H, et al. Protective effects of topical antimicrobials against neonatal tetanus. Int J Epidemiol 26:897–903, 1997.

557. Dhillon H, Menon PS. Active immunization of women in pregnancy with two injections of adsorbed tetanus toxoid for prevention of tetanus neonatorum in Punjab, India. Indian J Med Res 63:583–589, 1975.

558. Chen ST, Edsall G, Peel MM, Sinnathuray TA. Timing of antenatal tetanus immunization for effective protection of the neonate. Bull World Health Organ 61:159–163, 1983.

559. Owa JA, Makinde OO. Neonatal tetanus in babies of women immunized with tetanus toxoid during pregnancy. Trop Doct 20:156–157, 1990.

560. Ghosh JB. Prevention of tetanus neonatorum [letter]. Indian Pediatr 27:210, 1990.

561. Deivanayagam N, Nedunchelian K, Kamala KG. Neonatal tetanus: observations on antenatal immunization, natal and immediate postnatal factors. Indian J Pediatr 58:119–122, 1991.

562. Bjerregaard P, Steinglass R, Mutie DM, et al. Neonatal tetanus mortality in coastal Kenya: a community survey. Int J Epidemiol 22:163–169, 1993.

563. Gendrel D, Richard-Lenoble D, Massamba MB, et al. Placental transfer of tetanus antibodies and protection of the newborn. J Trop Pediatr 36:279–282, 1990.

564. Madico G, Salazar G, McDonald J, et al. Rates of tetanus protection and transplacental tetanus antibody transfer in pregnant women from different socioeconomic groups in Peru. Clin Diagn Lab Immunol 3:753–755, 1996.

565. van Geldermalsen AA. Misguided advice on vaccines, Cameroon. Lancet 338:1528, 1991.

566. Milstien J, Griffin PD, Lee J-W. Damage to immunisation programmes from misinformation on contraceptive vaccines. Reprod Health Matters 6:24–28, 1995.

567. Lim Tan M. All in the name of life. Reprod Health Matters 6:29–30, 1995.

568. Rey M, Guillaumont P, Majnoni d'Intignano B. Benefits of immunization versus risk factors in tetanus. Dev Biol Stand 43:15–23, 1979.

569. Carducci A, Avio CM, Bendinelli M. Cost-benefit analysis of tetanus prophylaxis by a mathematical model. Epidemiol Infect 102: 473–483, 1989.

570. Cvjetanovic B, Grab B, Uemura K, Bytchenko B. Epidemiologic model of tetanus and its use in the planning of immunization programmes. Int J Epidemiol 1:125–137, 1972.

571. Smucker CM, Swint JM, Simmons GB. Prevention of neonatal tetanus in India: a prospective cost-effectiveness analysis. J Trop Pediatr 30:227–236, 1984.

572. Berman P, Quinley J, Yusef B, et al. Maternal immunization in Aceh Province, Sumatra: the cost effectiveness of alternative strategies. Soc Sci Med 33:185–192, 1991.

Chapter 28

Varicella Vaccine

ANNE A. GERSHON • MICHIAKI TAKAHASHI • JANE SEWARD

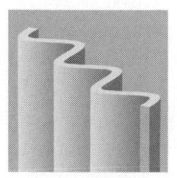 The varicella-zoster virus (VZV) causes two distinct diseases, varicella (chickenpox) and herpes zoster (HZ, shingles). Infection with VZV in temperate climates where vaccination is not used approaches 100% by the second decade of life. Whereas the disease may be mild in some individuals, more recent epidemiologic studies indicate that there is significant morbidity and some mortality with primary infection in previously healthy individuals. A live, attenuated VZV (Oka strain) vaccine has been in use for almost three decades in healthy and immunocompromised individuals and high-risk adults. The Oka strain of vaccine is now licensed for use in many countries for the prevention of primary infection in all healthy children and adults. Progress also has been made in the understanding of the pathogenesis of HZ, and definitive studies to determine the effectiveness of vaccination of the elderly for preventing or ameliorating HZ are now underway.

Historical Aspects

In the early medical literature, varicella and smallpox were often confused. The clinical differentiation was made by Heberden in 1767. Varicella was first proved to be an infectious disease in 1875 when Steiner transmitted the virus by inoculating volunteers with vesicular fluid from patients with varicella.[1] In 1892, von Bokay[2] reported that varicella occurred in individuals who were in close contact with persons with HZ, suggesting for the first time that the two diseases were caused by the same agent. It was not until the early part of the 20th century that this hypothesis was proven by inducing varicella in children who were inoculated with vesicular fluid from patients with HZ.[3,4] Garland, in 1943,[5] suggested that HZ might be due to reactivation of VZV acquired earlier in life. The causative virus was first isolated in cell culture by Weller and Stoddard in 1952[6] from samples of vesicular fluid from patients with varicella. Later studies by

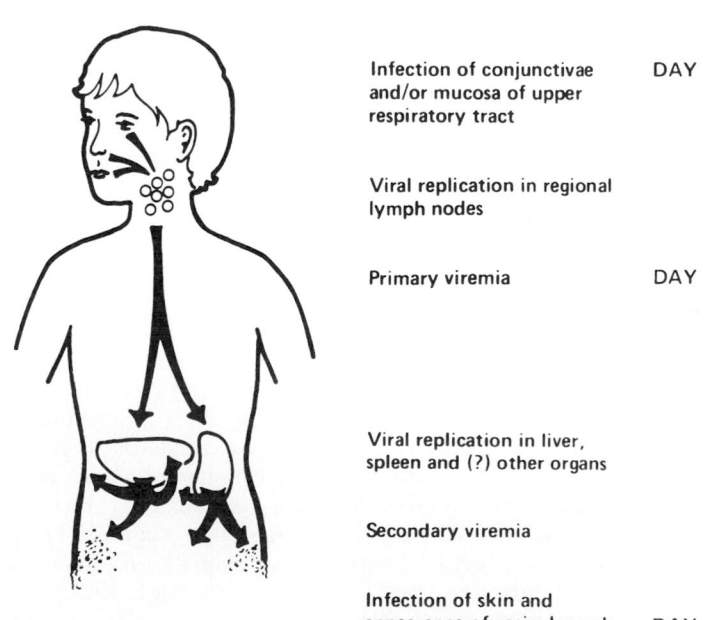

Infection of conjunctivae and/or mucosa of upper respiratory tract	DAY 0
Viral replication in regional lymph nodes	
Primary viremia	DAY 4-6
Viral replication in liver, spleen and (?) other organs	
Secondary viremia	
Infection of skin and appearance of vesicular rash	DAY 14

INCUBATION PERIOD

FIGURE 28–1 ■ Possible pathogenesis of chickenpox. (Adapted from Grose C. Variation on a theme by Fenner: the pathogenesis of chickenpox. Pediatrics 68:735, 1981.)

Weller and colleagues indicated that the viruses isolated from subjects with varicella and HZ were morphologically and serologically identical, and the name *varicella-zoster virus* was given to the agent.[7-9] In 1974, Takahashi and his colleagues at Osaka University produced a live VZV vaccine by attenuation of a wild-type strain by passage through various diploid cultures.[10] This attenuated VZV vaccine, the Oka strain, was suitable for human use and has been subsequently administered to millions of individuals for prevention of varicella. Molecular studies have shown the restriction endonuclease patterns of viral genomes of isolates from subjects with varicella and subsequent HZ,[11] as well as those from vaccine recipients with subsequent HZ,[12,13] to be identical, proving that HZ is due to reactivation of latent VZV. Therefore, clinical trials are now in progress to determine whether immunization of individuals with a prior history of varicella can prevent or modify HZ.

Background

Clinical Description

Varicella (Chickenpox)

The pathogenesis of varicella was conceptualized by Grose in 1981,[14] based on the pathogenesis of mouse pox, originally outlined by Fenner in 1948[15] (Fig. 28–1). VZV is transmitted from person to person by airborne droplets via the upper respiratory tract or from vesicular fluid of skin lesions. Although less readily transmitted than measles, it is highly contagious, with secondary attack rates in susceptible household contacts as high as 86%.[16,17] Varicella also can be transmitted to susceptible individuals from patients with HZ, although analysis of household contacts suggests the risk of viral transmission is less than that from varicella.

IMMUNOCOMPETENT CHILDREN AND ADULTS

In the exposed, susceptible immunocompetent individual, the virus replicates over the next 2 to 3 days in regional lymph nodes, followed by a primary viremia on days 4 to 6 after infection. The virus is thought to replicate in the liver and spleen and possibly other organs. A secondary viremia occurs about 10 to 14 days after infection, which is coincident with the appearance of the vesicular rash characteristic of varicella. In the infected host, there is either a short or absent prodromal period of malaise and fever for 1 or 2 days before the appearance of the characteristic rash. The rash appears in crops; each crop usually progresses within less than 24 hours from macules to papules, vesicles, pustules, and finally crusts. New lesions occur in crops over the next 5 to 6 days, with various stages of healing noted on the patient over the course of the illness. The lesions are pruritic and can scar if they become secondarily infected. In several published studies, the average number of vesicles ranges from 250 to 500 in otherwise healthy children.[17,18] The height of the fever usually parallels the extent of the rash, and the subject is usually ill for 5 to 7 days. The rash has a central distribution, with a concentration of lesions on the trunk, scalp,

and face. Second cases of varicella have been reported in immunocompetent persons but are unusual.[19-21] The explanation for second attacks remains unclear. One hypothesis is that the avidity of VZV antibodies is lower in persons who develop second cases than in those who do not.[22] Another possibility is that VZV is adept at immune evasion and can temporarily subvert the immune system.[23,24] There is evidence that subclinical reinfection with VZV is common.[25-27]

Varicella in otherwise healthy children has a wide variety of extracutaneous manifestations, which are, however, infrequent. These include pneumonia, encephalitis, cerebellar ataxia, arthritis, appendicitis, hepatitis, glomerulonephritis, pericarditis, and orchitis.[28-31] The most common complication in children is secondary bacterial infection of the skin.[30] Staphylococci or group A β-hemolytic streptococci are the usual causative pathogens. Group A streptococcal infections may be unusually severe and even fatal following varicella.[32-35] Acute cerebellar ataxia may develop prior to rash onset or up to 10 days afterward, with truncal ataxia often the only neurologic sign. Cerebellar ataxia in association with varicella is estimated to occur in 1 in 4000 cases among children less than 15 years of age and can result in hospitalization.[36] Varicella encephalitis is a much more serious and much less common complication (1 in 100,000 cases) than cerebellar ataxia, and carries a more guarded prognosis.

Adults with varicella have a significantly higher per case morbidity and mortality with primary VZV infection than do healthy children.[29,37,38] The height and duration of the febrile response are greater and rash is frequently more severe, with a greater number of lesions and increased time for clearing in comparison to children.[39,40] Constitutional symptoms such as malaise, myalgias, anorexia, and dehydration are of greater intensity in adults. Complications of varicella in the adult include encephalitis, which is seven times more common than in healthy children.

PREGNANT WOMEN AND NEWBORNS

There is increased morbidity of varicella in a varicella-susceptible woman and her fetus.[41] Varicella in the first trimester may cause damage to the fetal central nervous system, resulting in permanent scarring of the skin, shortening of the extremities, chorioretinitis, microphthalmia, optic atrophy, cataract, Horner's syndrome, blindness, mental retardation, and fetal demise. This constellation of problems in infants whose mothers had varicella in pregnancy is clinically diagnostic of the congenital varicella syndrome. There is a high correlation between the presence of limb abnormalities and serious central nervous system damage.[41] Although similar fetal abnormalities have been reported following maternal HZ infection, the congenital syndrome caused by HZ is exceedingly rare.[41] Patuszak et al. conducted a prospective case-control study of 106 pregnant women with varicella and performed a meta-analysis combining the results of this study with those of other published prospective studies.[42] They estimated a 2% risk of varicella embryopathy if infection occurred during the first 20 weeks of gestation. Enders et al. prospectively studied 1373 women with varicella and

366 with zoster during pregnancy. The risk of the fetal syndrome was 0.4% after maternal varicella in weeks 1 through 12, and 2% after maternal varicella in weeks 13 through 20.[43] Maternal zoster was not associated with fetal abnormalities.

Infection at any time during fetal life may result in latent infection that is poorly controlled by the host and subsequently reactivates as HZ early in life, in infancy or childhood.[41,44–46] Third-trimester infection may cause severe maternal infection, including pneumonia, as well as a life-threatening disseminated infection in the newborn. Maternal varicella that develops within 5 days before or 2 days after delivery is potentially the most serious for the newborn infant.[41] In the days immediately preceding delivery, protective maternal antibodies to VZV have not yet been formed or crossed the placenta, and after delivery, presumably because of the immaturity of cell-mediated immunity, the baby is at risk for development of an illness resembling varicella in a leukemic child. The infected infant may develop hemorrhagic skin lesions and primary varicella pneumonia, which can be avoided in many cases with prompt prophylactic administration of varicella-zoster immune globulin (VZIG) and judicious use of acyclovir (ACV).[41,46,47]

IMMUNOCOMPROMISED INDIVIDUALS

Varicella in an immunodeficient individual may lead to a more serious form of illness referred to as progressive varicella.[48] Individuals with malignant disease who are receiving chemotherapy, radiotherapy, or both—especially those with leukemia, those receiving high doses of steroids for any reason (i.e., organ transplantation, severe asthma), and those with congenital deficits in cell-mediated immunity—appear to be at greatest risk to develop severe varicella with complications. The association of a decreased immune response and severe varicella was first noted in the early 1950s.[49] In 1975, it was reported that 30% of children with leukemia with varicella developed disseminated infections, with 10% mortality.[50] By 1987, in the post–antiviral therapy era, morbidity and mortality had not changed substantially.[51] Complications from varicella have become more common as greater numbers of children are treated successfully for malignant disease,[50] are surviving transplantation,[52] and are receiving high doses of steroids for asthma.[53,54] Although severe and even fatal cases of varicella have been described in children with human immunodeficiency virus (HIV) infection, it appears that the magnitude of risk from varicella is not as great as for leukemic children.[55,56]

Herpes Zoster (Shingles)

During the primary infection with VZV, the virus migrates to the dorsal root and trigeminal ganglia, where it usually remains latent for the lifetime of the individual. It is hypothesized that the waning of cell-mediated immunity to VZV later in life or during immunosuppression resulting from a variety of causes enables the virus to reactivate, resulting in a unilateral, dermatomal, usually painful vesicular rash. The HZ rash may remain localized to one to three dermatomes, but in a minority of patients it disseminates outside the dermatomal area and causes widespread lesions

that resemble varicella. The rash begins as erythematous, maculopapular lesions that rapidly evolve into a vesicular rash. The vesicles may coalesce to form bullous lesions. In the immunocompetent host, these lesions continue to form over a period of 3 to 5 days, with the total duration of disease being 10 to 15 days. It may take as long as 1 month before the skin returns to normal. Occasional patients may develop dermatomal pain without cutaneous lesions (*zoster sine herpete*), which can be confirmed serologically to be HZ.

HZ may involve the eyelids when the first or second branch of the fifth cranial nerve is affected, but keratitis heralds a sight-threatening condition, herpes zoster ophthalmicus. Keratitis may be followed by severe iridocyclitis, secondary glaucoma, or neuroparalytic keratitis. When the geniculate ganglion is involved, the Ramsay Hunt syndrome may occur, with pain and vesicles in the external auditory meatus, loss of taste in the anterior two thirds of the tongue, and ipsilateral facial palsy. However, thoracic and lumbar dermatomes most commonly are involved. Motor paralysis can occur as a consequence of the involvement of the anterior horn cells in a manner similar to that encountered with polio. Neuromuscular disorders associated with HZ include Guillain-Barré syndrome, transverse myelitis, and myositis.[57–59]

The major risk factors for development of HZ are increasing age (>50 years), immunosuppression, and VZV infection acquired in utero or during the first year of life (possibly as a result of a poor cell-mediated immunity response to the virus at young ages).[44,45,60–62] In 1965, Hope-Simpson published estimates of incidence rates of 74 per 100,000 persons per year among children less than 10 years of age, increasing to 1010 per 100,000 persons per year among those 80 to 89 years of age.[63] Thus, if all persons were to live to the ninth decade, approximately 15% would develop HZ over their lifetime, with a sharp increase in the incidence of disease beginning at about age 50 years. In a more recent study by Schmader and colleagues, the lifetime incidence of HZ among African-Americans was half that reported by whites in a study of community-dwelling elderly residents of North Carolina.[64] After adjusting for age, cancer history, gender, education, and urban or rural residence, race remained a significant protective factor.

HZ is more common and more severe in immunocompromised than in immunologically normal individuals. Lesion formation continues for up to 2 weeks, and scabbing may not occur until 3 to 4 weeks into the disease course.[65] Immunosuppressed subjects are at risk for cutaneous dissemination and visceral involvement, including varicella pneumonitis, hepatitis, and meningoencephalitis. In leukemic children who have experienced varicella, a cumulative rate of HZ of about 15% has been observed.[66,67] As many as 30% of patients may develop HZ after bone marrow transplantation.[65] A similar percentage of adults with HIV infection may develop HZ.[68] Children who develop varicella after HIV infection has occurred are at even higher risk to develop HZ, especially if varicella occurs in the setting of a low CD4+ T-lymphocyte level, in which case the cumulative rate approaches 70%.[55] Chronic HZ has been reported in HIV-infected patients.[69] In these individuals, there is sustained new lesion formation with an absence of healing of the existing lesions. Many of these chronic syndromes have been associated with the isolation of VZV that is resistant to ACV.[70]

The most debilitating complication of HZ is postherpetic neuralgia. Postherpetic neuralgia is uncommon in young individuals, but may occur in 25% to 50% of patients developing zoster over the age of 50 years.[71–74] As many as 20% to 40% of patients over the age of 60 may experience postherpetic neuralgia of 3 months or longer. The case incidence of this complication is not known precisely because the definition of postherpetic neuralgia (including measures of severity and effect on quality of life) varies among studies.[74–77] Postherpetic neuralgia may cause constant pain in the involved dermatome or consist of intermittent stabbing pain. Pain is often reported to be worse at night or on exposure to temperature changes. In some patients, the pain is incapacitating.

Virology

VZV is a herpesvirus, a member of the subfamily Alphaherpesvirinae.[78] The virion is composed of approximately 125,000 base pairs, making it one of the smaller agents in the group. The entire genome has been sequenced.[79] The virus is characterized by (1) a linear genome of $80 \pm 3 \times 10^6$ Da with inverted terminal sequences present internally that result in two predominant isomeric DNA molecules,[80–82] (2) a relatively short replication cycle, (3) a host range limited to humans and some higher primates, and (4) frequent latent infection of sensory ganglia. The virions are round or polygonal with a central DNA core. The nucleocapsid is approximately 100 nm in diameter and consists of 162 hexagonal capsomeres organized as an icosahedron (20 sides) with a central axial hollow with 5:3:2 axial symmetry.[79] The capsid is surrounded by a tegument and an envelope derived in part from cellular membranes. The entire VZV particle is 180 to 200 nm in diameter. There are 70 open reading frames (ORFs) that encode for at least 68 viral gene products. VZV DNA is synthesized in a cascade of expression of immediate early (IE) or α regulatory genes, followed by expression of early

(E) or β genes that encode for regulatory and structural proteins, followed by expression of late (L) or γ genes that encode for structural proteins. Interruption of the cascade, particularly at the IE stage, can result in failure to synthesize infectious virus.[83]

At least 30 polypeptides, which are L gene products with different molecular weights, have been detected in VZV; at least 7 of these are glycosylated.[84,85] The known glycoproteins (gps) are termed B, C, E, H, I, K, and L (Fig. 28–2), corresponding to those of herpes simplex virus (HSV). There is, however, no equivalent of the major gp of HSV, gD, in VZV.[79] VZV gB is probably essential to infectivity, plays a role in fusion with other cells to facilitate infection, and is the target of neutralizing antibodies.[84–86] The major gp of VZV is gE, which is the most abundantly expressed gp and is highly immunogenic. It is linked to gI and with gI is an Fc receptor on infected cells.[87] It also binds to mannose 6-phosphate receptors, which may be critical to VZV infection, and it provides signal sequences that mediate assembly of viral proteins and envelopment in the trans-Golgi network.[88,89] gE and gI are thought to function as navigator gps, directing additional gps to the cell surface and trans-Golgi network, where final envelopment of virions takes place.[90–92] Recently, a new variant VZV virus lacking gE has been isolated from two individuals.[92a] Although the two viruses may be escape mutants arising from separate mutations, it is possible that there is a second serotype of VZV circulating in northern North America. The biological significance of this variant remains to be defined. VZV gH, when complexed with gL, is involved in cell-to-cell spread by inducing membrane fusion, and it is a target of neutralizing antibodies.[89,93–95] In addition to glycosylated proteins, some IE gene products of VZV are also immunogenic.[96] IE62 protein, which is encoded by VZV ORF 62, is closely related to the regulatory polypeptide Vmw175 (or ICP4) of HSV 1.[97] This protein was at one time thought to be purely nonstructural, as is ICP4 for HSV. However, IE62 protein has been identified as a major component of the VZV tegument[98] that is also highly immunogenic.[99] With regard to gene expression and regulation, IE62 protein is the initial transactivating protein of VZV. Other regulatory proteins of VZV are encoded by ORFs 4, 10, 61, and 63.[100–104]

During latent infection, several VZV genes are expressed in sensory ganglia; these are mostly IE genes (ORFs 4, 62, and 63). There is also some E gene expression (ORFs 21, 29), but L genes are not expressed.[83,105–107] This degree of gene expression during latency is considerably more extensive than that seen in latent infection with HSV and suggests that, even during latent VZV infection, a certain degree of viral replication is occurring. Although some investigators have localized latent VZV infection either to satellite cells[108] or to neurons,[109] others have demonstrated latent VZV in both neurons and satellite cells of sensory human ganglia.[110] It is thought, however, that latent infection occurs primarily in neurons.[111–113] Reactivation of VZV with production of infectious virions in human neurons in dorsal root ganglia has been visualized using in situ hybridization to identify VZV DNA in autopsy specimens.[110] Patients with impaired cell-mediated immunity have an increased incidence of HZ, which is consistent with the hypothesis that at least some aspects of suppression of

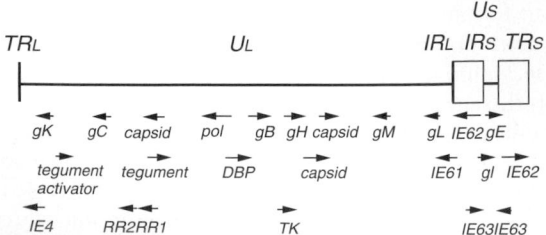

FIGURE 28–2 ■ Diagram of the structure of the VZV genome. The linear double-stranded DNA consists of a long unique segment (U$_L$) of approximately 199 kbp, flanked by terminal and internal repeats (TR$_L$ and IR$_L$), and a short unique sequence (U$_S$) of approximately 5.4 kbp, flanked by terminal and internal repeats of 6.8 kbp (TR$_S$ and IR$_S$). The direction of transcription (arrows) of some of the important gene products are indicated below the map.

VZV reactivation are under immunologic control.[28,66,114] An animal model of latent VZV infection in the rat has been developed that may help to clarify how latent infection with VZV is maintained.[115–117] An in vitro model of VZV latency in isolated sensory ganglia from guinea pigs that can be manipulated to reactivate also has been described.[118]

Growth of VZV in cell monolayer cultures is rather slow, with poor infectious yields and the absence of infectious virions in supernatant media. Viral spread occurs directly from an infected cell to another uninfected cell. Within the infected individual, VZV also spreads only from cell to cell, which is probably why cellular immunity is crucial in host defense. In order to obtain cell-free VZV in vitro, infectious virions must be released artificially by disruption of cells by methods such as sonication or freeze-thawing.[28] The cell-associated nature of the virus has tended to impede research on VZV and undoubtedly slowed vaccine development as well.

Pathogenesis as It Relates to Prevention

Varicella is a highly contagious disease. VZV spreads by the airborne route,[119,120] and infectivity is maximal in the early stages of the illness.[121] Infectivity is postulated to occur by droplet or aerosol of vesicular fluid from skin lesions, or from respiratory secretions from infected patients.[121–124] Studies of transmission of vaccine-type VZV in leukemic vaccinees have implicated skin lesions as the source of infectious virus.[124] In patients with varicella, virus isolation in cell culture from skin is easily accomplished, but it is extremely difficult to isolate VZV from respiratory secretions.[125] Limited epidemiologic data, however, suggest that respiratory spread can occur.[126] Data from polymerase chain reaction (PCR) studies of respiratory secretions have yielded differing results and have not clarified the issue of whether respiratory spread of VZV is significant. In one study, only 1 (3.3%) of 30 oropharyngeal samples was positive for VZV DNA during the first day of the rash of chickenpox,[123] but in another study 26% and 90% of samples were positive during the incubation period and after clinical onset, respectively.[122] In yet another study, VZV DNA was detected in the respiratory tract of 45 patients with varicella in 28 patients (62%) on day 1, in 50% on day 6, and in 22% after day 6.[127] The different rates of positivity obtained in various studies may reflect differences in primers used as well as differences in techniques for collection of respiratory secretions. The demonstration of VZV DNA, however, does not necessarily indicate the presence of infectious virus in respiratory secretions. There is more evidence that VZV is spread from skin lesions than that it is spread from the respiratory tract.

In infection, the site of host invasion of VZV appears to be the conjunctivae or the mucosa of the upper respiratory tract or both. Based on the mouse pox model of Fenner,[14] it is hypothesized that, in primary infection, VZV replicates locally in the lymph nodes for several days, causing a primary viremia of low magnitude that delivers the virus to the viscera, where further multiplication occurs. A demonstrable secondary viremia of greater magnitude subsequently results (see Fig. 28–2). Culture of mononuclear cells from 5 days before to 2 days after appearance of rash in patients with natural varicella (Table 28–1) has yielded VZV,[128–133]

TABLE 28–1 ■ Isolation of Varicella-Zoster Virus from Mononucleocytes of Children with Typical Courses of Varicella

	Day	VZV Isolation	Contact
Before rash (total 15 cases)	11	0/1	Family
	7	0/1	School
	6	0/1	Family
	5	1/2	Family
	4	1/2	Family
	2	4/4	Family
	1	4/4	Family
Rash	0	1/2	
After rash (total 9 cases)	1	3/4	
	2	0/2	
	3	0/1	

Adapted from Ozaki T, Ichikawa T, Matsui Y, et al. Viremic phase in nonimmunocompromised children with varicella. J Pediatr 104:85–87, 1984; and Asano Y, Itakura N, Hiroishi Y, et al. Viremia is present in the incubation period in nonimmunocompromised children with varicella. J Pediatr 106:69–71, 1985.

as has PCR.[127,134] The presence of VZV in CD4+ and CD8+ T lymphocytes also has been demonstrated by in situ hybridization during early varicella.[123] In a model of VZV infection in the SCID-hu mouse, VZV also could be detected in human T lymphocytes.[135] Viremia also has been demonstrated in patients with disseminated HZ using either virus isolation or PCR.[136–138]

Immune Response to VZV

The precise roles of humoral immunity and cell-mediated immunity in protection against VZV infection are not entirely understood but are summarized as follows (reviewed by Arvin and Gershon[52]).

Cell-Mediated Immunity

Both structural and regulatory proteins of VZV are recognized during varicella by T lymphocytes, which induce protection from further VZV infection. Immunity usually is maintained for decades and is mediated by both CD4+ and CD8+ T lymphocytes, which can be demonstrated by cell proliferation and cytokine production in vitro after antigenic stimulation. Memory T lymphocytes belong to the CD45RO+CCR7- phenotype.[139] Memory responses may be maintained in part because of periodic exogenous re-exposure to others with either varicella or HZ, as well as by endogenous re-exposure to the virus during subclinical reactivation of VZV. T lymphocytes from varicella-immune individuals produce cytokines of the Th1 type, such as interleukin-2 and interferon-γ, which potentiate clonal expansion of virus-specific T cells on exposure to VZV antigens.[28] CD4+ T lymphocytes provide help so that humoral responses to VZV antigens develop and are maintained following varicella.

Cell-mediated immunity to VZV is important in recovery from VZV infections in which cell-to-cell spread is occurring and also in prevention of development of clinical HZ. That cell-mediated immunity is required to maintain the balance between the host and latent VZV is suggested by the correlation between diminished cell-mediated immunity and an increased risk of HZ. Susceptibility of individuals to VZV reactivation is not related to diminished levels of VZV antibodies. Cell-mediated immunity appears to be the response of major importance in control of VZV by the host. This is seen most clearly from clinical observations that patients with isolated agammaglobulinemia have normal courses of varicella and are not subject to an increased incidence of HZ, while those with defects in cell-mediated immunity are at risk to develop disseminated and possibly fatal varicella.

Cell-mediated immunity to VZV after immunization has been determined mainly by lymphocyte transformation to VZV antigen, expressed as a stimulation index, and with an intradermal skin test. Cell-mediated immune responses measured by lymphocyte transformation and skin test are promptly detected after natural infection; peak activity occurs within 1 to 2 weeks and then gradually decreases to lower levels.[140-146] In vitro, cell-mediated immunity to VZV can be detected by stimulation of lymphocytes in vitro with VZV antigens,[66,114,147-150] and by specific lysis of histocompatible target cells by cytotoxic T cells stimulated with VZV antigen.[151-153] Natural killer cell and antibody-dependent cellular toxicity to VZV have also been reported.[154-156]

Cell-mediated immune responses develop within days after onset of clinical varicella and remain positive for many years; however declining cell-mediated immunity is noted with advancing age, beginning at about age 50 years.[149,157,158] Decreased cell-mediated immunity to VZV is a necessary but not sufficient requirement for development of HZ.[147] Patients with poor cell-mediated immune responses during varicella are also at risk to develop severe or fatal varicella.[147]

Cell-mediated immune responses of normal subjects with remote clinical evidence of varicella are characterized by occasional high activity in the absence of symptoms, suggesting either exposure to VZV with boosting of immunity or possibly subclinical reactivation of VZV.[159] Increases in cell-mediated immunity usually occur after HZ, even in immunocompromised patients, which probably accounts for the observation that second attacks of HZ are uncommon.[160] Subclinical viremia has been demonstrated in immunocompromised individuals following bone marrow transplantation.[161]

Class I restricted lysis of VZV-infected target cells has been described following immunization of elderly seropositive individuals. This cell-mediated immune response was more prominent in subjects who were immunized with live varicella vaccine compared with those who were given a similar dose of inactivated vaccine.[162]

Humoral Immunity

Serum Immunoglobulin M Antibody Response. After natural varicella, serum VZV immunoglobulin M (IgM) is detectable for days to weeks. This antibody is also detectable following zoster, so that its presence does not serve to differentiate between varicella and zoster (i.e., primary vs. secondary infection). As with many IgM tests, false-negative and false-positive reactions may occur.[26,163] The kinetics of humoral, nasopharyngeal, and cellular immunity in patients with clinical varicella are shown in Figure 28-3.

Serum Immunoglobulin G Antibody Response. After natural infection, VZV-specific immunoglobulin G (IgG) antibody, as measured by the fluorescent antibody to mem-

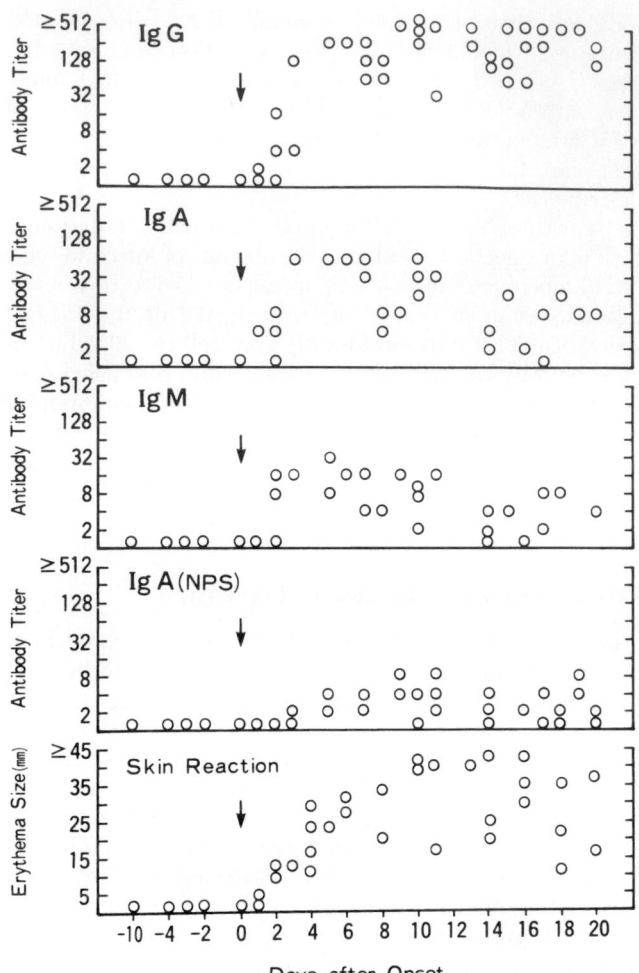

FIGURE 28-3 ■ The kinetics of appearance of humoral (blood), nasopharyngeal (NPS, secretory), and cellular (skin reactive) immunity in patients with clinical varicella. The antibody titers were measured by fluorescent antibody to membrane antibody. *Arrows* at day 0 indicate the onset of varicella infection. (From Baba K, Yabuuchi H, Takahashi M, et al. Seroepidemiologic behavior of varicella-zoster virus infection in semiclosed community after introduction of VZV vaccine. J Pediatr 105:712–716, 1984, with permission.)

brane antigen (FAMA) test, is detected in most patients within the first 4 days after the onset of rash and other symptoms.[142] Peak IgG levels are attained at 4 to 8 weeks, and levels usually remain high for up to 6 to 8 months, after which titers decline two- to threefold. Positive VZV FAMA titers have been detected in 100% of healthy adults for years to decades after clinical varicella.[27,164-167]

Serum Immunoglobulin A Antibody Responses. Serum immunoglobulin A (IgA) antibody responses to natural infection are detectable very early in the course of varicella, in most cases within the first 3 to 4 days after the onset of symptoms.[142] Serum IgA antibody responses attain peak levels by the fourth week of illness. Although levels subsequently decline, serum IgA antibody was detected in 44% of subjects up to 14 months after varicella.[142]

Nasopharyngeal Humoral Immune Response. Nasopharyngeal VZV-specific IgA antibody responses are detectable at the onset of clinical symptoms in patients with natural infections.[168] Nearly all patients exhibit IgA antibody responses within the first week. Maximum titers are attained at the third week of illness, and the IgA antibody activity declines subsequently.

Diagnosis

The diagnosis of varicella usually can be made clinically by the characteristic rash and epidemiologic factors such as age of the patient, lack of history of the illness, and exposure to individuals with varicella or HZ in the previous 2 to 3 weeks. HZ, however, may be confused with recurrent HSV infection, especially if the face or trunk is involved and there is no previous history of a similar rash.[169] When deemed necessary, laboratory diagnosis is best made either by demonstration of viral antigens in scrapings from skin vesicles, or by isolation of VZV from these lesions. Rapid diagnosis can be accomplished by direct immunofluorescence assay. This test is carried out by scraping a suspicious skin lesion, making a smear on a microscope slide, fixing with ethanol or acetone, and staining with commercially produced fluorescein-tagged monoclonal antibody to VZV gE.[125,170] This assay is widely available.

The virus may be isolated in human embryonic lung fibroblasts (HELF), with the appearance of cytopathic effect within 2 days to several weeks after inoculation. PCR has been employed successfully for diagnosis of VZV infection, utilizing vesicular fluid, respiratory secretions, and cerebrospinal fluid.[122,123,171–177] Although PCR is still primarily a research tool, it is now more clinically available than previously and is becoming more widely used. It appears to be more sensitive than either immunofluorescence or virus isolation for diagnosis of infection with this labile agent.[171,172,175,178]

Serologic tests for VZV-specific antibody permit documentation of immunity to varicella, and also diagnosis of varicella by a fourfold or greater rise in antibody titer following the illness. Serologic tests are of limited value for the diagnosis of HZ, however, because heterologous rises in VZV antibody titer may occur when HSV reactivates in an individual immune to varicella.[125] It is possible to make the diagnosis of active VZV infection on a single serum specimen by demonstration of specific antibody to VZV IgM; VZV IgM may be detected in HZ as well as in varicella.[125] The complement fixation (CF) test has largely been replaced by enzyme-linked immunosorbent assay (ELISA) for measurement of IgG antibodies to VZV. ELISA assays are fairly specific, but as many as 10% false-positive reactions in true susceptibles have been recorded.[179] Commercially available ELISA tests are also less sensitive than the FAMA test,[125,164,179,180] but ELISA tests have the advantage of being more adaptable to large-scale testing than the very sensitive but cumbersome FAMA test. An ELISA that uses gp of VZV for antigen has been reported to be highly sensitive,[181] but it is not commercially available. Moreover, positive antibody titers detected by this method in some 2-year-old children (and older children as well) prior to developing varicella suggest that the assay may be overly sensitive.[182] However, this assay has shown reproducibility when different batches of vaccine were used for immunization, and there was an excellent linear concordance when neutralizing antibody levels and gp ELISA titers were compared.[183]

An immune adherence hemagglutination (IAHA) assay has been described that has been utilized to analyze seroconversions to VZV, particularly in studies in Japan.[184,185] A latex agglutination (LA) assay based on the clumping of latex particles coated with VZV gps, observed in the presence of VZV antibody, combines the sensitivity of FAMA with the ease of performance of ELISA.[165,166] In addition, this assay can be performed within 15 minutes and requires no complicated equipment. There is a high degree of correlation between the presence of antibodies to VZV measured by FAMA and LA after close exposure to VZV, and protection from varicella after natural infection as well as after immunization.[165,166] Experience in reading the test is useful because the identification of agglutination is somewhat subjective. As with many serologic tests, moreover, occasional false-positive and false-negative reactions have been reported.[186] A reliable, sensitive, rapid means of identifying individuals who have immunity to VZV, particularly following immunization, continues to be needed.

Treatment and Prevention

Useful antiviral therapy for varicella and HZ first became available in the early 1970s. Antiviral therapy is helpful to speed recovery from varicella and HZ, especially in elderly and immunocompromised patients, but it does not decrease virus shedding or prevent latent infection. Vidarabine was the first successful antiviral drug to be used, but it was supplanted by ACV, a DNA chain terminator and an inhibitor of DNA polymerase that is less toxic than vidarabine.[187–189] Intravenous ACV speeds healing of varicella and HZ in immunocompromised patients, and orally administered ACV, at high doses, is used to treat patients with HZ, particularly those over 50 years of age.[187–191] Orally administered ACV may be used to treat otherwise healthy children with varicella, but the antiviral effect on varicella is minimal in part because of the poor absorption of the drug when given orally and the lower sensitivity of VZV to ACV, in comparison to that of HSV. A double-blind placebo-controlled study in which 102 healthy children were given ACV 40 to 80 mg/kg (or placebo) daily for 5 days, beginning within 24 hours of rash onset, revealed that the mean number of skin lesions was significantly reduced from over 500 to 336.[18] On average, there was 1 day less of fever, but children who were treated with ACV did not return to school any more rapidly than those who received placebo. A multicenter collaborative study involving 815 similarly treated children, given 80 mg/kg of ACV daily, yielded similar results.[192] The benefit to secondary household cases was not increased beyond that of primary cases. The modest benefit conferred by ACV therapy is not surprising in view of the self-limited nature of chickenpox in children. Studies in adolescents[193] and adults[194] have not indicated more striking antiviral effects, although ACV frequently is administered to these groups because they are at higher risk to develop severe varicella than healthy children. A study in otherwise healthy children with varicella indicated that 5 days of oral ACV was as effective as 7 days.[195]

The newer oral antiviral drug, valacyclovir (VCV), which is well absorbed from the gastrointestinal tract and is rapidly converted to ACV in the body, results in blood levels of ACV that are significantly higher than those achieved by administering ACV orally. Although VCV has efficacy for treatment of HZ,[196] no studies of varicella have been performed, nor have children participated in any clinical trials of this drug. Famciclovir (FCV), which is also administered orally, is rapidly converted to penciclovir in the body; penciclovir has an action similar to that of ACV. As is the case for VCV, FCV is useful for treatment of HZ but has not been studied for treatment of varicella.[197,198] The antiviral drug soruvidine[40] was not approved by the Food and Drug Administration (FDA) in the United States because of the lack of significant benefit over ACV and the potential for toxicity in patients being treated for cancer.

Postexposure prophylaxis with antiviral therapy for prevention of varicella has been tried and met with some success in small studies. Acyclovir was administered to 25 children following household exposure and prevented disease in most patients.[199] Of patients who have been studied, immunity appears to persist for several years even with no evidence of clinical disease.[200] Unfortunately, however, less than 85% of patients will develop antibodies to VZV after this form of prophylaxis, and therefore, to be assured of adequate future protection, VZV antibody titers must be determined some weeks afterward.[201] Alternatively, varicella vaccine subsequently may be administered. Although dosages and timing have varied, administration of ACV at a dose of 10 to 20 mg/kg four times a day between days 7 and 14 after exposure was most usually used. Prophylaxis administered earlier than 1 week after exposure does not seem to provide as good protection.[202] There are no published studies in which immunization and antiviral therapy have been combined. This approach also has not been studied in immunocompromised individuals, for whom prophylaxis with passive immunization is preferable (see *Varicella-Zoster Immune Globulin* below). In areas where passive immunization is not available, an alternative approach would be to treat immunocompromised patients who develop varicella with ACV at the very first sign of illness. Thus for control of varicella, and possibly of HZ, prevention of chickenpox by vaccination would seem to offer greater potential benefit.

Epidemiology

Incidence and Seroprevalence

Varicella is a highly contagious disease that occurs worldwide and, in the absence of a vaccination program, in most populations it affects nearly every person by mid-adulthood. HZ cases represent a method for regular exposure and introduction of VZV into communities that otherwise may not be large enough to sustain endemic transmission of VZV. The epidemiology of varicella differs between temperate and tropical climates; these differences may relate to climate, population density, and the risk of exposure.[203–206] In temperate climates, virtually all persons are infected by age 15 years, with the highest incidence of disease occurring among children 1 to 9 years of age.[207] In tropical climates, cases are acquired at older ages, with a higher proportion of cases and higher susceptibility among adults. In temperate climates, varicella shows a strong seasonal pattern with peak incidence in late winter and spring, and seasonality also has been described in many tropical climates, with peak incidence in the cooler, drier months.[206]

Prior to the national varicella vaccination program in the United States, annual varicella incidence measured from national household survey data was 15.0 to 16.0 cases per 1000 population.[206,207] These rates represent averaged rates over a decade; significant variations in incidence from year to year have been described from the United States and other countries.[29,208–214] In other temperate climates, reported incidence using different methods of data collection have been generally lower than U.S. rates. In the United Kingdom, surveillance data reported by physicians show average reported rates of disease of 5.0 (range 2.4 to 8.8) per 1000 total population,[211] notification rates in Scotland vary from 4.8 to 7.9 per 1000 total population,[208] and in France, reported rates vary from 10 to 13.5 cases per 1000 total population.[209] Lower disease incidence from hospital- and physician-based surveillance probably reflects incomplete levels of reporting and the fact that not all varicella cases are seen by a physician or nurse.[29,206] Higher rates are likely to reflect data collection during epidemic disease years.

Before introduction of varicella vaccine in the United States in 1995, varicella age-specific incidence had shifted to earlier ages, with children in the preschool and early elementary school years (approximately ages 3 to 7 years) having the highest age-specific incidence; one regional study showed peak diseases incidence as early as 2 years.[215,216] These data are consistent with findings in France, where the highest age-specific incidence in the 1990s was reported in preschool-age children (1 to 4 years)[209]; in Italy, where national disease reporting during 1991 to 1996 showed the highest rate of varicella notifications among children 0 to 4 years of age[217] and where a sentinel physician study showed the highest varicella incidence among children 3 to 5 years of age[218]; in England and Wales, where an increase in reported cases among children less than 5 years old and changes in age-related VZV seroprevalence have occurred over the past 25 years[219,220]; and in Scotland, where there has been an increase in incidence among 1- to 4-year-old children from 1981 to 1998.[208] In Slovenia, during the last 10 years, the highest incidence of reported varicella has occurred among children 1 to 2 years of age, followed by children 2 to 3 years of age.[212]

VZV seroprevalence data reflect age-specific disease incidence. Seroprevalence data from a nationally representative population-based survey in the United States with 18,000 persons tested in the prevaccine era (1988 to 1994) demonstrated a high VZV seroprevalence in the U.S. population: 86% for 6- to 11-year-olds, 93% for 12- to 19-year-olds, 95.5 % for 20- to 29-year-olds, and 99% or greater for adults 30 years and older.[221] More than 90% of adolescents or young adults are VZV seropositive in Germany, Spain, Japan, Switzerland, Czechoslovakia, Brazil, and the United Kingdom,[213,219,222–226] with lower seroprevalence reported in Italy among 10- to 14-year-old children (82.1%) and 15- to 19-year-olds (~ 85%),[217] and in Australia, where 78% of 14- to 19-year-old women attending antenatal clinics were seropositive.[227] Differences in seroprevalence have been described by race, gender, country of origin, and number of siblings in the household.[221,222,228–231]

In tropical climates, VZV seroprevalence reflects a higher mean age of infection than in temperate climates,[203,232–235] with higher susceptibility among adults. In such countries, seroprevalence among adolescents or young adults has ranged from 10% to 20% in St. Lucia (an island community) to 80% to 100% in Taiwan and urban Calcutta, India.[203,206,234,236–248] In a study in Thailand, differences in VZV seroprevalence were described according to climate, with significantly higher age-adjusted seroprevalence in the cooler than in the warmer regions.[204] In the warmer regions only, the age-specific seroprevalence was significantly higher in the urban population than the rural population, as was also described in India.[205] In contrast, high seroprevalence among women of child-bearing age has been described from tropical areas in Australia,[249] and, in Eritrea, VZV seroprevalence among an isolated adult population was 44% compared with other adult groups in the same areas, among whom immunity ranged from 91% to 96%.[250]

Significance as a Public Health Problem

In countries that have achieved control or elimination of other vaccine-preventable diseases using vaccines recommended for routine use in childhood (including those for polio, diphtheria/pertussis/tetanus, measles, mumps, rubella, *Haemophilus influenzae* type b, and hepatitis B), understanding the health burden and costs that result from varicella and HZ, as well as the costs and benefits of various vaccination strategies, is important for considering a varicella vaccination program. In the immediate prevaccine era in the United States, there were an average of 4 million cases of varicella each year (15.0 to 16.0 cases per 1000 population) that resulted in an average of 10,500 hospitalizations (4.1 hospitalizations per 100,000 population) and 100 deaths every year (0.4 per million population).[38,207,251,252] In 2002, the global annual disease burden resulting from varicella can be estimated as 75 million cases using an incidence rate of 15 cases per 1000 population per year applied to the global population of approximately 5 billion. Despite the lower population incidence of HZ, the health burden resulting from this condition is considerable.[227,253–255]

In developed countries where data on mortality have been reported, overall varicella mortality has ranged from 0.20 to 0.65 per million population in the United States, with similar mortality rates reported from Australia and the United Kingdom[38,227,254,256] Population-based case-fatality data have been described only from developed countries; in both the United States and the United Kingdom, the highest risk of death occurs in adults, with case-fatality rates of 20 per 100,000 cases, 20 to 25 times higher than case-fatality rates for preschool-age children (0.7 to 0.8 per 100,000 cases).[38,254,256] After deaths, hospitalizations caused by varicella provide the next best estimate of the burden of severe disease. These data are important for describing morbidity and for calculating the economic and social costs of varicella infection, which may now be prevented by vaccination. Various studies have described annual rates of varicella hospitalizations in the range of 4.0 to 4.5 per 100,000 population,[252,254,255] with lower hospitalization rates (2.6 to 3.2 per 100,000) reported from Spain[257] and higher rates (3.1 to 9.9) reported from Scotland.[208] The risk of hospitalization varies by age. Reflecting the high incidence among children, the majority of varicella hospitalizations (approximately two thirds) also occur among children; however, infants and adults are at significantly increased risk of severe disease and hospitalization compared with children 1 to 4 and 5 to 9 years of age.[36,207,252,254]

There are few data on the health burden of varicella in developing countries, in countries with high HIV seroprevalence, and in countries with tropical climates where a higher proportion of varicella cases may occur among adults. In these situations, varicella morbidity and mortality may be higher than described in developed countries.

Passive Immunization

Ordinary Immunoglobulin G

The first studies indicating that varicella could be modified by administration of human immune globulin (IG) following exposure to VZV were reported by Ross et al.[17] He and his co-workers demonstrated that varicella could be attenuated by giving IG to varicella-susceptible children within 72 hours after household exposure. Larger doses of IG produced decreasing numbers of skin lesions. However, no completely preventive effect of IG was noted at any dosage level.

Varicella-Zoster Immune Globulin

When globulin prepared from serum of patients recovering from HZ with high VZV antibody titers was given to children who had been exposed to varicella, chickenpox was prevented.[258] This material, termed *zoster immune globulin* (ZIG), was first tested in a double-blind controlled fashion in healthy children, for whom a dose of 2 mL, administered within 72 hours of exposure, prevented varicella. In a subsequent efficacy study, 15 children who were undergoing therapy for leukemia or other malignant disease who had household exposures to varicella were given a 5-mL dose of ZIG within 72 hours of exposure. Varicella was severe in one child, mild in nine, and subclinical in five. All children had persistence of antibodies to VZV for at least 2 years, suggesting that ZIG modified varicella in these high-risk children, although it did not prevent infection.[259]

It was subsequently determined that a high-potency globulin with titers equal to those in ZIG could be prepared by using outdated units of plasma with high VZV antibody titers.[260] This material was termed *varicella-zoster immune globulin*, and it was licensed and recommended for use in the United States in the early 1980s, with revised recommendations by the Centers for Disease Control and Prevention (CDC) in 1996.[261,262] It is estimated that VZIG contains more than 10 times the amount of antibody to VZV as does ordinary IG.

Zoster immune plasma (ZIP) has efficacy in preventing or modifying varicella in immunocompromised patients,[263,264] but treatment of immunocompromised patients with disseminated HZ with ZIP is not effective.[265] This is not surprising because HZ may occur in the face of high antibody titers to VZV.

Passive immunization is thus known to be effective against chickenpox. On occasion, however, varicella may be severe in passively immunized immunocompromised children, including newborns, despite use of the correct dose at the proper time.[51,259,265,266] Passive immunization, moreover is of limited use because an exposure to VZV must be recognized in order for it to be given.

Active Immunization

The KMcC Candidate Vaccine Strain

The Oka strain of VZV is the only vaccine strain that is currently available for use. Prior to clinical trials with this vaccine in the 1970s, however, another candidate vaccine strain (KMcC) was developed by serial passage of VZV in human diploid cells and underwent a few clinical trials.[267,268] It was tested at the 40th and 50th passage levels in healthy children; 26 children were given the passage-40 vaccine, and 17 were given passage-50 vaccine. The seroconversion rate for children in both groups was 100%. Papular skin lesions occurred in 31% of the passage-40 vaccinees but only in 6% of the passage-50 vaccinees.

A series of 10 clinical trials were performed in which either the Oka or one of the two passages of the KMcC strain of varicella vaccine was administered to 369 children.[140] Postimmunization clinical reactivity, mainly in the form of skin rash, was minimal with the Oka and the KMcC passage-50 vaccine, but was unacceptably high (31%) following the KMcC passage-40 vaccine. Immunogenicity of both KMcC strains was high: 93% to 100% of vaccinees seroconverted by the FAMA assay, and/or developed positive in vitro lymphocyte proliferation responses to VZV antigen. There were at least 281 known varicella exposures in vaccinees. A high degree of protection from or modification of varicella was observed 9 to 48 months after immunization with each strain. Five episodes of mild varicella, however, occurred in children who experienced a seroconversion after immunization. The KMcC passage-50 vaccine was judged unacceptable because all these episodes occurred in children who received passage-50, and thus it seemed insufficiently protective. Comparatively better immunogenicity of the Oka strain versus the KMcC strain also was noted in rhesus monkeys.[269] The passage-40 KMcC vaccine also was judged unacceptable because of its high rate of vaccine-associated rash. In summary, it did not seem possible to obtain a passage of the KMcC candidate vaccine strain with an acceptably low degree of reactogenicity that was sufficiently effective; the passage that was highly immunogenic was unacceptably reactogenic, whereas the one that was not reactogenic was also not strongly immunogenic.

The Oka Vaccine Strain

Description and Development

The Oka strain of varicella vaccine was developed as follows[10,270]: (1) fluid was taken from the vesicles of a 3-year-old boy (whose family name was Oka) who had typical chickenpox but who was otherwise healthy, and (2) VZV was isolated in primary HELF cell cultures. Attempts to obtain an attenuated strain of virus were made by serial cultivation 11 times at 34°C in HELF and 12 passages in guinea pig fibroblast cells (GPFC). Because GPFC are non-

primate cells in which VZV can be propagated, these cells were hypothesized to be suitable for obtaining a VZV variant that might become attenuated for the human host. Finally, there were two passages in WI-38 human diploid cells to prepare the master seed virus, followed by three passages in MRC-5 human diploid cells to prepare the seed virus. Vaccine pools usually were made after two to three additional passages in MRC-5 cells.

For vaccine preparation, infected tissue cultures were washed with phosphate-buffered saline, and infected cells were harvested in the presence of ethylenediaminetetra-acetic acid. The cell suspension in vaccine medium was then sonicated to obtain cell-free virus; a titer of 1500 to 5000 plaque-forming units (PFU) per milliliter of VZV usually was obtained. Initial safety testing of the vaccine included demonstration of lack of pathogenicity after parenteral and intracerebral inoculation of small animals and monkeys. The absence of C-type particles and latent viruses was confirmed morphologically and biochemically.

The Oka strain (parental and vaccine) and wild-type VZV (Dumas) have been sequenced. A number of sequence differences have been identified, particularly in ORF 62. However, it is not known which, if any, of these mutations are responsible for attenuation of the vaccine strain.[271–274]

Vaccine Virus Attributes

The vaccine virus has various biologic and biophysical attributes that can be used to distinguish it from wild-type viruses.[13,148,275–278] These include the following.

TEMPERATURE SENSITIVITIES

The vaccine strain is slightly temperature sensitive at 39°C, in comparison to wild-type strains. The foci of the vaccine strains are also smaller than those of wild-type strains at high temperatures but similar in size to the wild-type strains at lower temperatures.[13]

DIFFERENCE IN INFECTIVITY IN GUINEA PIG EMBRYO FIBROBLASTS AND HELF

The infectivities of the vaccine strain and wild-type strains are different by plaque titration assay on guinea pig embryo fibroblasts (GPEF) and HELF. The vaccine strain exhibits a ratio of infectivity in GPEF compared to HELF ranging from 10 to 50 times higher than that demonstrated with 12 wild-type strains, including the Oka parental wild-type strain. Presumably, this increased infectivity of the vaccine strain in guinea pig cell cultures is due to its prior adaptation in these cells during attenuation.[13,279] The immunogenicity of the vaccine virus is also far better than that of other wild-type viruses in guinea pigs,[278,280] which is also probably related to the difference in the capacity of the vaccine virus to replicate in cultured guinea pig cells.

DNA CLEAVAGE PROFILE

Differences in the migration patterns of DNA fragments of the vaccine-type virus and other wild-type strains can be demonstrated after cleavage of purified DNA obtained from viruses propagated in cell cultures, using restriction endonucleases. In a comparison of DNA from the vaccine-type virus and wild-type viruses, significantly different cleavage patterns were seen using HpaI, BamHI, BglI, and PstI enzymes.[275,277,279] In early studies in the United States employing *Bgl*I, it was noted that a novel restriction site in vaccine-type virus resulted in a different pattern of migration of fragments A through C in comparison with wild-type VZV[277] (Fig. 28–4). This distinction was attributed to differences between most but not all American and Japanese circulating wild-type viruses, rather than a marker of attenuation.[276] With *Pst*I, an additional cleavage site is present in wild-type virus (between the O and L fragments) that is not found in vaccine-type virus.[275,281]

A more practical approach that does not require virus isolation to distinguish between vaccine-type and wild-type VZV utilizes PCR and restriction endonuclease digestion of the resulting DNA fragments.[281] This method is based on the above-noted differences between wild-type VZV and the Oka strain. Two primer pairs are used, one that generates a 220-bp fragment flanking a novel *Bgl*I restriction site in vaccine-type virus and another that generates a 350-bp fragment that is cleaved in all wild-type VZVs. The resulting amplification products are subjected to digestion with *Bgl*I and *Pst*I restriction enzymes, and the fragments are separated by electrophoresis in a 4% agarose gel. By examining the number and sizes of the DNA fragments, wild- and vaccine-type viruses can be distinguished (Fig. 28–5). In a series of 19 VZV isolates, there was 100% correlation between standard analysis of VZV isolates by culture, purification of DNA, and restriction endonuclease digestion and

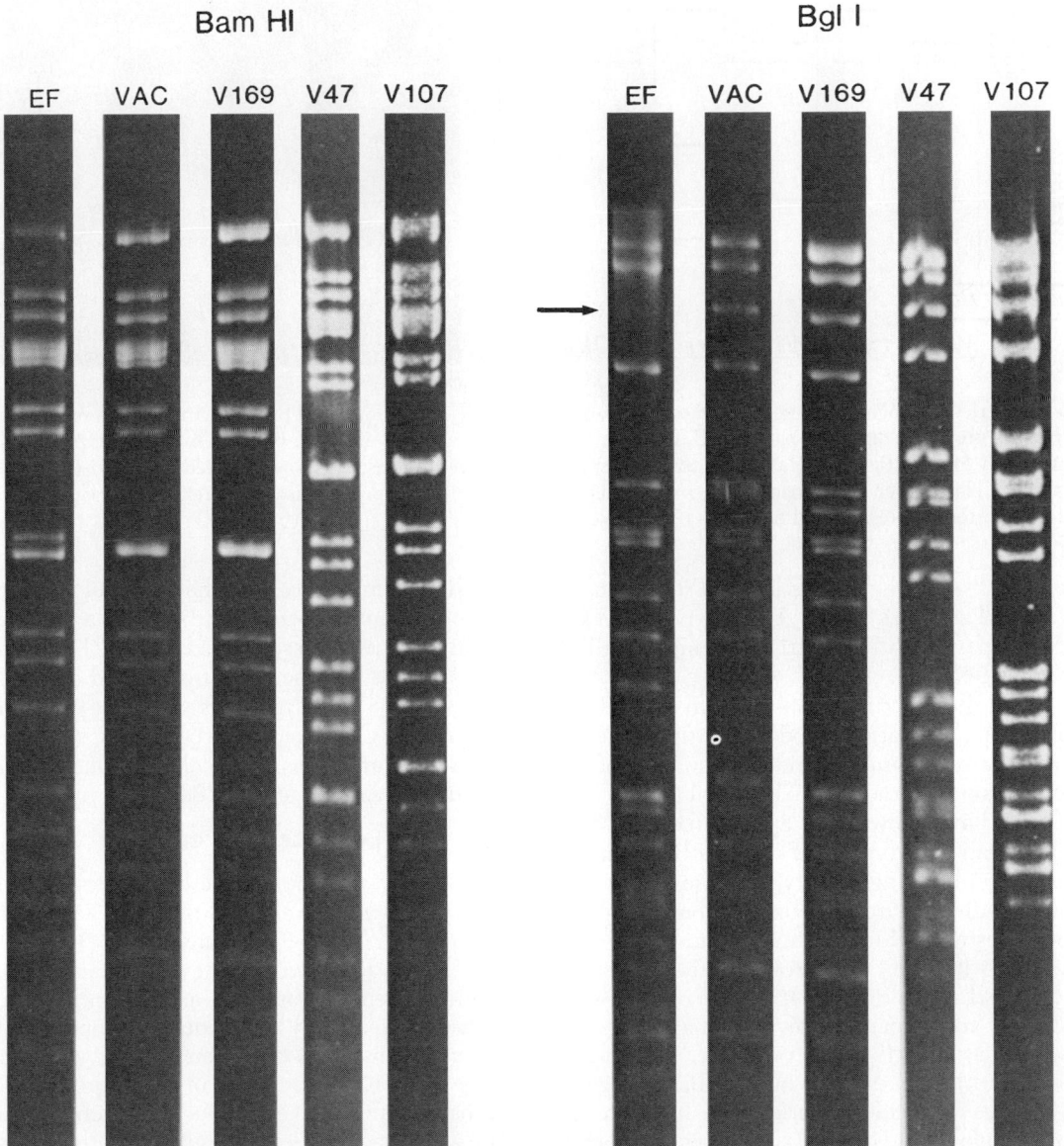

FIGURE 28–4 ■ Restriction endonuclease analysis of VZV isolates obtained from vaccinees with a rash after immunization (V47 and V107) and from a varicella-susceptible sibling (V169) exposed to a leukemic vaccinee with mild vaccine-associated rash. Strains studied here are all vaccine type. Viral DNA was digested with *Bam*HI or *Bgl*I, processed by electrophoresis through 0.8% agarose, and stained with ethidium bromide. EF is wild-type virus control, and VAC is Oka vaccine control. The illustration is a composite of several gels, causing apparent minor differences between isolates. The arrow points to *Bgl*I A, B, and C fragment migration characteristic of Oka vaccine strain. (From Gershon AA, Gelb L, LaRussa P. Live attenuated varicella vaccine: efficacy for children with leukemia in remission. JAMA 252:355–362, 1984, with permission. Copyright 1984, American Medical Association.)

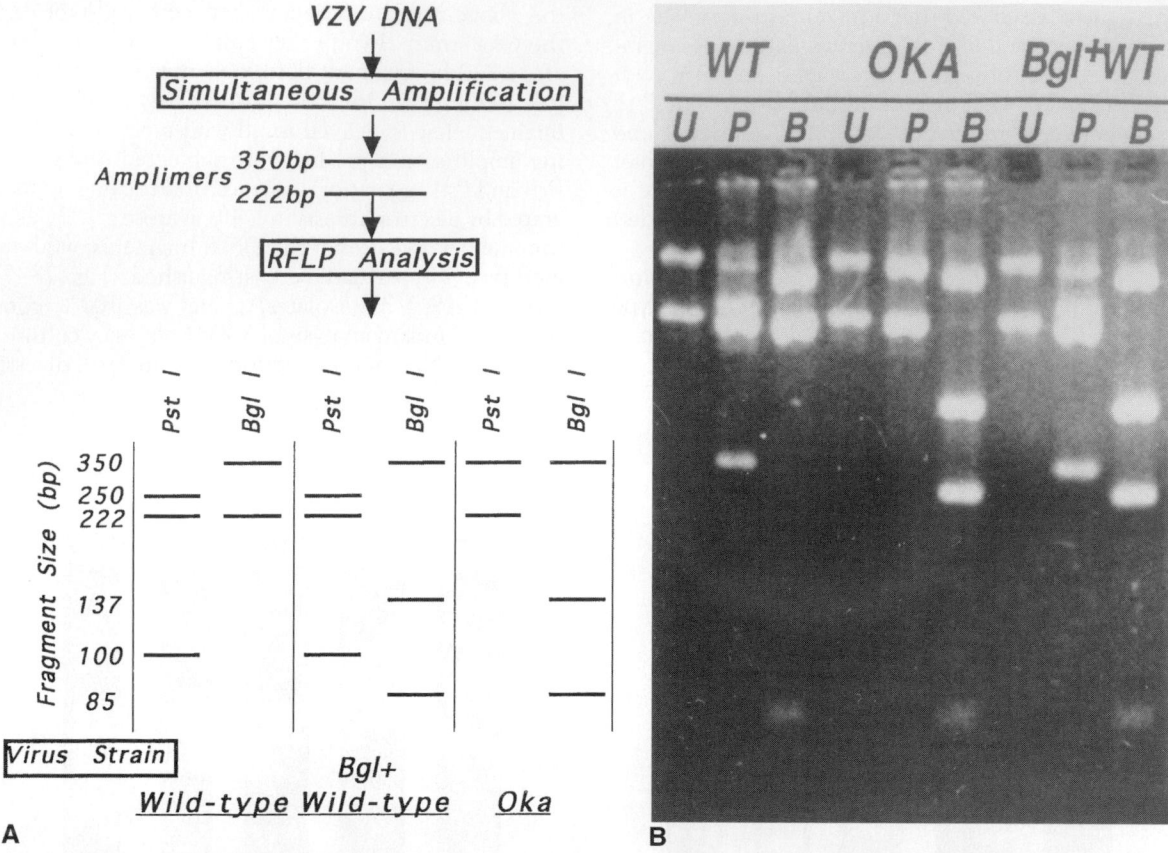

FIGURE 28–5 ■ Restriction fragment length polymorphism analysis of VZV DNA amplified by polymerase chain reaction. *A*, Schematic representation of the predicted digestion patterns. *B*, Representative examples of amplification products from wild-type (lanes 1 through 3), Oka (lanes 4 through 6), and Bgl+WT (lanes 7 through 9) strains that were undigested (U) or digested with *Pst*I (P) or *Bgl*I (B). (From LaRussa P, Lungu O, Hardy I, et al. Restriction fragment length polymorphisms of polymerase chain reaction products from vaccine and wild-type varicella-zoster isolates. J Virol 66:1016–1020, 1992, with permission.)

the PCR method.[281] All Oka strains lack a *Pst*I restriction site and have a *Bgl*I restriction site. All wild-type VZVs in the United States have a *Pst*I restriction site and most lack a *Bgl*I restriction site.

Studies utilizing the described amplification by PCR and treatment of the amplification products with restriction enzymes have confirmed and extended a number of the analyses described above. Studies of 92 clinical isolates from the United States have shown that approximately 20% of circulating American wild-type VZVs have a *Bgl*I cleavage site.[282] All of the circulating wild-type viruses had a *Pst*I restriction site. Studies of viruses obtained from New York, California, and Australia (113 specimens) did not identify circulating viruses with the DNA profile of the Oka strain (i.e., that lack a *Pst*I restriction site).[282] One of nine wild-type VZVs studied from Japan, however, had a *Pst*I restriction site as well as a *Bgl*I restriction site.[282] Thus, in countries other than Japan, the best marker for the vaccine strain is the absence of a *Pst*I restriction site. In Japan, the combination of single-strand conformational polymorphism profile after PCR amplification of the R2 terminal repeat (within *Hpa*I-K fragment, ORF 14) and analysis of the *Pst*I site is useful for distinguishing between Oka and other clinical isolates.[283] More recently, an *Sma*I restriction site was identified in ORF 62 that clearly discriminates between the Oka strain and all wild-type strains, including problematic Japanese strains.[271,284] This has been modified for use in a

rapid real-time PCR assay that is useful for identification of adverse events associated with varicella vaccine.[177] In 2001, a clinical specimen submitted to the CDC from Hawaii was identified as vaccine strain by *Pst*I and *Bgl*II, but was determined to be wild-type virus using the *Sma*I method, indicating that Oka-like wild-type strains, seen previously only in Japan, are also in circulation outside Japan (CDC, unpublished observations, 2001).

Molecular Evidence of Attenuation

Remarkable mutations have been identified in IE62 when the nucleotide sequences of the Oka vaccine and its parental VZV were compared.[272,273] As shown in Figure 28–6, the vaccine virus gene 62 contains a mixture of different sequences that have variations at 15 nucleotide positions, whereas only one sequence is present for the Oka parental virus gene 62. There were no nucleotide changes in genes 4, 10, 61, or 63, all of whose products are known to transregulate VZV genes. Nucleotide changes in gene 62 of the Oka vaccine strain resulted in the creation of new restriction sites that were recognized by *Bss*HII at position 107,136 and *Nae*I at position 107,256, resulting in three fragments (400, 267, and 114 bp), whereas that of Oka parental virus and 54 other clinical isolates had no cleavage sites for *Nae*I and *Bss*HII, resulting in one 781-bp fragment. Thus the Oka vaccine virus could be distinguished from the parental virus and other clinical isolates using a simplified

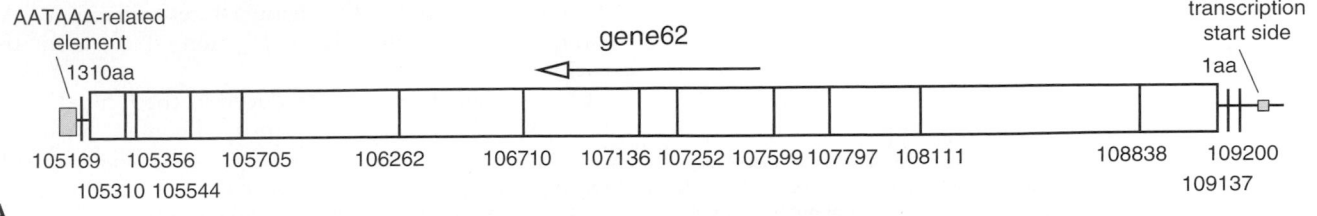

A

position(+100,000)		5169	5310	5356	5544	5705	6262	6710	7136	7252	7599	7797	8111	8838	9137	9200
Oka parental	all 9 clones	A	A(Leu)	T(Ile)	A(Val)	T(Ala)	T(Arg)	A(Ala)	T(Ala)	T(Ser)	A(Val)	A(Leu)	T(Pro)	A(Met)	A	A
Oka vaccine	clone 1	A	A	C(Val)	G(Ala)	C(Ala)	C(Gly)	G(Ala)	C(Ala)	C(Gly)	G(Ala)	A	C(Pro)	A	A	G
	clone 2	A	A	C	G	C	C	A	C	C	G	A	C	A	A	A
	clone 3	G	G(Ser)	C	G	C	C	A	C	C	A	G(Pro)	C	A	A	G
	clone 4	A	G	C	G	C	C	G	C	C	G	A	C	A	A	G
	clone 5	G	A	C	G	C	C	A	C	C	G	A	C	A	A	A
	clone 6	A	A	C	G	C	C	T(Ala)	C	C	A	A	C	A	A	G
	clone 7	G	A	C	G	C	C	A	C	C	G	A	C	A	A	A
	clone 8	G	A	C	G	C	C	A	C	C	G	A	C	G(Thr)	G	A
	clone 9	G	G	C	G	C	C	A	C	C	G	G	C	G	G	A

B

FIGURE 28–6 ■ Summary of sequence analysis of the distinct nine clones isolated from Oka vaccine virus and of the identical nine clones from Oka parental virus. A, Structure of gene 62. Amino acid residues (aa) are numbered from 1 to 1310 moving from the N- to the C-terminus. *Vertical lines* indicate the positions of nucleotide differences between Oka vaccine and its parental viruses. B, Sequence analysis of clones from Oka vaccine and its parental virus. All nine clones of parental virus had the same DNA sequence, whereas the vaccine virus was a mixture of at least eight different clones that had a variety of mutations at 15 positions. Nucleotide changes at eight positions caused amino acid conversions.

restriction-enzyme fragment length polymorphism analysis using *Nae*I and *Bss*HII.

The presence of nucleotide replacements that have accumulated in gene 62 of the Oka strain is not yet understood. Because the Oka vaccine virus was passaged at low temperature in human embryo fibroblasts and guinea pig embryo cells, mutant viruses may have been selected during the passages.

VZV gene 62 is present in large quantities in virion tegument,[98] and the yield of infectious virus generated by four overlapping cosmid clones is greatly improved when a gene 62–expressing plasmid is transfected.[285] Thus the mutation in Oka gene 62 may influence the replication of the virus and play a role in the attenuation of VZV. Studies of the regulatory activities of gene 62 in a transient transfection assay indicate that this gene in the vaccine virus has weaker transactivational activity than that of the wild-type virus in activating IE gene promotors (such as gene 4), E gene promotors (such as gene 28 for DNA polymerase and gene 29 for the major DNA binding protein), and L gene promoters (such as gene 68 for gE) (Fig. 28–7). These data also suggest that gene 62 may play an important role in the attenuation.[273]

Clinical Evidence of Attenuation

At present, the evidence of attenuation of varicella vaccine is mainly clinical. For example, the incidence of rash following subcutaneous injection of varicella vaccine is far lower than the incidence of rash in natural infection. This observation could be interpreted as suggestive of attenuation but not conclusive, however, because the virus is delivered by an unnatural route (i.e., by injection rather than inhalation).

There are, nevertheless, two further indications of attenuation in human studies. First, when the vaccine (800 to 2500 PFU) was administered to 19 healthy children by inhalation, the incidence of rash remained low.[168] Although the inoculating dose of virus under natural circumstances cannot be known and therefore cannot be compared with the dose of vaccine virus, these observations are highly suggestive of attenuation. Second, when rare, inadvertent transmission of vaccine virus to a healthy susceptible has occurred, the disease has been invariably mild or subclinical.[124,174,286,287] Moreover, the rate of transmissibility of the Oka strain in a household setting is far lower than that of wild-type VZV. In leukemic vaccinees, the rate of transmission was four to five times lower.[124]

The mildness of the clinical illness in children infected by the respiratory route with the Oka strain, the high rate of subclinical infection, and the low rate of transmissibility all provide evidence that the Oka strain is attenuated. Clinical evidence of reversion of the Oka strain to virulence has not been observed.

Additional evidence suggestive of attenuation is that, in contrast to natural infection, the Oka strain appears to be less likely to induce a demonstrable viremia following immunization. Viremia was not detected in 18 healthy or 10 immunocompromised vaccine recipients who had no clinical symptoms.[178] However, viremia resulting from vaccine virus was found in a leukemic child in remission for only 6 months when immunized, who had vesicles and fever to 104°F 20 days following vaccination.[288] These observations suggest that vaccine virus is attenuated because, in contrast

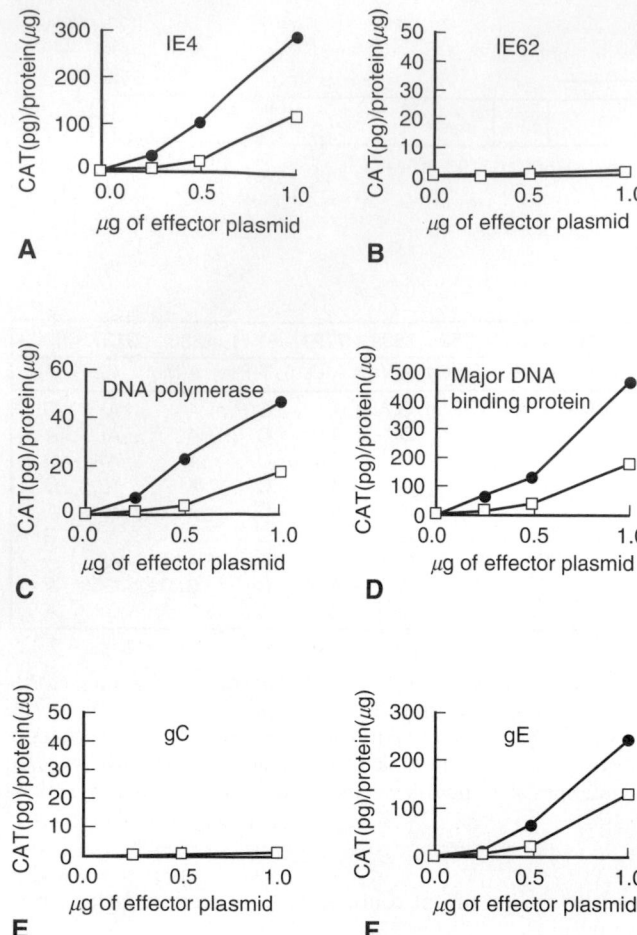

FIGURE 28–7 ■ Comparison of transactivational activity by the Oka vaccine(□) and its parental (●)IE62 on VZV gene promotors. CV1 cells were co-transfected with 0.25 (μg of a reporter plasmid and same amounts of either pVac-IE62 or pPar-IE62. The CAT concentrations were standardized to each protein concentration. All experiments were repeated at least three times independently. (From Gomi Y, Imagawa T, Takahashi M, Yamanishi K. Comparison of DNA sequence and transactivation activity of open reading frame 62 of Oka varicella vaccine and its parental viruses. Arch Virol Suppl 17:49–56, 2001, with permission.)

to natural varicella, development of viremia in healthy hosts has not been demonstrated. The Oka strain does, however, retain the ability to infect in animal model systems of VZV such as the guinea pig[28] and in the rat model of VZV latency.[289]

Constituents of Vaccine

For vaccine preparation, infected cells are harvested, suspended in the vaccine medium, and sonicated or exposed to a high-speed jet stream that shears the cells to obtain cell-free virus. Clinical studies indicate that the ratio of total viral antigen to total infectious viral particles is important in eliciting the appropriate immune response to vaccination.[290] Vaccine medium may vary according to the manufacturer; however, it generally contains sucrose and buffering salts. The vaccine is marketed in a lyophilized form to improve stability during prolonged storage. Reconstitution is accomplished with sterile distilled water

(0.5 mL) according to the manufacturer's directions. All manufacturers provide reconstitution fluid with the vaccine.

Oka varicella vaccine is produced in the United States (Varivax; Merck & Co., Inc), Belgium (Varilrix; GlaxoSmithKline), and Japan (OKAVAX; Biken, distributed by Aventis Pasteur). The vaccines vary in (1) passage number in human diploid cells, (2) virus dose (1000 to 10,000 PFU), (3) trace antibiotics added to ensure sterility during preparation, and (4) stabilizers and other minor constituents.

Seed lots of Oka vaccine have been prepared from virus passaged 11 times in HELF, 12 times in GPFC, and 5 times in human diploid cells. Manufacturers add from three to nine additional passages in human diploid cells to prepare enough vaccine to meet marketing needs. Lyophilized varicella vaccine can be stored at refrigerator temperatures (4° to 8° C) for up to 2 years. However, it is preferable to store the vaccine at freezer temperature (−15° C) for best preservation of the vaccine.

Results of Vaccination

Clinical trials with the Oka vaccine were initiated in Japan by Takahashi in 1974.[10] The vaccine was first given to 70 healthy children at doses ranging from 100 to 2000 PFU. The Oka strain was immunogenic at doses greater than 200 PFU, and no significant reactions were noted in the children. Initial protective efficacy was demonstrated by giving the vaccine to susceptible household contacts immediately after exposure.[291] Healthy children were vaccinated within 3 days of exposure. None of 18 vaccinated children developed varicella, whereas all of the 19 unvaccinated contacts developed typical varicella. Studies continued in Japan to include vaccination of children with malignant diseases where the severity of varicella was the greatest. The Oka strain was licensed to several other pharmaceutical companies (Merck & Co., Inc., Pasteur Mérieux, and SmithKline Beecham [now GlaxoSmithKline]), who later conducted clinical trials in Europe, the United States, and Canada.

Results in Children

Healthy Children

DOSE/ROUTE SELECTION

Clinical studies began in Japan in healthy adults and children before they progressed to the immunosuppressed population. After initial safety studies in healthy adults, children in Japan were given varying doses of the Oka strain to determine the minimum effective dose.[292–295] Seroconversion rates of more than 95% were obtained in normal children with 300 to 500 PFU when administered by subcutaneous injection. In another dose-response study using the Oka strain vaccine manufactured by SmithKline Beecham, seroconversion rates of 95.5% were induced with approximately 600 PFU.[296]

The Oka strain vaccine manufactured by Merck (Oka/Merck) has been tested in various dose titration studies during the development of the vaccine. Each time there was a change in the manufacturing process, dose titration studies were performed. The first study was conducted in 137 healthy children who were randomized to receive approximately 43, 435, 970, and 4350 PFU.[297] Of the 99 initially seronegative children who received doses of 435 PFU or greater, 94% of those assayed at 2 weeks and 100% of those assayed at 4 or 6 weeks seroconverted. Children who received only 43 PFU seroconverted more slowly than those who received higher doses. The geometric mean antibody titers (GMTs) at 6 weeks were similar for all vaccine doses. All vaccine dose levels were well tolerated, with no significant differences in the rate of clinical reactions by dose. The frequency of varicella-like rash was 3%, and all rashes were mild. Two additional studies were performed with later formulations of the vaccine.[298,299] In these studies, the vaccine was not diluted to obtain the lower PFU dose levels but was exposed to slightly elevated temperatures to accelerate the decay of infectious particles. This process mimics what would actually happen during prolonged storage of the vaccine (i.e., constant antigen with decreasing PFU in the injected dose). Doses lower than 500 PFU resulted in seroconversion rates greater than 90%; however, dose levels of 80 to 160 PFU and 439 PFU elicited significantly lower antibody titers compared to dose levels of 1125, 1770, and 3625 PFU.

A more recent comparison of the safety, tolerability, and immunogenicity in healthy children ages 12 to 24 months, using one dose of either Oka/Merck vaccine (50,000 or 16,000 PFU) or Varilrix (40,000 PFU), produced by GlaxoSmithKline, resulted in safety patterns that were similar. The proportion of children who seroconverted, as measured by gp ELISA, following each type of vaccine was 97.1%, 95.2%, and 85.6%, respectively.[300]

Administration of the vaccine using an inhalation method was tested in a small study in an institution in Osaka, Japan.[301] Oka strain virus at doses of 800 to 2500 PFU was well tolerated by the 23 children greater than 1 year of age enrolled in the study. All of the children seroconverted. During an outbreak of varicella in the institution 1.5 years after immunization, none of the vaccinees developed clinical varicella. In contrast, all 166 susceptible unvaccinated control children contracted clinical varicella. Unlike subcutaneous injection, however, the dose of vaccine virus is difficult to control by the inhalation method and the method itself is somewhat cumbersome.

SAFETY

The most common adverse events reported after varicella vaccination from two placebo-controlled studies were minor and included mild tenderness and redness at the injection site (~15% to 20% of vaccinees), fever (~14% of vaccinees), and mild rash (~4 % of vaccinees). In one double-blind, placebo-controlled clinical trial, the only complaint that occurred more often in vaccinated children compared to placebo recipients was pain and redness at the injection site ($P < 0.05$).[302] The rash usually consists of 10 or fewer lesions occurring from 7 to 21 days following vaccination. A similar percentage of children reported a rash at the injection site, usually consisting of two to four lesions. It is difficult to culture vaccine-type virus from a healthy child with a vaccine-associated rash, but it has been reported.[303] Vaccinated healthy children who develop more than 30 lesions after vaccination, particularly within the first 2 weeks after the injection, would be suspect for intercurrent infection with wild-type strain (see below).

Following the licensure of the Merck varicella vaccine in the United States in 1995, investigators at Merck and Columbia University undertook a postlicensure safety study of varicella vaccine. Medical personnel and consumers were invited to submit information on possible adverse reactions to varicella vaccine to Merck's Worldwide Adverse Experience System (WAES), a database that can be described as a passive, voluntary, and of necessity incomplete reporting system. Nevertheless, there was the potential with WAES to learn much about possible adverse events temporally or otherwise apparently associated with varicella immunization. These vaccinees included children and adults who were presumed by their health care professionals to be otherwise healthy, but who were thought to have experienced possible adverse reactions to varicella vaccine. The WAES reports were by law also submitted to the FDA's Vaccine Adverse Event Reporting System (VAERS). In WAES, clinical data and if possible laboratory specimens were submitted. Clinical information was sent to Merck investigators, and laboratory specimens, mostly for PCR analysis,[171] were sent in coded fashion to investigators at Columbia University.[174] In particular, the study was probing for the following events: rashes of over 50 lesions within 42 days following immunization; possible instances of secondary transmission of the Oka strain to others; varicella and zoster occurring after vaccination; and neurologic, dermatologic, and other possible complications of VZV infection after immunization. Between May 1, 1995, and April 30, 1999, 16.1 million doses of varicella vaccine were distributed in the United States, and 7963 adverse events were reported to WAES. Rashes identified as caused by Oka strain occurred from 5 to 42 days after vaccination (median 21 days) and ranged from 1 to 500 skin lesions (median 51). Rashes identified as caused by wild-type VZV occurred between 1 and 24 days after immunization (median 8 days), with 10 to 1000 reported skin lesions (median 51). Transmission was associated with wild-type VZV with some frequency but occurred only three times with Oka strain (see above).

Complications of VZV Oka strain were proven in fewer than 10 vaccinees. Most of these patients were immunocompromised or had other serious medical conditions that were undiagnosed at the time of immunization.[174] They included a 19-year-old with cholangitis, a 38-year-old asplenic man, a toddler with HIV infection and virtually no CD4 lymphocytes,[304] a child with adenosine deaminase deficiency,[305] and a 5-year-old with multiple developmental disorders and reactive airway disease for which he was receiving steroids. A vaccinated nurse developed 300 skin lesions with low-grade fever caused by Oka strain. All of these patients recovered, although at least half of them were treated with ACV.

There were 19 reports of encephalitis from 4 to 365 days (median 20) and 24 reports of ataxia 1 to 61 days (median 16) after vaccination; in none was Oka strain implicated, although the wild-type virus was identified in two.[174] There were 20 reports of self-limited erythema multiforme, 15 of thrombocytopenia, and 7 of anaphylaxis temporally related to vaccination but not shown to be due to Oka strain VZV. In summary, this postlicensure investigation of vaccine safety[174] as well as that reported by VAERS on essentially the same population[306] indicated that the vaccine is extremely safe when administered to millions of individuals. Of 14 fatalities temporally associated with varicella vaccination, none were proven to be due to the Oka strain, although 2 were associated with wild-type VZV.[306] An additional study of almost 90,000 children immunized in Northern California between 1995 and 1996 found no increased risk for serious events that are well-recognized complications of natural varicella, including ataxia, encephalitis, or bleeding disorders following varicella vaccination.[307]

CONTACT SPREAD OF VACCINE VIRUS

In leukemic vaccinees, the chance of transmission was reported to be directly proportional to the number of skin lesions in the vaccinee.[124] Of 93 siblings exposed to a leukemic vaccinee with a vaccine-associated rash, 21 (23%) seroconverted. Of these children, 5 of 21 (24%) never developed a rash. In comparison, the normal expected subclinical attack rate of wild-type varicella is about 5%.[17] In exposed siblings who developed a rash, the average number of skin lesions was 38 (median 12; range 1 to 200).[286] In comparison, children with wild-type varicella have on average 300 to 500 skin lesions.[17] There was only one report of tertiary spread in the collaborative study, further suggesting that the vaccine virus has limited ability for transmission.[124] The low transmission rate is of importance because it has potential implications concerning the spread of vaccine-type VZV from healthy vaccinees, such as health care workers, to other susceptibles. If a healthy vaccinee has no rash, the opportunity for spread of the virus has never been proven and thus seems close to nonexistent. Even with a rash, the chance of spread from a healthy vaccinated individual seems almost negligible. No spread was found in 112 siblings exposed to a leukemic vaccinee who did not have a vaccine-associated rash. Rash therefore seems to be crucial for potential transmission to occur. There was concern during the first few years after licensure in the United States that healthy children with rash might also transmit the Oka strain to others.

Transmission of the Oka strain had been addressed in two clinical studies in healthy children using the Merck vaccine prior to licensure.[302,308] In one study, children in a household were randomized to receive either vaccine or placebo.[302] In that study, there were no reports of transmission of clinical disease such as rash. However, 3 of the 439 initially seronegative placebo recipients exposed to vaccinees seroconverted to VZV without symptoms. No rash was reported in the vaccine recipients to whom they had been exposed. In view of the importance of rash in transmission, it seems that these results are more likely to be the result of serologic errors rather than actual transmission of VZV. In the second study, siblings of susceptible immunocompromised children (most with a diagnosis of leukemia) were vaccinated.[308] There was no evidence of clinical or serologic transmission of the Oka virus following vaccination in the approximately 30 families studied.

In healthy vaccinees, transmission has been exceedingly rare, with only three documented occurrences despite the distribution of over 30 million doses of vaccine in the United States between 1995 and 2002. In contrast, the usual rate of transmission of the wild-type virus under similar circumstances (i.e., family contact) is about 90%.[17] In each instance there was a vaccine-associated rash.[174] Persons to whom transmission of Oka virus was proven from a healthy vaccinee were a 4-month-old sibling of a vaccinee, the healthy father of a vaccinee, and a pregnant mother.[174,309] Based on the estimated annual childhood risk of developing varicella of 9% and the high degree of transmissibility of the wild-type virus, the risk from natural disease to a susceptible pregnant woman with young children is calculated to be greater than the potential risk resulting from vaccination of the child.[310] Thus children 12 months of age or older should receive varicella vaccine even if there is a varicella-susceptible pregnant woman living in their household. There has been one additional recorded instance of transmission involving the child of a parent who was immunized with an Oka vaccine not licensed for use in the United States that was being employed in a research protocol.[311] These few contact cases have been uniformly mild. In view of the distribution of over 20 million doses of varicella vaccine in the United States at the time of these occurrences, such a transmission event is exceedingly rare.

IMMUNOGENICITY

After immunization with at least 500 PFU of the Oka strain, serum IgG antibody responses are easily detected within 1 month after vaccination, and antibody can be detected for months to years in most individuals. However, the individual and mean IgG antibody titers may be 10 to 30 times lower after vaccination than after natural infection, depending on the dose of vaccine virus administered and the age at immunization.[27,290,291,312,313] However, titers of antibodies to VZV have often been observed to increase with time. Presumably as a result of exposure to the wild-type virus, subclinical boosting of the immune response occurs, eventually resulting in IgG titers that are similar to those after natural infection.[314,315] Serum IgA antibody is detectable only occasionally and at low levels in vaccinees immunized by inhalation, and VZV serum IgA is virtually undetectable in subjects immunized subcutaneously.[168] In contradistinction to the response after varicella, secretory IgA antibody responses to VZV have not been demonstrated after immunization, regardless of the route or dose of administration of vaccine.[168] However, it should be pointed out that, as for many vaccines, immune correlates of protection against VZV infection are not entirely delineated. It is not known what level of IgG is protective or if IgA at mucosal sites offers protection against infection.

In the 3303 children immunized in the United States in clinical trials during the late 1980s, VZV antibody titers were determined with the VZV gp ELISA assay 6 weeks following immunization.[316] Their seroconversion rate was 96%, with a GMT of about 1:12. It was noted, however, that the seroconversion rate in adolescents ages 13 to 17 years was only 79%; moreover, their GMT was 1:6, half the levels seen in healthy children. During prelicensure clinical trials conducted by Merck from 1982 to 1991 in the United States, a clear relationship between the dose of vaccine administered and the antibody titer measured by gp ELISA was observed.[315]

A more recent update concerning 8429 healthy children from Japan, where 1.39 million healthy children were vaccinated between 1987 and 1993, continued to indicate the highly immunogenic behavior of the vaccine. Using IAHA, seroconversion to VZV was found in 2347 of 2565 children (91.5%), with a GMT of 1:12, 1 month later.[317] There are no published data on the use of commercially available VZV antibody tests to determine seroconversion rates in healthy children. Presumably, however, because these tests are less sensitive than the gp ELISA assay, many children will have undetectable antibodies when commercial tests are used, despite successful immunization. Although quantitative information is not available, failure to detect antibodies by commercial ELISA tests was reported to the WAES after vaccination.[174]

In vaccinated healthy children, the skin test became positive as early as 4 days after immunization in about half the children (Fig. 28–8), 7 to 9 days prior to detection of neutralizing antibodies.[141] Similarly, in another study, lymphocyte transformation became positive about 1 week before neutralizing antibodies were detected.[318] The stimulation index against VZV antigen in 74 healthy American children 6 weeks after immunization was 58.6 (± 6.5).[319]

Immunocompromised Children: Safety and Immunogenicity

In Japan in the mid-1970s, a group of 39 children with underlying diseases such as nephrosis, nephritis, asthma, and hepatitis, about one third of whom were receiving steroids, were immunized. They were given a dose of 1000 to 2000 PFU of the Oka vaccine manufactured by Biken

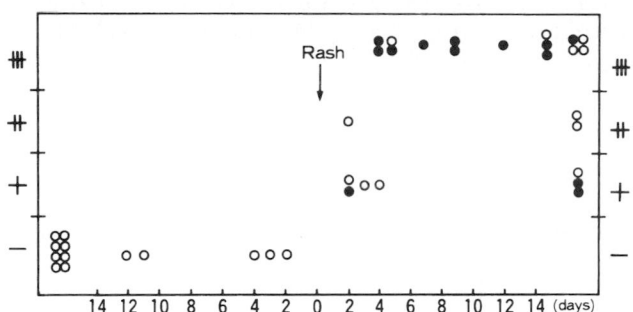

Skin test was done on 22 children

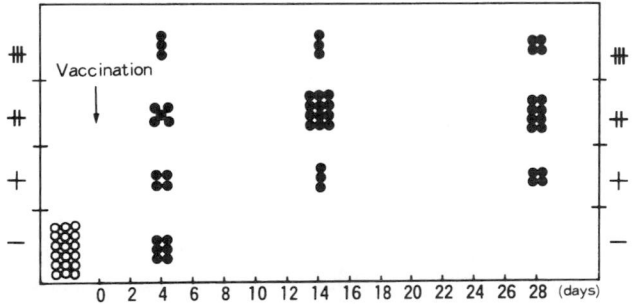

Skin test was done 4 times in all the 18 vaccinated children

o indicates the first skin test
● indicates the 2nd, 3rd, 4th skin tests

FIGURE 28–8 ■ Comparison of the time of conversion of the varicella skin reaction in children after natural varicella infection (*top*) or vaccination (*bottom*). (From Takahashi M, Baba K. A live varicella vaccine. In de la Maza LM, Peterson EM [eds]. Medical Virology III. New York, Elsevier, 1984, p 255, with permission.)

(Oka/Biken). All of these children developed VZV antibodies as determined by CF.[10,270]

A major departure in immunization with live virus vaccines occurred when children with leukemia and other malignancies were vaccinated.[320] Prior to this time, live vaccines were considered to be contraindicated for use in immunocompromised children. Given the high risk from natural varicella, however, 11 children with leukemia and 6 with solid tumors who were in remission from their malignant disease were immunized in Japan. Their chemotherapy, 6-mercaptopurine (6MP) and methotrexate (MTX), was empirically withheld for 1 week before and 1 week after immunization.[320–324] In these studies, the seroconversion rate for antibodies against VZV, measured by CF or IAHA, approached 100%. Subsequently, a report of 326 leukemic children who were immunized in Japan was published, confirming and extending these data.[295] Most of these children seroconverted to VZV after immunization as determined by FAMA or IAHA.

In the late 1970s in the United States, in children with leukemia and varicella, a chickenpox dissemination rate of 30% with 7% mortality was reported.[50] Based on the successful studies of immunization of leukemic children in Japan, open-label clinical trials in children with acute lymphoblastic leukemia in remission were begun in the United States and Canada in 1979. These studies first brought varicella vaccine to the United States.

The largest clinical trial in leukemic children was conducted by the Varicella Vaccine Collaborative Study Group, sponsored by the National Institute of Allergy and Infectious Diseases (NIAID), which was organized to conduct these trials.[66,148,286,325–330] At the time of immunization, children had to meet the following criteria: be in continuous remission from leukemia for at least 1 year, have no detectable antibodies to VZV by FAMA, have a positive response to mitogens in vitro, and have more than 700/mm³ circulating lymphocytes. Over a decade, 64 children whose chemotherapy for leukemia had been completed, and 511 children whose chemotherapy was suspended for 2 weeks, were immunized.[329,331] Chemotherapy for most of these children was daily 6MP, weekly MTX, and monthly pulses of prednisone and vincristine, regimens that were more intense than those given to Japanese children in earlier studies. By the late 1980s in the United States, higher doses of MTX, prednisone, and cyclophosphamide were being administered. Although it was initially planned to administer one dose of vaccine, because of a failure of seroconversion as measured by FAMA after one dose in about 15% and loss of detectable VZV FAMA antibody after a year in about 5% of leukemic vaccinees, two doses of vaccine given 3 months apart were recommended. In this study, a seroconversion to VZV occurred in 82% of leukemic children after one dose of vaccine and in 95% after two doses of vaccine.[148,327–329] In general, about 80% of vaccinees tested developed positive cell-mediated immune responses after one dose of vaccine and 90% after two doses, mirroring the experience with humoral immune responses.

Rash developed in 5% of leukemic children no longer receiving chemotherapy and in about 50% of those still receiving maintenance chemotherapy, about 1 month after the first dose of vaccine.[329] Rashes were less common after the second dose of vaccine, occurring in only 10% of children still receiving maintenance chemotherapy. The rash following vaccination in children with acute lymphoblastic leukemia is usually maculopapular and vesicular and can resemble a mild form of varicella. About 40% of children receiving chemotherapy who developed rash were treated with high oral doses (900 mg/m² four times a day) of ACV (particularly those with more than 50 skin lesions or with rash that lasted more than 7 days).[329] Children with more severe rashes (usually those with >200 lesions) were treated with intravenous ACV at a standard dosage. Oka strain VZV is sensitive to ACV, and ACV therapy did not appear to interfere with the development of the immune response.[329]

A retrospective analysis of rash after immunization led to the recommendation that children not be given steroids for at least 2 weeks after immunization.[332] There was no increase in the rate of relapse of leukemia in vaccinated leukemic children compared to children who had natural varicella either in the United States or in Japan.[328,332,333]

In two other smaller studies conducted in the United States in immunocompromised patients, 84 leukemic children were immunized.[334,335] The seroconversion rates were similar to those observed in the collaborative study. Twenty-two children with solid tumors (Wilms' tumor and rhabdomyosarcoma) also were immunized in the collaborative study (Gershon et al., unpublished results, 1980–1990). After two doses of vaccine, 77% seroconverted as determined by FAMA assay. Thirty-two percent of these children had minor vaccine-associated rashes.

In Japan, five cases of severe reactions to varicella vaccine, consisting of extensive skin rash and high fever, have been reported.[295] All of these children were receiving high doses of immunosuppressive medications that were not withheld before immunization. None of these children suffered permanent sequelae, and all recovered. In the United States, a few severe reactions to vaccine have been reported in leukemic children who received a lot of vaccine that is no longer being used and that had a significantly lower antigen-to-infectivity ratio than other varicella vaccines.[327,336] In postlicensure safety studies, several children with immunodeficiency diseases (who were already discussed above) were diagnosed when they developed complications from Merck varicella immunization.[174]

There are additional reports of immunization of small numbers of immunocompromised children. In a study of 23 uremic children, vaccine was given at least 2 months prior to renal transplantation. The vaccine was well tolerated, with an 87% seroconversion rate after one dose of vaccine.[337] In another study in Spain, 34 children, half on dialysis and half after transplantation, were immunized. Their seroconversion rate, as measured by ELISA, was 85% after one dose; 10% had a mild vaccine-associated rash.[338]

In a larger report of immunization of children with renal failure, a group of 212 French children were immunized prior to renal transplantation and followed between 1980 and 1994. They were compared with a group of 49 similar children with no history of vaccination or chickenpox and 415 similar children who had previous varicella. Antibodies to VZV were measured by FAMA and by ELISA. One year after immunization, 62% were VZV antibody positive.[339]

Studies are ongoing to evaluate the immunization of children with HIV infection in the Pediatric AIDS Clinical Trials Group (PACTG). In a small study involving 41 HIV-infected children whose CD4+ T lymphocyte levels were relatively normal (greater than 25%) and who were asymptomatic or only mildly symptomatic (CDC stage N1 or A1) with regard to their HIV infection, 85% developed evidence of an immune response to VZV after two doses of vaccine. Antibodies were detectable by FAMA in 60% and a positive stimulation index developed in 83% The rate of vaccine-associated rash was similar to that seen in healthy vaccinees (5%), and, unlike leukemic vaccinees, none required treatment with an antiviral drug to control symptoms following vaccination. Although there are no efficacy data for these children, none developed documented VZV infections during the study period, although one child had a mild rash that was clinically diagnosed as mild varicella.[340] Based on this study, the CDC's Advisory Committee on Immunization Practices (ACIP) has recommended that varicella vaccine be considered to be given to HIV-infected children who are mildly symptomatic.[341] Two doses, 3 months apart, are recommended. In the PACTG, HIV-infected children with lower CD4 lymphocyte levels and who are symptomatic are now being immunized, but no safety data are yet available for these children.

Further studies in immunocompromised children are sparse. An additional trial in children with renal failure was reported in which 31 children were immunized with two doses of vaccine and developed an immune response without adverse effects.[342] In Thailand, 29 children with chronic liver disease were given one dose of varicella vaccine, with 100% seroconversion and no serious adverse events.[342a] There is a report of a small clinical trial in which 11 children, ranging in age from 5.5 months to 7 years 9 months (median age 10 months) were given one dose of varicella vaccine prior to liver transplantation (median interval 95 days, range 40 to 289 days). Only three of the children responded serologically to immunization. Administration of varicella vaccine did not affect the management of subsequent VZV exposures in that, after an exposure, passive immunization was still given.[343]

Vaccination of immunocompromised individuals proved to be useful for evaluating the relationship between immunization and development of HZ, because immunocompromised individuals are at high risk to develop HZ if they have had previous varicella infection.[67] A lower incidence of HZ in vaccinees was noted in uncontrolled studies[13,344,345] and in controlled trials in children with leukemia[66,330] (see *Herpes Zoster in Vaccinated Individuals* below). This lower incidence again suggests the attenuation of the Oka strain. In these studies, there was a direct correlation between the risk of HZ and prior presence of VZV on the skin. It is hypothesized that VZV reaches nerve ganglia from skin infection and then becomes latent.[346] One could extrapolate to the hypothesis that, because healthy vaccinees have a low incidence of VZV rash, they may be at a lower risk to develop HZ later in life. Definitive information, however, will take another three to four decades of observation. However, zoster in healthy vaccinees is, thus far, unusual (see below).

Efficacy and Effectiveness

In general, varicella vaccination has been found to be highly effective in preventing disease. There have generally been three types of efficacy and effectiveness studies: double-blind, placebo-controlled; case-control; and open-label studies in which protection after household exposure has been examined. In the first published study of varicella vaccine, immunization was used to terminate a potential outbreak of nosocomial chickenpox.[10] All of the healthy children who were immunized developed specific antibodies, and no further cases of varicella occurred. The vaccinated children were protected after four subsequent hospital exposures to varicella.[312] Although this was not a classical efficacy study, these data strongly suggested that live, attenuated varicella vaccine would be effective in preventing disease.

DOUBLE-BLIND, PLACEBO-CONTROLLED STUDIES (EFFICACY)

Two double-blind, placebo-controlled efficacy studies, both performed in healthy children, have been published. The first was conducted in the early 1980s using Merck's Oka vaccine in the suburbs of Philadelphia.[302] In this study, 468 children were immunized with one dose of varicella vaccine containing approximately17,000 PFU (the original report of 8700 PFU was erroneous) and 446 were given placebo. Over the following 9 months there were 39 cases of varicella, all in the placebo recipients, resulting in a calculated vaccine efficacy of 100%. During the second year of follow-up, one vaccinated child developed modified varicella consisting of 17 lesions after exposure to wild-type varicella, resulting in an efficacy of 98%. During a 7-year follow-up, 95% of these vaccinees were estimated to have remained free of varicella.[347] These data are somewhat difficult to compare with those of subsequent studies in the United States, however, because these children received the highest dose of vaccine ever used in the United States, and this dose is not currently available or under consideration for future use.[315]

A second controlled study was performed in Finland, using vaccine produced by SmithKline Beecham (now GlaxoSmithKline). This study included 513 healthy children ages 10 to 30 months. They were divided into three groups: those who were given a high dose of vaccine (10,000 or 15,850 PFU), those who were given a low dose (1260 or 630 PFU), and those who were given placebo. There was a seroconversion rate approaching 100% in vaccinees, as determined by FAMA. Children were observed for 29 months on average. During this time there were 65 serologically confirmed cases of varicella: 5 in the high-dose group (3% attack rate), 19 in the low-dose group (11.4% attack rate), and 41 (25.5% attack rate) in the placebo group. The differences in protection were significant for each group, compared with each other and with controls. The breakthrough varicella in vaccinees was a very minor illness with on average less than 30 skin lesions.[348]

POSTLICENSURE EFFECTIVENESS STUDIES

In the postlicensure period, monitoring vaccine performance is essential to assess effectiveness of the licensed vaccine product under conditions of community storage and handling. Vaccine effectiveness may be studied by a variety of methods, including investigation of outbreaks, prospective and retrospective cohort studies, case-control studies, and household secondary attack rate studies. In the United States, where a national childhood vaccination program was implemented in 1995, the majority of postlicensure varicella vaccine studies have provided effectiveness esti-

mates in the same range as described before licensure, 71% to 100%, with greater than 95% protection against moderate and/or severe disease.[349] Case definitions for varicella and for moderate and severe disease may vary between studies, and this may affect vaccine effectiveness; studies using a clinical case definition are more likely to underestimate vaccine effectiveness, whereas those with a laboratory confirmed case definition are more likely to overestimate effectiveness.[350] Severe varicella disease has been defined as more than 300 lesions in some studies and more than 500 lesions in others.

Outbreaks provide an excellent opportunity to study vaccine performance; because of the high clinical attack rate of chickenpox, the majority of unvaccinated children are likely to become cases, especially in settings where repeated exposures occur. In an outbreak in a day care setting involving 148 eligible children, 81 children (55%) developed varicella over a 15-week time period. By the end of the outbreak, the cumulative attack rate in unvaccinated children was 88% (72 of 82) compared with 14% (9 of 66) among vaccinated children.[351] Varicella vaccine effectiveness against all disease was 86% (95% confidence interval [CI], 73% to 92%), with 100% effectiveness (95% CI, 96% to 100%) in preventing moderate and severe varicella. Varicella in vaccinated children was milder than in unvaccinated children. This study raised the question of whether children with underlying reactive airway disease are as well protected as healthy children; this question has not yet been resolved.

Other outbreaks have described vaccine effectiveness predominantly in the range of 70% to 100%, with several lower estimates of 44% (95% CI, 6.9% to 66.3%) against all disease and 86% (95% CI, 38.7% to 96.8%) against moderate/severe disease in a child care setting, and 59% (95% CI, −1% to 84%) against all disease in an elementary school setting.[352–355] One possible explanation for the low vaccine effectiveness estimates in these settings is that outbreaks that come to public health attention are more likely to represent situations where the vaccine failed and may therefore represent extreme estimates of vaccine effectiveness.[356] Situations where the vaccine has performed well do not come to public health attention. Nevertheless, our understanding of vaccine performance is enhanced by studying effectiveness in different population and age group settings and using a variety of different methods. Several outbreak investigations have raised issues for further study, including earlier age at vaccination and time since vaccination as risk factors for lower vaccine effectiveness.[354]

In a prospective cohort study of children from birth to 6 years of age attending 11 day care centers in North Carolina, varicella vaccine was 83% (95% CI, 69% to 91%) effective in preventing varicella disease and was 100% effective in preventing moderate to severe varicella.[357] These investigators found in a subsequent study that there was evidence of herd immunity because the decrease of varicella occurred in unvaccinated children as well as vaccinated children.[358]

A case-control study was carried out in private practice settings in Connecticut between 1997 and 2000.[175] There were 202 children with varicella confirmed by PCR and 389 practice-matched controls who did not have clinical varicella. Twenty-three percent of the children with varicella had received varicella vaccine compared with 61% of children with no varicella. This study showed a vaccine effectiveness of 85% (95% CI, 78% to 90%). The vaccine was 97% effective in preventing severe varicella (95% CI, 93% to 99%). In vaccinated children, 86% had mild disease, and 48% of the unvaccinated children had mild disease (P < 0.001); thus, for children who developed varicella despite immunization, the illness was highly likely to be modified.

EFFICACY IN IMMUNOCOMPROMISED VACCINEES

Significant information on efficacy in immunocompromised leukemic children in the United States and Canada was gathered from the NIAID collaborative study. In this group, there were 123 household exposures to varicella over a decade, with 17 cases of breakthrough chickenpox, for a rate of protection of 86%.[66,327-329] Varicella occurred in a total of 39 vaccinated children, most of whom did not have household exposures to chickenpox; this was generally a modified illness, with an average of 96 skin lesions (range 1 to 640). None of these leukemic children with breakthrough varicella required treatment with antiviral drugs.

The protective efficacy of vaccine was also examined in 212 French children who were immunized prior to renal transplantation. They were compared with a group of 49 similar children with no history of vaccination or chickenpox and 415 similar children who had previous varicella. The incidence of varicella was significantly lower in vaccinees (26 of 212, or 12%) than in those who were not vaccinated (22 of 49, or 45%). The disease was also less severe in the vaccinated children, with no deaths; there were three deaths from varicella in the unvaccinated group. Varicella occurred only in vaccinees who lost detectable VZV antibodies after vaccination; no cases of varicella were observed in those who remained antibody positive. Four (1%) of the 415 patients with a history of past varicella developed a second attack, which was similar to the attack rate in vaccinees.[339] The calculated vaccine efficacy in this study was 73%.

POSTEXPOSURE EFFECTIVENESS

In the 1970s and early 1980s, postexposure use of different formulations of varicella vaccine was extensively studied by Japanese researchers, who administered vaccine from 1 to more than 5 days following exposure, to healthy and ill susceptible children in hospital, community, and household settings[10,293,312,359-362] (Fig. 28–9). These studies used attack rates from historical controls to calculate vaccine effectiveness, which ranged from 60% among children who received a very low-dose vaccine to 100% in children who received vaccine similar to the licensed U.S. product. Asano and colleagues conducted two household postexposure effectiveness studies of healthy seronegative children comparing vaccinated and unvaccinated exposed children. In one study, 0 of 18 exposed children who were vaccinated 0 to 3 days following exposure developed varicella compared with 19 of 19 children who did not receive vaccine (Oka/Biken vaccine, 800 to 1000 PFU); vaccine effectiveness was therefore 100%.[291] In the other study (Oka/Biken vaccine, ≥ 500 PFU), in which 34 children were vaccinated within 3 days of exposure and 24 children were not vaccinated, vaccine effectiveness was 94.2% in preventing all disease.[363] Both studies found the vaccine to be 100% effective in preventing moderate or severe disease if administered within 3 days

of exposure. The only double-blind, placebo-controlled trial was conducted in the United States administering an Oka/Merck vaccine with 4350 PFU (similar to the U.S. licensed vaccine) 1 to 5 days postexposure to healthy seronegative children exposed within households.[364] For prevention of all disease, the vaccine was 90% effective if administered within 3 days of exposure and 67% effective when administered within 5 days. If administered within 5 days, the vaccine was 100% effective in preventing moderate or severe disease.

In the United States, postexposure prophylaxis was not originally recommended after licensure because the vaccine that was approved for routine use had not actually been used in postexposure trials. However, a small study carried out in the United States with the licensed vaccine in 1997 indicated that this approach was highly effective in preventing severe varicella. Ten children under the age of 13 years, who were exposed to their siblings with varicella, were immunized within 3 days of the exposure. Five developed no illness and five had very mild varicella, with only one child having more than 20 skin lesions.[365]

Another postexposure effectiveness assessment occurred in a shelter for homeless people in Philadelphia in 1998, when a young mother and her 11-month-old child in the shelter developed varicella.[366] Forty-two children with no history of varicella were immunized within the next 3 days. There were two cases of mild varicella about 2 weeks later. One case of moderately severe chickenpox occurred in a child who had not been vaccinated as a result of an erroneous disease history. Using either of two methods to calculate vaccine effectiveness (100% attack rate in the one

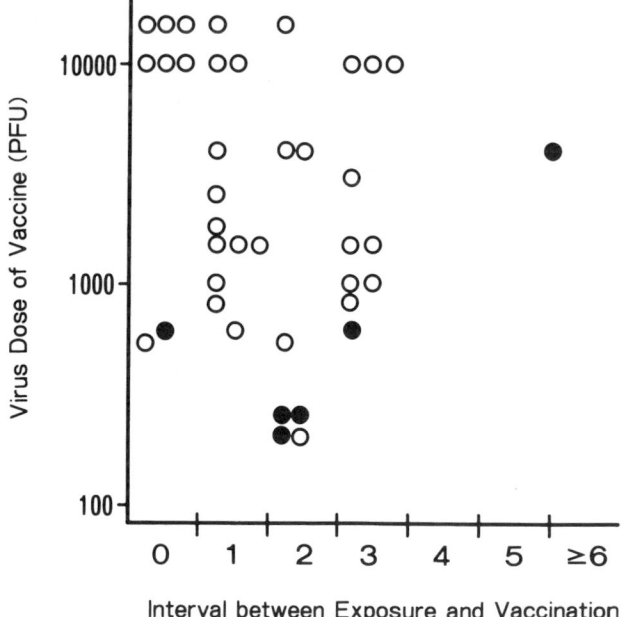

FIGURE 28–9 ■ The protective effect of inoculation with live varicella vaccine in household contacts with regard to the dose of virus and the time between exposure and vaccination. ○ no varicella, ● varicella (Adapted from Asano Y, Hirose S, Iwayama S, et al. Protective effect of immediate innoculation of a live varicella vaccine in household contacts in relation to the viral dose and interval between exposure and vaccination. Biken J 25:43–45, 1982.)

unvaccinated case or historical attack rates in unvaccinated children), postexposure vaccination was 95% effective in preventing varicella and 100% effective in preventing severe varicella in these children. Although this study was limited by several factors, including lack of serologic or virologic data and an unknown natural attack rate in homeless shelters, the effectiveness of the vaccine seems convincing. This shelter was closed for 6 weeks, while a similar shelter with no postexposure intervention experienced 63 cases of varicella and was closed for 6 months.[366] After reviewing data from all postexposure studies, including those conducted with the licensed U.S. vaccine, in 1999, postexposure use of varicella vaccine was recommended in the United States.[341]

BREAKTHROUGH VARICELLA

This phenomenon is described as varicella developing more than 42 days after immunization. During the late 1980s, 3303 children in the United States were immunized in clinical trials with one of five production lots of Oka/Merck vaccine, at a dose of 1000 to 1625 PFU.[316] There were 82 subsequent household exposures to varicella, and 12% developed breakthrough disease. Breakthrough infections were very mild, with about 1/10th the number of expected skin lesions. These observations are consistent with those of many other investigators who have also reported cases of mild breakthrough varicella in vaccinated healthy children.[140,175,314,351,357,364,367-372] Prospective experience from Japan in 2454 healthy children vaccinated between 1991 and 1993 indicated breakthrough varicella in 151 (6.2%) during the first year after vaccination, when breakthrough varicella was most frequent. Most cases were clearly attenuated. Earlier, retrospective data in Japanese children immunized between 1987 and 1990, indicated an attack rate of about 12% in the 6 to 36 months after vaccination, again with generally mild breakthrough infections.[317]

Most cases of breakthrough varicella consist of a skin rash of fewer than 50 lesions, unaccompanied by fever. The rate and severity of breakthrough varicella do not appear to increase over time after vaccination. Very few serious complications have been reported in previously vaccinated individuals in association with breakthrough varicella. Presumably those cases with the most severe problems occurred in persons who did not develop an immune response after vaccination. One Japanese child received the Oka strain vaccine manufactured in Japan at the age of 24 months. The child had a documented seroconversion to VZV determined by IAHA 4 weeks after vaccination. At 45 months of age, he developed aseptic meningitis along with an episode of wild-type varicella. Varicella infection was confirmed by the presence of viral DNA in cerebrospinal fluid by PCR with Southern blot hybridization. The child recovered without sequelae.[373] An adult who had no detectable protective antibodies after one dose of vaccine developed varicella complicated by renal involvement about 2 years after immunization.[374] In a Merck postmarketing safety study, after over 16 million doses of varicella vaccine had been distributed in the United States, 1424 cases of breakthrough varicella were reported.[174] Of 236 cases in which the number of skin lesions was reported, the median number was 49. Among these individuals, 56% had fewer than 50 skin lesions, 33% had between 50 and 300,

and 11% had over 300. Eleven patients were hospitalized, mostly for complications of varicella such as bacterial superinfection or neurologic problems. There was one death, in a 9-year-old girl with a history of asthma who was receiving steroids when she developed the breakthrough infection.

In contrast to the rarity of transmission of the Oka strain from person to person, there is little information on how frequently a vaccinated individual with breakthrough varicella transmits the wild-type virus. There has been one report of transmission of wild-type varicella from a vaccinated adult to a varicella-susceptible person, in which a vaccinated adult in Cincinnati, Ohio, developed breakthrough varicella and transmitted what was presumably wild-type infection to another adult.[375] The frequency with which spread of wild-type VZV from healthy vaccinees to others occurs is still unclear. Vigorous spread of wild-type VZV from vaccinated children in day care has been observed, although some of these cases may have been the result of primary vaccine failure.[355] During the prelicensure clinical trials, the rate of spread of wild-type VZV from children with breakthrough disease to their vaccinated household contacts was reported to be 12%.[372] More information concerning this phenomenon should become available in the future.

Overall it appears that varicella vaccine is highly protective in preventing severe disease and moderately effective in preventing all disease. It may be that the routine use of two doses of vaccine even for healthy children will decrease the rate of breakthrough disease. However, even in the minority of vaccinees who develop a breakthrough infection, there is evidence of partial immunity. It must be remembered that even immunity resulting from natural varicella may not be complete in all individuals, with resultant second cases of varicella in some persons and development of HZ in others. Possibly, imperfect immunity against VZV may offer an advantage, because it allows an opportunity for boosting of immune responses through exposure to VZV. One theoretical reason to decrease the rate of breakthrough varicella, however, is to prevent the wild-type virus from establishing latent infection, which has the potential to reactivate subsequently and cause zoster.

Results in Adolescents and Adults

Safety and Immunogenicity

Adults who have been immunized have lower seroconversion rates than healthy children. Small early studies suggested that the vaccine was more immunogenic in adults than it is now recognized to be. In 1985, in Switzerland, 32 healthy seronegative adults, mainly medical personnel, were given an Oka strain vaccine manufactured by RIT (Oka/RIT), with a reported 90% seroconversion rate.[376] At a similar time, in the United Kingdom, 34 seronegative nurses were immunized with Oka/RIT, and 94% seroconverted as determined by several serologic tests, including ELISA and immunofluorescence.[377] After 3 years, however, only 66% remained seropositive. In studies conducted by Alter et al.[378] and Arbeter et al.,[364] 89% to 94% of 53 adults seroconverted after one dose of vaccine as determined by FAMA.

In the NIAID collaborative study, during roughly 1980 to 1990, 268 healthy adults whose average age was 27 years were immunized.[27,329,379] Most were given two doses of vaccine 3 months apart; their seroconversion rate was 82% after one dose and 90% after two doses, as determined by FAMA. This experience is also consistent with the experience with rates of seroconversion in 79 vaccinated adolescents following one dose of vaccine.[316] In the NIAID study, the rate of mild vaccine-associated rash (average of nine skin lesions) was 10%, and, although it was possible to isolate vaccine-type VZV from a few vaccinated individuals, there was no recognition of spread to others.

Larger studies in adults using vaccine produced by Merck have indicated that adults require two doses of vaccine to achieve a seroconversion rate greater than 90%.[380] As for children, there are no data on seroconversions in healthy adults using commercially available tests. However, it would not be surprising, given the insensitivity of commercial tests, to find that many seroconversions in vaccinated adults cannot be detected by these methods. In one comparative study of LA, FAMA, and a commercial ELISA in 48 adults 1 to 3 years after immunization, positive VZV antibody levels were detected in 52%, 69%, and 36%, respectively.[165]

Positive VZV cell-mediated immune responses, including cytotoxic T lymphocytes, also have been observed in vaccinated adults in studies in the United States.[153] A cytotoxic T-cell response in 23 adult vaccinees was found to be similar to that observed in adults with past natural varicella.[153] The cell-mediated immune responses of adults to varicella vaccine are, however, lower than those observed in children.[381]

Efficacy

In the NIAID collaborative study, 57 adults were reported to have experienced household exposures to varicella, with 15 resultant breakthrough cases of chickenpox, an attack rate of 26%. This attack rate appeared to be higher than that seen in children who had been given similar lots and dosages of vaccine. Only adults who lost detectable VZV antibodies by FAMA and/or LA developed breakthrough varicella. However, only 50% of adults who had undetectable antibodies within the previous year developed clinical varicella after a household exposure. Most experienced a modified form of varicella.[27,329,379]

A follow-up study of a group of 120 vaccinated adult American or Canadian health care workers, some of whom were from the NIAID collaborative study and received Merck vaccine (82%) and others of whom received GlaxoSmithKline (18%) vaccine in different clinical trials, revealed the following[179]: after as long as 20 years (mean 4.6 years), 12 (10%) developed varicella 6 months to 8.4 years after vaccination, with a mean of 40 skin lesions. A seroconversion to VZV was documented by FAMA in 96%, but even vaccinees who failed to seroconvert and subsequently developed varicella had mild infections. In comparison to FAMA, LA and ELISA were 82% and 74% sensitive and 94% and 89% specific, respectively, in these vaccinees.

Duration of Immunity Following Vaccination

Persistence of immunity can be examined by following antibody titers over time and also by assessing the breakthrough rate of varicella and its mildness or severity with time.

Healthy Children

Several studies indicate that humoral, cellular, and protective immunity lasts for many years after immunization in healthy children. In Japan, a 5-year follow-up study of 26 healthy immunized children revealed that 100% had detectable neutralizing antibodies and 96% had positive FAMA titers.[314] None of these children developed breakthrough chickenpox, although many had been exposed to VZV. In a subsequent study of 106 Japanese children, 14 of whom had been receiving steroid therapy when they were immunized, there were five cases of breakthrough chickenpox.[367] Four of the cases developed in the first year after immunization. There were 147 recognized occasions when these children were exposed to VZV. Serum specimens were available from 38 children; FAMA antibody titers were 1:4 or greater in 37 (97%), with a GMT of 1:9. In 29 control children who had experienced natural varicella, FAMA titers were 1:4 or greater in 100%, with a GMT of 1:10. The VZV skin test was positive in 97% of each group. Because the average VZV antibody titer following immunization is lower than that following natural varicella, these results indicate that a boost in antibody titer had occurred in vaccinees, probably as a result of subclinical reinfection following exposure to exogenous virus.

A 10-year follow-up as well as a subsequent 20-year follow-up after immunization in Japan showed that 25 of 25 young adults remained seropositive and 26 of 26 retained positive cell-mediated immune responses as indicated by positive skin tests.[317,367,382]

A follow-up of 87 American vaccinees who were given approximately 17,000 PFU of vaccine revealed that 97% retained positive VZV immune responses (measured by gp ELISA and lymphocyte stimulation) 5 to 6 years after immunization.[383] In other American studies, in which most of 127 vaccinees received doses of vaccine of roughly 1000 to 3000 PFU, 95% remained seropositive for up to 6 years.[383] Persistence of antibodies for 2 years after vaccination was 94% in a study of 36 immunized toddlers in Ohio.[370] Of over 500 healthy additional children who were immunized in various studies in America, for whom there is a follow-up of as long as 6 years, over 95% remained seropositive by gp ELISA.[347,369,384] Another group of 603 vaccinated children showed over 89% persistence of varicella antibodies 6 years after vaccination. Compared with historical rates of varicella, the effectiveness of vaccination was about 90%.[384a] In a study of 53 vaccinated children whose FAMA antibody titers were measured for as long as 10 years after immunization, most remained VZV antibody positive.[371] Humoral immune responses against VZV, as measured by FAMA, appear to be more durable in healthy children than in immunized adults or leukemic children.[179,329] It is of the utmost importance to continue to follow healthy children who were immunized for persistence of immunity, particularly after the time when there is widespread use of varicella vaccine and little opportunity for boosting of immunity through exposure to natural infection. Toward this goal, the FDA has mandated that long-term studies of immunity following varicella vaccination be carried out.[315]

Most published studies of long-term follow-up of vaccinated children report that, annually, from 1% to 3% have developed breakthrough chickenpox after significant exposure to wild-type varicella.[182,316,347,348,368,369] Studies of the rate of breakthrough varicella in vaccinated American children for as long as 10 years following vaccination in prelicensure clinical trials indicated a rate of breakthrough varicella from 0% to 4% per year; lower rates of illness were associated with higher doses of vaccine[315] (see Table 28–2). Two recent reports have suggested that vaccination of children when they are less than 15 months old is associated with an increased rate of breakthrough varicella.[354,385]

The cumulative rate of breakthrough varicella has been reported in a number of long-term studies. In the study in which 17,000 PFU was given, 95% of children remained varicella free 7 years after vaccination.[383] Protection after this dose of varicella vaccine was higher than that seen in other studies in which lower dosages were administered. For example, in the study of Johnson et al. (N = 280, dose of 950 to 3250 PFU), 17% developed varicella after 10 years[371]; in that of Clements et al. (N = 465; dose of 950 to 3250 PFU), 19% had varicella after 5 years[369]; and in that of Takayama et al. (N = 459; dose of 1000 PFU),[386] 34% had varicella after 7 years. These breakthrough rates seem to be higher than optimal, and it is possible that administration of a second dose to children would decrease this rate. Whether these breakthrough cases represent waning immunity remains unclear. Importantly, however, most of the observed breakthrough cases of varicella were mild, and severe varicella was not seen in any of these studies.

There is a correlation between protection from varicella and the height of the gp ELISA titer 6 weeks following immunization. Optical density values of over 10 units at 6 weeks are associated with a lower chance of development of future breakthrough varicella.[182,369,387] In order to achieve high levels of VZV antibodies following immunization, which might be associated with better overall protection, studies utilizing two doses of varicella vaccine 4 to 8 weeks apart have been conducted in healthy children. These studies have indicated that this approach is safe, but whether two doses will offer greater protection than one dose for healthy children has not been examined.[319,388] A 10-fold increase in antibody titer was observed after the second dose of vaccine,[319] however, which suggests that two doses of vaccine would offer better protection than one.

Immune correlates of protection against varicella have been studied but need further clarification and development. A positive FAMA titer or skin test following natural varicella, at the time of close exposure to VZV, is highly predictive of protection against disease.[145,165,389] A positive FAMA after vaccination, at the time of intimate exposure to the virus, also correlates strongly with protection from disease.[179] However, neither the FAMA test nor the skin test is widely available. A gp ELISA titer of 5 units or greater 6 weeks after vaccination is reported to be an "approximate correlate of protection for individual vaccines."[387] However, the gp ELISA assay is available only on a research basis. Moreover, the protection seen after a positive gp ELISA test does not seem to be as effective as that following a positive FAMA test. A positive VZV skin test

TABLE 28–2 ■ Long-Term Clinical Follow-up of Varivax Recipients: Breakthrough Incidence and Number of Vaccinees Studied per Year[*]

Interval After Immunization	Vaccine Manufacturing Campaign				
	1982 Lot (17,430 PFU)	1982 Lot (950 PFU)	1984 Lot (2460–14,000 PFU)	1987 Lot (1000–1625 PFU)	1991 Lot (2900–9000 PFU)
ACTIVE AND PASSIVE FOLLOW-UP COMBINED					
1[†]	0.2% (487)	0.4% (908)	0.3% (1154)	2.1% (3537)	0.2% (1011)
2	0.0% (543)	1.2% (1021)	0.9% (1294)	2.9% (3842)	0.8% (1134)
3	0.6% (534)	2.1% (1004)	0.6% (1279)	3.3% (3713)	1.0% (682)
4	1.3% (528)	1.2% (989)	0.7% (1271)	3.6% (3563)	
5	1.9% (518)	2.1% (971)	0.8% (1261)	3.3% (3371)	
6	1.0% (513)	0.9% (956)	0.9% (1247)	3.0% (2831)	
7	0.6% (508)	0.3% (951)	0.9% (1076)		
8	0.0% (506)	0.4% (943)			
9	0.2% (505)	0.5% (938)			
10	0.0% (504)	0.0% (917)			
ACTIVE FOLLOW-UP ALONE					
1	0.2% (401)	0.8% (615)		3.0% (2994)	0.6% (955)
2	‡	1.2% (417)		3.3% (2415)	0.8% (717)
3	‡	2.4% (123)		4.4% (911)	‡
4	‡	1.8% (111)		4.3% (538)	
5	‡	1.9% (108)		4.5% (376)	

[*]For each follow-up interval, the annual incidence (%) of breakthrough varicella and the number of children (in parentheses) included in the study population are shown. When *active and passive follow-up periods* were combined, calculations assumed that all breakthrough cases that occurred in vaccinated individuals were reported. The 12-month follow-up intervals started 6 weeks after initial vaccination in this population. In *active follow-up alone*, only those subjects contacted for information on breakthrough disease within the previous interval were included. Individuals reimmunized with vaccine were excluded from further analysis.

[†]Excludes infections occurring within 6 weeks of vaccination.

[‡]Fewer than 100 subjects actively observed during preceding 12-month interval.

From Krause P, Klinman DM. Efficacy, immunogenicity, safety, and use of live attenuated chickenpox vaccine. J Pediatr 127:518–529, 1995, with permission.

after an exposure is also highly correlated with protection against disease and/or a positive VZV antibody titer.[145,389]

A major question exists as to whether vaccine-induced immunity to VZV will remain positive when exposures to VZV become unusual in the postvaccine era. It was possible to assess whether exposure and consequent boosting are required to maintain positive VZV antibody titers after vaccination in a small group of handicapped institutionalized children who had no exposures to VZV for 5 years after being immunized.[390] The 16 vaccinated children, as well as 7 children who had experienced natural varicella, maintained positive VZV antibody titers for 5 years. Skin test reactions also remained positive in 14 of 16 vaccinees. Six VZV-seronegative children remained seronegative during this 5-year period, indicating that no VZV was circulating in this isolated population during this interval. Thus humoral and cellular immunity conferred by vaccine lasted at least 5 years, without boosting by natural infection. It is possible, although difficult to prove, that subclinical reactivation of latent VZV may serve to stimulate immunity so that exogenous exposure to VZV may not be required to preserve immunologic memory.

Immunocompromised Patients

There has been a high degree of persistence of antibodies to VZV in vaccinated leukemics, although the rate of persistence is lower than that in healthy children. Over an 11-year interval, 13% of vaccinees who originally seroconverted become seronegative by FAMA or LA.[329] Many of these children were exposed to varicella but did not become ill. After a re-seroconversion, titers in leukemic children usually remain detectable, and in a number of patients who re-seroconverted without symptoms, the Western blot antibody pattern was characteristic of an anamnestic response.[327,391] Furthermore, the attack rate of clinical varicella among leukemic vaccinees who had again become seronegative and who had household exposures was only 30%, not the 80% to 90% that would be expected in varicella-susceptible individuals.[327] Neither the incidence nor the severity of breakthrough varicella in leukemic vaccines increased with time, even as many of these vaccinees became young adults.[329] The meaning of loss of a detectable antibody titer years after immunization is difficult to interpret but may represent some waning of immunity. At present, however, no booster immunizations are recommended.

The only other group of immunocompromised patients for whom there is long-term follow-up are those who received renal transplants. Antibody persistence was determined in French children who had been immunized prior to renal transplantation. After 10 years, 42% were seropositive by ELISA, a test that usually has low sensitivity.[339] It is possible that, had a more sensitive test to measure antibodies been used, the rate of antibody persistence would have been greater.

Healthy Adults

Studies on American adults vaccinated in the NIAID collaborative study have indicated that 60% to 90% are seropositive by FAMA and/or LA antibody tests as long as 13 years after vaccination[329,392] (Table 28–3). The incidence and severity of varicella did not seem to increase with time in these vaccinated adults (Fig. 28–10).[329]

TABLE 28–3 ■ Varicella Vaccine in Healthy Adults[*]

Year	Number	Number with Varicella (%)	Percentage Seronegative
1	343	8 (2)	34
2	234	8 (3)	33
3	174	2 (1)	40
4	115	5 (4)	10
5	68	4 (6)	30
6	45	2 (4)	10
7–13	40	2 (5)	18

[*]Long-term follow-up with regard to breakthrough illness and antibody loss with time. During 13 years of followup, breakthrough varicella developed in 9%.

From Gershon A. Varicella-zoster virus: prospects for control. Adv Pediatr Infect Dis 101:93–104, 1995, with permission.

In more recent follow-up studies of a subset of these vaccinees (120 health care workers), 31% lost detectable FAMA antibodies after, on average, 8 years. Twelve (10%) developed varicella; all had mild infections, despite loss of detectable VZV antibodies.[179] In another study from this group of investigators, 9% of almost 500 adult vaccinees developed chickenpox, with follow-up for some individuals as long as 21 years. Eighteen (21%) developed varicella after household exposure (n = 85). Neither the severity of breakthrough varicella nor the attack rate after household exposure increased with time.[393]

In the Merck postlicensure studies of vaccine safety, which included adults and children, breakthrough varicella was very rarely severe.[174] There were 11 reports of breakthrough varicella that was thought to be severe after the distribution of over 16 million doses of vaccine. Presumably most of these cases occurred in individuals who did not respond immunologically to the vaccine.

Summary

In summary, all data thus far support long-term persistence of humoral or cellular immunity in most healthy vaccinees, both children and adults. Although loss of detectable antibodies may occur, usually complete, and at least partial,

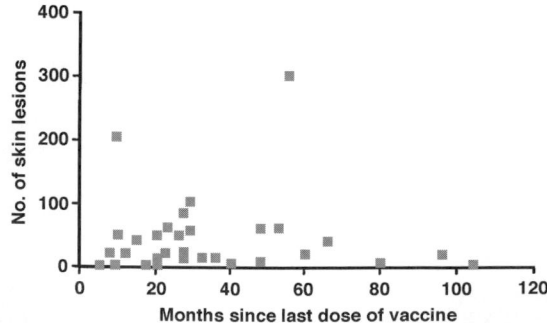

FIGURE 28–10 ■ Number of skin lesions in 31 vaccinated adults with breakthrough varicella months to years later with respect to the time since the last dose of varicella vaccine was given. Note that the severity of illness did not increase with an increasing interval (in months) since immunization. The average number of skin lesions was 43. (From Gershon A. Varicella-zoster virus: prospects for control. Adv Pediatr Infect Dis 10:93–124, 1995, with permission.)

immunity to VZV persists. Boosting of immunity through exposure to VZV occurs, but whether it is required for long-term persistence of immunity is not yet known. The only somewhat troubling finding thus far is the reported high cumulative rate of breakthrough varicella in some healthy vaccinees, which may have been dose related. However, these breakthrough cases usually have been mild.

Herpes Zoster in Vaccinated Individuals

A major question concerning the varicella vaccine has been whether the vaccine virus can establish latency, potentially resulting in later development of HZ. A long-term follow-up of vaccinated, healthy children will be required to answer this question definitively, but it is doubtful that such a study, spanning over 5 decades, can ever be practically performed. Nevertheless, it is possible to obtain some significant information on the issue. In U.S. studies, the incidence of HZ has not been increased in healthy immunized children.[394,395] Table 28–4 outlines the cases of HZ reported in clinical trials.

The reported incidence of HZ in healthy young vaccinated children is 13 cases per 100,000 person-years of observation.[396] In children ages 5 to 9 years who experienced natural varicella, it was 30 cases per 100,000 person-years of observation.[61] Specimens from rashes clinically diagnosed as HZ were investigated in 56 vaccinees in the Merck post-

marketing safety study.[174] The Oka strain was identified in 22 and wild-type VZV in 10. It should be recalled that this safety information pertained to over 16 million doses of vaccine that had been distributed. It is not possible to calculate the incidence of HZ from this information, but it is clear that HZ remains a rare occurrence in healthy vaccinated children.

Comparative information on the frequency of development of HZ in immunized immunocompromised children and those who had natural varicella is available. This is because children with leukemia who have had natural chickenpox develop HZ at a much higher rate than healthy children.[67] Vaccinated leukemic children were therefore followed closely for development of HZ and compared to leukemic children who had natural varicella. In Japan, one study found HZ in 8 (15%) of 52 vaccinated children and in 11 (18%) of 63 children with a history of varicella.[397] In the United States, none of 34 vaccinated leukemics but 15 (21%) of 73 leukemics with a history of varicella developed HZ ($P = 0.017$),[344] also suggesting that HZ would be less common after immunization than natural infection. In the NIAID collaborative study, the rate of HZ was 2% in vaccinees and 15% in controls with a history of varicella. A subset of these vaccinees were prospectively matched, according to chemotherapeutic protocol, with 96 leukemic children who had experienced natural varicella. A life table analysis revealed that the incidence of HZ was significantly

TABLE 28–4 ■ Cases of Herpes Zoster (HZ) Reported After Vaccination with Oka/Merck

Age (yr)	Interval Since Vaccination (yr)	Vaccine Dose (PFU)	VZV-Like Rash After Vaccination	Culture Results	Serology Results*	Description of Cases
8	4.2	87	No	Negative	Acute = 1448	10 papular and 25 vesicular lesions on back over right scapula and right arm; no other complaints
6	3.6	872	No	None	Acute = 2750	~9 erythematous patches, ranging in size from 2 × 2 mm to 15 × 9 mm, each composed of clusters of papulovesicular lesions; lesions were located along the right T6 dermatome; some upper airway congestion, itching
7	5.8	950	Chickenpox 1.5 yr before onset of HZ	Negative	Acute = 34.4 Conv = 2155	Vesicular rash on chest, arms (73 vesicles along C8, T1, T2 dermatomes); minimal itching, painful and burning sensation 1 week before onset
4	2.4	1460	Yes—injection site rash	None	Conv = 247.2	"Few" papular lesions in sacral area; no complaints
12	1.8	1460	No	Negative	Acute = 20	22 zoster-like lesions, papules and vesicles with surrounding erythema on left arm–hand; pruritus, local irritation: stinging before onset of lesion
2	1.8	3010	No	Positive; wild type	Acute = 112.2 Conv = 1551.9	Zoster-like lesions in the path of right ulnar nerve, right buttocks, right shoulder; restless; lesions painful to touch
6	3.3	5880	Non–injection site rash	None	Acute = 115 Conv = 2025	1 vesicular chain from upper chest to upper left arm; itching
2	1.2	5850	No	Negative	No sample	5 papular, 6 vesicular, 5 macular lesions on left upper arm and fourth and fifth digit of left hand; minor discomfort on lesions

*Glycoprotein-based enzyme-linked immunosorbent assay; conv, convalescent.
From White CJ. Clinical trials of varicella vaccine in healthy children. Infect Dis Clin North Am 10:595–608, 1996, with permission.

lower in vaccinees than in the matched leukemics who had experienced natural varicella[66,330] (Fig. 28–11).

Similar results were found in vaccinated children who underwent renal transplantation. In the study of vaccination of French children prior to renal transplantation, over 10 years, the rate of HZ was 7% in vaccinees, 13% in those with varicella before transplantation, and 38% in those who developed varicella after grafting.[339]

There are several possibilities, which are not mutually exclusive, as to why HZ may be less common after vaccination than after natural infection. One is that the virus is attenuated and less able to reactivate than the wild-type virus. Another is that the vaccine strain may have less frequent access to sensory nerves if there is a lower incidence of viremia and infection of the skin, as is frequently the case after vaccination.

It was first observed in Japan that HZ occurred far more frequently in children who had a vaccine-associated rash (16% of 83) than in those with no rash after immunization (2% of 249) (Collaborative Study Group of Varicella Vaccine, Ministry of Health and Welfare, Japan, unpublished data, 1974 to 1983). This observation was confirmed and extended in the NIAID collaborative study.[66,330] Of 13 vaccinated leukemic children who developed HZ, 11 (85%) had a prior history of a VZV-related rash, either vaccine associated (8 children) or breakthrough varicella (3 children). Both children with no history of rash developed HZ at the injection site of the vaccine. In the 268 vaccinees who had any type of previous VZV-related rash, the chance of subsequent development of HZ was more than six times greater than in the 280 vaccinees who had no VZV-associated rash. In the NIAID collaborative study, it was possible to

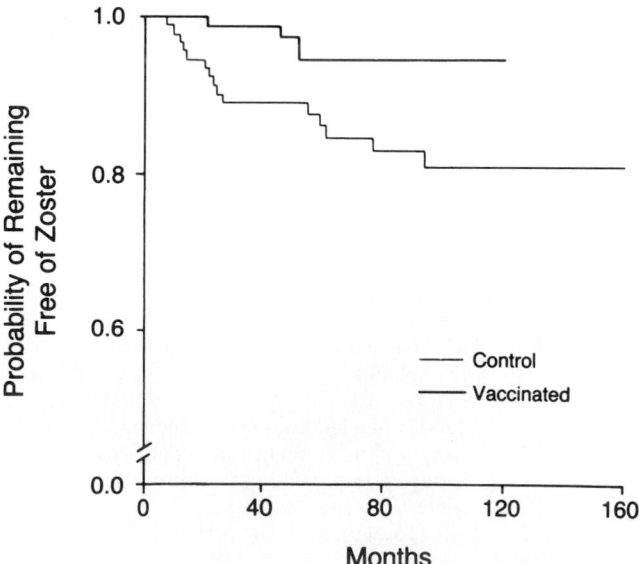

FIGURE 28–11 ▪ Kaplan-Meier product-limit analysis of the probability of remaining free of zoster in 96 children with leukemia who received varicella vaccine and 96 children with leukemia who had naturally acquired chickenpox before or after the diagnosis of leukemia. (From Hardy IB, Gershon A, Steinberg S, et al. The incidence of zoster after immunization with live attenuated varicella vaccine: a study in children with leukemia. N Engl J Med 325:1545–1550, 1991, with permission of the *New England Journal of Medicine*.)

type four of the viruses causing HZ. Two were due to vaccine-type virus and two were caused by wild-type VZV.[329] Because a vaccine-associated rash is unusual in healthy vaccinated children or adults, and breakthrough varicella is also unusual, it is expected that the incidence of HZ will be lower in healthy vaccinees than in those who have had the natural infection.[346]

In the NIAID collaborative study, only 1 adult of 268 has developed HZ. This physician vaccinee had seroconverted after vaccination, but she lost detectable VZV antibodies after 1 year. She was exposed to a patient with varicella, after which she again seroconverted without any symptoms. About 1 year later she developed thoracic HZ from which wild-type VZV was cultured.[398] Although the cell-mediated immune response to VZV has been found to be low in vaccinated adults and this is known to predispose to HZ, the incidence of HZ appears to be low in adult vaccinees. Thus there is a single report of HZ in an adult vaccinee, although not caused by the vaccine-type virus, as mentioned above. There are no reports of the Oka strain causing zoster in an adult.

Studies of Simultaneous Administration of Varicella Vaccine with Other Vaccines

Studies have been performed in children to evaluate the safety and immunogenicity of varicella given with measles-mumps-rubella (MMR) vaccine.[399,400] In the study reported by Englund et al.,[399] seroconversion rates were greater than 95% for all four viral components whether given concomitantly at separate anatomic sites using two syringes, or separated by 6 weeks. The varicella vaccine used in that study contained approximately 3450 PFU. All vaccines were well tolerated whether given simultaneously or 6 weeks apart. In the study reported by Just et al.,[400] there were no statistical differences in seroconversion rates to varicella in children who received the varicella vaccine alone (either ~6000 or ~12,000 PFU) or simultaneously with MMR vaccine. If the two vaccines were mixed together in the same syringe, however, approximately 20% of the children did not seroconvert to varicella.

More recent studies using the Oka vaccine manufactured by Merck, containing approximately 3000 PFU and given concomitantly at separate sites with MMR vaccine, indicated no significant interactions[401] (Table 28–5). Children 12 to 23 months of age were randomized to receive either MMR followed by the varicella vaccine 6 weeks later or the two vaccines concomitantly. Seroconversion rates were more than 98% to all four components in both groups, and the GMTs were similar.

Clinical studies evaluating the safety and immunogenicity when varicella vaccine manufactured by Merck is administered concomitantly with oral poliovirus vaccine (OPV), *Haemophilus influenzae* type b (Hib) vaccine, MMR vaccine, and diphtheria and tetanus toxoids and acellular and whole-cell pertussis (DTaP and DTwP) vaccines have been completed. All vaccines were well tolerated whether given concomitantly or separately from varicella vaccine. In one study, children 12 to 23 months of age were randomized to receive OPV, DTwP-Hib, MMR, and varicella vaccines concomitantly or varicella vaccine given 6 weeks later.[402] Titers to VZV were significantly lower ($P \leq 0.001$)

TABLE 28–5 ■ Concomitant Use Study: MMR II and Oka/Merck Varicella Vaccine Seroconversion Rates and Geometric Mean Titers*

	Group A	Group B	Geometric Mean Fold Difference, Group A/Group B (95% CI)
Viral component	MMR II and Varivax given concomitantly	MMR II and Varivax given 6 wk apart	
Measles			
Seroconversion rate	98% (247/252)	98.2% (224/228)	0.98 (0.85, 1.13)
GMTs	131.0	133.3	
Mumps			
Seroconversion rate	99.6% (239/240)	99.1% (216/218)	1.03 (0.85, 1.25)
GMTs	82.5	80.0	
Rubella			
Seroconversion rate	98.4% (247/251)	100% (225/225)	1.02 (0.88, 1.18)
GMTs	154.8	151.8	
Varicella			
Seroconversion rate	99.5% (199/200)	100% (174/174)	0.74 (0.63, 0.87)
GMTs	13.2	17.9	

*Six weeks after vaccination.
CI, confidence interval; GMTs, geometric mean titers.
From White CJ. Clinical trials of varicella vaccine in healthy children. Infect Dis Clin North Am 10:595–608, 1996, with permission.

in the group that received all vaccines concomitantly (11.2 vs. 15.2 by gp ELISA), but seroconversion rates to VZV were greater than 95% in both groups. One year after vaccination, the GMTs to VZV were similar between the groups (28.2 vs. 27.3). In another study, varicella vaccine was given concomitantly or 6 weeks after DTaP, Hib, and OPV. Results showed similar safety and immunogenicity for all antigens tested (Dr. Joel Ward, University of California at Los Angeles, personal communication, 1998).

A combination MMR-varicella vaccine has been difficult to develop because titers to the varicella component are unacceptably low.[401,403–405] It is hoped, however, that eventually such a product will become available, in which case two doses of varicella vaccine may become standard.

Indications for Vaccination

Healthy Children

The Oka vaccine manufactured by Biken was licensed in the late 1980s for use in healthy children in Japan and Korea. The Oka vaccine manufactured by Merck was licensed in the United States in 1995. Following licensure, the vaccine was recommended for universal use by the American Academy of Pediatrics[406–408] and the ACIP[262,341] for healthy, varicella-susceptible children 12 months to 12 years of age. Only one dose (administered subcutaneously) is recommended at present; ongoing surveillance and studies are being conducted to determine the need for a two-dose vaccine policy in children, similar to the policy recommendations for MMR vaccines. Oka vaccines manufactured by GlaxoSmithKline and Merck were later licensed for use in healthy children in several European countries such as Germany and Spain. Oka vaccines manufactured by Biken, GlaxoSmithKline, and Merck were later licensed in several countries in the Far East, Southeast Asia, and Central and South America, including the Philippines, Australia, Hong Kong, Singapore, Thailand, Brazil, and Mexico. It is expected that many of the other developed countries worldwide will license the vaccine for use in healthy children over the next few years. In 2002, the United States was the only country where universal childhood vaccination programs are being implemented.

On the basis of available data on postexposure effectiveness of varicella vaccine, in the United States, varicella vaccine is recommended for postexposure use and also for outbreak control in healthy children and adults.[341]

Immunocompromised Children

Varicella vaccine is licensed for use in immunocompromised children in Japan, Korea, and some European countries. In the United States, the FDA allows the vaccine to be used in leukemic children in remission for at least 1 year on an individual, compassionate-use basis. Vaccination for this purpose can be arranged by contacting the Varivax Coordinating Center at Bio-Pharm Clinical Services, Inc. (4 Valley Square, Blue Bell, PA 19422; telephone 215-283-0897). The following guidelines are suggested for vaccination of leukemic children in the United States:

1. The child must be in full remission from leukemia for at least 1 year.
2. The child must have a total peripheral lymphocyte count of 700 cells/mm³ or more on the day the vaccine is administered.
3. Tests for cell-mediated immunity, such as stimulation of peripheral blood lymphocytes with mitogens or antigens, prior to immunization are optional.
4. Antileukemic chemotherapy should be withheld for 1 week before immunization and 1 week afterward. In addition, steroid therapy should not be given for a total of 2 weeks after vaccination.[332] It is only necessary to withhold chemotherapy for the first dose of vaccine.
5. Two doses of vaccine, 3 months apart are given. It is desirable to document a seroconversion to VZV by a sensitive, reliable test such as FAMA or LA in leukemic vaccinees. Most commercially available ELISA tests are not sensitive enough for this purpose,

and experience with other ELISA tests may be too limited to be used to indicate immunity in these high-risk children.[409] The sensitive LA antibody assay is currently the best widely available test for this purpose.

6. Close follow-up after vaccination is recommended for possible adverse effects. Children who develop more than 50 skin lesions should be given ACV. Usually this can be given orally, at a dose of 900 mg/kg per dose 4 times a day. Children who appear ill or toxic or who have extensive skin rashes (over 200 lesions) should receive ACV intravenously at the usual dosage for varicella (1500 mg/m²/day).

Children who are somewhat immunocompromised, such as those with asthma or nephrosis who are receiving low doses of steroids, have been safely immunized in Japan.[295] No data are available from the United States; however, based on Japanese studies, the vaccine is recommended for use in these children.[262,341,406,407] The American Academy of Pediatrics recommends that children receiving more than 2 mg/kg/day of prednisone (or its equivalent) not be immunized until they have not taken steroids for at least 3 months. Limited data from a clinical trial in which two doses of varicella vaccine were administered to 41 asymptomatic or mildly symptomatic HIV-infected children (CDC class N1 or A1, age-specific CD4+ T-lymphocyte count of ≥25%) indicated that the vaccine was immunogenic and safe.[340] Based on these data, the ACIP has stated that, after weighing potential risks and benefits, varicella vaccine should be considered for use in HIV-infected children who are asymptomatic and have more than 25% CD4 lymphocytes[341] because children infected with HIV are at increased risk for morbidity from varicella and herpes zoster (i.e., shingles) compared with healthy children. Eligible children should receive two doses of varicella vaccine with a 3-month interval between doses. There are no published recommendations in the United States for immunization of children with renal failure prior to transplantation.

Adults

Because healthy adults are at increased risk to develop severe varicella, it is highly desirable that they be immunized if they are susceptible to chickenpox. It is particularly important to immunize those who are likely to be exposed to VZV, such as persons who live or work in environments where transmission of VZV is likely (e.g., teachers of young children, day care employees, and residents and staff members in institutional settings); persons who live and work in environments where transmission can occur (e.g., college students, inmates and staff members of correctional institutions, and military personnel); nonpregnant women of child-bearing age; adolescents and adults living in households with children; and international travelers. In the United States, vaccine is recommended for susceptible healthy adults. Susceptibility can be determined by absence of history of varicella or on the basis of negative serology. Two doses of vaccine are given 4 to 8 weeks apart. It is desirable to perform serologic testing for susceptibility to varicella by ELISA or LA before vaccination, particularly for women of child-bearing age and hospital personnel. Following immunization, LA could be used as a practical test to confirm a seroconversion because ELISA lacks sensitivity. If it not possible to perform serologic testing prior to immunization, then vaccination of adults with no history of varicella can be carried out, but at least 70% of these adults will have pre-existing immunity to varicella.[145,410] A study done in India documented annual outbreaks of varicella among health care workers, and the authors recommended systematic vaccination of susceptible persons to avoid nosocomial transmission.[410a]

Studies for Prevention of Herpes Zoster

Many healthy adults ages 55 to 65 years with a past history of varicella and detectable humoral immunity to VZV have negative cell-mediated immune responses to VZV.[157,158] Because it is now apparent that low cell-mediated immunity to VZV predisposes to development of HZ, there is interest in immunizing elderly individuals with varicella vaccine. In one open-label study, 33 healthy individuals in this age group were immunized with live, attenuated vaccine, and, in 28 (85%), vaccination induced a change from negative to positive VZV cell-mediated immunity as measured by lymphocyte transformation.[411] An increase in antibody titer also was observed in over 75% of the vaccinees. Retesting of a few of the vaccinees showed that the increase in cell-mediated immunity persisted for at least 1 year. In another study, 11 of 11 vaccinated elderly adults manifested a cell-mediated immune response, including increased responder cell frequency levels, that was similar to that seen in elderly adults following HZ, indicating that immunization can elicit a T-cell response in this group.[160]

In a study in Japan, individuals 50 years old or older were screened for VZV antibodies by IAHA and were skin tested for cell-mediated immunity to VZV. All were seropositive, but eight were skin test negative.[412] A high-titered vaccine (3.0×10^4 PFU) was administered. After immunization, the skin test reaction showed increased positivity, with a change in score from (−) to (+ or ++) in 7 of 8 subjects, from (+) to (++ or +++) in 3 of 5 subjects, and from (++) to (+++) in 6 of 10 subjects. Enhancement of VZV antibody titers (defined as a twofold or greater increase) was observed in all vaccine recipients. This boost in antibody titer occurred in 15 of 15 subjects with a prevaccination titer of 1:16 or less, and in 19 of 24 subjects with a prevaccination titer of 32 or greater. These results also indicate that administration of live varicella vaccine can boost immunity to VZV in the elderly (Table 28–6).

TABLE 28–6 ■ Enhancement of VZV Skin Test Reaction and Antibody Response in the Elderly by Giving Live Varicella Vaccine*

VZV skin test			
(−)	→	(+)	7/8
(+)	→	(++)	3/5
(++)	→	(+++)	6/10
Antibody response		15/15	(prevaccination titer ≤ 16)
(2-fold or greater increase)		19/24	(prevaccination titer = 32)

*Four to 6 weeks after giving one dose of VZV vaccination to the elderly (≥50 to 65 years old), VZV skin test was done and blood specimen was collected. Antibody assay (IAHA) was performed simultaneously for pre- and postvaccination sera.

From Takahashi M, Kamiya H, Asano Y, et al. Immunization of the elderly to boost immunity against varicella-zoster virus (VZV) as assessed by VZV skin test reaction. Arch Virol Suppl 17:161–172, 2001, with permission.

Clinical studies also have suggested the possible efficacy of boosting of immunity to prevent or modify zoster. The incidence of HZ was lower in children who received two doses of vaccine than in those who received one dose among leukemic children vaccinated in the NIAID collaborative study, suggesting that immunization of individuals who may already have latent infection can prevent HZ.[331] In this same study, a household exposure to varicella also was associated with protection against zoster. In an uncontrolled study of 202 individuals ages 55 to over 87 years, there was an increase in cell-mediated immunity to VZV, as determined by an increase in responder cell frequency in a lymphocyte transformation assay with VZV as the antigen, that lasted as long as 4 years. Although, mainly because of the small study size, the incidence of HZ was not clearly decreased, all presumed cases of zoster were exceedingly mild and of short duration, with very little pain.[413] In a small ($N = 200$) double-blind controlled study in healthy older individuals, a significant increase in cell-mediated immunity to VZV was observed after vaccination. However, this study was not large enough to examine whether zoster could be prevented or modified by immunization.[414] A double-blind, placebo-controlled efficacy study involving over 30,000 individuals over age 50 years is currently in progress, which should determine definitively whether immunization will prevent or modify HZ.[415]

The potential for the ability of an inactivated form of varicella vaccine to prevent zoster in bone marrow transplant patients has been explored.[416,417] These studies indicate that this approach can be successful in preventing zoster in these high-risk patients. In a group of patients who received four doses of heat-inactivated vaccine containing 6115 PFU, one dose prior to autologous transplant and three doses afterward, 7 (13%) of 53 vaccines and 19 (33%) of 58 unvaccinated controls developed zoster ($P = 0.01$).[416]

Contraindications and Precautions

Contraindications and precautions to vaccination as recommended by the ACIP in the United States are summarized below. Information in the package insert should also be reviewed carefully before administration of varicella vaccine.

Allergy to Vaccine Components

Vaccination is contraindicated for persons who have a history of anaphylactic reaction to any component of the vaccine, including gelatin. Varicella vaccine does not contain preservatives or egg protein—substances that have caused hypersensitive reactions to other vaccines. Varicella vaccine should not be administered to persons who have a history of anaphylactic reaction to neomycin.

Illness

Vaccination of persons who have severe illness should be postponed until recovery. Vaccine can be administered to susceptible children who have mild illnesses with or without low-grade fever (e.g., diarrhea or upper respiratory tract infection).[418] Although no data exist regarding whether either varicella or varicella vaccine exacerbates tuberculosis, vaccination is not recommended for persons who have untreated, active tuberculosis.

Altered Immunity

In the United States, use of varicella vaccine is contraindicated in persons with cellular immune deficiencies, including blood dyscrasias, leukemia (except under a research protocol as described above), lymphomas of any type, and other malignant neoplasms affecting the bone marrow or lymphatic systems. Updated recommendations for use of varicella vaccine state that persons with impaired humoral immunity may now be vaccinated and that some HIV-infected children may now be considered for vaccination (see above).[262,341]

Persons Who Have Conditions That Require Steroid Therapy

Susceptible persons who are receiving systemic steroids for certain conditions (e.g., asthma) and who are not otherwise immunocompromised can be vaccinated if they are receiving less than 2 mg/kg of body weight or a total of 20 mg/day of prednisone or its equivalent. Antibody status should be assessed 6 weeks postvaccination, and persons who have not seroconverted should be revaccinated. Some experts suggest withholding steroids for 2 to 3 weeks following vaccination when possible.

No data have been published concerning whether susceptible children receiving only inhaled doses of steroids can be vaccinated safely. However, most experts concur, on the basis of clinical experience, that vaccination of these children is safe (CDC, unpublished data, 1999).

Use of Salicylates

No adverse events associated with the use of salicylates after varicella vaccination have been reported. However, the vaccine manufacturer recommends that vaccine recipients avoid using salicylates for 6 weeks after receiving varicella virus vaccine because of the association between aspirin use and Reye's syndrome following varicella. Vaccination with subsequent close monitoring should be considered for children who have rheumatoid arthritis or other conditions requiring therapeutic aspirin because the risk for serious complications associated with aspirin is likely to be greater in children in whom natural varicella disease develops than in children who receive the vaccine containing attenuated VZV.

Recent Administration of Blood, Plasma, or Immune Globulin

Because the vaccine is a live, attenuated virus, it should not be given concurrently with IG. The effect of the administration of IG on the response to varicella vaccine is unknown. However, because of the potential inhibition of the response to varicella vaccination by passively transferred antibodies, varicella vaccine should not be administered for at least 5 months after administration of blood (except washed red blood cells), plasma, IG, or VZIG. In addition, IG and VZIG should not be administered for 3 weeks after vaccination unless the benefits exceed those of vaccination. In such cases, the vaccinee should either be revaccinated 5 months later or tested for immunity 6 months later and then revaccinated if seronegative.

Exposure of Immunocompromised Persons to Vaccinees

Healthy persons in whom varicella-like rash develops following vaccination appear to have a minimal risk for transmission of vaccine virus to their close contacts (e.g., family members). Only four cases have been documented of transmission from healthy persons to immunocompetent household members (see *Contact Spread of Vaccine Virus* above). Vaccinees in whom vaccine-related rash develops, particularly health care workers and household contacts of immunocompromised persons, should avoid contact with susceptible persons who are at high risk for severe complications. If a susceptible, immunocompromised person is inadvertently exposed to a person who has a vaccine-related rash, VZIG need not be administered because disease associated with this type of transmission is expected to be mild. For susceptible persons, having an immunocompromised household member is not a contraindication to vaccination.

Pregnant Women and Nursing Mothers

Although no infants with the congenital varicella syndrome secondary to vaccine-type virus have been reported, vaccination in pregnancy is contraindicated. If a woman inadvertently receives varicella vaccination 3 months before or at any time during pregnancy, it should be reported to the Varivax Pregnancy Registry (1-800-986-8999) to monitor the maternal-fetal outcomes.[419] Published data from this registry indicate that 92 women known to be seronegative to varicella have been inadvertently vaccinated; 58 of them received the first dose of vaccine during the first or second trimester. No cases of the congenital varicella syndrome were identified among 56 live births.[420] For susceptible persons, having a pregnant household member is not a contraindication to vaccination.

Whether attenuated vaccine VZV is excreted in human milk and, if so, whether the infant could be infected are not known. Most live vaccines have not been demonstrated to be secreted in breast milk. Therefore, the ACIP considers that varicella vaccine may be considered for a nursing mother. A study is in progress to provide data on this issue.

Public Health Considerations

Goals and Cost Effectiveness of Vaccination

The goal of varicella vaccination is to prevent severe illness and death resulting from varicella. Monitoring the effects of the varicella vaccination program should include both vaccine (safety, coverage, and effectiveness) and disease monitoring. To assess the impact of the varicella vaccination program, monitoring trends in both varicella and HZ are needed. Although varicella vaccine has been available in Japan for 20 years, it is not a routinely recommended childhood vaccine there under the national vaccination program, hence use has been limited and coverage has remained low, well below 50%. The greatest amount of experience with implementation of a national vaccination program is from the United States. Varicella vaccine was added to the routine childhood vaccination program in 1995, and, by December 2001, vaccine coverage among children 19 to 35 months was 76%.[421]

In the United States, monitoring occurrence of infectious diseases is most commonly conducted using a nationally notifiable disease surveillance system. However,

because varicella was not a nationally notifiable disease at the start of the vaccination program, active varicella surveillance was established in 1995 in three communities with a combined population of 1.2 million persons. By 2000, in these communities, vaccine coverage among children 19 to 35 months had reached 74% to 84% and reported varicella cases and hospitalizations had declined dramatically (Fig. 28–12 and Table 28–7). From 1995 to 2000, varicella cases declined 71%, 84%, and 79% in the three communities.[422] Cases declined to the greatest extent among children 1 to 4 years of age, but cases declined in all age groups, including infants and adults, indicating herd immunity effects. From 1995 to 2000, among adults 20 years of age or older, reported cases per 1000 population declined from 0.8 to 0.2, and, in infants less than 12 months, reported cases declined from 19.7 to 4.8 per 1000 population. In the combined surveillance areas, varicella-related hospitalizations declined from a range of 2.7 to 4.2 per 100,000 population from 1995 to 1998 to 0.6 and 1.5 per 100,000 population in 1999 and 2000, respectively.[422] In the United States, surveillance for varicella and HZ is being conducted in larger population settings, with no change noted thus far in the incidence of HZ in any age group as varicella incidence declined markedly in all age groups (CDC, unpublished data, 2001).

Depending on the goals of a vaccination program, options for other countries to consider include universal vaccination of children between 12 and 18 months of age

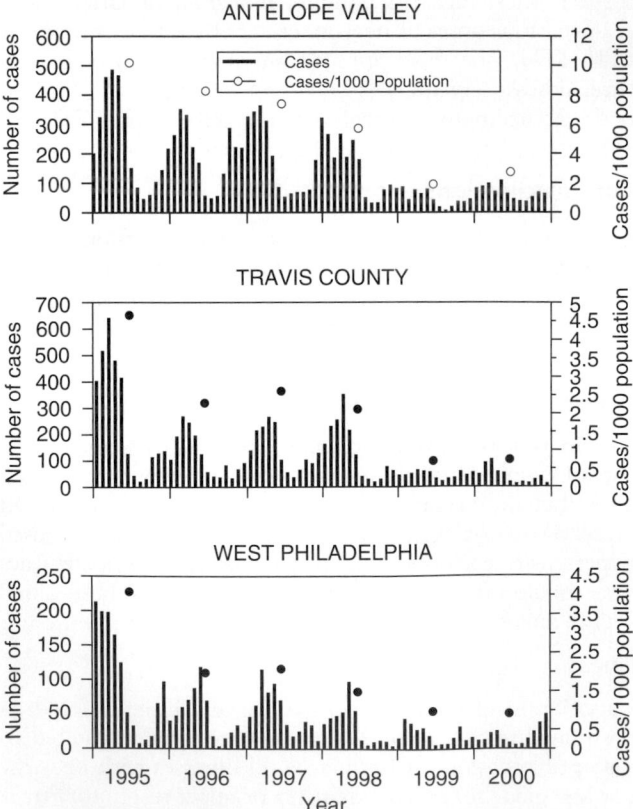

FIGURE 28–12 ▪ Reported varicella cases by month and annual rates of reported cases per 1000 population in three surveillance areas, 1995–2000.

TABLE 28–7 ▪ Percent Reduction of Reported Varicella Cases in 2000 Compared to 1995 in Three Surveillance Areas in the United States

Age	Antelope Valley, CA (%)	Travis County, TX (%)	West Philadelphia, PA (%)
<1	69	81	68
1–4	83	90	83
5–9	63	77	77
10–14	65	75	80
15–19	85	83	81
≥20	66	64	68
Total	71	84	79

From Seward JF, Watson BM, Peterson CL, et al. Varicella disease after introduction of varicella vaccine in the United States, 1995–2000. JAMA 287:606–611, 2002.

with or without catch-up vaccination of older children and adolescents. Other possibilities include selective vaccination of adolescents and/or adults, including women of child-bearing age, or targeted vaccination of high-risk groups, including children with leukemia, HIV infection, and candidates for organ transplantation; health care workers; and family contacts of immunocompromised persons.

Several published studies on the significance of varicella as a public health problem were considered when varicella vaccine was added to the childhood immunization schedule in the United States.[30,423–425] Additional studies providing data on costs of varicella, as well as cost-benefit and cost-effectiveness studies providing economic evaluations of childhood vaccination programs and selective vaccination programs among adolescents, adults, women of child-bearing age, military recruits, health care workers, and pediatric liver and kidney transplant recipients, have since been published from the United States, France, Germany, Spain, Australia, New Zealand, and Canada.[426–445] The majority of these articles are summarized in a review of economic evaluations of varicella vaccination programs.[446] There is general agreement that universal vaccination of 15-month-old children is beneficial from a societal perspective mainly because of savings from prevented lost workdays for the parents. From the health care payer perspective, a universal childhood vaccination program will not provide savings at the current price of vaccine.

Several studies have concluded that, from a purely economic viewpoint, vaccination of susceptible adolescents is the optimal approach.[426,427] However, because the major burden of disease caused by varicella occurs in children, vaccination of adolescents would have limited impact on reducing overall disease burden.

Results from several studies examining whether it is cost effective to conduct serologic testing prior to vaccination of adolescents or adults with negative or uncertain varicella histories have been conflicting. Two studies found that serologic testing was more cost effective than routinely vaccinating all those with negative or uncertain disease histories,[447,448] whereas one study did not.[449]

The costs and public health impact of varicella disease in hospital settings have been well documented with regard to such factors as work furloughs, serologic testing, patient isolation, administration of VZIG, wages paid to replacement health care workers, and infection control staff time.[431,432,434,440,445,450] Studies of vaccination programs aimed at preventing nosocomial VZV exposure and transmission to high-risk patients by vaccinating health care workers have confirmed that these programs generate savings from an employer's perspective.[431,432,434,440,445,450] Factors that affect the results the most are vaccine price and accuracy of screening of disease history as it relates to true susceptibility. In the United States, health care workers are designated as a priority group for vaccination because of their risk of close contact with persons at high risk for severe disease. Because nosocomial VZV problems are likely to be universal and the problem may be greater in populations where a higher proportion of adult health care workers are susceptible, protection of health care workers through vaccination should be strongly considered even in countries where a childhood vaccination program is not a high priority.

Effect of Vaccination on Herpes Zoster Incidence

The effect that varicella may have on the incidence of HZ is poorly understood. It is recognized that the risk of acquiring HZ is related to loss of cell-mediated immunity to VZV. Whether exposure to varicella disease throughout life maintains immunity to VZV through external boosting is uncertain. Several studies have attempted to take into account the effect that a varicella vaccination program may have on HZ using mathematical modeling of VZV transmission, with assumptions of external boosting of VZV immunity and the duration of the boost in immunity to estimate the incidence of HZ. These studies predict that, if exposure to varicella is an important mechanism for preventing reactivation of VZV, a short- to medium-term increase in HZ cases may occur after implementation of a varicella vaccination program, although, in the long term, a reduction in zoster cases is expected to occur provided that vaccine recipients have a lower risk of developing zoster than persons who acquire natural infection.[451,452] Evidence that exposure to varicella may affect the risk of developing HZ was provided by a study that reported a lower age-specific incidence of HZ among persons who lived in households with children less than 16 years of age, considered a surrogate for risk of exposure to varicella.[453] Administration of varicella vaccine has been shown to boost cell-mediated immunity to VZV in the elderly,[411,412,415] and a study among adults to determine whether vaccination prevents or modifies HZ is in progress in the United States.[415] Ongoing surveillance for changes in the epidemiology of both varicella and HZ are underway in the United States.

Potential for Eradication

Because VZV is able to establish latency, and because breakthrough varicella occurs, it is not expected that a universal immunization program with a live, attenuated VZV vaccine will completely eliminate circulation of the virus. Thus varicella presents unique and challenging issues with regard to eventual eradication of the disease. Nevertheless, the widespread use of varicella vaccine will improve the health of many children, adolescents, and adults who will no longer have to suffer with varicella and in the future perhaps HZ.

Acknowledgments

Work on this chapter was supported in part by Grants AI24021 and AI127187 from the National Institutes of Health.

REFERENCES

1. Takahashi M. Chickenpox virus. Adv Virus Res 29:285–356, 1983.
2. von Bokay J. Uber den aetiologischen zusammenhang der varizellen mit gewissen fallen von herpes zoster. Wien Klin Wochenschr 22:1323–1326, 1909.
3. Bruusgaard E. The mutual relation between zoster and varicella. Br J Dermatol Syph 44:1–24, 1932.
4. Kundratitz K. Experimentelle Ubertragung von Herpes Zoster auf den Mensschen und die Beziehungen von Herpes Zoster zu Varicellen. Monatsschr Kinderheilkd 29:516–523, 1925.
5. Garland J. Varicella following exposure to herpes zoster. N Engl J Med 228:336–337, 1943.
6. Weller T, Stoddard MB. Intranuclear inclusion bodies in cultures of human tissue inoculated with varicella vesicle fluid. J Immunol 68:311–319, 1952.
7. Weller TH. Serial propagation in vitro of agents producing inclusion bodies derived from varicella and herpes zoster. Proc Soc Exp Biol Med 83:340–346, 1953.
8. Weller TH, Coons AH. Fluorescent antibody studies with agents of varicella and herpes zoster propagated in vitro. Proc Soc Exp Biol Med 86:789, 1954.
9. Weller TH, Witton HM. The etiologic agents of varicella and herpes zoster: serological studies with the viruses as propagated in vitro. J Exp Med 108:869–890, 1958.
10. Takahashi M, Otsuka T, Okuno Y, et al. Live vaccine used to prevent the spread of varicella in children in hospital. Lancet 2:1288–1290, 1974.
11. Straus SE, Reinhold W, Smith HA, et al. Endonuclease analysis of viral DNA from varicella and subsequent zoster infections in the same patient. N Engl J Med 311:1362–1364, 1984.
12. Williams DL, Gershon A, Gelb LD, et al. Herpes zoster following varicella vaccine in a child with acute lymphocytic leukemia. J Pediatr 106:259–261, 1985.
13. Hayakawa Y, Torigoe S, Shiraki K, et al. Biologic and biophysical markers of a live varicella vaccine strain (Oka): identification of clinical isolates from vaccine recipients. J Infect Dis 149:956–963, 1984.
14. Grose CH. Variation on a theme by Fenner. Pediatrics 68:735–737, 1981.
15. Fenner F. The pathogenesis of the acute exanthems: an interpretation based on experimental investigations with mousepox (infectious ectromelia of mice). Lancet 2:915–920, 1948.
16. Hope-Simpson RE. Infectiousness of communicable diseases in the household (measles, mumps, and chickenpox). Lancet 2:549, 1952.
17. Ross AH, Lencher E, Reitman G. Modification of chickenpox in family contacts by administration of gamma globulin. N Engl J Med 267:369–376, 1962.
18. Balfour HH, Kelly JM, Suarez CS, et al. Acyclovir treatment of varicella in otherwise healthy children. J Pediatr 116:633–639, 1990.
19. Gershon AA, Steinberg S, Gelb L, for the NIAID Collaborative Varicella Vaccine Study Group. Clinical reinfection with varicella-zoster virus. J Infect Dis 149:137–142, 1984.
20. Junker AK, Angus E, Thomas E. Recurrent varicella-zoster virus infections in apparently immunocompetent children. Pediatr Infect Dis J 10:569–575, 1991.
21. Terada K, Kawano S, Shimada Y, et al. Recurrent chickenpox after natural infection. Pediatr Infect Dis J 15:179–181, 1996.
22. Junker AK, Tilley P. Varicella-zoster virus antibody avidity and IgG-subclass patterns in children with recurrent chickenpox. J Med Virol 43:119–124, 1994.
23. Abendroth A, Arvin AM. Immune evasion as a pathogenic mechanism of varicella zoster virus. Semin Immunol 13:27–39, 2001.
24. Farrell HE, Davis-Poynter NJ. From sabotage to camouflage: viral evasion of cytotoxic T lymphocyte and natural killer cell-mediated immunity. Cell Dev Biol 9:369–378, 1998.
25. Arvin A, Koropchak CM, Wittek AE. Immunologic evidence of reinfection with varicella-zoster virus. J Infect Dis 148:200–205, 1983.
26. Gershon A, Steinberg S, Borkowsky W, et al. IgM to varicella-zoster virus: demonstration in patients with and without clinical zoster. Pediatr Infect Dis J 1:164–167, 1982.
27. Gershon AA, Steinberg S, for the NIAID Collaborative Varicella Vaccine Study Group. Live attenuated varicella vaccine: protection in healthy adults in comparison to leukemic children. J Infect Dis 161:661–666, 1990.
28. Arvin A, Gershon A. Live attenuated varicella vaccine. Annu Rev Microbiol 50:59–100, 1996.
29. Choo PW, Donahue JG, Manson JE, Platt R. The epidemiology of varicella and its complications. J Infect Dis 172:706–712, 1995.
30. Preblud SR. Varicella: complications and costs. Pediatrics 76(suppl):728–735, 1986.
31. Quintero-del-Rio AI, Fink CW. Varicella arthritis in childhood. Pediatr Infect Dis J 16:241–243, 1997.
32. Centers for Disease Control and Prevention. Outbreak of invasive group A streptococcus associated with varicella in a childcare center—Boston, MA, 1997. MMWR Morb Mortal Wkly Rep 46:944–948, 1997.
33. Davies HD, McGeer A, Schwarts B, et al. Invasive group A streptococcal infections in Ontario, Canada. N Engl J Med 335:547–553, 1996.
34. Laupland KB, Davies HD, Low DE, et al. Invasive group A streptococcal disease in children and association with varicella-zoster virus infection. Ontario Group A Streptococcal Study Group. Pediatrics 105:E60, 2000.
35. Wilson G, Talkington D, Gruber W, et al. Group A streptococcal necrotizing fasciitis following varicella in children: case reports and review. Clin Infect Dis 20:1333–1338, 1995.
36. Guess HA, Broughton DD, Melton LJ, Kurland L. Population-based studies of varicella complications. Pediatrics 78(suppl):723–727, 1986.
37. Gogos CA, Bassaris HP, Vagenakis AG. Varicella pneumonia in adults: a review of pulmonary manifestations, risk factors, and treatment. Respiration 59:339–343, 1992.
38. Meyer P, Seward JF, Jumaan AO, Wharton M. Varicella mortality: trends before vaccine licensure in the United States, 1970–1994. J Infect Dis 182:383–390, 2000.
39. Wallace MR, Woelfl I, Bowler WA, et al. Tumor necrosis factor, interleukin-2, and interferon-gamma in adult varicella. J Med Virol 43:69–71, 1994.
40. Wallace MR, Chamberlin CJ, Sawyer MH, et al. Treatment of adult varicella with sorivudine: a randomized, placebo controlled trial. J Infect Dis 174:249–255, 1996.
41. Gershon A. Chickenpox, measles, and mumps. In Remington J, Klein J (eds). Infections of the Fetus and Newborn Infant (5th ed). Philadelphia, WB Saunders, 2001, pp 683–732.
42. Pastuszak A, Levy M, Schick B, et al. Outcome after maternal varicella infection in the first 20 weeks of pregnancy. N Engl J Med 330:901–905, 1994.
43. Enders G, Miller E, Cradock-Watson J, et al. Consequences of varicella and herpes zoster in pregnancy: prospective study of 1739 cases. Lancet 343:1548–1551, 1994.
44. Brunell PA, Kotchmar GSJ. Zoster in infancy: failure to maintain virus latency following intrauterine infection. J Pediatr 98:71–73, 1981.
45. Dworsky M, Whitely R, Alford C. Herpes zoster in early infancy. Am J Dis Child 134:618–619, 1980.
46. Hanngren K, Grandien M, Granstrom G. Effect of zoster immunoglobulin for varicella prophylaxis in the newborn. Scand J Infect Dis 17:343–347, 1985.
47. Meyers J. Congenital varicella in term infants: risk reconsidered. J Infect Dis 129:215–217, 1974.
48. Gershon A, Silverstein S. Varicella-zoster virus. In Richman D, Whitley R, Hayden F (eds). Clinical Virology. Washington, DC, ASM Press, 2002, pp 413–432.
49. Cheatham WJ, Weller TH, Dolan TF, Dower JC. Varicella: report of two fatal cases with necropsy, virus isolation, and serologic studies. Am J Pathol 32:1015–1035, 1956.
50. Feldman S, Hughes W, Daniel C. Varicella in children with cancer: 77 cases. Pediatrics 80:388–397, 1975.

51. Feldman S, Lott L. Varicella in children with cancer: impact of antiviral therapy and prophylaxis. Pediatrics 80:465–472, 1987.

52. Lynfield R, Herrin JT, Rubin RH. Varicella in pediatric renal transplant patients. Pediatrics 90:216–220, 1992.

53. Lanter R, Rockoff JB, DeMasi J, et al. Fatal varicella in a corticosteroid-dependent asthmatic receiving troleandomycin. Allergy Proc 11:83–87, 1990.

54. Silk H, Guay-Woodford L, Perez-Atayde A, et al. Fatal varicella in steroid-dependent asthma. J Allergy Clin Immunol 81:47–51, 1988.

55. Gershon A, Mervish N, LaRussa P, et al. Varicella-zoster virus infection in children with underlying HIV infection. J Infect Dis 176:1496–1500, 1997.

56. Jura E, Chadwick E, Josephs SH, et al. Varicella-zoster virus infections in children infected with human immunodeficiency virus. Pediatr Infect Dis J 8:586–590, 1989.

57. Hogan EL, Krigman MR. Herpes zoster myelitis. Arch Neurol 29:309–313, 1973.

58. Norris FH, Dramov B, Calder CD, et al. Virus-like particles in myositis accompanying herpes zoster. Arch Neurol 21:25–31, 1969.

59. Rubin D, Fusfeld RD. Muscle paralysis in herpes zoster. Calif Med 103:261–266, 1965.

60. Baba K, Yabuuchi H, Takahashi M, Ogra P. Increased incidence of herpes zoster in normal children infected with varicella-zoster virus during infancy: community-based follow up study. J Pediatr 108:372–377, 1986.

61. Guess H, Broughton DD, Melton LJ, Kurland L. Epidemiology of herpes zoster in children and adolescents: a population-based study. Pediatrics 76:512–517, 1985.

62. Terada K, Kawano S, Yoshihiro K, Morita T. Varicella-zoster virus (VZV) reactivation is related to the low response of VZV-specific immunity after chickenpox in infancy. J Infect Dis 169:650–652, 1994.

63. Hope-Simpson RE. The nature of herpes zoster: a long term study and a new hypothesis. Proc R Soc Med 58:9–20, 1965.

64. Schmader K, George LK, Burchett GM, et al. Racial differences in the occurrence of herpes zoster. J Infect Dis 171:701–704, 1995.

65. Whitley RJ. Varicella-zoster infections. In Mandell GL, Bennett JE, Dolin R (eds). Principles and Practice of Infectious Diseases. Philadelphia, Churchill Livingstone, 2000, pp 1580–1586.

66. Hardy IB, Gershon A, Steinberg S, et al. The incidence of zoster after immunization with live attenuated varicella vaccine: a study in children with leukemia. N Engl J Med 325:1545–1550, 1991.

67. Feldman S, Hughes WT, Kim HY. Herpes zoster in children with cancer. Am J Dis Child 126:178–184, 1973.

68. Veenstra J, Krol A, van Praag R, et al. Herpes zoster, immunological deterioration and disease progression in HIV-1 infection. AIDS 9:1153–1158, 1995.

69. Gnann JW, Whitley RJ. Natural history and treatment of varicella-zoster in high risk populations. J Hosp Infect 18:317–329, 1991.

70. Jacobson MA, Berger TG, Fikrig S. Acyclovir-resistant varicella-zoster virus infection after chronic oral acyclovir therapy in patients with the acquired immunodeficiency syndrome. Ann Intern Med 112:187–191, 1990.

71. Esiri M, Tomlinson A. Herpes zoster: demonstration of virus in trigeminal nerve and ganglion by immunofluorescence and electron microscopy. J Neurol Sci 15:35–48, 1972.

72. Gilden D. Herpes zoster with postherpetic neuralgia—persisting pain and frustration. N Engl J Med 330:932–934, 1994.

73. Gilden DH, Kleinschmidt-DeMasters BK, LaGuardia JJ, et al. Neurologic complications of the reactivation of varicella-zoster virus. N Engl J Med 342:635–645, 2000.

74. Watson CPN, Gershon A. Herpes Zoster and Postherpetic Neuralgia. Amsterdam, Elsevier, 2001.

75. Hope-Simpson RE. Postherpetic neuralgia. J R Coll Gen Pract 25:571–575, 1975.

76. McKendrick MW, McGill JI, Wood MJ, et al. Lack of effect of acyclovir on postherpetic neuralgia. BMJ 298:431, 1989.

77. Wood MJ. Herpes zoster and pain. Scand J Infect Dis 78:53–61, 1991.

78. Roizman B, Carmichael LE, Deinhardt W, et al. Herpesviridae: definition, provisional nomenclature and taxonomy. Intervirology 16:201–217, 1981.

79. Davison AJ, Scott JE. The complete DNA sequence of varicella-zoster virus. J Gen Virol 67:1759–1816, 1986.

80. Dumas AH, Geelen JLMC, Weststrate MW, et al. XbaI, PstI, and BglII restriction enzyme maps of the two orientations of the varicella-zoster virus genome. J Virol 39:390–400, 1981.

81. Ecker JR, Hyman RW. Varicella zoster virus DNA exists as two isomers. Proc Natl Acad Sci U S A 79:156–160, 1982.

82. Straus SE, Aulakh HS, Ruyechan WT, et al. Structure of varicella-zoster virus DNA. J Virol 40:516–526, 1981.

83. Hay J, Ruyechan WT. Varicella-zoster virus: a different kind of herpesvirus latency? Semin Virol 5:241–248, 1994.

84. Grose C. Glycoproteins encoded by varicella-zoster virus: biosynthesis, phosphorylation, and intracellular trafficking. Annu Rev Microbiol 44:59–80, 1990.

85. Grose C. Glycoproteins of varicella-zoster virus and their herpes simplex virus homologs. Rev Infect Dis 13(suppl):S960–S963, 1991.

86. Keller PM, Neff B, Ellis RW. Three major glycoprotein genes of varicella-zoster virus whose products have neutralization epitopes. J Virol 52:293–297, 1984.

87. Yao Z, Grose C. Unusual phosphorylation sequence in the gpIV (gI) component of the varicella-zoster virus gpI-gpIV glycoprotein complex (VZV gE-gI complex). J Virol 68:4204–4211, 1994.

88. Zhu Z, Gershon MD, Hao Y, et al. Envelopment of varicella zoster virus (VZV): targeting of viral glycoproteins to the trans-Golgi network. J Virol 69:7951–7959, 1995.

89. Zhu Z, Hao Y, Gershon MD, et al. Targeting of glycoprotein I (gE) of varicella-zoster virus to the trans-Golgi network by a signal sequence (AYRV) and patch in the cytosolic domain of the molecule. J Virol 70:6563–6575, 1996.

90. Wang Z, Gershon MD, Lungu O, et al. Intracellular transport of varicella-zoster glycoproteins. J Infect Dis 178(suppl):S7–S12, 1998.

91. Wang Z-H, Gershon MD, Lungu O, et al. Trafficking of varicella-zoster virus glycoprotein gI: T338-dependent retention in the trans-Golgi network, secretion, and mannose 6-phosphate-inhibitable uptake of the ectodomain. J Virol 174:6600–6613, 2000.

92. Wang Z-H, Gershon MD, Lungu O, et al. Essential role played by the C-terminal domain of glycoprotein I in envelopment of varicella-zoster virus in the trans-Golgi network: interactions of glycoproteins with tegument. J Virol 75:323–340, 2001.

92a. Tipples GA, Stephens GM, Sherlock C, et al. New variant of varicella-zoster virus. Emerg Inf Dis 8:1504–1505, 2002.

93. Forghani B, Grose C. Neutralization epitope of the varicella-zoster virus gH:gL glycoprotein complex. Virology 199:458–462, 1994.

94. Rodriquez JE, Monninger T, Grose C. Entry and egress of varicella virus blocked by same anti-gH monoclonal antibody. Virology 196:840–844, 1993.

95. Maresova L, Pasieka TJ, Grose C. Varicella-zoster virus gB and gE coexpression, but not gB or gE alone, leads to abundant fusion and syncytium formation equivalent to those from gH and gL coexpression. J Virol 75:9483–9492, 2001.

96. Bergen RE, Sharp M, Sanchez A, et al. Human T cells recognize multiple epitopes of an immediate early/tegument protein (IE 62) and glycoprotein I of varicella-zoster virus. Viral Immunol 4:151–166, 1991.

97. Disney GH, Everett RD. A herpes simplex virus type 1 recombinant with both copies of the Vmw175 coding sequences replaced by the homologous varicella-zoster open reading frame. J Gen Virol 71:2681–2689, 1990.

98. Kinchington PR, Hougland J, Arvin A, et al. The varicella-zoster virus immediate-early protein IE62 is a major component of virus particles. J Virol 66:359–366, 1992.

99. Sabella C, Lowry P, Abbruzzi G, et al. Immunization with immediate-early tegument protein (open reading frame 62) of varicella-zoster virus protects guinea pigs against virus challenge. J Virol 67:7673–7676, 1993.

100. Cohen J, Seidel KE. Varicella-zoster virus (VZV) open reading frame (ORF) 10 protein, the homologue of the essential herpes simplex virus protein VP16, is dispensable for VZV replication in vitro. J Virol 68:7850–7858, 1994.

101. Debrus S, Sadzot-Delvaux C, Nikkels AF, et al. Varicella-zoster virus gene 63 encodes an immediate-early protein that is abundantly expressed during latency. J Virol 69:3240–3245, 1995.

102. Kinchington PR, Bookey D, Turse SE. The transcriptional regulatory proteins encoded by varicella-zoster virus open reading frames (ORFs) 4 and 63, but not ORF 61, are associated with purified virus particles. J Virol 69:4274–4282, 1995.

103. Moriuchi H, Moriuchi M, Smith HA, Cohen JI. Varicella-zoster virus open reading frame 4 is functionally distinct from and does not complement its herpes simplex virus type 1 homolog, ICP27. J Virol 68:1987–1992, 1994.

104. Perera LP, Kaushal S, Kinchington PR, et al. Varicella-zoster virus open reading frame 4 encodes a transcriptional activator that is functionally distinct from that of herpes simplex virus homology ICP27. J Virol 68:2468–2477, 1994.

105. Cohrs RJ, Barbour M, Gilden DH. Varicella-zoster virus (VZV) transcription during latency in human ganglia: detection of transcripts to genes 21, 29, 62, and 63 in a cDNA library enriched for VZV RNA. J Virol 70:2789–2796, 1996.

106. Lungu O, Panagiotidis C, Annunziato P, et al. Aberrant intracellular localization of varicella-zoster virus regulatory proteins during latency. Proc Nat Acad Sci U S A 95:7080–7085, 1998.

107. Mahalingham R, Wellish M, Cohrs R, et al. Expression of protein encoded by varicella-zoster virus open reading frame 63 in latently infected human ganglionic neurons. Proc Nat Acad Sci U S A 93:2122–2124, 1996.

108. Croen KD, Ostrove JM, Dragovic LY, Straus SE. Patterns of gene expression and sites of latency in human ganglia are different for varicella-zoster and herpes simplex viruses. Proc Soc Nat Acad Sci U S A 85:9773–9777, 1988.

109. Mahalingham R, Wellish M, Dueland AN, et al. Localization of herpes simplex virus and varicella zoster virus DNA in human ganglia. Ann Neurol 31:444–448, 1992.

110. Lungu O, Annunziato P, Gershon A, et al. Reactivated and latent varicella-zoster virus in human dorsal root ganglia. Proc Nat Acad Sci U S A 92:10980–10984, 1995.

111. Kennedy P, Grinfield E, Gow JW. Latent varicella-zoster virus is located predominantly in neurons in human trigeminal ganglia. Proc Nat Acad Sci U S A 95:4658–4662, 1998.

112. Kennedy P, Grinfeld E, Gow JW. Latent varicella-zoster virus in human dorsal root ganglia. Virology 258:451–454, 1999.

113. Kennedy PGE, Grinfeld E, Bell JE. Varicella-zoster virus gene expression in latently infected and explanted human ganglia. J Virol 74:11893–11898, 2000.

114. Arvin AM, Pollard RB, Rasmussen L, Merigan T. Selective impairment in lymphocyte reactivity to varicella-zoster antigen among untreated lymphoma patients. J Infect Dis 137:531–540, 1978.

115. Annunziato PW, Lungu O, Panagiotidis C. Varicella zoster virus in human and rat tissue specimens. Arch Virol Suppl 17:135–142, 2001.

116. Merville-Louis M-P, Sadzot-Delvaux C, Delree P, et al. Varicella-zoster virus infection of adult rat sensory neurons in vitro. J Virol 63:3155–3160, 1989.

117. Rentier B, Debrus S, Sadzot-Delvaux C, et al. Varicella-zoster virus latency in the nervous system of rats and humans is accompanied by the abundant expression of an immediate-early protein that is also present in acute infection. Presented at the Keystone Symposium on Virus Entry, Replication, and Pathogenesis, Santa Fe, NM, February 10–16, 1996.

118. Chen J, Gershon A, Silverstein SJ, et al. Latent and lytic infection of isolated guinea pig enteric and dorsal root ganglia by varicella zoster virus. J Med Virol March, 2003.

119. Gustafson TL, Lavely GB, Brauner ER, et al. An outbreak of nosocomial varicella. Pediatrics 70:550–556, 1982.

120. Leclair JM, Zaia J, Levin MJ, et al. Airborne transmission of chickenpox in a hospital. N Engl J Med 302:450–453, 1980.

121. Moore DA, Hopkins RS. Assessment of a school exclusion policy during a chickenpox outbreak. Am J Epidemiol 133:1161–1167, 1991.

122. Kido S, Ozaki T, Asada H, et al. Detection of varicella-zoster virus (VZV) DNA in clinical samples from patients with VZV by the polymerase chain reaction. J Clin Microbiol 29:76–79, 1991.

123. Koropchak C, Graham G, Palmer J, et al. Investigation of varicella-zoster virus infection by polymerase chain reaction in the immunocompetent host with acute varicella. J Infect Dis 163:1016–1022, 1991.

124. Tsolia M, Gershon A, Steinberg S, Gelb L. Live attenuated varicella vaccine: evidence that the virus is attenuated and the importance of skin lesions in transmission of varicella-zoster virus. J Pediatr 116:184–189, 1990.

125. Gershon A, Forghani B. Varicella-zoster virus. In Lennette E (ed). Diagnostic Procedures for Viral, Rickettsial, and Chlamydial Infections. Washington, DC, American Public Health Association, 1995, pp 601–613.

126. Brunell PA. Transmission of chickenpox in a school setting prior to the observed exanthem. Am J Dis Child 143:1451–1452, 1989.

127. Sawyer MH, Wu YN, Chamberlin CJ, et al. Detection of varicella-zoster virus DNA in the oropharynx and blood of patients with varicella. J Infect Dis 166:885–888, 1992.

128. Asano Y, Itakura N, Hiroishi Y, et al. Viremia is present in incubation period in nonimmunocompromised children with varicella. J Pediatr 106:69–71, 1985.

129. Asano Y, Itakura N, Kajita Y, et al. Severity of viremia and clinical findings in children with varicella. J Infect Dis 161:1095–1098, 1990.

130. Feldman S, Epp E. Isolation of varicella-zoster virus from blood. J Pediatr 88:265–267, 1976.

131. Feldman S, Epp E. Detection of viremia during incubation period of varicella. J Pediatr 94:746–748, 1979.

132. Myers MG. Viremia caused by varicella-zoster virus: association with malignant progressive varicella. J Infect Dis 140:229–233, 1979.

133. Ozaki T, Ichikawa T, Matsui Y, et al. Viremic phase in nonimmunocompromised children with varicella. J Pediatr 104:85–87, 1984.

134. Ozaki T, Kajita Y, Asano Y, et al. Detection of varicella-zoster virus DNA in blood of children with varicella. J Med Virol 44:263–265, 1994.

135. Moffat JF, Stein MD, Kaneshima H, Arvin AM. Tropism of varicella-zoster virus for human CD4+ and CD8+ T lymphocytes and epidermal cells in SCID-hu mice. J Virol 69:5236–5242, 1995.

136. Feldman S, Chaudhary S, Ossi M, Epp E. A viremic phase for herpes zoster in children with cancer. J Pediatr 91:597–600, 1977.

137. Gershon A, Steinberg S, Silber R. Varicella-zoster viremia. J Pediatr 92:1033–1034, 1978.

138. Ito M, Nishihara H, Mizutani K, et al. Detection of varicella zoster virus (VZV) DNA in throat swabs and peripheral blood mononuclear cells of immunocompromised patients with herpes zoster by polymerase chain reaction. Clin Diagn Virol 4:105–112, 1995.

139. Fearon DT, Manders P, Wagner SD. Arrested differentiation, the self-renewing memory lymphocyte, and vaccination. Science 293:248–250, 2001.

140. Arbeter AM, Starr SE, Preblud S, et al. Varicella vaccine trials in healthy children: a summary of comparative follow-up studies. Am J Dis Child 138:434–438, 1984.

141. Baba K, Yabuuchi H, Okuni H, Takahashi M. Studies with live varicella vaccine and inactivated skin test antigen: protective effect of the vaccine and clinical application of the skin test. Pediatrics 61:550–555, 1978.

142. Baba K, Yabuuchi H, Takahashi M, et al. Seroepidemiologic behavior of varicella zoster virus infection in a semiclosed community after introduction of VZV vaccine. J Pediatr 105:712–716, 1984.

143. Kamiya H, Ihara T, Hattori A, et al. Diagnostic skin test reactions with varicella virus antigen and clinical application of the test. J Infect Dis 136:784–788, 1977.

144. Kumagai T, Chiba Y, Wataya Y, et al. Development and characteristics of the cellular immune response to infection with varicella-zoster virus after natural or vaccine-induced infection. J Infect Dis 141:1–13, 1980.

145. LaRussa P, Steinberg S, Seeman MD, Gershon AA. Determination of immunity to varicella by means of an intradermal skin test. J Infect Dis 152:869–875, 1985.

146. Shiraki K, Yamanishi K, Takahashi M. Biological and immunological characterization of the soluble skin test antigen of varicella-zoster virus. J Infect Dis 149:501–504, 1983.

147. Arvin AM. Varicella-zoster virus. In Fields BN (ed). Virology. New York, Raven Press, 1995, pp 2547–2586.

148. Gershon AA, Steinberg S, Gelb L, and the NIAID Collaborative Varicella Vaccine Study Group. Live attenuated varicella vaccine: efficacy for children with leukemia in remission. JAMA 252:355–362, 1984.

149. Hayward A, Herberger M. Lymphocyte responses to varicella-zoster virus in the elderly. J Clin Immunol 7:174–178, 1987.

150. Zaia JA, Leary PL, Levin MJ. Specificity of the blastogenic response of human mononuclear cells to herpes antigens. Infect Immun 20:646–651, 1978.

151. Arvin A, Koropchak C, Sharp M, et al. The T-lymphocyte response to varicella-zoster viral proteins. Adv Exp Med Biol 278:71–83, 1990.

152. Arvin AM. Varicella-zoster virus: molecular virology and virus-host interactions. Curr Opin Microbiol 4:442–449, 2001.

153. Sharp M, Terada K, Wilson A, et al. Kinetics and viral protein specificity of the cytotoxic T lymphocyte response in healthy adults immunized with live attenuated varicella vaccine. J Infect Dis 165:852–858, 1992.

154. Ihara T, Starr S, Ito M, et al. Human polymorphonuclear leukocyte-mediated cytotoxicity against varicella-zoster virus-infected fibroblasts. J Virol 51:110–116, 1984.

155. Ihara T, Ito M, Starr SE. Human lymphocyte, monocyte and polymorphonuclear leucocyte mediated antibody-dependent cellular cytotoxicity against varicella-zoster virus-infected targets. Clin Exp Immunol 63:179–187, 1986.

156. Kamiya H, Starr S, Arbeter A, Plotkin S. Antibody dependent cell-mediated cytotoxicity against varicella-zoster virus infected targets. Infect Immun 38:554–557, 1982.

157. Berger R, Florent G, Just M. Decrease of the lympho-proliferative response to varicella-zoster virus antigen in the aged. Infect Immun 32:24–27, 1981.

158. Burke BL, Steele RW, Beard OW, et al. Immune responses to varicella-zoster in the aged. Arch Intern Med 142:291–293, 1982.

159. Luby J, Ramirez-Ronda C, Rinner S, et al. A longitudinal study of varicella zoster virus infections in renal transplant recipients. J Infect Dis 135:659–663, 1977.

160. Hayward A, Levin M, Wolf W, et al. Varicella-zoster virus-specific immunity after herpes zoster. J Infect Dis 163:873–875, 1991.

161. Wilson A, Sharp M, Koropchak C, et al. Subclinical varicella-zoster virus viremia, herpes zoster, and T lymphocyte immunity to varicella-zoster viral antigens after bone marrow transplantation. J Infect Dis 165:119–126, 1992.

162. Hayward A, Buda K, Jones M, et al. Varicella-zoster virus-specific cytotoxicity following secondary immunization with live or killed vaccine. Viral Immunol 9:241–245, 1996.

163. Gershon A, LaRussa P, Steinberg S. Varicella-zoster virus. In Murray PR (ed). Manual of Clinical Microbiology (7th ed). Washington, DC, ASM Press, 1999, pp 900–918.

164. Williams V, Gershon A, Brunell P. Serologic response to varicella-zoster membrane antigens measured by indirect immunofluorescence. J Infect Dis 130:669–672, 1974.

165. Gershon A, Steinberg S, LaRussa P. Detection of antibodies to varicella-zoster virus by latex agglutination. Clin Diagn Virol 2:271–277, 1994.

166. Steinberg S, Gershon A. Measurement of antibodies to varicella-zoster virus by using a latex agglutination test. J Clin Microbiol 29:1527–1529, 1991.

167. Gershon A, Steinberg S. Antibody responses to varicella-zoster virus and the role of antibody in host defense. Am J Med Sci 282:12–17, 1981.

168. Bogger-Goren S, Baba K, Hurley P, et al. Antibody response to varicella-zoster virus after natural or vaccine-induced infection. J Infect Dis 146:260–265, 1982.

169. Kalman CM, Laskin OL. Herpes zoster and zosteriform herpes simplex virus infections in immunocompetent adults. Am J Med 81:775–778, 1986.

170. Coffin SE, Hodinka RL. Utility of direct immunofluorescence and virus culture for detection of varicella-zoster virus in skin lesions. J Clin Microbiol 33:2792–2795, 1995.

171. LaRussa P, Hughes P, Pearce J, et al. Use of polymerase chain reaction (PCR) assay to identify and type varicella zoster virus. Presented at the Society for Pediatric Research Annual Meeting, Washington, DC, May 6, 1993.

172. LaRussa P, Steinberg S, Gershon A. Diagnosis and typing of varicella-zoster virus (VZV) in clinical specimens by polymerase chain reaction (PCR). In Program and Abstracts of the 34th Interscience Conference on Antimicrobial Agents and Chemotherapy, Orlando, FL, October 4–7. Washington, DC, ASM Press, 1994.

173. Puchhammer-Stockl E, Popow-Kraupp T, Heinz F, et al. Detection of varicella-zoster virus DNA by polymerase chain reaction in the cerebrospinal fluid of patients suffering from neurological complications associated with chicken pox or herpes zoster. J Clin Microbiol 29:1513–1516, 1991.

174. Sharrar RG, LaRussa P, Galea S, et al. The postmarketing safety profile of varicella vaccine. Vaccine 19:916–923, 2000.

175. Vazquez M, LaRussa P, Gershon A, et al. The effectiveness of the varicella vaccine in clinical practice. N Engl J Med 344:955–960, 2001.

176. Espy M, Teo R, Ross T, et al. Diagnosis of varicella-zoster virus infections in the clinical laboratory by LightCycler PCR. J Clin Microbiol 38:3187–3189, 2000.

177. Loparev VN, McCaustland K, Holloway B, et al. Rapid genotyping of varicella-zoster virus vaccine and wild type strains with fluorophore-labeled hybridization probes. J Clin Microbiol 38:4315–4319, 2000.

178. Asano Y, Itakura N, Hiroishi Y, et al. Viral replication and immunologic responses in children naturally infected with varicella-zoster virus and in varicella vaccine. J Infect Dis 152:863–868, 1985.

179. Saiman L, LaRussa P, Steinberg S, et al. Persistence of immunity to varicella-zoster virus vaccination among health care workers. Infect Control Hosp Epidemiol 22:279–283, 2001.

180. Demmler G, Steinberg S, Blum G, Gershon A. Rapid enzyme-linked immunosorbent assay for detecting antibody to varicella-zoster virus. J Infect Dis 157:211–212, 1988.

181. Wasmuth EH, Miller WJ. Sensitive enzyme-linked immunosorbent assay for antibody to varicella-zoster virus using purified VZV glycoprotein antigen. J Med Virol 32:189–193, 1990.

182. White CJ, Kuter BJ, Ngai A, et al. Modified cases of chickenpox after varicella vaccination: correlation of protection with antibody response. Pediatr Infect Dis J 11:19–22, 1992.

183. Krah DL, Cho I, Schofield T, Ellis RW. Comparison of gpELISA and neutralizing antibody responses to Oka/Merck live varicella vaccine (Varivax®) in children and adults. Vaccine 15:61–64, 1997.

184. Forghani B, Schmidt N, Dennis J. Antibody assays for varicella-zoster virus: comparison of enzyme immunoassay with neutralization, immune adherence hemagglutination, and complement fixation. J Clin Microbiol 8:545–552, 1978.

185. Gershon A, Kalter Z, Steinberg S. Detection of antibody to varicella-zoster virus by immune adherence hemagglutination. Proc Soc Exp Biol Med 151:762–765, 1976.

186. Landry ML, Ferguson D. Comparison of latex agglutination test with enzyme-linked immunosorbent assay for detection of antibody to varicella-zoster virus. J Clin Microbiol 31:3031–3033, 1993.

187. Whitley RJ, Gnann J, Hinthorn D, et al. Disseminated herpes zoster in the immunocompromised host: a comparative trial of acyclovir and ganciclovir. J Infect Dis 165:450–455, 1992.

188. Whitley R. Therapeutic approaches to varicella-zoster virus infections. J Infect Dis 166(suppl):S51–S57, 1992.

189. Whitley RJ, Gnann JW. Acyclovir: a decade later. N Engl J Med 327:782–789, 1992.

190. Wood MJ, Kay R, Dworkin RH, et al. Oral acyclovir therapy accelerates pain resolution in patients with herpes zoster: a meta analysis of placebo controlled trials. Clin Infect Dis 22:341–347, 1996.

191. Wood MJ. Current experience with antiviral therapy for acute herpes zoster. Ann Neurol 35(suppl):S65–S68, 1994.

192. Dunkel L, Arvin A, Whitley R, et al. A controlled trial of oral acyclovir for chickenpox in normal children. N Engl J Med 325:1539–1544, 1991.

193. Balfour HH, Rotbart H, Feldman S, et al. Acyclovir treatment of varicella in otherwise healthy adolescents. J Pediatr 120:627–633, 1992.

194. Wallace MR, Bowler WA, Murray NB, et al. Treatment of adult varicella with oral acyclovir: a randomized, placebo-controlled trial. Ann Intern Med 117:358–363, 1992.

195. Balfour HH, Edelman CK, Andeerson RS, et al. Controlled trial of acyclovir for chickenpox evaluating time of initiation and duration of therapy and viral resistance. Pediatr Infect Dis J 20:919–926, 2001.

196. Beutner KR, Friedman DJ, Forszpaniak C, et al. Valacyclovir compared with acyclovir for improved therapy for herpes zoster in immunocompetent adults. Antimicrob Agents Chemother 39:1546–1553, 1995.

197. Tyring S, Barbarash RA, Nahlik JE, et al. Famciclovir for the treatment of acute herpes zoster: effects on acute disease and post herpetic neuralgia. Ann Intern Med 123:89–96, 1995.

198. Tyring S, Belanger R, Bezwoda W, et al. A randomized, double-blind trial of famciclovir versus acyclovir for the treatment of localized dermatomal herpes zoster in immunocompromised patients. Cancer Invest 19:13–22, 2001.

199. Asano Y, Yoshikawa T, Suga S, et al. Postexposure prophylaxis of varicella in family contact by oral acyclovir. Pediatrics 92:219–222, 1993.

200. Yoshikawa T, Suga S, Kozawa T, et al. Persistence of protective immunity after postexposure prophylaxis of varicella with oral acyclovir in the family setting. Arch Dis Child 78:61–63, 1998.

201. Huang Y-C, Lin T-Y, Chiu C-H. Acyclovir prophylaxis of varicella after household exposure. Pediatr Infect Dis J 14:152–154, 1995.

202. Suga S, Yoshikawa T, Ozaki T, Asano Y. Effect of oral acyclovir against primary and secondary viraemia in incubation period of varicella. Arch Dis Child 69:639–643, 1993.

203. Garnett GP, Cox MJ, Bundy DAP, et al. The age of infection with varicella-zoster virus in St. Lucia, West Indies. Epidemiol Infect 110:361–372, 1993.

204. Lolekha S, Tanthiphabha W, Sornchai P, et al. Effect of climatic factors and population density on varicella zoster virus epidemiology within a tropical country. Am J Trop Med Hyg 64:131–136, 2001.

205. Mandal BK, Mukherjee PP, Murphy C, et al. Adult susceptibility to varicella in the tropics is a rural phenomenon due to the lack of previous exposure. J Infect Dis 178(suppl):S52-S54, 1998.

206. Seward J, Wharton M. Epidemiology of varicella. In Arvin A, Gershon A (eds). Varicella-Zoster Virus. Cambridge, UK, Cambridge University Press, 2000, pp 187–205.

207. Wharton M. The epidemiology of varicella-zoster virus infections. Infect Dis Clin North Am 10:571–581, 1996.

208. Bramley JC, Jones IG. Epidemiology of chickenpox in Scotland: 1981 to 1998. Commun Dis Public Health 3:282–287, 2000.

209. Degeun S, Chau NP, Flahault A. Epidemiology of chickenpox in France (1991–1995). J Epidemiol Community Health 52 (suppl):46S–98S, 1998.

210. Gordon JE. Chickenpox: an epidemiologic review. Am J Med Sci 244:362–389, 1962.

211. Joseph CA, Noah ND. Epidemiology of chickenpox in England and Wales 1967–1985. Br Med J 296:673–676, 1988.

212. Socan M, Kraigher A, Pahor L. Epidemiology of varicella in Slovenia over a 20-year period (1979–1998). Epidemiol Infect 126:279–283, 2001.

213. Trlifajova J, Svandova E, Havrlantova M, et al. Varicella morbidity in Czechoslovakia. J Hyg Epidemiol Microbiol Immunol 24:192–199, 1980.

214. Varughese PV. Chickenpox in Canada. Can Med J 138:133–134, 1988.

215. Finger R, Hughes JP, Meade BJ, et al. Age-specific incidence of chickenpox. Pub Health Reps 190:750–755, 1994.

216. Yawn BP, Yawn RA, Lydick E. Community impact of childhood varicella infections. J Pediatr 130:759–765, 1997.

217. Gabutti G, Penna C, Rossi M, et al. The seroepidemiology of varicella in Italy. Epidemiol Infect 126:433–440, 2001.

218. Fornaro P, Gandini F, Marin M, et al. Epidemiology and cost analysis of varicella in Italy: results of a sentinel study in the pediatric practice. Pediatr J Infect Dis 18:414–419, 1999.

219. Kudesia G, Partridge S, Farrington CP, Soltanpoor N. Changes in age related seroprevalence of antibody to varicella zoster virus: impact on vaccine strategy. J Clin Pathol 55:154–155, 2002.

220. Ross AM, Fleming DM. Chickenpox increasingly affects preschool children. Commun Dis Public Health 3:213–215, 2000.

221. Kilgore PE, Kruszon-Moran D, Seward J, et al. Varicella in Americans from NHANES III: implications for control through routine immunization. J Med Virol March, 2003.

222. Heininger U, Braun-Fahrlander C, Desgrandchamps D, et al. Seroprevalence of varicella-zoster virus immunoglobulin G antibodies in Swiss adolescents and risk factor analysis for seronegativity. Pediatr Infect Dis J 20:775–778, 2001.

223. Salleras L, Dominguez A, Vidal J, et al. Seroepidemiology of varicella-zoster virus infection in Catalonia (Spain): rationale for universal vaccination programmes. Vaccine 19:183–188, 2000.

224. Taylor-Weidmann J, Yamashita K, Miyamura K, Yamazaki S. Varicella-zoster virus prevalence in Japan: no significant change in a decade. Jpn J Med Sci Biol 42:1–11, 1989.

225. Wutzler P, Farber I, Wagenpfeil S, et al. Seroprevalence of varicella-zoster in the German population. Vaccine 20:121–124, 2002.

226. Yu AL, Costa JM, Amaku M, et al. Three year seroepidemiological study of varicella-zoster virus in Sao Paulo, Brazil. Rev Inst Med Trop Sao Paulo 42:125–128, 2000.

227. Chant KG, Sullivan EA, Burgess MA, et al. Varicella-zoster virus infection in Australia. Aust N Z J Public Health 22:413–418, 1998.

228. Gershon A, Raker R, Steinberg S, et al. Antibody to varicella-zoster virus in parturient women and their offspring during the first year of life. Pediatrics 58:692–696, 1976.

229. Jerant AF, DeGaetano JS, Epperly TD, et al. Varicella susceptibility and vaccination strategies in young adults. J Am Board Fam Pract 11:296–306, 1998.

230. Kelley PW, Petruccelli BP, Stehr-Green P, et al. The susceptibility of young adult Americans to vaccine-preventable infections: a national serosurvey of US Army recruits. JAMA 266:2724–2729, 1991.

231. Struewing JP, Hyams KC, Tueller JE, Gray GC. The risk of measles, mumps, and varicella among young adults: a serosurvey of US Navy and Marine Corps recruits. Am J Public Health 83:1717–1720, 1993.

232. Balraj V, John TJ. An epidemic of varicella in rural southern India. J Trop Med Hyg 97:113–116, 1994.

233. Sinha DP. Chickenpox—a disease predominantly affecting adults in rural west Bengal, India. Int J Epidemiol 5:367–374, 1976.

234. Venkitaraman AR, Seigneurin JM, Lenoir GM, John TJ. Infections due to the human herpesviruses in southern India: a seroepidemiological survey. Int J Epidemiol 15:561–566, 1986.

235. White E. Chickenpox in Kerala. Indian J Public Health 22:141–151, 1978.

236. Akram DS, Qureshi H, Mahmud A, et al. Seroepidemiology of varicella-zoster in Pakistan. Southeast Asian J Trop Med Public Health 31:646–649, 2000.

237. Barzaga NG, Roxas JR, Florese RH. Varicella-zoster virus prevalence in metro Manila, Philippines. JAMA (SE Asia) 274(suppl): S633–S635, 1994.

238. Bhattarakosol P, Chantarabul S, Pittayathikhun K, et al. Prevalence of anti-varicella zoster IgG antibody in undergraduate students. Asian Pac J Allergy Immunol 14:129–131, 1996.

239. Juffrie M, Graham RR, Tan RI, et al. Seroprevalence of hepatitis A virus and varicella zoster antibodies in a Javanese community (Yogyakarta, Indonesia). Southeast Asian J Trop Med Public Health 31:21–24, 2000.

240. Lee BW. Review of varicella zoster epidemiology in India and Southeast Asia. Trop Med Int Health 3:886–890, 1998.

241. Lin YJ, Huang LM, Lee CY, et al. A seroepidemiological study of varicella-zoster virus in Taipei City. Zhonghua Min Guo Xiao Er Ke Yi Xue Hui Za Zhi 37:11–15, 1996.

242. Longfield JN, Winn RE, Gibson RL, et al. Varicella outbreaks in army recruits from Puerto Rico. Arch Intern Med 150:970–973, 1990.

243. Migasena S, Simasathien S, Desakorn V, et al. Seroprevalence of varicella-zoster virus antibody in Thailand. Int J Infect Dis 2:26–30, 1997.

244. Nassar NT, Touma HC. Brief report: susceptibility of Filipino nurses to the varicella-zoster virus. Infect Control 7:71–72, 1986.

245. Ooi PL, Goh KT, Doraisingham S, Ling AE. Prevalence of varicella-zoster virus infection in Singapore. Southeast Asian J Trop Med Public Health 23:22–25, 1992.

246. Venkitaraman AR, John TJ. The epidemiology of varicella in staff and students of a hospital in the tropics. Int J Epidemiol 13:502–505, 1984.

247. Venkitaraman AR, Seigneurin JM, Baccard M, et al. Measurement of antibodies to varicella-zoster virus in a tropical population by enzyme-linked immunosorbent assay. J Clin Microbiol 20:582–583, 1984.

248. Withers BG, Kelley PW, Pang LW, et al. Vaccine-preventable disease susceptibility in a young adult Micronesian population. Southeast Asian J Trop Med Public Health 25:569–574, 1994.

249. O'Grady KA, Merianos A, Patel M, Gilbert L. High seroprevalence of antibodies to varicella zoster virus in adult women in a tropical climate. Trop Med Int Health 5:732–736, 2000.

250. Ghebrekidan H, Ruden U, Cox S, et al. Prevalence of herpes simplex virus types 1 and 2, cytomegalovirus, and varicella-zoster virus infections in Eritrea. J Clin Virol 12:53–64, 1999.

251. Centers for Disease Control and Prevention. Varicella-related deaths among children, United States, 1997. MMWR Morb Mortal Wkly Rep 47:365–368, 1998.

252. Galil K, Brown C, Lin F, Seward J. Hospitalizations for varicella in the United States, 1988–1999. Pediatr Infect Dis J 221:931–935, 2002.

253. Edmunds WJ, Brisson M, Rose JD. The epidemiology of herpes zoster and potential cost-effectiveness of vaccination in England and Wales. Vaccine 19:3076–3090, 2001.

254. Fairley CK, Miller E. Varicella-zoster virus epidemiology—a changing scene? J Infect Dis 174(Supp 3): 314–319, 1996.

255. Liu F, Hadler JL. Epidemiology of primary varicella and herpes zoster hospitalizations: the pre-varicella vaccine era. J Infect Dis 181:1897–1905, 2000.

256. Rawson H, Crampin A, Noah N. Deaths from chickenpox in England and Wales 1995–7: analysis of routine mortality data. BMJ 323:1091–1093, 2001.

257. Gil A, Oyaguez I, Carrasco P, Gonzalez A. Epidemiology of primary varicella hospitalizations in Spain. Vaccine 20:295–298, 2001.

258. Brunell P, Ross A, Miller L, Kuo B. Prevention of varicella by zoster immune globulin. N Engl J Med 280:1191–1194, 1969.

259. Gershon A, Steinberg S, Brunell P. Zoster immune globulin: a further assessment. N Engl J Med 290:243–245, 1974.

260. Zaia J, Levin M, Preblud S, et al. Evaluation of varicella-zoster immune globulin: protection of immunosuppressed children after household exposure to varicella. J Infect Dis 147:737–743, 1983.

261. Centers for Disease Control. Varicella-zoster immune globulin for the prevention of chickenpox. MMWR Morb Mortal Wkly Rep 33:84–100, 1984.

262. Centers for Disease Control and Prevention. Prevention of varicella: recommendations of the Advisory Committee on Immunization Practices (ACIP). MMWR Morb Mortal Wkly Rep 45:1–36, 1996.

263. Balfour HH, Groth KE, McCullough J, et al. Prevention or modification of varicella using zoster immune plasma. Am J Dis Child 131:693–696, 1977.

264. Balfour HH, Groth KE. Zoster immune plasma prophylaxis of varicella: a follow up report. J Pediatr 94:743–746, 1979.

265. Groth KE, McCullough J, Marker S, et al. Evaluation of zoster immune plasma: treatment of herpes zoster in patients with cancer. JAMA 239:1877–1879, 1978.

266. Bakshi S, Miller TC, Kaplan M, et al. Failure of VZIG in modification of severe congenital varicella. Pediatr Infect Dis 5:699–702, 1986.

267. Arbeter AM, Starr SE, Weibel RE, et al. Live attenuated varicella vaccine: the KMcC strain in healthy children. Pediatrics 71:307–312, 1983.

268. Neff BJ, Weibel RE, Villerajos VM, et al. Clinical and laboratory studies of KMcC strain of live attenuated varicella virus. Proc Soc Exp Biol Med 166:339–347, 1981.

269. Asano Y, Albrecht P, Behr DF, et al. Immunogenicity of wild and attenuated varicella zoster virus strains in rhesus monkeys. J Med Virol 14:305–312, 1984.

270. Takahashi M, Okuno Y, Otsuka T, et al. Development of a live attenuated varicella vaccine. Biken J 18:25–33, 1975.

271. Argaw T, Cohen J, Klutch M, et al. Nucleotide sequences that distinguish Oka vaccine from parental Oka and other varicella-zoster virus isolates. J Infect Dis 181:1153–1157, 2000.

272. Gomi Y, Imagawa T, Takahashi M, Yamanishi K. Comparison of DNA sequence and transactivation activity of open reading frame 62 of Oka varicella vaccine and its parental viruses. Arch Virol Suppl 17:49–56, 2001.

273. Gomi Y, Imagawa T, Takahashi M, Yamanishi K. Oka varicella vaccine is distinguishable from its parental virus in DNA sequence of open reading frame 62 and its transactivation activity. J Med Virol 61:497–503, 2000.

274. Lim SM, Song SW, Kim SL, et al. Comparison of the attenuated BR-Oka and the wild type strain of varicella zoster virus (VZV) on the DNA level. Arch Pharm Res 23:418–423, 2000.

275. Brunell P, Geiser C, Novelli V, et al. Varicella-like illness caused by live varicella vaccine in children with acute lymphocytic leukemia. Pediatrics 79:922–927, 1987.

276. Gelb LD, Dohner DE, Gershon AA, et al. Molecular epidemiology of live, attenuated varicella virus vaccine in children and in normal adults. J Infect Dis 155:633–640, 1987.

277. Martin JH, Dohner D, Wellinghoff WJ, Gelb LD. Restriction endonuclease analysis of varicella-zoster vaccine virus and wild type DNAs. J Med Virol 9:69–76, 1982.

278. Takahashi M, Asano Y, Kamiya H, Baba K. Varicella vaccine: case studies. Microbiol Sci 2:249–254, 1985.

279. Takahashi M, Hayakawa Y, Shiraki K, et al. Attenuation and laboratory markers of the Oka-strain varicella-zoster virus. Postgrad Med 61:37–46, 1985.

280. Myers M, Duer HL, Haulser CK. Experimental infection of guinea pigs with varicella-zoster virus. J Infect Dis 142:414–420, 1980.

281. LaRussa P, Lungu O, Hardy I, et al. Restriction fragment length polymorphism of polymerase chain reaction products from vaccine and wild-type varicella-zoster virus isolates. J Virol 66:1016–1020, 1992.

282. LaRussa P, Steinberg S, Arvin A, et al. PCR and RFLP analysis of VZV isolates from the USA and other parts of the world. J Infect Dis 178(suppl):S64–S66, 1998.

283. Mori T, Takahara R, Toriyama T, et al. Identification of the Oka strain of the live attenuated varicella vaccine from other clinical isolates by molecular epidemiological analysis. J Infect Dis 178:35–38, 1998.

284. Loparev VN, Argaw T, Krause P, et al. Improved identification and differentiation of varicella-zoster virus (VZV) wild type strains and an attenuated varicella vaccine strain using a VZV open reading frame 62-based PCR. J Clin Microbiol 38:3156–3160, 2000.

285. Moriuchi M, Moriuchi H, Straus SE, Cohen JR. Varicella-zoster virus (VZV) virion-associated transactivator open reading frame 62 protein enhances the infectivity of VZV DNA. Virology 200:297–300, 1994.

286. Gershon A, LaRussa P, Steinberg S. Varicella vaccine: use in immunocompromised patients. Infect Dis Clin North Am 10:583–594, 1996.

287. Hughes P, LaRussa PS, Pearce JM, et al. Transmission of varicella-zoster virus from a vaccinee with underlying leukemia, demonstrated by polymerase chain reaction. J Pediatr 124:932–935, 1994.

288. Ihara T, Kamiya H, Torigoe S, et al. Viremic phase in a leukemic child after live varicella vaccination. Pediatrics 89:147–149, 1992.

289. Annunziato P, LaRussa P, Lee P, et al. Evidence of latent VZV infection in rat dorsal root ganglia. J Infect Dis 178(suppl):S48–S51, 1998.

290. Bergen RE, Diaz P, Arvin A. The immunogenicity of Oka/Merck varicella vaccine in relation to infectious varicella-zoster virus and relative viral antigen content. J Infect Dis 162:1049–1054, 1990.

291. Asano Y, Nakayama H, Yazaki T, et al. Protection against varicella in family contacts by immediate inoculation with live varicella vaccine. Pediatrics 59:3–7, 1977.

292. Horiuchi K. Chickenpox vaccination of healthy children: immunological and clinical responses and protective effect in 1978–1982. Biken J 27:37–38, 1984.

293. Naganuma Y, Osawa S, Takahashi R. Clinical application of a live varicella vaccine (Oka strain) in a hospital. Biken J 27:59–61, 1984.

294. Ozaki T, Ichikawa T, Asano Y, et al. Clinical trial of the Oka strain of live attenuated varicella vaccine on healthy children. Biken J 27:39–42, 1984.

295. Takahashi M, Kamiya H, Baba K, et al. Clinical experience with Oka live varicella vaccine in Japan. Postgrad Med 61:61–67, 1985.

296. Andre F. Summary of clinical studies with the Oka live varicella vaccine produced by Smith Kline-RIT. Biken J 27:89–98, 1984.

297. Weibel R, Kuter B, Neff B, et al. Live Oka/Merck varicella vaccine in healthy children: further clinical and laboratory assessment. JAMA 245:2435–2439, 1985.

298. Rothstein EP, Bernstein H, Penridge P, et al. Dose titration study of live attenuated varicella vaccine in healthy children. J Infect Dis 175:444–447, 1997.

299. Watson B, Piercy S, Soppas D, et al. The effect of decreasing amounts of live virus, while antigen content remains constant, on immunogenicity of Oka/Merck varicella vaccine. J Infect Dis 168:1356–1360, 1993.

300. Lau YL, Vessey SJ, Chan IS, et al. A comparison of safety, tolerability and immunogenicity of Oka/Merck varicella vaccine and VARILRIX in healthy children. Vaccine 20:2942–2949, 2002.

301. Baba K, Yabuuchi H, Takahashi M, Ogra P. Live attenuated varicella vaccine: efficacy trial in an institution. Presented at the 18th International Congress of Pediatrics, Washington, DC, 1986.

302. Weibel R, Neff BJ, Kuter BJ, et al. Live attenuated varicella virus vaccine: efficacy trial in healthy children. N Engl J Med 310:1409–1415, 1984.

303. Chartrand S, Madison BG, Steinberg S, Gershon A. Varicella vaccine in day care centers. In Program and Abstracts of the 25th Interscience Conference on Antimicrobial Agents and Chemotherapy, Minneapolis, MN, September 29–October 2. Washington, DC, ASM Press, 1985.

304. Kramer JM, LaRussa P, Tsai WC, et al. Disseminated vaccine strain varicella as the acquired immunodeficiency syndrome-defining illness in a previously undiagnosed child. Pediatrics 108:E39, 2001.

305. Ghaffar F, Carrick K, Rogers BB, et al. Disseminated infection with varicella-zoster virus vaccine strain presenting as hepatitis in a child with adenosine deaminase deficiency. Pediatr Infect Dis J 19:764–765, 2000.

306. Wise RP, Salive ME, Braun MM, et al. Postlicensure safety surveillance for varicella vaccine. JAMA 284:1271–1279, 2000.
307. Black S, Shinefield H, Ray P, et al. Post marketing evaluation of the safety and effectiveness of varicella vaccine. Pediatr Infect Dis 18:1041–1046, 1999.
308. Diaz PS, Au D, Smith S, et al. Lack of transmission of the live attenuated varicella vaccine virus to immunocompromised children after immunization of their siblings. Pediatrics 87:166–170, 1991.
309. Salzman MB, Sharrar R, Steinberg S, LaRussa P. Transmission of varicella-vaccine virus from a healthy 12 month old child to his pregnant mother. J Pediatr 131:151–154, 1997.
310. Long S. Toddler-to-mother transmission of varicella-vaccine virus: how bad is that? J Pediatr 131:10–12, 1997.
311. LaRussa P, Steinberg S, Meurice F, Gershon A. Transmission of vaccine strain varicella-zoster virus from a healthy adult with vaccine-associated rash to susceptible household contacts. J Infect Dis 176:1072–1075, 1997.
312. Asano Y, Nakayama H, Yazaki T, et al. Protective efficacy of vaccination in children in four episodes of natural varicella and zoster in the ward. Pediatrics 59:8–12, 1977.
313. LaRussa PL, Gershon AA, Steinberg S, Chartrand S. Antibodies to varicella-zoster virus glycoproteins I, II, and III in leukemic and healthy children. J Infect Dis 162:627–633, 1990.
314. Asano Y, Albrecht P, Vujcic LK, et al. Five-year follow-up study of recipients of live varicella vaccine using enhanced neutralization and fluorescent antibody membrane antigen assays. Pediatrics 72:291–294, 1983.
315. Krause P, Klinman DM. Efficacy, immunogenicity, safety, and use of live attenuated chickenpox vaccine. J Pediatr 127:518–525, 1995.
316. White CJ, Kuter BJ, Hildebrand CS, et al. Varicella vaccine (VARI-VAX) in healthy children and adolescents: results from clinical trials, 1987 to 1989. Pediatrics 87:604–610, 1991.
317. Asano Y. Varicella vaccine: the Japanese experience. J Infect Dis 174(suppl):S310–S313, 1996.
318. Kumagai T, Chiba Y, Fujiyama M, et al. Humoral and cellular immune response to varicella-zoster virus in children inoculated with live attenuated varicella vaccine. Biken J 23:135–141, 1980.
319. Watson B, Boardman C, Laufer D, et al. Humoral and cell-mediated immune responses in healthy children after one or two doses of varicella vaccine. Clin Infect Dis 20:316–319, 1995.
320. Izawa T, Ihara T, Hattori A, et al. Application of a live varicella vaccine in children with acute leukemia or other malignant diseases. Pediatrics 60:805–809, 1977.
321. Ha K, Baba K, Ikeda T, et al. Application of a live varicella vaccine in children with acute leukemia or other malignancies without suspension of anticancer therapy. Pediatrics 65:346–350, 1980.
322. Konno T, Yamaguchi Y, Minegishi M, et al. A clinical trial of live attenuated varicella vaccine (Biken) in children with malignant diseases. Biken J 27:73–75, 1984.
323. Nunoue T. Clinical observations on varicella-zoster virus vaccinees treated with immunosuppressants for a malignancy. Biken J 27:115–118, 1984.
324. Sato Y, Miyano T, Kawauchi K, Yokoyama M. Use of live varicella vaccine in acute leukemia and malignant lymphoma. Biken J 27:111–113, 1984.
325. Gershon A. Immunoprophylaxis of varicella-zoster infections. Am J Med 76:672–677, 1984.
326. Gershon A, Steinberg S, Gelb L, for the NIAID Collaborative Varicella Vaccine Study Group. Live attenuated varicella vaccine: use in immunocompromised children and adults. Pediatrics 78 (suppl):757–762, 1986.
327. Gershon AA, Steinberg S, for the NIAID Collaborative Varicella Vaccine Study Group. Persistence of immunity to varicella in children with leukemia immunized with live attenuated varicella vaccine. N Engl J Med 320:892–897, 1989.
328. Gershon AA, LaRussa P, Steinberg S. Live attenuated varicella vaccine: current status and future uses. Semin Pediatr Infect Dis 2:171–177, 1991.
329. Gershon A. Varicella-zoster virus: prospects for control. Adv Pediatr Infect Dis 10:93–124, 1995.
330. Lawrence R, Gershon A, Holzman R, et al for the NIAID Varicella Vaccine Collaborative Study Group. The risk of zoster after varicella vaccination in children with leukemia. N Engl J Med 318:543–548, 1988.
331. Gershon A, LaRussa P, Steinberg S, et al. The protective effect of immunologic boosting against zoster: an analysis in leukemic children who were vaccinated against chickenpox. J Infect Dis 173:450–453, 1996.
332. Lydick E, Kuter BJ, Zajac B, Guess H for the NIAID Collaborative Varicella Vaccine Study Group. Association of steroid therapy with vaccine-associated rashes in children with acute lymphocytic leukaemia who received Oka/Merck varicella vaccine. Vaccine 7:549–553, 1989.
333. Takahashi M, Gershon A. Live attenuated varicella vaccine. In Levine M, Woodrow GC, Kaper JB, Cobon GS (eds). New Generation Vaccines. New York, Marcel Dekker, 1997, pp 647–658.
334. Arbeter A, Granowetter L, Starr S, et al. Immunization of children with acute lymphoblastic leukemia with live attenuated varicella vaccine without complete suspension of chemotherapy. Pediatrics 85:338–344, 1990.
335. Brunell PA, Shehab Z, Geiser C, Waugh JE. Administration of live varicella vaccine to children with leukemia. Lancet 2:1069–1073, 1982.
336. Marwick C. Lengthy tale of varicella vaccine development finally nears a clinically useful conclusion. JAMA 273:833–835, 1995.
337. Broyer M, Boudailliez B. Prevention of varicella infection in renal transplanted children by previous immunization with a live attenuated varicella vaccine. Transplant Proc 17:151–152, 1985.
338. Zamora I, Simon JM, Da Silva ME, Piqueras AI. Attenuated varicella vaccine in children with renal transplants. Pediatr Nephrol 8:190–192, 1994.
339. Broyer M, Tete MT, Guest G, et al. Varicella and zoster in children after kidney transplantation: long term results of vaccination. Pediatrics 99:35–39, 1997.
340. Levin MJ, Gershon AA, Weinberg A, et al. Immunization of HIV-infected children with varicella vaccine. J Pediatr 139:305–310, 2001.
341. Centers for Disease Control and Prevention. Prevention of varicella. MMWR Morb Mortal Wkly Rep 48:1–6, 1999.
342. Webb NJ, Fitzpatrick MM, Hughes DA, et al. Immunisation against varicella in end stage and pre-end stage renal failure. Trans-Pennine Paediatric Nephrology Study Group. Arch Dis Child 82:141–143, 2000.
342a. Nithichalyo C, Chongsrisawat V, Hutagalung T, et al. Immunogenicity and adverse a\effects of live attenuated varicella vaccine (Oka-strain) in children with chronic liver diease. Asian Pacific J Allergy Immunol 19:101–105, 2001.
343. Donati M, Zuckerman M, Dhawan A, et al. Response to varicella immunization in pediatric liver transplant recipients. Transplantation 70:1401–1404, 2000.
344. Brunell PA, Taylor-Wiedeman J, Geiser CF, et al. Risk of herpes zoster in children with leukemia: varicella vaccine compared with history of chickenpox. Pediatrics 77:53–56, 1986.
345. Hayakawa Y, Yamamoto T, Yamanishi K, Takahashi M. Analysis of varicella zoster virus (VZV) DNAs of clinical isolates by endonuclease HpaI. J Gen Virol 67:1817–1829, 1986.
346. Hardy IB, Gershon A, Steinberg S, et al. Incidence of zoster after live attenuated varicella vaccine. In Program and Abstracts of the 31st International Conference on Antimicrobial Agents and Chemotherapy, Chicago, IL, September 29–October 2. Washington, DC, ASM Press, 1991.
347. Kuter BJ, Weibel RE, Guess HA, et al. Oka/Merck varicella vaccine in healthy children: final report of a 2-year efficacy study and 7-year follow-up studies. Vaccine 9:643–647, 1991.
348. Varis T, Vesikari T. Efficacy of high titer live attenuated varicella vaccine in healthy young children. J Infect Dis 174(suppl): S330–S334, 1996.
349. Seward JF. Update on varicella. Pediatr Infect Dis J 20:619–621, 2001.
350. Schlesselman JJ. Case-Control Studies: Design, Conduct, Analysis. New York, Oxford University Press, 1982, pp 137–138.
351. Izurieta H, Strebel P, Blake P. Post-licensure effectiveness of varicella vaccine during an outbreak in a child care center. JAMA 278:1495–1498, 1997.
352. Berrios-Torres SI, Raymond D, Blythe D, et al. Evaluation of Varicella zoster virus (VZV) vaccine effectiveness in an elementary school outbreak. 39th Meeting of the Infectious Diseases Society of America, San Francisco, 2002.

353. Buchholz U, Moolenaar R, Peterson C, Mascola L. Varicella outbreaks after vaccine licensure: should they make you chicken? Pediatrics 104:561–563, 1999.
354. Galil K, Fair E, Mountcastle N, Britz P, Seward J. Younger age at vaccination may increase risk of varicella vaccine failure. J Infect Dis 186:102–105, 2002.
355. Galil K, Lee B, Strine T, et al. Outbreak of varicella at a day-care center despite vaccination. NEJM 347:1909–1915.
356. Fine PE, Zell ER. Outbreaks in highly vaccinated populations: implications for studies of vaccine performance. Am J Epidemiol 139:77–90, 1994.
357. Clements D, Moreira SP, Coplan P, et al. Postlicensure study of varicella vaccine effectiveness in a day-care setting. Pediatr Infect Dis J 18:1047–1050, 1999.
358. Clements DA, Zaref JI, Bland CL, et al. Partial uptake of varicella vaccine and the epidemiological effect on varicella disease in 11 day-care centers in North Carolina. Arch Pediatr Adolesc Med 155:433–461, 2001.
359. Asano Y, Yazaki T, Miyata T, et al. Application of a live attenuated varicella vaccine to hospitalized children and its protective effect on spread of varicella infection. Biken J 18:35–40, 1975.
360. Asano Y, Iwayama S, Miyata T, et al. Spread of varicella in hospitalized children having no direct contact with an indicator zoster case and its prevention by a live vaccine. Biken J 23:157–161, 1980.
361. Katsushima N, Yazaki N, Sakamoto M, et al. Application of a live varicella vaccine to hospitalized children and its follow-up study. Biken J 25:29–42, 1982.
362. Katsushima N, Yazaki N, Sakamoto M, et al. Effect and follow up on varicella vaccine. Biken J 27:51–58, 1984.
363. Asano Y, Hirose S, Iwayama S, et al. Protective effect of immediate inoculation of a live varicella vaccine in household contacts in relation to the viral dose and interval between exposure and vaccination. Biken J 25:43–45, 1982.
364. Arbeter A, Starr SE, Plotkin SA. Varicella vaccine studies in healthy children and adults. Pediatrics 78(suppl):748–756, 1986.
365. Salzman MB, Garcia C. Postexposure varicella vaccination in siblings of children with active varicella. Pediatr Infect Dis J 17:256–257, 1998.
366. Watson B, Seward J, Yang A, et al. Post exposure effectiveness of varicella vaccine. Pediatrics 105:84–88, 2000.
367. Asano Y, Nagai T, Miyata T, et al. Long-term protective immunity of recipients of the Oka strain of live varicella vaccine. Pediatrics 75:667–671, 1985.
368. Bernstein HH, Rothstein EP, Watson BM, et al. Clinical survey of natural varicella compared with breakthrough varicella after immunization with live attenuated Oka/Merck varicella vaccine. Pediatrics 92:833–837, 1993.
369. Clements DA, Armstrong CB, Ursano AM, et al. Over five-year follow-up of Oka/Merck varicella vaccine recipients in 465 infants and adolescents. Pediatr Infect Dis J 14:874–879, 1995.
370. Johnson C, Rome L, Stancin T, Kumar M. Humoral immunity and clinical reinfections following varicella vaccine in healthy children. Pediatrics 84:418–421, 1989.
371. Johnson C, Stancin T, Fattlar D, et al. A long-term prospective study of varicella vaccine in healthy children. Pediatrics 100:761–766, 1997.
372. Watson BM, Piercy SA, Plotkin SA, Starr SE. Modified chickenpox in children immunized with the Oka/Merck varicella vaccine. Pediatrics 91:17–22, 1993.
373. Naruse H, Minwata H, Ozaki T, et al. Varicella infection complicated with meningitis after immunization: case report. Acta Pediatr Jpn 35:345–347, 1993.
374. Pillai JJ, Gaughan WJ, Watson B, et al. Renal involvement in association with postvaccination varicella. Clin Infect Dis 17:1079–1080, 1993.
375. Kacica MA, Connelly BL, Myers MG. Communicable varicella in a health care worker 21 months following successful vaccination with live attenuated varicella vaccine. In Program and Abstracts of the 28th Interscience Conference on Antimicrobial Agents and Chemotherapy, Los Angeles, October 23–26. Washington, DC, ASM Press, 1988.
376. Just M, Borger R, Leuscher D. Live varicella vaccine in healthy individuals. Postgrad Med J 61:129–132, 1985.
377. Ndumbe PM, Cradock-Watson JE, MacQueen S, et al. Immunisation of nurses with a live varicella vaccine. Lancet 1:1144–1147, 1985.
378. Alter SJ, McVey CJ, Jenski L, Myers M. Varicella live virus vaccine in normal susceptible adults at high risk for exposure. In Program and Abstracts of the 25th Interscience Conference on Antimicrobial Agents and Chemotherapy, Minneapolis, MN, September 29–October 2. Washington, DC, ASM Press, 1985.
379. Gershon AA, Steinberg S, LaRussa P, et al for the NIAID Collaborative Varicella Vaccine Study Group. Immunization of healthy adults with live attenuated varicella vaccine. J Infect Dis 158:132–137, 1988.
380. Kuter BJ, Ngai A, Patterson CM, et al. Safety, tolerability, and immunogenicity of two regimens of Oka/Merck varicella vaccine (Varivax ®) in healthy adolescents and adults. Vaccine 13:967–972, 1995.
381. Nader S, Bergen R, Sharp M, Arvin A. Comparison of cell-mediated immunity (CMI) to varicella-zoster virus (VZV) in children and adults immunized with live attenuated varicella vaccine. J Infect Dis 171:13–17, 1995.
382. Asano Y, Suga S, Yoshikawa T, et al. Experience and reason: twenty year follow up of protective immunity of the Oka live varicella vaccine. Pediatrics 94:524–526, 1994.
383. Watson B, Gupta R, Randall T, Starr S. Persistence of cell-mediated and humoral immune responses in healthy children immunized with live attenuated varicella vaccine. J Infect Dis 169:197–199, 1994.
384. Zerboni L, Nader S, Aoki K, Arvin AM. Analysis of the persistence of humoral and cellular immunity in children and adults immunized with varicella vaccine. J Infect Dis 177:1701–1704, 1998.
384a. Shinefield HR, Black SB, Staehle BO, et al. Vaccination with measles, mumps and rubella vaccine and varicella vaccine: safety, tolerability, immunogenicity, persistence of antibody and duration of protection against varicella in healthy children. Pediatr Infect Dis J 21:555–561, 2002.
385. Dworkin MS, Jennings CE, Roth-Thomas J, et al. An outbreak of varicella among children attending preschool and elementary school in Illinois. Clin Infect Dis 35:102–104, 2002.
386. Takayama N, Minamitani M, Takayama M. High incidence of breakthrough varicella observed in healthy Japanese children immunized with live varicella vaccine (Oka strain). Acta Paediatr Jpn 39:663–668, 1997.
387. Li S, Chan I, Matthews H, et al. Inverse relationship between six week postvaccination varicella antibody response to vaccine and likelihood of long term breakthrough infection. Pediatr Infect Dis J 21:337–342, 2002.
388. Ngai A, Stahele BO, Kuter BJ, et al. Safety and immunogenicity of one vs. two injections of Oka/Merck varicella vaccine in healthy children. Pediatr Infect Dis J 15:49–54, 1996.
389. Somekh E, Bujanover Y, Tal G, et al. An intradermal skin test for determination of immunity to varicella. Arch Dis Child 85:484–486, 2001.
390. Ueda K, Tokugawa K, Nakashima F, Takahashi M. A five-year immunological follow-up study of the institutionalized handicapped children vaccinated with live varicella vaccine or infected with natural varicella. Biken J 27:119–122, 1984.
391. Dubey L, Steinberg S, LaRussa P, et al. Western blot analysis of antibody to varicella-zoster virus. J Infect Dis 157:882–888, 1988.
392. Hardy I, Gershon A. Prospects for use of a varicella vaccine in adults. Infect Dis Clin North Am 4:160–173, 1990.
393. Ampofo K, Saiman L, LaRussa P, et al. Persistence of immunity to live attenuated varicella vaccine in healthy adults. Clin Infect Dis 34:774–779, 2002.
394. Plotkin SA, Starr S, Connor K, Morton D. Zoster in normal children after varicella vaccine. J Infect Dis 159:1000–1001, 1989.
395. White CJ. Clinical trials of varicella vaccine in healthy children. Infect Dis Clin North Am 10:595–608, 1996.
396. White CJ. Letter to the Editor. Pediatrics 89:354, 1992.
397. Kamiya H, Kato T, Isaji M, et al. Immunization of acute leukemic children with a live varicella vaccine (Oka strain). Biken J 27:99–102, 1984.
398. Hammerschlag MR, Gershon A, Steinberg S, et al. Herpes zoster in an adult recipient of live attenuated varicella vaccine. J Infect Dis 160:535–537, 1989.

399. Englund JA, Suarez CS, Kelly J, et al. Placebo-controlled trial of varicella vaccine given with or after measles-mumps-rubella vaccine. J Pediatr 114:37–44, 1989.

400. Just M, Berger R, Just V. Evaluation of a combined measles-mumps-rubella-chickenpox vaccine. Dev Biol Stand 65:85–88, 1986.

401. White CJ, Stinson D, Staehle B, et al. Measles, mumps, rubella, and varicella combination vaccine: safety and immunogenicity alone and in combination with other vaccines given to children. Clin Infect Dis 24:925–931, 1997.

402. Shinefield HR, Black S, Morozumi P, et al. Safety and immunogenicity of concomitant separate administration of MMRII, Tetramune (Wyeth Lederle DPT & HbOC) and Varivax (Oka/Merck Varicella Vaccine) vs concomitant injections of MMRII, and Tetramune with Varivax given six weeks later. Presented at the Washington, DC, Society for Pediatric Research, 1996.

403. Brunell PA, Novelli VM, Lipton SV, Pollock B. Combined vaccine against measles, mumps, rubella, and varicella. Pediatrics 81:779–784, 1988.

404. Reuman PD, Sawyer MH, Kuter BJ, Matthews H, for the MMRV Study Group. Safety and immunogenicity of concurrent administration of measles-mumps-rubella-varicella vaccine and PedvaxHIB® vaccines in healthy children twelve to eighteen months old. Pediatr Infect Dis J 16:662–667, 1997.

405. Watson B, Laufer D, Kuter B, et al. Safety and immunogenicity of a combined live attenuated measles, mumps, rubella, and varicella vaccine (RRR$_{II}$V) in healthy children. J Infect Dis 173:731–734, 1996.

406. Committee on Infectious Diseases. Live attenuated varicella vaccine. Pediatrics 95:791–796, 1995.

407. Committee on Infectious Diseases. Varicella vaccine update. Pediatrics 105:136–141, 2000.

408. Pickering LK (ed). Red Book: Report of the Committee on Infectious Diseases (25th ed). Elk Grove Village, IL, American Academy of Pediatrics, 2000.

409. Provost PJ, Krah DL, Kuter BJ, et al. Antibody assays suitable for assessing immune responses to live varicella vaccine. Vaccine 9:111–116, 1991.

410. LaRussa P, Steinberg S, Waithe E, et al. Comparison of five assays for antibody to varicella-zoster virus and the fluorescent-antibody-to-membrane-antigen test. J Clin Microbiol 25:2059–2062, 1987.

410a. Richard VS, John TJ, Kenneth J, et al. Should health care workers in the tropics be immunized against varicella? J Hosp Infect 47:243–245, 2001.

411. Berger R, Luescher D, Just M. Enhancement of varicella-zoster-specific immune responses in the elderly by boosting with varicella vaccine. J Infect Dis 149:647, 1984.

412. Takahashi M, Kamiya H, Asano Y, et al. Immunization of the elderly to boost immunity against varicella-zoster virus (VZV) as assessed by VZV skin test reaction. Arch Virol Suppl 17:161–172, 2001.

413. Levin M, Murray M, Zerbe G, et al. Immune responses of elderly persons 4 years after receiving a live attenuated varicella vaccine. J Infect Dis 170:522–526, 1994.

414. Trannoy E, Berger R, Hollander G, et al. Vaccination of immunocompetent elderly subjects with a live attenuated Oka strain of varicella-zoster virus: a randomized, controlled, dose-response trial. Vaccine 18:1700–1706, 2000.

415. Levin MJ. Use of varicella vaccines to prevent herpes zoster in older individuals. Arch Virol Suppl 17:151–160, 2001.

416. Hata A, Asanuma H, Rinki M, et al. Use of an inactivated varicella vaccine in recipients of hematopoietic cell transplants. N Engl J Med 347:26–34, 2002.

417. Redman R, Nader S, Zerboni L, et al. Early reconstitution of immunity and decreased severity of herpes zoster in bone marrow transplant recipients immunized with inactivated varicella vaccine. J Infect Dis 176:578–585, 1997.

418. Dennehy PH, Saracen CL, Peter G. Seroconversion rates to combined measles-mumps-rubella-varicella vaccine of children with upper respiratory infection. Pediatrics 94:514–516, 1994.

419. Centers for Disease Control and Prevention. Varivax pregnancy registry established. MMWR Morb Mortal Wkly Rep 45:20–21, 1997.

420. Shields KE, Galil K, Seward J, et al. Varicella vaccine exposure during pregnancy: data from the first 5 years of the pregnancy registry (1). Obstet Gynecol 98:14–19, 2001.

421. Centers for Disease Control and Prevention. Estimated vaccination coverage with individual vaccines and selected vaccination series among children 19–35 months by state, US National Immunization Survey. MMWR Morb Mortal Wkly Rep 51:664–666, 2002.

422. Seward JF, Watson BM, Peterson CL, et al. Varicella disease after introduction of varicella vaccine in the United States, 1995–2000. JAMA 287:606–611, 2002.

423. Huse DM, Meissner C, Lacey MJ, Oster G. Childhood vaccination against chickenpox: an analysis of benefits and costs. J Pediatr 124:869–874, 1994.

424. Lieu T, Cochi S, Black S, et al. Cost-effectiveness of a routine varicella vaccination program for U.S. children. JAMA 271:375–381, 1994.

425. Preblud SR, Orenstein WA, Koplan JP, et al. A benefit-cost analysis of a childhood vaccination programme. Postgrad Med J 61:17–22, 1985.

426. Beutels P, Clara R, Tormans G, et al. Costs and benefits of routine varicella vaccination in German children. J Infect Dis 174(suppl): S335–S341, 1996.

427. Brisson M, Edmunds WJ. The cost-effectiveness of varicella vaccination in Canada. Vaccine 20:1113–1125, 2002.

428. Burnham BR, Wells TS, Riddle JR. A cost-benefit analysis of a routine varicella vaccination program for United States Air Force Academy cadets. Mil Med 163:631–634, 1998.

429. Coudeville L, Paree F, Lebrun T, Sailly J. The value of varicella vaccination in healthy children: cost-benefit analysis of the situation in France. Vaccine 17:142–151, 1999.

430. Diez Domingo J, Ridao M, Latour J, et al. A cost benefit analysis of routine varicella vaccination in Spain. Vaccine 17:1306–1311, 1999.

431. Faoagali JL, Darcy D. Chickenpox outbreak among the staff of a large, urban adult hospital: costs of monitoring and control. Am J Infect Control 23:247–250, 1995.

432. Gayman J. A cost-effectiveness model for analyzing two varicella vaccination strategies. Am J Health Syst Pharm 55(suppl):S4–S8, 1998.

433. Glantz JC, Mushlin AI. Cost-effectiveness of routine antenatal varicella screening. Obstet Gynecol 91:519–528, 1998.

434. Gray AM, Fenn P, Weinberg J, et al. An economic analysis of varicella vaccination for health care workers. Epidemiol Infect 119:209–220, 1997.

435. Howell MR, Lee T, Gaydos CA, Nang RN. The cost-effectiveness of varicella screening and vaccination in U.S. Army recruits. Mil Med 165:309–315, 2000.

436. Kitai IC, King S, Gafni A. An economic evaluation of varicella vaccine for pediatric liver and kidney transplant recipients. Clin Infect Dis 17:441–447, 1993.

437. Law B, Fitzsimon C, Ford-Jones L, et al. Cost of chickenpox in Canada: part I. Cost of uncomplicated cases. Pediatrics 104:1–6, 1999.

438. Law B, Fitzsimon C, Ford-Jones L, et al. Cost of chickenpox in Canada: part II. Cost of complicated cases and total economic impact. The Immunization Monitoring Program-Active (IMPACT). Pediatrics 104:7–14, 1999.

439. Lieu T, Black SB, Rieser N, et al. The cost of childhood chickenpox: parents' perspective. Pediatr Infect Dis J 13:173–177, 1994.

440. Nettleman MD, Schmid M. Controlling varicella in the healthcare setting: the cost effectiveness of using varicella vaccine in healthcare workers. Infect Control Hosp Epidemiol 18:504–508, 1997.

441. Rothberg M, Bennish ML, Kao JS, Wong JB. Do the benefits of varicella vaccination outweigh the long-term risks? A decision-analytic model for policymakers and pediatricians. Clin Infect Dis 34:885–894, 2002.

442. Scuffham P, Devlin N, Eberhart-Phillips J, Wilson-Salt R. The cost-effectiveness of introducing a varicella vaccine to the New Zealand immunisation schedule. Soc Sci Med 49:763–779, 1999.

443. Scuffham PA, Lowin AV, Burgess MA. The cost-effectiveness of varicella vaccine programs for Australia. Vaccine 18:407–415, 1999.

444. Smith WJ, Jackson LA, Watts DH, Koepsell TD. Prevention of chickenpox in reproductive-age women: cost-effectiveness of routine prenatal screening with postpartum vaccination of susceptibles. Obstet Gynecol 92:535–545, 1998.

445. Tennenberg A, Brassard JE, Van Lieu J, Drusin L. Varicella vaccination for healthcare workers at a university hospital: an analysis of costs and benefits. Infect Control Hosp Epidemiol 18:405–411, 1997.

446. Thiry N, Beutels P, Van Damme P, Doorslaer E. Economic evaluation of varicella vaccination programmes: a review of the literature. PharmacoEconomics 121:13–38, 2003.

447. Ronan K, Wallace MR. The utility of serologic testing for varicella in an adolescent population. Vaccine 19:4700–4702, 2001.

448. Smith KJ, Roberts MS. Cost effectiveness of vaccination strategies in adults without a history of chickenpox. Am J Med 108:723–729, 2000.

449. Lieu T, Finkler LJ, Sorel M, et al. Cost-effectiveness of varicella serotyping versus presumptive vaccination of school-age children and adolescents. Pediatrics 95:632–638, 1995.

450. Weber DJ, Rotala WA, Parham C. Impact and costs of varicella prevention in a university hospital. Am J Public Health 78:19–23, 1988.

451. Brisson M, Edmunds WJ, Gay NJ, et al. Modeling the impact of immunization on the epidemiology of varicella-zoster virus. Epidemiol Infect 125:651–669, 2000.

452. Garnett GP, Ferguson NM. Predicting the effect of varicella vaccine on subsequent cases of zoster and varicella. Rev Med Virol 6:151–161, 1996.

453. Brisson M, Gay N, Edmunds WJ, Andrews NJ. Exposure to varicella boosts immunity to herpes-zoster: implications for mass vaccination against chickenpox. Vaccine 20:2500–2507, 2002.

Chapter 29

Combination Vaccines

MICHAEL D. DECKER • KATHRYN M. EDWARDS •
HUGUES H. BOGAERTS

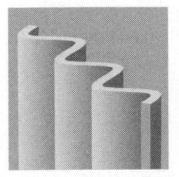

The continuing increase in the number of effective vaccines suitable for use in infancy and early childhood has posed substantial economic and logistic difficulties. Providing these vaccines as separate injections not only is expensive but also requires multiple needle sticks, distressing parents, providers, and patients alike. Scheduling additional vaccination visits to reduce the number of injections per visit increases costs, burdens staff, and jeopardizes the entire immunization program by increasing the likelihood of missed vaccinations. The shipping, handling, and storage of a plethora of vaccines are burdensome and expensive and increase the possibility of error. These problems have stimulated continuing efforts to develop new combination vaccines. However, the development and evaluation of combination vaccines can pose complex issues, many of which were reviewed by scientists from academia, government, and industry at a workshop convened by the U.S. Food and Drug Administration (FDA) in 1993 and at a symposium at the U.S. National Institutes of Health in 2000. The proceedings of those meetings provide useful references.[1,2]

The combining of multiple related or unrelated antigens into a single vaccine is not a new concept; combination vaccines have long been a bedrock of our pediatric and adult immunization programs. Those combination vaccines in common use include diphtheria and tetanus toxoids, available alone (DT or Td) or with whole-cell (DTwP) or acellular (DTaP) pertussis vaccine; inactivated (IPV) or live oral (OPV) trivalent poliovirus vaccine; and measles and rubella vaccine, available alone (MR) or with mumps vaccine (MMR).

The first combination vaccine licensed in the United States was trivalent influenza vaccine, approved in November 1945, and the second was a hexavalent pneumococcal vaccine, licensed in 1947.[3] DTwP, although developed in 1943, was not licensed until March 1948. IPV was licensed in 1955, and the individual OPV serotypes were licensed from 1961 to 1962. Efforts to overcome the interference seen with simultaneous administration of three live vaccines delayed the licensure of trivalent OPV until June 1963. MMR and MR were licensed in April 1971, and quadrivalent meningococcal vaccine in 1978. Only brief

mention is made in this chapter of these traditional combination vaccines, which are discussed in their own chapters elsewhere in this text.

As the number of safe and effective pediatric vaccines has grown, efforts have intensified to develop increasingly complex combination vaccines. Most such pediatric combination vaccines begin with a DTwP or DTaP vaccine and add such antigens as IPV, conjugate *Haemophilus influenzae* type b (Hib), and hepatitis B (HepB). As development efforts for the DT(a)P-based combinations have matured, some manufacturers have turned their efforts toward developing so-called second-shot combinations that incorporate conjugate pneumococcal (PnC) and conjugate meningococcal (MnC) antigens. A third developmental stream has been directed toward combination vaccines targeted principally at travelers, typically based on HepB or hepatitis A (HepA) components.

Our primary focus will be on the newer combination vaccines that merge products such as IPV, HepB, or Hib vaccine with each other or with one or more of the aforementioned traditional combination vaccines. We will identify issues that complicate the development, evaluation, and licensure of combination vaccines and then review, group by group, various combination vaccines with particular reference to clinical data regarding their immunogenicity, reactogenicity, and efficacy. Table 29–1 outlines the current status of the newer combination vaccines, and Table 29–2 provides further details concerning those that are licensed.

Terminology

The vaccine industry has undergone dramatic consolidation over the past 20 years; both long-established companies and new biotechnology start-ups have been acquired or merged. These changes render nomenclature problematic. For vaccines currently marketed, we will use the name of the current manufacturer, even when describing studies conducted by a predecessor company. For products not presently marketed, we will use the name of the company that produced them, even if that company now is owned by or operates under a successor name. To further assist the reader, Table 21–6 lists most current major vaccine manufacturers, along

TABLE 29–1 ■ Combination Vaccines Presently Licensed or Under Development*

Vaccines Combined†	Combination Has Been Licensed			Clinical Trials Conducted
	In Europe or Canada	In USA	In Other Countries	
Td/IPV	AP-MSD, AvP-Ca			
DT/IPV	AP-MSD, AvP-Ca			
DTwP/IPV	AP-MSD, AvP-Ca		AvP-Fr	
DTwP/Hib	AP-MSD, AvP-Ca, GSK, Wyeth, Chiron		AvP-Ca, AvP-Fr, Chiron	
DTwP/Hib/IPV	AP-MSD, AvP-Ca		AvP-Ca, AvP-Fr	
DTwP/HepB	GSK		GSK	
DTwP/HepB/Hib	GSK		GSK	Merck
DTwP/HepB/MnC/Hib				GSK
DTaP/IPV	AP-MSD, AvP-Ca, BL, GSK, SSI		AvP-Ca, AvP-Fr, GSK	
DTaP/Hib	AvP-Ca, GSK	AvP-US‡	AvP-Fr, GSK	
DTaP/IPV/Hib	AP-MSD, AvP-Ca, GSK, SSI		AvP-Ca, GSK	BL
DTaP/HepB	GSK		GSK	
DTaP/IPV/HepB	GSK	GSK	GSK	
DTaP/Hib/HepB	GSK		GSK	
DTaP/Hib/IPV/HepB	AP-MSD, GSK		GSK, AvP-Fr	AvP-US, Merck
DTap/Hib/IPV/HepB/MNC				GSK
Tdap/IPV	AP-MSD			
HepB/Hib	AP-MSD	Merck		
HepB/HepA	GSK	GSK	GSK	
HepA/typhoid	AP-MSD; GSK			
MMRV				GSK, Merck
MnC/Hib				GSK, Wyeth
PnC/MnC				Wyeth
PnC/MnC/Hib				Wyeth

*Products combining only multiple serotypes of a single pathogen are excluded, as are DT, DTP, DTaP, OPV, IPV, and MMR. Only those manufacturers who distribute their products internationally are listed; other manufacturers may produce some products (e.g., DTP/IPV) for local or regional use. Some products represent components derived from, or joint efforts of, more than one manufacturer; in such cases, their principal distributor is shown.

†No discrimination is made between products distributed in combined form and those distributed in separate containers, for combination at the time of use.

‡Licensed for the fourth (booster) dose only.

aP, acellular pertussis vaccine (infant formulation); ap, acellular pertussis vaccine (adolescent/adult formulation); AP-MSD, Aventis Pasteur MSD; AvP, Aventis Pasteur (CA, Canada; Fr, France; US, United States); BL, Baxter Laboratories; D, diphtheria toxoid vaccine (infant formulation); d, diphtheria toxoid vaccine (adolescent/adult formulation); GSK, GlaxoSmithKline; HepA, hepatitis A vaccine; HepB, hepatitis B vaccine; Hib, conjugate *Haemophilus influenzae* type b vaccine; IPV, enhanced inactivated trivalent poliovirus vaccine; MMRV, measles, mumps, rubella, and varicella vaccine; MnC, meningococcal conjugate vaccine (serotype C initially, additional serotypes subsequently); PnC, pneumococcal conjugate vaccine (7-valent initially, 9- or 11-valent subsequently); SSI, Statens Seruminstitut; T, tetanus toxoid vaccine; WP, whole-cell pertussis vaccine. See Table 21–6 for information on prior names of pharmaceutical companies.

with the names of predecessor, component, or acquired companies.

In this chapter, the use of a virgule to coordinate the names of two vaccines (e.g., DTwP/IPV) indicates a combination of those two vaccines; a plus sign (e.g., DTwP + IPV) indicates their concurrent but separate administration.

Because so many different combination vaccines are available within some classes (e.g., DTaP/Hib) and simple, unambiguous generic names do not exist for the various products, trade names are used herein to refer to specific combination vaccines whenever possible.

Principles of Combined Vaccines

Simultaneous Vaccines

A combination vaccine consists of two or more separate immunogens that have been physically combined in a single preparation. This concept differs from that of simultaneous vaccines, which, although administered concurrently, are physically separate (i.e., injected at separate sites or delivered by separate limbs). Although some studies have shown altered immune responses to various vaccines when they are given concurrently with other vaccines but at separate sites, there is no evidence that the efficacy of any vaccine recommended for routine use in childhood is materially altered by concurrent administration with any other vaccines recommended for administration at the same age.[4] Similarly, adverse events after concurrent administration of multiple vaccines generally are increased only modestly, if at all, compared with events after the administration of the most reactogenic vaccine alone. Thus we do not review the many studies that have evaluated simultaneous administration, except to the extent that they provide reference data against which results from combined vaccines can be compared.

Combination Vaccines and the Immune System

Antibodies recognize conformationally determined epitopes on protein or polysaccharide antigens. Modification of an antigen's B-cell epitopes during vaccine preparation may reduce the ability of vaccine-induced antibody to bind to the pathogen. Consequently, the techniques used to produce an antigen may have important implications for the

TABLE 29–2 ■ Characteristics of Combination Vaccines Presently Available in Canada, Europe, or the United States*

Combination	Trade Name	Source	Each 0.5-mL Dose Is Formulated to Contain:†
CANADA			
DT/IPV	DT Polio Adsorbed	AvP	25 Lf D, 5 Lf T, poliomyelitis vaccine types 1 (Mahoney, 40D), 2 (MEF-1, 8D), and 3 (Saukett, 32D), 1.5 mg Al_3PO_4, trace polymyxin B and neomycin, 27 ppm formaldehyde, and 0.5% 2-PE
Td/IPV	Td Polio Adsorbed	AvP	2 Lf D, 5 Lf T, poliomyelitis vaccine types 1 (Mahoney, 40D), 2 (MEF-1, 8D), and 3 (Saukett, 32D), 1.5 mg Al_3PO_4, trace polymyxin B and neomycin, 27 ppm formaldehyde, and 0.5% 2-PE
DTaP/IPV	QUADRACEL	AvP	20 µg PT, 20 µg FHA, 3 µg PRN, 5 µg FIM types 2 and 3, 15 Lf D, 5 Lf T, poliomyelitis vaccine types 1 (Mahoney, 40D), 2 (MEF-1, 8D), and 3 (Saukett, 32D), 0.6% ± 0.1% (v/v) 2-PE, 1.5 mg Al_3PO_4, trace polymyxin B and neomycin
DTaP/IPV/Hib	PENTACEL PEDIACEL	AvP AvP	*Quadracel* packaged with, and used to reconstitute, *ActHIB* (10 µg PRP conjugated to 24 µg T) 20 µg PT, 20 µg FHA, 3 µg PRN, 5 µg FIM types 2 and 3, 15 Lf D, 5 Lf T, poliomyelitis vaccine types 1 (Mahoney, 40D), 2 (MEF-1, 8D), and 3 (Saukett, 32D), 10 µg PRP conjugated to 20 µg T, 0.6% ± 0.1% (v/v) 2-PE, 1.5 mg Al_3PO_4; trace streptomycin, polymyxin B, and neomycin may be present
HB/HA	Twinrix Pediatric	GSK	Not less than 360 EU inactivated HA virus and 10 µg of recombinant HBsAg protein; 0.025 mg $Al(OH)_3$, 0.2 mg Al_3PO_4, 2.5 mg 2-PE
	Twinrix Adult	GSK	A **1-mL** dose contains not less than 720 EU inactivated HA virus and 20 µg of recombinant HBsAg protein; 0.05 mg $Al(OH)_3$, 0.4 mg Al_3PO_4, 5.0 mg 2-PE
EUROPE			
DT/IPV	DT-Polio	AvP	1 immunization dose of D, 1 immunization dose of T, 1 immunization dose of inactivated type 1 polio, 1 immunization dose of inactivated type 2 polio, 1 immunization dose of inactivated type 3 polio; max 0.5 µl 2-PE, max. 100 µg formaldehyde
Td-IPV	Revaxis	AvP	At least 2 IU D, 20 IU T, and poliomyelitis vaccine types 1 (Mahoney, 40D), 2 (MEF-1, 8D), and 3 (Saukett, 32D); $Al(OH)_3$, 2-PE
DTwP-IPV	Terracoq	AvP	At least 30 IU D, 60 IU T, 4 IU wP, and poliomyelitis vaccine types 1 (Mahoney, 40D), 2 (MEF-1, 8D), and 3 (Saukett, 32D); 0.65 mg $Al(OH)_3$, 2.5 µl 2-PE, 12.5 µg formaldehyde
DTwP/Hib	QuattVaxem	Chiron	At least 30 IU D, 60 IU T, 2 IU wP, 10 µg PRP conjugated to 25 µg CRM_{197}, 1.36 mg Al_3PO_4, 0.05 mg thimerosal

Continued

TABLE 29–2 ■ Characteristics of Combination Vaccines Presently Available in Canada, Europe, or the United States*—cont'd

Combination	Trade Name	Source	Each 0.5-mL Dose Is Formulated to Contain:†
			EUROPE
DTwP-HB	TETRAct-Hib	AvP	At least 30 IU D, 60 IU T, 4 IU wP, and 10 μg PRP conjugated to 20 μg T; 0.65 mg Al(OH)$_3$, 2.5 μl 2-PE, 12.5 μg formaldehyde
DTwP-HB	Tritanrix Hep B	GSK	At least 30 IU D, 60 IU T, 4 IU wP, and 10 μg recombinant HBsAg protein; 0.63 mg Al(OH)$_3$, 0.63 mg Al$_3$PO$_4$, 0.5 mg 2-PE, 0.025 mg thimerosal
DTwP-HB/Hib	Tritanrix Hep B Hib	GSK	At least 30 IU D, 60 IU T, 4 IU wP, 10 μg recombinant HBsAg protein, and 10 μg of PRP conjugated to T; 0.63 mg Al(OH), 0.63 mg Al$_3$PO$_4$, 0.5 mg 2-PE, 0.025 mg thimerosal
DTwP/IPV/Hib	PENTAct-Hib (also Pentacoq, PentHIBest)	AvP	At least 30 IU D, 60 IU T, 4 IU wP, 10 μg PRP conjugated to 20 μg T, and poliomyelitis vaccine types 1 (Mahoney, 40D), 2 (M.E.F.1, 8D), and 3 (Saukett, 32D); 0.65 mg Al(OH)$_3$, 2.5, μl 2-PE, 12.5 μg formaldehyde
DTaP/IPV	Certiva IPV	Baxter	40 μg PT, 15 Lf D, 6 Lf T, trivalent eIPV
DTaP/IPV	DiTeKiPol	SSI	At least 30 IU (25 Lf) D, at least 40 IU (7 Lf) TT, 40 μg P, and at least 60% of the following poliovirus amounts: type 1 (Brunhilde), 40 D; type 2 (MEF-1), 8 D; type 3 (Saukett), 32 D; 1 mg aluminum (as hydroxide), 0.3 mg sodium dihydrogen phosphate dihydrate, <25 μg formaldehyde, <0.2 μg neomycin, trace phenolsulfonphthalein
	Infanrix IPV (also Infanrix Tetra, Infanrix Quinta, Cinquerix)	GSK	At least 30 IU D, at least 40 IU T, 25 μg PT, 25 μg FHA, 8 μg PRN, poliomyelitis vaccine types 1 (Mahoney, 40D), 2 (MEF-1, 8D), and 3 (Saukett, 32D); 0.5 mg Al(OH)$_3$, 2.5 mg 2-PE
	Tetravac	AvP	At least 30 IU D, at least 40 IU T, 25 μg PT, 25 μg FHA, poliomyelitis vaccine types 1 (Mahoney, 40D), 2 (MEF-1, 8D), and 3 (Saukett, 32D); 0.3 mg Al(OH), 2.5 μl 2-PE, 12.5 μg formaldehyde
Tdap/IPV	Repevax	AvP	2 Lf D, 5 Lf T, 2.5 μg PT, 5 μg FHA, 3 μg PRN, 5 μg FIM types 2 and 3, poliomyelitis vaccine types 1 (Mahoney, 40D), 2 (MEF-1, 8D), and 3 (Saukett, 32D); 0.6% ± 0.1% (v/v) 2-PE, 1.5 mg Al$_3$PO$_4$, trace polymyxin B and neomycin
DTaP/Hib	Infanrix Hib	GSK	At least 30 IU D, at least 40 IU T, 25 μg PT, 25 μg FHA, 8 μg PRN, and 10 μg PRP conjugated to T; 0.5 mg Al(OH)$_3$, 2.5 mg 2-PE
DTaP/HepB	Infanrix Hep B	GSK	At least 30 IU D, at least 40 IU T, 25 μg PT, 25 μg FHA, 8 μg PRN, and 10 μg recombinant HBsAg protein; 0.5 mg Al(OH)$_3$, 0.2 mg Al$_3$PO$_4$, 2.5 mg 2-PE

DTaP/IPV/Hib	*DiTeKiPol/ActHiB*	SSI	At least 30 IU (25 Lf) D, at least 40 IU (7 Lf) T, 40 μg PT, at least 60% of the following poliovirus amounts: type 1 (Brunhilde), 40 D; type 2 (MEF-1), 8 D; type 3 (Saukett), 32 DU, and 10 μg PRP conjugated to TT; 1 mg aluminum (as hydroxide), 0.3 mg sodium dihydrogen phosphate dihydrate, <25 μg formaldehyde, <0.2 μg neomycin, trace phenolsulfonphthalein, trometamol
	Infanrix IPV Hib	GSK	At least 30 IU T, at least 40 IU D, at least 40 IU PT, 25 μg FHA, 8 μg PRN, poliomyelitis vaccine types 1 (Mahoney, 40D), 2 (MEF-1, 8D), and 3 (Saukett, 32D), and 10 μg of PRP conjugated to TT; 0.5 mg Al(OH)$_3$, 2.5 mg 2-PE
	Pentavac Pentaxim	AvP	At least 30 IU D, at least 40 IU T, 25 μg PT, 25 μg FHA, poliomyelitis vaccine types 1 (Mahoney, 40D), 2 (MEF-1, 8D), and 3 (Saukett, 32D), and 10 μg PRP conjugated to T; 0.3 mg Al(OH)$_3$, 2.5 μl 2-PE, 12.5 μg formaldehyde
DTaP/HepB/Hib	*Infanrix Hep B Hib*	GSK	At least 30 IU D, at least 40 IU T, 25 μg PT, 25 μg FHA, 8 μg PRN, 10 μg recombinant HBsAg protein and 10 μg PRP conjugated to T; 0.5 mg Al(OH)$_3$, 0.2 mg Al$_3$PO$_4$, 2.5 mg 2-PE
DTaP/HepB/IPV	*Infanrix PeNTa*	GSK	At least 30 IU D, at least 40 IU T, 25 μg PT, 25 μg FHA, 8 μg PRN, poliomyelitis vaccine types 1 (Mahoney, 40D), 2 (MEF-1, 8D), and 3 (Saukett, 32D), and 10 μg recombinant HBsAg protein; 0.5 mg Al(OH)$_3$, 0.2 mg Al$_3$PO$_4$, 2.5 mg 2-PE
DTaP/HepB/IPV/Hib	*Hexavac*	AvP	At least 30 IU D, at least 40 IU T, 25 μg PT, 25 μg FHA, poliomyelitis vaccine types 1 (Mahoney, 40D), 2 (MEF-1, 8D), and 3 (Saukett, 32D), 10 μg recombinant HBsAg protein, and 10 μg PRP conjugated to T; 0.3 mg Al(OH)$_3$, 2.5 μl 2-PE, 12.5 μg formaldehyde
	Infanrix Hexa	GSK	At least 30 IU DT, at least 40 IU T, 25 μg PT, 25 μg FHA, 8 μg PRN, poliomyelitis vaccine types 1 (Mahoney, 40D), 2 (MEF-1, 8D), and 3 (Saukett, 32D), 10 μg recombinant HBsAg protein, and 10 μg PRP conjugated to T; 0.5 mg Al(OH)3, 0.32 mg Al3PO4, 2.5 mg 2-PE
HepB/HepA	*Twinrix pediatric*	GSK	Not less than 360 EU inactivated HA virus and 10 μg recombinant HBsAg protein; 0.025 mg Al(OH), 0.2 mg Al$_3$PO$_4$, 2.5 mg 2-PE
	Twinrix adult	GSK	A **1-mL dose** contains not less than 720 EU inactivated HA virus and 20 μg recombinant HBsAg protein; 0.05 mg Al(OH)$_3$, 0.4 mg Al$_3$PO$_4$, 5.0 mg 2-PE
HepA/typhoid	*Hepatyrix*	GSK	A **1-mL dose** contains 25 μg of the Vi polysaccharide of *Salmonella typhi* and not less than 1440 ELISA units of inactivated hepatitis A viral antigen; 0.5 mg Al(OH)$_3$, 5.0 mg 2-PE
	ViATIM Vivaxim	AvP	A **1-mL dose** contains 25 μg of the Vi polysaccharide of *Salmonella typhi* and 160 antigen units of inactivated hepatitis A viral antigen

Continued

TABLE 29–2 ■ Characteristics of Combination Vaccines Presently Available in Canada, Europe, or the United States*—cont'd

Combination	Trade Name	Source	Each 0.5-mL Dose Is Formulated to Contain:[†]
			UNITED STATES
DTaP/Hib	*TriHIBit*	AvP	6.7 Lf D, 5 Lf TT, 46.8 μg pertussis antigens (approximately 23.4 μg inactivated PT and 23.4 μg FHA), 10 μg PRP conjugated to 24 μg TT, not more than 0.170 mg aluminum, 0.01% thimerosal, not more than 100 μg (0.02%) residual formaldehyde, and trace amounts of formaldehyde (<0.3 μg mercury/dose), gelatin, and polysorbate 80
DTaP/HepB/IPV	*Pediarix*	GSK	25 Lf D, 10 Lf T, 25 μg PT, 25 μg FHA, 8 μg PRN, poliomyelitis vaccine types 1 (Mahoney, 40D), 2 (MEF-1, 8D), and 3 (Saukett, 32D), and 10 μg recombinant HBsAg protein; 0.5 mg Al(OH)$_3$, 0.2 mg Al$_3$PO$_4$, 2.5 mg 2-PE
HepB/Hib	*Comvax*	Merck	7.5 μg PRP, conjugated to PRP 125 μg OMP, 5 μg HBsAg, approximately 225 μg aluminum hydroxide, 35 μg sodium borate (decahydrate) as a pH stabilizer, and 0.9% sodium chloride.
HepB/HepA	*Ambirix, Twinrix* (2-dose series)	GSK	A **1-mL dose** contains not less than 720 EU inactivated HA virus and 20 μg recombinant HBsAg protein, 0.45 mg aluminum (as hydroxide and phosphate), 5 mg 2-PE, and trace thimerosal (<1 μg mercury), formalin (not more than 0.1 mg), MRC-5 proteins (not more than 2.5 μg), amino acids, yeast proteins, neomycin, and polysorbate 20

*Products combining only multiple serotypes of a single pathogen are excluded, as are DT, DTP, DTaP, OPV, IPV, and MMR. Excludes products that are licensed but not distributed. Only those manufacturers who distribute their products internationally are listed; other manufacturers may produce some products (e.g., DTP/IPV) for local or regional use. No discrimination is made between products distributed in combined form and those distributed in separate containers, for combination at the time of use.

[†]D (in the context of poliovirus potency); D, antigen units; E4, Elisa Units; FHA, filamentous hemagglutinin; FIM, fimbriae agglutinogens; HA, hepatitis A; HBsAg, hepatitis B surface antigen; Lf, limit of flocculation units; OMPC, outer membrane protein complex of *Nesseria meningitidis*; 2-PE, 2-phenoxyethanol; PRN, pertactin; PRP, polyribosylribitol phosphate; PT, pertussis toxoid; TT, tetanus toxoid.

aP, acellular pertussis vaccine (infant formulation); ap, acellular pertussis vaccine (adolescent/adult formulation); AvP, Aventis Pasteur; D, diphtheria toxoid vaccine (infant formulation); d, diphtheria toxoid vaccine (adolescent/adult formulation); GSK, GlaxoSmithKline; HepA, hepatitis A vaccine; HepB, hepatitis B vaccine; Hib, conjugate *Haemophilus influenzae* type b vaccine; IPV, enhanced inactivated trivalent poliovirus vaccine; PnC, pneumococcal conjugate vaccine; PRP, polyribosylribitol phosphate; SSI, Statens Seruminstitut; T, tetanus toxoid vaccine; wP, whole-cell pertussis vaccine. See Table 21–6 for information on prior names of pharmaceutical companies.

immunogenicity (and, presumably, the efficacy) of a vaccine containing that antigen.[5] This principle is illustrated by the results from the Multicenter Acellular Pertussis Trial, which compared 13 acellular pertussis (aP) vaccines and found that levels of antibody to pertussis toxin correlated poorly with the quantity of toxoided pertussis toxin present in the vaccines.[6] For example, one of the acellular vaccines contained a genetically inactivated pertussis toxin produced by recombinant technology. This vaccine produced markedly higher antibody responses per microgram than did the remainder of the evaluated vaccines, whose pertussis toxin components were inactivated chemically (e.g., with formaldehyde or glutaraldehyde) rather than genetically.[6]

Carrier-Induced Epitopic Suppression

The remarkable success of the polysaccharide-protein conjugate Hib vaccines in virtually eliminating Hib disease is testimony to the utility and effectiveness of the conjugate vaccine approach. However, some bacterial pathogens, such as *Streptococcus pneumoniae*, have many serotypes that cause disease, requiring that numerous conjugates be combined into one vaccine. Theories regarding the human immune response and vaccine studies in animals and humans suggest that simultaneous exposure to multiple conjugate antigens (as with a polyvalent conjugate vaccine) can result in either enhanced or diminished immune responses.[7–11]

The phenomenon of carrier-induced epitope-specific suppression is one in which antibody responses to haptens presented on a carrier are inhibited by prior immunization with the specific carrier. Studies in animals have shown that the dose, route, choice of carrier protein, and presence of adjuvant contribute to determining whether epitopic suppression or enhancement of the immune response occurs. Suppression more frequently occurs when large amounts of carrier protein are used for priming and high anticarrier antibody titers are achieved.[12] Concurrent administration of two conjugate vaccines employing the same carrier also may lead to interference. For example, a study among infants given a combination vaccine containing Hib capsular polysaccharide (polyribosylribitol phosphate [PRP]) conjugated to tetanus toxoid (PRP-T) plus a quadrivalent pneumococcal vaccine conjugated to either tetanus or diphtheria toxoid found reduced Hib antibodies among those infants whose pneumococcal vaccine was conjugated to tetanus toxoid rather than diphtheria toxoid.[13] These data make it clear that the effect of prior or concomitant administration of proteins used in conjugate vaccines is unpredictable and must be evaluated for each vaccine combination.

Other Issues Affecting Immune Responses

Chemical or physical interactions among the vaccine components being combined can result in an alteration of the immune response to vaccine.[12] Adjuvants such as aluminum hydroxide and aluminum phosphate bind to inactivated vaccines by noncovalent ionic binding. The combination of one vaccine that is generally administered with adjuvant with another vaccine that is not administered with adjuvant may lead to displacement of the adjuvant and reduced immunogenicity of the first vaccine. Furthermore, the adjuvant might combine with the second antigen and thereby alter the immune response to the second vaccine as well.

Buffers, stabilizers, excipients, and similar components included in one vaccine may interfere with the components of another vaccine (e.g., thimerosal can destroy the potency of IPV). Although such vaccines cannot be mixed in the vial, distribution of the two vaccines in a dual-chambered syringe can circumvent this problem.

Live vaccines can interfere immunologically with each other. For example, one vaccine might stimulate immune responses, such as interferon production, that inhibit replication of another virus.

Correlates of Protection

Immune responses to vaccines traditionally have been assessed by measuring humoral antibodies to the vaccine antigens. For some antigens, studies of vaccine efficacy and immunogenicity have identified correlations between levels of antibody and protection from disease. Identifying such serologic *correlates of protection* provides important benefits. For example, these correlates enable attention to be focused on clinically pertinent performance rather than on numerical differences that may be statistically significant but are clinically irrelevant (e.g., if a combination vaccine produced serologic results for a particular antigen that were significantly lower than those seen in the comparison arm but were nonetheless greater than the level known to provide clinical protection throughout the period of risk, then the diminished immunogenicity would not alter the acceptability of the combination vaccine.) Furthermore, such correlates permit the licensure of a new vaccine based on clinical studies that compare its immunogenicity to that of prior vaccines of proven efficacy. The identification of correlates is of sufficient importance that it should be an explicit objective of any efficacy study of an antigen for which such correlates are not yet determined with confidence.

Correlates of protection can take a number of forms. The most useful are those that identify an individual level of antibody that directly predicts protection: persons with at least this much antibody are considered protected; as antibody levels decline below the protective level, risk increases. Correlates of this kind have been identified for several common vaccine antigens, including measles virus, poliovirus, and tetanus toxoid. For some other antigens, such as diphtheria, a direct relation has been shown between a certain mean level of antibody in the population and protection of that population from outbreaks of the disease in question, but an individual with that level of antibody is not necessarily protected.

For some antigens, levels of personal antibody have been identified that are considered to assure protection, but it is not necessarily true that persons with progressively less antibody are at correspondingly greater risk. Depending on such factors as the nature of the exposure and the incubation period of the disease in question, anamnestic immune responses may provide protection even when pre-exposure antibody levels are low or undetectable. For example, for HepB there is growing evidence that anyone who ever seroconverted and established immune memory is protected from clinical disease, even if their antibody levels subsequently drop below the lower limit of detection.[14,15] The same concept also may be applicable to Hib.[16]

Finally, there are some antigens, particularly including pertussis, for which correlations between antibody levels and protection are uncertain. The lack of clear correlates poses problems for the licensure of new aP vaccines[17-19] and has stimulated the pursuit of more sophisticated analyses in the hopes of identifying useful correlations. As detailed in Chapter 21, a number of such analyses have been completed for various pertussis vaccines, with at least partial success.[20,21]

These issues have focused increasing attention in recent years on the role of the cellular immune system in determining protection (particularly long term) following vaccination. For example, it has been shown[22] that pertussis vaccines induce T-cell responses specific for the vaccine components that increase progressively over the course of the vaccination schedule. After completion of the primary series and before the toddler booster, cell-mediated immune responses persist, whereas antibody levels decline markedly.

Murine challenge models also have proven useful to evaluate the protective efficacy of pertussis-containing vaccines, for which randomized efficacy trials are no longer feasible, given the high uptake of recommended infant pertussis vaccination in nearly all countries. Typically, infant mice are immunized with the equivalent of a human dose, followed by a respiratory challenge with *Bordetella pertussis*. Over succeeding days, animals are sacrificed and clearance of bacteria from the lungs is measured as an indication of the degree of protection induced by the vaccine, compared to unvaccinated control animals. Using this model, it has been possible to replicate the clinical protection observed in efficacy studies conducted in human infants,[23,24] demonstrate differences in performance of various pertussis vaccines,[25] and evaluate the efficacy of different pertussis vaccines against variant B. *pertussis* strains.[26,27]

Other Impediments to the Development of Combination Vaccines

Combination vaccines can present difficult issues with respect to investment of the funds necessary for clinical development. Typically, at the moment of commercial introduction of a new combination vaccine, its component vaccines already are available and could continue to be used instead of the combination, should the combination's price exceed the premium buyers are willing to pay for the convenience the combination represents. The price of the combination thus is effectively capped, and its costs of development must be expected to be recoverable within that cap or the combination will not be developed.

Patent and other proprietary issues also complicate the generation of combination vaccines. Vaccine manufacturers cannot market vaccines that contain antigens they do not own or license. The best possible combination vaccine might be one that incorporated components from two or more manufacturers, but, absent agreement between the companies, this combination will not become available. Although the dramatic consolidation in recent years among vaccine manufacturers has eased this problem, as have cross-licensing agreements, it has not disappeared.

Basic Design Concepts for Combination Vaccine Trials

The Challenges

Combining multiple antigens into one injection requires demonstration in clinical trials that the combination will

not materially reduce the safety or immunogenicity of the component vaccines and, in some instances, that efficacy is retained.[28-30]

Combination vaccine trials should be prospective, randomized, and double blinded and should have appropriate comparison (control) groups. Defining the comparison groups can be problematic when evaluating a multicomponent vaccine. If no pertinent data are available and if one wishes to be able to detect reduced immunogenicity of any component in the combination vaccine, the number of study arms required for the complete evaluation of an n-component vaccine is 2^n, based on the possible combinations alone. Other factors may further increase the number of study arms needed. For example, the sequence of administration of certain antigens may play an important role in immunogenicity. As is discussed later, it has been shown that the response to some Hib vaccines may depend on previous or concurrent administration of diphtheria and tetanus toxoids and pertussis vaccine (DTP). Evaluation of such interactions may require study arms that receive the implicated antigens in different sequences.

Another complicating factor is that reduced antibody responses to one component of a combination could be due to immunologic interference that would occur even if the antigens were injected at different sites during the same visit or, alternatively, to chemical or physical inactivation that occurs only when the antigens are combined in a single injection. The need to differentiate these two possibilities would require additional study arms. Ethical concerns also complicate study design, because vaccines that are recommended for routine use in the study population cannot be withheld in order to study vaccine interactions (although they can be administered at intercalated visits).

Some Solutions

With all these factors serving to complicate the development of combination vaccines, what tactics could be used in response? Most commonly, the new combination is evaluated against each of its components given alone, deferring study of the subcombinations in the hope that no interference will be observed. Sometimes, earlier studies have evaluated predecessor vaccines that differ from the new combination by lacking only a single component; the new combination can then be compared to its predecessor plus the new component, given separately.

Multicenter studies allow larger enrollments—and thus more arms—than are possible at a single institution. A multicenter trial that is well designed with standardized protocols can be an effective means of evaluating multiple vaccines or multicomponent products, as was shown by the Multicenter Acellular Pertussis Trial.[6] The Swedish and Italian DTaP efficacy trials, with their coordinated protocols and control vaccines, are other pertinent examples.[31,32]

It may be possible to simplify study of a combination vaccine by administering to one of the comparison arms a similar, previously studied vaccine, thereby allowing comparison of the current results to those obtained in other arms of the prior study. This *bridging technique* was employed in the Swedish aP efficacy trials to compare the results from each trial.[31,33,34] The methodologic risks of this approach can be reduced through coordinated efforts to enhance the comparability of serologic and reaction data gathered for similar vaccines in independent studies. With adequate standardization, incorporation of a prior study arm as a comparison arm in the current study could allow comparison with the results obtained in the other arms of the prior study.

Licensure of Combination Vaccines

To be licensed, vaccines must be demonstrated to be safe and effective. When the components are well characterized (as is usually the case), this typically is accomplished through clinical trials that compare the combination with its components given separately to a similar combination that already is licensed, or, occasionally, with another standard of care.

Most licensing authorities have similar criteria for the evaluation of these parameters. For example, U.S. law states that a combination pharmaceutical product may be licensed when "combining of the active ingredients does not decrease the purity, potency, safety, or effectiveness of any of the individual active components" [21 CFR 601.25(d)(4)].

Evaluating Effectiveness

It is uncommon to require an efficacy trial for a vaccine that combines components previously proven efficacious; instead, demonstration of adequate immunogenicity is required. However, defining "adequate" can be problematic. Determining equivalent potency is reasonably straightforward when applied to drugs, for which effects typically vary directly with dose, but is much more difficult to interpret with respect to vaccines. Vaccines cannot provide more than 100% protection, no matter how high the antibody response; for many antigens, seroprotective antibody levels are either unknown or disputed; and for some antigens, achievement of a particular serum antibody response may be irrelevant, as long as immune memory is established.

The FDA must follow the applicable law, but has flexibility in determining the criteria that define "equivalence." For components with known seroprotective antibody levels, the FDA has required that there be no more than a 10% difference in the seroprotection rates of the combination and its separately administered components (although the FDA has authority to alter this requirement, they have done so only rarely and slightly; e.g., the upper 95% confidence limit on the difference in proportions of infants achieving Hib antibody levels of 1 μg/mL with Comvax versus PedvaxHIB is 11%, according to the package insert). If seroprotective levels are not well established, then typically the FDA will put more focus on seroconversion rates and geometric mean antibody titers (GMTs), applying the 10% test to the former and allowing a 1.5-fold range for the latter.

In a Guidance Document[35] regarding combination vaccines, the FDA noted that "If antibody concentrations induced by the combination vaccine are lower than those induced by the component vaccines, a 'protective' antibody level might still be attained." Although appropriate, this principle can prove difficult to apply in practice because of uncertainty regarding such factors as the correct protective concentration to use; whether any particular antibody concentration is necessary if immune memory has been established; whether there is a minimum seroconversion rate required for population protection; and whether achieving antibody concentrations that substantially exceed the minimum necessary to confer personal protection provides any further benefit (e.g., by suppressing colonization and thereby reducing transmission). Indeed, the importance of humoral antibody itself may be unclear; for at least some vaccines, humoral antibody may be a surrogate for other, more important components of the immune response, particularly cell-mediated immunity.

Evaluating Safety

As a general rule, systemic adverse events are increased only modestly, if at all, after concurrent administration of multiple vaccines compared with events after the administration of the most reactogenic vaccine alone. Local adverse events often are somewhat more common and more severe at the site of injection of the combination, but this increase usually is offset by the absence of injections—and consequently the absence of local reactions—in other limbs. So far, no combination vaccine has elicited a new type of reaction not previously seen with its components.

For a combination vaccine based on well-characterized components (as is nearly always the case), demonstration of safety is straightforward: the combination is compared to its components given separately or to another licensed combination and the rates and severities of adverse events are compared. Although noninferiority (or superiority) is desired, a modest increase in minor adverse reactions is often considered acceptable, recognizing that there has been a concomitant decrease in the number of sites experiencing local reactions.

Recent years have seen an increase in prelicensure safety study sample size requirements from licensing authorities in general and from the FDA in particular. In addition, many authorities expect some (or most) of the safety data to be obtained among subjects from their own countries. Both trends slow licensure without necessarily providing any commensurate benefits. There is little evidence that populations differ materially in the nature or rates of vaccine-associated adverse events, and large increases in sample size require large increases in resources but yield only small increases in statistical power. These issues particularly impact combination vaccines, which commonly do not provide new antigens but merely a more convenient presentation, and whose uptake therefore is sensitive to price, as discussed earlier.

The Question of Multiple Antigens and Immune Overload

Some parents' groups concerned with vaccine-associated adverse reactions have been critical of the administration of multiple vaccine antigens simultaneously and have suggested that doing so is unsafe. However, reviews of the reactions associated with simultaneous administration of multiple antigens have demonstrated a remarkable safety record.[36]

Despite being repeatedly debunked, the assertion continues to circulate—particularly on the Internet—that the normal infant immune system is capable of becoming "overloaded," and that vaccination can induce such overload.

There is no evidence to support such an assertion, and much evidence to refute it[37-39] (see Chapter 62). Indeed, it may be true that the infant immune system requires fairly intensive challenge to develop normally, and that insufficient stimulation leads to an increased risk of autoimmune disorders.[40,41]

A concern that infant immune systems may be "overwhelmed" by simultaneous exposure to several antigens is difficult to entertain when one considers the thousands of antigens to which a newborn is naturally exposed in the first few months of life. Moreover, although more vaccines are administered today, far fewer antigens are delivered than in the past, when DTwP and vaccinia were used routinely.

The Institute of Medicine recently addressed this issue, among others, in its report entitled *Immunization Safety Review: Multiple Immunizations and Immune Dysfunction*, and concluded that the evidence favored rejection of a causal relationship between multiple immunizations and an increased risk of type 1 diabetes or heterologous infections, and was inadequate to accept or reject a causal relationship with allergic disease, particularly asthma.[42]

Postmarketing Surveillance

Before administering a subsequent dose of any vaccine, practitioners should inquire about adverse events associated with the previous vaccination. Unexpected events occurring soon after vaccination, especially if severe enough to require medical attention, should always be reported. For example, in the U.S. the National Childhood Vaccine Injury Act requires health care providers and manufacturers to report serious adverse events after vaccination to the Vaccine Adverse Event Reporting System (VAERS),[43] established to provide a single system for collection and analysis of reports of all adverse events associated with vaccines. The VAERS report is designed to permit description of the adverse event, the type of vaccine received, the timing of the vaccination and the adverse event, demographic information about the recipient, concurrent medical illnesses or medication, and the prior history of adverse events following vaccine. The data are monitored continually to detect clusters of events by vaccine type, manufacturer, and lot of vaccine. Reports may trigger additional investigation. Unfortunately, because the VAERS reports are nonrandom clinical reports, they are useful for generating hypotheses but not for testing them. Large, linked databases may be able to provide the data needed to test hypotheses of causation after an association is noted by VAERS. Health care providers perform an important function by reporting all clinically significant adverse events to VAERS (*www.vaers.com*), particularly as they relate to new combination vaccine products.

Postmarketing surveillance in an increasing number of countries (e.g., the United States, the United Kingdom, Canada) is being facilitated by the use of large databases linking information sources such as pharmacies, health care providers, hospitals, and commercial health care organizations. The integrated data information systems maintained by some governments for their publicly financed medical care or hospitalization programs also have been used for this purpose.

The Traditional Combined Vaccines: DTwP, IPV, OPV, and MMR

As noted earlier, DTwP was developed in 1943 and licensed in the United States in 1948. Its component antigens had long been available separately: the first pertussis vaccine (see Chapter 21) was licensed to the Massachusetts Public Health Biological Laboratories in 1914; mixtures of diphtheria toxin and antitoxin came into use the same year; alum-precipitated diphtheria toxoid (see Chapter 13) was licensed in 1926; and adsorbed tetanus toxoid (see Chapter 27) was licensed in 1937.[3] Pertussis vaccine is a potent adjuvant, and the combining of the three antigens in DTwP actually improved the immunogenicity of the toxoids as compared to separate administration.[44,45] Adsorption of the vaccines with aluminum further improved immunogenicity while decreasing the severity of adverse reactions associated with pertussis vaccine.[46]

MMR vaccines are produced in many countries (see Chapters 19, 20, and 26, respectively). Multiple strains of each vaccine have been used, although three MMR formulations currently predominate worldwide (from Aventis Pasteur [AvP], GlaxoSmithKline [GSK], and Merck & Co.). Rates of adverse reactions after the administration of MMR are only modestly higher than those seen with the individual component products, and seroconversion rates are essentially unchanged.[47-51] The various MMR vaccines all appear to be highly immunogenic.[52-54]

Advances in tissue culture techniques permitted the development of trivalent IPV (see Chapter 24), which underwent extensive field trials in 1954. These trials found 90% efficacy against poliovirus types 2 and 3 but only about 70% efficacy against type 1.[55] Investigation revealed that the preservative thimerosal inactivated the vaccine virus, with relatively greater effect on type 1 poliovirus than on types 2 and 3; in response, other preservatives were substituted. Further improvements in production techniques in the late 1970s allowed the introduction of enhanced-potency IPV, which provides substantially higher immunogenicity.[56-58] There is no evidence of interference between the inactivated vaccine strains themselves, unlike the situation with trivalent OPV (see Chapter 25). Because enteroviruses can compete with each other in the gut, concerns about such interference initially prompted immunization at three separate visits with the monovalent Sabin OPVs, which were licensed from 1961 to 1962. However, it was soon found that adequate immunogenicity could be obtained by adjusting the relative concentrations of the three strains in the trivalent vaccine and employing a three-dose series, and trivalent OPV became licensed in June 1963.

Combinations Based on DTwP (or Its Components)

Overview

In general, currently available combinations of DTwP with IPV, HepB, and/or Hib do not manifest clinically important interference among their components and do not result in adverse reactions that materially exceed, in frequency or severity, those seen with the same DTwP vaccine given alone. The DTwP-based combinations in international distribution that are most widely used are those from AvP (DTwP/IPV, DTwP/Hib, and DTwP/IPV/Hib) and GSK (DTwP/HepB and DTwP/HepB/Hib).

DTwP/IPV, DT/IPV, and Td/IPV

Overview

Although reduced antibody responses to IPV have been shown for some obsolete DTwP/IPV combinations, clinically important interference among the diphtheria, tetanus, whole-cell pertussis (wP), and IPV components has not been demonstrated for currently available combinations incorporating those antigens. In those studies in which combination recipients showed reduced antibody responses to diphtheria and tetanus, all or nearly all nonetheless achieved seroprotective levels. Similarly, pertussis and poliovirus seroconversion rates and absolute antibody levels remained high even with combined vaccine, and the clinical importance of any reduction in mean antibody levels, for either polio or pertussis, is unknown.

The Studies

In 1960, Bordt and colleagues compared IPV, DTwP, and DTwP/IPV among 192 previously unimmunized children ranging in age from 1 month to 6 years.[59] Compared to separate vaccines, the combined vaccine showed higher poliovirus, diphtheria, and tetanus neutralizing antibody responses and pertussis agglutinating antibodies for infants (1 to 5 months), toddlers (6 months to 2 years), and older children (3 to 6 years).

In the late 1980s, investigators in Pakistan compared DTwP/IPV with DTwP + OPV and found good poliovirus immunogenicity in both groups.[60] A 1996 study comparing DTwP (Connaught USA) + IPV (IPOL) versus DTwP/IPV reported that 96% to 100% of recipients in both groups had neutralizing antibody to all three poliovirus serotypes at 6 months of age.[61]

None of these studies found material reductions in responses to the DTwP components. A comparison of DTwP and DTwP/IPV in Scandinavian children found enhanced DTwP antibody responses in the group given the combination vaccine,[62] and a noncomparative study in Burkina Faso found that two doses of a DTwP/IPV vaccine produced good poliovirus and tetanus antibody responses.[63] Antibody responses to diphtheria were lower than those for poliovirus and tetanus, although 98% of children were primed.

The first report clearly documenting reduced antibody responses to the pertussis component of a DTwP/IPV vaccine was that of Baker and colleagues,[64] who compared serologic responses to DTwP and IPV (both produced by Connaught Laboratories Ltd., Ontario, Canada), given combined or separately, versus DTwP + OPV. Unexpectedly, whether the products were administered separately or combined into a single injection, IPV recipients demonstrated significantly lower pertussis antibody responses, for both pertussis toxin and filamentous hemagglutinin, than did OPV recipients.[64] Halperin and colleagues more recently conducted a follow-up study comparing DTwP + IPV with DTwP/IPV and found significantly lower pertussis antibody

responses with the combined than with the separate vaccines.[65] Neither of these reports included data concerning the immunogenicity of the IPV component.

Most studies conducted more recently have evaluated DTwP/IPV combinations that also include Hib, HepB, or both, and these studies generally have focused on comparing the responses for the latter components, not DTwP or IPV. However, the mean diphtheria, tetanus, pertussis, and poliovirus antibody levels reported in these studies appear unremarkable, and seroprotection or seroresponse rates typically are 100% for these antigens.

A Td/IPV preparation (Revaxis; AvP) is available in Europe and has been evaluated as a booster in children ages 6 to 9 years,[66] in young adults,[67] and in older adults (two-dose schedule).[67] The combination induced protective antibody responses in all children, 99.6% of young adults, and 94% of older adults; adverse reactions were temporary and generally mild.

DTwP/Hib (With or Without IPV)

Overview

Many studies have shown that administering DTwP and Hib in combination results in reduced mean PRP antibody levels compared to giving the same components separately. However, even in those studies with statistically significant reductions,[68–70] antibody levels still were high (albeit not as high as with separate administration) and at least 90% of children (typically, >95%) developed greater than 1 μg/mL of antibody to PRP. Thus, reduced immunogenicity of Hib when given in combination with DTwP appears to be of no clinical importance.

The Studies

A number of studies have evaluated vaccines that combine DTwP with conjugate Hib vaccine (and, in some instances, also with IPV). The first such studies compared the separate or combined administration of AvP's PRP-T (ActHIB) and DTwP in Israeli infants.[71] No increase in adverse events or interference with DTwP antibody responses was detected. The study contained no comparison group given PRP-T alone, but PRP antibody responses appeared consistent with those seen in prior studies. A Canadian study comparing a combination of DTwP (Connaught Canada) and PRP conjugated to diphtheria toxoid (PRP-D) with DTwP + PRP-D as boosters at 18 months of age found no differences in antibody responses to the PRP, tetanus, or diphtheria components and found a slight reduction in pertussis agglutinins in the combined group.[72]

Concern soon was raised by a series of studies conducted in Chile and Canada (Vancouver) that evaluated the performance of PRP-T given separately or combined with French (AvP), Canadian (Connaught Canada), or U.S. (Connaught USA) DTwP vaccines.[68,69,73–75] As shown in Table 29–3, with each DTwP, combined versus separate administration produced a significant difference in antibody response for at least one antigen.[68–70,73–92]

Not surprisingly, these findings sparked additional studies of DTwP/PRP-T combination vaccines (with or without IPV).[70,76–84,93–101] For most antigens, differences in GMTs between the combined and separately administered vaccines were inconsistent, with few achieving statistical significance (see Table 29–3). The only clear trend has been for antibody to PRP, which commonly was reduced for combined compared to separate administration of PRP-T. Nonetheless, nearly all children receiving the combination vaccines developed antibody levels considered protective (e.g., >1.0 μg/mL for PRP or >0.01 IU/mL for diphtheria or tetanus), suggesting that these reductions in mean antibody levels are of no clinical importance. It is uncertain what role is played by individual DTwP vaccines, or their specific components, in determining the nature of any interactions with a combined Hib vaccine.

Surveillance data provide further reassurance that use of the combined DTwP/PRP-T does not reduce efficacy in comparison to DTwP and PRP-T administered separately. In Chile, surveillance for pertussis in matched areas that used either DTwP alone or DTwP/PRP-T found no significant difference in the rates of pertussis in the two areas.[102] In the area using DTwP/PRP-T, efficacy against invasive Hib disease was more than 90%. Surveillance in Canada found a continued low rate of invasive Hib disease after the licensure and widespread use of DTwP/PRP-T in that country, with no change in the extremely low rates of vaccine failure.[103,104] Similarly, there was no increase in invasive Hib disease in the United States after the 1993 licensure of DTwP/PRP-T and a similar product, DTwP/PRP–H. influenzae type b oligosaccharide conjugate (HbOC) (Tetramune; Wyeth Lederle Vaccines & Pediatrics).[105]

The studies shown in Table 29–3 involved lyophilized PRP-T reconstituted with DTwP. More recently, a fluid preparation of PRP-T combined with DTwP has been prepared. A comparative trial found no difference in the immunogenicity and reactogenicity of the two preparations.[99]

Some studies have evaluated the use of a dual-chambered syringe to separate the DTwP or DTwP/IPV components from the Hib component until the moment of injection.[70,83,98] Although the reductions in HiB antibody responses that are seen with fully liquid or manually mixed combinations are mitigated, this approach has not been commercialized.

DTwP combinations with the conjugate Hib vaccines PRP–outer membrane protein (OMP) (PedvaxHIB; Merck & Co.), PRP-HbOC (HibTITER; Wyeth Lederle Vaccines & Pediatrics), or PRP-CRM$_{197}$ (QuattVaxem; Chiron Vaccines) have been studied.[85–92] The data do not suggest that combining these vaccines materially interferes with the immunogenicity of any components (see Table 29–3); indeed, improved immunogenicity was seen more often than interference.

None of the combinations that include DTwP and any conjugate Hib vaccine has been shown to be associated with materially increased adverse reactions. Typically, adverse reactions were slightly greater with the combinations than with the DTwP alone; however, they were less than the aggregate of local reactions seen when separate vaccines were given at separate injection sites.

DTwP/HepB (With or Without Hib)

A number of studies have evaluated combination vaccines that incorporate DTwP, HepB, and, more recently, Hib components (Table 29–4).[106–117] For all studies but one,[106]

both the DTwP (Tritanrix) and the PRP-T (Hiberix) were manufactured by GSK. In general, the addition of HepB to DTwP resulted in significantly increased mean HepB antibody levels and unchanged DTwP responses; the further addition of Hib to the combination resulted in no consistent changes in antibody responses. In one study,[106] the Hib component was a PRP-T (ActHIB) manufactured by AvP and the DTwP component was sourced from the Michigan Department of Public Health; all measured responses were enhanced with the combination.

Two studies[110,117] have evaluated the effect of a booster dose of DTwP/HepB/Hib given at 18 months of age to subjects who received DTwP/HepB + Hib or DTwP/HepB/Hib for the primary series. Both groups had high antibody responses to the booster; mean levels tended to be higher in the group primed with DTwP/HepB/Hib and were significantly so for antibody to PRP. Another study evaluated an Australian DTwP (Commonwealth Serum Laboratories) with Merck's Hib and HepB vaccines and found good antibody responses after booster administration.[118]

DTwP/Measles

In 1973, Mérieux and colleagues administered lyophilized measles vaccine reconstituted with DTwP/IPV to 20 seronegative children and found good responses to the measles and polio components.[119] From 1970 to 1978, public health nurses working in the Marshall Islands routinely drew up DTwP and measles vaccine in the same syringe. Surveillance during a measles epidemic in 1978 revealed no significant difference in protection between those immunized with the combined vaccines (measles attack rate, 16.1%) or with the measles vaccine alone (attack rate, 17.9%).[120] Encouraged by these reports, John and colleagues conducted a series of experiments[121–123] involving the administration of DTwP or DTwP/IPV combined in the same syringe with measles vaccine. They found no significant difference in adverse reactions, measles antibody titers, or measles seroconversion rates.[123]

Combinations Based on Acellular Pertussis Vaccine

Overview

The development of numerous effective aP vaccines (see Chapter 21) and their licensure in combination with diphtheria and tetanus toxoids (DTaP) represented an important advance that quickly stimulated efforts to combine DTaP with other routine vaccines of infancy, such as Hib, IPV, and HepB. Building on the experience with DTwP combination vaccines, efforts turned first to evaluating combinations of DTaP and conjugate Hib vaccines, in light of their similar schedules, universal use in developed countries, and lack of orally administered alternatives. It was soon found that combining DTaP with Hib tended to reduce, often markedly, the Hib antibody response. This discovery slowed development of combinations based on DTaP/Hib and stimulated development of alternative combinations such as DTaP/IPV, DTaP/HepB, and DTaP/IPV/HepB. It also prompted research into the clinical relevance of the reduced response, which has

TABLE 29–3 ■ Studies Comparing Combined or Simultaneous Administration of DTwP/IPV, DTwP/Hib, and DTwP/IPV/Hib Vaccines for Primary Immunization of Infants

| Place | Ages (Mo) | Vaccines | Ratio of Antibody Levels with Combined Vaccine to Levels with Separate Vaccines* | | | | | | | | |
| | | | | | | | | | Polioviruses | | |
			PRP	D	T	PT	FHA	AGG	1	2	3
Chile[68,69]	2, 4, 6	DTwPf/PRP-T1, DTwPf + PRP-T1	0.43†	1.00	0.85	0.97	1.07	0.62‡			
Vancouver[74]	2, 4, 6	DTwPc/PRP-T1 (Lot 1), DTwPc + PRP-T1	1.16	1.33	1.00	0.80	1.00	0.88			
Vancouver[74]	2, 4, 6	DTwPc/PRP-T1 (Lot2), DTwPc + PRP-T1	1.03	1.33	0.78	0.80	0.75	0.68†			
Vancouver[75]	2, 4, 6	DTwPc/IPV/PRP-T1, DTwPc/IPV + PRP-T1	0.75	1.02	0.66	0.78	0.9	0.79			
Chile[73]	2, 4, 6	DTwPu/PRP-T1, DTwPu + PRP-T1	0.70	1.32†	0.78	1.10	0.86	1.41			
USA[76]	2, 4, 6	DTwPu/PRP-T1, DTwPu + PRP-T1	0.88	1.09	0.94	1.01	1.00				
USA[77]	2, 4, 6	DTwPu/PRP-T1, DTwPu + PRP-T1	1.60	1.14	0.96	1.44	0.69		1.55	1.38	0.79
UK[78]	2, 3, 4	DTwPe/PRP-T1, DTwPe + PRP-T1	0.75	1.01	1.83†	1.68	1.11	1.12			
Chile[79]	2, 4, 6	DTwP/PRP-T, DTwP				1.12	0.94	0.96			
Israel[80]	2, 4, 6	DTwPf/IPV/PRP-T1, DTwPf/IPV	0.96	0.86	0.65†			0.70†	1.01	0.78	1.29
The Gambia[81]	2, 3, 4	DTwPf/PRP-T1, DTwPf + PRP-T1	0.73	1.11	1.16	0.91	0.77	§			
UK[82]	2, 3, 4	DTwPf/PRP-T1, DTwPf + PRP-T1‖	0.25†	0.78							
Belgium[70]	3, 4, 5	DTwPf/PRP-T1 (DCS), DTwPf + PRP-T1	0.61†	1.08	0.79			0.70			
Belgium[70]	3, 4, 5	DTwPf/PRP-T1, DTwPf + PRP-T1	0.37†	0.84	0.99			1.07			
Chile[70]	3, 4, 5, 6	DTwPf/PRP-T1 (DCS), DTwPf + PRP-T1	0.79†	0.89	1.01			0.99			
Chile[70]	3, 4, 5, 6	DTwPf/PRP-T1, DTwPf + PRP-T1	0.64		0.97			1.01			
France[83]	2, 3, 4	DTwPf/IPV/PRP-T1, DTwPf/IPV + PRP-T1	1.41†	0.48	0.15†			1.14	1.03	0.95	0.82
France[83]	2, 3, 4	DTwPf/IPV/PRP-T1 (DCS), DTwPf/IPV + PRP-T1	0.62	0.33	0.11†			0.74†	0.79	0.88	0.72
Brazil[84]	2, 4, 6	DTwPf/PRP-T1, DTwPf + PRP-T1	0.79			0.83					
Brazil[84]	2, 4, 6	DTwPf/IPV/PRP-T1, DTwPf/IPV + PRP-T1				0.75					
USA[85]	2, 4, 6	DTwPu/PRP (unconjugated), DTwPu						1.41			
Finland[86]	3, 4, 6	DTwP/PRP-D, DTwP		1.17	0.99						
The Gambia[87]	2, 3, 4	DTwP/PRP-OMP, DTwP + PRP-OMP	1.03	.80	.71			0.88			
USA[88,89]	2, 4, 6	DTwPw/PRP-HbOC, DTwPw + PRP-HbOC	1.51†	1.78†	1.82†			2.22†			
USA[90]	2, 4, 6	DTwPw/PRP-HbOC, DTwPw + PRP-HbOC	¶	¶	¶			¶			
UK[78]	2, 3, 4	DTwPe/PRP-HbOC, DTwPe + HbOC	1.30	0.93	1.48†	1.06	1.39	1.10			
UK[91]	2, 3, 4	DTwPe/PRP-T, DTwPe + PRP-T2	0.51†	1.73†	0.75	1.20	0.97	0.78			
Spain[92]	2, 3, 4	DTwPg/PRP-HbOC, DTwPg + PRP-HbOC	1.86	1.26	1.16	0.88	**				

* A ratio less than 1 indicates that mean antibody levels were lower with the combined vaccine than with separate injections; a ratio higher than 1, that levels were higher with combined than separate injections. A blank cell indicates that the comparison was not possible or is not available.

† Difference significant at $P \leq 0.05$.

‡ P value not available.

§ Agglutinin titers were not determined. However, the rate of seroconversion (AGG ≥ 320) was significantly lower ($P < 0.05$) in the combined group (79% vs. 92%). Combined vaccine group was compared to UK historical controls, who received the same PRP-T on the same schedule, but a different DTwP.

¶ Serologic assays were performed only for the DTwP/PRP-HbOC group (PRP, 8.20 μg/mL; D, 0.92 IU/mL; T, 7.52 U/mL; AGG, 110.1/dilution), and were said to be "comparable to values reported . . . in other series."

** Pertactin, 0.56.

AGG, pertussis agglutinins; D, diphtheria toxin; DCS, dual-chamber syringe; DTwP, diphtheria and tetanus toxoids and whole-cell pertussis vaccine; DTwPb, DTwP produced by GlaxoSmithKline (Belgium); DTwPc, DTwP produced by Connaught Laboratories (Canada); DTwPe, DTwP produced by Wellcome Laboratories (England); DTwPf, DTwP produced by Aventis Pasteur (France); DTwPg, DTwP produced by Chiron Vaccines, Marburg, Germany; DTwPu, DTwP produced by Connaught Laboratories (USA); DTwPw, DTwP produced by Wyeth Laboratories (USA); EU, ELISA units; FHA, filamentous hemagglutinin; IPV, inactivated poliovirus vaccine; PRP, polyribosylribitol phosphate; PRP-D, PRP–diphtheria toxoid conjugate vaccine; PRP-HbOC, PRP–diphtheria CRM$_{197}$ protein conjugate vaccine; PRP-OMP, PRP–meningococcal outer membrane protein conjugate vaccine; PRP-T$_1$ (ActHIB; Aventis Pasteur) and PRP-T$_2$ (Hiberix; GlaxoSmithKline), PRP–tetanus toxoid protein conjugate vaccine (lyophilized and reconstituted at time of use with diluent or DTwP, unless indicated as DCS); PT, pertussis toxin; T, tetanus toxin.

TABLE 29–4 ■ Studies Comparing Combined or Simultaneous Administration of Vaccines Containing GSK DTwP and Hepatitis B Components, With or Without Hib Components, for Primary Immunization of Infants

Place	Ages (Mo)	Vaccines	Ratio of Antibody Levels with Combined Vaccine to Levels with Separate Vaccines*				
			PRP	D	T	WBP	HBs
Spain[116]	3, 5, 7	DTwP/HepB, DTwP		0.79	0.70	0.79	
USA[106]	2, 4, 6	DTwP/HepB/PRP-T, DTwP/HepB+PRP-T[†]		1.63[‡]	1.08[‡]	1.47[‡]	2.02
Chile[112,117]	2, 4, 6	DTwP/HepB/PRP-T, DTwP/HepB+PRP-T[§]	0.70	0.95	0.98	0.86	0.94
Myanmar[109]	1.5, 3, 5	DTwP/HepB/PRP-T, DTwP/HepB+PRP-T[§]	1.07	0.74[‡]	2.23[‡]	0.95	1.00[‖]

*A ratio less than 1 indicates that mean antibody levels were lower with the combined vaccine than with separate injections; a ratio higher than 1, that levels were higher with combined than separate injections. A blank cell indicates that the comparison was not possible or is not available.
[†]OmniHIB, SmithKline Beecham (produced by Pasteur Mérieux Connaught and identical to ActHIB).
[‡]Difference significant at $P \leq 0.05$.
[§]Hiberix, GlaxoSmithKline.
[‖]Including only those subjects seronegative at birth.
D, diphtheria toxin; DTwP, diphtheria and tetanus toxoids and whole-cell pertussis vaccine; HBs, hepatitis B surface antigen; HepB, hepatitis B vaccine (SmithKline Beecham); PRP, polyribosylribitol phosphate; PRP-T, PRP–tetanus toxoid protein conjugate vaccine; T, tetanus toxin; WBP, whole Bordetella pertussis (a mixture of serotypes 1, 2, and 3 used in a solid-phase immunoassay).

resulted in Hib-containing pentavalent and hexavalent (DTaP/IPV/Hib/HepB) combinations becoming accepted in Europe and some other jurisdictions despite reduced Hib responses. In contrast, attention in North America has focused on DTaP/IPV/HepB and on DTaP/Hib-based combinations built on the Canadian five-component DTaP, which appears not to interfere materially with Hib responses.

The DTaP-based combinations most widely available worldwide are produced by AvP and GSK. AvP markets products based on the French DTaP2 (Pentavac, Hexavac, etc.) in Europe and elsewhere, and products based on the

Canadian DTaP5 (Quadracel, Pentacel, Pediacel, etc.) in the Western Hemisphere, Asia, and elsewhere. GSK markets the full range of Infanrix (DTaP3)-based combinations worldwide, including a hexavalent and various pentavalent and quadrivalent combinations. Statens Seruminstitut (SSI) markets in Europe DTaP1/IPV and DTaP1/IPV/Hib combinations based on the same monocomponent aP used in Certiva, the U.S. DTaP1. Baxter is developing similar products for the United States, and a DTaP2/Hib combination (TriHIBit) based on the U.S./Japanese DTaP2 is marketed in the United States. No combinations based on the

TABLE 29–5 ■ Studies Evaluating Combined or Simultaneous Administration of DTaP and IPV Vaccines

Place	Ages (Mo)	Vaccines[†]	PRP Antibody Levels (µg/mL)	
			% >1.0	GMC
Canada[126]	17–19	DTaP5/IPV, DTaP5 + IPV (MRC-5 cell line)		
Canada[126]	17–19	DTaP5/IPV, DTaP5 + IPV (Vero cell line)		
France[127]	3, 4, 5	DTaP2/IPV, DTwP/IPV		
Chile[128,129]	3, 5, 7[§]	DTaP2/IPV+PRP-T$_1$, DTaP2+IPV+PRP-T$_1$	98, 95	19.0, 21.7
Chile[128,129]	2, 4, 6	DTaP2/IPV+PRP-T$_1$, DTaP2+IPV+PRP-T$_1$	97, 96	7.46, 14.1
Finland[130]	(2), 4, 6	DTaP3/PRP-T$_2$/IPV, DTaP3/PRP-T$_2$ + IPV	48, 19[‡]	0.56, 0.38

*A ratio less than 1 indicates that mean antibody levels were lower with the combined vaccine than with separate injections; a ratio higher than 1, that levels were higher with combined than separate injections. A blank cell indicates that the comparison was not possible or is not available.
[†]aP2, French two-component aP (e.g., Triavax, or similar); aP3, Infanrix; aP5, Tripacel (see Chapter 21 for details of vaccines). PRP-T$_1$, ActHIB (Aventis Pasteur); PRP-T$_2$, Hiberix (GlaxoSmithKline).
[‡]Difference significant at $P \leq 0.05$.
[§]DTaP and IPV were given at 2, 4, and 6 months; PRP-T was given at 3, 5, and 7 months. Polio antibody levels estimated from figures

U.S./Japanese DTaP4 (Acel-IMUNE; Wyeth) or the Italian DTaP3 (Triacelluvax; Chiron) are available.

Adding IPV to DTaP or to DTaP/Hib

Overview

Combining IPV with DTaP or with DTaP/Hib has no consistent effect on antibody responses to the DTaP and IPV components, with few differences achieving statistical significance. Ongoing surveillance in Sweden has shown continued reductions in pertussis incidence among the vaccinated population, concomitant with the transition from DTaP to DTaP/IPV and DTaP/IPV/Hib.[124,125]

The Studies

Although Tables 29–5 through 29–9 attempt to separate data regarding DTaP/IPV, DTaP/Hib, DTaP/HepB, DTaP/HepB/HIB, and DTaP/IPV/Hib combinations, in fact most of the relevant studies have evaluated several of these combinations simultaneously. Within the few that have looked only at DTaP/IPV (Table 29–5), pertussis responses tend to be maintained or enhanced with the combination.[126–130] Poliovirus responses appear to vary by serotype, with antibodies to types 1 and 2 somewhat enhanced and type 3 somewhat reduced; few of these variations achieved statistical significance. French infants immunized at 3, 4, and 5 months of age had better responses to DTaP2/IPV than to DTwP/IPV.[127] A comparison of two different IPVs, given at 17 to 19 months separately or combined with the Canadian DTaP5, showed that the combined vaccines generally produced higher poliovirus and pertussis antibody levels than did vaccination with DTaP5 plus separate IPV or OPV (Table 29–5).[126]

A number of key issues were illustrated by one of the first published studies comparing combined versus separate administration of DTaP, IPV, and Hib. Finnish infants were immunized at 2 months with DTaP3 and then at 4 and 6 months with DTaP3, IPV, and PRP-T given either all separately, all combined, with the DTaP3 and IPV combined, or with the DTaP3 and PRP-T combined.[130] As shown in Table 29–6, PRP antibody responses were markedly reduced among infants receiving PRP-T in combination (whether or not IPV was included in the combination), but not if the PRP-T were given separately (whether or not the IPV was given separately). Pertussis responses varied little (see Table 29–5); poliovirus responses were reduced with the combination. The extent to which any of these results was due to the nontraditional schedule, which included only two Hib doses, is unclear. In a follow-up study, available participants were given a booster with DTaP3 and PRP-T at 24 months of age. Vaccines were given separately to those who had been primed with separate vaccines; those who had been primed with combination vaccines were randomized to be given a booster with separate or combined vaccines.[131] Despite the large difference in PRP antibody levels at 7 months of age, there was little difference in levels prior to the booster dose at 24 months of age. After receiving a booster dose, all groups showed strong responses, which were about twice as high among those primed with separate vaccines. The groups primed with combined vaccine had roughly equal responses to the booster dose, whether they were given combined or separate vaccines as booster doses.

In addition to the DTaP/IPV combinations presented in Table 29–5, the aP component of Baxter's Certiva (a DTaP1 whose pertussis component consists solely of pertussis toxin; see Chapter 21) has been combined with DT and IPV from SSI as DiTeKiPol.[132–134] A comparison of this DTaP1/IPV at 3, 5, and 12 months of age versus DT/IPV at 5, 6, and 15 months plus wP at 5 and 9 weeks and 10 months found that the combination achieved protective antibody levels for diphtheria, tetanus, and the polio serotypes as well as significantly better pertussis responses[134]; strong cell-mediated immunity was demonstrated for the pertussis component.[133]

							Poliovirus Serotypes		
PRP	D	T	PT	FHA	PRN	FIM	1	2	3
	1.28	0.98	1.23	0.96	2.05‡	1.61	1.17	1.61‡	0.80
	0.90	1.01	1.08	0.96	1.41‡	1.14	1.17	1.30	0.74
	2.47‡	1.14‡					1.79‡	1.24	1.43
0.88	0.72	0.74‡				1.6‡	0.5‡	0.4§	
0.53‡			0.89	0.87			1.1	1.2	1.0
1.47	1.09	1.44	1.02	1.09	1.13		0.34‡	0.49	0.61

*Ratio of Antibody Levels with Combined Vaccine to Levels with Separate Vaccines

‖Only DTaP was given at 2 months, without IPV or PRP-T.

Note: In those studies incorporating Hib, the Hib administration was not different between study groups (i.e., Hib either was given separately to all subjects or was part of the combination for all subjects). aP, acellular pertussis vaccine; D, diphtheria toxin; DTaP, diphtheria and tetanus toxoids and acellular pertussis vaccine; DTwP, diphtheria and tetanus toxoids and whole-cell pertussis vaccine; FHA, filamentous hemagglutinin; FIM, fimbrae; GMC, geometric mean concentration of antibody; Hib, *Haemophilus influenzae* type b; IPV, inactivated poliovirus vaccine; PRN, pertactin; PRP, polyribosylribitol phosphate; PRP-T, PRP-tetanus toxoid protein conjugate vaccine; PT, pertussis toxin; T, tetanus toxin.

TABLE 29–6 ■ Antibody to PRP Among 120 Infants Given DTAP at 2 Months, Then DTAP, IPV, and Conjugate Hib Vaccine, Separately or Together, at 4 and 6 Months

	Primary Series GMC (μg/ml)	
Vaccines Given at 4 and 6 Months	6 Mo (No.)	7 Mo (No.)
DTaP3, IPV, and PRP-T$_2$, all separate	0.19 (30)	3.94 (30)
DTaP3 and IPV mixed, PRP-T$_2$ separate	0.18 (28)	3.10 (30)
DTaP3 and PRP-T$_2$ mixed, IPV separate	0.10 (29)	0.38 (30)
DTaP3, IPV, and PRP-T$_2$ all mixed	0.09 (27)	0.56 (30)

DTaP3, diphtheria and tetanus toxoids and acellular pertussis vaccine (*Infanrix*; GlaxoSmithKline); GMC, geometric mean concentration of antibody; Hib, *Haemophilus influenzae* type b; IPV, inactivated poliovirus vaccine; No., number of subjects providing serum samples for assay; PRP, polyribosyl-ribitol phosphate; PRP-T$_2$, PRP–tetanus toxoid protein conjugate vaccine (*Hiberix*, GlaxoSmithKline).
Data from Eskola et al.[130,131]

Adverse reactions were similar for the DTaP1/IPV and DT/IPV groups. This combination was used routinely in Denmark from 1997 through mid-2002 and is also licensed in Finland, Sweden, Germany, and Austria.

An adult-formulation tetanus and diphtheria toxoids and acellular pertussis (Tdap5)/IPV combination (Repevax; AvP) has been licensed in Europe for use as a booster among persons aged 5 years and over. The combination produced generally lower antibody responses in adults than adolescents; generally lower responses than separately administered TD and aP; and generally higher responses than separately administered IPV. Nonetheless, tetanus, diphtheria, and IPV responses exceeded protective levels and aP responses exceeded those typically seen in infants following the primary series; reaction rates did not differ between separate and combined administration.[135] SSI is also develop-ing a Tdap1/IPV combination vaccine, which has been evaluated in a clinical trial in Göteborg, Sweden and is anticipated to be implemented in Denmark in July 2004 for use as a booster at 5 years of age.

Although it is generally true that vaccines given simultaneously at separate injection sites do not interfere with each other, such interactions are occasionally noted. Among subjects given DTaP2/PRP-T (TriHIBit) along with IPV, sequential IPV-IPV-OPV, or OPV at 2, 4, and 6 months, Rennels et al. found that both the GMTs (1.2, 1.3, and 3.1 μg/mL, respectively) and the proportions achieving PRP antibody responses of 1.0 μg/mL or greater (54%, 55%, and 79%, respectively) were reduced by coadministration of IPV.[136] In contrast, Daum et al. found that PRP antibody responses to the same DTaP2/PRP-T combination did not significantly differ among groups coadminis-

TABLE 29–7 ■ Studies Evaluating Combined or Simultaneous Administration of DTaP3 and HepB Vaccines

Place	Ages (Mo)	Vaccines[†]	Comment
Turkey[138]	3, 4, 5	DTaP3/HepB	Group 1
	3, 4, 5	DTaP3 + HepB	Group 2
	3, 4, 5	DTaP3	Group 3
Lithuania[139]	3, 4.5, 6	DTaP3/HepB	Mixed in vial
	3, 4.5, 6	DTaP3/HepB	Mixed at time of injection
	3, 4.5, 6	DTaP3 + HepB	
Italy[140]	2, 4, 6	DTaP3/HepB	Group 1
	3, 5	DTaP3/HepB	Group 2, after first 2 injections
	3, 5, 11	DTaP3/HepB	Group 2, after third injection
USA[141]	2, 4, 6	DTaP3/HepB	
	2, 4, 6	DTaP3 + HepB	HepB given at birth, 1, and 6 mo
Not stated[142]	2, 4, 6	DTaP3/HepB	
	2, 4, 6	DTaP3	
	2, 4, 6	HepB	
USA[143]	2, 4, 6	DTaP3/HepB	Group C
	2, 4, 6	DTaP3 + HepB	Group D

*Units: HB, mIU/mL; pertussis components, EU; diphtheria and tetanus, IU. A blank cell indicates that data are not available.
[†]All vaccines produced by GlaxoSmithKline.
‡ Difference significant at *P* ≤0.05.
D, diphtheria; DTaP3, GSK diphtheria and tetanus toxoids and acellular pertussis vaccine; EU, ELISA units; FHA, filamentous hemagglutinin; HB, hepatitis B; HepB, hepatitis B vaccine; PRN, pertactin; PT, pertussis toxin; T, tetanus toxin.

tered OPV or IPV at 2 and 4 months (GMTs, 4.0 vs. 3.4 µg/mL; proportions ≥1.0 µg/mL, 77% vs. 74%).[137] The difference in results of these two studies remains unexplained.

Adding HepB to DTaP or to DTaP/IPV

Overview

Combining HepB with DTaP or with DTaP/IPV generally produces somewhat higher DTap and polio antibody responses than are achieved with the same components given separately on the same schedule. However, the HepB responses following the combinations typically are lower than seen with monovalent HepB, not because of interference, but because administration schedules for combinations typically are more closely spaced than are schedules for monovalent HepB. The magnitude of HepB antibody responses is directly correlated with the time between doses. Accordingly, HepB responses are lower if the HepB is administered (whether separately or in a combination) at, for example, 2, 4, and 6 months or 3, 4, and 5 months rather than at, for example, 0, 1, and 6 months or 3, 5, and 11 months.

The Studies

GSK has obtained licensure throughout Europe and in many other countries of a DTaP3/HepB combination vaccine. Table 29–7 summarizes studies comparing the performance of this vaccine with the separately administered components and also comparing various administration schedules.[138–143] The combination vaccine retains the immunogenicity profile of the separate components and stimulates antibody concentrations associated with protection with a variety of schedules.

A comparison of combined vaccine at ages 2, 4, and 6 months versus a currently recommended schedule in the United States—HepB at birth and 1 and 6 months of age and DTaP3 at 2, 4, and 6 months of age—found significantly higher antibody responses for combined vaccine for every component except HepB, which was significantly lower.[141] However, the mean HepB antibody with combined vaccine was nonetheless high (1280 mIU/mL), and 98% of subjects had levels greater than 10 mIU/mL, the level considered protective.

Table 29–7 reveals a clear-cut correlation between dosing interval and HepB response of the combination. Progressively compressing the schedule from 2-4-6 through 3-4.5-6 to 3-4-5 months leads to progressively reduced HepB responses, whether given separately or in combination; in each case, results are somewhat higher with the combination. An Italian study[140] that evaluated a 3-5-11 schedule recorded very high HepB responses following the third dose, again suggesting that increasing the dosing interval is associated with an enhanced immune response.

GSK's DTaP3/IPV/HepB combination vaccine (Infanrix Penta; PEDIARIX) has been evaluated in a variety of schedules and compared with its components given separately, with DTwP-based combinations, and as a control vaccine in studies of the GSK hexavalent combination (see below).

In a randomized U.S. study, the response rates following DTaP3/HepB/IPV vaccine at 2, 4, and 6 months of age were shown to be noninferior (indeed, often superior) to U.S.-licensed DTaP3, HepB, OPV, and IPV vaccines administered separately on the same schedule.[143] In a study in Moldova, 320 eligible infants given a birth dose of HepB were randomized to receive DTaP3/HepB/IPV + Hib or DTwP/IPV/Hib +

Mean Antibody Levels 1 Month After Last Injection[*]					
HB	D	T	PT	FHA	PRN
343	2.05	4.35	56	89	129
275	1.88	4.38	52	114	159
6	1.59	4.03	47	89	125
667	1.40	2.21	47.9	184	170
518	1.06	2.00	46.7	131	124
438	1.10	1.76	46.7	158	148
949	0.19		56.1	153	240
572	0.11		31.8	86	113
5554	1.71		65.3	232	372
1280[‡]	1.93	3.82	72.3	459	195
4620[‡]	1.00	2.11	52.2	334	138
929	1.96	3.08	66.5	285	233
	1.88	2.22	60.0	220	170
1895					
919	1.2	3.1	72.8[‡]	234[‡]	155
805	0.8	2.3	47.5[‡]	153[‡]	109

TABLE 29–8 ■ Studies Evaluating Combined or Simultaneous Administration of DTaP and Hib Vaccines

Place	Ages (Mo)	Vaccines†
USA[150]	18	DTaP2u/PRP-D, DTaP2 + PRP-D
USA[151]	15–20	DTaP2u/PRP-T$_1$, DTaP2 + PRP-T$_1$
USA[152]	15–21	DTaP4/HbOC, DTaP4 + HbOC
USA[153]	12–15	DTaP4/HbOC, DTaP4 + HbOC
USA[153]	15–18	DTaP4/HbOC, DTaP4 + HbOC
Germany[154]	2, 3, 4	DTaP2u/PRP-D, DTaP2 + PRP-D
Germany[155]	2, 3, 4	DTaP2u/PRP-T$_1$, DTaP2 + PRP-T$_1$
Belgium[156]	3, 4, 5	DTaP2u/PRP-T$_1$, DTaP2 + PRP-T$_1$
Turkey[156]	3, 4, 5	DTaP2u/PRP-T$_1$, DTaP2 + PRP-T$_1$
USA[157]	2, 4, 6	DTaP2u/PRP-T$_1$, DTaP2 + PRP-T$_1$
USA[136]	2, 4, 6	DTaP2u/PRP-T$_1$ + OPV, DTaP2 + PRP-T$_1$ + OPV
Germany[158,159]	3, 4, 5	DTaP3/PRP-T$_2$, DTaP3 + PRP-T$_2$
Germany[158,159]	3, 4, 5	DTaP3/PRP-T$_1$, DTaP3 + PRP-T$_1$
USA[160]	2, 4, 6	DTaP4/HbOC, DTaP4 + HbOC
Taiwan[161]	2, 4, 6	DTaP5/PRP-T$_1$, DTaP5 + PRP-T$_1$

*A ratio less than 1 indicates that mean antibody levels were lower with the combined vaccine than with separate injections; a ratio higher than 1, that levels were higher with combined than separate injections. A blank cell indicates that the comparison was not possible or is not available.

†aP2, French two-component aP (e.g., *Triavax* or similar); aP2u, *Tripedia*; aP3, *Infanrix*; aP4, *ACEL-IMUNE* or similar Takeda-type aP vaccine; aP5, *Tripacel* or equivalent five-component aP vaccine (see Chapter 21 for details of vaccines). PRP-T$_1$, *ActHiB* (Aventis Pasteur); PRP-T$_2$, *Hiberix* (GlaxoSmithKline).

HepB at 6, 10, and 14 weeks of age.[99] After the primary vaccination course, both groups showed equivalently high seroprotection rates and mean antibody levels. The HepB seroprotection rate in the DTaP3/HepB/IPV + Hib group was greater than 98.6% immediately before the third dose (14 weeks of age), compared to 88.7% in the DTwP/IPV/Hib + HepB group.

Several studies have evaluated coadministration of DTaP3/IPV/HepB with various Hib vaccines (PRP-OMP, PRP-HbOC, and two PRP-Ts [GSK and AvP]) and found no interference.[143,144] Five different booster options for children primed with the pentavalent vaccine have been investigated,[145,146] with all regimens resulting in high rates of seroprotection or seropositivity and marked increases in GMTs or concentrations.

Safety data, based on over 20,000 doses, showed the low rates of minor local reactions typical of aP-based vaccines, with somewhat lower rates among combination recipients for most reactions.[147] A rectal temperature of 38°C (100.4°F) or greater was more common in subjects who received DTaP3/HepB/IPV and Hib concomitantly than in those who received DTaP3 and Hib concomitantly, perhaps because of the additional antigens delivered in the combination. The incidence of temperature greater than 39.5°C (103.1°F), although higher with the combination, nonetheless was low in both the DTaP3/HepB/IPV + Hib vaccine group (1.4%) and the control group (0.8%). A similar comparative pattern of adverse reactions was found in the booster phase of the same study.[148]

In conjunction with the licensure of PEDIARIX in the United States, a further study is being conducted to compare PEDIARIX versus separately administered DTaP3, HepB, and IPV; both groups also receive conjugate pneumococcal and Hib vaccines. By virtue of administering IPV to the control group, rather than OPV as in the preceding studies, this new study provides a more appropriate comparison of the DTaP3/HepB/IPV combination versus its separate components. Results are presented in the PEDIARIX package insert[149] for the percentage of infants, within 4 days of dose 1 at 2 months of age, who had fever of at least: 38°C (100.4°F); 38.5°C (101.3°F); 39°C (102.2°F); and 39.5°C (103.1°F). For each of these comparisons, fever was experienced by a higher proportion of the PEDIARIX group than the separate-vaccine group. The study also collected data on unplanned visits to seek medical care following immunization; medical attention was sought for fever within 4 days following vaccination by 1.2% of PEDIARIX recipients versus no recipients of the separate vaccines.

Adding Hib to DTaP or to DTaP/IPV

Overview

Numerous studies[94,101,128,129,136,150–189] have evaluated various DTaP/Hib and DTaP/IPV/Hib combinations and have produced remarkably consistent results. All combinations are highly immunogenic when used to boost previously primed children. When used for primary immunization, responses to the components other than Hib have been generally similar to those obtained with separate administration. The combi-

PRP Antibody Levels (µg/mL)		Ratio of Antibody Levels with Combined Vaccine to Levels with Separate Vaccines*						
%>1.0	GMC	PRP	D	T	PT	FHA	PRN	FIM
53, 76								
100, 100								
	26.9, 32.4	0.83						
98, 100	37.9, 48.4	0.78	0.71		0.55‡	0.93	0.96	1.00
98, 96	50.2, 43.3	1.16	0.94		0.79	1.32	1.04	1.00
	0.58, 0.44	1.34						
91, 99	2.83, 4.3	0.66‡						
	1.78, 6.19	0.29‡						
	5.02, 11.7	0.43‡						
85, 100‡	4.29, 7.0	0.61‡	1.67‡	0.79‡	1.00	1.29‡		
	3.17, 4.43	0.72	0.80	1.45	0.97	0.86		
72, 88	2.02, 7.20	0.28‡	0.92	0.85‡	0.89‡	0.77‡	0.81‡	
N/A, 88	2.75, 5.44	0.51‡						
55, 94‡	1.15, 16.4	0.07‡						
95, 99	11.8, 13.0	0.91			1.25	1.00	1.31	1.30

‡Difference significant at P ≤0.05.

aP, acellular pertussis vaccine; D, diphtheria toxin; DTaP, diphtheria and tetanus toxoids and acellular pertussis vaccine; FHA, filamentous hemagglutinin; FIM, fimbrae; GMC, geometric mean concentration of antibody; HbOC, PRP–diphtheria CRM$_{197}$ protein conjugate vaccine; OPV, oral poliovirus vaccine; PRN, pertactin; PRP, polyribosylribitol phosphate; PRP-D, PRP–diphtheria toxoid conjugate vaccine; PRP-T, PRP–tetanus toxoid protein conjugate vaccine; PT, pertussis toxin; T, tetanus toxin.

nation vaccines (other than those containing the weak immunogen PRP-D) also stimulate good Hib responses, with GMTs typically in the range of 2 to 5 µg/mL, but these responses almost always are substantially lower than the high responses obtained with PRP-T or HbOC when given separately.[194–196] The clinical relevance of this reduction in Hib immunogenicity, which has impeded licensure of these combinations in some jurisdictions, particularly including the United States, is discussed in detail below.

Adverse events following primary and booster immunization generally are similar to those seen with the separate vaccines; a modest increase in rates of low-grade fever or minor local reactions is not uncommon and is offset by the absence of local reactions at sites spared injection because a combination was used.

The Studies

A combination consisting of a Biken-type DTaP2 plus PRP-D (see Chapter 14) was used as a booster dose in toddlers primed with DTwP. Pertussis antibody responses were comparable after combined or separate vaccines. PRP antibody responses were low, as expected with PRP-D, but were materially lower in the combined vaccine group.[150] However, when used to immunize infants at 2, 3, and 4 months of age, the combined vaccine produced somewhat better Hib responses than did PRP-D given separately.[154]

A DTaP4/Hib combination composed of Acel-IMUNE and PRP-HbOC was evaluated first as a booster for toddlers primed with HbOC plus DTwP or DTaP4 and then as a three-dose primary series.[152,153,160,174] Adverse reactions were mild, although somewhat more common after boosting with the combined product.[152] Antibody responses after booster immunization at 12 to 21 months of age did not differ significantly between the combined and separate vaccines (Table 29–8).[152,153] In contrast, there was a markedly reduced antibody response to Hib after primary immunization with the combined product.[160]

TriHIBit, the combination of Tripedia and PRP-T (ActHIB), is licensed in the United States for use as a booster in children 15 to 18 months of age, in whom it produces Hib antibody levels comparable to those seen with the separate vaccines.[151] When used for primary immunization of infants, TriHIBit produced responses to the DTaP components that equaled or exceeded those of Tripedia; mean PRP antibody levels were significantly lower with the combined vaccine (4.3 µg/mL) than with the separate vaccines (7.0 µg/mL).[155,157]

Another study showed that the magnitude of reduction in PRP antibody associated with giving DTaP2 and PRP-T in combination rather than separately in the primary series depended on the number of times the vaccines were administered in combination, and that administration of separate vaccines for the third dose of the primary series could not overcome the impaired immune response associated with prior use of the interfering combination. Infants were given either TriHIBit at 2, 4, and 6 months; the combination at 2 and 4 months but separate vaccines at 6 months; or the combination at 2 months but separate vaccines at 4 and 6 months. GMTs at 7 months were 2.7, 3.3, and 5.25 µg/mL, respectively; proportions achieving 1.0 µg/mL were 75%, 86%, and 92%, respectively.[177]

DTaP2/Hib or DTaP2/IPV/Hib vaccines produced by AvP using their French two-component aP vaccine (Triavax; see Chapter 21) have been evaluated in many populations. Combination with ActHIB has been evaluated in British,[176] Belgian,[156] and Turkish[156] infants, among others (see Table 29–8). The British infants developed low levels of antibody to PRP (mean, 0.48 µg/mL) after primary immunization at 2, 3, and 4 months of age,[163] but they developed high levels (mean, 36.8 µg/mL) after a booster dose of PRP-T at 13 months of age.[163] Although the Belgian and Turkish infants, immunized at 3, 4, and 5 months of age, had markedly better mean PRP antibody levels than the British infants after primary immunization with combined vaccine, their responses were substantially higher with separate vaccines.[156]

Lagos and colleagues compared DTaP2/IPV, DTaP2 + IPV, and DTaP2 + OPV given at 2, 4, and 6 months of age, all groups receiving PRP-T at 3, 5, and 7 months of age, with DTaP2/IPV/PRP-T and DTaP2/IPV + PRP-T given at 2, 4, and 6 months of age (Tables 29–5 and 29–9).[128,129] All groups had poliovirus seroconversion rates of 99% or 100%, with higher antibody levels among the groups receiving IPV in combination than in the groups receiving separate IPV or OPV. Responses to pertussis toxin, filamentous hemagglutinin, and PRP were substantial in all groups but were superior in those receiving separate injections. Whether PRP-T was given combined or separately, PRP antibody levels were markedly higher in study subjects receiving PRP-T at 3, 5, and 7 months of age than in those receiving all antigens at 2, 4, and 6 months of age, despite the fact that levels were determined at 7 months of age (and thus did not reflect the effect of the third injection in the former groups). It is not known whether this result was caused by age, carrier priming, or immunologic interference. When a booster dose of DTaP2/PRP-T was given at 12 months, all groups had strong PRP antibody responses (mean levels, 48.6 to 95.2 µg/mL), but significantly higher antibody levels were seen in the groups primed at 3, 5, and 7 months of age.[128,129]

Other studies also suggest that immunization at an earlier age might worsen the problem of reduced antibody responses to Hib when given in combination with DTaP. In a French study in which PRP-T was administered at 2, 3, and 4 months of age, combined with or separately from DTaP2/IPV, PRP antibody levels were 1.95 µg/mL with the combined vaccine and 5.18 µg/mL with separate vaccines (see Table 29–9).[166,167] Another French study compared administration of DTaP2/IPV/PRP-T at ages 2, 3, and 4 months or 2, 4, and 6 months and found higher mean antibody levels for all antigens in the group immunized later.[167,178,179] Responses to PRP differed significantly, both for the proportions exceeding 1 µg/mL (70% vs. 89%) and for mean antibody levels (1.7 vs. 4.7 µg/mL).[167] However, when given a booster at 15 months of age, both groups responded equally well to all antigens (PRP antibody levels were 36.8 and 31.8 µg/mL for 2-3-4 and 2-4-6, respectively).[167,179] Similar results have been obtained among Swedish children immunized at ages 3, 5, and 12 months or 2, 4, 6, and 13 months. Not surprisingly, antibody levels were higher after primary immunization with the 2-4-6 schedule than the 3-5 schedule, although there was no significant difference in the proportion that achieved defined protective levels or had fourfold rises in antibody titer.[180]

Following booster immunization at 12 or 13 months of age, antibody levels were virtually identical in the two groups.

Premature birth also has been shown to accentuate the reduction in antibody responses to Hib when given in combination with DTaP. A study comparing antibody responses to DTaP3/PRP-T of infants born at less than 32 weeks' gestation and full-term infants found markedly reduced Hib GMTs (0.27 vs. 0.81 µg/mL) and proportions achieving 1 µg/mL (21 vs. 46%) among the premature infants.[181]

Schmitt and colleagues used Infanrix (GSK) to reconstitute two similar PRP-T vaccines, ActHIB (AvP) and Hiberix (GSK). PRP antibody levels and seroconversion rates with the two Hib vaccines were reasonably comparable, and were higher with separate than combined vaccine.[158,159] Both the combined and separate vaccines produced high levels of antibody to the DTaP3 components; all antibody levels were slightly lower with the combined vaccine.[158,159] Available subjects were given a booster at 18 to 19 months of age with Hiberix, ActHIB, or Hiberix vaccine mixed with Infanrix. PRP antibody levels after the booster dose were high: 24 to 40 µg/mL for those boosted with the Infanrix/Hiberix combination and 85 to 137 µg/mL for those primed and boosted with the separately administered Hib vaccines.[159] Assessment of T-lymphocyte proliferative responses and cytokine production after priming and before and after the booster dose found no differences between combined and separate vaccines.[182,183]

Combined or separate administration of GSK's DTaP3/IPV and AvP's PRP-T was evaluated among children ages 15 to 24 months; combining the PRP-T with the DTaP3/IPV did not materially alter antibody responses (see Table 29–9).[162] Dagan and colleagues compared DTaP3/IPV/PRP-T with DTwP/IPV/PRP-T (Pentacoq; AvP) given at 2, 4, 6, and 12 months of age and found strong antibody responses to all components after both the primary series and the booster dose.[185,186] Polio antibody levels after primary immunization and PRP antibody levels after the booster dose were significantly higher with the DTaP than the DTwP combination. Another study comparing GSK's DTaP3/IPV and PRP-T, given combined or separately at 2, 4, and 6 months of age, found good responses to all components in both groups.[186] Antibody levels were similar with combined vaccine or separate administration for diphtheria toxoid, the three pertussis antigens, and the three poliovirus types. Anti–tetanus toxoid titer was higher with the combined vaccine, whereas the mean PRP antibody response was reduced by half with the combined product. PRP antibody levels no longer differed between the two groups before and 1 month after the booster dose given at 18 months of age. Following the fourth dose, all children in both groups had antibody levels above 1 µg/mL; GMTs were 32.9 and 47.8 µg/ms for the combined and separate groups respectively. To further evaluate the question of priming by PRP-T given in combination with DTaP3, a study was conducted in Israel in which children vaccinated with DTaP3/IPV/Hib at 2, 4, and 6 months were boosted at 10 or 12 months with unconjugated PRP antigen.[187] The plain PRP elicited an increase in antibody titers within 7 to 10 days, achieving levels above those reported in several trials conducted in unprimed children vaccinated with the unconjugated vaccine at the same age. These findings demonstrate priming of the PRP response.

TABLE 29–9 ■ Studies Evaluating Administration of Pentavalent or Hexavalent DTaP-Based Combinations Versus Separate Administration of One or More Contained Components

Place	Ages (Mo)	Vaccines†	PRP Antibody Levels (IgG, µg/mL)		Ratio of Antibody Levels with Combined Vaccine to Levels with Separate Vaccines*								Poliovirus Serotypes		
			%>1.0	GMC	PRP	HB	D	T	PT	FHA	PRN	FIM	1	2	3
France[162]	15–24	DTaP3/IPV/PRP-T₁, DTaP3/IPV + PRP-T₁	100, 97	60.4, 60.0	1.01		1.19	0.84	1.15	1.11	1.03		0.89	0.74	1.05
Canada[163,164]	17–19	DTaP5/IPV/PRP-T₁,‡ DTaP5/IPV + PRP-T₁	99, 100	32.5, 26.9	1.21										
Sweden[165]	3, 5	DTaP1/IPV/PRP-T₁, DTaP1/IPV + PRP-T₁	27, 26	0.4, 0.6	0.67		0.57§	1.86§	1.04				0.80	0.92	0.75
Sweden[164]	3, 5, 12	DTaP1/IPV/PRP-T₁, DTaP1/IPV + PRP-T₁	92, 92	6.9, 11.3	0.61§		0.77§	156§	1.11				0.94	1.00	0.89
France[166,167]	2, 3, 4	DTaP2/IPV/PRP-T₁, DTaP2/IPV + PRP-T₁	71,88§	1.9, 5.2	0.36§		1.03	0.81	0.98	0.84			0.73	0.76	0.58
Chile[128,129]	2, 4, 6‖	DTaP2/IPV/PRP-T₁, DTaP2 + IPV+PRP-T₁	97, 98	7.5, 22	0.34§		0.42§	0.41§	0.73§	0.78			1.72§	1.88§	2.37§
France[168]	2, 4, 6	DTaP2/IPV/HepB/PRP-T₁, DTaP2/IPV/PRP-T₁ + HepB		2.1, 3.7	0.56§	0.44§	0.98	1.25§	0.74§	1.19§			1.37	1.60§	1.20
USA[143]	2, 4, 6	DTaP3/HepB/IPV + PRP-T₁, DTaP3/HepB + IPV + PRP-T₁	94, 98	6.2, 7.1	0.87	1.81	1.08	1.19	1.33§	0.51§	0.97		1.95§	1.56	4.0§
USA[143]	2, 4, 6	DTaP3/HepB/IPV + PRP-T₁, DTaP3 + HepB + OPV + PRP-T₁	94, 95	6.2, 7.8	0.79	2.06§	1.63§	1.61§	2.04§	0.78§	1.38		0.51§	0.41§	3.82§
Germany[169]	3, 4, 5	DTaP3/HepB/IPV/PRP-T₂, DTaP3/IPV/PRP-T₂ + HepB		2.2, 1.8	1.22	1.14	1.56	1.23	1.23	1.14	1.13		1.48	1.41	1.36
Germany[169]	3, 4, 5	DTaP3/HepB/IPV/PRP-T₂, DTaP3/HepB/IPV + PRP-T₂		2.2, 5.6	0.39§	0.83	1.00	1.23	0.95	1.00	0.93		1.19	1.22	1.00
Germany[169]	3, 4, 5	DTaP3/HepB/IPV + PRP-T₂, DTaP3/IPV/PRP-T₂ + HepB		5.6, 1.8	3.11§	1.38	1.56§	1.00	1.29§	1.14	1.21		1.24	1.16	1.37
USA[170]	2, 4, 6	DTaP3/HepB/IPV/PRP-T₂, DTaP3 + HepB + OPV + PRP-T₁	84, 92	2.65, 5.53	0.48§	1.33	1.40	1.33	1.60	0.92	1.25		0.41§	0.33§	4.19§

Continued

TABLE 29–9 ■ Studies Evaluating Administration of Pentavalent or Hexavalent DTaP-Based Combinations Versus Separate Administration of One or More Contained—cont'd

Place	Ages (Mo)	Vaccines†	PRP Antibody Levels (IgG, µg/mL)		Ratio of Antibody Levels with Combined Vaccine to Levels with Separate Vaccines*								Poliovirus Serotypes		
			%>1.0	GMC	PRP	HB	D	T	PT	FHA	PRN	FIM	1	2	3
Germany[171]	3, 4, 5	DTaP3/HepB/IPV/PRP-T₂, DTaP3/HepB/IPV + PRP-T₂	77, 89	2.62, 4.45	0.59§	0.75	0.94	0.78	0.91	0.98	0.95		0.82	0.97	0.75
France[178]	2, 3, 4	DTaP3/HepB/IPV/PRP-T₂, DTaP3/HepB/IPV + PRP-T₂	62, 63	1.5, 1.6	0.97	0.78	1.13	0.9	1.02	1.07	1.11		1.38	1.03	1.50
Slovakia[173]	3, 5, 11	DTaP3/HepB/IPV/PRP-T₂, DTaP3/HepB/IPV + PRP-T₂		19.1, 18.9	1.01	1.34	0.97	0.89	1.37	1.14	0.82		0.82	0.90	0.73
Italy, Germany[169]	3, 5, 11	DTaP3/HepB/IPV/PRP-T₂, DTaP3/HepB/IPV + PRP-T₂		38, 32	1.19	0.78	1.03	1.06	0.92	0.87	1.13		1.14	1.33	1.18
Canada[94, 161, 164]	2, 4, 6	DTaP5/IPV/PRP-T₁[¶], DTaP5/IPV + PRP-T₁	85, 89	5.04, 3.83	1.32		0.67§	0.61§	1.20	1.06	1.16	0.83	0.90	0.85	1.17
Canada[94, 163, 164]	2, 4, 6	DTaP5/IPV/PRP-T₁[‡], DTaP5/IPV + PRP-T₁	89, 89	4.86, 3.83	1.27		0.81	0.68	0.84	0.94	1.37	0.83	0.88	0.92	0.69

*A ratio less than 1 indicates that mean antibody levels were lower with the combined vaccine than with separate injections; a ratio higher than 1, that levels were higher with combined than separate injections. A blank cell indicates that the comparison was not possible or is not available.

†aP1, Monocomponent aP containing PT only (Certiva or equivalent); aP2, French two component aP (e.g., Triavax or similar); aP3, Infanrix; aP4, ACEL-IMUNE or similar Takeda-type aP vaccine; aP5, Tripacel or equivalent five-component aP vaccine (see Chapter 21 for details of vaccines). PRP-T₁, ActHiB (Aventis Pasteur); PRP-T₂, Hiberix (GlaxoSmithKline).

‡DTaP5/IPV/PRP-T combined, fully liquid, in vial.

§Difference significant at P ≤ 0.05.

‖DTaP and IPV were given at 2, 4, and 6 months; PRP-T was given at 3, 5, and 7 months. Polio antibody levels estimated from figures.

¶DTaP5/IPV used to reconstitute lyophilized PRP-T.

aP, acellular pertussis vaccine; D, diphtheria toxin; DTaP, diphtheria and tetanus toxoids and acellular pertussis vaccine; FHA, filamentous hemagglutinin; FIM, fimbrae; GMC, geometric mean concentration of antibody; HB, hepatitis B; HepB, hepatitis B vaccine; IPV, inactivated poliovirus vaccine; OPV, oral poliovirus vaccine; PRN, pertactin; PRP, polyribosylribitol phosphate; PRP-T, PRP–tetanus toxoid protein conjugate vaccine; PT, pertussis toxin; T, tetanus toxin.

In addition to the previously discussed DTaP5/IPV (Quadracel), combination vaccines based on the Canadian five-component aP vaccine, such as DTaP5/Hib (Actacel) and DTaP5/IPV/Hib (Pentacel and Pediacel) have been evaluated in various locales. In a comparative trial in Taiwan of the DTaP5/Hib combination versus the separate components, 95% of combination recipients achieved at least 1 μg/mL of antibody to PRP. Geometric mean pertussis and Hib antibody levels did not differ between combined and separate administration (see Table 29–8).[161] Another comparative trial examined vaccination at 2, 4, 6, and 18 months of age with (1) DTaP5/IPV used to reconstitute lyophilized PRP-T (Pentacel), (2) a fully liquid DTaP5/IPV/PRP-T (Pediacel), or (3) DTaP5/IPV and PRP-T given separately.[94,163,164] All three groups responded well after primary and booster immunization (see Table 29–9). The liquid and lyophilized combinations performed similarly[163]; antibody responses with the liquid combination did not differ significantly from those of the separate vaccines for any antigen.[94,163,164]

The SSI DTaP1/IPV combination (DiTeKiPol) is also available packaged with ActHIB for reconstitution as a DTaP1/IPV/PRP-T combination (DiTeKiPol-ActHIB); this latter combination has been used routinely in Denmark since July 2002. A study compared DiTeKiPol and ActHIB given combined or separately at 3, 5, and 12 months. Following both the second and the third injection, Hib GMTs were lower with the combination but the proportions achieving levels of 1.0 μg/mL or higher were equal (27% after the second and 92% after the third injection; see Table 29–9).[165]

Clinical Relevance of Reduced Hib Responses in DTaP-Based Combinations

The observation that most combinations incorporating both DTaP and Hib produced reduced Hib antibody responses, as compared to concomitant administration at separate sites of the same vaccines, raised concern over the appropriateness of such combinations for general vaccination programs. Will these reduced antibody responses result in impaired protection of either the individual or the community?

The essential characteristic of Hib is its PRP capsule, which is a major virulence factor and a target for antibodies that mediate protection against the disease. The immature immune systems of infants are unable to mount a satisfactory immune response to a polysaccharide antigen but do respond well to protein antigens. A vaccine containing PRP conjugated to a protein stimulates a brisk antibody response not only to the carrier protein but also to the polysaccharide.[197] This T-cell–dependent response also produces immunologic memory, with the capacity for boosting of antibody following subsequent exposure (either natural or by way of booster vaccination). The use of conjugated Hib vaccines has resulted in almost complete control of Hib disease in countries employing them as part of universal childhood vaccination programs.[198–200]

The historically recognized serologic correlates of protection for Hib were developed from studies of the first-generation, unconjugated, plain polysaccharide Hib vaccines (i.e., those consisting of PRP alone). Based on antibody levels among study children who did or did not develop invasive Hib disease, it was estimated that it was necessary to have 0.10 μg/mL[201] or 0.15 μg/mL[202] of antibody at the time of Hib exposure to be protected from invasive Hib disease. Given the demonstrated waning of antibody levels over time, it was suggested that a postimmunization level of 1 μg/mL was required for long-term protection, that is, to ensure a minimal level of 0.10 μg/mL for a second year.[202]

It is increasingly questioned, however, whether these benchmark levels, derived from studies of unconjugated PRP vaccines, are equally applicable to the antibody responses produced by conjugated vaccines. Not only do the conjugated vaccines stimulate higher antibody responses, but there is an associated maturation of the immune response (i.e., increased functional capacity of the antibodies) that results in increased avidity of the antibodies, both prior to and after booster challenge. Moreover, the levels obtained with the DTaP-based Hib combinations are still within the broad range of antibody titers achieved with other licensed Hib conjugates administered separately.[16] Perhaps most importantly, the conjugated vaccines induce B-cell memory that leads to a rapid anamnestic response after Hib exposure,[16,188] and consequently protection may not depend solely on pre-infection levels of circulating antibody.

A panel of experts considered these issues[16] and commented that "with the proviso that careful clinical surveillance of Hib disease is maintained, we encourage the introduction of DTaP-Hib combinations. . . ." Indeed, combination vaccines that manifest reduced Hib antibody responses have been approved by European and other authorities. Hospital- and laboratory-based surveillance of Hib disease in Germany (where DTaP/Hib, DTaP/IPV/Hib, and DTaP/IPV/HepB/Hib combination vaccines were progressively introduced starting in 1996) has not detected any increase thus far in invasive Hib disease, and incidence rates continue to fall.[189–191]

Unfortunately, the situation is not simple. Ongoing surveillance of Hib disease in the United Kingdom has detected an increase in invasive Hib disease that appears to be associated with a recent reduction in population immunity to Hib.[192] Suggested explanations include waning of the effect of the original UK catch-up campaign, fewer opportunities for natural boosting, or a reduced vaccine immunogenicity. The latter possibility takes on special significance in light of a companion report that documents a seven- to eight-fold higher risk of invasive Hib disease among recipients of the DTaP3/Hib combination vaccine introduced in January 1999.[193] Even if this report is substantiated, however, the issue may be of relevance only in the context of an immunization schedule as unusual as has been employed in the UK, which has attempted to protect the population through administration of Hib-containing vaccine at 2, 3, and 4 months with no subsequent booster.

As noted, although some licensing authorities have been willing to license DTaP/Hib combinations with reduced Hib immunogenicity without requiring an efficacy trial to prove the combination's efficacy against Hib, others have not. For example, no such combination is licensed for primary immunization in the United States or Canada, nor is the FDA likely to approve such a combination in the proximate future.

The applicability to conjugate vaccines of the benchmark antibody levels (0.15 and 1.0 μg/mL) derived from polysaccharide vaccines clearly is questionable, but no more pertinent benchmarks have been established. The induction of immune memory by the conjugate vaccines is undeniable, but the extent to which memory alone is sufficient for protection from invasive Hib disease, independent of any particular level of circulating antibody, is not known. Moreover, the heterogeneity of the U.S. population, which includes groups at distinctly elevated risk, may justify a higher standard on the part of U.S. regulators than is felt necessary in Europe. For example, PRP-D (Prohibit) was proven in an efficacy trial to be inadequate to protect an Alaskan population,[203] whereas it has proven perfectly capable of protecting Scandinavian populations,[204,205] probably because disease occurs later in the latter. The unambiguous solution would be to conduct efficacy trials of the vaccines in question in appropriate populations, but the costs, ethical concerns regarding withholding immunization in the control groups, and enormous difficulty of conducting such trials, now that use of conjugate Hib vaccines is widespread, effectively rule out that solution.

Finally, the herd immunity that is so important in abolition of Hib disease within a population depends in large measure on the abolition of colonization, which appears to require higher levels of antibody than are required for personal protection,[206,207] and thus may be more sensitive to reduced or delayed immunogenicity.[208] Unlike the U.K. data, the German surveillance data appear to be reassuring in this regard, but, inasmuch as a substantial proportion of the children under 5 years of age in the surveillance population[188] had been immunized with monocomponent Hib vaccines, full confidence that the observed interference is of no clinical importance will require several more years of surveillance of cohorts of infants immunized solely with the vaccines in question.

DTaP/HepB/Hib and DTaP/IPV/HepB/Hib Combinations

A number of studies have evaluated GSK's DTaP3/HepB/PRP-T combination vaccine.[209–215] As seen with most of the DTaP3/Hib and DTaP3/IPV/Hib combinations previously described, DTaP3/Hib-based combinations tend to produce lower PRP antibody levels than are obtained with separate administration of the Hib component. For example, among children randomized at 2, 4, and 6 months of age to receive DTaP3/HepB/PRP-T, DTaP3/HepB + PRP-T, or DTaP3 + HepB + PRP-T, mean PRP antibody levels at 7 months of age were 1.5, 6.9, and 6.4 μg/mL, and the proportions achieving 1 μg/mL were 68%, 91%, and 90%, respectively.[209,210] No interference was seen in the antibody responses to the other components. Children whose 7-month PRP antibody levels were below 1.0 μg/mL were administered a booster dose at 11 to 15 months of age, resulting in mean PRP antibody levels of 5.1 μg/mL for the combined group and 3.0 μg/mL for the other two groups.[211]

A different study also found comparable responses with combined and separate administration for all antigens except PRP-T. PRP antibody levels were 1.2 and 5.5 μg/mL, and proportions achieving 1 μg/mL were 58% and 88% for the combined and separate groups, respectively.[211] Children with low antibody responses to primary immunization again had excellent responses when given booster doses. The same PRP results were found in a German study in which infants were immunized at 3, 4, and 5 months of age; mean PRP antibody levels were 1.2 and 5.5 μg/mL, respectively, for DTaP3/HepB/PRP-T and DTaP3/HepB + PRP-T.[212] Zepp and colleagues gave unconjugated PRP to children at 12 months of age who had been immunized at 3, 4, and 5 months of age with DTaP3/HepB/PRP-T. The children developed good antibody responses to PRP promptly after the booster immunization, demonstrating that the combination vaccine had successfully primed the immune system.[213] A consistency study with three lots of DTaP3/HepB mixed with three lots of PRP-T found Hib antibody levels of 0.15 μg/mL or greater in 100% and 1 μg/mL or greater in 85% of subjects; the GMT was 4.05 μg/mL.[214]

Hexavalent (DTaP/HepB/IPV/Hib) vaccines from GSK and AvP have now been licensed in Europe and elsewhere. The AvP product (Hexavac) is fully liquid, whereas the GSK product (Infanrix Hexa) consists of the liquid DTaP3/HepB/IPV used to reconstitute the lyophilized PRP-T. Both products have been extensively studied to characterize their immunogenicity, safety, and adaptability to a variety of primary and booster schedules.[145,146,168,171,173,216–226] As would be expected based on the results from their quadrivalent and pentavalent predecessors, both products show good immunogenicity for their included antigens, producing seroprotection or seroconversion rates and GMTs similar to those seen with separate injections, except that Hib responses are somewhat lower than seen with separate administration (see Table 29–9). The incidences of local and systemic adverse events following administration of the hexavalent combined vaccines appear thus far to be comparable to those seen with other licensed DTaP-based vaccines.

From a programmatic point of view, it is important that these vaccines can be safely and effectively coadministered with the 7-valent pneumococcal conjugate vaccine (Prevnar) and the meningococcal C conjugate vaccines that are indicated for use according to the same infant schedule, particularly because at least one study showed markedly reduced antibody responses to tetanus-conjugated serotypes in an experimental 7-valent conjugated pneumococcal vaccine, when administered concomitantly with a DtaP2/IPV/PRP-T combination vaccine.[227]

For each of the hexavalent vaccines, a separate open randomized study compared their administration alone or concomitantly with the CRM_{127}-conjugated Prevnar.[228,229] For both Infanrix Hexa and Hexavac, the concomitant-administration groups showed significant antibody rises to all PnC antigens, whereas PnC antibodies declined in the control groups, and predefined seroprotective antibody concentrations against the hexavalent antigens were achieved by an equally large proportion of infants in the concomitant and control groups. In the Hexavac study, antibody responses following the third dose were higher in the concomitant-vaccine group for diphtheria whereas for HepB they were higher in the control group (89% vs. 94%). Rates of adverse reactions did not differ between study groups in either study, except that low-grade fever (38–39°C) was most common in the groups receiving concomitant *Prevnar*.

A subsequent study evaluating *Infanrix Hexa* given alone or concomitantly with *Prevnar* at 3, 4, and 5 months found no significant differences between groups in the antibody responses to the *Infanrix Hexa* components.[230] The proportions achieving pneumococcal antibody levels of 0.05 µg/mL or greater were 100% for all serotypes except 6B (97.2%) and 23F (98.6%). Once again, fever between 38°C and 39°C was more common in the group receiving concomitant *Prevnar* (42%) than in the group receiving only *Infanrix Hexa* (23%). A companion study compared safety of the same regimens at the fourth consecutive dose, given at 12 to 23 months, and found fever between 38.5°C and 39.5°C in 22% of the concomitant-vaccine group versus 12.3% of the *Infanrix Hexa*-only group.[231] Fever greater than 39.5°C was uncommon, being seen in only 2.8% of the concomitant and 1.6% of the comparison groups.

A comparison of the administration of a conjugate meningococcal C vaccine (*Meningitec*, Wyeth Lederle) given simultaneously with *Infanrix Hexa* at 2, 4, and 6 months or separately at 3, 5, and 7 months found no material differences in proportions seroprotected or rates of adverse reactions.[232] A comparison of *Hexavac* given alone or simultaneously with a different conjugate meningococcal vaccine (NeisVac-C, Baxter BioScience) found that the meningococcal vaccine did not appear to influence the immune response to the hepatitis B, IPV, or pertussis components of *Hexavac* nor did *Hexavac* appear to influence the immune responses to the meningococcal vaccine.[233]

A direct comparison of *Infanrix Hexa* versus *Hexavac* found immune response rates and GMTs to be higher with *Infanrix Hexa* for diphtheria, polio, and hepatitis B and similar following both vaccines for Hib, tetanus, and pertussis (pertussis toxin and filamentous hemagglutinin). The incidences of clinically relevant adverse events were low in both groups.[234]

Taken together, these studies raise the possibility that the two hexavalent vaccines might differ with respect to their hepatitis B immune responses. Additional clinical trials that directly compare the two hexavalent vaccines, including their interactions with concomitant conjugate vaccines, will be helpful in elucidating such questions

Combinations Based on Hepatitis Vaccine, Without DT(A)P

HepB/Hib Combinations

Comvax (Merck & Co; marketed by Aventis Pasteur MSD in Europe as Procomvax and other trade names) is a licensed combination of HepB vaccine (Recombivax, 5 µg) and PRP-OMP conjugate Hib vaccine (PedvaxHIB, 7.5 µg). A study comparing Comvax and its constituent components given at 2, 4, and 12 to 15 months of age found no material difference in antibody responses.[235–237] Mean PRP antibody levels for the combined and separate products (2.5 and 2.8 µg/mL, respectively) and proportions exceeding 1.0 µg/mL at 6 months of age (72% and 76%, respectively) were in the usual range for PedvaxHIB (see Chapter 14). When infants were given a booster dose at 12 to 15 months of age, the corresponding values were 9.5 and 10.2 µg/mL and 92% and 93%, respectively. Responses to the HepB component also were as expected, with 92% and 98% of subjects in the respective groups achieving protective levels of antibody (≥10 mIU/mL) at 6 months of age, and with 98% and 100%, respectively, achieving these levels after boosting.

HepB/HepA Combinations

A combination incorporating HepA and HepB antigens (Twinrix; GSK) is available in the United States, Canada, Europe, and elsewhere. The combined vaccine is available in an adult formulation that contains 720 EU of inactivated hepatitis A antigen and 20 µg of recombinant hepatitis B antigen, and in a pediatric formulation that contains half these amounts.

A comparative trial in adults of Twinrix versus its individual components (Havrix and Engerix-B) given separately at 0, 1, and 6 months found excellent antibody responses, with 100% of combined-vaccine recipients achieving protective levels of both antibodies before the 6-month injection.[238] Another comparative trial[239] confirmed the equivalence of Twinrix and its component vaccines given separately at 0, 1, and 6 months: 99.6% of 264 Twinrix vaccinees developed antibodies against hepatitis A (GMT, 4756 mIU/mL) versus 99.3% of 269 recipients of the monovalent vaccines (GMT, 2948 mIU/mL); for hepatitis B, 95.1% of the Twinrix vaccinees achieved protective titers (GMT, 2099 mIU/mL) versus 92.2% (GMT, 1871 mIU/mL) of the subjects receiving monovalent vaccines. Other studies have provided comparable data.[240,241]

A comparative trial of Twinrix versus its components given in an accelerated 0-, 7-, and 21-day schedule, developed for those individuals (e.g., travelers) in need of rapid protection against hepatitis A and B, found that 99% of the vaccinees in both groups were positive 1 month later for anti–hepatitis A antibodies (GMT, 845 mIU/mL for the combined vaccine versus 512 mIU/mL for the separate) and 82% of the Twinrix vaccinees were protected against hepatitis B (vs. 84% in the monovalent group; GMTs, 65 mIU/mL and 98 mIU/mL, respectively). In all studies, Twinrix was well tolerated, with no increased reactogenicity compared to its monovalent components.

A long-term follow-up study[242] found that, at month 72 following vaccination, 100% of 87 adult subjects still had antibodies against hepatitis A and 89% were still seroprotected against hepatitis B. Of 81 children evaluated at month 60, all retained their antibodies against hepatitis A and 95% remained seroprotected against hepatitis B. The combined vaccine and separate vaccine groups did not differ in spontaneously reported adverse events.[242]

A two-dose Twinrix schedule also has been evaluated.[243–245] In these studies, children were given two doses of the adult formulation of Twinrix (720 EU of inactivated hepatitis A antigen and 20 mg of hepatitis B surface antigen). In one study, 237 children ages 1 to 11 years were vaccinated at 0 and 6 months; at month 7, all had seroconverted to hepatitis A (GMT, 11,543 mIU/mL) and 98.5% were seroprotected against hepatitis B (GMT, 8056 mIU/mL).[244] A second study among children ages 12 to 15 years compared the adult formulation given at 0 and 6 months versus the pediatric formulation given at 0, 1, and 6 months and found them equivalent.[245] A third study found equivalence for vaccination with Twinrix at 0 and 6 months or at 0 and 12 months.[246] Therefore, the adult formulation of Twinrix can be administered to children and adolescents in a two-dose schedule, with the second dose following the first by 6 to 12 months. In Europe, the adult formulation licensed for use in this indication and schedule is known as Ambirix.

HepA/Typhoid Combinations

Vaccines composed of *Salmonella typhi* capsular polysaccharide Vi (Vi vaccine) have proven safe and effective in prevention of typhoid fever. The combination of Vi with HepA offers an attractive option for travelers or others who need protection from both diseases, given that typhoid fever and hepatitis A are among the most common vaccine-preventable diseases in travelers and share overlapping areas of endemicity. Two such vaccines are available, Hepatyrix (GSK) and ViATIM (AvP). Hepatyrix is provided as a fully liquid preparation, whereas ViATIM is presented in a dual-chambered syringe that mixes the two components at the moment of injection.

The proof of concept for these combinations was obtained in a preliminary study that found similar GMTs following Havrix administered concomitantly with Typherix versus the two combined.[247] Subsequently the new combined formulation was tested against each single vaccine alone or the two given concomitantly; GMTs did not significantly differ, and seroconversion rates were greater than 94% for Vi and greater than 97% for HepA.[247] A lot consistency study among 465 persons ages 15 to 50 years found that greater than 95% of subjects had seroconverted for anti-Vi antibodies and greater than 86% for hepatitis A antibody by day 14 following Hepatyrix, rising to 96% and 100%, respectively, after 1 month.[248] After a booster dose of Havrix, all vaccinees were seropositive against hepatitis A, with a 7.5-fold increase in GMT. No increase in reactogenicity was seen compared to the single vaccines.

ViATIM was evaluated in a study that compared separate administration of Typhim Vi and Avaxim versus single injection using the dual-chambered syringe. Seroconversion rates at 14 days for combined and separate administration were 86.4% and 88.2%, respectively, for Vi and 95.6% and 94.2%, respectively, for HepA; at 28 days, Vi rates were essentially unchanged but HepA rates had risen to 98.7% and 100%, respectively (because of differing definitions of seroconversion, these rates cannot be directly compared to those cited for Hepatyrix in the preceding paragraph).[249] A subsequent study evaluated three lots of ViATIM and found a fourfold or greater rise in Vi antibodies for 92.1% of subjects; all previously seronegative subjects seroconverted for HepA.[250]

More recently, a direct comparison of ViATIM versus Hepatyrix found statistically higher Vi and HepA serocon-

version rates and GMTs at 14 and 28 days after ViATIM, whereas systemic and local reactions (mainly pain at the injection site) were lower after Hepatyrix.[251]

Combinations Based on Measles or MMR Vaccine

MMR Combined with Varicella Vaccine

Merck and GSK have had active MMR/varicella vaccine (MMRV) development efforts underway for some years, which are hoped to reach fruition by the middle of the present decade. Each company's MMRV incorporates a different measles strain but the same rubella strain (see Chapters 19 and 26) plus each company's derivative of the Jeryl-Lynn mumps strain and of the Oka varicella strain (see Chapters 20 and 28). As shown in Table 29–10, a variety of formulations have been evaluated. It has proven difficult to balance the components so as to preserve the high seroconversion rates and antibody levels achieved when giving MMR and varicella vaccine separately.[53,54,252-262]

The development by GSK of a new MMR vaccine (Priorix) and of a refrigerator-stable formulation of varicella vaccine (Varilrix) prompted the starting of a new MMRV clinical development program by that manufacturer. The new combination (see Table 29–10) has been shown to elicit seroconversion rates of 95.7% or greater for each component,[254] with similar lymphocyte stimulation indices following combined or separate administration.[262] Fever and rash appear to be somewhat more common with MMRV than MMR.[265]

Merck's latest formulation of MMRV (ProQuad), which incorporates "process upgrade varicella vaccine" (PUVV), was evaluated as a two-dose regimen at three different dose levels of the varicella component (2495, 6750, or 14,350 PFU/0.5 mL), compared to single doses of M-M-R II and PUVV administered concomitantly at separate sites. Antibody responses were measured after each dose. Only the formulation containing the highest varicella concentration induced a varicella immune response similar to that of separate vaccines after the first dose; all three two-dose regimens induced significantly higher varicella seroconversion rates and GMTs. For measles, mumps, and rubella, all four single-dose regimens were equally immunogenic; the three two-dose regimens produced significantly higher GMTs (see Table 29–10).[261]

Obsolete Combinations

Combinations of Yellow Fever, Smallpox, and/or Measles Vaccines

The use of combination smallpox/yellow fever vaccines began in 1939, when investigators at the Pasteur Institute of Dakar began to study coadministration of these vaccines through a single scarification site.[263] After successful animal and human studies, mass vaccination campaigns were conducted in French West Africa, with more than 14 million people receiving the combined vaccine (containing the yellow fever strain adapted to mouse brain) between 1939 and

TABLE 29–10 ■ Studies Evaluating Combined or Simultaneous Administration of Vaccines Containing Measles, Mumps, Rubella, and Varicella Components

Place	Ages (Mo)	Vaccines	Potency* MMR, V	Percent Seroconversion, Combined Minus Separate†				Ratio of Antibody Levels with Combined Vaccine to Levels with Separate Vaccines‡				
				V	Me	Mu	Ru	V	Me	Mu	Ru	PRP
GLAXOSMITHKLINE (EARLIER FORMULATIONS)												
Switzerland[252]	15–24	MMRV, MMR + V	Std, Low	−35§	−4	0	0					
Switzerland[252]	15–24	MMRV, MMR + V	Std, High	−18§	3	−3	−3					
Finland[253]	12–18	MMRV, MMR + V	Std, High	−12§	0	−2	−1					
Finland[253]	12–18	MMRV, MMR + V	Low, Low	−20	−4	−3	0					
GLAXOSMITHKLINE (NEW FORMULATION)												
Europe[254]	12–24	MMRV, MMR + V	Std, High	−2	−1	−2	−3	0.63	1.49	1.18	0.84	
MERCK & CO (EARLIER FORMULATIONS)												
USA[255,256]	15–17	MMRV, MMR + V	Std, Low	0	0	−6	0	1.07	1.10	1.15	1.33	
USA[257]	15	MMRV, MMR + V	Std?, Low	+16§	0	+3	−1	1.27	1.00	1.47	0.94	
USA[258]	12–19	MMRV, MMR + V	Std, High	0	0	0	0	0.46§	1.23	1.00	1.25	
USA[259]	12–30	MMRV, MMR + V	Std, High	−3	0	−1	0	0.49§	1.27	1.13	1.14	
USA[259]	12–30	MMRV + DTaP4 + OPV, MMR + V + DTaP4 + OPV	Std, High	−1	−4§	−2	−1	0.58§	0.95	0.82	1.08	
USA[260]	12–18	MMR + Hib, MMR + V + Hib	Std, High	−2	−1	−2	0	0.71§	1.39	0.94	1.18	1.03
MERCK & CO (NEW FORMULATIONS)												
USA[261]	12–23	MMRV (one dose), MMR + V (one dose)	Std, Low	−29§	−1	0	0	0.31§	0.99	1.05	1.02	
USA[261]	12–23	MMRV (one dose), MMR + V (one dose)	Std, Middle	−13§	−1	−1	0	0.57§	1.22§	1.08	0.97	
USA[261]	12–23	MMRV (one dose), MMR + V (one dose)	Std, High	−4	0	−1	0	0.64§	1.24§	1.18	0.91	
USA[261]	12–23	MMRV (two doses), MMR + V (one dose)	Std, Low	+7§	0	0	0	9.06§	2.17§	2.85§	2.08§	
USA[261]	12–23	MMRV (two doses), MMR + V (one dose)	Std, Middle	+7§	0	0	0	20.6§	3.09§	2.51§	1.82§	
USA[261]	12–23	MMRV (two doses), MMR + V (one dose)	Std, High	+6§	0	0	0	25.4§	2.95§	2.87§	2.01§	

*Relative potency of MMR and V components. For MMR, comparison is to standard product (std). For V, "low" is 950 to 2300 PFU; "high" is greater than 2300 PFU.
†Seroconversion rate (in percent) among those receiving combined vaccine, minus those receiving separate vaccines; a positive number indicates higher seroconversion with the combined vaccine, and a negative number indicates lower seroconversion with combined vaccine.
‡A ratio less than 1 indicates that mean antibody levels were lower with the combined vaccine than with separate injections; a ratio higher than 1, that levels were higher with combined than separate injections. A blank cell indicates that the comparison was not possible or is not available.
§Difference significant at P ≤0.05.
DTaP4, ACEL-IMUNE brand of diphtheria and tetanus toxoids and acellular pertussis vaccine; Hib, Haemophilus influenzae type b; Me, measles; MMR, measles-mumps-rubella vaccine; Mu, mumps; OPV, oral poliovirus vaccine; PFU, plaque-forming units; PRP, polyribosylribitol phosphate; Ru, rubella; V, varicella.

1945 alone.[264,266] Smallpox/yellow fever combination vaccines using the safer, although less immunogenic, 17D chick embryo strain, appeared to be safe and highly immunogenic in pilot studies and were readily manufactured and stored.[266] Subsequent studies in British East Africa found only about 70% seroconversion to yellow fever under field conditions, leading investigators to recommend simultaneous rather than combined immunization.[267–269]

Soon after measles vaccine became available, researchers from the U.S. National Institutes of Health studied its use in combination with smallpox and yellow fever vaccines in Burkina Faso (previously Upper Volta).[270–274] Neutralizing antibody responses to measles, vaccinia, and yellow fever vaccines were materially lower in the combined-vaccine groups. The ability of measles and yellow fever vaccines, but not vaccinia vaccine, to induce circulating interferon might explain the apparent interference found in the groups receiving combinations containing measles and yellow fever vaccines.[272]

Good results were obtained with a measles/smallpox vaccine in which the components were combined before lyophilization,[273] and with a combination vaccine using a high-dose tetanus toxoid vaccine combined at the time of administration with measles vaccine.[274]

More recently, investigators in at least four African countries have evaluated the use of a combined measles/yellow fever vaccine.[275–277] In a randomized study in Côte d'Ivoire, infants (ages 6 to 9 months) had comparable seroresponse rates to measles vaccine, yellow fever vaccine, or the combined vaccine.[275] Similar results were obtained in Mali for both infants (ages 4 to 8 months) and toddlers (ages 12 to 24 months).[276] Investigators in Cameroon found higher seroconversion rates with the combined than with the separate vaccines, as well as significantly higher yellow fever antibody levels 30 days after immunization in the group given combined vaccine.[277] A trial in Nigeria similarly found that antibody levels and seroconversion rates were higher with combined than separate vaccines.[278]

Many other obsolete combination vaccines of historical relevance have not been mentioned.[279,280]

Future Combinations

Wyeth Lederle is conducting clinical trials of PnC/Hib, PnC/MnC, and PnC/MnC/Hib combinations. A comparison of 7-valent (7v) PnC and HbOC, given combined or separately, found significantly lower antibody concentrations for five of the seven pneumococcal serotypes. Hib responses did not differ with respect to the proportions achieving 0.15 μg/mL (97% vs. 98%) or 1.0 μg/mL (80% vs. 82%); GMTs were reduced with the combination (3.52 vs. 4.79 μg/mL), but this difference did not achieve significance.[281] In contrast, a study comparing 7vPnC/MnC/HbOC with the separate administration of HbOC plus either 7vPnC or 9vPnC/MnC found that GMTs and seroresponse rates in the combination vaccine groups met the statistical criteria for noninferiority for the pneumococcal antigens, but the PRP antibody response to the PnC/MnC/HbOC combination was inferior to that of separately administered HbOC (GMTs of 4.5, 12.0, and 16.0,

respectively).[282] This reduced Hib responsiveness, thought possibly to represent antigen overload with the carrier protein, may prevent inclusion of that component in future PnC/MnC combinations. Meanwhile, development of 9vPnC/MnC (serotype C) continues, to be followed by 9vPnC/MnC (quadrivalent) toward the end of the decade. Additionally, Wyeth or others may develop DTwP/PnC combinations.

The Program for Appropriate Technology in Health (PATH; www.path.org) and the World Health Organization, with support from the Gates Foundation, have launched the Meningitis Vaccine Project to develop affordable conjugate meningococcal vaccines directed toward the needs of sub-Saharan Africa and other impacted, impoverished areas. PATH also has announced a project, in collaboration with GSK, to develop a heptavalent DTwP-HB-Hib-conjugate meningococcus serotypes A/C vaccine.

One abstract has reported development by GSK of a heptavalent combination vaccine; DTaP/HepB/IPV was used to reconstitute Hib/MnC. Three different formulations of this heptavalent combination were compared to *Infanrix Hexa*. One formulation was said to be non-inferior to the hexavalent control with respect to Hib responses; other immunogenicity and safety comparisons were said to be satisfactory.[285]

There are also a host of other new combination vaccines under development that incorporate multiple serotypes of a single antigen, which are well described in other chapters. Among these potentially important combination vaccines are trivalent influenza vaccines, including those of novel modes of delivery (see Chapters 17 and 18); polyvalent pneumococcal vaccines (see Chapters 22 and 23) and meningococcal vaccines (see Chapter 34), especially the conjugate products presently under development; and polyvalent rotavirus vaccine (see Chapter 51). Other targets for combination vaccines include tick-borne infections, arboviruses, and additional agents of diarrheal diseases.

Practical Issues in the Use of Combination Vaccines

Choice of Combination Versus Separate Component Vaccines

In their joint statement on combination vaccines, the major advisory groups have stated that "The use of licensed combination vaccines is preferred over separate injection of their equivalent component vaccines."[283] The 2000 *Red Book* additionally commented, "Combination vaccine products may be given whenever any component of the combination is indicated and its other components are not contraindicated, provided they are approved by the FDA for the child's age."[284]

Although slightly different, these recommendations are not inconsistent. When the combination consists of the same components that the practitioner would have given separately at the same visit, it is clear that the combination is preferred. In other circumstances (e.g., the combination does not incorporate the same components that the practitioner would have given; the components are the same, but the practitioner would have given one or more on a different schedule; the patient does not need one or more of the components, but receipt is not contraindicated), use of the combination is acceptable but not necessarily preferred.

Not addressed in these recommendations are cost and reimbursement issues (see below).

Administration of Superfluous Antigens

As a variety of vaccines become available that combine different antigens, physicians will increasingly find that the simplest (and even, perhaps, the least expensive) alternative will be use of a combination vaccine that includes an antigen that the patient does not need, having already received that antigen in the recommended quantity and timing. Some antigens are known to be associated with increased adverse effects when administered too frequently (e.g., diphtheria toxoid), but these are few. Fortunately, it has been shown for many vaccine antigens that an extra dose may be given without adverse consequence. In particular, the low reactogenicity of Hib, IPV, and HepB vaccines makes it unlikely that an extra dose of any of these antigens would cause a problem.

Interchangeability

When multiple combination vaccines are available from several different manufacturers, practitioners will question whether the vaccines can be used interchangeably. This question can be difficult to answer even for monocomponent vaccines, and there is little hope of definitive answers for multicomponent vaccines. Consider, for example, a study performed to evaluate the interchangeability of the three conjugate Hib vaccines indicated for the infant primary series.[286] Of the 27 theoretically possible permutations of three vaccines and three injections, 5 were evaluated. Once there are multiple, distinct DTaP, DTaP/Hib, DTaP/Hib/IPV (and so on) combination vaccines, there will be little likelihood that any particular substitution will have been studied.

The Advisory Committee on Immunization Practices has recognized certain vaccines as interchangeable: DTwP (and its individual components), IPV, OPV, Hib (as long as three doses are given), and HepB.[4] For those vaccines for which there are no data on the interchangeability of licensed products from various manufacturers (e.g., DTaP[287] and the newer combination vaccines[283]), the Advisory Committee on Immunization Practices has recommended that the same product be used throughout the primary series. However, if the identity of the product previously used is not known or if the product is not available at the time of the child's visit, then any licensed product appropriate to the child's immunization status and requirements may be used. As the Centers for Disease Control and Prevention noted, "Providers should not miss the opportunity to administer a dose of acellular pertussis vaccine for which the child is eligible if the vaccine used for the earlier doses is not available."[288]

In this day of bulk vaccine purchase through competitive bidding by large health maintenance organizations and the government, it is unrealistic to presume that the same vaccine will always be available for each child at the time of each vaccination. The situation is further complicated by the fact that 25% of U.S. children see at least two different health care providers for their vaccination series and that the average time for a child to remain in a publicly funded health care plan is 10 months. Different practitioners are likely to stock different combination vaccines. Because the need to interchange vaccines will arise so often, it is reassuring to know that interchange of one brand of vaccine for another has never been shown to result in performance that is outside the range expected for the vaccines in question.

Ad Hoc Combinations

Providers should not create their own ad hoc combinations by mixing separate vaccines in the same syringe unless there is evidence establishing the stability, safety, and immunogenicity of the resultant combination, as reflected in the package inserts.

Public Health Considerations

Cost Issues

Whether the combination vaccine purchaser is a government, a health maintenance organization or some other intermediary, or the practitioner and patient, it must be expected that economic factors will influence decisions. It is obvious that premium pricing of the combination or reduced provider reimbursement (as a result of administration of fewer injections) may inhibit use of the combination. Less obvious, but equally important, are the economic benefits that flow from use of a combination: savings resulting from simplified vaccine purchase, storage, and handling; reduced costs for labor and supplies; elimination of the need for scheduling several vaccination visits to avoid multiple injections; and, of course, increased patient satisfaction and greater compliance with vaccination recommendations.

Many of the newer vaccines, such as DTaP, conjugate Hib, and complex combinations, are substantially more expensive to produce than DTwP, OPV, and other traditional combination vaccines. Certainly, cost considerations will constrain the use of some of these vaccines in parts of the world. DTwP, for example, is produced locally at low cost in many countries, and its replacement with DTaP must be weighed against other health care expenditures. Some other relatively expensive vaccines, such as HepB or Hib, offer such clear benefits that they are being used in many developing countries. Once a country has committed to using HepB or conjugate Hib vaccine, for example, it is likely to find that combinations that also provide such antigens as DTP or IPV can be purchased for less than the cost of purchasing, storing, shipping, tracking, and injecting the separate component vaccines.

Tracking of Vaccinations

The increasing variety of alternative vaccines, including those with multiple antigens, that might be used to satisfy childhood vaccination requirements makes it unlikely that a practitioner will be able to deduce the precise vaccination history of a new patient. Although legislation has mandated since March 1988 that medical records of vaccination should contain the identity of the vaccine manufacturer, the date of administration, and the lot number of the vaccine given, such practitioner-based records are not commonly automated or retrievable by others. Immunization registries are confidential, population-based, computerized information systems that collect vaccination data about all children within a geographic area. Registries can elucidate uncertain vaccination histories, identify children who are due or late for vaccinations, generate reminder and recall notices to ensure that children are vaccinated appropriately, identify provider sites and geographic areas with low vaccination coverage, and provide denominator information for outbreak investigations. One of the national health objectives for 2010 is to increase to 95% the proportion of children less than 6 years of age who participate in fully operational, population-based immunization registries. Currently, approximately half of U.S. children less than 6 years of age are participating in a registry.[289,290] Efforts should continue to increase the percentage of children participating in registries.

Methods also are needed to improve the accuracy and convenience of recording and transferring vaccine information from the vaccine vial to the medical record. One solution currently being pursued by manufacturers and the FDA is to include machine-readable bar codes or stickers with vaccines to facilitate the electronic transfer of information.

REFERENCES

1. Williams JC, Goldenthal KL, Burns DL, et al (eds). Combined vaccines and simultaneous administration: current issues and perspectives. Ann N Y Acad Sci 754:xi–404, 1995.
2. Breiman R, Goldenthal K (eds). International Symposium on Combination Vaccines: Proceedings of a Symposium Organized and Sponsored by the National Vaccine Program Office and Held at the National Institutes of Health, 2–4 February 2000. Clin Infect Dis 33(suppl 4):S271–S375, 2001.
3. Grabenstein JD. Immunofacts: Vaccines and Immunologic Drugs. St. Louis, Facts and Comparisons, 1995.
4. Centers for Disease Control and Prevention. General recommendations on immunization: recommendations of the Advisory Committee on Immunization Practices (ACIP). MMWR 51(RR-2):1–44, 2002.
5. Arnon R, Van Regenmortel MHV. Structural basis of antigenic specificity and design of new vaccines. FASEB J 6:3265–3274, 1992.
6. Edwards KM, Meade BD, Decker MD, et al. Comparison of 13 acellular pertussis vaccines: overview and serologic response. Pediatrics 96:548–557, 1995.
7. Chu C, Schneerson R, Robbins JB, et al. Further studies on the immunogenicity of Haemophilus influenzae type b and pneumococcal type 6A polysaccharide-protein conjugates. Infect Immun 40:245–256, 1983.
8. Castillo de Febres O, Decker MD, Estopinan M, et al. Enhanced antibody response in Venezuelan infants immunized with Haemophilus influenzae type b–tetanus toxoid conjugate vaccine. Pediatr Infect Dis J 13:635–639, 1994.
9. Schneerson R, Robbins JB, Chu C, et al. Serum antibody responses of juvenile and infant rhesus monkeys injected with Haemophilus influenzae type b and pneumococcus type 6A capsular polysaccharide-protein conjugates. Infect Immun 45:582–591, 1984.
10. Anderson P, Pichichero M, Edwards K. Priming and induction of Haemophilus influenzae type b capsular antibodies in early infancy by Dpo20, an oligosaccharide-protein conjugate vaccine. J Pediatr 111:644–650, 1987.
11. Barington T, Skettrup M, Juul L, et al. Non-specific suppression of the antibody response to Haemophilus influenzae type b conjugate vaccines by preimmunization with vaccine components. Infect Immun 61:432–438, 1993.
12. Insel RA. Potential alterations in immunogenicity by combining or simultaneously administering vaccine components. Ann N Y Acad Sci 754:35–47, 1995.
13. Dagan R, Eskola J, Leclerc C, et al. Reduced response to multiple vaccines sharing common protein epitopes that are administered simultaneously to infants. Infect Immun 66:2093–2098, 1998.
14. Banatvala J, Van Damme P, Oehen S. Lifelong protection against hepatitis B: the role of vaccine immunogenicity in immune memory. Vaccine 19:877–885, 2000.
15. European Consensus Group on Hepatitis B Immunity. Are booster immunisations needed for lifelong hepatitis B immunity? Lancet 355:561–565, 2000.
16. Eskola J, Ward J, Dagan R, et al. Combined vaccination of Haemophilus influenzae type b conjugate and diphtheria-tetanus-pertussis containing acellular pertussis. Lancet 354:2063–2068, 1999.
17. Granoff DM, Rappuoli R. Are serological responses to acellular pertussis antigens sufficient criteria to ensure that new combination vaccines are effective for prevention of disease? Dev Biol Stand 89:379–389, 1997.
18. Granoff DM. Challenges for licensure of new diphtheria, tetanus, acellular pertussis (DTaP) combination vaccines: point. Pediatr Infect Dis J 15:1069–1070, 1996.
19. Edwards KM, Decker MD. Challenges for licensure of new diphtheria, tetanus toxoid, acellular pertussis (DTaP) combination vaccines: counterpoint. Pediatr Infect Dis J 15:1070–1073, 1996.
20. Storsaeter J, Hallander HO, Gustafsson L, et al. Levels of antipertussis related to protection after household exposure to Bordetella pertussis. Vaccine 16:1907–1916, 1998.
21. Cherry JD, Gornbein J, Heininger U, et al. A search for serologic correlates of immunity to Bordetella pertussis cough illnesses. Vaccine 16:1901–1906, 1998.
22. Zepp F, Knuf M, Habermehl P, et al. Pertussis-specific cell-mediated immunity in infants after vaccination with a tricomponent acellular pertussis vaccine. Infect Immun 64:4078–4084, 1996.
23. Guiso N, Capiau C, Carletti G, et al. Intranasal murine model of Bordetella pertussis infection, I: prediction of protection in human infants by acellular vaccines. Vaccine 17:2366–2376, 1999.
24. Mills KH, Ryan M, Ryan E, et al. A murine model in which protection correlates with pertussis vaccine efficacy in children reveals complementary roles for humoral and cell-mediated immunity in protection against Bordetella pertussis. Infect Immun 66:594–602, 1998.
25. Poolman J. Comparison of seven licensed Pa vaccines in a mouse respiratory model [abstr 233]. In Abstracts of the 39th Interscience Conference on Antimicrobial Agents and Chemotherapy, San Francisco, September 24–27, 1999, p 356.
26. Poolman J. Efficacy of Infanrix in promoting lung clearance of B. pertussis strains expressing pertactin antigenic variants in a mouse respiratory model [abstr 234]. In Abstracts of the 39th Interscience Conference on Antimicrobial Agents and Chemotherapy, San Francisco, September 24–27, 1999, p 356.
27. Boursaux-Eude C, Thiberge S, Carletti G, et al. Intranasal murine model of Bordetella pertussis infection, II: sequence variation and protection induced by a tricomponent acellular vaccine. Vaccine 17:2651–2660, 1999.
28. Edwards KM, Decker MD. Combination vaccines: hopes and challenges. Pediatr Infect Dis J 13:345–347, 1994.
29. Decker MD, Edwards KM. Issues in design of clinical trials of combination vaccines. Ann N Y Acad Sci 754:234–240, 1995.
30. Edwards KM, Decker MD. Combination vaccines consisting of acellular pertussis vaccines. Pediatr Infect Dis J 16(suppl 4):S97–S102, 1997.
31. Gustafsson L, Hallander HO, Olin P, et al. A controlled trial of a two-component acellular, a five-component acellular, and a whole-cell pertussis vaccine. N Engl J Med 334:349–355, 1996.
32. Greco D, Salmaso S, Mastrantonio P, et al. A controlled trial of two acellular vaccines and one whole-cell vaccine against pertussis. N Engl J Med 334:341–348, 1996.
33. Ad Hoc Group for the Study of Pertussis Vaccines. Placebo-controlled trial of two acellular pertussis vaccines in Sweden—protective efficacy and adverse events. Lancet 1:955–960, 1988.
34. Olin P, Rasmussen F, Gustafsson L, et al. Randomised controlled trial of two-component, three-component, and five-component acellular pertussis vaccines compared with whole-cell pertussis vaccine. Lancet 350:1569–1577, 1997.

35. Guidance for Industry for the Evaluation of Combination Vaccines for Preventable Diseases: Production, Testing and Clinical Studies (Docket No 97N–0029). Rockville, MD, U.S. Food and Drug Administration, 1997.

36. King GE, Hadler SC. Simultaneous administration of childhood vaccines: an important public health policy that is safe and efficacious. Pediatr Infect Dis 13:394–407, 1994.

37. Offit PA, Quarles J, Gerber MA, et al. Addressing parents' concerns: do multiple vaccines overwhelm or weaken the infant's immune system? Pediatrics 109:124–129, 2002.

38. Halsey NA. Combination vaccines: defining and addressing current safety concerns. Clin Infect Dis 33(suppl):S312–S318, 2001.

39. Halsey NA. Safety of combination vaccines: perception versus reality. Pediatr Infect Dis J 20(suppl):S40–S44, 2001.

40. Bach J-F. The effect of infections on susceptibility to autoimmune and allergic diseases. N Engl J Med 347:911–920, 2002.

41. Weiss ST. Eat dirt—the hygiene hypothesis and allergic diseases. N Engl J Med 347:930–931, 2002.

42. Stratton K, Wilson CV, McCormick MC (eds). Immunization Safety Review: Multiple Immunizations and Immune Dysfunction. Immunization Safety Review Committee, Board on Health Promotion and Disease Prevention, Institute of Medicine. Washington, DC, National Academy Press, 2002.

43. Chen RT, Rastogi SC, Mullen JR, et al. The Vaccine Adverse Event Reporting System (VAERS). Vaccine 12:542–550, 1994.

44. Greenberg L, Fleming DS. The immunizing efficacy of diphtheria toxoid when combined with various antigens. Can J Public Health 39:131–135, 1948.

45. Spiller V, Barnes JM, Holt LB, et al. Immunization against diphtheria and whooping-cough: combined versus separate inoculations. BMJ 2:639–642, 1955.

46. Aprile MA, Wardlaw AC. Aluminum compounds as adjuvants for vaccines and toxoids in man: a review. Can J Public Health 57:343–354, 1966.

47. Lerman SJ, Bollinger M, Brunken JM. Clinical and serologic evaluation of measles, mumps, and rubella (HPV-77:DE5 and RA 27/3) virus vaccines, singly and in combination. Pediatrics 68:18–22, 1981.

48. Berger R, Just M, Gluck R. Interference between strains in live virus vaccines, I: combined vaccination with measles, mumps and rubella vaccine. J Biol Stand 16:269–273, 1988.

49. Weibel RE, Carlson AJ Jr, Villarejos VM, et al. Clinical and laboratory studies of combined live measles, mumps, and rubella vaccines using the RA 27/3 rubella virus. Proc Soc Exp Biol Med 165:323–326, 1980.

50. Beck M, Smerdel S, Dedic I, et al. Immune response to Edmonston-Zagreb measles virus strain in monovalent and combined MMR vaccine. Dev Biol Stand 65:95–100, 1986.

51. Buynak EB, Weibel RE, Whitman JE Jr, et al. Combined live measles, mumps, and rubella virus vaccines. JAMA 207:2259–2262, 1969.

52. Schwarz AJ, Jackson JE, Ehrenkranz NJ, et al. Clinical evaluation of a new measles-mumps-rubella vaccine. Am J Dis Child 129:1408–1412, 1975.

53. Just M, Berger R, Gluck R, et al. Evaluation of a combined vaccine against measles-mumps-rubella produced on human diploid cells. Dev Biol Stand 65:25–27, 1986.

54. Berger R, Just M. Interference between strains in live virus vaccines. II: combined vaccination with varicella and measles-mumps-rubella vaccine. J Biol Stand 16:275–279, 1988.

55. Francis TM Jr, Napier JA, Voight RB, et al. Evaluation of the 1954 Field Trial of Poliomyelitis Vaccine (Final Report). Ann Arbor, University of Michigan, 1957.

56. Cohen H, Nagel J. Two injections of diphtheria-tetanus-pertussis-polio vaccine as the backbone of a simplified immunization schedule in developing countries. Rev Infect Dis 6(suppl):S350–S351, 1984.

57. van Wezel AL, van Steenis G, van der Marel P, et al. Inactivated poliovirus vaccine: current production methods and new developments. Rev Infect Dis 6(suppl):S335–S340, 1984.

58. Salk J. One-dose immunization against paralytic poliomyelitis using a noninfectious vaccine. Rev Infect Dis 6(suppl):S444–S450, 1984.

59. Bordt DE, Whalen JW, Boyer PA, et al. Poliomyelitis component in quadruple antigen. JAMA 174:1166–1169, 1960.

60. Qureshi AW, Zulfiqar I, Raza A, et al. Comparison of immunogenicity of combined DPT-inactivated injectable polio vaccine (DPT-IPV) and association of DPT and attenuated oral polio vaccine (DPT + OPV) in Pakistani children. J Pak Med Assoc 39:31–35, 1989.

61. Meschievitz C, Blatter M, Starr S, et al. Safety and immunogenicity of IPV only or a sequential schedule of IPV (given separately or in combination with DTP) followed by OPV [abstr H089]. In Abstracts of the 36th Interscience Conference on Antimicrobial Agents and Chemotherapy, New Orleans, September 15–18, 1996.

62. Ruuskanen O, Viljanen MK, Salmi TT, et al. DTP and DTP-inactivated polio vaccines: comparison of adverse reactions and IgG, IgM and IgA antibody responses to DTP. Acta Paediatr Scand 69:177–182, 1980.

63. Rumke HC, Schlumberger M, Floury B, et al. Serological evaluation of a simplified immunization schedule using quadruple DPT-polio vaccine in Burkina Faso. Vaccine 11:1113–1118, 1993.

64. Baker JD, Halperin SA, Edwards K, et al. Antibody response to Bordetella pertussis antigens after immunization with American and Canadian whole-cell vaccines. J Pediatr 121:523–527, 1992.

65. Halperin SA, Langley JM, Eastwood BJ. Effect of inactivated poliovirus vaccine on the antibody response to Bordetella pertussis antigens when combined with diphtheria-pertussis-tetanus vaccine. Clin Infect Dis 22:59–62, 1996.

66. Stojanov S, Liese JG, Bendjenana H, et al. Immunogenicity and safety of a trivalent tetanus, low-dose diphtheria, inactivated poliomyelitis booster compared with a standard tetanus, low-dose diphtheria booster at six to nine years of age. Pediatr Infect Dis J 19:516–521, 2000.

67. Laroche P, Barrand M, Wood SC, et al. The immunogenicity and safety of a new combined diphtheria, tetanus and poliomyelitis booster vaccine (Td-eIPV). Infection 27:49–56, 1999.

68. Ferreccio C, Clemens J, Avendano A, et al. The clinical and immunologic response of Chilean infants to Haemophilus influenzae type b polysaccharide-tetanus protein conjugate vaccine coadministered in the same syringe with diphtheria-tetanus toxoids-pertussis vaccine at two, four, and six months of age. Pediatr Infect Dis J 10:764–771, 1991.

69. Clemens JD, Ferreccio C, Levine M, et al. Impact of Haemophilus influenzae type b polysaccharide-tetanus conjugate vaccine on responses to concurrently administered diphtheria-tetanus-pertussis vaccine. JAMA 267:673–678, 1992.

70. Hoppenbrouwers K, Lagos R, Swennen B, et al. Safety and immunogenicity of an Haemophilus influenzae type b–tetanus toxoid conjugate (PRP-T) and diphtheria–tetanus–pertussis (DTP) combination vaccine administered in a dual-chamber syringe to infants in Belgium and Chile. Vaccine 16:921–927, 1998.

71. Watemberg N, Dagan R, Arbelli Y, et al. Safety and immunogenicity of Haemophilus type b–tetanus protein conjugate vaccine, mixed in the same syringe with diphtheria-tetanus-pertussis vaccine in young infants. Pediatr Infect Dis J 10:758–763, 1991.

72. Scheifele D, Bjornson G, Barreto L, et al. Controlled trial of Haemophilus influenzae type b diphtheria toxoid conjugate combined with diphtheria, tetanus, and pertussis vaccines, in 18-month-old children, including comparison of arm versus thigh injection. Vaccine 10:455–460, 1992.

73. Avendano A, Ferreccio C, Lagos R, et al. Haemophilus influenzae type b polysaccharide-tetanus protein conjugate vaccine does not depress serologic responses to diphtheria, tetanus, or pertussis antigens when coadministered in the same syringe with diphtheria-tetanus-pertussis vaccine at two, four, and six months of age. Pediatr Infect Dis J 12:638–643, 1993.

74. Scheifele D, Barreto L, Meekison W, et al. Can Haemophilus influenzae type b–tetanus toxoid conjugate vaccine be combined with diphtheria toxoid–pertussis vaccine–tetanus toxoid? Can Med Assoc J 149:1105–1112, 1993.

75. Gold R, Scheifele D, Barreto L, et al. Safety and immunogenicity of Haemophilus influenzae vaccine (tetanus toxoid conjugate) administered concurrently or combined with diphtheria and tetanus toxoids, pertussis vaccine and inactivated poliomyelitis vaccine to healthy infants at two, four, and six months of age. Pediatr Infect Dis J 13:348–355, 1994.

76. Kaplan SL, Lauer BA, Ward MA, et al. Immunogenicity and safety of Haemophilus influenzae type b–tetanus protein conjugate vaccine alone or mixed with diphtheria-tetanus-pertussis vaccine in infants. J Pediatr 124:323–327, 1994.

77. Miller MA, Meschievitz CK, Ballanco GA, et al. Safety and immunogenicity of PRP-T combined with DTP: excretion of capsular polysaccharide and antibody response in the immediate post-vaccination period. Pediatrics 95:522–527, 1995.

78. Begg NT, Miller E, Fairley CK, et al. Antibody responses and symptoms after DTP and either tetanus or diphtheria Haemophilus influenzae type b conjugate vaccines given for primary immunisation by separate or mixed injection. Vaccine 13:1547–1550, 1995.

79. Levine OS, Lagos R, Losonsky GA, et al. No adverse impact on protection against pertussis from combined administration of *Haemophilus influenzae* type b conjugate and diphtheria–tetanus toxoid–pertussis vaccines in the same syringe. J Infect Dis 174:1341–1344, 1996.

80. Dagan R, Botujansky C, Watemberg N, et al. Safety and immunogenicity in young infants of *Haemophilus* b–tetanus protein conjugate vaccine, mixed in the same syringe with diphtheria-tetanus-pertussis–enhanced inactivated poliovirus vaccine. Pediatr Infect Dis J 13:356–362, 1994.

81. Mulholland EK, Hoestermann A, Ward JI, et al. The use of *Haemophilus influenzae* type b–tetanus toxoid conjugate vaccine mixed with diphtheria-tetanus-pertussis vaccine in Gambian infants. Vaccine 14:905–909, 1996.

82. Bell F, Martin A, Blondeau C, et al. Combined diphtheria, tetanus, pertussis, and *Haemophilus influenzae* type b vaccines for primary immunisation. Arch Dis Child 75:298–303, 1996.

83. Langue J, Ethevenaux C, Champsaur A, et al. Safety and immunogenicity of *Haemophilus influenzae* type b–tetanus toxoid conjugate, presented in a dual-chamber syringe with diphtheria–tetanus–pertussis and inactivated poliomyelitis combination vaccine. Eur J Pediatr 158:717–722, 1999.

84. Araujo OO, Forleo-Neto E, Vespa GN. Associated or combined vaccination of Brazilian infants with a conjugate *Haemophilus influenzae* type b (Hib) vaccine, a diphtheria ± tetanus ± whole-cell pertussis vaccine and IPV or OPV elicits protective levels of antibodies against Hib. Vaccine 19:367–375, 2001.

85. Coulehan JL, Hallowell C, Michaels RH, et al. Immunogenicity of a *Haemophilus influenzae* type b vaccine in combination with diphtheria-pertussis-tetanus vaccine in infants. J Infect Dis 148:530–534, 1983.

86. Eskola J, Kayhty H, Gordon LK, et al. Simultaneous administration of *Haemophilus influenzae* type b capsular polysaccharide-diphtheria toxoid conjugate vaccine with routine diphtheria-tetanus-pertussis and inactivated poliovirus vaccinations of childhood. Pediatr Infect Dis J 7:480–484, 1988.

87. Mulholland EK, Ahonkhai VI, Greenwood AM, et al. Safety and immunogenicity of *Haemophilus influenzae* type b–*Neisseria meningitidis* group B outer membrane protein complex conjugate vaccine mixed in the syringe with diphtheria-tetanus-pertussis vaccine in young Gambian infants. Pediatr Infect Dis J 12:632–637, 1993.

88. Paradiso PR, Hogerman DA, Madore DV, et al. Safety and immunogenicity of a combined diphtheria, tetanus, pertussis and *Haemophilus influenzae* type b vaccine in young infants. Pediatrics 92:827–832, 1993.

89. Paradiso PR. Combination vaccines for diphtheria, tetanus, pertussis, and *Haemophilus influenzae* type b. Ann N Y Acad Sci 754:108–113, 1995.

90. Black SB, Shinefield HR, Ray P, et al. Safety of combined oligosaccharide conjugate *Haemophilus influenzae* type b (HbOC) and whole cell diphtheria-tetanus toxoids-pertussis vaccine in infancy. Pediatr Infect Dis J 12:981–985, 1993.

91. Jones IG, Tyrrell H, Hill A, et al. Randomised controlled trial of combined diphtheria, tetanus, whole-cell pertussis vaccine administered in the same syringe and separately with *Haemophilus influenzae* type b vaccine at two, three, and four months of age. Vaccine 16:109–113, 1998.

92. Asensi-Botet F, Viviani S, Veronese A, et al. Safety, tolerability, and immunogenicity of a combined DTPHIB (diphtheria, tetanus, pertussis, *Haemophilus influenzae* type B-CRM$_{197}$ conjugate full liquid) vaccine [poster 12-PT291]. Presented at the 23rd International Congress of Pediatrics, Beijing, China, September 2001.

93. Carlsson RM, Claesson BA, Iwarson S, et al. Studies on a Hib conjugate vaccine (PRP-T): the effects of coadministered tetanus toxoid vaccine, combined administration with injectable polio vaccine, and administration route [abstr G74]. *In* Abstracts of the 35th Interscience Conference on Antimicrobial Agents and Chemotherapy, San Francisco, September 17–20, 1995.

94. Mills E, Gold R, Thipphawong J, et al. Safety and immunogenicity of a combined five-component pertussis-diphtheria-tetanus-inactivated poliomyelitis-*Haemophilus* b conjugate vaccine administered to infants at two, four, and six months of age. Vaccine 16:576–585, 1998.

95. Amir J, Melamed R, Bader J, et al. Immunogenicity and safety of a liquid combination of DT-PRP-T versus lyophilized PRP-T reconstituted with DTP. Vaccine 15:149–154, 1997.

96. Scheifele DW, Meekison W, Guasparini R, et al. Evaluation of booster doses of *Haemophilus influenzae* type b–tetanus toxoid conjugate vaccine in 18-month-old children. Vaccine 13:104–108, 1995.

97. Langue J, Fritzell B, Preziozi MP, et al. Evaluation de la vaccination des enfants de 3 mois avec le polyoside capsulaire d'Haemophilus influenzae type B (Hib) conjugé à la toxine tétanique (PRP-T). Pediatrie 46:821–824, 1991.

98. Kanra G, Yurdakok K, Ceyhan M, et al. Immunogenicity and safety of *Haemophilus influenzae* type b capsular polysaccharide tetanus conjugate vaccine (PRP-T) presented in a dual-chamber syringe with DTP. Acta Paediatr Jpn 39:676–678, 1997.

99. Gylca R, Gylca V, Benes O. A new DTPa-HBV-IPV vaccine co-administered with Hib, compared to a commercially available DTPw-IPV:Hib vaccine co-administered with HBV, given at 6, 10, and 14 weeks following HBV at birth. Vaccine 19:825–833, 2001.

100. Hoppenbrouwers K, Roelants M, Ethevenaux C, et al. The effect of reconstitution of an *Haemophilus influenzae* type b-tetanus toxoid conjugate (PRP-T) vaccine on the immune responses to a diphtheria-tetanus-whole cell pertussis (DTwP) vaccine: a five-year follow-up. Vaccine 17:2588–2598, 1999.

101. Vidor E, Hoffenbach A, Fletcher MA. *Haemophilus influenzae* type b vaccine: reconstitution of lyophilised PRP-T vaccine with a pertussis-containing paediatric combination vaccine, or a change in the primary series immunisation schedule, may modify the serum anti-PRP antibody responses. Curr Med Res Opin 17:197–209, 2001.

102. Lagos R, Horwitz I, Toro J, et al. Large scale, postlicensure, selective vaccination of Chilean infants with PRP-T conjugate vaccine: practicality and effectiveness in preventing invasive *Haemophilus influenzae* type b infections. Pediatr Infect Dis J 15:216–222, 1996.

103. Scheifele DW. Recent trends in pediatric *Haemophilus influenzae* type b infections in Canada. Immunization Monitoring Program, Active (IMPACT) of the Canadian Paediatric Society and the Laboratory Centre for Disease Control. Can Med Assoc J 154:1041–1047, 1996.

104. Scheifele D, Gold R, Marchessault V, et al. Failures after immunization with *Haemophilus influenzae* type b vaccines—1991–1995. Can Commun Dis Rep 22:17–20, 1996.

105. Centers for Disease Control and Prevention. Summary of notifiable diseases, United States, 1996. MMWR 45:73, 1996.

106. Black S, Shinefield H, Ray P, et al. Safety and immunogenicity of combined DTP-hepatitis B-PRP-T vaccine (DTPHH) (SmithKline Beecham) in infants [abstr G73]. *In* Abstracts of the 35th Interscience Conference on Antimicrobial Agents and Chemotherapy, San Francisco, September 17–20, 1995.

107. Poovorawan Y, Theamboonlers A, Sanpavat S, et al. Comparison study of combined DTPw-HB vaccines and separate administration of DTPw and HB vaccines in Thai children. Asian Pac J Allergy Immunol 17:113–120, 1999.

108. Prikazsky V, Bock HL. Higher anti-hepatitis b response with combined DTPw-HBV vaccine compared with separate administration in healthy infants at 3, 4, and 5 months of age in Slovakia. Int J Clin Pract 55:156–161, 2001.

109. Win KM, Aye M, Htay-Htay H, et al. Comparison of separate and mixed administration of DTPw-HBV and Hib vaccines: immunogenicity and reactogenicity profiles. Int J Infect Dis 2:79–84, 1997.

110. Santos JI, Martin A, De Leon T, et al. DTPw-HB and Hib primary and booster vaccination: combined versus separate administration to Latin American children. Vaccine 20:1887–1893, 2002.

111. Ramkissoon A, Coovadia HM, Jugnundan P, et al. Antibody responses and safety following a pentavalent vaccine: combined DTP-hepatitis B–*Haemophilus influenzae* type b (Hib) at 2, 4, and 6 months of age [abstract]. *In* Abstracts of the Seventh International Congress for Infectious Diseases, Hong Kong, June 10–13, 1996, p 72.

112. Riedemann S, Reinhardt G, Jara J, et al. Reactogenicity and immunogenicity of a diphtheria-tetanus-pertussis-hepatitis B and *Haemophilus influenzae* type B vaccine (DTPw-HBV-Hib) versus separately administered DTPw-HBV and Hib vaccines in infants [abstract]. J Paediatr Child Health 33(suppl 1):S121, 1997.

113. Papaevangelou G, Karvelis E, Alexiou D, et al. Evaluation of a combined tetravalent diphtheria, tetanus, whole-cell pertussis and hepatitis B candidate vaccine administered to healthy infants according to a three-dose vaccination schedule. Vaccine 13:175–178, 1995.

114. Usonis V, Bakasenas V, Taylor D, Vandepapeliere P. Immunogenicity and reactogenicity of a combined DTPw-hepatitis B vaccine in Lithuanian infants. Eur J Pediatr 155:189–193, 1996.

115. Aristegui J, Garrote E, Gonzalez A, et al. Immune response to a combined hepatitis B, diphtheria, tetanus and whole-cell pertussis

vaccine administered to infants at 2, 4, and 6 months of age. Vaccine 15:7–9, 1997.

116. Diez-Delgado J, Dal-Re R, Llorente M, et al. Hepatitis B component does not interfere with the immune response to diphtheria, tetanus, and whole-cell *Bordetella pertussis* components of a quadrivalent (DTPw-HB) vaccine: a controlled trial in healthy infants. Vaccine 15:1418–1422, 1997.

117. Riedemann S, Reinhardt G, Jara J, et al. Immunogenicity and reactogenicity of combined versus separately administered DTPw-HBV and Hib vaccines given to healthy infants at 2, 4, and 6 months of age, with a booster at 18 months. Int J Infect Dis 6:215–222, 2002.

118. Nolan T, Hogg G, Darcy M-A, et al. 18m booster immunogenicity and reactogenicity in infants immunised with a combination DTPw-Hib-hepatitis B vaccine [abstr 751]. *In* Abstracts of the 1997 Pediatric Academic Societies' Annual Meeting, Washington, DC, May 1997.

119. Mérieux C, Triau R, Ajjan N, et al. Vaccination quintuple: association du vaccin rougeole hyperattenue (Schwarz) avec le vaccin antidiphtherique, antitetanique, anticoquelucheux adsorbe et antipoliomyelitique inactive. Rev Pediatr 9:79–84, 1973.

120. McIntyre RC, Preblud SR, Polloi A, et al. Measles and measles vaccine efficacy in a remote island population. Bull World Health Organ 60:767–775, 1982.

121. John TJ, Selvakumar R. Mixing measles vaccine with DPT and DPTP. Lancet 1:1154, 1985.

122. John TJ, Selvakumar R, Balrai V, et al. Antibody response to measles vaccine with DTPP. Am J Dis Child 141:14, 1987.

123. Simoes EAF, Balraj V, Selvakumar R, et al. Antibody response of children to measles vaccine mixed with diphtheria-pertussis-tetanus or diphtheria-pertussis-tetanus-poliomyelitis vaccine. Am J Dis Child 142:309–311, 1988.

124. Olin P. Whooping cough is declining, but the risk for small infants has not been reduced. Smittskydd 8:8–9, 2002.

125. Storsaeter J. DTPa vaccination: continued high field effectiveness in Sweden [abstr S-11]. *In* Abstracts of the 18th Annual Meeting of the European Society for Paediatr Infectious Diseases, Noordwijk, the Netherlands, May 3–5, 2000.

126. Halperin SA, Davies HD, Barreto L, et al. Safety and immunogenicity of two inactivated poliovirus vaccines in combination with an acellular pertussis vaccine and diphtheria and tetanus toxoids in seventeen- to nineteen-month-old infants. J Pediatr 130:525–531, 1997.

127. David T, Cadoz M, Gobert P, et al. Acellular pertussis vaccine combined with diphtheria and tetanus toxoids and inactivated polio vaccine (AcPDT IPV): comparison to a DTP-IPV with a whole cell pertussis component (WcPDT IPV) in infants [abstr 60]. *In* Abstracts of the 31st Interscience Conference on Antimicrobial Agents and Chemotherapy, Chicago, September 29–October 2, 1991.

128. Lagos R, Kotloff K, Hoffenbach A, et al. Clinical response to pentavalent parenteral diphtheria, tetanus, acellular pertussis (DTaP), inactivated polio (eIPV) and *Haemophilus influenzae* b (Hib) conjugate vaccine in 2, 4, and 6 month old Chilean infants [abstr 609]. *In* Abstracts of the 35th Annual Meeting of the Infectious Diseases Society of America, San Francisco, September, 1997.

129. Lagos R, Kotloff K, Hoffenbach A, et al. Clinical acceptability and immunogenicity of a pentavalent parenteral combination vaccine containing diphtheria, tetanus, acellular pertussis, inactivated poliomyelitis, and *Haemophilus influenzae* type b conjugate antigens in two-, four-, and six-month-old Chilean infants. Pediatr Infect Dis J 17:294–304, 1998.

130. Eskola J, Olander RM, Hovi T, et al. Randomised trial of the effect of co-administration with acellular pertussis DTP vaccine on immunogenicity of *Haemophilus influenzae* type b conjugate vaccine. Lancet 348:1688–1692, 1996.

131. Eskola J, Litmanen L, Saarinen L, et al. Responses at 24 months to a combined DTaP-Hib conjugate vaccine in children vaccinated with the same vaccines at 4 and 6 months [abstr G060]. *In* Abstracts of the 36th Interscience Conference on Antimicrobial Agents and Chemotherapy, New Orleans, September 15–18, 1996.

132. Hronowski L, Rohrbaugh J, Prebula R, et al. Immunogenicity of a new *Haemophilus influenzae* type b polysaccharide–tetanus toxoid (Hib-TT) conjugate vaccine and the immunogenicities of the individual components in the pentavalent Hib-TT + DTaP + IPV vaccine [abstr E78]. *In* Abstracts of the 93rd General Meeting of the American Society for Microbiology, Washington, DC, 1993.

133. Gyhrs AG, Olsen A, Petersen JV, et al. T-cell immunity in children vaccinated with hydrogen peroxide detoxified PT in a DTaP-IPV combination vaccine [abstr E92]. *In* Abstracts of the 95th General Meeting of the American Society for Microbiology, San Francisco, September 1995.

134. Gyhrs A, Lyngholm E, Larsen SO, et al. Safety and immunogenicity of a tetravalent diphtheria-tetanus-acellular pertussis-inactivated poliovirus vaccine. Scand J Infect Dis 31:579–585, 1999.

135. Halperin SA, Smith B, Russell M, et al. Adult formulation of a five component acellular pertussis vaccine combined with diphtheria and tetanus toxoids and inactivated poliovirus vaccine is safe and immunogenic in adolescents and adults. Pediatr Infect Dis J 19:276–283, 2000.

136. Rennels MB, Englund JA, Bernstein DI, et al. Diminution of the anti-polyribosylribitol phosphate response to a combined diphtheria-tetanus-acellular pertussis *Haemophilus influenzae* type b vaccine by concurrent inactivated poliovirus vaccination. Pediatr Infect Dis J 19:417–423, 2000.

137. Daum RS, Zenko CE, Given GZ, et al. Absence of a significant interaction between a *Haemophilus influenzae* conjugate vaccine combined with a diphtheria toxoid, tetanus toxoid and acellular pertussis vaccine in the same syringe and inactivated polio vaccine. Pediatr Infect Dis J 19:710–717, 2000.

138. Kanra G, Ceyhan M, Ecevit Z, et al. Primary vaccination of infants with a combined diphtheria-tetanus-acellular pertussis-hepatitis B vaccine. Pediatr Infect Dis J 14:998–1000, 1995.

139. Usonis V, Bakasenas V, Willems P, et al. Feasibility study of a combined diphtheria-tetanus-acellular pertussis-hepatitis B (DTPa-HBV) vaccine, and comparison of clinical reactions and immune responses with diphtheria-tetanus-acellular pertussis (DTPa) and hepatitis B vaccines applied as mixed or injected into separate limbs. Vaccine 15:1680–1686, 1997.

140. Giammanco G, Moiraghi A, Zotti C, et al. Safety and immunogenicity of a combined diphtheria-tetanus-acellular pertussis-hepatitis B vaccine administered according to two different primary vaccination schedules. Vaccine 16:722–726, 1998.

141. Greenberg DP, Wong VK, Partridge S, et al. Safety and immunogenicity of a combination diphtheria-tetanus toxoids-acellular pertussis-hepatitis B vaccine administered at two, four, and six months of age compared with monovalent hepatitis B vaccine administered at birth, one month, and six months of age. Pediatr Infect Dis J 21:769–777, 2002.

142. Andre F. The way forward—combined vaccines [abstr SD5]. *In* Extended Abstracts from the 9th Triennial International Symposium on Viral Hepatitis and Liver Disease, Rome, 1996.

143. Yeh SH, Ward JI, Partridge S, et al. Safety and immunogenicity of a pentavalent diphtheria, tetanus, pertussis, hepatitis B, and polio combination vaccine in infants. Pediatr Infect Dis J 20:973–980, 2001.

144. Usonis V, Bakasenas V. Does concomitant injections of a combined diphtheria-tetanus-acellular pertussis-hepatitis B, virus-inactivated polio virus vaccine influence the reactogenicity and immunogenicity of commercial *Haemophilus influenzae* type b conjugate vaccine? Eur J Pediatr 158:398–402, 1999.

145. Schmitt HJ, Knuf M, Beutel K, et al. Antibody persistence, PRP-specific immune memory and booster response in children primed with a new combination vaccine DTPa-HBV-IPV given as either a mixed or separate injection [abstract]. *In* Abstracts of the 18th Annual Meeting of the European Society for Paediatric Infectious Diseases, Noordwijk, the Netherlands, May 3–5, 2000, pp 37–38.

146. Infanrix Hexa: European Public Assessment Report, Revision 1. London, European Agency for the Evaluation of Medicinal Products, January 15, 2002. Available at *www.eudra.org/human-docs/humans/EPAR/Infanrixhexa/infanrixhexa*.

147. Zepp F, Schuind A, Meyer C, et al. Reactogenicity of a new pentavalent combination, DTPa-HBV-IPV administered with Hib vaccine, in comparison with widely used commercial vaccines, in 5,472 subjects [abstract]. *In* Abstracts of the 17th Annual Meeting of the European Society for Paediatric Infectious Diseases, Crete, Greece, May 1999, p 72.

148. Zepp F, Knuf M, Schuerman L, et al. A combined DTPa-HBV-IPV for use (as a fourth dose) in the second year of life [abstract]. *In* Proceedings of the 37th Annual Meeting of the Infectious Diseases Society of America, Philadelphia, November 18–21, 1999, p 155.

149. PEDIARIX Prescribing Information. Philadelphia: SmithKline Beecham Pharmaceuticals, December 2002, pp 17–18.

150. Kovel A, Wald ER, Guerra N, et al. Safety and immunogenicity of acellular diphtheria-tetanus-pertussis and *Haemophilus* conjugate vaccines given in combination or at separate injection sites. J Pediatr 120:84–87, 1992.

151. Product Information: TriHIBit. *In* Physician's Desk Reference. Montvale, NJ, Medical Economics, 1998, pp 2138–2142.

152. Shinefield H, Black S, Adelman T, et al. Safety and immunogenicity of DTaP-HbOC—a combined oligosaccharide conjugate (HbOC, HibTITER) *Haemophilus influenzae* type b and acellular DTP vaccine (DTaP) in toddlers [abstr 306]. *In* Abstracts of the 32nd Interscience Conference on Antimicrobial Agents and Chemotherapy, Anaheim, CA, October 11–14, 1992.

153. Rennels M, Hohenboken M, Reisinger K, et al. Comparison of acellular pertussis-diphtheria-tetanus toxoids and *Haemophilus influenzae* type b vaccines administered separately versus combined in younger versus older toddlers. Ped Infect Dis J 17:164–166, 1998.

154. Liese JG, Harzer E, Hosbach P, et al. Immunogenicity of a combined DTaP-PRP-D conjugate vaccine compared to separate injections in infants [abstr G106]. *In* Abstracts of the 36th Interscience Conference on Antimicrobial Agents and Chemotherapy, New Orleans, September 15–18, 1996.

155. Liese JG, Harzer E, Hosbach P, et al. Hib antibody response of a combined DTaP-PRP-T conjugate vaccine compared to separate injections in infants [abstr G105]. *In* Abstracts of the 36th Interscience Conference on Antimicrobial Agents and Chemotherapy, New Orleans, September 15–18, 1996.

156. Hoppenbrouwers K, Kanra G, Silier T, et al. Priming effect of the combined DTaP/Act-HIB vaccine [abstr 73]. *In* Abstracts of the 15th Annual Meeting of the European Society for Paediatric Infectious Diseases, Paris, May 1997.

157. Pichichero ME, Latiolais T, Bernstein DI, et al. Vaccine antigen interactions after a combination diphtheria–tetanus toxoid–acellular pertussis/purified capsular polysaccharide of *Haemophilus influenzae* type b–tetanus toxoid vaccine in two-, four-, and six-month-old infants. Pediatr Infect Dis J 16:863–870, 1997.

158. Schmitt HJ. Immunogenicity and reactogenicity of 2 Hib tetanus conjugate vaccines administered by reconstituting with DTaP or given as separate injections [abstr G63]. *In* Abstracts of the 35th Interscience Conference on Antimicrobial Agents and Chemotherapy, San Francisco, September 17–20, 1995.

159. Schmitt HJ, Zepp F, Muschenborn S, et al. Immunogenicity and reactogenicity of a *Haemophilus influenzae* type b tetanus conjugate vaccine when administered separately or mixed with concomitant DTPa primary and booster immunizations. Eur J Pediatr 157:208–214, 1998.

160. Shinefield H, Black S, Ray P, et al. Safety of combined acellular pertussis DTaP-HbOC vaccine (Lederle-Praxis) in infants [abstr G72]. *In* Abstracts of the 36th Interscience Conference on Antimicrobial Agents and Chemotherapy, New Orleans, September 15–18, 1996.

161. Lee CY, Thipphawong J, Huang LM, et al. An evaluation of the safety and immunogenicity of a five-component acellular pertussis, diphtheria, and tetanus toxoid vaccine (DTaP) when combined with a *Haemophilus influenzae* type b–tetanus toxoid conjugate vaccine (PRP-T) in Taiwanese infants. Pediatrics 103:25–30, 1999.

162. Begue P, Stagnara J, Vie-Le-Sage F, et al. Immunogenicity and reactogenicity of a booster dose of diphtheria, tetanus, acellular pertussis and inactivated poliomyelitis vaccines given concurrently with *Haemophilus* type b conjugate vaccine or as pentavalent vaccine. Pediatr Infect Dis J 16:787–794, 1997.

163. Thipphawong J, Baretto L, Mills E, et al. A fully-liquid, acellular pertussis vaccine combined with IPV and Hib vaccines (DTaP-IPV-PRP-T) is safe and immunogenic without significant interactions (Workshop W3E). *In* Abstracts of the International Conference on Acute Respiratory Infections, Canberra, Australia, July 7–10, 1997.

164. Mills E, Russell M, Cunning L, et al. A fully liquid acellular pertussis vaccine combined with IPV and Hib vaccines (DTaP-IPV-PRP-T) is safe and immunogenic without significant interaction [abstr G95]. *In* Abstracts of the 37th Interscience Conference on Antimicrobial Agents and Chemotherapy, Toronto, September 28–October 1, 1997.

165. Knutsson N, Trollfors B, Taranger J, et al. Immunogenicity and reactogenicity of diphtheria, tetanus, and pertussis toxoids combined with inactivated polio vaccine, when administered concomitantly with or as a diluent for a Hib conjugate vaccine. Vaccine 19:4396–4403, 2001.

166. Langue J, David T, Roussel F, et al. Safety and immunogenicity of DTaP-IPV and Act-HIB vaccines administered either combined or separately to infants at 2, 3, and 4 months of age [abstr 79]. *In* Abstracts of the 15th Annual Meeting of the European Society for Paediatric Infectious Diseases, Paris, May 1997.

167. Hoffenbach A, Langue J, Mallet E, et al. Influence of combining DTaP-IPV and Act-HIB vaccines and of changing the primary immunization schedule on the antibody response to *Haemophilus influenzae* type b [abstr 80]. In Abstracts of the 15th Annual Meeting of the European Society for Paediatric Infectious Diseases, Paris, May 1997.

168. Mallet E, Fabre P, Pines E, et al. Immunogenicity and safety of a new liquid hexavalent combined vaccine compared with separate administration of reference licensed vaccines in infants. Pediatr Infect Dis J 19:1119–1127, 2000.

169. Zepp F, Schuind A, Habermehl P, et al. Evolution of combination vaccines: comparison of two candidate vaccines with licensed vaccine [abstract]. *In* Abstracts of the 18th Annual Meeting of the European Society for Pediatric Infectious Diseases, Noordwijk, the Netherlands, May 3–5, 2000, pp 38–39.

170. Blatter MM, Reisinger KS, Terwelp DR, et al. Immunogenicity of a combined diphtheria, tetanus, acellular pertussis (DT-tricomponent Pa)–hepatitis B (HB)–inactivated poliovirus (IPV) admixed with *Haemophilus influenzae* type B (Hib) vaccine in infants. Pediatr Res 43(4, pt 2):141A, 1998.

171. Schmitt HJ, Knuf M, Ortiz E, et al. Primary vaccination of infants with diphtheria-tetanus-acellular pertussis-hepatitis B virus-inactivated polio virus and *Haemophilus influenzae* type b vaccines given as either separate or mixed injections. J Pediatr 137:304–312, 2000.

172. Cohen R, Ortiz E, Wollaert L, et al. Final Study Report for Clinical Trial 217744/025: DTPa-HBV-IPV-025. Rixensart, Belgium, GlaxoSmithKline Biologicals, 1999.

173. Avdicova M, Prikazsky V, Willems P, et al. A novel DTPa-HBV-IPV/Hib combined vaccine compared to concomitant administration of licensed vaccines given at 3, 5, 11 months of age: antibody persistence and response to final dose [abstract]. *In* Abstracts of the 18th Annual Meeting of the European Society for Pediatric Infectious Diseases, Noordwijk, the Netherlands, May 3–5, 2000, pp 36–37.

174. Hogerman D, Malinoski FJ, Madore DV, et al. Safety and immunogenicity of DTaP-HbOC in toddlers primed by DTP and HbOC as separate injections or DTP-HbOC combination vaccine. Pediatr Res 33:171A, 1993.

175. Daum RS, Zenko CE, Given GZ, et al. Magnitude of interference after diphtheria-tetanus toxoids–acellular pertussis/*Haemophilus influenzae* type b capsular polysaccharide–tetanus vaccination is related to the number of doses administered. J Infect Dis 184:1293–1299, 2001.

176. Bell F, Heath P, Shackley F, et al. Effect of reconstitution with an acellular pertussis, diphtheria, tetanus vaccine on antibody response to Hib vaccine (PRP-T) [abstr 69]. In Abstracts of the 15th Annual Meeting of the European Society for Paediatric Infectious Diseases, Paris, May 1997.

177. Bell F, Heath P, Shackley F, et al. Immunological memory to Hib following combined acellular pertussis, diphtheria, tetanus/Hib vaccine. Presented at the Paediatric Research Society Meeting, Sheffield, England, September 1997.

178. Mallet E, Hoffenbach A, Salomon H, et al. Primary immunization with combined, acellular DTaP-IPV-Act-HIB vaccine given at 2-3-4 or 2-4-6 months of age [abstr 19]. *In* Abstracts of the 14th Annual Meeting of the European Society for Paediatric Infectious Diseases, Elsinore, Denmark, May 1996.

179. Mallet E, Hoffenbach A, Pines E, et al. Immunogenicity of the fourth dose of a combined DTaP-IPV/Act-HIB vaccine administered at 15 months of age to children primed either at 2, 3, and 4 or at 2, 4, and 6 months of age [abstr 81]. *In* Abstracts of the 15th Annual Meeting of the European Society for Paediatric Infectious Diseases, Paris, May 1997.

180. Carlsson RM, Claesson BA, Selstam U, et al. Safety and immunogenicity of a combined diphtheria-tetanus-acellular pertussis-inactivated polio vaccine–*Haemophilus influenzae* type b vaccine administered at 2-4-6-13 or 3-5-12 months of age. Pediatr Infect Dis J 17(11):1026–1033, 1998.

181. Slack MH, Schapira D, Thwaites RJ, et al. Immune response of premature infants to meningococcal serogroup C and combined diphtheria-tetanus toxoids-acellular pertussis–*Haemophilus influenzae* type b conjugate vaccine. J Infect Dis 184:1617–1620, 2001.

182. Meyer CU, Schmidtke P, Habermehl P, et al. Mixed administration of DTaP/Hib vaccine has no impact on the generation of pertussis-specific cell-mediated immune (CMI) responses [abstr 585]. *In* Abstracts of the 35th Annual Meeting of the Infectious Diseases Society of America, San Francisco, September 17–20, 1997.

183. Zepp F, Meyer CU, Schmidtke P, et al. Established pertussis-specific T-cellular immune responses remain stable after vaccination with multivalent DTPa-Hib combination vaccines [abstr 699 Fr]. *In* Abstracts of the 36th Annual Meeting of the Infectious Diseases Society of America, Denver, 1998.

184. Dagan R, Agbaria K, Piglansky L, et al. Immunogenicity of a combined diphtheria, tetanus, acellular pertussis, inactivated poliovirus and *H. influenzae* type b–tetanus conjugate vaccine (DTPa-IPV-Hib) in infants [abstr G59]. *In* Abstracts of the 36th Interscience Conference on Antimicrobial Agents and Chemotherapy, New Orleans, September 15–18, 1996.

185. Dagan R, Igbaria K, Piglansky L, et al. Safety and immunogenicity of a combined pentavalent diphtheria, tetanus, acellular pertussis, inactivated poliovirus and *Haemophilus influenzae* type b–tetanus conjugate vaccine in infants, compared with a whole cell pertussis pentavalent vaccine. Pediatr Infect Dis J 16:1113–1121, 1997.

186. Halperin SA, King J, Law B, et al. Safety and immunogenicity of *Haemophilus influenzae*–tetanus toxoid conjugate vaccine given separately or in combination with three-component acellular pertussis vaccine combined with diphtheria and tetanus toxoids and inactivated poliovirus vaccine for the first four doses. Clin Infect Dis 28:995–1001, 1999.

187. Dagan R, Amir J, Ashkenazi S, et al. Early response to nonconjugated polyribosylribitol phospate challenge as evidence of immune memory after combined diphtheria-tetanus-pertussis-polio-*Haemophilus influenzae* type b primary vaccination. Pediatr Infect Dis J 20:587–592, 2001.

188. Zepp F, Meyer CU, Kowalzol F, et al. Evaluation of the immunological memory induced by primary vaccination with *Haemophilus influenzae* type b (Hib) tetanus conjugate vaccine co-administered with various DTPa-based vaccines [abstract]. *In* Abstracts of the 39th Interscience Conference on Antimicrobial Agents and Chemotherapy, San Francisco, September 26–29, 1999.

189. Schmitt HJ, Von Kries R, Hassenpflug B, et al. *Haemophilus influenzae* type b disease: impact and effectiveness of diphtheria-tetanus toxoids-acellular pertussis (-inactivated poliovirus)/*H. influenzae* type b combination vaccines. Pediatr Infect Dis J 20:767–774, 2001.

190. Kalies H, Meyer N, Siedler A, Schmitt HJ, von Kries R. Effectiveness of DTPa/HIB and DTPa-IPV/HIB combination vaccines in Germany: four-year follow-up. 21st Annual Meeting of the European Society for Paediatric Infectious Diseases (ESPID), April 2003, Taormina, Sicily, Abstract 298.

191. Kalies H, Heinrich B, Weissmann B, Siedler A, Schmitt HJ, von Kries R. No increase of systemic *Haemophilus influenzae* type b (Hib) infections in Germany after the introduction of hexavalent DTaP-IPV-HB combination vaccines. 21st Annual Meeting of the European Society for Paediatric Infectious Diseases (ESPID), April 2003, Taormina, Sicily, Abstract 190.

192. Trotter CL, McVernon J, Andrews NJ, et al. Antibody to *Haemophilus influenzae* type b after routine and catch-up vaccination. Lancet 361:1523–1524, 2003.

193. McVernon J, Andrews N, Slack MPE, Ramsay ME. Risk of vaccine failure after *Haemophilus influenzae* type b (Hib) combination vaccines with acellular pertussis. Lancet 361:1521–1523, 2003.

194. Decker MD, Edwards KM, Bradley R, et al. Comparative trial in infants of four conjugate *Haemophilus influenzae* type b vaccines. J Pediatr 120:184–189, 1992.

195. Greenberg DP, Lieberman JM, Marcy SM, et al. Enhanced antibody responses in infants given different sequences of heterogeneous *Haemophilus influenzae* type b conjugate vaccines. J Pediatr 126:206–211, 1995.

196. Capeding MR, Nohynek H, Pascual LG, et al. The immunogenicity of three *Haemophilus influenzae* type b conjugate vaccines after a primary vaccination series in Philippine infants. Am J Trop Med Hyg 55:516–520, 1996.

197. Kayhty H, Eskola J, Peltola H, et al. Antibody response to four *Haemophilus influenzae* type b conjugate vaccines. Am J Dis Child 145:223–227, 1991.

198. Peltola H. *Haemophilus influenzae* type b disease and vaccination in Europe: lessons learned. Pediatr Infect Dis J 17(9 suppl):S126–132, 1998.

199. *Haemophilus influenzae* type b disease control using Pentacel, Canada, 1998–1999. Can Commun Dis Rep 26:93–96, 2000.

200. Progress toward elimination of *Haemophilus influenzae* type b invasive disease among infants and children—United States, 1998–2000. MMWR 51:234–237, 2002.

201. Kayhty H, Peltola H, Karanko V, et al. The protective level of serum antibodies to the capsular polysaccharide of *Haemophilus influenzae* type b. J Infect Dis 147:1100, 1983.

202. Anderson P. The protective level of serum antibodies to the capsular polysaccharide of *Haemophilus influenzae* type b. J Infect Dis 149:1034, 1984.

203. Ward J, Brenneman G, Letson GW, et al. Limited efficacy of a *Haemophilus influenzae* type b conjugate vaccine in Alaska Native infants. The Alaska *H. influenzae* Vaccine Study Group. N Engl J Med 323:1393–1401, 1990.

204. Jonsdottir KE, Steingrimsson O, Olaffsson O. Immunisation of infants in Iceland against *Haemophilus influenzae* type b. Lancet 340:252–253, 1992.

205. Peltola H, Aavitsland P, Hansen KG, et al. Perspective: a five-country analysis of the impact of four different *Haemophilus influenzae* type b conjugates and vaccination strategies in Scandinavia. J Infect Dis 179:223–229, 1999.

206. Fernandez J, Levine OS, Sanchez J, et al. Prevention of *Haemophilus influenzae* type b colonization by vaccination: correlation with serum anti-capsular IgG concentration. J Infect Dis 182:1553–1556, 2000.

207. Kauppi M, Eskola J, Kayhty H. Anti-capsular polysaccharide antibody concentrations in saliva after immunization with *Haemophilus influenzae* type b conjugate vaccines. Pediatr Infect Dis J 14:286–294, 1995.

208. Galil K, Singleton R, Levine OS, et al. Reemergence of invasive *Haemophilus influenzae* type b disease in a well-vaccinated population in remote Alaska. J Infect Dis 179:101–106, 1999.

209. Greenberg DP, Wong VK, Partridge S, et al. Evaluation of a new combination vaccine that incorporates diphtheria-tetanus-acellular pertussis (DTaP), hepatitis B (HB) and *Haemophilus influenzae* type b (Hib) conjugate (PRP-T) vaccines [abstr G70]. *In* Abstracts of the 35th Interscience Conference on Antimicrobial Agents and Chemotherapy, San Francisco, September 17–20, 1995.

210. Greenberg DP, Wong VK, Partridge S, et al. Immunogenicity of a booster dose of Hib conjugate vaccine in children with impaired immune responses following primary vaccination with DTaP-Hep B-PRP-T vaccine [abstr G061]. *In* Abstracts of the 36th Interscience Conference on Antimicrobial Agents and Chemotherapy, New Orleans, September 15–18, 1996.

211. Pichichero ME, Passador S. Administration of combined diphtheria and tetanus toxoids and pertussis vaccine, hepatitis B vaccine, and *Haemophilus influenzae* type b (Hib) vaccine to infants and response to a booster dose of Hib conjugate vaccine. Clin Infect Dis 25:1378–1384, 1997.

212. Schmitt HJ, Bock H, Bogaerts H, et al. Single injection of a combined DTPa-Hep B and Hib tetanus conjugate vaccine: a feasibility study [abstr G64]. *In* Abstracts of the 35th Interscience Conference on Antimicrobial Agents and Chemotherapy, San Francisco, September 17–20, 1995.

213. Zepp F, Schmitt HJ, Kaufhold A, et al. Evidence for induction of polysaccharide specific B-cell-memory in the 1st year of life: plain *Haemophilus influenzae* type b-PRP (Hib) boosts children primed with a tetanus-conjugate Hib-DTPa-HBV combined vaccine. Eur J Pediatr 156:18–24, 1997.

214. Aristégui J, Dal-Ré R, Garrote E, et al. Assessment of the immunogenicity and reactogenicity of a quadrivalent diphtheria, tetanus, acellular pertussis and hepatitis B (DTPa-HBV) vaccine administered in a single injection with *Haemophilus influenzae* type b conjugate vaccine, to infants at 2, 4, and 6 months of age. Vaccine 16:1976–1981, 1998.

215. Omeñaca F, Dal-Ré R, D'Apuzzo V et al. Reactogenicity of DTPa-HBV/Hib vaccine administered as a single injection vs DTPa-HBV and Hib vaccines administered simultaneously at separate sites, to infants at 2, 4, and 6 months of age. Vaccine 19:4260–4266, 2001.

216. Heininger U, Schuerman L. Evidence for pre-booster antibody persistence in an open randomised study on infants primed with DTPa-HBV-IPV/Hib or DTPa-IPV/Hib + HBV vaccines at 3, 4, 5 months of age [abstract]. *In* Abstracts of the 19th Annual Meeting of the European Society for Paediatric Infectious Diseases, Istanbul, Turkey, March 2001, p 10.

217. Product Information: Infanrix® Hexa. Rixensart, Belgium, SmithKline Beecham, 2001.

218. Blatter M, Pichichero M, Harrison C, et al. A combination DTPa-HepB-IPV/Hib vaccine administered to infants at 2,4, and 6 months of age with or without a hepatitis B vaccine birth dose [abstract]. *In* Abstracts of the 38th Annual Meeting of the Infectious Disease Society of America, New Orleans, September 2000, p 321.

219. Pichichero ME, Blatter MM, Reisinger KS, et al. Impact of a birth dose of hepatitis B vaccine on the reactogenicity and immunogenicity of diphtheria-tetanus-acellular pertussis-hepatitis B-inactivated poliovirus–*Haemophilus influenzae* type b combination vaccination. Pediatr Infect Dis J 21:854–859, 2002.

220. Cohen R, Schuerman L. Reactogenicity of a new DTPa-HBV-IPV (+&-Hib) vaccine after the primary and booster doses [abstract]. *In* Abstracts of the 18th Annual Meeting of the European Society for Paediatric Infectious Diseases, Noordwijk, the Netherlands, May 3–5, 2000, p 39.

221. Lagos R, Muñoz A, Fabre P, et al. Immunogenicity and safety of a new liquid hexavalent vaccine given at 2, 4, and 6 months of age [abstract]. *In* Abstracts of the 37th Annual Meeting of the Infectious Diseases Society of America, Philadelphia, November 18–21, 1999.

222. Liese JG, Stojanov S, Berut F, et al. Large scale safety study of a liquid hexavalent vaccine (D-T-acP-IPV-PRPT-HBs) given at 2, 4, 6, and 12 to 14 months of age. Vaccine 20:448–454, 2002.

223. Flodmark CE, Schödel L, Hessel L. Immunogenicity and safety of Hexavac administered to healthy Swedish infants at 3, 5, and 12 months of age. Presented at the Pediatric Infectious Diseases Society Conference, Monterey, CA, October 28–30, 2001.

224. Carriere JP, Giard P, Muller JM, et al. Safety and reactogenicity of a liquid hexavalent combined vaccine administered to healthy toddlers aged 16–20 months [abstract]. *In* Abstracts of the European Society for Paediatric Infectious Diseases, Noordwijk, the Netherlands, May 3–5, 2000.

225. Stojanov S, Liese JG, Barrand M, et al. Safety profile of a liquid hexavalent vaccine given at 2, 4, and 6 months of age [abstract]. *In* Abstracts of the 37th Annual Meeting of the Infectious Diseases Society of America, Philadelphia, November 18–21, 1999.

226. Crovari P, Zepp F, Dentico P, et al. Immunogenicity and reactogenicity of combined DTPa-HBV-IPV/Hib vaccine compared to concomitant administered DTPa-HBV-IPV and Hib vaccines given at 3, 5, and 11 months of age [abstract]. *In* Abstracts of the 19th Annual Meeting of the European Society for Paediatric Infectious Diseases, Istanbul, Turkey, March 2001, p 88.

227. Dagan R, Yaich M, Maleckar J, Eskola J. Reduction in antibody responses to an 11-valent pneumococcal vaccine (PncT/D) when coadministered with a vaccine containing acellular pertussis (aP) [abstr G-1069]. *In* Abstracts of the 42nd Interscience Conference on Antimicrobial Agents and Chemotherapy, San Diego, September 27–30, 2002.

228. Schmitt HJ, Petersen G, Corsaro B. Immunogenicity and safety of a 7-valent pneumococcal conjugate vaccine (Prevnar) coadministered with a DTaP-IPV-HBV/Hib vaccine (Infanrix Hexa) [abstr G-835]. *In* Abstracts of the 42nd Interscience Conference on Antimicrobial Agents and Chemotherapy, San Diego, September 27–30, 2002.

229. Olivier C, Liese JG, Stojanov S, et al. Immunogenicity and safety of the 7-valent pneumococcal conjugate vaccine (7VPnC-Prevenar) coadministered with a hexavalent DTaP-IPV-HBV/Hib vaccine (Hexavac) [abstr G-836]. *In* Abstracts of the 42nd Interscience Conference on Antimicrobial Agents and Chemotherapy, San Diego, September 27–30, 2002.

230. Saenger R, Dobbelaere K, Schuerman L. Immunogenicity and safety of DTPa-HBV-IPV/Hib coadministered with 7-valent pneumococcal conjugate vaccine. Third World Congress of Pediatric Infectious Diseases (WSPID), Santiago, Chile, November 2002, Abstract 259.

231. Saenger R, Maechler G, Schuerman L. Safety of a booster dose of DTPa-HBV-IPV/HIB compared to concomitant administration of DTPa-IPV/HIB and HBV vaccines. 21st Annual Meeting of the European Society for Paediatric Infectious Diseases (ESPID), April 2003, Taormina, Sicily, Abstract 257.

232. Tejedor JC, Omenaca F, Garcia-Sicilia F, et al. The Spanish 076 Study Group. Co-administration of diphtheria-tetanus-acellular pertussis-HBV-IPV/Hib with meningococcal C conjugate vaccine. 21st Annual Meeting of the European Society for Paediatric Infectious Diseases (ESPID), April 2003, Taormina, Sicily, Abstract 175.

233. Poellabauer EM, Himly C, Loew-Baselli A, et al. Group C meningococcal TT conjugate vaccine (NeisVac-C^R)-absence of immunological interference with hepatitis B, IPV, and acellular pertussis (AP).

234. Saenger R, The German 086-study group, Meurice F, Schuerman L. Comparison of the immunogenicity of diphtheria-tetanus-acellular pertussis-IPV-HBV/Hib compared to diphtheria-tetanus-acellular pertussis-HBV-IPV-Hib given as a primary vaccination course at 2, 4, and 6 months of age. 21st Annual Meeting of the European Society for Paediatric Infectious Diseases (ESPID), April 2003, Taormina, Sicily, Abstract 211.

235. West DJ, Hesley TM, Jonas LC, et al. Safety and immunogenicity of a bivalent *Haemophilus influenzae* type b/hepatitis B vaccine in healthy infants. Pediatr Infect Dis J 16:593–599, 1997.

236. Petersen K, Bulkow L, McMahon B, et al. Immunogenicity of a combined hepatitis B and *Haemophilus influenzae* type b conjugate vaccine in Alaska Native infants. Int J Circumpolar Health 57:285–292, 1998.

237. West DJ, Rabalais GP, Watson B, et al. Antibody responses of healthy infants to concurrent administration of a bivalent *Haemophilus influenzae* type b–hepatitis B vaccine with diphtheria-tetanus-pertussis, polio and measles-mumps-rubella vaccines. BioDrugs 15:413–418, 2001.

238. Ambrosch F, Wiedermann G, Andre FE, et al. Clinical and immunological investigation of a new combined hepatitis A and hepatitis B vaccine. J Med Virol 44:452–456, 1994.

239. Joines RW, Blatter M, Abraham B, et al. A prospective, randomized, comparative US trial of a combination hepatitis A and B vaccine (Twinrix®) with corresponding monovalent vaccines (Havrix® and Engerix-B®) in adults. Vaccine 19:4710–4719, 2001.

240. Thoelen S, Van Damme P, Leentvaar-Kuypers A, et al. The first combined vaccine against hepatitis A and B: an overview. Vaccine 17:1657–1662, 1999.

241. Abraham B, Baine Y, De Clercq N, et al. Magnitude and quality of antibody response to a combination hepatitis A and hepatitis B vaccine. Antiviral Res 53:63–73, 2002.

242. Van Damme P, Leroux-Roels G, Law B, et al. Long-term persistence (5–6 years) of antibodies induced by vaccination and safety follow-up, with the first combined vaccine against hepatitis A and B in children and adults. J Med Virol 65:6–13, 2001.

243. Nothdurft HD, Dietrich M, Zuckerman JN, et al. A new accelerated vaccination schedule for rapid protection against hepatitis A and B. Vaccine 20:1157–1162, 2002.

244. Van der Wielen M, Van Damme P, Collard F. A two-dose schedule for combined hepatitis A and hepatitis B vaccination in children ages one to eleven years. Pediatr Infect Dis J 19:848–853, 2000.

245. Van Damme P, Van der Wielen M. Combining hepatitis A and B vaccination in children and adolescents. Vaccine 19:2407–2412, 2001.

246. Burgess M, Rodger A, Waite S, Collard F. Comparative immunogenicity and safety of two dosing schedules of a combined hepatitis A and B vaccine in healthy adolescent volunteers: an open, randomised study. Vaccine 19:4835–4841, 2001.

247. Van Hoecke C, Lebaccq E, Beran J, et al. Concomitant vaccination against hepatitis A and typhoid fever. J Travel Med 5:1116–1120, 1998.

248. Beran, J, Beutels M, Levie K, et al. A single dose, combined vaccine against typhoid fever and hepatitis A: consistency, immunogenicity and reactogenicity. J Travel Med 7:246–252, 2000.

249. Overbosch D, Peyron F, Picot N, Varichon JP. Immunogenicity and safety of a combined typhoid fever and hepatitis A vaccine: a comparison of a combined vaccine in a dual-chamber syringe versus the monovalent vaccines [abstr FC07.03]. *In* Abstracts of the Seventh Conference of the International Society of Travel Medicine, Innsbruck, Austria, May 27–31, 2001.

250. Loebermann M, Kollaritsch H, Chappey O, et al. Immunogenicity and safety of a combined typhoid fever and hepatitis A vaccine in healthy adults [abstr PO02.16]. *In* Abstracts of the Seventh Conference of the International Society of Travel Medicine, Innsbruck, Austria, May 27–31, 2001.

251. Beeching NJ, Clarke P, Walker E, et al. A comparison of two combined vaccines against typhoid fever and hepatitis A: ViATIM™ and Hepatyrix™ [abstract]. *In* Abstracts of the Fourth Scientific Conference of the British Travel Health Association, London, UK, March 2, 2002.

252. Just M, Berger R, Just V. Evaluation of a combined measles-mumps-rubella-chickenpox vaccine. Dev Biol Stand 65:85–88, 1986.

253. Vesikari T, Ohrling A, Baer M, et al. Evaluation of live attenuated varicella vaccine (Oka-RIT strain) and combined varicella and MMR vaccination in 13–17-month-old children. Acta Paediatr Scand 80:1051–1057, 1991.

254. André FE, Steens JM, Zepp F. A combined measles, mumps, rubella and varicella candidate vaccine [abstr 26]. In Proceedings of the Fourth International Conference on Varicella, Herpes Zoster & Post-Herpetic Neuralgia, La Jolla, CA, 2001.

255. Arbeter AM, Baker L, Starr SE, et al. The combination measles, mumps, rubella and varicella vaccine in healthy children. Dev Biol Stand 65:89–93, 1986.

256. Arbeter AM, Baker L, Starr SE, et al. Combination measles, mumps, rubella and varicella vaccine. Pediatrics 78(4 pt 2):742–747, 1986.

257. Brunell PA, Novelli VM, Lipton SV, et al. Combined vaccine against measles, mumps, rubella, and varicella. Pediatrics 81:779–784, 1988.

258. Watson BM, Laufer DS, Kuter BJ, et al. Safety and immunogenicity of a combined live attenuated measles, mumps, rubella, and varicella vaccine (MMR$_{II}$V) in healthy children. J Infect Dis 173:731–734, 1996.

259. White CJ, Stinson D, Staehle B, et al. Measles, mumps, rubella, and varicella combination vaccine: safety and immunogenicity alone and in combination with other vaccines given to children. Clin Infect Dis 24:925–931, 1997.

260. Reuman PD, Sawyer MH, Kuter BJ, et al. Safety and immunogenicity of concurrent administration of measles-mumps-rubella-varicella vaccine and PedvaxHIB vaccines to healthy children twelve to eighteen months old. The MMRV Study Group. Pediatr Infect Dis J 16:662–667, 1997.

261. Shinefield H, Black S, Marchant C, et al. A dose selection study in healthy children comparing measles, mumps, rubella, and varicella (ProQuad) vaccine to M-M-R II given concomitantly with process upgrade varicella vaccine (PUVV) in separate injections [abstract]. In Abstracts of the 20th Annual Meeting of the European Society for Paediatric Infectious Diseases, Vilnius, Lithuania, May 2002.

262. Zepp F, Meyer CU, Habermehl P, et al. Cellular immune response to varicella in healthy subjects 12 to 22 months old receiving either a combined measles-mumps-rubella-varicella vaccine or separate measles-mumps-rubella and varicella vaccines [abstr G-1560]. In Abstracts of the 41st Interscience Conference on Antimicrobial Agents and Chemotherapy, Chicago, December 16–19, 2001.

263. Peltier M, Durieux C, Jonchere H, et al. Pénétration du virus amaril neurotrope par voie cutanée: vaccination mixte contre la fièvre jaune et la variole [note préliminaire]. Bull Acad Natl Med (Paris) 17:657, 1939.

264. Peltier M. Yellow fever vaccination, simple or associated with vaccination against smallpox, of the populations of French West Africa by the method of the Pasteur Institute of Dakar. Am J Public Health 37:1026–1032, 1947.

265. Nolan T, McIntyre P, Roberton D, Descamps D. Reactogenicity and immunogenicity of a live attenuated tetravalent measles-mumps-rubella-varicella (MMRV) vaccine. Vaccine 21:281–289, 2002.

266. Hahn RG. A combined yellow fever–smallpox vaccine for cutaneous application. Am J Hyg 54:50–70, 1951.

267. Dick GWA, Horgan ES. Vaccination by scarification with a combined 17D yellow fever and vaccinia vaccine. J Hyg (Camb) 50:376–383, 1952.

268. Meers PD. Combined smallpox–17D yellow fever vaccine for scratch vaccination. Trans R Soc Trop Med Hyg 53:196–201, 1959.

269. Meers PD. Further observations on 17D–yellow fever vaccination by scarification, with and without simultaneous smallpox vaccination. Trans R Soc Trop Med Hyg 54:493–501, 1960.

270. Meyer HM, Hostetler DD Jr, Bernheim BC, et al. Response of Volta children to jet inoculation of combined live measles, smallpox, and yellow fever vaccines. Bull World Health Organ 30:783–794, 1964.

271. Meyer HM Jr. Field experience with combined live measles, smallpox, and yellow fever vaccines. Arch Ges Virusforsch 16:365–366, 1965.

272. Meyer HM, Hopps HE, Bernheim BC, Douglas RD. Combined measles-smallpox and other vaccines. In First International Conference on Vaccines Against Viral and Rickettsial Diseases in Man (Pan American Health Organization Scientific Publ No 147). Washington, DC, Pan American Health Organization, 1967, pp 336–342.

273. Weibel RE, Stokes J Jr, Buynak EB, et al. Clinical-laboratory experiences with combined dried live measles-smallpox vaccine. Pediatrics 37:913–920, 1966.

274. Gateff C, Relyveld EH, Le Gonidec G, et al. Étude d'une nouvelle association vaccinal quintuple. Ann Microbiol (Paris) 124:387–409, 1973.

275. L'huillier M, Mazzariol MJ, Zadi S, et al. Study of combined vaccination against yellow fever and measles in infants from six to nine months. J Biol Stand 17:9–15, 1989.

276. Mouchon D, Pignon D, Vicens R, et al. The combined measles–yellow fever vaccination in African infants aged 6 to 10 months. Bull Soc Pathol Exot 83:537–551, 1990.

277. Soula G, Sylla A, Pichard E, et al. A new combined vaccine against yellow fever and measles in infants aged 6 to 24 months in Mali. Bull Soc Pathol Exot 84(5 pt 5):885–897, 1991.

278. Adu FD, Omotade OO, Oyedele OI, et al. Field trial of combined yellow fever and measles vaccines among children in Nigeria. East Afr Med J 73:579–582, 1996.

279. Lery L, Rotivel Y, Trabaud MA, et al. Combined tetanus-rabies vaccination. Dev Biol Stand 65:209–220, 1986.

280. Ambrosch F, Fritzell B, Gregor J, et al. Combined vaccination against yellow fever and typhoid fever: a comparative trial. Vaccine 12:625–628, 1994.

281. Choo S, Seymour L, Morris R, et al. Immunogenicity and reactogenicity of a pneumococcal conjugate vaccine administered combined with a Haemophilus influenzae type b conjugate vaccine in United Kingdom infants. Pediatr Infect Dis J 19:854–862, 2000.

282. Rennels M, Reisinger K, Rathore M, et al. Safety and immunogenicity of combined conjugate 9-valent S. pneumoniae-meningococcal group C (9vPnC-MnCC) and H. influenzae b-9vPnC-MnCC (HbOC-9vPnC-MnCC) vaccine [abstr G-2039]. In Abstracts of the 41st Interscience Conference on Antimicrobial Agents and Chemotherapy, Chicago, December 16–19, 2001.

283. Centers for Disease Control and Prevention. Combination vaccines for childhood immunization: recommendations of the Advisory Committee on Immunization Practices (ACIP), the American Academy of Pediatrics (AAP), and the American Academy of Family Physicians (AAFP). MMWR 48(RR-5), 1999.

284. American Academy of Pediatrics. Scheduling immunizations. In Pickering LK (ed). 2000 Red Book: Report of the Committee on Infectious Diseases (25th ed). Elk Grove Village, IL, American Academy of Pediatrics, pp. 20–26, 2000.

285. Schmitt HJ, Leroux-Roels G, Lebacq E, Saenger R, Boutriau D. Combination diphtheria-tetanus-acellular pertussis-hepatitis b-inactivated polio and Haemophilus influenzae type b-meningococcal C conjugate vaccine. 21st Annual Meeting of the European Society for Paediatric Infectious Diseases (ESPID), April 2003, Taormina, Sicily, Abstract 293.

286. Anderson EL, Decker MD, Englund JA, et al. Interchangeability of conjugated Haemophilus influenzae type b vaccines in infants. JAMA 273:849–853, 1995.

287. Centers for Disease Control and Prevention. Pertussis vaccination: use of acellular pertussis vaccines among infants and young children. Recommendations of the Advisory Committee on Immunization Practices (ACIP). MMWR 46:19, 1997.

288. Pertussis. In Atkinson W, Wolfe C (eds). Epidemiology and Prevention of Vaccine-Preventable Diseases (7th ed). Atlanta, Centers for Disease Control and Prevention, 2002.

289. Centers for Disease Control and Prevention. Development of community- and state-based immunization registries: CDC response to a report from the National Vaccine Advisory Committee. MMWR 50(RR-17):1–28, 2001.

290. Centers for Disease Control and Prevention. Immunization registry progress—United States, 2002. MMWR 51:760–762, 2002.

Chapter 30

Adenovirus Vaccine

CHARLOTTE A. GAYDOS • JOEL C. GAYDOS

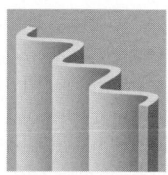

Introduction

Adenoviruses have been associated with many clinical syndromes, particularly with a variety of infections that affect the respiratory tract, the gastrointestinal (GI) system, and the eye. The virus, which was recovered from surgically removed human adenoids, was first isolated by Rowe el al. as "adenoid degeneration agent" in 1953.[1] Hilleman and Werner independently reported the isolation of "respiratory illness agents" from an acute respiratory disease (ARD) epidemic at Fort Leonard Wood, Missouri.[2] References to clinical keratoconjunctivitis and "shipyard eye" probably caused by adenoviruses were made as early as 1889 and in the 1940s.[3,4] These agents comprised a related group of viruses, being associated with several clinical syndromes such as ARD, pharyngitis, conjunctivitis, pneumonitis, and atypical pneumonia.[5] They were named adenoviruses by a committee chaired by Enders.[6] Certain types of adenoviruses soon became identified as causes of severe epidemics of ARD in military recruit populations.[7,8]

Adenovirus infections can be fatal in immunocompromised patients and a cause of serious infection and pneumonia in children, especially infants.[9–14] They have also been associated with infections in acquired immunodeficiency syndrome (AIDS) and bone marrow transplant patients.[15,16] Acute hemorrhagic cystitis and other infections in patients with immune deficiencies are major problems because these infections are often fatal.[12,16] Adenovirus infections are responsible for approximately 10% of pneumonia cases in hospitalized children and cause up to 15% of cases of gastroenteritis in infants and children.[9,17,18] Epidemic keratoconjunctivitis, usually caused by adenovirus (ADV) type 8 or 37, is a severe eye disease that may lead to subepithelial corneal keratitis.[19,20]

By the 1960s, adenoviruses were recognized as causes of significant respiratory illness in military populations.[7,8,21] Up to 80% of recruits developed adenovirus infections and 20% required hospitalization.[8,22] Median attack rates for new recruits ranged from 6 to 16.7 per 100 per month at the most affected northern and midwestern military posts and from 2.3 to 2.6 per 100 per month for posts in the south and west.[21] The search for vaccines for adenoviruses was stimulated by the

significant morbidity, disruption to training and the medical care system, and economic loss at military training centers. In one outbreak, up to 40% of the men in a training unit were lost to illness within a 2-week period, and many who were hospitalized had to restart training.[23] The costs associated with excessive hospitalizations, additional medical personnel, and retraining created an economic burden.[23] In addition to the economic loss and severe morbidity suffered by military trainees, several pneumonia deaths associated with ADV type 7 have been recorded for young, previously healthy trainees undergoing basic training.[24–27] One recent case demonstrated central nervous system involvement.[27]

As the 20th century came to a close, two significant changes occurred in the epidemiology of the adenoviruses. Beginning in 1971, military recruits routinely received live, oral enteric-coated vaccines for ADV types 4 and 7, which were safe and effective.[28] In 1994, the sole manufacturer announced that vaccine production would be terminated permanently. The U.S. Department of Defense supply of vaccines against ADV types 4 and 7 diminished, and adenovirus-associated ARD re-emerged in military training populations.[29–31] All vaccine stocks were depleted in 1999. The second significant change was in the geographic distribution of type 7: ADV 7d2 and 7h were found to have undergone extensive geographic spread from previously restricted areas.[32,33]

Background

Clinical Description

A variety of clinical syndromes have been described associated with the 51 serotypes of human adenoviruses that have been described (Table 30–1). Excellent reviews describing the most common serotypes associated with particular diseases have been published.[34–37]

Endemic Respiratory Adenovirus in Children

Although most children become infected with some of the common adenoviruses early in life, only about 50% of these infections result in disease.[34,38,39] Up to 80% of children acquire antibodies to ADV types 1, 2, and 5.[39–41] Isolation studies indicate ADV types 1, 2, 5, 3, and 6 are most

TABLE 30–1 ■ Clinical Syndromes Associated with Adenovirus Infections

Clinical Syndrome	Subgenus	Common Serotypes	Population at Risk
Endemic respiratory	B, C	1, 2, 3, 5, 6, 7	Infants, children
Epidemic respiratory	B, C	5, 7	Children (day care)
Acute respiratory disease	B, E	3, 4, 7, 14, 21	Military recruits
Pharyngoconjunctival fever	B, C, E	1, 3, 4, 7, 14	School-age children, young adults
Keratoconjunctivitis	B, D	8, 11, 19, 37	All age groups
Hemorrhagic cystitis	B	11, 21, 34, 35	Immunocompromised patients, children
Infantile gastroenteritis	F, G	40, 41	Children
Other syndromes	B, C, E, D	2, 4, 7, 12, 19, 32, 37	Children, adults
Immune deficiency	B, D	34, 35, 43–49	Transplant, AIDS, and immunocompromised patients

AIDS, acquired immunodeficiency syndrome.

common, in that order.[34] The syndromes of ill children include pharyngitis, bronchitis, bronchiolitis, croup, and pneumonia.[11,42] Occasionally pneumonia may be fatal, especially when it is associated with ADV type 7.[9,43–45] The incidence of diseases caused by adenoviruses is higher in late winter, spring, and early summer, and both sexes are equally affected.[38,46] The mode of transmission in children is thought to be primarily fecal-oral.[39]

Epidemic Respiratory Adenovirus in Children

Occasionally, epidemics occur in day care facilities and orphanages, especially with ADV types 5 and 7, but also with other types.[47–49] In addition to causing outbreaks in closed populations, ADV type 7a can cause large epidemics affecting children in open communities.[50]

Acute Respiratory Disease of Military Recruits

In young adults who live in closed communities such as boarding schools and military recruit camps, adenoviruses may cause epidemics of illnesses similar to influenza, including tracheobronchitis and pneumonia severe enough to require hospitalization.[2,7,51,52] The incubation period of the disease is 4 to 5 days.[52] Prior to the use of vaccines in the U.S. military, ADV types 4 and 7 accounted for 60% of all respiratory illnesses in recruits who were hospitalized, while types 3, 14, and 21 were less frequently observed.[21] At some northern basic training posts, rates of 6 to 8 per 100 men per week translated into 600 to 800 ARD hospitalized admissions per week.[23]

Typical ARD is a febrile disease with symptoms of sore throat, fever, cough, coryza, rhinorrhea, headache, and chest pain.[2,34,52] Physical examinations reveal rales and rhonchi with little evidence of consolidation, and chest radiographs show patchy interstitial infiltrates, principally in the lower lung fields.[2,37,52] Symptoms last 3 to 10 days.[34] The infection is characteristically self-limited, no specific therapy exists, and superinfection and death are rare but do occur.[2,24] Routes of transmission are reported to be airborne or aerosolized virus inhaled into the lung. The virus has been isolated for more than 2 weeks after exposure.[2,53] Seven to 10% of pneumonia cases in military recruits have been demonstrated to be caused by adenoviruses.[8,54] Hilleman reported that about 15% of soldiers hospitalized during outbreaks of adenovirus-associated respiratory illness developed radiographic evidence of pulmonary involvement.[22] During a 1997 outbreak of ADV 4–caused ARD at a large training center, hospitalized recruits were febrile and usually had headache and sore throat.[55] The average period for hospitalization was 7.8 days.[55] Women sol-

diers were ill for a longer period, but waited longer than men to seek medical care.[55] Women recruits have been reported to be at lower risk for hospitalization than men, but this is not a consistent finding.[23,28,30,31]

Pharyngoconjunctival Fever

This syndrome is characterized by pharyngitis, conjunctivitis, and spiking fever.[56] First described in the 1920s as associated with swimming, the cause subsequently has been linked to insufficient chlorination.[57–59] Either one or both eyes are affected, and diarrhea, coryza, tonsillar exudate, and lymphadenopathy may be observed. The most frequent association has been with ADV types 3 and 7, but other types such as 1, 4, and 14 have been observed.[56] The disease is associated with summer camps, swimming pools, and lakes, and occurs in children and young adults, often spreading to other family members.[56,59,60] The incubation period is 6 to 9 days, and the virus may be isolated from pool water.[56,58] There is little bacterial superinfection and no permanent damage to the eye.[37]

Keratoconjunctivitis

Epidemics of conjunctivitis in adults caused by adenoviruses were first described by German investigators and later by Jawetz et al. as "shipyard eye."[4,61] The disease was observed at industrial settings where shipbuilding took place and was probably transmitted because of inadequate infection control practices when workers sought care for chemical irritation and minor trauma from paint and rust chips.[4] The disease, with an incubation time of 8 to 10 days, is characterized by conjunctivitis, edema of the eye, pain, photophobia, and lacrimation. Superficial erosions as well as subepithelial infiltrates of the cornea may occur.[34] Preauricular lymph gland swelling and involvement of cervical and submaxillary lymph glands may be observed.[34]

The disease has been associated with ADV types 8, 19, and 37 and rarely other types.[62–66] Additionally, ADV types 19 and 37 have been isolated from the genital tract of young adults with epidemic keratoconjunctivitis, and the possibility of sexual transmission has been considered.[67,68] Many epidemics of keratoconjunctivitis have been reported to be associated with ophthalmology practices, where spread from contaminated ophthalmic solutions, fingers, and instruments has been implicated.[62,63,65,69,70]

Hemorrhagic Cystitis

Hemorrhagic cystitis syndrome in children has been shown to be caused by adenovirus infections in 23% to 51% of cases in America and Japan.[71] Although the route of spread is unknown, types 11 and 21 (group B adenoviruses), which are uncommon in respiratory infections, were isolated most frequently.[71] Boys were two to three times more commonly affected than girls. Clinical findings included gross hematuria of 3 days' duration. Dysuria, microscopic hematuria, and urinary frequency lasted a few days longer.[71,72] No viremia or structural abnormalities were found. Adenoviral antigen in exfoliated bladder epithelial cells can be demonstrated by immunofluorescence.[71] Cases of acute hemorrhagic cystitis after renal and bone marrow transplantation have been increasingly reported.[73–75] Adenovirus types 34 and 35, also group B adenoviruses, were first isolated from renal transplant patients, but neither was associated with symptoms of hemorrhagic cystitis.[76] Tubulointerstitial nephritis caused by ADV type 11 in adults and children receiving bone marrow transplants has been described.[77]

Infantile Gastroenteritis

Adenoviruses were first visualized by electron microscopy as etiologic agents of diarrhea, but they could not be grown on standard tissue culture cells. These adenoviruses are defective and require transformed human embryonic kidney (HEK) cells or Chang's conjunctival cells for isolation. They can be detected by enzyme immunoassay (EIA).[78–80] Numerous outbreaks have been described, and adenoviruses may account for up to 12% of all infant diarrhea.[81–83] The diarrhea is watery, usually associated with fever, and may last 1 to 2 weeks.[37] The etiologic serotypes, 40 and 41, are related serologically and belong to subgenus F.

Other Syndromes Associated with Adenoviral Infections

Encephalitis as well as meningoencephalitis cases associated with adenoviruses have occurred occasionally.[27,84,85] A fatal case of cerebral edema caused by adenovirus type 5 was reported in a previously healthy 18-month-old infant.[86] Fatal neonatal disseminated infections with ADV types 4, 7, 12, and 32 have been reported.[87] A pertussis-like syndrome, as well as a relationship between pertussis and infections with adenoviruses, have also been described.[76,88–91] Persistent adenoviral infection has also been associated with chronic airway obstruction in children.[92] ADV types 2, 19, and 37 have been isolated from genital lesions and have been associated with orchitis, urethritis, and cervicitis.[36] Nosocomial transmission to susceptible health care workers and other patients has been reported, probably related to the long periods that the virus is secreted in the stool, the possible aerosolization of the virus, and fomite transmission.[36] Recently, a target sequence of the adenoviral capsid gene was present in increasing frequency in infants with bronchopulmonary dysplasia, an association deserving of further investigation.[93]

Association with Immunocompromised Patients

Adenoviruses have been implicated as opportunistic agents in patients with immune deficiency states, such as those with AIDS, receiving cancer chemotherapy, having bone marrow transplants, or undergoing renal and lung transplantation.[14,15,74,94–98] These patients are prone to pneumonia and disseminated adenoviral infection. ADV type 35 has been associated with urinary tract disease in people with AIDS.[99] Some of the newer types, such as 43 through 49, have been discovered in AIDS patients.[99,100] Adenoviruses have also been described as a cause of parotitis in patients with AIDS.[101]

A review of 201 bone marrow recipients over 4 years indicated that adenovirus infections occurred in 20.9% of patients, with a higher incidence in pediatric patients than in adult patients (31.3% vs. 13.6%; $P = 0.003$).[102] Type 35 was the most common serotype identified.[102] Thirty-one percent of patients (13 of 42) with isolates had adenovirus disease, and 7 patients died.[102] An excellent review of adenoviruses in the immunocompromised host was done by Hierholzer in 1992.[12] Adenovirus infections in these patients were associated with case-fatality rates as high as 60% in those with pneumonia, compared to only 15% in immunocompetent hosts with pneumonia. Radiographs often demonstrate patchy interstitial infiltrates, usually in the lower lung fields.[103] Figure 30–1 shows the chest radiograph, which was obtained on day 45 post-transplant, of a 20-year-old recipient of an autologous bone marrow transplant for diffuse large cell lymphoma (B-cell type) with systemic ADV type 11 infection. He expired on day 80. Adenovirus was recovered from conjunctival, urine, and bronchoalveolar lavage cultures. Similarly, a case fatality rate of 50% occurred in immunocompromised people with hepatitis and associated adenovirus infections, compared to 10% in similarly infected immunocompetent patients with hepatitis.[12] Positive serum polymerase chain reaction (PCR) for adenovirus has been reported to predict severe disseminated adenovirus infection in immunocompromised patients.[104]

Study of 532 hematopoietic stem cell transplant recipients during 1986 to 1997 found a 12% incidence of adenovirus infections, with pediatric patients being more likely than adults to have a positive culture (23% vs. 9%).[105]

Virology

Human adenoviruses are double-stranded, nonenveloped DNA viruses belonging to the genus *Mastadenovirus* (from

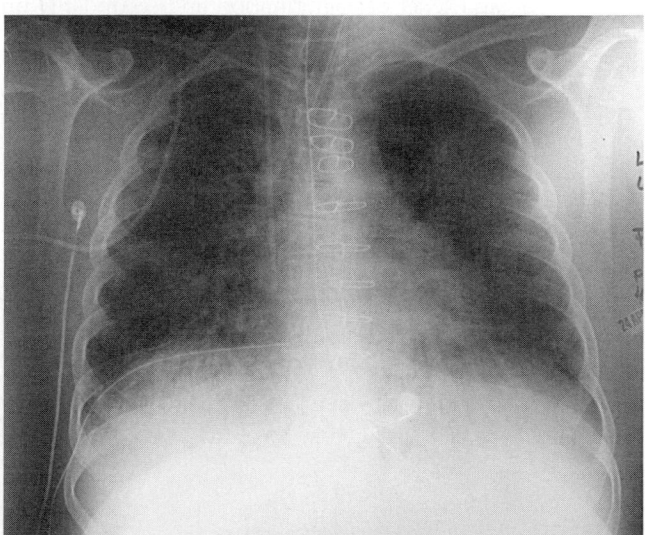

FIGURE 30–1 ■ Pneumonia caused by adenovirus type 11 in a 20-year-old recipient of an autologous bone marrow transplant. (Courtesy of Stuart Ray, M.D., Johns Hopkins University, Baltimore, MD.)

the Greek *mastos*, for *breast*, infecting mammals only), family *Adenoviridae*.[106] The other genus is *Aviadenovirus* (from the Latin *avis*, for *bird*), which is serologically distinct from *Mastadenovirus* and has a different genomic organization.[106] The capsid of the human adenoviruses demonstrates icosahedral symmetry and contains 252 capsomeres. The capsomeres consist of 240 hexons and 12 pentons with a projecting fiber on each of the pentons (Fig. 30–2). The pentons and hexons are each derived from different viral polypeptides. The fibers, which are responsible for type-specific antibodies, vary in length among human strains and sometimes are absent in some animal strains.[107–111] The hexons are both type-specific and group-specific antigens, primarily inducing group-specific complement-fixing antibodies, whereas the pentons are especially active in hemagglutination.[112] The virions are 70 to 90 nm in diameter and composed of 10 structural proteins with molecular weights of 5000 to 120,000.[36] In cesium chloride, they have a buoyant density of 1.33 to 1.34 g/cm³ and a molecular weight of 170×10^6 to 175×10^6 by sedimentation coefficient.[36] There is a single molecule of linear, double-stranded DNA of 26×10^6 to 45×10^6 molecular weight inside the capsid, and the G + C base compositions of the human virus genomes range from 47% to 60%.[102,106,112]

Adenoviruses are unusually stable in the presence of physical and chemical agents, as well as adverse pH, and thus survive for long periods of time outside the host, making them available for transmission to others. They can be destroyed by heat at 56°C for 30 minutes, ultraviolet irradiation, 0.25% sodium dodecyl sulfate, chlorine at 0.5 μ/mL, and formalin, but are resistant to ether and chloroform. These viruses replicate in the cell nucleus, tending to be host specific. By determination with reference horse antisera, there are 51 serotypes of human adenoviruses now described, and these have been grouped into subgenera A through F.[113] Historically, hemagglutination properties have also allowed a separation of the human adenoviruses into the subgenuses A through F, with the scheme being based primarily on complete agglutination of monkey or rat erythrocytes, partial agglutination of rat erythrocytes, and level of agglutination and secondarily on complete agglutination of human, chicken, and other erythrocytes[36,37] (Table 30–2).

In addition to the human adenoviruses, the genus *Mastadenovirus* also contains bovine, canine, equine, murine, ovine, porcine, and tree shrew adenovirus species.[106] Tentative additional species in the genus include caprine, guinea pig, ovine C, and simian adenoviruses.[106] Species designation now depends on at least two of the following characteristics[106]:

- Calculated phylogenetic distance based on matrix analysis of the protease, pVIII, hexon, and DNA polymerase amino acid sequence comparisons
- DNA hybridization
- Restriction enzyme fragmentation
- Percentage of genomic G + C
- Oncogenicity in rodents
- Growth characteristics
- Host range
- Cross-neutralization
- Possibility of recombination
- Hemagglutination
- Genetic organization of the E3 region

Some adenovirus serotypes have been determined to be oncogenic in animals and to transform cell lines, but oncogenicity has not been observed in humans. This potential, as well as other viral properties noted above, appear to support the historically used serotyping and hemagglutination scheme (see Table 30–2).[106,112–116] Use of restriction endonucleases has also demonstrated that variants of the same serotype can occur.[117] For example, ADV type 7 isolates from five continents have been subdivided into more than 15 different genotypes.[118] Similarly, restriction endonuclease typing has been applied to ADV types 3 and 4, as well as types 3 and 7 from pneumonia cases.[119–122] Hybridization or genetic recombination of viruses may occur in vivo, and types 34 and 35 may be recombinants with type 7.[96,97]

Pathogenesis

Depending on the route of inoculation, the serotype, and the immune state of the host, adenoviruses can cause diseases or asymptomatic infections in the respiratory tract and in other sites. Respiratory infection is presumed to result

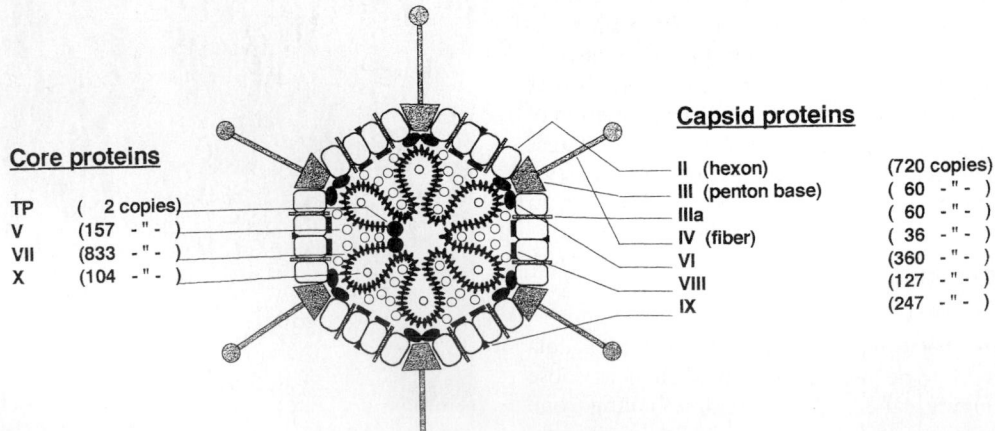

Core proteins

TP	(2 copies)
V	(157 -"-)
VII	(833 -"-)
X	(104 -"-)

Capsid proteins

II (hexon)	(720 copies)
III (penton base)	(60 -"-)
IIIa	(60 -"-)
IV (fiber)	(36 -"-)
VI	(360 -"-)
VIII	(127 -"-)
IX	(247 -"-)

FIGURE 30–2 ▪ Schematic model illustrating the adenovirus particle. The tentative location and copy number of peptides are indicated for the core and capsid proteins. (From Russkanen O, Meurman O, Kusjavi A. Adenoviruses. *In* Richman DD, Whitley RJ, Hayden FG [eds]. Clinical Virology. New York, Churchill Livingstone, 1997, pp 525–547, with permission.)

TABLE 30–2 ■ Classification Schemes for Adenoviruses of Humans

Subgenus	Hemagglutination Group	Serotypes	Potential for Tumors in Animals	Transforming Potential	Percentage of G + C in DNA
A	Rat (incomplete)	12, 18, 31	High	Moderate	48–49
B	Monkey (complete)	3, 7, 11, 14, 16, 21, 34, 35, 50	Moderate	Moderate	50–52
C	Rat (incomplete)	1, 2, 5, 6	Low or none	Low	57–59
D	Rat (complete)	8, 9, 10, 13, 15, 17, 19, 20, 22–30, 32, 33, 36–39, 42–49, 51	Low or none	Moderate	57–61
E	Rat (incomplete)	4	Low or none	Low	57–59
F	Rat (atypical)	40, 41	None	None	Not done

Adapted from Baum SG. Adenovirus. *In* Mandel GL, Bennett JE, Dolin R (eds). Principles and Practices of Infectious Diseases. New York, Churchill Livingstone, 2000, pp 1624–1630.

from inhalation of aerosolized virus, whereas ocular infection, gastroenteritis, and nosocomial infections may arise from fomites, water, or fecal-oral contamination. Reactivation of the latent virus is believed to occur.[52] Some 50% of tonsils removed surgically may have adenoviruses isolated from the tissue, suggesting that these viruses may stay in a latent state for long periods.[123] Virus has been also isolated from lymphocytes, kidney, blood, cerebrospinal fluid, and most body organs.[12,14,15,43,44,85,96,124–126] Extensive pathology has been found in the lungs, with microscopic necrosis of the tracheal and bronchial epithelium.[34] Acidophilic intranuclear inclusions are seen in bronchial epithelial cells in addition to basophilic masses of cells surrounded by clear halos, which may indicate aggregations of viral material.[43] A mononuclear infiltrate, rosette formation, and focal necrosis of mucous glands characteristically are seen.[34]

Three types of interaction of virus with infected cells may occur. A lytic infection may take place during which the virus completes an entire replicative cycle.[37] From 10^5 to 10^6 progeny viruses per cell may be produced, of which only 1% to 5% are actually infectious.[37] The second type of interaction is the chronic, inapparent, or latent infection, where small numbers of virus may be produced, and an inapparent infection results. Viral shedding from the GI tract may occur for years.[34] In addition to aerosolization, intestinal shedding of respiratory virus is an important factor to consider in the prevention of nosocomial spread in hospitals and chronic care homes.[34,127,128] Persistent infection has been reported in epithelial cells from monkeys.[129] Lymphoid cells are thought to be the reservoir for these persistent infections.[130,131] The third type of interaction is oncogenic transformation, whereby the viral DNA is integrated into the host genome, where it is replicated with the cellular host DNA, but only the early steps in the viral cycle occur and no infectious virions are produced.[132]

The genes from adenoviruses are expressed in the cell nucleus in two phases: "early" (E), which precedes viral DNA replication, and "late."[130] Early genes encode proteins that function to counteract immunosurveillance, especially those from the E3 transcription unit.[130] The "late" genes primarily encode viral structural proteins. The functions of the E1 proteins include the induction of DNA synthesis in quiescent cells, immortalization of primary cells in cooperation with activated *ras* or with the E1B proteins, transactivation of delayed early genes, induction or repression of several cellular genes, and induction of apoptosis. These proteins are responsible for inducing sensitivity to tumor necrosis factor (TNF), a key inflammatory cytokine with antiviral properties.[130] None of the E3 genes is required for adenovirus replication in cultured cells, but several of the E3-coded proteins (10.4K, 14.5K, and 14.7K) inhibit TNF cytolysis.[130,133] Because a major function of TNF may be to prevent viral replication, the inhibition of TNF by these viral proteins may be a significant mechanism of pathogenesis.

Another significant E3-coded protein is Gp 19K. This glycoprotein is located in the endoplasmic reticulum and forms a complex with class I antigens of the major histocompatibility complex (MHC), preventing cells from being killed by cytotoxic T lymphocytes (CTLs).[130] A cotton rat animal model was used by Ginsberg et al. to study the pathogenesis of ADV types 2 and 5, which cause a pneumonia similar to that seen in humans.[133,134] Two phases of infection were seen, the initial phase, characterized by the infiltration of monocytes and neutrophils, and a later phase associated with the infiltration of lymphocytes. The pathology appeared to reflect the response by host immune defenses to viral infection. Gp 19K markedly reduced the transport of the class I MHC to the surface of the infected cells and therefore the attack of CTLs.[134] In support of this mechanism of pathogenesis is the finding that mutants lacking Gp 19K are more pathogenic than wild-type virus because the mutants do not block the CTL response or the synthesis of cytokines associated with this CTL response.[130,133] It is now known that only the early genes are required to induce the complete pathogenesis of adenovirus infection in cotton rats.[134] Although several cytokines, such as TNF-α, interleukin-1, and interleukin-6, were elaborated during the first 2 to 3 days of the infection in the cotton rat model, only TNF-α played a major role in pathogenesis.[134] Steroids almost completely eliminated the pneumonic inflammatory response to infection.[134]

Pathology caused by latent infection with adenoviruses has been linked to chronic obstructive pulmonary disease (COPD).[131,135] Some have suggested that childhood viral diseases represent an independent risk factor for COPD.[136] The adenoviral E1A proteins can stimulate the transcription of many heterologous viral and cellular genes. These proteins possess the ability to interact with the DNA-binding domains of several cellular transcription factors and activate a wide variety of genes.[137,138] The adenoviral genome has been found to be present in the lungs of more patients with COPD than in controls.[139] E1A proteins are expressed in epithelial cells of human lung tissue, and, by increasing the expression of several genes important in controlling the inflammatory process, these may contribute to the pathogenesis of COPD. The events described above may amplify the airway inflammation associated with cigarette smoking.[135]

The recent isolation and cloning of a 46-kDa protein adenovirus receptor, which mediates attachment and infection, may facilitate the development of new strategies to limit diseases caused by adenoviruses.[140] This protein has been identified as the receptor for the Coxsackie B virus and ADV types 2 and 5 and has been referred to as CAR.

Diagnosis

Adenoviral infections generally cannot be diagnosed on clinical grounds alone because the clinical pictures of these infections resemble those caused by other microorganisms and are variable.[92] In military epidemics however, severe febrile upper respiratory illness (URI), mild febrile URI, and afebrile URI were studied to determine if a differential characteristic might exist. In the recruits studied, 36% of those with afebrile and mild febrile URI versus 79.2% of those with severe febrile disease had an adenovirus identified.[141] Traditionally, laboratory support and qualified personnel are necessary in order to diagnose adenoviruses in clinical specimens or to perform serologic assays. Detailed diagnostic procedures have been outlined.[35,36,76] Considerations include specimen type; collection; storage procedures; types of laboratory tests, including serologic assays; and availability of newer types of diagnostic assays.

Specimen Types

The optimal specimen depends on the clinical picture, as well as the suspected serotype.[92] Adenoviruses can be isolated from a variety of specimens, including throat swabs, nasal washes, conjunctival scrapings and swabs, stool, blood, cerebrospinal fluid, and biopsied tissue specimens. Because they are relatively stable viruses, adenoviruses can be recovered if properly transported to the laboratory. Specimens for viral isolation should be collected early in the illness and shipped promptly to the local laboratory at 4°C or frozen at −70°C for shipment to a reference laboratory. Swab and tissue specimens must be transported in viral transport media containing antibiotics and 0.5% gelatin or bovine serum albumin.[35,36,76,92] Freezing specimens at −70°C is recommended if immediate culture inoculation is not possible. Guidelines issued by the virology laboratory should be followed.

Urine specimens (20 mL) should be fresh and should be sedimented at 2000 × g for 5 minutes to pellet exfoliated cells, and both the pellet and supernatant should be cultured.[35,36] Urine, stool, and cerebrospinal fluid should be transported in clean containers and not in transport media. Stool suspensions give better yield than rectal swabs.[34] Blood should be collected in preservative-free heparin and fractionated on Ficoll-Hypaque gradient centrifuges.[36]

Serologic diagnosis requires paired blood samples. The first (acute) specimen should be collected as early as possible in the illness and the second (convalescent) specimen should be collected 2 to 4 weeks later. Stored sera should be kept at −20°C until testing.

Cell Culture

Because adenoviruses are host specific, isolation is most easily accomplished in human cells.[92] Even though the best isolation sensitivity is achieved in HEK cells, which are difficult to obtain, other continuous cell lines such as A549, HeLa, Hep-2, KB, and MRC-5 are in common use today. All serotypes of adenoviruses grow well and produce typical cytopathic effect, except ADV types 40 and 41.[36] Types 40 and 41 require the Graham-293 adenovirus type 5-transformed secondary HEK cell line, but may grow in A549 cells or tertiary cynomolgus monkey kidney cells.[35,36] Specimen preparation before inoculation is extremely important with regard to centrifugation, treatment with antibiotics, and homogenization, and is described in detail by Hierholzer.[36] Typical cytopathic effect may be relatively slow and characteristically begins at the periphery on the monolayer. Infected cells become rounded, enlarged, and refractile; are intranuclear; and aggregate into clusters that are irregular.[36] A 4-week incubation with blind passage is recommended.[36] Isolation is still the gold standard and most sensitive (85% to 100%) for adenovirus diagnosis, except for gastroenteritis.[92] An improved culture technique for adenovirus isolation using centrifugation of 24-well plates and needing only 48 hours' incubation has been reported to enhance sensitivity of culture.[142]

Identification of Isolated Viruses

Subsequent identification of isolated viruses as adenoviruses can be made by immunofluorescence using monoclonal antibodies (IFA), complement fixation (CF), EIA, time-resolved fluoroimmunoassay (TR-FIA), DNA hybridization assays, counterimmunoelectrophoresis, and latex agglutination.[36,143–146] In general IFA, EIA, TR-FIA, and CF are used to classify a viral isolate to genus level as an adenovirus. Agglutination with monkey, human, and rat erythrocytes is employed to assign the virus to a subgroup, and further hemagglutination inhibition and serum neutralization (SN) tests are used to serotype the isolate.[36] A rapid diagnostic procedure is the shell vial culture modification, whereby monolayers are inoculated with the clinical specimen using centrifugation and, after several days' incubation, are stained with monoclonal antibodies to the hexon protein.[144]

Typing Tests

SN assays have been the gold standard method used to type adenoviruses.[36] Hemagglutination inhibition is convenient, but requires fresh rat and monkey erythrocytes. Reference antisera may be available from the American Type Culture Collection (Manassas, VA). Three types of SN tests have been described: conventional 7-day assays using Hep-2, A549, HeLa, HEK, or Graham-293 cells; the 3-day test in primary rhesus monkey kidney cells; and microneutralization tests in secondary monkey kidney cells, Vero cells, and Hep-2 cells.[36]

Restriction enzyme analysis can be used for the separation of a serotype into multiple genotypes.[115,117] The genomic variability of the ADV type 3 and type 7 genome types has been investigated extensively using a panel of 12 restriction enzymes.[118,119,122] In addition, type 4 isolates have been genotyped by use of restriction enzymes.[120,121] These analyses have been applied mainly for molecular epidemiology studies, but may be useful in outbreak investigations. A nomenclature system has been suggested and described in detail, with a recommended protocol for the designation of new genome types.[118,122]

Rapid subgenera typing of human adenoviruses has been reported by restriction endonuclease analysis following PCR amplification of virus DNA from highly conserved sequences and by using degenerate consensus primers.[147,148] This method is useful when rapid typing of clinical samples is desirable and correlates well with serotyping by the neutralization test and traditional restriction enzyme analysis of full-length adenovirus DNA.[147,148]

A molecular epidemiologic study of ADV type 7 isolates from 1966 to 2000 was performed.[32] Using restriction enzyme analyses, most (65%) of 166 strains were demonstrated to be Ad7b. However, two new genomes also were identified that were previously undocumented in North America: Ad7d2 (28%), appearing through the Midwest, the Northeast, and Canada; and Ad7h (2%), appearing only in the Southwest of the United States. Ad7d2 has been the cause of several civilian outbreaks and the cause of a large respiratory disease outbreak at a military recruit training center.[29,32,149]

Molecular sequencing has been used to study strain variation in serotypes 4 and 7, with respect to determining the suitability of vaccine strains that were used to develop military vaccines in the 1960s.[150] Sequencing of a 1500-base-pair region of the adenovirus neutralization epitope from the prototype vaccine viruses, community acquired viruses, and recent wild-type strains from military personnel with respiratory disease was performed. There was no significant strain variation in the epitope studied for type 7, but for type 4 there was continuous genetic drift with replacement by a new variant. The new strain has been in circulation since 1995 and is different than the ADV type 4 prototype strain used for the original vaccine.[150]

Direct Detection

Electron microscopy and immunoelectron microscopy have been used in the past as the principal direct detection methods for identifying adenoviruses in clinical material, especially biopsy and autopsy specimens, as well as for the detection of these agents as causes of gastroenteritis.[36,151–153] Immunofluorescence can be useful for rapid identification of cells from unfrozen specimens using monoclonal and polyclonal antibodies against the hexon antigen, which is group specific. The antibodies are commercially available.[143,154] EIA and TR-FIA can both be used to detect antigenic proteins in clinical specimens, as can latex agglutination.[145,146,155,156] The sensitivity of EIA was 84.8% in one large series.[155] A commercial EIA used for the diagnosis of conjunctivitis had a sensitivity of only 62.3% compared to culture, however.[157]

Nucleic Acid Hybridization and Polymerase Chain Reaction

Nucleic acid hybridization using dot-blot, sandwich, and in situ techniques has also been used for diagnosis, but has not been adopted for routine use in clinical laboratories.[158–163]

PCR assays have been developed for the diagnosis of adenoviruses, especially for types 40 and 41, because they are difficult to grow.[164–169] Allard et al. first developed a set of primers with homology to the conserved sequences of the hexon gene, which would amplify adenovirus strains from all six subgenera, A through F.[166,168] Their second pair of primers detected only the enteric types 40 and 41, while a third set was specific for type 40, thus differentiating types 40 and 41. PCR with restriction fragment length polymorphism (RFLP) analysis has been used to detect and also differentiate types 40 and 41.[170] The combination of PCR amplification with liquid-phase hybridization quantitated by time-resolved fluorometry has been used by Hierholzer et al. to identify adenoviruses from a variety of clinical specimens, including urine, stool, and tissue suspensions.[164] Procedures for the performance of PCR assays have been well described.[165,167,169] Primers published by Allard et al., useful for some types of adenoviruses, failed to detect the ADV type 11 from the patient shown in Figure 30–1.[166,168] Newly designed primers, HEX3/HEX4, were used successfully to amplify DNA from the specimens from this patient.[171]

PCR has been used with myocardial tissue samples for the diagnosis of adenovirus infection.[172,173] Right ventricular endomyocardial biopsies from pediatric patients with rejection after transplantation were positive for adenoviruses in 14 (10.8%) of 129 samples.[172] Adenoviruses were diagnosed by PCR in 15 (39.4%) of 38 right ventricular biopsy samples from 34 pediatric patients with acute myocarditis.[173]

PCR for adenovirus detection has been used with success on formalin-fixed, paraffin-embedded autopsy specimens from children with viral pneumonitis and disseminated adenovirus infection.[174,175] Adenoviral DNA was demonstrated by PCR in 3 (6.8%) of 44 lung tissue samples from immunocompromised patients with pneumonia.[161]

Adenoviruses from throat, nasopharyngeal, and ocular specimens have also been diagnosed by PCR, offering improved sensitivity over immunoassay and greater speed of diagnosis over culture.[167,176–178] The combination of PCR with RFLP analysis was used to detect and type adenoviruses from conjunctival specimens.[179] The PCR was 100% sensitive compared to culture with 127 specimens, and the positives were further classified as to types 37, 3, 11, 8, and 4 by RFLP.[179] Only three restriction endonucleases (EcoT141, HaeIII, and HinfI) were required to differentiate 14 prototypes. PCR with rapid subgenus identification using one-step RFLP with three endonucleases has been described.[180] The use of a multiplex PCR assay for detection of both adenoviruses and herpes simplex viruses in eye swabs has the potential to rapidly detect more than one pathogen with one assay.[181] Additionally, PCR has been used to detect adenoviruses in polluted waters.[182]

A rapid, type-specific, hexon-based quantitative fluorogenic PCR for ADV type 4 has been developed that could be used successfully for clinical samples.[183] PCR also has been successfully used to identify culture-negative environmental samples during an adenovirus-associated respiratory disease outbreak.[184] However, at the present time there is no commercially available PCR assay.

Serology

Acute adenovirus infection can be diagnosed by significant (fourfold) titer rises in response to the hexon antigen by testing acute and convalescent sera with one of several methods. The CF method, measuring group-specific antibodies, is the most widely used and best standardized.[36] The sensitivity is about 50% to 70%.[92,185] Complement-fixing antibody production in infants and young children may be poor, and the CF test can be falsely negative, whereas in adults complement-fixing antibodies from previous infections may cause difficulty in diagnosing a new infection.[34] EIA, also measuring group-specific antibodies, is more sensitive than the CF test and has the added advantage that it can be automated.[36] Sensitivity of the EIA assay has been reported to be 73% to 87%.[92,185] Hemagglutination inhibition and SN assays are more sensitive than CF, but, because they measure type-specific antibodies, these assays are not suitable for routine diagnosis and most reagents are not commercially available. They are described by Hierholzer.[36] A colorimetric microneutralization assay, described by Crawford-Miksza and Schnurr, automates the reading and interpretation of viral infectivity and neutralization and is useful for testing large numbers of specimens.[186]

Treatment

The effect of gamma globulin on ARD was studied in military recruits in the 1960s; protection against adenoviruses was not observed.[187] Topical human fibroblast (β-) interferon has been reported to have a beneficial effect on epidemic keratoconjunctivitis.[188] Nucleoside analogues have been demonstrated to have a potent, nontoxic inhibitory effect on replication of adenoviruses in human embryonic fibroblasts cultures.[189]

Although ribavirin is active against adenoviruses in vitro, no specific antiviral treatment for adenoviral infections is presently recommended.[92] Nebulized ribavirin was used with some success for two children with pneumonia caused by adenovirus.[190] Intravenous ribavirin reportedly has been used in immunocompromised patients, as well as in patients with hemorrhagic cystitis and disseminated disease.[191–195] Intravenous ribavirin was given to 12 adult blood and marrow transplant recipients without appreciable benefit.[196] Successful clearance of adenoviral hepatitis with intravenous ribavirin therapy was also reported in a pediatric liver transplant recipient.[197,198]

The activities of ganciclovir and acyclovir were tested in cell culture and in cotton rat eyes against ADV type 5, which is known to cause severe eye disease.[199] The 50% inhibitory dose was determined by plaque reduction assays in human cells to be 47 and 604 μM for ganciclovir and acyclovir, respectively. When cottontail rabbits were inoculated with 10^5 plaque-forming units per eye, topical treatment for 21 days with 3%, 1%, or 0.3% formulations demonstrated that only the highest dose of 3% reduced the incidence, duration, and titer of virus shed. The differences were not statistically significant, but the observed trend suggested that the 3% dose had a suppressive effect on some disease parameters.[199]

Epidemiology

Incidence and Prevalence

The epidemic characteristics of the adenoviruses vary somewhat among the subgenera.[34] The reason for the tissue tropism exhibited by various types is unknown.[200] However, there are many similar characteristics among the adenoviruses. They are all transmitted by direct contact, aerosolized virus, the fecal-oral route, or water. Those in subgenus C (types 1, 2, 5, and 6) are usually endemic and acquired in early childhood.[34] Many of the other types occur either sporadically or in epidemics. Many adenovirus infections are subclinical or asymptomatic, especially those in subgenera A and D. Conversely, the types (especially 4, 7, and 21) in subgenera B and D usually cause symptomatic respiratory disease.[34] The enteric adenoviruses (types 40 and 41) of subgenus F cause gastroenteritis. The highest incidence of infection for the most common adenoviruses (types 1, 2, 5, and 6) occurs in children less than 2 years of age.

Because only about 50% of childhood adenovirus infections result in disease, prevalence as detected by antibody studies is high.[39–41] By school age, most children have been exposed to several types of adenoviruses. Infections caused by ADV types 4, 7, 14, and 21 may occur at a later age.

Geographically, most types of adenoviruses have been recovered from all areas of the world.[46] From approximately 25,000 isolation reports to the World Health Organization, a periodicity over 10 years was noted for the incidence of ADV types 7, 8, and 19 and less so for types 3 and 4.[46] Age predilections were highly significant for infants for subgenus A (types 12, 18, and 31); for infants and small children for subgenus C (types 1, 2, 5, and 6); for schoolchildren for type 3; for schoolchildren and adults for type 7; and for adults for types 4, 8, and other species of subgenera B, D, and E.[46] A predilection for males was observed for all types in subgenera B and C, and for types 4 and 19.[46]

A national surveillance report for 1982 to 1993 from Japan indicated that illnesses associated with adenoviruses were most common for URI (51% of 17,265 patients), followed by conjunctivitis (32%), and gastroenteritis (18%).[201] ADV type 3 was the most frequently isolated; yearly fluctuations were observed for types 3 and 4; and very few isolates occurred for type 7, which is considered to cause severe pneumonia in many countries.[201]

Study of 166 isolates of human ADV type 7 obtained from the United States and eastern Ontario, Canada, during 1966 to 2000 identified two genome types previously undocumented in North America, types 7d2 and 7h.[32] Since 1996, adenovirus type 7d2 has caused several civilian outbreaks and a large respiratory disease outbreak at a military training center.[29]

Significance as a Public Health Problem

The site of transmission for adenoviruses for most endemic infections has been considered to be the home. Transmission rates are higher in children's institutions and day care centers, as well as in lower socioeconomic groups.[17,18] Enteric adenoviruses may be an important pathogen in the day care setting.[202] Epidemics associated with ADV type 3 often occur in association with swimming activities.[60] Type 8 adenoviruses have been associated with transmission in physicians offices.[61]

Nosocomial outbreaks of adenovirus keratoconjunctivitis have been reported from the accident and emergency department of a major eye hospital in the United Kingdom.[162,203,204] Nosocomial conjunctivitis, pharyngitis, and pneumonia caused by adenoviruses have been noted in hospital intensive care units.[17,205,206]

In current hospital practice, there are increasing numbers of immunocompromised patients, and a growing problem with adenoviral disease is that of severe infection among the immunocompromised.[12] The epidemiologic concern relates to acquisition from a nosocomial perspective, because these patients may be hospitalized for long periods of time. Additionally, reactivation of a latent infection could possibly initiate a nosocomial outbreak. Persons with deficient cell-mediated immunity are at greatest risk for adverse outcomes.[34] Bone marrow transplant patients are especially susceptible to adenovirus infections.[74,102] Immunodeficient patients with pneumonia may experience fatality rates as high as 60%.[12]

Chronic diarrhea in AIDS patients is often a diagnostic problem. A prospective study using extensive diagnostic techniques, such as duodenal, jejunal, and rectal biopsies, demonstrated that 6.5% of such patients were diagnosed with adenovirus infections.[207]

Acute Respiratory Disease of Military Recruits

The epidemic nature of certain adenovirus strains in military recruits has been particularly well documented.[7] Prior to the use of vaccines in the U.S. military, serotypes 4 and 7 accounted for 60% of all ARD in recruits who were hospitalized, while serotypes 3, 14, and 21 were less frequently observed.[21] Up to 80% of recruits became infected, while seasoned military personnel experienced lower rates.[7] Patterns of infections in Dutch military recruits demonstrated that ADV types 4, 7, and 21 were the prevalent types, with attack rates of 20% to 60% and with 7% to 14% of recruits requiring hospital admission.[208]

Extensive studies in unimmunized U.S. Marine Corps personnel showed three different patterns of disease.[209] In contrast to U.S. Army recruits, in whom adenovirus infections were prevalent throughout the year with peaks in fall and winter, Marines experienced sharply demarcated winter epidemics in both advanced recruits and more experienced soldiers. Most of the isolates were type 4, except for a few type 7 isolates. Over 85% of febrile illnesses were associated with adenovirus disease.[210]

Although the civilian experience has not established a requirement for a vaccine, the epidemic nature and extensive morbidity suffered by military recruits during the 1960s demonstrated an overwhelming need for adenovirus vaccines for military use. One well-studied and typical epidemic at Fort Dix, New Jersey, exemplified this requirement.[23] A platoon of 48 men was followed prospectively for their 8 weeks of basic training. Of 92 episodes of respiratory illness, 24 required hospitalization. The documented hospitalization rate for ARD caused by ADV type 4 was 5 per 100 soldiers per week.[23] At large basic training posts, this rate translated to approximately 500 to 800 ARD admissions per week, which had a devastating impact on military hospitals.[23,28] Excess medical costs and the fact that soldiers had to be recycled because of lost training time resulted in significant economic loss to the military. Serious disruptions to training schedules led to administrative attempts to control epidemics, such as sleeping head-to-foot and keeping military units separated (cohorting).[28] Beginning in 1971, live, enteric-coated, oral vaccines for ADV types 4 and 7 were routinely administered.[28]

In 1994, the Department of Defense was notified that the sole producer of ADV types 4 and 7 vaccines, Wyeth Laboratories, would stop production permanently. Beginning in 1984, Wyeth repeatedly notified the Department of Defense of the need to negotiate a contract that would take into consideration the renovation of the existing vaccine production facility; however, the contract was not renegotiated.[211] Bulk vaccine production ceased in 1995, and all vaccine was placed in tablet form in 1996. Through requests for extensions of expiration dates and use of vaccines only during September through March, rather than year round, the military attempted to obtain maximum benefit from the remaining supply. By 1999, all vaccine supplies were depleted.

Since the loss of manufacture of the ADV types 4 and 7 vaccines, there have been many documented outbreaks of ARD caused by adenoviruses in military training centers. The first recorded epidemic took place during April and May of 1995, at Fort Jackson, South Carolina, during a lapse of vaccine administration that occurred because of a logistical error that temporarily interrupted vaccine production.[30] ADV type 4 was identified as the etiologic agent in unvaccinated soldiers, who experienced hospitalization rates of 11.6% during basic training.[30] In 1997, shortly after the manufacturer ceased vaccine production completely, another epidemic of ADV type 4 persisted at Fort Jackson from May until December, during which more than 1000 male and female recruits were hospitalized, with more than 66% having an ADV type 4 isolated.[31] Evaluation of the epidemic, clinical, and immunologic risk factors for adenovirus infection was performed for a subset of patients, demonstrating that anti-adenovirus type 4 immunity was low in new recruits, risk of illness was higher in smokers, and 81% of patients from whom paired sera were collected demonstrated a fourfold or higher increase in serum anti–type 4 adenovirus titer after infection.[55] Results of a nationwide seroprevalence survey among unimmunized U.S. Army trainees confirmed the lack of protective neutralization antibodies to ADV types 4 and 7, with nearly 90% being susceptible to at least one serotype.[212]

The ADV type 4 epidemic appeared to spread from the Army basic training population at Fort Jackson to Fort Gordon, Georgia, where type 4 virus was isolated from 50% of 147 soldiers undergoing advanced training who were hospitalized with ARD.[213] Of the whole advanced training cohort, 80% came to Fort Gordon from Fort Jackson between August and December 1997. Clinically, these soldiers demonstrated a mean oral temperature of 101.9°F; 9% of male patients had a lumbar puncture performed, and 18.3% had radiographic evidence of pneumonia.[214]

Another ADV type 4 outbreak occurred in the basic trainee population at Lackland Air Force Base, Texas, in the fall and winter of 1999–2000. Attack rates ranged from 6 to 19 per 1000, with weekly hospitalizations of 19 to 69 patients per week, with an average length of stay of 5 days.[215] A total of 786 admissions during the 4.5-month period required a dedicated hospital ward and provider team, costing the facility an estimated $2,693,779.[215]

The Navy also experienced outbreaks in the postvaccine era. The largest epidemic in recent history of respiratory illness caused by ADV types 7 and 3 was reported at the Navy's sole basic training center.[29] There were 541 cases of adenovirus infection with 378 cases caused by type 7 and 132 caused by type 3. During one week, the overall rate of respiratory illness reached 52 cases per 1000 recruits per week.[29]

Gray et al. provided a concise overview of population-based surveillance for respiratory disease at four U.S. military training centers as the last of the stores of vaccines were depleted.[149] Between October 1996 and June 1998, 53.1% of 1814 throat cultures from symptomatic trainees yielded adenoviruses.[149] ADV types 4, 7, 3, and 21 accounted for 57%, 25%, 9%, and 7% of the isolates, respectively.[149]

Respiratory diseases will probably always present some problems for the U.S. military, but much of the morbidity caused by adenoviruses, the main problem among recruits, could be alleviated by the reacquisition and use of the vaccines.[216] Since the initial disruption in the supply of an adenovirus vaccine and the subsequent loss of all vaccine stocks, increased respiratory disease rates have been observed at Army, Navy, Marine Corps, Air Force, and Coast Guard training sites (Figs. 30–3 and 30–4). ADV type 4 has been the primary cause, with a large type 7 outbreak occurring in Navy recruits.[29] Efforts to quickly establish a new producer for the adenovirus vaccines have been encouraged and supported by many members of the military and civilian medical communities. [217–221]

A very high rate for adenovirus infections has been reported for military conscripts in Finland.[220] Recent reports of outbreaks from other militaries are lacking. We do not know if this is because outbreaks are not occurring or because outbreaks are not being identified and reported. Differences in geographic locations of training sites, weather conditions, degrees of crowding, stress of training regimens, and sizes of training units may influence the occurrence or severity of adenovirus-associated respiratory disease. In 1997, an ARD outbreak caused by ADV type 11 occurred in a civilian job

Febrile Respiratory Illness (FRI) and Adenovirus (ADV) Morbidity Among Symptomatic Trainees at Eight Military Training Centers

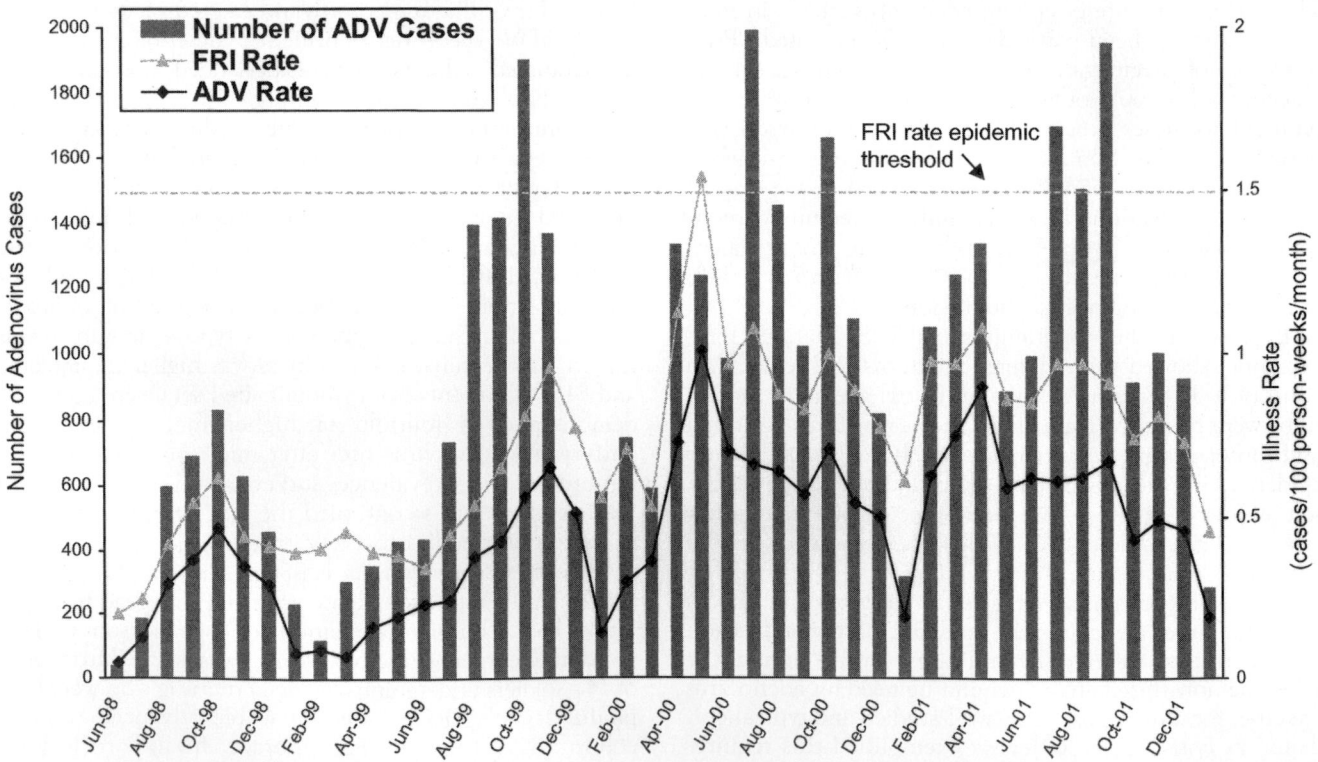

FIGURE 30–3 ▪ Febrile respiratory illness (FRI) rate per 100 person-weeks per month, adenovirus (ADV)-associated FRI rate per 100 person-weeks per month, and number of ADV-associated FRI cases at eight basic (initial entry) training sites for military recruits, June 1998 through January, 2002. During the period September 1998 through March 1999, any unexpired adenovirus vaccine stocks that were available were used; all vaccine stocks were depleted in early 1999. The FRI rate epidemic threshold of 1.5 cases per 100 person-weeks per month is an arbitrary threshold used to identify sites for detailed epidemiologic investigations or interventions. (Courtesy of Anthony Hawksworth, The Department of Defense Center for Deployment Health Research at the Naval Health Research Center, San Diego, CA.)

Adenovirus Infection Rates at Basic Training Centers

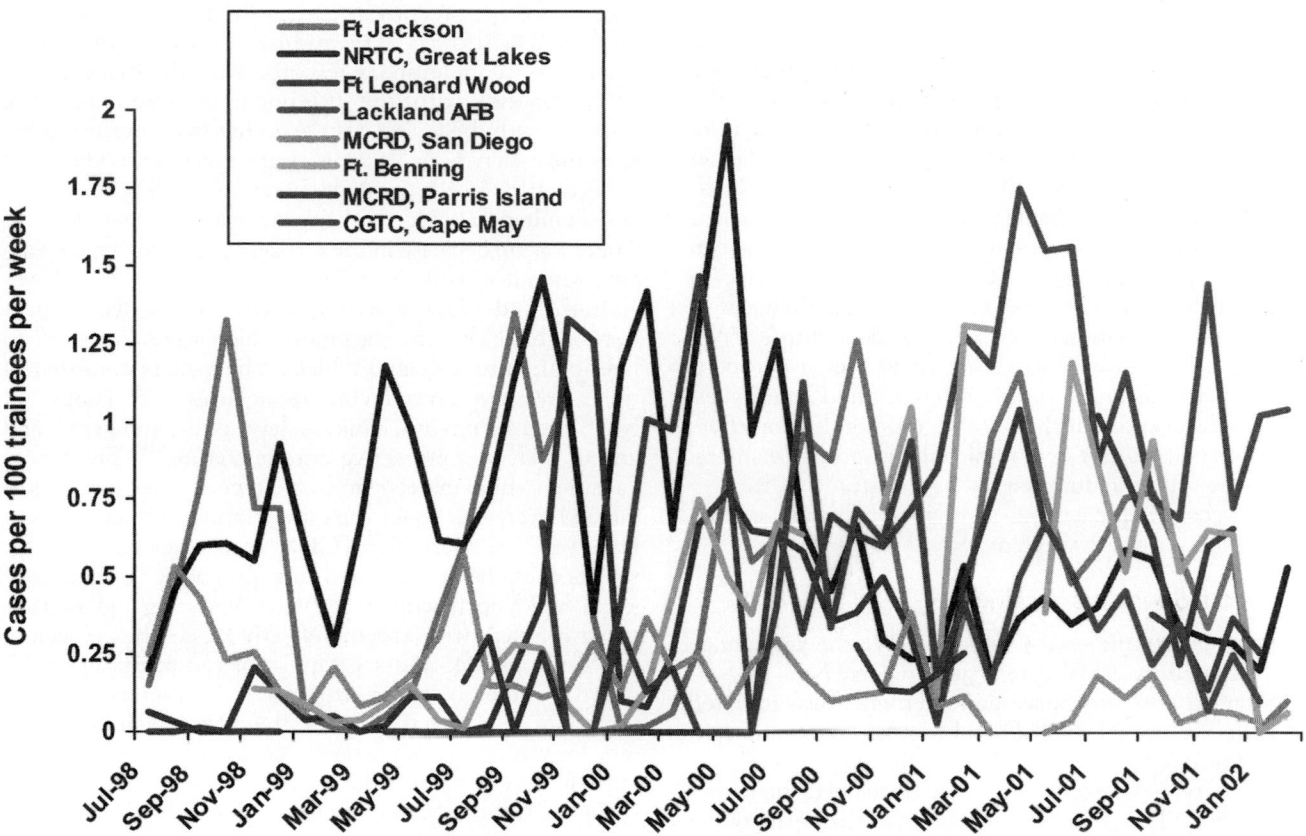

FIGURE 30–4 ■ Febrile respiratory illness rates at eight training centers, July 1998 through January 2002, as reported by the Naval Health Research Center, San Diego, CA, as part of the Department of Defense Global Emerging Infections Surveillance and Response System. Participating training centers were U.S. Army Fort (Ft) Jackson (SC), Ft Leonard Wood (MO), and Ft Benning (GA); Marine Corps Recruit Depot (MCRD), San Diego (CA) and MCRD Parris Island (SC); Naval Recruit Training Center (NRTC), Great Lakes (IL); Lackland Air Force Base (AFB) (TX); and the US Coast Guard Training Center (CGTC), Cape May (NJ). All stocks of adenovirus vaccines were depleted in early 1999. (Courtesy of Anthony Hawksworth, The Department of Defense Center for Deployment Health Research at the Naval Health Research Center, San Diego, CA.)

corps training center in an environment similar to that of a military training center.[221] Increased availability of more sensitive laboratory tests for viral respiratory disease agents may identify more adenovirus-associated respiratory disease outbreaks, perhaps even in civilian colleges.

Passive Immunization

There have been no attempts to passively protect people against adenovirus-associated disease outside of the research setting.[187]

Active Immunization

Prior Approaches That Have Been Abandoned

The first adenovirus vaccine, which was bivalent for types 4 and 7, was grown in monkey kidney cells and formalin inac-

tivated.[28] After safety tests, a small trial in 1957 reduced admissions for adenoviruses by 98% and a large trial of 8238 soldiers was 90% effective in reducing hospitalization.[222,223] A trivalent vaccine, which also included type 3, was also tested.[224] Large-scale production of vaccine lots led to variation in antigenicity, resulting in a loss of protection rates, with only a 52% reduction in hospital illnesses resulting from adenoviruses.[225] Even this low rate of protection was reported in 1965 to have saved the Army about $5 million per year.[225] Adenovirus seed lots were found to be contaminated with simian virus 40, an oncogenic virus, in 1963 and the license for the vaccine was rescinded.[23]

Development of the Current Vaccine

Early Vaccines

Use of a live vaccine for ARD caused by ADV type 7 was investigated, and oral administration was reported in 1960 to induce high antibody levels.[226] Chanock and colleagues demonstrated that some adenoviruses infect the GI tract but do not produce symptoms in adults. This led to the administration of the virus as a vaccine in an enteric-coated capsule, which produced an asymptomatic, intestinal infection.[227,228] Many safety studies were performed in human volunteers, including the administration of the ADV type 4 and type 7 vaccines separately, and the simultaneous administration of both the type 4 and type 7 vaccines.[227] Neutralizing titers were observed and asymptomatic infections were evidenced by the recovery of virus from rectal specimens. Initial vaccine work using HEK cells was later modified to use human diploid fibroblast strains WI-26 and WI-38, because the primary cells were not suitable for large-scale production and there was fear of contamination of the primary lines with other human pathogens.[228] Because some adenoviruses are oncogenic in animals, much attention was paid to safety studies in hamsters and to the transformation of cell lines by adenoviruses.[229,230]

Additional field trials for ADV type 4 vaccine were conducted at Parris Island, South Carolina, and Great Lakes, Illinois, and showed that the vaccine was highly protective, safe, antigenic, and not communicable in military trainees. Vaccine use led to reductions in ARD rates of 50%.[231,232] Intrinsic vaccine efficacy was as high as 82% and specific disease reduction was as high as 69%.[232]

Combined Adenovirus Vaccines

Use of the monotypic type 4 vaccine led to the appearance of ARD caused by ADV type 7 at Fort Dix, New Jersey.[23] The Army Adenovirus Surveillance Program was initiated to identify the agents of ARD and to assess fluctuations in disease patterns.[21]

Before a type 7 vaccine could be developed, numerous studies addressed the oncogenicity potential to humans of the type 7 virus.[233-236] A trial for ADV type 7 vaccine demonstrated safety, infectivity, antigenicity, and lack of communicability similar to that observed for the type 4 vaccine.[237] Additional trials indicated that, when the types 4 and 7 vaccines were given simultaneously, no decrease in antigenicity occurred, and with mass immunization there was 95% suppression of type 7-associated disease.[237-240] Numerous appearances and outbreaks of ADV type 21 in military populations in the United States and in Europe led to the initiation of studies using a type 21 prototype vaccine in safety and immunogenicity trials.[241-245] Because of the absence of prolonged outbreaks associated with ADV type 21, the type 21 vaccine was never licensed or tested for efficacy.[28]

Producers

The sole supplier for the ADV types 4 and 7 vaccines was Wyeth Laboratories Incorporated (Marietta, PA). Wyeth ceased production of the vaccine in 1996, and all vaccine stocks were depleted in 1999. The Wyeth vaccines were routinely administered to military trainees from 1971 until the depletion of supplies. These were the last adenovirus vaccines manufactured for use in the U.S. military with Food and Drug Administration approval, and are described below. For more recent developments, see the section on Future vaccines.

Dosage, Route, and Preparations

Original trials for ADV type 7 vaccine were conducted using 0.05 mL of a 1:10 dilution of the ADV type 7 pool (10^6 median tissue culture infective doses [$TCID_{50}$]) within a hard gelatin capsule and given orally.[227] Time of disintegration within the intestine was assayed radiographically using a barium sulfate-containing capsule and varied between 1 and 5 hours.[227] Dosage studies using the Wyeth vaccine for type 7 virus in clinical trials used three doses: $10^{6.8}$ $TCID_{50}$, $10^{4.8}$ $TCID_{50}$, and less than 10 $TCID_{50}$.[237,238] There was 100% antibody response with the highest dose, 95% response with the intermediate dose, and 56% response with the lowest dose. Another study evaluated the response when both vaccines were given individually at doses of $10^{5.4}$ $TCID_{50}$ for type 7 and 10^4 $TCID_{50}$ for type 4, and simultaneously for both vaccines at the same doses.[237] There was no decrease in the antigenicity of the type 4 vaccine when it was given with the type 7 vaccine.[238]

In the mid-1960s, Wyeth Laboratories took over production of the adenovirus vaccines, which were converted to live, oral, enteric-coated tablets. The tablets consisted of three layers: a central core of at least 10^5 $TCID_{50}$ of lyophilized adenovirus, a middle layer of inert material, and an outer layer of protective enteric coating.[239] The type 4 vaccine (white tablets) and the type 7 vaccine (yellow tablets) were packaged separately, and each tablet contained no less than $10^{4.5}$ $TCID_{50}$ of live adenovirus. The tablets could be administered simultaneously but had to be swallowed quickly without chewing. Vomiting and diarrhea could interfere with vaccine effectiveness. These vaccines were indicated for military populations shown to be at risk of ARD caused by the specific adenovirus serotypes represented in the tablets. Use of the vaccines in pregnant females was not recommended because the possible effects on fetal development had not been studied.

In 1971, the U.S. military began routinely administering both vaccines to males reporting to recruit training centers, but only during the winter months.[23] The incoming recruits were given the vaccines within hours of arrival at a training center in order to obtain protection as early as possible in the training program. Initially, women were not given the vaccines because ARD outbreaks caused by adenoviruses had never been documented among military women, and there was concern about the possibility of administering the vaccines to women who were pregnant.[28]

The program of administering the vaccines only during the high-risk winter months was directed at control, rather than eradication, of ARD caused by adenoviruses.[23] With this schedule, late spring and early fall outbreaks occurred. These outbreaks prompted the U.S. Army and the U.S. Navy to adopt a policy of year-round administration of both adenovirus vaccines in 1983.[28] Taking a different course, the U.S. Air Force stopped the administration of adenovirus vaccines at its only recruit training center in Texas in the mid-1980s and adopted a program of surveillance with use of the vaccines only as indicated.[28]

When the military started immunizations to protect against ARD caused by adenoviruses, training programs were segregated by gender. These separate training programs have since been combined, leading to concern that the risk for ARD caused by adenoviruses would be the same for both men and women. The U.S. military regulations for immunizations required that, based on risk, ADV types 4 and 7 vaccines be administered simultaneously and only once to Army, Navy, and Marine Corps recruits.[246] In the Air Force and Coast Guard, the vaccines were administered when directed by the appropriate authority.[246] The same regulation described precautions to be taken to avoid unintentional administration of the vaccines during pregnancy and instructions regarding counseling against the possibility of pregnancy for 3 months following immunization.[246]

In response to the cessation of adenovirus vaccine production in 1996, the Army, Navy, and Marine Corps modified their policy of year-round vaccine administration in order to conserve the remaining vaccine for use in higher risk months only. The modified policy directed that the vaccines be given to arriving military recruits only during the period of September 1 through March 31 until all vaccine stocks had been used. All existing vaccine stocks were exhausted in 1999.

Constituents

The vaccine tablets contained live viruses, materials added for the growth and maintenance of viruses and cells, and other pharmaceutical materials. Human diploid fibroblast cells (strain WI-38) were used for virus preparation, and growth was maintained in minimum essential medium, Eagle's solution, antibiotics (neomycin sulfate, gentamicin sulfate, and amphotericin B), fetal calf serum, and sodium bicarbonate. After harvesting, the viral growth was freed of particulate material by filtration and dried by lyophilization. During drying, additives including human serum albumin, plasdone, sucrose, d-mannose, d-fructose, dextrose, potassium phosphate, and monosodium glutamate were used to preserve viability. Before processing into tablets, the virus preparation was diluted with lactose powder.[247] The vaccine tablets also contained cellulose acetate, phthalate, alcohol, acetone, castor oil, magnesium stearate, and Amberlite. The type 7 vaccine tablets could be distinguished from the type 4 tablets by their yellow color. The color was produced by FD&C Yellow No. 5 (tartrazine), which could cause allergic-type reactions.

Vaccine Stability

Problems occurred with stability of the Wyeth vaccines in the early 1970s, with disease control being less than desired. The loss of potency was traced to a several-fold log decrease in the virus titer a few months postmanufacture, which was due to contamination of the vaccine viruses in the core by the solvent used in the enteric coating process.[23] The problem was resolved by adequate ventilation of the solvent during production.[23]

The license under which Wyeth produced the vaccines allowed for a 12-month cold storage period after packaging of the vaccines. This equated to annual shipments to the military of products that were dated to expire in 1 year. The vaccines were stored at between 2° and 8°C, but not frozen.

Results of Vaccination

Immune Responses

Oral adenovirus vaccine recipients could shed virus fecally after about 4 days, and could continue to do so for an additional 7 to 8 days, and possibly to 6 weeks.[243,248] Vaccinees

developed neutralizing humoral antibody (immunoglobulin [Ig] G, IgM, and IgA).[243] In soldiers who were free of pre-existing antibody, an average of 80% to 95% developed a neutralizing antibody level of 1:8, while less than 50% demonstrated complement-fixing antibody.[238,249] Neutralizing antibody responses developed in 2 to 3 weeks. In general, antibody titers were less than those achieved after natural infection.[250,251] Local secretory IgA antibody was not induced by the oral vaccine, and reinfection of the respiratory tract was possible, but usually mild or asymptomatic.[252] Because viremia and viruria could occur in patients with febrile disease, invasiveness beyond mucosal surfaces could be important in the pathogenesis of the disease and infection.[253] The serum neutralizing antibody produced as a result of vaccination may have prevented the typical febrile disease associated with natural infection.[249] Local IgA antibody could be produced experimentally by the intranasal inoculation of an ADV type 4 vaccine in liquid.[252]

Results of Controlled Trials of Protection Against Disease

Military recruits who received ADV type 4 vaccine exhibited increased resistance to respiratory disease caused by this virus.[228,231,254] A number of major well-controlled studies of military personnel were performed from 1963 to 1966, in which over 42,000 soldiers were studied.[255] Use of the vaccine reduced ARD by 50% on average and adenovirus infection in recruits by over 90%. Table 30–3 shows the summary results of some of the clinical trials for type 4 vaccine.

Field trials began in 1969 for the ADV type 7 vaccine and indicated protection against disease in susceptible individuals.[238,240,256] Additionally, the two vaccines for types 4 and 7 could be administered simultaneously without interference or loss of efficacy.[238,240,257] As a result of using the vaccines at one large Air Force base over a 9-year period, ARD caused by adenovirus disappeared.[258] The Adenovirus Surveillance Program demonstrated that the combination

TABLE 30–3 ■ Summary of Clinical Trials Using Enteric-Coated Oral Adenovirus Vaccines

Study[*]	Total Vaccinated	Reduction in Hospitalization (%)	Reduction in Adenovirus ARD (%)
1	125	Not done	100
2	339	Not done	100
3	6,883	Not done	96
4	386	46	69
5	23,015	50	Not done
6	607	69	94
7	10,863	47	95
8	4,364	Not done	98
9	3,867	Not done	95

[*]Studies 1 to 7, ADV type 4 vaccine was administered. Studies 8 and 9, ADV types 4 and 7 vaccines were administered.
ARD, acute respiratory disease.
Adapted from Lee SG, Hung PP. Vaccines for control of respiratory disease caused by adenoviruses. Med Virol 209:209–216, 1993.

of the two adenovirus vaccines were highly effective in controlling epidemic ARD.[21] Table 30–3 summarizes some of the clinical trials performed for the type 7 vaccine. From 1971 to 1999, the live, enteric-coated adenovirus vaccines for types 4 and 7 were administered to new military recruits, and successfully controlled ARD caused by adenoviruses.

Other Evidence of Effectiveness

The successful impact of the adenovirus vaccination program can be seen in Figure 30–5, which demonstrates the median weekly ARD rate per 100 men at one large Army basic training post, Fort Dix, New Jersey. No herd immunity can be assumed, because the new recruit cohort changed with every new basic trainee group. Except for the loss of vaccine potency that occurred in the 1970s with solvent contamination,[23] there has never been a reported outbreak of ARD in the U.S. military caused by ADV type 4 or type 7 in groups receiving these vaccines.

The excess morbidity caused by ARD and associated costs are of significant concern to the military. A cost-benefit analysis was performed by Collis et al., which estimated that the use of the vaccines for ADV types 4 and 7 in 1970–1971 saved $7.53 million.[259] The costs of the vaccines produced by a new manufacturer are expected to increase, but a cost-effectiveness analysis for the continued use of the vaccines in Army recruits indicated that use of these vaccines is still expected to be cost effective, having the potential to save approximately $1.5 million annually over no vaccination.[260] A cost-effectiveness analysis was also performed for the Navy, demonstrating that, compared to no vaccination, seasonal vaccination could prevent 4015 cases of adenovirus infections, saving $2.9 million; year-round vaccination would prevent 4555 cases, saving $2.6 million.[261] These analyses support the fact that the military could save millions of dollars by reacquiring and using the adenovirus vaccines for military recruits, in addition to alleviating significant future morbidity and possibly death in recruits.[27,219]

Duration of Immunity

The duration of immunity and persistence of circulating antibody following immunization have never been deter-

mined. The adenovirus vaccines were developed to protect new members of the military (recruits) against ARD caused by ADV types 4 and 7 during training required on entry in the services, which consists of elementary military training (basic training) and training to develop special military skills. The adenovirus vaccines were very effective in accomplishing the outcome for which they were intended, and there was never a need to determine the duration of protection against disease or the persistence of circulating antibodies over time.

Adverse Events

In 1973, a Navy trainee was hospitalized with fever, malaise, and dyspnea for 11 days after receiving the ADV type 4 and type 7 vaccines.[26] The patient died on the 10th hospital day with the diagnosis of ADV type 7 pneumonia, based on the isolation of the virus by cell culture. It was not possible to determine whether his infection was due to a wild-type 7 adenovirus prior to the development of vaccine-induced immunity or to a vaccine strain.[26]

Adverse reactions following the oral administration of the types 4 and 7 vaccines have not been reported. Four study groups were followed for inpatient and outpatient episodes of illness during vaccine safety and immunogenicity trials at Lackland Air Force Base, Texas, in 1976. In addition to the placebo group, one group received three vaccines simultaneously (types 4, 7, and 21), another group received two vaccines simultaneously (types 4 and 7), and the last group received the type 21 vaccine only.[245] No appreciable differences were noted in the inpatient or outpatient experiences of the different groups.[245] Of 146 soldiers who received vaccines to ADV types 4 and 7, there were 2 hospitalizations (1.4%) for ARD, 2 (1.4%) for GI disease, and 3 (2%) for other illnesses.[245] Compared to 101 soldiers in the placebo group, who had hospitalizations of 3 (3%), 2 (2.0%), and 1 (1.0%) for the same categories, respectively, the rates were not different.[245] The outpatient episodes recorded for the same categories of illness also did not differ: ARD, 14.4% for vaccinees compared to 19.8% for placebo group; GI disease, 5.5% compared to 4.0%; and other illnesses, 24% compared to 31.7%.

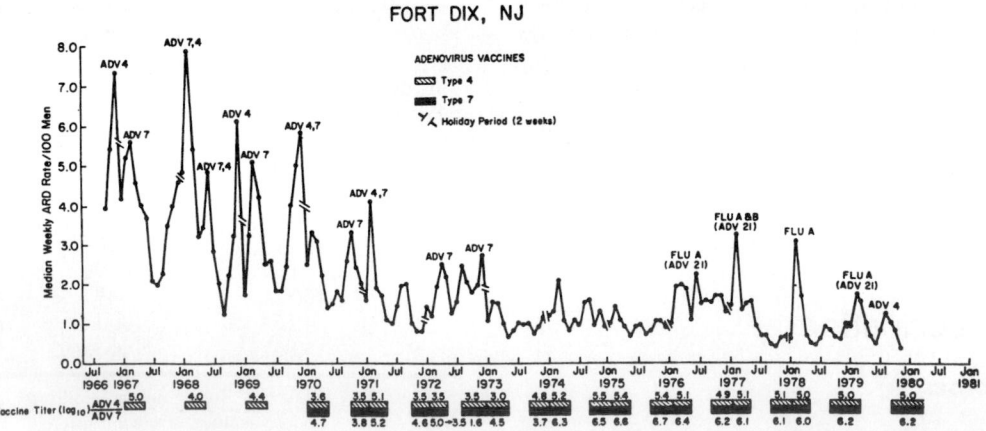

FIGURE 30–5 ■ The median weekly acute respiratory disease (ARD) rate per 100 men at Fort Dix, New Jersey, during the years 1966 to 1980, demonstrating the impact of ADV type 4 and type 7 vaccines. The vaccine titer is listed for each year across the bottom of the graph. (Courtesy of Colonel William H. Bancroft, U.S. Army Headquarters Medical Research and Material Command, Fort Detrick, MD.)

Spread to sites outside the GI tract has not been reported in vaccine recipients.[249] Because the virus is shed fecally for up to 6 weeks, the virus may be spread to family members or very close contacts by fecal-oral transmission.[248]

Indications for Vaccines

Wyeth adenovirus vaccines were indicated for the prevention and control of specific adenovirus-associated ARD in populations with a high risk of exposure, a high level of susceptibility, and a high risk of subsequent infection and disease. In 1976, 42% of Army recruits tested lacked neutralizing antibody to ADV types 4 or 7,[245] and the initial analysis of data from a seroprevalence study of more current recruits supported a continuing high level of susceptibility.[212] In 1995, an outbreak of ADV type 4 was reported in Army basic trainees at Fort Jackson, South Carolina who had not been immunized. The attack rate for the most affected unit at the height of the outbreak was 11.6% per week.[30] In a study of military trainees with ARD, Gray et al. found that unvaccinated trainees were much more likely than vaccinated trainees to be culture positive for ADV types 4 and 7 (odds ratio = 28.1; 95% confidence interval, 20.2 to 39.3).[149] Therefore, the vaccines were indicated for use in selected military populations undergoing their initial military training. The vaccines were not recommended for use in other populations.

Contraindications and Precautions

Gentamicin sulfate, neomycin sulfate, and amphotericin B were used in the vaccine manufacturing process, and traces could be found in the final product. People with known sensitivity to any of these antibiotics were not to receive the vaccines. The FD&C Yellow No. 5 (tartrazine) in the type 7 tablets could cause bronchial asthma or other allergic-type reactions in susceptible people. Sensitivity to this substance occurs infrequently but is often seen in people with aspirin hypersensitivity.

The live, oral adenovirus vaccines were never subjected to animal reproduction studies. Therefore, it is not known if these vaccines had the potential to cause fetal damage if given to a pregnant woman or to affect reproductive capacity. Administration of the vaccines to pregnant women was to be avoided.

Adenoviruses have caused severe, overwhelming, and often fatal infections in immunocompromised individuals. Concern about potentially severe adverse effects if an adenovirus vaccine were given to such an individual prompted a study of recruits who had early human immunodeficiency virus (HIV) infection and received the standard vaccines required for military induction, including the adenovirus vaccines.[262] Although significantly fewer (P < 0.03) HIV-positive subjects responded to the ADV type 4 vaccine than did normal soldiers, no clinically apparent adverse reactions were detected.[262] Response to the type 7 vaccine was difficult to define because many vaccine recipients in both groups had high neutralizing antibody titers at the time of vaccination.[262] More severely immunocompromised individuals, who might inadvertently be infected through fecal shedding from normal vaccine recipients, have not been studied.

Simultaneous Vaccination with Other Vaccines

The adenovirus vaccines were routinely given to military recruits with many other vaccines in the first 8 days after induction into the military. Table 30–4 shows an example of an immunization schedule for military trainees.[262] Type-specific neutralizing antibodies to the adenovirus vaccines were produced in the vaccinated trainees and were associated with protection against ARD. Interference with immune responses when the adenovirus vaccines were given with other vaccines has not been identified.[262]

Future Vaccines

Resuming Vaccine Production for the Military

To prevent adenovirus-related morbidity and mortality following the loss of the adenovirus vaccines, and with the encouragement and support of the Institute of Medicine and the Armed Forces Epidemiological Board, the Department of Defense awarded a contract for production of the adenovirus vaccines on September 25, 2001.[27,200,213,220,263,264] Barr Laboratories (Pomona, NY) received a $17.4 million 3-year contract to resume manufacturing ADV types 4 and 7 vaccines.[211] The vaccines are expected to be similar to the discontinued Wyeth products. The initial contract requires an Investigational New Drug application, sponsored by the Army Office of the Surgeon General, and completion of Phase I clinical trials. Following successful completion of the Phase I trials, an option for $18 million is expected to be approved to support Phase II and III trials and Food and Drug Administration approval.[211] The license will be held by the manufacturer, and the vaccines are expected to be available in 2008.[211] Challenges in meeting projected target dates could be related to ensuring that acetone is appropriately used in the manufacturing, the availability of viable cGMP WI-38 human diploid fibroblast cells, and addressing concerns about transmissible bovine

TABLE 30–4 ■ **Example of an Immunization Schedule for Military Trainees**

Day 0 (arrival)	Adenovirus, live, oral, types 4 and 7
Day 1	Influenza, zonal purified, formaldehyde inactivated, whole virion for intramuscular injection
	Meningococcal polysaccharide vaccine, groups A, C, Y, and WI-135 combined for subcutaneous injection
Day 3	Tetanus and diphtheria toxoids adsorbed for intramuscular injection
Day 8	Poliovirus vaccine, live, oral, types 1, 2, and 3
	Measles virus, live for subcutaneous administration
	Rubella virus, live for subcutaneous injection, given only if the recruit is not immune by enzyme-linked immunoassay

Adapted from Rhodes JL, Birx DL, Wright C, et al. Safety and immunogenicity of multiple conventional immunizations administered during early HIV infection. J Acquir Immune Defic Syndr 4:724–731, 1991.

spongiform encephalopathy agents from fetal calf serum contaminating virus seeds.

Subunit Vaccine

In 1963, soluble viral subunit antigens were found to be highly immunogenic on parenteral administration in animals.[249,264] Crystalline hexon and fiber antigens from ADV type 5 have been shown to induce neutralizing antibody and protection in human volunteers who were challenged.[265] There has been no additional development of these antigens as potential vaccines. However, adenovirus vaccines consisting of soluble viral subunit antigens would be free of DNA and could alleviate fear of the oncogenic potential of adenoviruses.[249]

Recombinant Vaccines

Advances in molecular biology have permitted in vivo and in vitro gene transfer into mammalian cells. Genetically engineered adenoviruses, which are deficient in genes noted for oncogenicity, have been altered to carry heterologous genes from other pathogens.[239] Use of adenoviruses as multiple carrier vaccines could induce immunity to a number of other pathogens, as well as to adenoviruses.[249] Because of their nonpathogenicity compared to ADV types 4 and 7, serotypes 2 and 5 have been used mostly for the development of recombinant vaccines.[266] The adenovirus recombinants have been generated using a variety of strategies. The cloning into the E1 region of a transgene uses a bacterial plasmid carrying the foreign DNA flanked by two subsegments of the wild-type viral genome, which provide the nucleotide sequences for the recombination. The chimeric plasmid is co-transfected with the wild-type adenovirus genome into E1 transcomplementing Graham-293 cells.[266] The recombinant viruses are produced by in vivo homologous recombination between the two input DNA molecules and are defective for the E1A and E1B genes and require Graham-293 cells for growth.[266] Another strategy uses in vitro ligation between plasmid DNA and viral DNA to make up the complete recombinant DNA before transfection.[266] The expression of the hepatitis B surface antigen in the adenovirus E3 gene region has been reported to induce antibody in animals.[267-269]

Studies have investigated the immunogenicity of recombinant adenovirus vaccines (type 4-, 5-, and 7-vectored) carrying the *env* or *gag*-protease genes of the HIV virus.[270-272] Chimpanzees responded with type-specific neutralizing anti-HIV antibodies at secretory sites and cell-mediated immune responses to both Gag and Env antigens.[271,272] Adenoviruses have been also used to express DNA inserts from other viruses, such as human cytomegalovirus, bovine herpesvirus, pseudorabies virus, rabies virus, Epstein-Barr virus, human parainfluenza virus, respiratory syncytial virus, and rotavirus.[266,273,274] Some of these have been tested in a variety of animals, including dogs and chimpanzees, as well as a variety of laboratory animals.[266,275] Some of the advantages and disadvantages of the potential use of adenovirus-vectored vaccines and the safety issues, as well as foreseen obstacles related to their future use, have been addressed.[266,276-278] Imler reviewed the desired characteristics of the second-generation adenovirus-vectored vaccines.[276]

Genetically engineered adenoviruses also have been investigated as gene transfer vectors for such genes as the cystic fibrosis gene and α_1-antitrypsin in preclinical experiments.[279-281] Early genes that are required for viral replication are deleted, rendering the adenoviruses nonreplicative and potentially efficient agents of gene transfer.[279-281] Inefficient gene transfer has also been reported.[282] Dose-dependent inflammatory lung infiltrates resulting from use of such constructs may prove to be a problem.[281] However, one investigation provided data that do not support a role for the production of cytokines by bronchial epithelial cells in the pathogenesis of such inflammation.[283] Others have reported that a similar E1/E3-deficient vector induced increased interleukin-8 production in A549 alveolar epithelial cells.[282] Future uses of adenovirus vaccines as carriers of genes from other pathogens and as gene transfer agents for genetic diseases await safety and efficacy trials in both animals and human subjects. Uses of adenoviruses as vectors for vaccines and for gene therapy of cancer have been reviewed.[284,285]

Public Health Considerations

Epidemiologic Results of Vaccination

In the prevaccine era, ARD caused by adenoviruses caused significant morbidity at military training centers. These outbreaks were extremely costly in terms of medical care requirements and time lost from training.[28] The routine administration of the type 4 and type 7 adenovirus vaccines, which began in 1971, resulted in an extremely efficacious, cost-effective, and safe immunization program.[28,259-261] Initially, the vaccines were administered only during the high-risk winter months. The occurrence of spring and fall outbreaks prompted a modification of the program to administration of the vaccines year round.[28] From 1971 to 1999, with the exception of a period in the 1970s when defective vaccines contaminated with solvent were used,[23] there has never been a reported outbreak of ARD caused by ADV type 4 or type 7 in U.S. military units that received the vaccines. Outbreaks of ARD caused by ADV type 21 have occurred, but these have been sporadic.[28,245]

A problem in the administrative system used to procure vaccines for the U.S. military resulted in an adenovirus vaccine production delay that began in the spring of 1994 and lasted until late February 1995.[28] There was only one outbreak of ARD caused by adenoviruses reported in conjunction with that production delay.[30] When Wyeth Laboratories announced in 1994 that it would no longer produce the adenovirus vaccines, many within the Department of Defense and the different military services asked if the vaccines were still needed. Some thought that improved military barracks with modern heating, ventilation, and air-conditioning systems may have significantly reduced the risk of transmission of the adenoviruses and subsequent disease in susceptible people. The assessment of current risk was hampered by an absence of data on the prevalence of antibodies to adenoviruses in recruits and an absence of studies to assess carriage, transmission, infection, and disease associated with adenoviruses when the vaccines were not given. Because of the success of the vaccines in controlling ARD, the military lost the capability to do serologic studies and had no incentive to study the behavior of adenoviruses in Air Force recruits who had not been routinely receiving the vaccine, but did not have outbreaks. Unfortunately, with the loss of the vaccines, adenovirus-associated ARD increased in all uniformed services, including the Air Force.

Interest in ARD caused by adenoviruses in military populations increased greatly, outbreaks flourished, and several studies were initiated to develop current data and information. The Department of Defense faces several winters without the vaccines until the new manufacturer is in a production mode, possibly in 2008.[211] The decision to resume production was based on a continuing low prevalence of antibodies to ADV types 4 and 7 in people coming into the military,[212] the occurrence of documented outbreaks when the vaccines were not given,[29–31,149,213,286] and almost 30 years of experience of not having ARD outbreaks when potent adenovirus vaccines were being administered.[28]

Disease Control Strategies Now and in the Future

Adenovirus vaccines types 4 and 7 were the primary means for controlling ARD caused by adenoviruses in the U.S. military. Other means consisted of administrative measures and adherence to industry-accepted standards for heating, air conditioning, and ventilation systems. The administrative measures, such as providing each trainee a minimum amount of floor space and enforcing other practices (e.g., cohorting), were aimed at reducing contact and transmission among the trainees.[287,288] Cohorting is a practice whereby military training units are formed into cohorts at the beginning of the training period and contact between people in different cohorts is kept to a minimum during the training period. Within the military barracks, in a line of beds, the recruits could be required to sleep in an alternating head-to-foot pattern, rather than having all heads at the same end of the bed. This is done to increase the distance between breathing zones during the night. Additionally, recruits sleeping in an open area may be required to hang sheets from the ceiling to provide physical barriers between beds. Personal hygiene practices, to include using a handkerchief when sneezing or coughing and hand washing, are supposed to be stressed at all times.[287,288] Even for the best-studied nonvaccine interventions, hand washing and bunk spacing, there is only limited evidence supporting effectiveness.[287,289]

Standards for environmental variables address indoor air temperature, humidity, contaminants, and air exchanges per hour. These standards are intended to define minimum criteria for indoor air quality that will be acceptable to human occupants. Any association between the standards and the risk of acquiring ARD caused by adenoviruses is weak or empirical. However, these are the only standards available and are recommended for use in military buildings.[290]

Recommended Use

Adenovirus vaccines were recommended for use in military populations at risk of developing ARD caused by adenoviruses. Use of these vaccines was not recommended for other populations. Current and future studies of virus transmission and disease occurrence in pediatric populations, chronic care and other civilian institutional settings, high-level health care organizations, and colleges may identify other markets for adenovirus vaccines. The development of adenovirus vaccines for children will require dosage forms other than enteric-coated tablets or the use of further attenuated virus strains.

Acknowledgments

The authors thank Leonard N. Binn, Ph.D., Department of Virus Diseases, Walter Reed Army Institute of Research, Silver Spring, MD; and Gregory C. Gray, M.D., M.P.H., Department of Epidemiology, College of Public Health, University of Iowa, Iowa City, IA, for their review of this chapter and their thoughtful suggestions.

REFERENCES

1. Rowe WP, Huebner RJ, Gilmore LK. Isolation of a cytopathogenic agent from human adenoids undergoing spontaneous degeneration in tissue culture. Proc Soc Exp Biol Med 84:570–573, 1953.
2. Hilleman MR, Werner JH. Recovery of new agent from patients with acute respiratory illness. Proc Soc Exp Biol Med 85:183–188, 1954.
3. Adler H. Keratitis subepithelialis. Zentralbl Prakt Augenhelkd 16:289–294, 1889.
4. Jawetz E. The story of shipyard eye. Br Med J 1:873–878, 1959.
5. Huebner RJ, Rowe WP, Ward TJ. Adenoidal-pharyngeal-conjunctival agents. N Engl J Med 251:1077–1087, 1954.
6. Enders JF, Bell JA, Dingle J. Adenoviruses group name proposed for new respiratory tract viruses. Science 124:119–120, 1956.
7. Dingle JH, Langmuir AD. Epidemiology of acute respiratory disease in military recruits. Am Rev Respir Dis 97(suppl):1–65, 1968.
8. Hilleman MR, Gauld RL, Butler RL. Appraisal of occurrence of adenovirus caused respiratory illness in military populations. Am J Hyg 66:29–51, 1957.
9. Chang C, Lepine P, Lelong M, Le-Tan-Vinn SP. Severe and fatal pneumonia in infants associated with adenovirus infections. Am J Hyg 67:367–378, 1958.
10. Johanson ME, Brown M, Hierholzer JC. Genome analysis of adenovirus type 31 from immunocompromised and immunocompetent patients. J Infect Dis 163:293–299, 1991.
11. Brandt CD, Kim HW, Vargosko AJ, et al. Infections in 18,000 infants and children in a controlled study of respiratory tract disease. I. Adenovirus pathogenicity in relation to serologic type and illness syndrome. Am J Epidemiol 90:484–500, 1969.
12. Hierholzer JC. Adenoviruses in the immunocompromised host. Clin Microbiol Rev 5:262–274, 1992.
13. Pinto A, Beck R, Jadavji T. Fatal neonatal pneumonia caused by adenovirus type 35. Arch Pathol Lab Med 116:95–99, 1992.
14. Stalder H, Hierholzer JC, Oxman MN. New human adenovirus candidate (adenovirus type 35) causing fatal disseminated infection in a renal transplant recipient. J Clin Microbiol 6:257–265, 1977.
15. Hierholzer JC, Wigand R, Anderson IJ, et al. Adenoviruses from patients with AIDS: a plethora of serotypes and a description of five new serotypes of subgenus D types 43–47. J Infect Dis 158:804–813, 1988.
16. Ambinder RF, Burns W, Forman M, et al. Hemorrhagic cystitis associated with adenovirus infection in bone marrow transplantation. Arch Intern Med 146:1400–1401, 1986.
17. Pingleton SK, Pingleton WW, Hill RH, et al. Type 3 adenoviral pneumonia occurring in a respiratory intensive care unit. Chest 73:554–555, 1978.
18. Albert MJ. Enteric adenoviruses. Arch Virol 88:1–17, 1986.
19. Warren D, Nelson KE, Farrar JA, et al. A large outbreak of epidemic keratoconjunctivitis—problems in controlling nosocomial spread. J Infect Dis 160:938–943, 1989.
20. Wishart PK, James C, Wishart MS, Darougar S. Prevalence of acute conjunctivitis caused by chlamydia, adenovirus, and herpes simplex virus in an ophthalmic casualty department. Br J Ophthalmol 68:653–655, 1984.

21. Dudding BA, Top FH, Winter P. Acute respiratory disease in military trainees: the adenovirus surveillance program 1966–1971. Am J Epidemiol 97:187–198, 1973.

22. Hilleman MR. Epidemiology of adenovirus respiratory infections in military recruit populations. Ann N Y Acad Sci 67:262–272, 1967.

23. Top HR Jr. Control of adenovirus acute respiratory disease in U.S. Army trainees. Yale J Biol Med 48:185–195, 1975.

24. Dudding BA, Wagner SC, Zeller JA. Fatal pneumonia associated with adenovirus type 7 in three military recruits. N Engl J Med 286:1289–1292, 1972.

25. Levin S, Dietrich J, Guillory J. Fatal nonbacterial pneumonia associated with adenovirus type 4: occurrence in an adult. JAMA 201:155–157, 1967.

26. Loker EF, Hodges GR, Kelly DJ. Fatal adenovirus pneumonia in a young adult associated with ADV-7 vaccine. Chest 66:197–199, 1974.

27. Two fatal cases of adenovirus-related illness in previously healthy young adults—Illinois, 2000. MMWR Morb Mortal Wkly Rep 50:553–555, 2001.

28. Gaydos CA, Gaydos JC. Adenovirus vaccines in the U.S. military. Mil Med 160:300–304, 1995.

29. Ryan MAK, Gray GC, Smith B, et al. Large epidemic of respiratory adenovirus types 7 and 3 in healthy young adults. Clin Infect Dis 34:577–582, 2002.

30. Barraza EM, Ludwig SL, Gaydos CA, Brundage JF. Reemergence of adenovirus type 4 acute respiratory disease (ARD) in military trainees: report of an outbreak during a lapse in vaccination. J Infect Dis 179:1531–1533, 1999.

31. McNeill KM, Hendrix RM, Lindner JL, et al. Large, persistent epidemic of adenovirus type 4-associated acute respiratory disease in US army trainees. Emerg Infect Dis 5:798–801, 1999.

32. Erdman DD, Xu W, Gerber SI, et al. Molecular epidemiology of adenovirus type 7 in the United States, 1966–2000. Emerg Infect Dis 8:269–277, 2002.

33. Hashido M, Mukouyama A, Sakae K, et al. Molecular and serological characterization of adenovirus genome type 7h isolated in Japan. Epidemiol Infect 122:281–286, 1999.

34. Foy HM. Adenoviruses. In Evans AS (ed). Viral Infections of Humans. New York, Plenum Press, 1989, pp 77–89.

35. Rubin BA. Clinical picture and epidemiology of adenovirus infections. Acta Microbiol Hung 40:303–323, 1993.

36. Hierholzer JC. Adenoviruses. In Murray PR, Baron EJ, Pfaller MA, et al (eds). Manual of Clinical Microbiology (6th ed). Washington, DC, ASM Press, 1997, pp 947–953.

37. Baum SG. Adenovirus. In Mandell GL, Bennett JE, Dolin R (eds). Principles and Practice of Infectious Diseases. New York, Churchill Livingstone, 1995, pp 1382–1387.

38. Brandt CD, Kim HW, Jeffries BC, et al. Infections in 18,000 infants and children in a controlled study of respiratory tract disease: variation in adenovirus infections by year and season. Am J Epidemiol 95:218–227, 1972.

39. Fox JP, Brandt CD, Wassermann FE, et al. The virus watch program: a continuing surveillance of viral infections in metropolitan New York families. VI. Observations of adenovirus infections: virus excretion patterns, antibody response, efficiency of surveillance, patterns of infection and relation to illness. Am J Epidemiol 89:25–50, 1969.

40. Cooney MK, Hall CE, Fox JP. The Seattle virus watch: evaluation of isolation methods and summary of infections detected by virus isolations. Am J Epidemiol 96:286–305, 1972.

41. Hall CE, Brandt CD, Frothingham TE, et al. The virus watch program: a continuing surveillance of viral infections in metropolitan New York families. IX. A comparison of infections with several respiratory pathogens in New York and New Orleans families. Am J Epidemiol 94:367–385, 1971.

42. Foy HM, Cooney MK, McMahan R, Grayston JT. Viral and mycoplasmal pneumonia in a prepaid medical care group during an eight-year period. Am J Epidemiol 161:123–126, 1973.

43. Benyesh-Melnick M, Rosenberg HS. The isolation of adenovirus type 7 from a fatal case of pneumonia and disseminated disease. J Pediatr Gastroenterol 64:83–87, 1964.

44. Simla S, Ylikorkala O, Wasz-Hockert O. Type 7 adenovirus vaccine in volunteers: clinical and immunological responses. J Pediatr 79:605–611, 1971.

45. Straube RC, Thompson MA, Van Dyke RB, et al. Adenovirus type 7b in a children's hospital. J Infect Dis 147:814–819, 1983.

46. Schmitz H, Wigand R, Heinrich W. Worldwide epidemiology of human adenovirus infections. Am J Epidemiol 117:455–466, 1983.

47. Pacini DL, Collier AM, Henderson FW. Adenovirus infections and respiratory illnesses in children in group day care. J Infect Dis 156:920–927, 1987.

48. Cole RM, Mastrota FM, Floyd TM, Chanock RM. Illness and microbial experiences of nursery children at Junior Village. Am J Hyg 74:267–292, 1961.

49. Gerber SI, Erdman DD, Pur SL, et al. Outbreak of adenovirus genome type 7d2 infection in a pediatric chronic-care facility and tertiary-care hospital. Clin Infect Dis 32:694–700, 2001.

50. Mitchell LS, Taylor B, Reimels W, et al. Adenovirus 7a: a community-acquired outbreak in a children's hospital. Pediatr Infect Dis 19:996–1000, 2000.

51. Commission on Acute Respiratory Disease. Experimental transmission of minor respiratory illness to human volunteers by filter-passing agents: demonstration of two types of illness characterized by long and short incubation periods and different clinical features. J Clin Invest 26:957–973, 1947.

52. Baum SG. Adenoviruses. In Gorbach SL, Bartlett JB, Blacklow NB (eds). Infectious Diseases. Philadelphia, WB Saunders, 1992, pp 1663–1667.

53. Couch RB, Cate TR, Dougla RJ. Effects of route of inoculation on experimental respiratory viral disease in volunteers and evidence for airborne transmission. Bacteriol Rev 30:517–531, 1966.

54. Amundson DE, Weiss PJ. Pneumonia in military recruits. Mil Med 159:629–631, 1994.

55. Sanchez JL, Binn LN, Innis BL, et al. Epidemic of adenovirus-induced respiratory illness among US military recruits: epidemiologic and immunologic risk factors in healthy, young adults. J Med Virol 65:710–718, 2001.

56. Bell JA, Rowe WP, Engler JI, et al. Pharyngoconjunctival fever: epidemiological studies of a recently recognized disease entity. JAMA 157:1083–1092, 1955.

57. Bahn C. Swimming bath conjunctivitis. New Orleans Med Sci J 79:586–590, 1927.

58. D'Angelo LJ, Hierholzer JC, Keenlyside RA, et al. Pharyngoconjunctival fever caused by adenovirus type 4: report of a swimming pool-related outbreak with recovery of virus from pool water. J Infect Dis 140:42–47, 1979.

59. Parrott RH, Rowe WP, Huebner RJ, et al. Outbreak of febrile pharyngitis and conjunctivitis associated with type 3 adenoidal-pharyngeal-conjunctival virus infection. N Engl J Med 251:1087–1090, 1954.

60. Foy HM, Cooney MK, Hatlen JB. Adenovirus type 3 epidemic associated with intermittent chlorination of a swimming pool. Arch Environ Health 17:795–802, 1968.

61. Hogan MJ, Crawford JW. Epidemic keratoconjunctivitis superficial punctate keratitis, keratitis sub-epithelialis, keratitis maculosa, keratitis nummularis. Am J Ophthalmol 25:1057–1078, 1942.

62. D'Angelo LJ, Hierholzer JC, Holman RC, Smith JD. Epidemic keratoconjunctivitis caused by adenovirus type 8: epidemiologic and laboratory aspects of a large outbreak. Am J Epidemiol 113:44–49, 1981.

63. Darougar S, Grey RHB, Thaker U, McSwiggan DA. Clinical and epidemiological features of adenovirus keratoconjunctivitis in London. Br J Ophthalmol 67:1–7, 1983.

64. Guyer B, O'Day DM, Hierholzer JC, Schafner W. Epidemic keratoconjunctivitis: a community outbreak of mixed adenovirus type 8 and type 19 infection. J Infect Dis 132:142–150, 1975.

65. Kemp MC, Hierholzer JC, Cabradilla CP, Obijeski JF. The changing etiology of epidemic keratoconjunctivitis: antigenic and restriction enzyme analyses of adenovirus type 19 and 37 isolated over a 10-year period. Acta Paediatr Scand 148:24–33, 1983.

66. Darougar S, Walpita P, Thaker U, et al. Adenovirus serotype isolated from ocular infections in London. Br J Ophthalmol 67:111–114, 1983.

67. Muzerie CJ, Wermenbol AG, Schaap GJP. Adenovirus 37: identification and characterization of a medically important new adenovirus type of subgroup D. J Med Virol 7:105–118, 1981.

68. Harnett GB, Newnham WA. Isolation of adenovirus type 19 from the male and female genital tracts. Br J Vener Dis 57:55–57, 1981.

69. Sprague JB, Hierholzer JC, Currier RW II, et al. Epidemic keratoconjunctivitis: a severe industrial outbreak due to adenovirus type 8. N Engl J Med 289:1341–1346, 1973.

70. Keenlyside RA, Hierholzer JC, D'Angelo LJ. Keratoconjunctivitis associated with adenovirus type 37—an extended outbreak in an ophthalomologist office. J Infect Dis 147–191, 1983.

71. Mufson MA, Belshe RB. A review of adenoviruses in the etiology of acute hemorrhagic cystitis. J Urol 115:191, 1976.

72. Numazaki Y, Kimasaka T, Yano N, et al. Further study of acute hemorrhagic cystis due to adenovirus type 11. N Engl J Med 289:344–347, 1973.

73. Koga S, Shindo K, Matsuya F, et al. Acute hemorrhagic cystitis caused by adenovirus following renal transplantation: review of the literature. J Urol 149:838–839, 1993.

74. Londergan TA, Walzak MP. Hemorrhagic cystitis due to adenovirus infection following bone marrow transplantation. J Urol 151:1013–1014, 1994.

75. Echavarria MS, Ray SC, Ambinder R, et al. PCR detection of adenovirus in a bone marrow transplant recipient: hemorrhagic cystitis as a presenting manifestation of disseminated disease. J Clin Microbiol 37:686–689, 1999.

76. Horwitz MS. Adenoviridae and their replication. In Fields BN, Knipe DM, Chanock RM, et al (eds). Virology. New York, Raven Press, 1990, pp 1679–1721.

77. Ito M, Hirabayashi N, Uno Y. Necrotizing tubulointerstitial nephritis associated with adenovirus infection. Hum Pathol 22:1225–1231, 1991.

78. Koc J, Wigand R, Weil M. The efficacy of various laboratory methods for the diagnosis of adenovirus conjunctivitis. Zentralbl Bakteriol Mikrobiol Hyg 263:607–615, 1987.

79. Yolken RH, Lawrence F. Gastroenteritis associated with enteric type adenovirus in hospitalized infants. J Pediatr Gastroenterol 101:21–26, 1982.

80. Brandt CD, Kim HW, Rodriguez WJ, et al. Comparison of direct electron microscopy, immune electron microscopy, and rotavirus enzyme linked immunosorbent assay for detection of gastroenteritis viruses in children. J Clin Microbiol 13:976–981, 1981.

81. Chiba S, Nakatq S, Nakamuba I, et al. Outbreak of infantile gastroenteritis due to type 40 adenovirus. Lancet 2:954–957, 1983.

82. Rodriguez WJ, Kim HW, Brandt CD, et al. Fecal adenoviruses from a longitudinal study of families in metropolitan Washington D.C.: laboratory clinical and epidemiologic observations. J Pediatr Gastroenterol 107:514–520, 1985.

83. Uhnoo I, Wadell G, Svensson L, Johansson ME. Importance of enteric adenoviruses 40 and 41 in acute gastroenteritis in infants and young children. J Clin Microbiol 20:365–372, 1984.

84. Simila S, Jouppila R, Salmi A. Encephalomeningitis in children associated with an adenovirus type 7 epidemic. Acta Paediatr Scand 59:310, 1970.

85. Kelsey DS. Adenovirus meningoencephalitis. Pediatrics 61:291–293, 1978.

86. Chatterjee NK. Isolation and characterization of adenovirus 5 from the brain of an infant with fatal cerebral edema. Clin Infect Dis 31:830–833, 2000.

87. Abzug ML, Levine MJ. Neonatal adenovirus infection: four patients and review of the literature. Pediatrics 87:890–896, 1991.

88. Connor JD. Evidence for an etiologic role of adenoviral infection in pertussis syndrome. N Engl J Med 283:390–394, 1970.

89. Klenk EL, Gwaltney JM, Bass JW. Bacteriologically proved pertussis and adenovirus infection. Am J Dis Child 124:203–207, 1972.

90. Sturdy PM, Court SD, Gardner PS. Viruses and whooping-cough. Lancet 2:978–979, 1971.

91. Nelson KE, Gavitt F, Batt MD, et al. The role of adenoviruses in the pertussis syndrome. J Pediatr Gastroenterol 86:335–341, 1975.

92. Russkanen O, Meurman O, Kusjavi A. Adenoviruses. In Richman DD, Whitley RJ, Hayden FG (eds). Clinical Virology. New York, Churchill Livingstone, 1997, pp 525–547.

93. Couroucli XI, Welty SE, Ramsay PL, et al. Detection of microorganisms in the tracheal aspirates of preterm infants by polymerase chain reaction: association of adenovirus infection with bronchopulmonary dysplasia. Pediatr Res 47:225–232, 2000.

94. Shields AF, Hackman RC, Fife KH, et al. Adenovirus infections in patients undergoing bone-marrow transplantation. N Engl J Med 312:529–533, 1985.

95. Carmichael GPJ, Zahradnick JM, Moyer GH, Porter DD. Adenovirus hepatitis in an immunosuppressed adult patient. Clin Pathol 71:352–355, 1979.

96. DeJong PJ, Valderrama G, Spigland I, Horwitz MS. Adenovirus isolates from urine of patients with acquired immunodeficiency syndrome. Lancet 1:1293–1296, 1983.

97. Horwitz MS, Valderrama G, Korn R, Spigland I. Adenovirus isolates from the urines of AIDS patients: characterization of group B

recombinants. In Gottlieb MS, Groopman JE (eds). Acquired Immune Deficiency Syndrome (UCLA Symposia on Molecular and Cellular Biology). New York, Alan R Liss, 1984, pp 187–207.

98. Ohori NP, Michaels MG, Jaffe R, et al. Adenovirus pneumonia in lung transplant recipients. Hum Pathol 26:1073–1079, 1995.

99. Flomenberg PR, Chen M, Munk G. Molecular epidemiology of adenovirus type 35 infections in immunocompromise host. J Infect Dis 155:1127–1134, 1987.

100. Schnurr D, Dondero ME. Two new candidate adenovirus serotypes. Intervirology 36:79–83, 1993.

101. Gelfand MS, Cleveland KO, Lancaster D, et al. Adenovirus parotitis in patients with AIDS. Clin Infect Dis 19:1045–1048, 1994.

102. Flomenberg P, Babbitt J, Drobyski WR, et al. Increasing incidence of adenovirus disease in bone marrow transplant recipients. J Infect Dis 169:775–781, 1994.

103. Dolin R. Viral pneumonia. In Gorbach SL, Bartlett JB, Blacklow NB (eds). Infectious Diseases. Philadelphia, WB Saunders, 1992, pp 485–490.

104. Echavarria M, Forman M, van Tol MJD, et al. Prediction of severe disseminated adenovirus infection by serum PCR. Lancet 358:384–385, 2001.

105. Howard DS, Phillips IGL, Reece DE, et al. Adenovirus infections in hematopoietic stem cell transplant recipients. Clin Infect Dis 29:1494–1501, 1999.

106. Benko M, Harrach B, Russell WC. Family Adenoviridae. In van Regenmortel MHV, Fauquet CM, Bishop DHL et al (eds). Virus Taxonomy. San Diego, Academic Press, 2000, pp 227–238.

107. Ginsberg HS, Pereira HG, Valentine RC, Wilcox WC. A proposed terminology for the adenovirus antigens and virion morphological subunits. Virology 28:782–783, 1966.

108. Horne RW, Bonner S, Waterson AP. The icosohedral form of an adenovirus. J Mol Biol 1:84–86, 1956.

109. Maizel JV Jr, White DO, Scharff MD. The polypeptides of adenovirus: evidence for multiple protein components in the virion and a comparison of types 2, 7A and 12. Virology 36:115–125, 1968.

110. Van Oostrum J, Burnett RM. Molecular composition of the adenovirus type 2 virion. J Virol 56:439–488, 1985.

111. Philipson J, Peterson U, Lindberg U. Molecular biology of adenoviruses. Virol Monogr 14:1–115, 1975.

112. Wadell G. Adenoviridae: the adenoviruses. In Lennett EH, Halonen P, Murphy FA (eds). Laboratory Diagnosis of Infectious Disease: Principles and Practice. New York, Springer Verlag, 1988, pp 284–300.

113. Hierholzer JC, Stone YO, Broderson JR. Antigenic relationships among the 47 human adenoviruses determined in reference horse antisera. Arch Virol 121:179–197, 1991.

114. Hierholzer JC, Wigand R, De Jong JC. Evaluation of human adenoviruses 38, 39, 40 and 41 as new serotypes. Intervirology 29:1–10, 1988.

115. Wadell G. Molecular epidemiology of human adenoviruses. Curr Top Microbiol Immunol 110:191–220, 1984.

116. Adrian T, Wadell G, Hierholzer JC, Wigand R. DNA restriction analysis of adenovirus prototypes 1 to 41. Arch Virol 91:277–290, 1986.

117. Adrian T, Becker M, Hierholzer JC, Wigand R. Molecular epidemiology and restriction site mapping of adenovirus 7 genome types. Arch Virol 106:73–84, 1989.

118. Li Q-G, Wadell G. Analysis of 15 different genome types of adenovirus type 7 isolated on five continents. J Virol 60:331–335, 1986.

119. Li Q-G, Wadell G. Comparison of 17 genome types of adenovirus type 3 identified among strains recovered from six continents. J Clin Microbiol 20:1009–1015, 1988.

120. Adrian T. Genome type analysis of adenovirus type 4. Intervirology 34:180–183, 1992.

121. Cooper RJ, Bailey AS, Killough R, Richmond SJ. Genome analysis of adenovirus 4 isolated over a six year period. J Med Virol 39:62–66, 1993.

122. Li Q-G, Zheng Q, Liu Y, Wadell G. Molecular epidemiology of adenovirus type 3 and 7 isolated from children with pneumonia in Beijing. J Med Virol 49:170–177, 1996.

123. Evans AS. Latent adenovirus infections of the human respiratory tract. Am J Hyg 67:256–266, 1958.

124. Andiman WA, Miller G. Persistent infection with adenovirus type 5 and 6 in lymphoid cells from humans and wooly monkeys. J Infect Dis 145:83–88, 1982.

125. Zahradnik JM, Spencer MJ, Porter DD. Adenovirus infection in the immunocompromised patient. Am J Med 68:725–732, 1980.
126. Yolken RH, Bishop CA, Townsend TR. Infectious gastroenteritis in bone-marrow transplant recipients. N Engl J Med 306:1009–1012, 1982.
127. Brummitt CF, Cherrington JM, Katzenstein DA. Nosocomial adenovirus infections: molecular epidemiology of an outbreak due to adenovirus. J Infect Dis 158:423–432, 1988.
128. Reid JA, Breckon D, Hunter PR. Infection of staff during an outbreak of viral gastroenteritis in an elderly person's home. J Hosp Infect 16:81–85, 1990.
129. Baum SG. Persistent adenovirus infections of nonpermissive monkey cells. J Virol 23:412, 1977.
130. Wold WSM. Adenovirus genes that modulate the sensitivity of virus-infected cells to lysis by TNF. J Cell Biochem 53:329–335, 1993.
131. Horvath J, Palkonyay L, Weber J. Group C adenovirus DNA sequences in human lymphoid cells. J Virol 59:189–192, 1986.
132. Huebner RJ, Rowe WP, Lane WT. Oncogenic effects in hamsters of human adenoviruses types 12 and 18. Proc Natl Acad Sci U S A 48:2051, 1962.
133. Ginsberg HS, Lundholm-Beauchamp U, Horswood RL, et al. Role of early region 3 (E3) in pathogenesis of adenovirus disease. Proc Natl Acad Sci U S A 86:3823–3827, 1989.
134. Ginsberg HS, Prince GA. The molecular basis of adenovirus pathogenesis. Infect Agents Dis 3:1–8, 1994.
135. Elliott WM, Hayashi S, Hogg JC. Immunodetection of adenoviral E1A proteins in human lung tissue. Am J Respir Cell Mol Biol 12:642–648, 1995.
136. Gold DR, Tager IB, Weiss ST, et al. Acute lower respiratory illness in childhood as predictor of lung function and chronic respiratory symptoms. Am Rev Respir Dis 140:877–884, 1989.
137. Liu F, Green MR. Promoter targeting by adenovirus E1a through interaction with different cellular DNA binding domains. Nature 368:520–525, 1994.
138. Shenk T, Flint J. Transcriptional and transforming activities of the adenovirus E1a proteins. Adv Cancer Res 57:47–85, 1991.
139. Matsuse T, Hayashi S, Kuwano K, et al. Latent adenoviral infection in the pathogenesis of chronic airways obstruction. Am Rev Respir Dis 146:177–184, 1992.
140. Bergelson JM, Cunningham JA, Droguett G, et al. Isolation of a common receptor for Coxsackie b viruses and adenoviruses 2 and 5. Science 275:1320–1323, 1997.
141. Buescher EL. Respiratory disease and the adenoviruses. Med Clin North Am 51:769–779, 1967.
142. Durepaire N, Ranger-Rogez S, Denis F. Evaluation of rapid culture centrifugation method for adenovirus detection in stool. Diagn Microbiol Infect Dis 24:25–29, 1996.
143. Hierholzer J, Schmidt I, Emmons NJ. Diagnostic Procedures for Viral, Rickettsial, and Chlamydial Infections (6th ed). Washington, DC, American Public Health Association, 1989, pp 219–264.
144. Rabalais GP, Stout GG, Ladd KL, Cost KM. Rapid diagnosis of respiratory viral infections by using a shell vial assay and monoclonal antibody pool. J Clin Microbiol 30:1505–1508, 1992.
145. Thomas EE, Roscoe DL. The utility of latex agglutination assays in the diagnosis of pediatric viral gastroenteritis. Am J Clin Pathol 101:742–746, 1994.
146. Hierholzer JC, Johansson KH, Anderson LJ, et al. Comparison of monoclonal time-resolved fluoroimmunoassay with monoclonal capture biotinylated detector enzyme immunoassay for adenovirus antigen detection. J Clin Microbiol 25:1662–1667, 1987.
147. Elnifro EM, Cooper RJ, Klapper PE, Bailey AS. PCR and restriction endonuclease analysis for rapid identification of human adenovirus subgenera. J Clin Microbiol 38:2055–2061, 2000.
148. Allard A, Albinsson B, Wadell G. Rapid typing of human adenoviruses by a general PCR combined with restriction endonuclease analysis. J Clin Microbiol 39:498–505, 2000.
149. Gray GC, Goswami PR, Malasig M, et al. Adult adenovirus infections: loss of orphaned vaccines precipitates military respiratory disease epidemics. Clin Infect Dis 31:663–670, 2000.
150. Crawford-Miksza LK, Nang RN, Schnurr DP. Strain variation in adenovirus serotypes 4 and 7a causing acute respiratory disease. J Clin Microbiol 37:1107–1112, 1999.
151. Madeley CR. The emerging role of adenoviruses as inducers of gastroenteritis. Pediatr Infect Dis 5:S63–S74, 1986.
152. Brown M, Petric M, Middleton PJ. Diagnosis of fastidious enteric adenoviruses 40 and 41 in stool specimens. J Clin Microbiol 20:334–338, 1984.
153. Wolfgang S, Schneider T, Heise W, et al. Stool viruses coinfections and diarrhea in HIV-infected patients. J Acquir Immune Defic Syndr Hum Retrovirol 13:33–38, 1996.
154. Wood DJ, Bijlsma K, De-Jong JC, Tonkin C. Evaluation of a commercial monoclonal antibody-based enzyme immunoassay for detection of adenovirus types 40 and 41 in stool specimens. J Clin Microbiol 27:1155–1158, 1989.
155. Kok T, Mickan LD, Burrell CJ. Routine diagnosis of seven respiratory viruses and Mycoplasma pneumoniae by enzyme immunoassay. J Virol 50:87–100, 1994.
156. Wood SR, Sharp IR, De-Jong JC, Uijterwaal-Verweij MW. Development and preliminary evaluation of an enzyme immunosorbent assay for the detection of adenovirus type 8. J Med Virol 44:348–352, 1994.
157. Bryden AS, Bertrand J. Diagnosis of adenovirus conjunctivitis by enzyme immunoassay. Br J Biomed Sci 53:182–184, 1996.
158. Hyypia T. Detection of adenovirus in nasopharyngeal specimens by radioactive and nonradioactive DNA probes. J Clin Microbiol 21:730–733, 1985.
159. Ranki M, Virtanen M, Palva A. Nucleic acid sandwich hybridization in adenovirus diagnosis. Curr Top Microbiol Immunol 104:307–318, 1983.
160. Bateman ED, Hayashi S, Kuwano K. Latent adenoviral infection in follicular bronchiectasis. Am J Respir Crit Care Med 151:170–176, 1995.
161. Nuovo MA, Nuovo GJ, Becker J, et al. Correlation of viral infection histology and mortality in immunocompromised patients with pneumonia. Diagn Mol Pathol 2:200–209, 1993.
162. Ankers HE, Klapper PE, Cleator GM, et al. The role of a rapid diagnostic test adenovirus immune dot blot in the control of an outbreak of adenovirus type 8 keratoconjunctivitis. Eye 7(suppl):15–17, 1993.
163. Wiley LA, Roba LA, Kowalski RP, et al. A 5 year evaluation of the adenoclone test for the rapid diagnosis of adenovirus from conjunctival swabs. Cornea 15:363–367, 1996.
164. Hierholzer JC, Halonen PE, Dahlen PO, et al. Detection of adenovirus in clinical specimens by polymerase chain reaction and liquid phase hybridization quantitated by time resolved fluorometry. J Clin Microbiol 31:1886–1891, 1993.
165. McDonough M, Ruuskanen O, Sarkkinen H. PCR detection of human adenoviruses. Diagn Mol Microbiol 2:389–393, 1993.
166. Allard A, Girones R, Juto P, Wadell G. Polymerase chain reaction for detection of adenoviruses in stool samples. J Clin Microbiol 28:2659–2667, 1990.
167. Hussain MAS, Costelli P, Morris DJ, et al. Comparison of primer sets for detection of fecal and ocular adenovirus infection using the polymerase chain reaction. J Med Virol 49:187–194, 1996.
168. Allard A, Albinsson B, Wadell G. Detection of adenoviruses in stool from healthy persons and patients with diarrhoea by two-step polymerase chain reaction. J Med Virol 37:149–157, 1992.
169. Arthur R. PCR based methods for the detection of adenoviruses. In Ehrlich GD, Greenberg SJ (eds). PCR Based Diagnostics in Infectious Disease. Boston, Blackwell Scientific, 1994, pp 447–454.
170. Timessen CT, Nell MJ. Detection and typing of subgroup F adenoviruses using the polymerase chain reaction. J Virol 59:73–82, 1996.
171. Echavarria M, Forman M, Ticehurst J, et al. PCR method for detection of adenovirus in urine of healthy and human immunodeficiency virus-infected individuals. J Clin Microbiol 36:3323–3326, 1998.
172. Schowengerdt KO, Ni J, Denfield SW, et al. Diagnosis, surveillance, and epidemiologic evaluation of viral infections in pediatric cardiac transplant recipients with the use of the polymerase chain reaction. J Heart Lung Transplant 15:111–123, 1996.
173. Martin AB, Webber S, Fricker J, et al. Acute myocarditis: rapid diagnosis by PCR in children. Circulation 90:330–339, 1994.
174. Akhtar N, Ni J, Langston C, et al. PCR diagnosis of viral pneumonitis from fixed-lung tissue in children. Biochem Mol Med 58:66–76, 1996.
175. Turner PC, Bailey AS, Cooper RJ, Morris DJ. The polymerase chain reaction for detecting adenovirus DNA in formalin fixed paraffin embedded tissue obtained post mortem. J Infect Dis 27:43–48, 1993.

176. Kinchington PR, Turse SE, Kowalski RP, Jerold GY. Use of polymerase chain amplification reaction for the detection of adenoviruses in ocular swab specimens. Invest Ophthalmol Vis Sci 35:4126–4134, 1994.

177. Morris DJ, Cooper RJ, Barr T, Bailey AS. Polymerase chain reaction for rapid diagnosis of respiratory adenovirus infection. J Infect Dis 32:113–117, 1996.

178. Morris DJ, Bailey AS, Cooper RJ, et al. Polymerase chain reaction for rapid detection of ocular adenovirus infection. J Med Virol 46:126–132, 1995.

179. Saitoh-Inagawa W, Oshima A, Aoki K, et al. Rapid diagnosis of adenoviral conjunctivitis by PCR and restriction fragment length polymorphism analysis. J Clin Microbiol 34:2113–2116, 1997.

180. Kidd AH, Jonsson M, Garwicz D, et al. Rapid subgenus identification in human adenovirus isolates by a general PCR. J Clin Microbiol 34:622–627, 1996.

181. Jackson R, Morris DJ, Cooper RJ, et al. Multiplex polymerase chain reaction for adenovirus and herpes simplex virus in eye swabs. J Virol Methods 56:41–49, 1996.

182. Puig M, Jofre J, Lucena F, et al. Detection of adenoviruses and enteroviruses in polluted waters by nested PCR amplification. Appl Environ Microbiol 60:2963–2970, 1994.

183. Houng HS, Liang S, Chen CM, et al. Rapid type-specific diagnosis of adenovirus type 4 infection using a hexon-based quantitative fluorogenic PCR. Diagn Microbiol Infect Dis 42:227–236, 2002.

184. Echavarria M, Kolavic SA, Cersovsky S, et al. Detection of adenoviruses (AdV) in culture-negative environmental samples by PCR during an AdV-associated respiratory disease outbreak. J Clin Microbiol 38:2982–2984, 2000.

185. Meurman O, Ruuskanen O, Sarkkinen H. Immunoassay diagnosis of adenovirus infections in children. J Clin Microbiol 18:1190–1195, 1983.

186. Crawford-Miksza LK, Schnurr DP. Quantitative colorimetric microneutralization assay for characterization of adenoviruses. J Clin Microbiol 32:2331–2334, 1994.

187. Chin J, Stallones RA, Lennett E. The effect of gamma globulin on acute respiratory illness in military recruits. Am J Epidemiol 86:193–198, 1966.

188. Ramano A, Ladizenski E, Guarari-Rotman D, Revel M. Clinical effect of human fibroblast derived interferon in treatment of adenovirus epidemic keratoconjunctivitis and its complications. Tex Rep Biol Med 41:559–565, 1981.

189. Baba M, Mori S, Shigeta S, DeClerco E. Selective inhibitory effects of (s)-9-3(3-hydroxy-2-phosphonylmethoxypropyl) adenine and 2'-nor-cyclic GMP on adenovirus replication in vitro. Antimicrob Agents Chemother 31:337–339, 1987.

190. Buchdall RM, Taylor P, Warner JO. Nebulised ribavirin for adenovirus pneumonia. Lancet 2:1070–1071, 1985.

191. Cassano WF. Intravenous ribavirin therapy for adenovirus cystis after allogeneic bone marrow transplantation. Bone Marrow Transplant 7:247–248, 1991.

192. Murphy GF, Wood DP, McRoberts JW, Henslee-Downey PJ. Adenovirus associated hemorrhagic cystitis treated with intravenous ribavirin. J Urol 149:565–566, 1993.

193. McCarthy AJ, Bergin M, DeSilva LM, Stevens M. Intravenous ribavirin therapy for disseminated adenovirus infection. Pediatr Infect Dis 14:1003–1004, 1995.

194. Kapelunshnik J, Delukina M. Intravenous ribavirin therapy for adenovirus gastroenteritis after bone marrow transplantation. J Pediatr Gastroenterol 21:110–112, 1995.

195. Sabroe I, McHale J, Tait DR. Treatment of adenoviral pneumonitis with intravenous ribavirin and immunoglobulin. Thorax 50:1219–1220, 1995.

196. La Rosa AM, Champlin RE, Mirza N, et al. Adenovirus infections in adult recipients of blood and marrow transplants. Clin Infect Dis 32:871–876, 2001.

197. Arav-Boger R, Echavarria M, Forman M, et al. Clearance of adenoviral hepatitis with ribavirin therapy in a pediatric liver transplant recipient. Pediatr Infect Dis J 19:1097–1100, 2000.

198. Prevention/minimization of adenovirus infection (memorandum [November 23]). Falls Church, VA, Department of Defense Armed Forces Epidemiological Board, 2001.

199. Trousdale MD, Goldschmidt PL, Nobrega R. Activity of ganciclovir against human adenovirus type 5 infection in cell culture and cotton rat eyes. Cornea 13:435–439, 1994.

200. Wright PF. Respiratory disease. In Viral Pathogenesis. Nathanson N. (ed.) Philadelphia, Lippincott-Raven, 1997, pp 703–711.

201. Yamadera S, Yamashita K, Akatsuka M, et al. Adenovirus surveillance. Jpn J Med Sci Biol 48:199–210, 1995.

202. Prado V, O'Ryan ML. Acute gastroenteritis in Latin America. Dis Latin Am 8:77–106, 1994.

203. Klapper PE, Cleator GM. Adenovirus cross-infection: a continuing problem. J Hosp Infect 30:262–267, 1995.

204. Richmond SJ, Burman R, Crosdale E. A large outbreak of keratoconjunctivitis due to adenovirus type 8. J Hyg 93:285–291, 1984.

205. Holladay RC, Campbell DG. Nosocomial viral pneumonia in the intensive care unit. Clin Chest Med 16:121–133, 1995.

206. Larsen RA, Jacobson JT, Jacobson JA. Hospital associated epidemic of pharyngitis and conjunctivitis caused by adenovirus. J Infect Dis 154:706–709, 1986.

207. Blanshard C, Francis N, Gazzard BG. Investigation of chronic diarrhoea in acquired immunodeficiency syndrome: a prospective study of 155 patients. Gut 39:824–832, 1996.

208. Van der Veen J, Oki KG, Abarbanel MFW. Patterns of infection with adenovirus types 4, 7, and 21 in military recruits during a 9-year survey. J Hyg 67:255–268, 1969.

209. Bloom HH, Forsyth BR, Johnson KM. Patterns of adenovirus infections in Marine Corp personnel. I. A 42-month survey in recruit and non recruit populations. Am J Hyg 80:328–342, 1964.

210. Forsyth BR, Bloom HH, Johnson KM, Chanock RM. Patterns of adenovirus infections in Marine Corps personnel. II. Longitudinal study of successive advanced recruit training companies. Am J Hyg 80:343–356, 1964.

211. Lee T, Miller R. Remanufacture of adenovirus vaccines type 4 and 7. Presented at the Department of Defense Recruit and Trainee Healthcare Symposium, Poster Presentation (Abstract) Towson, MD, April 15–18, 2002.

212. Ludwig SL, Brundage JF, Kelley PW, et al. Prevalence of antibodies to adenovirus serotypes 4 and 7 among unimmunized US army trainees: results of a retrospective nationwide seroprevalence survey. J Infect Dis 78:1776–1778, 1998.

213. McNeill KM, Benton FR, Monteith SC, et al. Epidemic spread of adenovirus type 4-associated acute respiratory disease between US army installations. Emerg Infect Dis 6:415–419, 2000.

214. McNeill KM, Gaydos JC, Watts BL, et al. Clinical presentations of otherwise healthy young soldiers with reemergent adenovirus type 4-associated acute respiratory disease [abstr 88]. In Abstracts of the International Conference on Emerging Infectious Diseases, Atlanta 2000.

215. Dewitt CC, Laural VL, Walter EA, et al. Adenovirus type 4 outbreak in military basic trainees: reemergence of disease due to lack of vaccine availability [abstr 51]. In Abstracts of the Meeting of the Infectious Diseases Society of America, New Orleans, 2000.

216. Gray GG, Callahan JD, Hawksworth AW, et al. Respiratory diseases among US military personnel: countering emerging threats. Emerg Infect Dis 5:379–387, 1999.

217. Katz SL. A tale of two vaccines. Clin Infect Dis 31:671–672, 2000.

218. Urgent attention needed to restore lapsed adenovirus vaccine availability (report [November 6]). Washington, DC, Institute of Medicine, 2000.

219. Russell PK. Adenovirus infection is not trivial. U S Med Nov:32, 1998.

220. Raty R, Kleemola M, Melen K, et al. Efficacy of PCR and other diagnostic methods for the detection of respiratory adenoviral infections. J Med Virol 59:66–72, 1999.

221. Centers for Disease Control and Prevention. Civilian outbreak of adenovirus acute respiratory disease—South Dakota, 1997. MMWR Morb Mortal Wkly Rep 47:567–570, 1998.

222. Stallones RA, Hilleman MR, Gauld RL. Adenovirus vaccine for prevention of acute respiratory illness. J Am Med Assoc 163:9–15, 1957.

223. Hilleman MR, Greenberg JH, Warfield MS. Second field evaluation of bivalent types 4 and 7 adenovirus vaccine. Arch Intern Med 102:428–436, 1958.

224. Culver JO, Lennetti EH, Flintjer JD. Adenovirus vaccine: a field evaluation of protective capacity against respiratory disease. Am J Hyg 69:120–126, 1959.

225. Sherwood RW, Buescher EL, Nitz RE. Effect of adenovirus vaccine on acute respiratory disease in U.S. Army recruits. JAMA 178:1115–1127, 1961.

226. Hitchcock G, Tyrell DA, Bynol ML. Vaccination of man with attenuated live adenovirus. J Hyg (Camb) 58:288–292, 1960.

227. Couch RB, Chanock RM, Cate TR. Immunization with types 4 and 7 adenovirus by selective infection of the intestinal tract. Am Rev Respir Dis 88:394–403, 1963.

228. Chanock RM, Ludwig W, Huebner RJ. Immunization by selective infection with type 4 adenovirus, grown in human diploid tissue culture. I. Safety and lack of oncogenicity and tests for potency in volunteers. JAMA 195:445–452, 1966.

229. Trentin JJ, Van Hoosier JL, Samper L. The oncogenicity of human adenoviruses in hamsters. Proc Soc Exp Biol Med 127:683–689, 1968.

230. McBride WD, Wiener A. In vitro transformation of hamster kidney cells by human adenovirus type 12. Proc Soc Exp Biol Med 115:870–874, 1964.

231. Edmonson WP, Purcell RH, Gundelfinger BF. Immunization by selective infection with type 4 adenovirus, grown in human diploid tissue culture. II. Specific protective effect against epidemic disease. JAMA 195:453–459, 1966.

232. Pierce WE, Rosenbaum MJ, Edwards EA. Live and inactivated adenovirus vaccines for the prevention of acute respiratory illness in naval recruits. Am J Epidemiol 87:237–246, 1968.

233. Huebner RJ. The problem of oncogenicity of adenoviruses. In First International Conference on Vaccines Against Viral and Rickettsial Diseases of Man. Washington, DC, Pan American Health Organization, 1967, p 1.

234. Gilden RV, Kern J, Lee YK. Serologic surveys of human cancer patients for antibody to adenovirus T antigens. Am J Epidemiol 91:500–509, 1970.

235. McAllister RM, Gliden RV, Green M. Adenoviruses in human cancer. Lancet 1:831–833, 1972.

236. National Cancer Institute. The Virus Cancer Program. Bethesda, MD, National Cancer Institute, Viral Oncology Area, Division of Cancer Cause and Prevention, 1974, p 1.

237. Top FH, Grossman RA, Bartelloni PJ. Immunization with live types 7 and 4 adenovirus vaccine: safety, infectivity and potency of adenovirus type 7 vaccine in humans. J Infect Dis 124:148–154, 1971.

238. Top FH, Buescher EL, Bancroft WH. Immunization with live types 7 and 4 adenovirus vaccines: antibody response and protective effect against acute respiratory disease due to adenovirus type 7. J Infect Dis 124:155–160, 1971.

239. Rubin BA, Rorke LB. Adenovirus vaccines. In Plotkin SA, Mortimer EA (eds). Vaccines (2nd ed). Philadelphia, WB Saunders, 1994, pp 475–502.

240. Top FH, Dudding BA, Russell PK. Control of respiratory disease in recruits with types 4 and 7 adenovirus vaccines. Am J Epidemiol 94:142–146, 1971.

241. Van der Veen J, Dykman JH. Association of type 21 adenovirus with acute respiratory illness in military recruits. Am J Hyg 76:149–159, 1962.

242. Dudding BA, Bartelloni PJ, Scott RM. Enteric immunization with live adenovirus type 21 vaccine: tests for safety, infectivity, immunogenicity, and potency in volunteers. Infect Immun 5:295–299, 1972.

243. Scott RM, Dudding BA, Romano SV. Enteric immunization with live adenovirus type 21 vaccine: systemic and local immune responses following immunization. Infect Immun 5:300–304, 1972.

244. Top FH, Brandt WE, Russell PK. Adenovirus ARD in basic combat trainees. In Research in Biological and Medical Sciences, Annual Progress Report. Washington, DC, Walter Reed Army Institute of Research, 1976, pp 462–465.

245. Takafuji ET, Gaydos JC, Allen RG, Top FH Jr. Simultaneous administration of live enteric-coated adenoviruses type 4, 7 and 21 vaccines: safety and immunogenicity. J Infect Dis 140:48–53, 1979.

246. Departments of the Army (AR40-562 TNB61), the Navy (BUMEDINST 6230.15), the Air Force (Joint Instruction 48-110), and Transportation (CG COMDTINST M623.4E). Immunizations and Chemoprophylaxis (publ no 1996-404-611, November 1). Washington, DC, U.S. Government Printing Office, 1995, p 20059.

247. Tint H, Stone JL, Minecci LC, Rubin BA. Type 4 adenovirus vaccine, live, prepared in human diploid cell for oral administration. Progr Immunobiol Stand 3:113–122, 1969.

248. Stanley ED, Jackson GG. Spread of enteric live adenovirus type 4 vaccine in married couples. J Infect Dis 119:51–59, 1969.

249. Lee SG, Hung PP. Vaccines for control of respiratory disease caused by adenoviruses. Rev Med Virol 3:209–216, 1993.

250. Bellanti JA, Artenstein BC, Brand BS, et al. Immunoglobin responses in serum and nasal secretions after natural adenovirus infections. J Immunol 103:891–898, 1969.

251. Rosenbaum MJ, De Berry P, Sullivan EJ. Characteristics of vaccine-induced and natural infection with adenovirus type 4 in naval recruits. Am J Epidemiol 88:45–54, 1997.

252. Smith T, McCown WA, McCown JW. Experimental respiratory infection with type 4 adenovirus vaccine in volunteers: clinical and immunological responses. J Infect Dis 122:239–248, 1970.

253. Gutekunst RR, Heggie AD. Viremia and viruria in adenovirus infection. N Engl J Med 261:374–378, 1961.

254. Van der Veen J, Abarbanel NFW, Oki KG. Vaccination with live type 4 adenovirus: evaluation of antibody responses and protective efficacy. J Hyg (Camb) 66:499–511, 1968.

255. Peckinpaugh RO, Pierce WE, Rosenbaum MJ, et al. Mass enteric live adenovirus vaccination during epidemic ARD. JAMA 205:75–80, 1968.

256. Rosenbaum MJ, Edwards EA, Hoeffler DF, et al. Recent experiences with live adenovirus vaccines in navy recruits. Mil Med 4:251–257, 1975.

257. Gooch WM, Mogabgab WJ. Simultaneous oral administration of live adenovirus types 4 and 7 vaccine. Arch Environ Health 25:388–394, 1972.

258. Meiklejohn G. Viral respiratory disease at Lowry Air Force Base in Denver 1952–1982. J Infect Dis 148:775–784, 1983.

259. Collis PB, Dudding BA, Winter PE, et al. Adenovirus vaccines in military recruit populations: A cost benefit analysis. J Infect Dis 128:745–752, 1973.

260. Howell MR, Nang RN, Gaydos CA, Gaydos JC. Prevention of adenoviral acute respiratory disease in army recruits: cost-effectiveness of a military vaccination policy. Am J Prev Med 14:168–175, 1998.

261. Hyer RN, Howell MR, Ryan MAK, Gaydos JC. Cost-effectiveness of reacquiring and using adenovirus types 4 and 7 vaccines in naval recruits. Am J Trop Med 62:613–618, 2000.

262. Rhoads JL, Birx DL, Wright DC, et al. Safety and immunogenicity of multiple conventional immunizations administered during early HIV infections. J Acquir Immune Defic Syndr Hum Retrovirol 4:724–731, 1991.

263. Recommendation for the use of adenovirus vaccine (memorandum [January 9]). Falls Church, VA, Department of Defense Armed Forces Epidemiological Board, 1998.

264. Wilcox WC, Ginsber HS. Production of specific neutralizing antibody with soluble antigens of type 5 adenovirus. Proc Soc Exp Biol Med 114:37–42, 1963.

265. Couch RB, Kasel JA, Pereira HG, et al. Induction of immunity in man by crystalline adenovirus type 5 capsid antigens. Proc Soc Exp Biol Med 143:905–910, 1973.

266. Randrianarison-Jewtoukoff V, Perricaudet M. Recombinant adenoviruses and vaccines. Biologicals 23:145–157, 1995.

267. Chengalvala M, Lubeck MD, Davis AR. Evaluation of adenovirus type 4 and 7 recombinant hepatitis b vaccines in dogs. Vaccine 9:485–490, 1991.

268. Morin JE, Lubeck MD, Barton JE. Recombinant adenovirus induces antibody response to hepatitis B virus surface antigen in hamsters. Proc Natl Acad Sci U S A 84:4626–4630, 1987.

269. Morin JE, Lubeck MD, Mason BB. Recombinant adenovirus vaccines for hepatitis B virus. In Woodrow GC, Levine MM (eds). New Generation Vaccines. New York, Marcel Dekker, 1990, pp 448–457.

270. Prevec I, Bhristie BS, Laurie KE. Immune response to HIV-1 gag antigens induced by recombinant adenovirus vectors in mice and rhesus macaque monkeys. J Acquir Immune Defic Syndr Hum Retrovirol 4:568–576, 1991.

271. Natuk RJ, Lubeck MD, Chanda PK, et al. Immunogenicity of recombinant human adenovirus-human immunodeficiency virus vaccines in chimpanzees. AIDS Res Hum Retroviruses 9:395–404, 1993.

272. Lubeck MD, Natuk RJ, Chengalvala M, et al. Immunogenicity of recombinant adenovirus-human immunodeficiency virus vaccines in chimpanzees following intranasal administration. AIDS Res Hum Retroviruses 10:1443–1449, 1994.

273. Lutze-Wallace C, Sapp T, Sidhu M, Wandeler A. In vitro assessment of the genetic stability of a live recombinant human adenovirus vaccine against rabies. Can J Vet Res 59:157–160, 1995.

274. Xiang ZQ, Yang Y, Wilson JM, Ertl HCJ. A replication defective human adenovirus recombinant serves as a highly efficacious vaccine carrier. Virology 219:220–227, 1996.

275. Natuk RJ, Davis AR, Chanda PK, et al. Adenovirus vectored vaccines. Dev Biol Stand 82:71–77, 1994.
276. Imler JL. Adenovirus vectors as recombinant viral vaccines. Vaccine 13:1143–1151, 1995.
277. Ginsberg HS. The ups and downs of adenovirus vectors. Bull N Y Acad Med 1:53–58, 1996.
278. Limbach KJ, Paoletti E. Nonreplicating expression vectors: application in vaccine development and gene therapy. Epidemiol Infect 116:241–256, 1996.
279. Lemarchand P, Jaffe HA, Daniel C, et al. Adenovirus mediated transfer of a recombinant human cx 1-antitrypsin cDNA to human endothelial cells. Proc Natl Acad Sci U S A 89:6482–6486, 1992.
280. Rosenthal W, Dalemans M, Fukayama M, et al. In vivo transfer of the human cystic fibrosis transmembrane conductance regulator gene to the airway epithelium. Cell 68:143–155, 1992.
281. Crystal RG, McElvaney NG, Rosenfeld MA, et al. Administration of an adenovirus containing the human CFTR cDNA to the respiratory tract of individuals with cystic fibrosis. Nat Genet 8:42–51, 1994.
282. Grubb BR, Pickles RJ, Ye H, et al. Inefficient gene transfer by adenovirus vector to cystic fibrosis airway epithelia of mice and humans. Nature 371:802–806, 1994.
283. Noah TL, Wortman IA, Hu PC, et al. Cytokine production by cultured human bronchial epithelial cells infected with a replication-deficient adenoviral gene transfer vector or wild-type adenovirus type 5. Am J Respir Cell Mol Biol 14:417–424, 1996.
284. Babiuk LA, Tikoo SK. Adenoviruses as vectors for delivering vaccines to mucosal surfaces. J Biotechnol 83:105–113, 2000.
285. Zhang WW. Development and application of adenoviral vectors for gene therapy of cancer. Cancer Gene Ther 6:113–138, 1999.
286. Barraza EM. Adenovirus outbreak—basic trainees, Fort Jackson, SC. Medical Surveillance Monthly Report (U.S. Army Center for Health Promotion and Preventive Medicine, Aberdeen Proving Ground, MD) 1(June):9–10, 1995.
287. Ryan MAK, Christian RS, Wohlrabe J. Handwashing and respiratory illness among young adults in military training. Am J Prev Med 21:79–83, 2001.
288. Gaydos JC. Returning to the past: respiratory illness, vaccines, and handwashing. Am J Prev Med 21:150–151, 2001.
289. Brodkey C, Gaydos JC. United States Army guidelines for troop living space: a historical review. Mil Med 145:418–421, 1980.
290. American Society of Heating, Refrigerating and Air-Conditioning Engineers (ASHRAE). Ventilation for acceptable indoor air quality: standard 62, 2001. Available at *www.ashrae.org/STANDARDS/intp-std.htm*

Chapter 31

Anthrax Vaccine

PHILIP S. BRACHMAN • ARTHUR M. FRIEDLANDER • JOHN D. GRABENSTEIN

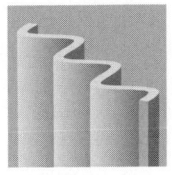

Anthrax, a zoonotic disease caused by *Bacillus anthracis*, has three forms: cutaneous, inhalational, and gastrointestinal. Mortality in untreated cutaneous cases is about 20%, and less than 1% if antibiotics are given. Inhalational anthrax is almost 100% fatal if untreated, and gastrointestinal cases have an untreated mortality rate of 25% to 75%. Meningitis may be a complication of any of the three forms. Natural cases primarily are associated with industrial, agricultural, or laboratory exposure. The natural disease is not a major public health problem in the world today, although occasional epidemics do occur. However, the intentional use of *B. anthracis* as a bioterrorist weapon in the fall of 2001 irrevocably altered our views of public health, not just for anthrax but also for many other infections.

Historically, anthrax is considered to have been the fifth and sixth plagues described in Exodus (circa 1491 BC). Hippocrates described the disease in approximately 300 BC. Europeans recorded epizootics and epidemics in the 16th century. Between 1750 and 1850, the disease in humans and animals was described in detail, and the organism was characterized.

In the 1870s, Koch cultured *B. anthracis* on artificial media and demonstrated definitively for the first time the microbial etiology of an infectious disease. In 1881, Pasteur attenuated the organism and conducted a successful field test of his vaccine for livestock. Greenfield performed similar work at the same time.[1] In the late 1800s and early 1900s, cases of cutaneous and inhalational industrial anthrax involved rag pickers in Germany and wool sorters in England.[2] The term *woolsorters' disease* referred to inhalational anthrax. Because of the large number of reported cases in England, Britons established a wool disinfection station in Liverpool.[3] All incoming wool and other animal fibers were disinfected using formaldehyde baths before being further processed. Subsequently, the number of cases of anthrax among these workers decreased significantly.

Cases of human anthrax have been reported from almost every country. However, the actual number of cases in the world is at best an estimate. In 1958, Glassman estimated the annual worldwide incidence at 20,000 to 100,000 cases.[4] In the 1980s and 1990s, the global total decreased to an estimated 2000 cases annually.

Industrial cases occurred primarily in European and North American countries, associated with the processing of animal materials, such as hair, wool, hides, and bones. Agricultural cases occur primarily in Asian and African countries and result from contact with diseased domestic animals or their products, such as hair, wool, hides, bones, and carcasses, including meat.

In the United States, the earliest reports of animal anthrax came in the early 1700s from what is now Louisiana. Sporadic animal cases were reported later from almost every state. Areas with more regularly reported cases are now called anthrax districts and primarily include the Great Plains states. Human anthrax was first reported from Kentucky in 1824. Human cases subsequently occurred throughout the United States, with the majority reported from industrialized states in the Northeast. However, as the textile industry moved to other parts of the country, human cases arose in the new locations.

Several unusual epidemics have been reported since the late 1970s. The largest epidemic in modern times occurred in Zimbabwe, with approximately 10,000 human cases reported between 1979 and 1985, including approximately 7000 cases occurring in 1979 and 1980.[5-7] Most of the affected people had cutaneous lesions, but some gastrointestinal cases also were reported. The source of infections was infected cattle.

Another unusual epidemic occurred in Sverdlovsk, Russia, in 1979. After an accidental release of spores from a military microbiology facility, at least 77 human cases of inhalational anthrax with at least 66 deaths occurred among people exposed to an aerosol containing *B. anthracis* organisms.[8,9] Some cases also occurred in sheep and cattle grazing up to 50 km downwind from the facility, possibly as a result of the same release, although natural anthrax outbreaks previously had been reported from the region. Iraq's admission to the United Nations that it produced weapons containing anthrax spores and was prepared to launch them during the 1991 Persian Gulf War confirmed fears of the potential use of *B. anthracis* as a biologic weapon.[10]

In late September 2001, a Florida man developed inhalational anthrax, the first case in the United States since 1976. He subsequently died.[11] Initially thought to be an isolated case, he was the first diagnosed case among 11 confirmed inhalational cases and 7 confirmed and 4 suspected cutaneous

887

cases of anthrax reported from Florida, New York, New Jersey, the District of Columbia, and Connecticut.[12-14] Exposure to contaminated mail was the confirmed or apparent source of infection in all patients.[12-15] Among cutaneous cases, lesions developed on the forearm, neck, chest, or fingers.[16] Of the 11 inhalational cases, the median age was 56 years (range 43 to 94 years). The average incubation from known exposure to symptoms was 4 days (range 4 to 6 days).[14]

The incidence of human anthrax in the developed world is extremely low. The only impetus for the development of an improved human vaccine is the threat of *B. anthracis* used as a biologic weapon. This horrendous possibility was unfortunately given credence by the 1979 Sverdlovsk incident and the 1991 Iraqi experience. These events prompted the U.S. Department of Defense to begin anthrax vaccinations for some members of the Armed Forces. The 2001 bioterrorist-related anthrax outbreaks in the eastern United States confirmed our fears and heightened interest in the effort to develop new vaccines. The specter of anthrax used as a bioterrorist weapon against civilian populations on a larger scale than that yet experienced poses possible catastrophic consequences.[17] Given that spores can persist in experimentally infected animals after treatment with antibiotics for more than 30 days,[18-21] the major efforts in public health management of such an event focus on early diagnosis and postexposure prophylaxis with both antibiotics and vaccination.

Background

Clinical Description

There are three primary forms of anthrax: cutaneous, inhalational, and gastrointestinal.[22,23] Secondary meningitis can occur with all three forms of anthrax. Rarely, a case of anthrax meningitis has been reported in which the primary site was not identified. In the United States, approximately 95% of reported cases have been cutaneous and 5% inhalational. There have been no confirmed gastrointestinal cases in the United States.

Cutaneous Anthrax

The incubation period for cutaneous anthrax is 1 to 7 days (usually 2 to 5 days). The lesion is first noted as a small, pruritic papule. Within several days, the papule develops into a vesicle that may be 1 to 2 cm in diameter. Occasionally, the initial papule is surrounded by a ring of vesicles, which then coalesce to form a large vesicle. The vesicular fluid is clear or serous colored and contains numerous *B. anthracis* organisms and a paucity of leukocytes. Nonpitting edema and erythema may develop around the lesion. Pain is not present unless there is secondary infection. The vesicle may enlarge to 2 to 3 cm in diameter, sometimes becoming hemorrhagic. Systemic symptoms are usually mild and can include malaise and low-grade fever. There may be regional lymphangitis and lymphadenopathy. Approximately 5 to 7 days after the onset of disease, the vesicle ruptures, revealing a straight-edged, depressed ulcer crater that develops a typical black eschar. Over a period of 2 to 3 weeks, the eschar loosens and falls off, most often without scar formation. The evolution of the lesion is not affected by antibiotic treatment.

The lesion most often occurs on an exposed part of the body, such as the face, neck, or arm. Large, irregularly shaped cutaneous lesions have been seen in some industrial cases that developed when many organisms were rubbed into the skin. Occasionally, a lesion involving the ocular area is more extensive. The orbit may become involved, with subsequent damage to the lids and ductal system.

More severe cutaneous involvement occasionally occurs that is referred to as *malignant edema*, in which multiple bullae surround the site of the initial lesion and extensive local edema, induration, and toxemia are present. At times the edema may be massive, extending from a primary lesion on the neck to the groin.

Rarely, multiple cutaneous lesions have occurred that probably represent multiple inoculations of spores through the skin. Reinfections have been reported very rarely but not confirmed.

Inhalational Anthrax

One to 5 days after inhaling an infectious dose of *B. anthracis* organisms, nonspecific symptoms develop that include malaise, fatigue, myalgia, slight temperature elevation, and minimal nonproductive cough. Symptoms similar to an upper respiratory infection are characteristically absent. There may be a feeling of precordial oppression. Auscultation of the chest may reveal rhonchi. A slight improvement may occur within 2 to 4 days, but then severe respiratory distress develops suddenly, including dyspnea, cyanosis, stridor, and profuse diaphoresis. In some cases, subcutaneous edema of the neck and chest may be present. Physical examination reveals a patient with toxic symptoms who has an elevated pulse, respiratory rate, and temperature. Physical exam may reveal signs of a pleural effusion. Widening of the mediastinum on radiographic examination of the chest is frequently seen, as are pleural effusions. The leukocyte count may be elevated moderately. Shock may develop, and death usually occurs within 24 hours of the onset of the acute phase. Death likely is caused by lymphatic/vascular obstruction in the mediastinum, with pulmonary hemorrhage and edema associated with large pleural effusions and toxicity. The clinical courses of five patients in a goat hair epidemic are shown in Figure 31–1.[24]

The patients treated in 2001 frequently reported chills, prolonged fatigue, nausea or vomiting, and chest discomfort.[14] None had an initially normal chest radiograph[13] (Table 31–1). They frequently manifested paratracheal fullness, hilar fullness, and pleural effusions or infiltrates or both; in some patients these initial findings were subtle. Among all eight patients who had not received antibiotics before diagnosis, *B. anthracis* grew in blood cultures drawn at initial examination. Six of the 11 (55%) survived with aggressive supportive care and multidrug antibiotic regimens.[13,14] All four individuals who exhibited fulminant signs of illness, with severe respiratory distress or hypotension or meningitis when they presented, died despite receiving antibiotics active against *B. anthracis*.[13]

Anthrax meningitis has been reported to occur in approximately 50% of inhalational anthrax cases, but it can develop after bacteremia secondary to the other forms and, very rarely without an obvious primary source. Clinically, it resembles other meningitides, although it is frequently hemorrhagic.

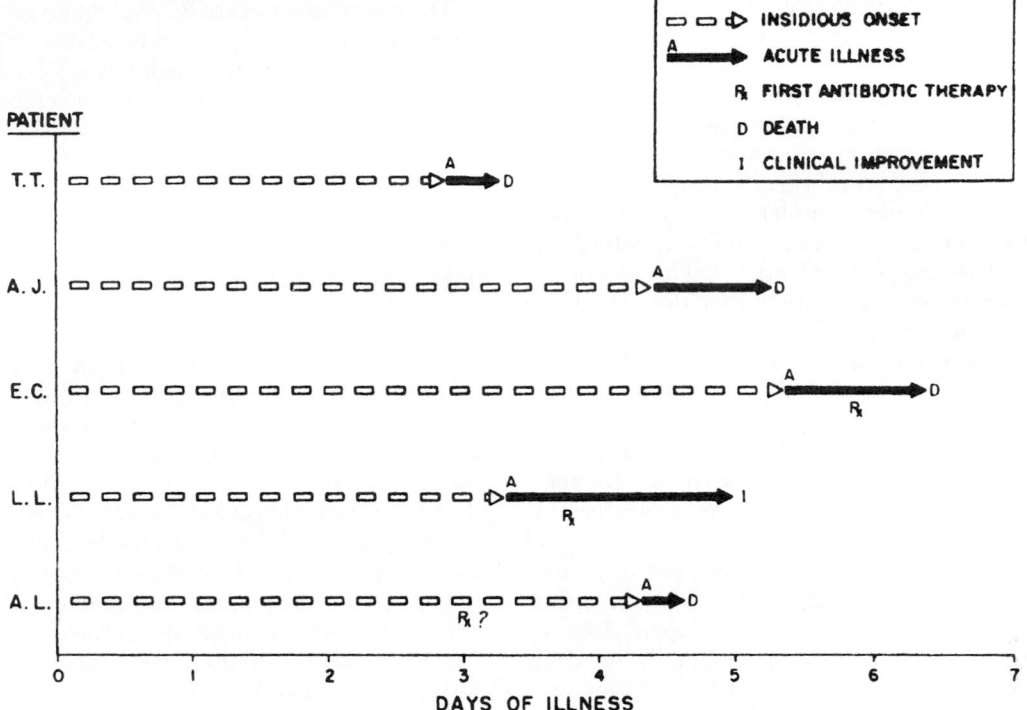

FIGURE 31–1 ■ Diagrammatic representation of the two stages of inhalation anthrax exemplified by the Manchester patients: insidious onset (→) and acute toxemia (A→). The occurrence of first antibiotic treatment (Rx) and death (D) or improvement (I) is shown in temporal relationship to these stages.[24]

Gastrointestinal Anthrax

Symptoms of gastrointestinal anthrax develop 2 to 5 days after the ingestion of contaminated meat. The initial symptoms of disease consist of nausea, vomiting, anorexia, and fever followed by abdominal pain and diarrhea, which may be bloody. Hematemesis, possibly severe, may develop. In some cases, the presentation is that of an acute abdomen and has prompted surgical exploration of the abdomen. Physical examination reveals an elevated temperature, pulse, and respiratory rate. Sepsis with toxemia, shock, and death may develop.

Oral-oropharyngeal anthrax occurs when ingested organisms gain entrance to the subcutaneous tissues through the oral or oropharyngeal tissue. In these cases, local ulcers, fever, anorexia, cervical or submandibular lymphadenopathy, or edema may develop.

Bacteriology

B. anthracis, the causative agent of anthrax, is a large, grampositive, spore-forming, nonmotile bacillus (1.0 to 1.5 × 3

TABLE 31–1 ■ Initial Clinical Findings in 10 Patients with Bioterrorism-Related Inhalational Anthrax, October through November, 2001

Chest radiography findings	
Any abnormality	10/10
Mediastinal widening	7/10
Infiltrates/consolidation	7/10
Pleural effusion	8/10
Chest computed tomography findings	
Any abnormality	8/8

to 10 μm). The organism grows readily on sheep blood agar aerobically and is nonhemolytic under these conditions. The colonies are large, rough, and gray-white, with irregular, tapered, curving outgrowths that cause the typical "Medusa head" appearance. A loop drawn up through a colony makes the disturbed part of the colony stand upright like whipped egg white. In the presence of high concentrations of carbon dioxide, the organisms form antiphagocytic capsules, and colonies are smooth and mucoid. In tissue, the bacteria are encapsulated and appear singly or in chains of two or three bacilli. Bacterial identification is confirmed by the production of toxin antigen; lysis by a specific gamma bacteriophage; the presence of a capsule and cell wall polysaccharide, as determined by fluorescent antibody testing; and virulence for mice and guinea pigs. Polymerase chain reaction tests for toxin and capsule genes are also confirmatory. Genetic analyses of different isolates reveal that *B. anthracis* is one of the most monomorphic, homogeneous bacterial species known.[25,26]

The spores are quite resistant to environmental extremes, and may survive for decades in certain soil conditions. Viable spores were reported to persist for weeks to months within the lungs of rhesus monkeys after inhalation, at which time they are still capable of germinating and causing fatal infection.[18–21]

Pathogenesis

The known virulence determinants of *B. anthracis* important in pathogenesis are the capsule and two protein exotoxins. The importance of the capsule was appreciated early in this century when Bail demonstrated that organisms that lost the ability to produce capsule were avirulent.[27]

Extensive studies by Sterne[28] and others in the 1930s expanded this idea and further showed that such nonencapsulated strains could induce immunity to anthrax, thus demonstrating that the capsule is not necessary to induce protective immunity. The strains developed by Sterne have proved remarkably effective as live vaccines for domesticated animals and are used worldwide.[29]

As is true for many bacterial virulence factors, the genes encoding the anthrax capsule are carried on an extrachromosomal 96-kilobase plasmid (pX02).[30,31] This discovery allowed more definitive confirmation that the capsule is necessary for virulence. Anthrax strains lacking the capsule plasmid failed to produce capsule and were attenuated.[32] The capsule, a protein composed of poly-D-glutamic acid, enhances virulence by making the organism resistant to phagocytosis and also may protect the bacilli from lysis by cationic proteins in serum.[33] Although the capsule is a necessary virulence factor, it is not an effective immunogen in most experimental animals.

A role for toxins in anthrax pathogenesis was suspected from the earliest studies of Koch,[34] but it was not firmly established until 1954, when Smith and Keppie demonstrated that sterile plasma from experimentally infected guinea pigs was lethal after being injected into other animals.[35] Evans and Shoesmith showed that *B. anthracis* culture filtrates produce edema after injection into the skin of rabbits.[36] Much work was done in the 1950s and 1960s to study the role of toxins in disease and immunity.[37,38] Although since the mid-1980s there have been great advances in our understanding of the molecular biology of the toxins,[39] their exact role in pathogenesis remains less well defined. Anthrax has been characterized as being due to a large bacterium that produces a feeble toxin.[40] Although it is clear that anthrax is an invasive disease and that the lethal toxin, when given intravenously, is relatively impotent compared with other bacterial toxins, both the lethal and edema toxins are thought to be important in the establishment of disease by impairing host defenses.

The anthrax toxins, like many bacterial toxins (e.g., diphtheria, tetanus, botulinum), possess a binding domain by which they bind to target cell receptors and an active domain that is responsible for the biochemical and usually enzymatic activity of the toxin. The anthrax toxins are unusual in that the binding and active domains are present on two distinct proteins, and the two toxins share the same binding protein. This binding protein is called protective antigen (PA). PA combined with a second protein called lethal factor (LF) constitutes the anthrax lethal toxin, which is lethal when injected into experimental animals.[41,42] The same PA combined with a third protein, edema factor (EF), constitutes the edema toxin, which causes edema when injected into experimental animals.[41,42] The edema toxin is undoubtedly responsible for the massive edema that may be present in cases of anthrax, especially inhalational anthrax. The 89-kDa EF is a calmodulin-dependent adenylate cyclase that raises intracellular cyclic AMP levels.[43] The 85-kDa LF has been shown to be a zinc metalloprotease that inactivates mitogen-activated protein kinase kinases,[44,45] although the exact cellular target responsible for its biologic effect remains unknown. Consistent with this model, each of the individual proteins alone lacks biologic activity.

The crystal structures of PA,[46] LF,[47] and EF[48] have all been determined. The current model based on in vitro cell culture studies suggests that the PA molecule first binds to a host cell anthrax toxin receptor.[49] The PA molecule then is cleaved by a cell-surface protease, releasing a 20-kDa amino-terminal fragment. The cell-bound 63-kDa carboxy-terminal fragment heptamerizes and creates a second binding domain to which either or both of the active proteins (i.e., the lethal or edema factor) binds. The complex then enters the cell through endocytosis and exerts its toxic effect within the cytosol.

The genes for the toxin proteins are carried on a second 182-kilobase plasmid (pX01).[50] The pathogenic role of the toxins was demonstrated clearly when strains deleted from the plasmid coding for the toxin genes but still encapsulated were shown to be attenuated.[32,50] Of historical significance, it appears that the veterinary vaccine strains produced by Pasteur by passage at high temperature do not contain the plasmid for the toxin genes.[50] This characteristic explains the lack of virulence of these vaccines. Further work has shown that deleting the PA gene alone eliminates the organism's virulence,[51] thus confirming the central role of PA in the activity of the two toxins as well as their role in virulence.

Early studies showed that crude toxin preparations or combinations of edema and lethal toxins inhibited neutrophil killing,[52] chemotaxis,[53] or phagocytosis.[33] More recent work has shown that the edema toxin inhibits neutrophil phagocytosis[54] and priming of the respiratory burst of neutrophils.[55] Evidence exists that, at low concentrations, lethal and edema toxins may block the production of proinflammatory cytokines,[56,57] and so interfere with the early protective inflammatory response. Some evidence also suggests that the lethal toxin acts on macrophages to release the cytokines interleukin-1β and tumor necrosis factor-α,[23,58] whereas, at higher concentrations, it is specifically cytolytic for these cells.[59] In terms of pathogenesis, the greater importance of lethal toxin versus edema toxin was demonstrated with a mouse model in which an anthrax strain containing the lethal toxin alone retained some virulence, whereas a strain containing only the edema toxin was avirulent when compared with the parent strain containing both toxins.[60]

Infection begins when the spore is introduced through the skin or mucosa. At the local site, the spore germinates into the vegetative bacillus with production of the antiphagocytic capsule. The edema and lethal toxins produced by the organism impair leukocyte function and contribute to the distinctive findings of tissue necrosis, edema, and relative absence of leukocytes. If not contained, the bacilli spread to the draining regional lymph nodes, thereby leading to the further production of toxins and the induction of the typical hemorrhagic, edematous, and necrotic lymphadenitis. From the lymph nodes, the bacteria multiply further and enter the blood stream to produce a systemic infection.

In inhalational anthrax, spores are ingested by alveolar macrophages and are transported to the tracheobronchial and mediastinal lymph nodes, where they germinate.[61] Local production of toxins by extracellular bacilli leads to the massive hemorrhagic, edematous, and necrotic lymphadenitis and mediastinitis that is so characteristic of this form of the disease. The bacilli then spread through the blood, causing septicemia and, at times, hemorrhagic meningitis. Late in the disease, toxin is present in the blood at high concentrations,[37] with the lethal toxin occurring as a complex of PA and LF.[62]

The site of action and the role of lethal toxin in the mechanism of death from infection remain obscure, but the uncontrolled release of cytokines and other possible mediators from macrophages may be involved. Death is due to respiratory failure with overwhelming bacteremia that is often associated with meningitis and subarachnoid hemorrhage.

Diagnosis

A diagnosis of cutaneous anthrax should be considered after the appearance of a painless, pruritic papule that develops into a vesicle, revealing a black eschar at the base of a shallow ulcer. Examination by Gram's stain or culture of the vesicular fluid should confirm the diagnosis, but prior antibiotic therapy quickly renders the infected site culture negative. Biopsy at the lesion edge, examined by Gram's stain, immunohistology, and polymerase chain reaction, may be useful in people treated with antibiotics. In addition, there should be a history of exposure to materials that have been contaminated with B. anthracis.

The diagnosis of inhalational anthrax is difficult, but it should be suspected in cases with a history of exposure to an aerosol that contains B. anthracis, followed by an initial phase during which the symptoms of inhalational anthrax are nonspecific, as described previously. Once the acute stage has developed, a widened mediastinum seen on a chest radiograph, often with pleural effusions, should suggest the diagnosis. In untreated cases, culture of blood and pleural effusions will readily establish the diagnosis. In cases previously treated with antibiotics, polymerase chain reaction of blood and pleural fluid, as well as immunohistochemical examination of pleural fluid or transbronchial biopsy specimens, are of value, as demonstrated in the recent outbreak.[13,14,16] Because primary pneumonia is not usually a feature of inhalational anthrax, sputum examinations do not aid diagnosis. The radiographic differential diagnosis should include histoplasmosis, sarcoidosis, tuberculosis, and lymphoma. A computed tomography scan of the chest may be helpful to detect mediastinal hemorrhagic lymphadenopathy and edema, peribronchial thickening, and pleural effusions.

Gastrointestinal anthrax is difficult to diagnose because of its rarity and similarity to other more common severe gastrointestinal diseases. An epidemiologic history of ingesting contaminated meat, particularly in association with other similar cases, should suggest the diagnosis. Microbiologic cultures are not helpful in confirming the diagnosis unless bacteremia is present. The diagnosis of oral-oropharyngeal anthrax can be made from the clinical and physical findings. Adequate data are not available to assess the value of bacteriologic cultures in confirming the diagnosis.

Treatment and Prevention with Antibiotics

Mild cases of cutaneous anthrax may be treated effectively orally with a penicillin, a tetracycline, or another antibiotic, depending on antimicrobial resistance. If spreading infection or prominent systemic symptoms are present, then high-dose parenteral therapy should be given as for inhalational anthrax until there is a clinical response. Effective therapy reduces the edema and systemic symptoms but does not change the evolution of the skin lesion itself.

Treatment of inhalational or gastrointestinal anthrax requires high-dose intravenous therapy with two or more antibiotics, to include a fluoroquinolone or doxycycline.[13,14,21,63–66] Limited animal data suggest that the addition of an aminoglycoside to penicillin treatment would provide additional benefit. Regimens should be altered based on susceptibility testing and clinical status. The successful treatment of 6 of the 11 inhalational cases in the 2001 bioterrorist attacks suggests that, with rapid treatment with effective antibiotics and modern supportive care, including aggressive management of pleural effusions, mortality is similar to that of other causes of sepsis.

Prophylactic treatment to prevent anthrax after exposure to an infectious spore aerosol should include oral antibiotics for 30 to 60 days or more, depending on individual circumstances (e.g., extent of exposure, vaccination status).[66–68] The Food and Drug Administration confirms the evidence for safety and efficacy of ciprofloxacin, doxycycline, and penicillin G procaine for this indication,[65] with amoxicillin recommended for children and pregnant or lactating women, depending on microbial resistance.[14,63,64,66,69] Pre- or postexposure vaccination may enable shorter courses of antibiotics.[66,70] Postexposure vaccination alone would not be expected to be effective.[21]

Epidemiology

Several theories explain the ecology of soil infected with B. anthracis. One theory suggests that B. anthracis spores can persist for many years in some types of soil under certain conditions. These conditions are a soil rich in nitrogen and organic material and with adequate calcium, a pH greater than 6.0, and an ambient temperature greater than 15.5°C. It remains unclear whether there are cycles of germination and replication within the soil or if amplification within mammalian hosts serves to maintain the population in the soil between outbreaks in animals.

Animal anthrax results from animals ingesting B. anthracis spores, either from eating contaminated feed or while grazing on pastures. Soil becomes contaminated from contaminated fertilizer or contaminated feed spread on the ground or from diseased animals that contaminate the soil with their secretions before or after death.[71]

The number of reported human anthrax cases in the United States has declined steadily since adequate surveillance data have been available. Between 1916 and 1925, the annual average number of cases was 127; between 1948 and 1957, 44 cases; between 1978 and 1987, 0.9 case; and between 1988 and 2000, 0.25 case. Of the 235 human cases reported from 1955 to 2000, 20 were fatal (Fig. 31–2).[72,73] Among these cases, 224 had cutaneous lesions (118 on an arm, 65 on the head or neck, 11 on the trunk, 8 on a leg, and 22 at an unknown site) and 11 were inhalational cases.

The traditional classification of cases is related to the source of infection, that is, whether it is acquired in an industrial, an agricultural, or a laboratory setting. The basic epidemiologic principles are the same in developing and developed countries. Agricultural anthrax is a more significant problem in developing countries, and industrial anthrax occurs more commonly in developed countries. Industrial anthrax results from the exposure of susceptible

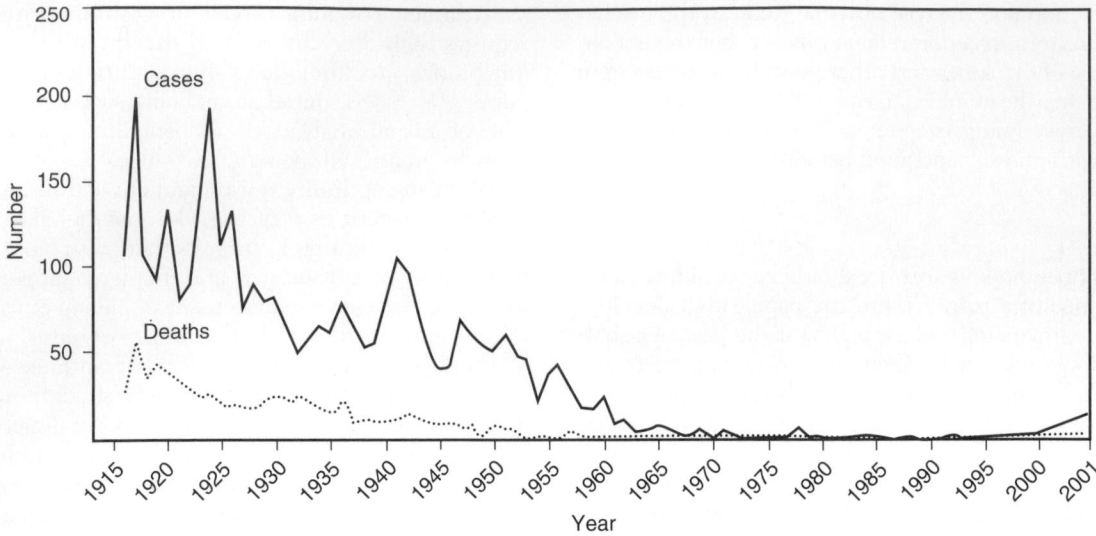

FIGURE 31–2 ▪ Number of cases of anthrax and deaths caused by anthrax in humans, United States, 1916 to 2001. (Data from the Centers for Disease Control and Prevention. [72,73])

individuals to contaminated animal products that include wool, goat hair, hides, or bones. These materials come from animals that either were infected with B. anthracis before death or are contaminated after death (e.g., from contaminated soil with which the carcass or animal products came into contact). The wool and hair from infected animals may be clipped from live animals or pulled from carcasses. A hide may be obtained from an animal that has died of anthrax. Bones can be collected from grazing areas on which animals die or from rendering plants that may handle carcasses of animals that have died from anthrax.

Wool and goat hair are processed into yarn that is used in the textile and carpet industries or in the preparation of other cloth-like materials. Hides are processed into leather goods. Bones are used in preparing bone meal, gelatin, and fertilizer. In industrial cases, cutaneous anthrax results from spores that gain entrance through the skin by entering pre-existing wounds or by being rubbed through the skin or on a hair fiber that may penetrate the skin. At times, the processing of goat hair and wool creates infectious aerosols that may result in inhalational anthrax when inhaled. A rendering plant is another source of potential infection.

Cases associated with agricultural settings result from contact with diseased animals or with the products of animals that have died of anthrax. Affected individuals are primarily agricultural workers, veterinarians, or individuals who kill and butcher infected animals or butcher the carcasses

of animals that have died of anthrax. This contact results in cutaneous anthrax or, if the infected meat is ingested, gastrointestinal or oral-oropharyngeal anthrax.

Laboratory-associated cases of anthrax are rare. These are essentially all cutaneous, although a few inhalational cases have occurred. Rarely, cases have been reported after contact with contaminated clothing, such as woolen coats or pilots' leather helmets. Table 31–2 presents the sources of infection of the 257 cases reported in the United States from 1955 to 2001. The two vaccine-associated cases of agricultural anthrax resulted from the inadvertent injection of animal vaccine into the hand of the vaccinator.

Exposures related to bioterrorist events represent a new category. The anthrax terror attacks of fall 2001 resulted in 11 confirmed inhalational cases and 7 confirmed and 4 suspected cutaneous cases of anthrax reported from Florida, New York, New Jersey, the District of Columbia, and Connecticut.[12–14] Exposure to contaminated mail was the confirmed or apparent source of infection in all patients.[14,15] More than 32,000 people received short courses of prophylactic antibiotics while potential exposures were evaluated,[67] and among these more than 10,000 people received 60 days or more of antibiotics with or without postexposure vaccination as prophylaxis.[68,74] Exposures may have resulted from opening contaminated letters or packages, from working in buildings with high-speed automated mail-sorting machines, or through contact

TABLE 31–2 ▪ Sources of Infection in 257 Cases of Human Anthrax in the United States, 1955 to 2001

Industrial (No.)	Agricultural (No.)	Terrorism (No.)
Goat hair (113)	Animal (42)	Inhalational
Wool (34)	Vaccine (2)	Working in mail-processing facility (7)
Goat skin (16)	Unknown (8)	Receiving mail (confirmed or presumptive) (4)
Meat (3)	**Total**: 52	Cutaneous
Bone (4)		Working in mail-processing facility (7)
Unknown (13)		Receiving mail (confirmed or presumptive) (4)
Total: 183		**Total**: 22 (18 confirmed and 4 suspected)

with cross-contaminated pieces of mail or environments contaminated with spores.

Passive Immunization

In the era before antibiotics, animal antisera were common therapeutic products.[75] One of the first was anthrax antiserum, developed in France by Marchoux and in Italy by Sclavo in 1895.[76,77] Although it was used initially for prophylaxis and treatment of anthrax among livestock, Sclavo later used his product to treat human disease, either cutaneous or septicemic. He reported 10 deaths among 164 treated patients (6% mortality, compared to the Italian case-fatality rate of 24%). Sclavo injected 30 to 40 mL of antiserum subcutaneously, repeated 24 hours later. In severe cases, he also injected 10 mL or more intravenously.

Between the 1910s and 1940s, clinicians in Europe and the Americas treated patients with anthrax antiserum using 25 to 300 mL daily for 5 days, sometimes in combination with arsenicals.[75–86] One patient with severe cutaneous anthrax recovered after receiving 2265 mL of antiserum.[87] No controlled studies were performed to demonstrate efficacy. Anthrax antiserum for therapy of cutaneous anthrax was superseded by therapy with sulfanilamide, followed by penicillin and other antibiotics.[85,88]

Equine anthrax antiserum produced by live-spore vaccination has been licensed in China,[89] the Soviet Union, and later Russia for decades, and its use continues, although the magnitude or frequency of use is unclear. In recent years, the Lanzhou Institute of Biological Products in China developed a lyophilized anti-anthrax $F(ab)_2$ formulation of equine immunoglobulin G (IgG) fragments, for human use by intracutaneous, intramuscular, or intravenous administration, but it is little used (Dong Shulin, personal communication, 2002).

Experimental evidence indicates that passive immunization with equine antibody produced against attenuated Sterne veterinary vaccine strains or against crude toxins prevents disease in animals when given before or shortly after spore challenge.[18,90] Rhesus monkeys could be protected with one or two doses of equine anti-anthrax spore hyperimmune serum when begun 1 day after low-dose aerosol challenge. Forty-five percent of immune serum–treated animals survived, compared to 10% of controls.

More recent studies by Little et al. showed efficacy of anti-PA antiserum prophylaxis against an intramuscular challenge in animals.[91] The anti-PA polyclonal antibody protected against death and anti-PA monoclonal antibody significantly delayed mortality. Reuveny and colleagues similarly found in passive immunization studies of guinea pigs that polyclonal anti-PA antisera conferred protection against an intradermal challenge dose of 40 median lethal doses (LD_{50}).[92]

Kobiler and colleagues challenged guinea pigs intranasally with a 25 LD_{50} dose of spores.[93] The animals were then treated with anti-PA, anti-LF, or anti–Sterne vaccine antibodies. Intraperitoneal administration of rabbit anti-PA serum 24 hours after infection protected 90% of infected animals, with lesser efficacy seen with anti-Sterne and anti-LF antibodies. Beedham and colleagues demonstrated that mice could be protected against challenge with a vaccine strain using serum but not spleen lymphocytes from PA-vaccinated animals, supporting the long-standing evidence that antibody is the major mechanism of vaccine-induced immunity.[94]

Although the importance of anthrax toxins in pathogenesis suggests that antiserum may play a role in treatment, modern western interest in such products for human use was not rekindled until the anthrax bioterrorism attacks in the fall of 2001.[95] The need for therapeutic tools other than antibiotics may be especially great in the case of antibiotic-resistant strains of B. anthracis, although there remains no definitive evidence to date of efficacy in humans.

Active Immunization

History of Vaccine Development

Although there is great historical interest in Pasteur's development of the first effective live bacterial vaccine, and live, attenuated veterinary vaccines are still used, human vaccines against anthrax consist of proteins purified from anthrax cultures, except as indicated in the following discussion. Early human anthrax vaccines (presumably live) were used in the 1910s but found little favor.[77] Sterne developed live, attenuated strains in the 1930s, which led to worldwide use for domesticated animals.[29] Russian investigators developed similar vaccines for both animal and human use. In 1946, Gladstone identified the PA component of cultures of B. anthracis.[96] Belton and Strange increased the yields of PA to allow large-scale production,[90] leading to the current British vaccine. Wright and colleagues used similar techniques to develop the precursors to the American vaccine.[97–99]

There has been confusion in the older literature over the use of the term protective antigen. Before the identification of the anthrax toxins, this term was applied to uncharacterized material derived from sterile extracts of experimental anthrax lesions[100,101] or from crude culture supernatants,[96] which were effective immunogens in experimental animals. Protective antigen is the term also applied to one of the toxin proteins, which is the plasmid-encoded binding component of the anthrax toxins described previously. It has become clear that these terms apply to the same protein. The major effective immunogen in culture supernatants is the PA component of the toxins, although smaller amounts of LF and EF may be present; their contribution to protective immunity has remained controversial.[37] In older studies, EF enhanced the protective efficacy of PA in some experimental animals.[102,103] The results of these studies are difficult to interpret because the preparations used may not have been pure and free from cross-contamination. Studies using the PA gene cloned into B. subtilis demonstrated conclusively that PA alone, in the absence of EF, LF, or other B. anthracis proteins, protects animals against experimental infection.[104] Although other experiments have shown that purer preparations of PA, free of immunologically detectable LF or EF,[105] or recombinant PA,[106] can protect experimental animals, it remains unknown whether adding EF or LF enhances the vaccine efficacy of PA.

Description of Vaccines

The human anthrax vaccine licensed in the United States, Anthrax Vaccine Adsorbed (AVA), is produced by the

BioPort Corporation (Lansing, MI) from sterile filtrates of microaerophilic cultures of an attenuated, unencapsulated nonproteolytic strain (V770-NP1-R) of *B. anthracis*. The cell-free culture filtrate, thought to contain predominantly PA, is adsorbed to aluminum hydroxide, and the final product contains no more than 2.4 mg of aluminum hydroxide per 0.5-mL dose. Formaldehyde, in a final concentration of no more than 0.02%, and 0.0025% benzethonium chloride are present as preservatives. Current product-content standards require 5 to 20 μg/mL of total protein, of which at least 35% is the 83-kDa PA protein, measured by densitometric analysis on sodium dodecyl sulfate–polyacrylamide gel electrophoresis after pooling 12 sublots.[107] It is unknown whether the PA is biologically active.

Some lots produced in Lansing in the 1980s appeared to contain small amounts of LF and lesser amounts of EF, as determined by induction of antibody responses in animal recipients,[32,105,108,109] although this has not been reported in the limited observations in human vaccinees.[109] Analysis found no detectable EF by Western blotting. Enzyme-linked immunosorbent assay (ELISA) studies found LF to be present in the range of 10 to 30 ng/mL of fermentation filtrate before adsorption.[107] Analysis by mouse macrophage cytotoxicity assay suggested that LF is present in a biologically inactive form.[107] Although it is clear that PA by itself is an effective immunogen, it remains unresolved whether the small amounts of LF or EF that may be present in some lots of the vaccine contribute to the vaccine's protective efficacy.

Potency testing of the BioPort vaccine is performed by assessing biologic activity after parenterally challenging guinea pigs. The vaccine is stored at 2° to 8°C. The recommended schedule for vaccination is 0.5 mL given subcutaneously at 0, 2, and 4 weeks, followed by 0.5-mL boosters at 6, 12, and 18 months. Studies of immunogenicity with intramuscular administration and fewer doses are underway. With continued exposure, additional yearly boosters are recommended. The vaccine is stable for 3 years after a successful potency test.

Anthrax Vaccine Precipitated, a similar vaccine from the Centre for Applied Microbiological Research (Porton Down, Salisbury, Wiltshire) was developed in the United Kingdom, first administered to humans in the early 1950s, and licensed in 1979.[110–114] This vaccine is made by precipitating the sterile cell-free culture filtrate of a derivative of the attenuated, noncapsulating Sterne strain 34F$_2$ with aluminum potassium sulfate.[113] LF and EF are present in this vaccine at levels higher than believed to be found in lots of the U.S. vaccine from the 1980s.[109,115] The vaccine contains thimerosal as a preservative. The British vaccine is administered intramuscularly in a regimen of three 0.5-mL doses at 0, 3, and 6 weeks, with a booster dose 6 months after the third dose. Subsequent booster doses are given annually.[1]

A vaccine consisting of a suspension of live spores, named STI-1 for the Sanitary-Technical Institute, has been used for humans in the Soviet Union and its subsequent independent republics since 1953.[71,116] This strain, similar to the Sterne strain used in veterinary vaccines, is unencapsulated.[116] Although this vaccine has a reputation for causing substantial side effects, its developers assert that it is reasonably well tolerated and shows some degree of protective efficacy.[116–118] This vaccine, manufactured by the Tbilisi Scientific Research Institute of Vaccines & Serums (Tbilisi, Georgia), the Institute of Microbiology (Kirov [Viatka], Russian Federation), and

perhaps other locations, is given by scarification through a 10- to 20-μL drop of vaccine containing 1.3 to 4×10^8 spores or subcutaneously.[1,71,114,116,118–121] The initial dose is followed by a second dose 21 days later, with yearly boosters.

Another live spore human vaccine given by scarification has been manufactured by the Lanzhou Institute of Biological Products (Lanzhou, Gansu, People's Republic of China) since the 1960s, based on avirulent strain A16R.[71,89] A single dose contains 1.6 to 2.4×10^8 colony-forming units. A single booster dose is given 6 to 12 months after the first vaccination (Dong Shulin, personal communication, 2002).

Immunogenicity of Vaccine

The results of two studies indicated that immunization with the licensed U.S. vaccine induced an immune response (as measured by indirect hemagglutination) to PA in 83% of vaccinees 2 weeks after the first three doses,[122] and in 91% of those tested after receiving two or more doses.[123] The titers fell over time, but 100% of vaccinees responded with an anamnestic response to the annual booster dose. This hemagglutination assay correlated with results obtained by using an ELISA against PA,[124] which is the current test of choice. Analysis using a more sensitive ELISA against PA demonstrated that seroconversion occurs in 96% to 100% of vaccinees after the second dose.[125]

Using a more sensitive validated ELISA assay, Pittman found that one dose of Anthrax Vaccine Adsorbed evoked detectable anti-PA IgG antibodies in 60% to 84% of vaccinees.[126] After two doses, 95% to 100% of vaccinees developed anti-PA antibodies. The kinetics of anti-PA IgG response by this ELISA appear in Figure 31–3.[126] Prolonging the interval between the first two doses by a few weeks beyond the licensed 2-week interval increased antibody responses.[125,127] More extended intervals did not impair booster responses among Persian Gulf War troops given anthrax and botulinum vaccines after gaps of 18 to 24 months.[128] A preliminary study comparing subcutaneous and intramuscular administration of anthrax vaccine revealed higher titers to PA when a four week interval between the first two doses was compared to two weeks, and better tolerance of the vaccine by the IM route.[125] If confirmed by a larger study now in course, both the route of vaccination and the schedule of anthrax vaccine are likely to be improved.

Cellular Responses

Soviet scientists developed a skin-test antigenic reagent known as anthraxin in 1957, derived from the edematous fluid of infected animals given an unencapsulated *B. anthracis* strain.[121] Licensed in 1962, the skin test product is an autoclaved liquid composed of an undefined heat-stable polysaccharide-protein–nucleic acid complex, without anthrax capsular or toxigenic material.[121,129] A positive skin test after 0.1 mL intradermal injection is defined as erythema ≥8 mm with local induration persisting for 48 hours.[121] Anthraxin demonstrated utility in identifying cases of anthrax[116,130] and identifying STI-1 vaccine–induced immunity in guinea pigs, sheep, and humans.[116] Experimental data show that guinea pigs vaccinated against anthrax that developed a positive anthraxin skin test were immune to a subsequent parenteral challenge.[121] Positive and negative predictive values of individual test results have not been published. There is limited

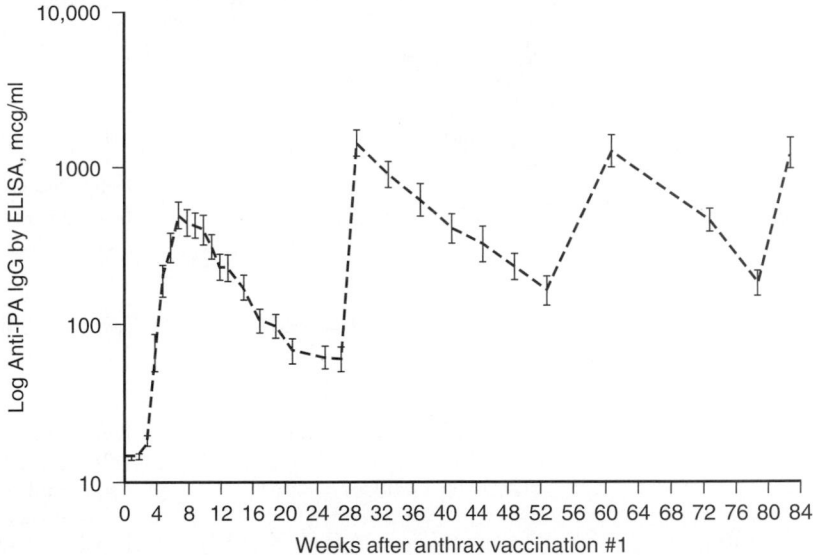

HUMAN ANTIBODY KINETICS AFTER ANTHRAX VACCINATION,
SUBCUTANEOUS, 0-2-4 WEEK–6-12-18 MONTH SCHEDULE

FIGURE 31–3 ■ Anti-PA IgG antibody kinetics using the Food and Drug Administration–licensed dosing schedule. (Data from Pittman PR. Comparative Study to Determine the Best Two-Dose Schedule and Route of Administration of Human Anthrax Vaccine: Final Study Report to the Food & Drug Administration. Fort Detrick, MD, U.S. Army Medical Research Institute of Infectious Diseases, 2000.)

experience with the skin test antigen in humans in western countries, and its utility in predicting immunity in humans remains unknown.

Correlates of Protection

After a naturally acquired infection, antibody to PA develops in 68% to 93% of cases as reported in different series, depending on the time when samples are drawn.[115,123,124,131] Antibody to LF occurs in 42% to 55% of cases, whereas antibody to EF is less frequently observed.[115,124] Antibody to the anthrax capsule occurs in 67% to 94% of cases.[124,131] This reaction contrasts with that of vaccinees, in which no response to capsule is expected because the vaccine strain is nonencapsulated. In the 2001 epidemic of inhalational anthrax, antibody to PA was detected in all confirmed survivors.

In experimental animals, there is generally a correlation between immunity and antibody titer to PA after immunization with the human vaccine.[132] However, the live veterinary vaccine provides significantly greater protection against anthrax in experimental animals than does the human vaccine, even though it often induces lower levels of antibody to PA,[105,108,109] suggesting that other antigens may be involved in protection. Thus the relationship between antibody to PA, as measured in these assays, and immunity remains obscure.

More recent studies using both live and protein-based vaccines have demonstrated a strong correlation between antibodies to PA and immunity. Barnard and Friedlander showed, for the first time using live vaccines producing varying amounts of PA, that protection was strongly correlated with antibody titers to PA,[133] a finding subsequently confirmed by Cohen and colleagues.[134] Pitt and colleagues, using the licensed human vaccine, found a similar in vitro correlation of immunity with antibody to PA, measured by ELISA and toxin neutralization, in a rabbit model of

inhalational anthrax.[132] Reuveny and colleagues, using a PA vaccine to protect guinea pigs against an intradermal challenge, found that toxin neutralizing antibodies correlated better with survival than did antibodies measured by ELISA.[92] Further analysis of the antibody response to different epitopes on PA will further our knowledge of the nature of the protective antibodies.

Efficacy of Vaccine

The protective efficacy of different experimental PA-based vaccines that were derived from culture filtrates of *B. anthracis* was clearly demonstrated with the use of various animal models and routes of challenge.[101,113] A comprehensive, peer-reviewed evaluation by the National Academy of Sciences reported that "The committee finds that the available evidence from studies with humans and animals, coupled with reasonable assumptions of analogy, shows that AVA as licensed is an effective vaccine for the protection of humans against anthrax, including inhalational anthrax, caused by all known or plausible engineered strains of *B. anthracis*."[107]

A controlled clinical trial was conducted with a less potent vaccine similar to the currently licensed U.S. vaccine.[135] This field-tested vaccine was composed of an alum-precipitated, cell-free culture supernatant from an attenuated, unencapsulated, nonproteolytic strain of *B. anthracis*. This strain differed slightly from that used to produce the licensed vaccine and was grown under aerobic rather than microaerophilic conditions.[98] The study was conducted in a susceptible population working in four mills in the northeastern United States, where raw imported goat hair contaminated with *B. anthracis* was used. The results indicated that vaccination, compared with inoculation with a placebo, provided 92.5% protection against anthrax, combining the cutaneous and inhalational cases (95% confidence interval, 65% to 100%). No isolated assessment of

TABLE 31–3 ■ Efficacy of Anthrax Vaccines Against Inhalational Challenge in Rhesus Macaques

Reference	Vaccine Product	Vaccination
Wright et al. (1954)[98]	Alum-precipitated "preparation 138"	Two 1-mL SC doses 16 days apart
Darlow et al. (1956)[110]	Alum-precipitated vaccine	Two 1.25-mL SC doses 10 days apart
Ivins et al. (1996)[136]	Anthrax Vaccine Adsorbed	Two 0.5-mL IM doses 2 weeks apart
Pitt et al. (1996)[137]	Anthrax Vaccine Adsorbed	Two 0.5-mL IM doses 28 days apart
	rPA 50 μg + Al(OH)$_3$	Two 0.5-mL IM doses 28 days apart
Pitt et al. (1999)[138, *]	Anthrax Vaccine Adsorbed	Two 0.5-mL IM doses 28 days apart
Ivins et al. (1998)[106]	Anthrax Vaccine Adsorbed	One 0.5-mL IM dose
	rPA 50 μg + various adjuvants	One 0.5-mL IM dose
Fellows et al. (2001)[139]	Anthrax Vaccine Adsorbed	Two 0.5-mL IM doses 4 weeks apart

*Additional data from IM, intramuscular; LD$_{50}$, median lethal dose; rPA, recombinant protective antigen; SC, subcutaneous. (MLM Pitt, personal communication, 2002.)

the effectiveness of the vaccine against inhalational anthrax could be made because there were too few cases, although the only inhalational cases observed occurred in nonvaccinated individuals. This same vaccine previously was shown to protect rhesus monkeys against an aerosol exposure to anthrax spores.[21,107,118] A review of the methods and results of the trial noted above, as well as results of a trial with the live spore vaccine developed in the former Soviet Union, concluded that both products were effective.[118]

There have been no controlled clinical trials in humans of the efficacy of the currently licensed U.S. vaccine, although the differences between the BioPort vaccine and the PA-based vaccine used in the Brachman et al. study[135] are minor from a regulatory perspective.[107] The BioPort vaccine has been tested extensively in animals and has protected guinea pigs against both an intramuscular[108,109] and an aerosol[105] challenge. More recent experiments show that this vaccine also protected rhesus monkeys against a lethal aerosol challenge with anthrax spores.[106,136–139] Inhalational challenge studies in nonhuman primates vaccinated with either the licensed human vaccine or a recombinant PA vaccine are summarized in Table 31–3.

Duration of Immunity

The duration of immunity induced by vaccination has not been clearly established. In the field trials that evaluated a vaccine similar to the currently licensed U.S. vaccine, one case of cutaneous anthrax occurred 5 months after the initial three-dose series and just before the scheduled 6-month boosting dose.[135] Although data are insufficient to support any firm

conclusions, this observation suggests that the immunity induced by the initial series of three doses of the current vaccine may not be long lasting and that the recommended schedule of annual boosters is necessary. Ongoing studies of clinical correlates of protection that involve reducing the total number of vaccine doses by using longer intervals between booster doses, and using an intramuscular rather than subcutaneous route of injection, will help clarify this point.[135a]

Postexposure Prophylaxis with Vaccination

Postexposure vaccination by itself is unlikely to be of any benefit because of the short incubation period and the rapid course of the disease. Animal studies support this conclusion.[21] However, vaccination combined with antibiotic prophylaxis before the onset of clinical illness may offer the best possible protection against inhalational anthrax after an aerosol exposure. This is because of the unusual propensity of anthrax spores to persist in the host for long periods and possibly germinate after antibiotics have been discontinued.[18–21] Vaccination will allow for the development of an immune response during the period of antibiotic prophylaxis. Thus postexposure vaccination may shorten the period of antibiotic prophylaxis required for protection.

This recommendation is supported by a National Academy of Sciences report that concluded that

these limited data suggest that the use of vaccine in combination with an appropriate antibiotic for 30 days could provide excellent postexposure protection against inhalational anthrax. Although the additional benefit from receiving the vaccine after a prolonged period of antibiotic use is not

Challenge Dose	Challenge Strain	Vaccination to Challenge	Time from Last Survival	
			Vaccinated Animals	Unvaccinated Animals
39,000–82,000 spores	Vollum	16 days	3/4	0/4
890,000 to 3 million spores	Vollum	34 days	4/4	0/2
10–15 LD_{50}	M.36 Vollum	7 days	10/10	0/10
10–15 LD_{50}	M.36 Vollum	1 yr	10/10	0/10
10–15 LD_{50}	M.36 Vollum	2 yr	6/7	1/9
255–760 LD_{50}	Ames	8 wk	10/10	0/5
161–247 LD_{50}	Ames	38 wk	3/3	
239–535 LD_{50}	Ames	100 wk	7/8	0/2
899 ± 62 LD_{50}	Ames	3 mo	9/9	0/2
899 ± 62 LD_{50}	Ames	3 mo	9/10	
133 ± 43 LD_{50}	Ames	3 mo	5/5	0/6
74.4 LD_{50}	Ames	6 wk	10/10	0/3
78–117 LD_{50}	Ames	6 wk	28/29	
398 LD_{50} (Ames equivalent)	ASIL K7978-Namibia	6 wk	10/10	0/2
1004 LD_{50} (Ames equivalent)	ASIL K9729-Turkey	6 wk	8/10	0/2

proven, reliance on the vaccine alone after exposure is clearly insufficient, as some protection is needed during the time required for an immune response to develop.[107]

Vaccine Safety

Common Adverse Effects

Studies of an earlier PA-based vaccine used in the human field trial showed that, during the initial series of three subcutaneous injections, the incidences of systemic and of significant local reactions were 0.7% and 2.4%, respectively.[98,135] An increase to 1.3% and 2.7%, respectively, was noted with the booster doses. A more detailed study showed that local reactions increased in frequency up to the fifth inoculation and then declined.[135] In this study, there was a 0.2% incidence of systemic reactions and a 2.8% overall incidence of significant local reactions. Systemic reactions include mild generalized myalgia, slight headache, and mild to moderate malaise for 1 to 2 days. Most local reactions are mild, consisting of 1 to 2 cm of erythema and slight local tenderness appearing the first day and disappearing within 1 to 2 days. Significant local reactions consist of induration, erythema greater than 5 cm in diameter, edema, pruritus, local warmth, and tenderness. These reactions are maximal at 1 to 2 days after vaccination and usually disappear over 2 to 3 days. Very rarely, the edema may be extensive and extend from the deltoid to the forearm. A small, painless nodule at the injection site, persisting for several weeks, also has been observed, but only rarely. Severe local reactions were observed in individuals with a history of cutaneous anthrax

who were inadvertently immunized.[98] All local reactions resolved without complication.

The licensed aluminum hydroxide–adsorbed PA vaccine, when first used, gave an incidence of local reactions similar to that of the alum-precipitated vaccine, although no detailed observations were reported.[99] In an open-label study from 1966 to 1971 with the licensed vaccine, approximately 7000 textile employees, laboratory workers, and other at-risk individuals received 15,907 doses.[140,141] There were 24 reports (0.15% of doses) of severe local reactions (defined as edema or induration >120 mm in diameter or marked limitation of arm motion or axillary node tenderness). There were 150 reports (0.9%) of moderate local reactions (edema or induration 30 to 120 mm in diameter) and 1373 reports (8.6%) of mild local reactions (erythema only or induration <30 mm in diameter). Four cases of systemic reactions (<0.06%), reported as transient, included fever, chills, nausea, and general body aches.

The U.S. Army Medical Research Institute of Infectious Diseases (USAMRIID) assessed the safety of the licensed anthrax vaccine as part of a randomized clinical study between 1996 and 1999.[125] A total of 28 volunteers received subcutaneous doses according to the licensed schedule. Each volunteer was observed for 30 minutes after administration of AVA and scheduled for follow-up evaluations at 1 to 3 days, 1 week, and 1 month after vaccination. Four volunteers reported seven acute adverse events within 30 minutes after subcutaneous administration. These included erythema (3), headache (2), fever (1), and elevated temperature (1). Of these events, a single patient reported simultaneous occurrence of headache, fever, and elevated temperature (100.7°F). The most common local reactions reported were tenderness, erythema, subcutaneous nodule, induration, warmth, local pruritus, limited arm motion, and edema. Local reactions were found to occur more often in women. No abscess or necrosis was observed at the injection site. Systemic reactions included malaise, headache, myalgia, fever, anorexia, respiratory difficulty, and nausea or vomiting (4%). All local and systemic adverse events reported in this study were transient in nature. There was one report of a delayed-type hypersensitivity reaction beginning with lesions 3 days after the first dose.

USAMRIID also analyzed the occupational health records of 1583 workers (1249 men and 334 women) who reported adverse events after receiving 10,722 doses of the licensed anthrax vaccine from 32 separate vaccine lots.[142] Of this group, 273 people received 10 or more doses and 46 people received 20 or more doses. With regard to injection-site reactions, 3.6% of doses were reported to produce redness, induration, itching, or edema. Most people who reported a reaction received subsequent doses without problems, but the subset of people who reported an injection-site reaction were more likely to report a local reaction to a later dose. Systemic events of headache, fever, chills, malaise, and muscle or joint aches were reported after 1% of doses. The most common of these were headache (0.4%), malaise (0.4%), and fever (0.1%). Women noted both local (i.e., erythema, induration, edema, swollen lymph nodes, lumps) and systemic (i.e., headache, fever, dizziness, hives) events more commonly than men. Vaccine recipients less than 40 years old reported adverse events more often than those 40 years or older.

Two uncontrolled case series used self-administered surveys to assess anthrax vaccine safety. Among 601 health care workers at an Army hospital in Honolulu,[107,143] women reported more localized itching (56% to 68%) than did men (24% to 31%). Women developed more subcutaneous nodules (81% to 93%) than did men (56% to 65%). Moderate to large injection-site reactions (erythema >10 cm) were more common among women (40% to 51%) than men (17% to 32%). Women reported more swelling of the lower arm (8% to 15%) than did men (7% to 10%). About 20% of men and women reported symptoms that they personally judged could be ignored; 15% reported symptoms that affected their activity for a short time, but did not limit their ability to perform duties; 8% reported symptoms that affected their activity for a short time that were relieved by self-treatment with nonprescription medication; and less than 2% reported symptoms unrelieved by medication, with their ability to perform duties limited for a short time. From 1.5% to 2.7% of women and from 1.2% to 2.1% of men reported systemic events leading to limitation of performing duties. Events in both genders were similar in resolving on their own over the course of a few days without residual consequences.

The other uncontrolled case series was at a U.S. Army base in South Korea.[107,143] Participants included 2214 men and 610 women given the licensed anthrax vaccine. Women reported subcutaneous nodules more frequently (50% to 62%) than men (21% to 29%). Erythema greater than 12 cm in diameter was self-reported by 2% to 4% of women and 0.4% to 1% of men. Women experienced more itching at the local site (20% to 37% vs. 6% to 8%); fever (2% to 4% vs. 1%), chills (3% to 6% vs. 1% to 2%), and malaise (8% to 15% vs. 4% to 7%) than did men. Overall,

0% to 1.9% reported that their work activity had been limited to some extent or were placed on limited duty. From 0% to 1.1% reported losing 1 or more days of duty; 0.4% to 1.7% consulted a clinic for the reaction. Regardless of gender, almost all reported events were localized or minor and self-limited and did not lead to impairment of work performance.

Rare Adverse Effects

The best evidence evaluating the overall safety of the licensed vaccine comes from database studies from the Army Medical Surveillance Activity and the Naval Health Research Center.[107,144] These studies established that anthrax-vaccinated and unvaccinated personnel of either gender are hospitalized and visit outpatient clinics at the same rates overall for each of 14 major categories within the International Classification of Diseases, and for each of several specific diagnoses with speculative association with anthrax vaccination. For example, 1 per 35 anthrax-vaccinated people is hospitalized each year, compared to 1 per 28 unvaccinated people being hospitalized per year.

Three reports described the long-term health of 99 male laboratory workers who received a variety of licensed and investigational vaccines (volume range, 52 to 134 mL), including both the early and the current formulation of anthrax vaccine.[145-147] The third study included a small control group. Although there were elevations in liver and kidney function tests and white blood cell counts in some of these men, none developed any unusual diseases or unexplained symptoms that the authors attributed to repeated doses of multiple vaccines.

All reports to the Vaccine Adverse Event Reporting System (VAERS) involving the licensed anthrax vaccine were evaluated by the Anthrax Vaccine Expert Committee (AVEC), composed of civilian physicians.[148] The AVEC evaluated 1857 VAERS reports and additional medical records corresponding to 1793 recipients of the licensed anthrax vaccine between March 1998 and February 2002. The 1857 adverse event reports can be grouped into three main categories, based on effect on the vaccine recipient's functional status: hospitalization, inability to work for 24 hours or more, and "other." Sixty-four of the 1857 reports involved hospitalization. The civilian panel found that 11 of the 64 "very likely/certainly" or "probably" were caused by anthrax vaccine. All 11 involved allergic or inflammatory reactions at the injection site. Another 172 reports involved inability to work for 24 hours or more (but did not involve hospitalization); 94 of the 172 certainly or probably were caused by anthrax vaccine. These 94 reports primarily described injection-site reactions, various rashes, acute allergic reactions, and viral-like symptoms. The balance of the 1857 reports, 1621, involved neither hospitalization nor time off work for 24 hours or more. All were reviewed by the AVEC, which found no patterns of unexpected adverse events.

Two cases of optic neuritis were reported in soldiers subsequent to anthrax vaccination. Optic nerve antibodies were found in one case, but no epitopes were found in common between optic nerve and the anthrax organism.[148a]

A cohort study involving 4092 active-duty women in the U.S. Army assessed the effect of the licensed anthrax vaccine on pregnancy and childbirth.[149] This cohort contrasted 3135 women vaccinated against anthrax and 957 unvaccinated women, with 39,519 person-months of follow-up. The anthrax-vaccinated and unvaccinated women had an equivalent likelihood of becoming pregnant, as well as giving birth. The study found no differences in birth outcomes between the two groups, but the study did not have adequate statistical power to rule out a small effect of vaccination on adverse birth outcome, given the low number of adverse outcomes.

These and other safety studies of anthrax vaccine, some still in the peer-review process before publication, were critically reviewed by the expert committee convened by the National Academy of Sciences.[107] This comprehensive, peer-reviewed report concluded that the licensed anthrax vaccine has a side effect profile similar to that of other adult vaccines. According to the reviewers,

> The committee found no evidence that people face an increased risk of experiencing life-threatening or permanently disabling adverse events immediately after receiving AVA, when compared with the general population. Nor did it find any convincing evidence that people face elevated risk of developing adverse health effects over the longer term, although data are limited in this regard (as they are for all vaccines)."[107]

A list of studies showing the safety of AVA are given in Table 31–4.

Indications for Vaccination

Routine immunizations are recommended for industrial workers who handle potentially contaminated animal products, including wool, goat hair, hides, and bones imported from countries in which animal anthrax continues to occur. These countries are primarily in Asia and Africa but are occasionally in South America or the Caribbean. A veterinarian or agricultural worker who has contact with potentially infected animals should be immunized, as should laboratory workers who work with B. anthracis.[70]

Special circumstances that warrant vaccination with anthrax vaccine include a threat of biologic warfare or terrorism. The U.S. Armed Forces began vaccinating some service members in 1998 to protect against anthrax arising from the use of B. anthracis as a biologic weapon.

Contraindications and Precautions

A contraindication to being vaccinated is a hypersensitivity reaction to the vaccine. This is uncommon, but several individuals who have received the initial dose or doses developed moderately severe local reactions with some systemic response. If it is necessary to immunize such individuals, pretreatment with antihistamines and nonsteroidal anti-inflammatory drugs may be of value, although this has not been evaluated scientifically.[70]

Public Health Considerations

The use of the anthrax vaccine in industrialized populations had a significant impact on the reduction of natural anthrax cases among industrial workers and is one of the main methods by which industrial anthrax was controlled. Improvements in the industrial environment, with better manufacturing equipment and environmental control, also have helped reduce the industrial risks of naturally occurring anthrax. Additionally, replacement of animal products (primarily goat hair) with synthetic fibers has had a favorable impact on the occurrence of anthrax infection. It is ironic that mail-processing machines replaced wool-processing machines as a source of industrial risk in the 2001 anthrax bioterrorism attacks.

Agricultural cases have been reduced by control of the disease in animals through the use of animal vaccines. The routine immunization of animals in areas with continuing cases of animal anthrax and the immunization of appropriate humans agriculturally and industrially exposed to B. anthracis will serve to reduce the number of naturally occurring human cases.

Future Vaccines

Current acellular vaccines against anthrax are less than ideal for several reasons. These vaccines are composed of an incompletely defined culture supernatant adsorbed to aluminum hydroxide. There is only partial quantification of

TABLE 31–4 ■ Anthrax Vaccine Safety Studies

Study	Number of subjects
Brachman (1962)[135]	379
CDC observational study, review by FDA, advisors[140]	6986
Fort Detrick multidose, multivaccine safety studies[145–147]	99
Fort Detrick special immunization program (2001)[142]	1583
Fort Bragg booster study (after Persian Gulf War)[128]	281
USAMRIID reduced-dose/route-change study (2001)[125]	173
Canadian Forces safety survey[107]	576
TAMC-600 survey (Tripler Army Medical Center)[107,143]	603
U.S. Forces Korea records (2000)[107,143]	2824
USAF visual acuity study[107]	958
USAF Air Combat Command study, Langley Air Force Base[163]	5187
VAERS review by Anthrax Vaccine Expert Committee (2002)[148]	1793
Inpatient/Outpatient cohort study[107,144,164]	350,296 person-yr

CDC, Centers for Disease Control and Prevention; FDA, Food and Drug Administration; USAF, U.S. Air Force; USAMRIID, U.S. Army Medical Research Institute of Infectious Diseases; VAERS, Vaccine Adverse Event Reporting System.

the PA content of the vaccine or other constituents, so the degree of purity is not fully known. Standardization is determined by biologic activity in an animal potency test. Studies in progress will determine the extent to which administering this aluminum-adsorbed vaccine subcutaneously (rather than intramuscularly) is responsible for the observed rate of injection-site reactions. The currently licensed schedule is less than optimal, in that six doses are required over 18 months, followed by annual boosters. A simpler vaccination schedule with fewer doses is also being evaluated. Although there is evidence that the efficacy of the vaccine against parenteral challenge of rodents may be less against some strains of anthrax than others,[108,109,115] the vaccine protected rhesus monkeys against a more rigorous aerosol challenge with all strains tested, including those overcoming resistance in rodents.[136,139] Clearly, the ideal anthrax vaccine would be more completely defined and less reactogenic, and able to produce long-lasting immunity within 30 days.[107]

Further understanding of the molecular pathogenesis of anthrax and of the structure of the PA and its interaction with LF and EF can be expected to lead to significant progress toward the development of improved vaccines. For example, genetically defined mutations in the receptor-binding domain,[150,151] the protease-sensitive domain,[152] or other parts of the molecule[153] may generate a less toxic PA preparation to be used either alone or as a complex with edema or lethal factor. Similarly, mutations in either the edema or lethal toxin may allow evaluation of nontoxic complexes with PA. Evidence in experimental animals suggests that adjuvants other than aluminum may increase the protective efficacy of PA substantially even after a single dose,[154,155] and that new formulations using microcapsules also may be of value.[156]

Several vaccine candidates based on recombinant PA protected rhesus monkeys from inhalational challenge.[104,106,157,158] These vaccines are in the most advanced stages of development and are undergoing final preclinical testing before beginning Phase I human trials.

Another approach has been to develop live vaccines for human use, because several reports demonstrated that a live vaccine protects experimental animals better than does the licensed human PA vaccine.[105,108,109,157] The precedent exists for using such a vaccine in humans in Russia and the former Soviet republics. Live vaccines that are known to protect experimental animals against anthrax include aromatic compound–dependent, toxigenic, nonencapsulated strains of B. anthracis,[155] as well as B. anthracis,[133] B. subtilis,[157] Salmonella,[159] and vaccinia,[160] each constructed to contain the cloned PA gene. Finally, other approaches using PA or LF have included nonreplicating DNA vaccines[161] (C Schmaljohn, personal communication, 2002) and viral replicons (JL Lee, personal communication, 2002).

Attempts to identify antigens other than the PA of the toxin that may contribute to protection are also underway. Spore components[134,162] and the capsule (AM Friedlander, personal communication, 2002) have been shown to offer additional protection in some small-animal models. In addition, the forthcoming completion of the B. anthracis genome is anticipated to advance the search for new vaccine candidates as well as therapeutic targets.

Although these efforts are in the experimental stage, they may lead to the production of a vaccine that is less reactogenic, requires fewer doses, and provides more effective and long-lasting immunity.

REFERENCES

1. Turnbull PCB. Anthrax vaccines: past, present and future. Vaccine 9:533–539, 1991.
2. LaForce FM. Woolsorters' disease, England. Bull N Y Acad Med 54:956–963, 1978.
3. Wool disinfection and anthrax: a year's working of the model station. Lancet 2:1295–1296, 1922.
4. Glassman HN. World incidence of anthrax in man. Public Health Rep 73:22–24, 1958.
5. Davies JCA. A major epidemic of anthrax in Zimbabwe. Part 1. Cent Afr J Med 28:291–298, 1982.
6. Davies JCA. A major epidemic of anthrax in Zimbabwe. Part 2. Cent Afr J Med 29:8–12, 1983.
7. Davies JCA. A major epidemic of anthrax in Zimbabwe. Part 3. Cent Afr J Med 31:176–180, 1985.
8. Abramova FA, Grinberg IM, Yampolskaya OV, Walker DH. Pathology of inhalational anthrax in 42 cases from the Sverdlovsk outbreak in 1979. Proc Natl Acad Sci U S A 90:2291–2294, 1993.
9. Meselson M, Guillemin J, Hugh-Jones M, et al. The Sverdlovsk anthrax outbreak of 1979. Science 266:1202–1208, 1994.
10. Zilinskas RA. Iraq's biological weapons: the past as future? JAMA 278:418–424, 1997.
11. Centers for Disease Control and Prevention. Ongoing investigation of anthrax—Florida, October 2001. MMWR 50:877, 2001.
12. Centers for Disease Control and Prevention. Update: investigation of bioterrorism-related anthrax—Connecticut, 2001. MMWR 50:1077–1079, 2001.
13. Jernigan JA, Stephens DS, Ashford DA, et al, for the Anthrax Bioterrorism Investigation Team. Bioterrorism-related inhalational anthrax: the first 10 cases reported in the United States. Emerg Infect Dis 7:933–944, 2001.
14. Bell DM, Kozarsky PE, Stephens DS. Clinical issues in the prophylaxis, diagnosis, and treatment of anthrax. Emerg Infect Dis 8:222–225, 2002.
15. Centers for Disease Control and Prevention. Evaluation of Bacillus anthracis contamination inside the Brentwood mail processing and distribution center—District of Columbia, October 2001. MMWR 50:1129–1132, 2001.
16. Centers for Disease Control and Prevention. Update: investigation of bioterrorism-related anthrax and interim guidelines for clinical evaluation of persons with possible anthrax. MMWR 50:941–948, 2001. (published errata in MMWR 50:991, 2001).
17. Kaufman AF, Meltzer MI, Schmid GE. The economic impact of a bioterrorist attack: are prevention and postattack intervention programs justifiable? Emerg Infect Dis 3:83–94, 1997.
18. Henderson DW, Peacock S, Belton FC. Observations on the prophylaxis of experimental pulmonary anthrax in the monkey. J Hyg 54:28–36, 1956.
19. Gochenour WS Jr, Sawyer WD, Henderson JE, et al. On the recognition and therapy of Simian woolsorter's disease. J Hyg (Camb) 61:317–325, 1963.
20. Glassman HN. Industrial inhalation anthrax: discussion. Bacteriol Rev 30:657–659, 1966.
21. Friedlander AM, Welkos SL, Pitt MLM, et al. Postexposure prophylaxis against experimental inhalation anthrax. J Infect Dis 167:1239–1243, 1993.
22. Dixon TC, Meselson M, Guillemin J, Hanna PC. Anthrax. N Engl J Med 341:815–826, 1999.
23. Schwartz MN. Recognition and management of anthrax—an update. N Engl J Med 345:1621–1626, 2001.
24. Plotkin SA, Brachman PS, Utell M, et al. An epidemic of inhalation anthrax, the first in the twentieth century: I. Clinical features. Am J Med 29:992–1001, 1960.
25. Price LB, Hugh-Jones M, Jackson PJ, Keim P. Genetic diversity in the protective antigen gene of Bacillus anthracis. J Bacteriol 181:2358–2362, 1999.
26. Keim P, Price LB, Klevytska AM, et al. Multiple-locus variable-number tandem repeat analysis reveals genetic relationships within Bacillus anthracis. J Bacteriol 182:2928–2936, 2000.

27. Bail O. Cited in Sterne M. Anthrax. *In* Stableforth AW, Galloway IA (eds). Infectious Diseases of Animals. Vol. 1. London, Butterworth Scientific Publications, 1959, p 22.

28. Sterne M. Anthrax. *In* Stableforth AW, Galloway IA (eds). Infectious Diseases of Animals. Vol. 1. London, Butterworth Scientific Publications, 1959, pp 16–52.

29. Sterne M. Distribution and economic importance of anthrax. Fed Proc 26:1493–1495, 1967.

30. Green BD, Battisti L, Koehler TM, Thorne GB. Demonstration of a capsule plasmid in *Bacillus anthracis*. Infect Immun 49:291–297, 1985.

31. Uchida I, Sekizaki T, Hashimoto K, Terkado N. Association of the encapsulation of *Bacillus anthracis* with a 60 megadalton plasmid. J Gen Microbiol 131:363–367, 1985.

32. Ivins BE, Ezzell JW Jr, Jemski J, et al. Immunization studies with attenuated strains of *Bacillus anthracis*. Infect Immun 52:454–458, 1986.

33. Keppie J, Harris-Smith PW, Smith H. The chemical basis of the virulence of *Bacillus anthracis*. IX. Its aggressions and their mode of action. Br J Exp Pathol 44:446–453, 1963.

34. Koch R. Beitrage zur Biologie der Pflanzen. Med Classics 2:787–820, 1938.

35. Smith H, Keppie J. Observations on experimental anthrax: demonstration of a specific lethal factor produced in vivo by *Bacillus anthracis*. Nature 173:869–870, 1954.

36. Evans DG, Shoesmith JG. Production of toxin by *Bacillus anthracis*. Lancet 1:136, 1954.

37. Lincoln RE, Fish DC. Anthrax toxin. *In* Montie TG, Kadis S, Ajl SJ (eds). Microbial Toxins. Vol. 3. New York, Academic Press, 1970, pp 361–414.

38. Stephen J. Anthrax toxin. *In* Domer F, Drews J (eds). Pharmacology of Bacterial Toxins. Oxford, Pergamon Press, 1986, pp 381–395.

39. Leppla SH. The anthrax toxin complex. *In* Alouf JE, Freer JH (eds). Sourcebook of Bacterial Protein Toxins. London, Academic Press, 1991, pp 277–302.

40. Dalldorf FGF, Kaufmann AF, Brachman PS. Woolsorters' disease: an experimental model. Arch Pathol 92:418–426, 1971.

41. Stanley JL, Smith H. Purification of factor I and recognition of a third factor of the anthrax toxin. J Gen Microbiol 26:49–66, 1961.

42. Beall FA, Taylor MJ, Thorne GB. Rapid lethal effects in rats of a third component found upon fractionating the toxin of *Bacillus anthracis*. J Bacteriol 83:1274–1280, 1962.

43. Leppla SH. Anthrax toxin edema factor: a bacterial adenylate cyclase that increases cyclic AMP concentrations of eukaryotic cells. Proc Natl Acad Sci U S A 79:3162–3166, 1982.

44. Hammond SE, Hanna PG. Lethal factor active-site mutations affect catalytic activity in vitro. Infect Immun 66:2374–2378, 1998.

45. Duesbury NS, Webb CP, Leppla SH, et al. Proteolytic inactivation of MAP-kinase-kinase by anthrax lethal factor. Science 280:734–737, 1998.

46. Petosa C, Collier RJ, Klimpel KR, et al. Crystal structure of the anthrax toxin protective antigen. Nature 385:833–838, 1997.

47. Pannifer AD, Wong TY, Schwarzenbacher R, et al. Crystal structure of the anthrax lethal factor. Nature 414:229–233, 2001.

48. Drum CL, Yan S-Z, Bard J, et al. Structural basis for the activation of anthrax adenylyl cyclase exotoxin by calmodulin. Nature 415:396–402, 2002.

49. Bradley KA, Mogridge J, Mourez M, et al. Identification of the cellular receptor for anthrax toxin. Nature 414:225–229, 2001.

50. Mikesell P, Ivins BE, Ristroph JD, Dreier TM. Evidence for plasmid-mediated toxin production in *Bacillus anthracis*. Infect Immun 39:371–376, 1983.

51. Cataldi A, Labruyere F, Mock M. Construction and characterization of a protective antigen-deficient *Bacillus anthracis* strain. Mol Microbiol 4:1111–1117, 1990.

52. Bail O, Weil F. Beitrage zum Studium der Milzbrandinfektion. Arch Hyg Bakteriol 73:218–264, 1911.

53. Kashiba S, Motishima T, Kato K, et al. Leucotoxic substance produced by *Bacillus anthracis*. Biken J 2:97–104, 1959.

54. O'Brien J, Friedlander A, Dreier T, et al. Effects of anthrax toxin components on human neutrophils. Infect Immun 47:306–310, 1985.

55. Wright GG, Read PW, Mandell GL. Lipopolysaccharide releases a priming substance from platelets that augments the oxidative response of polymorphonuclear neutrophils to chemotactic peptide. J Infect Dis 157:690–696, 1988.

56. Hoover DL, Friedlander AM, Rogers LC, et al. Anthrax edema toxin differentially regulates lipopolysaccharide-induced monocyte production of tumor necrosis factor alpha and interleukin-6 by increasing intracellular cyclic AMP. Infect Immun 62:4432–4439, 1994.

57. Pellizzari R, Guidi-Rontani C, Vitale G, et al. Anthrax lethal factor cleaves MKK3 in macrophages and inhibits the LPS/IFN-gamma-induced release of NO and TNFalpha. FEBS Lett 462:199–204, 1999.

58. Hanna PC, Acosta D, Collier RJ. On the role of macrophages in anthrax. Proc Natl Acad Sci U S A 90:10198–10201, 1993.

59. Friedlander AM. Macrophages are sensitive to anthrax lethal toxin through an acid-dependent process. J Biol Chem 261:7123–7126, 1986.

60. Pezard G, Berche P, Mock M. Contribution of individual toxin components to virulence of *Bacillus anthracis*. Infect Immun 59:3472–3477, 1991.

61. Ross JM. The pathogenesis of anthrax following the administration of spores by the respiratory route. J Pathol Bacteriol 73:485–494, 1957.

62. Ezzell JW Jr, Abshire TG. Serum protease cleavage of *Bacillus anthracis* protective antigen. J Gen Microbiol 138:543–549, 1992.

63. Centers for Disease Control and Prevention. Update: investigation of bioterrorism-related anthrax and interim guidelines for exposure management and antimicrobial therapy, October 2001. MMWR 50:909–919, 2001. (published errata in MMWR 50:962, 2001)

64. Centers for Disease Control and Prevention. Update: interim recommendations for antimicrobial prophylaxis for children and breastfeeding mothers and treatment of children with anthrax. MMWR 50:1014–1016, 2001.

65. Food and Drug Administration. Prescription drug products: doxycycline and penicillin G procaine administration for inhalational anthrax (post-exposure). Fed Reg 66:55679–55682, 2001.

66. Inglesby TV, O'Toole T, Henderson DA, et al, for the Working Group on Civilian Biodefense. Anthrax as a biological weapon, 2002: updated recommendations for management. JAMA 287:2236–2252, 2002.

67. Centers for Disease Control and Prevention. Update: investigation of bioterrorism-related anthrax and adverse events from antimicrobial prophylaxis. MMWR 50:973–976, 2001.

68. Centers for Disease Control and Prevention. Update: adverse events associated with anthrax prophylaxis among postal employees—New Jersey, New York City, and the District of Columbia metropolitan area, 2001. MMWR 50:1051–1054, 2001.

69. Centers for Disease Control and Prevention. Updated recommendations for antimicrobial prophylaxis among asymptomatic pregnant women after exposure to *Bacillus anthracis*. MMWR 50:960, 2001.

70. Advisory Committee on Immunization Practices. Use of anthrax vaccine in the United States. MMWR 49(RR-15):1–20, 2000.

71. Turnbull PCB. Guidelines for the Surveillance and Control of Anthrax in Humans and Animals (3rd ed) (report no WHO/EMC/ZDI/98.6). Geneva, World Health Organization, 1998.

72. Summary of notifiable diseases, United States—1999. MMWR 48:1–94, 1999.

73. Centers for Disease Control and Prevention. Human anthrax associated with an epizootic among livestock—North Dakota, 2000. MMWR 50:677–680, 2001.

74. Centers for Disease Control & Prevention. Evaluation of postexposure antibiotic prophylaxis to prevent anthrax. MMWR 51:59, 2002.

75. Parish HJ. A History of Immunizations. Edinburgh, E&S Livingstone Ltd, 1965, pp 42–50.

76. Sclavo A. Serum treatment of anthrax in man. Riv Ital Igine 14:161–175, 1954.

77. Regan JC. The advantage of serum therapy as shown by a comparison of various methods of treatment of anthrax. Am J Med Sci 162:406–423, 1921.

78. Reinle GG, Archibald RA. A case of anthrax. J Infect Dis 19:718–720, 1916.

79. Ludy JB, Rice EC. Anthrax at Camp Hancock, Ga. JAMA 71:1133–1136, 1918.

80. Regan JC. The local and general serum treatment of cutaneous anthrax. JAMA 77:1944–1948, 1921.

81. Fleming A, Petrie GE. Recent Advances in Vaccine and Serum Therapy. Philadelphia, P. Blakiston's Son & Co, 1934, pp 152–156.

82. Lucchesi PF. Serum treatment of 19 cases of anthrax including one of external, internal and bacteremic type. Am J Med Sci 183:795–802, 1932.

83. Eurich FW. Some notes on industrial anthrax: its diagnosis and treatment. Br Med J 2:50–53, 1933.

84. Ivanovics G. The standardization of anti-anthrax sera. Bull Health Org League Nations 7:836–844, 1938.

85. Lucchesi PE, Gildersleeve N. Treatment of anthrax. JAMA 116:1506–1508, 1941.

86. Grabar P, Staub A-M. Fractionation of horse anti-anthrax serum. Ann Inst Pasteur 68:355–360, 1942.

87. Hodgson AE. Cutaneous anthrax. Lancet 1:811–813, 1941.

88. Gold H. Anthrax: a report of one hundred seventeen cases. Arch Intern Med 96:387–396, 1955.

89. Dong SL. Progress in the control and research of anthrax in China. Salisbury Med Bull Suppl 68:104–105, 1990.

90. Belton FG, Strange RE. Studies on a protective antigen produced in vitro from Bacillus anthracis: medium and methods of production. Br J Exp Pathol 37:144–152, 1954.

91. Little SF, Ivins BE, Fellows PF, Friedlander AM. Passive protection by polyclonal antibodies against Bacillus anthracis infection in guinea pigs. Infect Immun 65:5171–5175, 1997.

92. Reuveny S, White MD, Adar YY, et al. Search for correlates of protective immunity conferred by anthrax vaccine. Infect Immun 69:2888–2893, 2001.

93. Kobiler D, Gozes Y, Rosenberg H, et al. Efficiency of protection of guinea pigs against infection with Bacillus anthracis spores by passive immunization. Infect Immun 70:544–560, 2002.

94. Beedham RJ, Turnbull PCB, Williamson ED. Passive transfer of protection against Bacillus anthracis infection in a murine model. Vaccine 19:4409–4416, 2001.

95. Enserink M. Anthrax: 'borrowed immunity' may save future victims. Science 295:777, 2002.

96. Gladstone GP. Immunity to anthrax: protective antigen present in cell-free culture filtrates. Br J Exp Pathol 27:394–418, 1946.

97. Wright GG, Puziss M, Neely WB. Studies on immunity in anthrax. IX. Effect of variations in cultural conditions on elaboration of protective antigen by strains of Bacillus anthracis. J Bacteriol 83:515–522, 1962.

98. Wright GG, Green TW, Kanode RG. Studies on immunity in anthrax. V. Immunizing activity of alum-precipitated protective antigen. J Immunol 73:387–391, 1954.

99. Puziss M, Wright GG. Studies on immunity in anthrax. X. Gel-adsorbed protective antigen for immunization of man. J Bacteriol 85:230–236, 1963.

100. Bail O. Untersuchungen über naturliche und kunstliche Milzbrandimmunitat. Zentralbl Bakteriol I Abt Orig 37:270–280, 1904.

101. Cromartie WJ, Watson DW, Bloom WL, Heckly RJ. Studies on infection with Bacillus anthracis. II. The immunological and tissue damaging properties of extracts prepared from lesions of B. anthracis infection. J Infect Dis 80:14–27, 1947.

102. Stanley JL, Smith H. The three factors of anthrax toxin: their immunogenicity and lack of demonstrable enzymic activity. J Gen Microbiol 31:329–337, 1963.

103. Mahlandt BG, Klein F, Lincoln RE, et al. Immunologic studies of anthrax. IV. Evaluation of the immunogenicity of three components of anthrax toxin. J Immunol 96:727–733, 1966.

104. Ivins BE, Welkos SL. Cloning and expression of the Bacillus anthracis protective antigen gene in Bacillus subtilis. Infect Immun 54:537–542, 1986.

105. Ivins BE, Welkos SL. Recent advances in the development of an improved, human anthrax vaccine. Eur J Epidemiol 4:12–19, 1988.

106. Ivins BE, Pitt MLM, Fellows PF, et al. Comparative efficacy of experimental anthrax vaccine candidates against inhalation anthrax in rhesus macaques. Vaccine 16:1141–1148, 1998.

107. Joellenbeck LM, Zwanziger L, Durch JS, Strom BL (eds). The Anthrax Vaccine: Is It Safe? Does It Work? Washington, DC, National Academy Press, 2002.

108. Little SF, Knudson GB. Comparative efficacy of Bacillus anthracis live spore vaccine and protective antigen vaccine against anthrax in the guinea pig. Infect Immun 52:509–512, 1986.

109. Turnbull PCB, Broster MG, Carman JA, et al. Development of antibodies to protective antigen and lethal factor components of anthrax toxin in humans and guinea pigs and their relevance to protective immunity. Infect Immun 52:356–363, 1986.

110. Darlow HM, Belton FC, Henderson DW. The use of anthrax antigen to immunise man and monkey. Lancet 2:476–479, 1956.

111. Vaccine against anthrax. Br Med J 2:717–718, 1965.

112. Darlow HM. Vaccination against anthrax. In Silver IH (ed). Aerobiology. London, Academic Press, 1970, p 199.

113. Hambleton P, Carman JA, Melling J. Anthrax: the disease in relation to vaccines. Vaccine 2:125–132, 1984.

114. Turnbull PCB. Current status of immunization against anthrax: old vaccines may be here to stay for a while. Curr Opin Infect Dis 13:113–120, 2000.

115. Turnbull PCB, Leppla SH, Broster MG, et al. Antibodies to anthrax toxin in humans and guinea pigs and their relevance to protective immunity. Med Microbiol Immunol 177:293–303, 1988.

116. Shlyakhov EN, Rubinstein E. Human live anthrax vaccine in the former USSR. Vaccine 12:727–730, 1994.

117. Shuylak VP. Epidemiological efficacy of anthrax STI vaccine in Tadjik SSR [in Russian]. Zh Mikrobiol Epidemiol Immunobiol 47:117–120, 1970.

118. Demicheli V, Rivetti D, Decks JJ, et al. The effectiveness and safety of vaccines against human anthrax: a systematic review. Vaccine 16:880–884, 1998.

119. Hambleton P, Turnbull PCB. Anthrax vaccine development: a continuing story. Adv Biotechnol Processes 13:105–122, 1990.

120. Stepanov AV, Marinin LI, Pomerantsev AP, Staritsin NA. Development of novel vaccines against anthrax in man. J Biotechnol 44:155–160, 1996.

121. Shlyakhov E, Rubinstein E, Novikov I. Anthrax post-vaccinal cell-mediated immunity in humans: kinetics pattern. Vaccine 15:631–636, 1997.

122. Johnson-Winegar A. Comparison of enzyme-linked immunosorbent and hemagglutination assays for determining anthrax antibodies. J Clin Microbiol 20:357–361, 1984.

123. Buchanan TM, Feeley JG, Hayes PS, Brachman PS. Anthrax indirect microhemagglutination test. J Immunol 107:1631–1636, 1971.

124. Sirisanthana T, Nelson KE, Ezzell J, Abshire TG. Serological studies of patients with cutaneous and oral-oropharyngeal anthrax from northern Thailand. Am J Trop Med Hyg 39:575–581, 1988.

125. Pittman PR, Kim-Ahn G, Pifat DY, et al. Anthrax vaccine: safety and immunogenicity of a dose-reduction, route comparison study in humans. Vaccine 20:1412–1420, 2002.

126. Pittman PR. Comparative Study to Determine the Best Two-Dose Schedule and Route of Administration of Human Anthrax Vaccine: Final Study Report to the Food & Drug Administration. Fort Detrick, MD, U.S. Army Medical Research Institute of Infectious Diseases, 2000.

127. Pittman PR, Mangiafico JA, Rossi CA, et al. Anthrax vaccine: increasing intervals between the first two doses enhances antibody response in humans. Vaccine 18:213–216, 2000.

128. Pittman PR, Hack D, Mangiafico J, et al. Antibody response to a delayed booster dose of anthrax vaccine and botulinum toxoid. Vaccine 20:2107–2115, 2002.

129. Shlyakhov E. Anthraxin—a skin test for early and retrospective diagnosis of anthrax and anthrax vaccination assessment. Salisbury Med Bull Suppl 87:109–110, 1996.

130. Pfisterer RM. Retrospective verification of the diagnosis of anthrax by means of the intracutaneous skin test with the Russian allergen "anthraxin" in a recent epidemic in Switzerland. Salisbury Med Bull Suppl 68:80, 1990.

131. Harrison LH, Ezzell JW, Abshire TG, et al. Evaluation of serologic tests for diagnosis of anthrax after an outbreak of cutaneous anthrax in Paraguay. J Infect Dis 160:706–710, 1989.

132. Pitt MLM, Little SF, Ivins BE, et al. In vitro correlation of immunity in a rabbit model of inhalational anthrax. Vaccine 19:4768–4773, 2001.

133. Barnard JP, Friedlander AM. Vaccination against anthrax with attenuated recombinant strains of Bacillus anthracis that produce protective antigen. Infect Immun 67:562–567, 1999.

134. Cohen S, Mendelson I, Altboum Z, et al. Attenuated nontoxinogenic and nonencapsulated recombinant Bacillus anthracis spore vaccines protect against anthrax. Infect Immun 68:4549–4558, 2000.

135. Brachman PS, Gold H, Plotkin SA, et al. Field evaluation of a human anthrax vaccine. Am J Public Health 52:632–645, 1962.

135a. Institute of Medicine. An assessment of the CDC anthrax vaccine safety and efficacy research program. Washington, DC: National Academy Press, 2002.

136. Ivins BE, Fellows PF, Pitt MLM, et al. Efficacy of a standard human anthrax vaccine against *Bacillus anthracis* aerosol spore challenge in rhesus monkeys. Salisbury Med Bull Suppl 87:125–126, 1996.

137. Pitt MLM, Ivins BE, Estep JE, et al. Comparison of the efficacy of purified protective antigen and MDPH to protect non-human primates from inhalation anthrax. Salisbury Med Bull Suppl 87:130, 1996.

138. Friedlander AM, Pittman PR, Parker GW. Anthrax vaccine: evidence for safety and efficacy against inhalational anthrax. JAMA 282:2104–2106, 1999.

139. Fellows PF, Linscott MK, Ivins BE, et al. Efficacy of a human anthrax vaccine in guinea pigs, rabbits, and rhesus macaques against challenge by *Bacillus anthracis* isolates of diverse geographical origin. Vaccine 19:3241–3247, 2001.

140. Food and Drug Administration. Biological products; bacterial vaccines and toxoids; implementation of efficacy review. Fed Reg 50:51002–51117, 1985.

141. Product information: BioThrax, Anthrax Vaccine Adsorbed. Lansing, MI, BioPort Corporation, January 31, 2002.

142. Pittman PR, Gibbs PH, Cannon TL, Friedlander AM. Anthrax vaccine: short-term safety experience in humans. Vaccine 20:972–978, 2001.

143. Centers for Disease Control and Prevention. Surveillance for adverse events associated with anthrax vaccination—U.S. Department of Defense, 1998–2000. MMWR 49:341–345, 2000.

144. Sato PA, Reed RJ, Smith TC, Wang LZ. DoD-wide medical surveillance for potential long-term adverse events associated with anthrax immunization: hospitalizations. Vaccine 20:2369–2375, 2002.

145. Peeler RN, Cluff LE, Trever RW. Hyper-immunization of man. Bull Johns Hopkins Hosp 103:183–198, 1958.

146. Peeler RN, Kadull PJ, Cluff LE. Intensive immunization of man: evaluation of possible adverse consequences. Ann Intern Med 63:44–57, 1965.

147. White III CS, Adler WH, McGann VG. Repeated immunization: possible adverse effects. Reevaluation of human subjects at 25 years. Ann Intern Med 81:594–600, 1974.

148. Sever JL, Brenner AI, Gale AD, et al. Safety of anthrax vaccine: a review by the Anthrax Vaccine Expert Committee (AVEC) of adverse events reported to the Vaccine Adverse Event Reporting System (VAERS). Pharmacoepidemiol Drug Safety 11:189–202, 2002.

148a. Kerrison JB, Lounsbury D, Thirkill CE, et al. Optic neuritis after anthrax vaccination. Ophthalmology 109:99–104, 2002.

149. Wiesen AR, Littell CT. Relationship between prepregnancy anthrax vaccination and pregnancy and birth outcomes among US Army women. JAMA 287:1556–1560, 2002.

150. Singh Y, Klimpel KR, Quinn CP, et al. The carboxy-terminal end of protective antigen is required for receptor binding and anthrax toxin activity. J Biol Chem 266:15493–15497, 1991.

151. Little SE, Lowe JR. Location of receptor-binding region of protective antigen from *Bacillus anthracis*. Biochem Biophys Res Commun 180:531–537, 1991.

152. Singh Y, Chaudhary VK, Leppla SH. A deleted variant of *Bacillus anthracis* protective antigen is non-toxic and blocks anthrax toxin action in vivo. J Biol Chem 264:19103–19107, 1989.

153. Novak JM, Stein MP, Little SE, et al. Functional characterization of protease-treated *Bacillus anthracis* protective antigen. J Biol Chem 267:17186–17193, 1992.

154. Ivins BE, Welkos SL, Little SE, et al. Immunization against anthrax with *Bacillus anthracis* protective antigen combined with adjuvants. Infect Immun 60:662–668, 1992.

155. Turnbull PCB, Quinn CP, Hewron R, et al. Protection conferred by microbially-supplemented UK and purified PA vaccines. Salisbury Med Bull 68:89–91, 1990.

156. Flick-Smith HC, Eyles JE, Hebdon R, et al. Mucosal or parenteral administration of microsphere-associated *Bacillus anthracis* protective antigen protects against anthrax infection in mice. Infect Immun 70:2022–2028, 2002.

157. Ivins BE, Welkos SL, Knudson GB, Little SF. Immunization against anthrax with aromatic compound-dependent (aro-) mutants of *Bacillus anthracis* and with recombinant strains of *Bacillus subtilis* that produce anthrax protective antigen. Infect Immun 58:303–308, 1990.

158. McBride BW, Mogg A, Telfer JL, et al. Protective efficacy of a recombinant protective antigen against *Bacillus anthracis* challenge and assessment of immunological markers. Vaccine 16:810–817, 1998.

159. Coulson NM, Fulop M, Titball RM. *Bacillus anthracis* protective antigen, expressed in *Salmonella typhimurium* SL3261, affords protection against anthrax spore challenge. Vaccine 12:1395–1401, 1994.

160. Iacono-Connors LC, Welkos SL, Ivins BE, Dalrymple JM. Protection against anthrax with recombinant-virus-expressed protective antigen in experimental animals. Infect Immun 59:1961–1965, 1991.

161. Price BM, Liner AL, Park S, et al. Protection against anthrax lethal toxin challenge by genetic immunization with a plasmid encoding the lethal factor protein. Infect Immun 69:4509–4515, 2001.

162. Brossier F, Levy M, Mock M. Anthrax spores make an essential contribution to vaccine efficacy. Infect Immun 70:661–664, 2002.

163. Rehme PA, Williams R, Grabenstein JD. Ambulatory medical visits among anthrax-vaccinated and unvaccinated personnel after return from southwest Asia. Military Medicine 167: 205–210, 2002.

164. Lange JL, Lesikar SE, Brundage JF, Rubertone MV. Comprehensive systematic surveillance for adverse effects of anthrax vaccine adsorbed, US Armed Forces, 1998–2000. Vaccine 21: [in press], 2003.

Chapter 32

Cholera Vaccines

DAVID A. SACK • DENNIS R. LANG

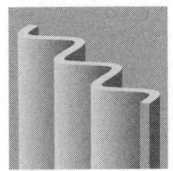

Cholera is an acutely dehydrating, watery diarrheal disease caused by intestinal infection with the bacterium *Vibrio cholerae* serogroups O1 and, more recently, O139. Cholera has probably existed on the Indian subcontinent for thousands of years. Ancient manuscripts describe the physical symptoms of what we now recognize as cholera gravis: rapid-onset vomiting, abdominal pain, explosive diarrhea, dehydration, and death. It is one of the dreaded epidemic and pandemic diseases that have had the power to alter history. Cholera has the unusual ability to spread rapidly to large numbers of people, to spread internationally, and to kill a high proportion of those affected. Before the development of effective rehydration therapy with intravenous and oral fluids, cholera epidemics were associated with case-fatality rates that exceeded 40% and led to tens of thousands of deaths in single outbreaks. John Snow is credited with understanding the importance of water as a key vehicle for the spread of the disease,[1,2] but it was not until the early 1880s that Robert Koch recovered the causative agent from the fecal specimen of a patient with the disease.[3]

History of Vaccine Development

Preparations of killed parenteral whole-cell cholera vaccine began being produced shortly after Koch's discovery.[4] Although later controlled studies showed the injectable vaccine to have limited public health usefulness, it apparently had some short-term efficacy. In 1884 in Spain, Ferran produced a killed bacterial vaccine and inoculated thousands of people with it in an area experiencing an epidemic at the time. Of those inoculated, 1.3% came down with cholera compared with 7.7% of those who were not vaccinated.[5]

Shortly after Ferran, Haffkine began working on a cholera vaccine. His work was stimulated by the cholera epidemics in his native Russia; however, he was not able to return to his homeland, so instead he went to India, where he began giving vaccine to large numbers of persons living in the Delhi and Calcutta areas. He became convinced of the success of his vaccine in 1894 when none of the 116 immunized persons in a Calcutta slum developed cholera, whereas nine cases were reported among 84 unimmunized controls.[5,6]

The popularity of the vaccine grew during the early part of the 1900s as the cholera problem continued and no effective therapy existed to combat it. Notable is the account of Russell, who carried out large-scale trials of injectable cholera vaccines in the 1920s.[7] When vaccine efficacy was assessed in a trial in which more than 8000 persons received two doses and 17,000 received one dose of the parenteral vaccine and 25,000 persons were not immunized, the vaccines were associated with a protective efficacy of about 80% during a 3-month follow-up period. Similarly, in further studies involving up to 3 million persons in (uncontrolled) trials in India, the injectable vaccine appeared to show excellent efficacy.[8] There were numerous anecdotal reports concerning the effectiveness of the parenteral vaccine.[9]

A killed oral cholera vaccine was also tested by Russell in the 1920s in India.[7] In retrospect, this is an especially interesting vaccine because of later developments in the 1980s with a "new" killed oral cholera vaccine (described later in the chapter). This vaccine, termed *Bezredka's bili-vaccine* because it was developed at the Pasteur Institute by Bezredka and contained bile salts in addition to killed *V. cholerae*, was tested in India along with the parenteral vaccine described earlier. The oral vaccine provided protection that was approximately equal (82%) to that of the injectable vaccine and appeared to be highly protective against cholera-related deaths. Because of the bile salts, the vaccine also caused diarrhea in some persons, and thus it was not acceptable to potential recipients who feared the vaccine teams were in fact spreading cholera. Unfortunately, this apparent success with an oral cholera vaccine was not to be followed up for more than 50 years.

Because of the apparent efficacy of vaccine from these early but poorly controlled studies, the panic that accompanied cholera epidemics, and the lack of consistently effective treatment, the parenteral vaccine became widely used. For expatriates, such as colonists living in areas that were endemic for cholera, this was wise at the time, especially in the absence of safe water and refrigeration. The requirement to receive booster doses every 6 months was not a serious constraint for these expatriates because cholera was an ever-present risk, and the vaccine, without doubt, prevented many cases during this early colonial period. With the accompanying panic stimulated by cholera epidemics, many countries began requiring proof of vaccination for travelers crossing international boundaries in the (mistaken) belief that vaccination would prevent the international traveler from spreading the bacterium between countries.

Although the killed parenteral whole-cell cholera vaccine is still the only one available commercially in the United States, it is not recommended for any indication by the World Health Organization (WHO). This vaccine fell from favor for several reasons. First, during the 1960s several controlled studies from East Pakistan (now Bangladesh), India, the Philippines, and Indonesia showed that the vaccine had only limited efficacy (approximately 50%) and that protection lasted only about 6 months.[10] Some vaccine preparations were associated with higher efficacy, but these tended to be associated with higher rates of side effects. More important, however, each of the injectable vaccines needed to be given frequently (every 6 to 12 months) to maintain clinically significant protection. Resources for intensive vaccination programs were not available in areas that are endemic for cholera and, if mobilized, would have distracted resources from other more effective interventions.

Other factors were also important. For example, the risk of cholera declined substantially for the expatriates and upper classes residing in cholera-endemic areas. This decline was due to the improvement in water and food quality associated with the boiling and chlorination of water and the more hygienic preparation of food. Similarly, the risk of cholera among soldiers also decreased because of improved standards for water and food in military settings.

Furthermore, other methods were found to be more useful in managing cholera epidemics than parenteral vaccination, for example, provision of safe food and water and effective case management of cholera cases as they occur. Also important was the development of effective rehydration fluid therapy, using standardized intravenous and oral solutions, that lowered case-fatality rates to less than 1% (for those who had access to treatment), making cholera much less feared than it had been previously.

Hence the upper classes and expatriates did not need cholera vaccination, and it was not cost effective for the lower socioeconomic groups. Unfortunately however, large population groups in Asia, Africa, and South America remain without safe water or food and are also without access to medical care; thus, they have a serious risk from cholera and need an alternative effective cholera vaccine.[11]

Why the Disease Is Important

Disease caused by V. cholerae O1 or O139 continues as a serious threat to human health, particularly in the developing countries of Asia, Africa, and South and Central America. In addition to the threat posed to residents of these regions, the disease is also a threat to travelers to these areas of the world. Indeed, the cases of cholera reported to occur in developed countries are almost always acquired during foreign travel.[12,13] Although accurate figures are impossible to obtain as a result of under-reporting,[14] it is estimated that more than 100,000 deaths caused by cholera occur each year in the world.[15]

Background

Clinical Description

Severe cholera (cholera gravis) is characterized by acute diarrhea and usually vomiting, which leads rapidly (within 4 to 18 hours) to moderate and frequently profound dehydration. Typically, a previously healthy individual is suddenly stricken with watery diarrhea and copious projectile vomiting. Ten and more voluminous stools may be passed within a few hours, at first liquid in consistency and then becoming like rice water. The complications from cholera arise from the loss of fluid volume and electrolytes, especially sodium, potassium, and bicarbonate, in the stool and vomitus. These losses result in hypovolemia, metabolic acidosis, and potassium deficiency.[16,17]

Secondary complications may arise from the hypovolemia or from inadequate or inappropriate fluid and electrolyte replacement. Complications can include renal failure, hypokalemia, arterial occlusions (especially in the elderly), pulmonary edema, and premature delivery or abortion. Most patients experience a decrease in blood glucose levels during treatment, but some young children experience profound hypoglycemia and seizures.[18,19] The cause of severe hypoglycemia is not known.

Not all patients with cholera experience the severe cholera gravis syndrome just described. In fact, most infected people have only mild diarrhea or may be asymptomatic. The case-to-infection ratio (number of symptomatic cases per asymptomatic people infected) has ranged from 1:3 to 1:100 depending on the geographical region, biotype, phase of epidemic, and size of inoculum.[20] The nature of the epidemic appears to affect the case-to-infection ratio, because explosive epidemics tend to have more severe cases, probably because of higher inoculum sizes resulting from the large number of infected persons contaminating the environment.

Bacteriology

Formerly, it was thought that epidemic cholera could be caused only by toxigenic strains of V. cholerae serogroup O1. However, another serogroup, O139, has emerged as a cause of epidemic cholera in Asia, with a clinical syndrome and epidemiologic spread identical to those caused by serogroup O1.[26,27] Thus, there are now two serogroups of V. cholerae that can cause epidemic cholera, O1 and O139.

There are other serogroups of V. cholerae that can cause sporadic cases of diarrhea, or they may cause systemic infections, but they do not cause epidemic disease. These are called non O1-non O139 V. cholerae (formerly, called nonagglutinating or NAG vibrios because they did not agglutinate with the O1 antiserum). Some strains of O1 or O139 V. cholerae, especially those found in the environment, do not produce toxin. These also do not cause epidemic disease. Thus the epidemic strains always belong to either O1 or O139 and also produce toxin.

The serogroup O1 V. cholerae is subdivided into two serotypes based on specific antigens in the O antigen:

Ogawa and Inaba. It is also divided into two biotypes based on biochemical reactions: classical and El Tor. More recently, genetic markers for the classical and El Tor strains have been identified. Classical strains appear to have disappeared in recent years because the last case was detected in Bangladesh in the mid 1990s. The current (seventh) pandemic strain is an El Tor biotype, but it switches back and forth between Ogawa and Inaba. Strains of serogroup O139 need not be further subdivided in the clinical laboratory.

Phage types formerly were used to further classify strains, but molecular methods are increasingly being used.[23,24] Multilocus enzyme electrophoresis can distinguish between classical and El Tor strains[25,26] and has grouped the toxigenic El Tor biotype strains into four major clonal groups or electrophoretic types (ETs) representing broad geographic areas. These include the Australian clone (ET1), the Gulf Coast clone (ET2), the seventh pandemic clone (ET3), and the Latin American clone (ET4).[24,27,28] In addition, a standardized ribotyping scheme for V. cholerae O1[29] and for O139[23] can distinguish 7 different ribotypes among classical strains, 20 ribotypes and subtypes among El Tor strains, and 6 distinct ribotypes among O139 strains. These latter molecular methods are useful for molecular epidemiology, but are not needed in the clinical laboratory.

Pathogenesis as It Relates to Prevention

Crucial steps in the pathogenesis of cholera include colonization of the small intestinal mucosa and the elaboration of the enterotoxin (cholera toxin [CT]), as shown in Figure 32–1. Both host and bacterial factors affect the likelihood of colonization. People with low levels of gastric acid are more susceptible to colonization and severe disease, because gastric acid normally kills a large proportion of these acid-sensitive bacteria. Lack of gastric acid, on the other hand, allows a higher proportion of the bacteria to survive transit through the stomach to reach the intestine, where colonization can occur. Colonization occurs more readily in people with type O blood, at least for El Tor strains, but it is inhibited in persons with intestinal antibody to the bacteria.

Bacterial factors that facilitate colonization are also important. Bacterial motility allows the bacteria to penetrate the mucous lining of the mucosa and come into close association with the epithelium. Colonization is also dependent on production of the pilus structures such as the toxin-coregulated pilus and the mannose-sensitive pilus.[30,31] Lee and colleagues presented a thorough discussion of the temporal expression of the virulence factors of V. cholerae and their role in pathogenesis.[32] If the bacteria colonize the mucosa in sufficient numbers, they are able to secrete quantities of CT close to the mucosa and thereby cause disease. However, intestinal antitoxin, if present in high concentrations, can block the CT from binding and is therefore protective.

CT, a protein with a molecular weight of 84,000, has a subunit structure consisting of a central active subunit (A subunit) and a surrounding pentomeric binding subunit (B subunit [CTB]) (Fig. 32–2).[33,34] The A subunit is responsible for the physiologic and toxic activity of the toxin, and the B subunit is responsible for the characteristic tight binding to the GM_1 ganglioside on the intestinal epithelial cell surface.[35] After attachment to the surface of the cells, CT stimulates the enzyme adenylate cyclase, which initiates a cascade of bio-

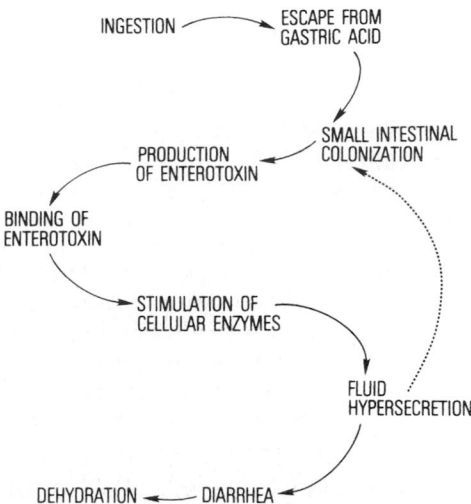

SUMMARY OF PATHOPHYSIOLOGIC EVENTS
OF ENTEROTOXIN–MEDIATED DIARRHEA

FIGURE 32–1 ■ Essential steps in the pathophysiology of cholera. After bacteria are ingested, they must escape gastric acid and move into the small intestine. The vibrios then colonize the mucosal cells of the small intestine, using motility (flagella) and colonizing pili, such as toxin-coregulated pili. Toxin secreted by the vibrio attaches to the receptor (GM_1 ganglioside), whereupon the A subunit enters the cell and stimulates intracellular enzymes, leading to hypersecretion of water and salts. The fluid secretion exceeds the capacity of the intestinal cells for reabsorption and is passed as watery diarrheal stool, leading to severe and rapid dehydration. The composition of the diarrheal fluid may facilitate further growth of the vibrio.

chemical events that lead to hypersecretion of fluid and electrolytes far in excess of the absorptive capacity of the gut.[36] The excess fluid is thus passed out as diarrheal fluid. In cholera, the activity of CT is limited to the intestinal mucosa because CT is not absorbed. If CT were to enter the blood stream, it would have major systemic effects in many tissues of

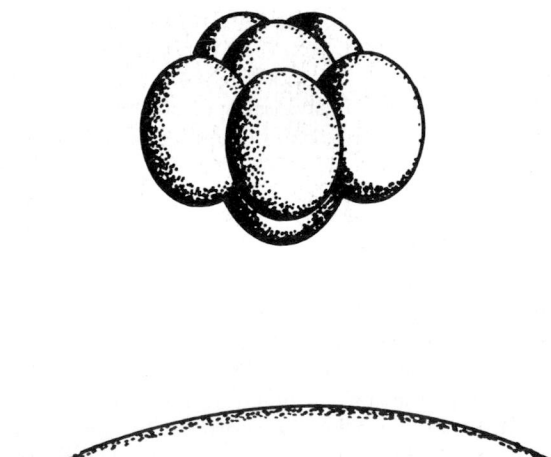

FIGURE 32–2 ■ Model of the cholera toxin, which is composed of five binding (B) subunits surrounding a central active (A) subunit. The binding subunits bind specifically to GM_1 ganglioside and are the immunodominant portion of the toxin but stimulate no physiologic activity. The A subunit is responsible for the toxic activity.

the body,[37] because the receptor (GM$_1$ ganglioside) and enzyme system (cyclic AMP) are present in all mammalian cells; however, systemic effects from CT are not seen clinically because toxin is not absorbed.

Diagnosis

The diagnosis of cholera can be suspected clinically but is confirmed by culturing the organism from a fecal culture. V. cholerae is preserved well in routine fecal transport media, although Cary-Blair medium is preferred. Primary bacteriologic plates should include selective media such as thiosulfate-citrate–bile salts–sucrose (TCBS) or taurocholate-tellurite-gelatin agar (TTGA).[38,39] Bacteriologic confirmation of initial cases in a region is essential because of the epidemic implications, but during major epidemics, laboratory confirmation is not needed except on a sample basis. Rapid immunologic diagnostic tests have been developed for both O1 and O139 V. cholerae strains, and these allow for diagnosis within a few minutes of collecting the stool sample.[40] The rapid tests are based on detection of the O antigen (lipopolysaccharide [LPS]) of the cells using monoclonal, gold-labeled antibodies on a solid matrix. Newer tests are being developed that use a dipstick format. Clinical management of the individual case, however, does not depend on laboratory confirmation, because treatment is aimed at rehydration and only secondarily toward eradicating the bacteria.

Acute and convalescent sera can be tested for vibriocidal or agglutinating antibodies to confirm the diagnosis of cholera caused by serogroup O1; a fourfold rise in titer is diagnostic of recent cholera infection.[41] A similar assay is possible for serogroup O139 but is more difficult, because the capsule found on this strain makes it less sensitive to complement-mediated killing, and the assay is performed in only a few research laboratories. The O139 vibriocidal assay generally uses a mutant strain lacking the capsule as the target strain in the assay. Antitoxin antibodies are also stimulated during infection and can be measured; however, this measurement is not completely specific, because other vibrios as well as Escherichia coli can produce an immunologically similar cholera-like toxin and stimulate antitoxin responses. In general, acute and convalescent sera are not needed to diagnose an individual patient; however, the measurement of serum titers can be helpful during epidemiologic evaluations.

Case Management

Oral rehydration salt solution should be considered as the first treatment for cholera, although intravenous fluids with a polyelectrolyte solution (e.g. Ringer's lactate) are needed in cases of severe dehydration or shock.[42] The most important therapy is the rapid replacement of fluids to correct the dehydration, replacing a base to correct the acidosis and providing potassium to correct the potassium deficiency. With proper treatment, no patient should die of cholera, but if treatment is delayed, is given too slowly, or is inappropriate, case fatality rates exceed 5% even today.

In severe cholera cases such as those coming to the hospital, an effective antibiotic will reduce the volume of diarrhea and the length of time the organism is excreted in the stool. Doxycycline or tetracycline is the antibiotic of choice for sensitive strains, but resistance to this class of drug may occur.[42] Thus one must monitor antibiotic resistance during cholera epidemics in order to choose another antibiotic when necessary. Other clinically effective antibiotics include ciprofloxacin, cotrimoxazole, erythromycin, chloramphenicol, azithromycin, and furazolidone. Prophylactic antibiotics should not be used for prevention.

Epidemiology

The global annual number of cholera cases caused by serogroups O1 and O139 is not known because of considerable under-reporting, but it probably exceeds 1 million. More than 1 million cases occurred in Latin America during the first 3 years of the 1991 epidemic, causing about 9000 deaths. Most cases of cholera occur in Asia, but these generally are not reported to the WHO. Rates of illness in the Ganges delta area are approximately 1 to 4 cases per 1000 population. Estimates of global cholera-specific mortality are believed to be 100,000 to 130,000 deaths per year, with most of the cholera deaths occurring in Asia and Africa. In addition to the endemic and epidemic cases occurring in developing countries, sporadic cases occur along the U.S. Gulf Coast and are almost always associated with undercooked shellfish, especially crabs.[43] Most other cases in the United States and other developed countries arise as a consequence of travel to endemic areas.[44]

Most cholera cases occur in older children or adults, although in endemic areas the highest age-specific rates of disease occur between 2 and 5 years of age.[45] An exception is Latin America, where rates have been highest in adult men, probably as a result of their eating food outside the home. Cholera is less common in children younger than 2 years and is especially rare in breast-fed children. V. cholerae O139 has tended to occur predominantly in adults even in South Asia, where serotype O1 has higher rates in children.[22]

Transmission occurs through consumption of contaminated water or food and is often the result of combined contamination. Contaminated water, for example, is often used to "wash" fresh food, and thus the food becomes contaminated, becoming the vehicle of transmission. Contaminated food, if kept at room temperature, supports the growth of V. cholerae and may lead to common-source outbreaks.[46,47]

Although the vibrio is generally thought to spread by the fecal-oral route, it can also persist in environmental waters without continued contamination with human feces.[48] During epidemics, environmental waters may become heavily contaminated with V. cholerae from infected human feces, and this contamination further spreads the epidemic. Once the surface waters become contaminated, an environmental reservoir can maintain the bacterium without further fecal contamination if appropriate conditions of salinity, temperature, and the like exist. As demonstrated in Louisiana, the environmental reservoir can lead to additional sporadic primary cases from contaminated seafood, but, if sanitation is adequate, secondary cases do not occur. If sanitation is poor, the sporadic cases may be followed by additional secondary cases and may lead to another epidemic through amplification of the inoculum and further contamination of the waters.[48]

In the environment, the vibrio associates with certain plankton, chitinous shelled animals (e.g., crabs), and vegetation.[49-54] These associations appear to be crucial for the vibrio's long-term survival. Furthermore, the association with chitinous shells increases the risk of transmission via crabs, shrimp, and other shellfish, many of which are eaten only partially cooked. In some cultures, raw fish may also become a vehicle of transmission. Unfortunately, even if the fish are caught in uncontaminated waters, they may become contaminated when washed in harbor water as the catch is brought to market, and cooked food may become re-contaminated in the kitchen with utensils exposed to uncooked food.

In addition to the consumption of specific high-risk foods, other risk factors for cholera include low socioeconomic status, which correlates with the use of impure water, poor sanitation, and poverty; hypochlorhydria[55-58]; lack of breast-feeding (in infants)[59,60]; and having type O blood (for El Tor biotype).[61-64] Among people living in the cholera-endemic area of the Ganges delta region, the proportion of people with type O blood is relatively low compared with that of other areas of the world. Some researchers have speculated that this unusual distribution of blood groups is associated with cholera-related pressure against people with type O blood.[65] The protection infants receive from breast-feeding may be due to antibodies in the breast milk but also may be due to less exposure to contaminated food and liquids.

Recent Changes in the Epidemiology of Cholera

The recent years have been especially notable for cholera because of the occurrence of three major epidemiologic events. First, this organism, which formerly was universally susceptible to tetracycline, has during the last 20 years developed antibiotic resistance such that susceptibility testing must now be included in the surveillance for cholera. Unlike many other enteric organisms, the predominant strains often loose their resistance and revert to being sensitive again, so antibiotic resistance is a characteristic that varies from time to time and place to place.[66,67]

The second event was the entry, in 1991, of El Tor biotype V. cholerae O1 into Latin America.[68] This was the first time cholera had invaded the Americas in more than 100 years. It has since spread throughout South and Central America and thus has invaded all regions of the world. Because conditions seemed favorable for cholera to spread to Latin America much sooner, the fact that cholera had not appeared in these countries provided hope that it would not reach this region. These hopes were unfounded, however, and an explosive epidemic occurred in Peru and other Andean countries, spreading to neighboring countries of South and Central America in a stepwise manner. Since the initial peak, rates have decreased in the region. The decline may be due in part to control measures, but it also may be due to changes in acquired immunity among susceptible people or to ecologic changes. Because a high proportion of people in Latin America have type O blood,[69] the epidemic was likely heightened, especially among Native American populations, who also had less access to treatment than did other groups.

The third, and very worrisome, event of the 1990s was the epidemic caused by a new strain of cholera, beginning in India and Bangladesh.[22,70] All previous epidemics of cholera had been associated with serogroup O1 V. cholerae, but this epidemic was caused by the new serogroup O139. Because of its origins in the region around the Bay of Bengal, the new strain has been termed V. cholerae Bengal. Although the illness is clinically indistinguishable from cholera caused by serogroup O1, the new serogroup is especially important for vaccine development because immunity to serogroup O1 vibrio does not confer immunity to serogroup O139.[71] This suggests that new cholera vaccines will need to protect against the O139 serotype as well as the O1 type. Since its first recognition in Bangladesh and India, V. cholerae Bengal has spread to other countries in Asia but not outside this region. Within India and Bangladesh, the strain continues to be isolated, with variations in the proportion of cases caused by this strain depending on the season and location. During some seasons, the O139 has been more common than the O1 serotype. It is not possible to know if this strain represents the next pandemic strain or if it will remain localized in the area around the Bay of Bengal, but it has established an endemic focus in this region, and it seems highly probable that this will become the eighth pandemic strain. Sporadic cases have appeared in other areas among travelers from Asia to other parts of the world, including the United States, but there have been no secondary cases in these other areas.

Cholera in Refugee Settings

Cholera is a major risk for refugee camps, with about 75% of such camps in Africa having an outbreak at some point.[72] This is not surprising because of the poor sanitation conditions and lack of potable water in these settings. The severity of an outbreak among refugees was illustrated by the epidemic that occurred in 1994 among Rwandan refugees in Zaire, killing about 40,000 people in a few weeks.[73] Thus refugee camps are one target for new cholera vaccines, and the use of vaccines in this setting appears to be cost effective if the vaccine can be provided at a reasonably low cost. Displaced refugees not living in camps may be at even higher risk because they lack health services in the event of cholera outbreaks.[74]

Immunity from Natural Exposure

Persons who have been infected with V. cholerae develop a protective immune response. This conclusion is based on both volunteers who were challenged 5 years following an original challenge with virulent cholera[75] and on analysis of cohorts from endemic areas of Bangladesh.[76] There is some evidence that classical strains may induce a more solid immunity than El Tor strains, although this is confounded by differences in serotype in which Inaba appears to better immunize than Ogawa.[77]

The basis for the immune protection appears to be due to local intestinal immunoglobulin A (IgA) antibody against the bacterial cells, although antibody to the toxin also contributes to protection.[78,79]

Passive Immunization

Passive immunization against cholera has not been employed. Protection using passive immunization (injected immune globulin) is theoretically possible because very high titers of serum antibody can protect, as shown by the short-lived protection seen after parenteral immunization and as demonstrated in animal studies in which dogs were protected by injected immune globulin.[80] From a practical standpoint, however, sustaining the high levels of antibody required is not possible with passive immunization. By contrast, passive immunity for infants through the ingestion of breast milk is feasible and likely to be critically important. Protection of breast-feeding infants appears to be partially mediated by antibody, although other factors also may be important.[60,81]

Active Immunization

Whole-Cell Injectable Vaccine

This vaccine is not recommended, but it is available commercially in some countries. The vaccine consists of killed *V. cholerae* and contains both Ogawa (usually classical strain NIH 41) and Inaba (usually classical strain NIH 35A3) serotypes. The strains are grown on trypticase soy agar, harvested with isotonic sodium chloride solution, and killed and preserved with 0.5% phenol. Using optical density measurements, the vaccine contains 4 billion organisms of each serotype per milliliter.

Primary immunization consists of two doses, 1 week to 1 month apart. For adults and children older than 10 years, the dosage is 0.5 mL. For children from 6 months to 4 years, the dosage is 0.2 mL, and for children from 5 to 10 years, the dosage is 0.3 mL. Booster doses with the same volume are given at 6-month intervals. The vaccine is not recommended for children younger than 6 months.

Results of Immunization

Approximately 90% of those persons immunized with the killed whole-cell parenteral vaccine develop a serologic response as measured by vibriocidal titer rise.[82] In endemic areas, older children (5 to 14 years) and adults usually respond after a single dose, but, for those younger than 5 years, two doses may be needed. Older individuals (older than 5 years) generally start with a higher titer before immunization because of natural exposure, and the geometric mean peak titer following immunization is about twice as high as that seen in children younger than 5 years. Titer rises are relatively short lived, with significant falls in titer occurring within 6 months.

In controlled trials with the commercial vaccine, vaccine efficacy has been approximately 50% for about 6 months. Protection from the vaccine usually correlates with vibriocidal titer.[83] Some studies have suggested that a doubling of titer decreases the risk by approximately 50%; however, there are exceptions to this general finding. Specifically, when a monovalent Ogawa vaccine was given in Bangladesh, the vaccine induced a rise in both Inaba and Ogawa vibriocidal titers but only protected against the homologous serotype, suggesting that the antibody in the serum is not the protective factor.[84] Also, there is no "protective titer" such that a certain titer correlates with a high degree of protection. It seems that persons with higher titers can develop disease if a high inoculum is ingested.

Injectable cholera vaccine should not be given simultaneously with yellow fever vaccine because it has been observed to decrease the immune response to this other more important vaccine.

Adverse Events

Side effects from parenteral whole-cell cholera vaccine are similar to those from killed whole-cell typhoid vaccine, although perhaps somewhat less severe.[82] Approximately 50% of vaccinees develop a soreness and inflammation at the site, and from 10% to 30% develop generalized symptoms of fever and malaise. Approximately 1% to 5% stay in bed for a day or two. Symptoms usually last for 1 to 3 days, although some individuals experience a delayed reaction, with a sore arm developing between days 4 and 7. Life-threatening reactions have been extremely rare, but allergic anaphylactic reactions are possible.

Indications

There are no indications for administering parenteral whole-cell cholera vaccine to any person of any age. However, persons who might benefit from the vaccine are those who are able to receive the vaccine on a regular basis (i.e., boosters at 6-month intervals), who are at very high risk for cholera, and who have no access to medical care should cholera occur. Persons fitting this description are extremely few and certainly do not include the usual tourists to cholera-endemic areas.

Contraindications

Because whole-cell cholera vaccine is a killed vaccine, there is no specific contraindication for persons with immunosuppression. Data are lacking on safety during pregnancy. Simultaneous vaccination for yellow fever is a contraindication because the cholera vaccine has been reported to interfere with immune responses to yellow fever vaccine.

Active Immunization with New Oral Vaccines

Two vaccines are currently available and licensed in certain countries of the world, although neither is available in the United States. They include a whole-cell killed vaccine and a live oral vaccine, as summarized in the following sections. The WHO now recommends the killed oral vaccine for refugee areas where the risk of cholera is high.[11]

Both of the new licensed vaccines are given orally. An oral vaccine is attractive for several reasons. It is easy to administer, and it has no risk of needle-borne infections. Furthermore, it stimulates the local immune system of the intestine in a manner that is more similar to the immune response induced by naturally occurring disease. Natural infections are known to be protective against subsequent infection. Both of these vaccines are designed for protection against serogroup O1, but neither protects against serogroup O139.

Defining serologic correlates of protection is not straightforward. The most commonly used correlate is the serum vibriocidal antibody, and this appears to be useful following vaccination with live oral vaccines or following naturally occurring disease. Following immunization with a killed oral vaccine, there is a vibriocidal response, but it is much lower in magnitude, is short lived, and does not correlate with protection. The previously used whole-cell injectable vaccines also stimulated high vibriocidal titers, but these titers did not correlate with long-lasting protection. Thus vibriocidal titers are useful when comparing serologic results within the same type of vaccine, but probably not between different types of vaccines.

Whole-Cell Killed Vaccine + CTB (Dukoral)

The vaccine contains a mixture of four batches of killed different strains of *V. cholerae* O1 to represent both serogroups (Inaba and Ogawa) and biotypes (El Tor and classical), as well as CTB. Two of the batches are heat killed to express the LPS antigens and two are formalin killed to better preserve the protein antigens. The CTB is produced by a genetically engineered *V. cholerae* strain that hyperproduces this antigen. The vaccine is free from any A subunit, so it has no biologic activity associated with CT. The recombinant CTB retains its ability to bind to the GM_1 ganglioside of the cell membrane. Because the heat-labile toxin of *E. coli* cross-reacts with CT, this antigen provides cross-protection against enterotoxigenic *E. coli*. Because this killed vaccine is given orally, there are no known serious side effects, and there is no chance of reversion. CTB is acid sensitive, so the vaccine is given with a buffer to protect this antigen from stomach acid. The whole-cell antigens, and especially LPS, are not acid sensitive.

Two doses are needed to immunize (three doses in children). Because it is a killed product, the entire antigenic dose is delivered to the patient, and there is no requirement for the vaccine to multiply in the host to be immunogenic, as is required for the live oral vaccine.

CONSTITUENTS OF THE VACCINE

Dukoral is prepared as a liquid formulation, and comes as a whitish 3-mL suspension in a single-dose glass vial. Each dose of the vaccine consists of a total dose of 10^{11} killed bacteria along with 1 mg of recombinant CTB. The vaccine vial comes with a sachet of buffer salts consisting of sodium hydrogen carbonate, citric acid, sodium carbonate, saccharin, sodium citrate, and raspberry flavor. The buffer is supplied as white effervescent granules and is to be dissolved in a glass of water to which the vaccine is added, and then drunk.

MANUFACTURE OF THE VACCINE

Batches of *V. cholerae* strains are grown in large fermenters. The harvested bacteria are then killed with either formalin or heat and the different batches are then combined to make a mixture of the batches in equal concentrations of bacteria. All fermentation, harvesting, and mixing and all transfers between these steps are performed within a closed, steam-sterilizable system to facilitate processing and eliminate the risk of contamination. The CTB is prepared from a strain of *V. cholerae* that is genetically engineered to produce this antigen, but it lacks the genes for producing cholera A subunit. Following fermentation, CTB is purified and then added to the whole-cell vaccine.

PRODUCER AND PREPARATIONS, DOSAGE AND ROUTE

Dukoral is produced by SBL Vaccin AB (Stockholm) and is packaged in a two-dose package with two unit-dose vials of vaccine and two sachets with buffer. Dukoral is registered in Scandinavian countries, and registration in other countries is in process. It remains experimental in the United States.

For adults, the vaccine is given as two oral doses to be given at an interval of 1 to 6 weeks. Children 2 to 6 years of age should receive three doses with an interval of 1 to 6 weeks between doses. For persons at continued risk of cholera, booster doses should be given to adults every 2 years and to children every 6 months.

VACCINE STABILITY

The vaccine should be kept refrigerated (2° to 8°C) and it should not be frozen.

SAFETY

The vaccine has been well tolerated and is considered safe even in young children. The package insert states: "Gastrointestinal side effects (upset stomach) may occur occasionally." The package insert also states that the vaccine "may be administered during pregnancy and lactation."

INDICATIONS

The vaccine is indicated for travelers to a developing country where cholera is endemic The vaccine is recommended for persons living in developing countries who are high risk for cholera, and it is especially recommended for refugees where cholera is known to be a risk, though cost considerations continue to limit its use.

CONTRAINDICATIONS AND PRECAUTIONS

There are no known contraindications to the vaccine.

Live Oral Vaccine (Orochol)

Live, attenuated oral vaccines are attractive because of the likelihood that one dose will be sufficient to induce a maximum immune response. Attempts have been made to develop such vaccines by creating attenuated mutants that do not produce CT and are not virulent. Such a mutant should stimulate antibacterial immunity (and antitoxic immunity if CTB is expressed) in a manner similar to that of natural infection but without the symptoms associated with naturally acquired *V. cholerae* infection. CVD103-HgR is the vaccine strain used in Orochol Berna and Orochol E Berna.[85,86] The strain has been engineered to express CTB but not the enzymatically active A subunit, and it is mercury resistant (to serve as a marker of the vaccine strain). The parent of CVD103-HgR, classical Inaba 569B, does not produce Shiga-like toxin, and the resulting mutant appears to be safe when given in doses up to 5×10^9 per dose. The safety profile of this vaccine is likely due, in part, to the relatively poor colonization within the human gut. Because the vaccine strain is live, the viability of the bacteria must be preserved while in storage (maintenance of a cold chain), and the bacteria must be protected from stomach acid, which is accomplished by formulating and packaging of the vaccine with a buffer.

CONSTITUENTS OF THE VACCINE

Orochol and Orochol E vaccines are consumed as a liquid to facilitate use in children and to enhance vaccine efficacy. The external container consists of a double-chambered aluminum foil sachet. One chamber contains 2.0 g of bacterial lyophilizate mixed with excipients (to facilitate handling by expanding the volume), 300 mg of sucrose, 2.1 g of lactose, and aspartame, ascorbic acid, and casein hydrolysate, while the other chamber contains a neutralized sodium bicarbonate buffer (2.65 g of sodium bicarbonate and 1.65 g of ascorbic acid). The vaccine is reconstituted by mixing the contents of both chambers in 100 mL of water. Each dose of vaccine contains 2×10^8 colony-forming units (CFU) or more of CVD103-HgR (Orochol Berna) for developed areas of the world or 2×10^9 CFU or more of CVD103-HgR for developing areas of the world (Orochol E Berna).

MANUFACTURE OF THE VACCINE

Vibrio cholerae CVD103-HgR is fermented in CF medium. The bacterial suspension is harvested by tangential flow filtration to preserve cell appendages. The bacterial concentrates are mixed with stabilizers composed of various sugars, amino acids, and antioxidants. The stabilized suspensions are lyophilized and the freeze-dried bacterial concentrates harvested, milled into a fine powder, and stored at −20°C. All fermentation, harvesting, and mixing and all transfers between these steps are performed within a closed, steam-sterilizable system to facilitate processing and eliminate the risk of contamination. All subsequent handling (lyophilization, formulation, etc.) is done in gas-tight, sterile areas or clean rooms.

PRODUCER AND PREPARATIONS, DOSAGE AND ROUTE

Orochol and Orochol E are produced by Berna Biotech Ltd. (Berne, Switzerland) and packaged in a two-compartment sachet. One compartment contains a single dose of either 2×10^8 (Orochol Berna) or 2×10^9 (Orochol E Berna) CFU. Orochol is registered in Canada, Switzerland, Australia, and New Zealand. The formulation for endemic areas of the world, Orochol E, is registered in Argentina, Bolivia, Colombia, Ecuador, El Salvador, Guatemala, Honduras, Panama, Peru, the Philippines, Sri Lanka, Switzerland, and Venezuela. It remains experimental in the United States.

The vaccine is given as a single oral dose along with a buffer salt to neutralize stomach acidity. The effective dose of live organisms in persons not living in developing countries is 2×10^8 (dose present in Orochol), whereas in developing countries, a dose of 2×10^9 live organisms was required to generate a good immune response (the dose present in Orochol E). The reason that persons in developing countries require a higher dose is not known.

VACCINE STABILITY

The vaccine contains freeze-dried live bacteria; therefore, a cold chain is needed to preserve the vaccine's potency up to the point of reconstitution. The vaccine is to be administered immediately following reconstitution.

SAFETY

The vaccine has been well tolerated and is considered safe even in young children. The package insert states: "In the course of clinical trials, the following side effects and their incidence have been recorded: diarrhea in more than 10% of cases; abdominal cramps, headache, nausea, fatigue, skin eruption, discomfort, gurgling gastrointestinal sounds, raised temperature (≤38°C), loss of appetite in 1 to 10% of cases. Flatulence in <1% of patients." A study by Perry and co-workers has indicated that the vaccine is safe in human

immunodeficiency virus–positive patients, although the subjects in this study were not severely immunodeficient.[87] Data are not available as to safety in pregnancy.

INDICATIONS

The vaccine is indicated in travelers to a developing country where cholera is endemic. The vaccine is not yet licensed for this purpose in the United States.

CONTRAINDICATIONS AND PRECAUTIONS

There are no known contraindications to the vaccine. Because it is a live bacterial vaccine, it should be used with caution in persons with immunodeficiency or in persons who are pregnant.

Future Vaccines

Killed Oral Vaccines

A killed whole-cell vaccine for oral immunization is produced in Vietnam.[88] Although it is similar to Dukoral, it does not contain any CTB, and thus provides no antitoxic immunity. Without CTB, it does not require any antacid buffer and is therefore easier to administer. It does include the whole cells of *V. cholerae* O139, but the protective efficacy against this serogroup is not known. The product is not recommended by the WHO outside Vietnam because it is not yet being produced according to Good Manufacturing Practices (GMPs), but it is a very inexpensive vaccine that has promise for developing countries.[89,90] Other killed whole-cell vaccines (without CTB) that are similar to the Vietnam vaccine but produced under GMP conditions are under development.

Live Oral Vaccines

Other live, attenuated strains have been tested in human volunteers in the United States. Among these is Peru 15, being developed by Avant Immunotherapeutics, Inc. (Needham, MA). This vaccine is derived by attenuating an O1 El Tor Inaba strain isolated in Peru in 1991. The attenuating mutations have deleted the entire CT cassette, including flanking recombination sites, and inactivated the *recA* gene by inserting the coding region for CTB under control of a heat shock promoter, thereby making it incapable of incorporating homologous DNA by recombination while providing the CTB antigen. The strain is also motility deficient. The vaccine was first tested using freshly harvested organisms and then as a lyophilized vaccine.[91,92] More recently, a GMP-produced lyophilized formulation proved safe and highly efficacious.[93] Further trials in the United States and in endemic regions are planned for the near future.

A vaccine named Bengal 15 is also being developed by Avant Immunotherapeutics. This vaccine is similar in its method of attenuation to Peru 15, but was produced from a strain of the O139 serotype. Early trials of freshly harvested vaccine organisms appeared to be safe and efficacious in small numbers of U.S. volunteers.[94] Additional live, attenuated strains have been produced and tested at the University of Maryland. Among these vaccine candidates are CVD 111,[95] an El Tor serotype O1 strain, and CVD 112, an El Tor serotype O139 strain.[96]

Parenteral Vaccines

A parenteral vaccine for cholera was developed and tested in Phase I studies. The vaccine is a polysaccharide conjugate vaccine and does stimulate high titers of vibriocidal antibodies. It is not known if this approach will be protective.[97]

Results of Vaccination

Whole-Cell Killed Vaccine + LTB (Dukoral)

Efficacy and Effectiveness

The efficacy of Dukoral was established in a large field trial in Bangladesh in 1985.[45,98] The study involved 89,596 persons who were randomized to receive at least one dose of one of three preparations: the whole-cell–CTB vaccine, a whole-cell vaccine without CTB, and a killed *E. coli* placebo. Of these, 62,285 persons took all three scheduled doses and were included in the efficacy analysis. In this trial, the whole-cell–CTB subunit vaccine was found to protect adults for 3 years and to protect children under age 5 years for 6 to 12 months. For adults and older children, the efficacy during the first year was 78%, and for the second year it was 63%. Adults who received two doses of the vaccine, but did not take the third dose, had a similar efficacy when compared to those who received two doses of placebo. For children 2 to 5 years of age, vaccine efficacy fell from high-grade protection (estimated at 100% during the first 6 months) to 21% during the second 6 months. A total of 283 cases of cholera occurred in the placebo group during the 5 years of follow-up, allowing for a high degree of statistical power.

The vaccine's efficacy was confirmed in a study in the Peruvian military in which 1426 subjects were randomized to receive two doses of vaccine or placebo 1 to 2 weeks apart.[99] After vaccination, of the 16 cases of cholera detected, 14 occurred in the placebo group (protective efficacy of 86%). In another study in Peru carried out over a 2-year period, surveillance was carried out using both active (household) and passive (hospital) surveillance. During the first year following two doses of vaccine, there were few hospital cases and nearly all cases were mild, being detected through active surveillance. During this first year, there was no evidence of protection. A booster dose was given a year after the first immunizations, and, during the subsequent year, the cholera epidemic was more severe, with most cases being detected in the hospital. During this second year, the vaccine did show high-grade protection.[100]

Immunogenicity

ANTIBODIES

Vaccination stimulates the development of both vibriocidal and anti-toxin antibodies in the serum and also stimulates IgA intestinal antibodies.[101] Titers of serum vibriocidal antibodies are lower and less frequent with the killed oral vaccine than with the live oral vaccine, but the local intestinal immune response is comparable to that seen with naturally occurring cholera.[78] Rises in serum immunoglobulin G and IgA antitoxin titers as measured by enzyme-linked immunosorbent assay are seen in most vaccinees.

CELLULAR RESPONSES

The CTB stimulates γ-interferon in mucosal tissues following immunization, although it is not known if this relates to protection.[102]

CORRELATES OF PROTECTION

Although Dukoral stimulates protective immunity, there is no good serologic correlate of protection that would be considered quantitative.[103] The serum vibriocidal and antitoxin assays can be used to compare and validate the immunogenicity of different lots of the killed vaccine or to compare adequacy of buffering, but these measures are not useful in determining degree or duration of protection.

DURATION OF IMMUNITY AND PROTECTION

Protection has been demonstrated to last for 3 years in Bangladesh in adults and older children but to wane after 6 months in children under age 5 years.[45] The onset of protection is not known but is likely to occur within 10 days of the second dose.

HERD IMMUNITY

Because Dukoral is a killed vaccine, there is no chance of passing the vaccine to others in the community as could theoretically happen with a live vaccine. Studies indicate, however, that the vaccine may protect against asymptomatic infection as well as disease, and thus it could interrupt transmission within a community.[104] The vaccine afforded protection to children of immunized mothers. Even though the children were not immunized, they were protected, and the most likely mechanism of protection was the protection afforded to the mothers who then did not pass the infection on to their children.[81]

POSTEXPOSURE PROPHYLAXIS AND THERAPEUTIC VACCINATION

No postexposure prophylaxis has been demonstrated nor would it be expected.

Live Oral Vaccine (Orochol)

Efficacy and Effectiveness

In a recent double-blind, controlled challenge study for efficacy done in the United States, 85 volunteers received a single oral dose of Orochol of between 2 and 8×10^8 vaccine organisms or placebo.[105] The vaccine was well tolerated. Three months later, 51 volunteers returned to undergo challenge with virulent, frozen *V. cholerae* N16961, an O1 El Tor strain that was developed as a standard challenge strain[106] and has been completely sequenced.[107] Efficacy against all diarrhea was 80% and against severe diarrhea was 91%. These results indicate that this vaccine provides good protection in immunologically naïve persons for up to 3 months and would be useful as a vaccine for travelers to endemic regions.

In a large Phase III trial conducted in 67,000 volunteers in Indonesia, Orochol failed to demonstrate efficacy in this endemic region.[108] The reason for the apparent high efficacy in North American volunteers and the low efficacy in this cholera-endemic area is not understood. Further studies in endemic areas thus are needed to understand the efficacy of the vaccine in these different settings.

Immunogenicity

ANTIBODIES

Following oral vaccination with a live oral vaccine, the serum vibriocidal response is the best correlate of protection for *V. cholerae* and the best measure of successful stimulation of antibacterial immunity. High serum vibriocidal as well as anti-LPS antibodies are stimulated in most vaccinees given CVD103-HgR. Intestinal IgA antibodies are also produced against the LPS antigen. Individuals who have not been previously exposed to cholera (naïve volunteers) respond well (fourfold or greater rise in vibriocidal antibody titers) to a dose of 10^8 organisms,[105,109,110] whereas volunteers from endemic areas required a higher dose of 10^9 organisms to stimulate an equivalent response.[111,112] Antitoxin responses are seen in many volunteers, but the titer rises are less consistent and of lower magnitude than the antibodies directed against the bacterial cell wall antigens.[109]

CELLULAR RESPONSES

No cellular responses to Orochol or Orochol E have been determined.

CORRELATES OF PROTECTION

The recognized correlate of protection for Orochol (and following natural infection) is the serum vibriocidal antibodies. This is likely not the mechanism of protection, however.

HERD IMMUNITY

No studies have been done to test the induction of herd immunity, but herd immunity is theoretically possible. This might occur through transmission of the live vaccine strain to others who have not received the vaccine directly. Alternatively, herd immunity might occur as a result of protecting vaccinees from asymptomatic infection, thereby reducing contamination of the environment with virulent *V. cholerae*. It should be noted that a small minority of those immunized excrete the strain and that the strain has been intentionally weakened (attenuated); its survival in the environment is not expected to be long. Whether the widespread use of any attenuated cholera vaccine in an endemic area has the ability to induce herd immunity through secondary infection of others must await such use and evaluation.

DURATION OF IMMUNITY AND PROTECTION

Protection has been demonstrated to last for up to 6 months following vaccination of naïve volunteers. Significant efficacy was induced within 8 days of vaccination.[113]

POSTEXPOSURE PROPHYLAXIS AND THERAPEUTIC VACCINATION

No postexposure prophylaxis has been demonstrated nor would it be expected.

Public Health Considerations

The WHO recommends the use of the killed oral vaccine for use in refugee settings at high risk for cholera and has suggested that a stockpile be available for emergency use.[114] The vaccine has been distributed in such settings and appears to be useful in protecting against outbreaks of cholera.[115,116] The usefulness and cost effectiveness of either the killed or live, attenuated oral vaccines in endemic areas have yet to be determined, although it would seem that these vaccines could significantly reduce the rates of cholera in these areas. In addition to reducing rates of illness, vaccination should also reduce costs associated with hospitalization. Vaccines would be especially useful if epidemics could be predicted in time to implement a vaccine program prior to the outbreak.

Some have argued that providing vaccine is less cost effective than providing other cholera control interventions (water or sanitation improvements) or providing treatment for those who develop the disease. In fact, these different strategies are not alternatives, but should be considered complementary in the control of cholera. Provision of improved hygiene will lessen the size of the inoculum consumed, making the vaccines more effective, and use of the vaccines will decrease the numbers of persons contaminating the environment.

Relying entirely on provision of water and sanitation and on good case management also raises the issue of equity, with poor people (e.g., those most likely to get cholera) being the ones who are less likely to have improved sanitation or access to good case management. By contrast, a vaccine may be given to rich and poor alike and could prevent the life-threatening illness that might require high-level medical care. Vaccines are generally more equitable than provision of case management, and this is likely true for cholera as well.

The rationale for recommending cholera vaccine for travelers and military personnel is similar to that for other travelers' vaccines, that is, prevention of an unlikely but severe illness. Because the vaccines are safe and are given orally, most travelers are likely to welcome the vaccines, especially because the vaccine (at least those versions that stimulate antitoxic immunity) may prevent some cases of enterotoxigenic *E. coli* diarrhea as well. Unfortunately, the risk of cholera in travelers is not known because such cases occurring during overseas travel are not reported, but the risk is not negligible.

The currently available vaccines are suitable for travelers, but they have limitations for more general public health use. Future vaccines should include antigens for *V. cholerae* O139 because it seems likely that this will be the next pandemic strain. They should be convenient to give quickly to large numbers of people with a minimum of supervision, as may be needed in refugee settings or prior to an expected epidemic. A requirement for a cold chain is a constraint unless the vaccine can be given through routine services such as the Expanded Program on Immunisation, but, if special programs are needed, the vaccine should be stable at room temperature to minimize the need for an expensive infrastructure. It seems likely that booster doses will be needed at some interval (perhaps 2-year intervals), so an over-the-counter formulation may fit best with the public health constraints. Finally, the vaccines for cholera will need to be very inexpensive (likely less than $1 per dose) if they are to have wide public health application in developing countries.

Fortunately, a number of new experimental vaccines are under study.[117] Including CVD112 and Bengal 15, both attenuated strains of serogroup O139, and attenuated strains of *Salmonella typhi* expressing O antigens. In addition, injectable vaccines consisting of O antigens coupled to the carrier protein pseudomonas exotoxin A are also under development.

REFERENCES

1. Snow J, Frost WH, Richardson BW. Snow on cholera, being a reprint of two papers by John Snow, M.D. New York, Commonwealth Fund, 1936.
2. Howard-Jones N, Robert Koch and the cholera vibrio: a centenary. Br Med J (Clin Res Ed) 288:379–381, 1984.
3. Koch R. An address on cholera and its bacillus. Br Med J 2:453–459, 1884.
4. Lutzker E, Jochnowitz C. Waldermar Haffkine: pioneer of cholera vaccine. ASM News 7:366–369, 1987.
5. Bornside GH. Waldemar Haffkine's cholera vaccines and the Ferran-Haffkine priority dispute. J Hist Med Allied Sci 37:399–422, 1982.
6. Cited in Pollitzer R. Cholera. World Health Organization, Geneva. 1959, pp 324–326.
7. Chandr Sekar C. Statistical assessment of the efficacy of anti-cholera inoculation from the data of 63 cheris in south Srcot district. Indian J Med Res 35:153, 1947.
8. Pollitzer R. Cholera. Geneva, World Health Organization, 1959.
9. Mosley WH, Bart KJ, Sommer A. An epidemiological assessment of cholera control programs in rural East Pakistan. Int J Epidemiol 1:5–11, 1972.
10. Sack DA. Underestimating the cholera problem and the potential for vaccination—a case for accelerating use of cholera vaccines. Bull Inst Pasteur 93:1–7, 1995.
11. Synder JD, Blake PA. Is cholera a problem for US travelers? JAMA 247:2268–2269, 1982.
12. Mahon BE, Mintz ED, Greene KD, et al. Reported cholera in the United States, 1992–1994: a reflection of global changes in cholera epidemiology. JAMA 276:307–312, 1996.
13. Siddique AK, Zaman K, Baqui AH, et al. Cholera epidemics in Bangladesh: 1985–1991. J Diarrhoeal Dis Res 10:79–86, 1992.
14. Committee on Issues and Priorities for New Vaccine Development. The prospects for immunizing against *Vibrio cholerae*. In New Vaccine Development: Establishing Priorities. Vol. II. Diseases of Importance in Developing Countries. Washington, DC, National Academy Press, 1986, pp 376–389.
15. Zaman K, Yunus M, Rahman A, et al. Efficacy of a packaged rice oral rehydration solution among children with cholera and cholera-like illness. Acta Paediatr 90:505–510, 2001.
16. Carpenter CC. Cholera: diagnosis and treatment. Bull N Y Acad Med 47:1192–1203, 1971.
17. Sack DA, Islam S, Brown KH, et al. Oral therapy in children with cholera: a comparison of sucrose and glucose electrolyte solutions. J Pediatr 96:20–25, 1980.
18. Butler T, Arnold M, Islam M. Depletion of hepatic glycogen in the hypoglycaemia of fatal childhood diarrhoeal illnesses. Trans R Soc Trop Med Hyg 83:839–843, 1989.
19. Khan M, Shahidullah M. Cholera due to the El Tor biotype equals the classical biotype in severity and attack rates. J Trop Med Hyg 83:35–39, 1980.
20. Garg S, Saha PK, Ramamurthy T, et al. Nationwide prevalence of the new epidemic strain of *Vibrio cholerae* O139 Bengal in India. J Infect 27:108–109, 1993.
21. Cholera Working Group. Large epidemic of cholera-like disease in Bangladesh caused by Vibrio cholerae O139 synonym Bengal. Lancet 342:387–390, 1993.
22. Faruque SM, Saha MN, Asadulghani, et al. The O139 serogroup of *Vibrio cholerae* comprises diverse clones of epidemic and nonepidemic strains derived from multiple *V. cholerae* O1 or non-O1 progenitors. J Infect Dis 182:1161–1168, 2000.
23. Wachsmuth IK, Evins GM, Fields PI, et al. The molecular epidemiology of cholera in Latin America. J Infect Dis 167:621–626, 1993.
24. Momen H, Salles CA. Enzyme markers for *Vibrio cholerae*: identification of classical, El Tor and environmental strains. Trans R Soc Trop Med Hyg 79:773–776, 1985.
25. Cameron DN, Khambaty FM, Wachsmuth IK, et al. Molecular characterization of *Vibrio cholerae* O1 strains by pulsed-field gel electrophoresis. J Clin Microbiol 32:1685–1690, 1994.
26. Muthing J, Neumann U. Selective detection of terminally alpha 2-3 and alpha 2-6 sialylated neolacto-series gangliosides by immunostaining on thin layer chromatograms. Biomed Chromatogr 7:158–161, 1993.
27. Chen F, Evins GM, Cook WL, et al. Genetic diversity among toxigenic and nontoxigenic *Vibrio cholerae* O1 isolated from the Western Hemisphere. Epidemiol Infect 107:225–233, 1991.
28. Popovic T, Bopp C, Olsvik O, Wachsmuth K. Epidemiologic application of a standardized ribotype scheme for *Vibrio cholerae* O1. J Clin Microbiol 31:2474–2482, 1993.
29. Taylor RK, Miller VL, Furlong DB, Mekalanos JJ. Use of phoA gene fusions to identify a pilus colonization factor coordinately regulated with cholera toxin. Proc Natl Acad Sci U S A 84:2833–2837, 1987.
30. Jonson G, Holmgren J, Svennerholm AM. Identification of a mannose-binding pilus on *Vibrio cholerae* El Tor. Microb Pathog 11:433–441, 1991.
31. Lee SH, Hava DL, Waldor MK, Camilli A. Regulation and temporal expression patterns of *Vibrio cholerae* virulence genes during infection. Cell 99:625–634, 1999.
32. Holmgren J, Lonnroth I, Ouchterlony O. Identification and characterization of cholera exotoxin in culture filtrates of *V. cholerae*. Acta Pathol Microbiol Scand [B] Microbiol Immunol 79:448, 1971.
33. Lonnroth I, Holmgren J. Subunit structure of cholera toxin. J Gen Microbiol 76:417–427, 1973.
34. Holmgren J, Lonnroth I, Svennerholm L. Fixation and inactivation of cholera toxin by GM1 ganglioside. Scand J Infect Dis 5:77–78, 1973.
35. Kimberg DV, Field M, Johnson J, et al. Stimulation of intestinal mucosal adenyl cyclase by cholera enterotoxin and prostaglandins. J Clin Invest 50:1218–1230, 1971.
36. Pierce NF, Graybill JR, Kaplan MM, Bouwman DL. Systemic effects of parenteral cholera enterotoxin in dogs. J Lab Clin Med 79:145–156, 1972.
37. Rennels MB, Levine MM, Daya V, et al. Selective vs. nonselective media and direct plating vs. enrichment technique in isolation of *Vibrio cholerae*: recommendations for clinical laboratories. J Infect Dis 142:328–331, 1980.
38. O'Brien M, Colwell R. Modified taurocholate-tellurite-gelatin agar for improved differentiation of *Vibrio* species. J Clin Microbiol 22:1011–1013, 1985.
39. Qadri F, Hasan JA, Hossain J, et al. Evaluation of the monoclonal antibody-based kit Bengal SMART for rapid detection of *Vibrio cholerae* O139 synonym Bengal in stool samples. J Clin Microbiol 33:732–734, 1995.
40. Benenson AS, Saad A, Mosley WH. Serological studies in cholera. 2. The vibriocidal antibody response of cholera patients determined by a microtechnique. Bull World Health Organ 38:277–285, 1968.
41. World Health Organization and Global Task Force on Cholera Control. Guidelines for Cholera Control. Geneva, World Health Organization, 1994.
42. Lowry PW, Pavia AT, McFarland LM, et al. Cholera in Louisiana: widening spectrum of seafood vehicles. Arch Intern Med 149:2079–2084, 1989.
43. Steinberg EB, Greene KD, Bopp CA, et al. Cholera in the United States, 1995–2000: trends at the end of the twentieth century. J Infect Dis 184:799–802, 2001.
44. van Loon FP, Clemens JD, Chakraborty J, et al. Field trial of inactivated oral cholera vaccines in Bangladesh: results from 5 years of follow-up. Vaccine 14:162–166, 1996.
45. Rabbani GH, Greenough WB III. Food as a vehicle of transmission of cholera. J Diarrhoeal Dis Res 17:1–9, 1999.
46. Weber JT, Mintz ED, Canizares R, et al. Epidemic cholera in Ecuador: multidrug-resistance and transmission by water and seafood. Epidemiol Infect 112:1–11, 1994.
47. Blake PA, Allegra DT, Snyder JD, et al. Cholera—a possible endemic focus in the United States. N Engl J Med 302:305–309, 1980.
48. Nalin DR. Cholera, copepods, and chitinase. Lancet 2:958, 1976.
49. Huq A, Huq SA, Grimes DJ, et al. Colonization of the gut of the blue crab (Callinectes sapidus) by *Vibrio cholerae*. Appl Environ Microbiol 52:586–588, 1986.
50. Epstein PR. Algal blooms in the spread and persistence of cholera. Biosystems 31:209–221, 1993.

51. Islam MS, Drasar BS, Bradley DJ. Attachment of toxigenic *Vibrio cholerae* O1 to various freshwater plants and survival with a filamentous green alga, *Rhizoclonium fontanum*. J Trop Med Hyg 92:396–401, 1989.

52. Huq A, Small EB, West PA, et al. Ecological relationships between *Vibrio cholerae* and planktonic crustacean copepods. Appl Environ Microbiol 45:275–283, 1983.

53. Huq A, West PA, Small EB, et al. Influence of water temperature, salinity, and pH on survival and growth of toxigenic *Vibrio cholerae* serovar O1 associated with live copepods in laboratory microcosms. Appl Environ Microbiol 48:420–424, 1984.

54. Nalin DR, Levine MM, Rhead J, et al. Cannabis, hypochlorhydria, and cholera. Lancet 2:859–862, 1978.

55. Sack GH Jr, Pierce NF, Hennessey KN, et al. Gastric acidity in cholera and noncholera diarrhoea. Bull World Health Organ 47:31–36, 1972.

56. Merrell DS, Camilli A. Acid tolerance of gastrointestinal pathogens. Curr Opin Microbiol 5:51–55, 2002.

57. van Loon FP, Clemens JD, Shahrier M, et al. Low gastric acid as a risk factor for cholera transmission: application of a new non-invasive gastric acid field test. J Clin Epidemiol 43:1361–1367, 1990.

58. Clemens JD, Sack DA, Harris JR, et al. Breast feeding and the risk of severe cholera in rural Bangladeshi children. Am J Epidemiol 131:400–411, 1990.

59. Glass RI, Svennerholm AM, Stoll BJ, et al. Protection against cholera in breast-fed children by antibodies in breast milk. N Engl J Med 308:1389–1392, 1983.

60. Sircar BK, Dutta P, De SP, et al. ABO blood group distributions in diarrhoea cases including cholera in Calcutta. Ann Hum Biol 8:289–291, 1981.

61. Black RE, Levine MM, Clements ML, et al. Association between O blood group and occurrence and severity of diarrhoea due to *Escherichia coli*. Trans R Soc Trop Med Hyg 81:120–123, 1987.

62. Clemens JD, Sack DA, Harris JR, et al. ABO blood groups and cholera: new observations on specificity of risk and modification of vaccine efficacy. J Infect Dis 159:770–773, 1989.

63. Holmgren J, Lindblad M, Fredman P, et al. Comparison of receptors for cholera and *Escherichia coli* enterotoxins in human intestine. Gastroenterology 89:27–35, 1985.

64. Glass RI, Holmgren J, Haley CE, et al. Predisposition for cholera of individuals with O blood group: possible evolutionary significance. Am J Epidemiol 121:791–796, 1985.

65. Glass RI, Huq I, Alim AR, Yunus M. Emergence of multiply antibiotic-resistant *Vibrio cholerae* in Bangladesh. J Infect Dis 142:939–942, 1980.

66. Mhalu FS, Mmari PW, Ijumba J. Rapid emergence of El Tor *Vibrio cholerae* resistant to antimicrobial agents during first six months of fourth cholera epidemic in Tanzania. Lancet 1:345–347, 1979.

67. Tauxe RV, Blake PA. Epidemic cholera in Latin America. JAMA 267:1388–1390, 1992.

68. Swerdlow DL, Mintz ED, Rodriguez M, et al. Severe life-threatening cholera associated with blood group O in Peru: implications for the Latin American epidemic. J Infect Dis 170:468–472, 1994.

69. Bhattacharya SK, Bhattacharya MK, Nair GB, et al. Clinical profile of acute diarrhoea cases infected with the new epidemic strain of *Vibrio cholerae* O139: designation of the disease as cholera. J Infect 27:11–15, 1993.

70. Albert MJ, Alam K, Rahman AS, et al. Lack of cross-protection against diarrhea due to *Vibrio cholerae* O1 after oral immunization of rabbits with *V. cholerae* O139 Bengal. J Infect Dis 169:709–710, 1994.

71. Naficy A, Rao MR, Paquet C, et al. Treatment and vaccination strategies to control cholera in sub-Saharan refugee settings: a cost-effectiveness analysis. JAMA 279:521–525, 1998.

72. Siddique AK, Salam A, Islam MS, et al. Why treatment centres failed to prevent cholera deaths among Rwandan refugees in Goma, Zaire. Lancet 345:359–361, 1995.

73. Sack DA. Cholera vaccine in refugee settings. JAMA 280:600–602, 1998.

74. Cash RA, Music SI, Libonati JP, et al. Response of man to infection with *Vibrio cholerae*. II. Protection from illness afforded by previous disease and vaccine. J Infect Dis 130:325–333, 1974.

75. Clemens JD, van Loon F, Sack DA, et al. Biotype as determinant of natural immunising effect of cholera. Lancet 337:883–884, 1991.

76. Longini IM Jr, Yunus M, Zaman K, et al. Epidemic and endemic cholera trends over a 33-year period in Bangladesh. J Infect Dis, 86:246–251, 2002.

77. Svennerholm AM, Jertborn M, Gothefors L, et al. Mucosal antitoxic and antibacterial immunity after cholera disease and after immunization with a combined B subunit-whole cell vaccine. J Infect Dis 149:884–893, 1984.

78. Svennerholm AM, Holmgren J. Synergistic protective effect in rabbits of immunization with *Vibrio cholerae* lipopolysaccharide and toxin/toxoid. Infect Immun 13:735–740, 1976.

79. Pierce NF, Reynolds HY. Immunity to experimental cholera. I. Protective effect of humoral IgG antitoxin demonstrated by passive immunization. J Immunol 113:1017–1023, 1974.

80. Clemens JD, Sack DA, Chakraborty J, et al. Field trial of oral cholera vaccines in Bangladesh: evaluation of anti-bacterial and anti-toxic breast-milk immunity in response to ingestion of the vaccines. Vaccine 8:469–472, 1990.

81. Benenson AS, Joseph PR, Oseasohn RO. Cholera vaccine field trials in east Pakistan. 1. Reaction and antigenicity studies. Bull World Health Organ 38:347–357, 1968.

82. Mosley WH, McCormack WM, Ahmed A, et al. Report of the 1966–67 cholera vaccine field trial in rural East Pakistan. 2. Results of the serological surveys in the study population—the relationship of case rate to antibody titre and an estimate of the inapparent infection rate with *Vibrio cholerae*. Bull World Health Organ 40:187–197, 1969.

83. Mosley WH, Aziz KM, Rahman AS, et al. Field trials of monovalent Ogawa and Inaba cholera vaccines in rural Bangladesh—three years of observation. Bull World Health Organ 49:381–387, 1973.

84. Kaper JB, Levine MM. Recombinant attenuated *Vibrio cholerae* strains used as live oral vaccines. Res Microbiol 141:901–906, 1990.

85. Cryz SJ Jr, Kaper J, Tacket C, et al. *Vibrio cholerae* CVD103-HgR live oral attenuated vaccine: construction, safety, immunogenicity, excretion and non-target effects. Dev Biol Stand 84:237–244, 1995.

86. Perry RT, Plowe CV, Koumare B, et al. A single dose of live oral cholera vaccine CVD 103-HgR is safe and immunogenic in HIV-infected and HIV-noninfected adults in Mali. Bull World Health Organ 76:63–71, 1998.

87. Trach DD, Clemens JD, Ke NT, et al. Field trial of a locally produced, killed, oral cholera vaccine in Vietnam. Lancet 349:231–235, 1997.

88. Naficy AB, Trach DD, Ke NT, et al. Cost of immunization with a locally produced, oral cholera vaccine in Viet Nam. Vaccine 19:3720–3725, 2001.

89. Trach DD, Cam PD, Ke NT, et al. Investigations into the safety and immunogenicity of a killed oral cholera vaccine developed in Viet Nam. Bull World Health Organ 80:2–8, 2002.

90. Sack DA, Shimko J, Sack RB, et al. Comparison of alternative buffers for use with a new live oral cholera vaccine, Peru-15, in outpatient volunteers. Infect Immun 65:2107–2111, 1997.

91. Sack DA, Sack RB, Shimko J, et al. Evaluation of Peru-15, a new live oral vaccine for cholera, in volunteers. J Infect Dis 176:201–205, 1997.

92. Cohen MB, Giannella RA, Bean J, et al. Randomized, controlled human challenge study of the safety, immunogenicity, and protective efficacy of a single dose of Peru-15, a live attenuated oral cholera vaccine. Infect Immun 70:1965–1970, 2002.

93. Coster TS, Killeen KP, Waldor MK, et al. Safety, immunogenicity, and efficacy of live attenuated *Vibrio cholerae* O139 vaccine prototype. Lancet 345:949–952, 1995.

94. Tacket CO, Kotloff KL, Losonsky G, et al. Volunteer studies investigating the safety and efficacy of live oral El Tor *Vibrio cholerae* O1 vaccine strain CVD 111. Am J Trop Med Hyg 56:533–537, 1997.

95. Tacket CO, Losonsky G, Nataro JP, et al. Initial clinical studies of CVD 112 *Vibrio cholerae* O139 live oral vaccine: safety and efficacy against experimental challenge. J Infect Dis 172:883–886, 1995.

96. Gupta RK, Taylor DN, Bryla DA, et al. Phase 1 evaluation of *Vibrio cholerae* O1, serotype Inaba, polysaccharide-cholera toxin conjugates in adult volunteers. Infect Immun 66:3095–3099, 1998.

97. Clemens JD, Sack DA, Harris JR, et al. Field trial of oral cholera vaccines in Bangladesh. Lancet 2:124–127, 1986.

98. Sanchez JL, Vasquez B, Begue RE, et al. Protective efficacy of oral whole-cell/recombinant-B-subunit cholera vaccine in Peruvian military recruits. Lancet 344:1273–1276, 1994.

99. Taylor DN, Cárdenas V, Sanchez JL, et al. Two-year study of the protective efficacy of the oral whole cell plus recombinant B subunit cholera vaccine in Peru. J Infect Dis 181:1667–1673, 2000.

100. Sack DA, Clemens JD, Huda S, et al. Antibody responses after immunization with killed oral cholera vaccines during the 1985 vaccine field trial in Bangladesh. J Infect Dis 164:407–411, 1991.
102. Kilhamn J, Brevinge H, Quiding-Jarbrink M, et al. Induction and distribution of intestinal immune responses after administration of recombinant cholera toxin B subunit in the ileal pouches of colectomized patients. Infect Immun 69:3466–3471, 2001.
103. Clemens JD, van Loon F, Sack DA, et al. Field trial of oral cholera vaccines in Bangladesh: serum vibriocidal and antitoxic antibodies as markers of the risk of cholera. J Infect Dis 163:1235–1242, 1991.
104. Clemens JD, Sack DA, Rao MR, et al. Evidence that inactivated oral cholera vaccines both prevent and mitigate *Vibrio cholerae* O1 infections in a cholera-endemic area. J Infect Dis 166:1029–1034, 1992.
104. Tacket CO, Cohen MB, Wasserman SS, et al. Randomized, double-blind, placebo-controlled, multicentered trial of the efficacy of a single dose of live oral cholera vaccine CVD 103-HgR in preventing cholera following challenge with *Vibrio cholerae* O1 El Tor Inaba three months after vaccination. Infect Immun 67:6341–6345, 1999.
105. Sack DA, Tacket CO, Cohen MB, et al. Validation of a volunteer model of cholera with frozen bacteria as the challenge. Infect Immun 66:1968–1972, 1998.
106. Heidelberg JF, Eisen JA, Nelson WC, et al. DNA sequence of both chromosomes of the cholera pathogen *Vibrio cholerae*. Nature 406:477–483, 2000.
107. Richie EE, Punjabi NH, Sidharta YY, et al. Efficacy trial of single-dose live oral cholera vaccine CVD 103-HgR in North Jakarta, Indonesia, a cholera-endemic area. Vaccine 18:2399–2410, 2000.
108. Cryz SJ Jr, Levine MM, Kaper JB, et al. Randomized double-blind placebo controlled trial to evaluate the safety and immunogenicity of the live oral cholera vaccine strain CVD 103-HgR in Swiss adults. Vaccine 8:577–580, 1990.
109. Kotloff KL, Wasserman SS, O'Donnell S, et al. Safety and immunogenicity in North Americans of a single dose of live oral cholera vaccine CVD 103-HgR: results of a randomized, placebo-controlled, double-blind crossover trial. Infect Immun 60:4430–4432, 1992.
110. Suharyonom, Simanjuntak C, Witham N, et al. Safety and immunogenicity of single-dose live oral cholera vaccine CVD 103-HgR in 5-9-year-old Indonesian children. Lancet 340:689–694, 1992.
111. Su-Arehawaratana P, Singharaj P, Taylor DN, et al. Safety and immunogenicity of different immunization regimens of CVD 103-HgR live oral cholera vaccine in soldiers and civilians in Thailand. J Infect Dis 165:1042–1048, 1992.
112. Tacket CO, Losonsky G, Nataro JP, et al. Onset and duration of protective immunity in challenged volunteers after vaccination with live oral cholera vaccine CVD 103-HgR. J Infect Dis 166:837–841, 1992.
113. World Health Organization. Potential Use of Oral Cholera Vaccines in Emergency Situations. (Report of a WHO meeting, Geneva, Switzerland, 12–13 May 1999 [WHO/CDS/CSR/EDC/99.4]). Geneva, World Health Organization, 1999.
114. Legros D, Paquet C, Perea W, et al. Mass vaccination with a two-dose oral cholera vaccine in a refugee camp. Bull World Health Organ 77:837–842, 1999.
115. Dorlencourt F, Legros D, Paquet C, et al. Effectiveness of mass vaccination with WC/rBS cholera vaccine during an epidemic in Adjumani district, Uganda. Bull World Health Organ 77:949–950, 1999.
116. Ivanoff B. Choléra: les vaccins actuels et futurs. Méd Trop 61:245–248, 2001.

Chapter 33

Japanese Encephalitis Vaccines

SCOTT B. HALSTEAD • THEODORE F. TSAI

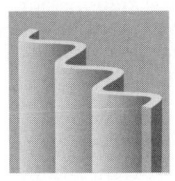

Japanese encephalitis (JE), a mosquito-borne flaviviral infection, is the leading recognized cause of childhood encephalitis in Asia. Approximately 20,000 cases and 6000 deaths are reported annually, but in many locations the disease is not under systematic surveillance, and official reports undoubtedly underestimate the true number of cases (Fig. 33–1).[1-3] Although the disease is transmitted only in Asia, because the region contains more than 3 billion people and 60% of the world's population, regional JE-associated morbidity may exceed worldwide morbidity from herpes encephalitis, the latter estimated at 5 cases per 1 million population per year, or approximately 30,000 cases worldwide.[4,5] With the near-eradication of poliomyelitis, JE now is the continent's leading cause of childhood viral neurologic infection. By any standard, JE is a major public health problem that potentially can be controlled by proven effective vaccines.

History of Disease

Summer-fall encephalitis outbreaks consistent with JE were recorded in Japan as early as 1871, the largest of which, in 1924, led to more than 6000 cases, 60% of them fatal.[6] A filterable agent from human brain tissue was isolated in rabbits that year, and, in 1934, Hayashi transmitted the disease experimentally to monkeys.[7] Soon after, the availability of JE and related St. Louis encephalitis (StLE) viral isolates made possible serologic confirmation of encephalitis cases occurring elsewhere in the region, including a cluster of cases occurring in 1934 through 1935 in Beijing.[8] The virus initially was called Japanese B encephalitis (the modifying "B" has since fallen into disuse) to distinguish the disease from Von Economo's type A encephalitis, which had different clinical and epidemiologic characteristics. The mosquito-borne mode of JE transmission was elucidated with the isolation of JE virus from *Culex tritaeniorhynchus* mosquitoes in 1938, and subsequent field studies established the role of aquatic birds and pigs in the viral enzootic cycle. Viruses isolated from human cases in Japan in 1935 and in Beijing in 1949 provided the prototype Nakayama and

Beijing and P3 strains, respectively, that are in principal use in vaccine production today.

During the first half of this century, JE was recognized principally in temperate areas of Asia in the form of perennial outbreaks in Japan, Korea, and China.[1] Annual outbreaks of several thousand cases recurred in Japan until as recently as 1966, with a public health impact that was magnified further by the concentration of these outbreaks during the summer season. In Korea, after 5616 cases and 2729 deaths were recorded in 1949, epidemics continued every 2 or 3 years, culminating in an unprecedented 6897 cases in 1958 (Fig. 33–2).[9] However, China has accounted for the majority of cases in the region; between 1965 and 1975, more than 1 million cases were reported, 175,000 in 1971 alone (Fig. 33–3).[10] Public health efforts that placed a great emphasis on vaccination produced a dramatic decline in cases; however, coverage remains low in many provinces, and in recent years incidence in the rural population has remained stable. In Japan, Korea, and Taiwan, the introduction of national immunization programs after 1965 led to the near-elimination of the disease; however, the absence of reported cases is disarming because enzootic transmission of the virus in its enzootic cycle continues in these locations[11] (Fig. 33–4), and periodic outbreaks, as in Korea in 1982 (see Fig. 33–2), have occurred.

Although sporadic viral encephalitis cases had been noted in northern Thailand, JE was not recognized as a major public health problem in Southeast Asia until 1969, when an epidemic of 685 cases was reported from the Chiang Mai Valley.[12] Yearly outbreaks producing thousands of cases and hundreds of deaths followed in the northern region, and JE became recognized as a leading cause of childhood mortality and disability (Fig. 33–5).[13] Subsequently, in 1974, the first of several epidemics was recorded in an area of Myanmar (Burma) adjacent to the Chiang Mai Valley.[14] In Vietnam, since reinstatement of notification in 1979, several thousand JE cases have been reported annually, and the disease has been recognized as a public health threat in the densely populated deltas of the Mekong and Red Rivers.[15] Incidence rates exceeding 20 per 100,000 have been reported from areas of the northern delta near Hanoi. The disease probably occurs with equal

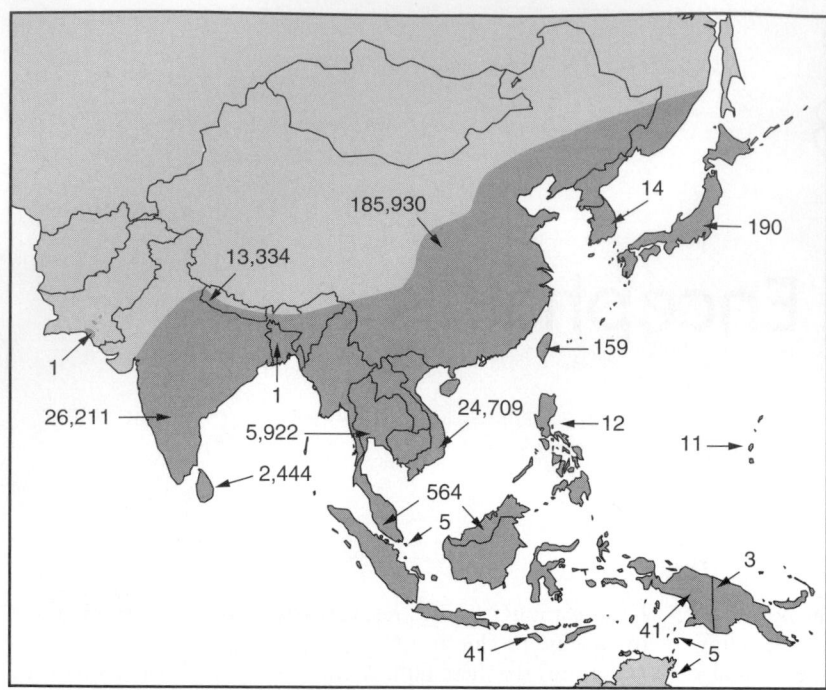

FIGURE 33–1 ▪ Reported cases of Japanese encephalitis, 1986 to 2000, and areas with proven or suspected enzootic viral transmission. (Data from World Health Organization and other reports; see Table 33–20 for updated geographic distribution.)

frequency in epidemiologically similar Cambodia, where clinically compatible cases have been observed, but outbreaks have not been reported. Recent studies in Penang, Malaysia, and Bali, Indonesia, indicate that 40% to 50% of hospitalized encephalitis cases are caused by JE, thereby underscoring the inadequacy of public health surveillance, because few cases previously had been reported from these locations, and even the occurrence of JE had been questioned.[16,17] The continued public health impact of JE in the region has led to efforts in Thailand and, more recently, in Vietnam to implement programs of childhood immunization and vaccine production.[15,18]

JE transmission was first recognized in Southwest Asia after an outbreak occurred in 1948 in Sri Lanka. Sporadic cases and later epidemics were recognized on the Indian subcontinent around Vellore.[19,20] Outbreaks were documented only in southern India until 1973, when JE epidemics were reported in the north in the Burdwan and Bankura districts of West Bengal and afterward in Bihar and

Uttar Pradesh. Large outbreaks of JE, often involving adults, subsequently were reported from various states, and the disease is currently considered hyperendemic in northern India and southern Nepal, central India (Andra Pradesh), and southern India (Goa, Karnataka, and Tamil Nadu) (Fig. 32–6). JE recently has been shown to occur as far west as the Indus valley in Pakistan.[21] The apparent spread to or amplification of JE in new areas has been correlated with agricultural development and intensive rice cultivation supported by irrigation schemes.[22] In Sri Lanka and southern Nepal, hyperendemic transmission of malaria and JE were documented to have followed deforestation and development in the Mahaweli River Valley and Terai, respectively.[23,24] The potential spread of JE is being watched closely in Irian Jaya, Indonesia, the irrigated Thar desert of Rajasthan, as well as other places under development where conditions receptive to viral transmission and amplification recently have been created. Recent novel introductions leading to outbreaks on Saipan and the Torres Strait islands between New Guinea and northern Australia, and a sporadic case on the Cape York peninsula of mainland Australia, illustrate the potential for JE virus to be transferred over significant distances, possibly by viremic migratory birds or by windblown mosquitoes.[25,26] Although development has led to the near-elimination of JE in economically advanced Asian countries (Japan, Korea, Taiwan, and Singapore), early investments in agricultural development in Southeast and South Asia, emphasizing new crops and animal husbandry, seem to have increased JE transmission.

Background

Clinical Illness

The great majority of infections are not apparent, and only 1 in approximately 250 infections results in symptomatic

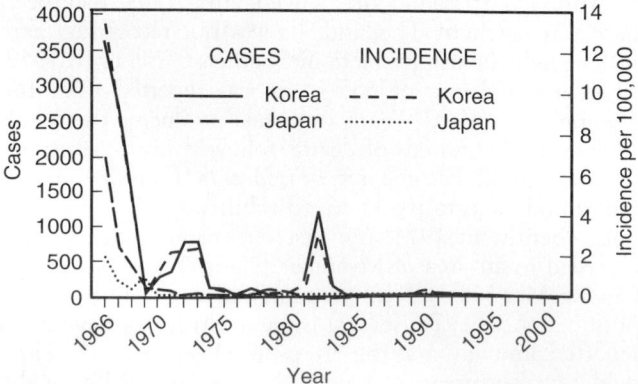

FIGURE 33–2 ▪ Reported Japanese encephalitis cases and incidence, Japan and Korea, 1966 to 1995. (Data from World Health Organization reports.)

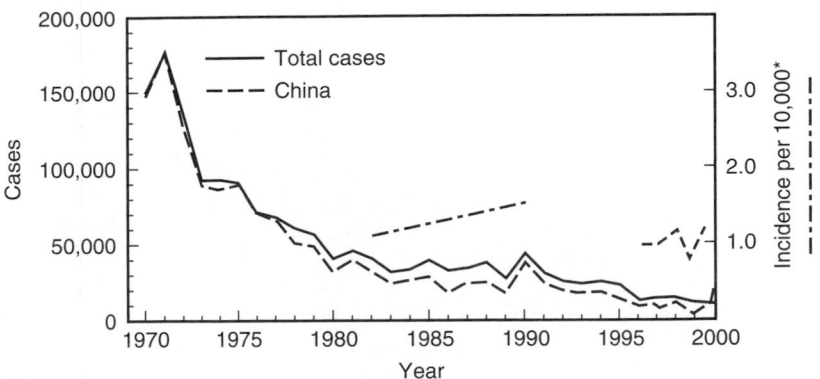

* For China, rural population, children <15 years: denominator available for 1982 and 1990 only

A

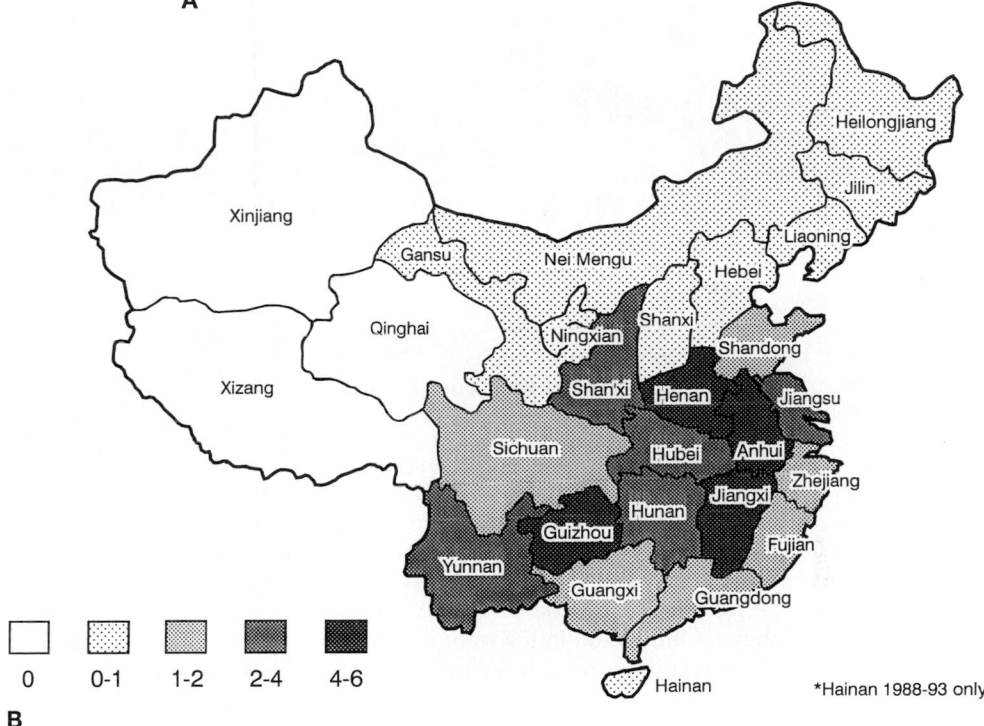

FIGURE 33–3 ■ *A,* Reported cases of Japanese encephalitis (JE) for Asian countries and for China only, 1970 to 2000 (Data from World Health Organization reports). Incidence rates for China are based on enumerated rural populations of children younger than 15 years in 1982 and 1990. *B,* Incidence of JE per 100,000 population by province, China, 1983 to 1993. (*B* from Yu YX. Japanese encephalitis in China. Southeast Asian J Trop Med Public Health 26S3:17–21, 1995, with permission.)

| 0 | 0-1 | 1-2 | 2-4 | 4-6 |

*Hainan 1988-93 only

B

illness in susceptible Asians.[27,28] The principal clinical manifestation of illness is encephalitis. Milder clinical presentations, such as aseptic meningitis and simple febrile illness with headache, may sometimes occur but usually escape recognition.[29–38] The incubation period is 5 to 15 days. Illness usually begins with abrupt onset of high fever, change in mental status, gastrointestinal symptoms, and headache, followed gradually by disturbances in speech or gait or other motor dysfunction. Irritability, vomiting, and diarrhea or an acute convulsion may be the earliest signs of illness in an infant or child. Seizures occur in more than 75% of pediatric patients and less frequently in adults. Conversely, presentation with headache and meningism is more common in adults than in children.

A progressive decline in alertness eventually leads to stupor and coma. A substantial proportion of patients become totally unresponsive and require ventilatory assistance. Generalized weakness and changes in muscle tone, especially hypertonia and hyperreflexia, are common, but focal motor deficits—including paresis, hemiplegia, or tetraple-

gia; cranial nerve palsies (especially central facial palsy); and abnormal reflexes—also may be present. Sensory disturbances are seen less frequently. Central hyperpnea, hypertension, pulmonary edema, and urinary retention may complicate the illness. Although symptoms suggest elevated intracranial pressure in many cases, papilledema and other signs of increased intracranial pressure are rarely seen. In a controlled trial, dexamethasone therapy did not improve outcome.[39] Signs of extrapyramidal involvement, including tremor, mask-like facies, rigidity, and choreoathetoid movements, are characteristic of JE, but these signs may be obscured initially by generalized weakness.

Clinical laboratory examination discloses a moderate peripheral leukocytosis with neutrophilia and mild anemia. Hyponatremia, reflecting inappropriate antidiuretic hormone secretion, is a frequent complication. Cerebrospinal fluid (CSF) pressure is usually normal. Pleocytosis ranges from a few to several hundred cells per cubic millimeter, with a lymphocytic predominance; neutrophils may be seen in early samples.[40] CSF protein is moderately elevated in about

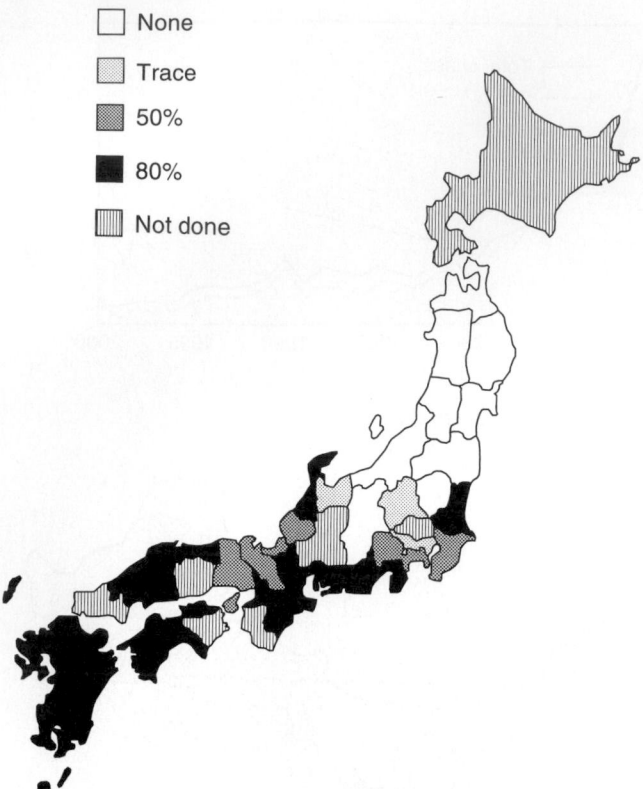

None
Trace
50%
80%
Not done

FIGURE 33–4 ■ Japanese encephalitis seroprevalence in swine by district, Japan, October 1996. The absence of reported human cases belies continued transmission of the virus in its enzootic cycle, as demonstrated by high rates of pig infections. (From Taniguchi K, Matsunaga Y. National epidemiologic surveillance of vaccine-preventable diseases, Japan, October 1995, with permission.)

50% of cases. Reduced levels of CSF monoamines (homovanillic and 5-hydroxyindoleacetic acids) have been found in the acute phase of illness and in recovery, but these reductions have not correlated consistently with clinical parkinsonism.[41]

Computed tomography (CT) and magnetic resonance imaging (MRI) scans reveal low-density areas and abnormal signal intensities, respectively, in the thalamus, basal ganglia, pons, and putamen.[42–46] Acute changes in the thalamus may be a helpful differentiating feature: When compared with encephalitis cases resulting from other causes, in JE cases, T_2-weighted MRI images more frequently disclose bilateral thalamic high-intensity lesions representing hemorrhages, while single-photon emission CT more often shows increased activity in the thalami and putamina.[45] MRI abnormalities may be seen in the spinal cord, underscoring that JE is an encephalomyelitis. Electromyographic changes reflecting anterior horn cell degeneration are detected, especially in patients with clinical wasting. However, abnormalities in somatosensory evoked potentials are rare, which is consistent with the infrequency of clinical sensory deficits. Delays in central motor conductance time reflect widespread involvement of white matter, thalamus, brain stem, and spinal cord.[46] Electroencephalography (EEG) tracings typically show diffuse δ wave activity, but α coma also may be seen. Imaging and neurophysiologic abnormalities indicative of thalamic damage correlate with several of the clinical manifestations typifying the acute phase of illness.

Five to 30% of cases are fatal, with some deaths occurring after a brief prodrome and fulminant course lasting a few days and others occurring after a more protracted course with persistent coma. Young children (<10 years) are more likely than adults to die, and, if they survive, they are more likely to have residual neurologic deficits. Overall, approximately one third of surviving patients exhibit serious residual neurologic disability.[30,47–52] Principal sequelae include memory loss, impaired cognition, behavioral disturbances, convulsions, motor weakness or paralysis, and abnormalities of tone and coordination. In children, motor abnormalities frequently improve or eventually resolve, but behavioral changes and psychological deficits have been detected 2 to 5 years after recovery in up to 75% of pediatric cases; EEG abnormalities also may persist in the absence of detectable clinical signs.[47,48] Evidence of previous dengue immunity is associated with better outcome.[53]

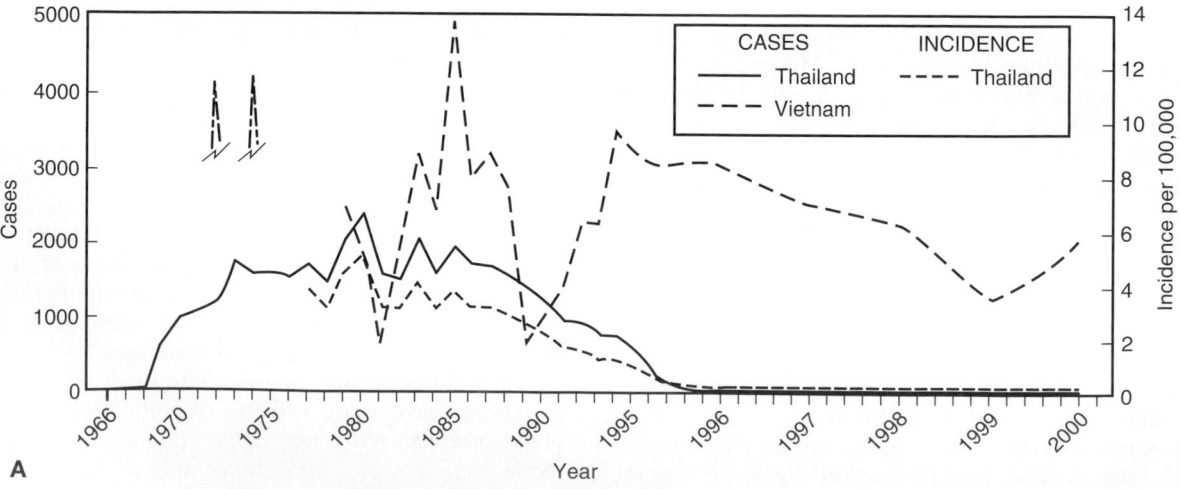

FIGURE 33–5 ■ *Top*, Reported Japanese encephalitis cases and incidence, Thailand and Vietnam, 1966 to 2000. *Lower left*, Incidence per 100,000 by province, Thailand, 1993. *Lower right*, Incidence per 100,000 by province, Vietnam, 1993. (Thai data from Chunsuttiwat S, Warachit P. Japanese encephalitis in Thailand. Southeast Asian J Trop Med Public Health 26[suppl 3]:43–46, 1995. Vietnamese data from Nguyen HT, Nguyen TY. Japanese encephalitis in Vietnam 1985–93. Southeast Asian J Trop Med Public Health 26[suppl 3]:47–50, 1995.)

Continued

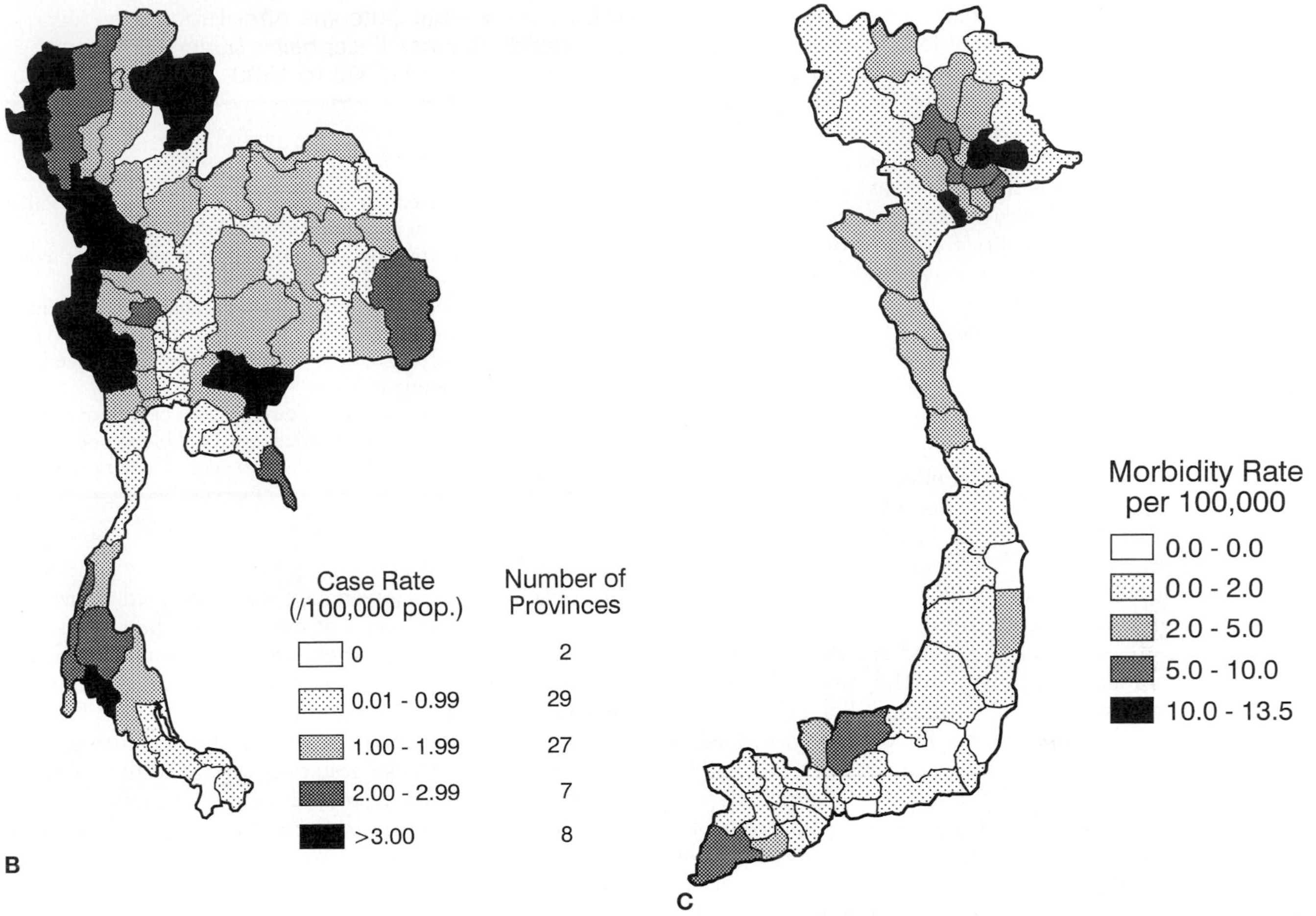

Case Rate
(/100,000 pop.)
Number of
Provinces
0 2
0.01 - 0.99 29
1.00 - 1.99 27
2.00 - 2.99 7
>3.00 8
B
Morbidity Rate
per 100,000
0.0 - 0.0
0.0 - 2.0
2.0 - 5.0
5.0 - 10.0
10.0 - 13.5
C

FIGURE 33–5 ▪ **Cont'd**

Poor prognosis has been associated with a short prodromal interval, clinical presentation in deep obtundation, respiratory dysfunction, prolonged fever, focal presentation, status epilepticus, and the presence of extrapyramidal signs or pathologic reflexes.[47,54–58] In some locations concurrent neurocysticercosis has been reported in more than one third of JE cases, with evidence of increased mortality in coinfected patients (see later discussion).[59]

Anecdotal observations suggest that infection may fail to clear in certain individuals, with the possibility of clinical relapse several months after resolution of the acute illness.[60] In several cases symptoms recurred, and virus was recovered from persistently infected peripheral lymphocytes despite circulating antibody. Other recovered patients who were studied months after recovery had apparently asymptomatic viremias. The possibility of subacute or persisting infection

CASES
India
Nepal
Sri Lanka
Cases
8000
7000
6000
5000
4000
3000
2000
1000
0
1966 1970 1975 1980 1985 1990 1995 1996 1997 1998 1999 2000
Year

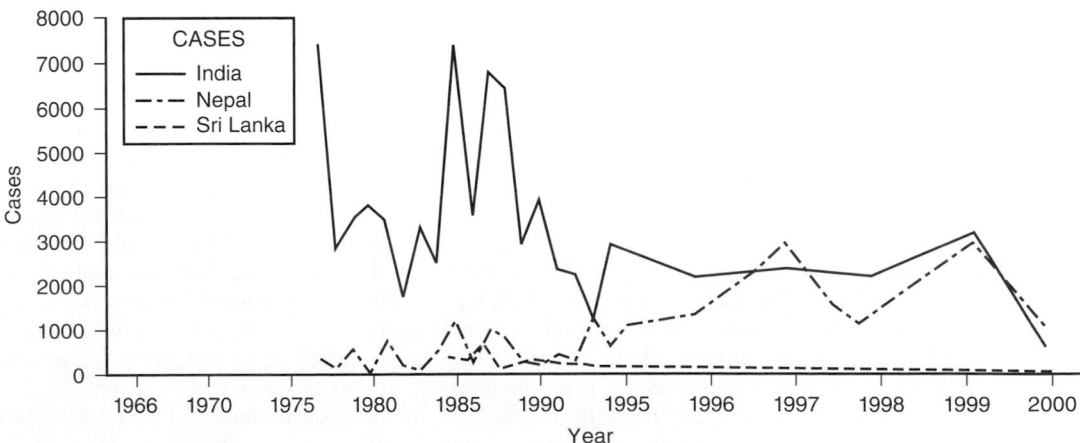

FIGURE 33–6 ▪ Reported Japanese encephalitis cases, India, Nepal, and Sri Lanka, 1977 to 2000. (Data from World Health Organization reports.)

in the central nervous system (CNS) was demonstrated in 5% of patients whose CSF contained virus or viral antigen for 3 weeks or who had intrathecal immunoglobulin M (IgM) antibodies 50 to 180 days after onset.[60,61] The clinical significance of these observations and conditions under which JE virus persists in humans are unclear.

No specific therapy is available, but supportive treatment can reduce morbidity and mortality significantly. Mannitol and other modalities to control intracerebral pressure often are needed. Trihexyphenidyl hydrochloride and central dopamine agonists have been used to treat acute extrapyramidal symptoms.[62] Neutralizing murine monoclonal antibodies, developed in China, have been reported to improve clinical outcome in small controlled clinical trials, and licensure in that country has been sought.[63] Experimental studies in mice and monkeys also suggest the potentially beneficial effect of interferon, and, in an uncontrolled series of 14 patients treated with recombinant interferon-α, 13 survived; however, further studies have not been undertaken.[64,65] A number of antiviral compounds, including ribavirin, exhibit activity in vitro but have not been evaluated clinically.

Pathologic abnormalities are found chiefly in the CNS; however, inflammatory changes in the myocardium and lung and hyperplasia of reticuloendothelial cells in the spleen, liver, and lymph nodes have been described.[66] Cerebral edema and congested leptomeninges are visible on gross examination of the brain, and "punched-out" necrolytic lesions in the gray matter may be conspicuous.[66-72] Histopathologic examination discloses a pattern of diffuse microglial proliferation with nodular formation around dead or degenerating neurons, in which viral antigen can be demonstrated by immunohistochemical staining.[40,68,72] Viral antigen is distributed principally in the thalamus, midbrain, hippocampus, and temporal cortex, but also in Purkinje and granular cells of the cerebellum and in the brain stem reticular formation. However, viral antigen also has been demonstrated in well-preserved neurons independent of glial reaction—in some cases, well after the acute phase of illness, suggesting intracellular viral persistence. Gliomesenchymal nodules are seen in a parallel distribution within the brain and anterior horn of the spinal cord. In patients dying with residual neurologic impairment several years after resolution of the acute illness, scarred rarified foci are found in a characteristic distribution in the thalamus, substantia nigra, and hippocampus.[73]

Congenital Infection

Relatively little is known of the risks of JE acquired in pregnancy and the consequences of intrauterine infection. In areas where the disease is endemic, children are exposed and become immune at an early age. Consequently, few women of child-bearing age are at risk for the disease. Although the virus is an established cause of abortions and abnormal births in pigs,[74] the first associations of JE with adverse events in human pregnancy were not reported until as late as 1980.[75-76] In a series of outbreaks in Uttar Pradesh, India, JE infections were documented in nine pregnant women (Table 33–1). Four who acquired JE in the first or second trimester miscarried, and the virus was recovered from products of conception in two cases. In five women who acquired the illness in the third trimester, no

TABLE 33–1 ■ Fetal Outcome After Laboratory-Confirmed Japanese Encephalitis During Pregnancy, Uttar Pradesh, India, 1978 to 1980

Weeks of Gestation	Outcome
8	Aborted; Japanese encephalitis (JE) virus isolated from placenta and fetal brain
10	Aborted; no virus isolated from placenta or fetal brain
20	Aborted; cord blood and products of conception not tested
22	Aborted; JE virus isolated from placenta, fetal brain, and liver
28 (2 cases)	Normal full-term delivery; cord blood not tested
30 (2 cases)	Normal full-term delivery; cord blood not tested
36	Normal full-term delivery; cord blood not tested

adverse outcomes of pregnancy were observed. However, JE virus–specific IgM was not measured in the infants, and it is unknown whether they were congenitally infected. Experimental data also suggest that risk of congenital infection may be related to gestational age. Human placental organ cultures, obtained from medically terminated pregnancies at 8 to 12 weeks' gestation, supported JE viral replication, but tissues from full-term pregnancies were resistant to infection.[77] Experimental studies have shown that JE viral neurotropism is related to neuronal immaturity.[78,79]

The spectrum of adverse outcomes associated with congenital JE viral infections is undefined. It is unknown whether congenital infection causes fetal malformation or asymptomatic infection during pregnancy leads to fetal infection or adverse outcome.

Virology

JE virus is one of 70 viruses in the *Flavivirus* genus of the Flaviviridae family.[80,81] The complete genomic sequences of JE virus and several other flaviviruses have been determined, including yellow fever (YF) virus, the prototype virus in the family. Morphologically, flaviviruses are spherical, approximately 40 to 50 nm in diameter, with a lipid membrane enclosing an isometric 30-nm-diameter nucleocapsid core comprising a capsid (C) protein and a single-stranded messenger (positive)-sense viral RNA.[82] Membrane surface projections are composed of a glycosylated envelope (E) and membrane (M) protein, a mature form of the premembrane (prM) protein. JE viral RNA, 10,976 bases in length, encodes an uninterrupted open reading frame (ORF), flanked by 95- and 585-base untranslated regions at the 5′ and 3′ ends, respectively.[83,84] Protein translation at the first encountered AUG codon near the 5′ end yields a polyprotein precursor of 3432 amino acids that is co- or post-translationally processed by a virus-specific nonstructural (NS) protease complex, NS2B-NS3, host cell signal peptidase, or unidentified host cell–specific protease into at least 10 mature viral proteins (Fig. 33–7). The order of proteins encoded in the JE virus ORF, as with other flaviviruses, is 5′-C-prM-E-NS1-NS2A-NS2B-NS3-NS4A-NS4B-NS5-3′.

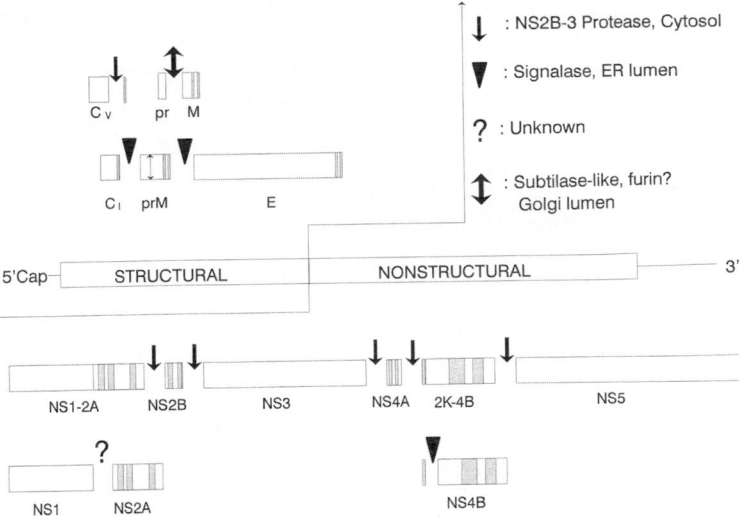

FIGURE 33–7 ■ Schematic representation of flaviviral polyprotein processing. The middle region outlines the viral genome: *line regions*, the 5′ and 3′ nontranslated regions; *boxed region*, open reading frame for structural and nonstructural proteins. Co-translational cleavage by host cell–encoded signalase separating structural and nonstructural proteins occurs at the E protein C-terminus. A subtilase-like cellular enzyme, furin, may be responsible for prM cleavage. Potential transmembrane regions of the viral polyprotein are indicated by shaded areas.

Flaviviruses replicate in a variety of cultured cells of vertebrate and arthropod origin. Viral entry occurs by receptor-mediated endocytosis, with the formation of coated vesicles, or by direct fusion with plasma membranes.[85–87] The nucleocapsid is uncoated by acid-dependent fusion of viral and endosomal membranes, releasing genomic RNA into the cytoplasm, where viral replication continues with immediate translation of the uncoated viral genome.[85] The translated polyprotein then is processed and assembled into a virus-specific replication complex.

Extensive proliferation of membranous organelles in the perinuclear region may be a unique feature of flavivirus-infected cells.[84,87] Ultrastructural examination discloses convoluted membranes (CMs), paracrystalline structures (PCs), proliferating endoplasmic reticulum (ER), spherical smooth structures (SMSs) of about 100 nm in diameter found adjacent to other induced membranes, and vesicle packets (VPs).[88] Membranous structures are partially surrounded by virus particles, many in aggregates within smooth membranes continuous with paired ER membranes.[89] In Kunjin virus–infected cells, RNA synthesis and RNA polymerase activity are not detected until 8 hours after infection, after which smooth membrane–associated VPs are seen. NS3 and NS5 proteins, functioning as a helicase or an RNA-dependent RNA polymerase, respectively, are directed to VP membranes through an interaction with NS1 to assemble the flavivirus replication complex. Subsequently, PCs and SMSs develop, and an interconversion of PCs to CMs appears.[87,88] The collection of induced membranes may represent virus factories in which translation, RNA synthesis, and virus assembly occur.

Of the two viral membrane-associated proteins, the 53-kDa surface protein E exhibits the most important biologic properties, including viral attachment to cellular receptors, specific membrane fusion, and elicitation of virus-neutralizing, hemagglutination-inhibiting, and anti-fusion antibodies.[81] Immature intracellular virions contain prM, the glycosylated precursor of the 7- to 8-kDa M protein. Cotransport of prM-E protein heterodimers through an exocytic pathway is essential for maturation and biosynthesis of authentic E protein; prM prevents low-pH-induced rearrangements of E, acting as a chaperone for its efficient secretion and proper folding.[90–92] Before release from the cell, the prM protein is cleaved by a putative subtilase-like enzyme associated with the *trans*-Golgi membrane, leaving only M protein associated with the mature virion.[93]

The hydrophobic carboxyl terminus of the E protein provides a membrane-associated anchor, while an extensive ectodomain, stabilized by disulfide bridging, is folded into three antigenic domains (A, B, and C) that are variably related to (1) determinants representing flaviviral group-, subgroup-, and virus-specific epitopes and (2) biologic functions.[94] Crystallographic examination of the tick-borne encephalitis (TBE) viral E protein reveals it to be a homodimer lying parallel to the viral surface. The monomers fold into three distinct structural domains—I, II, and III—corresponding to the antigenic domains C, A, and B, respectively.[95] Domain III contains an immunoglobulin-like module extending perpendicular to the viral surface that is likely to be involved in receptor binding. Binding of JE virions to certain cells of CNS lineage may be associated with the presence of specific neurotransmitter receptors.[96] Dengue-2 virus selectively binds cellular heparan sulfates of the glycosaminoglycan (GAG) family via E protein GAG-binding motifs within the carboxyl terminal and externally accessible regions of domains I and III.[97–98] Similar mechanisms may apply to JE and other flaviviruses.[99]

Virus-specific and cross-reactive neutralizing epitopes have been mapped to specific regions of the flavivirus E glycoprotein.[94–100] Comprehensive cross-neutralization studies indicate the close antigenic relationship of JE virus to StLE, West Nile, Koutango, and Usutu viruses and several flaviviruses found in Australia (e.g., Murray Valley encephalitis and Kunjin, Alfuy, Stratford, and Kokobera viruses) and their classification into a single antigenic complex.[101,102] No serologic cross-reactions with hepatitis C virus have been observed.[103]

The biochemical, antigenic, and genetic relationships of JE viruses isolated from different geographic regions and at various times have been compared by using polyclonal and monoclonal antibodies, two-dimensional gel electrophoresis of T1 ribonuclease-digested virion RNA, and genomic sequencing.[104,105] The molecular phylogeny of JE viruses, based on the 240-base nucleotide sequence of viral prM, divides JE isolates into five distinct genotypes, with a

TABLE 33–2 ■ Geographic Distribution of Japanese Encephalitis Viruses by Genotype

Genotype	Country or Region (Year of Isolation)
1	Japan (1935, 1955, 1957, 1959, 1979, 1982)
	China (1949, 1960)
	Korea (1982, 1987, 1991, 1994)
	Okinawa (1968–1992)
	Taiwan (1972, 1987)
	Philippines (1977, 1984)
	Vietnam (1964–1988)
	Nepal (1985)
	India (1963, 1970, 1972, 1975, 1978–1980, 1982, 1985)
	Sri Lanka (1969, 1987)
2	Thailand (1979, 1982–1985, 1992, 1993)
	Cambodia (1969)
3	Indonesia (1970, 1978, 1979, 1981)
	Thailand (1983)
	Malaysia (1970)
	Sarawak (1968)
	Australia (1995)
4	Indonesia (1981)
5	Singapore (1994)

Data from Chen et al.,[106,107] Huong et al.,[108] Ma et al.,[109] Ritchie et al.,[110] Chung et al.,[111] and Uchil and Satchidanandam.[112]

maximum divergence of 21% among the isolates (Table 33–2).[106–112] The largest genotype consists of viruses from Japan, Okinawa, China, Taiwan, Vietnam, the Philippines, Sri Lanka, India, and Nepal. A second genotype comprises isolates from northern Thailand and Cambodia, and a third comprises isolates from southern Thailand, Malaysia, Sarawak, Australia, and Indonesia. Five Indonesian isolates—two from Java, two from Bali, and one from Flores—similar to each other and distinct from other Indonesian isolates, form the fourth genotype. Co-circulation of multiple genotypes was observed only in Thailand and Indonesia. An antigenic analysis using five virus-specific monoclonal antibodies classified strains into four antigenic types, without correspondence to the genotypes above.

JE virus isolates from the same region but from different years show a high degree of nucleotide similarity. Sixteen Vietnam and 23 Okinawa strains of JE virus isolated between 1964 and 1988 and between 1968 and 1992 differed by only 3.2% and 4%, respectively.[107,109] However, viruses could be distinguished chronologically before and after 1986 in Okinawa and before and after 1975 in Vietnam. Genetic drift appears to be the main mechanism by which JE virus continuously evolves, although novel viral introductions have been documented, indicating the potential for genotypic displacement.[25,110] However, when 92 genomes with complete envelope sequences in the GeneBank were analyzed, the level of inter-genotypic diversity was less than observed across poliovirus or dengue serotypes. This genetic analysis supports the contention that all known JE virus isolates comprise a single serotype.[113]

Pathogenesis

After an infectious mosquito bite, viral replication occurs locally and in regional lymph nodes. Virions disseminate to secondary sites, where further replication contributes to a viremia. Invasion of the CNS probably occurs from the blood by antipodal transport of virions through vascular endothelial cells.[40,114] Infection in the CNS spreads by viral dissemination through the extracellular space or by direct intercellular spread.[115] Sensitized T-helper (Th) cells stimulate an inflammatory response by recruiting macrophages and lymphocytes to the perivascular space, parenchyma and CNS, where the inflammatory response clears infected neurons, with subsequent formation of glial nodules.[40,66–68,116] The predominant cell type in the CSF and in the parenchyma is helper/inducer (CD4+) T cells, with B lymphocytes confined chiefly to the perivascular space.[116,117]

Why only one in several hundred infections in nonimmune indigenous humans develops into symptomatic neuroinvasive disease is unclear. Factors that contribute to neuroinvasion include age and, based on work in laboratory animals, genetic acquired host factors.[27,78,79,118–120] Selection of genetic resistance to infection in humans with long exposure to a fatal viral infection may explain the observed differences in case-infection ratios in foreigners of limited residence versus indigenous Asian populations.[27] Macrophages are important in the nonspecific clearance of virus, and their depletion leads to extended viremia, CNS invasion, and death in experimentally infected mice.[121] However, circulating antibody plays a critical role in modulating infection by limiting viremia in the preneuroinvasive phase. Both JE virus–specific and heterologous (e.g., dengue) antibodies contribute to protection, and low levels of neutralizing antibody may be sufficient to prevent viremia.[53,122–125] Guinea pigs or mice that had been previously immunized with attenuated JE vaccine and that no longer had detectable neutralizing antibodies (<1:4) were protected against intraperitoneal challenge infection, and, moreover, their serum passively protected mice.[126] Experimentally infected monkeys immunosuppressed with cyclophosphamide have no measurable antibody response and exhibit an increased susceptibility to paralytic encephalitis and a diminished CNS inflammatory reaction.[127] Conversely, passive transfer of specific monoclonal antibodies can enhance neurovirulence in intracerebrally challenged mice.[128]

Clinically, high CSF interferon-α levels and low CSF virus-specific IgM and immunoglobulin G antibodies have been associated with a fatal outcome, suggesting that delayed or poor local antibody response and uninhibited CNS virus proliferation determines outcome.[129,130] The reactivities of intrathecal and serum antibodies differ in Western blot analyses, but the relationship of these response patterns to outcome is unknown. Recovered patients develop antibodies to both structural and NS proteins and exhibit CD4+ and CD8+ T-cell proliferative responses to JE viral lysate, in favor of an antigen containing structural E and prM/M proteins only.[131] In a large clinical study, only 24% of patients developed a T-lymphocyte response to whole virus or viral E protein (structural proteins), and response was not correlated with survival.[132]

Other studies suggest an important role for immunopathology in pathogenesis of JE. Whereas intrathecal IgM or neutralizing antibodies did not correlate with outcome, antibodies to neural antigens (neurofilament and myelin basic protein) were associated with death, suggesting that neural damage resulted in a destructive autoimmune response.[72,129,133,134] CSF viral immune complex formation also was associated with mortality, further implicating the possibility of autoimmune injury.

Cell-mediated immune mechanisms have been described in athymic nude mice, which, in contrast to normal adult mice, die or develop an extended illness with secondary viremias after peripheral inoculation.[135,136] Antibodies did not appear in nude mice, indicating the functional importance of Th cells. Interestingly, although virus replicated to high titers in brain tissue, histopathologic evidence of encephalitis was absent, indicating that T cells are required in mediating pathologic changes. Mice immunosuppressed with cyclophosphamide and then immunized with live, attenuated vaccine but not inactivated vaccine, are able to resist experimental challenge. Specific JE viral immunity can be transferred passively with spleen cells from immune mice, including animals immunized with live, attenuated JE vaccine, but not from those immunized with inactivated vaccine.[126,137–138] Both Lyt2.2+ and L3T4+ cells are needed to protect adult mice against intracerebral challenge, and direct intracerebral introduction of the effector cells is required, suggesting the importance of local T-cell enhancement of antibody production in the CNS.

The role of cytokines in recovery and pathogenesis has not been investigated extensively. Complementing the limited experience with interferon, experimental prophylaxis with a combination of interferon-α and interleukin-12 protected mice challenged with related StLE virus; however, interferon had no effect after infection was established.[139-140] Nitric oxide (NO) has been shown to inhibit JE viral replication in vitro. However, in experimental TBE virus infection, NO had no effect on viral replication and exacerbated the infection.[141,142] A viral-induced macrophage-derived chemotactic factor that modulates neutrophil activity and increases capillary permeability in mice also has been described: Its action to increase blood-brain barrier permeability was implicated in increasing viral neuroinvasion.[143]

Conditions that compromise the integrity of the blood-brain barrier have been suspected to increase risk for neuroinvasion and neurodissemination. Several observations suggest that dual infection with another infectious agent, especially *Taenia solium* in neurocysticercosis, is a risk factor.[59,69,144–146] The incidental finding of cysts in a disproportionate number of JE cases at autopsy has indicated their potential contribution to a fatal outcome.[69,144,145] There is anecdotal observations of dual herpes and JE viral infections in autopsied human JE cases.[146] The mechanisms by which dual infections apparently augment the risk of symptomatic illness are unclear, but increased CNS dissemination of JE virus was shown experimentally in mice infected with both JE and herpes.[146] Other physiologic or structural conditions that compromise the integrity of the cerebrovasculature or the blood-brain barrier also may contribute to risk. Atherosclerotic and hypertensive cerebrovascular diseases are suspected risk factors for StLE, and foreign bodies (e.g., ventricular shunts) have predisposed patients to poliovirus neuroinvasion.[147] Experimental disruption of the blood-brain barrier by microwave irradiation was shown to predispose mice to JE viral neuroinvasion.[148]

The impact of human immunodeficiency virus (HIV) infection and acquired immunodeficiency syndrome on the outcome of JE has not been reported; however, in several StLE outbreaks, HIV infection appeared to increase the risk for developing overt encephalitis after infection.[149]

Diagnosis

Although a history of exposure to an endemic area and certain clinical features may suggest JE, clinical diagnosis is unreliable, and laboratory confirmation, usually by serologic tests, is necessary. JE virus occasionally can be recovered from blood in the preneuroinvasive phase (up to 3 to 7 days after onset), but patients presenting with encephalitis usually are no longer viremic.[2,29,55,150] Virus has been recovered from CSF in 68% of patients when the highly sensitive system of isolation in *Toxorhynchites splendens* mosquitoes was used.[151] Viral antigen often can be demonstrated in brain tissue when no virus can be isolated from the same specimen and when viral antibodies are undetectable. JE virus produces cytopathic effects in Vero, LLCMK$_2$, and PS cells and kills suckling mice inoculated intracerebrally. C6/36 and AP61 mosquito cell lines and *T. splendens*, inoculated intrathoracically, also are sensitive systems for viral isolation. Infection is silent in C6/36 cells, so inoculated cultures must be examined for viral antigen by immunofluorescent (IF) antibody or other techniques. Viral isolates are readily identified by IF techniques using virus-specific monoclonal antibodies or by neutralization.

The most widely used diagnostic method is IgM-capture enzyme-linked immunosorbent assay (ELISA).[57,152] Specific IgM can be detected in CSF, serum, or both in approximately 75% of patients within the first 4 days after illness onset, and nearly all patients are positive 7 days after onset. Both fluids should be tested to maximize sensitivity. Rapid membrane-based systems for bedside serologic diagnosis are in development.

In approximately 30% of cases, antigen-bearing infected cells can be identified in CSF by IF antibody before intrathecal IgM is detected, yielding a specific diagnosis within hours of a lumbar puncture. However, the procedure's sensitivity (58%) was lower than that of combined IgM-capture ELISA testing of acute serum and CSF (84%).[151] In preliminary studies, JE viral genomic sequences have been detected in CSF by polymerase chain reaction; however, detection of CSF IgM by ELISA was more sensitive.[153] Additional comparative evaluations are needed, particularly of acute-phase serum samples, which may provide a better yield than CSF.[29,57]

A specific diagnosis also can be confirmed by demonstrating fourfold or greater changes in antibody titer by conventional serologic procedures (e.g., hemagglutination inhibition, complement fixation, IF antibody, ELISA, or neutralization). Heterologous flaviviral antibodies (e.g., to dengue and West Nile viruses) are a potential source of false-positive reactions. These infections can be differentiated by epitope-blocking ELISA or by obtaining ELISA absorbance ratios to the respective antigens.[154] Synthetic antigens, including recombinant virus-like particles expressing the viral E protein, are a potential source of standardized antigen with improved specificity.[155]

Epidemiology

Endemic Areas in Asia

JE is transmitted in epidemics or in an endemic pattern, or both, in virtually every country of Asia (see Fig. 33–1; see also Table 33–20). Officially reported cases significantly underestimate the magnitude and geographic extent of risk because of under-reporting and, in some countries, widespread immunization. Transmission is seasonal, occurring approximately from May to September in temperate areas of China, Korea, Japan, and far eastern Russia. Farther south, the transmission season is somewhat longer, extending from March through October (Fig. 32–8). In tropical areas of Southeast Asia and India, seasonal transmission is particular to local patterns of monsoon rains and bird migration, with the possibility of two transmission intervals in a calendar year. The virus is transmitted throughout the year in some sites.

JE is principally a disease of rural areas in which vector mosquitoes proliferate in close association with birds and pigs, which serve as vertebrate amplifying hosts (Fig. 33–9).[1,2,29,156,157] Humans and horses may become ill after infection, but such infections contribute minimally to the transmission cycle.[158,159] Experimental observations and field studies indicate that the virus overwinters in infected adult mosquitoes.[157] Vertical infection of mosquitoes may contribute to virus survival.[156,157] Long-term persistence in tissues and blood of JEV-infected vertebrate hosts, such as bats and reptiles, has been demonstrated. Introduction of the virus by viremic migratory birds or by windblown mosquitoes also may occur.[156,160] Self-limited outbreaks on Western Pacific islands—Guam in 1947, Saipan in 1990, and the Australian Torres Strait islands in 1995 and 1998—were examples of viral introductions possibly by migratory birds or, in the last case, by windblown mosquitoes.[25,26,161,162]

Culex tritaeniorhynchus is the principal JE vector in most areas of Asia, but various other ground pool– and rice paddy–breeding species, including *C. vishnui, C. pseudovis nuri, C. gelidus, C. fuscocephala, C. bitaeniorhynchus, C. infula, C. whitmorei,* and *C. annulus,* are also important locally.[156,157] JE virus has been recovered from *C. pipiens*

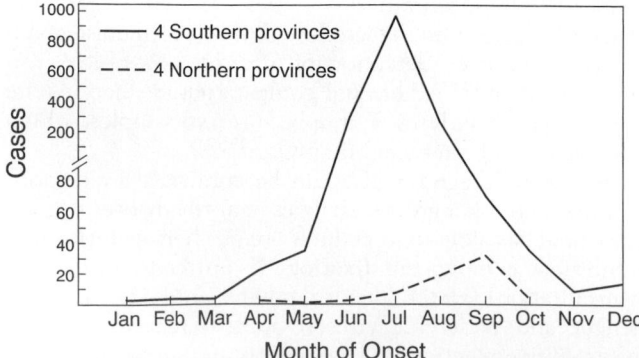

FIGURE 33–8 ■ Seasonal distribution of Japanese encephalitis cases in four southern and four northern provinces, China, 1993. (From Yu YX. Japanese encephalitis in China. Southeast Asian J Trop Med Public Health 26[suppl 3]:17–21, 1995, with permission.)

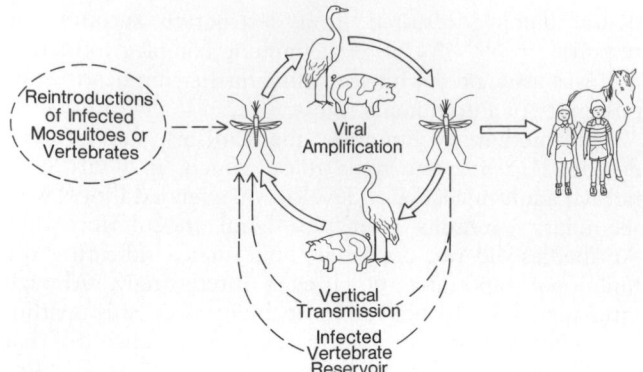

FIGURE 33–9 ■ Transmission cycle of Japanese encephalitis (JE) virus. The *open arrows* indicate known portions of the cycle, and the *dashed arrows* indicate speculative portions. Infections and clinical illnesses in humans and horses are incidental to the transmission cycle. The overwintering mechanism for JE virus is undefined, but experimental and field observations suggest a role for vertical transmission in vector mosquitoes.

pallens and *C. quinquefasciatus* in urban locations. In addition, *C. annulirostris* has been identified as a vector in the Western Pacific, *Aedes togoi* in sylvatic locations in Siberia, and members of the *Anopheles hyrcanus* group in northeastern India.[20,110] Although vector abundance and risk for human infection are associated with rainfall, with the introduction of wet rice cultivation, paddy flooding schedules have come to influence vector bionomics. Single paddies can produce more than 30,000 adult mosquitoes in a day. Collectively, these artificial breeding sites overpower the impact of natural sources. In these circumstances, mosquito abundance fluctuates with periodic rice field flooding and can peak at any time of the year, including the dry season.[163,164]

In temperate regions, vector mosquitoes emerge in May, and, after several initial rounds of viral amplification, high rates of pig seroconversion are detected. This is followed almost immediately by the onset of human cases, typically in July and August. By virtue of high levels and lengthy periods of viremia after infection and their prevalence as domestic animals, pigs are the key hosts for viral amplification. Infections in adult pigs are asymptomatic, but infection during pregnancy frequently results in abortions and stillbirths, with significant economic losses. In some locations, enzootic transmission of the virus is initiated among aquatic birds, and, in well-characterized outbreaks in which pigs were absent, such birds have served as epidemic amplifying hosts.[165] Other domesticated animals, such as cattle, dogs, sheep, cows, and chickens, and peridomestic rodents may become infected, but these fail to develop a sufficient viremia to support further viral amplification.[166] JE mosquito vectors are zoophilic; consequently, cows and certain other animals can reduce risk to humans by diverting vector mosquitoes (zooprophylaxis).[167] Immunization of pigs prevents abortion and stillbirths and also may reduce viral transmission by nullifying the role of pigs as viral amplifiers.[167-169] Experimental immunization of nearly the entire pig inventory on one island led to a significant reduction in human cases.[167]

In rural villages, all elements of the enzootic transmission cycle are found in proximity to human residences and

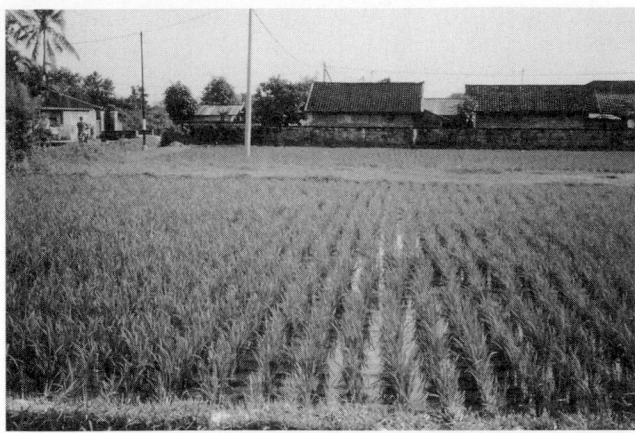

FIGURE 33-10 ■ In Indonesia, flooded rice paddies are the principal breeding sites for larval stages of Japanese encephalitis virus mosquito vectors. The disease is transmitted chiefly in rural areas, especially in those employing irrigation schemes, where vector mosquitoes and pigs, the principal vertebrate amplifying host, are abundant near human residences.

activities (Fig. 33–10). Consequently, exposure and infection occur at an early age. In areas where transmission is hyperendemic, half of all cases occur in children younger than 4 years of age, and nearly all cases are found in children younger than 10 years (Fig. 33–11). Usually cases in males exceed those in females, possibly reflecting greater outdoor exposure in boys. Typical incidence rates in those younger than 19 years range from 1 to more than 10 per 10,000 population per year. For example, in Tamil Nadu (southern India) and in the Changmai Valley (northern Thailand), rates were 6 and 4 per 10,000 population, respectively. Seroprevalence studies disclose nearly universal infection by early adulthood, and, in areas where enzootic viral transmission is particularly intense, seroprevalence rates may increase by 25% per year during childhood. By one estimate, the minimum probability of an

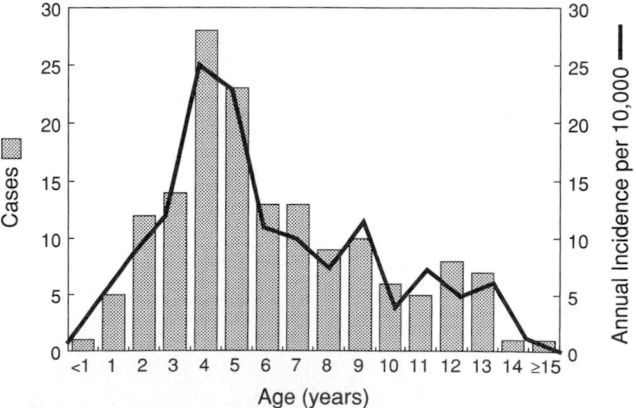

FIGURE 33-11 ■ Reported Japanese encephalitis cases and age-specific incidence, Nallur Primary Health Centre, South Arcot District, Tamil Nadu, India, 1986 to 1990. (Adapted with permission from Gajanana A, Thenmozi V, Samuel P, Reuben R. A community-based study of subclinical flavivirus infections in children in an area of Tamil Nadu, India, where Japanese encephalitis is endemic. Bull World Health Organ 73:237–244, 1995.)

infectious mosquito bite in Tamil Nadu was 0.47 to 0.77 per year.[28,170]

Behavioral and other factors associated with the risk of acquiring JE vary regionally. Household crowding, religion, ethnicity, exposure to domestic animals, and lack of air conditioning were detected as risk factors in some studies.[6,25,171] Use of permethrin-impregnated mosquito nets, but not untreated nets, is protective.[172] Although risk for acquiring JE is greatest in rural areas, conditions that permit enzootic viral transmission exist within or at the periphery of many Asian cities. For example, JE cases in Taiwan are reported principally from areas surrounding Taipei; in Vietnam, JE incidence is highest in and near Hanoi; and in India, urban outbreaks have occurred in Lucknow. Cases frequently are reported from suburban areas of major cities such as Bangkok, Beijing, and Shanghai. In a study to determine the causes of childhood encephalitis cases hospitalized in Beijing, JE was the etiology in 5% of cases, herpes virus in 2%, mumps in 7%, and enteroviruses in 15%.[173] The relative frequency of JE cases is notable because the disease is not considered to be endemic in northern China and immunization coverage in Beijing is high. Sporadic reports of cases from Hong Kong and, previously, Singapore (vide infra) attest to the possibility of enzootic viral transmission near highly developed urban areas.

In developed Asian countries (e.g., Japan and Korea), JE incidence has decreased over several decades to fewer than 5 cases annually (see Fig. 33–2). A number of factors other than immunization have contributed to the decline, including secular trends toward a higher standard of living, a reduction in land under cultivation, widespread use of agricultural pesticides, and centralized pig production. The impact of economic development and secular factors has been demonstrated most clearly in Singapore, which has no national immunization program. Although JE previously was endemic on the island, no indigenous cases have been detected since 1992, and serosurveys have shown no antibodies in children younger than 12 years of age, indicating the near-elimination of viral transmission through indirect modern urban infrastructure, mosquito control, and complete prohibition of pig rearing on the island.[174] Although imported pigs are held briefly in quarantine, their segregation from the human population probably has had a major impact on viral amplification.

In countries where childhood cases have been prevented by immunization, the age distribution of cases has shifted toward adults, and particularly to the elderly. In Japan the previous bimodal age distribution of cases, with peaks in young children and in the elderly, has shifted toward a predominance of cases in adults (Fig. 33–12).[11,175] A similar pattern holds in Korea and has emerged in developed municipalities of China. An analysis of age-specific incidence by decade in an area of Shanghai showed that, since 1961, case rates declined most dramatically in children, reflecting the impact of immunization; however, rates also declined in other age groups, reflecting a secular decrease in risk (Fig. 33–13). The result is that incidence rates are similar in both adults and children.

In Taiwan, age-specific incidence is highest in adults 20 to 39 years old, probably because this cohort is too old to have been immunized fully when mass vaccinations began in 1968 and too young to have acquired infections naturally

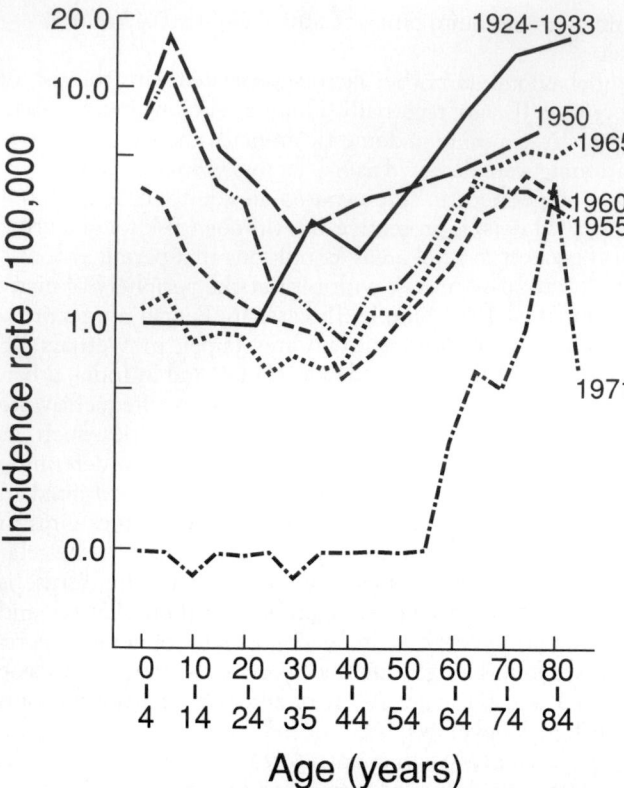

FIGURE 33–12 ■ Age-specific incidence of Japanese encephalitis in Japan, 1924 to 1971. Although Japanese encephalitis is most visible as a childhood disease, the age-specific incidence is bimodal, with elevated risk in children and the elderly. As a result of universal childhood immunization, sporadic cases now occur almost exclusively in the elderly. The causes of increased risk with advanced age are unknown. (Adapted from Oya A. Epidemiology of Japanese encephalitis, Rinsho to Biseibutsu. Clin Diagn Microbiol 16:5–9, 1989.)

in a developing society. The loss of vaccine-derived immunity can be inferred from declining JE antibody prevalence rates, from 49% in primary school to 38% in junior high school, 34% in junior college, and 29% in university students.[176] A similar trend also has been seen in Japan, where the induction and maintenance of immunity, presumably by immunization, through the first decade of life is followed by a subsequent decline, reflecting loss of vaccine-induced

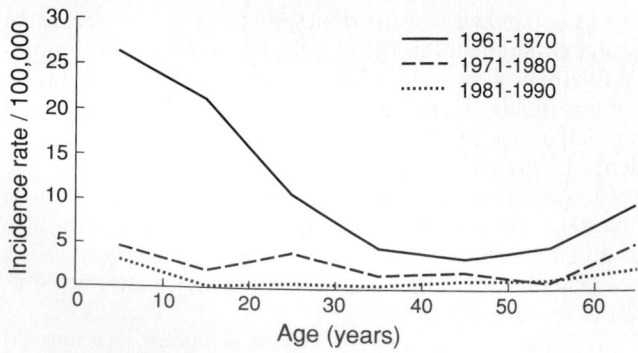

FIGURE 33–13 ■ Age-specific incidence of Japanese encephalitis, Nanshi District, Shanghai, by decade. (Data from ZY Xu, personal communication, 1997.)

antibodies (Fig. 33–14). The subsequent rise in antibody rates in people older than 35 probably represents naturally acquired immunity in cohorts born before national JE immunization was established in the 1960s.

Waning vaccine-induced immunity, age-related host factors, and reduced opportunities for natural exposure and "boosting" infections in an increasingly urban population may contribute to increased risk of acquiring JE in adults, even those who presumably had been infected naturally earlier in life.[177] The relative importance of JE in adults has yet to be addressed as a public health priority. Surveillance to measure JE incidence in adults and to detect cases of secondary vaccine failure should be undertaken to determine the need for booster doses after childhood.

Travelers and Expatriates

Although JE vaccine is used principally in Asia to protect local populations, the vaccine also is marketed in developed countries for travelers to Asia, expatriates, and especially military personnel. (For the purposes of this discussion, *expatriates* are defined as residents through a transmission season.) Sporadic cases have been reported in travelers from North America, Europe, Russia, Israel, and Australia and, paradoxically, in Japanese and Taiwanese tourists to other endemic areas of Asia.[178-182]

Data on cases in travelers have not been collected systematically. Informal surveys of diagnostic laboratories suggest that risk is low. Among 24 JE cases reported to the Centers for Disease Control and Prevention (CDC) from 1978 through 1992, 11 occurred in expatriates, 8 of whom were U.S. military personnel or their dependents. Among other reported cases in Americans, only one was in a tourist, one was in a summer student, and in one case the exposure history was unknown. U.S. Department of Transportation statistics indicate that 2 to 3 million U.S. citizens travel by air to Asia each year; however, these figures are not the population at risk; most travelers have brief itineraries without outdoor, nighttime exposure in at-risk

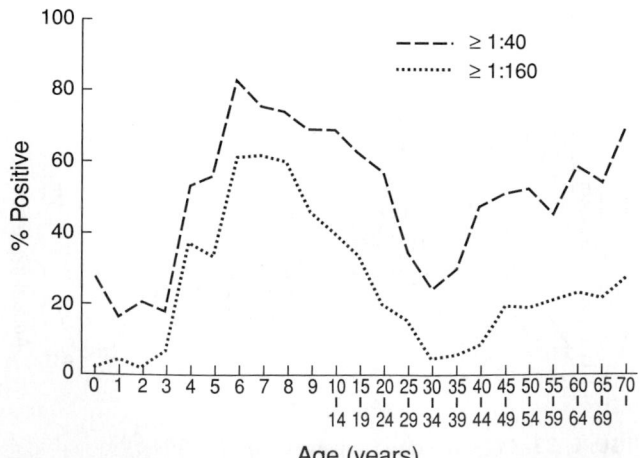

FIGURE 33–14 ■ Age-specific seroprevalence of Japanese encephalitis neutralizing antibodies, Japan, 1994; age-balanced random sample of 10 prefectures (N = 2027). (From Taniguchi K, Matsunaga Y. National epidemiologic surveillance of vaccine-preventable diseases, Japan, October 1995, with permission.)

TABLE 33–3 ■ Japanese Encephalitis in Nonimmunized American and Other Western Military Personnel, 1945 to 1991

Location	Year	No. of Cases	Approximate Population at Risk	Rate/ 10,000/W	Reference
Okinawa	1991	3	19,000	0.1*	183
Thailand	1972	9	2500	2.1†	32
Vietnam‡	1966–1967	2	2000	0.9§	184
Korea	1958	3	860	1.6§	27
Korea‖	1950	103	114,813	0.4§	188
Korea	1946	3	1500	0.9§	187
Okinawa	1945	11	77,000¶	0.05*	201

*Rate based on exposure during a 6-month transmission season.
†Rate based on exposure during 4 months.
‡Australian personnel.
§Rate based on exposure during a 5-month transmission season.
‖American and British personnel.
¶Partially immunized population.

areas. A few may have been immunized. Annual incidence in American travelers can be estimated roughly at under 1 per 1 million population.

Risk also can be extrapolated from attack rates in unimmunized American, Australian, and British soldiers exposed in Asia. Rates have ranged from 0.05 to 2.1 per 10,000 population per week in soldiers who were exposed intensely under field conditions, in some instances during epidemics (Table 33–3).[27,32,183–188] These rates are similar to those among children residing in hyperendemic areas, where annual reported incidence rates typically are in the range of 0.1 to 1 per 10,000 population. Accepting the high estimate and recognizing that transmission is limited to about a 5-month period in most areas, the monthly risk can be estimated as 1 per 50,000 population per month, or 1 per 200,000 population per week.

The risk for acquiring JE after a single mosquito bite can be appreciated by considering the following probabilities of infection and illness:

1. Only bites of vector species are potentially infectious.
2. Even in epidemic circumstances, viral infection rates in vector mosquitoes rarely exceed 3%.
3. If a nonindigenous individual is infected, symptomatic neuroinvasive illness may occur at a rate of 1 per 30 to 50 infections.[27]

Further reducing the risk of an infectious bite, *C. tritaeniorhynchus* and other JE vectors are chiefly zoophilic and prefer animal rather than human hosts. They feed chiefly in the evening and during the crepuscular (twilight) periods at dawn and dusk, and, though they may enter houses to feed, they principally are exophilic and seek hosts outdoors. Travelers can reduce risk by wearing mosquito repellant and long-sleeved shirts and trousers, by avoiding outdoor activities in the evening, and by sleeping under permethrin-impregnated mosquito nets or in screened or air-conditioned rooms.[189,190]

Risk for acquiring JE during travel is highly variable and depends on the destination and season of travel and the activities of the individual (Table 33–4). Although travelers who remain in rural areas for extended periods are at greatest risk, well-publicized cases have been reported in

travelers with brief itineraries in resorts or urban locations.[179–181] For example, in 1996, three cases were reported among travelers to Bali, perhaps a unique situation that may reflect the proximity of local tourist hotels and beaches to areas with intense enzootic viral transmission.

Immunization

Passive Immunization

JE immune plasma and immune globulin are not commercially available. Experimental data in mice, goats, and rhesus monkeys indicate a prophylactic and therapeutic potential for polyclonal antibodies or a mixture of JE monoclonal antibodies, although combined peripheral and either intraspinal or subdural administration was required for maximum effect with the latter.[63,191–193] A small controlled trial in humans suggested a potential therapeutic benefit of passive immunization with the antibody combination (see *Clinical Illness* above).[63] However, experience with prophylaxis of TBE using human TBE-specific immune globulin indicates that antibody must be administered within a short period after tick exposure to be effective and that late administration (i.e., after 4 days) may

TABLE 33–4 ■ Risk Factors for Acquiring Japanese Encephalitis During Travel to Asia

Risk factors
  Travel to developing country
  Travel during transmission season
  Travel to rural areas
  Extended period of travel or residence
  Outdoor activities, especially in twilight period and evenings
  Advanced age
  Pregnancy (risk to developing fetus)
Protective factors
  Repellents
  Protective clothing
  Residence in air-conditioned or well-screened areas
  Permethrin-treated mosquito nets

worsen outcome.[194] Although there are few data, early treatment with interferon alfa, perhaps in combination with immune plasma, may be an effective approach to prophylaxis of illness after known exposure, such as in a laboratory accident.[29,64,140] Information on availability of immune plasma can be obtained from the U.S. Army Medical Research Institute for Infectious Diseases, Frederick, MD, or the Walter Reed Army Medical Center, Silver Spring, MD.

Active Immunization

Worldwide, three JE vaccines are in widespread production and use (Table 33–5); however, only inactivated JE vaccine produced in mouse brain is distributed commercially and is available internationally.[195] Inactivated JE vaccine and live, attenuated JE vaccine, both grown in primary hamster kidney (PHK) cells, are manufactured and distributed exclusively in the People's Republic of China (PRC).[196] Despite an apparently limited pattern of domestic distribution, more than 70 million doses of inactivated PHK vaccine and 60 million doses of live, attenuated vaccine are produced and distributed annually in the PRC, whereas all manufacturers in Japan produce approximately 11 million doses of mouse brain–derived vaccine for domestic use in Japan. Biken, the principal Japanese manufacturer of inactivated mouse brain vaccine, distributes about 2 million doses abroad by arrangement through Connaught Pasteur Mérieux. The vaccine is licensed as JE-VAX in the United States, Canada, Israel, and several Asian countries, but is still distributed under special exemptions in most European countries.

Inactivated Mouse Brain–Derived Japanese Encephalitis Vaccine

Inactivated mouse brain–derived JE vaccines were produced in Russia and Japan in the 1930s, and the former was shown to be efficacious against Russian autumnal encephalitis (a synonym for JE).[197] During World War II, a simple uncentrifuged 10% suspension of infected mouse brain, inactivated with formalin, was produced in the United States as a vaccine for the military. The vaccine was variably immunogenic, but efficacy field trials could not be completed.[198–201]

A more stable inactivated chick embryo–derived vaccine, also developed by the U.S. military, had an 80% efficacy in children given a combination of mouse brain– and chick embryo–derived vaccines.[202–206] However, the latter vaccine was less immunogenic in adults, and its efficacy in soldiers never could be evaluated. Although this vaccine was given to all U.S. soldiers assigned to Asia from 1948 to 1951, use was discontinued in 1952 after review of available data failed to produce convincing evidence of immunogenicity and efficacy.[184–188]

Successive refinements of the mouse brain vaccine were introduced by research institutes in Japan, leading to the current purified vaccine (Fig. 33–15).[196,207,208] Mouse brain–derived vaccines are produced in Japan and elsewhere using a similar sequence of centrifugation, ultrafiltration, protamine sulfate precipitation, and formalin inactivation in the cold, followed by further purification by ultrafiltration, ammonium sulfate precipitation, and continuous zonal centrifugation on sucrose density gradients. National standards in Japan specify minimal immunogenicity and potency in mice (compared with a vaccine standard) and maximal total protein (80 μg/mL) and myelin basic protein (MBP) content (2 ng/mL), among other specifications. Bulk vaccine is diluted with medium 199 and phosphate buffer to meet a potency standard.[209,210] Although the quantity of JE E protein is not controlled, in one study a dose was estimated to contain approximately 50 μg. The vaccine is stabilized with gelatin and sodium glutamate and preserved with thimerosal. In Japan, the vaccine is distributed principally in liquid form; for international distribution, it is lyophilized and reconstituted with sterile water.

VACCINE STABILITY AND STORAGE

Lyophilized Biken vaccine is stable at 4°C for at least 1 year and retains more than 90% of its potency after 28 weeks at 22°C. At 37°C, lyophilized vaccine retains 95% of its original potency after 4 weeks.[208] After reconstitution, a JE vaccine made in India is stable at 22°C for at least 2 weeks, but at 37°C, potency declines to 85%.[211]

TABLE 33–5 ■ Japanese Encephalitis Vaccines

Vaccine Type	Substrate	Viral Strains	Manufacturers
Inactivated	Mouse brain	Nakayama, Beijing-1 (P1)	*India*: Central Research Institute (currently inactive) *Japan*: Biken (Research Foundation for Microbial Disease of Osaka University), Chiba, Denka-Seiken Co., Ltd., Chemo-Sero Therapeutic Research Institute, Kitasato Institute, Saikin-Kagaku Institute, Takeda *Korea*: Green Cross *Taiwan*: National Institute of Preventive Medicine, Guo-Guang *Thailand*: Government Pharmaceutical Organization *Vietnam*: National Institute of Hygiene
Inactivated	Primary hamster kidney cells	P3	*People's Republic of China*: Beijing, Shanghai, and Changchun Institutes of Biological Products
Live, attenuated	Primary hamster kidney cells	SA14-14-2	*People's Republic of China*: Chengdu, Wuhan Institutes of Biological Products

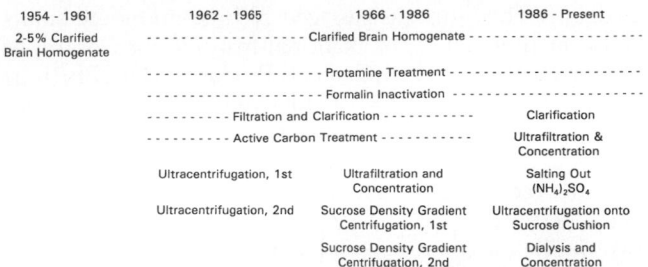

| 1954 - 1961 | 1962 - 1965 | 1966 - 1986 | 1986 - Present |

FIGURE 33–15 ■ Evolution of purification procedure for inactivated Japanese encephalitis vaccine derived from infected mouse brain. (Adapted from Oya A. Japanese encephalitis vaccine. *In* Fukumi H [ed]. Vaccination Theory and Practice. Tokyo, International Medical Foundation of Japan, 1975, pp 69–82; and Oya A. Japanese encephalitis vaccine. Acta Pediatr Jpn 30:175–184, 1988.)

A field study in Thailand showed that seroconversion rates were higher after immunization with lyophilized vaccine than after immunization with liquid vaccine. A moderate loss of potency was demonstrated after liquid vaccine was exposed to simulated field conditions.[212]

VIRAL STRAINS

The Nakayama strain of JE virus, isolated from the CSF of a patient in 1935 and maintained by continuous mouse brain passage, has been the principal strain used in mouse brain–derived vaccines produced throughout Asia.[195] The strain was chosen because of good propagation characteristics and because it provided cross-protection against other JE viral strains in mice. Cross-immunization studies in mice with strains from diverse areas of Asia indicated that strains of the JaGAr01/Beijing type (e.g., Beijing-1, known as P1 in China, and the equivalent P3 strain; see later discussion) confer a broader neutralizing antibody response against various JE viral isolates than does the Nakayama strain (Fig. 33–16).[213–217] The Beijing-1 strain grows to higher titer and

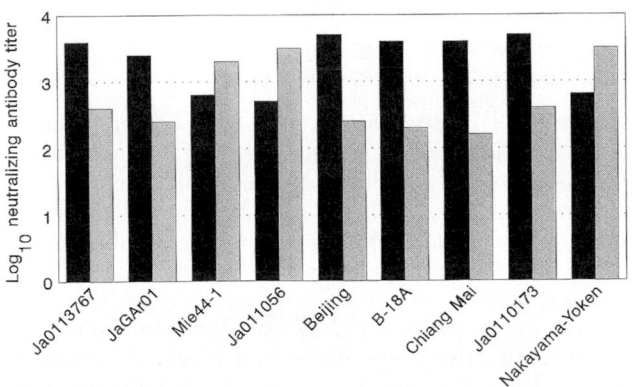

FIGURE 33–16 ■ Neutralizing antibody response to various Japanese encephalitis (JE) viral strains in mice immunized with inactivated Nakayama or Beijing strains of JE vaccines. The latter conferred a broader heterologous response in immunized mice, but evidence of better protective efficacy in humans is lacking. (Adapted from Japanese encephalitis vaccine lyophilized, "Biken." Unpublished report, Research Foundation for Microbial Diseases of Osaka University, Osaka, Japan, 1991, pp 1–149.)

the vaccine produces higher heterologous antibody titers in immunized mice than does the Nakayama strain vaccine. Although vaccine produced from either strain meets standardized mouse protection tests for potency, the Beijing-1 vaccine is formulated in half the volume. Biken, the principal Japanese manufacturer of JE vaccine, has used the Beijing-1 strain since 1989 in vaccine produced for domestic consumption, whereas the Nakayama strain is used in vaccines distributed internationally.

A natural diversity of JE viral strains has been demonstrated in minor antigenic differences and in biologic characteristics such as growth in cell culture and neuroinvasiveness in experimentally infected mice. However, there is no evidence of corresponding differences in human pathogenicity and no evidence that immunity to one strain would not protect against disease caused by another.[113,218,219]

DOSAGE AND ROUTE OF ADMINISTRATION

In most areas of Asia, vaccine produced from the Nakayama strain is given subcutaneously in two 0.5-mL doses 1 to 4 weeks apart (1.0 mL for people >3 years of age) usually beginning at the age of 12 to 36 months, with a booster dose at 1 year and additional booster doses thereafter at 1- to 3-year intervals.[195] In practice, immunization schedules are quite variable. The Biken package insert recommends an interval of 1 to 2 weeks for primary immunization; however, many immunogenicity studies have used a 4-week interval. Primary vaccination is recommended at 18 months of age in Thailand, at 15 to 27 months of age in Taiwan, at 3 years of age in Korea, and at 6 to 90 months of age (usually 36 months) in Japan. With no evidence from efficacy studies, boosters are recommended to be given 1 year later and, in Taiwan, once again at school entry; in Korea, booster doses were given annually until 15 years of age, but now a revised schedule of triennial boosters is recommended. Boosters are given at 4 years, 9 to 12 years, and 14 to 15 years of age in Japan. Beijing-1 strain–derived vaccine is formulated with a higher antigen concentration, and the recommended dose is 0.5 mL (0.25 mL for children under 3 years of age).[217,220]

The primary series has been administered to infants (with diphtheria and tetanus toxoids and pertussis [DTP] vaccine) as early as 2 months of age in clinical trials, but, because JE rarely occurs in infants younger than 1 year, there is no need to begin immunization at that age other than to save administration costs.[221]

Immunogenicity studies in subjects from areas without endemic transmission (western countries and areas of India) indicate that three doses are necessary for an adequate antibody response (see later discussion).[182,222–224] The CDC's Advisory Committee on Immunization Practices recommends three doses, on days 0, 7, and 30 (Table 33–6).[225] An abbreviated schedule in which doses are administered on days 0, 7, and 14 also results in uniform seroconversion; however, neutralizing antibody titers are significantly lower. Although approximately 80% of vaccinees respond after two doses, this schedule is not recommended.[182] Recommendations for booster doses are based on limited data. Neutralizing antibody titers were maintained for 3 years in 37 of 39 U.S. Army vaccinees given the Biken vaccine; however, field studies indicate greater variability in antibody persistence.[222] Until further data become available, a booster dose is recommended 2 years after the

TABLE 33–6 ▪ Recommended Immunization Schedule for Inactivated Japanese Encephalitis Vaccine

Vaccines	Primary*	Booster*
Adults and children ≥3 yr	1.0 mL given on days 0, 7, and 30†	1.0 mL given at 2 yr of age and thereafter at intervals of 3 yr or as determined by serologic testing
Children >6 mo and <3 yr	0.5 mL in schedule as above	0.5 mL in schedule as above

*All doses given subcutaneously.
†An abbreviated schedule of immunization on days 0, 7, and 14 should be used only when the recommended schedule cannot be followed.

primary series and thereafter as determined by serologic monitoring.[225]

In a study of infants 15 months of age, simultaneous administration of inactivated JE vaccine with measles, mumps, and rubella vaccine did not result in reduced immunogenicity or increased side effects.[226] Under Thailand's Expanded Program of Immunization, JE vaccine is given concurrently with the fourth dose of DTP and oral poliovirus vaccine at 18 months.[221] A comparison of administration routes in adults showed that a 0.1-mL intradermal dose may be as immunogenic as the standard administration of 1.0 mL subcutaneously, at least when given as a booster.[227] It is unknown whether malaria prophylaxis with chloroquine or mefloquine adversely affects the immune response to JE vaccine in a way similar to the effect on inactivated rabies and live oral cholera vaccines.

Inactivated Primary Hamster Kidney Cell–Derived Japanese Encephalitis Vaccine

Inactivated JE vaccine prepared from the P3 strain in PHK cells is produced exclusively in the PRC and has been that country's principal JE vaccine since 1968.[196] Approximately 70 million doses are distributed annually, making this the most widely used JE vaccine worldwide. The PRC previously had relied on a succession of inactivated mouse brain– and whole chick embryo–derived vaccines, as described earlier. Attempts to produce a cell culture–derived JE vaccine were motivated by concerns about potential contaminating neural antigens and allergic reactions associated with the crude vaccines, and also by the desire to improve immunogenicity and ease of production. Among the numerous primary and continuous cell culture systems that were examined, PHK cells were discovered to produce the highest infectious yield.[228]

Vaccine is prepared in primary cell cultures derived from kidneys of golden Syrian hamsters. Monolayers are washed of growth medium and infected with JE virus. One day later, infected monolayers are washed and refed. The supernatant cell culture fluid is inactivated with 0.05% formalin, stabilized with 0.1% human albumin, and tested for residual infectivity and potency. Liquid vaccine retains potency for more than 2 years at 4°C to 8°C.

VIRAL STRAIN

The P3 strain of JE virus was recovered in 1949 from the brain of a human patient during the P1 (Beijing-1) strain

epidemic. The virus was passaged 70 times in mouse brains and is maintained at the National Institute for Control of Pharmaceutical and Biological Products (NICPBP) in Beijing. Inactivated PHK cell–derived vaccine made from the P3 strain is more immunogenic, produces a better heterologous antibody response (to Nakayama virus), and confers greater cross-protection in mice than the mouse brain–derived Nakayama strain vaccine manufactured by Biken. The inclusion of both P3 and Nakayama strains in a bivalent inactivated PHK cell culture vaccine was synergistic in mouse protection tests.[196] This experimental formulation has not been evaluated in humans.

DOSAGE AND ROUTE OF ADMINISTRATION

JE vaccine is given seasonally in early spring without concurrent administration of other vaccines. Vaccination schedules vary locally. In the officially recommended schedule, the vaccine is administered subcutaneously in two 0.5-mL doses, 1 week apart, to children 12 months of age. Three booster doses are given 1 year later (0.5 mL) and at 6 years of age and again at 10 years of age (1.0 mL). In some provinces, boosters are given annually until age 10. In Hunan province, where JE cases were occurring at a young age, primary immunization with two doses was begun at 6 months, with four subsequent boosters—the so-called 6-6 schedule.

Because vaccine is given only during annual spring campaigns rather than at a specific chronologic age in childhood, children who miss the annual opportunity for vaccination remain unprotected through the transmission season.

In one study, concurrent administration with bacille Calmette-Guérin (BCG), measles, or DTP vaccine at 6 to 10 months of age was not associated with increased adverse events and, compared with JE vaccine administered alone, led to higher JE ELISA antibodies in the first two groups and to no change in the last. Concurrent JE vaccine administration did not lead to significant changes in responses to measles or DTP antibody titers or in the size of BCG reactions.[229]

ENHANCED INACTIVATED JAPANESE ENCEPHALITIS VACCINE PRODUCED IN PRIMARY HAMSTER KIDNEY CELLS

Experimental inactivated vaccines with higher potencies were formulated by concentrating the standard inactivated PHK cell–derived vaccine through an ultrafilter (10-fold concentrated vaccine), followed by ultracentrifugation (purified virion vaccine). In a field trial, one subcutaneous 1.0-mL dose of enhanced-potency vaccine produced uniform seroconversion to homologous P3 antigen and levels of heterologous antibody to Nakayama virus similar to those obtained with two doses of standard vaccine.[196] Efforts to develop these vaccines further have been discontinued, because of the complexity and expense of the purification procedures.

Live, Attenuated Japanese Encephalitis Vaccine

Attenuated JE viral strains have been sought by passaging wild strains serially in various cell culture systems, including PHK, chick embryo, and embryo mouse skin cells.[230–233] Loss of neurovirulence in mice, hamsters, or pigs, or any combination of the three, initially suggested the possibility of safe use in humans. Attenuation may be correlated with decreased binding to mouse brain cell receptors.[234] Typical of many laboratory-attenuated viruses, OCT-541, a temperature-dependent strain obtained by serial PHK cell passage, was overattenuated, with a loss of infectivity in horses and in humans. Workers at the NICPBP in Beijing pursued attenuation of JE virus in PHK cells and derived strain SA14-14-2, which proved to be safe and immunogenic in animals and humans (see Table 33–5).[235–239] The vaccine's efficacy was demonstrated in field trials and the vaccine was licensed in the PRC in 1988. Currently, 60 million doses are distributed annually in southwestern and western China.

Several hundred ampules of seed virus, prepared from the sixth passage level of SA14-14-2 virus, are maintained at the NICPBP in Beijing. Lyophilized seed virus (PHK5) is provided to the production institute, where it is passaged once for the production seed (PHK6). PHK cells are obtained from 10- to 12-day-old golden Syrian hamsters maintained in colonies at the Chengdu and Wuhan Production Institutes. Monolayers are inoculated with diluted virus, and cells are fed with minimal essential medium containing human albumin, gentamicin, and kanamycin. Infected cell culture fluid with an infectious titer of approximately $10^{7.2}$ plaque-forming units (PFU)/mL is harvested at 78 to 96 hours and coarsely filtered, and the resulting liquid vaccine is lyophilized. Gelatin (1%) and sucrose (5%) are added as stabilizers. Lyophilized vaccine is reconstituted and diluted with sterile water for injection.[240]

Vaccine must meet standards for absence of neurovirulence in adult mice, stability for reversion to neurovirulence after intracerebral passage in suckling mice, and freedom from adventitious agents, including retroviruses. A highly sensitive product-enhanced reverse transcriptase (PERT) assay could not detect any reverse transcriptase activity in finished or bulk vaccine. A co-cultivation assay on production cell culture using human cell lines followed by PERT assay that allowed an expanded opportunity of detecting cross-species infection of retroviruses into human cells did not show any reverse transcriptase activity in PHK cells. The finished vaccine must have an infectious titer exceeding $10^{5.7}$ PFU/mL.

VACCINE STABILITY AND STORAGE

The infectious titer of lyophilized vaccine is not appreciably changed after storage at 37°C for 7 to 10 days, at room temperature for 4 months, or at 2°C to 8°C for at least 1.5 years. After reconstitution with sterile saline or distilled water and storage at 23°C, the vaccine's infectious titer is stable for 2 to 4 hours or 2 hours, respectively.[240]

VIRAL STRAIN

The vaccine parent strain, SA14, was isolated in 1954 from *C. pipiens* larvae collected in Xian (Table 33–7). After isolation and 11 serial passages in weanling mice, the virus was attenuated through 100 passages in PHK cells at 36°C to 37°C. Neurovirulence in monkeys had been lost at this passage level. Further plaque selection and cloning in chick embryo cells and subpassages in mice and hamsters by peripheral and oral infection were performed resulting in a stable non-neurovirulent virus. The resulting SA14-5-3 and SA14-14-2 strains no longer reverted to an established criterion of neurovirulence after intracerebral passage in suckling mice while remaining potent in mouse immunization-challenge studies.[235–239,241–246]

SA14-5-3 virus did not kill 3-week-old mice by either subcutaneous or direct intracerebral inoculation. Direct intrathalamic and intraspinal inoculation of the virus in monkeys resulted in no mortality or morbidity and a minimal degree of CNS inflammation, limited to areas around the injection sites. Histopathologic changes were characterized by perivascular lymphocytic cuffs and focal mononuclear cell infiltration, with rare direct neuronal degeneration or necrosis.

SA14-5-3 vaccine was shown to be safe in humans, and field trials in endemic areas disclosed seroconversion rates greater than 85%. However, rates of only 61% were obtained in subjects from nonendemic areas.[235] Expanded field trials in southern China involving more than 200,000 immunized children confirmed the vaccine's safety and yielded efficacies ranging from 88% to 96% over 5 years (Table 33–8).[247] However, the vaccine's poor immunogenicity in flavivirus-naive subjects from nonendemic areas suggested that SA14-5-3 virus, like previous live JE virus candidate vaccines, had been overattenuated and did not replicate uniformly in humans. To increase immunogenicity, SA14-5-3 virus was serially passaged five times by subcutaneous inoculation of suckling mice, using skin, subcutaneous tissue, and local peripheral lymph nodes as the passage material.[236] After plaque selection and cloning twice in PHK cells, the SA14-14-2 strain was obtained. SA14-14-2 virus was equally attenuated but more immunogenic in mice, pigs, and humans, producing seroconversion rates greater than 90% in nonimmune subjects.[238,239]

TABLE 33–7 ▪ Passage History of Japanese Encephalitis SA14-14-2 Virus

• SA 14 virus isolated from pool of *Culex pipiens* larvae	Parent
• One hundred serial passages in primary hamster kidney (PHK) cells; three plaque purifications in CE cells	Clone 12-1-7
• Two × plaque purification in CE cells	Clone 17-4
• One mouse IP passage; spleen harvested for CE cell plaque passage	Clone 2
• Three × plaque purification in CE cells	Clone 9
• One mouse SC passage; skin harvested for one CE cell plaque passage	Clone 9-7
• Six hamster PO passages; spleens harvested for 2 × plaque purification in PHK cells	Clone 5-3
• Five suckling mouse SC passages (using skin and peripheral lymph node inocula); 2 × PHK cell plaque purifications	Clone 14-2

IP, intraperitoneal; PO, per os; SC, subcutaneous.

TABLE 33–8 ■ Efficacy of SA14-5-3 Attenuated Japanese Encephalitis Vaccine, Guangtong, People's Republic of China

Year	Vaccinated		Unvaccinated		Efficacy (95% CI) (%)
	Total	JE Cases	Total	JE Cases	
1973	205,359	58	26,180	63	88 (85–92)
1974	205,301	12	26,117	22	93 (90–97)
1975	205,289	8	26,095	7	85 (70–95)
1976	205,281	7	26,088	13	93 (88–97)
1977	205,274	3	26,075	9	96 (92–99)

CI, confidence interval; JE, Japanese encephalitis.
Data from Regional Antiepidemic Station, Hueyang, Guangtong. Preliminary observations on epidemiological effectiveness of JE live vaccine. Bull Biol Prod 7:111–114, 1978.

The reduced neurovirulence of the SA14-14-2 strain was confirmed in 3-week-old mice and monkeys (Table 33–9). Compared with the parent SA14 strain, which killed weanling mice by subcutaneous or intracerebral inoculation with median lethal doses (LD_{50}) in the range of $10^{5.5}$ to $10^{8.3}$ LD_{50}/mL, respectively, SA14-14-2 virus produced no mortality and only minor clinical signs in a few intracerebrally inoculated animals. Combined intrathalamic and intraspinal inoculation of rhesus monkeys produced no clinical illness and only minor inflammatory reactions in the substantia nigra and cervical spinal cord. Mice were more sensitive than monkeys to intracerebral infection, with some animals showing mild neuronal lesions in the cerebral cortex, hippocampus, or basal ganglia.[248] Compared with histopathologic lesions produced by the parent SA14 virus, the inflammatory reaction to SA14-14-2 virus was greater and neuronal necrosis was significantly less. In 5-week-old mice inoculated intracerebrally with the virus pair, ultrastructural studies showed that the parent virus produced cytopathologic changes in the majority of neurons, particularly in the rough ER and Golgi apparatus of the neuronal secretory system, while it could not be confirmed that the vaccine strain replicated at all and neurons appeared normal.[244]

Further evidence of the strain's reduced neurotropism comes from experimental studies in athymic nude mice. No deaths or histopathologic abnormalities were observed after intraperitoneal or subcutaneous inoculation of a viral dose greater than 10^7 median tissue culture infective doses ($TCID_{50}$), and virus could not be recovered from brain tissue.[137] Although cyclophosphamide increases susceptibility of mice (and also of monkeys, as discussed earlier) to virulent JE virus, immunosuppression with cyclophosphamide did not lead to encephalitis in mice inoculated peripherally with SA14-14-2 virus.[138,139] The strain also did not kill intracerebrally inoculated weanling hamsters. Phenotypic characteristics of the vaccine strain (PHK_8), such as small plaque size, reduced mouse neurovirulence, and genetic properties, were stable through at least 10 additional PHK cell culture passages.[245]

Compared with two doses of inactivated P3 vaccine, a single dose of live vaccine is more immunogenic and potent in protecting mice and guinea pigs against challenge, as measured by survival after intraperitoneal inoculation and

TABLE 33–9 ■ Comparative Neurovirulence of Attenuated SA14-14-2 and Parent SA14 Japanese Encephalitis Viruses in 3-Week-Old Mice and Adult Rhesus Monkeys

Virus Strain (Virus Titer, PFU/mL)	Inoculation Route	Mice			Rhesus Monkeys	
		Dilution	Died/Tested	Histopathologic Score (Neuronal Lesions)*	Died/Tested	Histopathologic Score (Neuronal Lesions)*†
SA14 parent (6.15×10^8)	IC	10^{-1}	ND	ND	2/2	2–4
		10^{-4}	8/8	2–4	0/1	2–3
		10^{-5}	ND	ND	2/2	2–4
		10^{-6}	8/8	2–3	2/2	2–4
		10^{-7}	8/8	2–4	2/2	2–4
		10^{-8}	8/8	2–4	ND	ND
	SC	10^{-1}	30/30	2–4 (day 5)	ND	ND
SA14-14-2 (8×10^6)	IC	1:5	0/30³	0–2	0/4	0–1
	SC	1:5	0/30‡	0(1)§	ND	ND

*0 = No lesion; 1 = ≤5%, 2 = 6% to 20%, 3 = 21% to 50%, and 4 = > 50% of neurons died.
†Inoculation in thalami bilaterally (each 0.5 mL) and lumbar spinal cord (0.2 mL).
‡No clinical illness in mice inoculated subcutaneously; only a few minor clinical signs in intracerebrally inoculated mice.
§One mouse showed a few dead nerve cells.
IC, intracerebral; ND, no data; SC, subcutaneous.
Data from Ling JP, Zhu YG, Du GZ, et al. Comparative susceptibilities of rhesus monkeys and mice to Japanese encephalitis virus. Unpublished report, Institute for Control of Pharmaceutical and Biological Products, Beijing, China, 1996.

suppression of viremia, respectively. Six months after immunization, when neutralizing antibody titers declined to low levels (1:5), mice receiving attenuated vaccine were protected at higher rates (100%) than mice receiving inactivated vaccine (33%). Adoptive immunity, obtained by transfer of immune spleen cells from immunized mice (50% protection vs. 10%), and passive protection from immune serum (80% vs. 33%) were better in mice immunized with live vaccine.[249] Induction of cellular immunity also was shown by higher levels of protection in cyclophosphamide-suppressed immunized mice (see earlier discussion). Attenuated vaccine provided more effective protection than inactivated P3 vaccine against a spectrum of JE strains isolated in China.[241]

Attenuation of SA14-14-2 virus was produced empirically by serial cell culture passage, and the underlying molecular basis of its neuroattenuation still is under active investigation. The nucleotide sequence of the neurovirulent parent SA14 virus differs from that of SA14-14-2 and two other attenuated SA14-2–derived vaccine viruses in only seven amino acid substitutions found in all three attenuated strains. Four were in the envelope protein (E138, E176, E315, and E439), one was in NS protein 2B (NS2B63), one was in NS3 (NS3105), and one was in NS4B (NS4B106).[250–252] Studies of other attenuated JE viral strains have shown the spectrum of mutations associated with phenotypical attenuation. ML-17, a pig vaccine strain derived by serial passage in primary monkey kidney cells, contains six amino acid changes in the protein coding region and one nucleotide change within the 3′ noncoding region (nt-10512) (GJ Chang, unpublished results, 1997). An amino acid change at E-138, also present in SA14-14-2 virus, was shown to be sufficient for mouse neuroattenuation when introduced into a JE complementary DNA (cDNA) infectious clone. The other five changes are unique in ML-17 virus: E-146, NS3-192, NS4A-72, NS4B-274, and NS4B-315. Only six passages of virulent Nakayama and 826309 viruses in HeLa cells (HeLa p6) resulted in significantly reduced neuroinvasiveness and neurovirulence for mice and altered receptor-binding activity.[96] Nucleotide sequences of their structural protein genes revealed that the viruses differed by eight and nine amino acid mutations, respectively. Attenuated viruses also have been obtained by selecting neutralization escape variants. Attenuation was associated with single base changes resulting in single E protein amino acid changes and was linked with altered early virus–cell interactions but not with replication.[253,254] Manipulations of infectious cDNA will be essential to analyze the contribution of individual mutations in JE viral neuroattenuation.

SA14-14-2 virus also is propagated in BHK-21 cells as a swine vaccine that has been shown to protect against JE virus–associated abortions. SA14-14-2 and the 2-8 strain, obtained from further attenuation of the 12-1-7 strain (see Table 33–7), also are manufactured into effective equine vaccines distributed in China.[255,256] Other attenuated viruses, such as the "m" and ML-17 strains, are used in swine vaccines in Japan and other Asian countries.

Inferences from several studies indicate a negligible potential for mosquito transmission of attenuated JE viruses from a vaccinated pig or human; however, more definitive experiments are needed. 255 SA14-14-2 virus can be isolated from blood of vaccinees, but it is present at infectious titers below the usual oral infection threshold of mosquitoes. Attenuated JE 2-8 virus, which has a pedigree similar to that of SA14-14-2 virus, replicates in intrathoracically inoculated *C. tritaeniorhyncus* mosquitoes; however, infected mosquitoes failed to transmit the virus, and infection rates after oral feeding were low. The virus did not revert to a neurovirulent phenotype after mosquito passage.[255] Transmission experiments with the SA14-14-2 strain itself are needed.

DOSAGE AND ROUTE OF ADMINISTRATION

In China, the vaccine is licensed for 0.5-mL dose to be administered subcutaneously to children at 1 year of age and again at 2 years. In some areas, a booster dose is given at 6 years. No other vaccines are given concurrently. Like the inactivated PHK cell–derived vaccine, SA14-14-2 vaccine is distributed in annual spring campaigns rather than according to an age-based schedule. There are no data on combined administration with other vaccines.

A more conventional administration schedule in which the two primary doses were given at intervals of 1 or 2.5 months was shown to produce immunity in 94% to 100% of immunized school-age children.[257] If similar results can be shown in infants, it may be possible to administer the vaccine with other immunogens, such as measles, according to an age-based immunization schedule.

Experimental Vaccines

Several candidate JE vaccines are in various stages of clinical and preclinical development or research.[258,259] Recombinant vaccine candidates engineered by inserting four JE viral genes—prM, E, NS1, and NS2a—into vaccinia (NYVAC) or canarypox (ALVAC) viruses have been extensively evaluated. Both recombinants expressed the encoded JE structural and NS gene products and stimulated JE protective antibodies in mice; two doses of the former also protected rhesus monkeys against lethal viral challenge. In a Phase I human trial, the vaccines were somewhat more reactogenic than mouse brain vaccine but were otherwise safe. Two doses of the NYVAC-JE recombinant were nearly as immunogenic as three doses of inactivated mouse brain JE vaccine, but only in vaccinia-naive volunteers. JE neutralizing antibodies were elicited in all five non–vaccinia-immune recipients but in none of five vaccinia-immune volunteers. Antibody responses were observed in only 1 of 10 ALVAC-JE vaccinees.[260] Although the NYVAC-JE recombinant virus proved safe and potent in vaccinia-nonimmune subjects, the apparent failure to replicate in vaccinia-immune subjects places some limits on utility.

Several groups have produced experimental inactivated whole-virion vaccines from infected Vero cell cultures. Cell culture medium with high viral infectious titers, harvested continuously from microcarrier cultures, inactivated with formalin, and further concentrated, has yielded candidate vaccine meeting mouse protection potency standards established for the inactivated mouse brain vaccine. Phase I clinical trials are scheduled in the near term. Inactivated vaccines produced by similar means for polio and rabies have been safe, highly immunogenic, and compatible with

DTP vaccines given to infants. A similarly potent inactivated JE vaccine that could be given in a conventional immunization schedule would lower administration costs and improve JE vaccine coverage in the region.[259]

The potential for adventitious agents in the PHK cell substrate of attenuated SA14-14-2 vaccine has stimulated attempts to adapt the virus to more conventional cell systems. The strain was adapted to primary dog kidney (PDK) cells and, after passing monkey neurovirulence and other safety tests, was produced under Good Manufacturing Practices conditions in its ninth PDK cell passage by the Walter Reed Army Institute of Research as a candidate vaccine.[246] The Investigational New Drug vaccine, containing an infectious titer of more than $10^{5.5}$ PFU/mL, was given safely to adults and children in Phase I human trials, but neutralizing antibody responses to a single dose were detected in only 2 of 4 and 14 of 45 vaccinees (31%), respectively, with geometric mean antibody titers (GMTs) ranging from 7 to 40 (YX Yu, personal communication, 1997). In view of the apparently low antibody responses, the PDK-passaged strain was considered overattenuated, and development was discontinued. Subsequently the virus was adapted to Vero cells, and its potential either as a live virus or inactivated whole-virion vaccine is currently under investigation.[261]

Neuroattenuated JE virus was produced by introducing defined nucleotide substitutions into the E gene. Virions and virion subunits derived from cDNA protected mice from death following challenge.[262,263] JE viral subunit proteins produced in various expression systems, including *Spondoptera frugiperda*, *Escherichia coli*, *Saccharomyces cerevisiae*, and *Drosophila* Schneider 2 cells, have had variable success in eliciting mouse immunogenicity and protective potency, depending on the expressed epitopes and their conformation.[263-266] The identification of peptides mimicking the conformation of viral epitopes may be expedited by screening pentapeptide libraries against monoclonal antibodies with previously defined specificity.[267] A vaccinia-JE virus recombinant that releases extracellular particles (EPs) composed of JE, prM, and E proteins resulted in an apparently more authentic configuration than when presented as simple peptides.[268] When given without adjuvant, EPs induced long-lasting antibody and memory T cells in immunized mice. Immunogenic subviral particles containing JE E protein also have been produced in other systems, including an alphaviral recombinant virus.[269,270] Novel delivery systems and adjuvants have been explored as a means to improve immunogenicity, to direct the Th1 or Th2 response, or to improve the convenience of immunization (e.g., the inactivated mouse brain vaccine has been microencapsulated in glycolide and lactide polymer microspheres designed to degrade at specific intervals).[271]

Another approach being explored is the intramuscular or intracutaneous injection of naked DNA plasmids encoding viral prM and E genes under the control of a cytomegalovirus immediate early promotor. Using JE plasmids, immunized mice were protected against challenge with wild-type viruses.[272-275]

By far the most promising genetic approach has been the construction of flavivirus chimeras in which the YF 17D genome contributes NS genes and SA14-14-2 contributes prM and E genes. The resultant infectious clone has the neurovirulence properties of SA14-14-2, but Vero cell growth characteristics of 17D.[276,277] The YF/JE chimera has proved to be highly immunogenic in rhesus monkeys and protects against intracerebral and intranasal challenge using a wild virus strain.[278,279] The chimera cannot be transmitted by mosquito vectors of JE or YF viruses.[280] Importantly, when inoculated into six susceptible and six YF-immune human volunteers, both high- and low-dose formulations raised high levels of JE neutralizing antibodies without significant adverse effects.[281]

Results of Vaccination

Protective Effects of Immunization

Inactivated Mouse Brain–Derived Japanese Encephalitis Vaccine

A neutralizing antibody titer of more than 1:10 generally is accepted as evidence of protection and postvaccination seroconversion. Passively immunized mice that acquire this level of neutralizing antibody are protected against challenge from 10^5 LD_{50} of JE virus, a typical dose transmitted by an infectious mosquito bite. Indirect observations from human trials have associated efficacy with this criterion.[175] Although individual laboratories employ test procedures of varying sensitivity to measure neutralizing antibody, results are surprisingly robust. Plaque reduction neutralization tests are used most frequently, and procedural differences, such as choice of challenge virus strain, cell systems, addition of exogenous complement, and choice of endpoints (ranging from 50% to 90% plaque reduction in serum dilution tests), affect test sensitivity. Some laboratories still employ $\log_{10}$ neutralization indices (LNIs) in tests using a single serum dilution. However, despite procedural differences, neutralizing antibody titers in three laboratories (the U.S. CDC, Japan's National Institutes of Health, and the Yale Arbovirus Research Unit) were shown to be highly correlated (R. DeFraites, unpublished observations, 1998). No international standard for protective antibody units has been established.

IMMUNOGENICITY

Among Asian children immunized with two doses of Nakayama strain– or Beijing-1 strain–derived vaccines, neutralizing antibody responses to the respective homologous vaccine strains are in the range of 94% to 99%;[258,259,282-284] responses to strains representing a heterologous antigenic group are lower (results of selected studies are shown in Table 33–10). The proportion of vaccinees retaining detectable neutralizing antibodies and their GMTs declined rapidly in the year after the primary two-dose series, so that only 78% to 89% of Nakayama vaccine recipients and 88% to 100% of Beijing-1 vaccine recipients still had detectable levels before the scheduled 1-year booster. Antibody persistence was greater among Beijing-1 vaccine recipients. After booster immunization (third vaccine dose), antibody response rates were uniformly high (100%).

Immunogenicity studies in Asian subjects should be interpreted in light of the immunologic background of vaccinees. Although some studies have been carried out in nonendemic areas and in subjects without JE viral antibod-

TABLE 33–10 ■ Homologous and Heterologous Neutralizing Antibody Responses in Children Immunized with Inactivated Nakayama or Beijing Strain Japanese Encephalitis Vaccines

Vaccine Strain	Challenge Virus in Neutralizing Antibody Determination	After Second Dose		1 Yr After Primary Series		After Third Dose (1-yr Booster)	
		No.	% Response (GMT)	No.	% Response (GMT)	No.	% Response (GMT)
Nakayama	Nakayama*	186	99	123	89§	107	100
	Nakayama†	93	94§ (120)	40	78 (35)	40	100 (562)
	Beijing†	93	74§ (43)	40	35 (26)	40	95 (190)
	Nakayama‡	329	97 (63)	311	79 (20)	—	
Beijing	Beijing*	196	99	141	100§	114	100
	Nakayama†	93	82‖ (42)	40	52§ (34)	40	100 (501)
	Beijing†	93	94‖ (79)	40	88§ (66)	40	100 (2754)
	Nakayama‡	59	80‖ (20)	58	55§ (13)	—	
	Beijing‡	54	94‖ (79)	51	92§ (63)	—	

*Data from Konishi E, Kurane I, Mason PW, et al. Induction of Japanese encephalitis virus–specific cytotoxic T lymphocytes in humans by poxvirus-based JE vaccine candidates. Vaccine 16:842–849, 1998.

†Data from Fu DW, Zhand PF. Establishment and characterization of Japanese B encephalitis virus persistent infection in the Sf9 cell line. Biologicals 24:225–233, 1996.

‡Data from Chambers TJ, Tsai TF, Pervikov Y, Monath TP. Vaccine development against dengue and Japanese encephalitis: report of a World Health Organization meeting. Vaccine 15:1494–1502, 1997.

§$P < 0.001$.

‖$P < 0.03$.

GMT, geometric mean antibody titer.

ies, in other studies, undetected exposures to JE, dengue, and other flaviviruses prevalent in Asia may have resulted in an augmented antibody response after immunization and apparently better immune responses. Where the influence of previous flaviviral infections was unlikely, vaccinees receiving two doses produced lower seroconversion rates and lower GMTs (Table 33–11 and Fig. 33–17A).[18,182,222–224] Moreover, as rapidly as 6 to 12 months after primary immunization with two doses, neutralizing antibody titers declined below 1:8 in 90% of vaccinees (Fig. 33–17B).[182] A three-dose primary schedule was more immunogenic, resulting in seroconversion rates exceeding 90% and significantly higher neutralizing antibody titers.[20,182,222–224] A comparison of long (days 0, 7, and 30) and short (days 0, 7, and 14) three-dose schedules disclosed uniform seroconversion in all subjects but significantly higher neutralizing antibody

titers in vaccinees immunized over the longer period (30 days).

Vaccine prepared from the Beijing-1 strain appears to be more immunogenic, despite its smaller delivered volume, yielding higher seroconversion rates and higher antibody titers to heterologous Nakayama virus (see Table 33–10).[282–287] Similar but more marked differences were seen in comparative neutralization of field viral strains from Taiwan, paralleling those in experimentally immunized mice (see Fig. 33–16).[288] The clinical importance of these differences in strain reactivity is uncertain. Results of the efficacy trial comparing a monovalent Nakayama strain vaccine with a bivalent vaccine also containing Beijing-1 antigen showed that the two were equally efficacious (see later discussion).[289] JE vaccines produced locally in Thailand, India, Vietnam, and Taiwan all employ the

TABLE 33–11 ■ Immunogenicity of Nakayama Strain Inactivated Japanese Encephalitis Virus Mouse Brain–Derived Vaccine in Subjects from Nonendemic Areas After Two or Three Doses

Study Group	Two-Dose Series			Three-Dose Series		
	No.	Seroconversion Rate (%)	GMT	No.	Seroconversion Rate (%)	GMT
United States (1984–1987)[182]	118	77	28	72	98	141
United Kingdom (1983)[223]	27	33	31–61	94	88	146–214
United States (1990)[224]	20	80		25	100*	
United States (1990)[222]				526	100	140/692†
Kolhapur, India (1990)‡	250	50		242	95	
Bagalore, India (1990)‡	184	73		184	98	

*Dose 3 at week 26.

†Day 60 serum; short and long three-dose schedules, $P < 0.0001$.

‡Children, 7 to 14 years old.

Data from Banerjee K. Japanese encephalitis in India (a country report). In Proceedings of a Regional Workshop on Control Strategies for Japanese Encephalitis, Department of Medical Sciences, Ministry of Public Health, Nonthaburi, Thailand, October 4–6, 1994.

GMT, geometric mean antibody titer.

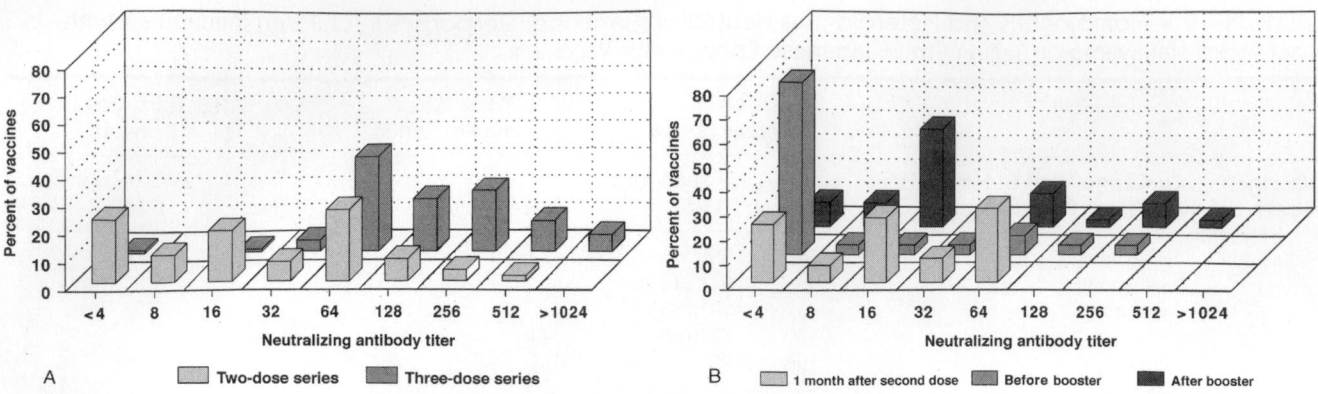

FIGURE 33–17 ▪ *A,* Antibody response to inactivated mouse brain–derived Japanese encephalitis vaccine in a trial among U.S. citizens. Only 77% of vaccinees who received two doses seroconverted, compared with 99% of vaccinees who received three doses. Geometric mean antibody titers also were higher in the latter group (28 vs. 141). (Adapted from Poland JD, Cropp CB, Craven RB, Monath TP. Evaluation of the potency and safety of inactivated Japanese encephalitis vaccine in US inhabitants. J Infect Dis 161:878–882, 1990.) *B,* Six to 12 months after primary immunization, only 10% of vaccinees who were given two doses retained protective levels of neutralizing antibody. Booster immunization led to a greater than 90% response.

Nakayama strain, and no field observations have suggested a geographic pattern of vaccine failure. Neutralizing activity may be present below the threshold of detection in in vitro assays, and T-cell memory may have been established in vaccinees who appear to be seronegative, providing sufficient help to clear infections on re-exposure.

Although previous exposures to dengue and certain other flaviviruses probably enhance the immune response to JE vaccine, antibody responses did not differ in people with a history of YF vaccination, unlike the accelerated response to inactivated TBE vaccine seen among YF-vaccinated individuals.[290]

Vaccinees are exposed only to viral structural proteins, and, in contrast to recovered patients, they do not produce radioprecipitating antibodies to viral NS proteins. Their memory T-cell proliferative responses to a viral-like particle containing only structural proteins also differ from those of recovered patients, whose CD4+ and CD8+ cell responses also include viral NS proteins.[131] The implications of these immune response differences are uncertain.

Impaired responses to vaccination were observed in infants with vertically acquired HIV infection when compared with control seroreverting infants born to HIV-infected women: 5 (36%) of 14 HIV-infected children and 18 (67%) of 27 control children developed JE antibodies after immunization (odds ratio [OR] 0.3; *P* = 0.06); among those with positive titers, the GMT of HIV-infected children also was lower (15.1 vs. 23.8; *P* = 0.17).[291] The response to additional doses beyond the primary two doses was not studied. Immune response in other immunocompromised states has not been studied systematically.[292]

EFFICACY

Efficacy of the Nakayama vaccine has been evaluated in two masked, randomized, placebo-(tetanus toxoid–) controlled field trials. In the first evaluation, a prototype of the current vaccine was field-tested in 1965 in Taiwan; two doses yielded an 80% efficacy in the first year after immunization (Table 33–12).[293-295] A subsequent masked, randomized, placebo-controlled field trial in Thailand compared the efficacies of the currently produced monovalent Nakayama vaccine with a specially formulated bivalent vaccine also containing Beijing-1 antigen (see Table 33–12).[289] Two doses of vaccine or placebo were given 1 week apart to children 1 year of age and older. After a 2-year observation period, efficacies of the monovalent and bivalent vaccines were identical, with an overall efficacy of 91%. Lower risks of dengue and dengue hemorrhagic fever also were observed in the JE-vaccinated groups, although the differences were not significant. Experimental studies in monkeys suggest that immunization against JE might provide cross-protection against West Nile virus.[125]

TABLE 33–12 ▪ Efficacy of Inactivated Mouse Brain–Derived Japanese Encephalitis Vaccine*

Country	Study Group	No. at Risk	Case Rate/100,000	Efficacy (95% CI) (%)
Taiwan, 1965[293,295]	Total vaccinated	133,943	4.48	76 (63–90)
	1 dose	22,194	9.01	50 (26–88)
	2 doses	111,749	3.58	80 (71–93)
	Placebo	131,865	18.20	—
	Nonvaccinated	140,514	24.91	—
Thailand, 1984–1985[289]	Total vaccinated	43,708	4.60	91 (70–97)
	Monovalent	21,628	4.60	91 (54–98)
	Bivalent	22,080	4.50	91 (54–98)
	Placebo	21,516	51.10	—

*Two doses of Nakayama or bivalent Nakayama/Beijing mouse brain–derived vaccines.
CI, confidence interval.

PERSISTENCE OF IMMUNITY AND PROTECTION

Studies in Asia to determine the persistence of vaccine-derived immunity are complicated by natural infections with dengue, West Nile virus, or other flaviviruses and re-exposure to JE virus itself, all of which act to reinforce and broaden vaccine-derived immunity to JE virus.[101,102,122–124] Even with the potential for these reinforcing infections, several studies in Asian and in Western subjects (see previous discussion) indicate a progressive decline in antibody levels in the first year after primary immunization with two doses (see Fig. 33–17 and Table 33–10).[182,207] Cross-sectional serosurveys in Japan and Taiwan (see earlier discussion; see also Fig. 33–14) indicate a rapid decline of antibody levels in childhood. Observations of vaccine efficacy in the Taiwan field trial parallel these results: In the second year after immunization, protective efficacy declined from 80% to 55% (95% confidence interval [CI] = 39% to 75%).[294] In the Thailand field trial of the current vaccine formulation, efficacy was shown through 2 years of observation. Further follow-up data are not available.

These and other data (see Table 33–11) indicate the need for boosters after a two-dose primary immunization series. A third dose generally has been given at 1 year and subsequently at intervals of 1 to 3 years (Fig. 33–18). Booster doses are followed by significant increases in neutralizing antibody titer and uniform anamnestic responses in subjects who had reverted to seronegative. A small study of vaccinees receiving an Indian-manufactured JE vaccine found that 34 (97%) of 35 retained neutralizing antibodies 3 years after a primary series of three doses, and 31 (91%) of 34 retained antibodies at 4.5 years, with GMTs of 71 and 32, respectively. However, the boosting effect of naturally acquired flaviviral infections in these subjects cannot be ruled out.[296]

Flavivirus-naive U.S. Army soldiers who received a three-dose primary immunization series retained protective neutralizing antibody titers for at least 1 year (GMT = 76). Antibody titers at 12 months were unchanged from those observed 3 months after immunization (GMT = 78). A booster dose given at 12 months was followed by a significant anamnestic response (GMT = 1117). In a limited number of subjects studied 3 years after the primary series, 16 (94%) of 17 who had neither traveled to Asia nor received a booster retained neutralizing antibody titers of greater than 1:10, and their GMTs at 6 months and at 3 years after primary immunization were unchanged.[222] Although these observations suggest that the first booster immunization is needed no sooner than 2 to 3 years after primary immunization, the interval for subsequent boosters has not been established.

Inactivated Primary Hamster Kidney Cell–Derived Japanese Encephalitis Vaccine

Two doses of inactivated PHK cell–derived vaccine, given 1 week apart, produced an LNI greater than 50 in only 60% to 68% of children who had no prevaccination JE viral antibodies (Table 33–13).[297–300] Immunity wanes rapidly after primary immunization with two doses, and 1 year later only 10% of vaccinees have an LNI greater than 50. The rapid decline in antibody provides some justification for the vaccine's administration in spring campaigns before the onset of the transmission season. A booster dose results in an anamnestic response in 93% to 100% of recipients. After 3 to 4 years, seropositivity is maintained at an LNI of greater than 50 in 64% of vaccinees, and a subsequent booster dose is followed by 100% seroconversion.[196,301] Extensive randomized field trials among 480,000 children have demonstrated vaccine efficacies in the range of 76% to 95% (Table 33–14).[195,300]

Although regional trials in Wuxi and Nanjing disclosed partial protection against acquiring JE (efficacies of 85% to 87%), more detailed clinical studies showed that cases in vaccinated children were milder than those in unvaccinated children. None of the 6 cases in immunized children resulted in death or neurologic sequelae, whereas 3 of the 25 cases in unimmunized children were fatal, and 3 led to

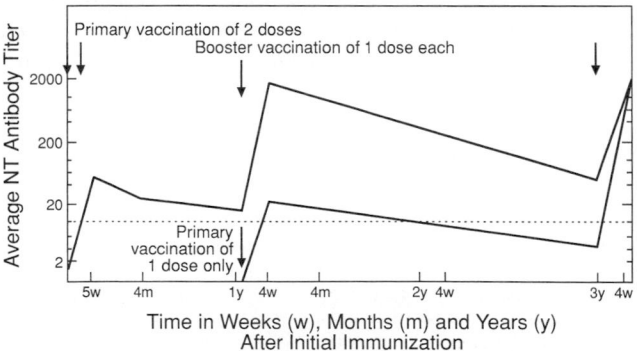

FIGURE 33–18 ▪ A schematic of the antibody response to two doses of inactivated mouse brain–derived Japanese encephalitis (JE) vaccine and of booster doses. Antibody levels declined to subprotective levels within 1 year after primary immunization. Protective levels recovered after booster immunization and declined after 3 to 4 years. Although this study was carried out in an area of Japan where JE transmission is limited, the effects of natural infection on antibody response and persistence of immunity cannot be ruled out. NT, Neutralizing. (Adapted from Kanamitsu M, Hashimoto N, Urasawa S, et al. A field trial with an improved Japanese encephalitis vaccine in a nonendemic area of the disease. Biken J 13:313–328, 1970.)

TABLE 33–13 ▪ **Neutralizing Antibody Response to Inactivated P3 Japanese Encephalitis Vaccine, Yanji, Jilin, China**

Year	Vaccination	Interval Between Vaccination and Bleeding	Proportion Seropositive (%)
1973	Dose 1	1 mo	15/25 (60)
	Dose 2	3 mo	8/28 (29)
		1 yr	3/29 (10)
1974	Booster	1 mo	27/29 (93)
1975		1 yr	50/63 (79)
1976		2 yr	32/47 (68)
1977		3 yr	42/64 (64)
1978		4 yr	40/62 (64)
1978	Booster 2	1 mo	62/62 (100)

Data from National Vaccine and Serum Institute, An Yang Municipal Health Station, Jiangsu Provincial Health Station, et al.[297]; Wang et al.[298]; National Serum and Biologics Institute, Jiling Yang Gi Health Station[299]; and Ren.[300]

TABLE 33–14 ■ Efficacy of Inactivated P3 Japanese Encephalitis Vaccine, People's Republic of China

Year	Region	Study Group	No. of Subjects	Cases of Japanese Encephalitis	Incidence Rate/100,000	Efficacy (95% CI) (%)
1967	Wuxi	Vaccinated*	38,482	3	7.8	84 (75–95)
		Nonvaccinated	34,182	17	52.8	
1968	Nanjing	Vaccinated	52,004	3	5.8	87 (73–96)
		Nonvaccinated	18,584	8	43.0	
1968	Hunan	Vaccinated	75,083	7	9.3	76 (63–90)
		Nonvaccinated	48,543	19	39.1	
1969	Beijing	Vaccinated	86,847	3	3.5	87 (81–96)
		Nonvaccinated	76,260	21	27.5	
1973	Guangxi	Vaccinated	58,211	2	3.4	95 (90–100)
		Nonvaccinated	10,165	7	68.9	

*Two doses with an interval of 1 week.
CI, confidence interval.
Data from Gu and Ding[195] and Ren.[300]

sequelae. These observations suggest that clinical efficacy is better than the reported protective efficacy.[196] A case-control study measuring vaccine effectiveness in Henan province, China, found that full immunization (two primary doses and annual boosters until age 10) was 78% effective (95% CI = 16% to 94%) in preventing the disease, and partial immunization was 68% effective (95% CI = 29% to 92%). The relative risk of acquiring JE was 4.54 in unimmunized children and 3.12 in partially immunized children.[301]

The aggregated data indicate that the inactivated P3 vaccine has some utility in preventing the disease; however, the need for repeated booster doses and its relatively low efficacy limit its use.

Immune responses to single doses of concentrated or purified inactivated PHK cell vaccines (see previous discussion) were similar to those observed after two doses of the standard vaccine. All subjects seroconverted, and respective GMTs were 45, 72, and 46.[196] No data on efficacy or persistence of immunity are available, and further work has been discontinued.

Live, Attenuated Japanese Encephalitis Vaccine

A comparison of vaccines derived from SA14-5-3 and SA14-14-2 showed that the former was less immunogenic, producing seroconversion in only 61% of 13 vaccinees and having a neutralizing GMT of 5, compared with a 92.3% seroconversion rate in subjects receiving a similar infectious dose of SA14-14-2 vaccine.[238] Several small immunogenicity studies of the SA14-14-2 vaccine have been reported, with variable results. After a single dose, antibody responses are produced in 85% to 100% of nonimmune 1- to 12-year-old children, with a response gradient that parallels progressive vaccine dilution (Table 33–15).[238,239,257,302,303] Lower seroconversion rates were obtained with vaccine dilutions that had infectious titers less than $10^{6.7}$ $TCID_{50}/mL$, which has been established as the minimal standard of vaccine infectivity.

Because of variable immune response rates after one dose, SA14-14-2 vaccine is given in a schedule of two doses separated by a year, according to the custom of administering JE vaccines in annual spring campaigns. The immuno-

genicity of two doses given at intervals of either 1 or 2.5 months was shown in 12- to 15-year-old children. Response rates were similar: 75% to 100% after one dose and 94% to 100% after two doses (two vaccine lots were compared), but there was a trend toward better seroconversion with the longer interval, and GMTs were approximately twofold higher (65 to 89 vs. 115 to 158, respectively). If these results can be confirmed in infants, the SA14-14-2 vaccine could be integrated into a routine childhood immunization schedule, potentially improving vaccine coverage.[257] The effect of maternal immunity on antibody response in infants has not been examined.[303]

Efficacy trials in children 1 to 10 years old have consistently yielded high protection rates, above 98% (Table 33–16).[247,304,305] In the 1991 Yunnan field study, neither of the two cases in vaccinated children produced serious illness, but three deaths occurred in the unvaccinated cohort, and more than 50% of the remaining cases were considered severe. In the Guizhou study, equally good protection was observed through a second year after a booster dose was given. Efficacy was shown with the more attenuated proto-

TABLE 33–15 ■ Immune Response to One Dose of SA14-14-2 Attenuated Japanese Encephalitis Vaccine by Vaccine Infectious Titer

Year	Vaccine Titer*	Seroconversion Rate (%)†	GMT	Reference
1979	6.7	12/13 (92)	29	238
	5.7	12/17 (71)	10	
	4.7	10/16 (62)	10	
1985	>7.0	23/23 (100)	>32	239
	6.0	10/12 (83)	23	
1987	7.0	33/39 (85)	23	303
1992	6.0–6.5‡	18/19 (95)	25	
1994	6.8‡	29/29 (100)	31	
	6.5‡	24/26 (92)	27	

*Log_{10} median tissue culture infective dose ($TCID_{50}$) per milliliter.
†Greater than 1:10 neutralizing antibody titer.
‡Log (plaque-forming units/milliliter).
GMT, geometric mean antibody titer.

TABLE 33–16 ■ Protective Efficacy of SA14-14-2 Attenuated Japanese Encephalitis Vaccine, China

Province	Year	Study Group	No. of Subjects	Cases of Japanese Encephalitis	Incidence/ 100,000	Efficacy (95% CI) (%)
Guizhou	1988	Vaccinated*	86,132	1	1.16	98.0 (96–100)
		Nonvaccinated	21,149	12	56.7	
	1989	Vaccinated†	86,933†	0	2.30	100
		Nonvaccinated	16,869	12	71.1	100
Jiang-Xi	1989	Vaccinated*	64,027	2	3.12	98.4 (97–100)
		Nonvaccinated	4546	9	198.0	
	1990	Vaccinated†	63,927	1	1.56	99.8 (98–100)
		Nonvaccinated	5784	37	639.6	
	1991–1993	Vaccinated†	~65,000	0		100
		Nonvaccinated	~7000	24 (3 yr)	~109.6	
Yunnan	1991	Vaccinated‡	29,639	2	6.75	95.7 (94–99)
		Nonvaccinated	29,006	46	158.6	
Anhui	1992	Vaccinated	145,758	2	1.37	99.3 (99–100)
		Nonvaccinated	11,264	22	195.3	

*Children 1 to 10 years old immunized with single primary dose.

†Combination of 1- to 10-year-old children immunized in previous year(s), 1-year-old children given primary dose, and 2-year-old children given booster dose.

‡Children 1 to 7 years old immunized with single primary dose only.

CI, confidence interval.

Data from Hueyang Antiepidemic Station,[247] Chendu Biologics Institute[304] and Wang et al.[305]

type SA14-5-3 vaccine, although protection was lower than that achieved with the SA14-14-2 vaccine (see Table 33–8).[247,304,305]

A study measuring the effectiveness of the SA14-14-2 vaccine, using case-control methods, disclosed protection levels similar to those estimated by previous efficacy studies. When immunization histories were compared among 56 hospitalized laboratory-confirmed JE cases and 1299 age-matched village controls, the vaccine's effectiveness was 80% for one dose (95% CI = 44% to 93%) and 98% for two doses (95% CI = 86% to 99.6%).[306] Because of uncertainties about the methodologic approach of earlier efficacy studies, the consistency of this result with previous estimates was reassuring. Furthermore, effectiveness is a measure of the vaccine's performance under the usual circumstances of health care delivery rather than the artificial conditions of a study, which is additional evidence of the vaccine's robustness.

In a field trial in Nepal in 1999, involving more than 160,000 subjects 1 to 15 years of age, the efficacy of a single dose of SA14-14-2 vaccine given just a few days prior to the onset of a large JE outbreak was 99.3%. Vaccine in this study contained $10^{5.8}$ PFU/0.5 mL. In the case-control study, no JE cases had received vaccine compared with nearly 58% of age- and sex-matched village controls.[307] The efficacy of a single dose in preventing JE cases in the next year, 2000, continued to be greater than 98% (YM Sohn, HC Ohrr, SH Shin, personal communication, 2001). The study provides evidence that SA14-14-2 will be useful to combat epidemics. Although the vaccine lot used in this field trial was made for export, vaccine having been packaged in individual 1-mL syringes, this study clearly demonstrates that, under supervised administration, SA14-14-2 vaccine can be highly protective after just one dose. Consideration should be given to revising dosage recommendations in China.

Side Effects of Immunization

Inactivated Mouse Brain–Derived Japanese Encephalitis Vaccine

LOCAL AND NONSPECIFIC ADVERSE EVENTS

Local tenderness, redness, or swelling at the injection site occurs in approximately 20% of individuals immunized with inactivated mouse brain–derived vaccines. Mild systemic symptoms, chiefly headache, low-grade fever, myalgias, malaise, and gastrointestinal symptoms, are reported by 10% to 30% of vaccinees (Table 33–17).[182,223,224,282]

NEUROLOGIC ADVERSE EVENTS

The vaccine's neural tissue substrate has raised concern about the possibility of postvaccination neurologic side effects.[308] The manufacturing process purifies the infected mouse brain suspension extensively, and MBP content is controlled below 2 ng/mL, well below the dose considered to have an encephalitogenic effect in a guinea pig test system. However, measurements of other acute disseminated encephalomyelitis (ADE)–associated neural proteins (e.g., proteolipid protein, myelin-oligodendrocyte glycoprotein) have not been reported. Experimental immunization of guinea pigs and *Cynomolgus* monkeys with adjuvant and 50 times the normal dose of vaccine did not result in clinical or histopathologic evidence of encephalomyelitis.[309,310]

In 1945, in one of the first mass uses of mouse brain–derived JE vaccine, 53,000 American soldiers on Okinawa were immunized with a crude inactivated mouse brain suspension after a JE outbreak occurred on the island.[201] Acute vaccine-associated side effects, including the occurrence of acute neurologic events, were monitored. Eight neurologic reactions, principally polyneuritis, were observed. However, similar cases were reported concurrently in nonvaccinated individuals, and it is unclear

TABLE 33–17 ■ Reported Side Effects of Inactivated Mouse Brain–Derived Japanese Encephalitis Vaccine

Country	Subjects	Local Side Effects (%)*	Systemic Side Effects (%)†	Reference
Thailand	490	<1	1.7–2.9	289
United States	59	18	9	182
United States	1328	12	2	
	526			
	1st dose	20	5	224
	2nd dose	12	2	
	3rd dose	11	1	
United States	3573	23	10–13	224
Thailand	448	2	1.3–1.8	289

*Local tenderness, redness, swelling, itching, and numbness.
†Chiefly fever, headache, malaise, rash; also chills, dizziness, myalgia, nausea, vomiting, abdominal pain, diarrhea, sore throat, blurred vision, increased salivation and taste, difficulty concentrating, and emotional instability.

whether the illnesses were vaccine related. One case of Guillain-Barré syndrome, temporally related to JE immunization, was reported among approximately 20,000 American soldiers immunized with the vaccine prior to U.S. licensure.

An early prospective study in Japan to detect vaccine-associated adverse events (AEs) found no neurologic complications occurring within 1 month after vaccination in 38,384 subjects receiving crude or purified vaccine.[308] A country-wide study to detect neurologic complications found 26 temporally related cases (meningitis, convulsions, demyelinating disease, polyneuritis) between 1957 and 1966, but rates and comparisons with nonimmunized controls were not available. Passive surveillance of vaccine-related AEs in Japan is conducted through sentinel hospitals, clinics, and pharmacies and through manufacturers. Surveillance data on JE vaccine AEs come principally from the manufacturers (Biken and others). Few neurologic complications temporally related to JE vaccination have been reported, but denominators of vaccinees were not available in all years, and the sensitivity of this passive surveillance system is unknown (Table 33–18).[217,309,311]

In 1992, two anecdotal cases of temporally related vaccine-associated ADE in Japan prompted a survey of 162 Japanese medical institutions to solicit additional cases.[312]

TABLE 33–18 ■ Reported Neurologic Manifestations Temporally Associated with Japanese Encephalitis Vaccination, Japan

Years	No. of Cases	Estimated Rate
1965–1970	75	$1/10^6$
1971–1978	?	$2.3/10^{6†}$
1979–1980	6	—
1981–1982	3	—
1983–1986	?	—
1987–1989	2	—

*Inactivated mouse brain–derived vaccine.
†1971 to 1973 data from Tokyo only: two cases per 883,373 vaccinees.
Data from Japanese encephalitis vaccine lyophilized, "Biken,"[217] Egashira et al.[309] and Okinaka et al.[311]

Five more cases spanning 22 years were reported, including two with elevated CSF MBP levels.[313] Neither the numerator of cases nor the denominator of vaccinees was defined rigorously, but the authors estimated that ADE occurred in fewer than 1 in 1 million vaccinees. In an unrelated report, there were 2 deaths due to anaphylactic shock and four ADE cases (two fatal) temporally related to vaccination were reported in Korea in 1994; one, also fatal, was reported in 1996. An additional fatal case of acute encephalopathy occurred in a 15-year-old girl who received her ninth dose of JE vaccine and her third dose of hantaviral vaccine (also made in mouse brain) 4 and 2 weeks, respectively, before onset of stupor and seizures (YM Sohn, unpublished observations, 2002).

An additional report of vaccination-associated ADE cases in Danish travelers, unprompted by previous reports from Japan and Korea, suggests that the issue of neurologic complications should be reinvestigated.[314] After a vaccinee developed ADE in 1995, a review of the national database disclosed two similar temporally related cases in 1983 and 1989, all in adults. Because JE vaccine distribution in Denmark is controlled, the denominator of vaccinees and a rate for AEs could be estimated. The rate of temporally related ADE, 1 in 50,000 to 75,000 vaccinees, is far above previous estimates of all neurologic complications and in the same range as JE incidence in countries where the disease is endemic. In the United States, a postmarketing study revealed that no serious neurologic AEs were temporally associated with JE vaccine between January 1993 and June 1999, while in Japan, 17 vaccine-related neurologic disorders were reported from April 1996 to October 1998.[315]

These reports and the high rate of serious events in the Danish study suggest the need for continuing postmarketing surveillance. In Korea, where no naturally acquired JE case has occurred in recent years, public objections to neurologic AEs associated with vaccine have led to a widely held belief that there is greater risk from the vaccine than from the disease itself.

Although the bovine spongiform encephalopathy outbreak has raised concern over the potential for contamination of biologicals with prions from animal sources, there has been little discussion about risks of the JE vaccine mouse brain substrate. Factors mitigating against such a risk are (1) the low, if any, natural incidence of a mouse-transmissible spongiform encephalopathy; (2) the vaccine purification process that removes certain proteins from the final product; and (3) the species barrier. In the absence of a naturally occurring murine spongiform encephalopathy, the principal concern is co-mixing of mice designated for vaccine production with mice infected in a research project. Although this seems unlikely, mice used in vaccine production are supplied by multiple subcontractors whose facilities may be difficult to monitor. The vaccine formalin inactivation process does not inactivate and potentially could stabilize contaminating prions. However, on balance it seems highly unlikely that the vaccine poses a risk for transmission of a spongiform encephalopathy agent.

HYPERSENSITIVITY REACTIONS

Vaccine-related allergic AEs not reported previously from Asia were recognized after 1989 in Australia and several European and North American countries as the vaccine became used widely in travelers.[182,183,316-322] Hypersensitivity reactions have consisted principally of generalized urticaria, angioedema, or both, which in a few patients were potentially life threatening. These reactions generally have responded to oral antihistamines or corticosteroids, but recalcitrant cases have required hospitalization and parenteral steroid therapy. A temporally related death was reported in a man with multiple hypersensitivities who also had received plague vaccine.[183] Numerous lots and different manufacturers have been implicated.[319] In retrospect, allergic side effects, including urticaria, angioedema, and moderate dyspnea, were observed in recipients of the crude mouse brain vaccine administered on Okinawa in 1945.[201]

An important feature of the reactions is the potential for delayed onset, particularly after a second dose. In a prospective study of 14,249 U.S. Marines, the median interval between immunization and onset was 18 to 24 hours after the first dose, with 74% of reactions occurring within 48 hours.[182,183,317] Among reactors to a second dose, there was a greater delay, with a median interval of 96 hours and a range of 20 to 336 hours. Reactions have developed after a second or third dose when previous doses were given uneventfully. A nested case-control study found an elevated risk with history of various allergic disorders (e.g., urticaria: OR 11.4 [95% CI = 2.4 to 62.1]; allergic rhinitis: OR 9.2 [95% CI = 2.8 to 23.1]; asthma, rhinitis, or both: OR 6.5 [95% CI = 2.1 to 20.8]; and any allergy: OR 5.7 [95% CI = 1.8 to 18.1]).[183] Another small study also implicated alcohol

consumption and receipt of another vaccine 1 to 9 days previously, as opposed to simultaneously, as risk factors.[323]

Reported rates have varied according to the approach to ascertainment (Table 33-19). Recent prospective or retrospective studies have found risk of an allergic AE, usually defined as objective urticaria or angioedema, in the range of 18 to 64 per 10,000 vaccinees.[316,318,322-325] A large postmarketing study in the United States and Japan determined the AE rate to be 2.8 and 15.0 per 100,000 doses in Japan and the United States, respectively.[315] Hypersensitivity rates were 0.8 and 6.3 per 100,000 doses, respectively. A cluster of two deaths resulting from anaphylactic shock in children receiving JE vaccine was reported in Korea in 1994. In a follow-up study to measure the incidence of JE vaccine-related AEs, one case of anaphylactic shock with syncope and collapse, three cases of generalized urticaria, and three cases of severe erythema were found in 15,487 Korean children immunized between May 15 and June 30, 1995. The rate of 0.03% was lower than that observed in adult travelers, which could reflect either biologic differences in reactivity or the sensitivity of surveillance (YM Sohn, unpublished observations, 1996).

Although the pathogenesis of the hypersensitivity reactions is not proven, in three Japanese children experiencing systemic reactions, immunoglobulin E (IgE) antibodies to gelatin were demonstrated, suggesting that gelatin, which is added as a vaccine stabilizer, may be a provoking antigen.[326] Further analysis of reactions showed two patterns: One was a combination of urticarial rash and wheezing, which was associated with the presence of antigelatin IgE in the serum, and the second was a cardiovascular collapse syndrome apparently caused by another mechanism.[327] A similar syndrome has been described in recipients of diploid cell-derived rabies vaccine in whom symptoms developed after a delay of as long as 1 week after booster immunization.[328] Immunologic studies demonstrated IgE antibodies to human albumin, which is added to the vaccine as a stabilizer and chemically altered by the inactivating agent β-propiolactone.[329] Allergic reactions in recipients of crude mouse brain vaccine in Okinawa were attributed to formalin-altered proteins. In a Danish case-control study, about one third of allergic reactions could be attributed to an allergic predisposition in the vaccinees. The main risk factors were young age, female gender, previous allergic skin reactions or hayfever, skin reactivity to nickel, and hyperresponsiveness to mosquito bites.[330]

TABLE 33-19 ■ Hypersensitivity Reactions* After Immunization with Inactivated Mouse Brain–Derived Japanese Encephalitis Virus Vaccine

Country	Cases/Vaccinees	Rate/10,000 Vaccinees	95% CI (%)	Reference
Denmark	68/≈175,150	1–17†	—	317
United Kingdom	2/314	64	8–200	321
Australia (Torres Strait)	10/3511	28	14–500	325
United States (postmarketing surveillance, travelers)	4/767	52	14–130	324
Active duty military (Okinawa)	26	18	11–25	183

*Generalized urticaria or angioedema.
†Rates varied by vaccine lot.
CI, confidence interval.

Inactivated Primary Hamster Kidney Cell–Derived Japanese Encephalitis Vaccine

Few adverse reactions have been reported in connection with the P3 inactivated vaccine. Local reactions, including swelling at the injection site, are observed in about 4% of vaccinees, and mild systemic symptoms, such as headache and dizziness, are reported by fewer than 1% of vaccinees. Fever higher than 38°C previously was a complication in 12% of vaccinees, but, after a reduction in bovine serum in the currently formulated vaccine, febrile reactions have been halved. A urticarial allergic reaction was observed in only 1 of nearly 15,000 vaccinees surveyed.[289] Recent clusters of reactions temporally related to vaccination and consisting of acute asthenia, syncope, and disorientation have been reported from disparate areas of the country. Some features of the reactions suggest that they may be outbreaks of hysteria, but their consistency and occurrence in a widespread geographic distribution are difficult to explain.

Live, Attenuated Japanese Encephalitis Vaccine

An estimated 100 million children have been immunized with the live, attenuated vaccine without apparent complication. Clinical monitoring of experimentally immunized subjects has documented the absence of local or systemic symptoms after immunization; specifically, headache and symptoms that might be associated with neuroinvasive infection as well as fever and signs and symptoms of systemic infection have not been observed after immunization. In a study of 867 children in whom fever was monitored over a 21-day period after immunization, temperatures above 37.6°C were recorded in fewer than 0.5% of vaccinees, and fever-onset days were distributed throughout the observation interval, mitigating against a vaccine-related febrile illness after a specific incubation period. In the same study, symptoms were recorded from 588,512 other vaccinees; fever was reported in 0.046% of subjects, rash in 0.01%, dizziness in 0.0003%, and nausea in 0.0003%, but these rates are difficult to interpret in the absence of similar observations in controls.[239,331]

A block-randomized cohort study of 13,266 vaccinated and 12,951 nonvaccinated 1- to 2-year-old children followed prospectively for 30 days confirmed the vaccine's safety. No cases of encephalitis or meningitis were detected in either group, and rates of hospitalization, new onset of seizures, fever lasting more than 3 days, and allergic, respiratory, and gastrointestinal symptoms were similar in the two groups. The observations excluded a vaccination-related encephalitis risk above 1 in 3400.[332]

The rates of clinical encephalitis among children vaccinated in field trials (see Table 33–16) provide additional reassurance that the SA14-14-2 virus does not itself cause encephalitis at a detectable rate. Rates of clinical encephalitis in children receiving SA14-14-2 vaccine—1.16 to 6.75 per 100,000 population—are lower than reported population-based incidence rates of childhood encephalitis (15 to 30 per 100,000 population).

No observations on the vaccine's safety in pregnant women or in immunocompromised individuals, specifically those with HIV infection, have been reported.

Indications for Immunization

Endemic Areas

In rural areas of Asia, intense JE virus transmission in the enzootic cycle leads to a high risk of exposure at an early age. Universal primary immunization is indicated for children between 1 and 2 years of age. The peak risk of infection is in children between 1 and 4 years of age, which may reflect the waning protective effects of maternal immunity and patterns of outdoor activity that place young children at risk. However, cases occur in children through the first decade of life, and, in most areas with risk of enzootic transmission, immunity should be maintained by boosters through the age of 10 years.

Although incidence may vary regionally in countries at risk, universal childhood immunization is desirable because, even in economically advanced countries, viral transmission cannot be eliminated, and the cumulative risk of acquiring the illness over a lifetime of exposure probably justifies universal protection. Furthermore, conditions leading to epidemic transmission are unpredictable, and, at intervals, outbreaks may lead to large numbers of cases even in urban areas. Hong Kong and Singapore may be special cases in which, despite the absence of a national immunization policy, the possibility of enzootic viral transmission is limited by the exclusively urban environment.[174] For the most part, stepwise implementation of national JE vaccination programs, initially in epidemic foci and in areas with hyperendemic transmission, has been necessary because of economic considerations.[18,333]

Expatriates

JE vaccine is recommended for expatriates whose principal residence is in an area where JE is endemic or epidemic. Risk of acquiring JE among expatriates is variable and depends principally on the specific location of intended residence, housing conditions, nature of activities, and the possibility of unanticipated exposure to high-risk areas (see *Travelers* below). Risk varies regionally and within specific countries. Viral transmission is seasonal in most areas and can fluctuate from year to year in a given location. Figure 33–1 and Table 33–20 summarize and extrapolate available data on locations and seasonality of risk by country. Patterns of viral transmission may change, and physicians and travelers are cautioned to consult public health officials for current data and trends.

Travelers

JE vaccine is recommended for selected travelers to Asia and should not be considered a routine immunization. Risk of acquiring JE during travel is extremely low (see earlier discussion), and the vast majority of visitors to Asia on business or in tours are at low risk and need not be immunized. In addition, the vaccine is costly; the average wholesale price of three doses in the United States is $147. Because JE viral transmission is confined to certain seasons and occurs principally in rural areas, only visitors with such a travel itinerary have a high risk of acquiring the disease. Travelers and their physicians should weigh individual risk factors and disease risk in the area and season of anticipated travel in light of the potential for vaccine side effects (see Fig. 33–1 and Tables 33–4 and 33–20).[189,190,319,334,334a]

TABLE 33–20 ■ Risk of Japanese Encephalitis by Country, Region, and Season*

Country	Affected Areas/Jurisdictions	Transmission Season	Comments
Bangladesh	Few data, probably widespread	Possibly July–December, as in northern India	Outbreak reported from Tangail district, Dacca division; sporadic cases in Rajshahi division
Bhutan	No data	No data	
Brunei	Presumed to be sporadic-endemic, as in Malaysia	Presumed year-round transmission	
Cambodia	Probably endemic-hyperendemic country-wide	Presumed to be May–October	Cases from Phnom Penh recognized
India	Reported cases from all states except Arunachal, Dadra, Daman, Diu, Gujarat, Himachal, Jammu, Kashmir, Lakshadweep, Meghalaya, Nagar Haveli, Orissa, Punjab, Rajasthan, and Sikkim	South India: May–October in Goa; October–January in Tamil Nadu; August–December in Karnataka; second peak, April–June in Mandya district Andhra Pradesh: September–December North India: July–December	Outbreaks in West Bengal, Bihar, Karnataka, Tamil Nadu, Andhra Pradesh, Assam, Uttar Pradesh, Manipure, Maharashtra, and Goa; urban cases reported (e.g., Lucknow)
Indonesia	Kalimantan, Bali, Nusa Tenggara, Sulawesi, Mollucas, West Irian, Java, Lombok	Probably year-round risk; varies by island; peak risks associated with rainfall, rice cultivation, and presence of pigs; peak period of risk: November–March; June–July in some years	Hyperendemic on Bali; sporadic cases recognized elsewhere; vaccine not recommended if travel is to major cities only
Japan†	Rare-sporadic cases on all islands, except Hokkaido	June–September except Ryukyu Islands (Okinawa), April–October	Vaccine not routinely recommended if travel is to major cities only; enzootic transmission without human cases observed on Hokkaido
Korea†	North Korea: no data	July–October	Last major outbreaks in 1982–1983; vaccine not recommended if travel is to major cities only
	South Korea: rare sporadic cases		
Laos	Presumed to be endemic-hyperendemic country-wide	Presumed to be May–October	No data
Malaysia	Sporadic-endemic in all states of Peninsula, Sarawak, and probably Sabah	No seasonal pattern; year-round transmission	Vaccine not recommended if travel is to major cities only
Myanmar	Presumed to be endemic-hyperendemic country-wide	Presumed to be May–October	Repeated outbreaks in Shan State in Chiang Mai Valley
Nepal	Hyperendemic in southern lowlands (Terai); sporadic cases now recognized in Kathmandu Valley	July–December	Vaccine recommended for travelers to lowlands
Pakistan	May be transmitted in central deltas	Presumed to be June–January	Cases reported near Karachi; endemic areas overlap those for West Nile virus
Papua–New Guinea	Sporadic cases (1956 and 1997–1998) reported from Western, Gulf, and South Highland Provinces	Unknown	Vaccine not routinely recommended

Continued

TABLE 33-20 ■ Risk of Japanese Encephalitis by Country, Region, and Season*—cont'd

Country	Affected Areas/Jurisdictions	Transmission Season	Comments
People's Republic of China	Cases in all provinces except Xizang (Tibet), Xinjiang, and Qinghai; hyperendemic in southern China; endemic–periodically epidemic in temperate areas; Hong Kong: rare cases in New Territories	*Northern China:* May–September *Southern China:* April–October (Guangshi, Yunnan, Gwangdong, and Southern Fujian, Szechuan, Guizhou, Hunan, and Jiangsi provinces)	Vaccine not routinely recommended for travelers to major cities only (including Hong Kong)
Philippines	Presumed to be endemic on all islands	Uncertain; speculations based on locations and agroecosystems *West Luzon, Mindoro, Negro Palowan:* April–November *Elsewhere:* year-round; greatest risk, April–January	Outbreaks described in Nueva Ecija, Luzon, and Manila
Russia	Far Eastern maritime areas south of Khabarousk	Peak period, July–September	Rare human cases reported
Singapore	Rare cases—last indigenous case in 1992	Year-round transmission not detected recently	Vaccine not routinely recommended
Sri Lanka	Endemic in all but mountainous areas; periodically epidemic in northern and central provinces	October–January; secondary peak of enzootic transmission, May–June	Recent outbreaks in central (Anuradhapura) and northwestern provinces
Taiwan[†]	Sporadic cases except in central mountains	April–October; June peak	Cases in and around Taipei
Thailand	Hyperendemic in north; sporadic-endemic in south	May–October	Annual outbreaks in Chiang Mai Valley; sporadic cases in Bangkok suburbs
Vietnam	Endemic-hyperendemic in all provinces	May–October	Highest rates in and near Hanoi
Western Pacific and Australia	Discrete epidemics reported on Guam, Saipan (northern Mariana Islands); sporadic cases in Torres Strait and Cape York peninsula, Australia	Uncertain; possibly September–January in the Pacific; February–April in far northern Australia	Enzootic cycle may not be sustainable; epidemics may follow introductions of virus; single case reported on Australian mainland (Cape York peninsula) in 1998

Notes:

1. Assessments are based on publications, surveillance reports, and personal correspondence.
2. Extrapolations have been made from available data.
3. Transmission patterns may change.
4. Consult the Centers for Disease Control and Prevention (telephone 1-970-221-6400) or other public health authorities for the latest trends.

[†]Reported human cases may not accurately reflect risks to nonimmune visitors because of high immunization rates in local populations. Humans are incidental to the transmission cycle. High levels of viral transmission may occur in the absence of human disease.

Immunization is recommended for visitors to epidemic or endemic areas during the transmission season, especially when there will be an extended period of exposure (more than 30 days) or the individual is at high risk of exposure to vectors because of the nature of his or her activities or housing. For example, bicyclists on tours and workers on field projects in rural areas may have greater outdoor exposure to vector mosquitoes. In addition, advanced age and pregnancy may affect risk and outcome of JE. Repellents and other protective measures are recommended in any case, because other vector-borne diseases may be transmitted in the same areas. General precautions are especially important to travelers in whom vaccine is contraindicated, who are unable to complete immunization because of departures on short notice, or who do not choose to be immunized because their visits to high-risk areas are brief or carry an equivocal risk.

Because allergic reactions to mouse brain–derived JE vaccine may be delayed for 1 week after immunization, and to allow protective antibody levels to develop, vaccinees ideally should defer travel until 7 days after receiving the last vaccine dose. Travelers should remain in areas accessible to medical care for 7 days after immunization.

Research Laboratory Workers

There have been 22 cases of laboratory-acquired JE virus, principally in research settings where infectious JE virus was used.[335] Infection can be transmitted by percutaneous or mucous membrane exposures and potentially by aerosols, especially from preparations containing high viral concentrations, which occur during viral purification. Immunization presumably protects against percutaneous exposures; however, it is unknown whether vaccine-derived immunity, especially from inactivated vaccine, protects against aerosol infection. Immunization is advised for all research laboratory personnel who potentially may be exposed to field or virulent strains of the virus. Although no formal biosafety recommendations have been issued for work with the attenuated vaccine SA14-14-2 strain, sufficient data are available on its attenuation such that immunized workers should be permitted to handle that virus under Biosafety Level 2 conditions, paralleling recommendations for the attenuated vaccine strains of YF, Junin, Rift Valley fever, chikungunya, and Venezuelan equine encephalitis viruses.[319]

Contraindications to Immunization

Mouse brain–derived JE vaccine is contraindicated in people who have had an allergic reaction to the vaccine, to gelatin, or to other rodent-derived products, including previous doses of JE vaccine. Other biologicals made in rodent tissue include vaccines against rabies, the hantaviral agents of hemorrhagic fever with renal syndrome, Hantaan and Seoul viruses, products derived from Chinese hamster ovary cells, and murine monoclonal antibodies. Hantaan virus vaccine made in mouse brain and purified by methods similar to those used in JE vaccine manufacture is produced in Korea and is under evaluation in China. A hantaviral vaccine produced in primary gerbil (*Meriones unguiculatus*) kidney cells also has limited distribution in China. YF vaccine made from the French neurotropic strain previously was produced in mouse brain, but production was discontinued in 1982.

Anecdotal reports of ADE occurring in temporal relationship to vaccination suggest that the mouse brain–derived vaccine should not be used in individuals who have recovered from ADE or Guillain-Barré syndrome or who have multiple sclerosis or other demyelinating disorders.

Hypersensitivity reactions to mouse brain–derived JE vaccine are more common in individuals with allergic conditions (e.g., asthma; allergic rhinitis; drug or Hymenoptera venom sensitivity; and food allergy, especially to gelatin-containing foods [see earlier discussion]). If these individuals are offered JE vaccine, they should be advised of the potential for vaccine-related angioedema and generalized urticaria. Hypersensitivity to a protein found in mouse urine is common in animal caretakers and certain laboratorians. It is unknown whether this sensitivity carries a specific risk in recipients of JE vaccine.

There are no specific contraindications to the use of PHK-derived inactivated JE vaccine except history of allergic reaction to a previous dose.

JE vaccines pose a theoretical risk to the developing fetus. No adverse outcomes of pregnancy have been associated directly with JE vaccine. Travelers and their physicians must balance the theoretical risks of JE vaccine in pregnancy against the potential risks of acquiring JE and the adverse outcome of the disease.

There are few data on the safety and efficacy of inactivated JE vaccines in immunocompromised individuals. A small study of children with various chronic diseases, including some oncology patients, disclosed no difference in immunogenicity or reactogenicity in recipients of mouse brain–derived vaccine.[282] Infants vertically infected with HIV responded less well to the vaccine (see earlier discussion), but no unusual AEs were recorded.[281]

Live, attenuated JE vaccine potentially carries an additional risk in pregnant women and immunocompromised patients. Although experimental data suggest that JE SA14-14-2 virus may not be neurotropic in immunosuppressed animals, there are no data on the vaccine's safety in immunocompromised individuals, specifically HIV-infected patients. When JE vaccine must be given to pregnant women or to immunocompromised patients, available inactivated JE vaccine should be used rather than live vaccine.

Public Health Considerations

Although a secular trend toward declining JE incidence has been observed with widespread use of JE vaccine, coincident socioeconomic changes also may have contributed to falling disease incidence (Fig. 33–19). In Thailand, for example, encephalitis incidence had begun a steady decline since the mid-1970s, nearly two decades before the national JE immunization program was instituted in 1990 (see Fig. 33–5), and in Singapore, reductions in disease incidence and viral transmission have been attributed solely to factors other than vaccination (see earlier discussion).[13,174] The most important have been (1) improved agricultural productivity and increasing urbanization, resulting in fewer rural dwellers at risk; (2) a decline in land area under rice

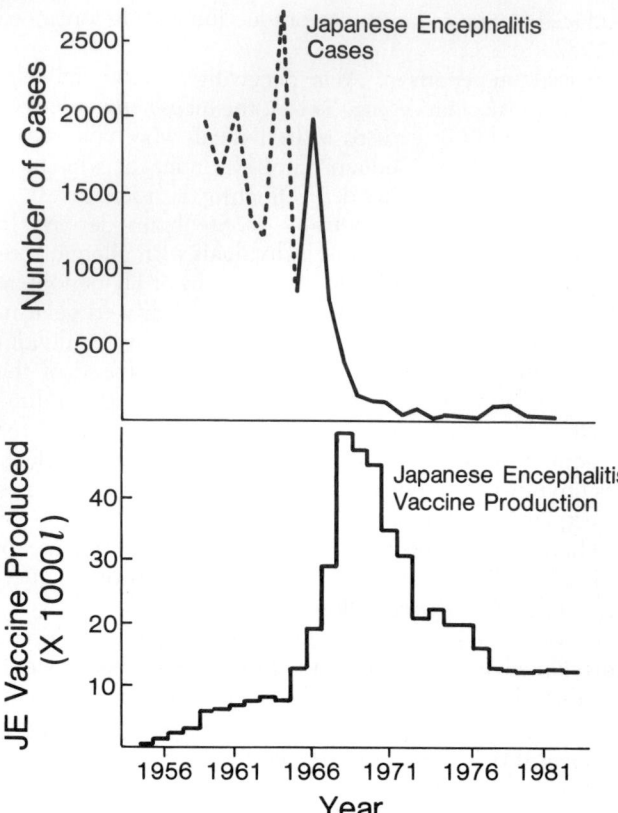

FIGURE 33–19 ■ Incidence of Japanese encephalitis (JE) in relationship to vaccine distribution in Japan, 1956 to 1981. *Dotted line*, reported cases; *solid line*, confirmed cases since 1965. (Adapted from Oya A. Japanese encephalitis vaccine. Acta Pediatr Jpn 30:175–184, 1988.)

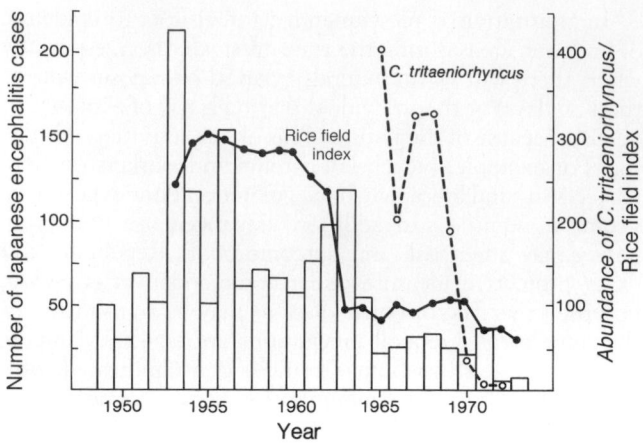

FIGURE 33–20 ■ The relationship of reduced land area in rice paddies, declining abundance of vector *Culex tritaeniorhyncus* mosquitoes, and reported Japanese encephalitis (JE) cases on Okinawa, 1949 to 1973. JE vaccine was licensed in Japan in 1954, but, in addition to immunization, incidental factors associated with development may have contributed to the decline in reported cases. The rice field index is expressed as a percentage of area cultivated in 1964 (100%). (Data from T. Fukunaga, personal communication, 1994.)

cultivation; and (3) increased use of agricultural pesticides, which have reduced numbers of vector mosquitoes (Fig. 33–20).[321] Although pig inventories actually have increased, changes in husbandry practices, especially centralized rearing, probably have resulted in an overall reduction of infected vectors in areas where people are active. Improvements in the general standard of living and, in specific locations, vector control programs have further reduced risk of exposure and infection.

Observations from the PRC, where development has been less extensive, are somewhat clearer in demonstrating the impact of immunization. JE incidence rates in Beijing and in other areas of China where high immunization rates are maintained have declined dramatically and have remained low (Figs. 33–13 and 33–21 and Table 33–21).[10,195] Although vaccine coverage is high in cities and in prosperous districts, coverage remains low in many rural locations, often in the very places with greatest risk. The principal barriers to immunization include the cost of the vaccine, which must be borne by families because JE vaccine is not government subsidized as a childhood vaccine, and inaccessibility to the health care system.

As a zoonotic disease with natural viral reservoirs, JE never can be eliminated. Although its transmission can be modulated by factors mentioned earlier, these approaches alone or in combination cannot be relied on to reduce disease incidence as effectively as human vaccination.

Successful control of JE by universal immunization in at least three countries in the region suggests that an extension of these efforts throughout the continent could lead to the near-elimination of the disease. However, for all of the approved vaccines, unresolved issues potentially limit their acceptability as a solution for region-wide control of the disease.

The inactivated mouse brain–derived vaccine is troubled by safety and other issues. Moreover, the vaccine's 91% efficacy, when extrapolated to the entire cohort of children younger than 15 years in Asia—approximately 1 billion children—yields an absolute number of primary vaccine failures of questionable acceptability. Assuming a JE incidence rate of 1 per 10,000 population in children younger than 15 years, approximately 100,000 cases would occur in the absence of any immunization. If every child was immu-

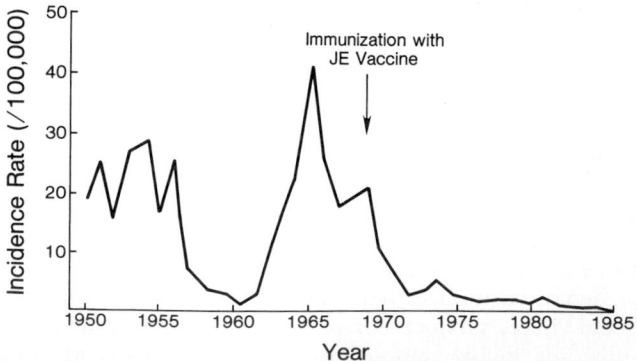

FIGURE 33–21 ■ Declining incidence of Japanese encephalitis (JE) in Beijing and association with mass immunization, 1950 to 1985. (Adapted from Gu PW, Ding ZF. Inactivated Japanese encephalitis [JE] vaccine made from hamster cell culture [review]. Jpn Encephalitis Hemorrhagic Fever Renal Syndr Bull 2:15–26, 1987.)

TABLE 33–21 ■ Japanese Encephalitis Immunization Coverage and Incidence, Liaoning

District	Population of 1- to 10-Yr-Olds	No. of Children Immunized	% Immunized	Incidence in 1- to 10-Yr-Olds
Zhuang Ho	237,457	33,637	14.2	35.0
Fu Hsien	187,414	161,491	86.7	6.5
Xin Chin	135,754	120,839	89.0	3.6

From Huang CH. Studies of Japanese encephalitis in China. Adv Virus Res 27:71–101, 1982.

nized but only 91% were protected, 9000 residual cases would occur annually as a result of primary vaccine failure. Although additional booster doses presumably would improve efficacy, the strategy also would lead to increased costs for a vaccine that already is considered costly and of marginal benefit for the cost.

A study of the vaccine's benefits and costs in Thailand showed that a national immunization program of 18-month-old infants had an effectiveness of $15,715 per case prevented and a benefit-cost ratio of 4.6:1 at the current Thai domestic production cost of $2.16 for two 0.5-mL doses.[322] A sensitivity analysis based on varying JE incidence rates showed that the program no longer was economical (where the ratio fell below 1:1) at an incidence rate of 3 per 100,000 population. In less developed countries where the prevention of lost productivity would yield lower savings, national vaccination programs would be uneconomical at higher incidence rates. Whether vaccine cost could be reduced further by economies of scale is uncertain because, unlike viral vaccines produced in cell cultures, scaling up production involves considerable labor in the rearing, inoculation, and harvesting of mice, as well as an extensive purification process.

The SA14-14-2 vaccine, produced under government subsidy in China, "costs" $0.30 per dose; however, under internationally accepted manufacturing standards, its production cost per dose will be in the same range as the inactivated mouse brain vaccine. Fewer doses are required for long-term protection, which reduces the overall costs per child protected. The vaccine is licensed in Korea and may be manufactured for international distribution in the future.[9] The principal concerns for its broader acceptance are regulatory, potential PHK adventitious agents, manufacture in GMP facilities, and safety, if administered to HIV infected persons.

REFERENCES

1. Igarashi A. Epidemiology and control of Japanese encephalitis. World Health Stat Q 45:299–305, 1992.
2. Burke DS, Leake CJ. Japanese encephalitis. In Monath TP (ed). The Arboviruses: Epidemiology and Ecology. Vol. 3. Boca Raton, FL, CRC Press, 1988, pp 63–92.
3. Umenai T, Krzysko R, Bektimirov TA, Assaad FA. Japanese encephalitis: current worldwide status. Bull World Health Organ 63:625–631, 1985.
4. Whitley RJ. Herpes simplex virus. In Fields BN, Knipe DM (eds). Virology. New York, Raven Press, 1990, pp 1843–1997.
5. Nicolosi A, Hauser VA, Beghi E, Kurland LT. Epidemiology of central nervous system infection in Olmsted County, Minnesota, 1950–1981. J Infect Dis 154:399–408, 1986.
6. Hiroyama T. Epidemiology of Japanese encephalitis [in Japanese]. Saishin-Igaku 17:1272–1280, 1962.
7. Inada R. Compte rendu des recherches sur l'encephalite epidemique au Japon. Off Int Hyg Pub Bull Mens 29:1389–1401, 1937.
8. Kuttner AG, T'sun T. Encephalitis in north China: results obtained with neutralization tests. J Clin Invest 15:525–530, 1936.
9. Sohn YM. Japanese encephalitis immunization in Korea: past, present, and future. Emerg Infect Dis 6:17–24, 2000.
10. Yu YX. Japanese encephalitis in China. Southeast Asian J Trop Med Public Health 26(suppl 3):17–21, 1995.
11. Wu YC, Chien LJ, Lin TL, et al. The epidemiology of Japanese encephalitis on Taiwan during 1966–1997. Am J Trop Med Hyg 61:78–84, 1999.
12. Grossman RA, Edelman R, Willhight M, et al. Study of Japanese encephalitis virus in Chiang Mai Valley, Thailand. Am J Epidemiol 98:133–149, 1973.
13. Chunsuttiwat S, Warachit P. Japanese encephalitis in Thailand. Southeast Asian J Trop Med Public Health 26(suppl 3):43–46, 1995.
14. Thein S, Aung H, Sebastian AA. Study of vector, amplifier, and human infection with Japanese encephalitis virus in a Rangoon community. Am J Epidemiol 128:1376–1382, 1988.
15. Nguyen HT, Nguyen TY. Japanese encephalitis in Vietnam 1985–1993. Southeast Asian J Trop Med Public Health 26(suppl 3):47–50, 1995.
16. Kari IK, Suharyono W, Jennings GB. Clinical aspects of Japanese encephalitis. Unpublished observations, Denpasar, Indonesia, 1990–1995.
17. Cardosa MJ, Hooi TP, Kaur P. Japanese encephalitis virus is an important cause of encephalitis among children in Penang. Southeast Asian J Trop Med Public Health 26:272–275, 1995.
18. Vasakarava S. Japanese encephalitis vaccine implementation in Thailand. Southeast Asian J Trop Med Public Health 26(suppl 3):54–56, 1995.
19. Carey DE, Myers RM, Reuben R, Webb JKG. Japanese encephalitis in South India: a summary of recent knowledge. J Indian Med Assoc 52:10–15, 1969.
20. Sunish IP, Reuben R. Factors influencing the abundance of Japanese encephalitis vectors in ricefields of India. I. Abiotic. Med Vet Entomol 15:381–392, 2001.
21. Igarashi A, Tanaka M, Morita K, et al. Detection of West Nile and Japanese encephalitis viral genome sequences in cerebrospinal fluid from acute encephalitis cases in Karachi, Pakistan. Microbiol Immunol 38:827–830, 1994.
22. Service MW. Agricultural development and arthropod-borne disease—a review. Revista Saúde Publica 25:165–178, 1991.
23. Joshi DD. Current status of Japanese encephalitis in Nepal. Southeast Asian J Trop Med Public Health 26:34–40, 1995.
24. Peiris JSM, Amerasinghe FP, Amerasinghe PH, et al. Japanese encephalitis in Sri Lanka: I. The study of an epidemic—vector incrimination, porcine infection, and human disease. Trans R Soc Trop Med Hyg 86:307–323, 1992.
25. Paul WS, Moore PS, Karabatsos N, et al. Outbreak of Japanese encephalitis on the island of Saipan, 1990. J Infect Dis 167:1053–1058, 1993.
26. Hanna JN, Ritchie SA, Phillips DA, et al. An outbreak of Japanese encephalitis in the Torres Strait, Australia, 1995. Med J Aust 165:256–260, 1996.
27. Halstead SB, Grosz CR. Subclinical Japanese encephalitis. I. Infection of Americans with limited residence in Korea. Am J Hyg 75:190–201, 1962.

28. Gajanana A, Thenmozhi V, Samuel P, Reuben R. A community-based study of subclinical flavivirus infections in children in an area of Tamil Nadu, India, where Japanese encephalitis is endemic. Bull World Health Organ 73:237–244, 1995.

29. Innis B. Japanese encephalitis. In Porterfield J (ed). Exotic Viral Infections. Oxford, Chapman & Hall, 1995, pp 147–174.

30. Kalayanarooj S. Japanese encephalitis: clinical manifestations, outcome and management. Southeast Asian J Trop Med Public Health 26(suppl 3):9–10, 1995.

31. Lincoln AF, Sivertson SE. Acute phase of Japanese B encephalitis: two hundred and one cases in American soldiers, Korea, 1950. JAMA 150:268–273, 1952.

32. Benenson MW, Top FH, Gresso W, et al. The virulence of Japanese B encephalitis virus in Thailand. Am J Trop Med Hyg 24:974–980, 1975.

33. Bu'lock FA. Japanese B virus encephalitis in India—a growing problem. Q J Med 233:825–836, 1986.

34. Misra UK, Kalita J. Movement disorders in Japanese encephalitis. J Neurol 244:299–303, 1997.

35. Kamala CS, Venkatwshwara Rao M, George S, Prasanna NY. Japanese encephalitis in children in Bellary Karnataka. Indian Pediatr 26:445–452, 1989.

36. Rathi AK, Kushwaha KP, Singh YD, et al. JE virus encephalitis: 1988 epidemic at Gorakhpur. Indian Pediatr 30:325–333, 1993.

37. Kumar R, Mathur A, Singh KB, et al. Clinical sequelae of Japanese encephalitis in children. Indian J Med Res 97:9–13, 1993.

38. Kumar R, Mathur A, Kumar A, et al. Clinical features and prognostic indicators of Japanese encephalitis in children in Lucknow (India). Indian J Med Res 91:321–327, 1990.

39. Hoke CH, Vaughn DW, Nisalak A, et al. Effect of high-dose dexamethasone on the outcome of acute encephalitis due to Japanese encephalitis virus. J Infect Dis 165:631–637, 1992.

40. Johnson RT, Burke DS, Elwell M, et al. Japanese encephalitis: immunocytochemical studies of viral antigen and inflammatory cells in fatal cases. Ann Neurol 18:567–573, 1985.

41. Kusuhara T, Ayabe M, Hino H, et al. Cerebrospinal fluid levels of monoamines in patients with Japanese encephalitis. Eur Neurol 36:236–237, 1996.

42. Misra UK, Kalita J. Encephalopathy with bilateral thalamotegmental lesions? Japanese encephalitis. AJNR Am J Neuroradiol 17:192–193, 1996.

43. Koelfen W, Freund M, Guckel F, et al. MRI of encephalitis in children: comparison of CT and MRI in the acute stage with long-term follow-up. Paediatr Neuroradiol 38:73–79, 1996.

44. Misra UK, Kalita J, Jain SK, Mathur A. Radiological and neurophysiological changes in Japanese encephalitis. J Neurol Neurosurg Psychiatry 57:1484–1487, 1994.

45. Kimura K, Dosaka A, Hashimoto Y, et al. Single-photon emission CT findings in acute Japanese encephalitis. AJNR Am J Neuroradiol 18:465–469, 1997.

46. Kumar R, Misra UK, Kalita J, et al. MRI in Japanese encephalitis. Neuroradiology 39:180–184, 1997.

47. Kumar R, Mathur A, Singh KB, et al. Clinical sequelae of Japanese encephalitis in children. Indian J Med Res [A] 97:9–13, 1993.

48. Schneider RJ, Firestone MH, Edelman R, et al. Clinical sequelae after Japanese encephalitis: a one-year follow-up study in Thailand. Southeast Asian J Trop Med Public Health 5:560–568, 1974.

49. Huang PJ, Huang YH, Wu PH, et al. A survey of clinical sequelae of Japanese encephalitis. Epidemiol Bull 12:19–26, 1996.

50. Weaver OM. Japanese encephalitis: clinical features. Neurology 8:887–889, 1958.

51. Pieper SJL, Kurland LT. Sequelae of Japanese B and mumps encephalitis: recent follow-up of patients affected in 1947–1948 epidemic on Guam. Am J Trop Med Hyg 7:481–490, 1958.

52. Simpson TW, Meiklejohn G. Sequelae of Japanese B encephalitis. Am J Trop Med 27:727–731, 1947.

53. Edelman R, Schneider RJ, Chieowanich P, et al. The effect of dengue virus infection on the clinical sequelae of Japanese encephalitis: a one-year follow-up study in Thailand. Southeast Asian J Trop Med Public Health 6:308–315, 1975.

54. Kumar R, Selvan AS, Sharma S, et al. Clinical predictors of Japanese encephalitis. Neuroepidemiology 13:97–102, 1994.

55. Burke DS, Lorsomrudee W, Leake CJ, et al. Fatal outcome in Japanese encephalitis. Am J Trop Med Hyg 34:1203–1210, 1985.

56. Burke DS, Morrill JC. Levels of interferon in the plasma and cerebrospinal fluid of patients with acute Japanese encephalitis. J Infect Dis 155:797–799, 1987.

57. Burke DS, Nisalak A, Ussery MA, et al. Kinetics of IgM and IgG responses to Japanese encephalitis virus in human serum and cerebrospinal fluid. J Infect Dis 151:1093–1099, 1985.

58. Ravi V, Parida S, Desai A, et al. Correlation of tumor necrosis factor levels in the serum and cerebrospinal fluid with clinical outcome in Japanese encephalitis. J Med Virol 51:132–136, 1997.

59. Desai A, Shankar SK, Jayakumar PN, et al. Co-existence of cerebral cysticercosis with Japanese encephalitis: a prognostic indicator. Epidemiol Infect 118:165–171, 1997.

60. Sharma S, Mathur A, Prakash R, et al. Japanese encephalitis virus latency in peripheral blood lymphocytes and recurrence of infection in children. Clin Exp Immunol 85:85–89, 1991.

61. Ravi V, Desai A, Shenoy PK, et al. Persistence of Japanese encephalitis virus in the human nervous system. J Med Virol 40:326–329, 1993.

62. Huy BV, Tu HC, Luan TV, Lindqvist R. Early mental and neurological sequelae after Japanese B encephalitis. Southeast Asian J Trop Med Public Health 25:549–553, 1994.

63. Ma WY, Jiang SZ, Zhang MJ, et al. Preliminary observations on treatment of patients with Japanese B encephalitis with monoclonal antibody. J Med Coll PLA 7:299–302, 1992.

64. Harinasuta C, Nimmanitya S, Titsyakorn U. The effect of interferon alpha A on two cases of Japanese encephalitis in Thailand. Southeast Asian J Trop Med Public Health 16:332–336, 1985.

65. Harrington DG, Hilmas DE, Elwell MR, et al. Intranasal infection of monkeys with Japanese encephalitis virus: clinical response and treatment with a nuclease-resistant derivative of poly(I)-poly(C). Am J Trop Med Hyg 26:1191–1198, 1977.

66. Hiyake M. The pathology of Japanese encephalitis. Bull World Health Organ 30:153–160, 1964.

67. Esiri MM, Reading MC, Squier MV, Hughes JT. Immunocytochemical characterization of the macrophage and lymphocyte infiltrate in the brain in six cases of human encephalitis of varied aetiology. Neuropathol Appl Neurobiol 15:289–305, 1989.

68. Li ZS, Hong SF, Gong NL. Immunohistochemical study of Japanese B encephalitis. Chin Med J 101:768–771, 1988.

69. Shankar SK, Rao TV, Mruthyunjayanna BP, et al. Autopsy study of brains during an epidemic of Japanese encephalitis in Karnataka. Indian J Med Res 78:431–440, 1983.

70. Zimmerman HM. The pathology of Japanese B encephalitis. Am J Pathol 22:965–991, 1946.

71. Haymaker W, Sabin AB. Topographic distribution of lesions in central nervous system in Japanese B encephalitis. Arch Neurol Psychiatry 57:673–692, 1947.

72. Desai A, Shankar SK, Ravi V, et al. Japanese encephalitis virus antigen in the human brain and its topographic distribution. Acta Neuropathol 89:368–373, 1995.

73. Ishii T, Matsushita M, Hamada S. Characteristic residual neuropathological features of Japanese B encephalitis. Acta Neuropathol (Berl) 38:181–186, 1977.

74. Burns KF. Congenital Japanese B encephalitis infection of swine. Proc Soc Exp Biol Med 75:621–625, 1950.

75. Chaturvedi UC, Mathur A, Chandra A, et al. Transplacental infection with Japanese encephalitis virus. J Infect Dis 141:712–715, 1980.

76. Mathur A, Tandon HO, Mathur KR, et al. Japanese encephalitis infection during pregnancy. Indian J Med Res 81:9–12, 1985.

77. Bhonde RR, Wagh UV. Susceptibility of human placenta to Japanese encephalitis virus in vitro. Indian J Med Res 82:371–373, 1985.

78. Ogata A, Nagashima K, Hall WW, et al. Japanese encephalitis virus neurotropism is dependent on the degree of neuronal maturity. J Virol 65:880–886, 1991.

79. Kimura-Kuroda J, Ichikawa M, Ogata A, et al. Specific tropism of Japanese encephalitis virus for developing neurons in primary rat brain culture. Arch Virol 130:477–484, 1993.

80. Kuno G, Chang G-JJ, Tsuchiya KR, et al. Phylogeny of the genus Flavivirus. J Virol 72:73–83, 1998.

81. Chambers TJ, Hahn CS, Galler R, Rice CM. Flaviviruses genome organization, expression and replication. Annu Rev Microbiol 44:649–688, 1990.

82. Murphy FA. Togavirus morphology and morphogenesis. In Schlesinger RW (ed). The Togaviruses: Biology, Structure and Replication. New York, Academic Press, 1980, pp 241–316.

83. Sumiyoshi H, Mori C, Fuke I, et al. Complete nucleotide sequence of the Japanese encephalitis virus genome RNA. Virology 161:497–510, 1987.

84. Nitayaphan S, Grant JA, Chang GJ, Trent DW. Nucleotide sequence of the virulent SA-14 strain of Japanese encephalitis virus and its attenuated vaccine derivative, SA-14-14-2. Virology 177:541–552, 1990.

85. Gollins SW, Porterfield JS. Flavivirus infection enhancement in macrophages: an electron microscopic study of viral cellular entry. J Gen Virol 66:1969–1982, 1985.

86. Hase T, Summers PL, Dubois DR. Ultrastructural changes of mouse brain neurons infected with Japanese encephalitis virus. Int J Exp Pathol 71:493–505, 1990.

87. Ng ML, Hong SS. Flavivirus infection: essential ultrastructural changes and association of Kunjin virus NS3 protein with microtubules. Arch Virol 106:103–120, 1989.

88. Westaway EG, Mackenzie JM, Kenney MT, et al. Ultrastructure of Kunjin virus–infected cells: colocalization of NS1 and NS3 with double-stranded RNA, and of NS2B with NS3, in virus-induced membrane structures. J Virol 71:6650–6661, 1997.

89. Mackenzie JM, Jones MK, Young PR. Immunolocalization of the dengue virus nonstructural glycoprotein NS1 suggests a role in viral RNA replication. Virology 220:232–240, 1996.

90. Konishi E, Mason P. Proper maturation of the Japanese encephalitis virus envelope glycoprotein requires cosynthesis with the premembrane protein. J Virol 67:1672–1675, 1993.

91. Allison SL, Stadler K, Mandl CW, et al. Synthesis and secretion of recombinant tick-borne encephalitis virus protein E in soluble and particulate form. J Virol 69:5816–5820, 1995.

92. Heinz FX, Stadler K, Püschner-Auer G, et al. Structural changes and functional control of the tick-borne encephalitis virus glycoprotein E by the heterodimeric association with protein prM. Virology 198:109–117, 1994.

93. Stadler K, Allison S, Schalich J, Heinz FX. Proteolytic activation of tick-borne encephalitis virus by furin. J Virol 71:8475–8481, 1997.

94. Mandl CW, Guirakhoo FG, Holzmann H, et al. Antigenic structure of the flavivirus envelope protein E at the molecular level, using tick-borne encephalitis virus as a model. J Virol 63:564–571, 1989.

95. Rey FA, Heinz FX, Mandl C, et al. The envelope glycoprotein from tick-borne encephalitis virus at 2 Å resolution. Nature 375:291–298, 1995.

96. Cao JX, Ni H, Wills MR, et al. Passage of Japanese encephalitis virus in HeLa cells results in attenuation of virulence in mice. J Gen Virol 76:757–764, 1995.

97. Chen Y, Maguire T, Marks RM. Demonstration of binding of dengue virus envelope protein to target cells. J Virol 70:8765–8772, 1996.

98. Chen Y, Maguire T, Hileman RE, et al. Dengue virus infectivity depends on envelope protein binding to target cell heparan sulfate. Nat Med 3:866–871, 1997.

99. Kimura T, Kimura-Kuroda J, Nagashina K, Yasui K. Analysis of virus-cell binding characteristics on the determination of Japanese encephalitis virus susceptibility. Arch Virol 139:239–251, 1994.

100. Becker Y. Computer analysis of antigenic domains and RDG-like sequences (RCW6) in the E glycoprotein of flaviviruses: an approach to vaccine development. Virus Genes 4:267–282, 1990.

101. Calisher CH, Karabatsos N, Dalrymple JM, et al. Antigenic relationships among flaviviruses as determined by cross-neutralization tests with polyclonal antisera. J Gen Virol 70:37–43, 1989.

102. Porterfield JS. The flaviviruses (group B arboviruses): a cross-neutralization study. J Gen Virol 23:91–96, 1974.

103. Wu JS, Lu CF, Lin SY. Prevalence of antibody to hepatitis C virus (anti-HVC) in different populations in Taiwan. Chung Hua Min Kuo Weishong Wu Chi Mein J Hsueh Tsa Chih 24:55–60, 1991.

104. Poidinger M, Hall RA, Mackenzie JS. Molecular characterization of the Japanese encephalitis serocomplex of the flavivirus genus. Virology 218:417–421, 1996.

105. Hasegawa T, Yoshida M, Kobayashi Y, Fujita S. Antigenic analysis of Japanese encephalitis viruses in Asian by using monoclonal antibodies. Vaccine 13:1713–1721, 1995.

106. Chen WR, Tesh RB, Rico-Hesse R. Genetic variation of Japanese encephalitis virus in nature. J Gen Virol 71:2915–2920, 1990.

107. Chen WR, Rico-Hesse R, Tesh RB. A new genotype of Japanese encephalitis virus from Indonesia. Am J Trop Med Hyg 47:61–69, 1992.

108. Huong VT, Ha QDQ, Deubel V. Genetic study of Japanese encephalitis viruses from Vietnam. Am J Trop Med Hyg 49:538–544, 1993.

109. Ma SP, Arakaki S, Makino Y, Fukunaga T. Molecular epidemiology of Japanese encephalitis virus in Okinawa. Microbiol Immunol 40:847–855, 1996.

110. Ritchie SA, Phillips D, Broom A, et al. Isolation of Japanese encephalitis virus from Culex annulirostris in Australia. Am J Trop Med Hyg 56:80–84, 1997.

111. Chung YJ, Nam JH, Ban SJ, Cho HW. Antigenic and genetic analysis of Japanese encephalitis viruses isolated from Korea. Am J Trop Med Hyg 55:91–97, 1996.

112. Uchil PD, Satchidanandam V. Phylogenetic analysis of Japanese encephalitis virus: envelope gene based analysis reveals a fifth genotype, geographic clustering, and multiple introductions of the virus into the Indian subcontinent. Am J Trop Med Hyg 65:242–251, 2001.

113. Tsarev SA, Sanders ML, Vaughn DW, Innis BL. Phylogenetic analysis suggests only one serotype of Japanese encephalitis virus. Vaccine 18(suppl 2):36–43, 2000.

114. Dropulic B, Masters CL. Entry of neurotropic arboviruses into the central nervous system: an in vitro study using mouse brain endothelium. J Infect Dis 161:685–691, 1990.

115. Hase T, Summers PL, Ray P. Entry and replication of Japanese encephalitis virus in cultured neurogenic cells. J Virol Methods 30:205–214, 1990.

116. Johnson RT, Intralawan P, Puapanwatton S. Japanese encephalitis: identification of inflammatory cells in cerebrospinal fluid. Ann Neurol 20:691–695, 1986.

117. Iwasaki Y, Sako K, Tsunoda I, Ohara Y. Phenotypes of mononuclear cell infiltrates in human central nervous system. Acta Neuropathol (Berl) 85:653–657, 1993.

118. Kiura K, Onodera T, Nishida A, et al. A single gene controls resistance to Japanese encephalitis virus in mice. Arch Virol 112:261–270, 1990.

119. Miura K, Goto N, Suzuki H, Fujisaki Y. Strain difference of mouse in susceptibility to Japanese encephalitis virus infection. Exp Anim 37:365–373, 1988.

120. Wills MR, Singh BK, Debnath NC, Barrett AD. Immunogenicity of wild-type and vaccine strains of Japanese encephalitis virus and the effect of haplotype restriction on murine immune responses. Vaccine 11:761–766, 1993.

121. Ben-Nathon D, Huitinga I, Lustig S, et al. West Nile virus neuroinvasion and encephalitis induced by macrophage depletion in mice. Arch Virol 141:459–469, 1996.

122. Sather GE, Hammon WM. Protection against St. Louis encephalitis and West Nile arboviruses by previous dengue virus (types 1–4) infection. Proc Soc Exp Biol Med 135:573–578, 1970.

123. Tarr GC, Hammon WM. Cross-protection between group B arboviruses: resistance in mice to Japanese B encephalitis and St. Louis encephalitis viruses induced by dengue virus immunization. Infect Immunol 9:909–915, 1974.

124. Edelman R, Nisalak A, Pariyanonda A, et al. Immunoglobulin response and viremia in dengue-vaccinated gibbons repeatedly challenged with Japanese encephalitis virus. Am J Epidemiol 97:208–218, 1973.

125. Goverdhan MK, Kulkarni AB, Gupta AK, et al. Two-way cross protection between West Nile and Japanese encephalitis viruses in bonnet macaques. Acta Virol 36:277–283, 1992.

126. Jia LL, Zheng Z, Yu YX. Study on the immune mechanism of JE attenuated live vaccine (SA-14-14-2 strain). Chin J Immunol Microbiol 12:364–366, 1992.

127. Nathanson N, Cole GA. Fatal Japanese encephalitis virus infection in immunosuppressed spider monkeys. Clin Exp Immunol 6:161–166, 1970.

128. Gould EA, Buckley A. Antibody-dependent enhancement of yellow fever and Japanese encephalitis virus neurovirulence. J Gen Virol 70:1605–1608, 1989.

129. Ghosh SN, Prasad SR, Thakare JP, et al. Evidence for synthesis of immunoglobulins within central nervous system of Japanese encephalitis cases. Indian J Med Res 86:276–283, 1987.

130. Burke DS, Nisalak A, Lorsomrudee W, et al. Virus-specific antibody-producing cells in blood and cerebrospinal fluid in acute Japanese encephalitis. J Med Virol 17:283–292, 1985.

131. Konishi E, Kurane I, Mason PW, et al. Japanese encephalitis virus-specific proliferative responses of human peripheral blood T lymphocytes. Am J Trop Med Hyg 53:278–283, 1995.

132. Desai A, Ravi V, Chandramuki A, Gourie-Devi M. Proliferative response of human peripheral blood mononuclear cells to Japanese encephalitis virus. Microbiol Immunol 39:269–273, 1995.

133. Desai A, Ravi V, Guru SC, et al. Detection of autoantibodies to neural antigens in the CSF of Japanese encephalitis patients and correlation of findings with the outcome. J Neurol Sci 122:109–116, 1994.

134. Desai A, Ravi V, Chandremuki A, Gourie-Devi M. Detection of immune complexes in the CSF of Japanese encephalitis patients: correlation of findings with outcome. Intervirology 37:352–355, 1994.

135. Lad VJ, Gupta AK, Goverdhan MK, et al. Susceptibility of BL6 nude (congenitally athymic) mice to Japanese encephalitis virus by the peripheral route. Acta Virol 37:232–240, 1993.

136. Murali-Krishna K, Ravi V, Manjunath R. Protection of adult but not newborn mice against lethal intracerebral challenge with Japanese encephalitis virus by adoptively transferred virus-specific cytotoxic T lymphocytes: requirement for L3T4+ cells. J Gen Virol 77:705–714, 1996.

137. Yu YX, Wang JF, Zheng GM, Li HM. Response of normal and athymic mice to infection by virulent and attenuated Japanese encephalitis viruses. Chin J Virol 1:203–209, 1985.

138. Jia LL, Zheng Z, Yu YX. Pathogenicity and immunogenicity of attenuated Japanese encephalitis vaccine (SA14-14-2) in immune-inhibited mice. Virol Sinica 8:20–24, 1993.

139. Monath TP, Borden EC. Effects of thorotrast on humoral antibody, viral multiplication and interferon during infections with St. Louis encephalitis virus in mice. J Infect Dis 123:297–300, 1971.

140. Brooks TJ, Phillpotts RJ. Interferon-alpha protects mice against lethal infection with St. Louis encephalitis virus delivered by aerosol and subcutaneous routes. Antiviral Res 41:57–64, 1999.

141. Lin Y, Huang Y, Ma S, et al. Inhibition of Japanese encephalitis virus infection by nitric oxide: antiviral effect of nitric oxide on RNA virus replication. J Virol 71:5227–5235, 1997.

142. Kreil T, Eibl MM. Nitric oxide and viral infection: no antiviral activity against a flavivirus in vitro, and evidence for contribution to pathogenesis in experimental infection in vivo. Virology 219:304–306, 1996.

143. Khanna N, Mathur A, Chaturvedi UC. Regulation of vascular permeability by macrophage-derived chemotactic factor produced in Japanese encephalitis. Immunol Cell Biol 72:200–204, 1994.

144. Liu YF, Teng CL, Liu K. Cerebral cysticercosis as a factor aggravating Japanese B encephalitis. Chin Med J 75:1010–1017, 1957.

145. Das SK, Nityanand S, Sood K. Japanese B encephalitis with neurocysticercosis. J Assoc Physicians India 39:643–644, 1991.

146. Hayashi K, Arita T. Experimental double infection of Japanese encephalitis virus and herpes simplex virus in mouse brain. Jpn J Exp Med 47:9–13, 1977.

147. Gutierrez K, Abzug MJ. Vaccine-associated poliovirus meningitis in children with ventriculoperitoneal shunts. J Pediatr 117:424–427, 1990.

148. Lange DG, Sedmak J. Japanese encephalitis virus (JEV): potentiation of lethality in mice by microwave radiation. Bioelectromagnetics 12:335–348, 1991.

149. Okhuysen PC, Crane JK, Pappas J. St. Louis encephalitis in patients with human immunodeficiency virus infection. Clin Infect Dis 17:140–141, 1993.

150. Kedarnath N, Prasad SR, Dandawate CN, et al. Isolation of Japanese encephalitis and West Nile viruses from peripheral blood of encephalitis patients. Indian J Med Res 79:1–7, 1984.

151. Gajanana A, Samuel PP, Thenmozhi V, Rajendran R. An appraisal of some recent diagnostic assays for Japanese encephalitis. Southeast Asian J Trop Med Public Health 27:673–679, 1996.

152. Innis BL, Nisalak A, Nimmannitya S, et al. An enzyme-linked immunosorbent assay to characterize dengue infections where dengue and Japanese encephalitis cocirculate. Am J Trop Med Hyg 40:418–427, 1989.

153. Meiyu F, Huosheng C, Cuihua C, et al. Detection of flaviviruses by reverse transcriptase-polymerase chain reaction with the universal primer set. Microbiol Immunol 41:209–213, 1997.

154. Burke DS, Nisalak A, Gentry MK. Detection of flavivirus antibodies in human serum by epitope-blocking immunoassay. J Med Virol 23:165–173, 1987.

155. Konishi E, Mason PW, Shope RE. Enzyme-linked immunosorbent assay using recombinant antigens for serodiagnosis of Japanese encephalitis. J Med Virol 48:76–79, 1996.

156. Rosen L. The natural history of Japanese encephalitis virus. Annu Rev Microbiol 40:395–414, 1986.

157. Scherer WF, Buescher EL. Ecologic studies of Japanese encephalitis virus in Japan. I. Introduction. Am J Trop Med Hyg 8:644–650, 1959.

158. Gould DJ, Byrne RJ, Hayes DE. Experimental infection of horses with Japanese encephalitis virus by mosquito bite. Am J Trop Med Hyg 13:742–746, 1964.

159. Wang YJ, Gu PW, Liu PS. Japanese B encephalitis virus infection of horses during the first epidemic season following entry into an infected area. Chin Med J 95:63–66, 1982.

160. Min JG, Xue M. Progress in studies on the overwintering of the mosquito Culex tritaeniorhynchus. Southeast Asian J Trop Med Public Health 27:810–817, 1996.

161. Hammon WM, Tigertt WD, Sather GE. Epidemiologic studies of concurrent "virgin" epidemics of Japanese B encephalitis and of mumps on Guam, 1947–1948, with subsequent observations including dengue, through 1957. Am J Trop Med Hyg 7:441–467, 1958.

162. Ritchie SA, Rochester W. Wind-blown mosquitoes and introduction of Japanese encephalitis. Emerging Infect Dis 7:900–903, 2001.

163. Olson JG, Atmosoedjono S, Lee VH, Ksiazek TG. Correlation between population indices of Culex tritaeniorhynchus and Cx. gelidus (Diptera: Culicidae) and rainfall in Kapuk, Indonesia. J Med Entomol 20:108–109, 1983.

164. Phanthumachinda B. Ecology and biology of Japanese encephalitis. Southeast Asian J Trop Med Public Health 2653:11–16, 1995.

165. Soman RS, Rodrigues FM, Guttikar SN, Guru PY. Experimental viraemia and transmission of Japanese encephalitis virus by mosquitoes in ardeid birds. Indian J Med Res 66:709–718, 1977.

166. Ilkal MA, Dhanda V, Rao BU, et al. Absence of viraemia in cattle after experimental infection with Japanese encephalitis. Trans R Soc Trop Med Hyg 82:628–631, 1988.

167. Takahashi K, Matsuo R, Kuma M, et al. Use of vaccine in pigs. A. Effect of immunization of swine upon the ecological cycle of Japanese encephalitis virus. In Hammon WM, Kitaoka M, Downs WG (eds). Immunization for Japanese Encephalitis. Amsterdam, Excerpta Medica, 1972, pp 292–303.

168. Sasaki O, Karoji Y, Kuroda A, et al. Protection of pigs against mosquito-borne Japanese encephalitis virus by immunization with a live attenuated vaccine. Antiviral Res 2:355–360, 1982.

169. Vaughn DW, Hoke CH. The epidemiology of Japanese encephalitis: prospects for prevention. Epidemiol Rev 14:197–221, 1992.

170. Gajanana A, Rajendran R, Samuel PP, et al. Japanese encephalitis in south Arcot District, Tamil Nadu: a three-year longitudinal study of vector density and vector infection frequency. J Med Entomol 34:651–659, 1997.

171. Chaudhuri N, Shaw BP, Mondal KC, Maity CR. Epidemiology of Japanese encephalitis. Indian Pediatr 297:861–865, 1992.

172. Dapeng L, Konghua Z, Jinduo S, et al. The protective effects of bed nets impregnated with pyrethroid insecticide and vaccination against Japanese encephalitis. Trans R Soc Trop Med Hyg 88:632–634, 1994.

173. Xu YH, Zhaori GT, Vene S, et al. Viral etiology of acute childhood encephalitis in Beijing diagnosed by analysis of single samples. Pediatr Infect Dis J 15:1018–1024, 1996.

174. Goh KT. Vaccines for Japanese encephalitis. Lancet 348:340, 1996.

175. Oya A. Epidemiology of Japanese encephalitis. Rinsho to Biseibutsu 16:5–9, 1989.

176. Chang KY, Tseng TC. Seroepidemiological investigation on Japanese encephalitis in Taiwan. Chin J Microbiol Immunol 26:25–37, 1993.

177. Matsuda S. An epidemiologic study of Japanese B encephalitis with special reference to the effectiveness of vaccination. Bull Inst Public Health 11:173–190, 1962.

178. Tsai TF, Chang G-JJ, Yu XY, et al. Japanese Encephalitis. In Plotkin SA, Orenstein WA (eds). Vaccines (3rd ed). Philadelphia, WB Saunders, 1999.

179. Buhl MR, Black FT, Andersen PL, Laursen A. Fatal Japanese encephalitis in a Danish tourist visiting Bali for 12 days. Scand J Infect Dis 28:189, 1996.

180. MacDonald WBG, Tink AR, Ouvrier RA, et al. Japanese encephalitis after a two-week holiday in Bali. Med J Aust 150:334–336, 1989.

181. Rose MR, Hughes SM, Gatus BJ. A case of Japanese B encephalitis imported into the United Kingdom. J Infect 6:261–265, 1983.

182. Poland JD, Cropp CB, Craven RB, Monath TP. Evaluation of the potency and safety of inactivated Japanese encephalitis vaccine in U.S. inhabitants. J Infect Dis 161:878–882, 1990.

183. Berg SW, Mitchell BS, Hanson RK, et al. Systemic reactions in US Marine Corps personnel who received Japanese encephalitis vaccine. J Infect Dis 24:265–266, 1997.

184. Ognibene AJ. Japanese B encephalitis. *In* Ognibene AJ, Barrett O (eds). Internal Medicine in Vietnam: General Medicine and Infectious Diseases. Washington, DC, U.S. Army Office of the Surgeon General and Center for Military History, 1982, pp 534–551.

185. Pond WL, Smadel JE. Neurotropic viral diseases in the Far East during the Korean War (Army Medical Science Graduate School Medical Science Publ No 4). Recent Adv Med Surg 2:219–233, 1954.

186. Sabin AB. Encephalitis. U.S. Army Med Dept Bull 7:9–21, 1947.

187. Sabin AB, Schlesinger RW, Ginder DR, Matumoto M. Japanese B encephalitis in American Soldiers in Korea. Am J Hyg 46:356–375, 1947.

188. Long AP, Hullinghorst RL, Gauld RL. Japanese B encephalitis—Korea 1950 (Army Medical Science Graduate School Medical Science Publ No 4). Recent Adv Med Surg 2:317–329, 1954.

189. Tsai TF, Niklasson B, Goujon C. Arboviruses and zoonotic viruses. *In* Dupont HL, Steffen R (eds). Textbook of Travel Medicine and Health. Hamilton, Ontario, Canada, BC Decker, 1997, pp 200–214.

190. Centers for Disease Control and Prevention. CDC Health Information for International Travel, 1996–1997. Atlanta, Centers for Disease Control and Prevention, 1996, pp 112–116.

191. Zhang M, Wang M, Jiang S, Ma W. Passive protection of mice, goats, and monkeys against Japanese encephalitis with monoclonal antibodies. J Med Virol 29:133–138, 1989.

192. Ohyama A, Ishiga A, Fujita N, et al. Effect of human gamma globulin upon encephalitis viruses. Jpn J Microbiol 3:159–169, 1959.

193. Lubiniecki AS, Cypess RH, Hammon WM. Passive immunity of arbovirus infection. II. Quantitative aspects of naturally and artificially acquired protection in mice for Japanese (B) encephalitis virus. Am J Trop Med Hyg 22:535–542, 1973.

194. Waldvogel K, Bossart W, Huisman T, et al. Severe tickborne encephalitis following passive immunization. Eur J Pediatr 155:775–779, 1996.

195. Oya A. Japanese encephalitis vaccine. Acta Pediatr Jpn 30:175–184, 1988.

196. Gu PW, Ding ZF. Inactivated Japanese encephalitis (JE) vaccine made from hamster cell culture [review]. JE HFRS Bull 2:15–26, 1987.

197. Smorodintsev AA, Shubladse AK, Neustroer VD. Etiology of autumn encephalitis in the Far East of the USSR. Arch Ges Virus Forsch 1:549–559, 1940.

198. Sabin AB, Duffy CE. Antibody response of human beings to centrifuged, lyophilized Japanese B encephalitis vaccine. Proc Soc Exp Med Biol 65:123–126, 1947.

199. Sabin AB. Antibody response of people of different ages to two doses of uncentrifuged, Japanese B encephalitis vaccine. Proc Soc Exp Med Biol 65:127–135, 1947.

200. Sabin AB, Ginder DR, Matumoto M, Schlesinger RW. Serological response of Japanese children and old people to Japanese B encephalitis mouse brain vaccine. Proc Soc Exp Med Biol 65:135–139, 1947.

201. Sabin AB. Epidemic encephalitis in military personnel: isolation of Japanese B virus on Okinawa in 1945, serologic diagnosis, clinical manifestations, epidemiologic aspects, and use of mouse brain vaccine. JAMA 133:281–293, 1947.

202. Smadel JE, Randall R, Warren J. Preparation of Japanese encephalitis vaccine. U.S. Army Med Dept Bull 7:963–973, 1947.

203. Sabin AB, Tigertt WD. Evaluation of Japanese B encephalitis vaccine. I. General background and methods. Am J Hyg 63:217–227, 1956.

204. Ando K, Satterwhite JP. Evaluation of Japanese B encephalitis vaccine. III. Okayama field trial, 1946–1949. Am J Hyg 63:230–237, 1956.

205. Tigertt WD, Hammon WM, Berge TO, et al. Japanese B encephalitis: a complete review of experience on Okinawa 1945–1949. Am J Trop Med 30:689–722, 1950.

206. Tigertt WD, Berge TO, Burns KF, Satterwhite JP. Evaluation of Japanese B encephalitis vaccine. IV. Pattern of serologic response to vaccination over a five-year period in an endemic area (Okayama, Japan). Am J Hyg 63:238–249, 1956.

207. Kanamitsu M, Hashimoto N, Urasawa S, et al. A field trial with an improved Japanese encephalitis vaccine in a nonendemic area of the disease. Biken J 13:313–328, 1970.

208. Takaku K, Yamashita T, Osanai T, et al. Japanese encephalitis purified vaccine. Biken J 11:25–39, 1968.

209. Shope RE. The potency test for inactivated Japanese encephalitis (JE) vaccines. JE HFRS Bull 2:27–32, 1987.

210. World Health Organization. Requirements for Japanese encephalitis vaccine (inactivated) for human use. World Health Organ Tech Rep Ser 77:1133–1156, 1988.

211. Gowal D, Singh G, Rao Bhau LN, Saxena SN. Thermostability of Japanese encephalitis vaccine produced in India. Biologicals 19:37–40, 1990.

212. Fukunaga T, Rojanasuphot S, Wungkorbkiat S, et al. Japanese encephalitis vaccination in Thailand. Biken J 17:21–31, 1974.

213. Kobayashi Y, Hasegawa H, Oyama T, et al. Antigenic analysis of Japanese encephalitis virus by using monoclonal antibodies. Infect Immunol 44:117–123, 1984.

214. Hashimoto H, Nomoto A, Watanabe K, et al. Molecular cloning and complete nucleotide sequence of the genome of Japanese encephalitis virus Beijing-1 strain. Virus Genes 1:305–317, 1988.

215. Kitano T, Yabe S, Kobayashi M, et al. Immunogenicity of JE Nakayama and Beijing-1 vaccines. JE HFRS Bull 1:37–41, 1986.

216. Kitano T. Immunogenicity and field trial of Beijing-1 vaccine. Osaka, Japan, Working Group on Vaccine Development and Vaccination Strategies for Japanese Encephalitis, 1985, pp 1–8.

217. Japanese encephalitis vaccine lyophilized, "Biken." Unpublished report, Research Foundation for Microbial Diseases of Osaka University, Osaka, Japan, 1991, pp 1–149.

218. Huang CH. Studies of virus factors as causes of inapparent infection in Japanese B encephalitis: virus strains, viraemia, stability to heat and infective dosage. Acta Virol 1:36–45, 1957.

219. Huang CH. Studies of Japanese encephalitis in China. Adv Virus Res 27:71–101, 1982.

220. Kitano T. Field trial of inactivated JE Beijing vaccine in Japan. Osaka, Japan, Working Group on Japanese Encephalitis Vaccines, 1987, pp 1–5.

221. Rojanasuphot S, Nachiangmai P, Srijaggrawalong A, Nimmannitya S. Implementation of simultaneous Japanese encephalitis vaccine in the expanded program of immunization of infants. Mosquito-Borne Dis Bull 9:86–92, 1992.

222. Gambel JM, DeFraites R, Hoke C, et al. Japanese encephalitis vaccine: persistence of antibody up to 3 years after a three-dose primary series. J Infect Dis 171:1074, 1995.

223. Henderson A. Immunization against Japanese encephalitis in Nepal: experience of 1152 subjects. J R Army Med Corps 130:188–191, 1984.

224. Sanchez JL, Hoke CH, McCowan J, et al. Further experience with Japanese encephalitis vaccine. Lancet 335:972–973, 1990.

225. Inactivated Japanese encephalitis virus vaccine: recommendations of the Immunization Practices Advisory Committee (ACIP). MMWR 42(RR-1):1–15, 1993.

226. Tseng CY, Hwang KP, Lin KH, et al. Comparison of immunogenicity of simultaneous and nonsimultaneous vaccination with MMR and JE vaccine among 15-month-old children. Acta Paediatr Sin 40:162–165, 1999.

227. Intralawan P, Paupunwatana S. Immunogenicity of low dose Japanese encephalitis vaccine (BIKEN) administered by the intradermal route: preliminary data. Asian Pacific J Allergy Immunol 11:79–83, 1993.

228. Lee CYG, Grayston JT, Kenny GE. Growth of Japanese encephalitis virus in cell culture. J Infect Dis 115:321–329, 1965.

229. Zhang XC, Nie SX, Din CS, Wang MJ. Observations on the efficacy of inactivated Japanese encephalitis vaccine in combination with other vaccines. Chin J Public Health 6:203, 1990.

230. Inoue YK. An attenuated mutant of Japanese encephalitis virus. Bull World Health Organ 30:181–185, 1964.

231. Yoshida I, Takagi M, Inokuma E, et al. Establishment of an attenuated ML-17 strain of Japanese encephalitis virus. Biken J 24:47–67, 1981.

232. Kodama K, Sasaki N, Inoue YK. Studies of live attenuated Japanese encephalitis vaccine in swine. J Immunol 100:194–200, 1968.

233. Hammon WM, Darwish MA, Rhim JS, et al. Studies on Japanese B encephalitis virus vaccines from tissue culture. V. Response of man to live, attenuated strain of OCT541 virus vaccine. J Immunol 96:518–524, 1966.

234. Ni H, Barrett A. Attenuation of Japanese encephalitis virus by selection of its mouse brain membrane receptor preparation escape variants. Virology 241:30–36, 1998.

235. Yu YX, Ao J, Chu YG, et al. Studies on variation of JE virus V. Biological characteristics of the attenuated vaccine strain. Acta Microbiol Sin 13:16–24, 1973.

236. Yu YX, Fang C, Wu PF, Li HM. Studies on the variation of JE virus VI. The changes in virulence and immunity after passaging subcutaneously in suckling mice. Acta Microbiol Sin 15:133–138, 1975.

237. Yu YX, Wu PF, Ao J, et al. Selection of a better immunogenic and highly attenuated live vaccine virus strain of JE. I. Some biological characteristics of SA14-14-2 mutant. Chin J Microbiol Immunol 1:77–84, 1981.

238. Ao J, Yu Y, Tang YS, et al. Selection of a better immunogenic and highly attenuated live vaccine strain of Japanese encephalitis. II. Safety and immunogenicity of live JBE vaccine SA14-14-2 observed in inoculated children. Chin J Microbiol Immunol 3:245–248, 1983.

239. Yu YX, Zhang GM, Guo YP, et al. Safety of a live-attenuated Japanese encephalitis virus vaccine (SA14-14-2) for children. Am J Trop Med Hyg 39:214–217, 1988.

240. Wang SG, Yang HJ, Den YY, et al. Studies on the production of SA14-2 Japanese encephalitis live vaccine. Chin J Virol 6:38–43, 1990.

241. Yu YX, Zhang GM, Zheng Z. Studies on the immunogenicity of live and killed Japanese encephalitis (JE) vaccines to challenge with different Japanese encephalitis virus strains. Chin J Virol 5:106–110, 1989.

242. Wills MR, Sil BK, Cao JX, et al. Antigenic characterization of the live attenuated Japanese encephalitis vaccine virus SA14-14-2: a comparison with isolates of the virus covering a wide geographic area. Vaccine 10:861–872, 1992.

243. Sil BK, Wills MR, Cao JX. Immunogenicity of experimental live attenuated Japanese encephalitis vaccine viruses and comparison with wild-type strains using monoclonal and polyclonal antibodies. Vaccine 10:329–333, 1992.

244. Hase T, Dubois DR, Summers PL, et al. Comparison of replication rates and pathogenicities between the SA14 parent and SA14-14-2 vaccine strains of Japanese encephalitis virus in mouse brain neurons. Arch Virol 130:131–143, 1993.

245. Jia LL, Zhong Z, Yu YX. Study on the stability of viral strains of live-attenuated Japanese encephalitis vaccine. Chin J Biol 5:174–176, 1992.

246. Eckels KH, Yu XY, Dubois DR, et al. Japanese encephalitis virus live-attenuated vaccine, Chinese strain SA14-14-2: adaptation to primary canine kidney cell cultures and preparation of a vaccine for human use. Vaccine 6:513–518, 1988.

247. Regional Antiepidemic Station, Hueyang, Guangtong. Preliminary observation on epidemiological effectiveness of JE live vaccine. Bull Biol Prod 7:111–114, 1978.

248. Ling JP, Zhu YG, Du GZ, et al. Comparative susceptibilities of rhesus monkeys and mice to Japanese encephalitis virus. Unpublished report, Institute for Control of Pharmaceutical and Biological Products, Beijing, China, 1996.

249. Jia LL, Zheng Z, Wang SW, Yu YX. Protective effects and antibody responses in guinea pigs immunized with Japanese encephalitis live-attenuated vaccine SA14-14-2 after challenge with virulent JE virus. Prog Microbiol Immunol (China) 23:73–75, 1995.

250. Ni H, Chang GJ, Xie H, et al. Molecular basis of attenuation of neurovirulence of wild-type Japanese encephalitis virus strain SA14. J Gen Virol 76:409–413, 1995.

251. Ni HL, Barrett ADT. Molecular differences between wild-type Japanese encephalitis virus strains of high and low mouse neuroinvasiveness. J Gen Virol 77:1449–1455, 1996.

252. Aihara S, Rao CM, Yu YX. Identification of mutations that occurred on the genome of Japanese encephalitis virus during the attenuation process. Virus Genes 5:95–109, 1991.

253. Cecilia D, Gould EA. Nucleotide changes responsible for loss of neuroinvasiveness in Japanese encephalitis virus neutralization-resistant mutants. Virology 181:707, 1991.

254. Hasegawa H, Yoshida M, Shiosaka T, et al. Mutations in the envelope protein of Japanese encephalitis virus affect entry into cultured cells and virulence in mice. Virology 191:158–165, 1992.

255. Chen BQ, Beaty BJ. Japanese encephalitis vaccine (28 strain) and parent (SA 14 strain) viruses in Culex tritaeniorhynchus mosquitoes. Am J Trop Med Hyg 31:403–407, 1982.

256. Ao J, Yu YX, Wu PF, Zhang GM. Further observations on JBE attenuated live vaccines used for prevention of stillbirths in swine. Acta Microbiol Sin 21:174–179, 1981.

257. Tsai TF, Yu YX, Jia LL, et al. Immunogenicity of live attenuated SA14-14-2 Japanese encephalitis vaccine—a comparison of 1- and 3-month immunization schedules. J Infect Dis 177:221–223, 1998.

258. Chambers TJ, Tsai TF, Pervikov Y, Monath TP. Vaccine development against dengue and Japanese encephalitis: report of a World Health Organization meeting. Vaccine 15:1494–1502, 1997.

259. Tsai TF. New initiatives for the control of Japanese encephalitis by vaccination: minutes of a WHO/CVI meeting, Bangkok, Thailand, 13–15 October 1998. Vaccine 18(suppl):1–25, 2000.

260. Kanesa-thasan N, Smucny JJ, Hoke CH, et al. Safety and immunogenicity of NYVAC-JEV and ALVAC-JEV attenuated recombinant Japanese encephalitis virus-poxvirus vaccines in vaccinia-nonimmune and vaccinia-immune humans. Vaccine 19:483–491, 2000.

261. Srivastava AK, Putnak JR, Lee SH, et al. A purified inactivated Japanese encephalitis virus vaccine made in Vero cells. Vaccine 19:4557–4465, 2001.

262. Sumiyoshi H, Tignor GH, Shope RE. Characterization of a highly attenuated Japanese encephalitis virus generated from molecularly cloned cDNA. J Infect Dis 171:1144–1151, 1995.

263. Fuijta H, Sumiyoshi H, Mori C, et al. Studies in the development of Japanese encephalitis vaccine: expression of virus envelope glycoprotein V3 (E) gene in yeast. Bull World Health Organ 65:303–308, 1987.

264. McCown J, Cochran M, Putnak R, et al. Protection of mice against lethal Japanese encephalitis with a recombinant baculovirus vaccine. Am J Trop Med Hyg 42:491–499, 1990.

265. Srivastava AK, Morita K, Igarishi A. Immunogenicity of Japanese encephalitis virus envelope glycoprotein E prepared by four different methods. Trop Med 32:103–113, 1990.

266. Jan LR, Yang CS, Henchal LS, et al. Increased immunogenicity and protective efficacy in outbred and inbred mice by strategic carboxyl-terminal truncation of Japanese encephalitis virus envelope glycoprotein. Am J Trop Med Hyg 48:412–423, 1993.

267. Hirabayashi Y, Fukuda H, Kimura J, et al. Identification of peptides mimicking the antigenicity and immunogenicity on Japanese encephalitis virus protein using synthetic peptide libraries. J Virol Methods 61:23–26, 1996.

268. Konishi E, Win KS, Kurane I, et al. Particulate vaccine candidate for Japanese encephalitis induces long-lasting virus-specific memory T lymphocytes in mice. Vaccine 15:281–286, 1997.

269. Pugachev K, Mason PW, Frey TK. Sindbis vectors suppress secretion of subviral particles of Japanese encephalitis virus from mammalian cells infected with SIN-JEV recombinants. Virology 209:155–166, 1995.

270. Yeolekar LR, Banerjee K. Immunogenicity of immunostimulating complexes of Japanese encephalitis virus in experimental animals. Acta Virol 40:245–250, 1996.

271. Eldridge JH, Hammond CJ, Meulbroek HA, et al. Controlled vaccine release in the gut-associated lymphoid tissues. I. Orally administered biodegradable microspheres target the Peyer's patches. J Controlled Release 11:205–214, 1990.

272. Barrett AD. Current status of flavivirus vaccines. Ann N Y Acad Sci 951:262–271, 2001.

273. Chen HW, Pan CH, Liau MY, et al. Screening of protective antigens of Japanese encephalitis virus by DNA immunization: a comparative study with conventional viral vaccines. J Virol 73:10137–10145, 1999.

274. Ashok MS, Rangarajam PN. Evaluation of the potency of BIKEN inactivated Japanese encephalitis vaccine and DNA vaccines in an intracerebral Japanese encephalitis virus challenge. Vaccine 15:155–157, 2000.

275. Chang JG, Hunt AR, Davis B. A single intramuscular injection of recombinant plasmid DNA induces protective immunity and prevents Japanese encephalitis in mice. J Virol 74:4244–4252, 2000.

276. Monath TP, Soike K, Levenbook I, et al. Recombinant, chimeric live attenuated vaccine (ChimeriVax) incorporating the envelope genes of Japanese encephalitis (SA14-14-2) virus and the capsid and nonstructural genes of yellow fever (17D) virus is safe, immunogenic and protective in non-human primates. Vaccine 17:1869–1882, 1999.

277. Arroyo J, Guirakhoo F, Fenner S, et al. Molecular basis for attenuation of neurovirulence of a yellow fever virus/Japanese encephalitis virus chimera vaccine (ChimeriVax-JE). J Virol 75:934–942, 2001.

278. Monath TP, Levenbook I, Soike K, et al. Chimeric yellow fever virus 17D-Japanese encephalitis virus vaccine: dose response effectiveness and extended safety testing in rhesus monkeys. J Virol 74:1742–1751, 2000.

279. Raengsakulrach B, Nisalak A, Gettayacamin M, et al. An intranasal challenge model for testing Japanese encephalitis vaccines in rhesus monkeys. Am J Trop Med Hyg 60:329–337, 1999.

280. Bhatt TR, Crabtree MB, Guirakhoo F, et al. Growth characteristics of the chimeric Japanese encephalitis virus vaccine candidate, ChimeriVax JE (YF/JE SA 14-14-2), in Culex tritaeniorhynchus, Aedes albopictus and Aedes aegypti mosquitoes. Am J Trop Med Hyg 62:480–484, 2000.

281. Monath TP, McCarthy K, Bedford P, et al. Clinical proof of principle for ChimeriVax: recombinant, live attenuated vaccines against flavivirus infections. Vaccine 20:1004–1018, 2002.

282. Rojanasuphot S, Charoensook OA, Ungchusak K, et al. A field trial on inactivated mouse brain Japanese encephalitis vaccines produced in Thailand. Mosquito-Borne Dis Bull 8:11–16, 1991.

283. Wu YC. Neutralizing antibody responses to Nakayama and Beijing strain JE vaccine in children of Taipei City, 1993–1994. Unpublished report, National Institute of Preventive Medicine, Taipei, Taiwan, 1994.

284. Nimmannitya S, Hutami S, Kalayanarooj S, Rojanasuphot S. A field study on Nakayama and Beijing strains of Japanese encephalitis vaccines. Southeast Asian J Trop Med Public Health 26:689–693, 1995.

285. Susilowati S, Okuno Y, Fukunaga T, et al. Neutralization antibody responses induced by Japanese encephalitis virus vaccine. Biken J 24:137–145, 1981.

286. Okuno Y, Okamoto Y, Yamada A, et al. Effect of current Japanese encephalitis vaccine on different strains of Japanese encephalitis virus. Vaccine 5:128–132, 1987.

287. Juang RF, Okuno Y, Fukunaga T, et al. Neutralizing antibody responses to Japanese encephalitis vaccine in children. Biken J 26:25–34, 1983.

288. Ku CC, King CC, Lin DY, et al. Homologous and heterologous neutralization antibody responses after immunization with Japanese encephalitis vaccine among Taiwan children. Med Virol 44:122–131, 1994.

289. Hoke CH, Nisalak A, Sangawhipa N, et al. Protection against Japanese encephalitis by inactivated vaccines. N Engl J Med 319:608–614, 1988.

290. Kayser M, Klein H, Paasch I, et al. Human antibody response to immunization with 17D yellow fever and inactivated TBE vaccine. J Med Virol 17:35–45, 1985.

291. Rojanasuphot S, Shaffer N, Chotpitayasunondh T, et al. Response to Japanese encephalitis vaccine among HIV-infected children, Bangkok, Thailand. Southeast Asian J Trop Med Public Health 29:443–450, 1998.

292. Yamada A, Imanishi J, Juang RF, et al. Trial of inactivated Japanese encephalitis vaccine in children with underlying diseases. Vaccine 4:32–34, 1986.

293. Hsu TC, Chow LP, Wei HY, et al. A controlled field trial for an evaluation of effectiveness of mouse-brain Japanese encephalitis vaccine. J Formosa Med Assoc 70:55–61, 1971.

294. Okuno T, Tseng PT, Hsu ST, et al. Japanese encephalitis surveillance in China (province of Taiwan) during 1958–1971. II. Age-specific incidence in connection with Japanese encephalitis vaccination program. Jpn J Med Sci Biol 28:255–267, 1975.

295. Hsu TC, Chow LP, Wei HY, et al. A completed field trial for an evaluation of the effectiveness of mouse-brain Japanese encephalitis vaccine. In Hammon WMcD, Kitaoka M, Downs WG (eds). Immunization for Japanese Encephalitis. Amsterdam, Excerpta Medica, 1972, pp 285–291.

296. Gowal D, Tahlan AK. Evaluation of effectiveness of mouse brain inactivated Japanese encephalitis vaccine produced in India. Indian J Med Res 102:267–271, 1995.

297. National Vaccine and Serum Institute, An Yang Municipal Health Station, Jiangsu Provincial Health Station, et al. Effectiveness of the Japanese B encephalitis inactivated vaccine of hamster kidney cell culture type. Acta Microbiol Sin 16:48–53, 1976.

298. Wang SG, Yang HJ, Den YY, et al. Improved inactivated Japanese encephalitis vaccine produced in primary hamster kidney cells.

299. National Serum and Biologics Institute, Hebei Health Station, Funien County Health Station. Biol Prod Comm 8:283–285, 1979.

299. National Serum and Biologics Institute, Jiling Yang Gi Health Station. Studies on immunization schedules for Japanese encephalitis vaccine. Chin J Prev Med 6:360–363, 1981.

300. Ren YL. Biol Prod Comm (Chinese) 7:111, 1978. Cited in Huang CH. Studies of Japanese encephalitis in China. Adv Virus Res 27:72–101, 1982.

301. Luo DP, Yin HJ, Liu XL, et al. The efficacy of Japanese encephalitis vaccine in Henan, China: a case-control study. Southeast Asian J Trop Med Public Health 25:643–646, 1994.

302. Ao G, Yu YX, Wu PF, et al. Studies on mutation of Japanese B encephalitis virus. VII. An observation of persistence of immunity in children inoculated with JBE attenuated live vaccine (SA-14-5-3 mutant). Acta Microbiol Sin 21:501–505, 1981.

303. Jia LL, Yu YX, Zheng Z. Neutralizing antibody response of Japanese encephalitis live vaccine in children residing in JE endemic area. Chin J Zoonoses 11:343–344, 1995.

304. Report on epidemiologic results of lyophilized Japanese encephalitis vaccine. Unpublished report, Chengdu Biologics Institute, Chengdu, PRC,1991.

305. Wang JL, Na JC, Zhao SS, et al. An epidemiologic study of the efficacy of live Japanese encephalitis vaccine. Chin J Biol 6:36–37, 1993.

306. Hennessy S, Liu ZL, Tsai TF, et al. Effectiveness of live-attenuated Japanese encephalitis vaccine (SA14-14-2): a case-control study. Lancet 347:1583–1586, 1996.

307. Bista MB, Banerjee MK, Shin SH, et al. Efficacy of single-dose SA 14-14-2 vaccine against Japanese encephalitis: a case-control study. Lancet 358:791–795, 2001.

308. Kitaoka M. Follow-up on use of vaccine in children in Japan. In Hammon WMcD, Kitaoka M, Downs WG (eds). Immunization for Japanese Encephalitis. Amsterdam, Excerpta Medica, 1972, pp 275–277.

309. Egashira Y, Okawa T, Oya A, et al. Allergic encephalitis in guinea pigs and monkeys with special reference to the relationship between the properties of the antigen and the reaction of the host. Proc Comm Jpn Encephal Vaccine 1:66–70, 1966.

310. Shiraki H. Etiological study of demyelinating disease. Proc Comm Jpn Encephal Vaccine 1:70–71, 1966.

311. Okinaka S, Toyokura Y, Tsukagoshi H, et al. Physical reactions following vaccination against Japanese B encephalitis with special reference to neurological complications. Adv Neurol Sci 11:410–424, 1965.

312. Ohtaki E, Murakami Y, Komori H, et al. Acute disseminated encephalomyelitis after Japanese B encephalitis vaccination. Pediatr Neurol 8:137–139, 1992.

313. Ohtaki E, Matsuishi T, Hirano Y, Maekawa K. Acute disseminated encephalomyelitis after treatment with Japanese B encephalitis vaccine (Nakayama-Yoken and Beijing strains). J Neurol Neurosurg Psychiatry 59:316–317, 1995.

314. Plesner A, Soborg PA, Herning M. Neurological complications and Japanese encephalitis vaccination. Lancet 348:202–203, 1996.

315. Takahashi H, Pool V, Tsai TF, et al. Adverse events after Japanese encephalitis vaccination: a review of post-marketing surveillance data from Japan and the United States. Vaccine 18:2963–2969, 2000.

316. Andersen MM, Ronne T. Side effects with Japanese encephalitis vaccine. Lancet 337:1044, 1991.

317. Plesner AM, Ronne T. Allergic mucocutaneous reactions to Japanese encephalitis vaccine. Vaccine 15:1239–1243, 1997.

318. Ruff TA, Eisen D, Fuller A, Kass R. Adverse reactions to Japanese encephalitis vaccine. Lancet 338:881–882, 1991.

319. Tsai TF. Inactivated Japanese encephalitis virus vaccine: recommendations of the Advisory Committee on Immunization Practices (ACIP). MMWR 42(RR-1):1–15, 1993.

320. Beecham HJ III, Pock AR, May LA, Tsai TF. A cluster of severe reactions following improperly administered Takeda Japanese encephalitis vaccine. J Travel Med 4:8–10, 1997.

321. Nothdurft HD, Jelinek T, Marschang A, et al. Adverse reactions to Japanese encephalitis in travellers. J Infect 32:119–122, 1996.

322. Nazareth B, Levin J, Johnson H, Begg N. Systemic allergic reactions to Japanese encephalitis vaccine. Vaccine 12:666, 1994.

323. Robinson P, Ruff T, Kass R. Australian case-control study of adverse reactions to Japanese encephalitis. J Travel Med 2:159–164, 1995.

324. Froeschle J. Unpublished report. Swiftwater, PA, Pasteur Mérieux Connaught, 1994.

325. Hanna J, Barnett D, Ewald D. Vaccination against Japanese encephalitis in the Torres Strait. Commun Dis Intell 20:188–190, 1996.

326. Sakaguchi M, Yoshida M, Kuroda W, et al. Systemic immediate-type reactions to gelatin included in Japanese encephalitis vaccines. Vaccine 15:121–122, 1997.

327. Sakaguchi M, Inouye S. Two patterns of systemic immediate-type reactions to Japanese encephalitis vaccines. Vaccine 16:68–69, 1998.

328. Dressen DW, Bernard KW, Parker RA, et al. Immune complex–like disease in 23 persons following a booster dose of rabies diploid cell vaccine. Vaccine 4:45–49, 1986.

329. Anderson MC, Baer H, Frazier DJ, Quinnan GV. The role of specific IgE and beta-propiolactone in reactions resulting from booster doses of human diploid cell rabies vaccine. J Allergy Clin Immunol 80:861–868, 1987.

330. Plesner A-M, Tonne T, Wachmann H. Case-control study of allergic reactions to Japanese encephalitis vaccine. Vaccine 18:1830–1836, 2000.

331. Ma X, Yu YX, Wang SG. Observations on safety and serological efficacy from a large-scale field trial of Japanese encephalitis vaccine. Chin J Biol 6:188–191, 1993.

332. Liu ZL, Hennessy S, Strom BL, et al. Short-term safety of live-attenuated Japanese encephalitis vaccine (SA14-14-2): results of a 26,239-subject randomized trial. J Infect Dis 176:1366–1369, 1997.

333. Siraprapasiri T, Sawaddiwudhipong W, Rojanasuphot S. Cost benefit analysis of Japanese encephalitis vaccination program in Thailand. Southeast Asian J Trop Med Public Health 28:143–148, 1997.

334. Ruff TA. Japanese B encephalitis vaccine—time for a reappraisal? Med J Aust 161:511, 1994.

334a. Shlim DR, Solomon T. Japanese encephalitis vaccine for the travelers: exploring the limits of risk. Clin Infect Dis 35:183–188, 2002.

335. U.S. Public Health Service, Centers for Disease Control, and National Institutes of Health. Biosafety in Microbiological and Biomedical Laboratories. Washington, DC, U.S. Public Health Service, 1988, pp 82–92.

Chapter 34

Meningococcal Vaccines

DAN M. GRANOFF* • IAN M. FEAVERS • RAY BORROW

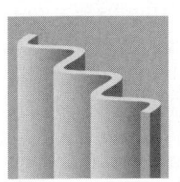

History

Meningococci (*Neisseria meningitidis*) are fastidious gram-negative endotoxin-containing organisms. The pathogen is unique among causes of bacterial meningitis for its ability to cause epidemic disease. Epidemics of meningococcal meningitis were first described in Geneva, Switzerland, by Vieusseux in 1805,[1] and in Medfield, Massachusetts, by Danielson and Mann in 1806.[2] Weichselbaum was the first to culture meningococcus from patients with meningitis in 1887.[3] Meningococcal epidemics in sub-Saharan Africa have been recognized for more than 100 years.[4]

Importance of Meningococcal Disease

Meningococci cause serious disease worldwide. In sub-Saharan Africa, large epidemics occur every 5 to 10 years. In the United States and Europe, the last major meningococcal epidemics were in the 1940s. However, the organism remains the most common cause of bacterial meningitis in children and young adults. Each year there are approximately 3000 cases of meningococcal disease reported in the United States[5] and 7700 cases in Western Europe.[6] Approximately half of the cases are meningitis. In New Zealand, an epidemic of group B meningococcal disease has been ongoing for more than a decade.[7]

Before the advent of antibiotics, the mortality rate from meningococcal disease was 70% to 85%. Specific antiserum therapy was introduced early in the 20th century and lowered the risk of death to approximately 30%. Today, despite an increased understanding of the pathogenesis of meningococcal disease and the availability of appropriate treatments, the overall mortality rate remains at 10% to 15%.[5,8]

Recent research is increasing our understanding of why some individuals who acquire the organism develop invasive meningococcal disease, whereas hundreds of others acquiring the same organism do not.[9] However, much remains to be learned about the complex interactions between the organism and the host that affect the development and outcome of meningococcal infection. Other baffling questions relate to the geographic distribution of strains causing disease in different populations. Why are group A strains responsible for most epidemic disease in sub-Saharan Africa, and what factors have led to the virtual disappearance of group A strains from the United States and Europe for more than 50 years? Also, what factors have led to the emergence of group Y disease in the United States or group B disease in New Zealand in the 1990s, or to group W135 strains in Sub-Saharan Africa in 2001 and 2002?[10,11]

Background

Clinical Description and Presentation

The dominant clinical features of meningococcal disease are fever, rash, and meningitis, but the initial signs and symptoms may be indistinguishable from those of other severe bacterial, rickettsial, or viral infections. Sixty percent of patients with meningococcal disease will have experienced symptoms for less than 24 hours when they present to the hospital.

The most common clinical presentation is acute bacterial meningitis. Older children and adults typically present with abrupt onset of fever, headache, photophobia, and complaints of aching all over. Seizures occur in approximately 20% of patients. Signs of altered consciousness (hyperactivity or lethargy) are prominent. Nuchal rigidity is a common sign except in infants, in whom a more gradual onset of fever, poor feeding, and lethargy are the typical presenting complaints, and a bulging fontanel may be the major clue of central nervous system involvement. A rash is present in the majority of cases of meningococcal disease, consisting of typical petechiae or larger purpuric lesions that usually are most apparent on the chest, upper arms, and axillae.[8] Maculopapular rashes also are common and may occur in the absence of petechiae.

Ten to 20% of patients with meningococcal disease present with severe sepsis or meningococcemia ("purpura fulminans"). Meningitis may be absent, but the organism is

*D.M.G. was supported, in part, by grants RO1 AI 45642 and AI46464 from the National Institutes of Allergy and Infectious Disease, National Institutes of Health. This chapter incorporates some material written by Martha Lepow, Bradly Perkins, Patricia Hughes, and Jan Poolman, authors of the chapter on meningococcal vaccines that appeared in the third edition of *Vaccines*.

widely disseminated in the bloodstream and in multiple other organs. Signs and symptoms of septicemia are heralded by spreading purpura. Progression of disease is rapid, with onset of hypotension and signs of multiple organ failure. White blood cell counts may be very high or low, but c reactive protein is usually elevated.[11a] At the time of autopsy, acute adrenal hemorrhage may be present (Waterhouse-Friderichsen syndrome).

Up to 15% of patients with meningococcal disease may present with pneumonia.[8] In the absence of a characteristic rash, the cause of the pneumonia may go unrecognized because the clinical microbiology laboratory may not report isolation of *N. meningitidis* in sputum cultures. Much less common manifestations of meningococcal disease include myocarditis, endocarditis, or pericarditis; arthritis; conjunctivitis; urethritis; pharyngitis; and cervicitis. Late in the course of treated disease, arthritis or pericarditis may occur as a result of immune complex formation.

Many patients with severe meningococcemia respond poorly to treatment with antimicrobial agents, steroids, or vasopressor agents, and death may occur within hours of onset. In most case series, the mortality rate from severe meningococcemia remains at approximately 40%. More commonly, the course of meningococcal disease is less fulminant, and therapeutic interventions with antimicrobial agents and supportive treatments are successful.

Complications of Meningococcal Disease

Approximately 10% to 20% of patients with meningococcal disease develop permanent sequelae. The risk is not uniform, and patients with certain genetic polymorphisms are at greatly increased risk of dying or developing permanent sequelae[9] (see below). These sequelae include deforming limb loss from gangrene, extensive skin scarring requiring grafting, or cerebral infarction. Patients with meningococcal meningitis who do not develop septic shock are much less likely to die or develop these sequelae (<10%), but they are at risk of developing neurosensory hearing loss, mild to moderate cognitive deficits, or seizure disorders.[12–15] The risk of these neurologic complications with meningococcal meningitis appears to be lower than that of patients with meningitis caused by other bacterial agents such as *Haemophilus influenzae* or *Streptococcus pneumoniae*.[16,17]

Bacteriology

Neisseria meningitidis is a gram-negative, encapsulated, aerobic diplococcus.[18] The organism is usually grown on chocolate agar or Mueller-Hinton media in an atmosphere containing 5% to 10% carbon dioxide. Catlin-6 medium[19] and Frantz medium[20] also have been used as defined and partially defined liquid culture media, respectively. At least 13 serologically distinct meningococcal groups have been defined on the basis of the immunochemistry of the capsular polysaccharide.[21,22] The meningococcus only infects humans, with organisms of groups A, B, C, W135, and Y responsible for almost all cases of disease. For epidemiologic purposes, meningococci have been further classified into serotypes and serosubtypes on the basis of the immunologic reactivity of the PorB and PorA outer membrane proteins, respectively.[23–27] The accepted nomenclature lists the capsular group, the PorB serotype, and the

PorA subtype, each separated by a colon. The VR1-(loop 2) and VR2-(loop 4) encoded epitopes of PorA are given in order after the prefix P1., separated from one another by a comma (e.g., B:4:P1.7,4).[28,29] Meningococci also can be divided into immunotypes on the basis of variation in the lipo-oligosaccharide structure, but for epidemiologic studies this classification system is less frequently used to characterize isolates.[30]

The meningococcus is naturally competent from transformation with DNA, which provides a mechanism for the horizontal exchange of genetic material.[31] As a consequence, the organism has a more panmictic population structure than many bacterial species[32] and has been shown to exchange the genes encoding key antigens that are used both in the serologic characterization of isolates and as vaccine components.[33–35] Thus the characterization of *N. meningitidis* strains based on the products of single genetic loci does not provide a reliable reflection of the underlying genetic relationships between isolates. Multilocus enzyme electrophoresis was for a long time the method of choice for genotyping meningococci and has been used to identify genetically related isolates designated as subgroups (in case of group A isolates) or electrophoretic types (ET) (for other capsular groups).[36] This technique has been superseded by the determination of the genetic relationships among isolates by multilocus sequence typing, which capitalizes on recent developments in high-throughput nucleotide sequence analysis to index variation based on sequence polymorphisms in housekeeping genes.[37] Multilocus typing approaches have been used to monitor the global epidemiology of meningococcal disease, to determine the relationships between isolates in localized outbreaks, and to provide evidence for capsular switching among meningococci. Because the protection offered by currently licensed meningococcal vaccines is capsular group specific, the facility to exchange capsule genes has potential ramifications for choice of vaccine formulations and vaccination policy.[38]

The complete nucleotide sequences of the genomes of two meningococcal isolates, the group A (subgroup IV) isolate Z2491[39] and the group B (ET-5 complex) isolate MC58,[40] have been determined. The genome sequence of a third isolate, group C (ET-37 complex) FAM18, is nearing completion (see *www.sanger.ac.uk/Projects/N_meningitidis/seroC.shtml*). These genomic data provide insights into the biochemistry of *N. meningitidis* in both its commensal and virulent lifestyles. The most notable features of the meningococcal genome are the unprecedented number of repetitive elements, presumed to contribute to genome fluidity, and the large number of genes that have the potential to undergo phase variation. These features make an important contribution to the antigenic variability and phenotypic adaptability of the organism.

Pathogenesis as It Relates to Prevention

The meningococcus only colonizes the nasopharynx of humans and has no other known environmental niche. The organism occurs frequently as a harmless commensal and typically is carried at any one time by more than 10% of the population. Meningococci are transmitted from person to person by aerosol droplets or contact with respiratory secretions (e.g., kissing or sharing a glass). Viral respiratory infections[41] and exposure to tobacco smoke[42,43] or indoor firewood stoves[44] are associated with increased rates of meningococcal carriage or disease. The higher carriage probably results from alterations in the mucosal surface that enhances binding of the bacteria or decreases the ability of the host to clear the organism from the nasopharynx. Studies of the population biology of the meningococcus indicate that most invasive disease is caused by bacteria from a limited number of hypervirulent lineages. Carriage isolates, in contrast, belong to diverse lineages, many of which have never been associated with disease.[45] The implication of these observations is that certain meningococci are genetically predisposed to cause disease.

Following attachment to nasopharyngeal mucosal cells, the organism replicates and establishes a carrier state. Pili appear to be the most important adhesin, and two opacity-associated proteins (Opa and Opc) also function as adhesins.[46] Attachment to epithelial cells is mediated by specific receptors such as CD46.[46] Attachment initiates loss of piliation by the bacteria as well as cytoskeletal rearrangements in the host cell that result in internalization of the bacteria within membrane-bound vesicles by endocytosis. Once the organism has established a carrier state, the likelihood of acquiring invasive meningococcal disease depends on the virulence of the particular organism, host factors affecting innate susceptibility,[9] and the presence or absence of serum antibodies capable of activating complement-mediated bacteriolysis and clearing the organism from the blood stream.[47] Once meningococci enter the bloodstream, the spleen also is important for clearance of the bacteria. Because of impaired clearance, patients with asplenia or hyposplenic function are at increased risk of acquiring severe meningococcal disease.[48]

Goldschneider et al. reported on the importance of serum bactericidal antibodies in protection against disease in 1969 in their study of military recruits.[47] These investigators obtained baseline serum samples at the beginning of basic training. Group C bactericidal antibodies were present in sera of approximately 80% of the recruits. Those with detectable serum bactericidal antibody frequently became meningococcal carriers but did not develop disease, while virtually all individuals acquiring meningococcal disease lacked serum bactericidal activity. Recruits who lacked serum bactericidal antibody and in whom group C carriage was documented had meningococcal disease attack rates as high as 38.5%.

The complement cascade is activated by serum antibodies via the classical pathway, which results in both opsonization and bacteriolysis of meningococci. In the absence of specific anti-meningococcal antibodies, these complement-mediated functions can be activated by the alternative pathway.[49] Given the central role of complement proteins in host defenses against invasive N. meningitidis disease, it is not surprising that persons with underlying deficiencies of properdin,[50-55] C3, or the late complement components (C5 through C9), are at greatly increased risk of acquiring meningococcal disease. Although complement deficiencies only account for 1% of patients with meningococcal disease overall, they should be considered in patients with recurrent meningococcal disease, or with disease caused by organisms with unusual capsular groups such as X, Z, W135, or 29E.[51,52] An increased risk of meningococcal disease also has been associated with the presence of structural variants of mannose-binding lectin,[56,57] a constituent of serum that

binds to meningococci and activates the complement cascade.[49,58,59] In contrast to deficiencies of complement proteins, the prevalence of polymorphisms of mannose-binding lectin is much greater in the general population. Therefore, as compared to complement deficiencies, these structural variants of manonose-binding lectin may play a more important role (i.e., high attributable risk) in susceptibility of the general population to meningococcal disease, particularly in children and adolescents who have not yet acquired serum bactericidal antibodies.

A variety of other genetic polymorphisms appear to influence the severity of disease without affecting the risk of acquiring meningococcal disease.[9] These include a receptor on neutrophils for immunoglobulin G (IgG)2 or IgG3, termed *Fc gamma receptor IIA* (FcγRIIA), which affects the ability of the phagocytic cell to clear opsonized bacteria from the bloodstream.[60-63] Several studies have found an association between the FcγRIIA-R131 polymorphism, which binds IgG2 poorly, and an increased risk of severe forms of meningococcal disease.[60-64] Patients homozygous for a genetic polymorphism associated with high expression of interleukin (IL)-10[65] or altered production of tumor necrosis factor-α (TNF-α)[65,66] are reported to be at higher risk of severe disease. Patients with a genotype associated with high plasma concentrations of plasminogen activator inhibitor-1,[67] a procoagulant that inhibits fibrinolysis and may promote intravascular fibrin deposition, are also at increased risk. Taken together, the accumulating data support a strong genetic component of altered host responses in otherwise healthy individuals that underlies the dramatic disparity in clinical outcomes of patients infected with meningococci.

Diagnosis

Diagnosis of meningococcal disease is achieved through conventional cultures of blood, cerebrospinal fluid, hemorrhagic skin lesions, or other infected sites. Gram staining for demonstration of the organism also remains an important diagnostic tool. Latex agglutination test for detection of meningococcal capsular polysaccharides in serum or cerebrospinal fluid also is widely utilized, but false-negative results are common, particularly for group B organisms. False-positive results for group B organisms also may occur in patients receiving sustained life support as a result of detection of cross-reactive polysialyic acid[68] released from damaged brain (unpublished observations of D.M.G.). Serodiagnosis also is available for confirmation of diagnosis, but the results are retrospective and often inconclusive.[69]

In the United Kingdom, detection of meningococcal DNA by polymerase chain reaction (PCR) has become widely available through use of a centralized reference laboratory. Some of the first meningococcal PCR assays were based on detection of the meningococcal insertion sequence (IS) element IS1106, but the results lacked satisfactory specificity because of inherent genetic mobility of these elements between species and genera. Second-generation PCR tests target different meningococcal sequences consisting of conserved regions of the capsular transport gene (*ctrA* gene). For initial screening of test samples, these sequences can be amplified to identify all clinically significant meningococcal capsular groups. Confirmation of capsular group–specific sequences within the sialyltransferase (*siaD*) gene is then used to discriminate between capsular group B, C, Y, or W135 organisms.[70] For diagnosis of group A isolates, PCR amplification targets *orf 2* sequences within the gene cassette required for the synthesis of the capsule for group A.[71] One advantage of PCR is that it can detect DNA sequences from clinical samples containing organisms that cannot be isolated by conventional culture methods, particularly from patients who have received antimicrobial therapy.[72] The increased use of PCR diagnosis in the United Kingdom has resulted in greatly enhanced case detection (43% of all cases diagnosed in 2001 were based on a clinically compatible illness and positive PCR only[73]).

Treatment and Prevention

Antibiotics

Many antimicrobial agents, including intravenously administered aqueous penicillin, are effective for treatment of patients with meningococcal disease. Early initiation of antibiotic therapy of patients suspected of having meningococcal infection and arranging for rapid admission to the hospital may help decrease mortality and morbidity.[74,75] Intramuscular administration may be used for the first dose if there are difficulties obtaining intravenous access. Because the clinical presentation of meningococcal disease can overlap that of bacterial meningitis or sepsis caused by other organisms, depending on the age of the patient, clinical presentation, exposure history, and the presence or absence of other epidemiologic risk factors, broader empirical therapy should be considered before the diagnosis is confirmed.[8] Appropriate broader treatments include cefotaxime or ceftriaxone given by the intravenous or intramuscular route. In patients with meningitis, vancomycin should be added empirically as a second drug because of concerns about penicillin- or cephalosporin-resistant *S. pneumoniae*. For treatment of meningococcal disease, chloramphenicol also is effective, although resistance to this drug has been reported in some countries.[76] Antibiotic treatment for 5 to 7 days is adequate therapy for most systemic meningococcal illnesses.

Other Therapies

In the preantibiotic era, the mortality rate from meningococcal disease averaged 85%. With the advent of sulfonamide therapy, the overall mortality rate fell to 12% to 15%, where it has remained despite the availability of newer antibiotics, sophisticated fluid therapy, steroid therapy, and vasodilators. Patients presenting with purpura fulminans continue to have the highest mortality rates (up to 50%). This syndrome is a result of a massive release of proinflammatory mediators[77] and development of shock and disseminated intravascular coagulation with local accumulation of thrombi in small and large arterial vessels from a procoagulant state.

Activated protein C is an endogenous anticoagulant that suppresses excessive thrombosis and fibrin formation.[78,79] The molecule also has a dual anti-inflammatory role,[78] down-regulating TNF-α and IL-1-β production in animal models of sepsis, and decreasing levels of IL-6 in patients with sepsis. Decreased levels of protein C are pres-

ent in most patients with meningococcal sepsis,[80,81] and patients with the lowest levels have the worse prognosis. The results of two open-label studies suggested that treatment of patients with meningococcemia with protein C concentrate prepared from human plasma improved mortality and morbidity, as compared to that of historical controls.[82,83] The results of a large, prospective randomized trial in patients with severe sepsis caused by a variety of gram-positive or gram-negative bacteria or fungi indicated that treatment with recombinant human activated protein C (drotrecogin alfa [activated]) decreased the 28-day mortality rate by 19.4%, as compared to that of patients treated with placebo (95% confidence interval [CI], 6.6% to 30.5%; $P = 0.005$).[79] The main adverse event associated with drotrecogin alfa [activated] therapy in this study was an excess of serious bleeding (3.5% vs. 2.0%; $P = 0.06$).

The Food and Drug Administration recently approved the use of drotrecogin alfa [activated] (Xigris, Eli Lilly) for adjunctive therapy in patients with septic shock.[84] The randomized trial demonstrating improved survival with this therapy included few if any patients infected with *N. meningitidis*. Thus the benefit of drotrecogin alfa [activated] treatment of patients with meningococcemia has not been formally demonstrated, and the safety and effectiveness have not been established in children. Nevertheless, given the similarities in the underlying pathology of septicemia caused by *N. meningitidis* and other gram-negative bacteria, and the poor prognosis of patients with meningococcemia, adjunctive therapy with drotrecogin alfa [activated] should be considered for patients having a relatively high risk of death.

Other antiendotoxic or anticytokine therapies remain experimental. These include bactericidal permeability–increasing protein (BPI), which neutralizes endotoxin and has bactericidal activity against *N. meningitidis*. In a randomized Phase III trial, children with meningococcal disease treated with a recombinant N-terminal fragment of BPI had lower morbidity than patients given placebo as adjunctive therapy, but there was no statistically significant difference in mortality, the primary endpoint of the trial.[85] However, because of a low mortality rate in the controls, this trial was underpowered to detect a significant difference for this endpoint.[86] Other experimental treatments for meningococcemia include plasmapheresis, which anecdotally is reported to be successful under some circumstances.

Dexamethasone therapy for 4 days, with the first dose given before the initiation of antibiotic therapy, is reported to decrease the rate of neurosensory deafness in patients with meningitis caused by *H. influenzae* type b. The benefit of steroid therapy in meningitis patients infected with *N. meningitidis* or *S. pneumoniae* remains unproven, but some experts recommend its use.[87]

Chemoprophylaxis

Close contacts of a patient with meningococcal disease are at greatly increased risk of acquiring disease. The source of infection can be either the index patient or another close contact who is an asymptomatic carrier. The risk of acquiring disease is greatest in household contacts and in other close contacts who are exposed to oral secretions through kissing or sharing of eating utensils or glasses. The risk of transmission of the organism to health care workers is low, but persons performing mouth-to-mouth resuscitation or unprotected health care workers exposed during management of endotracheal tubes are at increased risk.[88] Rifampin, ceftriaxone, and ciprofloxacin all have been demonstrated to eradicate nasopharyngeal *N. meningitidis* colonization, and these agents are recommended for chemoprophylaxis of close contacts.[8,88] Chemoprophylaxis should be offered to household members, and to other persons with a history of prolonged close contact within the 7 days before onset of disease in the index patient. Prophylaxis of day care contacts and staff is recommended in the United States[88] but not routinely in the United Kingdom.[75] Because the risk of disease in contacts is highest in the first week after onset of disease in the index patient, prophylaxis should be administered to contacts as soon as possible, preferably within 24 hours of identification of the index patient. Penicillin therapy does not reliably eradicate nasopharyngeal colonization.[89] Therefore, prophylaxis is also recommended at the time of hospital discharge for eradication of colonization of index patients treated with penicillin.[88]

Chemoprophylaxis given to large populations in response to outbreaks of meningococcal disease has not been demonstrated to be efficacious in lowering the risk of disease and increases the likelihood of emergence of antimicrobial resistance. In small school-based outbreaks, chemoprophylaxis to all people within the population may be considered. If undertaken, the medication should be administered to all members at the same time.

Epidemiology

Incidence, Prevalence, and Public Health Burden

Meningococcal disease is a global problem that occurs in all countries. Group A meningococci are particularly noted for their ability to cause large-scale epidemics, which without doubt represent the most serious public health issue caused by *N. meningitidis*.[4] Since the Second World War, epidemic meningococcal disease caused by group A organisms has been largely confined to developing countries, especially the so-called "meningitis belt" of sub-Saharan Africa, where disease can spread rapidly over large geographic regions, resulting in a pandemic outbreak within a very short period.

In the United States and Europe, most cases of meningococcal disease are sporadic. The burden of endemic meningococcal disease varies among countries. Countries with high incidence rates (>3 per 100,000 population per year) include Iceland, Malta, the Netherlands, Ireland, Spain, and the United Kingdom.[6] Compared with rates in these countries, the United States has a relatively low incidence of disease (approximately 1 per 100,000[88]). The incidence of meningococcal disease in the United States between 1971 and 2001 is shown in Figure 34–1.

The age-specific incidence of meningococcal disease is related to the degree of prevailing immunity in the population and, therefore, disease is most common among the very young, who have not yet acquired natural immunity. The highest age-specific incidence of disease in the United States is in infants less than 1 year of age, with a peak of 15.9 per 100,000 population in 4- to 5-month-old infants.[5] The corresponding rate in U.K. infants age 6 months is 50

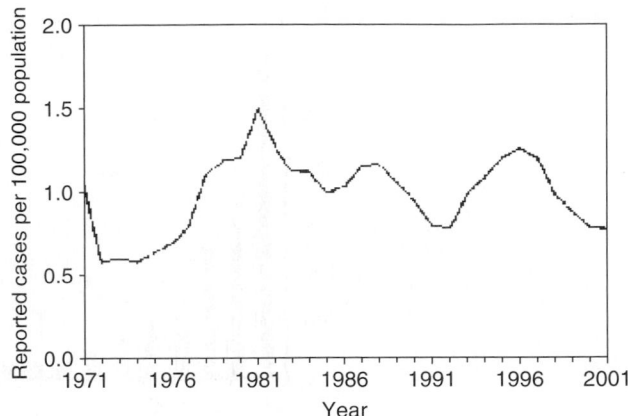

FIGURE 34–1 ▪ Incidence of meningococcal disease in the United States, 1971 to 2001. (CDC data courtesy of Drs. B. Perkins and N. Rosenstein.)

per 100,000 population.[90] By 4 years of age, the annual attack rates in the United Kingdom and the United States fall to approximately 5 and 2.5 per 100,000 population, respectively.[91] In most developed countries, meningococcal disease remains one of the leading infectious causes of death in childhood.

In both the United States and the United Kingdom, there are small peaks in incidence among teenagers and certain college student groups (particularly freshmen), which may be related to the increased contact in dormatories and residence halls, as well as other social activities in this age group. The age distribution of cases in the United Kingdom is shown in Figure 34–2A, which illustrates the increase in cases among teenagers. The corresponding number of deaths at each age is shown in Figure 34–2B. The fatality rate among teenagers also is disproportionately higher than that in infants and children, particularly for disease caused by group C strains.

In temperate climates, rates of meningococcal infections peak during the winter months, irrespective of age. This association may be a result of closer personal contact during the winter months, lack of ventilation, or an increase in catarrhal infections, all factors that increase the transmission of the organism.

Meningococcal Group A Disease

Group A isolates are the major cause of endemic meningococcal disease in the meningitis belt of Sub-Saharan Africa,[92] but these strains rarely (<0.3% of cases) cause disease in the United States[5] or in Europe.[6] Notable exceptions were an outbreak in the United States in the Pacific Northwest in the 1970s among people living on skid row,[93] and more recently in Moscow, Russia, where group A isolates accounted for more than 10% of cases.[94]

The annual incidence of disease during group A epidemics in sub-Saharan Africa can on occasion exceed 1000 per 100,000 population. A map of the meningitis belt is shown in Figure 34–3. The case fatality rate during group A epidemics in Africa is usually between 10% and 15%.[4] Genotypic analyses of epidemiologically defined group A isolates indicate that pandemic outbreaks of group A

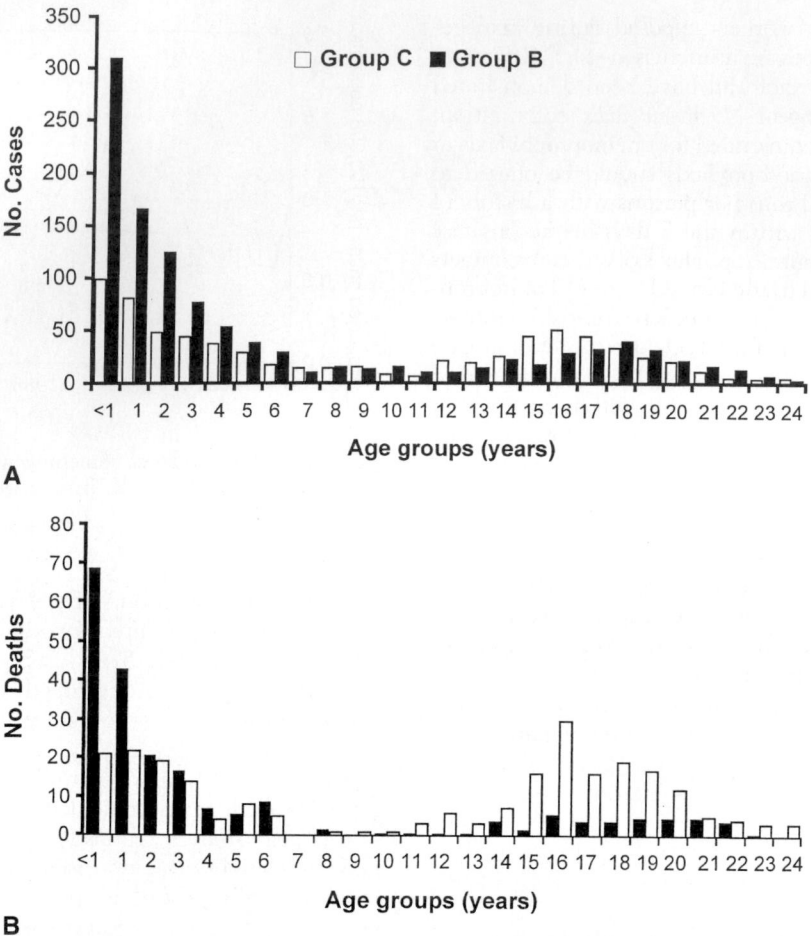

FIGURE 34–2 ■ Group B and C meningococcal disease in England and Wales, April 1998 to March 1999, by age group, prior to the introduction of group C conjugate vaccine. A, Number of cases. B, Number of deaths.

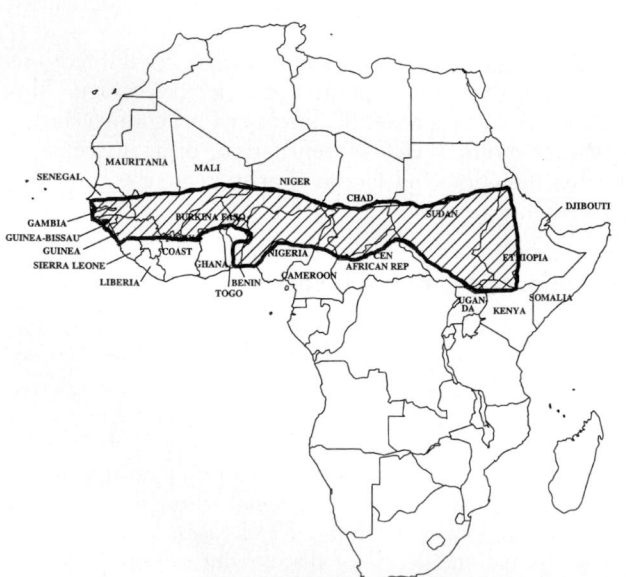

FIGURE 34–3 ■ The sub-Saharan African meningitis belt. (From Control and prevention of meningococcal disease and control and prevention of serogroup C, meningococcal disease: Evaluation and management of suspected outbreaks. Recommendations of the Advisory Committee on Immunization Practices [ACIP]. MMWR 46[RR–5], 1–21, 1997.)

disease are caused by the global spread of specific clonal lineages.[92] Work by Achtman and colleagues has demonstrated how the lineage known as subgroup III was responsible for two global pandemics during the latter half of the 20th century.[95] The first started with large epidemics in China in the mid-1960s and subsequently spread, causing epidemics in Moscow (1969 to 1971),[96] Norway (1973), Finland (1975), and, finally, Brazil in the mid-1970s. After a gap of about 10 years, subgroup III bacteria then re-emerged, causing new outbreaks in China, Nepal, and, in 1987, among pilgrims to the Hajj. Subgroup III epidemics followed in Sudan, Chad, Ethiopia, Kenya, and Tanzania[97] and spread into Zambia and the Central African Republic by the mid-1990s.[98]

Meningococcal Group B Disease

Group B disease is the most important cause of endemic disease in developed countries, accounting for up to 80% of sporadic meningococcal cases in certain European countries, and approximately 30% to 40% of cases in the United States.[5] Group B strains also can cause epidemic disease.[36] As compared with group A epidemics, group B epidemics begin more slowly, are associated with lower rates of disease, and may last a decade or longer. Group B epidemic disease also is associated with emergence of hypervirulent strains.

For example, in the 1970s an increase in the incidence of disease caused by ET-5 complex group B strains was noted in Norway (B:15:P1.7,16) and Spain (B:4:P1.19,15).[36] A severe epidemic in Cuba in the 1980s was caused by group B strains with ET-5 complex (B:4:P1.19,15) and led to increased disease in the Saõ Paulo region of Brazil in the late 1980s.[36] Group B meningococci strains from the ET-5 complex become established in Canada in the 1990s, and substantial increases in incidence also were noted in the United States in Oregon and Washington State (B:15:P1.7,16).[99] In the early 1990s, an epidemic of disease caused by lineage III (B:4:P1.7–2,4) isolates was identified in New Zealand that was especially associated with increased disease rates in the Pacific Islanders and Maori populations.[7] This epidemic has persisted for more than a decade.

Meningococcal Group C Disease

The percentage of group C isolates responsible for endemic meningococcal disease varies by country. In the United States, group C isolates accounted for approximately 25% to 30% of disease during the 1990s. Iceland, Northern Ireland, Russia (Moscow), the Slovak Republic, Spain, and Switzerland report 40% or more of recent disease caused by group C isolates.[6]

Group C outbreaks occurred in the 1960s in U.S. Army recruits[100] and in the 1970s in an urban setting in Saõ Paulo, Brazil,[101] and were caused by ET-37 complex strains.[35] In the 1990s, Spain suffered a large outbreak of group C disease, with the most common phenotype being C:2b:P1.5,2 (ET-3).[102] ET-3 is closely related to the ET-37 complex. The ET-15 clone of the ET-37 complex arose and caused a large group C outbreak in Canada in the 1990s[103,104] before spreading worldwide.[105] ET-15 meningococci tend to be more virulent than other members of the ET-37 complex, and attack rates, fatality rates, and the proportion of sequelae in patients infected with ET-15 strains have been reported to exceed the respective rates observed for disease caused by isolates that are other members of the ET-37 complex.[13,105] The increase of group C disease in the United Kingdom in the 1990s was caused by ET-15 isolates of the ET-37 complex, which caused outbreaks in universities and was associated with high fatality rates.[106]

Meningococcal Groups Y and W135 Disease

Until the 1990s, disease caused by strains with capsular groups Y or W135 was associated mainly with patients with complement deficiencies.[107] However, in the United States, the proportion of disease caused by group Y strains rose from 2% of disease in 1989 to 1991[108] to 10.6% in 1992, to 32.6% in 1996.[5] Group Y disease currently affects all age groups in the United States, including infants, whereas in other areas of the world disease caused by group Y strains remains rare and disproportionately affects older age groups. Patients with group Y disease also are more likely to have pneumonia than patients with disease caused by strains with other capsular groups.[109,110]

Large numbers of pilgrims from the meningitis belt of Africa congregate at the Hajj, and a fatal case of group W135 disease was reported in a pilgrim in 1995.[111] In 2000 and 2001, outbreaks of group W135 disease during Hajj pilgrimages were reported in Saudi Arabia. W135 was shown to spread from pilgrims to contacts in their home countries.[111a] Group W135 isolates belonging to the ET-37 complex also have been isolated from otherwise healthy patients with meningococcal disease in Mali in 1994,[112] in The Gambia[112] and Cameroon in 1995, and in Chad in 1996.[113] In 2002, more than 10,000 cases caused by group W135 isolates were reported from Burkina Faso.[11] Control of emerging epidemics of W135 disease in sub-Saharan Africa poses a new challenge because the available bivalent meningococcal polysaccharide vaccine does not contain group W135 polysaccharide. Also, the tetravalent vaccine, which contains W135 polysaccharide, is more expensive and is in short supply worldwide.[11]

Group W135 bacteria remain an infrequent cause of disease in the United States or Europe. However, in England and Wales, 51 cases, including eight fatalities, of disease caused by W135 ET-37 complex strains were reported following Hajj 2000, while in the first 12 days following the start of Hajj 2001, 33 cases, including nine fatalities, were reported. Of these 33 cases, 6 were in Hajj pilgrims, 16 were secondary cases, and 11 had no identifiable Hajj association.[114]

Mechanisms of Immunity to Meningococcal Disease

Natural Acquisition of Meningococcal Humoral Immunity

Many newborns have serum bactericidal antibodies that are acquired transplacentally from their mothers and persist in the infant for a few months. Thereafter, natural acquisition of serum bactericidal antibodies to *N. meningitidis* is inversely related to age. Low levels of bactericidal antibodies are present below 2 years, which corresponds to the age group at greatest risk of acquiring meningococcal disease. Between 2 and 12 years of age there is a progressive increase in the prevalence of serum antibody, which coincides with a decrease in the incidence of disease. Depending on the strain tested, approximately 60% to 80% of young adults have detectable serum meningococcal bactericidal antibodies.[47,115]

Naturally acquired serum bactericidal antibodies to *N. meningitidis* result from asymptomatic carriage of pathogenic and nonpathogenic meningococci,[115] as well as carriage of the antigenically related species, *Neisseria lactamica*.[49] Robbins and co-workers in the late 1960s postulated that naturally acquired group A bactericidal antibodies resulted from acquisition of cross-reactive meningococcal group A anti-capsular antibodies that are stimulated by colonization by *Escherichia coli* or *Bacillus pumilus* strains that express group A cross-reacting polysaccharide.[116–119] However, adsorption studies of pooled γ-globulin fractions suggested that these cross-reacting anticapsular antibodies may play only a minor role in naturally acquired serum bactericidal antibody to group A strains.[47] In contrast, the majority of naturally acquired serum bactericidal antibodies to group C strains is directed at the group C polysaccharide.[47]

In children, most naturally acquired serum bactericidal antibodies to group B meningococci appear to be directed against noncapsular antigens.[49] In adults, naturally acquired immunoglobulin M (IgM) group B anticapsular antibodies may contribute to serum bactericidal activity. Although serum IgG antibodies to the group B capsule are reported to be prevalent in adults,[120] these antibodies may be nonspecific because their binding in an enzyme-linked immunosorbent assay (ELISA) is not inhibited by soluble group B polysaccharide.[121] Also, compared to IgM anti-capsular antibody, IgG group B anti-capsular antibodies have poor complement bactericidal activity,[122,123] and are poorly protective in an animal model.[122] Therefore, the contribution of naturally occurring IgG antibodies to group B polysaccharide to protective immunity is questionable.

Active Immunization

History of Meningococcal Vaccine Development

Vaccines offering protection against meningococcal disease have been available for more than 30 years, but, even in 2002, there is no formulation that offers comprehensive protection against strains from all of the pathogenic capsular groups. With the benefit of hindsight, the development of meningococcal vaccines has been hampered by the biology of N. meningitidis and its unique relationship with the human host. The organism has evolved an array of sophisticated mechanisms to evade host defenses, which confound attempts to produce a truly comprehensive vaccine. These mechanisms include the production of poorly immunogenic polysaccharide capsules and lipopolysaccharides, some of which mimic glycosylated structures on human tissue. Surface-exposed proteins that elicit immune response exhibit variability in both their antigenic structure and expression. In addition, the meningococcus is naturally able to accept DNA, providing the organism with a mechanism for genetic exchange and almost endless possibilities for the reassortment of nucleic acid sequences, including those encoding its principal antigens. Only recently, with the detailed analyses of the meningococcal genome, has the real extent of these mechanisms become fully appreciated.[39,40,124,125]

Early attempts to develop meningococcal vaccines were based on using killed whole bacterial cells.[126–128] Between 1900 and 1940, several trials were conducted using killed whole cells, but the studies were poorly controlled and in most instances it was impossible to tell whether the vaccines tested conferred protective immunity.[129] Further pursuit of a whole-cell vaccine was curtailed by the excessive reactogenicity of such preparations. Following the successful development of tetanus and diphtheria toxoid vaccines in the1930s, the protective potential of crude meningococcal culture filtrates containing inactivated exotoxin was explored.[130,131] Perhaps not surprisingly, these preparations proved to be immunogenic, but they would have certainly been contaminated with capsular polysaccharide antigen, outer membranes, and lipopolysaccharides. Subsequently, enthusiasm for the development of meningococcal vaccines waned in the face of overwhelming optimism surrounding early successes with treatment and prevention of disease with antibiotics, most notably the sulfonamides. However, by the early 1960s sulfonamide-resistant isolates of N. meningitidis were widespread and represented an important problem among military personnel recruited at the time of the war in Vietnam, which promoted renewed interest in meningococcal vaccine development.[100,132]

During the early 1940s, Scherp and Rake demonstrated that serum from horses immunized with group-specific capsular polysaccharides protected mice against lethal challenge with N. meningitidis,[133] but purified preparations of capsular polysaccharide failed to elicit antibody responses in humans.[134,135] In retrospect, the poor immunogenicity of these preparations can be attributed to the relatively low molecular size of the polysaccharide, because subsequent studies showed that only polysaccharide antigens of high molecular weight induce antibody responses in humans.[136] By the end of the 1960s, Gotschlich and his colleagues, working at the Walter Reed Army Institute, had developed an alternative approach for the purification of high-molecular-weight meningococcal polysaccharides that were safe and immunogenic in humans.[137,138] Meningococcal capsular polysaccharides purified in this way form the basis of the currently licensed bivalent (A and C) and tetravalent (A, C, W135, and Y) vaccines, while the determination of the molecular size of the polysaccharide components remains a critical feature of the quality control of these products.

As described below, the principal limitation of polysaccharide vaccines is that they do not induce T-cell–dependent immunity. This property has profound implications for the poor effectiveness of these vaccines in children, as well as the inability of polysaccharide vaccines to elicit long-term immunologic memory.[139–141] The chemical conjugation of polysaccharides to protein carrier molecules ensures that a T-cell–dependent immune response is induced,[142] and the success of this approach in immunization programs was first demonstrated in humans with the H. influenzae type b vaccine in the 1980s.[143–145] Subsequently, similar conjugate vaccines based on the group A and C polysaccharides of the meningococcus were developed.[146] Monovalent group C conjugates were tested extensively in clinical studies during the 1990s, and proved to be safe and capable of inducing highly bactericidal and boostable immune responses in infants and children.[147–150] As described below, group C conjugate vaccines were introduced in the United Kingdom in late 1999 and are now widely used in other European countries as a result of the mutual recognition process, which expedites the licensure of a vaccine in other European Union countries once it has been accepted by the licensing authority of one member country. Vaccine manufacturers are currently developing multivalent meningococcal polysaccharide-protein conjugate vaccines that contain capsular groups A, C, Y, and W135. The prospect for a comprehensive vaccine that will also offer protection against group B meningococci is more remote at present, although a number of promising candidate group B vaccines are under consideration (reviewed by Morley and Pollard[151] and Jodar et al.[152]).

Composition of Meningococcal Vaccines

POLYSACCHARIDE VACCINES

Meningococcal polysaccharide vaccines (Table 34–1) are available in bivalent (groups A and C) and tetravalent (groups A, C, W135, and Y) formulations. The vaccines consist of freeze-dried meningococcal polysaccharides together

TABLE 34–1 ■ Meningococcal Polysaccharide Vaccines*

Manufacturer	Vaccine	Active Constituents	Other Excipients	Diluent
Aventis Pasteur	Mengivac™	Group A polysaccharide Group C polysaccharide	Lactose (2 mg)	Phosphate-buffered saline solution
	Menomune™*	Group A polysaccharide Group C polysaccharide Group W135 polysaccharide Group Y polysaccharide	Lactose (2.5–5.0 mg) Sodium chloride (4.25–4.75 mg)	Pyrogen-free water
GSK Biologicals	AC Vax™	Group A polysaccharide Group C polysaccharide	Lactose (12.6 mg)	Saline solution
	ACWY Vax™	Group A polysaccharide Group C polysaccharide Group W135 polysaccharide Group Y polysaccharide	Lactose (12.6 mg)	Saline solution

*All vaccines shown are licensed in European countries. Menomune is available in the United States and Canada and is sold in other countries under the trade name Menomune-A/C/Y/W-135. All vaccines contain 50 µg of each of the capsular polysaccharides shown and are lyophilized, requiring reconstitution with preservative-free diluent. For multidose vials, the diluent used to reconstitute Menomune contains thimerosal (mercury derivative) 1:10,000 as a preservative.

with lactose as the lyophilization excipient and are supplied with diluent in which they are reconstituted. In the case of multidose vials manufactured by Aventis Pasteur, the diluent contains thimerosal as a preservative. No adjuvant is included with meningococcal polysaccharide vaccines. The vaccines are stable while freeze-dried, with shelf lives of several years when stored between 2° and 8°C.

All commercially available meningococcal polysaccharide vaccines contain 50 µg per dose of each component polysaccharide as lyophilized powders (Table 34–1). The vaccine should be stored at 2° to 8°C. When reconstituted with diluent provided by the manufacturers, the vaccines are administered subcutaneously as a 0.5-mL dose. (Mengivac, which is licensed in Europe, can also be given intramuscularly). In the United States, a tetravalent A, C, Y, and W135 vaccine is produced and marketed as Menomune by Aventis Pasteur (Swiftwater, PA). It is available in single-dose and 10-dose vials. This vaccine is available in other countries as "Menomune-A/C/Y/W-135." The single-dose vials should be administered within 30 minutes after reconstitution. Reconstituted multidose vials should be stored at 2° to 8°C, and unused vaccine should be discarded after 10 days. Menomune and another tetravalent vaccine, ACWY Vax (GSK Biologicals), as well as two bivalent A and C vaccines,

Mengivac (Aventis Pasteur) and AC Vax (GSK Biologicals), are available in Europe, generally as single-dose vials. These vaccines should be administered as soon as possible after reconstitution, no later than 1 hour.

CONJUGATE VACCINES

Three monovalent group C conjugate vaccines (Table 34–2) are currently licensed in European countries and in Canada; two are based on oligosaccharides derived from group C capsular polysaccharide that are conjugated to the nontoxic CRM_{197} derivative of diphtheria toxin, and the third consists of de-O-acetylated group C polysaccharide conjugated to tetanus toxoid. Despite the differences between them, all three vaccines elicit boostable bactericidal antibody responses against meningococci, whether the test organisms in the assay express O-acetylated or de-O-acetylated group C capsule.

Meningitec (Wyeth Vaccines) is prepared by the controlled treatment of group C polysaccharide with sodium periodate, followed by the separation of the resulting oligosaccharides from high-molecular-weight saccharide and conjugation to CRM_{197} by reductive amination. Although Menjugate (Chiron Vaccines) is also composed of group C oligosaccharide conjugated to CRM_{197}, its manufacture differs

TABLE 34–2 ■ Meningococcal Group C Conjugate Vaccines*

Manufacturer	Vaccine	Active Constituents per Dose	Adjuvant	Other Excipients	Presentation
Wyeth Vaccines	Meningitec™	10 µg O-acetylated group C oligosaccharide conjugated to approximately 15 µg CRM_{197}	$AlPO_4$	Sodium chloride	Single dose, liquid suspension, vial
Chiron Vaccines	Menjugate®	10 µg O-acetylated group C oligosaccharide conjugated to 11–25 µg CRM_{197}	$Al(OH)_3$	Mannitol, sodium phosphate buffer	Single dose, freeze-dried, vial reconstituted with diluent
Baxter Immuno	NeisVac-C™	10 µg de-O-acetylated group C polysaccharide conjugated to 10–20 µg tetanus toxoid	$Al(OH)_3$	Sodium chloride	Single dose, pre-filled syringe

*All vaccines shown are preservative free.

from that of Meningitec. Menjugate is manufactured from group C polysaccharide that has been partially hydrolyzed at low pH and size fractionated before being conjugated to CRM_{197} through a bis-N-hydroxysuccinamide ester of adipic acid.[146] In the manufacture of NeisVac-C (Baxter Immuno), the group C polysaccharide is first de-acetylated with sodium hydroxide but, because N-acetyl groups are part of the protective epitopes, the amino groups are then re-acetylated with acetic anhydride.[153] Following limited depolymerization with sodium periodate and size fractionation, the de-O-acetylated oligosaccharide is conjugated directly to the tetanus toxoid by reductive amination. The single dose formulations of all three vaccines do not contain any form of preservative, although phenoxyethanol was used as a preservative in the multidose vials prepared by Chiron Vaccine and used for the mass immunization program in the United Kingdom.

Group C conjugate vaccines are stable at the recommended storage temperature (2° to 8°C). Studies in which the conjugate vaccines have been stored at higher temperatures, or subjected to repeated cycles of freeze-thawing, indicated that the structural stability of the oligosaccharide chains and of the protein carrier was related to the conjugation chemistry or formulation of the vaccine.[154] However, the immunogenicity of the vaccines in mice was only affected by incubation of the vaccines under more extreme conditions that resulted in the release of a substantial proportion of free saccharide.[155]

Methods of Determining Immunogenicity

The principal assays used to assess meningococcal vaccine immunogenicity are an ELISA to measure serum anticapsular antibody concentrations[156] and a bactericidal assay to measure serum antibody functional activity.[157] Both assays have been standardized to yield reproducible data, and the results provide important information on vaccine performance.

The bactericidal assay measures the interaction of antibody and complement at the bacterial surface, which results in bacterial death. Although opsonization as a result of binding of IgG and C3 to the bacteria is likely to be an important protective mechanism, complement-mediated serum bactericidal activity is a critical immune mechanism by which serum antibody confers protection to the host against developing meningococcal disease. The original study demonstrating a correlation between serum bactericidal activity and protection against developing meningococcal disease used human complement in the assay.[47] However, it is difficult to find sufficient amounts of human sera that lack antimeningococcal antibodies to serve as a source of exogenous complement. Therefore, most laboratories today use infant rabbit serum as an exogenous source of complement in the assay because suitable infant rabbit sera are widely available and can be shared among laboratories for standardization of the assay.[158] Rabbit serum also is recommended by the World Health Organization (WHO) as a source of complement for assessing human bactericidal responses to meningococcal polysaccharide vaccines as part of biologic standardization.[159]

Bactericidal titers measured with rabbit complement are higher than those measured with human complement.[123,160,161] Thus the source of complement in the assay needs to be taken into consideration in interpreting bactericidal antibody responses. When measured with human complement, a bactericidal titer of 1:4 or 1:8 or greater is generally considered protective. With rabbit complement, the "protective" threshold is controversial.[158,161,162] Studies have found that titers as high as 1:128 to 1:256 are needed when measured with rabbit complement to assure that a titer of 1:4 or 1:8 is present if measured with human complement.[161,162] Titers between 1:8 and 1:64 measured with rabbit complement are uncertain as a measure of protective immune response to vaccination, and further serologic data should be generated.

For licensure of group C conjugate vaccines in the United Kingdom, a combination of additional indicators was used to assess immune responses.[162] These included (1) evidence of a fourfold rise in bactericidal antibody titer between pre- and 1 month post–primary immunization sera; or (2) demonstration of induction of immunologic memory based on a "booster" bactericidal antibody response to a 10-μg challenge dose of meningococcal polysaccharide vaccine administered at least 6 months following the primary series, as compared to the response of a naïve cohort of similar age immunized with polysaccharide vaccine for the first time. Evidence of induction of immunologic memory by the conjugate vaccination also may be supported by an increase in avidity indices of group C–specific IgG antibody, comparing sera obtained 1 month to 6 or more months after the primary series.[162]

The results of the standardized ELISA for measurement of groups A or C serum anticapsular antibody concentrations do not distinguish between bactericidal and nonbactericidal anticapsular antibodies.[163,164] This problem is heightened when assaying heterogeneous anticapsular antibody populations. These include naturally induced anticapsular antibodies or anticapsular antibodies elicited at different ages by meningococcal polysaccharide vaccine[163] (Fig. 34–4). Additional settings associated with heterogeneous anticapsular antibody populations include young children immunized with polysaccharide or conjugate vaccines,[164–166] or the antibody responses of infants given a first dose of conjugate vaccine as compared to the second. A modified ELISA has been described that incorporates a fixed concentration of a chaotropic agent in the serum diluting buffer to minimize detection of low-avidity anticapsular antibodies.[167] When assaying heterogeneous antibody populations, serum anticapsular antibody concentrations measured by this modified ELISA correlated better with the magnitude of the respective group C bactericidal titers than do anticapsular antibody concentrations measured by the standard ELISA. Other assays that have been used to assess vaccine immunogenicity include a radioantigen binding assay (RABA).[168] This assay as well as the ELISA also can be adapted to provide information on antibody avidity.[169–171]

Results with Meningococcal Polysaccharide Vaccine

Immunogenicity of Meningococcal Polysaccharide Vaccine

Unconjugated capsular polysaccharide vaccines elicit serum antibody responses largely in the absence of T-cell help

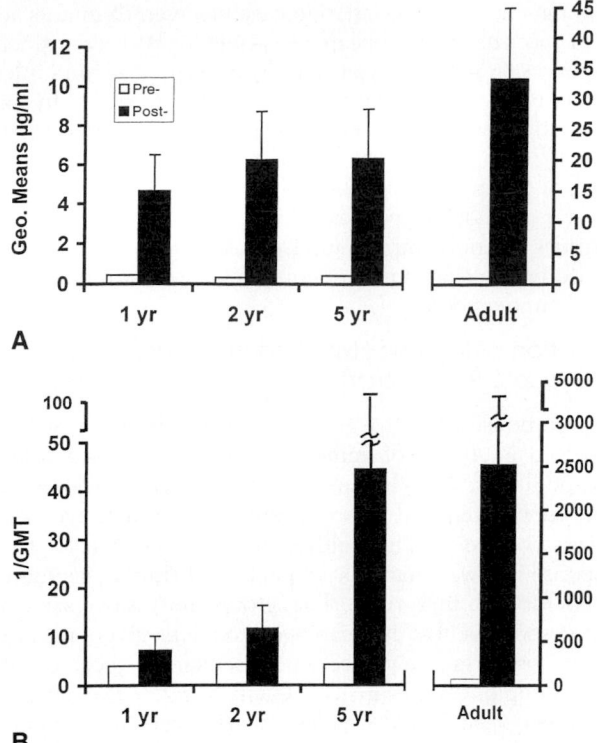

A

B

FIGURE 34–4 ■ Age-dependent group C antibody responses to meningococcal polysaccharide vaccine (A, C, Y, and W135). A, ELISA measuring total anticapsular antibody concentrations. B, Bactericidal titers measured with rabbit complement. Note that axes for the adult responses on both panels (*right side*) are shown on different scales than the corresponding axes showing the responses of the children (*left side*). (Adapted from Maslanka SE, Tappero JW, Plikaytis BD, et al. Age-dependent *Neisseria meningitidis* serogroup C class-specific antibody concentrations and bactericidal titers in sera from young children from Montana immunized with a licensed polysaccharide vaccine. Infect Immun 66:2453–2459, 1998.)

(so-called T-cell–independent [TI] antigens). TI antigens are immunogenic in older children and adults but typically are poorly immunogenic in infants, and repeated injections do not elicit antibody boosting at any age. The ability of older children and adults to produce serum antibodies in response to capsular polysaccharides is considered to be an indicator of intrinsic B-cell maturation. However, there is growing evidence that acquisition of antibody responsiveness, at least in adults, also reflects natural priming and generation of anticapsular B-cell populations in the memory state, because anticapsular antibodies elicited by capsular polysaccharide vaccination are isotype-switched and hypermutated, features indicative of a secondary antibody response.[172,173] Consistent with this mechanism is the relatively high group C anticapsular antibody avidity elicited in adults by meningococcal polysaccharide vaccine,[173a] albeit possibly lower than that elicited in adults by a group C conjugate vaccine.[174a]

Age-Related Immunogenicity

There is an age-related increase in antibody responsiveness to meningococcal groups A and C polysaccharide vaccine. However, immunized infants and children can mount serum anticapsular antibody responses.[163,166,174,176] Representative group C anticapsular antibody responses as measured by ELISA in sera of children of different ages and in adults are

shown in Figure 34–4A. At age 5 years, the magnitude of the geometric mean anticapsular antibody response is approximately 20% of that of an immunized adult. Note that the corresponding geometric mean bactericidal antibody titer (GMT) of children immunized at age 5 years is less than 2% of that of adults (Fig. 34–4B).

The serum anticapsular antibody responses of children under age 2 years given a single injection of group A polysaccharide vaccine are lower than those to group C polysaccharide vaccine.[174,175] However, infants immunized at 7 to 18 months of age with group A polysaccharide vaccine paradoxically show booster responses to a second injection of vaccine, which are not observed after a second injection of group C polysaccharide vaccine (see *Response to Booster Immunization* below).

The relationship between serum anticapsular antibody concentrations as measured by ELISA or RABA and protection from developing meningococcal disease is unknown. In sera from immunized infants, there may be no detectable bactericidal activity in the presence of relatively high group A or C anticapsular antibody concentrations.[164a,165,166] Complement-mediated bactericidal activity of groups A and C anticapsular antibodies elicited by meningococcal polysaccharide vaccination of children also is disproportionately lower than that of anticapsular antibodies elicited by vaccination of older children and adults.[163,164a,166] (For representative data for group C responses, compare the ELISA results in Figure 34–4A to the bactericidal titers in Figure 34–4B.[163]) Thus, depending on the age of the person, meningococcal polysaccharide vaccination can elicit either protective or nonprotective anticapsular antibodies. This disparity implies distinct age-related antibody repertoires that result in differences in antibody avidity or fine antigenic specificity, both of which appear to affect the functional activity of the antibody against the bacteria.[164a] These age-related differences in antibody bactericidal activity also underscore the difficulties in establishing a single threshold concentration of serum anticapsular antibody that is sufficient for predicting protection from disease.[177] Given these uncertainties, the results of bactericidal assays, albeit imperfect, are preferable for predicting protection after vaccination than are anti-capsular antibody concentrations.[158]

Much less information is available on the immunogenicity of groups Y and W135 polysaccharides contained in tetravalent meningococcal polysaccharide vaccines.[178–181] The available data indicate that children and adults given a single injection of tetravalent vaccine develop fourfold or greater serum bactericidal antibody responses to each of the capsular groups contained in the vaccine. These responses are presumed to confer protective immunity.

Kinetics and Persistence of Bactericidal Antibody

Most adults develop protective bactericidal antibody levels within 7 to 10 days after meningococcal polysaccharide vaccination, which peak at approximately 2 to 4 weeks after immunization. Serum bactericidal titers then decline over 2 years to plateau at approximately 5% of their respective peak values and remain above baseline preimmunization levels for at least 10 years (Fig. 34–5).[182] In contrast, bactericidal antibody responses of children decline more rapidly. In one study, the group C bactericidal antibody responses of children immunized with meningococcal polysaccharide

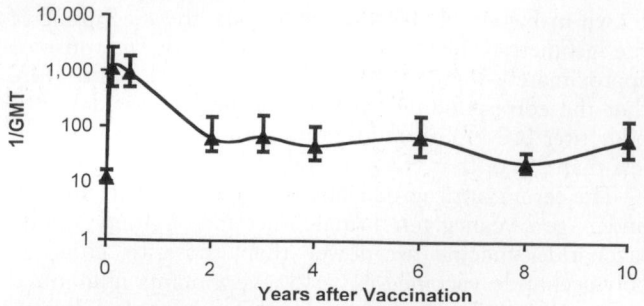

FIGURE 34–5 ■ Group C bactericidal antibody titers of U.S. military personnel after immunization with meningococcal polysaccharide vaccine (A, C, Y, and W135). Each time point represents the geometric mean bactericidal antibody titer (GMT) of approximately 40 individuals. (Adapted from Zangwill KM, Stout RW, Carlone GM, et al. Duration of antibody response after meningococcal polysaccharide vaccination in US Air Force personnel. J Infect Dis 169:847–852, 1994.)

vaccine at ages 18 months to 5 years declined to baseline within 1 year.[183] In another study, infants immunized in The Gambia with two doses of meningococcal bivalent A and C polysaccharide vaccine at 3 and 6 months of age had group A and C serum bactericidal titers at 18 to 23 months of age that were indistinguishable from those of unimmunized control children.[139] The Gambian children were given a third dose of polysaccharide vaccine at 18 to 23 months. Their serum bactericidal antibody titers at age 5 years were indistinguishable from those of unimmunized control children.[184]

Response to Booster Immunization.

As shown in Table 34–3, an injection of group A meningococcal polysaccharide vaccine given at 3 months of age primed infants for the ability to mount booster antibody responses to a second injection of group A polysaccharide vaccine given at 12 months of age.[185] Booster antibody responses to unconjugated polysaccharides, which are considered TI antigens, are very atypical. For example, in the same study an injection of group C polysaccharide vaccine given at 3 months of age resulted in lower group C antibody responses to a second immunization given at 12 months, as compared to the magnitude of the group C antibody responses of 12-month-olds immunized for the first time (Table 34–3) (so-called immune hyporesponsiveness; see below). In another study, an injection of tetravalent

meningococcal polysaccharide vaccine given to infants at 6 to 11 months of age appeared to prime for booster antibody responses to W135 polysaccharide following a second injection of tetravalent vaccine given 12 months later.[181] In contrast, there was no evidence of a booster response to the group Y component. The disparity between repeated injections of group A or, possibly, W135 polysaccharide to elicit booster antibody responses, while groups C and Y polysaccharides do not, implies fundamental differences in their respective mechanism(s) of immunogenicity, which remain poorly understood.

Induction of Immune Hyporesponsiveness to Group C Polysaccharide

Hyporesponsiveness to group C polysaccharide has been observed in studies of immunized infants,[139,174] toddlers,[147] and adults.[140,186,187] Immunized persons with hyporesponsiveness can respond to revaccination with meningococcal polysaccharide vaccine, although the magnitude of their response is lower than that of persons of similar age immunized for the first time. The group most susceptible to hyporesponsiveness is infants or toddlers given repeated injections of meningococcal polysaccharide vaccine.[139,147] For example, infants in The Gambia given two doses of meningococcal A and C polysaccharide vaccine at 3 and 6 months of age were re-immunized with polysaccharide vaccine at mean age of 19.7 months. The group C bactericidal titers measured in serum samples obtained 10 to 14 days later were nearly 10-fold lower than those of control children immunized for the first time (GMTs of 1:26 vs. 1:239, respectively).[139] In contrast, there was no evidence of induction of hyporesponsiveness to group A polysaccharide. Indeed, there was a suggestion of priming to group A polysaccharide because the postimmunization group A GMT was 1:1783 in the group that previously received the polysaccharide vaccine versus 1:338 in control children of similar ages immunized for the first time.[139]

Hyporesponsiveness to group C polysaccharide also has been observed 4 years after a single dose of meningococcal polysaccharide vaccine given to adults,[140] and can persist in immunized children for as long as 4 to 5 years.[184] Although there are conflicting data,[184] as noted above, hyporesponsiveness to group A polysaccharide appears to be less of a problem in immunized infants or children than with group C polysaccharide[139,174] (see also Table 34–2).

The clinical importance of vaccine-induced hyporesponsiveness to group C polysaccharide is unknown. Because of

TABLE 34–3 ■ Anticapsular Antibody Responses at 12 Months of Age in Relation to Previous Meningococcal Polysaccharide Vaccination at 3 Months of Age

Antibody Tested	No. Tested	Prior Vaccine at 3 Mo.	Vaccine at 12 Mo.	Antibody Conc. at 13 Mo.*	
				Geometric Mean (µg/mL)	%>1 (µg/mL)
Group A	14	Group A	Group A	4.00	79
	28	Group C	Group A	0.87	40
Group C	41	Group C	Group C	0.83	30
	38	Group A	Group C	2.10	89

*Antibody concentrations measured by a radioantigen binding assay.
Adapted from Gold R, Lepow ML, Goldschneider I, et al. Kinetics of antibody production to group A and group C meningococcal polysaccharide vaccines administered during the first six years of life: prospects for routine immunization of infants and children. J Infect Dis 140: 690–697, 1979.

impaired ability to develop a group C serum anticapsular antibody response, persons with hyporesponsiveness whose serum anticapsular antibody concentrations have declined to below protective levels may, in theory, be at increased risk of acquiring meningococcal disease if they are exposed to a pathogenic group C *N. meningitidis* strain. This theoretical concern, however, is not substantiated by clinical experience. Meningococcal polysaccharide vaccine has been used extensively in the military for more than two decades, and has been given to large populations during mass immunization campaigns[188,190] without evidence of an increased risk of later acquiring group C meningococcal disease.

Efficacy of Group C Polysaccharide Vaccine

Two large-scale field trials of group C vaccine were undertaken in 1969 and 1970 among U.S. military recruits at high risk of acquiring meningococcal disease.[191,192] A total of 28,245 recruits in both trials were randomized to receive meningococcal C vaccination and 114,481 unimmunized men served as controls. During the 8 weeks of follow-up, 73 culture-confirmed cases occurred among the controls (an attack rate of 0.637 per 1000) as compared to 3 cases among the vaccinated (an attack rate of 0.106/1000, which includes one case occurring 9 days after vaccination that was excluded from the original analysis). Vaccine efficacy from the combined data set was 83% if the case at 9 days (a period when a protective antibody response might be expected) is included, or 89% if this case is excluded. The protection induced by the vaccine was group specific. In the first trial, the attack rate of group B meningococcal disease was fivefold higher in the vaccinated group than in the control group, but the difference in the respective incidence rates was not statistically significant. In the second trial, there were no cases of group B disease in the vaccinated or control groups. Since October 1972, meningococcal polysaccharide vaccine has been administered to all incoming recruits, and meningococcal disease caused by strains with capsular groups contained in the vaccine has been eliminated as an important health problem in the U.S. Army. Routine immunization of Italian military personnel with meningococcal polysaccharide vaccine also has resulted in good control of disease.[193]

The efficacy of group C polysaccharide vaccine in young children was evaluated in a prospective field trial conducted in 1974 during a major group C epidemic in São Paulo, Brazil.[194] Approximately 67,000 children ages 6 to 36 months were randomized to receive either a dose of group C vaccine or, as a control, diphtheria and tetanus toxoids. During the 17 months of follow-up, there were 31 culture- or serology-confirmed cases among the vaccinated group and 45 cases among the controls (efficacy = 31%; 95% CI, –11% to 58%). For children ages 6 to 23 months, vaccine efficacy was 12% (95% CI, –55 to 62%). For children 24 to 36 months, vaccine efficacy was 55% (95% CI, –4% to 72%). Children age 2 years in this study showed significant anticapsular antibody responses to vaccination.[195] The low observed efficacy in this trial, however, has been attributed to the possibility that the vaccine used was suboptimal.[196]

The efficacy of meningococcal vaccine also has been estimated as part of postlicensure studies. In response to an outbreak of group C meningococcal disease in Gregg County Texas, the State Department of Health vaccinated approximately 36,000 residents, 2 to 29 years of age.[189] The results of a case-control study found group C efficacy rates of 85% among 2- to 29-year olds, and 93% for children 2 to 5 years. The 95% CIs for both estimates were wide (27% to 97% and 16% to 99%, respectively).

In Quebec, Canada, approximately 1.6 million doses of meningococcal polysaccharide vaccine were administered to persons ages 6 months to 20 years in response to an increase in the incidence of meningococcal disease caused by a virulent clone of *N. meningitidis* group C. The investigators compared the incidence rates of group C disease among vaccinated and unvaccinated populations.[188] For children less than 2 years, there were eight cases in the vaccinated group and none in the unvaccinated group ($P = 0.38$). Vaccine efficacy estimated for this age group, therefore, was negative, but the 95% CI was large. In children ages 2 to 9 years, vaccine efficacy was 41% (95% CI, –106% to 79%). Among persons 5 to 20 years, vaccine efficacy was 65% during the first 2 years of follow-up (95% CI, 20% to 84%), and 0% between 3 and 5 years after vaccination (95% CI, –5% to 65%). The surveillance data from Canada also were used to estimate vaccine efficacy by a method based on the distribution of vaccine capsular group and non-vaccine capsular group cases occurring in vaccinated and unvaccinated individuals[188a]. Among 54 cases caused by group C strains, 38 occurred in vaccinated individuals. The authors estimated vaccine effectiveness to be 71% (95% CI, 21% to 89%), with lower effectiveness in children less than 2 to 9 years of age (50%; 95% CI, –65% to 85%) and higher in adults (83%; 95% CI, 39% to 96%). In this analysis, efficacy appeared to persist between 2 and 5 years after vaccination. This report also underscores that a vaccine can be efficacious even when a high proportion of group C cases occurs in vaccinated persons[221].

In summary, the immunogenicity and efficacy of group C polysaccharide vaccine are clearly age related, being high in adults and low or negligible in infants and young children. The exact age when children develop protective efficacy remains poorly defined. The duration of protection in immunized adults is also poorly defined. The Canadian study described above is unique in its long duration of follow-up, but the lack of efficacy found during years 3 to 5 after vaccination is an imprecise estimate because of the small number of cases in both the vaccinated and unvaccinated populations. Duration of protection after vaccination, therefore, has been inferred from studies of persistence of serum bactericidal antibody after vaccination. However, these studies used rabbit complement to measure the titers, so it is uncertain whether the magnitude of the serum antibody levels is sufficient to confer protection in the absence of induction of immunologic memory (see *Methods of Determining Immunogenicity*, above). If the serum bactericidal titers present at 2 to 3 years after vaccination are sufficient to confer protection, then the data suggest that protection should remain unchanged for up to 10 years (Fig. 34–5). Alternatively, protection may be conferred only during the first 2 years after vaccination, when titers are substantially higher. In children ages 2 to 5 years, the decline in group C serum bactericidal antibody titers is much more rapid than in adults and, in contrast to adults, the antibody titers of children usually return to preimmunization levels within a year.[183]

TABLE 34–4 ■ Summary of Seven Controlled Trials Measuring the Efficacy of Group A Meningococcal Polysaccharide Vaccine

Location (Reference)	Study No.	Age Group (yr)	Follow-Up (mo)
Egypt (Wahdan et al., 1973)[267]	1	6–15	6
Egypt (Wahdan et al., 1977)[199]	2	6–15	12
			13–23
Sudan (Erwa et al., 1973)[268]	3	1 to >21	4
Mali (Saliou et al., 1978)[200]	4	0.5–6	36
Nigeria (Greenwood et al., 1978)[213]	5	All	2
Finland (Peltola et al., 1977)[269]	6	0.25–5	12
Finland (Makela et al., 1975)[270]	7	Military recruits	9

*For purposes of the table, the 95% confidence intervals for the percent efficacy shown for each of the studies were calculated from the respective incidence rates in the vaccinated subjects and controls.

Efficacy of Group A Polysaccharide Vaccine

Table 34–4 summarizes the results of seven controlled field trials measuring the efficacy of meningococcal group A polysaccharide vaccine. In most of the studies, the small number of cases and short duration of observation limit interpretation of the data. Consistently, however, high levels of vaccine efficacy were observed in all age groups, including infants.

The efficacy of group A polysaccharide vaccine also has been confirmed by observational studies conducted during mass immunization campaigns. In one such study, approximately two thirds of an estimated 671,000 population of Bamako Mali were immunized in 1981 with meningococcal polysaccharide vaccine in response to a group A epidemic.[197] Vaccination was targeted at the age group 1 to 30 years. During the 5 weeks between completing the vaccination campaign and the end of the epidemic, the attack rate among vaccinated persons (0.7/10,000) was significantly lower than that among unvaccinated persons (4.7/10,000; vaccine efficacy 85%; 95% CI, 80% to 90%). In another study in New Zealand,[198] over 130,000 doses of meningococcal polysaccharide vaccine were administered to children 3 months to 13 years of age during an epidemic of group A disease. No cases of group A disease were observed among children given a single injection of vaccine at 18 months of age or older (100% efficacy). However, there were seven cases in children immunized between 3 and 18 months. Vaccine efficacy for this age group during the first year of follow-up was 52% (95% CI, –330% to 95%), which fell to 16% (95% CI, –538% to 90%) after 1 year. None of the children ages 3 to 17 months who developed disease received the booster dose of vaccine recommended for this age group.

There are only limited data on the duration of protection against group A disease. One controlled field trial (Study 2, Table 34–4) followed children ages 6 to 15 years in Egypt for 24 months after vaccination.[199] There was high efficacy for the first 12 months but no efficacy between 13 and 24 months. Interpretation of the lack of efficacy in the second

year is limited by the suboptimal low molecular size of the vaccine used in that study. The efficacy study in Mali (Study 4, Table 34–4) included follow-up for 3 years, but there were too few cases in the unimmunized controls in years 2 and 3 of the study to obtain an estimate of the duration of protection.[200]

In a retrospective study in Burkina Faso, approximately 103,000 infants and children ages 3 months to 16 years were vaccinated in response to a group A epidemic.[201] The results of case-control studies conducted 1, 2, and 3 years after vaccination indicated overall efficacy of 87% for year 1, 70% for year 2, and 54% for year 3. Age had no effect on the efficacy rate observed in the first year, but, by the third year, vaccine efficacy was only 8% for children immunized below 4 years of age, as compared to 67% for children immunized at 4 to 16 years of age.

In summary, the high efficacy of group A polysaccharide vaccine in infants and young children is virtually unique among unconjugated bacterial polysaccharide vaccines. However, two doses of group A polysaccharide vaccine appear to be needed below 18 months of age, and serum bactericidal titers decline rapidly in immunized infants and young children. The anticapsular antibody responses of immunized infants also have lower complement-mediated bactericidal activity than that of anticapsular antibodies induced by vaccination of adults.

No studies have evaluated the efficacy of prevention of group A meningococcal disease in Africa by a vaccination regimen of two or more doses given to infants or other age groups. However, the data described above (see also *Kinetics and Persistence of Bactericidal Antibody* above) indicate that even multiple doses of meningococcal polysaccharide vaccine given in the first 2 years of life are unlikely to result in sustained protection against group A disease. Also, if bivalent or tetravalent meningococcal polysaccharide vaccines are used for routine prevention of group A disease, the vaccinated infants and toddlers would be expected to develop hyporesponsiveness to group C polysaccharide (see *Induction of Immune Hyporesponsiveness to Group C Polysaccharide* above), which could persist for up to 4 years.[140,184] As noted

| No. Cases/No. Persons | | Efficacy (%) | |
Vaccinated	Controls	(95% CI*)	Comments
0/62,295	8/62,054	100 (41% to 100%)	
1/88,263	9/88,383	89 (19% to 99%)	Molecular weight of vaccine
3/88,263	3/88,383	0 (−650% to 87%)	lower than optimal
0/10,891	7/10,749	100 (30% to 100%)	Same vaccine used as in study 2
0/16,395	6/21,957	100 (−16% to 100%)	All 6 cases in controls occurred within 2 years
1/520	8/523	88 (6% to 99%)	Household contact study
0/49,295	6/48,977	100 (15% to 100%)	Infants <18 mo received 2 doses
1/16,458	11/20,748	89 (20% to 99%)	

above, the clinical importance of hyporesponsiveness is unknown, but theoretically it could increase their risk of acquiring group C disease, should the children be exposed to the organism. Therefore, if meningococcal polysaccharide vaccine is used for routine prevention of group A disease, it would be preferable to employ a monovalent group A vaccine.

To date, meningococcal polysaccharide vaccine has been used mainly for prevention of group A disease under emergency conditions of outbreaks. To ensure effective control of outbreaks, an outbreak has to be recognized early, and mobilization for mass immunization must be rapid. An emergency response plan has been prepared by the World Health Organization and the Centers for Disease Control and Prevention that outlines necessary steps for identifying and responding to outbreaks.[202] However, even with optimal rapid response, less than 60% of outbreak-related cases will be prevented and, under real-life circumstances, substantially lower percentages of cases are actually prevented. For these reasons, Robbins and colleagues have recommended that the entire population of the sub-Saharan meningitis belt receive group A vaccine in a mass program.[203,204] Thereafter, they propose routine immunization with one dose of group A vaccine at 2 years of age and another at 5 years of age for elimination of group A disease in the region. Although a recent theoretical modeling analysis suggests that such an approach is cost-effective, many questions remain about the effectiveness of this approach.[204a] These include the duration of protection, the effect of vaccination on interruption of transmission of the organism (see below), or the ability to implement multiple doses of vaccine in children living in one of the poorest areas of the world. Given these concerns, further data are needed from pilot programs conducted in sub-Saharan Africa to determine the effectiveness of this approach.

For control of epidemic meningococcal disease in sub-Saharan Africa, an improved meningococcal vaccine is needed. Ideally such a vaccine will elicit protective serum antibody concentrations at all ages, preferably after a single dose, and will also induce long-term immunologic memory

so that protection can be sustained when serum anticapsular antibody concentrations have declined to subprotective levels. The ideal vaccine also should interrupt transmission of the organism in the population. Polysaccharide-protein conjugate vaccines offer the prospect of both eliciting longer-term protective immunity at all ages and also decreasing transmission of the pathogen in the population (Table 34–5). In 2001, the Bill and Melinda Gates foundation awarded a grant of $70 million to the World Health Organization and a nongovernmental organization, Program for Applied Technology in Health (PATH), to develop and implement a meningococcal conjugate vaccine for use in sub-Saharan Africa.[204b] For the first time funding is available to develop a new vaccine targeted against a strain of pathogen that is largely confined to a poor region of the world. One challenge for this program will be to license and produce sufficient quantities of a low-cost conjugate vaccine in a short time period. A second challenge

TABLE 34–5 ■ Properties of Meninogococcal Polysaccharide and Conjugate Vaccines

Property	Polysaccharide	Conjugate
Immunogenicity		
Adults	High	High
Young children	Poor	High
Quality of antibody in children		
Avidity	Low	High
Bactericidal activity	Low	High
Response to booster	Poor*	High
Induction of immunologic memory	No	High
Effect of colonization	+/−	Yes†

*Repeated immunization of infants and toddlers elicits booster antibody responses to group A polysaccharide vaccine, whereas hyporesponsiveness is observed to group C polysaccharide (see text).
†Demonstrated for *Haemophilus influenzae* type b and for *Streptococcus pneumoniae* conjugate vaccines. Data also indicate that group C *Neisseria meningitidis* conjugate vaccination lowers carriage.[227]

will be to implement an effective vaccination program for control of epidemics in sub-Saharan Africa under logistically difficult conditions.

Efficacy of Groups Y and W135 Polysaccharide Vaccine

There are no data on the efficacy of groups Y and W135 polysaccharides. For licensure of the tetravalent meningococcal polysaccharide vaccines, the efficacy of the group Y and W135 components was inferred based on fourfold or greater bactericidal antibody responses measured with rabbit complement.

Effect of Meningococcal Polysaccharide Vaccination on Colonization and Herd Immunity

The ideal vaccine both protects the host from developing disease and interrupts transmission of the organism in the community by diminishing colonization. There are conflicting data on the effect of meningococcal polysaccharide vaccination on colonization. Studies conducted in military populations exposed to rapid spread of group C organisms indicated decreased acquisition rates of group C organisms within a few weeks to months after vaccination.[138,191,205-207] These studies also provided evidence for the replacement of the prevailing group C isolate with meningococci of other groups. Similar studies carried out in the Finnish military showed trends toward decreased carriage of group A meningococci 7 to 16 weeks after immunization with bivalent vaccine.[208] However, a number of studies among school-age children in Africa failed to demonstrate a consistent or sustained effect of polysaccharide vaccination on colonization with group A meningococci.[199,209-211] Also, group A carriage rates of 12% to 35% have been reported following vaccination.[212,213] Taken together, the data indicate that polysaccharide vaccination provides only transient and incomplete protection against nasopharyngeal carriage, with the effect being largest in enclosed populations such as military recruits and lowest in open populations of children.

Safety of Meningococcal Polysaccharide Vaccines

Meningococcal polysaccharide vaccines (bivalent A and C, or tetravalent A, C, Y, and W135) have been administered to millions of persons, including the military, civilians as part of mass vaccination programs, and travelers to areas of the world with endemic disease.[88] The vaccines are considered to be safe and well tolerated.[213a] Pain and redness at the injection site are the most commonly reported adverse events (up to 40%). These local reactions are typically of mild severity and last 1 to 2 days. Transient low-grade fever is reported in less than 5% of adults. Higher fevers (>38.4°C) occur in less than 1% of immunized persons. Severe reactions are uncommon, consisting of wheezing or urticaria in an estimated 1 per 1,000,000 doses, or anaphylaxis in less than 1 per 1,000,000 doses. There are also rare reports of Guillain-Barré syndrome or other neurologic disorders such as optic neuritis, paresthesia, or convulsions with onset temporally associated with vaccination. In most of the reported instances, multiple injections were given to the patients, so the role of meningococcal vaccination was uncertain.[88]

Results with Meningococcal Polysaccharide-Protein Conjugate Vaccines

Immunogenicity of Meningococcal Polysaccharide-Protein Conjugate Vaccines

The development of protein-polysaccharide conjugate vaccines has overcome the limitations of polysaccharide vaccines by presenting the polysaccharide moiety of the vaccine covalently coupled to a carrier protein. B cells recognizing the polysaccharide process the protein carrier and present peptide epitopes to CD4-positive T cells. These carrier-specific T cells provide help to the B cell and result in increased immunogenicity of the polysaccharide component in individuals unresponsive to unconjugated polysaccharide, such as young infants. The resulting conjugate vaccines have many desirable properties that result in more effective vaccines than the corresponding unconjugated polysaccharide vaccines (Table 34–5).

The quality of the antibody of the anticapsular antibody elicited by conjugate vaccines is superior to that elicited by unconjugated polysaccharide vaccines with respect to higher avidity or the ability to elicit complement-mediated bactericidal activity. This is especially true in children but also has been observed in immunized adults.[174b] Conjugate vaccines also induce a population of long-lasting memory B cells capable of responding to unconjugated polysaccharide, which results in generation of immunologic memory. The characteristics of a memory response include an IgG antibody response to a subsequent challenge with unconjugated polysaccharide that is of higher magnitude than that of a person immunized for the first time; higher antibody avidity (from somatic mutation of the immunoglobulin variable region genes encoding the hypervariable or complementary determining regions of the anti-capsular antibody) and, possibly, more rapid induction of the antibody response.

Age-Related Immunogenicity

Complement-mediated bactericidal antibody responses remain the best serologic correlate of protective immunity. However, as described in the section on *Methods of Determining Immunogenicity* above, interpretation of the results is confounded by the different assay methods used to measure bactericidal antibody, particularly the choice of exogenous human or rabbit complement. Nevertheless, substantial evidence indicates that all three group C conjugate vaccines licensed in the United Kingdom are highly immunogenic after two or three doses given in the first 6 months of life. In one study, over 95% of infants immunized with the Chiron group C conjugate vaccine developed serum bactericidal titers of 1:8 or greater as measured with human complement[150] (a threshold titer estimated to be twofold higher than that necessary for protection[47]). In other studies of the Wyeth or Baxter conjugate vaccines, similar high percentages of infants given two or three doses of the respective conjugate vaccines developed bactericidal titers of 128 or higher when measured with rabbit complement (a threshold predictive of a titer of 4 or higher when measured with human complement).[161,162] The magnitude of the responses of the infants in these studies is similar to that elicited by a dose of unconjugated meningococcal polysaccharide vaccine given to young adults (Fig. 34–6), an age group known to be highly protected by group C polysaccharide vaccination. Based on these immunogenicity data, the efficacy of these conjugate vaccines in infants was inferred, which formed the basis of their registration in Europe.

Up to a quarter of children 12 months to 5 years of age given a single dose of the Chiron or Wyeth conjugate vaccines develop serum bactericidal antibody titers that are in the equivocal range of 1:8 to 1:64 when measured with rabbit complement.[162] (Representative data for the Wyeth vaccine are shown in Table 34–6.) The clinical importance of these equivocal bactericidal titers after one dose of vaccine is unknown because virtually all of the immunized children in this age group show evidence of induction of immunologic memory.[171] Also, as described below, preliminary estimates of efficacy after introduction of group C meningococcal conjugate vaccine in the United Kingdom indicate high efficacy after a single dose of vaccine in toddlers ages 12 to 14 months.

There are only limited comparative immunogenicity data available from prospective, randomized studies of the three group C conjugate vaccines licensed in the United Kingdom. In one study, toddlers immunized with a single dose of the Baxter vaccine at 12 to 18 months of age had higher GMTs than did those given the Chiron or Wyeth vaccines[171] (Fig. 34–7). The reasons for the higher responses to the Baxter vaccine are unknown. They could result from the use of tetanus toxoid as the carrier protein or de-O-acetylated capsular polysaccharide in the Baxter vaccine, as opposed to CRM_{197} protein and O-acetylated capsular polysaccharide in the two vaccines made by the other manufacturers. Because all three vaccines are highly immunogenic and induce memory, the clinical importance of the higher titers after one dose of the Baxter vaccine with respect to protection against disease also is unknown.

As compared with group C conjugate vaccines, much less information is available on the immunogenicity of group A–containing conjugate vaccines. In one study of a

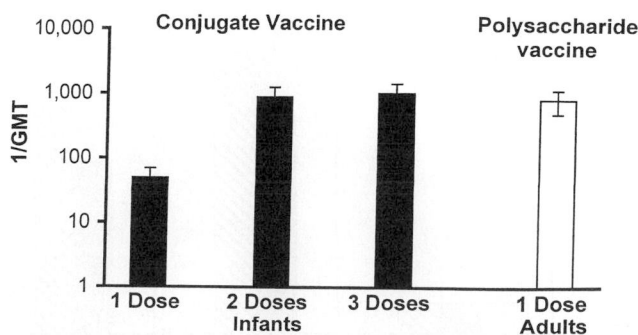

FIGURE 34–6 ■ Serum bactericidal antibody responses of U.K. infants immunized with the Wyeth group C conjugate vaccine at 2, 3, and 4 months of age.[148] For comparison, serum group C bactericidal antibody responses of young adults immunized with meningococcal polysaccharide vaccine are shown.[187] Titers were measured with rabbit complement.

bivalent A and C conjugate vaccine prepared by Aventis Pasteur, infants in Niger given three injections at 6, 10, and 14 weeks of age developed group A serum bactericidal antibody responses that were substantially greater than those observed in control infants immunized with meningococcal polysaccharide vaccine or *H. influenzae* type b conjugate vaccine.[166] In a study in the United Kingdom of a bivalent conjugate vaccine prepared by Chiron, infants immunized at 2, 3, and 4 months of age also developed serum group A bactericidal antibody responses.[214]

Anticapsular Antibody Kinetics and Persistence

Following a single dose of group C conjugate vaccine in adults, group C–specific IgG and bactericidal titers did not decline (or increase) in the 4 days following vaccination.[215] By day 10, antibody levels had risen significantly. In infants immunized at 2, 3, and 4 months of age, high antibody concentrations are present 1 month after the third dose but then decline markedly during the first year of life. At 12 months of age, antibody titers are still above preimmunization concentrations.[148,150]

Only limited data are available on persistence of serum antibodies after completing the three-dose schedule in infancy with no booster doses of polysaccharide or conjugate vaccine,[216] the currently recommended immunization

TABLE 34–6 ■ Serum Bactericidal Antibody Titers 4 Weeks After Vaccination with a Single Dose of Meningococcal C Conjugate Vaccine (Meningitec, Wyeth Vaccines)

			4 Wk Postvaccination Bactericidal Titer*					
			Titer ≤4		Titer 8–64		Titer ≥128	
Age	No.	GMT	No.	(%)	No.	(%)	No.	(%)
2 mo	50	33	16	(32)	15	(30)	19	(38)
12–14 mo	71	141	6	(8)	17	(24)	48	(68)
3–4 y	87	908	1	(1)	10	(11)	76	(88)
14–17 y	81	3890	0	(0)	0	(0)	81	(100)
18–26 y	86	1425	0	(0)	6	(7)	80	(93)

*Titers were measured at the Public Health Laboratory Service Reference Laboratory, Manchester, UK, using baby rabbit complement.[148,187,271,272]

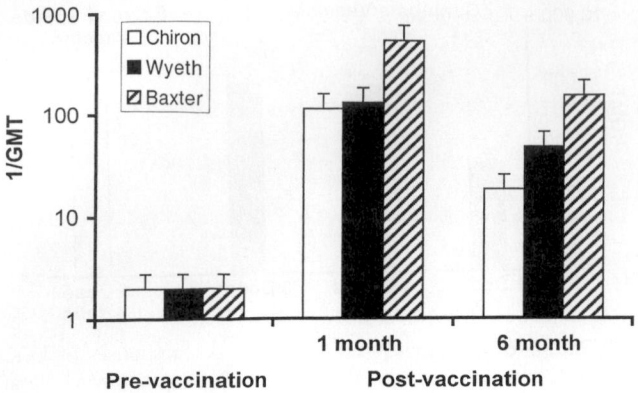

FIGURE 34-7 ▪ Serum bactericidal antibody responses in toddlers 1 and 6 months after a dose of meningococcal group C conjugate vaccine. Figure prepared from data from a randomized study of vaccine produced by three different manufacturers.[171]

schedule in the United Kingdom. In one study, group C–specific IgG and serum bactericidal antibody titers had declined to prevaccination levels by age 4 years.[216]

Immunologic Memory

Evidence for the induction of group C immunologic memory by conjugate vaccination has been reported in studies conducted 6 months to 4 years following primary immunization in infants[139,148,150,217] or adults.[140] Immunologic memory to the group A portion of bivalent A and C conjugate vaccines has been demonstrated for candidate bivalent conjugate vaccines prepared by Aventis Pasteur[166] or Chiron Vaccines.[217,218] However, in a study done in The Gambia, the group A portion of the Chiron vaccine did not prime for immunologic memory, although a group C memory response was observed.[139]

Evidence suggests that immunization with larger quantities of polysaccharide antigen per dose of conjugate vaccine results in higher postprimary serum bactericidal antibody levels than does a lower dose of antigen.[166] Also, giving two or three doses of conjugate vaccine to infants in the first 6 months of life elicits higher serum antibody responses than does one dose (Fig. 34-4). In contrast, use of lower doses of antigen[166,219] or fewer numbers of doses[220] appears to prime for higher memory antibody responses to a subsequent challenge with unconjugated polysaccharide vaccine. The relative importance of vaccine-induced serum antibody concentrations as opposed to induction of immunologic memory in conferring protection against invasive disease caused by encapsulated bacteria is a subject of considerable debate.[221] Nevertheless, these observations on the disparity between the dose of antigen or the number of injections and induction of serum antibody levels as opposed to immunologic memory may have important implications for the design of future meningococcal conjugate vaccines if ongoing studies demonstrate the importance of immunologic memory in protection against meningococcal disease.

Effect of Prior Polysaccharide Vaccination

Immunization with unconjugated meningococcal vaccine induces hyporesponsiveness to group C polysaccharide (see above). Whether or not this hyporesponsiveness can be overcome by group C conjugate vaccination therefore is of

considerable interest. Children randomized to a schedule of two doses of polysaccharide vaccine at 15 to 23 months of age, followed by a third dose of polysaccharide vaccine given a year later, had evidence of lower anticapsular and bactericidal antibody responses to a subsequent dose of a group C conjugate vaccine given at an average age of 50 months, when compared with antibody responses to conjugate vaccine of control children given one previous dose of polysaccharide vaccine in the second year of life.[222] However, the magnitude of the bactericidal responses of both groups to the conjugate vaccination would be expected to be sufficient to confer protection. In another study, infants given a single dose of meningococcal polysaccharide vaccine under the age of 1 year had a fourfold lower GMT in response to a subsequent dose of group C conjugate vaccine given at 12 to 18 months of age, as compared to that of children immunized for the first time (respective GMTs of 1:30 and 1:140).[223] In the same study, a single dose of meningococcal polysaccharide given after 24 months of age did not interfere with the responses to a subsequent dose of group C conjugate vaccine (respective GMTs of 1:277 and 1:309). In both age groups, prior exposure to polysaccharide vaccine did not appear to interfere with the avidity of the antibody elicited by the dose of conjugate vaccine (considered evidence of induction of immunologic memory). Therefore, the children previously exposed to polysaccharide vaccine below 1 year of age may still have been protected by the conjugate vaccination, despite their lower antibody responses.

Adults who have been given a prior dose of meningococcal polysaccharide vaccine have lower bactericidal antibody responses to a subsequent dose of group C conjugate vaccine than adults immunized with the conjugate vaccine for the first time.[215] There also was a suggestion that the effect of the prior polysaccharide vaccination may be dose dependent in that adults given two prior doses of polysaccharide vaccine had lower bactericidal antibody responses following conjugate vaccination than those given a single prior dose. However, the proportion of those with bactericidal responses above the putative threshold for protection was not altered by the prior exposure to one or two doses of the polysaccharide vaccine.

Effectiveness of Meningococcal C Conjugate Vaccine

Incidence of Disease

The relatively low incidence of group C disease in the United Kingdom meant that randomized controlled trials to measure protective efficacy of the new group C conjugate vaccines were impractical. However, efficacy of these vaccines was inferred on the basis of the immunogenicity data and extrapolating from the success of conjugate vaccine technology in decreasing *H. influenzae* type b disease. In England and Wales, group C disease had risen from 26% of cases in 1994 to 34% in 1998. Enhanced surveillance was initiated in 1999 throughout England and Wales, and the total number of group C cases for this year was estimated at 1500, with at least 150 deaths.

In November 1999, group C conjugate vaccination was introduced in the 15- to 17-year-old age group, and in infants who were vaccinated at 2, 3, and 4 months of age along with their routine primary immunization. From mid-

January 2000 onward, catch-up immunization with one dose of vaccine was done in toddlers ages 12 to 23 months, and in infants ages 5 to 11 months who received two doses of vaccine. Vaccination of 2- to 15-year-olds with a single dose was completed by late 2000. Population-based active surveillance monitored age-specific and capsular group-specific incidences of disease and estimated vaccine coverage.[224] Within 12 to 18 months of vaccine introduction, a marked decline was observed in the number of cases and number of deaths caused by group C disease in the age groups targeted for immunization.[152,224,225] Formal estimates of age-specific vaccine efficacy in England up to September 2001 using the screening method[226] are approximately 90% or above for all vaccinated age groups.[224,225] The dramatic decline in group C disease in the overall population is illustrated in Figure 34–8. During this period, there was no appreciable change in the pattern of group B disease. Surveillance of meningococcal disease continues in the United Kingdom.[226a] This follow-up will be important because, in the absence of booster doses of vaccine, there will be declining serum antibodies in the population and efficacy will rely on a combination of herd immunity and the ability of individuals to mount memory antibody responses on encountering the bacterium.

Carriage of *Neisseria meningitidis* and Herd Immunity

A large carriage study was undertaken in the United Kingdom before and after introduction of group C conjugate vaccines to measure the effectiveness of vaccination on carriage of meningococci. Comparison of carried meningococci isolated from 14,064 students ages 15 to 17 years, prior to introduction of group C conjugate vaccination in 1999, with culture results obtained from 16,583 age-matched students surveyed in 2000 after introduction of vaccination indicated a 66% decrease in the carriage of encapsulated group C meningococci.[227] The was no evidence of an increase in carriage by group B isolates or other capsular groups.

Herd immunity following introduction of the group C conjugate vaccine in England also has been estimated.[228] The age-specific attack rates among unvaccinated persons from January to September 2001, after introduction of group C conjugate vaccine, were compared to the historical attack rates of the respective cohorts for the period January to September 1999,

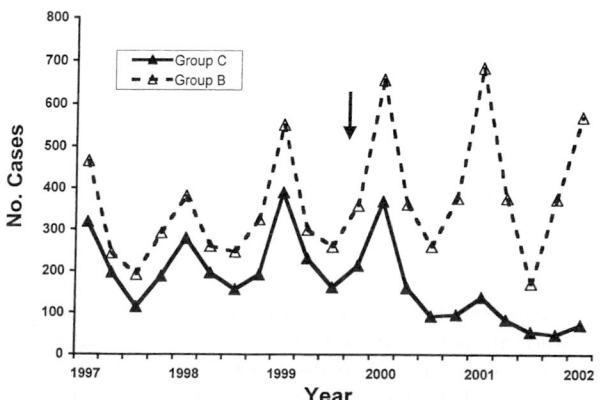

FIGURE 34–8 ■ Laboratory-confirmed cases of group B and C meningococcal disease (by quarter), England and Wales, 1997 to 2002. The *arrow* shows when group C conjugate vaccination was introduced.

before conjugate vaccination was introduced. Evidence of herd immunity is apparent (Table 34–7).[228] Although not shown in Table 34–7, there was no effect of the vaccination campaign on the incidence of group C disease in persons too old to have received vaccine. This result may not be surprising given the high carriage rates in young adults ages 20 to 24 years who did not receive vaccine.[229]

During the immunization campaign, concerns were raised that capsular switching from group C to group B strains might result from pressure exerted by antibodies induced in the population by meningococcal C conjugate vaccination.[38] To investigate this possibility, surveillance was established to monitor molecular markers of meningococcal organisms isolated from patients with invasive disease. The predominant group C strains in the United Kingdom are from the ET-37 complex and express the outer membrane PorB serotype 2a, which is rarely found among group B strains. Therefore, expression of PorB serotype 2a, together with multilocus sequence typing data, have been used to monitor for capsular switching from group C to group B cases (B:2a being presumptive evidence of capsular switch mutants). Since the introduction of the group C conjugate vaccines in the United Kingdom, the number of B:2a cases has not risen above historical levels. Thus, to date, there is no evidence in the United Kingdom of an increase in group B disease caused by strains that have undergone capsular switching from group C to group B.

Safety of Meningococcal C Conjugate Vaccine in the United Kingdom

From prelicensure U.K. safety studies in which nearly 3000 children were vaccinated in eight schools (four primary and four secondary), transient headache of mild to moderate severity was the most commonly reported adverse event, with the highest rate (12%) in the first 3 days after vaccination. Headache was reported more frequently in secondary school than in primary school children and more frequently in girls than boys. Local reactions at the injection site consisted of pain, tenderness, and occasional redness. These tended to be of mild to moderate severity, were maximal on the third postvaccination day, and typically resolved within a day (E. Miller, personal communication).

Postlicensure surveillance of adverse vaccine events through passive reports from health professionals in the United Kingdom to the Medicines Control Agency/Committee on Safety of Medicines indicate a rate of one adverse event per 2875 doses of meningococcal group C vaccine distributed in the first 10 months of the U.K. campaign.[230] Nearly all of these adverse events were not serious, consisting of transient headache, local reactions, pyrexia, or dizziness. Anaphylaxis was reported at a rate of 1 per 500,000 doses distributed.

Recommendations for the Use of Meningococcal Polysaccharide Vaccines

Meningococcal A, C, Y, and W135 polysaccharide vaccine is currently administered to military recruits in the

Vaccination Against Group B Meningococci

There are no vaccines currently licensed in the United States or Europe for prevention of disease caused by group B strains. One commercially available vaccine is produced in Cuba by the Finlay Institute and is licensed in 19 countries, mainly in Latin America. This vaccine is prepared from strain CU385 (B:4,7:19,15) and consists of outer membrane vesicles (OMVs) that are noncovalently complexed with group C polysaccharide. The Finlay OMV vaccine without group C polysaccharide also is being developed in partnership with GlaxoSmithKline for use in Europe and the United States. A similar OMV vaccine prepared from strain H44/76 (B:15:7,16) also is under development by the Norwegian Institute of Public Health in partnership with Chiron Vaccines. OMV vaccines have been used in large numbers of people without notable serious safety concerns, although local reactions at the injection site and transient malaise and fever are common.[243,244] In field trials undertaken in Cuba, Brazil, Chile, and Norway, the efficacies of these vaccines in older children and adults ranged from 57% to 83% but, when tested in children less than 4 years of age, there was no significant protection (reviewed by Jodar et al.[152]). The protective immunity induced by OMV vaccine is principally directed against the highly variable, immunodominant outer membrane proteins.[245] As a result, these vaccines do not elicit serum bactericidal antibody against many heterologous meningococcal strains, although broader immune responses may be detected by the more sensitive whole-blood bactericidal assay.[246] Because OMV vaccines also do not offer good protection in children less than 4 years of age,[152] the applicability of these vaccines for routine immunization programs to decrease endemic group B meningococcal disease caused by antigenically diverse meningococci is questionable. These vaccines may, nevertheless, play an important role as an intervention to disrupt outbreaks of disease caused by a single meningococcal clone. For example, for more than a decade New Zealand has experienced an epidemic of group B disease caused by a lineage III, P1.7,4 strain.[7] In response to a request from the New Zealand Ministry of Health, Chiron Vaccines has agreed to produce an OMV vaccine based on the outbreak strain.[152] The vaccine is expected to be available by 2004.

New Directions

Development of Conjugate Vaccines for Prevention of Disease Caused by Groups A, Y, and W135

A multivalent pneumococcal conjugate vaccine that also contains conjugated group C meningococcal polysaccharide is under clinical development by Wyeth Vaccines for use in infants. Multivalent meningococcal conjugate vaccines containing groups A, C, Y, and W135 are also in clinical development by Aventis Pasteur, Chiron Vaccines, and GlaxoSmithKline Biologicals. Introduction of these vaccines into routine infant and/or toddler immunization programs could have a substantial effect on the incidence of meningococcal disease. The use of a multivalent conjugate vaccine in older high school or college students also offers the prospect of decreasing the risk of meningococcal disease and transmission in these age groups without the concern of inducing immune hyporesponsiveness, which is observed after group C meningococcal polysaccharide vaccination.

Prospects for Control of Disease Caused by Group B Strains

In contrast to the situation with groups A, C, Y, and W135 strains of meningococci, there is no vaccine available in the United States or Europe for prevention of disease caused by group B meningococci. Native group B polysaccharide is a poor candidate because it contains epitopes that cross-react with sialylated proteins in human tissue. A promising conjugate vaccine, based on a chemically modified group B polysaccharide that is less cross-reactive with human antigens than native group B polysaccharide, is at an early stage of clinical evaluation. In laboratory animals, this conjugate elicits anticapsular antibodies with complement-mediated bactericidal activity, which confer passive protection in animal models of bacteremia.[247–249] However, a subset of the antibodies elicited by this vaccine have autoantibody activity.[249,250] There is no direct evidence that these autoantibodies are harmful, but it will be a difficult and lengthy process to prove that such a vaccine is safe for widespread use in humans. The possibility of conjugate vaccines based on conserved meningococcal lipopolysaccharide epitopes that do not cross-react with host antigens is also under consideration,[251–253] although such vaccines have not yet been tested in humans.

Two recent review articles summarize development of meningococcal vaccines targeted to prevention of Group B strains.[152,254] The most advanced approaches employ recombinant membrane proteins or improved outer membrane protein vesicles. A hexavalent PorA-based vesicle vaccine was developed in the Netherlands at the National Institute of Public Health and the Environment (RIVM) using OMVs prepared from two N. meningitidis strains that each express three different PorA proteins. The hexavalent PorA OMV vaccine has been evaluated in adults, children, and infants.[255–257] In infants, the bacterial antibody responses after a primary three-dose series were only modest. Also, as compared to the antibody responses elicited by the corresponding monovalent vesicle vaccine, interference was observed in the immunogenicity between certain serotype antigens contained in the multivalent vaccine. After a fourth dose in toddlers, higher serum bactericidal antibody responses were observed, a result suggesting that such a vaccine might be efficacious. One example of a purified recombinant protein vaccine is Neisserial surface protein A (NspA),[258] a membrane protein of unknown function being developed as a meningococcal vaccine by Shire Pharmaceuticals (formerly, BioChem Vaccins in Canada). Immunization of experimental animals with recombinant NspA (rNspA) elicits serum bactericidal antibodies that confer passive protection in animal models of group B meningococcal bacteremia.[259–261] The results of Phase I trials with rNspA have not been made public. Two major challenges to developing an effective rNspA vaccine will be to understand the mechanism for why some strains are susceptible to anti-NspA complement-mediated bacteriolysis while others are resistant, and to develop vaccine formulations that are more immunogenic than natural infection.[262]

Developments in meningococcal genomics and proteomics have provided alternative approaches to the identification of candidate vaccine antigens,[263,264] and the term *reverse vaccinology* has been adopted for antigens first identified by computer analysis of the genome.[265] A number of promising vaccine candidates have been identified from "genome mining."[152,263,266] Clinical evaluation of such antigens is just beginning.

REFERENCES

1. Vieusseux M. Memoire sur le maladie qui a regne a Geneva au printemps de 1805. J Med Clin Pharm 11:163–182, 1805.
2. Danielson L, Mann E. A history of a singular and very noted disease, which lately made its appearance in Medfield. Med Agricultural Reg 1:65–69, 1806.
3. Weichselbaum A. Ueber die aetiologie der akuten meningitis cerebrospinal. Fortschr Med 5:573–583, 620–626, 1887.
4. Greenwood B. Manson Lecture: Meningococcal meningitis in Africa. Trans R Soc Trop Med Hyg 93:341–353, 1999.
5. Rosenstein NE, Perkins BA, Stephens DS, et al. The changing epidemiology of meningococcal disease in the United States, 1992–1996. J Infect Dis 180:1894–1901, 1999.
6. Cartwright K, Noah N, Peltola H. Meningococcal disease in Europe: epidemiology, mortality, and prevention with conjugate vaccines. Report of a European advisory board meeting Vienna, Austria, 6–8 October, 2000. Vaccine 19:4347–4356, 2001.
7. Martin DR, Walker SJ, Baker MG, Lennon DR. New Zealand epidemic of meningococcal disease identified by a strain with phenotype B:4:P1.4. J Infect Dis 177:497–500, 1998.
8. Rosenstein NE, Perkins BA, Stephens DS, et al. Meningococcal disease. N Engl J Med 344:1378–1388, 2001.
9. Sparling PF. A plethora of host factors that determine the outcome of meningococcal infection. Am J Med 112:72–74, 2002.
10. Meningococcal disease, serogroup W135 (update). Wkly Epidemiol Rec 76:213–214, 2001.
11. Meningococcal disease, serogroup W135, Burkina Faso: preliminary report, 2002. Wkly Epidemiol Rec 77:152–155, 2002.
11a. Wells LC, Smith JC, Weston VC, et al. The child with a non-blanching rash: how likely is meningococcal disease? Arch Dis Child 85:218–222, 2001.
12. Fellick JM, Sills JA, Marzouk O, et al. Neurodevelopmental outcome in meningococcal disease: a case-control study. Arch Dis Child 85:6–11, 2001.
13. Erickson L, De Wals P. Complications and sequelae of meningococcal disease in Quebec, Canada, 1990–1994. Clin Infect Dis 26:1159–1164, 1998.
14. Erickson LJ, De Wals P, McMahon J, Heim S. Complications of meningococcal disease in college students. Clin Infect Dis 33:737–739, 2001.
15. Edwards MS, Baker CJ. Complications and sequelae of meningococcal infections in children. J Pediatr 99:540–545, 1981.
16. Dodge PR, Davis H, Feigin RD, et al. Prospective evaluation of hearing impairment as a sequela of acute bacterial meningitis. N Engl J Med 311:869–874, 1984.
17. Dodge PR, Scaer M, Holmes SJ, et al. Psychometric testing in bacterial meningitis: results of a long-term prospective study of infants and children treated between 1973 and 1977. J Child Neurol 16:854–857, 2001.
18. Vedros NA. Genus I. *Neisseria*. *In* Krieg NR, Holt JG (eds). Bergey's Manual of Systematic Bacteriology. Baltimore, Williams & Wilkins, 1984, pp 290–296.
19. Fu J, Bailey FJ, King JJ, et al. Recent advances in the large scale fermentation of *Neisseria meningitidis* group B for the production of an outer membrane protein complex. Biotechnology (NY) 13:170–174, 1995.
20. Frantz ID. Growth requirements of the meningococcus. J Bacteriol 43:757–761, 1942.
21. Branham SE. Serological relationships among meningococci. Bact Rev 17:175–188, 1953.
22. Vedros NA. Development of meningococcal serogroups. *In* Vedros NA (ed). Evolution of Meningococcal Disease. Boca Raton, FL, CRC Press, 1987, pp 33–37.
23. Tsai CM, Frasch CE, Mocca LF. Five structural classes of major outer membrane proteins in *Neisseria meningitidis*. J Bacteriol 146:69–78, 1981.
24. Frasch CE, Zollinger WD, Poolman JT. Serotype antigens of *Neisseria meningitidis* and a proposed scheme for designation of serotypes. Rev Infect Dis 7:504–510, 1985.
25. Abdillahi H, Poolman JT. Typing of group-B *Neisseria meningitidis* with monoclonal antibodies in the whole-cell ELISA. J Med Microbiol 26:177–180, 1988.
26. Abdillahi H, Poolman JT. *Neisseria meningitidis* group B serosubtyping using monoclonal antibodies in whole-cell ELISA. Microb Pathog 4:27–32, 1988.
27. Abdillahi H, Poolman JT. Definition of meningococcal class 1 OMP subtyping antigens by monoclonal antibodies. FEMS Microbiol Immunol 1:139–144, 1988.
28. Maiden MC, Feavers IM. Meningococcal typing. J Med Microbiol 40:157–158, 1994.
29. Maiden MC, Russell J, Suker J, Feavers IM. *Neisseria meningitidis* subtype nomenclature. Clin Diagn Lab Immunol 6:771–772, 1999.
30. Scholten RJ, Kuipers B, Valkenburg HA, et al. Lipo-oligosaccharide immunotyping of *Neisseria meningitidis* by a whole-cell ELISA with monoclonal antibodies. J Med Microbiol 41:236–243, 1994.
31. Smith JM, Dowson CG, Spratt BG. Localized sex in bacteria. Nature 349:29–31, 1991.
32. Maiden MCJ, Feavers IM. Population genetics and global epidemiology of the human pathogen *Neisseria meningitidis*. *In* Baumberg S, Young JPW, Saunders JR, Wellington EMH (eds). Population Genetics of Bacteria. Cambridge, UK: Cambridge University Press, 1995, pp 269–293.
33. Caugant DA, Mocca LF, Frasch CE, et al. Genetic structure of *Neisseria meningitidis* populations in relation to serogroup, serotype, and outer membrane protein pattern. J Bacteriol 169:2781–2792, 1987.
34. Feavers IM, Heath AB, Bygraves JA, Maiden MC. Role of horizontal genetic exchange in the antigenic variation of the class 1 outer membrane protein of *Neisseria meningitidis*. Mol Microbiol 6:489–495, 1992.
35. Wang JF, Caugant DA, Morelli G, et al. Antigenic and epidemiologic properties of the ET-37 complex of *Neisseria meningitidis*. J Infect Dis 167:1320–1329, 1993.
36. Caugant DA, Froholm LO, Bovre K, et al. Intercontinental spread of a genetically distinctive complex of clones of *Neisseria meningitidis* causing epidemic disease. Proc Natl Acad Sci U S A 83:4927–4931, 1986.
37. Maiden MC, Bygraves JA, Feil E, et al. Multilocus sequence typing: a portable approach to the identification of clones within populations of pathogenic microorganisms. Proc Natl Acad Sci U S A 95:3140–3145, 1998.
38. Maiden MC, Spratt BG. Meningococcal conjugate vaccines: new opportunities and new challenges. Lancet 354:615–616, 1999.
39. Parkhill J, Achtman M, James KD, et al. Complete DNA sequence of a serogroup A strain of *Neisseria meningitidis* Z2491. Nature 404:502–506, 2000.
40. Tettelin H, Saunders NJ, Heidelberg J, et al. Complete genome sequence of *Neisseria meningitidis* serogroup B strain MC58. Science 287:1809–1815, 2000.
41. Cartwright KA, Jones DM, Smith AJ, et al. Influenza A and meningococcal disease. Lancet 338:554–557, 1991.
42. Blackwell CC, Weir DM, James VS, et al. Secretor status, smoking and carriage of *Neisseria meningitidis*. Epidemiol Infect 104:203–209, 1990.
43. Fischer M, Hedberg K, Cardosi P, et al. Tobacco smoke as a risk factor for meningococcal disease. Pediatr Infect Dis J 16:979–983, 1997.
44. Hodgson A, Smith T, Gagneux S, et al. Risk factors for meningococcal meningitis in northern Ghana. Trans R Soc Trop Med Hyg 95:477–480, 2001.
45. Jolley KA, Kalmusova J, Feil EJ, et al. Carried meningococci in the Czech Republic: a diverse recombining population. J Clin Microbiol 38:4492–4498, 2000.

46. Nassif X. Interaction mechanisms of encapsulated meningococci with eucaryotic cells: what does this tell us about the crossing of the blood-brain barrier by *Neisseria meningitidis*? Curr Opin Microbiol 2:71–77, 1999.

47. Goldschneider I, Gotschlich EC, Artenstein MS. Human immunity to the meningococcus. I. The role of humoral antibodies. J Exp Med 129:1307–1326, 1969.

48. Condon RJ, Riley TV, Kelly H. Invasive meningococcal infection after splenectomy. BMJ 308:792–793, 1994.

49. Pollard AJ, Frasch C. Development of natural immunity to *Neisseria meningitidis*. Vaccine 19:1327–1346, 2001.

50. Schlesinger M, Nave Z, Levy Y, et al. Prevalence of hereditary properdin, C7 and C8 deficiencies in patients with meningococcal infections. Clin Exp Immunol 81:423–427, 1990.

51. Fijen CA, Kuijper EJ, Hannema AJ, et al. Complement deficiencies in patients over ten years old with meningococcal disease due to uncommon serogroups. Lancet 2:585–588, 1989.

52. Fijen CA, Kuijper EJ, te Bulte MT, et al. Assessment of complement deficiency in patients with meningococcal disease in the Netherlands. Clin Infect Dis 28:98–105, 1999.

53. Linton SM, Morgan BP. Properdin deficiency and meningococcal disease—identifying those most at risk. Clin Exp Immunol 118:189–191, 1999.

54. Nicholson A, Lepow IH. Host defense against *Neisseria meningitidis* requires a complement-dependent bactericidal activity. Science 205:298–299, 1979.

55. Nielsen HE, Koch C, Magnussen P, Lind I. Complement deficiencies in selected groups of patients with meningococcal disease. Scand J Infect Dis 21:389–396, 1989.

56. Bax WA, Cluysenaer OJ, Bartelink AK, et al. Association of familial deficiency of mannose-binding lectin and meningococcal disease. Lancet 354:1094–1095, 1999.

57. Hibberd ML, Sumiya M, Summerfield JA, et al. Association of variants of the gene for mannose-binding lectin with susceptibility to meningococcal disease. Meningococcal Research Group. Lancet 353:1049–1053, 1999.

58. Jack DL, Dodds AW, Anwar N, et al. Activation of complement by mannose-binding lectin on isogenic mutants of *Neisseria meningitidis* serogroup B. J Immunol 160:1346–1353, 1998.

59. Jack DL, Jarvis GA, Booth CL, et al. Mannose-binding lectin accelerates complement activation and increases serum killing of *Neisseria meningitidis* serogroup C. J Infect Dis 184:836–845, 2001.

60. Platonov AE, Shipulin GA, Vershinina IV, et al. Association of human Fc gamma RIIa (CD32) polymorphism with susceptibility to and severity of meningococcal disease. Clin Infect Dis 27:746–750, 1998.

61. Fijen CA, Bredius RG, Kuijper EJ, et al. The role of Fc gamma receptor polymorphisms and C3 in the immune defence against *Neisseria meningitidis* in complement-deficient individuals. Clin Exp Immunol 120:338–345, 2000.

62. van der Pol WL, Huizinga TW, Vidarsson G, et al. Relevance of Fc gamma receptor and interleukin-10 polymorphisms for meningococcal disease. J Infect Dis 184:1548–1555, 2001.

63. Domingo P, Muniz-Diaz E, Baraldes MA, et al. Associations between Fc gamma receptor IIA polymorphisms and the risk and prognosis of meningococcal disease. Am J Med 112:19–25, 2002.

64. Platonov AE, Kuijper EJ, Vershinina IV, et al. Meningococcal disease and polymorphism of Fc gammaRIIa (CD32) in late complement component-deficient individuals. Clin Exp Immunol 111:97–101, 1998.

65. Westendorp RG, Langermans JA, Huizinga TW, et al. Genetic influence on cytokine production and fatal meningococcal disease. Lancet 349:170–173, 1997.

66. Nadel S, Newport MJ, Booy R, Levin M. Variation in the tumor necrosis factor-alpha gene promoter region may be associated with death from meningococcal disease. J Infect Dis 174:878–880, 1996.

67. Westendorp RG, Hottenga JJ, Slagboom PE. Variation in plasminogen-activator-inhibitor-1 gene and risk of meningococcal septic shock. Lancet 354:561–563, 1999.

68. Finne J, Leinonen M, Makela PH. Antigenic similarities between brain components and bacteria causing meningitis: implications for vaccine development and pathogenesis. Lancet 2:355–357, 1983.

69. Gray SJ, Borrow R, Kaczmarski E. Meningococcal serology. *In* Pollard AJ, Maiden MC (eds). Meningococcal Disease: Methods in Molecular Medicine. Totowa, NJ, Humana Press, 2001, pp 289–304.

70. Guiver M, Borrow R. PCR diagnosis. *In* Pollard AJ, Maiden MC (eds). Meningococcal Disease: Methods in Molecular Medicine. Totowa, NJ, Humana Press, 2001, pp 23–39.

71. Orvelid P, Backman A, Olcen P. PCR identification of the group A *Neisseria meningitidis* gene in cerebrospinal fluid. Scand J Infect Dis 31:481–483, 1999.

72. Hackett SJ, Guiver M, Marsh J, et al. Meningococcal bacterial DNA load at presentation correlates with disease severity. Arch Dis Child 86:44–46, 2002.

73. Hackett SJ, Guiven M, Marsh J, et al. Meningococcal bacterial DNA load at presentation correlates with disease severity. Arch Dis Child 86:44–46, 2002.

74. Jolly K, Stewart G. Epidemiology and diagnosis of meningitis: results of a five-year prospective, population-based study. Commun Dis Public Health 4:124–129, 2001.

75. Public Health Laboratory Service Meningococcus Forum. Guidelines for public health management of meningococcal disease in the U.K. Commun Dis Public Health 5:187–204, 2002.

76. Galimand M, Gerbaud G, Guibourdenche M, et al. High-level chloramphenicol resistance in *Neisseria meningitidis*. N Engl J Med 339:868–874, 1998.

77. Hackett SJ, Thomson AP, Hart CA. Cytokines, chemokines and other effector molecules involved in meningococcal disease. J Med Microbiol 50:847–859, 2001.

78. Alberio L, Lammle B, Esmon CT. Protein C replacement in severe meningococcemia: rationale and clinical experience. Clin Infect Dis 32:1338–1346, 2001.

79. Bernard GR, Vincent JL, Laterre PF, et al. Efficacy and safety of recombinant human activated protein C for severe sepsis. N Engl J Med 344:699–709, 2001.

80. Powars D, Larsen R, Johnson J, et al. Epidemic meningococcemia and purpura fulminans with induced protein C deficiency. Clin Infect Dis 17:254–261,1993.

81. Fijnvandraat K, Derkx B, Peters M, et al. Coagulation activation and tissue necrosis in meningococcal septic shock: severely reduced protein C levels predict a high mortality. Thromb Haemost 73:15–20, 1995.

82. White B, Livingstone W, Murphy C, et al. An open-label study of the role of adjuvant hemostatic support with protein C replacement therapy in purpura fulminans-associated meningococcemia. Blood 96:3719–3724, 2000.

83. Smith OP, White B, Vaughan D, et al. Use of protein-C concentrate, heparin, and haemodiafiltration in meningococcus-induced purpura fulminans. Lancet 350:1590–1593, 1997.

84. Schwetz BA. From the Food and Drug Administration. JAMA 287:33, 2002.

85. Levin M, Quint PA, Goldstein B, et al. Recombinant bactericidal/permeability-increasing protein (rBPI21) as adjunctive treatment for children with severe meningococcal sepsis: a randomised trial. rBPI21 Meningococcal Sepsis Study Group. Lancet 356:961–967, 2000.

86. Giroir BP, Scannon PJ, Levin M. Bactericidal/permeability-increasing protein—lessons learned from the Phase III, randomized, clinical trial of rBPI21 for adjunctive treatment of children with severe meningococcemia. Crit Care Med 29:S130–S135, 2001.

87. Schaad UB, Kaplan SL, McCracken GH Jr. Steroid therapy for bacterial meningitis. Clin Infect Dis 20:685–690, 1995.

88. Prevention and control of meningococcal disease. Recommendations of the Advisory Committee on Immunization Practices (ACIP). MMWR 49:1–10, 2000.

89. Abramson JS, Spika JS. Persistence of *Neisseria meningitidis* in the upper respiratory tract after intravenous antibiotic therapy for systemic meningococcal disease. J Infect Dis 151:370–371, 1985.

90. Jones D. Epidemiology of meningococcal disease in Europe and the USA. *In* Cartwright K (ed). Meningococcal Disease. New York, John Wiley & Sons, 1995, pp 147–175.

91. Pastor P, Medley FB, Murphy TV. Meningococcal disease in Dallas County, Texas: results of a six-year population-based study. Pediatr Infect Dis J 19:324–328, 2000.

92. Achtman M. Global epidemiology of meningococcal disease. *In* Cartwright K (ed). Meningococcal Disease. New York, John Wiley & Sons, 1995, pp 159–176.

93. Counts GW, Gregory DF, Spearman JG, et al. Group A meningococcal disease in the U.S. Pacific Northwest: epidemiology, clinical features, and effect of a vaccination control program. Rev Infect Dis 6:640–648, 1984.

94. Achtman M, van der Ende A, Zhu P, et al. Molecular epidemiology of serogroup A meningitis in Moscow, 1969 to 1997. Emerg Infect Dis 7:420–427, 2001.

95. Olyhoek T, Crowe BA, Achtman M. Clonal population structure of Neisseria meningitidis serogroup A isolated from epidemics and pandemics between 1915 and 1983. Rev Infect Dis 9:665–692, 1987.

96. Wang JF, Caugant DA, Li X, et al. Clonal and antigenic analysis of serogroup A Neisseria meningitidis with particular reference to epidemiological features of epidemic meningitis in the People's Republic of China. Infect Immun 60:5267–5282, 1992.

97. Bjorvatn B, Hassan-King M, Greenwood B, et al. DNA fingerprinting in the epidemiology of African serogroup A Neisseria meningitidis. Scand J Infect Dis 24:323–332, 1992.

98. Guibourdenche M, Hoiby EA, Riou JY, et al. Epidemics of serogroup A Neisseria meningitidis of subgroup III in Africa, 1989–94. Epidemiol Infect 116:115–120, 1996.

99. Centers for Disease Control and Prevention. Serogroup B meningococcal disease—Oregon, 1994. MMWR 44:121–124, 1995.

100. Artenstein MS, Schneider H, Tingley MD. Meningococcal infections. 1. Prevalence of serogroups causing disease in US Army personnel in 1964–70. Bull World Health Organ 45:275–278, 1971.

101. Souza de Morais J, Munford RS, Risi JB, et al. Epidemic disease due to serogroup C Neisseria meningitidis in Sao Paulo, Brazil. J Infect Dis 129:568–571, 1974.

102. Berron S, De La Fuente L, Martin E, Vazquez JA. Increasing incidence of meningococcal disease in Spain associated with a new variant of serogroup C. Eur J Clin Microbiol Infect Dis 17:85–89, 1998.

103. Ashton FE, Ryan JA, Borczyk A, et al. Emergence of a virulent clone of Neisseria meningitidis serotype 2a that is associated with meningococcal group C disease in Canada. J Clin Microbiol 29:2489–2493, 1991.

104. Whalen CM, Hockin JC, Ryan A, Ashton F. The changing epidemiology of invasive meningococcal disease in Canada, 1985 through 1992: emergence of a virulent clone of Neisseria meningitidis. JAMA 273.390–394, 1995.

105. Krizova P, Musilek M. Changing epidemiology of meningococcal invasive disease in the Czech Republic caused by new clone Neisseria meningitidis C:2a:P1.2(P1.5), ET-15/37. Cent Eur J Public Health 3:189–194, 1995.

106. Ramsay M, Kaczmarski E, Rush M, et al. Changing patterns of case ascertainment and trends in meningococcal disease in England and Wales. Commun Dis Rep CDR Rev 7:R49–R54, 1997.

107. Figueroa JE, Densen P. Infectious diseases associated with complement deficiencies. Clin Microbiol Rev 4:359–395, 1991.

108. Jackson LA, Wenger JD. Laboratory-based surveillance for meningococcal disease in selected areas, United States, 1989–1991. MMWR 42(SS-O):21–30, 1993.

109. Koppes GM, Ellenbogen C, Gebhart RJ. Group Y meningococcal disease in United States Air Force recruits. Am J Med 62:661–666, 1977.

110. Smilack JD. Group-Y meningococcal disease: twelve cases at an army training center. Ann Intern Med 81:740–745, 1974.

111. Yousuf M, Nadeem A. Fatal meningococcaemia due to group W135 amongst Hajj pilgrims: implications for future vaccination policy. Ann Trop Med Parasitol 89:321–322, 1995.

111a. Wilder-Smith A, Barkham TM, Earnest A, et al. Acquisition of W135 meningococcal carriage in Hajj pilgrims and transmission to household contacts: prospective study. BMJ 325:365–366, 2002.

112. Kwara A, Adegbola RA, Corrah PT, et al. Meningitis caused by a serogroup W135 clone of the ET-37 complex of Neisseria meningitidis in West Africa. Trop Med Int Health 3:742–746, 1998.

113. Guibourdenche M, Chippaux JP, Ouedraogo-Traore R, et al. Evolution of the second pandemic due to strains of Neisseria meningitidis A:4:P1.9/clone III-I. Survey in four African countries: Niger, Burkina Faso, Cameroon and Chad October 1995–May 1996. In Zollinger WD, Frasch CE, Deal CD (eds). 10th International Pathogenic Neisseria Conference. Bethesda, MD: National Institutes of Health, 1996, pp 523–524.

114. Hahne SJ, Gray SJ, Jean F, et al. W135 meningococcal disease in England and Wales associated with Hajj 2000 and 2001. Lancet 359:582–583, 2002.

115. Goldschneider I, Gotschlich EC, Artenstein MS. Human immunity to the meningococcus. II. Development of natural immunity. J Exp Med 129:1327–1348, 1969.

116. Myerowitz RL, Gordon RE, Robbins JB. Polysaccharides of the genus Bacillus cross-reactive with the capsular polysaccharides of Diplococcus pneumoniae type 3, Haemophilus influenzae type b, and Neisseria meningitidis group A. Infect Immun 8:896–900, 1973.

117. Robbins JB, Myerowitz L, Whisnant JK, et al. Enteric bacteria cross-reactive with Neisseria meningitidis groups A and C and Diplococcus pneumoniae types 1 and 3. Infect Immun 6:651–656, 1972.

118. Vann WF, Liu TY, Robbins JB. Bacillus pumilus polysaccharide cross-reactive with meningococcal group A polysaccharide. Infect Immun 13:1654–1662, 1976.

119. Guirguis N, Schneerson R, Bax A, et al. Escherichia coli K51 and K93 capsular polysaccharides are crossreactive with the group A capsular polysaccharide of Neisseria meningitidis: immunochemical, biological, and epidemiological studies. J Exp Med 162:1837–1851, 1985.

120. Devi SJ, Robbins JB, Schneerson R. Antibodies to poly[(2→8)-alpha-N-acetylneuraminic acid] and poly[(2→9)-alpha-N-acetylneuraminic acid] are elicited by immunization of mice with Escherichia coli K92 conjugates: potential vaccines for groups B and C meningococci and E. coli K1. Proc Natl Acad Sci U S A 88:7175–7179, 1991.

121. Granoff DM, Kelsey SK, Bijlmer HA, et al. Antibody responses to the capsular polysaccharide of Neisseria meningitidis serogroup B in patients with meningococcal disease. Clin Diagn Lab Immunol 2:574–582, 1995.

122. Raff HV, Bradley C, Brady W, et al. Comparison of functional activities between IgG1 and IgM class-switched human monoclonal antibodies reactive with group B streptococci or Escherichia coli K1. J Infect Dis 163:346–354, 1991.

123. Mandrell RE, Azmi FH, Granoff DM. Complement-mediated bactericidal activity of human antibodies to poly alpha 2→8 N-acetylneuraminic acid, the capsular polysaccharide of Neisseria meningitidis serogroup B. J Infect Dis 172:1279–1289, 1995.

124. Saunders NJ, Jeffries AC, Peden JF, et al. Repeat-associated phase variable genes in the complete genome sequence of Neisseria meningitidis strain MC58. Mol Microbiol 37:207–215, 2000.

125. Feavers IM. ABC of meningococcal diversity. Nature 404:451 452, 2000.

126. Sophian A, Black J. Prophylactic vaccination against epidemic meningitis. JAMA 59:527–532, 1912.

127. Greenwood M. The outbreak of cerebrospinal fever at Salisbury in 1914–15. Proc R Soc Med 10:44–60, 1916.

128. Gates FL. A report on antimeningitis vaccination and observations on agglutinins in the blood of chronic meningococcus carriers. J Exp Med 28:449–474, 1918.

129. Underwood EA. Recent knowledge of the incidence and control of cerebrospinal fever. Br Med J 1:757–763, 1940.

130. Ferry NS, Steele AH. Active immunization with meningococcus toxin. JAMA 104:983–984, 1935.

131. Kuhns D, Kisner P, Williams MP, Moorman PL. The control of meningococcic meningitis epidemics by active immunization with meningococcus soluble toxin: further studies. JAMA 110:484–487, 1938.

132. Miller JW, Siess EE, Feldman HA. In vivo and in vitro resistance to sulfadiazine in strains of Neisseria meningitidis. JAMA 186:139–141, 1963.

133. Scherp HW, Rake G. Studies on meningococcal infection. XIII: Correlation between antipolysaccharide and the antibody which protects mice against infection with type I meningococci. J Exp Med 81:85–92, 1945.

134. Kabat EA, Kaiser H, Sikorski H. Preparation of the type specific polysaccharide of the type I meningococcus and a study of its effectiveness as an antigen in human beings. J Exp Med 80:229–307, 1944.

135. Watson RG, Scherp HW. The specific hapten of serogroup C (group II alpha) meningococcus. I: Preparation and immunological behaviour. J Immunol 81:331–336, 1958.

136. Kabat EA, Bezer AE. The effect of variation on molecular weight on the antigenicity of dextran in man. Arch Biochem 78:306–313, 1958.

137. Gotschlich EC, Liu TY, Artenstein MS. Human immunity to the meningococcus. 3. Preparation and immunochemical properties of the group A, group B, and group C meningococcal polysaccharides. J Exp Med 129:1349–1365, 1969.

138. Gotschlich EC, Goldschneider I, Artenstein MS. Human immunity to the meningococcus. IV. Immunogenicity of group A and group C meningococcal polysaccharides in human volunteers. J Exp Med 129:1367–1384, 1969.

139. Leach A, Twumasi PA, Kumah S, et al. Induction of immunologic memory in Gambian children by vaccination in infancy with a group A plus group C meningococcal polysaccharide-protein conjugate vaccine. J Infect Dis 175:200–204, 1997.

140. Granoff DM, Gupta RK, Belshe RB, Anderson EL. Induction of immunologic refractoriness in adults by meningococcal C polysaccharide vaccination. J Infect Dis 178:870–874, 1998.

141. Goldblatt D. Immunisation and the maturation of infant immune responses. Dev Biol Stand 95:125–132, 1998.

142. Robbins JB, Schneerson R, Anderson P, Smith DH. The 1996 Albert Lasker Medical Research Awards. Prevention of systemic infections, especially meningitis, caused by Haemophilus influenzae type b: impact on public health and implications for other polysaccharide-based vaccines. JAMA 276:1181–1185, 1996.

143. Anderson P, Pichichero ME, Insel RA. Immunization of 2-month-old infants with protein-coupled oligosaccharides derived from the capsule of Haemophilus influenzae type b. J Pediatr 107:346–351, 1985.

144. Granoff DM, Boies EG, Munson RS Jr. Immunogenicity of Haemophilus influenzae type b polysaccharide–diphtheria toxoid conjugate vaccine in adults. J Pediatr 105:22–27, 1984.

145. Einhorn MS, Weinberg GA, Anderson EL, et al. Immunogenicity in infants of Haemophilus influenzae type B polysaccharide in a conjugate vaccine with Neisseria meningitidis outer-membrane protein. Lancet 2:299–302, 1986.

146. Costantino P, Viti S, Podda A, et al. Development and phase 1 clinical testing of a conjugate vaccine against meningococcus A and C. Vaccine 10:691–698, 1992.

147. MacDonald NE, Halperin SA, Law BJ, et al. Induction of immunologic memory by conjugated vs plain meningococcal C polysaccharide vaccine in toddlers: a randomized controlled trial. JAMA 280:1685–1689, 1998.

148. Richmond P, Borrow R, Miller E, et al. Meningococcal serogroup C conjugate vaccine is immunogenic in infancy and primes for memory. J Infect Dis 179:1569–1572, 1999.

149. Richmond P, Goldblatt D, Fusco PC, et al. Safety and immunogenicity of a new Neisseria meningitidis serogroup C-tetanus toxoid conjugate vaccine in healthy adults. Vaccine 18:641–646, 1999.

150. MacLennan JM, Shackley F, Heath PT, et al. Safety, immunogenicity, and induction of immunologic memory by a serogroup C meningococcal conjugate vaccine in infants: a randomized controlled trial. JAMA 283:2795–2801, 2000.

151. Morley SL, Pollard AJ. Vaccine prevention of meningococcal disease, coming soon? Vaccine 20:666–687, 2001.

152. Jodar L, Feavers I, Salisbury D, Granoff DM. Development of vaccines against meningococcal disease. Lancet 359:1499–1508, 2002.

153. Michon F, Huang CH, Farley EK, et al. Structure activity studies on group C meningococcal polysaccharide-protein conjugate vaccines: effect of O-acetylation on the nature of the protective epitope. Dev Biol (Basel) 103:151–160, 2000.

154. Ho MM, Bolgiano B, Corbel MJ. Assessment of the stability and immunogenicity of meningococcal oligosaccharide C-CRM197 conjugate vaccines. Vaccine 19:716–725, 2000.

155. Ho MM, Lemercinier X, Bolgiano B, Corbel MJ. Monitoring stability of meningococcal group C conjugate vaccines: correlation of physico-chemical methods and immunogenicity assays. Dev Biol (Basel) 103:139–150, 2000.

156. Gheesling LL, Carlone GM, Pais LB, et al. Multicenter comparison of Neisseria meningitidis serogroup C anticapsular polysaccharide antibody levels measured by a standardized enzyme-linked immunosorbent assay. J Clin Microbiol 32:1475–1482, 1994.

157. Maslanka SE, Gheesling LL, Libutti DE, et al. Standardization and a multilaboratory comparison of Neisseria meningitidis serogroup A and C serum bactericidal assays. The Multilaboratory Study Group. Clin Diagn Lab Immunol 4:156–167, 1997.

158. Jodar L, Cartwright K, Feavers IM. Standardisation and validation of serological assays for the evaluation of immune responses to Neisseria meningitidis serogroup A and C vaccines. Biologicals 28:193–197, 2000.

159. Wong KH, Barrera O, Sutton A, et al. Standardization and control of meningococcal vaccines, group A and group C polysaccharides. J Biol Stand 5:197–215, 1977.

160. Zollinger WD, Mandrell RE. Importance of complement source in bactericidal activity of human antibody and murine monoclonal antibody to meningococcal group B polysaccharide. Infect Immun 40:257–264, 1983.

161. Santos GF, Deck RR, Donnelly J, et al. Importance of complement source in measuring meningococcal bactericidal titers. Clin Diagn Lab Immunol 8:616–623, 2001.

162. Borrow R, Andrews N, Goldblatt D, Miller E. Serological basis for use of meningococcal serogroup C conjugate vaccines in the United Kingdom: reevaluation of correlates of protection. Infect Immun 69:1568–1573, 2001.

163. Maslanka SE, Tappero JW, Plikaytis BD, et al. Age-dependent Neisseria meningitidis serogroup C class-specific antibody concentrations and bactericidal titers in sera from young children from Montana immunized with a licensed polysaccharide vaccine. Infect Immun 66:2453–2459, 1998.

164. Granoff DM, Maslanka SE, Carlone GM, et al. A modified enzyme-linked immunosorbent assay for measurement of antibody responses to meningococcal C polysaccharide that correlate with bactericidal responses. Clin Diagn Lab Immunol 5:479–485, 1998.

164a. Harris SL, King WJ, Ferris W, Granoff DM. Age-related disparity in functional activities of human group C serum anticapsular antibodies elicited by meningococcal polysaccharide vaccine. Infect Immun 71:275–286, 2003.

165. Lieberman JM, Chiu SS, Wong VK, et al. Safety and immunogenicity of a serogroups A/C Neisseria meningitidis oligosaccharide-protein conjugate vaccine in young children: a randomized controlled trial. JAMA 275:1499–1503, 1996.

166. Campagne G, Garba A, Fabre P, et al. Safety and immunogenicity of three doses of a Neisseria meningitidis A + C diphtheria conjugate vaccine in infants from Niger. Pediatr Infect Dis J 19:144–150, 2000.

167. Granoff DM, Donnelly J. A modified ELISA for measurement of high avidity IgG antibodies to meningococcal serogroup C polysaccharide that correlate with bactericidal titers. In Pollard AJ, Maiden MC (eds). Meningococcal Disease: Methods in Molecular Medicine. Totowa, NJ, Humana Press, 2001, pp 305–316.

168. Gotschlich EC, Rey M, Triau R, Sparks KJ. Quantitative determination of the human immune response to immunization with meningococcal vaccines. J Clin Invest 51:89–96, 1972.

169. Schlesinger Y, Granoff DM. Avidity and bactericidal activity of antibody elicited by different Haemophilus influenzae type b conjugate vaccines. The Vaccine Study Group. JAMA 267:1489–1494, 1992.

170. Goldblatt D, Vaz AR, Miller E. Antibody avidity as a surrogate marker of successful priming by Haemophilus influenzae type b conjugate vaccines following infant immunization. J Infect Dis 177:1112–1115, 1998.

171. Richmond P, Borrow R, Goldblatt D, et al. Ability of 3 different meningococcal C conjugate vaccines to induce immunologic memory after a single dose in UK toddlers. J Infect Dis 183:160–163, 2001.

172. Barington T, Hougs L, Juul L, et al. The progeny of a single virgin B cell predominates the human recall B cell response to the capsular polysaccharide of Haemophilus influenzae type b. J Immunol 157:4016–4027, 1996.

173. Baxendale HE, Davis Z, White HN, et al. Immunogenetic analysis of the immune response to pneumococcal polysaccharide. Eur J Immunol 30:1214–1223, 2000.

173a. Goldblatt D, Borrow R, and Miller E. Natural and vaccine-induced immunity and immunologic memory to Neisseria meningitidis serogroup C in young adults. J Infect Dis 185:397–400, 2002.

174. Gold R, Lepow ML, Goldschneider I, et al. Clinical evaluation of group A and group C meningococcal polysaccharide vaccines in infants. J Clin Invest 56:1536–1547, 1975.

174a. Harris SL, Finn A, and Granoff DM. Disparity in functional activity between anticapsular antibodies induced in adults by immunization with an investigational group A and C Neisseria meningitidis diphtheria toxoid conjugate vaccine and by polysaccharide vaccine. Infect Immun 71:3402–3408, 2003.

175. Gold R, Lepow ML, Goldschneider I, Gotschlich EC. Immune response of human infants to polysaccharide vaccines of group A and C Neisseria meningitidis. J Infect Dis 136(suppl):S31–S35, 1977.

176. Kayhty H, Karanko V, Peltola H, et al. Serum antibodies to capsular polysaccharide vaccine of group A Neisseria meningitidis followed for three years in infants and children. J Infect Dis 142:861–868, 1980.

177. Granoff DM. Assessing efficacy of Haemophilus influenzae type b combination vaccines. Clin Infect Dis 33(suppl 4):S278–S287, 2001.

178. Hankins WA, Gwaltney JM Jr, Hendley JO, et al. Clinical and serological evaluation of a meningococcal polysaccharide vaccine groups A, C, Y, and W135. Proc Soc Exp Biol Med 169:54–57, 1982.

179. Cadoz M, Armand J, Arminjon F, et al. Tetravalent (A, C, Y, W 135) meningococcal vaccine in children: immunogenicity and safety. Vaccine 3:340–342, 1985.

180. Armand J, Arminjon F, Mynard MC, Lafaix C. Tetravalent meningococcal polysaccharide vaccine groups A, C, Y, W 135: clinical and serological evaluation. J Biol Stand 10:335–339, 1982.

181. Peltola H, Safary A, Kayhty H, et al. Evaluation of two tetravalent A, C, Y, and W135 meningococcal vaccines in infants and small children: a clinical study comparing immunogenicity of O-acetyl-negative and O-acetyl-positive group C polysaccharides. Pediatrics 76:91–96, 1985.

182. Zangwill KM, Stout RW, Carlone GM, et al. Duration of antibody response after meningococcal polysaccharide vaccination in US Air Force personnel. J Infect Dis 169:847–852, 1994.

183. Espin Rios I, Garcia-Fulgueiras A, Navarro Alonso JA, et al. Seroconversion and duration of immunity after vaccination against group C meningococcal infection in young children. Vaccine 18:2656–2660, 2000.

184. MacLennan J, Obaro S, Deeks J, et al. Immune response to revaccination with meningococcal A and C polysaccharides in Gambian children following repeated immunisation during early childhood. Vaccine 17:3086–3093, 1999.

185. Gold R, Lepow ML, Goldschneider I, et al. Kinetics of antibody production to group A and group C meningococcal polysaccharide vaccines administered during the first six years of life: prospects for routine immunization of infants and children. J Infect Dis 140:690–697, 1979.

186. Borrow R, Joseph H, Andrews N, et al. Reduced antibody response to revaccination with meningococcal serogroup A polysaccharide vaccine in adults. Vaccine 19:1129–1132, 2000.

187. Richmond P, Kaczmarski E, Borrow R, et al. Meningococcal C polysaccharide vaccine induces immunologic hyporesponsiveness in adults that is overcome by meningococcal C conjugate vaccine. J Infect Dis 181:761–764, 2000.

188. De Wals P, De Serres G, Niyonsenga T. Effectiveness of a mass immunization campaign against serogroup C meningococcal disease in Quebec. JAMA 285:177–181, 2001.

188a. Rivest P, Allard R. The effectiveness of serogroup C meningococcal vaccine estimated from routine surveillance data. Vaccine 20:2533–2536, 2002.

189. Rosenstein N, Levine O, Taylor JP, et al. Efficacy of meningococcal vaccine and barriers to vaccination. JAMA 279:435–439, 1998.

190. Jackson LA, Schuchat A, Reeves MW, Wenger JD. Serogroup C meningococcal outbreaks in the United States: an emerging threat. JAMA 273:383–389, 1995.

191. Artenstein MS, Gold R, Zimmerly JG, et al. Prevention of meningococcal disease by group C polysaccharide vaccine. N Engl J Med 282:417–420, 1970.

192. Gold R, Artenstein MS. Meningococcal infections. 2. Field trial of group C meningococcal polysaccharide vaccine in 1969–70. Bull World Health Organ 45:279–282, 1971.

193. Biselli R, Fattorossi A, Matricardi PM, et al. Dramatic reduction of meningococcal meningitis among military recruits in Italy after introduction of specific vaccination. Vaccine 11:578–581, 1993.

194. Taunay AE, Feldman HA, Bastos C, et al. Avaliacao do efeito protector de vacina polissacaridica antimeningococica do groupo C, em criancas de 6 A 36 meses. Rev Inst Adolfo Lutz 38:77–82, 1978.

195. Amato Neto V, Finger H, Gotschlich EC, et al. Serologic response to serogroup C meningococcal vaccine in Brazilian preschool children. Rev Inst Med Trop Sao Paulo 16:149–153, 1974.

196. Frasch CE. Meningococcal vaccines: past, present and future. In Cartwright K (ed). Meningococcal Disease. New York, John Wiley & Sons, 1995, pp 245–283.

197. Binkin N, Band J. Epidemic of meningococcal meningitis in Bamako, Mali: epidemiological features and analysis of vaccine efficacy. Lancet 2:315–318, 1982.

198. Lennon D, Gellin B, Hood D, et al. Successful intervention in a group A meningococcal outbreak in Auckland, New Zealand. Pediatr Infect Dis J 11:617–623, 1992.

199. Wahdan MH, Sallam SA, Hassan MN, et al. A second controlled field trial of a serogroup A meningococcal polysaccharide vaccine in Alexandria. Bull World Health Organ 55:645–651, 1977.

200. Saliou P, Stoeckel P, Lafaye A, et al. [Controlled tests of anti-meningococcal polysaccharide A vaccine in the African Sahel area (Upper Volta and Mali)]. Dev Biol Stand 41:97–108, 1978.

201. Reingold AL, Broome CV, Hightower AW, et al. Age-specific differences in duration of clinical protection after vaccination with meningococcal polysaccharide A vaccine. Lancet 2:114–118, 1985.

202. Miller MA, Wenger J, Rosenstein N, Perkins B. Evaluation of meningococcal meningitis vaccination strategies for the meningitis belt in Africa. Pediatr Infect Dis J 18:1051–1059, 1999.

203. Robbins JB, Schneerson R, Gotschlich EC. A rebuttal: epidemic and endemic meningococcal meningitis in sub-Saharan Africa can be prevented now by routine immunization with group A meningococcal capsular polysaccharide vaccine. Pediatr Infect Dis J 19:945–953, 2000.

204. Robbins JB, Towne DW, Gotschlich EC, Schneerson R. "Love's labours lost": failure to implement mass vaccination against group A meningococcal meningitis in sub-Saharan Africa. Lancet 350:880–882, 1997.

204a. Parent du Chantelet I, Gessner D, da Silva A. Comparison of cost-effectiveness of preventive and reactive mass immunization campaigns against meningococcal meningitis in West Africa: a theoretical modeling analysis. Vaccine 19:3420–3431, 2001.

204b. Jodar L, LaForce MF, Ceccarini C, et al. Meningococcal conjugate vaccine for Africa: A model for developing new vaccines for the poorest countries. The Lancet, 361:4997–4999, 2003.

205. Devine LF, Pierce WE, Floyd TM, et al. Evaluation of group C meningococcal polysaccharide vaccine in marine recruits, San Diego, California. Am J Epidemiol 92:25–32, 1970.

206. Stroffolini T, Angelini L, Galanti I, et al. The effect of meningococcal group A and C polysaccharide vaccine on nasopharyngeal carrier state. Microbiologica 13:225–229, 1990.

207. Di Martino M, Cali G, Astorre P, et al. Meningococcal carriage and vaccination in army recruits in Italy. Boll Ist Sieroter Milan 69:357–359, 1990.

208. Sivonen A. Effect of Neisseria meningitidis group A polysaccharide vaccine on nasopharyngeal carrier rates. J Infect 3:266–272, 1981.

209. Blakebrough IS, Greenwood BM, Whittle HC, et al. Failure of meningococcal vaccination to stop the transmission of meningococci in Nigerian schoolboys. Ann Trop Med Parasitol 77:175–178, 1983.

210. Hassan-King MK, Wall RA, Greenwood BM. Meningococcal carriage, meningococcal disease and vaccination. J Infect 16:55–59, 1988.

211. Moore PS, Harrison LH, Telzak EE, et al. Group A meningococcal carriage in travelers returning from Saudi Arabia. JAMA 260:2686–2689, 1988.

212. Schwartz B, Al-Tobaiqi A, Al-Ruwais A, et al. Comparative efficacy of ceftriaxone and rifampicin in eradicating pharyngeal carriage of group A Neisseria meningitidis. Lancet 1:1239–1242, 1988.

213. Greenwood BM, Hassan-King M, Whittle HC. Prevention of secondary cases of meningococcal disease in household contacts by vaccination. Br Med J 1:1317–1319, 1978.

213a. Bell R, Braun MM, Modtrey GT. Safety data on meningococcal polysacharaide vaccine from the vaccine adverse event reporting system. Clin Infect Dis 32:1273–1280, 2001.

214. Fairley CK, Begg N, Borrow R, et al. Conjugate meningococcal serogroup A and C vaccine: reactogenicity and immunogenicity in United Kingdom infants. J Infect Dis 174:1360–1363, 1996.

215. Borrow R, Southern J, Andrews N, et al. Comparison of antibody kinetics following meningococcal serogroup C conjugate vaccine between healthy adults previously vaccinated with meningococcal A/C polysaccharide vaccine and vaccine-naive controls. Vaccine 19:3043–3050, 2001.

216. Borrow R, Goldblatt D, Andrews N, et al. Antibody persistence and immunological memory at 4 years after meningococcal group C conjugate vaccination in children in the United Kingdom. J Infect Dis 186:1353–1357, 2002.

217. Borrow R, Fox AJ, Richmond PC, et al. Induction of immunological memory in UK infants by a meningococcal A/C conjugate vaccine. Epidemiol Infect 124:427–432, 2000.

218. Joseph H, Miller E, Dawson M, et al. Meningococcal serogroup A avidity indices as a surrogate marker of priming for the induction of immunologic memory after vaccination with a meningococcal A/C conjugate vaccine in infants in the United Kingdom. J Infect Dis 184:661–662, 2001.

219. Ahman H, Kayhty H, Vuorela A, et al. Dose dependency of antibody response in infants and children to pneumococcal polysaccharides conjugated to tetanus toxoid. Vaccine 17:2726–2732, 1999.

220. MacLennan J, Obaro S, Deeks J, et al. Immunologic memory 5 years after meningococcal A/C conjugate vaccination in infancy. J Infect Dis 183:97–104, 2001.

221. Lucas AH, Granoff DM. Imperfect memory and the development of *Haemophilus influenzae* type B disease. Pediatr Infect Dis J 20:235–239, 2001.

222. MacDonald NE, Halperin SA, Law BJ, et al. Can meningococcal C conjugate vaccine overcome immune hyporesponsiveness induced by previous administration of plain polysaccharide vaccine? JAMA 283:1826–1827, 2000.

223. Borrow R, Goldblatt D, Andrews N, et al. Influence of prior meningococcal C polysaccharide vaccination on the response and generation of memory after meningococcal C conjugate vaccination in young children. J Infect Dis 184:377–380, 2001.

224. Miller E, Salisbury D, Ramsay M. Planning, registration, and implementation of an immunisation campaign against meningococcal serogroup C disease in the UK: a success story. Vaccine 20(suppl 1):S58–S67, 2001.

225. Ramsay ME, Andrews N, Kaczmarski EB, Miller E. Efficacy of meningococcal serogroup C conjugate vaccine in teenagers and toddlers in England. Lancet 357:195–196, 2001.

226. Farrington CP. Estimation of vaccine effectiveness using the screening method. Int J Epidemiol 22:742–746, 1993.

226a. Shigematsu M, Davidson KL, Charlett A, et al. National enhanced surveillance of meningococcal disease in England and Northern Ireland, January 1999–June 2001. Epidemiol Infect 129:459–470, 2002.

227. Maiden M, Stuart J, for the United Kingdom Meningococcal Carriage Group. Reduced carriage of serogroup C meningococci in teenagers one year after the introduction of meningococcal C conjugate polysaccharide vaccine in the United Kingdom. Lancet 359:1829–1831, 2002.

228. Balmer P, Borrow R, Miller E. Impact of meningococcal C conjugate vaccine in the UK. J Med Microbiol 51:717–722, 2002.

229. Cartwright KA, Stuart JM, Jones DM, Noah ND. The Stonehouse survey: nasopharyngeal carriage of meningococci and *Neisseria lactamica*. Epidemiol Infect 99:591–601, 1987.

230. Medicines Control Agency/Committee on Safety of Medicines. Safety of meningococcal group C conjugate vaccines. Curr Probl Pharmacovigilance 26:14, 2000.

231. Laboratory-acquired meningococcal disease—United States, 2000. MMWR 51:141–144, 2002.

232. Boutet R, Stuart JM, Kaczmarski EB, et al. Risk of laboratory-acquired meningococcal disease. J Hosp Infect 49:282–284, 2001.

232a. Memish ZA. Meningococcal disease and travel. Clin Infect Dis. 34:84–90, 2002.

233. Harrison LH, Pass MA, Mendelsohn AB, et al. Invasive meningococcal disease in adolescents and young adults. JAMA 286:694–699, 2001.

234. Neal KR, Nguyen-Van-Tam J, Monk P, et al. Invasive meningococcal disease among university undergraduates: association with universities providing relatively large amounts of catered hall accommodation. Epidemiol Infect 122:351–357, 1999.

235. Harrison LH, Dwyer DM, Maples CT, Billmann L. Risk of meningococcal infection in college students. JAMA 281:1906–1910, 1999.

236. Bruce MG, Rosenstein NE, Capparella JM, et al. Risk factors for meningococcal disease in college students. JAMA 286:688–693, 2001.

237. Racoosin JA, Whitney CG, Conover CS, Diaz PS. Serogroup Y meningococcal disease in Chicago, 1991–1997. JAMA 280:2094–2098, 1998.

238. Meningococcal disease and college students. Recommendations of the Advisory Committee on Immunization Practices (ACIP). MMWR 49:13–20, 2000.

239. Control and prevention of serogroup C meningococcal disease: evaluation and management of suspected outbreaks. Recommendations of the Advisory Committee on Immunization Practices (ACIP). MMWR 46(RR-5):13–21, 1997

240. Chief Medical Officer, Chief Nursing Officer and the Chief Pharmacist. Current vaccine and immunisation issues (PL/CMO/2001/1, Pl.CNO/2001/1, PL/CPHO/2001/1). Department of Health, National Health Service, United Kingdom, accessed 2001. Available at *www.doh.gov.uk/cmo/plcmo2001-5.pdf*

241. Chief Medical Officer, Chief Nursing Officer and the Chief Pharmacist. Extending Meningitis C vaccine to 20–24 year olds: pneumococcal vaccine for at-risk under 2 year olds (PL/CMO/2002/1, PL/CNO/2002/1, PL/CPHO/2002/1). Department of Health, National Health Service, United Kingdom, accessed 2002, Available at *www.doh.gov.uk/meningitis-vaccine/index.htm*

242. Lingappa JR, Rosenstein N, Zell ER, et al. Surveillance for meningococcal disease and strategies for use of conjugate meningococcal vaccines in the United States. Vaccine 19:4566–4575, 2001.

243. Aavitsland P, Bjune G, Aasen S, Halvorsen S. Adverse events following vaccine or placebo injection in an efficacy trial of an outer membrane vesicle vaccine against group B meningococcal disease in Norwegian secondary schools 1988–1991. NIPH Ann 14:133–134; discussion 136–137, 1991.

244. Bjune G, Hoiby EA, Gronnesby JK, et al. Effect of outer membrane vesicle vaccine against group B meningococcal disease in Norway. Lancet 338:1093–1096, 1991.

245. Rosenqvist E, Hoiby EA, Wedege E, et al. Human antibody responses to meningococcal outer membrane antigens after three doses of the Norwegian group B meningococcal vaccine. Infect Immun 63:4642–4652, 1995.

246. Morley SL, Cole MJ, Ison CA, et al. Immunogenicity of a serogroup B meningococcal vaccine against multiple *Neisseria meningitidis* strains in infants. Pediatr Infect Dis J 20:1054–1061, 2001.

247. Jennings HJ, Roy R, Gamian A. Induction of meningococcal group B polysaccharide-specific IgG antibodies in mice by using an N-propionylated B polysaccharide-tetanus toxoid conjugate vaccine. J Immunol 137:1708–1713, 1986.

248. Ashton FE, Ryan JA, Michon F, Jennings HJ. Protective efficacy of mouse serum to the N-propionyl derivative of meningococcal group B polysaccharide. Microb Pathog 6:455–458, 1989.

249. Fusco PC, Michon F, Tai JY, Blake MS. Preclinical evaluation of a novel group B meningococcal conjugate vaccine that elicits bactericidal activity in both mice and nonhuman primates. J Infect Dis 175:364–372, 1997.

250. Granoff DM, Bartoloni A, Ricci S, et al. Bactericidal monoclonal antibodies that define unique meningococcal B polysaccharide epitopes that do not cross-react with human polysialic acid. J Immunol 160:5028–5036, 1998.

251. Gu XX, Tsai CM. Preparation, characterization, and immunogenicity of meningococcal lipooligosaccharide-derived oligosaccharide-protein conjugates. Infect Immun 61:1873–1880, 1993.

252. Verheul AF, Snippe H, Poolman JT. Meningococcal lipopolysaccharides: virulence factor and potential vaccine component. Microbiol Rev 57:34–49, 1993.

253. Moxon ER, Hood D, Richards J. Bacterial lipopolysaccharides: candidate vaccines to prevent *Neisseria meningitidis* and *Haemophilus influenzae* infections. Adv Exp Med Biol 435:237–243, 1998.

254. Morley SL, Pollard AJ. Vaccine prevention of meningococcal disease, coming soon? Vaccine 20:666–687, 2001.

255. Cartwright K, Morris R, Rumke H, et al. Immunogenicity and reactogenicity in UK infants of a novel meningococcal vesicle vaccine containing multiple class 1 (PorA) outer membrane proteins. Vaccine 17:2612–2619, 1999.

256. de Klejin ED, de Groot R, Labadie J, et al. Immunogenicity and safety of a hexavalent meningococcal outer-membrane-vesicle vaccine in children 2–3 and 7–8 years of age. Vaccine 18:1456–1466, 2000.

257. Longworth E, Borrow R, Goldblatt D, et al. Avidity maturation following vaccination with a meningococcal recombinant hexavalent PorA OMV vaccine in UK infants. Vaccine 20:2592–2596, 2002.

258. Martin D, Cadieux N, Hamel J, Brodeur BR. Highly conserved *Neisseria meningitidis* surface protein confers protection against experimental infection. J Exp Med 185:1173–1183, 1997.

259. Moe GR, Tan S, Granoff DM. Differences in surface expression of NspA among *Neisseria meningitidis* group B strains. Infect Immun 67:5664–5675, 1999.

260. Cadieux N, Plante M, Rioux CR, et al. Bactericidal and cross-protective activities of a monoclonal antibody directed against *Neisseria meningitidis* NspA outer membrane protein. Infect Immun 67:4955–4959, 1999.

261. Moe GR, Zuno-Mitchell P, Lee SS, et al. Functional activity of antineisserial surface protein A monoclonal antibodies against strains of *Neisseria meningitidis* serogroup B. Infect Immun 69:3762–3771, 2001.

262. Farrant JL, Kroll JS, Brodeur BR, Martin D. Detection of anti-NspA antibodies in sera from patients convalescent after meningococcal infection. *In* Abstracts of the Eleventh International Pathogenic Neisseria Conference. Nice, France, Editions E. D. K., 1998.
263. Pizza M, Scarlato V, Masignani V, et al. Identification of vaccine candidates against serogroup B meningococcus by whole-genome sequencing. Science 287:1816–1820, 2000.
264. Sun YH, Bakshi S, Chalmers R, Tang CM. Functional genomics of *Neisseria meningitidis* pathogenesis. Nat Med 6:1269–1273, 2000.
265. Rappuoli R. Reverse vaccinology, a genome-based approach to vaccine development. Vaccine 19:2688–2691, 2001.
266. Poolman J, Berthet FX. Alternative vaccine strategies to prevent serogroup B meningococcal diseases. Vaccine 20(suppl 1):S24–S26, 2001.
267. Wahdan MH, Rizk F, el-Akkad AM, et al. A controlled field trial of a serogroup A meningococcal polysaccharide vaccine. Bull World Health Organ 48:667–673, 1973.
268. Erwa HH, Haseeb MA, Idris AA, et al. A serogroup A meningococcal polysaccharide vaccine: studies in the Sudan to combat cerebrospinal meningitis caused by *Neisseria meningitidis* group A. Bull World Health Organ 49:301–305, 1973.
269. Peltola H, Makela H, Kayhty H, et al. Clinical efficacy of meningococcus group A capsular polysaccharide vaccine in children three months to five years of age. N Engl J Med 297:686–6891, 1977.
270. Makela PH, Kayhty H, Weckstrom P, et al. Effect of group-A meningococcal vaccine in army recruits in Finland. Lancet 2:883–886, 1975.
271. Bramley JC, Hall T, Finn A, et al. Safety and immunogenicity of three lots of meningococcal serogroup C conjugate vaccine administered at 2, 3 and 4 months of age. Vaccine 19:2924–2931, 2001.
272. Burrage M, Robinson A, Borrow R, et al. Effect of vaccination with carrier protein on response to meningococcal C conjugate vaccines and value of different immunoassays as predictors of protection. Infect Immun 70:4946–4954, 2002.

Chapter 35

Miscellaneous Limited-Use Vaccines

PHILLIP PITTMAN • STANLEY A. PLOTKIN

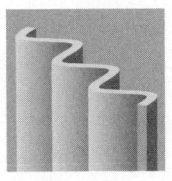

U.S. military personnel have the potential for exposure to many infectious agents as endemic diseases as well as in their unnatural form as biologic weapons. Increasingly, civilian populations may be targets for terrorist attacks using microorganisms (or their toxins), as was demonstrated by the purposeful dissemination of anthrax spores following ballistic attacks on the World Trade Center and the Pentagon in 2001. The U.S. Army has had a long-standing program to develop vaccines with which to combat these threats. Many of these vaccine products are currently in use at the U.S. Army Medical Research Institute of Infectious Diseases (USAMRIID) and elsewhere to protect laboratory researchers; meanwhile, advances in technology are being applied in developing the next generation of vaccines.

The principal organization responsible for medical countermeasures against biologic warfare agents within the Department of Defense (DOD) is the U.S. Army Medical Research and Materiel Command (MRMC) located at Fort Detrick, Maryland. The subordinate unit with current direct responsibility for this exclusively defensive mission is USAMRIID. Prior to 1969, when the United States maintained an offensive biologic weapons program, the U.S. Army Medical Unit (subordinate to the Walter Reed Army Institute of Research in Washington, DC) served in this capacity. Many of the biowarfare vaccines used today were conceived at the U.S. Army Medical Unit and then underwent further development and/or scale-up at the National Drug Laboratories, more recently known as The Salk Institute, Government Services Division (TSI-GSD), in Swiftwater, Pennsylvania, but which is now closed. The majority of vaccines developed at Fort Detrick have, for a variety of reasons, remained Investigational New Drugs (INDs). All of these vaccines underwent extensive preclinical testing and have been in Phase II trials for many years.

Table 35–1 presents all IND products developed and held at the MRMC/USAMRIID. The Candid #1 Junin (Argentine hemorrhagic fever [AHF]) vaccine, successful in a Phase III efficacy trial in Argentina, has been incorporated into that country's public health program and has been administered to over 10,000 at-risk people.

Venezuelan equine encephalitis (VEE) TC-83 vaccine, eastern equine encephalitis (EEE) vaccine, western equine encephalitis (WEE) vaccine, Tularemia LVS vaccine, Rift Valley fever (RVF) vaccine, and the whole-cell Q fever vaccine each have been administered to over 1000 volunteers, whereas RVF vaccine MP-12, Q fever CMR, Chikungunya, and Vaccinia/Hantaan each have been administered to a hundred volunteers or fewer.

Each of these vaccines is administered under an approved protocol, and all volunteers provide written informed consent prior to receipt. The protocols and consent forms are reviewed by the USAMRIID Scientific Review Committee and the USAMRIID Human Use Committee as well as the Army Surgeon General's Human Subjects Research Review Board before submission to the Food and Drug Administration (FDA). Protocols are conducted in accordance with the Declaration of Helsinki and applicable DOD and FDA regulations and guidelines. Many of these vaccines have been in use since the 1960s and 1970s, and all are subject to periodic potency and lot-release testing as required by the FDA.

Continuous monitoring for safety and immunogenicity is conducted through USAMRIID's Special Immunizations Program. To date, all vaccines have demonstrated an acceptable safety profile and reasonable immunogenicity (Table 35–2). The most reactogenic product is the live, attenuated VEE (TC-83) vaccine, which frequently induces a short-term systemic reaction. The inactivated vaccines, with the exception of the whole-cell Q fever vaccine, require multiple doses for priming and frequent periodic boosting in order to maintain acceptable levels of neutralizing antibody. All vaccines have been administered to both males and nonpregnant females, and the vaccines recipients have a broad age and ethnicity/race mix. With the exception of Junin vaccine (with which a Phase III trial was conducted), efficacy of these products is inferred by the absence of laboratory-acquired infection among recipients. However, because laboratory practices and engineering controls have evolved in concert with use of the vaccines, quantifying efficacy on a continuous basis is difficult.

Alphavirus Vaccines

The alphaviruses are a group of mosquito-borne, lipid-enveloped, positive-stranded RNA viruses belonging to

---

George R. French contributed to this chapter in prior editions.

TABLE 35–1 ■ Investigational New Drug, Limited-Use Vaccines: Characteristics and Administration

Name	Type	Dosage (mL)	Route	Schedule (days)	Boosters
VEE TC-83	Live, attenuated	0.5	SC	0	C84
VEE C-84	Inactivated	0.5	SC	0*	Yes
EEE	Inactivated	0.5	SC	0, 28	Yes
WEE	Inactivated	0.5	SC	0, 7, 28	Yes
RVF	Inactivated	1.0	SC	0, 7, 28	Yes
RVF ZH-548	Live, attenuated	1	SC	0	No
Junin	Live, attenuated	0.5	SC	0	No
Q fever	Inactivated	0.5	SC	0	No
Q fever CMR	Inactivated	0.5	SC	0	No
Tularemia LVS	Live, attenuated	0.06	Scarification	0	Yes
Vaccinia/Hantaan	Live, attenuated	0.06/0.5	Scarification/IM	0	
Botulinum	Inactivated	0.5	SC	0, 14, 84	Yes

*Given only after TC-83 and titer ≤ 1:20.
IM, intramuscular; SC, subcutaneous.

the family Togaviridae. Alphaviruses are responsible for two distinct clinical syndromes: fever, chills, headache, myalgias, vomiting, and encephalitis (e.g., VEE, EEE, WEE, etc.); and fever, rash, and polyarthralgias/arthritis (e.g., Chikungunya, Ross River virus, and O'nyong-nyong). Several excellent reviews are available on the classification, epidemiology, and clinical features of these agents.[1,2] Vaccines have been developed by the DOD against four alphaviruses: VEE, WEE, EEE, and Chikungunya.

Experience with sequential administration of alphavirus vaccines at USAMRIID has led to a number of interesting observations relating to immunologic interference. Prior immunization with inactivated EEE and/or

WEE vaccines decreases the ability to mount a neutralizing antibody response following receipt of live, attenuated VEE (TC-83) vaccine (PR Pittman, unpublished results). Similarly, interference occurs when two live, attenuated alphavirus vaccines, VEE TC-83 and Chikungunya, are administered sequentially.[3] Volunteers initially vaccinated against VEE TC-83 exhibited poor neutralizing antibody responses to live, attenuated Chikungunya virus vaccine (46% response rate). Among persons initially inoculated with either Chikungunya vaccine or placebo who then received live, attenuated VEE (TC-83) vaccines, geometric mean antibody titers to VEE virus by 80% plaque-reduction neutralization test ($PRNT_{80}$) were uniformly depressed in

TABLE 35–2 ■ Assessment of Efficacy and Safety of Selected Limited-Use Vaccines

Name	Tests of Effectiveness	Effective	Reactions Systemic	Local
VEE TC-83, live	Reduction in laboratory-associated infections	Yes	+++	+
VEE C-84, inactivated	Unknown	Probably	+	+
EEE, inactivated	Reduction in laboratory-associated infections	Probably	+	+
WEE, inactivated	Reduction in laboratory-associated infections	Probably	+	+
Chikungunya	Phase I testing	Probably	±	±
RVF, inactivated	Reduction in laboratory-associated infections	Yes	+	+
RVF ZH-548, live	In progress	To be determined	±	±
Junin, live	Formal Phase II field trial	Yes	±	±
Q fever, inactivated	Reduction in laboratory-associated infections	Probably	+	++
Q fever CMR, inactivated	In progress	To be determined	+	+
Tularemia LVS, live	Reduction in laboratory-associated infections	Yes	+	++++
Vaccinia/Hantaan, live	In progress	To be determined	+	±
Botulinum Toxoid Pentavalent (ABCDE)	Reduction in lab-associated infection	Yes	+	++

+/– = Unusual, + = Occasional, ++ = Mild or Low, +++ = Moderate, ++++ = Severe or Pronounced

Chikungunya vaccine recipients compared with placebo recipients.[3]

Venezuelan Equine Encephalitis Virus Vaccines

Two VEE vaccines are available for human use: a live, attenuated product (TC-83) and a formalin-inactivated product (C-84); both derive from the same lineage. Laboratory infections with epizootic VEE strains closely related to the parent essentially have been eliminated since introduction of these vaccines.

The live, attenuated TC-83 virus, as subtype I-AB strain, was isolated from a Trinidad donkey brain that was passaged 13 times in embryonated eggs.[4] The virus was attenuated by 78 passages in fetal guinea pig heart (FGPH) cell cultures, plaque-picked in chick embryo fibroblasts (CEFs), and then passaged four additional times in FGPH cell cultures.[5] The VEE TC-83 virus designation is a direct reference to the 83 passages in cell culture. VEE C-84 vaccine is formalin inactivated and is made from the TC-83 production seed, TC-82, that has undergone one additional passage in CEFs.[6] This C-84 production seed is passaged once more in CEFs to derive the C-84 vaccine, which is inactivated with 0.1% formalin and then freeze-dried. The inactivation procedure is based on that used by Salk et al. to inactivate the poliovirus.[7] TC-83 and C-84 contain streptomycin and neomycin, each at a concentration of 50 μg/mL.

At USAMRIID, immunologically naïve individuals at risk for exposure to VEE receive the live, attenuated TC-83 vaccine. The response rate ($PRNT_{80}$ titer >1:20) to TC-83 alone is 82%.[8] When TC-83 is followed by C-84, a combined response rate of well over 90% is observed. Female responders tend to have titers similar to male responders, but the frequency of nonresponders tends to be higher among females than males. The nature of this gender differential is not understood.

Approximately 23% of individuals receiving TC-83 sustain adverse reactions.[8] A subset of recipients suffer headache, sore throat, malaise, fatigue, myalgias, arthralgias, chills, and fever similar to that seen following natural VEE infection. The local reaction rate is less than 5%. C-84 has a local reaction rate of approximately 5% but has essentially no systemic reactions associated with its administration. Despite reports of diabetes mellitus, abortion, and teratogenesis related to natural wild-type VEE disease, there is no conclusive evidence of long-term adverse events related to the use of either of these vaccines. Before pregnancy testing became available, there were two cases of spontaneous abortion temporally related to the administration of TC-83. However, VEE virus was not recovered from culture of tissues in either case. Since the advent of pregnancy testing, great care is used to ensure that females are not pregnant before administration of TC-83. In addition, care is exercised to avoid vaccination of persons with a family history of diabetes mellitus.

The ideal VEE vaccine would have a high seroconversion rate (over 95%) and a low reaction rate (less than 5%). By these standards, TC-83 is reactogenic and has a moderate response rate as measured by neutralizing antibody. In addition, TC-83 does not protect adequately against distantly related VEE subtype I-AB variants or the other enzootic VEE subtypes II through VI. A new-generation vaccine candidate uses twin site-directed mutagenesis of the full-length complementary DNA clone of the virulent virus RNA.[9] There is a lethal deletion at the PE-2 cleavage signal site and a suppressor mutation at site 253 of the E1 glycoprotein. These two deletion mutations should prevent reversion to wild-type VEE virus. This promising vaccine candidate is undergoing preclinical testing.

Western Equine Encephalitis Virus Vaccine

An inactivated western equine encephalitis vaccine, TSI-GSD-210 (manufactured by The National Drug Company and its successor The Salk Institute, Government Services Division), has been used at Fort Detrick since the 1970s to immunize at-risk laboratory personnel. The WEE vaccine is a lyophilized product derived from supernatant fluids of primary CEF cell cultures infected with the attenuated CM4884 strain of WEE.[10,11] The supernatant fluid is harvested and filtered, the virus is inactivated with formalin, and the final product is lyophilized for storage at −20°C. The vaccine contains 50 μg/mL of neomycin.

In an analysis of 363 volunteers who received 0.5 mL of TSI-GSD-210 subcutaneously at 0, 7, and 28 days, 151 subjects (41.6%) responded with a $PRNT_{80}$ titer of 1:40 or greater, whereas 212 subjects (58.4%) failed to achieve this neutralizing antibody titer.[12] Seventy-six of 115 initial nonresponders (66%) were converted to responder status after a single booster. Kaplan-Meier plots showed that a regimen consisting of three initial doses and one booster induced protective levels of antibody ($PRNT_{80}$ >1:40) lasting for 1.6 years in 50% of initial responders. Local and systemic adverse events are uncommon with this vaccine. Among 363 vaccinees receiving three initial injections of the WEE vaccine, only 5 reported local or systemic reactions. There have been no instances of occupational WEE documented in laboratory workers who develop neutralizing antibody following vaccination. WEE vaccine continues to be administered as part of Phase II clinical trials; however, no efficacy trial has been conducted.

Eastern Equine Encephalitis Virus Vaccine

The EEE vaccine is a lyophilized product originating in primary CEF cell cultures infected with the attenuated PE-6 strain of EEE virus. The seed for the EEE virus is passaged twice in adult mice and twice in guinea pigs, then passaged nine times in embryonated eggs, followed by three passages in CEFs.[13] The supernatant fluid is harvested and filtered and contains 50 μg of neomycin and streptomycin, and 0.25% w/v of Human Serum Albumin, USP. The virus is then inactivated with 0.05% formalin. When inactivation is completed, the residual formalin is neutralized by treatment with sodium bisulfite. The final product is lyophilized for storage at −20°C.

Among 255 volunteers who received two primary vaccinations of EEE vaccine (TSI-GSD-104) between 1992 and 1998, 197 (77.3%) responded with a $PRNT_{80}$ titer of 1:40 or greater.[14] Sixty-six percent of initial nonresponders subsequently seroconverted following receipt of an intradermal EEE vaccine booster. Among initial responders whose titers waned over time, 98.6% responded to a booster dose of EEE vaccine. Local and systemic side effects are infrequent: less than 1% after the primary vaccine series and 3.7% after the first booster. Kaplan-Meier plots show that two primary and one intradermal booster of TSI-GSD-104 provide satisfactory neutralizing anti-EEE antibody in 50% of initial responders for up to 2.2 years.

Chikungunya Virus Vaccine

Chickungunya is an alphavirus that may cause an acute viral syndrome in humans characterized by fever, rash, and arthritis.[15] Some individuals who are human leukocyte antigen B27 positive may develop long-term joint involvement.[16] Although epidemics have been documented as occurring since the late 18th century, the virus was first isolated during the 1952–53 Tanzanian epidemic.[1] Several attempts were made to develop an efficacious inactivated vaccine using chick embryo cell cultures, suckling mice brain, and African green monkey kidney, with variable success.[17]

A live, attenuated vaccine was made from the seed of the last of these vaccines, CHIK strain 15561, isolated from an infected patient during a Chikungunya epidemic in Thailand in 1962.[17,18] The 11th African green monkey kidney passage of CHIK strain 15562, made at the Walter Reed Army Institute of Research, was transferred to USAMRIID and passaged in Medical Research Council (MRC)-5 cells. After 18 passages in MRC-5 cells, CHIK 181/clone 25 was selected as a vaccine seed strain based on biomarkers. CHIK 181/clone 25 was efficacious in a suckling mice model and in the nonhuman primate.[17]

A randomized, double-blind, placebo-controlled trial of the live, attenuated Chikungunya vaccine showed that alphavirus-naïve volunteers have a seroconversion rate of 98%.[18] At 1 year after immunization, 85% of vaccinees remained seropositive. Injection site and systemic symptoms, including flu-like symptoms, were similar in vaccine and placebo recipients. However, the vaccine was temporally associated with arthralgia in 8% of vaccinees. One volunteer in the vaccine group developed a pruritic, eczema-like rash at the injection site. Interference between Chikungunya vaccine and the live, attenuated VEE (TC-83) vaccine has been discussed earlier. This live, attenuated Chikungunya vaccine requires additional Phase II and Phase III clinical testing.

Ross River Virus

Epidemic polyarthritis was first recognized in Australia in 1928; however, Ross River virus (RRV), its causative agent, was first isolated in 1963 from a pool of mosquitoes.[19–21] Epidemic polyarthritis, or RRV, is essentially limited to Australia, Fiji, and the surrounding islands, including American Samoa and the Cook Islands, where several thousand cases occur per year.[22,23] This positive, single-stranded RNA virus belongs to the genus *Alphavirus*, family *Togaviridae*. In humans, polyarthritis may be followed by fever, rash, and lethargy. U.S. marines participating in Operation Tandem Thrust in Queensland, Australia, in 1997 had an infection rate of 1.5%; nine developed RRV disease.[24]

A vaccine candidate was derived from a virus isolate from a human case of classical epidemic polyarthritis using

the C6-36 cell line (*Aedes albopictus*).[25] The candidate underwent four serial passages in MRC-5 human fetal lung cells followed by two passages in Vero cells. Cell cultures contained penicillin (100 units/mL) and streptomycin (100 µg/mL). The virus was inactivated using binary ethyleneimine. The vaccine induced neutralizing antibody in mice and protected mice against viremia when challenged intravenously with live RRF virus.

Bunyavirus Vaccines

The Bunyaviridae are a large family of separated, lipid-enveloped, negative-stranded RNA viruses. Vaccines against human pathogens representing two of the five genera, RVF virus (*Phlebovirus* genus) and Hantaan virus (*Hantavirus* genus), have been developed at Fort Detrick.

Rift Valley Fever Vaccines

RVF is a mosquito-borne infection endemic to sub-Saharan Africa and affecting primarily ruminant animals. Under appropriate climatologic conditions, however, explosive epizootics among animals and epidemics in humans occur with considerable morbidity and mortality. In recent years, RVF has demonstrated its potential for spreading northward to Egypt and into Yemen and Saudi Arabia in the Asian continent. The consequences of further spread into naïve animal and human populations are potentially devastating.

The U.S. Army has developed two vaccines to combat this threat: an inactivated RVF vaccine (TSI-GSD-200) and, more recently, a live, attenuated product (RVF MP-12). The Entebbe strain of RVF, isolated from a mosquito pool in Bwamba County, Uganda, is the source for the inactivated vaccine.[26] The virus was passaged 184 times in adult mice, followed by two passages in fetal rhesus lung (FRhL) cells to form the production seed. Although the original vaccine was produced in primary African green monkey kidney cells, the current vaccine lots are produced in FRhL cells.[27,28] The vaccine is inactivated in 0.05% formalin. Following verification of viral inactivation, the residual formaldehyde is neutralized with sodium bisulfite to less than 0.01%. A study of the immunogenicity and safety of inactivated RVF vaccine in humans over a 12-year period showed the vaccine to be safe and immunogenic when the primary series and one booster are administered.[29] In this study, 540 of 598 volunteers (90%) administered three subcutaneous doses of 1.0 mL TSI-GSD-200 on days 0, 7, and 28 responded with a $PRNT_{80}$ titer of 1:40 or greater. Three fourths of the initial nonresponders developed $PRNT_{80}$ titer of 1:40 or greater after a single booster. However, about 10% of recipients require repeated boosting (PR Pittman, unpublished data).

An isolated RVF strain recovered from a nonfatal human case that occurred during the first Egyptian epidemic in 1977 was used to derive the live, attenuated RVF vaccine. The virus (ZH-548) was passaged twice in suckling mouse brain, then once in FRhL cells. It was then attenuated by 12 serial alternating passages in human lung cell cultures (MRC-5 cells, certified for vaccine use) by previously described methods[30] in the presence or absence of 5-fluorouracil. The resulting RVF MP12 vaccine is a lyophilized product originating from supernatant fluids harvested from the final mutagenesis passage. The vaccine has undergone extensive testing in several animal species: rodents, sheep (including pregnant ewes and naïve neonatal lambs), cattle (including in utero vaccinated bovids), and monkeys.[31–34]

RVF MP-12 has undergone clinical evaluation in human volunteers at USAMRIID. In a Phase II randomized, double-blinded, dose-escalation/route-seeking study, 56 healthy, nonpregnant subjects were randomly selected to receive RVF MP-12 ($10^{4.7}$ plaque-forming units [PFU] subcutaneously, $n = 10$; $10^{3.4}$ PFU intramuscularly, $n = 6$; or $10^{4.4}$ PFU intramuscularly, $n = 27$) or placebo ($n = 13$).[35] Only infrequent and minor side effects were seen among both placebo and MP-12 recipients. Six volunteers, all from the group receiving $10^{3.4}$ PFU intramuscularly, had transient low-titer viremia by amplification using an in situ enzyme-linked immunosorbent assay (ELISA). One of these volunteers had a titer of 1.3 log by direct plaquing in cell culture. Neutralizing antibodies (measured by $PRNT_{80}$ titer), as well as RVF-specific immunoglobulin M and immunoglobulin G, were observed in 40 of 43 vaccine recipients (93%). The highest peak geometric mean antibody titers were observed in the group receiving $10^{4.4}$ PFU intramuscularly. Overall, 28 (85%) of 34 RVF MP-12 recipients available for testing remained seropositive ($PRNT_{80}$ ≥1:20) at 1 year following inoculation.

Hantavirus Vaccines

Hantaviruses causing hemorrhagic fever with renal syndrome (HFRS) have been, and continue to be, significant endemic disease threats to U.S. military forces on the Korean peninsula and throughout Europe.[36] At least 14 distinct viral strains are distributed worldwide.[37] In addition to HFRS, hantaviruses are responsible for the recently described hantavirus pulmonary syndrome.[37,38] Humans become infected with hantavirus by inhalation of aerosolized rodent excreta.[39] The prototype hantavirus, Hantaan, was first isolated in Korea; the first vaccine also was developed there to protect against HFRS.[38,40,41] This vaccine, the ROK84/105 strain, harvested from suckling mouse brains, is concentrated by protamine sulfate precipitation and centrifugation. The concentrate is then exposed to formalin inactivation and purified by ultrafiltration and sucrose gradient ultracentrifugation. Aluminum hydroxide is added to the vaccine as an adjuvant, thimerosal as a preservative, and gelatin as a stabilizer. The final product reportedly has less than 0.01 ng/mL of myelin basic protein. The recommended regimen for this product, Hantavax, is two doses of 5120 ELISA units (0.5 mL) given 1 month apart by the subcutaneous or intramuscular routes.

Little has been published on the vaccine, but the manufacturer reports that tolerance is good, although allergic reactions occur, presumably as a result of mouse brain antigens. A serologic response measurable by indirect fluorescence is seen in nearly all vaccinees. Neutralizing antibodies are usually absent after one dose, but present in about 75% of subjects after the second dose.[42] They decrease to 16% at 12 months, at which time a booster is recommended. Although there are no placebo-controlled data on the efficacy of the vaccine, a similar vaccine made in North Korea reportedly showed 88% to 100% efficacy,

and Hantavax itself has been effective in uncontrolled epidemiologic studies done in South Korea and Yugoslavia.[43,44] Vaccines made in cell culture are available in China against both hantavirus and Seoul virus strains. The substrate is cell cultures of golden hamster kidney or Mongolian gerbil kidney. A bivalent vaccine is also licensed there. The efficacy of these vaccines is reportedly better than 90%.[43,44]

At USAMRIID, advances in technology fueled development of bioengineered hantavirus vaccines. Two experimental approaches studied to date include vaccinia-vectored hantavirus genes, and the same genes inserted into bacterial plasmids as DNA vaccines. The creation of a recombinant vaccinia-vectored Hantaan virus vaccine carrying envelope and nucleocapsid genes of the virus has been described.[45,46] The recombinant vaccinia-vectored Hantaan virus vaccine was efficacious in the hamster infectivity model; even if pre-existing immunity to vaccinia virus was present, it could be overcome by a second intramuscular injection of the vaccine candidate.[45] A double-blinded, placebo-controlled clinical trial involving 142 volunteers using two subcutaneous injections 4 weeks apart showed that, for vaccinia-naïve volunteers, neutralizing antibodies to Hantaan virus or vaccinia virus occurred in 72% or 98%, respectively, whereas neutralizing antibodies to Hantaan virus were detected in only 26% of vaccinia-immune volunteers.[46]

DNA plasmids, alphavirus replicons, baculovirus-produced proteins, and chimeric hepatitis B particles are all under study as additional hantavirus vaccine candidates.[44,47]

Arenavirus Vaccines

Several members of the arenavirus family of segmented negative-stranded RNA viruses are recognized as causative agents for viral hemorrhagic fever syndromes in humans. To date, efforts to develop protective immunogens against arenavirus have met with limited success.[48] During the 1980s, the first successful vaccine against an arenavirus, Junin virus, was developed through a collaboration between the government of Argentina and the U.S. Army.

Junin Virus Vaccine

Junin virus is the causative agent of AHF, endemic to the pampas of north-central Argentina. Humans become infected with Junin virus by inhalation of infected rodent secretions and excretions.[49–51] Death occurs in 15% to 30% of patients inflicted with AHF if untreated.

For several decades attempts were in made in Argentina to develop an efficacious vaccine against AHF. The resulting inactivated and live, attenuated vaccine candidates all failed for various reasons.[48] The product developed at USAMRIID, Candid #1, is a descendant of the prototype XJ strain Junin virus, isolated in guinea pig from a fatal AHF case. Following another passage in the guinea pig, the virus underwent 44 newborn mouse brain passages, then was cloned and passaged 19 times in certified FRhL cells.[48,52,53] Candid #1 proved effective in preventing disease in guinea pigs and rhesus macaques after lethal Junin virus challenge.[52,54,55] Phase I and II clinical testing in humans showed Candid #1 to be safe and immunogenic.[56,57]

Over 90% of volunteers developed antibodies against Junin virus, and 99% developed a Junin virus–specific cellular immune response. In a pivotal efficacy study, 3255 volunteers were randomized to receive the vaccine and 3245 were randomized to receive a placebo. During the trial, 23 volunteers developed an illness that met the clinical case definition for AHF.[58,59] Of these, 22 had received a placebo and 1 had received the vaccine; vaccine efficacy by intent-to-treat analysis was 95% (95% confidence interval, 82% to 99%; $P < 0.001$).

Junin vaccine is recommended for individuals exposed to the Junin virus because of occupational (agricultural or laboratory) exposure. Indeed, it continues to be used in Argentina to protect against AHF. The development of this vaccine represents a successful collaboration between USAMRIID and the Argentine Ministry of Health and Social Action, under the auspices of the United Nations Development Program and the Pan-American Health Organization.

Limited-Use Vaccines Against Rickettsial Disease

Q Fever

Q fever is a highly infectious zoonotic disease of humans usually caused by aerosol transmission of the rickettsia *Coxiella burnetii* from infected sheep or goats.[60] Fever and pneumonia are the most frequent clinical manifestations of Q fever, although hepatitis, endocarditis, and a variety of other complications may develop. Antibiotics are effective but may act slowly, and a chronic fatigue syndrome after Q fever has been reported, presumably as a result of cytokine dysregulation.[61]

Mechanisms of immunity to Q fever vaccine are complex. Although antibody is important to clear extracellular organisms, it is sensitization of lymphocytes to Q fever antigen and secretion of lymphokines that clears intracellular infection and provides immunologic memory.[62]

The agent of Q fever was adapted to growth in the chick embryo yolk sac, and an early vaccine was made by formalin inactivation of rickettsia produced in eggs.[63] This vaccine was effective in humans, including those subjected to experimental challenge, but it also gave occasional severe local reactions that sometimes progressed to abscess formation. Eventually it was shown that reactions were associated with pre-existing immunity to Q fever. Accordingly, the practice of screening prospective vaccinees for local induration after inoculation with a skin test antigen made from diluted vaccine was adopted.

Advances in rickettsial biology and vaccinology led to a new generation of immunogens. It was realized that only phase I Q fever rickettsia, analogous to smooth forms of bacteria, were protective, and that a transition to phase II (rough) would occur if the organism was passaged too many times in chick embryo. This led to the development of vaccines based on phase I organisms only.[64]

Additionally, it was recognized that purification to remove chicken protein and lipid and isolation of whole inactivated rickettsia by extraction, filtration, or centrifugation would result in a cleaner, less reactogenic, and highly immunogenic product. Two whole-cell vaccines came into use in high-risk subjects: an Australian vaccine made and licensed by Commonwealth Serum Laboratories[62,65] and a vaccine made and tested by the U.S. Army[66] but not licensed. Both are administered as a single subcutaneous injection of 30 µg. The Australian vaccine is purified using high concentrations of NaCl to remove nonprotective antigens. The U.S. Army vaccine is also extracted with NaCl, then subjected to ethanol–Freon 113 extraction, and finally purified further on a $CaHPO_4$ $2H_2O$ (brushite) column. Despite these purification processes, however, it was discovered that skin testing of prospective recipients remained necessary to prevent serious reactions in those who had experienced prior infection.

Whole-cell vaccines have undergone considerable clinical testing. In Australia, both a placebo-controlled trial[67] and an open trial in abattoir workers[68,69] showed efficacy approaching 100% (Table 35–3). The U.S. Army vaccine was subjected to a controlled challenge in volunteers; this trial also proved highly successful.[70]

In order to eliminate the problem of reactions, third-generation Q fever vaccines have been prepared in the United States[71,72] and Czechoslovakia.[73] These latter vaccines, extracted with chloroform-methanol or other lipid solvents to remove lipid A (thought to be the chief offending substance in the rickettsiae), have not yet been shown to be equivalent to whole-cell Q fever vaccine in protection of humans.

A live, attenuated Q fever vaccine produced in chick embryo yolk sac has been developed in Russia.

Limited-Use Vaccines Against Bacterial Diseases

Tularemia

Tularemia, a bacterial bioterrorism threat, can be a significant endemic and epidemic human disease. The causative bacterium of tularemia, *Francisella tularensis*, was isolated in

TABLE 35–3 ■ Protection by Q Fever Vaccines

| Vaccines | Type of Study | Number of Cases of Q Fever | | |
		Vaccinated	Unvaccinated	Protection
U.S.	Random, challenge	2/32	5/6	92%
Australian	Random placebo-controlled	0/98	7/102	100%
Australian	Observational	3*/2716	52/2012	96–100%

*Vaccinated during incubation period of Q fever.
Data from Ormsbee RA, Marmion BP. Prevention of *Coxiella burnetii* Infection: Vaccines and Guidelines for those at risk. In: Marne TJ, ed. The Disease, Vol. 1, Q fever. Chapter 12. CRC Press, Boca Raton, FL, 1990, pp 775–748.

1912, and in 1919 Edward Francis made the association with the human disease "deer fly fever."[74]

Many of the more than 200 cases of *F. tularensis* documented in the American medical literature resulting from laboratory exposure occurred in laboratory personnel who had received one or more injections of a phenol-killed vaccine and/or acetone-prepared vaccine.[75–78] One of these early inactivated products, the Foshay vaccine, showed incomplete protective efficacy against tularemia organisms introduced by the respiratory and intracutaneous routes.[79,80] Although circulating antibodies could be demonstrated following administration of these vaccines, the antibodies generated were not protective. It was concluded that the protective antigen of *F. tularemia* was destroyed in the inactivation procedures used to prepare the vaccines.

Partly on this basis, an effort to develop a live vaccine of *F. tularemia* was undertaken. By avoiding destruction of the protective antigen, live vaccines, which cause actual infection, are thought to produce an immunity closer to that caused by the disease itself than do killed vaccines, in particular by generating persistent antibodies and cellular immunity.

Soviet investigators initially developed a live tularemia vaccine in 1942.[81] Ampoules of this "viable" tularemia vaccine were brought to the United States from the Russian Institute of Epidemiology and Microbiology (Gamaleia Institute) by Shope in 1956.[82] Eigelsbach and Downs then derived a vaccine strain from an ampoule of this product, which they designated the live vaccine strain (LVS).[83]

Studies done at Fort Detrick in the early 1960s showed LVS to be protective for mice and guinea pigs in virulent challenge.[83] This protection was subsequently shown to be due to cell-mediated immunity when passively transferred spleen cells from immunized mice afforded protection to nonimmune recipients.[84] Similar immunization studies were done in monkeys, which also demonstrated a significant immune response to vaccination with LVS.[85]

LVS initially was given by scarification to volunteers at Fort Detrick in 1958.[86] The vaccination procedure appeared to be benign after clinical evaluations involving 29 individuals.[80] Only a pink scar remained 1 month postvaccination. Transient, axillary lymphadenitis was observed in approximately half of the individuals, but none of the 29 men exhibited fever or other systemic reactions following immunization with LVS. All persons showed bacterial agglutinin antibodies; peak titers were observed 29 to 59 days postvaccination and were sustained.[87]

At challenge doses up to 2500 organisms, a significant protective effect was seen in volunteers vaccinated with LVS; only 20% of vaccinated individuals showed clinical illness compared to 85% of the unvaccinated controls. None of the vaccinated individuals showing clinical illness had symptoms severe enough to require treatment. At higher challenge doses, however, immunity was overcome; with 25,000 organisms there was no significant protection in terms of occurrence of clinical illness, with 90% of the vaccinated individuals showing some symptomatology as compared to 85% of the controls. There was, however, some protection in terms of severity of illness. Only 60% of the vaccinated group had symptoms severe enough to require treatment, as compared to 100% of the control group.[87]

The efficacy of live tularemia vaccine when administered by aerosol has been tested.[88,89] In one study,[89] 6 of 16 individuals were protected against challenge with the virulent SCHU-S4 strain of *F. tularensis* by previous aerosol exposure to live tularemia vaccine. Serologic studies showed that all the protected individuals had measurable circulating antibody. Of the 10 individuals not protected, only one had circulating antibody.

LVS (NDBR-101) has been used since the mid-1960s and has been associated with a significant decline in the rate of laboratory-acquired infections at Fort Detrick.[90] The vaccine remains investigational and is administered only under protocol and written informed consent. The lots undergo required lot-release and potency tests as required by the FDA for IND products. Efforts are underway to develop new-generation vaccines against tularemia using modern technologies.

Brucellosis

Primarily a disease of animals, brucellosis first was described by military personnel in 1859 as Mediterranean gastric remittent fever or Malta fever.[91] The consumption of unpasteurized goat milk was found to be the source in the Malta epidemic.[92] Bruce isolated the etiologic agent in 1886 from a fatal case of Malta fever.[93] Initially named *Micrococcus melitensis*, the genus later was named for its discoverer and is currently known as *Brucella melitensis*. *Brucella* species are non–spore-forming gram-negative coccobacilli that exist worldwide. Several animal species become infected with *Brucella* species. Humans become infected on contact with infected animals, by consuming unpasteurized infected milk or other dairy products, and by working with the organism under laboratory conditions. Brucellosis presents with nonspecific flu-like symptoms that are often much more prominent than the gastrointestinal symptoms.

Effective vaccines for animals are available for *B. melitensis* and *B. abortus*. Use of these vaccines has led to a dramatic decrease in human disease in countries where animal disease is enzootic. Currently, there is no vaccine for human use.

Pseudomonas

Pseudomonas Vaccine

Pseudomonas aeruginosa is a nosocomial pathogen of some consequence, but in addition it causes life-threatening infections in cystic fibrosis patients owing to its production of a thick, mucoid capsule. Although antibodies to the lipopolysaccharide develop in cystic fibrosis patients after infection, they are of low affinity and do not protect. In contrast, artificial immunization with lipopolysaccharide from eight different strains coupled chemically with the pseudomonas exotoxin A elicited high affinity IgG antibodies.[94] Trials in CF patients showed freedom from pseudomonas colonization at four and ten year follow up, respectively, in 61% and 68% of vaccinees versus 39% and 28% of matched control patients.[95,96] The vaccine is being developed by Berna, and is in a Phase III efficacy trial.[97]

Botulism

Botulinum Pentavalent (ABCDE) Toxoid

Botulism is a neurologic intoxication caused by botulinum toxin, the most poisonous agent known to mankind. It is produced by the bacterium *Clostridium botulinum*. Seven toxin types (A through G) have been recognized, with all but G having caused human disease.[98] Botulinum neurotoxin is a significant biowarfare and bioterrorism threat. The neurotoxin causes a symmetric, descending flaccid paralysis with classical bulbar palsies characterized by diplopia, dysphonia, dysarthria, and dysphagia. As paralysis progresses, generalized weakness occurs, and, if untreated, death occurs from airway obstruction and diaphragmatic muscle paralysis. Interestingly, this toxin has many therapeutic uses as well, notably but not limited to, blepharospasm, strabismus, cervical torticollis, and various dystonias.[99–101]

Pentavalent (ABCDE) botulinum toxoid (PBT) has been available as a prophylactic countermeasure to botulism since the 1960s. The vaccine is investigational; as such, it is administered under protocol with written, informed consent. PBT, Aluminum Phosphate Adsorbed, is administered in 0.5-mL doses subcutaneously at weeks 0, 2, and 12 and a booster is given at 1 year. In 1963, Fiock et al. showed the vaccine to be immunogenic in humans.[102] The vaccine has been administered to over 10,000 persons, including approximately 8000 during the Gulf War of 1991.[103] Analysis of more than 5000 doses of PBT administered at USAMRIID has shown that the initial priming series is associated with a local reaction rate of about 5% and booster doses with a rate of about 12%. Females have a higher local reaction rate than males: 12% versus 4% for the primary series and 20% versus 10% for boosters. Systemic reactions following PBT administration occur in about 1% of injections (PR Pittman, unpublished data). Nonhuman primate data show the vaccine to be efficacious at preventing death in monkeys given a lethal aerosol challenge of botulinum toxin.[104]

Botulism Immune Globulin

The U.S. military has developed botulism immune globulin from two sources: an equine heptavalent (ABCDEFG) immune globulin [F(ab')$_2$] and a human pentavalent (ABCDE) immune globulin. Both are investigational and have been used successfully in humans.[105,106] A trivalent (ABE) antitoxin is also available from the Centers for Disease Control and Prevention.

REFERENCES

1. Johnston RE, Peters CJ. Alphaviruses. *In* Fields BN, Knipe DM, Howley PM, et al (eds). Fields' Virology (3rd ed). Philadelphia, Lippincott–Raven, 1996, pp 843–898.
2. Monath TP (ed). The Arborviruses: Epidemiology and Ecology. Vol. 4. Boca Raton, FL, CRC Press, 1988, pp 113–143.
3. McClain DJ, Pittman PR, Ramsburg HH, et al. Immunologic interference from sequential administration of live attenuated alphavirus vaccines. J Infect Dis 177.634–641, 1998.
4. Kubes V, Rios FA. The causative agent of infectious equine encephalitis in Venezuela. Science 90:20–21, 1939.
5. Berge TO, Banks IS, Tigerrt WD. Attenuation of Venezuelan encephalomyelitis virus by in vitro cultivation in guinea pig heart cells. Am J Hyg 73:209–218, 1961.
6. Cole FW, May SW, Eddy GA. Inactivated Venezuelan equine encephalomyelitis virus prepared from attenuated (TC-83) virus. Appl Microbiol 27:150–153, 1974.
7. Salk JE, Krech U, Youngner JS, et al. Formaldehyde treatment and safety testing of experimental poliomyelitis vaccines. Am J Public Health 44:563–570, 1954.
8. Pittman PR, Makuch RS, Mangiafico JA, et al. Long-term duration of detectable neutralizing antibodies after administration of live-attenuated VEE vaccine and following booster vaccination with inactivated VEE vaccine. Vaccine 14:337–343, 1996.
9. Davis NL, Brown KW, Greenwald GF, et al. Attenuated mutants of Venezuelan equine encephalitis virus containing lethal mutations in the PE2 cleavage signal combined with a second site suppressor mutation in E1. Virology 212:102–110, 1995.
10. Robinson DM, Berman S, Lowenthal JP, Hetrick FM. Western equine encephalitis vaccine produced in chick embryo cell cultures. Appl Microbiol 14:1011–1014, 1966.
11. Bartelloni PJ, McKinney RW, Calia FM, et al. Inactivated western equine encephalomyelitis vaccine propagated in chick embryo cell culture. Am J Trop Med Hyg 20:146–149, 1971.
12. Pittman PR. Immunization of persons at risk of exposure to western equine encephalitis virus: continued assessment of the safety and effectiveness of western equine encephalitis vaccine, inactivated, TSI-GSD 210 (Protocol No IND 2013:FY99-12). Ft. Detrick, MD, U.S. Army Medical Research Institute of Infectious Diseases, 1999.
13. Maire LF III, McKinney RW, Cole FE Jr. An inactivated eastern equine encephalomyelitis vaccine propagated in check-embryo cell culture. Am J Trop Med Hyg 19:119–122, 1970.
14. Pittman PR. Immunization of persons at risk of exposure to eastern equine encephalitis virus: continued assessment of the safety and effectiveness of eastern equine encephalitis vaccine, inactivated, TSI-GSD 104 (Protocol No IND 266:FY99-11). Ft. Detrick, MD, U.S. Army Medical Research Institute of Infectious Diseases, 1999.
15. Deller JJ, Russell PK. Chikungunya disease. Am J Trop Med Hyg 17:1007–1011, 1968.
16. Kennedy AC, Fleming J, Solomon L. Chikungunya viral arthropathy: a clinical description. J Rheumatol 7:231–236, 1980.
17. Levitt NH, Ramsburg HH, Hasty SE, et al. Development of an attenuated strain of chikungunya virus for use in vaccine production. Vaccine 4:179–184, 1986.
18. Edelman R, Tacket CO, Wasserman SS, et al. Phase II safety and immunogenicity study of live chikungunya virus vaccine TSI-GSD-218. Am J Trop Med Hyg 62:681–685, 2000.
19. Nimmo JR. An unusual epidemic. Med J Aust 1:549–550, 1928.
20. Doherty RL, Whitehead RH, Gorman BM, O'Gower AK. The isolation of a third group-A arbovirus in Australia, with preliminary observations on its relationship to epidemic polyarthritis. Aust J Sci 26:183–184, 1963.
21. Doherty RL, Gorman BM, Whitehead RH, Carley JG. Studies of epidemic polyarthritis: the significance of three group-A arboviruses isolated from mosquitoes in Queensland. Aust Annu Med 13:322–327, 1964.
22. Marshall ID, Miles JAR. Ross River virus and epidemic polyarthritis. *In* Harris KF (ed). Current Topics in Vector Research. Vol. 2. New York, Praeger, 1984, pp 31–56.
23. Harley D, Sleigh A, Ritchie S. Ross River virus transmission, infection and disease: a cross-disciplinary review. Clin Microbiol Rev 14:909–932, 2001.
24. Russell RC, Cope SE, Yung AJ, Hueston L. Combating the enemy—mosquitoes and Ross River virus in a joint military exercise in tropical Australia. Am J Trop Med Hyg 59:S307, 1998.
25. Yu S, Asakov JG. Development of a candidate vaccine against Ross River virus infection. Vaccine 12:1118–1124, 1994.
26. Smithburn KC. Rift Valley fever: the neurotropic adaptation of the virus and the experimental use as a vaccine. Br J Exp Pathol 30:1–16, 1949.
27. Kark JD, Aynor Y, Peters CJ. A Rift Valley fever vaccine trial. I. Side effects and serologic response of a six month follow-up. Am J Epidemiol 116:808–820, 1982.
28. Randall R, Gibbs CJ Jr., Aulisio CG, et al. The development of a formalin-killed Rift Valley fever virus vaccine for use in man. J Immunol 89:660–671, 1962.

29. Pittman PR, Liu CT, Cannon TL, et al. Immunogenicity of an inactivated Rift Valley fever vaccine in humans: a 12-year experience. Vaccine 18:181–189, 1999.

30. Caplen H, Peters CJ, Bishop DH. Mutagen directed attenuation of Rift Valley fever vaccine. J Gen Virol 66:2271–2277, 1985.

31. Morrill JC, Carpenter L, Taylor D, et al. Further evaluation of a mutagen-attenuated Rift Valley fever vaccine in sheep. Vaccine 9:35–41, 1991.

32. Baskerville A, Hubbard KA, Stephenson JR. Comparison of the pathogenicity for pregnant sheep of Rift Valley fever virus and a live attenuated vaccine. Res Vet Sci 52:307–311, 1992.

33. Morrill JC, Mebus CA, Peters CJ. Safety and efficacy of a mutagen-attenuated Rift Valley fever virus vaccine in cattle. Am J Vet Res 58:1104–1109, 1997.

34. Morrill JC, Mebus CA, Peters CJ. Safety of a mutagen-attenuated Rift Valley fever virus vaccine in fetal and neonatal bovids. Am J Vet Res 58:1110–1114, 1997.

35. Pittman PR. Evaluation of the safety and immunogenicity of Rift Valley fever vaccine [live, attenuated, mutagenized (ZH548 MP-12 TSI-GSD-223-Lot 7-2-88)] administered subcutaneously or intramuscularly: final report to the Food and Drug Administration. Ft. Detrick, MD, U.S. Army Medical Research Institute of Infectious Diseases, 1999.

36. Lee HW. Hemorrhagic fever with renal syndrome in Korea. Rev Infect Dis 11(suppl 4):S864–S876, 1989.

37. Schmaljohn C, Hjelle B. Hantaviruses: a global disease problem. Emerg Infect Dis 3:95–104, 1997.

38. Lee HW, Lee PW, Johnson KM. Isolation of the etiologic agent of Korean hemorrhagic fever. J Infect Dis 137:298–308, 1978.

39. Nichol ST, Spiropoulou CF, Morzunov S, et al. Genetic identification of a hantavirus associated with an outbreak of acute respiratory illness. Science 262:914–917, 1993.

40. Lee HW, Ahn CN. Field trial of an inactivated vaccine against HFRS in humans. Arch Virol Suppl 1:35–47, 1990.

41. A Major Breakthrough in Preventive Medicine: Hantavax (HFRS Vaccine, KGCC). Seoul, Korea, Korea Green Cross Corporation, 1997.

42. Cho HW, Howard CR. Antibody responses in humans to an inactivated hantavirus vaccine (Hantavax). Vaccine 17:2569–2575, 1999.

43. Kruger DH, Ulrich R, Lundkvist AA. Hantavirus infections and their prevention. Microbes Infect 3:1129–1144, 2001.

44. Hooper JW, Li D. Vaccines against hantaviruses. Curr Top Microbiol Immunol 256:171–191, 2001.

45. Schmaljohn C, Hasty S, Dalrymple J. Preparation of candidate vaccinia-vectored vaccines for haemorrhagic fever with renal syndrome. Vaccine 10:10–13, 1992.

46. McClain DJ, Summers PL, Harrison SA, et al. Clinical evaluation of a vaccinia-vectored Hantaan virus vaccine. J Med Virol 60:77–85, 2000.

47. Ulrich R, Koletzki D, Lachmann S, et al. New chimaeric hepatitis B virus core particles carrying hantavirus (serotype Puumala) epitopes: immunogenicity and protection against virus challenge. J Biotechnol 73:141–153, 1999.

48. Barrera Oro JG, McKee KT Jr, Spisso J, et al. A refined complement-enhanced neutralization test for detecting antibodies to Junin virus. J Virol Methods 29:71–80, 1990.

49. Maiztegui JI. Clinical and epidemiological patterns of Argentine hemorrhagic fever. Bull World Health Organ 52:567–575, 1975.

50. Mills JN, Ellis BA, McKee KT Jr, et al. Junin virus activity in rodents from endemic and nonendemic loci in central Argentina. Am J Trop Med Hyg 44:589–597, 1991.

51. Mills JN, Ellis BA, McKee KT Jr, et al. A longitudinal study of Junin virus activity in the rodent reservoir of Argentine hemorrhagic fever. Am J Trop Med Hyg 47:749–763, 1992.

52. Barrera Oro JG, Eddy G. Characteristics of candidate live attenuated Junin virus vaccine [abstr S4-10]. In Program and Abstracts of the 4th International Conference on Comparative Virology, Banff, Canada, 1982.

53. Whalen KH. Demonstration of inapparent heterogeneity in a population of an animal virus by single-burst analysis. Virology 20:230–234, 1963.

54. McKee KT Jr, Barrera Oro JG, Kuehne AI, et al. Candid no. 1 Argentine hemorrhagic fever vaccine protects against lethal Junin virus challenge in rhesus macaques. Intervirology 34:154–163, 1992.

55. McKee KT Jr, Barrera Oro JG, Kuehne AI, et al. Safety and immunogenicity of a live-attenuated Junin (Argentine hemorrhagic fever) vaccine in rhesus macaques. Am J Trop Med Hyg 48:403–411, 1993.

56. MacDonald C, McKee K, Peters C, et al. Initial assessment of humans inoculated with a live-attenuated Junin virus vaccine [abstr]. In Program and Abstracts of the 7th International Congress of Virology, Edmonton, Canada, 1987.

57. Maiztegui JI, McKee KT Jr. Inoculation of human volunteers with a vaccine against Argentine hemorrhagic fever [abstr]. In Program and Abstracts of the 6th International Conference on Comparative and Applied Virology, Banff, Canada, 1989.

58. Maiztegui JI, McKee KT Jr, Barrera Oro JG, et al. Protective efficacy of a live attenuated vaccine against Argentine hemorrhagic fever. AHF Study Group. J Infect Dis 177:277–283, 1998.

59. Harrison LH, Halsey NA, McKee KT Jr, et al. Clinical case definitions for Argentine hemorrhagic fever. Clin Infect Dis 28:1091–1094, 1999.

60. Milazzo A, Hall R, Storm PA, et al. Sexually transmitted Q fever. Clin Infect Dis 33:399–402, 2001.

61. Pentilla IA, Harris RJ, Storm P, et al. Cytokine dysregulation in the post-Q-fever fatigue syndrome. Q J Med 91:549–560, 1998.

62. Ormsbee RA, Marmion BP. Prevention of *Coxiella burnetii* Infection: Vaccines and Guidelines for those at risk. In: Marne TJ, ed. The Disease, Vol. 1. Q fever, Chapter 12. CRC Press, Boca Raton, FL, 1990, pp 225–248.

63. Smadel JE, Snyder MJ, Robbins FC. Vaccination against Q fever. Am J Hyg 47:71–81, 1948.

64. Spicer DC, De Sanctis AN. Preparation of Phase I Q fever antigen suitable for vaccine use. Appl Environ Microbiol 32:85, 1976.

65. Marmion BP. Development of Q-fever vaccines, 1937 to 1967. Med J Aust 2:1074–1078, 1967.

66. Luoto L, Bell JF, Casey M, Lackman DB. Q fever vaccination of human volunteers. I. The serologic and skin-test response following subcutaneous injections. Am J Hyg 78:1–15, 1963.

67. Shapiro RA, Siskind V, Schofield FD, et al. A randomized, controlled, double-blind, cross-over, clinical trial of Q fever vaccine in selected Queensland abattoirs. Epidemiol Infect 104:267–273, 1990.

68. Marmion BP, Ormsbee RA, Kyrkou M, et al. Vaccine prophylaxis of abattoir-associated Q fever. Lancet 2:1411–1414, 1984.

69. Ackland JR, Worswick DA, Marmion BP. Vaccine prophylaxis of Q fever: a follow-up study of the efficacy of Q-Vax (CSL) 1985–1990. Med J Aust 160:704–708, 1994.

70. Benenson AS. Q fever vaccine: efficacy and present status. In Smadel JE (ed). Symosium on Q Fever. Walter Reed Army Institute of Medicine Science Publication No 6. Washington, DC, Walter Reed Army Institute of Medicine, 1959, p 47.

71. Williams JC, Damrow TA, Waag DM, Amano KI. Characterization of a Phase I *Coxiella burnetii* chloroform-methanol residue vaccine that induces active immunity against Q fever in C57BL/10 ScN mice. Infect Immun 51:851–858, 1986.

72. Fries LF, Waag DM, Williams JC. Safety and immunogenicity in human volunteers of a chloroform-methanol residue vaccine for Q fever. Infect Immun 61:1251–1258, 1993.

73. Kazar J, Brezina R, Palanova A, et al. Immunogenicity and reactogenicity of a Q fever chemovaccine in persons professionally exposed to Q fever in Czechoslovakia. Bull World Health Organ 60:389–394, 1982.

74. Francis E. Deer-fly fever or Pahvant Valley plague: a disease of man of hitherto unknown etiology. Public Health Prev 34:2061–2062, 1919.

75. Van Metre TE Jr, Kadull PJ. Laboratory-acquired tularemia in vaccinated individuals: a report of 62 cases. Ann Intern Med 50:621–632, 1959.

76. Overholt EL, Tigerrt WD, Kadull PJ, et al. An analysis of forty-two cases of laboratory-acquired tularemia: treatment with broad spectrum antibiotics. Am J Med 30:785–806, 1961.

77. Foshay L, Hesselbrock WH, Wittenberg HJ, Rodenberg AH. Vaccine prophylaxis against tularemia in man. Am J Public Health 32:1131–1145, 1942.

78. Kadull PJ, Reames HR, Coriell LL, Foshay L. Studies on tularemia: immunization of man. J Immunol 65:425–435, 1950.

78. Saslaw S, Eigelsbach HT, Wilson HE, et al. Tularemia vaccine study. I. Intracutaneous challenge. Arch Intern Med 107:689–701, 1961.

80. Saslaw S, Eigelsbach HT, Prior JA, et al. Tularemia vaccine study. II. Respiratory challenge. Arch Intern Med 107:702–714, 1961.

81. Tigertt WD. Soviet viable *Pasteurella tularensis* vaccines: a review of selected articles. Bacteriol Rev 26:354–373, 1962.

82. Shope RE. An account of the observations made by the United States Medical Mission to the USSR. Mimeograph, Yale University, April 1956.

83. Eigelsbach HT, Downs CT. Prophylactic effectiveness of live and killed tularemia vaccines. I. Production of vaccine and evaluation in the white mouse and guinea pig. J Immunol 87:415–425, 1961.

84. Eigelsbach HT, Hunter DH, Janssen WA, et al. Murine model for study of cell-mediated immunity: protection against death from fully virulent *Francisella tularensis* infection. Infect Immun 12:999–1005, 1975.

85. Eigelsbach HT, Tulis JJ, McGavran MH, White JD. Live tularemia vaccine. I. Host-parasite relationship in monkeys vaccinated intracutaneously or aerogenically. J Bacteriol 84:1020–1027, 1962.

86. Hornick RB. Studies on *Pasteurella tularensis*: evaluation of a living vaccine for tularemia. *In* Annual Report. Fort Detrick, MD, U.S. Army Medical Unit, 1958, Section II, pp 1–5.

87. Saslaw S, Carhart S. Studies with tularemia vaccines in volunteers. III. Serologic aspects following intracutaneous or respiratory challenge in both vaccinated and nonvaccinated volunteers. Am J Med Sci 241:689–699, 1961.

88. McCrumb FR Jr. Commission on epidemiological survey. *In* Annual Report. Armed Forces Epidemiological Board, Office of the Surgeon General, United States Army, Washington, DC, 1962, pp 81–86.

89. Sawyer WD, Tigertt WD, Crozier D, et al. Annual Progress Report. Fort Detrick, MD, U.S. Army Medical Unit, 1962, p 153.

90. Burke DS. Immunization against tularemia: analysis of the effectiveness of live Francisella tularensis vaccine in prevention of laboratory-acquired tularemia. J Infect Dis 135:55–60, 1977.

91. Marston JA. Report on fever (Malta). Great Br Army Med Dept Rep 3:486–521, 1861.

92. Williams E. The Mediterranean Fever Commission: its origin and achievements. *In* Young EJ, Corbel MJ (eds). Brucellosis: Clinical and Laboratory Aspects. Boca Raton, FL, CRC Press, 1989, pp 11–23.

93. Bruce D. Note on the recovery of a microorganism in Malta fever. Practitioner 39:161, 1887.

94. Schaad UB, Lang AB, Wedgwood J, et al. Safety and immunogenicity of *Pseudomonas aeruginosa* conjugate A vaccine in cystic fibrosis. The Lancet 338:1236, 1991.

95. Lang AB, Schaad UB, Rudeberg A, et al. Effect of high-affinity anti-*Pseudomonas aeruginosa* lipopolysaccharide antibodies induced by immunization on the rate of *Pseudomonas aeruginosa* infection in patients with cystic fibrosis. J of Pediatr 127:711–717, 1995.

96. Lang AB, Metcalfe IC. Vaccination against *Pseudomonas aeruginosa*: clinical trial results. In Proceedings 25th Europ. Cystic Fibrosis Conf. Genova; Romano L, Manno G, and Galietta L JV (eds), Monduzzi Editore S.p.A., Bologna; 2002; pp.183–187.

97. Herzog C. Personal communication to Plotkin S. November 26, 2002.

98. Arnon SS. Botulism as an intestinal toxemia. *In* Blaser MJ, Smith PD, Ravdin JI, et al (eds). Infections of the Gastrointestinal Tract. New York, Raven Press, 1995, pp 257–271.

99. Scott AB. Botulinum toxin injection into extraocular muscles as an alternative to strabismus surgery. J Pediatr Ophthalmol Strabismus 17:21–25, 1980.

100. Schantz EJ, Johnson EA. Properties and use of botulinum toxin and other microbial neurotoxins in medicine. Microbiol Rev 56;80–99, 1992.

101. Jankovic J, Hallet M (eds). Therapy with Botulinum Toxin. New York, Marcel Dekker, 1994.

102. Fiock MA, Cardella MA, Gearinger NF. Studies on immunity to toxins of *Clostridium botulinum*. IX. Immunologic response of man to purified pentavalent ABCDE botulinum toxoid. J Immunol 90:697–702, 1963.

103. Pittman PR, Sgoren MH, Hack D, et al. Antibody response to a delayed booster dose of anthrax vaccine and botulinum toxoid. Vaccine 20:2107–2115, 2002.

104. Franz DR, Jahrling PB, Friedlander AM, et al. Clinical recognition and management of patients exposed to biological warfare agents. JAMA 278:399–411, 1997.

105. Weber JT, Hibbs RG Jr, Darwish A, et al. A massive outbreak of type E botulism associated with traditional salted fish in Cairo. J Infect Dis 167:451–454, 1993.

106. Hibbs RG, Weber JT, Corwin A, et al. Experience with the use of an investigational F(ab')₂ heptavalent botulism immune globulin of equine origin during an outbreak of type E botulism in Egypt. Clin Infect Dis 23:337–340, 1996.

Chapter 36

Plague

RICHARD W. TITBALL • E. DIANE WILLIAMSON •
DAVID T. DENNIS

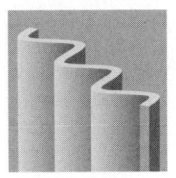 During the last two millennia, the bacterium *Yersinia pestis* has been responsible for social and economic devastation on a scale unmatched by other infectious diseases or armed conflicts. The first reliable reference is to the Justinian plague (AD 542–750), which originated in central Africa and spread throughout the Mediterranean Basin. The second pandemic, the Black Death, which started on the Eurasian border in the mid-14th century, may have caused 25 million deaths in Europe (25% to 30% of the population), persisted on the continental land mass for several centuries, and culminated in the Great Plague of London in 1665. The third pandemic started in China in the middle of the 19th century, spread east and west, and caused 10 million deaths in India alone. Credible estimates indicate that almost 200 million deaths could be attributed to plague,[1] which swept across Europe in these three major epidemics.[2] The disease occurred in both bubonic and pneumonic ("black death") forms. The bubonic form spreads as a result of transmission of the bacterium from rodents to humans via the bites of infective fleas (usually the rat flea, *Xenopsylla cheopsis*[2]). The close contact of humans with infected rats undoubtedly contributed to the spread of the disease by this route. In some instances, bacteremic spread of plague bacilli to the lungs leads to the development of the secondary pneumonic form of the disease; subsequent person-to-person transmission by respirable droplets can result in rapid epidemic spread of primary pneumonic plague.[3] It is the pneumonic form of the disease that is most feared and that is associated with a mortality rate approaching 100% when untreated.[4,5]

For reasons that are not fully understood, epidemics of urban plague have dramatically waned, but data from the World Health Organization indicate that plague is still a significant public health problem, especially in Africa, Asia, and South America (Fig. 36–1).[6,7] In plague-endemic areas of the world, vaccines may be useful in preventing plague in people at high risk. Such vaccines are also of use in protecting people who handle *Y. pestis* in research and diagnostic laboratories.

Background

Clinical Description

Bubonic Plague

Bubonic plague is the form of disease that typically occurs after a flea that has previously fed on an infected rodent then bites humans. In some circumstances, infection occurs via open wounds that are exposed to infected material through handling and other direct contact.[4] Within 2 to 6 days of infection, the patient develops a fever, headache, and chills.[8] Occasionally, lesions develop at the site of inoculation. The classical feature of bubonic plague is the development of swollen and tender lymph nodes called *buboes*, from the Greek *bubon*, meaning *groin*. (The buboes are often located in the inguinal and femoral lymph nodes, which drain the original site of infection on the lower extremities.[4]) Bacteremia is common in patients with bubonic plague, typically resulting in blood culture counts ranging from fewer than 10 to 4×10^7 colony-forming units (CFU)/mL.[4] In instances of high levels of bacteremia, there are often associated gastrointestinal symptoms or vomiting, nausea, abdominal pain, and diarrhea.[4] Early intervention during the course of disease with antibiotics such as streptomycin, gentamicin, tetracycline, or chloramphenicol usually leads to rapid recovery.[9]

Septicemic Plague

Primary septicemic plague is a clinical diagnosis in a patient who has acute toxic illness, large numbers of *Y. pestis* in the bloodstream, and no identifiable anatomic site of infection, such as a peripheral bubo.[8] Clinically, the disease appears similar to other gram-negative septicemias, with elevated temperature, chills, headache, malaise, and gastrointestinal disturbances. In the absence of aggressive treatment, life-threatening complications of the systemic inflammatory response syndrome occur, such as disseminated intravascular coagulation and bleeding, adult respiratory distress syndrome, shock, and organ failure. Owing to the absence of localizing signs, the diagnosis of primary plague sepsis may be delayed and result in a high case-fatality rate. The

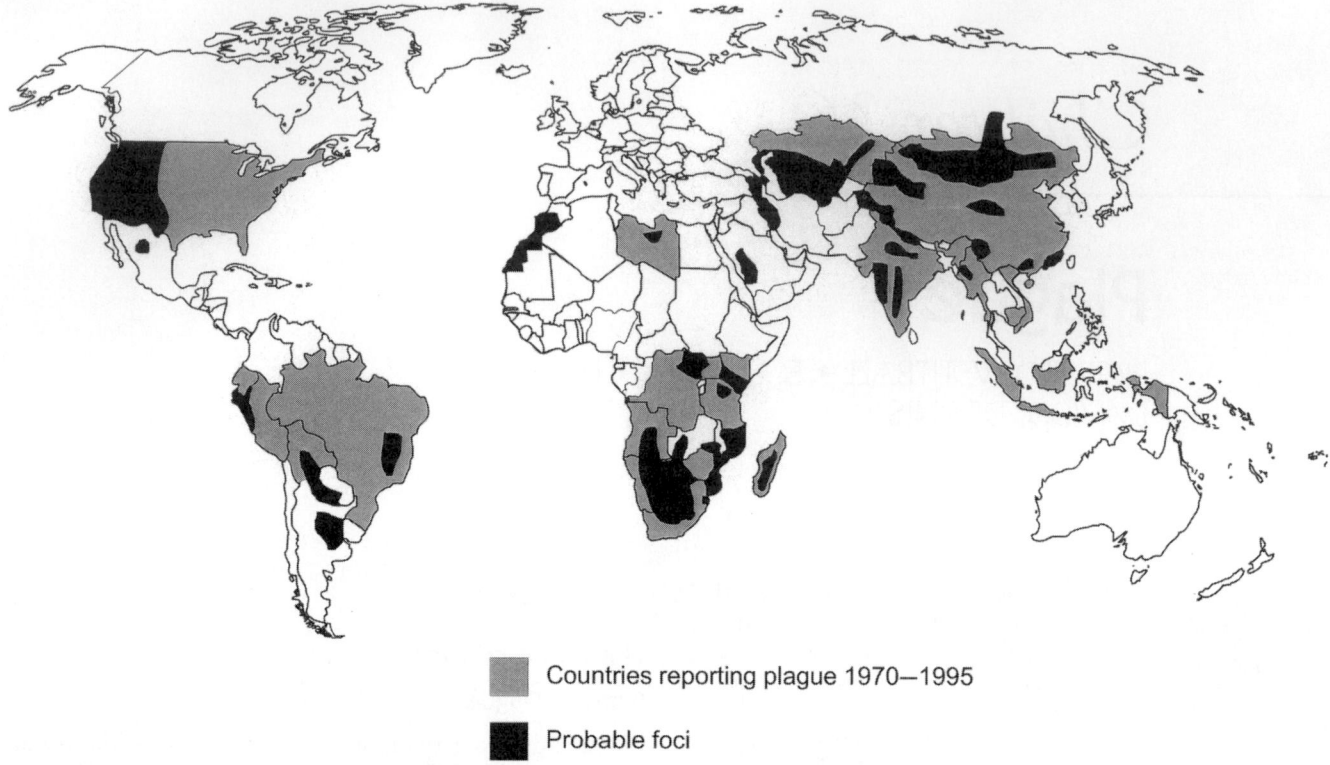

Countries reporting plague 1970–1995

Probable foci

FIGURE 36–1 ▪ Worldwide incidence of plague, 1970 to 1995. (Data from the World Health Organization, the Centers for Disease Control and Prevention, and country sources.)

overall case-fatality rate for persons with plague sepsis is in the range of 20% to 40%.

Pneumonic Plague

Some colonization of pulmonary tissues occurs in virtually all untreated fatal cases of plague, but most of these patients do not develop a transmissible plague pneumonia.[8] However, when there is colonization of the alveolar spaces after a respiratory exposure, a suppurative pneumonia develops, and during the terminal stages of disease there is coughing and the production of a highly infectious, watery, and bloody sputum. Pneumonic plague is the most widely feared form of the disease because it is proposed that Y. pestis can be spread from person to person as respiratory droplets formed during coughing.[10] Although explosive outbreaks of pneumonic plague involving large numbers of persons have not been recorded since the early part of the 20th century,[11,12] there is considerable evidence supporting the potential for the rapid spread of disease by this route. A number of experiments with animals (guinea pigs, lemurs, and nonhuman primates) have demonstrated the potential for the cross-infection of control animals from infected animals showing the symptoms of pneumonic disease.[13–17] More significantly, good evidence supporting the potential for the airborne spread of infection in humans has been derived from an analysis of an outbreak of pneumonic plague in Madagascar. In this outbreak, four cases of pneumonic plague were attributed to contact with one patient who had developed secondary pneumonic plague. These 4 infected individuals apparently then transmitted the disease to 11 others, one of whom transmitted the disease to 2 further individuals.[18] In total, 18 individuals contracted pneumonic plague, and 8 died.

The available evidence indicates that the inhalation of airborne droplets containing Y. pestis by susceptible individuals leads to the development of pneumonic plague within 1 to 3 days.[8] The rapidity with which the infection spreads between individuals, along with the relatively short incubation period, make control of the disease difficult, and antibiotic therapy may be ineffective after pulmonary symptoms have developed.[4,8,9] Primary pneumonic plague is now rare; in the United States, the few cases that do occur are often acquired by veterinarians and owners of cats that are experiencing a plague pneumonia.[4,5] Nevertheless, the potential for pneumonic plague to quickly spread in human populations is evident from the reports of the great plagues of the Middle Ages and of the large outbreaks of pneumonic plague in Manchuria in the early 20th century.

Bacteriology

The etiologic agent of plague is Y. pestis, a gram-negative bacterium that is a member of the family Enterobacteriaceae. The bacterium is able to grow at temperatures between 4° and 40°C and has nutritional requirements for L-isoleucine, L-valine, L-methionine, L-phenylalanine, and glycine. The species has been subdivided into three biovars (orientalis, mediaevalis, and antigua) on the basis of their ability to convert nitrate to nitrite and to ferment glycerol; however, all three biovars show similar virulence in animal models.[4] The genus Yersinia also includes Y. enterocolitica and Y. pseudotuberculosis species, both of which are pathogens of humans but rarely cause disease with a fatal outcome.[1,9]

Studies have shown that *Y. pestis* evolved from *Y. pseudotuberculosis* (most probably serotype 1b) between 1500 and 20,000 years ago[19] by the acquisition of virulence determinants and by the inactivation of a range of genes that are thought to be required for an enteric lifestyle.[20] The acquired virulence genes appear to be located primarily on two plasmids. Both *Y. pestis* and *Y. pseudotuberculosis* possess a 70-kilobase (kb) low calcium response (Lcr) plasmid that encodes a variety of *Yersinia* outer membrane peptides (Yops).[21,22] However, the 9.5-kb pesticin plasmid and the 100- to 110-kb Tox plasmids are present only in *Y. pestis*.[1] The *pla* gene on the pesticin plasmid encodes a surface-bound protease (plasminogen activator), which has potent fibrinolytic activity.[1] Post-translational processing of the *pla* gene product results in the formation of a coagulase enzyme. The Tox plasmid shows extensive sequence homology with a plasmid pHCM2, possessed by some strains of *Salmonella typhi*.[23] However, some regions of the Tox plasmid appear to be unique to *Y. pestis*, and one of these regions includes the *caf* operon encoding the F1 capsular antigen. The *caf* operon encodes the 17-kDa polypeptide F1 antigen (Caf1[24]); the Caf1M chaperone, which allows export from the cell[25]; and the Caf1A polypeptide, which anchors the F1 antigen into the outer membrane.[26] The Caf1R regulatory protein, which is responsible for the induction of F1 capsule production at 37°C, is also encoded by the *caf* operon.[27] It is possible that other virulence determinants, or genes required for the lifestyle of *Y. pestis*, also are encoded on the Tox plasmid (and also on the *S. typhi* pHCM2 plasmid). The identity and functions of these genes awaits a full investigation.

Pathogenesis

Plague is a zoonosis in which *Y. pestis* is transferred most commonly from its animal reservoir (rodents) to humans via fleas (Fig. 36–2). The flea ingests blood-borne bacteria from the infected rodent, and growth of the bacteria leads to blockage of the foregut. The hemin storage system is thought to play an important role in the formation of this blockage.[28] The blockage prevents digestion of the blood meal, and further ingestion of blood leads to regurgitation of bacteria-contaminated material.[29] Movement of the flea to a new rodent host leads to infection of the rodent, and it is thought that the bacterium persists in the environment as the result of a stable rodent-flea infection cycle. However, in situations in which humans and rodents are in close proximity or when the rodent population is reduced, either as a result of the disease or rodent control measures, humans and other warm-blooded mammals serve as alternative hosts. In this respect, *Y. pestis* differs from the other human pathogenic *Yersinia* species in that it is an obligate parasite. The organism circulates in a "sylvatic" form in wild rodent populations, typically causing a fatal disease in murines and sciurines and a milder, subclinical infection in gerbillines and dipodids.[30]

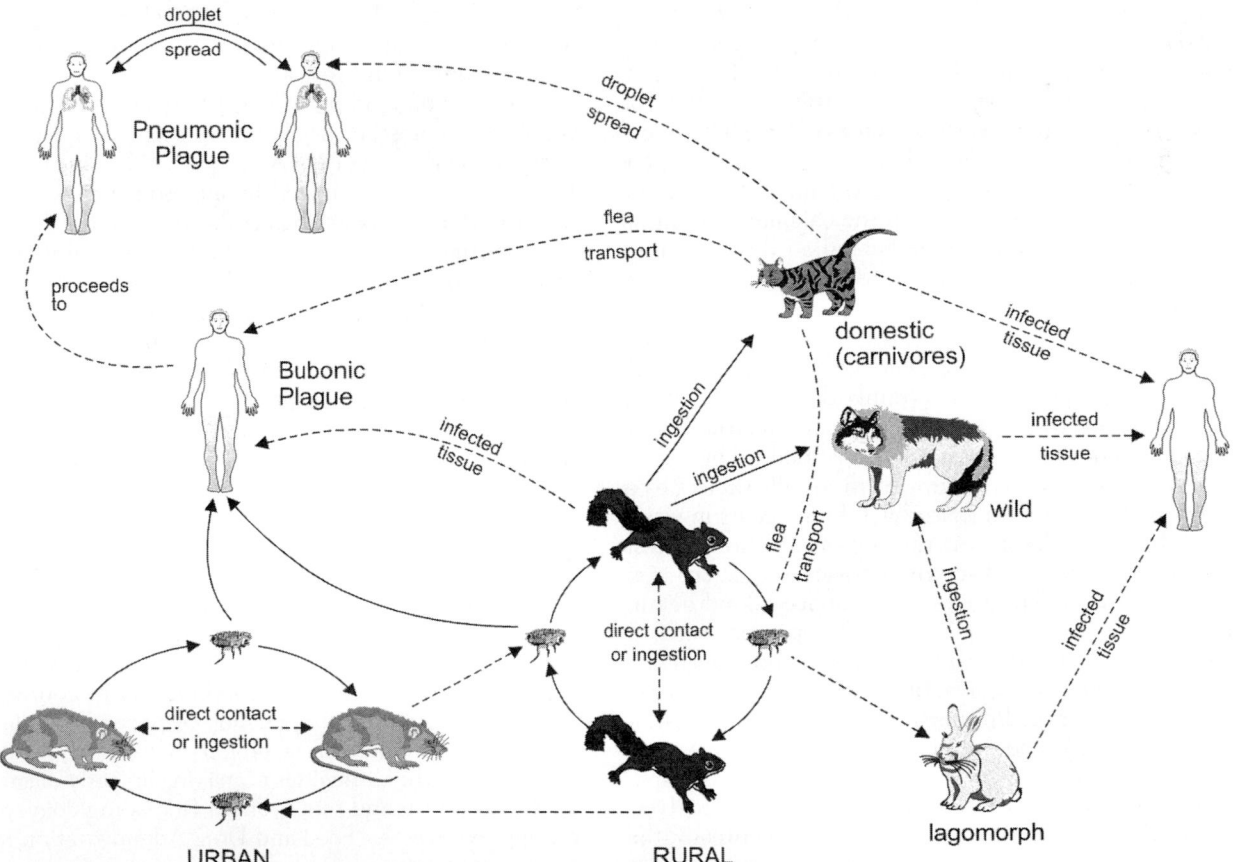

FIGURE 36–2 ■ Transmission routes of plague. *Solid lines* indicate the usual routes of transmission, and occasional routes are shown with *dashed lines*. (From Perry RD, Fetherston JD. *Yersinia pestis*—etiologic agent of plague. Clin Microbiol Rev 10:35–66, 1997, with permission.)

Infection of humans usually occurs as the result of a bite from an infected flea. It has been suggested that as many as 24,000 bacteria are delivered into the host with a single bite.[4] The expression of many of the virulence genes in *Y. pestis* is up-regulated at 37°C, and bacteria delivered by the flea, where they have been growing for several days at ambient temperatures of 28°C or less, do not express the F1 antigen or many of the Lcr plasmid products that are thought to allow the bacteria to resist phagocytosis. Therefore, many of the bacteria that are delivered into the host are easily phagocytosed by polymorphonuclear leukocytes or monocytes. The bacteria within polymorphonuclear leukocytes are destroyed, but those within monocytes survive and express various virulence determinants, thereby allowing growth and eventual release from the monocytes.[31] One such virulence determinant is the pH6 antigen, a fibrillar adhesin induced by low pH conditions such as those encountered in the phagosome, which has a pH of 4.5.[32] The expression of the pH6 antigen may facilitate entry into naïve monocytes or participate in the delivery of *Yersinia*-secreted proteins to monocytes and polymorphonuclear leukocytes. Bacteria released from monocytes are resistant to phagocytosis. The F1 capsule might be expected to play a key role in avoiding further phagocytosis.[33] However, mutants of *Y. pestis* that are unable to produce F1 antigen are still able to cause disease in the mouse, albeit in a more protracted form.[34] Other Yops might also play a role in killing phagocytic cells. For example, the YopE protein is a cytotoxin that is transferred into host cells after bacterial contact[22]; the YopH protein is a tyrosine phosphatase that has antiphagocytic cell activity[22]; and the V antigen that is exported from the bacterial cell has been reported to have a profound immunomodulatory effect on cells of the host immune system, by down-regulating the production of γ-interferon and tumor necrosis factor-α.[35,36] The expression of Yops is further regulated by the environmental calcium concentration, such that maximum expression of these proteins occurs at 37°C when the calcium concentration is below 2.5 mmol (the so-called low calcium response[1]). These are the conditions encountered within the phagosome, and intracellular V antigen is thought to play a key role in the regulation of this response.[37] However, under these conditions in vitro growth of the bacterium virtually ceases. Yop production certainly does occur in vivo, but, paradoxically, the bacteria are also able to grow. Either Yop expression in the mammalian host is induced by conditions yet to be identified, or growth in vivo is subject to a different regulatory system than that which occurs in vitro.

An ability to proliferate at the site of infection in host tissues indicates that the bacterium possesses efficient iron acquisition systems. The role of the surface-bound hemin storage proteins in iron acquisition is not proven, but it is known that the bacterium does have an iron-scavenging system based on the yersiniabactin siderophore.[4] The bacteria become disseminated from the site of primary infection into regional lymph nodes that drain these tissues. Within the lymph node, further growth of the bacteria, accompanied by a massive inflammatory reaction, leads to lymphadenopathy and the formation of buboes. Eventually, the bacteria can be disseminated by the lymphatic system, gain access to the bloodstream, and colonize pulmonary tissues, which may lead to development of the pneumonic form of

the disease. Untreated pneumonic plague is almost invariably fatal, but the precise mechanisms that lead to death of the host have not been identified. The bacterium does produce a soluble exotoxin,[4,38] but this exotoxin is reported to be active only in murines. Because an overwhelming septicemia is a feature of fatal plague infection, it seems likely that lipopolysaccharide is responsible for the systemic inflammatory response syndrome and its sequelae, such as disseminated intravascular coagulation in the terminal stages of the disease.

Diagnosis of Plague

An initial diagnosis of plague is based primarily on a clinical examination of the patient. This clinical diagnosis is usually supported by laboratory tests. Bacteriologic diagnosis of plague is usually made on the basis of the analysis of aspirates taken from a bubo, or from blood or sputum samples. The most straightforward analysis involves Gram or Wayson staining of air-dried smears on microscope slides.[39,40] After staining, *Y. pestis* cells appear as small gram-negative rods with a characteristic bipolar staining (safety pin appearance). The standard confirmatory test employs specific phage lysis of *Y. pestis* grown on standard solid media, such as sheep blood agar or MacConkey agar plates. Culture on Congo red agar, ideally at 26° to 28°C, results in so-called bull's-eye colonies, which have a red pigmented central region and paler margins.[40] However, culture methods are generally considered to be too slow (typically taking 48 hours) in the context of the rapid progression of the disease (and especially pneumonic or septicemic plague), and a presumptive diagnosis should be made and treatment begun before obtaining results of culture.

A variety of rapid tests for *Y. pestis* are available, including direct fluorescent antibody staining of the F1 capsular antigen and the use of DNA probes.[40-43] Passive hemagglutination and enzyme-linked immunosorbent assays can be used to detect serum antibodies directed against the F1 capsular antigen; however, antibodies typically are not detectable until about 1 week following onset of illness, and confirmation by observing a diagnostic rise in antibodies requires comparison of acute and convalescent serum titers. A new exciting development is the demonstration that an immunogold-chromatographic hand-held assay can be used for the direct detection of the F1 antigen in bubo aspirates, serum, or urine samples.[44] Conceivably such tests could be used at the patient's bedside for rapid, early diagnosis.

Treatment and Prevention with Antimicrobials

The successful treatment of plague is dependent on the commencement of therapy during the early stages of the disease. In cases of bubonic plague treated with antibiotics, the fatality rate is generally less than 5%. In contrast, the successful treatment of septicemic or pneumonic plague is more difficult because of the rapidity with which the disease develops and the difficulties of making an early diagnosis.

Streptomycin and tetracyclines (including doxycycline) are approved by the Food and Drug Administration for the treatment of plague.[39,45] For the treatment of plague meningitis, intravenously administered chloramphenicol is the antibiotic of choice because of its ability to cross the blood-brain barrier.[39,45] For all antibiotics, a 10-day course is recommended. In mice infected with *Y. pestis* by the airborne route, successful treatment of disease with ciprofloxacin was dependent on the commencement of antibiotic dosing within 24 hours of exposure to the pathogen.[46]

Improvement in the condition of patients suffering from bubonic plague is seen within 2 to 3 days, but buboes may remain for several weeks after successful treatment. A strain of *Y. pestis* showing plasmid-mediated resistance to tetracycline, streptomycin, chloramphenicol, and sulfonamides has been isolated from a case of bubonic plague in Madagascar.[47] Therefore, the failure of a patient to respond to antibiotic treatment should alert the clinician to the possibility of an antibiotic-resistant strain of *Y. pestis*.

Family members and other close contacts of individuals suffering from plague should be maintained under surveillance for at least 7 days after their last possible exposure to *Y. pestis*. It may be appropriate to use tetracycline or doxycycline prophylactically for 7 days in these individuals, especially if the primary case is pneumonic plague. The prophylactic use of antibiotics is recommended even in individuals who have been previously vaccinated with the killed whole-cell vaccines and who might have been exposed to airborne *Y. pestis*[5] because of the limited ability of this type of vaccine to provide protection against pneumonic disease.

Models of Disease and Protection

Y. pestis causes disease in a wide variety of laboratory animals,[4] and animal models of the disease in humans have been developed using mice, guinea pigs, and other primates. Most experimental work has been carried out with the mouse model of disease, which has been accepted as a meaningful indicator of the likely responses to infection and protection in humans. However, the disease in the mouse model may not faithfully mimic disease in humans because of the susceptibility of mice to the murine exotoxin.[38] Although this limitation might be resolved by using the guinea pig model of disease, the protracted nature of the disease in this species[4] suggests that the mouse model is a better indicator of the infection that occurs in animal reservoirs. In a comparative study with mice and guinea pigs, it was concluded that mice were more suitable for the evaluation of plague vaccines,[48] and this species is approved by the U.S. Public Health Service for the testing of plague vaccines. Disease arising from the delivery of *Y. pestis* by the subcutaneous route (median lethal dose [MLD], 1 to 2 CFU[49,50]) is considered to mimic bubonic plague, whereas the exposure of mice to the bacteria via aerosols inhaled through the nose results in the pneumonic form of the disease (MLD, 2×10^4 CFU[50]).

The efficacy of currently licensed plague vaccines is determined by measuring the ability of sera from immunized mice, guinea pigs, monkeys, or humans to protect mice passively against *Y. pestis*. Serum is injected intravenously into groups of 10 mice (0.5 mL serum per mouse), and the mice are then challenged subcutaneously with 100 MLD of *Y. pestis*.[51,52] The mouse protection index (MPI) is expressed as the percentage mortality of the group of mice (over 14 days) divided by the average time to death. MPI values of 10 or less are considered to be indicative of protection.[53] A similar test is being developed to demonstrate the efficacy of next-generation plague vaccines, based on a parallel line analysis for test and reference vaccines.

Epidemiology

Endemic foci of plague occur mainly in semiarid regions of the world (see Fig. 36–1). The main foci have been identified in the southwestern United States, the former Soviet Union, South America, South Africa, and Asia. Not surprisingly, these are the regions of the world that report the highest incidence of human plague. Data from the World Health Organization indicate that the average annual incidence of plague worldwide was 2544 cases from 1988 to 1999[6,7,54]; although the trend was downward until 1981, there has been an apparent increase in the incidence of disease during the 1990s. It is possible that this increase is the result of more efficient diagnosis and reporting of cases. However, the reported outbreak of plague in Surat, India, during 1994, although overstated by the press, serves as a reminder that the disease can reappear explosively. Serologic testing of individuals during this outbreak showed that there were 876 presumptive cases of plague and 54 fatalities.[4,55] Since 1990, the main plague activity in the world has been in Madagascar and southeastern Africa. In the United States, a new trend in plague epidemiology appears to be related to the residential encroachment on former rural areas that contain enzootic foci.[4] Inhabiting of such areas can lead to bites of humans by infected fleas or to infection as the result of close contact with infected wild rodents or other animals (e.g., domestic cats) that have become infected.

Potential Use as an Agent of Bioterrorism

Recently plague vaccines have also attracted considerable attention because of the potential for *Y. pestis* to be used as an agent of biologic warfare or bioterrorism.[39] It is likely that *Y. pestis* used in this way would be disseminated by the airborne route, and would cause pneumonic plague. A report by the World Health Organization in 1970[56] indicated that, in a worst-case scenario, the airborne release of 50 kg of *Y. pestis* over a city of 5 million would result in 150,000 cases of plague. Of these 36,000 would be expected to die. The released bacteria would remain viable for 1 hour. Disease that resulted from the deliberate release of *Y. pestis* in this way would appear within 1 to 6 days of exposure, and most probably within 2 to 4 days.[39] The initial symptoms would resemble other severe respiratory illnesses,[39] which might make early diagnosis (and optimal treatment) difficult. The indicators of an attack with *Y. pestis* would include the clustering of cases, the lack of prior deaths in rodents in the area, the incidence of disease in individuals without known risk factors, and disease in areas where plague is not known to be endemic.[39] The unpredictable nature of such attacks and the potential for such weapons to cover large areas, and consequently to infect large numbers of individuals, might pose requirements for vaccines and immunoprophylactics that rapidly provide protection against disease. These problems are considered later in this chapter.

Passive Immunization

Early studies showed that serum from human volunteers immunized with purified F1 antigen or with a killed whole-cell vaccine could be used in the passive protection of mice against a parenteral challenge with 100 MLD of Y. pestis.[52] Indeed, this is the basis of the MPI test that is used to evaluate the efficacy of killed vaccines. More recently, there have been several reports that the passive immunization of mice with antiserum against the V antigen provides protection against parenteral challenge with Y. pestis.[57–59] However, there is no licensed antiserum that can be used in humans to prevent or treat plague.

Active Immunization

Killed Whole-Cell Vaccines

Killed Y. pestis organisms have been used as a vaccine since 1897, when Waldemar Haffkine inoculated himself with an experimental vaccine. A killed vaccine for human use was first produced in the United States in 1946 (Army Vaccine). Improvements to this vaccine have led to the plague vaccine, which is produced from the virulent 195/P strain of Y. pestis.[60] During the 1990s, there have been several commercial suppliers of killed whole-cell vaccines against plague. Plague Vaccine USP, which contains formaldehyde-killed bacteria, was formerly manufactured by Cutter Laboratories and from 1994 was manufactured by Greer Laboratories Inc. Production of this vaccine was discontinued in 1999, and currently there is no licensed vaccine available for use in the United States.

An alternative killed vaccine is manufactured by the Commonwealth Serum Laboratories (Parkville, Australia). This vaccine contains heat-killed bacteria (Y. pestis strain 195/P) that are resuspended in saline containing 0.5% weight per volume of phenol to a concentration of 3×10^9 organisms per milliliter. The vaccine is given subcutaneously, and the initial course in adults is two 0.5-mL doses of vaccine at an interval of 1 to 4 weeks (Table 36–1). The vaccine can be administered to children using modified immunization schedules. For example, children 6 months to 2 years of age are given three 0.1-mL doses of vaccine at intervals of 1 to 4 weeks (Table 36–1). Six monthly booster doses of this vaccine are recommended.

Live, Attenuated Vaccines

Vaccination of humans also has been achieved using a live, attenuated vaccine strain of Y. pestis (strain EV76). This vaccine strain, which was derived from a fully virulent strain by in vitro passage,[61] has been used since 1908, especially in the former Soviet Union and the French colonies. At present, however, the vaccine is not commercially available or licensed for use in humans. The genetic lesion that results in attenuation has not been defined, but the strain is known to be a pigmentation (pgm) mutant. This mutation prevents the bacterium from assimilating hemin[4] and may also result in a change in surface properties of the bacterium.[28] The recommended dosing regimen for EV76 is to use 5.8×10^6 CFU as a priming dose and to boost with the killed whole-cell vaccine.[61,62]

Indications for Vaccine Use

The killed whole-cell vaccine has been recommended for use in individuals who are working with fully virulent strains of Y. pestis (e.g., researchers and laboratory workers). The vaccine may be considered for use in persons with regular contact with the wild hosts of plague or their fleas, in places where plague occurs. It also may be considered for use in personnel who are deployed to work in areas where the disease is endemic (e.g., military personnel, field workers, and agricultural consultants), especially if they may be exposed to epizootic plague.[5] Vaccination against plague is not a statutory requirement for travel to any country. The vaccination of populations in plague-endemic areas of the world is not routinely indicated, because the incidence of disease is relatively low and most cases of disease are of the bubonic form, which can be treated with antibiotics. Use of the vaccine in the indigenous population might be considered in areas where there is recurrent or intense plague activity that cannot be controlled by other measures. Because several months are required to complete the course of vaccination, however, the vaccine has a limited use in controlling sporadic plague epidemics. Use of the vaccine might be indicated in individuals who regularly come into contact with animals where enzootic plague foci are known to be present.[5]

A newer generation of plague vaccines against plague also might be of value in situations where Y. pestis is expected to be used, or has been used, as an agent of bioter-

TABLE 36–1 ■ Schedules and Dosages of the Commonwealth Serum Laboratories Killed Whole-Cell Vaccine

Age of Recipient	Volume Administered (mL)			
	First Dose	Second Dose*	Third Dose*	Booster Dose
6 mo–2 yr	0.1	0.1	0.1	0.1[†]
3–6 yr	0.2	0.2	0.2	0.2[†]
7–11 yr	0.3	0.3	0.3	0.3[†]
> 12 yr	0.5	0.5	—	0.3[‡]

*One to 4 weeks after previous dose.
[†]At 6-month intervals after dose 3.
[‡]At 6-month intervals after dose 2. Dose can be reduced to 0.1 mL intradermally for individuals who have reactions to previous doses of the vaccine.

rorism. Although antibiotics might also provide protection against disease, it is not clear if sufficient quantities could be stockpiled to allow the treatment of large populations for long periods of time. In addition, there is concern over the appropriateness of long courses of broad-spectrum antibiotics being used in large numbers of individuals. It seems likely that antibiotics will have a clear utility for the protection of relatively small numbers of individuals while vaccines would be required for the protection of entire populations. At the present time it seems unlikely that routine mass vaccination of entire populations, in the absence of any clear indication of an impending attack, would be undertaken. Therefore, vaccines for protection of the civilian population might need to be used at short notice and will need to induce a protective response rapidly, ideally after a single vaccine dose. In many ways these requirements are similar to those for vaccines that would be used to protect the armed forces against biologic weapons under battlefield conditions. In this respect, there is a clear opportunity to exploit military research to provide vaccines suitable for use in the civilian population, and some vaccines that meet these criteria are being developed.

Postexposure Prophylaxis

The currently available killed whole-cells vaccine is not suitable for postexposure use because several months are required to complete the primary vaccination schedule. The use of antibiotics should be considered in the case of possible exposure to Y. pestis, even in vaccinees who have completed the full vaccination schedule, because this vaccine offers poor protection against pneumonic plague.

Precautions and Contraindications

Killed whole-cell vaccines should not be used in individuals who have a history of hypersensitivity to any of the vaccine components (e.g., beef protein, soya, casein, sulfite, phenol, or formaldehyde). The safety and efficacy of the vaccine in people younger than 18 years or in pregnant women are not known.

Results of Vaccination

Immune Responses

Although Y. pestis produces a variety of potentially protective antigens (including F1 antigen, V antigen and other Yops, and lipopolysaccharide), most workers consider that antibody against the F1 antigen is the key protective response induced by killed whole-cell vaccines. Although the V antigen is known also to induce a protective response against Y. pestis, the level of V antigen is low or undetectable in killed whole-cell vaccines.[63] There is good experimental evidence that the titer of F1 antibody, determined by passive hemagglutination, does correlate with protection against plague in animal models.[62] Ninety percent of animals with anti-F1 passive hemagglutination titers of 128 survived challenge with 1×10^3 to 5×10^5 CFU of Y. pestis, whereas the proportions of animals with titers of 32 to 64 or 16 that survived were 46% and 6%, respectively. Passive

immunization studies with sera obtained from immunized animals[53] or humans[64] also suggest that anti-F1 passive hemagglutination titers of 1:128 or greater were protective. However, the accepted test for demonstrating the efficacy of vaccines involves passive immunization of mice with sera and the demonstration of an MPI of 10 or less. More recent trials with the Greer Laboratories' vaccine suggest that 55% to 58% of individuals develop an antibody response with an MPI of 10 after two vaccinations[5]; however, even after multiple (an average of five) vaccinations, 8% of individuals fail to develop any antibody response.

Protective Efficacy

None of the plague vaccines that have been developed have been subjected to a randomized, clinically controlled field study in humans.[65] Although controlled clinical studies are desirable, the sporadic and relatively low incidence of plague means that such studies would be difficult to conduct. Evidence for the efficacy of killed whole-cell vaccines is based mainly on studies in animals, on evidence that they induce antibody in humans that can passively protect animals, and on data obtained from Vietnam. From 1961 to 1971, many thousands of Vietnamese civilians developed plague (333 cases/10^6 person-years of exposure), but the incidence of disease in immunized U.S. troops based in Vietnam during this period was low. (The total of eight cases represents one case per 10^6 person-years of exposure.[5,66]) Although this difference in the incidence of disease might be attributed to different exposures of these populations to Y. pestis, it is worth noting that many military personnel developed murine typhus, which is also transmitted by X. cheopis.[5] Furthermore, serologic studies indicated that some immunized individuals were exposed to Y. pestis and developed subclinical infections.[66] The effectiveness of killed whole-cell vaccines against the pneumonic form of the disease is more questionable, however, and cases of pneumonic plague have been reported in vaccinated individuals.[55,67] In the murine model of disease, immunization with two doses of the killed whole-cell vaccine provided solid protection against a subcutaneous challenge with 5000 MLD of Y. pestis and partial protection (60% survival) against a subcutaneous challenge with 50,000 MLD of Y. pestis.[49] In contrast, when challenged with approximately 100 MLD of Y. pestis by the airborne route, none of the mice that had been immunized with two doses of the vaccine survived.[68] Although these data alone do not necessarily indicate the effectiveness of the vaccine in humans, when viewed alongside the reports previously cited, the overall evidence is that the vaccine is better able to protect against bubonic plague than against pneumonic plague. All of these studies, however, have been carried out using F1-positive strains of Y. pestis. However, because the main protective component of killed whole-cells vaccines appears to be the F1-negative antigen, the efficacy of this vaccine to provide protection against F1-negative strains of Y. pestis, which are rarely encountered in natural infections, has not been fully tested.

Immunization of mice with the EV76 live, attenuated vaccine strain does induce protection against both subcutaneous and inhalation challenges with virulent strains of Y. pestis,[49] and in this respect the performance of this vaccine is superior to the performance of the killed whole-cell vaccines. The enhanced protection offered by the live vaccine might be due to three factors: (1) it is known that the killed whole-cell vaccine does not contain immunogenic levels of several outer membrane proteins such as V antigen[63]; (2) it has been suggested that the chemical or heat inactivation of the bacterium results in structural changes in other surface components such as the F1 antigen[50]; and (3) local responses to vaccination with EV76 in mice suggest that a limited local infection is initiated and that the duration of exposure to the antigenic complement is therefore prolonged. The immune response induced by the live, attenuated vaccine may be more authentic than that induced by the killed whole-cell preparations.

Persistence of Immunity

Few studies have examined the duration of immunity to *Y. pestis* after immunization with killed whole-cell vaccines. However, it is generally considered that immunity is short lived. Booster immunizations may be needed at 6-month intervals to ensure that a protective response is maintained. The duration of immunity following immunization with live, attenuated vaccines is not known.

Safety

The killed whole-cell vaccines are known to be reactogenic in humans.[69,70] The manufacturer of the Cutter vaccine reported that reactions such as malaise, headaches, local erythema and induration, or mild lymphadenopathy occurred in approximately 10% of vaccinees; this frequency of side effects is reported by other workers.[61] Data provided by the manufacturer of the Greer vaccine suggest that more than 10% of vaccinees suffer side effects (Table 36–2). Allergic reactions induced by immunization with killed whole-cell vaccines, evidenced mainly as urticaria, occur

TABLE 36–2 ■ Percentage of Individuals Reporting Local or Systemic Side Effects within 48 Hours of Vaccination with the Greer Plague Vaccine*

Reaction	% of Recipients Reporting Reactions	
	After First Dose (*n* = 67)	After Second Dose (*n* = 59)
LOCAL		
Tenderness	71.6	18.6
Decreased arm motion	11.9	1.7
Erythema	4.5	0
Warmth	3.0	1.7
Edema	1.5	0
SYSTEMIC		
Headache	19.4	6.8
Nausea	13.4	3.4
Malaise	10.4	5.1
Dizziness	6.0	0
Chills	4.5	3.4
Joint pain	4.5	0
Muscle pain	4.5	0
Anorexia	1.5	0
Diarrhea	1.5	0
Vomiting	1.5	0

*Vaccinees received the second dose 30 days after the first dose.

infrequently.[69] One study found that the frequency of side effects was much greater in individuals who had previously been immunized with the live EV vaccine.[61]

The safety of the EV76 live, attenuated vaccine has been questioned by several workers. Meyer et al.[71] reviewed the use of live, attenuated vaccines, such as strain EV76, in humans. In one study in the former Soviet Union, a febrile response was reported in 20% of vaccinees, accompanied by headache, weakness, and malaise. Erythema surrounding the site of vaccination that could reach dimensions of 15 × 15 cm frequently was reported. Some severe systemic reactions required hospitalization. Numerous unsuccessful attempts were made to reduce the incidence of side effects by administering the vaccine by different routes, including by scarification, by the inhalational route, and even intraocularly.[71] Of equal concern is the finding that the EV76 strain is able to cause disease in some animal species. Russell and colleagues reported that immunization of mice with *Y. pestis* EV76 induced severe side effects and occasional (approximately 1%) fatalities,[49] and the vaccine is reported to cause fatal infections in vervets.[71]

Future Developments

Subunit Vaccines

Although the killed or attenuated vaccines just described have several shortcomings, they do indicate that protection against both the bubonic and pneumonic forms of plague is possible. Work toward the development of a subunit vaccine is supported by two observations. First, the major antibody response to *Y. pestis* (in sera from either vaccinated or convalescent individuals) is known to be directed against the F1 antigen.[72] Second, the V antigen has attracted attention as a component of a vaccine,[73] and the improved performance of live vaccines over killed vaccines might be explained by the ability of only the live vaccines to induce an antibody response to the V antigen.[63]

The F1 antigen can be produced from cultures of *Y. pestis*,[74,75] but recent studies have used recombinant F1 antigen produced by expressing the *caf* operon in *Escherichia coli* bacteria.[76-78] Intraperitoneal or intramuscular immunization with native F1 or recombinant F1 antigens adjuvanted with alum induced an immune response that protected mice against a subcutaneous challenge with as many as 10^5 CFU of virulent *Y. pestis*.[50,63] Although the F1 antigen also induced protection against inhalation challenge with 100 MLD of an F1-positive strain of *Y. pestis*,[50] there was concern that a vaccine based solely on the F1 antigen would not provide protection against naturally occurring but virulent F1-negative strains of *Y. pestis* (although only one such naturally occurring strain has been reported). The production of V antigen for vaccine studies has, until recently, been difficult. The V antigen is produced at low levels by *Y. pestis* and readily degrades during purification. As a result, difficulties in preparing the V antigen from this source precluded the evaluation of this antigen in active immunization studies. The fusion of the gene that encodes the V antigen (*lcrV*) with a carrier protein such as protein A or glutathione-*S*-transferase allows production of the V antigen in *E. coli* bacteria.[73] The V antigen can be cleaved from the carrier protein using a site-specific protease such as thrombin or factor X_a.[73] Immunization of mice intraperitoneally with either the fusion protein or the V antigen adjuvanted with alum induced protection against a subcutaneous challenge with 4×10^6 CFU of Y. pestis.[73] More recently, the expression of V antigen has been transferred into the pGEX-6P-2 system, which utilizes a recombinant enzyme to cleave rV from the GST fusion protein, making this expression system suitable for high-level production of the V antigen in a system suitable for vaccine manufacture.[78] A significant advantage over the F1 antigen is the ability of the V antigen to induce protection against virulent F1-negative strains of Y. pestis such as the Java 9 strain. Protection against 1000 or more MLD of either virulent F1 positive or F1-negative strains of Y. pestis given by the inhalation route has been reported.[79]

The protection afforded individually by the F1 and V antigens was defeated by very high subcutaneous challenge levels of 10^9 CFU of Y. pestis.[63] However, protection against this challenge was achieved after intraperitoneal immunization in multiple doses with a mixture of the F1 and V antigens.[63] The vaccine also protected mice against 100 MLD of Y. pestis given by the inhalation route (Table 36–3), suggesting that the vaccine would provide protection against pneumonic plague in humans.[68] The advantages of such a combined subunit vaccine lie not only with the enhanced level of protection afforded against disease but also with the ability of the vaccine to confer protection against both F1-positive and F1-negative strains of Y. pestis.

The mechanism by which this vaccine induces protective immunity has been the subject of considerable investigation during the past few years. The F1 capsule is thought to inhibit phagocytosis of the bacterium by preventing complement-mediated opsonization.[33,80] Therefore, it is possible that induced antibody against the F1 antigen opsonizes the bacterium and promotes antibody-dependent cellular cytotoxicity. Some vaccinated animals do appear to harbor the pathogen even in a mutated F1-negative form.[50] The killed whole-cell vaccines are less effective than purified F1 antigen in inducing high titers of antibody to F1.[50,63] Antibody against the V antigen may also be of overriding importance

in protection against plague, and immunization with V antigen has been shown to restore the ability of the host to produce tumor necrosis factor-α and γ-interferon in response to infection.[36] Therefore, immunization with the V antigen would enable the host to mount a normal inflammatory response and thereby enable the host phagocytes to clear bacteria opsonized by antibody against F1 antigen. Although protection against plague in the mouse model has been demonstrated to correlate with the specific immunoglobulin G (IgG) titer to the subunits (specifically of the IgG1 subclass in the mouse, in response to this alhydrogel-adjuvanted vaccine),[81] there is no doubt that the mechanism of protection following immunization with the F1+V proteins also involves T-cell memory, and this has been demonstrated in the mouse model.[81,82] In the mouse, the T-cell response to alhydrogel-adsorbed F1+V is biased toward Th2, and this response is highly protective. However, research has illustrated that, although delivery of the F1+V proteins formulated in the Ribi adjuvant system to IL4T mice (genetic knockouts for the interleukin-4 receptor) induced predominantly a Th1 response, the passive transfer of their antiserum into B-cell–deficient knockout mice, with no intrinsic antibody, protected the latter fully against live organism challenge.[83] Such experimental data suggest that protection against plague in the mouse can be afforded by either the Th1 or Th2 pathways and that optimum protection is expected from a balanced Th1/Th2 response.

The F1+V subunit vaccine is now in advanced development, having successfully completed preclinical safety and efficacy[84,85] testing and initial clinical trialing, and it shows good promise as the next-generation plague vaccine.

Mucosal Vaccine Formulations

Although systemic immunization with alhydrogel-adsorbed F1+V has been demonstrated in the mouse model to protect against aerosol challenge with plague, the observed protection was attributed primarily to the transudation of systemic IgG into the lungs.[68] The induction additionally of F1+V-specific immunoglobulin A, particularly in the upper respiratory tract, may enhance the protection expected from the vaccine against inhalational exposure to Y. pestis. This type of response could be induced by the mucosal delivery of the subunits. Although the oral delivery of purified F1 antigen did not induce an antibody response,[86] a considerable body of work has now been carried out on the polymeric microencapsulation of the F1 and V antigens and the mucosal delivery of microencapsulated formulations to achieve protective immunity. The first report of the successful individual encapsulation of the F1 and V antigens into poly L-lactide microspheres was made by Williamson et al.,[82] while Reddin et al. reported the encapsulation of F1 only.[87] Williamson et al.[82] demonstrated that, by combining the individual microsphere batches, an additive protective effect could be achieved. Subsequently, many refinements have been made to the formulation, the principal of which was the successful co-encapsulation of the subunits such that both retained immunogenicity[88] and protective efficacy.[89,90] Further refinements included the substitution of polymers conferring particular properties of stability and hydrophobicity and of approaches to controlling particle size and loading (reviewed by Titball and Williamson[91]). A

TABLE 36–3 ■ Protection Afforded by Killed Whole-Cell Vaccine, EV76 Vaccine, or F1- and V-Antigen Subunit Experimental Vaccine Against Parenteral or Inhalation Challenge with *Yersinia pestis* Strain GB

Vaccine	Protection (% Survival) Against Challenge (MLD)	
	Subcutaneous Route*	Inhalation Route
Control	0 (10^1)	0 (10^1)[†]
Killed whole-cell vaccine	60 (2×10^6)	50 (2×10^3)[†]
EV76	100 (2×10^9)	66 (8.5×10^3)[‡]
F1 + V	100 (2×10^9)	100 (4×10^4)[†]

*Tested in Balb/C-strain mice.
[†]Tested in CBA-strain mice.
[‡]Tested in Porton-strain outbred mice.
EV76, attenuated live vaccine strain of Y. pestis; F1 + V, subunit vaccine containing the F1- and V-antigens of Y. pestis; MLD, median lethal dose.

microsphere formulation suitable for nasal administration has been derived that is fully protective against an inhalational challenge with *Y. pestis* after only two immunizing doses in the mouse model,[92] and, because the nasal route of immunization effectively accesses both the mucosal and systemic immune systems,[93] there is every prospect of enhancing the nasal formulation further to achieve a protective single-dose vaccine. Liposomal encapsulation of the plague subunit vaccine offers an alternative approach to mucosal delivery.[87] The only approach to an oral vaccine for plague that has met with success to date is the use of *Salmonella typhimurium* expressing the F1-encoding operon, which induced a high level of protection against subcutaneous challenge with *Y. pestis*.[94,95]

Live, Attenuated Vaccines

The finding that the live EV76 vaccine induces protection against plague, although its use is accompanied by unacceptable local and systemic side effects,[71] has prompted some studies to develop rationally attenuated strains of *Y. pestis* as a vaccine. Work toward this goal has been based on the finding that other gram-negative pathogens can be attenuated by the introduction of mutations into genes essential for bacterial growth, virulence, or survival in the host, and that the nature of the attenuating mutation can influence the immunogenicity and reactogenicity of these vaccines. Strains of *Y. pestis* with mutations in the *aroA*, *phoP*, or *htrA* genes have been considered as candidate live, attenuated vaccines. Mutations within genes involved in aromatic amino acid biosynthesis have been shown to attenuate markedly a variety of pathogens, including *Y. enterocolitica*, *S. typhimurium*, and *S. typhi*. An *aroA* mutant of *Y. pestis* was not attenuated in mice but was attenuated in guinea pigs, and these animals subsequently developed antibodies to the F1 and V antigens.[96] Although these guinea pigs also were protected against a subsequent challenge with 10^7 CFU of virulent *Y. pestis*,[96] further work is needed to determine the reason for the species-dependent virulence of the *aroA* mutant before it can be considered for further studies. The mutation of the *phoP* gene, encoding the PhoP component of a two-component regulatory system, resulted in a derivative of *Y. pestis* that was only 75-fold attenuated in mice after subcutaneous challenge.[97] This level of attenuation does not compare well with the severe attenuation of a *S. typhimurium phoP* mutant[98] and might reflect the different lifestyles of these pathogens. Thus, in contrast to the *S. typhimurium phoP* mutant, a *Y. pestis phoP* mutant does not appear to be a candidate live vaccine for use in humans. Similarly, the degree of attenuation of an *htrA* mutant of *Y. pestis* was not sufficient to merit consideration of this mutant as a live, attenuated vaccine.[99] The completion of the *Y. pestis* genome sequence has identified a wide range of other genes that might be inactivated to yield a live, attenuated vaccine.[29] Therefore, this approach to vaccine development should not be discounted.

REFERENCES

1. Brubaker B. Factors promoting acute and chronic diseases caused by yersiniae. Clin Microbiol Rev 4:309–324, 1991.
2. Pollitzer R. Plague. World Health Organ Monogr Ser 22:1–698, 1954.
3. Butler T. Plague and Other *Yersinia* Infections. New York, Plenum Press, 1983.
4. Perry RD, Fetherston JD. *Yersinia pestis*—etiologic agent of plague. Clin Microbiol Rev 10:35–66, 1997.
5. Prevention of plague: Recommendations of the Advisory Committee on Immunization Practices (ACIP). MMWR Morb Mortal Wkly Rep 45(RR-14):1–15, 1996.
6. Human Plague in 1998 and 1999. World Health Organ Wkly Epidemiol Rec 75(42):337–344, 2000.
7. Human plague in 1994. Wkly Epidemiol Rec 22:165–168, 1996.
8. Poland JD, Barnes AM. Plague. *In* Steele JH, Stoenner H, Kaplan W, Torten M (eds). CRC Handbook Series in Zoonoses. Boca Raton, FL, CRC Press, 1979, pp 515–597.
9. Christie AB, Corbel MJ. Plague and other yersinial diseases. *In* Smith GR, Easmon CSF (eds). Topley and Wilson's Principles of Bacteriology, Virology and Immunity. Vol. 3. London, Edward Arnold, 1990, pp 399–410.
10. Meyer KF. Pneumonic plague. Bacteriol Rev 35:249–261, 1961.
11. Kellog WH. An epidemic of pneumonic plague. Am J Public Health 10:599–605, 1920.
12. Dickie W. Plague in California 1900–1925. Proc Conf State Prov Health Authorities North Am 21:30–78, 1926.
13. Druett HA, Robinson JM, Henderson DW, et al. Studies on respiratory infection. II. The influence of aerosol particle size on infection of the guinea pig with *Pasteurella pestis*. J Hyg 54:37–48, 1956.
14. Girard G, Robic J. Pneumonie pesteuse expérimentale. Arch Inst Pasteur Tananarive Année 8:32–34, 1940.
15. Robic J. Del' emploi du "Maki" comme animale d'expérience à Madagascar: son intérêt dans l'étude de la peste. Bull Soc Pathol Exotique 34:246–249, 1941.
16. Robic J. Peste expérimentale du Maki. Arch Inst Pasteur Tananarive Année 10:23–25, 1942.
17. Meyer KF, Larson A. The pathogenesis of cervical septicemic plague developing after exposure to pneumonic plague produced by intratracheal infection in primates. *In* Proceedings of the Symposium for the Diamond Jubilee of the Haffkine Institute, Bombay, India, January 10–14, 1959, 1960, pp 1–12.
18. Ratsitorahina M, Chanteau S, Rahalison L, et al. Epidemiological and diagnostic aspects of the outbreak of pneumonic plague in Madagascar. Lancet 355:111–113, 2000.
19. Achtman M, Zurth K, Morelli G, et al. *Yersinia pestis*, the cause of plague, is a recently emerged clone of *Yersinia pseudotuberculosis*. Proc Natl Acad Sci U S A 96:14043–14048, 1999.
20. Parkhill J, Wren BW, Thomson NR, et al. Genome sequence of *Yersinia pestis*, the causative agent of plague. Nature 413:523–527, 2001.
21. Cornelis GR, Biot T, Lambert de Rouvroit C, et al. The *Yersinia yop* regulon. Mol Microbiol 3:1455–1459, 1989.
22. Straley SC, Skrzypek E, Plano GV, et al. Yops of *Yersinia* spp. pathogenic for humans. Infect Immun 61:3105–3110, 1993.
23. Prentice MB, James KD, Parkhill J, et al. *Yersinia pestis* pFra shows biovar-specific differences and recent common ancestry with a *Salmonella enterica* serovar Typhi plasmid. J Bacteriol 183:2586–2594, 2001.
24. Galyov EE, Smirnov OY, Karlishev AV, et al. Nucleotide sequence of the *Yersinia pestis* gene encoding F1 antigen and the primary structure of the protein. FEBS Lett 277:230–232, 1990.
25. Galyov EE, Karlishev AV, Chernovskaya TV, et al. Expression of the envelope antigen F1 of *Yersinia pestis* is mediated by the product of *caf1M* gene having homology with the chaperone protein PapD of *Escherichia coli*. FEBS Lett 286:79–82, 1991.
26. Karlyshev AV, Galyov EE, Smirnov OY, et al. A new gene of the *f1* operon of *Y. pestis* involved in the capsule biogenesis. FEBS Lett 297:77–80, 1992.
27. Karlyshev AV, Galyov EE, Abramov VM, et al. *Caf1R* gene and its role in the regulation of capsule formation of *Y. pestis*. FEBS Lett 305:37–40, 1992.
28. Hinnesbusch BJ, Perry RD, Schwan TG. Role of the *Yersinia pestis* hemin storage (*hms*) locus in the transmission of plague by fleas. Science 273:367–370, 1996.
29. Cavanaugh DC. Specific effect of temperature upon transmission of the plague bacillus by the oriental rat flea, *Xenopsylla cheopis*. Am J Trop Med Hyg 20:264–272, 1971.
30. Van Zwanenberg D. The last epidemic of plague in England? Suffolk 1906–1918. Med Hist 14:63–74, 1970.
31. Cavanaugh DC, Randall R. The role of multiplication of *Pasteurella pestis* in mononuclear phagocytes in the pathogenesis of flea-borne plague. J Immunol 83:348–363, 1959.

32. Lindler LE, Klemper MS, Straley SC. *Yersinia pestis* pH 6 antigen: genetic, biochemical and virulence characterisation of a protein involved in the pathogenesis of bubonic plague. Infect Immun 58:2569–2577, 1990.

33. Williams RC, Gewurz H, Quie PG. Effects of fraction 1 from *Yersinia pestis* on phagocytosis in vitro. J Infect Dis 126:235–241, 1972.

34. Friedlander AM, Welkos SL, Worsham PL, et al. Relationship between virulence and immunity as revealed in recent studies of the F1 capsule of *Yersinia pestis*. Clin Infect Dis 21:S178–S181, 1995.

35. Nakajima R, Brubaker RR. Association between virulence of *Yersinia pestis* and suppression of gamma interferon and tumor necrosis factor alpha. Infect Immun 61:23–31, 1993.

36. Nakajima R, Motin VL, Brubaker RR. Suppression of cytokines in mice by protein A-V antigen fusion peptide and restoration of synthesis by active immunisation. Infect Immun 63:3021–3029, 1995.

37. Price SB, Cowan C, Perry RD, et al. The *Yersinia pestis* V antigen is a regulatory protein necessary for Ca^{2+}-dependent growth and maximal expression of low-Ca^{2+}-response virulence genes. J Bacteriol 173:2649–2657, 1991.

38. Montie TC, Montie DB. Protein toxins of *Pasteurella pestis*: subunit composition and acid binding. Biochemistry 10:2094–2100, 1971.

39. Inglesby TV, Dennis DT, Henderson DA, et al. Plague as a biological weapon: medical and public health management. JAMA 283:2281–2290, 2000.

40. Russell P, Nelson M, Whittington D, et al. Laboratory diagnosis of plague. Br J Biomed Sci 54:231–236, 1997.

41. Rahalison L, Vololonirina E, Ratsitorahina M, et al. Diagnosis of bubonic plague by PCR in Madagascar under field conditions. J Clin Microbiol 38:260–263, 2000.

42. Norkina OV, Kulichenko AN, Gintsburg AL, et al. Development of a diagnostic test for *Yersinia pestis* by the polymerase chain reaction. J Appl Bacteriol 76:240–245, 1994.

43. Neubauer H, Rahalison L, Brooks TJ, et al. Serodiagnosis of human plague by an anti-F1 capsular antigen specific IgG/IgM ELISA and immunoblot. Epidemiol Infect 125:593–597, 2000.

44. Chanteau S, Rahalison L, Ratsitorahina M, et al. Early diagnosis of bubonic plague using F1 antigen capture ELISA assay and rapid immunogold dipstick. Int J Med Microbiol 290:279–283, 2000.

45. Titball RW. Plague. *In* Rakel RE, Bope ET (eds). Conn's Current Therapy. Philadelphia, WB Saunders Company, 2002, pp 117–118.

46. Russell P, Eley SM, Green M, et al. Efficacy of doxycycline and ciprofloxacin against experimental *Yersinia pestis* infection. J Antimicrob Chem 41:301–305, 1998.

47. Galimand M, Guiyoule A, Gerbaud G, et al. Multidrug resistance in *Yersinia pestis* mediated by a transferable plasmid. N Engl J Med 337:677–680, 1997.

48. Von Metz E, Eisler DM, Hottle GA. Immunogenicity of plague vaccines in mice and guinea pigs. Appl Microbiol 22:84–88, 1971.

49. Russell P, Eley SM, Hibbs SE, et al. A comparison of plague vaccine, USP and EV76 vaccine induced protection against *Yersinia pestis* in a murine model. Vaccine 13:1551–1556, 1995.

50. Andrews GP, Heath DG, Anderson GW Jr, et al. Fraction 1 capsular antigen (F1) purification from *Yersinia pestis* CO92 and from an *Escherichia coli* recombinant strain and efficacy against lethal plague challenge. Infect Immun 64:2180–2187, 1996.

51. Bartelloni PJ, Marshall JD, Cavanaugh DC. Clinical and serological responses to plague vaccine. Mil Med 138:720–722, 1973.

52. Meyer KF, Foster LE. Measurement of protective serum antibodies in human volunteers inoculated with plague prophylactics. Stanford Med Bull 6:75–79, 1948.

53. Meyer KF. Effectiveness of live or killed plague vaccines in man. Bull World Health Organ 42:653–666, 1970.

54. WHO report on plague in 1973. World Health Organ Wkly Epidemiol Rec 49:253–254, 1974.

55. Barnes AM. Surveillance and control of bubonic plague in the United States. Symp Zool Soc Lond 50:237–270, 1982.

56. Anonymous. Medical and Public Health Effects of Attack with Chemical or Biological Weapons. *In* Health Aspects of Chemical and Biological Weapons. Geneva, World Health Organization, 1970, pp 98–112.

57. Lawton WD, Erdman RL, Surgalla MJ. Biosynthesis and purification of V and W antigens in *Pasteurella pestis*. J Immunol 91:179–184, 1963.

58. Motin VL, Nakajima R, Smirnov GB, et al. Passive immunity to yersiniae mediated by anti-recombinant V antigen and by protein A-V fusion peptide. Infect Immun 62:4192–4201, 1994.

59. Une T, Nakajima R, Brubaker RR. Roles of V antigen in promoting virulence in *Yersinia*. Contrib Microbiol Immunol 9:179–185, 1986.

60. Williams JE, Altieri PL, Berman S, et al. Potency of killed plague vaccines prepared from a virulent *Yersinia pestis*. Bull World Health Organ 58:753–756, 1980.

61. Meyer KF, Smith G, Foster LE, et al. Plague immunization. IV. Clinical reactions and serologic response to inoculations of Haffkine and freeze-dried plague vaccine. J Infect Dis 129:S30–S36, 1974.

62. Williams JE, Cavanaugh DC. Measuring the efficacy of vaccination in affording protection against plague. Bull World Health Organ 57:309–313, 1979.

63. Williamson ED, Eley SM, Griffin K, et al. A new improved sub-unit vaccine for plague: the basis of protection. FEMS Immunol Med Microbiol 12:223–230, 1995.

64. Marshall JD, Cavanaugh DC, Bartelloni PJ, et al. Plague immunization. III. Serologic response to multiple inoculations of vaccine. J Infect Dis 129:S26–S29, 1974.

65. Jefferson T, Demicheli V, Pratt M. Vaccines for preventing plague (Cochrane Review). *In* The Cochrane Library, Issue 3, 2002. Update Software Ltd, Oxford.

66. Cavanaugh DC, Elisberg BL, Llewellyn C, et al. Plague immunization. V. Indirect evidence for the efficacy of plague vaccine. J Infect Dis 129:S37–S40, 1974.

67. Cohen RJ, Stockard JL. Pneumonic plague in an untreated plague vaccinated individual. JAMA 202:365–366, 1967.

68. Williamson ED, Eley SM, Stagg AJ, et al. A sub-unit vaccine elicits IgG in serum, spleen cell cultures and bronchial washings and protects immunized animals against pneumonic plague. Vaccine 15:1079–1084, 1997.

69. Reisman RE. Allergic reactions due to plague vaccine. J Allergy 46:49–56, 1970.

70. Marshall JD, Bartelloni PJ, Cavanaugh DC, et al. Plague immunization. II. Relation of adverse clinical reactions to multiple immunizations with killed vaccine. J Infect Dis 129:S19–S25, 1974.

71. Meyer KF, Cavanaugh DC, Bartelloni PJ, et al. Plague immunization. I. Past and present trends. J Infect Dis 129:S13–S18, 1974.

72. Williams JE, Arntzen L, Tyndal GL, et al. Application of enzyme immunoassays for the confirmation of clinically suspect plague in Namibia, 1982. Bull World Health Organ 64:745–752, 1982.

73. Leary SEC, Williamson ED, Griffin KF, et al. Active immunization with V-antigen from *Yersinia pestis* protects against plague. Infect Immun 63:2854–2858, 1995.

74. Baker EE, Sommer H, Foster LE, et al. Studies on immunization against plague. I. The isolation and characterization of the soluble antigen of *Pasteurella pestis*. J Immunol 68:131–145, 1952.

75. Meyer KF, Hightower JA, McCrumb FR. Plague immunization. VI. Vaccination with the fraction 1 antigen of *Yersinia pestis*. J Infect Dis 129:S41–S45, 1974.

76. Simpson WJ, Thomas RE, Schwan TG. Recombinant capsular antigen (fraction 1) from *Yersinia pestis* induces a protective antibody response in BALB/C mice. Am J Trop Med Hyg 43:389–396, 1990.

77. Miller J, Williamson ED, Lakey JH, et al. Macromolecular organisation of recombinant *Yersinia pestis* F1 antigen and the effect of structure on immunogenicity. FEMS Immun Med Microbiol 21:213–221, 1998.

78. Carr S, Miller J, Leary SEC, et al. Expression of a recombinant form of the V antigen of *Yersinia pestis*, using three different expression systems. Vaccine 18:153–159, 2000.

79. Anderson GW, Leary SEC, Williamson ED, et al. Recombinant V antigen protects mice against pneumonic and bubonic plague caused by F1-capsule–positive and –negative strains of *Yersinia pestis*. Infect Immun 64:4580–4585, 1996.

80. Rodrigues CG, Carneiro CMM, Barbosa CFT, et al. Antigen F1 from *Yersinia pestis* forms aqueous channels in lipid bilayer membranes. Braz J Med Biol Res 25:75–79, 1992.

81. Williamson ED, Vesey PM, Gillhespy KJ, et al. An IgG1 titre to the F1 and V antigens correlates with protection against plague in the mouse model. Clin Exp Immunol 116:107–114, 1999.

82. Williamson ED, Sharpe GJE, Eley SM, et al. Local and systemic immune response to a microencapsulated sub-unit vaccine for plague. Vaccine 14:1613–1619, 1996.

83. Elvin SJ, Williamson ED. The F1 and V subunit vaccine protects against plague in the absence of IL-4 driven immune responses. Microb Pathog 29:223–230, 2000.

84. Williamson ED, Eley SM, Stagg AJ, et al. A single dose sub-unit vaccine protects against pneumonic plague. Vaccine 19:566–571, 2001.

85. Jones SM, Day F, Stagg AJ, et al. Protection conferred by a fully recombinant sub-unit vaccine against *Yersinia pestis* in male and female mice of four inbred strains. Vaccine 19:358–366, 2001.

86. Thomas RE, Simpson WJ, Perry LL, et al. Failure of intragastrically administered *Yersinia pestis* capsular antigen to protect mice against challenge with virulent plague: suppression of fraction 1–specific antibody response. Am J Trop Med Hyg 47:92–97, 1992.

87. Reddin KM, Easterbrook TJ, Eley SM, et al. Comparison of the immunological and protective responses elicited by microencapsulated formulations of the F1 antigen from *Yersinia pestis*. Vaccine 16:761–767, 1998.

88. Spiers ID, Alpar HO, Eyles JE, et al. Studies on the co-encapsulation, release and integrity of two sub-unit antigens: rV and rF1 from *Yersinia pestis*. J Pharm Pharmacol 51:991–997, 1999.

89. Eyles JE, Sharp GJE, Williamson ED, et al. Intranasal administration of poly (lactic acid) microsphere co-encapsulated *Yersinia pestis* sub-unit s confers protection from pneumonic plague in the mouse. Vaccine 16:698–707, 1998.

90. Eyles JE, Spiers ID, Williamson ED, et al. Analysis of local and systemic immunological responses to intra-tracheal, intra-nasal and intra-muscular administration of microsphere co-encapsulated *Yersinia pestis* sub-unit vaccines. Vaccine 16:2000–2009, 1998.

91. Titball RW, Williamson ED. Vaccination against bubonic and pneumonic plague. Vaccine 19:4175–4184, 2001.

92. Eyles JE, Williamson ED, Spiers ID, et al. Generation of protective immune responses to plague by mucosal administration of microsphere co-encapsulated recombinant sub-units. J Contr Rel 63:191–200, 2000.

93. Eyles JE, Bramwell VW, Williamson ED, et al. Microsphere translocation in systemic tissues following intranasal administration. Vaccine 19:4732–4742, 2001.

94. Oyston PCF, Williamson ED, Leary SEC, et al. Immunization with live recombinant *Salmonella typhimurium aroA* producing F1 antigen protects against plague. Infect Immun 63:563–568, 1995.

95. Titball RW, Howells AM, Oyston PCF, et al. Expression of the *Yersinia pestis* capsular antigen (F1 antigen) on the surface of an *aroA* mutant of *Salmonella typhimurium* induces high level protection against plague. Infect Immun 65:1926–1930, 1997.

96. Oyston PFC, Russell P, Williamson ED, et al. An *aroA* mutant of *Yersinia pestis* is attenuated in the guinea pig but virulent in mice. Microbiology 142:1847–1853, 1995.

97. Oyston PC, Dorrell N, Williams K, et al. The response regulator PhoP is important for survival under conditions of macrophage-induced stress and virulence in *Yersinia pestis*. Infect Immun 68:3419–3425, 2000.

98. Galan JE, Curtiss R 3rd. Virulence and vaccine potential of *phoP* mutants of *Salmonella typhimurium*. Microb Pathog 6:433–443, 1989.

99. Williams K, Oyston PC, Dorrell N, et al. Investigation into the role of the serine protease HtrA in *Yersinia pestis* pathogenesis. FEMS Microbiol Lett 186:281–286, 2000.

Chapter 37

Rabies Vaccine

STANLEY A. PLOTKIN • CHARLES E. RUPPRECHT •
HILARY KOPROWSKI

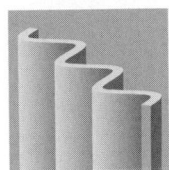

I have seen agony in death only once, in a patient with rabies; he remained acutely aware of every stage in the process of his own disintegration over a twenty-four-hour period, right up to his final moment.

LEWIS THOMAS. *THE LIVES OF A CELL.* NEW YORK, BANTAM BOOKS, 1974.

Background

Rabies is an acute viral encephalitis transmitted from animal to animal or from animal to human by exposure to saliva. Virus in saliva attaches to peripheral nerve endings and travels to the brain. In nature, rabies is a disease of mammals, involving the Canidae (dogs, wolves, foxes, coyotes, and jackals), Procyonidae (raccoons), Viverridae (mongooses), Mephitadae (skunks), and Chiroptera (bats) as reservoirs or vectors. All mammalian species are believed to be susceptible.

Human infection with rabies is nearly always secondary to animal bite, although exposures through the inhalation of virus or through the transplantation of infected corneas have occurred. In most of the world, the major reservoir for human rabies is the dog, responsible for an enormous incidence of bites. Although they do not function as reservoirs, cats are important vectors of the disease.

Historical Perspective

It has been suggested that rabies was known before 2300 BC, based on a description in the Mesopotamian Laws of Eshnunna.[1] Ancient texts from Egypt, China, Persia, Palestine, India, and China also appear to contain allusions to the disease.[2] The first certain references to rabies are from Greek literature. Homer, Democritus, and Aristotle referred to *lyssa* (Greek for rabies) in their writings, and in the first century AD, the Roman scholar Aulus Cornelius Celsus was perhaps the first to provide an accurate description of the disease and the wide range of species susceptible to infection. Rabies is frequently mentioned in western and

Arabic writings during the Middle Ages. In the 15th century AD, the Italian savant Girolamo Fracastoro established the principle of the incurable wound, that is, the disease is always lethal. The Talmud also mentions that one should not believe people who say that they were bitten by a rabid animal and survived.

Shortly after Cortez's exploration of the Americas, the first Bishop of Oceania described "small animals" that bit the toes of Spanish soldiers during the night. The soldiers later died of a disease that could have been rabies, and other Spanish sources describe vampire bats that even now play a major role in the transmission of rabies in Latin America. In fact, it is possible that terrestrial rabies was largely absent in the New World until introduced late in the 16th century.[2]

Early in the 19th century, a school of authors believed that rabies was purely a psychiatric disease. However, the dramatic symptoms and nearly 100% fatality rate of rabies attracted the curiosity of the first modern microbiologists, and, by the end of the 19th century, an effective vaccination procedure was developed.[3,4] Edgar Allan Poe may have died of rabies in Baltimore.[5]

Experimental transmission of rabies by inoculation of saliva was first demonstrated in 1804 by the German scientist Gottfried Zinke. In 1879 in Lyon, France, Pierre-Victor Galtier transmitted rabies from dog to rabbit and from rabbit to rabbit and used intravenous injections of rabid material to immunize sheep and goats. However, Galtier's work was to be overshadowed by that of his famed contemporary, Louis Pasteur. Obviously, much of the credit for rabies research belongs to Pasteur, but one must not overlook the contributions of his collaborators, Roux, Chamberland, and Thuillier. These three investigators carried out most of his laboratory manipulations, because Pasteur, more than 60 years old, was partially disabled by stroke.

The Pasteur group established in 1881 that the central nervous system is the principal site of rabies virus replication. They transmitted the disease by submeningeal inoculation into rabbits and were able to maintain the virus in this host for more than 100 passages. It was Roux who noticed originally that the virulence of rabies-infected spinal cords decreased rapidly when they were suspended in dry air and was extinguished completely in 15 days. From this observation, Pasteur developed a practical method of vaccination. Dogs injected subcutaneously with serial

An earlier contributor to this chapter was the late Tadeusz Wiktor.

suspensions of fragments of rabies virus–infected spinal cords, beginning with cord dried long enough to be avirulent and using successively less dried cords, resisted rabies when they were injected intracerebrally with a virulent virus.

Fifty dogs were protected this way. Although experiments performed to demonstrate that dogs can be made refractory to rabies by vaccination *after* they had been bitten by "mad" dogs were inconclusive, treatment of a human patient, Joseph Meister, was attempted on July 6, 1885, perhaps subsequent to other nonpublished attempts at human vaccination. Meister, who had been bitten 14 times by a rabid dog 60 hours previously, received a subcutaneous inoculation of spinal cord suspension derived from rabid rabbits and preserved in a flask of dry air for 15 days. Twelve successive inoculations were made with cords of increasing virulence, for a total of 13 inoculations during a 10-day period. The boy not only resisted natural rabies but also escaped large quantities of highly virulent virus that were contained in the last five doses of vaccine.

The Pasteur method of treatment aroused great interest in medical circles and, despite some disagreements, was rapidly accepted. The Pasteur Institute of Paris was founded in 1888, and within a decade there were Pasteur Institutes throughout the world.

Criticism, however, was forthcoming. The occasional failures raised questions about the safety of the vaccine, especially because virulent material was being inoculated into the patients at the end of the treatment. Also, there were obviously no controls for comparison to confirm the effectiveness of the method. Pasteur thought that vaccine failures could be attributed to prolonged delays in initiating treatment or to excessive bites on the face or head that resulted in a short incubation period.

Clinical Description

A comprehensive review of human rabies has been published by Hemachudha et al.[6] Reported incubation periods for rabies have been as short as 5 to 6 days, but, in the majority of cases, the incubation period is between 20 and 60 days.[7] Although incubation periods of longer than 6 months are reported in less than 1% of cases, identification of strains by monoclonal antibodies and genetic sequencing has permitted positive confirmation of periods as long as 6 years.[8] Incubation periods are usually shorter when the site of the bite is on the head rather than an extremity.[9] Without vaccination, the risk of death varies with the quantity of virus in the saliva of the biting animal, and the severity and location of the bite. Dog bites are associated with a mortality of 38% to 57%.[6]

Signs of rabies in animals are well known. After a nonspecific prodromal period, a variable proportion of animals develop aggressive or combative behavior, irritability, viciousness, and hyperreaction to external stimuli. In these cases, the clinical course is described as *furious* rabies. A paralytic phase then develops characterized by weakness of one or more limbs, jaw drop resulting from paralysis of muscles of the head and neck, and difficulty in phonation and respiration, leading ultimately to death. Alternatively, paralysis may predominate with no aggressive signs, described as "dumb" rabies.

Clinical rabies presents either in a furious form (two thirds of the cases) or in a paralytic form. Rabies transmitted from dogs is usually furious, whereas that transmitted from vampire bats is usually paralytic. The furious form is characterized by fluctuating consciousness, phobic spasms, and signs of autonomic dysfunction such as dilated pupils and hypersalivation. In the paralytic form, the patient is conscious but appears to have the Guillain-Barré syndrome. In distinction from the latter syndrome, rabies patients usually have fever, intact sensory function, percussion myoedema, and urinary incontinence. The clinical illness in humans may be divided into the following five stages: incubation period, prodrome, acute neurologic phase, coma, and death or rare recovery.[10]

During the incubation period, there are no symptoms and no means of diagnosis; clinical illness begins with the prodromal complaints of malaise, anorexia, fatigue, headache, and fever. Pain or paresthesia at or close to the site of exposure is reported in 50% to 80% of cases, and apprehension, anxiety, agitation, irritability, nervousness, insomnia, or depression may be prominent during this period. After a prodromal period that lasts 2 to 10 days, objective signs of nervous system involvement develop, including hyperactivity, disorientation, hallucinations, seizures, bizarre behavior, nuchal stiffness, and paralysis. As in animals, a period of hyperactivity lasting hours to days develops in a majority of cases. In humans, this hyperactivity is characteristically intermittent and consists of periods of agitation lasting 1 to 5 minutes. These hyperactive periods may occur spontaneously or may be precipitated by a variety of tactile, auditory, visual, or other stimuli.[11] Between these periods, the patient is usually cooperative and able to communicate. Hydrophobia (the fear of water) appears to develop in most cases of furious human rabies. Attempts to drink or eat may produce severe painful spasms of the pharynx and larynx and precipitate an episode of hyperactivity that is extremely frightening to the patient. Subsequently, simply the sight of liquids may precipitate episodes of pharyngeal spasms. Bright lights, loud noises, or air currents also may precipitate spasms.

Other abnormalities during the acute and neurologic phase include muscle fasciculation (particularly near the site of the exposure), hyperventilation, hypersalivation, focal or generalized convulsions, and, rarely, priapism or increased libido. Unless the patient dies abruptly, paralysis generally becomes the major problem. Paralysis may be symmetric; asymmetric with maximal involvement of the bitten extremity; or ascending, as in the Guillain-Barré syndrome.[12] Paralysis may be the presenting symptom, as seems often to be the case after bat bites.

In the acute neurologic phase, the mental status of the patient gradually deteriorates during a period of 2 to 12 days. This phase ends either with abrupt death from cardiac or respiratory arrest or with onset of coma. Coma may last for hours or months, depending on the intensity of care. Without supportive care, respiratory arrest usually develops shortly after the onset of coma and leads to death, within 5 days for furious rabies and 13 days for paralytic rabies.[13] With intensive medical support, respiratory arrest may not occur, and the patient may live with assisted ventilation for up to several months.

The differential clinical diagnosis is large, and rabies is often unsuspected.[14] Clinical laboratory determinations, including those done on cerebrospinal fluid (CSF), seldom show striking abnormalities. Electroencephalography, computerized tomography scans, and magnetic resonance imaging may show abnormalities in the thalamus and basal ganglia,[15] but do not help in the diagnosis.

To date, there are fewer than 10 cases of known survival among humans who showed signs of disease, all of whom recovered with sequelae and one with severe psychogenic disturbance.[16–21] All survivors had received either preexposure or postexposure rabies vaccination. Despite trials of steroids, interferon, and other antivirals, there is no therapy of proven value.[22]

Virology

Rabies virus belongs to the family Rhabdoviridae, genus *Lyssavirus*, consisting of genetically related enveloped viruses with a single, nonsegmented, negative-stranded RNA. The virus is shaped like a bullet, 200 nm long and 75 nm wide. The virus contains multiple copies of the following five structural proteins: virion transcriptase (L), glycoprotein (G), nucleoprotein (N), nucleocapsid phosphoprotein (NS or P), and matrix protein (M). The L, N, and NS proteins are noncovalently bound to the virion RNA, and the resulting ribonucleoprotein complex forms a helically coiled structure within the virion. The nucleocapsid complex is surrounded by a lipoprotein envelope consisting of the M protein, and the surface projection of the G proteins extends to the exterior of the virus.[23]

Like some other RNA viruses, rabies strains exist as quasi species.[23a,23b] Phylogenetic analyses suggest that rabies virus (lyssavirus type 1) originally may have been a virus of bats, spreading to terrestrial carnivores only between 500 and 1500 years ago.[24,25] According to this hypothesis, the earlier historical references mentioned above may have resulted from previous crossovers that became extinct.

The rabies virus G protein, which is a trimer of about 67 kDa, is the major antigen responsible for inducing production of virus-neutralizing antibodies (VNAs) and for conferring immunity against lethal infection with rabies virus.[26,27] It also contains determinants of virulence.[28,29] The G gene was the first rabies virus gene to be cloned and sequenced.[30] From the nucleotide sequence, a polypeptide 524 amino acids long was deduced, which included a signal sequence of 19 amino acids.[23] An arginine at position 333 appears necessary for virulence.[31]

The immunogenic activity of purified native G protein and of smaller fragments of G protein, both naturally occurring and derived by chemical cleavage of the rabies virus G protein, has been compared in a variety of ways to determine the structural basis of VNA production after immunization.[23] Although the role of the humoral immune response to rabies is debated,[32–34] evidence for the importance of VNAs in prevention of viral infection is convincing both in humans (see later) and in animals. With regard to a cellular response, T-helper cells are necessary for antibody induction, whereas cytolytic T cells directed against the nucleoprotein (N) induced by vaccination may be important to destroy infected cells before entry of virus into the central nervous system. Interestingly, the cytolytic T-cell response may be suppressed in natural infection.

Rabies-Related Viruses

Since the early 1970s, viruses have been isolated from animals and humans that are serologically related to rabies virus. Although members of this group showed some immunologic cross-reactivity with the rabies virus, they were sufficiently different to be originally classified as *rabies-related viruses*. The *Lyssavirus* genus is now considered to contain seven viruses.[35] Type 1 is the rabies virus itself as type species; type 2 is the Lagos bat virus, originally isolated from bats in Nigeria[36]; type 3 is the Mokola virus, isolated from a shrew in Nigeria[37]; type 4 is the Duvenhage virus, isolated from a human with a case of rabies-like illness in South Africa[37]; type 5 is European bat virus 1, isolated from a human case in Russia; type 6 is European bat virus 2, isolated from a human case in Finland[38]; and type 7 is a new isolate from Australian bats. At present, it is difficult to relate any human disease to type 2 virus. Mokola virus can cause lethal infection in rabies-vaccinated dogs and cats.[39,40] European bat *Lyssavirus* 1 has been isolated from bats captured in Poland, Denmark, Finland, and northern provinces of Germany.[37] Strains of *Lyssavirus* types 5 and 6 are apparently widely distributed in European bats.[41] Although tests in mice showed that human diploid cell rabies vaccine could protect against the European bat viruses,[42] and vaccination of exposed humans has so far been successful,[41] only 73% of vaccinated patients developed neutralizing antibodies to these viruses, usually when they had mounted a strong antibody response to the rabies vaccine virus.[43] The larger public health significance of the other rabies-related viruses remains to be determined.

Pathogenesis as It Relates to Prevention

When inoculated in a wound, rabies virus may take days or weeks to reach the central nervous system. It is this fact that makes postexposure prophylaxis possible. During this early period, the virus is susceptible to VNAs and even to mechanical removal by washing. There is some evidence that initial replication may occur in muscle cells surrounding the wound, providing an amplification of the original inoculum. However, experimental data show that central nervous system entry can occur without any prior replication in the muscle.[44] Another site proposed for possible persistence of rabies virus before entry into the central nervous system is the macrophage, from which the virus could reactivate to cause disease,[45] but the importance of replication in non-nerve cells to the pathogenesis of rabies remains controversial.[46] In any event, at some point in time, the virus attaches to receptors, which may include the nicotinic acetylcholine receptors of the neuromuscular junction or lipoproteins on the membrane (see later), and begins a passive journey to the cytosol, where it replicates and spreads within the central nervous system.[47,48] Dietzschold and colleagues[49] have demonstrated that the action of rabies VNAs is not exerted solely outside of the cell. In an animal model, the effectiveness of antibody was associated with entry into the cell by endocytosis and inhibition of viral transcription. Whether the antibody acts directly or by signal transduction to inhibit viral protein synthesis is unclear.[50]

The rabies virus G protein has sequences similar to certain neurotoxins and binds to the α-subunit of the acetylcholine receptor.[51–53] This receptor undoubtedly functions in the entry of virus into muscle, but other lipoprotein receptors function on the nerve cell.[54] Once in the neurons, the virus travels in the axons at a rate of 12 to 24 mm/day in rodents but perhaps faster in humans. In rodents, virus may reach the central nervous system in 3 to 5 days, where it causes a widespread encephalitis[55] progressing at 20 to 40 mm/day.

Once established in the neurons of the brain, the virus starts to move in the opposite direction, down the axons to replicate in peripheral tissues, most notably in the nerve plexus of the salivary glands, from which excretion in saliva permits transmission by bite to maintain the circuit of infection.[35] However, extraneural tissues also are infected, including heart, pancreas, adrenal glands, and gastrointestinal tract.[56,56a]

The pathophysiology of the fatal outcome is not completely understood. Although encephalitis is widespread, neuronal destruction is not. Nevertheless, some cells may die from an apoptotic process.[57] Death probably results from the involvement of brain centers controlling the cardiorespiratory system. In general, the histologic presence of Negri bodies parallels that of rabies virus antigen, although many infected cells do not have these inclusions. Rabies virus antigen is most prevalent in the periaqueductal gray matter and the Purkinje cells of the cerebellum.[58] Although the fatality rate in rabies is extremely elevated, rare documented recovery and even chronic persistent infection have been documented in dogs.[59]

Hemachudha and colleagues[6] have emphasized the role of cellular immunity in the course of rabies. They correlate strong T-cell responses and cytokine secretion (in particular interleukin-6) with early death and the encephalitic form of the disease, and weak T-cell responses with paralysis and longer survival.

Evidence of a serologic response to rabies virus can be demonstrated by a variety of laboratory techniques, including mouse neutralization, fluorescent focus inhibition, indirect fluorescent antibody, plaque neutralization, immunolysis of rabies-infected cells, and binding techniques using the radioimmunoassay or enzyme-linked immunosorbent assay procedures. Serum antibodies develop late after natural infection in humans. In individuals without history of vaccination, serum antibodies are first detected on about the 10th day of illness and thereafter rise rapidly to high levels. Antibodies are also present in CSF late in the clinical course. Antibody titers of CSF are much higher than would be expected from seepage into CSF from circulating blood. Because vaccination does not induce CSF antibodies, the presence of high CSF antibody titers supports the diagnosis of clinical rabies.[16,17]

The absence of detectable serum antibodies until around the second week of illness (if at all) and of CSF antibodies until approximately the third week of illness (when significant systemic and neurologic problems occur) raises the possibility that some of the clinical symptoms result from the interaction of host antibodies with rabies virus–infected cells.[47] In individuals who receive postexposure prophylaxis, but who nevertheless develop rabies, antibody titers after the onset of clinical illness rise more rapidly and to higher levels than in individuals who do not receive such immunization. In mouse experiments, both neutralizing antibodies and infiltration of cellular inflammatory cells were necessary to clear infection with an attenuated rabies from the central nervous system,[60] but this process occurs too late in the usual situation.

Diagnosis

Clinical diagnosis of rabies requires differentiation from a wide variety of diseases that can cause neurologic symptoms. Because laboratory diagnosis may not be possible during the first week of illness, presumptive diagnosis based on clinical symptoms is important. As noted previously, the clinical symptoms of rabies encephalitis that may distinguish it from other forms of encephalitis are as follows: pain and paresthesia near the site of exposure, hydrophobia, hypersalivation, hyperventilation, agitated behavior, asymmetric or ascending paralysis, and aerophobia—all developing during a 2- to 10-day period. Detection of lesions in the brainstem, hippocampus, and thalamus by magnetic resonance imaging is suggestive of rabies.[6] These symptoms, signs, and a history of exposure to a rabid animal strongly suggest the diagnosis of rabies. Other diagnoses that figure prominently in the differential diagnosis of furious rabies include porphyria, tetanus, and drug intoxication; for paralytic rabies, Guillain-Barré syndrome, poliomyelitis, and Japanese encephalitis should be considered.[14] More recently, West Nile virus, Enterovirus 71, and Nipah virus all must enter into the differential diagnosis.

Definitive diagnosis of rabies infection of humans and suspected animal vectors depends on the detection and identification in infected brain tissue of rabies virus antigen, of specific inclusions (Negri bodies); or of viral nucleic acid by the reverse transcriptase polymerase chain reaction (RT-PCR)[61]; on the presence of antibodies in the CSF; and on the isolation and identification of the virus from brain tissue or saliva. The standard diagnostic technique is to search for rabies antigen in brain by fluorescent antibody staining or by enzyme-linked immunosorbent assay. The thalamus provides the best samples.[62] Identification of viral nucleic acid by dot-blot hybridization or by RT-PCR is useful, particularly if specimens are in poor condition. Demonstration of Negri bodies has a variable sensitivity and is of only historical interest, whereas virus isolation is a procedure used for confirmation of other positive test results. Isolation can be accomplished in tissue culture or by intracerebral inoculation of suckling mice.[63] Although diagnostic procedures generally are initiated in tissue specimens collected post mortem, rabies infection also can be identified in vivo during the extended course of the disease. In those cases, the fluorescent antibody staining technique enables detection of viral antigen in impressions of cornea or in cryoscopic sections of skin biopsy samples from the hairline of the neck, where antigen can be detected in the nerves surrounding the hair follicles.[64]

In addition, as shown in Table 37–1, RT-PCR on saliva provides a rapid and sensitive test for rabies as early as 5 days after onset of symptoms.[65,66] Improved sensitivity was obtained when an RNA polymerase was included in the reaction and electrochemiluminescence was used for detection of product. This technique, called nucleic acid–based sequence amplification, detected the rabies genome in saliva, urine, and CSF as early as 2 or 3 days after symptoms.[67,68] Serial tests should be performed to increase sensitivity.[68] A latex agglutination test for viral antigen in dog saliva also has been developed.[69]

Between 1980 and 1996, 32 cases of rabies were diagnosed in the United States, but only 20 were diagnosed

TABLE 37–1 ■ Antemortem Diagnostic Test Results for 20 Human Patients with Rabies in the United States, 1980–1996*

Test	No. of Patients Positive for Rabies Virus/Total No. Tested (%)		Earliest Positive Result, Day of Illness
RT-PCR of saliva for rabies RNA	10/10	(100)	5
Rabies antigen in brain biopsy	3/3	(100)	8
Rabies antigen in nuchal skin	10/15†	(67)	5
Virus isolation from saliva	9/15‡	(60)	5
Serum antibody to rabies	10/18	(56)	5§
Rabies antigen in cornea	2/8	(25)	14
CSF antibody to rabies	2/13	(15)	15‖

*Data are from reverse transcriptase studies.
†Two patients had earlier skin biopsies that were negative, but became positive on subsequent biopsy.
‡One patient had an earlier test that was negative.
§Latest negative result on day 24; median to positive result was 10 days.
‖Latest negative result on day 24.
CSF, cerebrospinal fluid; RT-PCR, reverse transcriptase–polymerase chain reaction.
Data from Noah DL, Drenzek CL, Smith JS, et al. Epidemiology of human rabies in the United States, 1980 to 1996. Ann Intern Med 128:922–930, 1998.

before death, probably because only 7 had a known history of exposure to potentially rabid animals. This problem arose in large part because most of the patients had been infected with rabies virus variants from bats, presumably as a result of undocumented bat bites.[70]

Epizootiology and Epidemiology

Animals

Mammals

Rabies is a disease of both domestic and wild mammals, particularly dogs and related species, raccoons, mongooses, skunks, and bats. In areas in which animal control programs are not extensively developed, dogs and cats account for most of the rabid animals reported and cause the majority (90%) of human rabies exposures. After effective domestic animal rabies control programs in these areas, the numbers of rabid dogs and cats markedly decrease, as illustrated in the United States from the 1940s to the 1960s. Wildlife are then recognized as the main reservoir of rabies virus. In the United States since 1960, the majority of cases of animal rabies has been in wildlife species, and most of the human rabies cases have been secondary to bites by rabid wildlife, including bats.[12,71] Curiously, bats do not often transmit virus to dogs or cats.[72] The situation is similar in western Europe, where domestic species accounted for only 28% of 8155 reported rabid animals. Of the wild species, foxes accounted for 83% and raccoon dogs 11%.[73]

Figure 37–1 is a composite map of the United States showing the terrestrial animal reservoirs present in each region.[74,75] The salient features are that skunks are the important vectors for rabies in the western and central United States, whereas raccoon rabies exists in the east. The original focus of raccoon rabies was in the southeast, but a second developed in the northeast owing to importation of animals, and now raccoon rabies is contiguous from Maine to Florida and west to Ohio.[76] Foci of fox rabies are evident in the eastern states bordering Canada and in Alaska. Rabies control is costly: in New York State alone

the cost of rabies prevention in humans was calculated to be $2.3 million per year.[76a] Table 37–2 lists rabies cases by species for the United States in 2000.[75]

Table 37–3 lists the principal animal vectors of rabies throughout the world.[66] In western Europe foxes account for up to 80% of rabid animals.[77] Molecular analysis of European strains shows that rabies originated in dogs, but has since jumped to red foxes and raccoon dogs.[78] Infection in the latter animals has gradually spread from east to west. Canine rabies is still widespread in Asia, Africa, and parts of Latin America. However, vaccination of pet dogs can be an effective strategy for protection of humans and has eliminated terrestrial rabies in Great Britain, Iceland, Western Europe, Australia, Japan, and many other islands, as, for example, in the Caribbean and Oceania.[47,79] An immunization coverage of 60% to 70% is estimated to prevent canine rabies outbreaks.[80]

Foxes are important vectors in Canada, Alaska, and the former Union of Soviet Socialist Republics. Mongooses

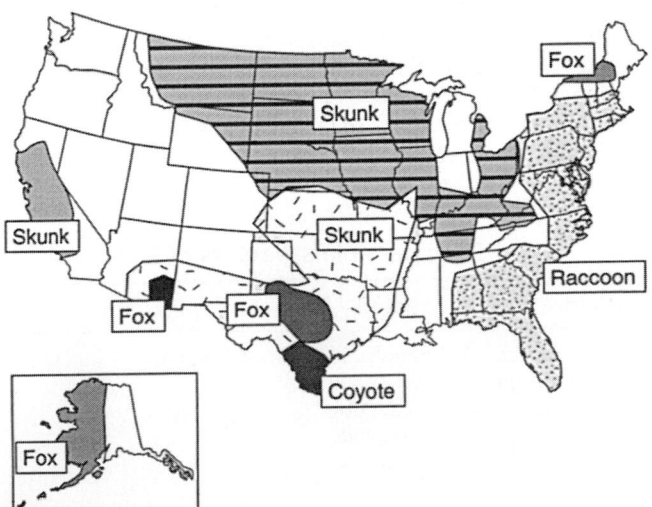

FIGURE 37–1 ■ Distribution of major terrestrial reservoirs of rabies in the United States.

TABLE 37–2 ■ Cases of Animal Rabies in the United States, 2001

	Number	Percent
WILD		
Raccoons	2787	37
Skunks	2282	31
Bats	1281	17
Foxes	432	6
Rodents/lagomorphs	56	0.8
Other	116	1.6
TOTAL	6939	93
DOMESTIC		
Cats	270	7.6
Dogs	89	1.2
Cattle	82	1.1
Horses/mules	51	0.9
Sheep/goats	3	0.04
Swine	2	0.03
Other	0	0.0
TOTAL	497	7

From Krebs JW, Noll HR, Rupprecht CE, Childs JE. Rabies surveillance in the United States during 2001. J Am Vet Med Assoc 221: 1690–1701, 2002, with permission.

imported into the Caribbean Islands now form a reservoir for rabies, and that animal plays the same role in southern Africa. The vampire bat is a major threat to cattle in Latin America and has been involved in many biting incidents in humans. Rabid cattle also may excrete rabies virus in saliva.[81] Like all mammals, rodents, squirrels, and voles are susceptible to infection[47] but are infrequently rabid, and human transmission of disease by these animals has not resulted. In Thailand, an Asian country in which rabies has been extensively studied, 95% of the animals involved in biting incidents are dogs, often less than 6 months of age,[82] with cats accounting for another 3%. The remaining 2% include monkeys, civets, tigers, and other animals, which testifies to the high infectiousness of rabies virus. Dogs randomly captured in Thailand developed rabies within 1 month in 3% to 4% of cases, and, interestingly, there was serologic evidence of prior rabies infection in 15% to 20% of dogs.[83]

Rabies in terrestrial animals (excluding bats) is now absent in many islands such as the United Kingdom, Australia, and Japan. Much of western Europe is also now rabies free, though rabies still occurs in central and eastern Europe, including

TABLE 37–3 ■ Principal Animal Vectors of Rabies

Location	Vectors
North America	Skunks, raccoons, foxes, bats
Western Europe	Foxes, bats
Eastern Europe	Foxes, dogs
Latin America	Dogs, bats
Caribbean	Mongooses
Africa	Dogs, jackals, mongooses, foxes
Asia	Dogs, cats, monkeys, mongooses, and arctic foxes

Germany. Most of the large Asian countries, Africa, the former Soviet Union, and large parts of South America still report considerable rabies in domestic animals.

Travelers are at risk, as confirmed by the report of seven cases of rabies in the United States acquired abroad between 1990 and 2001.[75] The risk of rabies exposure in Nepal was calculated to be 5.7 per 1000 person-years for expatriates and 1.9 per 1000 person-years for tourists.[84] The epidemiology of rabies has been revolutionized by the development of monoclonal antibodies.[85] Panels of these antibodies, directed against epitopes specific to isolates from different animal species and from different geographic locations, are used to identify viruses. Thus it is now possible to identify an isolate from humans or animals as to the source and to demonstrate that the infection was transmitted far away in time and place. Sequencing of the viral genome after RT-PCR amplification has supplemented our knowledge of strain variability.[86] Vaccine strains differ in sequence from wild strains by as much as 10% to 15% of nucleotides. Sequence data suggest that some strains in the Western Hemisphere and in South Africa were imported from Europe.[87,88]

Bats

Bats are not incidental vectors of rabies virus, but rather probably the original host of the virus, which in some distant past developed epizootiologic cycles in mammals.[24] Widespread infection of insectivorous bats throughout the United States was well documented in the 1950s. However, the importance of bat rabies, particularly from the silver-haired bat *Lasionycteris noctivagans*, to human transmission has become evident (see *Human Rabies* below) The eastern pipistrelle bat (*Pipistrellus subflavus*) is important in the East and Midwest. Although rabid bats are more likely to attack people,[89] an infected bat may act normally.[90,91] Moreover, infected bats may survive but continue to excrete virus.[91a] The rabies virus recovered from the silver-haired bat is a variant that appears to be able to replicate better in epidermal tissues.[92]

Although neutralizing titers are not always raised in humans against rabies-related viruses carried by bats,[43] there is good cross-neutralization of bat rabies virus strains by standard cell culture vaccines (CCVs).[93]

Nonbite Transmission

Nonbite transmission has been reviewed by Gibbons,[94] who found 27 well-documented cases of transmission by means other than bites, and 17 other less well-documented cases. Of the total 44 cases, 18 were caused by improperly inactivated vaccine in Brazil, 8 from corneal transplants, 8 from contamination of skin whose integrity had been impaired, 4 by aerosols created in laboratory or bat-infested caves, and 6 from human to human. Among the alleged causes of human-to-human transmission were transplacental passage, lactation, kissing, intercourse, and providing health care. Gibbons[94] also found three reports of transmission by human bites.

Aside from direct animal contact, aerosol and direct implantation of infected tissue may transmit rabies to humans. Infection by aerosol has been suspected in caves inhabited by millions of bats, and under laboratory conditions.[12,95] Unwitting corneal transplantation from patients deceased from rabies also has resulted in transmission.[12,96] Human-to-human transmission by bite is extremely rare, but transmission has been reported after kissing, intercourse, and maternal rabies.[94,97,98]

Human Rabies

The epidemiology of human rabies closely follows the epizootiology of animal rabies. The dog is the major global reservoir of rabies. In the United States alone, a million dog bites occur each year,[99] and the situation is worse in some other parts of the world.[100] Human rabies has been reported from all continents except Antarctica, but the majority of cases occur in countries where canine rabies is not well controlled. The World Health Organization (WHO) estimate of humans vaccinated for exposure to rabies exceeds 10 million annually.[101] The WHO also estimated between 35,000 and 50,000 human rabies cases in 1997, most of them in India.[102] The annual incidence of rabies deaths per 100,000 population has been calculated as 3 in India, 0.01 to 0.2 in Latin America, and an uncertain 0.0001 to 13 in Africa, respectively.[97] Human rabies is most common in people younger than 15 years, with about 40% of cases found in children 5 to 14 years, but all age groups are susceptible. The majority of rabies victims are male. In the United States, the highest incidence of human rabies postexposure prophylaxis occurs among rural boys, primarily during the summer months.[103]

In the United States, the recent salient fact has been the emergence of bats as the leading transmitter to humans. Between 1983 and 2000, bat-related variants were identified in 26 of 28 diagnosed human rabies cases of domestic origin.[104] There were also 12 imported cases during the same period. In 2000 there were five human rabies cases, four of which were from bats.[105] No history of contact with bats could be elicited in the majority of cases, and only two gave a definite history of a bite, suggesting that unperceived bites in sleeping individuals may have been responsible.[106–108] A similar situation exists in Canada.[98]

Passive Immunization

Antiserum alone will not prevent rabies and is not recommended except in combination with vaccine (see under *Serum and Vaccine Treatment* below).

Active Immunization

Prior Approaches

Table 37–4 summarizes the history of the development of rabies vaccines and lists currently available vaccines. Many different strains have been used for preparation of rabies vaccines. The history of some of these strains is given in Figure 37–2.

TABLE 37–4 ■ Important Past and Present Rabies Vaccines for Humans

Vaccine Name	Manufacturer	Type	Substrate	Remarks	Where Used
NERVE TISSUE					
Pasteur	None	Inactivated by drying	Rabbit spinal cord	Residual live virus	NLU
Fermi	None	Phenolized live virus	Sheep, goat, or rabbit brains	Contained nerve tissue, residual live virus?	NLU
Semple	Many	Phenol inactivated	Sheep, goat, or rabbit brains	Contains nerve tissue	Asia, Africa
Fuenzalida	Many	Inactivated	Suckling mouse brain	Decreased myelin content	South America
AVIAN					
PDEV	Berna	β-Propiolactone inactivated	Duck embryo	Purified by ultracentrifugation	Europe, ROW
DEV	None	Inactivated	Duck embryo	Allergy to avian antigens	NLU
CELL CULTURE					
HDCV	PMC, Berna, Chiron Behring	β-Propiolactone inactivated	Human cultured fibroblasts	Expensive, world standard for rabies vaccine	United States, Europe ROW
RVA	Michigan	β-Propiolactone inactivated	Fetal rhesus cell culture	Fewer allergic reactions	United States
PHKCV	Local	Formalin inactivated	Primary Syrian hamster kidney cell culture	Used in People's Republic of China	China, Russia
PCECV	Chiron Behring	β-Propiolactone inactivated	Chick embryo cell culture	Purified by ultracentrifugation	Germany, United States, ROW
PVRV	PMC	β-Propiolactone inactivated	Vero cell line	Purified by ultracentrifugation	France, ROW

Abbreviations for vaccines listed here are those used in the text. NLU, no longer used; ROW, rest of world; PMC, Pasteur Mérieux–Connaught.

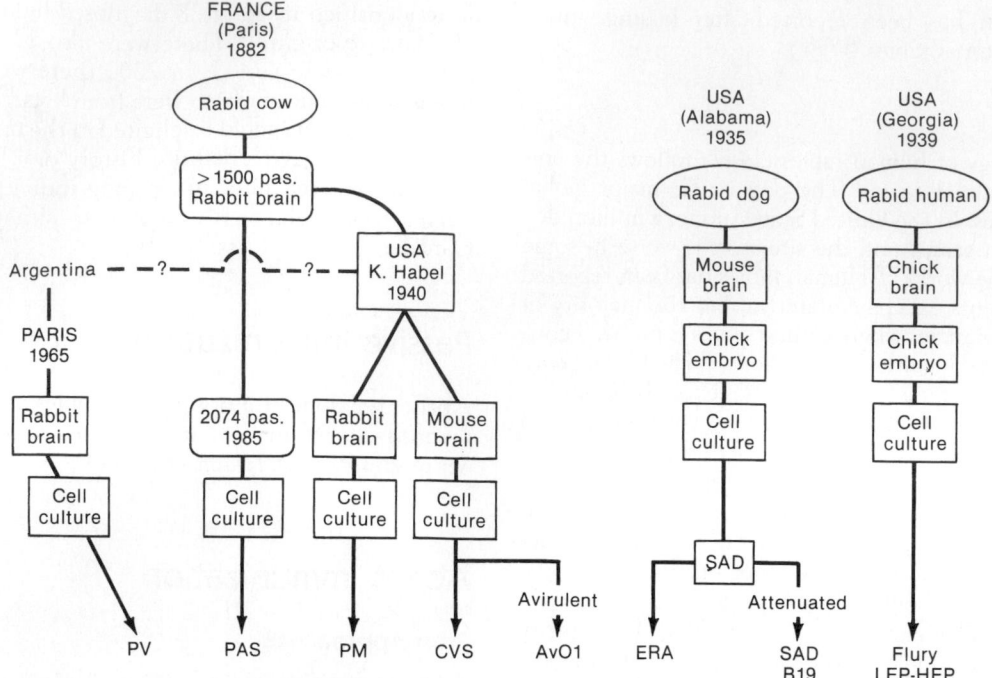

FIGURE 37–2 ▪ History of strains of rabies virus used as vaccine seeds. (From Sacramento D, Badrane H, Bourhy H, Tordo N. Molecular epidemiology of rabies virus in France: comparison with vaccine strains. J Gen Virol 73:1149–1158, 1992, with permission.)

For more than 70 years after Pasteur's original work, only vaccines containing nerve tissue were available. Major modifications in nerve tissue vaccine preparation were introduced by Fermi[109] and by Semple,[110] who used phenol to partially or completely inactivate virus. Adverse reactions to rabies vaccines containing brain tissue have been recognized since the time of Pasteur. In addition to neurologic complications attributed to the presence of myelinated tissue in the vaccine, fixed virus may be pathogenic for humans, contrary to the "Pasteurian dogma," although it took 75 years before it was proved that some cases of paralysis after vaccination were caused by imperfectly inactivated vaccine virus.

Myelin-free vaccines prepared from neonatal mouse brains were introduced by Fuenzalida and colleagues[111] in 1956 and are still widely used in South America and the former Soviet Union. Introduction of the duck embryo vaccine (DEV), prepared from virus propagated in embryonated duck eggs,[112] greatly reduced the number and severity of postvaccinal reactions; however, DEV was less immunogenic than the brain tissue vaccine. Fourteen to 23 daily inoculations were recommended for both these vaccines, but even this "heroic" dosage did not always protect against rabies after severe exposure. Thus there had long been a pressing need for a highly immunogenic antirabies vaccine that could be used safely and effectively at low doses, both for primary immunization and for treatment after exposure.

Cell Culture Rabies Vaccines

The solution to the problem of safety of rabies vaccines lay in the development of vaccines prepared from rabies virus grown in tissue culture free of neuronal tissue. The first attempts to develop a tissue culture vaccine were made by Kissling[113] in 1958 and by Fenje[114] in 1960. Both investigators used the primary hamster kidney cell for rabies virus production.

Human Diploid Cell Vaccine

In the early 1960s, workers at the Wistar Institute in Philadelphia selected the human diploid cell strain WI-38 for virus propagation to avoid the difficulties inherent in the use of primary tissue cultures, such as induction of allergy to animal proteins.[115,116] The vaccine thus developed, the human diploid cell vaccine (HDCV), containing concentrated and purified virus, evoked much better immune responses in experimental animals and in humans than did DEV, suckling brain, or adult brain tissue vaccines.[117,118] The technical advances leading to the development of the vaccine included the adaptation of the Pitman-Moore strain of virus to WI-38 cells,[119] the inactivation of cell-free virus by β-propiolactone, and the concentration of virus by ultrafiltration.[120]

Currently, HDCV is produced in MRC-5 human fibroblasts that are inoculated with the Pitman-Moore L503 3M strain. Virus-containing supernatants are harvested and concentrated 10 to 20 times by ultrafiltration or ultracentrifugation, reaching a titer of about 10^7 median lethal dose/mL before inactivation, which is done with 1:4000 β-propiolactone. Potency is assessed by the National Institutes of Health (NIH) test in mouse brain and is at least 2.5 IU/dose.

After 4 years of clinical studies in volunteers,[121] the vaccine was used in humans exposed to severe wounds by rabid dogs and wolves in Iran. All vaccinated people developed VNAs, survived, and remained free of rabies.[122] HDCV was first licensed in Europe for pre-exposure and postexposure immunization of humans in 1976. HDCV was licensed in the United States in June 1980. The results of 5 years of clinical experience in the United States with no failures to prevent rabies were summarized by Winkler.[123] An estimated 85% of doses are used for pre-exposure immunization and booster doses for maintenance of antibody; 15% are for postexposure immunization. It is estimated that more than 1.5 million people have been treated throughout the world.

HDCV is basically the concentrated supernatant of MRC-5 human embryo fibroblast cell cultures infected with rabies virus. Each dose of the vaccine sold in the United States contains rabies virus inactivated by β-propiolactone, 5% human albumin, phenolsulfonphthalein, and neomycin sulfate (<150 μg) as an antibiotic. The vaccine is lyophilized to a powder form and reconstituted in sterile water. The rabies antigen content is at least 2.5 IU/dose. The vaccine contains no preservative or stabilizer.

HDCV was formerly produced in the United States by Wyeth Laboratories, with use of N-tributylphosphate as the inactivating agent. As of 1984, all vaccine sold in the United States is manufactured by Aventis Pasteur (Lyon, France) according to the method above. Aventis Pasteur in Canada also produces an HDCV based on the Evelyn-Rokitnicki-Abelseth (ERA) strain of rabies virus. In Europe, Chiron Behring (Marburg, Germany) produces HDCV from the Pitman-Moore strain. Neither of the latter two HDCVs contains human albumin or phenolsulfonphthalein (See the section "Allergic Reactions").

Ideal storage conditions are 2° to 8°C, at which temperatures the vaccine is stable for at least 3.5 years.[124] However, vaccine stored for 1 month at 37°C was still potent.[125,126]

Vero Cell Vaccine

There have been intense efforts worldwide to produce vaccines at a lower cost that meet or improve on the levels of safety and efficacy achieved with HDCV. These new tissue culture vaccines are listed in Table 37–4. All CCVs must have a potency of at least 2.5 IU/dose as measured by the NIH test.

A continuous African green monkey kidney cell line, called *Vero*, has come into use as a cell substrate for viral vaccines, and a new *purified Vero cell culture rabies vaccine* (PVRV) based on growth of virus in that cell line has been developed and licensed by Aventis Pasteur in Europe and in many countries in the developing world.[127] An advantage of the Vero cell is that it can be grown and infected on microcarrier beads and cultivated in fermenters to produce large volumes of tissue culture fluid containing rabies virus.

The rabies virus strain in PVRV is the same as that used for HDCV production. It is inactivated with β-propiolactone and concentrated and purified by zonal centrifugation and ultrafiltration. Clinical studies have shown that the VNA responses after primary and booster injections are equivalent to those seen after pre-exposure or postexposure treatment with HDCV.[128] Postexposure protection after severe exposures has been demonstrated in Thailand[129] and China,[130] without unusual adverse reactions.

A *chromatographically purified Vero cell culture rabies vaccine* (CPRV) has been developed to reduce cellular DNA and foreign protein content. This vaccine is well tolerated and highly immunogenic, although slightly less so than HDCV, as shown in Table 37–5.[131–134] CPRV was used successfully in the Philippines to protect against severe rabies exposures.[135]

Chick Embryo Cell Culture

Purified chick embryo cell culture vaccine (PCECV), prepared by Chiron Behring, has been evaluated together with HDCV in postexposure protection of animals and humans.[136–139] No significant differences in protection between the two vaccines were observed. To prepare PCECV, the Flury low egg passage (LEP)-C25 strain is grown in primary chick embryo fibroblasts. The virus is inactivated by 0.025% β-propiolactone and then concentrated and purified by density gradient centrifugation. The lyophilized vaccine contains processed gelatin as stabilizer and traces of neomycin, chlortetracycline, and amphotericin B. PCECV is now registered worldwide, including in the United States, and about 20 million doses have been used. Reconstitution studies have shown that the rehydrated vaccine is stable for at least 1 week in the refrigerator.[140]

PCECV has been tested extensively in Croatia[141] and India.[142] Over a 10-year experience with PCECV in India, the vaccine was well tolerated, with only 4% of 1375 people reporting reactions, although some urticarial reactions have been seen.[143] Immunogenicity was also good, with geometric mean titers (GMTs) of neutralizing antibodies after postexposure treatment of about 4 IU and of less than 1 IU in only 0.9% of patients. A comparative study with

TABLE 37–5 ■ Geometric Mean RFFIT Titers (GMT) and Seroconversion After Primary Immunization with a Five-Dose Series of HDCV or CPRV and HRIG Administered on Day 0

Days After First Dose	CPRV (n = 18)		HDCV (n = 124)	
	GMT (IU/mL)	% Seropositive	GMT (IU/mL)	% Seropositive
0	0.025	0	0.025	0
7	0.17	1.7	0.18	4.03
14	6.9	100	10.3	100
28	14.6	100	20.5	100
42	16.9	100	29.4	100
90	7.8	100	15.4	100
180	3.4	98.3	7.2	99.2
365	1.6	92.2	3.7	98.3

RFFIT, rapid fluorescent focus inhibition test; CPRV, chromatically purified vero cell culture rabies vaccine; HRIG, human rabies immune globulin.
From Jones RL, Froeschle JE, Atmar RL, et al. Immunogenicity, safety and lot consitency in adults of a chromatographically purified Vero-cell rabies vaccine: a randomized, double-blind trial with human diploid cell rabies vaccine. Vaccine 19:4635–4643, 2001, with permission.

TABLE 37–6 ■ Rabies GMT in Humans After Intramuscular HDCV or PCECV

Day	HDCV	PCECV
0	<0.05 (n = 79)	<0.05 (n = 82)
28	12.0 (n = 79)	9.3 (n = 82)
49	25.8 (n = 79)	25.3 (n = 82)
387 (–3)	1.49 (n = 69)	2.92 (n = 67)

n, number of subjects.

From Briggs DJ, Dreeson DW, Nicolay U, et al. Purified Chick Embryo Cell Culture Rabies Vaccine: interchangeability with Human Diploid Cell Culture Rabies Vaccine and comparison of one- versus two-dose post-exposure booster regimen for previously immunized persons. Vaccine 19:1055–1060, 2000, with permission.

HDCV showed titers after PCECV to be slightly lower at 28 days after simulated exposure, but equal titers at 49 days, as shown in Table 37–6.[144]

PCECV is licensed in the United States under the trade name RabAvert®. Although not licensed for intradermal use in the United States, it is used by that route elsewhere (see *Schedules Employing the Intradermal Route* below). A similar type of vaccine (Flury high egg passage [HEP] strain) is produced in Japan with limited distribution.[145] PCECV vaccinees develop a positive skin test against yellow fever vaccine, probably because of chicken protein common to both vaccines, and the two should be administered with caution in egg-allergic patients.[146]

Hamster Kidney

Primary hamster kidney cell culture vaccine (PHKCV) is produced by the Institute of Poliomyelitis and Virus Encephalitides, Moscow, and by several institutes in China, including the Wuhan Institute of Biological Products. PHKCV was approved for use in China in 1980, where it has completely replaced the Semple-type rabies vaccine. The Chinese vaccine contains the Beijing strain, which is inactivated by formalin. The final material contains 0.01% thimerosal, 10 mg human albumin, and aluminum hydroxide. The vaccine is supplied as a freeze-dried concentrate and is administered on a five- or six-dose schedule in China.[147] PHKCV is reportedly well tolerated and protective against proven rabies exposures.[148]

Duck Embryo

The Swiss Serum and Vaccine Institute, Bern, introduced a *purified DEV (PDEV)* that uses the Pitman-Moore strain. No duck protein is detectable by immunodiffusion test. Concentration is achieved by density gradient ultracentrifugation. The virus is inactivated by β-propiolactone, and thimerosal is added as a preservative. Antigenic potency and antibody responses evoked in humans are comparable to those of HDCV.[149] Mild local reactions are noted that occur only slightly more frequently than with HDCV. PDEV differs from other CCVs in that, after reconstitution, it is a slightly turbid suspension. Its nucleoprotein content is higher than that of other vaccines.[150] If it is used intradermally, the dose must be 0.2 mL.[151,152]

Recently, production of PDEV has been transferred to Cadila Health Ltd., an Indian manufacturer.

Fetal Rhesus Lung

To provide an alternative to vaccine made in human cells, the Michigan State Health Department (now called Bioport) prepared a rhesus diploid cell culture vaccine (RVA). The Kissling-CVS rabies strain was adapted to DBS-FRHL-2 cell cultures (a fetal rhesus monkey lung fibroblast), inactivated with β-propiolactone, and then adjuvanted with alum phosphate.[153,154] It is given on the same pre-exposure schedules as HDCV and is considered to be equally safe and effective.[155] RVA is licensed in the United States and was once distributed by GlaxoSmithKline, but is now expected to be distributed by Bioport.

Despite the aforementioned developments, CCVs are still used far less throughout the world than are nerve tissue vaccines. For development of an even less expensive rabies vaccine, a baby hamster kidney cell line (BHK-21) is under study as a vaccine substrate.[156]

Immunization Schedules (Table 37–7)

Pre-exposure

The recommended pre-exposure immunization regimen in the United States is three doses of HDCV, RVA, or PCECV on days 0, 7, and 21 or 28. The dose is 1 mL administered intramuscularly (see *Schedules Employing the Intradermal Route* below). More than 50,000 people have received rabies pre-exposure immunization with HDCV in the United States; there have been no rabies cases in any of these individuals.

An attempt was made to use suckling mouse brain vaccine in a pre-exposure schedule of 0, 2, 4, and 30 days, but the results were unsatisfactory.[157]

Postexposure

The postexposure regimen recommended in the United States and by the WHO is rabies immune globulin (RIG) on day 0 and a cell culture vaccine on each of days 0, 3, 7, 14, and 28; 1 mL of vaccine is administered intramuscularly in the deltoid area only.[158] In Europe, a sixth dose used to be recommended at 90 days, but the sixth dose may not substantially raise titers beyond those obtained after five doses.[159]

Those who have received prior pre-exposure or postexposure treatment with a CCV, or who have proven VNAs to rabies after other vaccines, should receive an intramuscular injection on each of days 0 and 3, without RIG. Anamnestic responses are excellent.[157] Those who have received a nerve tissue vaccine without a documented VNA response must undergo the full postexposure regimen.

Alternative Vaccine Schedules

The application of rabies vaccination faces several practical problems, particularly in developing countries. These include the cost of the vaccine, the cost and the unavailability of antiserum, and the difficulty in getting patients to return a sufficient number of times to complete the series of injections. Therefore, alternative schedules have been suggested to decrease the number of visits, and the intradermal route rather than the intramuscular route of injection has been used to decrease the volume of vaccine and therefore the cost.

TABLE 37–7 ■ Regimens for Pre-Exposure and Postexposure Vaccination with Rabies Vaccines

Vaccination	Route	Days on Which Doses Are Given	Remarks
Pre-exposure	IM[†]	0, 7, 21, or 28	Standard U.S. regimen
	ID[‡]	0, 7, 21, or 28	Economical, but not to be used in those taking antimalarial medications. Unlicensed route in U.S.
Postexposure[*]	IM[†]	0, 3, 7, 14, 28	U.S. and WHO recommendation
	IM[†]	0 (2 doses), 7, 21	Used in some countries when RIG not indicated
		0, 3, 7 (2 doses each), 28, 90	Used in Thailand with PVRV, PCEC, or HDCV
	ID[‡]	0 (8 doses), 7 (4 doses), 28, 90	Used in developing countries with HDCV, PCEC, or PVRV cell culture vaccines
	ID[‡§]		
Booster	IM[†]	0, 3	Only after documented vaccination with cell culture vaccine[*‖]
(for re-exposure)	ID[‡]	0, 3	Only after documented vaccination with cell culture vaccine[*‖]

[*]Together with rabies immune globulin.
[†]Give 0.5 mL (PVRV) or 1.0 mL, depending on the vaccine, into the deltoid.
[‡]Give 0.1 or 0.2 mL, depending on the vaccine, over the deltoids.
[§]Give 0.1 mL at multiple sites (see text).
[*‖]Or demonstrated presence of VNAs after other vaccines.
ID, intradermal; IM, intramuscular.

SCHEDULES WITH FEWER VISITS

An alternative schedule developed in Yugoslavia and also extensively used in France is designated 2-1-1.[160,161] It consists of two injections of 1.0 mL intramuscularly on day 0 and one each on days 7 and 21. Suckling mouse brain vaccine also has been successfully employed according to this schedule.[162] However, if passive immunization is simultaneously given, some reports[163–165] show that the average antibody response and the persistence of antibody are compromised, whereas other reports[166,167] show no interference. Immunosuppression by human rabies immune globulin (HRIG) appears to be absent when HDCV is the vaccine used in the 2-1-1 schedule. However, a failure of the 2-1-1 schedule after a bite on the lip has been reported,[168] and in our opinion the use of the 2-1-1 schedule is best restricted to mild exposures and situations where patient compliance is poor.

SCHEDULES EMPLOYING THE INTRADERMAL ROUTE

The expense of a full regimen of intramuscular HDCV (about $600 in the United States for a five-dose regimen) led to attempts to reduce the cost by taking advantage of the intradermal route. Aoki, Turner, Nicholson, and their colleagues demonstrated that rapid antibody responses could be induced by various intradermal regimens, including multisite postexposure inoculations.[169–171] Although injection by the intramuscular and subcutaneous routes results in higher titers, intradermal administration for pre-exposure or booster vaccinations appears to be adequate.[99,172] Two intradermal doses of 0.1 mL successfully boosted titers in those previously given DEV.[99,173]

Intradermal postexposure regimens have now undergone extensive evaluations and are indicated in the circumstances of insufficient vaccine, insufficient funds, and the availability of staff experienced in intradermal injection technique.[174,175] The vaccines that may be used by this route are HDCV, PVRV, PCECV, and PDEV. The antigenic content of the rehydrated vaccine should always be at least 0.25 IU/0.1 mL. The injection should be given with use of a 1.0-mL syringe and a 25- or 27-gauge needle, with the needle introduced parallel to the skin into the epidermal layer. A papule should always be produced at the site of the injection.[176]

For *pre-exposure* immunization, three doses are necessary.[126] Intradermal injection has been widely used to immunize veterinary students and others at high risk of rabies exposure. Antibody titers are lower after intradermal than after intramuscular inoculation but still adequate (Fig. 37 3). Local reactions are annoying but tolerable after intradermal vaccination, and systemic reactions are virtually absent. However, the death in Kenya in 1983 of a Peace Corps volunteer who had been preimmunized with HDCV by the intradermal regimen raised questions regarding the efficacy of this route.[177] Intensive review of immunization records revealed that people vaccinated overseas, whether intramuscularly or intradermally, often had lower and shorter lived antibody responses than expected from observations made in people immunized in the United States. One factor shown to be significantly associated with lower immunologic responses is the concurrent administration of

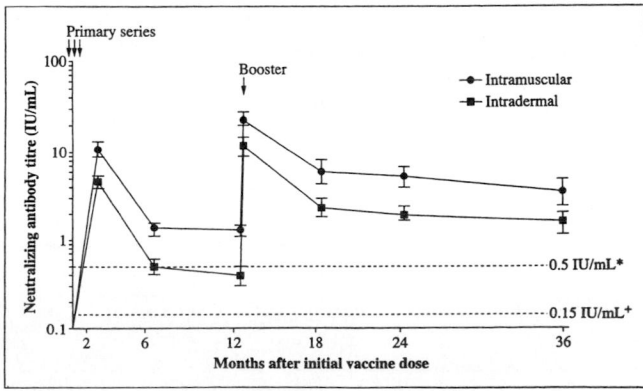

FIGURE 37–3 ■ Kinetics of neutralizing antibody response to purified Vero-cell rabies vaccine after two regimens of primary and booster pre-exposure immunization given intradermally or intramuscularly. *Minimally adequate titers defined by the World Health Organization. +Minimally adequate titers defined by the Centers for Disease Control and Prevention.

chloroquine for antimalarial chemoprophylaxis.[128] People receiving concurrent antimalarial chemoprophylaxis or other immunogens are now recommended to receive the intramuscular and not the intradermal regimen for antirabies pre-exposure immunization. Moreover, those who receive an intradermal pre-exposure regimen in developing countries should have titers checked after immunization.[178] The situation in the United States is now complicated by the removal of the intradermal formulation from the market. Whereas 0.1-mL intradermal doses can be withdrawn from vials containing the 1.0-mL intramuscular dose, this is an off-label use justified only when there are numerous persons to vaccinate on the same day.

However, *postexposure* intradermal immunization using vaccine from intramuscular vials is licensed in Thailand and is used in developing countries to make CCVs more readily available for rabies exposures. Warrell and colleagues[179,180] developed the concept of multiple intradermal vaccinations. In their scheme, which is often used in India, HDCV or PCECV is given intradermally at eight different sites (deltoid, suprascapular, thigh, and abdominal wall on day 0; four 0.1-mL doses over the deltoid and thigh on day 7; and single doses over the deltoid on days 28 and 91).[180a] However, antibodies are not induced any more rapidly by this regimen than by others, and concomitant antiserum is still indicated.[180b] Phanuphak and associates[181] developed another intradermal schedule that is now the standard regimen used in Thailand. PVRV, PCECV, or PDEV is given over both deltoids in a volume of 0.1 or 0.2 mL on days 0, 3, and 7, followed by single injections on days 30 and 90. The volume of injection in the Thai regimen is decided by the volume of reconstitution: 0.1 mL from a 0.5-mL vial (in practice, this is PVRV) and 0.2 mL from a 1.0-mL vial.[174] The two intradermal regimens were compared in India, where the eight-site regimen induced higher antibody titers, particularly at 7 days.[182] Intradermal vaccination is considerably less expensive than the full intramuscular use of HDCV and has been demonstrated to be protective in Thailand.[83,181,183,184] In Thai practice the vaccine is sometimes reconstituted and stored for a week under refrigeration in order to use the same vial for the first three injections of vaccine. So far, this practice has not resulted in treatment failures.[184a]

Neutralizing responses after intradermal vaccination with HDCV or PVRV were compared in Thailand.[183] All vaccinees in both groups were seropositive at day 14, whereas at day 90, adequate VNA levels were found in 95%

of PVRV recipients and 96% of HDCV recipients. A comparison of intradermal PVRV or PCECV with intramuscular PCECV showed no important differences in antibody responses (Table 37-8).[185] In addition, Thai workers simulated two-dose postexposure booster vaccination in subjects previously vaccinated intradermally or intramuscularly with PVRV. The subjects vaccinated and boosted intradermally all developed anamnestic responses, although these were slower and of lower magnitude than in the all-intramuscular group.[186] Conversely, a booster study done with a four-site intradermal regimen showed higher titers than after intramuscular immunization.[187]

Using the Thai regimen, PDEV was shown to be immunogenic by the intradermal route if the intradermal dose was 0.2 mL, as shown in Table 37-9.[151] PDEV given by either intramuscular or intradermal routes was studied in the Philippines.[186] By day 90, 94% of the intradermal vaccinees and 98% of the intramuscular vaccinees had antibodies above 0.5 IU, and the GMTs were about 3 IU in both groups.

PCECV was also studied in Thailand,[188] both with and without concomitant administration of HRIG. Neutralizing antibodies peaked at a GMT of about 10 IU in both groups, and there were no failures. About 40 patients exposed to rabies were all protected by PCECV. Thai workers keep the reconstituted vaccine at 4°C for 1 week in order to provide patients with the first three doses from the same vial.[140]

Currently in India, intradermal vaccination is practiced with the four WHO-approved vaccines, enabling a reduction in cost from $81 for the intramuscular regimen to about $13 for an intradermal regimen.[189]

Serum and Vaccine Treatment

The proper postexposure prevention of rabies always includes combined vaccination and passive antibody administration. This is true even when nerve tissue vaccine is employed. The use of antirabies serum in postexposure prophylaxis serum goes back many years; in 1891, Babes and Cerchez[190] treated people severely bitten by rabid wolves with whole blood from vaccinated humans and dogs. In Iran, Baltazard and Ghodssi[191] observed an overall mortality of 25% in patients bitten by confirmed rabid wolves and treated with nerve tissue vaccine, regardless of the severity and site of the wounds. Among individuals wounded in the head and face, mortality was 42%. When these results were compared with mortality rates observed in individuals

TABLE 37-8 ■ Rabies Geometric Mean Virus Neutralization Antibody Titers (GMTs) After Intradermal 2-2-2-0-1-4 Schedule or Intramuscular Postexposure Schedule (0, 3, 7, 14, 30 Days)

| Day | GMT (IU/mL) (range) | | |
	Intradermal PCECV (n = 58)	Intradermal PVRV (n = 59)	Intramuscular PCECV (n = 37)
7	0.34 (0.05–19.1)	0.32 (0.1–2.2)	0.29 (<0.05–19.1)
14	28.5 (1.1–1318.0)	28.9 (1.6–350.0)	12.3 (0.1–301.0)
30	10.9 (1.5–171.0)	10.9 (0.6–157.0)	18.5 (0.5–217.0)
90	3.0 (0.4–59.1)	2.7 (0.5–47.0)	4.7 (0.5–60.9)

From Briggs DJ, Banzhoff A, Nicolay U, et al. Antibody response of patients after postexposure rabies vaccination with small intradermal doses of purified chick embryo cell vaccine or purified Vero cell rabies vaccine. Bull World Health Organ 78:696, 2000, with permission.

TABLE 37–9 ■ Geometric Mean Titers (in IU) of Neutralizing Antibodies After Various Intradermal Regimens

Vaccine	Route*	Schedule†	N	Day 14	Day 28	N <0.5 IU
PDEV	IM	A	15	3.1	4.0	0
PVRV	ID	B	9	11.9	5.2	0
PDEV	ID (0.1 mL)	B	11	2.9	1.4	1
PDEV	ID (0.2 mL)	B	12	2.9	1.5	0
PDEV	ID (0.1 mL)	C	16	4.6	3.2	0
PDEV + ERIG	ID (0.2 mL)	B	15	3.0	1.1	0‡

*ID, intradermal; IM, intramuscular.
†A, one dose on days 0, 3, 7, 14, and 28; B, two doses on days 0, 3, and 7 and one dose on days 28 and 90; C, four doses on days 0, 3, and 7 and one dose on days 28 and 90.
‡One patient was negative at day 90.
Adapted from Khawplod P, Glueck R, Wilde H, et al. Immunogenicity of purified duck embryo rabies vaccine (Lyssavac-N) with use of the WHO; approved intradermal postexposure regimen. Clin Infect Dis 20:646–651, 1995.

exposed to rabid wolves but untreated for various reasons, it appeared that the postexposure treatment of severely exposed individuals with vaccine alone conferred insignificant protection.

The efficacy of the combined use of vaccine and rabies serum to improve these results was established through studies of the WHO Committee on Rabies. The superior results obtained experimentally by Habel and Koprowski[192] were confirmed in a field study in Iran in 1954.[193] Of 5 patients severely bitten by rabid wolves and treated with vaccine alone, 3 contracted rabies and died, whereas of 13 patients similarly bitten by the same wolf and treated with vaccine and serum, only 1 died. Cho and Lawson[194] performed an experiment on postexposure rabies vaccination. When dogs were inoculated in the femoral muscle, vaccine alone was not protective because of the short incubation period in this experimental system, whereas serum alone protected about 50% and serum together with vaccine protected 100%. Baer and Cleary[195] have shown that HRIG has synergistic activity with HDCV in a mouse challenge model. Thus these investigations demonstrated again the importance of rapid protection with antibodies and the synergy of serum with postexposure vaccination.

The intended purpose of RIG is to provide rabies antibody before an active response to the vaccine takes place. Isotyping of antibody after vaccination suggests that immunoglobulin (Ig) G antibody may not appear for 14 days.[149] Evidence that the need for simultaneous RIG and HDCV is not merely theoretical is provided by reports of rabies that occurred after administration of HDCV without RIG.[196,197]

The first commercially available rabies antisera were produced in horses, but approximately 40% of adult recipients developed serum sickness.[198,199] A purified and pepsin-treated equine rabies immune globulin (ERIG) was developed by the Swiss Serum Institute and Aventis Pasteur, and has been widely used in Asia, though not in the United States. It is associated with only a 1% rate of serum sickness reactions,[200] after a recommended dose of 40 IU/kg.

Wilde and co-workers[200,201] in Thailand have carefully studied the use of ERIG. In their experience, the risk of anaphylaxis is only 1 in 35,000 people, and only 1% to 1.6% of recipients develop serum sickness. Moreover, although a skin test with 0.02 mL of a 1:100 dilution of ERIG is rec-

ommended before use, and the response is positive in 5% to 10% of patients, a positive test response was not predictive of serum sickness. They consider a risk of anaphylaxis to be present only if there is a wheal of 10 mm or greater in diameter or if a wheal of 5 to 10 mm is accompanied by a flare of 20 mm or more. To assure safety from contaminating equine viruses, a new heat-treated and more purified ERIG has been developed, which should give fewer reactions.[202,203] Both the old and new ERIG contain F(ab')2 fragments rather than the whole globulin. In the process of substitution of new for old, ERIG supplies have diminished, creating shortages in some areas.[203a]

Human Rabies Immune Globulin was prepared originally by Bayer (formerly Cutter) and Aventis Pasteur from the plasma of volunteers immunized with HDCV to provide an antibody preparation that would not produce serum sickness. Berna, Bayer, and Aventis Behring (formerly Behringwerke AG and Centeon) now also produce an HRIG. The products sold in the United States currently are Imogam® Rabies–HT (Aventis Pasteur) and Bayrab® (Bayer Biological Products). Administration of RIG has not been associated with reactions other than occasional local pain and low-grade fever.[204] The dose is 20 IU/kg, with as much as possible of the volume instilled at the site of the bite, and the remainder, if any, given into the muscle at a distant site. This recommendation is new, because it has been determined (see later) that the VNA level after intramuscular administration of RIG is low and that local administration is therefore preferable. The recommended dose should not be exceeded, because too much passive antibody has a dampening effect on the active antibody responses.[205] For the same reason, the dose should not be repeated. However, if the RIG was not given immediately, it should still be given up to the seventh day after exposure, by which time an active response to vaccination should begin. After administration of HRIG, serum neutralizing antibodies can be detected within 24 hours, reach a level of about 0.1 IU at 3 days, and decay with a half-life of about 21 days.[206] The Thai group also studied patients who were started on vaccine up to 5 days before coming for RIG treatment, and found that this delay was not accompanied by suppression of the active immune response.[207]

Local infiltration of antibodies is crucial because serum levels of VNAs achieved after intramuscular administration alone may be low or negligible.[202,203] Local infiltration provides additional VNAs at the site of contamination with the virus. To have a sufficient volume for infiltration in the case of multiple bites, particularly in children, the RIG can be diluted in normal saline.[207,208] Rabies developed in five children in whom local infiltration was not performed as recommended.[209]

American recommendations now call for the local infiltration of the entire HRIG dose, if feasible. If not, the remainder should be given intramuscularly at a site distant from the vaccine injection. Where HRIG is not available, ERIG in its new chromatographically purified and heat-treated form should be employed.[210]

Results of Immunization

Immune Responses

Although nerve tissue vaccines are not optimal either with regard to safety or efficacy, a well-made Fermi vaccine is immunogenic, as shown in Ethiopia.[210a]

Extensive studies have been conducted of antibody responses to CCVs.[99,118,127–129,132,136–139,142,143,145,147,150–155,162,211–220] The essential points discovered during those studies are as follows:

1. The most important immune response to rabies vaccines is antibodies to the G protein of the viral envelope.[26,211] Antibody is normally measured by neutralization or inhibition of fluorescent foci induced by whole virus.
2. Antibodies appear by 7 to 14 days after the first dose.
3. Vaccine doses given during the first 14 days prime the immune system, but at least one dose at 21 days or later is necessary for high and persistent titers.
4. Three doses of CCV delivered over 21 to 28 days induce antibodies in 100% of individuals and can be used as a pre-exposure regimen.
5. With intramuscular vaccination, the primary regimen for postexposure use is four doses given in the first 2 weeks and a fifth dose given as a booster at day 28 or later.
6. Intradermal regimens use multiple sites (ranging from two to eight), administered on four or five occasions between days 0 and 90.
7. Antibody titers after vaccination with CCV are usually greater than 10 IU, significantly higher than obtained in individuals given nerve tissue vaccine.
8. It is not necessary to check rabies antibody titers after pre-exposure or postexposure immunization with CCV, unless the vaccinee is immunosuppressed (see below), has received chloroquine, or has undergone anesthesia.[221] HIV-infected patients may respond poorly to rabies vaccines[222] and should be monitored serologically.
9. Subjects older than 50 years respond less well than those younger, but all seroconvert after five doses.[223,223a]
10. The place of cellular immunity in protection remains uncertain. Although cellular responses of both the T-helper and the human leukocyte antigen (HLA)-restricted cytotoxic T-cell types clearly are produced, direct proof of a protective function is lacking, whereas antibodies are demonstrably effective.[31,224,225]
11. Vaccinees of HLA groups B7 and Dr2 show early and high antibody responses, whereas those of HLA group Dr3 respond late and with low levels.[150]
12. There is molecular mimicry of the nicotine receptor-binding motif between rabies G protein and human immunodeficiency virus (HIV) glycoprotein 120, which may induce antibodies to HIV in rabies vaccinees.[226,227] False-positive tests for antibodies to HIV have been reported after rabies vaccination,[228,229] but the phenomenon appears to be uncommon.[230]

The typical evolution of antibodies after vaccination is shown in Tables 37–5 and 37–8.[231]

Effectiveness

The efficacy of Semple-type nerve tissue vaccine has been estimated to be about 84% in India,[232] although protection may be lower after severe exposure. For CCVs, Nicholson[233] estimates a failure rate of 1 in 80,000 in developed countries and between 1 in 12,000 and 1 in 30,000 in developing countries.

During the development of HDCV, efficacy studies were carried out in Iran, Germany, and the United States. In Iran, 45 people exposed in eight different incidents to eight proven rabid wolves or dogs were given six doses of HDCV after exposure. Antirabies serum also was given with the first vaccine doses. The presence of rabies virus in the brain was confirmed for all eight animals. In four animals tested, high virus titers also were found in the salivary glands. All vaccinees developed antibodies, and none developed rabies.[122] In Germany, 63 individuals bitten by rabid animals were uniformly protected. The accumulated experience of the Centers for Disease Control and Prevention in the United States was summarized in 1980, at which time 90 people exposed to rabid animals had all survived after HDCV vaccination.[234]

The HDCV produced by Berna was subjected to trial in 100 Thai patients exposed to proven rabid animals. All patients were protected by the standard five-dose regimen, although the GMT of rabies VNAs at 90 days after the first vaccination was relatively low at 2.57 IU.[235] Understandably, there have been no placebo-controlled studies of the efficacy of rabies vaccines. The CCVs, including PVRV, PCECV, PDEV, and PHKCV, have been accepted based on the induction of VNAs and lack of failures after postexposure vaccination.[129,136–139,142,143,145,147, 150,151,153,154]

Protection studies in mice show that antibodies induced by the G protein contained in HDCV neutralized 17 different street rabies viruses.[236]

Persistence of Immunity and Booster Doses

Rabies VNAs do not stay at elevated levels for long periods after vaccination with the usual pre-exposure schedules. By 1 year, VNAs fall to geometric mean levels between 1 and 3.5 IU,[120,237,238] and by 2 years, they may fall below the minimum acceptable level of 0.5 IU in approximately 20% of subjects. Nevertheless, Thraenhart and colleagues[239] reported the presence of VNAs in the serum of 18 people vaccinated 2 to 14 years earlier. Antibodies reacting with many virus proteins were still present, in addition to lymphocyte proliferation responses to the same proteins.

Booster doses of vaccine are efficient in restoring VNAs, with 100% of subjects showing a fivefold rise by day 7.[237] Two booster doses enhance somewhat the speed of the booster response.[240] Therefore, previously immunized individuals who are again exposed to rabies should receive two booster doses 3 days apart, without RIG. Boosters can be given either intramuscularly or intradermally, although no preparation approved for intradermal use is available in the United States. Studies[140,241] have compared four-site intradermal inoculations with the standard two-dose intramuscular inoculations in previously vaccinated volunteers undergoing simulated re-exposure to rabies, and found that the intradermal group had better booster responses. When maintenance of protective antibodies is desired after pre-exposure vaccination, as in laboratory workers, a booster is given at 1 year after primary vaccination, which invariably produces an anamnestic response (see further discussion below under *Indications for Vaccination*). However, because of allergic reactions to the HDCV used in the United States (see *Reactions to Cell Culture Vaccines* later), routine boosters are not recommended in the absence of definite exposure. Laboratory workers who have continuous exposure to wild rabies virus should have antibody levels checked every 6 months and should receive a single booster immunization if the titer falls below 0.5 IU (or complete neutralization at a serum dilution of 1:5).

Vaccination of Immunosuppressed Persons

Briggs and Schwenke[242] compared the persistence of antibodies in civilians and in Peace Corps volunteers who receive chloroquine for prophylaxis of malaria. At 1.5 to 2 years after primary vaccination, adequate titers were found in 99% of civilians and 88% of Peace Corps volunteers who received the vaccine intramuscularly and in 93% of civilians and 64% of Peace Corps volunteers who received the vaccine intradermally, showing that chloroquine was immunosuppressive.

Numerous studies on HIV-infected patients have shown that, although rabies vaccination is safe,[243] those with CD4+ cell counts lower than 300/mm^3 or 15% of lymphocytes are unlikely to respond with antibodies.[243-247] Patients on immunosuppressive drugs and those with diabetes also should be monitored for antibody responses.[248,249] In contrast, pregnant women respond normally to rabies vaccine.[250]

Mechanism of Protection

Pre-exposure vaccination with potent rabies vaccines leads to the development of VNAs. Vaccination also induces production of cytotoxic T cells, which have been shown to protect vaccinated mice in the absence of neutralizing antibodies. A high level of cell-mediated cytotoxic activity can be maintained by repeated inoculations of vaccine, and the presence of VNAs does not interfere with the secondary stimulation of sensitized lymphocytes.

The exact mechanism of protection of humans through postexposure vaccination is still unknown, although VNAs play a major role. The fact that only monoclonal antibodies that interact with macrophages are effective in protection of mice against disease may indicate that a complex mechanism is involved in antibody protection after challenge.

Concentrated and inactivated rabies vaccine of tissue culture origin is able to induce high levels of circulating interferon a few hours after its administration and can protect animals from rabies infection if it is given shortly before or after challenge with virus. This interferon-induced protection, however, is not specific because similar protection can be obtained with concentrated vaccines produced from unrelated viruses, such as influenza and Kern Canyon. However, only the rabies vaccine can protect when it is given several days before challenge with rabies virus. The combined treatment with interferon or interferon inducers in addition to rabies vaccine is more efficacious than vaccine alone in experimental animals when treatment is initiated several hours after challenge.[251] The role of interferon in human prophylaxis is undefined.

Treatment Failures

Thraenhart and colleagues[150] reviewed 28 cases of rabies that developed despite postexposure treatment with modern vaccines. In 90% of cases, RIG had not been administered or had been administered incorrectly. Other errors included passive immunization more than 24 hours before vaccine, incorrect local wound cleansing, injection of vaccine into the buttocks instead of the deltoid, and late initiation of immunization. Only two patients, both of whom had severe facial injuries, could be considered true treatment failures.

A follow-up study of treatment failures after 15 million doses of PCECV reported 47 treatment failures. All had occurred in India and Thailand, and in no case were WHO treatment guidelines completely followed.[252]

Other failures also may relate to deviations from standard prophylaxis.[168,253,254] However, a bite on the face with a large inoculum of rabies virus may overwhelm postexposure vaccination.

Adverse Reactions

Reactions to Rabies Vaccines Containing Animal Brain Tissues[119]

GENERAL SYSTEMIC REACTIONS

The various minor disorders that may develop during or after a course of antirabies treatment include fever, headache, insomnia, palpitations, and diarrhea. Sensitization to proteins contained in older nerve tissue vaccines can cause a sudden shock-like collapse, usually toward the end of the course of treatment.

LOCAL REACTIONS

Erythematous patches may develop approximately 7 to 10 days after the beginning of antirabies treatment. Local erythems and swelling may also appear a few hours after vaccine injection and fade in 6 to 8 hours.

SEVERE AND FATAL REACTIONS

A patient may suffer from serious and often fatal illness after nerve tissue vaccine. These accidents are of two types:

(1) *rage de laboratoire*, a disease induced by the living "fixed virus" present in the old Pasteur vaccine, and (2) *neuroparalytic accidents*, which present the greatest danger from rabies vaccination. All types of vaccine containing adult mammalian nervous tissues exhibit similar capacities for inducing neuroparalytic reactions. The neuroparalytic accident usually develops between the 13th and 15th days of the treatment and may assume one of the following three forms:

1. *Landry type.* In this type of accident, the patient rapidly becomes pyrexial and suffers pain in the back. Flaccid paralysis of the legs begins, and within 1 day the arms become paralyzed. Later the paralysis spreads to the face, tongue, and other muscles. The fatality rate is about 30%; in the remaining 70%, recovery usually occurs rapidly. The incidence varies between 1 in 7000 and 1 in 42,000 recipients.[255]
2. *Dorsolumbar type.* Less severe than the Landry type, this is the most common form of neuroparalytic accident. Clinical features are explicable by the presence of dorsolumbar myelitis. The patient may be febrile and feel weak, with paralysis of the lower limbs, diminished sensation, and sphincter disturbances. The fatality rate does not exceed 5%.
3. *Neuritic type.* In this type of accident, the patient may be pyrexial and usually shows a temporary paralysis of the facial, oculomotor, glossopharyngeal, or vagus nerves.

Neuroparalytic accidents are caused by allergic "encephalomyelitis," attributable specifically to sensitization to adult nerve tissue antigen (myelin basic protein).[256] High-titered antibodies to human myelin proteins and to gangliosides often are detected in these patients.[257] The incidence of these reactions to nerve tissue vaccine varies widely from 0.017% (1:6000) to 0.44% (1:230) and is definitely lower in people receiving DEV (1:32,000) and in people receiving properly manufactured vaccine of newborn rodent brain (1:8000).

One study observed 1392 Tunisian adults who were given a Semple-type vaccine prepared by phenol inactivation of rabies virus–infected lamb brains.[258] Seven patients developed neurologic complications, including paralysis or paresis in five. Most of the patients had elevated cell counts in their CSF. A rate of one neurologic complication in 200 vaccinations is unacceptable and illustrates the desirability of replacing nerve tissue vaccines with CCVs.

Reactions to Cell Culture Vaccines

GENERAL REACTIONS

CCVs are widely accepted as well-tolerated rabies vaccines, although reported reaction rates to primary immunization have varied with the monitoring system. In a large-scale testing of the safety and immunogenicity of HDCV performed on American veterinary students, adverse reaction rates observed in more than 1770 volunteers were as follows: significantly sore arm (15% to 25%); headache (5% to 8%); malaise, nausea, or both (2% to 5%); and allergic edema (0.1%).[120] In another study of postexposure vaccination, 21% had local reactions, 3.6% had fever, 7% had headache, and 5% had nausea.[234] The most common local reactions are

erythema, pain, and induration. These results have been confirmed by more modern studies.[131] When HDCV is administered to children, in whom psychological overlay is presumably less than in adults, there are few complaints.

ALLERGIC REACTIONS

After licensure of HDCV in the United States and widespread use, allergic reactions began to be reported, principally after booster doses.[259,260] The overall incidence of reactions was 11 in 10,000 (0.11%) vaccinees, but, after boosters, the incidence rose to 6%.[261] Anaphylactic type 1 (IgE) reactions occurred in about 10% of the reported cases, all during the primary series (1 in 10,000 vaccinations), but the majority appeared to be type 3 hypersensitivity (IgG-IgM) reactions occurring 2 to 21 days after booster doses (Table 37–10). These reactions have been attributed to antigenicity conferred on human albumin used as stabilizer in the vaccine by the β-propiolactone used to inactivate the virus, which increases the capacity of the albumin to form immune complexes.[262–264]

Fortunately, respiratory symptoms are mild, and there have been no fatalities. Antihistamines, epinephrine, and occasionally steroids have been used in successful treatment of the reactions, which have resolved in 2 to 3 days.

The Aventis Pasteur, Berna, and Behring HDCVs are produced by use of additional purification steps to remove human albumin. Systemic reactions to booster doses are uncommon with these vaccines.[265,266] The manufacturers of PVRV and PCECV contend that allergic reactions are absent after primary or booster doses with those two CCVs.

NEUROLOGIC REACTIONS

Although five cases of central nervous system disease, including transient neuroparalytic illness of the Guillain-Barré type, have been reported among the millions of individuals given HDCV,[267–271] this rate is too low to be certainly related to vaccination, because the background incidence of such diseases is about 1 in 100,000 per year. The low incidence after HDCV compares with a neurologic complication

TABLE 37–10 ■ Signs and Symptoms in Three Cohorts Containing 255 Subjects Reporting Presumed Immune Complex–Type Hypersensitivity Reactions* After Booster Immunization with Human Diploid Cell Rabies Vaccine Given Intradermally (ID) or Intramuscularly (IM)

Number with any sign or symptom	29 (11.4%)
Pruritic rash	17 (59%)
Urticaria	24 (90%)
Edema	14 (48%)
Joint	4 (14%)
Fever	1 (3%)
Difficulty breathing	1 (3%)
Mean delay after booster before reaction	9.6 days
Range: ID	3–13 days
Range: IM	8–11 days

*Coombs and Gell type III.
From Centers for Disease Control and Prevention. Systemic allergic reactions following immunization with human diploid cell rabies vaccine. MMWR 33:185–188, 1984.

rate of 1 in 1600 people for nerve tissue vaccine, 1 in 8000 for suckling mouse brain vaccine, and 1 in 32,000 for DEV.

In Thailand, a switch from Semple-type vaccine to HDCV resulted in a drop in the rate of neurologic complications from 1 in 155 to less than 1 in 50,000 treatments. At the same time, the failure rate dropped from 1 in 2000 to 1 in 25,000 treatments without the use of RIG.[272] If reactions occur after one CCV, a switch can be made to another produced in a different cell substrate without danger.

Indications for Vaccination

Pre-Exposure Vaccination

All high-risk professionals, such as veterinarians, hunters, trappers, dog catchers, mail carriers, spelunkers, and laboratory workers contemplating working with rabies virus, should be prophylactically immunized against rabies. The recommended regimens are given in Table 37–7. After receiving the three-dose pre-exposure regimen, those who are repeatedly exposed to high concentrations of rabies virus in the laboratory should have VNA levels checked every 6 months and should be given a booster dose intramuscularly or intradermally if the titer is less than 0.5 IU. Veterinarians and others exposed to rabid animals should be similarly checked every 2 years.

Peace Corps workers, missionaries or others who remain for long periods in rabies-enzootic countries certainly deserve pre-exposure vaccination.[273] A survey of travelers revealed that, after an average of 17 days in Thailand, 1.3% and 8.9% had been bitten or licked by a dog, respectively, and 0.5% had required rabies vaccination.[274] Moreover, postexposure vaccination in developing countries is often complicated by problems of availability of potent vaccine and RIG.[275] However, a decision analysis concluded that routine pre-exposure vaccination would cost $275,000 per case averted and that it should be individualized according to the traveler's situation.[276] Our recommendation would be to vaccinate those who will be staying in remote areas for more than a few days, particularly children.

In countries where rabies is endemic and children are frequently exposed to rabid animals, one might contemplate prophylactic vaccination against rabies as part of pediatric immunization. Dog bites are a considerable problem in many areas of the world and accounted for more than 5% of visits to the emergency department of a Bangkok hospital, of which 55% were by children.[277] So far, prophylaxis has been restricted to the children of Westerners going to live in areas enzootic for rabies,[278] but clinical trials in children have been performed in developing countries.[279] A preliminary study was done with the PVRV vaccine in Thailand, where two doses were given intramuscularly in association with routine pediatric immunizations at 2 and 4 months of age.[280] Seroconversion to rabies occurred in 100% of infants, without significant interference with the other vaccines. A similar study was done with three doses of intradermal rabies vaccine at 2, 3, and 4 months of age, with an adequate immune response (GMT of 12 IU/mL).[281]

Pre-Exposure Booster Vaccination

After pre-exposure vaccination, antibodies decline sharply within the first year of vaccination. If a booster dose is given 1 year later, subjects segregate themselves into two groups: good responders, who develop a titer greater than 30 IU by 14 days after booster; and poor responders, whose titers are lower. The former, who represent 75% of subjects, may not need further booster vaccination for 10 years, whereas the latter may need more frequent boosters.[282] This strategy reduces costs.[283,284]

Primary vaccination by the intradermal route gives less sustained immunity, but the intradermal route is an effective means of giving a routine booster.[126]

Postexposure Treatment (Tables 37–11 through 37–13)

The essential triad of postexposure rabies prophylaxis is local treatment, vaccination, and antiserum administration. Local treatment of bites and scratches consists of vigorous washing with soap and water, followed, if possible, with 70% alcohol, 0.1% quaternary ammonium compound, or

TABLE 37–11 ■ Rabies Postexposure Prophylaxis Guide for the United States, 1999

Animal Type	Evaluation and Disposition of Animal	Postexposure Prophylaxis Recommendations
Dogs, cats, and ferrets	Healthy and available for 10 days' observation	Persons should not begin prophylaxis unless animal develops clinical signs of rabies.[*]
	Rabid or suspected rabid	Immediately vaccinate.
	Unknown (e.g., escaped)	Consult public health officials.
Skunks, raccoons, foxes, and most other carnivores; bats	Regarded as rabid unless animal proven negative by laboratory tests[†]	Consider immediate vaccination.
Livestock, small rodents, lagomorphs (rabbits and hares), large rodents (woodchucks and beavers), and other mammals	Consider individually	Consult public health officials. Bites of squirrels, hamsters, guinea pigs, gerbils, chipmunks, rats, mice and other small rodents, rabbits, and hares almost never require antirabies postexposure prophylaxis.

[*]During the 10-day observation period, begin postexposure prophylaxis at the first sign of rabies in a dog, cat, or ferret that has bitten someone. If the animal exhibits clinical signs of rabies, it should be euthanized immediately and tested.
[†]The animal should be euthanized and tested as soon as possible. Holding for observation is not recommended. Discontinue vaccine if immunofluorescence test results of the animal are negative.
From Centers for Disease Control and Prevention. Human rabies prevention—United States, 1999: recommendations of the Advisory committee on Immunization Practices (ACIP). MMWR 48(RR-1):7, 1999.

TABLE 37–12 ■ Rabies Postexposure Prophylaxis Schedule, United States, 1999

Vaccination Status	Treatment	Regimen*
Not previously vaccinated	Wound cleansing	All postexposure treatment should begin with immediate thorough cleansing of all wounds with soap and water. If available, a virucidal agent such as a povidone-iodine solution should be used to irrigate the wounds.
	HRIG	Administer 20 IU/kg body weight. If anatomically feasible, *the full dose* should be infiltrated around the wound(s), and any remaining volume should be administered intramuscularly (IM) at an anatomic site distant from vaccine administration. Also, RIG should not be administered in the same syringe as the vaccine. Because HRIG may partially suppress the active production of antibody, no more than the recommended dose should be given.
	Vaccine	HDCV, RVA, or PCECV, 1.0 mL, IM (deltoid area[†]), one each on days 0[‡], 3, 7, 14, and 28
Previously vaccinated[§]	Wound cleansing	All postexposure treatment should begin with immediate thorough cleansing of all wounds with soap and water. If available, a virucidal agent such as a povidone-iodine solution should be used to irrigate the wounds.
	RIG	RIG should *not* be administered
	Vaccine	HDCV, RVA, or PCEV, 1.0 mL, IM (deltoid area[†]), one each on days 0[**] and 3.

*These regimens are applicable for all age groups, including children.
[†]The deltoid area is the only acceptable site of vaccination for adults and older children. For younger children, the outer aspect of the thigh may be used. Vaccine should never be administered in the gluteal area.
[‡]Day 0 is the day the first dose of vaccine is administered.
[§]Any person with a history of pre-exposure vaccination with HDCV, RVA, or PCVEC; prior postexposure prophylaxis with HDCV, RVA, or PCECV; or previous vaccination with any other type of rabies vaccine and a documented history of antibody response to the prior vaccination.
From Centers for Disease Control and Prevention. Human Rabies Prevention—United States, 1999: Recommendations of the Advisory Committee on Immunization Practices (ACIP). MMWR, 48(RR-1):1–21, 1999.

povidone-iodine. Surgical suturing should be avoided for 7 days, but, in any case, RIG (see later) should always be administered before suturing.[285] Antibiotics and tetanus toxoid may be indicated to prevent other infections.[286]

A decision to give postexposure rabies vaccine should be based on consideration of the following issues[287,288]:

1. Was the patient's skin broken by the bite or scratch, or were mucous membranes contaminated? If not, no real exposure has occurred. The risk of rabies after bite by a rabid animal has been estimated at 5% to 80%, whereas the risk after scratches is much less (0.1% to 1%). The risk after mucous membrane contact is low.[289] However, see point 10 below relative to bat exposures.

2. If the bite was by a dog or cat, is domestic animal rabies found in the particular geographic area? Many areas of the world, such as Oceania, Antarctica, and the United Kingdom, are free of rabies in mammals. In many cities of the United States, even stray animals are unlikely to be rabid.

3. Was the dog or cat vaccinated against rabies? Vaccination diminishes the risk, but not completely. Proper vaccination of pets should not be accepted at face value. Documentation should be required to show at least two vaccinations with a potent vaccine; one dose of inactivated vaccines is insufficient to warrant efficacy.[285,290]

4. Is the biting animal a domestic dog or cat and available for observation? If yes, vaccination may be postponed. However, in rabies-enzootic areas, vaccination is advisable, even if the domestic animal appears normal, because of short incubation periods in humans and the frequent difficulty in being certain of the biting animal.[291]

TABLE 37–13 ■ WHO 1992 Recommendations for Rabies Postexposure Prophylaxis

Category	Type of Contact with a Suspect or Confirmed Rabid Animal	Recommended Treatment
I	Touching or feeding of animals	None if reliable case history is available.
	Licks on intact skin	Pre-exposure treatment may be offered.
II	Nibbling of uncovered skin	Administer vaccine immediately.
	Minor scratches or abrasions without bleeding	Stop treatment if animal remains healthy throughout an
	Licks on broken skin	observation period of 10 days or if animal is killed humanely and found to be negative for rabies by appropriate laboratory techniques.
III	Single or multiple transdermal bites or scratches	Administer rabies immune globulin and vaccine immediately.
	Contamination of mucous membrane with saliva (i.e., licks)	Stop treatment if animal remains healthy throughout an observation period of 10 days or if animal is killed humanely and found to be negative for rabies by appropriate laboratory techniques.

From WHO Expert Committee on Rabies. World Organization Tech. Rep Ser 824:1–84, 1992.

5. If the bite was inflicted by a wild animal, was it a species likely (e.g., skunk and raccoon) or unlikely (e.g., squirrel and rat) to be rabid? Local conditions must be taken into account; for example, in Thailand rabies has been reported in rats,[292] an unlikely finding elsewhere.

6. Was the bite provoked or unprovoked? This criterion is useful only in areas of low incidence and not where the incidence of rabies in dogs is elevated.[285] In Thailand, even when the animal's behavior appeared normal, an assessment of provocation did not correlate with the presence of rabies at autopsy of the animal.[293] Attempts to play with wild animals should be considered provocative.

7. If exposure was to a rabid human, use the same criteria for vaccination as with a biting animal. Only individuals who were bitten or scratched, who gave mouth-to-mouth resuscitation, or who were exposed to saliva or nerve tissues need to be vaccinated.[290]

8. RIG should always be given in combination with vaccine for transdermal or mucous membrane exposure (see *Serum and Vaccine Treatment* above). The dose of HRIG is 20 IU/kg, and that of ERIG 40 IU/kg. As much as possible of the RIG should be inoculated locally, diluted if necessary in saline to provide sufficient volume. If necessary, local anesthesia can be provided with procaine-type compounds.[294] The remainder of the RIG, if any, should be given in the deltoid or gluteus muscles.

9. The dose is the same regardless of age; children tolerate vaccination well and demonstrate excellent antibody response, as has been demonstrated in different ethnic groups.[219,295-297]

10. Rabies postexposure prophylaxis is recommended for all people with bite, scratch, or mucous membrane exposure to a bat, unless the bat is available for testing and is negative for evidence of rabies. The inability of care providers to elicit information surrounding potential exposures may be influenced by the limited injury inflicted by a bat bite (in comparison to lesions inflicted by terrestrial carnivores) or by circumstances that hinder accurate recall of events. Therefore, postexposure prophylaxis is also appropriate even in the absence of a demonstrable bite or scratch when there is reasonable probability that such contact occurred (e.g., a sleeping individual awakens to find a bat in the room, an adult witnesses a bat in the room with a previously unattended child, mentally deficient person, or intoxicated individual). Fortunately, tests of antibodies obtained from humans after vaccination with HDCV or PECECV show good neutralization of rabies virus from bats.[298]

Useless vaccination can be avoided if circumstances are found that make the chances of rabies exposure remote. When exposures occur to animals in whom rabies is not suspected, large numbers of people often receive vaccine.[299] A survey of practice in 11 university-associated urban emergency departments revealed that rabies prophylaxis was administered inappropriately in 40% of cases.[300] Tables 37–11 through 37–13 should be consulted as a guide for the selection of postexposure prophylaxis in the United States and elsewhere in the world.[290,301] Table 37–7 describes preexposure and postexposure regimens.

Postexposure Booster Vaccination

If an individual has been vaccinated with a CCV and later exposed again to rabies, two booster injections of a vaccine are recommended because one may not always be sufficient.[302] Patients who received vaccine intradermally for their primary series are particularly at risk of a slow response to booster.[303] Another suggestion from Thailand is to give four simultaneous intradermal vaccinations as a single booster.[304] However, subjects who previously received CCV uniformly have long-lasting immunologic memory,[305] and there is no evidence that more than two boosters are necessary. Patients who gave a history of vaccination with nerve tissue vaccines responded poorly to boosters in 18% of cases,[306] and they should therefore receive a full primary regimen unless antibodies were previously shown to be present.

Contraindications to Vaccination

Because rabies is a lethal disease, any contraindication to postexposure treatment should be considered carefully before disqualifying an individual for antirabies treatment.

Individuals with histories of severe allergies are more prone to develop allergic reactions to rabies vaccine. When those individuals are vaccinated, prophylactic antihistamines should be given and epinephrine should be available. If an allergic reaction occurs, one may give an alternative vaccine of different tissue origin, for example, PVRV or PCECV in the case of a reaction to HDCV. A similar strategy was applied in allergic individuals in whom brain tissue vaccine caused symptoms of central nervous system involvement during the course of injections. Administration of nerve tissue vaccine was interrupted immediately, and the series was completed with vaccine produced in tissue other than brain.

However, only severe reactions not controlled with premedication are grounds for interruption of rabies vaccination. Treatment with steroids may control allergy but may also inhibit VNA responses. Accordingly, antibody titers should be determined after the last dose if steroids has been used. Similarly, patients receiving immunosuppressive medications for other diseases should have VNA levels checked after immunization to verify an adequate response to the vaccine.[307]

Pregnancy is not a contraindication to rabies vaccination.[308,309] Follow-up of 202 Thai women vaccinated during pregnancy revealed no excess of medical complications or abnormal births.[310]

The "Fourth"-Generation Rabies Vaccines and Antibodies[311]

Recombinant poxvirus vaccines are being used extensively in animals (see under *Rabies Vaccination of Animals* below), and both vaccinia and canarypox vectors containing the rabies G protein have been prepared and tested in humans.[312–314] With both vectors, two injections at 1-month intervals raised levels of rabies VNAs, although less than two injections of HDCV given at the same interval. A third dose of the vectors gave striking booster effects, both to those who had received the vectors previously and to those who had received the HDCV previously.

Plasmid vaccines containing the complementary DNA of the gene for the rabies virus G glycoprotein have been constructed. Protection on challenge with wild virus was demonstrated in mice, dogs, cats, and monkeys.[315–319] Some DNA-vaccinated monkeys were protected against challenge 1 year after a single injection.[320]

The rabies virus N protein also may be important in protection.[321,322] Although the G protein alone is protective in experimental animals, so is the N protein, but without the induction of VNAs. After vaccination with CCV, antibodies appear to both N and G proteins.[323] The function of N may be to induce protective cellular immune responses, but it also appears to enhance antibody responses to G.[32,324] The N protein might be used to sensitize hosts to rabies proteins, so that subsequent injection of CCV would result in prompt development of high titers of VNAs. However, the N protein does not appear to broaden the neutralizing responses against rabies-related viruses.[325] The N protein can be produced in a baculovirus vector, which is a potential source of antigen for large-scale pre-exposure immunization of humans and animals.[326] Large amounts of G protein also can be produced by baculovirus vectors.[327] Synthetic peptides have been constructed that produce antibodies in laboratory animals, but none of the peptides has so far induced either development of VNAs or protection against rabies virus challenge. Anti-idiotypic antibodies as vaccines are still experimental.[328] It may be possible to genetically engineer attenuated rabies strains and to have them serve as vectors of foreign genes.[329] Engineering involving reverse genetics also may allow for the construction of species-specific rabies vaccines.

Monoclonal antibodies that neutralize rabies virus have been produced in human–mouse hybrid cells, and might be an alternative to the scarce HRIG.[330–332]

Public Health Considerations

Rabies Vaccination of Animals

From the beginning of his involvement with rabies, Pasteur recognized that, for the most part, protection of humans could be achieved effectively through the vaccination of dogs. Although dogs were used to obtain most of the experimental data on protection from 1884 to 1885, it was not until the early 1920s that a practical and successful canine vaccine was developed.

The first vaccine for mass vaccination of dogs was a modified Semple type prepared by Umeno and Doi[333] in Tokyo in 1921. It proved effective in controlling rabies in dogs in Japan and in other countries that produced and used this type of vaccine. The quality of vaccine improved greatly with Habel's introduction of a standard mouse potency test for the Semple-type vaccine, which ensured the potency of the vaccines in mass vaccination programs.[334]

In 1945, Johnson[335] demonstrated that a single dose of a potent, phenol-inactivated vaccine protected dogs against a challenge with street rabies virus for a period of more than 1 year. From 1945 on, this was virtually the only type of vaccine used for control of rabies in dogs, cats, and other domestic animals.

A modified live virus vaccine was introduced by Koprowski[336] in 1948. Successive passages of a strain of virus of human origin, first in 1-day-old chicks and then in embryonated hens' eggs, resulted in the loss of pathogenicity for dogs, providing an attenuated strain safe for dogs, called Flury LEP. Further passages of Flury LEP virus in embryonated hens' eggs resulted in a vaccine that was no longer effective for adult laboratory animals yet was lethal for newborn mice, called Flury HEP. Both Flury LEP and Flury HEP were given to many types of domestic animals in different parts of the world. However, the live, attenuated Flury virus vaccine was discontinued in the late 1970s.

Another attenuated strain of rabies virus, ERA, was introduced by Canadian workers in 1964.[337] The ERA vaccine was shown to provide excellent immunity, lasting for at least 3 years. However, several vaccine-induced cases of rabies in cats resulted in the cessation of its use.

Several inactivated rabies vaccines for animals prepared from brains of newborn mice or from virus of tissue culture origin were introduced in the 1980s and are now in general use in Europe and the Americas. However, only inactivated virus vaccines and live recombinant vaccines are licensed for domestic animals in the United States.

Oral vaccination of wildlife to prevent the spread of rabies in terrestrial animals such as foxes, raccoons, and coyotes has become possible. The Street Alabama Dufferin (SAD B19) attenuated strain has been put into fish and bone meal baits for the vaccination of foxes.[338] The virus is grown on a baby hamster kidney cell line and is stable even at high environmental temperatures. A dose of approximately 10^6 infectious units immunizes 100% of foxes, which has allowed its wide application in Germany and elsewhere in central Europe.[339] However, because the SAD B19 strain retains residual pathogenicity for rodents, a more attenuated strain called SAG2 has been developed.[340]

Genetic engineering has been applied to rabies immunization by the construction of a vaccinia virus recombinant containing the gene for the G protein (V-RG).[341] The recombinant is placed in baits, and, on ingestion by animals, it multiplies only in the tonsils and the buccal area. Extensive tests conducted in many species have confirmed the safety and efficacy of vaccination with this construct, and field tests in France, Belgium, and the United States have confirmed the promising laboratory results.[342–346] A human infection with the vaccinia recombinant produced local lesions but no lasting effect.[347] Widespread application of V-RG in Belgium starting in 1989 reduced fox rabies from 841 cases in that year to 2 cases in 1993. Concomitantly, a marked drop occurred in human exposures requiring vaccination.[348] The widespread use of these oral vaccines has changed the epizootiology of rabies in Europe, and vaccination with V-RG has begun in the United States, including New Jersey, New York, Massachusetts, Florida, Texas, Vermont, Ohio, Virginia, Pennsylvania, and West Virginia.

In the United States, two types of rabies vaccines are available for animals: inactivated virus vaccines and canarypox recombinant vaccines. Both types require boosters after 1 to 3 years.[349]

Rabies Vaccination of Humans

More than 4 million people are vaccinated each year after presumed exposure to rabies, particularly in Asia.[350] It is difficult to define precisely the effect of rabies vaccination on the incidence of human rabies, because the risk of the disease is variable. Nevertheless, when untreated patients who were bitten by proven rabid animals are followed, disease rates of between 3 and 80% are observed,[7,351] depending on the location and severity of bites.[352] In the United States, relatively few of the 30,000 to 40,000 people vaccinated annually are actually at risk of rabies. However, the paucity of cases of rabies in individuals given potent vaccines together with antiserum argues that many cases of rabies are being prevented. In Texas in 1989, 34% of the skunks, 19% of the foxes, and 15% of the bats involved in biting incidents were rabid, so there is risk to humans.[353]

Control of dog rabies is jointly responsible with vaccination of exposed humans for the current rarity of human rabies in North America and Europe. In developing countries, nerve tissue vaccine reduces the incidence of rabies in vaccinees,[351] but large numbers of exposed individuals turn to indiginous methods of rabies control and never receive vaccine.[353a] Thus need exists for inexpensive CCVs and for health education to aid in appropriate vaccine use. The availability of HRIG or ERIG in developing countries remains a problem.[354]

The majority of human and animal rabies cases could be prevented by control of the canine population through responsible pet ownership, contraception, capture of stray dogs, and vaccination. The last is a widely effective technique only in developed countries where the cost is acceptable, where booster vaccination of pets can be required, and where there is an adequate medical and veterinary infrastructure. In other areas, with different socioeconomic conditions, only the first three methods may be feasible, often with difficulty. A safe and effective oral vaccine for dogs would be a great advance in the control of rabies, and, as stressed earlier, oral vaccines for certain wildlife vectors already have had an impact on rabies epizootiology. Control of rabies in wild mammals, particularly bats, is not presently possible.

Pre-exposure vaccination with CCVs also could reduce the incidence of human rabies in high-risk areas and professions, as has been achieved among veterinarians and Peace Corps workers. Routine pre-exposure vaccination of children in areas where animal rabies is prevalent is under consideration. Elimination of rabies in dogs should receive major emphasis, which will serve to markedly reduce vaccination of humans. The production of recombinant rabies antigen vaccines produced in transgenic plants may be a consideration for rabies prevention and control in the new century.[355]

REFERENCES

1. Steele JH. History of rabies. *In* Baer GM (ed). The Natural History of Rabies. Vol. 1. New York, Academic Press, 1975, pp 1–29.
2. Theodorides J. Histoire de la Rage. Paris, Masson, 1986.
3. Wiktor T. Historical aspects of rabies treatment. *In* Koprowski H, Plotkin SA (eds). World's Debt to Pasteur. New York, Alan R. Liss, 1985, pp 141–151.
4. Pasteur L. Method pour prevenir la rage apres morsure. C R Acad Sci 101:765–772, 1885.
5. Benitez RM. A 39-year-old man with mental status change. Md Med J 45:765–769, 1996.
6. Hemachudha T, Laothamatas J, Rupprecht CE. Human rabies: a disease of complex neuropathogenetic mechanisms and diagnostic challenges. Lancet Neurol 1:101–109, 2002.
7. Hattwick MA. Human rabies. Public Health Rev 3:229–274, 1974.
8. Smith JS, Fishbein DB, Rupprecht CE, Clark K. Unexplained rabies in three immigrants in the United States: a virologic investigation. N Engl J Med 324:205–211, 1991.
9. Held JR, Tierkel ES, Steele JH. Rabies in man and animals in the United States, 1946–65. Public Health Rep 82:1009–1018, 1967.
10. Hemachudha T. Human rabies: clinical aspects, pathogenesis, and potential therapy. Curr Top Microbiol Immunol 187:121–143, 1994.
11. Warrell DA. The clinical picture of rabies in man. Trans R Soc Trop Med Hyg 70:188–195, 1976.
12. Anderson LJ, Nicholson KG, Tauxe RV, Winkler WG. Human rabies in the United States, 1960 to 1979: epidemiology, diagnosis, and prevention. Ann Intern Med 100:728–735, 1984.
13. Awasthi M, Parmar H, Patankar T, Castillo M. Imaging findings in rabies encephalitis. AJNR Am J Neuroradiol 22:677–680, 2001.
14. Dodet B, Meslin FX, Heseltine E (eds). Clinical Aspects of Human Rabies: Fourth International Symposium on Rabies Control in Asia, March 5–9, 2001, Hanoi, Viet Nam. Paris, World Health Organization, 2001.
15. Baevsky RH, Bartfield JM. Human rabies: a review. Am J Emerg Med 11:279–286, 1993.
16. Hattwick MA, Weis TT, Stechschulte CJ, et al. Recovery from rabies: a case report. Ann Intern Med 76:931–942, 1972.
17. Porras C, Barboza JJ, Fuenzalida E, et al. Recovery from rabies in man. Ann Intern Med 85:44–48, 1976.
18. Winkler WG, Fashinell TR, Leffingwell L, et al. Airborne rabies transmission in a laboratory worker. JAMA 226:1219–1221, 1973.
19. Gode GR, Saksena R, Batra RK, et al. Treatment of 54 clinically diagnosed rabies patients with two survivals. Indian J Med Res 88:564–566, 1988.
20. Alvarez L, Fajardo R, Lopez E, et al. Partial recovery from rabies in a nine-year-old boy. Pediatr Infect Dis J 13:1154–1155, 1994.
21. Madhusudana SN, Nagaraj D, Uday M, et al. Partial recovery from rabies in a six-year-old girl. Int J Infect Dis 6:85–86, 2002.
22. Dutta JK, Dutta TK. Treatment of clinical rabies in man: drug therapy and other measures. Int J Clin Pharmacol Ther 32:594–597, 1994.
23. Wunner WH, Dietzschold B, Wiktor T. Antigenic structure of rhabdoviruses. *In* Von Regenmortel MHV, Neurath AD (eds). Immunochemistry of Viruses: The Basis for Serodiagnosis and Vaccines. New York, Elsevier Science, 1985, pp 367–388.
23a. Kissi B, Badrane H, Audry L, et al. Dynamics of rabies virus quasispecies during serial passages in heterologous hosts. J Gen Virol 80 (Pt 8):2041–2050, 1999.
23b. Morimoto K, McGettigan JP, Foley HD, et al. Genetic engineering of live rabies vaccines. Vaccine 19 (25–26):3543–3551, 2001.
24. Badrane H, Tordo N. Host switching in *Lyssavirus* history from the Chiroptera to the Carnivora orders. J Virol 75:8096–8104, 2001.
25. Holmes EC, Woelk CH, Kassis R, Bourhy H. Genetic constraints and the adaptive evolution of rabies virus in nature. Virology 292:247–257, 2002.
26. Wiktor TJ, Gyorgy E, Schlumberger D, et al. Antigenic properties of rabies virus components. J Immunol 110:269–276, 1973.
27. Gaudin Y, Ruigrok RW, Tuffereau C, et al. Rabies virus glycoprotein is a trimer. Virology 187:627–632, 1992.
28. Ito N, Takayama M, Yamada K, et al. Rescue of rabies virus from cloned cDNA and identification of the pathogenicity-related gene: glycoprotein gene is associated with virulence for adult mice. J Virol 75:9121–9128, 2001.
29. Dietzschold B, Wunner WH, Wiktor T, et al. Characterization of an antigenic determinant of the glycoprotein which defines pathogenicity of fixed rabies virus strains. Proc Natl Acad Sci U S A 80:70–74, 1982.
30. Anilionis A, Wunner WH, Curtis PJ. Structure of the glycoprotein gene in rabies virus. Nature 294:275–278, 1981.
31. Wunner WH, Dietzschold B. Rabies virus infection: genetic mutations and the impact on viral pathogenicity and immunity. Contrib Microbiol Immunol 8:103–124, 1987.

32. Dietzschold B, Ertl HC. New developments in the pre- and post-exposure treatment of rabies. Crit Rev Immunol 10:427–439, 1991.

33. Nathanson N, Gonzalez-Scarano F. New developments in the pre- and post-exposure treatment of rabies. In Baer GM (ed). The Natural History of Rabies. Boca Raton, FL, CRC Press, 1991, pp 145–161.

34. Xiang ZQ, Knowles BB, McCarrick JW, Ertl HC. Immune effector mechanisms required for protection to rabies virus. Virology 214:398–404, 1995.

35. Smith JS. New aspects of rabies with emphasis on epidemiology, diagnosis, and prevention of the disease in the United States. Clin Microbiol Rev 9:166–176, 1996.

36. Crick J, Tignor GH, Moreno K. A new isolate of Lagos bat virus from the Republic of South Africa. Trans R Soc Trop Med Hyg 76:211–213, 1982.

37. Schneider LG, Barnard BJH, Schneider H. Application of monoclonal antibodies for epidemiological investigations and oral vaccine studies. I. African viruses. In Proceedings of an International Conference on Rabies Control in the Tropics, Institut Pasteur, Tunis, Algeria, October 3–6, 1983.

38. Lumio J, Hillbom M, Roine R, et al. Human rabies of bat origin in Europe. Lancet 1:378, 1986.

39. Foggin CM. Rabies in Africa with emphasis on rabies-related viruses. In Koprowski H, Plotkin SA (eds). World's Debt to Pasteur. New York, Alan R. Liss, 1985, pp 219–234.

40. Shope RE. Rabies virus antigenic relationships. In Baer GM (ed). The Natural History of Rabies. New York, Academic Press, 1975, pp 141–152.

41. Gardner SD. Bat rabies in Europe. J Infect 18:205–208, 1989.

42. Lafon M, Herzog M, Sureau P. Human rabies vaccines induce neutralising antibodies against the European bat rabies virus (Duvenhage). Lancet 2:515, 1986.

43. Herzog M, Fritzell C, Lafage M, et al. T and B cell human responses to European bat lyssavirus after post-exposure rabies vaccination. Clin Exp Immunol 85:224–230, 1991.

44. Shankar V, Dietzschold B, Koprowski H. Direct entry of rabies virus into the central nervous system without prior local replication. J Virol 65:2736–2738, 1991.

45. Ray NB, Ewalt LC, Lodmell DL. Rabies virus replication in primary murine bone marrow macrophages and in human and murine macrophage-like cell lines: implications for viral persistence. J Virol 69:764–772, 1995.

46. Charlton KM. The pathogenesis of rabies and other lyssaviral infections: recent studies. Curr Top Microbiol Immunol 187:95–119, 1994.

47. Clark HF, Prabhakar BS. Rabies. In Oslen RG, Krakowa S (eds). Comparative Pathobiology of Viral Diseases. Boca Raton, FL, CRC Press, 1985, pp 165–214.

48. Spriggs DR. Rabies pathogenesis: fast times at the neuromuscular junction. J Infect Dis 152:1362–1363, 1985.

49. Dietzschold B, Kao M, Zheng YM, et al. Delineation of putative mechanisms involved in antibody-mediated clearance of rabies virus from the central nervous system. Proc Natl Acad Sci U.S.A 89:7252–7256, 1992. [Published erratum appears in Proc Natl Acad Sci U S A 89:9365, 1992]

50. Dietzschold B, Morimoto K, Hooper DC. Mechanisms of virus-induced neuronal damage and the clearance of viruses from CNS. In Gosztonyi G (ed). The Mechanisms of Neuronal Damage in Virus Infections of the Nervous System. New York, Springer, 2001, pp 145–155.

51. Lentz TL, Wilson PT, Hawrot E, Speicher DW. Amino acid sequence similarity between rabies virus glycoprotein and snake venom curaremimetic neurotoxins. Science 226:847–848, 1984.

52. Bracci L, Antoni G, Cusi MG, et al. Antipeptide monoclonal antibodies inhibit the binding of rabies virus glycoprotein and alpha-bungarotoxin to the nicotinic acetylcholine receptor. Mol Immunol 25:881–888, 1988.

53. Gastka M, Horvath J, Lentz TL. Rabies virus binding to the nicotinic acetylcholine receptor alpha subunit demonstrated by virus overlay protein binding assay. J Gen Virol 77 (pt 10):2437–2440, 1996.

54. Tsiang H. An in vitro study of rabies pathogenesis. Bull Inst Pasteur 83:41–56, 1985.

55. Tsiang H. Pathophysiology of rabies virus infection of the nervous system. Adv Virus Res 42:375–412, 1993.

56. Jackson AC, Ye H, Phelan CC, et al. Extraneural organ involvement in human rabies. Lab Invest 79:945–951, 1999.

56a. Jogai S, Radotra BD, Banerjee AK. Rabies viral antigen in extracranial organs: a post-mortem study. Neuropathol Appl Neurobiol 28(4):334–338, 2002.

57. Jackson AC, Park H. Apoptotic cell death in experimental rabies in suckling mice. Acta Neuropathol (Berl) 95:159–164, 1998.

58. Jackson AC, Ye H, Ridaura-Sanz C, Lopez-Corella E. Quantitative study of the infection in brain neurons in human rabies. J Med Virol 65:614–618, 2001.

59. Fekadu M. Latency and aborted rabies. In Baer GM (ed). The Natural History of Rabies. Boca Raton, FL, CRC Press, 1991, pp 191–198.

60. Hooper DC, Morimoto K, Bette M, et al. Collaboration of antibody and inflammation in clearance of rabies virus from the central nervous system. J Virol 72:3711–3719, 1998.

61. Kamolvarin N, Tirawatnpong T, Rattanasiwamoke R, et al. Diagnosis of rabies by polymerase chain reaction with nested primers. J Infect Dis 167:207–210, 1993.

62. Bingham J, van der Merwe M. Distribution of rabies antigen in infected brain material: determining the reliability of different regions of the brain for the rabies fluorescent antibody test. J Virol Methods 101:85–94, 2002.

63. King AA, Turner GS. Rabies: a review. J Comp Pathol 108:1–39, 1993.

64. Matsumoto S. Electron microscopy of central nervous system infection. In Baer GM (ed). The Natural History of Rabies. New York, Academic Press, 1975, pp 33–61.

65. Noah DL, Drenzek CL, Smith JS, et al. Epidemiology of human rabies in the United States, 1980 to 1996. Ann Intern Med 128:922–930, 1998.

66. Plotkin SA. Rabies. Clin Infect Dis 30:4–12, 2000.

67. Wacharapluesadee S, Hemachudha T. Nucleic-acid sequence based amplification in the rapid diagnosis of rabies. Lancet 358:892–893, 2001.

68. Wacharapluesadee S, Hemachudha T. Urine samples for rabies RNA detection in the diagnosis of rabies in humans. Clin Infect Dis 34:874–875, 2002.

69. Kasempimolporn S, Saengseesom W, Lumlertdacha B, Sitprija V. Detection of rabies virus antigen in dog saliva using a latex agglutination test. J Clin Microbiol 38:3098–3099, 2000.

70. Sang E, Farr RW, Fisher MA, Hanna SD. Antemortem diagnosis of human rabies. J Fam Pract 43:83–87, 1996.

71. Centers for Disease Control. Annual Summary 1983: reported morbidity and mortality in the United States. Mor Mort Wkly Rep 32:46, 1984.

72. Sabcharoen A, Lang J, Attanath P, et al. A new Vero cell rabies vaccine: results of a comparative trial with human diploid cell rabies vaccine in children. Clin Infect Dis Jul;29(1):141–149, 1999.

73. Finnegan CJ, Brookes SM, Johnson N, et al. Rabies in North America and Europe. J R Soc Med 95:9–13, 2002.

74. Krebs JW, Strine TW, Smith JS, et al. Rabies surveillance in the United States during 1995. J Am Vet Med Assoc 209:2031–2044, 1996.

75. Krebs JW, Noll HR, Rupprecht CE, Childs JE. Rabies surveillance in the United States during 2001. J Am Vet Med Assoc 221(12):1690–1701, 2002.

76. Centers for Disease Control and Prevention. Update: raccoon rabies epizootic—United States, 1996. JAMA 277:282–283, 1997.

76a. Chang HG, Eidson M, Noonan-Toly C, et al. Public health impact of reemergence of rabies, New York. Emerg Infect Dis 8(9):909–913, 2002.

77. Steck F, Wandeler A. The epidemiology of fox rabies in Europe. Epidemiol Rev 2:71–96, 1980.

78. Bourhy H, Kissi B, Audry L, et al. Ecology and evolution of rabies virus in Europe. J Gen Virol 80(pt 10):2545–2557, 1999.

79. Takayama N. Rabies control in Japan. Jpn J Infect Dis 53:93–97, 2000.

80. Coleman PG, Dye C. Immunization coverage required to prevent outbreaks of dog rabies. Vaccine 14:185–186, 1996.

81. Delpietro HA, Larghi OP, Russo RG. Virus isolation from saliva and salivary glands of cattle naturally infected with paralytic rabies. Prev Vet Med 48:223–228, 2001.

82. Mitmoonpitak C, Tepsumethanon V, Wilde H. Rabies in Thailand. Epidemiol Infect 120:165–169, 1998.

83. Wilde H, Chutivongse S, Tepsumethanon W, et al. Rabies in Thailand: 1990. Rev Infect Dis 13:644–652, 1991.

84. Pandey P, Shlim DR, Cave W, Springer MF. Risk of possible exposure to rabies among tourists and foreign residents in Nepal. J Travel Med 9:127–131, 2002.

85. Dietzschold B, Rupprecht CE, Tollis M, et al. Antigenic diversity of the glycoprotein and nucleocapsid proteins of rabies and rabies-related viruses: implications for epidemiology and control of rabies. Rev Infect Dis 10(suppl 4):S785–S798, 1988.

86. Sacramento D, Badrane H, Bourhy H, Tordo N. Molecular epidemiology of rabies virus in France: comparison with vaccine strains. J Gen Virol 73(pt 5):1149–1158, 1992.

87. von Teichman BF, Thomson GR, Meredith CD, Nel LH. Molecular epidemiology of rabies virus in South Africa: evidence for two distinct virus groups. J Gen Virol 76(pt 1):73–82, 1995.

88. Smith JS, Orciari LA, Yager PA, et al. Epidemiologic and historical relationships among 87 rabies virus isolates as determined by limited sequence analysis. J Infect Dis 166:296–307, 1992.

89. Pape WJ, Fitzsimmons TD, Hoffman RE. Risk for rabies transmission from encounters with bats, Colorado, 1977–1996. Emerg Infect Dis 5:433–437, 1999.

90. Setien AA, Brochier B, Tordo N, et al. Experimental rabies infection and oral vaccination in vampire bats (Desmodus rotundus). Vaccine 16:1122–1126, 1998.

91. Ronsholt L, Sorensen KJ, Bruschke CJ, et al. Clinically silent rabies infection in (zoo) bats [see comments]. Vet Rec 142:519–520, 1998.

91a. Mc Coll KA, Tordo N, Setien AA. Bat lyssavirus infections. Rev Sci Tech Off Int Epiz 19:117–196, 2002.

92. Morimoto K, Patel M, Corisdeo S, et al. Characterization of a unique variant of bat rabies virus responsible for newly emerging human cases in North America. Proc Natl Acad Sci U S A 93:5653–5658, 1996.

93. Dietzschold B, Hooper DC. Human diploid cell culture rabies vaccine (HDCV) and purified chick embryo cell culture rabies vaccine (PCECV) both confer protective immunity against infection with the silver-haired bat rabies virus strain (SHBRV). Vaccine 16:1656–1659, 1998.

94. Gibbons RV. Cryptogenic rabies, bats, and the question of aerosol transmission. Ann Emerg Med 39:528–536, 2002.

95. Rabies prevention—United States, 1991: recommendations of the Immunization Practices Advisory Committee (ACIP). MMWR 40(RR-3):1–19, 1991.

96. World Health Organization. Sixth report of the Expert Committee on Rabies. World Health Organ Tech Rep Ser 523:1–55, 1973.

97. Remington PL, Shope T, Andrews J. A recommended approach to the evaluation of human rabies exposure in an acute-care hospital. JAMA 254:67–69, 1985.

98. Fekadu M, Endeshaw T, Alemu W, et al. Possible human-to-human transmission of rabies in Ethiopia. Ethiop Med J 34:123–127, 1996.

99. Brogan TV, Bratton SL, Dowd MD, Hegenbarth MA. Severe dog bites in children. Pediatrics 96(5 pt 1):947–950, 1995.

100. Wilde H. Managing facial dog bites. J Oral Maxillofac Surg 53:1368, 1995.

101. WHO recommendations on rabies post-exposure treatment and the correct technique of intradermal immunization against rabies (WHO/EMC/ZOO/96.6). Geneva, World Health Organization, 2002, p 1.

102. Varughese P. Human rabies in Canada—1994–2000. Can Commun Dis Rep 26(24):210–211, 2000.

103. Bernard KW, Roberts MA, Sumner J, et al. Human diploid cell rabies vaccine: effectiveness of immunization with small intradermal or subcutaneous doses. JAMA 247:1138–1142, 1982.

104. Messenger SL, Smith JS, Rupprects CE. Emerging epidemiology of bat-associated cryptic cases of rabies in humans in the United States. Clin Infect Dis 35:738–747, 2002.

105. Centers for Disease Control and Prevention. Human rabies—California, Georgia, Minnesota, New York and Wisconsin, 2000. JAMA 285:158–160, 2001.

106. Human rabies—California, 1995. MMWR 45:353–356, 1996.

107. Krebs JW, Smith JS, Rupprecht CE, Childs JE. Rabies surveillance in the United States during 1997. J Am Vet Med Assoc 213:1713–1728, 1998.

108. Warrell MJ. Human deaths from cryptic bat rabies in the USA. Lancet 346:65–66, 1995.

109. Fermi C. Uber die Immunisierung gegen Wutkrankheit. Z Hyg Infectionskrankh 58:233–276, 1908.

110. Semple D. The preparation of a safe and efficient antirabic vaccine. Sci Mem Med Sanit Dep India No 44, 1911.

111. Fuenzalida E, Palacios R, Borgono JM. Anti-rabies antibody response in man to vaccine made from infected suckling-mouse brains. Bull World Health Organ 30:431–436, 1964.

112. Peck FB, Powell HM, Culbertson CG. Duck-embryo rabies vaccine: study of fixed virus vaccine grown in embryonated duck eggs and killed with betapropiolactone. JAMA 162:1373–1376, 1956.

113. Kissling RE. Growth of rabies virus in non-nervous tissue culture. Proc Soc Exp Biol 98:223–225, 1958.

114. Fenje PA. A rabies vaccine from hamster kidney tissue cultures: preparation and evaluation in animals. Can J Microbiol 6:605–610, 1960.

115. Hayflick L, Moorehead PS. The serial cultivation of human diploid cell substrates. Exp Cell Res 25:585–621, 1961.

116. Plotkin SA. Vaccine production in human diploid cell strains. Am J Epidemiol 94:303–306, 1971.

117. Wiktor TJ, Sokol F, Kuwert E, Koprowski H. Immunogenicity of concentrated and purified rabies vaccine of tissue culture origin. Proc Soc Exp Biol Med 131:799–805, 1969.

118. Wiktor TJ, Plotkin SA, Grella DW. Human cell culture rabies vaccine: antibody response in man. JAMA 224:1170–1171, 1973.

119. Wiktor T. Virus vaccines and therapeutic approaches. In Bishop HDL (ed). Rhabdoviruses (3rd ed). Boca Raton, FL, CRC Press, 1980, pp 1–11.

120. Plotkin SA. Rabies vaccine prepared in human cell cultures: progress and perspectives. Rev Infect Dis 2:433–448, 1980.

121. Plotkin SA, Wiktor T. Rabies vaccination. Annu Rev Med 29:583–591, 1978.

122. Bahmanyar M, Fayaz A, Nour-Salehi S, et al. Successful protection of humans exposed to rabies infection: postexposure treatment with the new human diploid cell rabies vaccine and antirabies serum. JAMA 236:2751–2754, 1976.

123. Winkler WG. Current status of use of human diploid cell strain rabies vaccine in the United States, May 1984. In Vodopija I, Nicholson KG, Bijok U (eds). Improvements in Rabies Post-Exposure Treatment. Zagreb, Zagreb Institute of Public Health, 1985, pp 3–9.

124. Chippaux A, Chaniot S, Piat A, Netter R. Stability of freeze-dried tissue culture rabies vaccine. In Kuwert EK, Merieux C, Koprowski H, Bogel K (eds). Rabies in the Tropics. Berlin, Springer-Verlag, 1985, pp 322–324.

125. Nicholson KG, Burney MI, Ali S, Perkins FT. Stability of human diploid-cell-strain rabies vaccine at high ambient temperatures. Lancet 1:916–918, 1983.

126. Turner GS, Nicholson KG, Tyrrell DA, Aoki FY. Evaluation of a human diploid cell strain rabies vaccine: final report of a three year study of pre-exposure immunization. J Hyg (Lond) 89:101–110, 1982.

127. Montagnon BJ. Polio and rabies vaccines produced in continuous cell lines: a reality for Vero cell line. Dev Biol Stand 70:27–47, 1989.

128. Ajjan N, Pilet C. Comparative study of the safety and protective value, in pre-exposure use, of rabies vaccine cultivated on human diploid cells (HDCV) and of the new vaccine grown on Vero cells. Vaccine 7:125–128, 1989.

129. Suntharasamai P, Warrell MJ, Warrell DA, et al. New purified Vero-cell vaccine prevents rabies in patients bitten by rabid animals. Lancet 2:129–131, 1986.

130. Wang XJ, Lang J, Tao XR, et al. Immunogenicity and safety of purified Vero-cell rabies vaccine in severely rabies-exposed patients in China. Southeast Asian J Trop Med Public Health 31:287–294, 2000.

131. Lang J, Cetre JC, Picot N, et al. Immunogenicity and safety in adults of a new chromatographically purified Vero-cell rabies vaccine (CPRV): a randomized, double-blind trial with purified Vero-cell rabies vaccine (PVRV). Biologicals 26:299–308, 1998.

132. Hafkin B, Hattwick MA, Smith JS, et al. A comparison of a WI-38 vaccine and duck embryo vaccine for preexposure rabies prophylaxis. Am J Epidemiol 107:439–443, 1978.

133. Jones RL, Froeschle JE, Atmar RL, et al. Immunogenicity, safety and lot consistency in adults of a chromatographically purified Vero-cell rabies vaccine: a randomized, double-blind trial with human diploid cell rabies vaccine. Vaccine 19:4635–4643, 2001.

134. Picot N, Le Menet V, Rotivel Y, et al. Booster effect of a new chromatographically purified Vero-cell rabies vaccine (CPRV): immunogenicity and safety of a single or double injection. Trans R Soc Trop Med Hyg 95:342–344, 2001.

135. Quiambao BP, Lang J, Vital S, et al. Immunogenicity and effectiveness of post-exposure rabies prophylaxis with a new chromatographically purified Vero-cell rabies vaccine (CPRV): a two-stage randomised clinical trial in the Philippines. Acta Trop 75:39–52, 2000.

136. Bijok U, Vodopija I, Smerdel S, et al. Purified chick embryo cell (PCEC) rabies vaccine for human use: clinical trials. Behring Inst Mitt 76:155–164, 1984.

137. Scheiermann N, Baer J, Hilfenhaus J, et al. Reactogenicity and immunogenicity of the newly developed purified chick embryo cell (PCEC)-rabies vaccine in man. Zentralbl Bakteriol Mikrobiol Hyg A 265:439–450, 1987.

138. Nicholson KG, Farrow PR, Bijok U, Barth R. Pre-exposure studies with purified chick embryo cell culture rabies vaccine and human diploid cell vaccine: serological and clinical responses in man. Vaccine 5:208–210, 1987.

139. Dreesen DW, Fishbein DB, Kemp DT, Brown J. Two-year comparative trial on the immunogenicity and adverse effects of purified chick embryo cell rabies vaccine for pre-exposure immunization. Vaccine 7:397–400, 1989.

140. Khawplod P, Tantawichien T, Wilde H, et al. Use of rabies vaccines after reconstitution and storage. Clin Infect Dis 34:404–406, 2002.

141. Vodopija I, Baklaic Z, Vodopija R. Rabipur: a reliable vaccine for rabies protection. Vaccine 17:1739–1741, 1999.

142. Sehgal S, Bhattacharya D, Bhardwaj M. Ten year longitudinal study of efficacy and safety of purified chick embryo cell vaccine for pre- and post-exposure prophylaxis of rabies in Indian population. J Commun Dis 27:36–43, 1995.

143. Dutta JK. Adverse reactions to purified chick embryo cell rabies vaccine. Vaccine 12:1484, 1994.

144. Briggs DJ, Dreesen DW, Nicolay U, et al. Purified Chick Embryo Cell Culture Rabies Vaccine: interchangeability with Human Diploid Cell Culture Rabies Vaccine and comparison of one- versus two-dose post-exposure booster regimen for previously immunized persons. Vaccine 19:1055–1060, 2000.

145. Arai YT, Ogata T, Oya A. Studies on Japanese-produced chick embryo cell culture rabies vaccines. Am J Trop Med Hyg 44:131–134, 1991.

146. Chino F, Oshibuchi S, Ariga H, Okuno Y. Skin reaction to yellow fever vaccine after immunization with rabies vaccine of chick embryo cell culture origin. Jpn J Infect Dis 52:42–44, 1999.

147. Lin FT. The protective effect of the large-scale use of PHKC rabies vaccine in humans in China. Bull World Health Organ 68:449–454, 1990.

148. Lin FT, Na L. Developments in the production and application of rabies vaccine for human use in China. Trop Doct 30(1):14–16, 2000.

149. Glück R, Wegmann A, Germanier R, et al. Confirmation of need for rabies immunoglobulin as well as post-exposure vaccine. Lancet 2:1216–1217, 1984.

150. Thraenhart O, Marcus I, Kreuzfelder E. Current and future immunoprophylaxis against human rabies: reduction of treatment failures and errors. Curr Top Microbiol Immunol 187:173–194, 1994.

151. Khawplod P, Glück R, Wilde H, et al. Immunogenicity of purified duck embryo rabies vaccine (Lyssavac-N) with use of the WHO-approved intradermal postexposure regimen. Clin Infect Dis 20:646–651, 1995.

152. Rubin RH, Hattwick MA, Jones S, et al. Adverse reactions to duck embryo rabies vaccine: range and incidence. Ann Intern Med 78:643–649, 1973.

153. Berlin BS, Mitchell JR, Burgoyne GH, et al. Rhesus diploid rabies vaccine (adsorbed), a new rabies vaccine. II. Results of clinical studies simulating prophylactic therapy for rabies exposure. JAMA 249:2663–2665, 1983.

154. Burgoyne GH, Kajiya KD, Brown DW, Mitchell JR. Rhesus diploid rabies vaccine (adsorbed): a new rabies vaccine using FRhL-2 cells. J Infect Dis 152:204–210, 1985.

155. Berlin BS. Rabies Vaccine Adsorbed: neutralizing antibody titers after three-dose pre-exposure vaccination. Am J Public Health 80:476–477, 1990.

156. Perrin P, Madhusudana S, Gontier-Jallet C, et al. An experimental rabies vaccine produced with a new BHK-21 suspension cell culture process: use of serum-free medium and perfusion-reactor system. Vaccine 13:1244–1250, 1995.

157. Zanetti CR, Chaves LB, Silva AC, et al. Studies on human anti-rabies immunization in Brazil. I—Evaluation of the 3 + 1 pre-exposure vaccination schedule under field conditions. Rev Inst Med Trop Sao Paulo 37:349–352, 1995.

158. Fishbein DB, Sawyer LA, Reid-Sanden FL, Weir EH. Administration of human diploid-cell rabies vaccine in the gluteal area. N Engl J Med 318:124–125, 1988.

159. Hasbahceci M, Kiyan M, Eyol E, et al. Human diploid-cell rabies vaccine: efficacy of four doses. Lancet 347:976–977, 1996.

160. Vodopija I, Sureau P, Lafon M, et al. An evaluation of second generation tissue culture rabies vaccines for use in man: a four-vaccine comparative immunogenicity study using a pre-exposure vaccination schedule and an abbreviated 2-1-1 postexposure schedule. Vaccine 4:245–248, 1986.

161. Vodopija I. Current issues in human rabies immunization. Rev Infect Dis 10(suppl 4):S758–S763, 1988.

162. Zanetti CR, Lee LM, Chaves LB, et al. Studies on human anti-rabies immunization in Brazil. II—Preliminary evaluation of the 2-1-1 schedule for human pre-exposure anti-rabies immunization, employing suckling mouse brain vaccine. Rev Inst Med Trop Sao Paulo 37:353–356, 1995.

163. Chutivongse S, Wilde H, Fishbein DB, et al. One-year study of the 2-1-1 intramuscular postexposure rabies vaccine regimen in 100 severely exposed Thai patients using rabies immune globulin and Vero cell rabies vaccine. Vaccine 9:573–576, 1991.

164. Vodopija I, Sureau P, Smerdel S, et al. Interaction of rabies vaccine with human rabies immunoglobulin and reliability of a 2-1-1 schedule application for postexposure treatment. Vaccine 6:283–286, 1988.

165. Lang J, Simanjuntak GH, Soerjosembodo S, Koesharyono C. Suppressant effect of human or equine rabies immunoglobulins on the immunogenicity of post-exposure rabies vaccination under the 2-1-1 regimen: a field trial in Indonesia. MAS054 Clinical Investigator Group. Bull World Health Organ 76:491–495, 1998.

166. Vodopija I, Sureau P, Smerdel S, et al. Comparative study of two human diploid rabies vaccines administered with antirabies globulin. Vaccine 6:489–490, 1988.

167. Wasi C, Chaiprasithikul P, Auewarakul P, et al. The abbreviated 2-1-1 schedule of purified chick embryo cell rabies vaccination for rabies postexposure treatment. Southeast Asian J Trop Med Public Health 24:461–466, 1993.

168. Scrimgeour EM, Mehta FR. Rabies in Oman: failed postexposure vaccination in a lactating woman bitten by a fox. Int J Infect Dis 5:160–162, 2001.

169. Aoki FY, Tyrrell DA, Hill LE. Immunogenicity and acceptability of a human diploid-cell culture rabies vaccine in volunteers. Lancet 1:660–662, 1975.

170. Turner GS, Aoki FY, Nicholson KG, et al. Human diploid cell strain rabies vaccine: rapid prophylactic immunisation of volunteers with small doses. Lancet 1:1379–1381, 1976.

171. Nicholson KG, Prestage H, Cole PJ, et al. Multisite intradermal antirabies vaccination: immune responses in man and protection of rabbits against death from street virus by postexposure administration of human diploid-cell-strain rabies vaccine. Lancet 2:915–918, 1981.

172. Ajjan N, Soulebot JP, Triau R, Biron G. Intradermal immunization with rabies vaccine: inactivated Wistar strain cultivated in human diploid cells. JAMA 244:2528–2531, 1980.

173. Burridge MJ, Baer GM, Sumner JW, Sussman O. Intradermal immunization with human diploid cell rabies vaccine: serological and clinical responses of persons with and without prior vaccination with duck embryo vaccine. JAMA 248:1611–1614, 1982.

174. Report of a WHO Consultation on Intradermal Application of Human Rabies Vaccines [abstr]. Geneva, World Health Organization, 1995, p. 2.

175. Intradermal Application of Rabies Vaccines: Report of a WHO Consultation, Bangkok, Thailand. Geneva, World Health Organization, 2000.

176. Dreesen DW, Brown WJ, Kemp DT, et al. Pre-exposure rabies prophylaxis: efficacy of a new packaging and delivery system for intradermal administration of human diploid cell vaccine. Vaccine 2:185–188, 1984.

177. Human rabies—Kenya. MMWR 32:494–495, 1983.

178. Bernard KW, Fishbein DB, Miller KD, et al. Pre-exposure rabies immunization with human diploid cell vaccine: decreased antibody responses in persons immunized in developing countries. Am J Trop Med Hyg 34:633–647, 1985.

179. Warrell MJ, Suntharasamai P, Nicholson KG, et al. Multi-site intradermal and multi-site subcutaneous rabies vaccination: improved economical regimens. Lancet 1:874–876, 1984.

180. Warrell MJ, Nicholson KG, Warrell DA, et al. Economical multiple-site intradermal immunisation with human diploid-cell-strain vaccine is effective for post-exposure rabies prophylaxis. Lancet 1:1059–1062, 1985.

180a. Madhusudana SN, Anand NP, Shamsundar R. Evaluation of two intradermal vaccination regiments using purified chick embryo cell vaccine for post-exposure prophylaxis of rabies. Int J Infect Dis 6:210–214, 2002.

180b. Khawplod P, Wilde H, Tepsumethanon S, et al. Prospective immunogenicity study of multiple intradermal injections of rabies vaccine in an effort to obtain an early immune response without the use of immunoglobin. Clin Infect Dis 35(12):1562–1565, 2002.

181. Phanuphak P, Khawplod P, Sirivichayakul S, et al. Humoral and cell-mediated immune responses to various economical regimens of purified Vero cell rabies vaccine. Asian Pac J Allergy Immunol 5:33–37, 1987.

182. Madhusudana SN, Anand NP, Shamsundar R. Evaluation of two intradermal vaccination regimens using purified chick embryo cell vaccine for post-exposure prophylaxis of rabies. Natl Med J India 14:145–147, 2001.

183. Chutivongse S, Wilde H, Supich C, et al. Postexposure prophylaxis for rabies with antiserum and intradermal vaccination. Lancet 335:896–898, 1990.

184. Suntharasamai P. Clinical trials of rabies vaccines in Thailand. Southeast Asian J Trop Med Public Health 19:537–547, 1988.

184a. Kamoltham T, Khawplod P, Wilde H. Rabies intradermal post-exposure vaccination of humans using reconstituted and stored vaccine. Vaccine 20(27–28):3272–3276, 2002.

185. Briggs DJ, Banzhoff A, Nicolay U, et al. Antibody response of patients after postexposure rabies vaccination with small intradermal doses of purified chick embryo cell vaccine or purified Vero cell rabies vaccine. Bull World Health Organ 78:693–698, 2000.

186. Kositprapa C, Limsuwun K, Wilde H, et al. Immune response to simulated postexposure rabies booster vaccinations in volunteers who received preexposure vaccinations. Clin Infect Dis 25:614–616, 1997.

187. Tantawichien T, Benjavongkulchai M, Limsuwan K, et al. Antibody response after a four-site intradermal booster vaccination with cell-culture rabies vaccine. Clin Infect Dis 28:1100–1103, 1999.

188. Suntharasamai P, Chaiprasithikul P, Wasi C, et al. A simplified and economical intradermal regimen of purified chick embryo cell rabies vaccine for postexposure prophylaxis. Vaccine 12:508–512, 1994.

189. Dutta JK, Warrell MJ, Dutta TK. Intradermal rabies immunization for pre- and post-exposure prophylaxis. Natl Med J India 7:119–122, 1994.

190. Babes V, Cerchez T. Traite de la rage. Ann Inst Pasteur 10:625–702, 1891.

191. Saltazard M, Ghodssi M. Prevention de la rage humaine. Natl Med J India 17:366–367, 19535.

192. Habel K, Koprowski H. Laboratory data supporting the clinical trial of antirabies serum in persons bitten by a rabid wolf. Bull World Health Organ 13:773–779, 1955.

193. Baltazard M, Bahmanyar M. Essai pratique du serum antirabique chez les mordus par loups enrages. Bull World Health Organ 13:747–779, 1955.

194. Cho HC, Lawson KF. Protection of dogs against death from experimental rabies by postexposure administration of rabies vaccine and hyperimmune globulin (human). Can J Vet Res 53:434–437, 1989.

195. Baer GM, Cleary WF. A model in mice for the pathogenesis and treatment of rabies. J Infect Dis 125:520–527, 1972.

196. Devriendt J, Staroukine M, Costy F, Vanderhaeghen JJ. Fatal encephalitis apparently due to rabies: occurrence after treatment with human diploid cell vaccine but not rabies immune globulin. JAMA 248:2304–2306, 1982.

197. Wattanasri S, Boonthai P, Thongcharoen P. Human rabies after late administration of human diploid cell vaccine without hyperimmune serum. Lancet 2:870, 1982.

198. Rabies prevention—United States. MMWR 33:393–408, 1984.

199. Karliner JS. Incidence of reactions following administration of antirabies serum. JAMA 193:359–362, 1965.

200. Wilde H, Chomchey P, Punyaratabandhu P, et al. Purified equine rabies immune globulin: a safe and affordable alternative to human rabics immune globulin. Bull World Health Organ 67:731–736, 1989.

201. Tantawichien T, Benjavongkulchai M, Wilde H, et al. Value of skin testing for predicting reactions to equine rabies immune globulin. Clin Infect Dis 21:660–662, 1995.

202. Lang J, Gravenstein S, Briggs D, et al. Evaluation of the safety and immunogenicity of a new, heat-treated human rabies immune globulin using a sham, post-exposure prophylaxis of rabies. Biologicals 26:7–15, 1998.

203. Lang J, Attanath P, Quiambao B, et al. Evaluation of the safety, immunogenicity, and pharmacokinetic profile of a new, highly purified, heat-treated equine rabies immunoglobulin, administered either alone or in association with a purified, Vero-cell rabies vaccine. Acta Trop 70:317–333, 1998.

203a. Wilde H, Khawplod P, Hemachudha T, et al. Postexposure treatment of rabies infection: can it be done without immunoglobulin? Clin Infect Dis J 23:477–480, 2002.

204. Helmick CG, Johnstone C, Sumner J, et al. A clinical study of Merieux human rabies immune globulin. J Biol Stand 10:357–367, 1982.

205. Anderson JA, Daly FT Jr, Kidd JC. Human rabies after antiserum and vaccine postexposure treatment: case report and review. Ann Intern Med 64:1297–1302, 1966.

206. Loofbourow JC, Cabasso VJ, Roby RE, Anuskiewicz W. Rabies immune globulin (human): clinical trials and dose determination. JAMA 217:1825–1831, 1971.

207. Khawplod P, Wilde H, Chomchey P, et al. What is an acceptable delay in rabies immune globulin administration when vaccine alone had been given previously? Vaccine 14:389–391, 1996.

208. Wilde H, Khawplot P, Benjavongkulchai M, Sitprija V. Method of administration of rabies immune globulin. Vaccine 12:1150–1151, 1994.

209. Wilde H, Sirikawin S, Sabcharoen A, et al. Failure of postexposure treatment of rabies in children. Clin Infect Dis 22:228–232, 1996.

210. Wilde H, Khawplod P, Hemachudha T, Sitprija V. Postexposure treatment of rabies infection: can it be done without immunoglobulin? Clin Infect Dis 34:477–480, 2002.

210a. Ayele W, Fekadu M, Zewdi B, et al. Immunogenicity and efficacy of fermi-type nerve tissue rabies vaccine in mice and in humans undergoing post-exposure prophylaxis for rabies in Ethiopia. Ethiop Med J 39:313–321, 2001.

211. Turner GS. Immunoglobulin (IgG) and (IgM) antibody responses to rabies vaccine. J Gen Virol 40:595–604, 1978.

212. Cabasso VJ, Dobkin MB, Roby RE, Hammar AH. Antibody response to a human diploid cell rabies vaccine. Appl Microbiol 27:553–561, 1974.

213. Resultats serologiques d'immunization et de hyper-immunization de l'homme avec un nouveau vaccin antirabique obtenu sur cultures de cellules diploides humaines WI-38. In La Rage: Colloque, Paris, 1973.

214. Banmanyar M. Results of antibody profiles in man vaccinated with the HDCS vaccine with various schedules. Symp Series Immunol Stand 21:231–239, 1974.

215. Shah U, Jaswal GS, Mansharamani HJ, et al. Trial of human diploid cell rabies vaccine in human volunteers. Br Med J 1:997, 1976.

216. Kuwert EK, Marcus I, Werner J, et al. Post-exposure use of human diploid cell culture rabies vaccine. Dev Biol Stand 37:273–286, 1976.

217. Kuwert EK, Marcus I, Werner J, et al. Some experiences with human diploid cell strain-(HDCS) rabies vaccine in pre- and post-exposure vaccinated humans. Dev Biol Stand 40:79–88, 1978.

218. Cox JH, Klietmann W, Schneider LG. Human rabies immunoprophylaxis using HDC (MRC-5) vaccine. Dev Biol Stand 40:105–108, 1978.

219. Plotkin SA, Wiktor T. Vaccination of children with human cell culture rabies vaccine. Pediatrics 63:219–221, 1979.

220. Kuwert EK, Marcus I, Hoher PG. Neutralizing and complement-fixing antibody responses in pre- and post-exposure vaccinees to a rabies vaccine produced in human diploid cells. J Biol Stand 4:249–262, 1976.

221. Fescharek R, Franke V, Samuel MR. Do anaesthetics and surgical stress increase the risk of post-exposure rabies treatment failure? Vaccine 12:12–13, 1994.

222. Thisyakorn U, Pancharoen C, Ruxrungtham K, et al. Safety and immunogenicity of preexposure rabies immunization in HIV-infected children. In Abstracts of the Eighth International Congress on Infectious Diseases, Boston 1998, p 236.

223. Mastroeni I, Vescia N, Pompa MG, et al. Immune response of the elderly to rabies vaccines. Vaccine 12:518–520, 1994.

223a.Leder K, Weller PF, Wilso ME. Travel vaccines and elderly persons: review of vaccines available in the United States. Clin Infect Dis J 33:1553–1566, 2001.

224. Suss J, Sinnecker H. Immune reactions against rabies viruses—infection and vaccination. Exp Pathol 42:1–9, 1991.

225. Celis E, Wiktor TJ, Dietzschold B, Koprowski H. Amplification of rabies virus-induced stimulation of human T-cell lines and clones by antigen-specific antibodies. J Virol 56:426–433, 1985.

226. Bracci L, Ballas SK, Spreafico A, Neri P. Molecular mimicry between the rabies virus glycoprotein and human immunodeficiency virus-1 GP120: cross-reacting antibodies induced by rabies vaccination. Blood 90:3623–3628, 1997.

227. Bracci L, Neri P. Molecular mimicry between the rabies virus and human immunodeficiency virus. Arch Pathol Lab Med 119:391–393, 1995.

228. Pearlman ES, Ballas SK. False positive human immunodeficiency virus screening test related to rabies vaccination. Arch Pathol Lab Med 118:805–806, 1994.

229. Plotkin SA, Loupi E, Blondeau C. False-positive human immunodeficiency virus screening test related to rabies vaccination. Arch Pathol Lab Med 119:679, 1995.

230. Henderson S, Leibnitz G, Turnbull M, Palmer GH. False-positive human immunodeficiency virus seroconversion is not common following rabies vaccination. Clin Diagn Lab Immunol 9:942–943, 2002.

231. Persistence of antibodies in children after pre-exposure primary and booster immunizations with purified Vero cell rabies vaccine, chromatographically purified Vero cell rabies vaccine and human diploid cell vaccine. In Dodet B, Meslin FX, Heseltine E (eds). Clinical Aspects of Human Rabies: Fourth International Symposium on Rabies Control in Asia, March 5–9, 2001, Hanoi, Viet Nam. Paris, World Health Organization, 2001, p 29.

232. Veeraraghaven N, Subrahmanyan TP. The value of 5 percent Semple vaccine prepared in distilled water in human treatment: comparative mortality among the treated and untreated. Indian J Med Res 46:518–524, 1958.

233. Nicholson KG. Modern vaccines: rabies. Lancet 335:1201–1205, 1990.

234. Anderson LJ, Sikes RK, Langkop CW, et al. Postexposure trial of a human diploid cell strain rabies vaccine. J Infect Dis 142:133–138, 1980.

235. Wilde H, Glück R, Khawplod P, et al. Efficacy study of a new albumin-free human diploid cell rabies vaccine (Lyssavac-HDC, Berna) in 100 severely rabies-exposed Thai patients. Vaccine 13:593–596, 1995.

236. Lodmell DL, Smith JS, Esposito JJ, Ewalt LC. Cross-protection of mice against a global spectrum of rabies virus variants. J Virol 69:4957–4962, 1995.

237. Rosanoff E, Tint H. Responses to human diploid cell rabies vaccine: neutralizing antibody responses of vaccinees receiving booster doses of human diploid cell rabies vaccine. Am J Epidemiol 110:322–327, 1979.

238. Nicholson KG, Turner GS, Aoki FY. Immunization with a human diploid cell strain of rabies virus vaccine: two-year results. J Infect Dis 137:783–788, 1978.

239. Thraenhart O, Kreuzfelder E, Hillebrandt M, et al. Long-term humoral and cellular immunity after vaccination with cell culture rabies vaccines in man. Clin Immunol Immunopathol 71:287–292, 1994.

240. Fishbein DB, Bernard KW, Miller KD, et al. The early kinetics of the neutralizing antibody response after booster immunizations with human diploid cell rabies vaccine. Am J Trop Med Hyg 35:663–670, 1986.

241. Burridge MJ, Sumner JW, Baer GM. Intradermal immunization with human diploid cell rabies vaccine: serological and clinical responses of immunized persons to intradermal booster vaccination. Am J Public Health 74:503–505, 1984.

242. Briggs DJ, Schwenke JR. Longevity of rabies antibody titre in recipients of human diploid cell rabies vaccine. Vaccine 10:125–129, 1992.

243. Thisyakorn U, Pancharoen C, Wilde H. Immunologic and virologic evaluation of HIV-1-infected children after rabies vaccination. Vaccine 19:1534–1537, 2001.

244. Jaijaroensup W, Tantawichien T, Khawplod P, et al. Postexposure rabies vaccination in patients infected with human immunodeficiency virus. Clin Infect Dis 28:913–914, 1999.

245. Pancharoen C, Thisyakorn U, Tantawichien T, et al. Failure of pre- and postexposure rabies vaccinations in a child infected with HIV. Scand J Infect Dis 33:390–391, 2001.

246. Thisyakorn U, Pancharoen C, Ruxrungtham K, et al. Safety and immunogenicity of preexposure rabies vaccination in children infected with human immunodeficiency virus type 1. Clin Infect Dis 30:218, 2000.

247. Rabies Vaccination in Immunosuppressed Patients. Paris, Merieux Foundation/World Health Organization, 2001.

248. Post-exposure Treatment of Patients with Impaired or Suboptimal Immunity. Paris, Merieux Foundation/World Health Organization, 2001.

249. Deshmukh RA, Yemul VL. Fatal rabies encephalitis despite post-exposure vaccination in a diabetic patient: a need for use of rabies immune globulin in all post-exposure cases. J Assoc Physicians India 47:546–547, 1999.

250. Sudarshan MK, Madhusudana SN, Mahendra BJ. Post-exposure prophylaxis with purified Vero cell rabies vaccine during pregnancy—safety and immunogenicity. J Commun Dis 31:229–236, 1999.

251. Baer GM, Moore SA, Shaddock JH, Levy HB. An effective rabies treatment in exposed monkeys: a single dose of interferon inducer and vaccine. Bull World Health Organ 57:807–813, 1979.

252. What Can Be Learned from a Decade of Worldwide Postmarketing Surveillance? [abstr 6.07]. Paris, Institut Pasteur, 1997.

253. Gacouin A, Bourhy H, Renaud JC, et al. Human rabies despite post-exposure vaccination. Eur J Clin Microbiol Infect Dis 18:233–235, 1999.

254. Ki-Zerbo GA, Kyelem N, Ouattara Y, et al. Apropos of a case of rabies occurring despite vaccination after exposure. Med Trop (Mars) 60:67–69, 2000.

255. Udawat H, Chaudhary HR, Goyal RK, et al. Guillain-Barré syndrome following antirabies Semple vaccine—a report of six cases. J Assoc Physicians India 49:384–385, 2001.

256. Javier RS, Kunishita T, Koike F, Tabira T. Semple rabies vaccine: presence of myelin basic protein and proteolipid protein and its activity in experimental allergic encephalomyelitis. J Neurol Sci 93:221–230, 1989.

257. Laouini D, Kennou MF, Khoufi S, Dellagi K. Antibodies to human myelin proteins and gangliosides in patients with acute neuroparalytic accidents induced by brain-derived rabies vaccine. J Neuroimmunol 91:63–72, 1998.

258. Bahri F, Letaief A, Ernez M, et al. Neurological complications in adults following rabies vaccine prepared from animal brains. Presse Med 25:491–493, 1996.

259. Systemic allergic reactions following immunization with human diploid cell rabies vaccine. MMWR 33:185–188, 1984.

260. Dreesen DW, Bernard KW, Parker RA, et al. Immune complex-like disease in 23 persons following a booster dose of rabies human diploid cell vaccine. Vaccine 4:45–49, 1986.

261. Fishbein DB, Yenne KM, Dreesen DW, et al. Risk factors for systemic hypersensitivity reactions after booster vaccinations with human diploid cell rabies vaccine: a nationwide prospective study. Vaccine 11:1390–1394, 1993.

262. ACIP Rabies Prevention—United States, 1984. MMWR 33:393–407, 1984.

263. Anderson MC, Baer H, Frazier DJ, Quinnan GV. The role of specific IgE and beta-propiolactone in reactions resulting from booster doses of human diploid cell rabies vaccine. J Allergy Clin Immunol 80:861–868, 1987.

264. Swanson MC, Rosanoff E, Gurwith M, et al. IgE and IgG antibodies to beta-propiolactone and human serum albumin associated with urticarial reactions to rabies vaccine. J Infect Dis 155:909–913, 1987.

265. Fishbein DB, Dreesen DW, Holmes DF, et al. Human diploid cell rabies vaccine purified by zonal centrifugation: a controlled study of antibody response and side effects following primary and booster pre-exposure immunizations. Vaccine 7:437–442, 1989.

266. Briggs DJ, Dreesen DW, Morgan P, et al. Safety and immunogenicity of Lyssavac Berna human diploid cell rabies vaccine in healthy adults. Vaccine 14:1361–1365, 1996.

267. Bernard KW, Smith PW, Kader FJ, Moran MJ. Neuroparalytic illness and human diploid cell rabies vaccine. JAMA 248:3136–3138, 1982.

268. Boe E, Nyland H. Guillain-Barré syndrome after vaccination with human diploid cell rabies vaccine. Scand J Infect Dis 12:231–232, 1980.

269. Knittel T, Ramadori G, Mayet WJ, et al. Guillain-Barré syndrome and human diploid cell rabies vaccine. Lancet 1:1334–1335, 1989.

270. Tornatore CS, Richert JR. CNS demyelination associated with diploid cell rabies vaccine. Lancet 335:1346–1347, 1990.

271. Moulignier A, Richer A, Fritzell C, et al. Meningoradiculitis after injection of an antirabies vaccine: a vaccine from human diploid cell culture. Presse Med 20:1121–1123, 1991.
272. Thongcharoen P, Wasi C, Chavanich L, Sirikawin S. Rabies in Thailand. *In* Mackenzie JS (ed).Viral Disease in South-East Asia and Western Pacific. New York, Academic Press, 1982, p 606.
273. Arguin PM, Krebs JW, Mandel E, et al. Survey of rabies preexposure and postexposure prophylaxis among missionary personnel stationed outside the United States. J Travel Med 7:10–14, 2000.
274. Phanupak P, Ubolyam S, Sirivichayakul S. Should travellers in rabies endemic areas receive pre-exposure rabies immunization? Ann Med Interne (Paris) 145:409–411, 1994.
275. Wilde H. Preexposure rabies vaccination. J Travel Med 1:51–54, 1994.
276. LeGuerrier P, Pilon PA, Deshaies D, Allard R. Pre-exposure rabies prophylaxis for the international traveller: a decision analysis. Vaccine 14:167–176, 1996.
277. Fridell E, Grandien M, Johansson R. Pre-exposure prophylaxis against rabies in children by human diploid cell vaccine. Lancet 1:623, 1984.
278. Lumbiganon P, Chaiprasithikul P, Sookpranee T, et al. Pre-exposure vaccination with purified chick embryo cell rabies vaccines in children. Asian Pac J Allergy Immunol 7:99–101, 1989.
279. Bhanganada K, Wilde H, Sakolsataydorn P, Oonsombat P. Dog-bite injuries at a Bangkok teaching hospital. Acta Trop 55:249–255, 1993.
280. Lang J, Duong GH, Nguyen VG, et al. Randomised feasibility trial of pre-exposure rabies vaccination with DTP-IPV in infants. Lancet 349:1663–1665, 1997.
281. Lang J, Hoa DQ, Gioi NV, et al. Immunogenicity and safety of low-dose intradermal rabies vaccination given during an Expanded Programme on Immunization session in Viet Nam: results of a comparative randomized trial. Trans R Soc Trop Med Hyg 93:208–213, 1999.
282. Strady A, Lang J, Lienard M, et al. Antibody persistence following preexposure regimens of cell-culture rabies vaccines: 10-year follow-up and proposal for a new booster policy. J Infect Dis 177:1290–1295, 1998.
283. Strady C, Jaussaud R, Beguinot I, et al. Predictive factors for the neutralizing antibody response following pre-exposure rabies immunization: validation of a new booster dose strategy. Vaccine 18:2661–2667, 2000.
284. Strady C, Hung Nguyen V, Jaussaud R, et al. Pre-exposure rabies vaccination: strategies and cost-minimization study. Vaccine 19:1416–1424, 2001.
285. Wilde H. Rabies. Int J Infect Dis 1:135–142, 1996.
286. Fleisher GR. The management of bite wounds. N Engl J Med 340:138–140, 1999.
287. Plotkin SA, Clark HF. Rabies. *In* Feigin RD, Cherry JD (eds). Textbook of Pediatric Infectious Diseases. Philadelphia, WB Saunders, 1998, pp 2111–2125.
288. Mann JM. Systematic decision-making in rabies prophylaxis. Pediatr Infect Dis 2:162–167, 1983.
289. Fishbein DB, Robinson LE. Rabies. N Engl J Med 329:1632–1638, 1993.
290. Human rabies prevention—United States, 1999: recommendations of the Advisory Committee on Immunization Practices (ACIP). MMWR 48(RR-1):1–21, 1999.
291. Hemachudha T, Chutivongse S, Wilde H, Phanuphak P. Latent rabies (reply). N Engl J Med 324:1890–1891, 1991.
292. Dutta JK. Treatment after rodent exposure necessary to avoid death from rabies. Public Health 115:243, 2001.
293. Siwasontiwat D, Lumlertdacha B, Polsuwan C, et al. Rabies: is provocation of the biting dog relevant for risk assessment? Trans R Soc Trop Med Hyg 86:443, 1992.
294. Kaplan MM, Cohen D, Koprowski H. Studies on the local treatment of wounds for the prevention of rabies. Bull World Health Organ 26:765–775, 1962.
295. Ajjan N, Strady A, Roumiantzeff M, Xueref C. Effectiveness and tolerance of rabies post-exposure treatment with human diploid cell rabies vaccine in children. *In* Kuwert E, Merieux C, Koprowski H, Bogel K (eds). Rabies in the Tropics. Berlin, Springer-Verlag, 1985, pp 86–90.
296. Thongcharoen P, Wasi C, Chavanich L. Post-exposure prophylaxis against rabies in children with human diploid cell vaccine. Lancet 2:436–437, 1982.
297. Lang J, Plotkin SA. Rabies risk and immunoprophylaxis in children. Adv Pediatr Infect Dis 13:219–255, 1997.
198. Dietzschold B, Hooper DC. Efficacy of human rabies vaccines for a newly emerging rabies virus strain in North America [abstr 53.005]. *In* Abstracts of the Eighth International Congress on Infectious Diseases, Boston, 1998, p 158.
299. Rotz LD, Hensley JA, Rupprecht CE, Childs JE. Large-scale human exposures to rabid or presumed rabid animals in the United States: 22 cases (1990–1996). J Am Vet Med Assoc 212:1198–1200, 1998.
300. Moran GJ, Talan DA, Mower W, et al. Appropriateness of rabies postexposure prophylaxis treatment for animal exposures. Emergency ID Net Study Group. JAMA 284:1001–1007, 2000.
301. WHO Expert Committee on Rabies. World Health Organ Tech Rep Ser 824:1–84, 1992.
302. Gherardin AW, Scrimgeour DJ, Lau SC, et al. Early rabies antibody response to intramuscular booster in previously intradermally immunized travelers using human diploid cell rabies vaccine. J Travel Med 8:122–126, 2001.
303. Jaijaroensup W, Limusanno S, Khawplod P, et al. Immunogenicity of rabies postexposure booster injections in subjects who had previously received intradermal preexposure vaccination. J Travel Med 6:234–237, 1999.
304. Tantawichien T, Tantawichien T, Supit C, et al. Three-year experience with 4-site intradermal booster vaccination with rabies vaccine for postexposure prophylaxis. Clin Infect Dis 33:2085–2087, 2001.
305. Naraporn N, Khawplod P, Limsuwan K, et al. Immune response to rabies booster vaccination in subjects who had postexposure treatment more than 5 years previously. J Travel Med 6:134–136, 1999.
306. Khawplod P, Wilde H, Yenmuang W, et al. Immune response to tissue culture rabies vaccine in subjects who had previous postexposure treatment with Semple or suckling mouse brain vaccine. Vaccine 14:1549–1552, 1996.
307. Thongcharoen P, Wasi C. Possible factors influencing unsuccessful protection of post-exposure prophylaxis for rabies by human diploid cell vaccine. J Med Assoc Thai 68:386–387, 1985.
308. Chabala S, Williams M, Amenta R, Ognjan AF. Confirmed rabies exposure during pregnancy: treatment with human rabies immune globulin and human diploid cell vaccine. Am J Med 91:423–424, 1991.
309. Chutivongse S, Wilde H. Postexposure rabies vaccination during pregnancy: experience with 21 patients. Vaccine 7:546–548, 1989.
310. Chutivongse S, Wilde H, Benjavongkulchai M, et al. Postexposure rabies vaccination during pregnancy: effect on 202 women and their infants. Clin Infect Dis 20:818–820, 1995.
311. Paolazzi CC, Perez O, De Filippo J. Rabies vaccine: developments employing molecular biology methods. Mol Biotechnol 11:137–147, 1999.
312. Wiktor TJ, MacFarlane RI, Reagan KJ, et al. Protection from rabies by a vaccinia virus recombinant containing the rabies virus glycoprotein gene. 1984. Biotechnology 24:508–512, 1992.
313. Cadoz M, Strady A, Meignier B, et al. Immunisation with canarypox virus expressing rabies glycoprotein. Lancet 339:1429–1432, 1992.
314. Cadoz M, Strady A, Jaussaud R, et al. Tolerance et immunogenicite de deux vaccins antibiotiques recombinants: ALVAC-RG et NYVAC-RG. Paper presented at the International Rabies Meeting, Paris, Institute Pasteur, 1997.
315. Xiang ZQ, Spitalnik S, Tran M, et al. Vaccination with a plasmid vector carrying the rabies virus glycoprotein gene induces protective immunity against rabies virus. Virology 199:132–140, 1994.
316. Osorio JE, Tomlinson CC, Frank RS, et al. Immunization of dogs and cats with a DNA vaccine against rabies virus. Vaccine 17:1109–1116, 1999.
317. Perrin P, Jacob Y, Aguilar-Setien A, et al. Immunization of dogs with a DNA vaccine induces protection against rabies virus. Vaccine 18:479–486, 1999.
318. Lodmell DL, Ray NB, Parnell MJ, et al. DNA immunization protects nonhuman primates against rabies virus. Nat Med 4:949–952, 1998.
319. Lodmell DL, Ewalt LC. Post-exposure DNA vaccination protects mice against rabies virus. Vaccine 19:2468–2473, 2001.
320. Lodmell DL, Parnell MJ, Bailey JR, et al. One-time gene gun or intramuscular rabies DNA vaccination of non-human primates: comparison of neutralizing antibody responses and protection against rabies virus 1 year after vaccination. Vaccine 20:838–844, 2001.

321. Dietzschold B, Wang HH, Rupprecht CE, et al. Induction of protective immunity against rabies by immunization with rabies virus ribonucleoprotein. Proc Natl Acad Sci U S A 84:9165–9169, 1987.

322. Fekadu M, Sumner JW, Shaddock JH, et al. Sickness and recovery of dogs challenged with a street rabies virus after vaccination with a vaccinia virus recombinant expressing rabies virus N protein. J Virol 66:2601–2604, 1992.

323. Kasempimolporn S, Hemachudha T, Khawplod P, Manatsathit S. Human immune response to rabies nucleocapsid and glycoprotein antigens. Clin Exp Immunol 84:195–199, 1991.

324. Celis E, Rupprecht CE. New and improved vaccines against rabies. In Woodrow GC, Levine M (eds). New Generation Vaccines. New York, Marcel Dekker, 1990, pp 419–438.

325. Drings A, Jallet C, Chambert B, et al. Is there an advantage to including the nucleoprotein in a rabies glycoprotein subunit vaccine? Vaccine 17:1549–1557, 1999.

326. Fu ZF, Dietzschold B, Schumacher CL, et al. Rabies virus nucleoprotein expressed in and purified from insect cells is efficacious as a vaccine. Proc Natl Acad Sci U S A 88:2001–2005, 1991.

327. Prehaud C, Takehara K, Flamand A, Bishop DH. Immunogenic and protective properties of rabies virus glycoprotein expressed by baculovirus vectors. Virology 173:390–399, 1989.

328. Reagan KJ, Wunner WH, Wiktor TJ, Koprowski H. Anti-idiotypic antibodies induce neutralizing antibodies to rabies virus glycoprotein. J Virol 48:660–666, 1983.

329. Morimoto K, McGettigan JP, Foley HD, et al. Genetic engineering of live rabies vaccines. Vaccine 19:3543–3551, 2001.

330. Champion JM, Kean RB, Rupprecht CE, et al. The development of monoclonal human rabies virus-neutralizing antibodies as a substitute for pooled human immune globulin in the prophylactic treatment of rabies virus exposure. J Immunol Methods 235:81–90, 2000.

331. Hanlon CA, DeMattos CA, DeMattos CC, et al. Experimental utility of rabies virus-neutralizing human monoclonal antibodies in postexposure prophylaxis. Vaccine 19:3834–3842, 2001.

332. Hanlon CA, Niezgoda M, Morrill PA, Rupprecht CE. The incurable wound revisited: progress in human rabies prevention? Vaccine 19:2273–2279, 2001.

333. Umeno S, Doi Y. The study on the anti-rabic inoculation of dogs and the results of its practical application. Kitasato Arch Exp Med 4:89, 1921.

334. Habel K. Evaluation of a mouse test for the standardization of the immunizing power of antirabies vaccines. Public Health Rep 55:1473, 1940.

335. Johnson HN. In Proceedings of the 49th Annual Meeting of the United States Livestock Sanitary Association. Washington, DC, United States Livestock Sanitary Association, 1945.

336. Koprowski H. Studies on chick embryo adapted rabies virus. J Immunol 60:533–554, 1948.

337. Abelseth MK. An attenuated rabies vaccine for domestic animals produced in tissue cultures. Can Vet J 5:279–293, 1964.

338. Brochier B, Thomas I, Iokem A, et al. A field trial in Belgium to control fox rabies by oral immunisation. Vet Rec 123:618–621, 1988.

339. Schneider LG. Rabies virus vaccines. Dev Biol Stand 84:49–54, 1995.

340. Lafay F, Benejean J, Tuffereau C, et al. Vaccination against rabies: construction and characterization of SAG2, a double avirulent derivative of SADBern. Vaccine 12:317–320, 1994.

341. Wiktor T, MacFarlane RI, Dietzschold B, et al. Immunogenic properties of vaccinia recombinants expressing the rabies glycoprotein. Ann Inst Pasteur 136:405–411, 1985.

342. Koprowski H. Rabies oral immunization. Curr Top Microbiol Immunol 146:137–151, 1989.

343. Desmettre P, Languet B, Chappuis G, et al. Use of vaccinia rabies recombinant for oral vaccination of wildlife. Vet Microbiol 23:227–236, 1990.

344. Brochier B, Kieny MP, Costy F, et al. Large-scale eradication of rabies using recombinant vaccinia-rabies vaccine. Nature 354:520–522, 1991.

345. Roscoe DE, Holste WC, Sorhage FE, et al. Efficacy of an oral vaccinia-rabies glycoprotein recombinant vaccine in controlling epidemic raccoon rabies in New Jersey. J Wildl Dis 34:752–763, 1998.

346. Pastoret PP, Brochier B. Epidemiology and control of fox rabies in Europe. Vaccine 17:1750–1754, 1999.

347. Rupprecht CE, Blass L, Smith K, et al. Human infection due to recombinant vaccinia-rabies glycoprotein virus. N Engl J Med 345:582–586, 2001.

348. Brochier B, Boulanger D, Costy F, Pastoret PP. Towards rabies elimination in Belgium by fox vaccination using a vaccinia-rabies glycoprotein recombinant virus. Vaccine 12:1368–1371, 1994.

349. Compendium of Animal Rabies Prevention and Control, 2001. National Association of State Public Health Veterinarians, Inc. MMWR 50(RR-8):1–9, 2001.

350. Meslin FX, Fishbein DB, Matter HC. Rationale and prospects for rabies elimination in developing countries. Curr Top Microbiol Immunol 187:1–26, 1994.

351. Veeraraghaven N. Scientific report for 1968. Pasteur Institute of Southern India, Coonoor, India. 1969, p 36.

352. Hattwick MA, Gregg MB. The disease in man. In Baer GM (ed). The Natural History of Rabies. New York, Academic Press, 1975, pp 281–304.

353. Fishbein DB. Rabies. Infect Dis Clin North Am 5:53–71, 1991.

353a. Dutta JK. Disastrous results of indigenous methods of rabies prevention in developing countries. Int J Infect Dis 6:236–237, 2002.

354. Kositprapa C, Wimalratna O, Chomchey P, et al. Problems with rabies postexposure management: a survey of 499 public hospitals in Thailand. J Travel Med 5:30–32, 1998.

355. Modelska A, Dietzschold B, Sleysh N, et al. Immunization against rabies with plant-derived antigen. Proc Natl Acad Sci U S A 95:2481–2485, 1998.

Chapter 38

Tick-Borne Encephalitis Virus Vaccine

P. NOEL BARRETT • FRIEDRICH DORNER •
HARTMUT EHRLICH • STANLEY A. PLOTKIN

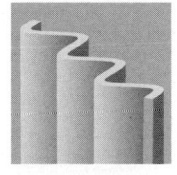

Tick-borne encephalitis (TBE) virus is a member of the family Flaviviridae,[1] which comprises approximately 70 different viruses that cause many serious diseases in a wide variety of vertebrates, including humans. These viruses are all serologically related as determined by hemagglutination-inhibition (HI) assays.[2] However, by cross-neutralization tests, flaviviruses can be divided into eight serologic subgroups, each containing more closely related viruses.[3,4] The first subgroup contains TBE virus, which was previously differentiated into a western and a far eastern subtype by using agar gel diffusion and antibody absorption tests[5] as well as peptide mapping and monoclonal antibodies.[6,7] More recent studies have demonstrated the existence of a third Siberian subtype,[8,9] but the degree of variation between strains within all subtypes was demonstrated to be low. A maximum difference of 5.6% at the amino acid level was found between the three subtypes, which is in the range of variation reported for other flaviviruses.[8]

TBE virus is one of the major human pathogenic flaviviruses. The far eastern subtype established itself in 1930 as a major public health problem in central Russia. The effects of the western subtype, which is prevalent in western, central, and eastern parts of Europe, were first described as early as 1931 by Schneider,[10] who reported a seasonal outbreak of meningitis cases in the district of Neunkirchen in Lower Austria. This was the first report of TBE in the literature. Shortly afterward, the disease was reported from the far eastern part of Russia and from 1939 onward also in its European part. In 1949, the virus was isolated for the first time outside of Russia. In subsequent years TBE has been identified in the majority of European countries. The name *tick-borne encephalitis* refers to the tick, its chief vector. The disease also has been referred to as *spring-summer meningoencephalitis, central European encephalitis, Far Eastern encephalitis, Taiga encephalitis,* or *Russian spring-summer encephalitis.*

Among the flaviviruses, TBE virus has one of the highest impacts as a human pathogen, as indicated by the disease prevalence in endemic areas (for review, see Monath and Heinz[11]). According to a study conducted in 1958, 56% of all viral central nervous system diseases in Austria were caused by TBE virus infection.[12] Thus, before the start of the vaccination program, it was the most important and most frequent disease of this type in adults, with several hundred hospitalization cases being reported each year.[13]

Background

Clinical Description

The clinical course of the disease is largely determined by the TBE virus subtype. Compared with the virus prevalent in Europe, the far eastern variety has proven to be more virulent and to lead to paresis far more often; its associated mortality is also higher.[14,15] The typical course of TBE is diphasic and can be outlined as follows. The incubation period, which is clinically silent, may last between 2 and 28 days,[16,17] but in most cases it is between 7 and 14 days. The first stage, which may last for 1 to 8 days, corresponds to the viremic phase. It is associated with nonspecific systemic signs and symptoms such as fatigue, headache, aching back and limbs, nausea, and general malaise, with temperatures rising to 38°C or higher in most cases. Sometimes exceptionally high initial temperatures may occur, rising above 40°C.[18]

An afebrile interval follows the first stage of TBE, and lasts 1 to 20 days. During this time, patients are usually free of symptoms. Another sudden rise of temperature marks the beginning of the second stage of the disease. Only about one third of those symptomatic with TBE virus infection proceed into the second phase of the disease. The clinical manifestations in this second febrile episode are far more serious. The patients run temperatures that are higher than the average temperatures in other forms of viral meningitis or meningoencephalitis. In the majority of cases, there is central nervous system involvement in the form of meningitis with lymphocytosis and elevated cerebrospinal fluid protein. About a third of cases have more severe disease with signs of encephalitis, including paralysis, stupor, and pyramidal tract signs.[19,20] In paralytic forms of the disease, paralysis, especially in the region of the shoulder girdle, develops 5 to 10 days after the remission of fever. Paralysis may progress up to 2 weeks, followed by a moderate tendency toward improvement.

Hospitalization varies between 3 and 40 weeks,[21,22] depending on the severity of the illness. In children and juveniles, meningitis is the predominant form of the disease; this is why the infection usually takes a milder course than that observed in adults. Pareses and lasting sequelae are rare in young patients. However, a few cases of severe TBE have been reported, even in young children.[23–25] After the approximate age of 40, patients affected by TBE increasingly develop the encephalitic form of the disease. In older patients, especially in persons older than 60, TBE increasingly takes a severe course, leading to paralysis and sometimes resulting in death.[24]

Not all persons infected with TBE run the entire course of the disease. In approximately 65% of cases the infection remains silent, although viremia can be demonstrated; or the patient shows the clinical picture of the initial phase of TBE, but the symptoms subside without developing into full-blown TBE. The remaining 35% of those infected develop the second phase of TBE, the majority of whom run the typical biphasic course. In the remainder, the infection is inapparent during the first stage and the onset of clinical illness coincides with the beginning of the second phase of the disease.[17,21] A clinical follow-up study recently reported from Lithuania involved 133 patients with TBE.[25a] Moderate or severe encephalitis occurred in 56% of the patients, with peripheral or cranial nerve paralysis in 9%. Although mortality was low, 31% of patients suffered permanent central nervous system sequelae. Steroids did not appear useful.

The course of disease with the far eastern variety differs clinically from the European form. The onset of illness is more often gradual than acute, with a prodromal phase including fever, headache, anorexia, nausea, vomiting, and photophobia. These symptoms are followed by stiff neck, sensorial changes, visual disturbances, and variable neurologic dysfunctions, including paresis, paralysis, sensory loss, and convulsions. In fatal cases, death occurs within the first week after onset. The case-fatality rate is approximately 20% compared to 1% to 2% for the European form,[26] but these figures may be biased by the different standards of medical treatment available in western Europe and eastern regions. In contrast to the European form, the disease caused by the far eastern variety is more severe in children than in adults. Neurologic sequelae occur in 30% to 80% of survivors, especially residual flaccid paralyses of the shoulder girdle and arms. Little information is available on the virulence of the recently described Siberian subtype with respect to the course of disease in humans. However, animal studies have demonstrated that the limited number of Siberian subtype strains studied have higher virulence in mice than do far eastern strains.

Virology

Electron microscopy of negatively stained TBE virus shows it to be spherical, with a diameter of about 50 nm, carrying a fringe of small projections on its surface. The virus particle consists of an electron-dense spherical nucleocapsid of approximately 30 nm in diameter that is surrounded by a lipid bilayer. In sucrose density gradients, purified virus sediments homogeneously at about 200S and bands after equilibrium centrifugation at a density of about 1.19 g/cm^3 (for review, see Monath and Heinz[11]). The virus genome consists of a single, positive-stranded RNA molecule of about 11,000 nucleotides in length. Mature virions are composed of three structural proteins termed envelope (E), core (C), and membrane (M) protein with molecular weights of 55,000, 15,000, and 8,000, respectively.[27,28] The envelope proteins E and M are type 1 membrane proteins embedded in the lipid bilayer by C-terminal hydrophobic anchors. In addition, a precursor of the membrane protein (prM) is present in immature intracellular virus particles. The M protein is derived by a furin-mediated cleavage from the glycosylated precursor protein prM. C is the only protein constituent of the isometric nucleocapsid that contains the virion RNA. The virus RNA also codes for seven nonstructural (NS) proteins that can be detected only in infected cells. The coding sequence of the positively stranded RNA is 5'-C-prM-E-NS1-NS2A-NS2B-NS3-NS4A-NS4B-NS5-3'. All viral proteins are encoded within a single open reading frame. The individual proteins are released from a precursor polyprotein by co-translational and post-translational cleavage.[29]

Glycoprotein E plays a central role in the biology of flaviviruses. It contains the important antigenic determinants responsible for HI and neutralization and is responsible for induction of immunologic responses in the infected host. Structural elements of the E protein determinants are known to be involved in the binding of virions to cell receptors and in intraendosomal fusion at low pH.[30]

At present, in addition to the glycoprotein E, only one other viral protein, the NS protein 1 (NS1), has been associated with a role in protective immunity. This is a glycoprotein with molecular weight of approximately 48,000[31] that is not present in the virion but is found on the surface of infected cells. It has been demonstrated that protective immunity can be elicited by immunization with NS1 from the flaviviruses yellow fever and dengue-2[32–34] and that monoclonal antibodies directed against the NS1 protein of yellow fever virus also can protect animals against infection with this virus.[32] This protection cannot be due to the neutralization of free virus but may result from antibody-dependent cell-mediated cytotoxicity or complement-fixing activity of the antibodies. However, because the NS1 protein is not a component of the successful inactivated whole-virus TBE vaccines, it is clearly not essential for the induction of protective immune responses in the TBE system.

Pathogenesis

The picture of manifest TBE depends on the virulence of the virus and the individual resistance of the patient.[18,35] After the bite of an infected tick, the virus usually replicates in the dermal cells at the site of the bite. From there the virus is transferred by afferent lymphatic vessels to the regional lymph nodes. After further replication in lymphoid tissue, the virus is spread via the lymphatic system and the bloodstream, and it invades other susceptible organs or tissues, especially the reticuloendothelial system. Massive virus replication takes place there, and only after this stage is it possible for the virus to reach the central nervous system. High production of virus in the primarily affected organs is a prerequisite for the virus to cross the blood-brain barrier, because the capillary endothelium is not easily infected. Once it has invaded these endothelial cells from the lumen, the virus replicates and enters the central nervous system by seeding through the capillary endothelium into the brain tissue. TBE virus also may spread along nerve fibers. This route may play a role in laboratory infections by aerosols. After infecting the neuroepithelial cells of the nasal mucous membrane, the virus directly enters the brain via the fila olfactoria. Considering the short incubation period and the often extremely severe course of aerosol infections, this route of entry seems likely.[36] However, in arthropod-borne infections, neural spread of the virus is of little importance.

Diagnosis

TBE can be diagnosed definitively only by means of laboratory techniques, because the clinical manifestations of the disease are not specific and are usually not sufficient for diagnosis. However, the laboratory results have no influence on the treatment of TBE and mainly serve for differential diagnosis, because similar symptoms also may be observed in other infections.

In the viremic phase of the initial stage of the disease, the virus can be identified by blood culture in a suitable cell line or in suckling mice.[37] With the onset of the second phase of the disease, the virus can be isolated only from the cerebrospinal fluid.[37,38]

Because the symptoms that affect the central nervous system usually are not observed until 2 to 4 weeks after the tick bite, antibodies against the virus are nearly always present at the time of admission to a hospital and can be detected readily by standard serologic tests. Initially, a recent infection with TBE virus was established by an increase of the titer in the HI test, neutralization test, or complement fixation test or by titer reduction in the HI test by 2-mercaptoethanol treatment in one serum.[37,39–41] These tests are now used mainly for confirmatory purposes and are being replaced by rapid, sensitive, and reliable enzyme-linked immunosorbent assay (ELISA) systems based on the detection of immunoglobulin M (IgM) antibodies in the early phase of TBE. A four-layer ELISA system for the detection of TBE virus–specific IgM has been developed that is extremely sensitive and that prevents interference when high-titer virus-specific immunoglobulin G (IgG) antibodies for TBE are present.[42] In this system, the solid phase is coated with μ chain–specific antiserum to human IgM. After incubation with the serum sample, purified TBE virus is added, followed by enzyme-labeled anti-TBE virus immunoglobulin. At an early stage after the onset of illness, anti-TBE virus IgM could be detected in serum dilutions up to 10^{-4}. A commercial development of this system (Immunozym FSME, Progen Biotechnik GmbH, Heidelberg) allows measurement of both IgM and IgG antibodies.

The value of quantitative IgG antibody determination by ELISA after vaccination against TBE virus has been investigated by examining the correlation between ELISA antibodies, neutralizing antibodies, and HI antibodies in postvaccination serum. Compared to hepatitis B or A virus, for which there is only one serotype, the problem is significantly more complex with TBE virus because it is related antigenically to several other viruses that infect humans, and the interference in ELISA of cross-reactive but non-neutralizing antibodies should be considered. However, an excellent and highly significant correlation was found between ELISA IgG units and the antibody titers obtained by the HI as well as the neutralization assay, provided there was no other exposure to flavivirus antigens except TBE vaccination.[43] Yellow fever vaccination and/or dengue virus infections induced significant levels of antibodies reactive in TBE ELISA and HI tests, which did not, however, exhibit neutralizing activity against TBE virus. It was concluded that the level of IgG antibodies as measured by ELISA is a good marker for predicting the presence of neutralizing antibodies after TBE vaccination, but only in the absence of flavivirus cross-reactive antibodies. Otherwise, a neutralization assay is necessary for assessing immunity.

Treatment

No specific therapy for TBE has been established so far.[18,35] The treatment of TBE patients with RNAse obtained from bovine pancreas[44] and with emetine[45] has not been generally accepted. Corticosteroids apparently lead to a rapid temperature decrease and an improvement of subjective symptoms[46] but at the same time seem to prolong the period of hospitalization as compared to patients receiving only symptomatic treatment.

Because there is no specific treatment targeting the virus itself, symptomatic treatment of patients with TBE is required. The most important measures that can be taken in the clinical management of patients are maintenance of water and electrolyte balance, provision of sufficient caloric intake, and the administration of analgesics, vitamins, and antipyretics.[13,35,47,48] Physiotherapy of paralyzed limbs is essential to prevent muscle atrophy. Because person-to-person transmission of the virus has never been observed, there is no need to isolate TBE patients.[49]

Epidemiology

Incidence and Prevalence Data

Ticks are the chief vectors and reservoir hosts of TBE virus in nature.[50] In Europe, eight species of ticks have been identified so far that are capable of transmitting TBE virus. *Ixodes ricinus*, the common castor bean tick, is the chief vector and thus is mainly responsible for the spread of the virus in western and central Europe and the European part of Russia.[51] The far eastern subtype of the virus is found in the eastern part of Russia, and its vector is primarily *Ixodes persulcatus*.[14,39] The virus can be transmitted to humans or other hosts by larvae, nymphs, or adult ticks (Fig. 38–1). TBE virus is transferred to the host with the saliva of the infected tick. On humans, ticks attach themselves to the hair-covered portion of the head, the ears, the arm and knee joints, and the hands and feet. The epidermis is punctured

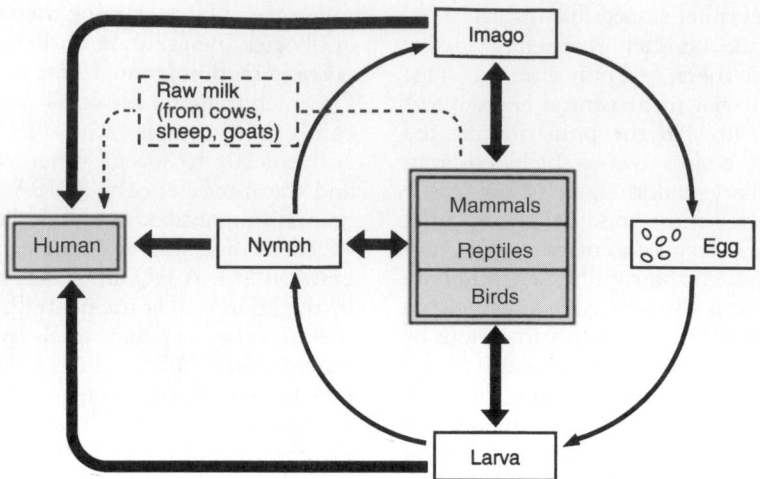

FIGURE 38–1 ■ Transmission cycle of the tick-borne encephalitis virus in a natural focus.

with the chelicerae, and the hypostome is inserted. Owing to the anesthetizing effect of the tick's saliva, the bite causes no pain and often passes unnoticed by the host. This may be the main reason why persons with manifest TBE sometimes cannot recall having been bitten by a tick.

Ticks parasitize more than 100 different species of mammals, reptiles, and birds. Infection of *I. ricinus* with TBE virus by a host harboring the virus is only possible during the viremic stage in the host, provided the virus titer in its blood is high enough to infect the vector. A long viremic stage, along with a high virus titer, is most likely to be observed in small vertebrates, such as the yellow-necked field mouse, the red-backed vole, the common vole, and the dormouse. In large mammals (e.g., roe, deer, goat), viremia is short-lived, and only low virus titers are reached. During the viremic stage, milk from goats, cows, and sheep may contain the virus and may be a source of infection for humans. Infection by the alimentary route as a result of the ingestion of raw milk has been reported from Poland and the former Yugoslavia,[38,52] and, in 1974, several cases of TBE occurred in Slovakia after the patients had eaten cheese made from raw sheep's milk.[53] However, this route of infection probably does not play any role in Western Europe. Laboratory infections have likewise been reported.[54] Although it has not been observed, human-to-human transmission is a theoretical possibility, for example, when blood from a viremic donor is transfused to a patient.

In Central Europe, two seasonal peaks of TBE are seen, one in June/July and the second in September/October, corresponding to two waves of feeding by larvae and nymphs.

The TBE virus is almost exclusively restricted to areas of Europe and Asia, with no incidence in other areas of the world. The distribution of the TBE virus covers almost the entire southern part of the nontropical Eurasian forest belt, from Alsace-Lorraine in the West to Vladivostok and northern and eastern regions of China in the East through to Hokkaido in Japan. Figure 38–2 shows the endemic areas in Europe and Asia. A recent review of TBE epidemiology showed the largest number of reported cases coming from Russia, but the Czech Republic, Latvia, Lithuania, and Estonia each reported more than 200 cases.[54a]

Considerable data also are available on the prevalence of TBE among inhabitants of endemic areas. In most endemic areas of Austria and southern Germany, TBE prevalence has been found to be 4% to 8%. In the most severely affected areas in the east and southeast of Austria, prevalence as high as 14% may be reached. Prevalence is also extremely high in Russia, followed by the Baltic States, Czech and Slovak republics, eastern Germany, Sweden, and Finland. Little is known about the rate of infection in China.

A much higher percentage of TBE antibody-positive persons has been observed among high-risk groups, such as persons working in agriculture and forestry, hikers, ramblers, people engaged in outdoor sports, and collectors of mushrooms and berries. However, a higher percentage of the populations appears to be joining the recognized high-risk groups with changes in human behavior that have brought more people into contact with infected ticks. Under forecast climate change scenarios, it is also predicted that enzootic cycles of TBE virus may not survive along the southern edge of their present range, where case numbers are indeed decreasing.[55] New foci are predicted, however, and have been observed in Scandinavia.[56]

Significance as a Public Health Problem

Table 38–1 gives the prevalence of antibodies to TBE found in those countries in which the disease is a public health issue and/or where infections have been reported for a long time. In many of those countries, morbidity has been increasing continually for years. This may partly be due to improved diagnosis of the disease. However, peaks of infection such as that observed in 1994 in Austria may be due to increased proliferation of small mammals after mild winters, and, as a consequence, also of ticks.

Passive Immunization

An immunoglobulin concentrate is available for pre- and postexposure prophylaxis of TBE. This is available as a 16% protein solution and contains specific gamma globulin against TBE virus, with an antibody titer of at least 1:640 as measured in an HI test. This product can be administered before exposure or up to 48 hours after a tick bite in an endemic area. However, a number of cases of suspected enhancement of infection were reported after use of TBE immunoglobulin in children.[57] Although there is certainly no direct evidence of enhancement of TBE virus infection

Vaccination against Tick-borne Encephalitis

Distribution map of Western and Eastern subtype of TBE virus

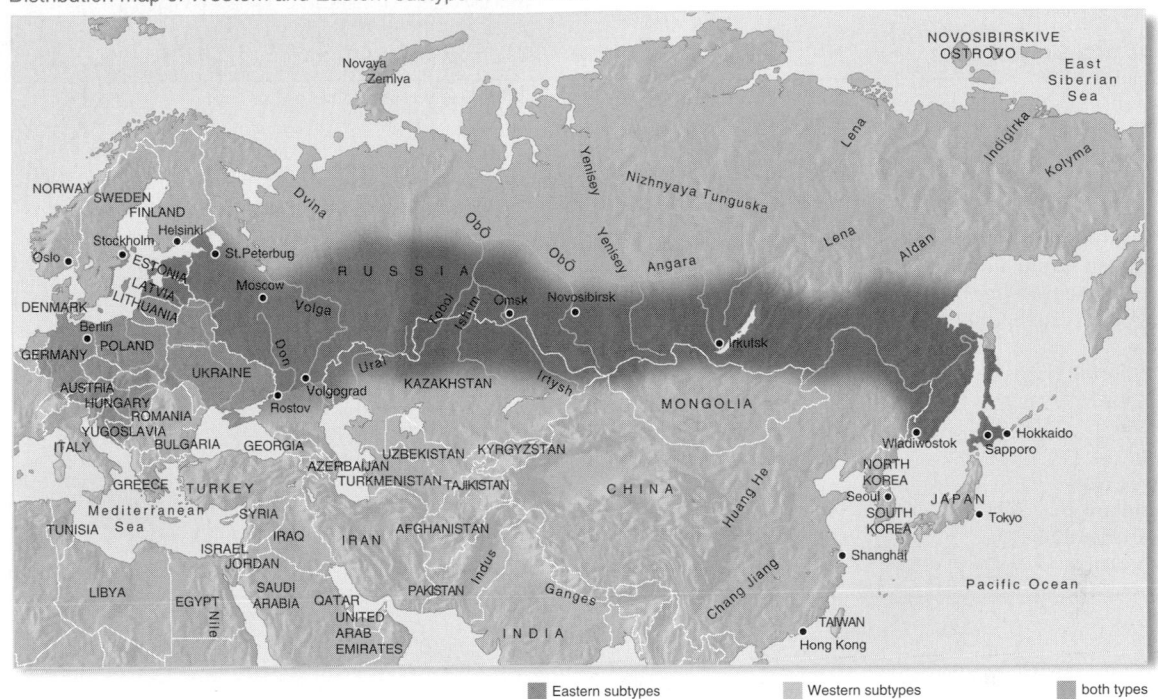

■ Eastern subtypes	■ Western subtypes	■ both types

FIGURE 38–2 ■ Distribution map of western and eastern subtype of TBE virus.

after correct use of immune globulins in humans, and such enhancement has been demonstrated not to occur in a mouse model,[58] the use of this product has been restricted for postexposure prophylaxis to persons 14 years of age and older. For postexposure prophylaxis, the product is administered at a dosage of 0.2 mL/kg body weight, and for preexposure prophylaxis at a dosage of 0.05 mL/kg body weight. Protection following pre-exposure usage is considered to be provided 24 hours after administration and to last approximately 4 weeks.

Active Immunization

History of Vaccine Development

Initial Approaches That Were Abandoned

In 1937, a few months after identifying the agent responsible for Russian spring-summer encephalitis, the far eastern subtype of TBE, vaccinations were carried out in the Russian Army with use of an inactivated suspension from infected mouse brain. This vaccine was the first flavivirus vaccine to be used in humans and was only the third human virus vaccine. Subsequent studies in the former Soviet Union with a similar formalin-inactivated preparation demonstrated the vaccine to be 90% effective in preventing disease.[59] However, the presence of myelin in this crude preparation resulted in an unacceptable level of allergic complications. At that time, attempts to remove the mouse brain component resulted in the loss of most of the viral antigen. Research was then directed toward attempts to produce the vaccine in cell culture, and at the present time two types of formalin-inactivated TBE vaccines derived

from chicken embryo cells are in use in the former Soviet Union, both using the Sofjin isolate of TBE virus. The first vaccine is manufactured from nonconcentrated, unpurified virus containing culture fluid.[60] This vaccine, however, contains residual chicken embryo cell impurities and requires a long vaccination schedule. The second vaccine, which is produced only in small quantities, is manufactured by 20- to 30-fold concentration of the initial culture fluid with simultaneous purification of the virus.[61] Although these procedures reduce the reactogenicity of the vaccine, they do not eliminate the problem, because comprehensive data from volunteers still indicate that the vaccine is moderately reactogenic.

First attempts to develop a vaccine against the western subtype of TBE virus were made in Czechoslovakia in the

TABLE 38–1 ■ Prevalence of Antibody to Tick-borne Encephalitis Virus in the Population of Endemic Areas

Country	Prevalence (%)
Austria	4–8
Former Czechoslovakia	2–38
Finland	0.4–39
Former GDR	7–42
Germany	4–8
Hungary	17
Italy	1.5
Sweden	7–29
Switzerland	1.4
Former USSR	30–100

TABLE 38–2 ■ Overview of Pharmaceutical Composition of Different TBE Vaccines from Baxter (Immuno AG)

Ingredients of a Single Dose	FSME-IMMUN® Until End of 1998	FSME-IMMUN® from 01/1999
Active substance: formaldehyde-inactivated, sucrose gradient purified, TBE virus antigen (µg)	1–3.5	2–3.5
Origin of production virus seed	Mouse brain suspension	Mouse brain suspension
Adjuvant: aluminum hydroxide (mg)	1	1
Stabilizer: human serum albumin (mg)	0.5	0.5
Preservative: thimerosal (mg)	0.05	—
Stabilizer of preservative: disodium EDTA (mg)	0.35	—
Buffer system		
Sodium chloride (mg)	3.45	3.45
$Na_2HPO_4 \cdot 2\,H_2O$ (mg)	0.22	0.22
KH_2PO_4 (mg)	0.045	0.045
Sucrose (mg)	Max. 15	Max. 15
Formaldehyde (µg)	Max. 5	Max. 5
Protamine sulfate	Trace	Trace
Neomycin and gentamycin	Trace	Trace
Water for injection	add 0.5 mL	add 0.5 mL

1960s.[62,63] This formalin-inactivated preparation was grown in primary avian fibroblast cultures. The vaccine was shown to be effective in a variety of laboratory animals and also in human volunteers.[64,65]

Description of Current Vaccines and History of Development

In 1971, a cooperative project for the development of an inactivated vaccine that could be produced commercially in large quantities was initiated between Professor Christian Kunz at the Institute of Virology in Vienna, Austria, and the Microbiological Research Establishment in Porton Down, United Kingdom. A vaccine was prepared using an Austrian tick virus isolate (Neudörfl), which was cloned in specific pathogen–free (SPF) chicken embryo cells. The vaccine was prepared by growing virus in suspensions of primary SPF chicken embryo cells, clarifying by centrifugation, and purifying by hydroxylapatite chromatography after inactivation with formalin. Aluminum hydroxide (Al[OH]₃) was added as an adjuvant. More than 400,000 people were vaccinated in Austria, and serologic tests revealed highly satisfactory seroconversion rates of more than 90% after two vaccinations, as measured in the HI test.[66] However, because antibodies tended to decline after the second dose, it was necessary to inject a third dose 9 to 12 months later. Also, despite its efficacy, local and systemic side effects such as headache, malaise, and pyrexia were common. There were reasons to assume that these side effects were caused by contaminating cellular proteins, and attempts were made to establish a more efficient purification procedure in a collaboration with Immuno AG (now Baxter Vaccine AG, Vienna, Austria). This was achieved by the use of

continuous-flow zonal centrifugation.[67] Calculated from the potency per microgram of protein, this zonally purified vaccine had a level of purity approximately 90 times higher than that of the previously used vaccine. Subsequent trials in human volunteers showed that the efficacy of this new vaccine was high, and the level of side effects had been reduced drastically.[68]

Following the introduction of zonal centrifugation in 1979, the basic manufacturing process and formulation of the vaccine remained unchanged for a number of years. Since 1999, the manufacturing process and the pharmaceutical composition have been subjected to a number of alterations (Table 38–2). In 1999, the preservative thiomersal was removed from the final formulation to fulfill the requirements of the European Pharmacopoeia. In the year 2000, significant changes were made to the manufacturing process and final formulation, which required licensure of the vaccine as a totally new development. This vaccine was referred to as TicoVac® and was free not only of thiomersal but also of human serum albumin. The manufacturing process also was changed to generate a production virus seed that was free of potential contaminating mouse brain protein. This was achieved by subjecting the master virus seed to two sequential passages in primary chick embryo cells in lieu of a passage in SPF baby mice as carried out for the original vaccine. The details of the chick-chick (CC) embryo cell culture–passaged production virus seed and original mouse brain (MB)–derived seed are described in Figure 38–3.

A comparison of the virus generated from this new CC-derived production virus and the MB-derived material was carried out by sequencing and epitope mapping studies. The full sequence of the two membrane proteins prM and

	TicoVac® from 2000	FSME-IMMUN® (New) from 2001	FSME-IMMUN (Junior)® from 2002
	2.7 (target) 2–3.5 (range)	2.4 (target) 2–2.75 (range)	1.2 (target) 1–1.375 (range)
	Supernatant from chick embryo cells	Supernatant from chick embryo cells	Supernatant from chick embryo cells
	1	1	0.5
	—	0.5	0.25
	—	—	—
	—	—	—
	Buffer system		
	3.75	3.45	1.725
	0.715	0.22	0.11
	0.136	0.045	0.0225
	Max. 15	Max. 15	Max. 7.5
	Max. 5	Max. 5	Max. 2.5
	Trace	Trace	Trace
	Trace	Trace	Trace
	add 0.5 mL	add 0.5 mL	add 0.25 mL

glycoprotein E were compared by reverse transcriptase–polymerase chain reaction analysis of the MB- and CC-derived virus. All sequenced regions were identical at the amino acid level and also were identical with the published sequence in the European Molecular Biology Laboratory data base.[69] The identity of the virus generated from this new CC-derived production virus with the MB-derived material also was demonstrated by epitope mapping of infectious and inactivated virus harvests using 18 different monoclonal antibodies. All data obtained demonstrated that all samples, both those from MB-derived production virus and those from CC-derived production virus, showed identical patterns of reactivity with the monoclonal antibodies used. These accumulated data emphasized that the additional passages in chick cells to produce the CC-derived virus did not result in any changes in the sequence or structure of the immunologically critical membrane proteins.

The removal of human serum albumin from the final formulation, however, led to an unexpected increase in reports of adverse drug reactions in TicoVac-vaccinated persons. There was a substantial increase in the rate of high fever in infants and small children, and a number of cases of febrile convulsions were observed in children up to 24 months of age. Subsequent analysis suggested that vaccine without albumin could induce tumor necrosis factor-α and interleukin-1β in whole blood samples from normal individuals.[70] Human albumin was subsequently reintroduced into the vaccine formulation for the year 2001, and there was a dramatic reduction in the rate of adverse drug reaction reports with this amended formulation (FSME-IMMUN® [new]) compared to TicoVac.

A second TBE vaccine, similar to FSME-IMMUN, was licensed in Germany in 1991 (Encepur™; Chiron Behring, Marburg, Germany) and was subsequently introduced to a number of other European countries. This vaccine was based on the K23 virus strain isolated in Southern Germany, which has a nucleic acid sequence close to that of the Neudörfl strain (A Goubeaud, personal communication, 2002). Like the original vaccine, the virus was grown on primary chick embryo cells, inactivated by formaldehyde, and purified by continuous-flow density-gradient centrifugation. The vaccine was stabilized with processed bovine gelatin and adsorbed onto $Al(OH)_3$.[71] Two formulations of vaccine were provided by Chiron Behring, one containing half the dose, which was recommended for children younger than 12 years (Encepur-K™).[72] However an accumulation of notifications of allergic reactions in children receiving Encepur-K resulted in a withdrawal of that product from the market. Both the adult and pediatric formulations have now been replaced with improved formulations that do not contain gelatin as a stabilizer.

Constituents

An overview of the pharmaceutical compositions of the four generations of Baxter TBE vaccines is presented in Table 38–2. The presently licensed vaccine, FSME-IMMUN® (strain Neudörfl), contains 2.4 μg TBE virus antigen, 1 mg $Al(OH)_3$, 0.5 mg human albumin, less than 0.005 mg formaldehyde, and less than 15 mg sucrose in a volume of 0.5 mL. Protamine sulfate, neomycin, and

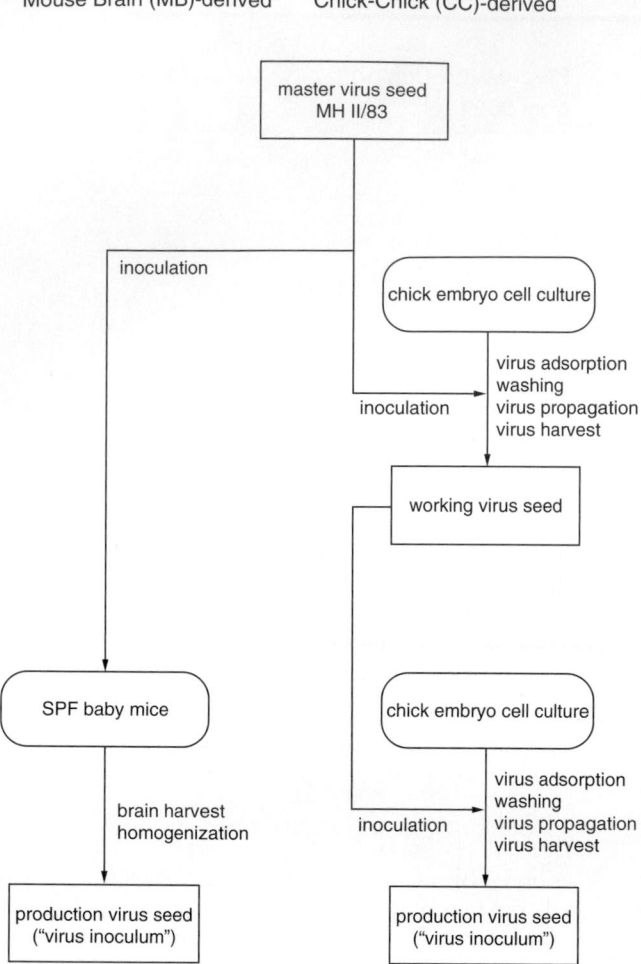

Mouse Brain (MB)-derived   Chick-Chick (CC)-derived

FIGURE 38–3 ▪ Scheme for generation of production virus seed from mouse brain (MB) and from chick-chick embryo cell culture (CC).

gentamicin are present only in trace amounts. The pediatric formulation, FSME-IMMUN (Junior)®, contains 1.2 µg virus antigen, 0.5 mg aluminum hydroxide, 0.25 mg human albumin, less than 0.0025 mg formaldehyde, and less than 7.5 mg sucrose in a final volume of 0.25 mL water for injection.

The currently licensed Chiron Behring vaccine, Encepur adults™, contains 1.5 µg TBE virus antigen (strain K23), 1 mg aluminum hydroxide, and a maximum of 0.005 mg formaldehyde with trace amounts of neomycin, gentamicin, and chlortetracycline in a total volume of 0.5 mL. The pediatric formulation, Encepur children™, contains 0.75 µg TBE virus antigen with 0.5 mg aluminum hydroxide, a maximum of 0.0025 mg formaldehyde, and trace amounts of neomycin, gentamicin, and chlortetracycline in a total volume of 0.25 mL. No details are provided about the concentration of sucrose in the Chiron Behring vaccine formulation.

Manufacture of Vaccine

A schematic diagram describing the manufacturing process for the Baxter vaccine is presented in Figure 38–4.

The master seed virus was prepared from one isolate made from a pool of five ticks in the area of Neudörfl in Austria (Fig. 38–5). This isolate was passaged once by intracerebral injection of SPF mice, and the virus recovered from the mouse brain suspension was cloned on primary chicken embryo cells. The cloned virus was then subjected to four further passages in SPF baby mice to make a master seed virus that consists of a 2% mouse brain suspension. For the latest generation of Baxter vaccine, this material is subjected to two further passages in chick embryo cells to generate the production virus seed as described in Figure 38–3. This virus seed is then used as an inoculum for a primary culture of chicken embryo cells derived from SPF eggs. This production cell culture is infected with the production virus and, after an adsorption period, the infected cells are washed and further incubated at 37°C for a period of 96 to 114 hours. The virus-containing supernatant is separated from the cells by centrifugation and then inactivated with formaldehyde at a concentration of 0.185 g/L for 33 hours at 37°C. The inactivated virus harvest is then treated with protamine sulfate to precipitate cell debris and further purified using sucrose density-gradient ultracentrifugation. The virus-containing sucrose fraction is then stored at −20°C before thawing and pooling of a number of different purified virus harvests to give the bulk vaccine preparation. The bulk vaccine is then diluted with a human albumin containing buffer to give the required virus antigen concentration. An aluminum hydroxide suspension is then added to this diluted pool to give an end concentration of 2 mg/mL. The final bulk vaccine is then filled into syringes before labeling and packaging.

Producers and Preparations

TBE vaccines are now produced commercially by two manufacturers: Baxter Vaccine AG and Chiron Behring. Both manufacturers use essentially the same process to produce the vaccine, the major differences being the use of different strains and the addition of a stabilizer, human serum albumin, by Baxter. The Chiron Behring formulation does not contain a stabilizer. Both manufacturers provide adult and pediatric formulations.

Dosage and Route

The immunization regimen for the Baxter vaccines consists of a first dose followed by a second dose 3 weeks to 3 months later, and a third dose 9 to 12 months after the second dose. According to present experience, the protection achieved by this immunization schedule persists for at least 3 years. A booster injection is recommended 3 years after the last immunization. The vaccine is administered by intramuscular injection, preferably into the upper arm. The basic immunization schedule for the Chiron Behring vaccine is also three injections, with a first dose followed by a second dose at 1 to 3 months after the first immunization, and a third dose 9 to 12 months after the first. A rapid immunization schedule is also available for those with immediate risk, with three injections on days 0, 7, and 21, followed by a fourth dose 12 to 18 months later. A booster

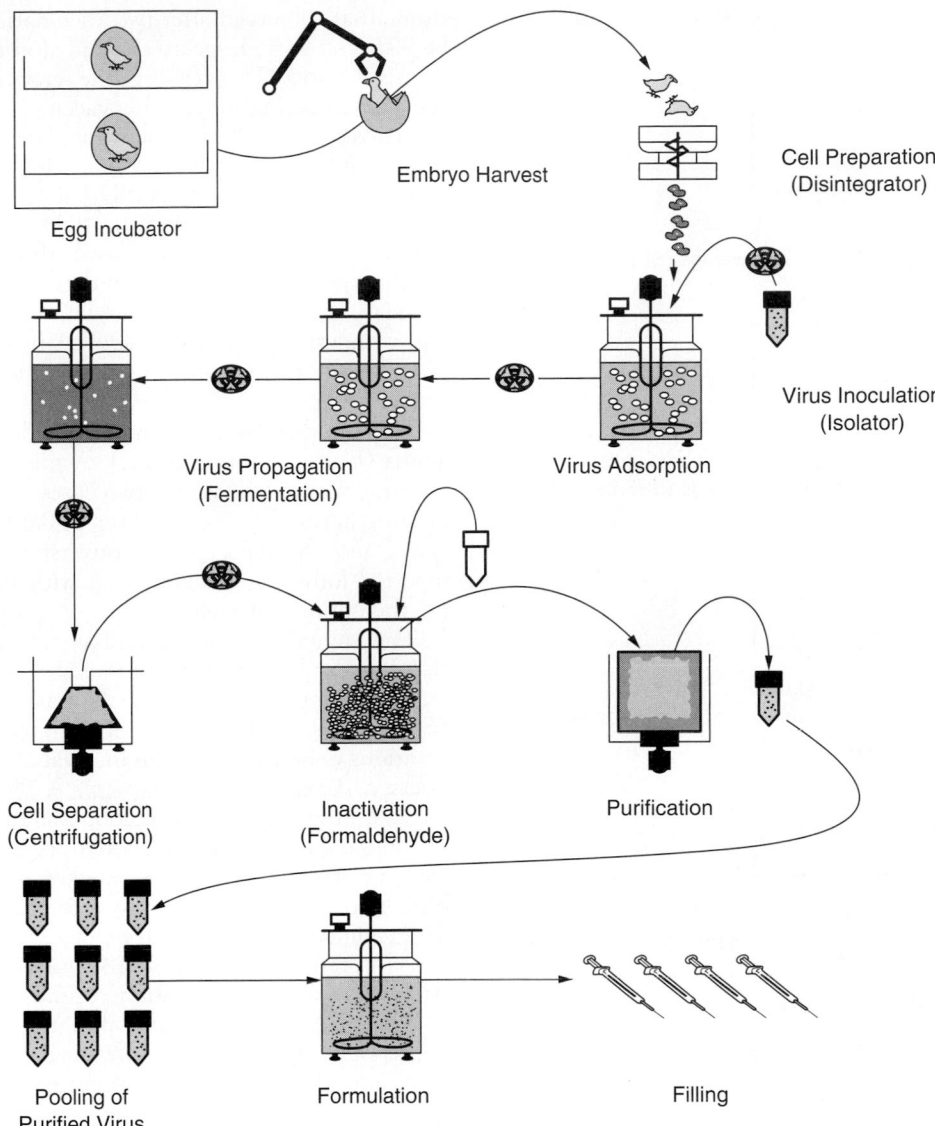

FIGURE 38–4 ▪ Schematic for TBE virus production.

injection after 3 years is also recommended for both adult and pediatric formulations.

Vaccine Stability and Storage

The Baxter vaccine may be stored at 2°C to 8°C for 24 months. Chiron Behring's vaccine has a shelf life of 15 months at this temperature. It is likely that both vaccines will have their shelf lives further extended as more stability data become available, because both vaccines were recently introduced to the market.

Results of Vaccination

Immunogenicity of Vaccine

Antibodies

TBE virus–specific IgG antibodies in serum samples are detected in a three-layer ELISA. The Neudörfl strain TBE virus is used by Baxter as a coating antigen, and test sera are used at a dilution of 1:100. Peroxidase-labeled goat antihuman IgG is used as a detecting antibody, and absorbance is measured at 450 nm. It has been demonstrated that the quantitative determination of specific IgG in TBE postvaccination sera by ELISA exhibits good correlation between HI and neutralization titers.[43] Chiron Behring uses the K23 strain in a similar format.

In a prospective, randomized, placebo-controlled, double-blind study in 1191 healthy adults who were seronegative for TBE antibodies at baseline, FSME-IMMUN produced with CC-derived virus seed with and without thiomersal was compared to FSME-IMMUN produced with MB-derived virus seed, and a placebo (Baxter, internal report). The study was stratified into part A, part B, and part C. Part A encompassed the first and second of three vaccinations, administered 28 to 35 days apart. The third vaccination, 8 to 10 months after the second vaccination, was administered in the context of study part B. In part C, those volunteers who received a placebo in parts A and B were randomized to receive three doses of one of the three vaccines. TBE antibody titers were determined

Preparation on Master Virus Seed MH II/83

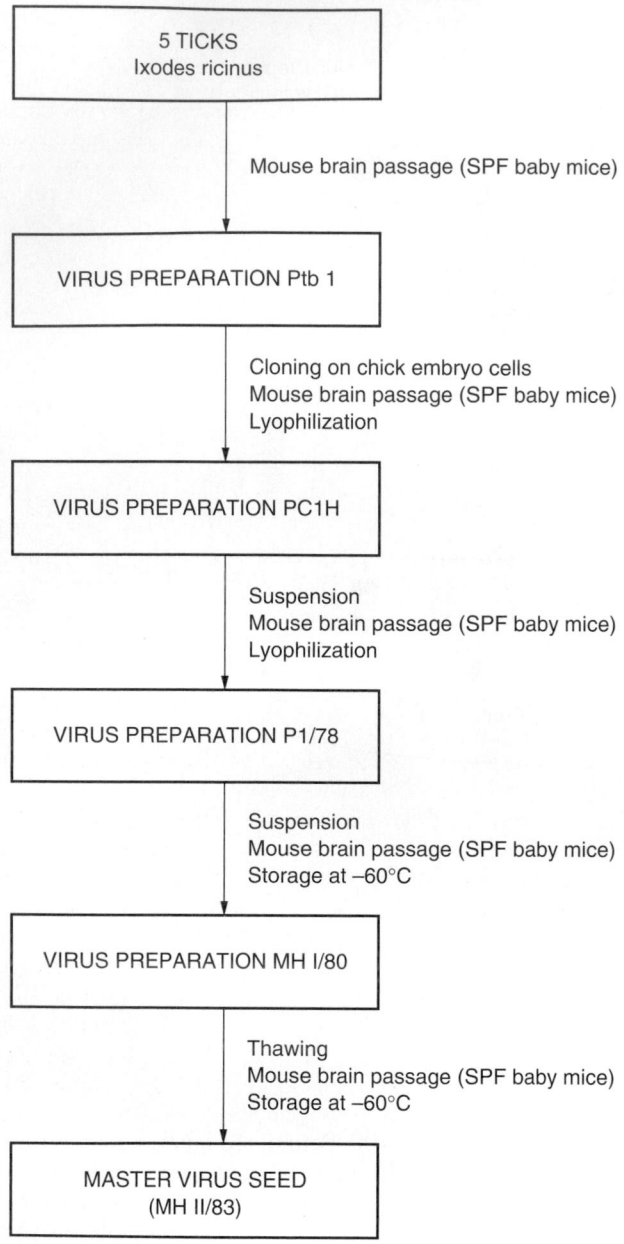

FIGURE 38–5 ■ Preparation of master seed virus MH II/83.

immediately before the first vaccination and 28 to 35 days after the second and third vaccinations. Blood samples were analyzed for the presence of TBE virus IgG antibodies by means of an ELISA and a neutralization test. For the latter, the titer resulting in 100% inhibition of virus growth was determined. Seroconversion was defined as a twofold geometric titer increase over baseline in the ELISA and/or neutralization test.

In this study, the seroconversion rates after two vaccinations with the FSME-IMMUN vaccine in Part A were found to be 98% and 93% for the formulations with and without thimerosal, respectively. In Part C, the seroconversion rates for both the vaccines (with and without

thimerosal) observed after two vaccinations were found to be 99% and 97%, respectively, and after the third vaccination 100% and 97%. In part B, the seroconversion rate after the third vaccination of the vaccine, with and without thimerosal, was 100% for both formulations. Data evaluated according to the ELISA results defining antibody responses above 126 Vienna Units [VIEU]/mL as positive, showed a seroconversion rate of 98% to 100%. The study showed that, in terms of immunogenicity, both the FSME-IMMUN vaccines produced according to the new method (with the production virus obtained from chick embryo cells), with and without thimerosal, are equivalent to the old vaccine produced by passage of the master virus seed in a mouse brain system.

These findings were confirmed in a dose-finding study in adults (Baxter, internal report). A total of 405 volunteers were randomized to receive two doses of either 2.4 μg (the existing licensed dosage), 1.2 μg, or 0.6 μg TBE virus antigen 1 month apart. A seroconversion rate of 97% was reported following immunization with two dosages of 2.4 μg, the optimal antigen dosage.

The immunogenicity of the half-dose pediatric formulation has also been tested in a number of trials. In the most recently completed study with the Baxter pediatric vaccine FSME-IMMUN (Junior), the immunogenicity of two vaccinations (administered at an interval of 14 to 32 days) was assessed (Baxter, internal report). A 99% seroconversion rate was observed after the second immunization.

Similar data have been reported for the Chiron Behring vaccines previously on the market. Seroconversion by ELISA to the Chiron Behring vaccine given by the standard regimen of three doses is reported to be 45%, 98%, and 100% at, respectively, 4, 6, and 45 weeks after the first dose. After the rapid immunization regimen, seroconversion is 91% and 99%, respectively, after the second and third doses. When measured by neutralization test, 100% of subjects are positive at the time points indicated.[73-76] Geometric mean antibody titers postimmunization were similar to those in convalescent sera.[73] The new Chiron Behring formulation free of gelatin is reported by the company to induce immune responses comparable to those of the previous formulation.[77]

Chiron Behring also performed a booster study, in which 100% of subjects preimmunized with Encepur and 74% of subjects preimmunized with FSME had fourfold increases in titers.[77]

No systematic studies of TBE vaccination in different types of immunosuppressed individuals have been done, but heart transplant patients under cyclosporine treatment responded poorly,[78] and it is likely that any immunosuppression will have a similar effect.

Cellular Responses

No data are available on the generation or role of T-cell responses in immunized individuals.

Correlates of Protection

Based on data generated from 20 years of field experience, a serologic correlate of protection for the vaccine has been established. Serum IgG levels of 127 VIEU/mL or greater are considered protective, and 63 to 126 VIEU/mL are borderline.

Herd Immunity

Herd immunity cannot be induced by immunization because the virus is not spread by person-to-person contact. Transmission is almost exclusively by the tick vector from an animal host.

Efficacy and Effectiveness of Vaccine

No controlled clinical trials have been carried out to demonstrate the efficacy of vaccination in protecting against disease. However, both commercially available western vaccines have been demonstrated to be highly effective in inducing seroconversion in a number of clinical trials (see *Antibodies* above) and in public health use (see *Public Health Considerations* below).

Although it is not widely used in Russia and Asia, cross-protection potency studies in mice showed that the TBE virus vaccines are effective not only against European strains but also against Russian and Asian strains of the virus.[70,79,80]

Duration of Immunity and Protection

Antibody persistence also has been evaluated in follow-up studies carried out with the different FSME-IMMUN formulations. It was demonstrated that, 42 months after the third immunization, 48% of volunteers had antibody titers lower than 127 VIEU/mL, the putative protective level. For this reason, a booster immunization is recommended 3 years after the third immunization. Nevertheless, when blood samples were drawn from vaccinees 3 to 6 years after the last immunization, a large proportion still had antibodies (Table 38–3).

Postexposure Prophylaxis and Therapeutic Vaccination

The vaccine is not recommended for use as postexposure prophylaxis or as a therapeutic vaccination. However, a trial of combined vaccination and immunoglobulin administration has been performed, and, although the passive antibody reduced the geometric mean antibody titer by half, 98% of subjects given the combined regimen did respond.[81] Thus combined passive and active immunization may be feasible after exposure.

Safety

As with all intramuscularly administered vaccines, occasional local reactions may occur, such as reddening and swelling around the injection site or swelling of the regional lymph nodes, as may general reactions such as fatigue, pain in a limb, nausea, and headache. On rare occasions after administration of the adult vaccine, short-lived fever, vomiting, or temporary rash may occur. In very rare cases, neuritis of a varying degree of severity may be present. After a single dose of vaccine, it was reported that a young woman developed inflammation of the nerves to the gravity muscles in the legs and feet,[82] and neurologic complications have also been reported after simultaneous immunization against TBE virus and tetanus.[83] Although there is no evidence for any association between immunization and aggravation of disease, it cannot be totally excluded that TBE vaccination, as for all vaccines, does not result in an aggravation of autoimmune diseases such as multiple sclerosis or iridocyclitis in some patients.

Studies carried out in adults for FSME-IMMUN (new) (see *Antibodies* above) provided valuable data on the safety of this formulation. A double-blind, randomized, dose-finding study was conducted in 405 healthy volunteers to determine the optimal dosage of the FSME-IMMUN (new) vaccine (0.6, 1.2, and 2.4 μg TBE antigen) (Baxter, internal report). At the optimal dose of 2.4 μg [AU4](97% seroconversion after two vaccinations), there was no fever (≥38.0°C) observed in any of the 132 volunteers randomized to this dose. A subsequent Phase III, single-blind, randomized, multicenter study was designed to investigate the safety of two vaccinations with the 2.4-μg dose of FSME-IMMUN (new) vaccine in 3966 healthy volunteers ages 16 to 65 years (Baxter, internal report). The Chiron Behring product Encepur (as marketed in 2001) was used as a control. Safety was assessed by means of body temperature measurements and adverse event reporting during the study. In general, no unexpected adverse events were observed during this clinical study. There were no vaccine-related serious adverse events reported after the first or the second vaccination with either vaccine. Fever (≥38.0°C) after the first vaccination occurred in 0.8% (95% confidence interval [CI]: 0.5% to 1.2%) in the FSME-IMMUN study group compared to 5.8% (95% CI: 4.3% to 7.3%) of volunteers in the Encepur study group. The distinct nature of the 95%

TABLE 38–3 ■ Rate of Seroconversion After Three or More Tick-Borne Encephalitis Virus Vaccinations

| Time After Third Vaccination | HI* | | ELISA* | |
	N	No. Positive (%)	N	No. Positive (%)
2 wk	1937	1899 (98)	1723	1714 (99.5)
3 yr	514	384 (74)	490	438 (89)
4 yr	160	126 (79)	145	138 (96)
5 yr	141	126 (88)	144	140 (97)
6 yr	90	73 (82)	88	80 (91)

*Antibody titer measured by hemagglutination inhibition (HI) and enzyme-linked immunosorbent assay (ELISA) tests.
Adapted from Kunz C. Epidemiology of tick-borne encephalitis and the impact of vaccination on the incidence of disease. *In* Eibl MM, Huber C, Peter HH, Wahn U (eds). Symposium in Immunology V. Berlin, Springer-Verlag, 1996, pp 143–149.

CIs indicates that the difference in fever rate between the study groups is significant. The fever cases were mainly mild in nature (38.0°C to 39°C), and only one moderate case (39.1°C to 40.0°C) was reported following vaccination with Encepur. Systemic reactions excluding fever were reported in 13.6% (95% CI: 12.4% to 14.9%) of volunteers who had been vaccinated with FSME-IMMUN and in 31.0% (95% CI: 28.2% to 34.0%) of vaccinees who received Encepur. Similarly, the 95% CIs show significant differences between the study groups.

The tolerability of FSME-IMMUN (Junior) has been evaluated in a large-scale postmarketing surveillance of 1899 healthy children at 110 medical centers in Austria.[83a] The rate of fever cases (>38°C) within 3 days of the first vaccination was determined in this survey. The probability of occurrence of fever after the first vaccination was shown to be 20.3%. The majority of these cases were mild (15.8% of the total surveillance population), with some moderate (4.3%) and a very small proportion of severe (0.3%) cases. Interestingly, the highest incidence of fever cases were reported in the winter months of February and March, with a subsequent drop in the number of fever cases in the months of April through July (Table 38–4). An explanation for this could be a higher frequency of undiagnosed infections during the winter and early spring, particularly in children in the 1- to 3-year age group, which was the most populous age group (63.1% of the total surveillance population). These data also indicate that clinical trials carried out in young children in the winter months may overestimate the rate of fever caused by vaccination. A recent dose response study of the new pediatric formulation (1.2 mcg protein) showed approximately 15% fever in children less than five years old, and approximately 3% in children six to 15 years.[83b] No placebo group was included.

The market experience during the vaccination season in 2001 confirms the positive results obtained in clinical trials. Because TicoVac was only marketed during the year 2000, and FSME-IMMUN (new) (2001 formulation) has been marketed since January 2001, a comparison of annual pharmacovigilance data from Austria constitutes, in effect, a comparison of data for the various vaccines. The adverse event incidence rates (per 100,000 population) with FSME-IMMUN (1999 formulation) and FSME-IMMUN (new) (2001 formulation) are comparable and considerably lower than those seen with TicoVac (Table 38–5). The slight increase in reporting in the year 2001 compared with the old formulation of FSME-IMMUN may be explained by the increased awareness of the possibility of fever cases, resulting from the experience with TicoVac.

Indications for Vaccine

Vaccination is warranted for persons living in endemic areas, people working under high-risk conditions (foresters, woodcutters, farmers, military personnel, laboratory workers), and tourists engaged in high-risk activities (e.g., field work, camping, hunting).

Contraindications and Precautions

Persons with acute disorders that require treatment should not be vaccinated until at least 2 weeks after full recovery. Allergies to components of the vaccines or severe reactions to egg ingestion constitute contraindications. In the case of a known or suspected autoimmune disease, an unfavorable influence of the vaccination on the autoimmune disease must be weighed against the risk of a TBE virus infection, although there is no evidence to support the hypothesis that vaccination can cause autoimmunity. The safety of both vaccines for use during pregnancy and lactation has not been established in controlled clinical trials, and therefore vaccines should be given only with caution after individual consideration of potential risks and benefits.

Administration with Other Vaccines

No studies have been carried out concerning concomitant use of TBE and other vaccines. It has been speculated that previous yellow fever infection or vaccination could affect TBE vaccination. Such problems are difficult to study because of cross-reactive flavivirus antibodies. However, it has been reported that TBE neutralizing antibodies could be induced only after the third vaccination in persons with pre-existing antibodies to yellow fever and infection with dengue type 1 virus,[43] indicating that there may be some negative effects of cross-reacting antibodies on TBE immunization.

Future Vaccines

Following the adverse event reports associated with the use of TicoVac and Encepur-K, new formulations of both adult and pediatric vaccines were successfully introduced by both companies in 2002, following extensive clinical trial programs. It is thus unlikely that major new developments can

TABLE 38–4 ■ Incidence of Fever Cases After First Vaccination with FSME-IMMUN Junior

Month	Number of Vaccinated Volunteers	Number (%) of Fever Cases Reported			
		Mild	Moderate	Severe	Total
January	11	—	—	—	—
February	311	65 (20.9)	17 (5.5)	1 (0.3)	83 (26.7)
March	853	159 (18.6)	49 (5.7)	2 (0.2)	210 (24.6)
April	388	46 (11.9)	10 (2.6)	1 (0.3)	57 (14.7)
May	241	21 (8.7)	5 (2.1)	1 (0.4)	27 (11.2)
June	60	7 (11.7)	—	—	7 (11.7)
July	36	2 (5.6)	—	—	2 (5.6)
August	3	—	—	—	—

TABLE 38–5 ■ Adverse Event Incidence Rates of TBE Vaccines from January 1, 1999, to December 31, 2001, in Austria

Year	TBE Vaccine	Doses Distributed	Number of Reports (Incidence [/100, 000])		
			Nonserious	Serious	Total
1999	FSME-IMMUN	1,965,109	46 (2.3)	6 (0.3)	52 (2.6)
2000	TicoVac	1,476,716	822 (55.7)	91 (6.2)	913 (61.9)
2001	FSME-IMMUN (new)	1,783,970	63 (3.5)	12 (0.7)	75 (4.2)

Source: Baxter, internal report.

be expected from either of these companies in the coming years. However, a number of promising experimental developments have been reported in the area of recombinant subunit and nucleic acid vaccines.

A number of recombinant experimental vaccines have been developed in which glycoprotein E was expressed in recombinant vaccinia virus or in mammalian cell lines.[84–87] Whereas soluble envelope glycoproteins were much less immunogenic than inactivated whole-virus particles, micellar aggregates of glycoprotein E or recombinant subviral particles were excellent immunogens and exhibited efficacies similar to those of inactivated virus vaccine with respect to antibody induction and protection against challenge in a mouse model.[87] These studies emphasize that major quantitative and possibly qualitative differences in the immune response are observed when the protein is presented in particulate or soluble form. The best candidate for a recombinant vaccine thus would appear to be particulate subviral particles, which consist of recombinant glycoprotein E in association with prM in dimer form and lipid.[88] DNA immunization studies also have demonstrated that a plasmid construct that encoded for such a subviral particle was capable of inducing complete protection in mice from challenge with 1000 median infective doses of a highly mouse-pathogenic TBE virus strain.[89]

There have been reports of the efficacy of a recombinant NS1 candidate vaccine in protecting mice from challenge with TBE virus.[90,91] It also has been reported that subneutralizing concentrations of antibodies to glycoprotein E of another flavivirus (i.e., dengue) can mediate antibody-dependent enhancement of infectivity, which has been implicated in the pathogenesis of dengue hemorrhagic fever and dengue shock syndrome.[92] It could therefore be argued that it would be advantageous to use NS1 as the only vaccine component and not to incorporate glycoprotein E in a vaccine preparation. However, there is no evidence for TBE vaccine-induced antibody enhancement in humans.

All inactivated and subunit vaccines suffer from the intrinsic disadvantage that booster injections may be required to maintain protective immunity. TBE vaccine booster injections are recommended at 3- to 5-year intervals after an initial immunization schedule of three vaccinations. The development of an attenuated live virus vaccine would provide major advantages with respect to generation of a long-lasting immunity without frequent booster injections. The large amount of information concerning neurovirulence of TBE virus generated by sequencing,[93] monoclonal antibody escape mutant studies,[94] and x-ray crystallography analysis[95] should facilitate the specific generation of stable attenuated live virus vaccines using infectious complementary DNA clone technology. It has

been reported that deletion mutants of the 3′ noncoding region of the TBE virus genome were four orders of magnitude less virulent than the wild-type TBE virus.[96] In spite of their high degree of attenuation, these mutants efficiently induced protective immune responses in mice even at low inoculation doses. Further attenuation could be achieved by introducing a mutation at a putative flavivirus receptor-binding site. The most significant attenuation in mice was achieved by mutagenesis of threonine 310. Combining this mutation with deletion mutations in the 3′ noncoding region yielded mutants that were highly attenuated but still conferred a solid protective immunity.[97]

Although live viral vaccines have in many cases proven to be an extremely effective tool for the prevention of disease, the production of conventional live vaccines in cell culture has many disadvantages. These include the potential for contamination with adventitious agents and genetic alterations during propagation, making it necessary to do extensive testing before release. A novel live, attenuated TBE virus vaccination strategy has been developed consisting of the application of in vitro–synthesized infectious RNA instead of the live virus itself. When administered using the GeneGun, less than 1 mg of RNA was required to initiate replication of virus that was attenuated by a specifically engineered mutation, and this induced a protective immunity in laboratory mice.[98] Because this approach uses RNA, it does not have the potential drawbacks of DNA vaccines and thus combines the advantages of conventional live viral vaccines with those of nucleic acid–based vaccines.

Public Health Considerations

Epidemiologic Results of Vaccination

The TBE vaccine is widely used in central Europe (approximately 35 million doses have been administered since 1980), and the vaccine has been a major success in preventing TBE infections in this region. Although the vaccine is not incorporated into routine pediatric immunization, a campaign of voluntary immunization has been instituted since 1980 by the Austrian Health Ministry, so that the majority of children older than 2 years are immunized. This campaign is carried out in early spring of each year, and the vaccine is often given simultaneously with other routine vaccines in children. Figure 38–6 shows that, since the beginning of this vaccination campaign in Austria, the number of cases of TBE has been reduced from a high of 677 in 1979 to a low of 41 in 1999. The extensive diagnostic service for TBE in Austria permits calculation of the protection rate of the vaccine using clinical and epidemiologic data from the Austrian population.

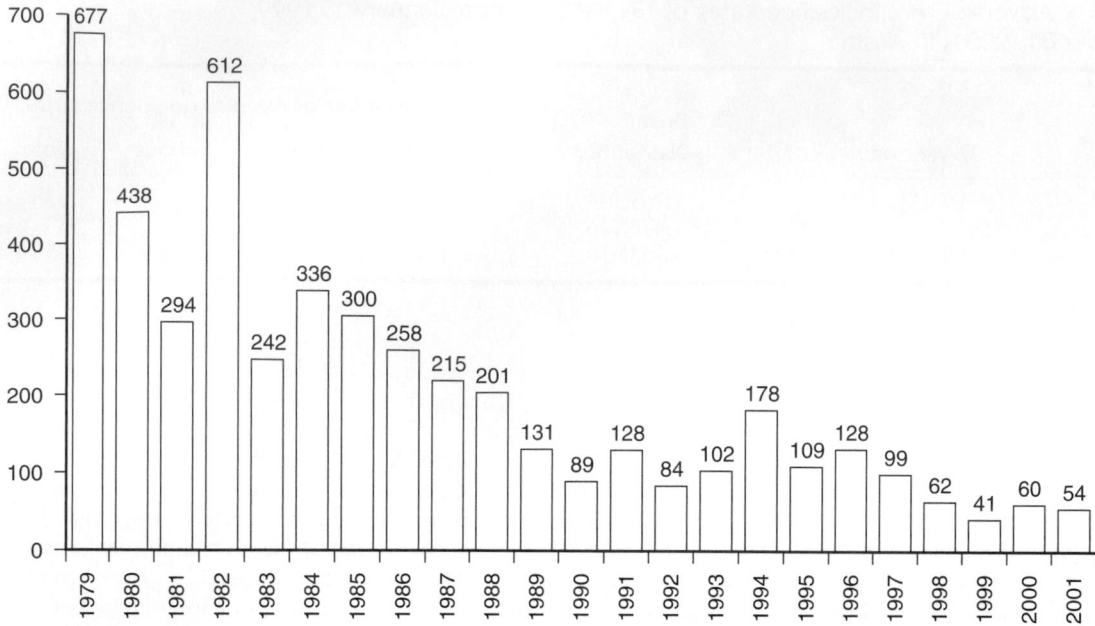

FIGURE 38–6 ▪ TBE cases in Austria, 1979 through 2001.

A calculation of the protection rates of the vaccine for the years 1994 to 1997 in Austria are presented in Table 38–6. Assuming that the total population of Austria (7.8 million) is exposed to the disease, and taking into account the number of TBE cases occurring in vaccinated and unvaccinated individuals, mean protection rates of 98% could be calculated after two or three immunizations for these 4 years. However, these calculations must be accepted with considerable reservation because the unvaccinated population may differ considerably in risk from the vaccinated population. The most that can be said reliably is that few cases of TBE have occurred after TBE vaccination with either of the two vaccines, while cases continue to occur in the unvaccinated population. More impressive, whereas the incidence of TBE in Austria has declined markedly since the advent of generalized vaccination, that of neighboring Czechoslovakia has actually increased.[98a]

Disease Control Strategies

Because ticks attach to any spot on the host and from there try to reach an uncovered part of the skin, adequate cloth-ing may help to make access to the skin more difficult for ticks. Protective clothes must be completely closed to be really effective, but this would be unacceptable to people spending their leisure time or holidays in endemic areas in the warm season.

In former Czechoslovakia, forestry workers were given protective clothing impregnated with dichlorodiphenyl-trichloroethane (DDT) and were regularly disinfested after work.[99] Furthermore, a variety of repellants were used, such as diethyltoluamide, indalone, dimethyl carbate, dimethyl phthalate, and benzyl benzoate. These preparations provided protection for only a few hours, however. Moreover, there have been reports from Russia of ticks becoming resistant to repellants.[100]

Eradication or Elimination

Efforts to eradicate the disease in the past were concentrated on the extermination of the tick population in TBE virus endemic areas. In former Czechoslovakia and USSR, large-scale eradication measures using tetrachlorvinphos, DDT, or hexachlor did not produce the desired effect. Because the virus persists not only in ticks but also in a large

TABLE 38–6 ▪ Calculation of the Effectiveness of TBE Virus Vaccination in Austria After Two or Three Vaccinations

| Year | Number of Cases / Exposed Population (×1000) | | | Protection Rate (%) | |
	Not Vaccinated	Two	Three or more	Two	Three or more
1994	165/2340	1/390	6/5070	96.4	98.3
1995	104/2110	1/460	4/5230	95.6	98.5
1996	118/2031	0/520	0/5121	100	97
1997	95/2161	0/390	4/5249	100	98.3
Median Protective Efficacy of FSME-IMMUN				98	98

number of wild animals, such measures are unlikely to eradicate or even control the disease. The most effective method to prevent infection is vaccination.

Acknowledgments

We would like to thank Ms. Sandra Schittengruber for her assistance in preparing the manuscript and Drs. Susanne Schober-Bendixen, Monika Fink, and Eric Busch-Petersen for helpful discussions and critical reading of the manuscript.

REFERENCES

1. Westway EG, Brinton MA, Gaidamovitch SY, et al. Flaviviridae. Intervirology 24:183–192, 1985.
2. Casals J. The arthropod-borne group of animal viruses. Trans N Y Acad Sci 19:219–235, 1957.
3. DeMadrid AT, Porterfield JS. The flaviviruses (group B arboviruses): a cross-neutralization study. J Gen Virol 23:91–96, 1974.
4. Calisher CH, Karabatsos N, Dalrymple JM, et al. Antigenic relationships between flaviviruses as determined by cross-neutralization tests with polyclonal antisera. J Gen Virol 70:37–43, 1989.
5. Clarke DH. Further studies on antigenic relationship among the viruses of the group B tick-borne complex. Bull World Health Organ 31:45–56, 1964.
6. Heinz FX, Kunz C. Homogeneity of the structural glycoprotein from European isolates of tick-borne encephalitis virus: comparison with other flaviviruses. J Gen Virol 57:263–274, 1981.
7. Heinz FX, Berger R, Tuma W, et al. A topological and functional model of epitopes of the structural glycoprotein of tick-borne encephalitis virus defined by monoclonal antibodies. Virology 126:525–537, 1983.
8. Ecker M, Allison SL, Meixner T, Heinz FX. Sequence analysis and genetic classification of tick-borne encephalitis viruses from Europe and Asia. J Gen Virol 80:179–185, 1999.
9. Lundkvist A, Vene S, Golovljova I, et al. Characterization of tick-borne encephalitis virus from Latvia: evidence for co-circulation of three distinct subtypes. J Med Virol 65:730–735, 2001.
10. Schneider H. Über epidemische akute "meningitis serosa." Wien Klin Wochenschr 44:350–352, 1931.
11. Monath TP, Heinz FX. Flaviviruses. In Fields BN, Knipe DM, Howley PM (eds). Fields Virology (3rd ed). Philadelphia, Lippincott–Raven, 1996, pp 961–1034.
12. Krausler J, Kraus P, Moritsch H. Klinische und virologisch-serologische Untersuchungsergebnisse bei Frühsommer-Meningoencephalitis und anderen Virusinfektionen des ZNS im Bezirk Neunkirchen. Wien Klin Wochenschr 70:634–637, 1958.
13. Radda A. Die Frühsommer-Meningoenzephalitis in Österreich. In Jusatz H (ed). Beiträge zur Geoökologie der Zentraleuropäischen Zecken-Encephalitis. Berlin, Springer-Verlag AO, 1978, pp 42–47.
14. Blaskovic D. Tick-borne encephalitis in Czechoslovakia. Arch Environ Health 21:453–461, 1970.
15. Grinschgl G, Richling E. Die Zentraleuropäische Enzephalomyelitis, eine "arthropod borne" Erkrankung vom Typ der Russischen Frühjahr-Sommer-Enzephalitis. Giorn Mal Infect Paras 9:3–15, 1957.
16. Duniewicz M. Klinisches Bild der Zentraleuropäischen Zeckenencephalitis. Münch Med Wochenschr 118:1609–1612, 1976.
17. Reisner H. Clinic and treatment of tick-borne encephalitis (TBE): introduction. In Kunz C (ed). Tick-Borne Encephalitis. Wien, Facultas Verlag, 1981, pp 1–5.
18. Conrads R, Plassmann E. Frühsommer-Meningoenzephalitis (FSME). Fortsch Med 100:799–801, 1982.
19. Koletzko B, Reinhardt D. Frühsommermeningoenzephalitis (FSME). Monatsschr Kinderheilkd 144:426–434, 1996.
20. Kaiser R, Vollmer H, Schmidtke K, et al. Follow-up and prognosis of early summer meningoencephalitis [in German]. Nervenarzt 68:324–330, 1997.
21. Ziebart-Schroth A. Frühsommermeningoenzephalitis (FSME): Klinik und besondere Verlaufsformen. Wien Klin Wochenschr 84:778–781, 1972.
22. Bodemann H, Hoppe-Seyler P, Blum H, et al. Schwere und ungünstige Verlaufsformen der Zeckenenzephalitis (FMSE) 1979 in Freiburg. Dtsch Med Wochenschr 105:921–942, 1980.
23. Kunz C. Die Frühsommer-Meningoenzephalitis. Pediatr Praxis 14:189–192, 1974.
24. Krausler J. 23 years of TBE in the district of Neunkirchen (Austria). In Kunz C (ed). Tick-Borne Encephalitis. Wien, Facultas Verlag, 1981, pp 6–12.
25. Messner H. Pediatric problems of TBE. In Kunz C (ed). Tick-Borne Encephalitis. Wien, Facultas Verlag, 1981, pp 25–27.
25a. Mickiene A, Laiskonis A, Gunther G, et al. Tick-borne encephalitis in an area of high endemicity in Lithuania: disease severity and long-term prognosis. Clin Infect Dis 35:650–658, 2002.
26. Gresikova M, Beran GW. Arboviral zoonoses in Central Europe, tick-borne encephalitis (TBE). In Beran GW (ed). CRC Handbook Series in Zoonoses, Section B: Viral Zoonoses. Vol. 1. Boca Raton, FL, CRC Press, 1981, pp 201–208.
27. Heinz FX, Kunz C. Characterization of TBEV and immunogenicity of its surface components in mice. Acta Virol 21:308–316, 1977.
28. Blaskovic DJ, Slavik J. Fine structure of tick-borne encephalitis virus. In Kunz C (ed). Tick-Borne Encephalitis. Wien, Facultas Verlag, 1981, pp 133–141.
29. Rice CM. Flaviviridae: the viruses and their replication. In Fields BN, Knipe DM, Howley PM (eds). Fields Virology (3rd ed). Philadelphia, Lippincott–Raven, 1996, pp 931–959.
30. Heinz FX. Epitope mapping of flavivirus glycoproteins. Adv Virus Res 31:103–168, 1986.
31. Lee JM, Crooks AJ, Stephenson JR. The synthesis and maturation of a non-structural extracellular antigen from tick-borne encephalitis virus and its relationship to the intracellular NS1 protein. J Gen Virol 70:335–343, 1989.
32. Schlesinger JJ, Brandris MW, Walsh EE. Protection against 17D yellow fever encephalitis in mice by passive transfer of monoclonal antibodies to the nonstructural glycoprotein gp 48 and by active immunization with gp 48. J Immunol 135:2805–2809, 1985.
33. Schlesinger JJ, Brandriss MW, Cropp CB, et al. Protection against yellow fever in monkeys by immunization with yellow fever virus non-structural protein NS1. J Virol 60:1153–1155, 1986.
34. Schlesinger JJ, Brandriss MW, Walsh EE. Protection of mice against dengue 2 virus encephalitis by immunization with the dengue 2 virus non-structural glycoprotein NS1. J Gen Virol 68:853–857, 1987.
35. Ackermann B, Rehse-Küpper B. Die zentraleuropäische Enzephalitis in der Bundesrepublik Deutschland. Fortschr Neurol Psychiat 47:103–122, 1979.
36. Hofmann H. Die unspezifische Abwehr bei neurotropen Arbovirusinfektionen. Zentralbl Bakteriol Hyg I Abt Orig A 223:143–163, 1973.
37. Hofmann H. Diagnosis of TBE in the virological routine laboratory. In Kunz C (ed). Tick-Borne Encephalitis. Wien, Facultas Verlag, 1981, pp 129–132.
38. Blessing J. Epidemiologie und Diagnose der Frühsommer-Meningoenzephalitis. Med Welt 32:1345–1347, 1981.
39. Ackermann R, Rehse-Küpper B, Löser R, et al. Neutralisierende Serumantikörper gegen das Virus der Zentraleuropäischen Enzephalitis bei der ländlichen Bevölkerung der Bundesrepublik Deutschland. Dtsch Med Wochenschr 93:1747–1754, 1968.
40. Kunz C, Hofmann H, Dippe H. Die Frühdiagnose der Frühsommer-Meningoenzephalitis (FSME) im Hämagglutinationshemmungstest durch Behandlung des Serums mit 2-Mercaptoäthanol. Zentralbl Bakteriol Hyg I Abt Orig A 218:273–279, 1971.
41. Kunz C, Krausler J. Bildung und Überdauern der komplementbindenden Antikörper nach Infektionen mit Frühsommer-Meningoencephalitis (tick-borne-encephalitis) Virus. Arch Ges Virusforsch 14:499–507, 1964.
42. Heinz F, Roggendorf M, Hofmann H, et al. Comparison of two different enzyme immunoassays for detection of immunoglobulin M antibodies against tick-borne encephalitis virus in serum and cerebrospinal fluid. J Clin Microbiol 14:141–146, 1981.
43. Holzmann H, Kundi M, Stiasny K, et al. Correlation between ELISA, hemagglutination inhibition, and neutralization tests after vaccination against tick-borne encephalitis. J Med Virol 48:102–107, 1996.
44. Glukhov N, Jerusalimsky A, Canter V, et al. Ribonuclease treatment of tick-borne encephalitis. Arch Neurol 33:598–603, 1976.

45. Synek P. Treatment of tick-borne meningoencephalitis with emetine. Rev Czechosl Med 20:29–33, 1974.

46. Duniewicz M, Kulkova H. Kortikoide in der Behandlung von Zecken und anderen Virus-Meningoenzephalitiden. Münch Med Wochenschr 124:63–64, 1982.

47. Duniewicz M. Klinisches Bild der Zentraleuropäischen Zeckenenzephalitis. Münch Med Wochenschr 118:1609–1612, 1976.

48. Kunz C. Die Prophylaxe der Frühsommer-Meningoenzephalitis (FSME) in der dermatologischen Praxis. Schrifttum Praxis 5:55–58, 1974.

49. Moritsch H, Krausler J. Die Frühsommer-Meningo-Enzephalitis in Niederösterreich 1956–1958. Epidemiologie und Klinik im Seuchengebiet Neunkirchen. Dtsch Med Wochenschr 84:1934–1939, 1959.

50. Jettmar HM. Über die Rolle der Zecken bei der Verbreitung der zweiwelligen Meningoenzephalitis in Österreich. Anzeig Schädlingsk 30:129–132, 1957.

51. Gresikova M, Kozuch O, Nosek J. Die Rolle von Ixodes ricinus als Vektor des Zeckenenzephalitisvirus in verschiedenen mitteleuropäischen Naturherden. Zentralbl Bakteriol Parasit 207:423–429, 1968.

52. Blaskovic D. Epidemiologische und immunologische Probleme bei der Zeckenencephalitis. Wien Klin Wochenschr 70:742–749, 1958.

53. Gresikova M, Sekeyova M, Stupalova S, et al. Sheep milk-borne epidemic of tick-borne encephalitis in Slovakia. Intervirology 5:57–61, 1975.

54. Bodemann H, Pausch J, Schmitz H, et al. Die Zeckenenzephalitis (FSME) als Labor-Infektion. Med Welt 28:1779–1781, 1977.

54a. Süss J. Epidemiology and ecology of TBE relevant to the production of effective vaccines. Vaccine 21:S1–S35, 2003.

55. Randolph SE. The shifting landscape of tick-borne zoonoses: tick-borne encephalitis and Lyme borreliosis in Europe. Philos Trans R Soc Lond B Biol Sci 356:1045–1056, 2001.

56. Lindgren E, Gustafson R. Tick-borne encephalitis in Sweden and climate change. Lancet 358:16–18, 2001.

57. Kluger G, Schöttler A, Waldvogel K, et al. Tick-borne encephalitis despite specific immunoglobulin prophylaxis. Lancet 346:1502, 1995.

58. Kreil TR, Eibl MM. Pre- and postexposure protection by passive immunoglobulin but no enhancement of infection with a flavivirus in a mouse model. J Virol 71:2921–2927, 1997.

59. Smorodintsev AA, Ilyenko VI. Results of laboratory and epidemiological study of vaccination against tick-borne encephalitis. In Livikova H (ed). Biology of Viruses of TBE Complex (Symposia of Czechoslovak Academy of Sciences. Vol. 3). New York, Academic Press, 1962, pp 332–343.

60. Lvov DK, Gagarina AV. Immunoprophylaxis of tick-borne encephalitis [in Russian]. In Chumakov MP (ed). Tick-Borne Encephalitis and Other Arboviral Diseases (Viruses and Viral Diseases. Vol. 1). Moscow, VNIIMI, pp 97–127, 1965.

61. Elbert LB, Krasilnikov IV, Drozdov SG, et al. Concentrated purified vaccine against tick-borne encephalitis produced by ultrafiltration and chromatography [in Russian]. Vopr Virusol 1:90–93, 1985.

62. Danes L, Benda R. Study of the possibility of preparing a vaccine against tick-borne encephalitis using tissue culture methods. I. Propagation of tick-borne encephalitis virus in tissue culture for vaccine preparation. Acta Virol 4:25, 1960.

63. Danes L, Benda R. Study of the possibility of preparing a vaccine against tick-borne encephalitis using tissue culture methods. II. The inactivation by formaldehyde of the tick-borne encephalitis virus in liquids prepared from tissue cultures: immunogenic properties. Acta Virol 4:32–36, 1960.

64. Benda R, Danes L. Study of the possibility of preparing a vaccine against tick-borne encephalitis using tissue culture methods. V. Experimental data for the evaluation of the efficiency of formol-treated vaccines in laboratory animals. Acta Virol 5:37–49, 1961.

65. Danes L, Benda R. Study of the possibility of preparing a vaccine against tick-borne encephalitis using tissue culture methods. IV. Immunization of humans with test samples of inactivated vaccine. Acta Virol 4:335–340, 1960.

66. Kunz C, Hofmann H, Stary A. Field studies with a new tick-borne encephalitis (TBE) vaccine. Zentralbl Bakteriol Hyg J Abt Orig A 243:141–144, 1976.

67. Heinz FX, Kunz C, Fauma H. Preparations of a highly purified vaccine against tick-borne encephalitis by continuous flow zonal ultracentrifugation. J Med Virol 6:213–221, 1980.

68. Kunz C, Heinz FX, Hofmann H. Immunogenicity and reactogenicity of a highly purified vaccine against tick-borne encephalitis. J Med Virol 6:103–109, 1980.

69. Mandl CW, Heinz FX, Kunz C. Sequence of the structural proteins of tick-borne encephalitis virus (western subtype) and comparative analysis with other flaviviruses. Virology 166:197–205, 1988.

70. Marth E, Kleinhappl B. Albumin is a necessary stabilizer of TBE-vaccine to avoid fever in children after vaccination. Vaccine 20:532–537, 2001.

71. Klockmann U, Krivanec K, Stephenson JR, Hilfenhaus J. Protection against European isolates of tick-borne encephalitis virus after vaccination with a new tick-borne encephalitis vaccine. Vaccine 9:210–212, 1991.

72. Girgsdies OE, Rosenkranz G. Tick-borne encephalitis: development of a paediatric vaccine. A controlled, randomized, double-blind, and multicentre study. Vaccine 14:1421–1428, 1996.

73. Klockmann U, Bock HL, Kwasny H, et al. Humoral immunity against tick-borne encephalitis virus following manifest disease and active immunization. Vaccine 9:42–46, 1991.

74. Harabacz I, Bock H, Jüngst C, et al. A randomized Phase II study of a new tick-borne encephalitis vaccine using three different doses and two immunization regimens. Vaccine 10:145–150, 1992.

75. Data on file. Marburg, Germany, Chiron Behring Laboratories, 1997.

76. Encepur New Drugs Statement. Marburg, Germany, Chiron Behring, 1999.

77. Product Information: Encepur(tm). Marburg, Germany, Chiron Behring, 2002.

78. Dengler TJ, Zimmermann R, Meyer J, et al. Vaccination against tick-borne encephalitis under therapeutic immunosuppression: reduced efficacy in heart transplant recipients. Vaccine 17:867–874, 1999.

79. Holzmann H, Vorobyova MS, Ladyzhenskaya IP, et al. Molecular epidemiology of tick-borne encephalitis virus: cross-protection between European and Far Eastern subtypes. Vaccine 10:345–349, 1992.

80. Hayasaka D, Goto A, Yoshii K, et al. Evaluation of European tick-borne encephalitis virus vaccine against recent Siberian and far-eastern subtype strains. Vaccine 19:4774–4779, 2001.

81. von Hedenstrom M, Heberle U, Theobald K. Vaccination against tick-borne encephalitis (TBE): influence of simultaneous application of TBE immunoglobulin on seroconversion and rate of adverse events. Vaccine 13:759–762, 1995.

82. Scholz E, Wiethölter H. Postvakzinale Schwerpunktneuritis nach prophylaktischer FSME-Impfung. Dtsch Med Wochenschr 112:544–546, 1987.

83. Schabet M, Wiethölter H, Grodd W, et al. Neurological complications after simultaneous immunization against tick-borne encephalitis and tetanus. Lancet 2:959–960, 1989.

83a. Pavlova BG, Loew-Baselli A, Fritsch S, et al. Tolerability of modified tick-borne encephalitis vaccine FSME-Immun "New" in children: results of post-marketing surveillance. Vaccine 21:742–745, 2003.

83b. Mai I, Fritsch S, Loew-Baselli A, et al. Safety and immunogenicity results of a modified TBE vaccine (FSME-IMMUN® "NEW") in children. Abstract 247. 21st Annual Meeting of the European Society for Paediatric Infectious Diseases (ESPID), Giardini Naxos, Taormina, Sicily, April 9–11, 2003.

84. Venugopal K, Gould EA. Towards a new generation of flavivirus vaccines. Vaccine 12:966–975, 1994.

85. Allison SL, Mandl CW, Kunz C, et al. Expression of cloned envelope protein genes from the flavivirus tick-borne encephalitis virus in mammalian cells and random mutagenesis by PCR. Virus Genes 8:187–198, 1994.

86. Allison SL, Stadler K, Mandl C, et al. Synthesis and secretion of recombinant tick-borne encephalitis virus protein E in soluble and particulate form. J Virol 69:5816–5820, 1995.

87. Heinz FX, Allison SL, Stiasny K, et al. Recombinant and virion-derived soluble and particulate immunogens for vaccination against tick-borne encephalitis. Vaccine 13:1636–1642, 1995.

88. Ferlenghi I, Clarke M, Ruttan T, et al. Molecular organization of a recombinant subviral particle from tick-borne encephalitis virus. Mol Cell 7:593–602, 2001.

89. Aberle JH, Aberle SW, Allison SL, et al. A DNA immunization model study with constructs expressing the tick-borne encephalitis virus envelope protein E in different physical forms. J Immunol 163:6756–6761, 1999.

90. Jacobs SC, Stephenson JR, Wilkinson GWG. High-level expression of the tick-borne encephalitis virus NS1 protein by using an adenovirus-based vector: protection elicited in a murine model. J Virol 66:2086–2095, 1992.

91. Jacobs SC, Stephenson JR, Wilkinson GWG. Protection elicited by a replication-defective adenovirus vector expressing the tick-borne encephalitis virus non-structural glycoprotein NS1. J Gen Virol 75:2399–2402, 1994.

92. Halstead SB. Antibody, macrophages, dengue virus infection, shock and hemorrhage: a pathogenetic cascade. Rev Infect Dis 11(suppl 4):830–839, 1989.

93. Wallner G, Mandl CW, Ecker M, et al. Characterization and complete genome sequences of high- and low-virulence variants of tick-borne encephalitis virus. J Gen Virol 77:1035–1042, 1996.

94. Holzmann H, Stiasny K, Ecker M, et al. Characterization of monoclonal antibody-escape mutants of tick-borne encephalitis virus with reduced neuroinvasiveness in mice. J Gen Virol 78:31–37, 1997.

95. Rey FA, Heinz FX, Mandl C, et al. The envelope glycoprotein from tick-borne encephalitis virus at 2 å resolution. Nature 375:291–298, 1995.

96. Mandl CW, Holzmann H, Meixner T, et al. Spontaneous and engineered deletions in the 3' noncoding region of tick-borne encephalitis virus: construction of highly attenuated mutants of a flavivirus. J Virol 72:2132–2140, 1998.

97. Mandl CW, Allison SL, Holzmann H, et al. Attenuation of tick-borne encephalitis virus by structure-based site-specific mutagenesis of a putative flavivirus receptor binding site. J Virol 74:9601–9609, 2000.

98. Mandl CW, Aberle JH, Aberle SW, et al. In vitro-synthesized infectious RNA as an attenuated live vaccine in a flavivirus model. Nat Med 4:1438–1440, 1998.

98a. Kunz C. TBE vaccination and the Austrian experience. Vaccine 21: S50–S55, 2003.

99. Heinz F, Asmera J, Januska J. Present activity in natural foci of tick-borne encephalitis in the CSSR. In Tick-Borne Encephalitis: Proceedings of the International Symposium, Baden/Vienna, 1979. Wien, Facultas Verlag, 1981, pp 279–281.

100. Hoffmann G. Zeckenprophylaxe und -bekämpfung. In Probleme der Insekten-und Zeckenbekämpfung: Ökologische, medizinische und rechtliche Aspekte. Berlin, Schmidt Verlag, 1978, pp 72–75.

Chapter 39

Typhoid Fever Vaccines

MYRON M. LEVINE

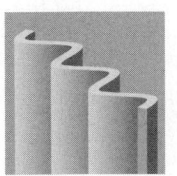

History

Typhoid fever is an acute generalized infection of the reticuloendothelial system, intestinal lymphoid tissue, and gallbladder caused by *Salmonella* Typhi. A broad spectrum of clinical illness can ensue, with more severe forms being characterized by persisting high fever, abdominal discomfort, malaise, and headache. In the preantibiotic era, the disease ran its course over several weeks and was accompanied by a case-fatality rate of approximately 10% to 20%.

Prior to the first quarter of the 19th century, typhoid fever was not recognized as a distinct clinical entity and often was confused with other prolonged febrile syndromes, particularly typhus fever of rickettsial origin. There is considerable debate over who first clearly differentiated typhus fever from typhoid (i.e., typhus-like) fever. Medical historians have argued over who should receive credit for this clinical clarification, and it has been variously bestowed on Huxham (1782),[1] Louis (1829),[2] Gerhard (1837),[3] and Schoenlein (1839).[4] Gerhard, in Philadelphia, argued that two similar, yet distinct, febrile illnesses existed that were clearly discernible from one another on the basis of pathologic findings; one (typhoid) manifested marked intestinal lesions. Schoenlein referred to two distinct forms of typhus: "exanthematicus" and "abdominalis." However, William Jenner is responsible for definitively dispelling controversy on the subject.[5,6] Jenner provided precise clinical descriptions and observations of pathologic conditions from postmortem examinations that allowed a clear-cut differentiation between the two illnesses. He argued that the pathologic lesions in Peyer's patches and mesenteric lymph nodes were peculiar to typhoid and were never seen with typhus. In 1847, the term *enteric fever* was introduced in an attempt to replace typhoid fever and avoid confusion with typhus.[7] Although this term is frequently used, it has by no means replaced the appellations *typhoid fever* and *paratyphoid fever* in common usage.

William Budd's book, *Typhoid Fever: Its Nature, Mode of Spreading and Prevention*, published in 1873,[8] was a milestone in epidemiology because it clearly described the contagious nature of the disease and incriminated transmission via fecally contaminated water sources years before the causative organism was identified. Eberth (1880)[9] visualized the causative bacilli in tissue sections from infected patients, and Gaffky (1884)[10] grew it in pure culture. Known in earlier years as *Bacillus typhosus*, *Eberthella typhosa*, *Salmonella typhi*, and *Salmonella typhosa*, it is currently referred to as *Salmonella enterica* serovar Typhi (*Salmonella* typhi).[11,12]

Salmonella Paratyphi A and B also cause enteric fever (paratyphoid fever), which in most instances is clinically indistinguishable from typhoid fever. In general, where enteric fever is endemic, typhoid accounts for approximately 90% of the clinical cases and paratyphoid for the rest.

Inactivated (heat-killed, phenol-preserved) S. Typhi were utilized as parenteral vaccines as far back as 1896 by Pfeiffer and Kolle[13] in Germany and Wright in England.[14] Wright administered his vaccine (three doses 2 weeks apart) to two medical officers in the Indian Army, one of whom thereafter ingested wild typhoid bacilli without developing illness. Wright then evaluated his vaccine in 2835 volunteers in the Indian Army.[15] Although local and generalized adverse reactions were common, results were considered to be sufficiently encouraging for a decision to be made to vaccinate troops embarking for the Boer War in South Africa. Outcry over the frequency of adverse reactions led to a suspension of vaccination. However, on Wright's insistence, a board of inquiry was established to review data on the reactogenicity and efficacy of the vaccine. The committee concluded that the vaccine was efficacious and that its value in preventing typhoid fever exceeded the price paid in adverse reactions. As a consequence, by World War I typhoid vaccination became virtually routine in the British Army.

Importance of Typhoid Fever

The transmission of typhoid fever is fostered where sanitation is primitive and water supplies are not treated and there exist chronic or short-term carriers of S. Typhi (who serve as a reservoir of infection). In such situations, human fecal material can contaminate water supplies. In endemic areas, the peak incidence of typhoid fever is typically observed among school-age children. Typhoid constitutes the main enteric disease threat faced by children in developing countries after they have survived the gauntlet of diarrheal and dysenteric infections encountered during the first 5 years of life.

Because the case-fatality rate in the preantibiotic era was 10% to 20%, typhoid fever was a much-feared disease. Following the discovery in 1948 that chloramphenicol (and subsequently certain other antibiotics) can successfully treat typhoid fever, dropping case fatality to well below 1%, the interest in typhoid vaccines thereafter historically become a weathervane for the prevalence of antibiotic-resistant strains of S. Typhi. Interest in vaccines waned as long as effective inexpensive oral antibiotics were available, only to resurge when resistant strains appeared and made treatment difficult. Beginning about 1990, strains of S. Typhi that exhibit plasmid-encoded resistance to all the oral antibiotics that were the mainstays of therapy in the 1970s and 1980s (chloramphenicol, trimethoprim-sulfamethoxazole, and amoxicillin) began to disseminate throughout Asia and northeast Africa.[16–22] This emergence of multiply antibiotic-resistant typhoid during the last decade of the 20th century has led to an increase in the incidence of severe cases, hospitalizations, and complications and an increase in typhoid mortality.[16–19,22]

Background

Clinical Description of Typhoid Fever and Its Most Frequent Complications

Typhoid fever exhibits a wide range of clinical severity. Classical full-blown cases begin with malaise, anorexia, myalgia, fever that increases in stepwise fashion to reach 39°C to 40°C, abdominal discomfort, and headaches.[23–25] A bronchitic cough is common in the early stage of illness. The fever often follows three stages. Initially it rises gradually, in stepwise fashion, by daily increments of 0.5°C to 1°C until, after 5 to 7 days, sustained fever of 39°C to 41°C is present. Without appropriate antimicrobial therapy, the fever remains at this level for approximately 10 to 14 days. With convalescence, the fever diminishes, also in stepwise fashion, over several days. During the period of sustained fever, approximately 20% of white patients manifest an exanthem (so-called rose spots) consisting of subtle, salmon-colored macules, 2 to 4 mm in size, which blanch with pressure. Rose spots are seen most often on the chest, abdomen, and back; S. Typhi can be cultured from rose spots.[26] Constipation is typical in older children and adults, whereas diarrhea may occur in young children with typhoid fever.

The peripheral leukocyte count in typhoid fever is often below 4500/mm³, which helps in the differential diagnosis. Thrombocytopenia is also common, with platelets dropping below 80,000/mm³. Liver dysfunction, as detected by mildly elevated serum transaminase values, is observed in most patients. Prior to the availability of fluoroquinolone antibiotics such as ciprofloxacin, approximately 10% of patients treated with earlier antimicrobials of choice, such as chloramphenicol, trimethoprim-sulfamethoxazole, or amoxicillin, manifested clinical relapses; notably, the clinical illness in relapse is much milder

Two of the most feared complications of typhoid fever, intestinal perforation and hemorrhage, are a consequence of the intestinal lesions that are so prominent in the pathology of S. Typhi infection. These complications occur in approximately 0.5% to 1.0% of cases and are more common in individuals who have been ill for several weeks without proper antibiotic therapy. Other uncommon complications of typhoid fever include typhoid hepatitis, empyema, osteomyelitis, and psychosis. More rarely, arthritis, meningitis, myocarditis, and empyema of the gallbladder can occur. In Indonesia, a particularly severe form of typhoid fever is commonly encountered in which cerebral dysfunction, including obtundation, delirium or coma, and shock are present.[27] Unless steroid therapy accompanies appropriate antimicrobial therapy in patients suffering from this form of the disease, the case-fatality rate exceeds 20%.[27]

Although infants may manifest severe clinical forms of typhoid fever, bacteremic S. Typhi infection in children younger than 2 years of age is often remarkably mild and is not recognized clinically as enteric fever.[28,29]

Approximately 2% to 5% of patients with typhoid fever, depending on age and sex, become chronic gallbladder carriers of the organism.[30,31] More rarely, chronic renal carriers occur.

Bacteriology

Taxonomy within the genus Salmonella continues to evolve and is a source of considerable confusion. Originally, speciation was based on association with distinct clinical syndromes. With the Kauffman-White serologic classification, each distinct O:H serotype was given species status, a situation that rather quickly became ponderous. In 1980, the Approved Lists described five species: S. enteritidis, S. typhi, S. typhimurium, S. cholerasuis, and S. arizonae.[32] The most recent classification and speciation, based on DNA relatedness and molecular analysis, reduces the genus Salmonella to two species, S. enterica and S. bongori. Salmonella enterica is further subdivided into subspecies designated with Roman numerals.[11,12,33] Serotypes within S. enterica subspecies I are still almost always referred to by their previous genus/species designations. Thus, for example, in order to avoid confusion, S. enterica serovar Typhi continues to be referred to in most international journals of microbiology, infectious diseases, epidemiology, and vaccinology as Salmonella typhi or Salmonella Typhi. Following the most current taxonomy, S. Typhi is the terminology that will be used in this chapter.

Serologically, S. Typhi falls into group D Salmonella on the basis of its lipopolysaccharide (LPS) O antigens 9 and 12.[34] Salmonella Typhi is motile, and its peritrichous flagella bear flagellar (H) antigen d, which is also encountered in approximately 80 other bioserotypes of Salmonella.[34] Occasional isolates from Indonesia have flagella that bear other antigens (j and z66).[35,36] Strains freshly isolated from patients express on their surface a polysaccharide capsule, the Vi (for virulence) antigen.[34,37–40] Vi consists of a homopolymer of N-acetyl-galacturonic acid[41–43]; the presence of Vi prevents O antibody from binding to the O antigen.[38] As is discussed subsequently, there is evidence that O, Vi, and H antigens each play a protective role with certain typhoid vaccines.

At the level of the clinical microbiology laboratory, S. Typhi exhibits a remarkable degree of homogeneity, in comparison with the other species of *Salmonella*. *Salmonella* Typhi rarely exhibits biochemical or serologic variability. One exception is found in Indonesia, where a few percent of isolates bear flagellar antigen j or z66 rather than d. Previously, only phage typing using Vi phages was helpful in differentiating strains from different geographic areas. More recently, several molecular epidemiologic techniques, including pulsed-field gel electrophoresis and ribotyping, have proven their worth in differentiating S. Typhi strains from diverse sources.[44-49]

Salmonella Typhi does not ferment lactose; it produces hydrogen sulfide (H_2S) but does not produce gas. As a consequence, suspicious colonies are evident on usual lactose-containing media such as *Salmonella-Shigella* agar or MacConkey's agar as lactose-negative colonies. The biochemical pattern in triple-sugar iron agar is rather characteristic, manifested by an acid butt without gas, an alkaline slant, and obvious H_2S production. Fresh isolates typically agglutinate with Vi but not necessarily with group D antiserum. However, if the bacteria are boiled to remove the Vi capsule, a reaction with group D antiserum is then readily seen.

The complete sequence of the 4,809,037-bp genome of multiple antibiotic-resistant S. Typhi strain CT 18 has been reported.[50] Approximately 70% to 80% of the genome shares a backbone containing genes similar in sequence and order to those in *Escherichia coli* and other salmonellae. Intermittently along this backbone are clusters of S. *enterica*–specific and S. Typhi–specific genes (i.e., genes not found in S. Typhimurium or other S. *enterica* serovars) and more than 200 pseudogenes (including several that play a role in virulence in S. Typhimurium). In addition to the 218,150-bp plasmid encoding antibiotic resistance, another 106,516-bp plasmid was found that shows common derivation with the pFra virulence plasmid of *Yersinia pestis*.[50,51]

Pathogenesis

Pathogenesis of Acute Typhoid Fever

Salmonella Typhi and S. Paratyphi A and B are highly invasive bacteria that pass through the intestinal mucosa of humans rapidly and efficiently to eventually reach the reticuloendothelial system, where, after an 8- to 14-day incubation period, they precipitate a systemic illness.[52] S. Typhi is a highly host-adapted pathogen; humans comprise the only natural host and reservoir of this infection.

Our comprehension of the steps involved in the pathogenesis of typhoid fever comes from four sources: (1) clinicopathologic observations in humans,[53,54] (2) volunteer studies,[55] (3) studies of a chimpanzee model,[56,57] and (4) analogies drawn from S. Typhimurium and S. Enteritidis infection in mice (the "mouse typhoid" model).[58,59] The probable steps in the pathogenesis of S. Typhi infection in humans are summarized in the following text.

Susceptible human hosts ingest the causative organisms in contaminated food and water. The inoculum size and the type of vehicle in which it is ingested greatly influence the attack rate for typhoid fever and also affect the incubation period. Doses of 10^9 and 10^8 pathogenic S. Typhi ingested by volunteers in 45 mL of skim milk induced clinical illness in 98% and 89% of individuals, respectively; doses of 10^5 organisms caused typhoid fever in 28% to 55% of vol-

unteers, whereas none of 14 subjects who ingested 10^3 organisms developed clinical illness.[55]

When the ingested typhoid bacilli pass through the pylorus and reach the small intestine, they rapidly penetrate the mucosal epithelium by one of two mechanisms to arrive in the lamina propria. One mechanism of invasion involves typhoid bacilli being actively taken up by M cells,[60-62] the dome-like epithelial cells that cover Peyer's patches and other organized lymphoid tissue of the gut. From here they enter mononuclear and dendritic cells in the underlying lymphoid tissue. In a second, quite distinct, invasive mechanism, bacilli are believed to be internalized by enterocytes, wherein they enter membrane-bound vacuoles that pass through the cell and ultimately release the bacteria at the basal portion of the cell without destroying the enterocyte. Takeuchi provided a highly descriptive electron-photomicrographic documentation of the analogous passage of S. Typhimurium through intestinal mucosa.[63] A third paracellular mode of entry also has been proposed.[64]

On reaching the lamina propria in the nonimmune host, typhoid bacilli elicit an influx of macrophages that ingest the organisms but are generally unable to kill them. Some bacilli apparently remain within macrophages of the small intestinal lymphoid tissue. Other typhoid bacilli are drained into mesenteric lymph nodes, where further multiplication and ingestion by macrophages take place. Shortly after invasion of the intestinal mucosa, a primary bacteremia is believed to take place in which S. Typhi organisms are filtered from the circulation by fixed phagocytic cells of the reticuloendothelial system. It is believed that the main route by which typhoid bacilli reach the bloodstream in this early stage is by lymph that drains from mesenteric nodes to eventually reach the thoracic duct and then the general blood circulation. It is conceivable that ingestion of a massive inoculum followed by widespread invasion of the intestinal mucosa could result in rapid and direct invasion of the bloodstream. As a result of this primary bacteremia, the pathogen rapidly attains an intracellular haven throughout the organs of the reticuloendothelial system, where it resides during the incubation period (usually 8 to 14 days) until the onset of clinical typhoid fever.

Clinical illness is accompanied by a fairly sustained "secondary" bacteremia. In their report of experimental S. Typhi challenge studies in volunteers, Hornick and colleagues described one volunteer who began a 7-day course of oral chloramphenicol only 1 day after ingesting pathogenic S. Typhi and who developed clinical typhoid fever 9 days after the antibiotic was discontinued.[55] This report provides evidence that the typhoid bacilli have attained their intracellular haven within 24 hours after ingestion.

The Vi antigen is a virulence property.[37,40,65] Felix and Pitt, who originally described the antigen and gave it its name, showed that Vi antigen enhanced the pathogenicity of S. Typhi for mice.[37,65] Virtually all strains freshly isolated from patients possess this polysaccharide capsule. Both epidemiologic observations and studies in volunteers support the contention that S. Typhi strains that possess Vi are more virulent than strains lacking this polysaccharide.[55]

Pathogenesis of the Chronic Typhoid Carrier State

During the primary bacteremia that follows ingestion of typhoid bacilli and seeds the reticuloendothelial system, organisms also reach the gallbladder, an organ for which S. Typhi has a remarkable predilection. Following intravenous inoculation, S. Typhi rapidly appear in the gallbladder of rabbits.[66,67] Salmonella Typhi can be readily cultured from bile or from bile-stained duodenal fluid in patients with acute typhoid fever.[68–70] In approximately 2% to 5% of patients, the gallbladder infection becomes chronic.[30,31] The proclivity to become a chronic carrier is greater in females and increases with age at the time of acute S. Typhi infection, thereby resembling the epidemiology of gallbladder disease. The infection tends to become chronic in individuals who have a pre-existing pathologic gallbladder condition at the time of acute S. Typhi infection.

Diagnosis

Bacteriologic Diagnosis

Confirmation of the diagnosis of typhoid fever requires recovery of S. Typhi from a suitable clinical specimen. Because of practicality and relative ease of access, multiple blood cultures should be obtained from patients in whom the diagnosis is suspected clinically. The rate of recovery of S. Typhi in blood cultures depends on many factors, including the volume cultured, the ratio of the volume of blood to the volume of culture broth in which it is inoculated (the ratio should be at least 1:8), the inclusion of anticomplementary substances in the medium (such as sodium polyanetholsulfonate or bile), and whether the patient has already received antibiotics to which the S. Typhi is sensitive. With the use of three 5-mL blood cultures, S. Typhi can be recovered from the blood in approximately 70% of suspect cases.

The gold standard of bacteriologic confirmation of typhoid fever is the bone marrow culture, which is positive in 85% to 96% of cases, even when the patient has received antibiotics.[26,71] In the 1980s, great interest was shown in the use of duodenal string devices to obtain bile-stained duodenal fluid for culture.[68–70,72] The combination of a duodenal string and two blood cultures generally provides a sensitivity of bacteriologic confirmation equal to that achieved with bone marrow cultures but without the invasiveness of the latter.[68]

Stool cultures lead to recovery of the organism in only 45% to 65% of cases. The yield tends to be somewhat higher in children.[70]

Serodiagnosis of Typhoid Fever

Serodiagnosis of typhoid fever has been attempted since the late 19th century, when Widal and Sicard (1896),[73] among others,[74,75] showed that the serum of patients with typhoid fever agglutinated typhoid bacilli. The Widal test, which is still practiced today in many areas, involves the search for agglutinins in the patient's serum and may be performed with antigen in tubes or on slides; the former is generally more accurate. By careful choice of antigen, both O and H antibodies can be selectively measured. By use of S. Typhi strain O901, which lacks flagellar and Vi antigens, S. Typhi O antibody can be selectively measured. To detect antibodies against the appropriate H antigen (d), a strain such as S. Virginia is selected that possesses the identical flagellar antigen (d) but shares no O somatic antigens with S. Typhi.[76] Most patients with typhoid fever have elevated levels of O and H antibody at the time of onset of clinical illness.[76,77]

Anderson[78,79] and Anderson and Gunnell[80] have emphasized the importance and usefulness of H titers in serodiagnosis of typhoid fever. However, some have reported that the prevalence of H antibodies in adults living in endemic areas is too high for the test to be useful in that age group.[76] Nevertheless, it can be helpful in diagnosing children younger than 10 years of age in endemic areas and persons of any age from nonendemic areas. A history of inoculation with parenteral killed whole-cell vaccines invalidates the use of the Widal test. Interest has reappeared in the use of the slide test for O agglutinins of S. Typhi, even for adults in endemic areas.[81] Several new relatively simple serodiagnostic kits also have appeared for detecting antibodies to S. Typhi O antigen and to a 50-kDa outer membrane protein antigen.[82–84]

Serologic tests to measure Vi antibody using highly purified Vi antigen are available.[85–87] Although this serology, including passive hemagglutination,[85] enzyme-linked immunosorbent assay (ELISA),[87] and radioimmunoassay, is practical for the detection of chronic S. Typhi carriers, most of whom have quite elevated levels of Vi antibody, it is of little help in diagnosing acute typhoid fever because only a minority of patients with acute infection manifest detectable Vi antibody.

Rapid Immunoassays

Over the years, many attempts have been made to develop tests that detect S. Typhi antigens or nucleic acid in blood, urine, or body fluids, thereby providing a rapid diagnostic test for typhoid fever.[88–99] With few exceptions, these tests have been disappointing and have failed to warrant the enthusiasm of the initial reports. The immunoassays are based on the detection of the O, Vi, or other antigens of S. Typhi in blood or urine using coagglutination, ELISA, or counter-current immunoelectrophoresis, whereas the polymerase chain reaction and DNA probe methods attempt to amplify S. Typhi genes and hybridize them with labeled specific gene probes. These assays aim to be more sensitive, practical, economical, and rapid than bacteriologic culture, yet comparably specific. Unfortunately, so far no assay has adequately accomplished these objectives, and a satisfactory test that might replace bacteriologic culture remains a laudable but elusive goal.

Epidemiology

Basic Epidemiologic Features

Humans are the sole reservoir of S. Typhi infection as well as the only natural host. The infection is transmitted when susceptible hosts ingest food or water that has been contaminated by fecal matter. In contrast, transmission from person to person by direct contact is exceedingly uncommon. As a consequence of these epidemiologic features, typhoid fever represents the quintessential infectious disease for which transmission is related to levels of sanitation and quality of water supply. Typhoid fever can abound wherever sanitation and food hygiene are primitive. The highest incidence usually occurs where water supplies serving large populations are contaminated by fecal matter. This situation existed at the end of the 19th century in most large cities in the United States and western Europe, where piped water supplies were available but the water was usually untreated.[100] The water sources (usually rivers) were also the repository for the discharged sewage of the cities. In this manner, the transmission of typhoid fever was amplified, causing the disease to be highly endemic in large cities throughout the United States and Europe. With the introduction of water treatment at the turn of the 20th century, including sand filtration and chlorination, the incidence of typhoid fever plummeted precipitously in the large cities of the United States despite the continued existence within those cities of many chronic carriers of S. Typhi.[100,101] Typhoid fever remains endemic in most of the less-developed areas of the world, where fecal contamination of water sources still occurs. This includes many countries in Africa, Asia, and Latin America.

Incidence and Prevalence

In endemic areas, a characteristic age-specific incidence of typhoid fever occurs, with a low incidence in children younger than 2 years of age, a peak incidence in school-age children (5 to 19 years), and a low incidence in adults older than 35 years. The apparent low incidence in young children in part relates to decreased exposure to vehicles of transmission. However, other evidence suggests that infection of children less than 2 years of age may be much more common than previously appreciated but the clinical consequence of S. Typhi infection in the infant host is often mild or atypical illness, even in the face of bacteremic infection.[28,29]

It is presumed that, in developing countries with primitive conditions of human waste disposal and widespread contamination of water supplies, water represents the most common vehicle of transmission and the number of organisms ingested is usually small. Thus multiple subclinical and mild infections are believed to occur for each full-blown clinical case. In contrast, in more developed countries with good sanitation, typhoid is transmitted when chronic carriers contaminate food vehicles through a breakdown in proper practices of personal and food hygiene. In these common-source food-borne outbreaks, the inocula ingested are presumably often relatively large, and high attack rates ensue; under these conditions, fewer subclinical cases occur.

It is difficult to quantify the magnitude of the typhoid fever problem worldwide because the clinical picture is confused with that of many other febrile infections, and the capacity for routine bacteriologic confirmation is absent in most areas of the less-developed world.[102–104] Nevertheless, in the course of several vaccine field trials carried out during the 1980s in Latin America, Asia, and Africa, it was possible to confirm the incidence of typhoid fever that occurred in the unimmunized control subjects during several years of surveillance. In these trials, high annual incidence rates were recorded, including 810 cases per 10^5 population in Indonesia, 653 per 10^5 in Nepal, 442 per 10^5 in South Africa, and 227 cases per 10^5 persons in Chile.[105–108]

Seroepidemiologic studies that have measured the prevalence of S. Typhi H antibody have been very useful in quantifying the prevalence of typhoid fever in different geographic areas.[76,102,109] However, this seroepidemiologic technique has not been widely applied.

Typhoid as a Public Health Problem

It has been estimated that each year more than 33 million cases and more than 500,000 deaths occur worldwide that are due to typhoid fever.[102,103,110] Surveillance data generated by quantifying the incidence of typhoid fever in placebo groups participating in large-scale field trials of typhoid vaccines show annual incidence rates from 227 to 810 cases per 10^5 population in typhoid-endemic areas.[105–108]

Three populations are at particularly high risk of developing typhoid fever and would benefit from immunoprophylaxis with a safe, effective, inexpensive, and practical vaccine. These include children in endemic areas,[28,76,111–113] travelers and military personnel from industrialized countries who visit endemic areas in less-developed countries,[114–117] and clinical microbiology technicians.[118–120]

Seroepidemiologic studies in Peru and Chile have shown that, by 15 to 19 years of age, 50% to 80% of teenagers have serologic evidence of past infection with S. Typhi.[76,102,109] In endemic areas, typhoid fever is a major cause of absenteeism from school and from employment. Direct expenditures for hospitalization and medication further raise the public health costs of this disease.[121] For areas in which it is unlikely that improved sanitation and treated water supplies will become a reality in the near future, a safe vaccine that provides long-term protection would be particularly beneficial in relation to its cost, because an initial investment in immunization provides many years of protection. Because typhoid fever exhibits its peak incidence in school-age children—a "captive" population in many countries—a school immunization program could target the high-risk population of schoolchildren.[122–124]

Travelers from industrialized countries who visit less-developed countries in which typhoid fever is endemic are at particular risk of developing the disease.[102,114–117] Travelers are probably at special risk in endemic areas because they do not have the background immunity that much of the indigenous population has acquired as a consequence of multiple subclinical infections. For U.S. travelers, South America and the Indian subcontinent have been the areas of highest risk.[115] Since 1990, isolates from Asia and northeast Africa have increasingly been resistant to many clinically relevant antibiotics, including chloramphenicol, amoxicillin, and trimethoprim-sulfamethoxazole.[21,103,125] Partial resistance to ciprofloxacin and other fluoroquinolones is also emerging in Southeast Asia and some other regions.[126]

In recent years it has become recognized that microbiology technicians in laboratories, particularly clinical laboratories, constitute a high-risk group for the development of typhoid fever. A review from the Centers for Disease Control and Prevention[120] revealed that 11.2% of the reported sporadic (i.e., not outbreak-associated) cases of typhoid fever in the United States in a 33-month period occurred in laboratory technicians. In the course of their work, these individuals process stool or blood cultures containing S. Typhi before it is recognized that the pathogen is present. The predilection for laboratory workers to develop typhoid fever suggests that, under these special conditions, the disease may be spread by aerosol or by direct contact. This observation is in contrast to the lack of contact spread of this infection under more natural conditions and may be related to the organism existing in pure culture in the laboratory.

Passive Immunization

Passive protection by means of antiserum or immunoglobulin is not used to prevent typhoid or paratyphoid fever.

Active Immunization

For historical as well as practical purposes, we can group the various typhoid vaccines that have been evaluated in clinical trials and the few that have been used as licensed vaccine products into three categories:

1. Vaccines that are no longer in use or that are no longer under investigation
2. Vaccines that are currently available in various countries as licensed products
3. Future vaccines that are under active clinical evaluation

The various past, present, and future typhoid vaccines can be considered to fall into five broad groups for review.

1. Inactivated whole-cell parenteral vaccines
2. Subunit parenteral or aerosolized vaccines
3. Inactivated whole-cell oral vaccine
4. Attenuated S. Typhi strains used as live oral vaccines
5. Parenteral polysaccharide–carrier protein conjugate vaccines

Early Vaccines Not Presently in Use

For a more detailed review of the early vaccines, readers are referred to the chapters on typhoid vaccine in the first two editions of this book.[127,128] A few of the vaccines mentioned in this section were licensed products that at one time were in fairly widespread use. Others among the vaccines cited did not progress beyond early clinical trials or large-scale field trials because of unsatisfactory safety profiles, poor immunogenicity, disappointing efficacy relative to other typhoid vaccines, or difficulty in manufacture (e.g., loss of potency following lyophilization).

Parenteral Inactivated Whole-Cell Vaccines

Alcohol-Inactivated Vaccine. The prototype alcohol-inactivated vaccine was prepared in the 1940s by Felix, who published experimental evidence contending that alcohol treatment of S. Typhi was superior in preserving the Vi antigen because it resulted in a vaccine that outperformed the heat-inactivated, phenol-preserved vaccine in the mouse protection assay.[129,130] For some years this vaccine replaced the heat-inactivated, phenol-preserved vaccine in routine use in the British Armed Forces.

Formalin-Inactivated, Phenol-Preserved Vaccine. This vaccine, which was evaluated for efficacy in a controlled field trial,[131] was prepared by inactivating S. Typhi with formalin and then preserving the vaccine in phenol.

Acetone-Inactivated and Dried Vaccine. This type of vaccine was prepared because of evidence showing that ace-

tone inactivation preserves the Vi antigen (thereby increasing potency in active mouse protection assays) and improves the stability of the vaccine on long-term storage.[132-134] In preparing acetone-inactivated and dried vaccine, S. Typhi are precipitated and inactivated with acetone and then air dried or lyophilized.[133] The manufacturing process required to prepare acetone-inactivated, dried vaccine is much more demanding than that for making heat-phenolized vaccine. For this reason, although there were some manufacturers of this vaccine up through the 1990s (including Wyeth, which made a lyophilized formulation for use by the U.S. military), it is no longer in active production.

Oral Inactivated Whole-Cell Vaccines

As early as the 1920s, Besredka[135,136] promulgated the use of killed S. Typhi or attenuated strains as oral vaccines to elicit "local immunity." In the 1960s and 1970s, several large-scale field trials[137-143] and experimental challenge studies in volunteers[144] were carried out to assess the efficacy of oral inactivated whole-cell vaccines, which at that time were widely sold and used in Europe. The oral killed vaccines that were evaluated in field trials or volunteer studies include acetone-inactivated vaccine and formalin-inactivated vaccine.

Parenteral or Aerosolized Subunit Vaccines

Many attempts were made to prepare extracts and sonicates of S. Typhi and to purify antigens for use as parenteral vaccines. The various subunit immunizing agents (which in the 1960s were referred to as "chemical" vaccines) that were evaluated for efficacy in controlled field trials (or in volunteer studies) include the following:

1. Freeze-and-thaw extract vaccines[145]
2. Trypsinized extract vaccines[146]
3. Purified LPS vaccines (hot water–phenol extraction method)[147]
4. Purified Vi polysaccharide vaccine prepared by denaturing conditions[148,149]

One chemical vaccine of the trypsinized extract variety also was evaluated for efficacy in a controlled field trial after administration by the aerosol route.[137]

Freeze-and-Thaw Extract Vaccines. A parenteral vaccine prepared by the method of Grasset[145] was assessed for efficacy in a controlled field trial in Poland.[150]

Trypsinized Extract Vaccines. Several trypsinized extract vaccines, prepared according to Topley and associates,[146] were subjected to field trials of efficacy in the Soviet Union and Poland.[131,150,151]

Purified Lipopolysaccharide Vaccines. Two parenteral vaccines consisting of S. Typhi LPS O antigen prepared by the hot water–phenol extraction method[147] were evaluated in controlled field trials in Poland[150] and the Soviet Union.[131]

Purified, Denatured Vi Polysaccharide. In the early 1950s, Landy and co-workers[148,152] isolated Vi antigen from *Citrobacter freundii* (previous designations of this bacterium include *Paracolon ballerup*, *Bethesda ballerup*, and *Escherichia coli 5396/38*) and S. Typhi for use as a parenteral vaccine.

Organisms grown on solid agar were inactivated with acetone, after which the dried, acetone-killed bacteria were submitted to multiple extractions with saline, ethanol, and acetic acid to separate Vi from protein, LPS, and nucleic acid. This early method of preparation of purified Vi antigen apparently denatured the polysaccharide, resulting in a complete loss of O-acetyl and a diminution of N-acetyl moieties.[40,153,154] Landy's denatured Vi vaccine was never evaluated for efficacy in field trials. However, in experimental challenge studies in volunteers, a single 25-μg parenteral dose conferred only modest (25% vaccine efficacy), insignificant protection.[55]

Attenuated Strains as Live Oral Vaccines

Attenuated *S.* Typhi strains that were evaluated in Phase I and II clinical trials but that were abandoned from further development include the following:

1. Streptomycin-dependent strains[155–157]
2. Vi-positive variant of *galE* mutant Ty21a[158]
3. *galE, via* (Vi-negative) recombinant mutant strain EX642 derived from wild-type strain Ty2[159]
4. G 2260 hybrid strain (carrying DNA from *E. coli* K-12 and *Shigella flexneri*)[160]
5. Δ*aroA*, Δ*purA* auxotrophic strain 541Ty derived from wild-type strain CDC10-80 (phage type A)[161]
6. 543Ty, Vi-negative derivative of auxotrophic strain 541Ty[161]
7. Δ*aroC*, Δ*aroD* double-mutant recombinant strain CVD 906 (derived from wild-type strain ISP 1820, phage type 46)[162,163]
8. Δ*cya,*Δ*crp* mutant strain χ3927 (derived from wild-type strain Ty2)[164,165]
9. Δ*aroA*, Δ*phoP/phoQ* strain Ty445 (derived from wild-type strain CDC10-80)[166]
10. Δ*aroA*, Δ*aroD* strain PBCC211 (derived from wild-type strain CDC10-80)[167]
11. Δ*aroA*, Δ*aroD*, Δ*htrA* strain PBCC222 (Δ*htrA* derivative of PBCC211)[167]

Streptomycin-Dependent Mutant Vaccines. The streptomycin-dependent strains of Reitman[155] and Mel and colleagues[156,157] were developed by repeated cultivation of pathogenic *S.* Typhi in the presence of streptomycin. These strains were unable to proliferate in the absence of streptomycin. However, the basis for their attenuation extends beyond dependency on streptomycin to maintain growth because these vaccine strains are innocuous even when administered orally along with streptomycin, which allows the organisms to proliferate.[157,168,169] In volunteer challenge studies, freshly harvested organisms of Reitman's streptomycin-dependent oral vaccine proved to be highly protective, whereas lyophilized preparations were not.[168,170]

Vi-Positive Variant of Ty21a. Cryz and associates[158] constructed a Vi-positive variant of strain Ty21a (see below) that was well tolerated and had immunogenicity comparable to that of Ty21a in Phase I clinical trials.[171] The protective efficacy of this attenuated strain was never evaluated in clinical trials.

Δ*galE, via* (Vi-Negative) Strain EX642. Using recombinant techniques, Hone and colleagues[159] deleted a 0.4-kb internal portion of *galE* from wild-type strain Ty2. A further mutant that lacked Vi antigen was selected and referred to as strain EX642. When this strain was fed to four adult volunteers in a dose of 7×10^8 colony-forming units (CFU) with buffer to neutralize gastric acid, two of the four volunteers developed typhoid fever.[159]

Strain G 2260. G 2260 is a hybrid strain of *S.* Typhi that has incorporated into its genome chromosomal segments from both *E. coli* K-12 (the *rha⁺ xyl⁺ fuc⁺* region) and *S. flexneri* 2a (the *pro⁺ his⁺* region).[160] This oral vaccine was well tolerated and modestly immunogenic in a small Phase I study. Seven vaccinees were challenged with 2×10^5 CFU of a virulent *S.* Typhi strain; two subjects shed the challenge strain and none developed illness.[160] Because no unimmunized control volunteers were concomitantly challenged, the stringency of the challenge model and the level of vaccine efficacy cannot be ascertained.

Δ*aroA*, Δ*purA* Mutant 541Ty. Vaccine strain 541Ty was derived from wild-type *S.* Typhi strain CDC10-80 by transducing deletions in two separate genes, each previously characterized in *S.* Typhimurium and affecting a different biosynthetic pathway. The mutations cause requirements for metabolites that are unavailable in adequate concentration in mammalian tissues.[161,172,173] The deletion mutation in *aroA* creates a requirement for aromatic compounds, including two (*para*-aminobenzoic acid and 2,3-dihydroxybenzoic acid) that are not available in adequate concentration in human tissues. The second deletion mutation, in *purA*, causes a specific requirement for adenine (or an assimilable compound such as adenosine).[161,174] These nutritional requirements render *S.* Typhi mutant 541Ty unable to sustain growth in mammalian tissues. A third mutation, in *hisG*, leads to a histidine requirement. Although the *hisG* mutation did not affect virulence, it provided an additional biochemical marker to clearly differentiate the vaccine strain from wild-type *S.* Typhi. In Phase I clinical trials, Ty541 was well tolerated but poorly immunogenic in eliciting serologic responses to *S.* Typhi antigens.[170]

Δ*aroA*, Δ*purA*, Vi-Negative Strain 543Ty. Strain 543Ty is a spontaneously derived mutant of 541Ty that lacks the Vi polysaccharide capsular antigen; in all other ways this Vi-negative variant was identical to 541Ty.[161] Like 541Ty, Ty543 was well tolerated but poorly immunogenic in eliciting serologic responses to *S.* Typhi antigens in Phase I clinical trials.[170] The protective efficacy of 541Ty and 543Ty was never examined in clinical trials.

Δ*aroC*, Δ*aroD* Recombinant Strain CVD 906. By recombinant techniques, precise deletions of 0.65 and 0.35 kb, respectively, were made in *aroC* and *aroD* of wild-type strain ISP1820 (phage type 46, isolated in 1983 from the blood culture of a Chilean school child with uncomplicated typhoid fever), resulting in vaccine strain CVD 906.[162] This strain was evaluated in Phase I clinical trials and was found to be highly immunogenic with a single oral dose but insufficiently attenuated. Febrile adverse reactions occurred in several vaccinees.[163,165]

Δ*cya*, Δ*crp* Strain χ3927. In *Salmonella* the products encoded by *cya* (adenylate cyclase) and *crp* (the cyclic AMP receptor protein) comprise a global regulatory system that regulates the transcription of multiple genes and operons.[164]

These include genes concerned with the transport and breakdown of catabolites; the expression of fimbriae, flagella, and one outer membrane protein; and the transport systems for carbon sources. Deletion mutations were made in *cya* and *crp* of S. Typhimurium by illegitimate excision of a transposon that had been inserted into each of these genes.[164] The Δ*cya* and Δ*crp* of S. Typhimurium were then moved into wild-type S. Typhi strain Ty2 by transduction with phage P22. The resultant S. Typhi vaccine strain was designated χ3927.[165,175]

When evaluated in Phase I dose-response clinical trials,[165] χ3927 was moderately immunogenic but caused unacceptable febrile reactions in some subjects, and so further clinical trials were discontinued.

Δ*aroA*, Δ*phoP*/*phoQ* Strain Ty445. Deletion mutations in *aroA* and *phoP*/*phoQ* were introduced into wild–type strain CDC10-80 to derive vaccine candidate Ty445. In a Phase I clinical trial, this vaccine strain was well tolerated but poorly immunogenic, leading to its abandonment from further development.[166]

Δ*aroA*, Δ*aroD* Strain PBCC211. Deletions were introduced in two genes (*aroA* and *aroD*) encoding enzymes in the aromatic amino acid biosynthesis pathway in wild-type strain CDC10-80. Three different formulations of this vaccine strain were tested in Phase I clinical trials. With two lyophilized formulations, some subjects developed fever. At the highest dosage levels tested, a proportion of vaccinees manifested silent, self-limited vaccinemias on days 4 to 5 after ingesting a single dose of vaccine.[167]

Δ*aroA*, Δ*aroD*, Δ*htrA* Strain PBCC222. A deletion in *htrA* was introduced into strain PBCC211 to derive vaccine strain PBCC222.[167] A definitive lyophilized formulation of this candidate contained in sachets was tested in Phase I clinical trials in subjects who received dosage levels of 10^7 to 10^9 CFU.[167] No vaccinemias were detected in recipients of this strain, but some who ingested the highest dosage level developed fever, chills, and headache, leading to abandonment of further clinical trials.

Currently Licensed, Available, and Used Vaccines

Currently licensed, used, and commercially available typhoid vaccines include

1. Heat-inactivated, phenol-preserved whole-cell parenteral vaccine (both liquid and lyophilized formulations and occasionally adsorbed to alum adjuvant)
2. Purified Vi polysaccharide parenteral vaccine
3. Attenuated *galE, via* (Vi-negative) strain Ty21a, used as a live oral vaccine

The results of the various clinical trials and field trials that established the safety, immunogenicity, and efficacy of the currently available typhoid vaccines are described in other sections of this chapter.

Parenteral Inactivated Whole-Cell Vaccines

Parenteral inactivated whole-cell vaccines to prevent typhoid fever have been used since the end of the 19th century. The experience with the early killed S. Typhi parenteral vaccines has been reviewed.[176] Not until the

mid-1950s were randomized, controlled field trials undertaken to assess the absolute and relative efficacy of more modern parenteral killed whole-cell typhoid vaccines.

HEAT-INACTIVATED, PHENOL-PRESERVED VACCINE

By far the most widely available and utilized parenteral killed whole-cell vaccine worldwide is the heat-inactivated, phenol-preserved vaccine, which is relatively easy to prepare and standardize and is produced in essentially the same manner as that originally reported by Pfeiffer and Kolle[13] and Wright and co-workers.[14,15,177] The heat-killed, phenol-preserved vaccine is made by heating agar- or broth-grown S. Typhi (usually to 56°C for 1 hour) and then suspending them in a 0.5% phenol solution, usually to a concentration of 10^9 organisms/mL.

Purified Vi Polysaccharide Vaccine

In a modern approach to purify Vi under nondenaturing conditions, Wong and co-workers[178] and Robbins and Robbins[40] treated S. Typhi with hexadecyltrimethylammonium bromide (Cetavlon®; Eastman Organic Chemicals), the detergent that was previously instrumental in the preparation of purified meningococcal polysaccharide vaccines.[179] This extraction method results in purified Vi that is not denatured and that preserves the O- and N-acetyl moieties, as opposed to the methods used by Landy and co-workers that yielded denatured Vi. The chemical structure of Vi polysaccharide is shown in Figure 39–1.

Scale-up of production of Vi to an industrial manufacturing process was worked out by scientists from the laboratory of John B. Robbins at the National Institute of Child Health and Human Development and Aventis Pasteur.[180] The Ty2 strain of S. Typhi is cultured in 1000-L fermenters, after which the bacteria are fixed with formaldehyde and Vi polysaccharide is extracted from supernatants using cetrimonium bromide. The Vi is further purified, dried, dissolved in a buffer solution, and filter sterilized. After appropriate controls of this material, it is filled into single-dose syringes.

Attenuated S. Typhi Strain Ty21a as a Live Oral Vaccine

Ty21a was derived from wild-type strain Ty2 by treatment with the mutagenic agent nitrosoguanidine.[181] A mutant was selected that exhibited a complete absence of activity of the enzyme uridine diphosphate (UDP)-galactose-4-epimerase and a reduction of approximately 80% in the activity

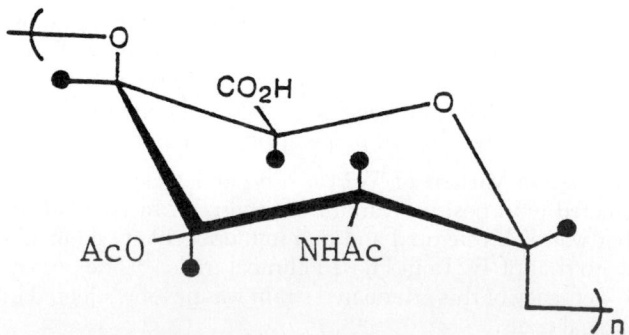

FIGURE 39–1 ■ The chemical composition of Vi polysaccharide, which is a homopolymer of $(1{\rightarrow}4)$-α-D-GalρANAc that is variably acetylated at carbon 3.

of two other Leloir enzymes, galactokinase and galactose-1-phosphate uridyl transferase. A further mutant was then selected that lacked the Vi antigen. This strain was designated Ty21a.[181]

Galactose residues are an important component of the smooth LPS O antigen in wild-type S. Typhi. The enzyme encoded by the *galE* gene, UDP-galactose-4-epimerase, isomerizes UDP-glucose to UDP-galactose and vice versa (Fig. 39–2). UDP-galactose provides galactose residues that can be incorporated into the smooth LPS O antigen of S. Typhi. When grown in the absence of galactose, Ty21a does not express smooth O antigen, because it has no source of UDP-galactose; in this state it is not immunogenic.[182] In contrast, when *galE* mutant Ty21a is grown in the presence of exogenous galactose, the two other Leloir pathway enzymes (see Fig. 39–2) allow this monosaccharide to be assimilated to UDP-galactose and utilized to synthesize smooth O antigen. However, because of the lack of epimerase, strain Ty21a (like other *galE* mutants) accumulates galactose-1 phosphate and UDP-galactose when grown in the presence of exogenous galactose (see Fig. 39–2). In vitro, it can be shown that accumulation of these intermediate products leads to bacterial death by lysis.[181]

For many years it was thought that the *galE* and Vi mutations together accounted for the impressive in vivo safety of Ty21a. In the light of more recent data, it is now recognized that the *galE* and Vi mutations in Ty21a do not by themselves explain the attenuation of this strain.[159] Other mutations within strain Ty21a that also were induced by the nonspecific chemical mutagenesis contribute importantly to the safety of this oral vaccine strain. One such mutation may be in *rpoS* (*katF*), which encodes an RNA polymerase sigma factor; this mutation diminishes the ability of the bacteria to survive various stress conditions, including nutrient deprivation.[183]

Producers of Currently Available Vaccines

Killed Whole-Cell Vaccine

The only United States manufacturer of parenteral inactivated whole-cell typhoid vaccine for civilian use in the 1990s, Wyeth-Lederle, which made a heat-inactivated, phenol-preserved whole-cell liquid product, has discontinued production. Up through the 1990s, Wyeth also produced a lyophilized, acetone-inactivated parenteral vaccine for the U.S. Armed Forces. The U.S. military has since switched to the use of Ty21a or Vi.

Elsewhere throughout the world there are some producers of heat-inactivated, phenol-preserved typhoid vaccines for parenteral use. The available products are published in the World Health Organization's *International List of Availability of Vaccines and Sera*.[184] In addition to commercial sources, government public health institutes in some countries in Asia, Latin America, and Africa manufacture their own typhoid vaccines.

Purified Vi Polysaccharide Parenteral Vaccine

There are presently two licensed Western manufacturers of purified Vi, Aventis Pasteur (TYPHIM Vi®, available in the United States and many European and other countries) and GlaxoSmithKline (Typherix®, available in several European countries). In addition, several vaccine manufacturers in Asia (e.g., China, Vietnam) and Russia make Vi products for local consumption.

Ty21a Live Oral Vaccine

Ty21a (Vivotif Berna®) is manufactured by Berna Biotech (previously called the Swiss Serum and Vaccine Institute). Under license, it is also distributed by a number of other vaccine distributors, such as Chiron in Italy and Chiron-Behring in Germany.

Dosage and Immunization Schedules

Parenteral Inactivated Whole-Cell Vaccines

The various parenteral killed whole-cell vaccines are usually administered subcutaneously with 0.5-mL injections containing approximately 5×10^8 bacteria; two doses are given 1 month apart. In an effort to diminish both local and systemic adverse reactions associated with these vaccines, some investigators have recommended the administration of 0.1 mL intradermally.[185-194] Although the antigenicity of vaccine given by the intradermal route has been compared with vaccine administered by the subcutaneous route, no controlled field trials of efficacy have been carried out to assess the protective value of intradermal immunization.

Subunit Vaccines

The modern nondenatured Vi vaccines are administered as a single subcutaneous or intramuscular injection containing 25 µg of purified polysaccharide.[106,107,180,195,196] Single doses

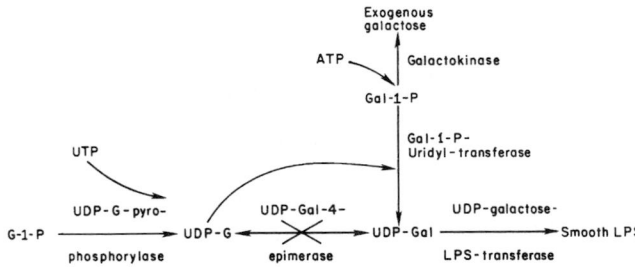

FIGURE 39–2 ■ The scheme of incorporation of exogenous galactose by *galE* mutant Ty21a; attenuated S. Typhi vaccine strain is shown. When grown in the absence of galactose, Ty21a does not produce smooth lipopolysaccharide (LPS) O antigen and is nonimmunogenic. Grown in the presence of exogenous galactose, this hexose sequentially is processed to become galactose-1 phosphate (Gal-1-P) and then uridine diphosphate–galactose (UDP-Gal). Because of the complete lack of UDP–Gal-4-epimerase in Ty21a, UDP-Gal cannot be converted to UDP-glucose (UDP-G), but it can be further incorporated into smooth LPS O antigen. However, the accumulation of UDP-Gal and Gal-1-P consequent to the block of UDP–Gal-4-epimerase activity results in bacteriolysis. (Adapted from Germanier R, Furer E. Immunity in experimental salmonellosis. II. Basis for the avirulence and protective capacity of *galE* mutants of *Salmonella* Typhimurium. Infect Immun 4:663–673, 1971.)

that contain 50 μg of purified polysaccharide were also studied in Phase II and III clinical trials.[106,197]

Ty21a Live Oral Vaccine

Irrespective of the formulation or whether a three-dose or four-dose oral immunization schedule is followed, each dose (capsule or sachet of lyophilized vaccine) contains 2 to 6 × 10^9 CFU of Ty21a.

With the enteric-coated capsule formulation, a four-dose oral immunization schedule is recommended in the United States and Canada, whereas in other countries throughout the world a three-dose regimen is used. Ty21a vaccine is administered with an interval of 1 day between doses. Increasing the interval between doses of enteric-coated vaccine to 21 days does not enhance protection.[123,198] One of the field trials with Ty21a carried out in Santiago, Chile, showed that immunization with four doses within an 8-day period provides significantly greater protection than three doses.[124] Based on results of this field trial, the U.S. Food and Drug Administration and the Canadian Drug Board licensed Ty21a as a four-dose immunization schedule, with a dose given every other day.

Two field trials, carried out in Chile[199] and Indonesia,[105] each directly compared the relative efficacy of three doses of Ty21a given in enteric-coated capsules versus vaccine administered as a liquid suspension (which is reconstituted by emptying a sachet containing lyophilized vaccine and a sachet containing buffer into 100 mL of water). The doses of vaccine were given every other day in the trial in Chile, whereas in Indonesia the doses were administered 1 week apart. In each of these trials, three doses of Ty21a in the liquid formulation provided better protection than the enteric-coated capsules. In the Chilean field trial, the difference in the level of efficacy conferred by the two formulations was highly significant.[199] Since 1997, the liquid formulation of Ty21a has been licensed by a number of countries with a three-dose immunization regimen that recommends an interval of 2 days between doses.

A practical question arises when a subject fails to complete the full course of immunization with three to four doses of Ty21a: Does one need simply to complete the number of doses, or must one complete the full schedule? A definitive answer is not available. However, as a rule of thumb, if less than 3 weeks have passed since the last dose, one may continue to complete the immunization with the missing doses. If more than 3 weeks have passed, the full regimen of this well-tolerated vaccine should be administered de novo.

Formulations Available

Parenteral Inactivated Whole-Cell Vaccine

The heat-inactivated, phenol-preserved vaccine is usually available as a liquid suspension containing 1 × 10^9 bacilli/mL.

Purified Vi Polysaccharide Parenteral Vaccine

Purified Vi is available as a solution containing 25 μg of Vi polysaccharide in 0.5 mL of phenolic isotonic buffer. Single-dose syringes are the usual formulation. By special order, 20-dose and 50-dose vials can be made available.

Ty21a Live Oral Vaccine

There have been three successive commercial formulations of Ty21a, each representing a notable improvement over the earlier versions. The initial commercial formulation of Ty21a (which was available for only a short time) consisted of gelatin-coated capsules containing either NaHCO$_3$ (0.4 to 0.5 g) or lyophilized vaccine (2 to 6 × 10^9 CFU/dose).[123,198,200,201] Vaccination with this initial formulation involved the ingestion of two gelatin capsules, each containing bicarbonate, followed by a third capsule containing vaccine; doses were ingested every other day for a total of three vaccine doses.

Field trials in Santiago, Chile, compared the efficacy of the gelatin capsule-NaHCO$_3$ formulation with a formulation consisting of lyophilized vaccine in enteric-coated capsules (2 to 6 × 10^9 CFU/capsule) that requires no pretreatment with buffer to neutralize gastric acid.[123,198] Following results of controlled field trials that demonstrated the superiority of the enteric-coated capsule formulation over the gelatin-coated capsule formulation, the latter was withdrawn and replaced with the enteric-coated capsule formulation. Enteric-coated capsules should be ingested on a fasting stomach with a little water.

Since 1997, the liquid suspension formulation of Ty21a has been licensed in several countries with a three-dose immunization regimen that recommends an interval of every other day between doses. This formulation comes as a double sachet, one sachet containing 2 to 10 × 10^9 CFU of lyophilized vaccine and the other containing buffer. The contents of the two sachets are added to 100 mL of water with stirring, resulting in the vaccine suspension.

Constituents

Parenteral Inactivated Whole-Cell Vaccine

Each dose of heat-inactivated, phenol-preserved vaccine typically contains 1 × 10^9 bacilli/mL. Phenol (0.5%) is added to the final product as preservative.

Purified Vi Polysaccharide Parenteral Vaccine

Purified Vi is available as a solution containing 25 μg of Vi polysaccharide in 0.5 mL of phenolic isotonic buffer. Each immunizing dose contains 25 μg of Vi polysaccharide, less than 1.25 mg of phenol in TYPHIM Vi and 1.1 mg in Typherix, and q.s. 0.5 mL of isotonic buffer (4.15 mg sodium chloride; 0.065 mg sodium dibasic phosphate, 2H$_2$O; 0.023 mg sodium monobasic phosphate, 2H$_2$O; and q.s. 0.5 mL water for injection).

Ty21a Live Oral Vaccine

ENTERIC-COATED CAPSULES

Gelatin capsules are coated with phthalate to render them resistant to acid. Each coated capsule contains 2 to 6 × 10^9 CFU of Ty21a, 5 to 50 × 10^9 nonviable Ty21a, 26 to 130 mg of sucrose, 1 to 5 mg of ascorbic acid, 1.4 to 7.0 mg of an amino acid mixture, 100 to 180 mg of lactose, and 3.6 to 4.4 mg of magnesium stearate.

LIQUID SUSPENSION FORMULATION

The vaccine sachet contains 2 to 10 × 10^9 CFU of Ty21a, 5 to 60 × 10^9 nonviable Ty21a, 15 to 250 mg of sucrose, 0.6

to 10 mg of ascorbic acid, 0.8 to 15 mg of an amino acid mixture, 1.5 g of lactose, and 20 to 30 mg of aspartame. The accompanying sachet of buffer contains 2.4 to 2.9 g of sodium bicarbonate, 1.5 to 1.8 g of ascorbic acid, and 0.18 to 0.22 g of lactose.

Vaccine Stability

Parenteral Inactivated Whole-Cell Vaccines

Driesens has shown that the stability of the pH of liquid formulations of acetone-inactivated vaccine is the major determinant of the vaccine's shelf life and that this stability is related to the type of glass vial.[202] Acetone-inactivated fluid vaccines stored in buffered saline solutions maintained potency for more than 30 months when stored at 4°C. By contrast, the same vaccine in unbuffered saline solution lost potency as the pH increased. Vaccines packaged in U.S. Pharmacopeia borosilicate glass vials retained stable pH and potency, whereas vaccines stored in type III U.S. Pharmacopeia soda-lime glass vials were less stable. If kept refrigerated, heat-inactivated, phenol-preserved vaccine has a shelf life of 18 months after leaving the manufacturer's cold storage.

Using the active mouse protection test as the measure of vaccine potency, Joo and Zsidai[203] systematically investigated the stability of fluid and lyophilized forms of heat-inactivated, phenol-preserved, and acetone-inactivated vaccines stored at 37°C or 4°C for 12 weeks. Their results showed that fluid vaccines must be maintained in the cold chain to maintain potency; the fluid vaccines lost significant potency within 2 weeks of storage at 37°C. By contrast, the lyophilized vaccine retained potency even after 12 weeks of storage at high temperature. The potency of lyophilized vaccine after long-term storage has been corroborated by Dimache and associates,[187] who showed that lyophilized vaccine was still antigenic and still gave acceptable results in the mouse protection test after 5 years of storage at 4°C. The shelf life of lyophilized typhoid vaccine is dependent on the residual moisture content of the lyophilate; the lower the residual moisture, the longer the shelf life.[203] Vaccines with moisture contents below 3% have a long shelf life.

Purified Vi Polysaccharide Parenteral Vaccine

The Vi polysaccharide vaccine is highly stable and in theory should not require a cold chain even in tropical conditions. The Vi polysaccharide retains its physicochemical characteristics after 6 months' storage at 37°C and after 2 years at 22°C. Nevertheless, the manufacturers recommend that the vaccine be stored in a refrigerator at 2°C to 8°C for up to 18 months, and they caution against freezing the products.

Ty21a Live Oral Vaccine

Long-term storage of Ty21a should be at 4°C. The shelf life of lyophilized Ty21a is dependent on residual moisture content and maintenance of a cold chain.[204,205]

The potency requirements of Ty21a dictate that the viable counts within each dose (enteric-coated capsule or packet of lyophilized vaccine) exceed 2×10^9 CFU. Prolonged storage for 7 days at room temperature (20°C to 25°C, or 73°F to 82°F) resulted in progressively lower viable counts over time. Nevertheless, after a 7-day test period, all 10 lots tested still met the minimum potency require-

ments.[206] Similarly, three separate lots of Ty21a maintained potency when stored at 37°C (98.6°F) for 12 hours.[206]

Laboratory Control of Vaccine Lots (Potency Assays)

Parenteral Inactivated Whole-Cell Vaccines

Many laboratory tests of typhoid vaccine "potency" were carried out in conjunction with the large-scale controlled field trials of vaccine efficacy sponsored by the World Health Organization in an attempt to identify a test, an animal model, or an assay that can predict vaccine potency in humans reliably.[207-223] These tests have consisted mainly of measurement of antibody responses in animals (and humans) and active protection assays in small laboratory animals. Unfortunately, no satisfactory laboratory test has been identified that clearly predicts the potency of all parenteral killed or extract typhoid vaccines or attenuated strains used as live oral vaccines.

The World Health Organization Expert Committee on typhoid vaccines concluded that no single potency test can be used to predict reliably the efficacy of typhoid vaccines in humans.[222] Nevertheless, two assays have shown sufficient correlation with field trial results of parenteral vaccines to have advocates: (1) an elicitation of H antibodies following parenteral immunization of rabbits and (2) an active mouse protection test.

In conjunction with field trials of the fluid alcohol-inactivated and heat-inactivated, phenol-preserved parenteral vaccines in Yugoslavia,[224] investigators in several laboratories found that the more effective heat-inactivated, phenol-preserved vaccine elicited significantly higher levels of H antibody in rabbits.[56,217,223] Similarly, in conjunction with the later field trials comparing the lyophilized heat-inactivated, phenol-preserved (L) and acetone-inactivated (K) reference vaccines,[131,150,225-228] the more effective K vaccine was again found to stimulate significantly higher H antibody titers in both rabbits and humans (Table 39-1).[209,210,216,218,225,229] Debate has raged as to whether this observation implies that protection is directly related to H antigens and mediated by H antibodies or whether the H agglutinins rather serve as a marker to denote that a gentler method of inactivation of S. Typhi has preserved other highly labile and uncharacterized protective antigens.[230]

S. Typhi is an impressively human host–adapted parasite. This fact has greatly impeded the development of a relevant and practical animal model for the testing of typhoid vaccines. Among primates, only chimpanzees develop an experimental infection with S. Typhi that in its pathogenesis rather closely resembles that found in humans. Furthermore, following inoculation by whatever route, no small laboratory animal species manifests a general infection that resembles human typhoid fever. Several types of active immunization of mice (subcutaneous or intraperitoneal) followed by intraperitoneal challenge with S. Typhi in saline or mucin have been evaluated in various laboratories.[207,210-213,215-221,223,228,229,231,232] The different techniques gave varying results; sometimes results from different laboratories were contradictory, despite ostensibly using essentially the same procedure with reference reagents. Nevertheless, several investigators have argued that active intraperitoneal immunization of mice followed 7 to 14 days later by intraperitoneal challenge with

TABLE 39–1 ■ Comparison of Acetone-Inactivated (K) and Heat and Phenol–Inactivated (L) Reference Vaccines: Ability to Stimulate Antibody, Activity in Mouse Protection Tests, and Efficacy in Field Trials

Test	Vaccine Group K	Vaccine Group L	Tetanus Toxoid Control
Agglutinins in humans*			
H	1008	720	16
O	13	17	2
Vi†	21	20	4
Agglutinins in rabbits			
H	320	40‡	—
O	320	640	—
Active mouse protection test			
Relative potency	3.6	1.0	—
Efficacy in controlled field trials			
Guyana (7 yr of surveillance)	88%	67%	—
Yugoslavia (2 ½ yr of surveillance)	79%	51%	—

*Geometric mean titer 2 weeks after second dose of vaccine.
†Measured by passive hemagglutination.
‡Geometric mean titer 7 days after fourth inoculation with vaccine diluted 1:100.

pathogenic S. Typhi in mucin represents the best potency test for typhoid vaccines, among the various alternatives. Results of this assay paralleled the results of the field trials of K and L vaccines (see Table 39–1). Much controversy surrounds the overall usefulness and applicability of this assay because it strongly favors vaccines that have a high Vi antigen content; vaccines that are potent in stimulating Vi antibody are highly protective in mice because Vi is a major virulence property in this species.[129,233–236] Because acetone inactivation of S. Typhi enhances the preservation of Vi,[132,235,236] the K vaccine performed particularly well in this assay when compared with the L vaccine, which preserves Vi less well.

The field trial in Egypt[237] of an acetone-inactivated typhoid vaccine prepared from a nonflagellated mutant (TNM1) of S. Typhi strain Ty2[79,80] provided the opportunity to evaluate which was more important: elicitation of H antibody or potency in the mouse protection test. This vaccine did not stimulate H antibody because it lacked flagella; however, it was as potent in mouse protection tests as the acetone-inactivated reference vaccine K. Nevertheless, in the field trial this vaccine was not protective,[237] suggesting that the active mouse protection test is not an adequate predictor of efficacy of typhoid vaccines in humans. Despite the controversy that surrounds it, the active mouse protection test was used in the United States to assay the potency of parenteral killed whole-cell typhoid vaccines.[238]

Purified Vi Polysaccharide Parenteral Vaccine

The active protection test in mice, as used for the inactivated whole-cell parenteral vaccines, can serve as a potency test for the Vi vaccine.

Ty21a and Other Live Oral Vaccines

At present, viable counts of vaccine organisms are used as the measure of potency of live oral vaccines. Until a more relevant potency test is developed, the active protection test in mice can also serve as a potency test for attenuated-strain vaccines; here the vaccine is also inoculated intraperitoneally in mice even though it is administered orally in humans.

Results of Vaccination

Immune Response

Because of the complex nature of the pathogenesis of S. Typhi clinical infection, a protective role is probably played by secretory intestinal antibody (in preventing mucosal invasion), circulating antibody (against bacteremic organisms), and cell-mediated immunity (to eliminate intracellular bacilli). With parenteral vaccines, the circulating antibody response is substantial and presumably provides the predominant protective effect. In contrast, with live, attenuated oral vaccines, the circulating antibody response may be modest, but vigorous secretory intestinal immunoglobulin A (IgA) and cell-mediated immune responses occur that are believed to be responsible for the protection conferred by that type of vaccine.

Unfortunately, with S. Typhi the critical antigens responsible for protection are not agreed on, and data are somewhat contradictory. With parenteral vaccines, elicitation of serum H (flagellar) antibodies in humans correlates with protection, whereas stimulation of O and Vi antibodies does not.[209,223,225,237] In contrast, with live oral vaccines the mucosal IgA and systemic cell-mediated immune responses appear in large part to be directed toward the O and H antigens but not to the Vi antigen.[123,163,165,170, 202,239–252] In fact, one attenuated strain (Ty21a) lacks Vi antigen[140] yet provides significant protection.[105,108,123, 198,199,253,254]

Parenteral Inactivated Whole-Cell Vaccines

SERUM ANTIBODY RESPONSE

Typically, in assessing the seroconversion after vaccination with a parenteral inactivated whole-cell typhoid vaccine, serum antibodies are measured to the O, H (d), and Vi antigens. O antibodies were formerly assayed by bacterial agglutination (Widal test),[209] but ELISA using purified LPS has become popular in recent years.[163,165,170,239,241–243,255] H antibody is measured by agglutination using an appropriate whole-cell antigen such as S. Virginia (which has the same d flagellar antigen as S. Typhi but lacks Vi and has distinct O antigens) or by ELISA using purified S. Typhi flagella.[170,239,241,242] Vi antibody can be measured by passive hemagglutination,[85,86,197] radioimmunoassay,[40,106,197,256] or ELISA.[87,107] It is important to utilize highly purified undenatured Vi antigen to avoid cross-reactions. For this reason, only since the 1980s has Vi serology become reliably specific.

The evidence suggesting that anti-H antibodies may play a role in protection has been discussed in part in the section on vaccine potency (see *Laboratory Control of Vaccine Lots*

[Potency Assays] above. In Yugoslavia, Poland, the Soviet Union, and Guyana, field trials of efficacy were carried out with several different well-characterized parenteral killed whole-cell vaccines, including alcohol-inactivated, heat-phenolized, and acetone-inactivated vaccines. Measurement of serologic responses to these vaccines in groups of vaccinees and in immunized laboratory animals allowed protective efficacy to be correlated with antibody response. Those killed whole-cell parenteral vaccines that were most protective in the field stimulated the highest levels of H antibody. A similar correlation between H titer and protection against typhoid fever was found in healthy young adult volunteers who in the 1960s and 1970s participated in experimental challenge studies to assess the efficacy of typhoid vaccines.[169,182,257] Control volunteers who had elevated H titers (presumably derived by natural infection or vaccination many years earlier during military service) were significantly protected against development of typhoid fever.

However, the most convincing evidence that H antibody is important comes from the field trial by Wahdan and colleagues[237] of an acetone-killed and dried vaccine prepared from a strain of S. Typhi that lacks H antigen. This vaccine, which did not elicit H antibodies, failed to confer significant protection.

Table 39–1 shows the serum antibody responses to S. Typhi O, H, and Vi antigens following vaccination of children with parenteral acetone-inactivated or heat-inactivated, phenol-preserved whole-cell vaccines.[208] These data from children in the Guyana field trial are representative of the serologic responses encountered with these types of vaccines.

O antibody that appears following inoculation with parenteral inactivated whole-cell typhoid vaccines is largely immunoglobulin M (IgM), whereas the H antibody response is initially IgM and then becomes immunoglobulin G (IgG).[249,258–262]

MUCOSAL IMMUNE RESPONSE

Not surprisingly, the few studies that have examined mucosal immunity after administration of parenteral inactivated whole-cell vaccine have reported minimal secretory IgA (sIgA) antibody or gut-derived IgA antibody-secreting cell (ASC) responses.[249,263–265]

CELL-MEDIATED IMMUNE RESPONSE

Some cell-mediated immune responses have been measured following vaccination with parenteral killed whole-cell vaccines.[244,250,266,267] The assays utilized have included lymphocyte replication or antibody-dependent mononuclear cell migration inhibition in the presence of soluble antigen or inhibition of growth of S. Typhi by mononuclear cells. The cell-mediated response after administration of these vaccines has not been prominent.

Purified Vi Polysaccharide Parenteral Vaccine

SERUM ANTIBODY

Parenteral Vi polysaccharide vaccine elicits serum IgG Vi antibody responses in approximately 85% to 95% of adults or children above 2 years of age. Table 39–2 shows the serum Vi and O antibody responses reported by Tacket et al.[197] following vaccination of young adults with one of two purified Vi antigen vaccines prepared from S. Typhi. The vaccines differed in their degree of purity; one Vi vaccine had 5% residual contamination with LPS, but the other was 99.8% pure. This difference was reflected in the serologic response. Although similar Vi antibody seroconversions occurred in approximately 90% of recipients of either preparation, those who received the more purified preparation had only a 26% seroconversion of O antibody versus 83% who seroconverted to O antigen following inoculation with the less purified vaccine.

The serologic responses of other groups of adults and children in nonendemic and endemic areas to the TYPHIM Vi vaccine are shown in Table 39–3.[106,107,180,256,268,269] In contrast with the strong responses in adults and older children, the Vi antibody response in toddlers in Indonesia was weak and short lived.[180] High seroconversion rates also have been reported among preschool children (99%),[270] school-age children 4 to 14 years of age (99.5%),[195] and

TABLE 39–2 ■ Immune Response to Two *Salmonella* Typhi Vi Polysaccharide Vaccine Candidates

	Vi Titers*			S. Typhi Lipopolysaccharide Titers (ELISA)		
	Geometric Mean Titer			Geometric Mean Tilter		
	Before	After	Seroconversions (%)[†]	Pre	Post	Seroconversions (%)[‡]
Vi Lot 53226						
Maryland students	0.17	2.57	100	0.11	0.78	83
Chilean recruits				0.15	0.77	83
Vi Lot IMS1569						
French volunteers	0.07	2.73	95	0.12	0.22	26[§]

*Measured by radioimmunoassay.
[†]Increase in antibody of 0.15 µg/mL.
[‡]Increase in net optical density of 0.15.
[§]χ^2 = 28.3; P< 0.0001 versus recipients of lot 53226.
Data from Tacket CO, Ferreccio C, Robbins JB, et al. Safety and characterization of the immune response to two *Salmonella typhi* Vi capsular polysaccharide vaccine candidates. J Infect Dis 154:342–345, 1986.

TABLE 39–3 ■ Serum Vi Antibody Responses Measured by Radioimmunoassay in Adults and Children Immunized with 25-μg Doses of a Liquid Formulation of Purified Vi Polysaccharide Vaccine

Location	Age Group (yr)	N	Vi Antibody		Rate of Seroconversion (%)[†]	Reference
			Geometric Mean Titler (μg/mL)			
			Pre	Post[*]		
United States	18–40	54	0.2	3.2	93	256
Nepal	45–55	8	0.5	4.4	63	106
	15–44	43	0.4	3.7	79	
	5–14	65	0.2	1.9	77	
Indonesia	>22	22	0.8	11.3	68	180
	5–12	80	0.3	5.0	88	
	2–4	54	0.2	5.8	96	
Kenya	5–15	97	0.3	2.0	76	269

[*]One month after immunization.
[†]Fourfold or greater rise in titer.

adolescents 11 to 18 years of age (99%)[196] immunized with the Typherix vaccine. Agglutinating antibody responses were also seen in 96% of adults.[270a]

Purified Vi polysaccharide behaves like a T-lymphocyte–independent antigen. The serum antibody response is not boosted by administration of additional doses of Vi vaccine.[256,268] A second dose of Vi given by Keitel et al.[256] 27 to 34 months after a primary inoculation stimulated fourfold rises in serum Vi antibody titer in 33% to 50% of subjects. However, the titers only returned to the levels achieved 1 month after the primary immunization. Titers of Vi antibody progressively fall over time.[256] Klugman et al.[271] proposed that a serum Vi antibody titer of 1.0 μg/mL or greater be considered a conservative estimate of the threshold required to confer protection.

As with other T-cell–independent purified polysaccharide vaccines, Vi is not a good immunogen in infants. Most infants do not respond; among those that do, the responses are meager and short lived.

There is one report in Belgian adults in which the serologic response was compared following a dose of TYPHIM Vi or a dose of Typherix.[272] At 28 days postimmunization, 94% of TYPHIM Vi and 95% of Typherix recipients had serum Vi antibodies. Measured again at 12 months postimmunization, 74% and 67%, respectively, still had elevated Vi titers; the geometric mean titers of recipients of the two vaccines were very similar at 28 days and 12 months following immunization.[272]

Ty21a Live Oral Vaccine

SERUM ANTIBODY RESPONSE

The serum antibody response has been extensively studied with Ty21a. Gilman and colleagues noted that Ty21a vaccine grown in the presence of galactose (which leads to organisms bearing smooth LPS O antigen) was highly protective, whereas vaccine grown in the absence of galactose (resulting in rough organisms) was not.[182] These investigators reported that recipients of vaccine grown in the presence of galactose experienced a significantly greater seroconversion of O antibody.

Using serum IgG O antibody measured by ELISA in Chilean 15- to 19-year-olds, Levine and associates showed a correlation between seroconversion to various dosage schedules and formulations and protective efficacy in field trials (Table 39–4).[123] With the currently licensed enteric-coated capsule formulation, there is a stepwise increase in the proportion of vaccinees who manifest significant rises in serum IgG O antibody depending on whether one, two, or three doses of vaccine are administered within 1 week. Although serum O antibody is not believed to be the operative mechanism of immunity elicited by attenuated strains, it clearly correlates with protection. Because measurement of serum IgG ELISA antibody to S. Typhi O antigen is a simple technique, it provides investigators with a practical tool for comparing immunization schedules and formulations and for evaluating new candidate live oral vaccines.

MUCOSAL IMMUNE RESPONSE

During the past decade, the intestinal mucosal immune response to Ty21a and several new live oral vaccines has been studied rather extensively. Most recipients of the usual three-dose oral regimen of Ty21a develop local antibody responses to O antigen.[245–249,252,264,265,273–276] Forrest reported that the propensity to develop a significant rise in intestinal sIgA O antibody following immunization with Ty21a is inversely correlated with the preimmunization baseline level of intestinal antibody.[277] Subjects who have elevated baseline titers of sIgA O antibody mount significantly lower-fold rises than those of vaccinees with absent or low titers. This inverse correlation between baseline titer and propensity to seroconvert also has been reported for the serum vibriocidal antibody response following immunization with live oral cholera vaccines[278] and with Ty21a expressing *Vibrio cholerae* O1 antigen.[279]

Following oral administration of antigen, activated lymphocytes in the Peyer's patches and other gut-associated lymphoid tissue migrate to local lymph nodes to mature. After maturation, they return to the lamina propria of the intestine as well as to other organs of the mucosal immune

TABLE 39–4 ■ Rates of Seroconversion of IgG-ELISA *S.* Typhi O Antibody After One to Three Oral Doses of Ty21a Live Oral Typhoid Vaccine Given Within 1 Week

Formulation	No. of Doses	Seroconversion Rate	%	Efficacy in Field Trials (%)
Enteric-coated capsules	3	61/96	64	67
	2	22/50	44	47
	1	9/50	18	18
Vaccine/NaHCO$_3$ in gelatin capsules	3	99/195	50	21

Serologic data from Levine MM, Ferreccio C, Black RE, et al. Progress in vaccines to prevent typhoid fever. Rev Infect Dis 11 (suppl 3):S552–S567, 1989. Field trial surveillance data are from the first 36 months of follow-up in field trials in Area Norte (Black RE, Levine MM, Ferreccio C, et al. Efficacy of one or two doses of Ty21a *Salmonella typhi* vaccine in enteric-coated capsules in a controlled field trial. Vaccine 8:81–84, 1990.) and Area Occidente (Levine MM, Ferreccio C, Black RE, et al. Large-scale field trial of Ty21a live oral typhoid vaccine in enteric-coated capsule formulation. Lancet 1:1049–1052, 1987.) Santiago, Chile.

system, such as the salivary glands, respiratory tract, genitourinary tract, and mammary glands. Kantele and co-workers[245–249,274,276] and Forrest[280] have shown that such gut-derived migrating cells can be detected in peripheral blood and that the ability of these cells to secrete specific IgA antibody in the presence of specific antigen can be quantified by means of the enzyme-linked immunospot assay (ELISPOT)[281] or similar techniques.[280] These IgA-producing migrating cells are only detectable during a few days after immunization. The peak detection of gut-derived IgA ASCs in peripheral blood following oral immunization occurs approximately 7 days after vaccination.[165,239,241,242,245–249,274]

Kantele immunized adult Finnish volunteers with different formulations and immunization schedules of Ty21a, attempting to parallel the different regimens that were used in field trials of the efficacy of Ty21a in Chile and Indonesia.[245] Kantele's results demonstrate that the gut-derived IgA ASC response closely correlates with the efficacy results recorded in field trials (Table 39–5). Thus three doses (taken every other day) of Ty21a in enteric-coated capsules are markedly more immunogenic than one dose, and Ty21a in a liquid suspension is more immunogenic than vaccine in enteric-coated capsules.

Forrest and associates studied the mucosal immune response when three doses of Ty21a are administered per rectum on days 0, 2, and 5.[282] Each dose of vaccine contained 2 × 10^{11} CFU, a 100-fold larger dose than is con-

tained in the commercial Ty21a preparation. These vaccinees showed a significant increase in sIgA anti–*S.* Typhi O antibody in jejunal fluid, serum, and saliva and in gut-derived IgA ASCs.[282]

CELL-MEDIATED IMMUNE RESPONSE

Cell-mediated immune responses have been measured following vaccination with Ty21a.[244,250,251,265,283–286] The assays utilized have included lymphocyte replication in the presence of soluble or particulate antigen,[283,284] inhibition of growth of S. Typhi by mononuclear cells in the presence of antibody, and detection of CD8$^+$ cytotoxic T lymphocytes (CTLs).[244,250,251,265,285] Newer live oral vaccines stimulate fairly potent cell-mediated immune responses.[240,287]

In their studies of the lymphocyte replication response to various S. Typhi antigens following oral immunization with Ty21a, Murphy and co-workers[283,284] observed that the most sensitive and specific antigen was heat-inactivated, phenol-preserved particulate S. Typhi. Sztein et al. have found purified flagella from S. Typhi also to be an excellent antigen for stimulation of immune lymphocytes.[240]

Tagliabue and co-workers described a potent anti-*Salmonella* immune response following oral immunization with Ty21a that involves peripheral blood mononuclear cells (PBMCs) and immune serum. Mixing PBMCs from a neutral donor with postimmunization sera from vaccinees results in marked inhibition of growth of S. Typhi.[244,250,251,265] Neither mononuclear cells by themselves nor post-

TABLE 39–5 ■ Magnitude of Trafficking, Gut-Derived IgA Antibody-Secreting Cell Response to *S.* Typhi O Antigen After Immunization with Different Formulations and Dosage Schedules of Live Oral Typhoid Vaccine Ty21a

Vaccine Strain	Formulation	No. of Doses	No. of Viable Organisms/Dose	IgA ASC Response % Responders	GMN[†]
Ty21a	Gelatin capsule/NaHCO$_3$	3*	2 × 10^9	7/10[‡]	6
Ty21a	Enteric-coated capsules	3*	2 × 10^9	18/20	23
Ty21a	Liquid suspension	3*	2 × 10^9	19/20	63
	Liquid suspension	2*	2 × 10^9	16/20	12
	Liquid suspension	1	2 × 10^9	10/20	3

*Every-other-day schedule.
[‡]Geometric mean number of IgA antibody-secreting cells (ASCs) per 10^6 peripheral blood mononuclear cells.
[†]Number of responders/number of subjects vaccinated.

vaccination serum alone had this effect. These investigators reported that the PBMC that mediates this effect is a CD4$^+$ lymphocyte and that the specific serum antibodies are of the IgA class. This group also showed that intestinal sIgA could substitute for serum IgA.

Salerno-Goncalves et al.[285] observed that immunization with Ty21a induced specific CTLs that could lyse S. Typhi–infected cells and secrete interferon-γ (IFN-γ), an important effector molecule against intracellular pathogens. Most Ty21a vaccinees exhibited consistently increased CD8-mediated lysis of target cells by postimmunization PBMCs compared to preimmunization levels. Using an IFN-γ ELISPOT assay that they developed to quantify the frequency of IFN-γ spot-forming cells (SFCs) in PBMCs from Ty21a vaccinees, Salerno-Goncalves et al. also detected significant increases in IFN-γ SFCs following immunization compared to preimmunization levels. IFN-γ was secreted predominantly by CD8$^+$ T cells. A strong correlation was recorded between the cytolytic activity of CTL lines and the frequency of IFN-γ SFC ($r^2 = 0.910$, $P < 0.001$).[285]

Lundin et al. corroborated that oral vaccination with three doses of Ty21a induces both CD4$^+$ and CD8$^+$ IFN-γ–producing cells and antigen-specific CD4$^+$ and CD8$^+$ memory T cells.[286] Moreover, Lundin et al. studied the homing characteristics of T-cell responses and found that almost all of the IFN-γ producing memory T cells express the gut-homing integrin β-7.[286]

COMPARISON WITH NATURAL INFECTION

The circulating, secretory, and cell-mediated immune responses are relatively strong following natural infection and include both prominent serum and cell-mediated components.[55,76,288–294] Parenteral killed whole-cell vaccines elicit a serum response equal to that of natural infection but not a comparable cell-mediated response. With live oral vaccines the opposite is true.

Murphy and associates[283,284] observed that the PBMCs from healthy adults living in typhoid-endemic areas who have no known history of acute typhoid fever often specifically proliferate when exposed to S. Typhi antigens. This corroborates results of antibody prevalence studies that indicate that considerable mild or subclinical infection occurs in such areas.

Results of Controlled Field Trials

Parenteral Inactivated Whole-Cell Vaccines

From the mid-1950s to the early 1970s, the World Health Organization sponsored a series of well-designed, randomized, controlled field trials in countries with endemic typhoid to assess the absolute and relative efficacy of various typhoid vaccines and their duration of protection. In these studies, only culture-confirmed cases were used in calculating incidence rates and vaccine efficacy. In the first trial, in Yugoslavia, the efficacy of two doses of alcohol-killed vaccine was compared with that of heat-inactivated, phenol-preserved vaccine, with tetanus toxoid serving as the control vaccine.[223,224,295] Both vaccines gave significant protection, but the heat-inactivated, phenol-preserved vaccine proved to be superior to the alcohol-killed vaccine (Table 39–6).

In the early 1950s, laboratory studies demonstrated that acetone-inactivated typhoid vaccine resulted in better preservation of the Vi antigen,[132] thus raising the question of whether such a vaccine might be superior to the heat-inactivated, phenol-preserved vaccine. The Walter Reed Army Institute of Research prepared for the World Health Organization large reference lots of acetone-inactivated and heat-inactivated, phenol-preserved vaccines,[133,134] designated vaccines K and L, respectively, for large-scale field trials to be carried out in Yugoslavia,[227] Guyana,[225,226] Poland,[150,228] and the Soviet Union.[131] The K and L vaccines and the methods for their production also served as international standards to prepare future lots of vaccines of these types for subsequent field trials. For example, in addition to the K and L reference vaccines themselves, two

TABLE 39–6 ■ Comparison of Heat-Inactivated, Phenol-Preserved and Alcohol-Killed, Alcohol-Preserved Fluid Parenteral Typhoid Vaccines Given as Two Primary Doses With or Without a Reinforcing Dose 1 Year Later (Yugoslavia, 1954–1960)

Vaccine Group	No. Vaccinated	Cases of Typhoid Per 10⁵*	Vaccine Efficacy (%)	Duration of Surveillance (yr)
Heat inactivated				
Two primary doses	11,503	61[a]	68	1
Two primary and booster doses	8595	81[b]	74	5[†]
Alcohol inactivated				
Two primary doses	12,017	141[c]	27	1
Two primary and booster doses	8913	157[d]	50	5[†]
Control (tetanus toxoid)				
Two primary doses	11,988	192[e]	—	5[†]
Two primary and booster doses	9002	311[f]	—	5[†]

*Significance:
a versus e; $P = 0.0086$.   b versus f; $P = 0.0012$.
a versus c; $P = 0.083$.   d versus f; $P = 0.048$.
c versus e; $P = 0.42$.   b versus d; $P = 0.22$.
†Period of surveillance after inoculation with booster dose.
Adapted from Yugoslav Typhoid Commission. A controlled field trial of the effectiveness of phenol and alcohol typhoid vaccines. Bull World Health Organ 26:357–369, 1962.

additional K-type vaccines have been tested in controlled field trials and have provided critical information. These include a K-type vaccine used in a randomized, controlled field trial in Tonga to directly compare the efficacy of one versus two doses of vaccine[296]; a K-type vaccine made from a nonflagellated S. Typhi strain, which was field tested for efficacy in Alexandria, Egypt[237]; and a K-type vaccine evaluated in a single dose against an alum-adsorbed, heat-inactivated, phenol-preserved vaccine.[297,298]

Results of the trials with K, L, and K-type vaccines are summarized in Table 39–7. The major conclusions that can be drawn are the following:

1. Both acetone-inactivated and heat-inactivated, phenol-preserved typhoid vaccines provide significant protection against typhoid fever after two subcutaneous doses, but the acetone-killed vaccine is somewhat superior (79% to 88% protection for the K vaccine versus 51% to 66% for the L vaccine).[131,150,226,227]

2. The efficacy of the reference K and L vaccines varied from one geographic site to another.

3. When directly compared in a randomized trial (Tonga), two doses of an acetone-inactivated vaccine gave significantly superior protection to that of a single dose.[296] Previously, in nonrandomized comparisons, little difference had been noted between the efficacy conferred by one or two doses.[226]

4. A K-type vaccine prepared from a nonflagellated S. Typhi strain failed to provide significant protection.[237]

5. A single dose of a K-type vaccine, without adjuvant, provided protection comparable to that of a single dose of an alum-adsorbed, heat-inactivated, phenol-preserved vaccine.[297,298]

The K and L vaccines also were evaluated for efficacy in experimental challenge studies in North American volunteers.[55] Perhaps the most important insight to come from these studies was the observation that protection conferred by the vaccines was relative to the number of pathogenic S. Typhi used for the experimental challenge (Table 39–8). When 10^5 pathogenic S. Typhi comprised the challenge inoculum, the K and L vaccines provided approximately 70% protection. However, when the challenge inoculum contained 10^7 bacilli, there was virtually no protection demonstrable (0% to 14% vaccine efficacy). Differences in inoculum size in nature may be responsible for some of the differences of vaccine efficacy encountered among different field sites and over time.

Purified Vi Polysaccharide Parenteral Vaccine

Two randomized, controlled field trials were carried out in Nepal[106] and South Africa[107] to investigate the efficacy of the first nondenatured purified Vi vaccine. A single 25-µg dose conferred 72% protection against typhoid fever in Nepal during 17 months of follow-up and 64% efficacy in South Africa over 21 months of surveillance (Table 39–9). The Nepal trial included all ages from preschool to adults, whereas the South African trial was performed in schoolchildren. A subsequent report from the South African trial showed that, over 3 years of follow-up, vaccine efficacy was 55% (see Table 39–9).[271]

A locally produced Vi vaccine prepared by the Shanghai Institute of Biological Products was evaluated in a randomized, placebo-controlled, double-blind trial in Guangxi, China.[299] In total, 65,287 subjects received a single 30-µg dose of Vi and 65,984 controls got a dose of saline; 92% of subjects were children 5 to 19 years of age at the time of vaccination.[299] During 19 months of follow-up, 7 cases of blood culture–confirmed typhoid fever were detected among the vaccinees versus 23 confirmed cases among the controls, demonstrating a vaccine efficacy of 69% (95% confidence interval [CI], 28% to 87%).[299] Confirmatory data on another outbreak have been reported.[376]

Vi-negative strains of S. Typhi are rare in nature, but such variants are capable of causing clinical typhoid fever.[55] Some have argued that, because the Vi vaccine is unlikely to protect against such strains, the widespread use of Vi may select for such strains.[300–302] However, thus far there has been no convincing evidence of the emergence of Vi-negative isolates of S. Typhi.

Ty21a Live Oral Vaccine

In early studies in adult volunteers, multiple doses of freshly harvested Ty21a organisms were found to be safe and to confer significant protection against experimental challenge.[182] Thereafter, a field trial of efficacy was carried out in Alexandria, Egypt, where approximately 16,000 school children 6 and 7 years of age were given three 10^9-organism doses of vaccine on Monday, Wednesday, and Friday of one week.[253,254] Lyophilized vaccine in glass vials was reconstituted with 30 mL of diluent and ingested by the children approximately 1 to 3 minutes after they chewed a tablet containing 1.0 g of $NaHCO_3$. Approximately 16,000 other children received placebo in this randomized, double-blind, controlled field trial. During 3 years of epidemiologic surveillance, only one culture-confirmed case of typhoid fever occurred among the vaccinees as opposed to 22 cases among the controls (96% protection) (Table 39–10).

Although this preliminary field trial with Ty21a provided highly encouraging results, considerable further work needed to be carried out to ascertain whether Ty21a could be a practical public health tool. The liquid formulation used in Egypt was not readily amenable to mass production, so alternate formulations had to be prepared and evaluated. It was necessary to determine whether fewer (one or two) doses could protect, to assess the duration of protection, to investigate the effect of increased spacing between vaccine doses, and to ascertain whether infants and young children could be immunized safely and successfully. Many of these questions were answered in a series of five randomized, controlled field trials carried out in Santiago, Chile (four trials), and Indonesia (one trial) under the auspices of the World Health Organization and the Pan American Health Organization.[108,122–124,198,199]

The four field trials in Chile involved approximately 550,000 children ages 6 to 19 years who were vaccinated in school-based programs, after which epidemiologic surveillance was maintained through the health centers of the National Health Service. Only culture-confirmed cases were used in the computation of incidence rates and vaccine efficacy.

In the field trial in the Western (Occidente) administrative area of Santiago,[198] the efficacy conferred by three

TABLE 39–7 ■ Results of Controlled Field Trials of Lyophilized Acetone-Inactivated and Heat and Phenol-Inactivated Reference Vaccines

Field Site, Dates	Age Groups	Vaccine (No. of Doses)	No. Vaccinated	Duration of Surveillance	Incidence of Typhoid per 10^5*	Vaccine Efficacy (%)	Reference
Yugoslavia 1960–1963	2–50 yr (mostly schoolchildren)	K (2)	5028	2 ½ yr	318[a]	79	227
		L (2)	5068	2 ½ yr	727[b]	51	
		Control (2)	5039	2 ½ yr	1488[c]	—	
Guyana 1960–1967	5–15 yr (schoolchildren)	K (2)	24,046	7 yr	67[d]	89	226
		L (2)	23,431	7 yr	209[e]	65	
		Control (2)	27,241	7 yr	602[f]	—	
Poland 1961–1964	5–14 yr (schoolchildren)	K (2)	81,534	3 yr	7[g]	85	150
		Control (2)	83,734	3 yr	47[h]	—	
Soviet Union 1962–1965	Schoolchildren and young adults (92 age 7–15 yr)	L (2)	36,112	2 ½ yr	55[i]	66	131
		Control (2)	36,999	2 ½ yr	162[j]	—	
Tonga 1966–1973	All ages (69 were <21 yr)	K-type† (2)	11,128	7 yr	288 (180)‡[k]	39 (56)†	296
		K-type† (1)	11,391	7 yr	500 (272)‡[l]	0 (34)†	
		Controls (2)	11,129	7 yr	476 (413)‡[m]	—	
Egypt 1978–1981	6–7 yr (schoolchildren)	Nonflagellated K-type (2)§	16,679	11 mo	114[m]	0	237
		Control (2)	16,650	11 mo	84[m]	—	
Soviet Union 1965	7–20 yr	K-type (1)‖	52,347	10 mo	21[n]	53	298
		Control (1)	52,816	10 mo	45[o]	—	

*Significance:

a versus c; $P = 0.00001$.	e versus f; $P < 0.03$.
b versus c; $P < 0.0004$.	d versus e; $P < 0.000046$.
a versus b; $P = 0.0064$.	g versus h; $P = 0.0000025$.
d versus f; $P < 0.000001$.	i versus j; $P = 0.000021$.

k versus m; $P < 0.03$.
l versus m; $P = 0.87$.
k versus l; $P = 0.015$.
n versus o; $P = 0.045$.

†A distinct lot of lyophilized acetone-inactivated vaccine made at the Walter Reed Army Institute of Research in a manner identical to their product of reference vaccine K.

‡Numbers in parentheses are results of the first 5 years of surveillance.

§A lyophilized acetone-inactivated vaccine prepared by the Lister Institute, London, from strain TNM1, a nonflagellated mutant of S. Typhi Ty2.

‖Lyophilized acetone-inactivated vaccine prepared at the Institute of Vaccines and Sera, Zagreb, according to methods for K vaccine Production (Walter Reed Army Institute of Research, 1964[134]).

TABLE 39–8 ■ Efficacy of Parenteral Acetone-Inactivated (K) and Heat and Phenol–Inactivated (L) Reference Vaccines and Vi Polysaccharide Vaccine in Experimental Challenge Studies in Volunteers: Effect of Size of Challenge Inoculum on Efficacy

| Vaccine Group | 10^5 *S. Typhi*[*] | | 10^7 *S. Typhi*[*] | |
	Attack Rate	Vaccine Efficacy	Attack Rate	Vaccine Efficacy
K[†]	4/43 (9%)	63%	12/28 (43%)	14%
L[†]	3/45 (7%)	71%	13/24 (54%)	0
Vi[‡]	3/17 (18%)	25%	10/14 (71%)	0
Control	28/104 (24%)	—	15/30 (50%)	—

[*]Inoculum of pathogenic *S. Typhi* ingested by volunteers.
[†]Three subcutaneous doses were administered.
[‡]One 50-µg subcutaneous dose of Landy's denatured Vi vaccine was given.
Data from Hornick RB, Greisman SE, Woodward TE, et al. Typhoid fever: pathogenesis and control. N Engl J Med 283:686–691, 739–746, 1970.

TABLE 39–9 ■ Results of Randomized, Controlled, Double-Blind Field Trials in Nepal and South Africa Assessing the Efficacy of a Single 25-µg Dose of Nondenatured Purified Vi Polysaccharide Subunit Vaccine in Preventing Culture-Confirmed Typhoid Fever

	Period of Follow-Up	Vi Vaccine	Control Vaccine
Nepal Trial[*]	17 mo		
No. of subjects		3457	3450
Cases		9	32
Incidence/10^5		260	928
Efficacy		72%	—
(95% CI)		(42%–86%)	—
South Africa Trial[†]	21 mo		
No. of subjects		5692	5692
Cases		16	44
Incidence 10^5		281	773
Efficacy		64%	—
(95% CI)		(36%–79%)	—
	36 mo		
Cases		30	66
Incidence/10^5		527	1160
Efficacy		55%	—
(95% CI)		(30%–71%)	—

[*]Participants were randomized to receive a 0.5-mL intramuscular inoculation containing either 25 µg of purified Vi or 23-valent pneumococcal polysaccharide. (Data from Acharya VL, Shrestha MB, Cadoz M, et al. Prevention of typhoid fever in Nepal with the Vi polysaccharide of *Salmonella typhi*: a preliminary report. N Engl J Med 317: 1101–1104, 1987.)
[†]Participants were randomized to receive a single 25-µg intramuscular dose of Vi or a 50-µg dose of meningococcal polysaccharide vaccine. (Data from Klugman K, Gilbertson IT, Koornhof HJ, et al: Protective activity of Vi polysaccharide vaccine against typhoid fever. Lancet 2:1165–1169, 1987; and Klugman KP, Koornhof HJ, Robbins JB, et al: Immunogenicity, efficacy and seriological correlate of protection of *Salmonella typhi* Vi capsular polysaccharide vaccine three years after immunization. Vaccine 14:435–438, 1996.)
CI, confidence interval.

doses of vaccine in enteric-coated capsules was compared with that provided by three doses of vaccine in the gelatin capsule–NaHCO₃ formulation. As seen in Table 39–11, over 3 years of surveillance the enteric-coated vaccine provided significantly superior protection. Over 7 years of follow-up, the regimen of three doses of Ty21a in enteric-coated capsules (every-other-day interval between doses) conferred 62% protection.[303]

A randomized, controlled, double-blind field trial in the Northern (Norte) area of Santiago showed that immunization with only one or two doses of Ty21a in enteric-coated capsules resulted in a moderate level of protection that was short lived (Table 39–12).[108] Although two doses of vaccine conferred 60% protection during the first 2 years of surveillance, efficacy dropped to insignificant levels during the third year and virtually disappeared by the fourth year of surveillance.

A very large trial involving more than 200,000 school children was carried out in the Southern (Sur) and Central administrative areas of Santiago to compare directly the protective effects of two, three, or four doses of Ty21a vaccine in enteric-coated capsules and to assess the use of Ty21a as a public health tool.[124] No placebo group was included in this trial. The salient feature of this trial is the observation that ingestion of four doses of vaccine resulted in a significantly lower incidence of typhoid than three doses (Table 39–13). The results of this trial formed the basis for the recommended four-dose immunization schedule following licensure of Ty21a in the United States and Canada (a three-dose regimen is used elsewhere).

In the mid-1980s, the Swiss Serum and Vaccine Institute succeeded in preparing a "liquid suspension" formulation of Ty21a for large-scale field trials that was amenable to large-scale manufacture. The new formulation consists of two packets, one containing a dose of lyophilized vaccine and the other containing buffer. Contents of the two packets are mixed in a cup containing 100 mL of water, and the suspension is then ingested by the subject to be vaccinated. Field trials were initiated in Santiago, Chile,[199] and in Plaju, Indonesia,[105] to directly compare this new liquid for-

mulation of Ty21a (that somewhat resembles what was used in the Alexandria, Egypt, field trial) with the enteric-coated capsule formulation. Results of these trials are summarized in Table 39–14. Vaccine administered as a liquid suspension was superior to vaccine in enteric-coated capsules. In the Santiago trial, the difference was highly significant. Ty21a given as a liquid suspension protected young children as well as older children.[199] In previous trials with enteric-coated vaccine, young children were not as well protected as older children.[198]

Vi Conjugate Vaccine

Szu and colleagues pursued a stepwise program to develop an optimal Vi conjugate vaccine that culminated in a candidate for clinical trials consisting of Vi polysaccharide conjugated to recombinant *Pseudomonas aeruginosa* exotoxin A.[268,304] After demonstration of the safety and immunogenicity of this conjugate,[304] the efficacy conferred by a two-dose (6 weeks apart) immunization schedule of the vaccine was evaluated in a large-scale, randomized, controlled field trial in Vietnam in children 2 to 5 years of

TABLE 39–10 ■ Field Trial of Efficacy of Three Doses of a Liquid Formulation of Ty21a Vaccine Given with NaHCO₃ to 6- and 7-Year-Old Schoolchildren in Alexandria, Egypt

Group*	Confirmed Cases of Typhoid Fever	Incidence per 10^5	Vaccine Efficacy (%)
Vaccinees n = 16,486	1	6.1	96 (77–99)†
Placebo n = 15,902	22	138.3	

*Period of observation: 1978 to 1981.
†95% confidence interval.
Adapted from Wahdan MH, Serie C, Cerisier Y, et al. A controlled field trial of live *Salmonella* typhi strain Ty21a oral vaccine against typhoid: three-year results. J Infect Dis 145:292–296, 1982.

age.[305] In total, 5525 children received two dose of Vi conjugate and 5566 received placebo. During 27 months of follow-up, active surveillance was carried out to detect cases of typhoid fever by visiting children weekly, eliciting a symptom history, and recording their axillary temperature. Subjects who had a temperature of 37.5°C or greater for at least 3 days were referred to a health center where 5 mL of blood was drawn for bacteriologic culture. Typhoid fever was diagnosed in 4 of 5525 vaccinees and 47 of 5566 controls, demonstrating an efficacy of 91.5% (95% CI, 77.1% to 96.6%) (Table 39–15).[305] The level of efficacy did not vary by year of age among these 2- to 5-year-olds, nor did it appear to wane during the second year of surveillance.

Duration of Vaccine-Derived Immunity

Parenteral Inactivated Whole-Cell Vaccines

The longest periods of surveillance (7 years) for efficacy of the parenteral killed whole-cell vaccines were carried out in the Guyana and Tonga field trials. In Guyana, two doses of the acetone-killed K vaccine conferred a high level of protection (88%) for 7 years.[226] In contrast, in Tonga, two doses of a K-type vaccine provided moderate protection for a period of only 5 years, after which protection was no longer demonstrable.[296] Two doses of the heat-inactivated, phenol-preserved vaccine (L) tested in Guyana showed moderate (77%) protection during the first 3 years, but this level fell to 47% protection during the last 4 years of surveillance. In several other field trials in which the period of surveillance was only 2 ½ years, the acetone-inactivated and heat-inactivated, phenol-preserved vaccines conferred significant protection for at least 30 months.[131,150,227]

Purified Vi Polysaccharide Parenteral Vaccine

In the South African field trial, surveillance was maintained for 3 years. During this 3-year period, the efficacy of the Vi vaccine was 55% (see Table 39–9).[271]

Ty21a Live Oral Vaccine

In the field trial in Alexandria, Egypt, three doses of a liquid formulation of vaccine conferred a high level of protection (96%) that persisted for 3 years, the point at which surveillance was discontinued.[253] Three doses of vaccine in enteric-coated capsules given at an interval of every other day conferred 67% protection over 3 years[198] and 62% protection over 7 years of follow-up in a field trial in Santiago, Chile[303]; fewer doses of vaccine in enteric-coated capsules in Santiago, Chile, conferred significant protection for only 2 years.

Three doses of Ty21a in a liquid formulation provided 77% protection for 3 years[199] and 79% protection during a fourth and fifth year of follow-up (78% protection over the 5 years of follow-up) in a field trial in Santiago.[303]

Comparison of Vaccine-Derived Immunity with Natural Immunity

Several sources of data suggest that the immunity that follows clinical infection with pathogenic S. Typhi is relative

TABLE 39–11 ■ Comparison of the Efficacy of Two Different Formulations of Ty21a Live Oral Vaccine Given by Two Different Immunization Schedules in Area Occidente, Santiago, Chile: Results of 36 Months of Follow-up (9/1983–8/1986)

	Enteric-Coated Capsules		Gelatin Capsules with NaHCO₃		Placebo
	Long Interval*	Short Interval†	Long Interval	Short Interval	
N	21,598	22,170	21,541	22,379	21,906
Cases	34	23	46	56	68
Incidence‡	157.4ᵃ	103.7ᵇ	213.5ᶜ	250.3ᵈ	310.4ᵉ
Efficacy	49% (24–66)§	67% (47–79)	31% (0–52)	19% (0–43)	—

*Three doses, 21 days between doses.
†Three doses, 1 to 2 days between doses.
‡Significance:
  a versus e; P = 0.0006.
  b versus e; P < 0.00001.
  c versus e; P = 0.0023.
  a + b vs. c + d; P = 0.001.
  d versus e; P = 0.21.
  a versus c; P = 0.23.
  b versus d; P = 0.00052.
§95% confidence interval.
Data from Levine MM, Ferreccio C, Black RE, et al. Large-scale field trial of Ty21a live oral typhoid vaccine in enteric-coated capsule formulation. Lancet 1:1049–1052, 1987.

TABLE 39–12 ▪ Comparison of the Efficacy of One Versus Two Doses of Ty21a Live Oral Typhoid Vaccine Given in Enteric-Coated Capsule Formulation: Results of a Randomized, Controlled, Double-Blind Trial in Area Norte, Santiago, Chile

	One Dose (N = 27,618)	Two Doses (N = 27,620)	Placebo (N = 27,305)
YEAR 1 (7/82–6/83)			
No. of cases	47	30	62
Incidence/10^5*	170.2[a]	108.6[b]	227.1[c]
Efficacy	25%	52%	—
YEAR 2 (7/83–6/84)			
No. of cases	25	11	38
Incidence/10^5	90.5	39.8	139.2
Efficacy	35%	71%	—
YEAR 3 (7/84–6/85)			
No. of cases	19	15	19
Incidence/10^5	68.8	54.3	69.6
Efficacy	0%	22%	—
YEAR 4 (7/85–6/86)			
No. of cases	30	23	28
Incidence/10^5	108.6	83.3	102.5
Efficacy	−6%	19%	—

*Significance:
 a versus c; $P = 0.42$.
 a versus b; $P = 0.037$.
 b versus c; $P = 0.0032$.
 Data from Black RE, Levine MM, Ferreccio C, et al. Efficacy of one or two doses of Ty21a *Salmonella* typhi vaccine in enteric-coated capsules in a controlled field trial. Vaccine 8:81–84, 1990.

and can be overcome. Marmion and colleagues[306] and others have reported successive outbreaks of typhoid fever in soldiers who, in the space of a few months, experienced two separate bouts of typhoid fever. In the volunteer studies carried out by Hornick and colleagues[55] and DuPont and associates,[144] two relevant observations were reported. The first is that immunity to typhoid fever is relative and can be overcome if a large infecting dose is ingested. Second, the protective effect of a prior clinical typhoid infection was only 33%; that is, 5 of 22 volunteers (23%) who recovered from an induced S. Typhi infection developed typhoid fever when re-challenged with pathogenic organisms, as opposed to 11 of 34 control volunteers ($P > 0.05$).

Based on these observations, it can be argued that Vi polysaccharide vaccine and Ty21a, as well as the parenteral killed whole-cell vaccines, stimulate rather credible immunity compared with natural immunity elicited by infection with wild-type S. Typhi. Undoubtedly, in endemic areas most individuals experience multiple subclinical S. Typhi infections, each serving to further boost the state of immunity; persons who develop overt disease represent a minority of all infected persons.

TABLE 39–13 ▪ Comparison of the Efficacy of Two, Three, and Four Doses of Ty21a Vaccine in Enteric-Coated Formulation: Results of a Randomized Field Trial in Area Sur and Area Central, Santiago, Chile

Surveillance from 11/1984 to 10/1987	Two Doses	Three Doses	Four Doses
No. of vaccinees	66,615	64,783	58,421
No. of cases	123	104	56
Incidence/10^5*	184.6[a]	160.5[b]	95.8[c]
95% confidence interval	152–271	130–191	71–121

*Significance:
 a versus c; $P = 0.0004$.
 b versus c; $P = 0.002$.
 a versus b; $P = 0.32$.
 Data from Ferreccio C, Levine MM, Rodriguez H, et al. Comparative efficacy of two, three, or four doses of Ty21a live oral typhoid vaccine in enteric-coated capsules: a field trial in an endemic area. J Infect Dis 159:766–769, 1989.

TABLE 39–14 ▪ Comparison of the Efficacy of Three Doses of Ty21a Administered in Enteric-Coated Capsules or as a Liquid Suspension of Vaccine Organisms: Results of Randomized, Placebo-Controlled Field Trials in Santiago, Chile, and Plaju, Indonesia

	Santiago, Chile			Plaju, Indonesia		
	Enteric-Coated Capsules	Liquid Suspension	Placebo	Enteric-Coated Capsules	Liquid Suspension	Placebo
No. of subjects	34,696	36,623	10,302	5209	5066	10,268
No. of cases of typhoid	63	23	28	61	48	208
Incidence/10^5	182	63	272	468	379	810
Efficacy	33%	77%	—	42%	53%	—
95% confidence interval	0–57%	60%–87%	—	23%–57%	36%–66%	—

Data from Levine M, Ferreccio C, Cryz S, Ortiz E. Comparison of enteric-coated capsules and liquid formulation of Ty21a typhoid vaccine in a random-ized controlled field trial. Lancet 336:891–894, 1990; and Simanjuntak C, Paleologo F, Punjabi N, et al. Oral immunisation against typhoid fever in Indonesia with Ty21a vaccine. Lancet 338:1055–1059, 1991.

Adverse Events

Parenteral Inactivated Whole-Cell Vaccines

COMMON

Although the parenteral killed whole-cell vaccines provide moderate to good protection, high rates of systemic and local adverse reactions make them unsatisfactory public health tools.[131,225,227,307–309] Table 39–16 summarizes the adverse reaction rates from several controlled, double-blind evalua-tions of parenteral killed whole-cell vaccines. The high rates of fever, malaise, local erythema, induration, and pain are obvious. Acetone-inactivated and heat-inactivated, phenol-preserved vaccines administered by jet gun cause higher rates of local adverse reactions than vaccine given by syringe.[310]

Many investigators have compared the reactogenicity and antigenicity of small intradermal doses of parenteral killed whole-cell vaccines with those of full subcutaneous doses. Most of these studies have shown that 0.1-mL intra-dermal doses elicit significantly fewer adverse reactions than full (0.5-mL) subcutaneous doses of vaccine, and the serologic response is only slightly diminished.[185–192] Nevertheless, the protective efficacy of intradermal vaccine has never been assessed in a field trial.

RARE

Rarely, more significant reactions have been attributed to vaccination with parenteral killed whole-cell typhoid vac-cines. These include thrombocytopenic purpura,[311,312]

acute renal disease,[313–317] dermatomyositis,[318] appendici-tis,[319] erythema nodosum,[320] multiple sclerosis,[321] and a syndrome of high fever, severe malaise, and toxemia,[308,309] sometimes accompanied by coagulopathy, thrombocytope-nia, hepatitis, and renal insufficiency.[322] Rarely, sudden death occurs following parenteral inoculation with inacti-vated whole-cell typhoid vaccine.[317] Among the above-mentioned rare severe adverse events, the syndrome of high fever and toxemia and the occurrence of sudden death have biologic plausibility based on abnormally potent responses of certain individuals to S. Typhi endo-toxin inoculated parenterally via whole-cell vaccine, lead-ing to cytokine release and a cascade of events ultimately resulting in shock and perhaps death.

Purified Vi Polysaccharide Parenteral Vaccine

When Vi vaccine is highly purified, it is well toler-ated.[180,195–197,256] As little as 5% impurity with LPS results in systemic adverse reactions in a proportion of recipients.[197] In controlled Phase II trials in U.S. adults, local reactions including pain and tenderness were the most common adverse events.[197,256] Passive surveillance carried out during field trials showed the Vi vaccine to be as well tolerated as the licensed (meningococcal and pneumococcal) polysac-charide vaccines that served as the control preparations in these trials.[106,107]

There is one study in which Belgian adults were ran-domly allocated to be inoculated with TYPHIM Vi or one

TABLE 39–15 ▪ Cases of Typhoid Fever in Pediatric Recipients* of Parenteral Vi Conjugate Vaccine or Placebo in a Randomized, Double-Blind Controlled, Field Trial in Vietnam

	Vi–Recombinant Exoprotein A Conjugate	Placebo	Vaccine Efficacy (95% CI)	P Value
Two-dose recipients	5525	5566		
Typhoid fever cases	4	47	91.5% (77.1%–96.6%)	<0.001
Cases/10^3 children	0.72	8.44		
All children	5991	6017		
Typhoid fever cases	5	56	91.1% (78.6%–96.5%)	<0.001

*Children were 2, 3, 4, or 5 years of age at the time of vaccination and were followed for 27 months thereafter.
Data from Lin FYC, Ho VA, Khiem HB, et al. The efficacy of a *Salmonella Typhi* Vi conjugate vaccine in two- to five-year-old children. N Engl J Med 344:1263–1269, 2001.

TABLE 39–16 ■ Frequency of Fever, Malaise, and Pain at the Injection Site Approximately 24 Hours After Subcutaneous Inoculation with Heat and Phenol–Inactivated (L) and Acetone-Inactivated (K) Whole-Cell Typhoid Vaccines or Tetanus Toxoid

Vaccine Group	No. of Vaccinees			Fever After Vaccination (%)			Inability to Work (%)	Local Pain (%)	
	Yugoslavia	Guyana	USSR	Yugoslavia*	Guyana†	USSR‡	Yugoslavia	Yugoslavia	Guyana
Heat and phenol–inactivated	343	86	1656	24	29	6.7	23	35	54
Acetone-inactivated	326	80	—	22	26	—	21	32	45
Tetanus toxoid	328	86	1757	3	7	2.4	5	4	—

*37°C.
†>37.8°C.
‡37.5°C.

Data from Yugoslav Typhoid Commission. A controlled field trial of the effectiveness of acetone-dried and inactivated and heat-phenol–inactivated typhoid vaccines in Yugoslavia. Bull World Health Organ 30:623–630, 1964; Ashcroft MT, Morrison-Ritchie J, Nicholson CC. Controlled field trial in British Guyana schoolchildren of heat-killed-phenolized and acetone-killed lyophilized typhoid vaccines. Am J Hyg 79:196–206, 1964; and Hejfec LB, Salmin LV, Lejtman MZ, et al. A controlled field trial and laboratory study of five typhoid vaccines in the USSR. Bull World Health Organ 34:321–339, 1966.

TABLE 39–17 ▪ Randomized, Placebo-Controlled, Double-Blind Clinical Trials of Three Doses of Ty21a in Enteric-Coated Capsules, in Milk with $NaHCO_3$, or in Buffer Suspension to Assess Reactogenicity of the Vaccine in Adults, School-Age Children, and Preschool-Age Children

	Adults, Chile		6- and 7-Year-Olds	
Adverse Reaction*	Enteric-Coated Vaccine (N = 385)	Placebo (N = 367)	Enteric-Coated Vaccine (N = 172)	Placebo (N = 172)
Diarrhea	1.8†	1.1	1.2	9.9
Vomiting	0.5	0.3	2.3	11.0
Fever	0.3	0.5	0.6	0.6
Rash	0.5	0.5	ND	ND

*No adverse reactions occurred significantly more frequently in vaccinees than in placebo controls in these clinical trials, all of which utilized active surveillance methods to detect adverse reactions.
†Percent of total subjects in the group with reactions.
ND, Not determined.
Data from Levine MM, Black RE, Ferreccio C, et al. The efficacy of attenuated *Salmonella typhi* oral vaccine strain Ty21a evaluated in controlled field trials. *In* Holmgren J, Lindberg A, Molly R (eds). Development of Vaccines and Drugs Against Diarrhea. Lund, Sweden, Studentlitteratur, 1986, pp 90–101; Black RE, Levine MM, Young C, et al. Immunogenicity of Ty21a attenuated *Salmonella typhi* given with sodium bicarbonate or in enteric-coated capsules. Dev Biol Stand 53:9–14, 1983; and Simanjuntak C, Paleologo F, Punjabi N, et al. Oral immunisation against typhoid fever in Indonesia with Ty21a vaccine. Lancet 338:1055–1059, 1991.

of three lots of Typherix and local and systemic reactogenicity was compared.[272] This was not a double-blind study. None of the recipients of either vaccine had high fever (≥39°C); 0% of TYPHIM Vi and 2% of Typherix recipients reported low-grade fever (<39°C). Local erythema, soreness, and swelling were reported significantly more often in the 100 recipients of TYPHIM Vi (21%, 33%, and 17%, respectively) than among the 300 subjects who got the lots of Typherix (3%, 8%, and 2%, respectively).

Ty21a Live Oral Vaccine

Ty21a provides significant protection without causing adverse reactions.[105,123,254,323–325] Results of three double-blind, placebo-controlled studies that utilized active surveillance methods to assess the reactogenicity of Ty21a in adults and children are shown in Table 39–17. The rates of adverse reactions in the vaccine recipients were not significantly higher than those for the placebo group for any symptom or sign. In large-scale field trials with Ty21a, involving approximately 550,000 schoolchildren in Chile and 32,000 in Egypt and approximately 20,000 subjects ranging in age from 3 years to adulthood in Indonesia, passive surveillance failed to identify vaccine-related adverse reactions.[105,108,198,199,254,326]

Indications

Populations for whom vaccine is indicated include the following:

1. Travelers to less-developed areas where typhoid is known or believed to be endemic

2. Military personnel (who represent a special group of travelers)
3. School-age children in areas in which typhoid is endemic, particularly where multiply antibiotic-resistant strains are prevalent
4. Microbiology technicians in clinical microbiology laboratories or in research laboratories in which S. Typhi is handled

Table 39–18 summarizes the immunization schedules and dosages, for different age groups, for the oral Ty21a and the parenteral Vi and heat-inactivated, phenol-preserved whole-cell vaccines.[122,327]

Typhoid vaccine is *not* generally indicated following floods, earthquakes, or other natural disasters during which the water and sewage systems may suffer structural damage.[328,329] Resources should rather be directed toward repairing the contaminated water sources, which, it is hoped, could be achieved long before a mass vaccination could be completed and the protective effect of vaccine initiated. Nevertheless, there are situations in which typhoid vaccines may serve as a helpful adjunct to other control measures. For example, if a major upheaval occurs in a region of a country where typhoid is endemic and formidable economic or political obstacles are expected to impede timely improvements in water supply quality and sanitation infrastructure, selective vaccination of high-risk groups may be helpful.[330]

It has been suggested by some that a period of increased risk of acquisition of typhoid fever occurs for approximately

	All Ages, Indonesia			
Enteric-Coated Vaccine (N = 311)	Liquid Suspension Placebo (N = 291)	Vaccine (N = 333)	Placebo (N = 255)
3.9	3.1	3.8	5.5
1.0	1.7	1.5	0.8
4.8	1.7	4.8	3.5
1.0	0.3	1.2	0.4

10 days after the administration of the first dose of parenteral killed whole-cell vaccine; this has been referred to as the "negative phase" after vaccination.[331–334] Such a phenomenon has not been described for Vi or Ty21a vaccines.

Contraindications

There are no contraindications to immunization with parenteral Vi polysaccharide vaccine other than known hypersensitivity to any component of the vaccine. Although there are no definitive contraindications to immunization with killed whole-cell vaccines, in view of the reactogenicity of this vaccine, it should not be given to persons who have experienced severe systemic reactions on previous inoculation with this vaccine. Moreover, it would be prudent to avoid giving this vaccine to debilitated or elderly persons with chronic health problems, such as patients with cardiac, renal, collagen vascular, or oncologic disease.

As a general rule, Ty21a should not be given to pregnant women, although adverse effects on the pregnant woman or fetus have not been reported. Similarly, caution should be taken before anyone with a known depression of cell-mediated immunity is given Ty21a. However, there would appear to be no risk for immunocompromised household contacts of Ty21a vaccinees because excretion of Ty21a has never been detected in any subject given the available formulations that contain 2 to 6×10^9 CFU per dose.

If immunocompromised individuals, including persons with human immunodeficiency virus (HIV) infection, must travel to endemic areas, Vi vaccine should be administered. It is important to immunize such travelers because studies of HIV-infected individuals in typhoid-endemic areas have revealed that they are at greatly increased risk of developing typhoid fever.[335]

Ty21a should not be administered to individuals who are taking antibiotics. Certain antimalarials, particularly mefloquine, exhibit activity against Ty21a in vitro.[206,336,337] In clinical trials, coadministration of chloroquine, mefloquine, or chloroquine plus pyrimethamine-sulfadoxine did not significantly suppress the IgG O antibody response following immunization with Ty21a,[338,339] whereas coadministration of proguanil did.[338] Based on these data, it has been proposed that Ty21a should not be taken with proguanil. However, it has since been shown in a randomized, double-blind, placebo-controlled clinical trial that daily administration of Malarone® (atovaquone plus proguanil) for 12 weeks did not diminish the serum IgG S. Typhi O antibody response in children (4 to 16 years of age) given three doses of the liquid formulation of Ty21a; notably, the first dose of Ty21a was coadministered with a dose of CVD103-HgR live oral cholera vaccine.[340] Ty21a may be taken with chloroquine, but one should wait 8 to 24 hours after administration of mefloquine before initiating immunization with Ty21a.

Simultaneous Administration of Typhoid Vaccines with Other Vaccines

Parenteral Inactivated Whole-Cell and Subunit Vaccines

Parenteral killed whole-cell and subunit typhoid vaccines have been administered concomitantly with Paratyphi A and B, *Shigella flexneri* or *Shigella sonnei*, or tetanus (toxoid) antigens in field trials[131]; the typhoid components remained immunogenic and protective. Typhoid vaccines also have been administered parenterally in combination

TABLE 39–18 ▪ Immunization Schedules for Ty21a, Vi, and Heat-Inactivated, Phenol-Preserved Typhoid Vaccines

Vaccine	Formulation
Ty21a live strain	
Primary	Enteric-coated capsules
	Reconstituted liquid suspension[†]
Booster	Enteric-coated capsules
	Reconstituted liquid suspension[†]
Vi capsular polysaccharide	
Primary	Liquid
Booster	Liquid
Heat-inactivated, phenol-preserved whole-cell[‡]	
Primary	Liquid
Booster	Liquid

[*]Four doses in the United States and Canada; three doses in all other countries.

[†]Liquid suspension is currently licensed in only a few countries.

[‡]Because of frequency of severe adverse reactions associated with this vaccine (e.g., fever, malaise), it is not recommended for routine use. Rather, Ty21a or Vi should be used.

with tetanus and diphtheria toxoids and inactivated *Bordetella pertussis* and *V. cholerae* with serologic assessment.[185,189,341–343]

Purified Vi Polysaccharide Parenteral Vaccine

Clinical studies also have been carried out in which purified Vi polysaccharide was coadministered along with other parenteral vaccines, including inactivated poliovirus vaccine, yellow fever vaccine,[344,345] hepatitis B vaccine, hepatitis A vaccine,[345] rabies vaccine,[346] diphtheria and tetanus toxoids, acellular pertussis vaccine, meningococcal vaccine,[347] and measles-mumps-rubella vaccine.

A combination typhoid–hepatitis A vaccine has been developed by GlaxoSmithKline for use in travelers.[348,349] This combination vaccine, which contains 25 µg of Vi and 1440 units of inactivated hepatitis A virus antigen adsorbed to 0.5 mg of alum adjuvant, stimulates seroconversion to the component vaccine antigen in a manner equivalent to monovalent Vi and hepatitis A vaccines. A combination Vi–hepatitis A vaccine also has been developed by Aventis Pasteur (VIATIM®).

Ty21a Live Oral Vaccine

Ty21a can be coadministered along with oral attenuated poliovirus or with parenteral 17D-strain yellow fever vaccine.[206,338] Several large Phase II clinical trials have examined the safety and immunogenicity of coadministering the first or the third dose of the liquid suspension formulation of Ty21a in a combination oral vaccine cocktail along with

single-dose live oral cholera vaccine CVD103-HgR (available under the trade name Orochol® in Europe, Asia, and Latin America and the name Mutacol® in North America).[338,350,351] These studies have shown that there is no diminution in either the serum IgG S. Typhi O antibody response or the vibriocidal antibody response when these vaccines are coadministered as a combined oral vaccine cocktail versus when they are administered alone.[350,352,353]

Future Vaccines

Vi Conjugates

Because purified Vi polysaccharide acts like a T-lymphocyte–independent antigen, the serum antibody response cannot be readily boosted by administration of additional doses of Vi vaccine. In contrast, when Vi is conjugated to carrier proteins, such as tetanus or diphtheria toxoids, cholera toxin, cholera toxin B subunit, or recombinant exotoxin A of *P. aeruginosa*, it behaves as a T-lymphocyte–dependent antigen.[43,268,354,355] In animal models, subsequent inoculations with Vi conjugate vaccine clearly boost the serum Vi antibody titer.[43,268,354,355] The molecular weight of the Vi polysaccharide that is conjugated to the carrier protein influences the magnitude of the serologic response. Native Vi was superior to a derivative of lower molecular weight.[354] Early conjugates that Szu et al.[268,355] prepared utilizing tetanus toxoid as the carrier protein met

Route	Age	No. of Doses	Interval Between Doses	Interval Until Next Booster
Oral	≥6 yr	3 or 4*	2 days	5 yr
Oral	≥2 yr	3	2 days	5 yr
Oral	≥6 yr	3 or 4	2 days	5 yr
Oral	≥6 yr	3	2 days	5 yr
Intramuscular (0.5 mL)	≥ 2 yr	1	—	3 yr
Intramuscular (0.5 mL)	≥2 yr	1	—	3 yr
Subcutaneous				
(0.25 mL)	6 mo–10 yr	2	4 wk	3 yr
(0.50 mL)	>10 yr	2	4 wk	3 yr
Subcutaneous				
(0.25 mL)	6 mo–10 yr	1	4 wk	3 yr
(0.50 mL)	>10 yr	1	4 wk	3 yr

*Four doses in the United States and Canada; three doses in all other countries.
†Liquid suspension is currently licensed in only a few countries.
‡Because of frequency of severe adverse reactions associated with this vaccine (e.g., fever, malaise), it is not recommended for routine use. Rather, Ty21a or Vi should be used.

with technical difficulties, apparently because of the large molecular mass of Vi and its rigidity, which led to poor solubility and low yields. One lot of Vi–tetanus toxoid conjugate depolymerized during storage and was poorly immunogenic in a safety/immunogenicity trial in North American adults.

Szu et al.[268] reported success when 15 µg of Vi was covalently conjugated to E. coli LT B subunit or to recombinant exoprotein A of P. aeruginosa. The conjugates were well tolerated and significantly more immunogenic than unconjugated purified Vi polysaccharide.[268] Further clinical studies carried out in adults, school-age children, and preschool children in Vietnam compared the immunogenicity of two formulations of Vi–exoprotein A conjugate prepared using two different methods of conjugation. The conjugate prepared by treating the carrier protein with adipic acid dihydrazide and binding to Vi in the presence of 1-ethyl-3-(3-dimethylaminopropyl)carbodiimide elicited significantly higher titers of serum IgG Vi antibody than the other Vi conjugate (and also higher than Vi polysaccharide alone), yet was well tolerated. The superior conjugate showed a high rate of seroconversion in all ages after a single injection (containing 24 µg of Vi and 21.5 µg of exoprotein A) but a gradation in geometric mean titer that decreased progressively from adults to toddlers. The group of subjects given a second dose of this conjugate 6 weeks later exhibited a clear booster response in IgG Vi antibody titers.

The conjugate utilized in a subsequent Phase III field trial of efficacy in Vietnam contained 22.5 µg of Vi and 22 µg of exoprotein A per each 0.5-mL dose of vaccine.[305] Based on the high level of efficacy (91.5%) conferred by two doses of this vaccine in the field trial (see Table 39–15),[305] it is expected that some manufacturer will undertake scale-up and bring this vaccine to licensure.

Pectin, a common polysaccharide of plants, has a homopolymer composition similar to Vi in its backbone. Szu et al. also have shown that the treatment of pectin with acetic anhydride results in O-acetylation of C2 and C3, resulting in a moiety that now reacts with Vi antibody (whereas untreated pectin does not).[356] Szu and co-workers are investigating conjugates in which O-acetylated pectin rather than Vi is linked to the protein carrier.[356]

New Recombinant S. Typhi Strains as Live Oral Vaccines

Various investigators have applied recombinant DNA technology to engineer new candidate vaccine strains of S. Typhi that will be as well tolerated as Ty21a but much more immunogenic, so that protective immunity can be elicited with a single dose. Toward that ambitious goal, putative attenuated vaccine strains have been prepared by inactivating genes encoding various biochemical pathways,[159,161,162,357] global regulatory systems,[164,175] stress proteins,[358] other regulatory genes,[359,360] and putative virulence properties.[357]

Among these various strains, based on results of completed Phase I clinical trials, five strains remain viable vaccine candidates and are in various stages of clinical development as live oral typhoid vaccines or as live vectors. At least one other strain is poised to enter clinical trials. The status of these vaccine strains is briefly summarized below.

ΔaroC, ΔaroD, ΔhtrA Strain CVD908-htrA

Chatfield et al.[358] observed that inactivation of *htrA*, a gene encoding a stress protein that functions as a serine protease, attenuates wild-type *S.* Typhimurium for mice and protects orally immunized mice against challenge with a lethal dose of wild-type *S.* Typhimurium. Based on these observations, a deletion in *htrA* was introduced into ΔaroC, ΔaroD strain CVD 908 to yield the further derivative CVD 908-htrA. In Phase I clinical trials, single doses of CVD 908-htrA ranging from 5×10^7 to 5×10^9 CFU were as well tolerated as the CVD 908 parent,[241] although 2 of the 22 subjects developed loose stools[241]; mild diarrhea had not been observed in any recipients of CVD 908 during Phase I studies.[165,239] CVD 908-htrA stimulated significant rises in serum IgG O antibody, gut-derived IgA antibody ASCs, and cell-mediated immune responses in 90% to 100% of vaccinees. CVD 908-htrA was subsequently tested in a Phase II trial in which 79 subjects ingested either a 10^7 or a 10^8 CFU dose reconstituted from a lyophilate.[361] The vaccine was again well tolerated and immunogenic.[361]

Strain χ4073 with Mutations in *cya, crp, cdt*

Curtiss and Kelly[164] showed that, in *Salmonella*, the genes *cya* (encoding adenylate cyclase) and *crp* (encoding cyclic AMP receptor protein) comprise a global regulatory system that affects many genes and operons. They reported that *S.* Typhimurium strains that harbor deletions in *cya* and *crp* are attenuated compared to their wild-type parent, and oral immunization with such mutants protects mice against challenge with virulent *S.* Typhimurium.

Curtiss and co-workers[175] constructed vaccine candidate strain χ3927, a *cya, crp* double mutant of *S.* Typhi strain Ty2. In Phase I clinical trials, Tacket et al.[165] demonstrated that χ3927 was insufficiently attenuated from wild type because occasional subjects developed high fever and typhoid-like symptoms. Several subjects also manifested vaccinemias.[165] To achieve a greater degree of attenuation, Curtiss et al.[175] introduced into χ3927 a deletion mutation in *cdt*, a gene that affects the dissemination of *Salmonella* from gut-associated lymphoid tissue to deeper organs of the reticuloendothelial system such as the liver, spleen, and bone marrow.[362] The resultant *cya, crp, cdt* triple-mutant strain, χ4073, which was fed to healthy adult North Americans, with buffer, in single doses containing 5×10^5, 5×10^6, 5×10^7, or 5×10^8 CFU, was well tolerated except for one individual who developed diarrhea.[242] No subjects manifested vaccinemia. Four of five subjects who ingested 5×10^8 CFU exhibited significant rises in serum IgG O antibody and had ASCs that made IgA O antibody.

Strain Ty800 with a Mutation in *phoP/phoQ*

Hohmann et al. constructed strain Ty800, a *phoP/phoQ* deletion mutant of Ty2. This strain was generally well tolerated and immunogenic when evaluated in dosage levels from 10^7 to 10^{10} CFU in a small Phase I clinical trial involving 11 subjects.[243] At the highest dosage level, one of three vaccinees developed diarrhea (10 loose stools). Ty800 stimulated vigorous IgA ASCs and serum O antibody responses.

ΔaroC, ΔssaV Strain ZH9

The SsaV protein forms part of the *S. enterica* type III secretion system that plays a role in virulence, including affecting systemic invasiveness (in a mouse model) and replication in macrophages.[357] Hindle et al. reported results of a small Phase I clinical trial with strain ZH9, a ΔaroC, ΔssaV mutant of wild-type strain Ty2. In this small trial the vaccine was well tolerated, minimally excreted, and moderately immunogenic.[357]

Strain CVD 909

A higher level of protection may be attainable if a live oral vaccine can stimulate Vi antibody (like Vi and Vi conjugate vaccines) in addition to the other humoral and cellular responses elicited by live oral vaccines like Ty21a.[123,285,286] Disappointingly, otherwise promising live oral vaccine strains CVD 908-htrA, Ty800, and χ4073, although they express Vi in vitro, have failed to consistently stimulate serum Vi antibodies or IgA Vi ASCs when administered as oral vaccines.[165,239,241–243,361] This is not surprising because only 20% of patients with acute typhoid fever develop serum Vi antibodies.[85,87] Conversely, chronic gallbladder carriers of *S.* Typhi typically manifest high titers of serum Vi antibody, demonstrating that infection with *S.* Typhi can stimulate serum Vi antibodies.[87,364] The fact that expression of Vi is highly regulated in relation to environmental signals such as osmolarity may explain these somewhat contradictory observations. Two separate two-component systems are involved in this regulation.[359,364] Vi expression ensues when typhoid bacilli reside in certain extracellular environments such as blood and bile to protect them from complement-mediated, O antibody–dependent bacterial killing[38,40,65,365] but is apparently turned off when the bacteria gain their intracellular niche within macrophages. It was hypothesized that, if Vi expression by a live oral vaccine can be rendered constitutive so that it is expressed continuously, this may allow the stimulation of serum IgG and mucosal IgA Vi antibodies in orally vaccinated subjects. The *viaB* locus of *S.* Typhi contains the genes required for synthesis, surface transport, and anchoring of Vi.[366,367] Wang et al. replaced the promoter of *tviA*, the most upstream gene in the *viaB* locus of CVD 908-htrA, with a strong constitutive promoter to derive strain CVD 909, which expresses Vi constitutively.[368] To test the hypothesis, Phase I clinical trials have been initiated with CVD 909.

ΔguaBA Strains CVD 915 and CVD 916

Strain CVD 915,[371] a ΔguaBA mutant of wild-type strain Ty2, is also poised to move into clinical trials based on its performance in preclinical studies. CVD 916 is a constitutive Vi-expressing variant of CVD 915.

Attenuated Recombinant *S.* Typhi Strains as Live Vector Vaccines

Attenuated *S.* Typhi strains can function as so-called live vectors to express critical genes of other organisms and deliver them to the host immune system.[272–274] The appealing features of *Salmonella* strains that make them attractive as live vectors include the following: (1) the vaccines can be given via mucosal (oral or nasal) immunization; (2)

Salmonella strains elicit a broad immune response that includes serum antibodies, mucosal SIgA antibodies, and different types of cell-mediated immune responses; and (3) considerable experience has been gained in recent years in genetically manipulating *Salmonella*. A few clinical trials with the new generation of attenuated S. Typhi carrying foreign antigens and serving as live vectors have been published.[242,370–372] In animal models, S. Typhi can serve as a mucosal delivery system for DNA vaccines.[373,374]

Public Health Aspects

Epidemiologic Results of Vaccination

Because of their reactogenicity, parenteral killed whole-cell vaccines have rarely been employed in a systematic fashion in public health programs in endemic areas. The one exception is Thailand, where in the 1980s school-based immunization programs utilized parenteral heat-inactivated, phenol-preserved vaccine to control endemic typhoid. A retrospective review suggested that the Thai control program was highly successful.[375]

The lack of adverse reactions associated with live oral vaccine Ty21a or with parenteral Vi polysaccharide vaccine renders them particularly suitable for public health use in schoolbased immunization programs. In a large effectiveness trial involving immunization of more than 200,000 schoolchildren in Santiago, Chile, with the enteric-coated capsule formulation of Ty21a, the vaccine was found to be quite practical for large-scale use in schools.[124]

There is epidemiologic evidence that the large-scale field trials in Santiago, Chile, with Ty21a have produced a "herd immunity" effect.[123] In children within the placebo group in the first field trial of Ty21a in Area Norte, Santiago, the incidence of typhoid progressively fell as each of three field trials was initiated in subsequent years in other administrative areas of the city.[123] The incidence rate in this group diminished by approximately 70% from the mean incidence in the 3 years before the field trials. These data suggest that systematic application of live oral typhoid vaccine, even with a formulation that provides only approximately 60% to 70% efficacy, can notably diminish the incidence of the disease in endemic areas.

Table 39–19 contains a summary of the salient features of the two typhoid vaccines that have become available in recent years, oral Ty21a and parenteral Vi polysaccharide.

Disease Control Strategies

Because the peak incidence of clinical typhoid fever in most endemic areas occurs in school-age children 5 to 19 years of age, and because this is a "captive" population, in theory it should be possible to design control programs to incorporate school-based immunization with well-tolerated Ty21a or Vi vaccines. Field trials have clearly demonstrated that both Ty21a and Vi confer a moderate level of protection that endures for several years. Moreover, field experiences with Ty21a support the logistical practicality of such an approach. Ferreccio et al.[124] reported the practicality of school-based immunization in an effectiveness trial in 230,000 schoolchildren that compared two-dose, three-

dose, and four-dose regimens (all doses given within 8 days) of Ty21a. Further encouragement for programmatic use of typhoid vaccines comes from the observation of Levine et al.[123] that a herd immunity effect was evident in geographically separate areas of Santiago following the large-scale use of typhoid vaccine in other areas. There is also a report of a school-based immunization of 441 students in the face of an epidemic of typhoid in Guangxi, China, in which the vaccine showed 71% effectiveness, although the confidence limits were wide.[376] More extensive community use of Vi is being considered in some regions in Asia where there is a heavy burden of antibiotic-resistant typhoid fever.

Unfortunately, heretofore, public health authorities in endemic areas have not enthusiastically embraced the use of Ty21a or Vi in school-based immunization programs. One reason that health authorities have heretofore declined to institute school-based immunization with Ty21a or Vi is the concern that such a program would deflect scarce resources from the Expanded Programme on Immunisation (EPI), which in developing countries focuses mainly on infants less than 12 months of age. This is a valid concern because in most developing countries the EPI infrastructure is fragile and personnel resources are meager. For this reason, as an alternative strategy, several national health authorities have expressed interest in the possible inclusion of a typhoid vaccine in the EPI for infants. Such a strategy would allow typhoid fever control to proceed without deflecting resources from the traditional infant-targeted EPI. Unfortunately, no data are currently available to demonstrate that, if either Ty21a or Vi is given to infants, the immunity elicited would endure and protect years later when the children reach the high-risk school-age years. Although Ty21a has been shown to be immunogenic in toddlers and preschool children 2 to 5 years of age,[324,325] there have been no published reports of studies in infants less than 12 months of age. Vi polysaccharide vaccine has stimulated seroconversions of antibody in the majority of inoculated toddlers, but the titers achieved were notably lower than the titers observed in older children and they fell after several months.[180] If public health authorities in endemic areas are insistent in demanding typhoid vaccines that are immunogenic and protective in infants so that they can be added to the EPI, it will be necessary to await the eventual licensure of the new generation of Vi conjugates and the improved attenuated live oral vaccine strains that are presently in clinical trials.

Eradication or Elimination

Whereas chronic carriers constitute the reservoir of S. Typhi, the maintenance of a high incidence of typhoid fever requires conditions that permit amplified transmission of S. Typhi to susceptibles. Usually this involves fecal contamination of water sources consumed by large numbers of individuals. In the late 19th and early 20th centuries, it was demonstrated in Europe and the United States that treatment of municipal water supplies caused the incidence of typhoid fever to plummet, despite the continued existence in the population of large numbers of chronic carriers. Over one to two decades this led to near-elimination of typhoid fever from many areas.[100]

TABLE 39–19 ■ Comparison of the Characteristics of Live Oral Vaccine Ty21a and Parenteral Vi Polysaccharide Vaccine

Characteristic	Ty21a	Ty21a	Vi
Formulation	Enteric-coated capsules	"Liquid suspension"*	Liquid
Type of vaccine	Live	Live	Subunit
Route of administration	Oral	Oral	Parenteral
Immunization schedule	3 or 4 doses†	3 doses†	1 dose
Cold chain required by manufacturer	Yes	Yes	Yes
Well tolerated	Yes	Yes	Yes
Range of efficacy	35%–67%	55%–96%	64%–72%
Duration of efficacy	62% for ≥7 yr	78% for ≥5 yr	55% for ≥3 yr
Herd immunity effect	Yes	Yes	?
Can interfere with use of serum Vi antibody as a screening test to detect chronic typhoid carriers	No	No	Yes

*Lyophilized vaccine that is added to 100 mL of water, along with a buffer parameter, resulting in a vaccine suspension.
†Given every other day.

It is not known if programmatic use of Ty21a or Vi could accomplish the same near-elimination of typhoid fever as a public health problem. However, it is not likely that these vaccines would be the lynch pin of elimination campaigns. Conversely, future typhoid vaccines currently under development, including several attenuated strains that may function as single-dose oral vaccines and Vi conjugates, may be amenable for this purpose. If these future vaccines are well tolerated, are highly immunogenic in infants, and confer a high level of long-lasting protection, they could serve as the basis of typhoid fever control programs. Aggressive control programs that achieved a high level of coverage might nearly eliminate typhoid fever in certain populations.

It is epidemiologically feasible that typhoid fever can someday be eradicated from the world. This would require a combination of treatment of water supplies and provision of sanitation to diminish transmission; systematic screening to detect chronic typhoid carriers and treatment of the carriers to diminish the reservoir of infection; and, finally, programmatic use of well-tolerated, highly effective future typhoid vaccines. However, other more pressing global priorities and the enormous costs involved keep typhoid eradication to the level of a theoretical concept.

REFERENCES

1. Huxham J. To which is now added a dissertation on the malignant, ulcerous sore throat. *In* An Essay on Fevers. London, SA Cumberledge, 1782, pp 72–125.
2. Louis PCA. Recherches Anatomiques, Pathologiques et Therapeutiques sur la Maladie Connue sous les Noms de Gastroentérite, Fièvre Putride, Adynamique, Ataxique, Typhoide, etc., Comparée avec les Maladies Aigues les Plus Ordinaires. Paris, In Bailliere, 1829.
3. Gerhard WW. On the typhus fever, which occurred at Philadelphia in the spring and summer of 1836; illustrated by clinical observations at the Philadelphia Hospital; showing the distinction between this form of disease and dothinenteritis or the typhoid fever with alteration of the follicles of the small intestine. Am J Med Sci 19:289–322, 1837.
4. Schoenlein J. Allgemaine und specielle Pathologie und Therapie. Freiburg, St. Gallen, 1839.
5. Jenner W. Monthly on typhoid fevers—an attempt to determine the question of their identity or non-identity, by an analysis of the symptoms, and of the appearances found after death in 66 cases observed at the London Fever Hospital from Jan. 1847–Feb. 1849. Monthly J Med Sci 9:663–680, 1849.
6. Jenner W. On the identity or non-identity of typhoid and typhus fevers. Monthly J Med Sci 9:1849–1850.
7. Ritchie C. Practical remarks on the continued fevers of Great Britain, and on the generic distinctions between enteric fever and typhus. Monthly J Med Sci 7:347–358, 1846.
8. Budd W. Typhoid Fever: Its Nature, Mode of Spreading and Prevention. London, Longmans, 1873.
9. Eberth C. Organismen in den Organen bei Typhus abdominalis. Virchows Arch Path Anat 81:58–74, 1880.
10. Gaffky G. Zur Aetiologie des Abdominaltyphus. Mittheilungen aus dem kaiserlichen Gesundheitsante. Berlin, Reichsgesundheitsamt, 1884, pp 372–420.
11. Reeves MW, Evins GM, Heiba AA, et al. Clonal nature of *Salmonella typhi* and its genetic relatedness to other salmonellae as shown by multilocus enzyme electrophoresis, and proposal of *Salmonella bongori* comb. nov. J Clin Microbiol 27:313–320, 1989.
12. Le Minor L, Popoff MY. Designation of *Salmonella enterica* sp. nov., nom. rev., as the type and only species of the Genus *Salmonella*. Int J Syst Bacteriol 37:465–468, 1987.
13. Pfeiffer R, Kolle W. Experimentelle Untersuchunger zur Frage der Schutzimpfung des Menschen gegen Typhus abdominalis. Dtsch Med Wochenschr 22:735–737, 1896.
14. Wright A. On the association of serous hemorrhages with conditions and defective blood coagulability. Lancet 2:807–809, 1896.
15. Wright A, Leishman W. Remarks on the results which have been obtained by the antityphoid inoculations and on the methods which have been employed in the preparation of the vaccine. Br Med J 1:122–129, 1900.
16. Anand AC, Kataria VK, Singh W, Chatterjee SK. Epidemic multiresistant enteric fever in eastern India [letter]. Lancet 335:352, 1990.
17. Bhutta ZA, Naqvi SH, Razzaq RA, Farooqui BJ. Multidrug-resistant typhoid in children: presentation and clinical features. Rev Infect Dis 13:832–836, 1991.
18. Bhutta ZA. Impact of age and drug resistance on mortality in typhoid fever. Arch Dis Child 75:214–217, 1996.
19. Gupta A. Multidrug-resistant typhoid fever in children: epidemiology and therapeutic approach. Pediatr Infect Dis 13:124–140, 1994.
20. Mikhail IA, Haberberger RL, Farid Z, et al. Antibiotic-multiresistant *Salmonella typhi* in Egypt. Trans R Soc Trop Med Hyg 83:120, 1989.
21. Rowe B, Ward LR, Threlfall EJ. Spread of multiresistant *Salmonella typhi*. Lancet 336:1065–1066, 1990.
22. Nguyen TA, Ha Ba K, Nguyen TD. Typhoid fever in South Vietnam, 1990–1993. Bull Soc Pathol Exot 86:476–478, 1993.
23. Osler W. Typhoid fever. *In* Osler W (ed): The Principles and Practice of Medicine. New York, D. Appleton, 1892, p 2.
24. Huckstep R. Typhoid Fever and the other *Salmonella* Infections. Edinburgh, E & S Livingstone, 1962.
25. Hoffman T, Ruiz C, Counts G, et al. Waterborne typhoid fever in Dade County, Florida. Am J Med 59:481–487, 1975.
26. Gilman R, Terminel M, Levine M, et al. Relative efficacy of blood, urine, rectal swab, bone-marrow, and rose-spot cultures for recovery of *Salmonella typhi* in typhoid fever. Lancet 1:1211–1213, 1975.

27. Hoffman S, Punjabi N, Kumala S, et al. Reduction of mortality in chloramphenicol-treated severe typhoid fever by high-dose dexamethasone. N Engl J Med 310:82–88, 1984.

28. Ferreccio C, Levine MM, Manterola A, et al. Benign bacteremia caused by Salmonella typhi and paratyphi in children younger than 2 years. J Pediatr 104:899–901, 1984.

29. Mahle WT, Levine MM. Salmonella typhi infection in children younger than five years of age. Pediatr Infect Dis J 12:627–631, 1993.

30. Ames W, Robins M. Age and sex as factors in the development of the typhoid carrier state and a method of estimating carrier prevalence. Am J Public Health 33:221–230, 1943.

31. Ledingham J, Arkwright J. The Carrier Problem in Infectious Diseases. London, Arnold, 1912.

32. Skerman VBD, McGowan V, Sneath PHA. Approved lists of bacterial names. Int J Syst Bacteriol 30:225–420, 1980.

33. Baumler AJ, Heffron F, Reissbrodt R. Rapid detection of Salmonella enterica with primers specific for iroB. J Clin Microbiol 35:1224–1230, 1997.

34. Edwards P, Ewing W. Identification of Enterobacteriaceae (3rd ed). Minneapolis, Burgess Publishing Co., 1972.

35. Frankel G, Newton S, Schoolnik G, Stocker B. Intragenic recombination in a flagellin gene: characterization of the H1-j gene of Salmonella typhi. EMBO J 8:3149–3152, 1989.

36. Guinee P, Jansen W, Maas W, et al. An unusual H antigen (z66) in strains of Salmonella typhi. Ann Microbiol 132:331–334, 1981.

37. Felix A, Pitt R. A new antigen of B. typhosus. Lancet 2:186–191, 1934.

38. Felix A, Pitt R. The pathogenic and immunogenic activities of Salmonella typhi in relation to its antigenic constituents. J Hyg (Camb) 49:92–109, 1951.

39. Felix A, Krikorian A, Reitler R. The occurrence of typhoid bacilli containing Vi antigen in cases of typhoid fever and of Vi-antibody in their sera. J Hyg 35:421–427, 1935.

40. Robbins JD, Robbins JB. Reexamination of the protective role of the capsular polysaccharide Vi antigen of Salmonella typhi. J Infect Dis 150:436–449, 1984.

41. Baker EE, Whiteside RE, Basch R, Derow MA. The Vi antigen of the Enterobacteriaceae, I. Purification and chemical properties. J Immunol 83:680–686, 1961.

42. Clark W, McLaughlin J, Webster M. An aminohexuronic acid as the principal hydrolytic component of the Vi antigen. J Biol Chem 230:81–89, 1958.

43. Szu SC, Stone AL, Robbins JD, et al. Vi capsular polysaccharide-protein conjugates for prevention of typhoid fever: preparation, characterization, and immunogenicity in laboratory animals. J Exp Med 166:1510–1524, 1987.

44. Navarro F, Llovet T, Echeita MA, et al. Molecular typing of Salmonella enterica serovar Typhi. J Clin Microbiol 34:2831–2834, 1996.

45. Thong KL, Passey M, Clegg A, et al. Molecular analysis of isolates of Salmonella typhi obtained from patients with fatal and nonfatal typhoid fever. J Clin Microbiol 34:1029–1033, 1996.

46. Thong KL, Cordano AM, Yassin RM, Pang T. Molecular analysis of environmental and human isolates of Salmonella typhi. Appl Environ Microbiol 62:271–274, 1996.

47. Thong KL, Puthucheary S, Yassin RM, et al. Analysis of Salmonella typhi isolates from Southeast Asia by pulsed-field gel electrophoresis. J Clin Microbiol 33:1938–1941, 1995.

48. Thong KL, Cheong YM, Puthucheary S, et al. Epidemiologic analysis of sporadic Salmonella typhi isolates and those from outbreaks by pulsed-field gel electrophoresis. J Clin Microbiol 32:1135–1141, 1994.

49. Fica AE, Prat-Miranda S, Fernandez-Ricci A, et al. Epidemic typhoid in Chile: analysis by molecular and conventional methods of Salmonella typhi strain diversity in epidemic (1977 and 1981) and nonepidemic (1990) years. J Clin Microbiol 34:1701–1707, 1996.

50. Parkhill J, Dougan G, James KD, et al. Complete genome sequence of a multiple drug resistant Salmonella enterica serovar Typhi CT18. Nature 413:848–852, 2001.

51. Kidgell C, Pickard D, Wain J, et al. Characterisation and distribution of a cryptic Salmonella typhi plasmid pHCM2. Plasmid 47:159–171, 2002.

52. Levine M, Kaper J, Black RE, Clements M. New knowledge on pathogenesis of bacterial enteric infections as applied to vaccine development. Microbiol Rev 47:510–550, 1983.

53. Mallory F. A historical study of typhoid fever. J Exp Med 3:611–638, 1898.

54. Salas M, Angulo O, Villegus J. Patología de la fiebre tifoida en los niños. Biol Med Hosp Mex 17:63–68, 1960.

55. Hornick RB, Greisman SE, Woodward TE, et al. Typhoid fever: pathogenesis and immunologic control. N Engl J Med 283:686–691, 739–746, 1970.

56. Edsall G, Gaines S, Landy M, et al. Studies on infection and immunity in experimental typhoid fever. J Exp Med 112:143–166, 1960.

57. Gaines S, Sprinz H, Tully J, Tigertt W. Studies on infection and immunity in experimental typhoid fever. VII. The distribution of Salmonella typhi in chimpanzee tissue following oral challenge and the relationship between the numbers of bacilli and morphologic lesions. J Infect Dis 118:293–306, 1968.

58. Carter P, Collins R. The route of enteric infection in normal mice. J Exp Med 139:1189–1203, 1974.

59. Collins F. Salmonellosis in orally infected specific pathogen-free C57B1 mice. Infect Immun 6:191–198, 1972.

60. Collazo CM, Zierler MK, Galan JE. Functional analysis of the Salmonella typhimurium invasion genes invI and invJ and identification of a target of the protein secretion apparatus encoded in the inv locus. Mol Microbiol 15:25–38, 1995.

61. Collazo CM, Galan JE. The invasion-associated type-III protein secretion system in Salmonella—a review. Gene 192:51–59, 1997.

62. Kohbata S, Yokoyama H, Yabuchi E. Cytopathogenic effect of Salmonella typhi GIFU 10007 on M cells of murine ileal Peyer's patches in ligated ileal loops: an ultrastructural study. Microbiol Immunol 30:1225–1237, 1986.

63. Takeuchi A. Electron microscope studies of experimental Salmonella infection. I. Penetrations into the intestinal epithelium by Salmonella typhimurium. Am J Pathol 50:109–136, 1967.

64. Kops SK, Lowe DK, Bement WM, West AB. Migration of Salmonella typhi through intestinal epithelial monolayers: an in vitro study. Microbiol Immunol 40:799–811, 1996.

65. Felix A, Pitt R. Virulence of B. typhosus and resistance to O antigen. J Pathol Bacteriol 38:409–420, 1934.

66. Meyer K, Neilson N, Feusier M. The mechanism of gallbladder infections in laboratory animals. V. Experimental typhoid-paratyphoid carriers. J Infect Dis 28:456–509, 1921.

67. Nichols H. Observations on experimental typhoid infection of the gallbladder in the rabbit. J Exp Med 20:573–581, 1914.

68. Avendãno A, Herrera P, Horwitz I, et al. Duodenal string cultures: practicality and sensitivity for diagnosing enteric fever in children. J Infect Dis 53:359–362, 1986.

69. Benavente L, Gotuzzo E, Guerra J, et al. Diagnosis of typhoid fever using a string capsule device. Trans R Soc Trop Med Hyg 78:404–406, 1984.

70. Vallenas C, Hernandez H, Day B, et al. Efficacy of bone marrow, blood, stool, and duodenal contents cultures for bacteriologic confirmation of typhoid fever in children. Pediatr Infect Dis J 4:496–498, 1985.

71. Guerra-Caceres J, Gotuzzo-Herencia E, Crosby-Dagnino E, et al. Diagnostic value of bone marrow culture in typhoid fever. Trans R Soc Trop Med Hyg 73:680–683, 1979.

72. Hoffman S, Punjabi N, Rockhill R, et al. Duodenal string-capsule culture compared with bone-marrow, blood and rectal swab cultures for diagnosing typhoid and paratyphoid fever. J Infect Dis 149:157–161, 1984.

73. Widal G, Sicard A. Recherches de la réaction agglutinate dans le sang et le sérum desséchés des typhiques et dans la serosité des vesications. Bull Soc Med Paris (3rd ser) 13:681–682, 1896.

74. Durham H. Note on the diagnostic value of the serum of typhoid fever patients. Lancet 2:1746–1747, 1896.

75. Grunbaum A. Preliminary note on the use of the agglutinative action of human serum for the diagnosis of enteric fever. Lancet 2:806–807, 1896.

76. Levine MM, Grados O, Gilman RH, et al. Diagnostic value of the Widal test in areas endemic for typhoid fever. Am J Trop Med Hyg 27:795–800, 1978.

77. Parry CM, Hoa NT, Diep TS, et al. Value of a single-tube Widal test in diagnosis of typhoid fever in Vietnam. J Clin Microbiol 37:2882–2886, 1999.

78. Anderson ES. Proposed use of a non-motile variant of Salmonella typhi for the preparation of vaccine against typhoid fever. Symp Ser Immunobiol Stand 15:79–86, 1971.

79. Anderson ES. Suggested adoption of a non-motile variant of strain Ty2 for vaccination against typhoid fever. Progr Immunobiol Stand 5:373–377, 1972.

80. Anderson ES, Gunnell A. A suggestion for a new antityphoid vaccine. Lancet 2:1196–1200, 1964.

81. Hoffman S, Flanigan TP, Klaucke D, et al. The Widal slide agglutination test, a valuable rapid diagnostic test in typhoid fever patients at the Infectious Diseases Hospital of Jakarta. Am J Epidemiol 123:869–875, 1986.

82. House D, Wain J, Ho VA, et al. Serology of typhoid fever in an area of endemicity and its relevance to diagnosis. J Clin Microbiol 39:1002–1007, 2001.

83. Choo KE, Oppenheimer SJ, Ismail AB, Ong KH. Rapid serodiagnosis of typhoid fever by dot enzyme immunoassay in an endemic area. Clin Infect Dis 19:172–176, 1994.

84. Bhutta ZA, Mansurali N. Rapid serologic diagnosis of pediatric typhoid fever in an endemic area: a prospective comparative evaluation of two dot-enzyme immunoassays and the Widal test. Am J Trop Med Hyg 61:654–657, 1999.

85. Lanata CF, Levine MM, Ristori C, et al. Vi serology in detection of chronic *Salmonella typhi* carriers in an endemic area. Lancet 2:441–443, 1983.

86. Nolan CM, Feeley JC, White PC Jr, et al. Evaluation of a new assay for Vi antibody in chronic carriers of *Salmonella typhi*. J Clin Microbiol 12:22–26, 1980.

87. Losonsky GA, Ferreccio C, Kotloff KL, et al. Development and evaluation of an enzyme-linked immunosorbent assay for serum Vi antibodies for detection of chronic *Salmonella typhi* carriers. J Clin Microbiol 25:2266–2269, 1987.

88. Barrett TJ, Snyder JD, Blake PA, Feeley JC. Enzyme-linked immunosorbent assay for detection of *Salmonella typhi* Vi antigen in urine from typhoid patients. J Clin Microbiol 15:235–237, 1982.

89. Gupta AK, Rao KM. Simultaneous detection of *Salmonella typhi* Vi antigen and antibody in serum by counter-immunoelectrophoresis for an early and rapid diagnosis of typhoid fever. J Immunol Methods 30:349–353, 1979.

90. John TJ, Sivasan K, Kurien B. Evaluation of passive bacterial agglutination for the diagnosis of typhoid fever. J Clin Microbiol 20:751–753, 1984.

91. Rockhill RC, Rumans LW, Lesmana M, Dennis DT. Detection of *Salmonella typhi* D, VI, and d antigens, by slide coagglutination in urine from patients with typhoid fever. J Clin Microbiol 11:213–216, 1980.

92. Shetty NP, Hiresave S, Bhat P. Coagglutination and counterimmunoelectrophoresis in the rapid diagnosis of typhoid fever. Am J Clin Pathol 84:80–84, 1985.

93. Sivadasan K, Kurien B, John TJ. Rapid diagnosis of typhoid fever by antigen detection. Lancet 1:134–135, 1984.

94. Sundaraj T, Hango B, Subramanian S. A study on the usefulness of counter immunoelectrophoresis for the detection of *Salmonella typhi* antigen in the sera of suspected cases of enteric fever. Trans R Soc Trop Med Hyg 77:194–197, 1983.

95. Taylor DN, Harris JR, Barrett TJ, et al. Detection of urinary Vi antigen as a diagnostic test for typhoid fever. J Clin Microbiol 18:872–876, 1983.

96. Tsang RW, Chau PY. Serological diagnosis of typhoid fever by counter immunoelectrophoresis. Br Med J 282:1505–1507, 1981.

97. Rubin FA, Kopecko DJ, Sack RB, et al. Evaluation of a DNA probe for identifying *Salmonella typhi* in Peruvian and Indonesian bacterial isolates. J Infect Dis 157:1051–1053, 1988.

98. Song JH, Cho H, Park MY, et al. Detection of *Salmonella typhi* in the blood of patients with typhoid fever by polymerase chain reaction. J Clin Microbiol 31:1439–1443, 1993.

99. Zhu Q, Lim CK, Chan YN. Detection of *Salmonella typhi* by polymerase chain reaction. J Appl Bacteriol 80:244–251, 1996.

100. Wolman A, Gorman A. The Significance of Waterborne Typhoid Fever Outbreaks. Baltimore, Williams & Wilkins, 1931.

101. Typhoid in the large cities of the United States in 1919. JAMA 74:672–675, 1920.

102. Edelman R, Levine MM. Summary of an international workshop on typhoid fever. Rev Infect Dis 8:329–349, 1986.

103. Ivanoff B, Levine MM. Typhoid fever: continuing challenges from a resilient bacterial foe. Bull Inst Pasteur 95:129–142, 1997.

104. Committee on Issues and Priorities for New Vaccine Development, Institute of Medicine. New Vaccine Development: Establishing Priorities. Vol. II. Diseases of Importance in Developing Countries. Washington, DC, National Academy Press, 1985.

105. Simanjuntak C, Paleologo F, Punjabi N, et al. Oral immunisation against typhoid fever in Indonesia with Ty21a vaccine. Lancet 338:1055–1059, 1991.

106. Acharya VI, Lowe CU, Thapa R, et al. Prevention of typhoid fever in Nepal with the Vi capsular polysaccharide of *Salmonella typhi*: a preliminary report. N Engl J Med 317:1101–1104, 1987.

107. Klugman K, Gilbertson IT, Kornhoff HJ, et al. Protective activity of Vi polysaccharide vaccine against typhoid fever. Lancet 2:1165–1169, 1987.

108. Black RE, Levine MM, Ferreccio C, et al. Efficacy of one or two doses of Ty21a *Salmonella typhi* vaccine in enteric-coated capsules in a controlled field trial. Chilean Typhoid Committee. Vaccine 8:81–84, 1990.

109. Levine MM, Black RE, Ferreccio C, et al. Interventions to control endemic typhoid fever: field studies in Santiago, Chile. *In* Control and Eradication of Infectious Diseases: An International Symposium (PAHO Copublication Series No 1). Washington, DC, Pan American Health Organization, 1986, pp 37–53.

110. Committee on Issues and Priorities for New Vaccine Development, Institute of Medicine. The burden of disease resulting from various diarrheal pathogens. *In* New Vaccine Development: Establishing Priorities. Vol. II. Diseases of Importance in Developing Countries. Washington, DC, National Academy Press, 1986.

111. Ashcroft MT. The morbidity and mortality of enteric fever in British Guyana. W Ind Med J 11:62–71, 1962.

112. Ashcroft MT. Typhoid and paratyphoid fever in the tropics. J Trop Med Hyg 67:185–189, 1964.

113. Kligler IJ, Bachi R. An analysis of the endemicity and epidemicity of typhoid fever in Palestine. Acta Med Orient 4:243–261, 1945.

114. Rice PA, Baine WB, Gangarosa EJ. *Salmonella typhi* infections in the United States, 1967–1972: increasing importance of international travelers. Am J Epidemiol 106:160–166, 1977.

115. Ryan CA, Hargrett-Bean NT, Blake PA. *Salmonella typhi* infections in the United States, 1975–1984: increasing role of foreign travel. Rev Infect Dis 11:1–8, 1989.

116. Ryder RW, Blake PA. Typhoid fever in the United States, 1975 and 1976. J Infect Dis 139:124–126, 1979.

117. Taylor DN, Pollard RA, Blake PA. Typhoid in the United States and risk to the international traveler. J Infect Dis 148:599–602, 1983.

118. Blaser MJ, Feldman RA. Acquisition of typhoid fever from proficiency-testing specimens [Correspondence]. JAMA 303:1481–1482, 1980.

119. Blaser MJ, Lofgren JP. Fatal salmonellosis originating in a clinical microbiology laboratory. J Clin Microbiol 13:855–858, 1981.

120. Blaser MJ, Hickman FW, Farmer JJ, et al. *Salmonella typhi*: the laboratory as a reservoir of infection. J Infect Dis 142:934–938, 1980.

121. Ferreccio C. Typhoid—policy quandaries about use of Ty21a in Chile. *In* Sack DA, Freij L (eds): Prospects for Public Health Benefits in Developing Countries from New Vaccines Against Enteric Infections. Stockholm, Gotab, 1990, pp 67–81.

122. Levine MM, Taylor DN, Ferreccio C. Typhoid vaccines come of age. Pediatr Infect Dis J 8:374–381, 1989.

123. Levine MM, Ferreccio C, Black RE, et al. Progress in vaccines against typhoid fever. Rev Infect Dis 11(suppl 3):S552–S567, 1989.

124. Ferreccio C, Levine MM, Rodriguez H, Contreras R. Comparative efficacy of two, three, or four doses of Ty21a live oral typhoid vaccine in enteric-coated capsules: a field trial in an endemic area. J Infect Dis 159:766–769, 1989.

125. Rowe B, Ward LR, Threlfall EJ. Multidrug-resistant *Salmonella typhi*: a worldwide epidemic. Clin Infect Dis 24(suppl 1):S106–S109, 1997.

126. Wain J, Hoa NT, Chinh NT, et al. Quinolone-resistant *Salmonella typhi* in Viet Nam: molecular basis of resistance and clinical response to treatment. Clin Infect Dis 25:1404–1410, 1997.

127. Levine MM. Typhoid fever vaccines. *In* Plotkin SA, Mortimer A Jr (eds). Vaccines. Philadelphia, WB Saunders, 1988, pp 333–361.

128. Levine MM. Typhoid fever vaccines. *In* Plotkin SA, Mortimer E Jr (eds). Vaccines (2nd ed). Philadelphia, WB Saunders, 1994, pp 597–633.

129. Felix A. New type of typhoid and paratyphoid vaccine. Br Med J 1:391–395, 1941.

130. Felix A, Rainsford SG, Stokes EJ. Antibody response and systemic reactions after inoculation of a new T.A.B.C. vaccine O. Br Med J 1:435–440, 1941.

131. Hejfec LB, Salmin LV, Lejtman MZ, et al. A controlled field trial and laboratory study of five typhoid vaccines in the USSR. Bull World Health Organ 34:321–339, 1966.

132. Landy M. Enhancement of the immunogenicity of typhoid vaccine by retention of the Vi antigen. Am J Hyg 58:148–164, 1953.

133. Walter Reed Army Institute of Research. Preparation of dried acetone-inactivated and heat-phenol-inactivated typhoid vaccines. Bull World Health Organ 30:635–646, 1964.
134. Walter Reed Army Institute of Research, International Laboratory for Biological Standards SS. Physical and chemical studies on two dried inactivated typhoid vaccines (vaccine K and L). Bull World Health Organ 30:647–652, 1964.
135. Besredka A. De la vaccination contre les états typhoides par voie buccale. Ann Inst Pasteur 33:882–890, 1919.
136. Besredka A. Local Immunization. Baltimore, Williams & Wilkins, 1927.
137. Hejfets LB, Levina IA, Salmin LV, et al. Assessment of effectivity of oral killed typhoid and paratyphoid B vaccines and aerosol chemical typhoid vaccine in controlled field trials. J Hyg Epidemiol Microbiol Immunol 20:292–299, 1976.
138. Borgoño JM, Corey G, Engelhardt H. Field trials with killed oral typhoid vaccines. Dev Biol Stand 33:80–84, 1976.
139. Chuttani CS. Controlled field trials of three different oral killed typhoid vaccines in India. Dev Biol Stand 33:98–101, 1976.
140. Chuttani DS, Prakash K, Gupta P, et al. Controlled field trial of a high dose oral killed typhoid vaccine in India. Bull World Health Organ 55:643–644, 1977.
141. Chuttani CS, Prakash K, Vergese A, et al. Ineffectiveness of an oral killed typhoid vaccine in a field trial. Bull World Health Organ 48:756–757, 1973.
142. Chuttani CS, Prakash K, Vergese A, et al. Effectiveness of oral killed typhoid vaccine. Bull World Health Organ 45:445–450, 1971.
143. Hejfec LB, Levina LA, Antanova AA, et al. Controlled field trials of killed oral typhoid and paratyphoid B vaccines and cell-free chemical aerosol typhoid vaccine. Dev Biol Stand 33:93–97, 1975.
144. DuPont LH, Hornick RB, Snyder MJ, et al. Studies of immunity in typhoid fever: protection induced by killed oral antigens or by primary infection. Bull World Health Organ 44:667–672, 1971.
145. Grasset E. L'endoanatoxine typho-paratyphique dans la prophylaxie des infections typhoidiques. Rev Immunol (Paris) 15:1–19, 1951.
146. Topley WWC, Raistrick H, Wilson J, et al. Immunising potency of antigenic components isolated from different strains of Bact. typhosum. Lancet 1:252–260, 1937.
147. Westphal O, Luderitz O, Bister F. Uber die Extraktion von Bakterienmit Phenol/Wasser. Z Naturforsch 7b:148–155, 1952.
148. Landy M. Studies on Vi antigen, VI. Immunization of human beings with purified Vi antigen. Am J Hyg 60:52–62, 1954.
149. Landy M, Gaines S, Seal JP, Whiteside JE. Antibody responses of man to three types of antityphoid immunizing agents. Am J Public Health 44:1572–1579, 1954.
150. Polish Typhoid Committee. Controlled field trial and laboratory studies on the effectiveness of typhoid vaccines in Poland 1961–1964. Bull World Health Organ 34:211–222, 1966.
151. Hejfec LB. Results of the study of typhoid vaccines in four controlled field trials in the USSR. Bull World Health Organ 32:1–14, 1965.
152. Webster ME, Landy M, Freeman ME. Studies on Vi antigen. II. Purification of Vi antigen from Escherichia coli 5396/38. J Immunol 69:135–142, 1952.
153. Landy M, Johnson AG, Webster ME. Studies on Vi antigen. VIII. Role of acetyl in antigenic activity. Am J Hyg 73:55–65, 1961.
154. Whiteside RE, Baker EE. The Vi antigens of the Enterobacteriaceae. V. serologic differences of Vi antigens revealed by deacetylation. J Immunol 86:538–542, 1961.
155. Reitman M. Infectivity and antigenicity of streptomycin-dependent Salmonella typhosa. J Infect Dis 117:101–107, 1967.
156. Cvjetanovic B, Mel DM, Felsenfeld O. Study of live typhoid vaccine in chimpanzees. Bull World Health Organ 42:499–507, 1970.
157. Mel DM, Arsic BL, Radovanovic ML, et al. Safety tests in adults and children with live oral typhoid vaccine. Acta Microbiol Acad Sci Hung 21:161–166, 1974.
158. Cryz SJ Jr, Furer E, Baron LS, et al. Construction and characterization of a Vi-positive variant of the Salmonella typhi live oral vaccine strain Ty21a. Infect Immun 57:3863–3868, 1989.
159. Hone DM, Attridge SR, Forrest B, et al. A galE via (Vi antigen-negative) mutant of Salmonella typhi Ty2 retains virulence in humans. Infect Immun 56:1326–1333, 1988.
160. Dima VF. Volunteer studies in the development of a live oral typhoid vaccine. Arch Roumaines Pathol Exp Microbiol 42:196–198, 1983.
161. Edwards MF, Stocker BAD. Construction of aroA his pur strains of Salmonella typhi. J Bacteriol 170:3991–3995, 1984.
162. Hone DM, Harris AM, Chatfield S, et al. Construction of genetically defined double aro mutants of Salmonella typhi. Vaccine 9:810–816, 1991.
163. Hone DM, Tacket C, Harris A, et al. Evaluation in volunteers of a candidate live oral attenuated S. typhi vector vaccine. J Clin Invest 90:1–9, 1992.
164. Curtiss R III, Kelly SM. Salmonella typhimurium deletion mutants lacking adenylate cyclase and cyclic AMP receptor protein are avirulent and immunogenic. Infect Immun 55:3035–3043, 1987.
165. Tacket CO, Hone DM, Curtiss RI, et al. Comparison of the safety and immunogenicity of aroC, aroD and cya, crp Salmonella typhi strains in adult volunteers. Infect Immun 60:536–541, 1992.
166. Hohmann EL, Oletta CA, Miller SL. Evaluation of a phoP/phoQ-deleted, aroA-deleted live oral Salmonella typhi vaccine strain in human volunteers. Vaccine 14:19–24, 1996.
167. Dilts DA, Riesenfeld-Orn I, Fulginiti JP, et al. Phase I clinical trials of aroA, aroD, and aroA, aroD, htrA attenuated S. typhi vaccines: effect of formulation on safety and immunogenicity. Vaccine 18:1473–1484, 2000.
168. DuPont HL, Hornick RB, Snyder MJ, et al. Immunity in typhoid fever: evaluation of live streptomycin-dependent vaccine. Antimicrob Agents Chemother 10:236–239, 1970.
169. Levine MM, DuPont LH, Hornick RE, et al. Attenuated streptomycin-dependent Salmonella typhi oral vaccine: potential deleterious effects of lyophilization. J Infect Dis 133:424–429, 1976.
170. Levine MM, Herrington D, Murphy JR, et al. Safety, infectivity, immunogenicity and in vivo stability of two attenuated auxotrophic mutant strains of Salmonella typhi, 541Ty and 543Ty, as live oral vaccines in man. J Clin Invest 79:888–902, 1987.
171. Tacket CO, Losonsky G, Taylor DN, et al. Lack of immune response to the Vi component of a Vi-positive variant of the Salmonella typhi live oral vaccine strain Ty21a in human studies. J Infect Dis 163:901–904, 1991.
172. Hoiseth S, Stocker BAD. Aromatic-dependent Salmonella typhimurium are non-virulent and effective as live vaccines. Nature 292:238–239, 1981.
173. Stocker BAD, Hoiseth SK, Smith BP. Aromatic-dependent "Salmonella sp" as live vaccine in mice and calves. Dev Biol Stand 53:47–54, 1983.
174. Bacon GA, Burrows TW, Yates M. The effects of biochemical mutation on the virulence of Bacterium typhosum: the loss of virulence of certain mutants. Br J Exp Pathol 32:85–96, 1951.
175. Curtiss R III, Kelly SM, Tinge SA, et al. Recombinant Salmonella vectors in vaccine development. Develop Biol Standard 82:23–33, 1994.
176. Groschel DHM, Hornick RB. Who introduced typhoid vaccination: Almoth Wright or Richard Pfeiffer? Rev Infect Dis 3:1251–1254, 1981.
177. Wright AE, Semple D. Remarks on vaccination against typhoid fever. Br Med J 1:256–258, 1897.
178. Wong KH, Feeley JC, Northrup RS, Forlines ME. Vi antigen from Salmonella typhosa and immunity against typhoid fever. I. Isolation and immunologic properties in animals. Infect Immun 9:348–353, 1974.
179. Gotschlich EC, Liu TY, Artenstein MS. Human immunity to the meningococcus. III. Preparation and immunochemical properties of the group A, group B, and group C meningococcal polysaccharides. Exp Med 129:1349–1365, 1969.
180. Plotkin SA, Bouveret-Le Cam N. A new typhoid vaccine composed of the Vi capsular polysaccharide. Arch Intern Med 155:2293–2299, 1995.
181. Germanier R, Furer E. Isolation and characterization of gal E mutant Ty21a of Salmonella typhi: a candidate strain for a live oral typhoid vaccine. J Infect Dis 141:553–558, 1975.
182. Gilman RH, Hornick RB, Woodard WE, et al. Evaluation of a UDP-glucose-4-epimeraseless mutant of Salmonella typhi as a live oral vaccine. J Infect Dis 136:717–723, 1977.
183. Robbe-Saule V, Coynault C, Norel F. The live oral typhoid vaccine Ty21a is an rpoS mutant and is susceptible to various environmental stresses. FEMS Microbiol Lett 126:171–176, 1995.
184. International List of Availability of Vaccines and Sera. Geneva, World Health Organization, 1997.
185. Barr M, Sayers MHP, Stamm WP. Intradermal T.A.B.T. vaccine for immunization against enteric fever. Lancet 1:816–817, 1959.
186. Dimache GL, Dimache V, Ciudin L, et al. Intradermal typhoid vaccination in men by jet-injection: immunological estimation by laboratory test. Arch Roumaines Pathol Exp Microbiol 36:227–232, 1977.

187. Dimache GL, Dimache V, Croitoru M. The immunization of a five-years-old dried typhoid vaccine. Arch Roumaines Pathol Exp Microbiol 40:55–59, 1981.
188. Iwarson S, Larsson P. Intradermal versus subcutaneous immunization with typhoid vaccine. J Hyg (Camb) 84:11–15, 1980.
189. Keen TEB, Batholomeusz C. Immunization with intradermal T.A.B. tetanus vaccine. Med J Aust 49:591–593, 1962.
190. Perry RM. Comparison of typhoid "O" and "H" agglutinin responses following intracutaneous and subcutaneous inoculation of typhoid, paratyphoid A and B vaccine. Am J Hyg 26:388–393, 1937.
191. Tuft L, Yagle ELM, Rogers S. Comparative study of the antibody response after various methods of administration of mixed typhoid vaccine. J Infect Dis 50:98–110, 1932.
192. Van Gelder DW, Fister S. Intradermal immunization. III. Typhoid fever. Am J Dis Child 62:93–98, 1941.
193. Vella W. On vaccines and vaccination: typhoid-paratyphoid fevers. Postgrad Med J 48:98–100, 1972.
194. Dimache GL, Dimache V, Paxel A, Croitoru M. Intradermal various subcutaneous typhoid vaccination. Arch Roumaines Pathol Exp Microbiol 40:143–147, 1965.
195. Pelser HH. Reactogenicity and immunogenicity of a single dose of typhoid Vi polysaccharide vaccine in children aged between 4 and 14 years. BioDrugs 15(suppl 1):13, 2001.
196. Ramkissoon A, Jugnundan P. Reactogenicity and immunogenicity of a single dose of a typhoid Vi polysaccharide vaccine in adolescents. BioDrugs 15(suppl 1):21, 2001
197. Tacket CO, Ferreccio C, Robbins JB, et al. Safety and immunogenicity of two *Salmonella typhi* Vi capsular polysaccharide vaccines. J Infect Dis 154:342–345, 1986.
198. Levine MM, Ferreccio C, Black RE, Germanier R, for the Chilean Typhoid Committee. Large-scale field trial of Ty21a live oral typhoid vaccine in enteric-coated capsule formulation. Lancet 1:1049–1052, 1987.
199. Levine MM, Ferreccio C, Cryz S, Ortiz E. Comparison of enteric-coated capsules and liquid formulation of Ty21a typhoid vaccine in randomised controlled field trial. Lancet 336:891–894, 1990.
200. Hirschel B, Wuthrich R, Somain B, Steffen R. Inefficacy of the commercial live oral Ty21a vaccine in the prevention of typhoid fever. Eur J Clin Microbiol 4:295–298, 1985.
201. Levine MM, Black RE, Ferreccio C, et al. The efficacy of attenuated *Salmonella typhi* oral vaccine strain Ty21a evaluated in controlled field trials. *In* Holmgren J, Lindberg A, Molly R (eds): Development of Vaccines and Drugs Against Diarrhea. Lund, Sweden, Studentlitteratur, 1986, pp 90–101.
202. Driesens RJ. Effect of glass on pH-dependent stability of typhoid vaccine. J Clin Microbiol 2:85–88, 1975.
203. Joo I, Zsidai J. Stability of cholera and typhoid vaccines. J Biol Stand 6:341–348, 1977.
204. Cryz SJ Jr, Pasteris O, Varallyay SJ, Furer E. Factors influencing the stability of live oral attenuated bacterial vaccines. Dev Biol Stand 87:277–281, 1996.
205. Corbel MJ. Reasons for instability of bacterial vaccines. Dev Biol Stand 87:113–124, 1996.
206. Cryz SJ Jr. Post-marketing experience with live oral Ty21a vaccine (Vivotif Berna®). Lancet 341:49–50, 1993.
207. Olitzki A. Causing organisms and host's reactions. *In* Enteric Fevers. Basel, S. Karger, 1972, pp 430–486.
208. Ashcroft MT, Morrison-Ritchie J, Nicholson CC, Stuart CA. Antibody responses to vaccination of British Guiana schoolchildren with heat-killed-phenolized and acetone-killed lyophilized vaccines. Am J Hyg 80:221–228, 1964.
209. Benenson AS. Serological responses of man to typhoid vaccines. Bull World Health Organ 30:653–662, 1964.
210. Cvjetanovic B. Standardization and assay of typhoid reference vaccines K and L. Progr Immunobiol Stand 1:196–203, 1965.
211. Edsall G, Carlson MC, Formal SB, Benenson AS. Laboratory tests of typhoid vaccines within a controlled field study. Bull World Health Organ 20:1017–1032, 1959.
212. Ikic D. Ten years of field trials and laboratory examinations of vaccine against typhoid given. Progr Immunobiol Stand 2:175–182, 1965.
213. Joo I, Pusztai ZS, Julasz VP. Mouse protective ability of the international reference preparations of typhoid vaccine. Z Immun-Forsch 135:365–387, 1968.
214. Karolcek JM, Rusinko M, Draskovicova M, et al. Attempts to elaborate a new laboratory test for evaluation of the immunogenic efficiency of typhoid vaccines. J Hyg Epidemiol Microbiol Immunol 10:47–60, 1966.
215. Melikova BN, Lesnjak SV. International reference preparations of typhoid vaccine: potency by the active mouse protection test with three different routes of immunization. Bull World Health Organ 37:575–579, 1967.
216. Pittman M, Bohner HJ. Laboratory assays of different types of field trial typhoid vaccines and relationships to efficacy in man. J Bacteriol 91:1713–1723, 1966.
217. Standfast AFB. A report on the laboratory assays carried out at the Lister Institute of Preventive Medicine on the typhoid vaccine used in the field study in Yugoslavia. Bull World Health Organ 23:37–45, 1960.
218. Standfast AFB. Some observations on typhoid vaccine assay in 1964. Progr Immunobiol Stand 2:190–195, 1965.
219. Sterne M, Frim G. Assay of typhoid vaccines in man. J Med Microbiol 7:197–203, 1970.
220. Sterne M, Frim G. The significance of protection tests in mice for evaluating typhoid vaccines. Progr Immunobiol Stand 5:382–388, 1972.
221. Ungar J, Addison IE. The comparison of the antigenic assay in mice with that of antibody titration of immune rabbit serum. Progr Immunobiol Stand 2:183–189, 1965.
222. World Health Organization Expert Committee on Biological Standardization. Typhoid vaccine. World Health Organ Tech Rep Ser 413:19–20, 1969.
223. Yugoslav Typhoid Commission. Field and laboratory studies with typhoid vaccines. Bull World Health Organ 16:897–910, 1957.
224. Yugoslav Typhoid Commission. A controlled field trial of the effectiveness of phenol and alcohol typhoid vaccines. Bull World Health Organ 26:357–369, 1962.
225. Ashcroft MT, Morrison-Ritchie J, Nicholson CC. Controlled field trial in British Guyana schoolchildren of heat-killed-phenolized and acetone-killed lyophilized typhoid vaccines. Am J Hyg 79:196–206, 1964.
226. Ashcroft MT, Nicholson CC, Balwant S, et al. A seven-year field trial of two typhoid vaccines in Guiana. Lancet 2:1056–1060, 1967.
227. Yugoslav Typhoid Commission. A controlled field trial of the effectiveness of acetone-dried and inactivated and heat-phenol-inactivated typhoid vaccines in Yugoslavia. Bull World Health Organ 30:623–630, 1964.
228. Polish Typhoid Committee. Evaluation of typhoid vaccines in the laboratory and in a controlled field trial in Poland. Bull World Health Organ 31:15–27, 1965.
229. Spaun J, Uemura K. International reference preparations of typhoid vaccine. Bull World Health Organ 31:761–791, 1964.
230. Tully JG, Gaines S, Tigertt WD. Studies on infection and immunity in experimental typhoid fever. IV. Role of H antigen in protection. J Infect Dis 112:118–124, 1963.
231. Carter PB, Collins FM. Assessment of typhoid vaccines by using the intraperitoneal route of challenge. Infect Immun 17:555–560, 1977.
232. Spaun J. Studies on the influence of the route of immunization in the active mouse protection test with intraperitoneal challenge for potency of typhoid vaccines. Bull World Health Organ 31:793–798, 1964.
233. Landy M. Studies of Vi antigen. VII. Characteristics of the immune response in the mouse. Am J Hyg 65:81–93, 1957.
234. Landy M, Lamb E. Estimation of Vi antibody employing erythrocytes treated with purified Vi antigen. Proc Soc Exp Biol Med 82:593–598, 1953.
235. Wong KH, Feeley JC, Pittman M. Effect of Vi-degrading enzyme on potency of typhoid vaccines in mice. J Infect Dis 125:360–366, 1972.
236. Wong KH, Feeley JC, Pittman M, et al. Adhesion of Vi antigen and toxicity in typhoid vaccines inactivated by acetone or by heat and phenol. J Infect Dis 129:501–506, 1974.
237. Wahdan MH, Sippel JE, Mikhail IA, et al. Controlled field trial of a typhoid vaccine prepared with nonmotile mutant of *Salmonella typhi* Ty2. Bull World Health Organ 52:69–73, 1975.
238. Code of Federal Regulations. Title 21: Food and Drugs. Point 620. Subpart B. Washington, DC, National Archives and Records Administration, 1986, pp 69–70.
239. Tacket CO, Hone DM, Losonsky GA, et al. Clinical acceptability and immunogenicity of CVD 908 *Salmonella typhi* vaccine strain. Vaccine 10:443–446, 1992.
240. Sztein MB, Wasserman SS, Tacket CO, et al. Cytokine production patterns and lymphoproliferative responses in volunteers orally immunized with attenuated vaccine strains of *Salmonella typhi*. J Infect Dis 170:1508–1517, 1994.

241. Tacket CO, Sztein MB, Losonsky GA, et al. Safety of live oral *Salmonella typhi* vaccine strains with deletions in *htrA* and *aroC aroD* and immune response in humans. Infect Immun 65:452–456, 1997.

242. Tacket CO, Kelly SM, Schodel F, et al. Safety and immunogenicity in humans of an attenuated *Salmonella typhi* vaccine vector strain expressing plasmid-encoded hepatitis B antigens stabilized by the ASD balanced lethal system. Infect Immun 65:3381–3385, 1997.

243. Hohmann EL, Oletta CA, Killeen KP, Miller SI. *phoP/phoQ*-deleted *Salmonella typhi* (Ty800) is a safe and immunogenic single-dose typhoid fever vaccine in volunteers. J Infect Dis 173:1408–1414, 1996.

244. D'Amelio R, Tagliabue A, Nencioni L, et al. Comparative analysis of immunological responses to oral (Ty21a) and parenteral (TAB) typhoid vaccines. Infect Immun 56:2731–2735, 1988.

245. Kantele A. Antibody-secreting cells in the evaluation of the immunogenicity of an oral vaccine. Vaccine 8:321–326, 1990.

246. Kantele A. Immune response to prolonged intestinal exposure to antigen. Scand J Immunol 33:225–229, 1991.

247. Kantele A, Makela PH. Different profiles of the human immune response to primary and secondary immunization with an oral *Salmonella typhi* Ty21a vaccine. Vaccine 9:423–427, 1991.

248. Kantele A, Arvilommi H, Jokinen I. Specific immunoglobulin-secreting human blood cells after peroral vaccination against *Salmonella typhi*. J Infect Dis 153:1126–1131, 1986.

249. Kantele A, Arvilommi H, Kantele JM, et al. Comparison of the human immune response to live oral, killed oral, or killed parenteral *Salmonella typhi* Ty21a vaccines. Microb Pathog 10:117–126, 1991.

250. Tagliabue A, Nencioni CA, Caffarena A, et al. Cellular immunity against *Salmonella typhi* after live oral vaccines. Clin Exp Immunol 62:242–247, 1985.

251. Tagliabue A, Villa L, De Magistiris MT, et al. IgA-driven T-cell-mediated antibacterial immunity in man after live oral Ty21a vaccine. J Immunol 137:1504–1510, 1986.

252. Panero C, Saletti M, DiTommaso I. The detection of intestinal IgA in children following oral typhoid vaccine. Progr Immunobiol Stand 5:369–372, 1972.

253. Wahdan MH, Serie C, Cerisier Y, et al. A controlled field trial of live *Salmonella typhi* strain Ty21a oral vaccine against typhoid: three-year results. J Infect Dis 145:292–296, 1982.

254. Wahdan MH, Serie C, Germanier R, et al. A controlled field trial of live oral typhoid vaccine Ty21a. Bull World Health Organ 58:469–474, 1980.

255. Ambrosch F, Hirschhl A, Kremsher P, et al. Investigations on the humoral immune response to oral live typhoid vaccination with strain Ty21a. Munchen Med Wochenschr 127:775–778, 1985.

256. Keitel WA, Bond NL, Zahradnik JM, et al. Clinical and serological responses following primary and booster immunization with *Salmonella typhi* Vi capsular polysaccharide vaccines. Vaccine 12:195–199, 1994.

257. Woodward WE. Volunteer studies of typhoid fever and vaccines. Trans R Soc Trop Med Hyg 74:553–556, 1980.

258. Altemeir WA, Bellanti JA, Buescher EL. The IgM response of children to *Salmonella typhosa* vaccine. II. Comparison of amounts of IgM specific for the somatic, flagellar, and Vi antigens. J Immunol 103:924–930, 1969.

259. Chernokhvostova E, Luxemburg KI, Starshinova V, et al. Study on the production of IgG, IgA, and IgM antibodies to somatic antigens of *Salmonella typhi* in humans. Clin Exp Immunol 4:407–421, 1969.

260. Kumar R, Malaviya AN, Murthy RGS, et al. Immunological study of typhoid: immunoglobulins, C3, antibodies, and leukocyte migration inhibition in patients with typhoid fever and TAB-vaccinated individuals. Infect Immun 10:1219–1225, 1974.

261. Lospallato J, Miller W, Dorward B, Fink CW. The formulation of microglobulin antibodies. I. Studies on adult human. J Clin Invest 41:1415–1421, 1962.

262. May RP, Barnett JA, Sanford JP. Characterization of the antibody response to acetone-killed typhoid vaccine. Public Health Rec 82:257–259, 1967.

263. Forrest BD, LaBrooy JT, Dearlove CE, Shearman DJC. The human humoral immune response to *Salmonella typhi* Ty21a. J Infect Dis 163:336–345, 1991.

264. Sarasombath S, Banchuin N, Sukosol T, et al. Systemic and intestinal immunities after different typhoid vaccinations. Asian Pacific J Allergy Immunol 5:53–61, 1987.

265. Nisini R, Biselli R, Matricardi PM, et al. Clinical and immunological response to typhoid vaccination with parenteral or oral vaccines in two groups of 30 recruits. Vaccine 11:582–586, 1993.

266. Nath TR, Malaviya AN, Kumar R, et al. A study of the efficacy of typhoid vaccine in inducing humoral and cell-mediated immune responses in human volunteers. Clin Exp Immunol 30:38–43, 1977.

267. Rajagopalan P, Kumar R, Malaviya N. A study of humoral and cell-mediated response following typhoid vaccination in human volunteers. Clin Exp Immunol 47:275–282, 1982.

268. Szu SC, Taylor DN, Trofa AC, et al. Laboratory and preliminary clinical characterization of Vi capsular polysaccharide-protein conjugate vaccines. Infect Immun 62:4440–4444, 1994.

269. Mirza NB, Wamola IA, Estambale BA, et al. Typhim Vi vaccine against typhoid fever: a clinical trial in Kenya. East Afr Med J 72:162–164, 1995.

270. Cordero-Yap L, Rivera RG, Dispo AP, Mallabo J. Evaluation of a new Vi polysaccharide typhoid vaccine in children aged 2–5 years. BioDrugs 15(suppl 1):27, 2001.

270a. Dizer U, Gorenek L, Guner O, et al. Assessment of the antibody response in 110 healthy individuals who have been subject to Vi capsular polysaccharide vaccine. Vaccine. 20:3052–3054, 2002.

271. Klugman KP, Koornhof HJ, Robbins JB, Le Cam NN. Immunogenicity, efficacy, and serological correlate of protection of *Salmonella typhi* Vi capsular polysaccharide vaccine three years after immunization. Vaccine 14:435–438, 1996.

272. Lebacq E. Comparative tolerability and immunogenicity of Typherix or Typhim Vi in healthy adults: 0, 12-month and 0, 24-month administration. BioDrugs 15(suppl 1):5, 2001.

273. Bartholomeusz RCA, LaBrooy JT, Johnson M, et al. Gut immunity to typhoid—the immune response to a live oral typhoid vaccine, Ty21a. J Gastroenterol Hepatol 1:61–67, 1986.

274. Kantele A, Kantele JM, Arvilommi H, Makela PH. Active immunity is seen as a reduction in the cell response to oral live vaccine. Vaccine 9:428–431, 1991.

275. Cancellieri V, Fara GM. Demonstration of specific IgA in human feces after immunization with line Ty21a *Salmonella typhi* vaccine. J Infect Dis 151:482–484, 1985.

276. Kantele A, Kantele JM, Savilahti E, et al. Homing potentials of circulating lymphocytes in humans depend on the site of activation: oral, but not parenteral, typhoid vaccination induces circulating antibody-secreting cells that all bear homing receptors directing them to the gut. J Immunol 158:574–579, 1997.

277. Forrest BD. Impairment of immunogenicity of *Salmonella typhi* Ty21a due to preexisting cross-reacting intestinal antibodies. J Infect Dis 166:210–212, 1992.

278. Su-Arehawaratana P, Singharaj P, Taylor DN, et al. Safety and immunogenicity of different immunization regimens of CVD 103-HgR live oral cholera vaccine in soldiers and civilians in Thailand. J Infect Dis 165:1042–1048, 1992.

279. Attridge S. Oral immunization with *Salmonella typhi* Ty21a-based clones expressing *Vibrio cholerae* O-antigen: serum bactericidal antibody responses in man in relation to preimmunization antibody levels. Vaccine 9:877–882, 1991.

280. Forrest BD. Identification of an intestinal immune response using peripheral blood lymphocytes. Lancet 1:81–83, 1988.

281. Czerkinsky CC, Prince SJ, Michalek SM, et al. IgA antibody-producing cells in peripheral blood after ingestion of antigen: evidence for a common mucosal immune system in humans. Proc Natl Acad Sci U S A 84:2449–2553, 1987.

282. Forrest BD, Shearman DJC, LaBrooy JT. Specific immune response in humans following rectal delivery of live typhoid vaccine. Vaccine 8:209–211, 1990.

283. Murphy JR, Baqar S, Munoz C, et al. Characteristics of humoral and cellular immunity to *Salmonella typhi* in residents of typhoid-endemic and typhoid-free regions. J Infect Dis 156:1005–1009, 1987.

284. Murphy JR, Wasserman SS, Baqar S, et al. Immunity to *Salmonella typhi*: considerations relevant to measurement of cellular immunity in typhoid-endemic regions. Clin Exp Immunol 75:228–233, 1989.

285. Salerno-Goncalves R, Pasetti MF, Sztein MB. Characterization of CD8(+) effector T cell responses in volunteers immunized with *Salmonella enterica* serovar Typhi strain Ty21a typhoid vaccine. J Immunol 169:2196–2203, 2002.

286. Lundin BS, Johansson C, Svennerholm AM. Oral immunization with a *Salmonella enterica* serovar Typhi vaccine induces specific circulating mucosa-homing CD4(+) and CD8(+) T cells in humans. Infect Immun 70:5622–5627, 2002.

287. Sztein MB, Tanner MK, Polotsky Y, et al. Cytotoxic T lymphocytes after oral immunization with attenuated vaccine strains of *Salmonella typhi* in humans. J Immunol 155:3987–3993, 1995.

288. Balakrishna-Sarma VN, Malaviya AN, Kumar R, et al. Development of immune response during typhoid fever in man. Clin Exp Immunol 28:35–39, 1977.

289. Mabel TJ, Paniker CKJ. The role of cell-mediated immunity in typhoid. Asian J Infect Dis 3:69–75, 1979.

290. Mogensen HH. *Salmonella typhi*–induced stimulation of blood lymphocytes from persons with previous typhoid fever. Acta Pathol Microbiol Scand [C] 87C:41–45, 1979.

291. Nyergeo G, Ferencz A, Funk O. Development of specific cellular immunoreactivity in typhoid fever. Acta Microbiol Acad Sci Hung 26:321–324, 1979.

292. Rajagopalan P, Kumar R, Malaviya N. Immunological studies in typhoid fever. II. Cell-mediated immune responses and lymphocyte subpopulations in patients with typhoid fever. Clin Exp Immunol 47:269–274, 1982.

293. Sarasombath S, Banchuin N, Sukosal T, et al. Systemic and intestinal immunities after natural typhoid infection. J Clin Microbiol 15:1088–1093, 1987.

294. Thevanesam V, Arseculertne SN, Weliange LV, Athauda PK. Cell-mediated and humoral immune responses in human typhoid fever. Trop Geogr Med 34:13–17, 1982.

295. Cvjetanovic B. Field trial of typhoid vaccines. Am J Public Health 47:578–585, 1957.

296. Tapa S, Cvjetanovic B. Controlled field trial on the effectiveness of one and two doses of acetone-inactivated and dried typhoid vaccine. Bull World Health Organ 52:75–80, 1975.

297. Hefjec LB. Duration of postvaccination antityphoid immunity according to the results of strictly controlled field trials. J Hyg Epidemiol Microbiol Immunol 13:154–165, 1969.

298. Hefjec LB, Levina LA, Kuz'minova ML, et al. A controlled field trial to evaluate the protective capacity of a single dose of acetone-killed agar-grown and heat-killed broth-grown typhoid vaccines. Bull World Health Organ 40:903–907, 1969.

299. Yang HH, Wu CG, Xie GZ, et al. Efficacy trial of Vi polysaccharide vaccine against typhoid fever in south-western China. Bull World Health Organ 79:625–631, 2001.

300. Mehta G, Arya SC. Capsular Vi polysaccharide antigen in *Salmonella enterica* serovar Typhi isolates. J Clin Microbiol 40:1127–1128, 2002.

301. Arya SC. *Salmonella typhi* Vi antigen-negative isolates in India and prophylactic typhoid immunization. Natl Med J India 13:220, 2000.

302. Arya SC. Efficacy of Vi polysaccharide vaccine against *Salmonella typhi*. Vaccine 17:1015–1016, 1999.

303. Levine MM, Ferreccio C, Abrego P, et al. Duration of efficacy of Ty21a, attenuated *Salmonella typhi* live oral vaccine. Vaccine 17(suppl 2):S22–S27, 1999.

304. Kossaczka Z, Lin FY, Ho VA, et al. Safety and immunogenicity of Vi conjugate vaccines for typhoid fever in adults, teenagers, and 2- to 4-year-old children in Vietnam. Infect Immun 67:5806–5810, 1999.

305. Lin FYC, Ho VA, Khiem HB, et al. The efficacy of a *Salmonella Typhi* Vi conjugate vaccine in two- to-five-year-old children. N Engl J Med 344:1263–1269, 2001.

306. Marmion DE, Naylor GRE, Stewart IO. Second attacks of typhoid fever. J Hyg (Camb) 53:260–267, 1953.

307. McAnally TP, Ten Eyck RP. Influenza-like syndrome following typhoid immunization. Mil Med 149:200–201, 1984.

308. Rone JK, Friedstrom S. Severe systemic reactions to typhoid vaccination: two cases and a review of the literature. Mil Med 155:272–274, 1990.

309. Hoyt RE, Herip DS. Severe systemic reactions attributed to the acetone-inactivated parenteral typhoid vaccine. Mil Med 161:339–341, 1996.

310. Edwards EA, Johnson DP, Pierce WE, Peckinpaugh RO. Reactions and serologic responses to monovalent acetone-inactivated typhoid vaccine and heat-killed T.A.B. vaccine when given by jet-injection. Bull World Health Organ 541:501–505, 1974.

311. Goel RA. Idiopathic thrombocytopenic purpura: precipitation of relapse with T.A.B. vaccine. Indian Pediatr 18:267, 1981.

312. Tewari SA, Khan CR, Khan AS. Symptomatic thrombocytopenic purpura due to T.A.B. vaccine. J Assoc Physicians India 27:461–462, 1979.

313. Eisinger AJ, Smith JG. Acute renal failure after T.A.B. and cholera vaccination. Br Med J 1:381–382, 1979.

314. Joekes AM, Gabriel JRJ, Goggin MJ. Renal disease following prophylactic inoculation. Nephron 9:162–170, 1972.

315. Khan RI. Anaphylactoid reaction to typhoid-paratyphoid A and B vaccine. Trop Geogr Med 23:115–116, 1971.

316. Mittermayer CH. Lethal complications of typhoid-cholera-vaccination: case report and review of the literature. Beitr Path Bd 158:212–224, 1976.

317. Pounder DJ. Sudden, unexpected death following typhoid-cholera vaccination. Forensic Sci Int 24:95–98, 1984.

318. Cotterkill JA, Shapiro H. Dermatomyositis after immunization. Lancet 1:1158–1159, 1978.

319. Bowers WF, Shupe I. Acute appendicitis: sequela of typhoid inoculation. Mil Surgeon 90:413, 1942.

320. Thomson BJ, Nuki G. Erythema nodosum following typhoid vaccination. Scott Med J 30:173, 1985.

321. Miller H, Candrowski W, Schapira K. Multiple sclerosis and vaccination. Br Med J 2:210–213, 1967.

322. Kelleher PC, Kelley LR, Rickman LS. Anaphylactoid reaction after typhoid vaccination [letter]. Am J Med 89:822–824, 1990.

323. Black R, Levine MM, Young C, et al. Immunogenicity of Ty21a attenuated "*Salmonella typhi*" given with sodium bicarbonate or in enteric-coated capsules. Dev Biol Stand 53:9–14, 1983.

324. Cryz SJ Jr, Vanprapar N, Thisyakorn U, et al. Safety and immunogenicity of *Salmonella typhi* Ty21a vaccine in young Thai children. Infect Immun 61:1149–1151, 1993.

325. Olanratmanee T, Levine MM, Losonsky G, et al. Safety and immunogenicity of *Salmonella typhi* Ty21a liquid formulation vaccine in 4- to 6-year old Thai children. J Infect Dis 166:451–452, 1992.

326. Levine MM. Field trials of efficacy of attenuated *Salmonella typhi* oral vaccine Ty21a. *In* Robbins J (ed): Bacterial Vaccines. New York, Praeger, 1987.

327. Centers for Disease Control and Prevention. Typhoid immunization: recommendations of the Advisory Committee on Immunization Practices. MMWR 43:1–7, 1994.

328. Bollag U. Practical evaluation of a pilot immunization campaign against typhoid fever in a Cambodian refugee camp. Int J Epidemiol 9:121–122, 1980.

329. Sunderbruch JH. The case against typhoid immunization during flood periods. J Iowa Med Soc 55:488–489, 1965.

330. Taylor DN, Levine MM, Kuppens L, Ivanoff B. Why are typhoid vaccines not recommended for epidemic typhoid fever? J Infect Dis 180:2089–2090, 1999.

331. Hejfec LB. On the negative phase of postvaccination immunity to typhoid with reference to the results of epidemiological studies. J Hyg Epidemiol Microbiol Immunol 15:393–401, 1971.

332. Joo I. Benefit versus risk factors in cholera and typhoid immunization. Dev Biol Stand 43:47–52, 1979.

333. Topley WCC. The role of active or passive immunization in the control of enteric infection. Lancet 1:181–186, 1938.

334. Wilson GS. The Hazards of Immunization. London, Anthone Press, 1967.

335. Gotuzzo E, Frisancho O, Sanchez J, et al. Association between the acquired immunodeficiency syndrome and infection with *Salmonella typhi* or *Salmonella paratyphi* in an endemic typhoid area. Arch Intern Med 151:381–382, 1991.

336. Brachman PS Jr, Metchock B, Kozarsky PE. Effects of antimalarial chemoprophylactic agents on the viability of the Ty21a typhoid vaccine strain. Clin Infect Dis 15:1057–1058, 1992.

337. Horowitz H, Carbonaro CA. Inhibition of the *Salmonella typhi* oral vaccine strain, Ty21a, by mefloquine and chloroquine. J Infect Dis 166:1462–1464, 1992.

338. Kollaritsch H, Que JU, Kunz C, et al. Safety and immunogenicity of live oral cholera and typhoid vaccines administered alone or in combination with antimalarial drugs, oral polio vaccine, or yellow fever vaccine. J Infect Dis 175:871–875, 1997.

339. Wolfe MS. Precautions with oral live typhoid (Ty21a) vaccine [letter]. Lancet 336:631–632, 1990.

340. Faucher JF, Binder R, Missinou MA, et al. Efficacy of atovaquone/proguanil for malaria prophylaxis in children and its effect on the immunogenicity of live oral typhoid and cholera vaccines. Clin Infect Dis 35:1147–1154, 2002.

341. Clasener HAL. Immunization of man with *Salmonella* vaccine and tetanus-diphtheria vaccine: dose-response relationship, secondary response and competition of antigens. J Hyg (Camb) 65:457–466, 1967.

342. Clasener HAL, Beunders BJW. Immunization of man with typhoid and cholera vaccine: agglutinating antibodies after intracutaneous and subcutaneous injections. J Hyg (Camb) 65:449–456, 1967.

343. Cvjetanovic B, Ikic D, Lane WR, et al. Studies of combined quadruple vaccines against diphtheria, pertussis, tetanus and typhoid fever: reactogenicity and antigenicity. Bull World Health Organ 46:47–52, 1972.

344. Ambrosch F, Fritzell B, Gregor J, et al. Combined vaccination against yellow fever and typhoid fever: a comparative trial. Vaccine 12:625–628, 1994.

345. Jong EC, Kaplan KM, Eves KA, et al. An open randomized study of inactivated hepatitis A vaccine administered concomitantly with typhoid fever and yellow fever vaccines. J Travel Med 9:66–70, 2002.

346. Fritzell C, Rollin PE, Touir M, et al. Safety and immunogenicity of combined rabies and typhoid fever immunization. Vaccine 10:299–300, 1992.

347. Khoo SH, St. Clair Roberts J, Mandal BK. Safety and efficacy of combined meningococcal and typhoid vaccine. BMJ 310:908–909, 1995.

348. Van Hoecke C, Lebacq E, Beran J, et al. Concomitant vaccination against hepatitis A and typhoid fever. J Travel Med 5:116–120, 1998.

349. Beran J, Beutels M, Levie K, et al. A single dose, combined vaccine against typhoid fever and hepatitis A: consistency, immunogenicity and reactogenicity. J Travel Med 7:246–252, 2000.

350. Cryz SJ Jr, Que JU, Levine MM, et al. Safety and immunogenicity of a live oral bivalent typhoid fever (*Salmonella typhi* Ty21a)-cholera (*Vibrio cholerae* CVD 103-HgR) vaccine in healthy adults. Infect Immun 63:1336–1339, 1995.

351. Kollaritsch H, Furer E, Herzog C, et al. Randomized, double-blind placebo-controlled trial to evaluate the safety and immunogenicity of combined *Salmonella typhi* Ty21a and *Vibrio cholerae* CVD 103-HgR live oral vaccines. Infect Immun 64:1454–1457, 1996.

352. McAleer WJ, Buynak EB, Maigetter RZ, et al. Human hepatitis B vaccine from recombinant yeast. Nature 307:178–180, 1984.

353. Hilleman MR, Ellis R. Vaccines made from recombinant yeast cells. Vaccine 4:75–76, 1986.

354. Szu SC, Li X, Schneerson R, et al. Comparative immunogenicities of Vi polysaccharide-protein conjugates composed of cholera toxin or its B subunit as a carrier bound to high- or low-molecular weight Vi. Infect Immun 57:3823–3827, 1989.

355. Szu SC, Li XR, Stone AL, Robbins JB. Relation between structure and immunologic properties of the Vi capsular polysaccharide. Infect Immun 59:4555–4561, 1991.

356. Szu SC, Bystricky S, Hinojosa-Ahumada M, et al. Synthesis and some immunologic properties of an O-acetyl pectin [poly(1→ 4)-alpha-D-Gal*p*A]-protein conjugate as a vaccine for typhoid fever. Infect Immun 62:5545–5549, 1994.

357. Hindle Z, Chatfield SN, Phillimore J, et al. Characterization of *Salmonella enterica* derivatives harboring defined *aroC* and *Salmonella* pathogenicity island 2 type III secretion system (*ssaV*) mutations by immunization of healthy volunteers. Infect Immun 70:3457–3467, 2002.

358. Chatfield SN, Strahan K, Pickard D, et al. Evaluation of *Salmonella typhimurium* strains harbouring defined mutations in *htrA* and *aroA* in the murine salmonellosis model. Microb Pathog 12:145–151, 1992.

359. Pickard D, Li J, Roberts M, et al. Characterization of defined *ompR* mutants of *Salmonella typhi*: *ompR* is involved in the regulation of Vi polysaccharide expression. Infect Immun 62:3984–3993, 1994.

360. Miller SI, Loomis WP, Alpuche-Aranda C, et al. The *PhoP* virulence regulon and live oral *Salmonella* vaccines. Vaccine 11:122–125, 1993.

361. Tacket CO, Sztein MB, Wasserman SS, et al. Phase 2 clinical trial of attenuated *Salmonella enterica* serovar Typhi oral live vector vaccine CVD 908-*htrA* in U.S. volunteers. Infect Immun 68:1196–1201, 2000.

362. Kelly SM, Bosecker BA, Curtiss R III. Characterization and protective properties of attenuated mutants of *Salmonella cholerasuis*. Infect Immun 60:4881–4890, 1992.

363. Levine MM, Black RE, Lanata C, for the Chilean Typhoid Committee. Precise estimation of the numbers of chronic carriers of *Salmonella typhi* in Santiago, Chile, an endemic area. J Infect Dis 146:724–726, 1982.

364. Arricau N, Hermant D, Waxin H, et al. The RcsB-RcsC regulatory system of *Salmonella typhi* differentially modulates the expression of invasion proteins, flagellin, and Vi antigen in response to osmolarity. Mol Microbiol 29:835–850, 1998.

365. Felix A, Bhatnagar SS. Further observations on the properties of the Vi antigen of *B. typhosus* and its corresponding antibody. Br J Exp Pathol 16:422, 1935.

366. Virlogeux I, Waxin H, Ecobichon C, Popoff MY. Role of the *viaB* locus in synthesis, transport, and expression of *Salmonella typhi* Vi antigen. Microbiology 141:3039–3047, 1995.

367. Virlogeux I, Waxin H, Ecobichon C, et al. Characterization of the *rcsA* and *rcsB* genes from *Salmonella typhi*: *rcsB* through *tviA* is involved in regulation of Vi antigen synthesis. J Bacteriol 178:1691–1698, 1996.

368. Wang JY, Noriega FR, Galen JE, et al. Constitutive expression of the Vi polysaccharide capsular antigen in attenuated *Salmonella enterica* serovar Typhi oral vaccine strain CVD 909. Infect Immun 68:4647–4652, 2000.

369. Wang JY, Pasetti MF, Noriega FR, et al. Construction, genotypic and phenotypic characterization, and immunogenicity of attenuated Delta *guaBA Salmonella enterica* serovar Typhi strain CVD 915. Infect Immun 69:4734–4741, 2001.

370. Gonzalez C, Hone D, Noriega F, et al. *Salmonella typhi* vaccine strain CVD 908 expressing the circumsporozoite protein of *Plasmodium falciparum*: strain construction and safety and immunogenicity in humans. J Infect Dis 169:927–931, 1994.

371. Tacket CO, Galen J, Sztein MB, et al. Safety and immune responses to attenuated *Salmonella enterica* serovar Typhi oral live vector vaccines expressing tetanus toxin fragment C. Clin Immunol 97:146–153, 2000.

372. DiPetrillo MD, Tibbetts T, Kleanthous H, et al. Safety and immunogenicity of *phoP/phoQ*-deleted *Salmonella typhi* expressing *Helicobacter pylori* urease in adult volunteers. Vaccine 18:449–459, 1999.

373. Darji A, Guzman CA, Gerstel B, et al. Oral somatic transgene vaccination using attenuated S. *typhimurium*. Cell 91:765–775, 1997.

374. Pasetti MF, Anderson RJ, Noriega FR, et al. Attenuated ΔguaBA *Salmonella typhi* vaccine strain CVD 915 as a live vector utilizing prokaryotic or eukaryotic expression systems to deliver foreign antigens and elicit immune responses. Clin Immunol 92:76–89, 1999.

375. Bodhidatta L, Taylor DN, Thisyakorn U, Echeverria P. Control of typhoid fever in Bangkok, Thailand, by annual immunization of schoolchildren with parenteral typhoid fever. Rev Infect Dis 9:841–845, 1987.

376. Yang HH, Kilgore PE, Yang LH, et al. An outbreak of typhoid fever, Xing-An County, People's Republic of China, 1999: estimation of the field effectiveness of Vi polysaccharide typhoid vaccine. J Infect Dis 183:1775–1780, 2001.

Chapter 40

Yellow Fever Vaccine

THOMAS P. MONATH

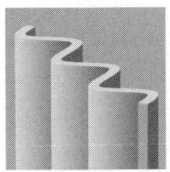

Yellow fever virus is the prototype member of the *Flavivirus* genus (from *flavus*, Latin for *yellow*), which includes 73 single-stranded RNA viruses, most of which are transmitted by mosquitoes or ticks. The disease caused by yellow fever virus is the original "viral hemorrhagic fever"—a systemic illness characterized by high viremia; hepatic, renal, and myocardial injury; hemorrhage; and high lethality. Sequence analysis of the envelope gene revealed that yellow fever virus diverged earlier than other mosquito-borne viruses from the ancestral flaviviral lineage, approximately 3000 years ago.[1]

History

The early history of yellow fever is uncertain because of the inexactness of clinical and epidemiologic descriptions. Carter[2] found the earliest record in a Mayan manuscript describing an epidemic with hematemesis (black vomit, or '*xekik*') in the Yucatan in 1648, and suggested that the virus and mosquito vector were introduced from Africa during the slave trade. The nosologic term *yellow fever* was first used in 1750 during an outbreak in Barbados.[3] Yellow fever became a major problem in the 18th century in colonial settlements in the Americas and West Africa. It was introduced repeatedly into seaports in the United States and Europe via sailing vessels infested with *Aedes aegypti* mosquitoes that sustained transmission among the crew. In 1793, for example, yellow fever appeared in Philadelphia, at the time the federal capital of the United States, killing 10% of the population.[4] Similar fates befell other cities throughout the 18th and 19th centuries.[5,6] In one of the worst medical disasters in the early history of the United States, yellow fever caused over 13,000 deaths in the lower Mississippi Valley in 1878.

Until the 20th century, yellow fever was widely believed to be an airborne "miasma" arising from filth, sewage, and rotting organic matter. Several physicians, most notably Carlos Findlay in Cuba,[7] suggested that yellow fever was transmitted by mosquitoes. Proof was not obtained until 1900, when Walter Reed and colleagues conducted experiments on human volunteers in Cuba demonstrating that the agent was a filterable virus transmitted by A. *aegypti* mosquitoes.[8] This led to successes in disease prevention through mosquito abatement during the first 20 years of this century. The last outbreak in the United States occurred in New Orleans in 1905, with 8399 cases and 908 deaths.

In 1925, the Rockefeller Foundation's West African Yellow Fever Commission laboratory in Yaba (Lagos), Nigeria, set out to determine the etiology of yellow fever, using imported monkeys for isolation of the causative agent. On June 30, 1927, the blood of a 28 year-old man named Asibi, a resident of the village of Kpeve, Ghana, that had been obtained 33 hours after the onset of mild yellow fever was inoculated into a rhesus monkey at the field laboratory in Accra. The animal was moribund 4 days later and had hepatic lesions consistent with yellow fever. Blood from this monkey was inoculated intraperitoneally into a second animal, which was transported during the incubation period to Yaba, where it developed clinical yellow fever the day after arrival. Stokes et al.[9] established the Asibi strain by continuous direct passage in monkeys and indirect passage through A. *aegypti* mosquitoes. Contemporary efforts at the Pasteur Institute in Dakar, Senegal, led to isolation of the French strain from a Syrian man (François Mayali) with mild yellow fever.[10] Isolation of the Asibi and French strains in 1927 enabled the development of vaccines, and research was initiated immediately in England, the United States, West Africa, and Brazil. Many years later, comparison of the genomes of the Asibi and French viruses confirmed that, despite differing passage histories, they were 99.8% identical at the sequence level, divergent at only 23 nucleotides and 9 amino acids.[11,12]

In 1928, Edward Hindle of the Wellcome Research Laboratories, London, described the first attempt to produce an inactivated vaccine.[13] This and subsequent efforts on inactivated yellow fever vaccines were, however, unsuccessful. In 1931, Sawyer et al.[14] at the Rockefeller Institute in New York first vaccinated humans with a live, attenuated virus (the neuroadapted French strain) mixed with immune serum. Vaccine development was spurred by a growing number of laboratory infections. In the 5 years following isolation of yellow fever virus, 32 cases (5 fatal) had occurred among laboratory workers.[15]

In 1932, Sellards and Laigret[16] tested the French mouse-brain virus without immune serum in humans, and, in 1934,

Mathis and co-workers[17] described the first field trial of this vaccine. Rejecting mouse brain tissue as a dangerous substrate, Theiler and Smith[18,19] at the Rockefeller Foundation developed a live vaccine (17D) attenuated by serial passage of the Asibi strain in cell cultures prepared from embryonated chicken eggs. In 1936, the 17D vaccine was tested in a small number of human volunteers in New York,[20] and it entered field trials in Brazil the following year.[21] By 1939, over 1 million Brazilians had received the 17D vaccine[22] and over 100,000 persons in French West Africa had received the French neurotropic vaccine (FNV).[23,24] During the 1940s, control of yellow fever at a population level was achieved in francophone Africa.[25] Immunization of laboratory workers, travelers, military personnel, and expatriate residents in endemic areas removed the threat of acquiring the disease, and the disease faded from public view, having been transformed from a major human plague to a medical curiosity by the end of World War II.

The availability of 17D—widely regarded as one of the safest and most effective viral vaccines ever developed—has not ensured adequate control of the disease. This represents a failure of public health policy and implementation of routine vaccination. In the past 15 years, there has been a resurgence of yellow fever[26,27] and a reappearance of the disease among unvaccinated tourists. Reinvasion of South America by A. aegypti (the vector responsible for interhuman transmission), the expansion of human populations in endemic regions, and increasing air travel raise concern about the reappearance of urban epidemics in the Americas, and increase the risk of introduction into Asia,[27] where yellow fever has never occurred.

Background

Clinical Description

The clinical spectrum of yellow fever is very broad, including truly subclinical infection, abortive infection with nonspecific grippe-like illness, and potentially lethal pansystemic disease with fever, jaundice, renal failure, and hemorrhage. This variability makes the clinical diagnosis of sporadic cases difficult, and is responsible for the underestimation of morbidity and inflation of case-fatality rates when only cases of full-blown yellow fever are enumerated. As for many other infections, this variability in response is due to intrinsic and acquired host resistance factors, and probably to differences in the pathogenicity of virus strains.

After an incubation period of 3 to 6 days, the onset is abrupt, with rigors and headache. The classical illness is characterized by three stages.[15,28–30] During the first "period of infection," lasting 3 to 4 days, virus is present in blood.[8,15,31] Fatal cases appear to have a longer duration of viremia than do cases in survivors. MacNamara[31] found peak viremias on day 2 to 3 of illness, with titers of up to 5.6 $\log_{10}$ mouse intracerebral median lethal dose (ICLD$_{50}$)/mL (Fig. 40–1). Nassar et al.[32] studied one patient on days 5 and 7 after onset; titers in whole blood were 4.6 and 2.7 $\log_{10}$ ICLD$_{50}$/mL, respectively.

The frequency of clinical symptoms and signs in yellow fever patients is shown in Figure 40–2. The period of infection is characterized by fever, malaise, prostration,

headache, photophobia, lumbosacral pain, pain in the lower extremities (particularly the knee joints), generalized myalgia, anorexia, nausea, vomiting, restlessness, irritability, and dizziness. On physical examination the patient appears toxic, with hyperemia of the skin; congestion of the conjunctivae, gums, and face; epigastric tenderness; and tenderness and enlargement of the liver. The tongue is characteristically small, pointed, and bright red at the tip and sides, with a white coating in the center. Early clinicians made much of this arcane sign, and it has stood the test of time. Initially the pulse rate is high, but by the second day there is a bradycardia relative to fever (Faget's sign). The average fever is 102° to 103° F and lasts 3.3 days, but temperature may rise as high as 105°F, a bad prognostic sign. Young children may experience febrile convulsions. Laboratory abnormalities include leukopenia (1.5 to 2.5 × 10^9/L) with a relative neutropenia. The leukopenia occurs precipitously, in concert with onset of illness.[15] Between 48 and 72 hours after onset, elevation of serum transaminase levels precedes the appearance of jaundice, with the levels often predicting the severity of hepatic dysfunction later in the illness.[32]

The period of infection may be followed by a distinct "period of remission" with abatement of fever and symptoms lasting up to 48 hours. The remission is often not obvious or very brief. In cases of abortive infection, the patient simply recovers at this stage. Such cases remain anicteric, and the nonspecificity of the syndrome makes it impossible to diagnose yellow fever clinically except during an epidemic. It is not known what proportion of patients infected with yellow fever virus develop truly subclinical infections versus abortive (anicteric) infection.

Approximately 15% of persons infected with yellow fever virus develop moderate or severe disease characterized by jaundice.[30,34] These patients enter the third stage of the disease, the "period of intoxication," on the third to sixth day after onset, with return of fever, relative bradycardia, nausea, vomiting, epigastric pain, jaundice, oliguria, and a hemorrhagic diathesis. Virus disappears from

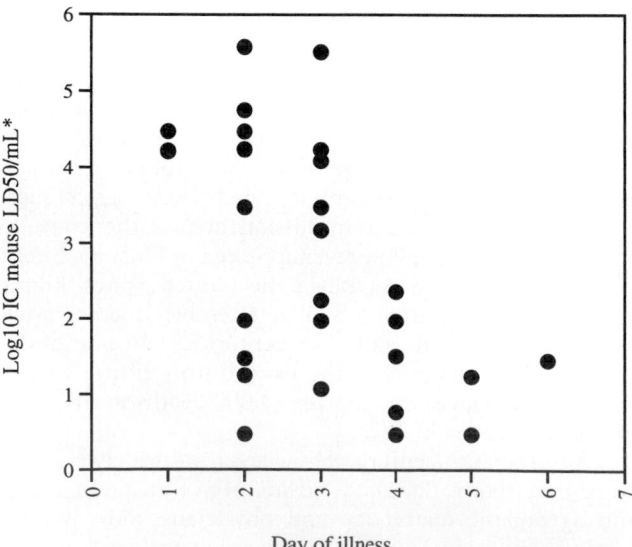

FIGURE 40–1 ■ Virus titers in blood of yellow fever patients, Nigeria, 1951 to 1953. *Minimal titer (endpoint not determined in all cases). (Data from MacNamara[31,34])

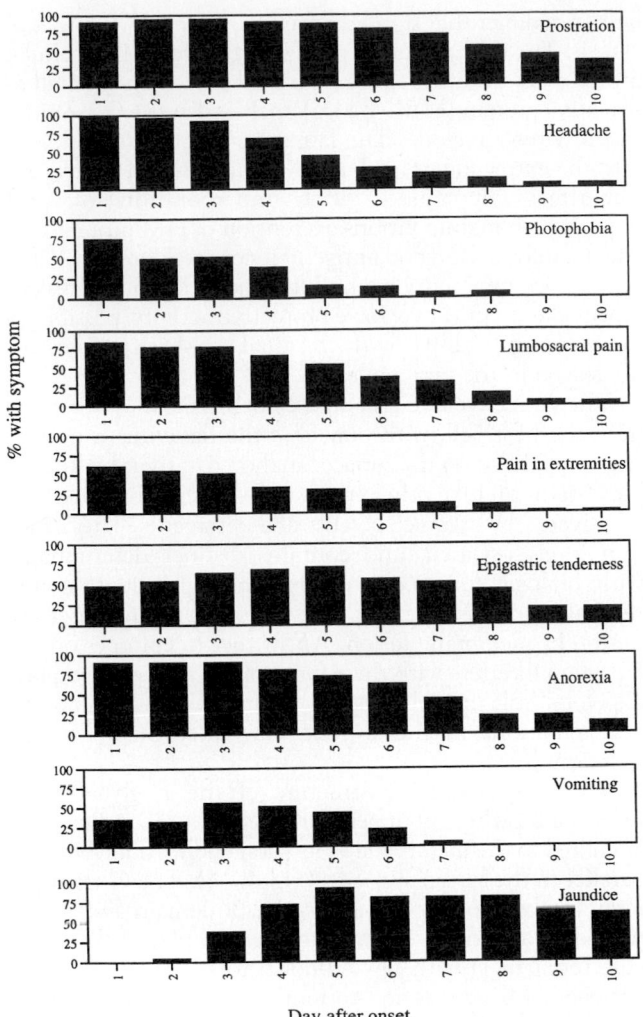

% with symptom

Prostration

Headache

Photophobia

Lumbosacral pain

Pain in extremities

Epigastric tenderness

Anorexia

Vomiting

Jaundice

Day after onset

FIGURE 40–2 ■ Proportion of cases of severe, nonfatal yellow fever with symptoms and signs by day of illness. (After Beeuwkes H. Clinical manifestations of yellow fever in the West African native as observed during four extensive epidemics of the disease in the Gold Coast and Nigeria. Trans R Soc Trop Med Hyg 1:61, 1936.)

blood and antibodies appear. The subsequent course reflects dysfunction of multiple organ systems, including the liver, kidneys, and cardiovascular system. Serum aspartate aminotransferase (AST) and alanine aminotransferase (ALT) peak early in the second week of illness and fall rapidly over a few days in patients who recover. AST levels typically exceed ALT, probably as a result of direct viral injury to myocardium and skeletal muscle or to injury of mitochondria. This distinguishes yellow fever from viral hepatitis, in which ALT levels typically exceed AST levels. Serum aminotransferase enzyme levels are proportional to disease severity. In one study, the mean AST and ALT levels in fatal cases were 2766 and 660 U, respectively, whereas in surviving patients with jaundice the mean levels were 929 and 351 U, respectively.[33] Alkaline phosphatase levels are normal or only slightly elevated. Direct bilirubin levels are typically between 5 and 10 mg/dL, with higher levels in fatal than nonfatal cases.[35]

Renal dysfunction is marked by an increase in albuminuria, reduction in urine output, and rising azotemia.

Albumin levels in the urine typically range between 3 and 5 g/L but may reach 20 g/L. Serum creatinine levels are three to eight times normal. In some patients who survive the hepatitis phase, renal failure predominates.[36] Death is preceded by virtually complete anuria. The hemorrhagic diathesis is manifested as coffee-grounds hematemesis, melena, hematuria, metrorrhagia, petechiae, ecchymoses, epistaxis, oozing of blood from the gums, and excessive bleeding at needle puncture sites. Laboratory correlates include thrombocytopenia, prolonged clotting and prothrombin times, and reductions in clotting factors synthesized by the liver (factors II, V, VII, IX, and X). Some patients have clotting abnormalities suggesting disseminated intravascular coagulation, including diminished fibrinogen and factor VIII and the presence of fibrin split products.[37,38]

The clinical significance of myocardial injury remains poorly understood. The electrocardiogram may show sinus bradycardia without conduction defects, as well as ST–T abnormalities, particularly elevated T waves, and extrasystoles,[15,39] presumably the result of virus replication and direct viral injury to the myocardium. Bradycardia may contribute to the physiologic decompensation associated with hypotension, reduced perfusion, and metabolic acidosis in severe cases. Acute cardiac enlargement may occur during the course of yellow fever infection.[15]

Central nervous system (CNS) signs include delirium, agitation, convulsions, stupor, and coma. In severe cases, the cerebrospinal fluid is under increased pressure, and may contain elevated protein but no cells. In one case, yellow fever virus was recovered from cerebrospinal fluid after death.[40] In patients dying of yellow fever, CNS signs appear to result from cerebral edema or metabolic factors, based on the virtual absence of inflammatory changes in brain tissue. Pathologic changes include petechiae (perivascular hemorrhages) and edema.[41] True yellow fever viral encephalitis is exceedingly rare, with few extant clinical case reports of paralysis, optic neuritis, and cranial nerve palsy suggesting neurologic infection, but without substantiating virologic evidence to differentiate encephalitis from encephalopathy.[42,43]

The critical phase of the illness occurs between the 5th and 10th days, at which point the patient either dies or rapidly recovers. Case-fatality rates vary widely, in part because of missed mild cases, but possibly reflect differences in virulence of viral strains. In recent investigations, the case-fatality rate in West African patients with jaundice approximated 20%.[44,45] Clinical severity and lethality of yellow fever is highest in older adults.[29,31,46–48] Events associated with a poor prognosis or imminent demise include leukocytosis, hypothermia, agitated delirium, intractable hiccups, seizures, hypoglycemia, hyperkalemia, metabolic acidosis, Cheyne-Stokes respirations, stupor, and coma.

In one series of 103 patients in Nigeria, the average stay in the hospital for surviving patients was 14 days (range 5 to 42 days) and the average duration of the acute illness was 17.8 days.[47] Although convalescence may be associated with weakness and fatigability lasting several weeks, healing of the liver and kidney is typically complete, without postnecrotic fibrosis. In some cases, jaundice and elevations in serum aminotransferases may persist for months after onset.[33,35,49] It is uncertain whether such atypical cases have had other underlying hematologic or hepatic diseases. In one study, the outcome of yellow fever in hepatitis B surface antigen–positive and –negative patients was similar.[50] Complications of yellow fever include superimposed bacterial pneumonia, parotitis, and sepsis associated with recovery from renal tubular necrosis. Late deaths during convalescence have been ascribed to myocarditis, arrhythmia, or heart failure,[48] but documentation of these events is poor.

Classification and Phylogenetic Relationships

Members of the genus *Flavivirus* are distinguished serologically by the neutralization test and were originally classified into eight antigenic complexes.[51,52] Yellow fever was found to be evolutionarily distant from other flaviviruses, as well as antigenically distinct, and did not fall within a complex. Yellow fever is also the most distantly related agent among mosquito-borne flaviviruses based on comparison of nucleotide sequences.[1,53] In a current taxonomic classification that synthesizes epidemiologic, antigenic, and genetic phylogeny, yellow fever virus is considered the type species in a complex that includes Wesselsbron, Sepik, Edge Hill, Bouboui, Uganda S, Banzi, Jugra, Saboya, and Potiskum viruses, Sepik virus being the closest relative.[54]

Virology

The principal focus here is on the molecular basis for attenuation of yellow fever 17D vaccine. For comprehensive reviews of flavivirus genome structure and replication, see Chambers and Monath[55] and Lindenbach and Rice.[56]

Genome Structure and Gene Products

Flaviviruses are small (40 to 60 nm) positive-sense, single-stranded RNA viruses. The genome of the prototype yellow fever virus contains 10,862 nucleotides, composed of a short 5' noncoding region (NCR), a single open reading frame (ORF) of 10,233 nucleotides, and a 3' NCR.[55,56] The 5' and 3' NCRs have conformational structure and interactive, complementary sequences important in cyclization of the viral genome during encapsidation and replication. The 3' and 5' NCRs function as promoters for negative and positive RNA strands, respectively, during replication, and mutations or deletions in these regions affect replication and virulence. The 3' NCR contains conserved consensus sequences (CSs) that pair with 5' NCR sequences during cyclization. The secondary structure of the 3' NCR forms pseudoknots.[57] Yellow fever virus strains have variable 3' NCR structures,[58] as discussed below (see *Geographic Variation in Virus Strains*). The ORF encodes three structural proteins at the 5' end (capsid [C], premembrane [prM], and envelope [E] proteins), followed downstream by seven nonstructural (NS) proteins. The proteins are encoded in the order C-prM-E-NS1-NS2A-NS2B-NS3-NS4A-NS4B-NS5 (Fig. 40–3). The structural proteins are included in the mature virion, whereas the NS proteins are responsible for replication and polypeptide processing. Virus proteins are cleaved after translation of the entire polyprotein at the rough endoplasmic reticulum (ER). Cell-associated virions form within the ER and are morphologically identical to extracellular particles.

The C protein (molecular weight [MW] ~11 kDa) interacts with genomic RNA to form the virion nucleocapsid. The prM glycoprotein (MW ~27 kDa) forms an intracellu-

lar heterodimer that stabilizes the E polypeptide during exocytosis. The prM protein is processed by a furin-like cellular protease before virus release from the cell, leaving a small M structural protein (MW ~8 kDa) anchored at the C-terminus in the virus envelope. The larger "pr" segment is released into the extracellular medium, although prM/M cleavage is sometimes incomplete, with incorporation of prM sequences in mature virions. Retention of prM protein may affect conformation and antigenicity of the E protein,[59] and may reduce infectivity by inhibiting acid-dependent fusion. Antibodies to prM may have protective activity, possibly by neutralizing virions with residual prM that remains uncleaved in the viral envelope.

The viral envelope is composed of a lipid bilayer derived from the host cell, with dimers of the flavivirus E protein (MW ~50 kDa) on the surface, anchored at their hydrophobic C-termini. Like other enveloped viruses, flaviviruses are inactivated by organic solvents and detergents. The E protein is glycosylated, and contains distinct determinants with biologic function, including hemagglutination and neutralization, attachment to cell receptors, and internalization by membrane fusion. Antibodies to epitopes on the E protein interfere with these functions. The E protein plays a pivotal role in cell tropism, virulence, and immunity, and mutations in the E gene may alter these biologic functions.[55,56]

The crystallographic structure of the E glycoprotein reveals a head-to-tail dimer composed of a 170 Å–long rod anchored to the membrane at its basal end with its long axis parallel to the virion surface[60] (Fig. 40–4). The C-terminus resembles an immunoglobulin constant domain and is connected by a flexible region to the central part of the molecule (domain I) with up-and-down topology having eight antiparallel β-strands and containing the N-terminus. Two

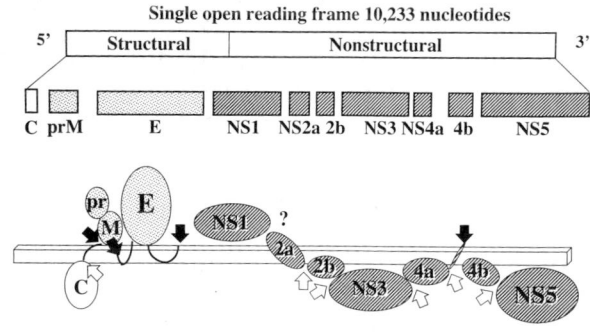

↑ Host signalase   ⇧ Ns2b/NS3 serine protease

FIGURE 40–3 ■ *Top*, Genome organization of flaviviruses, consisting of a single long open reading frame (ORF) of 10,862 nucleotides and flanking short nontranslated regions. The ORF encodes three structural genes at the 5' end (C-prM-E) and eight nonstructural genes encoding enzymes required for replication and post-translational processing of viral proteins. *Bottom*, Processing of the flavivirus proteins in relation to the endoplasmic reticular membrane in order of their synthesis, left to right. The enzymes involved in post-translational cleavage are derived from the host cell or from the viral NS2B/NS3 serine protease. (Adapted from Lindenbach BD, Rice CM. *Flaviviridae*: the viruses and their replication. *In* Knipe DM, Howley PM (eds). Fields' Virology. Vol. I. Philadelphia, Lippincott Williams & Wilkins, 2001, p 991.)

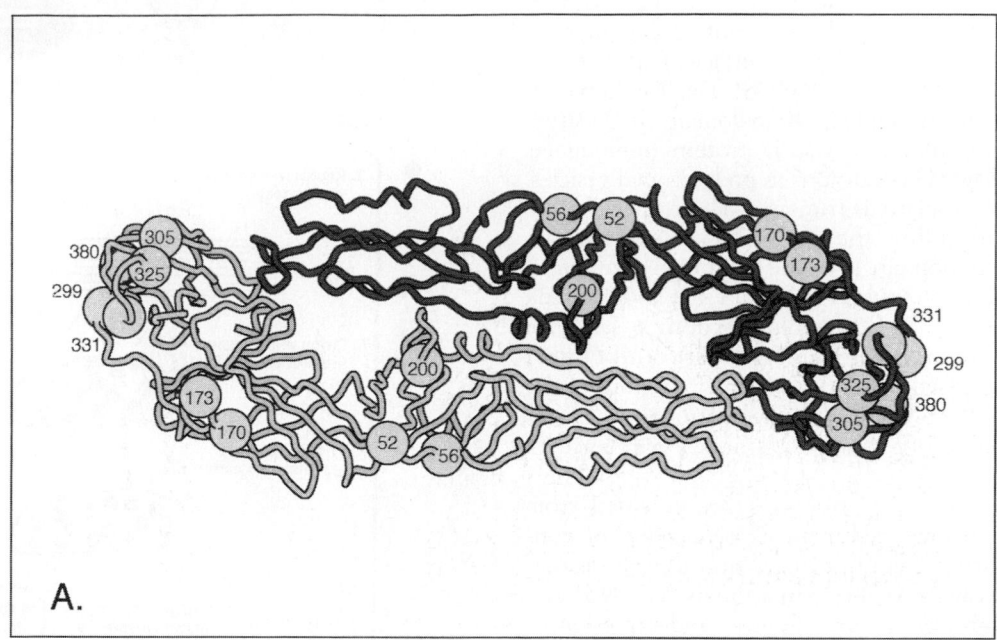

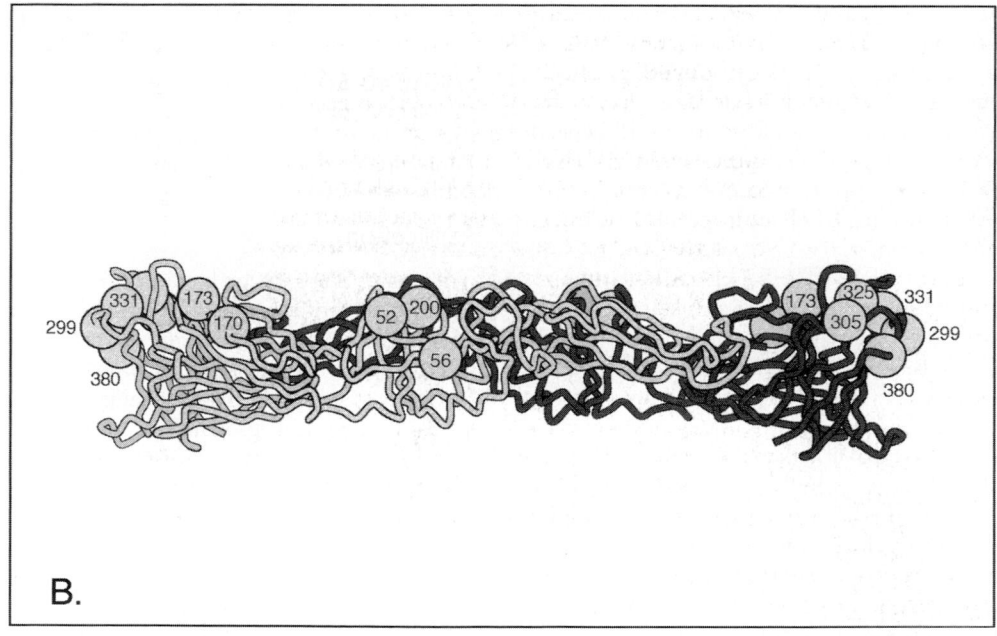

FIGURE 40–4 ■ Three-dimensional structure of the flavivirus envelope (E) glycoprotein, determined by crystallography. The E protein consists of a flat dimer parallel to the virus membrane, with each molecule having three domains. *A,* Top view of the molecule. *B,* Side view. Amino acid determinants that differ between yellow fever 17D vaccine and the parental Asibi virus are shown (circles with amino acid number); their possible functions are described in the text and in Table 40–2. (Adapted from Rey FA, Heinz FX, Mandl C, et al. The envelope glycoprotein from the tick-borne encephalitis virus at 2Å resolution. Nature 375:291, 1995; prepared by Dr. Stanley Watowich, Sealy Center for Structural Biology, based on data provided by Dr. Alan D. T. Barrett, both of the University of Texas Medical Branch, Galveston, TX.)

long loops (domain II) extending laterally are responsible for dimerization. A conserved stretch of 14 amino acids at the tip of one of the domain II loops constitutes the fusion domain responsible for internalization of nucleocapsids from endosomes into the cytoplasm of the infected cell.

Domain III contains ligands, including an RGD motif [Arg-Gly-Asp], presumptively involved in binding cell receptors. Mutations in this region of domain III often reduce infectivity and virulence. However, mutations that specifically disrupted the RGD motif–dependent integrin binding did not impair binding of the virus to insect or mammalian cells, indicating that integrin binding may not be critical to virus entry.[61] Neutralization determinants are conformational, and are scattered on the outer surface of all three flavivirus structural domains.[62,63] A CD8+ T-cell epitope has been described at position E332/340 in domain III.[64] During the early stage of infection, the E protein homodimers dissociate under low pH conditions in prelysosomal vesicles, and monomers reassociate as trimers.[65] The trimeric molecules extend outward from the virion surface, exposing the fusogenic region of domain II to the lysosomal membrane. This rearrangement is required for viral entry into the cell cytoplasm. The C-terminal membrane-spanning sequence of the E protein contains determinants that control trimer formation. As discussed below, mutations in regions of the E protein that affect low-pH conformational modifications during viral entry strongly influence virulence of flaviviruses.

Noninfectious subviral structures are released from infected cells. The slowly sedimenting hemagglutinin consists of 14-nm particles containing M and E proteins that are immunogenic and protective in animals. The NS1 glycoprotein is both released extracellularly and expressed on the surface of infected cells as a dimeric structure. The secreted form ("soluble complement-fixing" antigen) contains virus-specific and cross-reactive epitopes. Antibodies to NS1 do not neutralize virus infectivity, but provide protective immunity by complement-mediated lysis of infected cells containing NS1 on the cell surface.[66] Studies have demonstrated that NS1 is involved in flavivirus RNA replication. Mutations in the NS1 gene of yellow fever virus suppress RNA production.[67,68] NS1 interacts with NS4A and appears to control NS4A replicase activity.[69] A cytotoxic T-cell epitope also has been localized in NS1.[64]

NS2A is a small protein (MW ~22 kDa) that interacts with NS3, NS5, and 3' untranslated region sequences and appears to play an important role in RNA replication. Mutations in NS2A have been shown to impair yellow fever virus replication.[70,71] NS2A appears to play a critical role in assembly or release of virions. A dominant cytotoxic T-cell epitope has been localized at amino acid positions 110 to 118 of this protein.[64] NS3 (MW ~70 kDa) and NS2B (MW ~14 kDa) interact to form a complex with important enzymatic functions, including serine protease (responsible for post-translational cleavage of the virus polyprotein), RNA helicase, and RNA triphosphatase activities. The serine protease activity is located at the N-terminal one fourth of NS3, while the remaining three fourths contain the other enzymatic functions involved in RNA replication. Because of its critical functions, the NS3 gene sequence is highly conserved at the sequence level. The protein is also present in cell membranes, contains virus-specific T-cell epitopes, and is a target for attack by cytotoxic T cells.[64,72–74]

The NS4A (MW ~16 kDa) and NS4B (MW ~27 kDa) proteins are hydrophobic and membrane associated. Both proteins play a role in regulating RNA replication. The NS5 protein (MW ~103 kDa) is also highly conserved and functions both as the RNA-dependent RNA polymerase in virus replication and as a methyltransferase in 5' cap methylation.

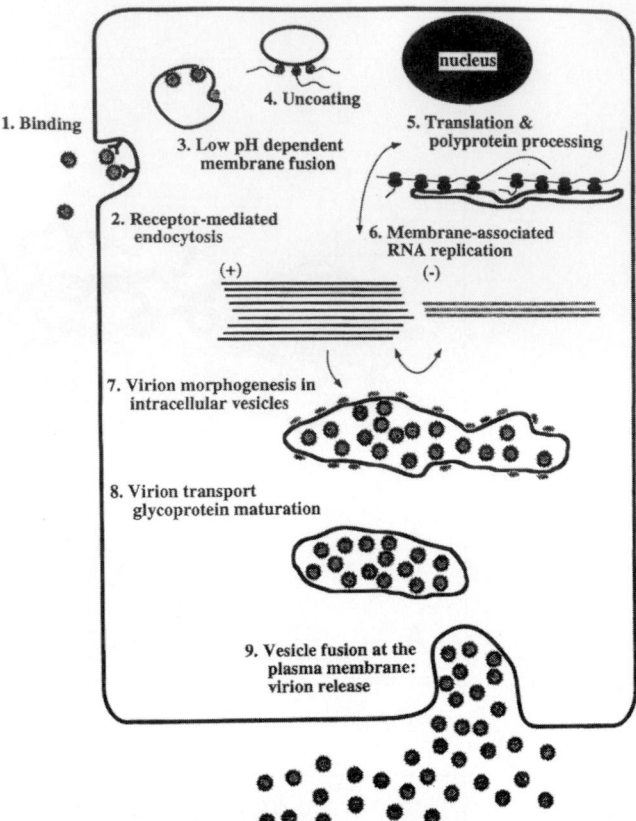

FIGURE 40–5 ■ Steps in replication cycle of flaviviruses. (From Lindenbach BD, Rice CM. *Flaviviridae*: the viruses and their replication. *In* Knipe DM, Howley PM (eds). Fields' Virology. Vol. I. Philadelphia, Lippincott Williams & Wilkins, 2001, p 991, with permission.)

Replication

The major steps in replication are shown in Figure 40–5. Flaviviruses enter cells by attachment to as-yet undefined receptors and are taken up in clathrin-coated vesicles. The nucleocapsids are released from prelysosomal vesicles into the cytoplasm by acid-mediated change in the configuration of domain II of the E protein, and fusion with the endosomal membrane. The positive-sense RNA is then translated to synthesize complementary negative RNA strands, which serve in turn as templates for progeny plus-strands. The message-sense RNA encodes replicase, helicase, and other enzymes required for continued replication; protease involved in post-translational processing; and structural proteins for virion assembly. Assembly of virus particles occurs in close association with ER. Virus particles are transported in intracellular vesicles to the plasma membrane, where they are exocytosed.

The translocation of flavivirus proteins across the ER membrane and proteolytic cleavages involved in post-translational processing of viral proteins are shown schematically in Figure 40–3. Mutations in signal sequences involved in cleavage of proteins may result in significant attenuation of infectivity and virulence.[75]

Molecular Determinants of Virulence

The entire genomes have been sequenced for the 17D and the French neurotropic vaccines and their wild-type progenitors, Asibi virus and the French viscerotropic virus.[12,76–78] Two substrains of 17D (17D-204 and 17DD) used for vaccine production and variants of 17D-204 virus (those manufactured in the United States [American Type Culture Collection, or ATCC], France, and the United Kingdom [Arilvax®; Evans Vaccines Ltd, Liverpool]; and the 17D-213 World Health Organization [WHO] vaccine seed) have also been partially or fully sequenced.[12,79–82] Because a large number of mutations occurred during the 230+ passages that separate vaccines from their parental strains, it is impossible to define those responsible for attenuation, nor is it clear which determinants encode viscerotropism and neurotropism. Sequence comparison of strains with different biologic properties has reduced the number of possibilities and allowed some educated guesses. Although some potentially important mutations have been identified, it is clear that virulence is multigenic, determined by nonstructural and structural genes of the virus. It is also important to note that nearly all studies on the molecular determinants of virulence have employed mouse models, which reveal only one of the two biologic properties of the virus (neurotropism). Hamsters were shown to be susceptible to a lethal disease with hepatic dysfunction and necrosis resembling wild-type yellow fever after infection with virus strains adapted by serial passage in hamster liver.[83,84] This model will permit dissection of the molecular determinants associated with viscerotropism (at least for the hamster).

The first comparison of nucleotide and amino acid differences between 17D-204 (ATCC) and Asibi virus was made by Hahn et al.[77] Of a total of 10,862 nucleotides, 67 changes (0.62%) were found, resulting in mutations in 31 (0.91%) of 3411 amino acids. The changes were not randomly distributed across the genome; the highest rates of change were in genes encoding E, NS2A, and NS2B and in the 3′ NCR. As additional sequences of 17D-204 and 17DD substrain vaccines became available, the number of amino acid differences between parental Asibi virus and attenuated viruses was reduced from 31 to 20, and the number of nucleotide differences in the 3′ NCR from 6 to 4 (Table 40–1).[54,55,60] Because of the functional importance of the E protein in attachment to and entry into cells, one or more of the eight amino acid differences that separate Asibi and the vaccine strains are likely to play a role in attenuation. The role of the E glycoprotein in neurovirulence of flaviviruses has been established by studies in which the E gene of a non-neurovirulent virus has been replaced by the corresponding gene of a virulent virus, resulting in a conversion to neurovirulent phenotype.[86]

Mutations in domains I, II, and III of the E protein have been associated with attenuation of flavivirus virulence. Such mutations may occur in functional regions responsible for structural changes of the protein during viral entry into cells. Studies of yellow fever and other flaviviruses have implicated three important clusters of mutations that promote attenuation, including the tip of the fusion domain (domain II), the hinge region between domains I and II, and the upper lateral surface of domain III that contains the putative receptor-binding site.[60,87] The locations of the eight amino acid differences between Asibi and 17D vaccines in the three-dimensional crystallographic structure of the E glycoprotein are shown in Figure 40–4 and Table 40–2. Four are nonconservative changes (E52 Gly→Arg; E200 Lys→Thr; E305 Ser→Phe; and E380 Thr→Arg). At

TABLE 40–1 ■ Amino Acid Differences Between Asibi Virus and Attenuated 17D Vaccines

Nucleotide	Gene	Amino Acid	Asibi	17D-204 and 17DD Vaccines
854	M	36	Leu	Phe
1127	E	52	Gly	Arg
1482		170	Ala	Val
1491		173	Thr	Ile
1572		200	Lys	Thr
1870		299	Met	Ile
1887		305	Ser	Phe
2112		380	Thr	Arg
2193		407	Ala	Val
3371	NS1	307	Ile	Val
3860	NS2A	61	Met	Val
4007		110	Thr	Ala
4022		115	Thr	Ala
4056		126	Ser	Phe
4505	NS2B	109	Ile	Leu
6023	NS3	485	Asp	Asn
6876	NS4A	146	Val	Ala
7171	NS4B	95	Ile	Met
10142	NS5	836	Glu	Lys
10338		900	Pro	Leu
10367	(3′ NCR)		U	C
10418			U	C
10800			G	A
10847			A	C

Data from Duarte dos Santos et al.[80] and Barrett.[85]

least three wild-type yellow fever strains with different passage histories or geographic origins (Asibi,[77] the French viscerotropic virus,[12] and a Peruvian strain 1899/81[88]) are identical at these amino acid residues, suggesting that the mutations in 17D play a role in attenuation.[80]

Amino acid residues E52 and E200 are located at the interface of domains I and II. Mutations in this region could affect acid-dependent conformational change in the endosome and virion internalization. Mutations at residue E52 also have been shown to attenuate another flavivirus (Japanese encephalitis) by altering virus entry into cells.[89] The conservative change at position E173 Thr→Ile corresponds to a site in tick-borne encephalitis virus at which a neutralization escape mutant had reduced neuroinvasiveness in mice[90]; mutations in this region also may interfere with the hinge function during acid-dependent fusion events.[91] Mutations in this region (residues E176/177) of yellow fever–Japanese encephalitis (YF/JE) chimeric virus also have been implicated in attenuation.[92] Neuroadaptation of yellow fever 17D virus by brain-brain passage resulted in an increase in neurovirulence of the virus and reversion (Ile→Thr) of the E173 residue.[93,94] Ryman et al. obtained further evidence for the importance of residue 173,[95] showing that it encodes an epitope recognized by wild-type specific monoclonal antibody (MAb) and that reversion at this site may have contributed to the neurovirulence phenotype of a variant [17D(wt+)] recovered from a 17D-204 vaccine. Mutations in the hinge region of Murray Valley encephalitis (MVE) also result in attenuation of neurovirulence.[96] The importance of this functional region to the viscerotropism

TABLE 40–2 ■ Location and Potential Function of Amino Acid Differences Between Asibi and 17D Vaccine Viruses in Three-Dimensional Structure of Flavivirus Envelope (E) Glycoprotein

Amino Acid	Asibi	17D	Domain	Potential Functional Role in Virulence/Attenuation
52	Gly	Arg	II	Hinge region between domains I and II; may affect fusion activation (low-pH conformational change)
170	Ala	Val	I	Outer surface of domain I, near known attenuating mutation in TBE virus
173	Thr	Ile	I	Outer surface of domain I, known attenuating mutation in TBE virus
200	Lys	Thr	II	Hinge region between domains I and II; may affect fusion activation (low-pH conformational change)
299	Met	Ile	I/III	Interface of domain I and III
305	Ser	Phe	III	External face of cell attachment domain
380	Thr	Arg	III	Cell attachment motif
407	Ala	Val	III	N-terminal part (helix I) of the stem-anchor region, role in structural integrity of E

TBE, tick-borne encephalitis.
Data from Rey et al.[60] and Mandl et al.[87]

of yellow fever virus also may be inferred from a study of an attenuated chimeric virus in which Japanese encephalitis prM-E genes were inserted into an infectious clone of 17D.[97] A reversion to the wild-type JE residue at E279 in the domain I-II interface resulted in a modest increase in neurovirulence but a significant decrease in viscerotropism for monkeys, assessed by measurement of viremia. This finding suggests that the two virulence measures of flaviviruses (neurotropism and viscerotropism) are not linked. A corollary is that the molecular determinants for mouse neurovirulence may have little relevance to viscerotropic virulence of yellow fever virus strains for humans. These observations are not surprising, because a successful human vaccine (FNV) was developed by serial passage and adaptation in mouse brains, resulting in a virus that was highly neurotropic but had lost its ability to cause hepatitis in monkeys and humans. Similarly, dengue virus adapted by passage in mouse brain was found to have reduced ability to cause systemic disease in humans.[98,99] Dissection of the 10–amino acid differences separating the parental and mouse-adapted dengue type 2 vaccine strain implicated a change from a negatively charged to a positively charged amino acid (Glu→Lys) at E126 within the hinge region of the E glycoprotein.[99,100] A separate experiment involving adaptation of dengue type 1 virus by mouse brain passage was associated with increased neurovirulence for mice and apoptotic cell death in neural cells but reduced apoptosis in human hepatocytes in culture.[101] These divergent effects on the induction of apoptosis in neural versus hepatic cells were associated with a mutation in functional regions of the genome affecting virus replication and assembly: the hinge region at E196 (Met→Val), the interface between domains I and III at E365 (Val→Ile), and two mutations in the proximal stem-anchor region (E405, Thr→Ile) and the NS3 helicase region.

In yellow fever 17D, the mutations at E299, E305, and E380 are located in domain III, which is proposed to contain the determinants involved in tropism and cell attachment. Residues E299 and 305 are located on the upper lateral surface of domain III and residue E380 is located in a highly conserved region in mosquito-borne flaviviruses implicated in cell receptor interactions and hemagglutination.[60] Changes in the cell attachment motif could alter neuro- or viscerotropism of the virus. Mutations in the

region E308/311 of tick-borne encephalitis virus resulted in significant attenuation.[87]

The change in 17D virus at residue E380 alters the sequence at the putative cell (integrin) attachment motif from Thr-Gly-Asp in Asibi virus to Arg-Gly-Asp (RGD) in 17D strains.[79] In one study of YF 17D, mutations in the RGD motif predicted to alter integrin binding did not interfere with virus replication.[61] Mutations in the RGD sequence of another flavivirus (Murray Valley encephalitis) resulted in attenuation of virulence for mice,[96,102] but the mutants were not significantly inhibited by heparin, indicating that alternate receptors (other that integrins) are responsible for interaction with virions. A mutation in tick-borne encephalitis at E384 resulted in attenuation.[103]

The mutation at position E407 in 17D virus occurs in the N-terminal part (helix I) of the stem-anchor region of the E protein. Mutations in the stem-anchor region of the protein can affect the structural integrity and spatial characteristics of the prM-E heterodimer,[104] and have been associated with attenuation of dengue,[99] Japanese encephalitis,[105] YF/JE chimeras,[92] and a tick-borne encephalitis group virus.[106] A neuroadapted strain of dengue-1 virus also contained a nonconservative mutation in the stem-anchor region (E405).[101] This region is involved in the dimer-trimer reconfiguration of the E protein during acid-induced fusogenic activity.[104,107] The potential importance of residue E305 in the attenuation phenotype of 17D vaccine was suggested by sequence analysis of virus recovered from the brain of a 3-year-old child in the United States who died of encephalitis following 17D immunization.[108] The brain virus differed from 17D vaccine at a locus in domain III located near the E305 residue (at E303 Glu→Lys), and was found to have increased neurovirulence for mice and monkeys.[109] Two other mutations (at E155 and NS4B72) were also present in the brain isolate; however, the mutation at E155 is less likely to be responsible because some attenuated vaccine strains have a wild-type residue at this locus,[79,109] and a neutralization escape mutant of 17D at E155 did not show any change in neurovirulence.[63]

The complexity of the genetic basis for virulence is underscored by studies of a 17D vaccine strain having increased neurovirulence as a result of multiple mouse-brain passages.[93,94] It has been shown repeatedly that 17D vaccine is not "fixed" with respect to neurovirulence, and that sequential mouse-brain passage of the vaccine results in increasing virulence.[110] The neuroadapted 17D virus reverted to the wild-type (Asibi) sequence at amino acid residues E52 and 173 and had other mutations, including one at the putative virulence determinant at residue E305 (Ser→Val). However, a chimera generated from an infectious clone of 17D virus and containing the E protein of the neuroadapted virus did not exhibit increased neurovirulence in the mouse model. In addition to mutations in the E gene, the neuroadapted virus also contained amino acid mutations in NS1, NS2A, NS4A, NS4B, and NS5. Introduction of all mutations in E and NS genes into the YF17D infectious clone resulted in reversion to virulence and higher viral loads in infected mice. These results illustrated the multigenic nature of virulence and suggested that one or more of the mutations in the NS proteins or the 3' noncoding region of the virus may contribute to neurovirulence. Studies with other flaviviruses have demonstrated that mutations in the NS coding region may reduce neurovirulence,[101,111] presumably by restricting the rate of viral RNA and protein production.

There are 11 amino acid changes in the nonstructural proteins of 17D viruses (see Table 40–1). One change occurs in the NS1 protein; four in NS2A; one each in NS2B, NS4A, and NS4B, and two in NS5. None of these mutations alters the hydrophobicity profile of the proteins, and thus they may not affect function. One change occurs in NS3 at residue 485, in a region of the protein with RNA helicase and triphosphatase activities involved in unwinding RNA during replication, and two mutations occur in the RNA polymerase (NS5). The latter changes may affect replication efficiency and may contribute to attenuation of 17D.

Several studies have illustrated the importance of the 3' NCR of flaviviruses to replication and virulence. The 3' NCR is divided into a proximal variable region that is variable in length among yellow fever virus strains and may contain specific repeat regions[112] and a 3' terminal region that contains a 90- to 120-nucleotide conserved region involved in folding into stem-loop secondary structure. The latter acts as a promoter for minus-strand synthesis during replication, and, depending on their location, mutations in the conserved stem-loop region may adversely affect replication.[113] Mutations or deletions in the proximal part of the conserved core region of tick-borne encephalitis virus caused attenuation without markedly perturbing replication, but when the deletions affected more distal parts of the core, replication was reduced or abolished.[114] The proximal, variable region of the 3' NCR does not appear to be critical to replication, and is tolerant of mutations and deletions. The latter may nevertheless markedly reduce virulence, a strategy used for construction of attenuated vaccines against dengue.[115] It is likely that one or more of the mutations in the 3' NCR of yellow fever 17D vaccine, which are found in the variable and the proximal conserved part of the structure, may contribute to the attenuated phenotype of the vaccine. However, the change at nucleotide 10,367 may possibly be dismissed because one 17D vaccine (Arilvax) contains a heterogeneous mixture, including the wild-type sequence.[82]

Although none of the specific differences in nonstructural genes of 17D viruses can be precisely implicated, other lines of evidence indicate the potential role in attenuation. A medium-sized plaque variant recovered from 17D-204 vaccine was shown to have reduced neurovirulence for mice.[116] A similar plaque variant purified from 17D-204 vaccine produced in South Africa had reduced mouse neurovirulence and differed from large plaque and uncloned vaccine at a single amino acid in NS5 (137 Pro→ Ser).[117] This mutation is in a region encoding the methyltransferase activity of NS5.

As pointed out above, little is known about the molecular basis of viscerotropism (the ability of wild-type yellow fever virus to replicate and damage non-neural tissue, particularly the liver), or the mutations responsible for loss of this trait in 17D vaccine. To approach this question, Wang et al.[78] compared the sequence of the French viscerotropic strain with that of the FNV, which was developed by over 100 sequential mouse-brain passages. The principal phenotypic change in FNV is loss of viscerotropism for monkeys and humans. Comparison of the parental and vaccine strains revealed 77 (0.7%) nucleotide and 35 (1%) amino acid changes scattered throughout the genome, with the highest frequency of mutations in the C, M, E, NS2A, and NS4B proteins. The large number of differences and lack of biologic data on the role of these mutations preclude speculations on the genetic basis of viscerotropism. Sequence comparison of FNV with 17DD and 17D–204 vaccines (both of which have markedly attenuated viscerotropism) revealed only two shared differences from the parental and other wild-type yellow fever viruses. These common differences, which evolved during the development of vaccine strains by completely distinct processes, were at amino acid residues in the M protein (35 Leu→Phe) and NS4B (95 Ile→Met). It is unclear which of these mutations is involved in loss of viscerotropism.

The development of a hamster model of viscerotropic yellow fever[83] provides a new approach to defining the molecular basis for viscerotropism. The model requires adaptation of wild-type virus strains by serial passage in hamsters. Asibi virus becomes virulent between the sixth and seventh hamster passage. A genomic analysis of the Asibi strain adapted to cause disease after seven hamster liver passages revealed 7 amino acid changes, 5 of which fell in the E gene at positions E27 (Gln→Trp), E28 (Asp→Gly), E155 (Asp→Ala), E323 (Lys→Arg), and E331 (Lys→Arg).[83a] Two of these changes (E323 and E331) fall within a functionally important region of the upper lateral surface of domain III involved in binding to cell receptors, and others are in the stem-anchor region. In another study, a mutation at E279 in the hinge 4 region of a YF/JE chimeric virus reduced viscerotropism of the virus in nonhuman primates,[97] demonstrating the divergent biologic properties of neuro- and viscerotropism and suggesting that mutations that occurred in the hinge region of the YF genome during derivation of 17D virus could be responsible for attenuation of viscerotropism. The Met→Lys mutation at position E279 in the YF/JE chimera, which is within the β-strand of the secondary structure, increases the net positive charge of the protein and results in a shortening of the β-strand secondary structure. Similarly, in a neuroadapted dengue type 2 vaccine, an increase in neurovirulence in mice and decrease in viscerotropism for humans also was due to a mutation from an acidic to a basic residue (Glu→Lys) at E126 within the hinge region.[99,100]

Several studies have shown that Asibi and FVV viruses lost both neurotropic and viscerotropic activities after a few passages in HeLa cells.[118,119] The HeLa-passaged virus rapidly accumulated mutations at 29 nucleotides and 10 amino acids, including 5 in the E protein, 1 in NS2A, and 3 in NS2B. The NS4B mutation (95 Ile→Met), associated with attenuation of Asibi to 17D in chicken embryo tissue and of FVV to FNV by passage in mouse brain, also appeared during HeLa cell passage, suggesting that it plays an important role in attenuation of yellow fever vaccines.[119] The changes are at E27, E155, E228, E331, and E390. A reversion at E155 was present in the virus recovered from a fatal case of postvaccinal encephalitis,[109] suggesting that this locus (possibly in concert with other mutations) may play a role in neurovirulence. Interestingly, passage of another wild-type virus (Dak1279) in HeLa cells did not result in attenuation.

Molecular Identification of Antigenic Determinants in Yellow Fever Virus and Vaccine Strains and Their Relationship to Virulence

Monoclonal antibodies recognize structurally distinct regions in the E protein of yellow fever virus,[120–126] including vaccine strain–specific epitopes, yellow fever virus–specific epitopes, and determinants cross-reactive with specific heterologous flaviviruses and with broad flavivirus group epitopes. Antibodies against vaccine strain–specific, virus-specific, and flavivirus group–reactive epitopes neutralize virus and may passively protect mice against intracerebral (IC) challenge. Interestingly, immunization with 17D virus generated MAbs that neutralized wild-type (Asibi) virus but not 17D,[120] and flavivirus group–reactive monoclonals generated after immunization with 17D,[120] Asibi,[124] or heterologous[125] flaviviruses neutralized wild-type virus. This multiplicity of neutralizing determinants helps to explain the broad protective immunity afforded by 17D vaccine against wild yellow fever virus strains, and the partial cross-protection by heterologous flaviviruses against yellow fever. Additional studies have defined epitopes that are substrain specific, differentiating 17D–204 vaccine from other yellow fever viruses, differentiating 17D–204 from 17DD vaccines, and even distinguishing between vaccines of the same substrain from different manufacturers.[125,127] Plaque-size variants purified from 17D vaccine also can be distinguished in neutralization and hemagglutination-inhibition (HI) tests.[126–128] Some monoclonals are specific for 17D and do not recognize wild-type virus.[120,129] The antigenic heterogeneity of 17D vaccine is due to the uncloned nature and different passage histories during manufacture and laboratory manipulation. At present, there is no recognized practical consequence, with respect to protective immunity, of the absence of some wild-type antigenic determinants in 17D vaccines.

Attenuation by passage of wild-type Asibi virus in HeLa cells was associated with acquisition of a vaccine-specific epitope recognized by MAb H5.[119] Gould et al.[130] identified a plaque variant in 17D vaccine that reacted with a monoclonal antibody specific for wild-type viruses and variants recovered from Asibi virus that reacted with a 17D–204 specific monoclonal, suggesting that 17D was

derived by a process of selection of subpopulations during serial passage.

Some neutralizing epitopes have been localized by sequencing escape mutants or wild-type antigenic variants recovered from 17D vaccine. An epitope at residue E173 is the only wild-type–specific antigenic determinant that has been localized[95]; as mentioned previously, this site is also a putative neurovirulence factor. A neutralization determinant in the E protein of both wild-type and 17D was identified at residues E71/72 in domain II of the E protein.[62,63] Ryman et al.[63] found an additional neutralizing epitope at either E155 or E158 in domain I. In a later analysis, Gould et al.[131] selected escape mutants from three 17D substrains with a monoclonal specific (MAb 864) for 17D–204 virus that had a number of functional activities, including neutralization, hemagglutination, and hemolytic and passive protection.[124,127,132] The escape mutants were characterized with respect to mouse neurovirulence and prM-E nucleotide sequence. One series of escape mutants had reduced neurovirulence for mice compared to the parental virus and had a Ser→Leu mutation at E325. E325 is the site of a Pro→Ser mutation that occurred in the derivation of 17D–204 from Asibi[77] but is not present in the 17DD substrain,[79] and thus is not considered to be relevant to the attenuated vaccine phenotype. In contrast, another neutralization escape mutant was neurovirulent for mice and contained an amino acid mutation at E305 (Phe→Ser), which is a conserved substitution across all 17D strains (see Table 40–1). This mutation represents a reversion to the wild-type residue at E305. The E305 and E325 residues are spatially close within domain III of the E glycoprotein and thus represent a conformational epitope[133] recognized by the MAb 864 used to generate the different escape mutants. The location of the epitope is consonant with the effector roles of antibody in blocking cell attachment and intracellular uncoating events. Clearly, this epitope also is critical to pathogenesis and neurovirulence. By Western blotting, the MAb864 recognizes both the prM and E proteins, suggesting that the E305/325 epitope is involved in the prM-E interaction during virus assembly.[59] Although an exhaustive search for neutralization and protective epitopes has not been made, it would appear that yellow fever viruses (like other flaviviruses) contain only a few (but more than one) such determinants in the E protein, which are structurally diverse. These epitopes must be conserved across wild-type strains, consistent with the broad protective activity of yellow fever vaccine against wild virus strains.

Antigenic determinants involved in cell-mediated immunity have been localized in yellow fever 17D virus, dengue virus,[73,134–137] and MVE viruses.[72,138] Yellow fever cytotoxic T lymphocyte determinants are found in the E proteins, and in multiple nonstructural proteins (NS1, NS2B, and NS3).[64] These T-cell epitopes are highly conserved, and probably contribute to the cross-protective activity of 17D vaccine against all geographic variants of wild-type yellow fever virus. In the case of yellow fever, cytotoxic T cells epitopes were found on E, NS1, NS2B, and NS3 proteins,[64] and these epitope sequences were conserved across multiple yellow fever strains. T-cell responses tend to be cross-reactive.[72,138] Cytotoxic T effector cells raised to MVE virus demonstrated significant cross-reactivity with target cells pulsed with yellow fever–derived NS3 peptides, despite the relative low sequence homology of the determinants.[139]

Pathogenesis

Virus-Cell Interactions

The first steps in infection involve the interaction of virus and host cell. Several mechanisms for cell infection have been described, including mammalian cell receptor–mediated endocytosis of yellow fever virus in clathrin-coated vesicles,[140,141] phagocytosis by monocyte-macrophages,[142,143] and fusion with the cell membrane and direct penetration as seen in mosquito cells.[143] The steps in the morphogenesis of new virions within the cell are shown diagrammatically in Figure 40–5. Yellow fever viral antigen in large amounts is found diffusely within the cytoplasm of infected cells,[144] representing accumulation of virions and viral proteins in the ER.

Pathogenesis in the Mosquito Vector

Infection of mosquitoes is initiated by ingestion of a blood meal containing a threshold concentration of virus (~3.5 $\log_{10}$/mL), resulting in infection of the midgut epithelium. The virus is released from the midgut into the hemolymph and spreads to other tissues, notably the reproductive tract and salivary glands. Seven to 10 days elapse between ingestion of virus and secretion in saliva (the so-called extrinsic incubation period [EIP]), at which point the vector is capable of transmitting virus when she refeeds on a susceptible host. Infection of reproductive tissues of the mosquito provides a mechanism for vertical transmission of yellow fever virus from the female mosquito to her progeny and from congenitally infected males to females during copulation.[145–147]

Mosquito infection is relevant to the subject of vaccines in the following ways.

Transmission of Live Vaccine Viruses. The use of a live vaccine might engender a risk of secondary spread by mosquitoes, and passage of vaccine virus could result in a reversion to a more virulent phenotype. This is unlikely for two reasons: (1) viremia following 17D vaccination is very low and below the threshold of oral infection of the vector[21,148,149] (with the proviso that viremia has not been measured in infants, who may sustain more active infections than adults, or in immunosuppressed individuals); and (2) 17D virus is poorly infectious for mosquitoes. Whitman[150] infected A. aegypti larvae with 17D virus after immersion in virus, but infected adult progeny were incapable of transmitting the virus. Bhatt et al.[151] reported that 17D vaccine virus inoculated by the intrathoracic route (thus bypassing the midgut barrier) replicated to a low level in A. aegypti and A. albopictus, but orally exposed mosquitoes contained no detectable virus after a 22-day EIP. Jennings et al.[109] showed that 45% of adult female A. aegypti that were fed on a high concentration of 17D vaccine in an artificial blood meal developed midgut infections, but no virus was detected in head tissue. In another study, only 1 of 32 A. aegypti orally exposed to 17D virus developed infection in head tissue, and none of the mosquitoes transmitted the virus.[152] Thus yellow fever 17D virus has lost its ability to be transmitted by A. aegypti, possibly as a result of an inability of the virus to cross the "midgut barrier."

At the molecular level, it has not been determined which mutations in 17D virus are responsible for restricted transmission by mosquitoes. However, it is of interest that Asibi virus passaged in HeLa cells lost mosquito competence[152] and that this change may have been associated with a mutation at NS4B.[119] In support of a role for nonstructural genes in determining mosquito competence, studies of chimeric viruses in which the prM-E genes of Japanese encephalitis,[151] West Nile, and dengue (B Johnson and BN Miller, personal communication, 2002) were inserted into a 17D infectious clone showed retention of the 17D phenotype in mosquitoes. The conclusion from these studies is that the inability to replicate efficiently in mosquitoes is determined by nonstructural genes of the virus.

Mode of Human Infection and Interaction with the Immune System. Approximately 10^3 virions are inoculated during mosquito feeding.[153] Salivary virus is deposited mainly in the extravascular tissues of the host during probing, because saliva that is injected intravascularly is apparently re-ingested by the mosquito during blood feeding.[154] Virus replication is initiated at the site of inoculation and spreads through lymphatic channels to regional lymph nodes. In the immunized host, the small inoculum would encounter antibodies in extracellular transudate and lymph. This suggests that a low level of immunity is sufficient to protect the host against disease. It is not known whether immunity is sufficient to sterilize the mosquito inoculum. However, under conditions of artificial inoculation of 17D vaccine to previously vaccinated subjects[149,155] or coadministration of vaccine viruses and immune serum,[14] sufficient virus replication occurs for a booster or primary immune response, respectively.

The expression of neutralization epitopes (determined with MAbs) may differ between yellow fever virus propagated in mosquito and mammalian cells.[125] The evolutionary and functional relevance of this observation are uncertain, but it may represent a means whereby mosquitoes infected with yellow fever virus would avoid the effects of neutralizing antibodies ingested in a blood meal. In terms of flavivirus vaccine development, host specificity of neutralization determinants suggests that certain arthropod cells may not yield effective inactivated or subunit immunogens for vertebrates.

Pathogenesis in the Vertebrate Host

Two biologic properties are inherent to all wild-type yellow fever viruses: *viscerotropism*, referring to the ability to cause viremia and to infect and damage the liver, spleen, heart, and kidneys; and *neurotropism*, the ability to infect the brain parenchyma and cause encephalitis. Wild-type yellow fever virus strains are predominantly viscerotropic in primate hosts.

Wild-type yellow fever virus has a relatively broad host range. In rodents (mice, hamsters, and guinea pigs), the virus is principally neurotropic, and the only extraneural organ showing significant virus replication is the adrenal gland.[156] Rodents develop encephalitis only after IC, intraocular, or intranasal inoculation. The time to death is typically 7 to 10 days, depending on strain and passage history (neuroadaptation). Adult mice infected by the peripheral route develop encephalitis if the blood-brain barrier is not completely developed (as in suckling mice up to 5 to 7 days of age) or is compromised by sham IC inoculation. The human correlate is the increased risk of very young human infants for neuroinvasion after vaccination with 17D vaccine, and of children for encephalitis following immunization with FNV. The basis for age-related resistance is uncertain. Zisman et al.[157] suggested that development of resistance was related to maturation of macrophages involved in yellow fever virus clearance.

Nonhuman primates and humans develop viscerotropic infections (hepatitis). Most nonhuman primate species develop viremic infections, and some New World and Asian monkeys develop lethal infections with fulminant hepatitis resembling the human disease.[158,159] Experimentally infected European hedgehogs (an insectivore) develop viscerotropic infection.[160] Tesh and colleagues developed a rodent model of viscerotropic yellow fever.[83,84] Hamsters (*Mesocricetus auratus*) sustained a viscerotropic disease resembling yellow fever when infected with wild-type virus strains that had been adapted by serial passages in hamster liver. The animals developed lethal infection characterized by high viremia, elevated serum aminotransferases, bilirubinemia, and hepatocellular necrosis and apoptosis. Adaptation of the Asibi strain also was found to be viscerotropic for hamsters after seven passages. The molecular changes associated with virus adaptation are discussed in the earlier section on *Molecular Determinants of Virulence*.

The pathophysiology of yellow fever in rhesus monkeys and humans is characterized by hepatic dysfunction, renal failure, coagulopathy, and shock[161–163]; monkeys develop a more fulminating illness than humans, lasting only 3 to 4 days. The median lethal dose (LD_{50}) of the Asibi strain in the monkey is 0.01 mouse $ICLD_{50}$, or approximately 0.2 Vero cell plaque-forming units (PFU). Higher virus doses shorten the incubation period but do not alter the duration or outcome of illness[164] (Table 40–3), implying that innate immune responses (e.g., natural killer [NK] cells) are insufficient to clear even a minimal infection. The susceptibility of human peripheral blood mononuclear cells to infection, and evidence from experimental animals,[162,163] suggest that lymphoid cells are important targets for early replication. After intraperitoneal inoculation of rhesus monkeys, Kupffer's cells in the liver were infected first (24 hours after inoculation). Virus was detectable on day 2 in serum and kidney and on day 3 in

bone marrow, spleen, and lymph nodes.[162] Early injury to Kupffer's cells also was noted after subcutaneous infection of monkeys.[163,165] Infection and degeneration of hepatocytes is a relatively late event, occurring in the last 24 to 48 hours before death in the monkey[162,163] and in the last phase of infection in humans. In fatal human cases, 5% to 100% (mean, 80%) of hepatocytes undergo coagulative necrosis.[166] The midzone of the liver lobule is principally affected, with sparing of cells bordering the central vein and portal tracts. The reason for this peculiar distribution of hepatic injury is unknown. Midzonal necrosis has been described in low-flow hypoxia, as a result of ATP depletion and oxidative stress of marginally oxygenated cells at the border between anoxic and normoxic cells,[167] and a similar mechanism might contribute to injury in yellow fever infection. However, yellow fever virus antigen and RNA have been observed principally in hepatocytes in the midzone,[168] suggesting a predilection of these cells to virus replication. Injury to hepatocytes is characterized by eosinophilic degeneration with condensed nuclear chromatin (Councilman's bodies), rather than by ballooning and rarefaction necrosis seen in virus hepatitis.[169]

The morphologic features suggest that chromatin fragmentation and apoptosis of Kupffer cells and liver cells are induced by yellow fever virus and are responsible for the characteristic eosinophilic degeneration of liver cells (Councilman's bodies). Apoptosis has been confirmed in liver tissue of fatal human cases of dengue hemorrhagic fever[170] and in dengue- and yellow fever–induced cell death of human hepatocyte cells in culture.[171,172] These viruses activate the transcription factor NF-κB, which in turn induces apoptosis. Induction by yellow fever virus is delayed compared to dengue, with induction of higher grade cytopathology before cell death occurs.[172] The apoptotic mode of cell death, rather than ballooning necrosis, may explain the virtual absence of inflammation in tissues affected by yellow fever. Other hepatic changes associated with yellow fever infection of the liver include microvesicular fat and ceroid/lipofuchsin deposits, and intranuclear (Torres) bodies. Because little inflammation occurs, the reticulin framework is preserved and complete healing occurs without residual fibrosis.

Renal pathology also is characterized by eosinophilic degeneration and fatty change of renal tubular epithelium without inflammation. These changes may represent

TABLE 40–3 ■ Experimental Yellow Fever in the Rhesus Monkey: Effect of Virus Dose on Incubation Period and Duration of Illness

Subcutaneous Dose (MICLD$_{50}$*)	Mortality (%)	Hours (mean)		
		Incubation Period	Duration of Illness	Time of Death
1000	100	60	40	100
10	100	67	44	111
1	100	90	40	130
0.1	100	186	43	224
0.01	67	182	39.5	222
0.001	0	—	—	—

*Mouse intracerebral median lethal dose.
Data from Spertzl RO, Kosch PC, Gilbertson SH, et al. Annual Progress Report. Fort Detrick, MD, U.S. Army Medical Research Institute of Infectious Diseases, 1972. Similar results were obtained in early studies (see Hindle[382]).

late-stage injury following shock. In monkeys, oliguria with maintenance of tubular function indicated prerenal failure associated with hypotension and the hepatorenal syndrome; acute tubular necrosis was a terminal event.[163] Yellow fever antigen was found in renal tubular cells of fatal human cases,[173] suggesting that direct viral injury is responsible. Glomerular lesions (Schiff-positive changes in basement membrane[174] and degeneration of cells lining Bowman's capsule) and yellow fever antigen in glomerulae 2 to 3 days after infection of monkeys (TP Monath, unpublished observations) have been observed, implying that direct viral injury accounts for the albuminuria observed in advance of renal failure.

Lymphocytic elements in the germinal centers of spleen, lymph nodes, tonsils, and Peyer's patches are depleted, and large mononuclear or histiocytic cells accumulate in the splenic follicles.[163,175] Necrosis of germinal centers is more striking in monkeys than in humans. It is unknown to what extent the lymphoid injury is the direct result of virus replication.

In addition to hepatic and renal dysfunction, the disease is characterized by hemorrhage and circulatory collapse. Decreased synthesis of vitamin K–dependent coagulation factors by the liver, and disseminated intravascular coagulation, contribute to the bleeding diathesis.[38,161] Platelet dysfunction, demonstrated by collagen- and ADP-stimulated aggregation, has been demonstrated in the monkey model (S Fisher-Hoch, J McCormick, and TP Monath, unpublished observations).

Direct virus injury to myocardial fibers, which show cloudy swelling and fatty changes[176,177] and viral antigen,[173] may contribute to shock. It is tempting to speculate that the circulatory shock seen in the terminal stage of yellow fever is mediated by cytokine dysregulation, as in the sepsis syndrome. Tumor necrosis factor-α (TNF-α) produced by infected/activated Kupffer's cells and splenic macrophages in response to virus injury might, together with interleukin (IL)-1, interferon-γ, platelet activating factor, and other cytokines, be responsible for cell injury, oxygen free radical formation, endothelial damage and microthrombosis, disseminated intravascular coagulation, tissue anoxia, oliguria, and shock. Patients dying of yellow fever show cerebral edema at autopsy, probably the result of microvascular dysfunction.

Immunopathologic Events

Neutralizing antibodies appear within 4 to 5 days after onset of natural infection with yellow fever virus (i.e., 7 to 8 days after infection).[15] Antibody and (presumably) cellular responses occur coincident with the clinical crisis ("period of intoxication"), and both free virions and hemagglutinating, complement-fixing (CF), or immunoprecipitating antigen[162,178] may be found in blood together with antibody at this time, suggesting that immune clearance of infected cells, associated with release of cytokines, might play a role in the pathogenesis of capillary leak and shock. Although there is no direct evidence to support the notion of an immunopathologic mechanism in acute yellow fever infection, this is an area for future investigation. In an artificial model, administration of MAbs to mice challenged intracerebrally with yellow fever virus caused enhanced perivascular inflammation and accelerated

death.[179,180] There is no known correlate of this phenomenon in humans.

Host Factors Affecting Susceptibility

Young age increases susceptibility to neuroinvasion of yellow fever vaccine strains. In some outbreaks, infection with viscerotropic strains was more lethal in infants than in older children,[46] and in adults over 50 than in younger persons.[29,31,46–48] Genetic determinants are known to affect the pathogenesis of flavivirus infections, and resistance to yellow fever virus in mice is determined by an autosomal dominant allele (*Flv*[r]).[181] Genetic background has been shown also to influence the immune response to flaviviruses in mice.[182] The role of genetic factors in human responses to yellow fever infection is uncertain. The older literature makes repeated reference to racial differences in the lethality of yellow fever, rates being lower in blacks than whites during outbreaks in West Africa,[46] tropical America,[183] and the United States.[184] It is uncertain whether the apparent increased resistance of blacks reflects acquired immunity or is due to genetic factors. Moreover, epidemics of yellow fever in Africa have been associated with high case-fatality rates. The question of racial differences in susceptibility to yellow fever will be resolved only by well-controlled epidemiologic and serologic studies in the setting of an outbreak affecting both races. In the case of the related flavivirus dengue, whites had a higher incidence of dengue hemorrhagic fever (DHF) than persons of the black race during an epidemic in Cuba, a finding that could not be explained on the basis of a racial difference in the background of immunity.[185,186] An association between human leukocyte antigen (HLA) haplotype and disease severity was found in patients with DHF.[187] It is unknown whether genetic factors associated with race determine the infection:illness ratio or a different degree of severity after appearance of symptoms. An anecdote of some interest with regard to genetic susceptibility is the report of two cases within a single family of the very rare severe viscerotropic syndrome following vaccination with 17DD vaccine in Brazil (unpublished data, Ministry of Health, Brazil).

Virus-Specified Factors

Wild-type yellow fever virus strains in Africa and South America have been classified into at least seven genotypes based on sequence analysis (see *Geographic Distribution* below), and there is microheterogeneity at the sequence level among strains within these groupings.[188] Because single mutations can affect the biologic behavior of yellow fever virus, it is not surprising that wild-type yellow fever virus strains differ with respect to neurovirulence for mice[189–191] or viscerotropism for monkeys.[192] Variation in virulence may explain differences in mortality rates observed in human epidemics, which have ranged from 3% to 20% in various outbreaks.[159] Despite the probable importance of virus-specified factors in pathogenesis of yellow fever, they remain poorly understood. Deubel et al.[193] found that South American strains were neuroinvasive for 8-day-old mice, whereas African viruses were not, and suggested that the higher case-fatality rates in South America could be due to strain differences in virulence. South American YF strains were more virulent than African strains in a neotropical primate, *Callithrix jacchus*.[156] In contrast, it was the impression of early workers that the South American viruses were less often lethal for rhesus monkeys.[156] Miller et al.[194] showed that the mosquito responsible for epidemic transmission in Nigeria had a low vector capacity, and proposed that the vector served as a genetic bottleneck for selection of a virulent virus strain able to elicit high viremias in humans.

Innate and Adaptive Immune Responses

Innate Immune Responses

NK cells and interferons appear during the early phase of virus replication, prior to the advent of virus-specific cytotoxic T cells and immunoglobulin. Sabin[195] demonstrated in humans that inoculation of dengue virus simultaneously or shortly after inoculation of yellow fever 17D vaccine delayed the onset and ameliorated dengue illness. Interference between yellow fever and an unrelated orbivirus, presumably mediated by innate immune responses, was demonstrated in a mouse model.[196] Monkeys given yellow fever 17D vaccine and challenged with virulent virus 1 to 3 days later (prior to the appearance of antibodies) were partially protected.[197] These interference phenomena were not due to adaptive immunity, and may have been mediated by interferons, other cytokines, NK cells, or other host resistance factors.

Peripheral blood mononuclear cells from yellow fever vaccinees demonstrated cytotoxicity against uninfected K562 cell targets, consistent with NK cell activity.[198] In vitro replication of yellow fever is inhibited by type I interferons, but yellow fever virus is 250 times less sensitive than vesicular stomatitis virus and more than 500 times less sensitive than alphaviruses (P Canonico, unpublished data). Nevertheless, monkeys treated with a potent inducer of interferon-γ [poly(I)-poly(C)] developed modestly elevated serum interferon levels and were protected against lethal yellow fever infection.[199] Vaccination of humans with 17D virus results a serum interferon response (Fig. 40–6). During the early phase of infection with 17D virus, elevated levels of the interferon-dependent enzyme 2′,5′-oligoadenylate

synthetase were found in T and B cells.[200] Because interferon appears shortly after viremia and may be effective if given shortly after infection,[201] it could play a role in recovery from natural infection.

Interferon-γ activates nonspecific antiviral host defense mechanisms, including NK cells and macrophages. Interferon-γ enhances antiviral activity of type I interferons, up-regulates major histocompatibility complex (MHC) classes I and II, Th1-dependent immunoglobulin G (IgG) 2a synthesis, and cytotoxic T cell activity. Dengue infection is characterized by activation of CD4$^+$ T cells that secrete interferon-γ,[202,203] and it is likely that interferon-γ exerts important immunoregulation in yellow fever. Administration of interferon-γ to monkeys inhibited yellow fever viremia and hepatic necrosis.[204] Interferon-γ knockout mice demonstrated deficient yellow fever viral clearance and reduced numbers of inflammatory cells after intracerebral inoculation, compared to parental mice.[205] A direct antiviral effect of interferon-γ also has been postulated.[206]

In addition to interferons, other proinflammatory cytokines and markers of T-cell activation have been measured in human subjects receiving yellow fever vaccine. Elevated levels of TNF-α, IL–1Ra,[207,208] neopterin and β_2-microglobulin, and circulating CD8$^+$ T cells, indicating T-cell activation, have been found during the early, viremic period following vaccination.[209]

Adaptive Immunity

Infection with yellow fever virus or vaccine is followed by a rapid specific immune response (see *Immune Responses* below). Neutralizing antibodies, cytolytic antibodies against viral proteins on the surface of infected cells, antibody-dependent cell-mediated cytotoxicity (ADCC) and cytotoxic T cells are presumed to mediate clearance of primary infection. However, there are few data on responses other than humoral immunity in yellow fever.

The humoral response to wild-type yellow fever virus is characterized by the appearance of immunoglobulin M (IgM) antibodies during the first week of illness.[210–212] IgM levels peak during the second week after onset and decline rapidly over 30 to 60 days. The magnitude of the IgM response in cases of primary yellow fever infection is significantly greater than in patients with prior flavivirus exposure, in whom the ratio of IgM to IgG is low. Antibodies with biologic activity (HI and neutralization) appear rapidly, typically by the fifth day of illness.[15,213,214] However, HI and neutralizing antibody responses are not linked in all cases, reflecting different HI and neutralization antigenic determinants on the viral envelope.[215] HI antibodies peak between 30 and 60 days after infection, and a significant decline in titer occurs during the succeeding 6 months. Neutralizing antibodies persist for many years, if not lifelong, after natural yellow fever infection, and provide complete protection against disease on re-exposure to the virus. Neutralizing antibodies have been documented as long as 78 years after illness.[216,217] No documented case of a second clinical yellow fever infection has been reported. CF antibodies appear during the second week after onset, rise during the convalescent period, and decline between 4 and 12 months after onset.

Antibody responses following primary yellow fever are specific for yellow fever antigen. Specificity declines with affinity maturation, and cross-reactions with related

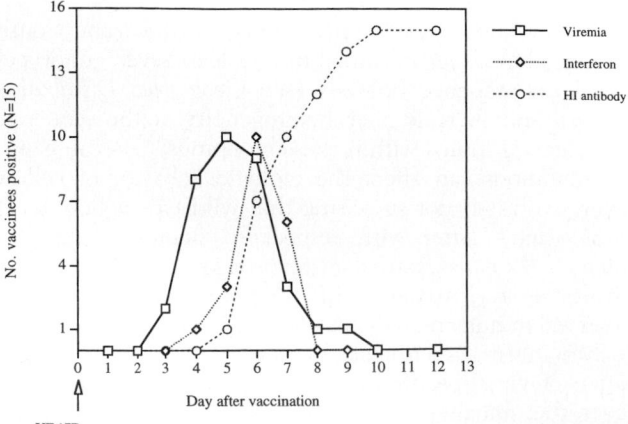

FIGURE 40–6 ▪ Circulating virus, interferon, and hemagglutination-inhibiting (HI) antibodies in adults inoculated with yellow fever 17D vaccine. (Modified from Wheelock EF, Sibley WA. Circulating virus, interferon and antibody after vaccination with the 17-D strain of yellow-fever virus. N Engl J Med 273:194–198, 1965.)

flaviviruses appear during the second week after onset.[213] Individuals with prior heterologous flavivirus immunity develop broadly cross-reactive antibody responses. The specificity of the immune response differs with the test used, with the HI test being least specific, CF being intermediate, and neutralization being most specific. The IgM antibody-capture enzyme-linked immunosorbent assay (ELISA) is specific in cases of primary infection, but cross-reactions develop over time and in cases with prior flavivirus experience. Because of the lower sensitivity of the indirect fluorescent antibody test, IgM antibodies were specific in patients with secondary infections.[212]

Cross-Protection

Previous infection with some flaviviruses may ameliorate the clinical severity of yellow fever. As early as 1923, dengue immunity was suggested as the basis for resistance to yellow fever in long-term residents of endemic areas,[218–220] and was later proposed as a barrier to introduction of yellow fever into Asia.[221–223] Early experiments indicated that passive transfer of dengue antibodies did not protect monkeys against challenge with yellow fever virus.[218] In contrast, monkeys *actively* immunized with dengue were relatively resistant to challenge with yellow fever virus, suggesting that cellular immunity played a role in cross-protection.[224] Monkeys actively immunized with two African flaviviruses (Zika and Wesselsbron), but not with West Nile or Banzi viruses, resisted challenge with yellow fever virus.[225] Humans with prior flavivirus immunity had a lower risk of severe disease during an epidemic than did individuals with primary yellow fever.[44] In another retrospective analysis in Ecuador, prior immunity to dengue appeared to reduce the clinical severity of yellow fever (R Izurieta et al., unpublished results, 2001).

There are very limited data on cross-protection or immune enhancement of dengue induced by yellow fever immunity (see *Antibody-Dependent Enhancement* below). Confirmation is a matter of considerable importance because dengue encroaches on the yellow fever–endemic region in the Americas. The hypothetical suggestion has been made that prior yellow fever immunization could enhance dengue infections, leading to an increased incidence of DHF/shock syndrome.[226]

Cross-protection is dependent on the virus causing primary infection, the interval between primary and secondary infection, and quantitative and qualitative aspects of the heterologous immune response. The importance of prior flavivirus immunity in vaccination is considered below in the section on *Immune Responses*.

Protein and Epitope Specificity and Functionality of Antibody Responses to Yellow Fever

The E protein of yellow fever viruses (and other flaviviruses) contains antigenic determinants responsible for neutralization and cytotoxic T-cell responses, and thus plays the principal role in protective immunity. This was demonstrated by active immunization of mice with recombinant vaccinia virus expressing the E protein[227] and by passive immunization of mice with anti-E Mabs.[131,228] Yellow fever–neutralizing epitopes are conformational (composed of discontinuous peptide sequences).[133,229] Yellow fever virus contains redundant neutralizing determinants, some

of which are conserved across strains.[62,63,132] Three discrete neutralization epitopes mapped at the genomic level by sequencing escape mutants are found at E71/72 [recognized by MAb 2E10), E155 (recognized by MAb B39), and E305/325 (recognized by MAb 864)]. The composite polyclonal immune response is therefore capable of protecting against multiple strains of virus that may differ at one (or several) but not all epitopes. This antigenic structure probably underlies the efficacy of vaccination with a single yellow fever strain (17D) against wild-type strains of yellow fever virus. Although vaccine and wild strains vary at other epitopes and neutralization titers in persons receiving 17D vaccine are higher against the homologous (vaccine virus) than against wild strains, antigenic conservation of neutralization epitopes is sufficient to ensure vaccine efficacy.

Neutralization is presumed to occur both as an extracellular event (in which antibody bound to virus interferes with virion attachment to as-yet undefined cell receptors) and intracellularly. Intracellular neutralization is mediated by antibodies inhibiting acid-dependent fusion of virions to the endosomal membrane, thus preventing release of viral RNA into the cytoplasm.[229] The importance of the Fc domain of neutralizing antibody was demonstrated by comparing the in vitro and in vivo activities of F(ab')$_2$ fragments of monoclonal antibodies.[230] F(ab')$_2$ fragments neutralized strongly in vitro but did not protect against yellow fever virus infection, whereas the full IgG molecule was protective. Presumably, the mediator of protection is complement or Fc-mediated ADCC, but alteration in reactivity of the hypervariable domain with antigenic determinants also could be involved.

Although the humoral immune responses to nonstructural yellow fever proteins have not been elucidated in human infections, their role has been partially explored experimentally. The NS1 protein is present in the cytoplasm and on the surface of infected cells, is secreted from infected cells, and contains determinants that elicit CF antibodies. MAb analysis of NS1 revealed the presence of both type-specific and cross-reactive epitopes, which are principally conformation dependent.[231] Mice and monkeys actively immunized with native or recombinant NS1 were protected against lethal yellow fever in the absence of neutralizing antibody,[232–234] the principal correlate of protection being complement-mediated cytolytic antibodies. Passive transfer of MAbs against NS1 having high CF activity, but not antibodies with low or no CF activity, afforded protection.[235] These studies suggested that antibodies recognizing cell membrane–bound NS1 may promote viral clearance by sensitizing infected cells to complement-mediated cytolysis. An intact Fc portion of the immunoglobulin molecule is required for protection by anti-NS1,[230,236] and antibody isotype-dependent differences in protective activities have been demonstrated.[57,235] The mechanism of protection by anti-NS1 and the role of Fc receptor–dependent effector functions, including CF, remain uncertain. Natural infection with yellow fever virus is associated with the presence of soluble CF antigen (NS1) in blood during the acute phase of infection[162] and is followed by strong CF antibody responses (presumably directed against NS1). However, because CF antibody responses occur late after infection, and vaccination with 17D virus does not induce a CF antibody response,[237,238] it is uncertain to what extent anti-NS1 plays a role in vivo in recovery or protection. Further studies in humans are needed to define the kinetics of the anti-NS1 response after natural infection and artificial immunization. There are no data on antibody responses to other nonstructural proteins of yellow fever.

Cytotoxic T cell epitopes have been localized in the E, NS1, NS2B, and NS3 proteins of yellow fever 17D and are conserved across wild-type strains.[64]

Antibody-Dependent Enhancement

Antibody-dependent enhancement of flavivirus replication in monocyte-macrophages has been demonstrated in vitro for a number of flaviviruses, including yellow fever. Schlesinger and Brandriss[239,240] demonstrated enhanced growth of yellow fever virus in U-937 cells in the presence of serum IgG from human subjects previously immunized with 17D vaccine. MAbs with yellow fever type-specific or flavivirus group reactivity also enhanced yellow fever infection in murine macrophage (P388D1) cells. Enhancement is typically mediated by non-neutralizing antibody-virus complexes that attach to cells via Fcγ type I or II receptors or complement receptors and increase virus internalization.[241–243] However, enhancement in macrophage-like cells occurred in the presence of neutralizing antibody, suggesting that cells bearing Fcγ receptors may facilitate infection after inoculation of yellow fever virus into an immune host, whereas other cells bearing other virus receptors are protected.[240] Active replication of immune complexes may explain the observation that persons re-immunized with 17D vaccine may develop increases in serum antibodies.[155,244]

Immune enhancement is believed to play a role in the pathogenesis of DHF in patients with non-neutralizing antibodies from a previous dengue infection who are infected with a new dengue serotype. The evidence for in vivo enhancement mediated by yellow fever antibodies is mixed. In one study, human volunteers previously immunized with yellow fever 17D had increased immune responses to live dengue-2 vaccine, possibly as a result of antibody-mediated enhancement of dengue virus replication[245,246] or rapid expansion of group-reactive memory T- and B-cell clones. An intriguing observation in a study of a live chimeric YF/JE vaccine in yellow fever–immune and nonimmune subjects was a tendency toward higher viremias in the immune subjects, suggesting the possibility of immune enhancement.[155] The effect was slight, but the sample size small. The chimeric virus system provides an ideal setting to test the immune enhancement hypothesis in humans.

There is no evidence that yellow fever vaccination increases the risk of DHF. This is a question of immense importance because dengue viruses are encroaching on yellow fever–endemic areas in South America, where routine 17D vaccination is performed. In one example, dengue type 4 struck Boa Vista (in the yellow fever–endemic Amazon region) in the early 1980s without the appearance of severe disease[247] although dengue type 4 is not a common cause of DHF. A watchful eye should be cast on the future epidemiology and clinical presentation of dengue as epidemics occur in areas where yellow fever vaccination is practiced, and serologic studies on individual cases of DHF should be performed to define the role of prior yellow fever immunity. In the case of Japanese encephalitis, pre-existing

immunity did not increase viremia following yellow fever 17D vaccination.[149]

Cellular Immunity

Little is known about the cellular responses to yellow fever. Only four human subjects vaccinated with 17D have been studied to date,[64] and there are no data on subjects infected with wild-type virus. Other data are drawn from studies on dengue.

Cytotoxic T lymphocytes mediate killing of flavivirus-infected cells and are an important effector mechanism of viral clearance during primary infection.[248] The kinetics of cytotoxic T cells with antiviral activity appear to be very rapid, occurring during the first 5 days after infection, and precede the appearance of antibodies.[246] In the mouse model of yellow fever encephalitis after direct IC challenge, studies with T- and B-cell knockouts have implicated both CD4+ cells and antibody as critical mediators of protection.[205] The protective role of CD4+ T cells may depend on their contribution to cytotoxic activity, antibody synthesis, or interferon-γ. Van der Most et al.[250] found interferon-γ–positive CD8+ T-cell frequencies of 1 in 700 in BALB/c mice immunized with a yellow fever/dengue chimeric virus. Depletion studies demonstrated that both CD4+ and CD8+ T cells were responsible for protection of mice immunized with the chimeric virus against dengue challenge.

Human dengue infection virus is associated with the appearance of activated peripheral blood mononuclear cells that proliferate on stimulation with dengue antigens. Both MHC class II restricted CD4+CD8− T-cell clones and class I restricted CD4−CD8+ T-cell clones from dengue immune donors have cytotoxic activities.[137,251,252] The majority of the T-cell clones studied target epitopes in nonstructural proteins, particularly NS3, and demonstrate both type specificity and various patterns of cross-reactivity. CD8+ T-cell reactive epitopes in the prM, E, NS3, and NS1-2A proteins also have been identified.[136,253]

Co et al.[64] studied the T-cell responses in four human subjects vaccinated with 17D. All four subjects responded by lymphoproliferation, cytotoxic T-cell, and interferon-γ ELISPOT assays. Antigen-specific responses by interferon-γ ELISPOT assay were observed at the earliest time point studied (14 days) and were detectable at 19 months after vaccination. CD8+ T-cell lines were established, the majority of which were HLA B35 restricted. CD8+ T-cell epitopes were recognized in viral proteins E, NS1, NS2B, and NS3. T-cell frequencies specific for these epitopes were in the range of 10^{-4}.

In persons with prior flavivirus experience, memory T helper and B cells reactive to specific and cross-reactive antigenic determinants contribute to the rapid anamnestic antibody response.

Diagnosis

The isolated case of yellow fever obviously presents a more difficult diagnostic challenge than a cluster of similar cases.[254] The pathognomonic picture of bi- or triphasic acute illness, conjunctival injection, the characteristic appearance of the tongue, jaundice, relative bradycardia, leukopenia, albuminuria, oliguria, and black vomit in an unvaccinated patient with a history of residence in or recent travel to a yellow fever–endemic zone presents little difficulty in clinical differentiation, but, in many patients, this full array of clinical signs is not present. Leptospirosis (Weil's syndrome) and louse-borne (*Borrelia recurrentis*) relapsing fever—characterized by jaundice, hemorrhage, disseminated intravascular coagulation, and a high case-fatality rate—closely resemble yellow fever.[122,193] Other diseases that must be differentiated clinically from yellow fever include viral hepatitis (especially hepatitis E in pregnancy and delta hepatitis), Q fever, West Nile virus hepatitis, Rift Valley fever, typhoid, and malaria. Malaria (blackwater fever) is usually distinguishable by the absence of proteinuria. Marburg disease, Ebola virus disease, DHF, and Lassa, Bolivian, Argentine, and Crimean-Congo hemorrhagic fevers are not usually associated with jaundice but may cause confusion. Mild yellow fever may resemble many other arboviral infections and influenza characterized by fever, headache, malaise, and myalgias.

Specific laboratory diagnosis is made by detection of virus or viral antigen in blood or by serology. Virus is readily isolated from blood during the first 4 days after onset, but isolations as late as 12 days or longer are recorded.[255] Of 90 cases confirmed during a yellow fever outbreak in the Ivory Coast in 1982, 27 (30%) were diagnosed by virus isolation from blood; all but 2 virus-positive patients were in the pre-icteric stage.[256] The virus also may be recovered from postmortem liver tissue.

Virus isolation is accomplished by intracerebral inoculation of suckling mice, intrathoracic inoculation of *Toxorhynchites* mosquitoes, or inoculation of cell cultures. Suckling mice develop encephalitis 7 to 14 days after inoculation; a virus-specific diagnosis may be made by immunofluorescence on impression slides of brain tissue or by serologic methods. Viral antigen is detected by immunofluorescence in head-squash preparations of inoculated mosquitoes after an incubation period of 10 to 12 days. *Aedes pseudoscutellaris* (AP61) cells are more sensitive than other in vitro methods for primary isolation of yellow fever virus,[257,258] and show cytopathic effects within 5 to 7 days after inoculation and viral antigen detectable by immunofluorescence in advance of cytopathic effects (e.g., day 3 after inoculation). *Aedes albopictus* (C6/36) cells, *Toxorhynchites amboinensis* cells, and mammalian cells (e.g., Vero, SW13) may be used, particularly if combined with reverse transcriptase–polymerase chain reaction (RT-PCR) or detection of viral antigen. RT-PCR employing primers spanning a conserved region of the E gene and a digoxigenin-labeled probe detected 10 PFU in cell cultures infected with most, but not all, strains of yellow fever virus.[259] RT-PCR has been used to detect the viral genome in clinical samples that were negative by virus isolation.[260] An analysis of viremia following 17D vaccination utilized a sensitive, semi-nested PCR and optimized procedures for serum sample processing.[209] The sensitivity of the method was 1.15 PFU/mL. Viral RNA was detectable in serum by this method when samples were negative by plaque assay in porcine kidney (PS) cells. Inspection of the time course of the viremia by RT-PCR suggested that the assay was able to detect infectious virus below the threshold of detection by plaquing. RT-PCR is coming into use as a routine rapid diagnostic tool for yellow fever, as illustrated in a recent case in a traveler.[261] The RT-PCR method requires further field testing but undoubtedly will gain acceptance for rapid identification of virus in original samples or early after inoculation of AP61 cells.

Rapid, early diagnosis is also possible by measurement of yellow fever antigen in serum by immunoassay.[258,262,263] The sensitivity of the assay for detection of virus in serum is approximately 3 $\log_{10}$ PFU/0.1 mL, significantly lower than that of RT-PCR. Under field conditions, antigen detection ELISA had a sensitivity of 69% and specificity of 100% compared to virus isolation in AP61 cell culture.[258] Samples for RT-PCR and ELISA do not need to be handled in a way that preserves infectivity; specimens also may be inactivated intentionally as a safety precaution where the diagnosis of dangerous pathogens (e.g., other viral hemorrhagic fevers) is considered.

Examination of the liver reveals the typical pathoanatomic features of yellow fever, including midzonal necrosis. *Liver biopsy during the illness should* never *be performed because fatal hemorrhage may ensue.* Histopathologic diagnosis may be difficult in patients who die after the second week of illness. Electron microscopy may reveal typical flavivirus particles in intracellular vacuoles.[264] Definitive postmortem diagnosis may be made by immunocytochemical staining for yellow fever antigen in the liver, heart, or kidney,[108,172,265,266] even in specimens stored for years at ambient temperature. The distribution of virus in the liver is midzonal, suggesting that hepatocytes bordering the central veins and portal tracts undergo less active virus replication. The viral genome also may be detected in formalin-fixed embedded tissues by RNA-RNA hybridization,[168] and it may be possible to utilize RT-PCR techniques to obtain yellow fever sequences from historical materials for epidemiologic and evolutionary studies.

Although older serologic methods for diagnosis (HI, CF, indirect immunofluorescence, and neutralization tests) are useful,[212–214] they have been replaced by the IgM-capture ELISA. The presence of IgM antibodies in a single sample provides a presumptive diagnosis, and confirmation is made by a rise in titer between paired acute and convalescent samples or a fall in titer between early and late convalescent samples. The specificity of the IgM ELISA is high in primary infections and in many cases of secondary infection.[211] However, cross-reactions complicate the diagnosis of yellow fever by all serologic methods, particularly in Africa, where multiple flaviviruses co-circulate. The phenomenon of "original antigenic sin" complicates flavivirus serologic investigations. Individuals with prior heterologous infection who develop yellow fever may have higher responses to the original virus, and those with prior yellow fever infection/vaccination who are subsequently infected with another flavivirus may have higher responses to yellow fever.[267]

Treatment

The management of patients with yellow fever has not been optimized because the disease occurs in remote areas with rudimentary medical services. An old saw, that may well be true, is that a patient with yellow fever (in the period of intoxication) does poorly with the stresses of being transported to the hospital, and it was long believed that it is better to treat a patient in situ. The fragility of patients with this disease should be considered in cases where long-range medical evacuation is contemplated.

An expert panel[30] recommended supportive care, including maintenance of nutrition and prevention of hypoglycemia; nasogastric suction to prevent gastric distention and aspiration; treatment of hypotension by fluid replacement and, if necessary, vasoactive drugs; administration of oxygen; correction of metabolic acidosis; treatment of bleeding with fresh frozen plasma; dialysis if indicated by renal failure; and treatment of secondary infections with antibiotics. Use of heparin to reverse disseminated intravascular coagulation is reserved for cases with documented consumption of clotting factors and activation of fibrinolytic mechanisms.

Antiserum to yellow fever produced in horses, monkeys, or chimpanzees protected rhesus monkeys against lethal yellow fever when given 1 to 3 days after challenge.[268,269] In contrast, treatment by administration of immune serum or by cross-circulation from an immune donor animal after clinical onset of yellow fever had no therapeutic effect.[270] There is little clinical experience in passive immunotherapy; in one case, mouse monoclonal neutralizing antibody was given as a "last resort" to a yellow fever patient in late-stage hepatorenal failure without any beneficial effect.[261] It is unlikely that antibody would be useful except in the setting of postexposure prophylaxis when given before onset of clinical disease.

Orthotopic liver transplantation would appear to be a viable clinical intervention in fulminant hepatitis caused by yellow fever. Because the patient is likely to have or to rapidly mount an effective immune response, it is unlikely that the transplanted liver would be adversely affected, but antibody could be administered at the time of transplantation. Another possible intervention is the use of extracorporeal support systems, such as the Molecular Adsorbent Recirculating System (MARS). The monkey model could be used to determine the feasibility of transplantation and of extracorporeal support systems.

Evidence for apoptotic cell death in yellow fever should stimulate clinical research on apoptosis mediators, including measurements of soluble Fas, Fas ligand, and TNF receptor. Ultimately it may be possible to inhibit apoptosis and spare liver injury. A role for endotoxin in shock and liver injury in yellow fever was suggested, based on the global damage to the reticuloendothelial system and the presence of lesions in the Peyer's patches of experimentally infected monkeys.[163] Therapeutic interventions based on this hypothesis have not been investigated.

Interferons have been investigated for the prevention and treatment of yellow fever in monkeys. Animals receiving 3.0 mg/kg of the interferon inducer poly (I)-poly(C) intravenously 8 hours before or 8 hours after challenge had low viremias and were significantly protected (71% to 75% survival) compared to untreated controls (0% survival), but those treated 24 hours after challenge were not protected.[199] Interferon-γ administered to monkeys 24 hours in advance of challenge and at daily intervals for 4 days reduced yellow fever viremia and significantly delayed hepatic dysfunction and death.[204] The requirement to administer interferons before infection or during the incubation period precludes their clinical use. In an individual with known exposure (e.g., in the case of an unimmunized laboratory worker with accidental infection), early postexposure prophylaxis with interferon-α, preferably with immune plasma, would be indicated.

Antiviral activity against yellow fever has been demonstrated in vivo for a number of nucleosides and plant-derived alkaloids.[271–273] Ribavirin is active against yellow fever virus in vitro, but at concentrations that are too high (9 to 10 mg/mL) for safe and effective treatment in vivo. Monkeys treated with ribavirin were not significantly protected against dengue[274] or yellow fever challenge (G Tignor, unpublished results, 1990), but dose and formulation may not have been optimized. In a mouse model of flavivirus encephalitis, ribavirin was ineffective (possibly because of its inability to cross the blood-brain barrier), whereas the prodrug ribavirin 2',3',5'-triacetate, showed antiviral activity.[275] Synergistic effects of ribavirin and related compounds, such as tiazofurin and selenazole, have been demonstrated in vitro but not investigated in vivo. A number of other nucleosides, including analogues of 6-azauridine, as well as natural plant alkaloids have shown in vitro activity but have not been tested in animals.[30]

Epidemiology*

Geographic Distribution

Yellow fever occurs in tropical South America and sub-Saharan Africa, where the enzootic transmission cycle involves tree hole–breeding mosquitoes and nonhuman primates. A detailed comprehension of the geography of yellow fever activity is critical to the proper utilization of yellow fever vaccine, in terms of both public health policy and protection of persons at risk of exposure during international travel. Yellow fever is one of three quarantinable diseases subject to International Health Regulations (the others are plague and cholera).

The first map of endemic regions—based on yellow fever immunity surveys conducted 50 to 60 years ago[276,277]—was prepared by the International Quarantine Commission and published by the United Nations Relief and Rehabilitation Administration (UNRRA) in 1946. This map has been modified from time to time based on new information[26,278,279] (the present version is shown in Fig. 40–7) but is still not an accurate reflection of yellow fever activity. The surveys on which it is based are out of date, and some areas (e.g., Somalia, Tanzania) are included based on scanty serologic data without there ever having been a notified human case. The artificial nature of the maps is emphasized by the demarcation along entire national borders and latitude lines.

Information on current yellow fever activity is published in the WHO's *Weekly Epidemiological Record* (WER), and by the Centers for Disease Control and Prevention (CDC), Division of Quarantine. Annual or biannual summaries of morbidity and epidemiologic trends also are published in the *WER*.[280–282] Current information also can be found on the CDC's Traveler's Health home page (*www.cdc.gov/travel/index.htm*). Although these materials have limitations,

---

*More extensive reviews of yellow fever epidemiology and ecology may be found in references 159 and 335 through 339.

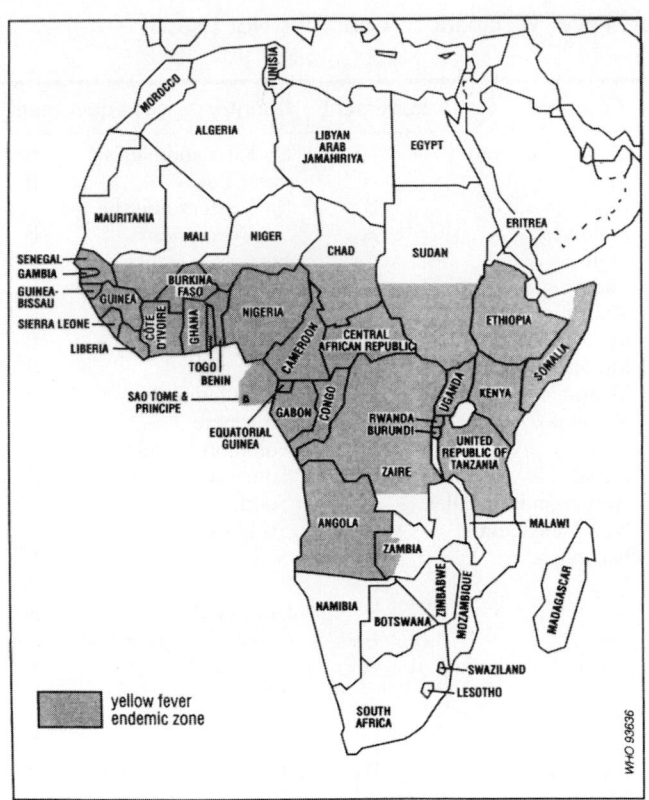
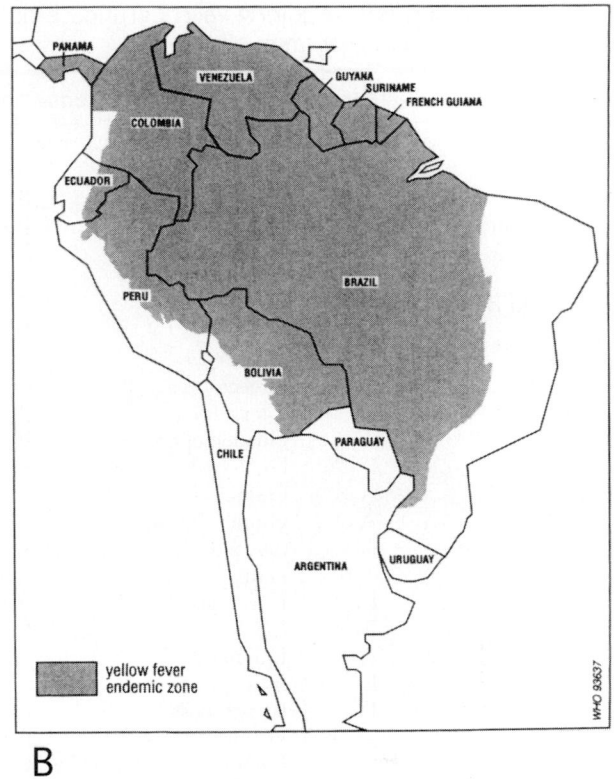

FIGURE 40–7 ■ Regions (*shaded*) of Africa and South America considered endemic for yellow fever. (Adapted from World Health Organization. International Travel and Health: Vaccination Requirements and Health Advice. Geneva, World Health Organization, 2002.)

they provide a picture of current "hot spots" of yellow fever activity. The user should keep in mind that endemic (and even epidemic) yellow fever occurs in areas that are silent with respect to official reports.

Most countries in receptive areas (in which yellow fever does not exist but where presence of the domiciliary vector, A. aegypti, would permit its development if introduced) require a valid yellow fever immunization certificate for entry from a yellow fever–endemic region. A current (2002) listing of receptive countries that require a valid certificate is provided in Monath et al.[212] and Theiler and Casals[213] and Table 40–4.

Areas at highest risk for introduction and secondary spread by A. aegypti are in the Americas, and include coastal regions and interior towns infested by this vector in Argentina, Brazil, Peru, Bolivia, Ecuador, Venezuela, Colombia, the Guianas, western Panama, Central America, the West Indies, Mexico, and the southern United States— areas historically affected by yellow fever in the past. Trinidad, Central America, and Mexico also have the capacity to sustain enzootic and epizootic transmission (jungle yellow fever). Between 1948 and 1954, the virus swept northward from Panama to Mexico in this fashion, causing multiple human outbreaks.[283] Jungle yellow fever has intermittently appeared on the island of Trinidad (e.g., 1954, 1959, 1978) with long silent interepidemic periods.[284]

Aedes aegypti–infested regions of southern Europe, the Middle East, Asia, Australia, and Oceania are also at risk of introduction of yellow fever. The virus has never been

recorded in India or other parts of Asia. The possible reasons for its absence include both demographic and biologic factors.[223] The most likely mode of introduction of yellow fever from endemic areas to Asia is by air travel of viremic humans, and all receptive areas can be reached by air from an endemic region within less than the incubation period of yellow fever.[27] However, yellow fever occurs in remote areas and affects individuals engaged in subsistence farming, who are infrequent international travelers. Biologic factors that limit the risk of introduction include cross-protection, principally by dengue, against which nearly all persons residing in Asia are immune. A third hypothesis is that A. aegypti strains in Asia have low vector competence for yellow fever virus.[285,286] It is likely that all three mechanisms combine to reduce the likelihood of introduction and spread of yellow fever virus in Asia.

Geographic Variation in Virus Strains

At least seven distinct genotypes have been found by sequencing wild-type yellow fever virus strains of different geographic origin. The database includes the entire genome sequences of the Asibi[63] and French viscerotropic[65] viruses (Ghana and Senegal, 1927), a 1979 Trinidad strain,[287] and a strain from the Ivory Coast,[288] and partial sequences of the prM-E genes, the 5′ and 3′ termini, and the NS4A-NS4B region of multiple isolates from South America and Africa isolated over a 60-year period.[58,88,188,289–294] These studies support the concept that yellow fever virus arose in Africa, with divergence of West and East African genotypes prior

TABLE 40–4 ▪ Countries Requiring Valid Certificate of Yellow Fever Vaccination (Countries Not Listed Have No Requirements for Immunization)

Country	Requirement	Country	Requirement	Country	Requirement	Country	Requirement
Afghanistan	A	Equatorial Guinea	A	Madagascar	J	St. Kitts and Nevis	B
Albania	B	Eritrea	A	Malawi	A	Saint Lucia	B
Algeria	B	Ethiopia	B	Malaysia	B†	St. Vincent and the	
American Samoa	B	Fiji	B*	Maldives	A	Grenadines	B
Angola	B	French Guiana	E	Mali	E	Samoa	B
Anguilla	B	French Polynesia	B	Malta	D*	Sao Tome and Principe	E
Antigua and Barbuda	B	Gabon	E	Mauritania	K	Saudi Arabia	L
Australia	C	Gambia	B	Mauritius	B†	Senegal	B
Bahamas	B	Ghana	H	Mozambique	B	Seychelles	C
Bangladesh	A*†	Greece	G	Myanmar	B	Sierra Leone	A
Barbados	B	Grenada	B	Namibia	B†	Singapore	C
Belize	A	Guadeloupe	B	Nauru	B	Solomon Islands	A
Benin	E	Guatemala	B	Nepal	A	Somalia	A
Bhutan	A	Guinea	B	Netherlands Antilles	G	South Africa	B†
Bolivia	A, F*	Guinea-Bissau	B*†	New Caledonia	B	Sri Lanka	B
Brazil	D*†	Guyana	A*†	Nicaragua	B	Sudan	B†
Brunei	C	Haiti	A	Niger	E	Suriname	A
Burkina Faso	E	Honduras	A	Nigeria	B	Swaziland	A
Burundi	B	India	I*	Niue	B	Syrian Arab Republic	A
Cambodia	A	Indonesia	A†	Oman	A	Tanzania	B†
Cameroon	E	Iraq	A	Pakistan	G*	Thailand	B†
Cape Verde	B*	Ivory Coast	E	Palau	B	Togo	E
Central African		Jamaica	B	Panama	F*	Tonga	B
Republic	E	Jordan	B	Papua New Guinea	B	Trinidad and Tobago	B
Chad	E	Kazakhstan	A	Paraguay	A*	Tunisia	B
China	A	Kenya	B	Peru	G, F*	Uganda	B
Colombia	F*	Kiribati	B	Philippines	B	Vietnam	B
Congo	E	Lao People's Democratic		Pitcairn	B	Yemen	B
Djibouti	B	Republic	A	Portugal (Azores and		Zaire	E
Dominica	B	Lebanon	A	Madeira only)	B*	Zimbabwe	A
Ecuador	B	Lesotho	A	Reunion	B		
Egypt	B*†	Liberia	E	Rwanda	E		
El Salvador	G	Libya	A	Saint Helena	B		

*See World Health Organization[279] for additional details regarding requirements from this country.
†Also includes travelers entering country from a country within the endemic zone.
A, Travelers entering country from infected area; B, travelers over 1 year of age entering country from infected area; C, travelers over 1 year of age who have been in or have been in transit through an infected area within 6 days (infected area is a country containing an area within the endemic zone); D, travelers over 9 months of age entering country from infected area; E, travelers over 1 year of age entering country; F, travelers going to specified sections of the country; G, travelers over 6 months of age entering country from infected area; H, all travelers entering country; I, travelers over 6 months of age who have been in or been in transit in an infected country; J, travelers who have been in or been intransit in an infected country; K, travelers over 1 year of age entering country except travelers arriving from a noninfected country and staying less than 2 weeks; L, all travelers from countries any part of which is infected.
Modified from World Health Organization. International Travel and Health: Vaccination Requirements and Health Advice. Geneva, World Health Organization, 2002.

to introduction of the virus into the Americas. The yellow fever virus genome has been relatively conserved, presumably because of restrictions imposed by host range. In a comparison of African strains belonging to five distinct genotypes, nucleotide substitutions varied from 0% to 25.8% and amino acid substitutions from 0% to 9.1%.[292] Yellow fever strains in Africa fall into five genotypes, West African type I (represented mainly by strains from western areas of the region, e.g., Nigeria) and genotype II (represented mainly by strains from the East, e.g., Senegal, Guinea-Bissau); the East/Central Africa genotype (Central African Republic, Ethiopia, Sudan, Zaire, Uganda); the East Africa genotype (Uganda, Kenya); and the Angola genotype (represented by a single strain from the 1971 outbreak). During a period of intense virus activity in 1987, West Africa I was active in the region in western Ivory Coast, Burkina Faso, Nigeria, and Cameroon, while West Africa genotype II circulated in eastern Ivory Coast, Senegal, Mali, and Mauritania. South American viruses fall into two phylogenetic groups with respect to the E, NS4A-NS4B, and 3′ NCR sequences.[58] The length of the 3′ NCR varied across genotypes based on the number of yellow fever–specific repeat sequences (RYFs). The West African I and II genotype viruses had three RYFs while the South American genotypes had a single RYF, and the Central/East Africa genotype had two RYFs. These data suggest that the ancestral yellow fever virus in Africa diverged into multiple genotypes before introduction of the virus into the New World (putatively from West Africa).[58,287] In contrast to the situation in Africa, one genotype is restricted to Peru and Bolivia and the other is found in all parts of tropical South America (JE Bryant and ADT Barrett, personal communication, 2002). The relatively high genetic stability of yellow fever viruses compared to many other RNA viruses is critical to the effectiveness of a single virus strain (17D) as a vaccine.

By cross-absorption with polyclonal antisera, African and New World yellow fever viruses can be distinguished serologically.[295] Slight differences were discerned between East and West African strains.[296] Wild-type strains vary with respect to reactivities with MAbs[127] but have not been classified as to geographic origin or genotype.[193]

Incidence

In Endemic/Epidemic Areas

Reviews of yellow fever epidemic activity in the intervals from 1950 to 1990 and from 1985 to 1994 are available in Monath[297] and Robertson et al.,[26] respectively. During the 15-year interval from 1985 to 1999, 25,846 cases and 7118 deaths were reported to the WHO (Table 40–5). The decade between 1986 and 1995 reflected a dramatic increase compared to previous and subsequent reporting intervals. In Africa, which accounted for 22,952 cases (89%), the annual incidence varied between 0 and 5000 cases, suggesting inconsistency of accurate reporting (Table 40–5, Fig. 40–8). Africa reported 5357 deaths, for a case-fatality rate of 23%. The frequency and intensity of epidemics in Africa are due to interhuman transmission by mosquito vectors present in high-density and high-human populations with low immunization coverage. In South America, yellow fever occurs in the Amazon region and contiguous areas. Between 1985 and 1999, 2894 cases and 1761 deaths were reported to the WHO (mean, 193 cases; range, 88 to 515 cases per year) (Table 40–5, Fig. 40–8). The annual incidence varies by country as a result of fluctuating epizootic activity. The lower incidence of yellow fever in South America than in Africa is due to transmission by enzootic vectors (principally from monkey to human), low densities of vectors, monkeys and human hosts, and relatively high vaccination coverage. The higher case-fatality rate (61%) in South America probably reflects surveillance based on death reports and the postmortem examination of livers, although it remains possible that the South American genotype(s) are more virulent than those in Africa.[193]

The recent resurgence of yellow fever is due to a series of epidemics in West Africa, particularly in Nigeria between 1986 and 1991.[45,298] Smaller outbreaks also have occurred in Benin (1996–1997), Cameroon (1990), the Ivory Coast (2001), Gabon (1994–95), Ghana (1993–94, 1996), Guinea (2001), Liberia (1995, 1998, 2000–01), Nigeria (1994–95), and Senegal (1995–96, 2002). In 1992, an epidemic was recognized in East Africa (Kenya) for the first time in 26 years.[299–301] In South America, Peru experienced an increased number of cases in the late 1980s and in 1995, reflecting the relatively low vaccine coverage in that country (between 30% and 50% of the at-risk population[302]) and migrations of nonimmunized laborers into forested regions. In 1995, the number of jungle yellow fever cases in Peru (492 cases, 192 deaths[280]) was the highest on record for any country in South America since 1927 (the earliest year for which statistics are available). An increase in the number of cases in Brazil in

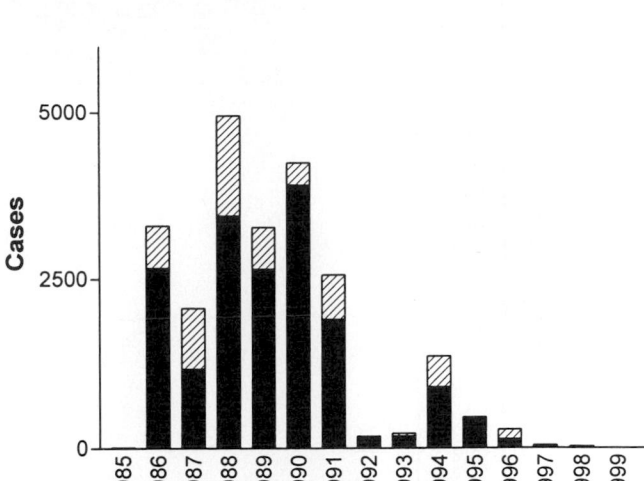

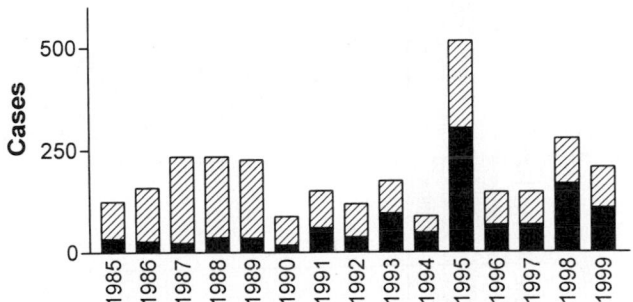

FIGURE 40–8 ■ Annual incidence of yellow fever cases and deaths in Africa and South America notified to the World Health Organization, 1985 through 1999. Note the difference in scale. The years 1986 through 1991 represented a period of major epidemic activity in Africa, and 1995 through 1999 a period of increased virus activity in South America.

1998 to 2000, and extensions of virus activity around Brasilia and into São Paulo, Goias, eastern Minas Gerais, and Santa Catarina states, prompted mass vaccination campaigns. Closer inspection of the fluctuations of yellow fever activity by country reveals only partial synchrony, indicating that epizootic waves occur as localized events (Fig. 40–9).[281] Increased virus transmission occurs with a periodicity of 7 to 10 years, in part because immunologically susceptible monkey populations are replenished at a slow rate after epizootics.

Only a small proportion of cases are typically notified because of occurrence of the disease in remote areas, late recognition of outbreaks, and lack of diagnostic facilities. Where specific investigations have been undertaken, the ratio of cases to official notifications varies between 1:1 and 311:1 (Table 40–6). In recent epidemics, case-finding and census data were used to estimate attack rates (Table 40–7). The incidence of disease in The Gambia (1978–79) was 44 per 1000 population, the mortality rate 8 per 1000, and the case-fatality rate 19.4%.[44] In Nigeria (1986), the incidence was 49 per

TABLE 40–5 ■ Incidence of Yellow Fever Based on Official Reports to the World Health Organization over 15-Year Interval (1986–1999)

	1985	1986	1987	1988	1989	1990	1991	1992	1993	1994	1995	1996	1997	1998	1999	TOTAL
AFRICA																
Angola				37												37
Benin												120	18			138
Burkina Faso	7													2		9
Cameroon						173				10						183
Equatorial Guinea																0
Gabon										28	16					44
Gambia																0
Ghana									39	79		27	6			151
Guinea			5													5
Ivory Coast													11			11
Liberia											360		1	25		386
Kenya								27	27	7	3					64
Mali			305													305
Mauritania			21													21
Niger																0
Nigeria	6	3291	1726	4920	3270	4075	2561	149	152	1227			7			21,384
Senegal											79	128				207
Sierra Leone											1					1
Togo			6													6
Zaire																0
Subtotal	*13*	*3291*	*2063*	*4957*	*3270*	*4248*	*2561*	*176*	*218*	*1351*	*459*	*275*	*43*	*27*	*0*	*22,952*
SOUTH AMERICA																
Bolivia	53	26	23	12	98	50	91	22	18	7	15	30	63	57	68	633
Brazil	7	9	16	21	9	2	15	12	66	18	4	15	3	34	75	306
Colombia	5	6	17	7		7	4	2	1	2	3	8	6	1	2	71
Ecuador	1					12	14	16	1		1	8	31	3	5	92
French Guiana														1		1
Panama																0
Paraguay																0
Peru	59	118	179	195	120	17	27	67	89	61	492	86	44	165	56	1775
Surinam																0
Trinidad & Tobago																0
Venezuela														15	1	16
Subtotal	*125*	*159*	*235*	*235*	*227*	*88*	*151*	*119*	*175*	*88*	*515*	*147*	*147*	*276*	*207*	*2894*
TOTAL	138	3450	2298	5192	3497	4336	2712	295	393	1439	974	422	190	303	207	25,846

1000, mortality 28 per 1000, and case-fatality rate 47%; of 200,000 residents in the affected region (Oju Local Government Area), 38,000 persons were infected, 10,000 developed jaundice, and 4700 died.[298] Based on serologic investigations, remarkably similar incidences of yellow fever infection were found in African outbreaks: 35% in Ethiopia (1960–62),[303] 44% in Senegal (1965),[304] 33% in The Gambia (1978–79),[44] 29% in the Ivory Coast (1982),[305] 31% in Burkina Faso (1983),[306] 19% in Nigeria (Oju region, 1986),[298] 21% in Nigeria (Oyo State, 1987),[45] 20% in Cameroon (1990),[307] and 20% in Nigeria (Imo State, 1994).[307a]

These serologic data provide a basis for estimating the ratio of illness to infection (see Table 40–7); in two West African outbreaks, the illness:infection ratio was 3.8:1 to 7.4:1. Because illness was defined by a case definition that included jaundice, the ratio would be lower if mild cases were included. In an epidemic of jungle yellow fever in Brazil, serologic evidence for recent infection was found more often in persons with a history of febrile illness than in those without fever (odds ratio 4.5; 95% confidence interval 2.3 to 8.5).

The evidence that prior heterologous flavivirus infection modified the incidence of yellow fever is conflicting. In The Gambia (1978–79), the infection:illness (jaundice) ratio was higher in persons with prior flavivirus exposure.[44] However, in Nigeria (Oju Region, 1986), jaundice rates were not significantly different for patients with primary yellow fever infection (14 of 84 cases, or 17%) and superinfections (13 of 53 cases, or 25%) (odds ratio 0.62, 95% confidence interval 0.24 to 1.56) (KM DeCock and TP Monath, unpublished data, 1987). The discrepancy could reflect differences in the specific heterologous flaviviruses responsible for prior immunity.

The burden of yellow fever in Africa has been estimated almost entirely in terms of epidemic disease, and only limited attempts have been made to define the incidence of *endemic* yellow fever infection. In Nigeria (1970–71), a laboratory diagnosis of yellow fever was made in 2 (1%) of 205 patients hospitalized with jaundice in areas without epidemic activity.[308] Using data from serologic surveys in Nigeria and an

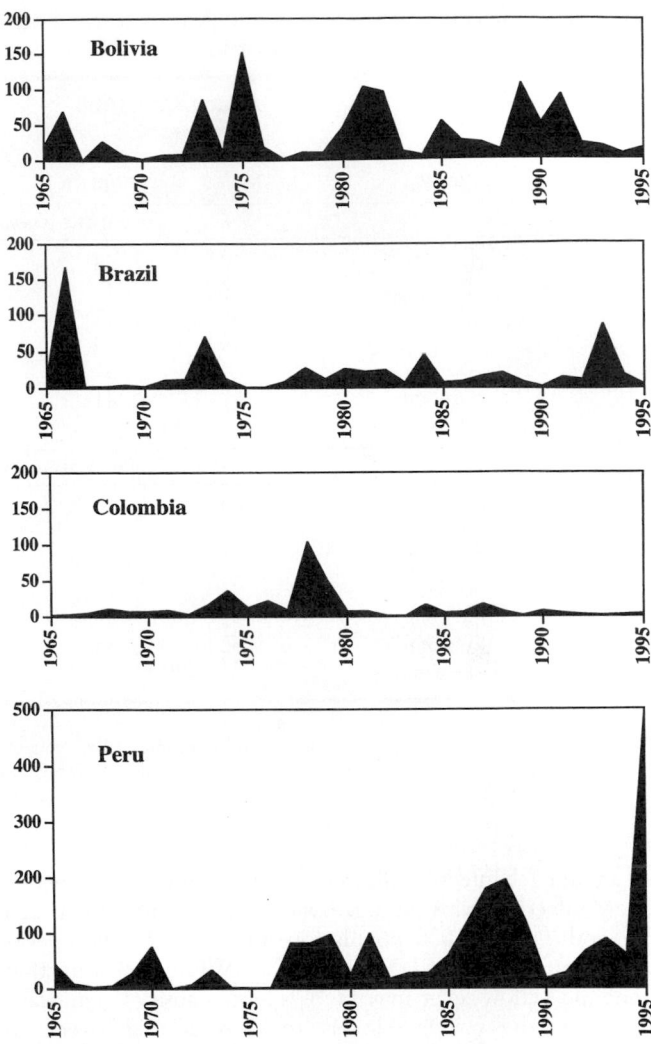

FIGURE 40–9 ■ Incidence of yellow fever in selected countries in South America, 1965 through 1995. Years of high incidence are not generally synchronous, indicating that epizootic activity occurs in discontinuous regions of the continent.

TABLE 40–6 ■ Epidemic Yellow Fever in Africa (Partial Listing): Officially Notified Cases and Estimated Actual Number of Cases Based on Epidemiologic Investigation

Country	Epidemic Year	Official Notification	Estimated by Direct Investigations	Ratio Actual: Reported	Reference
Ethiopia	1960–62	3010	100,000	33:1	303
Senegal	1965	243	2000–20,000	8:1–82:1	304
West Africa	1969	322	>100,000	311:1	593
Nigeria	1970	4	786	197:1	594
Ghana	1977–78	713	2400	3:1	595
Gambia	1978–79	30	8400	280:1	44
Mali	1987	305	1500	5:1	596
Nigeria	1986	1289	9100	7:1	298
Nigeria	1987	2676	120,000	45:1	45
Cameroon	1990	173	5000–20,000	29:1–116:1	597
Kenya	1992–93	54	55	1:1	333
Nigeria (Orsu LGA)	1994	120	775 in one community representing 22% of the total population	>6:1	598

TABLE 40–7 ■ Age- and Sex-Specific Attack Rates and Infection-to-Illness Ratios in Yellow Fever Epidemics in The Gambia and Nigeria

Age (yr)	Attack Rate/1000 Population		Infection Rate/1000 Population		Infection-Illness Ratio	
	Males	Females	Males	Females	Males	Females
I: THE GAMBIA (1978–1979)*						
0–9	70	63	528	333	7.5	5.3
10–19	56	43	395	387	7.1	9.0
20–29	39	27	441	238	11.3	8.8
30–39	49	19	105	394	2.1	20.7
40+	6	31	231	170	38.5	5.5
Subtotal	47	41	359	295	7.6	7.2
All ages, both genders	44		326		7.4	
II: NIGERIA (OJU REGION, 1986)†						
0–9	62	0	147	238	2.4	—
10–19	37	93	197	234	5.3	2.5
20–29	113	44	184	263	1.6	6.0
30–39	83	19	194	140	2.3	7.4
40+	33	39	114	156	3.5	4.0
Subtotal	62	35	166	211	2.7	6.0
All ages, both genders	49		187		3.8	

*Infection incidence based on complement fixation test.
†Infection incidence based on immunoglobulin M enzyme-linked immunosorbent assay.
Part I from Monath TP, Craven RB, Adjukiewicz, A. et al. Yellow fever in The Gambia, 1978–1979: epidemiologic aspects with observations on the occurrence of Orungo virus infections. Am J Trop Med Hyg 29:912, 1980. Part II from unpublished data, KM DeCock and TP Monath.

estimated 7:1 infection:illness ratio, the annual incidence of overt infection with jaundice was estimated to be between 1.1 and 2.4 per 1000 population and that of yellow fever death between 0.2 and 0.5 per 1000.[309] While indicating that endemic yellow fever may be a "silent" cause of significant morbidity, the incidence levels are 25- to 50-fold lower than those occurring during epidemics, and are thus below the threshold of detection by existing passive surveillance systems. It is likely that endemic yellow fever activity varies considerably from year to year, but that it causes thousands of unrecorded deaths annually in West Africa. This provides a strong rationale for preventive immunization.

Yellow Fever in Expatriate Residents, Travelers, and Military Personnel

In the prevaccine era, yellow fever was a major threat to expatriates living in and travelers to tropical America and Africa, including U.S. military personnel stationed overseas. Fourteen cases occurred in Navy personnel in Honduras and Nicaragua in 1919,[310] and a suspected case was reported in Brazil in 1929.[311] A single case (acquired in Fernando Po in 1938) was found among 2300 seamen of the Polish merchant fleet serving in the tropics.[312] Such cases became rare during World War II, after vaccination came into general use. A few cases among Europeans were reported during[48] and after[313] the 1941 outbreak in the Sudan, and among British forces in West Africa in 1942.[314] In 1952, a fatal case of yellow fever occurred in a previously vaccinated European working in Uganda.[315] In 1979, two fatal cases occurred in unvaccinated French tourists who visited an area of Senegal bordering The Gambia[316-318] (Table 40–8). These infections were acquired 1 year after a major outbreak in a region where the resident population had a high background of vaccine immunity.

TABLE 40–8 ■ Reported Yellow Fever Cases in Travelers, 1970–2002

Month, Year	Age/Sex	Vaccination Status	Residence	Exposure	Outcome	Reference
October 1979	42/M	No	France	Senegal	Died	316
October 1979	25/M	No	France	Senegal	Died	316
August 1985	27/F	No	Netherlands	Guinea-Bissau, Gambia, Senegal	Survived	320
October 1988	37/F	Yes	Spain	Niger, Mali, Burkina Faso, Mauritania	Survived	321
April 1996	53/M	No	Switzerland	Brazil (Amazonas)	Died	323
August 1996	42/M	No	United States	Brazil (Amazonas)	Died	322
August 1999	40/M	No	Germany	Ivory Coast	Died	282
September 1999	48/M	No	United States	Venezuela	Died	282
November 2001	47/F	No	Belgium	The Gambia	Died	261
March 2002	47/M	No	United States	Brazil (Amazonas)	Died	324

The French tourists returned to France during the early phase of illness and expired in a hospital in Paris. In 1979, a nonfatal case also occurred in a European resident of Dakar who visited the Gambian border,[317] and, in 1981, an unvaccinated Lebanese resident in Senegal died of yellow fever after visiting a camp near The Gambia.[319] In 1985, a nonfatal case of yellow fever occurred in the Netherlands in a female traveler to The Gambia, Senegal, and Guinea-Bissau.[320] In 1988, a vaccinated Spanish woman acquired yellow fever during travels through Mali, Burkina Faso, Niger, and Mauritania[321] 1 year after a widespread increase in yellow fever activity in West Africa. In 1996, two fatal cases occurred in unvaccinated American[322] and Swiss[323] tourists who had visited jungle areas near Manaus, Brazil and returned home during the early phase of illness and during the incubation period, respectively. These cases occurred during a period of increased yellow fever activity in the Amazon basin. In August 1999, a 40-year-old unvaccinated man became ill in Germany after a visit to the Ivory Coast and died 4 days later in the hospital.[282] In September 1999, a 48-year-old unvaccinated male U.S. citizen became ill on a trip to southern Venezuela; he returned to California on the 5th day of illness and died in the hospital on the 11th day after onset.[282] In November 2001, an unvaccinated Belgian tourist acquired yellow fever in The Gambia, returned home while ill, and died in the hospital,[261] and, in March 2002, an unvaccinated U.S. citizen acquired yellow fever while on a fishing trip on the Rio Negro (Amazonas, Brazil) and died in a Texas hospital.[324]

Risk of Acquiring Yellow Fever During Travel

The risk of acquiring yellow fever is determined by geographic location, season, duration of travel, activities that lead to exposure to mosquito bite, and the intensity of yellow fever virus transmission occurring at the time. Although reported cases of human disease are an important guide to yellow fever activity, they may be absent because of a high level of immunity in the resident population or not detected by surveillance. Based on estimates of attack rates (see *Incidence* above), it has been estimated that an unimmunized traveler to an *epidemic* area would have a risk of yellow fever illness and death of 1:267 and 1:1333, respectively, for a 2-week trip.[325]

During *interepidemic* periods in Africa, the incidence of overt disease is below the threshold of detection by existing surveillance. Such interepidemic conditions may last years or even decades in specific countries or regions. "Epidemiologic silence" may provide a sense of false security and lead to travel without the benefit of vaccination. The case in a Belgian traveler who spent 1 week in The Gambia is a case in point.[261] There was no evidence for yellow fever transmission at the time, and a high prevalence of vaccine immunity in the local population. Surveys in endemic areas of rural West Africa during "silent" periods indicate that the incidence of yellow fever illness approximates 1.1 to 2.4 per 1000 and yellow fever death 0.2 to 0.5 per 1000, below detection by existing surveillance.[27] In unvaccinated travelers to these areas, the risk of yellow fever illness may be esti-

mated at 1:1000 per month and yellow fever death 1:5000 (1:2000 risk of illness and 1:10,000 risk of death for a typical 2-week journey)[325] but varies considerably with season. These estimates, which are based on risk to local residents, may overestimate the risk to travelers who take precautions against mosquito bite and have less outdoor exposure than the indigenous population.

In South America, the incidence of disease is lower than in Africa. The risk of illness and death is probably 10 times lower than in rural West Africa (e.g., 1:20,000 illness risk and 1:100,000 death risk per 2-week journey) but varies greatly with specific location and season.[325] As in Africa, zoonotic virus transmission is often epidemiologically silent. The low reported incidence of yellow fever has diminished concern among travelers. In Brazil, for example, where the majority of the population lives in coastal regions outside the endemic zone, unimmunized recreational or vocational travelers to the interior are the usual victims of yellow fever. Four of the six cases among travelers from the United States and Europe between 1996 and 2002 were exposed in South America (see Table 40–8).

Cases Imported into Receptive Areas

Because the southern United States is infested with *A. aegypti*, importation of yellow fever has long been considered a significant threat.[326,327] The last outbreak resulting from introduction of the virus occurred in New Orleans in 1905. Between 1906 and 1996, 27 yellow fever cases (exclusive of laboratory infections) were reported in the United States, 23 of which were intercepted on ships arriving at Public Health Service Quarantine facilities.[327] The last imported case in the prevaccine era occurred in a Mexican immigrant who died in Texas in 1924. Since 1996, there have been six cases in unvaccinated tourists from the United States and Europe to South America and West Africa (see Table 40–8). In all cases, the affected individuals died after returning to their country of residence. Three patients acquired the infections in the Amazon region of Brazil; a river trip/fishing expedition on the Rio Negro (near Manaus) was the likely event leading to exposure in at least two cases.

Within countries affected by yellow fever, the disease may be acquired by unvaccinated residents who travel from an uninfected area to a region of endemic activity.[328] This is a recurring theme in South America, where unvaccinated migrant workers move from a coastal area or the Andean highlands into the Amazon region. In Brazil during the first half of 2000, 11 (14%) of 77 reported yellow fever cases were in tourists from coastal areas to the endemic part of the country.[329] In Africa, similar episodes undoubtedly are common but have been recorded infrequently and exclusively in expatriate residents, as noted above.

Risk Factors

The age, sex, and occupational distribution of yellow fever in Africa and South America differ. In South America, *Haemagogus* mosquitoes in the rainforest canopy transmit the virus; humans are infected by mosquitoes that previously fed on viremic monkeys ("jungle" yellow fever).[159,330]

Because human infection is linked to occupational activities, such as forest clearing, lumbering, and road construction, most patients are young adults and 70% to 90% are males (Fig. 40–10).[299,302,331] The prevalence of immunity in males exceeds that in females by 2.5- to 7.5-fold.[332] The age and sex distribution of jungle yellow fever cases differs from that observed in South America during *A. aegypti*–borne epidemics in the early 20th century. *Aedes aegypti* breeds in and around houses and sustains interhuman transmission of virus ("urban" yellow fever), with a high prevalence of infection in children and females.

In Africa, tree hole–breeding ("sylvatic") *Aedes* mosquitoes are responsible for yellow fever transmission between monkeys, from monkeys to humans, and between humans. During the rainy season, these vectors reach high densities in the moist savanna vegetational zone, and some species (*A. furcifer*, *A. africanus*) enter villages and houses. Yellow fever infection is endemic, and the prevalence of natural immunity accumulates rapidly with age, so that children are at highest risk (Table 40–9). A high attack rate in children (>70%) typically reflects an area where older individuals are protected by previous yellow fever vaccination campaigns (e.g., Senegal, 1965; Burkina Faso and Ghana, 1983; Mali, 1987). However, in some epidemics affecting populations without prior vaccination, the attack rate also has been higher in children (see Table 40–7). In The Gambia, the disease incidence in persons birth to 19 years was significantly higher than in older adults (*P* < 0.01), possibly as a result of naturally acquired yellow fever or heterologous flavivirus immunity in adults.[44] There are few data on the relationship between severity of illness and age. In the 1921 epidemic in Peru, the case-fatality rate was highest in infants and children birth to -5 years old and in older adults (Fig. 40–11).[46] Other authors[29,31,48,49] noted a higher case-fatality rate among the elderly, but lethality in infants was not assessed in these studies. Increased severity of illness in elderly individuals is known to occur in other flaviviral infections, notably Japanese encephalitis, St. Louis encephalitis, and West Nile encephalitis.

In Africa, a slight excess of cases among males has been observed during epidemics (see Table 40–9). This pattern was seen regardless of the role of domiciliary *A. aegypti* or sylvatic vectors, and is thus difficult to explain on the basis of differences in human behavior or exposure to mosquito bite. The higher proportion of male cases has been observed not only among notified or hospitalized patients, but also in population-based surveys, indicating that it is not due to reluctance of females to seek medical treatment. Serologic data have shown neither a consistently higher incidence of infection nor of susceptibility to illness among males (see Table 40–7), but small sample size and sampling biases in these surveys may preclude detection of small differences. Males were suspected to be more susceptible to yellow fever because cases of severe adverse events associated with 17D and FNV have been more frequent in males (see *Adverse Events* below). However, in the Kenyan outbreak (1992–93), female patients were 10.9 times more likely to die than male patients,[333] suggesting that males (with milder forms of illness) preferentially sought medical attention.

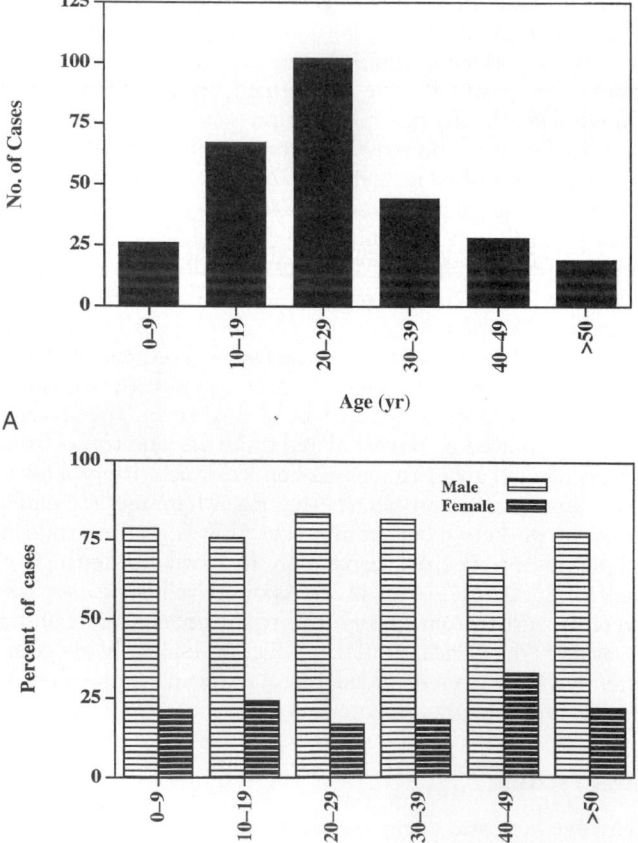

A

B

FIGURE 40–10 ■ Age (*A*) and sex (*B*) distribution of cases of yellow fever in South America, 1992 and 1993 (eight cases during this interval were of undetermined age). (Data from World Health Organization. Yellow fever in 1992 and 1993. Wkly Epidemiol Rec 70:65, 1995.)

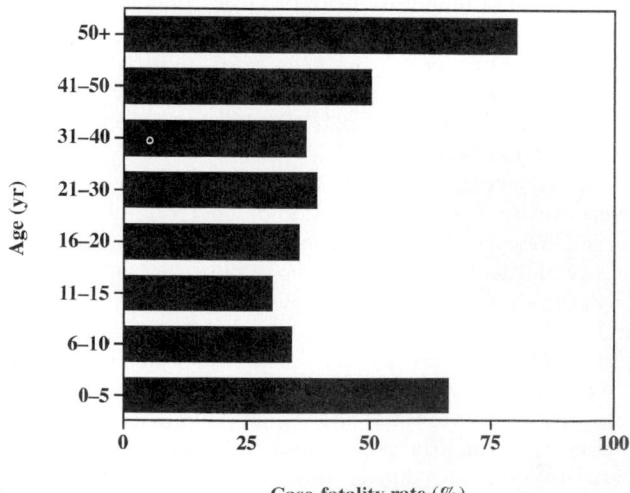

FIGURE 40–11 ■ Case-fatality rates by age group for 478 cases of yellow fever in Peru, 1921, suggesting a bimodal pattern of increased severity in the very young and the elderly. (Data from Hanson H. Observations on the age and sex incidence of deaths and recoveries in the yellow fever epidemic in the department of Lambayeque, Peru, in 1921. Am J Trop Med Hyg 9:233, 1929.)

TABLE 40-9 ■ Age and Sex Distribution of Yellow Fever Cases in Selected Epidemics in Africa, 1926–1994

Epidemic	No. Cases in Children/Total Cases (%)	Male:Female Ratio	Presumed Vectors	Reference
Ghana, Nigeria, 1926–28	32[‡]/122 (26)	2.3:1	? A. aegypti	29
Sudan (Nuba Mountains), 1940	110[‡]/306 (36)	1.7:1	A. aegypti, A. vittatus, other Sylvatic vectors	48
Senegal (Diourbel), 1965	86[‡]/89 (97)	—	A. aegypti	304
Nigeria (Jos Plateau area), 1969	38[‡]/209 (18)	2.5:1	A. luteocephalus	P. Brès, unpublished data
Ghana, 1969–70	99[†]/164 (60)	—	A. aegypti	594
Nigeria (Okwoga District), 1970	35[‡]/76 (46)	~1:1	A. africanus	593
Ivory Coast (Mbahiakro Subprefecture), 1982	43[†]/90 (48)	—	A. aegypti	256
Ghana (Volta and Eastern Regions), 1977–80	87[†]/294 (30)	—	A. aegypti	594
Burkina Faso (Manga and Fada N'Gourma Regions), 1983	40[†]/45 (89)	~1:1	A. furcifer	598, 599
Ghana (Northern Region), 1983	74[†]/87 (85)	—	A. aegypti	600
Nigeria (Oju LGA), 1986	20[‡]/39 (51)	2:1	A. africanus	298
Nigeria (Oyo State), 1987	72[‡]/102 (71)	1.4:1	A. aegypti	45
Mali (Kati Cercle), 1987	100[†]/143 (70)	2.1:1	A. furcifer, A. aegypti	601
Cameroon (Extreme North Province), 1990	91[*]/182 (73)	—	A. aegypti	307
Nigeria, 1991	1209[†]/2229 (54)	1.1:1	A. aegypti	602
Kenya (Baringo and Elgeyo Marakwet Districts), 1992–93	18[‡]/54 (33)	1.8:1	A. africanus	300, 333
Ghana (Upper Western Region), 1993–94	47[†]/69 (68)	2.0:1	?	603
Nigeria (Imo State), 1994	37[†]/116 (32)	1.3:1	? A. africanus	597

[*]0–9 years.
[†]0–15 years.
[‡]0–19 years.

Season and Climate

In South America, the incidence of yellow fever is highest during months of high rainfall, humidity, and temperature (January to May, with peak incidence in February and March), corresponding to the activity of *Haemagogus* mosquitoes, which breed in tree holes and thus are dependent on rainwater. Human exposure during agricultural activities is also increased at this time of the year. In the savanna zone of West Africa, cases appear during the mid-rainy season (August) and peak during the early dry season (October), corresponding to the period of maximum longevity of sylvatic mosquito vectors.[334] The domiciliary vector *A. aegypti* breeds in receptacles used by humans for water storage, and thus is less dependent on rainfall. Where this mosquito is involved in virus transmission, yellow fever may occur in the dry season in both rural areas and heavily settled urbanizations. Thus season is only a partially reliable guide to determining the risk of exposure and to making decisions on the need for immunization of travelers.

Fluctuations in rainfall profoundly affect mosquito vector abundance and the potential for yellow fever epidemics.[27,335–339] Surveillance of yellow fever in eastern Senegal has been actively maintained for over 20 years.[340] Enhanced virus activity in this region, reflected by virus isolations from mosquitoes, coincided with human epidemics over the entire West African region. This correlation may reflect prolonged rainfall or other undefined regional ecologic changes. The yellow fever outbreak in The Gambia in 1978 occurred after a period of 2 successive years of excess rainfall.[336] Similarly, excessive rainfall and prolongation of the rainy season, reflected by vegetational indices in satellite images, preceded the emergence of a sylvatic yellow fever epidemic in Nigeria in 1986.[339] In Brazil, excessive rainfall and abnormally high temperatures (resulting from an El Niño event) occurred during December 1999 and the first quarter of 2000, coinciding with the emergence of a large jungle yellow fever outbreak.[329]

Temperature influences yellow fever transmission rates.[341] The EIP of yellow fever virus in the mosquito vector is very sensitive to temperature, and an increase of a few degrees may shorten the EIP by days, resulting in a significantly increased rate of transmission.[342,343] Even brief exposure to high temperatures (e.g., in a sunlit forest clearing) can have this effect. Warm temperature also increases biting and reproductive rates of *A. aegypti*.[344] Thus long-term environmental change (global warming) may increase transmission rates of yellow fever.[345]

Transmission Cycles

The enzootic transmission cycle involves monkeys and diurnally active tree hole–breeding mosquitoes (*Haemagogus* species in South America and *A. africanus* in Africa) (Fig.

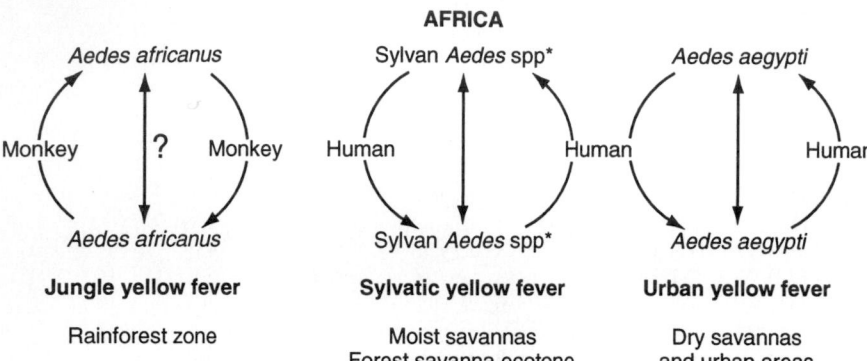

FIGURE 40–12 ■ Transmission cycles of yellow fever virus in South America (*top*) and Africa (*bottom*). In both continents, jungle yellow fever is transmitted through an enzootic cycle, whereas urban and sylvatic yellow fevers are transmitted through epidemic cycles. Transovarial transmission is indicated by *vertical arrows* showing virus transfer between mosquitoes, and may be an important mechanism for virus survival over the long dry season. *Species in West Africa: A. furcifer, A. taylori, A. luteocephalus, A. africanus, A. opok, A. vittatus, and A. metallicus;* in East Africa: *A. africanus and A. simpsoni (bromeliae).*

40–12). The density of vectors and human disease incidence are low, and human cases occur in a sporadic fashion. This transmission cycle accounts for "jungle yellow fever" cases in South America and in the rainforest zone of Africa.

Many species of nonhuman primates are susceptible to yellow fever infection (reviewed by Bugher,[158] Monath,[159] and Digoutte et al.[337]). The majority of African species have viremic infections sufficient to infect mosquitoes without developing clinical illness, whereas some neotropical species (e.g., howler monkeys) develop lethal infections. Depletion of vertebrate hosts through natural immunization and death during epizootic waves is a factor in the cyclic appearance of yellow fever activity. In many areas, deforestation and hunting pressure have markedly reduced monkey populations, and human beings serve as hosts in the yellow fever transmission cycle.[346] Although still debated, there is little evidence that nonprimate species are involved in enzootic transmission.[158,159,335,347]

The pattern of yellow fever activity in South America is characterized by intermittent "emergences" around the edges of the Amazon region. These outbreaks are preceded by evidence for increased virus transmission between monkeys and *Haemagogus* species within the Amazon basin, which moves in a circular fashion within the forest or along gallery forests of river courses. A detailed analysis of the patterns of virus activity preceding and during epidemics in Brazil is provided by Mondet.[348]

The ecology of yellow fever differs in areas bordering the rainforest block in Africa. A mosaic of savanna and forest in galleries along rivers characterizes this transitional vegetation zone. In this region and surrounding moist (Guinea) savanna, yellow fever transmission is effected by a wide variety of tree hole–breeding mosquito vectors.[159,334,335,337,338] In

West Africa, the principal vectors responsible for yellow fever transmission in the savanna zone include A. *furcifer*, A. *vittatus*, and A. *luteocephalus* as well as A. *africanus*. In East Africa, A. *africanus* and man-biting populations of the A. *simpsoni* complex play a similar role.[349,350] During the wet and early dry seasons, vector density reaches high levels. Vectors are active in plantation areas and in proximity to human dwellings and may enter houses.[338] Both humans and nonhuman primates may be involved as hosts in the transmission cycle, and the rate of virus transmission far exceeds that found in the rainforest zone. The savanna-forest ecotone and surrounding Guinea savanna has been described as the "zone of emergence" of yellow fever, and represents the region principally affected by epidemics.[335,337]

An epidemiologically distinct transmission cycle involves A. *aegypti*, which breeds in containers used to store water or in artificial containers that collect rainwater around human habitations. *Aedes aegypti* transmits yellow fever virus between humans, the sole viremic hosts in the cycle. The vector occurs in dry areas and heavily settled areas, but also is widely dispersed in settlements in rural areas. Urban outbreaks have followed introduction by viremic persons from areas of jungle yellow fever activity.[45,351] In the Americas, urban yellow fever outbreaks were common prior to the successful eradication of the vector.[330,352,353] Prior to a small cluster of cases in 1997 in Urban Santa Cruz, Bolivia, the last urban outbreak in continental South America occurred in western Brazil in 1942, and the last episode of A. *aegypti*–transmitted yellow fever in the Americas occurred in Trinidad in 1954.[353a,354] In contrast, Africa suffers many A. *aegypti*–borne epidemics, and the vector is prevalent in urban and rural areas. In dry areas (Sudan and Sahel savanna zones), where domiciliary A. *aegypti* may represent the only species capable of sustaining yellow fever transmission, outbreaks occur after introduction of the virus by viremic person(s). *Aedes aegypti*–borne epidemics in the past 30 years include those in Senegal in 1965; Angola in 1971; Ghana in 1969, 1977–80, and 1983; the Ivory Coast in 1982; and Nigeria between 1987 and 1991.[297]

Maintenance of Yellow Fever in Nature

The means of survival of yellow fever virus across the long dry season, when sylvatic mosquito vectors are virtually absent, remains incompletely understood. *Aedes* and *Haemagogus* eggs survive desiccation in tree holes and hatch with the return of rain. Experimental and field studies indicate that transovarial transmission is an important means of virus survival across the dry season.[143,147,355–357] Low-level horizontal transmission by drought-resistant vectors and alternative horizontal and vertical transmission cycles involving ticks[358] have been suggested as ancillary mechanisms. Persistent infection of experimentally infected nonhuman primates has been documented,[359,360] but such infections are probably not accompanied by viremias sufficient to infect vectors.

Prospects for Future Changes in Yellow Fever Epidemiology

The most alarming prospect for the future involves the re-emergence of urban (*A. aegypti*–borne) yellow fever in South America and the spread of yellow fever to heavily populated, *A. aegypti*–infested areas of the world that are currently free from the disease. These regions include both areas historically affected, such as the coastal regions of South America, the Caribbean, and North America, and regions that have not heretofore been reached by the dis-

ease but are considered receptive, including the Middle East, coastal East Africa, the Indian subcontinent, Asia, and Australia. Alterations in human demography and behavior, in virus activity, and in the distribution of *A. aegypti* underlie the potential for epidemiologic change. These alterations include

1. A recent upsurge of yellow fever virus activity and incidence of human infections, which increases the opportunity for geographic spread
2. The re-invasion of the South American continent by the domestic vector, *A. aegypti*[339,361] (Fig. 40–13)
3. Changes in human demography, principally the shifting balance of human populations from rural to urban residence, the expansion of internal communications, and opening of remote rural areas to commerce within countries in the yellow fever–endemic zone
4. Economic development and the growth of air travel, which have diminished the barriers to spread of yellow fever
5. Relaxation of regulations and enforcement of vaccination certification for travelers
6. Global warming

Spread of yellow fever outside its traditional boundaries and re-emergence of the urban disease in the Americas would greatly increase the demand for yellow fever vaccine.

Ecologic changes resulting from deforestation are also changing the landscape of sylvatic yellow fever. Destruction of habitat for nonhuman primates and certain vectors may reduce transmission in some areas, but in general such effects are counterbalanced by increased human encroachment into enzootic areas and opportunities for interhuman transmission of the virus.

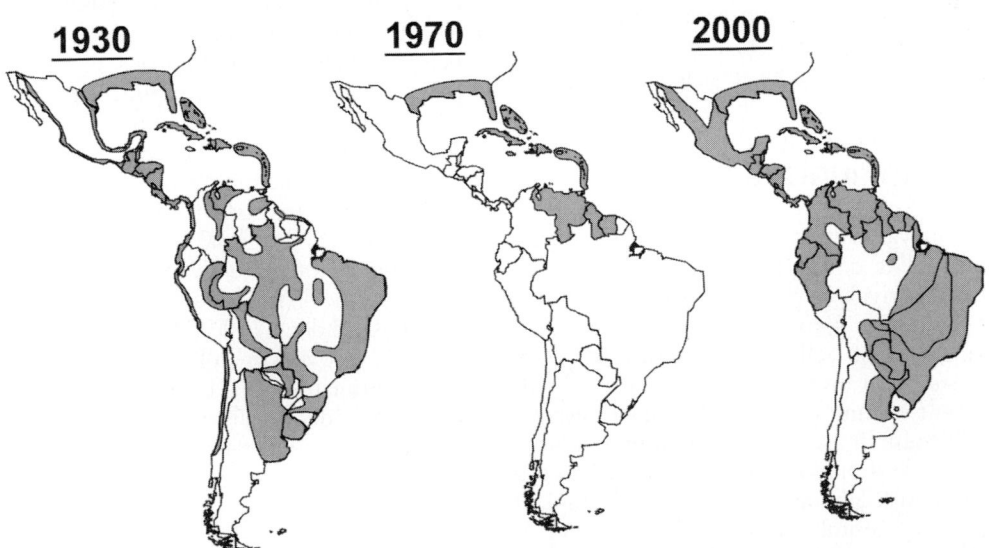

FIGURE 40–13 ■ Re-invasion of the South American continent by the urban vector of yellow fever, *A. aegypti*, during the period between 1930 and 2000. By 1970, the vector had been eliminated from many countries during intensive vector control efforts, under the leadership of the Pan-American Health Organization. The re-infestation led to the introduction and spread of epidemic dengue, and raises the risk of re-emergence of urban yellow fever.

Other Modes of Transmission

Laboratory infections with yellow fever were common in the prevaccine era and remain of concern today, particularly where unvaccinated clinical laboratory personnel encounter blood from patients during the early stage of illness. Some laboratory infections probably were acquired by the bite of mosquitoes experimentally infected in the laboratory or of wild mosquitoes infected after feeding on experimental animals; others were the result of direct contact with blood or aerosols of dried virus.[15,362,363] The stability of yellow fever virus is sufficient to permit transmission within short periods after generation of an infectious aerosol in the laboratory.[364] Under experimental conditions, a dose of only 10 MLD_{50} (LD_{50} determined by IC inoculation of mice 4 to 6 weeks of age) delivered by aerosol was sufficient to induce lethal infection in rhesus monkeys.[365] The absence of direct interhuman transmission indicates that virus is not shed in secreta or excreta at sufficiently high levels for transfer by contact or aerosols. There is no evidence that black vomit or urine is infectious. However, on multiple occasions, transmission has occurred between separately caged monkeys housed in a single room, possibly by aerosol spread.[156] Findlay and MacCallum[366] infected monkeys by a mucosal (intragastric) route, and Bauer and Hudson[367] transmitted yellow fever to monkeys by rubbing virus on unabraded skin. Some infections in laboratory workers may be explained by contact with viremic blood, but it remains unclear whether infection occurred via intact skin, abrasions, or contact with mucosal surfaces. The application of 17D vaccine by the intranasal route is discussed in the section entitled *Dose and Route of Administration*.

Yellow fever virus was extensively investigated in the U.S. biological weapons program. Whereas the virus could infect by the aerosol route, it was considered too unstable for successful weaponization. Instead, extensive studies were undertaken on the use of *A. aegypti* as an "entomologic weapon" capable of delivering the virus.[368,369]

Passive Immunization and Passive-Active Immunization

Passive immunization was utilized widely prior to the development of vaccines. The concept was established in the 19th century,[370] and convalescent serum was first used in the early 20th century.[371] Experimental validation was achieved after isolation of yellow fever virus. In 1928, Stokes et al.[9] reported that pretreatment with a small volume of convalescent serum protected monkeys against lethal challenge. Because of an increasing number of laboratory infections, standard practice was to administer convalescent serum to at-risk laboratory workers and to inject large amounts after accidental exposures. The potency of passive antibody and the schedule of immunization were not carefully controlled, and laboratory-acquired disease occurred in persons who had been previously immunized[372]; such cases were due to an inadequate dose of antibody and the long interval between transfer of serum and exposure.[164] In monkey studies, transfer of immune serum prior to challenge was protective, whereas immunization 24 hours after experimental challenge protected 55% of the animals, and

transfer at 48 or 72 hours protected only 15% to 20%.[373] Administration of antibody after clinical onset was ineffective.

Because of the difficulty in obtaining sufficient amounts of potent human serum, hyperimmune antibodies were prepared in nonhuman primates, horses, and goats.[374,375] Antibodies raised in monkeys and horses were shown to protect susceptible rhesus macaques. Heterologous antisera had limited usefulness for repeated administration to humans, but were applied together with partially attenuated virus to achieve active immunization. "Passive-active immunization" using an excess of human or animal serum mixed with partially attenuated virus (French neurotropic strain) elicited active immunity without untoward effects, and became standard practice.[14] However, it was a cumbersome method, requiring that the amount of immune serum be sufficient to protect against disease but not completely neutralize the virus and prevent active infection.[376] Use of heterologous serum was problematic because allergic reactions occurred in 85% of recipients of goat serum, and late reactions similar to abortive yellow fever infection were noted in some cases, possibly as a result of rapid clearance of the heterologous serum, allowing replication of the under-attenuated vaccines used in these studies (e.g., the 17E strain). The use of monkey serum was safer, but frequent failure to seroconvert was attributed to vaccine neutralization by the antiserum. Passive-active immunization was discontinued in 1936 with the advent of vaccines that could be administered safely without serum.[20]

A Recent Application of Passive Immunization

Commercial lots of serum immunoglobulin contain high titers of neutralizing antibodies to yellow fever,[377] presumably because 5% to 10% of plasma donors have been immunized during military service in the United States. There are no published reports of off-label use of intravenous immunoglobulin (IGIV) for passive immunoprophylaxis of persons with contraindications to active vaccination. A patient with chronic lymphocytic leukemia (CLL), in whom active vaccination was contraindicated, was planning a short trip to the Amazon region. Passive immunization with commercial IVIG was performed. The patient with CLL was treated with IVIG having a log_{10} neutralization index (LNI) of 3.0, to achieve a high initial passive titer and a protective level of antibody throughout several weeks of travel (R McMullen, TP Monath, and R Nichols, unpublished data, 2000). The level of antibody considered to be protective was an LNI of 0.7 based on studies in nonhuman primates.[378] Although this approach may have merit for certain individuals who cannot avoid travel to a high-risk area, it is expensive, requires monitoring of antibody levels in IGIV and the patient, and is not supported by clinical data on efficacy.

Maternal Antibody

Transplacental transfer of yellow fever neutralizing antibodies has been documented in monkeys[379] and humans,[380] and antibody has also been found in breast milk of immune mothers.[381] Because yellow fever 17D vaccine is not administered to infants prior to 6 months of age for safety reasons, maternal immunity does not pose an obstacle to effective immunization.

Active Immunization

Prior Approaches That Have Been Abandoned

Inactivated Vaccines

After isolation of the virus in 1927, attempts to develop an inactivated vaccine were made at the Wellcome Bureau of Scientific Research,[13,382] at the Oswaldo Cruz Institute in Brazil,[383] and at the Pasteur Institute in Paris.[268] The vaccines were prepared by phenol or formaldehyde treatment of infected monkey liver and/or spleen. Hindle inoculated rhesus monkeys with a single dose of inactivated liver tissue emulsion containing more than 10,000 monkey LD_{50}/g, and found that 80% of the immunized monkeys were protected against challenge.[382] However, his and others' studies were not controlled for residual live virus, nor were serologic studies performed. Subsequent studies in monkeys yielded erratic results,[384,385] and human trials in Brazil involving 25,000 persons were inconclusive.[268] Burke and Davis[372] reported yellow fever in an individual who had received inactivated liver tissue vaccine.

As virologic techniques improved, antigens were tested that were more suitable for vaccine production than infected monkey viscera. Gordon and Hughes[386] prepared vaccines from heat- or ultraviolet-inactivated tissue cultures (viscerotropic virus) or from mouse brain (neurotropic virus) containing known amounts of virus. Preparations containing residual live virus caused illness in monkeys, and survivors were immune to challenge. However, monkeys given various doses of fully inactivated vaccines did not develop antibodies and were not protected. It appeared that methods that fully inactivated virus also destroyed its antigenic properties. It should be noted, however, that all studies employed a single inoculum of antigen, a procedure that would not be expected to be very effective in the case of an inactivated vaccine. Sellards and Bennett[387] inoculated mice with multiple sequential doses of phenol-inactivated mouse brain and demonstrated protection against challenge, and rabbits immunized sequentially with inactivated virus developed neutralizing antibodies. However, prime-boost vaccination strategies were not used in monkeys or humans.

Obstacles to the development of inactivated vaccines included methodologic problems in antigen production, virus inactivation, and potency assays; ignorance about immunologic principles; and the lack of adjuvants. Given the growth characteristics of yellow fever virus, with titers of greater than 10^8 achievable in cell culture, and the success of inactivated vaccines against other flaviviruses, there is little doubt that a satisfactory product could be developed today. The failure of the early efforts to produce inactivated vaccines was certainly auspicious because success might have sidetracked development of live vaccines.

Passive-Active Immunization

This topic is discussed above in the section on *Passive Immunization and Passive-Active Immunization*.

French Neurotropic Vaccine

In 1930, Theiler showed that mice were susceptible to IC inoculation of yellow fever virus.[388] Following the lead of Pasteur, who had attenuated rabies virus by passage in rabbit brains, Theiler made a series of mouse brain passages of the French strain and showed that the adapted virus lost its viscerotropism for monkeys and protected them against challenge. However, in subsequent studies the neuroadapted virus caused fever, viremia, and lethal encephalitis after IC or intranasal inoculation, in a high proportion of monkeys, and even in individual animals after subcutaneous inoculation.[14,156,389–391] The virus was considered too dangerous without the coadministration of immune serum. The first human volunteers therefore were given immune human serum and neuroadapted virus (see *Passive Immunization and Passive-Active Immunization* above). This regimen resulted in the development of active immunity.[14]

In 1932, Sellards and Laigret reported the first human immunizations with the French strain in the absence of immune serum.[16,392] Systemic adverse reactions were attributed to underattenuation. To address this problem, a method was devised for "attenuating" the mouse brain virus by aging at room temperature. Subjects received three inoculations at intervals of 20 days with virus that had been aged for decreasing lengths of time.[393] Preliminary studies indicated that the regimen was well tolerated and that 90% seroconverted after the second dose. By 1934, 3196 persons in French West Africa had received this regimen, and 70% of those studied developed antibodies after the first dose.[17] One third of the recipients experienced a febrile reaction after the first dose, and there were two serious adverse events (myelitis, meningitis). In 1935, Nicolle and Laigret[394] simplified the method to a single inoculation of mouse-brain virus aged for 24 hours and treated with olive oil or egg yolk ostensibly to retard diffusion from the inoculation site. By 1939, over 20,000 persons in West Africa had received the single- or three-dose schedule. Concerns about reactogenicity decreased with vaccine use, despite occasional reports of postvaccinal encephalitis.[395,396] Careful follow-up studies were not routinely conducted, and the threat of natural infection superseded concerns about vaccine safety.

In 1939, Peltier et al. simplified yellow fever immunization by conversion from subcutaneous inoculation to the scarification technique used to deliver smallpox vaccine.[397] In 1939, nearly 100,000 persons were given FNV and smallpox vaccines simultaneously, without recognized adverse events. Of 1387 subjects followed up, 96.3% developed neutralizing antibodies 1 month after immunization. By 1941, FNV had been given via scarification to 1.9 million people in francophone Africa, and immunization was then made compulsory. By 1947, 14 million persons had been immunized.[398] In 1946, the UNRRA Standing Technical Committee on Health approved FNV, and the WHO granted similar approval in 1948.

FNV was prepared at the Pasteur Institute in Dakar, Senegal, by the IC inoculation of 2.5- to 3-month-old mice with approximately 20,000 LD_{50} of the French virus.[399] A seed lot system was not used, although passage level was restricted. Mice showing illness were killed and their brains aseptically removed and lyophilized. After sterility tests, brains from a batch were pooled, ground to powdered form, and again tested for sterility. The vaccine powder was filled into ampules containing 1/10th of a mouse brain (0.4 g), equivalent to 100 doses, and tested for sterility and potency. After reconstitution in 2 mL of gum arabic solution in phosphate buffer, the recommended minimum potency was 5000 LD_{50}/dose. The vaccine was quite stable and was stored at 4°C but shipped at ambient temperature. After reconstitution, a drop of the solution was placed on the skin and scarification performed with a vaccinostyle or similar instrument typically used to perform smallpox vaccinations. Gum Arabic in the vaccine dilvent provided a viscous medium facilitating percutaneous inoculation.

By 1953, 56 million doses had been delivered in francophone Africa (twice the population of the region).[24] As a result, the incidence of yellow fever declined in francophone countries (Fig. 40–14), but not in neighboring Nigeria and Ghana, where immunization was not practiced. Seroconversion rates were shown to exceed 95%,[400] and population surveys in French West Africa showed that the prevalence of immunity rose from approximately 20% before vaccination to 86% in 1952 to 1953.[401]

The safety of FNV was not evaluated carefully during the ramp-up to achieve full coverage. It was known that FNV

caused viremia in two thirds of subjects; that 10% to 15% experienced a "mild" reaction with fever, headache, and backache on days 4 to 6; and that rare cases of meningoencephalitis occurred 10 to 15 days after vaccination.[396,402–404] The incidence of encephalitis was initially estimated at between 1:3,000 and 1:10,000,[404] but its importance was minimized because full recovery was the rule, and because no serious reactions were noted during campaigns in French West Africa involving over 40 million persons.[398,405] However, contemporary reports described outbreaks of encephalitis and deaths following yellow fever immunization in French Equatorial Africa.[406] English and American workers considered FNV too dangerous for routine use, but, when epidemics struck Nigeria (1951–52) and Central America (1950–52), the danger of yellow fever exceeded vaccine-associated risks. In Nigeria, use of FNV was followed by an outbreak of encephalitis principally in children, with an incidence of 3% to 4% and case-fatality rate of 40%.[407,408] Autopsies showed lesions of encephalitis consistent with direct viral injury, and yellow fever virus was isolated from brain tissue, confirming that FNV and not an adventitious agent was responsible. In Costa Rica and Honduras, 10 definite and 5 possible cases of postvaccinal encephalitis occurred in children.[409]

The increased recognition of severe reactions in children led to a change in the policy for use of FNV. In 1959 and 1960, vaccination was restricted to persons over 10 years of age.[410] The distribution of vaccine decreased from approximately 8 million doses to 4 million doses per year. Within 5 years of cessation of routine immunization of children, epidemic yellow fever reappeared in Senegal for the fist time in 28 years.[304] The 1965 epidemic at Diourbel was the largest on record in West Africa, affecting up to 20,000 persons. Because of the high incidence of yellow fever in children and limited supplies of the safer 17D vaccine, the age limit for use of FNV was reduced to the original 2 years. Among 498,887 persons vaccinated with FNV vaccine, there were 231 cases of postvaccinal encephalitis.[411] The majority of cases occurred in children 2 to 11 years of age, in whom the incidence of encephalitis was approximately 1.4 per 1000 and the case-fatality rate 9%.[411,412] The clinical syndromes associated with acute encephalitis and the neuropsychiatric residua were described by Collomb et al.[413] This unfortunate episode confirmed the need both to provide a high rate of coverage of the childhood population in Africa and to utilize a safer method of immunization. In 1966, the Pasteur Institute, with the assistance of the WHO, expanded production of 17D vaccine at Dakar, Senegal, and by 1970 an official policy was established for use of 17D in persons under the age of 5 years.[414] Small amounts of FNV were used in regions with poor accessibility where use of the more thermolabile 17D vaccine was problematic, but in 1982 production of the vaccine was discontinued.

The potential contamination of FNV with murine viruses (e.g., lymphocytic choriomeningitis) has not been fully clarified. The isolation of yellow fever virus from brain tissue of fatal cases[407] and the absence of murine viruses in FNV lots[415] supports the hypothesis that the vaccine and not an adventitious agent was responsible for encephalitis. In addition to its inherent neurotropism, FNV appears to be genetically less stable than yellow fever 17D virus based on mutations and phenotypic changes occurring during labora-

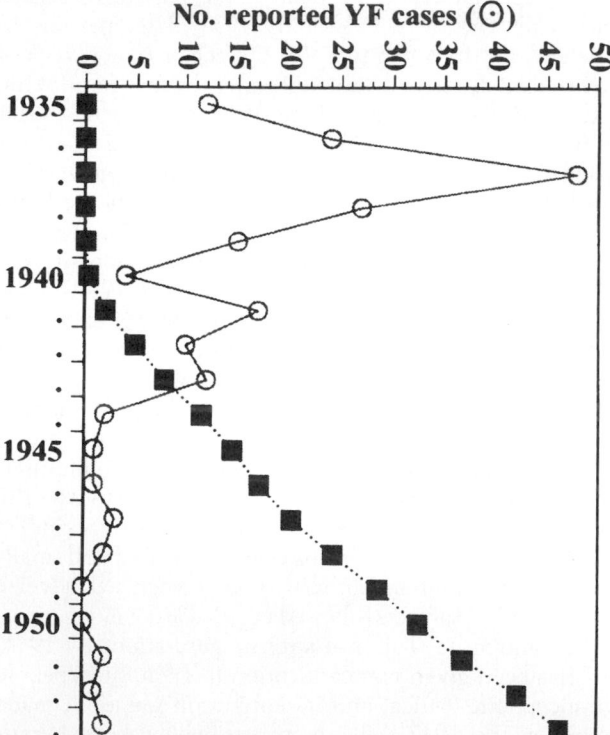

No. doses YF vaccinations (× 000,000) (■)

No. reported YF cases (☉)

FIGURE 40–14 ▪ Cumulative number of doses of FNV administered and incidence of yellow fever (YF) in French West Africa, 1935 through 1953. Compulsory vaccination of the indigenous population resulted in virtual disappearance of the disease. Neighboring anglophone countries, which did not practice immunization, continued to have epidemic yellow fever. (Data from Durieux C. Mass yellow fever vaccination in French Africa south of the Sahara. In Smithburn KC, Durieux C, Koerber R, et al (eds). Yellow Fever Vaccination (Monograph Ser No 30). Geneva, World Health Organization, 1956, pp 115–121. From Monath TP. Yellow fever vaccines: the success of empiricism, pitfalls of application, and transition to molecular vaccinology. In Plotkin S, Fantini M (eds). Vaccinia, Vaccination and Vaccinology: Jenner, Pasteur and Their Successors. Paris, Elsevier, 1996, pp 157–182, with permission.)

tory passage.[416] It is possible that some adverse reactions to the vaccine reflected genetic changes during manufacture or during replication of the vaccine in human hosts.

17D Vaccine Delivered by Scarification

In 1950, a decision was made in Nigeria to prepare 17D vaccine for immunization by scarification, to simplify and reduce the cost of delivery, and to permit use of formulations with less stringent requirements for sterility.[417] Beginning in 1951, trials were initiated using 17D vaccine alone, combined with smallpox vaccine, or combined with smallpox vaccine given at different sites.[417–421] The vaccine was prepared in eggs or by passage of the egg vaccine in mouse brain. Clinical trials revealed lack of seroconversion in up to 15% of those vaccinated with 17D alone and in 35% of those receiving combined yellow fever–smallpox immunization.[422] Revaccination with 17D at an interval of 14 days increased the seroconversion rate.[423] Studies in West Africa and Malaya suggested that vaccine failures might have been due to cross-protective heterologous flavivirus immunity.[424–427] A head-to-head comparison of 17D and FNV delivered by scarification showed a higher seroconversion rate in response to the French vaccine.[417] The apparent lower seroconversion rate of 17D applied by scarification probably was not due to vaccine titer differences,[423] but rather to the inherently higher capacity of FNV to replicate at the dose delivered by this method. Scarification was not adopted for routine delivery of 17D vaccine in anglophone Africa because of uncertainties about efficacy, lack of an efficient cold chain, absence of a public health policy for yellow fever vaccine production and immunization after independence from colonial rule, and the development of improved methods for vaccine delivery (the jet injector).

Yellow Fever 17D Vaccine

17D is the only strain currently used for human immunization against yellow fever.

Development and Early Clinical Testing

The original development of this vaccine, described by Lloyd et al.[428] and Theiler and Smith,[18] was achieved by empirical methods of sequential passage of the prototype Asibi virus in a substrate that was restrictive for growth. This process enhanced the selection of variants with altered biologic properties, without neuroadaptation by mouse brain passage as in the case of FNV. The first successful in vitro passages of Asibi virus were achieved in cultures of minced mouse-embryo tissues. After 18 subcultures, the virus was passed to cultures of minced whole chick embryo. After 58 passages, the virus, now designated as subculture series "17D," was propagated by subcultures in minced chick embryo cultures from which the brain and spinal cord had been removed. The final passage prior to human inoculation was in embryonated eggs.

A reduction in monkey neurovirulence and loss of viscerotropism occurred between the 89th and 114th passages, and reduction in mouse neurovirulence between the 114th and 176th passages. Monkeys inoculated by peripheral routes did not develop encephalitis; those inoculated intracerebrally developed histopathologic changes, but only 5% to 10% succumbed to encephalitis. The animals developed antibodies and resisted challenge with Asibi virus. Preclinical safety and efficacy were deemed sufficient to permit human studies. The initial trials using virus at the 227th and 229th passage levels were conducted in 1936, first in yellow fever–immune and then in nonimmune volunteers.[20,21] The trials showed acceptable tolerability and development of neutralizing antibodies. In early 1937, 17D vaccine was taken to Brazil, where it was used in trials of increasing size, leading to the establishment of local manufacturing and initiation of a mass vaccination campaign in 1938.[21,22,429] Between 1938 and 1941, over 2 million persons were immunized in Brazil.

Seed Lot System

During the initial phase of yellow fever vaccine production at the Rockefeller Foundation in New York and in Brazil between 1937 and 1941, a number of different substrains were used, representing independent parallel subculture lineages originating at about the 200th passage of the original 17D line (Fig. 40–15). Two main lineages (17D-204 and 17DD) were used for vaccine production.

Between 1938 and 1941, field trials and experimental studies revealed the importance of controlling passage level and virus substrain. Substrains 17DD high (305th to 395th passage levels) and $17D_2$ (passage 220) were found to be overattenuated, with poor seroconversion rates in humans and low viremias and poor immunogenicity in monkeys,[430,431] indicating that loss of immunogenicity could occur in as few as 20 passages in minced chicken embryo tissue cultures. More important, some substrains were associated with the appearance of encephalitis. In 1941, following an outbreak of postvaccinal encephalitis in Brazil, a survey of 55,073 persons who received different lots of the same substrain (NY17D-104) revealed the occurrence of 273 (0.5%) severe systemic reactions, including 199 (0.36%) with CNS signs and 1 fatal case of encephalitis.[432] A controlled study was performed in which over 19,000 individuals received different vaccine lots (including EP, $17D_3$, 17D-NY 310, and 17D-NY 104; see Fig. 40–15) that had been associated with the highest incidence of severe reactions or a control vaccine prepared from uninfected chick embryos. Children 5 to 14 years old sustained the highest incidence of encephalitis, with onset of CNS signs 9 to 12 days after immunization. The highest incidence of encephalitis (13 per 1000) was observed in recipients of the 17D-NY 104 vaccine. This substrain also was shown to produce the highest frequency of encephalitis in monkey neurovirulence tests. Other substrains (17D-NY310 and $17D_3$) associated with encephalitis in humans, but at a lower incidence than 17D-NY 104, caused early-onset and prolonged fever in monkeys.

Recognizing that continued serial passage could lead to unwanted alterations in the biologic properties of 17D vaccine, the Rio de Janeiro laboratory instituted a "seed-lot" system in 1941, in which primary seed and secondary seed lots were prepared, and the latter used to prepare multiple vaccine batches. The primary and secondary seeds were extensively characterized, and all vaccine lots were restricted to a single passage from the secondary seed. This system was utilized from 1942 onward by many manufacturers, and was formally established as a biologic standard by the UNRRA in 1945.[433] However, appropriate seed lots were not distributed to all manufacturers, and preparation

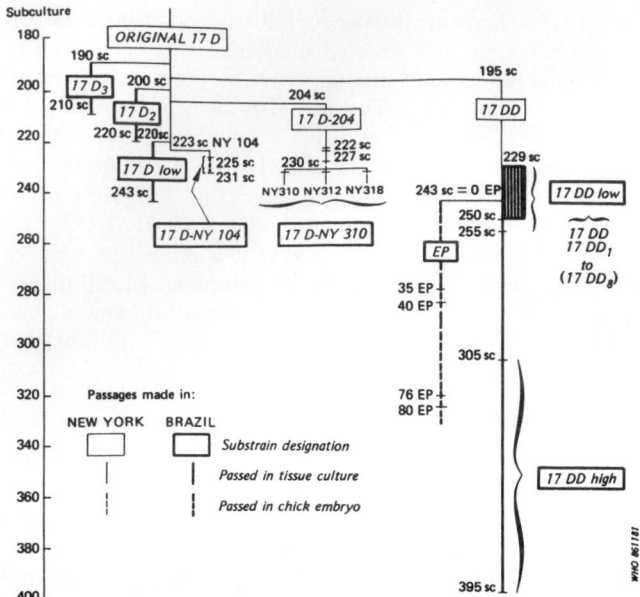

FIGURE 40–15 ■ Derivation of early vaccine lots from the original 17D virus, prior to the institution of a seed lot system (see text). (From Fox JP, Penna HA. Behavior of 17D yellow fever virus in rhesus monkeys: relation to substrain, dose and neural or extraneural inoculation. Am J Hyg 38:152, 1943; and Brès P, Koch M. Production and testing of the WHO yellow fever primary seed lot 213-77 and reference batch 168-73. Geneva, World Health Organ Tech Rep Ser 745(Annex 6):113, 1987, with permission.)

of vaccines by serial passage and without adequate neurovirulence testing continued in some countries in the 1950s. Several cases of encephalitis were reported following use of such vaccines at the Pasteur Institute during that time.[434] In 1957, publication of the WHO's "Requirements for Yellow Fever Vaccine" further standardized the seed-lot and manufacturing procedures.[435]

Vaccine Producers

Currently there are seven active manufacturers of yellow fever 17D vaccine (Table 40–10; N Dellepiane, WHO, personal communication, 2002). Three manufacturers in Brazil, France, and Senegal produce large amounts of vaccine for the Expanded Programme of Immunization (EPI) and mass vaccination campaigns during routine and emergency operations. Aventis Pasteur and Evans export vaccine

for the traveler's market. Global vaccine production is currently approximately 55 million doses. The number of manufacturers has decreased during the last 20 years, with facilities in the Netherlands, Australia, Nigeria, and South Africa no longer active. There are concerns about Good Manufacturing Practices standards at some of the current manufacturers, and it is likely that facility renovation and operational changes will be required to maintain WHO approval for continued production. Four manufacturers currently are approved by the WHO (Table 40–10).

All yellow fever vaccines are live, attenuated vaccines derived from the 17D strain, are produced in embryonated eggs, and meet WHO standards of safety and potency (see *Method of Manufacture, Control, and Lot Release Tests* below). Their biologic performance is presumed to be similar or identical with respect to seroconversion rate, quality of the immune response, durability of immunity, safety, and tolerability. Vaccines in current production differ, however, with respect to 17D substrain, passage level, formulation with stabilizers, thermostability, and contamination with avian leukosis virus. 17D vaccines are not biologically cloned and are heterogeneous mixtures of multiple virion subpopulations. Not surprisingly, differences have been found in plaque size,[116] oligonucleotide fingerprints,[436] and the nucleotide sequences of vaccines in current use.[80–82,85] There is no evidence to suggest that such variations affect safety or efficacy.

Substrains, Passage Histories, and Molecular Heterogeneity of 17D Vaccines in Current Use

Prior to initiating the attenuation process, Asibi virus was passaged sequentially 54 times in monkeys, either by direct injection of blood from the previous animal, or with an intervening passage in A. *aegypti* mosquitoes (Fig. 40–16). Throughout this passage history, the virus maintained its virulence for rhesus monkeys. Figures 40–15 through 40–18 show the virus passage history during the original development of 17D vaccines. In vitro cultivation began in December 1933 with the passage of the virulent Asibi strain in mouse embryo tissue culture and subsequently in chick embryo tissue culture to produce attenuated 17D vaccines (Fig. 40–17).[428] Two 17D substrains—17DD and 17D-204—currently used for vaccine manufacture represent independent subcultures performed at the Rockefeller Foundation, New York (see Fig. 40–15). The 17DD and 17D-204 substrains were derived from passage levels 195

TABLE 40–10 ■ Current Manufacturers of Yellow Fever 17D Vaccine

Country	Manufacturer	Qualified by WHO	Comment
United States	Aventis Pasteur (Swiftwater, PA)	No	Principally U.S. consumption, FDA-approved
Brazil	BioManguinhos (Rio de Janeiro)	Yes	
United Kingdom	Evans Vaccines (Speke, Liverpool)	Yes	
France	Aventis Pasteur (Marcy l'Etoile)	Yes	
India	Central Research Institute (Kisauli)	No	Local consumption
Colombia	Instituto Nacional de Salud (Bogota)	No	Local consumption
Russia	Institute of Poliomyelitis & Viral Encephalitides (Moscow)	No	Local consumption
Senegal	Pasteur Institute (Dakar)	Yes	
Switzerland	Berna (Bern)	No	Previous manufacturer Robert Koch Institute

FDA, Food and Drug Administration.

and 204, respectively, of the original 17D virus (see Figs. 40–15 and 40–17). 17DD virus was sent to Brazil at passage level 229, whereupon it was passed 14 times in minced chicken embryo tissue cultures and then, beginning at passage 243, in whole embryonated eggs (the "EP" lineage, see Fig. 40–15). Primary and secondary seeds were prepared in Brazil at passages 284 and 285, respectively, and the current vaccine is at passage 286 (Fig. 40–18). One of two 17DD primary seeds was transferred to the Pasteur Institute in Dakar, Senegal, and used to prepare new seed stocks for vaccine manufacture.

The 17D-204 substrain has been used by all other manufacturers. At passage level 222, the virus was propagated in embryonated eggs in order to prepare a vaccine lot (NY 75) (see Fig. 40–17). This vaccine was transferred to the Yellow Fever Laboratory in Bogota, Colombia, where additional egg passages were performed. Colombia No. 88 was returned to the Rockefeller Institute in 1940, whereupon a small number of passages in eggs were made at the Rockefeller Foundation or the Rocky Mountain Laboratory (National Institutes of Health) prior to the manufacture of primary seed stocks in France, the United States, Australia, the Netherlands, Germany, Colombia, South Africa, England, and India. The Pasteur Institute in Dakar switched from 17DD to 17D-204 virus for preparation of secondary seed free from avian leukosis virus. In 1977, the Robert Koch Institute in Berlin prepared for the WHO a primary seed free from avian leukosis virus, and maintains this as a refer-

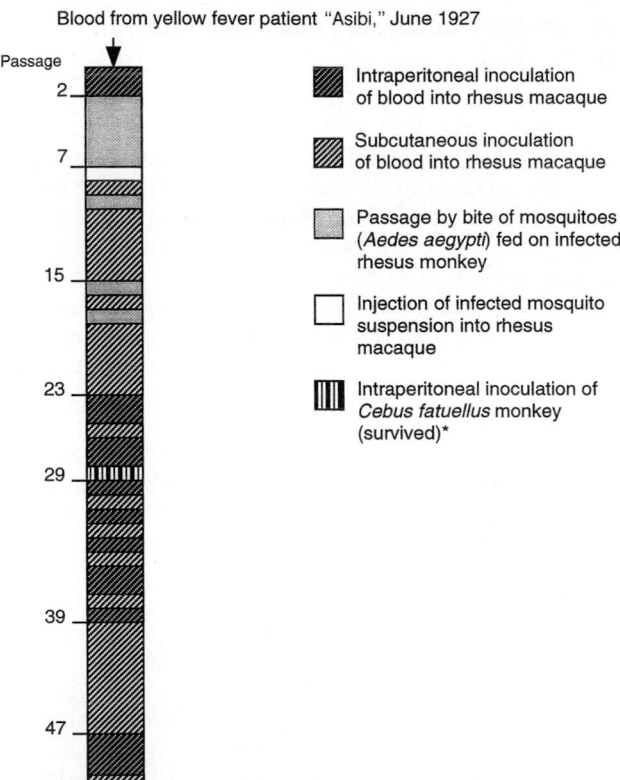

FIGURE 40–16 ■ Passage history of Asibi virus from original isolation to the initiation of in vitro culture for development of the 17D vaccine. *Not counted by authors but represents a passage in the history of Asibi virus before cultivation in vitro.

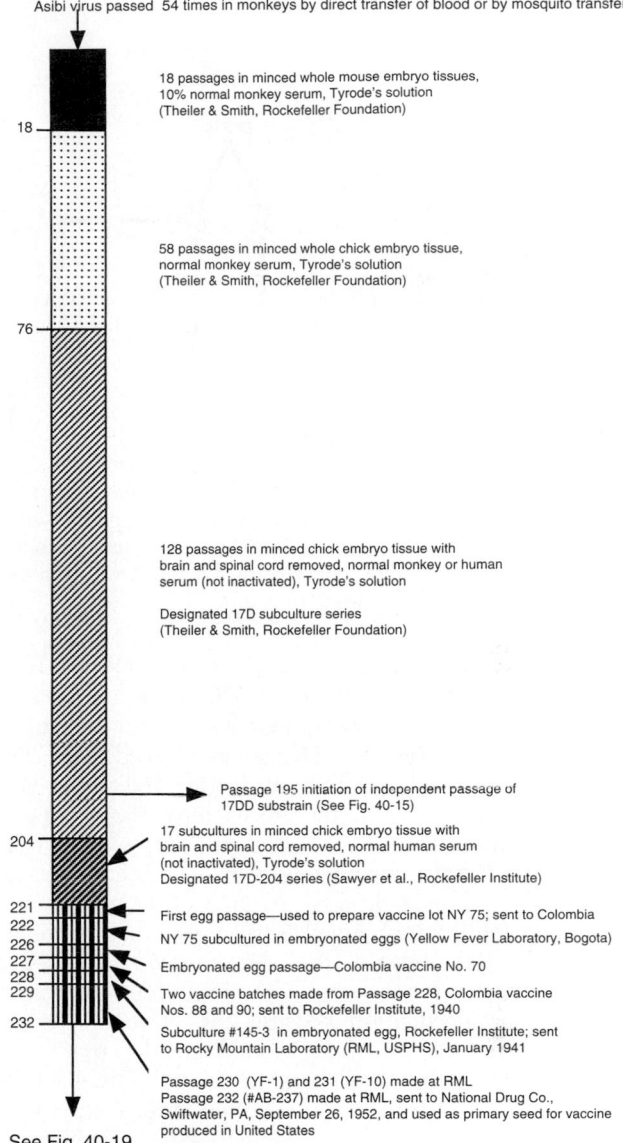

FIGURE 40–17 ■ Passage history of the seed virus used to prepare yellow fever vaccines. (Modified from Brès P, Koch M. Production and testing of the WHO yellow fever primary seed lot 213-77 and reference batch 168-73. Geneva, World Health Organ Tech Rep Ser 745(Annex 6):113, 1987.)

ence stock (designated 17D-213-77[437]) available to new manufacturers and as a source for emergency production. All current 17D-204 vaccines are produced at passage levels between 233 and 239.

The 17DD and 17D-204 substrains are distinguishable by MAb analysis, indicating variations in antigenic determinants on the E protein.[120,128,129,436,438] Antigenic differences also have been identified between vaccines produced from the 17D-204 substrain by different manufacturers.[128] Examination of yellow fever vaccines manufactured in 11 countries by T_1 oligonucleotide fingerprinting revealed a very high degree of genetic similarity.[436] The primary seed and vaccine produced in South Africa (Fig. 40–19) differed at one and two oligonucleotides, respectively. This difference was confirmed at the sequence level by Xie,[359] who found two changes in the 3' NCR. A comparison of the

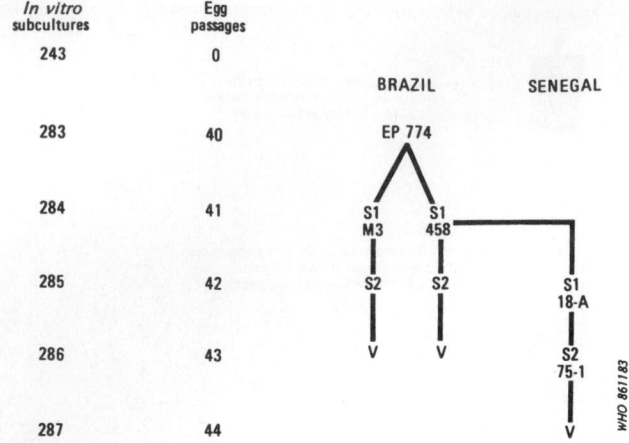

FIGURE 40–18 ■ Passage history of the 17DD substrain (derivation shown in Fig. 40–16) to prepare seed viruses and vaccines in Brazil and Senegal. (From Brès P, Koch M. Production and testing of the WHO yellow fever primary seed lot 213-77 and reference batch 168-73. Geneva, World Health Organ Tech Rep Ser 745(Annex 6):113, 1987, with permission.)

nucleotide and amino acid sequences of the 17DD substrain vaccine produced in Brazil, the WHO reference vaccine (17D-213), and 17D-204 strains manufactured in the United States, France, and the United Kingdom revealed that 17DD vaccine had accumulated fewer nucleotide and amino acid changes per passage during the process of development and attenuation than had 17D-204 vaccine viruses.[82,439] 17DD and 17D substrain vaccines differ at 10 amino acid residues[12,79,439] (Table 40–11). At five other amino acid residues, variability is observed between vaccines belonging to the 17D-204 substrain (including the WHO 17D-213 virus). These differences among vaccines do not appear to be related to attenuation because one or more vaccine strains has a residue at each position identical to that found in parental (virulent) Asibi virus (refer to Table 40–1 for shared differences between all vaccine strains and Asibi virus that may play a role in attenuation). An analysis of the United Kingdom vaccine (Arilvax) demonstrated con-

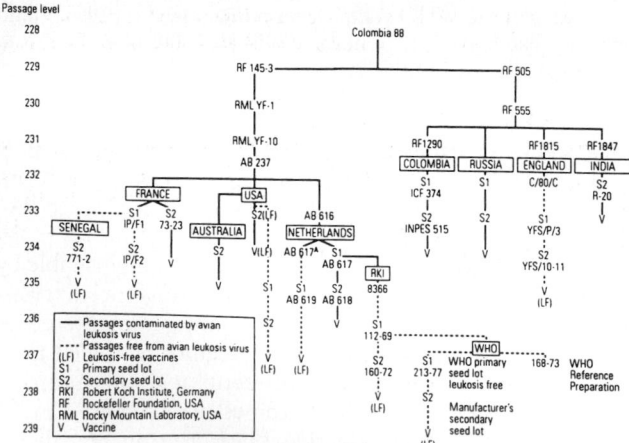

FIGURE 40–19 ■ Passage history of the 17D-204 substrain vaccines (derivation shown in Fig. 40–17) to prepare seed viruses and vaccines in various countries. (From Robertson SE, Hull BP, Tomori O, et al. Yellow fever: a decade of reemergence. JAMA 276:1157, 1996, with permission.)

sensus sequence heterogeneity at certain residues,[82] suggesting that more discriminating analytic methods and use of uncloned rather than plaque-purified viruses might reveal a slightly different picture of sequence differences among yellow fever strains.

The neurovirulence phenotypes of 17DD and 17D-204 substrains have been examined in mice[191] and monkeys.[440] Vaccines were compared with respect to average survival time and mortality after intranasal inoculation of young adult mice. 17DD substrain vaccines were neurovirulent after intranasal inoculation, whereas those derived from 17D-204 were not. In monkeys subjected to the WHO standard intracerebral neurovirulence test, slightly higher histopathologic lesion scores were found in the brains of animals inoculated with 17DD than with 17D-204 vaccines.[440] However, both 17DD and 17D-204 vaccines passed WHO standards and were well within the limits of acceptable safety in the monkey test. Overall, the data suggest that 17DD vaccine may be somewhat more neurovirulent than 17D-204 substrain vaccines as determined in animal models. Because both substrains have a long history of use in many millions of persons, and because all reported cases of postvaccinal encephalitis after stabilization of vaccine passage level have in fact involved 17D-204 substrain vaccines, there is no reason to suspect that the 17DD and 17D-204 substrains differ with respect to safety for humans. However, this conclusion eventually may require modification when surveillance for serious adverse events is intensified in Brazil, where 17DD vaccine is in routine use.

Method of Manufacture, Control, and Lot Release Tests

Biologic standards for yellow fever vaccines have been established by the WHO,[435] and all vaccines must comply with these basic standards and be produced according to Good Manufacturing Practices. National control authorities (e.g., the Food and Drug Administration in the United States) govern approval for use, and thus biologic standards differ somewhat from country to country. Manufacturers currently use seeds free from avian leukosis virus, but testing for other viral adventitious agents varies.

Primary (master) and secondary (manufacturer's working) seeds are tested for bacteria, fungi, mycoplasma, and adventitious viruses and are subjected to a standard safety and immunogenicity test in rhesus or cynomolgus monkeys,[435] A minimum of 10 monkeys are inoculated intracerebrally with 0.25 mL of virus containing 5000 to 50,000 MLD$_{50}$. Animals are monitored for clinical signs, viremia, antibody responses, and neuropathologic lesions (Table 40–12). For comparison, a reference control is inoculated into 10 other animals. Some authorities have advised using a reference vaccine that has failed the safety test (e.g., 17D Lot 6766).[440,441]

Vaccine is produced by aseptic inoculation of secondary seed into viable embryonated eggs.[442–444] Most manufacturers use eggs from closed, special pathogen-free flocks. The dose of secondary seed virus inoculated into 7- to 9-day-old embryonated eggs is 2000 to 5000 MLD$_{50}$ (or equivalent in plaque-forming units) in 0.1 mL. After incubation for 3 to 4 days, infected embryos are harvested aseptically. Embryos must be 12 days of age or less at the time of harvest. A single harvest is the pool of embryos inoculated together in a single production run. Methods for recovery of virus from infected embryos vary, but all include addition of sterile

TABLE 40–11 ■ Amino Acid Differences Between Yellow Fever 17D and 17DD Vaccine Substrain Viruses*

Nucleotide	Gene	Amino Acid	Asibi	17D-204 ATCC	17D-204 France	17D-204 [UK (Arilvax)]	17D-213 (WHO)	17DD (Brazil)
				AMINO ACID				
1140	E	56	A	V	V	V	V	A
1431		153	N	N	N	N	T	N
1436		155	D	D	D	D	D	S
1437		155	G	G	G	G	G	S
1946		325	P	S	S	S	S	P
2219		416	A	T	T	T	T	A
2220		416	T	T	T	T	T	V
4013	NS2A	112	L	F	F	F	F	L
5115	NS3	182	Q	Q	Q	Q	Q	R
5153		195	I	V	V	V/I	V	I
6758	NS4A	107	I	V	I	I	I	I
7319	NS4B	7	E	E	K	K	K	K
7701	NS5	22	Q	R	R	R	R	Q
8605		323	N	D	N	N	N	N
8808		391	N	N	N	N	N	S
				NUCLEOTIDE				
10367	3'NCR		T	C	C	C/T	C	C
10454			A	G	A	A	A	A
10550			T	C	C	C	C	T
10722			G	G	A	G	G	G

*These differences occurring between vaccine strains do not appear to play a role in attenuation because one or more vaccine strains have sequence identical to Asibi virus at the same amino acid residue. Nucleotide differences in the terminal noncoding regions (NCR) also are shown. Refer to Table 40–1 for differences between wild-type parental Asibi virus and 17D and 17DD vaccine substrains, which may play a role in attenuation. Data from Jennings et al.[12], Rice et al.[76], Dupuy et al.[81], Pugachev et al.[82], and Galler et al.[439]

water for injection (typically 1 to 2 mL/embryo), homogenization to "pulp," and clarification by centrifugation to yield supernatant fluid harvest. Individual harvests containing homogenate from a single pool of embryos are held frozen pending sterility tests. Sterility tests are performed at one or more steps prior to pooling single harvests into the final bulk, which may contain one or a pool of single harvests. The amount of final bulk prepared is determined principally by the volume capacity of the lyophilizer. The final bulk is diluted and blended with stabilizers (e.g., gelatin and sorbitol) based on potency (infectivity titer) to produce the drug product, filled into glass vials, and lyophilized. Sterile filtration is not performed because the consistency of the product renders filtration difficult and results in significant loss of titer. The manufacturing process thus is performed aseptically under Class 100 conditions. The target infectivity titer of the drug product is adjusted for a factor for losses expected across lyophilization and losses expected between release and end of shelf life. The release titer therefore exceeds the compendial minimum (1000 MLD_{50} or equivalent in PFU). In the case of YF-Vax® (Aventis Pasteur Inc., Swiftwater, PA) and Arilvax, the release titer is greater than 4.4 and greater than 5.0 $\log_{10}$ PFU/0.5 mL, respectively. The yield per embryo is typically in the range of 100 to 300 doses.

If a plaque assay is used for potency, the manufacturer must establish the relationship between MLD_{50} and plaque

TABLE 40–12 ■ Biologic Standards for Monkey Safety Tests* on 17D Vaccine Seeds[444]

Criterion	Test	Result
Viscerotropism	Viremia level on days 2, 4, and 6	Viremia < 500 MLD_{50}[†]/0.03 mL in all samples, and not greater than 100 MLD_{50} in more than one sample
Immunogenicity	Neutralizing antibody	>90% seroconversion on day 30
Neurotropism	Clinical observation daily for 30 days	Frequency of encephalitis and semiquantitative clinical score < reference seed
	Histologic evaluation (day 30)	Mean lesion scores < reference seed[‡]

*Ten nonimmune rhesus or cynomolgus monkeys are inoculated in the frontal lobe with 5000 to 50,000 MLD_{50} (or equivalent in plaque-forming units) and monitored for 30 days.

[†]Or equivalent in plaque-forming units.

[‡]Histologic grading performed on five levels of brain and six of cervical and lumbar spinal cord, using semiquantitative grading score of inflammation and neuronal degeneration. Areas of brain studied include "target" ares (areas that show more severe lesions irrespective of degree of neurovirulence of virus tested); "spared" areas; and "discriminator" areas that distinguish between vaccines of low and high neurovirulence. Mean group scores for target + discriminator areas combined and for discriminator areas alone are calculated.

From World Health Organization. Requirements for Yellow Fever Vaccine (Requirements for Biological Substances No. 3). Technical Report Series. Geneva, World Health Organization, 1997.

titer, since the WHO biologic standard is tied to the MLD_{50}. This relationship (approximately 50 $PFU{:}MLD_{50}$) has sometimes been difficult to establish, reflecting the variability of plaque titrations and/or the mouse assay.[444]

The final bulk is tested for absence of adventitious agents. Standards vary across national control authorities but include tests for bacteria, including *Mycobacterium avium*, fungi, and mycoplasma. Because yellow fever 17D vaccines were developed before the application of modern tests for adventitious viruses, the standards for testing may be less stringent than for new vaccines in some countries. Control (uninfected) eggs are routinely incubated along with eggs used for vaccine manufacture and are tested for viability and hemagglutinating viruses. The in vitro virus test in cell cultures and the in vivo virus test in mice, guinea pigs, and eggs may be required by some control authorities. These tests, which require subculture or blind passage) are complicated by the requirement to neutralize the test article (yellow fever 17D virus) in order to observe cultures or in vivo hosts for inapparent viruses. Neutralization requires a potent antiserum raised in a pathogen-free host against yellow fever antigen that has been produced in a host other than eggs. The neutralization procedure may be difficult, particularly when high-titer preparations must be tested in sensitive indicator cells or in suckling mice. Protein content before addition of stabilizers may not exceed 0.25 mg/dose. After filling, the final product is tested for identity by neutralization test, potency, thermostability, sterility, general safety in mice and guinea pigs, residual moisture, residual ovalbumin, and endotoxin. Some countries require that a monkey safety test be performed on each vaccine lot. As specified by the WHO standards,[435] potency must exceed 1000 MLD_{50} (or the equivalent in plaque titer) per dose. Typically, the dose in the final container exceeds the minimum specification by at least fivefold (0.7 log) to account for potential losses during storage.

Cost of Manufacture and Vaccine Price

The cost of manufacture of yellow fever vaccine is modest but highly dependent on local conditions (personnel wages, overhead, etc.) Price and sales margins vary by market segment. Current pricing (in 2002) for vaccine supplied to the WHO or the United Nations International Children's Emergency Fund (UNICEF) for use in emergencies or for the EPI is US$0.35 per dose (20-dose container) to $0.63 per dose (10-dose container), whereas the price for yellow fever vaccine sold to travelers in developed countries is as high as $55 per dose.

Adventitious Viruses

In 1966, yellow fever 17D vaccine was discovered to be contaminated with avian leukosis virus by Harris et al.[445] All vaccines produced at that time contained the agent because of the high prevalence of infection of chicken embryos. New seeds free of avian leukosis virus were developed in the 1970s, and all manufacturers now employ leukosis-free seeds as stipulated by WHO standards. Some current manufacturers use embryos contaminated with avian leukosis virus for vaccine production (a practice permitted by the WHO).[435] Although the presence of leukosis virus in yellow fever vaccine is certainly undesirable because of the possibility of insertion of leukosis virus oncogenes, there is no evidence to implicate the virus in human disease. The question was addressed by a retrospective survey of World War II veterans for cancer deaths.[446] The incidence of all cancers, lymphoma, and leukemia was not significantly different (and in fact was lower) in persons vaccinated 5 to 22 years previously with 17D vaccine than in those not vaccinated. Although not a WHO requirement, most manufacturers utilize eggs from specific pathogen-free flocks.

Vaccines manufactured in eggs, including yellow fever 17D, test positive by the product-enhanced reverse transcriptase (PERT) assay, reflecting the presence of defective particles containing endogenous avian leukosis or retrovirus sequences. No evidence has been found for infectious or inducible replication-competent retroviruses or for infection with avian leukosis or endogenous avian retrovirus in humans.[447,448] Tests for retroviral contamination by amplification in avian cell culture and quantitative PCR may be required for future regulatory approval of yellow fever vaccines made in eggs.

During the original formulation and early use of 17D vaccines, pooled human serum was used as a stabilizer. Vaccines were thereby contaminated with hepatitis B virus, resulting in outbreaks of jaundice (see *Adverse Events* below). Human serum was eliminated from yellow fever vaccines by 1942. Current vaccines carry no inherent risk of contamination with human hepatitis viruses.

Dose and Route of Administration

Yellow fever vaccine is given by the subcutaneous route in a volume of 0.5 mL. The usual site of inoculation is the upper arm; there are no data to suggest that anatomic site of inoculation is relevant to the immune response. Care is taken to avoid exposure of the live vaccine to alcohol or other skin disinfectants. The minimum dose requirement is 1000 MLD_{50}, or the equivalent in PFU. Although differences exist across laboratories, the ratio of $PFU{:}MLD_{50}$ is approximately 50:1. Because commercial vaccines contain an excess of virus to provide for losses during storage, the delivered dose is higher than the minimum standard. The actual dose contained in commercial vaccines varies, but at time of release ranges from 5 to 50 times the minimum. For example, the vaccine produced in the United States contains, 5.04 $\log_{10}$ PFUs/0.5 mL dose.

Recent attempts to immunize monkeys with 17D vaccine by the oral or intestinal route using acid-stable capsules were not successful (contrary to an earlier report[366]), whereas application of virus by intranasal spray resulted in uniform seroconversion.[449] Intranasal immunization has not been attempted in humans. The residual neurotropism of 17D virus raises safety concerns because of the possible exposure of olfactory neurons in the nasal cavity and potential for direct access to the brain via the ethmoid route.

Preparations Available, Including Combinations

All yellow fever vaccines in current use are live attenuated 17DD or 17D-204 substrain viruses, prepared in embryonated chicken eggs and formulated as lyophilized powder. Vaccines vary with respect to stabilizer additives and salt content. Some contain sodium chloride and buffer salts and are reconstituted with sterile water, while others are reconstituted with saline solution. Vaccines differ with respect to expiry date, but all require storage at point of use at 2° to 8°C, and must be discarded 1 hour after reconstitution.

Vaccines are supplied in single- and multiple-dose containers, the largest of which contains 100 doses for use in jet injectors. Vaccines produced in France (Stamaril®, Aventis Pasteur); England (Arilvax); Brazil (BioMinguinhos), and Senegal (Pasteur Institute) are exported for international use or supplied to the EPI through the UNICEF bid market. The vaccines produced elsewhere are used almost exclusively in-country for travelers and military personnel. Although certain combination vaccines have been tested clinically (including yellow fever–measles and yellow fever–typhoid), no products currently are commercialized.

Constituents, Including Antibiotics and Preservatives

There are no antibiotics or preservatives in yellow fever vaccines. For this reason, and because of instability of the virus after reconstitution, both single-dose and multidose vials must be used within a short interval of time, as specified on the package label (typically 1 hour). Salt, buffer, and stabilizer excipients vary by manufacturer.

Vaccine Thermostability

In 1987, the WHO published an addendum to the biologic standards, with a guideline (not a formal requirement) that vaccines meet a stability standard.[450] The specification included two criteria: the lyophilized vaccine held at 37°C for 14 days must (1) maintain minimum potency (>1000 MLD_{50} per 0.5-mL dose) and (2) show a mean loss of titer less than 1.0 log_{10} LD_{50}. Of the vaccines produced by the 12 approved manufacturers at that time, only five met the stability specifications.[451] Current WHO requirements for yellow fever vaccine[435] made the stability standard a requirement and also stipulate that the minimum vaccine expiry date shall be not less than 2 years after the last satisfactory potency test.

Without stabilizers, yellow fever vaccine loses 1.5 to 2.5 log_{10} LD_{50}/dose during 14 days at 37°C. Stabilized vaccines lose only 0.3 to 0.5 log_{10} LD_{50}/dose during this interval.[375] In one study, a stabilized lyophilized vaccine produced in Senegal met WHO standards after storage at 2° to 8°C for more than 3 years.[452,453] Storage at −20°C was superior to storage at 2° to 8°C. Stabilized yellow fever vaccine has a stability profile similar to or better than those of other thermolabile vaccines used in the EPI (including polio, measles, and pertussis vaccines). Thus, although the lyophilized vaccine requires proper storage and handling under cold chain conditions in the field, yellow fever vaccine is not the "weak link" in the EPI chain. Stabilizers differ by manufacturer. The vaccines produced in the United States and the United Kingdom use sorbitol and gelatin. The vaccine made in France employs sugars, amino acids, and divalent cations (lactose [4%], sorbitol [2%], histidine [0.01 M], and alanine [0.01 M] in phosphate-buffered saline containing Ca^{2+} and Mg^{2+}).[454,455] A disadvantage of yellow fever vaccine is its instability after reconstitution. The vaccine must be held on ice after reconstitution and is discarded after 1 hour. This instability leads to wastage under field conditions during mass immunization campaigns. Lopes et al.[456] found that vaccine maintained potency at 37°C for more than 3 hours in distilled water, whereas vaccine in phosphate buffer or saline with or without stabilizers lost potency. However, the water diluent was found to cause severe pain at the injection site, and its use has been discontinued.

Genetic Stability During Replication in the Host

17D vaccines are not plaque purified and contain heterogeneous subpopulations of plaque-size variants with differing mouse neurovirulence.[116,117,130] One variant recovered from 17D vaccine by plaque purification had a wild-type epitope and amino acid change at position E173.[63,95,130] The relative proportion of plaque size variants in 17D vaccines changes with passage.[116] Consensus sequencing of a 17D vaccine (Arilvax) revealed 12 nucleotide heterogeneities within structural and nonstructural genes and the 3′ NCR, indicating the quasi species nature of the vaccine.[82]

Given the safety record of 17D vaccines since stabilization of passage level, genotypic and phenotypic heterogeneity does not pose a safety problem, and in fact has been proposed to be a positive attribute of the vaccine.[85] No individual plaque variant of 17D virus has shown a neurovirulence phenotype that exceeds the vaccine itself, and thus changes in the relative proportion of variants on replication in humans might not alter virulence. Xie et al.[117] sequenced 17D virus strains isolated from the sera of six subjects given the 17D-204 vaccine produced in the United States. No mutations were found in the structural genes, and no more than two nucleotide changes were found in NS5 regions. Similarly, virus strains recovered from sera of monkeys 30 days after IC inoculation of 17D-204 vaccine contained no mutations or a single silent mutation in NS5.[117] These results indicate a high degree of genetic stability of 17D virus during in vivo replication. Mutations tend to accumulate at a significantly lower rate (10^{-5} to 10^{-6}) than expected for an RNA virus, and in a nonrandom fashion, principally in the NS5 gene. In addition, studies employing a truly clonal yellow fever 17D virus as a vector for foreign genes have been very successful,[155,457] indicating that the quasi species nature of 17D vaccine is not critical to safety and efficacy, and that it should be possible to develop a molecular (or biologic) clone of 17D as a vaccine.

Rare mutational events in 17D vaccine during replication in the host have been shown to alter pathogenicity. The first of two published fatal cases of encephalitis occurred in 1965 in a 3-year-old child who received 17D-204 vaccine.[108] Jennings et al.[109] defined the characteristics of the virus from brain tissue and commercial 17D vaccines at similar laboratory passage level. Compared to commercial vaccine, the brain isolate had higher neurovirulence for mice, caused severe encephalitis in a cynomolgus monkey, and reacted with a wild-type specific MAb. The brain isolate differed from 17D-204 at two residues in the E gene (E155 and E303) and one in NS4B. The potential role of these mutations in neurovirulence, particularly the change at position E303, has been discussed above in the section on *Virology*. A single mutation occurring during in vitro passage in the heterologous E protein of a chimeric yellow fever vaccine increased the neurovirulence of the virus.[97]

Results of Vaccination

Viremia Following 17D Vaccination

Whereas wild-type yellow fever virus causes high viremias in monkeys and humans, 17D vaccine induces minimal virus titers in circulating blood. A control test for the reduced viscerotropism of 17D vaccines is the measurement of viremia in monkeys on days 2, 4, and 6 following IC inoculation, which must not exceed 500 $MLD_{50}/0.03$ mL on any day and must not exceed 100 $MLD_{50}/0.03$ mL on more than 1 day.[435]

Viremia following 17D vaccination has been measured in adult humans. Smith et al.[21] found virus in serum of 13 (46%) of 28 subjects given 3 to 4 $\log_{10} MLD_{50}$ of 17D vaccine. The earliest onset of viremia occurred on day 4 and the latest on day 10. Of the 13 viremic individuals, 4 were viremic for 1 day, 5 for 2 days, and 4 for 3 days. The quantity of virus in blood was extremely small in all cases (<2 $MLD_{50}/0.03$ mL). Sweet et al.[149] measured viremias in subjects with and without prevaccination neutralizing antibodies to Japanese encephalitis virus. The 17D vaccine (National Drug Co., USA) contained approximately 6.4 $\log_{10}$ *suckling mouse* $ICLD_{50}$/dose (equivalent to approximately 5.3 to 5.8 $\log_{10} MLD_{50}$,[458] and thus substantially higher than the dose used by Smith et al.[21]). Viremia was measured by IC inoculation of infant mice with undiluted serum. Of 25 subjects without pre-existing flavivirus immunity, 15 (60%) had detectable viremia on 1 or more days during the 6-day sampling period (days 3 to 8 after vaccination). The highest incidence of viremia (48%) was on day 5, and the mean duration was 1.9 days. Titers were very low, because none of the sera caused 100% mortality in infant mice. There was no difference in the incidence or duration of viremia in subjects with pre-existing immunity to Japanese encephalitis virus.[149]

In a study of 15 young adults, Wheelock and Sibley[459] determined 17D viremia by a more sensitive method (inoculation of 0.1 mL of plasma into tube cultures of BHK-21 cells). Fourteen subjects (93.3%) had detectable viremia. The average time to onset of viremia was 4.4 days (range 3 to 6 days), and the mean duration was 2.5 days (range 1 to 5 days). Viremic days were sequential and continuous in most cases, but one individual had detectable viremia on days 4, 8, and 9. A rough estimation of the level of viremia was possible based on the detection in cell cultures inoculated with varying volumes of plasma. Virus titers were exceedingly low; in only 3 of 14 individuals was virus detected in cultures inoculated with 0.001 mL of plasma.

Actis and Sa Fleitas[460] studied 12 adults who received an unspecified dose of 17DD-EP vaccine produced in Brazil. The duration and level of viremia, detected by IC inoculation of weanling mice, were similar to those in previous studies, but a somewhat higher proportion of subjects were viremic than in other studies using mice for detection of viremia.

In two clinical trails of a chimeric YF/JE vaccine, yellow fever 17D (YF-Vax) was used as a control for safety in healthy adults 18 to 59 years of age[155] (also TP Monath et al., unpublished results, 2002). Viremia was measured by plaque assay in Vero cells. Nearly all subjects were viremic on 1 or more days. Approximately 30% to 60% of the subjects were viremic between days 4 and 6 after vaccination, with lower proportions at earlier and later time points (Fig. 40–20). The mean duration of viremia was approximately 2 days. Viremia levels were low (mean peak titers <20 PFU) and in no case exceeded 2 $\log_{10}$ PFU/mL. Six previously vaccinated subjects experienced no viremia after revaccination.

Similarly, Reinhardt et al.[209] inoculated 12 naïve and 5 previously vaccinated healthy adults 18 to 50 years of age

with the yellow fever 17D vaccine manufactured by the Robert Koch Institute. Viremia levels were measured by plaque assay in PS cells and by RT-PCR. The pattern and height of viremia were similar to those described above. There was no correlation between the level of viremia and the height of the neutralizing antibody response. The highest incidence of viremia by plaque assay was on days 5 (42%) and 6 (33%), the duration of viremia was 1 to 3 days, and the peak titer was 97 PFU/mL, with most values less than 20 PFU/mL. All 12 naïve subjects, including 5 who had no viremia by plaque assay, were positive by RT-PCR, and sera contained detectable viral RNA at least 1 day longer than by infectivity assay. None of the revaccinated subjects were positive by RT-PCR or plaque assay.

Taken together, these studies confirm that very low levels of virus are present in circulating blood for a brief period following 17D vaccination. Viremia occurs during the latter half of the first week after vaccination, and thus the incubation period and duration of viremia are not dissimilar to natural infection with yellow fever virus. Cessation of viremia corresponds to the time of appearance of neutralizing antibodies 8 to 9 days after immunization (see *Kinetics of the Immune Response* below). Titers of virus in blood are

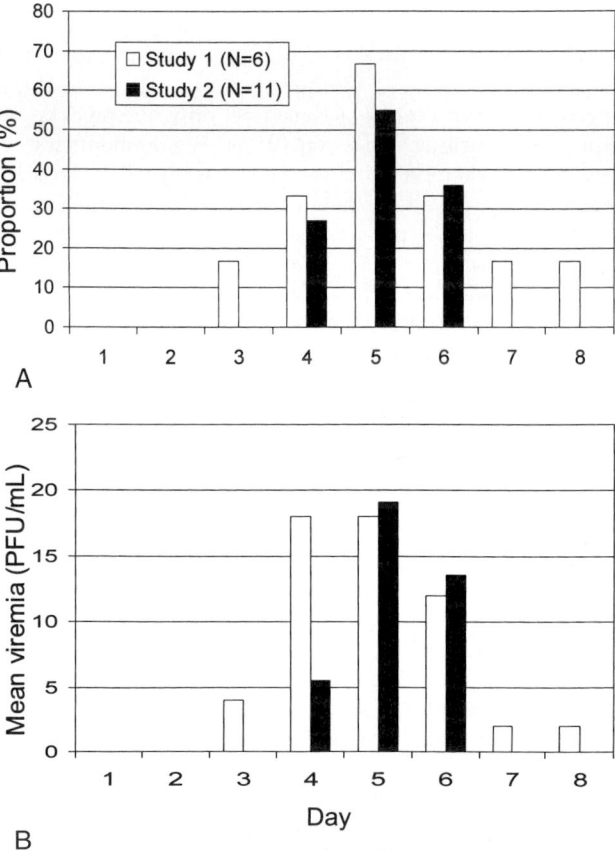

FIGURE 40–20 ■ *Top,* Proportion of healthy adults in two studies with viremia detectable by plaque-reduction assay following inoculation of yellow fever 17D vaccine (YF-Vax). *Bottom,* Mean viremia levels in the same studies. Viremia occurred principally between days 4 and 6 and did not exceed 2 $\log_{10}$ PFU/mL in any subject. (Data from Monath TP, McCarthy K, Bedford P, et al. Clinical proof of principle for ChimeriVax™: recombinant live, attenuated vaccines against flavivirus infections. Vaccine 20:1004, 2002, and an unpublished study.)

far below the infection threshold for mosquito vectors. The low viremia following 17D vaccine also may explain the apparent low risk of transmission of the virus to the fetus in women who have been immunized during pregnancy (see *Pregnancy and Lactation* below) and the low incidence of postvaccinal encephalitis. Detection of viremia is influenced by test methodology. PCR is more sensitive than infectivity assays, and might detect viral RNA in the absence of infectivity, for example, after the appearance of antibody.

There are no data on viremia levels in infants or children given 17D vaccine. The higher risk of postvaccinal encephalitis in young infants suggests the possibility that viremia levels may be higher or more prolonged (alternatively, susceptibility could reflect immaturity of the blood-brain barrier). No data are available on the height and duration of viremia in persons who are immunosuppressed.

Immune Responses

The neutralizing antibody response to 17D vaccine has been evaluated in numerous studies since development of the vaccine in the late 1930s. Theiler and Smith[20] and Smith et al.[21] demonstrated appearance of neutralizing antibodies within 1 to 2 weeks after immunization. In a field study in Brazil (1937–38), 94.1% of 882 vaccinees seroconverted after vaccination.[21] Subsequent clinical trials have confirmed the high immunogenicity of yellow fever 17D vaccine, with development of neutralizing antibodies exceeding 90% in nearly all studies (Table 40–13). Response rates have been similar for vaccines produced from the 17DD and 17D-204 substrains, for vaccines formulated with or without stabilizers, and for vaccines with and without avian leukosis virus. Although some early reports suggested that young children did not respond as well as older persons to 17D vaccine or lost immunity more rapidly,[461,462] this was not confirmed in other contemporary studies[463,464] or in more recent trials (Table 40–13). Race and gender do not appear to influence response rates, but specific studies are lacking.

Neutralizing antibody levels following immunization with 17D vaccine show individual variability. In the majority of cases, antibody titers are lower and their appearance is delayed compared to natural infection with yellow fever virus,[15,21,216] reflecting less virus replication and antigen expression by the attenuated strain. The minimal protective level of neutralizing antibodies induced by 17D vaccine has been estimated by dose-response studies in rhesus monkeys that were challenged after immunization with virulent yellow fever.[378,430,458] LNI values (measured by plaque reduction) of 0.7 or greater measured prechallenge (20 weeks after immunization) were strongly associated with protection (Table 40–14). Of 11 vaccinated monkeys that succumbed to challenge, 10 had a prechallenge LNI of 0.5 or less and one had an LNI of 0.9. Clinical trials of 17D vaccine have shown geometric mean LNI values of 2.2 or greater measured within a relatively brief interval (usually 1 month) after vaccination (see Table 40–13). As pointed out below, antibody titers measured by serum-dilution plaque reduction neutralization tests have been more variable, and no cutoff has been established correlating with protection.

Other experimental evidence supports the concept that minimal immunity is required for protection. Neutralizing antibodies appear in the sera of rhesus monkeys on day 6 to 7 after inoculation of 17D virus. However, some monkeys survive challenge performed after a shorter interval (1, 3, or 5 days) after vaccination, despite the absence of detectable antibodies.[18,197] Early protection may be mediated by a low-level specific antibody response (see *Kinetics of the Immune Response* below) or by innate immune responses.

Test Methods Affecting Interpretation of Antibody Responses

Various methods have been used to measure neutralizing antibodies, and these methods vary with respect to sensitivity (Table 40–15). Tests in mice were used through the 1950s and in some laboratories thereafter, but these tests were subject to considerable variability (reviewed by Smithburn[465]). The intraperitoneal neutralization test in newborn or 18- to 21-day-old mice was shown to be more sensitive for the detection of neutralizing antibodies than the IC neutralization test because of the higher and more rapid lethality of virus for mice inoculated by the latter route.[197,466]

Tissue culture neutralization tests have replaced tests in mice. These tests avoid the need for animals, are considerably more convenient and less costly, provide results in a shorter time (5 to 7 days versus 21 days in mice), and are more reliable and quantitative.[466,467] A standardized plaque-reduction test has been described.[466,468] A variety of continuous cell lines, including monkey kidney cells (MA-104, LLC-MK2, Vero), hamster kidney (BHK-21), and PS, as well as primary chick or duck embryo cells, may be used, and no clear differences in results have been found among these host cells. A comparative study showed that the intraperitoneal neutralization test performed in newborn mice was somewhat more sensitive for the assay of neutralizing antibodies than the constant serum–varying virus plaque-reduction test in MA-104 cells.[466] The cell culture test was, however, more sensitive than the IC suckling or adult mouse tests. Similarly, Poland et al.[469] showed that a constant virus–serum dilution plaque-reduction test in Vero cells was more sensitive than the IC adult mouse neutralization test.

Although differences in test sensitivity account for the variable geometric mean antibody responses noted in clinical trials (see Table 40–13), they do not appear to influence seroconversion rates, when seroconversion is measured relatively early (e.g., 1 month or several months) after vaccination. However, the determination of low antibody levels, for example, many years after vaccination may be problematic if an insensitive test is used. In a study of persons vaccinated 30 to 35 years earlier, Poland et al.[469] found that the IC adult mouse neutralization test had a 52% false-negative rate compared to plaque reduction, with the false-negative sera having low antibody titers.

As shown in Table 40–13, the serum-dilution plaque-reduction neutralization test has been used in recent years as the method of choice in clinical studies of yellow fever vaccines. However, a standardized assay was not used in these clinical trials. The sensitivity (reflected by geometric mean antibody titer) has varied considerably, presumably as a result of methodologic differences (use of accessory factor [complement]; agar overlay composition; plaque detection staining methods; and the endpoint [proportion of plaques

TABLE 40–13 ■ Seroconversion Rates and Neutralizing Antibody Responses to Yellow Fever 17D Vaccine in Clinical Trials

Study	Vaccine Manufacturer	Vaccine Specification	Dose (Log$_{10}$)*	Method†	Interval‡	Age	Study Site	N	Seroconversion (%)	Titer	Test Used§	Reference
1	National Drug Co. (USA)		6.1–6.4 SMLD$_{50}$	NSI	21 days	Adults	USA, Japan	41‖	100	>500	SDNT (IC, mice)	480
2	National Drug Co. (USA)		6.8 MLD$_{50}$	JI	3 wk	5–54 mo	Burkina Faso	72	97	NT	LNI (IC, mice)	566
3	Wellcome (UK)	ALV-contaminated	4.1–4.4 MLD$_{50}$	NSI	1 mo	Adults	England	38	97.4	1.6	LNI (IC, mice)	604
		ALV-free	4.1–4.4 MLD$_{50}$	NSI	1 mo	Adults	England	59	98.3	1.7		
4	National Drug Co. (USA)	ALV-contaminated	6.2–6.7 MLD$_{50}$	NSI or JI	28 days	Adults	USA	187	>99	2.2–3.5	LNI (cell culture)	471
		ALV-free	5.6–6.0 MLD$_{50}$	NSI	28 days	Adults	USA	187	>98	2.2–3.1	LNI (cell culture)	
5	National Drug Co. (USA)	Administered with or without smallpox vaccine at varied intervals	4.3–5.0 MLD$_{50}$	NSI	28 days	Adults	USA	483	99.8	2.2–2.6	LNI (cell culture)	605
6	Wellcome (UK)	Not stabilized	4.4 MLD$_{50}$	NSI	28 days	Adults	England	10	100	2.7	LNI (cell culture)	476
		Stabilized	4.2 MLD$_{50}$	NSI	28 days	Adults	England	20	100	2.9	LNI (cell culture)	
7	Institut Pasteur (Senegal)		ND	JI	25 days	Adults and children	Gambia	41	92.7	≥13.1	PRNT	238
8	Wellcome (UK)	ALV-free, stabilized	>3.0 MLD$_{50}$	NSI	2–11 wk	Adults	England	600	96.0	2.19	LNI (cell culture)	510
9	Connaught (USA)	ALV-free	3.7 PFU (LLC-MK2)	NSI	1 mo	Adults	USA	28¶	100	415	PRNT	606
10	Pasteur Mérieux (France)	Stabilized, ALV-free	5.3–5.4 PFU (PS)	NSI	1 mo	1–5 yr	Central African Republic	209	94	**	PRNT	607
11	Pasteur Mérieux (France)	Not stabilized	ND	NSI	1 mo +	Adults	France	143	99.3	14	PRNT	608
		Stabilized	ND	NSI	1 mo +	Adults	France	115	100	13	PRNT	
12	Institut Pasteur (Senegal)	Combined with DTP-polio, measles with or without HBV	ND	NSI	60 days	18–26 mo	Senegal	188	91.5–93.6	19.4–31.8	PRNT	567
13	FioCruz (Brazil)	17DD substrain; not stabilized	3.7 MLD$_{50}$	NSI	28 days	Adults	Brazil	15	100	1656	PRNT	477
		17DD substrain; stabilized	3.8 MLD$_{50}$	NSI	28 days	Adults	Brazil	31	100	1790	PRNT	
14	Pasteur Mérieux (France)	Stabilized, ALV-free	ND	NSI	45 days	6–7 mo	Ivory Coast	50	91	>1.5	PRNT	609
15	Pasteur Mérieux (France)	Stabilized, ALV-free	3.91 MLD$_{50}$	NSI	30 days	6–12 mo	Cameroon	68	92.6	22.63	PRNT	565
16	Pasteur Mérieux (France)	Stabilized, ALV-free	ND	NSI	195–240 days	4–8 mo	Mali	52	96.2	19.8	PRNT	610
		Stabilized, ALV-free	ND	NSI	195–240 days	12–24 mo	Mali	19	94.7	29.5	PRNT	
17	Connaught (USA)		ND	BJS	4–6 wk	Adults	USA	32	81	49.5	PRNT	611

	Manufacturer	Formulation	Virus content	†	Interval‡	Age	Country	No.	%	Titer	§	Ref.
18	Pasteur Mérieux (France)	Stabilized, ALV-free	ND	JI	2–4 wk	Adults	Nigeria	331‡	88.5	NT	PRNT	498
19	Pasteur Mérieux (France)	Stabilized, ALV-free	ND	NSI	45 days	Adults	France	36	100	NT	PRNT	614
20	Pasteur Mérieux (France)	Stabilized, ALV-free	3.9 TCID$_{50}$	NSI	35 days	Adults	Europe	41	100	26.6	PRNT	563
21	Pasteur Mérieux (France)	Combined with measles or HBV + measles	ND	NSI	30 days	9 mo	Senegal	172	96	16.8	PRNT	613
22	FioCruz (Brazil)	17DD substrain; stabilized	ND	JI	6 mo	>6 yr	Brazil	161	86.8	NT‡‡	PRNT	614
23	Pasteur Mérieux (France)	Combined with HAV and typhoid	ND	NSI	28 days	Adults	Switzerland	56	100	752	PRNT	615
24	Connaught (USA)	Stabilized, ALV-free	ND	NSI	28–30 days	Adults	USA	~35	Not specified	226.3	PRNT	564
25	Robert Koch (Germany)	Stabilized, ALV-free	ND	NSI	26 days	Adults	Germany	12	100	88	PRNT	209
26	Institut Pasteur (Senegal)	Stabilized, ALV-free	ND	NSI	3 mo	6 mo / 9 mo	Ghana	139 / 150	98.60 / 98.00	158.5 / 129.8	SDNT (Vero)	616
27	Pasteur Mérieux (France)	Stabilized, ALV-free	ND	NSI	10–14 and 28 days	Adults	England	93	Days 10–14: 86 Day 28:100	124 (day 28)	PRNT	482
	Evans Medical§§ (UK)	Stabilized, ALV-free	ND	NSI	10–14 and 28 days	Adults	England	92	Days 10–14: 88 Day 28:99	91 (day 28)	PRNT	
28	Aventis Pasteur|||| (USA)	Stabilized, ALV-free	ND	NSI	30 days	Adults	USA	291	99.30	2.21	LNI	470
	Evans Medical (UK)	Stabilized, ALV-free	ND	NSI	30 days	Adults	USA	283	98.60	2.06	LNI	

*MLD$_{50}$, mouse median lethal dose, performed per WHO requirements in 4- to 6-week-old animals; ND, not determined, but vaccine meets WHO standards (>1000 MDL$_{50}$); PFU, plaque-forming units, titration in cell culture (type specified); SMLD$_{50}$, suckling mouse median lethal dose; TCID$_{50}$, tissue culture median infective dose.

†BJS, Bioject system; JI, jet injector; NSI, needle and syringe injection.

‡Interval between vaccination and serologic testing.

§LNI, log neutralization index; PRNT, plaque-reduction neutralization test performed in cell culture; SDNT (IC mice), serum dilution–constant virus neutralization test (performed in suckling mice inoculated intracerebrally).

||Volunteers in the study with no pre-existing yellow fever immunity.

¶In this study, 17 of 28 subjects had previously received an experimental vaccine against dengue type 2.

**Seventy-eight percent of vaccinees had high neutralizing antibody titers (≥320).

††Includes all subjects in study except pregnant women.

‡‡Serum dilution–constant virus neutralization test in Vero cell cultures using cytopathic effect as the endpoint.

§§Vaccine bulk-manufactured by Wellcome and formulated for sale by Evans Medical.

||||Formerly Connaught, then Pasteur Mérieux Connaught.

ALV, avian leukosis virus; DTP, diphtheria-tetanus-pertussis; HAV, hepatitis A vaccine; HBV, hepatitis B vaccine; NT, not tested.

TABLE 40–14 ■ Neutralizing Antibody Response to Yellow Fever 17D Vaccine Correlates with Protection Against Challenge with 5.0 LOG_{10} LD_{50} of Virulent Asibi Virus

Log Neutralization Index (Plaque Reduction)	Protected	
	Yes	No
≥0.7	51/54 (94%)	1/11 (9%)
<0.7	3/54 (6%)	10/11 (91%)

Chi-square P <0.0001.
From Mason RA, Tauraso NM, Spertzel RO, et al. Yellow fever vaccine: direct challenge of monkeys given graded doses of 17D vaccine. Appl Microbiol 25:539, 1973, with permission.

reduced]). These variables make it impossible to compare immunogenicity in terms of antibody titers across different clinical trials. For these reasons, the constant serum–varying virus neutralization test is considered a preferable method for determination of the antibody response to yellow fever vaccine.[155,470] This method has been standardized, is reproducible, and has been compared rigorously to the mouse neutralization test.[466] The cutoff for a positive test (LNI of 0.7) has been established by protection studies in monkeys,[378] and the level of neutralization (quantity of virus neutralized) in undiluted or minimally diluted serum may be biologically more meaningful than a serum dilution endpoint titer. The test may, however, be slightly less sensitive than the constant virus–serum dilution plaque-reduction method. For measurement of the immune response in an individual, the difference in titer between pre- and postvaccination sera expressed as the LNI represents the neutralizing capacity of the serum. Because complement increases

the sensitivity of the yellow fever neutralization test, and because complement levels may be unstable in stored sera, it is preferable to heat-inactivate test samples and to add complement (or a standard source of fresh frozen serum) to the virus-serum mixture.

The HI and CF methods also have been used to measure responses to yellow fever vaccine.[426,464,466,471,472] The HI test is less sensitive than neutralization and is complicated by low specificity in persons with prior flavivirus exposure.[473] The choice of yellow fever antigen may affect results; use of 17D viral antigen provided a more sensitive assay for detecting vaccine-induced immunity than antigens prepared from FNV or a wild-type (JSS) strain.[472] Individuals without prior flavivirus exposure generally do not develop CF antibodies after administration of 17D vaccine.[237,238] The CF test therefore has been thought to distinguish recent infection with wild-type virus from vaccine-induced immunity. However, in one study, individuals with prior heterologous flavivirus immunity developed broadly cross-reactive CF antibodies to yellow fever following 17D vaccination.[237]

IgG ELISA is insensitive and unsatisfactory for the detection of seroconversion to 17D vaccine.[200,474] IgM antibody responses measured by ELISA are discussed in the section on *Antibody Subclass Response* below.

Vaccine Dose

The minimal potency requirements for yellow fever 17D vaccine are 3.0 log_{10} MLD_{50} (or the number of plaque-forming units in cell culture shown to be equivalent to that dose).[435] Vaccine potency of manufactured lots exceeds this minimal limit by at least fivefold to account for losses on storage.

A dose-response relationship was observed in rhesus monkeys inoculated intramuscularly with 17D vaccine[378,458] (Fig. 40–21). The dose at which 90% of the animals devel-

TABLE 40–15 ■ Methods Used to Measure Yellow Fever–Neutralizing Antibody Responses in Animals and Humans

Host (Age)	Description	Endpoint	Comment
Monkey (rhesus)	Simultaneous subcutaneous (SC) or intraperitoneal (IP) inoculation of test serum and virus	Death	Used in early studies before development of mouse model
Mouse (adult)	Intracerebral (IC) inoculation of preincubated mixture of serum with constant virus dose (100 LD_{50})	Survival ratio or survival time. Quantitative test (neutralization index*) measures difference in viral titer between test and control sera	In screening test, survival time endpoint more sensitive
Mouse (adult)	IC inoculation of starch followed by IP inoculation of serum-virus mixture	Survival ratio	Extensively employed in early serologic surveys
Mouse (18–21 days)	IP inoculation of serum-virus mixture	Survival ratio	More sensitive (higher serum antibody titers) than adult mouse tests
Mouse (newborn)	SC, IP, or IC inoculation of serum-virus mixtures	Survival ratio	More sensitive (higher serum antibody titers) than adult mouse tests
Cell culture	Constant serum–varying virus dilution	Neutralization index* determined by plaque reduction or CPE	Measures quantity of virus neutralized by neat or low dilution of serum
Cell culture	Constant virus–varying serum dilution	Highest serum dilution reducing a defined proportion of plaques	Sensitivity varies with endpoint selected (50%, 70%, 90% plaque reduction)

*Log_{10} neutralization index.
CPE, cytopathic effect.

oped a rise in LNI greater than 0.7 was approximately 1000 MLD_{50} (approximately equivalent to 4.7 to 5.0 $\log_{10}$ PFU[†]) and the 90% protective dose against lethal challenge was approximately 200 MLD_{50} (~4.0 to 4.3 $\log_{10}$ PFU). The 50% immunizing dose was approximately 2 MLD_{50} (~2.0 to 2.3 $\log_{10}$ PFU).

Dose response in humans was first determined by Fox et al. in 1943.[475] The minimal dose resulting in seroconversion was between 14 and 140 MLD_{50} (see above and footnote for conversion to PFU). At a dose of 14 MLD_{50}, 70% of the volunteers seroconverted. Large-scale field trials of various vaccine lots, some of which were of suboptimal potency, indicated that administration of doses in the range of 10 to 50 MLD_{50} immunized more than 85% of vaccinees. More recent dose-response studies (Table 40–16) indicate that doses of 100 to 200 PFU result in seroconversion of more than 90% of persons vaccinated. In addition, an unpublished study of Arilvax in the United Kingdom found that 13 (93%) of 15 subjects given 200 PFU seroconverted and that all subjects seroconverted at a dose of 2000 PFU or above. Thus the minimum potency requirements set by the WHO for yellow fever vaccines exceeds the 90% immunizing dose by 5- to 50-fold.

Interestingly, an inverse relationship between vaccine dose and antibody titer has been observed consistently.[427,430,476,477] Smith et al.[427] found significantly higher responses in subjects given doses of 5 to 50 MLD_{50} than in those given doses of 500 to 5000 MLD_{50}. In monkeys, inoculation of large doses of 17D virus resulted in earlier appearance of viremia, but viremia was inconsistent, lower in

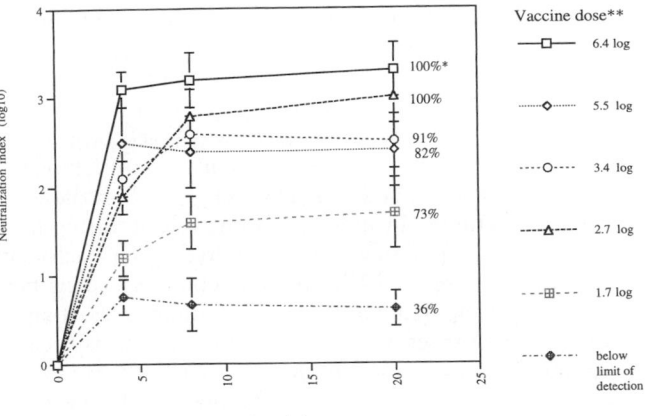

FIGURE 40–21 ▪ Neutralizing antibody responses (mean ± SE) in rhesus monkeys immunized with graded doses of yellow fever 17D vaccine. *Percent of monkeys positive (log neutralization index ≥0.7) 20 weeks after immunization. **Suckling mouse median lethal dose of 0.5 mL inoculum. (Data from Mason RA, Tauraso NM, Ginn RK. Yellow fever vaccine. V. Antibody response in monkeys inoculated with graded doses of the 17D vaccine. Appl Microbiol 23:908, 1972.)

magnitude, and briefer in duration than after inoculation of diluted virus.[430] Limited replication of the virus after the inoculation of very large doses may explain the lower magnitude of the immune response. This dose prozone effect is also clearly evident in mice (Fig. 40–22), and may be explained by the presence of interferon (produced in the infected egg), defective interfering particles, noninfectious antigen competing for cell receptors, or induction of a strong innate immune response by virus inoculated at the high dose range. Similar effects also have been noted with

---

[†]The PFU:MLD_{50} ratio is generally in the range of 50 to 100 but depends on multiple variables affecting sensitivity of test systems.

TABLE 40–16 ▪ Relationship Between Dose of Yellow Fever 17D Vaccine and Neutralizing Antibody Response

Vaccine Manufacturer	Dose	No. Subjects	Seroconversion Rate (%)	Mean Antibody Titer[*]	50% Immunizing Dose[†]	Reference
South African Institute for Medical Research	5000 MLD_{50}	4	100	1.55	~5 MLD_{50}	427
	500	7	100	1.80		
	50	8	100	3.04		
	5	8	62.5	2.80		
Wellcome (UK)	200,000 PFU	20	100	2.93–2.96	42 PFU (~7 MLD_{50})	476
	200	13	85	2.97		
	50	12	58	3.10		
	10	13	0	—		
BioManguinhos (Brazil)	2000 PFU[‡]	12	100	—	~20 PFU (~60 MLD_{50})	477
	1000–2000	34	100	—		
	500–1000	10	100	—		
	200–500	34	100	—		
	100–200	32	93.7	—		
	50–100	59	81.3	—		
	20–50	25	84.0	—		
	<20	53	41.5	—		

[*]Log neutralization index.
[†]LD_{50}/PFU ratio varies for different vaccines, based on differences between the sensitivity of the assays employed or (possibly) mouse virulence of the vaccines. The Wellcome vaccine (Freestone et al.[476]) had a MLD_{50}/PFU ratio of 0.17, whereas the FioCruz vaccine (Lopes et al.[477]) had a MLD_{50}/PFU ratio of 2.9.
[‡]Range of doses for volunteers receiving different vaccine lots tested in the study.
MLD_{50} mouse median lethal dose; PFU, plaque-forming units.

chimeric viruses utilizing yellow fever as a vector for the envelope genes of heterologous flaviviruses.[155]

Panthier[434] suggested that a low dose of 17D vaccine might cause a delay in antibody response and an increased risk of encephalitis. This hypothesis was based on a single case of encephalitis in a 4-week-old infant after pricking the skin with a needle dipped in 17D vaccine, and on the work of Fox and Penna[430] in monkeys. Low dose resulting from loss of vaccine potency was suggested as a factor in encephalitis caused by FNV in some epidemics. It is now known, however, that vaccination of infants less than 4 months of age carries a higher risk of encephalitis because of age susceptibility, not vaccine dose (see *Adverse Events* below). Moreover, application of low doses of 17D vaccine by scarification was not associated with adverse reactions.[417,418] Administration of small, intradermal doses of 17D vaccine is standard practice in persons with a history of egg allergy,[478,479] and there are no reports of an increased risk of encephalitis following this procedure. Finally, an epidemic of postvaccinal encephalitis occurred in Senegal in 1965,[411] when vaccine potency was not in question.

Antibody Responses Measured in a Large Clinical Trial

A randomized, double-blind outpatient study was conducted in 1440 healthy subjects, half of whom received the U.S. vaccine (YF-Vax) and half the vaccine manufactured in the United Kingdom (Arilvax).[470] A randomly selected subset of approximately 290 subjects in each treatment group was tested for neutralizing antibodies 30 days after vaccination. The primary efficacy endpoint was the proportion of subjects who developed an LNI of 0.7 or greater. Seroconversion occurred in 98.6% of subjects in the Arilvax group and 99.3% of subjects in the YF-Vax group

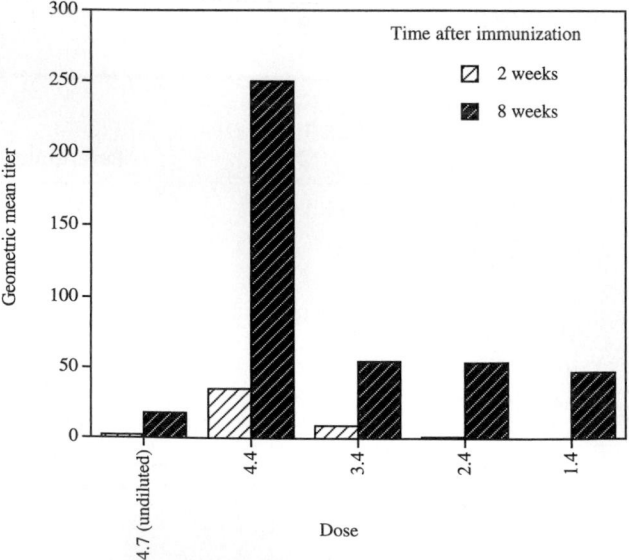

FIGURE 40–22 ▪ Neutralizing antibody response to yellow fever 17D vaccine in mice, showing the geometric mean titer of groups of five Swiss Webster mice inoculated subcutaneously with 0.1 mL of graded doses of commercial yellow fever 17D vaccine and tested 2 and 8 weeks after immunization. Antibody titers are geometric mean 50% plaque-reduction endpoints. A prozone was observed, with lower responses in mice given the highest virus dose. (Unpublished data from F Guirakhoo and TP Monath, 1997.)

(the vaccines were equivalent: $P < 0.001$). Both vaccines elicited mean antibody responses well above the minimal level (LNI of 0.7) protective against wild-type yellow fever virus. The mean LNI in the YF-Vax group was higher (2.21) than that in the Arilvax group (2.06; $P = 0.010$), possibly as a result of the higher dose contained in YF-Vax compared to Arilvax.

Kinetics of the Immune Response

Studies in rhesus monkeys established that neutralizing antibodies were detectable in serum on day 6 or 7 following inoculation of 17D virus, at which time the animals were completely refractory to challenge. Significant protection was present 1 to 2 days before the appearance of detectable neutralizing antibodies,[20,197,465] suggesting that very low levels of antibody were protective. Occasional animals survived challenge at even earlier times after 17D immunization, suggesting that interferon or other antiviral mechanisms also may play a role in protection.

Human immunization with 17D virus also is followed by the rapid appearance of neutralizing antibodies, detection of antibodies being dependent on the sensitivity of the neutralization assay. Early studies using the mouse protection test failed to detect antibodies 7 days after vaccination, but the majority of individuals had seroconverted on day 14.[20,21] Smithburn and Mahaffy[197] found neutralizing antibodies in 10% of a small group of subjects on day 7 and in 90% on day 10 after immunization. Wisseman et al.[480] found no evidence for immunity on day 6, but all subjects had seroconverted by day 14 after vaccination. In a more recent study, Lang et al.[481] found that 86% to 88% of adult subjects seroconverted by day 14, whereas 99% to 100% were seropositive on day 28 after vaccination. Similarly, Reinhardt et al.[209] showed that all subjects seroconverted between days 6 and 13 and that mean antibody titers increased slightly from 1:71 on day 13 to 1:88 on day 26 after vaccination. Monath et al.[155] found that 80% of subjects seroconverted by day 11 and 100% by day 31, with a marked increase in antibody level measured by LNI from 1.26 to 3.98. Based on human and monkey studies, Courtois[482] concluded that "man seems unable to form antibodies so early as the rhesus but by the 10th day his serum has a very high degree of protective activity. Judging from the studies carried out in monkeys, it seems probable that a protective mechanism begins to operate in man by the 8th or 9th day." This conclusion was incorporated into the International Health Regulations,[483] which stipulate that the vaccination certificate for yellow fever is valid 10 days after administration of 17D vaccine.

Studies employing more sensitive neutralization tests have demonstrated antibodies at earlier times following the administration of 17D vaccine. Monath[484] found the earliest evidence for neutralizing antibodies by plaque-reduction assay on day 4 in one of four volunteers, with all subjects seroconverting by day 8. Time to appearance of antibodies was not shortened by use of a kinetic neutralization test. Bonnevie-Nielsen et al.[200] found no antibodies by plaque-reduction neutralization test on day 4 after vaccination; 25% of subjects were immune on day 7 and 87.5% on day 12. Thus it seems that immunity to yellow fever may appear in a minority subset of individuals during the first week after immunization. Neutralizing antibody levels continue to increase during the first month after immunization, with peak titers found at 3 to 4 weeks.[480,484]

Antibody Subclass Response

The primary immune response is characterized by the appearance of neutralizing antibodies of the IgM class between days 4 and 7, several days before detection of IgG antibodies.[484] Titers of IgM neutralizing antibodies were 16- to 256-fold higher than those of IgG antibodies during the first 4 to 6 weeks after immunization, and IgM antibodies were found to persist for at least 18 months (the longest time examined). Prolonged synthesis of IgM antibodies may indicate persistence of antigen, possibly explaining the durability of yellow fever immunity (see *Duration of Immunity* below).

During a field study in Nigeria, 141 (36.6%) of 385 persons vaccinated with 17D seroconverted by IgM antibody-capture ELISA.[45] However, prior flavivirus exposure in this population was high, and this may have reduced IgM responses. In clinical studies in Europe, IgM antibodies measured by capture ELISA appeared in 83% of volunteers within 2 weeks after primary immunization.[200,209] However, IgM antibodies were not detected by this method in subjects tested 2 years after primary immunization.[200] The memory B-cell response after yellow fever revaccination was not associated with an IgM response in one study where the interval between primary vaccination and revaccination was relatively short (2 years),[200] whereas four of five subjects revaccinated with an interval greater than 10 years developed anti–yellow fever IgM in another study.[209]

Revaccination

According to International Health Regulations,[483] the yellow fever immunization certificate for international travel is valid for 10 years, whereupon revaccination is required. The regulation is conservative because vaccine immunity appears to last several decades if not for life.[469]

In some studies, prior immunity inhibited the response to revaccination, an expected finding for a live vaccine. In others, revaccination or vaccination of individuals with naturally acquired immunity was followed by a booster response in the majority of subjects, indicating that sufficient virus replication had occurred or that the antigenic mass of neutralized virus in the vaccine dose was sufficient to elicit a memory response. A booster response to revaccination was more likely in individuals with a low neutralizing antibody titer.[485]

Smith et al.[427] revaccinated eight subjects who had received 17D vaccine at least once (and up to five times) between 1 and 14 years previously, and who had LNIs of 2.1 to 3.6. Only one subject developed a significant rise in neutralizing antibodies. Wisseman and Sweet[244] revaccinated 11 adults 14 months after primary immunization. None had detectable viremia after revaccination, but all responded with a rise in neutralizing antibodies, and seven (64%) had greater than fourfold increases in titer (Fig. 40–23). The geometric mean titer rose from 121 to 576 after revaccination, but in most subjects the response was lower than to primary immunization. The dose of virus administered by the latter authors was 10- to 30-fold higher that that administered by Smith et al.[427]; this plus the lower number of prior immunizations may explain the difference between the

studies. Fox and Cabral[461] also concluded that a higher dose of 17D was required to boost individuals with pre-existing immunity.

Revaccination of 10 subjects 2 years after primary immunization was characterized by an increase in IgG antibodies detected by ELISA.[200] This response was greater than that observed in controls undergoing primary immunization, indicating a memory response resulting from prior sensitization. In another study, two individuals who were revaccinated 3 to 18 months after their last immunization had a rise in HI but not neutralizing antibody titers.[484] Reinhardt et al.[209] noted modest increases in neutralizing antibodies in five of five subjects revaccinated after an interval of greater than 10 years (Fig. 40–24), whereas Monath et al.[155] found that only three of six subjects revaccinated after a short interval (9 months) developed increases in neutralizing antibodies.

Immunization in Individuals with Prior Flavivirus Immunity

Yellow fever is distinct by neutralization test from other flaviviruses,[52] but it shares antigenic determinants detected by binding assays, HI, and CF.[213] Because of these cross-reactive determinants, the immune response to 17D vaccine is qualitatively different in naïve individuals and in those with prior heterologous immunity. The principal question is: Does pre-existing heterologous immunity reduce (by virtue of cross-protective antigens) or increase (through immune enhancement) the seroconversion rate, antibody titer, or antibody duration following 17D immunization? Conversely, does prior 17D vaccination modify the response to other flavivirus vaccines or natural infection?

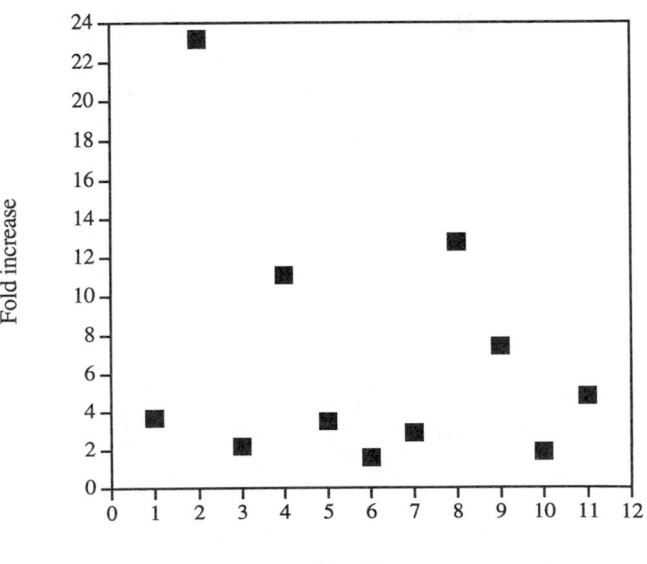

FIGURE 40–23 ■ Fold increase in neutralizing antibody titer in adults re-immunized with yellow fever 17D vaccine 14 months after primary immunization. Antibodies were measured by a serum dilution–constant virus test in weanling mice. (Data from Wisseman CL Jr, Sweet B. Immunological studies with group B arthropod-borne viruses. III. Response of human subjects to revaccination with 17D strain yellow fever vaccine. Am J Trop Med Hyg 11:570, 1962.)

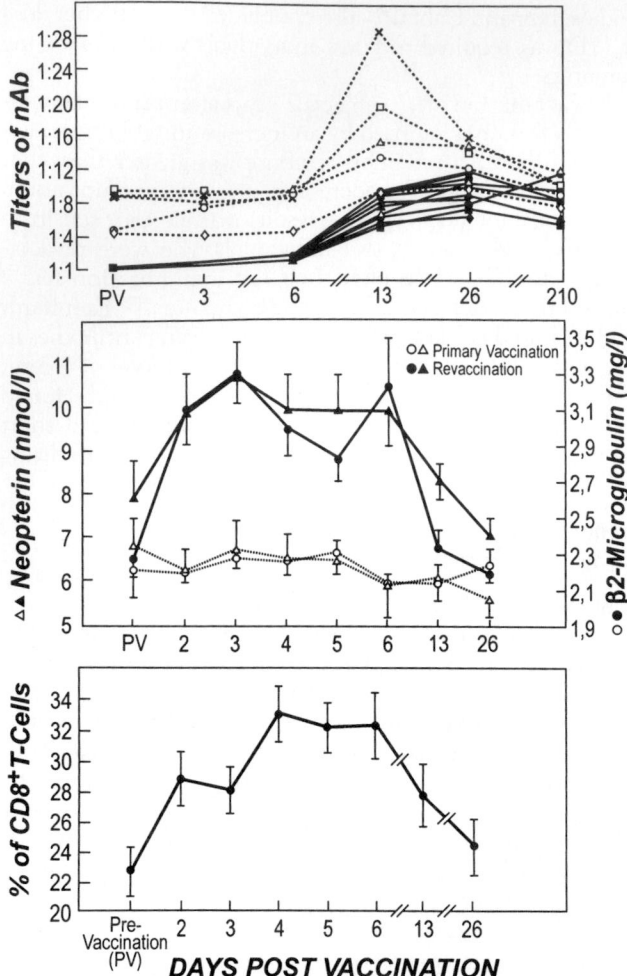

FIGURE 40–24 ■ *Top*, Kinetics of the neutralizing antibody (nAb) response to primary yellow fever vaccination (*solid lines*) and revaccination (*broken lines*) in individual subjects. *Middle*, Mean (± SE) neopterin (▲, Δ; nmol/L) and (β₂-microglobulin (●,○; mg/L) levels in serum after primary vaccination (*N* = 12, *solid lines*) and revaccination (*N* = 5, *broken lines*). *Bottom*, Mean (± SE) CD8⁺ T cell counts as percentage of total peripheral blood mononuclear cells after primary yellow fever vaccination (*N* = 12). (From Reinhardt B, Jaspert R, Niedrig M, et al. Development of viremia and humoral and cellular parameters of immune activation after vaccination with yellow fever virus strain 17D: a model of human flavivirus infection. J Med Virol 56:159, 1998, with permission.)

INTERFERENCE WITH 17D VACCINE CAUSED BY HETEROLOGOUS IMMUNITY

Interference by naturally acquired heterologous flavivirus immunity with the response to 17D vaccine is anticipated by experimental and field studies showing that heterologous immunity to dengue, Wesselsbron, and Zika viruses can cross-protect against infection with wild-type yellow fever virus.[44,224,225]

The evidence for interference with 17D vaccine in humans is conflicting, and discrepancies across studies may be due to the number of prior flavivirus infections, the breadth of the heterotypic response, or the identity of the viruses responsible for prior infection. Dengue immu-

nity appears to blunt the response to 17D vaccine in some studies, whereas prior infection with members of the Japanese encephalitis complex does not. Pond et al.[473] observed that persons with natural immunity to dengue, but not St. Louis encephalitis, had lower seroconversion rates to 17D vaccine. Individuals with monotypic neutralizing antibodies to Japanese encephalitis or with broad flavivirus cross-reactions had neutralizing antibody responses to 17D equivalent to those of immunologic virgins.[480] Moreover, viremic responses to 17D were not significantly different in persons with and without prior Japanese encephalitis immunity, indicating that replication of 17D virus was not reduced.[149] The results of these studies and those of Pond et al.[473] are consistent because St. Louis and Japanese encephalitis viruses are close antigenic relatives.

Naturally acquired yellow fever antibodies, resulting from infection with heterologous flaviviruses, significantly blunted the magnitude of the neutralizing antibody response to 17D vaccine.[238,427] Interference was particularly evident when 17D vaccine was given by scarification, presumably because of the lower dose of 17D administered by this route. Low response rates to 17D vaccine administered by scarification were associated with pre-existing heterologous flavivirus immunity in multiple studies in Africa.[423–425] In contrast, volunteers who had previously received a live, attenuated dengue vaccine and subsequently were given 17D vaccine had immune responses to yellow fever similar to those of dengue-nonimmune controls, suggesting no interference with yellow fever virus replication.[245] It is possible that the lack of interference was related to the attenuated properties of the dengue infection. In a study conducted in Nigeria, Omilabu et al.[486] found no restriction of neutralizing antibody responses to 17D vaccine in persons with various patterns of pre-existing flavivirus immunity.

There is no clear evidence that prior flavivirus immunity enhances replication of yellow fever 17D virus, or the immune response to 17D virus (see *Antibody-Dependent Enhancement* above).

HETEROLOGOUS IMMUNIZATION IN PERSONS IMMUNE TO YELLOW FEVER 17D

Live, attenuated dengue-2 vaccine was evaluated in persons with prior immunity to 17D vaccine.[246,487] In yellow fever–immune individuals, the response to dengue vaccine was independent of dose, and was of greater magnitude and duration than in nonimmune individuals.[246] The results suggested that cross-reactive non-neutralizing antibodies might have enhanced dengue virus replication in vivo.

Prior 17D immunization modulates the response to inactivated flavivirus vaccines through memory responses of IgG-producing B cells and restimulation of Th and follicular dendritic cells. In yellow fever–immune subjects receiving inactivated tick-borne encephalitis (TBE) vaccine, anti-TBE antibodies appeared earlier and in higher titers than in nonimmunes.[488] The anamnestic response also was characterized by the appearance of cross-reactive heterologous antibodies.

A chimeric Japanese encephalitis vaccine elicited a low-level yellow fever–specific response only in subjects who had been vaccinated previously with 17D and not in naïve subjects.[155]

SEROLOGIC SPECIFICITY

The primary neutralizing antibody response to 17D vaccine is highly specific, characterized by no or very low-titer antibodies to other flaviviruses.[480] Neutralizing antibodies in the IgG and IgM fractions of serum display similar specificity in primary vaccinees, whereas IgG (but not IgM) from an individual who had been vaccinated three times and was tested 18 months after the last immunization showed some flavivirus cross-reactivity.[484] The HI antibody response to primary immunization is also monotypic (type specific).[473] In contrast, persons with heterologous immunity respond to 17D vaccination with the development of a broadened response and appearance of both homologous (yellow fever) and heterologous neutralizing, HI, and CF antibodies.[238,480,484] Similarly, persons with prior 17D immunity respond to natural infection with heterologous flaviviruses with the development of a broadened flavivirus group response.[489]

The phenomenon of "original antigenic sin" has been noted in persons previously vaccinated with 17D virus and subsequently infected with another flavivirus. In such cases, an anamnestic response leads to a rapid rise in yellow fever antibodies, whereas the response to the current (heterologous) antigen is delayed. This phenomenon was observed in yellow fever–immune volunteers who were vaccinated with experimental dengue-2 vaccines.[245,487] Original antigenic sin may lead to diagnostic confusion in patients with clinical syndromes resembling naturally acquired yellow fever.[267]

Genetic Restriction

No studies have been reported on genetic restriction of immune responses to yellow fever. This is an area deserving study because studies in mice indicate that haplotype influences replication of flaviviruses[181] and the immune response to live viruses.[182]

Cytokine Responses and Markers of T-Cell Activation

In a study of adult volunteers given 17D vaccine, circulating interferon-α was detected in 10 of 15 subjects.[459] Interferon appeared and peaked 24 hours after viremia, in concert with the appearance of HI antibodies (see Fig. 40–6), and levels declined rapidly thereafter. These results are consistent with a subsequent study showing that 2′,5′-oligoadenylate synthetase activity in peripheral blood mononuclear cells increased by day 4 and peaked on day 7 after 17D immunization.[200] The role of interferon in clearance of 17D, and inhibition of replication of or immune response to coadministered vaccines, has not been clarified. It is likely that common side effects of 17D vaccine (headache, myalgia, asthenia) and the mild leukopenia associated with vaccination are related to release of interferon-α and other cytokines.[470] Increases in serum β_2-microglobulin, neopterin,[209] and TNF-α[208] have been found also during the first week after 17D vaccination (see Fig. 40–24) but not after revaccination. The increase in β_2-microglobulin reflects activation of T lymphocytes bearing MHC class I, and neopterin is released by monocyte-macrophages in response to interferon-γ released by activated T lymphocytes.

Cellular Immune Response

There are few data on the cellular immune response to 17D vaccine. Levels of circulating CD8+ cells have been found to increase following vaccination and precede the appearance of antibodies.[209] Four subjects vaccinated with 17D developed T-cell responses measured by lymphoproliferation, cytotoxic T-cell assay, and interferon-γ ELISPOT[64] (see *Cellular Immunity* above).

Evidence That Yellow Fever Vaccine Protects Against Disease

A large body of preclinical data in nonhuman primates has demonstrated the protective activity of yellow fever 17D vaccination against lethal challenge.[378,465] The development of neutralizing antibodies is strongly correlated with protection. The principal role of humoral antibodies in protection also was shown by transferring serum from immune monkeys before or shortly after challenge with virulent yellow fever.[164,373]

The effectiveness of 17D vaccine is based on preclinical observations and the demonstration of neutralizing antibodies in greater than 95% of persons who received the vaccine, but has never been tested in controlled clinical trials. However, several observations attest to the effectiveness of the vaccine:

1. Laboratory infections with yellow fever were commonplace prior to routine immunization but disappeared thereafter.
2. Observations over 50 years showed that jungle yellow fever in Brazil and other South American countries occurs only in persons who have not been immunized with 17D and that immunization during outbreaks resulted in rapid disappearance of cases.[352]
3. Yellow fever in francophone Africa virtually disappeared after the institution in 1941 of mandatory immunization with FNV[24] (see Fig. 40–14). A high rate of coverage of the population was followed by a marked reduction in the incidence of yellow fever, despite continued human exposure to the enzootic cycle. Yellow fever epidemics were reported during the 1940s and 1950s from neighboring anglophone countries, particularly Nigeria, in which routine vaccination was not practiced.

An assessment of the effectiveness of 17D vaccine was made during an epidemic in Nigeria in 1986 (KM DeCock and TP Monath, unpublished results). By determining vaccine coverage and the number of serologically confirmed yellow fever cases among vaccinated and unvaccinated subjects, vaccine efficacy was estimated to be 85%. The assessment was complicated by the simultaneous occurrence of natural infection and immunization in the population, by the potential for natural infection prior to onset of vaccine immunity, and by the reliance on historical data about disease and vaccination.

Because yellow fever vaccination is the standard of care, placebo-controlled efficacy trials cannot be performed today. New yellow fever vaccines will be licensed based on immunologic surrogates or, perhaps, comparability field trials. Further studies on the effectiveness of yellow fever vaccines, which could be done using case-control methodology, are nevertheless warranted, particularly in populations affected by human immunodeficiency virus (HIV) or malnutrition, in whom vaccine efficacy may be impaired.

Duration of Immunity

Immunity following 17D vaccination is remarkably durable, and it has been concluded that vaccination "confer(s) an immunity which . . . (is) almost life-long."[489] The yellow fever immunization certificate for international travel is valid for 10 years, an interval that was established based on published studies showing that neutralizing antibodies were present in 92% to 97% of persons 16 to 19 years after vaccination.[472,489] An analysis was performed in 1980, when World War II veterans were tested 30 to 35 years after a single dose of 17D vaccine.[469] Overall, 80.6% of the subjects were seropositive by plaque-reduction neutralization test. However, the service records used to determine immunization of some veteran groups were undependable; in a subset of 58 Navy and Air Corps veterans, 97% were seropositive. In one study, there was no significant change in neutralizing antibody levels between 1 and 7 months after vaccination,[209] and, in another, the authors found that 75% of subjects were seropositive 10 years after vaccination with a median neutralization titer of greater than 40.[474]

The basis of durable yellow fever immunity is a matter of speculation. Persistent infection of human cells in culture by yellow fever 17D virus has been described.[490] A human macrophage cell line and human peripheral blood mononuclear cells became persistently infected, with continued production of infectious virus without the appearance of cytopathic effects, in a fluctuating pattern suggesting a role for defective interfering particles.[240] Yellow fever virus was recovered from the brains of rhesus monkeys up to 159 days[360] and from sera 30 days[359] after IC inoculation. In addition, a variant virus recovered from a 17D vaccine pool caused persistent infection of mouse brain without overt disease.[130] These observations, as well as the prolonged synthesis of IgM antibodies in persons immunized with 17D virus,[484] suggest that chronic persistent infection or storage of antigen in vivo, possibly in follicular dendritic cells, may explain the durability of the human immune response.

Primary Vaccine Failure

A small minority of healthy individuals inoculated with 17D vaccine do not develop detectable neutralizing antibodies (see Table 40–13). Although there are few reports on this question, it appears that failure to mount a response on primary immunization does not represent an absolute refractoriness, because revaccination may be followed by development of neutralizing antibodies.[200]

Development of clinical yellow fever in persons with a history of 17D vaccination has been reported on rare occasions. Three cases (two fatal) occurred in British and Allied soldiers serving in West Africa during World War II.[314] In 1952, a fatal case of yellow fever occurred in a previously vaccinated European working in Uganda.[315] In 1988, a previously vaccinated Spanish woman acquired yellow fever during travels in West Africa.[321] It is uncertain whether these individuals had actually received 17D vaccine, had received vaccine that had deteriorated through improper storage or handling after reconstitution, or had simply failed to respond to the vaccine.

Host Factors Responsible for Vaccine Failures

MALNUTRITION

Protein-calorie malnutrition has been associated with failure to respond immunologically to 17D vaccine. In a study of eight children (mean age 2 years) with kwashiorkor, only one seroconverted after 17D vaccination, compared to five of six controls.[491] Further studies are required to assess the relevance of this finding to use of 17D vaccine in the EPI in Africa, particularly where covariates such as HIV infection may diminish immunoresponsiveness. Although there were no obvious adverse effects of immunization in the small series of kwashiorkor patients, the safety of yellow fever immunization in infants with malnutrition has not been fully assessed. Gandra and Scrimshaw[492] showed that 17D vaccine administered to children 4 to 11 years old recovering from malnutrition resulted in a significant catabolic effect lasting up to 12 days, in the absence of fever or other signs of increased metabolic rate. This suggests that 17D vaccine could result in a net loss of body nitrogen and aggravate the clinical effects of protein malnutrition. Further studies in fasted adults showed that metabolic changes and mobilization of protein associated with yellow fever immunization were related to dietary factors; a catabolic effect was not observed in subjects consuming a high-protein diet.[493,494]

PREGNANCY

In a field study conducted in Nigeria, the IgM ELISA and neutralizing antibody responses to 17D vaccine were statistically significantly impaired in pregnant women compared to nonpregnant females of child-bearing age, male students, and the general population.[495] Only 38.6% of the pregnant women developed neutralizing antibodies, compared to 81.5% to 93.7% of the other groups. The difference was attributed to the immunosuppression associated with pregnancy, emphasizing the need to re-immunize at-risk women who inadvertently have been vaccinated during pregnancy.

HUMAN IMMUNODEFICIENCY VIRUS INFECTION

HIV infection has been shown to reduce immunologic responsiveness to a number of nonreplicating and live childhood vaccines. In the case of inactivated flaviviral vaccines, HIV infection reduced the seroconversion rate to Japanese encephalitis[496] and diminished the humoral and T-cell responses to tick-borne encephalitis vaccine.[497] The number of subjects with HIV infection or immune suppression exposed to 17D is too small to assess safety, although no adverse events have been reported to date. Some case reports indicate that vaccination of HIV-infected subjects without severe immune suppression was followed by seroconversion.[498] However, when 17D vaccine was administered to 33 adult travelers with HIV infection and CD4+ counts greater than 200 cells/mm³,[499] only 70% percent responded by 1 month after vaccination, and one individual seroreverted between 1 and 3 months after vaccination. In another study, 10-month-old HIV-infected infants in the Ivory Coast were simultaneously immunized with 17D and measles vaccines.[500] Only 3 (17%) of 18 HIV-infected infants developed neutralizing antibodies 2 to 10 months after 17D vaccination, compared to 42 (74%) of 57 HIV-uninfected controls matched for age and nutritional status. These results indicate that HIV infection can impair the immune response to 17D vaccine, but the mechanism is uncertain. Because both HIV and 17D viruses exhibit tropism for human lymphoid cells,[501] it is possible that HIV infection interferes with replication of 17D vaccine. This question could be addressed by in vitro studies and clinical trials in which 17D viremia is compared across HIV-infected and -uninfected subjects.

Other Host-Specific Effects

Evaluation of neutralizing antibody responses in a large clinical trial revealed some heretofore unknown and subtle host effects on the immune response (Table 40–17).[470]

The antibody response was statistically significantly higher in males than in females. Naturally acquired yellow fever disease is more frequent in males, a finding that cannot be explained by epidemiologic factors (see *Risk Factors* above). Moreover, postvaccinal encephalitis caused by FNV was higher in males than in females, suggesting that males undergo a more active infection (see *Rare Adverse Events Caused by 17D Vaccine* below).

In this study, the race group with predominantly Caucasians had a higher mean antibody response than African-Americans and Hispanics. The lethality of wild-type yellow fever appears to be lower in blacks than whites. The trial data showing higher antibody responses in whites may reflect a higher level of susceptibility, virus replication, and antigen expression in this racial group.

The mean LNI was higher in smokers than nonsmokers. There are few studies on the interaction of smoking and the immune system, but most report a suppressive effect, for example, after hepatitis B vaccine.[502] In the case of 17D vaccine, it was postulated that the adaptive immune response might be enhanced by the suppression of innate immune responses (e.g., NK cell function) attributable to smoking.

Adverse Events

Yellow fever 17D has been widely acknowledged as one of the safest vaccines in use. Over 400 million persons have been immunized, with a long record of tolerability and safety.[503,504] However, within the past 5 years, a new syndrome (vaccine-associated viscerotropic adverse events) has been recognized to occur at a very low incidence, raising new concerns about the safety of 17D vaccines.

Historical Problems: Adverse Events Prior to Standardization of Vaccine Manufacture

Two significant events in the history of manufacture and use of 17D vaccine are of special interest. The first (described earlier in the section on *Seed Lot System*) was the occurrence of postvaccinal encephalitis associated with uncontrolled passage of 17D substrains during the early years of vaccine manufacture.[432] The problem was resolved when stabilization of passage level during vaccine manufacture was instituted in 1941. The second event, the development of acute hepatitis in persons who received 17D vaccine, was recognized as early as 1937 by Findlay and MacCallum.[505] Cases were reported in Brazil during the vaccination campaigns between 1938 and 1940 and, after careful study, were attributed to an adventitious agent in the vaccine rather than to viscerotropism of 17D virus.[506] In 1942, a massive outbreak of hepatitis appeared in U.S. military personnel immunized with 17D vaccine, resulting in approximately 28,000 cases and 62 deaths.[507] These reactions were due to the use of pooled human serum (contaminated with hepatitis virus) as a vaccine stabilizer. This practice was discontinued in Brazil in 1940 and in the United States in 1943,[508] with resolution of the problem. Subsequent retrospective serologic studies confirmed that the responsible agent was hepatitis B virus.[509]

TABLE 40–17 ■ Subtle Host Factor Effects on Log$_{10}$ Neutralization Index (LNI) in a Clinical Trial of Two Yellow Fever 17D Vaccines

Host Factor	Group	Parameter	Arilvax (N = 283)	YF-Vax (N = 291)	P Value (ANOVA) Host Effect
Gender	Male	No. tested	108	111	0.001
		Mean LNI	2.16	2.35	
	Female	No. tested	175	180	
		Mean LNI	1.99	2.12	
Race	Afro-American	No. tested	37	42	0.017
		Mean LNI	1.93	2.06	
	Hispanic	No. tested	15	15	
		Mean LNI	1.95	1.85	
	Other (Caucasian, Asian)	No. tested	231	234	
		Mean LNI	2.09	2.26	
Smoking	Yes	No. tested	54	73	0.017
		Mean LNI	2.26	2.27	
	No	No. tested	229	218	
		Mean LNI	2.01	2.19	

ANOVA, analysis of variance.
Data from Monath TP, Nichols R, Archambault WT, et al. Comparative safety and immunogenicity of two yellow fever 17D vaccines (ARILVAX™ and YF-VAX®) in a Phase III multicenter, double-blind clinical trial. Am J Trop Med Hyg 66:533–541, 2002.

Common Adverse Events Following Administration of 17D Vaccines

No placebo-controlled trial has ever been performed to assess adverse reactions associated with 17D vaccine. Fever, headache, and backache, described as mild in severity, were noted since the earliest studies of 17D vaccine.[20] During large-scale field trials in Brazil in 1937 to 1938, Soper et al.[431] noted mild systemic reactions in 5% to 8% of vaccinees. Among 2457 persons in Brazil from whom "reasonably accurate" clinical follow-up was obtained by Smith et al.,[21] 14.6% complained of headache for 1 to 2 days, 10.2% developed pains in the body (usually accompanied by headache), 1.4% missed time from work (usually only 1 day), and 0.16% spent one or more days in bed. These reactions, which generally were considered mild, occurred on the fifth to seventh day after immunization. Local reactions at the site of inoculation were not observed, and no systemic allergic reactions were noted.

Reactogenicity of 17D vaccine was monitored in 12 clinical trials conducted between 1953 and 2002 (Table 40–18). Self-limited and mild local reactions (erythema and pain at the inoculation site) and systemic reactions (headache, headache and fever, and fever without symptoms) occurred in a minority of subjects 5 to 7 days after immunization. The lack of placebo controls in all published reports makes interpretation of data on adverse events unreliable, although the lower incidence of adverse events in previously vaccinated subjects in one study suggests that these events are real. Reactogenicity in infants is no greater (or perhaps less) than in adults; this conclusion was also made during the early studies in Brazil in 1937 to 1938.[21]

Where subjects were under daily surveillance, a higher frequency of adverse events was detected. Moss-Blundell et al.[510] and Freestone et al.[476] determined adverse events in subjects in the United Kingdom who received stabilized 17D vaccine (Table 40–19). Assessment may have been biased by the characteristics of the study populations (military personnel and Wellcome employees, respectively). In Moss-Blundell et al.'s study, 514 adult military personnel were questioned for adverse events 2 and 11 weeks after vaccination, and a subset of 90 volunteers filled out a daily diary and took their temperatures for 10 days after vaccination. An interesting aspect of this trial was the determination of adverse events in those with and without pre-existing yellow fever immunity, providing a control for reactions caused by primary 17D virus replication versus the more limited replication following revaccination. Twenty (3.9%) of 514 seronegative and 1 (1.6%) of 64 seropositive vaccinees reported any adverse event at the routine follow-up visits. Of the 20 reactions in the seronegative group, 17 (85%) were local reactions (erythema and/or pain at the injection site noted immediately or within a few days after vaccination). The subset completing a daily diary reported a substantially higher rate of adverse reactions. Thirty-six (42%) of 86 seronegative subjects reported any adverse reaction (there were too few seropositives to draw a valid conclusion). Headache (10%) and local reactions (8%) were reported most frequently. In the study by Freestone et al.,[476] subjects completed diary cards for 8 days after vaccination. Mild reactions were noted in 10 (33%) of 30 subjects. A third study of 370 travelers followed by a telephone survey for 1 week provided similar data. Twenty-five percent of those immunized reported one or more reactions, generally mild, characterized by systemic flu-like symptoms (22%) or local reactions (5%, typically pain).[511]

Adverse events were monitored in a large clinical trial of approximately 1400 subjects, half of whom received YF-Vax and half Arilvax.[470] There were no serious adverse events attributable to either vaccine. Significantly more subjects in the YF-Vax group (71.9%) experienced one or more nonserious, drug-related adverse events than in the Arilvax group (65.3%; $P = 0.008$) (Table 40–20). The difference was due to a higher rate of local reactions of mild-moderate severity caused by YF-Vax. The most common systemic side effects were headache, asthenia, myalgia, malaise, fever, and chills. These were generally mild or moderate, but 7% to 8% of all treatment-emergent events were severe and interfered with normal activities. Rash was noted in approximately 3% of the subjects and urticaria in 0.3%. There were no cases of anaphylaxis, serum sickness, or other severe allergic reactions. The incidence of nonserious adverse events was lower in elderly persons than in younger subjects, and the difference was statistically significant for headache, malaise, injection site edema, and pain. Injection site reactions occurred between days 1 and 5. Systemic adverse events also occurred at highest incidence during this interval, but continued between days 6 and 11. As in the study by Moss-Blundell et al.,[510] the causal relationship between adverse events and 17D vaccines was suggested by the observation that asthenia, malaise, headache, fever, injection site inflammation, and injection site pain occurred at a significantly lower rate in subjects who were seropositive at baseline, indicating that these reactions were associated with active replication of vaccine virus. The systemic adverse events are presumably caused by T-lymphocyte activation and the release of cytokines, including interferons and TNF-α, during the viremic period.[148,208]

The mean white blood cell count decreased slightly between baseline and day 11, with a mild neutropenia. No subjects developed clinically significant thrombocytopenia ($<0.5 \times 10^5/\mu L$), 3.5% to 3.9% had elevations in AST, and 3.9% to 4.6% of subjects had an increase in ALT from normal to abnormal range between baseline and day 11. In most cases, levels were minimally elevated and returned to normal or had decreased by day 31. Subjects with elevated serum enzymes had no associated syndrome or constellation of other clinical laboratory abnormalities. There was no relationship between elevated serum enzymes and use of concomitant medications. Future placebo-controlled trials will be required to determine whether elevations in serum enzymes are nonspecific or are caused by 17D vaccine. However, the recent discovery (see following section) that 17D vaccines can cause rare cases of severe hepatitis suggested that the chemical hepatic dysfunction observed in this trial might represent a mild form of subclinical liver injury.

Rare Adverse Events Caused by 17D Vaccine

VACCINE-ASSOCIATED NEUROTROPIC ADVERSE EVENTS (POSTVACCINAL ENCEPHALITIS)

The 17D vaccine retains a degree of neurovirulence as demonstrated by IC inoculation of mice and monkeys and by the occurrence of rare cases of postvaccinal encephalitis in humans. These cases have occurred principally, but not exclusively, in very young infants. After institution of standardized manufacturing procedures in the early 1940s, no cases of meningoencephalitis temporally associated with 17D vaccine were reported for approximately 10 years.[512] In 1952 to 1953, five cases occurred among 1800 children

TABLE 40–18 ■ Adverse Events Noted in Clinical Trials of 17D Vaccines, Manufactured Using Standardized Methods, in Which Adverse Events Were Specifically Monitored

Trial	Vaccine	Placebo-Controlled?	Subjects (No. Tested)	Result
Kouwenaar (1953)[531]	Rocky Mountain Laboratory, USA	No	Adults, Netherlands (1130*)	4.5% with low-grade fever, 7.6% with mild headache, muscle ache, malaise lasting hours to 4 days
Tauraso et al. (1972)[471]	National Drug Co., USA	No	Adult prisoners, USA (1676)	"Low reactogenicity, minimal subjective and objective reactions"
Tauraso et al. (1972)[605]	National Drug Co., USA	No	Merchant Marine Cadets, USA (181†)	No local or generalized adverse reactions
Freestone et al. (1977)[476]	Wellcome, UK	No	Adults, UK (30‡)	33% with various symptoms (headache, fever, pain or redness at injection site [see text])
Moss-Blundell et al. (1981)[510]	Wellcome, UK	No	Adult male military, UK	
			514 seronegative§	3.9% reported any reaction; 0.2% headache only; 3.3% local reactions; 0.4% other (see text)
			64 seropositive§	1.6% reported local reaction (see text)
Roche et al. (1986)[608]	Pasteur Mérieux, France	No	Adult male military, France (297)	No adverse events attributable to vaccine
Lhuillier et al. (1989)[609]	Pasteur Mérieux, France	No	6–9-mo infants, Ivory Coast (74‖)	No adverse reactions
Mouchon et al. (1990)[565]	Pasteur Mérieux, France	No	6–12-mo infants, Cameroon (75‖)	No adverse reactions
Soula et al. (1991)[610]	Pasteur Mérieux, France	No	4–24-mo infants, Mali (115‖)	21% with fever >38°C; 2.6% with local induration; 1.7% with rash; 7% with conjunctivitis
Ambrosch et al. (1994)[563]	Pasteur Mérieux, France	No	Young adults, Austria (41)	2.4% with fever >38°C, 4.8% with malaise; short duration
Lang et al. (1999)[481]	Pasteur Mérieux, France, and Evans Medical, UK	No	Adults, UK (211)	Local reactions (15–16%); fever (0%); asthenia (8–11%); headache (12–13%); myalgia (6–9%)
Monath et al. (2002)[470]	Aventis Pasteur, USA, and Evans Medical, UK	No	Adults, USA (1440)	See Table 40–20

*Including 465 with a history of atopy or other allergic reactions.
†This was a study of sequential or simultaneous inoculation of smallpox and yellow fever 17D vaccines; in the group of 181 subjects included here, the vaccines were separated by 28 days.
‡Subjects receiving standard dose of 17D vaccine.
§Yellow fever neutralizing antibody status before 17D vaccination; numbers differ from those of Table 40–13 because not all subjects were interviewed for adverse events.
‖This was a study of combined or sequential vaccination; only subjects receiving yellow fever 17D vaccine alone are included in the table.

vaccinated at age less than 1 year at the Pasteur Institute in Paris. These cases (numbers 1 through 5 in Table 40–21) constitute the first evidence that 17D vaccine manufactured according to biologic standards and with restricted passage may be encephalitogenic in very young infants.‡ Over the years, an additional 20 cases have been reported, for a total of 25 published cases. Fifteen cases occurred during the 1950s, when there was no age restriction on use of the vaccine

in infants. Of the 15 cases, 13 (87%) occurred in infants 4 months of age or younger, and all were 7 months of age or younger. Recommendations for restriction of use of 17D vaccine to infants over 6 months of age[515] were followed by a reduction in incidence of encephalitis. Since 1960, only ten cases have been reported, one of which occurred in a 1-month-old infant in France, where the age limitation was not universally practiced.[516] Current recommendations for the

‡It is uncertain, however, whether these cases and several others reported subsequently at the Pasteur Institute by Panthier[434] could be due to variations in substrain and passage level of vaccine, which may not have been adequately controlled at the time. In his review, Stuart stated that the vaccine used in cases 1 through 5 was prepared by a single passage from seed virus supplied by the Rockefeller Foundation (New York) in 1946.

In addition to those cases described in Table 40–21, two fatal cases of possible encephalitis among 67,325 children between 6 months and 2 years of age who received 17D vaccine were noted during an emergency vaccination campaign in Senegal in 1965, for an incidence of 3 per 100,000.[411] The relationship of the reactions to 17D vaccine is in doubt because both had a

very short incubation time (1 and 4 days); one of the cases was ascribed to anaphylaxis.[412] In contrast, there were 231 cases of encephalitis among 498,887 persons given FNV, for an overall incidence of 46 per 100,000; however, the incidence in children ages 2 to 11 was 150 per 100,000.

Two other possible cases not included in the table have been mentioned in the literature. Dick and Horgan[513] make reference to a 6-year-old child in England given 17D vaccine 3 days after smallpox vaccination. The child developed encephalitis 11 days after 17D immunization, and made a full recovery. The administration of smallpox vaccine in this case makes the etiology uncertain. Thomson[514] cited the case of a 3-month-old child in England inoculated in 1954, in a personal reference from another physician.

TABLE 40–19 ■ Frequency of NonSerious Adverse Events After Yellow Fever 17D Vaccination*

Study; No. Subjects	Adverse Event	No. with AE	% with AE
Freestone et al. (1977)[476]	Any reaction	10	33%
	Headache only	1	3%
N = 30 (adult)	Headache and fever	2	7%
	Local reaction only[†]	2	7%
	Local reaction and headache	4	13%
	Lymphadenopathy	1	3%
Moss-Blundell et al. (1981)[510]	Any reaction	36	42%
	Headache only	9	10%
N = 86 (adult)	Fever only	7	8%
	Headache and fever	4	5%
	Local reaction only	1	1%
	Local reaction and headache	6	7%
	Other[‡]	9	10%
Pivetaud et al. (1986)[511]	Any reaction	94	25%
	Grippe-like systemic reaction	42	11%
N = 370 (age 1–84; majority 20–39 yr)	Fatigue, weakness	28	8%
	GI complaints, w/ or w/out vomiting	9	2%
	Headache only	5	1%
	Headache, fever, vomiting	1	0.3%
	Headache, dizziness	1	0.3%
	Local reaction[†]	17	5.0%
Lang et al. (1999)[481]	Percentage with ≥1 events		
	Systemic events	36	17.0%
N = 210 (106 received Stamaril® and 105 received Arilvax®)	Number of events		
	Fever only	0	
	Asthenia	19	
	Headache	25	
	Myalgia	15	
	Arthralgia	2	
	GI events	7	
	Local reactions[§]	33	16.0%
Monath et al. (2002)[470]	See Table 40–20		

*Results are from five studies in which subjects without pre-existing yellow fever immunity completed a daily diary or were actively followed up after vaccination. The trials were not blinded or placebo controlled.
[†]Pain and/or redness at site of inoculation.
[‡]Abdominal pain (1), nausea and vomiting (1), upper respiratory infection (6), rash (1).
[§]Pain, erythema, induration, or hematoma.
AE, adverse event; GI, gastrointestinal.

minimum age for vaccination differ, based on risk of exposure to natural infection with yellow fever (see *Contraindications and Precautions* below), but in no case should the vaccine be administered to infants 4 months old or younger.

The incidence of postvaccinal encephalitis in very young infants may be estimated at 0.5 to 4 per 1000 based on two reports that provide denominator data (Table 40–22). In contrast, the risk of developing encephalitis in persons over 9 months of age (the current minimum age recommended for routine immunization in the United States[478]) is extremely low. Only three such cases have been reported among travelers. In the United States, only one case has occurred between 1965 and 2001. As surveillance for serious adverse events improves, however, it is likely that additional cases of vaccine-associated neurotropic events in travelers will be recognized. Attempts by the CDC to intensify surveillance of vaccine-associated adverse events have identified cases of self-limited vaccine-associated neurotropic events in adults. Three suspected cases in adults were found during 2001 and 2002, raising concern as to whether neurotropic accidents are underestimated.

A report from Thailand describes the occurrence of fatal meningoencephalitis in an adult male with undiagnosed HIV and low CD4+ cell counts who received yellow fever vaccine.[517] This is the first report of a serious adverse event following yellow fever vaccination of a patient with immunosuppression. Presumably, a delayed or dampened immune response allowed neuroinvasion and unrestrained replication of the vaccine virus in the CNS.

The total number of yellow fever immunizations administered worldwide in the last 50 years approximates 400 million, the majority of which have been performed in developing countries. Surveillance for adverse events has been passive and insensitive to the discovery of rare events. In 1993, an active hospital-based surveillance system for postvaccinal encephalitis was established during a vaccination campaign in response to a yellow fever epidemic in Kenya (D Heymann, personal communication, 1997). Four encephalitis cases (one child of 2 years, three adults) were recorded, for an estimated incidence of 5.8 per 1 million vaccinees. Surprisingly, three of the four encephalitis cases had a fatal outcome. Although the population had a high prevalence of HIV infection, the rate

TABLE 40–20 ■ Frequencies of Adverse Events Occurring in a Clinical Trial Comparing Two Yellow Fever 17D Vaccines[*]

Body System/Preferred Term	Arilvax N (%)	YF-Vax N (%)	P Value[†]
Total Number of Subjects	715 (100.0)	725 (100.0)	
Subjects with no AE	214 (29.9)	180 (24.8)	**0.033**
Subjects with at least one AE	501 (70.1)	545 (75.2)	
Body as a Whole	459 (64.2)	510 (70.3)	**0.013**
Abdominal Pain	8 (1.1)	4 (0.6)	
Accidental Injury	13 (1.8)	9 (1.2)	
Asthenia	208 (29.1)	218 (30.1)	0.687
Back Pain	9 (1.3)	9 (1.2)	
Chills	76 (10.6)	74 (10.2)	0.797
Fever	102 (14.3)	110 (15.2)	0.656
Flu Syndrome	26 (3.6)	21 (2.9)	
Headache	229 (32.0)	236 (32.6)	0.866
Infection	34 (4.8)	36 (5.0)	0.903
Injection Site Edema	61 (8.5)	144 (19.9)	**<0.001**
Injection Site Inflammation	113 (15.8)	214 (29.5)	**<0.001**
Injection Site Pain	171 (23.9)	286 (39.4)	**<0.001**
Injection Site Reaction	27 (3.8)	43 (5.9)	**0.066**
Malaise	134 (18.7)	130 (17.9)	0.734
Pain	23 (3.2)	16 (2.2)	
Cardiovascular System	10 (1.4)	4 (0.6)	0.114
Digestive System	56 (7.8)	44 (6.1)	0.214
Diarrhea	12 (1.7)	8 (1.1)	
Dyspepsia	8 (1.1)	6 (0.8)	
Nausea	23 (3.2)	22 (3.0)	
Hemic and Lymphatic System	16 (2.2)	6 (0.8)	**0.032**
Leukopenia	8 (1.1)	3 (0.4)	
Eosinophilia	2 (0.3)	0	
Erythrocytes Abnormal	1 (0.1)	0	
Leukocytosis	3 (0.4)	2 (0.3)	
Lymphadenopathy	3 (0.4)	1 (0.1)	
Polycythemia	1 (0.1)	0	
WBC Abnormal	1 (0.1)	1 (0.1)	
Metabolic and Nutritional System	6 (0.8)	13 (1.8)	0.164
SGPT Increased	2 (0.3)	7 (1.0)	
Musculoskeletal System	174 (24.3)	188 (25.9)	0.504
Myalgia	171 (23.9)	185 (25.5)	0.502
Nervous System	37 (5.2)	37 (5.1)	1.000
Dizziness	13 (1.8)	10 (1.4)	
Respiratory System	61 (8.5)	47 (6.5)	0.161
Cough Increased	8 (1.1)	5 (0.7)	
Pharyngitis	19 (2.7)	14 (1.9)	
Rhinitis	24 (3.4)	18 (2.5)	
Sinusitis	13 (1.8)	9 (1.2)	
Skin and Appendages	32 (4.5)	37 (5.1)	0.623
Rash	22 (3.1)	24 (3.3)	
Special Senses	12 (1.7)	10 (1.4)	0.673
Urogenital System	17 (2.4)	24 (3.3)	0.342
Dysmenorrhea	4 (0.6)	8 (1.1)	
Pyuria	8 (1.1)	2 (0.3)	

[*]Adverse events occurring in 1% or more of subjects in a Phase III clinical trial comparing Arilvax and YF-Vax.
[†]P value is based on Fisher's exact test; bold type indicates statistically significant difference. Note: P value is provided for each adverse effect wherever the percentage for either treatment group is not less than 5%.
AE, adverse event; SGPT, serum glutamate pyruvate transaminase; WBC, white blood cell count.
From Monath TP, Nichols R, Archambault WT, et al. Comparative safety and immunogenicity of two yellow fever 17D vaccines (ARILVAX™ and YF-VAX®) in a Phase III multicenter, double-blind clinical trial. Am J Trop Med Hyg 66: 533–541, 2002, with permission.

of severe reactions to 17D vaccine was not significantly higher in HIV-infected than in noninfected persons. Further studies in large-scale campaigns, preferably using case-control methodology and application of laboratory techniques to establish etiology, are needed to clarify the risk of encephalitis following 17D vaccine.

The syndrome of 17D-associated encephalitis is characterized by onset 7 to 21 days after immunization of fever and variable neurologic signs, including meningismus, convulsions, obtundation, and paresis. The cerebrospinal fluid contains 100 to 500 cells (mixed polymorphonuclear and lymphocytic) and increased protein concentration. The clinical course has

TABLE 40–21 ■ Cases of Meningoencephalitis Temporally Associated with or Proved to Be Caused by Yellow Fever 17D Vaccine Manufactured According to Biologic Standards Established in 1945*

Case No.	Year	Location	Age	Sex	Incubation Period (days)	Outcome	Reference
1	1952–1953	France	7 mo	F	19	Survived	406
2	1952–1953	France	1.5 mo	M	11	Survived	406
3	1952–1953	France	1 mo	M	12	Survived	406
4	1952–1953	France	6 mo	M	12	Survived	406
5	1952–1953	France	4 mo	F	10	Survived	406
6	1952	South Africa/England[†,‡]	5 wk	M	21	Survived	618
7	1953	South Africa/England[†,‡]	4 mo	M	8	Survived	619
8	1953	Scotland[‡]	7 wk	M	17	Survived	515
9	1954	England	5 wk	F	9	Survived	620
10	1954	England	13 wk	?	~9	Survived	621
11	1954	Nigeria/England[†]	8 wk	M	~14[§]	Survived	622
12	1954	England	3 mo	M	8	Survived	623
13	1954	France	3 mo	M	8	Survived	624
14	1954	Portugal	6 wk	F	11	Survived	625
15	1959	United States	10 wk	F	12	Survived	626
16	1965	United States	3 yr	F	6	Died	108
17	1979	France	1 mo	M	13	Survived	517
18	1989	South Africa	13 yr	M	7	Survived	627
19	1990		19 yr	M	13	Survived	628
20	1990		59 yr	F	2[‖]	Survived	628
21	1991	Switzerland	29 yr	M	3 (18)[¶]	Survived	519
22	2001	United States	36 yr	M	13	Survived	628a
23	2001	United States	71 yr	M	13	Survived	628a
24	2002	United States	41 yr	M	16	Survived	628a
25	2002	United States	16 yr	M	23	Survived	628a

*There are less well substantiated but plausible records of other cases possibly caused by 17D vaccine (a 3-month-old child in England [Parrish, 1954, quoted in Thompson, 1955[515]] and a 6-year-old child who received 17D vaccine 3 days after smallpox vaccination [reported by Dick and Horgan in 1952[514]]).

†Country where immunized/where hospitalized, if different.

‡Vaccinated simultaneously or within a few days with smallpox (vaccination unsuccessful).

§Date of onset and hospitalization inaccurate in original publication (see Stuart).

‖Event occurred 2 days after revaccination with 17D (prior vaccination 10 years in the past).

¶Patient had biphasic illness starting 3 days after immunization, with partial remission and central nervous system signs developing 18 days after immunization.

typically been brief and recovery generally complete. One patient died[108] and a 29-year-old described by Merlo et al.[518] had residual mild ataxia 11 months after onset.

The basis for increased risk of encephalitis in young infants is unknown, but it parallels the increased susceptibility of neonatal mice to neuroinvasion and neurovirulence of yellow fever and other flaviviruses. Possibilities include (1) immaturity of the blood-brain barrier, (2) prolonged or higher viremia, and (3) immaturity of the immune system and delayed clearance of the infection. There are no data on 17D viremia levels or on the kinetics of the immune response in infants or children. The incidence of encephalitis following 17D vaccine has been more common in males (17 of 24 cases, or 71%) than in females. A slight excess of males (56%) was noted also in the cases of encephalitis following use of FNV,[411] and in epidemics of naturally acquired yellow fever, where no gender difference in exposure to the virus was evident (see *Risk Factors* above).

VACCINE-ASSOCIATED VISCEROTROPIC ADVERSE EVENTS

Such adverse events represent a newly recognized and apparently rare complication of 17D vaccines. Cases have been associated with vaccines manufactured in Brazil

TABLE 40–22 ■ Incidence of Encephalitis Associated with Administration of 17D Vaccine to Infants

Location	Years	Age	No. Vaccinations	No. Encephalitis Cases	Incidence/ 1000	Case-Fatality Rate (%)	Reference
France (Paris)	1952–1953	< 6 mo	1000	4	4	0	
		7–12 mo	800	1	1.25	0	
France (Lyon)	1958–1978	< 1 mo	1830	1	0.5	0	516

(17DD substrain), France, and the United States (17D-204 substrain). At least 13 cases (9 fatal) have been described of a syndrome closely resembling wild-type yellow fever; nine case histories have been published (Table 40–23).[519–522] Seven cases occurred in adults immunized for travel, and six were in children and young adults living in an endemic region. Five of six cases occurring in the United States were in elderly patients,[519] and four patients had a diversified and complex clinical presentation labeled "multi-organ failure." There was some uncertainty as to the role of 17D vaccine in direct viral injury, and postmortem evaluation to clarify pathogenesis was not performed. In contrast, virologic evidence in the cases occurring in Brazil and Australia and two cases in the U.S. supported the conclusion that an overwhelming infection with 17D virus was responsible.[520,521] In persons surviving long enough to assess the immune response, antibody titers to yellow fever were significantly higher than expected ($\geq$1:10,240),[519,628] consistent with an overwhelming infection (although a secondary response in the setting of prior heterologous flavivirus exposure was not ruled out). Similarities of the syndrome to wild-type yellow fever included rapid onset of fever and malaise within 3 to 5 days of vaccination, jaundice, oliguria, cardiovascular instability, hemorrhage, and midzonal necrosis of the liver at autopsy.[520,521] Large amounts of yellow fever viral antigen were found in the liver, heart, and other affected organs.

Similar cases undoubtedly have occurred but were missed or misdiagnosed throughout the history of use of yellow fever 17D vaccines. The recognition of viscerotropic adverse events is especially difficult in endemic areas, where the syndrome could be confused with wild-type yellow fever. The recent recognition in developed countries may be attributable to improved surveillance for vaccine-associated adverse events. Nevertheless, only 14 serious adverse events (not all of them resulting from viscerotropic accidents) were reported to the Vaccine Adverse Event Reporting System (VAERS) in the United States in 1990 to 1998, during which time period 1,443,686 doses of 17D vaccine were administered, a rate of 0.97 per 100,000.

Based on passive surveillance (reports to VAERS in the United States in 1990 to 1998) the incidence of vaccine-associated viscerotropic events was estimated at less than 1 per 400,000,[519] but the true incidence will remain unknown until prospective surveillance is applied to large populations undergoing primary vaccination. Since the syndrome was first described in 1996, at least 190 million doses of yellow fever vaccine have been distributed worldwide, with 13 reported cases. These serious adverse events are certainly rare. Vaccine-associated viscerotropic adverse events can occur only in the setting of primary vaccination of persons without pre-existing yellow fever immunity. One possible explanation for the occurrence of the syndrome in recent years is the discontinuation of administration of immune serum globulin for prevention of hepatitis A. Because commercial globulins contain yellow fever antibody, they may have protected against viscerotropic infection by coadministered 17D vaccine. Use of globulin has been supplanted by active vaccination against hepatitis A.

Vaccine-associated viscerotropic adverse events apparently are not caused by mutations arising in the virus, but appear to be related to individual host susceptibility.[519,523] Analyses of the vaccine lots and seed viruses associated with cases revealed no evidence for mutations in the vaccine that could explain the adverse events. The host factors responsible for increased susceptibility are unknown and are not identifiable by laboratory tests or medical history. A genetic basis is likely. Two cases (one confirmed) in a single family have been recorded in Brazil. Because the viscerotropic response to 17D is likely related to host genetics, it is advisable to ask travelers whether severe reactions to 17D vaccine have occurred in a family member and to avoid vaccinating someone with a family history of the adverse response.

The role of advanced age as a risk factor for serious adverse events has been the subject of concern in the United States.[519] A retrospective analysis of VAERS data revealed a higher incidence of serious adverse events (neurologic or multisystem involvement) to 17D vaccine in elderly persons, with persons older than 65 years having a risk 12 to 32 times higher than adults 25 to 44 years of age, suggesting that waning immunity with age may play a role (Table 40–24).[524] A similar conclusion was reached after analysis of postmarketing surveillance data for Arilvax in the United Kingdom (M Cetron and TP Monath, unpublished results). Although the cases of vaccine-associated viscerotropic events in Brazil were in children and young adults,[520] a predilection for severe reactions in the elderly would not be apparent in Brazil because older persons have been previously vaccinated. No clearly identifiable risk factors related to age and immunologic competence can be formulated at the present time.

As mentioned earlier in the section on *Common Adverse Events Following Administration of 17D Vaccines*, it is possible that the vaccine may induce a milder form of hepatic injury without overt clinical signs. Chemical hepatic dysfunction (elevations in ALT and AST) was noted in 3.5% to 4.6% of subjects 10 days after vaccination, with resolution thereafter.[470] Without a placebo group, it is uncertain whether the chemical hepatic dysfunction noted in this trial is related to the vaccine or has unrelated causes. If related to the vaccine, subclinical hepatic dysfunction is probably inconsequential because survivors of severe hepatitis caused by wild-type yellow fever virus have complete healing of the liver without postnecrotic cirrhosis. However, this marker could be used to study the genetic basis of susceptibility in humans.

The risk of acquiring yellow fever during travel to an endemic area probably exceeds the risk of vaccine-associated viscerotropic adverse events. Nevertheless, physicians should be aware of this serious complication of 17D vaccine, and that it may occur at higher frequency in primary vaccination of elderly persons. Special attention is drawn to the fact that, in two cases (see numbers 1 and 7 in Table 40–23), the intended travel destination was not within the yellow fever–endemic zone, and therefore vaccination was not necessary. Yellow fever vaccination should be employed only when justified by potential exposure to wild-type virus.

Patients with an undiagnosed febrile illness occurring within 10 days after vaccination should be investigated, and those with elevated liver enzyme levels should be hospitalized for observation. To provide much-needed data on causality, serial samples for quantitative viremia and antibody studies should be undertaken, and buffy coat cells or

TABLE 40–23 ■ Yellow Fever Vaccine-Associated Viscerotropic Adverse Events

Case	Year	Location	Travel Destination	Vaccine	Age/Sex/ Race	Pre-Existing Conditions	Days to Onset	Days to Hospitalization	Syndrome Initial
1	1998	US	Nepal, Thailand	YF-Vax*	76/M/W	Osteoarthritis, mild renal insufficiency, Crohn's (disease in remission)	4	7	Fever, headache, myalgia, fatigue
2	1998	US	Africa	YF-Vax	79/F/W	Hypothyroid, polymyalgia rheumatica, hypertension	2	3	Fever, myalgia, confusion, abdominal pain, diarrhea, cough, fatigue
3	1998	US	Amazon	YF-Vax	67/F/W	Ulcerative colitis, thymoma	5	6	Fever, myalgias, chills, nausea
4	1996	US	Africa	YF-Vax†	63/M/W	None	3	5	Fever, headache, myalgia, nausea, vomiting
5	1999	Brazil		BioMan-guinhos‡	5/F/W	Low birth weight, repeated episodes of bronchitis and diarrhea, aseptic meningitis	3	5	Fever, diarrhea, vomiting
6	2000	Brazil		BioMan-guinhos	22/F/B	None	4	8	Fever, headache, myalgia, sore throat
7	2001	Australia	Saudi Arabia	Stamaril§	56/M/W	None	2	5	Fever, rigors, nausea, vomiting, myalgia, arthralgia
8	2001	US	N. Africa, Turkey, Israel, Ecuador	YF-Vax	25/m/?	None	2	9	Fever, headache, lymphadenopathy, nausea, diarrhea
9	2002	US	Venezuela	YF-Vax	70/m/?	None	5	8	Fever, malaise, dyspnea, myalgia

*Oral typhoid vaccine administered 21 days before yellow fever vaccine.
§Concomitant meningococcal vaccine.
†Concomitant vaccination with oral polio, meningococcal vaccine; onset of nonspecific syndrome occurred 3 days after 17D vaccination, but symptoms subsided and, 2 days later (5 days after 17D), hepatitis A vaccine was administered. Severe syndrome onset followed hepatitis A vaccination by several hours.
‡Concomitant measles mumps rubella vaccine.

Evolving	Outcome	Clinical Lab Abnormalities		Virologic Findings	Histopathology (Liver)	Reference
		Initial	Peak			
Transient rash, hypotension, hypoxemia, dyspnea, agitation, confusion	Survived	AST 31 U/L; ALT 42 U/L; alk phos 41 U/L; bili 49.6 mmol/L; creat 362 mmol/L; plat 94,000/L	AST 122; ALT 122; alk phos 109; bili 99.2; creat 627.7; plat 67,000	17D virus isolated from serum (days 7 and 8) and CSF (day 10). PRNT antibody titer 1:20 (day 7), >10,240 (day 45)		519
Dyspnea, cardiac arrhythmia, hypotension, acidosis, hypoxemia, oliguria (requiring dialysis)	Died (day 21)	AST 40 U/L; ALT 27 U/L; alk phos 77 U/L; bili 8.6 mmol/L; creat 124 mmol/L; plat 154,000/L	AST 301; ALT 290; alk phos 310; bili 111; creat 265; plat 26,000	17D virus isolated from serum (day 7). PRNT antibody titer 1:640 (day 7), 10,240 (day 11)	Not done	519
Tachypnea, tachycardia, mechanical ventilation, hypotension	Died (day 9)	AST 85 U/L; alk phos 55 U/L: bili 32.5 mmol/L; creat 115 mmol/L; plat 194,000/L	AST 1638; alk phos 112; bili 32.5; creat 327; plat 7000	Not done	Not done	519
Transient rash, fever, rhabdomyolysis, myoglobinuria, oliguria (dialysis), epistaxis, hypotension, stupor	Died (day 30)	AST 113 U/L; ALT 109 U/L; alk phos 141 U/L; bili 94.1 mmol/L; creat 141 mmol/L; plat 121,000/L	AST 446; ALT 190; bili 133.4; creat 495; plat 25,000	Liver biopsy (day 28); YF antigen	Liver biopsy, minimal changes, not diagnostic	519
Respiratory distress, dehydration, hepatomegaly, jaundice, shock	Died (day 5)	AST 114 IU/L; ALT 160 IU/L; bili 18.8		17D virus isolated from blood, heart, liver, spleen at autopsy; large amounts of antigen in hepatocytes and Kupffer's cells	Midzonal necrosis, Councilman's bodies	520
Epigastric pain, jaundice, oliguria, hepatomegaly, edema, hypoxemia, respiratory distress, mechanical ventilation, hemothorax, hypotension	Died (day 10)	AST 430 U/L; ALT 190 U/L; creat 247.5 mmol/L; plat 54,000/L; proteinuria 1+	AST 511; ALT 91; alk phos 530; bili 194.9; creat 3447.6; plat 38,000	Anti-YF IgM (day 10); 17D virus isolated from blood, brain, liver, kidney, spleen, lung at autopsy; YF antigen in hepatocytes, Kupffer's cells	Midzonal necrosis, Councilman's bodies	520
Respiratory distress, oliguria, hypotension, hypoxemia, mechanical ventilation, acidosis	Died (day 10)	Normal	AST 6750 U/L; ALT 1550 U/L; creat 336	YF virus isolated and/or PCR positive serum, spleen, liver, muscle	Panlobular necrosis; steatosis; Councilman's bodies	521
Hepatic and renal failure, respiratory failure, hypotension	Survived		AST 436 U/L; ALT 362/ U/L; Bili 8.3 mg/dl; creat 10.4 mg/dl; creat kinase 789 U/L	Convalescent serum YF neutralizing antibody titer 1:640	N/A	628
Jaundice, respiratory failure, hypotension	Survived		AST 400 U/L; ALT 239 U/L; bili 1.4 mg/dl; creat 6.2 mg/dl	Serum on day 28 YF neutralizing antibody titer 1:1280	N/A	628

alk phos, alkaline phosphatase; ALT, alanine aminotransferase; AST, aspartate aminotransferase; B, black; bili, bilirubin; creat, creatinine; CSF, cerebrospinal fluid; F, female; IgM, immunoglobulin M; M, male; PCR, polymerase chain reaction; plat, platelets; PRNT, plaque-reduction neutralization test; W, white; YF, yellow fever.

TABLE 40–24 ▪ Incidence of Nonserious and Serious Adverse Events Reported to the VAERS, United States, 1990–1998*

Age (yr)	Vaccine Doses	Nonserious Adverse Events			Serious Adverse Events		
		Number	Rate/ 100,000	Relative Rate (95% CI)	Number	Rate/ 100,000	Relative Rate (95% CI)
15–24	189,991	12	6.32	1.8 (0.9–3.5)	2	1.05	3.7 (0.5–26)
25–44	702,783	25	3.56	Reference	2	0.29	Reference
45–64	442,605	15	3.39	1.0 (0.5–1.8)	5	1.13	4.0 (0.8–20)
65–74	86,222	3	3.48	1.0 (0.3–3.2)	3	3.48	12.3 (2.0–73)
>75	22,085	2	9.06	2.5 (0.6–10.7)	2	9.06	32 (4.5–226)
TOTAL	1,443,686	57	3.95		14	0.97	

*The 25 to 44-year age group served as the reference group for calculating relative rates (95% confidence intervals [CI]).
Data from Martin M, Weld LH, Tsai TF, et al. Advanced age is a risk factor for adverse events temporally associated with yellow fever vaccination. Emerg Infect Dis 7:945–951, 2001, with permission.

peripheral blood mononuclear cells frozen for future genetic studies. Such cases should be reported promptly to the VAERS (toll-free: 800-822-7967) and consultation sought with the CDC (Fort Collins, CO: 303-221-6428; Atlanta, GA: 404-417-8000).[522]

IMMEDIATE ALLERGIC REACTIONS TO EGG PROTEINS

Hypersensitivity reactions to egg proteins in yellow fever vaccine have been extremely infrequent. No such reactions were observed during initial use of the vaccine in over 2 million persons.[525] Guinea pig sensitization tests with 17D vaccine showed that anaphylactic reactions were reduced when the test vaccine was prepared from embryos less than 13 days old. For this reason, the age of embryos at time of harvest for production of 17D vaccine is 12 days or less.[442] Yellow fever vaccine contains multiple proteins derived from egg white and yolk.[526] In one study, 17D vaccine produced in the United States contained 7.8 μg ovalbumin per 0.5-mL dose.[527]

The first report of allergic phenomena associated with use of 17D vaccine was in 1942, during large-scale immunization of military personnel. Sulzberger and Asher[528] described three patients with a serum sickness syndrome (urticaria or erythema multiforme–like rash accompanied by malaise, fever, arthralgia, pruritus, nausea, and vomiting) with onset between 3 and 7 days after receipt of different lots of 17D vaccine. In 1943, Swartz[529] described a patient with a strong history of egg and other food allergies who developed anaphylaxis 5 minutes after receiving simultaneous injections of 17D and cholera vaccines. Skin testing revealed marked reactions to egg white and chicken meat and a moderate reaction to 17D (but not cholera) vaccine. Sprague and Barnard[530] reported a case of severe anaphylaxis occurring within 15 minutes after 17D vaccine in a man with known egg allergy.

The general consensus based on observations during the first 20 years of use of 17D vaccine was that allergic reactions are extremely rare, occurring at an incidence of less than 1 per 1 million, with reactions occurring principally in persons with known egg sensitivity. Reactions are typically mild, and thus may be under-reported. Kouwenaar[531] found the frequency of allergic reactions to yellow fever vaccine to be higher than expected, particularly in persons with a history of various allergies. He vaccinated 242 inoculated per-

sons having allergic histories with 0.1 mL of 17D vaccine by the intradermal route; if no reaction occurred within 45 minutes, the subjects received the remaining 0.4 mL subcutaneously. Nine (3.7%) of the subjects experienced allergic reactions, characterized clinically as exacerbations of known but dormant allergy (eczema, asthma, rhinitis) in four patients; urticaria occurring less than 3 days after vaccination in two cases; and "serum sickness–like disease" (urticaria or rash) occurring 6 to 14 days after vaccination in three cases. Of the nine subjects reacting to yellow fever vaccination, two had a known history of egg allergy and the others had various other food allergies, asthma, or hay fever. In a "control" group of 465 persons without a history of allergy, only 3 patients (0.6%) had a late reaction to yellow fever vaccine (facial erythema [2 cases] and urticaria [1 case]). In an additional group of 185 nonallergic individuals who were re-immunized with 17D vaccine, 1 (0.5%) experienced generalized urticaria. The skin test had a very low positive predictive value for the development of allergic response to yellow fever vaccine. There were insufficient data on the more important question of the negative predictive value of the skin test.

More recent and definitive data on the incidence of allergic reactions are few, principally because a prior history of intolerance or allergy to eggs or egg-based vaccines is considered a contraindication to the use of 17D vaccine, and few immunizations are given to such individuals. Guidelines for use of yellow fever and other egg-based vaccines recommend that egg-sensitive patients undergo scratch, prick, or needle puncture testing with 1:10 diluted vaccine and a negative and positive (histamine) control. If the test is negative, an intradermal test is performed with 0.02 mL of 1:100 vaccine.[479,532,533] Application of this skin test procedure in clinical practice was described by Mosimann et al.[534] In the case of a positive intradermal test (a wheal 5 mm or larger), and an established need for yellow fever vaccine, the patient may undergo a desensitization procedure consisting of increasing subcutaneous doses at 15- to 20-minute intervals under the supervision of an experienced physician.

In one study, 30,000 Navy and Marine Corps personnel were screened for a history of egg sensitivity, and 42 allergic patients underwent scratch and intradermal testing with crude egg white and a variety of egg-based vaccines, including yellow fever 17D; most patients also underwent oral egg challenge.[535] The study demonstrated that a history of egg allergy was not a strong contraindication to administration of egg-based vaccines because only 16% of the egg-sensitive subjects experienced any reaction, and these were mild in all cases. Skin tests were positive in 31% of the egg-sensitive subjects. Vaccination was performed in 39 subjects (excluding 3 subjects with strongly positive intradermal tests), using the egg-based vaccines causing the greatest reaginic activity. Intradermal skin testing with vaccine had reasonably high negative predictive value (0.80), but a lower positive predictive value (0.57) for an allergic reaction. However, the strength of positivity of the intradermal test appeared to correlate with severity of symptoms after vaccination.

Sensitization to egg-white protein by prior immunization with rabies vaccine produced in chick embryo cell culture was reported to cause a positive intradermal or scratch skin test in response to yellow fever vaccine.[536] No systemic allergic reactions have been noted in such cases. Similarly, prior yellow fever vaccination was reported to sensitize against a rabies vaccine manufactured in duck embryo cells.[537] There are no current precautions regarding sequential immunization with vaccines produced in chick tissue or cells, but few studies of egg/chick cell–based vaccine interactions have been performed. Influenza vaccine is manufactured in eggs but contains little residual egg protein, and can generally be safely given to egg-allergic persons,[538] and may not cross-sensitize to yellow fever vaccine. As noted below, gelatin (used as a vaccine stabilizer) must be considered in the evaluation of cross-sensitization to vaccines.

A case report of a woman who had no history of egg allergy and who suffered an anaphylactic reaction following yellow fever vaccine[539] is of interest. The patient had a history of intolerance to foods containing raw but not cooked eggs and had positive skin tests to raw egg antigen and 17D vaccine prepared from egg tissues without exposure to heat. Because few foods contain raw eggs and these are mixed with other ingredients, persons sensitized to raw eggs might not give an allergic history when queried prior to vaccination.

Since 1990, the CDC has enhanced procedures for reporting adverse events in response to vaccines.[540] Data collected between 1990 and 1997 revealed 45 cases of nonfatal hypersensitivity-type reactions (urticaria, angioedema, bronchospasm, anaphylaxis) temporally associated with yellow fever vaccine.[541] The incidence of allergic reactions cannot be established with accuracy. However, based on the number of vaccine doses distributed in the United States during the interval under study (5.2 million), and the assumptions that all reported events are caused by 17D vaccine and that the reporting sensitivity was 50%, the incidence of allergic reactions was estimated to be 1 in 58,000 doses. Although egg protein has been implicated in hypersensitivity reactions to yellow fever vaccine, other components also may play a role—for example, hydrolyzed porcine gelatin incorporated as a stabilizer by some manufacturers. Gelatin has been implicated in allergic reactions to measles, varicella, and Japanese encephalitis vaccines.[542,543]

OTHER RARE ADVERSE EVENTS TEMPORALLY RELATED TO 17D VACCINE

There are a number of individual case reports of adverse events possibly associated with yellow fever vaccination.

Although some are credible, such as the occurrence of ketoacidosis in an insulin-dependent diabetic patient 4 days after vaccination,[544] others (e.g., chronic lymphocytic leukemia,[545] malaria recrudescence,[546] multiple sclerosis,[547] and optic neuritis[548]) may represent chance associations in time. The absence of similar observations over the long history of use of yellow fever vaccine supports this view. Postmarketing surveillance by vaccine manufacturers, as well as the VAERS system, have accumulated cases of neurologic syndromes (Guillain-Barré syndrome, ataxia, Bell's palsy, mononeuritis) and bursitis, but the relationship of these events to vaccination is uncertain because they also occur as independent events in the population.

Mention is made in the literature of a favorable effect of yellow fever vaccine on reducing the incidence of recurrent herpes labialis in 11 patients,[549] but this observation has not been explored in controlled trials.

REACTIONS CAUSED BY IMPROPER HANDLING AND USE OF YELLOW FEVER VACCINE

Because yellow fever vaccine contains no preservative, improper handling of multiple-dose vials can lead to bacterial contamination, sometimes with serious consequences. Repeated use of the same needle and syringe, rubbing dirt or other materials into the inoculation site, and other practices also may contribute to infection. The author has personally observed a number of cases of superficial abscess formation at the site of jet injector immunization in Africa; the common practice of rubbing dirt, bark, balms, and native medicines or other materials onto the inoculation site was probably responsible.

Four known outbreaks of serious illness have been associated with contamination of yellow fever vaccine vials or inoculation equipment in Africa (Table 40–25). The clinical picture in all four episodes was similar, with marked swelling and pain of the vaccinated arm beginning hours after immunization, and progressing in the most severe cases to cardiovascular shock and death within hours to several days.[550–552] Some but not all cases had signs of necrotizing myositis (gangrene). In all episodes, known or potential problems with use of multiple-dose vaccine containers contaminated after reconstitution, improperly sterilized jet injector equipment, or reuse of syringes and needles were involved. Although no etiologic agent was implicated, *Clostridia* and group A or anaerobic *Streptococcus* were suspected.

Indications for Yellow Fever Vaccine

All inhabitants of countries, or areas within countries, endemic for yellow fever should be routinely immunized, preferably at 9 months of age. Areas endemic for yellow fever are shown in Figure 40–7. Within these countries, priorities may be established for immunization, related to risk of exposure to yellow fever virus. For example, residents in rural areas and areas of historical yellow fever epidemic activity are at higher risk than residents in large cities or areas in which yellow fever has not occurred in many years. Persons migrating from nonendemic to endemic areas are at high risk and should be immunized. Because such movements are difficult to control, and the potential exists for spread of yellow fever from rural to urban areas, a policy of universal immunization in countries within the endemic zone is favored.

TABLE 40–25 ▪ Episodes Involving Multiple Serious Adverse Events Characterized by Cellulitis or Necrotizing Myositis Associated with Probable Bacterial Contamination of 17D Vaccine After Reconstitution or Infection of Inoculation Site

Year	Location	No. Cases	No. Deaths (%)	Incidence*	Circumstances	Reference
1974	Ivory Coast	39	8 (20.5)	5.3/100,000 immunizations	Cases occurred at nine designated vaccinating centers; five-dose vials pooled to prepare 50–100 doses for jet injection	550
1982	Ghana	6	2 (33.3)		Cases occurred at single center; possible contaminated 50-dose vial or syringe	550
1984	Benin	31	11 (35.5)	4/10,000	Cases associated with one vaccinating team, six vaccinating sessions using multiple-dose vials, jet injectors	551
1987	Nigeria	25	5 (20)		Illegal clinics, unauthorized inoculators, reuse of syringes, multiple-dose vials	552

*Estimate, because number of persons vaccinated with vaccine vial(s) implicated in the contamination is unknown.

During epidemics of yellow fever, mass immunization should be instituted at the earliest possible stage of the outbreak. Priorities for immunizing population subsets according to geography or age group will be determined by local information on the progress of the outbreak and on the history of prior vaccination coverage.

Immigrants, travelers, and military personnel and dependents require immunization at least 10 days before arrival in endemic areas. As noted above in the section on *Incidence*, even a short stay in an area of virus transmission is dangerous. Because native inhabitants may be immune and the virus can circulate in a silent zoonotic cycle, the absence of recent notification of yellow fever in an area is not an indication that it is safe to enter without vaccination. Conversely, the notification of human cases within the past 1 to 2 years is an indication of high risk. Short-stay travelers to large cities within endemic areas, such as the coastal metropolises of West Africa (Accra, Lagos, Dakar, Abidjan, etc.) are at lower risk in the absence of a reported outbreak. However, cases of urban yellow fever currently (2002) are being reported within the city of Abidjan (the Ivory Coast), the first instance of yellow fever in a port city of the West African coast in decades. Clearly, visitors to this urban region currently require vaccination. Coastal areas of East Africa and most of South America are outside the area of yellow fever transmission.

Some countries in the endemic zones, and some countries outside the endemic zones but infested with A. *aegypti* and receptive to the introduction of yellow fever, require a valid certificate of immunization for travelers from endemic countries (see Table 40–4). A full listing is given in the WHO document "International Travel and Health"[279] (available from WHO Distribution and Sales, CH-1211 Geneva 27, Switzerland) and in the most current edition of the CDC's "Health Information for International Travel"[278] (available from the Superintendent of Documents, U.S. Government Printing Office, Washington, DC 20402; phone 202-512-1800). Some countries require a valid

immunization certificate even if the traveler has been in transit through an endemic country and even if the disembarking traveler is in transit. Controls at airports and borders are highly variable, but travelers respecting the regulations will avoid unnecessary delays. Persons with a contraindication to immunization (see below) should obtain a letter from their physician stating why immunization could not be performed.

Contraindications and Precautions

Age Restriction

Infants are at higher risk of postvaccinal encephalitis, and this risk is inversely proportional to age. Published guidelines differ somewhat on the minimum age for vaccination.[279,478,479,552,553] There is complete agreement, however, that the vaccine should never be administered to infants younger than 4 months of age, and that routine immunization may be performed at 9 months of age. Infants between the ages of 5 and 8 months should be immunized if there is a significant risk of natural infection (e.g., residence in or travel to a rural area in the yellow fever–endemic zone or in the context of an ongoing epidemic). Where the risk of exposure to yellow fever is very low (e.g., in large urban areas in endemic countries, especially in the context of brief visits by tourists), it is advisable to delay immunization until 12 months of age.

Pregnancy and Lactation

Initially, the use of yellow fever vaccine in pregnancy was not constrained, and many women were vaccinated without any reported adverse effects. In Paris, Stefanopoulo and Duvolon[512] immunized over 200 pregnant women between 1936 and 1946, and in Brazil, Smith et al.[21] vaccinated "a considerable number of women in all stages of pregnancy . . . with no untoward effects." Spontaneous abortion, stillbirth, and congenital malformation have not been observed in the aftermath of yellow fever epidemics. In one report of yellow fever death of a pregnant woman, there was no evidence that the fetus had developed hepatitis.[554] In another report, two women 2 and 5 months pregnant died of yellow fever; in neither case did the fetal livers show necrosis.[555]

The hypothetical risk of transplacental infection and the recognition that young infants (and thus, potentially, the unborn fetus) were susceptible to neuroinvasion by 17D virus led to the general recommendation that the vaccine not be administered during pregnancy unless clearly required, based on the judgment that a high risk of natural infection exists. Specific recommendations on this issue vary considerably. The position of the WHO is that vaccination is generally contraindicated in pregnancy but "is permitted after the sixth month of pregnancy when justified epidemiologically."[279] The American Committee on Immunization Practices does not specify a stage of pregnancy, but emphasizes the necessity of establishing a clear need for immunization.[478] Inadvertent immunization of women (generally in the early stages of pregnancy) is definitely not an indication for therapeutic abortion. Women should be cautioned that there is a hypothetical risk, but should be reassured that no harm to the fetus has ever been demonstrated. Fear of potential adverse effects may have led to an increase in therapeutic abortions during a vaccination campaign in Trinidad in 1977–78.[556]

More recent studies have addressed the risk of congenital infection in pregnant women who were inadvertently immunized with 17D vaccine during emergency vaccination campaigns. Nasidi et al.[495] studied 101 women who were immunized in Nigeria in 1986. Four women (4%) were immunized in the first trimester, 8 (8%) in the second trimester, and 89 (88%) in the third trimester. There were no adverse effects on fetuses or neonates attributable to vaccination among 40 infants who were carefully followed up. No evidence for transplacental infection was obtained in 40 babies whose cord blood samples were tested for IgM antibodies. The most important aspect of this study was the finding that women immunized during pregnancy had a significantly lower seroconversion rate (39%) compared to control groups immunized during the campaign. It was concluded that immunization of pregnant women might be justified in epidemic emergencies when there is a high risk of natural infection, but that response rates may be low as a result of the immunosuppression associated with pregnancy.

A second study was conducted following a vaccination campaign in Trinidad in 1989.[557] Approximately 400,000 persons were immunized, and 100 to 200 were estimated to have inadvertently received 17D vaccine during pregnancy. Forty-one cord blood samples were obtained from babies born to mothers who had received 17D vaccine during the first trimester. One infant (normal, full term) had IgM antibody in cord blood, suggesting that congenital infection with 17D virus may have occurred.

In a case-control study of 17D vaccination during early pregnancy, the relative risk of spontaneous abortion was estimated to be 2.3, but statistical power was low.[558]

Pregnant women who have received the vaccine should be reassured that there is no risk to themselves and very low risk to the fetus. These women should be followed to parturition, and, if fetal abnormality is noted, a cord blood sample should be obtained for IgM testing to determine whether congenital infection had occurred. Because the immune response to yellow fever vaccination during pregnancy is impaired, revaccination is indicated at an appropriate time after delivery. If vaccination during pregnancy is required because of a high risk of exposure during travel, it is advisable to determine whether successful immunization has been achieved by a test of neutralizing antibodies 10 to 14 days or more after vaccination. If seroconversion is not evident, revaccination should be considered, preferably after parturition.

Recommendations regarding use of 17D vaccine in breast-feeding mothers are absent or vary in different documents, and are purely hypothetical. A very large number of lactating women have been (appropriately) immunized during emergency vaccination campaigns, but no studies on subsequent effects on or vaccine virus transmission to infants have been conducted. Lactation is not considered a contraindication to 17D vaccination in the United States,[479] but is in the United Kingdom[553] because of the theoretical risk of transmission of 17D virus to the breast-fed infant. The theoretical concern is based in part on the knowledge that some tick-borne flaviviruses are secreted in milk of domesticated livestock, and that West Nile virus has been isolated from human milk.

Concurrent Infections, Medications, and Immunosuppression

Some national authorities recommend that vaccination be delayed in persons with acute concurrent infections.[553] Because of the theoretical risk of neuroinvasion and encephalitis, the vaccine is contraindicated in patients with known immunosuppression resulting from HIV infection or immunologic deficiency states (leukemia, lymphoma, generalized malignancy, other conditions affecting humoral and cellular immune responses, or treatment with immunosuppressive drugs, including high-dose corticosteroids). Low-dose corticosteroid treatment or intra-articular injections of corticosteroids do not pose a contraindication to yellow fever vaccination.[478,479] Asymptomatic HIV infection is not considered a contraindication in the United States[478,479] but is in the United Kingdom. As noted above, preliminary studies indicate that asymptomatic HIV infection may reduce the immune response to 17D vaccine. The report[517] of a healthy adult with low CD4+ cell counts as a result of HIV infection, who developed fatal encephalitis following yellow fever vaccination, is the first direct evidence for immunosuppression as a risk factor. This report supports the hypothetical precautions and cautions against vaccination of individuals with intrinsic or iatrogenic immune suppression.

Despite an earlier study to the contrary, yellow fever vaccine does not appear to depress tuberculin skin test sensitivity,[559] and is unlikely to adversely affect the course of active tuberculosis. However, there are no field studies of this question.

Blood, Bone Marrow, and Organ Donation

Blood donations should be delayed until 30 days after vaccination. There are no data on whether yellow fever vaccine may induce transient false-positive serologic tests for HIV or other blood-borne viruses, as has been reported for influenza vaccine.[560] No formal recommendations have been made on the suitability of persons who have received 17D vaccine at a remote point in time as organ or bone marrow donors. This issue has been raised because of the possibility that 17D virus causes a latent, persistent infection (reviewed in the section on *Duration of Immunity* above), which is contained and irrelevant in the immune host but might cause systemic infection in an immunosuppressed transplant recipient. The risk to recipients is purely hypothetical. Unless the vaccine changed its tropism and virulence during latency, the risk to the recipient, even if infected, would appear to be small. In a single report, bone marrow from a donor twin immunized 1 month previously with yellow fever 17D was grafted to an identical twin.[561] The recipient failed to develop yellow fever antibodies, indicating that no yellow fever B-cell clone had been transferred or that immunosuppressive therapy may have masked an immune response by the recipient to transferred virus. There were no untoward events attributable to the potential transfer of 17D virus.

Simultaneous and Combined Vaccination

Yellow fever vaccine has been given simultaneously at different sites or as a mixture, combined with a variety of other vaccines, including vaccinia, diphtheria-pertussis-tetanus, bacille Calmette-Guérin, measles, typhoid, cholera, hepatitis A, hepatitis B, and meningococcus A/C plus typhoid vaccines (Table 40–26). These studies are relevant to the use of 17D vaccine in routine childhood immunization programs, and to the immunization of travelers. In particular, the ability to coadminister or combine yellow fever and measles vaccines could reduce the cost and complexity of childhood immunization.

No increase in reactogenicity has been noted in studies of combined or simultaneous immunization, and, with few exceptions (noted below), there have been no alterations in reciprocal immune responses. On theoretical grounds alone, it is recommended that either live vaccines (such as measles) be given concurrently at different sites or the vaccinations be separated by 4 weeks; however, where this is impractical, the schedule may be modified. A study of yellow fever vaccine given at approximately weekly intervals after live measles vaccine showed no differences in immunogenicity.[562] Lipopolysaccharide is known to have adjuvant activity, and coadministration of the typhoid Vi vaccine appeared to enhance antibody titers to yellow fever, especially when the typhoid vaccine was combined with yellow fever.[563] However, in another study, no enhancement was observed when typhoid Vi and meningococcus A/C conjugate vaccines were coadministered with 17D.[564] An enhanced neutralizing antibody response to yellow fever was observed in a study of combined 17D-measles vaccine, perhaps as a result of cytokine induction by the unrelated virus.[565] Possible interference with yellow fever immune responses were noted when vaccinia and measles vaccine[566] or hepatitis B vaccine[567] were combined with 17D, but these results were not confirmed in other trials (see Table 40–26). An interesting observation, not relevant to current vaccination practices, was the mutual interference caused by simultaneous or sequential administration of 17D and inactivated parenteral whole-cell cholera vaccines.[568,569]

The interference induced by 17D vaccine with vibriocidal responses was not confirmed in another study,[570] and may not be real. The basis for interference is obscure because the interval between cholera and yellow fever immunization was as long as 4 weeks. Trials of combined yellow fever and live oral cholera vaccine (alone or with Ty21a live typhoid vaccine) showed no one-way interference with anticholera immunity or yellow fever antibody responses.[571,572]

Coadministration of Immune Serum Globulin and Yellow Fever Vaccine

Seroconversion rates and neutralizing antibody titers were not affected by the intramuscular administration of 5 mL of commercial pooled immune serum globulin containing high titers of yellow fever neutralizing antibodies 0 to 7 days before or at intervals after yellow fever 17D immunization[377]—a finding of practical importance prior to the advent of vaccines against hepatitis A. The results are not unexpected given the success of passive-active immunization and the observation that revaccination of individuals with neutralizing antibodies often results in a booster response.[244]

Yellow Fever Vaccine and Antimalarial Drugs

Chloroquine is known to inhibit the immune response to inactivated rabies vaccine and live oral cholera vaccine, and to interfere with flavivirus replication in vitro. In humans, there was no inhibitory effect of chloroquine at doses used for malaria prophylaxis on the response to yellow fever 17D.[573]

Future Yellow Fever Vaccines and Yellow Fever–Vectored Vaccines

Research sponsored by the WHO at the Oswaldo Cruz Foundation in Rio de Janeiro aimed at the development of a novel method for manufacturing 17D vaccine. The approach utilized a full-length complementary DNA (cDNA) clone of 17D-204 virus. The cDNA was reverse transcribed to full-length positive-strand RNA and transfected into primary chick embryo cells. The progeny virus was investigated as a vaccine candidate but was found to have a marginally acceptable neurovirulence profile.[440] Unlike current yellow fever vaccines, which are heterogeneous mixtures of virion subpopulations, the new vaccine is genetically homogeneous. It is likely that, with the introduction of some modifying mutations, a cDNA-based vaccine could be derived that would be safe and effective. The benefits of this approach are genetic homogeneity, reduced likelihood of selection of a subpopulation during replication in vitro or in vivo, manufacture of seed virus from bacterial plasmids (reducing the risk of adventitious viruses), and production of vaccine in a cell culture system.

An important aspect of the infectious clone work is that it set a precedent for novel, chimeric vaccines in which heterologous flavivirus prM-E genes (e.g., of Japanese encephalitis, West Nile, or dengue virus) have been inserted into the yellow fever 17D virus infectious clone.[92,155,457,574-577] The use of yellow fever 17D as a live vector is a promising approach for the development of new vaccines against other flaviviruses.[578] The virus also has been investigated as a vector for unrelated antigens, but significant size constraints exist on the insertion of heterologous genetic material. In one interesting example, a cytotoxic T-cell epitope was inserted between NS2B and NS3 for delivery of a tumor antigen.[579] Characterization of chimeric viruses has shown that the nonstructural genes of yellow fever 17D confer a highly attenuated phenotype on the vaccine candidates, including the restricted ability to replicate in mosquito vectors, while retaining the ability of the vaccines to efficiently immunize mice, monkeys, and humans. A full treatment of the subject of yellow fever–vectored vaccines is beyond the scope of this chapter (for a review, see Lai and Monath[580]).

Workers at BioManguinhos (Brazil) have produced a new seed stock and vaccines in primary chick embryo cell culture, rather than embryonated eggs. Manufacture in cell culture would be expected to increase vaccine virus yields significantly and thereby reduce costs. Although modernization of manufacture of 17D vaccine in cell culture has been a goal for many years, previous attempts have failed because of alterations in virulence phenotype during passage in cell culture (a problem avoided by a genetically uniform infectious clone) or poor yields resulting from in vitro interferon production. However, the tools of molecular biology were not available at that time to monitor genetic changes during cell culture propagation. The novel chimeric vaccines under development are being produced in Vero cell culture rather than primary chick embryo cells. Yields are very robust (7 to 8 $\log_{10}$ PFU/mL), and effective dose requirements are low.[155] The emerging data with chimeric yellow fever vaccines indicate that a similar approach could be used to manufacture yellow fever vaccines.

Combination vaccines are not being pursued actively by industry. Potential combinations of value might include yellow fever and measles vaccines for the EPI, and the combinations of 17D vaccine with inactivated vaccines (e.g., hepatitis A, typhoid) as a means of simplifying immunization regimens for travelers. Again, it is likely that the development of chimeric yellow fever–vectored vaccines will lead to combination vaccines against yellow fever and dengue, and against dengue and Japanese encephalitis; the combination of these vaccines with measles vaccines would be of interest for use in the EPI.

Public Health Considerations

Recommended Usage and Epidemiologic Results of Vaccination

South America

It is estimated that, of the total population in South America (258 million in 1997), 54 million (21%) inhabit the yellow fever–endemic zone. Yellow fever immunization has been implemented for decades in all countries with endemic yellow fever in South America, but vaccination coverage and strategies vary by country. Vaccination policy is changing, encouraged by the Pan-American Health Organization, toward implementation of yellow fever vaccination in the EPI and away from intermittent campaigns. Brazil has the largest population at risk and exemplifies the changing approach to vaccination. Until 1990, yellow fever

immunization had been conducted in mass campaigns every 5 years in the endemic area. In 1991, vaccination became the responsibility of permanent vaccination services in the endemic zone, and was conducted at fixed vaccination centers. In 1994, the responsibility passed to the National Program of Immunization (COPNI), and in 1998 routine yellow fever vaccine of infants was introduced into the EPI. In the endemic area, the vaccine is given at 6 months of age, whereas in the coastal area the vaccine is given at 9 months of age. Enhanced efforts to cover the population have occurred during periods of increased viral activity or geographic expansion. An example of the latter is the period between 1998 and 2000 when a large epizootic swept Brazil, causing 192 human cases and threatening densely populated areas on the fringe of the endemic zone. During that interval, over 35 million doses of vaccine were administered in mass campaigns, and consideration was given to introducing routine immunization in coastal areas outside the endemic zone.

Because jungle yellow fever affects principally adults in South America, there is less urgency to immunize young children than in Africa. In the mid 1980s, coverage rates in the "at-risk" population living in the endemic zone (see Fig. 40–7) varied considerably by country, with relatively high coverage (>70%) in Venezuela, Brazil, and Bolivia and low rates in some other countries, notably Ecuador and Peru (~30%).[302,581] The mass campaigns result in the unnecessary revaccination of large numbers of individuals; in Brazil, for example, 37 million doses were delivered in the endemic zone (population 17 million) between 1980 and 1988.[582] A chronic problem in South America is the movement of unimmunized persons from coastal regions, where immunization is not practiced, into the endemic zone. Improvements in roads, increased settlement within the Amazon region, and fluidity of human population movements hamper vaccination of immigrants and migrant workers.[302] Moreover, the re-invasion in South America by A. aegypti has increased the potential for urbanization of the disease and for introduction into coastal regions where immunization is not practiced. In addition to Brazil, other South American countries have officially accepted introduction of yellow fever vaccine into the routine EPI schedule, and implementation is currently underway in most countries.

The result of vaccination policies in South America is difficult to assess by historical comparisons with the prevaccine era because confounding events coincided with the introduction of wide-scale immunization, including the introduction of active surveillance (using viscerotomy, initiated in 1930) and the expansion of human settlements in endemic areas. Nevertheless, in countries such as Brazil, which instituted a program of immunization, the incidence of jungle yellow fever declined as vaccination coverage increased[582] (Fig. 40–25), whereas in other countries, where coverage has been low (e.g., Peru), large numbers of cases have occurred in recent years.

Africa

The increased incidence of epidemic yellow fever in Africa, beginning in the mid-1980s,[26,297,583] and the recognition that the disease predominantly affects children,[26,45] led to a reassessment of vaccination policy for Africa. In 1988, a joint UNICEF/WHO Technical Group on Immunization for the

TABLE 40–26 ■ Simultaneous and Combined Immunization with Yellow Fever 17D and Other Vaccines in Open-Label Trials

Vaccine Coadministered with 17D	Method	YF-Only Control Group?	Age Group
Vaccinia	Simultaneous	Yes	Adults
Vaccinia + measles seroconversion rate[†]	Combined	Yes	Children 5 mo–4.5 yr
Vaccinia + measles and vaccinia + measles + DPT	Simultaneous	No	Children 6 mo–2 yr
Vaccinia, measles, BCG, tetanus[*]	Simultaneous	No	Children 1–5 yr
Measles ($P < 0.05$)	Combined (not significant)	Yes	Infants
Measles	Combined	Yes	Infants
Measles	1–6/7–13/14–21/ 22–27; or >28 days after measles	No	Infants
Hepatitis B (plasma derived) unaffected but GMT lower ($P = 0.02$)	Simultaneous[‡]	Yes	Infants
Hepatitis B (plasma derived and recombinant)	Simultaneous[§]	Yes	Infants
Hepatitis A	Simultaneous	No	Adults
Hepatitis A	Simultaneous	Yes	Adults
Hepatitis A virosome seroconversion	Simultaneous	No	Adults
Hepatitis A	Simultaneous or within 4 wk	No	13–70 yr
Hepatitis A + typhoid Vi	Hepatitis A simultaneous with 17D + typhoid combined	No	Adults
Hepatitis A+/or typhoid Vi	Simultaneous 17D + hepatitis A + typhoid or 17D + typhoid; hepatitis A only control	No	Adults
Typhoid Vi	Combined or simultaneous	Yes	Adults
Cholera (whole cell, inactivated)[‖]	Simultaneous or 1 to >24 wk apart	Yes	Adults
Cholera (whole cell, inactivated)	Simultaneous or 4 wk apart	Yes	Children 2–5 yr
Cholera (whole cell, inactivated)	Simultaneous	Yes	Children (school age)
Cholera (live oral CVD 103 HgR)	Simultaneous	No	Adults
Cholera (live oral + live typhoid Ty21a)	Simultaneous	No	Adults
Cholera (live oral + live typhoid Ty21a)	Simultaneous		Adults
Meningococcus A/C + Typhoid Vi	Simultaneous	Yes	Adults

[*]In addition, an unpublished study showed that BCG could be successfully coadministered with 17D by jet injector, with appropriate responses to both vaccines (L Chambon et al., unpublished data, 1971).
[†]Seroconversion rate by survival time method 85% in combined group, 97% in 17D-only controls.
[‡]Subjects also received DTP-polio and measles vaccines at the same time that 17D or 17D and hepatitis B were administered.

Reactogenicity	Immunogenicity		Reference
	To Yellow Fever	To Other Vaccine	
Not altered	Not altered	Not altered	605
Not altered	Possible decrease in seroconversion rate[†]	Not altered	566
Not altered	Appropriate	Not altered	629
Not altered	No different than vaccinia + YF control	No significant decrease	630
Not altered	Enhanced GMT ($P < 0.05$)	Enhanced GMT (not significant)	567
Not altered	Not altered	Not altered	609
Not determined	No effect of interval between measles and yellow fever	Not applicable (only measles seroconverters included in study)	562
Not altered	Seroconversion rate unaffected but GMT lower ($P = 0.02$)	Not altered	567
Not altered	Not altered	Not determined	613
Not altered	Not determined	Not altered	631
Not altered	Not altered	Not altered	612
Not altered	Appropriate, 96% seroconversion	Not altered	632
Not determined	Appropriate, 100%	Not determined	633
Not altered	Appropriate	Not altered	615
Not altered	Appropriate (98.6–100% seroconversion, no difference in titer between groups)	Slight decrease in hepatitis A response when given with 17D + typoid	634
Not altered	Enhanced GMT ($P < 0.05$)	Not altered	563
No information provided	Decreased antibody titer when vaccines given 0–3 wk apart	Decreased antibody titer when vaccines given 0–3 weeks apart	568
Not determined	Decreased seroconversion rate and titer	Not determined	569
Not determined inactivated)	Not determined	Not altered (vibriocidal titers)	570
Not altered	Not determined	Not altered	571
Not altered	Not determined	Not altered	571
Not altered	Not altered	Not altered	572
Not altered	Not altered	Enhanced (meningococcal A and C significant)	564

[§]Subjects in all groups also received measles vaccine.
[ǁ]Some subjects also received vaccinia.
BCG, bacille Calmette-Guérin; DPT, diphtheria-tetanus-pertussis; GMT, geometric mean antibody titer; YF, yellow fever.

African Region and the EPI Global Advisory Group recommended that countries endemic for yellow fever incorporate 17D vaccine into the routine EPI schedule, either at 6 months of age or at 9 months of age together with measles vaccine.[584,585] In 1990, this recommendation was re-emphasized, with the additional suggestion that catch-up immunization of older children is needed in countries at high risk. Surveys conducted between 1987 and 1990 indicated coverage of approximately 80% of infants by 1 year of age in The Gambia, the Ivory Coast, and Senegal, but rates of only approximately 40% in Burkina Faso, Chad, Mauritania, and the Central African Republic. By 1991, 14[§] of 33 African countries at risk of yellow fever had officially incorporated 17D vaccine in the EPI, but uptake of the vaccine was poor in most countries, principally because of lack of donor funding for purchase of vaccine. In 1992 (13 countries reporting), the overall coverage was 19%; in 1993 (12 countries reporting) coverage was 14%; and in 1993 (11 countries reporting), coverage was 29%.[586] By 1995, rates were less than 50% in all countries (Fig. 40–26), excepting The Gambia, the Central African Republic, and Burkina Faso. The Gambia, which suffered a major outbreak in 1978–79[44] and responded with mass immu-

§Angola, Burkina Faso, Cameroon, Central African Republic, Chad, The Gambia, Ghana, the Ivory Coast, Mali, Mauritania, Niger, Nigeria, Senegal, and Togo.

nization of children and adults, followed by sustained high rates of coverage of infants in the EPI, is the only African country that is fully protected against yellow fever. Another technical consensus meeting was held at the WHO in 1998, at which time 17 of the 34 countries endemic for yellow fever had incorporated vaccine into the EPI, although coverage remained low. Of interest was the forecast for vaccine doses required under assumptions of increased coverage rates. In 1997, only 4 million doses of vaccine were supplied by UNICEF to African countries, whereas 24 million doses would be required to achieve 80% coverage of children living in high and moderate risk areas in the 34 affected countries, and 240 million doses would be required to undertake preventative mass campaigns. Demands for vaccine in response to outbreaks could severely stretch the capacity of manufacturers. These scenarios should be compared to the annual production capacity of approximately 30 million doses from manufacturers serving the African market. Shortages of vaccine for control of epidemics have been experienced, for example, during an outbreak in Guinea in 2000, leading to a recommendation for a strategic stockpile of 2 million doses to be held by UNICEF.[587]

Whereas a policy of routine immunization of infants in the EPI is an important goal, it should be emphasized that, even assuming the achievement of high coverage rates, it would take at least 15 years to create herd immunity sufficient to prevent epidemic spread without "catch-up" immunization of older children.[309] Because 17D vaccine induces lifelong immunity, as shown by

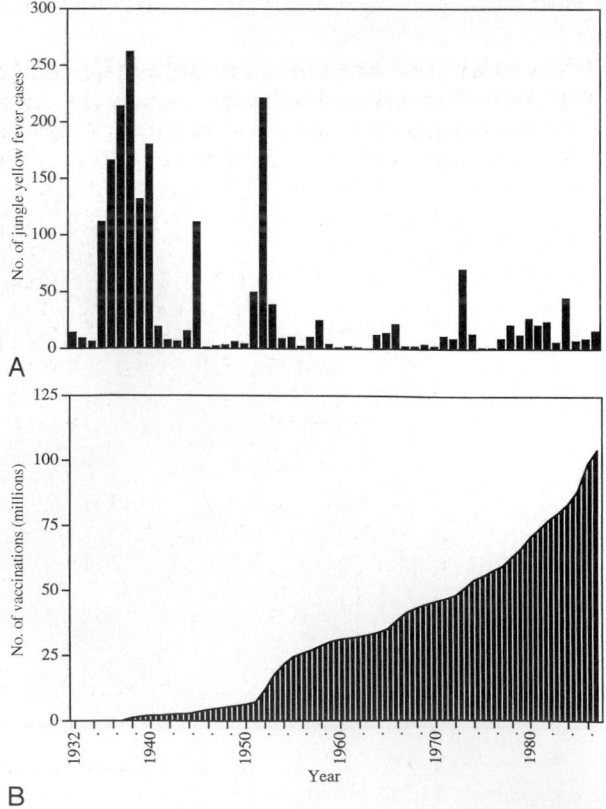

A

B

FIGURE 40–25 ■ Incidence of jungle yellow fever in Brazil (A) and the cumulative number of doses of 17D vaccine administered in the endemic area (B), 1932 through 1988. (Data from Calheiros LB. A febre amarela no Brasil. Simpósio Internacional sobre Febre Amarela e Dengue. Cinqüentenário da introdução da Cepa 17D no Brasil, Rio de Janeiro, Fundação Oswaldo Cruz, 1988, pp 74–85.)

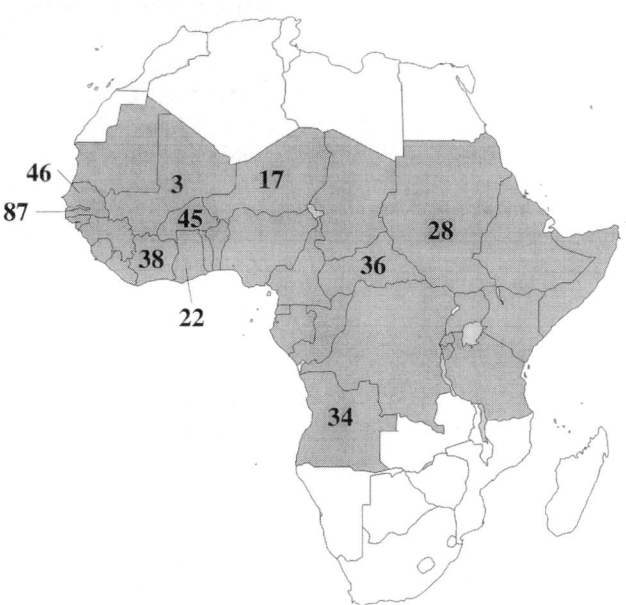

FIGURE 40–26 ■ Yellow fever vaccine coverage (%) of infants by 1 year of age, 1994, by country. Shaded countries are considered at risk of yellow fever. By 1997, coverage was only slightly improved; five countries provided a report to the WHO on yellow fever vaccine coverage: Niger (25%), Ghana (24%), the Ivory Coast (43%), the Central African Republic (53%), and Burkina Faso (55%). (Data from World Health Organization. Expanded Program of Immunization [Document WHO/EPI/GEN/97.02]. Geneva, World Health Organization, 1997.)

studies of populations that do not have an opportunity for boosting by natural exposure,[469] revaccination is unnecessary.

Cost-Benefit of Immunization

In an analysis of the benefit of immunization versus risk of yellow fever, Brès[504] concluded that a "fire-fighting" approach (emergency mass immunization in the face of outbreaks) was less costly than preventative immunization. Monath and Nasidi,[309] using a model in which routine yellow fever vaccination was hypothetically introduced into the EPI in Nigeria, explored this question. They concluded that 15 to 18 years would be required to achieve an effective immune barrier to epidemic spread, at which time routine immunization was seven- to eight-fold more efficient than emergency control in the number of cases and deaths prevented. The cost of routine immunization was estimated at $763/case and $3817/death prevented during epidemics, with lower costs if prevention of endemic disease was taken into account. These cost-effectiveness ratios compared favorably to those for other infections preventable by EPI vaccines in Africa.[588] The authors concluded that "The exceptional ability of a single dose of 17D vaccine to provide lifelong immunity is the keystone of its value in the EPI; an infant vaccinated . . . is fully protected over a 50-year lifetime for an investment of $0.01/year!"

Eradication or Elimination? The Level of Herd Immunity Required

Eradication of yellow fever by means of human vaccination is not feasible, since virus circulates independent of humans in nonhuman primates and mosquitoes.

Elimination of the disease is achievable by vaccination, but nearly 100% coverage would be necessary to prevent cases of jungle yellow fever acquired by exposure to enzootic vectors. Prevention of epidemics involving inter-human transmission by A. aegypti or sylvatic vectors in Africa or South America also would require a high prevalence of immunity. This was shown in the case of the severe epidemic in Senegal (1965), where the prevalence of immunity before the epidemic in children younger than 10 years (the age group affected during the outbreak) was estimated to have been 57%.[304] Brès[504] concluded that herd immunity must exceed 90% to preclude epidemic yellow fever. Mathematical models have been applied to the calculation of the proportion of human hosts susceptible to infection required to sustain an epidemic (reproductive rate of infection >1), but they require an understanding of the biting rate, probability of feeding on a human host, and transmission efficiency of the vector.[194,342,589] The effect of herd immunity on yellow fever transmission under different assumptions of vectorial capacity was explored by Monath and Nasidi.[309] The prevalence of immunity in a human population required to preclude an epidemic was estimated to be between 60% and 90% (Fig. 40–27). In a more recent and separate analysis, Massad et al.[589] reached a very similar conclusion, estimating that 58% to 88% yellow fever vaccination

coverage rates would be required to prevent urban yellow fever in São Paulo State, Brazil.

Distribution of Yellow Fever Vaccine to At-Risk Travelers

The International Sanitary Regulations specify that yellow fever vaccine be administered only by approved vaccinating centers, which are listed in a 1991 WHO publication[590] and updated in the WHO *WER*. This restriction provides assurances that the vaccine will be properly stored and delivered using aseptic technique within the specified time after reconstitution. A vaccination certificate, specifying the date of immunization and the vaccine lot number and signed by personnel at the vaccinating center, constitutes proof of valid immunization for the purposes of international travel.

In the United States, the CDC has the statutory authority to approve centers. This authority is delegated in turn to state health departments. There are currently approximately 3000 certified yellow fever vaccination centers in the United States (Fig. 40–28), concentrated principally in large metropolitan areas.[591]

Recent estimates of vaccine coverage in civilian travelers have shown low and declining coverage rates. In a model assessing immunization of travelers to high-risk regions within countries in the yellow fever zone, coverage declined steadily from 64% in 1992 to 31% in 1998.[325] If all travelers to endemic countries were considered, the coverage rate declined from 21% in 1992 to 10% in 1996. Travel appeared to increase without a concurrent increase in

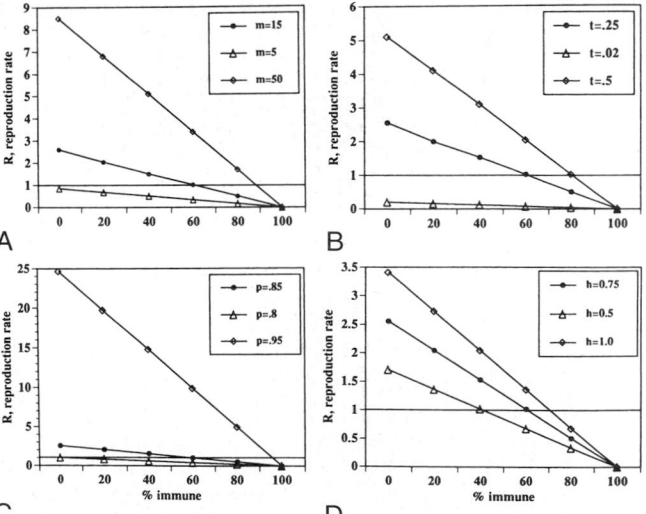

FIGURE 40–27 ■ Relationship between reproductive rate (R) of an epidemic and the prevalence of herd immunity in the host population under different assumptions of vectorial capacity. *A,* Effect of varying the number of mosquito bites per day (m). *B,* Effect of varying vector competence (t = proportion of mosquitoes transmitting the virus). *C,* Effect of varying the average daily survival time of the vector (p). *D,* Effect of varying the average proportion of vectors feeding on a human host (h). (From Monath TP, Nasidi A. Should yellow fever vaccine be included in the Expanded Program of Immunization in Africa? A cost-effectiveness analysis for Nigeria. Am J Trop Med Hyg 48:274, 1993, with permission.)

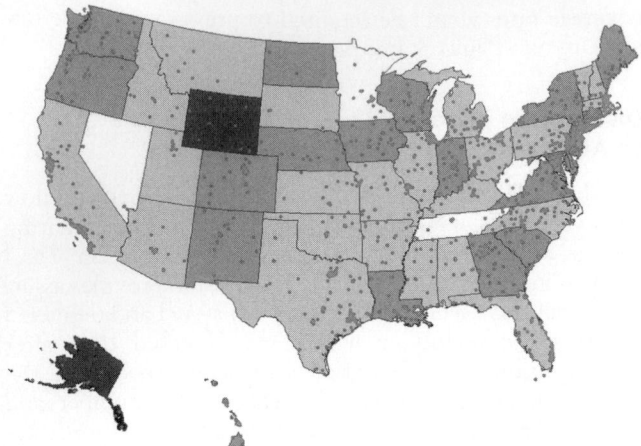

FIGURE 40–28 ■ Location of yellow fever vaccinating centers in the United States, showing concentration in metropolitan areas. (From Monath TP, Cetron M. Preventing yellow fever in travelers to the tropics. Clin Infect Dis 34:1369, 2002, with permission.)

vaccine doses administered. Fear of adverse events also may contribute to declining vaccine uptake in the future. The unfortunate result will be continued reports of fatal yellow fever among travelers.

REFERENCES

1. Zanotto PM, Gould EA, Gao GF, et al. Population dynamics of flaviviruses revealed by molecular phylogenies. Proc Natl Acad Sci USA 93;548, 1996.
2. Carter HR. Yellow Fever: An Epidemiological and Historical Study of Its Place of Origin. Baltimore, Williams & Wilkins, 1931.
3. Garrison FH. An Introduction to the History of Medicine with Medical Chronology, Suggestions for Study, and Bibliographical Data. Philadelphia, WB Saunders, 1929.
4. Powell JH. Bring Out Your Dead. Philadelphia, University of Pennsylvania Press, 1949.
5. Duffy J. Sword of Pestilence. Baton Rouge, LA, LSU Press, 1966.
6. Coleman W. Yellow Fever in the North. Madison, University of Wisconsin Press, 1987.
7. Finlay C. El mosquito hipoteticamente considerado como agente de transmision de la fiebre amarilla. Anal Real Acad Ciencias Med Fisicas Naturales 18:147, 1881.
8. Yellow Fever: A Compilation of Various Publications. Results of the Work of Maj. Walter Reed, Medical Corps, United States Army, and the Yellow Fever Commission (61st Congress Doc No 822). Washington, DC, Government Printing Office, 1911.
9. Stokes A, Bauer JH, Hudson NP. Experimental transmission of yellow fever to laboratory animals. Am J Trop Med Hyg 8:103, 1928.
10. Mathis C, Sellards AW, Laigret J. Sensibilité du *Macacus rhesus* au virus de la fièvre jaune. C R Acad Sci 186:604, 1928.
11. Deubel V, Ekue EK, Diop MM, et al. Introduction à l'analyse de la virulence du virus de la fièvre jaune (*Flaviviridae*): études génétiques, immunochimiques et biologiques comparatives entre les souches atténuées vaccinales et leurs souches parentales. Ann Inst Pasteur Virol 137E:191, 1986.
12. Jennings AD, Whitby JE, Minor PD, et al. Comparison of the nucleotide and deduced amino acid sequences of the structural protein genes of the yellow fever 17DD vaccine strain from Senegal with those of other yellow fever vaccine viruses. Vaccine 11:679, 1993.
13. Hindle E. A yellow fever vaccine. Br Med J 1:976, 1928.
14. Sawyer WA, Kitchen SF, Lloyd W. Vaccination against yellow fever with immune serum and virus fixed for mice. J Exp Med 55:945, 1932.
15. Berry GP, Kitchen SF. Yellow fever accidentally contracted in the laboratory: a study of seven cases. Am J Trop Med Hyg 11:365, 1931.
16. Sellards AW, Laigret J. Vaccination de l'homme contre la fièvre jaune. C R Acad Sci 194:1609, 1932.

17. Mathis C, Laigret J, Durieux C. Trois mille vaccinations contre la fièvre jaune Cen Afrique Occidentale Française au moyen du virus vivant souris, atténué par le vieillissment. C R Acad Sci 199:742, 1934.
18. Theiler M, Smith HH. The effect of prolonged cultivation in vitro upon the pathogenicity of yellow fever virus. J Exp Med 65:767, 1937.
19. Smith HH, Theiler M. The adaptation of unmodified strains of yellow fever virus to cultivation in vitro. J Exp Med 65:801, 1937.
20. Theiler M, Smith HH. The use of yellow fever virus modified by in vitro cultivation for human immunization. J Exp Med 65:787, 1937.
21. Smith HH, Penna HA, Paoliello A. Yellow fever vaccination with cultured virus (17D) without immune serum. Am J Trop Med Hyg 18:437, 1938.
22. Monath TP. Yellow fever vaccines: the success of empiricism, pitfalls of application, and transition to molecular vaccinology. *In* Plotkin S, Fantini M (eds). Vaccinia, Vaccination and Vaccinology: Jenner, Pasteur and Their Successors. Paris, Elsevier, 1996, pp 157–182.
23. Sorel F. La vaccination anti-amarile en Afrique occidentale française, mise en application du procédé de vaccination Sellards-Laigret. Bull Off Int Hyg Pub 28:1325, 1936.
24. Durieux C. Mass yellow fever vaccination in French Africa south of the Sahara. *In* Smithburn KC, Durieux C, Koerber R, et al (eds). Yellow Fever Vaccination (Monograph Ser No 30). Geneva, World Health Organization, 1956, pp 115–121.
25. Peltier M. Yellow fever vaccination, simple or associated with vaccination against smallpox, of the populations of French West Africa by the method of the Pasteur Institute of Dakar. Am J Public Health 37:1026, 1947.
26. Robertson SE, Hull BP, Tomori O, et al. Yellow fever: a decade of reemergence. JAMA 276:1157, 1996.
27. Monath TP. Epidemiology of yellow fever: current status and speculations on future trends. *In* Saluzzo J-F, Dodet B (eds). Factors in the Emergence of Arbovirus Diseases. Paris, Elsevier, 1997, pp 143–156.
28. Kerr JA. The clinical aspects and diagnosis of yellow fever. *In* Strode GK (ed). Yellow Fever. New York. McGraw-Hill, 1951, pp 385–426.
29. Beeuwkes H. Clinical manifestations of yellow fever in the West African native as observed during four extensive epidemics of the disease in the Gold Coast and Nigeria. Trans R Soc Trop Med Hyg 1:61, 1936.
30. Monath TP. Yellow fever: a medically neglected disease. Report on a seminar. Rev Infect Dis 9:165, 1987.
31. MacNamara FN. Man as the host of the yellow fever virus. MD thesis, Cambridge University, Cambridge, UK, 1955.
32. Nassar EDS, Chamelet ELB, Coimbra TLM. Jungle yellow fever: clinical and laboratorial studies emphasizing viremia on a human case. Rev Inst Med Trop São Paulo 37:337, 1995.
33. Oudart J-L, Rey M. Protéinurie, protéinémie et transaminasémies dans 23 cas de fièvre jaune confirmée. Bull World Health Organ 42:95, 1970.
34. MacNamara FN. A clinico-pathological study of yellow fever in Nigeria. W Afr Med J 6:137, 1957.
35. Elton NW, Romero A, Trejos A. Clinical pathology of yellow fever. Am J Clin Pathol 25:135, 1955.
36. Boulos M, Segurado AA, Shirome M. Severe yellow fever with 23-day survival. Trop Geogr Med 40:356, 1988.
37. Borges APA, Oliveira GSC, Almeida Netto JC. Estudo da coagulaçao sanguinea na febre amarela. Rev Patol Trop 2:143, 1973.
38. Santos F, Pereira Lima C, Paiva P, et al. Coagulaçao intravascular disseminada aguda na febre amarela: dosagem dos factores da coagulaçao. Brasilia Med 9:9, 1973.
39. Chagas E, De Freitas L. Electrocardiogramma na febre amarela. Mem Inst Oswaldo Cruz (Rio de Janeiro) Suppl 7:72, 1929.
40. Williams MC, Woodall JP, Simpson DIH. Yellow fever in central Uganda, 1964. III. Virus isolation from man and laboratory studies. Trans R Soc Trop Med Hyg 59:444, 1965.
41. Stevanson LD. Pathological changes in the central nervous system in yellow fever. Arch Pathol 27:249, 1939.
42. Stefanopoulo GJ, Mollaret P. Hémiplégie d'origine cérébrale et névrite optique au cours d'un cas de fièvre jaune. Bull Mém Soc Med Hôp Paris 50:1463, 1934.
43. Findlay GM, Stern RO. Essential neurotropism of yellow fever virus. J Pathol Bacteriol 41:431, 1935.
44. Monath TP, Craven RB, Adjukiewicz A, et al. Yellow fever in The Gambia, 1978–1979: epidemiologic aspects with observations on the occurrence of Orungo virus infections. Am J Trop Med Hyg 29:912, 1980.
45. Nasidi A, Monath TP, DeCock K. Urban yellow fever epidemic in western Nigeria 1987. Trans R Soc Trop Med Hyg 83:401, 1989.

46. Hanson H. Observations on the age and sex incidence of deaths and recoveries in the yellow fever epidemic in the department of Lambayeque, Peru, in 1921. Am J Trop Med Hyg 9:233, 1929.

47. Jones MM, Wilson DC. Clinical features of yellow fever cases at Vom Christian Hospital during the 1969 epidemic on the Jos Plateau, Nigeria. Bull World Health Organ 46:653, 1972.

48. Kirk R. Epidemic of yellow fever in Nuba Mountains, Anglo-Egyptian Sudan. Ann Trop Med Parasitol 35:67, 1941.

49. Klotz O, Simpson W. Jaundice and the liver lesions in West African yellow fever. Am J Trop Med Hyg 7:271, 1927.

50. Monath TP, Hadler SC. Type B hepatitis and yellow fever infections in West Africa. Trans R Soc Trop Med Hyg 81:172, 1987.

51. Porterfield JS. Antigenic characteristics and classification of Togaviridae. In Schlesinger RW (ed). The Togaviruses: Biology, Structure. New York, Academic Press, 1980, pp 13–46.

52. Calisher CH, Karabatsos N, Dalrymple JM, et al. Antigenic relationships among flaviviruses as determined by cross-neutralization tests with polyclonal antisera. J Gen Virol 70:37, 1989.

53. Kuno G, Chang G-J, Tsuchiya KR, et al. Phylogeny of the genus Flavivirus. J Virol 72:73, 1998.

54. Heinz FX, Collett MS, Purcell RH, et al. Family Flaviviridae. In Regenmortel MHV, Fauquet CM, Bishop DHL, et al (eds). Virus Taxonomy. 7th International Committee for the Taxonomy of Viruses. San Diego, Academic Press, 2000, pp 859–878.

55. Chambers TJ, Monath TP (eds). The Flaviviruses: Current Molecular Aspects of Evolution, Biology, and Disease Prevention. New York, Academic Press, 2003 [in press].

56. Lindenbach BD, Rice CM. Flaviviridae: the viruses and their replication. In Knipe DM, Howley PM (eds). Fields' Virology. Vol. I. Philadelphia, Lippincott Williams & Wilkins, 2001, p 991.

57. Olsthoorn RC, Bol JF. Sequence comparison and secondary structure analysis of the 3′ noncoding region of flavivirus genomes reveals multiple pseudoknots. RNA 7:1370, 2001.

58. Wang E, Weaver SC, Shope RE, et al. Genetic variation in yellow fever virus: duplication in the 3′ noncoding region of strains from Africa. Virology 225:274, 1996.

59. Guirakhoo F, Bolin RA, Roehrig JT. The Murray Valley encephalitis virus prM protein confers acid resistance to virus particles and alters the expression of epitopes within the R2 domain of E glycoprotein. Virology 191:921, 1992.

60. Rey FA, Heinz FX, Mandl C, et al. The envelope glycoprotein from the tick-borne encephalitis virus at 2Å resolution. Nature 375:291, 1995.

61. Van der Most RG, Corver J, Strauss JH. Mutagenesis of the RGD motif in the yellow fever virus 17D envelope protein. Virology 265:83, 1999.

62. Lobigs M, Dalgarno L, Schlesinger JJ, et al. Location of a neutralization determinant in the E protein of yellow fever virus (17D vaccine strain). Virology 161:474, 1987.

63. Ryman KD, Ledger TN, Weir RC Jr, et al. Yellow fever virus envelope protein has two discrete type-specific neutralizing epitopes. J Gen Virol 78:1353, 1997.

64. Co MD, Terajima M, Cruz J, et al. Human cytotoxic T lymphocyte responses to live attenuated 17D yellow fever vaccine: identification of HLA-B35-restricted CTL epitopes on nonstructural proteins NS1, NS2b, NS3, and the structural protein E. Virology 293:151–163, 2002.

65. Stiasny K, Allison SL, Marchler-Bauer A, et al. Structural requirements for low-pH-induced rearrangements in the envelope glycoprotein of tick-borne encephalitis virus. J Virol 70:8142, 1996.

66. Schlesinger JJ, Brandriss MW, Putnak JR, et al. Cell surface expression of yellow fever virus non-structural glycoprotein NS1: consequences of interaction with antibody. J Gen Virol 71:593, 1990.

67. Mulyaert IR, Galler RG, Rice CM. Mutagenesis of the N-linked glycosylation sites of the yellow fever NS1 protein: effects on virus replication and mouse neurovirulence. Virology 222:159, 1996.

68. Mulyaert IR, Galler RG, Rice CM. Genetic analysis of yellow fever virus NS1 protein: identification of a temperature-sensitive mutation which blocks RNA accumulation. J Virol 71:291, 1997.

69. Lindenbach BD, Rice CM. Genetic interaction of flavivirus nonstructural proteins NS1 and NS4A as a determinant of replicase function. J Virol 73:4611, 1999.

70. Nestorowicz A, Chambers TJ, Rice CM. Mutagenesis of the yellow fever virus NS2A/2B cleavage site: effects on proteolytic processing, viral replication and evidence for alternative processing of the NS2A protein. Virology 199:114, 1994.

71. Kümmerer BM, Rice CM. Mutations in the yellow fever virus nonstructural protein 2A selectively block production of infectious virus. J Virol 76:4773, 2002.

72. Mathews JH, Allan JE, Roehrig JR, et al. T-helper cell and associated antibody response to synthetic peptides of the E glycoprotein of Murray Valley encephalitis virus. J Virol 65:5141, 1991.

73. Rothman AL, Kurane I, Ennis FA. Multiple specificities in the murine CD4+ and CD8+ T-cell response to dengue virus. J Virol 70:6540, 1996.

74. Lobigs M, Arthur CE, Mullbacher A, et al. The flavivirus nonstructural protein NS3 is a dominant source of cytotoxic T cell peptide determinants. Virology 202:196, 1994.

75. Lee E, Stocks CE, Amberg SM, et al. Mutagenesis of the signal sequence of yellow fever virus prM protein: enhancement of signalase cleavage in vitro is lethal for virus production. J Virol 74:24, 2000.

76. Rice CM, Lenches EM, Eddy SR, et al. Nucleotide sequence of yellow fever virus: implications for flavivirus gene expression and evolution. Science 229:726, 1985.

77. Hahn CH, Dalrymple JM, Strauss JH, et al. Comparison of the virulent Asibi strain of yellow fever virus with the 17D vaccine strain derived from it. Proc Natl Acad Sci U S A 84:2019, 1987.

78. Wang E, Ryman KD, Jennings AD, et al. Comparison of the genomes of the wild-type French viscerotropic strain of yellow fever virus with its vaccine derivative French neurotropic vaccine. J Gen Virol 76:2749, 1995.

79. Post PR, Santos CND, Carvalho R, et al. Heterogeneity in envelope protein sequence and N-linked glycosylation among yellow fever virus vaccine strains. Virology 188:160, 1992.

80. Duarte dos Santos CN, Post PR, Carvalho R, et al: Complete nucleotide sequence of yellow fever virus vaccine strains 17DD and 17D-213. Virus Res 95:35, 1995.

81. Dupuy A, Despres P, Cahour A, et al. Nucleotide sequence comparison of the genome of two 7D-204 yellow fever vaccines. Nucleic Acids Res 17:2989, 1989.

82. Pugachev KV, Ocran SW, Guirakhoo F, et al. Heterogeneous nature of the genome of the ARILVAX yellow fever 17D vaccine revealed by consensus sequencing. Vaccine 20:996, 2002.

83. Tesh RB, Guzman H, da Rosa AP, et al. Experimental yellow fever virus infection in the golden hamster (Mesocricetus auratus) I. Virologic, bio chemical, and immunologic studies. J Infect Dis 183:1431, 2001.

83a. Mc Arthur MA, Suderman MT, Mutebi JP, et al. Molecular characterization of a hamster viscerotropic strain of yellow fever virus. J Virol 77:1462–1468, 2003.

84. Xiao SY, Zhang H, Guzman H, Tesh RB. Experimental yellow fever virus infection in the golden hamster (Mesocricetus auratus). II. Pathology. J Infect Dis 183:1437, 2001.

85. Barrett ADT. Yellow fever vaccine. Biologicals 25:17, 1997.

86. Pletnev AG, Bray M, Lai C-J. Chimeric tick-borne encephalitis and dengue type 4 viruses: effects of mutations on neurovirulence in mice. J Virol 67:4956, 1993.

87. Mandl CW, Allison SL, Holzmann H, et al. Attenuation of tick-borne encephalitis virus by structure-based site-specific mutagenesis of a putative flavivirus receptor binding site. J Virol 74:9601, 2000.

88. Ballinger-Crabtree M, Miller BR. Partial nucleotide sequence of South American yellow fever strain 1899/91: structural proteins and NS1. J Gen Virol 71:2115, 1990.

89. Hasegawa H, Yoshida M, Shiosaka T, et al. Mutations in the envelope protein of Japanese encephalitis virus affect entry into cultured cells and virulence in mice. Virology 191:158, 1992.

90. Holzmann H, Stiasny K, Ecker M, et al. Characterization of monoclonal antibody-escape mutants of tick-borne encephalitis virus with reduced neuroinvasiveness in mice. J Gen Virol 78:31, 1997.

91. Guirakhoo F, Heinz FX, Kunz C. Epitope model of tick-borne encephalitis virus envelope glycoprotein E: analysis of structural properties, role of carbohydrate side-chain, and conformational changes occurring at acidic pH. Virology 169:90, 1989.

92. Arroyo J, Guirakhoo F, Fenner S, et al. Molecular basis for attenuation of neurovirulence of a yellow fever virus/Japanese encephalitis virus chimera vaccine (ChimeriVax-JE). J Virol 75:934, 2001.

93. Schlesinger JJ, Chapman S, Nestorowicz A, et al. Replication of yellow fever virus in the mouse central nervous system: comparison of neuroadapted and nonneuroadapted virus and partial sequence analysis of the neuroadapted strain. J Gen Virol 77:1277, 1996.

94. Chambers TJ, Nickells M. Neuroadapted yellow fever virus 17D: genetic and biological characterization of a highly mouse-neurovirulent virus and its infectious molecular clone. J Virol 75:10912, 2001.

95. Ryman KD, Xie H, Ledger TN, et al. Short communication: antigenic variants of yellow fever virus with an altered neurovirulence phenotype in mice. Virology 230:376, 1997.

96. Hurrelbrink RJ, McMinn PC. Attenuation of Murray Valley encephalitis virus by site-directed mutagenesis of the hinge and putative receptor-binding regions of the envelope protein. J Virol 75:7692, 2001.

97. Monath TP, Arroyo J, Levenbook I, et al. Single mutation in the flavivirus envelope protein hinge region increases neurovirulence for mice and monkeys but decreases viscerotropism for monkeys: relevance to development and safety testing of live, attenuated vaccines. J Virol 76:1932, 2002.

98. Wisseman CL Jr, Sweet BH, Rosenzweig EC, et al. Attenuated living type 1 dengue vaccines. Am J Trop Med Hyg 12:377, 1963.

99. Bray M, Men R, Tokimatsu I, et al. Genetic determinants responsible for acquisition of dengue 2 virus mouse neurovirulence. J Virol 72:6433, 1998.

100. Gualano RC, Pryor MJ, Cauch MR, et al. Identification of a major determinant of mouse neurovirulence of dengue virus type 2 using stably cloned genomic-length cDNA. J Gen Virol 79:437, 1998.

101. Duarte dos Santos, Frenkiel M-P, Courageot M-P, et al. Determinants in the envelope E protein and viral RNA helicase NS3 that influence the induction of apoptosis in response to infection with dengue type 1 virus. Virology 274:292, 2000.

102. Lobigs M, Usha R, Nestorowicz A, et al. Host cell selection of Murray Valley encephalitis virus variants altered at the RGD sequence in the envelope protein and in mouse virulence. Virology 176:587, 1990.

103. Holzmann H, Heinz FX, Mandl CW, et al. A single amino acid substitution in envelope protein E of tick-borne encephalitis virus leads to attenuation in the mouse model. J Virol 64:5156, 1990.

104. Allison SL, Stiasny K, Stadler K, et al. Mapping of functional elements in the stem-anchor region of tick-borne encephalitis virus envelope protein E. J Virol 73:5605, 1999.

105. Ni H, Barrett ADT. Attenuation of Japanese encephalitis virus by selection of its mouse brain receptor preparation escape mutants. Virology 241:30, 1998.

106. Holbrook MR, Ni H, Shope RE, et al. Amino acid substitution(s) in the stem-anchor region of Langat virus envelope protein attenuates mouse neurovirulence. Virology 286:54, 2001.

107. Wang S, He R, Anderson R. prM- and cell-binding activities domains of the dengue virus E protein. J Virol 73:2547, 1999.

108. Fatal viral encephalitis following 17D yellow fever vaccine inoculation. JAMA 198:671, 1966.

109. Jennings AD, Gibson CA, Miller BR. Analysis of a yellow fever virus isolated from a fatal case of vaccine-associated human encephalitis. J Infect Dis 169:512, 1994.

110. Collier WA, De Roever-Bonnet H, Hoekstra J. A neurotropic variety of the vaccine strain 17D. Trop Geogr Med 11:80, 1959.

111. McMinn PC, Marshall ID, Dalgarno L. Neurovirulence and neuroinvasiveness of Murray Valley encephalitis virus mutants selected by passage in a monkey kidney cell line. J Gen Virol 76:865, 1995.

112. Wang E, Weaver SC, Shope RE, et al. Genetic variation in yellow fever virus: duplication in the 3' noncoding region of strains from Africa. Virology 225:274, 1996.

113. Zeng L, Falgout B, Markoff L. Identification of specific nucleotide sequences within the conserved 3'-SL in the dengue type 2 virus genome required for replication. J Virol 72:7510, 1998.

114. Mandl CW, Holzmann H, Meixner T, et al. Spontaneous and engineered deletions in the 3' noncoding region of tick-borne encephalitis virus: construction of highly attenuated mutants of a flavivirus. J Virol 72:2132, 1998.

115. Men R, Bray M, Clark D, et al. Dengue type 4 virus mutants containing deletions in the 3' noncoding region of the RNA genome: analysis of growth restriction in cell culture and altered viremia pattern and immunogenicity in rhesus monkeys. J Virol 70:3930, 1996.

116. Liprandi F. Isolation of plaque variants differing in virulence from the 17D strain of yellow fever virus. J Gen Virol 56:363, 1981.

117. Xie H, Ryman HD, Campbell GA, et al. Mutation in NS5 protein attenuates mouse neurovirulence of yellow fever 17D vaccine virus. J Gen Virol 79:1895, 1998.

118. Barrett ADT, Monath TP, Cropp CB, et al. Attenuation of wild-type yellow fever virus by passage in HeLa cells. J Gen Virol 71:2302, 1990.

119. Dunster LM, Wang H, Ryman KD, et al. Molecular and biological changes associated with HeLa cell attenuation of wild-type yellow fever virus. Virology 261:309, 1999.

120. Schlesinger JJ, Brandriss MW, Monath TP. Monoclonal antibodies distinguish between wild and vaccine strains of yellow fever virus by neutralization, hemagglutination inhibition, and immune precipitation of the virus envelope protein. Virology 125:8, 1983.

121. Schlesinger JJ, Walsh EE, Brandriss MW. Analysis of 17D yellow fever virus envelope protein epitopes using monoclonal antibodies. J Gen Virol 65:1637, 1984.

122. Monath TP, Schlesinger JJ, Brandriss MW, et al. Yellow fever monoclonal antibodies: type-specific and cross-reactive determinants identified by immunofluorescence. Am J Trop Med Hyg 33:695, 1984.

123. Geske T, Nichtila P, Seethaler H, et al. Establishment of hybridomas producing antibodies to viral surface epitopes related to pathogenic properties of yellow fever virus strains. Immunobiology 165:263, 1983.

124. Cammack N, Gould EA. Antigenic analysis of yellow fever virus glycoproteins: use of monoclonal antibodies in enzyme-linked immunosorbent assays. J Virol Methods 13:135, 1986.

125. Barrett ADT, Matthews JH, Miller BR, et al. Identification of monoclonal antibodies that distinguish between 17D-204 and other strains of yellow fever virus. J Gen Virol 71:13, 1990.

126. Barrett ADT, Pryde A, Medlen AR, et al. Examination of the envelope glycoprotein of yellow fever vaccine viruses with monoclonal antibodies. Vaccine 7:333, 1989.

127. Buckley A, Gould EA. Neutralization of yellow fever virus studied using monoclonal and polyclonal antibodies. J Gen Virol 66:2523, 1985.

128. Ledger TN, Sil BK, Wills MR. Variation in the biological function of envelope protein epitopes of yellow fever vaccine viruses detected with monoclonal antibodies. Biologicals 20:117, 1992.

129. Sil BK, Dunster LM, Ledger TN, et al. Identification of envelope protein epitopes that are important in the attenuation process of wild-type yellow fever virus. J Virol 66:4265, 1992.

130. Gould EA, Buckley A, Cane PA, et al. Use of a monoclonal antibody specific for wild-type yellow fever virus to identify a wild-type antigenic variant in 17D vaccine pools. J Gen Virol 70:1889, 1989.

131. Gould EA, Buckley A, Barrett ADT, et al. Neutralizing (54K) and non-neutralizing (54K and 58K) monoclonal antibodies against structural and non-structural yellow fever virus proteins confer immunity in mice. J Gen Virol 67:591, 1986.

132. Ryman KD, Ledger TN, Campbell GA, et al. Mutation in a 17D-204 vaccine substrain-specific envelope protein epitope alters the pathogenesis of yellow fever virus in mice. Virology 244:59, 1998.

133. Després P, Ruiz-Linares A, Cahour A, et al. The 15 amino acid residues preceding the amino terminus of the envelope protein of the yellow fever virus polyprotein precursor act as a signal peptide. Virus Res 16:59, 1990.

134. Gagnon SJ, Zeng W, Kurane I, et al. Identification of two epitopes on the dengue-4 virus capsid protein recognized by a serotype-specific and a panel of serotype-cross-reactive human $CD4^+$ cytotoxic T-lymphocyte clones. J Virol 70:141, 1996.

135. Roehrig JT, Risi PA, Bribaker JR, et al. T helper cell epitopes on the E glycoprotein of dengue-2 Jamaica virus. Virology 198:31, 1994.

136. Mathew A, Kurane I, Rothman A, et al. Dominant recognition by human $CD8^+$ cytotoxic T lymphocytes of dengue virus nonstructural proteins NS3 and NS2a. J Clin Invest 98:1684, 1996.

137. Kurane I, Brinton MA, Sampson AL, et al. Dengue virus-specific human $CD4^+CD8^-$ cytotoxic T-cell clones; multiple patterns of virus cross-reactivity by NS3-specific T-cell clones. J Virol 65:1823, 1991.

138. Hill AB, Mullbacher A, Parrish C, et al. Broad cross-reactivity with marked fine specificity in the cytotoxic T cell response to flaviviruses. J Gen Virol 73:1115, 1992.

139. Regner M, Lobigs M, Blanden R, et al. Antiviral cytotoxic T cells cross-reactively recognize disparate peptide determinants from related viruses but ignore more similar self- and foreign determinants. J Immunol 166:3820, 2001.

140. Ishak R, Tovey DG, Hovard T. Morphogenesis of yellow fever 17D in infected cell cultures. J Gen Virol 69:325, 1988.

141. Ng ML, Lau LC. Possible involvement of receptors in the entry of Kunjin virus into Vero cells. Arch Virol 104:129, 1989.

142. Gollins SW, Poterfield JS. Flavivirus infection enhancement in macrophages: an electron microscopic study of viral cellular entry. J Gen Virol 66:469, 1985.

143. Hase T, Summers PL, Eckels KH. Flavivirus entry into cultured mosquito cells and human peripheral blood monocytes. Arch Virol 104:129, 1989.

144. McGavran MH, White JD. Electron microscopic and immunofluorescent observations on monkey liver and tissue culture cells infected with the Asibi strain of yellow fever virus. Am J Pathol 45:501, 1964.

145. Cornet M, Robin Y, Héme G, et al. Une pousée épizootique de fièvre jaune selvatique au Sénégal oriental: isôlement du virus de lots de moustiques adultes et mâles et femelles. Méd Malad Infect 9:63, 1979.

146. Beaty BJ, Tesh RB, Aitken THG. Transovarial transmission of yellow fever virus in *Stegomyia* mosquitoes. Am J Trop Med Hyg 29:125, 1980.

147. Aitken THG, Tesh RB, Beaty B, et al. Transovarial transmission of yellow fever virus by mosquitoes (*Aedes aegypti*). Am J Trop Med Hyg 29:125, 1980.

148. Wheelock EF, Edelman R. Specific role of each human leukocyte type in viral infections. III. 17D yellow fever virus replication and interferon production in homogeneous leukocyte cultures treated with phytohemagglutinin. J Immunol 103:429, 1969.

149. Sweet BH, Wisseman CJ Jr, Kitaoka M. Immunological studies with group B arthropod-borne viruses. II. Effect of prior infection with Japanese encephalitis virus on the viremia in human subjects following administration of 17D yellow fever vaccine. Am J Trop Med Hyg 11:562, 1962.

150. Whitman L. Failure of *Aedes aegypti* to transmit yellow fever cultured virus (17D). Am J Trop Med Hyg19:19, 1939.

151. Bhatt TR, Crabtree MB, Guirakhoo F, et al. Growth characteristics of the chimeric Japanese encephalitis virus vaccine candidate, ChimeriVax™-JE (YF/JE SA14-14-2), in *Culex tritaeniorhynchus, Aedes albopictus* and *Aedes aegypti* mosquitoes. Am J Trop Med Hyg 62:480, 2001.

152. Miller BR, Adkins D. Biological characterization of plaque-size variants of yellow fever virus in mosquitoes and mice. Acta Virol 32:227, 1988.

153. Turell MJ. Horizontal and vertical transmission of viruses by insect and tick vectors. *In* Monath TP (ed). The Arboviruses: Epidemiology and Ecology. Vol. I. Boca Raton, FL, CRC Press, 1988, pp 127–152.

154. Turell MJ, Tammariello RF. Nonvascular delivery of St. Louis encephalitis and Venezuelan equine encephalitis by infected mosquitoes during feeding on a vertebrate host. Am J Trop Med Hyg 49:197, 1993.

155. Monath TP, McCarthy K, Bedford P, et al. Clinical proof of principle for ChimeriVax™: recombinant live, attenuated vaccines against flavivirus infections. Vaccine 20:1004, 2002.

156. Theiler M. The virus. *In* Strode GK (ed). Yellow Fever. New York, McGraw Hill, 1951, pp 46–136.

157. Zisman B, Wheelock EF, Allison AC: Role of macrophages and antibody in resistance of mice against yellow fever virus. J Immunol 107:236, 1971.

158. Bugher JC. The mammalian host in yellow fever. *In* Strode GK (ed). Yellow Fever. New York, McGraw-Hill, 1951, pp 299–384.

159. Monath TP. Yellow fever. *In* Monath TP (ed). The Arboviruses: Epidemiology and Ecology. Vol. V. Boca Raton, FL, CRC Press, 1988, pp 139–231.

160. Findlay GM, Clarke LP. Susceptibility of hedgehog to yellow fever: viscerotropic virus. Trans R Soc Trop Med Hyg 28:193, 1934.

161. Dennis LH, Reisberg BE, Crosbie J, et al. The original haemorrhagic fever: yellow fever. Br J Haematol 17:455, 1969.

162. Tigertt WD, Berge TO, Gochenour WS, et al. Experimental yellow fever. Trans N Y Acad Sci 22:323, 1960.

163. Monath TP, Brinker KR, Chandler FW, et al. Pathophysiologic correlations in a rhesus monkey model of yellow fever. Am J Trop Med Hyg 30:431, 1981.

164. Bauer JH. The duration of passive immunity in yellow fever. Am J Trop Med Hyg 11:451, 1931.

165. Bearcroft WGC. The histopathology of the liver of yellow fever infected rhesus monkey. J Pathol Bacteriol 74:295, 1957.

166. Klotz O, Belt TH. Pathology of the liver in yellow fever. Am J Pathol 6:663, 1930.

167. Marotto ME, Thurman RG, Lemasters JJ. Early midzonal cell death during low-flow hypoxia in the isolated, perfused rat liver: protection by allopurinol. Hepatology 8:585, 1988.

168. Monath TP, Ballinger ME, Miller BR, et al. Detection of yellow fever viral RNA by nucleic acid hybridization and viral antigen by immunocytochemistry in fixed human liver. Am J Trop Med Hyg 40:663, 1989.

169. Vieira WT, Gayotto LC, De Lima CP, et al. Histopathology of the human liver in yellow fever with special emphasis on the diagnostic role of the Councilman body. Histopathology 7:195, 1983.

170. Huerre MR, Lan NT, Marianneau P, et al. Liver histology and biological correlates in five cases of fatal dengue hemorrhagic fever in Vietnamese children. Virchows Arch 438:107, 2001.

171. Marianneau P, Cardona A, Edelman L, et al. Dengue virus replication in human hepatoma cells activates NF-kappa B which in turn induces apoptotic cell death. J Virol 71:3244, 1997.

172. Marianneau P, Steffan A-M, Royer C, et al. Differing infection patterns of dengue and yellow fever viruses in a human hepatoma cell line. J Infect Dis 178:1270, 1998.

173. De Brito T, Siqueira SAC, Santos RTM, et al. Human fatal yellow fever: immunohistochemical detection of viral antigens in the liver, kidney and heart. Pathol Res Pract 188:177, 1992.

174. Barbareschi G. Glomerulosi tossica in fiebre gialla. Rev Biol Trop 5:201, 1957.

175. Klotz O, Belt TH. Pathology in spleen in yellow fever. Am J Pathol 6:655, 1930.

176. Cannell DE. Myocardial degenerations in yellow fever. Am J Pathol 4:431, 1928.

177. Lloyd W. The myocardium in yellow fever. II. The myocardial lesions in experimental yellow fever. Am Heart J 6:504, 1931.

178. Hughes TP. Precipitin reaction in yellow fever. J Immunol 25:275, 1933.

179. Gould EA, Buckley A, Groeger BK, et al. Immune enhancement of yellow fever virus neurovirulence for mice: studies of mechanisms involved. J Gen Virol 68:3105, 1987.

180. Barrett ADT, Gould EA. Antibody-mediated early death *in vivo* after infection with yellow fever virus. J Gen Virol 67:2539, 1986.

181. Shellam GR, Sangster MY, Urosevic N. Genetic control of host resistance to flavivirus infection in animals. Rev Sci Tech 17:231–248, 1998.

182. Wills MR, Singh BK, Debnath NC, et al. Immunogenicity of wild-type and vaccine strains of Japanese encephalitis virus and the effect of haplotype restriction murine immune responses. Vaccine 7:761, 1993.

183. Elton NW. Sylvan yellow fever in Central America. Public Health Rep 67:426, 1952.

184. Matas R. Nursing in yellow fever and the duties of trained nurses in epidemics. Trained Nurse Hosp Rev Oct-Dec:3–24, 1905.

185. Bravo JR, Guzman MG, Kouri GP. Why dengue haemorrhagic fever in Cuba? I. Individual risk factors for dengue haemorrhagic fever/dengue shock syndrome. Trans R Soc Trop Med Hyg 81:816, 1987.

186. Guzman MG, Kouri GP, Bravo J, et al. Dengue haemorrhagic fever in Cuba: a retrospective seroepidemiologic study. Am J Trop Med Hyg 42:179, 1990.

187. Paradoa Perez ML, Trujillo Y, Basanta P. Association of dengue hemorrhagic fever with the HLA system. Hematologia 20:83, 1987.

188. Chang G-J, Cropp CB, Kinney RM, et al. Nucleotide sequence variation of the envelope protein gene identifies two distinct genotypes of yellow fever virus. J Virol 69:5773, 1995.

189. Fox JP. Non-fatal infection of mice following intracerebral inoculation of yellow fever virus. J Exp Med 77:507, 1943.

190. Fitzgeorge R, Bradish CJ. The *in vivo* differentiation of strains of yellow fever virus in mice. J Gen Virol 46:1, 1980.

191. Barrett ADT, Gould EA: Comparison of neurovirulence of different strains of yellow fever virus in mice. J Gen Virol 67:631, 1986.

192. Laemmert HW Jr. Susceptibility of marmosets to different strains of yellow fever virus. Am J Trop Med 24:71, 1944.

193. Deubel V, Schlesinger JJ, Digoutte J-P, et al. Comparative immunochemical and biological analysis of African and South American yellow fever viruses. Arch Virol 94:331, 1987.

194. Miller BR, Monath TP, Tabachnick WJ, et al. Epidemic yellow fever caused by an incompetent mosquito vector. Trop Med Parasitol 40:396–399, 1989.

195. Sabin A. Research on dengue during World War II. Am J Trop Med Hyg 1:30, 1952.

196. David-West TS. Concurrent and consecutive infection and immunization with yellow fever and UGMP-359 virus. Arch Virol 48:21, 1975.

197. Smithburn KC, Mahaffy AF. Immunization against yellow fever. Am J Trop Med 45:217, 1945.

198. Fagaeus A, Ehrnst A, Klein E, et al. Characterization of blood mononuclear cells reacting with K 562 cells after yellow fever vaccination. Cell Immunol 67:37, 1982.

199. Stephen EL, Sammons ML, Pannier WL, et al. Effect of a nuclease-resistant derivative of polyriboinosinic-polyribocytidylic acid complex on yellow fever in rhesus monkeys (*Macaca mulatta*). J Infect Dis 136:122, 1977.

200. Bonnevie-Nielsen V, Heron I, Monath TP, Calisher CH. Lymphocytic 2′, 5′-oligoadenylate synthetase activity increases prior to the appearance of neutralizing antibodies and immunoglobulin M and immunoglobulin G antibodies after primary and secondary immunization with yellow fever vaccine. Clin Diagn Lab Immunol 2:302, 1995.

201. Stephen EL, Scott SK, Eddy GA, et al. Effect of interferon on togavirus and arenavirus infections of animals. Texas Rep Biol Med 35:449, 1977.

202. Kurane I, Meager A, Ennis FA. Dengue virus-specific human T-cell clones: serotype cross-reactive proliferation, interferon-gamma production, cytotoxic activity. J Exp Med 170:763, 1989.

203. Kurane I, Innis BL, Nisalak A, et al. Human T cell responses to dengue antigens: proliferative responses and interferon-gamma production. J Clin Invest 83:506, 1989.

204. Arroyo JI, Apperson SA, Cropp CB, et al. Effect of human gamma interferon on yellow fever virus infection. Am J Trop Med Hyg 38:647, 1988.

205. Liu T, Chambers TJ. Yellow fever virus encephalitis: properties of the brain-associated T-cell response during virus clearance in normal and gamma interferon-deficient mice and requirement for CD4+ lymphocytes. J Virol 75:2107, 2001.

206. Kundig TM, Hengartner H, Zinkernagel RM. T-cell dependent interferon-γ exerts an antiviral effect in the central nervous system but not in peripheral solid organs. J Immunol 150:2316, 1993.

207. Hacker UT, Erhardt S, Tschop K, et al. Influence of the IL-1Ra gene polymorphism on in vivo synthesis of IL-1Ra and IL-1beta after live yellow fever vaccination. Clin Exp Immunol 125:465, 2001.

208. Hacker UT, Jelinek T, Erhardt S, et al. In vivo synthesis of tumor necrosis factor-alpha in healthy humans after live yellow fever vaccination. J Infect Dis 177:774, 1998.

209. Reinhardt B, Jaspert R, Niedrig M, et al. Development of viremia and humoral and cellular parameters of immune activation after vaccination with yellow fever virus strain 17D: a model of human flavivirus infection. J Med Virol 56:159, 1998.

210. Lhuillier M, Sarthou JL, Cordellier R, et al. Émergence endémique de la fièvre jaune en Côte d'Ivoire: place de la détection des IgM antiamariles dans la stratégie de surveillance. Bull World Health Organ 64:415, 1986.

211. Lhuillier M, Sarthou JL. Intérêt des IgM antiamariles dans le diagnostic et la surveillance épidémiologique de la fièvre jaune. Ann Virol (Inst Pasteur) 134E:349, 1983.

212. Monath TP, Cropp CP, Muth DJ. Indirect fluorescent antibody test for the diagnosis of yellow fever. Trans R Soc Trop Med Hyg 75:282, 1981.

213. Theiler M, Casals J. The serological reactions in yellow fever. Am J Trop Med Hyg 7:585, 1958.

214. Porterfield JS. The haemagglutination-inhibition test in the diagnosis of yellow fever in man. Trans R Soc Trop Med Hyg 48:261, 1954.

215. Heinz FX. Epitope mapping of flavivirus glycoproteins. Adv Virus Res 31:103, 1986.

216. Sawyer WA. Persistence of yellow fever immunity. J Prev Med 5:413, 1931.

217. Bauer JH, Hudson NP. Duration of immunity in human yellow fever as shown by protective power of serum. J Prev Med 4:177, 1930.

218. Snijders EP, Postmus S, Schüffner W. On the protective power of yellow fever sera and dengue sera against yellow fever virus. Am J Trop Med 14:519, 1934.

219. Frederiksen H. Historical evidence for interference between dengue and yellow fever. Am J Trop Med Hyg 4:483, 1955.

220. Ashcroft MT. Historical evidence of resistance to yellow fever acquired by residence in India. Trans R Soc Trop Med Hyg 73:247, 1979.

221. Dudley SF. Can yellow fever spread into Asia? An essay on the ecology of mosquito-borne disease. J Trop Med Hyg 37:273, 1934.

222. Downs WG. A new look at yellow fever and malaria. Am J Trop Med Hyg 30:516, 1981.

223. Monath TP. The absence of yellow fever from Asia: hypotheses. A cause for concern? Virus Info Exch Newsletter 6:106, 1989.

224. Theiler M, Anderson CR. The relative resistance of dengue-immune monkeys to yellow fever virus. Am J Trop Med Hyg 24:115, 1975.

225. Henderson BE, Cheshire PP, Kirya GB, et al. Immunologic studies with yellow fever and selected African group B arboviruses in rhesus and vervet monkeys. Am J Trop Med Hyg 19:110, 1970.

226. Guzman JR, Kron MA. Threat of dengue haemorrhagic fever after yellow fever vaccination. Lancet 319:1841, 1997.

227. Pincus S, Mason PW, Konishi E, et al. Recombinant vaccinia virus producing the prM and E proteins of yellow fever virus protects mice from lethal yellow fever encephalitis. Virology 187:290, 1992.

228. Brandriss MW, Schlesinger JJ, Walsh EE, et al. Lethal 17D yellow fever encephalitis in mice. I. Passive protection by monoclonal antibodies to the envelope proteins of 17D yellow fever and dengue 2 viruses. J Gen Virol 67:229, 1986.

229. Gollins SW, Porterfield JS. A new mechanism for the neutralization of enveloped viruses by antiviral antibody. Nature 321:244, 1986.

230. Schlesinger JJ, Chapman S. Neutralizing F(ab')2 fragments of protective monoclonal antibodies to yellow fever virus (YF) envelope

231. Falconar AKI, Young PR. Production of dimer-specific and dengue group cross-reactive mouse monoclonal antibodies to the dengue-2 virus non-structural glycoprotein NS1. J Gen Virol 72:961, 1991.

232. Schlesinger JJ, Brandriss MW, Cropp CB, et al. Protection against yellow fever in monkeys by immunization with yellow fever virus nonstructural protein NS1. J Virol 60:1153, 1986.

233. Putnak JR, Schlesinger JJ. Protection of mice against yellow fever virus encephalitis by immunization with a vaccinia virus recombinant encoding the yellow fever virus non-structural proteins, NS1, NS2a, and NS2b. J Gen Virol 71:1697, 1990.

234. Cane PA, Gould EA. Reduction of yellow fever virus mouse neurovirulence by immunization with a bacterially synthesized non-structural protein (NS1) fragment. J Gen Virol 69:1232, 1988.

235. Schlesinger JJ, Brandriss MW, Walsh EE. Protection against 17D yellow fever encephalitis in mice by passive transfer of monoclonal antibodies to the nonstructural glycoprotein gp48 and by active immunization with gp48. J Immunol 135:2805, 1985.

236. Schlesinger JJ, Foltzer M, Chapman S. The Fc portion of antibody to yellow fever virus NS1 is a determinant of protection against YF encephalitis in mice. Virology 192:132, 1993.

237. Lennette EH, Perlowagora A. Complement fixation test in the diagnosis of yellow fever: use of infectious mouse brain as antigen. Am J Trop Med 23:481, 1943.

238. Monath TP, Craven RB, Muth DJ. Limitations of the complement-fixation test for distinguishing naturally acquired from vaccine-induced yellow fever infection in flavivirus-hyperendemic areas. Am J Trop Med Hyg 29:624, 1980.

239. Schlesinger JJ, Brandriss MW. Antibody-mediated infection of macrophages and macrophage-like cell lines with 17D-yellow fever virus. J Med Virol 8:103, 1981.

240. Schlesinger JJ, Brandriss MW. Growth of 17D yellow fever virus in a macrophage-like cell line, U937: role of Fc and viral receptors in antibody-mediated infection. J Immunol 127:659, 1981.

241. Halstead SB, O'Rourke EJ. Dengue viruses and mononuclear phagocytes. I. Infection enhancement by non-neutralizing antibody. J Exp Med 146:201, 1977.

242. Gollins SW, Porterfield JS. Flavivirus infection enhancement in macrophages: radioactive and biological studies on the effect of antibody on viral fate. J Gen Virol 65:1261, 1984.

243. Cardosa MJ, Porterfield JS, Gordon S. Complement receptor mediates enhanced flavivirus replication in macrophages. J Exp Med 158:258, 1983.

244. Wisseman CL Jr, Sweet B. Immunological studies with group B arthropod-borne viruses. III. Response of human subjects to revaccination with 17D strain yellow fever vaccine. Am J Trop Med Hyg 11:570, 1962.

245. Bancroft WH Jr, Top FH Jr, Eckels KH, et al. Dengue-2 vaccine: virological, immunological, and clinical responses of six yellow fever immune recipients. Infect Immun 31:698, 1981.

246. Scott RMcN, Eckels KH, Bancroft WH. Dengue 2 vaccine: dose response in volunteers in relation to yellow fever immune status. J Infect Dis 148:1055, 1983.

247. Osanai CH, Travassos da Rosa AP, Tang AT, et al. Dengue outbreak in Boa Vista, Roraima. Rev Inst Med Trop Sao Paulo 25:53, 1983.

248. Liu Y, Blanden RV, Müllbacher A. Identification of cytolytic lymphocytes in West Nile-infected murine central nervous system. J Gen Virol 70:565, 1989.

249. Licon Luna RM, Lee E, Müllbacher A, et al. Lack of both Fas ligand and perforin protects from flavivirus-mediated encephalitis in mice. J Virol 76:3202, 2002.

250. Van der Most RG, Murati-Krishna K, Ahmed R, et al. Chimeric yellow fever/dengue virus as a candidate dengue vaccine: quantitation of the dengue-specific CD8 T-cell response. J Virol 74:8094, 2000.

251. Kurane I, Rothman AL, Bukowski JF, et al. T-lymphocyte responses to dengue viruses. In Brinton MA, Heinz FX (eds). New Aspects of Positive-Strand RNA Viruses. Washington, DC, ASM Press, 1990, pp 301–304.

252. Kurane I, Hebblewaite D, Brandt WE, et al. Lysis of dengue virus-infected cells by natural cell-mediated cytotoxicity and antibody-dependent cell mediated cytotoxicity. J Virol 52:223, 1984.

253. Bukowski JF, Kurane I, Lai C-J, et al. Dengue virus-specific cross-reactive CD8+ human cytotoxic T lymphocytes. J Virol 63:5086, 1989.

254. Findlay GM. Yellow fever and the Anglo-Egyptian Sudan. Ann Trop Med Parasitol 35:59, 1941.

255. Bensabath G, Pinheiro FP, Andrade AHP, et al. Exceptional achado em um caso humano de febre amarela: isolamento de vírus a partir do sangue no 12o dia de doença. Rev Serv Esp Saúde Pública 13:95, 1967.

256. Lhuillier M, Sarthou JL, Cordellier R, et al. Epidémie rurale de fièvre jaune avec transmission interhumaine en Côte d'Ivoire en 1982. Bull World Health Organ 63:527, 1985.

257. Varma MRG, Pudney M, Leake CL, et al. Isolations in a mosquito (*Aedes pseudoscutellaris*) cell line (Mos-61) of yellow fever virus strains from original field material. Intervirology 6:50, 1975.

258. Saluzzo JF, Monath TP, Cornet M, et al. Comparaison de différentes techniques pour la détection du virus de la fièvre jaune dans les prélièvements humains et les lots de moustiques: intérêt d'une méthode rapide de diagnostic par elisa. Ann Inst Pasteur Virol 136E:115, 1985.

259. Brown TM, Chang GJ, Cropp CB, et al. Detection of yellow fever virus by polymerase chain reaction. Clin Diagn Virol 2:41, 1994.

260. World Health Organization. Yellow fever—Kenya. Wkly Epidemiol Rec 70:175, 1995.

261. Colebunders R, Mariage J-L, Coche J-C, et al. A Belgian traveller who acquired yellow fever in The Gambia. Clin Infect Dis 35:113, 2002 [submitted for publication].

262. Monath TP, Hill LJ, Brown NV, et al. Sensitive and specific monoclonal immunoassay for detecting yellow fever virus in laboratory and clinical specimens. J Clin Microbiol 23:129, 1986.

263. Monath TP, Nystrom RR. Detection of yellow fever virus in serum by enzyme immunoassay. Am J Trop Med Hyg 33:151, 1984.

264. Piech KS, Shelburne JD, Connor DH, et al. An electron microscopic study of a human case of yellow fever. Lab Invest 42:143, 1980.

265. De La Monte SM, Linhares AL, Travassos Da Rosa APA, et al: Immunoperoxidase detection of yellow fever virus after natural and experimental infections. Trop Geogr Med 35:235, 1983.

266. Hall WC, Crowell TP, Watts DM, et al. Demonstration of yellow fever and dengue antigens in formalin-fixed paraffin-embedded human liver by immunohistochemical analysis. Am J Trop Med Hyg 45:408, 1991.

267. Filipe AR, Martins CMV, Rocha H. Laboratory infection with Zika virus after vaccination against yellow fever. Arch Ges Virusforsch 43:315, 1973.

268. Pettit A. Rapport sur la valeur immunisante des vaccins employés contre la fièvre jaune et la valeur thérapeutique du sérum antiamarile. Bull Acad Nat Méd 105:522, 1931.

269. Pettit A, Stefanopoulo GJ, Frasey X. Sérum anti-amaryllique. C R Soc Biol 99:541, 1928.

270. Spertzl RO, Kosch PC, Gilbertson SH, et al. Annual Progress Report. Fort Detrick, MD, U.S. Army Medical Research Institute of Infectious Diseases, 1972, p 246.

271. Gabrielsen B, Monath TP, Huggins JW, et al. Activity of selected amaryllidaceae constituents and related synthetic substances against medically important RNA viruses. *In* Chu CK, Cutler HG (eds). National Products as Antiviral Agents. New York, Plenum Press, 1992, pp 121–135.

272. Gabrielsen B, Monath TP, Huggins JW, et al. Antiviral (RNA) activity of selected amaryllidaceae isoquinoline constituents and synthesis of related substances. J Natural Products 55:1569, 1992.

273. Leyssen P, De Clerq E, Neyts J. Perspectives for the treatment of infections with *Flaviviridae*. Clin Microbiol Rev 13:67, 2000.

274. Malinoski FJ, Hasty SE, Ussery MA, et al. Prophylactic ribavirin treatment of dengue type 1 infection in rhesus monkeys. Antiviral Res 13:139, 1990.

275. Koff WC, Pratt RD, Elm JL Jr, et al. Treatment of intracranial dengue virus infections in mice with a lipophile derivative of ribavirin. Antimicrob Agents Chemother 24:134, 1983.

276. Sawyer WA, Whitman L. Yellow fever immunity survey of North, East and South Africa. Trans R Soc Trop Med Hyg 29:397, 1936.

277. Sawyer WA, Bauer JH, Whitman L. Distribution of yellow fever immunity in North America, Central America, West Indies, Europe, Asia and Australia, with special reference to the specificity of protection tests. Am J Trop Med 17:137, 1937.

278. Centers for Disease Control and Prevention. Health Information for International Travel 2001–2002. Atlanta, GA, Centers for Disease Control and Prevention, 2002.

279. World Health Organization. International Travel and Health: Vaccination Requirements and Health Advice. Geneva, World Health Organization, 2002.

280. World Health Organization. Yellow fever in 1994 and 1995. Wkly Epidemiol Rec 71:313, 1996.

281. World Health Organization. Yellow fever, 1996–1997. Wkly Epidemiol Rec 73:351 (Part I) and 73:370 (Part II), 1998.

282. World Health Organization. Yellow fever, 1998–1999. Wkly Epidemiol Rec 75:322, 2000.

283. Pan-American Health Organization. Yellow Fever Conference (PAHO Sci Publ No 19). Washington, DC, Pan-American Health Organization, 1955. (Reprinted from Am J Trop Med Hyg 4:571-6661, 1955.)

284. Tikasingh ES (ed). Studies on the Natural History of Yellow Fever in Trinidad (PAHO/WHO CAREC Monograph Series No 1). Washington, DC, Pan-American Health Organization, 1991.

285. Aitken THG, Downs WG, Shope RE. *Aedes aegypti* strain fitness for yellow fever transmission. Am J Trop Med Hyg 26:985–989, 1977.

286. Tabachnick WJ, Wallis GP, Aitken THG, et al. Oral infection of *Aëdes aegypti* with yellow fever virus: geographic variation and genetic considerations. Am J Trop Med Hyg 34:1219, 1985.

287. Pisano MR, Mercier V, Deubel V, et al. Complete nucleotide sequence and phylogeny of an American strain of yellow fever virus, TRINID79A. Arch Virol 144:1837, 1999.

288. Pisano MR, Nicoli J, Tolou H. Homogeneity of yellow fever virus strains isolated during an epidemic and a post-epidemic period in West Africa. Virus Genes 14:225, 1997.

289. Lepiniec L, Delgarno L, Huong VTQ, et al. Geographic distribution and evolution of yellow fever viruses based on direct sequencing of genomic cDNA fragments. J Gen Virol 75:417, 1994.

290. Deubel V, Digoutte J-P, Monath TP, et al. Genetic heterogeneity of yellow fever virus strains from Africa and the Americas. J Gen Virol 67:209, 1986.

291. Deubel V, Pailliez JP, Cornet M, et al. Homogeneity among Senegalese strains of yellow fever virus. Am J Trop Med Hyg 34:976, 1985.

292. Mutebi J-P, Wang H, Li L, et al. Phylogenetic and evolutionary relationships among yellow fever virus isolates in Africa. J Virol 75:6999, 2001.

293. Pisano MR, Durand JP, Tolou H. Partial genomic sequence determination of yellow fever virus strain associated with a recent epidemic in Gabon. Acta Virol 40:103, 1996.

294. Wang H, Jennings AD, Ryman KD, et al. Genetic variation among strains of wild-type yellow fever virus from Senegal. J Gen Virol 78:1349, 1997.

295. Clarke DH. Antigenic analysis of certain group B arthropod-borne viruses by antibody absorption. J Exp Med 111:21, 1960.

296. Theiler M, Downs WG. The Arthropod-Borne Viruses of Vertebrates. New Haven, CT, Yale University Press, 1973.

297. Monath TP. Yellow fever: Victor, Victoria? Conqueror, conquest? Epidemics and research in the last forty years and prospects for the future. Am J Trop Med Hyg 45:1, 1991.

298. DeCock KM, Monath TP, Nasidi A, et al. Epidemic yellow fever in Eastern Nigeria, 1986. Lancet 19:630, 1988.

299. World Health Organization. Yellow fever in 1992 and 1993. Wkly Epidemiol Rec 70:65, 1995.

300. World Health Organization. Yellow fever. Wkly Epidemiol Rec 68:159, 1993.

301. Sanders EJ, Borus P, Ademba G, et al. Sentinel surveillance for yellow fever in Kenya, 1993–1995. Emerg Infect Dis 2:236, 1996.

302. Pan-American Health Organization. Present status of yellow fever: memorandum from a PAHO meeting. Bull World Health Organ 64:511, 1986.

303. Sérié C, Casals J, Panthier R, et al. Études sur la fièvre jaune en Éthiopie. 2. Enquête sérologique sur la population humaine. Bull World Health Organ 38:843, 1968.

304. Brès P, Cornet M, Ly C, et al. Une epidemie de fièvre jaune au Senegal en 1965. I. Charactéristiques de l'épidémie. Bull World Health Organ 36:113, 1967.

305. World Health Organization. Yellow fever in 1982. Wkly Epidemiol Rec 41:313, 1983.

306. Roux J, Baudon D, Robert V, et al. L'épidémie de fièvre jaune du sud-est de la Haute Volta (Octobre-Decembre 1983): étude épidémiologique préliminaires. Méd Trop (Marseilles) 44:303, 1984.

307. Vicens R, Robert V, Pignon D, et al. L'épidémie de fièvre jaune de l'extrême nort du Cameroun en 1990: premier isôlement du virus amarile au Cameroun. Bull OMS 71:173, 1993.

307a. World Health Organization. Yellow fever—investigation of an epidemic in Imo State, Nigeria. Wkly Epidemiol Rec 70:107, 1995.

308. Monath TP, Smith EA, Onejeme SE, et al. Surveillance of yellow fever in Nigeria, 1970–71. Nigerian Med J 2:179, 1972.

309. Monath TP, Nasidi A. Should yellow fever vaccine be included in the expanded program of immunization in Africa? A cost-effectiveness analysis for Nigeria. Am J Trop Med Hyg 48:274, 1993.

310. Murdock FF. The American Legation Guard, Managua, Nicaragua. US Naval Med Bull 14:684, 1920.

311. Warner RA. A case of yellow fever among personnel attached to the United States Naval Mission to Brazil. US Naval Med Bull 27:786, 1929.

312. Tomaszunas S. Przypadki Chorob Tropikalnych Wsrod Pacjentow Instytutu Medycyny Morskiej. Bull Inst Marine Med Gdansk 14:239, 1963.

313. Kirk R, Bayoumi A. Notes on a fatal case of fellow fever. Ann Trop Med Parasitol 38:205, 1944.

314. Elliot M. Yellow fever in the recently inoculated. Trans R Soc Trop Med Hyg 38:231, 1944.

315. Ross RW, Haddow AJ, Raper AB, et al. A fatal case of yellow fever in a European in a Uganda. East Afr Med J 30:1, 1953.

316. Bendersky N, Carlet J, Ricomme JL, et al. Deux cas de fièvre jaune observés en France et contractés au Sénégal: aspects épidémiologiques et cliniques. Bull Soc Pathol Exot 73:54, 1980.

317. Digoutte JP, Plassart H, Salaun JJ, et al. À propos de trois cas de fièvre jaune contractée au Sènègal. Bull World Health Organ 59:759, 1981.

318. Rodhain F, Hannoun C, Jousset FX, et al. Isôlement du virus de la fièvre jaune à Paris à partir de deux cas humains importés. Bull Soc Path Exot 72:411, 1979.

319. World Health Organization. Yellow fever in 1981. Wkly Epidemiol Rec 39:297, 1982.

320. World Health Organization. Yellow fever in 1985. Wkly Epidemiol Rec 61:377, 1986.

321. Nolla-Salas J, Sadalls-Radresa J, Bada JL. Imported yellow fever in vaccinated tourist. Lancet 2:1275, 1989.

322. McFarland JM, Baddour LM, Nelson JE, et al. Imported yellow fever in a United States citizen. Clin Infect Dis 25:1143, 1997.

323. Barros ML, Boecken G. Jungle yellow fever in the central Amazon. Lancet 348:969, 1996.

324. Hall P, Fojtasek M, Pettigrove J, et al. Fatal yellow fever in a traveler returning from Amazonas, Brazil, 2002. MMWR Morb Mortal Wkly Rep 51:324, 2002.

325. Monath TP, Cetron M. Preventing yellow fever in travelers to the tropics. Clin Infect Dis 34:1369, 2002.

326. Sawyer WA. Public health implications of tropical and imported diseases: yellow fever and typhus and the possibility of their introduction into the United States. Am J Public Health 34:7, 1944.

327. Hughes JH, Porter JE. Measures against yellow fever entry into the United States. Public Health Rep 73:1101, 1958.

328. Coimbra TLM, Iversson LB, Spir M, et al. Investigação epidemiologica de casos de febre amarela na região noroeste do Esdade de São Paulo, Brasil. Rev Saude Publica 3:193, 1987.

329. Vasconcelos PF, Costa ZG, Travassos Da Rosa ES, et al. Epidemic of jungle yellow fever in Brazil, 2000: implications of climatic alterations in disease spread. J Med Virol 65:598, 2001.

330. Taylor RM. Epidemiology. In Strode GK (ed). Yellow Fever. New York, McGraw-Hill, 1951, pp 427–538.

331. Pinheiro FP, Travassos Da Rosa APA, Moraes MAP, et al. An epidemic of yellow fever in Central Brazil, 1972–1973. Am J Trop Med Hyg 27:125, 1978.

332. Soper FL. Present day methods for study and control of yellow fever. Am J Trop Med 17:655, 1937.

333. Sanders EJ, Marfin AA, Tukei PM, et al. First recorded outbreak of yellow fever in Kenya 1992–1993. I. Epidemiologic investigations. Am J Trop Med Hyg 59:644, 1998.

334. Cornet M, Chateau R, Valade M, et al. Données bioécologiques sur les vecteurs potentiels du virus amaril au Sénégal oriental: rôles des différents espèces dans la transmission du virus. Cah ORSTOM Sér Entomol Med Parasitol 16:315, 1978.

335. Germain M, Cornet M, Mouchet J, et al. La fièvre jaune en Afrique: données récentes et conceptions actuelles. Méd Trop (Marseilles) 41:31, 1981.

336. Germain M, Francy DB, Monath TP, et al. Yellow fever in The Gambia, 1978–1979: entomological aspects and epidemiological correlations. Am J Trop Med Hyg 30:929, 1980.

337. Digoutte J-P, Cornet M, Deubel V, et al. Yellow fever. In Porterfield JS (ed). Exotic Virus Infections. London, Chapman & Hall, 1995, pp 67–102.

338. Cordellier R. L'épidemiologie de la fièvre jaune en Afrique de l'Ouest. Bull World Health Organ 69:73, 1991.

339. Monath TP. Yellow fever and dengue—the interactions of virus, vector and host in the re-emergence of epidemic disease. Semin Virol 5:133, 1995.

340. World Health Organization. Yellow fever virus surveillance in Western Africa. Wkly Epidemiol Rec 69:93, 1994.

341. Reiter P. Weather, vector ecology and arboviral recrudescence. In Monath TP (ed). The Arboviruses: Ecology and Epidemiology. Vol. I. Boca Raton, FL, CRC Press, 1988, pp 245–255.

342. Smith CEG. Human and animal ecological concepts behind the distribution, behaviour and control of yellow fever. Bull Soc Pathol Exot 64:683, 1972.

343. Koopman JS, Prevots DR, Marin MAV, et al. Determinants and predictors of dengue infection in Mexico. Am J Epidemiol 133:1168, 1991.

344. Pant CP, Yasuno Y. Field studies on the gonotrophic cycle of Aedes aegypti in Bangkok, Thailand. J Med Entomol 10:219, 1973.

345. Patz JA, Epstein PR, Burke TA, et al. Global climate change and emerging infectious diseases. JAMA 275:217, 1996.

346. Monath TP, Kemp GE. The importance of non-human primates in yellow fever epidemiology in Nigeria. Trop Geogr Med 25:28, 1973.

347. Taufflieb R, Robin Y, Cornet M. Le virus amaril et la faune sauvage en Afrique. Cah ORSTOM Sér Entomol Med Parasitol 9:351, 1971.

348. Mondet B. Yellow fever epidemiology in Brazil. Bull Soc Pathol Exot 94:260, 2001.

349. Haddow AJ. The natural history of yellow fever in Africa. Proc R Soc Edinburgh 70:191, 1968.

350. Reiter P, Cordellier R. Ouma JO, et al. First recorded outbreak of yellow fever in Kenya, 1992–1993. II. Entomological investigations. Am J Trop Med Hyg 59:650, 1998.

351. Walcott AM, Cruz E, Paoliello A, et al. An epidemic of urban yellow fever which originated from a case contracted in the jungle. Am J Trop Med Hyg 17:677, 1937.

352. Soper FL. Yellow fever: present situation (October 1938) with special reference to South America. Trans R Soc Trop Med Hyg. 32:297, 1938.

353. Soper FL. The 1957 status of yellow fever in the Americas. Mosquito News 18:203, 1958.

353a. Van der Stuyft P, Gianella A, Pirard M, et al. Urbanization of yellow fever in Santa Cruz, Bolivia. Lancet 353:1558, 1999.

354. Downs WG. Epidemiological notes in connection with the 1954 outbreak of yellow fever in Trinidad, BWI. In Boshell JM, Bugher J, Downs W, et al (eds). Yellow Fever: A Symposium in Commemoration of Carlos Juan Finlay. Philadelphia, Jefferson Medical College, 1955, pp 71–78.

355. Dutary BE, Leduc JW. Transovarial transmission of yellow fever virus by a sylvatic vector, Haemagogus equinus. Trans R Soc Trop Med Hyg 75:128, 1981.

356. Fontenille D, Diallo M, Mondo M, et al. First evidence of natural vertical transmission of yellow fever virus in Aedes aegypti, its epidemic vector. Trans R Soc Trop Med Hyg 91:533, 1997.

357. Diallo M, Thonnon J, Fontenille D. Vertical transmission of the yellow fever virus by Aedes aegypti (Diptera, Culicidae): dynamics of infection in F1 adult progeny of orally infected females. Am J Trop Med Hyg 62:151, 2000.

358. Germain M, Saluzzo J-F, Cornet JP, et al. Isôlement du virus de la fièvre jaune à partir de la ponte et larves d'une tique, Amblyomma variegatum. C R Acad Sci Paris sér D 289:635, 1979.

359. Xie H. Mutations in the genome of yellow fever 17D-204 vaccine virus accumulate in the non-structural protein genes. PhD Dissertation, University of Texas Medical Branch, Galveston, TX, 1997.

360. Penna HA, Bittencourt A. Persistence of yellow fever virus in brains of monkeys immunized by cerebral inoculation. Science 97:448, 1943.

361. Gubler DJ. Dengue and dengue hemorrhagic fever: its history and resurgence as a global public health problem. In Gubler DJ, Kuno G (eds). Dengue and Dengue Hemorrhagic Fever. Wallingford, UK, CABI Publishing, 1997, pp 1–22.

362. Low CG, Fairley NH. Laboratory and hospital infections with yellow fever in England. Br Med J 125, 1931.

363. Cook GC. Fatal yellow fever contracted at the hospital for tropical diseases, London, UK in 1930. Trans R Soc Trop Med Hyg 88:712, 1994.

364. Miller WS, Demchak P, Rosenberger CR, et al. Stability and infectivity of airborne yellow fever and Rift Valley fever viruses. Am J Hyg 77:114, 1963.

365. Hearn HJ Jr, Chappell WA, Demchak P, et al. Attenuation of aerosolized yellow fever virus after passage in cell culture. Bacteriol Rev 30:615, 1966.

366. Findlay GM, MacCallum FO. Transmission of yellow fever virus to monkeys by mouth. J Pathol Bacteriol 49:53, 1939.

367. Bauer JH, Hudson NP. Passage of virus of yellow fever through skin. Am J Trop Med 8:371, 1928.

368. Hay A. A magic sword or a big itch: an historical look at the United States biological weapons programme. Med Conflict Surviv 15:215, 1999.

369. Hay A. Simulants, stimulants and diseases: evolution of the US biological warfare programme from 1945–1960. Med Conflict Surviv 15:198, 1999.

370. Sanarelli V. Immunity and serum therapy against yellow fever: third report. Ann Inst Pasteur 11:753, 1897.

371. Marchoux E, Salimbeni I, Simond P-L. La fièvre jaune. Ann Inst Pasteur 17:665, 1903.

372. Burke AW, Davis NC. Notes on laboratory infections with yellow fever. Am J Trop Med Hyg 10:419, 1930.

373. Davis NC. On the use of immune serum at various intervals after the inoculation of yellow fever virus into rhesus monkeys. J Immun 26:361, 1934.

374. Pettit A, Stefanopoulo GJ. Utilisation du sérum antiamarile d'origine animale pour la vaccination de l'homme. Bull Acad Nat Méd 110:67, 1933.

375. Theiler M, Smith HH. Use of hyperimmune monkey serum in human vaccination against yellow fever. Bull Off Int Hyg Pub 28:2354, 1936.

376. Theiler M, Whitman L. Quantitative studies of the virus and immune serum used in vaccination against yellow fever. Am J Trop Med Hyg 15:347, 1935.

377. Kaplan JE, Nelson DB, Schonberger LB, et al. The effect of immune globulin on the response to trivalent oral poliovirus and yellow fever vaccinations. Bull World Health Organ 62:585, 1984.

378. Mason RA, Tauraso NM, Spertzel RO, et al. Yellow fever vaccine: direct challenge of monkeys given graded doses of 17D vaccine. Appl Microbiol 25:539, 1973.

379. Hoskins M. Protective properties against yellow fever virus in the sera of the offspring of immune rhesus monkeys. J Immunol 26:391, 1934.

380. Soper FL, Beeuwkes H, Davis NC, et al. Transitory immunity to yellow fever in offspring of immune human and monkey mothers. Am J Hyg 19:549, 1938.

381. Stefanopoulo GJ, Laurent P, Wassermann R. Présence d'anticorps antiamariles dans le lait de femme immunisé contre la fièvre jaune. C R Soc Biol 122:915, 1936.

382. Hindle E. An experimental study of yellow fever. Trans R Soc Trop Med Hyg 22:405, 1928–1929.

383. Aragão H de B. Report upon some researches on yellow fever. Mem Oswaldo Cruz Inst Suppl 2:35, 1929.

384. Okell CC. Experiments with yellow fever vaccine in monkeys. Trans R Soc Trop Med Hyg 19:251, 1930.

385. Davis NC. Uso experimental de uma vaccina cloroformada contra a febre amarela. Brasil Med 45:368, 1931.

386. Gordon JE, Hughes TP. A study of inactivated yellow fever virus as immunizing agent. J Immunol 30:221, 1936.

387. Sellards AW, Bennett BL. Vaccination in yellow fever with non-infective virus. Ann Trop Med Parasitol 31:373, 1937.

388. Theiler M. The susceptibility of white mice to virus of yellow fever. Science 71:367, 1930.

389. Findlay GM, Clarke LP. Infection with neurotropic yellow fever virus following instillation into the nares and conjunctival sac. J Pathol Bacteriol 40:55, 1935.

390. Lloyd W, Penna HA. Studies on the pathogenesis of neurotropic yellow fever virus in Macaca rhesus. Am J Trop Med 13:1, 1933.

391. Sellards AW. Behavior of virus of yellow fever in monkeys and mice. Proc Natl Acad Sci U S A 17:339, 1931.

392. Laigret J. Recherches expérimentales sur la fièvre jaune. Arch Inst Pasteur Tunis 21:412, 1933.

393. Laigret J. Sur la vaccination contre la fièvre jaune par le virus de Max Theiler. Bull Off Int Hyg Pub 26:1078, 1934.

394. Nicolle C, Laigret J. La vaccination contre la fièvre jaune par le virus amaril vivant, desséché et enrobé. C R Acad Sci 201:312, 1935.

395. Laigret J. Au sujet des réactions nerveuses de la vaccination contre la fièvre jaune. Bull Soc Pathol Exot 29:823, 1936.

396. Sorel F. La vaccination anti-amarile en Afrique occidentale française, mise en application du procédé de vaccination Sellards-Laigret. Bull Off Int Hyg Pub 28:1325, 1936.

397. Peltier M, Durieux C, Jonchère H, Arquié E. Pénétration du virus amarile neurotrope par voie cutanée: vaccination contre la fièvre jaune et al variole, note préliminaire. Bull Acad Méd Paris 121:657, 1939.

398. Peltier M. Yellow fever vaccination, simple or associated with vaccination against smallpox, of the populations of French West Africa by the method of the Pasteur Institute of Dakar. Am J Public Health 37:1026, 1947.

399. Durieux C. Preparation of yellow fever vaccine at the Institut Pasteur, Dakar. In Smithburn KC, Durieux C, Koerber R, et al (eds). Yellow Fever Vaccination (Monograph Ser No 30). Geneva, World Health Organization, 1956, pp 31–39.

400. Durieux C, Koerber R. Post-vaccination immunity with yellow fever vaccine of the Institut Pasteur, Dakar. In Smithburn KC, Durieux C, Koerber R, et al (eds). Yellow Fever Vaccination (Monograph Ser No 30). Geneva, World Health Organization, 1956, pp 51–63.

401. Bonnel PH, Deutschman Z. La fièvre jaune en Afrique au cours des années récentes. Bull World Health Organ 11:325, 1957.

402. Kaplan M, Gluck AC. Méningo-encéphalite après vaccination anti-amarile. Soc Méd Hôp Paris 61:374, 1945.

403. Martin R, Rouesse G, Bonnefoi A. Cent cas de vaccination antiamarile (vaccin Laigret) pratiquée a l'Hôpital Pasteur. Bull Soc Pathol Exot 29:295, 1936.

404. Laigret J. Resultante de la vaccination contre la fièvre jaune après douze années de practique. Bull Acad Nat Méd 13:131, 1947.

405. Husson RA, Koerber R. Le vaccin contre la fièvre jaune préparé par l'Institut Pasteur de Dakar. Ann Inst Pasteur 85:735, 1953.

406. Stuart G. Reactions following vaccination against yellow fever. In Smithburn KC, Durieux C, Koerber R, et al (eds). Yellow Fever Vaccination (Monograph Ser No. 30). Geneva, World Health Organization, 1956, pp 143.

407. MacNamara FN. Reactions following neurotropic yellow fever vaccine given by scarification in Nigeria. Am J Trop Med Hyg 47:199, 1953.

408. Stones PB, MacNamara FN. Encephalitis following neurotropic yellow fever vaccine administered by scarification in Nigeria: epidemiological and laboratory studies. Trans R Soc Trop Med Hyg 49:176, 1955.

409. Eklund CM. Encefalitis infantil en Costa Rica y Honduras despues del empleo de la vacuna Dakar contra la fiebra amarilla. Bol San Panam 35:505, 1953.

410. Brès, P, Lacan A, Diop I, et al. Des campagnes de vaccination antiamarile en République du Sénégal. Bull Soc Pathol Exot 64:1038, 1963.

411. Rey M, Satge P, Collomb H, et al. Aspects épidémiologiques et cliniques des encéphalites consécutives à la vaccination antiamarile (d'après 248 cas observés dans quatre services hospitaliers de Dakar à la suite de la campagne 1965). Bull Soc Méd Afr Noire Langue Fr 11:560, 1966.

412. Sankalé M, Bourgeade A, Wade F, et al. Contribution à l'étude des réactions vaccinales observées en dehors de Dakar. Bull Soc Méd Afr Noire Langue Fr 11:617, 1966.

413. Collomb H, Rey M, Dumas M, et al. Syndromes neuro-psychiques au cours des encephalites postvaccinales. Bull Soc Med Afr Noire Langue Fr 3:575, 1966.

414. Ricosse JH, Albert JP. La vaccination antiamarile dats les états de l'OCCGE. Présenté à Conférence sur l'épidémiologie et le contrôle de la fièvre jaune en Afrique de l'Ouest, Bobo Dioulasso, March 20–23, 1971 (unpublished document No 266, OCCGE, Centre Muraz, Bobo Dioulasso, Haute Volta).

415. Brès, P, Robin Y. Étude virologique: considérations étiopathologéniques. Bull Soc Méd Afr Noire Langue Fr 11:610, 1966.

416. Holbrook MR, Li L, Suderman MT, et al. The French neurotropic vaccine strain of yellow fever virus accumulates mutations slowly during passage in cell culture. Virus Res 69:31, 2000.

417. Dick GWA. A preliminary evaluation of the immunizing power of chick-embryo 17D yellow fever vaccine inoculated by scarification. Am J Hyg 55-56:140, 1952.

418. Hahn RG. A combined yellow fever-smallpox vaccine for cutaneous application. Am J Hyg 53–54:50, 1951.

419. Cannon DA, Dewhurst F, Meers PD. Mass vaccination against yellow fever by scarification with 17D strain vaccine. Ann Trop Med Parasitol 51–52:256, 1957–1958.

420. Cannon DA, Dewhurst F. The preparation of 17D virus yellow fever vaccine in mouse brain. Ann Trop Med Parasitol 49:174, 1955.

421. Cannon DA, Dewhurst F. Vaccination by scarification with 17D yellow fever vaccine prepared at Yaba, Lagos, Nigeria. Ann Trop Med Parasitol 47:381, 1953.

422. Meers PD. Combined smallpox-17D yellow fever vaccine for scratch vaccination. Trans R Soc Trop Med Hyg 53:196, 1959.

423. Meers PD. Further observations on 17D-yellow fever vaccination by scarification, with and without simultaneous smallpox vaccination. Trans R Soc Trop Med Hyg 54:493, 1960.

424. Draper CC, Knott EG. Failure to respond to vaccination with 17D yellow fever virus by scarification and its significance. W Afr Med J April:78, 1964.

425. Fabiyi A, MacNamara FN. The effects of heterologous antibodies on the serological conversion rate after 17D yellow fever vaccination. Am J Trop Med Hyg 11:817, 1962.

426. Smith CEG, McMahon DA, Turner LH. Yellow fever vaccination in Malaya by subcutaneous injection and multiple puncture: haemagglutinin-inhibiting antibody responses in persons with and without pre-existing antibody. Bull World Health Organ 29:75, 1963.

427. Smith CEG, Turner LH, Armitage P. Yellow fever vaccination in Malaya by subcutaneous injection and multiple puncture: neutralizing antibody responses in persons with and without pre-existing antibody to related viruses. Bull World Health Organ 27:717, 1962.

428. Lloyd W, Theiler M, Ricci NI. Modification of the virulence of yellow fever virus by cultivation in tissues in vitro. Trans R Soc Trop Med Hyg 29:481, 1936.

429. Manso CdeS. Mass vaccination against yellow fever in Brazil 1937–54. In Smithburn KC, Durieux C, Koerber R, et al (eds). Yellow Fever Vaccination (Monograph Ser No 30). Geneva, World Health Organization, 1956, pp 123–140.

430. Fox JP, Penna HA. Behavior of 17D yellow fever virus in rhesus monkeys: relation to substrain, dose and neural or extraneural inoculation. Am J Hyg 38:152, 1943.

431. Soper FL, Smith HH, Penna HA. Yellow fever vaccination: field results as measured by the mouse protection test and epidemiological observations. In Proceedings of the Third International Congress on Microbiology, New York, September 2–9, 1939, pp 351–353.

432. Fox JP, Lennette EH, Manso C, et al. Encephalitis in man following vaccination with 17D yellow fever virus. Am J Hyg 36:117, 1942.

433. United Nations Relief and Rehabilitation Administration (UNRRA). Standards for the manufacture and control of yellow fever vaccine. Epidemiol Inform Bull 1:365, 1945.

434. Panthier R. À propos de quelques cas de réactions nerveuses tardives observées chez des nourrissons après vaccination antiamarile (17D). Bull Soc Pathol Exot 49:478, 1956.

435. World Health Organization. Requirements for yellow fever vaccine (Requirements for Biological Substances No 3, Revised 1995). World Health Organ Tech Rep Ser 872, 1998.

436. Monath TP, Kinney RM, Schlesinger JJ, et al. Ontogeny of yellow fever 17D vaccine: RNA oligonucleotide fingerprint and monoclonal antibody analyses of vaccines produced world-wide. J Gen Virol 64:627, 1983.

437. Brès P, Koch M. Production and testing of the WHO yellow fever primary seed lot 213-77 and reference batch 168-73. World Health Organ Tech Rep Ser 745(Annex 6):113, 1987.

438. Gould EA, Buckley A, Cane PA, et al. Examination of the immunological relationships between flaviviruses using monoclonal antibodies. J Gen Virol 66:1369, 1985.

439. Galler R, Post PR, Santos CN. Genetic variability among yellow fever 17D substrain vaccines. Vaccine 16:1024, 1998.

440. Marchevsky RS, Mariano J, Ferreira VS, et al: Phenotypic analysis of yellow fever virus derived from complementary DNA. Am J Trop Med Hyg 52:75–80, 1995.

441. Levenbook IS, Pelleu LJ, Elisberg BL. The monkey safety test for neurovirulence of yellow fever vaccines: the utility of quantitative clinical evaluation and historical examination. J Biol Stand 15:305, 1987.

442. Penna HA. Production of 17D yellow fever vaccine. In Smithburn KC, Durieux C, Koerber R, et al (eds). Yellow Fever Vaccination (Monograph Ser No 30). Geneva, World Health Organization, 1956, pp 67–90.

443. Tannock GA, Wark MC, Hair CG. The development of an improved experimental yellow fever vaccine. J Biol Stand 8:23, 1980.

444. Lopes O de Souza, de Almeida Guimarães SSD, de Carvalho R. Studies on yellow fever vaccine. I. Quality-control parameters. J Biol Stand 15:323, 1987.

445. Harris RJC, Dougherty RM, Biggs PM, et al. Contaminant viruses in two live virus vaccines produced in chick cells. J Hyg (Camb) 64:1, 1966.

446. Waters TD, Anderson PS Jr, Beebe GW, et al. Yellow fever vaccination, avian leukosis virus, and cancer risk in man. Science 177:76, 1972.

447. Weiss RA. Adventitious viral genomes in vaccines but not in vaccines. Emerg Infect Dis 7:153, 2001.

448. Hussain AI, Shanmugam V, Switzer WM, et al. Lack of evidence of endogenous avian leucosis virus and endogenous avian retrovirus transmission to measles, mumps, and rubella vaccine recipients. Emerg Infect Dis 7:66, 2001.

449. Niedrig M, Stolte N, Fuchs D, et al. Intra-nasal infection of macaques with yellow fever (YF) vaccine strain 17D: a novel and economical approach for YF vaccination in man. Vaccine 17:1206, 1999.

450. World Health Organization. Requirements for yellow fever vaccine: addendum 1987. World Health Organ Tech Rep Ser 771(Annex 9): 208, 1988.

451. World Health Organization. Yellow fever vaccines: thermostability of freeze-dried vaccine. Wkly Epidemiol Rec 62:181, 1987.

452. Monath TP. Stability of yellow fever vaccine. Dev Biol Stand 87:219, 1996.

453. Perrault R, Girault G, Moreau J-P. Stability-related studies on 17D yellow fever vaccine. Microbes Infect 2:33, 2000.

454. Barme M, Bronnaert C. Thermostabilisation du vaccin antiamarile 17D lyophilise. I Essai de substances protectrices. J Biol Stand 12:435, 1984.

455. Barme M, Vacher B, Ryhiner ML, et al. Thermostabilisation du vaccin antiamarile 17-D lyophilisé. II. Lots-pilotes prepares dans les conditions d'une production industrielle. J Biol Stand 15:67, 1987.

456. Lopes O de Souza, de Almeida Guimarães SSD, de Carvalho R. Studies on yellow fever vaccine. II. Stability of the reconstituted product. J Biol Stand 16:71, 1988.

457. Guirakhoo F, Arroyo J, Pugachev KV, et al. Construction, safety, and immunogenicity in non-human primates of a chimeric yellow fever-dengue tetravalent vaccine. J Virol 75:7290, 2001.

458. Mason RA, Tauraso NM, Ginn RK. Yellow fever vaccine. V. Antibody response in monkeys inoculated with graded doses of the 17D vaccine. Appl Microbiol 23:908, 1972.

459. Wheelock EF, Sibley WA. Circulating virus, interferon and antibody after vaccination with the 17-D strain of yellow-fever virus. N Engl J Med 273:194–198, 1965.

460. Actis DAS, Sa Fleitas MJ. Replaciones entre viremia y seroanticuerpos secundarios a la vacunacion antiamarilica de personsas vacunadas con "Cepa 17D -EP". Rev San Mil Argent 69:51, 1970.

461. Fox JP, Cabral AS. The duration of immunity following vaccination with the 17D strain of yellow fever virus. Am J Hyg 37:98, 1943.

462. Fox JP, Fonseca da Cunha J, Kossobudzki SL. Additional observations on duration of humoral immunity following vaccination with 17D strain of yellow fever virus. Am J Hyg 47:64, 1948.

463. Anderson CR, Gast Galvis A. Immunity to yellow fever five years after vaccination. Am J Hyg 45:302, 1947.

464. Dick GWA, Smithburn KC. Immunity to yellow fever six years after vaccination. Am J Trop Med 29:57, 1949.

465. Smithburn KC. Immunology of yellow fever. In Smithburn KC, Durieux C, Koerber R, et al (eds). Yellow Fever Vaccination (Monograph Ser No 30). Geneva, World Health Organization, 1956, pp 11–27.

466. Spector S, Tauraso NM. Yellow fever virus. I. Development and evaluation of a plaque neutralization test. Appl Microbiol 16:1770, 1968.

467. De Madrid AT, Porterfield JS. The flaviviruses (group B arboviruses): a cross-neutralization study. J Gen Virol 23:91, 1974.

468. Spector SL, Tauraso NM. Yellow fever virus. II. Factors affecting the plaque neutralization test. Appl Microbiol 18:736, 1969.

469. Poland JD, Calisher CH, Monath TP, et al. Persistence of neutralizing antibody 30–35 years after immunization with 17D yellow fever vaccine. Bull World Health Organ 59:895, 1981.

470. Monath TP, Nichols R, Archambault WT, et al. Comparative safety and immunogenicity of two yellow fever 17D vaccines (ARILVAX™ and YF-VAX®) in a Phase III multicenter, double-blind clinical trial. Am J Trop Med Hyg 66:533–541, 2002.

471. Tauraso NM, Coultrip RL, Legters LJ, et al. Yellow fever vaccine. IV. Reactogenicity and antibody response in volunteers inoculated with a vaccine free from contaminating avian leukosis viruses. Proc Soc Exp Biol Med 139:439, 1972.

472. Groot H, Ribeiro RB. Neutralizing and haemagglutination-inhibiting antibodies to yellow fever 17 years after vaccination with 17D vaccine. Bull World Health Organ 27:699, 1962.

473. Pond WL, Ehrenkranz NJ, Danauskas JX, et al. Heterotypic serologic responses after yellow fever vaccination: detection of persons with past St. Louis encephalitis or dengue. J Immunol 98:673, 1967.

474. Niedrig M, Lademann M, Emmerich P, Lafrenz M. Assessment of IgG antibodies against yellow fever virus after vaccination with 17D by different assays: neutralization test, haemagglutination inhibition test, immunofluorescence assay and ELISA. Trop Med Int Health 4:867, 1999.

475. Fox JP, Kossobudzki SL, Da Chuma JF. Field studies of the immune response to 17D yellow fever virus. Am J Hyg 38:132, 1943.

476. Freestone DS, Ferris RD, Weinberg A, et al. Stabilized 17D strain yellow fever vaccine: dose response studies, clinical reactions and effects on hepatic function. J Biol Stand 5:181, 1977.

477. Lopes O de Souza, de Almeida Guimaràes SSD, de Carvalho R. Studies on yellow fever vaccine. III. Dose response in volunteers. J Biol Stand 16:77, 1988.

478. Centers for Disease Control. Yellow fever vaccine. Recommendations of the Immunization Practices Advisory Committee (ACIP). MMWR Morb Mortal Wkly Rep 51(RR-17):1, 2002.

479. Package insert: YF-Vax® Yellow Fever Vaccine. Swiftwater, PA, Aventis Pasteur Inc., 1997.

480. Wisseman CL Jr, Sweet B, Kitaoka M, et al. Immunological studies with group B arthropod-borne viruses. I. Broadened neutralizing antibody spectrum induced by strain 17D yellow fever vaccine in human subjects previously infected with Japanese encephalitis virus. Am J Trop Med Hyg 11:550, 1962.

481. Lang J, Zuckerman J, Clarke P, et al. Comparison of the immunogenicity and safety of two 17D yellow fever vaccines. Am J Trop Med Hyg 60:1045, 1999.

482. Courtois G. Time of appearance and duration of immunity conferred by 17D vaccine. In Smithburn KC, Durieux C, Koerber R, et al (eds). Yellow Fever Vaccination (Monograph Ser No 30). Geneva, World Health Organization, 1956, pp 105–114.

483. World Health Organization. International Health Regulations (1969): Third Annotated Edition. Geneva, World Health Organization, 1983.

484. Monath TP. Neutralizing antibody responses in the major immunoglobulin classes to yellow fever 17D vaccination of humans. Am J Epidemiol 93:122, 1971.

485. Boiron H. De l'influence des revaccinations antiamariles sur le taux de l'immunité humorale. C R Soc Biol (Paris) 150:2219, 1956.

486. Omilabu SA, Adejumo JO, Olaleye OD, et al. Yellow fever haemagglutination-inhibiting, neutralising and IgM antibodies in vaccinated and unvaccinated residents of Ibadan, Nigeria. Comp Immun Microbiol Infect Dis 13:95, 1990.

487. Schlesinger RW, Gordon I, Frankel JW, et al. Clinical and serologic response of man to immunization with attenuated dengue and yellow fever viruses. J Immunol 77:352, 1956.

488. Kayser M, Klein H, Paasch I. Human antibody response to immunization with 17D yellow fever and inactivated TBE vaccine. J Med Virol 17:35, 1985.

489. Rosenzweig EC, Babione RW, Wisseman CL Jr. Immunological studies with group B arthropod-borne viruses. Am J Trop Med Hyg 12:232, 1963.

490. Doherty RL. Effects of yellow fever (17D) and West Nile viruses on the reactions of human appendix and conjunctiva cells to several other viruses. Virology 6:575, 1958.

491. Brown RE, Katz M. Failure of antibody production to yellow fever vaccine in children with kwashiorkor. Trop Geogr Med 18:125, 1966.

492. Gandra YR, Scrimshaw NS. Infection and nutritional status. Am J Clin Nutr 9:159, 1961.

493. Bistrian BR, Winterer JC, Blackburn GL, et al. Failure of yellow fever immunization to produce a catabolic response in individuals fully adapted to a protein-sparing modified fast. Am J Clin Nutr 30:1518, 1977.

494. Bistrian BR, George DT, Blackburn GL, et al. The metabolic response to yellow fever immunization: protein-sparing modified fast. Am J Clin Nutr 34:229, 1981.

495. Nasidi A, Monath TP, Vandenberg J, et al. Yellow fever vaccination and pregnancy: a four-year prospective study. Trans R Soc Trop Med Hyg 87:337, 1993.

496. Rojanasuphot S, Shaffer N, Chotpitayasunondh H, et al. Response to Japanese encephalitis vaccine among HIV-infected children. Southeast Asian J Trop Med Hyg 29:443, 1998.

497. Wolf HM, Pum M, Jager R, et al. Cellular and humoral immune responses in haemophiliacs after vaccination against tick-borne encephalitis. Br J Haematol 82:374, 1992.

498. Receveur MC, Thiebaut R, Vedy S, et al. Yellow fever vaccination of human immunodeficiency virus-infected patients: report of 2 cases. Clin Infect Dis 31:E7, 2000.

499. Goujon C, Tohr M, Feuillie V, et al. Good tolerance and efficacy of yellow fever vaccine among subjects who are carriers of human immunodeficiency virus (abstr). In Abstracts of the Fourth International Conference on Travel Medicine, Acapulco, Mexico, April 23–27, 1995.

500. Sibailly TS, Wiktor SZ, Tsai TF, et al. Poor antibody response to yellow fever vaccination in children infected with human immunodeficiency virus type 1. Pediatr Infect Dis J 16:1177, 1997.

501. Wheelock EF, Toy ST, Stjenerholm RL. Lymphocytes and yellow fever. I. Transient virus refractory state following vaccination of man with the 17-D strain. J Immunol 105:1304, 1970.

502. Roome AJ, Walsh SJ, Cartter ML, et al. Hepatitis B vaccine responsiveness in Connecticut public safety personnel. JAMA 270:2931, 1993.

503. Saenz AC. Yellow fever vaccines: achievements, problems, needs. In Proceedings of the International Conference on the Application of Vaccines Against Viral, Rickettsial, and Bacterial Diseases of Man. Section A. Arbovirus Diseases (Sci Pub No 226). Washington, DC, Pan-American Health Organization, 1971, p 31.

504. Brès P. Benefit versus risk factors in immunization against yellow fever. Dev Biol Stand 43:297, 1979.

505. Findlay GM, MacCallum FO. Hepatitis and jaundice associated with immunization against certain virus diseases. Proc R Soc Med 31:799, 1838.

506. Fox JP, Manso C, Penna HA, et al. Observations on the occurrence of icterus in Brazil following vaccination against yellow fever. Am J Hyg 36:68, 1942.

507. Sawyer WA, Meyer KF, Eaton MD, et al. Jaundice in Army personnel in western region of United States and its relation to vaccination against yellow fever. Am J Hyg 40:35, 1944.

508. Hargett MV, Burruss HW, Donovan A. Aqueous-base yellow fever vaccine. Public Health Rep 58:505, 1943.

509. Seeff LB, Beebe GW, Hoofnagle JH. A serologic follow-up of the 1942 epidemic of post-vaccination hepatitis in the US Army. N Engl J Med 316:965, 1987.

510. Moss-Blundell AJ, Bernstein S, Wilma M, et al. A clinical study of stabilized 17D strain live attenuated yellow fever vaccine. J Biol Stand 9:445, 1981.

511. Pivetaud JP, Raccurt CP, M'Bailara L, et al. Clinique: réactions post-vaccinales à la vaccination anti-amarile. Bull Soc Pathol Exot 79:772, 1986.

512. Stefanopoulo GJ, Duvolon S. Réactions observées au cours de la vaccination contre la fièvre jaune par virus atténué de culture (souche 17 D): à propos de 20.000 vaccinations pratiquées par ce procédé à l'Institut Pasteur de Paris (1936–1946). Bull Mém Soc Méd Hôp Paris 63:990, 1947.

513. Dick GWA, Horgan ES. Vaccination by scarification with a combined 17D yellow fever and vaccinia vaccine. J Hyg (Lond) 50:376, 1952.

514. Thomson WO. Encephalitis in infants following vaccination with 17D yellow fever virus: report of a further case. Br Med J 2:182, 1955.

515. Centers for Disease Control. Yellow fever vaccine. Recommendations of the Immunization Practices Advisory Committee. MMWR Morb Mortal Wkly Rep 18:189, 1969.

516. Louis JJ, Chopard P, Larbre F. Un cas d'encephalite après vaccination anti-amarile par la souche 17 D. Pédiatrie 36:539, 1981.

517. Kengsakul K, Sathirapongsasuti K, Punyagupta S. Fatal myeloencephalitis following yellow fever vaccination in a case with HIV infection. J Med Assoc Thai 85:131–134, 2002.

518. Merlo C, Steffen R, Landis T, et al. Possible association of encephalitis and 17D yellow fever vaccination in a 29-year-old traveler. Vaccine 11:691, 1993.

519. Martin M, Tsai TF, Cropp CB, et al. Multisystemic illness in elderly recipients of yellow fever vaccine: report of four cases. Lancet 358:98, 2001.

520. Vasconcelos PFC, Luna EJ, Galler R, et al. Serious adverse events associated with yellow fever 17DD vaccine in Brazil: report of two cases. Lancet 358:91, 2001.

521. Chan RC, Penney DJ, Litele D, et al. Hepatitis and death following vaccination with 17D-204 yellow fever vaccine. Lancet 358:121, 2001.

522. Centers for Disease Control and Prevention. Notice to readers: fever, jaundice, and multiple organ system failure associated with 17D-derived yellow fever vaccination, 1996–2001. MMWR Morb Mortal Wkly Rep 50:643, 2001.

523. Galler R, Pugachev KV, Santos CLS, et al. Phenotypic and molecular analyses of yellow fever 17DD vaccine virus associated with serious adverse events in Brazil. Virology 290:309, 2001.

524. Martin M, Weld LH, Tsai TF, et al. Advanced age is a risk factor for adverse events temporally associated with yellow fever vaccination. Emerg Infect Dis 7:945–951, 2001.

525. Berge TO, Hargett MV. Anaphylaxis in guinea pigs following sensitization with chick-embryo yellow fever vaccine and normal chick embryos. Public Health Rep 57:652, 1942.

526. Cohen SG, Mines SC. Variations in egg white and egg yolk components of virus and rickettsial vaccines. J Allergy 29:479, 1958.

527. O'Brien TC, Maloney CJ, Tauraso NM. Quantitation of residual host protein in chicken embryo-derived vaccines by radial immunodiffusion. Appl Microbiol 21:780, 1971.

528. Sulzberger MB, Asher C. Urticarial and erythema multiforme-like eruptions following injections of yellow fever vaccine. US Navy Med Bull 40:411, 1942.

529. Swartz H. Systemic allergic reaction induced by yellow fever vaccine. J Lab Clin Med 43:1663, 1943.

530. Sprague H, Barnard J. Egg allergy, significance in typhus and yellow fever immunization. US Naval Med Bull 45:71-74, 1945.

531. Kouwenaar W. The reaction to yellow fever vaccine (17D), particularly in allergic individuals. Doc Med Geogr Trop 5:75, 1953.

532. American Academy of Pediatrics. Report of the Committee on Immunization Practices (23rd ed). Elk Grove Village, IL, American Academy of Pediatrics, 1994.

533. Patterson R, DeSwarte RD, Greenberger PA, et al. Drug allergy and protocols for management of drug allergies. N Engl Reg Allergy Proc 7:325-342, 1986.

534. Mosimann B, Stoll B, Francillon C, et al. Yellow fever vaccine and egg allergy. J Allergy Clin Immunol 95:1064, 1995.

535. Miller JR, Orgel HA, Meltzer EO. The safety of egg-containing vaccines for egg-allergic patients. J. Allergy Clin Immunol 71:568, 1983.

536. Chino F, Oshibuchi S, Ariga H, et al. Skin reaction to yellow fever vaccine after immunization with rabies vaccine of chick embryo cell culture origin. Jpn J Infect Dis 52:42, 1999.

537. Cowdrey SC. Sensitization to duck embryo rabies vaccine produced by prior yellow-fever vaccination. N Engl J Med 274:1311, 1966.

538. James JM, Zeiger RS, Lester MR, et al. Safe administration of influenza vaccine to patients with egg allergy. J Pediatr 133:624, 1998.

539. Kelso J. Raw egg allergy—a potential issue in vaccine allergy. J Allergy Clin Immunol 106:990, 2000.

540. Centers for Disease Control. Vaccine Adverse Event Reporting System—United States. MMWR Morb Mortal Wkly Rep 39:730-733, 1990.

541. Kelso JM, Mootrey GT, Tsai TF. Anaphylaxis from yellow fever vaccine. J Allergy Clin Immunol 103:698, 1999.

542. Sakaguchi M, Nakayama T, Inoue S. Food allergy to gelatin in children with systemic immediate-type reactions, including anaphylaxis, to vaccines. J Allergy Clin Immunol 98:1058, 1996.

543. Sakaguchi M, Yoshida M, Kuroda W. Systemic immediate-type reactions to gelatin in Japanese encephalitis vaccines. Vaccine 15:121, 1997.

544. Receveur MC, Gabinski C, Le Bras M. Coma acidocétosique 4 jours après une vaccination antiamarile. Presse Méd (Paris) 24:41, 1995.

545. Martin L. Leucémie et vaccination antiamarile. Nouv Rev Franc Hematol 10:311, 1970.

546. Murgatroyd F, Findlay GM, MacCallum FO. Long-latent infection with Plasmodium ovale becoming manifest after yellow-fever vaccination. Lancet 1:1262, 1939.

547. Miller H, Cendrowski W, Schapira K. Multiple sclerosis and vaccination. Br Med J 2:210, 1967.

548. Voigt U, Baum U, Behrendt W, et al. Neuritis of the optic nerve after vaccinations against hepatitis A, hepatitis B and yellow fever. Klin Monatsbl Augenheilkd 218:688, 2001.

549. Neumann HH. Herpes simplex and yellow fever vaccine. Lancet 2:250, 1977.

550. World Health Organization. Prevention and Control of Yellow Fever in Africa. Geneva, World Health Organization, 1986.

551. World Health Organization. Informal Discussions on the Use of Yellow Fever Vaccine in Africa (Unofficial Report, May 10–11, 1985). Geneva, World Health Organization, 1985.

552. Oyelami SA, Oyaleye OD, Oyejide CO, et al. Severe post-vaccination reaction to 17D yellow fever vaccine in Nigeria. Rev Roum Virol 45:25, 1994.

553. Package insert: Arilvax® Yellow Fever Vaccine, Live BP. Liverpool, UK, Evans Medical Ltd., 1997.

554. Montenegro J. Gravidez e febre amarela. Rev Inst Adolfo Lutz 1:76, 1941.

555. Sicé A, Rodallec B. Manifestations hémorragiques de la fièvre jaune (typhus amarile): répercussions de l'infection maternelle sur l'organisme foetal. Bull Soc Pathol Exot 33:66, 1940.

556. Lewis MJ. Assessment of the yellow fever vaccination campaign in Trinidad, West Indies. In Tikasingh ES (ed), Studies on the Natural History of Yellow Fever in Trinidad (PAHO/WHO CAREC Monogr Ser 1). Washington, DC, Pan-American Health Organization, 1991, p 125.

557. Tsai TF, Paul R, Lynberg MC, et al. Congenital yellow fever virus infection after immunization in pregnancy. J Infect Dis 168:1520, 1993.

558. Nishioka S de A, Nunes-Araujo FR, Pires WP, et al. Yellow fever vaccination during pregnancy and spontaneous abortion: a case-control study. Trop Med Int Health 3:29, 1998.

559. Marvin JA, Zvolanek EE, Nowosiwsky T, et al. Tuberculin sensitivity (Tine) in apparently healthy subjects after yellow fever vaccination. Am Rev Respir Dis 98:703, 1968.

560. Simonsen L, Buffington J, Shapiro CN, et al. Multiple false reactions in viral antibody screening assays after influenza vaccination. Am J Epidemiol 141:1089, 1995.

561. Starling KA, Falletta JM, Fernbach DJ. Immunologic chimerism as evidence of bone marrow graft acceptance in an identical twin with acute lymphocytic leukemia. Exp Hematol 3:244, 1975.

562. Stefano I, Sato HK, Pannuti CS, et al. Recent immunization against measles does not interfere with the sero-response to yellow fever vaccine. Vaccine 17:1042, 1999.

563. Ambrosch F, Fritzell B, Gregor J, et al. Combined vaccination against yellow fever and typhoid fever: a comparative trial. Vaccine 12:625, 1994.

564. Dukes C, Froeschle J, George J, et al. Safety and immunogenicity of simultaneous administration of Typhim Vi (TV), YF-VAX (YF) and Menomune (MV) [abstr]. In Abstracts of the 36th Interscience Conference on Antimicrobial Agents and Chemotherapy, New Orleans, September 15–18, 1996.

565. Mouchon D, Pignon D, Vicens R, et al. Étude de la vaccination combinée rougeole-fièvre jaune chez l'enfant Africain agé de 6 à 10 mois. Bull Soc Pathol Exot 83:537, 1990.

566. Meyer HM Jr, Hostetler DD Jr, Bernheim BC, et al. Response of Volta children to jet inoculation of combined live measles, smallpox and yellow fever vaccines. Bull World Health Organ 30:783, 1964.

567. Yvonnet B, Coursaget P, Deubel V, et al. Simultaneous administration of hepatitis B and yellow fever vaccines. J Med Virol 19:307, 1986.

568. Felsenfeld O, Wolf RH, Gyr K, et al. Simultaneous vaccination against cholera and yellow fever. Lancet 1:457, 1973.

569. Gateff C, Le Gonidec G, Boche R, et al. Influence de la vaccination anticholérique sur l'immunisation antiamarile associée. Bull Soc Pathol Exot 66:266, 1973.

570. Gateff C, Dodlin A, Wiart J. Comparaison des réactions sérologiques induites par un vaccin anticholérique classique et une fraction vaccinante purifiée associés ou non au vaccin antiamarile. Ann Microbiol (Inst Pasteur) 126A:231, 1975.

571. Kollaritsch H, Que JU, Kunz C, et al. Safety and immunogenicity of live oral cholera and typhoid vaccines administered alone or in combination with antimalarial drugs, oral polio vaccine, or yellow fever vaccine. J Infect Dis 175:871, 1997.

572. Foster RH, Noble S. Bivalent cholera and typhoid vaccine. Drugs 58:91, 1999.

573. Tsai TF, Bolin RA, Lazuick JS, et al. Chloroquine does not adversely affect the antibody response to yellow fever vaccine. J Infect Dis 154:726–727, 1986.

574. Chambers TJ, Nestorowicz A, Mason PW, et al . Yellow fever/Japanese encephalitis chimeric viruses: construction and biological properties. J Virol 73.3095, 1999.

575. Guirakhoo F, Weltzin R, Chambers TJ, et al. Recombinant chimeric yellow fever-dengue type 2 virus is immunogenic and protective in nonhuman primates. J Virol 74:5477, 2000.

576. Monath TP, Soike K, Arroyo J, et al. Live, attenuated recombinant chimeric yellow fever-Japanese encephalitis vaccine: extended safety and immunogenicity studies in rhesus monkeys. J Virol 74:1742–1751, 2000.

577. Caufour PS, Motta MC, Yamamura AM, et al. Construction, characterization, and immunogenicity of recombinant yellow fever 17D-dengue type 2 virus. Virus Res 79:1, 2001.

578. Arroyo J, CA Miller, J Catalan, et al. Yellow fever vector live-virus vaccines: West Nile vaccine development. Trends Mol Med 7:329, 2001.

579. McAllister A, Arbetman AE, Mandl S, et al. Recombinant yellow fever viruses are effective therapeutic vaccines for treatment of murine experimental solid tumors and pulmonary metastases. J Virol 74:9197, 2000.

580. Lai C-J, Monath TP. Chimeric flaviviruses: novel vaccines against dengue fever, tick-borne encephalitis and Japanese encephalitis. *In* Chambers TJ, Monath TP (eds). The Flaviviruses: Current Molecular Aspects of Evolution, Biology, and Disease Prevention. New York, Academic Press, 2003 [in press].

581. Pan-American Health Organization. Yellow fever vaccination in the Americas. PAHO Epidemiol Bull 4:7, 1983.

582. Calheiros LB. A febre amarela no Brasil. *En* Simpósio Internacional sobre Febre Amarela e Dengue. Cinqüentenário da introdução da Cepa 17D no Brasil. Rio de Janeiro, Fundação Oswaldo Cruz, 1988, pp 74–85.

583. Tomori O. Impact of yellow fever on the developing world. Adv Virus Res 53:5, 1999.

584. Meegan JM. Yellow Fever Vaccine (Unofficial Report WHO/EPI/GEN/91.6). Geneva, World Health Organization, 1991.

585. Robertson SE. The Immunological Basis for Immunization. 8. Yellow Fever. (Document WHO/EPI/GEN/93.18). Geneva, World Health Organization, 1993.

586. World Health Organization. Expanded Programme of Immunization (Document WHO/EPI/GEN/97.02). Geneva, World Health Organization, 1997.

587. Nathan N, Barry M, Van Herp M, Zeller H. Shortage of vaccines during a yellow fever outbreak in Guinea. Lancet 358:2129, 2001.

588. Robertson RL, Foster SO, Hull HF, et al. Cost-effectiveness of immunization in The Gambia. Am J Trop Med Hyg 88:343, 1985.

589. Massad E, Coutinho FAB, Burattini MN, et al. The risk of yellow fever in a dengue-infested area. Trans R Soc Trop Med Hyg 95:370, 2001.

590. World Health Organization. Yellow-Fever Vaccinating Centres for International Travel. Geneva, World Health Organization, 1991.

591. Monath TP, Giesberg J, Fierros EG. Does restricted distribution limit access and coverage of yellow fever vaccine in the United States? Emerg Infect Dis, 5:488, 1999.

592. Carey DE, Kemp GE, Troup JM, et al. Epidemiological aspects of the 1969 yellow fever epidemic in Nigeria. Bull World Health Organ 46:645, 1972.

593. Monath TP, Wilson DC, Lee VH. The 1970 yellow fever epidemic in Okwoga District, Benue Plateau State, Nigeria. 1. Epidemiological observations. Bull World Health Organ 49:113, 1973.

594. Addy PAK, Minami K, Agadzi VK. Recent yellow fever epidemics in Ghana (1969–1983). East Afr Med J 63:422, 1986.

595. World Health Organization. Yellow fever in 1987. Wkly Epidemiol Rec 64:37, 1989.

596. World Health Organization. Yellow fever in 1989 and 1990. Wkly Epidemiol Rec 67:245, 1992.

597. World Health Organization. Yellow fever: investigation of an epidemic in Imo State, Nigeria. Wkly Epidemiol Rec 70:107, 1995.

598. Baudon D, Robert V, Roux J, et al. L'épidémie de fievre jaune au Burkina Faso en 1983. Bull World Health Organ 64:873, 1986.

599. Roux J, Baudon D, Robert V, et al. L'epidemie de fièvre jaune du Sud-Est De La Haute-Volta. Méd Trop (Marseilles) 44:304, 1984.

600. World Health Organization. Yellow fever in 1983. Wkly Epidemiol Rec 43:329, 1989.

601. Kurz X. Health Planning and Management for Epidemic Outbreaks: The Yellow Fever Epidemic in Mali, September–November 1987 (Unpublished Report). Geneva, World Health Organization, 1988.

602. World Health Organization. Yellow fever in 1991. Wkly Epidemiol Rec 68:209, 1993.

603. World Health Organization. Yellow fever. Wkly Epidemiol Rec 69:243, 1994.

604. Draper CC. A yellow fever vaccine free from avian leucosis viruses. J Hyg (Camb) 65:505, 1967.

605. Tauraso NM, Myers MG, Nau EV, et al. Effect of interval between inoculation of live smallpox and yellow-fever vaccines on antigenicity in man. J Infect Dis 126:362, 1972.

606. Bancroft WH Jr, Scott R McN, Eckels KH, et al. Dengue virus type 2 vaccine: reactogenicity and immunogenicity in soldiers. J Infect Dis 149:1005, 1984.

607. Georges AJ, Tible F, Meunier DMY, et al. Thermostability and efficacy in the field of a new, stabilized yellow fever virus vaccine. Vaccine 3:313, 1985.

608. Roche JC, Jouan A, Brisou B, et al. Comparative clinical study of a new 17D thermostable yellow fever vaccine. Vaccine 4:163, 1986.

609. Lhuillier M, Mazzariol MJ, Zadi S, et al. Study of combined vaccination against yellow fever and measles in infants from six to nine months. J Biol Stand 17:9, 1989.

610. Soula G, Sylla A, Pichard E. Ètude d'un nouveau vaccin combiné contre la fièvre jaune et la rougeole chez des enfants agés de 6 a 24 mois au Mali. Bull Soc Pathol Exot 84:885, 1991.

611. Jackson J, Dworkin R, Tsai T, et al. Bioject® injection vs. needle/syringe injection of yellow fever vaccine: comparison of antibody response [abstr]. *In* Abstracts of the 3rd International Conference on Travel Medicine, Paris, April 25–29, 1993.

612. Receveur MC, Quiniou JM, Delprat P, et al. Vaccination simultanée contre l'hepatite A et la fièvre jaune. Bull Soc Pathol Exot 86:406–409, 1993.

613. Coursaget P, Fritzell B, Blondeau C, et al. Simultaneous injection of plasma-derived or recombinant hepatitis B vaccines with yellow fever and killed polio vaccines. Vaccine 13:109, 1995.

614. Guerra HL, Sardinha TM, Travassos da Rosa APA, et al. Efetividade de vacina antiamarilica 17D: uma avaliação epidemiológica em serviços de saúde. Am J Public Health 2:115, 1997.

615. Dumas R, Forrat R, Lang J. Safety and immunogenicity of a new inactivated hepatitis A vaccine and concurrent administration with a typhoid fever vaccine or a typhoid fever + yellow fever vaccine. Adv Ther 14:160, 1997.

616. Osei-Kwasi M, Dunyo SK, Koram KA, et al. Antibody response to 17D yellow fever vaccine in Ghanaian infants. Bull World Health Organ 79:1056, 2001.

617. Swift S. Encephalitis after yellow fever vaccination. Br Med J 2:677, 1955.

618. Lartigaut M, Couteau M. Encéphalite bénigne après vaccination contre la fièvre jaune par le vaccine atténuée en tissu embryonnaire. J Med Bordeaux 121:506, 1954.

619. Smith JH. Encephalitis in an infant after vaccination with 17 D yellow fever virus. Br Med J 2:852, 1954.

620. Haas L. Encephalitis after yellow-fever vaccination. Br Med J 2:992, 1954.

621. Scott LG. Encephalitis after yellow fever vaccination. Br Med J 2:1108, 1954.

622. Beet EA. Encephalitis after yellow fever vaccination. Br Med J 1:226, 1955.

623. Lartigaut M, Lartigaut D. Encéphalite vaccinale du nourrisson après vaccination contre la fièvre jaune. J Med Bordeaux 131;1388, 1954.

624. de Castro Friere L. Meningoencephalite post vaccinação contra febre amarela. Rev Post Pediatr 18:65, 1955.

625. Feitel M, Watson EH, Cochran KW. Encephalitis after yellow fever vaccination. Pediatrics 78:956, 1960.

626. Schoub BD, Dommann CJ, Johnson S, et al. Encephalitis in a 13-year-old boy following 17D yellow fever vaccine. J Infect 21:105, 1990.

627. Drouet A, Chagnon A, Valence J, et al. Meningoencephalite après vaccination anti-amarile par la souche 17D: deux observations. Rev Med Interne 124:257, 1993.

628. Centers for Disease Control. Adverse events associated with 17D-derived yellow fever vaccination—United States 2001–2002. Morb Mortal Wkly Rep 51:989, 2002.

629. Ruben FL, Smith EA, Foster SO. Simultaneous administration of smallpox, measles, yellow fever, and diphtheria-pertussis-tetanus antigens to Nigerian children. Bull World Health Organ 48:175, 1973.

630. Gateff C, Relyveld EH, Le Gonidec G, et al. Étude d'une nouvelle association vaccinale quintuple. Ann Microbiol (Paris) 124B:387–409, 1973.

631. Gil A, González A, Dal-Ré R, et al. Interference assessment of yellow fever vaccine with the immune response to a single-dose inactivated hepatitis A vaccine (1440 E.U.): a controlled study in adults. Vaccine 14:1028, 1996.

632. Bovier PA, Althaus B, Glueck R, et al. Tolerance and immunogenicity of the simultaneous administration of virosome hepatitis A and yellow fever vaccines. J Travel Med 6:228, 1999.

633. Bock HL, Kruppenbacher JP, Bienzle U, et al. Does the concurrent administration of an inactivated hepatitis A vaccine influence the immune response to other travelers vaccines? J Travel Med 7:74, 2000.

634. Jong EC, Kaplan KM, Eves KA, et al. An open randomized study of inactivated hepatitis A vaccine administered concomitantly with typhoid fever and yellow fever vaccines. J Travel Med 9:66, 2002.

Chapter 41

Technologies for Making New Vaccines

RONALD W. ELLIS

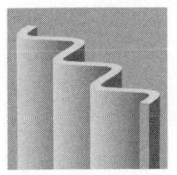 The number of technological approaches for making new vaccines has been growing rapidly for over 20 years. These developments stem from advances in a broad range of interrelated fields, including recombinant DNA (rDNA) and molecular biology, analytic biochemistry, protein and polysaccharide chemistry, fermentation, macromolecular purification, formulation, virology, bacteriology, and immunology. Most technical applications have been directed toward developing new vaccines for diseases not previously approachable by immunologic interventions. The vast majority of available vaccines have been directed to the prevention (prophylaxis) of infectious diseases rather than therapy of infected or diseased individuals. However, new technologies have extended this scope to vaccines for noninfectious diseases (e.g., autoimmune diseases and cancer) and therapeutic vaccines (e.g., certain infectious diseases, autoimmune diseases, cancer, and allergy). As a result, such successes are redefining the term *vaccine*.

There are two broad categories of vaccination, *active* and *passive*. Active vaccination stimulates the immune system to produce specific antibodies or cellular immune responses or both, which would protect against, ameliorate, or eliminate a disease. Passive vaccination utilizes a preparation of antibodies that neutralizes a pathogen or binds to a human cellular antigen and that is administered before or around the time of known or potential exposure or to a subject with disease or infection. References to the term *vaccine* generally refer to active vaccines, which are the subject of the great majority of research and development investigations in the field as well as the bulk of discussion in this chapter. Establishing lasting immunity through the administration of an active vaccine is a most important means of preventive medicine. Nevertheless, passive vaccination is desirable or essential in specific instances, particularly if no active vaccine is available or feasible, for immunocompromised individuals, for cancer treatment, or for the immediate efficacy of immunotherapy.

Vaccines are stored in solution (liquid or frozen) or in freeze-dried (lyophilized) form, depending on their stability and physical characteristics; the former are preferred for the convenience of the end user. Lyophilized vaccines are resuspended in diluent (resuspending fluid) at around the time of administration. The vaccine solution and diluent may contain the following additives: (1) preservatives or antibiotics to prevent bacterial growth; (2) stabilizers, including proteins or other organic compounds, to extend the dating period or shelf life for the product; (3) adjuvants for enhancing immune responses (see *Adjuvants* below); and (4) delivery systems for presenting the vaccine antigen(s) to appropriate cells of the immune system or preserving antigen(s) in vivo (see *Delivery Systems* below). The vaccine molecules and added components comprise the *vaccine formulation*.

This chapter summarizes the major technologies, key issues associated with their development, and immunologic objectives underlying different kinds of vaccines, with appropriate examples of specific vaccine types. The status of development of key vaccines made by each approach is identified, whether licensed or in clinical or preclinical evaluations (Table 41–1). Although most common licensed vaccines are discussed, not every possible approach is documented in this chapter. Most examples are for viruses and bacteria, but there also are licensed vaccines and noteworthy new developments for noninfectious diseases such as autoimmune diseases and cancer. The technologies and examples should provide the reader with a strong framework for appreciating the increasing diversity of approaches being taken to the research and development of vaccines for new targets that had not been approachable previously.

Active Vaccines

The protective immunity elicited by an active vaccine ideally would be lifelong and robust after a single or few doses with minimal side effects (reactogenicity). Available vaccines as well as those under development generally fall short of this ideal, which continues to stimulate new research initiatives in this field.

There are three general categories of active vaccines, whose salient features are outlined in Table 41–2. A *live*

TABLE 41–1 ■ Status of Development of Representative Human Vaccines Made by Different Technologies

Type of Vaccine[a]	Status of development[b]			Example[f]	Reference
	Preclinical Evaluation[c]	Clinical Evaluation[d]	Licensed Product[e]		
			ACTIVE		

Live
Classical virus

Type of Vaccine[a]	Preclinical Evaluation[c]	Clinical Evaluation[d]	Licensed Product[e]	Example[f]	Reference
Attenuation in cell culture			xx	Poliovirus	1
			xx	Measles virus	2
			xx	Mumps virus	3
			xx	Rubella virus	4
			x	Varicella-zoster virus (VZV)	5
Variants from other species			xx	Smallpox (vaccinia virus)	7
		x		Rotavirus	8
Reassorted genomes		x[g]		Rotavirus	9
		x		Influenza virus	11
Temperature-selected mutants		x		Influenza virus	13
		x		Respiratory syncytial virus (RSV)	14
Recombinant virus		x		Herpes simplex virus (HSV)	15, 16
Recombinant viral vector		x		Vaccinia virus[h]	18–20
		x		Adenovirus[i]	24, 138
Classical bacteria			xx	Tuberculosis (bacille Calmette-Guérin [BCG])	25
		x		Bladder cancer (BCG)	26
		x		Typhoid fever (Salmonella typhi)	27, 28
Recombinant bacteria		x		Cholera (Vibrio cholerae)	29
		x		Shigella	30
Recombinant bacterial vector		x		S. typhi[j]	31
		x		V. cholerae[j]	32
		x		Shigella flexneri[j]	33
		x		Streptococcus gordonii	37
	x			Listeria monocytogenes	34
	x			BCG	35
Dendritic cells		x		Melanoma	39
		x		Bladder cancer	40
	x			Autoimmunity	41

Inactivated/Subunit
Whole pathogen

Type of Vaccine[a]	Preclinical Evaluation[c]	Clinical Evaluation[d]	Licensed Product[e]	Example[f]	Reference
Inactivated bacteria			xx	Pertussis (Bordetella pertussis)	43
		x		Cholera	44
	xx			Enterotoxigenic Escherichia coli	45
Inactivated virus			xx	Poliovirus	46
			xx	Influenza virus	47
		x		Rabies virus	48
		x		Japanese encephalitis virus	49
			xx	Hepatitis A virus	42, 50
Whole cell		x		Melanoma	52
		x		Multiple myeloma	54
Protein based					
Natural			xx	Hepatitis B virus (HBV)	59
			xx	Pertussis	60–62
		x		Cancer	63
Chemically inactivated			xx	Tetanus (Clostridium tetani)	64
			xx	Diphtheria (Corynebacterium diphtheriae)	65
			xx	Pertussis	66
Genetically inactivated			x	Pertussis	67
		x		Diphtheria	68
Recombinant polypeptide			xx	HBV	69
		x		Lyme disease (Borrelia burgdorferi)	72
		x		Cholera	135
		xx		Human papillomavirus	71, 79
		xx		Human immunodeficiency virus (HIV)	73
		xx		HSV	74
		x		Allergy	75

TABLE 41–1 ■ Status of Development of Representative Human Vaccines Made by Different Technologies—Cont'd

Type of Vaccine[a]	Status of development[b] Preclinical Evaluation[c]	Clinical Evaluation[d]	Licensed Product[e]	Example[f]	Reference
ACTIVE					
		×		Diabetes	76, 77
	×			Fertility	78
Peptide based					
B-cell epitope					
Aggregate		×		Alzheimer's disease	81
Fusion protein		×		Malaria[k]	82
Conjugate		×		Malaria[l]	84
		×		Fertility[l]	85
		×		Pancreatic cancer[l]	86
		××		Non–small cell lung carcinoma[l]	87
Complex peptide	×			Malaria	89
Mimetopes	×			Cancer	91
	×			HIV	92
T-cell epitope					
CTL epitope		×		HBV	93
T-cell receptor			×	Multiple sclerosis	95
Carbohydrate and polysaccharide based					
Polysaccharide			×	*Haemophilus influenzae* type b (Hib)	96
			××	Meningococcal (*Neisseria meningitidis*)	97
			××	Pneumococcal (*Streptococcus pneumoniae*)	98
Polysaccharide conjugate			××	Hib[m]	99
			××	Pneumococcal[n]	100
		×		Group B streptococcal (*Streptococcus agalactiae*)[l]	102
Carbohydrate		×		Ovarian, breast cancer	103
		×		Melanoma	104
Anti-idiotype (antibodies)		×		Breast cancer	107
		×		Schistosome	108
Other		×		Cocaine	109
DNA-based					
Naked DNA		×		Influenza	112
		×		HIV	139
Facilitated DNA		×		HIV	116
		×		Metastatic renal cell carcinoma	117
	×			Influenza	114
Viral vector	×			Cancer	119
Viral delivery	×			Fowlpox virus[o]	120
		×		Canarypox virus[o]	121, 136
Bacterial delivery	×			*S. flexneri*	122
PASSIVE (ANTIBODIES)					
Polyclonal					
Human immune globulin (IG)			×	HBV (HBIG)	141
			×	VZV (VZIG)	142
			×	Cytomegalovirus (CMVIG)	143
			×	RSV (RSVIG)	144
			×	Tetanus (TIG)	146
Antibody fragment			×	Digoxin	145
Monoclonal					
Nonhuman		××		Ovarian cancer	150
Natural human		×		Cytomegalovirus	151
Cytomegalovirus		×		Melanoma	152
Recombinant human					
Human derived		×		HIV	153
		×		*Candida albicans*	155
Mouse derived		×		Colorectal and kidney cancer	157

Continued

TABLE 41–1 ■ Status of Development of Representative Human Vaccines Made by Different Technologies—Cont'd

Type of Vaccine[a]	Status of development[b]			Example[f]	Reference
	Preclinical Evaluation[c]	Clinical Evaluation[d]	Licensed Product[e]		
ACTIVE					
Recombinant humanized			×	RSV	160
			×	Breast cancer	147
		××		Allergy	161
Recombinant chimeric			×	Non-Hodgkin's lymphoma	148

[a]These categories are presented in the same order as in the text.
[b]This denotes the single most advanced status achieved by each example.
[c]Not yet evaluated in a human clinical trial.
[d]In clinical trial but not yet licensed; "××" denotes large-scale or Phase III trials on the path to licensure.
[e]Licensed in one or more major countries in the world; "××" denotes widespread use in multiple countries.
[f]These are representative examples for each vaccine strategy and not a comprehensive list of all examples, with key reference(s) illustrative of each example.
[g]Withdrawn post licensure.
[h]Expressing more than 50 different foreign polypeptides, especially including human immunodeficiency virus (HIV) and colorectal cancer.
[i]Expressing foreign polypeptides, including HIV-1 gag and env genes.
[j]Expressing foreign polypeptides include toxoids from Escherichia coli, Vibrio cholerae, and Clostridium tetani and cancer-specific antigens.
[k]Fusion partner is HBsAg.
[l]Conjugate carrier is TT.
[m]Conjugate carriers are TT, DT, CRM$_{197}$, and an outer membrane protein complex.
[n]Conjugate carrier is CRM$_{197}$.
[o]Expressing foreign polypeptides, especially including HIV.
CTL, cytotoxic T lymphocyte; DT, diphtheria toxin; HBsAg, hepatitis B surface antigen; TT, tetanus toxoid.

vaccine generally is a microorganism that can replicate on its own in the host or can infect cells and function as an immunogen without causing its natural disease; there also is a specialized example using live cells of the immune system. An *inactivated* or *subunit* vaccine is an immunogen that cannot replicate in the host. A *nucleic acid–based* vaccine (usually DNA), which likewise cannot replicate in humans, is taken up by cells, in which it directs the synthesis of the vaccine antigen(s). (The term *immunogen* refers to the property of eliciting an immune response, whereas the term *antigen* denotes the property of in vitro immunologic reactivity.)

The strategic choice for developing a live, inactivated/subunit, or DNA-based vaccine should take into account the pathogenesis, epidemiology, and immunobiology of the infection or disease in question as well as the technical feasibility of the various alternative vaccine designs. Epidemiology dictates the target population for the vaccine. The age and state of health of this population may favor certain designs as more appropriate for eliciting protective immunity. In the example of a vaccine intended for healthy infants, minimal reactogenicity is very important, and certain types of vaccines are useless because they do not

TABLE 41–2 ■ Comparative Properties of Active Vaccines

Characteristics	Advantages	Challenges
LIVE VACCINES		
• Able to replicate in the host • Attenuated in pathogenicity • Elicit antibodies and cell-mediated immunity	• May elicit broader immune responses • May require fewer doses • Generally longer lasting protection	• Uncertain window for attenuation • Uncertain safety before large-scale use • Stability • Analysis
SUBUNIT, INACTIVATED VACCINES		
• Unable to replicate in the host • Elicit mostly antibodies	• Cannot multiply or revert to pathogenicity • Generally less reactogenic • Nontransmissible to another person • Usually more feasible technically	• May require adjuvant • May require delivery system • Immunogenic potency • Variable efficacy
GENETIC VACCINES (DNA BASED)		
• Stimulate synthesis of antigens only in cells • Elicit mostly cell-mediated immunity	• Standardized method of production and analysis • Sustained immunologic stimulation	• Establishing proof-of-principal • Immunogenic potency

elicit protective immunity (see *Plain Polysaccharides* below). However, the degree of reactogenicity is far less important in the case of a therapeutic cancer vaccine. Populations at high risk for a given disease (e.g., drug addicts at risk for hepatitis B) may not be amenable to accepting or seeking vaccination; in such cases, an effective public health strategy has become the vaccination of groups (e.g., children) that are readily accessible to widespread vaccination. Knowledge of immunobiology should enable the identification of the type(s) of immunity that should be elicited by the vaccine; certain immune responses would be protective and others useless (even detrimental) to the prevention or treatment of a particular disease. The study of immunobiology is greatly facilitated (made possible in some cases) by developing an experimental animal model, the availability of which enables candidate vaccines to be tested and optimized for protective efficacy before bringing the best one(s) forward for clinical evaluation. Historically, only a limited range of technical designs has been feasible for a particular vaccine. Nevertheless, considering the expanding number of technical approaches, it should be possible in the foreseeable future to custom-design many vaccines for optimal efficacy and tolerability.

Live Vaccines

Some live vaccines are close to ideal in their capability to elicit lifelong protection in one or two doses with minimal reactogenicity. Such vaccines may be feasible in cases where the natural infection or disease confers lifelong protection on the host. Live vaccines (with the exception of dendritic cell vaccines; see *Dendritic Cells as Autologous Vaccines* below) consist of viruses or bacteria that replicate in the host in a fashion resembling that of the natural microorganism; hence the vaccine can elicit an immune response similar to that elicited by the natural infection. The live vaccine is attenuated, its disease-causing capacity having been virtually eliminated by biologic or technical manipulations. The live vaccine should be neither overattenuated (no longer infectious enough to function as a vaccine) nor underattenuated (retaining pathogenicity even to a limited extent). Live vaccines usually elicit both humoral immunity (antibodies) and cellular immunity (e.g., cytotoxic T-lymphocytes [CTLs]).

Although these attributes would appear to make it desirable that all active vaccines be live vaccines, this is not technically feasible for most vaccines under development. The balance between incomplete attenuation (and consequent disease-causing capability) and complete attenuation (inadequately immunogenic) is delicate and, for some viruses or bacteria, technically unachievable at present. Because a live vaccine can replicate, it may be possible for it to revert to its more naturally pathogenic form, unless there are multiple attenuating mutations. Moreover, some live vaccines can be transmitted from the vaccinee to a nonimmunized individual, which can be quite serious if the recipient has an immune deficiency (e.g., has acquired immunodeficiency syndrome or is undergoing cancer chemotherapy). In cases where the natural viral infection per se fails to induce a protective immune response, an attenuated virus would not be expected to produce a protective response. Finally, there have been two recent examples of licensed live vaccines having been withdrawn from distribution.

Classical Virus Vaccines

The term *classical* refers to technical strategies that do not utilize rDNA technology.

ATTENUATION IN CELL CULTURE

The production of live viral vaccines depends on efficiently propagating the virus in cell culture. The first classical strategy became possible during the 1950s with the advent of modern cell culture. The approach is empirical, in that the wild-type virus isolated from a natural human infection is passaged in vitro through one or more cell types that the virus ordinarily does not encounter in vivo, with the goal of attenuating its pathogenicity. In such cases, there may be competitive pressure to produce less damage to cells. (In contrast, a strategy to increase pathogenicity is to passage a viral or bacterial strain serially in vivo.) The mechanism by which mutation(s) are introduced during the course of attenuation is not always well understood or documented. In some cases (e.g., poliovirus[1]), it has been possible to demonstrate attenuation in a primate species, whereas in most cases attenuation has been proven only through the course of extensive clinical trials. The success of this empirical approach, which has been applied both to an oral vaccine (oral poliovirus vaccine[1]) and to injected (parenteral) vaccines (measles,[2] mumps,[3] rubella,[4] varicella[5]), has been borne out by the significant number of available licensed vaccines. The reactogenicity of such vaccines has been low enough that some of them (polio, measles) are broadly accepted worldwide for routine pediatric use. By means of intensive immunization programs with oral poliovirus vaccine, polio is approaching worldwide eradication. As a striking example of the challenge to proving attenuation, the Urabe strain of mumps virus was licensed after showing apparent safety in clinical trials. It then was observed, after several years of use in millions of children, that vaccination with this strain could cause aseptic meningitis at a rate of approximately 1 in 10,000 vaccinees[6]; given the availability of an alternative mumps vaccine without this effect, this strain was withdrawn from use in several countries.

VARIANTS FROM OTHER SPECIES

An animal virus that causes a veterinary disease similar to a human disease can be isolated and cultivated, anticipating that the animal virus will be attenuated for humans yet be sufficiently related to elicit protective immunity to the human virus. Smallpox, the first vaccine, is the prototype of this vaccine type. Two hundred years ago, Jenner first appreciated that individuals intentionally exposed to cowpox were resistant to smallpox, so he used the cowpox agent (vaccinia virus) for human vaccination against smallpox (caused by variola virus). The immunization program was applied worldwide using vaccinia virus[7] and resulted in the complete eradication of smallpox worldwide by the mid-1970s; this is the only infectious disease ever eradicated. This program is a tribute to the tireless efforts of countless individuals and to an effective control strategy. Unfortunately, the vaccine has had to re-enter production as a safeguard against the dissemination of variola virus as a weapon of bioterrorism.

Based on this model, first-generation vaccines for rotavirus consisted of nonreassortant animal viruses isolated from rhesus monkeys[8] and cows. However, such rotavirus vaccines were not reproducibly efficacious as human vaccines and were abandoned as development candidates.

REASSORTED GENOMES

A reassortant virus, which contains genes from two parental viruses, is derived following co-infection of a cell with two viruses with segmented genomes. To improve the efficacy of animal rotaviruses, reassortant rotaviruses were isolated that contained mostly animal rotavirus genes, which confer the attenuation phenotype for humans, as well as the gene(s) for human rotavirus surface protein(s) that elicit serotype-specific neutralizing antibodies for human rotavirus.[9,10] These reassortant rotaviruses have elicited higher efficacy rates as vaccine candidates than their non-reassortant parental animal viruses. The same approach has been applied to influenza vaccines, in which a virulent human influenza virus provides the genes that encode the immunogenic surface glycoproteins (hemagglutinin and neuraminidase), and an attenuated virus provides all other genes and, with them, the attenuation phenotype.[11]

The quadrivalent reassortant rhesus rotavirus vaccine[9] is another example of the challenge in establishing the attenuation profile of a live vaccine. After 1 year of commercial distribution in the United States, it was observed that the vaccine caused an increased incidence of intussusception of approximately 1 in 10,000 vaccinees immediately postvaccination. Although the overall risk/benefit ratio remained very high, the vaccine was withdrawn from distribution.

TEMPERATURE-SENSITIVE MUTANTS

Viral mutants can be selected according to their relative growth properties at different temperatures. Such viruses are called temperature-sensitive (ts), being unable to grow at elevated temperatures, or cold-adapted (ca), having been selected for growth in vitro at lower than physiologic (37°C) temperatures (i.e., down to 25°C). The strategy behind this approach is that ca or ts viruses will be less vigorous in their in vivo growth than their wild-type parental virus, hence less virulent and phenotypically attenuated. A ca influenza vaccine based on reassortants[11] has been evaluated extensively in clinical studies.[12] This vaccine is noteworthy in that it has been developed for intranasal administration. A ca influenza vaccine has been used widely in Russia,[13] and a double ts respiratory syncytial virus (RSV) vaccine has been tested clinically.[14] The use of a double mutant (i.e., one that contains two independent mutations) is an additional refinement resulting in a much lower frequency of reversion to wild-type virulence than for a single mutant.

Recombinant Virus Vaccines

Specific modifications or deletions can be made in viral genes so that the virus is more stably attenuated, that is, highly unlikely or unable to revert to virulence. The increased stability of the attenuation phenotype results from making the modification(s) extensive enough that reversion through back-mutation is impossible or highly unlikely. In contrast, attenuated viruses derived by classical strategies may have only point mutations and therefore

retain the capability to revert. Herpes simplex virus (HSV) has been genetically engineered[15] to be attenuated, to provide for antibody markers of vaccination that are differentiable from those of wild-type HSV infection, and to protect against both types 1 and 2 virus (HSV-1 and HSV-2). In another example, a particular HSV glycoprotein gene was deleted, resulting in an HSV strain that cannot replicate; this recombinant virus is produced in vitro in a cell line that supplies the deleted glycoprotein gene in trans, and the resultant virus can initiate infection in vivo without being able to replicate further.[16]

Recombinant Viral Vector Vaccines

rDNA technology also has been applied to developing novel live vaccines that have been engineered into carriers or vectors of foreign polypeptide antigens from other pathogens. The strategy in creating such vectors is to present the foreign antigen to the immune system in the context of a live virus infection in order to stimulate the immune system to respond to the antigen as a live immunogen, thereby developing broader immunity (humoral and cellular) to the corresponding human pathogen. The foreign polypeptide is expressed within the infected cell and either is transported to the cell surface to stimulate antibody production or is broken down into peptides, which are transported to the cell surface where they may elicit CTL responses. This strategy also has the potential advantage of amplification of the immunogenic signal when the live vector initiates multiple rounds of replication. If the vector virus is a commonly used vaccine, one could immunize simultaneously against the vector virus and another pathogen, ideally in a single dose. However, the immune response to the live viral vector per se ordinarily would limit the effectiveness of revaccination.[17]

The prototype viral vector is vaccinia virus, in which dozens of foreign polypeptides have been expressed.[18] Immunization of animals in at least 25 different animal infection models have protected against the pathogen encoding the foreign polypeptide. Recombinant vaccinia virus expressing human immunodeficiency virus type 1 (HIV-1) glycoprotein (gp) 160 has been tested clinically[19] for prophylactic and therapeutic applications. Recombinant vaccinia viruses expressing tumor antigens have been shown to be protective in rodent tumor model challenge studies, and a vector expressing carcinoembryonic antigen has been evaluated clinically for colorectal cancer.[20]

Given the known sequelae to immunization for smallpox (which are more serious in immunocompromised individuals) observed in the worldwide eradication program, vaccinia virus itself has been engineered to reduce its virulence without compromising its efficacy as a live viral vector.[21,22] Two other members of the poxvirus family, fowlpox and canarypox viruses, are being developed as naturally attenuated live virus vectors that can infect human cells but not produce infectious viral progeny. This inability to spread makes fowlpox and canarypox viral vectors classifiable as DNA-based vaccines (see Viral DNA Vaccine Delivery below).

Other mammalian viruses have been engineered into live vectors. Adenovirus, which has been used extensively in vaccines in military recruits to prevent acute respiratory disease, has been engineered to express foreign polypeptides and has elicited protective immunity in several viral challenge models in animals.[23] As described above, HSV also has been engineered into a live vector.[15] Optimizing foreign polypeptide expression for all these live viral vectors remains an important technical objective.

RNA viruses also can be engineered into vectors for expressing foreign polypeptides. Sindbis and other alphaviruses have received extensive attention because of their broad host range, ability to infect nondividing cells, and potential high-level expression per cell.[24] On this basis, Sindbis virus has been developed into a viral vector–based vaccine (see *Viral DNA Vector Vaccines* below).

Classical Bacterial Vaccines

It has been difficult to develop live, attenuated bacterial vaccines by classical strategies, because there has been relatively little success in culturing bacteria for attenuation while maintaining immunogenicity and because of reversion. There also may not be strong competitive or selective pressure for bacteria to become less virulent through genetic changes in vitro; bacteria could stop expressing virulence factors in vitro, then turn such expression back on in vivo. The one widely available live bacterial vaccine based on serial in vitro passage is for tuberculosis (TB) and cancer. This vaccine is a live, attenuated strain of *Mycobacterium bovis*, also known as bacille Calmette-Guérin (BCG).[25] Early in the 20th century, this bovine strain was attenuated by 231 successive in vitro subculturings over 13 years. There are many strains of BCG vaccine available worldwide that are derived from the original strain isolated in the early 20th century. These vaccines vary in terms of tolerability, immunogenicity, and rate of protective efficacy for TB in clinical trials (range of 0% to 80% protection) for reasons that may relate to the actual vaccine strains used or to differences in study populations. BCG vaccines have been inoculated into more than 3 billion people worldwide and have generally acceptable tolerability profiles. BCG vaccines also have been administered orally (see *Recombinant Bacterial Vector Vaccines* below). Following the observation that TB patients have reduced rates of cancer, BCG vaccine was developed into a vaccine for the treatment of superficial bladder cancer by intravesicular instillation.[26] BCG vaccine also has been employed as an adjuvant for the priming doses of a killed whole-cell melanoma vaccine (see *Whole Human Cell Vaccines* below).

Chemical mutagenesis followed by selection was employed to derive the attenuated Ty21a strain of *Salmonella typhi*.[27] This vaccine was licensed for preventing typhoid fever based on its record of safety and efficacy (~60% for several years) after a regimen of three to four doses.[28]

rDNA technology would be expected to be applied to attenuating any new bacterial strain that had promise as a live, attenuated vaccine. Therefore, it seems highly unlikely that a new live bacterial vaccine attenuated by a classical strategy alone will be developed.

Recombinant Bacterial Vaccines

The engineering of bacteria for attenuation is much more complex than the engineering of viruses because bacterial genomes are approximately 100-fold larger than those of viruses. The strategy for attenuation, like that for viruses, is to identify the gene(s) responsible for the virulence of the bacteria or for their ability to colonize and survive in particular tissue(s) in the host and to either eliminate the gene (preferred) or abolish or modulate its in vivo expression. As is the case for modification mutants of viruses, there usually is a balance between the virulence of a bacterial strain and its activity as a vaccine, which means that it is possible to overattenuate a bacterial strain to the point that it no longer replicates sufficiently in vivo to be effectively immunogenic.

Given that infection by *Vibrio cholerae* can protect against subsequent disease, *V. cholerae* strains have been developed as live cholera vaccines. Attenuation of these cholera strains has been accomplished by the rDNA-directed deletion of genes encoding virulence factors (e.g., cholera toxin [CT]).[29] Live, attenuated cholera vaccine candidates prepared in this fashion have been evaluated clinically, and one has been licensed. In order to assure attenuation by reducing the probability of reversion, it is desirable to delete at least two independent genes or genetic loci that contribute to virulence.

There have been attempts to develop *Shigella* strains into live vaccines by mutating particular chromosomal or plasmid-based genes in order to reduce pathogenicity.[30]

Recombinant Bacterial Vector Vaccines

Suitable strains of pathogenic bacteria have been engineered into live vectors for expressing foreign polypeptides. The most common development has been to engineer enteric pathogens for inducing mucosal immunity against the foreign polypeptide following oral delivery. *Salmonella typhi* vectors have been the most commonly developed strains in terms of immunology, molecular design, and clinical testing.[31] Strains of *V. cholerae*[32], *Shigella flexneri*[33] and *Listeria monocytogenes*[34] have been engineered likewise. The challenge for these vectors is to retain sufficient virulence for replication in the gut as well as to express appropriate levels of foreign polypeptides while achieving sufficient attenuation. The BCG vaccine strain also has been engineered as a live vector to express foreign polypeptides[35]; one aspect of the versatility of BCG is its efficacy in mice by different routes of administration (oral, intranasal, and intradermal).[36] The ability of some bacterial species to replicate intracellularly may augment the ability of expressed foreign polypeptides to elicit cellular immune responses against their respective pathogens.

Streptococcus gordonii, a Gram-positive commensal (nonpathogenic) bacteria, has been engineered to express foreign polypeptides on its surface by genetic fusion to attachment sequences of *S. gordonii* M protein.[37] One significant challenge is whether the foreign polypeptides will be sufficiently immunogenic, given that this bacterial species does not elicit an immune response that clears them naturally.

Dendritic Cells as Autologous Vaccines

Dendritic cells (DC) can be exploited as potent professional antigen-presenting cells for tumor-specific antigens. In this application, DCs are isolated from the patient and mixed ex vivo with tumor antigens. DCs ingest and process the antigens and re-express them on the DC surface. The cells then are reintroduced into the patient for antigen presentation and immune stimulation of T cells.[38] This approach has shown promise for melanoma[39] and bladder cancer.[40]

Because autoimmune diseases are characterized by the loss of immunologic tolerance to self-antigenic determinants, it may be possible to exploit DCs as antigen-presenting cells to achieve tolerance, as has been demonstrated in animal and in vitro models of diabetes, multiple sclerosis, and autoimmune encephalitis.[41]

Inactivated/Subunit Vaccines

Inactivated and subunit vaccines have certain advantages relating to their inability to multiply (see Table 41–2). Such vaccines are generally well tolerated, especially those that are purified to remove other macromolecules. Given the broad range of available approaches, it also is generally more technically feasible to produce an inactivated or subunit vaccine. The immunogenicity of such vaccines often is enhanced by administration with an adjuvant or delivery system (see *Formulation of Antigens* below). Nevertheless, any development program for this type of vaccine should acknowledge that multiple doses, often followed by booster doses, usually are necessary for attaining long-term protective immunity. In an exceptional case, short-term protection has been demonstrated following a single dose.[42] These vaccines usually function by stimulating humoral immune responses and by priming for immunologic memory. Such vaccines may stimulate CTL immunity when administered with certain adjuvants and delivery systems.

Whole-Pathogen Vaccines

The earliest technology in the 20th century was the only one technically feasible at that time, when there was little definition of specific antigens and their role in immunity. The inactivation of whole bacteria or whole viruses had the objective of eliciting the formation of antibodies to many antigens, from which some antibodies would neutralize the pathogen.

BACTERIAL

These vaccines are prepared by cultivating the bacteria (e.g., *Bordetella pertussis*), then collecting and inactivating the whole bacterial cells with heat or chemical agents (e.g., thimerosal or phenol).[43] The vaccine does not undergo further purification. Owing to their biochemically highly crude nature, the reactogenicity of such vaccines when given parenterally is usually greater than that of other types of vaccines. However, inactivated whole-cell *V. cholerae*[44] and enterotoxigenic *Escherichia coli* (ETEC)[45] vaccines have been well tolerated by the oral route. Even though the latter vaccine is now under active development, it seems less likely that new bacterial vaccines will be made in this fashion, given the number of alternative technologies available for preparing purified vaccines and the more exacting regulatory standards that have developed over time.

VIRAL

Inactivated viral vaccines likewise have been available for up to several decades, and are usually very well tolerated. Viruses generally are shed into cell culture media. Therefore, cell-free media from infected cultures are collected, and the large size of the virus particles relative to

other macromolecules in the media enables the particles to be enriched readily by simple purification techniques. Examples include poliovirus,[46] influenza virus,[47] rabies virus,[48] and Japanese encephalitis virus.[49] Alternatively, in the case of killed hepatitis A virus vaccine, infected cells are lysed, and virus particles are purified.[50] The virus particles are inactivated chemically, typically by treatment with formalin, and then may be adjuvanted by adsorption onto an aluminum salt. The key epitope(s) on the surface of many nonenveloped small viruses that elicit a protective immune response (protective epitope[s]) is often conformational, being formed by the highly ordered assembly of viral proteins into precise structures. For most of the viruses from which inactivated vaccines have been developed,[46–50] it may not be possible to mimic the conformation of such epitopes by other technologies (e.g., recombinant polypeptides). Inactivated viral vaccines tend to be highly potent immunogens. Thus this classical strategy, which has had an excellent track record of producing well-tolerated and efficacious vaccines, remains the technology of choice for many viral vaccines.

Whole Human Cell Vaccines

There are a variety of designs for cancer vaccines. Some of these are based on the use of individual tumor-specific antigens, either purified or expressed as part of a vector. A concern from using individual antigens in a vaccine is that the induced immune response following vaccination or administration of antibodies may stimulate antigenic modulation and diminished expression of the target antigen or loss of major histocompatibility complex class I expression or loss of other T-cell receptor–associated signaling, thereby reducing efficacy. The use of inactivated allogeneic whole tumor cells as a vaccine affords the opportunity to present a wide array of tumor-specific antigens to the immune system. Tumor cell lines are expanded in vitro, pooled (if more than one line is used), and inactivated. Vaccination with one such melanoma vaccine, pooled from three tumor cell lines and using BCG as adjuvant in its first two doses, significantly increases the survival of stage 3 and 4 melanoma patients,[51] and another such melanoma vaccine, pooled from two tumor cell lines and given with a synthetic adjuvant, has been licensed.[52]

Cells also can be genetically modified to express immunomodulators that may enhance antitumor immune responses. Irradiation of cells transduced with the recombinant vector renders them unable to proliferate yet still able to secrete the immunomodulator. Autologous melanoma cells were transduced with a recombinant adenovirus expressing granulocyte-macrophage colony-stimulating factor; cells then were irradiated and reinfused to melanoma patients, resulting in an antitumor effect.[53] Likewise, autologous plasma cells were transduced with recombinant adenovirus expressing interleukin-2; cells then were irradiated and reinfused to patients with multiple myeloma.[54]

Protein-Based Vaccines

Developing a (purified) protein-based vaccine is the favored strategy for many pathogens in which polypeptides contain protective epitopes, given the above-mentioned issues regarding inactivated bacterial vaccines and when an inactivated viral vaccine is technically unfeasible.

Protein-based approaches have relied on genetic, biochemical, and immunologic analyses to identify the specificity of protective antibodies and their corresponding polypeptides. More recently, genomics technology has enabled the identification of new vaccine antigens in lieu of prior available data. Once the complete sequence (or portions thereof) of the genomic DNA or RNA is available, open reading frames are identified. The derived amino acid sequence is inspected for features such as homologies with other proteins that are vaccine candidates or a hydrophobic N-terminal sequence, suggestive of surface localization. The genes are expressed in a recombinant host cell (typically *E. coli*), and the recombinant polypeptide is purified and used to immunize animals to derive polyclonal antibodies. Alternatively, the gene is injected into mice as a DNA vaccine (see *Nucleic Acid–Based Vaccines* below). The derived polyclonal antisera can be used in biologic assays (neutralization of viruses, opsonization of bacteria, binding to pathogen surface or cell surface) to see whether the protein may be an attractive vaccine candidate. The new protein also is used for immunization and challenge in an animal model. One of the earliest applications of genomics technology to viruses was to hepatitis C virus,[55] which was identified by means of cloning its viral genome. The DNA sequences of dozens of bacterial genomes have become available. For bacteria such as *Helicobacter pylori* that had been analyzed previously at the protein level for surface proteins that might be vaccine candidates, this analysis revealed new candidates antigens previously unrecognized.[56] The application of genomics to *Neisseria meningitidis* was accompanied by the analysis of more than 400 putative proteins, resulting in the identification of seven leading candidate vaccine antigens.[57]

Numerous discovery technologies have been used to identify human proteins (or carbohydrates) that are candidate cancer vaccine antigens, including unique tumor-specific antigens, tissue-specific antigens expressed both in tumors and the tissues from which the tumors arose, and shared antigens expressed in a range of tumors but not in normal adult tissues.[58] These antigens have been engineered and formulated into vaccines based on their polypeptides or peptides (or on their carbohydrates) by means of many of the technologies described here and in the sections on *Peptide-Based Vaccines* and *Carbohydrate- and Polysaccharide-Based Vaccines* below.

NATURAL ANTIGENS

The first protein-based vaccines relied on natural sources of antigens. In this regard, the first hepatitis B virus (HBV) vaccine is unique in utilizing a human source (plasma) for the vaccine antigen. Liver cells of individuals chronically infected with hepatitis B virus shed excess viral surface protein (i.e., hepatitis B surface antigen [HBsAg]). HBsAg was identified as a 22-nm lipoprotein particle antigen with protective epitopes. To develop a vaccine, plasma was harvested from long-term chronic HBV carriers, HBsAg was purified, and the final preparation was subjected to one to three inactivation techniques (depending on the manufacturer) to kill HBV and any other human agents possibly present in the starting plasma.[59] This vaccine has enjoyed widespread use and is well tolerated and highly efficacious.

Proteins purified from cultures of *B. pertussis* have been combined to formulate acellular pertussis vaccines, which eventually are expected to replace whole-cell pertussis vaccine for routine pediatric vaccinations in most developed countries. Depending on the number of different protein antigens, these licensed P_{ac} vaccines are referred to as one-, two-, three-, four-, or five-component vaccines.[60-62] These vaccines all contain pertussis toxoid (PT) as a component, the preparation of which is described below.

Proteins isolated from individual tumors have been used as cancer vaccines. In one application, individual tumors are isolated, the autologous gp96 heat-shock protein (hsp) is purified from each tumor, and the gp96 preparation is injected to the respective subject. Vaccination results in a stimulation of CTL responses.[63]

CHEMICAL INACTIVATION

Many bacteria produce protein toxins that are responsible for the pathogenesis of infection. The toxin molecules are purified from bacterial cultures (e.g., *B. pertussis*, *Clostridium tetani*, and *Corynebacterium diphtheriae*), and then detoxified by incubation with a chemical such as formalin or glutaraldehyde. Detoxified toxins, referred to as *toxoids*, thus represent two of the vaccines in the diphtheria, tetanus, and pertussis combination vaccine.[64,65] PT[66] combined with other pertussis antigens comprise the acellular pertussis vaccines.

GENETIC INACTIVATION

The chemical toxoiding procedure has the disadvantages of potential alteration of protective epitopes, with ensuing reduced immunogenicity, and the potential for reversion to a biologically active toxin. rDNA technology has been employed to produce a stable toxoid. As applied to pertussis, the toxin was mutated (twice to ensure the inability to revert) for reducing the enzymatic activity responsible for its toxicity. The altered gene was substituted for the native gene in *B. pertussis*, which then produces immunogenic but stably inactivated PT.[67] This double-mutant PT (which also is treated with formalin under milder conditions to improve its immunogenicity or stability) is a component of an acellular pertussis vaccine,[60] which is itself a mixed vaccine (see *Mixed Vaccines* below). A genetic approach to derive a diphtheria toxoid also was successful following the mutation of *C. diphtheriae* cultures and screening for enzymatically inactive yet antigenic toxin molecules. This genetic toxoid (CRM_{197})[68] is the protein carrier for a licensed *Haemophilus influenzae* type b (Hib) conjugate vaccine and pneumococcal conjugate vaccine (see *Conjugated Polysaccharides* below). This technology also has been applied to *V. cholerae* toxin and ETEC toxin to produce candidate mucosal adjuvants (see *Adjuvants* below).

RECOMBINANT POLYPEPTIDES

The expression of recombinant polypeptides as subunit vaccines arguably has been the most extensively used application of rDNA technology to the development of new vaccines. The first application of rDNA technology to the production of a vaccine was for HBV through the expression of the HBsAg gene in bakers' yeast (*Saccharomyces cerevisiae*),[69] which gave rise to 22-nm HBsAg particles; notably, expression of the HBsAg gene in *E. coli* gave rise to

HBsAg polypeptides but not HBsAg particles. HBsAg is a virus-like particle (VLP), in that its surface structure is highly similar to that of HBV virions. Purified yeast-derived HBsAg is adjuvanted with aluminum salts for formulation as vaccines, which have largely supplanted the equally efficacious and well-tolerated plasma-derived vaccine. With the goal of an edible vaccine, HBsAg also has been expressed in transgenic potato tubers; the purified HBsAg was immunogenic.[70]

Particles are almost always more immunogenic than individual polypeptides. Furthermore, particles (including VLPs) can elicit antibodies to conformational epitopes on the particle (and on the respective virus), whereas isolated surface polypeptides of the particle might not elicit the production of such antibodies. Examples of such particle immunogens are hepatitis A virus virions (immunogenic in humans at dosage levels as low as 50 ng) and HBsAg particles (VLPs). Another example of the effective use of VLPs is for human papillomavirus (HPV). The HPV virion is a highly ordered structure whose major protein is L1. Whereas *E. coli*-expressed L1 does not form particles, expression of L1 in eukaryotic cells results in the formation of VLPs (now in Phase III clinical trials) that elicit HPV-neutralizing antibodies.[71]

There are innumerable ongoing applications of rDNA technology to produce proteins as candidate vaccine antigens for viral, bacterial, and parasitic infections. The major *Borrelia burgdorferi* outer surface protein (OspA), expressed in *E. coli* as a recombinant lipoprotein,[72] has been licensed for the prevention of Lyme disease. Recombinant HIV-1 gp120 (rgp120) expressed in Chinese hamster ovary (CHO) cells[73] has been formulated into a vaccine that is in Phase III clinical studies. Similarly, recombinant HSV glycoproteins expressed in CHO cells were evaluated in Phase III clinical trials.[74]

Vaccine applications outside of infectious diseases have become increasingly diverse, for example, for allergy, oncology, autoimmunity, and fertility. Crude extracts from allergens such as ragweed can be used as therapeutic vaccines for ameliorating allergic symptoms. Therefore, an allergen-encoding gene is expressed in a heterologous host cell. A recombinant dust-mite allergen polypeptide has been further engineered to reduce its capacity to induce in vivo skin-test reactivity and in vitro histamine release from basophils of allergic patients while retaining essential T-cell epitopes.[75]

Before the clinical symptoms of type 1 diabetes develop, autoantibodies to pancreatic β-cell autoantigens (e.g., insulin) become detectable, following which β cells are destroyed by autoimmune attack. A range of recombinant autoantigens can prevent the development of type 1 diabetes in a mouse model. Clinical trials have shown that subcutaneous injection of recombinant *E. coli*–derived insulin into prediabetic patients resulted in a significant delay in the development of clinical type 1 diabetes.[76] Studies of the intranasal instillation of recombinant insulin have been further promising.[77]

Another novel application is in the field of human fertility. A protein on the surface of guinea pig sperm was purified, adjuvanted, and then injected into female guinea pigs. Vaccinated animals were rendered sterile, yet subsequently regained fertility after periods averaging 1 year following

vaccination.[78] This result enables the expression of the gene encoding the analogous human sperm protein for use as a reversible fertility vaccine. A peptide conjugate vaccine also has been developed as a fertility vaccine (see *B-Cell Epitopes* below).

Recombinant fusion proteins can be custom-designed for specific immunologic purposes. Based on the observation that microbial hsps can induce CD8+ CTLs, immunization of mice with a fusion of *M. bovis* BCG hsp65 with HPV-16 E7 protein was shown to induce CD8+ therapeutic efficacy against HPV E7+ tumor cells.[79] This fusion protein is in advanced clinical trials for treatment of HPV diseases.

Many host cells have been used for the expression of heterologous recombinant genes (Table 41–3). Expression systems have been developed for a range of bacterial and yeast species and for mammalian continuous cell lines (CCLs), such as CHO and African green monkey kidney (Vero) cells. Smaller proteins not requiring post-translational modifications generally can be expressed in immunogenic form in microbial expression systems. Other proteins produced in microbial expression systems have been developed and licensed for human therapeutic applications; such proteins include insulin, growth hormone, interferons, and interleukin-2. In contrast, polypeptides that require appropriate folding and post-translational modifications (e.g., glycosylation) for optimal immunogenicity or activity are expressed in mammalian CCLs. Licensed therapeutic proteins produced in mammalian CCLs include tissue plasminogen activator, erythropoietin, colony-stimulating factors, and monoclonal antibodies (MAbs). Whole animals and plants also can be employed as hosts for recombinant protein expression.

Peptide-Based Vaccines

B-cell epitopes against which neutralizing antibodies are directed (neutralization epitopes) can be precisely identified in a polypeptide. Some B-cell epitopes are conformational, being formed by the juxtaposition in three-dimensional space of amino acid residues from different portions of the polypeptide, meaning that such epitopes require the full

TABLE 41–3 ■ Hosts for Expression of Recombinant Proteins

Bacteria
  Escherichia coli
  Bordetella pertussis
  Vibrio cholerae
Yeast
  Saccharomyces cerevisiae
  Hansenula polymorpha
Mammalian cells
  Chinese hamster ovary
  African green monkey kidney
Mammals
  Goat
  Sheep
  Cow
Plants
  Tomato
  Potato
  Tobacco

polypeptide for proper immunogenicity. In contrast, other peptide epitopes are linear, being fully antigenic as sequences of approximately 6 to 20 amino acid residues. Many linear epitopes are weakly immunogenic when presented in the context of the full polypeptide, such that the full or partial polypeptide containing a neutralization epitope might not be an effective immunogen for that epitope. Furthermore, peptides would be effective vaccine antigens if they were rendered more immunogenic than they are as native peptides.

There are several technologies for increasing the immunogenicity of a linear B-cell neutralization epitope to make it a suitable vaccine antigen. A linear neutralization epitope has been defined for the malarial circumsporozoite (CS) protein (repetitive 4-amino-acid sequence).[80] The CS polypeptide contains a linear epitope that is recognized by neutralizing antibodies, yet the whole polypeptide elicits such antibodies only weakly. One might speculate that this represents a mechanism by which such pathogens have evolved to escape immunologic surveillance by rendering their neutralization epitopes naturally less immunogenic.

Several technologies have addressed the immunogenicity of peptides containing B-cell epitopes. There also have been approaches to the development of peptides with T-cell epitopes.

B-CELL EPITOPES

The application of the first four strategies discussed below—aggregate, fusion protein, conjugate, and complex peptide strategies—to weakly immunogenic peptides has resulted in immunogenic presentations that elicit substantially increased titers of neutralizing antibody compared with those elicited by the epitope presented either alone as a peptide or in the context of its natural full-length polypeptide. Nevertheless, the most effective strategy in terms of ultimate clinical utility is established on a case-by-case basis.

Aggregate. Some peptides have the ability, under appropriate incubation conditions, to form small or large aggregates that are more immunogenic. The Aβ protein is processed into a 42-amino-acid peptide that forms large fibrils and soluble aggregates in vivo, either or both of which may be associated with the development of Alzheimer's disease (AD). A candidate AD vaccine was formulated by incubating Aβ peptide (amino acids 1 to 42) into insoluble fibrils. This vaccine was shown to prevent the development of dementia in a transgenic mouse model of AD[81] and was tested clinically.

Fusion Protein. The immunogenicity of peptide epitopes can be increased by genetic fusion to a carrier protein particle. Two such fusion partners are HBsAg[82] and HBV core antigen,[83] a 28-nm HBV-encoded particle. The peptide fusion can be at the N- or C-terminus or at an internal sequence of the carrier protein, depending on which location affords the best immunogenic presentation while maintaining particle formation.

Conjugate. The peptide is synthesized with a reactive amino acid residue, through which it can be covalently linked or conjugated to a carrier protein. The most commonly used carrier proteins in conjugates are bacterial proteins that humans commonly encounter, such as tetanus toxoid (TT), for which a conjugate with the malarial CS epitope has been tested clinically.[84] Conjugation technology also has been applied to the formulation of a fertility vaccine based on human chorionic gonadotropin (hCG) or luteinizing hormone–releasing hormone (LH-RH). It has been demonstrated that antibodies to these peptide hormones inhibit fertilization; however, LH-RH and hCG per se are only weakly immunogenic. Conjugates of hCG or LH-RH to TT elicit antibodies that inhibit fertilization in laboratory animals; these conjugates have been evaluated clinically as fertility vaccines.[85] Furthermore, because hCG is expressed on pancreatic and prostate tumor cells, an hCG conjugate vaccine has been evaluated clinically as a therapeutic cancer vaccine.[86] A peptide from the tumor-specific antigen MUC-1 conjugated to keyhole-limpet hemocyanin is being evaluated for immunotherapy of non–small cell lung carcinoma.[87]

Complex Peptide. Multimers of the peptide sequence, such as multiple antigen peptides, can be synthesized for linkage in repeated arrays with resultant increase in peptide immunogenicity,[88] as applied to the malarial CS peptide epitopes.[89]

Mimetopes. By screening peptide libraries with antisera, peptides (mimetopes) can be identified that antigenically mimic the immunogen reactive with such antisera. This approach is a way to create an immunogen that cannot be produced readily by recombinant or synthetic methods. A peptide mimetope on the HBsAg S polypeptide, which reacts with anti-HBV surface antibodies, elicited anti-HBV surface antibodies when fused with a carrier protein.[90] The LeY antigen is a neolactoseries carbohydrate expressed on human tumor cells. Given the difficulty in isolating sufficient quantities of this carbohydrate for use as an immunogen, a peptide mimetope was isolated that mimics LeY; immunization of mice with a multiple antigen peptide mimetope of LeY reduces tumor growth in a mouse tumor model.[91] It also has been possible to use peptides that mimic carbohydrate epitopes on HIV-1 to elicit HIV-1 neutralizing antibodies.[92]

T-CELL EPITOPES

Effective immune prophylaxis or therapy for some diseases requires CTL or other T-cell immunity rather than neutralizing antibodies. T-cell epitopes elicit various T-cell immune functions and have been applied mostly to therapeutic vaccines.

CTL Epitopes. Peptide epitopes recognized by CTLs may be useful immunogens for HIV and *Mycobacterium tuberculosis* or immunotherapy for chronic diseases (e.g., hepatitis B). CTL peptide epitopes generally are poor immunogens. Thus, for an immunotherapeutic HBV vaccine, a CTL epitope from the HBV core protein was modified by covalent linkage to a T-helper (Th) epitope (from TT) as well as two palmitic acid molecules.[93] This vaccine was shown in clinical studies to be effective in eliciting HBV-specific CTLs and memory CTLs.

T-Cell Receptor. Therapy of autoimmune disease can involve *T-cell vaccination*,[94] for which the target antigen is the T-cell receptor and the goal is to reduce T-cell–mediated autoimmune activity. This approach has been applied successfully for glatiramer acetate,[95] a peptide copolymer of alanine, lysine, glutamic acid, and tyrosine that is licensed for the immunotherapy of multiple sclerosis (MS). It may function by inducing a shift from Th1 responses to glatiramer acetate–specific Th2 cells, which can mediate bystander suppression and thus ameliorate autoimmune antimyelin responses.

Carbohydrate- and Polysaccharide-Based Vaccines

Many bacteria have an outer polysaccharide capsule. Antibodies directed against capsular polysaccharides are protective for most encapsulated bacteria, thus establishing capsular polysaccharides as vaccine antigens. Components of lipopolysaccharide, another abundant surface molecule on Gram-negative bacteria, are used as vaccine antigens. Carbohydrates specific to the surface of certain types of cancer also have been used as vaccine antigens.

PLAIN POLYSACCHARIDES

The natural capsular polysaccharide contains up to hundreds of defined repeat units distinct for each bacterial species and antigenic subtype; each monomer consists of monosaccharides, phosphate groups, and other small organic moieties. The polysaccharide is shed by the organism during its growth and is harvested and enriched from the culture medium. These polysaccharide preparations are usually immunogenic in adults and children over 2 years of age. The polysaccharide elicits antibodies that may mediate bacteriolysis or opsonization of the organism, thereby protecting against infection. Polysaccharide vaccines have been licensed for Hib[96] (monovalent), *N. meningitidis*[97] (quadrivalent), and *Streptococcus pneumoniae*[98] (tridodecavalent). The shortcomings of these vaccines is that the polysaccharides, being T-cell–independent immunogens, are poorly immunogenic in children younger than 2 years owing to the immature status of their immune systems, and polysaccharides do not elicit immunologic memory in older children and adults.

CONJUGATED POLYSACCHARIDES

Infants and children younger than 2 years old do respond immunologically to T-cell–dependent immunogens (e.g., proteins). Conjugation of polysaccharide to a carrier protein converts the polysaccharide from a T-cell–independent to a T-cell–dependent immunogen. Consequently, polysaccharide conjugate vaccines can elicit protective immunoglobulin G (IgG) and immunologic memory in infants and young children. This strategy is important particularly for encapsulated bacteria such as Hib and *S. pneumoniae* (pneumococcal) owing to the preponderance of invasive diseases caused by these bacteria in children younger than 2 years old. The Hib bacteria are a single serotype ("b"). There are four licensed Hib conjugate vaccines,[99] all with different carrier proteins (TT, diphtheria toxoid, CRM_{197}, and an outer membrane protein complex from *N. meningitidis*) of different sizes and immunologic character, distinct polysaccharide chain lengths, and distinct conjugation chemistries. Thus these conjugate vaccines display one or more differences in the following properties: response of 2-month-old infants to the first dose of vaccine, responses of 4- and 6-month-old infants to the second and third doses, response of children older than 1 year to a booster dose, kinetics of

decay of antibody levels, peak antibody titer, and age at which protection first can be shown.

Pnemococcal bacteria consist of approximately 90 serotypes, as reflected in distinct capsular polysaccharide structures. For designing a pediatric pneumococcal conjugate vaccine, seven serotypes have been recognized as responsible for approximately 60% to 75% of the major pediatric pneumococcal diseases (acute otitis media, pneumonia, meningitis); a heptavalent pneumococcal conjugate vaccine has been licensed for pediatric use.[100] Other vaccines being tested in advanced clinical trials consist of mixtures of up to 11 individual pneumococcal polysaccharide conjugates.[101]

A conjugate of group B streptococcal polysaccharides can be used to immunize pregnant women[102] for the prevention of neonatal group B streptococcal meningitis (in contrast to Hib and pneumococcal invasive diseases, which are virtually absent from children younger than 1 to 2 months old). In this case, the polysaccharide conjugate vaccine would be advantageous over a polysaccharide vaccine in terms of eliciting high enough anti-polysaccharide antibody titers to enable sufficient protective IgG to cross the placenta to the fetus.

OTHER CARBOHYDRATES

Tumor cells have been shown to have specific carbohydrate structures either lacking or deficient in other cell types. Such carbohydrates may have utility as cancer vaccines. Examples include the use of sialyl-Tn carbohydrate for ovarian and breast cancer[103] and G_{M2} ganglioside for melanoma.[104] Such carbohydrates are rendered more immunogenic by conjugation to carrier proteins, as is done for capsular polysaccharides.

Anti-idiotypic Antibody Vaccines

The *idiotype* (Id; i.e., idiotypic determinant) is associated with the hypervariable region of the antibody (Ab) molecule and represents the unique antigenic determinants of that Ab. An antibody-1 (Ab-1) is defined as an antibody that recognizes a particular antigen (e.g., a vaccine candidate). The Id on Ab-1 itself can act as an immunogen that can elicit an immune response; the Abs that bind to the Id on Ab-1 are referred to as *anti-idiotypic antibodies* (anti-Id) or Ab-2. The *paratope* is the site on Ab-1 that binds to the particular antigen; thus the binding site of an anti-paratope antibody is a molecular mimic or mimetope of the antigen. If the Id and paratope represent the same or overlapping sites, then the particular antigen and anti-Id both bind at that site and have similar conformations and thus are mimics (Ab-1 is the image of the antigen and anti-Id). By virtue of the antibody-binding site of the anti-Id mimicking the conformation of the particular antigen (which may be a vaccine candidate), anti-Id molecules themselves can be used as vaccine candidates in which an epitope (mimicked by the Id) is presented on Ab-2, the carrier molecule. An excellent proof-of-principle that anti-Id represents an effective vaccine strategy comes from the demonstration that immunization of chimpanzees with anti-Id that mimicked HBsAg protected the animals from HBV infection.[105]

Numerous technologies exist for using an antigen as a vaccine candidate. Moreover, antibody molecules (Ab-2) are not necessarily a desirable carrier for an antigen (anti-Id)

Hence, the cases in which an anti-Id would be the preferred vaccine strategy are limited. Certain tumor antigens cannot be recognized immunologically by the host, because these antigens are self-antigens, often being expressed in low levels in the host. Nevertheless, the anti-Id that is the mimic of a tumor antigen, yet not identical in structure to the antigen (hence not a self-antigen), can elicit an immune response against the tumor antigen.[106] When the tumor antigen is a polysaccharide that cannot be isolated or synthesized in pharmaceutically useful quantities, an anti-Id of the mimic of the polysaccharide can be a cancer vaccine candidate. An anti-Id with specificity for the breast cancer–specific tumor antigen HMFG showed some indication of antitumor responses in subjects with metastatic breast cancer.[107] Similarly, an anti-Id for the parasite *Schistosoma mansoni* that mimics a schistosome carbohydrate epitope has shown promise as a vaccine candidate.[108] The degree to which the Ab-2 antigenic site can mimic the antigen in question to elicit a protective immune response needs to be established. To obtain the highest degree of specificity as a vaccine candidate, one would derive an MAb as an anti-Id and make it into a human or humanized MAb (see *Monoclonal Antibodies* below).

Other

A highly novel approach has been to develop a vaccine to counter addiction to cocaine. This is based on preclinical observations that antibodies can bind to and clear cocaine. A derivative of cocaine is conjugated to the B subunit of cholera toxin (CTB). This vaccine has been shown to induce anti-cocaine antibodies in cocaine abusers and in cocaine-abstinent subjects.[109]

Nucleic Acid–Based Vaccines

Another approach to a nonreplicating vaccine has been the use of DNA encoding a vaccine antigen, a technology that became very fashionable during the 1990s. The in vitro model for this technology lay in the transformation of cells in culture with a plasmid that directs the synthesis of a vaccine antigen. After cells in vivo take up DNA encoding vaccine antigen(s), the antigens can be secreted or associated with the cell surface in a way that would trigger a humoral or cellular immune response. DNA uptake can be facilitated by chemical formulation or delivery by a nonreplicating virus or bacteria; the latter approach fits the definition of a DNA-based vaccine (nonreplicating in vivo).

DNA immunization can be employed as a genomics technology, known as expression-library immunization.[110] In this technique, a microbial DNA genome is cloned as a library of DNA expression plasmids, mixtures of which are used to immunize an animal before challenge with the microorganism of interest. By successive fractionation and testing in the challenge model, protective plasmids (hence genes encoding protective antigens) can be identified.

Naked DNA Vaccines

The initial strategy has been to inject intramuscularly a solution of uncoated or *naked* DNA encoding a vaccine antigen.[111] Cells take up the DNA, transcribe its expression cassette, and synthesize the antigen, which may be processed similarly to a live viral infection. Humoral or cel-

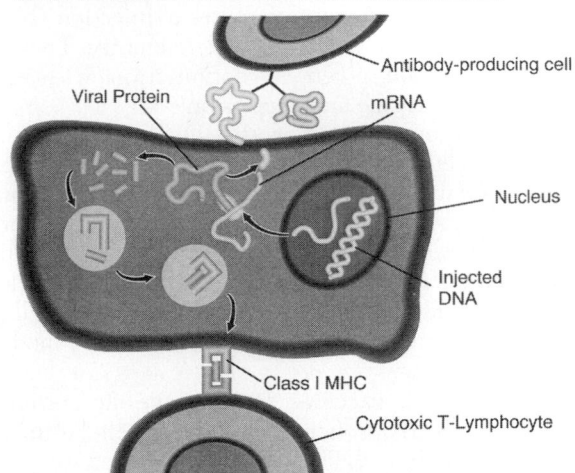

FIGURE 41–1 ■ Injection of DNA encoding a foreign protein can elicit antibodies and cytotoxic T lymphocytes. mRNA, messenger RNA.

lular immune responses to the encoded antigen are elicited (Fig. 41–1). The advantages of DNA vaccines are the relative technical ease of production and the ability to direct the synthesis of multiple copies of messenger RNA, hence the amplification of both antigen synthesis and immune responses. Such vaccines have been shown to be effective in many animal models of infection, especially virus models.[112]

Theoretical safety-related issues needed to be addressed for DNA vaccines as a novel technology. Preclinical studies showed that these vaccines did not induce detectable anti-DNA antibodies. Furthermore, the frequency of integration of plasmid DNA into chromosomal DNA was undetectable and calculated to be less than the rate of spontaneous integration events.

Clinical studies with DNA vaccines for influenza, HIV, and malaria have shown these vaccines to be well tolerated. This first generation of DNA vaccines were shown to elicit low and sporadic levels of specific antibodies, which did not provide for effective vaccination. Subjects receiving more than 1 mg of malaria DNA vaccine became positive for specific CTL activity. Beyond an excellent safety profile, these initial clinical data have suggested that the immunogenicity of naked DNA vaccines needed to be augmented, as discussed in the next section. These vaccines may have their best utility for inducing cell-mediated immune responses or as priming doses in prime-boost regimens (see *Mixed Regimens* below).

Facilitated DNA Vaccines

Facilitation can be at the level of cellular uptake of DNA, expression of messenger RNA, or immunologic activation. DNA has been incorporated into microprojectiles that then are "shot" directly into cells, which produce the encoded antigen that stimulates an immune response. This "gene gun" technique has been reported to be potent at eliciting immune responses[113]; it should be made more practical for broad clinical use. For increasing uptake, DNA has been coated with cationic lipids, lipospermines, or other molecules that neutralize its charge and have lipid groups for facilitating transfer across membranes.[114] Such formulations also are being investigated for alternate routes of injection (besides parenteral) that may elicit mucosal immunity. The anesthetic bupivacaine given in conjunction with DNA enhances DNA uptake and expression.[115]

The base composition of the DNA may affect its potency. Unmethylated CpG dinucleotides, which are present in bacterial but are greatly under-represented in mammalian DNA, represent structures that stimulate innate immunity in response to bacterial infection. As part of DNA vaccines or as adjuvants per se (see *Adjuvants* below), CpG dinucleotides have been shown to induce B-cell proliferation and immunoglobulin secretion, thereby modulating immunogenicity.[116]

Although DNA vaccines do elicit specific antibodies, they are particularly proficient at eliciting cellular immune responses, including CTLs. Therefore, naked (or facilitated) DNA vaccines may have utility for cancer immunotherapy, as is being investigated for a plasmid DNA–lipid complex for metastatic renal cell carcinoma.[117]

Viral DNA Vector Vaccines

A variation on the design of the expression plasmid is to use a virus-based DNA expression system that can amplify the level of RNA and protein expression as occurs in a live virus infection. Such a system has been developed based on Sindbis virus DNA vectors.[118]

Viral RNA Vector Vaccines

A self-replicating RNA encoding a tumor antigen can be used as a nucleic acid–based vaccine. A gene encoding the RNA replicase polyprotein of Semliki Forest virus in combination with the vaccine antigen is injected as RNA; immunization elicits both antibodies and CTL activity and protects mice from tumor challenge or prolongs survival when used therapeutically.[119] Efficacy correlates with apoptotic death of transfected cells, followed by DC uptake of dead cells, which could provide a mechanism for enhanced immunogenicity.

Viral DNA Vaccine Delivery

For DNA vaccine delivery by fowlpox or canarypox virus, the expression cassette for the recombinant protein is integrated into the viral genome. Although able to productively infect avian cells, these poxviruses can infect mammalian cells but do not produce infectious virus.[120,121] This single round of self-limiting infection may suffice to elicit broad immunity to a pathogen whose recombinant polypeptide is expressed by these avian poxviruses in infected cells, while reactogenicity would be less than that associated with vaccinia virus (given the inability of the avian poxviruses to spread). Canarypox virus (see *Recombinant Viral Vector Vaccines* above) expressing HIV-1 rgp160 or rgp120 has been used as part of a prime-boost HIV-1 vaccination regimen (see *Mixed Regimens* below).

Bacterial DNA Vaccine Delivery

Bacteria that replicate intracellularly can be engineered to deliver plasmid DNA into host cells for expressing vaccine antigens.[122] *Shigella flexneri* has been attenuated by a deletion mutant in the *asd* gene, an essential gene. Although such a strain can be propagated in vitro in the presence of diaminopimelic acid and can invade cells (as long as it maintains plasmid encoding invasion-associated polypeptides), it cannot replicate in vivo, where diaminopimelic acid is unavailable. A plasmid harboring a eukaryotic promoter and recombinant gene was transformed into this strain. The resultant recombinant *S. flexneri* strain was able to invade mammalian cells in vitro and to express the plasmid-encoded protein as a vaccine antigen. Because *S. flexneri* replicates in the intestine and stimulates mucosal immunity, this vector may be delivered orally and be effective for delivering DNA to cells where mucosal immunity is stimulated. Other bacterial species that can invade mammalian cells but not divide also may be able to deliver recombinant plasmids to different cell types for expressing recombinant proteins as vaccine antigens.

Formulation of Antigens

The immunogenicity of inactivated, subunit, and DNA-based vaccines may be enhanced by their *formulation*, which refers to the final form of the vaccine to be administered. In addition to the vaccine *active substance* (antigen or DNA), the formulation also may contain an adjuvant and/or delivery system. The adjuvant is a substance that stimulates an increased humoral and/or cell-mediated immune (CMI) response to a coadministered antigen. The delivery system is a vehicle for assuring the presentation of the vaccine in vivo to cells of the immune system or for stabilizing and releasing the antigen over an extended period of time. Adjuvants and delivery systems may overlap in structure and function. Many future vaccines are expected to contain new adjuvants and delivery systems. Reviews[123–125] with extensive bibliographies have been published for the wide variety of available experimental adjuvants and delivery systems. Some experimental adjuvants stimulate primarily antibody responses, while others stimulate primarily CMI responses, including CTLs.

A range of both benefits and challenges is associated with the use of novel adjuvants and delivery systems, as outlined in Table 41–4.

Adjuvants

Aluminum salts (hydroxide or phosphate) are the only adjuvants broadly licensed for human vaccines. These adjuvants have been used for decades in vaccines injected into more than 1 billion people worldwide. The vaccine antigen binds ionically to the aluminum salt, forming a macroscopic suspension.[126] This adjuvant preferentially promotes a Th2-type immune response (i.e., antibody-based) and thus is not

TABLE 41–4 ■ **Adjuvants and Delivery Systems**

Potential Benefits	Key Challenges
• Dosage level ↓	• Tolerability
• Number of doses ↓	• Long-term safety
• T-cell responses ↑	• Demonstrated need
• Antibody level ↑	• Analytic definition
• Antibody quality ↑	• Stability
• Responses ↑ for impaired individuals	• Pharmaceutical
• Mucosal immunity	• Formulation

useful for inducing a CMI response. Although aluminum salts have been useful for certain licensed vaccines (e.g., HBV, pertussis), they are not sufficiently potent for other vaccine antigens in eliciting optimally effective antibody responses.

The only new adjuvant that has been developed as part of a licensed vaccine is MF59, which is an oil-in-water emulsion. Inactivated split-virion influenza vaccine with MF59 has been shown to be more immunogenic than conventional influenza vaccine with an acceptable clinical tolerability.[127]

Given the need to improve on the adjuvanting properties of aluminum salts, many chemicals, biochemicals from natural sources, and proteins with immune-modulatory activity (cytokines) have been researched as potential adjuvants. The adjuvanticity of virtually all known formulations is associated with local or systemic side effects that may be mechanism based or nonspecific. The ideal adjuvant needs to achieve a balance between the degree of side effects and immune enhancement. The immunobiology of the particular vaccine application dictates whether one would prefer an adjuvant that would enhance antibody responses or CMI responses.

Certain bacterial toxins with ADP-ribosylating activity have been engineered as mucosal adjuvants. In particular, CT was shown to be active as a mucosal adjuvant for a coadministered antigen[128] when presented by the oral, nasal, vaginal, or rectal routes, as was shown subsequently for the heat-labile toxin (LT) of ETEC. These toxins are composed of a catalytic A subunit and a pentameric B subunit that binds to G_{M1} ganglioside on many cell types. CT and LT are toxic in humans, especially by the oral route (through which they induce diarrhea). There also has been concern about use of these adjuvants by the nasal route, given serious adverse events that have been observed in an influenza virosome vaccine containing LT.[129] Therefore, point mutations have been made to create toxoids with reduced or eliminated ADP-ribosylating activity, hence toxicity, while retaining adjuvanticity in mice.[130] An alternative approach has been to eliminate the B subunit of CT and substitute a synthetic dimeric peptide (DD) derived from *Staphylococcus aureus* protein A that binds to immunoglobulin (Ig). The fusion of the CTA subunit with the DD domain binds to Ig-positive cells, appears devoid of toxicity, retains ADP-ribosylating activity, and is active as an adjuvant in mice.[131] The tolerability and effectiveness of these engineered adjuvants needs to be validated in humans.

Delivery Systems

Besides presenting an antigen or DNA to its in vivo target cells, a delivery system may mediate other key activities. There may be a depot effect, whereby the antigen is maintained in an appropriate site for continual immune stimulation. There may be an enhancement of in vivo stability of DNA or antigen. The delivery system may enable efficient presentation of mucosally delivered vaccines for uptake by M cells, followed by transcytosis into Peyer's patches and presentation to lymphocytes for inducing mucosal immunity. Certain formulations may maintain the vaccine inside a physical structure for a significant in vivo time period, during which the vaccine is released slowly or in pulsatile fashion in order to function as a single-dose vaccine. No

delivery systems have been widely licensed yet. Gaining clinical and pharmaceutical experience with new delivery systems and adjuvants remains a key goal in the field.

A few specific viral and bacterial proteins have been shown to have adjuvanting and mucosal delivery properties in preclinical studies. A reovirus protein complexed with poly-L-lysine can adjuvant and present DNA for mucosal immune responses.[132] The *Streptococcus pyogenes* Sfp-1 protein also can provide for mucosal adjuvantation.[133]

The development of specific technologies for delivering vaccines by different routes of immunization (e.g., oral, nasal, transcutaneous) also has been a rapidly growing field. Many recombinant bacterial vectors (see *Recombinant Bacterial Vector Vaccines* above) are administered orally. Live *ca* influenza vaccine[12] is administered intranasally. The inactivated influenza virosome vaccine[129] also is administrated intranasally, although its use has been suspended (see *Adjuvants* above). Antigen mixed with CT, LT, or their toxoid derivatives and applied to the skin can stimulate transcutaneous immunization.[134]

Mixed Strategies

Vaccine development historically has employed the direct approach of a vaccine made by a single technology delivered in one or more doses. More recently, with increased appreciation of the immunobiology of particular infections and diseases, regimens have been developed that use either mixtures of vaccines made by different technologies (mixed vaccines) or different types of vaccines given during the overall dosing regimen (mixed regimens).

Mixed Vaccines

As discussed in the section on *Genetic Inactivation* above, the double mutant PT[67] is a component of an acellular pertussis vaccine.[59] As a consequence, this pertussis vaccine is a mix of recombinant and natural pertussis antigens.

Oral inactivated whole-cell cholera (WCC) vaccine, which lacks CT (and its toxic effects), has been shown to be well tolerated and to have a rate of efficacy of approximately 60% for 3 years.[44] In order to elicit CT-neutralizing antibodies, recombinant CTB is independently expressed, purified, and added back to the WCC vaccine. This combined WCC + recombinant CTB vaccine has been shown to have a higher rate of efficacy than WCC vaccine alone.[135] Because CTB is immunologically cross-reactive with the B subunit of LT, the combined vaccine also shows efficacy against ETEC.

Mixed Regimens

Immunization regimens with a sequence of different vaccines assess whether some vaccines are more efficient at priming and others at boosting immunologic memory; these mixed regimens have been evaluated, particularly for HIV-1 vaccines. Canarypox virus expressing recombinant HIV-1 rgp160 or rgp120 has been administered in two priming doses followed by boosting with rgp160 protein[136]; this regimen induced higher levels of neutralizing antibodies than immunizing with rgp160 alone. Likewise, clinical studies of two priming doses of rgp160 followed by boosting with a peptide from the major type-specific neutralization epitope of gp160 demonstrated the production of higher levels of HIV-1 neutralizing antibodies than those elicited by rgp160 alone.[137] Priming with adenovirus expressing HIV-1 gp160 followed by boosting with HIV-1 rgp120 elicited persistent titers of virus neutralizing antibodies and CTL activity and protected chimpanzees from HIV-1 challenge.[138] Priming with HIV-1 *gag* DNA vaccine followed by a dose of replication-defective adenovirus expressing HIV-1 *gag* was found to be effective at eliciting T-cell–based immune responses.[139]

Given the different kinetics of immune responses of infants to various Hib conjugate vaccines (see *Conjugated Polysaccharides* above), it was found that immunization at 2 months with an Hib conjugate vaccine followed by boosting with another at 4 and 6 months of age elicited higher anti-Hib polysaccharide antibody levels following each dose than immunization with either vaccine given separately in three doses.[140]

The above studies have demonstrated that using a vaccine with superior priming characteristics followed by boosting with the proper related vaccine may be an improved regimen for eliciting higher antibody titers. Such a regimen is more complicated to develop technically and clinically and to license than a one-vaccine regimen and thus would not be generally useful in a case where a one-vaccine regimen is effective (e.g., Hib conjugate vaccine). However, it may be useful for targets such as HIV-1 or malaria that have proven refractile to vaccine development to date.

Passive Vaccines

Antibody preparations, either monoclonal or polyclonal, are referred to as *passive vaccines*. Immediate immunologic activity may be necessary to prevent or treat an infectious disease, cancer, or other disease. Examples include (1) postexposure prophylaxis for known or suspected exposure to HBV[141] or varicella-zoster virus[142] in individuals who are unvaccinated and with no known prior exposure to the virus; (2) pre-exposure prophylaxis for at-risk individuals with an underlying pathology (transplantees infected with cytomegalovirus)[143] or infants with pulmonary pathologies and infected with RSV[144]; (3) administration to pregnant mothers who are viremic for cytomegalovirus[143] for the prevention of perinatal viral infection in newborns; and (4) treatment of toxicity resulting from digoxin.[145] The protective effect mediated by most of these antibody preparations is to (1) neutralize virus infectivity; (2) bind to bacteria, which then are destroyed by phagocytic cells; and (3) bind to and neutralize molecules such as toxins elaborated by the pathogen (e.g., tetanus[146]) or digoxin.[145]

Polyclonal antibodies can be processed for clinical use into F$_{ab}$, or antibody-binding fragments of the whole immunoglobulins.[145]

More recently, MAbs have been evaluated for cancer immunotherapy.[147,148] The underlying immunologic mechanisms for such MAbs would include antibody-dependent cytotoxicity, direct CTL activity, binding to tumor cells to mark them for attack and destruction by phagocytic cells, or stimulating apoptotic destruction.

Polyclonal Antibodies

The earliest preparations of antibody or immune globulin (IG) that were effective for antimicrobial therapy were made in species such as horses, which had been injected with bacterial toxoids. Although such antisera were therapeutically effective, the xenogeneic antibody elicited serious side effects (e.g., serum sickness) in recipients. A more recently developed product, equine rabies globulin, is widely used as a life-saving therapy in developing countries (giving <2% allergic reactions). Nevertheless, such IG preparations tend not to be used in humans, especially in developed countries, except in emergencies when no alternative therapy is available.

A range of human polyclonal IG products has been available for over 20 years. Depending on the IG under consideration, these products are prepared by pooling plasma from healthy volunteers (with known titers of the specific target antibody) who would have acquired high titers by vaccination or natural infection with possible silent boosting by the pathogen. The pooled plasma is fractionated with alcohol to enrich for antibody. The preparations are heat-treated under conditions that are known to destroy the infectivity of human pathogens (e.g., HIV-1). The final product usually is released on the basis of standardized specific antibody content. These products are generally efficacious.[141–144,146] However, the large injection volumes (normalized for body weight) and the high protein (antibody) content (as high as 1+ g) can result in adverse reactions in recipients.

Monoclonal Antibodies

The use of MAbs offers the prospects of avoiding human sources of IGs, improving the tolerability of passive vaccines by substantially reducing protein content and injection volume, and providing an antibody source of unlimited supply with unique specificity, absolute standardization, and high reproducibility. In some cases, a mixture of MAbs may be required to provide multiple epitope recognition akin to that of polyclonal sera. The invention of hybridoma technology in the mid-1970s provided for a source of murine MAbs (mMAbs) that required only the availability of the specific immunogen for mice.[149] Many developments in rDNA technology in the 1980s and 1990s have enabled the expression of high levels of recombinant MAbs in defined CCLs, the humanization or chimerization of mMAbs, the isolation of human MAbs (hMAbs) from transgenic mice, and the screening for specific hMAbs from a "library" of MAbs developed in lieu of having enough antigen for immunization.

Nonhuman

The first licensed therapeutic MAb of any type, which inhibits rejection of certain transplanted organs, was a mMAb with specificity for a T-cell surface molecule. Given the technologies available to produce human, humanized, or chimeric MAbs, and in light of issues regarding the tolerability of nonhuman antibodies, additional mMAbs are unlikely to become available for use as passive vaccines. A noteworthy exception to this principle is an mMAb that stimulates a tumor-directed anti-Ig immune response.[150]

Natural Human

The first-generation technology for making hMAbs was adopted from murine hybridoma technology.[151,152] B lymphocytes are harvested from individuals vaccinated for or recently infected with the desired pathogen; alternatively, B lymphocytes from healthy individuals are cultured in vitro in the presence of the desired pathogen or antigen. Such B lymphocytes are immortalized by transformation in vitro with Epstein-Barr virus or by fusion with a human or murine myeloma cell. The resultant cell population is cloned and screened for the hMAb of the desired specificity. The positive cells are single-cell cloned, expanded, and preserved. The immortalized cells can be adapted to the desired growth medium and expanded to the scale necessary to manufacture a product. Alternatively, the hMAb genes can be cloned and expressed to derive a recombinant MAb. Given the technical challenges of maintaining the stability and large-scale consistent growth characteristics of the hybridoma cells in contrast to the reliable expression levels and stability of recombinant MAbs secreted from defined CCLs, the recombinant route generally is preferred as a source of product.

Recombinant Human

HUMAN DERIVED

The genes for the hMAb heavy (H) and light (L) chains from such hybridoma cells[153] are cloned and coexpressed in a CCL (e.g., CHO or NS0 cells) with known capability for high levels of recombinant MAb expression. Alternatively, human B lymphocytes are harvested, and the variable (V) regions of the IgG L and H chains are cloned *en masse* to produce an *E. coli* combinatorial V-region expression library, in which all combinations of different H and L chains are coexpressed in individual *E. coli* cells.[154] This combinatorial expression library is screened for specific antigen binding. The identified V genes of interest are recloned, reassembled with constant (C) regions into complete human H- and L-chain genes, and then coexpressed in a CCL (per natural hMAbs). Alternatively, the identified V regions may be used as less-than-complete antibody molecules (e.g., Fab or single-chain F_v molecules). Such an MAb fragment is being investigated for therapy of *Candida albicans* infections.[155] The efficiency of the combinatorial approach offers the advantage of flexibility of soliciting human B-lymphocyte donors without the need for antigen for immunization as well as the ability to find antibodies of higher affinity than occur in nature.

MOUSE DERIVED

A more recent and versatile technology that has attracted widespread use is the *xenomouse*, which is a transgenic mouse into which transcriptionally active human Ig gene loci have replaced murine Ig loci.[156] MAbs derived from such mice through conventional hybridoma technology are fully hMAbs. Balancing the great versatility of deriving such hMAbs is the limitation that the human Ig gene repertoire in such xenomice is incomplete. Such MAbs are advancing in clinical development for indications such as colorectal and kidney cancer.[157]

Recombinant Humanized

An mMAb can be changed into a *humanized* MAb of the same antigenic specificity. The human immune system would not recognize the humanized MAb as foreign and

therefore would not produce antibodies against it (other than anti-Id). The V regions of H and L chains contain three hypervariable regions or complementarity determining regions (CDRs), each 5 to 18 amino acid residues in length. The six CDRs in an intact molecule come together in three-dimensional space to form the specific antigen-binding region of the antibody molecule (this region contains the Id and paratope, as discussed in the section on *Anti-idiotype Antibody Vaccines* above). The three CDRs in each chain fall in linear sequence in the midst of four V-region less-variable framework regions (FR). Humanization is accomplished by substituting on the DNA level the three CDRs from each murine H- and L-chain gene for the human CDRs in four human FRs from individual H- and L-chain genes.[158] Human FR domains with sequence homology to the murine FR domains are chosen for recombination. The substituted H- and L-chain V regions are reassembled with human H- and L-chain C regions, which are coexpressed in a CCL for scale-up and development as for any recombinant hMAb. The resultant humanized MAb contains only human-derived sequences except for the murine-derived CDRs and hence is nonimmunogenic, other than for an anti-Id response that may be elicited by any antibody.[159]

Humanized MAbs have been developed and licensed for applications in cancer, allergy, and infectious disease. Palivizumab, a humanized MAb that was developed based on its neutralizing activity, prevents RSV infections in at-risk newborns.[160] Trastuzumab, which is specific for the HER2 protein, is used for immunotherapy of HER2-positive breast tumors.[147] Omalizumab, which binds to immunoglobulin E (IgE), reduces symptoms of allergy by its ability to bind IgE and prevent IgE binding to mast cells and consequent histamine release.[161]

Recombinant Chimeric

There are potential technical limitations to being able to produce human or humanized MAbs, but chimeric MAbs have been easy to produce. The V-region genes from mMAb H and L chains are combined with human C-region H- and L-chain genes, which then are expressed in CCLs as chimeric MAbs. Such MAbs have more extensive murine-derived sequences than humanized MAbs. Nevertheless, such MAbs have been shown to be well tolerated and effective in a range of applications. Rituximab, a chimerized MAb specific for CD20, is used for immunotherapy of non-Hodgkin's lymphoma).[148]

Conclusion

Continued rapid technological developments over the past two decades have assured rapid expansion in the number of general strategies for making new vaccines. The number of approaches should continue to expand over the next decade, such that almost all antigens or epitopes can be presented in a highly immunogenic form in the context of a live or nonlive vaccine or be expressed through a DNA-based vaccine. Further understanding of gene function in viral and bacterial pathogens should enable live vaccines to be more stably and predictably attenuated as vaccines and as live vectors for vaccinating against other pathogens.

Adjuvant and delivery system technologies should provide formulations that are more potent than aluminum salts, yet as well tolerated, and enable oral delivery of purified proteins for immunization. Similarly, formulations of DNA may improve potency and the ability of DNA to be delivered by routes that elicit mucosal immunity. MAb technologies will provide for finer epitope specificity and for increased diversity of antigen recognition. There also should be significant further developments in applications to noninfectious diseases, such as cancer and autoimmune diseases, building on successes to date in the fields of multiple sclerosis, whole-cell vaccines for bladder cancer and melanoma, and MAbs for non-Hodgkin's lymphoma and breast cancer.

Beyond all these technological advances, the limiting factor in developing new vaccines for human use will continue to be a more comprehensive understanding of immunology. Some areas in which increased knowledge would have a practical payoff for vaccine development are the immunobiology of pathogens and of noninfectious diseases, the precise type and specificity of immune response required for solid and persistent protection against disease, the attainment of successful mucosal immunity, and the optimal vaccination strategy to achieve this protection.

REFERENCES

1. Sabin AB, Boulger LR. History of Sabin attenuated poliovirus vaccine. J Biol Stand 1:115–118, 1973.
2. Enders JF, Katz SL, Milovanovic MV, Holloway A. Studies on an attenuated measles-virus vaccine I. Development and preparation of the vaccine: technics for assay of effects of vaccination. N Engl J Med 263:153–159, 1960.
3. Buynak EB, Hilleman MR. Live attenuated mumps virus vaccine. I. Vaccine development. Proc Soc Exp Biol Med 123:768–775, 1966.
4. Plotkin SA, Farquhar JD, Katz M, Buser F. Attenuation of RA27/3 rubella virus in WI-38 human diploid cells. Am J Dis Child 118:178–185, 1969.
5. Takahashi M, Okuno Y, Otsuka T, et al. Development of a live attenuated varicella vaccine. Biken J 18:25–33, 1975.
6. Miller E, Goldacre M, Pugh S, et al. Risk of aseptic meningitis after measles, mumps, and rubella vaccine in UK children. Lancet 341:879–882, 1993.
7. Henderson DA. Smallpox eradication. Proc R Soc Lond 199:83–97, 1977.
8. Vesikari T, Kapikian AZ, Delem A, Zissis G. A comparative trial of rhesus monkey (RRV-1) and bovine (RIT 4237) oral rotavirus vaccines in young children. J Infect Dis 153:832–839, 1986.
9. Rennels MB, Glass RI, Dennehy PH, et al. Safety and efficacy of high-dose rhesus-human reassortant rotavirus vaccines—report of the national multicenter trial. Pediatrics 97:7–13, 1996.
10. Clark HF, Offit PA, Ellis RW, et al. The development of multivalent bovine rotavirus (strain WC3) reassortant vaccine for infants. J Infect Dis 174(suppl):S73–S80, 1996.
11. Maassab HF, DeBorde DC. Development and characterization of cold-adapted viruses for use as live virus vaccines. Vaccine 3:355–371, 1985.
12. Beyer WEP, Palache AM, de Jong JC, Osterhaus ADME. Cold-adapted live influenza vaccine versus inactivated vaccine: systemic vaccine reactions, local and systemic antibody response, and vaccine efficacy—a meta-analysis. Vaccine 20:1340–1353, 2002.
13. Ghendon YZ, Klimov AI, Alexandrova GI, Polezhaev FI. Analysis of genome composition and reactogenicity of recombinants of cold-adapted and virulent virus strains. J Gen Virol 53:215–224, 1981.
14. McKay E, Higgins P, Tyrrell D, Pringle C. Immunogenicity and pathogenicity of temperature-sensitive modified respiratory syncytial virus in adult volunteers. J Med Virol 25:411–421, 1988.
15. Meignier B, Longnecker R, Roizman B. In vivo behavior of genetically engineered herpes simplex viruses R7017 and R7020: construction and evaluation in rodents. J Infect Dis 158:602–614, 1988.
16. McLean CS, Challanain N, Duncan I, et al. Induction of a protective immune response by mucosal vaccination with a DISC HSV-1 vaccine. Vaccine 14:987–992, 1996.
17. Pincus S, Tartaglia J, Paoletti E. Poxvirus-based vectors as vaccine candidates. Biologicals 23:159–164, 1995.
18. Moss B. Vaccinia virus vectors. In Ellis R (ed). Vaccines: New Approaches to Immunological Problems. New York, Marcel Dekker, 1992, pp 345–357.
19. Perales MA, Schwartz DH, Fabry JA, Lieberman J. A vaccinia-gp160-based vaccine but not a gp160 vaccine elicits anti-gp160 cytotoxic T lymphocytes in some HIV-1 seronegative vaccinees. J Acquir Immune Defic Syndr Hum Retrovirol 10:27–35, 1995.
20. Marshall JL, Hoyer RJ, Toomey MA, et al. Phase I study in advanced cancer patients of a diversified prime-and-boost vaccination protocol using recombinant vaccinia virus and recombinant nonreplicating avipox virus to elicit anti-carcinoembryonic antigen immune responses. J Clin Oncol 18:3964–3973, 2000.
21. Lee MS, Roos JM, McGuigan LC, et al. Molecular attenuation of vaccinia virus: mutant generation and animal characterization. J Virol 66:2617–2630, 1992.
22. Tartaglia J, Perkus ME, Taylor J, et al. NYVAC: a highly attenuated strain of vaccinia virus. Virology 188:217–232, 1992.
23. Graham FL, Prevec L. Adenovirus-based expression vectors and recombinant vaccines. In Ellis R (ed). Vaccines: New Approaches to Immunological Problems. New York, Marcel Dekker, 1992, pp 363–390.
24. Schlesinger S. Alphaviruses—vectors for the expression of heterologous genes. Trends Biotechnol 11:18–22, 1993.
25. Bloom BR, Fine PEM. The BCG experience: implications for future vaccines against tuberculosis. In Bloom BR (ed). Tuberculosis: Pathogenesis, Prevention and Control. Washington, DC, ASM Press, 1994, pp 531–558.
26. Alexandroff AB, Jackson AM, O'Donnell MA, James K. BCG immunotherapy of bladder cancer: 20 years on. Lancet 353:1689–1694, 1999.
27. Germanier R, Furer E. Isolation and characterization of galE mutant Ty21a of Salmonella typhi: a candidate strain for a live, oral typhoid vaccine. J Infect Dis 131:553–558, 1975.
28. Levine MM, Black RE, Ferreccio C, et al for the Clinical Typhoid Committee. Large-scale field trial of Ty21a live oral typhoid vaccine in enteric-coated capsule formulation. Lancet 2:1049–1052, 1987.
29. Tacket CO, Losonsky G, Nataro JP, et al. Onset and duration of protective immunity in challenged volunteers after vaccination with live oral cholera vaccine CVD 103-HgR. J Infect Dis 166:837–841, 1992.
30. Kotloff KL, Taylor DN, Sztein MB, et al. Phase 1 evaluation of ΔvirG Shigella sonnei live, attenuated, oral vaccine strain WRSS1 in healthy adults. Infect Immun 70:2016–2021, 2002.
31. Gonzalez C, Hone D, Noriega FR, et al. Salmonella typhi vaccine strain CVD 908 expressing the circumsporozoite protein of Plasmodium falciparum: strain construction and safety and immunogenicity in humans. J Infect Dis 169:927–931, 1994.
32. Butterton JR, Beattie DT, Gardel CL, et al. Heterologous antigen expression in Vibrio cholerae vector strains. Infect Immunol 63:2689–2696, 1995.
33. Noriega FR, Losonsky G, Wang JY, et al. Further characterization of ΔaroA ΔvirG Shigella flexneri as a mucosal Shigella vaccine and a live-vector vaccine for delivering antigens of enterotoxigenic Escherichia coli. Infect Immunol 64:23–27, 1996.
34. Goosens PL, Montixi C, Saron M-F, et al. Listeria monocytogenes: a live vector able to deliver heterologous proteins within the cytosol and to drive a CD8-dependent T-cell response. Biologicals 23:135–143, 1995.
35. Stover CK, de la Cruz VF, Fuerst TR, et al. New use of BCG for recombinant vaccines. Nature 351:456–460, 1991.
36. Lagranderie M, Murray A, Gicquel B, et al. Oral immunization with recombinant BCG induces cellular and humoral immune responses against the foreign antigen. Vaccine 11:1283–1290, 1993.
37. Fischetti VA, Medaglini D, Pozzi G. Gram-positive bacteria for mucosal vaccine delivery. Curr Opin Biotechnol 7:659–666, 1996.
38. Timmerman JM, Levy R. Dendritic cell vaccines for cancer immunotherapy. Annu Rev Med 50:507–529, 1999.
39. Bancherau J, Palucka AK, Dhodapkar M, et al. Immune and clinical responses in patients with metastatic melanoma to CD34+ progenitor-derived dendritic cell vaccine. Cancer Res 61:6451–6458, 2001.
40. Nishiyama T, Tachibana M, Horiguchi Y, et al. Immunotherapy of bladder cancer using autologous dendritic cells pulsed with human

lymphocyte antigen-A24-specific MAGE-3 peptide. Clin Cancer Res 7:23–31, 2001.

41. Link H, Huang Y-M, Masterman T, Xiao B-G. Vaccination with autologous dendritic cells: from experimental autoimmune encephalitis to multiple sclerosis. J Neuroimmunol 114:1–7, 2001.

42. Werzberger WA, Mensch B, Kuter B, et al. A controlled trial of a formalin-inactivated hepatitis A vaccine in healthy children. N Engl J Med 327:453–457, 1992.

43. Cherry JD, Brunell PA, Golden GS, Karzon DT. Report of the Task Force on Pertussis and Pertussis Immunization—1988. Pediatrics 81:939, 1988.

44. Clemens JD, Sack DA, Harris JR, et al. Field trial of oral cholera vaccines in Bangladesh: results from three-year follow-up. Lancet 355:270–273, 1990.

45. Hall ER, Wierzba TF, Ahren C, et al. Induction of systemic antifimbria and antitoxin antibody responses in Egyptian children and adults by an oral, killed enterotoxigenic *Escherichia coli* plus cholera toxin B subunit vaccine. Infect Immun 69: 2853–2857, 2001.

46. Murdin AD, Barreto L, Plotkin S. Inactivated polio vaccines: past and present experience. Vaccine 14:735–746, 1996.

47. Crawford CR, Faiza AM, Mukhlis FA, et al. Use of zwitterionic detergent for the preparation of an influenza virus vaccine. 1. Preparation and characterization of disrupted virions. Vaccine 2:193–198, 1984.

48. Plotkin SA. Rabies vaccine prepared in human cell cultures: progress and perspectives. Rev Infect Dis 2:433–447, 1980.

49. Hoke CH, Nisalak A, Sangawhipa N. Protection against Japanese encephalitis by inactivated vaccines. N Engl J Med 319:608–614, 1988.

50. Provost PJ, Hughes JV, Miller WJ, et al. An inactivated hepatitis A viral vaccine of cell culture origin. J Med Virol 19:23–31, 1986.

51. Habal N, Gupta RK, Bilchik AJ, et al. CancerVax, an allogeneic tumor cell vaccine, induces specific humoral and cellular immune responses in advanced colon cancer. Ann Surg Oncol 8:389–401, 2001.

52. Mitchell MS. Perspective on allogeneic melanoma lysates in active specific immunotherapy. Semin Oncol 25:623–635, 1998.

53. Kusumoto M, Umeda S, Ikubo A, et al. Phase 1 clinical trial of irradiated autologous melanoma cells adenovirally transduced with human GM-CSF gene. Cancer Immunol Immunother 50:373–381, 2001.

54. Trudel S, Li Z, Dodgson C, et al. Adenovirus engineered interleukin-2 autologous plasma cell vaccination after high-dose chemotherapy for multiple myeloma—a Phase 1 study. Leukemia 15:846–854, 2001.

55. Choo QL, Kuo G, Weiner AJ, et al. Isolation of a cDNA clone from a blood-borne non-A, non-B viral hepatitis genome. Science 244:359–362, 1989.

56. Tomb J-F, White O, Kerlavage AR, et al. The complete genome sequence of the gastric pathogen *Helicobacter pylori*. Nature 388:539–547, 1997.

57. Pizza M, Scarlato V, Masignani V, et al. Identification of vaccine candidates against serogroup B meningococcus by whole-genome sequencing. Science 287:1816–1820, 2000.

58. Moingeon P. Cancer vaccines. Vaccine 19:1305–1326, 2001.

59. Hilleman MR, Bertland AU, Buynak EB, et al. Clinical and laboratory studies of HBsAg vaccine. *In* Vyas GN, Cohen SN, Schmid R (eds). Viral Hepatitis. Philadelphia, Franklin Institute Press, 1978, pp 525–541.

60. Greco D, Salmaso S, Mastrantonio P, et al. A controlled trial of two acellular vaccines and one whole-cell vaccine against pertussis. N Engl J Med 334:341–348, 1996.

61. Gustafson L, Hallander HO, Olin P, et al. A controlled trial of a two-component acellular, a five-component acellular, and a whole-cell pertussis vaccine. N Engl J Med 334:349–355, 1996.

62. Schmitt H-J, Wirsing von König, Neiss A, et al. Efficacy of acellular pertussis vaccine in early childhood after household exposure. JAMA 275:37–41, 1996.

63. Janetski S, Rosenhauer V, Lochs H, et al. Immunization of cancer patients with autologous cancer-derived heat-shock protein gp96 preparations: a pilot study. Int J Cancer 88:232–238, 2000.

64. Jones FG, Moss JM. Studies on tetanus toxoid. I. The antitoxic titer of human subject following immunization with tetanus toxoid and tetanus alum precipitated toxoid. J Immunol 30:115–125, 1936.

65. Ramon G. Sur le pouvoir floculant et sur les proprietes immunisantes d'une toxin diphterique rendue anatoxique (anatoxine). C R Acad Sci 177:1338–1340, 1923.

66. Chazono M, Yoshida I, Konobe T. The purification and characterization of an acellular pertussis vaccine. J Biol Stand 16:83–89, 1988.

67. Nencioni L, Pizza MG, Bugnoli M, et al. Characterization of genetically inactivated pertussis toxin mutants: candidates for a new vaccine against whooping cough. Infect Immunol 58:1308–1315, 1990.

68. Giannini G, Rappuoli R, Ratti G. The amino-acid sequence of two non-toxic mutants of diphtheria toxin: CRM_{45} and CRM_{197}. Nucleic Acids Res 12:4063–4069, 1984.

69. Valenzuela P, Medina A, Rutter WJ, et al. Synthesis and assembly of hepatitis-B virus surface-antigen particles in yeast. Nature 298:347–350, 1982.

70. Thanavala Y, Yang Y-F, Lyons P, et al. Immunogenicity of transgenic plant-derived hepatitis B surface antigen. Proc Natl Acad Sci U S A 92:3358–3361, 1995.

71. Jansen KU, Rosolowsky M, Schultz LD, et al. Vaccination with yeast-expressed cottontail rabbit papillomavirus (CRPV) virus-like particles protects rabbits from CRPV-induced papilloma formation. Vaccine 13:1509–1514, 1995.

72. Van Hoecke C, Comberbach M, De Grave D, et al. Evaluation of the safety, reactogenicity and immunogenicity of three recombinant outer surface protein (OspA) Lyme vaccines in healthy adults. Vaccine 14:1620–1626, 1996.

73. Berman PW, Gregory TJ, Riddle L, et al. Protection of chimpanzees from infection by HIV-1 after vaccination with recombinant glycoprotein gp120 but not gp160. Nature 345:622–625, 1990.

74. Langenburg AGM, Burke RL, Adair SF, et al. A recombinant glycoprotein vaccine for herpes simplex type 2: safety and efficacy. Ann Intern Med 122:889–898, 1995.

75. Takai T, Yokota T, Yasue M, et al. Engineering of the major house mite allergen Der f2 for allergen-specific immunotherapy. Nat Biotechnol 15:754–760, 1997.

76. Keller, RJ, Eisenbarth GS, Jackson RA. Insulin prophylaxis of individuals at risk of type-1 diabetes. Lancet 341:927–928, 1993.

77. Harrison LC. Risk assessment, prediction and prevention of type 1 diabetes. Pediatr Diabetes 2:71–82, 2001.

78. Primakoff P, Lathrop W, Woolman L, et al. Fully effective contraception in male and female guinea pigs immunized with the sperm protein PH20. Nature 335:543–546, 1988.

79. Chu NR, Wu HB, Wu T-C, et al. Immunotherapy of human papillomavirus (HPV) type 16 E7-expressing tumour by administration of fusion protein comprising *Mycobacterium bovis* bacille Calmette-Guérin (BCG) hsp65 and HPV 16 E7. Clin Exp Immunol 121:216–225, 2000.

80. Zavala F, Cochrane AH, Nardin EH, et al. Circumsporozoite proteins of malaria parasites contain a single immunodominant region with two or more identical epitopes. J Exp Med 157:1947–1957, 1983.

81. Schenk D, Barbour R, Dunn W, et al. Immunization with amyloid-β attenuates Alzheimer-disease-like pathology in the PDAPP mouse. Nature 400:173–177, 1999.

82. Vreden SG, Verhave JP, Oettinger T, et al. Phase I clinical trial of a recombinant malaria vaccine consisting of the circumsporozoite repeat region of *Plasmodium falciparum* coupled to hepatitis B surface antigen. Am J Trop Med Hyg 45:533–538, 1991.

83. Schodel F, Peterson D, Hughes J, et al. Hybrid hepatitis B virus core antigen as a vaccine carrier moiety. I. Presentation of foreign epitopes. J Biotechnol 44:91–96, 1996.

84. Herrington DA, Clyde DF, Losonsky G, et al. Safety and immunogenicity in man of a synthetic peptide in malaria vaccine against *Plasmodium falciparum* sporozoites. Nature 328:257–259, 1987.

85. Nash H, Talwar GP, Segal SJ, et al. Observations on the antigenicity and clinical effects of a candidate anti-pregnancy vaccine: beta-subunit of human chorionic gonadotropin linked to tetanus toxoid. Fertil Steril 34:328–335, 1980.

86. Talwar GP. Fertility regulating and immunotherapeutic vaccines reaching human trials stage. Hum Reprod Update 3:301–310, 1997.

87. Zhang S, Graeber LA, Helling F, et al. Augmenting the immunogenicity of synthetic MUC1 peptide vaccine in mice. Cancer Res 56:3315–3319, 1996.

88. Fehr T, Bachmann MF, Bucher E, et al. Role of repetitive antigen patterns for induction of antibodies against antibodies. J Exp Med 185:1785–1792, 1997.

89. Tam JP, Clavijo P, Lu Y-A, et al. Incorporation of T and B epitopes of the circumsporozoite protein in a chemically defined synthetic vaccine against malaria. J Exp Med 171:299–306, 1990.

90. Meola A, Delmastro P, Monaci P, et al. Derivation of vaccines from mimetopes: immunologic properties of human hepatitis B surface antigen mimetopes displayed on filamentous phage. J Immunol 154:3162–3172, 1995.

91. Kieber-Emmons T, Luo P, Qiu J, et al. Vaccination with carbohydrate peptide mimotopes promotes anti-tumor responses. Nat Biotechnol 17:660–665, 1999.

92. Agadjanyan M, Luo P, Westerink J, et al. Peptide mimicry of carbohydrate epitopes on human immunodeficiency virus. Nat Biotechnol 15:547–551, 1997.

93. Vitiello A, Ishioka G, Grey HM, et al. Development of a lipopeptide-based therapeutic vaccine to treat chronic hepatitis B infection. I. Induction of a primary cytotoxic T-lymphocyte response in humans. J Clin Invest 95:341–349, 1997.

94. Cohen IR. T-cell vaccination for autoimmune disease: a panorama. Vaccine 20:706–710, 2000.

95. Ge Y, Grossman RI, Udupa JK, et al. Glatiramer acetate (Copaxone) treatment in relapsing-remitting MS: quantitative MR assessment. Neurology 54:813–817, 2000.

96. Rodrigues LP, Schneerson R, Robbins JB. Immunity to *H. influenzae* type *b* I. The isolation, and some physicochemical, serologic and biologic properties of the capsular polysaccharide of *H. influenzae* type *b*. J Immunol 107:1071–1080, 1971.

97. Gotschlich EC, Liu TY, Artenstein MS. Human immunity to the meningococcus. III. Preparation and immunochemical properties of the group A, group B and group C meningococcal polysaccharides. J Exp Med 129:1349–1365, 1969.

98. Kass EG. Assessment of the pneumococcal polysaccharide vaccine. Rev Infect Dis 3(suppl):S1–S197, 1981.

99. Kniskern PJ, Marburg S, Ellis RW. *Haemophilus influenzae* type b conjugate vaccines. *In* Powell MF, Newman MJ (eds). Vaccine Design: The Subunit Approach. New York, Plenum Publishing Corporation, 1995, pp 673–694.

100. Black S, Shinefield H, Fireman B, et al for the Northern California Kaiser Permanente Vaccine Study Center Group. Efficacy, safety and immunogenicity of heptavalent pneumococcal conjugate vaccine in children. Pediatr Infect Dis J 19:187–195, 2000.

101. Wuorimaa T, Kayhty H, Leroy O, Eskola J. Tolerability and immunogenicity of an 11-valent pneumococcal conjugate vaccine in adults. Vaccine 19:1863–1869, 2001.

102. Wessels MR, Paoletti LC, Kasper DL, et al. Immunogenicity in animals of a polysaccharide-protein conjugate vaccine against type III group B streptococcus. J Clin Invest 86:1428–1433, 1990.

103. Sandmaier BM, Oparin DV, Holmberg LA, et al. Evidence of a cellular immune response against sialyl-Tn in breast and ovarian cancer patients after high-dose chemotherapy, stem cell rescue, and immunization with Theratope STn-KLH cancer vaccine. J Immunother 22:54–66, 1999.

104. Chapman PB, Morrissey DM, Panageas KS, et al. Induction of antibodies against GM2 ganglioside by immunizing melanoma patients using GM2-keyhole limpet hemocyanin + QS21 vaccine: a dose-response study. Clin Cancer Res 6:874–879, 2000.

105. Kennedy RC, Adler-Storthz K, Henkel RD, et al. Immune response to hepatitis B surface antigen: enhancement by prior injection of antibodies to the idiotype. Science 221:853–855, 1983.

106. Herlyn D, Wettendorff M, Iliopoulos D, et al. Modulation of cancer patients' immune responses by administration of anti-idiotypic antibodies. Viral Immunol 2:271–276, 1989.

107. Reece DE, Foon KA, Bhattacharya-Chatterjee M, et al. Use of the anti-idiotype antibody vaccine TriAb after autologous stem cell transplantation in patients with metastatic breast cancer. Bone Marrow Transplant 26:729–735, 2000.

108. Grzych JM, Capron M, Lambert PH, et al. An anti-idiotype vaccine against experimental schistosomiasis. Nature 316:74–76, 1985.

109. Kosten TR, Rosen M, Bond J, et al. Human therapeutic cocaine vaccine: safety and immunogenicity. Vaccine 20:1196–1204, 2002.

110. Barry MA, Wayne WC, Johnston SA. Protection against mycoplasma infection using expression-library immunization. Nature 377:632–635, 1995.

111. Wolff JA, Malone RW, Williams P, et al. Direct gene transfer into mouse muscle in vivo. Science 247:1465–1468, 1990.

112. Ulmer JB, Sadoff JC, Liu MA. DNA vaccines. Curr Opin Immunol 8:531–536, 1996.

113. Tacket CO, Roy MJ, Widera G, et al. Phase 1 safety and immune response studies of a DNA vaccine encoding hepatitis B surface antigen delivered by a gene delivery device. Vaccine 17:2826–2829, 1999.

114. Remy J-S, Sirlin C, Vierling P, Behr J-P. Gene transfer with a series of lipophilic DNA-binding molecules. Bioconjugate Chem 5:647–654, 1994.

115. Coney L, Wang B, Ugen KE, et al. Facilitated DNA inoculation induces anti-HIV-1 immunity in vivo. Vaccine 12:1545–1550, 1994.

116. Krieg AM, Yi A-K, Matson S, et al. CpG motifs in bacterial DNA trigger direct B-cell activation. Nature 374:546–549, 1995.

117. Thompson JA, Figlin R, Galanis E, et al. Phase II trial of plasmid DNA/lipid (leuvectin) immunotherapy in patients with metastatic renal cell carcinoma. Clin Cancer Res 6:517, 2000.

118. Dubensky TW, Driver DA, Polo JM, et al. Sindbis virus DNA-based expression vectors: utility for in vitro and in vivo gene transfer. J Virol 70:508–519, 1996.

119. Ying H, Zaks TZ, Wang R-F, et al. Cancer therapy using a self-replicating RNA vaccine. Nat Med 5:823–827, 1999.

120. Kent SJ, Stallard V, Corey L, et al. Analysis of cytotoxic T-lymphocyte responses to SIV proteins in SIV-infected macaques using antigen-specific stimulation with recombinant vaccinia and fowlpox viruses. AIDS Res Hum Retroviruses 10:551–560, 1994.

121. Fries LF, Tartaglia J, Taylor J, et al. Human safety and immunogenicity of a canarypox-rabies glycoprotein recombinant vaccine: an alternative poxvirus vector system. Vaccine 14:428–434, 1996.

122. Sizemore DR, Branstrom AA, Sadoff JC. Attenuated *Shigella* as a DNA delivery vehicle for DNA-mediated immunization. Science 270:299–302, 1996.

123. Gupta RK, Siber GS. Adjuvants for human vaccines—current status, problems and future prospects. Vaccine 13:1263–1276, 1995.

124. Vogel FR, Powell MF. A compendium of vaccine adjuvants and excipients. *In* Powell MF, Newman MJ (eds). Vaccine Design: The Subunit and Adjuvant Approach. New York, Plenum Press, 1996, pp 141–228.

125. Cox JC, Coulter AR. Adjuvants—a classification and review of modes of action. Vaccine 15:248–256, 1997.

126. Shirodkar S, Hutchinson RL, White JL, Hem SL. Aluminum compounds used as adjuvants in vaccines. Pharm Res 7:1282–1288, 1990.

127. De Donato S, Granoff D, Minutello M, et al. Safety and immunogenicity of MF59-adjuvanted influenza vaccine in the elderly. Vaccine 17:3094–3101, 1999.

128. Elson CD, Falding W. Generalized systemic and mucosal immunity in mice after mucosal stimulation with cholera toxin. J Immunol 132:2736–2744, 1984.

129. Gluck U, Gebbers J-O, Gluck R. Phase 1 evaluation of intranasal virosomal influenza vaccine with and without *Escherichia coli* heat-labile toxin in adult volunteers. J Virol 73:7780–7786, 1999.

130. Douce G, Turcottee C, Cropley I, et al. Mutants of *Escherichia coli* heat-labile toxin lacking ADP-ribosylating activity act as non-toxic mucosal adjuvants. Proc Natl Acad Sci U S A 92:1644–1648, 1995.

131. Agren LC, Ekman L, Lowendaler B, Lycke N. A genetically-engineered nontoxic vaccine adjuvant that combines B-cell targeting with immunomodulation by cholera toxin A1 subunit. J Immunol 158:3936–3946, 1997.

132. Wu Y, Wang X, Csencsits KL. M cell-targeted DNA vaccination. Proc Natl Acad Sci U S A 98:9318–9323, 2001.

133. Medina E, Talay SR, Chhatwal GS, Guzman CA. Fibronectin-binding protein 1 of *Streptococcus pyogenes* is a promising adjuvant for antigens delivered by mucosal route. Eur J Immunol 28:1069–1077, 1998.

134. Glenn GM, Scharton-Kersten T, Vassell R, et al. Transcutaneous immunization using bacterial ADP-ribosylating exotoxins as antigens and adjuvants. Infect Immun 67:1100–1106, 1999.

135. Clemens JD, Sack DA, Harris JR, et al. Impact of B subunit killed whole-cell and killed whole-cell-only oral vaccines against cholera upon treated diarrheal illness and mortality in an area endemic for cholera. Lancet 1:1375–1379, 1988.

136. Pialoux G, Excler J-L, Riviere Y, et al. A prime-boost approach to HIV preventive vaccine using recombinant canarypox virus expressing glycoprotein 160 (MN) followed by recombinant glycoprotein 160 (MN/LAI). AIDS Res Hum Retroviruses 11:373–381, 1995.

137. Salmon-Ceron D, Excler J-L, Sicard D, et al. Safety and immunogenicity of a recombinant HIV type 1 glycoprotein 160 boosted by a V3 synthetic peptide in HIV-negative volunteers. AIDS Res Hum Retroviruses 11:1479–1486, 1995.

138. Lubeck MD, Ntuk R, Myagkikh M, et al. Long-term protection of chimpanzees against high-dose HIV-1 challenge induced by immunization. Nat Med 3:651–658, 1997.

139. BioWorld Today March 4:3, 2002.

140. Anderson EL, Decker MD, Englund JA, et al. Interchangeability of conjugated *Haemophilus influenzae* type *b* vaccines in infants. JAMA 273:849–853, 1995.

141. Gerety RJ, Smallwood LA, Tabor E. Hepatitis B immune globulin and immune serum globulin. N Engl J Med 303:529–532, 1980.

142. Zaia JA, Levine MJ, Wright GG, Grady GF. A practical method for preparation of varicella-zoster immunoglobulin. J Infect Dis 137:601–608, 1978.

143. Snydman DR, Werner BG, Heinze-Lacey B, et al. Use of cytomegalovirus immune globulin to prevent cytomegalovirus disease in renal-transplant recipients. N Engl J Med 317:1049–1054, 1987.

144. DeVincenzo JP, Hirsch RL, Fuentes RJ, Top FH Jr. Respiratory syncytial virus immune globulin treatment of lower respiratory tract infection in pediatric patients undergoing bone marrow transplantation—a compassionate use experience. Bone Marrow Transplant 25:161–165, 2000.

145. Eddleston M, Rajapakse S, Rajakanthan, et al. Anti-digoxin Fab fragments in cardiotoxicity induced by ingestion of yellow oleander: a randomised controlled trial. Lancet 355:967–972, 2000.

146. Rubbo SD, Suri JC. Passive immunization against tetanus with human immune globulin. Br Med J 2:79–81, 1962.

147. Baselga J. Clinical trials of Herceptin (trastuzumab). Int J Cancer Suppl 15:S18–S24, 2001.

148. Grillo-Lopez AJ, White CA, Varns C, et al. Overview of the clinical development of rituximab: first monoclonal antibody approved for the treatment of lymphoma. Semin Oncol 26:66–73, 1999.

149. Kohler G, Milstein C. Continuous cultures of fused cells secreting antibody of predefined specificity. Nature 256:495–497, 1975.

150. Noujaim AA, Schultes BC, Baum RP, Madiyalakan R. Induction of CA125-specific B- and T-cell responses in patients injected with MAb-B43.13—evidence for antibody-mediated antigen processing and presentation of CA125 in vivo. Cancer Biother Radiopharm 16:187–203, 2000.

151. Matsumoto Y, Sugano T, Miyamoto C, Masuho Y. Generation of hybridomas producing human monoclonal antibodies against human cytomegalovirus. Biochem Biophys Res Commun 137:273–280, 1986.

152. Irie RF, Matsuki T, Morton DL. Human monoclonal antibody to ganglioside GM2 for melanoma treatment. Lancet 1:786–787, 1909.

153. Gorny MK, Xu J-Y, Gianakakos V, et al. Production of site-selected neutralizing human monoclonal antibodies against the third variable domain of the human immunodeficiency virus type 1 envelope glycoprotein. Proc Natl Acad Sci U S A 87:3238–3242, 1991.

154. Marks JD, Hoogenbaum HR, Bonnert TP, et al. By-passing immunization: human antibodies from V-gene libraries displayed on phage. J Mol Biol 222:581–597, 1991.

155. Matthews R, Hodgetts S, Burnie J. Preliminary assessment of a human recombinant antibody fragment to hsp90 in murine invasive candidiasis. J Infect Dis 171:1668–1671, 1995.

156. Mendez MJ, Green LL, Corvalan JRF, et al. Functional transplant of megabase human immunoglobulin loci recapitulates human antibody response in mice. Nat Genet 15:146–156, 1997.

157. Yang XD, Jia XC, Corvalan JR, et al. Development of ABX-EGF, a fully human anti-EGF receptor monoclonal antibody, for cancer therapy. Crit Rev Oncol Hematol 38:17–23, 2001.

158. Riechmann L, Clark M, Waldmann H, Winter G. Reshaping human antibodies for therapy. Nature 332:323–327, 1988.

159. Tempest PR, Bremner P, Lambert M, et al. Reshaping a human monoclonal antibody to inhibit human respiratory syncytial virus infection in vivo. Biotechnology 9:266–271, 1991.

160. Saez-Llorens X, Castano E, Null D, et al for the Medi-493 Study Group. Safety and pharmacokinetics of an intramuscular humanized monoclonal antibody to respiratory syncytial virus in premature infants and infants with bronchopulmonary dysplasia. Pediatr Infect Dis J 17:787–791, 1999.

161. Casale TB, Condemi J, Della Cioppa G, et al. Effect of omalizumab on symptoms of seasonal allergic rhinitis: a randomized controlled trial. JAMA 286:2956–2967, 2001.

Chapter 42

Cytomegalovirus and Herpes Simplex Vaccines

STANLEY A. PLOTKIN

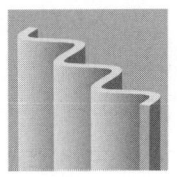 The human cytomegalovirus (CMV) is a pathogen for all seasons. For pregnant women it represents the most common intrauterine infection, leading to deafness and mental retardation in the newborn infant. It is also the second most common cause of the infectious mononucleosis syndrome when it infects young adults. In transplant patients, CMV may cause devastating disseminated infection and enhance graft rejection. For the immunosuppressed, particularly those with human immunodeficiency virus infection, CMV disease is a constant threat, held at bay by antivirals. Progress in vaccine development has been slow, but prospects are now better than ever.

Human CMV is in the Betaherpesvirinae virus group, and it replicates fully only in human cells.[1] Like other herpesviruses, it becomes latent after primary infection but may reactivate from the latent state. Primary infection and recrudescent infection may be either symptomatic or asymptomatic, depending on the viral load and the cellular immune status of the patient. Several antiviral drugs are available, including ganciclovir, cidofovir, and foscarnet, that are particularly useful to moderate the reactivated infection and disease that occurs in the setting of immunosuppression. They also are useful as a prophylactic in transplant recipients who are at high risk of CMV disease.

However, in terms of public health, the most important effect of CMV is the damage caused to a fetus when primary infection of the mother occurs during the first half of pregnancy. Approximately 1% (0.25%–2%, depending on the population studied) of all fetuses are infected in utero, regardless of the mother's serologic status. A key controversial point is the relative importance of disease in infants of mothers who were seronegative when infected versus disease in mothers who were seropositive when infected. Certainly the risk of fetal infection is different: about 40% transmission from seronegative mothers versus 1% from seropositive mothers. About 90% of infants infected during primary maternal infection and symptomatic at birth will suffer lasting damage, usually to the brain or organ of Corti.[2-5] However, in only about 10% of such cases is congenital CMV infection manifest at birth

in the form of microcephaly, hepatosplenomegaly, and other abnormalities. Overall, considering both symptomatic and asymptomatic newborns, about 20% will show late sequelae. Reinfection may occur in seropositive mothers and their infants and may be severe enough to cause disease. However, such infections are less likely to cause fetal damage.[2] The issue is just how much less likely? One answer given to that question is one third as likely, with less severe clinical manifestations.[6]

A study from the University of Alabama[7] concerned women with verified preconceptional immunity at the end of a previous pregnancy, whose progress was followed during a second pregnancy. They were compared with a group of pregnant women who had been seronegative at the end of the previous pregnancy but who had seroconverted in the interval. Congenital infection was demonstrated in 12.9% of the infants of mothers who had seroconverted. This percentage must be considered as the minimal risk for fetal transmission in pregnancy, because some of the women who seroconverted must have been infected before becoming pregnant the second time. Only 1.2% of the previously seroimmune mothers transmitted virus to their fetuses. Protection against infection of the infant afforded by prior seropositivity was calculated at 91%; protection against significant abnormality was even higher. For an excellent recent review of congenital infection, see Revello and Gerna.[7a]

Adler studied CMV infections acquired by seropositive and seronegative mothers in contact with children excreting CMV in day care centers.[8] Seropositivity after natural infection was unequivocally shown to protect against infection by contact with secretions. In contrast to the high rate of infection seen in seronegative mothers, infections in seropositive mothers were infrequent. Thus the induction of immunity equivalent to natural infection should protect against both CMV infection and disease.

The consequences of congenital CMV infection to society are enormous: an estimated $1 billion in health care costs alone.[9] For that reason, a report from the Institute of Medicine of the National Academy of Sciences placed CMV in its highest priority category for vaccine development, concluding that a vaccine would actually be cost saving.[10]

The possibility has been raised that CMV infection leads to atherosclerosis, presumably through endoarterial injury resulting from CMV replication.[11-14] A related complication of latent CMV infection may be the coronary artery restenosis that occurs with high frequency after endarterectomy.[15] Seropositive patients had a higher rate of restenosis than seronegative patients. The CMV IE2 protein has been shown to interact with the p53 tumor suppressor protein found in smooth muscle cells. According to one hypothesis, inactivation of p53 leads to smooth muscle hyperplasia and restenosis.[16]

The effects of human CMV on allograft recipients are dramatic. Seronegative kidney, liver, or heart transplant recipients are particularly likely to suffer severe disease or death when they receive kidneys from seropositive donors. Bone marrow transplant recipients are also prone to CMV disease, usually as a result of reactivation. CMV illness commonly takes the form of interstitial pneumonia, but hepatitis, nephritis, encephalitis, bone marrow depression, and potentiation of bacterial and fungal infections pose additional serious problems.[17-20]

Patients with human immunodeficiency virus infection are also commonly co-infected with CMV, and CMV-induced retinitis is one of the most common opportunistic infections in such patients.[21] Although several antiviral agents are available to treat CMV infections, toxicity and viral mutations leading to resistance complicate treatment.

Objectives of Vaccination

The first objective of a human CMV vaccine is to prevent primary infections in women during pregnancy—the infections that are most likely to lead to fetal disease.[2] The second objective is to convert susceptible patients to an immune status before they face the challenge of transplantation with CMV-bearing organs under conditions of immunosuppression.

A CMV vaccine might also have a third therapeutic objective if immune responses could be engendered to suppress reactivated infection. Infusion of donor lymphocytes capable of killing CMV-infected cells by CD8+ human leukocyte antigen (HLA)–restricted cytotoxic T lymphocytes (CTLs) protects bone marrow transplant patients against CMV pneumonia.[22,23] This suggests that induction of CTLs in donors by a vaccine could help control the infection in patients undergoing bone marrow transplant.[24]

Passive Immunization

Immune Globulin

Globulins containing high-titer antibodies to human CMV have been extensively used in transplant patients. The use of human CMV immune globulin (HCMV-IG) has become routine in solid organ transplant recipients, in whom good evidence for a preventive effect on CMV disease has been shown.[25-28] Licensed products are now available in the United States and are indicated for use in recipients of kidney, liver, and heart transplants who initially are seronegative.[28,29] Although the results have been controversial in bone marrow transplant patients,[30] some centers use HCMV-IG together with antivirals.[31]

Correlates of Protection

Considering that human CMV is a large and complex virus with at least 200 proteins, and considering its complicated natural history, it is not surprising that immune control involves more than one arm of the immune system. In addition to the evidence accrued with the use of immune globulins, other data from humans and animal models testify to the importance of antibody, at least in protection against primary infection.[32-35]

However, it is equally evident that inhibition of cellular immune responses, particularly but not solely CTLs, reduces the ability of the host to deal with an intracellular virus. The correlation between recovery of host cellular immunity and freedom from CMV disease has been apparent for many years.[23,36-39] Table 42–1 lists the human CMV proteins thought to be responsible for the induction of neutralizing antibodies and cellular immunity in the normal host.

Active Immunization

Currently there are seven approaches to CMV vaccine development being actively explored. These are listed in Table 42–2.

TABLE 42–1 ■ Cytomegalovirus Proteins That Might Be Included in a Subunit Vaccine

Proteins	Molecular Size (kDa)	Human Immune Responses	
		Neutralizing Antibody	Cytotoxic T Cells
Envelope glycoproteins			
gB (gcl)	55–130	+++	+
gH (gclll)	85–145	++	—
gN (gcll)	47–52	+	—
Structural proteins			
Lower matrix (pp65)	65–71	—	+++
Major nucleocapsid	150	—	+
28–32 kDa	28–32	—	—
Nonviron			
IE1	72	—	++

TABLE 42–2 ■ Current Strategies to Develop
a Vaccine Against Human Cytomegalovirus

Live, attenuated strain
Recombinants between wild and attenuated strains
Subunit glycoprotein B
Viral vectors containing CMV genes
Peptides containing Th and Tc epitopes
CMV DNA plasmids
Dense bodies

Live Virus Vaccines

The first approach to CMV vaccine development was that of live, attenuated strains. Elek and Stern[40] used the AD-169 laboratory strain to immunize normal adults, but the strain has not been further developed. Plotkin and colleagues[41] isolated a strain (Towne) from a congenitally infected infant and passaged it in human embryo fibroblasts until the 125th passage, with three clonings by plaque purification; pools were prepared at the 128th passage for vaccine trials.[42–44] Laboratory studies of the high-passage Towne virus indicated changes of in vitro markers that correlate with adaptation to cell culture.[42] Recently, Gerna et al.[42a] have shown that clinical isolates are transmitted to polymorphonuclear leukocytes and are able to grow in human endothelial cells, whereas Towne and other high passage isolates do not. This has been proposed as a marker of attenuation.

Initial clinical trials were performed in healthy adult volunteers.[44–46] When the vaccine was given subcutaneously or intramuscularly, seroconversion was seen in nearly 100% of volunteers (Fig. 42–1), but intranasal administration was not successful. During the second week after immunization, a local reaction consisting of erythema and induration appeared at the site of inoculation and lasted approximately 1 week, but systemic reactions were absent. Surprisingly, no virus was excreted in the pharynx or urine nor was any recovered from the blood. Routine clinical laboratory tests also showed normal results. Subsequent studies showed persistence of antibodies for at least several years in adult female pediatric nurses who were vaccinated with the Towne strain.[47]

Lymphocyte proliferation assays showed the important fact that cells had been sensitized to CMV antigens by vaccination. CD8+ cell–mediated HLA-restricted cytotoxicity of CMV-infected cells also was elicited in the Towne vaccinees.[48,49] Towne virus thus induced cellular as well as humoral immunity to CMV.[50] However, tests of lymphocyte subsets failed to show the increase in suppressor cells and decrease in the helper-to-suppressor cell ratio characteristic of acute CMV disease.[51]

In related studies, sera of vaccinees were tested for antibodies to early antigens (EAs) and immediate early antigens (IEAs) of the virus.[52,53] These are proteins not present in the virus particle and present only during replication. Most vaccinees developed IEA and EA antibodies, which signified limited replication of vaccine virus in the host. Biopsy and polymerase chain reaction studies revealed evidence of only transient production of virus.

Assessment of the data led to the conclusion that the Towne vaccine produces an abortive infection at the site of

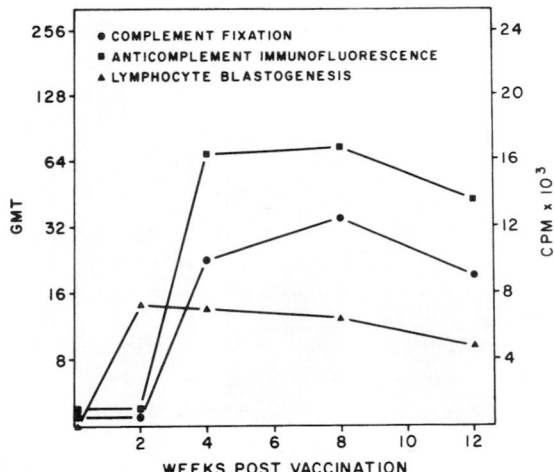

FIGURE 42–1 ■ Typical immune responses to the Towne strain of live, attenuated cytomegalovirus (CMV) vaccine showing the development of complement fixation antibodies, anticomplement immunofluorescence antibodies, and CMV-specific blastogenic responses. CPM, counts per minute; GMT, geometric mean antibody titer.

inoculation, which stimulates a similar range of antibody and cellular responses that are noted after natural infection, including delayed-type hypersensitivity that is expressed as the local reaction described previously. However, immune responses are lower than after natural infection, perhaps because no virus excretion or systemic reaction occurs after vaccination.[54]

Vaccine Efficacy in Transplant Patients

To demonstrate efficacy of Towne vaccine, advantage was taken of the high morbidity and mortality that CMV causes in seronegative renal transplant recipients who receive a kidney from a seropositive donor.[55–57] After a pilot study to demonstrate tolerance of the vaccine, controlled, double-blind trials were set up in prospective renal transplant recipients at the Hospital of the University of Pennsylvania and the Hospital of the University of Minnesota. The seronegative patients were randomized to receive vaccine or placebo subcutaneously. After 6 weeks had passed, the patients were added to the transplant list, and they received kidneys as they became available, over periods ranging from weeks to months. Once transplantation was done, the patients were observed clinically, virologically, and serologically for CMV-associated disease by individuals blind to the patients' vaccine status. Clinical evaluation included an arbitrary scoring system that enabled one to judge retrospectively the seriousness of the CMV disease.

The results are indicated in Figure 42–2.[58–60] Despite the induction of relatively poor antibody and cellular immune responses as a result of the patients' uremia and dialysis, the vaccine appeared to provide protection against severe CMV disease similar to that of prior natural infection. Two additional studies in renal transplant patients, one of which was multicentric, reached the same conclusion.[58,61]

Vaccine Virus Latency

Because immunosuppression reactivates latent natural CMV in seropositive individuals, it also should reactivate

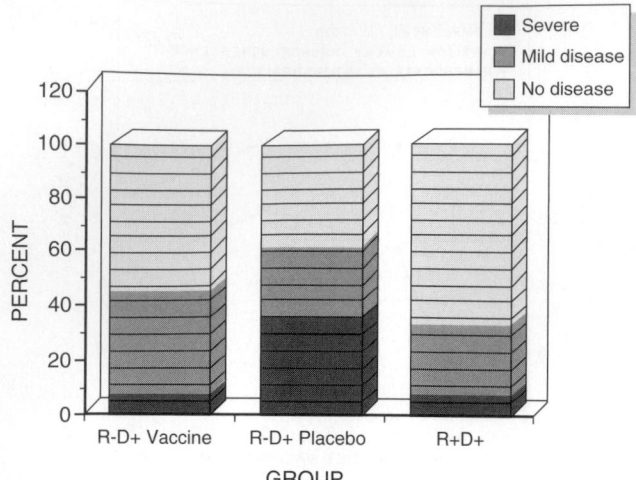

FIGURE 42–2 ■ Results of a double-blind, placebo-controlled trial of the Towne strain of live, attenuated cytomegalovirus (CMV) vaccine in renal transplant recipients. The *R–D+ Vaccine* column refers to the patients who originally were seronegative and who received kidneys from seropositive donors and had been vaccinated before the transplants. The *R–D+ Placebo* column refers to the control patients who received placebos before the transplants. The *R+D+* column represents the individuals who were naturally seropositive and received kidneys from seropositive donors. Thus the second column shows the risk of mild and severe CMV disease in seronegative individuals, the first column shows the protective effect of prior vaccination, and the third column shows the protective effect of prior natural immunity.

vaccine virus if it becomes latent in vaccinees. In fact, seronegative patients who received Towne vaccine followed by transplantation of a kidney from a seronegative donor did not excrete virus. Those who received kidneys from seropositive donors did excrete virus, but, when the strains were examined by DNA restriction-endonuclease assays, they were not Towne,[62] but rather strains that were latent in the donor kidneys that had been reactivated after transplantation.

Challenge of Normal Vaccinees

After this demonstration of safety and efficacy, volunteer Catholic priests who lived in a closed community and who were seronegative were vaccinated with Towne to see if they could be protected against an artificially administered challenge. One year later, in company with unvaccinated seronegative and naturally seropositive priests, they were challenged subcutaneously with varying doses of an unrelated wild CMV isolate called Toledo. A dose of 1000 plaque-forming units (PFU) caused illness, even in those who were naturally seropositive; therefore, this dose was not given to other groups.[63] At a 100-PFU dose, the challenge virus caused a mild infectious mononucleosis syndrome with virus excretion in seronegative individuals, but it did not affect naturally seropositive individuals.[64] Vaccinees also were protected against disease caused by 100 PFU, but about half transiently excreted virus without symptoms. After injection of 10 PFU, CMV infection and symptoms were obvious in the seronegative individuals, whereas both vaccinated and seropositive individuals resisted the challenge. Thus vaccination of normal individuals rendered

them resistant to an artificial parenteral challenge but somewhat less so than natural immunes. However, even natural immunity was imperfect if the challenge was large enough.

Despite the protection thus demonstrated against parenteral infection, Towne vaccine failed to prevent infection of seronegative mothers in contact with CMV-excreting children, although seropositive women were protected. A controlled trial conducted in a day care center showed no reduction in the infection rate of Towne-vaccinated mothers compared with placebo-inoculated mothers.[65] The authors speculated that the 20-fold lower neutralizing antibody levels induced by Towne vaccine in comparison with natural seropositivity accounted for the failure. Studies continue to try to improve the immunogenicity of the Towne virus.

Recombinants of Towne Vaccine

Scientists at Medimmune (formerly Aviron)[66] discovered that the Towne strain has genetic deletions in a particular part of its genome, called ULb'. A deletion of 13.5 kb was found in some lines of Towne virus. This region, present in all low-passage clinical isolates, contains at least 17 genes not found in the Towne strain. It was hypothesized that one or more of these genes code for proteins that would increase the replication and immunogenicity of the Towne strain in vivo. Four recombinant mutants of Towne and the low-passage virulent Toledo strain have been made in which different segments of Towne have been replaced by the analogous sequences of Toledo. Phase I trials of safety and immunogenicity of these recombinants have begun, first in seropositives at the insistence of the FDA, and subsequently in seronegatives.

Subunit Glycoprotein

As shown in Table 42–1, it is the glycoproteins in the envelope of CMV that induce neutralizing antibodies. Among the numerous glycoproteins present in the envelope, most attention has been directed toward the glycoprotein B (gB) protein (so called because of its analogy with the herpes simplex gB). The arguments for basing vaccine development on gB are given in Table 42–3. The gB protein appears to be immunodominant because 50% or more of neutralizing antibody in the sera of seropositive individuals is directed against this protein.[67,68] The glycoprotein analogous to gB has been purified from guinea pig CMV and shown to protect pups whose mother had been immunized before pregnancy and subsequently challenged during gestation.[69]

The gB protein initially was purified from the virus by immunoaffinity chromatography and inoculated into animals and then humans, with induction of neutralizing antibodies.[70–73] However, human CMV does not grow to sufficiently high titers to make native glycoprotein attractive as a vaccine source. Therefore, the gene for gB has been inserted into several expression vectors for use either for in vitro production of the protein or as a live vector. Chinese hamster ovary cells have been used to express whole or truncated gB.[74] Adenovirus 5, vaccinia, and canarypox deletion recombinants with the CMV gB gene inserted

TABLE 49–3 ■ Arguments for Glycoprotein gB as a Cytomegalovirus Vaccine

- gB bears neutralizing epitopes
- gB antibody accounts for about half of neutralizing activity in human convalescent sera
- Inoculation of gB elicits neutralizing antibody in animals and humans
- Proteins analogous to gB from mouse cytomegalovirus and guinea pig cytomegalovirus protect against acquired and transplacental infection

have been used in their living form to induce immune responses in animals, including neutralizing antibodies, lymphocyte proliferation to CMV virus, and human lymphocyte antigen–restricted T-cell cytotoxicity.[74–78]

Spaete and his colleagues at Chiron produced a truncated gB in Chinese hamster ovary cells, which was then purified and combined with an oil-in-water emulsion called MF59 for adjuvantation.[79] Inoculations of this material in concentrations of 20 to 100 µg induced anti-gB neutralizing antibodies after the third dose of a 0-, 1-, and 6-month schedule at a titer of approximately 1:60, similar to levels in natural seropositives.[80,81] A fourth dose at 12 months after the first boosted the titer to 1:115, falling back 6 months later to 1:67.[82,83] Toddlers also were vaccinated,[84] and, after three doses at 0, 1, and 6 months, they achieved titers averaging 1:638, higher than in adults.

Interestingly, both mucosal immunoglobulin G and secretory immunoglobulin A antibodies were induced in many of the vaccinees. Presence of the former in vaccinees was correlated with a serum neutralizing antibody titer of over 1:64.[80]

A potential problem with gB-based vaccines is antigenic variability, suggested by the discovery of four genotypes of this protein, based on sequencing of genomic DNA.[85] Although the genotypic differences do not appear to correlate with antigenic differences, there are weak associations of certain genotypes with specific clinical settings: type 1 is most common in congenital infection,[86] whereas types 3 and 4 are associated with serious disease in transplant patients.[82,87] Nevertheless, the demonstration that high levels of neutralizing antibodies can be reliably produced is an important step forward in CMV vaccine development.

Poxvirus Recombinants

Whether or not neutralizing antibodies will afford sufficient protection is debatable. The arguments in favor of the need for a CTL response have been mentioned above, and, in the mouse, protection against murine CMV infection has been shown to depend on a CD8+ cell–mediated CTL response directed against the IE1 protein of the virus.[88] The principal proteins of the human CMV that elicit CTLs are listed in Table 42–1. Although IE1 is also one of the important proteins for human CTLs, the lower matrix phosphoprotein, pp65, may be more important.[89–91]

Because viral vectors are particularly good at inducing CTL responses to the proteins coded by inserted foreign genes, both adenovirus[75] and canarypox recombinants containing CMV genes have been developed. Aventis Pasteur

has pursued the canarypox approach.[92] Canarypox gB and pp65 recombinants have been developed and tested.[93–95] The former did not appear to be as useful as subunit gB to induce antibody responses or to prime for antibody induction,[93, 96] but the pp65 recombinant gave excellent results, as shown in Figure 42–3. All 14 seronegative subjects given canarypox containing the gene for pp65 developed CTLs specific to CMV after two doses. The CTLs were CD8+ cell mediated and reached precursor frequencies similar to those found in naturally seropositive individuals.[94,95]

Peptides

Another method to induce CTLs has been developed by the Beckman Research Institute at the City of Hope (California).[97] Lipidated fusion peptides were constructed from multiple pp65 CTL epitopes, linked to a pan–HLA-DR T-helper cell epitope.[98] The epitopes cover the most prevalent HLA alleles in the Caucasian population, and have been shown to induce CTLs in mice transgenic for the human HLA2/DR1 allele.[99] Human trials are awaited.

DNA Plasmids

The recent discovery of DNA-based vaccination has been applied to CMV, with the demonstration in mice of antibody responses to gB and CTL responses to pp65.[100-104]

Future Considerations

New approaches to vaccination against cytomegalovirus are in development. Pepperl and Plachter[105] have purified dense bodies from CMV-infected cells and shown that they can induce antibodies and CTLs in mice transgenic for a

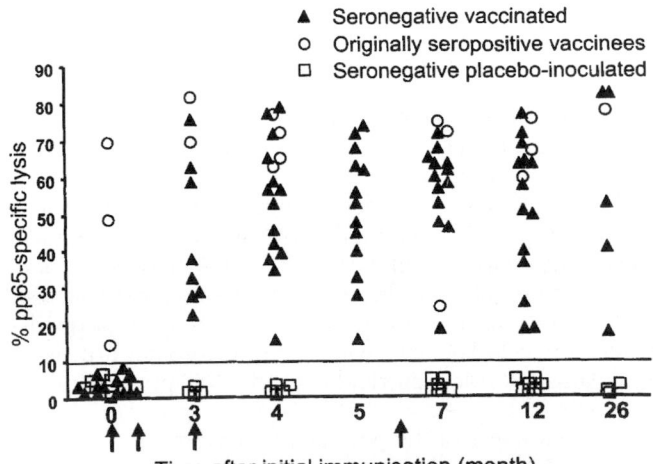

FIGURE 42–3 ■ Kinetics of pp65-specific CTL activity of 25 subjects after initial immunization with canarypox-CMV-pp65 Specific Lysis at E:T = 25:1 (E:T = 30:1 for subjects 9, 27, 32, 33, and 38 at M5) is shown at all time points. pp65-specific lysis is defined as significant at 10%. (From Gonczol E, Plotkin SA. Development of a cytomegalovirus vaccine: lessons from recent clinical trials. Exp Opin Biol Ther 1(3):401–412, 2001, with permission.)

TABLE 42–4 ■ Efficacy of Herpes gD in Alum/Monophosphoryl Lipid A Vaccine Against Newly Acquired Genital Herpes (Point Estimate and 95% Confidence Interval)

	Serologic Status at Entry		
		HSV-2/HSV-1 Negative[†]	
	HSV-2 Negative/HSV-1 Positive[*]	Study 1	Study 2
Men			
Disease	−10% (−127% to 47%)	−11% (−161% to 53%)	32% (−95% to 76%)
Infection	−17% (−91% to 27%)	−7% (−108% to 45%)	−19% (−128% to 38%)
Women			
Disease	42% (−31% to 74%)	73% (19% to 91%)	74% (9% to 93%)
Infection	25% (−11% to 49%)	46% (−2% to 71%)	39% (−6% to 65%)

[*]Approximately 930 subjects in each of vaccine and control groups.
[†]Approximately 700 subjects in each of vaccine and control groups.
From Stanberry LR, Spruance SL, Cunningham AL, et al. Glycoprotein-D-adjuvant vaccine to prevent genital herpes. N Engl J Med 347:1652–1661, 2002, with permission.

human HLA gene. In line with efforts to develop edible orally administered vaccines, CMV gB has been expressed in tobacco plants.[106]

For the immediate future, the most obvious strategy is to combine subunit gB with a vectored vaccine that produces protein targets of CTLs, in order to provide the vaccinee with both neutralizing antibodies and cellular immunity. The eventual success of one of these approaches to CMV vaccine is likely. Target groups for vaccination would be girls or women before they bear children and certain groups of seronegative transplant recipients or donors.[6,94,107,108,109]

Herpes Simplex

Herpes simplex virus (HSV) refers to two viruses, called type 1 and type 2, with similar genomic and morphologic structure, but with very different biologic and epidemiologic properties. Type 1 is transmitted by saliva and causes mainly oropharyngeal primary infection and labial recurrent infection, whereas type 2 is transmitted in genital secretions and causes primary and recurrent infection mainly on the vulva and penis.[110] Transmission of HSV-2 to newborns at the time of parturition may lead to devastating systemic and neurologic disease, and recurrent HSV-2 is a widespread venereal infection.

The correlates of protective immunity are not entirely understood. Passive maternal antibody seems important in preventing newborn infection, and CD4[+] lymphocytes of the Th1 type appear to be crucial to the immune response, but secretory antibodies, interferon-γ secretion, antibody-dependent cellular cytotoxicity, and cytotoxic T cells all may play a role, particularly in the prevention of recurrence.[111]

Vaccines against herpes have been sought for many years.[112] Although live mutant viruses have been tested clinically, and other approaches such as DNA vaccines are being explored,[113] the most advanced vaccines are based on adjuvanted glycoproteins.

Four double-blind, controlled, and randomized trials of two different glycoprotein vaccines have been reported. The Chiron Corporation developed a vaccine containing glycoproteins B and D of HSV-2 (each in a concentration of 30 μg) and the squalene oil–in-water adjuvant MF59. The vaccine schedule was three doses administered at 0, 1, and 6 months. One study was done in seronegative sexual partners of HSV-2–positive individuals, and the other in patients coming to a sexually transmitted disease clinic. The assessment of both studies revealed some degree of protection of female volunteers during a period of 6 months. However, protection did not persist, and male volunteers were not protected. HSV-1 seropositivity did not seem to affect the outcome.[114]

A second glycoprotein vaccine was developed by GlaxoSmithKline, containing 20 μg of the type 2 gD glycoprotein, also administered on a 0-, 1-, and 6-month schedule. The adjuvant used in the GlaxoSmithKline vaccine was alum (500 μg) plus 3-O-deacylated-monophosphoryl lipid A (50 μg). Trials were conducted in subjects seronegative for both HSV-1 and -2, or in subjects seronegative for HSV-2 only.[115] As shown in Table 42–4, the vaccine was over 70% efficacious in women who were seronegative for both HSV-1 and HSV-2. Remarkably, the vaccine was ineffective in women previously seropositive for HSV-1 and in men.

Although this suggests that HSV-1 immunity is protective against HSV-2, and that biologic factors render the vaccine efficacious in women but not in men, no completely satisfactory explanation of the results is available. Nevertheless, this vaccine is currently in Phase III trial in doubly seronegative women.

REFERENCES

1. Weller TH. The cytomegaloviruses: ubiquitous agents with protean clinical manifestations. N Engl J Med 285:267–274, 1971.
2. Fowler KB, Stagno S, Pass RF, et al. The outcome of congenital cytomegalovirus infection in relation to maternal antibody status. N Engl J Med 326:663–667, 1992.
3. Stagno S, Pass RF, Cloud G, et al. Primary cytomegalovirus infection in pregnancy: incidence, transmission to fetus, and clinical outcome. JAMA 256:1904–1908, 1986.
4. Williamson WD, Desmond MM, LaFevers N, et al. Symptomatic congenital cytomegalovirus: disorders of language, learning, and hearing. Am J Dis Child 136:902–905, 1982.
5. Hanshaw JB. Congenital cytomegalovirus infection: a fifteen year perspective. J Infect Dis 123:555–561, 1971.

6. Plotkin SA, Starr SE, Friedman HM, et al. Vaccines for the prevention of human cytomegalovirus infection. Rev Infect Dis 12(suppl 7): S827–S838, 1990.

7. Fowler KB, Stagno S, Pass RF. Congenital cytomegalovirus (CMV) infection risk in future pregnancies and maternal CMV immunity [abstr 191]. *In* Program and Abstracts of the 6th International Cytomegalovirus Workshop, Perdido Beach Resort, Orange Beach, AL, March 5, 1997.

7a. Revello MG, Gerna G. Diagnosis and management of human cytomegalovirus infection in the mother, fetus, and newborn infant. Clin Microbiol 14(4):680–715, 2002.

8. Adler SP. Current prospects for immunization against cytomegaloviral disease. Infect Agents Dis 5:29–35, 1996.

9. Porath A, McNutt RA, Smiley LM, Weigle KA. Effectiveness and cost benefit of a proposed live cytomegalovirus vaccine in the prevention of congenital disease. Rev Infect Dis 12:31–40, 1990.

10. Plotkin SA. Vaccines in the 21st century. Infect Dis Clin North Am 15:307–327, 2001.

11. Melnick JL, Adam E, DeBakey ME. Cytomegalovirus and atherosclerosis. BioEssays 17:899–903, 1995.

12. Nieto JF, Adam E, Sorlie P, et al. Cohort study of cytomegalovirus infection as a risk factor for carotid intimal-medial thickening, a measure of subclinical atherosclerosis. Circulation 94:922–927, 1996.

13. Persoons M, Daemen M, Bruning JH, Bruggeman C. Active cytomegalovirus infection of arterial smooth muscle cells in immunocompromised rats. Circ Res 75:214–220, 1994.

14. Berencsi K, Endresz V, Klurfeld D, et al. Early atherosclerotic plaques in the aorta following cytomegalovirus infection of mice. Cell Adhes Commun 5(1):39–47, 1998.

15. Zhou YF, Leon MB, Waclawiwq MA, et al. Association between prior cytomegalovirus infection and the risk of restenosis after coronary atherectomy. N Engl J Med 35:624–630, 1996.

16. Speir E, Modali R, Huang ES, et al. Potential role of human cytomegalovirus and p53 interaction in coronary restenosis. Science 265:391–394, 1994.

17. Glenn J. Cytomegalovirus infections following renal transplantation. Rev Infect Dis 3:1151–1178, 1981.

18. Falagas ME, Snydman DR, Griffith J, et al. Effect of cytomegalovirus infection status on first-year mortality rates among orthotopic liver transplant recipients. Ann Intern Med 126:275–279, 1997.

19. Winston DJ, Ho WG, Champlin RE. Cytomegalovirus infections after allogeneic bone marrow transplantation. Rev Infect Dis 12(suppl 7): S776–S792, 1990.

20. Zanten J, Leij L, Prop J, et al. Human cytomegalovirus: a viral complication in transplantation. Clin Transplant 12:145–158, 1998.

21. Mintz J, Leij L, Prop J. Cytomegalovirus infections in homosexual men. Ann Intern Med 99:326–329, 1983.

22. Riddell SR, Gilbert MJ, Li CR, et al. Reconstitution of protective CD8[†] cytotoxic T lymphocyte responses to human cytomegalovirus in immunodeficient humans by the adoptive transfer of T cell clones. *In* Michelson S, Plotkin SA (eds). Multidisciplinary Approach to Understanding Cytomegalovirus Disease. Paris, Elsevier Science Publications, pp 155–164, 1993.

23. Walter EA, Greenberg PD, Gilbert MJ, et al. Reconstitution of cellular immunity against cytomegalovirus in recipients of allogeneic bone marrow by transfer of T-cell clones from the donor [see comments]. N Engl J Med 333(16):1038–1044, 1995.

24. Riddell SR, Watanabe KS, Goodrich JM, et al. Restoration of viral immunity in immunodeficient humans by the adoptive transfer of T cell clones. Science 257:238–241, 1992.

25. Snydman DR, Werner BG, Heinze-Lacey B, et al. Use of cytomegalovirus immune globulin to prevent cytomegalovirus disease in renal transplant recipients. N Engl J Med 317:1049–1054, 1987.

26. Werner BG, Snydman DR, Freeman R, et al. Cytomegalovirus immune globulin for the prevention of primary CMV disease in renal transplant patients: analysis of usage under treatment IND status. Transplant Proc 25:1441–1443, 1993.

27. Snydman DR. Cytomegalovirus immunoglobulins in the prevention and treatment of cytomegalovirus disease. Rev Infect Dis 12(suppl 7): S839–S848, 1990.

28. Snydman DR. Prevention of cytomegalovirus-associated diseases with immunoglobulin. Transplant Proc 23(suppl 3):131–135, 1991.

29. Snydman DR, Werner BG, Dougherty NN, et al. Cytomegalovirus immune globulin prophylaxis in liver transplantation: a randomized, double-blind, placebo-controlled trial. Ann Intern Med 119:984–991, 1993.

30. Meyers JD. Critical evaluation of agents used in the treatment and prevention of cytomegalovirus infection in immunocompromised patients. Transplant Proc 23(3 suppl 3):139–142, discussion, 1991.

31. Emanuel D, Cunningham I, Jules-Elysee K, et al. Cytomegalovirus pneumonia after bone marrow transplantation successfully treated with the combination of ganciclovir and high-dose intravenous immune globulin. Ann Intern Med 109:777–782, 1988.

32. Yeager AS, Grumet FC, Hafleigh EB, et al. Prevention of transfusion-acquired cytomegalovirus infections in newborn infants. J Pediatr 98:281–287, 1981.

33. Adler SP, Chandrika T, Lawrence L, Baggett J. Cytomegalovirus infections in neonates acquired by blood transfusions. Pediatr Infect Dis 2:114–118, 1983.

34. Bratcher DF, Bourne N, Bravo FJ, et al. Effect of passive antibody on congenital cytomegalovirus infection in guinea pigs. J Infect Dis 172:944–950, 1995.

35. Chatterjee A, Harrison CJ, Britt WJ, Bewtra C. Modification of maternal and congenital cytomegalovirus infection by anti-glycoprotein b antibody transfer in guinea pigs. J Infect Dis 183:1547–1553, 2001.

36. Koszinowski UH, Del Val M, Reddehase MJ. Cellular and molecular basis of the protective immune response to cytomegalovirus infection. Curr Top Cell Regul 154:189–220, 1990.

37. Quinnan GV Jr, Kirmani N, Rook AH, et al. Cytotoxic T cells in cytomegalovirus infection: HLA-restricted T-lymphocyte and non-T-lymphocyte cytotoxic responses correlate with recovery from cytomegalovirus infection in bone-marrow-transplant recipients. N Engl J Med 307:7–13, 1982.

38. Reusser P, Ridell SR, Meyers JD, Greenberg D. Cytotoxic T-lymphocyte response to cytomegalovirus after human allogenic bone marrow transplantation: pattern of recovery and correlation with cytomegalovirus infection and disease. Blood 78:1373–1380, 1991.

39. Erlich KS, Mills J, Shanley JD. Effects of L3T4+ lymphocyte depletion on acute murine cytomegalovirus infection. J Gen Virol 70(pt 7): 1765–1771, 1989.

40. Elek SD, Stern H. Development of a vaccine against mental retardation caused by cytomegalovirus infection in utero. Lancet 1:1–5, 1974.

41. Plotkin SA, Furukawa T, Zygraich N, Huygelen C. Candidate cytomegalovirus strain for human vaccination. Infect Immun 12:521–527, 1975.

42. Plotkin SA, Huygelen C. Cytomegalovirus vaccine prepared in WI-38. Dev Biol Stand 37:301–305, 1976.

42a. Gerna G, Percivalle E, Baldanti F, et al. Lack of transmission to polymorphonuclear leukocytes and human umbilical vein endothelial cells as a marker of attenuation of human cytomegalovirus. J Med Virol 66:335–339, 2002.

43. Yamane Y, Furukawa T, Plotkin SA. Supernatant virus release as a differentiating marker between low passage and vaccine strains of human cytomegalovirus. Vaccine 1:23–25, 1983.

44. Plotkin SA, Farquhar J, Hornberger E. Clinical trials of immunization with the Towne 125 strain of human cytomegalovirus. J Infect Dis 134:470–475, 1976.

45. Plotkin SA. Vaccination against herpes group viruses, in particular, cytomegalovirus. Monogr Paediatr 11:58–74, 1979.

46. Just M, Buergin-Wolff A, Emoedi G, Hernandez R. Immunisation trials with live attenuated cytomegalovirus TOWNE 125. Infection 3:111–114, 1975.

47. Fleisher GR, Starr SE, Friedman HM, Plotkin SA. Vaccination of pediatric nurses with live attenuated cytomegalovirus. Am J Dis Child 136:294–296, 1982.

48. Quinnan GVJ, Delery M, Rook AH, et al. Comparative virulence and immunogenicity of the Towne strain and a nonattenuated strain of cytomegalovirus. Ann Intern Med 101:478–483, 1984.

49. Adler SP, Hempfling S, Starr S, et al. Safety and immunogenicity of the Towne strain cytomegalovirus vaccine. Pediatr Infect Dis J 17:200–206, 1998.

50. Starr SE, Glazer JP, Friedman HM, et al. Specific cellular and humoral immunity after immunization with live Towne strain cytomegalovirus vaccine. J Infect Dis 143:585–589, 1981.

51. Carney WP, Hirsch MS, Iacoviello VR, et al. T-lymphocyte subsets and proliferative responses following immunization with cytomegalovirus vaccine. J Infect Dis 147:958, 1983.

52. Friedman AD, Michelson S, Plotkin SA. Detection of antibodies to pre-early nuclear antigen and immediate-early antigens in patients immunized with cytomegalovirus vaccine. Infect Immun 38: 1068–1072, 1982.

53. Friedman AD, Furukawa T, Plotkin SA. Detection of antibody to cytomegalovirus early antigen in vaccinated, normal volunteers and renal transplant candidates. J Infect Dis 146:255–259, 1982.

54. Plotkin SA. CMV vaccines. Bull World Health Organ 5:96–109, 1984.

55. Pass RF, Long WK, Whitley RJ, et al. Productive infection with cytomegalovirus and herpes simplex virus in renal transplant recipients: role of source of kidney. J Infect Dis 137:556–563, 1978.

56. Burns RE, Brennan RB, Douglas RG, Talley TE. Clinical manifestations of renal allograft-derived primary cytomegalovirus infection. Am J Dis Child 131:759–763, 1977.

57. Suwansirikul S, Rao N, Dowling JN, Ho M. Primary and secondary cytomegalovirus infection. Arch Intern Med 137:1026–1029, 1977.

58. Balfour HH, Sach GW, Gehz RC, et al. Cytomegalovirus vaccine in renal transplant candidates: progress report of randomized placebo-controlled double-blind trial. In Michelson S, Pagano JS (eds). Cytomegalovirus: Pathogenesis and Prevention of Human Infection. New York, Alan R Liss, 1984, pp 289–304.

59. Plotkin SA, Smiley ML, Friedman HM, et al. Towne-vaccine-induced prevention of cytomegalovirus disease after renal transplants. Lancet 1:528–530, 1984.

60. Plotkin SA, Starr SE, Friedman HM, et al. Effect of Towne live virus vaccine on cytomegalovirus disease after renal transplant: a controlled trial. Ann Intern Med 114:525–531, 1991.

61. Plotkin SA, Higgins R, Kurtz JB, et al. Multicenter trial of Towne strain attenuated virus vaccine in seronegative renal transplant recipients. Transplantation 58:1176–1178, 1994.

62. Plotkin SA, Huang ES. Cytomegalovirus vaccine virus (Towne strain) does not induce latency. J Infect Dis 152:395–397, 1985.

63. Plotkin SA, Weibel RE, Alpert G, et al. Resistance of seropositive volunteers to subcutaneous challenge with low-passage human cytomegalovirus. J Infect Dis 151:737–739, 1985.

64. Plotkin SA, Starr SE, Friedman HM, et al. Protective effects of Towne cytomegalovirus vaccine against low-passage cytomegalovirus administered as a challenge. J Infect Dis 159:860–865, 1989.

65. Adler SP, Starr SE, Plotkin SA, et al. Immunity induced by primary human cytomegalovirus infection protects against secondary infection among women of childbearing age. J Infect Dis 171:26–32, 1995.

66. Cha TA, Edward T, Kemble W, et al. Human cytomegalovirus clinical isolates carry at least 19 genes not found in laboratory strains. J Virol 70:78–83, 1996.

67. Gonczol E, Plotkin SA. Development of a cytomegalovirus vaccine: lessons from recent clinical trials. Exp Opin Biol Ther 1:401–412, 2001.

68. Britt WJ, Vugler L, Butfiloski EJ, Stephens EB. Cell surface expression of human cytomegalovirus (HCMV) gp55-116 (gB): use of HCMV-recombinant vaccinia virus-infected cells in analysis of the human neutralizing antibody response. J Virol 64:1079–1085, 1990.

69. Harrison CJ, Britt WJ, Chapman NM, et al. Reduced congenital cytomegalovirus (CMV) infection after maternal immunization with a guinea pig CMV glycoprotein before gestational primary CMV infection in the guinea pig model. J Infect Dis 172:1212–1220, 1995.

70. Furukawa T, Gonczol E, Starr S, et al. HCMV envelope antigens induce both humoral and cellular immunity in guinea pigs. Proc Soc Exp Biol Med 175:243–250, 1984.

71. Hudecz F, Gonczol E, Plotkin SA. Preparation of highly purified human cytomegalovirus envelope antigen. Vaccine 3:300–304, 1985.

72. Gonczol E, Hudecz F, Ianacone J, et al. Immune responses to isolated human cytomegalovirus envelope proteins. J Virol 58:661–664, 1986.

73. Gonczol E, Ianacone J, Ho WZ, et al. Isolated gA/gB glycoprotein complex of human cytomegalovirus envelope induces humoral and cellular immune-responses in human volunteers. Vaccine 8:130–136, 1990.

74. Spaete RR. A recombinant subunit vaccine approach to HCMV vaccine development. Transplant Proc 23(suppl 3):90–96, 1991.

75. Marshall GS, Ricciardi RP, Rando RF, et al. An adenovirus recombinant that expresses the human cytomegalovirus major envelope glycoprotein and induces neutralizing antibodies. J Infect Dis 162:1177–1181, 1990.

76. Gonczol E, Berencsi K, Kauffman E, et al. Preclinical evaluation of an ALVAC (canarypox)-human cytomegalovirus glycoprotein B vaccine candidate: immune response elicited in a prime/boost protocol with the glycoprotein B subunit. Scand J Infect Dis Suppl 99:110–112, 1995.

77. Gonczol E, Berensci K, Pincus S, et al. Preclinical evaluation of an ALVAC (canarypox)–human cytomegalovirus glycoprotein B vaccine candidate. Vaccine 13:1080–1085, 1995.

78. Gonczol E, deTaisne C, Hirka G, et al. High expression of human cytomegalovirus (HCMV)-gB protein in cells infected with a vaccinia-gB recombinant: the importance of the gB protein in HCMV immunity. Vaccine 9:631–637, 1991.

79. Spaete RR, Saxena A, Scott PI, et al. Sequence requirements for proteolytic processing of glycoprotein B of human cytomegalovirus strain Towne. J Virol 64:2922–2931, 1990.

80. Wang JB, Adler SP, Hempfling S, et al. Mucosal antibodies to human cytomegalovirus glycoprotein B occur following both natural infection and immunization with human cytomegalovirus vaccines. J Infect Dis 174:387–392, 1996.

81. Pass RF, Duliège AM, Boppana S. Immunogenicity of a recombinant CMV gB vaccine. Pediatr Res 37:185A, 1995.

82. Torok-Storb B, Gooley T, Leisenring W, et al. Marrow allograft failure is associated with specific cytomegalovirus (CMV) genotypes [abstr 33]. In Program and Abstracts of the 6th International Cytomegalovirus Workshop, Perdido Beach Resort, Orange Beach, AL, March 5, 1996.

83. Pass R, Duliège AM, Sekulovich R, et al. Antibody response to a fourth dose of CMV gB vaccine in healthy adults [abstr 79]. In Program and Abstracts of the 6th International Cytomegalovirus Workshop, Perdido Beach Resort, Orange Beach, AL, March 5, 1997.

84. Mitchell D, Holmes SJ, Burke RL, et al. Immunogenicity of a recombinant human cytomegalovirus (CMV) gB vaccine in toddlers. Pediatr Res 41:127A, 1997.

85. Chou S, Dennison KM. Analysis of interstrain variation in cytomegalovirus glycoprotein B sequences encoding neutralization-related epitopes. J Infect Dis 163:1229–1234, 1991.

86. Bale JF, Petheram SJ, Miller JE, Murph JR. Cytomegalovirus (CMV) glycoprotein B (gB) genotypes in child care environments [abstr 188]. In Program and Abstracts of the 6th International Cytomegalovirus Workshop, Perdido Beach Resort, Orange Beach, AL, March 5, 1996.

87. Lo CY, Woo PCY, Lo SKF, et al. The frequency and distribution of CMV-enveloped glycoprotein genotypes in bone marrow and renal transplant recipients with CMV disease [abstr 126]. In Program and Abstracts of the 6th International Cytomegalovirus Workshop, Perdido Beach Resort, Orange Beach, AL, March 5, 1996.

88. Del Val M, Schlicht HJ, Wolkmer H, et al. Protection against lethal cytomegalovirus infection by a recombinant vaccine containing a single nonameric T-cell epitope. J Virol 65:3641–3646, 1991.

89. McLaughlin-Taylor E, Pande H, Forman SJ, et al. Identification of the major late human cytomegalovirus matrix protein pp65 as a target antigen for CD8+ virus-specific cytotoxic T lymphocytes. J Med Virol 43:103–110, 1994.

90. Wills MR, Carmichael AJ, Mynard K, et al. The human cytotoxic T-lymphocyte (CTL) response to cytomegalovirus is dominated by structural protein pp65: frequency, specificity, and T-cell receptor usage of pp65-specific CTL. J Virol 70:7569–7579, 1996.

91. Boppana SB, Britt WJ. Recognition of human cytomegalovirus gene products by HCMV-specific cytotoxic T cells. Virology 222:293–296, 1996.

92. Plotkin SA, Cadoz M, Meignier B, et al. The safety and use of canarypox vectored vaccines. Dev Biol Stand 84:165–170, 1995.

93. Adler SP, Plotkin SA, Gonczol E, et al. A canarypox vector expressing cytomegalovirus (CMV) glycoprotein B primes for antibody responses to a live attenuated CMV vaccine (Towne). J Infect Dis 180:843–846, 1999.

94. Gonczol E, Plotkin SA. Progress in vaccine development for prevention of human cytomegalovirus infection. Curr Top Cell Regul 154:255–274, 1990.

95. Berencsi K, Gyulai Z, Gonczol E, et al. A canarypox vector-expressing cytomegalovirus (CMV) phosphoprotein 65 induces long-lasting cytotoxic T cell responses in human CMV-seronegative subjects. J Infect Dis 183:1171–1179, 2001.

96. Bernstein DI, Schleiss MR, Berencsi K, et al. Effect of previous or simultaneous immunization with canarypox expressing cytomegalovirus (CMV) glycoprotein B (gB) on response to subunit gB vaccine plus MF59 in healthy CMV-seronegative adults. J Infect Dis 185:686–690, 2002.

97. Zaia JA, Sissons JG, Riddell S, et al. Status of cytomegalovirus prevention and treatment in 2000. Hematology (Am Soc Hematol Educ Program) 2000:339–355.

98. Diamond DJ, York J, Sun JY, et al. Development of a candidate HLA A*0201 restricted peptide based vaccine against human cytomegalovirus infection. Blood 90:1751–1767, 1997.

99. BenMohamed L, Krishnan R, Longmate J, et al. Induction of CTL response by a minimal epitope vaccine in HLA A*0201/DR1 transgenic mice: dependence on HLA class II restricted T(H) response. Hum Immunol 61:764–779, 2000.

100. Pande H, Campo K, Tanamachi B, et al. Direct DNA immunization of mice with plasmid DNA encoding the tegument protein pp65 (ppUL83) of human cytomegalovirus induces high levels of circulating antibody to the encoded protein. Scand J Infect Dis Suppl 99:117–120, 1995.

101. Endresz V, Kari L, Berencsi K, et al. Induction of human cytomegalovirus (HCMV)-glycoprotein B (gB)-specific neutralizing antibody and phosphoprotein 65 (pp65) specific cytotoxic T lymphocyte responses by naked DNA immunization. Vaccine 17:50–58, 1999.

102. Hwang ES, Kwon KB, Park JW, et al. Induction of neutralizing antibody against human cytomegalovirus (HCMV) with DNA-mediated immunization of HCMV glycoprotein B in mice. Microbiol Immunol 43:307–310, 1999.

103. Endresz V, Burian K, Berencsi K, et al. Optimization of DNA immunization against human cytomegalovirus. Vaccine 19:3972–3980, 2001.

104. Gonzalez Armas JC, Morello CS, Cranmer LD, Spector DH. DNA immunization confers protection against murine cytomegalovirus infection. J Virol 70:7921–7928, 1996.

105. Pepperl S, Plachter B. Dense bodies of human cytomegalovirus induce both humoral and cellular immune responses in the absence of viral gene expression [Abstract] (Publ No P-310). American Society of Virology, 2000.

106. Tackaberry ES, Dudani AK, Prior F, et al. Development of biopharmaceuticals in plant expression systems: cloning, expression and immunological reactivity of human cytomegalovirus glycoprotein B (UL55) in seeds of transgenic tobacco. Vaccine 17:3020–3029, 1999.

107. Britt WJ. Vaccines against human cytomegalovirus: time to test. Trends Microbiol 4:34–38, 1996.

108. Plotkin SA. Vaccination against cytomegalovirus, the changeling demon. Pediatr Infect Dis J 18:313–325, 1999.

109. Plotkin SA. Is there a formula for an effective CMV vaccine? J Clin Virol 25:S13–S21, 2002.

110. Whitley RJ, Roizman B. Herpes simplex virus infections. Lancet 357:1513–1518, 2001.

111. Whitley RJ, Miller RL. Immunologic approach to herpes simplex virus. Viral Immunol 14:111–118, 2001.

112. Stanberry LR, Cunningham AL, Mindel A, et al. Prospects for control of herpes simplex virus disease through immunization. Clin Infect Dis 30:549–566, 2000.

113. Baghian A, Chouljenko VN, Dauvergne O, et al. Protective immunity against lethal HSV-1 challenge in mice by nucleic acid-based immunisation with herpes simplex virus type-1 genes specifying glycoproteins gB and gD. J Med Microbiol 51:350–357, 2002.

114. Corey L, Langenberg AG, Ashley R, et al. Recombinant glycoprotein vaccine for the prevention of genital HSV-2 infection: two randomized controlled trials. Chiron HSV Vaccine Study Group [see comments]. JAMA 282:331–340, 1999.

115. Stanberry LR, Spruance SL, Cunningham AL, et al. Glycoprotein-D-adjuvant vaccine to prevent genital herpes. N Engl J Med 347:1652–1661, 2002.

Chapter 43

Diarrheal Disease Vaccines

JAMES P. NATARO • EILEEN M. BARRY

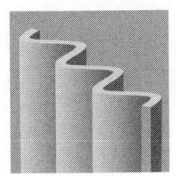

Bacterial enteric infections continue to take a heavy toll on the world's populations, particularly children living in the developing world. Despite the morbidity and mortality still attributed to these infectious diseases, the great diversity of enteric pathogens complicates vaccine development efforts enormously. Not only are there at least half a dozen different species or pathotypes that may account for most diarrheal disease in a particular area, but antigenic diversity among the strains of a given pathogen are the rule. In spite of these daunting obstacles, several enteric infections have been targeted for vaccine development, albeit with limited success. In this chapter, we consider the status of vaccine development efforts against *Escherichia coli*, *Shigella*, and *Campylobacter*, three of the most important diarrheal pathogens of humans.

Shiga Toxin–Producing *Escherichia coli*

Escherichia coli is the predominant facultative anaerobe in the human intestine and, as such, it engenders a significant degree of immune tolerance.[1] Within this massive microbial population of commensals, however, a variety of pathogenic subtypes of *E. coli* have evolved, and at least six distinct diarrheagenic pathotypes cause disease in humans.[2] Distinguishing these pathotypes from commensal flora in the laboratory has been a formidable challenge, but development of effective vaccines will require that the immune system learn to distinguish them as well. For these reasons, despite substantial research efforts, *E. coli* vaccine development has not been highly successful. Nevertheless, several promising avenues are currently being pursued.

Certain diarrheagenic *E. coli* strains have become lysogenized with phages encoding the Shiga toxin (Stx), first characterized in *Shigella dysenteriae*.[3] These organisms colonize the colonic mucosa and induce local damage without significant invasion. The most important Shiga toxin–producing *E. coli* (STEC) clone belongs to serotype O157:H7. In addition to Stx, this organism expresses an impressive array of virulence-related factors, including adherence factors and secreted host-damaging proteins

(reviewed by Nataro and Kaper[2]). Infection is accompanied by a watery diarrhea, frequently progressing to frank hemorrhagic colitis.[4,5] Systemic absorption of Stx leads to serious sequelae, including hemolytic uremic syndrome (HUS), which develops in up to 20% of pediatric patients infected with *E. coli* O157:H7. Other potentially fatal complications include intestinal perforation and cerebrovascular accident.

Identification of O157:H7 infection can be challenging because many patients present with nonspecific diarrheal illness, particularly during the early phase of illness. Once isolated in the lab, the bacterium can be identified by detection of its O (somatic) and H (flagellar) antigens. Often, however, the diagnosis is not suspected until the patient presents with the characteristic triad of HUS: thrombocytopenia, hemolytic anemia, and renal failure. There exist no effective means to prevent the development of HUS, even in the early stages of illness. Indeed, antibiotic therapy may exacerbate the illness and increase the likelihood that HUS will supervene.[6]

Epidemiology

Serotype O157:H7 is endemic in the United States. The ongoing FoodNet multicenter surveillance network has calculated a preliminary incidence of 2.1 cases per 100,000 population across all sites.[7] Infection is most common in the northern tier of U.S. states.

O157:H7 infection is acquired by ingestion of contaminated food or water or by person-to-person spread. Calculations from outbreak investigations have estimated the infectious dose of O157:H7 to be as low as 100 organisms, and perhaps less.[8] A natural reservoir for the pathogen exists in the intestines of cattle, including those maintained for beef production.[4] Several large outbreaks have been attributed to ingestion of contaminated meat and other foods, which are thought to be secondarily contaminated by bovine feces.[4] Although the organism is readily killed by high temperatures, inadequate cooking of beef or contamination of foods typically consumed uncooked can result in disease. Thus the difficulty in eliminating the organism from bovine populations presents significant challenges to control that may be best addressed via vaccination.

TABLE 43–1 ■ Approaches to Vaccination Against Shiga Toxin–Producing *E. coli* (STEC)

	Advantages	Disadvantages
ANTIGEN		
O157 polysaccharide	■ Represents most important capsular type ■ O antigen is immunogenic and possibly protective	■ Will not protect against all STECs
Shiga toxin	■ Responsible for all serious outcomes ■ Toxin can be inactivated via mutation	■ Optimal route of delivery not yet established ■ Inadvertent reactogenicity possible as a result of as yet uncharacterized toxic effects
Intimin outer membrane protein	■ Present on O157 and many other STECs ■ Immunogenic	■ Response may not be protective
MODE OF DELIVERY		
Oral	■ Protects at site of infection ■ Ease of administration ■ Potentially lower cost of production ■ Potential for convenient presentation of multiple antigens	■ Systemic response to antigens variable
Parenteral	■ No requirement for resistance to gastric acidity ■ May stimulate optimal systemic response to Stx ■ Ease of development	■ Administration more costly and complicated ■ Absence of mucosal protection

Shiga Toxin–Producing *Escherichia coli* Vaccine Candidates

A number of STEC vaccine approaches are under development (Table 43–1). Each approach has advantages and disadvantages, and neither the most effective antigen nor the optimal mode of delivery has been established.

Shiga Toxin Toxoids

All serious sequelae of STEC infection are due to the actions of Stx, an oligomeric toxin related to the toxin produced by *S. dysenteriae* 1 (reviewed by Sandvig[3]). Stx comprises a single catalytic A subunit of 32 kDa and five B subunits of 7.7 kDa each. The B subunits mediate binding to the cell via the glycolipid globotriaosylceramide (Gb3). The A subunit is an *N*-glycosidase that catalyzes the depurination of a single site in the 28S eukaryotic ribosomal RNA, thereby inhibiting protein synthesis and leading to the death of the target cell. The Stx family comprises two subgroups, Stx1 and Stx2, sharing 55% amino acid identity. Most cases of HUS are attributable to Stx2.

The importance of Stx in STEC disease has made it a natural target for immunization. Antibodies against the B subunit have been shown to prevent binding of the toxin to target cells.[9] However, the A-B complex is considerably more immunogenic than the B subunit alone, and thus both B and A-B toxoids have been examined as candidate vaccines. Despite the fact that the B subunit comprises the cell-binding moiety, it may not be completely devoid of cytotoxic effects,[10] and therefore its use as a vaccine may necessitate some degree of inactivation.

Keusch and colleagues have demonstrated that parenteral administration of Stx2 inactivated with formalin-lysine provided 100% protection to mice subsequently challenged intraperitoneally with 1000 median lethal doses of Stx2.[11] Human trials are pending. This approach has merit, and likely

will be tested first as a vaccine for *S. dysenteriae*, which is a more important pathogen than STEC worldwide.

Nasal immunization is a highly efficient route for the induction of mucosal responses. Byun et al.[12] immunized mice nasally with purified recombinant Stx1B with a cholera toxin adjuvant. Brisk serum immunoglobulin G (IgG) and mucosal immunoglobulin A (IgA) responses were observed, and the antibodies were able to block binding of Stx to its receptor. Like the oral route, the intranasal route of vaccination has the advantage of ease of administration, but an additional advantage is the lack of a requirement for acid stabilization of the antigen. Human trials of the Stx1B vaccine have not yet been reported.

O-Specific Polysaccharide Conjugate Vaccines

The *E. coli* O antigen represents the polysaccharide component of the gram-negative lipopolysaccharide (LPS). Because serogroup O157 is responsible for the large majority of severe STEC infections in the United States, immunity to the O157 O antigen is a reasonable objective of vaccination. Volunteers immunized with detoxified O157 polysaccharide conjugated to *Pseudomonas aeruginosa* recombinant exoprotein A mount excellent O antigen–specific responses after a single dose.[13] However, there is concern that such antibodies could lyse STEC in the human intestine and thereby promote release of Stx. For this reason, O157 LPS has been conjugated to the StxB1 subunit, to elicit simultaneous anti-toxic and anticapsular antibody responses. In young mice, this formulation induced both bactericidal antibodies to *E. coli* O157 and neutralizing antibodies to Stx.[14] This latter vaccine candidate is undergoing human trials.

Although an *E. coli* O157 polysaccharide-albumin conjugate elicited a strong serum antibody response on parenteral administration to mice, the vaccine did not protect the mice from intestinal colonization by *E. coli* O157.[15] These results raise some concerns that peripheral immunity may not be sufficient to protect against enteric infection. Similarly, mice orally vaccinated with a glycoconjugate vaccine containing the O157 antigen mixed with cholera toxin as adjuvant were not protected from colonization with O157:H7.[16] Finally, it should be noted that non-O157 serogroups are a significant cause of diarrhea and even HUS, especially outside of the United States.[2] Therefore, reliance on anti-O157 immunity may not provide complete protection against STEC disease.

Live, Attenuated Shiga Toxin–Producing *Escherichia coli* Vaccine Candidates

Several attenuated vector vaccines have been modified to express STEC antigens. Of these, only a few are being seriously considered as vaccine candidates. StxB has been coexpressed along with the outer membrane protein adhesin intimin in an attenuated *Vibrio cholerae* vector, Peru2. Intimin is a 94-kDa STEC protein whose binding to the enterocyte both facilitates colonization and initiates diarrheagenic signal transduction cascades. The intimin vaccine construct was tested in a rabbit model and found to elicit antibodies to StxB; one of two rabbits responded to intimin.[17]

An *E. coli* hemolysin-based system has been adapted to facilitate secretion of Stx2B across the outer membrane of a *Salmonella typhimurium aroA* auxotrophic vaccine vector.[18,19] This construct was shown to export the protein efficiently but has yet to be proven effective in humans.

Conlan et al. have found that orally administered *Salmonella landau*, a *Salmonella* strain that naturally expresses the O157 antigen, is able to elicit protection of mice from colonization by *E. coli* O157.[20] These results suggest that local exposure to the O157 antigen may induce resistance when delivered by *Salmonella*, although humans exposed to STEC do not generate highly protective O157 responses after natural infection.

Public Health Considerations and Indications for Vaccination

Because of the obstacles to control of STEC infection, there is appropriate interest in the development of safe and effective STEC vaccines. At the same time, there are significant policy issues regarding STEC vaccination of humans. Given the low incidence of serious infection and HUS, a vaccine would need to be highly effective and extraordinarily safe. Moreover, vaccination of cattle to prevent carriage of the organism is a viable alternative that is receiving increasing attention. Vaccination of cattle would not pose the same requirement for complete safety, but would presumably need to be economically feasible.

Enterotoxigenic *Escherichia coli*

Disease caused by enterotoxigenic *E. coli* (ETEC) is characterized by profuse watery diarrhea lasting several days. Infection is usually self-limited in a healthy individual but may lead to dehydration and malnutrition in young children, especially those in developing countries. Antibiotic treatment may shorten the duration of disease, but rehydration is usually considered sufficient. ETEC cause disease following ingestion of contaminated food or water by

attachment to the small bowel mucosa, followed by elaboration of heat-labile toxin (LT) and/or heat-stable toxin (ST). ETEC attach to specific enterocyte receptors by virtue of proteinaceous, hair-like fimbriae. Different strains of ETEC express antigenically distinct types of fimbriae, which have been named coli surface antigens (CSs) or colonization factor antigens (CFAs).[21] More than 20 types of fimbriae have been identified on human ETEC isolates, with seven types (CFA/I and CS1 through CS6) occurring most frequently. Immune responses mounted against these fimbriae are believed to be protective by inhibiting binding of bacteria to the gut epithelium.[21] Importantly, however, immune responses against one fimbrial type are not cross-protective against the other types. Therefore, a broadly effective vaccine would require inclusion of multiple fimbrial types.

Once attached to the intestinal epithelium, ETEC elaborate LT and/or ST enterotoxins, which induce the characteristic watery diarrhea. LT, highly homologous to cholera toxin, is composed of a single catalytic A subunit and five identical B subunits. Like Stx, the LT-B subunit comprises the cell-binding domain. Anti-LT responses are elicited in most people who have had diarrhea as a result of ETEC. Moreover, short-term protection against ETEC disease has been documented in individuals immunized with a cholera toxin B (CTB) subunit vaccine, as a result of immunologic cross-reactivity between cholera toxin and LT B subunits.[22]

ST is a small peptide toxin of only 18 to 19 amino acids that acts via stimulation of membrane-bound guanylate cyclase in target cells. In contrast to LT, ST is not immunogenic and is not considered a candidate immunogen.

Epidemiology

ETEC is the most commonly isolated enteropathogen in children under 5 years of age in developing countries, accounting for 200 million cases of diarrhea and several hundred thousand deaths each year.[23] The bacteria are also the number one cause of travelers' diarrhea, affecting individuals from industrialized countries traveling to developing regions of the world.

Vaccines Against Enterotoxigenic *Escherichia coli*

Several lines of evidence support the feasibility of an efficacious ETEC vaccine. Epidemiologic as well as volunteer studies have demonstrated homologous protection against re-infection by ETEC strains. This protection appears to be mediated by antibodies to adherence fimbriae. Numerous strategies have been employed in attempts to capitalize on the potential for ETEC immunity.

Whole-Cell Killed Vaccines

The most advanced ETEC vaccine candidate was developed by investigators at the University of Göteborg in Sweden, and consists of a killed whole-cell formulation plus recombinant CTB subunit (rCTB). The vaccine comprises five strains of formalin-killed ETEC, which collectively express the most prevalent fimbriae: CFA/I and CS1 through CS6. This vaccine has been found to be safe and immunogenic in adult volunteers as well as in children between 2 and 12 years of age.[24–26] Immune responses, as measured by intestinal lavage and antibody-secreting cells, were elicited against rCTB as well as each fimbrial type.[24] In addition, this vaccine has been found to be immunogenic when tested in endemic areas, including tests on adults and children in Bangladesh and Egypt.[25-28]

This work was prompted by the efficacy, albeit partial and brief, of a killed whole-cell cholera vaccine (plus CTB subunit) in prevention of ETEC disease in travelers.[22] The cholera-ETEC vaccine is indeed licensed for this application in 13 countries, though in neither the United States nor the United Kingdom.

Live, Attenuated Enterotoxigenic *Escherichia coli* Vaccine

Investigators at Acambis Ltd. in Cambridge, U.K., have developed two live, oral attenuated ETEC candidate strains that express CS1 and CS3. Introduction of mutations into the *aroC* and *ompR* genes or the *aroC*, *ompC*, *and ompF* genes of a nontoxigenic ETEC strain resulted in vaccine strains that were safe and generally well tolerated when fed to volunteers at doses of 10^7 to 10^9 colony-forming units (CFU) in a Phase I study.[29] Immune responses to the fimbrial components were recorded in volunteers ingesting the highest dose, with mild diarrhea occurring in approximately 15% of volunteers in this group. Interestingly, this result is similar to that found with the prototrophic version of the same strain previously tested in volunteers by Levine and co-workers.[30]

Live, Attenuated Bivalent Shigella–Enterotoxigenic *Escherichia coli* Vaccines

An alternative strategy pursued by investigators at the Center for Vaccine Development at the University of Maryland, Baltimore, involves presenting the ETEC fimbrial antigens in a live, attenuated *Shigella* vaccine strain. This approach utilizes a *Shigella* vaccine strain as a vector for the delivery of both ETEC fimbriae and LT toxoid. Preclinical animal studies have shown candidate vaccine formulations to be immunogenic in eliciting serum and mucosal immune responses to both the *Shigella* vector and the ETEC antigens.[31-33]

Purified Antigen Vaccines

Initial immunization attempts with purified fimbriae delivered by the oral route were not successful because of degradation of the antigens in the gastrointestinal tract.[30] Subsequently, investigators encapsulated CFA/II fimbriae in microspheres in an attempt to enhance uptake by gut-associated lymphoid tissue. Following delivery to volunteers, the CFA/II-microsphere vaccine was found to be modestly immunogenic but poorly protective against challenge with wild-type ETEC.[34]

Guerena-Burgueno et al. found that purified CS6 together with purified LT elicited both anti-CS6 and anti-LT responses in approximately half of the immunized volunteers when delivered by transcutaneous patch.[35] Interestingly, dermal patch immunization required the presence of LT as an adjuvant for stimulation of responses to the CS6 antigen. This approach could be highly promising, both in terms of ease of administration and as a mechanism for delivering multiple antigens simultaneously.

Subunit or Cross-Protective Peptide Vaccines

Although antigenically distinct, several of the fimbrial subunits share amino acid homology, especially CFA/I, CS1, CS2, and CS4. Based on this homology, it has been hypothesized that subunits or epitopes derived from the homologous regions might elicit cross-protective responses against ETEC bearing the related fimbriae. Several strategies have been employed to present fimbrial subunits or epitopes in an immunogenic fashion, including incorporation into the flagellar structure of *Salmonella*,[36] expression in edible plants,[37] or immunization with DNA vaccines.[38]

Public Health Considerations and Indications for Vaccination

Weanling infants in less industrialized countries comprise a reasonable target population for ETEC vaccination. Public health considerations are similar to those for rotavirus. However, the strength of the indication would rely on the efficacy of the vaccine against a broad array of ETEC adhesin types, as well as the ease of administration. It should be noted that mortality caused by ETEC is nearly always the result of dehydration, and so proper insititution of oral rehydration therapy would dramatically reduce mortality. Nevertheless, the high incidence of this infection makes vaccination a reasonable aim, especially if the vaccine also carried immunogens against other infections prevalent in the child's area. It should be noted also that an effective ETEC vaccine probably will produce only relatively short-lived protection and likely will not substantially reduce asymptomatic shedding. Thus ETEC vaccines may decrease the incidence of disease in the most vulnerable populations, but will not result in eradication of ETEC from developing countries.

In addition to weanling infants, travelers to developing countries are a target population for ETEC immunization. Although mortality is very low in this population, there could be economic incentive for development of such a vaccine. A drawback to this effort is that only a minority of all travelers' diarrhea cases are due to ETEC, so the traveler must be cognizant that even a perfectly protective ETEC vaccine does not provide license to violate the boundaries of good fecal-oral hygiene during foreign travel.

Shigella Species

Shigella species invade the colonic epithelium through M cells and then spread laterally from cell to cell (reviewed by Sansonetti[39]). The characteristic blood and mucus found in the stools of patients results from sloughing of contiguously invaded epithelial cells and the induction of inflammatory responses by the bacteria. This invasive ability, the major virulence characteristic of *Shigella*, is mediated by specialized factors encoded by a high-molecular-weight virulence plasmid. *Shigella dysenteriae* has an additional virulence factor, Stx, that inhibits protein synthesis in eukaryotic cells via inactivation of ribosomal RNA, leading to cell death. Stx is responsible for the sequelae, including HUS, associated with *S. dysenteriae* infection.

Epidemiology

Four species of *Shigella* cause significant disease in humans: *S. dysenteriae*, *S. flexneri*, *S. sonnei*, and *S. boydii*. *Shigella flexneri* is endemic in developing countries and is the most commonly isolated species worldwide. *Shigella sonnei* is the causative agent of most shigellosis in the United States as well as other highly industrialized countries, accounting for 77% of isolates in this environment, compared to 15% in less developed countries.[40] *Shigella dysenteriae* is not a common cause of endemic disease (with some exceptions) but can cause vicious outbreaks in confined populations, most notably during refugee situations. *Shigella boydii* remains a cause of infection in some less developed countries, but typically accounts for 6% or less of shigellosis cases.

Shigella species have no animal reservoir, so infection always results from contamination with human feces. Index cases typically result from ingestion of contaminated food or water. All *Shigella* species have a low infectious dose, so person-to-person transmission is common. Outbreaks in institutionalized populations typically feature predominantly person-to-person transmisssion cycles.

Like ETEC, *Shigella* is common among travelers and military personnel. Troops deployed to less industrialized countries or living in camp situations with less than optimal hygiene conditions are prime targets for *Shigella* outbreaks.

Vaccines Against *Shigella*

No licensed vaccine exists for *Shigella*. Research in many laboratories over the past 50 years has illuminated pathogenic mechanisms and has made inroads toward characterizing the requirements for a protective immune response. Epidemiologic and volunteer studies suggest that protective immunity is directed to the O-somatic antigen of the *Shigella* LPS polysaccharide and is type specific.[41,42] Although the four species of *Shigella* are divided into more than 47 serotypes, several specific types are considered the most important agents of human disease. An LPS-directed vaccine with broad-spectrum protective

efficacy would therefore necessitate inclusion of multiple serotypes.

Live, Attenuated Vaccines

Recent attempts at constructing live, attenuated oral strains have utilized molecular biology techniques to introduce well-defined mutations into wild-type *Shigella* strains (Table 43–2). Advances in the understanding of *Shigella* pathogenesis allow precise disruption of virulence genes without alteration in the invasive phenotype, which is believed to be required for a protective response.

Sansonetti and co-workers made a series of strains with mutations in the *virG* (*icsA*) gene, which is involved in cell-to-cell spread.[43] This approach was based on the theory that invasion could still occur but spread would be limited, thereby attenuating virulence. Double-mutant derivatives of strain *S. flexneri* 5a were produced containing mutations in *virG* and *ompB* or in *virG* and *iuc*, the gene encoding aerobactin.[44] In animal studies the *ompB*, *virG* strain was very safe but did not confer protection in 100% of the animals,[44] whereas the *virG*, *iuc* strain caused low-level side effects in some animals and 100% protection following challenge.[45] *Shigella flexneri* 2a strain SC602 was next engineered with the *virG*, *iuc* mutations. A dose-response clinical trial demonstrated that ingestion of 10^6 or 10^8 CFU caused symptoms of shigellosis in most volunteers, while a dose of 10^4 CFU caused only mild symptoms in a few volunteers.[46] Furthermore, volunteers ingesting a single dose of 10^4 CFU of SC602 were protected against challenge with wild-type *S. flexneri* 2a. This very promising study underscores the need for a broad range of safety associated with the use of a live vaccine strain.

A *virG*-deleted strain of *S. sonnei*, strain WRSS1, has been evaluated in a Phase I clinical study. A single dose of 10^3, 10^4, 10^5, or 10^6 CFU caused low-grade fever or mild diarrhea in 22% of recipients.[47] The vaccine was found to be highly immunogenic, generating robust levels of serum anti-LPS, and anti–LPS IgA antibody-secreting cells.[47]

TABLE 43–2 ▪ Efficacy and Tolerability of Live, Attenuated *Shigella* Vaccine Candidates

Organism or vaccine	Dose (CFU)	Adverse Reactions	% Anti-LPS Response (Geometric Mean)		Protective Efficacy*
			IgA Antibody-Secreting Cells	IgG Antibodies	
S. flexneri	10^2	43%	71% (18)	29%	Not tested
natural infection	10^3	92%	92% (239)	50%	70%
Streptomycin-dependent SmD[84]	10^{10}	0–15%	Not tested	38%	49%
EcSf2a-2[60]	10^9	0%	100% (59)	53%	48%
	10^8	10%	100% (16)	19%	27%
	10^9	17%	93% (21)	35%	0%
SC602[46]	10^4	13%	58% (18)	33%	52%
CVD 1203[50]	10^9	80%	100% (175)	46%	Not tested
	10^8	12%	91% (43)	45%	Not tested
	10^6	0%	60% (13)	30%	Not tested
CVD 1207[†]	10^{10}	20%	100% (35)	17%	Not tested
	10^9	8%	64% (9)	17%	Not tested
	10^8	0%	67% (5)	Not tested	Not tested
	10^7	0%	100% (6)	Not tested	Not tested
	10^6	0%	0% (0.1)	14%	Not tested

*Protective efficacy against experimental challenge.
[†]K. Kotloff, personal communication.
Courtesy of K. Kotloff (see text for details).

Based on the promising early work of Stocker and colleagues on auxotrophic *Salmonella* mutants,[48] Noriega and co-workers generated *S. flexneri* 2a vaccine strain CVD 1203 with mutations in *aroA* and *virG*.[49] This combination of mutations rendered the strain auxotrophic for aromatic amino acid biosynthesis and deficient in its ability to spread from cell to cell. In a Phase I study, volunteers ingesting CVD 1203 at doses of 10^8 or 10^9 CFU exhibited short-lived adverse reactions, including fever, diarrhea, and/or dysentery, in a dose-dependent manner.[50] However, a single dose of 10^6 CFU remained immunogenic, yet engendered no adverse reactions in any volunteer.

Further attempts at achieving the correct balance of immunogenicity and lack of reactogenicity led Noriega and co-workers to generate *S. flexneri* 2a strain CVD 1204, harboring a deletion in the *guaBA* operon.[51] This mutation rendered the bacteria auxotrophic for guanine and highly attenuated in the guinea pig model of keratoconjunctivitis. Two further derivatives of CVD 1204 carried additional mutations in one or both of two *Shigella* enterotoxins: ShET1, encoded by the *set* genes, and ShET2 encoded by the *sen* gene. Strain CVD 1209 contains mutations in *guaBA* and *set*, while CVD 1208 contains mutations in *guaBA*, *set*, and *sen*.[52] Human studies on this series of candidates are underway.

Combination Vaccines

The possibility that vaccination with a mixture of live, attenuated *Shigella* strains of distinct serotypes could engender protection against multiple types was suggested by Mel and co-workers in volunteer and field trials in the 1960s.[53] Using a molecular genetics approach, Klee and co-workers expressed the O-specific antigen from *S. dysenteriae* in a *S. flexneri* attenuated strain and were able to elicit both anti–*S. dysenteriae* and anti–*S. flexneri* responses in an animal model.[54–56] In a comprehensive strategy, Noriega and co-workers reasoned that inclusion of 3 of the 14 *S. flexneri* serotypes expressing all of the type- and group-specific antigens found on the other serotypes could engender cross-protection against all *S. flexneri* strains.[57] In animal studies, immunization with a combination of attenuated *S. flexneri* 2a and *S. flexneri* 3a conferred protection (ranging from 20% to 92%) against serotypes 1a, Y, 1b, 4b, 2b, and 5b.[57] These authors contend that addition of *S. flexneri* 6, *S. dysenteriae* type 1, and *S. sonnei* attenuated strains would provide protection against a majority of disease caused by *Shigella*. The above studies support the hypothesis that a multivalent vaccine is a realistic goal for providing broad-spectrum protection against *Shigella*.

Live Carrier Strains

An alternative method for engendering anti-*Shigella* LPS responses with a live vaccine is to use another bacterial species engineered to express *Shigella*-specific determinants. The *E. coli/Shigella* hybrid strain EcSf2a-2 comprises an *aroD*-deleted enteroinvasive *E. coli* strain expressing the LPS of *S. flexneri* 2a.[58] Volunteer studies differing in number and timing of doses demonstrated the vaccine to be generally well tolerated, with only mild symptoms in a few volunteers.[59,60] Although there was some degree of protection against challenge, this was not statistically significant. Subsequent field trials with EcSf2a-2 in an Israeli Defense

Force field site confirmed that the vaccine was well tolerated, but no efficacy data were generated as a result of the lack of disease caused by *S. flexneri* 2a during the course of the trial.[61]

Parenteral Shigella Vaccines

An alternative strategy for the generation of efficacious *Shigella* vaccines is based on the theory that parenteral O-specific IgG responses are protective against *Shigella* disease. Robbins and co-workers have produced conjugate vaccines consisting of purified *Shigella* LPS conjugated to a protein carrier.[62] Three conjugate vaccines have been tested, including *S. dysenteriae* type 1 LPS conjugated to tetanus toxoid, *S. flexneri* 2a LPS conjugated to recombinant *Pseudomonas* exoprotein A, and *S. sonnei* LPS conjugated to exoprotein A. These three candidates were shown to be immunogenic and efficacious against disease when tested in volunteer trials and field trials with the Israeli Defense Force.[62–65] Recent advances in conjugation chemistry, including the use of succinylated protein carriers, have resulted in improved immunogenicity of the *Shigella* LPS-protein conjugate vaccine.[66]

Public Health Considerations and Indications for Vaccination

Shigella vaccine development remains an active area of research, with both live, attenuated strains and LPS-protein conjugate strategies demonstrating promise. The availability of an efficacious vaccine would serve several populations in need, especially young children in developing countries where morbidity and mortality resulting from *Shigella* are highest and including military personnel and travelers to developing countries. In addition, such a vaccine would be an invaluable tool for combating the devastating morbidity and mortality resulting from explosive outbreaks of *Shigella*, especially *S. dysenteriae*.

Campylobacter jejuni

Campylobacter jejuni is a major cause of diarrheal disease in both industrialized and developing populations. The organism ranks as the most common bacterial cause of diarrhea in both the United States[67] and the United Kingdom.[68] In many developing countries, infection is nearly universal by early childhood, and in many cases asymptomatic reinfection and prolonged carriage are the rule.[69] Despite its frequent isolation in the United States, *Campylobacter* represents an important cause of travelers' diarrhea among Americans visiting developing countries; this is likely a function of the heterogeneous antigenic properties of clinical isolates. Perhaps of greater concern than its role in diarrheal disease is its association with many life-threatening cases of Guillain-Barré syndrome (GBS).[70] Vaccine development against *Campylobacter* thus constitutes a high priority for the military, travelers, and pediatric populations in the developing world, yet an effective vaccine is not yet available.

After an incubation period of 1 to 3 days, *Campylobacter* infection typically begins with a watery diarrhea phase. The infection commonly manifests with signs of inflammation:

fever, abdominal pain, and bloody diarrhea.[71] Infection in developing countries is more commonly watery in nature, without frank blood.[69] Untreated infection may subside after 3 to 7 days, but persistent disease is not uncommon.

GBS, a form of symmetric ascending paralysis with autoimmune etiology, may follow *Campylobacter* infection. GBS is usually self-limiting, but death may occur, especially if clinical management is not optimal.[70] The pathophysiology of *Campylobacter*-associated GBS is not fully elucidated, but, importantly, antibodies to the *C. jejuni* lipo-oligosaccharides (LOSs) have been shown to cross-react with human neural sheath gangliosides.[72,73]

Epidemiology

Campylobacter species are frequent commensals in the intestinal tracts of birds.[71] As such, they are commonly implicated in food-borne diarrheal illness, or as pathogens among populations in close contact with avian populations. Studies in industrialized countries estimate an overall disease incidence of approximately 1% per year,[67] and *Campylobacter* species have been implicated as the major cause of food-borne bacterial infection in the United States. In the United States, the mortality resulting from *Campylobacter* has been estimated at 200 to 700 deaths per year.[67]

In developing countries, *Campylobacter* may cause several infections per year per child, but the disease occurs almost exclusively in infants.[69] Estimates place the worldwide rate of *Campylobacter* infection at 400 million cases per year. In endemic areas, repeat infection is the rule, and typically repeated infections are milder. Children over the age of 5 years and adults are characteristically asymptomatic.[74]

Campylobacter is typically found to be the second most common cause of travelers' diarrhea after ETEC.[75] It frequently afflicts military populations, and may be responsible for large outbreaks during military exercises.[76] Some studies suggest that *Campylobacter*-associated cases of travelers' diarrhea may be more severe than those caused by other pathogens.[77] Although antibiotic therapy of *Campylobacter* infections may produce benefit if given early in the course of infection, antibiotic resistance is a growing concern.[78]

Transmission of *Campylobacter* generally occurs through consumption of contaminated water, milk, and raw meats, especially poultry.[67] Contact with animals and birds is a common source of infection. Person-to-person transmission is not efficient, and usually occurs from infant to parent.

Vaccines Against *Campylobacter*

Vaccine approaches to protect against *Campylobacter* infection are complicated by the organism's antigenic heterogeneity, and by the threat of GBS. Surface antigens of *Campylobacter* are highly diverse. Two antigenic typing systems are in use: the Lior system and the Penner system. The Lior typing scheme is based on a heat-labile surface antigen that is still not characterized[79]; 108 serotypes are recognized in this scheme. The Penner system recognizes over 60 serotypes and is based on LPS and LOS antigens.[80]

Immunity to *Campylobacter* is highly complex and not well understood. Immunity appears to be strain specific, and

the antigens conferring immunity are not well understood. Baqar et al. have reported severe clinical campylobacteriosis in an adult previously infected with *Campylobacter* in the course of a volunteer study.[81] For this patient, both strains were available to researchers, providing an unusual opportunity to examine the characteristics of the immune response. At the time of infection with the second *Campylobacter* strain, the patient had persisting antibodies against the first *Campylobacter* strain, and some of these antibodies cross-reacted with the second pathogen. Lymphocyte proliferative responses were observed to the first infecting strain early in the second infection, but not to the second strain; during the convalescence period, however, such responses were demonstrable to both strains. These data suggest that strain-specific cell-mediated responses may account for sterilizing immunity to *Campylobacter* infection.

Uncertainty regarding the mechanism of GBS is an obstacle to *Campylobacter* vaccine development. Thus vaccines that deliver whole bacteria, either viable or killed, must be generated and evaluated with extreme caution. Accordingly, the most intensively studied *Campylobacter* vaccine candidate comprises a mixture of heat- and formalin-killed whole bacteria derived from prototype strain 81-176, combined with *E. coli* LT as a mucosal adjuvant.[82] In mice, a single dose combined with LT provided homologous protection against intestinal colonization at an efficacy of 87%. Human studies are underway, but preliminary results suggest that the vaccine is well tolerated and efficacious, although multiple oral doses are required for protection. Data describing homologous and heterologous protection rates are not yet available.

Other vaccine strategies against *Campylobacter* are also being considered. The bacterial flagellin is an attractive candidate because of its relatively high antigenic conservation compared with surface LPS and LOS. A truncated recombinant flagellin subunit vaccine has been evaluated in mice.[83] When given in a single intranasal dose with LT, the flagellin induced anti-flagella antibody responses and over 80% protection against disease symptoms and colonization with a heterologous *C. jejuni* strain. As of this writing, this vaccine candidate has not yet been tested in humans. An advantage of the flagella-based vaccine strategy is that this molecule is not expected to elicit GBS.

Public Health Considerations and Indications for Vaccination

Campylobacter vaccination is a priority in developing countries, where infants experience a high burden of life-threatening diarrhea. It is important to note, however, that any effective *Campylobacter* vaccine would need to be deliverable and efficacious early in life. This requirement erects obstacles for delivery in developing nations, where many children do not have regular access to medical care.

Travelers to developing nations may benefit from *Campylobacter* vaccination, especially those traveling for prolonged periods and the military traveler. Although *Campylobacter* infection is less common than infection with *E. coli* and *Shigella*, the risk of GBS increases the risks of *Campylobacter* infection.

Widespread *Campylobacter* vaccination in developing nations would decrease the risk of death caused by infant diarrhea. Because of the presence of environmental reservoirs and the prevalence of asymptomatic excretion of the organism in immune individuals, it is unlikely that vaccination would substantially decrease the presence of the pathogen in the community. Indeed, vaccination may result in an upward shift in the age distribution of symptomatic infection. This effect could be beneficial because older children and adults are substantially more likely to survive campylobacteriosis.

REFERENCES

1. Bettelheim KA. *Escherichia coli* in the normal flora of humans and animals. *In* Sussman M (ed): *Escherichia coli*: Mechanisms of Virulence. Cambridge, UK, Cambridge University Press, 1997, pp 85–109.
2. Nataro JP, Kaper JB. Diarrheagenic *Escherichia coli*. Clin Microbiol Rev 11:142–201, 1998.
3. Sandvig K. Shiga toxins. Toxicon 39:1629–1635, 2001.
4. Slutsker L, Ries AA, Greene KD, et al. *Escherichia coli* O157:H7 diarrhea in the United States: clinical and epidemiologic features. Ann Intern Med 126:505–513, 1997.
5. Tarr PI, Neill MA. *Escherichia coli* O157:H7. Gastroenterol Clin North Am 30:735–751, 2001.
6. Wong CS, Jelacic S, Habeeb RL, et al. The risk of the hemolytic-uremic syndrome after antibiotic treatment of *Escherichia coli* O157:H7 infections. N Engl J Med 342:1930–1936, 2000.
7. Centers for Disease Control and Prevention. Preliminary FoodNet data on the incidence of foodborne illnesses—selected sites, United States, 2000. JAMA 285:2071–2073, 2001.
8. Tilden J Jr, Young W, McNamara AM, et al. A new route of transmission for *Escherichia coli*: infection from dry fermented salami. Am J Public Health 86:1142–1145, 1996.
9. Marcato P, Mulvey G, Read RJ, et al. Immunoprophylactic potential of cloned Shiga toxin 2 B subunit. J Infect Dis 183:435–443, 2001.
10. Marcato P, Mulvey G, Armstrong GD. Cloned Shiga toxin 2 B subunit induces apoptosis in Ramos Burkitt's lymphoma B cells. Infect Immun 70:1279–1286, 2002.
11. Keusch G, Acheson D, Marchant C, McIver J. Toxoid-based active and passive immunization to prevent and/or modulate hemolytic-uremic syndrome due to Shiga toxin-producing *Escherichia coli*. *In* Kaper J, O'Brien A (eds). *Escherichia coli* O157:H7 and Other Shiga Toxin-Producing *E. coli* Strains. Washington, DC, American Society for Microbiology, 1998, pp 409–418.
12. Byun Y, Ohmura M, Fujihashi K, et al. Nasal immunization with *E. coli* verotoxin 1 (VT1)-B subunit and a nontoxic mutant of cholera toxin elicits serum neutralizing antibodies. Vaccine 19:2061–2070, 2001.
13. Konadu EY, Parke JC Jr, Tran HT, et al. Investigational vaccine for *Escherichia coli* O157: phase 1 study of O157 O-specific polysaccharide-*Pseudomonas aeruginosa* recombinant exoprotein A conjugates in adults. J Infect Dis 177:383–387, 1998.
14. Konadu E, Donohue-Rolfe A, Calderwood SB, et al. Syntheses and immunologic properties of *Escherichia coli* O157 O-specific polysaccharide and Shiga toxin 1 B subunit conjugates in mice. Infect Immun 67:6191–6193, 1999.
15. Conlan JW, Cox AD, KuoLee R, et al. Parenteral immunization with a glycoconjugate vaccine containing the O157 antigen of *Escherichia coli* O157:H7 elicits a systemic humoral immune response in mice, but fails to prevent colonization by the pathogen. Can J Microbiol 45:279–286, 1999.
16. Conlan JW, KuoLee R, Webb A, et al. Oral immunization of mice with a glycoconjugate vaccine containing the O157 antigen of *Escherichia coli* O157:H7 admixed with cholera toxin fails to elicit protection against subsequent colonization by the pathogen. Can J Microbiol 46:283–290, 2000.
17. Butterton JR, Ryan ET, Acheson DW, Calderwood SB. Coexpression of the B subunit of Shiga toxin 1 and EaeA from enterohemorrhagic *Escherichia coli* in *Vibrio cholerae* vaccine strains. Infect Immun 65:2127–2135, 1997.
18. Tzschaschel BD, Guzman CA, Timmis KN, de Lorenzo V. An *Escherichia coli* hemolysin transport system based vector for the export of polypeptides: export of Shiga-like toxin IIeB subunit by *Salmonella typhimurium aroA*. Nat Biotechnol 14:765–769, 1996.
19. Tzschaschel BD, Klee SR, de Lorenzo V, et al. Towards a vaccine candidate against *Shigella dysenteriae* 1: expression of the Shiga toxin B-subunit in an attenuated *Shigella flexneri aroD* carrier strain. Microb Pathog 21:277–288, 1996.
20. Conlan JW, KuoLee R, Webb A, Perry MB. *Salmonella landau* as a live vaccine against *Escherichia coli* O157:H7 investigated in a mouse model of intestinal colonization. Can J Microbiol 45:723–731, 1999.
21. Levine M, Giron JA, Noriega F. Fimbrial vaccines. *In* Klemm P (ed). Fimbriae: Adhesion, Biogenics, Genetics, and Vaccines. Boca Raton, FL, CRC Press, 1994, pp 255–270.
22. Peltola H, Siitonen A, Kyronseppa H, et al. Prevention of travellers' diarrhoea by oral B-subunit/whole-cell cholera vaccine. Lancet 338:1285–1289, 1991.
23. Black RE. Epidemiology of diarrhoeal disease: implications for control by vaccines. Vaccine 11:100–106, 1993.
24. Jertborn M, Ahren C, Holmgren J, Svennerholm AM. Safety and immunogenicity of an oral inactivated enterotoxigenic *Escherichia coli* vaccine. Vaccine 16:255–260, 1998.
25. Savarino SJ, Brown FM, Hall E, et al. Safety and immunogenicity of an oral, killed enterotoxigenic *Escherichia coli*-cholera toxin B subunit vaccine in Egyptian adults. J Infect Dis 177:796–799, 1998.
26. Hall ER, Wierzba TF, Ahren C, et al. Induction of systemic antifimbria and antitoxin antibody responses in Egyptian children and adults by an oral, killed enterotoxigenic *Escherichia coli* plus cholera toxin B subunit vaccine. Infect Immun 69:2853–2857, 2001.
27. Savarino SJ, Hall ER, Bassily S, et al. Oral, inactivated, whole cell enterotoxigenic *Escherichia coli* plus cholera toxin B subunit vaccine: results of the initial evaluation in children. PRIDE Study Group. J Infect Dis 179:107–114, 1999.
28. Qadri F, Das SK, Faruque AS, et al. Prevalence of toxin types and colonization factors in enterotoxigenic *Escherichia coli* isolated during a 2-year period from diarrheal patients in Bangladesh. J Clin Microbiol 38:27–31, 2000.
29. Turner AK, Terry TD, Sack DA, et al. Construction and characterization of genetically defined aro omp mutants of enterotoxigenic *Escherichia coli* and preliminary studies of safety and immunogenicity in humans. Infect Immun 69:4969–4979, 2001.
30. Levine M, Black RE, Clements ML, et al. Prevention of enterotoxigenic *Escherichia coli* diarrheal infection by vaccines that stimulate antiadhesion (antipili) immunity. *In* Boedeker EC (ed): Attachment of Organisms to the Gut Mucosa. Boca Raton, FL, CRC Press, 1984, pp 223–244.
31. Altboum Z, Barry EM, Losonsky G, et al. Attenuated *Shigella flexneri* 2a Delta guaBA strain CVD 1204 expressing enterotoxigenic *Escherichia coli* (ETEC) CS2 and CS3 fimbriae as a live mucosal vaccine against Shigella and ETEC infection. Infect Immun 69:3150–3158, 2001.
32. Koprowski H 2nd, Levine MM, Anderson RJ, et al. Attenuated *Shigella flexneri* 2a vaccine strain CVD 1204 expressing colonization factor antigen I and mutant heat-labile enterotoxin of enterotoxigenic *Escherichia coli*. Infect Immun 68:4884–4892, 2000.
33. Noriega FR, Losonsky G, Lauderbaugh C, et al. Engineered deltaguaB-A deltavirG *Shigella flexneri* 2a strain CVD 1205: construction, safety, immunogenicity, and potential efficacy as a mucosal vaccine. Infect Immun 64:3055–3061, 1996.
34. Tacket CO, Reid RH, Boedeker EC, et al. Enteral immunization and challenge of volunteers given enterotoxigenic *E. coli* CFA/II encapsulated in biodegradable microspheres. Vaccine 12:1270–1274, 1994.
35. Guerena-Burgueno F, Hall ER, Taylor DN, et al. Safety and immunogenicity of a prototype enterotoxigenic *Escherichia coli* vaccine administered transcutaneously. Infect Immun 70:1874–1880, 2002.
36. Luna MG, Ferreira LC, Almeida DF, Rudin A. Peptides 14VIDLL18 and 96FEAAAL101 defined as epitopes of antibodies raised against amino acid sequences of enterotoxigenic *Escherichia coli* colonization factor antigen I fused to Salmonella flagellin. Microbiology 143:3201–3207, 1997.
37. Yu J, Langridge WH. A plant-based multicomponent vaccine protects mice from enteric diseases. Nat Biotechnol 19:548–552, 2001.
38. Alves AM, Lasaro MO, Almeida DF, Ferreira LC. DNA immunisation against the CFA/I fimbriae of enterotoxigenic *Escherichia coli* (ETEC). Vaccine 19:788–795, 2000.
39. Sansonetti PJ. Microbes and microbial toxins: paradigms for microbial-mucosal interactions III. Shigellosis: from symptoms to molecular

pathogenesis. Am J Physiol Gastrointest Liver Physiol 280: G319–G323, 2001.

40. Kotloff KL, Winickoff JP, Ivanoff B, et al. Global burden of Shigella infections: implications for vaccine development and implementation of control strategies. Bull World Health Organ 77:651–666, 1999.

41. Ferreccio C, Prado V, Ojeda A, et al. Epidemiologic patterns of acute diarrhea and endemic *Shigella* infections in children in a poor periurban setting in Santiago, Chile. Am J Epidemiol 134:614–627, 1991.

42. Tacket CO, Binion SB, Bostwick E, et al. Efficacy of bovine milk immunoglobulin concentrate in preventing illness after *Shigella flexneri* challenge. Am J Trop Med Hyg 47:276–283, 1992.

43. Bernardini ML, Mounier J, d'Hauteville H, et al. Identification of icsA, a plasmid locus of *Shigella flexneri* that governs bacterial intra- and intercellular spread through interaction with F-actin. Proc Natl Acad Sci U S A 86:3867–3871, 1989.

44. Sansonetti PJ, Arondel J, Fontaine A, et al. OmpB (osmo-regulation) and icsA (cell-to-cell spread) mutants of *Shigella flexneri*: vaccine candidates and probes to study the pathogenesis of shigellosis. Vaccine 9:416–422, 1991.

45. Sansonetti PJ, Arondel J. Construction and evaluation of a double mutant of *Shigella flexneri* as a candidate for oral vaccination against shigellosis. Vaccine 7:443–450, 1989.

46. Coster TS, Hoge CW, VanDeVerg LL, et al. Vaccination against shigellosis with attenuated *Shigella flexneri* 2a strain SC602. Infect Immun 67:3437–3443, 1999.

47. Kotloff KL, Taylor DN, Sztein MB, et al. Phase I evaluation of delta virG Shigella sonnei live, attenuated, oral vaccine strain WRSS1 in healthy adults. Infect Immun 70:2016–2021, 2002.

48. Hoiseth SK, Stocker BA. Aromatic-dependent *Salmonella typhimurium* are non-virulent and effective as live vaccines. Nature 291:238–239, 1981.

49. Noriega FR, Wang JY, Losonsky G, et al. Construction and characterization of attenuated delta aroA delta virG Shigella flexneri 2a strain CVD 1203, a prototype live oral vaccine. Infect Immun 62:5168–5172, 1994.

50. Kotloff KL, Noriega F, Losonsky GA, et al. Safety, immunogenicity, and transmissibility in humans of CVD 1203, a live oral *Shigella flexneri* 2a vaccine candidate attenuated by deletions in aroA and virG. Infect Immun 64:4542–4548, 1996.

51. Anderson RJ, Pasetti MF, Sztein MB, et al. DeltaguaBA attenuated *Shigella flexneri* 2a strain CVD 1204 as a *Shigella* vaccine and as a live mucosal delivery system for fragment C of tetanus toxin. Vaccine 18:2193–2202, 2000.

52. Kotloff KL, Noriega FR, Samandari T, et al. *Shigella flexneri* 2a strain CVD 1207, with specific deletions in virG, sen, set, and guaBA, is highly attenuated in humans. Infect Immun 68:1034–1039, 2000.

53. Mel DM, Arsic BL, Nikolic BD, Radovanic ML. Studies on vaccination against bacillary dysentery. 4. Oral immunization with live monotypic and combined vaccines. Bull World Health Organ 39:375–380, 1968.

54. Klee SR, Tzschaschel BD, Singh M, et al. Construction and characterization of genetically-marked bivalent anti-*Shigella dysenteriae* 1 and anti-*Shigella flexneri* Y live vaccine candidates. Microb Pathog 22:363–376, 1997.

55. Klee SR, Tzschaschel BD, Falt I, et al. Construction and characterization of a live attenuated vaccine candidate against *Shigella dysenteriae* type 1. Infect Immun 65:2112–2118, 1997.

56. Klee SR, Tzschaschel BD, Timmis KN, Guzman CA. Influence of different rol gene products on the chain length of *Shigella dysenteriae* type 1 lipopolysaccharide O antigen expressed by *Shigella flexneri* carrier strains. J Bacteriol 179:2421–2425, 1997.

57. Noriega FR, Liao FM, Maneval DR, et al. Strategy for cross-protection among *Shigella flexneri* serotypes. Infect Immun 67:782–788, 1999.

58. Newland JW, Hale TL, Formal SB. Genotypic and phenotypic characterization of an aroD deletion-attenuated *Escherichia coli* K12-*Shigella flexneri* hybrid vaccine expressing S. flexneri 2a somatic antigen. Vaccine 10:766–776, 1992.

59. Kotloff KL, Herrington DA, Hale TL, et al. Safety, immunogenicity, and efficacy in monkeys and humans of invasive *Escherichia coli* K-12 hybrid vaccine candidates expressing *Shigella flexneri* 2a somatic antigen. Infect Immun 60:2218–2224, 1992.

60. Kotloff KL, Losonsky GA, Nataro JP, et al. Evaluation of the safety, immunogenicity, and efficacy in healthy adults of four doses of live oral hybrid *Escherichia coli-Shigella flexneri* 2a vaccine strain EcSf2a-2. Vaccine 13:495–502, 1995.

61. Cohen D, Ashkenazi S, Green MS, et al. Safety and immunogenicity of the oral *E. coli* K12-*S. flexneri* 2a vaccine (EcSf2a-2) among Israeli soldiers. Vaccine 12:1436–1442, 1994.

62. Robbins J, Chu C, Schneerson R. Hypothesis for vaccine development: protective immunity to enteric diseases caused by nontyphoidal Salmonellae and Shigellae may be conferred by serum IgG antibodies to the O-specific polysaccharides of their lipopolysaccharides. Clin Infect Dis 15:346–351, 1992.

63. Chu CY, Liu BK, Watson D, et al. Preparation, characterization, and immunogenicity of conjugates composed of the O-specific polysaccharide of *Shigella dysenteriae* type 1 (Shiga's bacillus) bound to tetanus toxoid. Infect Immun 59:4450–4458, 1991.

64. Taylor DN, Trofa AC, Sadoff J, et al. Synthesis, characterization, and clinical evaluation of conjugate vaccines composed of the O-specific polysaccharides of *Shigella dysenteriae* type 1, *Shigella flexneri* type 2a, and *Shigella sonnei* (Plesiomonas shigelloides) bound to bacterial toxoids. Infect Immun 61:3678–3687, 1993.

65. Cohen D, Ashkenazi S, Green M, et al. Safety and immunogenicity of investigational *Shigella* conjugate vaccines in Israeli volunteers. Infect Immun 64:4074–4077, 1996.

66. Passwell JH, Harlev E, Ashkenazi S, et al. Safety and immunogenicity of improved *Shigella* O-specific polysaccharide-protein conjugate vaccines in adults in Israel. Infect Immun 69:1351–1357, 2001.

67. Tauxe R. Epidemiology of *Campylobacter jejuni* infections in the United States and other industrialized nations. In Nachamkin MB, Tompkins LS (eds): *Campylobacter jejuni*: Current Status and Future Trends. Washington, DC, ASM Press, 1992, pp 9–19.

68. Tompkins DS, Hudson MJ, Smith HR, et al. A study of infectious intestinal disease in England: microbiological findings in cases and controls. Commun Dis Public Health 2:108–113, 1999.

69. Coker A, Isokpehi R, Thomas B, et al. Human campylobacteriosis in developing countries. Emerg Infect Dis 8:237–243, 2002.

70. Lang D, Allos B, Blaser M. Workshop summary and recommendations regarding the development of Guillain-Barré syndrome following Campylobacter infection. J Infect Dis 176:S198–S200, 1997.

71. Skirrow M, Blaser M. *Campylobacter jejuni*. In Blaser M, Smith P, Ravdin J, et al. (eds). Infections of the Gastrointestinal Tract. New York, Raven Press, 1995, pp 825–848.

72. Yuki N. Infectious origins of, and molecular mimicry in, Guillain-Barré and Fisher syndromes. Lancet Infect Dis 1:29–37, 2001.

73. Ang CW, Laman JD, Willison HJ, et al. Structure of *Campylobacter jejuni* lipopolysaccharides determines antiganglioside specificity and clinical features of Guillain-Barré and Miller Fisher patients. Infect Immun 70:1202–1208, 2002.

74. Calva JJ, Ruiz-Palacios GM, Lopez-Vidal AB, et al. Cohort study of intestinal infection with *Campylobacter* in Mexican children. Lancet 1:503–506, 1988.

75. Farthing MJ. Travellers' diarrhoea. Br J Hosp Med 48:82–92, 1992.

76. Bourgeois AL, Gardiner CH, Thornton SA, et al. Etiology of acute diarrhea among United States military personnel deployed to South America and West Africa. Am J Trop Med Hyg 48:243–248, 1993.

77. Mattila L. Clinical features and duration of travelers' diarrhea in relation to its etiology. Clin Infect Dis 19:728–734, 1994.

78. Salazar-Lindo E, Sack RB, Chea-Woo E, et al. Early treatment with erythromycin of *Campylobacter jejuni*-associated dysentery in children. J Pediatr 109:355–360, 1986.

79. Lior H. New, extended biotyping scheme for *Campylobacter jejuni*, *Campylobacter coli*, and *Campylobacter laridis*. J Clin Microbiol 20:636–640, 1984.

80. Penner JL, Hennessy JN. Passive hemagglutination technique for serotyping *Campylobacter fetus* subsp. jejuni on the basis of soluble heat-stable antigens. J Clin Microbiol 12:732–737, 1980.

81. Baqar S, Rice B, Lee L, et al. *Campylobacter jejuni* enteritis. Clin Infect Dis 33:901–905, 2001.

82. Baqar S, Applebee LA, Bourgeois AL. Immunogenicity and protective efficacy of a prototype *Campylobacter* killed whole-cell vaccine in mice. Infect Immun 63:3731–3735, 1995.

83. Lee LH, Burg E 3rd, Baqar S, et al. Evaluation of a truncated recombinant flagellin subunit vaccine against *Campylobacter jejuni*. Infect Immun 67:5799–5805, 1999.

84. Mel D, Gangarosa EJ, Radovanovic ML, et al. Studies on vaccination against bacillary dysentery. 6. Protection of children by oral immunization with streptomycin-dependent *Shigella* strains. Bull World Health Organ 45:457–464, 1971.

Chapter 44

Human Immunodeficiency Virus

MARC P. GIRARD • TIMOTHY D. MASTRO • WAYNE KOFF

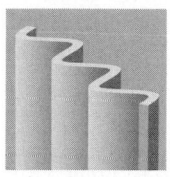

The acquired immunodeficiency syndrome (AIDS) was first described in 1981 as an outbreak of *Pneumocystis carinii* pneumonia among homosexual men in the United States.[1,2] Subsequent serologic and epidemiologic surveys showed that the disease rapidly spread to all countries in the world. Every day some 14,000 people, 90% of whom live in developing countries, become infected with human immunodeficiency virus (HIV).[3]

HIV is transmitted through contaminated blood or blood products, by use of contaminated needles or surgical instruments, or via sexual contact. The spread of the epidemic therefore could be stopped or slowed down through simple measures such as screening of blood donations, use of disposable syringes, and use of condoms. However, these measures often meet with profound behavioral resistance or ignorance on the part of the individuals at risk,[4] hence a vaccine that would prevent HIV infection and/or AIDS is urgently needed.

The development of effective HIV vaccines is hampered by the very properties of the virus[4a] (Table 44–1). These properties constitute major differences from "ordinary" viruses, which helps to explain why past successes in vaccine development cannot be duplicated easily in the case of HIV vaccines. Of particular concern is that HIV can persist in the host despite a vigorous and apparently normal immune response. In most individuals, HIV elicits a comprehensive cell-mediated immune response that includes natural killer (NK) cell activity and cytotoxic T-lymphocyte (CTL) activity targeted to cells expressing a variety of HIV antigens. In addition, CD8+ T lymphocytes are able to suppress the replication of HIV in vitro by a nonlytic mechanism[5,6] and to secrete β-chemokines that block the entry of macrophage-tropic HIV strains.[7,8] Most individuals infected with HIV eventually mount an antibody response that is capable of mediating antibody-dependent cell-mediated cytotoxicity (ADCC) and complement-dependent lysis of infected cells.[9] Neutralizing antibodies appear later in the course of the disease. Why these antiviral mechanisms fail to clear the virus is still unknown. It has been suggested that the enormous turnover of CD4+ T cells[10,11] eventually exhausts the immune system and that over-

whelming virus replication throughout the lymphoid system at the time of primary HIV infection leads to deletion or exhaustion of virus-specific CD8+ CTLs.[12] The rapid rate of replication of the virus, coupled with a high rate of mutations and recombinations, leads to accumulation of large numbers of mutant genomes, some of which are able to thrive as escape mutants that evade the immune response of the host.[13–18a] Other factors include the ability of HIV to remain incorporated as a latent provirus in the host cell DNA for long periods of time, and its ability to downregulate major histocompatibility complex (MHC) class I presentation of viral peptides at the surface of infected cells, making these cells immunologically "invisible."[19,20] Progression to AIDS may be accelerated by gradual impairment of cellular immunity.[21] Indeed, HIV-specific CTLs are blocked at an early differentiation stage, before the final perforin-rich, interferon (IFN)-γ–secreting effector stage, and thus may not exhibit full effector function.[22–25] Whether immune mechanisms would be more efficacious if induced in response to vaccination remains to be proven. In spite of some encouraging success in vaccine-induced protection from simian immunodeficiency virus (SIV) in macaques,[26–29] continuous efforts are still necessary before simple HIV vaccines can be made available for human use.[30–32]

Background

Clinical Disease

AIDS, a clinical syndrome associated with a progressive deterioration of the immune status of the individual, is characterized by the progressive depletion of the CD4+ T-lymphocyte population, which represents a major target of viral infection in vivo.[33–35] At the clinical level, this is characterized by a wide spectrum of clinical illnesses (lymphadenopathy, weight loss, chronic diarrhea, fevers, nephropathy, and neuropathies) and the occurrence of opportunistic infections, such as *P. carinii* pneumonia, tuberculosis, *Mycobacterium avium-intracellulare* infections, toxoplasmosis, candidiasis, cryptosporidiosis, severe viral infections (cytomegalovirus, hepatitis C, herpes simplex,

TABLE 44–1 ■ Obstacles to the Development of HIV Vaccines

Antigenic diversity and hypervariability of the virus
Transmission of disease by mucosal route
Transmission of the virus by infected cells
Resistance of wild-type virus to seroneutralization
Integration of the virus genome into the host cell chromosomes
Latency of the virus in resting memory T cells
Rapid emergence of viral escape mutants in the host
Down-regulation of MHC class I antigens
No spontaneous recovery from natural infection in spite of
    high-level immune responses of the host

MHC, major histocompatibility complex.

Epstein-Barr virus), and cancers (Kaposi's sarcoma and non-Hodgkin's B-cell lymphomas of Epstein-Barr virus origin).

Within 2 to 6 weeks after infection, the patient experiences an acute febrile phase with disseminated lymphadenopathy, rash, arthralgia, and myalgia, which is reminiscent of an episode of infectious mononucleosis. A transient decrease in the total lymphocyte count and an inversion of the CD4-to-CD8 ratio are observed. Primary infection is accompanied by p24 antigenemia and high plasma viral loads (Fig. 44–1), with HIV type 1 (HIV-1) RNA levels typically in the range of 2×10^6 to 2×10^7 copies/mL.[36–38] This burst of virus replication is accompanied by dissemination of the virus to lymphoid organs.[39,40] The patient is highly contagious at this phase but cannot be diagnosed by usual serologic procedures. Disappearance of clinical symptoms occurs within a few weeks together with down-regulation of viremia, as a consequence of the host's immune response, the major component of which consists of HIV-1–specific CD8[+] CTLs that are capable of eliminating a large number of virus-expressing cells.[41–44] A similar phenomenon has been observed in experimental SIV infection of rhesus monkeys.[45] The central role of CD8[+] T cells in controlling primary SIV infection in monkeys was unequivocally demonstrated through experimental deple-

tion of the CD8[+] T-cell compartment, showing that viremia persisted at high levels as long as the CD8[+] compartment remained depleted.[46] In humans, a marked oligoclonal expansion of certain Vβ subsets of CD8[+] T cells occurs,[41,44] but a significant number of HIV-specific CTL clones seem to rapidly disappear through clonal exhaustion.[12] A humoral immune response eventually follows,[9,47] and the patient becomes seropositive, except in rare cases.[48,49] Failure to seroconvert to viral antigens is observed in humans or macaques with extremely rapidly progressing HIV-1 or chimeric simian/human immunodeficiency virus (SHIV) infection with an X4 virus that results in massive loss of CD4[+] T-helper (Th) cells.[50–52]

A long asymptomatic period of clinical latency follows, during which a slow but steady decline in the CD4[+] cell number is observed. The patient is infectious because HIV-1 replication continues throughout the course of infection.[50,53,54] High antibody levels to all virus antigens (Env, Gag, and nonstructural virus proteins) are found in the patient's plasma together with circulating virions. It is estimated that 10^7 to 10^9 virions are produced per day, resulting in viral plasma loads of 10^4 to 10^6 RNA molecules per milliliter and in the destruction of approximately 2×10^9 CD4[+] T cells per day.[10,11,55,56]

Lymphoid organs tend to be the preferential site for replication as well as a reservoir of "trapped" extracellular virus on follicular dendritic cells.[39,40,57–59] Evidence suggests that, in addition to the short-lived infected CD4[+] T cells, which have a $t_{1/2}$ of a few days, long-lived infected cells with a $t_{1/2}$ of a few weeks, which might be macrophages, also make a significant contribution to plasma viremia.[60] Indeed, tissue macrophages seem to constitute the major source of increasing viremia that characterizes the last phase of HIV disease, and a variety of opportunistic infections can dramatically increase their production of virus.[61] Infectious HIV-1 also persists latently in a postintegrated form in resting memory CD4[+] lymphocytes. This reservoir is small, generally of less than a few thousand cells, with a $t_{1/2}$ of many months.[62,63a]

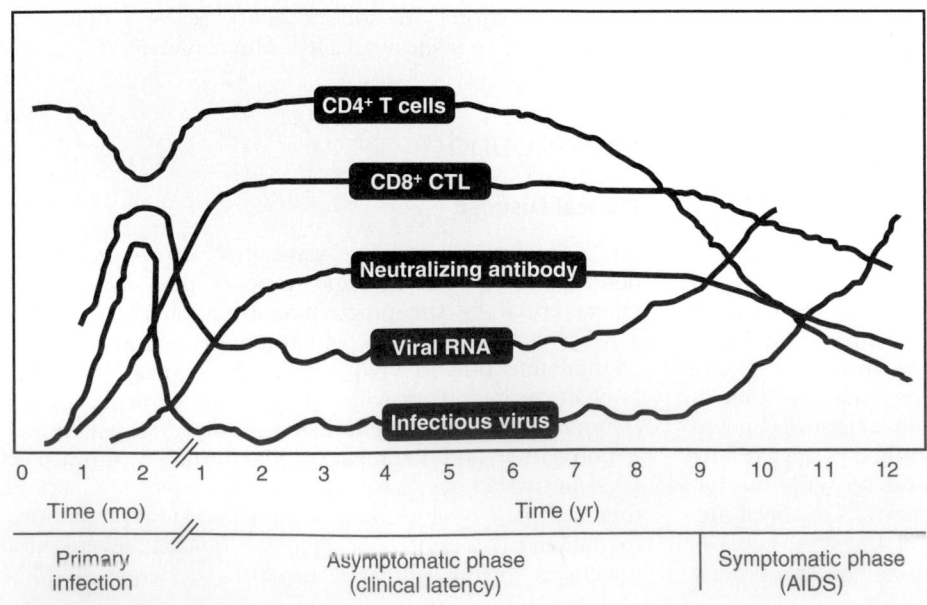

FIGURE 44–1 ■ Diagrammatic representation of the evolution of viral and immunologic markers during the course of a typical HIV-1 infection. CTL, cytotoxic T lymphocytes.

The asymptomatic phase can last from a few months to more than 20 years, after which symptoms appear. These have been classified according to severity and number[64] to define a series of successive stages in the evolution of the disease, such as the *lymphadenopathy syndrome,* the *AIDS-related complex,* and *full-blown AIDS.* The symptomatic phase of the disease is accompanied by p24 antigenemia, an accelerated decrease in the number of CD4+ T cells, a progressive loss of antibodies to Gag proteins and of HIV-specific CTLs, and a greatly increased virus load. Thus the number of peripheral T4-cells producing HIV-1 can reach 1 in 10 in the terminal stages of the disease, with production of up to 10^{10} virions per day.[10,11,55,56]

In industrialized countries, and before the advent of highly active antiretroviral therapy, death occurred with a median period of about 10 years, after the T4 cell number had dropped below 50 cells/mm^3, owing to fulgurant opportunistic infections. The survival time of adults and children with HIV infection is considerably shorter in sub-Saharan Africa, in part because of lack of adequate medical care but probably also because of persistent immune activation and high levels of cytokine secretion associated with chronic infections such as sexually transmitted and parasitic diseases.[33] Studies of HIV infections in West Africa indicate that HIV type 2 (HIV-2) induces a slower progression to disease than HIV-1.[65]

Infection with HIV also can manifest itself as a purely cachectic disease, to which the name *slim disease* has been given in Africa. It also can affect the brain directly, causing purely neurologic symptoms such as acute encephalitis or progressive dementia (*AIDS dementia complex*).

The rate of progression to disease among people infected with HIV is highly variable among individuals. The reason why long-term nonprogressors (LTNPs) remain devoid of symptoms more than 20 years after infection, whereas others (the rapid progressors) develop a fatal disease within 2 years, is unknown. These differences seem to depend on the age of the individual[66] and also on host and viral factors.[33,35] LTNPs typically show a polyclonal CTL response that is directed against multiple HIV-1 antigens and is maintained over time.[67] Survival analyses clearly show that disease progression is slower in Δccr5 heterozygotes[68,69] as well as in individuals with a mutation in CCR-2[70] (see *Virus-Cell Interactions* below) and can vary with human leukocyte antigen (HLA) alleles. Infections with parasites, bacteria (*Mycobacterium tuberculosis*), viruses (human herpesvirus [HHV]-6, cytomegalovirus, and human T-cell lymphotropic virus type I), or mycoplasmas (*M. fermentans, M. penetrans, M. pirum*)[71,72] have been implicated as cofactors of progression. There is also increasing evidence that the release of β-chemokines by primary peripheral blood mononuclear cells (PBMCs) activated in vitro correlates with slow or absent progression to HIV disease.[73,74]

The steady-state level of plasma viral load from about 6 months after infection strongly predicts how fast the disease will progress.[75-77] This is often referred to as the "set point." Patients with more than 10^5 HIV RNA copies/mL of plasma within 6 months of seroconversion are 10-fold more likely to progress to AIDS during the following 5 years than are those with less than 10^5 copies/mL, and maintenance of plasma RNA levels below 10,000/mL in early disease appears to be associated with decreased risk of progression to AIDS. The level of plasma viremia probably depends on the vigor of the individual's immune response to primary infection,[41-43] as reflected in the degree of diversity of the CD8+ Vβ repertoire that is mobilized in response to infection: T-cell receptor repertoire responses limited to only one or two Vβ families are associated with rapid disease progression, whereas broader CTL repertoire responses involving multiple Vβ families are associated with a clinically stable course and stable CD4+ T-cell counts.[78]

Patients with AIDS show increased levels of tumor necrosis factor-α (TNF-α); interleukin (IL)-1, -2, and -6; soluble IL-2 receptor; IFN-α and IFN-γ; β$_2$-microglobulin; and neopterin (an IL produced by macrophages in response to TNF-α). TNF-α, which acts through activation of nuclear transcription factor-κB (NF-κB), appears to be the most potent of the HIV-inducing cytokines.[79] The level of HIV replication in CD4+ T cells actually reflects the balance of the opposing effects of suppressive factors, such as β-chemokines RANTES (regulated on activation, normal T cell expressed and secreted) and macrophage inflammatory protein (MIP)-1α and -1β,[7,8] and HIV-1–inducing cytokines, such as TNF-α and IL-1β.[80] Another suppressor activity was identified by Walker and colleagues[5,6] in CD8+ T-cell culture supernatants. This activity is noncytotoxic and nonrestricted by MHC antigens, and is mediated by soluble factors distinct from known cytokines.[81-83]

CD4+ T cells are heterogeneous in their profiles of cytokine secretion, designated Th1, Th2, and Th0.[84] It has been observed that a shift from the Th1 to the Th2 cytokine profile,[85] or, rather, to the Th0 profile,[86] occurs during the course of HIV infection leading to AIDS. Th1 cells produce IL-2, TNF-β, and IFN-γ and promote cellular immunity (CTLs), whereas Th2 cells produce IL-4, IL-5, and IL-10; promote humoral immunity; and suppress CTL activity. T-tropic X4 HIV-1 strains proliferate preferentially in Th2- and Th0-type cell clones, which might explain why these strains become dominant when AIDS develops. The extended dominance of R5 viruses in HIV-infected LTNPs[87,88] argues strongly that host factors are important in controlling the virus population and that conditions favoring the replication of R5 rather than X4 strains must be prevalent in these individuals (see *Virus-Cell Interactions* below).

AIDS patients are anergic to recall antigens, as judged both by absence of delayed-type hypersensitivity (skin test) in vivo and by lack of Th cell proliferation in vitro. An important dysfunction observed in HIV-1-infected patients, but not in clinical nonprogressors, is the inability of HIV-1 specific CD4+ memory T cells to proliferate and produce IL-2 and IL-4 in response to HIV antigens.[88a] The unresponsiveness to recall antigens may also be the direct consequence of HIV infection on follicular dendritic cells, which severely impairs the ability of these cells to present antigens in vitro.[89] Engagement of T-cell receptors in the absence of a co-stimulatory signal, such as that provided by the B7-CD28 interaction at the contact between the antigen-presenting cell and the T cell, can lead to long-lived T-cell anergy. Anergy correlates with destruction of the lymph node follicles.[57-59,90]

A key dilemma in understanding the pathophysiology of AIDS is defining the mechanism responsible for the continuous decline in the number of CD4+ T cells.[90a]

Primary and secondary immune responses against persistent high-level viral replication lead to progressive depletion of CD4[+] effector and memory T cells. Peripheral depletion, in turn, triggers physiologic feedback responses resulting in accelerated production of new T cells. As long as the compensatory mechanisms are operative, the CD4[+] T-cell lineage is sustained. If and when these mechanisms falter, however, the T-cell compartment collapses.[91] The transition from mildly cytopathic R5 to broadly cytopathic X4-R5 or X4 virus strains seems to precede and possibly to drive the collapse of the CD4[+] T-cell count.

It is not clear, however, if direct killing of CD4[+] cells by HIV can explain the full spectrum of AIDS pathogenesis. Chimpanzee-adapted strains of HIV-1 are cytopathic for chimpanzee T cells, grow in chimpanzee macrophages-monocytes, and replicate efficiently in chimpanzees. However, these viruses do not induce AIDS in the animal,[92,93] with the exception of one reported case.[94] Specific mechanisms have been suggested to account for the depletion of CD4[+] cells in HIV-infected humans, such as cytolytic attack by HIV-specific CTLs of naive bystander CD4[+] cells that have bound virus-shed circulating glycoprotein (gp)120 molecules[95]; T-cell alloactivation, as in graft-versus-host disease, resulting from antigenic mimicry of the MHC by the gp120 molecule[96–98]; superantigen-mediated deletion of specific CD4[+] T-cell subsets[99]; apoptosis (programmed cell death),[100–102] perhaps induced by gp120[103] or, possibly, by the Tat protein[104]; and molecular mimicry between the ectodomain of gp41 and IL-2, leading to the induction of anti–IL-2 antibodies that block the interaction of the cytokine with its receptor.[105]

Apoptotic T lymphocytes can be observed early after HIV infection. Interestingly, no apoptotic lymphocytes can be found in HIV-infected chimpanzees or in SIV-infected African green monkeys, which do not develop disease in spite of persistent infection, whereas apoptotic lymphocytes are readily detected in SIV-infected rhesus macaques, which develop a typical AIDS disease.[101,102] In lymph nodes, apoptosis is found mostly in noninfected bystander cells and not in the productively infected cells, suggesting that apoptotic signals generated by the virus must be transmitted to uninfected cells.[4a,106] Apoptosis can be blocked in vitro by Th1 cytokines IL-2, IFN-α, and IL-12, whereas it is enhanced by Th2 cytokines IL-4 and IL-10.[107] The detailed mechanisms that trigger apoptosis still remain to be unraveled.

Kaposi's sarcoma is the leading neoplasm in AIDS patients. An enhancing effect of the HIV tat gene on the development of Kaposi's sarcoma has been reported,[108] perhaps as a result of synergism with Kaposi's sarcoma–associated herpesvirus/HHV-8 open reading frames 50 and 74. Tat is angiogenic and promotes malignancy.[109] It also alters the host immune response.[110]

Interest has been focused on the individuals who remain uninfected and seronegative in spite of definite exposure to HIV-1 and who, in contrast to the Δccr5 homozygotes,[111] have normal ccr5 genes. These individuals seem to have developed a cellular immune response, including Th cell proliferation and IL-2 secretion in response to Env peptides,[112] albeit in the absence of an antibody response. CTL activity has been detected against HIV-1 antigens in repeatedly exposed uninfected African commercial sex work-

ers[113–115a] as well as in uninfected children born to HIV-1–infected mothers[116] and in uninfected heterosexual partners of HIV-1–infected patients.[117–119] These findings are consistent with the hypothesis that these individuals experienced a silent HIV-1 infection that they were able to control through a Th1-type cellular immune response. Other mechanisms, such as increased secretion of β-chemokines by CD8[+] lymphocytes, cannot be excluded.[119,120] Finally, anti-HIV secretory immunoglobulin A has been found in the cervicovaginal secretions of seronegative uninfected heterosexual partners of HIV-infected men,[121] suggesting that a mucosally restricted B-cell response also could contribute to protective mucosal immunity against sexual transmission of HIV.[121a] It should, however, be emphasized that seropositivation to HIV and the development of overt HIV infection was observed in those Nairobi prostitutes who stopped being exposed to HIV. This suggests that the maintenance of their protective immunity required constantly repeated antigenic stimulations.[115a]

Virology

There are two well-defined etiologic agents of AIDS, HIV-1[122–124] and HIV-2,[125] both of which cause disease, but HIV-1 appears to be more aggressive and spreads more rapidly.[65] Both are nontransforming, cytopathic retroviruses belonging to the lentivirus subfamily. Lentiviruses produce characteristically slow, progressive infections, in which the virus causes disease after long periods of latency and persists in the host in spite of the host's active immune response.[126] Other lentiviruses are SIV, the feline immunodeficiency virus, the puma lentivirus, the bovine immunodeficiency virus, the Visna virus of sheep, the caprine arthritis-encephalitis virus, and the equine infectious anemia virus.

The HIV virion consists of an internal core particle built from 1200 molecules of capsid (p24gag) protein (Fig. 44–2) surrounded by a lipid envelope spiked with some 75 trimers of a highly glycosylated protein, gp160,[127] and wrapped around a scaffold made of the matrix (p17gag) protein.[128,129] The virus core contains two copies of the RNA genome; several molecules of an associated reverse transcriptase; and internal viral proteins such as p1, p2, p6, and the p7gag nucleocapsid[130,131] as well as cytoskeletal proteins such as cyclophilin A, actin, and moesin.[132] It also contains copies of viral proteins Vpr, Nef, and Vif, which play a role in early events in HIV replication. The gp160 Env molecules are made of two noncovalently linked polypeptide chains: the trans-membrane chain, gp41, anchors the spikes in the lipid bilayer of the envelope, maintains their trimeric structure,[133–137] and plays a major role in fusion of the virus and cell membranes[133,138–141]; and the external chain, gp120,[142–145] carries the important antigenic determinants of the virus and binds the CD4 receptor and co-receptors (see Virus-Cell Interactions, below). The 120-kDa gp120 molecule contains about 50 kDa of carbohydrate consisting of a mixture of high-mannose and complex sialic acid–containing carbohydrates.[143,146] Folding, assembly, disulfide bond formation, glycosylation, and transport of the envelope protein to the cell surface have been studied in detail.[147–149] There is evidence that the envelope of HIV-1 contains numerous molecules of type II HLA-DR and β$_2$-microglobulin borrowed from the host cell in which the

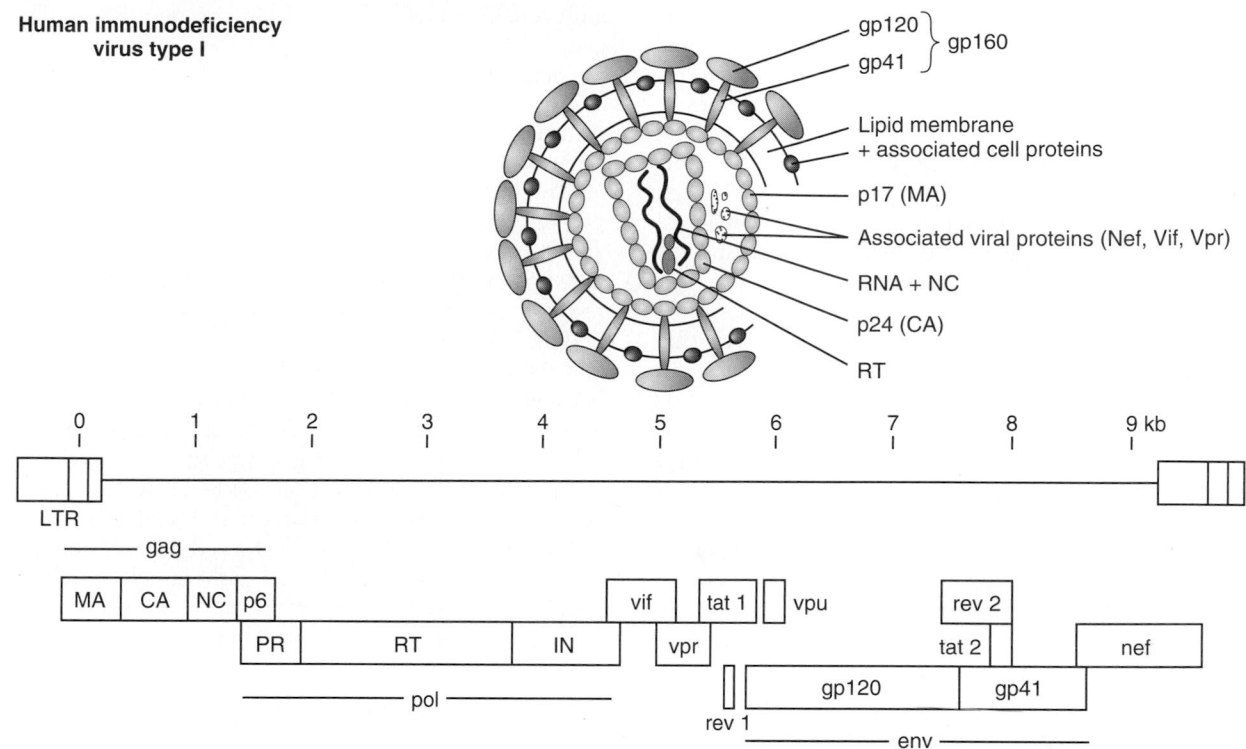

FIGURE 44–2 ▪ A schematic representation of the virion, depicting the viral envelope spiked with glycoprotein gp160 and associated cellular proteins and wrapped over a scaffold of matrix (MA) protein. The capsid, made of CA protein, encloses the dimeric genome RNA associated with the nucleocapsid (NC) protein, together with virion-associated proteins reverse transcriptase (RT), Vif, Vpr, and Nef. The diagram at the bottom represents the virus RNA as a straight line graded in kilobases (kb). The open boxes refer to the open reading frames (genes) on the RNA. IN, integrase; LTR, long terminal repeats; PR, protease.

virus last replicated,[150] together with cellular components such as CD43, CD44, CD55, CD59, CD63, CD71, intercellular adhesion molecule-1 (ICAM-1), and lymphocyte function-associated antigen-1 (LFA-1). This explains why the virus can be neutralized by antibodies to HLA-DR, LFA-1, β_2-microglobulin, or ICAM-1.[151]

The genome of HIV is a single-stranded RNA molecule, 9.5 kilobases in length.[152–154] It is flanked by two long terminal repeats (LTRs), each containing a transcription promoter and terminator, a polyadenylation signal, and regulatory elements that control the activity of the promoter and respond specifically to proteins from the host (Sp1, NF-κB, PRD-II factors). The RNA dimerizes through a "kissing loop" interaction involving a specific stem-loop element termed the *dimer linkage structure*.[155] The genetic variability of HIV, which is reflected at the molecular level by the variability of the nucleotide sequence of the RNA genome, is a major challenge in the development of a globally effective vaccine[156,157] (see below).

TABLE 44–2 ▪ Principal Roles of the HIV Accessory Proteins

Vpr	Together with matrix protein, targets the viral preintegration complex to the nucleus
	Arrests dividing cells in G_2 of the cell cycle
	Induces herniation of the nuclear membrane
	Enhances HIV replication in macrophages
Vpu	Down-regulates expression of CD4 molecules by targeting them to the proteasome, leading to their degradation in the endoplasmic reticulum
	Forms ion channels in the cell membrane, thus helping to promote the release of virions from infected cells
Vif	Plays a role in provirus formation and stabilizes newly synthesized DNA intermediates
	Associates with cytoskeleton intermediate filaments and helps transport incoming virions to the nucleus
	Neutralizes an innate antiviral mechanism
Nef	Associates with cellular protein kinases (PAK65, p56tck, p59Hck)
	Stimulates viral DNA synthesis and enhances virus infectivity in primary T cells and macrophages
	Enhances virus replication in vivo, contributing to high viral loads and pathogenesis
	Binds CD4 molecules at the plasma membrane and mediates their rapid endocytosis and lysosomal degradation
	Down-regulates cell surface expression of major histocompatibility complex class I antigens, a cytotoxic T-lymphocyte escape mechanism
	Activates the expression of Fas L, which induces apoptosis in bystander cells that express Fas

The genes of HIV-1 fall into three categories: the structural genes *gag* (core), *pol* (reverse transcriptase), and *env* (gp160), which are the basic genes found in all retroviruses; regulatory genes *tat* and *rev*, a unique feature of lentiviruses[158]; and "accessory" genes *nef*, *vpr*, *vpu*, and *vif*, the function of which is still little known[158-160] (Table 44–2). The mRNAs coding for the Gag-Pol, Env, Vif, Vpr, and Vpu proteins are unspliced or single spliced, whereas those coding for the regulatory proteins are multispliced. This property is used by the virus for the control of its expression.

The *tat* gene encodes a *trans*-activating protein that acts at the level of transcription by increasing viral messenger RNA (mRNA) production several hundred-fold through binding to a 59-residue stem-loop at the 5′ end of the nascent RNA molecules, called the Tat-responsive element. Tat prevents premature termination of mRNA transcription[161] through an interactive process that involves cyclin T1, cdk9, and RNA polymerase II. Tat also plays an important role in pathogenesis.[110]

The *rev* gene encodes a protein that activates the expression of the structural virus genes by allowing the nuclear export of unspliced or single-spliced HIV-1 mRNAs. These contain multiple nuclear retention sequences (also called *cis*-acting repression sequences) that prevent them from migrating from the nucleus to the cytoplasm.[162] The Rev protein binds to specific sequence elements on these RNAs, the Rev-responsive elements, and allows their migration from the nucleus to the cytoplasm by interacting with nuclear export factors. Rev thus controls the switch from an early phase of the virus cycle, when only regulatory viral proteins are synthesized, to a late phase, when structural proteins are made and virions assembled.[163]

The precise role and importance of *vif*, *vpu*, *vpr*, and *nef* are still not completely understood[159,160,164] (see Table 44–2). Vpr arrests dividing cells in G_2 of the cell cycle. Vpu is a membrane-spanning protein that plays a role in the release of virus particles from the infected cell. HIV-2 and SIV lack a *vpu* gene but carry another accessory gene, *vpx*, which seems to be a duplication of *vpr*. The *nef* gene, initially believed to code for a negative regulatory factor, appears to be a major virulence factor that contributes to the maintenance of high virus loads.[26,27,164-167] Transgenic mice expressing the SIV *nef* gene in their lymphocytes develop a disease very similar to human AIDS.[168] Nef decreases the expression of MHC class I antigens on the cell surface, thus providing the virus with a mechanism for evading the host cellular immune response.[19,20] Viruses expressing a fully functional *nef* gene have a strong growth advantage in vivo.[166]

Maturation of the core particle requires the proteolytic cleavage of the Gag precursor proteins Pr55*gag* and p160*gag-pol*, generating MA protein and an intermediate p40*gag* molecule, itself eventually cleaved to generate the CA, NC, p1, p2, and p6 internal proteins.[131,169] HIV-1 nucleocapsid NC, which is at all times tightly associated with the RNA genome, contains two zinc finger motifs that are necessary for packaging of genomic RNA and infectivity. Proteolytic cleavages take place after virion budding from the infected cell membrane and are catalyzed by the viral aspartyl proteinase encoded by the virus *pol* gene. The proteinase is a homodimer, each subunit contributing the

amino acid triplet DTG to form the active site. The *pol* gene also codes for other key enzymes: reverse transcriptase (associated with an RNase H activity) and an integrase that allows the integration of the virus complementary DNA into the host cell genome. These enzymes constitute prime targets for antiviral therapy.

The Gag polyprotein binds to cyclophilin A and incorporates this cellular peptidyl prolylisomerase into virions.[170] The HIV-1 Gag protein is transported to assembly sites on the inner leaflet of the plasma membrane, where it recruits the cellular machinery normally used to form multivesicular bodies. Virions emerge from the cell by budding. Assembly and budding often occur at sites of transient contact between the infected cell and other cell types. Thus HIV-1–specific effector T cells form "immunologic synapses" with HIV-1–infected cells through involvement of the T-cell receptor and adhesion molecules (LFA-1, ICAM-1, CD43). In this case, virus from the infected T cell is released in a polarized fashion at the site of the cell contact and directly spreads to the uninfected T cell without cell-to-cell fusion. Similar observations have been made when HIV-infected macrophages or T cells are placed in contact with epithelial cells.[171]

Virus-Cell Interactions

Entry of HIV-1 into cells is a multistep process in which the Env glycoprotein interacts with attachment factors, engages the CD4 receptor and then a co-receptor, and undergoes conformational changes that result in viral envelope–cell membrane fusion and virus entry. Among known attachment factors is DC-SIGN, a C-type lectin expressed on dendritic cells and macrophages that bind glycoproteins with high mannose content.[172] Dendritic cells can capture HIV virions through DC-SIGN attachment, internalize the virus transport it virus to lymphoid organs, and transmit it to T cells without becoming infected. DC-SIGN is abundant on dendritic cells in the intestinal mucosa but does not seem to be expressed on Langerhans' cells in the vaginal epithelium.[173]

With the exception of rare CD4-independent isolates, HIV-1, HIV-2, and SIV use as a receptor the CD4 (OK-T4) molecule, which is present on the surface of Th lymphocytes, monocytes-macrophages, lymph node follicular dendritic cells, Langerhans' cells in the skin, and microglia in the central nervous system.[174-176] The virus also can infect CD4⁻ cells, such as glial cells, mammary cells, NK cells, brain endothelial cells, and some gut epithelial cells in culture,[177,178] in which case the receptor molecule has been identified as a glycolipid, galactosylceramide.[179,180] Another HIV-1 receptor has been identified on human placenta; it belongs to the family of the C-type mannose-binding proteins but might simply be DC-SIGN.[181]

The CD4-binding domain of the gp120 molecule is a complex conformational motif. CD4 binds in a recessed pocket of gp120 flanked by variable regions exhibiting considerable glycosylation, and makes extensive contacts over about 800 Å of the gp120 surface.[143-145,182,183]

Binding of gp120 to CD4 triggers conformational changes that lead to the unmasking of the co-receptor binding site.[184] Binding to the co-receptor in turn triggers the exposure of the fusogenic domain located at the amino terminus of the gp41 molecule (Fig. 44–3A), allowing its interaction with the host cell membrane (see below).

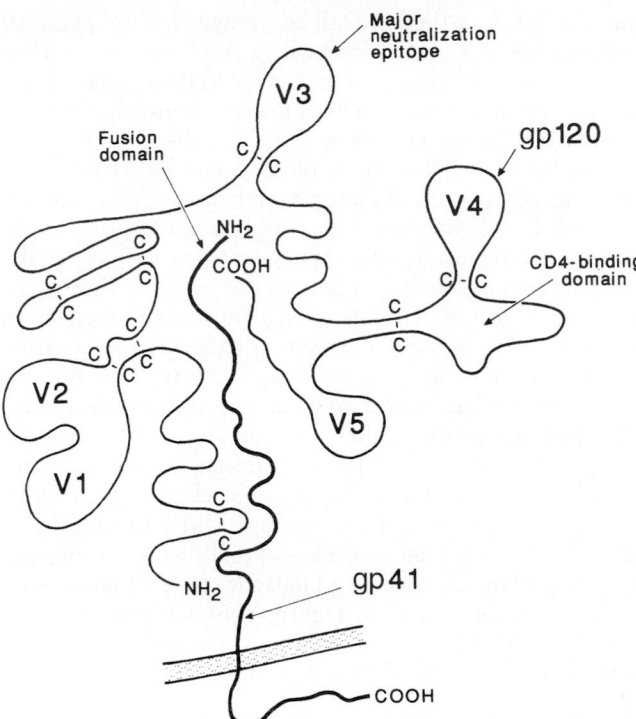

FIGURE 44–3 ■ A diagrammatic two-dimensional representation of the gp120 molecule indicating the position of the disulfide bridges (C–C) and the five hypervariable domains (V1 to V5). The gp41 molecule has been drawn as a thick wavy line but actually shows extensive folding.[135,136,139] (Modified from Leonard CK, Spellman MW, Riddle L, et al. Assignment of intra-chain disulfide bonds and characterization of potential glycosylation sites of the type 1 recombinant human immunodeficiency virus envelope glycoprotein (gp120) expressed in Chinese hamster ovary cells. J Biol Chem 265:1037–1038, 1990.)

Two distinct chemokine receptors, CXCR-4 (fusin) and CCR-5, act as co-receptors for the primate lentiviruses.[8,185–189] These receptors belong to the superfamily of G protein–coupled seven-transmembrane domain glycoproteins.

Most HIV isolates obtained at the time of primary infection and during the asymptomatic period of the disease are macrophage-tropic (M-tropic): They replicate in PBMCs but do not form syncytia in culture or infect CD4⁺-transformed T-cell lines.[190] They use CCR-5 as a co-receptor. Emerging later in infection, in association with CD4⁺ T-cell decline and progression to AIDS, are T lymphocyte–tropic (T-tropic) isolates.[50] These replicate in PBMCs as well as in immortalized T-cell lines and are syncytia inducing. A subset of T-tropic virus has been adapted to infect transformed CD4⁺ T-cell lines, generating T-cell line–adapted (TCLA) virus strains that have lost their ability to replicate efficiently in PBMCs. T-tropic strains use CXCR-4 as a co-receptor. The M-tropic and T-tropic phenotypes depend on specific envelope determinants located on the V3 loop of gp120,[191–196] which constitutes the "principal neutralization determinant" of HIV-1 TCLA strains.[197–200] Formation of syncytia by T-tropic virus strains depends on charged amino acids on the V3 loop[195,196,200,201] and can be aborted even after the CD4-binding step by V3-targeted neutralizing antibodies.[202] M tropism is also controlled by viral genes *vpr* and *vpu*.[159,160]

For simplicity, the CXCR-4–using viruses are called "X4" and the M-tropic, CCR-5–using viruses "R5." T-tropic primary isolates can use CXCR-4 as well as CCR-5, CCR-3, and CCR-2[203,204]; they are said to be dual-tropic ("X4-R5").[205,206] Unlike HIV-1, both M- and T-tropic SIV strains are R5.[207,208] Specific SIV co-receptors also have been identified.[209,210] Gp120 from X4 strains can form a trimolecular complex with CD4 and CXCR-4 in vitro, whereas gp120 from R5 isolates physically interacts with CD4 and CCR-5.[211–214] The affinity of gp120 for its co-receptor is greatly enhanced in the presence of CD4, suggesting that the latter not only provides a docking surface for gp120 but also triggers the exposure of the chemokine receptor–binding site, which is poorly exposed in the absence of CD4.[143,212,215]

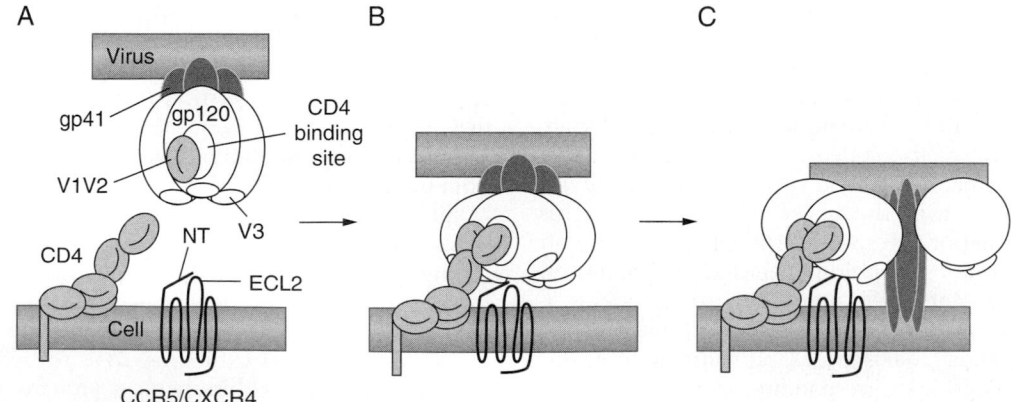

FIGURE 44–3B ■ A model for the interactions of the HIV envelope proteins (Env) with cell surface receptors (a) Schematic representation of the Env gp120/go41 trimer, and the CD4 cell and CCRS or CXCR4 chemokine receptors. NT, amino-terminal domain; ECL2, second extracellular loop. (b) Binding to domain 1 of CD4 cells induces conformational changes in gp120, unmasking a chemokine receptor binding site comprising a V3 loop and a conserved structure (c) Interaction with the chemokine receptor allows close apposition of the virus and cell membrane, and results in further conformational changes in the gp120/gp41 complex, eventually activating gp41 (i.e., allowing exposure its fusion peptide and insertion in the largest cell membrane.)

Interestingly, CD4-independent isolates of HIV-1, HIV-2, and SIV have been described that are able to interact directly with the co-receptors as a result of mutations in gp120 and/or gp41.[213,216] Thus the real virus receptors are actually the chemokine receptors, whereas the CD4 molecule can be viewed as a facilitator.

CC chemokines RANTES, MIP-1α, and MIP-1β, the three known CCR-5 ligands, potently inhibit the intracellular entry of R5 HIV-1 isolates[7,8,217,218] as well as the formation of CD4–gp120–CCR-5 trimolecular complexes in vitro,[212,213] whereas stromal cell–derived factor-1, a CXCR-4 ligand, blocks infection with X4 virus strains.[219,220]

Individuals who suffer a homozygous defect in the gene encoding CCR-5 show high resistance to HIV-1 infection in vivo.[111] The genetic defect, a 32–base pair deletion that results in a frameshift mutation and generates a nonfunctional CCR-5 receptor, renders PBMCs from these individuals highly resistant to infection by R5 isolates in vitro.[68,69,221] The mutation is present on chromosome 3p21 at a frequency of 9% to 10% in the white population (about 1% Δccr5/Δccr5 homozygotes) but is absent in African and Asian populations. A few individuals who are homozygous for the Δccr5 mutation nonetheless have been found to be infected with HIV-1[222]; it is hypothesized that they probably were infected with an X4 virus strain.

The conformation changes induced by the binding of CD4 to gp120 may cause gp120 to be "shed" from the virus surface, leaving the membrane-anchored gp41 subunit behind and inactivating the virus.[223] Alternatively, the binding of CD4 unmasks the co-receptor binding site on gp120 and allows the molecule to bind the relevant co-receptor. This, in turn, causes a new conformational change in the trimeric spikes that triggers the unfolding of the gp41 moiety, resulting in exposure of its hydrophobic, glycine-rich, N-terminal fusion peptide region (Fig. 44–3B).[138–140,184]

Crystallographic analysis of the core structure of gp41 has shown that it is a six-stranded helical bundle with an interior coiled-coil trimer of three parallel helices[133–137] corresponding to a leucine zipper domain,[134,141] also called "heptad repeat 1," around which three antiparallel helices forming "heptad repeat 2" pack in an oblique, antiparallel manner, in highly conserved, hydrophobic grooves on the surface of the trimer. The hydrophobic fusion peptide is immediately amino-terminal to the central three-stranded coiled-coil structure. This structure shows striking similarity to that of the low pH–induced conformation of the influenza HA2 subunit.[224] Activation of the envelope spike results in extension of the coiled-coil structure and exposure of the fusion peptide at the tip of the stalk, providing for easy contact with the target cell membrane. This prefusion conformation of gp41 is thought to mimic an "unsprung mousetrap."[225] Binding of gp41 to the target cell membrane triggers the gp41 mousetrap to snap closed, bringing into close proximity the viral and cell membranes, thus facilitating their coalescence and, ultimately, membrane fusion.[139] Peptides corresponding to the coiled-coil leucine zipper region of gp41 act as trans-dominant inhibitors of fusion.[141,226–227a]

After the entry of the virus core into the cytoplasm of susceptible cells, the genomic RNA is transcribed by reverse transcriptase into a single-stranded DNA intermediate, then a double-stranded circular DNA that is eventually inserted into the DNA of the host cell as a provirus.[167] In quiescent lymphocytes, this process occurs at a slow rate so that, for a few days, most of the virus is recovered in the cytoplasm as a labile, partial reverse transcript that eventually will be degraded.[228] There is evidence that T cells in culture can accumulate up to 80 copies of unintegrated HIV-1 DNA per cell as a consequence of multiple reinfections.[229] In contrast, infected T cells in vivo contain only a few copies of viral DNA.[230] Integration and subsequent expression of the provirus remain low-key as long as the host cell is not activated to begin differentiation or replication.[231] Activation can occur in response to mitogens or antigens or in response to specific interleukins such as TNF-α, granulocyte-macrophage colony-stimulating factor, or IL-6. At the molecular level, activation of the HIV-1 provirus results from the intervention of the cellular transcription activating factor NF-κB.[232] In resting cells, NF-κB is blocked in an inactive cytoplasmic complex with an inhibitor (IκB). On activation of the cell, the inhibitor is released and the factor migrates into the cell nucleus, where it binds the specific transcription activation sequences located upstream from the promoter on the HIV LTR. HIV thus uses for its own activation the very activation machinery of the host cell.[33,232,233]

Virus Variability

HIV exhibits a remarkable degree of genetic variability as a result of the error-prone nature of the viral reverse transcriptase (about 3×10^{-5} changes per replication cycle) and the high rate of virus production (up to 10^{10} virus particles per day).[10,234] Because of these factors, HIV-1 and HIV-2 evolve within an individual over time, yielding a swarm of related molecular clones that form a "quasispecies."[235–237] In general, genetic diversity among virus clones within an individual is about 2% to 3%. Selective pressure directs the evolution of the quasispecies.

Based on viral genetic sequences and phylogenetic analyses, HIV-1 strains have been classified into three distinct groups: M (main), N (new, or non-M, non-O), and O (outlier).[157,238,239] Each group is thought to have arisen from a separate cross-species transmission event.[240–242] The vast majority of the HIV-1 strains responsible for the global pandemic belong to group M. Group O was first described in Cameroon in 1990 and is highly divergent from group M, exhibiting only about 50% amino acid sequence identity to group M in the env gene.[243] Group O represents a small proportion (<5%) of HIV-1 infections in Cameroon.[244–246] Group N was identified in the late 1990s and is represented by a very small number of isolates from Cameroon.[247,248]

Since 1992, phylogenetic analyses of the env and gag genes have been used to classify the prevalent HIV-1 strains belonging to group M. These groupings are termed subtypes (also known as clades or genotypes) and are designated by letters A through K.[239] The group M subtypes are approximately equidistantly related, exhibiting 25% to 35% amino acid sequence difference within their env proteins and up to 20% difference within subtypes.[157,239] With improvements in genetic sequencing methods and more extensive genetic characterization of more viruses from around the world, it became clear that recombinant HIV-1 strains were relatively common.[154,156,249] By the mid-1990s, it was demonstrated that individuals could be dually infected with viruses from two

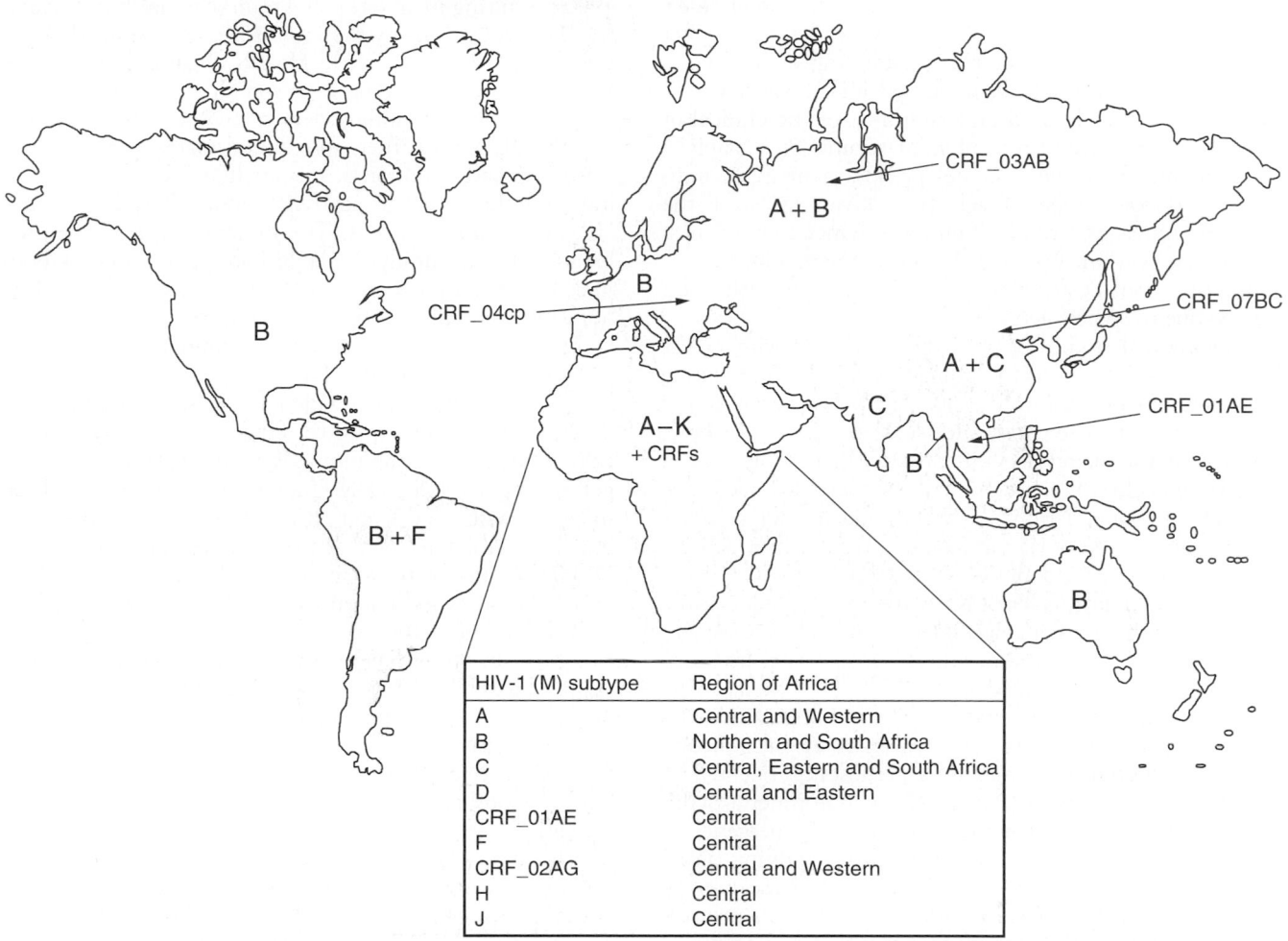

HIV-1 (M) subtype	Region of Africa
A	Central and Western
B	Northern and South Africa
C	Central, Eastern and South Africa
D	Central and Eastern
CRF_01AE	Central
F	Central
CRF_02AG	Central and Western
H	Central
J	Central

FIGURE 44–4 ■ Geographic distribution of HIV-1 major (M) group subtypes. For clarity, only the most prevalent subtypes are shown. CRF, circulating recombinant form. (After Tatt ID, Barlow KL, Nicoll A, Clewley JP. The public health significance of HIV-1 subtypes. AIDS (suppl 5): S59–S71, 2001.)

different subtypes.[239,250] Dual infection can result in recombinant viruses, often in complex mosaic forms. The term *circulating recombinant form* (CRF) was coined to describe viruses containing genetic material from more than one subtype that were circulating widely in a population.[157,238] In vitro, HIV-1 undergoes recombination at the extremely high rate of 2.8 crossovers per genome per cycle of replication, making it the most recombinogenic process observed in any mammalian-related system described so far.[250a]

The classification of HIV-1 strains into genetic subtypes has allowed for molecular epidemiologic studies to better characterize patterns of HIV transmission and spread.[251–253] The distribution of HIV-1 clades is shown in Figure 44–4. HIV-1 subtype B predominates in the epidemic in the industrialized countries of North America, Western Europe, Australia/New Zealand, parts of Latin America and the Caribbean, and some areas of Asia. However, other subtypes account for the global epidemic that is most severe in Africa and Asia.[157] HIV-1 subtype C accounts for a large proportion of infections in southern Africa, subtypes A and D are most common in eastern Africa, and in western Africa CRF02_AG (containing genetic material from subtypes A and G) predominates. Subtype B is rarely found in Africa, apart from persons who are epidemiologically linked to the Western epidemic. The heterosexual epidemic in

Thailand is overwhelmingly due to CRF01_AE.[254,255] The *env* region of these viruses clusters with a subtype designated E; however, a complete subtype E parental strain has not yet been identified. CRF01_AE also predominates in Cambodia, Vietnam, Southern China, and parts of Myanmar (Burma).[256–259] In China, the presence of subtypes B and C among populations of injection drug users (IDUs) in southern Yunnan Province yielded CRF07_BC and CRF08_BC, which subsequently became the predominant viruses as the HIV-1 epidemic spread to the north and the east.[260] The epidemic among IDUs in Kaliningrad, Russia, is due mainly to CRF03_AB.[261,262] In East Africa, studies have indicated that 30% to 40% of infections are with intersubtype recombinants.[157] Retrospective analysis of dried blood samples from northern Malawi has shown that in 1982 to 1986, subtypes A, C, and D were all present in small numbers, whereas by 1987 to 1989, 90% of the sequences were subtype C and AC, AD, or DC CRFs, indicative of explosive growth of subtype C in that area.[262a]

These data suggest that HIV-1 dual infection and the subsequent formation of recombinant viruses is not rare, and may be common. A prospective study of IDUs in Thailand documented two cases of sequential superinfection with two different subtypes, B and CRF01_AE.[263] In each case, the individual seroconverted to the primary subtype (B in one case and CRF01_AE in the other case), and later (1 to 6 months) became infected with the other subtype. Hopefully, a greater understanding of such cases will allow for the design of improved HIV-1 vaccines. To date, there is very limited understanding of the clinical or biologic significance of recombinant strains. Presumably, a recombinant virus that becomes predominant in an individual has some type of selective advantage over the parental strains, as a result of either enhanced viral fitness or immune evasion. When such a virus emerges as the predominant strain in an epidemic in a population, this also may be due to some selective advantage.

Longitudinal studies of individuals infected with HIV-1 show that, at the time of primary infection and during the asymptomatic stage of the disease, the virus clones that predominate in the host are slow-growing, M-tropic, non–syncytia-inducing R5 virus clones, whereas the onset of the terminal, clinical phase of the disease sees the emergence of rapidly growing, T-tropic, syncytia-inducing X4 viruses.[50] Sexual transmission of R5 viruses even in cases in which the donor harbored X4-R5 or X4 viruses has been well documented. Selection in favor of R5 viruses must operate at the time of infection in each newly infected individual. Owing to rapid diversification in the new host, virus isolates from two directly linked cases can vary by 4% to 5%.[264–266] Serial analysis of viral sequences from epidemiologically linked individuals revealed a different rate of evolution in the different individuals, suggesting that changes are host dependent.[267,268]

Selective pressures within the microenvironments of different anatomic compartments result in the emergence in various tissues of distinct, independently evolving quasispecies.[269] A large proportion of the virus clones seem to be replication defective but are propagated through complementation with replication-competent clones. Because of the sequence variation of the virus, one notes the emergence of escape mutants that arise as a consequence of immune selection and can escape either neutralizing antibodies[270,271,310,310a] or CTLs.[13–18a,272–274]

Nevertheless, HIV isolates from people with a common infection link, such as sex partners, mothers and their infants, or blood donors and recipients, show much closer genetic relatedness than do HIV isolates from people without a direct transmission link. Such genetic similarity can be used to investigate possible HIV transmission linkage, as was done in the case of transmission in a dental practice,[275] or in the hospital.[276]

Epidemiology

The evolution of the global HIV epidemic over the past decade is the most compelling argument for the need for a safe and effective preventive HIV vaccine. In the early 1990s, the modes of transmission of HIV were well defined and provided the basis for HIV prevention and control efforts. Global HIV prevention was based primarily on behavior change (to reduce the number of at-risk exposures to HIV), condom use (to reduce sexual HIV transmission) and the management of other sexually transmitted infections (STIs; to decrease the efficiency of sexual HIV transmission). Despite efforts to implement these control measures, the HIV epidemic doubled in size during the

1990s, resulting in an estimated total of 65 million cumulative HIV infections by the end of 2001. By early 2002, it was estimated by the World Health Organization and the Joint United Nations Programme on HIV/AIDS (UNAIDS) that there were 40 million persons living with HIV infection. In 2001 alone, there were an estimated 5 million new infections and 3 million deaths attributable to AIDS. This indicates that there are currently more than 14,000 new HIV infections every day. The difficulty of implementing broadly and sustaining available HIV prevention methods indicates that a preventive HIV vaccine may offer the best hope for eventual control of this pandemic.

The global epidemic is overwhelmingly the result of HIV-1, rather than HIV-2. HIV-2 is less transmissible than HIV-1 and causes immunodeficiency substantially more slowly.[65,277–279] Consequently, HIV-2 remains geographically limited, occurring primarily in West Africa or among persons epidemiologically linked to West Africa. Dual infection with HIV-1 and HIV-2 does occur[280]: The combined epidemiologic data do not support a protective effect of HIV-2 infection on incident HIV-1 infection,[281,282] although a study in Senegal suggested such protection.[283,284]

The burden of the HIV-1 epidemic is borne disproportionately by the developing world, especially Africa. Approximately 95% of new HIV-1 infections occur in the developing world, primarily among young adults in their most productive years. In sub-Saharan Africa in early 2002, there were 28 million persons living with HIV infection. The estimates for persons living with HIV were 1.4 million for Latin America, 0.9 million for North America, 0.4 million for the Caribbean, 0.6 million for Western Europe, 1 million for Eastern Europe and Central Asia, 0.4 million for North Africa and the Middle East, 6 million for South and Southeast Asia, and 1 million for East Asia and the Pacific.

HIV-1 transmission among adults and adolescents (horizontal) is primarily by sexual intercourse (vaginal, anal, or oral) and the exchange of blood or blood products, including via the reuse of needles and syringes. More than 90% of global HIV-1 infections among adults were due to sexual transmission.[285] Although a large proportion of STIs in developed Western countries early in the epidemic (which began expanding in the late 1970s) were among men who have sex with men (MSM), heterosexual transmission accounts for a very large proportion of infections in the developing countries of Africa, Asia, and Latin America, where the HIV/AIDS epidemic is most severe.[286] Sexual transmission of HIV-1 is facilitated by complex sexual networks, including those related to the commercial sex industry, and the presence of other STIs that increase the per-act probability of transmission.[285,287] There is a growing appreciation that male circumcision is a protective factor for HIV transmission; conversely, being uncircumcised is a risk factor for male acquisition of and transmission of HIV-1.[288,289] It is likely that recently infected persons who are in the process of seroconverting to HIV are more infectious to their sexual partners, because of a high level of HIV-1 in their blood and in genital secretions.[287,290,291]

Illicit injection drug use accounts for a varying proportion of HIV infections in various regions and locales in the world.[292,293] IDUs have experienced explosive epidemics of HIV-1 transmission in diverse parts of the world; HIV-1 prevalence rates often reach greater than 50% and can increase rapidly following the introduction of HIV-1 into existing networks.[294] Transmission in jails and prisons has facilitated rapid expansion of the epidemic in some cities.[295,296] HIV-1 transmission resulting from medical blood transfusions can be largely eliminated with effective screening of blood and blood products. However, in resource-poor settings blood safety is too often neglected, resulting in avoidable transmission events.[297,298] Also, the reuse of injection equipment in formal and informal medical settings in the developing world accounts for a poorly characterized proportion of transmission.

Mother-to-child (vertical) HIV-1 transmission accounts for most of the 800,000 annual new infections among children each year. Vertical transmission occurs prepartum, intrapartum, and postpartum via breast-feeding.[299–301] The largest proportion of vertical transmission occurs near the time of delivery; however, there is an increasing awareness of the proportion of transmission resulting from breast feeding in resource-poor areas where safe alternatives to breast feeding are not readily available. During the 1990s, great advances were made in the prevention of vertical transmission by use of antiretroviral drugs administered to the mother and infant.[302] Implementation of these interventions has dramatically decreased the incidence of perinatally acquired HIV infection in developed Western countries.

In Western countries, the incidence of new HIV infections generally leveled off or decreased during the 1990s. AIDS deaths dropped sharply following the introduction of highly active antiretroviral therapy in 1996. However, there is some evidence indicating a resurgence of risky sexual behavior resulting in increases in HIV and other STI transmission among some populations of MSM in these countries. It is hypothesized that this change in behavior is linked to optimism related to new and effective HIV/AIDS treatments.[303]

The HIV-1 epidemic in sub-Saharan Africa expanded at an alarming rate in the 1990s, especially in southern Africa. Social unrest, wars, large-scale population movements, rapid urbanization, newly established trucking routes, and grinding poverty have contributed to the conditions that facilitate HIV transmission. High rates of AIDS death have led to a growing population of orphans in Africa. One of the most useful measures of the extent of a generalized heterosexual epidemic is the HIV-1 prevalence among pregnant women attending antenatal care clinics. Such women reasonably represent the general, young adult female population and are accessible in clinics for HIV-1 seroprevalence surveys. HIV-1 seroprevalence among pregnant women varies greatly in Africa, from less than 5% in countries such as Senegal to more that 30% in Botswana, Zambia, and Zimbabwe. High rates of HIV infection among pregnant women have led to an epidemic of perinatal transmission and pediatric AIDS, reversing gains made in child survival in recent years. Efforts to implement HIV screening of pregnant women and prevent transmission with the use of zidovudine and/or nevirapine have made relatively little impact on this problem; these efforts will need to be redoubled in the future.[304] HIV prevention efforts in Uganda, led by high-level political leadership, are noteworthy for resulting in a decrease in HIV prevalence rates among pregnant women, and probably the adult population as a whole. The example of Uganda offers hope for African countries committed to stemming the epidemic.[305]

In Asia, the continent that is home to 60% of the world's population, extensive HIV transmission began only in the late 1980s. In 1988, there was an explosive epidemic of HIV-1 transmission among IDUs in Bangkok, Thailand; prevalence rates increased from less than 1% to greater than 40% within a year.[306] This was followed by a large epidemic of sexual transmission closely related to male patronage of female sex workers; HIV prevalence rates among brothel-based sex workers increased to greater than 50% in some cities by 1990. Thailand then mounted a successful multi-faceted HIV prevention campaign and was able to contain HIV-1 prevalence to less than 2% among the general adult population.[307] Injection drug use also has played a key part of the expansion of the epidemic in India, China, Vietnam, Myanmar (Burma), Malaysia, and Indonesia. The female commercial sex industry facilitates transmission in Thailand, Cambodia, India, Nepal, China, Vietnam, and several other countries. India now has probably the largest number of HIV infections among Asian countries.

Antigenic Determinants and Epitopes of Interest

The identification of neutralization epitopes and of epitopes recognized by Th cells and CTLs in HIV antigens is of major practical importance for the development of an HIV vaccine.[308]

Neutralizing Antibodies

Virus neutralization assays are designed to measure a reduction in virus infectious titer mediated by exposure to antibody. Infectivity of primary HIV-1 isolates is determined by infecting activated PBMCs in culture and assaying for p24 *gag* antigen or reverse transcriptase activity in extracellular medium. These assays involve several rounds of virus replication, and thus lack accuracy; they are labor intensive and time consuming. Assays that directly quantify single-round HIV-1 infection of PBMCs or transformed CD4+ CCR-5+ target cells have been developed.[309–310a] The precision and robustness of these new assays should facilitate the comparison of antibody responses to various HIV-1 immunogens and help revisit the issue of neutralizing antibodies.

The principal neutralizing antigenic determinant of HIV-1 TCLA strains has been mapped to the hypervariable V3 loop of gp120,[197,198,200] a continuous region of approximately 35 amino acids linked by a disulfide bond (see Fig. 44–3). Linear peptides with the sequence of the V3 loop elicit strain-specific neutralizing antibodies that do not interfere with CD4 binding but neutralize HIV-1 infectivity as a postbinding phenomenon by preventing fusion between virus envelope and cell membrane or between virus-infected and uninfected cells,[202] most probably by blocking interaction between gp120 and the CXCR-4 coreceptor. The conserved region that maps to the tip of the V3 loop (the GPGRAF motif in clade B viruses) induces neutralizing antibodies that cross-neutralize HIV-1 TCLA strains with homology in that region.[311,312] The V3 loop is highly immunodominant: Most HIV-1–infected or gp120/gp160-immunized individuals or animals produce antibodies to this epitope. V3-targeted neutralizing monoclonal antibodies (MAbs) have been demonstrated to protect chimpanzees passively from experimental infection with a TCLA strain of HIV-1.[313,314] Similarly, vaccine protection experiments against challenge with TCLA strains in chimpanzees have shown remarkable correlation between protection from infection and the titer of V3-targeted neutralizing antibodies in the animal.[315–320]

What is true of TCLA (X4) virus strains does not hold, however, for R5 viruses. Thus the V3 loop in primary HIV-1 isolates,[321–323] in HIV-2,[324] or in SIV[325] does not constitute a neutralization epitope. Primary HIV-1 isolates are relatively resistant both to sCD4 and to neutralizing antibodies, probably because of their three-dimensional envelope glycoprotein conformation and of its glycosylation. The neutralization resistance phenotype is associated with enhanced efficiency and speed of fusion after receptor and co-receptor engagement by the viral envelope.[326–328] Adaptation of primary HIV-1 to growth in permanent T-cell lines is accompanied by neutralization by both V3 MAbs and anti-gp120 immune sera,[329–331] whereas replacement of the V1-V2 or V3 loops of a TCLA strain with those of a primary isolate creates a neutralization-resistant virus. The V2 and V3 loops reside proximal to the chemokine receptor–binding site in gp120, which they probably shed from neutralizing antibodies while presenting potentially variable epitopes as a decoy to the immune system.[215] This question has, however, been recently revisited with the observation that six new human MAbs with specificities for conformation-dependent epitopes mapping to the V3 loop could recognize the V3 loop on the surface of native virions of primary isolates and displayed cross-clade neutralization activity against primary isolates from clades A, B, and F. Neutralization of some clade C and D viruses was also observed.[331a] This stands in sharp contrast to the type-specificity associated with anti-V3 antibodies derived from immunized animals.[321–323]

A second important cluster of HIV-1–neutralization epitopes has been identified in the V1/V2 region of gp120. MAbs for this region usually recognize conformational epitopes and can neutralize primary isolates as well as TCLA virus strains.[215,332–334] However, they show a restricted range of neutralization.

A third cluster of neutralization epitopes includes four relatively conserved epitopes defined by neutralizing human MAbs. These are MAb b12, directed against a conformational epitope overlapping the gp120 CD4-binding site[335–338]; MAb 2G12, targeted to a complex epitope formed by mannose residues contributed by the glycans attached to gp120 residues N295 and N332[339,340]; MAb 2F5, which has been mapped to a region overlapping the hexapeptide ELDKWA in the gp41 stem[341,342]; and MAbs Z13 and 4E10, directed against the sequence NWF(D/N)IT located carboxy-terminal to the 2F5 epitope.[343] These MAbs are able to neutralize a large number of primary HIV-1 isolates, irrespective of clade.[344] Passive immunization experiments using MAbs 2F5, 2G12, and b12 have shown that these antibodies can protect from HIV-1 or SHIV infections in hu-PBL severe combined immunodeficiency (SCID) mice (SCID mice grafted with human lymphocytes),[345] rhesus macaques,[346–349] or chimpanzees.[350] Remarkably, these MAbs can effectively protect from mucosal virus challenge when administered systemically.[351]

MAb b12 belongs to a group of MAbs with discontinuous epitopes that overlap part of the CD4-binding site[351a] and competitively inhibit CD4 binding to monomeric gp120.[352,353] They also inhibit gp120 binding to ccr5 and cell-to-cell fusion mediated by CD4-independent HIV-1 envelope glycoproteins, suggesting that they block the gp120 conformational transition that allows coreceptor binding.[353a] The b12 epitope is a major epitope on virions, as opposed to recombinant envelope gp160 or gp120 preparations,[354] suggesting that native envelope spikes from virions could have greater vaccine efficacy than recombinant Env molecules.[355] Similarly, the majority of well-recognized epitopes on monomeric gp120 are poorly presented on oligomeric gp120/gp141,[355–358] and neutralization of primary virus isolates correlates qualitatively with the affinity of the antibody for oligomeric but not for monomeric gp120.[358]

A last group of neutralizing MAbs[17b, 48d] have been termed CD4 induced (CD4i) because they bind with enhanced efficacy to gp120 when it is complexed with CD4.[359] Although they are potent neutralizers of TCLA viruses, the activity of these MAbs on primary virus isolates appears relatively weak but is greatly enhanced in the presence of CD4. The conserved CD4i epitopes are only transiently exposed after CD4i binding but prior to coreceptor interaction, limiting their accessibility to the corresponding antibodies.[359a]

It has been extremely difficult so far to present the envelope glycoprotein in a way that would stimulate a significant neutralizing antibody response to primary virus isolates. Immunization with gp120 elicits neutralizing antibodies against TCLA but not against primary HIV-1 isolates;[360,361] it is suspected that immunodominance in gp120 is for non-neutralization epitopes, whereas the more important conformational neutralization epitopes are poorly immunogenic.[357] Of major potential interest is the observation that vaccine preparations in which gp120 is complexed to CD4 show definite ability to induce neutralizing antibodies to primary HIV-1 isolates.[362–365] Conserved conformational neutralization epitopes also can be unmasked by deletion of the V2 loop (see *Subunit Vaccines* below).[366]

The possibility of classifying HIV-1 by neutralization serotypes has been tested in cross-neutralization studies using panels of virus isolates from different genetic clades and serum or plasmas from people infected with diverse HIV-1 subtypes. Data from several laboratories demonstrate that the pattern of neutralization of HIV-1 field isolates is not related to genetic subtype.[367–370]

About one third of the plasma samples show relatively broad, cross-clade neutralizing activity, whereas the other two thirds show a full spectrum of neutralizing activity. Similarly, some virus isolates appear to be sensitive to neutralization, whereas others show relative insensitivity. With use of serum pools rather than individual sera, the B subtype and CRF01_AE in Thailand could be distinguished as two distinct neutralization serotypes.[371] In another study, HIV-1 isolates could be grouped by multivariate analysis in a few neutralization clusters not correlated with genetic clades.[368] Of note is that sera from HIV-1 group M–infected individuals could neutralize HIV-1 group O isolates. There is also extensive cross-neutralization between HIV-1 and SIVcpz isolates, reflecting their evolutionary origins, but only infrequent and low titered cross-neutralization between HIV-1 and HIV-2.[372] Extensive cross-clade neutralization of HIV-1 primary isolates was observed with MAbs b12, 2F5, and 2G12.[373] This suggests that a vaccine, to be effective against multiple HIV-1 isolates, should induce 2F5-, 2G12-, and b12-like antibodies.

Synergism neutralization of HIV-1 TCLA isolates can be observed, at least to a certain degree, by mixing MAbs targeted to different neutralization epitopes,[374] or by mixing antibodies to CD4 and to the V2 and V3 loops.[375,376] Studies on primary isolates have shown less significant enhancement, except with triple or quadruple antibody combinations.[344,376]

In the course of HIV-1 infection, neutralizing antibodies to the autologous virus strain in the patient develop slowly, appearing on average only about 1 year after seroconversion, and titers remain low.[377] Heterologous neutralization of primary isolates seems to occur even later. Similar observations have been made in the case of macaques immunized with live, attenuated SIV vaccines or infected with SHIV,[378] demonstrating the existence of a complex and lengthy maturation of the antibody response during the first 6 to 8 months after infection, as reflected in progressive changes in antibody conformational dependence, avidity, and neutralization activity.[378–380] The use of sensitive, single-round viral infectivity assays has, however, revealed that autologous neutralizing antibodies can be detected as early as 72 days following seroconversion and progressively reach high titers.[310] The initial neutralization-sensitive virus is then replaced by successive populations of resistant escape viruses that contain mutations in env, many of which involve changes in N-linked glycosylation sites, suggesting an evolving "glycan shield" mechanism of neutralization escape.[310,310a] This is reminiscent of the equine infectious anemia virus infection, the recurrent virus cycles of which result from the sequential evolution of antigenic variants that escape serum antibody neutralization.[380a]

Antigenic determinants that might induce the production of enhancing antibodies are of potential concern for the development of vaccines.[381] In the case of HIV infection, enhancing antibodies can be evidenced by use of either of two in vitro systems: complement-mediated enhancement[382,383] and complement-independent enhancement.[384,385] Enhancing antibodies increase the infectivity of the virus for target cells by binding the virus to the Fc or the CR2 receptor at the cell surface. Human MAbs able to enhance HIV-1 infection in vitro were found to map to epitopes on gp41.[386] It also was observed that a V3 loop peptide from a given HIV-1 strain could elicit antibodies that enhanced infection by other HIV-1 strains.[387,388] Enhancing antibodies were found after virus challenge in SIV-vaccinated macaques that happened not to be protected. However, these animals did not develop a more severe or accelerated disease compared with their unvaccinated controls. The role that enhancing antibodies might play in facilitating infection with HIV or SIV or in aggravating disease therefore remains to be demonstrated.[389,390]

HIV-1 gp120 also has been identified as a major target for ADCC, which might contribute to protective immunity against HIV-1.[9,391–393] Cytolysis by ADCC is independent of MHC restriction and could lead to rapid destruction of HIV-infected cells that are transmitted at the time of infection.[9]

Cytotoxic T Lymphocytes

CD8+ CTL and CD4 helper T lymphocyte (HTL) responses play major roles in the containment of HIV and SIV. The appearance of CTLs in the acute phase of infection correlates with the initial control of primary viremia,[41–43,394] and depletion of CD8+ T cells prior to SIV infection results in an inability to control SIV.[46,395] Patients who maintain strong HIV-1–specific T-cell responses are better able to control virus replication.[396,397] Similarly, highly HIV-exposed female sex workers who remained persistently seronegative showed elevated levels of HIV-specific CD8+ T cells in PBMCs and cervical samples.[113–115] In rhesus macaques, mucosal SIV-specific CTLs correlated with control of virus replication following intraintestinal SIV challenge.[398] The ability of live, attenuated SIV to protect macaques against pathogenic challenge correlates with the induction and maintenance of strong CTL and HTL responses.[82,399]

CD8 T cells control viral infections through infected target cell lysis using a perforin/granzyme pathway (cytolytic activity) or through secretion of antiviral cytokines, such as IFN-γ[400] or β-chemokine. CD8+ T lymphocytes can also suppress HIV-1 replication by secreting β-chemokines[7,8] and/or soluble suppressive factors (SF).[5,6,81–83] SF can be up-regulated by immunization with viral antigens[401,402] or after alloimmunization.[403]

Our ability to measure T-cell responses to HIV or SIV has been extraordinarily improved of late by the advent of powerful new technologies such as tetramer-staining assays, which measure T-cell binding to peptides complexed to MHC molecules; enzyme-linked immunospot (ELISPOT) assays, which measure cytokine (IFN-γ) secretion in response to stimulations with overlapping peptide libraries; and intracellular cytokine staining assays.[404] Most data available to date have been obtained using the much less sensitive ^{51}Cr-release–based limiting dilution cytotoxic assays and therefore need to be re-evaluated. Also, the majority of CD8+ T-cell epitopes have been identified in the chronic phase of HIV infection, whereas recent evidence suggests that early responses to primary infection may target different epitopes.[16,405] Finally, the majority of HIV and SIV CTL epitopes studied have been those in the large viral structural proteins (Env, Gag, Pol) and in the Nef protein, neglecting the CTL epitopes in the small viral regulatory proteins Tat, Rev, Vif, and Vpr, whose importance has been outlined only recently.[16,406,407]

The HIV-1 Env glycoprotein can serve as a target antigen for CD8+ MHC class I–restricted CTLs, in association with HLA-A2, -A3, -B7, or -B17.[408] The V3 loop contains a CTL epitope that is restricted by HLA-A2. Several other CTL epitopes have been identified in gp160, many of which appear to be relatively well conserved and several of which overlap on the molecule.[409] Env-specific CD4+, MHC class II–restricted CTLs also have been evidenced in association with HLA-DR2 or HLA-DR4.[410]

Many HIV-1 CTL epitopes appear to be located in the Gag molecule, most particularly in conserved regions of p24gag (CA), as well as in several regions of the highly conserved Pol protein, and in the central and carboxy-terminal regions of Nef, in which a continuum of epitopes is recognized by CTL in association with a variety of histocompatibility antigens.[408,411] Of major importance for vaccine development is the observation that CTLs elicited in response to a clade B–based live recombinant canarypox HIV-1 vaccine were capable of recognizing primary HIV-1 isolates belonging to genetically diverse clades.[412]

Precursor CTL frequency in the blood of infected patients is usually as high as 1 per 10,000 and can reach up to 1% of T cells. Large numbers of SIV-specific CTLs also have been found within vaginal[413] and intestinal[414] intraepithelial lymphocytes in SIV-infected macaques.

Emergence and positive selection of CTL escape virus variants have been well documented[13–18a] (see *Virus Variability* above). Some escape variants can actually antagonize the activity of CTLs targeted to the wild-type epitopes, resulting in persistence of virus strains that otherwise would be recognized by the existing CTLs. This might explain why diversification of the virus quasispecies is often accompanied by maintenance of the original clones in the infected person.

Of major concern is the observation that a CTL response with only a single epitope specificity was unable to provide protective immunity against a live SIV challenge in macaques.[17,415] Similarly, administration to an HIV-1–seropositive individual of a large number of autologous CTLs to a single epitope in Nef resulted in the emergence of a variant viral strain missing that epitope.[273] Inclusion of several HIV-1 antigens in the same vaccine is therefore recommended to broaden the CTL response.

HIV antigens also have been studied for their ability to stimulate Th cell proliferation or IL-2 production in vitro. HTL epitopes have been mapped using sets of synthetic peptides. A major HTL epitope, *env*T1, was identified in gp120,[416] and several HTL epitopes have been mapped to p24*gag* and to the Nef protein.

Candidate HIV Vaccines

The development of an HIV vaccine is a formidable challenge. Most classical vaccines provide protection from disease but do not actually prevent infection; they allow a limited but controlled replication of the pathogen at the portal of entry. This raises the question of whether an HIV vaccine, if unable to prevent infection, could prevent development of disease. SIV-vaccinated and challenged macaques that became infected because of ineffective or insufficient immunization showed prolonged delay in the onset of disease and lived longer than unvaccinated control animals,[417] as a consequence of decreased virus loads. This suggests that an HIV vaccine, even if unable to provide sterilizing immunity, might prevent, or at least delay disease onset. Also, by reducing virus levels in blood and genital secretions, such a vaccine could reduce virus transmission.

As discussed below, classical vaccine strategies based on live, attenuated virus or whole inactivated virus have severe limitations. Most efforts to develop an HIV vaccine have therefore focused on newer vaccine approaches. Progress in antigen design and genetic manipulations of viral or bacterial vectors has considerably improved the diversity of antigen delivery systems. The following is a brief review of recent developments in the field.

Whole Inactivated Vaccines

Successful protection of macaques against pathogenic SIV challenge was observed in several experiments using whole inactivated SIV vaccines or formalin-inactivated SIV-infected cell extracts. The mechanism of protection unraveled when it was found that the relevant antigens in the vaccine preparations were not the SIV antigens but rather xenoantigens from the human cells used to grow the virus.[418] Monkeys also could be protected from challenge with SIV grown in human cells by immunization with purified HLA-DR,[419] raising the possibility of using alloimmunization to provide protection from HIV-1 infection in humans.

Whole inactivated HIV-1 vaccines have not been seriously considered as potential human vaccines, mostly because of safety considerations, also because of the difficulty of getting large quantities of the material, and in part because of failure of an early approach in chimpanzees.[420] The latter may have been due to the use of formalin in the inactivating procedure, which is most often highly damaging to protein structures. New, gentle inactivation methods have been developed, such as removal of essential Zn^{2+} ions from the Int and Gag proteins through the use of Aldithriol,[421] and ultraviolet inactivation of the viral RNA with the help of psoralen.[422] Combining these two methods results in an inactivated virus preparation with conserved envelope antigenicity whose immunogenicity is being evaluated. The number of envelope trimers per virion has been a subject of some controversy. One study shows that both X4 and R5 HIV-1 isolates have a Gag-to-Env ratio of approximately 60:1, which would correspond to only 7 to 14 trimeric envelope spikes per particle.[423] This low number might explain the virus's poor immunogenicity. An alternative is to use pseudovirions. These are viral particles without a genome; they include the Gag and Env structural proteins. In a test of the immunogenicity of pseudovirions with the Env component from a primary R5 virus isolate, HIV-1 BX08, the pseudoparticles induced neutralizing antibodies to the homologous HIV-1 BX08, but not to other HIV-1 isolates.[424]

Particulate vaccines made of hybrid particles expressing HIV-1 antigenic determinants on their surfaces also were tested. Thus the V3 loop of HIV-1 was expressed on the surface of poliovirus,[425] hepatitis B virus core particles,[426] hepatitis B surface antigen particles,[427] or the yeast retrotransposon virus-like particles (Ty-VLP).[428,429] These particles were found to be very immunogenic. A limitation of this approach, however, is the limited size of the determinant that can be inserted into the particle and the impossibility of mimicking complex conformation-dependent neutralization determinants.

Live, Attenuated Vaccines

Several studies have demonstrated vaccine protection against SIV infection using live, attenuated SIV vaccines. Rhesus monkeys infected with nonpathogenic molecular clones of SIVmac, such as 1A11 or BK28, developed persistent low-grade infection and were protected from superinfection with a low dose of pathogenic SIV and from disease, but not from superinfection with a high dose of SIV.[430] Protection was correlated with induction of a CTL response.[431,431a]

A live SIVmac vaccine, attenuated by deletion of the *nef* gene, demonstrated remarkable efficacy as a vaccine[26,28]: macaques challenged more than 2 years after immunization were protected against 1000 animal infectious doses of pathogenic SIVmac grown in monkey PBMCs. Deletion of *nef*, alone or in combination with deletions in *vpr* and in the LTR region,[379] showed no drastic effect on virus growth in cell culture.[432] These results were confirmed using two molecular clones of SIVmac: J5, a full-length pathogenic molecular clone, and C8, which is attenuated because of a 12-base pair deletion in the *nef* gene.[27,166] Immunization with C8 provided complete protection from infection with J5, including mucosal infection.[433]

However, SIVΔ*nef* establishes a state of indefinite persistence in the vaccinated host, could revert to full-size *nef* virulence in some animals,[166] and remained pathogenic to neonatal macaques, at least at a high dose.[434,435] It also caused disease in some adult monkeys.[436,436a] Efforts to render the virus safer and more efficacious have included the construction of replication-competent SIV Δ*nef* that expresses human IFN-γ[437] or the herpesvirus thymidine kinase.[438] Another approach has been the deletion of several accessory genes[439] or of the *rev* gene alone.[440] However, an inverse relationship has been demonstrated between the degree of virologic attenuation and induction of protective immune responses to SIV.[440a] Furthermore, even if attenuated SIV was proved to be safe in animals, the prospect of using a live, attenuated HIV-1 vaccine in humans would still meet with deep safety concerns, including the potential of promoting tumors through insertional oncogenesis. A few individuals harboring HIV for long periods of time without any sign of AIDS were shown to be infected with *nef*-deleted viruses,[441,442] but these persons experienced late decline in their CD4+ T-cell counts and slow evolution toward AIDS.[443–445]

Immunization of macaques with attenuated SIV provided protection from infection with genetically divergent SIV strains and with chimeric SHIV expressing an HIV-1 envelope against which no cross-neutralization activity could be detected.[29,433,446–448] A vigorous CTL response was

observed that arose early in infection and persisted for years after a single inoculation of virus.[82,399] Macaques immunized with attenuated SIVmac showed a high-level CTL response in iliac, mesenteric, and rectal lymph nodes[433] and were protected from mucosal challenge. Similarly, macaques previously exposed to subinfectious doses of HIV-2 demonstrated a virus-specific cellular immune response and were protected from SIV infection when challenged intrarectally, in spite of the absence of an SIV-specific antibody response.[449] Therefore, activation of the cell-mediated arm of the immune system only, without antibody formation, seems to be able to prevent mucosal SIV transmission in macaques.[450] Full protection from intravenous challenge may depend on the combination of high-avidity neutralizing antibodies with CTLs and other cellular immune mechanisms, including the secretion of β-chemokines.

Live Recombinant Vaccines

Live recombinant vaccines are made of a live, attenuated viral or bacterial strain used as a vector to carry the gene or genes that encode the appropriate antigens (Table 44-3). Live recombinant vaccines have a number of attractive features, including the ability to stimulate both humoral and cell-mediated immunity.

Vaccinia virus vectors expressing a variety of HIV and SIV genes have been tested in animals and, in some cases, humans.[451,452] The results indicate that HIV-specific T-cell responses could be induced, including CTLs, but anti-HIV antibody responses were usually weak and transient. The protective potential of recombinant vaccinia virus vaccines was demonstrated in the macaque/SIV model using a vaccinia virus expressing SIV Nef.[453] An inverse correlation was found between vaccine-induced *nef*-specific CTL precursor frequency and virus load measured after challenge with pathogenic SIVmac. In the animal with the strongest CTL response, virus was not detectable at any time.

The issue of lack of safety of vaccinia virus recombinants in immunocompromised people has led to prefer the use of attenuated vaccinia virus strains such as the NYVAC strain[454] or the modified vaccinia virus Ankara (MVA) strain,[455,456] a highly attenuated, host range–restricted strain of vaccinia virus that grows in chick embryo fibroblasts but is restricted at the stage of virion formation in mammalian cells. Another alternative is to replace vaccinia virus by canarypox (ALVAC) or avipox viruses.[457] The avian poxviruses do not replicate in mammalian cells and are therefore less immunogenic than vaccinia virus, but show none of the potential risks of vaccinia virus in humans. A prolonged and marked suppression of replication of HIV-2 was observed after immunization of rhesus macaques with NYVAC– or ALVAC–HIV-1 expressing HIV-1 Gag, Pol, or Env and boosting with HIV-1 antigens or peptides.[458] Quite remarkably, an NYVAC vector expressing the *gag*, *env*, and *pol* genes of SIV provided protection from infection with SIVmac by the rectal route but not by the intravenous route, despite total absence of neutralizing antibodies.[450] MVA recombinants were found to induce in nonhuman primates potent CTL responses able to partially control virus loads after challenge with pathogenic SHIVs or SIV.[459–462] Prime-boost combinations using a DNA vaccine for priming

TABLE 44–3 ■ Potential Vectors for Live Recombinant HIV-1 Vaccines

Viruses	Bacteria
Vaccinia virus	Bacillus Calmette-Guérin
Canarypox, fowlpox virus	*Salmonella*
Adenovirus AAV	*Lactobacillus*
Alphaviruses (VEEV, Sindbis, SFV)	*Streptococcus*
Flaviviruses (YFV)	*Listeria*
Rhabdoviruses (VSV, rabies virus)	
Myxovirus (influenza virus),	
Paramyxoviruses (Sendaï virus, measles virus)	
Picornavirus (poliovirus)	

AAV, adeno-associated virus; SFV, Semliki Forest virus; VEEV, Venezuelan equine encephalitis virus; VSV, vesicular stomatitis virus; YFV, yellow fever virus.

and recombinant MVA or fowlpox virus vaccines for boosting elicited the best CTL responses.[463,464] Immunized macaques showed lower virus loads and prolonged survival relative to controls following challenge with infectious virus, including pathogenic SHIVs[465] (see *HIV-1 Vaccine Studies in Animals* below).

Human adenovirus types 4, 5, and 7 offer several potential advantages as vectors for live recombinant vaccines. They can be administered orally, in the form of gelatin-coated tablets from which the virus is released in the intestine, or intranasally, and they can induce both systemic and mucosal immunity. Recombinant adenoviruses expressing the Env or Gag antigens from HIV-1 or SIV have been tested in animals and shown to induce long-lasting protective immunity in chimpanzees.[466-468] More recently, defective adenovirus type 5 (Ad5) vectors have been developed that bear a deletion of the E1 gene, which can be complemented using a packaging cell line that supplies the E1 gene product in *trans*. An Ad5 recombinant expressing HIV-1 Gag was found to successfully induce cellular immune responses in rhesus macaques and to attenuate infection and mitigate disease progression after challenge with a pathogenic SHIV.[469] A Phase I clinical study combining a DNA vaccine for priming and an Ad5 recombinant vaccine for boosting is underway.

Defective alphavirus "replicons" are attractive vectors because of the enormous amplification of the viral message that occurs after infection. Also, these viruses have the potential to target dendritic cells, resulting in efficacious antigen presentation. A major drawback is that they require transformed cells for the packaging system. The most developed replicon system is that of the Venezuelan equine encephalitis virus.[470] Sindbis virus[471] and Semliki Forest virus[472,473] replicons represent attractive alternatives.

Adeno-associated virus (AAV) can persist as an episome in the cell for extremely long periods of time. Recombinant HIV-AAV expresses relevant HIV antigens in a persistent manner,[474] which may be of great advantage for low-potency antigens.

Poliovirus can be used as a vector to express foreign antigenic determinants, such as the V3 loop, on the surface of its capsid, resulting in a chimeric virus particle.[425] A chimeric influenza virus was similarly engineered by inserting an epitope from the V3 loop into antigenic site B in the hemagglutinin.[475] An influenza virus recombinant expressing the 2F5 epitope was also engineered; it induced secretory antibody at the mucosal level but only low titers of circulating HIV-1–neutralizing antibodies.[476] A limitation of these chimeric virus systems is the small size of the HIV determinant that can be inserted into the virus particle without impairing stability.

Poliovirus replicons that encode HIV-1 Gag,[477] SIV Gag, or SIV Env SU[478] proteins have been shown to generate immune responses to HIV or SIV antigens in animals. Immunization of cynomolgus macaques by the nasal route with replicons of the attenuated Sabin vaccine strain expressing SIV gene fragments encompassing a large portion of the SIV genome resulted in protection of a majority of the animals from vaginal challenge with a pathogenic SIV.[479] However, the limited insertion capacity of the vector is a major obstacle to the eventual development of this approach.

Numerous other virus vector systems are being developed for the preparation of live recombinant HIV vaccines, such as the attenuated vaccine strains of measles or yellow fever viruses, rabies virus,[480,481] vesicular stomatitis virus,[482,483] or Sendaï virus,[484] to name only a few.

Live recombinant bacterial vaccines also have been developed using as a vector bacille Calmette-Guérin (BCG)[485-488] or *Salmonella* strains that have been attenuated by mutagenesis of genes involved in virulence and invasiveness.[489,490] *Listeria monocytogenes* and *Shigella* are other human bacterial pathogens from which attenuated strains have been derived that could be used as vaccine vectors.

A major potential problem with live recombinant viral or bacterial vaccines is their relative lack of efficacy in individuals previously exposed to the vector, as a result of residual immunity in the host. Such a restriction does not apply to the canarypox or avipox virus vectors but would apply to BCG, poliovirus, or adenovirus. It also applies to MVA and NYVAC in the population of persons born before 1970 and would apply to the whole population if vaccination against smallpox was to be resumed. This is also a potential issue for any vaccination regimen requiring booster injections, because successive immunizations with the same vector will induce potent immunity to the vector.

Successive immunizations with different vectors could overcome this problem. Evidence has been obtained that priming with a replication-defective Ad5 recombinant followed by boosting with a canary pox virus recombinant induced high levels of T-cell responses to HIV-1 antigens (E. Emili, unpublished observations, Keystone conference, April 2003).

Subunit Vaccines

Recombinant soluble HIV and SIV glycoproteins have been produced from yeast, insect cells, or mammalian cells to be used as subunit vaccines. The observation that HIV-1 gp160, gp140 (a soluble form of gp160 resulting from the deletion of the transmembrane and intracytoplasmic domains), or gp120 induced only a transient response in primates has prompted the search for strong adjuvants or special delivery formulations that would be suitable for human use. Thus experimental vaccines have been developed in which the antigens were either formulated into liposomes[491] or complexed under the form of immune-stimulating complexes (ISCOMs) with the saponin derivative Quil A.[492] These responses were not, however, sufficient to protect macaques from challenge with the virulent SIVmac.[493]

Recombinant HIV-1 gp140 or gp120 also has been used with newer adjuvant formulations such as water-in-oil emulsions with the saponin derivative QS21, enterobacteria cell wall derivatives, muramyl dipeptide derivatives, or specific adjuvant formulations such as SAF-1 or MF59.[494] These studies have underlined the importance of the conformational integrity of the envelope glycoprotein for the induction of neutralizing antibodies[495]: Current envelope vaccine candidates elicit high gp120-binding antibody titers with neutralizing activity against matched TCLA virus strains but not primary HIV-1 isolates. Antibodies elicited by gp120 are directed to linear epitopes exposed on denatured forms of the molecule. In contrast, oligomeric gp140 or gp160 elicits antibodies to native cell surface–expressed gp120/gp41 that are able to neutralize some primary HIV-1 isolates.[495] The antibodies induced by gp120 are usually incapable of neutralizing primary R5 isolates, even though they can neutralize the homologous X4 virus strain. They can therefore prevent infection if animals are challenged with a homologous X4 virus but not with a R5 virus strain.[496]

Several approaches have been undertaken to overcome these obstacles. Mixing gp120 from different virus strains, including primary isolates, may elicit a broader neutralizing antibody response.[497] It has been suggested than the envelope glycoproteins from certain virus strains may be significantly better at inducing broadly neutralizing antibodies than those from other strains.[498] Another approach has been to use soluble gp140 glycoprotein trimers. However, native trimers are too unstable to be purified intact.[499] Engineering the envelope protein to prevent cleavage into gp120 and gp41 yields soluble oligomeric forms of gp140, but these oligomers are not able to induce broadly neutralizing antibodies,[499,500] probably because they are not the native trimers.

In an attempt to make truly trimeric, stable molecules, the association between gp120 and gp41 was stabilized by the introduction of a covalent disulfide bond[501] or by strengthening the trimeric association between the gp41 subunit isoleucine zippers.[502] The resulting molecules showed enhanced immunogenic potency, but the improvement was far from optimal.[503]

Neutralization epitopes can be at least partially unmasked by removing glycosyl moieties from the envelope protein[504] or by deleting the second variable loop from the gp120 molecule.[505,506] Immunization with DNA expressing the ΔV2 form of the glycoprotein followed by boosting with the ΔV2 protein itself was shown to induce neutralizing antibodies to a number of primary isolates.[366] This vaccine regimen will presently be tested in human volunteers. Finally, in vitro–assembled gp120-CD4 receptor complexes have been used as immunogens and shown to induce broadly neutralizing antibodies.[362,363] The complex has been produced as a single-chain polypeptide, whereby gp120 is joined to the D1D2 domain of CD4 by an amino acid linker.[365,507] The single-chain polypeptide accurately mimics structural and antigenic features of the gp120-CD4 complex and was reported to induce broadly neutralizing antibodies.[507]

In spite of the above results, protection from SIV infection by gp160-based subunit vaccines has been observed in a few instances.[508–510] The possibility of using soluble antigens for mucosal immunization also has been investigated. Encapsulation of the antigens in microspheres made of copolymers of lactide and glycolide protects them from degradation by low pH and proteolytic enzymes and allows them to be targeted through M cells into the Peyer's patches.[511]

Subunit vaccines based on the accessory protein Tat also have been developed and have demonstrated at least partial protective efficacy in SHIV/macaque models.[512–514]

Synthetic Vaccines

Most initial attempts to use synthetic peptide immunogens have concentrated on the V3 loop. Sp10, a peptide with the sequence of part of the V3 loop from the HIV-1 MN strain, linked to that of envT1, a major Th determinant of gp120, elicited long-lasting anti-HIV neutralizing antibody and Th cell responses in a variety of animals without the need for coupling to a protein carrier.[515] The same peptide, linked to the sequence of the fusion domain of gp41, showed strong immune potency in goats and rabbits but was paradoxically tolerogenic in macaques and chimpanzees.

Linked to branched polylysine molecules as a multiple antigen peptide (MAP) system, V3 peptides induced a long-term, high-titer neutralizing antibody response to X4 viruses.[516] An octameric V3 MAP formulated in alum was found to be safe and immunogenic in human volunteers.[517] Adding a lipophilic membrane-anchoring moiety such as tripalmitoyl glyceryl cysteine (P3C) at the carboxyl terminus of MAP systems enabled their inclusion into liposomes. The hydrophobic P3C "foot" served as an adjuvant and provided the V3 peptide with the ability to prime CTLs in vivo. Although peptides and proteins usually do not induce a class I–restricted CD8+ response in vivo, lipopeptides have such a capacity[518,519] and may represent an interesting formulation for inducing or boosting the CTL immune response to HIV. Indeed, long lipopeptides with a fatty acid tail can induce broad cellular immune responses in humans as well as in animals.[520]

Naked DNA Vaccines

Injection into the muscle or the epidermis of an animal of a purified plasmid DNA that carries a gene encoding an antigen under the control of an appropriate mammalian transcription promoter leads to expression of the antigen in situ and triggers an immune response, mostly of the Th1 type.[521–524] The use of pure DNA offers many advantages, including ease of design, simplicity of preparation, and chemical stability. Studies of DNA vaccines in primates have been disappointing, however. Native HIV genes were found to be expressed with low efficiency as a result of unusual codon usage. Their replacement by synthetic HIV-1 genes with optimized codons allowed Rev-independent high-level expression of the gene products.[525] Further improvement in immunogenicity has come from combining DNA immunization with a Schiff base-forming drug,[526] or from physical presentation of the DNA, either on gold particles for dermal delivery, or adsorbed to polylactide/polyglycolide microparticles,[527] or adjuvanted with a nonionic copolymer adjuvant.[469] Delivery of genes for IL-2, IL-12, or granulocyte-macrophage stimulating factor along with a DNA vaccine resulted in augmented immune responses[528,529] and better control of infection following challenge of the immunized animals.[530]

Immunization with HIV-1 env DNA was substantially boosted with soluble gp120 or gp140.[531,532] Successful protection from SHIV challenge in macaques[531,533] and from HIV-1 challenge in chimpanzees[534] has been reported. Most often, however, DNA immunization was insufficient to provide protective levels of cell-mediated immune responses. This could be achieved by adding booster immunizations with a live recombinant vaccine, whether a poxvirus,[463–465,335–336] a Sendaï virus,[484] or a defective adenovirus recombinant.[469]

Result of Vaccination

HIV-1 Vaccine Studies in Animals

Primate models for AIDS vaccine development include the SIV/macaque model, the HIV-1/chimpanzee model, the HIV-2/macaque model, and the SHIV/macaque model.[537]

HIV-1 has been transmitted to chimpanzees[92,94,538] and pigtail macaques (Macaca nemestrina).[539] It also replicates in immunodeficient mice engrafted with human fetal lymphoid tissue (SCID-hu mice) or adult human peripheral blood leukocytes (hu-PBL-SCID mice).[540] Replication-competent chimeric viruses called SHIV that have the *gag, pol, vif,* and *nef* genes from SIVmac and the *env, tat,* and *rev* genes from HIV-1 replicate to high titers in cynomolgus and rhesus monkeys without causing disease.[541–543] Serial passages of the virus in macaques lead to the selection of pathogenic variants that induce CD4 lymphopenia and an AIDS-like disease in the animals.[544–548] Infection with pathogenic X4 SHIVs is usually followed by rapid and drastic loss of peripheral CD4+ T cells within 4 to 6 weeks after infection. In Indian rhesus macaques, death follows within a few months. It is therefore questionable whether these viruses make a valuable model for the study of HIV vaccines.[51] R5 SHIVs that induce a more progressive CD4+ T-cell decline have been developed.[549]

The testing of subunit vaccines in animals has been extensively pursued and has yielded different results depending on the model studied. In the SIV/macaque model, a partial protective immune response was elicited with SIVmne gp160 given as a booster immunization after priming the animals with live recombinant vaccinia virus expressing the SIVmne gp160.[508] No protection was obtained, however, when these experiments were repeated with the more virulent SIVmac. Protection of cynomolgus monkeys against HIV-2 was achieved using a detergent-disrupted whole HIV-2 preparation in incomplete Freund's adjuvant (IFA) or formulated in immunostimulating complexes and followed by boosting with V3 peptides.[509] The importance of humoral immunity in protection was clearly demonstrated by showing that HIV-2 infection could be prevented in naive recipients by passive immunization with serum from protected monkeys.[550]

Similarly, neonatal macaques were protected from oral SHIV challenge by pre- and postnatal treatment with a combination of the three broadly neutralizing MAbs (b12, 2F5, and 2G12),[351,551] and adult macaques were protected from SHIV challenge by passive immunization with 2F5, 2G12, and high-titer anti-HIV immunoglobulins.[346,347]

Several groups have shown that gp120- or gp140-based vaccines provide protection against experimental HIV-1 infection in chimpanzees with either cell-free or cell-associated HIV-1 IIIB (LAI).[315–318] Passive immunization of a chimpanzee with a V3-targeted, LAI-specific neutralizing monoclonal antibody protected the animal fully against challenge from cell-free HIV-1 LAI even when the antibody was administered after virus inoculation.[314] Neutralizing antibodies therefore represent a surrogate marker for vaccine efficacy in this experimental setting where the endpoint is infection with a TCLA strain.

Protection from infection with a heterologous X4 HIV-1 strain (HIV-1 SF2) was obtained by active immunization of chimpanzees with gp120 MN[320] and with hybrid gp140 MN/LAI and a V3 peptide derived from the MN strain.[319] Protection from HIV-1 SF2 was also obtained with a live adenovirus expressing gp160 MN followed by boosting with gp120 SF2[467] or with a naked DNA vaccine.[534] In contrast, two chimpanzees that were primed with a low dose of ALVAC–HIV vCP125, which expresses gp160 MN, and boosted with gp140 MN/LAI were not protected against challenge with SF2.[319] High neutralizing antibody titers against the MN and LAI HIV-1 strains were detected in the

protected chimpanzees compared with the unprotected ones. In the recombinant adenovirus-gp160 experiment, one chimpanzee with CTLs was protected from low-dose challenge in the absence of neutralizing antibodies, but protection against high-dose challenge occurred only in chimpanzees with high-titer neutralizing antibodies. HIV-1 SF2, however, is not virulent in chimpanzees, and no virus could be isolated from the control-immunized animals' PBMCs longer than 6 weeks after challenge, suggesting low virus burdens, even in control animals.

In the experiments by Girard et al.,[319] the protected chimpanzees were boosted again with gp140 MN/LAI and a V3 MN peptide, then challenged intravenously with a clade E (CRF01_AE) HIV-1. All animals became infected, in agreement with lack of antibody cross-neutralization and absence of V3 loop homology between HIV-1 MN and the E-CR412 strain used for challenge. Similarly, no cross-protection between HIV-1 LAI and HIV-1 DH012 could be observed in chimpanzees, although both are X4 strains and belong to clade B.[552] No neutralizing antibodies to DH012 were detected before challenge.

Female chimpanzees immunized repeatedly with ALVAC-HIV vCP250 by different routes (intramuscular, intranasal, vaginal, and rectal) could be protected from a cervicovaginal homologous challenge with HIV-1 IIIB (LAI) without a subunit booster. The observation was made in both female chimpanzees and in female macaques[553] that infection by the vaginal route with a low dose of virus was followed at times by transient viremia, but the infection never became established and seroconversion was not observed.

HIV-1 vaccines also have been studied in the SHIV/macaque model. Recombinant subunit vaccines were successfully tested for protection against nonpathogenic SHIVs derived from X4 HIV-1 strains. Thus vaccines based on gp120 were found to provide full protection from homologous SHIV challenge but not from a heterologous challenge with an SHIV based on another clade B strain.[554,555] Macaques immunized with HIV-1 SF2 gp120 formulated in ISCOMs were similarly protected from challenge with a SHIV based on a related strain.[556] Protection from infection with a nonpathogenic SHIV also was obtained using multiple homologous HIV-1 *env* DNA immunizations followed by booster immunizations with the envelope protein,[531] or by HIV-1 *env* and SIV *gag-pol* DNAs alone.[533]

There is as yet no report of successful protection of macaques against infection with a pathogenic SHIV following active immunization and challenge. The observation has been repeatedly made that immunized macaques nevertheless can be protected from CD4+ T-cell loss and induction of clinical AIDS following challenge with a pathogenic virus such as SHIV-89.6P.[465] Vaccination did not prevent infection, but the CTL response was associated with a significant decrease in virus load at the virus set point, and even, in some animals, by progressive decline of the set-point viral load to undetectable levels.[469,484] DNA vaccine regimens could be optimized by the addition of an IL-2 adjuvant[529,530] Control of viremia in the vaccinated animals was temporarily abolished upon CD8+ T-cell depletion in vivo, and progressively restored when the CD8 compartment replenished, clearly indicating that the control of the viral set point induced by the DNA–MVA vaccine was CD8 T-cell dependent (H.Robinson, unpublished observations,

Keystone conference, April 2003). Although the levels of viral DNA were not controlled in vaccinated animals, the viral DNA distinguished itself from that in the unvaccinated animals by consisting predominantly of unintegrated species, suggesting that the virus was suppressed or defective.[536a] These data are consistent with the premise that vaccines able to elicit HIV-specific CD8+ CTLs are likely to delay disease progression in HIV-infected persons.

However, contrary to these encouraging results in the SHIV-89.6P model, most rhesus macaques vaccinated with a DNA prime–MVA boost vaccine regimen and challenged with pathogenic SIVmac 239 experienced a gradual CD4 depletion and progressed to disease,[557,557a] thus raising the question of the validity of the results obtained with the SHIV model.[51]

Human Clinical Trials

Since 1987, when the first preventive HIV vaccine candidate entered clinical trials, more than 40 vaccine candidates have been evaluated in safety and immunogenicity trials, and one candidate has progressed to efficacy trials. In total, more than 10,000 HIV-uninfected volunteers have participated in clinical trials of HIV vaccines between 1987 and 2002. Databases of AIDS vaccines in human trials have now been established by the International AIDS Vaccine Initiative (*www.iavi.org*) and the National Institutes of Health (NIH) Vaccine Research Center (*www.vrc.nih.gov*), and provide details and references for the individual trials. Highlights and challenges ahead are summarized below.

HIV-1 Env-Based Subunit Vaccines

Initial clinical trials of candidate HIV vaccines in the late 1980s and early 1990s focused on the goal of stimulating neutralizing antibodies against HIV with recombinant subunits or synthetic peptide fragments of HIV env antigens. This was due in large part to attempts to mimic the successful development of subunit hepatitis B vaccines that utilized this strategy, and the hope that sexually transmitted and intravenously transmitted HIV would respond similarly to hepatitis B, and be preventable by induction of effective humoral immunity. This was also driven by preliminary chimpanzee protection studies demonstrating protection against HIV by vaccines inducing humoral immunity to HIV Env antigens.[315-320]

Initial trials tested envelope glycoproteins gp120 or gp140 derived from clade B TCLA HIV-1 strains IIIB, MN, or SF2 that were presented either in their soluble form or as related synthetic peptides (V3 loop) formulated with various adjuvants or expressed by live recombinant vectors (vaccinia virus, ALVAC) (Table 44-4). These envelope-based recombinant candidate vaccines were well tolerated, and to date there have been no consistently observed clinical or subclinical adverse immunologic or neurologic reactions among the volunteers.[558] Results from these early studies[559-561] have shown that soluble envelope glycoproteins or peptides are able to induce neutralizing antibodies against the homologous TCLA HIV-1 strain but not against primary HIV-1 isolates.[31,330,360,361] Branched V3 peptides (MAP) failed to improve the quality and magnitude of the humoral response induced by recombinant envelope

glycoproteins,[562] while formulation in adjuvants such as QS21 or oil-and-water emulsions containing QS21 + MPL, improved immune responses compared with alum.[554,563]

Initial candidate vaccines derived from the HIV-1 LAI strain were followed by vaccines based on HIV-1 MN and HIV-1 SF-2 strains, which at that time were believed to be more representative of virus circulating in the general population of the industrialized world. Emphasis was put on the use of mammalian cells for the production of recombinant envelope glycoproteins, to mimic natural glycosylation of the proteins, and for evaluation of new adjuvants, with the goal of improving immune responses both qualitatively and quantitatively. A recombinant envelope subunit vaccine, based on HIV-1 MN (MN gp120), induced antibodies that neutralized the homologous MN strain as well as other clade B TCLA virus strains (HIV-1 SF2 and LAI).[564] Maximum antibody levels were reached after three injections.

An SF2 gp120 candidate vaccine, combined with a novel adjuvant, MF59,[494] and administered with or without the immunomodulator muramyl tripeptide and dipalmitoyl phosphatidylethanolamine, induced gp120-binding antibodies that persisted for at least 24 weeks after the fourth injection. After three injections, all volunteers had developed neutralizing antibodies against the homologous HIV-1 SF2 strain, which in two thirds of them also cross-neutralized HIV-1 MN. A fully glycosylated HIV-1 LAI gp160 candidate vaccine, combined with alum and deoxycholate adjuvant, also resulted in a dose-related induction of neutralizing antibodies against the homologous HIV-1 LAI strain, although with lower titers than those observed with gp120.[565]

Finally, vaccination with a chimeric MN/LAI gp140 molecule, consisting of HIV-1 MN gp120 and truncated LAI gp41, and boosting with a linear V3-MN synthetic peptide, resulted in high levels of neutralizing antibodies against the homologous MN strain. In about half of the volunteers, these antibodies also neutralized HIV-1 SF2 but not HIV-1 LAI. Similarly, a gp120 envelope protein subunit derived from primary clade B isolate w61d induced type-specific neutralizing antibodies.[554]

Thus a number of mammalian-derived subunit recombinant envelope candidate vaccines and synthetic peptide vaccines have been shown to be well tolerated and to induce neutralizing antibodies against the homologous TCLA strains and occasionally against a few other strains from the B clade. However, these neutralizing antibodies were only active against TCLA-adapted strains and not against primary clinical HIV-1 isolates, and did not demonstrate breadth against globally diverse isolates. This spurred significant debate within the AIDS vaccine field in the early-mid 1990s as to whether the gp120 candidate should be evaluated in large-scale efficacy trials. These debates were further fueled by data from subjects who became HIV infected following immunization. Among the 2029 uninfected people enrolled by the AIDS Vaccine Evaluation Group (United States) in Phase I and II trials of candidate gp120 or gp160 AIDS vaccines between 1988 and 1996, 23 subjects were diagnosed with intercurrent HIV-1 infection. Thirteen had received a complete immunization schedule (three or more injections), six were partially immunized (two or fewer injections), and four were placebo recipients. They were enrolled in nine different protocols, including

TABLE 44–4 ■ HIV-1 Vaccine Candidates Tested in HIV-Uninfected Volunteers

Developer	Antigen	Adjuvant/Vehicle	Production Method
SUBUNITS			
MicroGeneSys	gp160 LAI	Alum	Baculovirus-insect cells
Immuno-AG	gp160 LAI	Alum + deoxycholate	Vaccinia/Vero cells
	gp160 MN	Alum + deoxycholate	Vaccinia/Vero cells
Aventis-Pasteur	gp140 MN/LAI	IFA or alum	Vaccinia/BHK21 cells
	gp140 TH023/LAI-DID (E)	Alum	Vaccinia/BHK21 cells
Chiron	Env-2-3 SF2	MF59+ MTPPE	CHO cells
	gp120 SF2	MF59 +/–MTPPE	CHO cells
	gp120 SF2	Comparison of adjuvants: alum, MF59, MF59 + MTPPE, SAF/2, SAF/2 + MDP, MPL, liposome MPL,	CHO cells
	p24	MF59	Yeast
	gp120 CM235 (E) + SF2(B)	MF59	CHO cells
Genentech/VaxGen	gp120 LAI	Alum	CHO cells
	gp120 MN	Alum	CHO cells
	gp120 MN	QS21	CHO cells
VaxGen	gp120 MN + GNE8 (B)	Alum	CHO cells
	gp120 MN + A244 (B/E)	Alum	CHO cells
GlaxoSmith Kline	gp120 w61D (B)	3D MPL + QS21 o/w emulsion	CHO cells
	gp120 w61D (B) + nef-tat	3D MPL + QS21 o/w emulsion	CHO cells
British Biotech	Ty p17/p24-LAI-VLP	None vs. alum	Yeast transposon
Italy/B. Ensoli	Tat-LAI	None	*Escherichia coli*
PEPTIDES			
United Biomedical	V3-octomeric MN	Alum	Chemical synthesis
	Gag-lipopeptide	Lipid conjugate	Chemical synthesis + lipid conjugation
	V3-ocotmeric MN	PLG microparticles	Chemical synthesis + PLG formulation
	V3-octomeric 15 strains	Alum	Chemical synthesis
Swiss Serum & Vaccine	V3-MN	PPD	Chemical synthesis
Wyeth	C4-V3-4 strains	IFA	Chemical synthesis
Cel-Sci	HGP-30–LAI	KLH	Chemical synthesis
Aventis Pasteur/ANRS	LIPO-5 or LIPO-6T Gag-pol-nef-lipopeptides (B)	Lipid conjugate ± tetanus toxoid	Chemical synthesis + lipid conjugation
ANRS	Gag-pol-nef-envlipopeptides (B)	Lipid conjugate ± QS21	
Aventis Pasteur/ANRS	V3 peptide MN	+ Alum??	Chemical synthesis
Aventis Pasteur/ANRS	CLTB-36; V3-p24 peptide	+ Alum or QS21	Chemical synthesis
CIGB-Cuba	V3 multiB peptides (6)		Chemical synthesis
RECOMBINANT VECTORS			
Bristol Myers Squibb	Env-LAI	NA	Recombinant vaccinia
Therion	Env-pol-gag-LAI	NA	Recombinant vaccinia
St. Jude's Hospital	Env-multiclade	NA	Recombinant vaccinia
Aventis Pasteur	Env-MN ALVAC-HIV (v-CP-125)	NA	ALVAC-canarypox
	Env-gag-pr-MN/LAI ALVAC-HIV (vCP-205)	NA	ALVAC-canarypox
	Env-gag-pr-epitopes in pol, nef ALVAC-HIV (vCP300)	NA	ALVAC-canarypox
	Env-gag-pr-epitopes in pol, nef ALVAC-HIV (vCP1433)	NA	ALVAC-canarypox
	Env-gag-pr-epitopes in nef-pol and vaccinia-derived genes E3L and K3L ALVAC HIV (vCP1452)	NA	ALVAC-canarypox
	Env-E-gag-pr (B/LAI) ALVAC-HIV (Vcp1521)	NA	ALVAC-canarypox
IAVI-MRC-UK-U. Nairobi-IDT	Gag + minigenes (A)	NA	Recombinant MVA
Merck	Gag (B)	NA	Replication-defective adenovirus type5
U. Maryland	gp120 LAI	NA	*Salmonella typhi*

Continued

TABLE 44–4 ■ HIV-1 Vaccine Candidates Tested in HIV-Uninfected Volunteers—cont'd

Developer	Antigen	Adjuvant/Vehicle	Production Method
DNA VACCINES			
Apollon/Wyeth	Env-rev (B)	Bupivacaine	Gene Vax plasmid
	Gag-pol (B)	Bupivacaine	Gene Vax plasmid
IAVI-MRC-UK-U. Nairobi-Cobra	Gag + minigenes (A)	None	pTHr plasmid
Merck	Gag (B)	None, alum, CRL1005 polaxamer	Plasmid
NIH Vaccine Research Center	Gag-pol-nef fusion (B)	Needle-less Biojector delivery	Plasmid
FIT (Finlands)	Nef (B)	None	Plasmid
Emory/GeoVex	Multigenes (B)	Gene-gun	Plasmid

MN rgp120 with alum or QS21, SF2 rgp120 in MF59 or MPL, LAI rgp160 and MN rgp160 with alum and deoxycholate, and recombinant vaccinia virus expressing LAI gp160. The incidence of HIV-1 infections in vaccine recipients was 0.38 per 100 person-years compared with 0.30 in placebo recipients. Virus load measured between 8 and 14 months after infection was lower in vaccine recipients than in nonvaccinated matched control subjects (7482 versus 16,696 RNA copies/mL, respectively), but this difference was not statistically significant. Syncytia-inducing viruses (X4) were isolated from two subjects who showed a rapid decline in CD4$^+$ lymphocyte counts, whereas the other 17 isolates obtained from the group were non–syncytia inducing (R5). The V3 loop amino acid sequence of the transmitted viruses was similar between vaccinees and control subjects. At 1 year after infection, CD4$^+$ lymphocyte counts were not significantly different between vaccine recipients and nonvaccinated matched control subjects (521 ± 249 versus 494 ± 236, respectively). The antibody responses before HIV infection in vaccinees were similar to those from the matched subjects who remained uninfected. In summary, there was no indication that the vaccine-induced immune response had any effect on the genotypic or phenotypic characteristics of the transmitted virus or on the early clinical course of HIV-1 infection.[566]

Two of the candidate vaccines discussed above (MN and SF2 gp120) were evaluated in a Phase II trial in the United States among 300 healthy volunteers, some of whom were at high risk of infection.[567] Finally, in 1998, a Phase III efficacy trial was launched in the United States, Canada, and the Netherlands by VaxGen, involving more than 5000 volunteers at high risk for sexually transmitted HIV infection. A similar study of more than 2500 IDU volunteers began in Thailand in mid-1999. The products being tested are HIV-1 gp120 from the MN clade B strain and from a clade B primary isolate (GNE8) for the U.S.-based trial, and gp120MN clade B supplemented by gp120 from a primary isolate of clade E (A244) for the Thai trial. The U.S. trials included mostly men who have sex with men and a few at-risk women, all whom were HIV negative when they joined the trial. During the 36-month double-blind, randomized trial, a total of seven injections of 300 µg gp120 were administered on a 6 month schedule over 30 months. The ratio of vaccine to placebo recipients was 2:1. The preliminary results of the study, announced in February 2003, indicated that the vaccine did not show a statistically significant reduction of HIV infection within the study population as a whole (protection of 3.8% with confidence intervals between −23% and 25%). Retrospectively, there was some indication of protection among African American and Asian volunteers who received the vaccine, amounting to a 67% efficacy level. Importantly, protection in the non-white subgroup appeared to correlate with a higher level of antibody to gp 120. However, this was based only on a small number of cases. Further trials obviously are necessary before firm conclusions are drawn.

Concurrently, a growing literature has suggested a significant role for cellular immunity and the need for multiple HIV genes in protection against AIDS, which has led to the view that complementary humoral and cellular immune responses might be elicited by using a prime-boost immunization regimen,[568] and that additional HIV gene fragments ought to be incorporated into the vaccine to elicit more comprehensive immune responses.[569,570] Strategies to stimulate cellular immunity are described below.

Nucleic Acid and Viral Vector Vaccines

As described earlier (see *Live, Attenuated Vaccines* above), studies in nonhuman primates suggested that live, attenuated (SIV) vaccines provided a significant level of protection against SIV infection in rhesus macaques.[26–29,433,446–448] This, coupled with natural history studies suggesting a role for CD8$^+$ T-cell responses in controlling HIV infection, led to the development of several strategies to try to mimic the efficacy of live, attenuated vaccines while concomitantly providing a greater level of safety. Among these strategies, several viral vectors and more recently nucleic acid vaccines containing multiple HIV genes were developed for evaluation in clinical trials.

The first viral vector vaccines were based on recombinant vaccinia,[571,572] and demonstrated that CD8$^+$ cytotoxic T cells could be stimulated in classical ^{51}Cr release assays. However, serious adverse effects have been reported in people given vaccinia virus for smallpox prevention, particularly in those with eczema or immunodeficiency.[573] Vaccinia virus caused severe local reaction and dissemination in an asymptomatic HIV-1–infected person.[574] In subjects immunized with a recombinant vaccinia virus expressing HIV-1 gp160 IIIB (HIVAC-1e), generalized malaise as well as local pain and tenderness developed 9 to 12 days after vaccination. Lymphadenitis was observed in 50% of the vaccinated subjects, and the median time for complete healing of the vaccinia lesion was 25 days.[452]

As a result, avian poxviruses such as canarypox[457] and attenuated poxviruses, such as MVA,[456] have been developed with the goal of providing greater safety. In addition, replication-defective recombinant adenoviruses have entered into clinical trials, after demonstrating induction of cellular immune responses in rhesus macaques and mitigation of disease progression when challenged with pathogenic SHIV.[469]

The use of a live canarypox vector (ALVAC) offers significant potential advantages over conventional vaccinia virus vectors with respect to safety.[575] Recombinant canarypox vaccines administered intramuscularly have been well tolerated in adult volunteers, including HIV-1–infected asymptomatic patients.[576] Results from several Phase I and II trials with recombinant canarypox vectors have demonstrated induction of CD8+ CTLs, but only in 15% to 30% of subjects at any given time point postimmunization.[577–581] Interestingly, however, the CTL responses generated by recombinant canarypox vectors were cross-clade,[412,582] and CTLs also have been demonstrated in rectal mucosa from vaccinated subjects (J. McElrath, unpublished observations, NIH-AIDS Vaccine Conference, September 2001), suggesting that subjects vaccinated parenterally may attain some level of anti-HIV immunity when exposed to HIV at mucosal surfaces via sexual transmission. This concept was tested in nonhuman primate studies, where recombinant canarypox vectors were shown to be capable of providing protection in neonatal monkeys exposed to mucosal challenge (M. Marthas, unpublished observations, Retrovirus Conference, February 2002).

MVA, a highly attenuated host range–restricted strain of vaccinia virus, has entered clinical trials under the form of a recombinant MVA expressing fragments of the HIV-1 Gag p24 (CA) and p17 (MA) antigens, and CTL epitopes from several HIV-1 antigens, based on HIV-1 subtype A prevalent in Eastern Africa.[582a] This clinical trial represents the first HIV vector vaccine trial with a product targeted to a strain of HIV that primarily circulates in Africa. Preliminary data (A. McMichael, unpublished observations, Keystone Conference, April 2002) utilizing IFN-γ ELISPOT assays, intracellular IFN-γ fluorescence-activated cell sorter assays, and tetramer staining of MHC-peptide complexes demonstrated the induction of HIV-specific CD8+ T cells in a subset of immunized subjects. Similar T-cell responses also were induced by recombinant defective adenovirus, expressing HIV-1 Gag subtype B (E. Emini, unpublished observations, Keystone Conference, April 2002).

DNA vaccines also have been evaluated in preliminary Phase I trials, with the general observation that naked DNA only stimulated transient cellular immune responses, even when doses as high as 5 mg of DNA were administered, suggesting that adjuvant formulations may be necessary for potentiating immunologic responses elicited by DNA vaccines.[583] Similarly, subunit vaccines in adjuvants designed to shift the immune responses to Th1 cellular immunity, and lipopeptides designed to stimulate cellular immune responses, are being evaluated in preliminary Phase I trials. Preliminary results from lipopeptide trials suggest that this vaccine strategy is also capable of eliciting CD8+ T-cell responses.[520,584]

In summary, several new viral vector, nucleic acid, and lipopeptide candidate HIV vaccines are currently being evaluated in Phase I clinical trials. The potential to combine these approaches with strategies to stimulate humoral immunity has led many groups to explore the prime-boost concept, that is, priming with one vaccine strategy and boosting with a different vaccine strategy, with the aim of stimulating a more comprehensive and long-lived immunity against HIV.

The Prime-Boost Concept

Preclinical studies in nonhuman primates have shown that priming with a viral vector or nucleic acid vaccine, followed by boosting with either another vector or subunit/peptide vaccine, provided advantages over immunization with single modalities. However, for this strategy to be commercially feasible, there would need to be significantly greater efficacy over single-modality vaccines to warrant the increased costs and complexities associated with developing two vaccines. The first HIV-1 vaccine prime-boost regimen tested in humans, which included priming with recombinant vaccinia virus expressing gp160 followed by boosting with paraformaldehyde-fixed recombinant vaccinia virus–infected PBMCs and soluble gp160,[451,571] was shown to induce both neutralizing antibodies to the homologous HIV-1 IIIB (LAI) strain and HIV-1–specific CTLs. A simplified regimen using only recombinant vaccinia virus and soluble gp160 or peptides (V3, p18, envT1) induced a transient neutralizing response after each booster, a long-lasting memory T-cell response (2-year follow-up), and memory CD8+, HLA class I–restricted Env-specific CTLs.[572] In a more systematic manner, vaccinia-naive volunteers first immunized with HIVAC-1e were subsequently boosted with baculovirus-derived gp160 IIIB in alum.[585] Neutralizing and fusion inhibition activities against the homologous strain as well as CD4-blocking antibodies were detected in about 50% of the subjects. Cross-reactive neutralization activity against HIV-1 MN was also detected. Seventy-five percent of the vaccinees demonstrated T-cell proliferative responses in vitro that were 3- to 10-fold higher than those induced by either vaccine alone and sustained for more than 18 months. Moreover, both CD8+ and CD4+ CTLs were detected.[586,587] Some vaccine-induced CD8+ CTL clones produced a soluble factor that inhibited HIV-1 replication in acutely infected autologous CD4+ blasts.[81,83,587,588] In a subsequent study, a longer interval between priming and boosting and two HIVAC-1e inoculations were associated with significantly higher neutralizing and fusion-inhibition antibody titers after boosting.[589]

A prime-boost regimen including priming with canarypox ALVAC–HIV vCP125, which expresses HIV-1 MN gp160, followed by two booster immunizations with recombinant hybrid gp140 MN/LAI in alum or IFA was well tolerated.[590] Antibodies to gp160 and to V3 were not detected after the two vCP125 injections but developed after the first booster immunization with gp140. After the second booster dose of gp140, neutralizing antibodies against HIV-1 MN were induced in 90% of the volunteers and against HIV-1 SF2 in 50% of them. Lymphoproliferation to gp140 was detected in only 25% of the subjects after the injections of vCP125 but in 100% after the first gp140 booster. An envelope-specific CTL activity also was observed cumulatively in 39% of the volunteers. This activity was mediated by MHC class I–restricted CD8+ T cells and was still present 2 years after the initial immunization in some subjects.[591] In contrast, three immunizations with gp140 MN/LAI alone elicited low-level neutralizing responses and lymphoproliferation to gp140 in 92% of the subjects but no CTL activity. Priming with gp140 MN/LAI followed by boosting with a synthetic V3 MN peptide induced high neutralizing antibody titers but no CTLs,[592] again emphasizing the essential role of priming with a live recombinant vector for the induction of a CTL response.

The prime-boost regimen next was tested in vaccinia-naive and vaccinia-immune volunteers using ALVAC–HIV-1 vCP125 at either 10^6 or 10^7 median tissue culture infective doses, followed by boosting with a Chinese hamster ovary–derived gp120 SF2 in MF59 adjuvant. High-titer neutralizing antibodies were elicited against both HIV-1 MN and HIV-1 SF2 in 100% of the volunteers. ADCC against both MN and SF2 also was detected in 70% of the subjects. Although the dose of ALVAC-HIV used for priming did not significantly influence the final neutralizing antibody titers, the higher dose of ALVAC apparently resulted in better priming of the cellular response, because Env-specific CD8+ CTLs were detected cumulatively in 40% of the subjects. In contrast with the prime-boost regimen involving HIVAC-1e and gp120, the prior vaccinia-immune status of the volunteers did not appear to impair the ability of the volunteers to respond to ALVAC-HIV and gp120.[593,594] Priming with a higher dose of ALVAC–HIV vCP205 and priming with ALVAC–HIV vCP300 and vCP1452 that express env and gag together with pol and nef CTL domains, followed by booster immunizations with gp120 SF2 in MF59, are being evaluated in HIV-uninfected adults according to various immunization schedules.

These studies demonstrate that clade B–based canarypox vaccines utilized as a prime can elicit, at least in some volunteers, a broad CTL reactivity capable of recognizing

TABLE 44–5 ■ Prime-Boost Candidates Tested in HIV-Uninfected Volunteers

Prime	Boost
Viral Vector Prime	
Vaccinia-gp160 LAI	gp160; gp120, V3
ALVAC-gp160 MN (vCP125)	gp140; gp120
ALVAC-env-gag-pr (vCP205)	CLTB-36, gp120; gp160, p24, lipopeptides, DNA
ALVAC-env-gag-pr-nef/pol epitopes (vCP300)	gp120, lipopeptides
ALVAC-env-gag-pr-nef-pol (vCP1433)	gp 160
ALVAC-env-gag-pr-nef-pol E3L/K3L (vCP1452)	gp 160, gp120, lipopeptides
ALVAC-env-gag-pr (E/B) (vCP1521)	gp120, gp160
Bacterial Vector Prime	
Salmonella typhi–gp120	gp120
DNA Vaccine Prime	
DNA gag-pol	vCP205; vCP1452
DNA env-rev	vCP205
DNA gag + minigenes (A)	MVA gag + minigenes (A)
DNA gag (B): naked, alum or CRL1005	Replication defective adeno–gag (B)
Subunit Prime	
gp140 MN/LAI	V3

viruses belonging to genetically diverse HIV-1 clades,[412,582] and reinforce the importance of including viral core antigens in the vaccine. The prime-boost concept, based on ALVAC vCP1521, the equivalent of ALVAC vCP 205, which expresses the gp120 gene from HIV-1 subtype E circulating in Thailand, along with the gag-pro genes from HIV-1 subtype B, combined with gp120 as a booster, was approved by the government of Thailand to begin Phase III efficacy trials in 16,000 volunteers to begin in late 2003, with data expected from these trials by 2008 to 2009. This trial will be undertaken as a collaboration between the governments of Thailand and the United States (WRAIR and the NIH), along with Aventis Pasteur (providing ALVAC) and VaxGen (providing gp120).

Preliminary studies also have been initiated with other prime-boost regimens to evaluate DNA priming followed by viral vector boosts, using either ALVAC, MVA,[595] or replication-defective adenovirus as the boosting immunogen. In addition, ALVAC prime followed by lipopeptide boosts has been evaluated in ongoing preliminary Phase I trials. Table 44–5 summarizes the prime-boost strategies that have been evaluated to date.

Postexposure Immunization

Because the progression of HIV disease appears to depend on the balance between viral replication and host immunity, either enhancement of host immunity or inhibition of viral replication could lead to long-term control of HIV disease. Studies of several candidate vaccines (envelope subunits, gp120-deleted inactivated HIV-1 preparations, and ALVAC-HIV expressing gp160 MN) have shown short-term safety but poor or limited immunogenicity in HIV-infected individuals, and no conclusive clinical benefit.[559,576,596,597] A beneficial effect of HIV vaccines on the immunologic and virologic markers of HIV disease progression in seropositive patients has not been observed consistently for the majority of patients under study and remains controversial. However, these immune-based strategies have been tested in the absence of or in association with suboptimal combinations of antiviral therapy. Thus it would be useful to evaluate the therapeutic potential of some of these candidates in the context of antiviral therapy, or in the context of structured treatment interruptions.

With regard to immune restoration in HIV-treated patients, the different immune-based strategies may have as objectives (1) the maintenance or potentiation of existing HIV-specific immune responses, (2) the restoration or potentiation of nonspecific immune responses, (3) the induction of de novo HIV-specific immune responses, or (4) the restoration of pre-existing HIV-specific immunity lost during HIV disease. Active anti-HIV immunization, especially designed to induce cell-mediated immune responses, might be seen as a complement of antiviral therapy and cytokine immunomodulation,[598,599] and deserves further clinical research. However, enthusiasm for such strategies needs to be tempered with the realization that, to date, clinical trials of candidate HIV vaccines used therapeutically have not demonstrated significant clinical benefit except, partially, when combined with highly active antiretroviral therapy.

Passive Immunotherapy

By analogy with the success of prophylactic and therapeutic regimens using passive immunization with specific hyperimmune globulin products derived from human plasma against blood-borne viral pathogens such as hepatitis B virus, the development of hyperimmune anti-HIV immune globulin preparations might be useful in prevention of HIV infection in laboratory workers and in newborns of HIV-infected mothers. Studies of possible correlations between levels and specificity of maternal HIV antibody and vertical transmission have shown conflicting results. It is currently unclear whether increased levels of maternal anti-HIV antibodies achieved either by passive administration of anti-HIV immune globulins or by active vaccination could interrupt vertical transmission. In addition, it is unknown whether maternally derived anti-HIV antibodies can have beneficial therapeutic properties (by reducing viral replication and delaying disease progression) for infants who become infected.[600] Studies have indicated a lower transmission rate from infected pregnant women with high-affinity/avidity antibody to conserved portions of HIV-1 gp41,[601] to the CD4 binding site,[602] or to the V3 loop of gp120.[603] Nontransmitting mothers frequently have neutralizing antibodies to their own virus; in contrast, transmitting mothers rarely have neutralizing antibody against their child's isolate. It has furthermore been reported that some mothers with autologous neutralizing antibody have antibodies that can neutralize some heterologous primary isolates.[604]

These data have prompted the search for human neutralizing MAbs. However, few of them have been found that are able to neutralize HIV-1 primary isolates in vitro. Those that do, such as MAbs 2F5,[341,342] b12,[335–338] 2G12,[339,340] and 4E10,[343] would certainly deserve further clinical studies.[376] As in the hepatitis B model, passive immunotherapy could conceivably be coupled with active immunization, as was suggested by the protection of newborns against SIV infection through vaccination of the mothers during pregnancy followed by passive immunization of the offspring at birth.[605] Hyperimmune anti–HIV-1 immune globulins in combination with MAbs 2F5 and 2G12 have shown additive or synergistic neutralization of primary HIV-1 isolates.[346,347,606] In addition, several of these monoclonals alone or in combination have protected rhesus macaques against challenge with pathogenic SHIV.[348,551,607] Using polyclonal IgG from HIV-infected chimpanzees for passive protection of pigtail macaques against a high-dose intravenous challenge with homologous SHIV-DH12, one could calculate that a fully protective dose corresponded to 150 mg IgG per kg body weight, i.e. an antibody titer of about 1:40 (M. Martin, personal communication, Cent Gardes Symposium, October 2002). IgG given 6 hours after challenge still blocked infection but their effect was limited by 24 hours. Polymeric 2F5, and 2G12 antibody of an IgI or IgM isotype seems to be several-fold more potent than the corresponding IgGs.[607a]

Improved Vaccine Concepts and Future Challenges

Several new candidate vaccines will be entering initial Phase I trials in the next 1 to 2 years, including novel vectors such as AAV, alphaviruses (Venezuelan equine encephalitis, Semliki Forest and Sindbis and VSV); multigenic vaccines incorporating structural and regulatory/accessory genes of HIV-1; novel formulations and adjuvants for immunopotentiation, including cytokines, microparticles, and co-stimulatory molecules; and bacterial delivery systems for oral immunization aimed at eliciting both systemic and mucosal immunity. In addition, many of these new candidates are based on genetic subtypes of HIV circulating in the developing world, where the epidemic is most severe, and offer the opportunity to test whether genetic variation of circulating viruses has a negative impact on the efficacy of candidate HIV vaccines.[608]

The challenges associated with eliciting broadly reactive cell-mediated immunity have been heightened by reports of escape from T-cell–mediated immune responses[13–18,557] and preliminary reports of superinfection.[609] These issues have led to increased focus on designing multigenic immunogens, along with candidates containing antigens across several genetic subtypes of HIV-1 or targeting conserved regions of HIV genes.

Antivector immunity is a potential challenge to the development of several viral vectors, as are manufacturing and regulatory issues associated with the development of such vectors. For example, anti-Ad5 neutralizing antibody prevalent in the population may limit the utility of this vector system, yet other strains of adenovirus not common to the population may overcome this issue, as may priming with DNA followed by boosting with adenovirus. Similarly, development of MVA vectors may need to be reassessed, particularly if immunization with smallpox vaccines as a biodefense measure becomes routine in the near future. In contrast, some vectors, such as alphavirus vectors, are not constrained by antivector immunity but face other challenges associated with large-scale development, such as the lack of packaging cell lines to facilitate large-scale manufacturing.

Another important question is that of protection at mucosal sites of entry. The most important mode of transmission of HIV is, by far, through sexual intercourse.[3,285–287] The facts that the overwhelming majority of new HIV infections worldwide are heterosexual and that women appear to have a greater risk of acquiring the infection through heterosexual transmission than do men suggest that vaccine-induced protection should be focused on sexual transmission and the potential need for mucosal immunity. A vaccine-induced barrier of mucosal immunity might play an important role in tipping the balance in favor of the host and preventing the establishment of HIV infection.[610] Although the role of secretory immunity to HIV is unclear,[611] induction of an immune response at the surface of the genital mucosa may be of added benefit in reducing HIV transmission.[121]

The observation that mucosal plasma cells can migrate to distant mucosal sites has generated the concept of a common mucosal immune system,[611] enabling the generation of an immune response at a mucosal surface distant from the mucosal site of antigen administration. It has been shown, for example, that not all the migrating lymphocytes that have been stimulated in Peyer's patches necessarily return to the intestinal mucosa. Certainly, the majority of these cells do recirculate to the intestine, but many also are found to colonize other mucosal surfaces, such as those of the respiratory and genital tracts. To stimulate optimal mucosal immunity, vaccines may need to be administered by a mucosal route, although observations have shown that protective mucosal immunity can be induced by other immunization routes,[612–613a] independent of immunization at mucosal surfaces. Thus, SIV-specific CD8[+] T-cells induced in response to immunization with a NYVAC recombinant were found in the mucosal tissues of all immunized animals regardless of whether the vaccine was administered by the intranasal or intrarectal route or systematically.[615a] Similarly, systemic immunization with plasmid DNA followed by MVA or defective adenovirus recombinants elicited high-frequency CTL responses in duodenal and distant colonic mucosal tissues.[613] Further studies comparing different vaccine strategies administered by different routes are needed to address this issue.[614]

Eliciting long-term protective immunity is the goal for any HIV vaccine, and perhaps the best eventual outcome for an HIV vaccine would be to mimic the protection observed with some live, attenuated SIV vaccines that provide long-term and durable immunity.[26–29,431–433] Recombinant AAV most closely mimics the persistence of immunity elicited by live, attenuated vaccines, because a single immunization with recombinant AAV elicits long-term cellular and humoral immunity (P. Johnson, unpublished observations, IAVI Meeting, September 2002), yet AAV also faces large-scale development challenges common to other viral vector systems.

Finally, it remains unclear which HIV antigens are required for protection against HIV, and which immune responses must be elicited to confer protective immunity. The need to develop vaccines including nonstructural HIV proteins Tat,[110,512–514] Rev,[615,616] and/or Nef[453] in addition to structural proteins Env and Gag-Pol, remains an open question. Although both the neutralizing antibody and the CTL arms of the immune response seem to be involved, other potential correlates are being investigated, such as secretion of chemokines,[7,8,120,617] cytokines,[400,618] and the HIV-1 viral suppressive factor.[5,6,81,83] Protection against AIDS also may include additional mechanisms associated with innate immunity.[619]

With respect to neutralizing antibodies,[582] the accessibility of gp120 to antibodies and its importance in early infection events have made it a key target for vaccine design. However, the question of how to induce antibodies able to neutralize primary HIV-1 isolates still remains unsolved. Neutralization epitopes in gp120 are not immunodominant, except in the TCLA HIV-1 strains that have been passaged multiple times through T-cell lines. These strains are extremely sensitive to neutralization in vitro by sera from seropositive individuals and gp120 vaccinees, in contrast with primary HIV-1 isolates. Antibodies that neutralize primary isolates have been mapped to a few distinct conformational epitopes, defined by MAbs b12, 2G12, 4E10, and 2F5, but induction of this type of antibodies by candidate vaccines has been unsuccessful to date[620] (see review in *Neutralizing Antibodies* and *Subunit Vaccines* sections above).

The use of complex vaccine preparations including Env and Gag proteins may render more difficult the differentiation between vaccinees and HIV-infected individuals, especially in countries where a high frequency of indeterminate Western blots is found. To address this problem, the HIV-1 envelope expressed by ALVAC–HIV vCP205 was deleted from the immunodominant region in the ectodomain of gp41, to which most HIV-1–infected subjects react. Sera of vCP205 vaccinees were negative in Western blots for the gp41 band and tested negative in a peptide–enzyme-linked immunosorbent assay based on the immunodominant region of gp41. However, because the ectodomain of gp41 is involved in folding and oligomerization of the gp120/gp41 complex, such a deletion might render the construct unable to induce conformation-dependent neutralizing antibodies, and deletion of this domain may delete other potentially important cellular immunity–focused epitopes.

The design of HIV-1 efficacy trials will have to address several critical scientific, ethical, and feasibility issues,[621] including but not limited to standards-of-care issues associated with treatment of HIV-infected subjects over the course of the trials, trials for adolescents, and licensing issues associated with selection of endpoints. Many of the biggest challenges in developing an AIDS vaccine still lie ahead, and there are many scientific unknowns.[551] To quote R. Zingernagel,[622] HIV is representative of little-cytopathic infectious agents whose disease-causing process involves immunopathology and that are never eliminated from the host, even under optimal conditions of long-term resistance and lasting immunity. Therefore, a vaccine against HIV combines the challenges that we have frustratingly experienced during the past 120 years for tuberculosis and leprosy. The aim at this time is a vaccine that shifts the overall immunopathologic disease kinetics toward later times by 10, 30, or 60 years. The different possible endpoints of an efficacy trial therefore will include protection against HIV-1 infection, protection against progression to disease, and reduction of the HIV transmission rate to others and to offspring by decreasing the viral load in the host. The mode of transmission (homosexual, intravenous, heterosexual) in the population in which the vaccine will be tested, the availability of efficacious viral drugs (especially in developed countries), and the modification of behavior of vaccinees during the study could substantially influence the interpretation of the vaccine efficacy results. These points will have to be addressed in due time, in the planning of the next set of efficacy trials.

There is no doubt that an effective AIDS vaccine would be a major tool in the global fight against HIV and AIDS. Unless we find a means to reverse the present trend, the AIDS pandemic will irreparably damage many societies.[3,623] With nearly 14,000 new HIV infections every day, along with nearly 8000 deaths attributable to AIDS every day, speed, collaboration, and multinational cooperation are essential. Collectively, these challenges suggest that a pragmatic approach, aimed at accelerating promising candidates through efficacy trials, developing better next-generation candidates, and addressing up-front vaccine licensure and deployment issues, represents the most effective strategy to shorten the time lines to eventual approval and delivery of safe and effective HIV vaccines.

Acknowledgments

The efficient and helpful assistance of Martine Bearth with the manuscript preparation is gratefully acknowledged.

REFERENCES

1. Gottlieb MS, Schroff R, Schanker HM, et al. *Pneumocystis carinii* pneumonia and mucosal candidiasis in previously healthy homosexual men. N Engl J Med 305:1425–1431, 1981.
2. Masur H, Michelis MA, Greene JB, et al. An outbreak of community acquired *Pneumocystis carinii* pneumonia: initial manifestation of cellular immune dysfunction. N Engl J Med 305:1431–1438, 1981.
3. Piot P. The science of AIDS: a tale of two worlds. Science 280:1844–1845, 1998.
4. Phaolcharoen W. HIV/AIDS prevention in Thailand: success and challenges. Science 280:1873–1874, 1998.
4a. Peterlin BM, Trono D. Hide. Shield and strike back: how HIV-infected-cells amid immune eradication. Nat Rev Immunol 3:97–67, 2003.
5. Walker CM, Moody DJ, Stites DP, Levy JA. CD8+ lymphocytes can control HIV infection in vitro by suppressing virus replication. Science 234:1563–1566, 1986.
6. Mackewicz C, Barker E, Levy JA. Role of beta-chemokines in suppressing HIV replication. Science 274:1393–1394, 1996.
7. Cocchi F, De Vico AL, Garzino Demo A, et al. Identification of RANTES, MIP-1 alpha and MIP-1 beta as the major HIV suppressive factors produced by CD8+ T cells. Science 270:1811–1815, 1995.
8. D'Souza MP, Harden VA. Chemokines and HIV-1 second receptors. Nat Med 2:1293–1300, 1996.
9. Forthal DN, Landucci G, Daar ES. Antibody from patients with acute human immunodeficiency virus (HIV) infection inhibits primary strains of HIV type 1 in the presence of natural-killer effector cells. J Virol 75:6952–6961, 2001.
10. Ho DD, Neumann AU, Perelson AS, et al. Rapid turnover of plasma virions and CD4 lymphocytes in HIV-1 infection. Nature 373:123–126, 1995.
11. Wei X, Gosh S, Taylor ME, et al. Viral dynamics in human immunodeficiency virus type 1 infection. Nature 373:117–122, 1995.
12. Pantaleo G, Soudeyns H, Demarest JF, et al. Evidence for rapid disappearance of initially expanded HIV-specific CD8+ T cell clones during primary HIV infection. Proc Natl Acad Sci U S A 94:9848–9853, 1997.
13. Borrow P, Lewicki H, Wei X, et al. Antiviral pressure-exerted by HIV-1 specific cytotoxic T lymphocytes (CTL) during primary infection demonstrated by rapid selection of CTL escape virus. Nat Med 3:205–211, 1997.
14. McMichael AJ, Phillips RE. Escape of human immunodeficiency virus from immune control. Annu Rev Immunol 15:271–296, 1997.
15. Evans DT, O'Connor DH, Jing P, et al. Virus specific cytotoxic T-lymphocyte responses select for amino-acid variation in simian immunodeficiency virus Env and Nef. Nat Med 5:1270–1276, 1999.
16. Allen TM, O'Connor DH, Jing P, et al. Tat-specific cytotoxic T lymphocytes select for SIV escape variants during resolution of primary viraemia. Nature 407:386–390, 2000.
17. Barouch DH, Kuntsman J, Kuroda MJ, et al. Eventual AIDS vaccine failure in a rhesus monkey by viral escape from cytotoxic T lymphocytes. Nature 415:335–339, 2002.
18. O'Connor DH, Allen TM, Vogel TV, et al. Acute phase cytotoxic T lymphocyte escape is a hallmark of simian immunodeficiency virus infection. Nat Med 8:493–499, 2002.
18a. Johnson WE, Desrosiers RC. Viral persistence: HIV's strategies of immune system evasion. Annu Rev Med 58:499–518, 2002.
19. Schwartz O, Maréchal V, Le Gall S, et al. Endocytosis of major histocompatibility complex class I molecules is induced by the HIV-1 Nef protein. Nat Med 2:338–342, 1996.
20. Collins KL, Chen BK, Kalams SA, et al. HIV-1 Nef protein protects infected primary cells against killing by cytotoxic T lymphocytes. Nature 391:397–401, 1998.
21. Miedema F, Klein MR. AIDS pathogenesis: a finite immune response to blame? Science 272:505–506, 1996.
22. Appay V, Nixon DF, Donahoe SM, et al. HIV-specific CD8+ T cells produce antiviral cytokines but are impaired in cytolytic function. J Exp Med 192:63–76, 2000.
23. Kostense S, Ogg GS, Mauting EM, et al. High viral burden in the presence of major HIV-specific CD8+ T cell expansions: evidence for impaired CTL effector function. Eur J Immunol 31:677–686, 2001.
24. Vogel TU, Allen TM, Altman JD, et al. Functional impairment of simian immunodeficiency virus-specific CD8+ T-cells during the chronic phase of infection. J Virol 75:2458–2461, 2001.
25. Appay V, Dunbar PR, Callan M, et al. Memory CD8+ T cells vary in differentiation phenotype in different persistent virus infections. Nat Med 8:379–385, 2002.
26. Daniel MD, Kirschhoff F, Czajak SC, et al. Protective effects of a live attenuated SIV vaccine with a deletion in the *nef* gene. Science 258:1938–1941, 1992.
27. Almond N, Kent K, Cranage M, et al. Protection by attenuated simian immunodeficiency virus in macaques against challenge with virus-infected cells. Lancet 345:1342–1344, 1995.
28. Wyand MS, Manson K, Montefiori DC, et al. Protection by live, attenuated simian immunodeficiency virus against heterologous challenge. J Virol 73:8356–8363, 1999.
29. Joag SV, Liu ZQ, Stephen EB, et al. Oral immunization of macaques with attenuated vaccine virus induces protection against vaginally transmitted AIDS. J Virol 72:9069–9078, 1998.
30. Letvin NL, Barouch DH, Montefiori DC. Prospects for vaccine protection against HIV-1 infection and AIDS. Annu Rev Immunol 20:73–99, 2002.
31. Burton DR, Moore JP. Why do we not have an HIV vaccine and how can we make one? Nat Med 4:495–498, 1998.
32. Girard M. Le long chemin du vaccin contre le SIDA. *In* Cohen G, Sansonetti P (eds). La Vaccinologie. Ann Inst Pasteur actu/Elsevier, Paris/Amsterdam, 2002, pp105–117.
33. Fauci AS. Immunodeficiency virus: infectivity and mechanisms of pathogenesis. Science 262:1011–1018, 1993.
34. McCune JM. HIV-1: the infective process in vivo. Cell 64:351–363, 1991.
35. Levy JA. Pathogenesis of human immunodeficiency virus infection. Microbiol Rev 57:183–289, 1993.
36. Daar ES, Mougdil T, Meyer RD, Ho DD. Transient high levels of viremia in patients with primary human immunodeficiency virus type 1 infection. N Engl J Med 324:961–964, 1991.
37. Clark SJ, Saag MS, Decker WD, et al. High titers of cytopathic virus in plasma of patients with symptomatic primary HIV-1 infection. N Engl J Med 324:954–960, 1991.
38. Graziosi C, Pantaleo G, Burini L, et al. Kinetics of human immunodeficiency virus type 1 (HIV-1) DNA and RNA synthesis during primary HIV-1 infection. Proc Natl Acad Sci U S A 90:6405–6409, 1993.
39. Pantaleo G, Graziosi C, Burini L, et al. Lymphoid organs function as major reservoirs for human immunodeficiency virus (HIV). Proc Natl Acad Sci U S A 88:9838–9842, 1991.
40. Haase AT. Quantitative image analysis of HIV-1 infection in lymphoid tissue. Science 274:985–989, 1996.
41. Pantaleo G, Demarest JF, Soudeyns HH, et al. Major expansion of CD8+ T cells with a predominant Vβ usage during the primary immune response to HIV. Nature 370:463–467, 1994.
42. Koup RA, Safrit JT, Cao Y, et al. Temporal association of cellular immune responses with the initial control of viremia in primary human immunodeficiency virus type 1 syndrome. J Virol 68:4650–4655, 1994.
43. Borrow P, Lewicki H, Hahn B, et al. Virus specific CD8+ cytotoxic T-lymphocyte activity associated with control of viremia in primary human immunodeficiency virus type 1 infection. J Virol 68:6103–6110, 1994.
44. Haynes BF, Pantaleo G, Fauci AS. Towards an understanding of the correlates of immune protective immunity of HIV infection. Science 271:324–328, 1996.
45. Chen ZW, Kou ZC, Lekutis C, et al. T cell receptor V beta repertoire in acute infection of rhesus monkeys with simian immunodeficiency viruses and a chimeric simian-human immunodeficiency virus. J Exp Med 182:21–32, 1995.
46. Schmitz JE, Kudora ML, Santra S, et al. Control of viremia in simian immunodeficiency virus infection by CD8+ lymphocytes. Science 283:857–860, 1999.
47. Moore JP, Cao Y, Ho DD, Koup RA. Development of the anti-gp120 antibody response during seroconversion to human immunodeficiency virus type 1. J Virol 68:5142–5155, 1994.
48. Imagawa DT, Lee MM, Wolinsky SM, et al. Human immunodeficiency virus type 1 infection in homosexual men who remain seronegative for prolonged periods. N Engl J Med 320:1458–1462, 1989.
49. Montagnier L, Brenner C, Chamaret S, et al. Human immunodeficiency virus infection and AIDS in a person with negative serology. J Infect Dis 175:955–959, 1997.
50. Schuitemaker H, Koot M, Kootstra NA, et al. Biological phenotype of human immunodeficiency virus type 1 clones at different stages of

infections: progression of disease is associated with a shift from mono-cytotropic to T-cell-tropic populations. J Virol 66:1354–1360, 1992.

51. Feinberg MB, Moore JB. AIDS vaccine models: challenging the challenge viruses. Nat Med 8:207–210, 2002.

52. Lu Y, Pauza CD, Lu X, et al. Rhesus macaques that become systematically infected with pathogenic SHIV 89.6-PD after intravenous, rectal, or vaginal inoculation and fail to make an antiviral antibody response rapidly develop AIDS. J Acquir Immune Defic Syndr Hum Retrovirol 19:6–18, 1998.

53. Ho DD, Moudgil T, Alam M. Quantitation of human immunodeficiency virus type 1 in the blood of infected persons. N Engl J Med 321:1621–1625, 1989.

54. Simmonds P, Balfe P, Pentherer JF, et al. Human immunodeficiency virus–infected individuals contain provirus in small numbers of peripheral blood mononuclear cells and at low copy number. J Virol 64:864–872, 1990.

55. Perelson AS, Neumann AU, Markowitz M, et al. HIV-1 dynamics in vivo: virion clearance rate, infected cell life-span, and viral generation time. Science 271:1582–1586, 1996.

56. Coffin J. HIV population dynamics in vivo: implications for genetic variation, pathogenesis, and therapy. Science 267:483–489, 1995.

57. Fox CH, Tenner-Racz K, Racz P, et al. Lymphoid germinal centers are reservoirs for HIV-1 RNA. J Infect Dis 164:1051–1057, 1991.

58. Pantaleo G, Graziosi C, Demarest JF, et al. HIV infection is active and progressive in lymphoid tissue during the clinically latent stage of disease. Nature 362:355–358, 1993.

59. Heath SL, Tew JG, Tew JG, et al. Follicular dendritic cells and human immunodeficiency virus infectivity. Nature 377:740–744, 1995.

60. Perelson AS, Essunger P, Cao Y, et al. Decay characteristics of HIV-infected compartments during combination therapy. Nature 387:188–191, 1997.

61. Orenstein JM, Fox C, Wahl SM. Macrophages as a source of HIV during opportunistic infections. Science 276:1857–1861, 1997.

62. Ho DD. Toward HIV eradication or revision: the tasks ahead. Science 280:1866–1867, 1998.

63. Chun T-W, Stuyver L, Mizell SB, et al. Presence of an inducible HIV-1 latent reservoir during highly active antiretroviral therapy. Proc Natl Acad Sci U S A 94:13193–13197, 1997.

63a. Persaud D, Zhou Y, Siliciano JM, Siliciano RF. Latency in human immunodeficiency virus type 1 infection: no easy answers. J Virol 77:1659–1665, 2003.

64. Centers for Disease Control. Revision of the CDC surveillance case definition for acquired immunodeficiency syndrome. MMWR 36(suppl):1S–15S, 1987.

65. Marlink R, Kanki P, Thior I, et al. Reduced rate of disease development after HIV-2 infection as compared to HIV-1. Science 265:1587–1595, 1994.

66. Philips AN, Lee CA, Elford J, et al. More rapid progression to AIDS in older HIV-infected people: the role of CD4+ T-cell count. J Acquir Immune Defic Syndr 4:970–975, 1991.

67. Lubaki NM, Ray SC, Dhruva B, et al. Characterization of a polyclonal cytolytic T lymphocyte response to human immunodeficiency virus in persons without clinical progression. J Infect Dis 175:1360–1367, 1997.

68. Dean M, Carrington M, Winkler C, et al. Genetic restriction of HIV-1 infection and progression to AIDS by a deletion allele of the CCR5 structural gene. Science 273:1856–1862, 1996.

69. Rana S, Besson G, Cook DG, et al. Role of CCR5 in infection of primary macrophages and lymphocytes by macrophage-tropic strains of human immunodeficiency virus: resistance to patient-derived and prototype isolates resulting from the Δccr5 mutation. J Virol 71:3219–3227, 1997.

70. Smith MW, Dean M, Carrington M, et al. Contrastic genetic influence of CCR2 and CCR5 variants on HIV-1 infection and disease progression. Science 277:959–965, 1997.

71. Lo SC, Tsai S, Benish JR, et al. Enhancement of HIV-1 cytocidal effects in CD4+ lymphocytes by the AIDS-associated mycoplasma. Science 251:1074–1076, 1991.

72. Lemaître M, Hénin Y, Destouesse F, et al. Role of mycoplasma infection in the cytopathic effect induced by human immunodeficiency virus type 1 in infected cell lines. Infect Immun 60:742–748, 1992.

73. Zagury D, Lachgar A, Chams V, et al. C-C chemokines, pivotal in protection against HIV type 1 infection. Proc Natl Acad Sci U S A 95:3857–3861, 1998.

74. Garzino-Demo A, DeVico AL, Cocchi F, Gallo RC. β-chemokines and protection from HIV type 1 disease. AIDS Res Hum Retroviruses 14(suppl 2):S177–S184, 1998.

75. Mellors JW, Rinaldo CR, Gupta P, et al. Prognosis in HIV-1 infection predicted by the quantity of virus in plasma. Science 272:1167–1170, 1996.

76. O'Brien WA, Hartigan PM, Martin D, et al. Changes of plasma HIV-RNA and CD4+ lymphocyte counts and the risk of progression to AIDS. N Engl J Med 334:426–431, 1996.

77. Watson A, Ranchalis J, Travis B, et al. Plasma viremia in macaques infected with simian immunodeficiency virus: plasma viral load early in infection predicts survival. J Virol 71:284–290, 1997.

78. Pantaleo G, Demarest JF, Schacker T, et al. The qualitative nature of the primary immune response to HIV infection is a prognosticator of disease progression independent of the initial level of plasma viremia. Proc Natl Acad Sci U S A 94:254–258, 1997.

79. Matsuyama T, Kobayashi N, Yamamoto N. Cytokines and HIV infection: is AIDS a tumor necrosis factor disease? AIDS 5:1405–1417, 1991.

80. Kinter A, Ostrowski M, Goletti D, et al. HIV replication in CD4+ T cells of HIV-infected individuals is regulated by a balance between the viral suppressive effects of endogenous β-chemokines and the viral inductive effects of other endogenous cytokines. Proc Natl Acad Sci U S A 93:14076–14081, 1996.

81. Levy JA, Mackewicz CE, Barker E. Controlling HIV pathogenesis: the role of the noncytotoxic anti-HIV response of CD8+ T cells. Immunol Today 17:217–224, 1996.

82. Gauduin MC, Glickmann RL, Ahmad S, et al. Immunization with live attenuated simian immunodeficiency virus induces strong type 1 T helper responses and betachemokine production. Proc Natl Acad Sci U S A 96:14031–14036, 1999.

83. Chang TL, Masoian A, Pine R, et al. A soluble factor(s) secreted from CD8+ T lymphocytes inhibits human immunodeficiency virus type 1 replication through STAT1 activation. J Virol 76:569–581, 2002.

84. Romagnani S. The Th1/Th2 paradigm. Immunol Today 18:263–266, 1997.

85. Clerici M, Shearer GM. A TH1 → TH2 switch is a critical step in the etiology of HIV infection. Immunol Today 14:107–111, 1993.

86. Maggi E, Mazzetti M, Ravina A, et al. Ability of HIV to promote a Th1 to Th0 shift and to replicate preferentially in Th2 and Th0 cells. Science 265:244–248, 1994.

87. Pantaleo G, Menzo S, Vaccarezzo M, et al. Studies in subjects with long-term nonprogressive human immunodeficiency virus infection. N Engl J Med 332:209–216, 1995.

88. Cao Y, Qin L, Zhang L, et al. Virologic and immunologic characterization of long-term survivors of human immunodeficiency virus type 1 infection. N Engl J Med 332:201–208, 1995.

88a. Imani N, Pires A, Hardy G, et al. A balanced typet 1 / type 2 response is associated with long-term nonprogressive human immunodeficiency virus type 1 infection. J Virol 76:9011–9023, 2002.

89. Borrow P, Evans CF, Oldstone MBA. Virus-induced immunosuppression: immune system–mediated destruction of virus-infected dendritic cells results in generalized immunosuppression. J Virol 69:1059–1070, 1995.

90. Odermatt B, Eppler M, Leist TP, et al. Virus-triggered acquired immunodeficiency by cytotoxic T-cell–dependent destruction of antigen-presenting cells with lymph follicle structure. Proc Natl Acad Sci U S A 88:8252–8256, 1991.

90a. Grossman Z, Meier-Schellersheim M, Souza AE, et al. CD4+ T-cell depletion in HIV infection: are we closer to understanding the cause? Nat Med 8:319–323, 2002.

91. McCure JM. The dynamics of CD4+ T cell depletion in HIV disease. Nature 410:974–979, 2001.

92. Wanatabe M, Ringler DJ, Fultz PN, et al. A chimpanzee-passaged human immunodeficiency virus isolate is cytopathic for chimpanzee cells but does not induce disease. J Virol 65:3344–3348, 1991.

93. Heeney J, Boggers W, Buijs L, et al. Immune strategies utilized by lentivirus-infected chimpanzees to resist progression to AIDS. Immunol Lett 51:45–52, 1996.

94. Novembre FJ, Saucier M, Anderson DC, et al. Development of AIDS in a chimpanzee infected with human immunodeficiency virus type 1. J Virol 71:4086–4091, 1997.

95. Siliciano RF, Lawton T, Knall C, et al. Analysis of host-virus interactions in AIDS with anti-gp120 T-cell clones: effect of HIV sequence variation and a mechanism for CD4+ depletion. Cell 54:561–575, 1988.

96. Habeshaw J, Hounsell E, Dalgleish A. Does the HIV envelope induce a chronic graft-versus-host–like disease? Immunol Today 13:207–210, 1992.

97. Zagury JF, Bernard J, Achour A, et al. Identification of CD4 as major histocompatibility complex functional peptide sites and their homology with oligopeptides from human immunodeficiency virus type 1

glycoprotein gp120: role in AIDS pathogenesis. Proc Natl Acad Sci U S A 90:7573–7577, 1993.

98. Dalgleish AG, Marriott JB, Souberbielle B, et al. The role of HIV gp120 in the destruction of the immune system. Immunol Lett 66:81–87, 1999.

99. Gougeon ML, Dadaglio G, Garcia S, et al. Is a dominant superantigen involved in AIDS pathogenesis? Lancet 342:50–51, 1993.

100. Ameisen JC, Capron A. Cell dysfunction and depletion in AIDS: the programmed cell death hypothesis. Immunol Today 12:102–105, 1991.

101. Gougeon ML, Garcia S, Heeney J, et al. Programmed cell death in AIDS-related HIV and SIV infections. AIDS Res Hum Retroviruses 9:553–563, 1993.

102. Estaquier J, Idziorek T, de Bels, et al. Programmed cell death and AIDS: significance of T-cell apoptosis in pathogenic and nonpathogenic primate lentiviral infections. Proc Natl Acad Sci U S A 91:9431–9435, 1994.

103. Laurent-Crawford AG, Krust B, Riviere Y, et al. Membrane expression of HIV envelope glycoproteins triggers apoptosis in CD4 cells. AIDS Res Hum Retroviruses 9:761–773, 1993.

104. Li CJ, Friedman DJ, Wang C, et al. Induction of apoptosis in uninfected lymphocytes by HIV-1 Tat protein. Science 268:429–431, 1995.

105. Serres P-F. AIDS: an immune response against the immune system. Role of a precise tridimensional molecular mimicry. J Autoimmun 16:287–291, 2001.

106. Finkel TH, Tudor-Williams G, Banda NK, et al. Apoptosis occurs predominantly in bystander cells and not in productively infected cells of HIV- and SIV-infected lymph nodes. Nat Med 1:129–134, 1995.

107. Clerici M, Sarin A, Coffman RL, et al. Type 1/type 2 cytokine modulation of T-cell programmed cell death as a model for human immunodeficiency virus pathogenesis. Proc Natl Acad Sci U S A 91:11811–11815, 1994.

108. Ensoli B, Barillari G, Salahuddin SZ, et al. Tat protein of HIV-1 stimulates growth of cells derived from Kaposi sarcoma lesions of AIDS patients. Nature 345:84–86, 1990.

109. Ensoli B, Buonaguro L, Bavillari G, et al. Release, uptake, and effects of extracellular human immunodeficiency virus type 1 Tat protein on cell growth and viral transactivation. J Virol 67:277–287, 1993.

110. Gallo RC. Tat as one key to HIV-induced immunopathogenesis and tat toxoid as an important component of a vaccine. Proc Natl Acad Sci USA 96:8324–8326, 1999.

111. Liu R, Paxton WA, Choe S, et al. Homozygous defect in HIV-1 coreceptor accounts for resistance of some multiply-exposed individuals to HIV-1 infection. Cell 86:367–377, 1996.

112. Clerici M, Giorgi JV, Chou C-C, et al. Cell-mediated immune response to human immunodeficiency virus (HIV) type 1 in seronegative homosexual men with recent sexual exposure to HIV-1. J Infect Dis 165:1012–1019, 1992.

113. Rowland-Jones S, Sutton J, Ariyoshi K, et al. HIV-specific cytotoxic T-cells in HIV-exposed but uninfected Gambian women. Nat Med 1:59–64, 1995.

114. Rowland-Jones S, Dong T, Fowke KR, et al. Cytotoxic T cell response to multiple conserved HIV epitopes in HIV-1 resistant prostitutes in Nairobi. J Clin Invest 102:1758–1765, 1998.

115. Kaul R, Plummer F, Kimani J, et al. HIV-1 specific mucosal CD8+ lymphocyte responses in the cervix of HIV-1-resistant prostitutes in Nairobi. J Immunol 164:1602–1611, 2000.

115a. Kaul R, Rowland-Jones SL, Kimani J, et al. Late seroconversion in HIV-resistant Nairobi prostitutes despite preexisting HIV-specific CD8+ responses. J Clin Invest 107:341–349, 2001.

116. Cheynier R, Langlade-Demoyen P, Marescot MR, et al. Cytotoxic T-lymphocyte response in the peripheral blood of children born to HIV-infected mothers. Eur J Immunol 22:2211–2217, 1992.

117. Langlade-Demoyen P, Ngo-Giang-Huang N, Ferchal F, Oskenhendler E. HIV nef-specific cytotoxic T lymphocytes in noninfected heterosexual contacts of HIV-infected patients. J Clin Invest 93:1293–1297, 1994.

118. Pinto LA, Sullivan J, Berzofsky JA, et al. ENV-specific cytotoxic T lymphocyte responses in HIV seronegative health care workers occupationally exposed to HIV-contaminated body fluids. J Clin Invest 96:867–876, 1995.

119. Skurnick JH, Palumbo P, Devico A, et al. Correlates of nontransmission in U.S. women at high risk of human immunodeficiency virus type 1 infection through sexual exposure. J Infect Dis 185:428–438, 2002.

120. Paxton WA, Martin SR, Yse D, et al. Relative resistance to HIV-1 infection of CD4 lymphocytes from persons who remain uninfected despite multiple high-risk sexual exposure. Nat Med 2:412–417, 1996.

121. Mazzoli S, Trabattoni D, Lo Capuco S, et al. HIV-1-specific mucosal and cellular immunity in HIV-seronegative partners of HIV-seropositive individuals. Nat Med 11:1250–1257, 1997.

121a. Clerici M, Barassi C, Devito C, et al. Serum IgA of HIV-exposed uninfected individuals inhibit HIV through recognition of a region within the α-helix of gp41. AIDS 16:1731–1791, 2002.

122. Barré-Sinoussi F, Chermann JC, Rey F, et al. Isolation of a T-lymphocytropic retrovirus from a patient at risk for acquired immune deficiency syndrome (AIDS). Science 220:868–871, 1983.

123. Popovic M, Sarngadharan MG, Read E, Gallo RC. Detection, isolation and continuous production of cytopathic retroviruses (HTLV-III) from patients with AIDS and pre-AIDS. Science 224:497–500, 1984.

124. Levy JA, Hoffman AD, Kramer S, et al. Isolation of lymphocytopathic retroviruses from San Francisco patients with AIDS. Science 225:840–842, 1984.

125. Clavel F, Mansiho K, Chamaret S, et al. Human immunodeficiency virus type 2 infection associated with AIDS in West Africa. N Engl J Med 316:1180–1185, 1987.

126. Narayan O, Clements JE. The biology and pathogenesis of lentiviruses. J Gen Virol 70:1617–1639, 1989.

127. Earl PL, Doms RW, Moss B. Oligomeric structure of the human immunodeficiency virus type 1 envelope glycoprotein. Proc Natl Acad Sci U S A 87:648–652, 1990.

128. Cosson P. Direct interaction between the envelope and matrix proteins of HIV-1. EMBO J 15:5783–5788, 1996.

129. Hill CP, Worthylake D, Bancroff DP, et al. Crystal structure of the trimeric human immunodeficiency virus type 1 matrix protein: implications for membrane association and assembly. Proc Natl Acad Sci U S A 33:3099–3104, 1996.

130. Henderson CE, Sourder RC, Copeland TD, et al. Gag precursors of HIV and SIV are cleaved into six proteins found in the mature virions. J Med Primatol 19:411–419, 1990.

131. Henderson CE, Bowers MA, Sourder RC, et al. Gag proteins of highly replicative MN strain of human immunodeficiency virus type 1: post-transcriptional modifications, proteolytic processing and complete amino acid sequences. J Virol 66:1856–1865, 1992.

132. Ott DE, Coren LV, Kane BP, et al. Cytoskeletal proteins inside human immunodeficiency virus type 1 virions. J Virol 70:7734–7743, 1996.

133. Lu M, Blacklow SC, Kim PS. A trimeric structural domain of the HIV-1 transmembrane glycoprotein. Nat Struct Biol 2:1075–1082, 1995.

134. Pombourios P, Wilson KA, Center RJ, et al. Human immunodeficiency virus type 1 envelope glycoprotein oligomerization requires the gp41 amphipathic alpha-helical/leucine zipper-like sequence. J Virol 71:2041–2049, 1997.

135. Chan DC, Fass D, Berger JM, Kim PS. Core structure of gp41 from the HIV-1 envelope glycoprotein. Cell 89:263–273, 1997.

136. Weissenhorn W, Dessen A, Marrison SC, et al. Atomic structure of the ectodomain from HIV-1 gp41. Nature 387:426–430, 1997.

137. Yang ZN, Mueser TC, Kaufman J, et al. The crystal structure of the SIV gp41 ectodomain at 1.47 Å resolution. J Struct Biol 126:131–144, 1999.

138. Bugge TH, Lindhardt BO, Hansen LL, et al. Characterization of the fusion domain of the human immunodeficiency virus type 1 envelope glycoprotein GP41. Proc Natl Acad Sci U S A 87:4650–4654, 1990.

139. Eckert DM, Kim PS. Mechanism of viral membrane fusion and its inhibition. Annu Rev Biochem 70:777–810, 2001.

140. Schaal H, Klein M, Gehrmann P, et al. Requirement of N-terminal amino acid residues of gp41 for human immunodeficiency virus type 1–mediated cell fusion. J Virol 69:3308–3314, 1995.

141. Shugars DC, Wild CT, Greenwell TK, Matthews TJ. Biophysical characterization of recombinant proteins expressing the leucine zipper-like domain of the human immunodeficiency virus type 1 transmembrane protein gp41. J Virol 70:2982–2991, 1996.

142. Leonard CK, Spellman MW, Riddle L, et al. Assignment of intrachain disulfide bonds and characterization of potential glycosylation sites of the type 1 recombinant human immunodeficiency virus envelope glycoprotein (gp120) expressed in Chinese hamster ovary cells. J Biol Chem 265:1037–1030, 1990.

143. Wyatt R, Sodroski J. The HIV-1 envelope glycoproteins: fusogens, antigens, and immunogens. Science 280:1884–1888, 1998.

144. Kwong PD, Wyatt R, Robinson J, et al. Structure of an HIV gp120 envelope glycoprotein in complex with the CD4 receptor and a neutralizing human antibody. Nature 393:648–659, 1998.

145. Wyatt R, Kwong PD, Desjardins E, et al. The antigenic structure of the HIV gp120 envelope glycoprotein. Nature 393:705–711, 1998.

146. Ratner L. Glucosidase inhibitors for treatment of HIV-1 infection. AIDS Res Hum Retroviruses 8:165–173, 1992.

147. Earl PL, Moss B, Doms RW. Folding, interaction with GRP78-BIP, assembly, and transport of the human immunodeficiency virus type 1 envelope protein. J Virol 65:2047–2055, 1991.

148. Otteken A, Earl PL, Moss B. Folding, assembly, and intracellular trafficking of the human immunodeficiency virus type 1 envelope glycoprotein analyzed with monoclonal antibodies recognizing maturational intermediates. J Virol 70:3407–3415, 1996.

149. Moore JP, Sattentau QJ, Wyatt R, Sodroski J. Probing the structure of the human immunodeficiency virus surface glycoprotein gp120 with a panel of monoclonal antibodies. J Virol 68:469–484, 1994.

150. Arthur LO, Bess JW Jr, Sowder RC, et al. Cellular proteins bound to immunodeficiency viruses: implications for pathogenesis and vaccines. Science 258:1935–1938, 1992.

151. Rizzuto CD, Sodroski JG. Contribution of virion ICAM-1 to human immunodeficiency virus infectivity and sensitivity to neutralization. J Virol 71:4847–4851, 1997.

152. Ratner L, Haseltine W, Patarca R, et al. Complete nucleotide sequence of the AIDS virus, HTLV-III. Nature 313:277–284, 1985.

153. Wain-Hobson S, Sonigo P, Danos O, et al. Nucleotide sequence of the AIDS virus, LAV. Cell 40:9–17, 1985.

154. Gao F, Robertson DL, Carruthers CD, et al. A comprehensive panel of near-full length clones and reference sequences for non-subtype B isolates of human immunodeficiency virus type 1. J Virol 72:5680–5698, 1998.

155. Paillart JC, Skripkin E, Ehresman B, et al. A loop "kissing" complex is the essential part of the dimer linkage of genomic HIV-1 RNA. Proc Natl Acad Sci U S A 92:5572–5577, 1996.

156. Robertson DL, Sharp P, McCutchan FE, Hahn BH. Recombination in HIV-1. Nature 374:124–126, 1995.

157. McCutchan FE. Understanding the genetic diversity of HIV-1. AIDS 14(suppl 3):S31–S44, 2000.

158. Jeang KR, Chang YN, Berkhout B, et al. Regulation of HIV expression: mechanisms of action of Tat and Rev. AIDS 5(suppl 2):S3–S14, 1991.

159. Trono D. HIV accessory proteins: leading roles for the supporting cast. Cell 82:189–192, 1995.

160. Emerman M, Malim MH. HIV-1 regulatory/accessory genes: keys to unraveling viral and host cell biology. Science 280:1880–1884, 1998.

161. Feinberg MB, Baltimore D, Frankel A. The role of Tat in the human immunodeficiency virus life cycle indicates a primary effect on transcriptional elongation. Proc Natl Acad Sci U S A 88:4045–4049, 1991.

162. Dayton AJ, Terwilliger EF, Potz J, et al. Cis-acting sequences responsive to the rev gene product of the human immunodeficiency virus. J Acquir Immune Defic Syndr 1:441–452, 1988.

163. Pomerantz RJ, Seshama T, Trono D. Efficient replication of human immunodeficiency virus type 1 requires a threshold level of Rev: potential implications for latency. J Virol 66:1809–1813, 1992.

164. Harris M. From negative factor to a critical role in virus pathogenesis: the changing fortunes of Nef. J Gen Virol 77:2379–2392, 1996.

165. Kestler HW, Ringler DH, Mori K, et al. Importance of the nef gene for maintenance of high virus loads and for development of AIDS. Cell 65:851–862, 1991.

166. Whatmore AM, Cook N, Hall GA, et al. Repair and evolution of Nef in vivo modulates simian immunodeficiency virus virulence. J Virol 69:5117–5123, 1995.

167. Greene WC, Peterlin BM. Charting HIV's remarkable voyage through the cell: basic science as a passport to future therapy. Nat Med 8:673–680, 2002.

168. Simard M-C, Chrobak P, Kay DG, et al. Expression of simian immunodeficiency virus nef in immune cells of transgenic mice leads to severe AIDS-like disease. J Virol 76:3981–3995, 2002.

169. Bryant M, Ratner L. Myristoylation-dependent replication and assembly of human immunodeficiency virus I. Proc Natl Acad Sci U S A 87:523–527, 1990.

170. Braaten D, Franke EK, Luban J. Cyclophilin A is required for the replication of group M human immunodeficiency virus type 1 (HIV-1) and simian immunodeficiency virus SIV (CP2) GAB but not group O HIV-1 or other primate immunodeficiency viruses. J Virol 70:4220–4227, 1996.

171. Johnson DC, Hubert MT. Directed egress of animal viruses promotes cell-to-cell spread. J Virol 76:1–8, 2002.

172. Geijtenbech TBH, Kwon DS, Torensman R, et al. DC-SIGN, a dendritic cell-specific HIV-1-binding protein that enhances trans-infection of T cells. Cell 100:587–597, 2000.

173. Jameson B, Baribaud F, Pöhlmann S, et al. Expression of DC-SIGN by dendritic cells of intestinal and genital mucosae in humans and rhesus macaques. J Virol 76:1866–1875, 2002.

174. Klatzmann D, Champagne E, Chamaret S, et al. T-lymphocyte T4 molecule behaves as the receptor for human retrovirus LAV. Nature 312:767–768, 1984.

175. Dalgleish AG, Beverley PCL, Clapham PR, et al. The CD4 (T4) antigen is an essential component of the receptor for the AIDS retrovirus. Nature 312:763–767, 1984.

176. Maddon PJ, Dalgleish AG, McDougal JS, et al. The T4 gene encodes the AIDS virus receptor and is expressed in the immune system and the brain. Cell 47:333–348, 1986.

177. Clapham P, Weber JM, Whitby D, et al. Soluble CD4 blocks the infectivity of diverse strains of HIV and SIV for T cells and monocytes but not for brain and muscle cells. Nature 337:388–390, 1989.

178. Clapham PR, McKnight A, Weiss RA. Human immunodeficiency virus type 2 infection and fusion of CD4-negative human cell lines: induction and enhancement by soluble CD4. J Virol 66:3531–3537, 1992.

179. Harouse JM, Bhat S, Spitalnik SL, et al. Inhibition of entry of HIV-1 in neural cell lines by antibodies against galactosyl ceramide. Science 253:320–323, 1991.

180. Fantini J, Cook DG, Nathanson N, et al. Infection of colonic epithelial cell lines by type 1 human immunodeficiency virus is associated with cell surface expression of galactosylceramide, a potential alternative gp120 receptor. Proc Natl Acad Sci U S A 90:2700–2704, 1993.

181. Curtis BM, Scharnowske S, Watson AJ. Sequence and expression of a membrane-associated C-type lectin that exhibits CD4-independent binding of human immunodeficiency virus envelope glycoprotein gp120. Proc Natl Acad Sci U S A 89:8356–8360, 1992.

182. Lasky LA, Nakamura G, Smith D. Delineation of a region of the human immunodeficiency virus type 1 gp120 glycoprotein critical for interaction with the CD4 receptor. Cell 50:975–985, 1987.

183. Olshevsky U, Helseth E, Furman C, et al. Identification of individual human immunodeficiency virus type 1 gp120 amino acids important for CD4 receptor binding. J Virol 64:5701–5707, 1990.

184. Sattentau QJ, Moore JP. Conformational changes in the human immunodeficiency virus envelope glycoproteins by soluble CD4 binding. J Exp Med 174:407–415, 1991.

185. Feng Y, Broder CC, Kennedy PE, Berger EA. HIV-1 entry co-factor: functional cDNA-cloning of a seven-transmembrane, G protein–coupled receptor. Science 272:872–877, 1996.

186. Dragic T, Litwin V, Allaway GP, et al. HIV entry into CD4+ cells is mediated by the chemokine receptor CC-CKR-5. Nature 381:667–673, 1996.

187. Deng HK, Choe S, Ellmeier W, et al. Identification of a major co-receptor for primary isolates of HIV-1. Nature 381:661–666, 1996.

188. Alkhatib G, Combadiere C, Broder CC, et al. CC-CKR5: a RANTES, MIP-1α, MIP-1β receptor as a fusion cofactor for macrophage-tropic HIV-1. Science 272:1955–1958, 1996.

189. Berger EA. HIV entry and tropism: the chemokine receptor connection. AIDS 11(suppl A):S3–S16, 1997.

190. Roos MT, Lange IM, de Goede RE, et al. Viral phenotype and immune response in primary human immunodeficiency virus type 1 infection. J Infect Dis 165:427–432, 1992.

191. Hwang SS, Boyle TJ, Lyerly HK, Cullen BR. Identification of the envelope V3 loop as the primary determinant of cell tropism in HIV-1. Science 253:71–74, 1991.

192. Grimaila RJ, Fuller BA, Rennert PD, et al. Mutations in the principal neutralization determinant of human immunodeficiency virus type 1 affect syncytium formation, virus infectivity, growth kinetics, and neutralization. J Virol 66:1875–1883, 1992.

193. Fouchier RA, Groenink M, Koostra NA, et al. Phenotype-associated sequence variation in the third variable domain of the human immunodeficiency virus type 1 gp120 molecule. J Virol 66:3183–3187, 1992.

194. Shioda T, Levy JA, Cheng-Mayer C. Small amino acid changes in the V3 hypervariable region of gp120 can affect the T-cell line and macrophage tropism of human immunodeficiency virus type 1. Proc Natl Acad Sci U S A 89:9434–9438, 1992.

195. Kuiken CL, de Jong J-J, Boan E. Evolution of the V3 envelope domain in proviral sequences and isolates of human immunodeficiency virus type 1 during transition of the viral biological phenotype. J Virol 66:4622–4627, 1992.

196. Harrowe G, Cheng-Mayer C. Amino acid substitutions in the V3 loop are responsible for adaptation to growth in transformed T cell–lines of a primary human immunodeficiency virus type 1. Virology 210:490–494, 1995.

197. Javaherian K, Langlois AJ, McDanal CB, et al. Principal neutralizing domain of the human immunodeficiency virus type 1 envelope protein. Proc Natl Acad Sci U S A 86:6768–6772, 1989.

198. LaRosa G, Davide JP, Weinhold K, et al. Conserved sequence and structural elements in the HIV-1 principal neutralizing domain. Science 249:932–935, 1990.

199. Freed EO, Myers DJ, Risser R. Identification of the principal neutralizing determinant of human immunodeficiency virus type 1 as a fusion domain. J Virol 65:190–194, 1991.

200. Moore JP, Nara PL. The role of the V3 loop of gp120 in HIV infection. AIDS 5(suppl 2):S21–S33, 1991.

201. Verrier F, Borman AM, Brand D, Girard M. Role of the HIV type 1 glycoprotein 120 V3 loop in determining coreceptor usage. AIDS Res Hum Retroviruses 15:731–743, 1999.

202. Nara PL. HIV-neutralization: evidence for rapid binding/post-binding neutralization from infected humans, chimpanzees, and gp120-vaccinated animals. Vaccine 89:137–144, 1989.

203. Choe H, Farzan M, Sun Y, et al. The β-chemokine receptors CCR-3 and CCR-5 facilitate infection by primary HIV-1 isolates. Cell 85:1135–1148, 1996.

204. Ross TM, Cullen BR. The ability of HIV type 1 to use CCR-3 as a coreceptor is controlled by envelope V1/V2 sequences acting in conjunction with a CCR-5 tropic V3 loop. Proc Natl Acad Sci U S A 95:7682–7686, 1998.

205. Simmons G, Wilkinson D, Reeves JD, et al. Primary, syncytium-inducing human immunodeficiency virus type 1 isolates are dual-tropic and most can use either Lestr or CCR5 as coreceptors for virus entry. J Virol 70:8355–8360, 1996.

206. Doranz BJ, Rucker J, Yi Y, et al. A dual-tropic primary HIV-1 isolate that uses fusin and the β-chemokine receptors CKR-5, CKR-3, and CKR-2b as fusion cofactors. Cell 85:1149–1158, 1996.

207. Edinger AL, Amédée A, Miller K, et al. Differential utilization of CCR5 by macrophage- and T cell–tropic simian immunodeficiency virus strains. Proc Natl Acad Sci U S A 94:4005–4010, 1997.

208. Marcon L, Choe H, Martin KA, et al. Utilization of C-C chemokine receptor 5 by the envelope glycoproteins of a pathogenic simian immunodeficiency virus, SIVmac239. J Virol 71:2522–2527, 1997.

209. Alkhatib G, Liao F, Berger EA, et al. A new SIV coreceptor, STRL33 [letter]. Nature 388:238, 1997.

210. Deng HK, Unutmaz D, Kewal Ramani VN, Littman DR. Expression cloning of new receptors used by simian and human immunodeficiency virus. Nature 388:296–300, 1997.

211. Lapham C, Ouyang J, Chandrasekhar B, et al. Evidence for cell-surface association between fusin and the CD4-gp120 complex in human cell lines. Science 274:602–605, 1996.

212. Wu L, Gerard NP, Wyatt R, et al. CD4-induced interaction of primary HIV-1 gp120 glycoprotein with the chemokine receptor CCR5. Nature 384:179–183, 1996.

213. Trkola A, Dragic T, Arthos J, et al. CD4-independent antibody-sensitive interactions between HIV-1 and its co-receptor CCR-5. Nature 384:184–187, 1996.

214. Verrier F, Charneau P, Altmeyer R, et al. Antibodies to several conformation-dependent epitopes of gp120/gp41 inhibit CCR5-dependent cell-to-cell fusion mediated by the native envelope glycoprotein of a primary macrophage-tropic HIV-1 isolate. Proc Natl Acad Sci U S A 94:9326–9331, 1997.

215. Wyatt R, Moore JP, Accola M, et al. Involvement of the V1/V2 variable loop structure in the exposure of human immunodeficiency virus type 1 gp120 epitopes induced by receptor binding. J Virol 69:5723–5733, 1995.

216. Endres MJ, Clapham PB, Marsh M, et al. CD4-independent infection by HIV-2 is mediated by fusin CXCR4. Cell 87:745–756, 1996.

217. Cocchi F, DeVico A, Garzino-Demo A, et al. The V3 domain of the HIV-1 gp120 envelope glycoprotein is critical for chemokine-mediated blockade of infection. Nat Med 2;1244–1747, 1996.

218. Jansson M, Popovic M, Karlsson A, et al. Sensitivity to inhibition by β-chemokines correlates with biological phenotype of primary HIV-1 isolates. Proc Natl Acad Sci U S A 93:15382–15387, 1996.

219. Bleul CC, Farzan M, Choe H, et al. The lymphocyte chemoattractant SDF-1 is a ligand for LESTR/fusin and blocks HIV-1 entry. Nature 382:829–833, 1996.

220. Oberlin E, Amara A, Bachelerie F, et al. The CXC chemokine SDF-1 is the ligand for LESTR/fusion and prevents infection by T-cell-line–adapted HIV-1. Nature 382:833–835, 1996.

221. Samson M, Libert F, Doranz BJ, et al. Resistance to HIV-1 infection in Caucasian individuals bearing mutant alleles of the CCR-5 chemokine receptor gene. Nature 382:722–725, 1996.

222. Biti R, French R, Young J, et al. HIV-infection in an individual homozygous for the CCR5 deletion allele. Nat Med 3:252–253, 1997.

223. Moore JP, McKeating JA, Weiss RA, Sattentau QJ. Dissociation of gp120 from HIV-1 virions induced by soluble CD4. Science 250:1139–1142, 1990.

224. Wiley DC, Skehel JJ. The structure and function of the hemagglutinin membrane glycoprotein of influenza virus. Annu Rev Biochem 56:365–394, 1987.

225. Binley J, Moore JP. The viral mousetrap. Nature 387:346–348, 1997.

226. Wild CT, Shugars DC, Greenwell TK, et al. Peptides corresponding to a predicted α-helical domain of human immunodeficiency virus type 1 gp41 are potent inhibitors of virus infection. Proc Natl Acad Sci U S A 91:9770–9774, 1994.

227. Chen C-H, Matthews TJ, McDanal CB, et al. A molecular clasp in the human immunodeficiency virus (HIV) type 1 TM protein determines the anti-HIV activity of gp41 derivatives: implications for viral fusion. J Virol 69:3771–3777, 1995.

227a. He Y, Vassell R, Zaitseva M, et al. Peptides trap the immunodeficiency virus type 1 envelope glycoprotein fusion intermediate at two sites. J Virol 77:1666–1671, 2003.

228. Stevenson M, Stanwick TT, Dempsey MP, Lamonica CA. HIV-1 replication is controlled at the level of T-cell activation and proviral integration. EMBO J 9:1551–1560, 1990.

229. Robinson HL, Zinkus DM. Accumulation of human immunodeficiency virus type 1 DNA in T cells: result of multiple infection events. J Virol 64:4836–4841, 1990.

230. Schnittman SM, Psallidopoulos MC, Lane HC, et al. The reservoir for HIV-1 in human peripheral blood is a T-cell that maintains expression of CD4. Science 245:305–308, 1989.

231. Kim S, Byrn R, Groopman J, Baltimore D. Temporal aspects of DNA and RNA synthesis during human immunodeficiency virus infection: evidence for differential gene expression. J Virol 63:3708–3713, 1989.

232. Leonardo MJ, Baltimore D. NF-KB: a pleiotropic mediator of inducible and tissue-specific gene control. Cell 58:227–229, 1989.

233. O'Brien W, Zack JA, Chen ISY. Molecular pathogenesis of HIV-1. AIDS 4(suppl 1):S41–S48, 1990.

234. Mansky LM, Temin HM. Lower in vivo mutation rate of human immunodeficiency virus type 1 than that predicted from the fidelity of purified reverse transcriptase. J Virol 69:5087–5094, 1995.

235. Hahn BH, Shaw GM, Taylor ME, et al. Genetic variation in HTLV-III/LAV over time in patients with AIDS or at risk for AIDS. Science 232:1548–1553, 1986.

236. Groenink M, Fouchier RA, de Goede RE, et al. Phenotypic heterogeneity in a panel of infectious molecular human immunodeficiency virus type 1 clones derived from a single individual. J Virol 65:1968–1975, 1991.

237. Eigen M. On the nature of virus quasispecies. Trends Microbiol 4:216–218, 1996.

238. Robertson DL, Anderson JP, Bradac JA, et al. HIV-1 nomenclature proposal. Science 288:55–57, 2000.

239. Peeters M, Sharp PM. Genetic diversity of HIV-1: the moving target. AIDS 14(suppl 3):S129–S140, 2000.

240. Gao F, Bailes E, Robertson DL, et al. Origin of HIV-1 in the chimpanzee Pan troglodytes troglodytes. Nature 397:436–441, 1999.

241. Korber B, Muldoon M, Theiler J, et al. Timing the ancestor of the HIV-1 pandemic strains. Science 288:1789–1796, 2000.

242. Peeters M, Courgnaud V, Abela B, et al. Risk to human health from a plethora of simian immunodeficiency viruses in primate bushmeat. Emerg Infect Dis 8:451–457, 2002.

243. De Leys R, Vanderborght B, Vanden Haesevelde M, et al. Isolation and partial characterization of an unusual human immunodeficiency

retrovirus from two persons of west-central African origin. J Virol 64:1207–1216, 1990.

244. Peeters M, Gueye A, Mboup S, et al. Geographical distribution of HIV-1 group O viruses in Africa. AIDS 11:493–498, 1997.

245. Zekeng L, Gurtler L, Afane ZE, et al. Prevalence of HIV-1 subtype O infection in Cameroon: preliminary results. AIDS 8:1626–1628, 1994.

246. Gurtler LG, Zekeng L, Tsague JM, et al. HIV-1 subtype O: epidemiology, pathogenesis, diagnosis, and perspectives of the evolution of HIV. Arch Virol Suppl 11:195–202, 1996.

247. Simon F, Mauclere P, Roques P, et al. Identification of a new human immunodeficiency virus type 1 distinct from group M and group O. Nat Med 4:1032–1037, 1998.

248. Ayouba A, Souquieres S, Njinku B, et al. HIV-1 group N among HIV-1-seropositive individuals in Cameroon. AIDS 14:2623–2625, 2000.

249. Nathanson N, Mathieson BJ. Biological considerations in the development of a human immunodeficiency virus vaccine. J Infect Dis 182:579–589, 2000.

250. Artenstein AW, VanCott TC, Mascola JR, et al. Dual infection with human immunodeficiency virus type 1 of distinct envelope subtypes in humans. J Infect Dis 171:805–810, 1995.

250a. Zhuang J, Jetzt AE, Sun G, et al. Human immunodeficiency virus type 1 recombination: rate, fidelity, and putative hot spots. J Virol 76:11273–11282, 2002.

251. Hu DJ, Dondero TJ, Rayfield MA, et al. The emerging genetic diversity of HIV: the importance of global surveillance for diagnostics, research, and prevention. JAMA 275:210–216, 1996.

252. Mastro TD, Kunanusont C, Dondero TJ, Wasi C. Why do HIV-1 subtypes segregate among persons with different risk behaviors in South Africa and Thailand? AIDS 11:113–116, 1997.

253. Beyrer C, Razak MH, Lisam K, et al. Overland heroin trafficking routes and HIV-1 spread in south and south-east Asia. AIDS 14:75–83, 2000.

254. Subbarao S, Limpakarnjanarat K, Mastro TD, et al. HIV type 1 in Thailand, 1994–1995: persistence of two subtypes with low genetic diversity. AIDS Res Hum Retroviruses 14:319–327, 1998.

255. Limpakarnjanarat K, Ungchusak K, Mastro TD, et al. The epidemiological evolution of HIV-1 subtypes B and E among heterosexuals and injecting drug users in Thailand, 1992–1997. AIDS 12:1108–1109, 1998.

256. Weniger BG, Takebe Y, Ou CY, Yamazaki S. The molecular epidemiology of HIV in Asia. AIDS 8(suppl 2):S13–S28, 1994.

257. Kusagawa S, Sato H, Watanabe S, et al. Genetic and serologic characterization of HIV type 1 prevailing in Myanmar (Burma). AIDS Res Hum Retroviruses 14:1379–1385, 1998.

258. Kusagawa S, Sato H, Kato K, et al. HIV type 1 env subtype E in Cambodia. AIDS Res Hum Retroviruses 15:91–94, 1999.

259. Kato K, Kusagawa S, Motomura K, et al. Closely related HIV-1 CRF01_AE variant among injecting drug users in northern Vietnam: evidence of HIV spread across the Vietnam-China border. AIDS Res Hum Retroviruses 17:113–123, 2001.

260. Motomura K, Kusagawa S, Kato K, et al. Emergence of new forms of human immunodeficiency virus type 1 intersubtype recombinants in central Myanmar. AIDS Res Hum Retroviruses 16:1831–1843, 2000.

261. Bobkov A, Kazennova E, Selimova L, et al. A sudden epidemic of HIV type 1 among injecting drug users in the former Soviet Union: identification of subtype A, subtype B, and novel gagA/envB recombinants. AIDS Res Hum Retroviruses 14:669–676, 1998.

262. Liitsola K, Tashkinova I, Laukkanen T, et al. HIV-1 genetic subtype A/B recombinant strain causing an explosive epidemic in injecting drug users in Kaliningrad. AIDS 12:1907–1919, 1998.

262a. McCormack GP, Glynn JR, Crampin AC, et al. Early evolution of the human immunodeficiency virus type 1 subtype C epidemic in rural Malawi. J Virol 76:12890–12899, 2002.

263. Ramos A, Hu DJ, Nguyen L, et al. Intersubtype human immunodeficiency virus type 1 superinfection following seroconversion to a primary infection in two injection drug users. J Virol 76:7444–7452, 2002.

264. McNearney T, Westervelt P, Thielan BJ, et al. Limited sequence heterogeneity among biologically distinct human immunodeficiency virus type 1 isolates from individuals involved in a clustered infection outbreak. Proc Natl Acad Sci U S A 87:1917–1921, 1990.

265. Burger H, Weiser B, Flaherty K, et al. Evolution of human immunodeficiency virus type 1 nucleotide sequence diversity among close contacts. Proc Natl Acad Sci U S A 88:11236–11240, 1991.

266. Wolfs TFW, Zwart G, Bakker M, Goudsmit J. HIV-1 genome RNA diversification following sexual and parenteral virus transmission. Virology 189:103–110, 1992.

267. McDonald RA, Mayers DL, Chung RC-Y, et al. Evolution of human immunodeficiency virus type 1 env sequence variation in patients with diverse rates of disease progression and T-cell function. J Virol 71:1871–1879, 1997.

268. Zhang L, Diaz RS, Ho DD, et al. Host-specific driving force in human immunodeficiency virus type 1 evolution in vivo. J Virol 71:2555–2561, 1997.

269. Wong JK, Ignacio CC, Torriani F, et al. In vivo compartmentalization of human immunodeficiency virus: evidence from the examination of pol sequences from autopsy tissues. J Virol 71:2059–2071, 1997.

270. Albert J, Abrahamson B, Nagy K, et al. Rapid development of isolate-specific neutralizing antibodies after primary HIV-1 infection and consequent emergence of virus variants which resist neutralization by autologous sera. AIDS 4:107–118, 1990.

271. Arendrup M, Nielsen C, Hansen J, et al. Autologous HIV-1 neutralizing antibodies: emergence of neutralization-resistant escape virus and subsequent development of escape virus neutralizing antibodies. J Acquir Immune Defic Syndr 5:303–307, 1992.

272. Phillips RE, Rowland-Jones S, Dixon DF, et al. Human immunodeficiency virus genetic variations that can escape cytotoxic T-cell recognition. Nature 354:453–459, 1991.

273. Koenig S, Conley AJ, Brewah YA, et al. Transfer of HIV-specific cytotoxic T lymphocytes to an AIDS patient leads to selection for mutant HIV variants and subsequent disease progression. Nat Med 1:330–336, 1995.

274. Price DA, Goulder PJR, Klenerman P, et al. Positive selection of HIV-1 cytotoxic lymphocyte escape variants during primary infection. Proc Natl Acad Sci U S A 97:1890–1895, 1997.

275. Ou CJ, Ciesielski CA, Myers G, et al. Molecular epidemiology of HIV transmission in a dental practice. Science 256:1165–1171, 1992.

276. Holmes EC, Zhang LQ, Smith Rogers A, Leigh Brown AJ. Molecular investigation of HIV infection in a patient of an HIV-infected surgeon. J Infect Dis 167:1411–1414, 1993.

277. Popper SJ, Sarr AD, Travers KU, et al. Lower human immunodeficiency virus (HIV) type 2 viral load reflects the difference in pathogenicity of HIV-1 and HIV-2. J Infect Dis 180:1116–1121, 1999.

278. Kanki PJ, Peeters M, Gueye-Ndiaye A. Virology of HIV-1 and HIV-2: implications for Africa. AIDS 11(suppl B):S33–S42, 1997.

279. Shanmugam V, Switzer WM, Nkengasong JN, et al. Lower HIV-2 plasma viral loads may explain differences between the natural histories of HIV-1 and HIV-2 infections. J Acquir Immune Defic Syndr 24:257–263, 2000.

280. Nkengasong JN, Kestens L, Ghys PD, et al. Dual infection with human immunodeficiency virus type 1 and type 2: impact on HIV type 1 viral load and immune activation markers in HIV-seropositive female sex workers in Abidjan, Ivory Coast. AIDS Res Hum Retroviruses 16:1371–1378, 2000.

281. Wiktor SZ, Nkengasong JN, Ekpini ER, et al. Lack of protection against HIV-1 infection among women with HIV-2 infection. AIDS 13:695–699, 1999.

282. Greenberg AE. Possible protective effect of HIV-2 against incident HIV-1 infection: review of available epidemiological and in vitro data. AIDS 15:2319–2321, 2001.

283. Travers K, Mboup S, Marlink R, et al. Natural protection against HIV-1 infection provided by HIV-2. Science 268:1612–1615, 1995.

284. Travers KU, Eisen GE, Marlink RG, et al. Protection from HIV-1 infection by HIV-2. AIDS 12:224–225, 1998.

285. Buve A, Carael M, Hayes RJ, et al. The multicentre study on factors determining the differential spread of HIV in four African cities: summary and conclusions. AIDS 15(suppl 4):S127–S131, 2001.

286. Lamptey PR. Reducing heterosexual transmission of HIV in poor countries. BMJ 324:207–211, 2002.

287. Mastro TD, Kitayaporn D. HIV type 1 transmission probabilities: estimates from epidemiological studies. AIDS Res Hum Retroviruses 14(suppl 3):S223–S227, 1998.

288. Halperin DT, Bailey RC. Male circumcision and HIV infection: 10 years and counting. Lancet 354:1813–1815, 1999.

289. Auvert B, Buve A, Lagarde E, et al. Male circumcision and HIV infection in four cities in sub-Saharan Africa. AIDS 15(suppl 4):S31–S40, 2001.

290. Mastro TD, Satten GA, Nopkesorn T, et al. Probability of female-to-male transmission of HIV-1 in Thailand. Lancet 343:204–207, 1994.

291. Hu DJ, Vanichseni S, Mastro TD, et al. Viral load differences in early infection with two HIV-1 subtypes. AIDS 15:683–691, 2001.

292. Des J. Structural interventions to reduce HIV transmission among injecting drug users. AIDS 14(suppl 1):S41–S46, 2000.

293. Des J, Dehne K, Casabona J. HIV surveillance among injecting drug users. AIDS 15(suppl 4):S13–S22, 2001.

294. Strathdee SA, van Ameijden EJ, Mesquita F, et al. Can HIV epidemics among injection drug users be prevented? AIDS 12(suppl A):S71–S79, 1998.

295. Vanichseni S, Kitayaporn D, Mastro TD, et al. Continued high HIV-1 incidence in a vaccine trial preparatory cohort of injection drug users in Bangkok, Thailand. AIDS 15:397–405, 2001.

296. Choopanya K, Des J, Vanichseni S, et al. Incarceration and risk for HIV infection among injection drug users in Bangkok. J Acquir Immune Defic Syndr 29:86–94, 2002.

297. Gisselquist D, Rothenberg R, Potterat J, Drucker E. Non-sexual transmission of HIV has been overlooked in developing countries. BMJ 324:235, 2002.

298. Drucker E, Alcabes PG, Marx PA. The injection century: massive unsterile injections and the emergence of human pathogens. Lancet 358:1989–1992, 2001.

299. Van de Perre P, Simon A, Hittimana DG, et al. Infective and anti-infective properties of breastmilk from HIV-1 infected women. Lancet 341:914–918, 1993.

300. Pitt J, Brambilla D, Reichelderfer P, et al. Maternal immunological and virologic factors for infant human immunodeficiency virus type 1 infection: findings from the Women and Infants Transmission Study. J Infect Dis 175:567–575, 1997.

301. Shaffer N, Roongpisuthipong A, Siriwasin W, et al. Maternal virus load and perinatal human immunodeficiency virus type 1 subtype E transmission, Thailand. Bangkok Collaborative Perinatal HIV Transmission Study Group. J Infect Dis 179:590–599, 1999.

302. De Cock KM, Fowler MG, Mercier E, et al. Prevention of mother-to-child HIV transmission in resource-poor countries: translating research into policy and practice. JAMA 283:1175–1182, 2000.

303. Katz MH, Schwarcz SK, Kellogg TA, et al. Impact of highly active antiretroviral treatment on HIV seroincidence among men who have sex with men: San Francisco. Am J Public Health 92:388–394, 2002.

304. Bulterys M, Fowler MG, Shaffer N, et al. Role of traditional birth attendants in preventing perinatal transmission of HIV. BMJ 324:222–224, 2002.

305. Ahmed S, Lutalo T, Wawer M, et al. HIV incidence and sexually transmitted disease prevalence associated with condom use: a population study in Rakai, Uganda. AIDS 15:2171–2179, 2001.

306. Weniger BG, Limpakarnjanarat K, Ungchusak K, et al. The epidemiology of HIV infection and AIDS in Thailand. AIDS 5(suppl 2):S71–S85, 1991.

307. Mastro TD, Limpakarnjanarat K. Condom use in Thailand: how much is it slowing the HIV/AIDS epidemic? AIDS 9:523–525, 1995.

308. Nixon DF, Brolinden K, Ogg G, Brolinden PA. Cellular and humoral antigenic epitopes in HIV and SIV. Immunology 76:515–534, 1992.

309. Mascola JR, Louder MK, Winter C, et al. Human immunodeficiency virus type 1 neutralization measured by flow cytometric quantitation of single-round infection of primary human T cells. J Virol 76:4810–4821, 2002.

310. Richman DD, Wrin TL, Little SJ, Petropoulos CJ. Rapid evolution of the neutralizing antibody response to human immunodeficiency virus (HIV) type 1 infection. Proc Nat Acad Sci USA, 100:4144–4149, 2003.

310a. Wei X, Decker JM, Wang S, et al. Antibody neutralization and escape by HIV-1. Nature, 422: 307–312, 2003

311. Ohno T, Terada M, Yoneda Y. A broadly neutralizing monoclonal antibody that recognizes the V3 region of human immunodeficiency virus type 1 glycoprotein gp120. Proc Natl Acad Sci U S A 88:10725–10729, 1991.

312. White-Sharf ME, Potts BJ, Smith LM, et al. Broadly neutralizing monoclonal antibodies to the V3 region of HIV-1 can be elicited by peptide immunization. Virology 192:197–206, 1993.

313. Emini EA, Nara PL, Schleif WA, et al. Antibody-mediated in vitro neutralization of human immunodeficiency virus type 1 abolishes infectivity for chimpanzees. J Virol 64:3674–3678, 1990.

314. Emini EA, Schleif WA, Numhong JM, et al. Prevention of HIV-1 infection in chimpanzees by gp120 V3 domain–specific monoclonal antibody. Nature 355:728–730, 1992.

315. Berman PW, Gregory TJ, Riddle L, et al. Protection of chimpanzees from infection by HIV-1 after vaccination with recombinant glycoprotein gp120 but not gp160. Nature 345:622–625, 1990.

316. Girard M, Kieny MP, Pinter A, et al. Immunization of chimpanzees confers protection against challenge with human immunodeficiency virus. Proc Natl Acad Sci U S A 88:542–546, 1991.

317. Fultz PN, Nara P, Barre-Sinoussi F, et al. Vaccine protection of chimpanzees against challenge with HIV-1 infected peripheral blood mononuclear cells. Science 256:1687–1690, 1992.

318. Bruck C, Thiriart C, Fabry L, et al. HIV-1 envelope-elicited neutralizing antibody titres correlate with protection and virus load in chimpanzees. Vaccine 12:1141–1148, 1994.

319. Girard M, Meignier B, Barré-Sinoussi F, et al. Vaccine-induced protection of chimpanzees against infection by a heterologous human immunodeficiency virus type 1. J Virol 69:6239–6248, 1995.

320. Berman PW, Murthy KK, Wrin T, et al. Protection of MN-gp120–immunized chimpanzees from heterologous infection with a primary isolate of human immunodeficiency virus type 1. J Infect Dis 173:52–59, 1996.

321. Bou-Habib DC, Roderiquez G, Ovarecz T, et al. Cryptic nature of envelope V3 region epitopes protects primary monocytotropic human immunodeficiency virus type 1 from antibody neutralization. J Virol 68:6006–6013, 1994.

322. Moore JP, Cao Y, Qing L, et al. Primary isolates of human immunodeficiency virus type 1 are relatively resistant to neutralization by monoclonal antibodies to gp120, and their neutralization is not predicted by studies with monomeric gp120. J Virol 69:101–109, 1995.

323. Vancott TC, Polonis VR, Loomis LD. Differential role of V3-specific antibodies in neutralization assays involving primary and laboratory-adapted isolates of HIV type 1. AIDS Res Hum Retroviruses 11:1379–1391, 1995.

324. Bjorling E, Broliden K, Bernardi D, et al. Hyperimmune sera against synthetic peptides representing the glycoprotein of human immunodeficiency virus type 2 can mediate neutralization and antibody-dependent cytotoxic activity. Proc Natl Acad Sci U S A 88:6082–6086, 1991.

325. Javaherian K, Langlois AJ, Schmidt S, et al. The principal neutralization determinant of simian immunodeficiency virus differs from that of human immunodeficiency virus type 1. Proc Natl Acad Sci U S A 89:1418–1422, 1992.

326. Park EJ, Quinnan GV. Both neutralization resistance and high infectivity phenotypes are caused by mutations of interacting residues in the human immunodeficiency virus type 1 gp 41 leucine zipper and the gp120 receptor- and coreceptor-binding domains. J Virol 73:5707–5713, 1999.

327. Park EJ, Zolla-Pasner S, Quinnan GV. Distinct mechanisms mediating enhanced infectivity and envelope conformational change determine global neutralization resistance phenotype of immunodeficiency virus type 1. J Virol 74:4183–4191, 2000.

328. Zhang PF, Bouma P, Park EJ, et al. A variable region 3 (V3) mutation determines a global neutralization phenotype and CD4-independent infectivity of a human immunodeficiency virus type 1 envelope associated with a broadly cross-reactive primary virus-neutralizing antibodies response. J Virol 76:644–655, 2002.

329. Sawyer LS, Wrin MT, Crawford-Miksza L, et al. Neutralization sensitivity of human immunodeficiency virus type 1 is determined in part by the cell in which the virus is propagated. J Virol 68:1342–1349, 1994.

330. Wrin T, Loh TP, Vennari JC, et al. Adaptation to persistent growth in the H9 cell line renders a primary isolate of human immunodeficiency virus type 1 sensitive to neutralization by vaccinee sera. J Virol 69:39–48, 1995.

331. Moore JP, Ho DD. HIV-1 neutralization: the consequences of viral adaptation to growth on transformed T cells. AIDS 9(suppl A):S117–S136, 1995.

331a. Gorny MK, Williams C, Volsky B, et al. Human monoclonal antibodies specific for conformation-sensitive epitopes of V3 neutralize human immunodeficiency virus type 1 primary isolates from various clades. J Virol 76:9035–9045, 2002.

332. McKeating JA, Shotton C, Cordell J, et al. Characterization of neutralizing monoclonal antibodies to linear and conformation-dependent epitopes within the first and second variable domains of human immunodeficiency virus type 1 gp120. J Virol 67:4937–4944, 1993.

333. Gorny MK, Moore JP, Conley AH, et al. Human anti-V2 monoclonal antibody that neutralizes primary but not laboratory isolates of human immunodeficiency virus type 1. J Virol 68:8312–8320, 1994.

334. Wu Z, Kayman SC, Honnen W, et al. Characterization of neutralization epitopes in the V2 region of human immunodeficiency virus type 1 gp120: role of glycosylation in the correct folding of the V1/V2 domain. J Virol 69:2271–2278, 1995.

335. Burton DR, Pyati J, Koduri R, et al. Efficient neutralization of primary isolates of HIV-1 by a recombinant human monoclonal antibody. Science 266:1024–1027, 1994.

336. Kessler JA II, McKenna PM, Emini EA, et al. Recombinant human monoclonal antibody IgG1b12 neutralizes diverse human immunodeficiency virus type 1 primary isolates. AIDS Res Hum Retroviruses 13:575–582, 1997.

337. Mo H, Stamamatos L, Ip JE, et al. Human immunodeficiency virus type 1 mutants that escape neutralization by human monoclonal antibody IgG1b12. J Virol 71:6869–6874, 1997.

338. Zwick MB, Bonnycastle LLC, Menendez A, et al. Identification and characterization of a peptide that specifically binds the human, broadly neutralizing anti-human immunodeficiency virus type 1 antibody b12. J Virol 75:6692–6699, 2001.

339. Trkola A, Purtscher M, Muster T, et al. Human monoclonal antibody 2G12 defines a distinctive neutralization epitope on the gp120 glycoprotein of human immunodeficiency virus type 1. J Virol 70:1100–1108, 1996.

340. Scanlan CN, Pantophlet R, Wormald MR, et al. The broadly neutralizing anti-human immunodeficiency virus type 1 antibody 2G12 recognizes a cluster of $\alpha1\rightarrow2$ mannose residues on the outer face of gp120. J Virol 76:7306–7321, 2002.

341. Muster T, Steindl F, Purtscher M, et al. A conserved neutralizing epitope on gp41 of human immunodeficiency virus type 1. J Virol 67:6642–6647, 1993.

342. Purtscher M, Trkola A, Gruber G, et al. A broadly neutralizing human monoclonal antibody against gp41 of human immunodeficiency virus type 1. AIDS Res Hum Retroviruses 10:1651–1658, 1994.

343. Zwick MB, Labrijn AF, Wang M, et al. Broadly neutralizing antibodies targeted to the membrane-proximal external region of human immunodeficiency virus type 1 glycoprotein gp41. J Virol 75:10892–10905, 2001.

344. Xu W, Smith-Franklin B, Li PL, et al. Potent neutralisation of primary human immunodeficiency virus clade C isolates with a synergistic combination of human monoclonal antibodies raised against clade B. J Hum Virol 4:55–61, 2001.

345. Gauduin MC, Parren PWHI, Weir R, Johnson RP. Passive immunization with a human monoclonal antibody protects hu-PBL-SCID mice against challenge by primary isolates of HIV-1. Nat Med 3:1389–1393, 1997.

346. Mascola JR, Lewis MG, Stiegler G, et al. Protection of macaques against pathogenic simian/human immunodeficiency virus 89.6PD by passive transfer of neutralizing antibodies. J Virol 73:4009–4018, 1999.

347. Mascola JR, Stiegler G, Van Cott TC, et al. Protection of macaques against vaginal transmission of a pathogenic HIV-1/SIV chimeric virus by passive infusion of neutralizing antibodies. Nat Med 6:207–210, 2000.

348. Parren PWHI, Marx PA, Hessel AJ, et al. Antibody protects macaques against vaginal challenge with a pathogenic R5 simian/human immunodeficiency virus at serum levels giving complete neutralization in vitro. J Virol 75:8340–8347, 2001.

349. Ruprecht RM, Hoffman-Lehmann R, Smith-Franklin BA, et al. Protection of neonatal macaques against experimental SHIV infection by human neutralizing monoclonal antibodies. Tranfus Clin Biol 8:350–358, 2001.

350. Conley AJ, Kessler JA II, Boots LJ, et al. The consequence of passive administration of an anti-human immunodeficiency virus type 1 neutralizing monoclonal antibody before challenge of chimpanzees with a primary virus isolate. J Virol 70:6751–6758, 1996.

351. Baba TW, Liska V, Hofmann-Lehmann R, et al. Human neutralizing monoclonal antibodies of the IgG1 subtype protect against mucosal simian-human immunodeficiency virus infection. Nat Med 6:200–206, 2000.

351a. Pantophlet R, Ollmann Saphire E, Poignard P, et al. Fine mapping of the interaction of neutralizing and nonneutralizing monoclonal antibodies with the CD4-binding site of human immunodeficiency virus type 1 gp120. J Virol 77:642–658, 2003.

352. Pinter A, Honnen WJ, Racho ME, Tilley SA. A potent, neutralizing monoclonal antibody against a unique epitope overlapping the CD4-binding site of HIV-1 gp120 that is broadly conserved across North American and African virus isolates. AIDS Res Hum Retroviruses 9:985–996, 1993.

353. Thali M, Furman C, Ho DD, et al. Discontinuous, conserved neutralization epitopes overlapping the CD4-binding region of human immunodeficiency virus type 1 gp120 envelope glycoprotein. J Virol 66:5635–5641, 1992.

353a. Raja A, Venturi M, Kwong P, Sodroski J. CD4 binding site antibodies inhibit human immunodeficiency virus gp120 envelope glycoprotein intersection with CCR5. J Virol 77:713–718, 2003.

354. Parren PWHI, Fisicaro P, Labrijn AF, et al. In vitro antigen challenge of human antibody libraries for vaccine evaluation: the human immunodeficiency virus type 1 envelope. J Virol 70:9046–9050, 1996.

355. Parren PWHI, Gauduin M-C, Koup RA, et al. Relevance of the antibody response against human immunodeficiency virus type 1 envelope to vaccine design. Immunol Lett 57:105–112, 1997.

356. Earl PL, Broder CC, Long D, et al. Native oligomeric human immunodeficiency virus type 1 envelope glycoprotein elicits diverse monoclonal antibody reactivities. J Virol 68:3015–3036, 1994.

357. Poignard P, Klasse PJ, Sattentau QJ. Antibody neutralization of HIV-1. Immunol Today 17:239–246, 1996.

358. Fouts TR, Binley JM, Trkola A, et al. Neutralization of the human immunodeficiency virus type 1 primary isolate JR-FL by human monoclonal antibodies correlates with antibody binding to the oligomeric form of the envelope glycoprotein complex. J Virol 71:2779–2785, 1997.

359. Thali M, Olshevsky U, Furman C, et al. Characterization of a discontinuous human immunodeficiency virus type 1 gp120 epitope recognized by a broadly reactive neutralizing human monoclonal antibody. J Virol 65:6188–6193, 1991.

359a. Dey B, Del Castillo CS, Berger EA. Neutralization of human immunodeficiency virus type 1 by CD4-17b, a single-chain chimeric protein based on sequential interaction of gp120 with CD4 and coreceptor. J Virol 77:2859–2865, 2003.

360. Van Cott TC, Bethke FR, Burke DS, et al. Lack of induction of antibodies specific for conserved, discontinuous epitopes of HIV-1 envelope glycoprotein by candidate AIDS vaccines. J Immunol 155:4100–4110, 1995.

361. Mascola JR, Snyder SW, Weislow OS, et al. Immunization with envelope subunit vaccine products elicits neutralizing antibodies against laboratory-adapted but not primary isolates of human immunodeficiency virus type 1. J Infect Dis 173:340–348, 1996.

362. Kang C-Y, Hariharan K, Nara PL, et al. Immunization with a soluble CD4-gp120 complex preferentially induces neutralizing anti–human immunodeficiency virus type 1 antibodies directed to conformation-dependent epitopes of gp120. J Virol 68:5854–5862, 1994.

363. DeVico A, Silver A, Thornton APM, et al. Covalently crosslinked complexes of human immunodeficiency virus type 1 (HIV-1) gp120 and CD4 receptors elicit a neutralizing immune response that includes antibodies selective for primary virus isolates. Virology 218:258–263, 1996.

364. Zhang W, Canziani G, Plugarin C, et al. Conformational changes of gp120 in epitopes near the CCR5-binding site are induced by CD4 and a CD4 miniproteomimetic. Biochemistry 38:9405–9413, 1999.

365. Fouts TR, Tuskan R, Godfrey K, et al. Expansion and characterization of a single-chain polypeptide analogue of the human immunodeficiency virus type 1 gp120-CD4 receptor complex. J Virol 74:11427–11436, 2000.

366. Barnett SW, Lu S, Srivastava I, et al. The ability of an oligomeric human immunodeficiency virus type I (HIV-1) envelope antigen to elicit neutralizing antibodies against primary HIV-1 isolates is improved following partial deletion of the second hypervariable region. J Virol 75:5526–5540, 2001.

367. Weber J, Fenyö E-M, Beddons S, et al. Neutralization serotypes of human immunodeficiency virus type 1 field isolates are not predicted by genetic subtype. J Virol 70:7827–7832, 1996.

368. Nyambi PN, Nkengasong J, Lewi P, et al. Multivariate analysis of human immunodeficiency virus type 1 neutralization data. J Virol 70:6235–6243, 1996.

369. Moore JP, Cao Y, Leu J, et al. Inter- and intraclade neutralization of human immunodeficiency virus type 1 genetic clades do not correspond to neutralization serotypes but partially correspond to gp120 antigenic serotypes. J Virol 70:427–444, 1996.

370. Kostrikis LG, Cao Y, Ngal H, et al. Quantitative analysis of serum neutralization of human immunodeficiency virus type 1 from subtypes A, B, C, D, E, F, and I: lack of direct correlation between neutralization epitopes and genetic subtypes and evidence for prevalent serum-dependent infectivity enhancement. J Virol 70:445–458, 1996.

371. Mascola JR, Louder MK, Surman SR, et al. Human immunodeficiency virus type 1 neutralizing antibody serotyping using serum pools and an infectivity reduction assay. AIDS Res Hum Retroviruses 12:1319–1328, 1996.

372. Nyambi MN, Willems B, Janssens W, et al. The neutralization relationship of HIV type 1, HIV type 2, and SIVcpz is reflected in the genetic diversity that distinguishes them. AIDS Res Hum Retroviruses 13:7–17, 1997.

373. Moore JP, McCutchan FE, Poon S-W, et al. Exploration of antigenic variation in gp120 from clades A through F of human immunodeficiency virus type 1 by using monoclonal antibodies. J Virol 68:8350–8364, 1994.

374. Laal S, Burda S, Gorny MK, et al. Synergistic neutralization of human immunodeficiency virus type 1 by combinations of human monoclonal antibodies. J Virol 68:4001–4008, 1994.

375. Tilley SA, Honnen WJ, Racho ME, et al. Synergistic neutralization of HIV-1 by human monoclonal antibodies against the V3 loop and the CD4-binding site of gp120. AIDS Res Hum Retroviruses 89:461–467, 1992.

376. Zwick MB, Wang M, Poignard P, et al. Neutralization synergy of human immunodeficiency virus type 1 primary isolates by cocktails of broadly neutralizing antibodies. J Virol 75:12198–12208, 2001.

377. Moog C, Fleury HJA, Pellegrin C, et al. Autologous and heterologous neutralizing antibody responses following initial seroconversion in human immunodeficiency virus type-1 infected individuals. J Virol 71:3734–3741, 1997.

378. Montefiori DC, Reimann KA, Wyand MS, et al. Neutralizing antibodies in sera from macaques infected with chimeric simian-human immunodeficiency virus containing the envelope glycoproteins of either a laboratory-adapted variant or a primary isolate of human immunodeficiency virus type 1. J Virol 72:3427–3431, 1998.

379. Wyand MS, Manson KH, Garcia-Moll M, et al. Vaccine protection by a triple deletion mutant of simian immunodeficiency virus. J Virol 70:3724–3733, 1996.

380. Cole KS, Rowles JL, Jagerski BA, et al. Evolution of envelope-specific antibody responses in monkeys experimentally infected or immunized with simian immunodeficiency virus and its association with the development of protective immunity. J Virol 71:5069–5079, 1997.

380a. Howe L, Leroux C, Issel CJ, Montelaro RC. Equine infectious anemia virus envelope evolution in vivo during persistent infection progressively increase resistance to in vitro serum antibody neutralization as a dominant phenotype. J Virol 76:10588–10597, 2002.

381. Homsy J, Meyer M, Levy JA. Serum enhancement of human immunodeficiency virus (HIV) infection correlates with disease in HIV-infected individuals. J Virol 64:1437–1440, 1990.

382. Robinson WE Jr, Montefiori DC, Mitchell WM. Complement-mediated antibody-dependent enhancement of HIV-1 infection requires CD4 and complement receptors. Virology 175:600–604, 1990.

383. Boyer V, Desgranges C, Travaud M, et al. Complement mediates human immunodeficiency virus type 1–infection of a human T cell line in a CD4- and antibody-independent fashion. J Exp Med 173:1151–1158, 1991.

384. Takeda A, Tuazon CV, Ennis FA. Antibody-enhanced infection by HIV-1 via Fc receptor–mediated entry. Science 242:580–583, 1988.

385. Jouault T, Chapuis F, Olivier R, et al. HIV infection of monocytic cells: role of antibody-mediated virus binding to Fc-gamma receptors. AIDS 3:125–131, 1989.

386. Robinson WE Jr, Kawamura T, Gorny MK, et al. Human monoclonal antibodies to the human immunodeficiency virus type 1 (HIV-1) transmembrane glycoprotein gp41 enhance HIV-infection in vitro. Proc Natl Acad Sci U S A 87:3185–3189, 1990.

387. Jiang S, Neurath AR. Potential risks of eliciting antibodies enhancing HIV-1 infection of monocytic cells by vaccination with V3 loops of unmatched HIV-1 isolates. AIDS 6:331–332, 1992.

388. Klikr SC, Shludo I, Haigwood NLO, Levy JA. V3 variability can influence the ability of an antibody to neutralize or to enhance infection by diverse strains of human immunodeficiency virus type 1. Proc Natl Acad Sci U S A 90:11518–11522, 1993.

389. Montefiori DC, Pantaleo G, Fink LM, et al. Neutralizing and infection-enhancing antibody responses to human immunodeficiency virus type 1 in long-term nonprogressors. J Infect Dis 173:60–67, 1996.

390. Verrier F, Moog C, Barré-Sinoussi F, et al. L'immunisation du macaque avec les virions purifiés d'un isolat primaire du virus de l'immunodéficience humaine de type 1 induit des anticorps facilitants. Bull Acad Natl Med 184:67–87, 1999.

391. Tyler DJ, Lyerly HK, Weinhold KJ. Anti–HIV-1 ADCC (mini-review). AIDS Res Hum Retroviruses 5:557–563, 1989.

392. Tanneau F, McChesney M, Lopez O, et al. Primary cytotoxicity against the envelope glycoprotein of human immunodeficiency virus-1: evidence for antibody-dependent cellular cytotoxicity in vivo. J Infect Dis 162:837–843, 1990.

393. Posner MR, Elboim HS, Cannon T, et al. Functional activity of an HIV-1 neutralizing IgG human monoclonal antibody: ADCC and complement-mediated lysis. AIDS Res Hum Retroviruses 8:553–558, 1992.

394. Kent SJ, Woodward A, Zhao A. Human immunodeficiency virus type 1 (HIV-1)–specific T cell responses correlate with control of acute HIV-1 infection in macaques. J Infect Dis 176:1188–1197, 1997.

395. Matana T, Shibata R, Siemon C, et al. Administration of an anti-CD8 monoclonal antibody interferes with the clearance of chimeric simian/human immunodeficiency viruses during primary infection of rhesus macaques. J Virol 72:164–169, 1998.

396. Harrer T, Harrer E, Kalams SA, et al. Cytotoxic T-lymphocytes in asymptomatic long-term nonprogressing HIV-1 infection. J Immunol 156:2616–2623, 1996.

397. Rosenberg ES, Billingoley JM, Caliendo AM, et al. Vigorous HIV-1-specific CD4+ T cell responses associated with control of viremia. Science 278:1447–1450, 1997.

398. Murphey-Corb M, Wilson LA, Trichel AM, et al. Selective induction of protective MHC class I-restricted CTL in the intestinal lamina propria of rhesus macaques by transient SIV infection of the colonic mucosa. J Immunol 162:540–549, 1999.

399. Johnson RP, Glickman RL, Young JQ, et al. Induction of vigorous cytotoxic T-lymphocyte responses by live attenuated simian immunodeficiency virus. J Virol 71:7711–7718, 1997.

400. Yang OO, Kalams SA, Trocha A, et al. Suppression of human immunodeficiency type 1 replication by CD8+ cells: evidence for HLA class I–restricted triggering of cytolytic and noncytolytic mechanisms. J Virol 71:3120–3128, 1997.

401. Aubertin AM, Le Grand R, Wang Y, et al. Generation of CD8+ T-cell-generated suppressor factor and beta-chemokines by targeted iliac lymph node immunization in rhesus monkeys challenged with SHIV-89.6P by the rectal route. AIDS Res Hum Retroviruses 16:381–392, 2000.

402. Wang Y, Tao L, Mitchell E, et al. Generation of CD8 suppressor factor and beta chemokines, induced by xenogeneic immunization, in the prevention of simian immunodeficiency virus infection in macaques. Proc Natl Acad Sci U S A 95:5223–5228, 1998.

403. Wang Y, Tao L, Mitchell E, et al. Allo-immunization elicits CD8+ T cell-derived chemokine HIV suppressor factors and resistance to HIV infection in women. Nat Med 5:1004–1009, 1999.

404. Allen TM, Watkins DI. New insights into evaluating effective T-cell responses to HIV. AIDS 15(suppl 5):S117–S126, 2001.

405. Goulder PJ, Altfeld M, Rosenberg ES, et al. Substantial differences in specificity of HIV-1 specific cytotoxic T cells in acute and chronic HIV infections. J Exp Med 193:181–193, 2001.

406. Addo MM, Altfeld M, Rosenberg ES, et al. The HIV-1 regulatory proteins Tat and Rev are frequently targeted by cytotoxic T lymphocytes derived from HIV-1-infected individuals. Proc Nat Acad Sci U S A 98:1781–1786, 2001.

407. Altfeld M, Addo MM, Elridge RL, et al. Vpr is preferentially targeted by CTL during HIV-1 infection. J Immunol 167:2743–2752, 2001.

408. Autran B, Levine NL. HIV epitopes recognized by cytotoxic T-lymphocytes. AIDS 5(suppl 2):S145–S150, 1991.

409. Wilson CC, Kalams SA, Wilkes BM, et al. Overlapping epitopes in human immunodeficiency virus type 1 gp120 presented by HLA-A, -B, and -C molecules: effects of viral variation on cytotoxic T-lymphocyte recognition. J Virol 71:1256–1264, 1997.

410. Stanhope PE, Clements ML, Siliciano RF. Human CD4+ cytotoxic T-lymphocyte responses to a human immunodeficiency virus type 1 gp160 subunit vaccine. J Infect Dis 168:92–100, 1993.

411. Koenig S, Fuerst TR, Wood L, et al. Mapping the fine specificity of cytolytic T-cell response to HIV-1 Nef protein. J Immunol 145:127–131, 1990.

412. Ferrari G, Humphrey W, McElrath MJ, et al. Clade B–based HIV-1 vaccines elicit cross-clade cytotoxic T-lymphocyte reactivites in uninfected volunteers. Proc Natl Acad Sci U S A 94:1396–1401, 1997.

413. Lohman BL, Miller CJ, McChesney MB. Antiviral cytotoxic T-lymphocytes in vaginal mucosa of simian immunodeficiency virus–infected rhesus macaques. J Immunol 155:5855–5860, 1995.

414. Couëdel-Courteille A, Le Grand R, Tulliez M, et al. Direct ex vivo simian immunodeficiency virus (SIV)–specific cytotoxic activity detected from small intestine intraepithelial lymphocytes of SIV-infected macaques at an advanced stage of infection. J Virol 71:1052–1057, 1997.

415. Yasutomi Y, Koenig S, Woods RM, et al. A vaccine-elicited, single viral epitope-specific cytotoxic T-lymphocyte response does not protect against intravenous, cell-free simian immunodeficiency virus challenge. J Virol 69:2279–2284, 1995.

416. Cease KB, Margalit H, Cornette JL, et al. Helper T-cell antigenic site identification in the acquired immunodeficiency syndrome virus gp120 envelope protein and induction of immunity in mice to the native protein using a 16 residue synthetic peptide. Proc Natl Acad Sci U S A 84:4249–4253, 1987.

417. Hirsch VM, Goldstein S, Hynes NA, et al. Prolonged clinical latency and survival of macaques given a whole inactivated simian immunodeficiency virus vaccine. J Infect Dis 170:51–59, 1994.

418. Stott EJ. Anti-cell antibody in macaques [letter]. Nature 253:393, 1991.

419. Arthur LO, Bess JW Jr, Urban RG, et al. Macaques immunized with HLA-DR are protected from challenge with simian immunodeficiency virus. J Virol 69:3117–3124, 1995.

420. Neidrig M, Gregerson JP, Fultz PN, et al. Immune responses of chimpanzees after immunization with the inactivated whole immunodeficiency virus (HIV-1), three different adjuvants and challenge. Vaccine 11:67–74, 1993.

421. Arthur LO, Bess JW Jr, Chertova EN, et al. Chemical inactivation of retroviral infectivity by targeting nucleocapsid protein zinc fingers: a candidate SIV vaccine. AIDS Res Hum Retrovirus 14(suppl 3):S311–S319, 1998.

422. Lin L, Cook DN, Wiesehahn GP, et al. Photochemical inactivation of viruses and bacteria in platelet concentrates by use of a novel psoralen and long-wavelength ultraviolet light. Transfusion 37:423–435, 1997.

423. Chertova E, Bess JW Jr, Crise BJ, et al. Envelope glycoprotein incorporation, not shedding of surface envelope glycoprotein (gp120/SU), is the primary determinant of SU content of purified human immunodeficiency virus type 1 and simian immunodeficiency virus. J Virol 76:5315–5325, 2002.

424. Montefiori DC, Safrit JT, Lydy SL, et al. Induction of neutralizing antibodies and gag-specific cellular immune responses to an R5 primary isolate of human immunodeficiency virus type 1 in rhesus macaques. J Virol 75:5879–5890, 2001.

425. Dedieu JF, Ronco J, van der Werf S, et al. Poliovirus chimaeras expressing sequences from the principal neutralization domain of human immunodeficiency virus type 1. J Virol 66:3161–3167, 1992.

426. Grene E, Mezule G, Borisova G, et al. Relationship between antigenicity and immunogenicity of chimeric hepatitis B virus core particles carrying HIV type 1 epitopes. AIDS Res Hum Retroviruses 13:41–51, 1997.

427. Schlienger K, Mancini M, Riviere Y, et al. Human immunodeficiency virus type 1 major neutralizing determinant exposed on hepatitis B surface antigen particles is highly immunogenic in primates. J Virol 66:2570–2576, 1991.

428. Adams SE, Dawson KM, Gull K, et al. The expression of hybrid HIV:Ty virus-like particles in yeast. Nature 329:68–70, 1987.

429. Layton GT, Harris SJ, Gearing AJH, et al. Induction of HIV-1-specific cytotoxic T lymphocytes in vivo with hybrid HIV-1 V3:Ty-virus-like particles. J Immunol 151:1097–1107, 1993.

430. Marthas ML, Sutjipto S, Higgins J, et al. Immunization with a live-attenuated simian immunodeficiency virus (SIV) prevents early disease but not infection in rhesus macaques challenged with pathogenic SIV. J Virol 64:3694–3700, 1990.

431. Lohman BL, McChesney MB, Miller CJ, et al. A partially attenuated simian immunodeficiency virus induces host immunity that correlates with resistance to pathogenic virus challenge. J Virol 68:7021–7029, 1994.

431a. Shacklett BL, Shaw KES, Adamson LA, et al. Live, attenuated simian immunodeficiency virus SIVmac-M4, with point mutations in the Env transmembrane protein intracytoplasmic domain, provides partial protection from mucosal challenge with pathogenic SIVmac251. J Virol 76:11365–11378, 2002.

432. Gibbs JS, Regier DA, Desrosiers RC. Construction and in vitro properties of SIVmac mutants with deletions in "nonessential" genes. AIDS Res Hum Retroviruses 10:607–616, 1994.

433. Cranage MP, Whatmore AM, Sharpe SA, et al. Macaques infected with live attenuated SIVmac are protected against superinfection via the rectal mucosa. Virology 229:143–154, 1997.

434. Baba TW, Liska V, Khimani AH, et al. Live attenuated, multiply deleted simian immunodeficiency virus causes AIDS in infant and adult macaques. Nat Med 5:194–203, 1999.

435. Wyand MS, Manson KH, Lackner AA, Desrosiers RC. Resistance of neonatal monkeys to live attenuated vaccine strains of simian immunodeficiency virus. Nat Med 3:32–36, 1997.

436. Cohen J. Weakened SIV vaccine still kills. Science 278:24–25, 1997.

436a. Hofmann-Lehmann R, Vlasak J, Williams AL, et al. Live attenuated, *nef*-deleted SIV is pathogenic in most adult macaques after prolonged observation. AIDS 17:157–166, 2003.

437. Giavedoni L, Ahmad S, Jones L, Yilma T. Expression of gamma interferon by simian immunodeficiency virus increases attenuation and reduces postchallenge virus load in vaccinated rhesus macaques. J Virol 71:866–872, 1997.

438. Chakrabarti BK, Maitra RK, Ma XZ, Kestler HW. A candidate live inactivatable attenuated vaccine for AIDS. Proc Natl Acad Sci U S A 93:9810–9815, 1996.

439. Guan Y, Whitney JB, Detorio M, Wainberg MA. Construction and in vitro properties of a series of attenuated simian immunodeficiency viruses with all accessory genes deleted. J Virol 75:4056–4067, 2001.

440. Von Gegerfelt AS, Liska V, Li PL, et al. Rev-independent SIV strains are nonpathogenic in neonatal macaques. J Virol 76:96–104, 2002.

440a. Johnson RP, Lifson JD, Czajak SC, et al. Highly attenuated vaccine strains of simian immunodeficiency virus protect against vaginal challenge inverse relationship of degree of protection with level of attenuation. J Virol 73:4952–4961, 1999.

441. Deacon NJ, Tsykin A, Solomon A, et al. Genomic structure of an attenuated quasi species of HIV-1 from a blood transfusion donor and recipients. Science 270:988–991, 1995.

442. Mariani R, Kirchhoff F, Greenough TC, et al. High frequency of defective *nef* alleles in a long-term survivor with nonprogressive human immunodeficiency virus type 1 infection. J Virol 70:7752–7764, 1996.

443. Greenough TC, Sullivan JL, Desrosiers RC. Declining CD4 T-cell counts in a person infected with nef-deleted HIV-1. N Engl J Med 340:236–237, 1999.

444. Learmont JC, Geczy AF, Mills J, et al. Immunological and virologic status after 14 to 18 years of infection with an attenuated strain of HIV-1. N Engl J Med 340:1715–1722, 1999.

445. Jekle A, Schramm B, Jayakumar P, et al. Coreceptor phenotype of natural human immunodeficiency virus with nef deleted evolves in vivo, leading to increased virulence. J Virol 76:6966–6973, 2002.

446. Clements JE, Montelaro RC, Zinc MC, et al. Cross-protective immune responses induced in rhesus macaque by immunization with attenuated macrophage-tropic simian immunodeficiency virus. J Virol 69:2737–2744, 1995.

447. Bogers WMJM, Niphuis H, ten Haaft P, et al. Protection from HIV-1 envelope bearing chimeric simian immunodeficiency virus (SHIV) in rhesus macaques infected with attenuated SIV: consequences of challenge. AIDS 9:F13–F18, 1995.

448. Shibata R, Siemon C, Czajak SC, et al. Live, attenuated simian immunodeficiency virus vaccines elicit potent resistance against a challenge with a human immunodeficiency virus type 1 chimeric virus. J Virol 71:8141–8148, 1997.

449. Putkonen P, Mäkitalo B, Böttiger D, et al. Protection of human immunodeficiency virus type 2–exposed seronegative macaques from mucosal simian immunodeficiency virus transmission. J Virol 71:4981–4984, 1997.

450. Benson J, Chougnet C, Robert-Guroff M, et al. Recombinant vaccine–induced protection against the highly pathogenic simian immunodeficiency virus SIV(mac251): dependence on route of challenge exposure. J Virol 72:4170–4182, 1998.

451. Zagury D, Bernard J, Cheynier R, et al. A group-specific anamnestic immune reaction against HIV-1 induced by a candidate vaccine against AIDS. Nature 332:728–731, 1988.

452. Graham BS, Belshe RB, Clements ML, et al. Vaccination of vaccinia-naive adults with human immunodeficiency virus type 1 gp160 recombinant vaccinia virus in a blinded, controlled, randomized clinical trial. J Infect Dis 166:244–252, 1992.

453. Gallimore A, Cranage M, Cook N, et al. Early suppression of SIV replication by CD8+ nef-specific cytotoxic T cells in vaccinated macaques. Nat Med 1:1167–1173, 1995.

454. Tartaglia J, Perkus ME, Taylor J, et al. NYVAC: a highly attenuated strain of vaccinia virus. Virology 188:217–232, 1992.

455. Meyer H, Sutter G, Mayr A. Mapping of deletions in the genome of the highly attenuated vaccinia virus MVA and their influence on virulence. J Gen Virol 72:1031–1038, 1991.

456. Moss B, Carroll MW, Wyatt LS, et al. Host-range restricted non-replicating vaccinia virus vectors as vaccine candidates. Adv Exp Med Biol 397:7–13, 1996.

457. Paoletti E, Taylor J, Meigner B, et al. Highly attenuated poxvirus vectors: Nyvac, Alvac, and Trovac. Dev Biol Stand 84:159–163, 1995.

458. Abimiku A, Franchini G, Tartaglia J, et al. HIV-1 recombinant poxvirus vaccine induces cross-protection against HIV-2 challenge in rhesus macaques. Nat Med 1:321–329, 1995.

459. Hirsch VM, Fuerst TR, Sutter G, et al. Patterns of viral replication correlate with outcome in simian immunodeficiency virus (SIV)–infected macaques: effect of prior immunization with a trivalent SIV vaccinia in modified vaccinia virus Ankara. J Virol 70:3741–3752, 1996.

460. Ourmanov I, Brown CR, Moss B, et al. Comparative efficacy of recombinant modified vaccinia virus Ankara expressing simian immunodeficiency virus (SIV) Gag-Pol and/or Env in macaques challenged with pathogenic SIV. J Virol 74:2740–2751, 2000.

461. Barouch DH, Santra S, Kuroda MJ, et al. Reduction of simian-human immunodeficiency virus 89.6P viremia in rhesus monkeys by recombinant modified vaccinia virus Ankara vaccination. J Virol 75:5151–5158, 2001.

462. Seth A, Ourmanov I, Schmitz JE, et al. Immunization with a modified vaccinia virus expressing simian immunodeficiency virus (SIV) Gag-Pol primes for an anamnestic Gag-specific cytotoxic T-lymphocyte response and is associated with reduction of viremia after SIV challenge. J Virol 74:2502–2509, 2000.

463. Kent SJ, Zhao A, Best SJ, et al. Enhanced T-cell immunogenicity and protective efficacy of a human immunodeficiency virus type 1 vaccine regimen consisting of consecutive priming with DNA and boosting with recombinant fowlpox virus. J Virol 72:10180–10188, 1998.

464. Robinson HL, Montefiori DC, Johnson RP, et al. Neutralizing antibody-independent containment of immunodeficiency virus challenge by DNA priming and recombinant pox virus booster immunization. Nat Med 5:526–534, 1999.

465. Robinson HL. New hope for an AIDS vaccine. Nat Rev Immunol 2:239–250, 2002.

466. Lubeck MD, Natuk RJ, Chengalvala M, et al. Immunogenicity of recombinant adenovirus–human immunodeficiency virus vaccines in chimpanzees following intranasal administration. AIDS Res Hum Retroviruses 10:1443–1449, 1994.

467. Lubeck MD, Natuk RJ, Myagkikh M, et al. Long-term protection of chimpanzees against high-dose HIV-1 challenge induced by immunization. Nat Med 3:651–658, 1997.

468. Buge SL, Richardson E, Alipanah S, et al. An adenovirus-simian immunodeficiency virus env vaccine elicits humoral, cellular, and mucosal immune responses in rhesus macaques and decreases viral burden following vaginal challenge. J Virol 71:8531–8541, 1997.

469. Shiver JW, Fu TM, Chen L, et al. Replication-incompetent adenoviral vaccine vector elicits effective anti-immunodeficiency-virus immunity. Nature 415:331–335, 2002.

470. Davis NL, Caley IJ, Brown KW, et al. Vaccination of macaques against pathogenic simian immunodeficiency virus with Venezuelan equine encephalitis virus replicon particles. J Virol 74:371–378, 2000.

471. Gardner JP, Frolov I, Perri S, et al. Infection of human dendritic cells by a Sindbis virus replicon vector is determined by a single amino acid substitution in the E2 glycoprotein. J Virol 74:11849–11857, 2000.

472. Tubukelas I, Berglund P, Fluton M, Liljeström P. Alphavirus expression vectors and their use as recombinant vaccines: a minimum. Gene 190:191–195, 1997.

473. Morris-Downes MM, Phenix KV, Smyth J, et al. Semliki Forest virus-based vaccines: persistence, distribution, and pathological analyses in two animal systems. Vaccine 19:1978–1988, 2001.

474. Liu XL, Clark KR, Johnson PR. Production of recombinant adeno-associated virus vectors using a packaging cell line and a hybrid recombinant adenovirus. Gene Ther 6:293–299, 1999.

475. Li S, Polonis V, Isobe H, et al. Chimeric influenza virus induces neutralizing antibodies and cytotoxic T cells against human immunodeficiency virus type 1. J Virol 67:6659–6666, 1993.

476. Muster T, Ferko B, Klima A, et al. Mucosal model of immunization against human immunodeficiency virus type 1 with a chimeric influenza virus. J Virol 69:6678–6686, 1995.

477. Morrow CD, Porter DC, Ansardi DC, et al. New approaches for mucosal vaccines for AIDS: encapsidation and serial passages of poliovirus replicons that express HIV-1 proteins on infection. AIDS Res Hum Retroviruses 10(suppl):S61–S66, 1994.

478. Anderson MJ, Porter DC, Moldovean Z, et al. Characterization of the expression and immunogenicity of poliovirus replicons that encode simian immunodeficiency virus SIVmac239 Gag or envelope SU proteins. AIDS Res Hum Retroviruses 13:53–62, 1997.

479. Crotty S, Miller CJ, Lohman BL, et al. Protection against simian immunodeficiency virus vaginal challenge by using Sabin poliovirus vectors. J Virol 75:7435–7452, 2001.

480. Schnell MJ, Foley MD, Silen CA. Recombinant rabies virus as potential live-viral vaccines for HIV-1. Proc Natl Acad Sci U S A 97:3544–3549, 2000.

481. McGettingan JP, Foley HD, Belyakov IM, et al. Rabies virus-based vectors expressing HIV-1 envelope protein induce a strong, cross-reactive cytotoxic T-lymphocyte response against envelope proteins from different HIV-isolates. J Virol 75:4430–4434, 2001.

482. Rose NF, Roberts A, Buonocore L, Rose JK. Glycoprotein exchange vectors based on vesicular stomatitis virus allow effective boosting and generation of neutralizing antibodies to a primary isolate of human immunodeficiency virus type 1. J Virol 74:10903–10910, 2000.

483. Rose NF, Marx PA, Luckay A, et al. An effective AIDS-vaccine based on live attenuated vesicular stomatitis virus recombinants. Cell 106:539–549, 2001.

484. Matano T, Kano M, Nakamura H, et al. Rapid appearance of secondary immune responses and protection from CD4 depletion after a highly pathogenic immunodeficiency virus challenge in macaques immunized with a DNA prime/Sendaï virus vector boost regimen. J Virol 75:11891–11896, 2001.

485. Méderlé I, Bourguin I, Ensergueix D, et al. Plasmidic versus integrative cloning of heterologous genes in Mycobacterum bovis BCG: impact on in vivo antigen persistence and immune responses. Infect Immun 70:303–314, 2002.

486. Aldovini A, Young RA. Humoral and cell-mediated immune responses to live recombinant BCG-HIV vaccines. Nature 351:479–482, 1991.

487. Lagranderie M, Balazuc AM, Gicquel B, Gheorghiu M. Oral immunization with recombinant Mycobacterium bovis BCG simian immunodeficiency virus nef induces local and systemic cytotoxic T-lymphocyte response in mice. J Virol 71:2302–2309, 1997.

488. Honda M, Matsuo K, Nakasone T, et al. Protective immune responses induced by secretion of a chimeric soluble protein from a recombinant Mycobacterium bovis bacillus Calmette-Guerin vector candidate vaccine for human immunodeficiency virus type 1 in small animals. Proc Natl Acad Sci U S A 92:10693–10697, 1995.

489. Fouts TR, Tuskan RG, Chada S, et al. Construction and immunogenicity of Salmonella typhimurium vaccine vectors that express HIV-1 gp120. Vaccine 13:1697–1705, 1995.

490. Steger KK, Pauza CD. Immunization of Macaca mulatta with AroA attenuated Salmonella typhimurium expressing the SIVp27 antigen. J Med Primatol 26:44–50, 1997.

491. Alvin CR. Liposomes as carriers of antigens and adjuvants. J Immunol Methods 140:1–13, 1991.

492. Browning M, Reid G, Osborne R, Jarrett O. Incorporation of soluble antigens into ISCOMs: HIV gp120 ISCOMs induce neutralizing antibodies. Vaccine 10:585–590, 1991.

493. Hulskotte EGJ, Geretti AM, Siebelink KHJ, et al. Vaccine-induced virus neutralizing antibodies and cytotoxic T-cells do not protect macaques from experimental infection with simian immunodeficiency virus SIVmac 1XH (JE). J Virol 69:6289–6296, 1995.

494. Van Nest GA, Steimer KS, Haigwood NH, et al. Advanced adjuvant formulations for use with recombinant subunit vaccines. In Chanock

RM, Lerner RA, Brown F, Ginsberg H (eds). Vaccines 92: Modern Approaches to New Vaccines. Cold Spring Harbor, NY, Cold Spring Harbor Laboratory, 1992, pp 57–62.

495. Van Cott TC, Mascola JR, Kaminski RW, et al. Antibodies with specificity for native gp120 and neutralization activity against primary human immunodeficiency virus type 1 isolates elicited by immunization with oligomeric gp160. J Virol 71:4319–4330, 1997.

496. Kumar A, Lifson JD, Silverstein PS, et al. Evaluation of immune responses induced by HIV-1 gp120 in rhesus macaques: effect of vaccination on challenge with pathogenic strains of homologous and heterologous simian human immunodeficiency viruses. Virology 274:149–164, 2000.

497. Cho MW, Kim YB, Lee MK, et al. Polyvalent envelope glycoprotein vaccine elicits a broader neutralizing antibody response but is unable to provide sterilizing immunity against heterologous simian/human immunodeficiency virus infection in pig-tailed macaques. J Virol 75:2224–2234, 2001.

498. Quinnan JV Jr, Zhang PF, Fu DW, et al. Expression and characterization of HIV type 1 envelope protein associated with a broadly reactive neutralizing antibody response. AIDS Res Hum Retroviruses 15:561–570, 1999.

499. Staropoli I, Chanel C, Girard M, Altmeyer R. Processing, stability and receptor binding properties of oligomeric envelope glycoprotein from a primary HIV-1 isolate. J Biol Chem 275:35137–35145, 2000.

500. Earl PL, Sugiura W, Montefiori DC, et al. Immunogenicity and protective efficacy of oligomeric human immunodeficiency virus type 1 gp140. J Virol 75:645–655, 2001.

501. Binley JM, Sanders RW, Clas B, et al. A recombinant immunodeficiency virus type 1 envelope glycoprotein complex stabilized by an intermolecular disulfide bond between the gp120 and gp41 subunits is an antigenic mimic of the trimeric virion-associated structure. J Virol 74:627–643, 2000.

502. Yang X, Wyatt R, Sodroski J. Improved elicitation of neutralizing antibodies against primary human immunodeficiency viruses by soluble stabilized envelope glycoprotein trimers. J Virol 75:1161–1171, 2001.

503. Stamatatos L, Davis D. New insights into protective humoral responses and HIV vaccines. AIDS 15(suppl 5):S105–S115, 2001.

504. Reitter JN, Desrosiers RC. Identification of replication-competent strains of simian immunodeficiency virus lacking multiple attachment sites for N-linked carbohydrates in variable regions 1 and 2 of the surface envelope protein. J Virol 72:5399–5407, 1998.

505. Stamatatos L, Cheng-Mayer C. An envelope modification that renders a primary neutralization-resistant clade B human immunodeficiency virus type 1 isolate highly susceptible to neutralization by sera from other clades. J Virol 72:7840–7845, 1999.

506. Cherpebis S, Srivastava I, Gettie A, et al. DNA vaccination with the human immunodeficiency virus type 1 SF262 delta V2 envelope elicits immune responses that offer partial protection from simian/human immunodeficiency virus infection to CD8+ T-cell-depleted rhesus macaques. J Virol 75:1547–1550, 2001.

507. Fouts T, Godfrey K, Boob K, et al. Cross-linked HIV-1 envelope-CD4 receptor complexes elicit broadly cross-reactive neutralizing antibodies in rhesus macaques. Proc Natl Acad Sci U S A 99:11842–11847, 2002.

508. Hu S-L, Abrams K, Barber GN, et al. Protection of macaques against SIV infection by subunit vaccines of SIV envelope glycoprotein gp160. Science 255:456–459, 1992.

509. Putkonen P, Bjorling E, Akerblom L, et al. Long-standing protection of macaques against cell-free HIV-2 with an HIV-2 ISCOM vaccine. J Acquir Immune Defic Syndr 7:551–559, 1994.

510. Stahl-Hennig C, Coulibaly C, Petry H, et al. Immunization with virion-derived glycoprotein 130 from HIV-2 or SIV protects macaques against challenge virus grown in human or simian cells or prepared ex vivo. AIDS Res Hum Retroviruses 10(suppl 2):S27–S32, 1994.

511. Eldridge J, Stoas JK, Meulbroek JA, et al. Biodegradable microspheres as a vaccine delivery system. Mol Immunol 28:287–294, 1991.

512. Cafaro A, Caputo A, Fracasso C, et al. Control of SHIV 89.6P infection of cynomologus monkeys by HIV-1 Tat protein vaccines. Nat Med 6:643–649, 1999.

513. Goldstein G, Mauson K, Tribbick G, Smith R. Minimization of chronic plasma viremia in rhesus macaques immunized with synthetic HIV-1 Tat peptides and infected with a chimeric simian/human immunodeficiency virus (SHIV 33). Vaccine 18:2789–2795, 2000.

514. Pauza DC, Trivedi P, Wallace M, et al. Vaccination with Tat toxoid attenuates disease in simian/HIV-challenged macaques. Proc Natl Acad Sci U S A 97:3515–3519, 2000.

515. Haynes BF, Torres JV, Langlois AJ, et al. Induction of HIV MN neutralizing antibodies in primates using a prime-boost regimen of hybrid synthetic gp120 envelope peptides. J Immunol 151:1646–1653, 1993.

516. Wang CY, Looney DJ, Li ML, et al. Long-term high-titer neutralizing activity induced by octameric synthetic HIV-1 antigen. Science 254:285–288, 1991.

517. Kelleher AD, Emery S, Cunningham P, et al. Safety and immunogenicity of UBI HIV-1 MN octameric V3 peptide vaccine administered by subcutaneous injection. AIDS Res Hum Retroviruses 13:29–32, 1997.

518. Deres K, Schild H, Wiesmüller KH, et al. In vivo priming of virus-specific cytotoxic T lymphocytes with synthetic lipopeptide vaccine. Nature 342:561–564, 1989.

519. Deprez B, Sauzet JP, Boutillon C, et al. Comparative efficiency of simple lipopeptide constructs for in vivo induction of virus-specific CTL. Vaccine 5:375–382, 1996.

520. Gahery-Segard H, Pialoux G, Charmeteau B, et al. Multi-epitopic B- and T-cell responses induced in humans by a human immunodeficiency virus type 1 lipopeptide vaccine. J Virol 74:1694–1703, 2000.

521. Wang B, Ugen KE, Srikantan V, et al. Gene inoculation generates immune response against human immunodeficiency virus type 1. Proc Natl Acad Sci U S A 90:4156–4160, 1993.

522. Wang B, Boyer J, Srikantan V, et al. Induction of humoral and cellular immune response to the human immunodeficiency type 1 virus in non-human primates by in vivo DNA inoculation. Virology 211:102–112, 1995.

523. Yasutomi Y, Robinson HL, Lu S, et al. Simian immunodeficiency virus–specific cytotoxic T lymphocyte induction through DNA vaccination of rhesus monkeys. J Virol 70:678–681, 1996.

524. Lu S, Arthos J, Montefiori DC, et al. Simian immunodeficiency virus DNA vaccination trial in macaques. J Virol 70:3978–3991, 1996.

525. Haas J, Park E-C, Seed B. Codon usage limitation in the expression of HIV-1 envelope glycoprotein. Curr Biol 6:315–324, 1996.

526. Charo J, Sundbäck M, Wasserman K, et al. Marked enhancement of the antigen-specific immune response by combining plasmid DNA-based immunization with a Schiff base-forming drug. Inf Immun 70:6652–6657, 2002.

527. O'Hagan D, Singh M, Ugozzoli M, et al. Induction of potent immune responses by cationic microparticles with adsorbed human immunodeficiency virus DNA vaccines. J Virol 75:9037–9043, 2001.

528. Kim JJ, Ayyavoo V, Bagarazzi ML, et al. In vivo engineering of a cellular immune response by coadministration of IL-12 expression vector with a DNA immunogen. J Immunol 158:816–826, 1997.

529. Barouch DH, Craiu A, Kuroda MJ, et al. Augmentation of immune responses to HIV-1 and SIV DNA vaccines by IL-2/Ig plasmid administration in rhesus monkeys. Proc Natl Acad Sci U S A 97:4192–4197, 2000.

530. Barouch DH, Santra S, Schmitz JE, et al. Control of viremia and prevention of clinical AIDS in rhesus monkeys by cytokine-augmented DNA vaccination. Science 290:486–492, 2000.

531. Letvin NL, Montefiori DC, Yasutomi Y, et al. Potent, protective anti-HIV immune responses generated by bimodal HIV envelope DNA plus protein vaccination. Proc Natl Acad Sci U S A 94:9378–9383, 1997.

532. Barnett SW, Rajasekar S, Legg H, et al. Vaccination with HIV-1 gp120 DNA induces immune responses that are boosted by a recombinant gp120 protein subunit. Vaccine 15:869–873, 1997.

533. Boyer JD, Wang B, Ugen KE, et al. In vivo protective anti-HIV immune responses in non-human primates through DNA immunization. J Med Primatol 25:242–250, 1996.

534. Boyer JD, Ugen KE, Wang B, et al. Protection of chimpanzees from high-dose heterologous HIV-1 challenge by DNA vaccination. Nat Med 3:526–532, 1997.

535. Hanke T, Samuel RV, Blanchard TJ, et al. Effective induction of simian immunodeficiency virus-specific cytotoxic T lymphocytes in macaques by using a multiepitope gene and DNA prime-modified vaccinia virus Ankara boost vaccination regimen. J Virol 73:7524–7532, 1999.

536. Amara RR, Villinger F, Altman JD, et al. Control of a mucosal challenge and prevention of AIDS in rhesus macaques by a multiprotein DNA/MVA vaccine. Science 292:69–74, 2001.

536a. Tang Y, Villinger F, Staprans SI, et al. Slowly declining levels of viral RNA and DNA in DNA/recombinant modified vaccinia virus Ankara-vaccinated macaques with controlled simian-human immunodeficiency virus SHIV-89.6P challenges. J Virol 76:10147–10154, 2002.

537. Heeney JL. Primate models for AIDS vaccine development. AIDS 10(suppl A):S115–S122, 1996.

538. Fultz PN, Sancier M, Anderson DC, et al. Development of AIDS in a chimpanzee infected with human immunodeficiency virus type 1. J Virol 71:4088–4091, 1997.

539. Agy MB, Frumkin LR, Corey L, et al. Infection of *Macaca nemestrina* by human immunodeficiency virus type 1. Science 257:103–106, 1992.

540. Mosier DE, Gulizia RJ, Baird SM, et al. Human immunodeficiency virus infection of human PBL-SCID mice. Science 251:791–794, 1991.

541. Li JT, Lord CI, Haseltine W, et al. Infection of cynomolgus monkeys with a chimeric HIV-1/SIVmac virus that expresses the HIV-1 envelope glycoproteins. J Acquir Immune Defic Syndr 5:639–646, 1992.

542. Li JT, Halloran M, Lord CI, et al. Persistent infection of macaques with simian human immunodeficiency virus. J Virol 69:7061–7071, 1995.

543. Reimann KA, Li JT, Voss G, et al. An *env* gene derived from a primary human immunodeficiency virus type 1 isolate confers high in vivo replicative capacity to a chimeric simian/human immunodeficiency virus in rhesus monkeys. J Virol 70:3198–3206, 1996.

544. Reimann KA, Li JT, Veazuy R, et al. A chimeric simian/human immunodeficiency virus expressing a primary patient human immunodeficiency virus type 1 isolate *env* causes an AIDS-like disease after in vivo passage in rhesus monkeys. J Virol 70:6922–6928, 1996.

545. Joag SV, Li Z, Foresman L, et al. Chimeric simian/human immunodeficiency virus that causes progressive loss of CD4$^+$ T cells and AIDS in pig-tailed macaques. J Virol 70:3189–3197, 1996.

546. Joag SV, Adamy I, Li Z, et al. Animal model of mucosally transmitted human immunodeficiency virus type 1 disease: intravaginal and oral deposition of simian/human immunodeficiency virus in macaques results in systemic infection, elimination of CD4$^+$ T cells, and AIDS. J Virol 71:4016–4023, 1997.

547. Lu Y, Salvato MS, Pauza CD, et al. Utility of SHIV for testing HIV-1 vaccine candidates in macaques. J Acquir Immune Defic Syndr Hum Retrovirol 12:99–106, 1996.

548. Karlsson GB, Halloran M, Li J, et al. Characterization of molecularly cloned simian-human immunodeficiency viruses causing rapid CD4$^+$ lymphocyte depletion in rhesus monkeys. J Virol 71:4218–4225, 1997.

549. Harouse JM, Agegnehu G, Tan RCH, et al. Distinct pathogenic sequela in rhesus macaques infected with CCR5 or CXCR4 utilizing SHIVs. Science 284:816–819, 1999.

550. Putkonen P, Thorstensson B, Ghavamzadeh L, et al. Prevention of HIV-2 and SIVsm infection by passive immunization in cynomolgus monkeys. Nature 352:436–438, 1991.

551. Hoffmann-Lehmann R, Vlasak I, Rasmussen RA, et al. Postnatal passive immunization of neonatal macaques with a triple combination of human monoclonal antibodies against oral simian human immunodeficiency virus challenge. J Virol 75:7470–7480, 2001.

552. Girard M, van der Ryst E, Barré-Sinoussi F, et al. Challenge of chimpanzees immunized with a recombinant canarypox–HIV-1 virus. Virology 239:98–104, 1997.

553. Miller CJ, Marthas M, Thorten J, et al. Intravaginal inoculation of rhesus macaques with cell-free simian immunodeficiency virus results in persistent or transient viremia. J Virol 68:6391–6400, 1994.

554. Mooij P, van der Kolk M, Bogers WMJM, et al. A clinically relevant HIV-1 subunit vaccine protects rhesus macaques from *in vivo* passaged simian-human immunodeficiency virus infection. AIDS 12:F15–F22, 1998.

555. Stott EJ, Almond N, Kent K, et al. Evaluation of candidate human immunodeficiency virus type 1 (HIV-1) vaccine in macaques: effect of vaccination with HIV-1 gp120 on subsequent challenge with heterologous simian immunodeficiency virus–HIV-1 chimeric virus. J Gen Virol 79:423–432, 1998.

556. Davis D, Morlein B, Åkerblom L, et al. A recombinant prime, peptide boost vaccination strategy can focus the immune response onto more than one epitope even though these may not be immunodominant in the complex immunogen. Vaccine 15:1661–1669, 1997.

557. Horton H, Vogel TV, Carter DK, et al. Immunization of rhesus macaques with a DNA prime/modified vaccinia virus Ankara boost

557a. Allen TM, Jing P, Calore B, et al. Effects of cytotoxic T lymphocytes (CTL) directed against a single simian immunodeficiency virus (SIV) Gag CTL epitope on the course of SIVmac239 infection. J Virol 76:10507–10511, 2002.

regimen induces broad simian immunodeficiency virus (SIV)-specific T-cell responses and reduces initial viral replication but does not prevent disease progression following challenge with pathogenic SIVmac239. J Virol 76:7187–7202, 2002.

558. Keefer MC, Wolff M, Gorse GJ, et al. Safety profile of Phase I and II preventive HIV type 1 envelope vaccination: experience of the NIAID AIDS Vaccine Evaluation Group. AIDS Res Hum Retroviruses 13:1163–1177, 1997.

559. Walker MC, Fast PE. Clinical trials of candidate AIDS vaccines. AIDS 8(suppl 1):S213–S236, 1994.

560. Graham BS, Wright PF. Candidate AIDS vaccines. N Engl J Med 333:1331–1339, 1995.

561. Dolin R. Human studies in the development of human immunodeficiency virus vaccine. J Infect Dis 172:1175–1183, 1995.

562. Gorse GJ, Keefer MC, Belshe RB, et al. A dose-ranging study of a prototype synthetic HIV-1MN V3 branched peptide vaccine. J Infect Dis 173:330–339, 1996.

563. Evans TG, McElrath MJ, Matthews T, et al. QS-21 promotes an adjuvant effect allowing for reduced antigen dose during HIV-1 envelope subunit immunization in humans. Vaccine 19:2080–2091, 2001.

564. Schwartz DH, Gorse G, Clements ML, et al. Induction of HIV-1-neutralising and syncytium-inhibiting antibodies in uninfected recipients of HIV-1$_{IIIB}$ rgp120 subunit vaccine. Lancet 342:69–73, 1993.

565. Belshe RB, Clements ML, Dolin R, et al. Safety and immunogenicity of a fully glycosylated recombinant gp160 human immunodeficiency virus type 1 vaccine in subjects at low risk of infection. J Infect Dis 168:1387–1395, 1993.

566. McElrath MJ, Corey L, Greenberg PD, et al. Human immunodeficiency virus type 1–infection despite prior immunization with a recombinant envelope vaccine regimen. Proc Natl Acad Sci U S A 93:3972–3977, 1996.

567. Graham BS, McElrath MJ, Connor RI, et al. Analysis of intercurrent HIV-1 infections in Phase I and II trials of candidate AIDS vaccines. J Infect Dis 177:310–319, 1998.

568. Excler JL, Plotkin S. The prime-boost concept applied to HIV preventive vaccines. AIDS 11(suppl A):S127–S137, 1997.

569. Amara RR, Smith JM, Staprans SI, et al. Critical role for Env as well as Gag-Pol in control of a simian-human immunodeficiency virus 89.6P challenge by a DNA prime-recombinant modified vaccinia virus Ankara vaccine. J Virol 76:6138–6146, 2002.

570. Voss G, Manson K, Montefiori D, et al. Prevention of disease induced by a partially heterologous AIDS virus in rhesus monkeys by using an adjuvanted multicomponent protein vaccine. J Virol 77:1049–1058, 2003.

571. Zagury D, Léonard R, Fouchard M, et al. Immunization against AIDS in humans. Nature 326:249–250, 1987.

572. Picard O, Achour A, Bernard J, et al. A 2-year follow-up of an anti-HIV immune reaction in HIV-1 gp160-immunized healthy seronegative humans: evidence for persistent cell-mediated immunity. J Acquir Immune Defic Syndr 5:539–546, 1992.

573. Goldstein JA, Neff JM, Lane JM, Koplan JP. Smallpox vaccination reactions, prophylaxis and therapy of complications. Pediatrics 55:342–347, 1975.

574. Redfield RR, Wright DC, James WD, et al. Disseminated vaccinia in a military recruit with human immunodeficiency virus (HIV) disease. N Engl J Med 316:673–676, 1987.

575. Plotkin SA, Cadoz M, Meignier B, et al. The safety and use of canarypox vectored vaccines. Dev Biol Stand 84:165–170, 1995.

576. Tubiana R, Gomard E, Fleury H, et al. Vaccine therapy in early HIV-1 infection using a recombinant canarypox virus expressing gp160 MN (ALVAC-HIV): a double-blind controlled randomized study of safety and immunogenicity. AIDS 11:819–841, 1997.

577. Belshe RB, Gorse GJ, Mulligan MJ, et al. Induction of immune responses to HIV-1 by canarypox (ALVAC) HIV-1 and gp120 SF2 recombinant vaccines in uninfected volunteers. AIDS 12:2401–2415, 1998.

578. Clements-Mann ML, Matthews TJ, Weinhold K, et al. HIV-1 immune responses induced by canarypox (ALVAC) gp160 MN, SF-2 rgp120 or both vaccines in seronegative adults. J Infect Dis 177:1230–1246, 1998.

579. Evans TG, Keefer MC, Weinhold K, et al. A canarypox vaccine expressing multiple HIV-1 genes given alone or with rgp120 elicits

broad and durable CD8+ CTL in seronegative volunteers. J. Infect Dis 180:290–298, 1999.

580. Salmon-Ceron D, Excler JL, Finkielasztejn L, et al. Safety and immunogenicity of a live recombinant canarypox virus expressing HIV-1 gp120 MN/tm/gag protease LAI (ALVAC-HIV, vCP205) followed by a p24-V3 synthetic peptide (CLTB-36) administered in healthy volunteers at low risk for HIV infection. AIDS Res Hum Retroviruses 15:633–645, 1999.

581. Belshe RB, Stevens C, Gorse GJ, et al. Safety and immunogenicity of a canarypox vectored HIV-1 vaccine with or without gp120: a Phase II study in higher and lower risk volunteers. J Infect Dis 183:1343–1352, 2001.

582. Graham BS. Clinical trials of HIV vaccines. Annu Rev Med 53:207–221, 2002.

582a.Hauke T, McMichael A. Design and construction of an experimental HIV-1 vaccine for a year-2000 clinical trial in Kenya. Nat Med 6:951–955, 2000.

583. Arrington J, Braun RP, Dong L, et al. Plasmid vectors encoding cholera toxin or the heat-labile enterotoxin from Escherichia coli are strong adjuvants for DNA vaccines. J Virol 76:4536–4546, 2002.

584. Pialoux G, Gahery-Segard H, Sermet S, et al. Lipopeptides induce cell mediated anti-HIV immune responses in seronegative volunteers. AIDS 15:1239–1249, 2001.

585. Graham BS, Matthews TJ, Belshe RB, et al. Augmentation of human immunodeficiency virus type 1 neutralizing antibody by priming with gp160 recombinant vaccinia and boosting with rgp160 in vaccinia-naive adults. J Infect Dis 167:533–537, 1993.

586. Cooney EL, McElrath MJ, Corey L, et al. Enhanced immunity to human immunodeficiency virus (HIV) envelope elicited by a combined vaccine regimen consisting of priming with a vaccinia recombinant expressing HIV envelope and boosting with gp160 protein. Proc Natl Acad Sci U S A 90:1882–1886, 1993.

587. Hammond SA, Bollinger RC, Stanhope PE, et al. Comparative clonal analysis of human immunodeficiency virus type 1 (HIV-1)–specific CD4+ and CD8+ cytolytic T lymphocytes isolated from seronegative humans immunized with candidate HIV-1 vaccines. J Exp Med 176:1531–1542, 1992.

588. Bollinger RC, Quinn TC, Liu AY, et al. Cytokines from vaccine-induced HIV-1 specific cytotoxic T lymphocytes: effects on viral replication. AIDS Res Hum Retroviruses 9:1067–1077, 1993.

589. Graham BS, Gorse GJ, Schwartz DH, et al. Determinants of antibody response after recombinant gp160 boosting in vaccinia-naive volunteers primed with gp160-recombinant vaccinia virus. J Infect Dis 170:782–786, 1994.

590. Pialoux G, Excler JL, Rivière Y, et al. A prime-boost approach to HIV preventive vaccine using a recombinant canarypox virus expressing glycoprotein 160 (MN) followed by a recombinant glycoprotein 160 (MN/LAI). AIDS Res Hum Retroviruses 11:373–381, 1995.

591. Fleury B, Janvier G, Pialoux G, et al. Memory cytotoxic T lymphocyte responses in human immunodeficiency virus type 1 (HIV-1)–negative volunteers immunized with a recombinant canarypox expressing gp160 of HIV-1 and boosted with a recombinant gp160. J Infect Dis 174:734–738, 1996.

592. Salmon-Ceron D, Excler JL, Sicard D, et al. Safety and immunogenicity of a recombinant HIV type 1 glycoprotein 160 boosted by a V3 synthetic peptide in HIV-negative volunteers. AIDS Res Hum Retroviruses 11:1479–1486, 1995.

593. Egan MA, Pavlat WA, Tartaglia J, et al. Induction of human immunodeficiency virus type 1 (HIV-1)–specific cytolytic T lymphocyte responses in seronegative adults by a nonreplicating, host-range restricted canarypox vector (ALVAC) carrying the HIV-1MN env gene. J Infect Dis 171:1623–1627, 1995.

594. Clements ML, Corey L, Weinhold K, et al. HIV immunity induced by priming with canarypox or vaccinia–gp 160 recombinants and boosting with rgp120 [abstr 166]. In Abstracts of the Annual Meeting of the Institute of Human Virology, Baltimore, MD, September 7–12, 1996.

595. Wee EG, Patel S, McMichael AJ, Hanke T. A DNA/MVA-based candidate human immunodeficiency virus vaccine for Kenya induces multi-specific T cell responses in rhesus macaques. J Gen Virol 83:75–80, 2002.

596. Eron JJ, Ashby MA, Giordano MF, et al. Randomised trial of MN gp120 HIV-1 vaccine in symptomless HIV-1 infection. Lancet 348:1547–1551, 1996.

597. Levine AM, Groshen S, Allen J, et al. Initial studies on active immunization of HIV-infected subjects using a gp120-depleted HIV-1 immunogen: long-term follow-up. J Acquir Immune Defic Syndr Hum Retrovirol 11:351–364, 1996.

598. Pantaleo G. How immune-based interventions can change HIV therapy. Nat Med 3:484–486, 1997.

599. Conors M, Kovacs JA, Krevat S, et al. HIV infection induces changes in CD4+ T cell phenotype and depletion within the CD4+ T-cell repertoire that are not immediately restored by antiviral or immune-based therapies. Nat Med 3:533–540, 1997.

600. Lambert JS, Mofenson LM, Fletcher CV, et al. Safety and pharmacokinetics of hyperimmune anti–human immunodeficiency virus (HIV) immunoglobulin administered to HIV-infected pregnant women and their newborns. J Infect Dis 175:283–293, 1997.

601. Ugen KE, Goedert JJ, Boyer J, et al. Vertical transmission of HIV infection: correlation with reactivity of maternal sera with glycoprotein 120 and gp41 peptides from HIV type 1. J Clin Invest 89:1923–1930, 1992.

602. Khouri YF, McIntosh K, Cavacini L, et al. Vertical transmission of HIV-1: correlation with maternal viral load and plasma levels of CD4 binding site anti-gp120 antibodies. J Clin Invest 95:732–737, 1995.

603. Rossi P, Moshese V, Broliden PA, et al. Presence of maternal antibodies to human immunodeficiency virus type 1 envelope glycoprotein gp120 epitopes correlates with the noninfective status of children born to seropositive mothers. Proc Natl Acad Sci U S A 86:8055–8058, 1989.

604. Scarlatti G, Albert J, Rossi P, et al. Mother-to-child transmission of human immunodeficiency virus type 1: correlation with neutralizing antibodies against primary isolates. J Infect Dis 168:207–210, 1993.

605. Van Rompay KKA, Otsyula MG, Tarara RP, et al. Vaccination of pregnant macaques protects newborns against mucosal simian immunodeficiency virus infection. J Infect Dis 173:1327–1335, 1996.

606. Mascola JR, Louder MK, van Cott TC, et al. Potent and synergistic neutralization of human immunodeficiency virus (HIV) type 1 primary isolates by hyperimmune anti-HIV immunoglobulin combined with monoclonal antibodies 2F5 and 2G12. J Virol 71:7198–7206, 1997.

607. Xu W, Hofmann-Lehmann R, McClure HM, Ruprecht RM. Passive immunization with human neutralizing monoclonal antibodies: correlates of protective immunity against HIV. Vaccine 20:1956–1960, 2002.

607a.Wolbank S, Kunert R, Stiegler G, katinger H. Characterization of human class-switched polymeric (Immunoglobulin M[IgM] and IgA) anti-human immunodeficiency virus type 1 antibodies 2F5 and 2G12. J virol 77(7):4095–4103, 2003.

608. Gashen B, Taylor J, Yusim K, et al. Diversity considerations in HIV-1 vaccine selection. Science 296:2354–2360, 2002.

609. Miller C, Gardner MB. AIDS and mucosal immunity: usefulness of the SIV macaque model of genital mucosal transmission. J Acquir Immune Defic Syndr 4:1169–1172, 1991.

610. Belec L, Georges AJ, Steenman G, Martin PM. Antibodies to human immunodeficiency virus in vaginal secretions of heterosexual women. J Infect Dis 160:385–391, 1989.

611. Mestecky J. The common mucosal immune system and current strategies for induction of immune responses in external secretions. J Clin Immunol 7:265–276, 1987.

612. Lehner T, Wang Y, Cranage M, et al. Protective mucosal immunity elicited by targeted iliac lymph node immunization with a subunit SIV envelope and core vaccine in macaques. Nat Med 2:767–775, 1996.

613. Baig J, Levy DB, McKay PF, et al. Elicitation of simian immunodeficiency virus-specific cytotoxic T lymphocytes in mucosal compartments of rhesus macaques by systemic vaccination. J Virol 76:11484–11490, 2002.

613a.Stevceva L, Alvarez X, Lackner AA, et al. Both mucosal and systemic routes of immunization with the live, attenuated NYVAC/simian immunodeficiency virus SIVgpc recombinant vaccine results in gag-specific CD8+ T-cell responses in mucosal tissues of macaques. J Virol 76:11659–11676, 2002.

614. Berzofsky JA, Ahlers JD, Belyakov IM. Strategies for designing and optimizing new generation vaccines. Nat Rev Immunol 1:209–219, 2001.

615. Osterhaus ADE, van Baalen CA, Gruter RA, et al. Vaccination with Rev and Tat against AIDS. Vaccine 17:2713–2714, 1999.

616. Verrier B, Le Grand R, Ataman-Önal Y, et al. Evaluation in rhesus macaques of Tal- and Rev-targeted immunization as a preventive vaccine against mucosal challenge with SMIV-BX08. DNA Cell Biol 21:653–658, 2002.

617. Garzino-Demo A, De Vico AL, Cocchi F, Gallo RC. Betachemokines and protection from HIV type 1 disease. AIDS Res Hum Retroviruses 14(suppl):S177–S188, 1998.

618. Zhou P, Goldstein S, Devadas K, et al. Human CD4+ cells transfected with IL-16 cDNA are resistant to HIV-1 infection: inhibition of mRNA expression. Nat Med 3:659–664, 1997.

619. Sasaki S, Amara RR, Yeow W-S, et al. Regulation of DNA-raised immune response by cotransfected interferon regulatory factors. J Virol 76:6652–6659, 2002.

620. Burton DR. A vaccine for HIV type 1: the antibody perspective. Proc Natl Acad Sci U S A 94:10018–10023, 1997.

621. Francis DP, Heyward WL, Popovic V, et al. Candidate HIV/AIDS vaccines: lessons learned from the world's first phase III efficacy trials. AIDS 17:147–156, 2003.

622. Zingernagel RM. Immunity, immunopathology and vaccines against HIV? Vaccine 20:1913–1917, 2002.

623. Mann JM. AIDS—the second decade: a global perspective. J Infect Dis 165:245–250, 1992.

Chapter 45

Human Papillomavirus Vaccines for Cervical Cancer Prevention

JOHN T. SCHILLER • DOUGLAS R. LOWY

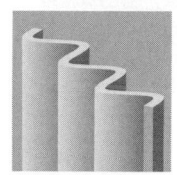

Cervical Cancer Basics

Cervical cancer is the second or third leading cause of cancer deaths in women. Worldwide, there are an estimated 450,000 cases and 200,000 deaths annually as a result of cervical cancer.[1] In comparison to most cancers, it tends to strike relatively young women. In most countries, there is a steady rise in incidence from the mid 20s to the mid 50s, after which the rates tend to remain relatively constant. Cervical cancers almost always occur at the junction between the columnar epithelium of the endocervix and the squamous epithelium of the ectocervix, called the transition zone.[2] They arise from well-documented premalignant neoplastic lesions that most often present first as mild dysplastic lesions that in a minority of cases then progress to high-grade dysplasias and carcinoma in situ before becoming malignant. The entire process usually takes decades (Fig. 45–1). Low-grade cervical dysplasias are common, and most regress spontaneously. In contrast, the minority of lesions that progress to high-grade dysplasias tend to persist and/or progress to cancers.[3]

Current cervical cancer prevention measures rely on identification of premalignant lesions by Papanicolaou (Pap) screening.[4] This test involves the microscopic identification of abnormal cells scraped from the cervical os. Visual inspection of the cervix by colposcopy, followed by histologic examination of colposcopy-directed biopsy specimens, is used to confirm the diagnosis. Women with high-grade lesions routinely undergo surgical ablation of their cervical transition zone.[5] Pap screening is certainly one of the most successful cancer prevention strategies ever devised, and cervical cancer rates tend to be much lower in the more developed countries that have the resources to implement organized Pap screening programs.[1] However, Pap screening is far from an ideal cancer prevention strategy. It is costly, with an estimated $5 to $6 billion annually spent on cervical cancer prevention in the United States alone.[6] It is too expensive to implement in most developing countries, and consequently cervical cancer is the leading cause of cancer deaths in women in many of them.[7] In addition, the test suffers from rather high false-negative rates and rather low compliance rates in some groups of women.[8] Finally, although surgical removal of premalignant lesions is generally well tolerated and greatly reduces a woman's risk of cervical cancer, it is not entirely without morbidity.

Human Papillomavirus and Cervical Cancer

It has been known for many years that cervical cancer has a risk factor profile consistent with that of a sexually transmitted disease.[9] However, a strong association with a specific infectious agent was not obtained until the early 1980s, when human papillomavirus (HPV) type 16 (HPV16) DNA was detected in the cells of approximately one half of cervical cancer biopsy specimens.[10] In the last 20 years, a remarkably strong and consistent causal association has been established between cervical cancer and prior persistent infection with a subset of the many HPVs that infect the human female genital tract.[11] In a recent worldwide survey, more than 99% of technically adequate cervical carcinoma and adenocarcinoma specimens contained HPV DNA, raising the possibility that HPV infection is the first necessary cause of cancer to be identified.[12] HPV infection also has been causally associated with a proportion of anal, vulvar, vaginal, and oral cancers.[13,14]

Neoplastic changes in cervical epithelium now can be understood in light of the HPV infections that cause them.[3] The low-grade cervical dysplasias identified in Pap screening tests are simply productive HPV infections. Most infections regress spontaneously. In contrast, high-grade dysplasias and cancers, which are the infrequent outcome of persistent infections, do not produce virions because viral gene expression usually is limited to two viral oncogenes, E6 and E7 (see Fig. 45–1). Malignant progression is thought to be due to the direct action of E6 and E7, which inactivate

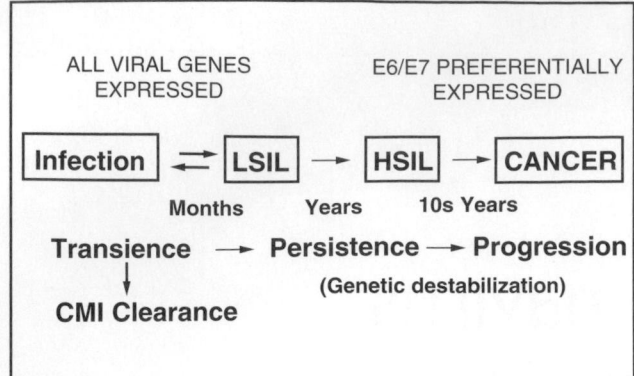

FIGURE 45–1 ■ HPV infection and cervical carcinogenesis. CMI = cell-mediated immunity; HSIL, high-grade squamous intraepithelial lesion; LSIL, low-grade squamous intraepithelial lesion. LSIL and HSIL are the cytologic counterparts of low-grade dysplasia and high-grade dysplasia, respectively.

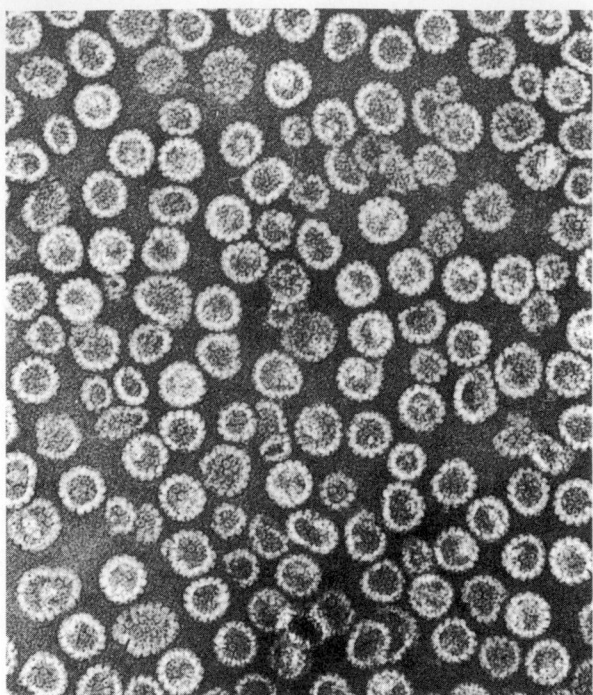

FIGURE 45–2 ■ Transmission electron micrograph of HPV 16 L1 virus-like particles purified from recombinant baculovirus–infected insect cell cultures (original magnification ×36,000).

the tumor suppressor proteins p53 and pRb, respectively, coupled with indirect effects of the genetic instability induced by the viral oncogenes.[15]

The usual regression of low-grade lesions is almost certainly the result of cell-mediated immune responses to the viral proteins.[16,17] However, the principal effector mechanisms and target antigens involved in immune-mediated regression of benign papillomavirus-induced lesions are not well understood. In part, this is because papillomavirus infections are remarkably species restricted. Because a domestic mouse papillomavirus has not been identified, the power of mouse immunology cannot readily be brought to bear on the subject. High-grade dysplasias and cancers infrequently regress. Several mechanisms could contribute to the persistence of advanced lesions despite the continued expression of viral antigens. First, E6 and E7 are expressed at relatively low levels, and viral infection does not induce cell lysis or other inducers of inflammation.[18] In addition, E6 and E7 can interfere with activation of interferon response genes.[19] These factors would favor a state of immune ignorance. Prolonged low-level epithelial expression in the absence of inflammation also might induce specific T-cell tolerance to E6 and E7.[20] Finally, advanced lesions generally have defects in class I antigen presentation, which would make them unlikely to induce cytotoxic T-lymphocyte (CTL) responses to the viral proteins.[21]

Prophylactic Vaccines

The identification of a virus as the primary cause of a major human cancer provides an exceptional opportunity for cancer prevention through vaccination. However, certain aspects of papillomavirus biology and its relationship to cervical cancer have placed challenges to the development of effective vaccines. Prophylactic vaccines based on live, attenuated or inactivated virions have proven to be very successful for other viruses, such as polio and measles.[22] This strategy could not be adopted for HPV vaccines for two reasons. First, difficulties in propagating the viruses preclude their large-scale production.[23] Second, the viral genomes contain oncogenes.[15] The theoretical possibility of vaccine-induced carcinogenesis by a live or inactivated HPV vaccine would be considered too great for a vaccine designed for use in healthy young people, the vast majority of whom are not destined to acquire cervical cancer in the absence of vaccination. Therefore, the design of prophylactic HPV vaccines has centered on subunit approaches.

The most well-developed and promising approach for immunoprophylaxis involves noninfectious virus-like particles (VLPs), which self-assemble spontaneously from 72 pentamers of the L1 major capsid protein (Fig. 45–2) (see papers by Frazer,[24] Galloway,[25] and Schiller[26] for reviews). Papillomavirus VLPs can be produced in a variety of cells, and clinical-grade VLPs are being produced in baculovirus-infected insect cells and *Saccharomyces cerevisiae*. They induce high titers of virion neutralizing antibodies after low-dose parenteral vaccination, even in the absence of adjuvant. In contrast, denatured monomeric L1 does not induce neutralizing antibodies. Studies with animal papillomavirus types in rabbits, dogs, and cattle demonstrated excellent protection from homologous virus challenge after VLP vaccination.[27–29] Protection could be transferred passively via serum, indicating that neutralizing antibodies are sufficient to confer protection. Although certainly encouraging, the relevance of these results for human vaccine development is limited by the fact that protection mediated by HPV VLP vaccination cannot be assessed directly because HPVs do not replicate or produce disease in animals. Also, none of the animal challenge models involve venereal transmission, the route by which the HPV infections that cause cancer are acquired.

Mice or rabbits vaccinated with HPV VLPs produce high titers of antibodies that prevent infection of cultured cells. However, HPV genotypes appear to be distinct serotypes, in that the neutralizing activity of the VLP antibodies is almost entirely genotype specific.[30–32] This is unfortunate because more than a dozen HPV types are associated with cervical

TABLE 45–1 ■ Efficacy Analyses of a Human Papillomavirus Type 16 (HPV-16) LI Virus-like-particle Vaccine

End Point	HPV-16 Vaccine				Placebo				Observed Efficacy (95% CI)*
	No. of women	Cases of infection	Woman-yr. at risk	Infection rate per 100 woman-yr. at risk %	No. of women	Cases of Infection	Woman-yr at risk	Infection rate per 100 woman-yr at risk %	%
Persistent HPV-16 infection	768	0	1084.0	0	765	41	1076.9	3.8	100 (90–100)
Transient or persistent HPV-16 infection	768	6	1084.0	0.6	765	68	1076.9	6.3	91.2 (80–97)

*CI denotes confidence interval.
From Koutsky KA, Ault KA, Wheeler CM, et al. A controlled trial of human papillomavirus type 16 vaccine. N Engl J Med 347:1649, 2002.

cancer. Worldwide, HPV16 and -18 are found in 50% to 60% and 10% to 20% of cervical cancers, respectively.[12] No other type is detected in more than a few percent of cancers.

A series of early-phase clinical trials of HPV VLP vaccines have been completed. L1 VLPs of four HPV types have been examined: the major oncogenic types, HPV16 and -18, as well as HPV6 and -11, which are nononcogenic but cause most external genital warts. Published studies and meeting presentations uniformly have reported high immunogenicity and low reactogenicity after three intramuscular injection of HPV VLPs in the 10- to 100-μg range.[33–35] Most studies have used a 0-, 1-, and 4- to 6-month vaccination schedule, based on previous findings with the hepatitis B particle vaccine. After vaccination without adjuvant, serum HPV16 VLP immunoglobulin G (IgG) titers were 40-fold higher than the titers measured after natural infection.[33] High titers of serum antibodies also were obtained when the VLPs were formulated in alum-based or MF59 (squalene emulsion) adjuvants.

The HPV infections involved in cervical carcinogenesis are confined to the epithelia of the genital tract and do not produce viremic dissemination.[18] Therefore, only antibodies in the genital tract mucosa would be mediators of protection from infection. Fortunately, cervical mucus secretions in women contain large amounts IgG, much of which is appar-

ently transudated from the serum.[36] An unpublished meeting report supports previous studies in monkeys[37] in finding substantial levels of VLP-specific IgG in the cervical secretions of women after intramuscular VLP vaccination. An encouraging pilot efficacy trial of an HPV16 L1 VLP vaccine was recently published.[38] After a mean follow-up of 17 months, none of the 768 VLP vaccinated young women acquired persistent HPV16 infection, whereas 41 of the 765 placebo recipients became persistently infected with HPV16 (Table 45–1).

Three large efficacy trials of HPV VLP vaccines either have begun or are in the final planning stage (Table 45–2). Each trial will involve vaccination of several thousand young women who are negative for genital tract HPV DNA. Because protection is expected to be restricted to the HPV types included in the vaccine, women will be monitored over the course of several years for type-specific acquisition of cervical HPV DNA. In addition, they will be periodically examined for HPV-induced premalignant lesions using standard Pap screening, colposcopy, and histology. For ethical reasons, cervical cancer cannot be used as the final endpoint in trials with active follow-up, and it would take decades to accrue enough cases to demonstrate protection. It is likely that demonstration of type-specific protection from high- and intermediate-grade cervical dysplasias ultimately will be needed to win

TABLE 45–2 ■ HPV VLP efficacy trials

Sponsor*	Production	Types	Site(s)
NIH	Insect cells	HPV 16	Costa Rica
GSK	Insect cells	HPV 16, −18	Multicentric†
Merck & Co.	Yeast	HPV 6, −11, −16, −18	Multicentric†

*NIH, National Institutes of Health; GSK, GlaxoSmithKline.
†North America, South America, and Europe.

regulatory approval for general distribution of the vaccine.[39] It is quite possible that this type of data may become available within the next 5 years.

Several interesting implementation questions will arise if a licensed prophylactic HPV vaccine were to become available. First, would it be preferable to vaccinate both young men and young women or to concentrate efforts on coverage of women? Although HPV-associated penile, anal, and oral cancers do occur in men, the incidence of these cancers is much lower than the incidence of cervical cancer in women. So, with the exception of a vaccine that contains the VLPs of the HPV types that cause genital warts (which afflict men and women to similar extents), young men would take the vaccine primarily to prevent cervical cancer in their future sex partners. One might suspect that vaccinating both sexes would substantially increase herd immunity, but the dynamics of venereal HPV transmission are too poorly characterized to draw firm conclusions on the impact of vaccinating men.[40] However, there are no indications that efficacy trials involving men are being planned. Second, would vaccination of adolescent girls (and boys) against a sexually transmitted disease be generally accepted by the public? It might be preferable to emphasize the cancer prevention aspects of the vaccine program in public awareness initiatives.[41] However, it will be difficult to promote administration of a cervical cancer vaccine to boys without stressing the sexually transmitted nature of the disease.

Third, how would availability of a vaccine influence Pap screening programs?[42] If the vaccines are type specific as expected, then they will not protect against the 10% to 20% of cervical cancers that are caused by types other than HPV16 and -18. Therefore, it is difficult to know how, or if, a successful vaccine against HPV16 and -18 would influence national recommendations for Pap screening intervals. In addition, vaccinated women might have lower rates of compliance with existing Pap screening programs because of the misconception that they are fully protected from developing cervical cancer. It may be difficult to develop a sufficiently balanced public awareness initiative that encourages women to accept both vaccination and periodic Pap testing. This might be especially true if the campaigns are financed by the vaccine manufacturers.

Finally, how would a prophylactic HPV vaccine be delivered to the poorer women of the world, who are most in need of it because they lack access to adequate Pap screening?[22] The current purified VLP-based vaccines are ill suited for widespread use in developing countries. Manufacture requires extensive purification from cultured cell extracts, making them expensive to produce. Their administration likely will involve three intramuscular injections of adolescents over a 6-month period, making the vaccine difficult and expensive to deliver. Efforts are underway to develop alternative prophylactic vaccine strategies that overcome these manufacturing and distribution liabilities. However, clinical trials of alternative approaches have not been reported.

Therapeutic Vaccines

Because it usually takes many years for initial HPV infection to progress to cervical cancer, there is a further opportunity to prevent cervical cancer via vaccine-induced regression of premalignant lesions. Although this type of vaccine is pro-

phylactic from the point of view of cancer, it normally would be considered therapeutic because its aim is to eliminate a persistent viral infection. In theory, any stage of HPV infection/premalignant cervical neoplasia could be targeted. In practice, most therapeutic vaccine development programs are likely to target high-grade dysplasias. Although asymptomatic and low-grade dysplasias have the theoretical advantage of having more potential viral antigen targets and may be less efficient at immune evasion, they have a high rate of spontaneous regression and usually are not treated. By contrast, high-grade dysplasias tend to persist and require surgical treatment.[5] Vaccines against high-grade cervical dysplasias are receiving increasing interest among tumor immunologists, in part because this disease has several advantageous characteristics for testing tumor immunotherapies. The viral E6 and E7 oncoproteins are attractive tumor-specific antigen targets because they are selectively retained and expressed during malignant progression, and as foreign antigens they have not been subject to embryologic tolerance. Large numbers of potential vaccinees routinely are identified in Pap screening programs. In addition, the course of disease is well understood, it can be followed noninvasively by colposcopy, and existing treatments are definitive. The extent to which high-grade dysplasia patients have developed T-cell tolerance to E6 and E7, and whether a substantial proportion of premalignant lesions, like cancers, have defects in class I restricted antigen presentation, are important questions that are currently under investigation.[43,44]

Cell-mediated immune responses have been generated against E6 and E7 of HPV16 and other oncogenic HPVs by a variety of strategies. Most investigations have concentrated on the generation of CTL responses to the viral proteins and have tested efficacy in transplantable HPV-expressing mouse tumor models. A variety of approaches based on peptides, fusion proteins, naked DNA, viral or bacterial vectors, or whole cells have been successful in protecting mice from transplanted tumor cell challenge (see papers by Frazer,[24] Ling et al.,[45] and Da Silva et al.[46] for reviews). Some vaccines also have induced regression of established mouse tumors. In a perhaps more biologically relevant model, naked DNA and *Listeria*-based vaccines induced cell-mediated immunity (CMI) to nonstructural cottontail rabbit papillomavirus (CRPV) proteins that prevented formation of cutaneous papillomas after CRPV challenge of domestic rabbits.[47,48] It has been more difficult to induce regression of established cutaneous warts in this model. However, a combination of the antiviral compound cidofovir and naked DNA vaccination against multiple viral proteins did induce regression in a proportion of established CRPV papillomas.[49] Also, the DNA vaccine alone was able to reduce the frequency of spontaneously progression of the papillomas to carcinomas.[50]

Two therapeutic vaccine strategies have been tested in early-phase clinical trials of high-grade HPV-induced anogenital dysplasia. One trial involved vaccination of HPV16-positive high-grade cervical and vulvar dysplasia patients with HPV16 E7 peptide-based vaccines.[51] The other trial involved vaccination of cervical or anal dysplasia patients with a mycobacterium heat shock protein 65–HPV16 E7 fusion protein.[52] The vaccines in both studies generated measurable cell-mediated immune responses to E7. Clinical improvement was noted in some patients, but

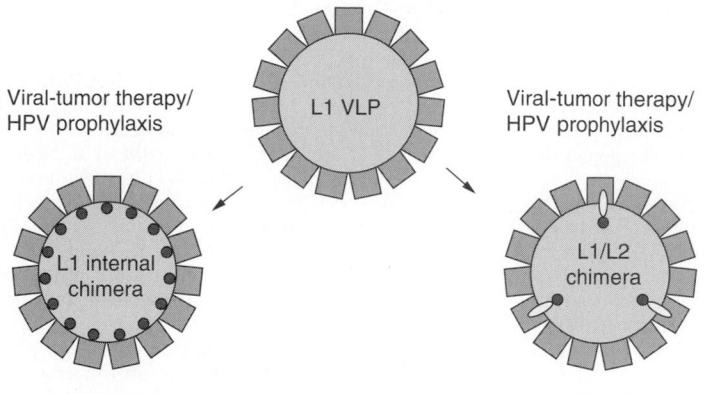

FIGURE 45–3 ■ Variations on VLP-based vaccines.

the trials were small and not designed to determine clinical efficacy. Additional and larger clinical studies of these and other therapeutic vaccine candidates are likely to follow.

Combined Prophylactic/ Therapeutic Vaccines

A vaccine that could both prevent infection in unexposed individuals and induce regression of genital lesions in at least a portion of the millions of women who are currently HPV infected certainly would be desirable. This is especially true in low-resource settings where infected women do not have the benefit of Pap screening to reduce their cervical cancer risk. Also, in deciding how to distribute limited health care resources, it may be difficult for many developing countries to adopt a strictly prophylactic HPV vaccination program because it would take many years to realize the intended public health benefit, reduction in the cervical cancer death rates. A combined vaccine might both decrease cervical cancer rates in this generation of women and provide maximum protection for the next generation.

It is very doubtful that the L1 VLP vaccines will act therapeutically. This is because L1 expression is undetectable in the proliferating cells of the epithelium in which the viral infection is maintained.[18] It is possible that a vaccine that induces CMI to the nonstructural viral proteins could act both as a prophylactic and a therapeutic vaccine, as suggested by the CRPV studies noted above. However, induction of neutralizing antibodies appears to be an important component of licensed viral vaccines.[53] Therefore, the most attractive combined vaccine candidates would induce both neutralizing antibodies and CMI to nonstructural viral proteins that are expressed in the proliferating cells of the lesions.

Currently, the most developed candidates with these characteristics are chimeric VLPs (Fig. 45–3).[54] They are VLPs in which nonstructural viral polypeptides are incorporated as fusions either to the end of L1 or to the L2 minor capsid protein, which is then incorporated into the VLPs during intracellular assembly.[55–58] In mouse models, they retain the ability to induce neutralizing antibodies but also can induce strong CTL responses to the incorporated polypeptide, usually E7. The ability of papillomavirus VLPs to induce acute phenotypic

and functional activation of dendritic cells is likely an important factor in the induction of potent antitumor responses after low-dose inoculation of chimeric VLPs in the absence of adjuvant or T-cell help.[59,60] Chimeric VLPs likely will be tested in both prophylactic and therapeutic clinical trials in the near future. There are other possibilities for a combined vaccine as well. For instance, CMI targets could be incorporated into the VLPs as DNA to form an HPV pseudovirus vaccine.[61] Alternatively, VLPs could be coadministered with one of the many strictly therapeutic vaccine candidates discussed above. These approaches are in early stages of development, and clinical trials do not appear to be imminent.

Conclusions

The establishment of the causal link between cervical cancer and infection by specific HPVs provides an exceptional opportunity to prevent this common cancer in women through vaccination. Both prophylactic and therapeutic vaccine candidates against the major oncogenic HPV types almost certainly will undergo extensive clinical testing in the immediate future. Within the next 5 years, there should be a good indication of whether these vaccines are likely to be broadly successful in preventing cervical cancer. The most effective candidates could well be licensed for general distribution by then. Licensure of a prophylactic vaccine could raise a host of implementation issues. Given the general optimism regarding the ultimate success of the prophylactic HPV vaccines, it may be reasonable to begin serious consideration of these issues.

REFERENCES

1. Parkin DM, Bray F, Ferlay J, Pisani P. Estimating the world cancer burden: Globocan 2000. Int J Cancer 94:153–156, 2001.
2. Eifel PJ, Berek JT, Thigpen JT. Cancer of the cervix, vagina, and vulva. *In* DeVita VT, Hellman S, Rosenberg SA (eds). Cancer Principles & Practice of Oncology (6th ed). Philadelphia, Lippincott Williams & Wilkins, 2001, pp 1526–1572.
3. Schiffman MH, Brinton LA. The epidemiology of cervical carcinogenesis. Cancer 76:1888–1901, 1995.
4. Schneider V, Henry MR, Jimenez-Ayala M, et al. Cervical cancer screening, screening errors and reporting. Acta Cytol 45:493–498, 2001.
5. Wright TC Jr, Cox JT, Massad LS, et al. 2001 Consensus Guidelines for the management of women with cervical cytological abnormalities. JAMA 287:2120–2129, 2002.

6. American Social Health Association, National HPV & Cervical Cancer Prevention Resource Center. HPV background information. Available at *www.ashastd.org/hpvccrc/background.html*

7. Sankaranarayanan R, Budukh AM, Rajkumar R. Effective screening programmes for cervical cancer in low- and middle-income developing countries. Bull World Health Organ 79:954–962, 2001.

8. Koss LG. The Papanicolaou test for cervical cancer detection: a triumph and a tragedy. JAMA 261:737–743, 1989.

9. Brinton LA. Epidemiology of cervical cancer—overview. *In* Munoz N, Bosch FX, Shah KV, Meheus A (eds). The Epidemiology of Human Papillomavirus and Cervical Cancer. Lyon, International Agency for Research on Cancer, 1992.

10. Dürst M, Gissmann L, Ikenberg H, zur Hausen H. A papillomavirus DNA from a cervical carcinoma and its prevalence in cancer biopsy samples from different geographic regions. Proc Natl Acad Sci U S A 80:3812–3815, 1983.

11. Bosch FX, Lorincz A, Munoz N, et al. The causal relation between human papillomavirus and cervical cancer. J Clin Pathol 55:244–265, 2002.

12. Walboomers JM, Jacobs MC, Manos MM, et al. Human papillomavirus is a necessary cause of invasive cervical cancer worldwide. J Pathol 189:12–19, 1999.

13. Zur Hausen H. Papillomaviruses in human cancers. Proc Assoc Am Physicians 111:581–587, 1999.

14. Gillison ML, Koch WM, Capone RB, et al. Evidence for a causal association between human papillomavirus and a subset of head and neck cancers. J Natl Cancer Inst 92:709–720, 2000.

15. Zur Hausen H. Immortalization of human cells and their malignant conversion by high risk human papillomavirus genotypes. Semin Cancer Biol 9:405–411, 1999.

16. Stern PL, Brown M, Stacey SN, et al. Natural HPV immunity and vaccination strategies. J Clin Virol 19:57–66, 2000.

17. Stanley MA. Immunobiology of papillomavirus infections. J Reprod Immunol 52:45–59, 2001.

18. Stubenrauch F, Laimins LA. Human papillomavirus life cycle: active and latent phases. Semin Cancer Biol 9:379–386, 1999.

19. Koromilas AE, Li S, Matlashewski G. Control of interferon signaling in human papillomavirus infection. Cytokine Growth Factor Rev 12:157–170, 2001.

20. Tindle RW. Immune evasion in human papillomavirus-associated cervical cancer. Natl Rev Cancer 2:59–65, 2002.

21. Brady CS, Bartholomew JS, Burt DJ, et al. Multiple mechanisms underlie HLA dysregulation in cervical cancer. Tissue Antigens 55:401–411, 2000.

22. Ulmer JB, Liu MA. Ethical issues for vaccines and immunization. Natl Rev Immunol 2:291–296, 2002.

23. Hagensee M, Galloway D. Growing human papillomaviruses and virus-like particles in the laboratory. Papillomavirus Rep 4:121–124, 1993.

24. Frazer I. Strategies for immunoprophylaxis and immunotherapy of papillomaviruses. Clin Dermatol 15:285–297, 1997.

25. Galloway DA. Is vaccination against human papillomavirus a possibility? Lancet 351:22–24, 1998.

26. Schiller JT. Papillomavirus-like particle vaccines for cervical cancer. Mol Med Today 5:209–215, 1999.

27. Suzich JA, Ghim S, Palmer-Hill FJ, et al. Systemic immunization with papillomavirus L1 protein completely prevents the development of viral mucosal papillomas. Proc Natl Acad Sci U S A 92:11553–11557, 1995.

28. Breitburd F, Kirnbauer R, Hubbert NL, et al. Immunization with virus-like particles from cottontail rabbit papillomavirus (CRPV) can protect against experimental CRPV infection. J Virol 69:3959–3963, 1995.

29. Kirnbauer R, Chandrachud L, O'Neil B, et al. Virus-like particles of bovine papillomavirus type 4 in prophylactic and therapeutic immunization. Virology 219:37–44, 1996.

30. Roden RBS, Greenstone HL, Kirnbauer R, et al. *In vitro* generation and type-specific neutralization of a human papillomavirus type 16 virion pseudotype. J Virol 70:5875–5883, 1996.

31. Unckell F, Streeck RE, Sapp M. Generation and neutralization of pseudovirions of human papillomavirus type 33. J Virol 71:2934–2939, 1997.

32. Giroglou T, Sapp M, Lane C, et al. Immunological analyses of human papillomavirus capsids. Vaccine 19:1783–1793, 2001.

33. Harro CD, Pang YY, Roden RB, et al. Safety and immunogenicity trial in adult volunteers of a human papillomavirus 16 L1 virus-like particle vaccine. J Natl Cancer Inst 93:284–292, 2001.

34. Evans TG, Bonnez W, Rose RC, et al. A Phase 1 study of a recombinant viruslike particle vaccine against human papillomavirus type 11 in healthy adult volunteers. J Infect Dis 183:1485–1493, 2001.

35. Brown DR, Bryan JT, Schroeder JM, et al. Neutralization of human papillomavirus type 11 (HPV-11) by serum from women vaccinated with yeast-derived HPV-11 L1 virus-like particles: correlation with competitive radioimmunoassay titer. J Infect Dis 184:1183–1186, 2001.

36. Mestecky J, Russell MW. Induction of mucosal immune responses in the human genital tract. FEMS Immunol Med Microbiol 27:351–355, 2000.

37. Lowe RS, Brown DR, Bryan JT, et al. Human papillomavirus type 11 (HPV11) neutralizing antibodies in the serum and genital mucosal secretions of African green monkeys immunized with HPV-11 virus-like particles expressed in yeast. J Infect Dis 176:1141–1145, 1997.

38. Koutsky KA, Ault KA, Wheeler CM, et al. A controlled trial of human papillomavirus type 16 vaccine. N Engl J Med 347:1645–1651, 2002.

39. Vaccines & Related Biological Products Advisory Committee. Transcript of the open session of the Vaccines & Related Biological Products Advisory Committee, November 28, 2001, on vaccine for the prevention of human papilloma virus. Available at *www.FDA.gov/ohrms/dockets/ac/01/transcripts/3805t1.htm*

40. Garnett GP, Waddell HC. Public health paradoxes and the epidemiological impact of an HPV vaccine. J Clin Virol 19:101–111, 2000.

41. Zimet GD, Mays RM, Winston Y, et al. Acceptability of human papillomavirus immunization. J Womens Health Gend Based Med 9:47–50, 2000.

42. Mays RM, Zimet GD, Winston Y, et al. Human papillomavirus, genital warts, Pap smears, and cervical cancer: knowledge and beliefs of adolescent and adult women. Health Care Women Int 21:361–374, 2000.

43. Doan T, Herd K, Street M, et al. Human papillomavirus type 16 E7 oncoprotein expressed in peripheral epithelium tolerizes E7-directed cytotoxic T-lymphocyte precursors restricted through human (and mouse) major histocompatibility complex class I alleles. J Virol 73:6166–6170, 1999.

44. Abdel-Hady ES, Martin-Hirsch P, Duggan-Keen M, et al. Immunological and viral factors associated with the response of vulval intraepithelial neoplasia to photodynamic therapy. Cancer Res 61:192–196, 2001.

45. Ling M, Kanayama M, Roden R, Wu TC. Preventive and therapeutic vaccines for human papillomavirus-associated cervical cancers. J Biomed Sci 7:341–356, 2000.

46. Da Silva DM, Eiben GL, Fausch SC, et al. Cervical cancer vaccines: emerging concepts and developments. J Cell Physiol 186:169–182, 2001.

47. Jensen ER, Shen H, Wettstein FO, et al. Recombinant *Listeria* monocytogenes as a live vaccine vehicle and a probe for studying cell-mediated immunity. Immunol Rev 158:147–157, 1997.

48. Leachman SA, Tigelaar RE, Shlyankevich M, et al. Granulocyte-macrophage colony-stimulating factor priming plus papillomavirus E6 DNA vaccination: effects on papilloma formation and regression in the cottontail rabbit papillomavirus-rabbit model. J Virol 74:8700–8708, 2000.

49. Christensen ND, Han R, Cladel NM, Pickel MD. Combination treatment with intralesional cidofovir and viral-DNA vaccination cures large cottontail rabbit papillomavirus-induced papillomas and reduces recurrences. Antimicrob Agents Chemother 45:1201–1209, 2001.

50. Han R, Cladel NM, Reed CA, et al. DNA vaccination prevents and/or delays carcinoma development of papillomavirus-induced skin papillomas on rabbits. J Virol 74:9712–9716, 2000.

51. Muderspach L, Wilczynski S, Roman L, et al. A phase I trial of a human papillomavirus (HPV) peptide vaccine for women with high-grade cervical and vulvar intraepithelial neoplasia who are HPV 16 positive. Clin Cancer Res 6:3406–3416, 2000.

52. Stressgen Biotechnologies. Stressgen announces robust HPV data from multiple Phase II clinical trials. November 27, 2001. Available at *www.stressgen.com/news/pr-011129-PhaseIIData.pdf* (for a summary of the results, go to *www.stressgen.com/product/phase2.htm*)

53. Robbins JB, Schneerson R, Szu SC. Hypothesis: serum IgG antibody is sufficient to confer protection against infectious diseases by inactivating the inoculum. J Infect Dis 171:1387–1398, 1995.

54. Da Silva DM, Velders MP, Rudolf MP, et al. Papillomavirus virus-like particles as anticancer vaccines. Curr Opin Mol Ther 1:82–88, 1999.

55. Muller M, Zhou J, Reed TD, et al. Chimeric papillomavirus-like particles. Virology 234:93–111, 1997.

56. Peng S, Frazer IH, Fernando GJ, Zhou J. Papillomavirus virus-like particles can deliver defined CTL epitopes to the MHC class I pathway. Virology 240:147–157, 1998.

57. Greenstone HL, Nieland JD, de Visser KE, et al. Chimeric papillomavirus virus-like particles elicit antitumor immunity against the E7 oncoprotein in an HPV16 tumor model. Proc Natl Acad Sci U S A 95:1800–1805, 1998.

58. Jochmus I, Schafer K, Faath S, et al. Chimeric virus-like particles of the human papillomavirus type 16 (HPV 16) as a prophylactic and therapeutic vaccine. Arch Med Res 30:269–274, 1999.

59. Lenz P, Day PM, Pang YS, et al. Papillomavirus-like particles induce acute activation of dendritic cells. J Immunol 166:5346–5355, 2001.

60. Rudolf MP, Fausch SC, Da Silva DM, Kast WM. Human dendritic cells are activated by chimeric human papillomavirus type-16 virus-like particles and induce epitope-specific human T cell responses in vitro. J Immunol 166:5917–5924, 2001.

61. Shi W, Liu J, Huang Y, Qiao L. Papillomavirus pseudovirus: a novel vaccine to induce mucosal and systemic cytotoxic T-lymphocyte responses. J Virol 75:10139–10148, 2001.

Chapter 46

Lyme Disease Vaccine

ALLEN C. STEERE

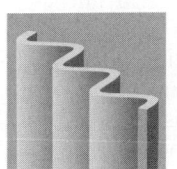

History of Lyme Disease

Lyme disease was described as a separate entity in 1976 because of geographic clustering of children in Lyme, Connecticut, who were thought to have juvenile rheumatoid arthritis.[1] The rural setting of the case clusters and the identification of an expanding skin lesion, erythema migrans, as a feature of the illness suggested that the disorder was transmitted by an arthropod. It soon became apparent that Lyme disease was a multisystem illness that affected primarily the skin, nervous system, heart, and joints.[2] Epidemiologic studies of patients with erythema migrans implicated certain ixodid ticks as vectors of the disease.[3]

In addition to providing clues about the cause of the illness, the initial expanding skin lesion linked Lyme disease in the United States with certain syndromes in Europe (erythema migrans, meningopolyneuritis, and acrodermatitis chronica atrophicans) that were described in the early and mid-20th century.[4–6] Lyme disease and these various syndromes were brought together conclusively in 1982, when Burgdorfer and Barbour isolated a previously unrecognized spirochete, now called *Borrelia burgdorferi*, from *Ixodes dammini* (also called *Ixodes scapularis*) ticks.[7] The spirochete then was recovered from patients with Lyme disease in the United States[8,9] and from those with erythema migrans, meningopolyneuritis, or acrodermatitis in Europe,[10–12] and the patients' immune responses were linked conclusively with this organism.[8]

Later, *B. burgdorferi* sensu lato (*B. burgdorferi* in the general sense) was divided into three pathogenic groups.[13] To date, all North American strains have belonged to the first group, *B. burgdorferi* sensu stricto (*B. burgdorferi* in the strict sense). Although all three groups have been found in Europe, most isolates there have been group 2 (*Borrelia garinii*) or group 3 (*Borrelia afzelii*) strains, and only the latter two groups have been found in Asia.

Lyme disease (or Lyme borreliosis) is now the most common vector-borne disease in the United States.[14] The infection is endemic in more than 15 states and has been responsible for focal outbreaks in some eastern coastal areas. If not recognized and treated appropriately, the spirochete may cause chronic, debilitating illness for a period of years. Because of the small size of nymphal *I. scapularis*, which is primarily responsible for transmission of the infection, efforts to prevent tick bites have been largely ineffective. Therefore, vaccination is an attractive strategy for prevention of the illness.

Background

Clinical Description

Lyme disease occurs in stages, with different manifestations at each stage. Early infection consists of localized erythema migrans (stage 1), followed within days to weeks by dissemination of the spirochete (stage 2), particularly to the nervous system, heart, or joints; this is followed within weeks to months by persistent infection (stage 3).[15] A patient may have one or all of the stages, and the infection may not become symptomatic until stage 2 or 3.

In 70% to 80% of patients in the United States, Lyme disease begins with a characteristic expanding skin lesion, erythema migrans (stage 1), which occurs at the site of the tick bite.[16,17] After an incubation period of 3 to 32 days, redness forms around the site and expands slowly. During the first several days, the lesion often has a homogeneous red appearance.[18] Later, as the lesion expands more, it frequently develops a red outer border with partial central clearing (Fig. 46–1). Within days to weeks, *B. burgdorferi* often disseminates hematogenously (stage 2). During this period, patients often have influenza-like symptoms such as malaise and fatigue, headache, neck pain, arthralgias, myalgias, fever, or regional lymphadenopathy. In addition, secondary annular skin lesions may develop that are similar to initial erythema migrans lesions but that lack indurated centers and are not associated with previous tick bites.

Within weeks, during or shortly after the period of early, disseminated infection, objective signs of acute neuroborreliosis develop in about 15% of untreated patients.[19,20] Possible manifestations include lymphocytic meningitis with episodic headache and neck stiffness, subtle encephalitis with difficulty with mentation, cranial neuropathy (particularly unilateral or bilateral facial palsy), motor or sensory radiculoneuritis, mononeuritis multiplex, cerebellar

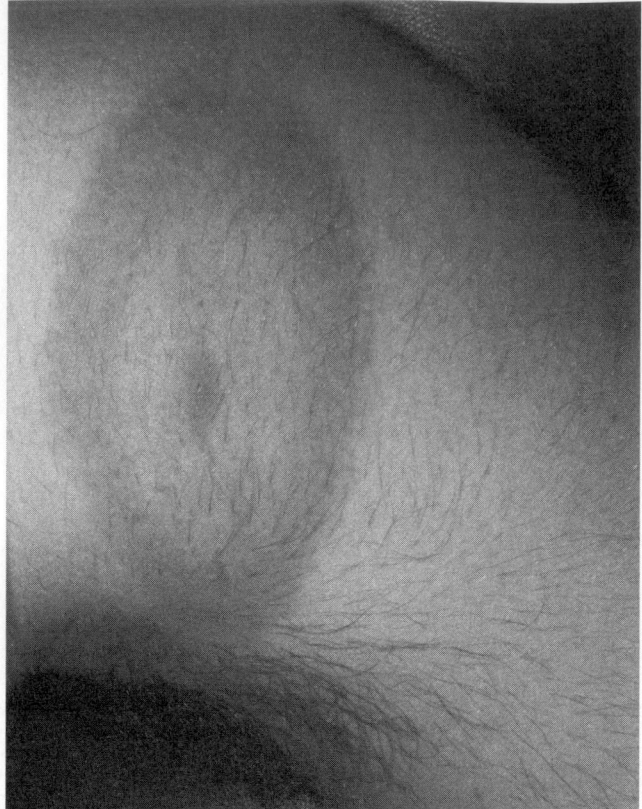

FIGURE 46–1 ■ A classic erythema migrans skin lesion (9 cm in diameter) is seen near the axilla. The lesion has partial central clearing, a bright red outer border, and a target center. (From Steere AC. Lyme disease. N Engl J Med 345:115, 2001, with permission. Copyright© 2001, Massachusetts Medical Society, All rights reserved. Photo courtesy of Dr. Vijay K. Sikand, East Lyme, Connecticut.)

ataxia, or myelitis. During this same period, about 5% of untreated patients have acute cardiac involvement—most commonly fluctuating degrees of atrioventricular block, occasionally acute myopericarditis, and rarely cardiomegaly or fatal pancarditis.[21,22] Even without antibiotic therapy, heart block or acute neurologic involvement usually resolves within weeks or months.

Months after the onset of illness (stage 3), about 60% of untreated patients in the United States begin to have intermittent attacks of oligoarticular arthritis, usually in one or a few large joints at a time, especially the knee.[23] Knees often become very swollen, and the swelling is out of proportion to the pain. By the time that arthritis is present, the infection often seems localized to affected joints, and systemic symptoms are minimal. In about 10% of patients, arthritis in the knees becomes chronic, defined as 1 year or more of continuous joint inflammation. The synovial tissue in such patients, which shows synovial hypertrophy, vascular proliferation, and a marked infiltration of mononuclear cells, is typical of that seen in all forms of chronic inflammatory arthritis, including rheumatoid arthritis.[24,25] However, even in untreated patients, intermittent or chronic Lyme arthritis usually resolves completely within several years.

Months to several years after disease onset, usually following the period of oligoarticular arthritis, up to 5% of untreated patients in the United States experience chronic neurologic manifestations of Lyme disease.[26] A mild

encephalopathy may develop, manifested primarily by subtle disturbances in memory.[26,27] Although inflammatory changes are not found in cerebrospinal fluid, intrathecal antibody production to the spirochete often can be demonstrated by antibody-capture enzyme immunoassay.[28] In addition, a chronic axonal polyneuropathy may develop, manifested primarily as spinal radicular pain or distal paresthesias.[29,30] Electromyograms in these patients typically show diffuse involvement of both proximal and distal nerve segments.

The basic outlines of Lyme borreliosis are similar worldwide, but there are regional variations, primarily between the illness found in America and that in Europe or Asia.[31] In North America, where the infection is caused by B. burgdorferi, widely disseminated early disease and subsequent arthritis are prominent features of the illness. In Europe, B. garinii may cause chronic encephalomyelitis, characterized by spastic paraparesis, cranial neuropathy, or cognitive impairment with marked intrathecal antibody production to the spirochete.[32] In addition, B. afzelii may cause acrodermatitis chronica atrophicans, in which inflammation and then atrophy of the skin occurs over many years or decades.[33] The spirochete has been cultured from such lesions as long as 10 years after their onset.[12]

Bacteriology

The structure of Borrelia species, including B. burgdorferi, is similar to that of all spirochetes: a protoplasmic cylinder surrounded by periplasm containing the flagella, which is surrounded, in turn, by an outer membrane (Fig. 46–2).[34] The genome of B. burgdorferi is quite small (approximately 1.5 Mb) and consists of a highly unusual linear chromosome of 950 kb as well as 9 linear and 12 circular plasmids.[35,36] The remarkable aspect of the B. burgdorferi genome is its large number of sequences for predicted or known lipoproteins, including plasmid-encoded outer surface proteins (Osps) A through F. In addition, during early, disseminated infection, a surface-exposed lipoprotein, called VlsE, undergoes extensive antigenic variation.[37] The only known virulence factors of B. burgdorferi are surface proteins, which allow the spirochete to attach to a variety of mammalian cells.

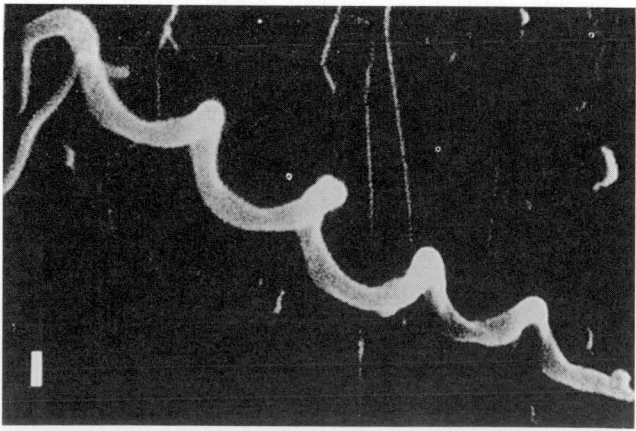

FIGURE 46–2 ■ Scanning electron micrograph of Borrelia burgdorferi, the causative agent of Lyme disease. Of the Borrelia species, B. burgdorferi is the longest (20 to 30 μm) and narrowest (0.2 to 0.3 μm), and it has fewer flagella (7 to 11). (From Johnson RC, Hyde RW, Rumpel CM. Taxonomy of the Lyme disease spirochetes. Yale J Biol Med 57:529, 1984, with permission.)

Pathogenesis

To maintain its complex enzootic cycle, B. burgdorferi must adapt to two markedly different environments, the tick and the mammalian host.[38] In the midgut of the tick, the spirochete expresses OspA and OspB.[39] When a blood meal is taken, these two proteins are down-regulated and OspC is up-regulated as the spirochete traverses to the tick salivary gland and to the mammalian host.[40]

After injection into the skin, B. burgdorferi usually first multiplies locally in the skin at the site of the tick bite. Several days later, the spirochete begins to spread in the skin, and, within days to weeks, it may disseminate to many sites. A number of mechanisms may aid in dissemination. For example, the sequences of OspC vary considerably among strains, and only a few groups of sequences are associated with disseminated disease.[41] Spreading through the skin and other tissue matrices may be facilitated by the binding of human plasminogen and its activators to the surface of the spirochete.[42] During dissemination and homing to specific sites, the organism attaches to certain host integrins,[43,44] matrix glycosaminoglycans,[45] and extracellular matrix proteins.[46] Borrelia decorin-binding proteins (Dbps) A and B bind decorin,[47] a glycosaminoglycan on collagen fibrils, which may explain why the organism is commonly aligned with collagen fibrils in the extracellular matrix in the heart, nervous system, or joints.

As shown definitively in mice, inflammatory innate immune responses are critical in the control of early, disseminated infection.[48,49] Spirochetal lipoproteins, which bind the CD14 molecule and toll-like receptor 2 on macrophages,[50] are potent activators of the innate immune response, leading to the production of macrophage-derived proinflammatory cytokines. In addition, type 1 T-helper (Th1) cells, which are part of the adaptive immune response, are prominent early in the infection.[51] Particularly in disseminated infection, adaptive T-cell and B-cell responses in lymph nodes lead to the production of antibody against many components of the spirochete.[52] Despite these innate and adaptive immune responses, the organism sometimes may survive in selected niches for years. In histologic sections, B. burgdorferi has been seen only extracellularly[53]; it has not been shown to survive intracellularly for prolonged periods.

In rodent models of B. burgdorferi infection, antibody responses to a number of Osps, including OspA, B, C, and F, and to DbpA,[54-57] have been shown to provide some degree of protective immunity against infection. In human patients with erythema migrans who are treated with antibiotic therapy, the antibody response does not develop fully, and such patients may become reinfected.[18] However, among patients with Lyme arthritis, a late manifestation of the disease, reinfection has not been noted, which suggests that the natural infection may induce long-term protective immunity. The specific responses that are responsible for protective immunity in the natural infection are not known.

Diagnosis

Borrelia burgdorferi may be cultured in a complex liquid medium called Barbour-Stoenner-Kelly medium.[8,9]

However, except for a few cases, positive cultures have been obtained only early in the illness, primarily from skin biopsy specimens of erythema migrans lesions,[58] less often from plasma samples,[59] and only occasionally from cerebrospinal fluid samples in patients with meningitis.[60] Later in the infection, polymerase chain reaction (PCR) testing has been valuable for the detection of B. burgdorferi DNA in joint fluid,[61,62] but it is not often positive with samples from other sites late in the illness.[63] Thus the diagnosis of Lyme disease usually is based on recognition of a characteristic clinical picture, exposure in an endemic area, and, except in patients with erythema migrans, a positive antibody response to B. burgdorferi by enzyme-linked immunosorbent assay (ELISA) and Western blot,[64] interpreted according to the criteria of the Centers for Disease Control and Prevention and the Association of State and Territorial Public Health Laboratory Directors.[65] In Europe, where there is less expansion of the antibody response, no single set of criteria for the interpretation of immunoblots results in high levels of sensitivity and specificity in all countries.[66]

During the first several weeks of infection, when most patients have erythema migrans, serodiagnostic tests are insensitive, and they depend primarily on the detection of an immunoglobulin M (IgM) response to the spirochete.[67,68] However, after 4 weeks of infection, when most patients in the United States have disseminated infection, the sensitivity and specificity of the immunoglobulin G (IgG) response to the spirochete are both very high, in the range of 95% to 99% as determined by the two-test approach of ELISA and Western blot.[68] A positive IgG blot requires reactivity with at least 5 of the following 10 bands (18, 23, 28, 30, 39, 41, 45, 58, 66, or 93 kDa).[65] In persons who have been ill for longer than 1 month, a positive IgM test alone is likely to represent a false-positive result; therefore, such a response should not be used to support the diagnosis of Lyme disease after the first month of infection.

Several caveats are important to keep in mind in the interpretation of serologic tests. First, antibody titers fall slowly after antibiotic treatment, but IgG and even IgM responses may persist for many years after treatment.[69] Thus current serologic tests demonstrate exposure to the spirochete, but they cannot distinguish between past or active infection. Second, B. burgdorferi may cause asymptomatic infection. In the SmithKline Beecham Lyme disease vaccine trial in the United States, in which participants were followed prospectively for 20 months, asymptomatic IgG seroconversion was demonstrated by Western blotting in about 10% of subjects with Lyme disease.[70] Finally, in tests that use whole, sonicated spirochetes as the antigen preparation, vaccination for Lyme disease may cause positive IgG results by ELISA.[71] However, vaccine-induced antibody responses, which are directed against the 31-kDa OspA protein, usually may be differentiated from infection-induced responses by Western blotting.[70] Thus, in each of these instances, care must be taken in the interpretation of serologic results.

Treatment and Prevention with Antimicrobials

Evidence-based treatment recommendations for Lyme disease have been published by the Infectious Diseases Society of America (Table 46–1).[72] For early localized or

TABLE 46–1 ■ Antibiotic Treatment Regimens for Lyme Disease*

EARLY INFECTION (LOCAL OR DISSEMINATED)

Adults
Doxycycline, 100 mg orally twice daily for 14–21 days
Amoxicillin, 500 mg orally 3 times daily for 14–21 days
Alternatives in case of doxycycline or amoxicillin allergy:
Cefuroxime axetil, 500 mg orally twice daily for 14–21 days
Erythromycin, 250 mg orally 4 times a day for 14–21 days

Children (Age 8 or less)
Amoxicillin, 250 mg orally 3 times a day or 50 mg/kg per day in 3 divided doses for 14–21 days
Alternatives in case of penicillin allergy:
Cefuroxime axetil, 125 mg orally twice daily or 30 mg/kg per day in 2 divided doses for 14–21 days
Erythromycin, 250 mg orally 3 times a day or 30 mg/kg per day in 3 divided doses for 14–21 days

NEUROLOGIC ABNORMALITIES (EARLY OR LATE)

Adults
Ceftriaxone 2 g IV once a day for 14–28 days
Cefotaxime, 2 g IV every 8 h for 14–28 days
Na penicillin G, 20 million U IV in 6 divided doses every 4 h for 14–28 days
Alternative in case of ceftriaxone or penicillin allergy:
Doxycycline, 100 mg orally 3 times a day for 30 days; this regimen may be ineffective for
   late neuroborreliosis
Facial palsy alone:
Oral regimens may be adequate

Children (Age 8 or younger)
Ceftriaxone, 75–100 mg/kg per day (maximum, 2 g) IV once a day for 14–28 days
Cefotaxime, 150 mg/kg per day in 3 or 4 divided doses (maximum, 6 g) for 14–28 days
Na penicillin G, 200,000–400,000 U/kg per day in 6 divided doses for 14–28 days

ARTHRITIS (INTERMITTENT OR CHRONIC)

Oral regimens listed above for 30–60 days *or*
IV regimens listed above for 14–28 days

CARDIAC ABNORMALITIES

First-degree AV block: oral regimens, as for early infection
High-degree AV block (P-R interval >0.3 s): IV regimens and cardiac monitoring; once the patient
   has stabilized, the course may be completed with oral therapy

PREGNANT WOMEN

Standard therapy for manifestation of the illness; avoid doxycycline

*Antibiotic recommendations are based on the guidelines from the Infectious Diseases Society of America.[72]
AV, atrioventricular; IV, intravenous.

disseminated infection, doxycycline 100 mg twice daily for 14 to 21 days is recommended in persons age 8 or older, except for pregnant women.[73,74] Amoxicillin 500 mg three times daily, the second-choice alternative, should be used in children or pregnant women.[73,74] In case of allergy or other contraindication to doxycycline or amoxicillin, cefuroxime axetil 500 mg twice daily is a third-choice alternative.[75] Erythromycin 250 mg four times daily or its congeners, which are fourth-choice alternatives, are recommended only for patients who are unable to take doxycycline, amoxicillin, or cefuroxime axetil.[74]

For patients with objective neurologic abnormalities, 2- to 4-week courses of intravenous ceftriaxone 2 g once a day are given most commonly.[26,76,77] Parenteral therapy with cefotaxime or penicillin G may be a satisfactory alternative. The signs and symptoms of acute neuroborreliosis usually resolve within weeks, but those of chronic neuroborreliosis improve only slowly, over a period of months. Objective evidence of relapse is rare after a 4-week course of therapy. In patients with high-degree atrioventricular

nodal block, intravenous therapy for at least part of the course and cardiac monitoring are recommended, but insertion of a permanent pacemaker is not necessary.

Either oral or intravenous regimens are usually effective for the treatment of Lyme arthritis.[77,78] Despite treatment with either oral or intravenous antibiotic therapy, about 10% of patients in the United States have persistent joint inflammation for months or even several years after 2 or more months of oral antibiotics or 1 or more months of intravenous antibiotics. If patients have persistent arthritis despite this treatment and if the results of PCR testing of joint fluid are negative, such patients may be treated with anti-inflammatory agents or arthroscopic synovectomy.

Should *I. scapularis* tick bites be treated with antibiotic prophylaxis? In studies, the frequency of Lyme disease after a recognized tick bite has been only about 1%,[79] perhaps because at least 24 hours of tick attachment seems to be necessary for transmission to occur.[80] Thus persons should remove an attached tick as soon as possible, and no other treatment is usually necessary. However, if the tick is engorged, indicating a longer duration of attachment, a single 200-mg dose of doxycycline effectively prevents Lyme disease when given within 72 hours after the tick bite.[81]

Epidemiology

Incidence and Prevalence Data

Lyme disease occurs primarily in three distinct foci in the United States: in the Northeast from Maine to Maryland, in the Midwest in Wisconsin and Minnesota, and to a lesser degree in the West, primarily in northern California (Fig. 46–3)[14,82]. However, sporadic cases have been reported in many states. In Europe, Lyme borreliosis is widely established in forested areas. The highest reported frequencies of the disease are in middle Europe and Scandinavia, particularly in Germany, Austria, Slovenia, and Sweden.[83,84] The infection also is found in Russia, China, and Japan.

Since surveillance for Lyme disease was begun in the United States in 1982, the number of cases reported to the Centers for Disease Control and Prevention has increased dramatically (Fig. 46–4). In recent years, about 15,000 to 18,000 cases have been reported yearly, accounting for more than 95% of all reported cases of vector-borne illness in the United States.[14] Persons of all ages are susceptible, but the highest reported rates occur in children less than 15 years of age and in adults 30 to 59 years of age.[14] The proliferation

of deer, which are the preferred host of the adult *I. scapularis*, was a major factor in the emergence of epidemic Lyme disease in the northeastern United States during the late 20th century.[85]

The risk of Lyme disease in a given area depends largely on the density of ixodid ticks as well as their feeding habits and animal hosts, which have evolved differently in different geographic locations. In the northeastern and north-central United States, *I. scapularis* ticks are abundant, and a highly efficient cycle of *B. burgdorferi* transmission occurs between immature larval and nymphal *I. scapularis* and white-footed mice.[86] This cycle results in high infection rates in nymphal ticks and a high frequency of human Lyme disease during the late spring and summer months.[14] Even within these regions, the disease is highly focal; almost 90% of the cases in the nation were reported in only 140 counties.[87] For example, in Connecticut, the state with the highest reported frequency of Lyme disease, the average annual incidence of the infection from 1992 to 1998 was 68 cases per 100,000 residents.[14] However, nearly half of the reported cases occurred in two counties in the southeastern part of the state where the township of Lyme is located. In the SmithKline Beecham Phase III Lyme disease vaccine trial, the yearly incidence of the disease in participants from hyperendemic areas was over 1%, and in some regions the seroprevalence of antibody to *B. burgdorferi* was as high as 5%.[70]

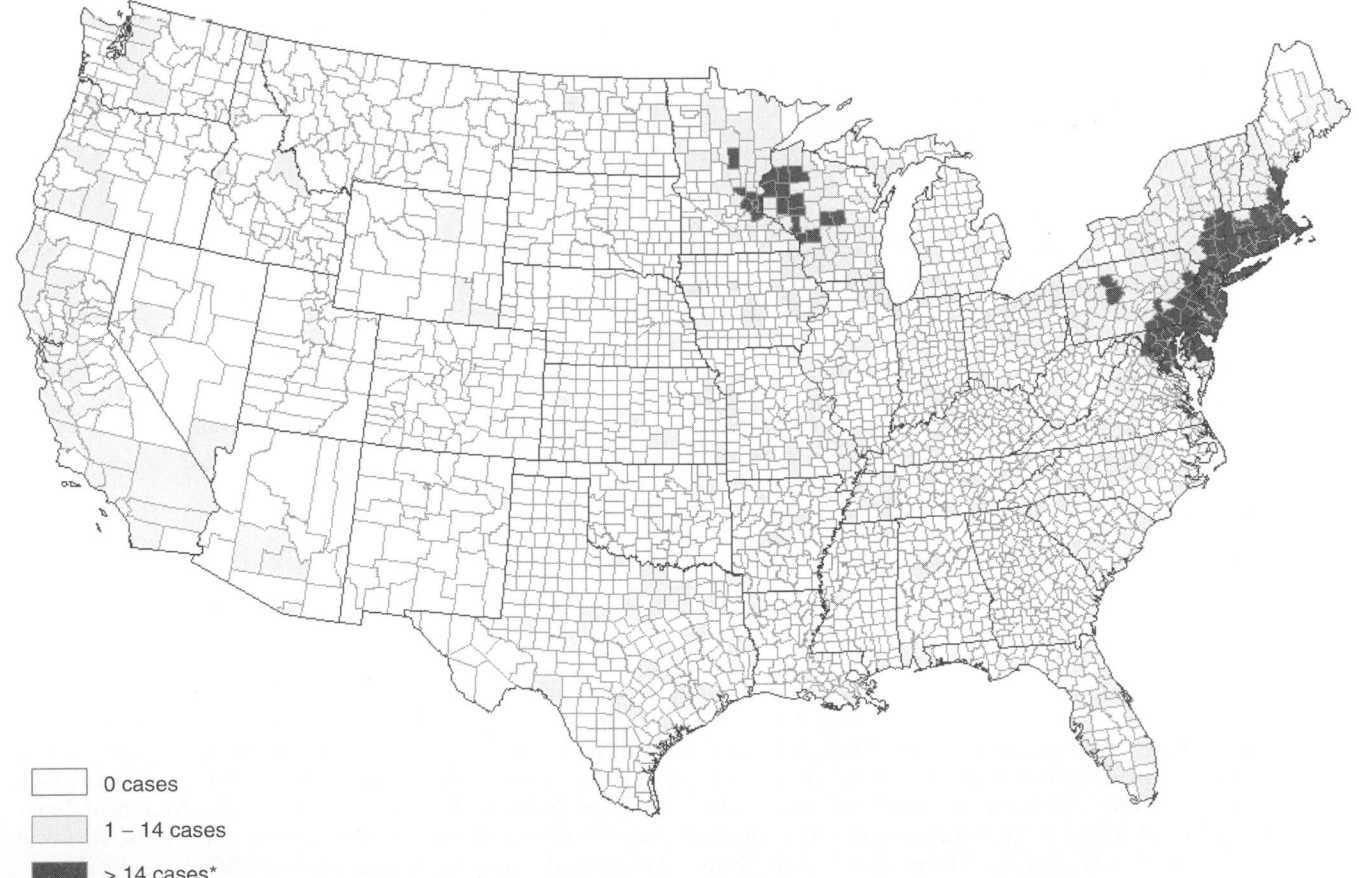

☐ 0 cases

▨ 1 – 14 cases

■ > 14 cases*

FIGURE 46–3 ■ Number of cases of Lyme disease in the United States, by county, reported to the Centers for Disease Control and Prevention in 2000. Approximately 90% of the cases were reported from only 140 counties in northeastern and upper midwestern states. (From Centers for Disease Control and Prevention. Lyme disease—United States, 2000. MMWR 51:29, 2002.)

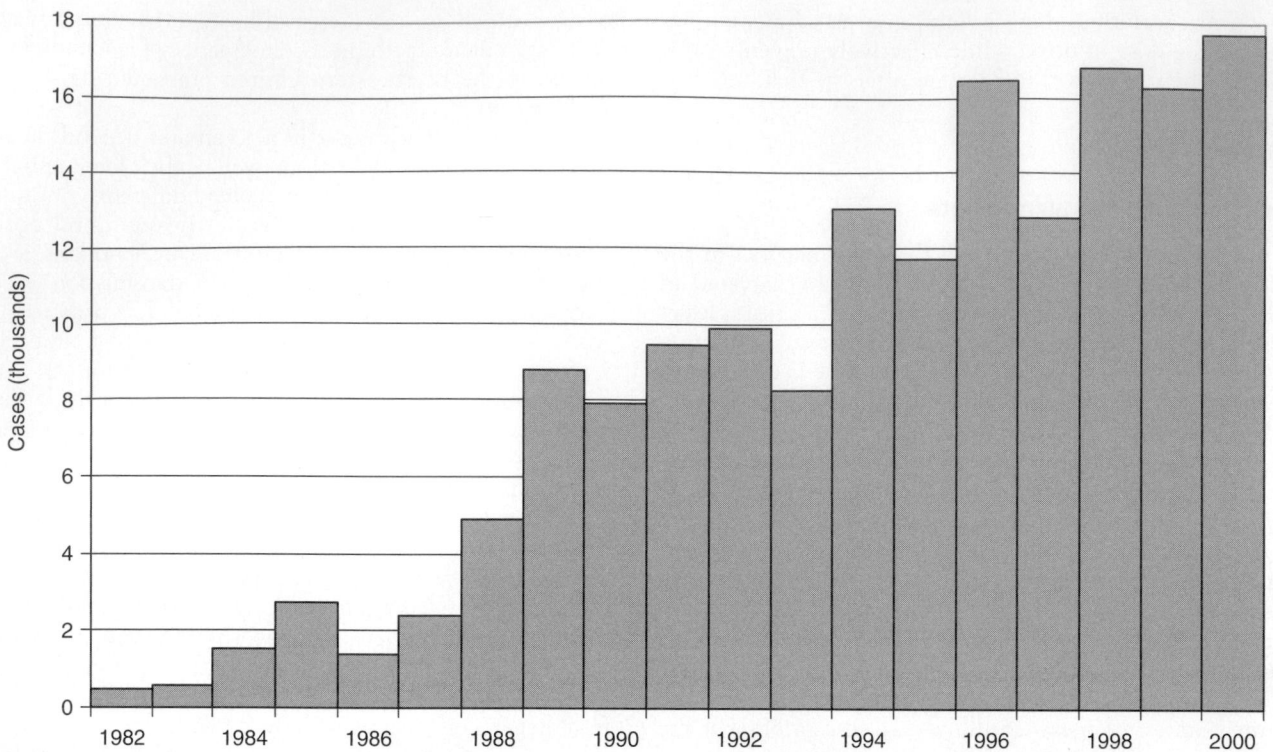

FIGURE 46–4 ■ Number of cases of Lyme disease in the United States, by year, reported to the Centers for Disease Control and Prevention from 1982 through 2000. Since surveillance was begun in 1982, the number of reported cases has increased dramatically. In 2000, nearly 18,000 cases were reported. (From Centers for Disease Control and Prevention. Lyme disease—United States, 2000. MMWR 51:29, 2002.)

The vector ecology of *B. burgdorferi* is quite different on the West coast in northern California, where the incidence of Lyme disease is low.[14] There, two intersecting cycles are necessary for disease transmission, one involving the dusky-footed wood rat and *Ixodes neotomae* ticks, which do not bite humans, and the other involving *I. pacificus* ticks, which do.[88] Because nymphal *I. pacificus* prefer to feed on lizards, which are not susceptible to *B. burgdorferi* infection, only the relatively few nymphal *I. pacificus* that previously fed on infected wood rats in the larval stage are responsible for spirochetal transmission to humans. Similarly, in the southeastern United States, nymphal *I. scapularis* feed primarily on lizards rather than rodents, and *B. burgdorferi* infection occurs rarely, if at all, in that part of the country.

Significance as a Public Health Problem

Even though the occurrence of Lyme disease is highly focal, certain locations, primarily in the northeastern United States, have been greatly affected.[14] Such areas have included suburban locations near Boston, New York, and Philadelphia, which are some of the most heavily populated parts of the country.[89] In addition, *I. scapularis* ticks continue to spread. In 1985, these ticks and Lyme disease were found in only 4 of the 58 counties in New York State.[90] By 2002, the ticks had spread to all but one of the 62 counties in the state (D. White and D. Morse, New York State Health Department, personal communication, January 16, 2003). Whereas personal preventive measures such as heavy clothing, tick repellants, and inspection after exposure have been advocated, their efficacy is limited.[90a] Although the limits of spread are not known, one can anticipate that epidemics of Lyme disease will continue to occur in new locations in the United States.

Passive Immunization

Passive immunization is not thought to be an important factor in protective immunity in Lyme disease. The spirochete is transmitted only by tick bite; person-to-person transmission has not been noted. Most patients have symptoms of the infection for months before protective immunity develops.

Active Immunization

History of Vaccine Development

In 1986, Johnson and his colleagues reported that Syrian hamsters could be immunized successfully against homologous strains of *B. burgdorferi* using a formalin-inactivated, whole-cell lysate of the spirochete.[91,92] These seminal studies showed that vaccination against Lyme disease was feasible. However, cross-protection among strains was limited. Immunization with European strains did not provide protection against U.S. strains and vice versa. Moreover, hamsters inoculated with a Northeast coast strain were not protected from infection with a West Coast strain. Subsequently, an inactivated whole-cell vaccine with a proprietary polymer-based adjuvant, called *Borrelia burgdorferi* bacterin (Fort Dodge Laboratories, Fort Dodge, IA) and a bivalent whole-cell killed vaccine (Solway Animal Health, Mendota Heights, MN) were licensed in the United States for use in dogs. However, little information is available regarding the safety and efficacy of these vaccines.[93,94] There was concern that vaccination of humans with inactivated whole-cell vaccines would be too reactogenic, and subunit vaccines consisting of a single recombinant protein were sought.

In 1990, Fikrig and his colleagues in the United States reported that immunization with a recombinant OspA protein of *B. burgdorferi* protected mice from challenge with several strains of the spirochete.[95] At the same time, Schaible and his colleagues in Germany showed that injection of a monoclonal antibody to OspA provided protection in a murine model of the infection.[96] Protection was afforded by the development of high-titered antibody to a conformational antibody epitope, called LA-2, in the C-terminal portion of the protein.[97] Because *B. burgdorferi* expresses OspA primarily in the midgut of the tick, spirochetal killing was accomplished mainly in the tick before transmission to the human host.[98] Immunization with the lipid component of the protein was important in the induction of the primary immune response.[99] In addition to mice, protective immunity to OspA was demonstrated in hamsters,[100] dogs,[101] and monkeys.[102,103] As with whole-cell lysates, immunization with OspA was highly protective when the challenge isolate was either identical or closely related to the one from which the protein was derived.[104,105] However, protection from more diverse isolates was more limited.[104,106]

At the same time, other approaches to vaccination were studied. In one study, a recombinant bacille Calmette-Guérin vaccine expressing an OspA lipoprotein protected mice against intradermal challenge with *B. burgdorferi*.[107] In addition, antibody responses to other Osps of *B. burgdorferi*, including OspB,[54] OspC,[55] OspF,[56] and DbpA,[57] afforded some degree of protective immunity in animal model systems, but not the complete protection observed with OspA (Table 46–2). In contrast, antibody reactivity with OspE or the flagellar protein of the spirochete did not provide protective immunity.[54]

TABLE 46–2 ■ Protection of Experimental Animals from *Borrelia burgdorferi* Infection*

Immunization	Challenge	Protection†
B. burgdorferi	*B. burgdorferi*	+++++
OspA	*B. burgdorferi*	+++++
OspB	*B. burgdorferi*	++++
OspC	*B. burgdorferi*	+++
OspE	*B. burgdorferi*	−
OspF	*B. burgdorferi*	+
P35 and P37	*B. burgdorferi*	++++
Flagellin	*B. burgdorferi*	−
P39	*B. burgdorferi*	+
P66	*B. burgdorferi*	+
DbpA	*B. burgdorferi*	++

*The data reflect the authors' interpretation of published studies.
†The degree of protection is graded on a scale from (−) to (+++++). (−) represents no protection and (+++++) represents substantial (nearly complete) protection. Intermediate grades reflect mild to moderate protection.
DbpA, decorin-binding protein A; Osp, outer surface protein.

In the early 1990s, two companies, Pasteur Mérieux Connaught (now Aventis Pasteur) and SmithKline Beecham (now GlaxoSmithKline) began the development of recombinant OspA vaccines for human use.[108,109] The vaccine made by GlaxoSmithKline was a recombinant OspA lipoprotein with adjuvant,[109] whereas the Aventis Pasteur vaccine was a recombinant OspA lipoprotein without adjuvant.[108] In December 1998, the vaccine made by GlaxoSmithKline, called LYMErix, was licensed and sold commercially until February 2002. Several review articles were written about Lyme disease vaccination.[110–115]

Constituents of the Vaccine

LYMErix contained lipidized OspA adsorbed onto aluminum hydroxide adjuvant in phosphate-buffered saline with phenoxyethanol as a preservative (pH 6.5 to 7.1).[70,109]

Manufacture of the Vaccine

LYMErix was produced using recombinant DNA technology. The OspA gene from the ZS7 strain of *B. burgdorferi* sensu stricto was placed in the pOA15 plasmid vector and grown in *Escherichia coli* strain AR58.[70,109] The OspA lipoprotein produced was a single polypeptide chain of 257 amino acids; the lipid moiety was covalently bonded to the N-terminus after translation.

Producers

LYMErix was produced by GlaxoSmithKline.

Preparations

LYMErix was available from December 1998 through February 2002. It was not formulated in combination with other vaccines.

Dosage and Route of Administration

Each 0.5-mL dose of LYMErix contained 30 μg of lipidized OspA with adjuvant, which was administered intramuscularly, usually in the deltoid muscle.[70] For primary immunization, it was recommended that three injections be given: one at the first visit, the second 1 month later, and the third at 12 months. However, equivalent antibody levels could be achieved by giving the third injection at either 2 or 6 months rather than at 12 months.[116,117] The important point was that the third injection should be in April to provide maximum levels of protection during May through July, the questing period for nymphal *I. scapularis* ticks.

Vaccine Stability

The recommendation was to refrigerate LYMErix at 2°C to 8°C. With refrigeration, the vaccine had an expiration date that was 24 months after the date of manufacture. The vaccine was stable at room temperature for up to 4 days. If freezing occurred, the vaccine was to be discarded.

Results of Vaccination

Immunogenicity of the Vaccine

Antibody Responses

Lyme disease vaccine induced an IgG antibody response to OspA, including reactivity with the protective conformational epitope, called LA-2, in the C-terminal portion of the protein.[97] Because the mechanism of the vaccine was antibody-mediated killing of the spirochete in the tick,[98] OspA antibody titers were the critical factor in vaccine efficacy. The levels of LA-2 equivalent antibodies were determined in a competitive-inhibition enzyme immunoassay in which a murine monoclonal antibody (called LA-2) competed for binding with the patient's LA-2 equivalent anti-OspA antibodies.[96,109] An alternative assay was the determination of IgG antibody titers to full-length OspA by indirect ELISA.[118] This assay measured not only the amount of antibody to the protective antibody epitope of OspA, but that to other OspA epitopes. For this reason, full-length OspA levels were not as accurate in predicting protection as were LA-2 equivalent antibody levels.

In the immunogenicity portion of the SmithKline Beecham Phase III trial, 95% of the 938 vaccine recipients tested from one site had LA-2 equivalent OspA antibody levels of 100 ng/mL or greater at month 2, 1 month after the second injection (Fig. 46–5).[70] Ten months later, the mean titer had declined markedly. At month 13, 1 month after the third injection, a marked anamnestic response was seen, and 99% had levels of 100 ng/mL or greater. At month 20, the mean titer had again declined. Thus, after three injections, most vaccine recipients developed high levels of LA-2 equivalent OspA antibody, but the antibody levels waned rather rapidly.

In the vaccine study, seven individuals were identified with very low antibody titers after vaccination.[119] The macrophages of these individuals produced less TNF-α and IL-6 after OspA stimulation, and had lower expression of Toll-like receptor (TLR)1 as compared with normal cells. TLR1 and TLR2 are required for lippoprotein recognition and defects in the TLR1/2 signaling pathway may account for hyporesponsiveness to OspA vaccination.

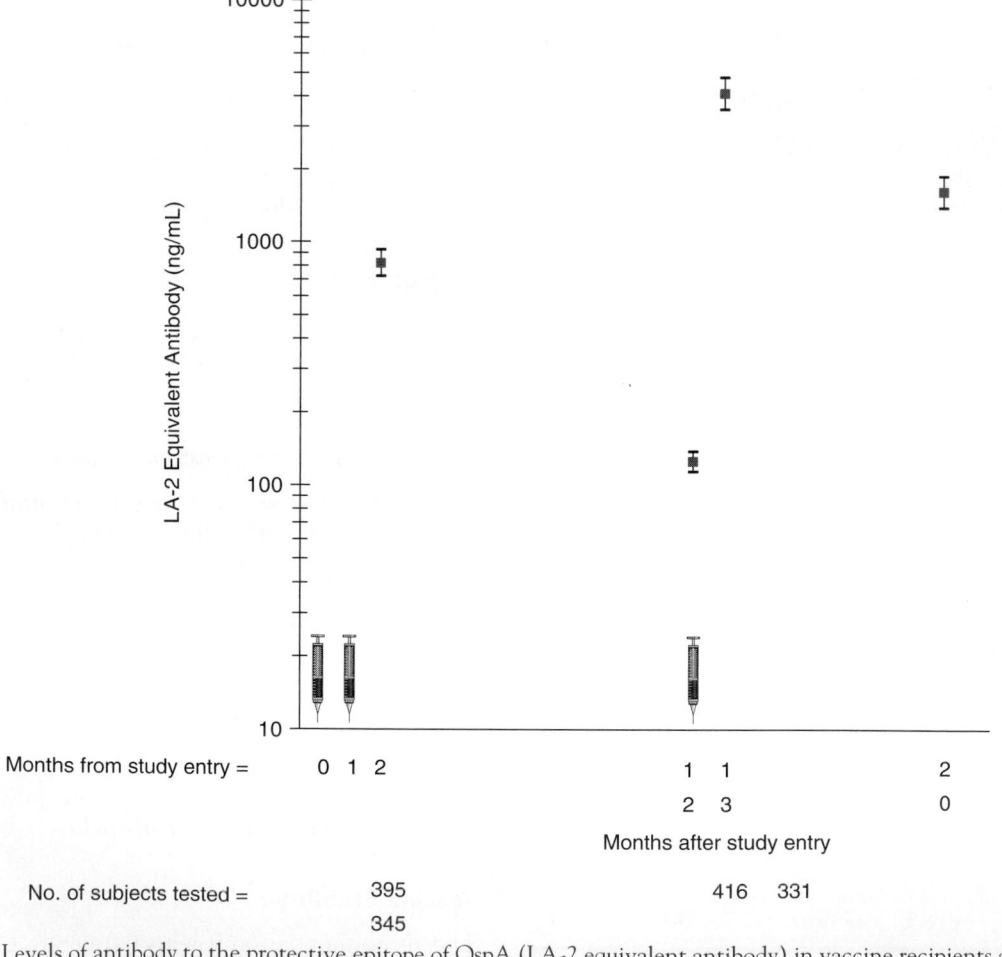

FIGURE 46–5 ■ Levels of antibody to the protective epitope of OspA (LA-2 equivalent antibody) in vaccine recipients at one study site. At month 2, 1 month after the second injection, the geometric mean antibody titer was 816 ng/mL. Ten months later, the mean titer had declined. At month 13, 1 month after the third injection, a marked anamnestic response was seen and the mean value was 4127 ng/mL. At month 20, the mean response had again declined, but was still twice as high as at month 2. The vertical bars indicate 95% confidence intervals. (From Steere AC, Sikand VK, Meurice F, et al. Vaccination against Lyme disease with recombinant *Borrelia burgdorferi* outer-surface lipoprotein A with adjuvant. N Engl J Med 339:209, 1998, with permission. Copyright © 1998, Massachusetts Medical Society, All rights reserved.)

Cellular Immune Responses

In the SmithKline Beecham Phase III trial, T-cell proliferative responses were determined to full-length OspA and to 20 overlapping OspA peptides in 41 vaccine and 44 placebo recipients from one site. Although the strength of the responses was often quite low, reactivity in the 41 vaccine recipients was significantly greater to full-length OspA and to peptide 8 than in placebo recipients (Fig. 46–6). This peptide contains the immunodominant T-cell epitope of OspA recognized by individuals with the human leukocyte antigen (HLA)-DRB1*0401 or other related alleles. Although a T-cell response may be important in priming B cells to produce antibody to OspA, vaccine-induced cellular immunity was not thought to play a direct role in spirochetal killing.

Correlates of Protection

In animal models, the levels of LA-2 equivalent antibodies, which were directed against the protective antibody epitope of OspA, accurately predicted the probability of becoming infected with B. burgdorferi.[101] In the SmithKline Beecham Phase III vaccine trial, the antibody titers were significantly lower in vaccinated subjects with breakthrough cases of Lyme disease than in subjects in two comparison groups ($P < 0.01$ for each comparison) (Fig. 46–7).[70] Later, these serum samples were used to determine the IgG antibody titers to full-length OspA by indirect ELISA. Titers of 700 to 1400 ELISA units(EL.U.)/mL provided 70% to 95% sensitivity to discriminate between vaccine success and failure.[118] After three injections, 90% of the adults tested and 100% of children attained levels of 1400 EL.U./mL.[120]

Herd Immunity

B. burgdorferi survives in a horizontal cycle of transmission between ticks and mice[15]; human infection is a dead end in the spirochetal life cycle. Therefore, herd immunity in human populations does not influence the frequency of infected ticks or the enzootic cycle of infection.

Vaccine Efficacy

The efficacy of recombinant OspA vaccines was determined in two Phase III trials, one sponsored by SmithKline Beecham[70] and the other sponsored by Pasteur Mérieux Connaught.[121] The SmithKline Beecham study involved 10,936 subjects, ages 15 to 70, who lived in 10 states endemic for Lyme disease. Participants received an injection of either recombinant B. burgdorferi OspA lipoprotein with adjuvant or placebo at enrollment and 1 and 12 months later. In cases of suspected Lyme disease, culture of skin lesions, PCR testing, or serologic testing was done, and serologic testing was performed in all study participants 12 and 20 months after study entry to detect asymptomatic infection.

In the first year, after two injections, 22 subjects in the vaccine group and 43 in the placebo group contracted definite Lyme disease ($P = 0.009$); the point estimate of vaccine efficacy was 49% (95% confidence interval, 15% to 69%).[70] In the second year, after the third injection, 16 vaccine recipients and 66 placebo recipients contracted definite Lyme disease ($P < 0.001$); the point estimate of vaccine effi-

cacy was 76% (95% confidence interval, 58% to 86%). Except for one participant each year who presented with Lyme arthritis, all definite cases in vaccine recipients had erythema migrans. Moreover, the arthritis case in year 1 most likely acquired the infection in the year prior to enrollment. During the first year, 2 subjects in the vaccine group and 13 in the placebo group had asymptomatic IgG seroconversion to B. burgdorferi ($P = 0.004$). In the second year, all 15 subjects with asymptomatic seroconversion were in the placebo group ($P = 0.001$). Thus the efficacy of the vaccine in preventing asymptomatic infection was 83% in the first year and 100% in the second year.

In the trial sponsored by Pasteur Mérieux Connaught,[121] 10,305 subjects 18 years of age or older were recruited. The first two injections were administered 1 month apart, and some patients received a booster dose at 12 months. The primary endpoint was the number of new clinically and serologically confirmed cases of Lyme disease. The efficacy of the vaccine was 68% in the first year and 92% in the second year among the 3475 subjects who received the third injection. Thus both studies showed that three injections of a recombinant OspA vaccine were quite effective in the prevention of Lyme disease for at least one tick transmission season.

Duration of Immunity and Protection

Although vaccinated subjects usually developed high levels of antibody to the protective epitope of OspA after three injections, the response declined rather rapidly.[70] If the correlate of protection was defined as 1400 EL.U./mL, a level with 95% sensitivity to discriminate vaccine success or failure,[118] a fourth injection probably would have been needed in most subjects the following year. Although long-term immunogenicity studies were not completed, it was anticipated that additional booster injections would have been needed in adults approximately every other year to maintain antibody titers at this level.

Postexposure Prophylaxis and Therapeutic Vaccination

There was no role for postexposure prophylaxis or therapeutic vaccination with recombinant OspA vaccines. Because B. burgdorferi down-regulates OspA expression during transmission to the human host,[39] an antibody response to this protein does not afford protection once the spirochete is transmitted to the human host.

Safety

Common Side Effects

During both Phase III clinical trials, pain and tenderness at the vaccination site were the most commonly reported adverse events.[70,121] In the SmithKline Beecham Phase III trial, approximately 24% of vaccine recipients noted pain at the injection site compared with 7% of placebo recipients ($P < 0.001$) (Table 46–3).[70] In addition, about 3% of vaccine recipients reported systemic symptoms of myalgias, achiness, fever, and chills, a significantly higher percentage than in placebo recipients. These reactions usually

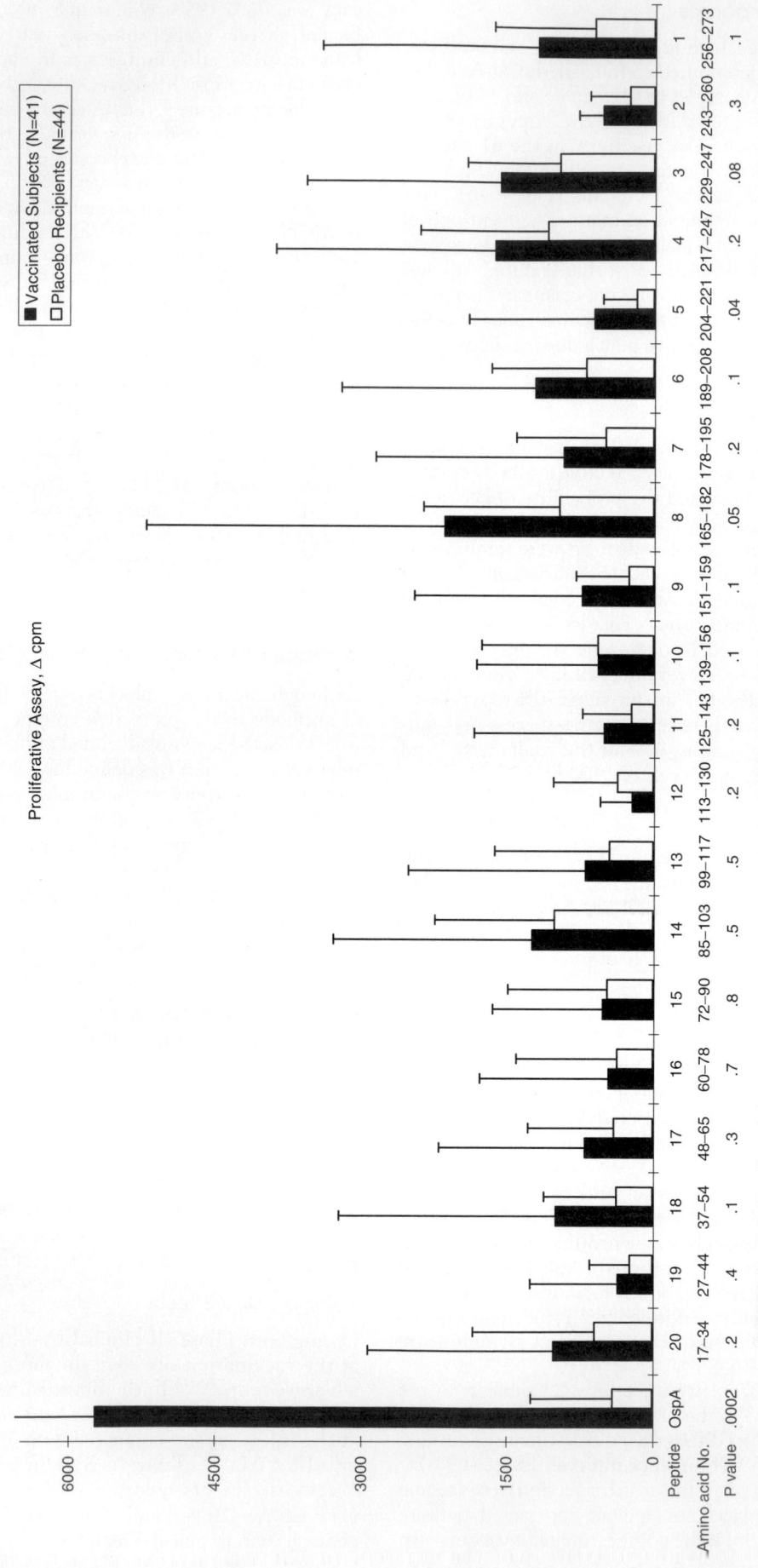

FIGURE 46–6 ▪ T-cell proliferative responses to full-length OspA and to 20 overlapping OspA peptides in 41 vaccine and 44 placebo recipients at one study site. Compared with placebo recipients, the responses in vaccine recipients were greater to full-length OspA and to epitopes contained within peptides 18, 14, 8, 4, 3, and 1. Significant differences between vaccine and placebo recipients were in the responses to full-length OspA ($P = 0.0002$) and peptide 8 ($P = 0.05$) as determined by t-test.

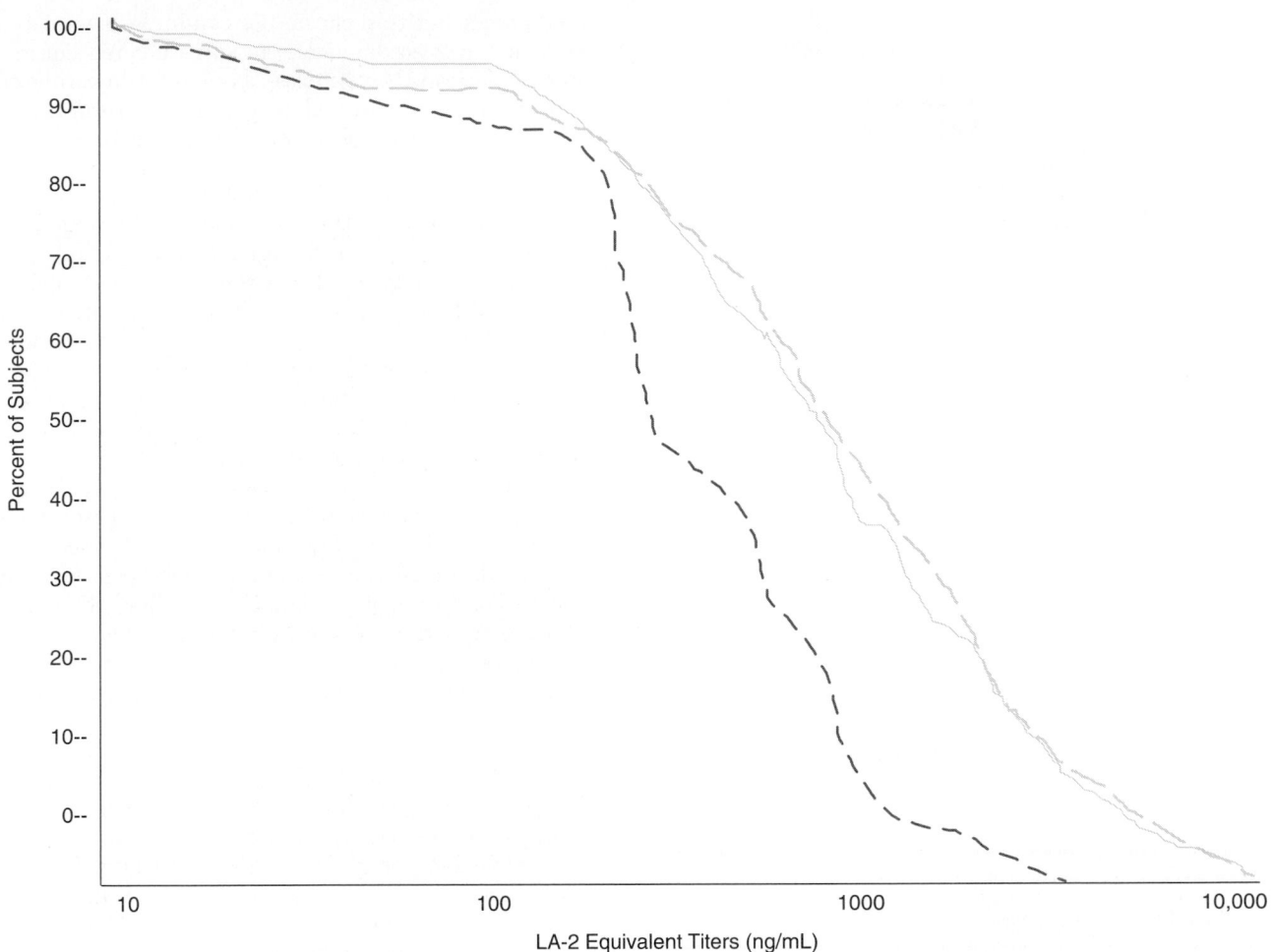

FIGURE 46-7 ■ Reverse cumulative curve of LA-2 equivalent OspA antibody levels at month 2 in 20 vaccinated subjects with break-through cases of definite Lyme disease, 512 vaccinated subjects evaluated for Lyme disease during year 1 in whom the diagnosis was not confirmed, and 395 vaccinated subjects from one study site. At month 2, 1 month after the second injection, the titers were significantly lower in vaccinated subjects with breakthrough cases of Lyme disease than in the other two comparison groups ($P \leq 0.01$ for each comparison). (From Steere AC, Sikand VK, Meurice F, et al. Vaccination against Lyme disease with recombinant *Borrelia burgdorferi* outer-surface lipoprotein A with adjuvant. N Engl J Med 339:209, 1998, with permission.)

occurred within 48 hours after vaccination and lasted for a median duration of 3 days. They were usually mild or moderate in severity, and the severity usually did not increase with subsequent injections. At one site, where information was solicited about fever, no patient reported a temperature above 39°C. No hypersensitivity reactions were noted. Eleven percent of participants had a past history of Lyme disease, and 2.3% were seropositive for *B. burgdorferi* at study entry.[70] These individuals were not different from the rest of the subjects in the safety profile of the vaccine.[70]

Similarly, in a study of safety and immunogenicity of LYMErix in 4087 children ages 4 to 18 years, higher incidences of local injection site reactions as well as systemic symptoms of fever, headache, fatigue, and arthralgia were noted in vaccine compared with placebo recipients.[119] In the vaccine group, 20.4% had these symptoms at a grade 3 level compared with 5.9% of the placebo recipients ($P = 0.001$). However, most reactions lasted a mean duration of only 2 to 3 days, and were mild or moderate in severity.

Rare Reactions

In the natural infection, about 10% of patients with Lyme arthritis, especially those with HLA-DRB1*0401 or related

alleles, have persistent arthritis for months or even several years after the apparent eradication of *B. burgdorferi* from the joint with antibiotic therapy.[78] During the 1990s, it was shown that patients with antibiotic treatment-resistant or antibiotic-responsive arthritis differ primarily in the cellular and humoral immune responses to OspA.[122–125] In 1998, the immunodominant T-cell epitope of OspA ($OspA_{165-173}$) presented by the 0401 molecule was identified.[125] In epitope mapping studies, 15 of 16 patients with treatment-resistant arthritis had reactivity with this OspA epitope compared with 1 of 5 patients with treatment-responsive arthritis ($P = 0.004$).[125] Thus it was postulated that autoimmunity may develop within the proinflammatory milieu of the joint in genetically susceptible patients because of molecular mimicry between a dominant T cell epitope of OspA and a homologous sequence in a host protein.

A search of the human protein database for homologous sequences to $OspA_{165-173}$ identified a similar sequence in human lymphocyte function-associated antigen-1 (LFA-$1\alpha_{L332-340}$) that was predicted to be presented by the DRB1*0401 molecule.[126] As determined by an ElisaSpot assay, 10 of the 11 treatment-resistant patients tested had Th1 responses in synovial fluid to OspA, LFA-1,

TABLE 46–3 ■ Percentage of Subjects with Symptoms (Overall Incidence ≥1%) Classified as Related, Possibly Related, or Unrelated to Vaccination*

Symptoms	Vaccine	Placebo	P Value
RELATED OR POSSIBLY RELATED			
Local Injection Site			
Soreness	24.1	7.6	<0.001
Redness	1.8	0.5	<0.001
Swelling	0.9	0.2	<0.001
Systemic			
Early (≤30 days)			
Arthralgia	3.9	3.5	0.34
Headache	3.0	2.5	0.14
Myalgias	3.2	1.8	<0.001
Fatigue	2.3	2.0	0.37
Achiness	2.0	1.4	0.01
Flu-like symptoms	2.0	1.1	<0.001
Fever	2.0	0.8	<0.001
Chills	1.8	0.5	<0.001
Upper respiratory tract infection	1.0	1.1	0.69
TOTAL	19.4	15.1	<0.001
Late (>30 days)			
Arthralgia	1.3	1.2	0.54
TOTAL	4.1	3.4	0.06
UNRELATED TO VACCINATION			
Early	27.1	27.9	0.37
Late	53.3	52.6	0.48

*Totals include all early or late, related or possibly related systemic events, not just those with a frequency of 1% or greater.

From Steere AC, Sikand VK, Meurice F, et al. Vaccination against Lyme disease with recombinant *Borrelia burgdorferi* outer-surface lipoprotein A with adjuvant. N Engl J Med 339:209, 1998, with permission.

or, in most instances, both.[126] It was subsequently shown that LFA-1α$_{L332-340}$ is only a weak partial agonist for OspA$_{165-173}$ reactive T cells,[127] and that the DRB1* 0101 molecule, which is implicated in treatment-resistant arthritis, does not bind the LFA-1 peptide.[128] Although OspA$_{165-173}$ is still strongly implicated in treatment-resistant Lyme arthritis, it seems unlikely that LFA-1 could serve as an autoantigen in this illness.

Because of these observations, the question arose of whether vaccination with recombinant OspA might exacerbate Lyme arthritis or induce autoimmune arthritis in genetically susceptible individuals. In the Phase III vaccine trials, however, vaccination with OspA was not associated with arthritis, neurologic abnormalities, or any other late syndrome 30 days or more after vaccination.[70,121] Although several subjects in the SmithKline Beecham Phase III trial developed inflammatory polyarthritis during the study and three subjects developed Lyme arthritis, these individuals were found in both the vaccine and placebo groups. In the Pasteur Mérieux Connaught trial, subjects with prior Lyme arthritis did not develop arthritis after vaccination.[121] Moreover, in a separate study of 30 patients with previous Lyme disease, those with a previous history of Lyme arthritis did not have a recurrence of arthritis after vaccination.[129] In the pediatric safety and immunogenicity study, one child had transient ankle swelling after dose 2, which resolved and did not recur after dose 3.[120] Thus vaccination

would appear not to replicate the conditions necessary for the induction of autoimmunity in joints as can occur in the natural infection. Nevertheless, because of lingering concerns about the theoretical potential for arthritogenicity, several publications urged caution with Lyme disease vaccination, particularly in individuals with arthritis.[130,131]

As with any vaccine trial, rare side effects may not be recognized in comparisons of vaccine and placebo groups. Thus the question remained: Might vaccination with OspA induce arthritis but at a frequency below the level of detectability in vaccine trials? In 2001, a case series of four patients were reported who developed arthritis after OspA vaccination.[132] In one of the patients, B. burgdorferi infection probably was acquired prior to vaccination, but joint swelling became manifest months after vaccination. The arthritis resolved with antibiotic therapy. This phenomenon was observed in three patients in the SmithKline Beecham Phase III trial, two in the vaccine group and one in the placebo group.[70] Three months after the third injection of vaccine, the second patient developed a moderate effusion of a knee, which lasted for several months. The third patient developed swelling of the finger and toe joints within 24 hours after the second injection, and his symptoms improved over the next 5 days. The final patient developed synovitis of multiple proximal interphalangeal joints 24 hours after the second vaccination, which lasted about 7 weeks.

In 2002, the Centers for Disease Control and Prevention and the Food and Drug Administration published the reports relating to Lyme disease vaccination from their Vaccine Adverse Event Reporting System (VAERS). From December 1996 through August 2000, during the first 19 months after licensure, approximately 1.4 million doses of LYMErix were distributed, and, during this period, 905 adverse events (0.06%) were reported to the VAERS.[133] The most common reports were of arthralgias (250 reports) or myalgias (195 reports) occurring after the first dose. These frequencies were consistent with the events observed in the clinical trials. In addition, arthritis was reported to have developed in 59 patients, arthrosis in 34 patients, and rheumatoid arthritis in 9 patients, usually after the second or third dose.[133] This frequency of arthritis was thought to be below the expected background incidence of arthritis occurring during this time period in an unvaccinated population.

Immunosuppressed Individuals

Lyme disease vaccines were not tested in immunosuppressed patients, and thus no information is available about the effectiveness of vaccination in such individuals.

Spread to Contacts

Because Lyme disease vaccines consisted of only a recombinant OspA protein, there was no risk of spread to contacts.

Indications for Vaccine

Most B. burgdorferi infections result from periresidential exposure to infected ticks during property maintenance, recreation, or leisure activities.[87] Thus persons who live or work in residential areas surrounded by woods or overgrown brush infested with vector ticks are at risk of acquiring Lyme disease. However, cost-effectiveness analyses concluded that vaccination for Lyme disease was economically attractive only for individuals who have a seasonal probability of

B. burgdorferi infection of greater than 1%.[134-136] Only a relatively small number of highly endemic areas in the northeastern and north-central United States have estimated annual incidences of the disease in this range. Moreover, the risk of Lyme disease differs not only between regions, states, and counties but also within counties and townships.

The Advisory Committee on Immunization Practices of the Centers for Disease Control and Prevention advised that vaccination should be considered by persons 15 to 70 years old who live in and visit high-risk areas and have frequent and prolonged exposure to *I. scapularis* ticks.[87] Vaccination was not recommended for persons with minimal or no exposure to such ticks.

Contraindications and Precautions

Recombinant OspA vaccines were tested only in normal individuals. Therefore, safety information was not available about vaccine use among patients with other diseases or in pregnant woman. Moreover, these vaccines were not licensed for use in children. Finally, because of the association of immunity to OspA and antibiodic treatment-resistant Lyme arthritis, it was recommended that the vaccine not be given to individuals with this form of arthritis.

Non-Immunologic Prevention

Protective measures for the prevention of Lyme disease may include the avoidance of tick-infected areas, the use of protective clothing, the use of repellants and acaricides, tick checks, and modifications of landscapes in or near residential areas.[87] However, these methods of prevention have not been shown to lower the incidence of Lyme disease,[137] presumably because people have trouble maintaining these tick prevention efforts throughout the entire tick-transmission season.

Future Considerations

In February 2002, GlaxoSmithKline discontinued the production of LYMErix because of poor sales. Several factors were probably contributory. First, Lyme disease is highly focal, and consideration of vaccination was recommended only for individuals in high-risk areas who had frequent exposure to ticks. Second, although children often were affected, the vaccine was approved for use only in adults. Third, immunity to OspA waned rather rapidly, and therefore it was anticipated that booster injections would be needed every 1 to 3 years. Finally, although never proven, there were lingering concerns regarding whether, in rare instances, vaccination with OspA may induce arthritis.

Several companies have worked on the development of other Lyme disease vaccines. Medimmune in Gaithersburg, Maryland, has researched a vaccine consisting of both a recombinant OspA lipoprotein and a recombinant DbpA. The hope was that these two proteins would induce protection in a larger percentage of subjects than OspA alone. The development of a Lyme disease vaccine for use in Europe has been more difficult than in the United States because all three pathogenic species of *B. burgdorferi* sensu lato cause the infection there. In an effort to provide protection against the range of European strains, Baxter Bioscience in Vienna, Austria, has researched a 14-valent recombinant OspC vaccine, and is now researching an altered OspA vaccine. These vaccines are not commercially available.

The OspA Lyme disease vaccines developed in the 1990s should be considered first-generation vaccines.[131] If future vaccines are developed, a goal should be to provide longer term protection and perhaps broader protection against variant strains of *B. burgdorferi*. If OspA is a component of the vaccine, alteration of the immunodominant T-cell epitope presented by the DRB1*0401 molecule may be desirable. If Lyme disease continues to spread in the United States and if more hyperendemic foci develop, vaccination may again become a priority. Experience gained in the last 10 years has proven the feasibility of vaccination for the prevention of this complex, tick-borne infection.

REFERENCES

1. Steere AC, Malawista SE, Snydman DR, et al. Lyme arthritis: an epidemic of oligoarticular arthritis in children and adults in three Connecticut communities. Arthritis Rheum 20:7, 1977.
2. Steere AC, Malawista SE, Hardin JA, et al. Erythema chronicum migrans and Lyme arthritis: the enlarging clinical spectrum. Ann Intern Med 86:685, 1977.
3. Steere AC, Broderick TF, Malawista SE. Erythema chronicum migrans and Lyme arthritis: epidemiologic evidence for a tick vector. Am J Epidemiol 108:312, 1978.
4. Afzelius A. Erythema chronicum migrans. Acta Derm Venereol (Stockh) 2:120, 1921.
5. Bannwarth A. Zur Klinik und Pathogenese der "chronischen lymphocytaren Meningitis." Arch Psychiatr Nervenkrankh 117:161,1944.
6. Herxheimer K, Hartmann K. Ueber Acrodermatitis chronica atrophicans. Arch Dermatol Syph 61:57, 255, 1902.
7. Burgdorfer W, Barbour AG, Hayes SF, et al. Lyme disease—a tick-borne spirochetosis? Science 216:1317, 1982.
8. Steere AC, Grodzicki RL, Kornblatt AN, et al. The spirochetal etiology of Lyme disease. N Engl J Med 308:733, 1983.
9. Benach JL, Bosler EM, Hanrahan JP, et al. Spirochetes isolated from the blood of two patients with Lyme disease. N Engl J Med 308:740, 1983.
10. Ackermann R, Kabatzki J, Boisten HP, et al. Spirochaten-Atiologie der Erythema-chronicum-migrans-Krankheit. Dtsch Med Wochenschr 109:92, 1984.
11. Preac-Mursic V, Wilske B, Schierz G, et al. Repeated isolation of spirochetes from the cerebrospinal fluid of a patient with meningoradiculitis Bannwarth. Eur J Clin Microbiol 3:564, 1984.
12. Asbrink E, Hovmark A. Successful cultivation of spirochetes from skin lesions of patients with erythema chronica migrans afzelius and acrodermatitis chronica atrophicans. Acta Pathol Microbiol Immunol Scand 93:161, 1985.
13. Baranton G, Assous M, Postic D. Three bacterial species associated with Lyme borreliosis: clinical and diagnostic implications. Bull Acad Natl Med 176:1075, 1992.
14. Centers for Disease Control and Prevention. Lyme disease—United States, 2000. MMWR 51:29, 2002.
15. Steere AC. Lyme disease. N Engl J Med 321:586, 1989.
16. Steere AC, Bartenhagen NH, Craft JE, et al. The early clinical manifestations of Lyme disease. Ann Intern Med 99:76, 1983.
17. Nadelman RB, Nowakowski J, Forseter G, et al. The clinical spectrum of early Lyme borreliosis in patients with culture-confirmed erythema migrans. Am J Med 100:502, 1996.
18. Smith RP, Schoen RT, Rahn DW, et al. Clinical characteristics and treatment outcome of early Lyme disease in patients with microbiologically confirmed erythema migrans. Ann Intern Med 136:421, 2002.
19. Reik L, Steere AC, Bartenhagen NH, et al. Neurologic abnormalities of Lyme disease. Medicine (Baltimore) 58:281, 1979.
20. Pachner AR, Steere AC. The triad of neurologic manifestations of Lyme disease: meningitis, cranial neuritis, and radiculoneuritis. Neurology 35:47, 1985.

21. Steere AC, Batsford WP, Weinberg M, et al. Lyme carditis: cardiac abnormalities of Lyme disease. Ann Intern Med 93:8, 1980.
22. Marcus LC, Steere AC, Duray PH, et al. Fatal pancarditis in a patient with coexistent Lyme disease and babesiosis: demonstration of spirochetes in the myocardium. Ann Intern Med 103:374, 1985.
23. Steere AC, Schoen RT, Taylor E. The clinical evolution of Lyme arthritis. Ann Intern Med 107:725, 1987.
24. Johnston YE, Duray PH, Steere AC, et al. Lyme arthritis: spirochetes found in synovial microangiopathic lesions. Am J Pathol 118:26, 1985.
25. Steere AC, Duray PH, Butcher EC. Spirochetal antigens and lymphoid cell surface markers in Lyme synovitis: comparison with rheumatoid synovium and tonsillar lymphoid tissue. Arthritis Rheum 31:487, 1988.
26. Logigian EL, Kaplan RF, Steere AC. Chronic neurologic manifestations of Lyme disease. N Engl J Med 323:1438, 1990.
27. Halperin JJ, Volkman DJ, Wu P. Central nervous system abnormalities in Lyme neuroborreliosis. Neurology 41:1571, 1991.
28. Steere AC, Berardi VP, Weeks KE, et al. Evaluation of the intrathecal antibody response to Borrelia burgdorferi as a diagnostic test for Lyme neuroborreliosis. J Infect Dis 161:1203, 1990.
29. Halperin JJ, Little BW, Coyle PK, et al. Lyme disease: cause of a treatable peripheral neuropathy. Neurology 37:1700, 1987.
30. Logigian EL, Steere AC. Clinical and electrophysiologic findings in chronic neuropathy of Lyme disease. Neurology 42:303, 1992.
31. Steere AC. Lyme disease. N Engl J Med 345:115, 2001.
32. Ackermann R, Rehse-Kupper B, Gollmer E, et al. Chronic neurologic manifestations of erythema migrans borreliosis. Ann N Y Acad Sci 539:16, 1988.
33. Asbrink E, Brehmer-Anderson E, Hovmark A. Acrodermatitis chronica atrophicans—a spirochetosis. Am J Dermatopathol 8:209, 1986.
34. Barbour AG, Hayes SF. Biology of Borrelia species. Microbiol Rev 50:381, 1986.
35. Fraser CM, Casjens S, Huang WM, et al. Genomic sequence of a Lyme disease spirochete, Borrelia burgdorferi. Nature 390:580, 1997.
36. Casjens S, Palmer N, Van Vugt R, et al. A bacterial genome in flux: the twelve linear and nine circular extrachromosomal DNAs in an infectious isolate of the Lyme disease spirochete Borrelia burgdorferi. Mol Microbiol 35:490, 2000.
37. Zhang J-R, Norris SJ. Genetic variation of the Borrelia burgdorferi gene vlsE involves cassettes-specific, segmental gene conversation. Infect Immun 66:3698, 1998.
38. de Silva AM, Fikrig E. Arthropod- and host-specific gene expression by Borrelia burgdorferi. J Clin Invest 100(suppl):S3, 1997.
39. Montgomery RR, Malawista SE, Feen KJM, et al. Direct demonstration of antigenic substitution of Borrelia burgdorferi ex vivo: exploration of the paradox of the early immune response to outer surface proteins A and C in Lyme disease. J Exp Med 183:261, 1996.
40. Schwan TG, Piesman J, Golde WT, et al. Induction of an outer surface protein on Borrelia burgdorferi during tick feeding. Proc Natl Acad Sci U S A 92:2909, 1995.
41. Seinost G, Dykhuizen DE, Dattwyler RJ, et al. Four clones of Borrelia burgdorferi sensu stricto cause invasive infection in humans. Infect Immun 67:3518, 1999.
42. Coleman JL, Gebbia JA, Pieman J, et al. Plasminogen is required for efficient dissemination of B. burgdorferi in ticks and for enhancement of spirochetemia in mice. Cell 89:1111, 1997.
43. Coburn J, Leong JM, Erban JK. Integrin αIIbβ3 mediates binding of the Lyme disease agent Borrelia burgdorferi to human platelets. Proc Natl Acad Sci U S A 90:7059, 1993.
44. Coburn J, Magoun L, Bodary SC, et al. Integrins αvβ3 and α5β1 mediate attachment of Lyme disease spirochetes to human cells. Infect Immun 66:1946, 1998.
45. Leong JM, Robbins D, Rosenfeld L, et al. Structural requirements for glycosaminoglycan recognition by the Lyme disease spirochete, Borrelia burgdorferi. Infect Immun 66:6045, 1998.
46. Probert WS, Johnson BJB. Identification of a 47kDa fibronectin-binding protein expressed by Borrelia burgdorferi isolate B32. Mol Microbiol 30:1003, 1998.
47. Guo BP, Brown EL, Dorward DW, et al. Decorin-binding adhesins from Borrelia burgdorferi. Mol Microbiol 30:711, 1998.
48. Weis JJ, McCracken BA, Ma Y, et al. Identification of quantitative trait loci governing arthritis severity and humoral responses in the murine model of Lyme disease. J Immunol 162:948, 1999.
49. Barthold SW, DeSouza M. Exacerbation of Lyme arthritis in beige mice. J Infect Dis 172:778, 1995.

50. Hirschfeld M, Kirschning CJ, Schwandner R, et al. Inflammatory signaling by Borrelia burgdorferi lipoproteins is mediated by toll-like receptor 2. J Immunol 163:2382, 1999.
51. Kang I, Barthold SW, Persing DH, et al. T-helper-cell cytokines in the early evolution of murine Lyme arthritis. Infect Immun 65:3107, 1997.
52. Vaz A, Glickstein L, Field JA, et al. Cellular and humoral immune responses to Borrelia burgdorferi antigens in patients with culture-positive early Lyme disease. Infect Immun 69:7437, 2001.
53. Duray PH. The surgical pathology of human Lyme disease: an enlarging picture. Am J Surg Pathol 11:47, 1987.
54. Fikrig E, Barthold SW, Marcantonio N, et al. Roles of OspA, OspB, and flagellin in protective immunity to Lyme borreliosis in laboratory mice. Infect Immun 60:657, 1992.
55. Preac-Mursic V, Wilske B, Patsouris E, et al. Active immunization with pC protein of Borrelia burgdorferi protects gerbils against B. burgdorferi infection. Infection 20:342, 1992.
56. Nguyen TP, Lam TT, Barthold SW, et al. Partial destruction of Borrelia burgdorferi within ticks that engorged on OspE- or OspF-immunized mice. Infect Immun 62:2079,1994.
57. Hanson MS, Cassatt DR, Guo BP, et al. Active and passive immunity against Borrelia burgdorferi decorin binding protein A (DbpA) protects against infection. Infect Immun 66:2143, 1998.
58. Berger BW, Johnson RC, Kodner C, et al. Cultivation of Borrelia burgdorferi from erythema migrans lesions and perilesional skin. J Clin Microbiol 30:359, 1992.
59. Wormser GP, Bittker S, Cooper D, et al. Comparison of the yields of blood cultures using serum or plasma from patients with early Lyme disease. J Clin Microbiol 38:1648, 2000.
60. Coyle PK, Goodman JL, Krupp LB, et al. Lyme disease: continuum. Lifelong Learning in Neurology. Vol. 5, No. 4, Part A. Philadelphia, Lippincott Williams & Wilkins, 1999.
61. Nocton JJ, Dressler F, Rutledge BJ, et al. Detection of Borrelia burgdorferi DNA by polymerase chain reaction in synovial fluid in Lyme arthritis. N Engl J Med 330:229, 1994.
62. Bradley JF, Johnson RC, Goodman JL. The persistence of spirochetal nucleic acids in active Lyme arthritis. Ann Intern Med 120:487, 1994.
63. Nocton JJ, Bloom BJ, Rutledge BJ, et al. Detection of Borrelia burgdorferi DNA by polymerase chain reaction in cerebrospinal fluid in patients with Lyme neuroborreliosis. J Infect Dis 174:623, 1996.
64. Centers for Disease Control. Case definitions for public health surveillance. MMWR 39(RR-13):1, 1990.
65. Centers for Disease Control and Prevention. Recommendations for test performance and interpretation from the Second International Conference on Serologic Diagnosis of Lyme Disease. MMWR 44:1, 1995.
66. Robertson J, Guy E, Andrews N, et al. A European multicenter study of immunoblotting in serodiagnosis of Lyme borreliosis. J Clin Microbiol 38:2097, 2000.
67. Engstrom SM, Shoop E, Johnson RC. Immunoblot interpretation criteria for serodiagnosis of early Lyme disease. J Clin Microbiol 33:419, 1995.
68. Dressler F, Whalen JA, Reinhardt BN, et al. Western blotting in the serodiagnosis of Lyme disease. J Infect Dis 167:392, 1993.
69. Kalish RA, McHugh G, Granquist J, et al. Persistence of immunoglobulin M or immunoglobulin G antibody responses to Borrelia burgdorferi 10–20 years after active Lyme disease. Clin Infect Dis 33:780, 2001.
70. Steere AC, Sikand VK, Meurice F, et al. Vaccination against Lyme disease with recombinant Borrelia burgdorferi outer-surface lipoprotein A with adjuvant. N Engl J Med 339:209, 1998.
71. Zhang YQ, Mathiesen D, Kolbert CP, et al. Borrelia burgdorferi enzyme-linked immunosorbent assay for discrimination of OspA vaccination from spirochete infection. J Clin Microbiol 35:233, 1997.
72. Wormser GP, Nadelman RB, Dattwyler RJ, et al. Practice guidelines for the treatment of Lyme disease. Clin Infect Dis 31(suppl):S1, 2000.
73. Dattwyler RJ, Volkman DJ, Conaty SM, et al. Amoxicillin plus probenecid versus doxycycline for treatment of erythema migrans borreliosis. Lancet 336:1404, 1990.
74. Massarotti EM, Luger SW, Rahn DW, et al. Treatment of early Lyme disease. Am J Med 92:396, 1992.
75. Nadelman RB, Luger SW, Frank E, et al. Comparison of cefuroxime axetil and doxycycline in the treatment of early Lyme disease. Ann Intern Med 117:273, 1992.

76. Logigian EL, Kaplan RF, Steere AC. Successful treatment of Lyme encephalopathy with intravenous ceftriaxone. J Infect Dis 180:377, 1999.

77. Dattwyler RJ, Halperin JJ, Volkman DJ, et al. Treatment of late Lyme borreliosis—randomized comparison of ceftriaxone and penicillin. Lancet 1:1191, 1988.

78. Steere AC, Levin RE, Molloy PJ, et al. Treatment of Lyme arthritis. Arthritis Rheum 37:878, 1994.

79. Shapiro ED, Gerber MA, Holabird NB, et al. A controlled trial of antimicrobial prophylaxis for Lyme disease after deer tick bites. N Engl J Med 327:1769, 1992.

80. Piesman J. Dynamics of Borrelia burgdorferi transmission by nymphal Ixodes dammini ticks. J Infect Dis 167:1082, 1993.

81. Nadelman RB, Nowakowski J, Fish D, et al. Prophylaxis with single-dose doxycycline for the prevention of Lyme disease after an Ixodes scapularis tick bite. N Engl J Med 345:79, 2001.

82. Steere AC, Malawista SE. Cases of Lyme disease in the United States: locations correlated with distribution of Ixodes dammini. Ann Intern Med 91:730, 1979.

83. Stanek G, Pletschette M, Flamm H, et al. European Lyme borreliosis. Ann N Y Acad Sci 539:274, 1988.

84. Berglund J, Eitrem R, Ornstein K, et al. An epidemiologic study of Lyme disease in southern Sweden. N Engl J Med 333:1319, 1995.

85. Matuschka FR, Spielman A. The emergence of Lyme disease in a changing environment in North America and central Europe. Exp Appl Acarol 2:337, 1986.

86. Spielman A. The emergence of Lyme disease and human babesiosis in a changing environment. Ann N Y Acad Sci 740:146, 1994.

87. Centers for Disease Control and Prevention. Recommendations for the use of the Lyme disease vaccine. MMWR 48:1, 1999.

88. Brown RN, Lane RS. Lyme disease in California: a novel enzootic transmission cycle of Borrelia burgdorferi. Science 256:1439, 1992.

89. Steere AC. Lyme disease: a growing threat to urban populations. Proc Natl Acad Sci U S A 91:2378, 1994.

90. White DJ, Chang HG, Benach JL, et al. The geographic spread and temporal increase of the Lyme disease epidemic. JAMA 266:1230, 1991.

90a. Vazquez M, Cartter ML, Shapiro ED. Effectiveness of personal preventive measures for lyme disease. [Abstr, 1866] Pediatric Societies' Annual Meeting, Seattle, May 3–6, 2003.

91. Johnson RC, Kodner C, Russell M. Passive immunization of hamsters against experimental infection with Borrelia burgdorferi. Infect Immun 53:713, 1986.

92. Johnson RC, Kodner C, Russell M. Active immunization of hamsters against experimental infection with Borrelia burgdorferi. Infect Immun 54:887, 1986.

93. Chu HJ, Chavez LGJ, Blumer BM, et al. Immunogenicity and efficacy study of a commercial Borrelia burgdorferi bacterin. J Am Vet Med Assoc 201:403, 1992.

94. Levy SA, Lissman BA, Ficke CM. Performance of a Borrelia burgdorferi bacterin in borreliosis-endemic areas. J Am Vet Med Assoc 202:1834, 1993.

95. Fikrig E, Barthold SW, Kantor FS, et al. Protection of mice against the Lyme disease agent by immunizing with recombinant OspA. Science 250:553, 1990.

96. Schaible UE, Kramer MD, Eichmann K, et al. Monoclonal antibodies specific for the outer surface protein A (OspA) of Borrelia burgdorferi prevent Lyme borreliosis in severe combined immunodeficiency (scid) mice. Proc Natl Acad Sci U S A 87:3768, 1990.

97. Sears JE, Fikrig E, Nakagawa TY, et al. Molecular mapping of Osp-A mediated immunity against Borrelia burgdorferi, the agent of Lyme disease. J Immunol 147:1995, 1991.

98. Fikrig E, Telford III SR, Barthold SW, et al. Elimination of Borrelia burgdorferi from vector ticks feeding on OspA-immunized mice. Proc Natl Acad Sci U S A 89:5418, 1992.

99. Erdile LF, Brandt MA, Warakomski DJ, et al. Role of attached lipid in immunogenicity of Borrelia burgdorferi OspA. Infect Immun 61:81, 1993.

100. Roehrig JT, Piesman J, Hunt AR, et al. The hamster immune response to tick-transmitted Borrelia burgdorferi differs from the response to needle-inoculated, cultured organisms. J Immunol 149:3648, 1992.

101. Golde WT, Piesman J, Dolan MC, et al. Reactivity with a specific epitope of outer surface protein A predicts for protection from infection with the Lyme disease spirochete, Borrelia burgdorferi. Infect Immun 65:882, 1997.

102. Philipp MT, Lobet Y, Bohm RP, et al. The outer surface protein A (OspA) vaccine against Lyme disease: efficacy in the rhesus monkey. Vaccine 15:1872, 1997.

103. Philipp MT, Lobet Y, Bohm RPJ, et al. Safety and immunogenicity of recombinant outer surface protein A (OspA) vaccine formulations in the rhesus monkey. J Spirochetal Tick-borne Dis 3:1, 1996.

104. Fikrig E, Barthold SW, Persing DH, et al. Borrelia burgdorferi strain 25015: characterization of outer surface protein A and vaccination against infection. J Immunol 148:2256, 1992.

105. Fikrig E, Telford III SR, Wallich R, et al. Vaccination against Lyme disease caused by diverse Borrelia burgdorferi. J Exp Med 181:215, 1995.

106. Dykhuizen DE, Polin DS, Dunn JJ, et al. Borrelia burgdorferi is clonal: implications for taxonomy and vaccine development. Proc Natl Acad Sci U S A 90:10163, 1993.

107. Stover CK, Bansal GP, Hanson MS, et al. Protective immunity elicited by recombinant bacille Calmette-Guerin (BCG) expressing outer surface protein A (OspA) lipoprotein: a candidate Lyme disease vaccine. J Exp Med 178:197, 1993.

108. Keller D, Koster FT, Marks DH, et al. Safety and immunogenicity of a recombinant outer surface protein A Lyme vaccine. JAMA 271:1764, 1994.

109. Van Hoecke C, Comberbach M, De Grave D, et al. Evaluation of the safety, reactogenicity, and immunogenicity of three recombinant outer surface protein (OspA) Lyme vaccines in healthy adults. Vaccine 14:1620, 1996.

110. Wormser GP. A vaccine against Lyme disease? Ann Intern Med 123:627, 1995.

111. Meurice F, Parenti D, Fu D, et al. Specific issues in the design and implementation of an efficacy trial for a Lyme disease vaccine. Clin Infect Dis 25(suppl):S71, 1997.

112. American Society of Health-System Pharmacists. I: Lyme Disease Vaccine. In AHFS Drug Information 1999. Vol. 80. Bethesda, MD, American Society of Health-System Pharmacists, 1999, p 12.

113. Thanassi WT, Schoen RT. The Lyme disease vaccine: conception, development, and implementation. Ann Intern Med 132:661, 2000.

114. Rahn DW. Lyme vaccine: issues and controversies. Infect Dis Clin North Am 15:171, 2001.

115. Poland GA. Prevention of Lyme disease: a review of the evidence. Mayo Clin Proc 76:713, 2001.

116. Parenti D, Schoen R, Sikand V, et al. Evaluation of reactogenicity and immunogenicity of LYMErix, recombinant L-OspA vaccine against Lyme disease, administered on two different schedules [abstract]. In Abstracts of the annual meeting of the Infectious Diseases Society of America, Denver, CO, 1998, p 705.

117. Van Hoecke C, Lebacq E, Beran J, et al. Alternative vaccination schedules (0, 1, and 6 months versus 0, 1, and 12 months) for a recombinant OspA Lyme disease vaccine. Clin Infect Dis 28:1260, 1999.

118. Parenti D, Gillet M, Sennewald E, et al. Correlate of protection for Lyme disease (LD) using LYMErix recombinant adjuvanted Borrelia burgdorferi outer surface lipoprotein A (L-OspA) vaccine [abstract]. In Abstracts of the annual meeting of the Infectious Diseases Society of America, Denver, CO, 1998, p 704.

119. Alexopoulou L, Thomas V, Schmare M, et al. Hyporesponsiveness to vaccination with Bosselia burgdorferi in humans and in TLR1- and TLR2-deficient mice. Nat Med 8:878, 2002.

120. Sikand VK, Halsey N, Krause PJ, et al. Safety and immunogenicity of a recombinant Borrelia burgdorferi outer surface protein A vaccine against Lyme disease in healthy children and adolescents: a randomized controlled trial. Pediatrics 108:123, 2001.

121. Sigal LH, Zahradnik JM, Lavin P, et al. A vaccine consisting of recombinant Borrelia burgdorferi outer-surface protein A to prevent Lyme disease. Recombinant Outer-Surface Protein A Lyme Disease Vaccine Study Consortium [see comments]. N Engl J Med 339:216, 1998. (published erratum appears in N Engl J Med 339:571, 1998)

122. Kalish RA, Leong JM, Steere AC. Association of treatment resistant chronic Lyme arthritis with HLA-DR4 and antibody reactivity to OspA and OspB of Borrelia burgdorferi. Infect Immun 61:2774, 1993.

123. Akin E, McHugh GL, Flavell RA, et al. The immunoglobulin G (IgG) antibody response to OspA and OspB correlates with severe and prolonged Lyme arthritis and the IgG response to P35 correlates with mild and brief arthritis. Infect Immun 67:173, 1999.

124. Lengl-Janssen B, Strauss AF, Steere AC, et al. The T helper cell response in Lyme arthritis: differential recognition of *Borrelia burgdorferi* outer surface protein A (OspA) in patients with treatment-resistant or treatment-responsive Lyme arthritis. J Exp Med 180:2069, 1994.

125. Chen J, Field JA, Glickstein L, et al. Association of antibiotic treatment-resistant Lyme arthritis with T cell responses to dominant epitopes of outer-surface protein A (OspA) of *Borrelia burgdorferi*. Arthritis Rheum 42:1813, 1999.

126. Gross DM, Forsthuber T, Tary-Lehman M, et al. Identification of LFA-1 as a candidate autoantigen in treatment-resistant Lyme arthritis. Science 281:703, 1998.

127. Trollmo C, Meyer AL, Steere AC, et al. Molecular mimicry in Lyme arthritis demonstrated at the single cell level: LFA-1α is a partial agonist for outer-surface protein A-reactive T cells. J Immunol 166:5286, 2001.

128. Steere AC, Falk B, Drouin EE, et al. Binding of outer surface protein A and human lymphocyte Function-associated 1 peptides to HLA-DR molecules associated with antibiotic treatment-resistant Lyme arthristis. Arthritis Rheum 48:534, 2003.

129. Schoen RT, Meurice F, Brunet CM, et al. Safety and immunogenicity of an outer surface protein A vaccine in subjects with previous Lyme disease. J Infect Dis 172:1324, 1995.

130. Lyme disease vaccine. Med Lett Drugs Ther 41:29, 1999.

131. Gardner P. Lyme disease vaccines. Ann Intern Med 129:583, 1998.

132. Rose CD, Fawcett PT, Gibney KM. Arthritis following recombinant outer surface protein A vaccination for Lyme disease. J Rheumatol 28:2555, 2001.

133. Lathrop SL, Ball R, Haber P, et al. Adverse event reports following vaccination for Lyme disease: December 1998—July 2000. Vaccine 20:1603, 2002.

134. Maes E, Lecomte P, Ray N. A cost-of-illness study of Lyme disease in the United States. Clin Ther 20:993, 1998.

135. Meltzer MI, Dennis DT, Orloski KA. The cost effectiveness of vaccinating against Lyme disease. Emerg Infect Dis 5:1, 1999.

136. Shadick NA, Liang MH, Phillips C, et al. The cost-effectiveness of vaccination against Lyme disease. Arch Intern Med 161:554, 2001.

137. Poland GA, Prevention of Lyme Disease: A review of the evidence. Mayo Clin Proc 76:713–724, 2001.

Chapter 47

Malaria Vaccines

FILIP DUBOVSKY • N. REGINA RABINOVICH

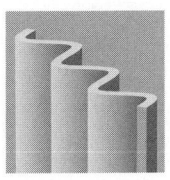

Human malaria is caused by four species of the protozoan *Plasmodium*: *P. falciparum*, *P. vivax*, *P. ovale*, and *P. malariae*. The life cycle and parasite-host interaction of each species determines the severity, pathogenesis, chronicity, and chronology of clinical disease.[1,2] *Plasmodium falciparum* causes the greatest number of deaths, and *P. vivax* has the greatest geographic distribution.[3] Malaria can thrive where the environment supports one of the 50 species of *Anopheles* mosquitoes that serve as the vector for transmission.[3,4] As recently as the early 1900s, malaria was endemic across every continent except Antarctica. Malaria elimination and control programs, primarily relying on insecticides and environmental control, led to the control of malaria in the United States, Europe, and Australia by the 1950s.[1] Over the past decade, malaria control programs have used a multifaceted strategy including environmental control, insecticides, bed nets, and chemotherapy.[5]

Background

All strains of the malaria parasite have a complex life cycle that begins in humans when the female mosquito deposits sporozoites subcutaneously during a blood meal. The sporozoites enter the bloodstream (Fig. 47–1A) and, in minutes, migrate to the liver and invade hepatocytes (Fig. 47–1B). Within this relatively immunoprotected intracellular environment, each sporozoite develops over a period of 6 to 16 days into tens of thousands of merozoites. *Plasmodium vivax* and *P. ovale* can develop into hypnozoites, which might remain quiescent in the liver for months to years. It is only after the parasites erupt from the hepatocytes that symptoms of clinical disease are apparent. In the bloodstream, the merozoites invade erythrocytes, multiply, mature over 24 to 72 hours, and finally lyse the red blood cells (Fig. 47–1C), proceeding immediately to invade new erythrocytes. Some of the merozoites develop into sexual-stage gametocytes, typically about 10 days after *P. falciparum* enters the blood stage (3 days for *P. vivax*). When these are taken up during an anopheline mosquito's blood meal, they can sexually combine and develop into sporozoites (10 to 22 days), restarting the cycle (Fig. 47–1D).

The classical signs and symptoms of malaria—acute febrile episodes and rigors that occur every 48 to 72 hours—coincide with the synchronized lysis of erythrocytes by newly matured merozoites. Systemic signs and symptoms associated with *P. falciparum* and *P. vivax* include fever, malaise, headache, photophobia, muscle aches, anorexia, nausea, and vomiting.[6] Severe disease occurs most frequently with *P. falciparum* because of its ability to infect a greater percentage of erythrocytes and to cytoadhere to capillary walls.[2,6] Clinical sequelae (such as acute renal failure, anemia, hypoglycemia, cerebral malaria, and pulmonary edema) occur most commonly in populations that are relatively immunonaïve, such as children and travelers.[7] Pregnant women are at special risk for severe disease and sequelae, indicating a unique mechanism of pathogenesis.[8]

Epidemiology and Burden of Disease

Quantification of the burden of malaria in affected populations is imprecise, impacted by access to diagnostic and therapeutic health centers, species prevalence, case definition, and low specificity of diagnosis.[9,10] It is thought that there are 300 to 500 million clinical cases per year globally, about 25% of which are caused by *P. vivax*. Estimated annual malaria-attributable deaths vary from 1.4 to 2.7 million,[9,11] with the majority of deaths occurring in children in Africa.[11] This translates into 39 million disability-adjusted life years lost annually[12] as one measure of malaria's economic and social disruption to developing nations.[13–15]

The number of malaria cases diagnosed within the United States has been stable at approximately 1000 to 1500 per year over the past decade, with the vast majority of cases reported by travelers and military personnel overseas. The United States has a very small number of congenital, blood-transfusion, and locally acquired cases.[16,17] Europe has a much higher rate of malaria, with 37,000 autochthonous and 13,000 imported cases reported in 1999.[18]

Vaccinology

Multiple lines of evidence suggest that a malaria vaccine for humans is feasible. Immunization of humans with irradiated

A

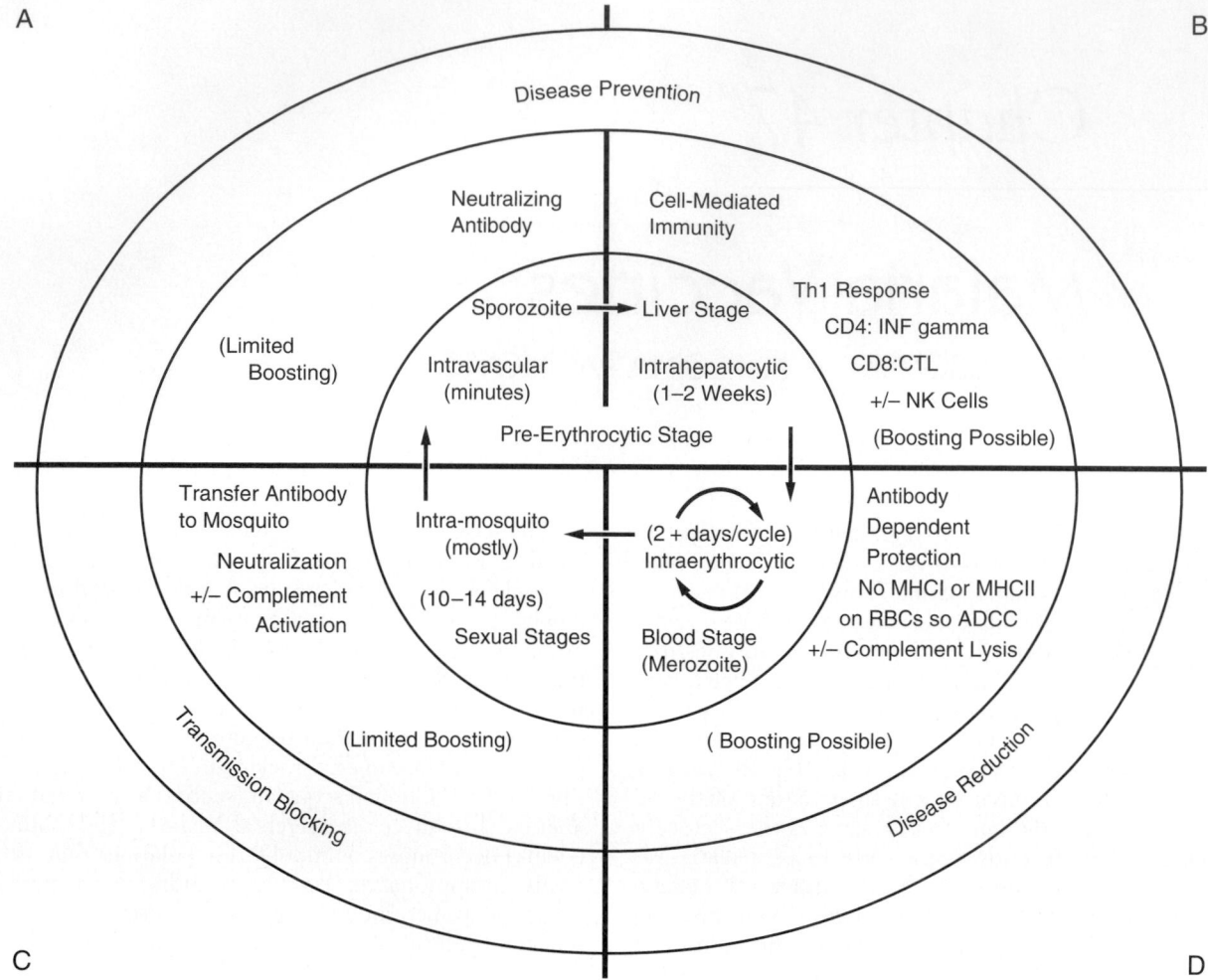

FIGURE 47–1 ■ The inner circle represents the *Plasmodium* life cycle, the middle circle the likely human immune response, and the outer circle the potential effect of a malaria vaccine targeting that stage of the parasite's life cycle. ADCC, antibody-dependent cell-mediated cytotoxicity; INF, interferon; MHCI, major histocompatibility complex class I; MHCII, major histocompatibility complex class II; NK, natural killer; RBCs, red blood cells; Th1, T-helper cell type 1.

(and thus attenuated) sporozoites confers sterile protection in roughly 90% of naïve volunteers when they are subsequently exposed to malaria.[19–21] Because this model requires each volunteer to be bitten by hundreds of mosquitoes over a period of several months, it is not a practical vaccination strategy but is useful in probing immune responses.[22] Naturally acquired clinical immunity occurs during the first two decades of life in people living in malaria-endemic countries.[23,24] In general, this immunity is imperfect, can wane rapidly, appears to be linked to intensity of exposure, and primarily impacts the severity of clinical disease.[25–28] Additionally, protection can be mimicked by the passive transfer of hyperimmune immunoglobulin into human volunteers.[29]

The immunologic correlate for clinical protection has yet to be identified. Through its complex life cycle, the malaria parasite exists in various immunologic "compartments." It is therefore possible to infer, in a stage-specific manner, the nature of the immune response that might impact the parasite. Furthermore, it is possible to extrapolate from other malaria intervention studies how the various stage-specific vaccines might work. Ultimately, it might

be necessary to combine antigens from different stages of the plasmodial life cycle into a single vaccine.

Pre-Erythrocytic Vaccines

Vaccine strategies targeting the sporozoite aim to generate a humoral immune response to neutralize the sporozoite and prevent it from invading the hepatocyte. The passive transfer of antibody specific to the sporozoite is protective in the murine ortholog model systems.[30] These models rely on vaccinating and protecting mice against the relevant plasmodial species (*P. yoelii* and *P. berghei*). Once the sporozoite has entered the relative immunoprotected intracellular environment of a hepatocyte, a successful vaccine strategy would harness cell-mediated immunity (CMI) (Fig. 47–1B).[31] Experiments in ortholog model systems and irradiated sporozoite challenge studies have implicated CD4+, CD8+, natural killer T, and γδ T cells in the inhibition of intrahepatic parasites.[32–38] A successful pre-erythrocytic vaccine could either induce an immune response that would prevent the sporozoite from entering the hepatocytes or destroy it once it invaded the hepatocytes. This would lead to sterile immunity, as was seen with irradiated sporozoites, and consequently be a disease-preventing vaccine (Fig. 47–1A and B). This type of vaccine would be ideal as a traveler's vaccine because it would prevent clinical disease. However, even a partially effective pre-erythrocytic vaccine could have large public health impact in the field if it behaved like other malarial interventions that target the pre-erythrocytic stage (insecticide-treated bed nets, intermittent drug therapy).[39–41]

Blood-Stage Vaccines

Merozoites enter the bloodstream after erupting from the hepatocyte. Within seconds they invade red blood cells, where they mature within cells that do not express major histocompatibility complex molecules. For this reason, the vaccine strategy has classically been considered antibody-dependent, either by inactivating the merozoites in the brief time they spend in the extracellular milieu or by targeting malarial antigens expressed on the red blood cell surface to antibody-dependent cellular inhibition (or possibly complement lysis).[36,42–44] Ortholog malaria models have implicated CD4+ T cells, nitric oxide, and γδ T cells in helping control blood-stage parasites,[36,45] and there is increasing evidence CMI can play a role in human protection.[46] Vaccines developed against this stage would serve as disease-reduction vaccines, mimicking naturally acquired immunity by suppressing the exponential multiplication of merozoites.[47,48]

Transmission-Blocking Vaccines

Transmission-blocking vaccines rely on the mosquito imbibing both antibody and complement along with the parasite during a blood meal. Within the mosquito, the antigens become exposed to antibodies during the parasite's maturation, thus neutralizing the sexual stages.[49–51] This type of vaccine would not prevent illness or infection in the vaccinated individual, but would prevent the further spread of malaria by mosquitoes feeding from the vaccinated host.[52,53] Such a vaccine could be useful in areas of low endemicity to halt transmission or as an important component of a multiantigen vaccine.

Clinical Experience

Currently, there are no registered malaria vaccines. However, a number of malaria vaccine candidates have been tested in clinical trials and have demonstrated variable safety and immunogenicity (Table 47–1). Historically, these vaccines have relied on antigens discovered by purifying proteins from various plasmodia species and by probing the immune response of exposed animals and individuals. It is unclear how the sequencing of the P. falciparum genome will impact future selection of antigens.

The pre-erythrocytic vaccines have focused largely on the circumsporozoite protein (CSP) that is a major surface protein of the sporozoite. This protein contains two major B-cell epitopes consisting of tandem repeats Asn-Ala-Asn-Pro and Asn-Val-Asp-Pro that several constructs have

included. Sporozoite Surface Protein 2 (SSP2)is another antigen that is exposed on the sporozoite and within the liver. Liver-Stage Antigen (LSA1) and Exported Protein (EXP1) are both expressed within the liver, but EXP1 also appears in the blood stage.

The blood-stage vaccines have focused on two proteins identified on the surface of the merozoite called Merozoite Surface Protein 1 (MSP1) and merozoite Surface Protein 2 (MSP2). Blood-stage antigens not associated with the merozoite surface also have been tried, such as Apical Membrane Antigen (AMA1), associated with the parasite rhoptry; Ring-stage–infected Erythrocyte Surface Antigen (RESA), associated with dense granules; and serine repeat antigen, associated with trophozoite and schizont stage.

Several vaccine candidates using these antigens have shown promise in artificial malaria challenge trials (Phase IIa) and endemic field trials (Phase IIb).

The SPf66 vaccine candidate was a synthetic multiepitope, multistage peptide vaccine tested in several Phase III trials involving tens of thousands of people. The reported efficacy of the various formulations tested was not sufficient to continue development;[54] reformulation with alternate adjuvant systems continues.[55,56]

The RTS,S vaccine candidate is a chimeric virus-like particle based on hepatitis B surface antigen. It has demonstrated protective efficacy of 30% to 80% against artificial sporozoite challenges in adults.[57,58] In a Phase IIb trial in semi-immune Gambian adults, RTS,S demonstrated a 72% protection efficacy against infection for the first 9 weeks, with efficacy waning rapidly thereafter.[59] The vaccine is currently in pediatric trials in Africa.

Combination B is a mixture of three blood-stage antigens delivered in a water-in-oil emulsion. In a small Phase IIb trial in Papua New Guinea, the vaccine reduced parasite density by 62% in children not pretreated with antimalarial medications.[60] Furthermore, there appeared to be vaccine-induced selection of parasite strains that were not targeted by the vaccine. A vaccine with multiple allelic forms of the putative effective component of Combination B is being developed for further trials.

Future Efforts

A number of vaccine candidates currently in early development are expected to be in field trials within the next 5 years. A variety of approaches is being developed, such as long synthetic peptides (with the CSP, MSP2/3, LSA3, and glutomate-rich protein [GLURP] antigens), recombinant proteins (with the MSP1/2/3/4/5, rhoptry-associated protein-[RAP2], AMA1, and Duffy-binding protein [PvRII] antigens), virus-like particles (with the CSP, AMA1, and MSP1 antigens), DNA vaccination (multiple pre-erythrocytic and blood-stage antigens), and viral-vectored vaccines using agents such as vaccinia, alphavirus, and adenovirus (multiple pre-erythrocytic and blood-stage antigens). In addition, both recombinant protein and DNA approaches have been used to create epitope-based vaccines. Many of the constructs under development can be formulated with a variety of immunoenhancers and adjuvants, thereby generating many possible vaccine candidates. As data on the performance

TABLE 47–1 ■ Malaria Vaccine Candidates Evaluated in Clinical Trials

Vaccine	Construct	Antigen	Phase	Trial Location	Ref.
SPf66	Multiepitope multistage synthetic peptide on alum	3 blood-stage epitopes linked by an immunodominant pre-erythrocytic epitope (NANP)	Multiple Phase I and Phase IIb	Tanzania, Ecuador, Venezuela, Colombia, Kenya, The Gambia, Thailand	61–83
FSV1 (R32tet$_{32}$)	NANP and NVDP CSP repeats on alum	NANP & NVPD, two immuno-dominant B-cell epitopes in CSP, a pre-erythrocytic sporozoite surface protein	Phase I/IIa	USA	84
R32ToxA	NANP and NVDP CSP repeats with *Pseudomonas* toxin A	See FSV1 above	Phase I/IIa Phase IIb	USA Kenya, Thailand	85 86, 87
R32NS1$_{81}$	NANP and NVDP CSP repeats with MPL, squalane, and mycobacterial cell wall	See FSV1 above	Phase I/IIa	USA	88
RTS,S	Chimeric hepatitis B surface VLP with CSP with MPL, QS-21 in emulsion (also tried with other adjuvants)	CSP, the major surface protein on the sporozoite; pre-erythrocytic	Phase I/IIa Phase I/IIb	USA, Belgium The Gambia	57,58, 89–91 92, 93
RLF	N-terminal and C-terminal portion of CSP in liposomes with MPL and alum	See RTS,S above	Phase I/IIa	USA	94
VaxSyn PfCSA	Baculovirus-expressed CSP on alum	See RTS,S above	Phase I	USA	95
Combi-nation A	Mixture of CSP and MSP2 on alum	CSP (see RTS,S above) and MSP2, a blood-stage protein located on the surface of the merozoite	Phase I/IIa	Switzerland	96
Comb-ination B	Mixture of MSP2, MSP1, L190, RESA in Montanide ISA 720	MSP1 and MSP2, two blood-stage proteins located on the surface of the merozoites; RESA, a blood-stage antigen associated with dense bodies within the parasite	Phase I/IIa Phase I/IIb	Australia Papua New Guinea	97, 98 60, 99
CVD 908-rCSP	CSP expressed in attenuated *Salmonella*	See RTS,S above	Phase I	USA	100
RPvCS	Yeast-expressed vivax CSP on alum	See RTS,S above	Phase I	USA	101
MSP1 P30P2	2 allelic forms of MSP1 with tetanus helper epitope on alum	MSP1, a blood-stage protein found on the surface of the merozoite	Phase I	USA	102
PfCSP DNA	Naked DNA vaccine coding for CSP	See RTS,S above	Phase I	USA	103,104
PfCSP 282–383	Long synthetic peptide of CSP with alum or Montanide ISA 720	See RTS,S above	Phase I	Switzerland	105,106
(T1B)$_4$MAP	Multiple antigenic peptide of CSP repeat with alum and QS-21	B-cell and T-cell epitopes from CSP, the major sporozoite surface protein; pre-erythrocytic	Phase I	USA	107
(T1BT*)$_4$ P3C	Polyoxime multiple antigenic peptide of CSP with Pam3Cys	B-cell and T-cell epitopes from CSP, the major sporozoite surface protein; pre-erythrocytic antigen	Phase I	USA	108
NYVAC-Pf7	Attenuated vaccinia bearing CSP, SSP2, LSA1, MSP1, SERA, AMA1	CSP, see RTS,S above; MSP1, see MSP1 P30P2 above; LSA1, a pre-erythrocytic antigen; SERA, a blood-stage antigen; AMA1, a blood-stage antigen; SSP2, a pre-erythrocytic antigen	Phase I/IIa	USA	109
P104/ P109-DT	MSP1 conjugated to DT and MSP2 conjugated to DT	See Combination B above	Phase I	Sri Lanka	110

Continued

TABLE 47-1 ■ Malaria Vaccine Candidates Evaluated in Clinical Trials—cont'd

Vaccine	Construct	Antigen	Phase	Trial Location	Ref.
NANP19-5.1	Fusion of 19 tandem NANP repeats with EXP1 on alum	NANP, see FSV1 above; EXP1, a liver-stage and blood-stage protein associated with the parasitophorous vacuole	Phase I/IIa Phase IIb	Switzerland Nigeria	111 112
R16HbsAg	16 tandem NANP repeats fused to HBsAg with alum	See FSV1 above	Phase I	Netherlands	113
(NANP)$_3$-TT	3 Tandem NANP repeats conjugated to TT with and without interferon-α	See FSV1 above	Phase I	Switzerland	114, 115

Alum, aluminum hydroxide; AMA, apical membrane antigen; CSP, circumsporozoite protein; DT, diphtheria toxoid; MPL, monophosphoryl lipid A; Montanide ISA 720, water-in-oil emulsion; MSP, merozoite surface protein; NANP, Asn-Ala-Asn-Pro pre-erythrocyte epitope; NVDP, Asn-Val-Asp-Pro pre-erythrocyte epitope; Pam3Cys, synthetic lipopeptide; HBsAg, hepatitis B surface antigen; L190, a portion of merozotite surface protein 1; LSA, liver-stage antigen; QS-21, a purified saponin derivative; RESA, ring-stage–infected erythrocyte surface antigen; SERA, serine repeat antigen; squaline, a metabolizable oil; SSP, sporozoite surface protein; TT, tetanus toxoid; VLP, virus-like particle.

of these products are generated in humans, it will be possible to look for immunologic correlates of protection and to validate the ortholog model systems as well as functional in vitro assays. Once these systems are developed, a less empirical approach to malaria vaccine development can be taken, allowing for focused product development of a few leading candidates.

REFERENCES

1. Gilles HM, Warrell DA (eds). Bruce-Chwatt's Essential Malariology (3rd ed). London, Edward Arnold, 1993.
2. Miller LH, Baruch DI, Marsh K, et al. The pathogenic basis of malaria. Nature 415:673–679, 2002.
3. Sherman IW (ed). Malaria: Parasite Biology, Pathogenesis, and Protection. Washington, DC, ASM Press, 1998.
4. Subbarao SK, Sharma VP. Anopheline species complexes and malaria control. Indian J Med Res 106:164–173, 1997.
5. World Health Organization. The World Health Report 1999: Making a Difference. Geneva, World Health Organization, 1999, pp 49–63.
6. Markell EK, Voge M, John DT. Medical Parasitology (7th ed). Philadelphia, WB Saunders, 1992.
7. Chen Q, Schlichtherle M, Wahlgren M. Molecular aspects of severe malaria. Clin Microbiol Rev 13:439–450, 2000.
8. Reeder JC. Malaria in pregnancy: getting to grips with a sticky problem. PNG Med J 42(3-4):73–76, 1999.
9. Breman J. The ears of the hippopotamus: manifestations, determinants, and estimates of the malaria burden. Am J Trop Med Hyg 64:1–11, 2001.
10. Murphy SC, Breman JG. Gaps in the childhood malaria burden in Africa: cerebral malaria, neurological sequelae, anemia, respiratory distress, hypoglycemia, and complications of pregnancy. Am J Trop Med Hyg 64(suppl):57–67, 2001.
11. Snow RW, Craig M, Diechmann U, et al. Estimating mortality, morbidity, and disability due to malaria among Africa's non-pregnant population. Bull World Health Organ 77:624–640, 1999.
12. World Health Organization. Annex Table 4: Leading causes of mortality and burden of disease, estimates for 1998. In The World Health Report 1999: Making a Difference. Geneva, World Health Organization, 1999, p 110.
13. Gallup JL, Sachs JD. The economic burden of malaria. Am J Trop Med Hyg 64(suppl):85–96, 2001.
14. Sachs J, Malaney P. The economic and social burden of malaria. Nature 415:680–685, 2002.
15. Sachs, J. Macroeconomics and Health: Investing in Health for Economic Development. World Health Organization, Geneva Switzerland, 2000.
16. Holtz TH, Katchur SP, MacArthur JR, et al. Malaria surveillance—United States, 1998. Mor Mortal Wkly Rep CDC Surveill Summ 50(5):1–18, 2001.
17. Sunstrum J, Elliott LJ, Barat LM, et al. Probable autochthonous Plasmodium vivax malaria transmission in Michigan: case report and epidemiological investigation. Am J Trop Med Hyg 65:949–953, 2001.
18. Sabatinelli G, Ejov M, Joergensen P. Malaria in the WHO European Region (1971–1999). Euro Surveill 6:61–65, 2001.
19. Clyde D. Immunity to falciparum and vivax malaria induced by irradiated sporozoites: a review of the University of Maryland studies, 1971–75. Bull World Health Organ 68(suppl):9–12, 1990.
20. Egan J. Humoral immune responses in volunteers immunized with irradiated Plasmodium falciparum sporozoites. Am J Trop Med Hyg 49:166–173, 1993.
21. Rieckmann KH, Beaudoin RL, Cassells JS. Use of attenuated sporozoites in the immunization of human volunteers against falciparum malaria. Bull World Health Organ 57(suppl 1):261–265, 1979.
22. Hoffman SL, Goh LM, Luke TC, et al. Protection of humans against malaria by immunization with radiation-attenuated Plasmodium falciparum sporozoites. J Infect Dis 185:1155–1164, 2002.
23. Trape JF, Rogier C, Konate L, et al. The Dielmo project: a longitudinal study of natural malaria infection and the mechanisms of protective immunity in a community living in holoendemic area of Senegal. Am J Trop Med Hyg 51:123–137, 1994.
24. Baird JK, Jones TR, Danudirgo EW, et al. Age-dependent acquired protection against Plasmodium falciparum in people having two-year exposure to hyperendemic malaria. Am J Trop Med Hyg 45:65–76, 1991.
25. Day KP, Marsh K. Naturally acquired immunity to Plasmodium falciparum. Immunol Today 12(3):A68–A71, 1991.
26. Baird J. Age-dependent characteristics of protection v. susceptibility to Plasmodium falciparum. Ann Trop Med Parasitol 92:367–390, 1998.
27. Hogh B. Clinical and parasitologic studies on immunity to Plasmodium falciparum malaria in children. Scand J Infect Dis 102(suppl):1–53, 1996.
28. Smith TA, Leunberger R, Lengeler C. Child mortality and malaria transmission intensity in Africa. Trends Parasitol 17:145–149, 2001.
29. Sabcharoen A, Burnouf T, Ouattara D, et al. Parasitologic and clinical human response to immunoglobulin administration in falciparum malaria. Am J Trop Med Hyg 45:297–308, 1991.
30. Marussig M, Renia L, Motard A, et al. Linear and multiple antigen peptides containing defined T and B epitopes of the Plasmodium yoelii circumsporozoite protein: antibody-mediated protection and boosting by sporozoite infection. Int Immunol 9:1817–1824, 1997.
31. Doolan DL, Hoffman SL. The complexity of protective immunity against liver-stage malaria. J Immunol 165:1453–1462, 2000.
32. Gonzalez-Aseguinolaza G, de Oliveira C, Tomaska M, et al. α-Galactosylceramide-activated Va14 natural killer T cells mediate protection against murine malaria. Proc Natl Acad Sci U S A 97:8461–8466, 2000.

33. Nardin EH, Nussenzweig R. T cell response to pre-erythrocytic stages of malaria: role in protection and vaccine development against pre-erythrocytic stages. Annu Rev Immunol 11:687–727, 1993.

34. Tsuji M, Romero P, Nussenzweig RS, et al. CD4+ cytolytic T cell clone confers protection against murine malaria. J Exp Med 172:1353–1357, 1990.

35. Tsuji M, Momobaerts P, Lefrancois L, et al. Gamma delta T cells contribute to immunity against the liver stages of malaria in alpha beta T-cell-deficient mice. Proc Natl Acad Sci U S A 91:345–349, 1994.

36. Good M, Doolan DL. Immune effector mechanism in malaria. Curr Opin Immunol 11:412–419, 1999.

37. Doolan DL, Hoffman SL. Pre-erythrocytic-stage immune effector mechanisms in Plasmodium spp. infections. Philos Trans R Soc Lond B Biol Sci 352:1361–1367, 1997.

38. Nardin E, Zavala F, Nussenzweig V, et al. Pre-erythrocytic malaria vaccine: mechanisms of protective immunity and human vaccine trials. Parassitologia 41:397–402, 1999.

39. Lengeler C. Insecticide-treated bednets and curtains for preventing malaria (Cochrane Review). In The Cochrane Library (Issue 3). Oxford, Update Software, 2002.

40. Saul A. Minimal efficacy requirements for malarial vaccines to significantly lower transmission in epidemic or seasonal malaria. Acta Trop 52:283–296, 1993.

41. Schellenberg D, Menendez C, Kahigwa E, et al. Intermittent treatment for malaria and anaemia control at time of routine vaccinations in Tanzanian infants: a randomised, placebo-controlled trial. Lancet 357:1471–1477, 2001.

42. Bouharoun-Tayoun H, Oeuvray C, Lunel F, et al. Mechanisms underlying the monocyte-mediated antibody-dependent killing of Plasmodium falciparum asexual blood stages. J Exp Med 182:409–418, 1995.

43. Long C. Immunity to blood stages of malaria. Curr Opin Immunol 5:548–556, 1993.

44. Holder AA, Guevara Patino JA, Uthaipibull C, et al. Merozoite surface protein 1, immune evasion, and vaccines against asexual blood-stage malaria. Parassitologia 41:409–414, 1999.

45. Good M. Towards a blood-stage vaccine for malaria: are we following all the leads? Nat Rev 1:117–125, 2001.

46. Plombo D, Lawrence G, Hirunpetcharat C, et al. Immunity to malaria following administration of ultra-low doses of Plasmodium falciparum-infected red cells. Lancet 360:610, 2002.

47. Tsuji M, Rodrigues E, Nussenzweig S. Progress toward a malaria vaccine: efficient induction of protective anti-malaria immunity. Biol Chem 382:553–570, 2001.

48. Richie TL, Saul A. Progress and challenges for malaria vaccines. Nature 415:694–701, 2002.

49. Kaslow D. Transmission-blocking immunity against malaria and other vector-borne diseases. Curr Opin Immunol 5:557–565, 1993.

50. Lobo CA, Dhar R, Kumar N. Immunization of mice with DNA-based Pfs-25 elicits potent malaria transmission-blocking antibodies. Infect Immun 67:1688–1693, 1999.

51. Hisaeda H, Stowers AW, Tsuboi T, et al. Antibody to malaria vaccine candidates Pvs25 and Pvs28 completely blocks the ability of Plasmodium vivax to infect mosquitoes. Infect Immun 68:6618–6623, 2000.

52. Kaslow D. Transmission-blocking vaccines: use and current status of development. Int J Parasitol 27:183–189, 1997.

53. Stowers A, Carter R. Current developments in malaria transmission-blocking vaccines. Expert Opin Biol Ther 1:619–628, 2001.

54. Graves P, Gelband H. Vaccines for preventing malaria (Cochrane Review). In The Cochrane Library (Issue 3). Oxford, Update Software, 2002.

55. Rosas JE, Pedraz JL, Hernandez RM, et al. Remarkably high antibody levels and protection against P. falciparum malaria in Aotus monkeys after a single immunization of SPf66 encapsulated in PLGA microspheres. Vaccine 20:1707–1710, 2002.

56. Potl-Frank F, Zurbrigen R, Helg A, et al. Use of reconstituted influenza virosomes as an immunopotentiating delivery system for a peptide-based vaccine. Clin Exp Immunol 117:496–503, 1999.

57. Kester KE, McKinney DA, Tornieporth N, et al. Efficacy of recombinant circumsporozoite protein vaccine regimens against experimental Plasmodium falciparum malaria. J Infect Dis 183:640–647, 2001.

58. Stoute JA, Slaoui M, Heppner DG, et al. A preliminary evaluation of a recombinant circumsporozoite protein vaccine against Plasmodium falciparum malaria. RTS,S Malaria Vaccine Evaluation Group. N Engl J Med 336:86–91, 1997.

59. Bojang KA, Obaro SK, D'Alessandro U, et al. An efficacy trial of the malaria vaccine SPf66 in Gambian infants—second year of follow-up. Vaccine 16:62–67, 1998.

60. Genton B, Betuela I, Felger I, et al. Related Articles: A recombinant blood-stage malaria vaccine reduces Plasmodium falciparum density and exerts selective pressure on parasite populations in a Phase 1-2b trial in Papua New Guinea. J Infect Dis 185:820–827, 2002.

61. Alonso PL, Smith T, Schellenberg JR, et al. Randomised trial of efficacy of SPf66 vaccine against Plasmodium falciparum malaria in children in southern Tanzania. Lancet 344:1175–1181, 1994.

62. Teuscher T, Schellenberg JR, Bastos de Azevedo I, et al. SPf66, a chemically synthesized subunit malaria vaccine, is safe and immunogenic in Tanzanians exposed to intense malaria transmission. Vaccine 12:328–336, 1994.

63. Alonso PL, Smith TA, Armstrong-Schellenberg JR, et al. Duration of protection and age-dependence of the effects of the SPf66 malaria vaccine in African children exposed to intense transmission of Plasmodium falciparum. J Infect Dis 174:367–372, 1996.

64. Beck HP, Felger I, Huber W, et al. Analysis of multiple Plasmodium falciparum infections in Tanzanian children during the Phase III trial of the malaria vaccine SPf66. J Infect Dis 175:921–926, 1997.

65. Acosta CJ, Galindo CM, Schellenberg D, et al. Evaluation of the SPf66 vaccine for malaria control when delivered through the EPI scheme in Tanzania. Trop Med Int Health 4:368–376, 1999.

66. Galindo CM, Acosta CJ, Schellenberg D, et al. Humoral immune responses during a malaria vaccine trial in Tanzanian infants. Parasite Immunol 22:437–443, 2000.

67. Schellenberg DM, Acosta CJ, Galindo CM, et al. Safety in infants of SPf66, a synthetic malaria vaccine, delivered alongside the EPI. Trop Med Int Health 4:377–382, 1999.

68. Sempertegui F, Estrella B, Moscoso J, et al. Safety, immunogenicity and protective effect of the SPf66 malaria synthetic vaccine against Plasmodium falciparum infection in a randomized, double-blind, placebo-controlled field trial in an endemic area of Ecuador. Vaccine 12:337–342, 1994.

69. Urdaneta M, Prata A, Struchiner CJ, et al. Evaluation of SPf66 malaria vaccine efficacy in Brazil. Am J Trop Med Hyg 58:378–385, 1998.

70. Noya O, Gabaldon Berti Y, Alarcon de Noya B, et al. A population-based clinical trial with the SPf66 synthetic Plasmodium falciparum malaria vaccine in Venezuela. J Infect Dis 170:396–402, 1994.

71. Patarroyo G, Franco L, Amador R, et al. Study of the safety and immunogenicity of the synthetic malaria SPf66 vaccine in children aged 1–14 years. Vaccine 10:175–178, 1992.

72. Amador R, Moreno A, Murillo LA, et al. Safety and immunogenicity of the synthetic malaria vaccine SPf66 in a large field trial. J Infect Dis 166:139–144, 1992.

73. Amador R, Moreno A, Valero V, et al. The first field trials of the chemically synthesized malaria vaccine SPf66: safety, immunogenicity, and protectivity. Vaccine 10:179–184, 1992.

74. Lopera TM, Restrepo M, Blair S, et al. Humoral immune response to the anti-malaria vaccine SPf66 in the Colombian Atrato River region. Mem Inst Oswaldo Cruz 93:495–500, 1998.

75. Valero MV, Amador LR, Galindo C, et al. Vaccination with SPf66, a chemically synthesised vaccine, against Plasmodium falciparum malaria in Colombia. Lancet 341:705–710, 1993.

76. Valero MV, Amador R, Aponte JJ, et al. Evaluation of SPf66 malaria vaccine during a 22-month follow-up field trial in the Pacific coast of Colombia. Vaccine 14:1466–1470, 1996.

77. Masinde GL, Krogstad DJ, Gordon DM, et al. Immunization with SPf66 and subsequent infection with homologous and heterologous Plasmodium falciparum parasites. Am J Trop Med Hyg 59:600–605, 1998.

78. Leach A, Drakeley CJ, D'Alessandro U, et al. A pilot safety and immunogenicity study of the malaria vaccine SPf66 in Gambian infants. Parasite Immunol 17:441–444, 1995.

79. D'Alessandro U. An efficacy trial of a malaria vaccine in Gambian infants and comparison with insecticide-treated bednets. Ann Trop Med Parasitol 90:373–378, 1996.

80. D'Alessandro U, Leach A, Drakeley CJ, et al. Efficacy trial of malaria vaccine SPf66 in Gambian infants. Lancet 346:462–467, 1995.

81. Migasena S, Heppner DG, Kyle DE, et al. SPf66 malaria vaccine is safe and immunogenic in malaria-naive adults in Thailand. Acta Trop 67:215–227, 1997.

82. Nosten F, Luxemberger C, Kyle DE, et al. Randomised, double-blind, placebo-controlled trial of SPf66 malaria vaccine in children in north-

western Thailand. Shoklo SPf66 Malaria Vaccine Trial Group. Lancet 348:701–707, 1996.

83. Nosten F, Luxemberger C, Kyle DE, et al. Phase I trial of the SPf66 malaria vaccine in a malaria-experienced population in Southeast Asia. Am J Trop Med Hyg 56:526–532, 1997.

84. Ballou WR, Luxemberger C, Kyle DE, et al. Safety and efficacy of a recombinant DNA *Plasmodium falciparum* sporozoite vaccine. Lancet 1:1277–1281, 1987.

85. Fries LF, Gordon DM, Schneider I, et al. Safety, immunogenicity, and efficacy of a *Plasmodium falciparum* vaccine comprising a circumsporozoite protein repeat region peptide conjugated to *Pseudomonas aeruginosa* toxin A. Infect Immun 60:1834–1839, 1992.

86. Sherwood JA, Copeland RS, Taylor KA, et al. *Plasmodium falciparum* circumsporozoite vaccine immunogenicity and efficacy trial with natural challenge quantitation in an area of endemic human malaria of Kenya. Vaccine 14:817–827, 1996.

87. Brown AE, Singharaj P, Webster HK, et al. Safety, immunogenicity, and limited efficacy study of a recombinant *Plasmodium falciparum* circumsporozoite vaccine in Thai soldiers. Vaccine 12:102–108, 1994.

88. Hoffman SL, Edelman R, Bryan JP, et al. Safety, immunogenicity, and efficacy of a malaria sporozoite vaccine administered with monophosphoryl lipid A, cell wall skeleton of mycobacteria, and squalene as adjuvant. Am J Trop Med Hyg 51:603–612, 1994.

89. Stoute JA, Kester KE, Krzych U, et al. Long-term efficacy and immune responses following immunization with the RTS,S malaria vaccine. J Infect Dis 178:1139–1144, 1998.

90. Lalvani A, Moris P, Voss G, et al. Potent induction of focused Th1-type cellular and humoral immune responses by RTS,S/SBAS2, a recombinant *Plasmodium falciparum* malaria vaccine. J Infect Dis 180:1656–1664, 1999.

91. Gordon DM, McGovern TW, Krzych U, et al. Safety, immunogenicity, and efficacy of a recombinantly produced *Plasmodium falciparum* circumsporozoite protein-hepatitis B surface antigen subunit vaccine. J Infect Dis 171:1576–1585, 1995.

92. Doherty JF, Pinder M, Tornieporth N, et al. A Phase I safety and immunogenicity trial with the candidate malaria vaccine RTS,S/SBAS2 in semi-immune adults in The Gambia. Am J Trop Med Hyg 61:865–868, 1999.

93. Bojang KA, Milligan PJ, Pinder M, et al. Efficacy of RTS,S/ASO2 malaria vaccine against *Plasmodium falciparum* infection in semi-immune adult men in The Gambia: a randomised trial. Lancet 358:1927–1934, 2001.

94. Heppner DG, Gordon DM, Gross M, et al. Safety, immunogenicity, and efficacy of *Plasmodium falciparum* repeatless circumsporozoite protein vaccine encapsulated in liposomes. J Infect Dis 174:361–366, 1996.

95. Herrington DA, Losonsky GA, Smith G, et al. Safety and immunogenicity in volunteers of a recombinant *Plasmodium falciparum* circumsporozoite protein malaria vaccine produced in Lepidopteran cells. Vaccine 10:841–846, 1992.

96. Sturchler D, Berger R, Rudin C, et al. Safety, immunogenicity, and pilot efficacy of *Plasmodium falciparum* sporozoite and asexual blood-stage combination vaccine in Swiss adults. Am J Trop Med Hyg 53:423–431, 1995.

97. Saul A, Lawrence G, Smillie A, et al. Human Phase I vaccine trials of 3 recombinant asexual stage malaria antigens with Montanide ISA720 adjuvant. Vaccine 17:3145–3159, 1999.

98. Lawrence G, Cheng QQ, Reed C, et al. Effect of vaccination with 3 recombinant asexual-stage malaria antigens on initial growth rates of *Plasmodium falciparum* in non-immune volunteers. Vaccine 18:1925–1931, 2000.

99. Genton B, Al-Yaman F, Anders R, et al. Safety and immunogenicity of a three-component blood-stage malaria vaccine in adults living in an endemic area of Papua New Guinea. Vaccine 18:2504–2511, 2000.

100. Gonzalez C, Hone D, Noriega FR, et al. Salmonella typhi vaccine strain CVD 908 expressing the circumsporozoite protein of *Plasmodium falciparum*: strain construction and safety and immunogenicity in humans. J Infect Dis 169:927–931, 1994.

101. Herrington DA, Nardin EH, Losonsky G, et al. Safety and immunogenicity of a recombinant sporozoite malaria vaccine against *Plasmodium vivax*. Am J Trop Med Hyg 45:695–701, 1991.

102. Keitel WA, Kester KE, Atmar RL, et al. Phase I trial of two recombinant vaccines containing the 19kd carboxy terminal fragment of *Plasmodium falciparum* merozoite surface protein 1 (msp-1(19)) and T helper epitopes of tetanus toxoid. Vaccine 18:531–539, 1999.

103. Le TP, Coonan KM, Hedstrom RC, et al. Safety, tolerability, and humoral immune responses after intramuscular administration of a malaria DNA vaccine to healthy adult volunteers. Vaccine 18:1893–1901, 2000.

104. Wang R, Doolan DL, Le TP, et al. Induction of antigen-specific cytotoxic T lymphocytes in humans by a malaria DNA vaccine. Science 282:476–480, 1998.

105. Lopez JA, Weilenman C, Audran R, et al. A synthetic malaria vaccine elicits a potent CD8(+) and CD4(+) T lymphocyte immune response in humans: implications for vaccination strategies. Eur J Immunol 31:1989–1998, 2001.

106. Roggero MA, Weilenmann C, Bonelo A, et al. *Plasmodium falciparum* CS C-terminal fragment: preclinical evaluation and Phase I clinical studies. Parassitologia 41:421–424, 1999.

107. Nardin EH, Oliveira GA, Calvo-Calle JM, et al. Synthetic malaria peptide vaccine elicits high levels of antibodies in vaccinees of defined HLA genotypes. J Infect Dis 182:1486–1496, 2000.

108. Nardin EH, Calvo-Calle JM, Oliveira GA, et al. A totally synthetic polyoxime malaria vaccine containing *Plasmodium falciparum* B cell and universal T cell epitopes elicits immune responses in volunteers of diverse HLA types. J Immunol 166:481–489, 2001.

109. Ockenhouse CF, Sun PF, Lanar DE, et al. Phase I/IIa safety, immunogenicity, and efficacy trial of NYVAC-Pf7, a pox-vectored, multiantigen, multistage vaccine candidate for *Plasmodium falciparum* malaria. J Infect Dis 177:1664–1673, 1998.

110. Ramasamy R, Wijesundere DA, Nagendran K, et al. Antibody and clinical responses in volunteers to immunization with malaria peptide-diphtheria toxoid conjugates. Clin Exp Immunol 99:168–174, 1995.

111. Sturchler D, Just M, Berger R, et al. Evaluation of 5.1-NANP19, a recombinant *Plasmodium falciparum* vaccine candidate, in adults. Trop Geogr Med 44(1-2):9–14, 1992.

112. Reber-Liske R, Salako LA, Matile H, et al. NANP19-5.1: a malaria vaccine field trial in Nigerian children. Trop Geogr Med 47(2):61–63, 1995.

113. Vreden SG, Verhave JP, Oettinger T, et al. Phase I clinical trial of a recombinant malaria vaccine consisting of the circumsporozoite repeat region of *Plasmodium falciparum* coupled to hepatitis B surface antigen. Am J Trop Med Hyg 45:533–538, 1991.

114. Sturchler D, Zimmer G, Berger R, et al. Interferon-alpha and synthetic peptide malaria sporozoite vaccine in non-immune adults: antibody response after 40 weeks. Bull World Health Organ 68(suppl):38–41, 1990.

115. Etlinger HM, F.A., Gillessen D, Heimer EP, et al. Assessment in humans of a synthetic peptide-based vaccine against sporozoite stage of the human malaria parasite, *Plasmodium falciparum*. J Immunol 120:626–633, 1988.

Chapter 48

Parasitic Disease Vaccines

PETER J. HOTEZ • JEFFREY M. BETHONY

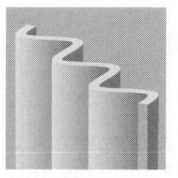

Parasitic diseases caused by helminths and unicellular eukaryotes (protozoa) are major causes of human disease and misery in the less-developed nations of the tropics. Attempts to develop vaccines against these organisms have been hampered by the difficulties in maintaining the organisms in the laboratory. With a few exceptions, in vitro culture methods have not been adequate; frequently laboratory animals such as dogs and nonhuman primates have been necessary to propagate their complex life cycles. This problem has thwarted efforts to scale up production of large numbers of parasites in order to develop attenuated or killed vaccines. Within the last decade, investigators in academic and government laboratories have started to apply modern biotechnology to the study of parasitic helminths and protozoa, resulting in the cloning and expression of some promising recombinant protective antigens. However, there has been little commercial interest in the development of these protective antigens as human vaccines. Lack of enthusiasm for parasitic disease vaccines among the traditional large vaccine manufacturers has resulted from concerns about their markets in developing economies, as well as their scientific and technological complexities.[1] Infusion of new funds from private philanthropies such as the Bill and Melinda Gates Foundation have re-energized attempts to manufacture public-sector vaccines for parasitic diseases.[2]

Anthelmintic Vaccines

Helminth infections are among the most prevalent infections of humans. Up to 2 billion individuals worldwide harbor one or more of the soil-transmitted nematodes *Ascaris lumbricoides*, *Trichuris trichiura*, and hookworms in their intestines. Hundreds of millions of people are infected with schistosomes (*Schistosoma mansoni*, *S. japonicum*, and *S. haematobium*). The World Health Organization (WHO) estimates that, together, the soil-transmitted helminths and schistosomes account for 40% of the global morbidity resulting from infection, exclusive of malaria (antimalaria vaccines are discussed in Chapter 47). In much of the developing world, *Ascaris*, *Trichuris*, and *Schistosoma* infec-

tions exhibit their highest prevalence and intensity among children and teenagers. Children who are chronically infected with heavy worm burdens develop deficits in physical, intellectual, and cognitive growth. In contrast to the other soil-transmitted helminths, hookworm burdens are highest in both adults and children. In South China, for instance, hookworm is considered an important problem among geriatric populations.[3,4]

Among the global efforts to control soil-transmitted helminth infections and schistosomiasis are concerted efforts to administer albendazole and praziquantel, respectively, on a yearly or twice-yearly basis. Because *Ascaris*, *Trichuris*, and the schistosomes primarily affect school-age children, these anthelmintic drugs often are administered as part of school-based health and education efforts. However, although albendazole and praziquantel are effective at temporarily reducing worm burden, children usually will reacquire their helminth infections several months after treatment.[5] This limits the usefulness of anthelmintic agents as a school-based public health control measure and does not address hookworm burdens among adult populations. As an alternative approach to control, efforts are now underway to develop anthelmintic vaccines.

The goals of anthelmintic vaccination are different from those of conventional antiviral and antibacterial vaccination. For instance, it is not likely that immunization with defined antigens will elicit sterilizing immunity against complex metazoan organisms. Instead, the most important goal is to reduce the worm burden below the disease-causing threshold. The essential concept of anthelmintic vaccines is to attempt to immunize against *disease* rather than *infection*. Examples of this idea would be to reduce the hookworm burden below the threshold that results in significant intestinal blood loss or to reduce the schistosome burden below the threshold that results in significant egg deposition and subsequent granuloma formation in the liver, intestines, and bladder. Still another approach to antidisease vaccination would be to directly block the action of parasite-induced pathogenic processes. In the case of hookworm, this would require blocking parasite-derived virulence factors that cause blood loss, and for schistosomiasis, blocking egg deposition. It is likely that anthelmintic vaccination will not be used in isolation, but rather will be in conjunction with other control efforts, including conventional chemotherapy.[6,7]

Hookworm Disease

Human hookworm infection is a leading cause of anemia and malnutrition among children in developing countries. An estimated 194 million cases occur in China alone.[8] There are two major species, *Necator americanus* and *Ancylostoma duodenale*, with the former the predominant hookworm worldwide. Humans become infected when third-stage larvae either penetrate through the skin (*N. americanus* and *A. duodenale*) or are ingested (*A. duodenale* only). On host entry, the larvae undergo extraintestinal migration in the vasculature and reach the heart and lungs. Hookworm larval lung migration is associated with a mild pneumonitis; the larvae ascend the airways and reach the larynx before they are coughed and swallowed. The larvae molt twice in the intestine to become adult hookworms that invade tissue and cause blood loss.

Early attempts at developing a hookworm vaccine relied on the observation that numerous small doses of living third-stage infective larvae (L3) could confer resistance against challenge hookworm infections. Resistance was measured by reductions in the worm burden, the worms' size, and the worms' fecundity. Immunity was seldom sterilizing. Later it was noted that larger doses of living L3 could be administered over shorter time periods if they were first damaged by ionizing radiation. This provided the basis for commercial radiation-attenuated hookworm L3 vaccines that could be administered to dogs in two doses. The canine hookworm vaccine was marketed first in Florida and later in the eastern United States during the 1970s, but ultimately it failed as a commercial veterinary product.[9] Among the reasons for its lack of commercial success were the high production costs in harvesting living L3, the limited shelf life of the product, and the misperceptions on the part of pet owners and veterinarians regarding an antidisease vaccine that reduced the worm burden but did not usually elicit sterilizing immunity.

It is not feasible to develop human antihookworm vaccines that use living L3, damaged or otherwise. However, studies are in progress to identify vaccine antigens from L3 that can reproduce the reduction in worm burdens afforded by the live vaccines.[10] One class of antigens under investigations is the *Ancylostoma*-secreted proteins (ASPs), which are released by host-stimulated infective hookworm larvae and contain amino acid sequences homologous to those of the major antigens from insect venoms.[11] Immunization of mice with an alum precipitate of recombinant ASP-1, a 45-kDa protein, reduces the number of hookworms that enter into the lung after oral infection,[12,13] while immunization with a baculovirus-expressed recombinant ASP homologous protein elicits high levels of protection in guinea pigs after challenge infections with sheep trichostrongyle nematodes. Another approach to vaccination takes advantage of the fact that adult hookworms ingest blood. Recently, two different adult-stage proteolytic enzymes were shown to align the brush border membrane of the hookworm gastrointestinal tract.[14] Parallel studies conducted with blood-feeding trichostrongyle nematodes of sheep and cattle

suggest that similar gut membrane-bound proteases are promising vaccine targets.

Critical to the success of vaccination is the requirement to express the enzymes in catalytically active conformations, which so far has required eukaryotic expression in either yeast (*Pichia pastoris*) or baculovirus. To date, hookworm burden reductions through vaccination with chemically defined antigens depend on high titers of host antigen-specific antibody (especially of the type 2 T-helper cell [Th2] type) that cross-reacts to the native antigen. This achievement requires antigen expression in eukaryotic systems and subsequent antigen formulation with either alum or alhydrogel. Because of its high yield and lower costs, *Pichia pastoris* is likely to emerge as the expression vector of choice for further process development and pilot manufacture. Human clinical trials with L3-derived ASPs and adult hookworm–derived proteases are in the early planning stages pending the outcome of process development and pilot manufacture.

Schistosomiasis

Schistosomes are snail-transmitted, water-borne parasitic platyhelminths (order *Trematoda*). High rates of infection occur near bodies of fresh water such as tributaries of the Nile River in Egypt and the Dongting and Boyang lakes in China.[15–17] The three major species groups of schistosomes, *Schistosoma mansoni*, *S. haematobium*, and the *S. japonicum* complex (including *S. japonicum* and *S. mekongi*), typically are distinguished by their unique snail vectors, location within the host vasculature, and egg morphology. Members of the *S. japonicum* complex also have important domestic animal reservoir hosts (pigs, cattle, water buffaloes). Asexual reproduction of the parasites occurs in freshwater snail intermediate hosts that release large numbers of free-swimming infective larval schistosomes, known as *cercariae*, into the water. The cercariae are attracted to linoleic acid and other skin components, causing them to attach and penetrate percutaneously with the aid of proteases. On host entry, the cercariae lose their characteristic tail and the resulting schistosomulae spend the next few weeks migrating through the blood stream and lungs until they reach the liver. Here they differentiate into male and female schistosomes. Male and female worm pairs migrate through the portal vasculature until they reach their final destination in the mesenteric or bladder venules. The worm pairs release eggs, which exit from the body in feces or urine and then hatch in fresh water. Freshly hatched miracidia swim via the action of their cilia. They are pluripotent and potentially can give rise to thousands of progeny on their entry into a suitable snail host.

Most of the morbidity associated with schistosomiasis occurs when the eggs fail to exit from the definitive human host. Trapped in the intestinal or bladder wall, or in the liver as they are swept up by the portal circulation, the eggs elicit granulomas and host fibrosis. In the liver, the so-called Symmer's pipestem fibrosis leads to portal hypertension and hepatosplenomegaly. Because of the location and greater numbers of eggs produced by *S. japonicum*, schistosomiasis japonica tends to be the most severe form. In addition, children with chronic schistosomiasis japonica (and possibly other forms as well) have deficits in physical growth.

A number of different approaches have been taken to design antischistosomal vaccines. As in other systems, the administration of radiation-attenuated cercariae results in the best protection to date. The mechanisms of resistance associated with the live cercarial vaccine have been worked out over the last 10 years using a mouse model.[18] Briefly, the damaged cercariae successfully penetrate the skin and become schistosomulae, whereupon they enter skin-draining lymph nodes (SLNs). Antigens released by the damaged cercariae in the SLNs stimulate the proliferation of helper T cells with type 1 (Th1) features, including the release of interferon-γ (IFN-γ) as a predominant cytokine. After induction of the primary immune response in the SLNs, lymphocytes mediating delayed-type hypersensitivity responses appear in the circulation. A proportion of attenuated parasites migrate from the skin to the lungs, the major site of immune elimination and parasite attrition. The arrival of schistosomula in the lungs provokes an infiltration of T lymphocytes, recruited from SLNs. Challenge of the vaccinated laboratory animals results in a second recruitment into the lungs of IFN-γ– and interleukin-3–secreting effector-memory T cells that have the capacity to block parasite migration. Thus the mononuclear cell infiltrate triggered by the arrival of challenge parasites in the lungs aggregates into a dense pulmonary focus of cells that prevents worm migration. IFN-γ is a key cytokine in this process because its neutralization results in a looser pulmonary focus that cannot impede the invading parasites. New evidence indicates that redundant immunologic pathways also may mediate vaccine protection from irradiated cercariae. High levels of antibodies and active Th2 immunity also may replicate the worm burden reductions afforded by Th1 immunity, especially after multiple doses of the vaccine. This observation has led Wilson and Coulson[18] to propose that, when vaccination achieves a significant deflection of the Th response in either a Th1 or Th2 direction, it will produce a measure of protection. The extreme bias toward one or the other pole will result in higher levels of protection, whereas intermediate responses (Th0) will result in successful establishment of parasitism.

In part based on this paradigm, vigorous attention has been focused on potential vaccine antigens from the schistosomula stages. Vaccination with stage-specific schistosomula surface antigens has resulted in disappointing protection, usually less than 40%.[16] Somewhat better protection has been achieved using antigens shared between schistosomula and adult schistosomes, including parasite-derived myosin (63 kDa), paramyosin (97 kDa), triose phosphate isomerase (28 kDa), glutathione-S-transferases (GSTs; 26 and 28 kDa), a fatty acid–binding protein (14 kDa), and a 23-kDa surface protein. To date, most of the vaccine studies are conducted in mice challenged with either S. mansoni or S. japonicum. However, because Asian schistosomiasis is associated with significant animal reservoirs, including cattle, water buffalo, and pigs, several veterinary vaccine trials have been conducted in China in these hosts.[17,19,20] To date, the recombinant antigen-based vaccine trials have been conducted with numerous adjuvants, including Freund's complete adjuvant, alum, bacille Calmette-Guérin (BCG), saponin, Quil A, and Bordetella pertussis. Because of the suggested role of IFN-γ and Th1 cellular immune responses in mediating protection, there have been some efforts to bias the host cytokine profile at the time of vaccination. Some success has been reported in this regard using interleukin-12 (IL-12) as an adjuvant as well as with DNA immunizations. The molecular basis of immunity with the schistosomula antigens is largely unstudied, except for new evidence that paramyosin may function as an Fc receptor for the parasite, so that antiparamyosin immune responses may somehow interfere with the parasite's immune escape mechanisms.[21]

A second approach to vaccination against schistosomiasis has been to target the fecundity of female adult schistosomes in order to diminish egg excretion into target host organs. Success with this approach has been reported by immunizing mice and large-animal reservoir hosts, including pigs and water buffaloes, with S. japonicum 26-kDa GST and paramyosin.[16,17] The possibility remains that, if levels of egg excretion can be reduced by vaccination of animal reservoir hosts, this approach might be sufficient to reduce schistosomiasis japonica transmission. Alternatively, it has been proposed that egg deposition and granuloma formation in the human host can be manipulated by immunotherapy because granuloma formation around the schistosome egg depends heavily on host cytokines, including tumor necrosis factor and Th2-associated cytokines.

An independent trial of candidate antigens for an S. mansoni vaccine was completed in the late 1990s under the auspices of the WHO's Special Programme for Research and Training in Tropical Diseases (WHO/TDR). Six vaccine candidate S. mansoni antigens were selected for independent testing:

1. The 28-kDa GST noted above.[22]
2. A 97-kDa paramyosin.[23] Paramyosin was first identified in sera from mice immunized with S. mansoni adult worm antigen in association with Mycobacterium bovis BCG. Immunization promoted 39% protection in mice, and the protein was recognized by sera from putative resistant subjects from areas where S. mansoni is endemic.
3. An irradiated larvae-associated vaccine antigen, the 62-kDa IrV-5[24], that is a derivative of a 200-kDa molecule with extensive homology with human myosin. The gene encoding IrV-5 was cloned from a complementary DNA library using an antibody (IrV-3) from immunized mice that was not present in sera from infected animals. The IrV-5 recombinant protein induced 75% protection in mice and 25% protection in baboons.
4. A 28-kDa triose phosphate isomerase (TPI).[25] TPI is an enzyme from the glycolytic pathway, identified by a monoclonal antibody that is capable of passively immunizing naïve mice against infection. The enzyme itself induces 30% to 60% protection in mice.
5. A 23-kDa integral membrane antigen (Sm-23)[26] that is part of a superfamily of proteins that includes CD9 and TAPA-1, first described in hematopoietic cells. Sm-23 gives 40% to 50% protection in mice.
6. A 14-kDa fatty acid–binding protein that also was thought to have protective immune cross-reactivity with Fasciola hepatica.[27] A recombinant form of Sm-14 protected mice by up to 67% against challenge with S. mansoni cercariae in the absence of adjuvant.

The same antigen provided complete protection against challenge with *F. hepatica* metacercariae in the same animal model.

None of the above candidate proteins reached the obligatory requirement of generating a 40% or better reduction in challenge-derived worm burdens relative to nonimmunized controls.[28] However, it was recommended that work should continue on these antigens, including progression to clinical or veterinary trials.

Previously, the development of a schistosomiasis vaccine depended on the acquisition of immunity noted in adult humans living in endemic areas. Indeed, a principal reason for selecting the molecules tested by WHO/TDR was their immunogenicity, or the capacity to induce the synthesis of specific antibody or to generate any other immune response. It has been suggested that, rather than examining parasite antigens recognized by infected animals and patients as potential vaccine immunogens, we should focus on the molecules against which little or no immune response is directed.[28] The logic of this suggestion is based on the fact that schistosomes and many other parasites are relatively long lived, and any of their antigens that induce strong immune responses are thus unlikely to be important in the context of vaccination because the organisms' survival is apparently unaffected by such immunity. Progress in development of vaccines for use against other organisms such as *Haemonchus contortus*[9] and *Boophilus microplus*[29] has been made by targeting "hidden" antigens that do not stimulate strong immune responses during the normal course of parasitization. A major goal of a human schistosomiasis vaccine will be to accelerate this process through either immunization with a cocktail of recombinant antigens, DNA immunizations, or host cytokine manipulation through bioimmunotherapy.

Antiprotozoan Vaccines

Significant progress has been made over the past 5 years in the development of first- and second-generation vaccines for malaria, leishmaniasis, and amebiasis. In contrast, vaccine development efforts for Chagas' disease (American trypanosomiasis) has been curtailed because of new successful efforts to control infection through vector control, while the phenomenon of antigenic variation has largely thwarted vaccine development for African sleeping sickness (African trypanosomiasis). Antimalaria vaccines are treated separately in Chapter 47.

Leishmaniasis

Leishmania species are flagellated kinetoplastid protozoan parasites transmitted by the bite of a female sandfly. There are cutaneous (CL), mucocutaneous (MCL), and visceralizing (VL) forms of human leishmaniasis. CL and MCL in the Western Hemisphere (predominantly Central and South America) are caused by members of the *L. mexicana* and *L. braziliensis* complex, whereas CL in the Eastern Hemisphere (predominantly India, central Asia, and parts of Africa and the Middle East) is caused by members of the *L. tropica* and *L. major* complex. VL, also known as *kala-azar*, is caused by *L. donovani* in India, Bangladesh, Nepal, and China; *L. infantum* in central Asia, north Africa, and southern Europe; and *L. chagasi* in Latin America. Members of the *L. donovani* complex are important emerging opportunistic pathogens in patients with acquired immunodeficiency disease.

Leishmanization, the ancient Middle Eastern and central Asian practice of injecting live *Leishmania* parasites as a means to actively immunize against disease, predates vaccination and may be as old as variolation. It relies on inoculating a person with live parasites using a thorn or other sharp instrument in order to artificially create a cutaneous lesion. The procedure causes mild disease (typically 1 to 2 cm in size) at an unexposed site, frequently the arm or buttocks, that heals over a period of 3 to 4 months. Successful leishmanization prevents the possibility that a cosmetically disfiguring lesion ("Delhi boil" or "oriental sore") might appear on the face. It is still practiced widely in Uzbekistan and possibly elsewhere in central Asia. In the 1980s, leishmanization was reintroduced as an emergency public health measure during the Iran-Iraq war when approximately 2 million people were inoculated.[30] The Iranian leishmanization program was subsequently halted when it was learned that up to 3% of the induced lesions lasted for more than a year; in some instances, the lesions never healed even with subsequent antiparasitic antimonial chemotherapy.[30]

In an effort to establish a safer anti-*Leishmania* immunization procedure, Iran launched a national vaccine development program during the early 1990s. A first-generation vaccine comprising killed *Leishmania* parasites was prepared under Good Manufacturing Practices by the Razi Vaccine and Serum Research Institute (Hessarak, Iran). The cell bank for the vaccine was derived from the identical strain of *L. major* used previously for the wartime leishmanization program. The *L. major* parasites were killed by autoclaving and then subsequently formulated with BCG. In a randomized, double-blind trial, the safety and efficacy of a single injection of the vaccine was compared with a BCG control among 3637 schoolchildren.[30] Children with a prior history of CL or those with a positive skin test reaction against leishmanial antigen were excluded from the study. The Iranian trial demonstrated the vaccine's safety, although its efficacy was not apparent until 6 months following the injection. It has been suggested that there was some protective effect from BCG in the immediate postvaccination period. Also of interest was the observation that protection was demonstrated better among boys who, because of Iranian dress and customs, presumably are exposed to a greater number of sandfly bites than girls.[30] Based on these results, additional trials are underway to evaluate multiple injections of the killed vaccine, as well as new formulations with alum and IL-12. A trial to evaluate the killed vaccine against *L. donovani* is also underway in Sudan. In South America, killed *L. amazonensis* and *L. mexicana* vaccines are being produced by BIOBRAS (Brazil) and Instituto de Biomedicina (Venezuela), respectively.

The partial success of autoclaved-killed *Leishmania* vaccines has stimulated efforts by several laboratories to reproduce vaccine protection using second-generation recombinant subunit antigens. To date, a number of lead candidates have shown promise in mice, particularly when formulated with IL-12 or other co-stimulators of Th1 immunity. In some cases, vaccination with plasmid DNAs encoding the antigens, either alone or in combination, elicits more potent and durable immunity. Budaro and colleagues[31] reported that a cocktail of recombinant *Leishmania* antigens coadministered with granulocyte-macrophage colony-stimulating factor worked as a therapeutic vaccine in 10 Brazilian patients with disfiguring ML. These individuals were refractory to chemotherapy with antimonial drugs. The likelihood is high that a range of new preventative and therapeutic vaccines for CL, ML, and VL will come on line within the next 3 years. In addition, new evidence indicates that protein antigens derived from the salivary glands of the sandfly vector also offer promise as vaccines.[32]

Amebiasis

Amebiasis secondary to intestinal and hepatic infection with *Entamoeba histolytica* is prevalent throughout the developing nations of the tropics. Human infection occurs through the ingestion of parasite cysts and subsequent invasion by trophozoites. Amebic colitis results from ulcerating mucosal lesions that result from chemical invasion caused by the release of parasite-derived proteases and hyaluronidases. Metastatic spread to the liver occurs when the trophozoites gain access to the afferent circulation that drains the colon into the portal vein.

New evidence from a cohort of Bangladeshi children suggests that mucosal immunoglobulin A antibody directed against the major 170-kDa amebic adherence lectin correlates with resistance to reinfection by *E. histolytica*.[33] The observation provides a human correlate to the finding that a peptide epitope of the amebic lectin elicits protection in laboratory animals and offers promise as a first-generation vaccine.[34-36]

REFERENCES

1. Hall BF. Vaccines for parasitic diseases of humans. *In* Ostiker R, Savage L (eds). Vaccines: New Advances in Technologies and Applications. Southborough, MA, IBC Biomedical Library, 1996, pp 6.4.1–6.4.16.
2. Hotez PJ. Vaccines as instruments of foreign policy: the new vaccines for tropical infectious diseases may have unanticipated uses beyond fighting diseases. EMBO Rep 2:862–868, 2001.
3. Gandhi NS, Jizhang C, Khoshnood K, et al. Epidemiology of *Necator americanus* hookworm infections in Xiulongkan Village, Hainan Province, China: high prevalence and intensity among middle-aged and elderly residents. J Parasitol 87:739–743, 2001.
4. Hotez PJ. China's hookworms. China Q 172:1029–1041,2002.
5. Albonico M, Smith PG, Ercole E, et al. Rate of reinfection with intestinal nematodes after treatment of children with mebendazole or albendazole in a highly endemic area. Trans R Soc Trop Med Hyg 89:538–541, 1995.
6. Bergquist NR, Hall BF, James SL. Schistosomiasis vaccine development. Immunologist 2(4):131–134, 1994.
7. McCarthy JS, Nutman TB. Perspective: prospects for development of vaccines against human helminth infections. J Infect Dis 174:1384–1390, 1996.
8. Hotez PJ, Zheng F, Long-qi X, et al. Emerging and reemerging helminthiases and the public health of China. Emerg Infect Dis 3:303–310, 1997.
9. Miller TA. Industrial development and field use of the canine hookworm vaccine. Adv Parasitol 16:333–342, 1978.
10. Hotez PJ, Hawdon JM, Cappello M, et al. Molecular approaches to vaccinating against hookworm disease. Pediatr Res 40:515–521, 1996.
11. Hotez PJ, Ghosh K, Hawdon JM, et al. Experimental approaches to the development of a recombinant hookworm vaccine. Immunol Rev 171:163–171, 1999.
12. Ghosh K, Hotez PJ. Antibody-dependent reductions in mouse hookworm burden after vaccination with *Ancylostoma caninum* secreted protein 1. J Infect Dis 180:1674–1681, 1999.
13. Liu S, Gosh K, Zhan B, et al. Hookworm burden reductions in BALB/c mice vaccinated with *Ancyclostoma* secreted protein 1 (ASP-1) from *Ancylostoma duodenale*, *A. caninum*, and *Necator americanus*. Vaccine 18:1096–1102, 2000.
14. Jones BF, Hotez PJ. Molecular cloning and characterization of Ac-mep-1, a developmentally regulated gut luminal metalloendopeptidase from adult *Ancylostoma caninum* hookworms. Mol Biochem Parasitol 119:107–116, 2002.
15. McManus DP. The search for a vaccine against schistosomiasis—a difficult path but an achievable goal. Immunol Rev 171:149–161, 1999.
16. McManus DP. A vaccine against Asian schistosomiasis: the story unfolds. Int J Parasitol 30:265–271, 2000.
17. McManus D. The *Schistosoma japonicum* angle on vaccine research. Parasitol Today 16:357–358, 2000.
18. Wilson RA, Coulson PS. Strategies for a schistosome vaccine: can we manipulate the immune response effectively? Microbes Infect 1:535–543, 1999.
19. Liu SX, Song GC, Xu YX, et al. Anti-fecundity immunity induced in pigs vaccinated with recombinant *Schistosoma japonicum* 26kDa glutathione-S-transferase. Parasite Immunol 17:335–340, 1995.
20. Liu SX, Song GC, Xu YX. Progress in the development of a vaccine against schistosomiasis in China. Int J Infect Dis 2:176–180, 1998.
21. Loukas A, Jones MK, King LT, et al. Receptor for Fc on the surfaces of schistosomes. Infect Immun 69:3646–3651, 2001.
22. Taylor JB, Vidal A, Torpier G, et al. The glutathione transferase activity and tissue distribution of a cloned Mr28K protective antigen of *Schistosoma mansoni*. EMBO J 7:465–472, 1988.
23. Pearce EJ, James SL, Hieny S, et al. Induction of protective immunity against *Schistosoma mansoni* by vaccination with schistosome paramyosin (Sm97), a nonsurface parasite antigen. Proc Natl Acad Sci U S A 85:5678–5682, 1988.
24. Soisson LM, Masterson CP, Tom TD, et al. Induction of protective immunity in mice using a 62-kDa recombinant fragment of a *Schistosoma mansoni* surface antigen. J Immunol 149:3612–3620, 1992.
25. Shoemaker C, Gross A, Gebremichael A, Harn D. cDNA cloning and functional expression of the *Schistosoma mansoni* protective antigen triose-phosphate isomerase. Proc Natl Acad Sci U S A 89:1842–1846, 1992.
26. Reynolds SR, Shoemaker CB, Harn DA. T and B cell epitope mapping of SM23, an integral membrane protein of *Schistosoma mansoni*. J Immunol 149:3995–4001, 1992.
27. Tendler M, Brito CA, Vilar MM, et al. A *Schistosoma mansoni* fatty acid-binding protein, Sm14, is the potential basis of a dual-purpose anti-helminth vaccine. Proc Natl Acad Sci U S A 93:269–273, 1996.
28. Doenhoff M. A vaccine for schistosomiasis: alternative approaches. Parasitol Today 14:105–109, 1998.
29. Willadsen P, Bird P, Cobon GS, Hungerford J. Commercialisation of a recombinant vaccine against *Boophilus microplus*. Parasitology 110(suppl):S43–S50, 1995.
30. Modabber F. First generation leishmaniasis vaccines in clinical development: moving, but what next? Curr Opin Anti-Infect Invest Drugs 2:35–39, 2000.
31. Budaro R, Lobo I, Campos-Neto A, et al. Successful treatment of mucosal leishmaniasis with recombinant based subunit vaccine [abstr 36]. *In* Abstracts of the Second World Congress on Leishmaniasis, Hersonisso, Certe, Greece, May 20–24, 2001.
32. Reed SG. Leishmaniasis vaccination: targeting the source of infection. J Exp Med 194:F7–F9, 2001.
33. Haque R, Ali IM, Sack RB, et al. Amebiasis and mucosal IgA antibody against *Entamoeba* adherence lectin in Bangladeshi children. J Infect Dis 183:1787–1793, 2001.
34. Petri WA Jr, Ravdin JI. Protection of gerbils from amebic liver abscess by immunization with the galactose-specific adherence lectin of *Entamoeba histolytica*. Infect Immun 59:97–101, 1991.
35. Lotter H, Zhang T, Seydel KB, et al. Identification of an epitope on the *Entamoeba histolytica* 170-kD lectin conferring antibody-mediated protection against invasive amebiasis. J Exp Med 185:1793–1801, 1997.
36. Stanley SL Jr. Protective immunity to amebiasis: new insights and new challenges. J Infect Dis 184:504–506, 2001.

Chapter 49

Poxviruses as Immunization Vehicles

DEVENDER SINGH SANDHU • JIM TARTAGLIA

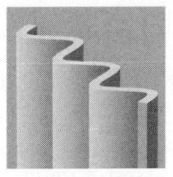

Since the initial reports illustrating the utility of vaccinia virus (VV) as a eukaryotic expression vector,[1,2] poxviruses have provided the scientific community with valuable reagents to achieve high-level expression of polypeptides, to address questions of structure-function relationship of polypeptides, to investigate the immunobiology of specific pathogens, and to develop recombinant vaccine candidates. This last application has received special attention for its potential to address vaccine needs in human and veterinary medicine.[3–20] Several advantages in using recombinant poxviruses as eukaryotic vectors for immunization purposes have provided the impetus for such investigation and are highlighted in Table 49–1.

Early examples of poxvirus-based vaccine candidates were based on conventional VV strains that were used during the Smallpox Eradication Program. Safety issues observed when using such vaccinia vaccine strains to vaccinate against smallpox[21–24] and the potential to reintroduce vaccinia as an immunizing agent led to the development of highly attenuated strains of VV and avipoxvirus as immunization vehicles (Table 49–2). This chapter focuses on the utility of such novel, highly attenuated poxvirus strains and refinements to enhance their effectiveness as immunization vehicles.

Highly Attenuated Vaccinia Virus Vector Strains—MVA and NYVAC

Near the end of the Smallpox Eradication Program, a number of highly attenuated VV strains were developed by the classical technique of passaging virus in laboratory animals and/or on tissue culture substrates.[1,25–27] One such virus strain, modified Vaccinia Ankara (MVA), was developed by passaging the Ankara strain about 500 times on primary chicken embryo fibroblasts (CEFs). This resulted in the inability of the virus to replicate on nonavian cells because of multiple genomic deletions and an abortive-late phenotype in most mammalian cells.[8,28–30] MVA can, however,

replicate efficiently on primary CEFs,[31,32] rabbit kidney cells,[33] the quail cell line, QT6 cells, and the baby hamster kidney cell line BHK21.[4] At least two genes affecting the host range of MVA have been identified.[34] Despite its highly attenuated phenotype, MVA has been shown to retain the ability to achieve efficient expression of recombinant gene products. Furthermore, MVA was assessed as a smallpox vaccine in over 120,000 recipients without significant adverse reactions (see section on Smallpox Vaccination, below).[35]

Another attenuated VV strain, NYVAC (for New York vaccinia strain), was developed using a genetic engineering approach. In this development, 18 open reading frames encoding gene products associated with virulence and host ranges were deleted from the Copenhagen strain.[36–39] NYVAC was found to be highly attenuated in a series of studies in animal models,[36] as well as displaying a favorable safety and immunogenicity profile in both animals and humans.[7,9,38] Replication of NYVAC is blocked at an early stage in numerous human cell lines, consistent with the deletion of host range genes, whereas productive infection is observed in African green monkey kidney (Vero) cells and primary CEFs.

Avipox Vectors—ALVAC/ FPV/CPV

Avipoxviruses initially were developed as potential vaccine vectors for poultry applications, but subsequently were found to have utility as immunization vehicles for mammalian species.[9,40] Fowlpox virus (FPV) and canarypox virus (CPV), as members of the *Avipoxvirus* genus, are known to be host restricted for replication to avian species.[41] FPV and CPV undergo abortive replication in mammalian cells, suggesting their use as host range–restricted mammalian expression vectors.[42,43] The stage at which *Avipoxvirus* replication is blocked varies for different nonavian cell lines, and both early and some late gene expression has been observed.[44] Analysis of the complete FPV and CPV genomic sequence reveals that that these genomes contain rearrangements in the conserved co-linear core of genes

TABLE 49–1 ■ Advantages Associated with Poxvirus-Based Vectors

- Capacity for multiple foreign gene inserts
- Simple method of in vitro recombination
- Cytoplasmic replication
- Authentic gene expression
- Robust production process
- Good stability profile
- Pancytotropic

present in VV.[45] Despite an abortive infection, the transcription and translation of appropriately engineered foreign genes results in the presentation of de novo synthesized proteins and their presentation to the immune system.[9,22,36] Replication restriction also provides for an exquisite safety barrier against vaccine-induced and vaccine-associated complications.

ALVAC represents a plaque-purified virus isolated after four rounds of plaque purification from the existing CPV vaccine strain, Kanapox.[46] ALVAC was found to efficiently express inserted transgenes in eukaryotic cells[47] and was found to display an excellent safety profile and to be immunogenic in a number of preclinical and clinical trials.[7–9,48–50] More recently, a second-generation ALVAC vector [ALVAC(2)] was developed to enhance virus-specified gene expression in cells of human origin.[15,48] However, it has not yet been established whether enhanced expression in vitro translates into a more robust immune response in humans.

Poxvirus Vector Development and Recombinant Virus Production

The generation of recombinant poxviruses has been well documented.[25,51–53] Poxviruses replicate in the cytoplasm, thereby requiring the use of poxvirus-specific transcription systems and promoters for expression of foreign genes. Therefore, initial steps in the generation of recombinants involve the cloning of a foreign gene of interest into a poxvirus promoter-regulated expression cassette, flanked by poxvirus sequences that direct recombination to the desired locus (Fig. 49–1). The early/late (E/L) H6 promoter has been used extensively for driving poxvirus-borne expression of foreign gene products,[20] and several other VV donor vectors are available with P7.5, P11, and synthetic E/L promoters.[54] Recombinant VV genomes with unique sites to

TABLE 49–2 ■ Poxvirus Strains Used as Immunization Vehicles

Vaccinia Virus
Existing vaccinia strains
NYVAC (18 ORFs deleted)
MVA (adapted to CEF)
Avipoxvirus
Fowlpox—FPV/TROVAC
Canarypox—CPV/ALVAC (adapted to CEF)
Canarypox—ALVAC (2) (+ E3L and K3L genes)

CEF, chick embryo fibroblasts; ORFs, open reading frames.

facilitate cloning and expression also have been developed.[55] In another approach, in vitro ligation of a foreign gene into the VV genome provides an alternative to homologous recombination,[8] allowing very large DNA fragments or even libraries of DNA fragments to be inserted directly into the VV genome.

Following the incorporation of the heterologous gene into the virus genome by in vitro recombination within permissive cell substrates infected with virus and transfected with a donor vector (Fig. 49–2), the chimeric genomes are packaged as infectious progeny virus. Several selection methods for recombinant poxviruses have been developed by taking advantage of the virus host range genes C7L and K1L.[56–58] In addition, a number of alternative methods have been defined for propagation and selection of recombinant viruses[59] and their large-scale production and purification.[10] Several reporter genes, such as *TK*, *Lac Z*, and/or *Ecogpt*, have been used in such selection systems.[60–67]

Poxvirus-Based Veterinary Vaccines

The applicability and commercial viability of poxvirus-based vaccines has been clearly evident in the veterinary area. Numerous examples (Table 49–3) exist demonstrating protective immunization of animals against diseases of veterinary importance,[7–9] and several poxvirus-based products have been registered for veterinary use (Table 49–4). Properties of these vaccines that enabled their development and licensure are (1) their safety in target species; (2) their ability to be incorporated into currently used combination vaccine formulations (vaccine logistics); (3) their ability to be integrated into a marketing strategy; and (4) their ability to meet protection standards regardless of immunologic readouts. In fact, a number of other ALVAC-based vaccine candidates are in the later stages of product development in the veterinary vaccine field.

Poxvirus-Based Human Vaccines

Poxviruses have been developed as human vaccine candidates for several diseases including acquired immunodeficiency disease (AIDS) and cancer. None are licensed at the present stage but many have entered clinical trials (Table 49–5). Recombinant poxviruses have been shown to be immunogenic, and there are several examples where protective efficacy has been established in animal models of infectious diseases.[5,7–9] The salient properties of poxvirus-based approaches demonstrated by extensive preclinical and clinical assessment are summarized below. These poxvirus-based approaches are described in more detail in the discussion of further progress within the fields of AIDS and cancer.

Poxviruses Are Safe and Effective Immunization Vehicles

There are numerous examples (see Table 49–5) of clinical trials describing the use of poxviruses as safe immunization

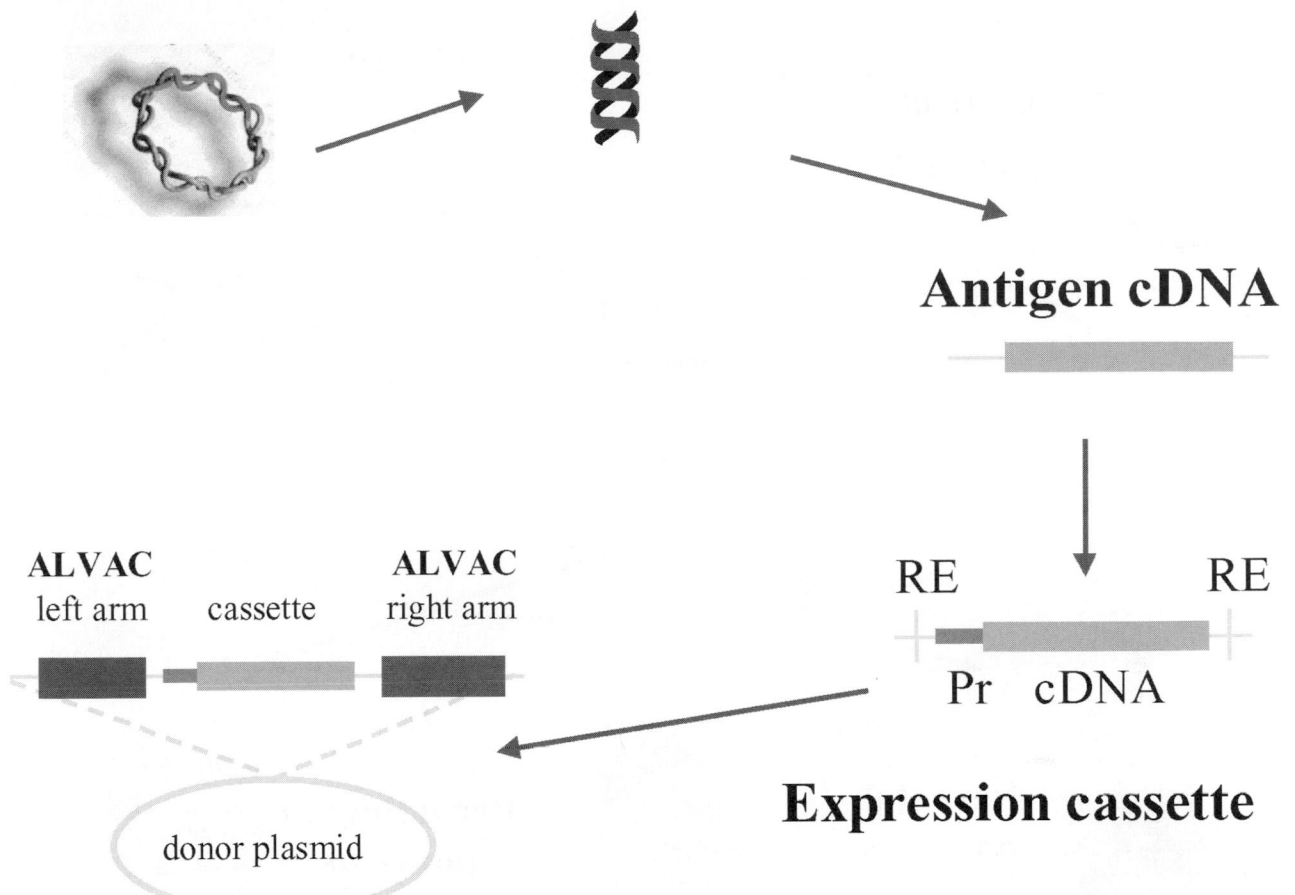

Antigen cDNA

ALVAC
left arm   cassette   ALVAC
right arm

RE   RE

Pr   cDNA

Expression cassette

donor plasmid

FIGURE 49–1 ■ Construction of the recombinant donor plasmid. A complementary DNA (cDNA) encoding the antigen of interest is cloned into an expression cassette in a donor plasmid. The expression cassette contains a promoter (Pr) and restriction endonuclease (RE) sites for insertion of foreign DNA. The cassette is flanked on either side by ALVAC DNA sequences (left arm and right arm) that direct homologous recombination with the insertion into the poxvirus genome, resulting in insertion of the gene of interest into the genome under control of the promoter.

vehicles.[3–9,12–20,38,274] Both MVA and NYVAC have been shown to be effective as safe immunization vehicles.[7,36,80,88] It should be noted that the in vitro properties of MVA appear quite similar to those of NYVAC. MVA- and NYVAC-based vectors were investigated in immune-suppressed macaques and were not found to induce any clinical, hematologic, or pathologic abnormalities.[274] No serious toxicities were observed in the 49 patients vaccinated with one or two vaccinations in Phase I studies with VV expressing HPV 16 and 18 E6/E7 genes.[103] Both NYVAC- and ALVAC-based vaccines have demonstrated an excellent safety profile in Phase I trials. ALVAC-based recombinants have been the most studied in human clinical trials, and local and systemic reactions have been recorded as minor and transient in nature.[7,179] Among pox vectors, ALVAC in particular has already proven to be a safe delivery vehicle and has been investigated in thousands of patients for vaccination against several diseases (Table 49–6).

Immunogenicity and Efficiency of Immunization Vehicles Cannot Be Generalized Across Species or Even Between Immunogens

Immunogenicity and efficiency may or may not differ between the same recombinant subunit encoded by different poxvirus vectors or by the same poxvirus vector tested in different species. Although an FPV-rabies recombinant expressing the rabies glycoprotein (RG) protected mice, cats, and dogs from lethal rabies challenge,[7,40] a similar CPV-based RG recombinant was found to be 100 times more efficacious than the FPV-based recombinant in protecting mice.[77] An ALVAC-RG recombinant elicited significant neutralizing antibody (NAb), whereas an ALVAC recombinant encoding human immunodeficiency virus (HIV) envelope proteins elicited no significant antibody responses.[49,218] ALVAC encoding measles virus (MV) proteins hemagglutinin and F antigens (ALVAC-MV), when inoculated in dogs, elicited NAbs and also protected the dogs from lethal canine distemper virus (CDV), which is closely related to MV.[43] The replication-incompetent CPV-MV recombinants elicited the same level of NAbs and protection to CDV challenge as were seen with replicating VV-MV recombinants.[43,77] Similarly, recombinant MVA (MVA–MV-H) encoding MV hemagglutinin protected against infection in mice and rats,[260] and NYVAC (K1L)-HA, also encoding MV hemagglutinin, elicited T-helper cell type 1 (Th1) antibody and cytotoxic T lymphocyte (CTL) responses against measles in mice.[262] Macaques vaccinated with MVA-FH encoding MV F antigens and hemagglutinin were effectively protected from measles

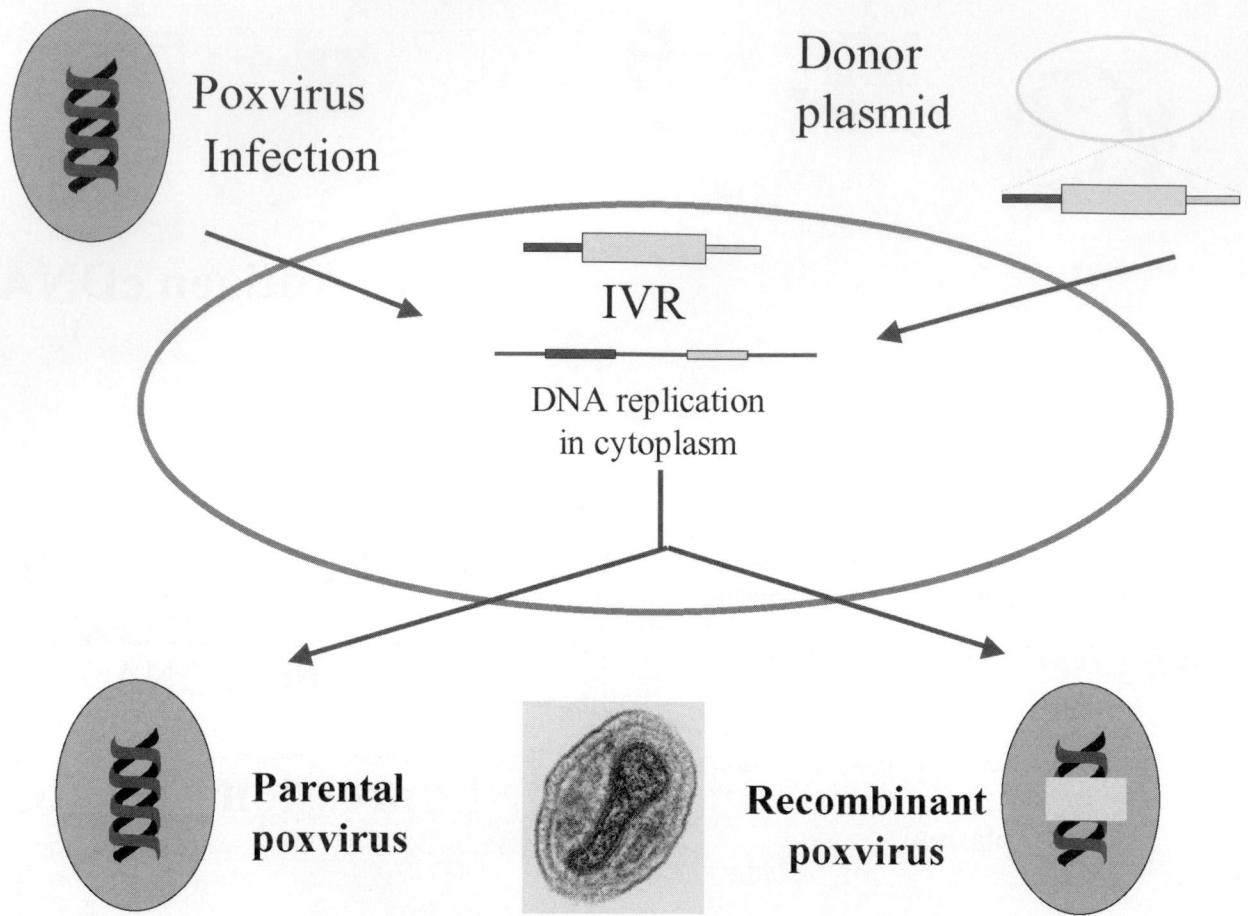

Poxvirus Infection

Donor plasmid

IVR

DNA replication in cytoplasm

Parental poxvirus

Recombinant poxvirus

FIGURE 49–2 ▪ Generation of ALVAC recombinants. Cells are infected with poxvirus and then transfected with the donor plasmid. In vitro recombination (IVR) results in the formation of a stable recombinant ALVAC virus. Different selection techniques are used to isolate recombinant poxviruses from the background population of parental poxviruses.

challenge, suggesting that MVA-FH could be tested as an alternative to the current measles vaccine for infants.[261] Furthermore, an ALVAC-measles trial with ALVAC-MV (vCP82) showed an immune response and clinical tolerance to a high-dose immunization (10^6 PFU) that was comparable to the reference Schwarz vaccine (P Saliou, J Tartaglia, D Singh-Sandhu, et al., unpublished observations, 2002). An ALVAC recombinant encoding a phosphoprotein-65 (pp65) of cytomegalovirus (CMV) was able to elicit a CMV-specific CD8+ CTL response in humans.[158] In fact, pp65-specific CTLs were elicited after two administrations of ALVAC-CMV pp65 in all immunized subjects and persisted for at least 26 months. Furthermore, the pp65 elicited a pp65-specific CD8+ response found at levels approaching those observed in CMV-seropositive individuals. These results contrast greatly with those observed with ALVAC-HIV, where cumulative HIV-specific CD8+ CTL responses have been observed in 40% to 60% of human volunteers.[218]

Highly Attenuated Poxvirus Vector Strains Are as Effective as Immunization Vehicles as Replication-Competent Vaccinia Vaccine Strains

Several examples have demonstrated the effectiveness of highly attenuated poxvirus strains when compared to replication-competent vaccinia strains.[7,8,15] MVA and ALVAC have proven to be as efficacious at inducing therapeutic or

protective immune responses as replication-competent VV strains in several infectious diseases[88,175,230–232,275] and tumor immunotherapy models.[276,277] Similar efficacy profiles also were observed with NYVAC and ALVAC viruses encoding RG or Japanese encephalitis virus (JEV) antigens.[7,9,241,266]

Vector-Specific Immunity Can Be an Issue, Especially for Vaccinia-Based Candidates

Once again generalizations cannot necessarily be made across species, immunogens, and experimental readouts.[5] Pre-existing immunity to the VV vectors exists in a large proportion of the human population. Vaccinia-based HIV-1 envelope recombinants in Phase I trials have elicited low HIV-specific humoral immunity and cell-mediated immunity (CMI),[195] and immune responses were more pronounced in vaccinia-naïve than vaccinia-experienced individuals. Some reports suggested that pre-existing immunity against VV could be overcome by using a mucosal delivery route for the recombinant virus,[278] but, regardless of this, the safety concerns in HIV trials and the fact that immunosuppression has been a contraindication for vaccination with vaccinia make it highly unlikely that vaccinia recombinants based on existing strains such as Wyeth or New York City Board of Health (NYCBH) would be used in HIV-endemic and other high-risk populations. Increasingly, vaccine development efforts have focused on highly attenuated poxvirus strains such as MVA, NYVAC, and ALVAC

TABLE 49–3 ■ Poxvirus-Based Protective Recombinant Veterinary Vaccines

Disease/Virus	Poxvirus	Reference
Avian influenza virus (AIV)	VV, FPV	68, 69
Bovine leukemia virus (BLV)	VV	70, 71
Bovine papillomavirus (BPV)	VV	72
Caprine arthritis encephalitis virus	VV	73, 74
Canine distemper virus (CDV)	NYVAC and ALVAC	75, 76
	VV	75, 77
Equine herpesvirus type 1 (EHV-1)	ALVAC	78, 79
Feline leukemia virus (FeLV)	ALVAC	80
Feline immunodeficiency virus (FIV)	ALVAC	81
Foot-and-mouth disease virus (FMDV)	VV	82
Infectious bursal disease virus	VV and FPV	83–85
Influenza virus	VV, MVA, FPV	86–88
Infectious bronchitis virus (IBV)	FPV	89
Marek's disease virus	FPV	90
Newcastle disease virus	VV and FPV	91
Neospora caninum (NC)	VV	92, 93
Rabies	VV and ALVAC	94–97
Rinderpest virus	VV	98–100
Venezuelan equine encephalitis virus	VV	101
Vesicular stomatitis virus	VV	102

ALVAC seems to be a promising vector because of its safety and its exclusive efficiency as an immunization vehicle in vaccinia-experienced individuals.[15] It should be noted that prior exposure to vaccinia or ALVAC, itself, has not led to a dampening effect on ALVAC-based candidates in veterinary species and humans.[132, 224, unpublished results] Human safety trials conducted with ALVAC RG[266,267] encoding RG found that reactogenicity was minimal and that immunization elicited functional antibodies to rabies glycoprotein. In the NYVAC trial, average anti-vaccinia antibody titers were much higher in vaccinia-immunized vaccinees in comparison to the vaccinia-naïve vaccinees. In trials of candidate JEV vaccines, safety and immunogenicity studies with NYVAC-JEV and ALVAC-JEV encoding JEV antigens were conducted in vaccinia-nonimmune and vaccinia-immune humans.[241,242] Both vaccines were safe and immunogenic and elicited antibody responses to JEV antigens, but NAb responses were observed only in VV-naïve recipients after immunization with NYVAC-JEV.

Poxvirus-Based Vaccine Candidates Can Adequately Elicit CD8+ Responses to Foreign Gene Products

Priming the immune system with a live recombinant poxvirus vector aims to elicit effector functions, such as

TABLE 49–4 ■ Poxvirus-Based Licensed Veterinary Vaccines (1990 to 2002)

Vaccina Virus
Raboral (rabies; Merial)
Fowlpox Virus
FPV/NDV (Newcastle; Merial)
FPV/NDV (Newcastle; Syntrovet)
FPV/AIV H5 + H7 (avian influenza; Merial)
ALVAC
Recombitek (CDV; Merial)
Purevax (rabies G; Merial)
Eurifel FELV (Merial)

serum NAbs or CTL targeted to the encoded antigen. Phase I clinical trials of several ALVAC-HIV recombinants, differing in their level of expression of various HIV components, clearly showed their priming potential for subsequent boosting with a recombinant envelope preparation, in addition to their ability to elicit CD8+ CTL responses.[218,224] The expression of multiple HIV components in poxvirus-based immunizations increased the breadth of the CD8+ CTL response.[228,229] In tumor model studies, immunization with VV expressing either human papillomavirus antigen E6 or antigen E7 protected mice from tumor challenge, and, moreover, protection was mediated by CD8+ lymphocytes.[170,171] Recombinant poxvirus vectors expressing hepatitis B virus surface antigen[166] and respiratory syncytial virus G protein[270] have been shown to elicit T-cell responses and to be protective in preclinical studies. Similarly, as discussed earlier, ALVAC CMVpp65 is the first recombinant vaccine to elicit CMV-specific responses with phenotype CD8 (+).

Prime-Boost Approaches Could Overcome Vector-Specific Immunity and Enhance the Immunogenicity of Foreign Genes Expressed by Modified Vectors

Several prime-boost strategies have been suggested to overcome limitations resulting from repeated use of poxvirus-based vaccine candidates, maximize immunologic priming, and enhance the boosting of humoral and CMI responses.[48,169,247,279,280] Such regimens have been used in combination with alternative viral vectors, naked DNA, and peptide-protein preparations.[120,252,253,281] It has been shown that immunization with MVA- or DNA-based malaria vaccine candidates alone does not induce complete protection in rodent models.[248–250,252] However, DNA/MVA prime-boost regimens, including regimens in which reduced doses of DNA were delivered by gene gun, were shown to induce CD8+ T cells and also confer significant protection against both malaria[250,252] and influenza.[234] NYVAC–simian immunodeficiency virus (SIV) and

TABLE 49-5 ■ Poxvirus Based Human Vaccine Candidates

Vaccine Target	Poxvirus Vector Used for Expression of Associated Genes or Subunits	Trial Stage	References
Cancer (several tumor-associated antigens)	VV, NYVAC, ALVAC, FPV	Preclinical, Phase I/II	14, 17, 39, 103–157
Cytomegalovirus	ALVAC (gB, pp65)	Phase I	158
Dengue fever	VV	Preclinical, Phase I	159, 160
Ebola virus	VV, MVA	Preclinical, Phase I	161
Epstein-Barr virus (EBV)	VV	Phase I	162, 163
Hantaan virus	VV	Phase II	164
Hepatitis delta virus (HDV)	VV	Preclinical	165
Hepatitis B virus (HBV)	VV	Preclinical	166, 167
Hepatitis C virus (HCV)	ALVAC	Preclinical	168
Herpes simplex virus types 1 and 2	VV	Preclinical	169
Human papillomavirus	VV	Preclinical	170–172
Human parainfluenza virus	VV, MVA	Preclinical	173–175
Human immunodeficiency virus types 1 and 2 (HIV-1/-2)	VV, attenuated VV, MVA, FPV, ALVAC	Preclinical, Phase I/II	48, 176–233
Influenza virus	VV	Preclinical	88, 234–240
Japanese encephalitis virus	VV, NYVAC, ALVAC, MVA	Preclinical, Phase I	46, 241–243
Lassa fever virus	VV	Preclinical	244
Leishmania infantum	VV	Preclinical	245
Malaria (Plasmodium falciparum/berghei/Knowlesi)	VV, ALVAC, FPV, MVA, NYVAC	Preclinical, Phase I	234, 246–258
Measles virus	VV, MVA, ALVAC, NYVAC	Phase I	259–262*
Mycobacterium tuberculosis	VV, MVA	Preclinical	263–265
Rabies	VV, ALVAC, FPV, NYVAC	Phase II/III	49, 97, 266, 267
Respiratory syncytial virus	VV	Preclinical	268–271
Varicella-zoster virus	VV	Basic R & D	272, 273

*Saliou P, Tartaglia J, Singh-Sandhu D, et al., unpublished observations, 2002.

MVA-SIV recombinants used alone or as part of prime-boost regimens have induced significant levels of protection against the highly virulent SIV$_{MAC251}$ isolate.[275,282] Other prime-boost examples that demonstrate high levels of T-cell responses and effective protection are shown in Table 49-7. These studies highlight the rapid advances in the development of effective prime-boost regimens for using poxvirus vectors to induce CMI and humoral immunity against infectious diseases and cancers.[7,17,218]

Use of Immunomodulators Could Enhance the Immunogenicity of Foreign Genes Expressed by Poxvirus-Based Vectors

Immunomodulators such as interleukin-12 (IL-12) have been shown to expand CD8$^+$ T-cell populations and to con-

TABLE 49-6 ■ ALVAC-Based Vaccines Tested in Humans

ALVAC Vector	No. of Volunteers
Rabies glycoprotein G	285
Measles glycoprotein F and HA	65
Cytomegalovirus gB	30
Cytomegalovirus pp65	40
Japanese encephalitis virus PrM, M, E, and NS1	12
HIV (various subunits)	>1700
Cancer antigens/co-stimulatory molecules	>180

trol experimental infections.[193] Specific anti–HIV-1 env, cellular responses were enhanced 20 times by using IL-12 during DNA prime–recombinant VV (rVV) boost regimens in comparison to a single rVVenv inoculation. However, cytokine doses, schedule of administration, and inoculation routes are some of the critical parameters to consider in such approaches because they can significantly influence the results of immunization.[191–193]

Acquired Immunodeficiency Syndrome

HIV-1[283,284] and HIV-2[285] are members of the lentivirus family and have been implicated as the cause of AIDS. Other members of the lentivirus family include SIV and feline immunodeficiency virus. Nonhuman primate models for AIDS vaccine development[286,287] include the macaque and chimpanzee models. Selected chimpanzee-passaged HIV-1 isolates can replicate to high levels and induce AIDS in chimpanzees, but this model has not been used frequently mainly for ethical reasons.[288] Although SIV does not cause any disease in its natural host species, some SIV isolates can induce AIDS in Asian monkeys, thereby providing an excellent model for vaccine studies.[289,290] However, there has been restricted use of the SIV/macaque model for HIV-1–based vaccines because of the differences in the envelope sequences of SIV and HIV-1. This has led to the

TABLE 49–7 ■ Vaccinia Recombinants Used in Prime-Boost Immunization Regimens Against Infectious Diseases

Pathogen/Disease	Prime	Boost	Immunity (Ab, CMI, Protection)	Reference
Malaria	DNA	MVA	High-level T-cell responses	253, 254
	Adenovirus	MVA	Complete protective efficacy (CD8+ T-cell responses)	247
	DNA	ALVAC	Partial protection and lower mean parasitemia	255
Hepatitis C virus	DNA	CPV	Enhanced antibody and T-cell responses	168
Leishmania infantum p36/LACK protein (VVp36) and IL-12 (VVp36-IL12)	p36 VVp36IL-12 VVp36	VVp36IL-12 P36 VVp36	P36/VVp36 IL-12 induced 52% reduction in lesion size and 2-log reduction in parasite load	245

development of chimeric viral isolates called simian/human immunodeficiency viruses (SHIV) that contain HIV-1 envelope proteins on an SIV backbone. Pathogenic SHIV isolates can cause death from AIDS in nonhuman primates[291–295] and therefore have been used in several trials. Several nonpathogenic SHIV strains can replicate to high titers in rhesus and cynomolgus monkeys without causing disease.[291,292,294]

Properties of HIV Gene Products Expressed by Poxvirus-Based Vectors

The biochemical, functional, and immunologic properties of several HIV gene products expressed by poxvirus-based vectors have been evaluated (Table 49–8). Poxviruses expressing a variety of HIV and SIV genes have been tested in animals and in some cases in humans.[13,194,200,218,295,296] The results suggest that HIV-specific T-cell responses and CTL responses could be induced by such candidates. However, in general, poxvirus-based lentivirus vaccine candidates elicit weak anti-HIV antibody responses. Currently, HIV vaccine candidates have only demonstrated partial protection and have not been shown to induce cross-NAbs against primary field isolates. Poxvirus-based HIV candidate vaccines are in various stages of development, and numerous approaches have been undertaken with different poxvirus vectors, including vaccinia,[180,206,207,214–216,297–299] NYVAC,[178,199,219,300] and ALVAC.[178,204,208,219,230,300–302] The following properties have been explored in the preclinical

studies to determine the immunogenicity of poxvirus-based vaccines expressing HIV-antigens.

Ability to Induce HIV-Specific CD8+ Major Histocompatibility Complex Class I–Restricted CTL Responses and Protective Efficacy

HIV-specific cellular and humoral immunity can be elicited in nonhuman primates with recombinant vaccinia constructs.[215,303] However, because of the inability of immunocompromised individuals to control systemic dissemination of the virus,[24] efforts have been focused on the use of attenuated poxviruses. Recombinant MVA constructs were found to be immunogenic and could induce CTL responses that were able to contain virus replication and to protect monkeys from SIV- and SHIV-induced disease.[180,216,275,304] Strong CD8+ CTL responses were elicited by vaccination with ALVAC and NYVAC encoding HIV glycoprotein (gp) 120[301] and by ALVAC encoding SIV *gag*, *pol*, and *env* (*gpe*).[305] ALVAC–SIV *gpe* also elicited low-frequency but durable memory CTL populations. In another study, protection of one of two chimpanzees was observed following immunization with ALVAC–HIV-1 (vCP250) expressing HIV-1 IIIB LAI, gp120/TM, *gag*, and *protease* (*pro*) gene products.[186] However, 5 months after challenge, booster inoculation, and a rechallenge, neither NAbs nor protection from a heterologous challenge with HIV-1$_{DH12}$ was observed.[186] NAb and protective immune responses were observed following vaccination of macaques with envelope

TABLE 49–8 ■ HIV-1 Antigens Expressed in Poxviruses

Antigen	Possible Function(s)	Poxvirus
Envelope Proteins		
Env (gp160)	Epitopes that elicit immune responses Highly glycosylated protein gp120 + gp41	ALVAC, FPV, MVA, VV
gp120	Binds the CD4 receptor and co-receptors	ALVAC, VV
Structural Proteins		
Gag	Involved in viral assembly	ALVAC, FPV, MVA, VV
Pol (RT)	Codes for PR, RT, and integrase	ALVAC, FPV, VV
Regulatory Proteins		
Tat	Transcriptional activation and increases the levels of viral RNA by several hundredfold	ALVAC, NYVAC, VV
Nef	Early events in replication, CD4 and MHC-I down-regulation	ALVAC, FPV

proteins derived from single or multiple viral isolates.[306] NYVAC-SIV *gpe* provided protection from infection with SIV$_{MAC251}$ by the rectal route.[282] In another approach, chimeras between HIV-1 (*env*) and VV immunogen proteins p14 (A27L gene) and p39 (A4L gene) resulted in levels of CD8$^+$ T-cell–specific responses to Env similar to those following immunization with the entire Env protein.[227]

Prime-Boost Approach to Induce Cell-Mediated and Humoral Immunity Against HIV

Several prime-boost approaches have been undertaken for HIV preventive vaccination as well as to maximize immunologic profiles with subunit immunogens.[218,307,308] Recombinant vaccinia immunization in combination with a protein boost protected monkeys from infection with some SIV isolates.[309] In a rhesus macaque model, DNA priming followed by a recombinant MVA booster expressing multiple HIV proteins effectively controlled a highly pathogenic immunodeficiency virus challenge via the intrarectal route.[177] Prime-boost regimens in the HIV-2/macaque challenge system using NYVAC– and ALVAC–HIV-2 recombinant viruses expressing the HIV-2 *env*, *gag*, and *pol* (*egp*) genes, or NYVAC expressing the HIV-2 envelope protein or gp120 moiety, have been investigated.[7,217,310] The majority of animals (seven of eight) were protected from challenge with HIV-2$_{SBL6669}$ parental virus and furthermore remained protected (five of seven) after a second challenge. These results were significant because 75% (three of four) and 100% (three of three) of control animals became infected after the first and second challenges, respectively. Several other strategies that exhibit partial control of viral replication as well as protections have been described (Table 49–9). Significant levels of protection against the virulent SIV$_{MAC251}$ isolate were observed with NYVAC-SIV[282] and MVA-SIV[275] used alone or as part of prime-boost regimens. Partial protection was observed in animals immunized with NYVAC–HIV-1 (*egp*) and NYVAC–HIV-2 (*egp*) and challenged with HIV-2$_{SBL6669}$. However, no protection was observed in NYVAC–HIV-2 immunized/SHIV$_{HXB2}$-challenged rhesus macaques, although NYVAC–HIV-1 immunization resulted in significantly lower viral burdens.[209] Interestingly, NAbs were observed only in NYVAC–HIV-2 immunized macaques, whereas both groups displayed cross-reactive CTLs against HIV-1 and HIV-2. In raising protective immunity against SHIV challenges, DNA priming and recombinant poxvirus boosting was more effective than DNA alone or DNA prime–protein boost.[311] Recently, prime-boost studies have been initiated with epitope-based poxvirus vaccine candidates.[176,196]

Enhancement of Cellular Immunity with Immunomodulators

Use of recombinant FPV (rFPV) (HIV-1 *gag/pol*–interferon-γ [IFN-γ]) in macaques infected with HIV-1 resulted in enhanced CTL responses in comparison to rFPV (HIV-1 *gag/pol*).[202] Similarly, immunization with rFPV vaccines (HIV *gag/pol*–IFN-γ) enhanced HIV-specific IFN-γ secretion following ex vivo stimulation of whole blood in macaques compared to vaccination with FPV *gag/pol* with-

out IFN-γ[312] A rVV (HIV-1 *env*) with IL-12 elicited enhanced anti-*env* CMI responses in mice.[191] In a related study, a prime-boost regimen with a DNA vector expressing HIV1 *env* with interleukin-2 IL-2 followed by rVV *env* also triggered enhanced CMI response.[192]

HIV Clinical Trials

Several clinical trials have been initiated to test prophylactic and therapeutic AIDS vaccine candidates. VV recombinants encoding HIV-1 genes have been shown to elicit humoral and CMI responses in humans. Among HIV-1 antigens, gp160 and gp120 have so far been studied extensively in different clinical trials. Other HIV antigens such as *gag* and *gag/pol*, which are highly immunogenic, currently are being investigated in Phase I/II trials. In several Phase I clinical trials, vaccinees were primed with recombinant VV encoding gp160 and subsequently boosted with recombinant gp (rgp)160 or rgp120. Low HIV-specific humoral and CMI responses were elicited by rgp160 or VV-gp160 immunization alone, whereas the prime-boost strategy elicited NAb and *env*-specific CTLs in the majority of cases.[170,182,195,205,222,313,314] A prime-boost regimen consisting of priming with HIVacle (VV encoding HIV-1 IIIB *env* glycoprotein) and boosting with adjuvanted rgp160 resulted in significantly higher and more sustained immune responses.[195,225] The combination regimen resulted in HIV-specific CD4$^+$ and CD8$^+$ CTL reactivities, whereas the individual immunogens elicited only CD4$^+$ CTL responses to HIVacle. As expected, immune responses were more evident in vaccinia-naïve than vaccinia-experienced individuals. Recombinant VVs expressing *env*, *gag*, and *pol* are currently being used in clinical trials.[315,317] Considering the safety concerns mentioned earlier and the fact that immunosuppression has been a contraindication for vaccination with vaccinia, it is more appropriate to use highly attenuated novel poxvirus strains MVA, NYVAC, and ALVAC as the vector of choice for expressing HIV recombinants. Because of these observations as well as the extensive safety and immunogenicity studies that have been undertaken, much attention has been given to ALVAC-HIV, which has demonstrated an equivalent immunological profile in VV-naïve and VV-experienced individuals.

In numerous safety and immunogenicity Phase I clinical studies, ALVAC constructs containing several HIV genes induced CTL responses in 50% to 70% of vaccinees.[166,205,210,218,224,228,230] Completed trials have shown durable anti–HIV-1 CD8$^+$ CTL responses generated by ALVAC–HIV-1 *env*, *gag*, and *pro* (vCP205) alone.[189] Interestingly, broader cytokine responses (Th1 and Th2 cytokines) were elicited by a prime-boost regimen using vCP205 with HIV1$_{SF2}$ rgp120.[190] A safety and immunogenicity trial conducted in vaccinia-immune and vaccinia-naïve HIV-uninfected adults resulted in the detection of HIV$_{MN}$ and HIV$_{SF2}$ NAbs in 100% of ALVAC-gp160/rgp120 recipients in comparison to less than 65% of recipients of ALVAC-gp160 alone or 89% of recipients of ALVAC-rgp120 alone.[224] The ALVAC-based recombinants (vCP205 and vCP300) were evaluated for their capacity to induce ex vivo activation and expansion of HIV-specific CD8$^+$ CTL precursors obtained from HIV-1–infected donors.[316] VCP205 elicited only *env* and *gag*

TABLE 49–9 ■ Poxvirus Recombinants Encoding HIV/SIV Genes Used in Pre-Clinical Studies

Gene/Subunit	Prime	Boost	Challenge	Immunity	Reference
SIV*Nef*	rVV and rDNA	rProtein	SIV$_{MAC J5}$	Anti-*Nef* antibodies (4/4), no protection	339
SIV *env, gag-pol, nef, rev* and *tat*	MVA	SFV	—	SIV-specific humoral and cellular responses.	206
SIV regulatory/accessory genes	rVV	—	—	SIV-specific CTL developed in 100% (4/4) macaques.	214
SIV-mac251/32H/J5	rMVA	—	Pathogenic SIV	All vaccinated monkeys infected, but viral replication was partially controlled.	207
HIV-2 *env, gag* or *pol* genes	NYVAC	ALVAC	HIV-2$_{SBL6669}$	rNYVAC – no CTL but +NAb titres. rALVAC— exhibited low/none NAb titres. All macaques were infected.	310
HIV2 *env*-gp 125 or HIV-2 V3 synthetic peptides	ALVAC	HIV-2 gp 125 or V3 peptides	Homologous cell-free HIV-2	No protection (4/4 monkeys) without boost. 40% protection (4/10) with prime/boost	178
Live HIV-2 vaccine	ALVAC and purified gp125	HIV-2 (IV) + pathoSI Vsm (IR)	—	Monkeys protected (3/5) and remaining were SIV-infected with limited viral replication.	219
SIV-*gpe* vs SIV-*gag-env* vaccine	DNA-SIV-*gag-env* vaccine	NYVA C-SIV gpe	SIV$_{mac251}$ virus T cell response.	Increased CD8+	199–200
Env, gag, pol	MVA	Oligomeric protein	Pathogenic SHIV	Significant control of viremia and delayed progress of disease macaques.	299
HIV-1 *gag, pro, env* (ALVAC and virus-like particle)	DNA DNA VLP	VLP ALVAC —	— — —	NAbs and Gag-specific CD8+ responses were detected in macaques with only these three P/B strategies.	204
SIV$_{MAC239}$ *gag, pol* and HIV-1$_{89.6}$ *env*	MVA	—	Pathogenic SHIV$_{89.6}$	High frequency of CTL, high titer SHIV$_{89.6}$ specific NAb and no evidence of clinical disease for 168 days in macaques.	180
SIV *gag* CTL epitopes	DNA	MVA	—	Ex-vivo SIV specific CD8+ CTL activity in PBMC from 5/6 vaccinated animals.	176
HIV derived epitopes	DNA	MVA	—	Induced cellular responses	221

CTLs, whereas vCP300 elicited broad reactivities against *env, gag, pol,* and *nef* determinants. Two rounds of in vitro stimulation with vCP300 resulted in eightfold expansion of CD8+ lymphocytes over a 35-day period. These studies suggest that HIV recombinants represent powerful polyvalent stimuli for activation and expansion of CD8+ lymphocyte responses.

The genetic diversity of HIV-1 is a significant issue affecting the development of an HIV-1 vaccine. ALVAC-HIV recombinants elicited HIV-specific CTL activity as measured against autologous targets infected with vaccinia-HIV recombinants expressing components from prototypic HIV-1 isolates, peptide-pulsed targets, and targets infected with prototypic clade B HIV-1 strains as well as with primary isolates from clades A through F.[302] HIV-1 interclade (B-LAI) versus B (MN) *env* gp160-specific CTL reactivity was investigated in HIV-1 clade B–infected individuals.[220] The majority of HIV-1–seropositive subjects (13 of 19) had significant clade B gp160 LAI CD8+ CTL responses and CTL cross-reactivity against clade C92BR025 *env* gp160 after vaccination. The ability to generate cross-clade T cells for cross-neutralization among diverse primary isolates is an important observation for the development of an HIV-1 vaccine.

A safety and immunogenicity study with ALVAC–HIV-1 and rgp120 SF2 vaccines was conducted in healthy adults who were at low risk of acquiring HIV infection and were also HIV seronegative.[183] CD8+ CTLs were induced in 64% of volunteers by the live recombinant ALVAC–HIV-1 vaccine, which also primed for a vigorous NAb response on boosting with the subunit gp120 vaccine. In a Phase II study, ALVAC–HIV-1 (vCP205) was evaluated with or without gp120 in 435 volunteers.[233] NAbs to the MN strain were elicited in 94% of volunteers who received vCP205 and gp120 compared to 56% of volunteers who received vCP205 alone.

Seronegative volunteers were given an ALVAC expressing gp120, gp41, *gag* and *pro* gene, and *nef* and *pol* CTL epitopes either simultaneously with or followed by rgp120 SF2.[228] CD8+ CTLs were detected in 61% of volunteers at some time during the trial. Gene-specific responses to *gag* (32%), *env* (22%), *nef* (16%), and *pol* (19%) were observed for at least 6 months after the last immunization. Canarypox *gag-env-pro* elicited in vitro CD8+ T-cell responses in approximately 62% of vaccinees (26 of 42) who received it.[179] Prime-boost immunization with canarypox *gag-pro-env* vector and rgp120 resulted in NAbs in 91% and CD8+ T-cell responses in 62% of vaccinated HIV-seronegative volunteers. Importantly, the frequency of CD8+ CTLs was similar between vaccinia-naïve and vaccinia-immune individuals.

These studies, including National Institutes of Health HIV Vaccines Trials Network (AVEG) and Thai/Walter Reed Army Institute of Research ALVAC-HIV Phase I/II clinical trials, have demonstrated the safety of the ALVAC–HIV-1 recombinants and also proven that ALVAC–HIV-1 is well tolerated in prime-boost combination with subunit antigen preparations and can elicit NAbs, cellular proliferative responses, CD8+ CTL responses, cross-clade reactivity, and antibody-dependent cellular cytotoxicity. Additional immunizations increase the CTL responses. Equivalent responses were observed in both vaccinia-experienced and vaccinia-naïve individuals. These studies also suggest that prime-boost regimens using ALVAC–HIV-1 vaccine candidates may elicit vigorous HIV-specific polyepitopic CD8+ CTL response and NAbs, which will be important in achieving protection against primary, transmitted viruses. Around 60 Phase I and II trials of 30 candidate vaccines have been conducted with different approaches, with promising results.[317–320] ALVAC–HIV-1 vaccines have been tested in more than 1700 volunteers/patients and have a safety profile acceptable for the initiation of Phase III studies.

Cancer

The last few years have seen tremendous growth in the development of cancer vaccines based on tumor-associated antigens (TAAs) and tumor-specific antigens that have been identified using technologies such as microarrays, serologic screening of complementary DNA expression libraries (SEREX), immunohistochemistry, reverse transcriptase–polymerase chain reaction, in-situ hybridization, reverse immunology, and laser capture microscopy[321–332] that enable the monitoring of differentially expressed gene

products. TAAs are antigens differentially expressed or overexpressed by tumor cells and specific to one or more cancers. For example, carcinoembryonic antigen (CEA) is overexpressed in colorectal, breast, and lung cancers. Several delivery systems that express TAAs, such as DNA or viruses, are being explored as therapeutic vaccines for human cancers and have been shown to break immune tolerance of TAAs.[333] CMI and humoral immune responses have been demonstrated against a variety of TAAs, including HER2/neu, CEA, p53, MAGE1, and MUC1, in different cancer vaccine studies. Poxvirus-based vaccine candidates can be more potent in the initiation of tumor-specific T-cell responses with the help of prime-boost regimens than vaccines employing other approaches.[334] Tumor cells can be rendered more immunogenic by inserting transgenes encoding T-cell co-stimulatory molecules such as B7.1 or cytokines such as IFN-γ, IL-2, and granulocyte-macrophage colony-stimulating factor, which may help in eliciting Th-1–type responses. Several cancer antigens and co-stimulatory molecules are being investigated in the poxvirus-based immunization studies (Table 49–10). ALVAC-mediated gene transfer in cancer immunotherapy[39,120–122,130,335–337] can induce CMI and humoral immune responses.[156,218,301,316] Several clinical trials have been completed or are in progress using recombinant poxvirus–based immunization strategies for the therapy of different cancers.[340–342]

Attenuated Poxviruses for Smallpox Vaccination

Recently there has been an increased likelihood of the premeditated introduction of smallpox and therefore it is imperative to develop new vaccines and vaccination strategies to protect the community.[343–345] Both targeted vaccination of health care workers and wider-scale vaccination programs have been considered.[345–346] Presently, the only commercially approved smallpox vaccine in the United States is Wyeth Dryvax, which is a lyophilized preparation of live VV derived from the New York City Board of Health (NYCBH) strain of VV. A primary vaccination confers full immunity to smallpox for 5 to 10 years and subsequent revaccination probably provides protection for another 10 years or more.[21] However, complications and adverse events specific to dermatologic and central nervous system disorders have been observed with the NYCBH vaccine and deaths have also been reported at a rate of 1 or 2 deaths per million primary vacinees.[23,347]

Due to the adverse events associated with VV vaccination, second generation attenuated vaccine viruses such as MVA, LC16m8 and NYVAC have been suggested as safer vaccines.[344,348] Two of these strains (LC16m8 and MVA) have been developed and tested for possible use as a smallpox vaccine.[348] LC16m8 caused few side effects when tested in 50,000 children in the 1970s[349] and MVA was assessed as a smallpox vaccine in over 120,000 recipients without significant adverse reactions.[35] Recently a Phase I trial of an MVA-based vaccine was completed in 100 subjects without any vaccine-associated serious adverse events being observed.[350] The development of a pock-mark and a neu-

TABLE 49–10 ■ Cancer Antigens and Co-Stimulatory Molecules Used in Poxvirus-Based Preclinical and Clinical Trials

Cancer Antigen	Pox Vector	Co-stimulatory Molecule	Pox Vector
PSA	FPV, VV	IL-2	ALVAC, VV
MAGE1	VV	IL-12	ALVAC
MAGE 1/3	ALVAC	GM-CSF	ALVAC, VV
DF3/Muc1	VV	CEA-B7.1	ALVAC
Muc-1	VV	CEA-TRICOM*	FPV, VV
HPV E6/E7	VV	B7.1(CD80)	ALVAC, FPV, VV
HPV E7/LLO	VV	ICAM-I (CD54)	VV
gp100	ALVAC, FPV	LFA-3 (CD58)	VV
p53(WT)	ALVAC, NYVAC	CD70	VV
Tyrosinase	FPV, VV	IFN-γ	VV
CEA	ALVAC, FPV NYVAC, VV	TFN-α	VV

*TRICOM-B7.1, ICAM-I, and LFA-3.[338]

tralizing antibody response, the currently accepted indication of protective immunogenicity, were observed in 99% and 96% of the subjects respectively. However, the field efficacy of these strains cannot be tested due to the absence of endemic smallpox disease and consequently there is no certainty that these vaccines could prevent smallpox. As a safety precaution and as an immediate contingency plan, the Dryvax and MVA vaccines are being generated and stockpiled worldwide.

Some other potential attenuated vaccine strains have also been evaluated. An initial immunization with CVI-78, a highly attenuated vaccinia virus (CVI-78) followed by a dose of VV was found to reduce the rate of side effects.[351] Studies with a replication-deficient Lister/Elstree strain of VV showed that it could induce levels of antibody and CTL responses comparable to those induced by MVA.[352] Studies are being continued to consolidate and compile safety and efficacy data for Dryvax, MVA, and other vaccine strains.

In future it will be important to explore the development of new smallpox vaccines and vaccination strategies using either attenuated VV or cross-protective recombinant viral antigens. With respect to the subject of this chapter, the implications of widespread smallpox vaccination with VV-based vaccines is unknown, since pre-existing immunity to VV is known to dampen immune responses to VV-derived immunization vehicles. It will be necessary to take account of this as novel vaccines are developed using poxvirus vectors.

Conclusion

Use of poxvirus-based vectors as immunization vehicles for the delivery of vaccines since 1982 has been both informative and exciting. New technologies aimed at enhancing the versatility of poxvirus-based vaccine candidates coupled to data emerging from current clinical trials point to a promising future for the use of the poxvirus immunization vehicles for prevention and treatment of infectious diseases

and cancer. Furthermore, novel vaccine approaches using poxvirus-based immunization vehicles have provided valuable groundwork for vector-based vaccines at the scientific, regulatory, and industrial levels. Poxvirus-based vectors have been validated in multiple preclinical and clinical studies. Results from several ongoing clinical studies will be critical in designing and refining new strategies to enhance both the safety and immunogenicity of poxvirus-based vaccines for different diseases, including cancer and AIDS. Future innovations in the development of adjuvants, inoculation regimens, and the design of the vector backbone could further improve the efficacy of poxvirus vectors (Table 49–11). For instance, carbomer-formulated ALVAC encoding equine herpesvirus type 1 (EHV-1) proteins induced high levels of neutralizing antibody and protection against EHV-1 infection in horses.[78,79] Similarly, use of a gelatin sponge matrix to encapsulate ALVAC–β-gal resulted in a greater distribution of gene expression on injection into solid tumors than injections of virus in the aqueous phase.[336,337] The next few years can confidently be predicted to bring further confirmation of the safety and efficacy of poxvirus-based vaccines, together with significantly improved methods for their use.

Acknowledgments

The authors wish to thank Andrew Murdin for critically reviewing this manuscript, Davinder Chawla for her advice and comments, and Carmela Care for her invaluable assistance and support.

TABLE 49–11 ■ Potential Avenues for Improvements to Poxvirus-Based Vaccine Candidates

Vector backbone
  Vector design
  Immunogen design
  Co-stimulatory molecules
  Detection and removal of immune inhibitory functions
Formulations
Regimen/delivery

REFERENCES

1. Mackett M, Smith GL, Moss B. Vaccinia virus: a selectable eukaryotic cloning and expression vector. Proc Natl Acad Sci U S A 79:7415–7419, 1982.
2. Panicali D, Paoletti E. Construction of poxviruses as cloning vectors: insertion of the thymidine kinase gene from herpes simplex virus into the DNA of infectious vaccinia virus. Proc Natl Acad Sci U S A 79:4927–4931, 1982.
3. Cox WI, Tartaglia J, Paoletti E, et al. Poxvirus recombinants as live vaccines. In Binns MM, Smith GL (eds): Recombinant Poxviruses. Boca Raton, FL, CRC Press, 1992, pp 123–162.
4. Carroll MW, Moss B. Host range and cytopathogenicity of the highly attenuated MVA strain of vaccinia virus: propagation and generation of recombinant viruses in a nonhuman mammalian cell line. Virology 238:198–211, 1997.
5. Flexner C, Moss B. New generation vaccines. In Levine MM, Woodrow GC, Kasper JB, Cobon GS (eds). New Generation Vaccines. New York, Marcel Dekker, 1997, pp 297–314.
6. Piccini A, Paoletti E. Vaccinia: virus, vector, vaccine. Adv Virus Res 34:43–64, 1988.
7. Perkus ME, Tartaglia J, Paoletti E. Poxvirus-based vaccine candidates for cancer, AIDS, and other infectious diseases. J Leukoc Biol 58:1–13, 1995.
8. Moss B. Genetically engineered poxviruses for recombinant gene expression, vaccination, and safety. Proc Natl Acad Sci U S A 93:11341–11348, 1996.
9. Paoletti E. Applications of poxvirus vectors to vaccination: an update. Proc Natl Acad Sci U S A 93:11349–11353, 1996.
10. Talavera A, Rodriguez JM. Vaccinia virus as an expression vector. Methods Mol Biol 8:219–233, 1991.
11. Moss B. Vaccinia virus: a tool for research and vaccine development. Science 252:1662–1667, 1991.
12. Karacostas V, Nagashima K, Gonda MA, et al. Human immunodeficiency virus-like particles produced by a vaccinia virus expression vector. Proc Natl Acad Sci U S A 86:8964–8967, 1989.
13. Tartaglia J, Pincus S, Paoletti E. Poxvirus-based vectors as vaccine candidates. Crit Rev Immunol 10:13–30, 1990.
14. Tartaglia J, Bonnet MC, Berinstein N, et al. Therapeutic vaccines against melanoma and colorectal cancer. Vaccine 19:2571–2575, 2001.
15. Tartaglia J. Recombinant poxvirus vaccine candidates: update and perspectives. Res Immunol 149:79–82, 1998.
16. Tsang KY, Zaremba S, Nieroda CA, et al. Generation of human cytotoxic T cells specific for human CEA epitopes from patients immunized with recombinant vaccinia-CEA vaccine. J Natl Cancer Inst 87:982–990, 1995.
17. Berinstein N. Carcinoembryonic antigen as a target for therapeutic anti-cancer vaccines: a review. J Clin Oncol 20:2197–2207, 2002.
18. Smith GL, Moss B. Infectious poxvirus vectors have capacity for at least 25,000 base pairs of foreign DNA. Gene 25:21–28, 1983.
19. Perkus ME, Piccini A, Lipinskas BR, et al. Recombinant vaccinia virus: immunization against multiple pathogens. Science 229:981–984, 1985.
20. Perkus ME, Limbach K, Paoletti E. Cloning and expression of foreign genes in vaccinia virus, using a host range selection system. J Virol 63:3829–3836, 1989.
21. Fenner F, Henderson DA, Arita I, et al. Smallpox and Its Eradication. Geneva, World Health Organization, 1988.
22. Perkus ME, Taylor J, Tartaglia J, et al. Live attenuated vaccinia and other poxviruses as delivery systems: public health issues. Ann N Y Acad Sci 754:222–233, 1995.
23. Lane JM, Ruben FL, Neff JM, et al. Complications of smallpox vaccination, 1968. N Engl J Med 281:1201–1208, 1969.
24. Redfield RR, Wright DC, James WD, et al. Disseminated vaccinia in a military recruit with human immunodeficiency virus (HIV) disease. N Engl J Med 316:673–676, 1987.
25. Mackett M, Smith GL, Moss B. General method for production and selection of infectious vaccinia virus recombinants expressing foreign genes. J Virol 49:857–864, 1984.
26. Panicali D, Davis SW, Mercer SR, et al. Two major DNA variants present in serially propagated stocks of the WR strain of vaccinia virus. J Virol 37:1000–1010, 1981.
27. Moss B, Smith GL, Mackett M. Use of vaccinia virus as an infectious molecular cloning and expression vector. Gene Amplif Anal 3:201–213, 1983.
28. Meyer H, Sutter G, Mayr A. Mapping of deletions in the genome of the highly attenuated vaccinia virus MVA and their influence on virulence. J Gen Virol 72:1031–1038, 1991.
29. Hochstein-Mintzel V, Hanichen T, Huber HC, et al. An attenuated strain of vaccinia virus (MVA): successful intramuscular immunization against vaccinia and variola. Zentralbl Bakteriol (A) 230:283–297, 1975.
30. Mayr A, Stickl H, Muller HK, et al. The smallpox vaccination strain MVA: marker, genetic structure, experience gained with the parenteral vaccination and behavior in organisms with a debilitated defence mechanism. Zentralbl Bakteriol (B) 167:375–390, 1978.
31. Drexler I, Heller K, Wahren B, et al. Highly attenuated modified vaccinia virus Ankara replicates in baby hamster kidney cells, a potential host for virus propagation, but not in various human transformed and primary cells. J Gen Virol 79(pt 2):347–352, 1998.
32. Moss B. Poxviridae and their replication. In Fields BN, Knipe DM, Chanock RM, et al (eds). Virology. New York, Raven Press, 1990, pp 2079–2111.
33. Staib C, Drexler I, Ohlmann M, et al. Transient host range selection for genetic engineering of modified vaccinia virus Ankara. Biotechniques 28:1137–1142, 1144–1146, 1148, 2000.
34. Wyatt LS, Carroll MW, Czerny CP, et al. Marker rescue of the host range restriction defects of modified vaccinia virus Ankara. Virology 251:334–342, 1998.
35. Mayr A, Hochstein-Mintzel V, Stickl H. Abstammung, Eigenschaften und Verwendung des attenuierten Vaccinia-stammes MVA. Infection 3:6–14, 1975.
36. Tartaglia J, Perkus ME, Taylor J, et al. NYVAC: a highly attenuated strain of vaccinia virus. Virology 188:217–232, 1992.
37. Pincus S, Tartaglia J, Paoletti E. Poxvirus-based vectors as vaccine candidates. Biologicals 23:159–164, 1995.
38. Tartaglia J, Cox WI, Pincus S, et al. Safety and immunogenicity of recombinants based on the genetically engineered vaccinia strain, NYVAC. Dev Biol Stand 82:125–129, 1994.
39. Roth J, Dittmer D, Rea D, et al. p53 as a target for cancer vaccines: recombinant canarypox virus vectors expressing p53 protect mice against lethal tumor cell challenge. Proc Natl Acad Sci U S A 93:4781–4786, 1996.
40. Taylor J, Weinberg R, Languet B, et al. Recombinant fowlpox virus inducing protective immunity in non-avian species. Vaccine 6:497–503, 1988.
41. Esposito JJ. Poxviridae. In Francki RIB, Fauquet CM, Knudson DL, Brown F (eds). Classification and Nomenclature of Viruses. New York, Springer-Verlag, 1991, pp 91–102.
42. Taylor J, Paoletti E. Fowlpox virus as a vector in non-avian species. Vaccine 6:466–468, 1988.
43. Taylor J, Weinberg R, Tartaglia J, et al. Nonreplicating viral vectors as potential vaccines: recombinant canarypox virus expressing measles virus fusion (F) and hemagglutinin (HA) glycoproteins. Virology 187:321–328, 1992.
44. Somogyi P, Frazier J, Skinner MA. Fowlpox virus host range restriction: gene expression, DNA replication, and morphogenesis in nonpermissive mammalian cells. Virology 197:439–444, 1993.
45. Afonso CL, Tulman ER, Lu Z, et al. The genome of Fowlpox virus. J Virol 74:3815–3831, 2000.
46. Tartaglia J, Cox WI, Taylor J, et al. Highly attenuated poxvirus vectors. AIDS Res Hum Retroviruses 8:1445–1447, 1992.
47. Paoletti E, Tartaglia J, Cox WI. Immunotherapeutic strategies for cancer using poxvirus vectors. Ann N Y Acad Sci 690:292–300, 1993.
48. Tartaglia J, Excler JL, El Habib R, et al. Canarypox virus-based vaccines: prime-boost strategies to induce cell-mediated and humoral immunity against HIV. AIDS Res Hum Retroviruses 14(suppl 3): S291–S298, 1998.
49. Cadoz M, Strady A, Meignier B, et al. Immunization with canarypox virus expressing rabies glycoprotein. Lancet 339:1429–1432, 1992.
50. Tubiana R, Gomard E, Fleury H, et al. Vaccine therapy in early HIV-1 infection using a recombinant canarypox virus expressing gp160MN (ALVAC-HIV): a double-blind, controlled, randomized study of safety and immunogenicity. AIDS 11:819–820, 1997.
51. Piccini A, Perkus ME, Paoletti E. Vaccinia virus as an expression vector. Methods Enzymol 153:545–563, 1987.
52. Macket M. Manipulation of vaccinia virus vectors. Methods Mol Biol 7:129–146, 1991.
53. Taylor J, Tartaglia J, Riviere M, et al. Applications of canarypox (ALVAC) vectors in human and veterinary vaccination. Dev Biol Stand 82:131–135, 1994.

54. Broder CC, Earl PL. Recombinant vaccinia viruses: design, generation, and isolation. Mol Biotechnol 13:223–245, 1999.

55. Pfleiderer M, Falkner FG, Dorner F. A novel vaccinia virus expression system allowing construction of recombinants without the need for selection markers, plasmids and bacterial hosts. J Gen Virol 76:2957–2962, 1995.

56. Gillard S, Spehner D, Drillien R, et al. Localization and sequence of a vaccinia virus gene required for multiplication in human cells. Proc Natl Acad Sci U S A 83:5573–5577, 1986.

57. Perkus ME, Goebel SJ, Davis SW, et al. Vaccinia virus host range genes. Virology 179:276–286, 1990.

58. Goebel SL, Johnson GP, Perkus ME, et al. The complete DNA sequence of vaccinia virus. Virology 179:247–266, 1990.

59. Smith GL. Vaccinia virus vectors for gene expression. Current Opin Biotechnol 2:713–717, 1991.

60. Earl PL, Moss B. Generation of recombinant vaccinia viruses. *In* Ausubel FM, Brent R, Kingston RE, et al (eds). Current Protocols in Molecular Biology. New York, Greene Publishing Associates/Wiley Interscience, 1991, pp 16–27.

61. Falkner FG, Moss B. *Escherichia coli gpt* gene provides selection for vaccinia virus open reading frame expression vectors. J Virol 62:1849–1854, 1988.

62. Falkner FG, Moss B. Transient dominant selection of recombinant vaccinia viruses. J Virol 64:3108–3111, 1990.

63. Boyle DB, Coupar BE. Construction of recombinant fowlpox viruses as vectors for poultry vaccines. Virus Res 10:343–356, 1988.

64. Boyle DB, Coupar BEH. A dominant selectable marker for the construction of recombinant poxviruses. Gene 65:123–128, 1988.

65. Chakrabarti S, Brechling K, Moss B. Vaccinia virus expression vector: coexpression of β-gal provides visual screening of recombinant virus plaques. Mol Cell Biol 5:3403–3409, 1985.

66. Panicali D, Grzelecki A, Huang C. Vaccinia virus vectors utilizing the β-gal assay for rapid selection of recombinant viruses and measurement of gene expression. Gene 47:193–199, 1986.

67. Spehner D, Drillien R, Lecocq JP. Construction of fowl poxvirus vectors with intergenic insertions: expression of the β-galactosidase gene and the measles virus fusion gene. J Virol 64:527–533, 1990.

68. Boyle DB, Selleck P, Heine HG. Vaccinating chickens against avian influenza virus. Aust Vet J 78:44–48, 2000.

69. De BK, Shaw MW, Rota PA, et al. Protection against virulent H5 avian influenza virus infection in chickens by an inactivated vaccine produced with recombinant vaccinia virus. Vaccine 6:257–261, 1988.

70. Portetelle D, Limbach K, Burny A, et al. Recombinant vaccine virus expression of the bovine leukemia virus envelope gene and protection of immunized sheep against infection. Vaccine 9:194–200, 1991.

71. Gatei MH, Naif HM, Kumar S, et al. Protection of sheep against bovine leukemia virus (BLV) infection by vaccination with rVV expressing BLV envelope glycoproteins. J Virol 67:1803–1810, 1993.

72. Meneguzzi G, Kieny MP, Lecocq X, et al. Vaccinia recombinant expressing early bovine papilloma virus (BPV) proteins: retardation of BPV1 tumour development. Vaccine 8:199–204, 1990.

73. Beyer JC, Chebloune Y, Mselli-Lakhal L, et al. Immunization with plasmid DNA expressing the caprine arthritis-encephalitis virus envelope gene: quantitative and qualitative aspects of antibody response to viral surface glycoprotein. Vaccine 19:1643–1651, 2001.

74. Cheevers WP, Hotzel I, Beyer JC, et al. Immune response to caprine arthritis-encephalitis virus surface protein induced by coimmunization with recombinant vaccinia viruses expressing the caprine arthritis-encephalitis virus envelope gene and caprine interleukin-12. Vaccine 18:2494–2503, 2000.

75. Welter J, Taylor J, Tartaglia J, et al. Mucosal vaccination with recombinant poxvirus vaccines protects ferrets against symptomatic CDV infection. Vaccine 17:308–318, 1999.

76. Welter J, Taylor J, Tartaglia J, et al. Vaccination against canine distemper virus infection in infant ferrets with and without maternal antibody protection, using recombinant attenuated poxvirus vaccines. J Virol 74:6358–6367, 2000.

77. Taylor J, Pincus S, Tartaglia J, et al. Vaccinia virus recombinants expressing either the measles virus fusion or hemagglutinin glycoprotein protect dogs against canine distemper virus challenge. J Virol 65:4263–4274, 1991.

78. Audonnet JC, Mumford JA, Jessett D, et al. Safety and efficacy of a canarypox-EHV recombinant vaccine in horses. *In* Wernery U, Wade JF, Mumford JA, Kaaden O-R (eds). Proceeding of the Eighth International Conference on Equine Infectious Diseases. Newmarket, R&W Publications Limited, 1998, pp 418–419.

79. Minke JM, Audonnet JC, Jessett D, et al. Canarypox as a vector for influenza and EHV-1 genes: challenges and rewards. *In* Proceedings of the 2nd International Veterinary Vaccines and Diagnostic Conference, Oxford, 2000.

80. Tartaglia J, Jarrett O, Neil JC, et al. Protection of cats against feline leukemia virus by vaccination with a canarypox virus recombinant, ALVAC-FL. J Virol 67:2370–2375, 1993.

81. Tellier MC, Pu R, Pollock D, et al. Efficacy evaluation of prime-boost protocol: canarypoxvirus-based feline immunodeficiency virus (FIV) vaccine and inactivated FIV-infected cell vaccine against heterologous FIV challenge in cats. AIDS 12:11–18, 1998.

82. Berinstein A, Tami C, Taboga O, et al. Protective immunity against foot-and-mouth disease virus induced by a recombinant vaccinia virus. Vaccine 18:2231–2238, 2000.

83. Bayliss CD, Peters RW, Cook JKA, et al. A recombinant fowlpox virus that expresses the VP2 antigen of infectious bursal disease virus induces protection against mortality caused by the virus. Arch Virol 120:193–205, 1991.

84. Shaw I, Davison TF. Protection from IBDV-induced bursal damage by a recombinant fowlpox vaccine, fpIBD1, is dependent on the titre of challenge virus and chicken genotype. Vaccine 18:3230–3241, 2000.

85. Tsukamoto K, Sato T, Saito S, et al. Dual-viral vector approach induced strong and long-lasting protective immunity against very virulent infectious bursal disease virus. Virology 269:257–267, 2000.

86. Chambers TM, Kawaoka Y, Webster RG. Protection of chickens from lethal influenza infection by vaccinia-expressed hemagglutinin. Virology 167:414–421, 1988.

87. Webster RG, Kawaoka Y, Taylor J, et al. Efficacy of nucleoprotein and haemagglutinin antigens expressed in fowlpox virus as vaccine for influenza in chickens. Vaccine 9:303–308, 1991.

88. Sutter G, Wyatt LS, Foley PL, et al. A recombinant vector derived from the host range-restricted and highly attenuated MVA strain of vaccinia virus stimulates protective immunity in mice to influenza virus. Vaccine 12:1032–1040, 1994.

89. Yu L, Liu W, Schnitzlein WM, et al. Study of protection by recombinant fowl poxvirus expressing C-terminal nucleocapsid protein of infectious bronchitis virus against challenge. Avian Dis 45:340–348, 2001.

90. Nazerian K, Lee LF, Yanagida N, et al. Protection against Marek's disease by a Fowl Pox Virus recombinant expressing the glycoprotein B of Marek's disease virus. J Virol 66:1409–1413, 1992.

91. Boursnell ME, Green PF, Samson AC, et al. A recombinant fowlpox virus expressing the hemagglutinin-neuraminidase gene of Newcastle disease virus (NDV) protects chickens against challenge by NDV. Virology 178:297–300, 1990.

92. Nishikawa Y, Xuan X, Nagasawa H, et al. Prevention of vertical transmission of *Neospora caninum*. Vaccine 19:1710–1716, 2001.

93. Nishikawa Y, Inoue N, Xuan X, et al. Protective efficacy of vaccination by recombinant vaccinia virus against *Neospora caninum* infection. Vaccine 19:1381–1390, 2001.

94. Brochier BM, Languet B, Blancou J, et al. Use of recombinant vaccinia-rabies virus for oral vaccination of fox cubs (*Vulpes vulpes*, L.) Vet Microbiol 18:103–108, 1988.

95. Brochier B, Kieny MP, Costy F, et al. Large-scale eradication of rabies using recombinant vaccinia-rabies vaccine. Nature 354:520–522, 1991.

96. Brochier B, Costy F, Pastoret PP. Elimination of fox rabies from Belgium using a recombinant vaccinia-rabies vaccine: an update. Vet Microbiol 46:269–279, 1995.

97. Taylor J, Meignier B, Tartaglia J, et al. Biological and immunogenic properties of a canarypox-rabies recombinant, ALVAC-RG (vCP65) in non-avian species. Vaccine 13:539–549, 1995.

98. Giavedoni L, Jones L, Mebus C, et al. A vaccinia virus double recombinant expressing the F and H genes of rinderpest virus protects cattle against rinderpest and causes no pock lesions. Proc Natl Acad Sci U S A 88:8011–8015, 1991.

99. Verardi PH, Aziz FH, Ahmad S, et al. Long-term sterilizing immunity to rinderpest in cattle vaccinated with a recombinant vaccinia virus expressing high levels of the fusion and hemagglutinin glycoproteins. J Virol 76:484–491, 2002.

100. Ohishi K, Inui K, Barrett T, et al. Long-term protective immunity to rinderpest in cattle following a single vaccination with a recombinant vaccinia virus expressing the virus haemagglutinin protein. J Gen Virol 81(pt 6):1439–1446, 2000.

101. Phillpotts RJ, Lescott TL, Jacobs SC. Vaccinia virus recombinants encoding the truncated structural gene region of Venezuelan equine encephalitis virus (VEEV) give solid protection against peripheral challenge but only partial protection against airborne challenge with virulent VEEV. Acta Virol 44:233–239, 2000.

102. Mackett M, Yilma T, Rose JK, et al. Vaccinia virus recombinants: expression of VSV genes and protective immunization of mice and cattle. Science 227:433–435, 1985.

103. Adams M, Borysiewicz L, Fiander A, et al. Clinical studies of human papilloma vaccines in pre-invasive and invasive cancer. Vaccine 19:2549–2556, 2001.

104. Akagi J, Hodge JW, McLaughlin JP, et al. Therapeutic antitumor response after immunization with an admixture of recombinant vaccinia viruses expressing a modified MUC1 gene and the murine T-cell costimulatory molecule B7. J Immunother 20:38–47, 1997.

105. Borysiewicz LK, Fiander A, Nimako M, et al. A recombinant vaccinia virus encoding papillomavirus types 16 and 18, E6 and E7 proteins as immunotherapy for cervical cancer. Lancet 347:1523–1527, 1996.

106. Charles LG, Xie YC, Restifo NP, et al. Antitumor efficacy of tumor-antigen-encoding recombinant poxvirus immunization in Dunning rat prostate cancer: implications for clinical genetic vaccine development. World J Urol 18:136–142, 2000.

107. Conry RM, Khazaeli MB, Saleh MN, et al. Phase I trial of a recombinant vaccinia virus encoding carcinoembryonic antigen in metastatic adenocarcinoma: comparison of intradermal versus subcutaneous administration. Clin Cancer Res 5:2330–2337, 1999.

108. Cole DJ, Wilson MC, Baron PL, et al. Phase I study of recombinant CEA vaccinia virus vaccine with post vaccination CEA peptide challenge. Hum Gene Ther 7:1381–1394, 1996.

109. Doehn C, Jocham D. Technology evaluation: TG-1031, Transgene SA. Curr Opin Mol Ther 2:106–111, 2000.

110. Drexler I, Antunes E, Schmitz M, et al. Modified vaccinia virus Ankara for delivery of human tyrosinase as melanoma-associated antigen: induction of tyrosinase- and melanoma-specific human leukocyte antigen A*0201-restricted cytotoxic T cells in vitro and in vivo. Cancer Res 59:4955–4963, 1999.

111. Elzey BD, Siemens DR, Ratliff TL, et al. Immunization with type 5 adenovirus recombinant for a tumor antigen in combination with recombinant canarypox virus (ALVAC) cytokine gene delivery induces destruction of established prostate tumors. Int J Cancer 94:842–849, 2001.

112. Flexner C, Moss B, London WT, et al. Attenuation and immunogenicity in primates of vaccinia virus recombinants expressing human interleukin-2. Vaccine 8:17–22, 1990.

113. Freund YR, Mirsalis JC, Fairchild DG, et al. Vaccination with a recombinant vaccinia vaccine containing the B7-1 co-stimulatory molecule causes no significant toxicity and enhances T cell-mediated cytotoxicity. Int J Cancer 85:508–517, 2000.

114. Gitelson E, Ghose A, Buckstein R, et al. ALVAC-mediated gene transfer is efficient in lymphoid malignancies of T- and early B-cell origin, but not in tumors arising from mature B-cells. Cancer Immunol Immunother 50:345–355, 2001.

115. Griffith TS, Kawakita M, Tian J, et al. Inhibition of murine prostate tumor growth and activation of immunoregulatory cells with recombinant canarypox viruses. J Natl Cancer Inst 93:998–1007, 2001.

116. He Z, Wlazlo AP, Kowalczyk DW, et al. Viral recombinant vaccines to the E6 and E7 antigens of HPV-16. Virology 270:146–161, 2000.

117. Horig H, Lee DS, Conkright W. Phase I clinical trial of a recombinant canarypoxvirus (ALVAC) vaccine expressing human carcinoembryonic antigen and the B7.1 co-stimulatory molecule. Cancer Immunol Immunother 49:504–514, 2000.

118. Hodge JW, McLaughlin JP, Abrams SI, et al. Admixture of a recombinant vaccinia virus containing the gene for the costimulatory molecule B7 and a recombinant vaccinia virus containing a tumor-associated antigen gene results in enhanced specific T-cell responses and antitumor immunity. Cancer Res 55:3598–3603, 1995.

119. Hodge JW, Schlom J, Donohue SJ, et al. A recombinant vaccinia virus expressing human prostate-specific antigen (PSA): safety and immunogenicity in a non-human primate. Int J Cancer 63:231–237, 1995.

120. Hodge JW, McLaughlin JP, Kantor JA, et al. Diversified prime and boost protocols using recombinant vaccinia virus and recombinant non-replicating avian poxvirus to enhance T-cell immunity and antitumor responses. Vaccine 15:759–768, 1997.

121. Hodge JW, Sabzevari H, Yafal AG, et al. A triad of costimulatory molecules synergize to amplify T-cell activation. Cancer Res 59:5800–5807, 1999.

122. Hodge JW, Schlom J. Comparative studies of a retrovirus versus a poxvirus vector in whole tumor-cell vaccines. Cancer Res 59:5106–5111, 1999.

123. Hodge JW, Grosenbach DW, Rad AN, et al. Enhancing the potency of peptide-pulsed antigen presenting cells by vector-driven hyper-expression of a triad of costimulatory molecules. Vaccine 19:3552–3567, 2001.

124. Hwang C, Sanda MG. Prospects and limitations of recombinant poxviruses for prostate cancer immunotherapy. Curr Opin Mol Ther 1:471–479, 1999.

125. Kass E, Schlom J, Thompson J, et al. Induction of protective host immunity to carcinoembryonic antigen (CEA), a self-antigen in CEA transgenic mice, by immunizing with a recombinant vaccinia-CEA virus. Cancer Res 59:676–683, 1999.

126. Kass E, Parker J, Schlom J, et al. Comparative studies of the effects of recombinant GM-CSF and GM-CSF administered via a poxvirus to enhance the concentration of antigen-presenting cells in regional lymph nodes. Cytokine 12:960–971, 2000.

127. Kass E, Panicali DL, Mazzara G, et al. Granulocyte/macrophage-colony stimulating factor produced by recombinant avian poxviruses enriches the regional lymph nodes with antigen-presenting cells and acts as an immunoadjuvant. Cancer Res 61:206–214, 2001.

128. Karupiah G, Blanden RV, Ramshaw IA. Interferon gamma is involved in the recovery of athymic nude mice from recombinant vaccinia virus/interleukin 2 infection. J Exp Med 172:1495–1503, 1990.

129. Karupiah G, Coupar BEH, Andrew ME, et al. Elevated natural killer cell responses in mice infected with recombinant vaccinia virus encoding murine IL-2. J Immunol 144:290–298, 1990.

130. Kawakita M, Rao GS, Ritchey JK, et al. Effect of canarypox virus (ALVAC)-mediated cytokine expression on murine prostate tumor growth. J Natl Cancer Inst 89:428–436, 1997.

131. Marshall JL, Hawkins MJ, Tsang KY, et al. Phase I study in cancer patients of a replication-defective avipox recombinant vaccine that expresses human carcinoembryonic antigen. J Clin Oncol 17:332–337, 1999.

132. Marshall JL, Hoyer RJ, Toomey MA, et al. Phase I study in advanced cancer patients of a diversified prime-and-boost vaccination protocol using recombinant vaccinia virus and recombinant nonreplicating avipox virus to elicit anti-carcinoembryonic antigen immune responses. J Clin Oncol 18:3964–3973, 2000.

133. McLaughlin JP, Schlom J, Kantor JA, et al. Improved immunotherapy of a recombinant carcinoembryonic antigen vaccinia vaccine when given in combination with interleukin-2. Cancer Res 56:2361–2367, 1996.

134. Motta I, Andre F, Lim A, et al. Cross-presentation by dendritic cells of tumor antigen expressed in apoptotic recombinant canarypox virus-infected dendritic cells. J Immunol 167:1795–1802, 2001.

135. Lamikanra A, Pan ZK, Isaacs SN, et al. Regression of established human papillomavirus type 16 (HPV-16) immortalized tumors in vivo by vaccinia viruses expressing different forms of HPV-16 E7 correlates with enhanced CD8(+) T-cell responses that are home to the tumor site. J Virol 75:9654–9664, 2001.

136. Lorenz MG, Kantor JA, Schlom J, et al. Induction of anti-tumor immunity elicited by tumor cells expressing a murine LFA-3 analog via a recombinant vaccinia virus. Hum Gene Ther 10:623–631, 1999.

137. Lorenz MG, Kantor JA, Schlom J, et al. Anti-tumor immunity elicited by a recombinant vaccinia virus expressing CD70 (CD27L). Hum Gene Ther 10:1095–1103, 1999.

138. Puisieux I, Odin L, Poujol D, et al. Canarypox virus-mediated interleukin 12 gene transfer into murine mammary adenocarcinoma induces tumor suppression and long-term antitumoral immunity. Hum Gene Ther 9:2481–2492, 1998.

139. Odin L, Favrot M, Poujol D, et al. Canarypox virus expressing wild type p53 for gene therapy in murine tumors mutated in p53. Cancer Gene Ther 8:87–98, 2001.

140. Qin H, Valentino J, Manna S, et al. Gene therapy for head and neck cancer using vaccinia virus expressing IL-2 in a murine model, with evidence of immune suppression. Mol Ther 4:551–558, 2001.

141. Ratliff TL, Kawakita M, Tartaglia J, et al. Canary-pox (ALVAC) virus-mediated cytokine gene therapy induces tumor specific and non-specific immunity against mouse prostate tumor. Acta Urol Belg 64:85, 1996.

142. Rosenwirth B, Kuhn EM, Heeney JL, et al. Safety and immunogenicity of ALVAC wild-type human p53 (vCP207) by the intravenous route in rhesus macaques. Vaccine 19:1661–1670, 2001.

143. Sanda MG, Smith DC, Charles LG, et al. Recombinant vaccinia-PSA (PROSTVAC) can induce a prostate-specific immune response in androgen-modulated human prostate cancer. Urology 53:260–266, 1999.

144. Scholl SM, Balloul JM, Le Goc G, et al. Recombinant vaccinia virus encoding human MUC1 and IL2 as immunotherapy in patients with breast cancer. J Immunother 23:570–580, 2000.

145. Schlom J, Kantor J, Abrams S, et al. Strategies for the development of recombinant vaccines for the immunotherapy of breast cancer. Breast Cancer Res Treat 38:27–39, 1996.

146. Schlom J, Tsang KY, Kantor JA, et al. Strategies in the development of recombinant vaccines for colon cancer. Semin Oncol 26:672–682, 1999.

147. Schutz A, Oertli D, Marti WR, et al. Immunogenicity of nonreplicating recombinant vaccinia expressing HLA-A201 targeted or complete MART-1/Melan-A antigen. Cancer Gene Ther 8:655–661, 2001.

148. Shankar P, Schlom J, Hodge JW. Enhanced activation of rhesus T cells by vectors encoding a triad of costimulatory molecules (B7-1, ICAM-1, LFA-3). Vaccine 20:744–755, 2001.

149. Spagnoli GC, Zajac P, Marti WR, et al. Cytotoxic T-cell induction in metastatic melanoma patients undergoing recombinant vaccinia virus-based immuno-gene therapy. Recent Results Cancer Res 160:195–201, 2002.

150. Toso JF, Oei C, Oshidari F, et al. MAGE-1-specific precursor cytotoxic T-lymphocytes present among tumor-infiltrating lymphocytes from a patient with breast cancer: characterization and antigen-specific activation. Cancer Res 56:16–20, 1996.

151. Tsang KY, Zhu M, Even J, et al. The infection of human dendritic cells with recombinant avipox vectors expressing a costimulatory molecule transgene (CD80) to enhance the activation of antigen-specific cytolytic T cells. Cancer Res 61:7568–7576, 2001.

152. Uzendoski K, Kantor JA, Abrams SI, et al. Construction and characterization of a recombinant vaccinia virus expressing murine intercellular adhesion molecule-1: induction and potentiation of antitumor responses. Hum Gene Ther 8:851–860, 1997.

153. von Mehren M, Arlen P, Tsang KY, et al. Pilot study of a dual gene recombinant avipox vaccine containing both carcinoembryonic antigen (CEA) and B7.1 transgenes in patients with recurrent CEA-expressing adenocarcinomas. Clin Cancer Res 6:2219–2228, 2000.

154. von Mehren M, Arlen P, Gulley J, et al. The influence of granulocyte macrophage colony-stimulating factor and prior chemotherapy on the immunological response to a vaccine (ALVAC-CEA B7.1) in patients with metastatic carcinoma. Clin Cancer Res 7:1181–1191, 2001.

155. Zajac P, Oertli D, Marti WR, et al. Melanoma specific immunotherapy with recombinant vaccinia [abstr 220]. In Abstracts of the Keystone Symposia—Gene-Based Vaccines: Mechanisms, Delivery Systems and Efficacy, Breckenridge, CO, April 10–15, 2002.

156. Zhu MZ, Marshall J, Cole D, et al. Specific cytolytic T-cell responses to human CEA from patients immunized with recombinant avipox-CEA vaccine. Clin Cancer Res 6:24–33, 2000.

157. Zhu M, Terasawa H, Gulley J, et al. Enhanced activation of human T cells via avipox vector-mediated hyperexpression of a triad of co-stimulatory molecules in human dendritic cells. Cancer Res 61:3725–3734, 2001.

158. Berencsi K, Gyulai Z, Gonczol E, et al. A canarypox vector-expressing cytomegalovirus (CMV) phosphoprotein 65 induces long-lasting cytotoxic T cell responses in human CMV-seronegative subjects. J Infect Dis 183:1171–1179, 2001.

159. Bray M, Zhao B, Markoff L, et al. Mice immunized with recombinant vaccinia virus expressing dengue 4 virus structural proteins with or without nonstructural protein NS1 are protected against fatal dengue 4 virus encephalitis. J Virol 63:2853–2856, 1989.

160. Falgout B, Bray M, Schlesinger JJ, et al. Immunization of mice with recombinant vaccinia virus expressing authentic dengue virus nonstructural protein NS1 protects against lethal dengue virus encephalitis. Virology 64:4356–4363, 1990.

161. Geisbert TW, Pushko P, Anderson K, et al. Evaluation in nonhuman primates of vaccines against Ebola virus. Emerg Infect Dis 8:503–507, 2002.

162. Morgan AJ, Mackett M, Finerty S, et al. Recombinant vaccinia virus expressing Epstein-Barr virus glycoprotein gp340 protects cottontop tamarins against virus-induced malignant lymphomas. J Med Virol 25:189–195, 1988.

163. Gu SY, Huang TM, Ruan L, et al. First EBV vaccine trial in humans using recombinant vaccinia virus expressing the major membrane antigen. Dev Biol Stand 84:171–177, 1995.

164. McClain DJ, Summers PL, Harrison SA, et al. Clinical evaluation of a vaccinia-vectored Hantaan virus vaccine. J Med Virol 60:77–85, 2000.

165. Fiedler M, Roggendorf M. Vaccination against hepatitis delta virus infection: studies in the woodchuck (Marmota monax) model. Intervirology 44:154–161, 2001.

166. Moss B, Smith GL, Gerin JL, et al. Live recombinant vaccinia virus protects chimpanzees against hepatitis B. Nature 311:67–69, 1984.

167. Roh S, Lee YK, Ahn BY, et al. Induction of CTL responses and identification of a novel epitope of hepatitis B virus surface antigens in C57BL/6 mice immunized with recombinant vaccinia viruses. Virus Res 73:17–26, 2001.

168. Pancholi P, Liu Q, Tricoche N, et al. DNA prime-canarypox boost with polycistronic hepatitis C virus (HCV) genes generates potent immune responses to HCV structural and nonstructural proteins. J Infect Dis 182:18–27, 2000.

169. Eo SK, Gierynska M, Kamar AA, et al. Prime-boost immunization with DNA vaccine: mucosal route of administration changes the rules. J Immunol 166:5473–5479, 2001.

170. Chen L, Thomas EK, Hu SL, et al. Human papillomavirus type 16 nucleoprotein E7 is a tumor rejection antigen. Proc Natl Acad Sci U S A 88:110–114, 1991.

171. Chen L, Mizuno MT, Singhal MC. Induction of cytotoxic T lymphocytes specific for syngeneic tumour expressing the E6 oncoprotein of human papillomavirus type 16. J Immunol 148:2617–2621, 1992.

172. Meneguzzi G, Cerni C, Kieny MP, et al. Immunization against human papillomavirus type 16 tumor cells with recombinant vaccinia viruses expressing E6 and E7. Virology 181:62–69, 1991.

173. Durbin AP, Cho CJ, Elkins WR. Comparison of the immunogenicity and efficacy of a replication-defective vaccinia virus expressing antigens of human parainfluenza virus type 3 (HPIV3) with those of a live attenuated HPIV3 vaccine candidate in rhesus monkeys passively immunized with PIV3 antibodies. J Infect Dis 179:1345–1351, 1999.

174. Spriggs MK, Collins PL, Tierney E, et al. Immunization with vaccinia virus recombinants that express the surface glycoproteins of human parainfluenza type 3 (PIV3) protects monkeys against PIV3 infection. J Virol 62:1293–1296, 1988.

175. Wyatt LS, Shors ST, Murphy BR, et al. Development of a replication-deficient recombinant vaccinia virus vaccine effective against parainfluenza virus 3 infection in an animal model. Vaccine 14:1451–1458, 1996.

176. Allen TM, Vogel TU, Fuller DH, et al. Induction of AIDS virus-specific CTL activity in fresh, unstimulated peripheral blood lymphocytes from rhesus macaques vaccinated with a DNA prime/modified vaccinia virus Ankara boost regimen. J Immunol 164:4968–4978, 2000.

177. Amara RR, Villinger F, Altman JD, et al. Control of a mucosal challenge and prevention of AIDS by a multiprotein DNA/MVA vaccine. Science 292:69–74, 2001.

178. Andersson S, Makitalo B, Thorstensson R, et al. Immunogenicity and protective efficacy of a human immunodeficiency virus type 2 recombinant canarypox (ALVAC) vaccine candidate in cynomolgus monkeys. Infect Dis 174:977–985, 1996.

179. AIDS Vaccine Evaluation Group 022 Protocol Team. Cellular and humoral immune responses to a canarypox vaccine containing human immunodeficiency virus type 1 Env, Gag, and Pro in combination with rgp120. J Infect Dis 183:563–570, 2001.

180. Barouch DH, Santra S, Kuroda MJ, et al. Reduction of simian-human immunodeficiency virus 89.6P viremia in rhesus monkeys by recombinant modified vaccinia virus Ankara vaccination. J Virol 75:5151–5158, 2001.

181. Boudet F, Chevalier M, Jourdier TM, et al. Modulation of the antibody response to the HIV envelope subunit by co-administration of infectious or heat-inactivated canarypoxvirus (ALVAC) preparations. Vaccine 19:4267–4275, 2001.

182. Belshe RB, Clements ML, Dolin R, et al. Safety and immunogenicity of a fully glycosylated recombinant gp160 human immunodeficiency virus type I vaccine in subjects at low risk of infection. J Infect Dis 168:1387–1395, 1993.

183. Belshe RB, Gorse GJ, Mulligan MJ, et al. Rapid induction of HIV-1 immune responses by canarypox (ALVAC) HIV-1 and gp120 SF2 recombinant vaccines in uninfected volunteers. AIDS 12:2407–2415, 1998.

184. Egan MA, Pavlat WA, Tartaglia J, et al. Induction of human immunodeficiency virus type 1 (HIV-1)-specific cytolytic T lymphocyte responses in seronegative adults by a nonreplicating, host-range-restricted canarypox vector (ALVAC) carrying the HIV-1MN env gene. J Infect Dis 171:1623–1627, 1995.

185. Girard M, Yue L, Barre-Sinoussi F, et al. Failure of a human immunodeficiency virus type 1 (HIV-1) subtype B-derived vaccine to prevent infection of chimpanzees by an HIV-1 subtype E strain. J Virol 70:8229–8230, 1996.

186. Girard M, van der Ryst E, Barre-Sinoussi F, et al. Challenge of chimpanzees immunized with a recombinant canarypox-HIV-1 virus. Virology 232:98–104, 1997.

187. Girard M, Meignier B, Barre-Sinoussi F, et al. Vaccine-induced protection of chimpanzees against infection by a heterologous human immunodeficiency virus type 1. J Virol 69:6239–6248, 1995.

188. Girard M. Antiviral vaccines. Med Trop 59:522–526, 1999.

189. Gorse GJ, Patel GB, Belshe RB. HIV type 1 vaccine-induced T cell memory and cytotoxic T lymphocyte responses in HIV type 1-uninfected volunteers. AIDS Res Hum Retroviruses 17:1175–1189, 2001.

190. Gorse GJ, Patel GB, Mandava MD, et al. Cytokine responses to human immunodeficiency virus type 1 (HIV-1) induced by immunization with live recombinant canarypox virus vaccine expressing HIV-1 genes boosted by HIV-1 (SF-2) recombinant GP120. Vaccine 19:1806–1819, 2001.

191. Gherardi MM, Ramirez JC, Rodriguez D, et al. IL-12 delivery from recombinant vaccinia virus attenuates the vector and enhances the cellular immune response against HIV-1 Env in a dose-dependent manner. J Immunol 162:6724–6733, 1999.

192. Gherardi MM, Ramirez JC, Esteban M. Interleukin-12 (IL-12) enhancement of the cellular immune response against human immunodeficiency virus type 1 env antigen in a DNA prime/vaccinia virus boost vaccine regimen is time and dose dependent: suppressive effects of IL-12 boost are mediated by nitric oxide. J Virol 74:6278–6286, 2000.

193. Gherardi MM, Ramirez JC, Esteban M. Towards a new generation of vaccines: the cytokine IL-12 as an adjuvant to enhance cellular immune responses to pathogens during prime-booster vaccination regimens. Histol Histopathol 16:655–667, 2001.

194. Graham BS, Belshe RB, Clements ML, et al. Vaccination of vaccinia-naive adults with human immunodeficiency virus type-1 gp160 recombinant vaccinia virus in a blinded, controlled, randomized clinical trial. J Infect Dis 166:244–252, 1992.

195. Graham BS, Matthews TJ, Belshe RB, et al. Augmentation of human immunodeficiency virus type-1 neutralizing antibody by priming with gp160 recombinant vaccinia and boosting with rgpl60 in vaccinia-naive adults. J Infect Dis 167:533–537, 1993.

196. Hanke T, McMichael AJ. Design and construction of an experimental HIV-1 vaccine for a year-2000 clinical trial in Kenya. Nat Med 6:951–955, 2000.

197. Hurpin C, Rotarioa C, Bisceglia H, et al. The mode of presentation and route of administration are critical for the induction of immune responses to p53 and antitumor immunity. Vaccine 16:208–215, 1998.

198. Hel Z, Venzon D, Poudyal M, et al. Viremia control following antiretroviral treatment and therapeutic immunization during primary SIV251 infection of macaques. Nat Med 6:1140–1146, 2000.

199. Hel Z, Tsai WP, Thornton A, et al. Potentiation of simian immunodeficiency virus (SIV)-specific CD4(+) and CD8(+) T cell responses by a DNA-SIV and NYVAC-SIV prime/boost regimen. J Immunol 167:7180–7191, 2001.

200. Hel ZK, Nacsa J, Tryniszewska E, et al. Containment of simian immunodeficiency virus infection in vaccinated macaques: correlation with the magnitude of virus-specific pre- and postchallenge CD4+ and CD8+ T cell responses. J Immunol 169:4778–4787, 2002.

201. Kaslow RA, Rivers C, Tang J, et al. Polymorphisms in HLA class I genes associated with both favorable prognosis of human immunodeficiency virus (HIV) type 1 infection and positive cytotoxic T-lymphocyte responses to ALVAC-HIV recombinant canarypox vaccines. J Virol 75:8681–8689, 2001.

202. Kent SJ, Zhao A, Dale CJ, et al. A recombinant avipoxvirus HIV-1 vaccine expressing interferon-gamma is safe and immunogenic in macaques. Vaccine 18:2250–2256, 2000.

203. Kent SJ, Zhao A, Best SJ, et al. Enhanced T-cell immunogenicity and protective efficacy of a human immunodeficiency virus type 1 vaccine regimen consisting of consecutive priming with DNA and boosting with recombinant fowlpox virus. J Virol 72:10180–10188, 1998.

204. Montefiori DC, Safrit JT, Lydy SL, et al. Induction of neutralizing antibodies and gag-specific cellular immune responses to an R5 primary isolate of human immunodeficiency virus type 1 in rhesus macaques. J Virol 75:5879–5890, 2001.

205. Pialoux G, Excler JL, Riviere Y, et al. A prime-boost approach to HIV preventive vaccine using a recombinant canarypox virus expressing glycoprotein 160 (MN) followed by a recombinant glycoprotein 160 (MN/LAI). AIDS Res Hum Retroviruses 11:373–381, 1995.

206. Nilsson C, Makitalo B, Berglund P, et al. Enhanced simian immunodeficiency virus-specific immune responses in macaques induced by priming with recombinant Semliki Forest virus and boosting with modified vaccinia virus Ankara. Vaccine 19:3526–3536, 2001.

207. Negri DR, Baroncelli S, Michelini Z, et al. Effect of vaccination with recombinant modified vaccinia virus Ankara expressing structural and regulatory genes of SIV(macJ5) on the kinetics of SIV replication in cynomolgus monkeys. J Med Primatol 30:197–206, 2001.

208. Pal R, Venzon D, Letvin NL, et al. ALVAC-SIV-gag-pol-env-based vaccination and macaque major histocompatibility complex class I (A*01) delay simian immunodeficiency virus SIVmac-induced immunodeficiency. J Virol 76:292–302, 2002.

209. Patterson LJ, Peng B, Abimiku AG, et al. Cross-protection in NYVAC-HIV-1-immunized/HIV-2-challenged but not in NYVAC-HIV-2-immunized/SHIV-challenged rhesus macaques. AIDS 14:2445–2455, 2000.

210. Salmon-Ceron D, Excler JL, Finkielsztejn L, et al. Safety and immunogenicity of a live recombinant canarypox virus expressing HIV type 1 gp120 MN160/Mntm/gag/protease (ALVAC-HIV, vCP205) followed by a p24E-V3MN synthetic peptide (CLTB-36) administered in healthy volunteers at low risk of HIV infection. AIDS Res Hum Retroviruses 15:633–645, 1999.

211. Salmon-Ceron D, Excler JL, Sicard D, et al. Safety and immunogenicity of a recombinant HIV type 1 glycoprotein 160 boosted by a V3 synthetic peptide in HIV-negative volunteers. AIDS Res Hum Retroviruses 11:1479–1486, 1995.

212. Salmon-Ceron D, Pialoux G, Excler JL, et al. Immunogenicity of booster injections of recombinant canarypox vectors or peptide in volunteers pre-immunized in HIV-1 Phase I trials [abstr 111]. In Abstracts of the Conference on Advances in AIDS Vaccine Development, Bethesda, MD, 1997.

213. Salmon D, Excler JL, Finkielsztejn L, et al. Immunogenicity of a live recombinant canarypoxvirus expressing gp120TM-MN/gag/protease–LAI (vCP205) boosted with a p24e/V3-MN peptide (CLTB36) in HIV-negative volunteers (ANRS Vac 03) [abstr Mo.A.155]. In Abstracts of the XIth International Conference on AIDS, Vancouver, July 1996.

214. Sharpe S, Polyanskaya N, Dennis M, et al. Induction of simian immunodeficiency virus (SIV)-specific CTL in rhesus macaques by vaccination with modified vaccinia virus Ankara expressing SIV transgenes: influence of pre-existing anti-vector immunity. J Gen Virol 82:2215–2223, 2001.

215. Shen L, Chen ZW, Miller MD, et al. Recombinant virus vaccine-induced SIV-specific CD8+ cytotoxic T lymphocytes. Science 252:440–443, 1991.

216. Seth A, Ourmanov I, Schmitz JE, et al. Immunization with a modified vaccinia virus expressing simian immunodeficiency virus (SIV) Gag-Pol primes for an anamnestic Gag-specific cytotoxic T-lymphocyte response and is associated with reduction of viremia after SIV challenge. J Virol 74:2502–2509, 2000.

217. Tartaglia J, Franchini G, Robert-Guroff M, et al. Highly attenuated poxvirus strains, NYVAC and ALVAC, in retrovirus vaccine development. In Girard M, Valette L (eds). Retroviruses of Human AIDS and Related Animal Diseases (Huitieme Colloque des Cent Gardes, Mardes-La-Coquette, Paris, France). Paris, Pasteur Merieux Serums et Vaccins/ANRS, 1994, pp 293–298.

218. Tartaglia J, Benson J, Cornet B, et al. Potential improvement for poxvirus-based immunizations vehicles. In Girard M, Dodet B (eds). Retroviruses of Human AIDS and Related Animal Disease (11th Colloque des Cent Gardes). Marnes-La-Coquelte, Elsevier, 1998, pp 187–197.

219. Walther-Jallow L, Nilsson C, Soderlund J, et al. Cross-protection against mucosal simian immunodeficiency virus (SIVsm) challenge in human immunodeficiency virus type 2-vaccinated cynomolgus monkeys. J Gen Virol 82(pt 7):1601–1612, 2001.

220. Wilson SE, Pedersen SL, Kunich JC, et al. Cross-clade envelope glycoprotein 160-specific CD8+ cytotoxic T lymphocyte responses in early HIV type 1 clade B infection. AIDS Res Hum Retroviruses 14:925–937, 1998.

221. Wee EG, Patel S, McMichael AJ, et al. A DNA/MVA-based candidate human immunodeficiency virus vaccine for Kenya induces multi-specific T cell responses in rhesus macaques. J Gen Virol 83(pt 1):75–80, 2002.

222. Zheng R. Technology evaluation: HIVAC-1e. Curr Opin Mol Ther 1:121–125, 1999.

223. Bures R, Gaitan A, Zhu T, et al. Immunization with recombinant canarypox vectors expressing membrane-anchored glycoprotein 120 followed by glycoprotein 160 boosting fails to generate antibodies that neutralize R5 primary isolates of human immunodeficiency virus type 1. AIDS Res Hum Retroviruses 16:2019–2035, 2000.

224. Clements-Mann ML, Weinhold K, Matthews TJ, et al. Immune responses to human immunodeficiency virus (HIV) type 1 induced by canarypox expressing HIV-1MN gp120, HIV-1SF2 recombinant gp120, or both vaccines in seronegative adults. NIAID AIDS Vaccine Evaluation Group. J Infect Dis 177:1230–1246, 1998.

225. Cooney EL, McElrath MJ, Corey L, et al. Enhanced immunity to human immunodeficiency virus (HIV) envelope elicited by a combined vaccine regimen consisting of priming with a vaccinia recombinant expressing HIV envelope and boosting with gp160-protein. Proc Natl Acad Sci U S A 90:1882–1886, 1993.

226. Coeffier E, Excler JL, Kieny MP, et al. Restricted specificity of anti-V3 antibodies induced in humans by HIV candidate vaccines. AIDS Res Hum Retroviruses 13:1471–1485, 1997.

227. Collado M, Rodriguez D, Rodriguez JR, et al. Chimeras between the human immunodeficiency virus (HIV-1) Env and vaccinia virus immunogenic proteins p14 and p39 generate in mice broadly reactive antibodies and specific activation of CD8+ T cell responses to Env. Vaccine 18:3123–3133, 2000.

228. Evans TG, Keefer MC, Weinhold KJ, et al. A canarypox vaccine expressing multiple human immunodeficiency virus type 1 genes given alone or with rgp120 elicits broad and durable CD8+ cytotoxic T lymphocyte responses in seronegative volunteers. J Infect Dis 180:290–298, 1999.

229. Evans T, Corey L, Clements-Mann ML, et al. CD8+ CTL induced in AIDS Vaccine Evaluation Group Phase I trials using canarypox vectors (ALVAC) encoding multiple HIV gene products (vCP125,vCP205, vCP300) given with or without subunit boost [abstr 495/21192]. AIDS 12:277, 1998.

230. Fleury B, Janvier G, Pialoux G, et al. Memory cytotoxic T lymphocyte responses in human immunodeficiency virus type 1 (HIV-1)-negative volunteers immunized with a recombinant canarypox expressing gp160 of HIV-1 and boosted with a recombinant gp160. J Infect Dis 174:734–738, 1996.

231. Franchini G, Benson J, Gallo R, et al. Attenuated poxvirus vectors as carriers in vaccines against human T cell leukemia-lymphoma virus type I. AIDS Res Hum Retroviruses 12:407–408, 1996.

232. Abimiku AG, Franchini G, Tartaglia J, et al. HIV-1 recombinant poxvirus vaccine induces cross-protection against HIV-2 challenge in rhesus macaques. Nat Med 1:321–329, 1995.

233. Belshe RB, Stevens C, Gorse GJ, et al. Safety and immunogenicity of a canarypox-vectored HIV-1 vaccine with or without gp120:a phase 2 study in higher-and- lower risk volunteers. J Infect Dis 183(9):1343–1352, 2001.

234. Degano P, Schneider J, Hannan CM, et al. Gene gun intradermal DNA immunization followed by boosting with modified vaccinia virus Ankara: enhanced CD8+ T cell immunogenicity and protective efficacy in the influenza and malaria models. Vaccine 18:623–632, 1999.

235. Sambhara S, Kurich A, Miranda R, et al. Severe impairment of primary but not memory responses to influenza viral antigens in aged mice: costimulation in vivo partially reverses impaired primary immune responses. Cell Immunol 210:1–4, 2001.

236. Swayne DE, Beck JR, Kinney N. Failure of a recombinant fowl poxvirus vaccine containing an avian influenza hemagglutinin gene to provide consistent protection against influenza in chickens preimmunized with a fowl pox vaccine. Avian Dis 44:132–137, 2000.

237. Ulmer JB, Donnelly JJ, Parker SE, et al. Heterologous protection against influenza by injection of DNA encoding a viral protein. Science 259:1745–1749, 1993.

238. Yewdell JW, Bennink JR, Smith GL, et al. Influenza A virus nucleoprotein is a major target for cross-reactive anti-influenza virus cytotoxic T lymphocytes. Proc Natl Acad Sci U S A 82:1785–1789, 1985.

239. Lawson CM, Bennink JR, Restifo NP, et al. Primary pulmonary cytotoxic T lymphocytes induced by immunization with a vaccinia virus recombinant expressing influenza A virus nucleoprotein peptide do not protect mice against challenge. J Virol 68:3505–3511, 1994.

240. Stitz L, Schmitz C, Binder D, et al. Characterization and immunological properties of influenza A virus nucleoprotein (NP): cell-associated NP isolated from infected cells or viral NP expressed by vaccinia recombinant virus do not confer protection. J Gen Virol 71:1169–1179, 1990.

241. Konishi E, Pincus S, Paoletti E, et al. A highly attenuated host range-restricted vaccinia virus strain, NYVAC, encoding the prM, E, and NS1 genes of Japanese encephalitis virus prevents JEV viremia in swine. Virology 190:454–458, 1992.

242. Kanesa-thasan N, Smucny JJ, Hoke CH, et al. Safety and immunogenicity of NYVAC-JEV and ALVAC-JEV attenuated recombinant Japanese encephalitis virus–poxvirus vaccines in vaccinia-nonimmune and vaccinia-immune humans. Vaccine 19:483–491, 2000.

243. Nam JH, Cha SL, Cho HW. Immunogenicity of a recombinant MVA and a DNA vaccine for Japanese encephalitis virus in swine. Microbiol Immunol 46:23–28, 2002.

244. Djavani M, Yin C, Lukashevich IS, et al. Mucosal immunization with Salmonella typhimurium expressing Lassa virus nucleocapsid protein cross-protects mice from lethal challenge with lymphocytic choriomeningitis virus. J Hum Virol 4:103–108, 2001.

245. Gonzalo RM, Rodriguez JR, Rodriguez D, et al. Protective immune response against cutaneous leishmaniasis by prime/booster immunization regimens with vaccinia virus recombinants expressing Leishmania infantum p36/LACK and IL-12 in combination with purified p36. Microbes Infect 3:701–711, 2001.

246. Aguiar JC, Hedstrom RC, Rogers WO, et al. Enhancement of the immune response in rabbits to a malaria DNA vaccine by immunization with a needle-free jet device. Vaccine 20:275–280, 2001.

247. Gilbert SC, Schneider J, Hannan CM, et al. Enhanced CD8 T cell immunogenicity and protective efficacy in a mouse malaria model using a recombinant adenoviral vaccine in heterologous prime-boost immunisation regimes. Vaccine 20:1039–1045, 2002.

248. Doolan DL, Sedegah M, Hedstrom RC, et al. Circumventing genetic restriction of protection against malaria with multigene DNA immunization: CD8+ cell-, interferon gamma-, and nitric oxide-dependent immunity. J Exp Med 183:1739–1746, 1996.

249. Doolan DL, Hoffmann SL. Multi-gene vaccination against malaria: a multi-stage, multi-immune response approach. Parasitol Today 13:171–178, 1997.

250. Sedegah M, Hedstrom R, Hobart P, et al. Protection against malaria by immunization with plasmid DNA encoding circumsporozoite protein. Proc Natl Acad Sci U S A 91:9866–9870, 1994.

251. Sedegah M, Jones TR, Kaur M, et al. Boosting with recombinant vaccinia increases immunogenicity and protective efficacy of malaria DNA vaccine. Proc Natl Acad Sci U S A 95:7648–7653, 1998.

252. Schneider J, Gilbert SC, Blanchard TJ, et al. Enhanced immunogenicity for CD8+ T cell induction and complete protective efficacy of malaria DNA vaccination by boosting with modified vaccinia virus Ankara. Nat Med 4:397–402, 1998.

253. Schneider J, Langermans JA, Gilbert SC, et al. A prime-boost immunisation regimen using DNA followed by recombinant modified vaccinia virus Ankara induces strong cellular immune responses against the Plasmodium falciparum TRAP antigen in chimpanzees. Vaccine 19:4595–4602, 2001.

254. Hill AV, Reece W, Gothard P, et al. DNA-based vaccines for malaria: a heterologous prime-boost immunisation strategy. Dev Biol (Basel) 104:171–179, 2000.

255. Rogers WO, Baird JK, Kumar A, et al. Multistage multiantigen heterologous prime boost vaccine for Plasmodium knowlesi malaria provides partial protection in rhesus macaques. Infect Immun 69:5565–5572, 2001.

256. Dong W, Li M, Bi H, et al. Assessment of a vaccinia virus vectored multi-epitope live vaccine candidate for Plasmodium falciparum. Int J Parasitol 31:57–62, 2001.

257. Hoffman SL, Doolan DL. Can malaria DNA vaccines on their own be as immunogenic and protective as prime-boost approaches to immunization? Dev Biol (Basel) 104:121–132, 2000.

258. Langford DJ, Edwards SJ, Smith GL, et al. Anchoring a secreted plasmodium antigen on the surface of recombinant vaccinia virus infected cells increases its immunogenicity. Mol. Cell. Biol. 6:3191–3199, 1986.

259. Zhu Y, Rota P, Wyatt L, et al. Evaluation of recombinant vaccinia virus–measles vaccines in infant rhesus macaques with preexisting measles antibody. Virology 276:202–213, 2000.

260. Weidinger G, Ohlmann M, Schlereth B, et al. Vaccination with recombinant modified vaccinia virus Ankara protects against measles virus infection in the mouse and cotton rat model. Vaccine 19:2764–2768, 2001.

261. Stittelaar KJ, Wyatt LS, de Swart RL, et al. Protective immunity in macaques vaccinated with a modified vaccinia virus Ankara-based measles virus vaccine in the presence of passively acquired antibodies. J Virol 74:4236–4243, 2000.

262. Kovarik J, Gaillard M, Martinez X, et al. Induction of adult-like antibody, Th1, and CTL responses to measles hemagglutinin by early life murine immunization with an attenuated vaccinia-derived NYVAC(K1L) viral vector. Virology 285:12–20, 2001.

263. Malin AS, Huygen K, Content J, et al. Vaccinia expression of Mycobacterium tuberculosis-secreted proteins: tissue plasminogen activator signal sequence enhances expression and immunogenicity of M. tuberculosis Ag85. Microbes Infect 2:1677–1685, 2000.

264. Feng CG, Blanchard TJ, Smith GL, et al. Induction of CD8⁺ T-lymphocyte responses to a secreted antigen of Mycobacterium tuberculosis by an attenuated vaccinia virus. Immunol Cell Biol 79:569–575, 2001.

265. McShane H, Behboudi S, Goonetilleke N, et al. Protective immunity against Mycobacterium tuberculosis induced by dendritic cells pulsed with both CD8(+)- and CD4(+)-T-cell epitopes from antigen 85A. Infect Immun 70:1623–1626, 2002.

266. Fries LF, Tartaglia J, Taylor J, et al. Human safety and immunogenicity of a canarypox-rabies glycoprotein recombinant vaccine: an alternative poxvirus vector system. Vaccine 14:428–434, 1996.

267. Tartaglia J, Singh-Sandhu D, Strady A, et al. Safety of NYVAC-Rabies (vP879) a live attenuated recombinant vaccine in healthy adult volunteers: Phase I clinical trial. Unpublished manuscript, Aventis Pasteur, Toronto (Canada), 2002.

268. Connors M, Kulkarni AB, Collins PL, et al. Resistance to respiratory syncytial virus (RSV) challenge induced by infection with a vaccinia virus recombinant expressing the RSV M2 protein (VacM2) is mediated by CD8⁺ T cells, while that induced by Vac-F or Vat-G recombinants is mediated by antibodies. J Virol 66:1277–1281, 1992.

269. Feldman SA, Crim RL, Audet SA, et al. Human respiratory syncytial virus surface glycoproteins F, G, and SH form an oligomeric complex. Arch Virol 146:2369–2383, 2001.

270. Johnson TR, Fischer JE, Graham BS. Construction and characterization of recombinant vaccinia viruses co-expressing a respiratory syncytial virus protein and a cytokine. J Gen Virol 82(pt 9):2107–2116, 2001.

271. Olmsted RA, Elango N, Prince GA, et al. Expression of the F glycoprotein of respiratory syncytial virus by a recombinant vaccinia virus: comparison of the individual contributions of the F and G glycoproteins to host immunity. Proc Natl Acad Sci U S A 83:7462–7466, 1986.

272. Maresova L, Pasieka TJ, Grose C. Varicella-zoster virus gB and gE coexpression, but not gB or gE alone, leads to abundant fusion and syncytium formation equivalent to those from gH and gL coexpression. J Virol 75:9483–9492, 2001.

273. Kutinova L, Hainz P, Ludvikova V, et al. Immune response to vaccinia virus recombinants expressing glycoproteins gE, gB, gH, and gL of Varicella-zoster virus. Virology 280:211–220, 2001.

274. Stittelaar KJ, Kuiken T, de Swart RL, et al. Safety of modified vaccinia virus Ankara (MVA) in immune-suppressed macaques. Vaccine 19:3700–3709, 2001.

275. Hirsch VM, Fuerst TR, Sutter G, et al. Patterns of viral replication correlate with outcome in simian immunodeficiency virus (SIV)-infected macaques: effect of prior immunization with a trivalent SIV vaccine in modified vaccinia virus Ankara. J Virol 70:3741–3752, 1996.

276. Carroll MW, Overwijk WW, Chamberlain RS, et al. Highly attenuated modified vaccinia virus Ankara (MVA) as an effective recombinant vector: a murine tumor model. Vaccine 15:387–394, 1997.

277. Caroll MW, Restifo MW. Poxviruses as vectors for cancer immunotherapy. In Stern PL, Beverley PLC, and Carroll MW (eds). Cancer Vaccines and Immunotherapy. Cambridge, Cambridge University Press, 2000, pp 47–62.

278. Belyakov IM, Moss B, Strober W, et al. Mucosal vaccination overcomes the barrier to recombinant vaccinia immunization caused by preexisting poxvirus immunity. Proc Natl Acad Sci U S A 96:4512–4517, 1999.

279. Ramshaw IA, Ramsay AJ. The prime-boost strategy: exciting prospects for improved vaccination. Immunol Today 21:163–165, 2000.

280. Ramirez JC, Gherardi MM, Rodriguez D, et al. Attenuated modified vaccinia virus Ankara can be used as an immunizing agent under conditions of preexisting immunity to the vector. J Virol 74:7651–7655, 2000.

281. Estcourt MJ, Ramsay AJ, Brooks A, et al. Prime-boost immunization generates a high frequency, high-avidity CD8(+) cytotoxic T lymphocyte population. Int Immunol 14:31–37, 2002.

282. Benson J, Chougnet C, Robert-Guroff M, et al. Recombinant vaccine-induced protection against the highly pathogenic simian immunodeficiency virus SIV(mac251): dependence on route of challenge exposure. J Virol 72:4170–4182, 1998.

283. Coffin J, Haase A, Levy JA, et al. What to call the AIDS virus? Nature 321:10, 1986.

284. Barre-Sinoussi F, Chermann JC, Rey F, et al. Isolation of a T-lymphotropic retrovirus from a patient at risk for acquired immune deficiency syndrome (AIDS). Science 220:868–871, 1983.

285. Clavel F, Mansiho K, Chamaret S, et al. HIV type 2 infection associated with AIDS in West Africa. N Engl J Med 316:1180–1185, 1987.

286. Heeney JL. Primate models for AIDS vaccine development. AIDS 10(suppl A):S115–S122, 1996.

287. Feinberg MB, Moore JP. AIDS vaccine models: challenging challenge viruses. Nat Med 8:207–210, 2002.

288. Novembre FJ, Saucier M, Anderson DC, et al. Development of AIDS in a chimpanzee infected with human immunodeficiency virus type I. J Virol 71:4086–4091, 1997.

289. Hirsch VM, Johnson PR. Pathogenic diversity of simian immunodeficiency viruses. Virus Res 32:183–203, 1994.

290. Letvin NL, King NW. Immunologic and pathologic manifestations of the infection of rhesus monkeys with simian immunodeficiency virus of macaques. J Acquir Immune Defic Syndr 3:1023–1040, 1990.

291. Li JT, Lord CI, Haseltine W, et al. Infection of cynomolgus monkeys with a chimeric HIV-1/SIVmac virus that expresses the HIV-1 envelope glycoproteins. J Acquir Immune Defic Syndr 5:639–646, 1992.

292. Li JT, Halloran M, Lord CI, et al. Persistent infection of macaques with simian-human immunodeficiency viruses. J Virol 69:7061–7067, 1995.

293. Luciw PA, Pratt-Lowe E, Shaw KE, et al. Persistent infection of rhesus macaques with T-cell line-tropic and macrophage-tropic clones of simian/human immunodeficiency viruses (SHIV). Proc Natl Acad Sci U S A 92:7490–7494, 1995.

294. Reimann KA, Li JT, Veazey R, et al. A chimeric simian/human immunodeficiency virus expressing a primary patient human immunodeficiency virus type I isolate env causes an AIDS-like disease after in vivo passage in rhesus monkeys. J Virol 70:6922–6928, 1996.

295. Zagury D, Bernard J, Cheynier R, et al. A group specific anamnestic immune reaction against HIV-1 induced by a candidate vaccine against AIDS. Nature 332:728–731, 1988.

296. Lockey TD, Slobod KS, Caver TE, et al. Multi-envelope HIV vaccine safety and immunogenicity in small animals and chimpanzees. Immunol Res 21:7–21, 2000.

297. Barrett N, Mitterer A, Mundt W, et al. Large-scale production and purification of a vaccinia recombinant-derived HIV-1 gp160 and analysis of its immunogenicity. AIDS Res Hum Retroviruses 5:159–171, 1989.

298. Earl PL, Hugin AW, Moss B. Removal of cryptic poxvirus transcription termination signals from the human immunodeficiency virus type 1 envelope gene enhances expression and immunogenicity of a recombinant vaccinia virus. J Virol 64:2448–2451, 1990.

299. Earl PL, Wyatt LS, Montefiori DC, et al. Comparison of vaccine strategies using recombinant env-gag-pol MVA with or without an oligomeric Env protein boost in the SHIV rhesus macaque model. Virology 294:278–281, 2002.

300. Engelmayer J, Larsson M, Lee A, et al. Mature dendritic cells infected with canarypox virus elicit strong anti-human immunodeficiency virus CD8+ and CD4+ T-cell responses from chronically infected individuals. J Virol 75:2142–2153, 2001.

301. Cox WI, Tartaglia J, Paoletti E. Induction of cytotoxic T lymphocytes by recombinant canarypox (ALVAC) and attenuated vaccinia (NYVAC) viruses expressing the HIV-1 envelope glycoprotein. Virology 195:845–850, 1993.

302. Ferrari G, Humphrey W, McElrath MJ, et al. Clade B-based HIV-1 vaccinees elicit cross-clade cytotoxic T lymphocyte reactivities in uninfected volunteers. Proc Natl Acad Sci U S A 94:1396–1401, 1997.

303. Hu SL, Fultz PN, McClure HM, et al. Effect of immunization with a vaccinia-HIV env recombinant on HIV infection of chimpanzees. Nature 328:721–723, 1987.

304. Ourmanov I, Brown CR, Moss B, et al. Comparative efficacy of recombinant modified vaccinia virus Ankara expressing simian immunodeficiency virus (SIV) Gag-Pol and/or Env in macaques challenged with pathogenic SIV. J Virol 74:2740–2751, 2000.

305. Santra S, Schmitz JE, Kuroda MJ, et al. Recombinant canarypox vaccine-elicited CTL specific for dominant and subdominant simian immunodeficiency virus epitopes in rhesus monkeys. J Immunol 168:1847–1853, 2002.

306. Cho MW, Kim YB, Lee MK, et al. Polyvalent envelope glycoprotein vaccine elicits a broader neutralizing antibody response but is unable to provide sterilizing protection against heterologous simian/human immunodeficiency virus infection in pigtailed macaques. J Virol 75:2224–2234, 2001.

307. Exceler JL, Plotkin S. The prime-boost concept applied to HIV preventive vaccines. AIDS 11(suppl A):127–137, 1997.

308. Newman MJ. Heterologous prime-boost vaccination strategies for HIV-1: augmenting cellular immune responses. Curr Opin Invest Drugs 3:374–378, 2002.

309. Hu SL, Abrams K, Barber GN, et al. Protection of macaques against SIV infection by subunit vaccines of SIV envelope glycoprotein gp160. Science 255:456–459, 1992.

310. Myagkikh M, Alipanah S, Markham PD, et al. Multiple immunizations with attenuated poxvirus HIV type 2 recombinants and subunit boosts required for protection of rhesus macaques. AIDS Res Hum Retroviruses 12:985–992, 1996.

311. Robinson HL. Multiprotein DNA priming and recombinant poxvirus boosting for an AIDS vaccine [abstr 005]. In Abstracts of the Keystone Symposia—Gene-Based Vaccines: Mechanisms, Delivery Systems and Efficacy, Breckenridge, CO, April 10–15, 2002.

312. Dale CJ, Zhao A, Jones SL, et al. Induction of HIV-1-specific T-helper responses and type 1 cytokine secretion following therapeutic vaccination of macaques with a recombinant fowlpoxvirus co-expressing interferon-gamma. J Med Primatol 29:240–247, 2000.

313. Corey L, McElrath MJ, Weinhold K, et al, for the AIDS Vaccine Evaluation Group. Cytotoxic T cell and neutralising antibody responses to human immunodeficiency virus type 1 envelope with a combination vaccine regime. J Infect Dis 177:301–309, 1998.

314. Fast P, Walker MC, Ketter N, et al. Evaluation of candidate HIV-1 prophylactic vaccines in phase I/II trials. In Retroviruses of Human AIDS and related Animal Diseases (M Girard and L Valette, eds.), Huitieme Collque des Cent Gardes, Marnes-La-Coquette, Paris, Pasteur Merieux Serums et Vaccins/ANRS, Paris, 271–279, 1994.

315. Esparaza J. Twenty years into the HIV/AIDS epidemic, and the hope of a preventive vaccine. Sixth European Conference on Experimental AIDS Research, Edinburgh, UK, 2001.

316. Ferrari G, Berend C, Ottinger J, et al. Replication-defective canarypox (ALVAC) vectors effectively activate anti-human immunodeficiency virus-1 cytotoxic T lymphocytes present in infected patients: implications for antigen-specific immunotherapy. Blood 15: 90(6):2406–2416, 1997.

317. Bojak A, Deml L, Wagner R. The past, present, and future of HIV-vaccine development: a critical view. Drug Discov Today 7(1):36–46, 2002.

318. McMichael A, Hanke T. The quest for an AIDS vaccine: is the CD8+ T-cell approach feasible. Nat Rev Immunol 2:283–291, 2002.

319. Robinson HL. New hope for an AIDS vaccine. Nat Rev Immunol 2:239–250, 2002.

320. Letvin NL, Barouch DH, Montefiori D. Prospects for vaccine protection against HIV-1 infection and AIDS. Annu Rev Immunol 20:73–99, 2002.

321. Ghadersohi, A, Chitta, K, Greco WR, et al. Tumour antigens and markers for breast and ovarian cancers. Front Biosci 7:48–57, 2002.

322. Rosenberg SA. A new era for cancer immunotherapy based on the genes that encode cancer antigens. Immunity 10:281–287, 1999.

323. Sgroi DC, Teng S, Robinson G, et al. In vivo gene expression profile analysis of human cancer progression. Cancer Res 59:5656–5661, 1999.

324. Schena M, Shalon D, Davis RW, et al. Quantitative monitoring of gene expression with a cDNA microarray. Science 270:467–470, 1995.

325. Offringa R, van der Burg SH, Ossendorp F, et al. Design and evaluation of antigen-specific vaccination strategies against cancer. Curr Opin Immunol 12:576–582, 2000.

326. De Plaen E, Lurquin C, Lethe B, et al. Identification of genes coding for tumour antigens recognized by cytolytic T lymphocytes. Methods 12:125–142, 1997.

327. Boon T, Coulie PG, Eynde BVD. Tumour cells recognized by T cells. Immunol Today 18:267–268, 1997.

328. Sidransky D. Emerging molecular markers of cancer. Nat Rev 2:210–219, 2002.

329. Scanlan MJ, Jager D. Challenges to the development of antigen-specific breast cancer vaccines. Breast Cancer Res 3:95–98, 2001.

330. Rosenberg SA. Cancer vaccines based on the identification of genes encoding cancer regression antigens. Immunol Today 18:175–182, 1997.

331. Eder JP, Kantoff PW, Roper K, et al. A Phase I trial of a recombinant vaccinia virus expressing prostate-specific antigen in advanced prostate cancer. Clin Cancer Res 6:1632–1638, 2000.

332. Huang EH, Kaufman HL. CEA-based vaccines. Expert Rev Vaccines 1:49–63, 2002.

333. Bonnet MC, Tartaglia J, Verdier F, et al. Recombinant viruses as a tool for therapeutic vaccination against human cancers. Immunol Lett 74:11–25, 2000.

334. Palmowski MJ, Choi EML, Hermans IF, et al. Competition between CTL narrows the immune response induced by prime-boost vaccination protocols. J Immunol 168:4391–4398, 2002.

335. Ghose A, Iakhnina E, Spaner D, et al. Immunogenicity of whole-cell tumor preparations infected with the ALVAC viral vector. Hum Gene Ther 11:1289–1301, 2000.

336. Siemens DR, Iwasawa T, Austin JC, et al. Biomarker distribution after injection into the canine prostate: implications for gene therapy. BJU Int 86:1076–1083, 2000.

337. Siemens DR, Austin JC, Hedican SP, et al. Viral vector delivery in solid-state vehicles: gene expression in a murine prostate cancer model. J Natl Cancer Inst 92:403–412, 2000.

338. Morse MA. Technology evaluation: CEA-TRICOM, Therion Biologics Corp. Curr Opin Mol Ther 3(4):407–412, 2001.

339. Wade-Evans AM, Atott J, Hanke T, et al. Specific proliferative T cell responses and antibodies elicited by vaccination with simian immunodeficiency virus Nef do not confer protection against virus challenge. AIDS Res. Hum. Retroviruses 17(16):1517–1526, 2001.

340. Wallack MK, Sivanandham M, Balch CM, et al. Surgical adjuvant active specific immunotherapy for patients with stage III melanoma: the final analysis of data from a phase III, randomized, double-blind, multicenter vaccinia melanoma oncolysate trial. J Am Coll Surg 187(1):69–77, 1998.

341. McAneny D, Ryan C, Beazley R, et al. Results of a phase I clinical trial using a recombinant vaccinia-carcinoembryonic antigen (CEA) vaccine in patients with advanced colorectal cancer. Ann Surg Oncol 3(5):495–500, 1996.

342. Kwak H, Hong H, Kaufman HL. Poxviruses as vectors for cancer immunotherapy. Curr Opin Drug Discov Devel 6(2): 161–168, 2003.

343. Breeman JG, Henderson DA. Diagnosis and management of smallpox. NEJM, 346:1300–1308, 2002.

344. Cono J, Casey CG, Bell DM. Smallpox vaccination and adverse reactions. Guidance for clinicians MMWR 52(RR):1–28, 2003.

345. Smith GL, McFadden G. Smallpox: anything to declare? Nature Reviews Immunology 2:521–527, 2002.

346. Hallaron ME, Longini Jr. IM, Nizam A, et al. Containing Bioterrorist Smallpox. Science, 298:1428–1432, 2002.

347. Lane JM, Ruben FL, Abrutyn E, et al. Deaths attributable to smallpox vaccination, 1959 to 1966, and 1968. JAMA 212: 441–444, 1970.

348. Rosenthal SR, Merchlinsky M, Keppinger C, et al. Developing new smallpox vaccines. Emerging Infect Dis 7:920–926, 2001.

349. Cohen J. Looking for vaccines that pack a Wallop without the side effects. Science 298:2314, 2002

350. Acambis Press Release (*http://www.acambis.com/default.asp?id=486'* Accessed on 25th March 2003.

351. Kempe CH, Fulginiti V, Minamitani M, et al. Small pox vaccination of eczema patients with a strain of attenuated live vaccine (CVI-78). Pediatrics 42:980–985, 1968.

352. Ober BT, Bruhl P, Schmidt M, et al. Immunogenicity and safety of defective vaccinia virus Lister: Comparison with modified Vaccinia Virus Ankara. J Virol 76:7713–7723, 2002.

Chapter 50

Respiratory Syncytial Virus Vaccine

RUTH A. KARRON

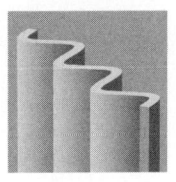

Respiratory syncytial virus (RSV) is the most important cause of viral lower respiratory tract illness (LRI) in infants and children worldwide.[1,2] In the United States, it is estimated that approximately 70,000 to 126,000 infants are hospitalized annually with RSV pneumonia or bronchiolitis, and that the rate of hospitalization for bronchiolitis has increased since 1980.[3] Though traditionally regarded as a pediatric pathogen, RSV also can cause life-threatening pulmonary disease in bone marrow transplant (BMT) recipients.[4] The elderly are also at risk for severe RSV disease,[5–8] and 14,000 to 62,000 RSV-associated hospitalizations of the elderly occur annually in the United States.[6]

Although the importance of RSV as a respiratory pathogen has been recognized for over 40 years, a vaccine is not yet available because of several problems inherent in RSV vaccine development. The peak of severe disease and mortality associated with pediatric RSV infection occurs in infants less than 3 months of age, who often have high titers of RSV maternally derived antibody. These young infants may not respond adequately to vaccination because of immunologic immaturity and/or suppression of the immune response by maternally derived antibody.[1,9–11] An RSV vaccine also will need to protect against the antigenically divergent groups A and B (see *The Virus* below). Most importantly, the vaccine must not potentiate naturally occurring RSV disease, as was observed with the formalin-inactivated RSV (FI-RSV) vaccine[12–14] (see *Past Experience: Formalin-Inactivated Respiratory Syncytial Virus Vaccine* below). Because serious RSV disease can occur in high-risk individuals who have experienced previous RSV infection as well as RSV-naive infants, it is likely that more than one type of RSV vaccine will be needed to immunize all of those who would benefit from vaccination. This chapter describes recent efforts to develop safe and effective RSV vaccines for the various populations at risk.

Background

Clinical Disease

Reinfection with RSV occurs throughout life, though disease manifestations differ. In young children, RSV infection is associated with a spectrum of respiratory illness, ranging from mild upper respiratory illness (URI) to life-threatening bronchiolitis and pneumonia. RSV is also the principal cause of viral otitis media in children.[17] In infants less than 6 weeks old, poor feeding and lethargy may predominate, and apnea may occur in the absence of other respiratory signs or symptoms.[18] In children hospitalized with RSV, mortality is estimated to be approximately 1%, though it is severalfold higher in infants who are premature[19,20] or who have chronic lung disease,[21] congenital heart disease,[22] or primary immunodeficiency disorders.[23,24] RSV is the leading viral cause of hospitalization and reduction in pulmonary function for children with cystic fibrosis.[16,25,26] In the United States, human immunodeficiency virus (HIV)–infected children often shed RSV for prolonged periods, but do not usually have more severe disease than their non–HIV infected counterparts[27]; however, more severe RSV disease may occur in HIV-infected children in developing countries.[28]

The potential link between RSV infection in early childhood and subsequent development of reactive airway disease remains an open question. Infants hospitalized with RSV infection frequently have demonstrable abnormalities in pulmonary function for years after the initial event, though they may ultimately become symptom free.[29] However, it is not clear whether RSV causes abnormal airway function, or is only one of many triggers in susceptible individuals.[29,30] Ultimately, an intervention that minimizes the severity of RSV disease (such as universal use of an RSV vaccine in infancy) may help to resolve this issue.

In healthy young adults, RSV infection generally is associated with mild URI.[31] Elderly adults attending adult day care or in long-term care facilities who are infected with RSV may have rhinorrhea (67% to 92%), cough (90% to 97%), fever (20% to 56%), and/or wheezing (6% to 35%).[8] Pneumonia occurs in up to 10% of these individuals.[32]

Immunocompromised patients, particularly those with hematologic malignancies and those undergoing BMT, are at high risk for severe RSV disease.[33] In these patients, URI precedes LRI, and the presence of rhinorrhea, sinusitis, and/or otalgia are clinical features that may help to distinguish between RSV and cytomegalovirus pneumonia.[4,8,16,34–36] The severity of disease depends on the magnitude of immunosuppression, with rates of pneumonia up to 75% in leukemic patients[37] and 79% in BMT patients.[38] For BMT recipients, infection that occurs pre-engraftment is associated with the highest risk of pneumonia and death, but mortality is still high (50% to 70%) in those who develop pneumonia postengraftment.[38]

The Virus

RSV is a member of the genus *Pneumovirus* of the family Paramyxoviridae. This virus has a genome comprised of a single strand of negative-sense RNA that is tightly associated with viral protein to form the nucleocapsid. The viral envelope is composed of a plasma membrane–derived lipid bilayer that contains virally encoded transmembrane proteins. A viral polymerase is packaged within the virion that transcribes genomic RNA into messenger RNA. RSV is composed of 15,222 nucleotides that encode three transmembrane surface proteins (F, G, and SH), two matrix proteins (M and M2), three nucleocapsid proteins (N, P, and L), and two nonstructural proteins (NS1 and NS2). The surface fusion (F) and attachment (G) glycoproteins are the only viral components that induce RSV neutralizing antibody and therefore are important targets of vaccine development. The F protein, in combination with proteins G and SH, is responsible for fusion of the viral envelope with the host cell membranes and for the characteristic syncytium formation in cell culture. Its genome is highly conserved between RSV groups. The G protein mediates attachment to the host cell surface, and is largely responsible for the antigenic diversity observed between RSV groups (see below). A secreted form of the G protein that lacks the N-terminal signal/anchor region also is produced, and it is reported that up to 80% of the G glycoprotein released from cells 24 hours after infection is in this secreted form.[39] The function of the secreted G protein is not known, though it may serve as a decoy for RSV neutralizing antibody.[40]

Cross-neutralization studies have shown that RSV isolates can be classified into two groups, designated A and B.[41] Although RSV A and B strains differ in all 10 viral proteins, the G glycoprotein shows the greatest divergence between groups, with only 53% amino acid homology between prototype RSV A and B viruses.[42] Group A RSV infection may cause more severe disease than group B RSV, though this has not been definitively established.[43,44] The impact of this antigenic dimorphism is not completely understood, but young children experiencing their second RSV infection frequently are reinfected with virus from the same group.[45]

Epidemiology

By 2 years of age, almost all children will have been infected with RSV, and approximately 50% will have been infected twice.[46] Reinfection can occur throughout life and is usually symptomatic; however, RSV infection generally does not cause LRI in immunocompetent adults and healthy older children.[31]

RSV epidemics occur yearly during winter and early spring in temperate climates and in the rainy season in some but not all tropical climates.[47,48] RSV group A and group B viruses co-circulate during epidemics, though one may predominate.[49–52] Humans are the only known reservoir for RSV. Spread of this highly contagious virus from contaminated nasal secretions occurs via large droplets rather than small-particle aerosols, so close contact with an infected individual or contaminated environmental surface is required for transmission.[53] RSV can persist as a fomite on hard surfaces for several hours,[54,55] and for this reason is an important cause of nosocomial respiratory illness, particularly on pediatric wards.[55]

Mechanisms of Immunity and Correlates of Protection

Virus-specific immune responses are largely responsible for protection against RSV-associated LRI and recovery from RSV infection. Immunity to RSV is mediated via humoral and cellular effectors, including serum antibody (acquired as a result of infection or maternally derived in young infants), secretory antibody, and major histocompatibility complex class I–restricted cytotoxic T lymphocytes. The RSV F glycoprotein also may elicit innate immune responses via toll-like receptors and CD14.[56,57] Natural immunity to RSV is incomplete and reinfection occurs throughout life, as has been demonstrated by epidemiologic studies,[46,58] and challenge studies in healthy young adults.[59] Healthy older children and adults, however, usually are protected against RSV-associated LRI. In general, humoral immune responses (secretory and serum antibodies) appear to protect against infection of the upper and lower respiratory tract, respectively, while cell-mediated responses directed against internal proteins appear to terminate infection. Although the adoptive transfer of primed T cells will halt RSV replication in immunodeficient mice, the adoptive transfer of RSV-specific cytotoxic T lymphocytes also may potentiate disease,[60] suggesting that there may be an immune component to RSV illness.

The role of local immunity in the protection of the upper respiratory tract against RSV is suggested by experimental data from studies in cotton rats,[61–63] and adult volunteers,[64] and by observational data from infants.[65] In adults, the presence of secretory neutralizing antibody, but not serum antibody, correlated with protection of the upper respiratory tract against RSV infection.[64] In infants, the development of immunoglobulin A (IgA) in nasal secretions correlated temporally with viral clearance following natural infection.[65]

RSV replicates exclusively in the respiratory epithelium. For this reason, serum neutralizing antibody does not prevent infection, as it does for pathogens that produce viremia, such as measles and varicella. However, high titers of RSV serum neutralizing antibody protect the lower respiratory tract against RSV infection, as has been demonstrated by animal studies,[61–63] epidemiologic observations in infants and young children,[66–68] and clinical trials of RSV hyperimmune globulin and monoclonal antibody in high-risk infants (see *Passive Immunization* below).

Primary infection with RSV does not always elicit an immune response that will protect the lower respiratory tract, because RSV-associated LRI can occur in young children experiencing their second episode of RSV.[46,68] Young infants develop levels of neutralizing antibody and F and G glycoprotein antibodies to RSV that are only 15% to 25% of those observed in older children.[69] The suboptimal response of young infants to primary infection with RSV has important implications for vaccine development because it suggests that more than one dose of vaccine likely will be needed to induce adequate levels of RSV serum neutralizing antibody in this population.

The immunologic requirements for protection against severe RSV disease are not clearly defined. Although it is known that a high level of serum neutralizing antibody (titer >1:200, as measured in a plaque reduction neutralization assay) is sufficient,[70,71] it is not known whether it is necessary. In adults and older children who have been previously infected with RSV, it is reasonable to expect that an effective RSV vaccine will boost levels of serum neutralizing antibodies. However, it is conceivable that vaccination may protect young RSV-naïve infants against severe RSV, even if high titers of neutralizing antibodies are not induced. In these infants, "challenge" with a second dose of a live, attenuated vaccine may help to predict whether some protection has been conferred by the first dose[72] (see *Biologically Derived Live, Attenuated Vaccines* below). Ultimately, correlates of protection against severe disease in young infants will have to be evaluated in the context of efficacy trials.

Passive Immunization

Based on experimental data in animals[61–63] and epidemiologic data in humans[68] suggesting that RSV neutralizing antibody protected against LRI, two products containing high titers of RSV neutralizing antibody were developed for clinical administration. The first of these, RSV Immune Globulin Intravenous (RSV-IGIV; RespiGam™), led to significant reductions in the rate and severity of LRI when administered to high-risk infants at doses of 750 mg/kg.[70] The titer of RSV neutralizing antibody achieved in infants who received this dose of RSV-IGIV was comparable to that demonstrated to protect the lungs of cotton rats against RSV infection in earlier studies.[70,71] The protective effect of RSV-IGIV in these young infants was confirmed by a subsequent placebo-controlled trial.[73] More recently, a monoclonal neutralizing antibody directed against the RSV F glycoprotein (palivizumab; Synagis™) also was shown to reduce the risk of hospitalization for RSV disease in premature infants and infants with chronic lung disease.[74] Because palivizumab is 50- to 100-fold more potent than RSV-IGIV, it can be administered intramuscularly in monthly doses. In infants with cyanotic heart disease, RSV-IGIV was associated with an increased incidence of adverse events,[70,75,76] but a recent Phase III study demonstrated that palivizumab was safe and effective in preventing hospitalizations for RSV in children with congenital heart disease.[77] Currently, the American Academy of Pediatrics recommends that high-risk infants receive prophylaxis during the RSV season.[76] Phase I trials also showed that palivizumab was well tolerated in a small number of BMT recipients.[78] Although the prophylactic efficacy of RSV-IGIV and palivizumab have been established, neither appears to ameliorate RSV disease when given therapeutically.[79,80]

Vaccine Development

General Considerations

A successful RSV vaccine should prevent serious RSV-associated LRI in those at risk. The primary target populations for RSV vaccines are very young infants and the elderly, though older high-risk children also would benefit from RSV immunization. It is likely that different vaccines will be needed for the various target populations: nonreplicating vaccines may be useful in the elderly, in high-risk older children, and for maternal immunization, but live virus vaccines are likely to be required for RSV-naïve infants.

Past Experience: Formalin-Inactivated Respiratory Syncytial Virus Vaccine

In the early 1960s, an FI-RSV was prepared and tested in infants and children. This vaccine, designated lot 100, was administered as 2 or 3 intramuscular doses separated by 1 to 3 months to infants and children between 2 months and 7 years of age.[12–14,81] Lot 100 not only failed to protect against wild-type (wt) RSV disease, but induced an exaggerated clinical response to wt RSV infection in infants who were RSV naïve prior to vaccination. Many vaccinees were hospitalized with LRI; in one study, the hospitalization rate of vaccinees approached 80% compared to 5% in controls.[12] Tragically, two infants who received lot 100 died following wt RSV infection, one at 14 months and the second at 16 months of age.[12] RSV was readily isolated from the lower respiratory tracts of these infants.

The mechanisms responsible for the FI-RSV vaccine-associated disease enhancement are still not completely understood. However, data obtained from lot 100 recipients[81–83] and from studies in rodent models[84–87] have led to the hypothesis that children vaccinated with FI-RSV remained susceptible to infection with wt RSV because vaccination produced inadequate levels of serum neutralizing antibodies and did not induce local immunity. Once infected with wt RSV, virus was not readily cleared because FI-RSV did not prime for a CD8+ cytotoxic T-cell response, and the viral infection produced a direct cytopathic effect in the lower respiratory tracts of these infants. In addition, immunization with FI-RSV primed for a type 2 helper T-cell–like response, with increased local production of interleukin (IL)-4, IL-5, and IL-10; an influx of lymphocytes and eosinophils; the possible release of additional mediators;

and resultant inflammation and bronchoconstriction.[88–91] Recently, we showed that immune complexes play a role in enhanced RSV disease through studies in mice and by demonstration of complement activation in the lungs of children who received lot 100 and died following wt RSV infection.[92]

The clinical experience with FI-RSV and the information gleaned from animal models of disease enhancement suggest key features of an RSV vaccine for seronegative infants. The vaccine should induce protective levels of neutralizing antibody, as well as CD8[+] RSV-specific cytotoxic T cells, and a pattern of CD4 response like that evoked by wt RSV. Although a live, attenuated vaccine is most likely to exhibit these characteristics,[9,89] it is possible that novel immunization strategies that combine nonreplicating vaccines with cytokines or new adjuvants might achieve these goals.[88,91]

Live Attenuated Respiratory Syncytial Virus Vaccines

Live attenuated vaccines may offer several advantages over nonreplicating vaccines, especially for RSV-naïve infants and young children. Intranasal immunization with a live, attenuated vaccine should induce both systemic and local immunity and therefore protect against URI as well as LRI. Also, the immune response to a live vaccine should closely resemble the response to natural infection and therefore not produce enhanced disease on exposure to wt virus.[9] Like other live attenuated intranasal respiratory virus vaccine candidates,[10,11] a live intranasal RSV vaccine candidate has been shown to replicate in young infants in the presence of maternally acquired antibody.[72] This feature will be critical for the success of a live attenuated RSV vaccine in young infants. A live attenuated RSV vaccine probably will need to be administered in multiple doses to young infants.

Biologically Derived Live, Attenuated Vaccines

Several strategies for the development of a live attenuated vaccine were originally explored, including the creation of host-range mutants, cold-passaged (cp) mutants, and temperature-sensitive (ts) mutants (which are unable to grow at high temperatures). Based on previous experience with live attenuated influenza vaccines,[93,94] growth of the cp and ts mutants in vivo was expected to be restricted, particularly in the lower respiratory tract (at core body temperature). The clinical evaluation of mutants developed between 1968 and 1976 that were either cp or ts (designated cpRSV [lot 3131], RSV ts-1, and RSV ts-2) has been extensively summarized elsewhere.[9,90,95] In brief, these vaccine candidates were either underattenuated (cpRSV and RSV ts-1) or overattenuated (RSV ts-2), and reversion to a wt (ts+) phenotype was observed in viral isolates obtained from infants and children who received the RSV ts-1 mutant. Transmission of the ts-1 mutant from vaccinated children to placebo recipients also occurred.[96,97] Importantly, enhanced disease was not observed when infants who received RSV ts-1 or cpRSV were naturally infected with wt RSV.[96,98] Although these early attempts to develop a live, attenuated RSV vaccine were unsuccessful, they established the use of placebo-controlled, double-blind trials with postvaccination surveillance through RSV epidemics as the model for future evaluation of live, attenuated RSV vaccines in children. In addition, cpRSV is the progenitor of the cptsRSV vaccines recently evaluated in children (Table 50–1; see below).

Investigators in the United Kingdom developed three ts mutants of RSV A, which were derived from the RSS-2 strain by chemical mutagenesis of virus grown in the MRC-5 human diploid cell line[99,100] (see Table 50–1). Though attenuated in comparison to wt RSV, two of these mutants caused URI in adults and therefore were not sufficiently attenuated for further evaluation in children.[99] Replication of the third mutant was not associated with illness in adults,[100] but this candidate has not been evaluated in children.

A series of live attenuated RSV A cpts candidate vaccines were derived from further attenuation of cpRSV through chemical mutagenesis. This process generated ts candidate vaccines with a range of shutoff temperatures (35° to 37°C) that displayed a spectrum of attenuation in

TABLE 50–1 ■ RSV Vaccines Evaluated in Clinical Trials Since 1990

Vaccine	Composition	Manufacturer	Subjects	Status
	SUBUNIT			
PFP-1, -2, -3	Purified F protein	Wyeth	Adults, children[*]	Active
BBG2Na	RSV G peptide-BB[†]	Pierre Fabre	Adults[‡]	Inactive
RSV A subunit	Co-purified F, G, M proteins	Aventis Pasteur	Adults	Active
FG	Recombinant FG fusion protein	SmithKline Beecham	Adults	Inactive
	LIVE, ATTENUATED			
ts-1A, B, C	RSV A ts mutants	MRC	Adults	Inactive
cp or cpts[§]	Serially passaged derivatives of cpRSV A2	NIH or Wyeth/NIH	Adults,[‡] children, infants	Inactive
Recombinant RSV	Recombinant derivatives of cpRSV A2[‖]	Wyeth/NIH	Adults, children, infants	Active

[*]Includes healthy adults, the elderly, pregnant women, and healthy and high-risk RSV-seropositive children.
[†]BB is the albumin-binding domain of streptococcal protein G, and functions as a carrier protein.
[‡]Healthy adults and the elderly.
[§]Includes cpRSV, which was evaluated in adults, and cpts248/955, cpts530/1009, cpts530/1030, and cpts248/404, each of which was evaluated in RSV-naïve children as young as 6 months. The cpts248/404 vaccine was evaluated in infants as young as 1 month of age.
[‖]Includes mutants with multiple ts mutations and/or deletions of nonessential genes.

rodents and nonhuman primates.[101–104] Each of these candidate vaccines was shown to protect chimpanzees against challenge with wt RSV.[101,102,105] Candidate vaccine viruses recovered from chimpanzees and nude mice showed greater stability of the *ts* phenotype than had previously been observed with the *ts*-1 virus.[90]

Several of these candidate intranasally administered vaccines were evaluated in Phase I clinical trials[72,105] (see Table 50–1). The *cpts*248/955 and 530/1009 vaccines were evaluated sequentially in adults, RSV-seropositive children, and RSV-seronegative children as young as 6 months. Although both *cpts*248/955 and 530/1009 were attenuated in adults and seropositive children, neither was sufficiently attenuated in seronegative children to permit evaluation in very young infants.[105] However, the *cpts*248/404 vaccine was subsequently evaluated in children and infants as young as 1 month old. The *cpts*248/404 vaccine was highly attenuated in these infants but caused nasal congestion that in some instances interfered with feeding and sleeping.[72] The *cpts* 248/404 vaccine also induced serum neutralizing antibody and RSV immunoglobulin G and IgA responses in children over 6 months of age, whereas predominantly IgA responses were observed in the younger infants.[72] Surveillance conducted in the RSV season following vaccination did not demonstrate disease enhancement but provided preliminary evidence of protection against symptomatic RSV infection.[72] Ninety-eight percent (173 of 176) of the isolates maintained the full *ts* phenotype; 3 isolates from a single subject showed an alteration in phenotype accompanied by a nucleotide substitution at the 404 site.

Although the *cpts*248/404 vaccine was not sufficiently attenuated for young infants, evaluation of this vaccine candidate provided important information regarding replication and immunogenicity of a live attenuated RSV vaccine in the presence of maternal antibodies, phenotypic stability of a *cpts* vaccine, and preliminary evidence of protection against illness following wt RSV infection.[72]

Genetically Engineered (Complementary DNA–Derived) Live, Attenuated Vaccines

The ability to recover infectious virus from complementary DNA (cDNA) clones of RSV[106] (Fig. 50–1) has provided insight into the genetic basis of attenuation of biologically derived vaccines and hastened the development of additional live, attenuated RSV vaccine candidates through the use of recombinant technology.[40,107] Mutations present in *cp*RSV and six of its *ts* derivatives were inserted into wt RSV singly and in combination, and the majority of attenuating mutations were found to occur in the polymerase gene, with a notable exception being the 404 mutation in the M gene start signal (Fig. 50–2).[40,107–109] Using this information, attenuating mutations from biologically derived vaccines have been combined to produce further attenuated vaccine candidates.[40,107,110] Deletion of a nonessential gene (SH, NS1, NS2, or M2-2[111]) in combination with known attenuating *cp* and *ts* mutations might also produce a highly attenuated, genetically stable vaccine (see Fig. 50–2).[112,113] Recombinant RSV vaccines containing *cp*, *ts*, and deletion mutations currently are being evaluated in clinical trials.[114] Foreign genes also can be inserted into a recombinant RSV genome,[115] so that a cDNA-derived bivalent RSV vaccine might be developed that contained the G genes from RSV

A and B.[115–117] Alternatively, immunomodulating genes (e.g., granulocyte-macrophage colony-stimulating factor) might be introduced in an effort to enhance immunogenicity in young infants.[115,118–120]

Recombinant technology also provides the opportunity for creation of chimeric viruses containing the RSV F and G surface glycoproteins, with one or more internal genes provided by related respiratory viruses. For example, a chimeric vaccine containing the bovine parainfluenza virus type 3 (PIV-3) backbone, human PIV-3 surface glycoproteins, and RSV F and G glycoproteins induced an immune response to both human PIV-3 and RSV in rhesus monkeys.[121] Chimeric viruses containing genes from human and bovine RSV also have been created.[40,122] Although native bovine RSV does not protect chimpanzees against human RSV challenge,[123] recombinant human/bovine chimeric vaccines may prove more successful.[40,122]

Subunit Vaccines

RSV F and G, the viral glycoproteins that induce neutralizing and protective antibodies (reviewed by Collins et al.[1]), have been evaluated as potential candidate vaccines. Subunit vaccines are most likely to be useful for immunization of the elderly and high-risk children, and might also be used for maternal immunization. Vaccines that have

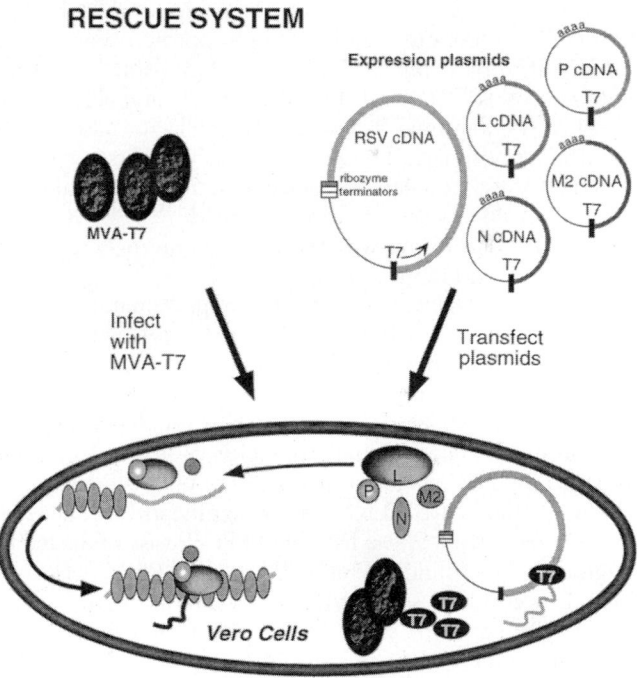

FIGURE 50–1 ■ Recombinant strains of RSV have been generated using genomic rescue technology.[104] A plasmid containing the full-length RSV antigenome cDNA and four "helper" plasmids containing the RSV L, N, P, and M2 (open reading frame 1) genes are transfected into Vero cells. The RSV antigenome and helper genes, under control of the bacteriophage T7 RNA polymerase promoter, are expressed following infection with MVA-T7 pol virus. Infectious RSV is recovered, amplified, and then biologically cloned by terminal dilution. The cloned virus is amplified in Vero cells to make Good Manufacturing Practices vaccine lots for use in Phase I clinical trials. (Courtesy of Drs. Valerie Randolph and Christopher Park, Wyeth Vaccines, Pearl River, NY).

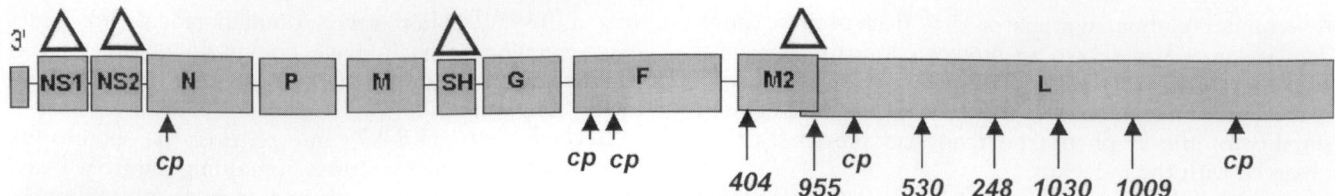

FIGURE 50–2 ■ Schematic of the RSV genome, showing the location of 11 attenuating mutations identified by genetic characterization of biologically derived attenuated virus strains: 5 *cp* mutations (in the N, F, and L genes), 5 *ts* mutations in the polymerase (L) gene (248, 955, 530, 1009, and 1030), and 1 *ts* mutation in the M2 gene start sequence (404). In addition, four attenuating "nonessential" gene deletions (ΔM2-2, ΔNS1, ΔNS2, and ΔSH) were identified by animal growth studies using recombinant RSV gene deletion mutants. These genes are not required for viral replication, and each attenuates wt RSV in primates. (Courtesy of Drs. Valerie Randolph and Christopher Park, Wyeth Vaccines, Pearl River, NY).

recently been evaluated in clinical trials include purified F glycoproteins[124–131]; co-purified F, G, and M proteins[132]; and BBG2Na, a peptide from the G glycoprotein conjugated to the albumin-binding domain of streptococcal protein G[133–136] (see Table 50–1). A chimeric RSV FG fusion protein vaccine was evaluated in Phase I trials in adults but is not being pursued further (S Holmes, personal communication, February, 2002).

RSV F subunit vaccines have been evaluated in healthy adults, in children over 12 months with and without chronic underlying pulmonary disease (chronic lung disease of prematurity or cystic fibrosis), in institutionalized and ambulatory elderly subjects, and in pregnant women.[125–131,137] These vaccines, designated purified F protein (PFP)-1, PFP-2, and PFP-3, contain the RSV F glycoprotein purified by immunoaffinity column (PFP-1) or ion exchange chromatography (PFP-2 and PFP-3). PFP-1 and PFP-2 are adsorbed to aluminum hydroxide, and PFP-3 is adsorbed to aluminum phosphate. The PFP vaccines have been well tolerated in these populations: acute reactions were minimal and enhanced disease was not observed.[125–131,137] In addition, 50 μg of vaccine was the most immunogenic of the doses tested, and fourfold or greater rises in RSV neutralizing antibody titers were observed in approximately 50% to 75% of the vaccinees, depending on the levels of preimmunization neutralizing antibodies. A meta-analysis of PFP-1 and PFP-2 studies in adults and children concluded that these vaccines appeared to reduce the incidence of RSV infections, though the heterogeneity of the populations studied raised doubts about the validity of this conclusion. The incidence of RSV LRI was not significantly reduced.[138]

Most recently, a Phase I study of PFP-2 was conducted in pregnant women and a Phase III study of PFP-3 was conducted in children with cystic fibrosis. Thirty-five women in the 30th to 34th week of uncomplicated pregnancies were randomized to receive either 50 μg of PFP-2 vaccine or saline placebo. PFP-2 was well tolerated and immunogenic in these women. All 35 infants were born healthy, and there was no difference in neonatal and perinatal outcomes between vaccine and placebo recipients. During RSV season, there was no increase in the frequency or morbidity associated with respiratory illness in infants of vaccine recipients. The geometric mean titers of RSV F antibody were fourfold higher in the children born of immunized mothers than those born of placebo recipients at birth, 2 months, and 6 months after delivery. Levels of RSV neutralizing antibody were not described.[131]

The efficacy trial of PFP-3 vaccine in children with cystic fibrosis was conducted based on previous studies that demonstrated reduction in numbers of LRI episodes (though not in episodes of RSV infection) in 34 children with cystic fibrosis who received PFP-2 vaccine or placebo.[139] In the Phase III trial, 298 children 1 to 12 years of age with cystic fibrosis were immunized with 30 μg of PFP-3/aluminum phosphate vaccine or aluminum phosphate alone. The vaccine was safe, well tolerated, and immunogenic, with 67% of subjects showing a fourfold rise in neutralizing antibody titer to RSV-A and 55% to RSV-B. However, there were no statistically significant differences in the frequency of LRI episodes in vaccine or placebo recipients (V LaPosta, personal communication, January, 2002).

A subunit vaccine consisting of co-purified F, G, and M proteins from RSV A has been administered intramuscularly to healthy adults with either alum or polydicarboxylatophenoxy-phosphazene (PCPP) as an adjuvant[132] (see Table 50–1). Both formulations of the vaccine were well tolerated and comparably immunogenic, with twofold and fourfold increases in neutralizing antibody titers detected in 96% to 100% and 76% to 83% of vaccinees, respectively. In this previously primed population, neutralizing antibody responses to RSV A and RSV B were detected with comparable frequency. Follow-up studies 1 year after the initial vaccination demonstrated that neutralizing antibody titers had waned but could be boosted by revaccination, suggesting that annual immunization with this vaccine will be necessary. Studies of this vaccine in other populations are in progress.

BBG2Na is a prokaryotically expressed fusion protein that consists of the central conserved region of the G glycoprotein from the RSV A long strain (residues 130 to 230) fused to the albumin-binding domain of streptococcal protein G, which acts as a carrier protein.[133–135,140,141] Residues 158 to 190 are conserved among RSV A isolates, and 163 to 174 are conserved among RSV A and B isolates.[142] Despite induction of only modest levels of RSV neutralizing antibody,[135] BBG2Na protected rodents against challenge with RSV, and sera from RSV-seropositive individuals was found to react with peptides derived from this region.[143] In Phase I trials, 10-, 100-, or 300-μg doses of BBG2Na in alum were well tolerated in healthy young adults.[136] Four weeks after immunization, the 100- and 300-μg doses of vaccine induced twofold or greater increases in neutralizing antibody in 33% to 71% of vaccinees.[136] In Phase II trials, two episodes of type 3 hypersensitivity reactions (purpura) were observed. An efficacy trial of BBG2Na in the elderly is in progress.

Conclusions

In the past decade, tremendous progress has been made in the development of RSV vaccines. Currently, two types of candidate vaccines are being evaluated in clinical trials: subunit vaccines for immunization of the elderly, RSV-seropositive children at high risk for severe RSV disease, and pregnant women; and live attenuated vaccines that would be used primarily for immunization of young infants, and possibly for immunization of the elderly. It is possible that combinations of different types of vaccines might be needed for certain populations: for example, optimal immune responses in the elderly might result from simultaneous administration of a live and a nonreplicating RSV vaccine.[137] The availability of recombinant technology should allow further refinement of existing live, attenuated candidate vaccines to produce engineered vaccines that are satisfactorily attenuated, immunogenic, and phenotypically stable.

REFERENCES

1. Collins PL, McIntosh K, Chanock RM. Respiratory syncytial virus. In Fields BN (ed). Fields Virology. New York, Raven Press, 1996, pp 1313–1351.
2. Hall CB. Prospects for a respiratory syncytial virus vaccine. Science 265:1393–1394, 1994.
3. Shay DK, Holman RC, Newman RD, et al. Bronchiolitis-associated hospitalizations among US children, 1980–1996. JAMA 282:1440–1446, 1999.
4. Fouillard L, Mouthon L, Laporte JP, et al. Severe respiratory syncytial virus pneumonia after autologous bone marrow transplantation: a report of three cases and review. Bone Marrow Transplant 9:97–100, 1992.
5. Falsey AR, Treanor JJ, Betts RF, Walsh EE. Viral respiratory infections in the institutionalized elderly: clinical and epidemiologic findings. J Am Geriatr Soc 40:115–119, 1992.
6. Han LL, Alexander JP, Anderson LJ. Respiratory syncytial virus pneumonia among the elderly: an assessment of disease burden. J Infect Dis 179:25–30, 1999.
7. Falsey AR. Respiratory syncytial virus infection in older persons. Vaccine 16:1775–1778, 1998.
8. Falsey AR, Walsh EE. Respiratory syncytial virus infection in adults. Clin Microbiol Rev 13:371–384, 2000.
9. Murphy BR, Hall SL, Kulkarni AB, et al. An update on approaches to the development of respiratory syncytial virus (RSV) and parainfluenza virus type 3 (PIV3) vaccines. Virus Res 32:13–36, 1994.
10. Clements ML, Makhene MK, Karron RA, et al. Effective immunization with live attenuated influenza A virus can be achieved in early infancy. J Infect Dis 173:44–51, 1996.
11. Karron RA, Steinhoff MC, Subbarao EK, et al. Safety and immunogenicity of a cold-adapted influenza A (H1N1) reassortant virus vaccine administered to infants less than six months of age. Pediatr Infect Dis J 14:10–16, 1995.
12. Kim HW, Canchola JG, Brandt CD, et al. Respiratory syncytial virus disease in infants despite prior administration of antigenic inactivated vaccine. Am J Epidemiol 89:422–434, 1969.
13. Kapikian AZ, Mitchell RH, Chanock RM, et al. An epidemiologic study of altered clinical reactivity to respiratory syncytial (RS) virus infection in children previously vaccinated with an inactivated RS virus vaccine. Am J Epidemiol 89:405–421, 1969.
14. Fulginiti VA, Eller JJ, Sieber OF, et al. Respiratory virus immunization. I. A field trial of two inactivated respiratory virus vaccines: an aqueous trivalent parainfluenza virus vaccine and an alum-precipitated respiratory syncytial virus vaccine. Am J Epidemiol 89:435–448, 1969.
15. Hall CB. Respiratory syncytial virus: a continuing culprit and conundrum. J Pediatr 135(suppl):S2–S7, 1999.
16. Hall CB. Respiratory syncytial virus and parainfluenza virus. N Engl J Med 344:1917–1928, 2001.
17. Heikkinen T, Thint M, Chonmaitree T. Prevalence of various respiratory viruses in the middle ear during acute otitis media. N Engl J Med 340:260–264, 1999.
18. Hall CB, Kopelman AE, Douglas RG Jr, et al. Neonatal respiratory syncytial virus infection. N Engl J Med 300:393–396, 1979.
19. Cunningham CK, McMillan JA, Gross SJ. Rehospitalization for respiratory illness in infants of less than 32 weeks' gestation. Pediatrics 88:527–532, 1991.
20. Berkovich S. Acute respiratory illness in the premature nursery associated with respiratory syncytial virus infections. Pediatrics 34:753–760, 1964.
21. Groothuis JR, Gutierrez KM, Lauer BA. Respiratory syncytial virus infection in children with bronchopulmonary dysplasia. Pediatrics 82:199–203, 1988.
22. MacDonald NE, Hall CB, Suffin SC, et al. Respiratory syncytial viral infection in infants with congenital heart disease. N Engl J Med 307:397–400, 1982.
23. Fishaut M, Tubergen D, McIntosh K. Cellular response to respiratory viruses with particular reference to children with disorders of cell-mediated immunity. J Pediatr 96:179–186, 1980.
24. McIntosh K, Kurachek SC, Cairns LM, et al. Treatment of respiratory viral infection in an immunodeficient infant with ribavirin aerosol. Am J Dis Child 138:305–308, 1984.
25. Hiatt PW, Grace SC, Kozinetz CA, et al. Effects of viral lower respiratory tract infection on lung function in infants with cystic fibrosis. Pediatrics 103:619–626, 1999.
26. Armstrong D, Grimwood K, Carlin JB, et al. Severe viral respiratory infections in infants with cystic fibrosis. Pediatr Pulmonol 26:371–379, 1998.
27. King JC Jr, Burke AR, Clemens JD, et al. Respiratory syncytial virus illnesses in human immunodeficiency virus and noninfected children. Pediatr Infect Dis J 12:733–739, 1993.
28. Madhi SA, Venter M, Madhi A, et al. Differing manifestations of respiratory syncytial virus-associated severe lower respiratory tract infections in human immunodeficiency virus type 1-infected and uninfected children. Pediatr Infect Dis J 20:164–170, 2001.
29. Martinez FD, Wright AL, Taussig LM, et al for the Group Health Med Associates. Asthma and wheezing in the first six years of life. N Engl J Med 332:133–136, 1995.
30. Kattan M. Epidemiologic evidence of increased airway reactivity in children with a history of bronchiolitis. J Pediatr 135(suppl):S8–S13, 1999.
31. Hall CB, Geiman JM, Biggar R, et al. Respiratory syncytial virus infections within families. N Engl J Med 294:414–419, 1976.
32. Falsey AR, Cunningham CK, Barker WH, et al. Respiratory syncytial virus and influenza A infections in the hospitalized elderly. J Infect Dis 172:389–394, 1995.
33. Whimbey E, Ghosh S. Respiratory syncytial virus infections in immunocompromised adults. Curr Clin Top Infect Dis 20:232–255, 2000.
34. Englund JA, Sullivan CJ, Jordan MC, et al. Respiratory syncytial virus infection in immunocompromised adults. Ann Intern Med 109:203–208, 1988.
35. Whimbey E, Champlin RE, Couch RB, et al. Community respiratory virus infections among hospitalized adult bone marrow transplant recipients. Clin Infect Dis 22:778–782, 1996.
36. Hertz MI, Englund JA, Snover D, et al. Respiratory syncytial virus induced acute lung injury in adult patients with bone marrow transplants: a clinical approach and review of the literature. Medicine 68:269–281, 1989.
37. Whimbey E, Couch RB, Englund JA, et al. Respiratory syncytial virus pneumonia in hospitalized adult patients with leukemia. Clin Infect Dis 21:376–379, 1995.
38. Harrington RD, Hooton TM, Hackman RC, et al. An outbreak of respiratory syncytial virus in a bone marrow transplant center. J Infect Dis 165:987–993, 1992.
39. Hendricks DA, McIntosh K, Patterson JL. Further characterization of the soluble form of the G glycoprotein of respiratory syncytial virus. J Virol 62:2228–2233, 1988.
40. Collins PL, Chanock RM, Murphy B. Respiratory syncytial virus. In Fields BN, Knipe DM, Howley PM (eds). Fields Virology (4th ed). Philadelphia, Lippincott Williams & Wilkins, 2001, pp 1443–1485.
41. Coates HV, Alling DW, Chanock RM. An antigenic analysis of respiratory syncytial virus isolates by a plaque reduction neutralization test. Am J Epidemiol 83:299–313, 1966.

42. Johnson PR Jr, Olmsted RA, Prince GA, et al. Antigenic relatedness between glycoproteins of human respiratory syncytial virus subgroups A and B: evaluation of the contributions of F and G glycoproteins to immunity. J Virol 61:3163–3166, 1987.

43. Taylor CE, Morrow S, Scott M, et al. Comparative virulence of respiratory syncytial virus subgroups A and B. Lancet 1:777–778, 1989.

44. McConnochie KM, Hall CB, Walsh EE, Roghmann KJ. Variation in severity of respiratory syncytial virus infections with subtype. J Pediatr 117:52–62, 1990.

45. Mufson MA, Belshe RB, Orvell C, Norrby E. Subgroup characteristics of respiratory syncytial virus strains recovered from children with two consecutive infections. J Clin Microbiol 25:1535–1539, 1987.

46. Henderson FW, Collier AM, Clyde WA Jr, Denny FW. Respiratory-syncytial-virus infections, reinfections and immunity: a prospective, longitudinal study in young children. N Engl J Med 300:530–534, 1979.

47. Mufson MA, Levin MJ, Wash RE, et al. Epidemiology of respiratory syncytial virus infection among infants and children in Chicago. Am J Epidemiol 98:88–95, 1973.

48. Spence L, Barratt N. Respiratory syncytial virus associated with acute respiratory infections in Trinidadian patients. Am J Epidemiol 88:257–266, 1968.

49. Hendry RM, Burns JC, Walsh EE, et al. Strain-specific serum antibody responses in infants undergoing primary infection with respiratory syncytial virus. J Infect Dis 157:640–647, 1988.

50. Hendry RM, Pierik LT, McIntosh K. Prevalence of respiratory syncytial virus subgroups over six consecutive outbreaks: 1981–1987. J Infect Dis 160:185–190, 1989.

51. Mufson MA, Belshe RB, Orvell C, Norrby E. Respiratory syncytial virus epidemics: variable dominance of subgroups A and B strains among children, 1981–1986. J Infect Dis 157:143–148, 1988.

52. Akerlind B, Norrby E. Occurrence of respiratory syncytial virus subtypes A and B strains in Sweden. J Med Virol 19:241–247, 1986.

53. Hall CB, Douglas RG. Modes of transmission of respiratory syncytial virus. J Pediatr 99:100–103, 1981.

54. Hall CB, Douglas RG Jr, Schnabel KC, Geiman JM. Infectivity of respiratory syncytial virus by various routes of inoculation. Infect Immun 33:779–783, 1981.

55. Hall CB. Nosocomial respiratory syncytial virus infections: the "Cold War" has not ended. Clin Infect Dis 31:590–596, 2000.

56. Haynes LM, Moore DD, Kurt-Jones EA, et al. Involvement of toll-like receptor 4 in innate immunity to respiratory syncytial virus. J Virol 75:10730–10737, 2001.

57. Kurt-Jones EA, Popova L, Kwinn L, et al. Pattern recognition receptors TLR4 and CD14 mediate response to respiratory syncytial virus. Nat Immunol 1:398–401, 2000.

58. Beem M. Repeated infections with respiratory syncytial virus. J Immunol 98:1115–1122, 1987.

59. Hall CB, Walsh EE, Long CE, Schnabel KC. Immunity to and frequency of reinfection with respiratory syncytial virus. J Infect Dis 163:693–698, 1991.

60. Cannon MJ, Openshaw PJM, Askonas BA. Cytotoxic T cells clear virus but augment lung pathology in mice infected with respiratory syncytial virus. J Exp Med 168:1163–1168, 1988.

61. Prince GA, Horswood RL, Camargo E, et al. Mechanisms of immunity to respiratory syncytial virus in cotton rats. Infect Immun 42:81–87, 1983.

62. Walsh EE, Schlesinger JJ, Brandriss MW. Protection from respiratory syncytial virus infection in cotton rats by passive transfer of monoclonal antibodies. Infect Immun 43:756–758, 1984.

63. Prince GA, Horswood RL, Chanock RM. Quantitative aspects of passive immunity to respiratory syncytial virus infection in infant cotton rats. J Virol 55:517–520, 1985.

64. Mills VJ, Van Kirk JE, Wright PF, Chanock RM. Experimental respiratory syncytial virus infection of adults. J Immunol 107:123–130, 1971.

65. McIntosh K, Masters HB, Orr I, et al. The immunologic response to infection with respiratory syncytial virus in infants. J Infect Dis 138:24–32, 1978.

66. Glezen WP, Paredes A, Allison JE, et al. Risk of respiratory syncytial virus infection for infants from low-income families in relationship to age, sex, ethnic group, and maternal antibody level. J Pediatr 98:708–715, 1981.

67. Holberg CJ, Wright AL, Martinez FD, et al. Risk factors for respiratory syncytial virus-associated lower respiratory illnesses in the first year of life. Am J Epidemiol 133:1135–1151, 1991.

68. Glezen WP, Taber LH, Frank AL, Kasel JA. Risk of primary infection and reinfection with respiratory syncytial virus. Am J Dis Child 140:543–546, 1986.

69. Murphy BR, Alling DW, Snyder MH, et al. Effect of age and preexisting antibody on serum antibody response of infants and children to the F and G glycoproteins during respiratory syncytial virus infection. J Clin Microbiol 24:894–898, 1986.

70. Groothuis JR, Simoes EAF, Levin MJ, et al. Prophylactic administration of respiratory syncytial virus immune globulin to high-risk infants and young children. N Engl J Med 329:1524–1530, 1993.

71. Hemming VG, Prince GA, Groothuis JR, Siber GR. Hyperimmune globulins in prevention and treatment of respiratory syncytial virus infections. Clin Microbiol Rev 8:22–33, 1995.

72. Wright PF, Karron RA, Belshe RB, et al. Evaluation of a live, cold-passaged, temperature-sensitive, respiratory syncytial virus vaccine candidate in infancy. J Infect Dis 182:1331–1342, 2000.

73. Prevent Study Group. Reduction of respiratory syncytial virus hospitalization among premature infants and infants with bronchopulmonary dysplasia using respiratory syncytial virus immune globulin prophylaxis. Pediatrics 99:93–99, 1997.

74. IMpact-RSV Study Group. Palivizumab, a humanized respiratory syncytial virus monoclonal antibody, reduces hospitalization from respiratory syncytial virus infection in high-risk infants. Pediatrics 102:531–537, 1998.

75. American Academy of Pediatrics, Committee on Infectious Diseases. Respiratory syncytial virus immune globulin intravenous: indications for use. Pediatrics 99:645–650, 1997.

76. American Academy of Pediatrics, Committee on Infectious Diseases. Prevention of respiratory syncytial virus infections: indications for the use of palivizumab and update on the use of RSV-IGIV. Pediatrics 102(3 pt 1):531–537, 1998.

77. Sondheimer HM, Cabalka AK, Feltes TF, Piazza FM, Connor EM. Palivizumab prevents hospitalization due to respiratory syncytial virus in young children with serious congenital heart disease. Pediatric Cardiology 23(6):664, 2002.

78. Boeckh M, Berrey MM, Bowden RA, et al. Phase 1 evaluation of the respiratory syncytial virus-specific monoclonal antibody palivizumab in recipients of hematopoietic stem cell transplants. J Infect Dis 184:350–354, 2001.

79. Rodriguez WJ, Gruber WC, Welliver RC, et al. Respiratory syncytial virus (RSV) immune globulin intravenous therapy for RSV lower respiratory tract infection in infants and young children at high risk for severe RSV infections. Respiratory Syncytial Virus Immune Globulin Study Group. Pediatrics 99:454–461, 1997.

80. Malley R, Devincenzo J, Ramilo O, et al. Reduction of respiratory syncytial virus (RSV) in tracheal aspirates in intubated infants by use of humanized monoclonal antibody to RSV F protein. J Infect Dis 178:1555–1561, 1998.

81. Chin J, Magoffin RL, Shearer LA, et al. Field evaluation of a respiratory syncytial virus vaccine and a trivalent parainfluenza virus vaccine in a pediatric population. Am J Epidemiol 89:449–463, 1969.

82. Murphy BR, Prince GA, Walsh EE, et al. Dissociation between serum neutralizing and glycoprotein antibody responses of infants and children who received inactivated respiratory syncytial virus vaccine. J Clin Microbiol 24:197–202, 1986.

83. Kim HW, Leikin SL, Arrobio J, et al. Cell-mediated immunity to respiratory syncytial virus induced by inactivated vaccine or by infection. Pediatr Res 10:75–78, 1976.

84. Graham BS, Henderson GS, Tang Y-W, et al. Priming immunization determines T helper cytokine mRNA expression patterns in lungs of mice challenged with respiratory syncytial virus. J Immunol 151:2032–2040, 1993.

85. Waris ME, Tsou C, Erdman DD, et al. Respiratory syncytial virus infection in BALB/c mice previously immunized with formalin-inactivated virus induces enhanced pulmonary inflammatory response with a predominant Th2-like cytokine pattern. J Virol 70:2852–2860, 1996.

86. Connors M, Kulkarni AB, Firestone C-Y, et al. Pulmonary histopathology induced by respiratory syncytial virus (RSV) challenge of formalin-inactivated RSV-immunized BALB/c mice is abrogated by depletion of CD4+ T cells. J Virol 66:7444–7451, 1992.

87. Hussell T, Baldwin CJ, O'Garra A, Openshaw PJM. CD8+ T cells control Th2-driven pathology during pulmonary respiratory syncytial virus infection. Eur J Immunol 27:3341–3349, 1997.

88. Tang Y-W, Neuzil KM, Fischer JE, et al. Determinants and kinetics of cytokine expression patterns in lungs of vaccinated mice challenged with respiratory syncytial virus. Vaccine 15:597–602, 1997.

89. Neuzil KM, Johnson JE, Tang Y-W, et al. Adjuvants influence the quantitative and qualitative immune response in BALB/c mice immunized with respiratory syncytial virus FG subunit vaccine. Vaccine 15:525–532, 1997.

90. Crowe JE Jr, Collins PL, Chanock RM, Murphy BR. Vaccines against respiratory syncytial virus and parainfluenza virus type 3. *In* Levin MM, Woodrow GC, Kaper JB, Cobon GS (eds). New Generation Vaccines. New York, Marcel Dekker, 1997, pp 711–725.

91. Tang YW, Graham GS. Interleukin-12 treatment during immunization elicits a T helper cell type 1-like immune response in mice challenged with respiratory syncytial virus and improves vaccine immunogenicity. J Infect Dis 172:734–738, 1995.

92. Polack FP, Teng MN, Collins PL, et al. A role for immune complexes in enhanced respiratory syncytial virus disease. J Exp Med 196:859–865, 2002.

93. Wright PF, Karzon DT. Live attenuated influenza vaccines. Prog Med Virol 34:70–88, 1987.

94. Maassab HF, DeBorde DC. Development and characterization of cold-adapted viruses for use as live virus vaccines. Vaccine 3:355–369, 1985.

95. Chanock RM, Murphy BM. Past efforts to develop safe and effective RSV vaccines. *In* Meignier B, et al. (eds). Animal Models of Respiratory Syncytial Virus Infections. Mérieux Foundation Publication, Mérieux, France, 1991, pp 35–42.

96. McIntosh K, Arbeter AM, Stahl MK, et al. Attenuated respiratory syncytial virus vaccines in asthmatic children. Pediatr Res 8:689–696, 1974.

97. Kim HW, Arrobio JO, Brandt CD, et al. Safety and antigenicity of temperature-sensitive (ts) mutant respiratory syncytial virus (RSV) in infants and children. Pediatrics 52:56–63, 1973.

98. Wright PF, Shinozaki T, Fleet W, et al. Evaluation of a live, attenuated respiratory syncytial virus vaccine in infants. J Pediatr 88:931–936, 1976.

99. McKay E, Higgins P, Tyrrell D, Pringle C. Immunogenicity and pathogenicity of temperature-sensitive modified respiratory syncytial virus in adult volunteers. J Med Virol 25:411–421, 1988.

100. Pringle CR, Filipiuk AH, Robinson BS, et al. Immunogenicity and pathogenicity of a triple temperature-sensitive modified respiratory syncytial virus in adult volunteers. Vaccine 11:473–478, 1993.

101. Crowe JE Jr, Bui PT, Siber GR, et al. Cold-passaged, temperature-sensitive mutants of human respiratory syncytial virus (RSV) are highly attenuated, immunogenic, and protective in seronegative chimpanzees, even when RSV antibodies are infused shortly before immunization. Vaccine 13:847–855, 1995.

102. Crowe JE Jr, Bui PT, Davis AR, et al. A further attenuated derivative of a cold-passaged temperature-sensitive mutant of human respiratory syncytial virus (RSV cpts-248) retains immunogenicity and protective efficacy against wild-type challenge in seronegative chimpanzees. Vaccine 12:783–790, 1994.

103. Crowe JE Jr, Bui PT, London WT, et al. Satisfactorily attenuated and protective mutants derived from a partially attenuated cold-passaged respiratory syncytial virus mutant by introduction of additional attenuating mutations during chemical mutagenesis. Vaccine 12:691–709, 1994.

104. Crowe JE Jr, Collins PL, London WT, et al. A comparison in chimpanzees of the immunogenicity and efficacy of live attenuated respiratory syncytial virus (RSV) temperature-sensitive mutant vaccines and vaccinia virus recombinants that express the surface glycoproteins of RSV. Vaccine 11:1395–1404, 1993.

105. Karron RA, Wright PF, Crowe JE Jr, et al. Evaluation of two live, cold-passaged, temperature-sensitive respiratory syncytial virus vaccines in chimpanzees and in human adults, infants and children. J Infect Dis 176:1428–1436, 1997.

106. Collins PL, Hill MG, Camargo E, et al. Production of infectious human respiratory syncytial virus from cloned cDNA confirms an essential role for the transcription elongation factor from the 5' proximal open reading frame of the M2 mRNA in gene expression and provides a capability for vaccine development. Proc Natl Acad Sci U S A 92:11563–11567, 1995.

107. Collins PL, Whitehead SS, Bukreyev A, et al. Rational design of live-attenuated recombinant vaccine virus for human respiratory syncytial virus by reverse genetics. Adv Virus Res 54:423–451, 1999.

108. Juhasz K, Whitehead SS, Boulanger CA, et al. The two amino acid substitutions in the L protein of cpts530/1009, a live-attenuated respiratory syncytial virus candidate vaccine, are independent temperature-sensitive and attenuation mutations. Vaccine 17:1416–1424, 1999.

109. Whitehead SS, Firestone C-Y, Collins PL, Murphy BR. A single nucleotide substitution in the transcription start signal of the M2 gene of respiratory syncytial virus vaccine candidate cpts248/404 is the major determinant of the temperature-sensitive and attenuation phenotypes. Virology 247:232–239, 1998.

110. Whitehead SS, Firestone CY, Karron RA, et al. Addition of a missense mutation present in the L gene of respiratory syncytial virus (RSV) cpts530/1030 to RSV vaccine candidate cpts248/404 increases its attenuation and temperature sensitivity. J Virol 73:871–877, 1999.

111. Jin H, Zhou H, Cheng X, et al. Recombinant respiratory syncytial viruses with deletions in the NS1, NS2, SH, and M2-2 genes are attenuated in vitro and in vivo. Virology 273:210–218, 2000.

112. Bukreyev A, Whitehead SS, Murphy BR, Collins PL. Recombinant respiratory syncytial virus from which the entire SH gene has been deleted grows efficiently in cell culture and exhibits site-specific attenuation in the respiratory tract of the mouse. J Virology 71:8973–8982, 1997.

113. Whitehead SS, Bukreyev A, Teng MN, et al. Recombinant respiratory syncytial virus bearing a deletion of either the NS2 or SH gene is attenuated in chimpanzees. J Virol 73:3438–3442, 1999.

114. Karron RA, Wright PF, Belshe RB, et al. Evaluation of live rRSV A2 vaccines in infants and children [abstr 5.2]. *In* Abstracts of the RSV After 45 Years meeting, Segovia, Spain, 2001.

115. Bukreyev A, Camargo E, Collins PL. Recovery of infectious respiratory syncytial virus expressing an additional, foreign gene. J Virol 70:6634–6641, 1996.

116. Whitehead SS, Hill MG, Firestone CY, et al. Replacement of the F and G proteins of respiratory syncytial virus (RSV) subgroup A with those of subgroup B generates chimeric live attenuated RSV. J Virol 73:9773–9780, 1999.

117. Jin H, Clarke D, Zhou H, et al. Recombinant human respiratory syncytial virus (RSV) from cDNA and construction of subgroup A and B chimeric RSV. Virology 251:206–214, 1998.

118. Bukreyev A, Whitehead SS, Murphy BR, Collins PL. Interferon gamma expressed by a recombinant respiratory syncytial virus attenuates virus replication in mice without compromising immunogenicity. Proc Natl Acad Sci U S A 96:2367–2372, 1999.

119. Bukreyev A, Whitehead SS, Prussin C, et al. Effect of coexpression of interleukin-2 by recombinant respiratory syncytial virus on virus replication, immunogenicity, and production of other cytokines. J Virol 74:7151–7157, 2000.

120. Bukreyev A, Belyakov IM, Berzofsky JA, et al. Granulocyte-macrophage colony-stimulating factor expressed by recombinant respiratory syncytial virus attenuates viral replication and increases the level of pulmonary antigen-presenting cells. J Virol 75:12128–12140, 2001.

121. Schmidt AC, Wenzke DR, McAuliffe JM, et al. Mucosal immunization of rhesus monkeys against respiratory syncytial virus subgroups A and B and human parainfluenza virus type 3 by using a live cDNA-derived vaccine based on a host range-attenuated bovine parainfluenza virus type 3 vector backbone. J Virol 76:1089–1099, 2002.

122. Buchholz UJ, Granzow H, Schuldt K, et al. Chimeric bovine respiratory syncytial virus with glycoprotein gene substitutions from human respiratory syncytial virus (HRSV): effects on host range and evaluation as a live-attenuated HRSV vaccine. J Virol 74:1187–1199, 2000.

123. Crowe JE Jr. Current approaches to the development of vaccines against disease caused by respiratory syncytial virus (RSV) and parainfluenza virus (PIV): a meeting report of the WHO Programme for Vaccine Development. Vaccine 13:415–421, 1995.

124. Falsey AR, Walsh EE. Safety and immunogenicity of a respiratory syncytial virus subunit vaccine (PFP-2) in ambulatory adults over age 60. Vaccine 14:1214–1218, 1996.

125. Falsey AR, Walsh EE. Safety and immunogenicity of a respiratory syncytial virus subunit vaccine (PFP-2) in the institutionalized elderly. Vaccine 15:1130–1132, 1997.

126. Belshe RB. Immunogenicity of purified F glycoprotein of respiratory syncytial virus: clinical and immune responses to subsequent natural infection in children. J Infect Dis 168:1024–1029, 1993.

127. Paradiso PR, Hildreth SW, Hogerman DA, et al. Safety and immunogenicity of a subunit respiratory syncytial virus vaccine in children 24 to 48 months old. Pediatr Infect Dis J 13:792–798, 1994.

128. Tristram DA, Welliver RC, Mohar CK, et al. Immunogenicity and safety of respiratory syncytial virus subunit vaccine in seropositive children 18–36 months old. J Infect Dis 167:191–195, 1993.

129. Piedra PA, Grace S, Jewell A, et al. Purified fusion protein vaccine protects against lower respiratory tract illness during respiratory syncytial virus season in children with cystic fibrosis. Pediatr Infect Dis J 15:23–31, 1996.

130. Groothuis JR, King SJ, Hogerman DA, et al. Safety and immunogenicity of a purified F protein respiratory syncytial virus (PFP-2) vaccine in seropositive children with bronchopulmonary dysplasia. J Infect Dis 177:467–469, 1998.

131. Munoz FM, Piedra PA, Maccato M, et al. Respiratory syncytial virus purified fusion protein-2 (RSV-PFP-2) vaccine in pregnancy [abstract]. *In* Abstracts of the RSV After 45 Years meeting, Segovia, Spain (unpublished) 2001.

132. Sales V, Goldwater R, Warren JT, et al. Safety and immunogenicity of a respiratory syncytial virus subtype A vaccine in adults—two Phase I studies [abstract]. *In* Abstracts of the 4th International Symposium on Respiratory Viral Infections, Curacao, Netherlands Antilles (unpublished) 2001.

133. Plotnicky-Gilquin H, Robert A, Chevalet L, et al. CD4+ T-cell-mediated antiviral protection of the upper respiratory tract in BALB/c mice following parenteral immunization with a recombinant respiratory syncytial virus G protein fragment. J Virol 74:3455–3463, 2000.

134. Plotnicky-Gilquin H, Huss T, Aubrey J-P, et al. Absence of lung immunopathology following respiratory syncytial virus (RSV) challenge in mice immunized with a recombinant RSV G protein fragment. Virology 258:128–140, 1999.

135. Power UF, Plotnicky-Gilquin H, Huss T, et al. Induction of protective immunity in rodents by vaccination with a prokaryotically expressed recombinant fusion protein containing a respiratory syncytial virus G protein fragment. Virology 230:155–166, 1997.

136. Power UF, Nguyen TN, Rietveld E, et al. Safety and immunogenicity of a novel recombinant subunit respiratory syncytial virus vaccine (BBG2Na) in healthy young adults. J Infect Dis 184:1456–1460, 2001.

137. Gonzalez IM, Karron RA, Eichelberger M, et al. Evaluation of the live attenuated cpts 248/404 RSV vaccine in combination with a subunit RSV vaccine (PFP-2) in healthy young and older adults. Vaccine 18:1763–1772, 2000.

138. Simoes EA, Tan DH, Ohlsson A, et al. Respiratory syncytial virus vaccine: a systematic overview with emphasis on respiratory syncytial virus subunit vaccines. Vaccine 20:954–960, 2001.

139. Piedra PA, Grace S, Jewell A, et al. Sequential annual administration of purified fusion protein vaccine against respiratory syncytial virus in children with cystic fibrosis. Pediatr Infect Dis J 17:217–224, 1998.

140. Brandt C, Power UF, Plotnicky-Gilquin H, et al. Protective immunity against respiratory syncytial virus in early life after murine maternal or neonatal vaccination with the recombinant G fusion protein BBG2Na. J Infect Dis 176:884–891, 1997.

141. Plotnicky-Gilquin H, Goetsch L, Huss T, et al. Identification of multiple protective epitopes (Protectopes) in the central conserved domain of a prototype human respiratory syncytial virus G protein. J Virol 73:5637–5645, 1999.

142. Power UF, Plotnicky-Gilquin H, Goetsch L, et al. Identification and characterisation of multiple linear B cell protectopes in the respiratory syncytial virus G protein. Vaccine 19:2345–2351, 2001.

143. Norrby E, Mufson MA, Alexander H, et al. Site-directed serology with synthetic peptides representing the large glycoprotein G of respiratory syncytial virus. Proc Natl Acad Sci U S A 84:6572–6576, 1987.

Chapter 51

Rotavirus Vaccines

H. FRED CLARK • PAUL A. OFFIT • ROGER I. GLASS • RICHARD L. WARD

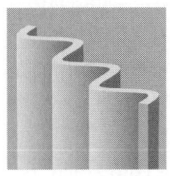

Rotaviruses are the leading cause of severe dehydrating diarrhea in infants and young children throughout the world. Virtually all children are infected by the time they reach 2 to 3 years of age.[1,2] Even in developed nations, where standards of hygiene are high, rotavirus is the most common cause of infant diarrhea.[3]

In the United States, rotavirus accounts for about 500,000 physician visits, 50,000 hospitalizations, and 20 to 40 deaths each year,[4,5] and the economic burden of disease is estimated to exceed $1 billion each year in medical and indirect costs.[4,6,7] In less developed countries, rotaviruses rank highest among the multiple microbial causes of severe gastroenteritis in children and contribute disproportionately to the mortality associated with the disease.[8-10] Worldwide, rotavirus is estimated to cause 450,000 to 600,000 deaths in children each year, which is approximately 20% of the estimated 2.4 to 3.2 million annual deaths from diarrhea.[11-14] Extensive global efforts to disseminate oral rehydration therapy in the developing world undoubtedly have contributed to a decline in diarrhea deaths.[15] However, the continuing mortality associated with rotavirus, 1200 to 1600 deaths per day, suggests that prevention through universal application of a safe, economical, and efficacious vaccine would be preferable. Because rotaviruses remain the most common cause of severe diarrhea in children in regions with high standards of health and sanitation, a rotavirus vaccine would have universal application as part of childhood immunization programs.

The first rotavirus vaccine (Rotashield; Wyeth-Lederle) was licensed by the U.S. Food and Drug Administration on August 31, 1998. In July 1999, after the vaccine had been administered to about 1 million children, Rotashield was temporarily suspended and eventually withdrawn from use when it was found to be a rare cause of intussusception. This review provides a description of Rotashield vaccine and other candidate vaccines.

Background

Clinical Disease

Evaluation of children admitted to the hospital with rotavirus infection reveals a consistent pattern. The disease is characterized by the sudden onset of watery diarrhea, fever, and vomiting.[16-19] Most disease is mild, but about 1 of every 75 children infected with rotavirus[4,5] will develop dehydration associated with severe loss of sodium and chloride in the stools and a compensated metabolic acidosis. In children admitted to the hospital with dehydration, fever and vomiting usually persist for 2 to 3 days and diarrhea persists for 4 to 5 days.[16-19]

The Virus

Rotavirus infection has been detected in most common species of domestic animals and in many species of wild mammals and birds. Whereas the great majority of human and animal rotaviruses share common group antigens (group A rotaviruses),[20] animal rotaviruses generally can be distinguished from human strains on the basis of type-specific surface antigens. Animals appear to be neither a reservoir for human strains nor a common source for transmission of rotaviruses to humans.

Certain rotaviruses of bovine or simian origin were propagated in cell culture to high titer before the more recent development of methods to propagate strains from humans.[21,22] Thus the molecular structure of rotavirus was largely determined by studies of the bovine strain, Nebraska calf diarrhea virus,[23] and the simian strain, SA11.[24]

Rotaviruses are 70-nm icosahedral viruses that constitute a distinct genus of the family *Reoviridae*.[20] The virus is composed of three shells (an outer and inner capsid and a core) that encase the genome of 11 segments of double-stranded RNA.[20] For the most part, each gene segment codes for a single protein. Gene segments can be separated on the basis of their molecular weight by polyacrylamide gel electrophoresis.[20] When mixed infections with distinct rotavirus strains occur under experimental conditions or in nature, the gene segments may reassort independently, producing progeny virus of mixed parentage. Analysis of such "reassortant" rotaviruses has led to identification of the gene segments encoding each of the structural polypeptides. This identification, in turn, has made possible techniques to intentionally reassort rotavirus strains and prepare candidate vaccine strains that incorporate desirable phenotypic characteristics of different parent strains.[25-27]

TABLE 51–1 ■ Biologically Significant Structural and Nonstructural Rotavirus Proteins

Designation	Product of Gene Segment	Approximate Molecular Weight (kDa)	Virion Localization	Biological Significance
VP4*	4	88,000	Outer capsid	Type-specific antigen, hemagglutinin
VP6	6	44,000	Inner capsid	Major subgroup antigen
VP7	7, 8, or 9	38,000	Outer capsid	Type-specific antigen
NSP4	10	28,000	Nonstructural	Enterotoxin

*Trypsin treatment of virion leads to production of VP4 cleavage products designated VP5 (MW 60,000) and VP8 (MW 27,000).
Data from Estes MK, Cohen J. Rotavirus gene structure and function. Microbiol Rev 53:410–449, 1989; Bellamy AR, Both GW. Molecular biology of rotaviruses. Adv Virus Res 38:1–43, 1990; and Ball JM, Tian P, Zeng CQY, et al. Age-dependent diarrhea induced by a rotaviral nonstructural glycoprotein. Science 272:101–104, 1996.

Four major structural and nonstructural proteins of rotavirus are of interest in vaccine development (Table 51–1). The outer shell of rotavirus contains two distinct proteins: VP4 and VP7.[16] Each of these proteins bears type-specific antigenic determinants, elicits serotype-specific neutralizing antibodies, and induces serotype-specific protective immune responses in vivo.[28–31] Protein VP7 is coded by gene segment 7, 8, or 9 in different rotavirus strains; protein VP4 is coded by gene segment 4.[20] The most highly represented viral structural protein is VP6, which is found in the internal capsid and bears group-specific antigenic determinants.[32] The nonstructural protein NSP4 was shown to be an enterotoxin.[33] Three structural proteins (VP1, VP2, and VP3) form the viral core, and four other nonstructural proteins (NSP1, NSP2, NSP3, and NSP5) are made during infection.[20]

Both of the surface proteins, VP4 and VP7, elicit distinct serotype-specific neutralizing antibodies as well as, in certain circumstances, cross-reactive neutralizing antibodies.[34–40] The VP7 protein is glycosylated, and serotypes determined by this protein are termed G types; 14 rotavirus G serotypes have been identified.[20] The VP4 protein is cleaved by the protease trypsin, and serotypes determined by this protein are termed P types.[20] The P protein presents in the form of 60 protein dimer spikes (the hemagglutinin) that extend beyond the VP7 surface of the virion while also penetrating through the outer capsid to interact with VP6 on the inner capsid.[20] Because of extensive cross-reactivity among different P types, it has not been possible to classify all P types by use of polyclonal hyperimmune antisera or monoclonal antibodies alone; however, the major human rotavirus P serotypes have been established. This led to development of an additional system of P typing into "genotypes" identified by nucleic acid hybridization and nucleic acid sequencing studies.[41]

Because of the above phenomena, a complex binomial nomenclature has been developed. A complete rotavirus serotype is described using an upper case letter for the P serotype, followed by a number in brackets that represents the P genotype. This is followed by the G type designation. For example, the most common human rotavirus is classified as P1A[8]G1. Following this nomenclature, the most common human serotypes (described through 2002) are listed in Table 51–2. This list is based primarily on studies of community infections.

Pathogenesis

Studies of rotavirus pathology and pathophysiology in animals and humans focus on four important questions:

1. In which intestinal and nonintestinal tissues do rotaviruses replicate and induce disease?
2. By what mechanism does rotavirus induce gastroenteritis?
3. Why is rotavirus-induced gastroenteritis primarily a disease of the young?
4. What factors of the host determine why rotavirus disease is more severe in developing than in developed countries?

Studies of natural rotavirus infection indicate that rotavirus replication is restricted to mature villous epithelial cells in the mucosal surface of the small intestine.[42–47] Replication progresses from the proximal to the distal small intestine.[45,48] Rotaviruses do not appear to replicate in immature epithelial cells of the villous crypt or in M cells overlying Peyer's patches.[49] In addition, rotaviruses have never been detected consistently in the blood or sites distant to the intestine. Although simian rotaviruses replicate in hepatic epithelial cells of inbred mice,[50] the relevance of these findings to human infection remains unclear.

Rotavirus replication in intestinal epithelial cells causes several physiologic and morphologic changes. Infected animals have a decreased capacity to absorb sodium, glucose, and water and have decreased levels of intestinal lactase, alkaline phosphatase, and sucrase.[51,52] These findings are consistent with an absorptive abnormality associated with an accelerated migration of immature epithelial cells toward the villous tip. Because no inflammatory changes occur in the lamina propria, in Peyer's patches, or at the intestinal mucosal surface,[42–47] it is unlikely that intestinal epithelial cell damage is mediated by the host immune response.

One of the rotavirus nonstructural proteins (NSP4) acts as a viral enterotoxin.[33] Exposure of intestinal epithelial cells to NSP4 induces diarrhea in suckling mice in an age-dependent, dose-dependent, and specific manner. Disease is caused by excess chloride secretion by a calcium-dependent signaling pathway. This finding is consistent with studies

TABLE 51–2 ■ The Most Common Human Group A Rotavirus Serotypes Worldwide in 2002

VP4 Serotype [Genotype]	Most Common VP7 Type Associates
P1A[8]	G1, G3, G4, G9
P1B[4]	G2
P2[6]	G9

using reassortant rotaviruses generated from pathogenic and nonpathogenic strains,[53] indicating that the genes that encoded pathogenic VP3, VP4, VP7, and NSP4 all were required to reconstitute virulence. Because virus replication is required for generation of nonstructural proteins, it is not surprising that attenuation of rotavirus virulence can occur in the absence of attenuating NSP4.[54]

Rotavirus infections are more likely to be severe in children 3 to 24 months of age than in younger infants or older children and adults.[55–58] Several studies have offered possible explanations for these differences in age susceptibility. First, children of increasing age may be protected by a virus-specific immune response generated by repeated natural infections.[59] Protection of young infants may be mediated by passively transferred, transplacental, maternal antibodies. Breast-feeding clearly protects against rotavirus disease.[60] Second, infant mice have a larger percentage of intestinal epithelial cells with putative rotavirus-binding proteins on the surface than do older mice[61]—an observation that correlates directly with the age susceptibility to disease. Last, rotavirus entry into target cells is facilitated by cleavage of VP4,[62,63] which occurs in the presence of trypsin, elastase, or pancreatin.[64] Quantities of these exopeptidases are decreased in intestinal fluid secretions of newborn infants compared with older infants and young children.[65]

Children in developing countries are more susceptible to severe rotavirus disease than those in developed countries. This is probably due to poor medical access, poor nutrition, and concomitant infections with other viruses and enteropathogenic bacteria.[66] Several studies in animals support the hypotheses that poor nutrition,[67,68] or associated bacterial infections, may enhance the severity of rotavirus-induced enteritis.[49,69,70]

Immunologic Factors Associated with Protection Against Disease

Protection against reinfection with rotavirus centers on two important questions: (1) Which effector function or functions of the immune response mediate protection? and (2) What is the importance of including different rotavirus serotypes in an optimal vaccine?

In 1983, the role of immunity to rotavirus was demonstrated by studies of natural infection in neonates.[71] Neonates infected in the first month of life were not protected against rotavirus reinfection but were protected against moderate to severe disease on reinfection. Conversely, neonates not infected with rotavirus during the first month of life were fully susceptible to diarrheal disease associated with the first rotavirus infection. Since then, studies of natural infection in infants and young children indicated that first infections protect against severe disease on reinfection.[72,73] For example, in Guinea-Bissau, a primary infection with rotavirus conferred 52% protection against subsequent rotavirus disease.[73a] Protection is mediated by the presence of virus-specific immunoglobulin A (IgA) at the intestinal mucosal surface[74,75] and is predicted by the presence of virus-specific IgA in the serum or feces.[74–76]

Although natural rotavirus infection protects against moderate to severe disease caused by reinfection, some children experience repeated episodes of diarrhea with the same serotype during the following rotavirus season,[77–88] and a small number of children develop symptomatic rotavirus infection twice within the same season.[74] These observations are consistent with the fact that effector functions at mucosal surfaces, such as production of virus-specific secretory IgA (sIgA), are usually short lived and that rotavirus-specific sIgA often is not detected at the intestinal mucosal surface within 1 year of symptomatic infection.[74,75] Modification of the severity of rotavirus disease caused by reinfection is most likely mediated by production of virus-specific sIgA by memory rotavirus-specific B cells in the intestinal lamina propria.[89]

The presence of rotavirus-specific sIgA at the intestinal mucosal surface (as reflected in the feces) and in serum is predictive of protection against disease in studies of natural infection but not in vaccine trials. Virus-specific IgA in feces or serum did not predict protection against disease after immunization of infants with simian-human reassortant rotaviruses.[90–92] Several explanations for this phenomenon have been posited. First, the absence of rotavirus-specific sIgA in feces does not necessarily predict the absence of rotavirus-specific memory B cells in the intestinal lamina propria.[89] The presence of rotavirus-specific memory B cells in the lamina propria could only be determined by intestinal biopsy. Second, protection against disease after immunization with animal rotaviruses may be mediated in part by virus-specific cytotoxic T lymphocytes (CTLs). Whereas the role of rotavirus-specific CTLs in protection against human disease is unknown, some evidence supports their importance in protection against disease in animals.[93–96] Alternatively, after immunization, cytokines with antiviral activity, which are produced by activated CD4+ T cells, may be generated either earlier or in greater quantities than they are after primary infection. Studies have found that rotavirus-specific CD4+ T cells alone mediated protection against challenge in experimental animals.[97,98] Several cytokines have been found to block rotavirus replication in vitro.[99]

A number of studies found that natural infection or immunization of children with one rotavirus serotype induced protection against challenge with a different serotype (heterotypic protection).[100,101] Heterotypic protection may be mediated by antibodies directed against cross-reactive epitopes on outer capsid proteins VP4 and VP7,[36] antigenically conserved inner capsid proteins that are actively transported through rotavirus-infected villous epithelial cells,[102] rotavirus-specific CTLs that broadly cross-react with cells infected with different rotavirus serotypes,[103] or antiviral cytokines generated by activated CD4+ T cells.[97,98]

The relative importance of including all common human P and G types in a rotavirus vaccine remains undetermined. However, it is clear that, after a primary, natural rotavirus infection, infants develop virus-specific neutralizing antibodies in serum directed against the infecting G type at levels greater than those directed against other G types.[104–108] In a similar manner, children are more likely to be protected against disease after reinfection with a G type to which they have already been exposed.[76,101] For these reasons, it may be of value for a rotavirus vaccine to contain all G types to which the child is likely to be exposed.

Diagnosis

Electron microscopy, which once served as the reference standard for diagnosis of rotavirus infections, has now been replaced by enzyme-linked immunosorbent assays (ELISAs). ELISA, which uses either polyclonal or monoclonal antibody preparations directed against the antigenically conserved inner capsid protein VP6, is as sensitive as electron microscopy but easier and less expensive to use.[109,110] However, false-positive ELISA results have been reported.[111]

More rapid detection of rotavirus antigens in fecal samples can be achieved by a latex agglutination assay.[112,113] Latex agglutination can be completed in several minutes and does not require the use of special equipment. However, latex agglutination is less sensitive than ELISA.

The detection of rotavirus by polyacrylamide gel electrophoresis, although not commercially available, offers several advantages over the ELISA and latex agglutination assays. Polyacrylamide gel electrophoresis is absolutely specific for the presence of rotavirus. In addition, detection of specific migration patterns of segmented double-stranded RNA (electropherotypes) is of value in determining specific strains associated with community outbreaks or nosocomial infections.

Epidemiology

Rotavirus is a universal infection in young children.[2] All children are exposed to rotavirus and acquire antibodies by 3 to 5 years of age, and most rotavirus diarrhea occurs during the first 3 years of life. In the first 3 months of life, infections are generally asymptomatic.[71] First infections after 3 months of age are generally associated with diarrhea that can be mild or severe, whereas subsequent exposures lead to milder illness or asymptomatic infections.[59,72,73,114] The observation that all children throughout the world are infected early in life suggests that rotavirus is not transmitted (like other bacterial and parasitic pathogens) through fecally contaminated water or food. Therefore, improvements in water, sanitation, and hygiene are unlikely to alter the incidence of disease. The priority placed on prevention of rotavirus by vaccination is predicated on the great global disease burden of rotavirus,[1,115] the recognition that natural immunity is protective, and the expectation that alternative public health measures, including the provision of clean food and water, are unlikely to prevent disease.

Little is known about the exact mode of transmission of rotavirus. Spread by airborne droplets or person-to-person contact is most likely. In a mouse model, airborne spread of epidemic diarrhea by a murine strain has been identified.[116] Furthermore, the disease has a distinct winter seasonality in temperate climates that is similar to that seen for viruses spread by the respiratory route, such as influenza and measles. Annual epidemics in the United States begin in the Southwest and spread to the North and East (Fig. 51–1). Humans are believed to be the only reservoir of human strains, and consistent transmission of animal strains to humans seems unlikely. Nevertheless, although classical epidemiology has failed to identify transmission of virus from animals to humans, reassortant strains composed of genomic segments from both human and animal rotaviruses have been identified. The presence of wild-type animal-human reassortants indicates that some mixing of strains must occur in nature and that this reassortment might be important for virus evolution.[117–119]

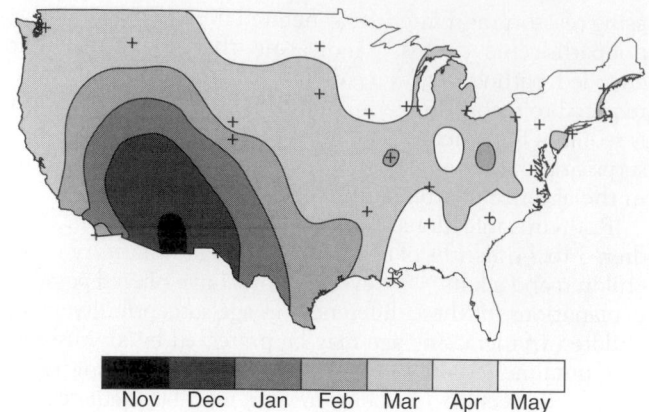

FIGURE 51–1 ■ Month of peak rotavirus activity—United States, July 1996 to June 1997, plus participating NREVSS laboratories. (From Laboratory-based surveillance for rotavirus—United States, July 1996–June 1997. MMWR 46:1092–1094, 1997, with permission.)

Certain clues about immunity and transmission of rotavirus can be gained from epidemic investigations and special studies. Whereas immunity is believed to protect adults from disease, parents and caretakers of children with rotavirus diarrhea can get mild disease, perhaps because practices such as diaper changing expose them to a large infectious dose.[120] Outbreaks in day care centers and hospitals can spread rapidly among nonimmune infants and young children, presumably because of person-to-person contact, airborne or droplet spread, or contact with contaminated toys.[121–123] In the elderly, outbreaks have been described that may be linked to waning immunity. Of note, many of these outbreaks have been associated with G2 strains that are antigenically distinct from the other common rotavirus serotypes. In adults traveling from developed to developing countries (i.e., persons who would be expected to be immune to rotavirus), the virus has been identified as a cause of diarrhea, perhaps because the mode of transmission is different or the inoculum size is greater.[124] In addition, people immunocompromised by human immunodeficiency virus infection,[125] hereditary immunodeficiency,[126,127] immunosuppression for organ transplantation,[128] or chemotherapy can develop rotavirus diarrhea with virus shedding that can persist for months.

Several differences in the epidemiology of rotavirus diarrhea between developed and developing countries may have an impact on future considerations concerning the use of vaccines. The distinct winter seasonality of rotavirus hospitalizations in temperate climates stands in contrast to the year-round exposure seen in tropical settings.[10] This means that a child born in a temperate climate after the rotavirus season will have to wait a full year until the next exposure, whereas a child born in a tropical setting could be exposed any day of the year. Consequently, the average age at first infection is younger in developing countries in tropical areas, and most rotavirus diarrhea in such sites occurs during a child's first year of life, compared with the first 2 or 3 years of life in developed countries. Therefore, an effective vaccine program in a developing country may require earlier and higher levels of coverage than programs in developed countries. In the laboratory, fecal specimens from children from developed countries have a simpler virologic picture, typically with a single strain of virus drawn from one of several common serotypes found globally.[129,130] In developing countries, the rate of mixed infections with two or more strains can reach 30%, and the viruses can include uncommon serotypes not found in other parts of the world.[131-135]

The burden of rotavirus diarrhea for children in developing countries became evident when the first diagnostic tests were used to study the etiology of diarrhea in hospitalized children (Table 51–3). In more than 100 studies conducted around the world among children younger than 5 years hospitalized for diarrhea, rotavirus was the most common cause of diarrhea (detected in 20% to 60% of cases). It has been estimated that between 450,000 and 600,000 children die each year of rotavirus diarrhea.[1,115] Longitudinal studies of children observed from birth to 2 years of age suggest that the incidence of rotavirus diarrhea varies directly with the intensity of surveillance. These studies indicate that most children (i.e., 1 in 1.2 to 1.3) will have an episode of rotavirus diarrhea in their first 3 to 5 years of life and, depending on the locale,[136-138] require medical attention or treatment. For example, in Vietnam, 605 per 1000 children die of rotavirus disease before 5 years of age.[138a]

In developed countries, rotavirus was long considered to cause a mild diarrheal illness of children that was rarely, if ever, severe and never fatal. Whereas early studies documented a clear winter peak of hospitalizations (accounting for as much as 80% of cases), no child in the United States was known to have died with a diagnosis of rotavirus diarrhea. These findings suggested that rotavirus disease was more a nuisance than a severe problem.[3] However, a series of studies examining the national profile of diarrheal hospitalizations and deaths in the United States put national data in a different light.[6,139,140] No *International Classification of Diseases* code specific for rotavirus diarrhea existed before 1993; however, the distinct winter peak in both hospitalizations and deaths for diarrhea among children 4 to 23 months of age was consistent with their being caused by rotavirus. Furthermore, in the United States, these peaks had a unique pattern that began in the Southwest in November and moved northeast, reaching New England in March or April. When laboratories were surveyed, rotavirus detections demonstrated the same temporal and geographic patterns.[141-143] On the basis of these data, the Centers for Disease Control and Prevention (CDC) developed national estimates for rotavirus diarrhea. These estimates indicate that each year 60% to 80% of the entire birth cohort of children will develop a mild diarrheal illness (~2.7 million episodes per year), 1 in 6.5 will seek medical attention, 1 in 72 (60,000 patients) will be hospitalized, and 1 in 200,000 (20 children) will die of rotavirus.[4] These data were similar to those developed by Matson and Estes for the United States[144] and are lower than similar estimates made for the United Kingdom,[145] Australia,[146] Ireland,[147] Venezuela,[148] and Finland. The cost of medical care in the United States was estimated to be more than $400 million; indirect costs are estimated to be in excess of $1 billion.[7] However, because rotavirus can cause vomiting and fever in the absence of diarrhea,[149] estimates of disease burden from medical records that include a code for diarrhea alone may underestimate the actual incidence of disease.

Passive Immunization

Passive immunization with rotavirus-specific antibodies ameliorates acute rotavirus infection in infants.[150-153] Past sources of rotavirus-specific antibodies were pooled commercial preparations of human serum immune globulin or colostrum from cows parenterally immunized with rotavirus. In both immunocompetent and immunocompromised children, oral inoculation with rotavirus-specific antibodies caused a decrease in the number of days with diarrhea as well as a decrease in the length of hospital stay. Nonetheless, no commercial preparation is currently available in the United States and the use of such a preparation would be limited.

Active Immunization

Nonhuman Rotaviruses

Two bovine-origin rotaviruses and one simian rotavirus strain were extensively investigated as potential candidates as oral vaccines for humans. In each case, promising early clinical trials characterized by low pathogenicity and impressive protective efficacy were followed by more extensive trials yielding inconsistent results. These vaccine viruses are currently of interest only to the extent that they contributed to the genome background for reassortant rotaviruses containing genes for human rotavirus surface

TABLE 51–3 ■ Estimated Disease Burden of Rotavirus Gastroenteritis in the United States and Worldwide

Parameter	United States		Worldwide	
	Total	Risk per Child	Total	Risk per Child
Births	3.9 million	—	130 million	—
Episodes of rotavirus gastroenteritis	2.7 million	1 in 1.4*	100 million	1 in 1.3
Physician or emergency department visits	600,000	1 in 65	—	—
Hospitalizations	60,000	1 in 72	—	—
Moderate to severe disease	—	—	16 million	1 in 8
Deaths	20	1 in 200,000	450,000–600,000	1 in 225
Medical costs	$300 million	—	—	—
Indirect and direct costs	$ 1 billion	—	—	—

*Meaning 1 of every 1.4 children born in the United States will have at least one episode of symptomatic rotavirus infection.

proteins. They are described briefly below because many of their phenotypic characteristics are retained to some extent in reassortant vaccines.

A single animal rotavirus strain of lamb origin is currently available in China.

Bovine Strain RIT4237

The first rotavirus vaccine to be evaluated in humans was the bovine strain Nebraska calf diarrhea virus (P6[1]G6),[23] which was named RIT4237 for use in human trials.[154] This virus was highly attenuated by approximately 200 passages in bovine cell culture and most often was administered to infants at a dose of 10^8 median tissue culture infective doses. Induction of immunity was associated with minimal replication; shedding of vaccine virus was noted in up to 20% of vaccine recipients.[155] Between 50% and 70% of vaccine recipients had a humoral immune response measured by rotavirus-specific ELISA for serum immunoglobulin G (IgG) or IgA or by virus neutralization.[155–157] No adverse clinical effects were noted in infants as young as 2 weeks of age.

In two initial efficacy trials of RIT4237 in 6- to 12-month-old Finnish infants, 50% and 58% were protected against all rotavirus diarrhea, and 88% and 82% were protected against "clinically significant" disease.[157,158] The natural challenge was serotype P1A[8]G1 human rotavirus. In subsequent efficacy trials performed in The Gambia and Rwanda and on a Native American reservation in the southwestern United States, little or no protection was observed.[159–161] Therefore, RIT4237 was withdrawn from further development. This action may have been premature because subsequent review of these trials indicated substantial epidemiologic pitfalls (i.e., immunizing older children who were already immune and not having adequate surveillance during follow-up to identify positive results) that would have biased against assessment of efficacy.

Several principles generally applicable to oral rotavirus vaccines in infants were established with RIT4237:

1. A live, attenuated oral vaccine could protect children.
2. The highest rates of immune response were achieved in infants 5 to 12 months of age, a time when prevaccination serum antibody titers (reflecting passively transferred maternal antibodies) were minimal.[155,157,162]
3. The specificity of serum virus neutralizing antibody responses was primarily restricted to the homologous (G6) serotype, but heterotypic immunity could protect children against human strains.[163,164]
4. Administration of infant formulas to buffer stomach acids before giving vaccine-enhanced virus-specific immune responses.[165,166]
5. Coadministration of rotavirus vaccine with oral poliovirus vaccine (OPV) had the potential to inhibit rotavirus-specific immune responses.[167]
6. Protection against severe rotavirus disease was always more efficient than protection against all rotavirus disease.

Bovine Strain WC3

Another bovine rotavirus vaccine strain, WC3 (P7[5]G6), was evaluated as a vaccine after only 12 cell-culture passages.[168] Like RIT4237, WC3 vaccine was given at high titers (10^7 plaque-forming units [PFU] per child), was shed infrequently (up to 30% incidence) in feces, and caused no adverse reactions.[168,169] Serum virus neutralizing antibody responses occurred in 71% to 100% of infants in trials in the United States and were primarily homotypic.[168]

In an initial double-blinded, placebo-controlled, efficacy trial performed in suburban Philadelphia, WC3 vaccine was associated with a 76% reduction in total rotavirus morbidity and 100% protection against moderate to severe rotavirus diarrhea when the natural challenge strain was P1A[8]G1.[100] Virus neutralizing antibodies did not correlate with protection from rotavirus illness. In a subsequent efficacy trial of WC3 conducted in Cincinnati, 100% of infant vaccine recipients developed WC3-specific neutralizing antibodies in serum but were not protected against (G1) rotavirus disease.[170] However, after immunization with WC3 vaccine, infants with evidence of prior infection with G1 rotavirus exhibited major booster responses in serum antibody titers to G1, G2, G3, and G4.[171] In an efficacy trial in Bangui, Central African Republic,[172] only 60% of infants developed homotypic virus neutralizing antibody responses, and there was little protection against rotavirus disease. Infants in Shanghai given WC3 experienced a 50% decrease in cases of rotavirus diarrhea (Guo et al., personal communication, 1991). Because of its inconsistent capacity to protect against disease, WC3 was not considered further as a potential vaccine candidate.

Simian Strain RRV

The third animal-origin rotavirus tested in infants was the rhesus rotavirus vaccine RRV (P5[3]G3), which was isolated from a young monkey with diarrhea[173] and tested as a vaccine candidate in the 16th cell-culture passage.[173] Although RRV is type G3,[174] the G protein is not identical with human G3.[175]

RRV was safe and immunogenic in children 2 to 12 years of age,[173] but, in infants 5 to 20 months of age, a clustering of febrile responses was noted 3 to 4 days after inoculation.[176] In Finnish infants 6 to 8 months of age, significant sequelae were associated with administration of RRV in a titer of 10^5 PFU.[177] In the same study, infants administered RIT4237 vaccine exhibited a lower rate of serum antibody responses but had no adverse reactions.[177]

The increased incidence of fevers was frequently absent in RRV vaccine recipients in developing countries,[178] and in younger infants (4 months of age or younger) inoculated with a lower dose of vaccine. Immunogenicity was less at lower doses (i.e., 10^4 PFU) and in children who were breast-feeding or did not receive a buffer before vaccination.[178–180] RRV at a dose of 10^4 PFU was nonreactogenic in newborn Venezuelan infants.[181] Coadministration of RRV and OPV did not appear to lead to significant inhibition of serum antibody responses to either vaccine.[181,182]

Results of clinical efficacy trials of RRV varied. Infants were given a single dose of 10^4 PFU between 2 and 12 months of age. Trials in Finland and Sweden identified modest protection (38% and 48%, respectively) against all cases of rotavirus diarrhea but greater efficacy against severe rotavirus diarrhea (67% and 80%, respectively).[183,184] However, in three trials in the United States, no protection was observed in New York or Arizona,[185,186] and only 29% protection was demonstrated in Maryland.[187] In all of these trials, the natural challenge viruses were predominantly G1.

The greatest efficacy of RRV was observed in Venezuela: The vaccine protected 65% of children from all rotavirus disease and 100% of children from severe disease.[188] The natural challenge rotavirus was predominately serotype G3. Vaccine-associated reduction in cases identified as G1, G2, or G4 (67%) was similar to the efficacy against G3 (70%).[189]

Lamb Strain LLR

The only licensed vaccine in use today is the Lanzhou Lamb Rotavirus Vaccine (LLR) developed at the Lanzhou Institute of Biological Products.[190] This live oral vaccine, which was derived from an ovine rotavirus isolated in 1985 and characterized as P[10]G12, was passaged 42 times in calf kidney cells. The vaccine is a liquid formulation with buffer containing $10^{5.5}$ infectious particles per dose in a volume of 3 mL and is given as a single dose between 2 and 24 months of age. In an efficacy trial, two cases of rotavirus diarrhea occurred among 1506 vaccine recipients, and eight cases occurred among 1583 placebo recipients (73% efficacy). The rates of mild reactions were similar in the vaccine and placebo groups. The vaccine was licensed in China in 2000 and currently is being sold in a number of provinces. Further studies are planned.

Animal × Human Reassortant Rotaviruses

Because protection against rotavirus disease by animal rotavirus strains was inconsistent, vaccine researchers focused efforts on recombinant (reassortant) rotaviruses. In vitro–derived reassortants were constructed bearing a human VP7 protein (to evoke human G type-specific neutralizing antibodies) and the remaining genes of an animal rotavirus (to attenuate rotavirus virulence for infants).[53,191] Such reassortant strains were prepared by using simian (RRV) or bovine (WC3 or UK) rotaviruses. In addition, naturally occurring bovine-human reassortants ("Indian strains") currently are being tested as vaccines.

The first generation of reassortants, including those in the first licensed vaccine (Rotashield), were designed to contain the gene coding for VP7 of a human virus and 10 genes of the animal virus. To prepare a reassortant, susceptible cell cultures, usually derived from African green monkeys, were co-infected with a human virus and an animal virus (Fig. 51–2). Reassortment of viral gene segments occurred by chance, and a virus containing the desired VP7 was selected by suppressing the VP7 of animal origin with a monotypic antiserum against that protein. Only viruses with human VP7 "broke through," and those also containing 10 genes from the animal virus were identified by gels showing the genomic segments of the reassortants. In some cases, additional confirmation was obtained by sequencing the viral genome.

Simian (Strain RRV)–Human Reassortant Rotaviruses (the First Licensed Rotavirus Vaccine)

The reassortant rotavirus vaccine candidates that were subjected to the earliest clinical testing consisted of simian-human rotavirus reassortants that contained a single human gene (i.e., that coding for VP7) and the remaining 10 genes were from RRV. These reassortant viruses were prepared by the Laboratory of Infectious Diseases at the National Institutes of Health.[192] The vaccine (Rotashield), produced by Wyeth-Lederle, contained RRV (P5BG3) and three simian-human reassortants of G types 1, 2, and 4 in a virus containing all the other genes of RRV. The type 1 human virus was the D strain, and the reassortant was designated RRV-G1; the type 2 virus was DS-1, and the reassortant was designated RRV-G2; and the type 4 virus was ST-3, and the reassortant was designated RRV-G4.

DOSAGE AND ROUTE

Field trials of the quadrivalent RRV-human reassortant vaccine were initiated at an inoculum of 10^4 PFU of each of the

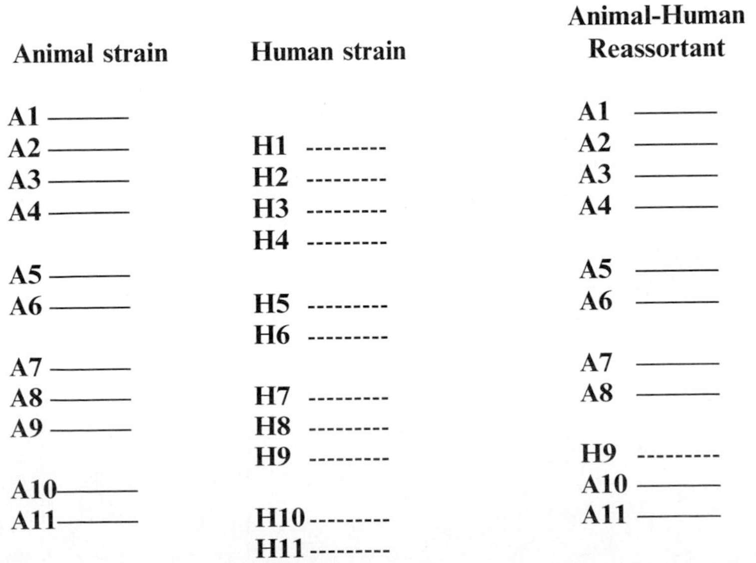

Animal strain	Human strain	Animal-Human Reassortant
A1 ———		A1 ———
A2 ———	H1 ---------	A2 ———
A3 ———	H2 ---------	A3 ———
A4 ———	H3 ---------	A4 ———
	H4 ---------	
A5 ———		A5 ———
A6 ———	H5 ---------	A6 ———
	H6 ---------	
A7 ———		A7 ———
A8 ———	H7 ---------	A8 ———
A9 ———	H8 ---------	
	H9 ---------	H9 ---------
A10———		A10———
A11———	H10---------	A11———
	H11---------	

FIGURE 51–2 ■ The rotavirus genome consists of 11 individual segments of double-stranded RNA (dsRNA). Segments can be distinguished by their pattern of migration in polyacrylamide gel electrophoresis. Progeny virions resulting from co-infection of monkey kidney cells with an animal and a human rotavirus strain often contain gene segments from each parent. The animal-human reassortant rotavirus strain shown has 10 dsRNA segments from the animal strain and 1 segment (gene segment 9) from the human strain. This was the strategy used to make the first rotavirus vaccine, Rotashield.

four viruses (i.e., 4×10^4 PFU) and completed at a dose of 1×10^5 PFU per strain (4×10^5 PFU total), the dose of the licensed vaccine.[192] In each of these trials, vaccine was administered orally in three doses, immunizations were separated by at least 3 weeks, and dosing was completed by the time a child was 6 to 7 months old. Outcomes included either episodes of rotavirus diarrhea reported through active surveillance by field workers during the rotavirus season or passive "catchment" surveillance of children attending a clinic or hospitalized for diarrhea confirmed to be caused by rotavirus. In the United States, two separate but comparable multicenter trials using the low (10^4 PFU per strain) and high (10^5 PFU per strain) doses did not demonstrate a significant difference in efficacy.[193,194] However, in Latin America, two trials conducted in Peru[195] and Brazil[196] with the lower dose of vaccine each demonstrated a lower efficacy against severe disease than a trial with the same low dose in the United States and a trial with the higher dose conducted in Venezuela.[197]

STABILITY

Rotashield was stable for 24 months between 20°C and 25°C in its lyophilized state and for 60 minutes at room temperature or 4 hours in a refrigerator after reconstitution.[198]

IMMUNOGENICITY

Rotashield was developed with the hope that children would develop serotype-specific immunity to the four most common G types of rotavirus in global circulation at that time (G1, G2, G3, and G4). Whereas more than 90% of children developed an immune response, as measured by the presence of virus-specific serum IgA or virus neutralizing antibodies directed against RRV, few children (<50%) developed serotype-specific neutralizing antibodies to each of the four human G serotypes. (Table 51–4 summarizes the immunogenicity data from one of the Rotashield studies performed in the United States.[194]) Nonetheless, studies of efficacy of Rotashield outperformed those using a single RRV-human reassortant (containing human G1) in seasons when strains other than G1 were circulating. This finding indicated that the strategy of using Rotashield to afford broad protection against several serotypes was correct even if there was not an adequate immunologic marker to predict protection against challenge or a complete understanding of the mechanism of this protection.[193,194,199]

EFFICACY

Seven efficacy trials of RRV-human vaccine were conducted, three using the vaccine in the lower dose and four using the vaccine in the higher dose (Table 51–5). In all of these trials, infants were enrolled for immunization between 6 weeks and 2 months of age, and three doses were given by mouth. Efficacy was greater against severe disease than against mild disease, and, in trials lasting 2 years, protection endured for both years.[199]

In general, the efficacy of the simian-human reassortant vaccine was lower in developing countries, an observation that has not been fully confirmed or completely explained. The protective efficacy of the low-dose vaccine was poorest in Peru,[195] intermediate in Brazil,[196] and best in the United States.[193] In a similar manner, the higher-dose preparations performed least well among Native Americans,[185] better among Venezuelans[197] and Americans,[199] and best among Finns.[200]

In trials using high-dose vaccine (Rotashield), efficacy ranged from 48% to 68% against any rotavirus disease and from 64% to 91% against severe disease (see Table 51–5). Of particular note, the efficacy reported in Venezuela (48% for mild disease and 88% for severe disease) was not significantly different from that reported in the multicenter trial in the United States (57% and 82%), suggesting that Rotashield might be well suited for use in developing countries. Furthermore, the observation that the higher dose worked in Venezuela, when a lower dose did not work in Peru or Brazil, suggested that in developing countries vaccine dose may be critical. Only two trials were large enough to examine protection against hospitalization. In the trial in Finland, all 22 children hospitalized for rotavirus diarrhea were in the placebo group,[200] and, in Venezuela, efficacy against hospitalization was 70%.[197]

A post-licensure effectiveness trial in Cincinnati showed 97% protection against hospitalization.[200a]

ADVERSE REACTIONS

A significant increase in mild fevers was observed 3 to 5 days after immunization with Rotashield. Low-grade fevers (temperature >38°C and <39°C) were most common (up to 15%) after the first dose, and a small group of children (1% to 2%) had higher temperatures (>39°C).[193,194,199,200] In the Finnish trial, fever was associated with diarrhea and abdominal cramping in about 3% of children.[201] No increase in

TABLE 51–4 ■ Geometric Mean Antibody Titers and Rates of Seroconversion from a Large-Scale Consistency Lot Study and an Efficacy Trial of Rotashield Vaccine (Rhesus Rotavirus [RRV]-Human Reassortants)

	Anti-Rotaviral Serum IgA	Serum Neutralization Antibody Assays*				
		RRV	G1	G2	G3	G4
Geometric mean antibody titer						
Rotashield (n = 142)	82.6	691.5	20.4	21.6	29.0	10.8
Placebo (n = 108)	17.7	7.1	10.4	6.6	7.6	6.3
Percent with fourfold rise in antibody titer†						
Rotashield (n = 185)	56	90	14	31	29	14
Placebo (n = 195)	2	2	1	0	1	2

*Reference strains used to determine serotype specificities evoked after oral inoculation of infants with Rotashield included rhesus rotavirus serotype G3 (RRV-3) and human rotavirus serotypes G1 (Wa), G2 (DS-1), G3 (P), and G4 (ST-3).
†All comparisons between vaccine and placebo recipients are statistically significant.
Data from Rennels MB, Glass RI, Dennehy PH, et al. Safety and efficacy of high-dose rhesus-human reassortant rotavirus vaccines: report of the National multicenter trial. Pediatrics 97:7–13, 1996.

TABLE 51–5 ■ Efficacy of RRV-Human Reassortant Vaccine

Dose (PFU), Country	Age Groups	N	Circulating Strains	% Efficacy (95% CI) Against Rotavirus Disease	
				All Disease	Severe Disease
4×10^4					
United States[91]	4–26 wk	662	G1, G3	57 (29–74)	82 (–9–97)
Peru[195]	2–4 mo	428	G1, G2	24	60
Brazil[196]	1–5 mo	540	G1, G2	57	NC
4×10^5					
United States[194]	5–25 wk	803	G1, G3	49 (31–63)	80 (56–91)
Finland[200]	3–5 mo	2398	G1, G2	68 (57–76)	91 (82–96)
Venezuela[197]	8–18 wk	2207	G1	48	88
United States[199]	6–24 wk	695	G3	50 (26–67)	69 (29–88)

CI, confidence interval; NC, not comparable.

the incidence of vomiting was associated with vaccination in the first 6 months of life. However, in earlier studies with RRV only, older children in Sweden did have an increased incidence of loose stools and fever, suggesting that replication of the virus in older children could lead to mild symptoms of diarrhea.[202] In Bangladesh, Rotashield caused fever in 15% of vaccinees, compared to 2% in placebo recipients. In addition, vaccine strain virus was isolated from some of the latter, indicating contact spread from vaccinees.[202a]

Table 51–6 summarizes adverse events reported during placebo-controlled trials of Rotashield.[198] Low-grade fever was the most prominent reaction.

Prior to licensure, intussusception was found in 5 of approximately 11,000 children who received RRV-human reassortant rotaviruses, which compared with 1 of approximately 4500 children who received placebo.[198] Intussusception was not found after the first dose in any child but was observed within 7 days after receiving the second or third dose of vaccine in 3 of the 5 affected children. Differences in rates of intussusception between vaccine and placebo recipients were not found to be statistically significant, and the incidence of intussusception in vaccine recipients was not greater than estimated background rates. However, both the CDC and the American Academy of Pediatrics warned in their recommendations for use of Rotashield vaccine that intussusception may be an adverse event associated with vaccination.[198,203] In addition, the relationship between Rotashield vaccine and intussusception was noted in the product insert.

In July 1999, after Rotashield vaccine had been given to about 1 million children, 15 cases of intussusception following administration of Rotashield were reported to the Vaccine Adverse Event Reporting System (VAERS).[204,205] Although approximately 2000 cases of intussusception occur each year in the United States, these 15 cases were greater than what would have been predicted given the general underreporting to VAERS. Following these reports, Rotashield vaccine was temporarily suspended from use[204] pending results of a case-controlled analysis by the CDC.

In October 1999, the CDC completed their analysis and found that the relative risk 3 to 7 days after receipt of the first or second dose of Rotashield was 37.27 (P < 0.001) and 3.8 (P = 0.05), respectively (Table 51–7).[206] Using case-control series and case-control analysis, the population-attributable risk was initially estimated to be about 1 case of intussusception per 10,000 children immunized.[206,207] Following results of the CDC analysis, Rotashield vaccine was discontinued for use.

Subsequent ecologic studies using hospital discharge diagnoses estimated that the attributable risk of intussusception following administration of Rotashield might be much smaller than initial estimates.[208,209]

POSSIBLE ETIOLOGIES OF INTUSSUSCEPTION FOLLOWING ADMINISTRATION OF ROTASHIELD VACCINE

Intussusception is not clearly a consequence of natural rotavirus infection.[210] Therefore, possible etiologies of intussusception must focus on differences between immunization

TABLE 51–6 ■ Summary of Adverse Reactions During Placebo-Controlled Trials of Rotashield Vaccine*

Symptom	Dose 1		Dose 2		Dose 3	
	Rotashield	Placebo	Rotashield	Placebo	Rotashield	Placebo
Temperature (>38°C)	461/2153 (21)†	124/2164 (6)	218/1983 (11)‡	181/2002 (9)	273/1918 (14)	250/1920 (13)
Temperature (>39°C)	37/2153 (2)†	12/2164 (1)	22/1983 (1)	14/2002 (1)	42/1918 (2)	28/1920 (1)
Decreased appetite	375/2181 (17)†	238/2191 (11)	226/2017 (11)	236/2038 (12)	269/1954 (14)	236/1965 (12)
Irritability	541/1317 (41)†	428/1336 (32)	486/1272 (38)	507/1292 (39)	466/1232 (36)	433/1262 (35)
Decreased activity	436/2179 (20)†	292/2190 (13)	238/2018 (12)	244/2036 (12)	203/1952 (10)	212/1965 (11)

*Includes summary data provided by Wyeth-Lederle Vaccines and Pediatrics. The data represent solicited symptoms per total number vaccinated (%) observed at least once within 5 days after each dose.
†P < 0.01.
‡P < 0.05.

TABLE 51–7 ■ Risk of Intussusception Following Administration of Simian-Human Reassortant Rotavirus Vaccine (Rotashield)

Dose	Risk Period (days)	Adjusted Odds Ratio (95% CI)	P Value
All	3–7	14.4 (7.0–29.6)	<0.001
	8–14	5.3 (2.1–13.9)	0.001
	15–21	1.1 (0.3–3.3)	0.91
First	3–7	37.2 (12.6–110.1)	<0.001
	8–14	8.2 (2.4–27.6)	0.001
	15–21	1.1 (0.2–5.4)	0.87
Second	3–7	3.8 (1.0–14.0)	0.05
	8–14	1.8 (0.4–9.5)	0.47
	15–21	0.9 (0.1–8.6)	0.94

CI, confidence interval.
Adapted from Murphy T, Gargiullo P, Massoudi M, et al. Intussusception among infants given an oral rotavirus vaccine. N Engl J Med 344:564–572, 2001.

with Rotashield and natural infection with wild-type human rotaviruses.

Three possible etiologies have been proposed. The first is the "unique strain" hypothesis, which proposes that a strain or strains of rotavirus contained in Rotashield vaccine may be pathogenic in a manner different from that caused by natural infection. Virus contained in Rotashield vaccine may be taken up at an intestinal site or processed by antigen-presenting cells in a manner different from that found after natural infection. Antigen-presenting cells involved following Rotashield administration may produce a panel of cytokines different from those with natural infection; blockage of specific cytokines has been found to be associated with ablation of transient intussusception in experimental animals.[211,212] The most likely candidate for the "unique strain" contained in Rotashield is simian strain RRV. Two biologic features of RRV are unique: (1) RRV is one of the few rotavirus strains that cause diarrhea across a number of species,[213] and (2) RRV is the only known rotavirus strain that causes severe and occasionally fatal hepatitis when orally inoculated into immunodeficient and immunocompetent strains of inbred mice.[50] Which, if any, of these unique biologic features are predictive of intussusception in children remains to be determined. In addition, shedding of RRV at greater levels than RRV-human reassortant viruses after the first and second doses of Rotashield vaccine (indicating an increased adaptation of RRV to grow in the infant intestine) parallels the increased risk of intussusception observed after the first and second doses.[214]

The second proposed etiology is the "bolus dose" hypothesis, which centers on the fact that Rotashield vaccine is probably given in a dose larger than that normally encountered after natural infection. Under natural conditions of infection, small quantities of human rotavirus are ingested and amplification of virus occurs after multiple cycles of replication in the small intestine.[45,48] Immunization, however, presents large quantities of virus to the small intestine in one bolus. The third possible etiology for intussusception following use of Rotashield vaccine is the "heterologous host virus" hypothesis. It is based on the fact that, although cross-species infection does occur to a limited extent in nature, children are not normally infected with heterologous host viruses.

The etiology of intussusception following administration of Rotashield vaccine remains unclear. However, two vaccines currently under the most intensive study (bovine-human rotavirus reassortants and an attenuated human strain) each employ a strategy distinct from RRV-human reassortants. If intussusception following Rotashield was due to a unique biologic feature of RRV, then neither bovine-human reassortants nor attenuated human strains are likely to cause intussusception. If intussusception following Rotashield was due to the fact that RRV is not typically encountered in nature (i.e., is a heterologous host virus), then bovine-human reassortants but not attenuated human strains may cause intussusception. Large-scale clinical studies of these different candidate vaccines are likely to provide some information about the cause or causes of intussusception with RRV-containing vaccine.

Bovine (Strain WC3)–Human Reassortant Rotaviruses

Type G1, G2, G3, and G4 reassortants have been created containing at least the VP7 gene of a human rotavirus on a predominantly bovine WC3 rotavirus genome background. In a similar manner, a P1A-containing virus has been constructed in a reassortant with 10 genes from WC3. Reassortants of G1, G2, G3, and G4 specificity have been administered individually to infants and demonstrated to be as safe as WC3 and, like WC3, to be shed in feces in low incidence (<10%) and at low concentration.[215-218] Therefore, WC3-containing vaccine is much less well adapted to growth at the infant intestinal mucosal surface than are RRV-containing vaccines.

IMMUNOGENICITY

Relative Capacity of VP4 and VP7 to Evoke Neutralizing Antibodies. Infants given one or two oral doses of the univalent G1 or G2 reassortant vaccine tended to have a more efficient neutralizing antibody response in serum to WC3 (the VP4 antigen in the reassortant) than to, respectively, G1 or G2 (the VP7 antigen in the reassortant).[215,218,219] This led to an early opinion that, unlike the response to parentally inoculated rotavirus, the neutralizing antibody response to VP4 predominated following oral administration. (This phenomenon also had been observed repeatedly in clinical trials with RRV-human reassortant rotaviruses.)

However, when a WC3 reassortant was constructed with a human P1A (VP4) and administered orally to infants, the serum neutralizing antibody responses after two doses were predominately to the WC3 VP7 surface G6 component (76% serum neutralizing antibody response to WC3 [VP7] and only 28% response to the P1A [VP4] surface component).[220] When two doses of a mixture of equal concentrations of the G1 (VP7) and P1A (VP4) single gene reassortants of WC3 were administered to infants, an excellent neutralizing antibody response in serum was obtained to both the P1AG1 parent (78%) and the WC3 P7G6 parent (100%).[220] Conversely, less than 35% of infants developed neutralizing antibodies to either WC3 or the human P1AG1 parent after oral inoculation with two doses of one double reassortant (a single virus containing both P1A and G1 on a WC3 background).[217,220]

Importance of Dose. It was later determined in two separate clinical trials that, compared with two doses, three doses of the univalent G1 reassortant resulted in higher rates of neutralizing antibody responses in serum (threefold increase in neutralizing antibody titers) to both the WC3 and the P1AG1 parent viruses (93% to 95% [WC3] and 70% to 78% [P1AG1]) (H.F. Clark, The Children's Hospital of Philadelphia, 1993, unpublished data). In infants from whom blood samples were obtained after each of three doses of the G1 reassortant, it was determined that neutralizing antibody responses to the WC3 and the P1AG1 parent rotaviruses occurred in different sequences (unpublished data). Most infants developed neutralizing antibodies to WC3 after the first dose, a few developed them after the second dose, and almost none developed them after the third dose. In contrast, a minority of infants responded to P1AG1 rotavirus after the first dose, but many more responded to the second and third doses. No infant responded after all three consecutive doses to either virus specificity (i.e., instead of consecutive boosting of titers with consecutive inoculations, a vigorous response to one dose appeared to inhibit a response of the same specificity to the following dose). Infants with neutralizing antibodies to P1AG1 virus prior to the first dose were less likely to develop an antibody response of that specificity after the first dose, but, after three doses, they exhibited response rates similar to those of originally seronegative infants (unpublished data).

EFFICACY TRIALS

In a pilot efficacy trial of the WC3 G1 reassortant involving 77 infants given two doses, complete protection against rotavirus disease was observed. Cases of disease in the placebo cohort were caused by either serotype G1 or G3.[219] A subsequent efficacy trial employed three doses of the G1 reassortant administered to 312 infants in either New York or Philadelphia. The vaccine provided 64% protection against all episodes of rotavirus disease and 84% protection against moderate to severe rotavirus disease (i.e., a score of >8 on a clinical severity scoring system scale of 2 to 24).[216] The predominant wild-type challenge rotavirus was serotype G1. No adverse effects followed administration of any dose of this vaccine.

Because of the success of the G1 univalent WC3 reassortant vaccine in situations of primarily G1 challenge, additional WC3 reassortants of the other traditionally most

common serotypes (i.e., G2, G3, and G4) were constructed. Each was individually evaluated in infants and found to be safe and immunogenic.

Prior to the availability of the G4 reassortant, the principle of using a multivalent WC3 reassortant vaccine was evaluated in an efficacy trial of WC3-human reassortant vaccine containing human G1, G2, G3, and P1A.[221,222] Quadrivalent WC3-human reassortant vaccine containing G1, G2, G3, and P1A, given in three doses and containing 10^7 PFU of each reassortant, was safe, immunogenic, and protective in a trial involving 439 infants in 10 different U.S. sites. Rates of vaccine virus shedding in feces were less than 10%. There was no significant excess of fever, diarrhea, or vomiting in vaccine recipients. The vaccine provided 74.6% protection against all rotavirus disease and 100% protection against severe rotavirus disease (i.e., a clinical score >16).

In the clinical trial of quadrivalent WC3-human reassortant vaccine containing G1, G2, G3, and P1A, a rotavirus-specific serum IgA antibody response occurred in 88% of vaccine recipients, and a fecal rotavirus-specific IgA antibody response occurred in 65% of vaccine recipients.[221,222] The incidence of children who developed virus neutralizing antibodies to serotype G1 was 57%. Similar rates of neutralizing antibody responses specific to types G3, G6, and P1A were observed; the neutralizing antibody response to G2 was slightly lower. The predominant wild-type rotavirus challenge strains as found in placebo cases of rotavirus disease were G1 (26 of 39 episodes [67%]) and G3 (10 of 39 episodes [26%]), while G2 and G4 were associated with two cases and one case, respectively. The "breakthrough" cases of rotavirus disease seen in quadrivalent rotavirus vaccine–immunized infants were predominately G1 (10 of 11 cases [91%]); the other breakthrough case was G2.

Following the clinical success of a quadrivalent WC3-human reassortant vaccine containing G1, G2, G3, and P1A, a pentavalent WC3 reassortant rotavirus vaccine was developed including an added G4 reassortant of WC3. This pentavalent vaccine (G1, G2, G3, G4, and P1A on a WC3 background) was tested in a much larger number of infants in Finland; preliminary results suggest that it too will be highly protective and immunogenic (H.F. Clark, T.A. Offit, The Children's Hospital of Philadelphia, 2002, unpublished data).

Because rotaviruses are highly acid labile, all of the above-mentioned clinical trials involved prefeeding of vaccine recipients with infant formula or Maalox. These trials also involved a frozen product thawed immediately before use. Because prebuffering and use of a frozen product are impractical, a vaccine diluent formulation was developed that contained both buffer and stabilizing components that permitted storage of viable vaccine refrigerated in liquid form. In a clinical trial of bivalent (types G1 and G2) reassortant vaccine, vaccine suspended in the buffer-stabilizer given without a previous oral buffer was compared with traditionally prepared vaccine given after a separate administration of buffer.[223] No adverse effects were observed. Although the trial was not designed to demonstrate efficacy, immune responses in infants given vaccine in the new formulation without prebuffering were excellent and equal to those of the prebuffered vaccine cohort (e.g., following administration of the vaccine in the buffer-stabilizer formulation, serum neutralizing antibody responses to G1 were 67% to 73% and rotavirus-specific IgA antibody responses were 84% to 91% in serum and 77% to 88% in feces).

Because of the initial results with the pentavalent bovine-human reassortant vaccine containing G1, G2, G3, G4, and P1A, extended clinical safety and efficacy trials are now in progress using the new buffer-stabilizer formulation. A brief summary of the results of clinical trials of WC3 reassortant rotavirus vaccines is presented in Table 51–8.

Bovine (Strain UK) × Human Reassortant Rotaviruses

Bovine-human reassortant rotaviruses also have been generated incorporating the genes for VP7 of either Gl, G2, G3, or G4 human serotypes and 10 genes from the bovine UK strain rotavirus, which (like strain WC3) is serotype P7G6.[224–226] These reassortants are serotypically (i.e., P and G types) identical to the G1, G2, G3, and G4 reassortants of bovine rotavirus WC3. Phase I studies were performed on each of the four UK reassortants individually in small numbers of infants (11 to 20 per G serotype) at doses up to $10^{5.8}$ PFU per strain. The vaccine was well tolerated and was shed in feces at rates ranging from 10% to 64% per group. Serum neutralizing antibody responses to the human parent rotaviruses (representing G types 1, 2, 3, and 4) ranged from 0% to 30% per serotype, but the neutralizing antibody responses to the corresponding UK parent virus were higher (30% to 82%). Only 50% of a group of 14 infants given a G1 reassortant developed evidence of any immune response (serum neutralizing antibodies or serum IgA or IgG detected by ELISA). However, following a second dose, all exhibited evidence of an immune response.

Subsequently a quadrivalent vaccine containing G1, G2, G3, and G4 reassortants of UK was administered in three doses to 20 infants.[226] Statistically significant evidence of adverse responses to vaccine was not noted. Nineteen (95%) of the infants developed neutralizing antibodies to UK bovine rotavirus; neutralizing antibody response rates to human rotaviruses of serotypes G1 through G4 ranged from 28% to 37%.[226]

Natural Bovine-Human Reassortant Rotaviruses

Naturally occurring bovine human reassortant rotaviruses were isolated in two sites in India—New Delhi (the 116E strain)[227] and Bangalore (the I321 strain).[228] Newborns infected with the 116E strain were found to be protected against severe disease on reinfection.[229] 116E strain is a human G9 isolate reassortant with a single VP4 gene segment from a bovine strain, giving a final designation P[10]G9. The I321 strain P[11]G10 has a bovine backbone with two segments coding nonstructural proteins NSP1 and NSP3 from human strains. Both of these strains are being developed for clinical trials.

Attenuated Human Rotaviruses

Newborn Rotavirus Strain M37

"Newborn strains" have been studied as potential vaccines because (1) infants in neonatal nurseries in several locales worldwide have been found to be infected with rotavirus with high prevalence but with little gastroenteritis[230]; (2) in neonatal nurseries in Melbourne and New Delhi, infants who were infected in the nursery experienced fewer and less severe subsequent episodes of rotavirus disease than did babies who escaped infection in the nursery[71]; and (3) a subclass of newborn rotavirus isolates obtained from nurseries in different countries was found to share the same antigenic phenotype of VP4 despite the fact that VP7 specificities were either G types 1, 2, 3, or 4.[35,230]

Type G1 newborn strain M37, isolated in Venezuela,[230] has been given in doses of 10^4 PFU to infants as young as 1.5 months old. An increased incidence of fevers 3 to 4 days after administration was observed in Venezuela[231] and Finland[232] but not in Maryland.[233] Serum antibody response rates to rotavirus measured by ELISA (IgG or IgA) ranged from 50% to 74%. Virus neutralizing antibody responses in serum to the immunizing M37 rotavirus ranged from 36% to 71%. However, G type 1–specific antibody responses were observed in only 10% to 27% of vaccine recipients.[231–233]

In an efficacy trial of M37, administration of 10^4 PFU per dose was associated with no protection against rotavirus diarrhea when the natural challenge virus was predominantly G1.[232]

Neonatal Rotavirus Strain RV3

Natural infection with RV3 (P6G3) in a neonatal nursery was reported by Bishop and colleagues[71] to protect infants from subsequent severe rotavirus disease. The virus was propagated in African green monkey kidney (AGMK) cell

TABLE 51–8 ■ Clinical Studies of WC3-Human Reassortant Rotavirus Vaccine: Placebo-Controlled Trials, Phases I and II

Vaccine (N)	Site(s)	Doses	Circulating Strains	Antibody Reponse (%)			Protective Efficacy (%) Against Rotavirus Disease		
				Serum IgA	Fecal IgA	NAb G1	All Disease	Disease Score >8*	Disease Score >16*
G1 (77)	Philadelphia[219]	2	G1, G3	ND	ND	22	100	—	—
G1 (312)	Philadelphia[216]								
	New York[216]	3	G1	ND	ND	70	64	87	ND
G1–G3, P1 (439)	Multicenter[222]	3	G1, G3	88	65	57	75	ND	100
G1, G2 (731)	Multicenter[223]	3	ND	89	83	70	ND†	ND	ND

NAb, neutralizing antibodies.
*Score of 8 or higher is moderate or severe disease, score of 16 or higher is severe disease.
†Infants vaccinated throughout the year to evaluate vaccine formulation, trial not designed (ND) to evaluate efficacy.

culture and evaluated as an oral vaccine in 3-month-old infants.[234] Strain RV3 appeared to be safe, and fecal shedding of vaccine virus was not detected by ELISA. Rotavirus-specific serum antibody responses were not detected, but coproantibody responses were detected in some vaccinees. Protective efficacy data are not yet available.

Strain 89-12

A rotavirus vaccine also has been developed from a human strain that was circulating in the community and associated with rotavirus illnesses. Attenuation of specific genes of wild-type human rotaviruses in vitro is limited by two considerations. First, animal model studies of the genetics of rotavirus virulence may not be predictive of virulence in infants.[53,235] Second, although available for several other viruses, the technology for gene rescue for rotaviruses has not yet been developed. As a result of these limitations, attenuation has been attempted by the historically proven method of serial passage in cell culture.

STRAIN CHARACTERISTICS

Symptomatic or asymptomatic infection of young children with a single circulating wild-type strain (serotype P1AG1) in Cincinnati provided 100% protection against subsequent rotavirus disease over a 2-year period.[72] A vaccine of this strain (i.e., 89-12) was developed after 33 passages of the virus in primary or serially passaged AGMK cells.[236] Initial safety and immunogenicity studies with this vaccine candidate indicated it was relatively safe and immunogenic in children less than 4 months of age.[236] Furthermore, nearly every child developed an immune response to the vaccine virus after two doses.

IMMUNOGENICITY

Limited comparisons of the effects of dose on the immunogenicity of the 89-12 candidate vaccine have been conducted.[236] Two of six infants orally inoculated with two doses of 10^4 focus-forming units (FFU) of strain 89-12 developed rotavirus-specific antibody responses in either serum or stool. However, 19 of 20 inoculated with two doses of 10^5 FFU of 89-12 developed rotavirus-specific antibodies, and 16 did so after the first dose.

EFFICACY TRIAL

The 89-12 vaccine candidate was evaluated in an efficacy trial in healthy 10- to 16-week-old infants at four centers in the United States. Two doses of 10^5 FFU or placebo were administered to 108 or 107 subjects, respectively.[237] Low-grade fever after the first dose was the only side effect more common in vaccine than placebo recipients (21 vs. 5 subjects, respectively; $P = 0.001$). An immune response to rotavirus was detected in 94% of vaccinees and in only 4% of the placebo recipients. During the first rotavirus season, rotavirus disease was detected in 18 placebo recipients and 2 vaccine recipients (efficacy of 89%). Ten placebo recipients but no vaccine recipients presented for medical care necessitated by rotavirus disease. In the second year, efficacy decreased to 59%, but only 1 case of severe rotavirus gastroenteritis occurred in vaccine recipients, while 10 severe cases occurred in placebo recipients. Vaccine efficacy for 2 years was 76% against any rotavirus gastroenteritis, 84% against severe disease, and 100% against very severe disease. Because G1 rotaviruses predominated during both years, the efficacy against heterotypic rotaviruses was not determinable.

RIX 4414 (Higher-Passaged Strain 89-12)

In order to produce a more homogeneous vaccine, strain 89-12 (33 passages in AGMK cells) was purified by endpoint dilution, and the new preparation is currently being evaluated in large trials in countries where non-G1 community strains typically are isolated.

Interestingly, the purified preparation of strain 89-12 (RIX 4414) produced no detectable illness in infants 6 to 12 weeks of age.[238] Oral inoculation of infants with RIX 4414 induced an immune response similar to that found after inoculation with the 33-passage strain.[238] Specifically, 16 (73%) of 22 six- to 12-week-old children developed serum rotavirus IgA responses after two doses of 10^4 FFU; 22 (85%) of 26 and 25 (96%) of 26 developed these responses after two doses of 10^5 and of 10^6 FFU, respectively. On the basis of these results, current safety and efficacy trials of RIX 4414 will use at least 10^5 FFU per dose.

Limits of Present Candidate Vaccines and Approaches to Improved Vaccines

After either natural infection or immunization, production of rotavirus-specific sIgA by small intestinal lymphocytes in the lamina propria is usually short lived. Therefore, one goal for future vaccines would be to prolong effector B-cell responses at the intestinal mucosal surface. Microencapsulation of rotaviruses, using a combination of aqueous anionic polymers (e.g., alginate or chondroitin sulfate) and aqueous amines (e.g., spermine), has been shown to enhance and prolong virus-specific IgA responses at the intestinal mucosal surface[239-241] and to enhance protection against challenge in mice.[242]

Another problem with using oral immunization of infectious virus to induce protection against challenge is the potential inhibitory effect of antibodies in breast milk and colostrum. There are two possible solutions to this problem. First, intramuscular immunization with rotavirus induces virus-specific antibodies in gut-associated lymphoid tissue and protection against challenge in animal studies.[243,244] Second, microencapsulation negates the inhibitory effects of passively transferred virus-specific antibodies in breast milk after oral inoculation of reovirus.[245]

Possible problems associated with the use of live, attenuated virus vaccines may be obviated by the use of virus-like particles,[246] purified rotavirus proteins,[98] or rotavirus-specific naked DNA.[247]

Future Directions and Public Health Considerations

A great deal has been learned from the initial experience with the simian-human reassortant rotavirus vaccine, Rotashield. First and foremost, the experience with Rotashield demonstrated that live oral vaccines can be effective in preventing rotavirus diarrhea in children. Second, despite its high cost (US$38/dose), the vaccine was rapidly embraced by the U.S. public, and, within 9 months, 17% of infants were immunized, primarily in the private sector and before any public sector purchases of the vaccine had been completed. Third, in the buildup to launch this vaccine, the public health community in the United States and abroad came to recognize rotavirus diarrhea as an important public health problem and to anticipate the vaccine as an important means to prevent rotavirus diarrhea in children. However, the rapid disappearance of Rotashield with the unanticipated identification of intussusception has left the health community with a 4-year gap until clinical testing of the next vaccines can be completed. Perhaps a lesson from this experience is not to count on the development of a single vaccine to address a major public health problem, because rare adverse events can never be anticipated. At the same time, the rare identification of intussusception will require that all new rotavirus vaccines licensed in the United States have a level of safety that is substantially improved over the level of safety achieved with Rotashield. Clinical trials will need to enroll in excess of 50,000 children in order to ensure that the rate of intussusception is not higher than the background rate. Both the WC-3 bovine rotavirus vaccine developed by Merck and the RIX 4414 strain developed by GlaxoSmithKline are now in large scale placebo-controlled safety and efficacy trails each encompassing 60,000 infants, including some in developing countries. Last, public health communities in the developing world were anticipating rotavirus vaccines as a major new addition to programs for child survival. With the disappearance of Rotashield, many local vaccine makers in China, India, Indonesia, and other settings have begun their own programs for rotavirus vaccine development and introduction. The methods for rotavirus vaccine development rely on classic cell-culture attenuation techniques that are available in many countries that produce OPV. Future vaccines ultimately could be quite affordable, safe, and effective.

Despite the disappointments from the loss of Rotashield, several positive benefits have emerged. When Rotashield was the only vaccine available, competitors were not aggressive in developing their own strains. Once Rotashield was removed, competition to fill the void increased, with both multinational and local producers striving to accelerate rotavirus vaccine development and testing. Furthermore, when Rotashield was the recommended vaccine for routine childhood rotavirus immunization, it would have been ethically difficult to test new vaccines in the United States and in other countries where Rotashield was universally recommended. With the withdrawal of this recommendation, new vaccines now can be tested in the United States and in Europe without having to conduct head-to-head comparisons with Rotashield.

Those who lost the most from the removal of Rotashield were children in developing countries, where this vaccine likely would have been a lifesaver. Although some argued that it was unethical not to use a vaccine that would have saved many lives in developing countries, the political acceptability of using Rotashield elsewhere was lost once the vaccine was withdrawn from the U.S. market.

Future development and introduction of rotavirus vaccines will require substantial input from the international donor community, including the World Health Organization,[248] the Global Alliance for Vaccines and Immunizations, and the Bill and Melinda Gates Children's Vaccine Program, which all have identified rotavirus vaccine development and introduc-

tion as a high priority. To expedite introduction, surveillance activities will need to be conducted early on to demonstrate the importance of rotavirus as a major cause of disease in each country where the vaccine will be considered. Then, clinical trials of new vaccines will be required to ensure that the vaccines work as well in populations in the developing world as they do in industrialized countries. Issues such as the effect of breast-feeding and administration of OPV on the immunogenicity of candidate vaccines will need to be determined. (Although neither breast-feeding nor concomitant administration of OPV substantially reduced the immunogenicity of Rotashield, studies will need to be repeated for future candidate vaccine strains.[249,250]) Safety will be a primary concern in these trials, and it will be expected that future trials also will need to be done to monitor intussusception as part of the improved safety profile of the next generation of vaccines. It is anticipated that these vaccines would be available for use by 2005 to 2007.

Rotavirus disease occurs commonly in regions with either high or low standards of sanitation. A rotavirus vaccine therefore would be most effective as part of a routine immunization program for infants. The development of safe and effective rotavirus vaccines within the next several years will allow much of the world's population to be protected against the severe and often devastating consequences of rotavirus infection.

REFERENCES

1. de Zoysa I, Feachem RG. Interventions for the control of diarrhoeal diseases among young children: rotavirus and cholera immunization. Bull World Health Organ 63:569–583, 1985.
2. Kapikian AZ, Hoshino Y, Chanock RM. Rotaviruses. In Fields BN, Knipe DM, Howley PM (eds). Fields Virology (4th ed). Vol. 2. Philadelphia, Lippincott–Raven, 2001, pp 1787–1833.
3. Brandt CD, Kim HW, Rodriguez JO, et al. Pediatric viral gastroenteritis during eight years of study. J Clin Microbiol 18:71–78, 1983.
4. Glass RI, Kilgore PE, Holman RC, et al. The epidemiology of rotavirus diarrhea in the United States: surveillance and estimates of disease burden. J Infect Dis 174(suppl 1):S5–S11, 1996.
5. Kilgore PE, Holman RC, Clarke MJ, Glass RI. Trends of diarrheal disease–associated mortality in U.S. children, 1968 through 1991. JAMA 274:1143–1148, 1995.
6. Jin S, Kilgore PK, Holman RC, et al. Trends in hospitalizations for diarrhea in United States children from 1979–1992: estimates of the morbidity associated with rotavirus. Pediatr Infect Dis J 15:397–404, 1996.
7. Smith J, Haddix A, Teutsch S, Glass RI. Cost effectiveness analysis of a rotavirus immunization program for the United States. Pediatrics 96:609–615, 1995.
8. Huilan S, Zhen LG, Mathan MM, et al. Etiology of acute diarrhoea among children in developing countries: a multicentre study in five countries. Bull World Health Organ 69:549–555, 1991.
9. Levine MM, Losonsky G, Herrington D, et al. Pediatric diarrhea: the challenge of prevention. Pediatr Infect Dis 5(suppl):S29–S43, 1986.
10. Cook SM, Glass RI, LeBaron CW, Ho M-S. Global seasonality of rotavirus infections. Bull World Health Organ 68:171–177, 1990.
11. Bern C, Martines J, de Zoysa I, Glass RI. The magnitude of the global problem of diarrhoeal disease: a ten-year update. Bull World Health Organ 70:705–714, 1992.
12. Murray CJ, Lopez AD. Global mortality, disability, and the contribution of risk factors: Global Burden of Disease Study. Lancet 349:1436–1442, 1997.
13. Walsh JA, Warren KS. Selective primary health care: an interim strategy for disease control in developing countries. N Engl J Med 301:967–974, 1979.
14. Snyder JD, Merson MH. The magnitude of the global problem of acute diarrhoeal disease: a review of active surveillance data. Bull World Health Organ 60:605–613, 1982.

15. Oral Rehydration Therapy: An Annotated Bibliography (Scientific Publication No 445). Washington, DC, Pan-American Health Organization, 1983.

16. Tallett S, MacKenzie C, Middleton P, et al. Clinical, laboratory, and epidemiologic features of a viral gastroenteritis in infants and children. Pediatrics 60:217–222, 1977.

17. Carr M, McKendrick D, Spyridakis T. The clinical features of infantile gastroenteritis due to rotavirus. Scand J Infect Dis 8:241–243, 1978.

18. Kovacs A, Chan L, Hotrakitya C, et al. Rotavirus gastroenteritis: clinical and laboratory features and use of the Rotazyme test. Am J Dis Child 141:161–166, 1987.

19. Rodriguez W, Kim H, Arrobio J, et al. Clinical features of acute gastroenteritis associated with human reovirus-like agent in infants and young children. J Pediatr 91:188–193, 1977.

20. Estes M. Rotaviruses and their replication. In Fields BN, Knipe DM, Howley PM (eds). Fields Virology (4th ed). Vol. 2. Philadelphia, Lippincott–Raven, 2001, pp 1747–1786.

21. Sato K, Inaba Y, Shinozaki T, et al. Isolation of human rotavirus in cell cultures. Arch Virol 69:155–160, 1981.

22. Urasawa T, Urasawa S, Taniguchi K. Sequential passages of human rotavirus in MA-104 cells. Microbiol Immunol 25:1025–1035, 1981.

23. Mebus CA, Kono M, Underdahl NR, Twiehaus MJ. Cell culture propagation of neonatal calf diarrhea (scours) virus. Can Vet J 12:69–72, 1971.

24. Malherbe HH, Strickland-Cholmley M. Simian virus SA11 and the related O agent. Arch Ges Virusforsch 22:235–245, 1969.

25. Midthun K, Greenberg HB, Hoshino Y, et al. Reassortant rotaviruses as potential live rotavirus vaccine candidates. J Virol 53:949–954, 1985.

26. Clark HF, Offit PA, Dolan KT, et al. Response of adult human volunteers to oral administration of bovine and bovine/human reassortant rotaviruses. Vaccine 4:25–31, 1986.

27. Midthun K, Hoshino Y, Kapikian AZ, Chanock RM. Single gene substitution rotavirus reassortants containing the major neutralization protein (VP7) of human rotavirus serotype 4. J Clin Microbiol 24:822–826, 1986.

28. Hoshino Y, Sereno MM, Midthun K, et al. Independent segregation of two antigenic specificities (VP3 and VP7) involved in neutralization of rotavirus infectivity. Proc Natl Acad Sci U S A 82:8701–8704, 1985.

29. Offit PA, Blavat G. Identification of the two rotavirus genes determining neutralization specificities. J Virol 57:376–378, 1986.

30. Offit PA, Clark HF, Blavat G, Greenberg HB. Reassortant rotaviruses containing structural proteins VP3 and VP7 from different parents induce antibodies protective against each parental serotype. J Virol 60:491–496, 1986.

31. Sabara M, Gilchrist JE, Hudson GR, Babiuk LA. Preliminary characterization of an epitope involved in neutralization and cell attachment that is located on the major bovine rotavirus glycoprotein. J Virol 53:58–66, 1985.

32. Kalica AR, Greenberg HB, Wyatt RG, et al. Genes of human (strain WA) and bovine (strain UK) rotaviruses that code for neutralization and subgroup antigens. Virology 112:385–390, 1981.

33. Ball JM, Tian P, Zeng CQY, et al. Age-dependent diarrhea induced by a rotaviral nonstructural glycoprotein. Science 272:101–104, 1996.

34. Larralde G, Li B, Kapikian AZ, Gorziglia M. Serotype-specific epitopes present on the VP 8 subunit of rotavirus VP 4 protein. J Virol 65:3213–3218, 1991.

35. Gorziglia MKY, Green K, Nishikawa K, et al. Sequence of the fourth gene of human rotaviruses recovered from asymptomatic or symptomatic infections. J Virol 62:2979–2984, 1988.

36. Hoshino Y, Wyatt RG, Greenberg HB. Serotypic similarity and diversity of rotaviruses of mammalian and avian origin as studied by plaque reduction neutralization. J Infect Dis 149:694–702, 1984.

37. Svensson L, Sheshbaradaran H, Visikari T, et al. Immune response to rotavirus polypeptides after vaccination with heterologous rotavirus vaccines (RIT 4237, RRV-1). J Gen Virol 68:1993–1999, 1987.

38. Ward RL, Knowlton DR, Schiff GM, et al. Relative concentrations of serum neutralizing antibody to VP 3 and VP 7 proteins in adults infected with a human rotavirus. J Virol 62:1543–1549, 1989.

39. Ward RL, Knowlton DR, Greenberg HG, et al. Serum-neutralizing antibody to VP 4 and VP 7 proteins in infants following vaccination with WC3 bovine rotavirus. J Virol 64:2687–2691, 1990.

40. Matsui S, Mackow E, Greenberg H. Molecular determinants of rotavirus neutralization and protection. Adv Virus Res 36:181–214, 1989.

41. Estes MK, Cohen J. Rotavirus gene structure and function. Microbiol Rev 53:410–449, 1989.

42. Mebus CA, Stair EL, Underdahl NR, Twiehaus MJ. Pathology of neonatal calf diarrhea induced by a reo-like virus. Vet Pathol 8:490–505, 1974.

43. Pearson GR, McNulty MS. Pathological changes in the small intestine of neonatal pigs infected with a pig reovirus-like agent (rotavirus). J Comp Pathol 87:363–375, 1977.

44. Snodgrass DR, Ferguson A, Allan F, et al. Small intestinal morphology and epithelial cell kinetics in lamb rotavirus infections. Gastroenterology 76:477–481, 1979.

45. Starkey WG, Collins J, Wallis TS, et al. Kinetics, tissue specificity and pathological changes in murine rotavirus infection of mice. J Gen Virol 67:2625–2634, 1986.

46. Holmes IH, Ruck BJ, Bishop RF, Davidson GP. Infantile enteritis viruses: morphogenesis and morphology. J Virol 16:937–943, 1975.

47. Suzuki H, Konno T. Reovirus-like particles in jejunal mucosa of a Japanese infant with acute infectious non-bacterial gastroenteritis. Tohoku J Exp Med 115:199–211, 1975.

48. Sheridan JF, Eydelloth RS, Vonderfecht SL, Aurelian L. Virus-specific immunity in neonatal and adult mouse rotavirus infection. Infect Immun 39:917–927, 1983.

49. Torres-Medina A. Effect of rotavirus and/or Escherichia coli infection on the aggregated lymphoid follicles in the small intestine of neonatal gnotobiotic calves. Am J Vet Res 45:652–660, 1984.

50. Uhnoo I, Riepenhoff-Talty M, Dharakul T, et al. Extramucosal spread and development of hepatitis with rhesus rotavirus in immunodeficient and normal mice. J Virol 64:361–368, 1990.

51. Davidson GP, Gall DG, Petric M, et al. Human rotavirus enteritis induced in conventional piglets: intestinal structure and transport. J Clin Invest 60:1402–1409, 1977.

52. Graham DY, Sackman JW, Estes MK. Pathogenesis of rotavirus-induced diarrhea: preliminary studies in miniature swine piglet. Dig Dis Sci 29:1028–1035, 1984.

53. Hoshino Y, Sereno MM, Kapikian AZ, et al. Genetic determinants of rotavirus virulence studied in gnotobiotic piglets. In Vaccines 93. Cold Spring Harbor, NY, Cold Spring Harbor Laboratory Press, 1993, pp 277–282.

54. Ward RL, Mason BB, Bernstein DI, et al. Attenuation of a human rotavirus vaccine candidate did not correlate with mutations in the NSP4 protein gene. J Virol 71:6267–6270, 1997.

55. Kapikian AZ, Wha H, Wyatt RG, et al. Human reovirus-like agent as the major pathogen associated with "winter" gastroenteritis in hospitalized infants and young children. N Engl J Med 294:965–972, 1976.

56. Perez-Schael I, Daoud G, White L, et al. Rotavirus shedding by newborn children. J Med Virol 14:127–136, 1984.

57. Chrystie IL, Totterdell BM, Banatvala JE. Asymptomatic endemic rotavirus infections in the newborn. Lancet 1:1176–1178, 1978.

58. Wenman WM, Hinde D, Feltham S, Gurwith M. Rotavirus infection in adults: results of a prospective family study. N Engl J Med 301:303–306, 1979.

59. Velazquez FR, Matson DO, Calva JJ, et al. Rotavirus infection in infants as protection against subsequent infections. N Engl J Med 335:1022–1028, 1996.

60. Matson DO, Velazquez R, Morrow AL, et al. Protective effect of breastfeeding upon first rotavirus infection and illness in a cohort of Mexican children. Pediatr Res 37:128, 1995.

61. Riepenhoff-Talty M, Lee PC, Carmody PJ, et al. Age-dependent rotavirus-enterocyte interactions. Proc Soc Exp Biol Med 170:146–154, 1982.

62. Fukuhara N, Yoshie O, Kitaoka S, Konno T. Role of VP 3 in human rotavirus internalization after target cell attachment via VP 7. J Virol 62:2209–2218, 1988.

63. Kaljot KT, Shaw RD, Rubin DH, Greenberg HB. Infectious rotavirus enters cells by direct cell membrane penetration, not by endocytosis. J Virol 62:1136–1144, 1988.

64. Estes MK, Graham DY, Mason BB. Proteolytic enhancement of rotavirus infectivity: molecular mechanisms. J Virol 39:879–888, 1981.

65. Lebenthal E, Lee PC. Development of functional response in human exocrine pancreas. Pediatrics 66:556–560, 1980.

66. Black REM, Merson MH, Rahman ASSM, et al. A two-year study of bacterial, viral, and parasitic agents associated with diarrhea in rural Bangladesh. J Infect Dis 142:660–664, 1980.

67. Noble RL, Sidwell RW, Mahoney AW, et al. Influence of malnutrition and alterations in dietary protein on murine rotavirus disease. Proc Soc Exp Biol Med 173:417–426, 1983.

68. Morrey JD, Sidwell RW, Noble RL, et al. Effects of folic acid malnutrition on rotaviral infection in mice. Proc Soc Exp Biol Med 176:77–83, 1984.

69. Newsome PM, Coney KA. Synergistic rotavirus and *Escherichia coli* diarrheal infection of mice. Infect Immun 47:573–574, 1985.

70. Tzipori S, Makin T, Smith M, Krautil F. Enteritis in foals induced by rotavirus and enterotoxigenic *Escherichia coli*. Aust Vet J 58:20–23, 1982.

71. Bishop R, Barnes G, Cipriani E, Lund J. Clinical immunity after neonatal rotavirus infection: a prospective longitudinal study in young children. N Engl J Med 309:72–76, 1983.

72. Bernstein DI, Sander DS, Smith VE, et al. Protection from rotavirus reinfection: 2-year prospective study. J Infect Dis 164:277–283, 1991.

73. Ward RL, Bernstein D. Protection against rotavirus disease after natural infection. J Infect Dis 169:900–904, 1994.

73a. Fisher TK, Valentiner-Branth P, Steinsland H, et al. Protective immunity after natural rotavirus infection: a community cohort study of newborn children in Guinea-Bissau, West Africa. J Infect Dis 186:593–597, 2002.

74. Matson DO, O'Ryan ML, Herrera I, et al. Fecal antibody responses to symptomatic and asymptomatic rotavirus infections. J Infect Dis 167:577–583, 1993.

75. Coulson B, Grimwood K, Hudson I, et al. Role of coproantibody in clinical protection of children during reinfection with rotavirus. J Clin Microbiol 30:1678–1684, 1992.

76. O'Ryan ML, Matson DO, Estes MK, Pickering LK. Anti-rotavirus G type-specific and isotype-specific antibodies in children with natural rotavirus infection. J Infect Dis 169:504–511, 1994.

77. Yolken R, Wyatt R, Zissis G. Epidemiology of human rotavirus types 1 and 2 as studied by enzyme-linked immunosorbent assay. N Engl J Med 299:1156–1161, 1978.

78. Black R, Greenberg H, Kapikian A, et al. Acquisition of serum antibody to Norwalk virus and rotavirus in relation to diarrhea in a longitudinal study of young children in rural Bangladesh. J Infect Dis 145:483–489, 1982.

79. Bishop R, Barnes G, Cipriani E, Lund J. Clinical immunity after neonatal rotavirus infection: a prospective longitudinal study in young children. N Engl J Med 309:72–76, 1983.

80. Mata L, Simhon A, Urratia J, et al. Epidemiology of rotaviruses in a cohort of 45 Guatemalan Mayan Indian children observed from birth to the age of three years. J Infect Dis 148:452–461, 1983.

81. Chiba S, Nakata S, Urasawa T, et al. Protective effect of naturally acquired homotypic and heterotypic rotavirus antibodies. Lancet 1:417–421, 1986.

82. Linhares A, Gabbay Y, Mascarenhas J, et al. Epidemiology of rotavirus subgroups and serotypes in Belem, Brazil: a three-year study. Ann Inst Pasteur (Virol) 139:89–99, 1988.

83. Georges-Courbot M, Monges J, Beraud-Cassel A, et al. Prospective longitudinal study of rotavirus infections in children from birth to two years of age in Central Africa. Ann Inst Pasteur (Virol) 139:421–428, 1988.

84. Friedman M, Gaul A, Sarov B, et al. Two sequential outbreaks of rotavirus gastroenteritis: evidence for symptomatic and asymptomatic reinfection. J Infect Dis 158:814–822, 1988.

85. Grinstein S, Gomez J, Bercovich J, Biscorn E. Epidemiology of rotavirus infection and gastroenteritis in prospectively monitored Argentine families with young children. Am J Epidemiol 130:300–308, 1989.

86. Reves R, Hossain M, Midthun K, et al. An observational study of naturally acquired immunity in a cohort of 363 Egyptian children. Am J Epidemiol 130:981–988, 1989.

87. O'Ryan M, Matson D, Estes M, et al. Molecular epidemiology of rotavirus in young children attending day care centers in Houston. J Infect Dis 162:810–816, 1990.

88. DeChamps C, Laveran H, Peigue-Lafeville J, et al. Sequential rotavirus infections: characterization of serotypes and electropherotypes. Res Virol 142:39–45, 1991.

89. Moser CA, Coffin SE, Cookinham S, Offit PA. Relative importance of rotavirus-specific effector and memory B cell responses in protection against challenge. J Virol 72:1108–1114, 1998.

90. Madore H, Christy C, Pichichero M, et al. Field trial of rhesus rotavirus or human-rhesus rotavirus reassortant vaccine of VP7 serotype 3 or 1 specificity in infants. J Infect Dis 166:235–243, 1992.

91. Bernstein D, Glass R, Rodgers G, et al. Evaluation of rhesus rotavirus monovalent and tetravalent reassortant vaccines in U.S. children. JAMA 273:1191–1196, 1995.

92. Ward R, Bernstein D. Lack of correlation between serum rotavirus antibody titers and protection following vaccination with reassortant RRV vaccines. Vaccine 13:1226–1252, 1995.

93. Offit PA, Dudzik KI. Rotavirus-specific cytotoxic T lymphocytes appear at the intestinal mucosal surface after rotavirus infection. J Virol 63:3507–3512, 1989.

94. Offit PA, Dudzik KI. Rotavirus-specific cytotoxic T lymphocytes passively protect against gastroenteritis in suckling mice. J Virol 64:6325–6328, 1990.

95. Dharakul T, Rott L, Greenberg HB. Recovery from chronic rotavirus infection in mice with severe combined immunodeficiency: virus clearance mediated by adoptive transfer of immune CD8+ T lymphocytes. J Virol 64:4375–4382, 1990.

96. Franco M, Tin C, Greenberg H. CD8+ T cells can mediate complete short-term and partial long-term protection against reinfection by rotavirus. J Virol 71:4165–4170, 1997.

97. Kushnir N, Bos NA, Zuercher AW, et al. B2 but not B1 B cells can contribute to CD4+ T cell-mediated clearance of rotavirus in SCID mice. J Virol 75:5482–5490, 2001.

98. McNeal MM, VanCott JL, Choi AH, et al. CD4 T cells are the only lymphocytes needed to protect mice against rotavirus shedding after intranasal immunization with a chimeric VP6 protein and the adjuvant LT (R192G). J Virol 76:560–568, 2002.

99. Bass DM. Interferon gamma and interleukin 1, but not interferon alpha, inhibit rotavirus entry into human intestinal cell lines. Gastroenterology 113:81–89, 1997.

100. Clark HF, Borian FE, Bell LM, et al. Protective effect of WC3 vaccine against rotavirus diarrhea in infants during a predominantly serotype 1 rotavirus season. J Infect Dis 158:570–587, 1988.

101. Chiba S, Nakata S, Urasawa T, et al. Protective effect of naturally acquired homotypic and heterotypic rotavirus antibodies. Lancet 1:417–421, 1986.

102. Burns J, Siadet-Pajouh M, Krishnaney A, Greenberg HB. Novel anti-viral effect against murine rotavirus by an anti-VP6 IgA monoclonal antibody that lacks conventional in vitro neutralizing activity. Science 272:104–107, 1996.

103. Offit PA, Dudzik KI. Rotavirus-specific cytotoxic T lymphocytes cross-react with target cells infected with different rotavirus serotypes. J Virol 62:127–131, 1988.

104. Matson D, O'Ryan M, Pickering L, et al. Characterization of serum antibody responses to natural rotavirus infections in children by VP7-specific epitope-blocking assays. J Clin Microbiol 30:1056–1061, 1992.

105. Zheng B, Han S, Yan Y, et al. Development of neutralizing antibodies and group A common antibodies against natural infections with human rotavirus. J Clin Microbiol 26:1506–1512, 1988.

106. Puerto F, Padilla-Noriega L, Zamora-Chavez A, et al. Prevalent patterns of serotype-specific seroconversion in Mexican children infected with rotavirus. J Clin Microbiol 25:960–963, 1987.

107. Gerna G, Sarasini A, Torsellini M, et al. Group- and type-specific serologic response in infants and children with primary rotavirus infections and gastroenteritis caused by a strain of known serotype. J Infect Dis 161:1105–1111, 1990.

108. Clark H, Dolan K, Horton-Slight P, et al. Diverse serologic response to rotavirus infection of infants in a single epidemic. Pediatr Infect Dis 4:626–631, 1985.

109. Brandt CD, Kim HW, Rodriguez WJ, et al. Comparison of direct electron microscopy, immune electron microscopy and rotavirus enzyme-linked immunosorbent assay for detection of gastroenteritis viruses in children. J Clin Microbiol 13:976–981, 1981.

110. Rubenstein AS, Miller MF. Comparison of enzyme immunoassay with electron microscopy procedures for detecting rotavirus. J Clin Microbiol 15:938–944, 1982.

111. Chrystie IL, Totterdell BM, Banatvala JE. False positive Rotazyme tests on faecal samples from babies [letter]. Lancet 2:1028, 1983.

112. Doern GV, Herrman JE, Henderson P, et al. Detection of rotavirus with a new polyclonal antibody enzyme immunoassay (Rotazyme II) and commercial latex agglutination test (Rotalex): comparison with a monoclonal antibody enzyme immunoassay. J Clin Microbiol 23:226–229, 1986.

113. Sanders RC, Campbell AD, Jenkins AF. Routine detection of human rotavirus by latex agglutination: comparison with latex agglutination, electron microscopy and polyacrylamide gel electrophoresis. J Virol Methods 13:285–290, 1986.

114. Bhan MK, Lew JF, Sazawal S, et al. Protection conferred by neonatal rotavirus infection against subsequent diarrhea. J Infect Dis 168:282–287, 1993.

115. Institute of Medicine. The prospects of immunizing against rotavirus. *In* New Vaccine Development: Diseases of Importance in Developing Countries. Vol. 2. Washington, DC, National Academy Press, 1986, pp D13-1–D13-12.

116. Kraft LM. Studies on the etiology and transmission of epidemic diarrhea of infant mice. J Exp Med 106:743–755, 1957.

117. Alfieri AA, Leite JPG, Nakagomi O, et al. Characterization of human rotavirus genotype P[8]G5 from Brazil by probe-hybridization and sequence. Arch Virol 141:2353–2364, 1996.

118. Gentsch J, Das BK, Jiang B, et al. Similarity of the VP4 protein of human rotavirus strain 116E to that of the bovine B223 strain. Virology 194:424–430, 1993.

119. Nakagomi T, Nakagomi O. RNA-RNA hybridization identifies a human rotavirus that is genetically related to feline rotavirus. J Virol 63:1431–1434, 1989.

120. Hrdy D. Epidemiology of rotaviral infection in adults. Rev Infect Dis 9:461–469, 1987.

121. Bartlett AV, Reves RR, Pickering LK. Rotavirus in infant-toddler day care centers: epidemiology relevant to disease control strategies. J Pediatr 113:435–441, 1988.

122. Pickering LK, Bartlett AV, Reves RR, Morrow A. Asymptomatic excretion of rotavirus before and after rotavirus diarrhea in children in day care centers. J Pediatr 112:361–365, 1988.

123. Pickering LK, Evans DG, DuPont HL. Diarrhea caused by *Shigella*, rotavirus, and *Giardia* in day care centers: prospective study. J Pediatr 99:51–56, 1981.

124. DuPont HL, Ericsson CD. Prevention and treatment of traveler's diarrhea. N Engl J Med 328:1821–1827, 1993.

125. Cunningham AL, Grohmann GS, Harkness J, et al. Gastrointestinal viral infections in homosexual men who were symptomatic and seropositive for human immunodeficiency virus. J Infect Dis 158:386–391, 1988.

126. Hindley F, McIntyre M, Clark B, et al. Heterogeneity of genome rearrangements in rotaviruses isolated from a chronically infected immunodeficient child. J Virol 61:3365–3372, 1987.

127. Saulsbury FT, Winkelstein JA, Yolken RH. Chronic rotavirus infection in immunodeficiency. J Pediatr 97:61–65, 1980.

128. Yolken RJ, Bishop CA, Towsend R. Infectious gastroenteritis in bone marrow transplant recipients. N Engl J Med 306:1009–1012, 1982.

129. Gentsch JR, Woods PA, Ramachandran M, et al. Review of G and P typing results from a global collection of strains: implications for vaccine development. J Infect Dis 174(suppl 1):S30–S36, 1996.

130. Griffin DD, Fletcher M, Levy ME, et al. Outbreaks of adult gastroenteritis traced to a single rotavirus genotype. J Infect Dis 185:1502–1505, 2002.

131. Hoshino Y, Kapikian AZ. Rotavirus vaccine development for the prevention of severe diarrhea in infants and young children. Trends Microbiol 2:242–249, 1994.

132. Ramachandran M, Das BK, Vij A, et al. Unusual diversity of human rotavirus G and P genotypes in India. J Clin Microbiol 34:436–439, 1996.

133. Timenetsky M do C, Santos N, Gouvea V. Survey of rotavirus G and P types associated with human gastroenteritis in São Paulo, Brazil, from 1986 to 1992. J Clin Microbiol 32:2622–2624, 1994.

134. Cunliffe NA, Gondwe JS, Broadhead RL, et al. Rotavirus G and P types in children with acute diarrhea in Blantyre, Malawi, from 1997 to 1998: predominance of novel P[6]G8 strains. J Med Virol 57:308–312, 1999.

135. Nakata S, Gatheru Z, Ukae S, et al. Epidemiological study of the G serotype distribution of group A rotaviruses in Kenya from 1991 to 1994. J Med Virol 58:296–303, 1999.

136. Gurwith M, Wenman W, Gurwith D, et al. Diarrhea among infants and young children in Canada: a longitudinal study in three northern communities. J Infect Dis 147:685–692, 1983.

137. Koopman JS, Turkish VJ, Monto AS, et al. Patterns and etiology of diarrhea in three clinical settings. Am J Epidemiol 119:114–123, 1984.

138. Rodriguez WJ, Kim HW, Brandt CD, et al. Longitudinal study of rotavirus infection and gastroenteritis in families served by a pediatric medical practice: clinical and epidemiologic observations. Pediatr Infect Dis J 6:170–176, 1987.

138a. Van Man N, Van Trang N, Phuong Lien H, et al. The epidemiology and disease burden of rotavirus in Vietnam: sentinel surveillance at 6 hospitals. J Infect Dis 183: 1707–1712, 2001.

139. Ho M-S, Glass RI, Pinsky PF, Anderson LJ. Rotavirus as a cause of diarrheal morbidity and mortality in the United States. J Infect Dis 158:1112–1116, 1988.

140. Ho M-S, Glass RI, Pinsky PF, et al. Diarrheal deaths in American children: are they preventable? JAMA 260:3281–3285, 1988.

141. Ing D, Glass RI, LeBaron CW, Lew JF. Laboratory-based surveillance for rotavirus in the United States, January 1989–May 1991. MMWR CDC Surveill Summ 41:47–56, 1992.

142. LeBaron CW, Lew J, Glass RI, et al, for the Rotavirus Study Group. Annual rotavirus epidemic patterns in North America: results of a five-year retrospective survey of 88 centers in Canada, Mexico, and the United States. JAMA 264:983–988, 1990.

143. Torok TJ, Clarke MJ, Holman RC, Glass RI. Visualizing geographic and temporal trends in rotavirus activity in the United States, 1991–1996. Pediatr Infect Dis J 16:941–946, 1997.

144. Matson DO, Estes MK. Impact of rotavirus infection at a large pediatric hospital. J Infect Dis 162:598–604, 1990.

145. Ryan MJ, Ramsay M, Brown D, et al. Hospital admissions attributable to rotavirus infection in England and Wales. J Infect Dis 174(suppl 1):S12–S18, 1996.

146. Ferson MJ. Hospitalizations for rotavirus gastroenteritis among children under five years of age in New South Wales. Med J Aust 164:273–276, 1996.

147. Lynch M, O'Halloran F, Whyte D, et al. Rotavirus in Ireland: national estimates of diseases burden, 1997 to 1998. Pediatr Infect Dis J 20:693–698, 2001.

148. Perez-Schael I. The impact of rotavirus disease in Venezuela. J Infect Dis 174(suppl 1):S19–S21, 1996.

149. Staat MA, Azimi PH, Berke T, et al. Clinical presentations of rotavirus infection among hospitalized children. Pediatr Infect Dis J 21:221–227, 2002.

150. Guarino A, Russo S, Castaldo A, et al. Passive immunotherapy for rotavirus-induced diarrhoea in children with HIV infection. AIDS 10:1176–1177, 1996.

151. Guarino A, Canani R, Russo S, et al. Oral immunoglobulins for treatment of acute rotaviral gastroenteritis. Pediatrics 93:12–16, 1994.

152. Guarino A, Guandalini S, Albano F, et al. Enteral immunoglobulins for treatment of protracted rotaviral diarrhea. Pediatr Infect Dis J 10:612–614, 1991.

153. Turner R, Kelsey D. Passive immunization for prevention of rotavirus illness in healthy infants. Pediatr Infect Dis J 12:718–722, 1993.

154. Delem A, Lobmann M, Zygraich N. A bovine rotavirus developed as a candidate vaccine for use in humans. J Biol Stand 12:443–445, 1984.

155. Vesikari T, Isolauri E, Delem A, et al. Immunogenicity and safety of live oral attenuated bovine rotavirus vaccine strain RIT 4237 in adults and young children. Lancet 2:807–811, 1983.

156. Mebus CA, White RG, Bass EP, Twiehaus MJ. Immunity to neonatal calf diarrhea virus. J Am Vet Med Assoc 163:880–883, 1973.

157. Vesikari T, Isolauri E, Delem A, et al. Clinical efficacy of the RIT 4237 live attenuated bovine rotavirus vaccine in infants vaccinated before a rotavirus epidemic. J Pediatr 107:189–194, 1985.

158. Vesikari T, Isolauri E, D'Hondt E, et al. Protection of infants against rotavirus diarrhoea by RIT 4237 attenuated bovine rotavirus strain vaccine. Lancet 1:977–980, 1984.

159. De Mol P, Zissis G, Butzler JP, et al. Failure of live, attenuated rotavirus vaccine [letter]. Lancet 2:108, 1986.

160. Hanlon P, Hanlon K, Marsh V, et al. Trial of an attenuated bovine rotavirus vaccine (RIT 4237) in Gambian infants. Lancet 1:1342–1345, 1987.

161. Santosham M, Letson GW, Wolff M, et al. A field study of the safety and efficacy of two candidate rotavirus vaccines in a Native American population. J Infect Dis 163:483–487, 1991.

162. Maldonado Y, Hestvik L, Wilson M, et al. Safety and immunogenicity of bovine rotavirus vaccine RIT 4237 in 3-month-old infants. J Pediatr 109:931–935, 1986.

163. Lanata CF, Black RE, deAguila R, et al. Protection of Peruvian children against rotavirus diarrhea of specific serotypes by one, two, or three doses of the RIT 4237 attenuated bovine rotavirus vaccine. J Infect Dis 159:452–459, 1989.

164. Vesikari T, Ruuska T, Delem A, et al. Efficacy of two doses of RIT 4237 bovine rotavirus vaccine for prevention of rotavirus diarrhea. Acta Paediatr Scand 80:173–180, 1991.

165. Vesikari T, Isolauri E, D'Hondt E, et al. Increased "take" rate of oral rotavirus vaccine in infants after milk feeding [letter]. Lancet 2:700, 1984.

166. Vesikari T, Ruuska T, Bogaerts H, et al. Dose-response study of RIT 4237 oral rotavirus vaccine in breast-fed and formula-fed infants. Pediatr Infect Dis J 4:622–625, 1985.

167. Vodopija I, Baklaic Z, Vlatkovic R, et al. Combined vaccination with live oral polio vaccine and the bovine rotavirus RIT 4237. Vaccine 4:233–236, 1986.

168. Clark HF, Furukawa T, Bell LM, et al. Immune response of infants and children to low-passage bovine rotavirus (strain WC3). Am J Dis Child 140:350–356, 1986.

169. Garbag-Chenon A, Fontaine J-L, Lasfargues G, et al. Reactogenicity and immunogenicity of rotavirus WC3 vaccine in 5–12-month-old infants. Res Virol 140:207–217, 1989.

170. Bernstein DI, Smith VE, Sander DS, et al. Evaluation of WC3 rotavirus vaccine and correlates of protection in healthy infants. J Infect Dis 162:1055–1062, 1990.

171. Ward RL, Sander DS, Schiff GM, Bernstein DI. Effect of vaccination on serotype-specific antibody responses in infants administered WC3 bovine rotavirus before or after a natural rotavirus infection. J Infect Dis 162:1298–1303, 1990.

172. Georges-Courbot MC, Monges J, Siopathis MR, et al. Evaluation of the efficacy of a low-passage bovine rotavirus (strain WC3) vaccine in children in Central Africa. Res Virol 142:405–411, 1991.

173. Kapikian AZ, Midthun K, Hoshino Y, et al. Rhesus rotavirus: a candidate vaccine for prevention of human rotavirus disease. In Lerner RA, Chanock RM, Brown F (eds). Molecular and Chemical Basis of Resistance to Parasitic, Bacterial, and Viral Diseases. Cold Spring Harbor, NY, Cold Spring Harbor Laboratory Press, 1985, pp 357–367.

174. Stuker G, Oshiro LS, Schmidt NH. Antigenic comparisons of two new rotaviruses from rhesus monkeys. J Clin Microbiol 11:202–203, 1980.

175. Nishikawa K, Hoshino Y, Taniguchi K, et al. Rotavirus v.p. 7 neutralization epitopes of serotype 3 strains. Virology 171:503–515, 1989.

176. Losonsky GA, Rennels MB, Kapikian AZ, et al. Safety, infectivity, transmissibility and immunogenicity of rhesus rotavirus vaccine (MMU18006) in infants. Pediatr Infect Dis 5:25–29, 1986.

177. Vesikari T, Kapikian AZ, Delem A, Zissis G. A comparative trial of rhesus monkey (RRV-1) and bovine (RIT 4237) oral rotavirus vaccines in young children. J Infect Dis 153:832–839, 1986.

178. Perez-Schael I, Gonzalez M, Daoud N, et al. Reactogenicity and antigenicity of the rhesus rotavirus vaccine in Venezuelan children. J Infect Dis 155:334–338, 1987.

179. Pichichero ME, Losonsky GA, Rennels MB, et al. Effect of dose and comparison of measures of vaccine taken for oral rhesus rotavirus vaccine. Pediatr Infect Dis J 9:339–344, 1990.

180. Pichichero ME. Effect of breast-feeding on oral rhesus rotavirus vaccine seroconversion: a metaanalysis. J Infect Dis 162:753–755, 1990.

181. Flores J, Daud D, Daud N, et al. Reactogenicity and antigenicity of rhesus rotavirus vaccine (MMV-18006) in newborn infants in Venezuela. Pediatr Infect Dis J 6:260–264, 1988.

182. Jalil F, Zaman S, Carlsson B, et al. Immunogenicity and reactogenicity of rhesus rotavirus vaccine given in combination with oral or inactivated poliovirus vaccines and diphtheria-tetanus-pertussis vaccine. Trans R Soc Trop Med Hyg 85:292–296, 1991.

183. Vesikari T, Rautanen T, Varis T, et al. Rhesus rotavirus candidate vaccine: clinical trial in children vaccinated between 2 and 5 months of age. Am J Dis Child 144:285–289, 1990.

184. Gothefors L, Wadell G, Juto P, et al. Prolonged efficacy of rhesus rotavirus vaccine in Swedish children. J Infect Dis 159:753–757, 1989.

185. Santosham M, Letson GW, Wolff M, et al. A field study of the safety and efficacy of two candidate rotavirus vaccines in a Native American population. J Infect Dis 163:483–487, 1991.

186. Christy C, Madore HP, Pichichero ME, et al. Field trial of rhesus rotavirus vaccine in infants. Pediatr Infect Dis J 7:645–650, 1988.

187. Rennels MB, Losonsky GA, Young AE, et al. An efficacy trial of the rhesus rotavirus vaccine in Maryland. Am J Dis Child 144:601–604, 1990.

188. Flores J, Perez-Schael I, Gonzalez M, et al. Protection against severe rotavirus diarrhea by rhesus rotavirus vaccine in Venezuelan children. Lancet 1:882–884, 1987.

189. Perez-Schael I, Garcia D, Gonzalez M, et al. A prospective study of diarrheal diseases in Venezuelan children to evaluate the efficacy of rhesus rotavirus vaccine. J Med Virol 30:219–229, 1990.

190. Global Alliance for Vaccines and Immunization. Rotavirus vaccine development and introduction in developing countries: preparing a global agenda. World Health Organization. May 14–15, 2001.

191. Burke B, Desselberger U. Rotavirus pathogenicity. Virology 218:299–305, 1996.

192. Kapikian AZ, Hoshino Y, Chanock RM, Perez-Schael I. Efficacy of a quadrivalent rhesus rotavirus–based human rotavirus vaccine aimed at preventing severe rotavirus diarrhea in infants and young children. J Infect Dis 174(suppl 1):S65–S72, 1996.

193. Bernstein DI, Glass RI, Rodgers G, et al. Evaluation of rhesus rotavirus monovalent and tetravalent reassortant vaccines in U.S. children. JAMA 273:1191–1196, 1995.

194. Rennels MB, Glass RI, Dennehy PH, et al. Safety and efficacy of high-dose rhesus-human reassortant rotavirus vaccines: report of the national multicenter trial. Pediatrics 97:7–13, 1996.

195. Lanata CF, Midthun K, Black RE, et al. Safety, immunogenicity, and protective efficacy of one and three doses of the tetravalent rhesus rotavirus vaccine in infants in Lima, Peru. J Infect Dis 174:268–275, 1996.

196. Linhares AC, Gabbay YB, Mascarenhas JDP, et al. Immunogenicity, safety, and efficacy of tetravalent rhesus-human, reassortant rotavirus vaccine in Belem, Brazil. Bull World Health Organ 74:491–500, 1996.

197. Perez-Schael I, Guntinas MJ, Perez M, et al. Efficacy of the rhesus-rotavirus based quadrivalent vaccine in infants and young children in Venezuela. N Engl J Med 337:1181–1187, 1997.

198. Centers for Disease Control and Prevention. Rotavirus vaccine for the prevention of rotavirus gastroenteritis among children: recommendations of the Advisory Committee on Immunization Practices. MMWR 48:1–23, 1999.

199. Santosham M, Moulton LH, Reid R, et al. Efficacy and safety of high-dose rhesus-human reassortant rotavirus vaccine in Native American populations. J Pediatr 131:632–638, 1997.

200. Joensuu J, Koskenniemi E, Pang XL, et al. Randomized placebo-controlled trial of rhesus-human reassortant rotavirus vaccine for prevention of severe rotavirus gastroenteritis. Lancet 350:1205–1209, 1997.

200a. Staat M, Roberts N, Bernstein D, et al. Effectiveness of Rotashield in preventing severe rotavirus (RV) disease requiring hospitalization. Pediatric Res 51: 278A, 2002.

201. Joensuu J, Koskenniemi E, Vesikari T. Clinical symptoms associated with rhesus-human reassortant rotavirus vaccine in Finland. Pediatr Infect Dis J 17:334–340, 1998.

202. Gothefors L, Wadell G, Juto P, et al. Prolonged efficacy of rhesus rotavirus vaccine in Swedish children. J Infect Dis 159:753–757, 1989.

202a. Breese JS, Arifeen SE, Azim T, et al. Safety and immunogenicity of tetravalent rhesus-based rotavirus vaccine in Bangladesh. Pediatr Infect Dis J 20:1136–1143, 2001.

203. Committee on Infectious Diseases, American Academy of Pediatrics. Prevention of rotavirus disease: guidelines for use of rotavirus vaccine. Pediatrics 102:1483–1491, 1998.

204. Centers for Disease Control and Prevention. Intussusception among recipients of rotavirus vaccine—United States, 1998–1999. MMWR 48:577–581, 1999.

205. Committee on Infectious Diseases, American Academy of Pediatrics. Possible association of intussusception with rotavirus vaccination. Pediatrics 104:575, 1999.

206. Murphy TV, Garguillo PM, Massoudi MS, et al. Intussusception among infants given an oral rotavirus vaccine. N Engl J Med 344:564–572, 2001.

207. Kramarz P, France EK, Destefano F, et al. Population-based study of rotavirus vaccination and intussusception. Pediatr Infect Dis J 20:410–416, 2001.

208. Chang H-G, Smith PF, Ackelsberg J, et al. Intussusception, rotavirus diarrhea, and rotavirus vaccine use among children in New York State. Pediatrics 108:54–60, 2001.

209. Simonsen L, Morens DM, Elixhauser A, et al. Effect of rotavirus vaccination programme on trends in admission of infants to hospital for intussusception. Lancet 358:1224–1229, 2001.

210. Chang E, Zangwill KM, Lee H, Ward JI. Lack of association between rotavirus infection and intussusception: implications for use of attenuated rotavirus vaccines. Pediatr Infect Dis J 21:97–102, 2002.

211. Lin Z, Cohen P, Nissan A, et al. Bacterial wall lipopolysaccharide as a cause of intussusception in mice. J Pediatr Gastroenterol Nutr 27:301–305, 1998.

212. Nissan A, Zhang J, Lin Z, et al. The contribution of inflammatory mediators and nitric oxide to lipopolysaccharide-induced intussusception in mice. J Surg Res 69:205–207, 1997.

213. Ciarlet M, Estes MK, Conner ME. Simian rhesus rotavirus is a unique heterologous (non-lapine) rotavirus strain capable of productive replication and horizontal transmission in rabbits. J Gen Virol 81:1237–1249, 2000.

214. Ward RL, Dinsmore AM, Goldbery G, et al. Shedding of rotavirus after administration of the tetravalent rhesus rotavirus vaccine. Pediatr Infect Dis J 17:386–390, 1998.

215. Clark HF, Borian FE, Modesto K, Plotkin SA. Serotype l reassortant of bovine rotavirus WC3, strain Wl79–9, induces a polytypic antibody response in infants. Vaccine 8:327–332, 1990.

216. Treanor J, Clark HF, Pichichero M, et al. Evaluation of the protective efficacy of a serotype l human-bovine rotavirus reassortant vaccine in infants. Pediatr Infect Dis J 14:301–307, 1995.

217. Clark HF, Offit PA, Ellis RW, et al. WC3 reassortant vaccines in children: brief review. Arch Virol Suppl 12:187–198, 1996.

218. Clark HF, Offit PA, Ellis RW, et al. The development of multivalent bovine rotavirus (strain WC3) reassortant vaccine for infants. J Infect Dis 174(suppl l):S73–S80, 1996.

219. Clark HF, Borian FE, Plotkin SA. Immune protection of infants against rotavirus gastroenteritis by a serotype 1 reassortant of bovine rotavirus WC3. J Infect Dis 161:1099–1104, 1990.

220. Clark HF, Welsko D, Offit PA. Infant responses to bovine WC3 reassortants containing human rotavirus VP7, VP4, or VP7 and VP4 [abstr]. In Abstracts of the 32nd Interscience Conference on Antimicrobial Agents and Chemotherapy, Anaheim, CA, October 11–14, 1992, p 343.

221. Clark HF, White CJ, Offit PA, et al, for the OHBRV Study Group. Preliminary evaluation of safety and efficacy of quadrivalent human-bovine reassortant rotavirus vaccine. Pediatr Res 37:172A, 1995.

222. Clark HF, Offit PA, Ward RL, et al. Safety, immunogenicity, and efficacy of a quadrivalent reassortant rotavirus vaccine (QRV). Pediatr Res 51:282A, 2002.

223. Clark HF, Burke CJ, Volkin DB, et al. Safety and immunogenicity in healthy infants of G1 and G2 human reassortant rotavirus (HRV) vaccine in new stabilizer/buffer (S/B) liquid formulation [abstr]. In Abstracts of the 44th Interscience Conference on Antimicrobial Agents and Chemotherapy, San Diego, CA, September 27–30, 2002.

224. Makhene M, Midthun K, Karron R, et al. Safety and immunogenicity of human–UK bovine rotavirus reassortants in adults and pediatric subjects [abstr SV39]. In Program and Abstracts of the Fifth Rotavirus Vaccine Workshop, Atlanta, GA, October 16–17, 1995.

225. Clements-Mann ML, Dudas R, Hoshino Y, et al. Safety and immunogenicity of live attenuated quadrivalent human-bovine (UK) reassortant rotavirus vaccine administered with childhood vaccines to infants. Vaccine 19:4676–4684, 2001.

226. Clements-Mann ML, Makhene MK, Mrukowicz J, et al. Safety and immunogenicity of live attenuated human-bovine (UK) reassortant rotavirus vaccines with VP7-specificity for serotypes 1, 2, 3, 4 in adults, children, and infants. Vaccine 17:2715–2725, 1999.

227. Das BK, Gentsch JR, Hoshino Y, et al. Characterization of the G serotype and genogroup of New Delhi newborn rotavirus strain 116E. Virology 197:99–107, 1993.

228. Dunn SJ, Greenberg HB, Ward RL, et al. Serotypic and genotypic characterization of human serotype 10 rotaviruses from asymptomatic neonates. J Clin Microbiol 31:165–169, 1993.

229. Bhan MK, Lew JF, Sazawal S, et al. Protection conferred by neonatal rotavirus infection against subsequent diarrhea. J Infect Dis 168:282–287, 1993.

230. Hoshino Y, Wyatt RG, Flores J, et al. Serotypic characterization of rotaviruses derived from asymptomatic human neonatal infections. J Clin Microbiol 21:425–430, 1985.

231. Flores J, Perez-Schael I, Blanco M, et al. Comparison of reactogenicity and antigenicity of M37 rotavirus vaccine and rhesus-rotavirus–based quadrivalent vaccine. Lancet 2:330–334, 1990.

232. Vesikari T, Ruuska T, Koivu H-P, et al. Evaluation of the M37 human rotavirus vaccine in 2- to 6-month-old infants. Pediatr Infect Dis J 10:912–917, 1991.

233. Midthun K, Halsey NA, Jett-Goheen M, et al. Safety and immunogenicity of human rotavirus vaccine strain M37 in adults, children, and infants. J Infect Dis 164:792–796, 1991.

234. Barnes G, Bishop R, Lund J, et al. Phase 1 trial of a neonatal strain (RV3) rotavirus vaccine candidate [abstr SV33]. In Program and Abstracts of the Fifth Rotavirus Vaccine Workshop, Atlanta, GA, October 16–17, 1995.

235. Offit PA, Blavat G, Greenberg HB, Clark HF. Molecular basis of rotavirus virulence: role of gene segment 4. J Virol 57:46–49, 1986.

236. Bernstein DI, Smith DE, Sherwood JR, et al. Safety and immunogenicity of live, attenuated human rotavirus vaccine 89-12. Vaccine 16:381–387, 1998.

237. Bernstein DI, Sack DA, Rothstein E, et al. Efficacy of live, attenuated human rotavirus vaccine 89-12 in infants: a randomised placebo-controlled trial. Lancet 354:287–290, 1999.

238. Vesikari T, Karvonen A, Espo M, et al. Reactogenicity and immunogenicity of a human rotavirus vaccine (HRV), given as primary vaccination to healthy infants aged 6–12 weeks. Presented at the Conference on Vaccines for Enteric Diseases VED 2001, Tampere, Finland, September 12–14, 2001.

239. Offit PA, Khoury CA, Moser CH, et al. Enhancement of rotavirus immunogenicity by microencapsulation. Virology 203:134–143, 1994.

240. Brown KA, Moser CA, Khoury CA, et al. Enhancement by microencapsulation of rotavirus-specific intestinal immune responses in mice assessed by enzyme-linked immunospot assay and intestinal fragment culture. J Infect Dis 171:1334–1338, 1995.

241. Khoury CA, Moser CA, Speaker TJ, Offit PA. Oral inoculation of mice with low doses of microencapsulated, noninfectious rotavirus induces virus-specific antibodies in gut-associated lymphoid tissue. J Infect Dis 172:870–874, 1995.

242. Moser CA, Speaker TJ, Offit PA. Effect of water-based microencapsulation on protection against EDIM rotavirus challenge in mice. J Virol 72:3859–3862, 1998.

243. Coffin SE, Klinek M, Offit PA. Induction of virus-specific antibody production by lamina propria lymphocytes following intramuscular inoculation with rotavirus. J Infect Dis 172:874–878, 1995.

244. Conner M, Crawford S, Barone C, Estes M. Rotavirus vaccine administered parenterally induces protective immunity. J Virol 67:6633–6641, 1993.

245. Periwal SB, Speaker TJ, Cebra JJ. Orally administered microencapsulated reovirus can bypass suckled, neutralizing maternal antibody that inhibits active immunization of neonates. J Virol 71:2844–2850, 1997.

246. Estes MK, Crawford SE, Penadanda ME, et al. Synthesis and immunogenicity of the rotavirus major capsid antigen using a baculovirus expression system. J Virol 61:1488–1494, 1987.

247. Herrmann JE, Chen SC, Fynan EF, et al. Protection against rotavirus infections by DNA vaccination. J Infect Dis 174(suppl):S93–S97, 1996.

248. World Health Organization. Report of the Meeting on Future Directions for Rotavirus Vaccine Research in Developing Countries, Geneva, 9–11 February 2000 (WHO/V&B 00.23). Geneva, World Health Organization, 2000.

249. Migasena S, Simasathien S, Samakoses R, et al. Simultaneous administration of oral rhesus-human reassortant tetravalent (RRV-TV) rotavirus vaccine and oral poliovirus vaccine (OPV) in Thai infants. Vaccine 13:168–174, 1995.

250. Rennels M. Influence of breast-feeding and oral poliovirus vaccine on the immunogenicity and efficacy of rotavirus vaccines. J Infect Dis 174(suppl 1):S107–S111, 1996.

Chapter 52

Staphylococcus aureus Vaccine

ANNE GREGERSON • ROBERT S. DAUM

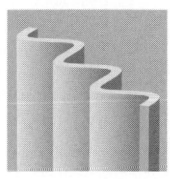 More than a century ago, the Scottish surgeon Alexander Ogdson first noticed an association between skin abscesses and an organism that formed structures resembling clusters of grapes when seen by light microscopy. The organism he saw, *Staphylococcus aureus*, is now known to be responsible for many serious community- and nosocomially acquired infections and several more recently recognized toxin-mediated diseases. It is also the most frequently isolated bacterial pathogen from patients with hospital-acquired infections. The defining characteristic of this species is the production of the extracellular enzyme coagulase and protein A. Staphylococci lacking coagulase are grouped under the designation coagulase-negative staphylococci (CoNS). Once thought to be nonpathogenic constituents of human bacterial flora, the approximately 15 species of CoNS are now also known to cause nosocomial and urinary tract infections in children. Catheter-related infections, prosthetic joint infections, endocarditis, and septic episodes in premature infants and other immunocompromised hosts are also important clinical manifestations of CoNS infections. Although they can be important pathogens in certain settings, vaccine development has been focused primarily on *S. aureus*, which is therefore the subject of this chapter.

Ecology

Staphylococci usually have a symbiotic relationship with their human hosts. Asymptomatic *S. aureus* colonization occurs intermittently in children and adults: 10% to 40% are asymptomatically colonized,[1–5] most commonly in the moist, sheltered anterior nasal vestibule. Additionally, the skin, hair, nails, axillae, perineum, and vagina (in about 10% of menstruating women) may be colonized.[6] Children have somewhat higher colonization rates than adults. *Staphylococcus aureus* colonization is usually transient or temporary, with carriage typically persisting for weeks to months. Hospital personnel and individuals with chronic skin conditions or implanted medical devices have a higher rate of asymptomatic *S. aureus* colonization than do individuals in the community.[7] Persistent chronic colonization occurs in a few individuals. Unlike *S. aureus*, CoNS isolates colonize human skin universally,[8,9] and multiple strains may be isolated from the same individual.

The Clinical Burden

Staphylococcus aureus is a major cause of morbidity and mortality in patients. It is the most virulent pathogen of the genus *Staphylococcus*. Unlike other members of the genus, *S. aureus* is well endowed with DNA elements that encode a variety of virulence factors (Fig. 52–1).

Superficial and invasive *S. aureus* infections occur in previously healthy individuals. Infections of the skin range from impetigo to abscess formation, cellulitis, or lymphadenitis, particularly of the cervical lymph nodes in children or adjacent to an infectious focus. *Staphylococcus aureus* also may cause several important ocular infections, including conjunctivitis, preseptal cellulitis, and endophthalmitis. *Staphylococcus aureus* is an infrequent cause of endocarditis; its clinical manifestations may be particularly severe. Pericarditis may be an isolated syndrome or may accompany endocarditis. Hematogenous seeding of a bone or joint may result in osteomyelitis, septic arthritis, or even bursitis on occasion. *Staphylococcus aureus* is a cause of several respiratory tract infections, including, rarely, otitis media or pneumonia. The latter may be a severe, necrotizing process with high mortality. Central nervous system (CNS) infections are infrequent and usually involve an assisted portal of entry for the organism, such as extension from an infected sinus, a dermal sinus, or a meningomyelocele. CNS Infectious syndromes may also include subdural or epidural empyemas. A spinal epidural abscess adjacent to the dura also may be caused by *S. aureus*. *Staphylococcus aureus* may rarely infect the urinary tract and be recovered from the urine of someone with high-grade bacteremia or a renal abscess.

Staphylococcus aureus (and CoNS as well) frequently complicate medical interventions where indwelling foreign

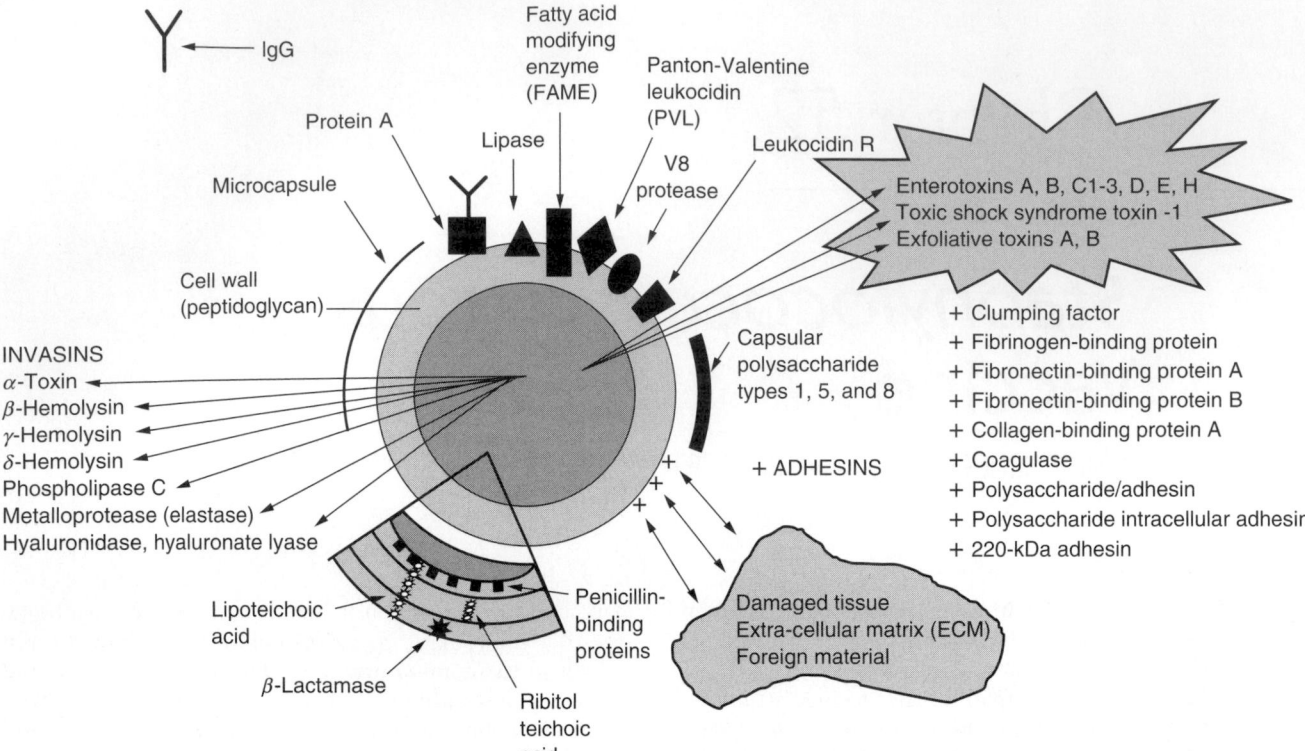

FIGURE 52–1 ■ Diagram of virulence factors of *Staphylococcus aureus*. (Modified from Figure 2, "Virulence Determinants of *Staphylococcus aureus*" in Todar K. Staphylococcus lecture. *In* Bacteriology 330: Host-Parasite Interactions. University of Wisconsin–Madison, 2002. Available at *www.bact.wisc.edu/Bact330/lecturestaph*; and Figure 1, "Structure of *S. aureus*" in Lowy FD. *Staphylococcus aureus* infections. N Engl J Med 339:520–532, 1998.)

bodies are employed in management. The insertion of plastic, metal, or Gore-Tex devices provides an opportunity for *S. aureus* to persistently adhere. Success in removing the organisms from the inserted device has posed a great challenge, even when the isolate is susceptible to the antibiotic in use. Thus certain patients, such as those needing hemodialysis, indwelling venous catheterization, indwelling intravascular Gore-Tex patches, artificial prostheses, or cerebrospinal fluid–flow diversionary devices, are at high risk for *S. aureus* infections.

Staphylococcus aureus is also the cause of a number of toxinoses whose clinical manifestations are associated with the effects of one or more elaboration and release exotoxins. Examples include toxic shock syndrome (TSS), scalded skin syndrome, food poisoning, and necrotizing pneumonia. A variety of veterinary infections are caused by *S. aureus* as well. For example, mastitis in cows is an economically important disease in dairy ruminants. For this reason, *S. aureus* has been a subject for investigation and veterinary vaccine development as well as a vaccine to prevent disease in patients.

The Problem of Antimicrobial Resistance in *S. aureus*

Before the introduction of antimicrobials in the early 1940s, the mortality rate of invasive *S. aureus* infections was about 90%; this rate decreased markedly following the introduction of penicillin G into clinical practice.[10] Almost

immediately, however, a few *S. aureus* isolates were noted to be resistant to penicillin.[11-13] By the end of the 1940s, most strains isolated from hospitalized patients were penicillin resistant[14]; currently, resistance rates exceed 90%, rendering penicillin virtually ineffective in treating *S. aureus* infections. The mechanism of resistance is the elaboration of a ß-lactamase, usually encoded by a transposon borne on a plasmid; there is cross-resistance with other ß-lactams that are susceptible to ß-lactamase digestion.

In the early 1960s, methicillin, representative of a new class of semisynthetic ß-lactam antibiotics that are relatively resistant to hydrolysis by staphylococcal ß-lactamases, was marketed. However, resistance to it was immediately recognized.[15,16] Such resistance is still referred to by the acronym MRSA (methicillin-resistant *S. aureus*), although methicillin is no longer in clinical use. MRSA isolates survive ß-lactam exposure by elaborating a peptidoglycan-synthesizing enzyme called penicillin-binding protein 2a that allows peptidoglycan synthesis despite the presence of a ß-lactam compound. This resistance mechanism conveys cross-resistance to all other ß-lactam antibiotics, including cephalosporins. Since their recognition, the prevalence of MRSA isolates has been slowly but relentlessly increasing,[17-19] and has not yet plateaued. Institutional prevalence rates of 25% to 45% are not uncommon.[20] A new development has been the recent recognition of community-acquired MRSA infections in patients who lack frequent contact with health care facilities.[21] The MRSA isolates responsible for these infections usually are resistant only to ß-lactam antibiotics; evidence is accumulating that these isolates are not related to their hospital counterparts and contain a novel, smaller chromosomal element called SCC*mec* IV [22,23] that may be more transposable than the larger SCC*mec* elements found in hospital MRSA isolates. This is of concern because it brings the potential to allow a more rapid increase in the prevalence of MRSA isolates.

Vancomycin, a glycopeptide antibiotic, until recently had been the only agent to which MRSA isolates had remained uniformly susceptible. This certainty eroded, however, with the recognition of glycopeptide intermediate–resistant *S. aureus* (GISA) (minimal inhibitory concentration [MIC] of vancomycin, ~8 to 12 μg/mL) isolates in Japan,[24] the United States,[25–28] and several other countries.[29–34] Often, patients with GISA isolates have been receiving dialysis and therefore have prolonged low-level serum vancomycin levels, an in vivo environment similar to that used to select for vancomycin-resistant mutants in the laboratory,[35,36] and have failed vancomycin treatment. More recently, vancomycin-resistant *S. aureus* isolates have been isolated from patients in Michigan and Pennsylvania[37a] with MICs of vancomycin greater than or equal to 32 μg/mL. These isolates bear genes from a vancomycin-resistant *Enterococcus faecalis* strain that effect a structurally altered peptidoglycan precursor that does not bind vancomycin. The occurrence of these isolates are important events that will greatly impact health care throughout the world.[37] The ever-evolving resistance mechanisms in *S. aureus* suggests that no antimicrobial therapy strategy will be unmet with a resistance strategy response by the staphylococci. The situation with antibiotic resistance in *S. aureus* is certainly one issue that has spurred vaccine development.

Microbiology and Pathogenesis

Staphylococci are hardy aerobic or facultatively anaerobic gram-positive bacteria that can persist in distressed environments such as acidic conditions, high sodium concentrations, and wide temperature variations; they can survive on fomites, in dust, or on clothing from several days to more than a week. Once staphylococcal infection is established, local and systemic effects result from direct invasion, hematogenous dissemination, and/or toxin release.

Though previously thought to be nonencapsulated, it is now clear that nearly all clinical *S. aureus* isolates and at least some CoNS isolates have a polysaccharide capsule, often called a microcapsule because of its thinness and adherence to the bacterial cell surface. The prevalence of two capsular polysaccharide types (5 and 8) in nearly all collections of clinically important human and veterinary isolates suggests an important role for these polysaccharides in pathogenesis, although, to date, its nature is uncertain. The cell wall of *S. aureus* is composed of peptidoglycan, ribitol, teichoic acid, and protein A, a surface protein to which the Fc region of the immunoglobulin G (IgG) molecule binds.[38–41] IgG antibody binding to the staphylococcal cell surface in this nonphysiologic manner decreases the efficiency by which *S. aureus* are opsonized and phagocytosed.[42–45]

The virulence of *S. aureus* is due to a combination of many elaborated virulence proteins that include extracellular products, such as α-,[46] β-,[47] γ-,[48] and δ-[49] hemolysins;

leukocidins[50]; proteases[51]; lipase[52]; deoxyribonuclease; a fatty acid–modifying enzyme[53]; and hyaluronidase.[54] Coagulase is an extracellular protein that binds host prothrombin to form staphylothrombin; this in turn activates thrombin, and thereby results in the formation of fibrin from fibrinogen.[55] A small amount of coagulase remains cell bound. Clumping factor is a distinct cell surface protein that binds fibrinogen, thereby producing the typical clusters of staphylococci when mixed with plasma.[56] The pathogenic roles of both coagulase and clumping factor have been uncertain; they may protect against host defenses by causing localized clotting, and clumping factor may aid in adherence to traumatized skin, endothelial structures, and foreign surfaces. Recognition of this role for *S. aureus* clumping factor has prompted investigation into its use as a vaccine antigen, as reviewed below.

α-Hemolysin, the best studied of the exotoxins, hemolyzes erythrocytes, necroses skin, and causes the release of cytokines and eicosanoids that may produce shock. It is lethal when injected into animals,[57] and mutants lacking α-toxin are less virulent.[58] However, pathogenic *S. aureus* isolates that do not produce α-hemolysin have been identified. ß-Toxin is a sphingomyelinase that damages membranes rich in this lipid, but its role in pathogenesis is uncertain. Although most human isolates do not express β-toxin, its elaboration by a majority of isolates associated with mastitis in cows suggests a potentially important pathogenic role, at least in that entity.[59] δ-Toxin and leukocidins are synergohymenotropic toxins that damage membranes of certain cells as a result of in-concert action by several elaborated proteins. Interestingly, the transcription of the individual protein components is separate.[48,60] The high percentage of γ-leukocidin–producing isolates from necrotizing skin infections suggests the importance of this toxin in the production of dermonecrosis. *Staphylococcus aureus* Panton-Valentine leukocidin recently has been indicted in cases of severe community-acquired pneumonia in children; the majority of those incidences were fatal and all were marked by hemorrhagic necrosis.[61]

Other toxins are produced by specific *S. aureus* isolates that mediate certain clinical syndromes. For example, epidermolytic (exfoliative) toxins A and B cause sloughing of skin that occurs in staphylococcal scalded skin syndrome.[62] The mechanism of epidermal splitting is unknown, although the toxins do have esterase and, possibly, protease activity.[63] The clinical characteristics of TSS can be attributed to the actions of two different types of toxins: toxic shock syndrome toxin-1 (TSST-1) and enterotoxins. TSST-1 is elaborated by *S. aureus* and is responsible for most TSS cases and nearly all of those associated with menses; antibody to TSST-1 is protective,[64] but patients with TSS often do not make antibody during convalescence from TSS. The family of *S. aureus* enterotoxins may cause vomiting and diarrhea when ingested and is responsible for staphylococcal food poisoning; these enterotoxins also may cause TSS when their entry is via a nongastrointestinal route. The enterotoxins B and C account for about half the TSS cases not associated with menses. The enterotoxins and TSST-1 have superantigen activity, that is, they can stimulate T cells nonspecifically, without normal antigen recognition.[65] This nonspecific antigen T-cell stimulation results in release of immunomodulators, particularly cytokines, an event that produces the clinical picture of TSS. Super-antigens bind to class II major histocompatibility complex receptors but only recognize the Vß element of the receptor, resulting in nonspecific polyclonal T-cell activation.[66]

Locally, the organisms may invade or necrose tissue and evoke a potent inflammatory response, which is largely mediated by the action of polymorphonuclear leukocytes. Abscess formation is common, with a necrotic center consisting of pus and a fibrin wall that makes penetration by antibiotics difficult. The infection may spread locally by the formation of sinus tracts and secondary abscesses. Hematogenous dissemination and infection of distant bones, joints, cardiac valves, or other tissues may result.

CoNS readily adhere to foreign bodies and cause infections that are difficult to eradicate without removal of the prosthetic material. Like S. aureus, CoNS have a cell wall composed of peptidoglycan and teichoic acid but with a glycerol backbone. The teichoic acid and surface proteins play a role in adhering to plastic and other foreign material.[67] In addition, secretion of material commonly called "slime" is thought to be important in the pathogenesis of infection because it coats foreign bodies, thereby insulating the organism; this in turn makes penetration by antibiotics and phagocytosis by host cells difficult. It has been surmised that S. epidermidis isolates may be more likely than those of other CoNS species to produce slime.[68]

Do We Need a Staphylococcal Vaccine?

Although all would agree that S. aureus is an important pathogen with protean clinical manifestations, substantial controversy exists as to whether S. aureus infections can be prevented by a vaccination approach, and, if so, which patients should be targeted to receive this preventive strategy. Various vaccine approaches have been employed with varying levels of promise and success. Interpretation of the data should be done with an understanding of whether the relevant vaccine antigen was chosen, what immune response was measured, what clinical endpoint was sought, if the work was performed in an animal, and whether the animal disease pathophysiology was relevant to a model of human disease. With these thoughts in mind, the available data regarding vaccine development in S. aureus are reviewed below.

Vaccine Development

Live Whole-Cell Vaccines

Several investigators have employed whole-cell vaccines with varying success at preventing certain S. aureus syndromes. A live, attenuated vaccine has been used to prevent bovine mastitis after attenuation of a bovine mastitis S. aureus isolate by mutation with nitrosoguanidine. The mutant also was selected for its ability to grow well at low temperatures, such as those found in breast tissue, and to replicate poorly at 37°C. The vaccine was injected into the mammary gland of pregnant or lactating mice, which produced an immunoglobulin A and IgG antibody response in

milk and serum as measured by an enzyme-linked immunosorbent assay in which killed S. aureus was the antigen. The vaccine also induced primed CD4 and CD8 lymphocyte populations capable of responding to staphylococcal antigens during in vitro stimulation and in vivo challenge.[69] Immunized mice had a 2-log$_{10}$ decrease in the quantity of S. aureus recovered from milk after challenge. A similar decrease was not observed when the vaccine was given parenterally.[70] Thus this whole-cell vaccine, injected locally, provided some protection against an infection whose pathogenesis involves access by the microorganism to the breast from the exterior.

Killed Whole-Cell Vaccines

In contrast, insignificant protection was found when a formalin-killed whole-cell vaccine prepared from one of two clinical S. aureus isolates from patients was used.[71,72] Their vaccine was given parenterally to rabbits prior to S. aureus challenge in a model of experimental endocarditis. Following immunization, antibodies to protein A and S. aureus bacterial agglutination titers were detected in serum at high levels. However, on intravenous challenge, the incidence of endocarditis, concentration of bacteria in infective vegetations, incidence of renal abscess, and the concentration of bacteria in infected kidneys[72] were all insignificantly different from data from unimmunized control animals. Thus systemic immunity after a parenteral challenge versus an invasive bacteremic disease syndrome was not achieved by systemic immunization with this whole-cell vaccine.

This experience was echoed by an interesting chapter in S. aureus vaccine development that concerned the development of a commercially available S. aureus vaccine called Staphypan™, which consisted of a killed suspension of S. aureus cells combined with a toxoided α-hemolysin (α toxin). The effectiveness of Staphypan was assessed in patients undergoing continuous ambulatory peritoneal dialysis who received a complex immunization series consisting of 10 injections. Among these patients, Staphypan was immunogenic with good serum antibody response against the α-hemolysin and to S. aureus cells in the dialysate of vaccine recipients. However, vaccine recipients had rates of peritonitis, catheter-associated infection, and S. aureus asymptomatic carriage that did not differ significantly from a saline-immunized control group.[73] Although this patient population may have posed challenges for the demonstration of vaccine efficacy and, possibly, raised issues regarding choice of outcome parameters, the failure of this vaccine reinforces the difficulties faced in the choice of vaccine components. Put simply, if the whole-cell vaccine had poor efficacy, how does one proceed to selection of components for a component vaccine?

Component Protein Vaccine Antigens

The choice of a relevant S. aureus protein as a component vaccine has obvious advantages over a whole-cell vaccine, particularly in an era of enhanced concern about issues regarding vaccine safety. Investigators have attempted to identify one or more protective antigens among the many toxins or "virulence factors" elaborated by S. aureus as foci for vaccine development (Table 52–1). Substantial effort spanning many years has suggested that a single protective antigen is not likely to be lurking among the many candidate compounds. Thus efficacy of a candidate vaccine antigen often is measured by decreases in disease severity without preventing infection per se. For example, immunization with purified α-toxoid or ß-toxoid vaccine using an experimental model of mastitis in lactating rabbits as an endpoint[74] indicated that both vaccines were immunogenic. In this model, mastitis, typified by abscesses at or near one or more teats, occasionally was complicated by a rapidly fatal, edematous, hemorrhagic mastitis with systemic manifestations termed "blue breast." Three clinically relevant S. aureus isolates were used for challenge of immunized animals. For two of the three isolates, α-toxoid prevented blue breast but not mastitis. The ß-toxoid vaccine had no apparent efficacy against either clinical outcome.[74]

Staphylococcal protein A, the dominant cell wall protein in S. aureus, is present in more than 95% of isolates and comprises about 75% of the S. aureus cell wall mass.[75] It has

TABLE 52–1 ■ Virulence Factors as Potential Targets for Vaccine Development

Factor	Gene
Virulence Factors Involved in Attachment	
Clumping factor	clfA
Fibrinogen-binding protein	fbpA
Fibronectin-binding protein A	fnbA
Fibronectin-binding protein B	fnbB
Collagen-binding protein	cna
Coagulase	cga
Polysaccharide/adhesin	ica locus
Polysaccharide intracellular adhesin	ica locus
220-kDa adhesin	
Virulence Factors Involved in Evasion of Host Defenses	
Enterotoxins A, B, C1–3, D, E, H	sea-h or entA-H
Toxic shock syndrome toxin-1	tst
Exfoliative toxins A, B	eta, etb
Protein A	spa
Lipase	geh
V8 protease	sasP
Fatty acid–modifying enzyme (FAME)	
Panton-Valentine leukocidin	lukF-PV, lukS-PV
Leukocidin R	luk-F-R, lukS-R
Capsular polysaccharide type 1	cap1 locus
Capsular polysaccharide type 5	cap5 locus
Capsular polysaccharide type 8	cap8 locus
Staphylokinase	sak
Virulence Factors Involved in Invasion/Tissue Penetration	
α-Toxin	hla
β-Hemolysin	hlb
γ-Hemolysin	hlgA, hlgB, hlgC
δ-Hemolysin	hld
Phospholipase C	plc
Metalloprotease (elastase)	sepA
Hyaluronidase, hyaluronate lyase	hysA

Modified from Projan SJ, Novick RP. The molecular basis of Pathogenicity. *In* Crossley KB, Archer GL (eds). The Staphylococci in Human Disease. New York, Churchill Livingstone, 57, 1997.

been known for many years that protein A is an antiphagocytic agent that binds immunoglobulin molecules of many mammalian species via its Fc reactive sites. It has been presumed that this biologically ineffectual binding precludes more productive immunoglobulin binding to the cell surface and thereby inhibits opsonophagocytosis. A reasonable question, therefore, has been whether protein A–specific antibodies could protect against S. aureus invasive disease. Unfortunately, using an infant rat model of S. aureus bacteremia in which organisms were injected subcutaneously, antibody to protein A provided passively had no effect on the rate of bacteremia, the rate of metastatic infection in lung or liver, or mortality.[75]

Recent interest has highlighted bacteria–host cell adhesion as a target for staphylococcal vaccine development. In the 1980s, the results of several studies indicated that S. aureus adhered to certain components of the host extracellular matrix (ECM).[76–79] Substantial effort has been invested in the identification of externally expressed bacterial proteins that mediate bacterial binding to host ECM. The proteins are collectively referred to as microbial surface components recognizing adhesive matrix molecules (MSCRAMMs) and mediate S. aureus binding to molecules such as fibronectin, fibrinogen/fibrin, elastin, vitronectin, collagen, laminin, elastin, decorin, and heparan sulfate–containing proteoglycans.[80] Many believe that identifying S. aureus proteins mediating adherence and then incorporating them into vaccine formulations constitutes an important direction for active or passive vaccine development.

For example, a recombinant collagen adhesin fragment was used to immunize mice. Subsequent experimental intravenous challenge with S. aureus decreased mortality from 87% to 13%.[81] Immunization with another MSCRAMM, fibronectin-binding protein, effected a 2-log (99%) decrease in bacterial density in vegetations on heart valves in experimental endocarditis.[82] Similarly, a fusion protein vaccine consisting of the fibrinogen-binding domain of fibrinogen-binding protein A effected a 99.9% decrease in S. aureus recovered from the mammary glands of experimentally challenged mice following immunization with this material.[83]

Recent attention has been focused on another MSCRAMM, clumping factor A (ClfA), a surface protein that binds fibrinogen and fibrin.[84,85] Some have confused ClfA with the S. aureus species-defining protein coagulase, which also binds fibrinogen. ClfA promotes clumping of bacterial cells (the defining staphylococcal morphology of clusters) and bacterial adherence to blood clots and to plasma-conditioned biomaterials as well as catheter-damaged heart valves. In a mouse model of S. aureus arthritis, the severity of arthritis was decreased after challenge with an S. aureus ClfA mutant. Moreover, mice immunized with purified recombinant ClfA and subsequently challenged with S. aureus developed less severe arthritis; passive immunization with anti-ClfA antibodies was protective against experimental septic arthritis and death.[86] Thus ClfA seems to be an important MSCRAMM that has protected or at least partially protected against experimental invasive S. aureus infections. Additional trials employing passive immunization with antibody to ClfA are underway. A donor-selected polyclonal anti-ClfA antibody is in a Phase II trial in low-birth-weight infants that is scheduled for completion in late

2003. A humanized anti-ClfA monoclonal antibody will receive a Phase I evaluation beginning in mid-2003 (J. Patti, personal communication, January 2003).

Carbohydrate Surface Molecules as Vaccine Candidates

Two lines of investigation have suggested that polysaccharides elaborated by S. aureus may be important, and perhaps protective, antigens. One group has examined an in vivo-expressed[87] polysaccharide poly-N-succinyl-β-1-6-glucosamine (PNSG). This intercellular adhesin was first recognized among strains of CoNS.[87] However, S. aureus isolates obtained from the lungs and sputum of cystic fibrosis patients reacted with anti-rabbit anti-PNSG antibody as well. Additional study revealed that eight examined isolates all had the icaADBC locus whose gene products synthesized PNSG among CoNS isolates. It was also appreciated that S. aureus strains can elaborate PNSG in vivo; in vitro expression is minimal or undetectable. Rabbits immunized with purified PNSG produced high-titer IgG anti-PNSG antibody. Passive immunization of mice with these rabbit anti-PNSG antibodies significantly decreased or eliminated bacterial persistence after experimentally induced kidney infection.[87] Active PNSG immunization of mice produced similar results.[88]

PNSG is structurally distinct from the prevalent type 5 and 8 S. aureus capsular polysaccharides. Interestingly, the elaboration of the type 5 or type 8 capsules was found to be inversely related to the expression of PNSG, suggesting that staphylococci may choose to preferentially express PNSG in vivo. The isolates that had in vivo expression of PNSG elaborated little capsular polysaccharide antigen. Moreover, trypticase soy broth cultivation of the S. aureus isolates under aerobic conditions resulted in a reversal of antigen expression: high capsular polysaccharide expression occurred and PNSG expression decreased. Although most clinical strains of S. aureus did not express this PNSG in vitro,[87,88] data from a follow-up study revealed that in vitro PNSG expression could be induced by growing the bacteria in a very rich medium, brain-heart infusion broth supplemented by 0.25% or greater glucose.[88]

Recognition of the crucial role of the polysaccharide capsule in the virulence of Streptococcus pneumoniae and Haemophilus influenzae type b has led to the development and deployment of highly successful pre-exposure preventive vaccine strategies currently in use in the United States and other industrialized countries. These vaccines rely on the notion that antibody to the capsular polysaccharide is opsonic and, thus, counter the antiphagocytic properties imparted by the capsular polysaccharide. The possibility that the S. aureus capsular polysaccharide is similarly a protective antigen that can greatly decrease the incidence of clinical disease to mirror the successes of the H. influenzae type b and S. pneumoniae conjugate vaccine programs seems unlikely from the available data, but substantial controversy exists regarding this question.

More than 90% of S. aureus isolates produce capsular polysaccharide. Four of these, types 1, 2, 5, and 8, have been chemically characterized. Isolates encapsulated by the type 1 and 2 polysaccharides are heavily encapsulated with mucoid colony morphology; such isolates are rarely encountered among clinical isolates. However, most clinical isolates are microencapsulated. The colonies produced by these organisms are not mucoid, unlike the situation with pathogens such as H. influenzae type b and S. pneumoniae, which shed capsular polysaccharide into the surrounding environment. In contrast, S. aureus capsular polysaccharide is shed only minimally if at all. There are 12 known types of S. aureus capsular polysaccharides. Two of these, types 5 and 8 account for 85% of isolates from patients. Because it had been shown that antibody to the types 5 and 8 capsular polysaccharides provided type-specific opsonophagocytosis[89] and conferred protection in animals,[90,91] although conflicting data exist,[92] a vaccine was prepared consisting of the type 5 and 8 capsular polysaccharides bound to recombinant Pseudomonas aeruginosa exotoxin A expressed in Escherichia coli. Because this trial goes to the heart of addressing the controversial question of whether the capsule is in fact a protective antigen, it is reviewed in some detail here.[93]

The trial participants were adult (mean age 58.3 years) hemodialysis patients, a population at high risk for invasive S. aureus infections. The trial was conducted in 1998 to 1999 among 73 hemodialysis centers. 1804 patients were randomized to receive an S. aureus capsular polysaccharide–protein conjugate vaccine or placebo. The vaccine consisted of 100 µg of the type 5 and 8 polysaccharides. Twenty-two percent of the participants were asymptomatic S. aureus carriers. The primary endpoint for the study was the occurrence of S. aureus bacteremia at any time in the first year after immunization beginning 2 or more weeks after immunization. Efficacy was estimated at various time points after immunization by counting bacteremic episodes that occurred.

The efficacy estimates provide a confusing picture. No statistically significant efficacy was observed 2 to 20 weeks after immunization. Twenty-eight episodes of S. aureus bacteremia occurred during this time. Ten of these were among the vaccinees. Data gathered at the 30-week and 40-week postimmunization time point revealed modest efficacy (63%; 95% confidence interval, 14% to 86%, and 57%; 95% confidence interval, 10% to 81%, respectively). However, this efficacy dissipated when observed at the 50-, 54-, or 91-week postimmunization time points. At these times, the vaccine efficacy estimates were 25% to 26% and insignificantly different from zero. The investigators interpreted these data to indicate that the vaccine had provided some protection for about 40 weeks after immunization.

Analysis of anticapsular antibody responses following immunization yielded several surprises. First, the geometric mean serum anticapsular antibody concentration in vaccinees was 80 µg/mL, a value vastly exceeding concentrations believed to be protective against other encapsulated bacteria such as H. influenzae type b and S. pneumoniae. Second, there were no discernible differences between the peak antibody levels in bacteremic vaccinees and controls. Third, the antibody concentrations peaked 6 weeks after immunization and declined thereafter, although significant protection was not observed until some time later. An additional surprising finding was the prevalence of serotype 336 among S. aureus isolates obtained from vaccinees and controls that accounted for about 20% of all the blood isolates. Of concern is that multiple surveys of serotypes of S. aureus isolates from patients had not identified this serotype before, or any other serotype accounting for such a large minority of clinical isolates. This finding also suggests that other serotypes will have to be targeted in addition to types 5 and 8 for a successful anticapsular-based vaccination program. More promising is the generally good safety profile among the vaccinees. Certainty about the protective role of a capsular polysaccharide conjugate vaccine will require additional evaluation. A second clinical trial with this capsular polysaccharide-protein conjugate vaccine is in the planning stage.

Epilogue

Many questions remain. Is the S. aureus disease burden sufficient in the general population to justify development of a universal vaccine approach? Can an antibody-eliciting vaccine protect against S. aureus disease syndromes whose pathogenesis is opportunism after a breach in the integument? Can an active immunization strategy be relied on for immunocompromised individuals at high risk for S. aureus invasive disease? Can a passive vaccination approach be delivered with sufficient regularity to be helpful to patients like those at a reasonable cost? What is the protective antigen for an active or a passive immunization strategy? Could a cocktail of antigens yield better protection than a single antigen-based vaccine? What is the role of the polysaccharide capsule? Its constant presence suggests that it may have an important biologic role, but is antibody to it protective? Identification of the protective antigen or a combination of protective antigens remains an unsolved problem despite intensive investigation, although several of the approaches described in this chapter do hold promise. An additional problem is understanding immunity to S. aureus, an organism that interacts with most if not all of us but causes invasive disease in only a small subset of patients. Is there an immunologic gap in such patients that can be traversed with a vaccine? Despite extensive investigation, we do not know the answer to many of these questions. Staphylococcus aureus remains the evasive, secretive pathogen that persists.

REFERENCES

1. Fekety FR, Buchbinder L, Shaffer EL, et al. Control of an outbreak of staphylococcal infections among mothers and infants in a suburban hospital. Am J Public Health 48:298–310, 1958.
2. Georgopapadakou NH, Dix BA, Mauriz YR. Possible physiological functions of penicillin-binding proteins in Staphylococcus aureus. Antimicrob Agents Chemother 29:333–336, 1986.
3. Shaffer TE, Baldwin JN, Rheins MS, Sylvester RF. Staphylococcal infections in newborn infants. I. Study of an epidemic among infants and nursing mothers. Pediatrics 18:750–761, 1956.
4. Millian SJ, Baldwin JN, Rheins MS, Weiser HH. Studies on the incidence of coagulase-positive staphylococci in a normal unconfined population. Am J Public Health 50:791–798, 1960.
5. Tuazon CU, Sheagren JN. Increased rate of carriage of Staphylococcus aureus among narcotic addicts. J Infect Dis 129:725–727, 1974.
6. Kloos WE, Bannerman TL. Update on clinical significance of coagulase-negative staphylococci. Clin Microbiol Rev 7:117–140, 1994.
7. John JF, Grieshop TJ, Atkins LM, Platt CG. Widespread colonization of personnel at a Veterans Affairs medical center by methicillin-resistant, coagulase-negative staphylococcus. Clin Infect Dis 17:380–388, 1993.
8. D'Angio CT, McGowan KL, Baumgart S, et al. Surface colonization with coagulase-negative staphylococci in premature neonates. J Pediatr 114:1029–1034, 1989.
9. Sidebottom DG, Freeman J, Platt R, et al. Fifteen-year experience with bloodstream isolates of coagulase-negative staphylococci in neonatal intensive care. J Clin Microbiol 26:713–718, 1988.
10. Smith IM, Vickers AB. Natural history of 338 treated and untreated patients with staphylococcal septicaemia. Lancet 1:1318–1322, 1960.
11. Fleming A. In-vitro tests of penicillin potency. Lancet 1:732–733, 1942.
12. Hobby GL, Meyer K, Chaffee E. Activity of penicillin in vitro. Proc Soc Exp Biol 50:277–280, 1942.
13. Rammelkamp CH, Maxon T. Resistance of Staphylococcus aureus to the action of penicillin. Proc Soc Exp Biol 51:386–389, 1942.
14. Barrett FF, Casey JI, Wilcox C, Finland M. Bacteriophage types and antibiotic susceptibility of Staphylococcus aureus: Boston City Hospital, 1967. Arch Intern Med 125:867–873, 1970.
15. Barber M. Methicillin-resistant staphylococci. J Clin Pathol 14:385–393, 1961.
16. Jevons MP. "Celbenin"-resistant staphylococci. Br Med J 1:124–125, 1961.
17. Haley RW, Hightower AW, Khabbaz RF, et al. The emergence of methicillin-resistant Staphylococcus aureus infections in United States hospitals: possible role of the house staff–patient transfer circuit. Ann Intern Med 97:297–308, 1982.
18. Jarvis WR, Thornsberry C, Boyce J, Hughes JM. Methicillin-resistant Staphylococcus aureus at children's hospitals in the United States. Pediatr Infect Dis J 4:651–655, 1985.
19. Thompson RL, Cabezudo I, Wenzel RP. Epidemiology of nosocomial infections caused by methicillin-resistant Staphylococcus aureus. Ann Intern Med 97:309–317, 1963.
20. Voss A, Liatovic D, Wallrauch-Schwarz C, et al. Methicillin-resistant Staphylococcus aureus in Europe. Eur J Clin Microbiol Infect Dis 13:50–55, 1994.
21. Herold BC, Immergluck LC, Maranan MC, et al. Community-acquired methicillin-resistant Staphylococcus aureus infections in children without traditional risk factors for infection. JAMA 279:593–598, 1998.
22. Ma XX, Ito T, Tiensasitorn C, et al. A novel type of staphylococcal cassette chromosome mec (SCCmec) identified in community-acquired methicillin-resistant Staphylococcus aureus strains. Antimicrob Agents Chemother 46:1147–1152, 2002.
23. Daum RS, Ito T, Hiramatsu K, et al. A novel staphylococcal chromosomal cassette containing mec is present in community-acquired methicillin-resistant Staphylococcus aureus isolates in Chicago. J Infect Dis 186:1344–1347, 2002.
24. Hiramatsu K, Hanaki H, Ino T, et al. Methicillin-resistant Staphylococcus aureus clinical strain with reduced vancomycin susceptibility. J Antimicrob Chemother 40:135–136, 1997.
25. Centers for Disease Control and Prevention. Staphylococcus aureus with reduced susceptibility to vancomycin—Illinois, 1999. MMWR 48:1165–1167, 2000.
26. Rotun SS, McMath V, Schoonmaker DJ, et al. Staphylococcus aureus with reduced susceptibility to vancomycin isolated from a patient with fatal bacteremia. Emerg Infect Dis. 5:147–149, 1999.
27. Sieradzki K, Roberts RB, Haber SW, Tomasz A. The development of vancomycin resistance in a patient with methicillin-resistant Staphylococcus aureus infection. N Engl J Med 340:517–523, 1999.
28. Smith TL, Pearson ML, Wilcox KR, et al. Emergence of vancomycin resistance in Staphylococcus aureus. N Engl J Med 340:493–501, 1999.
29. Ploy MC, Grelaud C, Martin C, et al. First clinical isolate of vancomycin-intermediate Staphylococcus aureus in a French hospital. Lancet 351:1212, 1998.
30. Bierbaum GK, Fuchs W, Lenz C, et al. Presence of Staphylococcus aureus with reduced susceptibility to vancomycin in Germany. Eur J Clin Microbiol Infect Dis 18:691–696, 1999.
31. Geisel R, Schmitz FJ, Thomas L, et al. Emergence of heterogeneous intermediate vancomycin resistance in Staphylococcus aureus isolates in the Dusseldorf area. J Antimicrob Chemother 43:846–848, 1999.
32. Ferraz V, Duse AG, Kassel M, et al Vancomycin-resistant Staphylococcus aureus occurs in South Africa. S Afr Med J 90:1113, 2000.
33. Trakulsomboon S, Danchaivijitr S, Rongrungruang Y, et al. First report of methicillin-resistant Staphylococcus aureus with reduced susceptibility to vancomycin in Thailand. J Clin Microbiol 39:591–595, 2001.

34. Wong SSY, Ho PL, Woo CY, Yuen KY. Bacteremia caused by staphylococci with inducible vancomycin heteroresistance Clin Infect Dis 29:760–767, 1999.

35. Daum RS, Gupta S, Sabbagh R, Milewski WM. Characterization of Staphylococcus aureus isolates with decreased susceptibility to vancomycin and teicoplanin: isolation and purification of a constitutively produced protein associated with decreased susceptibility. J Infect Dis 166:1066–1072, 1992.

36. Boyle-Vavra S, Carey R, Daum RS. Development of vancomycin and lysostaphin resistance in a methicillin-resistant Staphylococcus aureus isolate. J Antimicrob Chemother 48:617–625, 2001.

37. Centers for Disease Control and Prevention. Staphylococcus aureus resistant to vancomycin. MMWR 51:565–567, 2002.

37a. Centers for Disease Control and Prevention. Public health dispatch:vancomycin-resistant Staphylococcus aureus. MMWR 51:902, 2002.

38. Schleifer KH, Kroppenstedt RM. Chemical and molecular classification of staphylococci. J Appl Bacteriol (Soc Appl Bacteriol Symp Ser) 19:9S–24S, 1990.

39. Archibald AR. The chemistry of staphylococcal cell walls. In Cohen JO (ed): The Staphylococci. New York, Wiley-Interscience, 1972, p 75.

40. Chatterjee AN. Use of bacteriophage-resistant mutants to study the nature of the bacteriophage receptor site of Staphylococcus aureus. J Bacteriol 98:519–527, 1969.

41. Cheung AL, Bayer AS, Peters J, Ward JI. Analysis by gel electrophoresis, Western blot, and peptide mapping of protein A heterogeneity in Staphylococcus aureus strains. Infect Immun 55:843–847, 1987.

42. Verhoef J, Peterson PK, Verbrugh HA. Host-parasite relationship in staphylococcal infections: the role of the staphylococcal cell wall during the process of phagocytosis. Antonie Van Leeuwenhoek 45:49–53, 1979.

43. Peterson PK, Verhoef J, Sabath LD, Quie PG. Effect of protein A on staphylococcal opsonization. Infect Immun 15:760–764, 1977.

44. Verbrugh HA, Van Dijk WC, Peters R, et al. The role of S. aureus cell wall peptidoglycan, teichoic acid, and protein A in the process of complement activation and opsonization. Immunology 37:615–621, 1979.

45. Spika JS, Verbrugh HA, Verhoef J. Protein A effect on alternative pathway complement activation and opsonization of S. aureus. Infect Immun 34:455–460, 1981.

46. Bhakdi S, Tranum-Jensen J. Alpha-toxin of Staphylococcus aureus. Microbiol Rev 55:733–751, 1991.

47. Wadstrom T, Mollby R. Studies on extracellular proteins from Staphylococcus aureus. VII. Studies on beta-hemolysin. Biochim Biophys Acta 242:308–320, 1971.

48. Finck-Barbancon V, Duportail G, Meunier O, Colin DA. Pore formation by a two-component leukocidin from Staphylococcus aureus within the membrane of human polymorphonuclear leukocytes. Biochim Biophys Acta 1182:275–282, 1993.

49. Scheifele DW, Bjornson GL. Delta toxin activity in coagulase-negative staphylococci from the bowels of neonates. J Clin Microbiol 26:279–282, 1988.

50. Mortensen JE, Shryock TR, Kapral FA. Modification of bacteriocidal fatty acids by an enzyme of Staphylococcus aureus. J Med Microbiol 36:293–298, 1992.

51. Goguen JD, Hoe NP, Subrahmanyam YV. Proteases and bacterial virulence, a view from the trenches. Infect Agents Dis 4:47–54, 1995.

52. Lee CY, Iandolo JJ. Lysogenic conversion of staphylococcal lipase is caused by insertion of the bacteriophage L54a genome into the lipase structural gene. J Bacteriol 166:385–391, 1986.

53. Kapral FA, Smith S, Lal D. The esterification of fatty acids by Staphylococcus aureus fatty acid modifying enzyme (FAME) and its inhibition by glycerides. J Med Microbiol 37:235–237, 1992.

54. McClean D. Methods of assay of hyaluronidase and their correlation with skin diffusing activity. Biochem J 37:169–177, 1943.

55. Cheung AL, Projan SJ, Edelstein RE, Fischetti VA. Cloning, expression, and nucleotide sequence of Staphylococcus aureus gene (fbpa) encoding a fibrinogen-binding protein. Infect Immun 63:1914–1920, 1995.

56. McDevitt D, Francois P, Vaudaux P, Foster TJ. Molecular characterization of the clumping factor (fibrinogen receptor) of Staphylococcus aureus. Mol Microbiol 11:237–248, 1994.

57. Rogolsky M. Nonenteric toxins of Staphylococcus aureus. Microbiol Rev 43:320–360, 1979.

58. O'Reilly M, de Azavedo JC, Kennedy S, Foster TJ. Inactivation of the alpha-haemolysin gene of Staphylococcus aureus 8325-4 by site-directed mutagenesis and studies on the expression of its haemolysins. Microb Pathog 1:125–138, 1986.

59. Naidu TG, Newbould FH. Significance of beta-hemolytic Staphylococcus aureus as a pathogen to the bovine mammary gland. Zentralbl Veterinarmed [B] 22:308–317, 1975.

60. Guid-Rontani C, Fouque F, Alouf JE. Bifactorial versus monofactorial molecular status of Staphylococcus aureus gamma-toxin. Microb Pathog 16:1–14, 1994.

61. Gillet Y, Issartel B, Vanhems P, et al. Association between Staphylococcus aureus strains carrying gene for Panton-Valentine leukocidin and highly lethal necrotising pneumonia in young immunocompetent patients. Lancet 359:753–759, 2002.

62. Gemmell CG. Staphylococcal scalded skin syndrome. J Med Microbiol 43:318–327, 1995.

63. Rago JV, Vath GM, Bohach GA, et al. Mutational analysis of the superantigen staphylococcal exfoliative toxin A (ETA). J Immunol 164:2207–2213, 2000.

64. Garbe PL, Arko RJ, Reingold AL, et al. Staphylococcus aureus isolates from patients with non-menstrual toxic shock syndrome: evidence for additional toxins. JAMA 253:2538–2542, 1985.

65. Choi Y, Lafferty JA, Clements JR, et al. Selective expansion of T cells expressing V beta 2 in toxic-shock syndrome. J Exp Med 172:981–984, 1990.

66. Kotb M. Bacterial pyrogenic exotoxins as superantigens. Clin Microbiol Rev 8:411–426, 1995.

67. Hogt AH, Dankert J, Hulstaert CE, Feijen J. Cell surface characteristics of coagulase-negative staphylococci and their adherence to fluorinated poly(ethylenepropylene). Infect Immun 51:294–301, 1986.

68. Jones JW, Scott RJ, Morgan J, Pether JV. A study of coagulase-negative staphylococci with reference to slime production, adherence, antibiotic resistance patterns and clinical significance. J Hosp Infect 22:217–227, 1992.

69. Gomez MI, Sordelli DO, Buzzola FR, Garcia VE. Induction of cell-mediated immunity to Staphylococcus aureus in the mouse mammary gland by local immunization with a live attenuated mutant. Infect Immun 70:4254–4260, 2002.

70. Garcia VE, Gomez MI, Sanjuan N, et al. Intramammary immunization with live-attenuated Staphylococcus aureus: microbiological and immunological studies in a mouse mastitis model. FEMS Immunol Med Microbiol 14:45–51, 1996.

71. Lee JC. The prospects for developing a vaccine against Staphylococcus aureus. Trends Microbiol 4:162–166, 1996.

72. Greenberg DP, Ward JI, Bayer AS. Influence of Staphylococcus aureus antibody on experimental endocarditis in rabbits. Infect Immun 55:3030–3034, 1987.

73. Poole-Warren LA, Hallett MD, Hone PW, et al. Vaccination for prevention of CAPD-associated staphylococcal infection: results of a prospective multicentre clinical trial. Clin Nephrol 35:198–206, 1991.

74. Adlam C, Ward PD, McCartney AC, et al. Effect of immunization with highly purified alpha- and beta-toxins on staphylococcal mastitis in rabbits. Infect Immun 17:259–, 1977.

75. Greenberg DP, Bayer AS, Cheung AL, Ward JI. Protective efficacy of protein A-specific antibody against bacteremic infection due to Staphylococcus aureus in an infant rat model. Infect Immun 57:1113–1118, 1989.

76. Hawiger J, Timmons S, Strong DD, et al. Identification of a region of human fibrinogen interacting with staphylococcal clumping factor. Biochemistry 21:1407–1413, 1982.

77. Kuusela P. Fibronectin binds to Staphylococcus aureus. Nature 276:718–720, 1978.

78. Chhatwal GS, Preissner KT, Muller-Berghaus G, Blobel H. Specific binding of the human S protein (vitronectin) to streptococci, Staphylococcus aureus, and Escherichia coli. Infect Immun 55:1878–1883, 1987.

79. Speziale P, Raucci G, Visai L, et al. Binding of collagen to Staphylococcus aureus Cowan 1. J Bacteriol 167:77–81, 1986.

80. Joh D, Wann E, Kreikemeyer B, et al. Role of fibronectin-binding MSCRAMMs in bacterial adherence and entry into mammalian cells. Matrix Biol 18:211–223, 1999.

81. Nilsson IM, Patti JM, Bremell T, et al. Vaccination with a recombinant fragment of collagen adhesion provides protection against Staphylococcus aureus-mediated septic death. J Clin Invest 101:2640–2649, 1998.

82. Schennings T, Heimdahl A, Coster K, Flock JI. Immunization with fibronectin-binding protein from *Staphylococcus aureus* protects against experimental endocarditis in rats. Microb Pathogen 15:227–236, 1993.

83. Mamo W, Jonsson P, Flock JI, et al. Vaccination against *Staphylococcus aureus* mastitis: immunologic response of mice vaccinated with fibronectin-binding protein (FnBP-A) to challenge with *S. aureus*. Vaccine 12:988–992, 1994.

84. Foster T, Hook M. Surface protein adhesins of *Staphylococcus aureus*. Trends Microbiol 6:484–488, 1998.

85. Josefsson E, Hartford O, O'Brien L, et al. Protection against experimental *Staphylococcus aureus* arthritis by vaccination with clumping factor A, a novel virulence determinant. J Infect Dis 184:1572–1580, 2001.

86. Vastag B. New vaccine decreases rate of nosocomial infections. JAMA 285:1565–1566, 2001.

87. McKenney D, Pouliot KL, Wang Y, et al. Broadly protective vaccine for *Staphylococcus aureus* based on an in vivo-expressed antigen. Science 284:1523–1527, 1999.

88. McKenney D, Pouliot KL, Wang Y, et al. Vaccine potential of poly-1-6 β-D-*N*-succinylglucosamine, an immunoprotective surface polysaccharide of *Staphylococcus aureus* and *Staphylococcus epidermidis*. J Biotechnol 83:37–44, 2000.

89. Karakawa WW, Sutton A, Schneerson R, et al. Capsular antibodies induce type-specific phagocytosis of capsulated *Staphylococcus aureus* by human polymorphonuclear leukocytes. Infect Immun 56:1090–1095, 1988.

90. Lee JC, Park JS, Shepherd SE, et al. Protective efficacy of antibodies to the *Staphylococcus aureus* type 5 capsular polysaccharide in a modified model of endocarditis in rats. Infect Immun 65:4146–4151, 1997.

91. Fattom AL, Sarwar J, Ortiz A, Naso R. *Staphylococcus aureus* capsular polysaccharide vaccine and CP-specific antibodies protect mice against bacterial challenge. Infect Immun 64: 1659–1665, 1996.

92. Nemeth J, Lee JC. Antibodies to capsular polysaccharides are not protective against experimental *Staphylococcus aureus* endocarditis. Infect Immun 63:375–380, 1995.

93. Shinefield H, Black S, Fattom A, et al. Use of a *Staphylococcus aureus* conjugate vaccine in patients receiving hemodialysis. N Engl J Med 346:491–496, 2002.

Chapter 53

Immunization in the United States

WALTER A. ORENSTEIN • LANCE E. RODEWALD • ALAN R. HINMAN

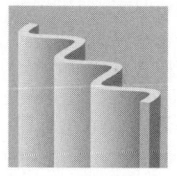

Vaccines represent some of the most important tools available for the prevention of disease. In addition to protecting the vaccinated individual from developing a potentially serious disease, they help protect the community by reducing the spread of infectious agents. For diseases spread from person to person, if a high enough proportion of the population is immunized, transmission may be interrupted in the community, thus providing protection to those who are not themselves immunized. This indirect protection is often called *community* or *herd immunity* (see Chapter 56).[1,2] From both theoretical and practical perspectives, disease usually disappears before immunization levels reach 100%, as has been seen with smallpox and poliomyelitis.[3–10]

With no intervention, the occurrence of a disease is affected only by the traditional considerations of host, agent, and environment. As a vaccine is introduced into a population, the incidence of the disease decreases, reaching an acceptable level of control (Fig. 53–1). Further application of the intervention may lead to interruption of transmission of the agent and disappearance of the agent from the area under consideration, but with a threat of reintroduction large enough that continued application of the intervention is required. This stage, *elimination*, describes the current goals for measles and rubella in the United States. If enough areas achieve elimination, *regional elimination* may be achieved. However, regional elimination is inherently unstable in this era of global transportation and is merely a way station on the road to true *eradication*, in which transmission of the agent has been halted throughout the world and continuation of the intervention may no longer be necessary.[11,12]

In 1980, the world was declared free of smallpox, ending the centuries of disease and death brought about by that disease (see Chapter 9).[13] Eradication of smallpox was possible because there was a highly effective vaccine, no nonhuman reservoir to perpetuate circulation of virus, and no long-term carrier state to perpetuate potential spread. Eradication was made simpler by the relatively low communicability of smallpox and by the fact that both disease and vaccine gave a readily visible marker of immunity, the scar. Eradication of smallpox has raised the possibility that other diseases might also be eradicated.[12,14–22] The United States has set goals for elimination of a number of diseases, including measles and rubella.

Immunization Recommendations

The development of vaccine schedules and recommendations begins with prelicensure evaluation of a vaccine (see discussion by the Center for Biologics Evaluation and Research at *www.fda.gov/cber*). Prelicensure trials of vaccines typically are performed in controlled settings with relatively small numbers (i.e., thousands) of individuals involved. These trials provide important information on seroconversion following vaccination, on clinical efficacy of the vaccine in preventing disease after exposure, and about common adverse events following vaccination and contraindications to the use of the vaccines. Prelicensure evaluation also provides information on the number of doses required to achieve protection and may give an indication of the duration of immunity following vaccination. If the prelicensure trials indicate that the vaccine is safe and effective, it may be licensed for use in a particular population group. Information about the safety and efficacy of administering a specific vaccine simultaneously with other vaccines may be obtained either before or after licensure of that vaccine, but information about the safety and efficacy of combining vaccines is obtained before combinations are licensed.

Recommendations for use of a vaccine depend on the balance of benefits of vaccination (including duration of protection), risks of disease, and risks of vaccination. This balance must be assessed periodically and when new information is available. As experience is gained with a particular vaccine, recommendations may need to be modified, as was the case with the withdrawal of the recommendation for rotavirus vaccine.[23,24] Since the mid-1960s, recommendations in the United States about vaccination of children traditionally

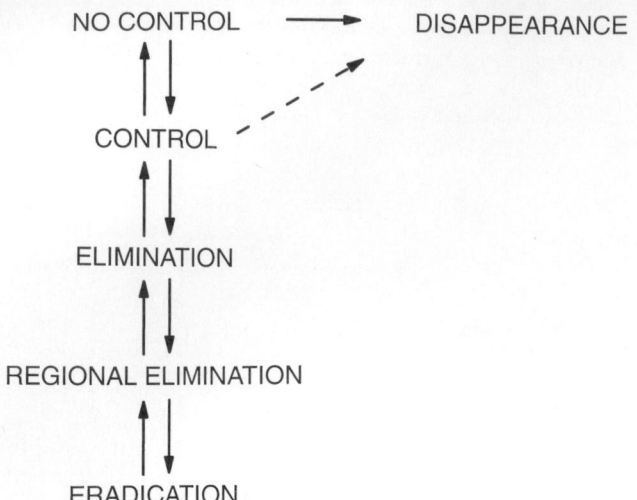

FIGURE 53-1 ▪ Spectrum of disease incidence.

have been developed by two advisory bodies: (1) the Advisory Committee on Immunization Practices (ACIP) of the Public Health Service and (2) the American Academy of Pediatrics Committee on Infectious Diseases (the *Red Book* Committee).[25] The ACIP recommendations, which originally were intended primarily for providers in the public sector, have in recent years addressed the needs of providers in public and private sectors. The *Red Book* recommendations are directed mainly toward children served by pediatricians. Since 1995, the ACIP, the American Academy of Pediatrics, and the American Academy of Family Physicians have collaborated to issue a single childhood immunization schedule, which is published annually in the journals *Morbidity and Mortality Weekly Report, Pediatrics,* and *American Family Physician.*[26,27] A continuously updated version of the harmonized schedule is available at *www.aap.org/family/parents/immunize.htm* or *www.cdc.gov/nip.*

Recommendations of the ACIP are published in the "Recommendations and Reports" supplement of the *Morbidity and Mortality Weekly Report;* those of the *Red Book* Committee are published in the *Report of the Committee on Infectious Diseases* (the *Red Book*), which is revised every 2 to 4 years. New or revised recommendations of the *Red Book* Committee developed between editions of the *Red Book* are published as issued in *Pediatrics.* Appendix 1 of this text lists the published recommendations of the ACIP as of April 2003. The American College of Physicians and the Infectious Diseases Society of America have formed the Task Force on Adult Immunization, which has issued guidelines for adult immunization.[28] Recommendations for immunization of Armed Services personnel are developed by the Armed Forces Epidemiological Board. In October 2002, the Advisory Committee on Immunization Practices issued an adult immunization schedule that was accepted by both the American Academy of Family Physicians and the American College of Obstetricians and Gynecologists.[28a]

The National Childhood Vaccine Injury Act of 1986 established a National Vaccine Program to coordinate all aspects of vaccine research, development, production, and use in both the private and the public sectors.[29] It also established a National Vaccine Advisory Committee (NVAC) to bring outside recommendations and advice to the National Vaccine Program.[30] Three important publications of the NVAC have been the "measles white paper,"[31] the report on adult immunization,[32] and the report on the status of United States vaccine research.[33] In addition, the NVAC played a critical role in the development of the "Standards for Child and Adolescent Immunization Practices."[34] The NVAC focuses most on programmatic policies and strategies, in contrast to the ACIP, which deals primarily with technical recommendations for vaccine use.

Sources of Information

Sources of information about immunization recommendations include the following:

1. *Official package circular.* Manufacturers provide product-specific information with each vaccine; some of these circulars are reproduced in their entirety in the *Physicians' Desk Reference* (a new edition is published annually by Thompson Medical Economics Company, Five Paragon Drive, Montvale, NJ 07645-1742; *www.medec.com*).

2. *Morbidity and Mortality Weekly Report.* This report is published weekly by the Centers for Disease Control and Prevention (CDC). ACIP statements are usually published in separate Recommendations and Reports supplements to the weekly publication. Current and back issues are available at *www.cdc.gov/mmwr.* Free electronic subscriptions are available by sending an e-mail message to *listserv@listserv.cdc.gov* with the body of the message reading: SUBscribe mmwr-toc. Paper subscriptions are available through the Superintendent of Documents, U.S. Government Printing Office, Washington, DC 20402-9235.

3. *Red Book: Report of the Committee on Infectious Diseases of the American Academy of Pediatrics.* The full report containing recommendations on all licensed vaccines is usually updated every 2 to 4 years. At the time this chapter went to press, the next edition of the *Red Book* was scheduled to be published in 2003. It may be ordered from American Academy of Pediatrics, PO Box 927, Elk Grove Village, IL 60007.

4. *Red Book Update.* The Committee on Infectious Diseases of the American Academy of Pediatrics publishes its recent positions and specific recommendations in *Pediatrics,* the journal of the Academy. It may be ordered from American Academy of Pediatrics, PO Box 927, Elk Grove Village, IL 60009-0927. Academy policy statements are also available at *www.aap.org/policy.*

5. *Guide for Adult Immunization.* This report was issued by the American College of Physicians in 1994 and can be ordered by calling 1-800-523-1546, extension 2600; or from Subscriber Services, American College of Physicians, Independence Mall West, Sixth Street at Race, Philadelphia, PA, 19106-1572; order online at *www.acponline.org/catalog/books/guide_imm.htm.* An updated version is due for publication in 2003.

6. *Health Information for International Travel (the Yellow Book).* This booklet is published annually by the

CDC as a guide to requirements and recommendations for specific immunizations and health practices for travel to various countries.[35] It can be obtained from the Superintendent of Documents, U.S. Government Printing Office, Washington, DC 20402-9235. A comprehensive and continuously updated resource for travel information is available at *www.cdc.gov/travel*. This site includes the Yellow Book, the Blue Sheet of summary international travel information, and the Green Sheet of summary information for cruise ships.

7. *Advisory memoranda for international travel.* Memoranda are published when necessary by the CDC to advise international travelers or those who provide information to travelers about specific outbreaks of communicable diseases abroad. These memoranda include health information for prevention and specific recommendations for immunization. They may be obtained from the Division of Quarantine, Centers for Disease Control and Prevention, Atlanta, GA 30333; or at *www.cdc.gov/travel*; or by telephone at 1-888-232-3228.

8. *Control of Communicable Diseases Manual.*[36] This manual is published by the American Public Health Association at approximately 5-year intervals; the 17th edition (2000) is currently available. The manual contains valuable information concerning infectious diseases, their occurrence worldwide, immunization, diagnostic and therapeutic issues, and up-to-date recommendations on isolation and other control measures for each disease presented. It may be ordered from The American Public Health Association, 1015 Fifteenth Street NW, Washington, DC 20005.

9. *State and local health departments, medical schools, and large hospitals.* Many of these agencies or institutions provide routine immunizations, immunization cards, and schedules to patients. They may also send out routine reports of disease incidence.

10. *The Task Force on Community Preventive Services* (*www.thecommunityguide.org*) has published structured reviews of evidence for interventions to improve public health. One of their reviews is universally recommended immunizations for children and adults, and the Task Force is conducting reviews of immunization recommendations for selected children and adults.

The CDC National Immunization Program has established toll-free numbers for answering questions from both the general public and providers: 1-800-232-2522 (English) and 1-800-232-0233 (Spanish). Inquiries can also be addressed to the CDC by e-mail (*nipinfo@cdc.gov*). The National Immunization Program operates an Internet site (*www.cdc.gov/nip*) that provides information for the general public, health departments, researchers, and providers.

Current Immunization Schedules

The information in this section primarily addresses vaccines recommended for universal or widespread use in the United States. Selection of the age at which a vaccine should be administered depends on the ability of the vaccinee to respond to the vaccine, the risk of exposure to disease, and the age distribution of disease morbidity.[37–39] In general, the approach is to administer vaccine at the earliest possible age at which the vaccine is reliably effective. Sometimes, it is necessary to compromise if the risk of disease is great in young infants; for example, during the 1989 to 1991 measles resurgence, the recommended age for vaccination was temporarily lowered to 6 months in areas with a high measles incidence.[40]

Figure 53–2 shows the recommended immunization schedule for infants, children, and adolescents in the United States for 2003.[27] As of March 2003, depending on the combination of vaccines used, a child fully immunized against 11 vaccine preventable diseases required 13 to 20 doses of vaccines by 18 months of age and 17 to 24 doses by 16 years of age, all by injection.[27] The United States schedule typically involves five to six vaccination visits in the first 2 years of life. Chapter 54 discusses the schedules for European countries, and Chapter 55, for developing countries. Figure 53–3 summarizes recommendations for routine antigens for use in adults and outlines some recommendations for vaccine use in adults belonging to groups in the United States who are at particular risk because of lifestyle, occupation, or environment.[28a,35,41–44] Individual chapters on each of the vaccines should be consulted for detailed information. Up-to-date versions of the childhood and adult schedules are available at *www.cdc.gov/nip*.

Special Groups for Whom Immunization Is Indicated

Certain groups of people are at increased risk for exposure to disease or for complications from disease and are therefore particularly in need of immunization. In general, these concerns are addressed in the chapters on individual vaccines (see also Chapter 8); some issues are summarized in Figure 53–3. Other groups require special consideration because of concern that their response to vaccines may be abnormal or that they may have unusually severe adverse events after immunization.

The United States Immunization Program

History

In the United States, immunizations are provided through both the private and the public sectors. The public sector consists primarily of health departments but also includes other clinics, such as community and migrant health centers and public hospital–based clinics supported by public funds. The federal government has provided support to state and local health departments for maternal and child health programs since the 1920s, and some of that funding has been used to support immunizations.[45] However, there was no specific federal involvement in immunization activities until 1955, when the inactivated polio vaccine was licensed. Through the Polio Vaccination Assistance Act, Congress appropriated funds in 1955 and 1956 to the Communicable Disease Center (now the CDC) to help states and local communities buy and administer vaccine. There was no further federal involvement until 1960, when

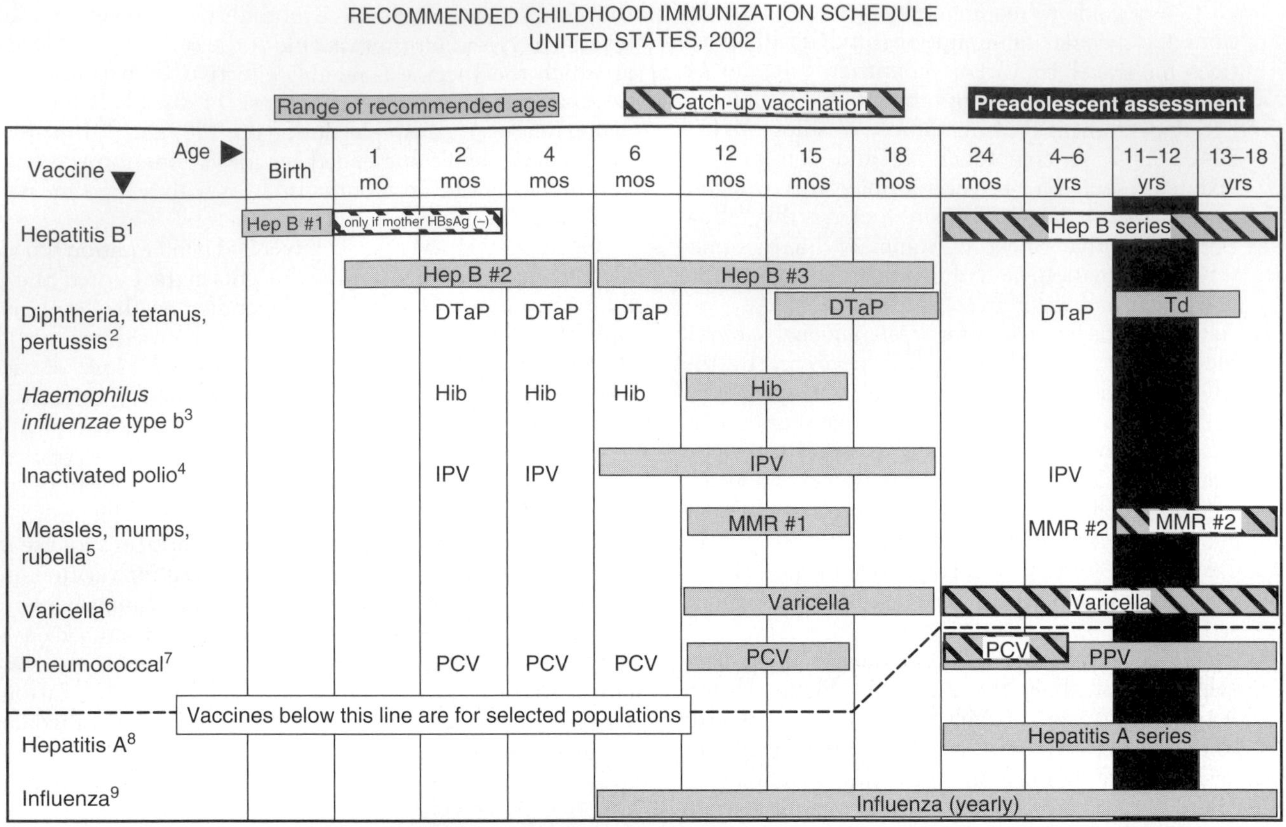

RECOMMENDED CHILDHOOD IMMUNIZATION SCHEDULE
UNITED STATES, 2002

Range of recommended ages	Catch-up vaccination	Preadolescent assessment

Vaccine ▼ Age ▶	Birth	1 mo	2 mos	4 mos	6 mos	12 mos	15 mos	18 mos	24 mos	4–6 yrs	11–12 yrs	13–18 yrs
Hepatitis B[1]	Hep B #1	only if mother HBsAg (−)								Hep B series		
			Hep B #2			Hep B #3						
Diphtheria, tetanus, pertussis[2]			DTaP	DTaP	DTaP		DTaP			DTaP	Td	
Haemophilus influenzae type b[3]			Hib	Hib	Hib	Hib						
Inactivated polio[4]			IPV	IPV		IPV				IPV		
Measles, mumps, rubella[5]						MMR #1				MMR #2	MMR #2	
Varicella[6]						Varicella				Varicella		
Pneumococcal[7]			PCV	PCV	PCV	PCV				PCV	PPV	
Vaccines below this line are for selected populations												
Hepatitis A[8]										Hepatitis A series		
Influenza[9]					Influenza (yearly)							

This schedule indicates the recommended ages for routine administration of currently licensed childhood vaccines, as of December 1, 2001, for children through age 18 years. Any dose not given at the recommended age should be given at any subsequent visit when indicated and feasible. ▨▨ Indicates age groups that warrant special effort to administer those vaccines not previously given. Additional vaccines may be licensed and recommended during the year. Licensed combination vaccines may be used whenever any components of the combination are indicated and the vaccine's other components are not contraindicated. Providers should consult the manufacturers' package inserts for detailed recommendations.

FIGURE 53–2 ▪ Childhood immunization schedule.

Congress made a one-time appropriation of $1 million for a stockpile of oral polio vaccine to be used in combating epidemics. This was quickly exhausted.

In 1962, President John F. Kennedy signed into law the Vaccination Assistance Act. The central thrust of this legislation was to allow the CDC to support mass immunization campaigns and to initiate maintenance programs, but no provision was made for a continuing program of support for immunizations. Two other important aspects of the bill were that it provided for vaccine instead of cash to be furnished directly to state and local health departments, and it also provided that personnel instead of cash could be furnished to grantees. These personnel were public health advisors and epidemiologists, who worked primarily in program coordination and surveillance. Direct delivery of immunization services (e.g., salaries of nurses, clinic supplies, expenses for increasing clinic hours) was not supported until 1992.

The first grants, authorized under section 317 of the Public Health Service Act, were made in June 1963. During the intervening 40 years since the Vaccination Assistance Act was signed into law, this grant program has thrived. There are now 64 grantees under what has become known as the "317" Immunization Grant Program: all 50 states, six large cities (including the District of Columbia), and eight territories and former territories. The level of grant funding has varied greatly over the years. When the grant program began in 1963, the only vaccines available were diphtheria and tetanus toxoids and whole-cell pertussis (DTP), polio, and smallpox. Since that time, funding has been expanded to cover all vaccines routinely recommended for children.

During the 1960s and 1970s, grant funding fluctuated substantially. In 1966, a national effort to eradicate measles began.[15] By 1968, measles incidence had decreased by more than 90% compared with prevaccine-era levels. With the licensure of the rubella vaccine in 1969 and the threat of a new epidemic of rubella, all federal funding for measles was shifted to rubella. A resurgence of measles occurred, peaking in 1971. In 1972, Congress appropriated additional funds that allowed the CDC to purchase vaccines other than rubella. Measles incidence decreased, reaching a low of 22,000 cases in 1974. During the mid-1970s, the overall budget for immunization grants decreased dramatically from the $8 to $10 million provided annually from 1963 to 1969 and the 1970 peak of $17 million to a low of only $5 million in 1976. A second resurgence of measles followed.[17,18]

In 1976, a national election took place that led to significant changes in the immunization program. In the early 1970s, immunization programs around the country were in varying states of effectiveness. In Arkansas, it was apparent that much remained to be done. Mrs. Betty Bumpers, wife

Footnotes
Recommended Childhood Immunization Schedule
United States, 2002

1. Hepatitis B vaccine (Hep B). All infants should receive the first dose of hepatitis B vaccine soon after birth and before hospital discharge; the first dose may also be given by age 2 months if the infant's mother is HBsAg-negative. Only monovalent hepatitis B vaccine can be used for the birth dose. Monovalent or combination vaccine containing Hep B may be used to complete the series; four doses of vaccine may be administered if combination vaccine is used. The second dose should be given at least 4 weeks after the first dose, except for Hib-containing vaccine which cannot be administered before age 6 weeks. The third dose should be given at least 16 weeks after the first dose and at least 8 weeks after the second dose. The last dose in the vaccination series (third or fourth dose) should not be administered before age 6 months.

Infants born to HBsAg-positive mothers should receive hepatitis B vaccine and 0.5 mL hepatitis B immune globulin (HBIG) within 12 hours of birth at separate sites. The second dose is recommended at age 1-2 months and the vaccination series should be completed (third or fourth dose) at age 6 months.

Infants born to mothers whose HBsAg status is unknown should receive the first dose of the hepatitis B vaccine series within 12 hours of birth. Maternal blood should be drawn at the time of delivery to determine the mother's HBsAg status; if the HBsAg test is positive, the infant should receive HBIG as soon as possible (no later than age 1 week).

2. Diphtheria and tetanus toxoids and acellular pertussis vaccine (DTaP). The fourth dose of DTaP may be administered as early as age 12 months, provided 6 months have elapsed since the third dose and the child is unlikely to return at age 15-18 months. **Tetanus and diphtheria toxoids (Td)** is recommended at age 11-12 years if at least 5 years have elapsed since the last dose of tetanus and diphtheria toxoid-containing vaccine. Subsequent routine Td boosters are recommended every 10 years.

3. *Haemophilus influenzae* type b (Hib) conjugate vaccine. Three Hib conjugate vaccines are licensed for infant use. If PRP-OMP (PedvaxHIB® or ComVax® [Merck]) is administered at ages 2 and 4 months, a dose at age 6 months is not required. DTaP/Hib combination products should not be used for primary immunization in infants at ages 2, 4 or 6 months, but can be used as boosters following any Hib vaccine.

4. Inactivated polio vaccine (IPV). An all-IPV schedule is recommended for routine childhood polio vaccination in the United States. All children should receive four doses of IPV at ages 2 months, 4 months, 6-18 months, and 4-6 years.

5. Measles, mumps, and rubella vaccine (MMR). The second dose of MMR is recommended routinely at age 4-6 years but may be administered during any visit, provided at least 4 weeks have elapsed since the first dose and that both doses are administered beginning at or after age 12 months. Those who have not previously received the second dose should complete the schedule by the 11-12 year old visit.

6. Varicella vaccine. Varicella vaccine is recommended at any visit at or after age 12 months for susceptible children, i.e. those who lack a reliable history of chickenpox. Susceptible persons aged $\geq$ 13 years should receive two doses, given at least 4 weeks apart.

7. Pneumococcal vaccine. The heptavalent **pneumococcal conjugate vaccine (PCV)** is recommended for all children age 2-23 months. It is also recommended for certain children age 24-59 months. **Pneumococcal polysaccharide vaccine (PPV)** is recommended in addition to PCV for certain high-risk groups. See *MMWR* 2000;49(RR-9);1-35.

8. Hepatitis A vaccine. Hepatitis A vaccine is recommended for use in selected states and regions, and for certain high-risk groups; consult your local public health authority. See *MMWR* 1999;48(RR-12);1-37.

9. Influenza vaccine. Influenza vaccine is recommended annually for children age $\geq$ 6 months with certain risk factors (including but not limited to asthma, cardiac disease, sickle cell disease, HIV, diabetes; see *MMWR* 2001;50(RR-4);1-44), and can be administered to all others wishing to obtain immunity. Children aged ≤12 years should receive vaccine in a dosage appropriate for their age (0.25 mL if age 6-35 months or 0.5 mL if aged ≥ 3 years). Children aged ≤ 8 years who are receiving influenza vaccine for the first time should receive two doses separated by at least 4 weeks.

For additional information about vaccines, vaccine supply, and contraindications for immunization, please visit the National Immunization Program Website at www.cdc.gov/nip or call the National Immunization Hotline at 800-232-2522 (English) or 800-232-0233 (Spanish).

Approved by the Advisory Committee on Immunization Practices (www.cdc.gov/nip/acip), the American Academy of Pediatrics (www.aap.org), and the American Academy of Family Physicians (www.aafp.org).

FIGURE 53-2 ▪ cont'd

---

of the Governor, became personally interested in immunizations and succeeded in getting increased support for immunizations and improved immunization levels in Arkansas. Her husband, Dale Bumpers, was then elected to the U.S. Senate and became an important leader on immunization in Congress. In November of 1976, Jimmy Carter was elected president. Subsequently, Mrs. Bumpers contacted the new administration and explained the deficiencies in the childhood immunization program in the United States and urged that something be done to improve the situation. As a result, in 1977, a national childhood immunization initiative was announced with two goals[46]:

1. Attainment of immunization levels of 90% in the nation's children by October 1979
2. Establishment of a permanent system to provide comprehensive immunization services to the 3 million children born in America each year

At the time, it was estimated that nearly 20 million American children were in need of at least one dose of a vaccine in order to be fully protected. The poor and the minority populations were disproportionately represented among those needing protection. Joseph A. Califano, Jr., the Secretary of the Department of Health, Education, and Welfare (now Health and Human Services) outlined a broad-based program involving increased federal support for immunizations, increased involvement of volunteers in all aspects of immunization activities, increased public awareness/public education activities, and increased cooperation between governmental agencies.[47]

Immunization grant funds increased dramatically from $5 million in 1976 to $17 million in 1977, $23 million in 1978, and $35 million in 1979. Intensive efforts began, concentrating on school-age children who experienced outbreaks of measles. A major effort was placed on reviewing immunization records of schoolchildren—in a 2-year period, more than 28 million records were reviewed, and children in need were immunized. Efforts also were expended to enact school immunization requirements in states that did not have them, and to enforce those already in existence. As a result of these efforts, all 50 states soon had, and were enforcing, school entry immunization laws. Since 1981, 95% or more of children entering school have had documented immunization. Given these levels, even with lower levels in preschoolers, the overall immunization level in children of all ages in this country was 90% or greater. Thus the first goal of the initiative was met. Unfortunately, the second goal of the 1977 initiative was not met.

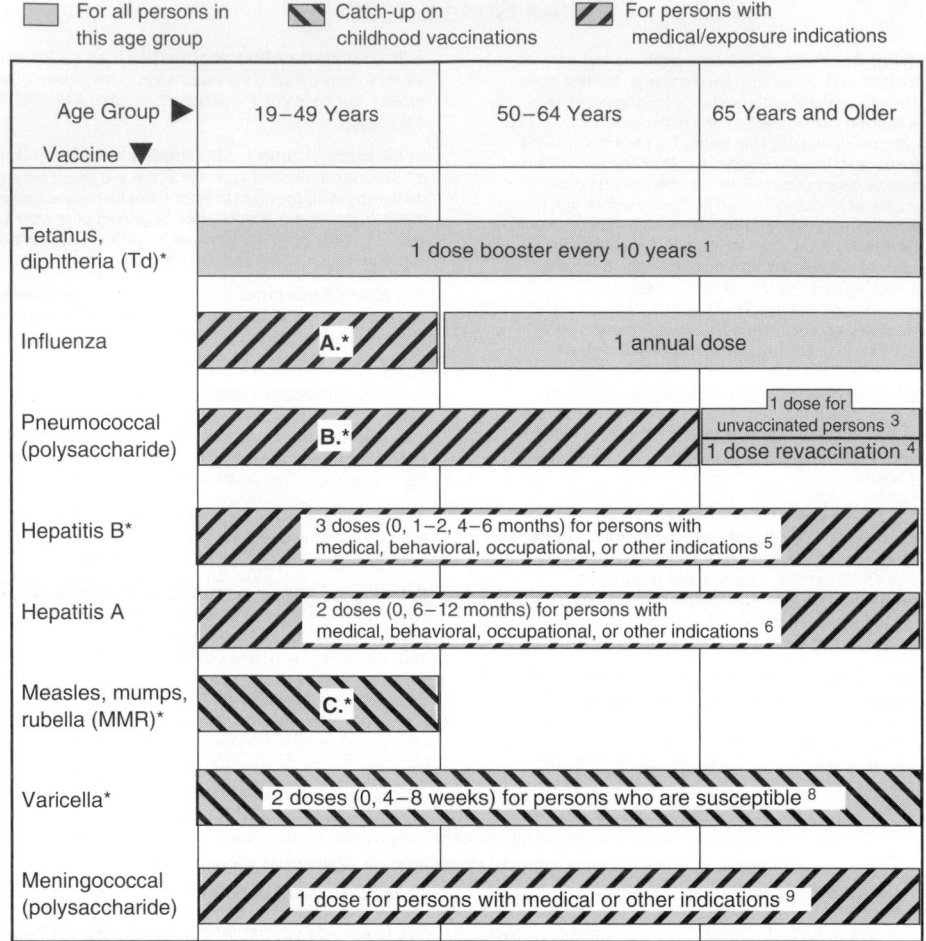

RECOMMENDED ADULT IMMUNIZATION SCHEDULE,
UNITED STATES, 2002–2003

☐ For all persons in this age group   ◪ Catch-up on childhood vaccinations   ▨ For persons with medical/exposure indications

Age Group ▶ Vaccine ▼	19–49 Years	50–64 Years	65 Years and Older
Tetanus, diphtheria (Td)*	1 dose booster every 10 years [1]		
Influenza	A.*	1 annual dose	
Pneumococcal (polysaccharide)	B.*		1 dose for unvaccinated persons [3] 1 dose revaccination [4]
Hepatitis B*	3 doses (0, 1–2, 4–6 months) for persons with medical, behavioral, occupational, or other indications [5]		
Hepatitis A	2 doses (0, 6–12 months) for persons with medical, behavioral, occupational, or other indications [6]		
Measles, mumps, rubella (MMR)*	C.*		
Varicella*	2 doses (0, 4–8 weeks) for persons who are susceptible [8]		
Meningococcal (polysaccharide)	1 dose for persons with medical or other indications [9]		

*A. 1 dose annually for persons with medical or occupational indications, or household contacts of persons with indications [2]

*B. 1 dose for persons with medical or other indications. (1 dose revaccination for immunosuppressive conditions) [3,4]

*C. 1 dose if measles, mumps or rubella vaccination history is unreliable; 2 doses for persons with occupational or other indications [7]

See footnotes for Recommended Adult Immunization Schedule, United States, 2002–2003 on.

*Covered by the Vaccine Injury Compensation Program. For information on how to file a claim call 800-338-2382. Please also visit www.hrsa.osp.gov/vicp. To file a claim for vaccine injury write: U.S. Court of Federal Claims, 717 Madison Place, N.W. Washington D.C., 20005. (202) 219-9657.

This schedule indicates the recommended age groups for routine administration of currently licensed vaccines for persons 19 years of age and older. Licensed combination vaccines may be used whenever any components of the combination are indicated and the vaccine's other components are not contraindicated. Providers should consult the manufacturers' package inserts for detailed recommendations.

Report all clinically significant post-vaccination reactions to the Vaccine Adverse Event Reporting System (VAERS). Reporting forms and instructions on filing a VAERS report are available by calling 800-822-7967 or from the VAERS website at www.vaers.org.

For additional information about the vaccines listed above and contraindications for immunization, visit the National Immunization Program Website at www.cdc.gov/nip/ or call the National Immunization Hotline at 800-232-2522 (English) or 800-232-0233 (Spanish).

Approved by the Advisory Committee on Immunization Practices (ACIP), and accepted by the American College of Obstetricians and Gynecologists (ACOG) and the American Academy of Family Physicians (AAFP)

FIGURE 53–3 ■ Adult immunization schedule. The first page is the schedule by age group; the second page is the schedule by medical condition; and the third page is the footnotes. (From Centers for Disease Control and Prevention. Adult immunization schedule: recommendations of the Advisory Committee on Immunization Practices [ACIP]. MMWR 51:904–908, 2002.)

Although the overall level of support for immunization grants rose rapidly in the late 1970s and throughout the 1980s (reaching $126.8 million in 1989), almost all of the increase was to meet the increasing cost of vaccines or the addition of new vaccines or additional doses of existing vaccines. In the 1980s, the level of federal support to grantees to carry out maintenance elements did not increase significantly, averaging $15.9 million but fluctuating between a low of $5 million in 1988 and a high of $26.1 million in 1989. Over the years, the federal government provided

RECOMMENDED IMMUNIZATIONS FOR ADULTS WITH MEDICAL CONDITIONS, UNITED STATES, 2002—2003

Legend: For all persons in this age group | Catch-up on childhood vaccinations | For persons with medical / exposure indications | Contraindicated

Medical Conditions ▼ / Vaccine ▶	Tetanus-Diphtheria (Td)*	Influenza	Pneumo-coccal (polysacch-aride)	Hepatitis B*	Hepatitis A	Measles, Mumps, Rubella (MMR)*	Varicella*
Pregnancy	For all persons in this age group	For all persons in this age group; A	For persons with medical / exposure indications	For persons with medical / exposure indications	For persons with medical / exposure indications	Contraindicated	Contraindicated
Diabetes, heart disease, chronic pulmonary disease, chronic liver disease, including chronic alcoholism	For all persons in this age group	For all persons in this age group; B	For all persons in this age group; C	For persons with medical / exposure indications; D	For persons with medical / exposure indications	Catch-up on childhood vaccinations	Catch-up on childhood vaccinations
Congenital immunodeficiency, leukemia, lymphoma, generalized malignancy, therapy with alkylating agents, antimetabolites, radiation or large amounts of corticosteroids	For all persons in this age group	For all persons in this age group	For all persons in this age group; E	For persons with medical / exposure indications	For persons with medical / exposure indications	Contraindicated	Contraindicated; F
Renal failure/end stage renal disease, recipients of hemodialysis or clotting factor concentrates	For all persons in this age group	For all persons in this age group	For all persons in this age group; E	For all persons in this age group; G	For persons with medical / exposure indications	Catch-up on childhood vaccinations	Catch-up on childhood vaccinations
Asplenia including elective splenectomy and terminal complement component deficiencies	For all persons in this age group	For all persons in this age group	For all persons in this age group; E, H, I	For persons with medical / exposure indications	For persons with medical / exposure indications	Catch-up on childhood vaccinations	Catch-up on childhood vaccinations
HIV infection	For all persons in this age group	For all persons in this age group	For all persons in this age group; E, J	For all persons in this age group	For persons with medical / exposure indications	Catch-up on childhood vaccinations; K	Contraindicated

A. If pregnancy is at 2nd or 3rd trimester during influenza season.

B. Although chronic liver disease and alcoholism are not indicator conditions for influenza vaccination, give 1 dose annually if the patient is ≥ 50 years, has other indications for influenza vaccine, or if the patient requests vaccination.

C. Asthma is an indicator condition for influenza but not for pneumococcal vaccination.

D. For all persons with chronic liver disease.

E. Revaccinate once after 5 years or more have elapsed since initi al vaccination.

F. Persons with impaired humoral but not cellular immunity may be vaccinated. *MMWR* 1999;48 (RR-06): 1–5.

G. Hemodialysis patient: Use special formulation of vaccine (40 ug/mL) or two 1.0 mL 20 ug doses given at one site. Vaccinate early in the courseof renal disease. Assess antibody titers to hep B surface antigen (anti-HBs) levels annually. Administer additional doses if anti-HBs levels decline to < 10 milliinternational units (mIU)/mL.

H. Also administer meningococcal vaccine.

I. Elective splenectomy: vaccinate at least 2 weeks before surgery.

J. Vaccinate as close to diagnosis as possible when CD4 cell counts are highest.

K. Withhold MMR or other measles containing vaccines from HIV-infected persons with evidence of severe immunsuppression. *MMWR* 1996; 45: 603–606, *MMWR* 1992; 41 (RR-17): 1–19.

FIGURE 53–3 ▪ cont'd

more of the same vaccines, as well as new ones, to a delivery system that was remaining static (at best) in the face of demands that were increasing. Investigations of the measles epidemics of 1989 to 1991, which especially affected unvaccinated preschool children, made it clear that the public sector delivery system was unequal to the challenge and that it required substantial assistance.

A part of the problem was that policies permitted immunization grant funds to be used to purchase vaccines and to carry out surveillance, investigation, education, and coordination but did not permit these funds to be used to support the delivery of vaccines (e.g., salaries of nurses, clinic supplies, expenses associated with increasing clinic hours). In 1991, President George Bush announced the federal government's support to accomplish a major health goal—namely, to raise immunization levels by the year 2000 so that 90% or more of the nation's children routinely completed their basic series of vaccinations by their second

Footnotes for
Recommended Adult Immunization Schedule, United States, 2002-2003

1. Tetanus and diphtheria (Td)—A primary series for adults is 3 doses: the first 2 doses given at least 4 weeks apart and the 3rd dose, 6-12 months after the second. Administer 1 dose if the person had received the primary series and the last vaccination was 10 years ago or longer. *MMWR* 1991; 40 (RR-10): 1-21. The ACP Task Force on Adult Immunization supports a second option: a single Td booster at age 50 years for persons who have completed the full pediatric series, including the teenage/young adult booster. *Guide for Adult Immunization.* 3rd ed. ACP 1994: 20.

2. Influenza vaccination—Medical indications: chronic disorders of the cardiovascular or pulmonary systems including asthma; chronic metabolic diseases including diabetes mellitus, renal dysfunction, hemoglobinopathies, immunosuppression (including immunosuppression caused by medications or by human immunodeficiency virus [HIV]), requiring regular medical follow-up or hospitalization during the preceding year; women who will be in the second or third trimester of pregnancy during the influenza season. Occupational indications: health-care workers. Other indications: residents of nursing homes and other long-term care facilities; persons likely to transmit influenza to persons at high-risk (in-home care givers to persons with medical indications, household contacts and out-of-home caregivers of children birth to 23 months of age, or children with asthma or other indicator conditions for influenza vaccination, household members and care givers of elderly and adults with high-risk conditions); and anyone who wishes to be vaccinated. *MMWR* 2002; 51 (RR-3): 1-31.

3. Pneumococcal polysaccharide vaccination—Medical indications: chronic disorders of the pulmonary system (excluding asthma), cardiovascular diseases, diabetes mellitus, chronic liver diseases including liver disease as a result of alcohol abuse (e.g., cirrhosis), chronic renal failure or nephrotic syndrome, functional or anatomic asplenia (e.g., sickle cell disease or splenectomy), immunosuppressive conditions (e.g., congenital immunodeficiency, HIV infection, leukemia, lymphoma, multiple myeloma, Hodgkins disease, generalized malignancy, organ or bone marrow transplantation), chemotherapy with alkylating agents, anti-metabolites, or long-term systemic corticosteroids. Geographic/other indications: Alaskan Natives and certain American Indian populations. Other indications: residents of nursing homes and other long-term care facilities. *MMWR* 1997; 47 (RR-8): 1-24.

4. Revaccination with pneumococcal polysaccharide vaccine—One time revaccination after 5 years for persons with chronic renal failure or nephrotic syndrome, functional or anatomic asplenia (e.g., sickle cell disease or splenectomy), immunosuppressive conditions (e.g., congenital immunodeficiency, HIV infection, leukemia, lymphoma, multiple myeloma, Hodgkins disease, generalized malignancy, organ or bone marrow transplantation), chemotherapy with alkylating agents, anti-metabolites, or long-term systemic corticosteroids. For persons 65 and older, one-time revaccination if they were vaccinated 5 or more years previously and were aged less than 65 years at the time of primary vaccination. *MMWR* 1997; 47 (RR-8): 1-24.

5. Hepatitis B vaccination—Medical indications: hemodialysis patients, patients who receive clotting-factor concentrates. Occupational indications: health-care workers and public-safety workers who have exposure to blood in the workplace, persons in training in schools of medicine, dentistry, nursing, laboratory technology, and other allied health professions. Behavioral indications: injecting drug users, persons with more than one sex partner in the previous 6 months, persons with a recently acquired sexually-transmitted disease (STD), all clients in STD clinics, men who have sex with men. Other indications: household contacts and sex partners of persons with chronic HBV infection, clients and staff of institutions for the developmentally disabled, international travelers who will be in countries with high or intermediate prevalence of chronic HBV infection for more than 6 months, inmates of correctional facilities. *MMWR* 1991; 40 (RR-13): 1-25. (www.cdc.gov/travel/diseases/hbv.htm)

6. Hepatitis A vaccination—For the combined HepA-HepB vaccine use 3 doses at 0, 1, 6 months). Medical indications: persons with clotting-factor disorders or chronic liver disease. Behavioral indications: men who have sex with men, users of injecting and noninjecting illegal drugs. Occupational indications: persons working with HAV-infected primates or with HAV in a research laboratory setting. Other indications: persons traveling to or working in countries that have high or intermediate endemicity of hepatitis A. *MMWR* 1999; 48 (RR-12): 1-37. (www.cdc.gov/travel/diseases/hav.htm)

7. Measles, Mumps, Rubella vaccination (MMR)—Measles component: Adults born before 1957 may be considered immune to measles. Adults born in or after 1957 should receive at least one dose of MMR unless they have a medical contraindication, documentation of at least one dose or other acceptable evidence of immunity. A second dose of MMR is recommended for adults who:
- are recently exposed to measles or in an outbreak setting
- were previously vaccinated with killed measles vaccine
- were vaccinated with an unknown vaccine between 1963 and 1967
- are students in post-secondary educational institutions
- work in health care facilities
- plan to travel internationally

Mumps component: 1 dose of MMR should be adequate for protection. Rubella component: Give 1 dose of MMR to women whose rubella vaccination history is unreliable and counsel women to avoid becoming pregnant for 4 weeks after vaccination. For women of child-bearing age, regardless of birth year, routinely determine rubella immunity and counsel women regarding congenital rubella syndrome. Do not vaccinate pregnant women or those planning to become pregnant in the next 4 weeks. If pregnant and susceptible, vaccinate as early in postpartum period as possible. *MMWR* 1998; 47 (RR-8): 1-57.

8. Varicella vaccination—Recommended for all persons who do not have reliable clinical history of varicella infection, or serological evidence of varicella zoster virus (VZV) infection; health-care workers and family contacts of immunocompromised persons, those who live or work in environments where transmission is likely (e.g., teachers of young children, day care employees, and residents and staff members in institutional settings), persons who live or work in environments where VZV transmission can occur (e.g., college students, inmates and staff members of correctional institutions, and military personnel), adolescents and adults living in households with children, women who are not pregnant but who may become pregnant in the future, international travelers who are not immune to infection. Note: Greater than 90% of U.S. born adults are immune to VZV. Do not vaccinate pregnant women or those planning to become pregnant in the next 4 weeks. If pregnant and susceptible, vaccinate as early in postpartum period as possible. *MMWR* 1996; 45 (RR-11): 1-36, *MMWR* 1999; 48 (RR-6): 1-5.

9. Meningococcal vaccine (quadrivalent polysaccharide for serogroups A, C, Y, and W-135)—Consider vaccination for persons with medical indications: adults with terminal complement component deficiencies, with anatomic or functional asplenia. Other indications: travelers to countries in which disease is hyperendemic or epidemic ("meningitis belt" of sub-Saharan Africa, Mecca, Saudi Arabia for Hajj). Revaccination at 3-5 years may be indicated for persons at high risk for infection (e.g., persons residing in areas in which disease is epidemic). Counsel college freshmen, especially those who live in dormitories, regarding meningococcal disease and the vaccine so that they can make an educated decision about receiving the vaccination. *MMWR* 2000; 49 (RR-7): 1-20. Note: The AAFP recommends that colleges should take the lead on providing education on meningococcal infection and vaccination and offer it to those who are interested. Physicians need not initiate discussion of the meningococcal quadrivalent polysaccharide vaccine as part of routine medical care.

FIGURE 53–3 ■ cont'd

---

birthday.[48] The President announced that model immunization plans would be developed in several areas of the country as a beginning for the national effort to ensure adequate and timely immunization of infants and young children. This began a process that ultimately resulted in the preparation of Immunization Action Plans by all 50 states and 28 metropolitan areas. Although there was great variation in needs reported from around the country, one theme common to virtually all plans was the need to increase the availability of immunization services. Consequently, for the first time, federal immunization grant funds were allowed to be used for the actual provision of immunization services.

President Bill Clinton's announcement of a Childhood Immunization Initiative (CII) in 1993[49–51] and the leadership and major infusion of funds associated with that initiative have brought the country to the point that it is now,

finally, achieving 90% coverage in preschool children.[52] Grant support for immunization programs, including service delivery (but excluding vaccine purchase), rose to a peak of $237.3 million in 1995. The five components of the CII included (1) improving the quality and quantity of vaccination delivery services; (2) expanding access to vaccines, particularly for poor children; (3) enhancing community involvement, education, and building partnerships; (4) improving the measurement of immunization coverage and the detection of vaccine preventable diseases; and (5) simplifying the immunization schedule and improving vaccines.[53]

Following successful completion of the 1996 CII goals, funding for the Section 317 program declined 43% between the peak funding year of 1995 and 1999. Concerned about the adequacy of immunization infrastructure in the United

States, Congress requested that the Institute of Medicine (IOM) conduct a study on the level of need for federal infrastructure support. The IOM recognized the damaging impact that the ebb and flow of infrastructure funding was having on the nation's immunization system, and recommended a combined, 5-year investment of $1.5 billion, shared between federal and state resources. Between the publication of the IOM's report in 2000,[54] and 2003, federal infrastructure funding was increased by $60 million per year, and approximates the peak base funding.[55]

Roles of the U.S. Immunization Program

The 2000 IOM publication "Calling the Shots" provided a useful conceptual framework for understanding the complex array of roles conducted by federal, state, and local immunization programs in collaboration with the nation's health care delivery system (Fig. 53–4). The IOM identified five key roles: (1) assure purchase of vaccine, (2) assure service delivery, (3) control and prevent infectious diseases, (4) conduct surveillance of vaccine coverage and safety, and (5) sustain and improve immunization coverage levels. The roles are displayed by the IOM as a solved puzzle in which the center piece is the control and prevention of infectious diseases, and the five roles are supported by a base of immunization finance policies and practices.[54]

Although vaccines are given in both private and public sectors, other important components of immunization programs as outlined by the IOM are coordinated primarily by health departments and other public sector agencies, including surveillance and investigation of disease, outbreak control, promotion of immunization, adverse-events

monitoring, assessment of immunization levels, and implementation of regulations and laws regarding immunization.[56,57]

Assure Purchase of Vaccine

The U.S. immunization program is a collaborative effort of public and private sectors. Public efforts have focused primarily on childhood immunizations. Based on 2001 data from the Biologics Surveillance System (CDC, unpublished data), approximately 56% of vaccines routinely recommended for children are purchased with public funds through federal contracts negotiated by the CDC with vaccine manufacturers. These contracts allow state and local immunization programs to obtain vaccines at reduced prices. The typical discount in 2002 was approximately 50% off the published catalog prices (Table 53–1). Reasons for the reduced prices have included (1) the ability to ship large quantities of vaccines to only a limited number of sites within a state, with states taking responsibility for shipment to individual clinics and providers; (2) the absence of return privileges for expired or unneeded vaccines, a privilege common in contracts with the private sector; and (3) an interest on the part of manufacturers to provide vaccines at lower cost for poorer children, who tend to be served by the public sector.

Funds for purchase through the contracts are provided through the federal government and may be supplemented by funds from each of the 64 federal immunization grant recipients. There are two major sources of federal funds: (1) the Vaccines for Children (VFC) program and (2) the federal 317 grant program. The VFC program supplies vaccines to participating providers for children 18 years of age or younger who are (1) eligible for Medicaid, (2) without any health insurance, or (3) Native American/ Alaska Native.[35,58,59] In addition, children who receive their immunizations at federally qualified health centers and who have commercial health insurance that does not include an immunization benefit (underinsured) can receive free vaccines through the VFC program. Federally qualified health centers are health care provider sites determined to be eligible by the Health Resources and Services Administration, and include community, migrant, and rural health centers (see *www.bphc.hrsa.gov*).

Funds for the VFC program are provided through the Medicaid Trust Fund, maintained by the Centers for Medicare & Medicaid Services (CMS). The VFC is an entitlement program that assures funds are available for eligible children each year. The ACIP establishes which vaccines are covered, the appropriate number of doses, and the schedule. An ACIP vote to include a vaccine in the VFC program or to increase the number of doses of a vaccine already in the program leads to rapid financing, once a federal contract has been obtained for the vaccine.

The 317 grant program provides federal funds for vaccines for children who are not eligible for the VFC program but who receive vaccines in state and local health department clinics, as well as for children served by private providers (in some states). Funds available under the 317 program must be appropriated each year by the Congress. In contrast, the law establishing the VFC program provides for financing on the basis of ACIP recommendations without

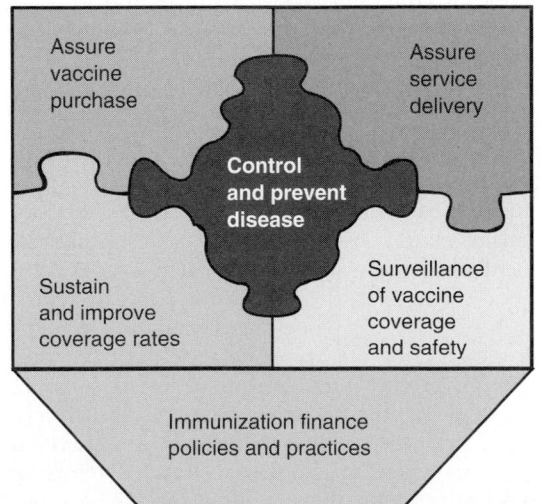

SIX ROLES OF THE NATION'S
IMMUNIZATION SYSTEM

Assure vaccine purchase

Assure service delivery

Control and prevent disease

Sustain and improve coverage rates

Surveillance of vaccine coverage and safety

Immunization finance policies and practices

FIGURE 53–4 ▪ Six roles of the nation's immunization system. (From Institute of Medicine. Calling the Shots: Immunization Finance Policies and Practices. Washington, DC, National Academy Press, 2000, p 7, with permission.)

TABLE 53–1 ▪ Changes in Vaccine Costs for Childhood Immunization, United States, 1987 to 2002*

1987			2002†		
Vaccines	CDC	Catalog	Vaccines	CDC	Catalog
4 OPV	$5.72 ($1.43)‡	$34.68 ($8.67)	4 IPV	$35.20 ($8.80)	$90.12–$93.24 ($22.53–$23.31)
5 DTP	$15.05 ($3.01)	$56.10 ($11.22)	5 DTaP	$58.75–$63.75§ ($11.75–$12.75)	$98.25–$103.20 ($19.65–$20.64)
1 MMR	$10.67	$17.88	2 MMR	$31.28 ($15.64)	$66.66 ($33.33)
1 Hib	$2.17	$6.68	3 Hib product	$24.96 ($8.32)	$61.89 ($20.63)
			4 Hib product	$29.00–$29.32 ($7.25–$7.33)	$63.52–$87.12 ($15.88–$21.78)
			3 Hepatitis B	$27.00–$27.75 ($9.00–$9.25)	$69.60–$72.60 ($23.20–$24.20)
1 Td	$0.09	$0.65	1 Td	$7.91 ($7.91)	$7.91 ($7.91)
			1 Varicella	$41.44 ($41.44)	$54.61 ($54.61)
			4 PCV7	$183.96($45.99)	$235.00 ($58.75)
Total	$33.70	$115.99	Total	$410.50–$420.61 ‖	$684.04–$720.34

*Prices as of February 23, 1987, and November 12, 2002.
†Representative series; other choices are possible. Excise tax of $0.75 per dose per disease prevented (e.g., IPV = $0.75, DTaP = $2.25) is included. When similar vaccines were available with different prices, the lowest price was used.
‡Figures in parentheses are costs per dose.
§Range, taking all the higher-priced individual vaccines versus all the lowest-priced individual vaccines when there is more than one manufacturer for a product.
‖The ranges in the Totals row indicate the minimum and maximum sums of the prices of vaccines needed to fully vaccinate a child using the routine schedule.
CDC, Centers for Disease Control and Prevention; DTaP, diphtheria and tetanus toxoids and acellular pertussis; DTP, tetanus and diphtheria toxoids and whole-cell pertussis; Hib, *Haemophilus influenzae* type b; IPV, inactivated poliovirus vaccine; MMR, measles-mumps-rubella; OPV, oral poliovirus vaccine; PCV7, 7-valent pneumococcal conjugate vaccine; Td, tetanus and diphtheria toxoids.

going through the annual congressional appropriations process. Funds for the VFC program, however, must be approved by the Department of Health and Human Services and the Office of Management and Budget.

State and local immunization grantees have the option to purchase vaccines through federal contracts with their own appropriated funds. Providers cannot charge parents or guardians for vaccines purchased through a federal contract, regardless of the funding source. Providers are permitted to charge a small administration fee; however, no one can be denied vaccines because of inability to pay the fee.

Approximately 44% of vaccines are purchased through the private sector. Managed care plans generally provide recommended vaccines without charge beyond standard premiums for all covered services.[31,60] In contrast, many traditional indemnity plans either do not cover routine childhood immunizations or cover them only after deductibles are paid. Vaccines not covered by insurance plans are usually purchased by parents or guardians.

The federal role in purchasing vaccines for adults is more limited. Medicare part B covers pneumococcal and influenza vaccination services for all persons 65 years of age and older who participate in part B (approximately 95% of all persons ≥65 years). State Medicaid programs, supported by federal contributions, may cover recommended vaccines for younger adults enrolled in Medicaid. State and local health departments may purchase limited quantities of influenza and pneumococcal vaccines with their own funds. The NVAC estimated in 1994 that public funds for vaccinations through health departments accounted for less than 10% of the financing of adult immunizations.[32] In 2002, public immunization grant programs reported purchasing

less than 5% of all influenza and pneumococcal vaccines sold in the United States (CDC, unpublished data, 2002).

Assure Service Delivery

Most vaccines for children are administered by private sector providers. Data from the 2001 National Immunization Survey of children 19 to 35 months of age (median age, 27 months) show that 57% of children received all vaccines from a single private health care provider, 14% received all vaccines from a health department clinic, and 29% received vaccines from a combination of sources or another type of provider (*www.cdc.gov/nip/coverage*).

Vaccination delivery in the public sector is primarily a responsibility of state and local governments. Since 1992, federal 317 grant funds have been used to support delivery, such as hiring of nurses and other clinic staff, vaccine promotion and education, and other delivery-related functions. In addition, federal funds that are part of state Medicaid resources and federal block grants to states can help support delivery.

Several changes in the U.S. health care system should lead to increases in the percentage of children served by the private sector. The VFC program provides free vaccine to participating private providers in order to serve eligible children. Before this program, parents of such children often had to pay for vaccines themselves or were referred to public clinics where vaccines were free.[61] Parental preference has been to have their children receive vaccines from their usual source of care.[62] Surveys have shown that providers enrolled in the VFC program are substantially more likely to immunize eligible children in their practices than are nonenrolled providers.[63]

A significant proportion of children enrolled in Medicaid are in private managed care plans that cover all services for children, including vaccination.[64] In 1997, the new Title XXI of the Social Security Act, called the State Children's Health Insurance Program, was created and administered by the CMS (see *www.cms.gov/schip*). This program allows states to provide health benefits for uninsured children of low-income families through expansion of the Medicaid program, through establishment of a separate child health care coverage program, or through provision of coverage with a combination of the Medicaid program and a new state program. Thus, through Medicaid or the State Children's Health Insurance Program, the CMS together with state funding will provide health benefits to children of parents with incomes up to 200% of the poverty level. As of 2001, approximately 4.6 million children have been enrolled, approximately 25% of whom were less than 6 years of age (see *www.cms.gov/schip*). Providing full coverage for vaccination services, including administration costs, to previously uninsured children has been shown in one state to decrease health department clinic use by 67%, to increase primary care provider use by 27%, and to increase vaccination coverage levels by 5%.[65] Thus the combination of the VFC program, managed Medicaid, and the State Children's Health Insurance Program is likely to result in fewer children being served in public clinics.

Control and Prevent Infectious Diseases

The desired outcome of immunization is disease reduction or elimination. Reports of the occurrence of vaccine-preventable diseases are the major means of evaluating the impact of most of the vaccine-preventable disease programs.[66,67] The Council of State and Territorial Epidemiologists, in consultation with the CDC, establishes the list of nationally notifiable diseases. In the United States, most of the 11 vaccine-preventable diseases of childhood are reported to the National Notifiable Disease Surveillance System. Information is obtained through state health departments, which have authority for mandating reporting of selected diseases to the state level by physicians and other health care providers.[68]

Data collected weekly include date of report and county of residence for all notifiable diseases. In addition, for many of the vaccine-preventable diseases, supplemental information (e.g., date of onset, age, sex, race/ethnicity, vaccination status, whether the case was confirmed by a laboratory, and disease complications) is forwarded to the CDC. For many of the vaccine-preventable diseases, reports by state of cases notified that week as well as the cumulative total for the year are published weekly in the *Morbidity and Mortality Weekly Report*. Case definitions have been established with Council of State and Territorial Epidemiologists that detail criteria for confirmation of a given illness as a case of a vaccine-preventable disease (see Appendix 4 of this text).[69]

The National Notifiable Disease Surveillance System is supplemented by other surveillance systems operated by the CDC.[67] For example, a registry is maintained for congenital rubella syndrome; this registry collects comprehensive information on the clinical status of the baby, complications, laboratory data, vaccination status of the mother, and other information. The paralytic polio surveillance system collects extensive data on the clinical characteristics of suspected cases; these data are reviewed by experts to determine whether the illness is polio. Diphtheria surveillance is enhanced through monitoring requests to the CDC for antiserum, which the CDC has responsibility for distributing. Efforts to collect data beyond the National Notifiable Disease Surveillance System are made for measles, pertussis, tetanus, *Haemophilus influenzae* type b, hepatitis B, and varicella. Laboratory-based surveillance systems are used to monitor causes of bacterial meningitis, including *H. influenzae* type b and pneumococcal disease.[70] Other laboratory-based systems, as well as death certificate data, are utilized for influenza surveillance.

Where data are not available nationally, special sentinel surveillance systems in selected states and communities may be established.[66] Examples include the sentinel counties surveillance system for hepatitis B, and a special varicella surveillance project in three sites (Antelope Valley, CA; Travis County, TX; and Philadelphia, PA).[71-74]

Reporting sensitivity for each of the surveillance systems varies. An evaluation of measles surveillance during an outbreak revealed that 45% of cases seen and diagnosed at hospitals were reported.[75] Capture-recapture methods have been used to estimate the completeness of reporting for many different surveillance systems. A capture-recapture evaluation of the completeness of reporting of diagnosed cases of vaccine-associated polio found that 81% of cases were reported during the period 1980 to 1991.[76] The congenital rubella syndrome registry was estimated to receive reports on about 20% of cases in the past,[77] while only about 32% of pertussis hospitalizations were reported during the late 1980s.[78] Completeness of reporting varies by source of report and type of disease, with more complete reporting from hospitals and laboratories than from physicians for diseases such as *H. influenzae* type b.[79] In one varicella active surveillance project, there was more complete reporting by schools than by providers.[72]

Surveillance data are analyzed to determine whether expected reductions of disease occur with increasing vaccine coverage; to evaluate potential changing epidemiology of disease, such as a shift to a predominance of adult cases where there had been a childhood focus; and to determine whether cases are a result of failure of vaccine or of failure to vaccinate.[66]

Vaccine Effectiveness

When a substantial proportion of cases of vaccine-preventable disease occur in persons with a history of prior vaccination, an investigation is often undertaken to determine whether the rates of vaccine failure are within expected ranges. *Vaccine effectiveness* is the term used for these observational studies, to contrast with *vaccine efficacy*, which is usually measured prospectively in randomized, double-blind, placebo-controlled trials. Several methods are used to evaluate vaccine effectiveness in the postlicensure setting, including cohort, case-control, secondary attack rates in families, and other techniques.[80] Vaccine effectiveness is calculated as

$$(1 - ARV/ARU) \times 100$$

where ARV is the attack rate in the vaccinated and ARU is the attack rate in the unvaccinated. When case-control studies are employed, the odds ratio is used to approximate the relative risk (ARV/ARU).

Of particular note has been a screening technique to help determine whether a new methodologically rigorous investigation of vaccine effectiveness is warranted.[80] The screening analysis requires data on the vaccination status of cases and the vaccination status of the populations from which the cases are drawn, often obtained from existing population-based estimates from surveillance and other methods. Data must always be broken down into dichotomous variables, with persons having received zero doses compared with those in a single vaccinated group. For example, for a vaccine recommended in three doses, the population of cases that are vaccinated must be calculated excluding persons who received only one or two doses. Similar adjustments must be made for coverage assessment. Figure 53–5 allows approximation of vaccine effectiveness using a graph.

When vaccine effectiveness is within expected limits yet disease transmission persists, new immunization strategies may be considered. For example, investigations showed that measles transmission could persist despite a vaccine effectiveness of greater than 90% and high levels of coverage with a single dose of vaccine.[40] This information was critical in the decision to recommend universally a second dose of measles vaccine. When vaccine effectiveness is lower than expected, investigations also are triggered into such causes as failure to maintain vaccine at the proper temperature (the "cold chain").

When most cases occur in unvaccinated persons, investigations can identify geographic and demographic characteristics to help guide future vaccination efforts. For example, a resurgence of measles in the United States during 1989 to 1991 was found to be caused by a failure to vaccinate young preschool children and led to a major national initiative to improve coverage.[31,50,51,53]

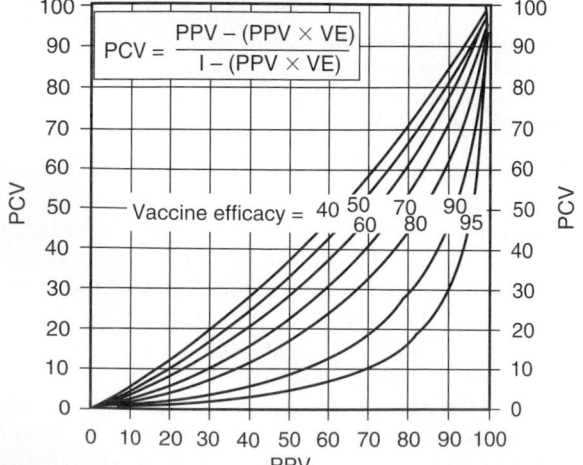

FIGURE 53–5 ▪ Percentage of cases vaccinated (PCV) per percentage of population vaccinated (PPV), for seven values of vaccine efficacy (VE). (From Orenstein WA, Bernier RH, Dondero TJ, et al. Field evaluation of vaccine efficacy. Bull World Health Organ 63:1055–1068, 1985, with permission.)

Conduct Surveillance for Immunization Coverage and Safety

Immunization coverage has been measured since 1960, with the exception of the 4 years immediately prior to the 1989 resurgence of measles.[81] Since 1994, immunization of preschool children has been measured through the National Immunization Survey,[52] which consists of 78 random telephone surveys measuring immunization coverage of 19- to 35-month-old children (median age, 27 months). Approximately 1 million households are sampled annually to obtain data on about 34,000 children.[82,83] The National Immunization Survey provides a national estimate of coverage, usually with 95% confidence intervals within plus or minus 1 percentage point of the point estimate, as well as comparable, statistically valid estimates for each of the 50 states and 28 of the largest urban areas. The survey is adjusted for households without telephones.[83] Attempts are made to collect immunization records from identified vaccine providers of each participant. Parental responses are adjusted on the basis of provider validation data. Further adjustments are made on the basis of demographic variables to give statistically valid estimates. The National Immunization Survey provides estimates by poverty status as well as by major racial and ethnic minority groups, including African-Americans, Hispanics, Asians and Pacific Islanders, and Native Americans/ Alaska Natives (*www.cdc.gov/nip/coverage*).[84–87]

A variety of techniques has been used to assess immunization coverage at the local level; these are primarily based on some form of cluster sample survey.[88–94] The least expensive and easiest-to-perform surveys are retrospective. School immunization records of kindergarten or first-grade students (5 to 6 years of age) are reviewed, and immunization status is determined retroactive to the second birthday.[94] Because these data are 3 to 4 years out of date (the interval between the time the children were 2 years of age and the time they entered school), such retrospective surveys offer little help in monitoring ongoing immunization performance. Surveys of current preschool children are more difficult to perform and are usually costly.

Parental histories are frequently found to be inaccurate, particularly as the immunization schedule has gotten more complex.[95] When asked if immunizations for a given child are up to date, parents tend to overestimate coverage.[96–98] They tend to underestimate the number of doses received when asked about specific vaccines that are recommended to be given in multiple doses (e.g., diphtheria and tetanus toxoids and acellular pertussis [DTaP] vaccine) and tend to overestimate coverage for vaccines recommended in a single dose for preschool children (e.g., measles-mumps-rubella [MMR] vaccine). On the basis of provider validation for the National Health Interview Survey, estimates for DTaP and polio vaccines had to be adjusted upward, and estimates for measles-containing vaccines had to be adjusted downward.[99] Requiring provider validation for local surveys increases the complexity and cost, but the accuracy is greatly improved.

Techniques have been developed for measuring the performance of individual providers and clinics. The Clinic Assessment Software Application (CASA) allows calculation of the coverage of children served by a given provider and can provide diagnostic information on reasons for low coverage, such as missed opportunities to provide all needed vaccines simultaneously. CASA can be obtained through the Clinic Assessment Software Application Support Team, Mailstop E-62, National Immunization Program, Centers for Disease Control and Prevention, Atlanta, GA 30333, or at *www.cdc.gov/nip*. The most valid samples are taken randomly from all records, although limited data suggest that the immunization coverage of consecutive age-eligible children seen in a given practice, regardless of the reason for a visit, also gives a valid measure of coverage.[100]

The National Committee on Quality Assurance (*www.ncqa.org*) has established immunization performance measures for managed care organizations in the Health Plan Employer Data and Information Set (HEDIS). HEDIS 2003 estimates immunization coverage for children who reached 2 years of age during the reporting year who were continuously enrolled in a specific managed care plan for the 12-month period preceding the second birthday (including members who have had no more than one break in enrollment of up to 45 days during the 12 months preceding the second birthday, or, for Medicaid plans, no more than one break of up to 1 month in duration).[101] Separate calculations are made for children enrolled in a plan covered by private funds and those covered by Medicaid.

The immunizations assessed through HEDIS 2003 are shown in Table 53–2. For preschool immunization, coverage is assessed for each of the vaccines listed and for two progressively inclusive combinations of vaccinations. Coverage is estimated by the use of (1) claims or encounter data on individual children in the numerator and the entire plan membership in the denominator or (2) a random sample of 411 commercial and 411 Medicaid children, with chart review to determine their immunization status. HEDIS 2003 also measures vaccination coverage levels for adolescents (MMR, hepatitis B, and varicella vaccines), adults 50 to 64 years of age (influenza vaccine), and older (≥65 years) adults (influenza and pneumococcal polysaccharide vaccines) among plan members who were continuously enrolled for the previous 12 months (see Table 53–2).[101–103]

Measurement of childhood immunization coverage levels continues to be an active area of research.[95,104–108] The IOM recognized the strong influence that measurement technique has on estimated coverage at the clinic level and the population level, and recommended a harmonization of measurement techniques.[54] A particularly challenging issue in the United States has been the lack of centralized records, leading to a scattering of immunization histories across multiple immunization providers for individual children.[109,110] Immunization registries hold promise to alleviate this measurement difficulty (see *Immunization Registries* below).

National immunization coverage estimates for influenza and pneumococcal vaccinations and receipt of tetanus toxoid among adults are obtained from the National Health Interview Survey.[111] State-specific data for influenza and pneumococcal vaccinations are collected through the Behavioral Risk Factor Surveillance System, a state-based telephone survey of the civilian, noninstitutionalized, adult (≥18 years of age) population.[112] In 2002, the system consisted of independent telephone surveys of all 50 states in which similar methods were used. Data are based on recall of the respondent.

Underimmunization in Children

Since the 1989 to 1991 measles resurgence, a great deal of research has been conducted to understand barriers that prevent timely immunization of preschool children. Several potential barriers were determined *not* to be significant when they were examined closely. First, many investigators have speculated that parental attitudes toward vaccination can explain underimmunization; however, the evidence shows otherwise—most parents are very supportive of protecting their children through vaccination.[113] Second, attitudes of providers have remained very positive toward routine vaccination. Third, most preschool children have access to an immunization provider. For example, according to the 1993 National Health Interview Survey, 93% of undervaccinated children who were 19 to 35 months of age had a usual source of primary care.[114] Having access to a primary care provider and using services are not the same, however.

TABLE 53–2 ■ HEDIS 2003 Immunization Performance Measures for Preschool Children, Adolescents, and Adults*

2-Yr-Olds	Adolescents (13 yr)	Adults ≥65 Yr
4 doses of DTaP or DT	Second dose of MMR	1 dose of influenza vaccine
3 doses of IPV	3 doses of hepatitis B	1 dose of pneumococcal poly-
1 dose of MMR during the second year of life	1 dose of varicella	saccharide vaccine
3 doses of Hib, with at least 1 during the second year of life	Combination 1: 1 MMR and 3 hepatitis B	
3 doses of hepatitis B with at least one of them after 6 months of age	Combination 2: Combination 1 plus 1 dose of varicella	
1 dose of varicella during the second year of life		
Combination 1: 4 DTaP, 3 IPV, 1 MMR, 3 Hib, and 3 hepatitis B		
Combination 2: Combination 1 plus 1 dose of varicella		

*Varicella includes either documented vaccination with varicella vaccine or a history of chickenpox.
DTaP, diphtheria and tetanus toxoids and acellular pertussis; DT, diphtheria and tetanus toxoids for use in children; Hib, *Haemophilus influenzae* type b; IPV, inactivated poliovirus vaccine; MMR, measles-mumps-rubella.
From National Committee for Quality Assurance. Effectiveness of care. In HEDIS 2003—The Health Plan Employer Data and Information Set. Washington, DC, National Committee for Quality Assurance, 2002, pp 61–71.

PARENTAL FACTORS

Many risk factors have been associated with low immunization coverage; these factors are primarily poverty related and include low educational level of parents,[85] large family size, low socioeconomic status, nonwhite race or ethnicity, young parental age, lack of prenatal care, use of public clinics as a primary source of immunizations, and late start of the immunization series.[84,115-123]

Some religious groups have opposed immunization, and a small percentage of parents have philosophical objections to immunizations. Although outbreaks of disease have been reported among persons who object to or claim exemption from immunization,[124,125] particularly because they may cluster in groups, persons opposed to immunization account for a small proportion of the population.[126-129] A survey of the United States showed that 42 states had less than 1% of the population claim any exemption between 1994 and 1996, including a medical contraindication under the school law.[130] Of the remaining states, none exceeded 2.5% exemptions, and their average was only slightly greater than 1%.

Older studies tended to associate lower coverage with reliance on public clinics for immunization. However, data from the 2001 National Immunization Survey show that children vaccinated by health department clinics are within 3 percentage points of those vaccinated by private providers (75% vs. 78%; see *www.cdc/gov/nip/coverage*).

Although children who are late in starting the immunization series often account for less than 50% of underimmunized children, almost all studies have shown that the failure to obtain any immunizations by 3 months of age has been associated with some of the highest relative risks of underimmunization at 24 months of age.[121,123,131-135] A child who appears at a vaccine provider at 3 months of age or older with no prior immunizations should be singled out for special tracking to ensure that the full series is completed before the second birthday. Furthermore, the information supports efforts to link every child with a vaccine provider at birth.

Parental health beliefs do not necessarily correlate with the immunization status of their children.[136] For example, Bates and co-workers queried low-income mothers of urban infants in Indianapolis about their attitudes concerning vaccines and vaccine-preventable diseases 48 to 72 hours after they gave birth and evaluated the relationship of those beliefs to their child's immunization status at 7 months of age.[122] There were no significant differences in immunization status of children between parents who perceived that vaccine-preventable diseases were serious and those who did not (28% vs. 32%) or between those who perceived that their child was likely to be susceptible to disease and those who did not (30% vs. 29%). Paradoxically, children born to parents who believed there was great benefit to preventing disease were less likely to be immunized than those who saw less benefits from prevention (23% vs. 34%). Immunization levels were low in all groups. The lack of correlation of parental beliefs and immunization status of children has also been found in other studies.[118,137,138]

Most parents lack knowledge about the complexity of the immunization schedule and tend to overestimate coverage when asked if their child's immunizations are up to date. For example, Goldstein and colleagues found that more than one third of the children whose parents claimed that their child had received the recommended immunizations for his or her age were underimmunized according to clinic records.[96] Parents of more than half of all of the underimmunized children in the study thought their children's immunizations were up to date. These data and others suggest that immunization messages targeted to parents that stress the importance of early childhood immunization may not have great impact on improving immunization levels, because many parents of underimmunized children believe that they have already adequately immunized their child. Few parents understand the complexity of the schedule and the fact that 13 to 20 doses of vaccines are recommended by 18 months of age to fully immunize a preschool child in the United States.

Several studies of parents have identified factors that parents believe contribute to underimmunization, such as long waiting times at clinics, difficulties obtaining appointments, lack of adequate transportation, and lack of understanding of the immunization schedule.[120,139-141] However, the precise role of these factors in contributing to underimmunization is not clear. Some studies have shown that children with appointments for well-child care, including immunization, have high "no-show rates," particularly if parents are poor, which can lead to failure to obtain timely immunization.[119,142,143] Employer practices that make it difficult for parents to get time off from work to get their children immunized may contribute to failure to obtain immunizations.[120] Parental beliefs that children with minor illnesses, such as upper respiratory illnesses, should not be vaccinated, even though the illnesses are not true contraindications, also may contribute to failure to keep appointments.[144]

The data taken together show that providers play a major, if not *the* major, role in the immunization status of their patients. Parents tend to want their children immunized, to look to their provider for guidance on immunization, and to rely on the provider for reminders about the schedule. Parents identify barriers in provider practices, such as long waits, that tend to discourage immunization.

PROVIDER FACTORS

Underimmunized children appear to have substantially more access to the health care system than was previously assumed. Mustin and associates reported that 60% of infants who were not adequately vaccinated by 8 months of age had had at least three well-child visits.[145] Almost all children have had at least one immunization by 2 years of age (*www.cdc.gov/nip/coverage*).[133,134] Opportunities for immunization are being missed when children who are eligible for immunization visit health care providers but are not vaccinated.[146,147]

Missed opportunities can be divided into two major categories: (1) a child seeks care in a setting in which immunizations are normally offered (e.g., well-child care) but is not adequately immunized, and (2) a child seeks care in a setting in which immunizations are not normally offered (e.g., an emergency department, an acute care clinic). The former generally occur because all needed immunizations are not offered simultaneously when they could be or because invalid contraindications are invoked to defer immunization. This type of missed opportunity also occurs if a child is not vaccinated at his or her usual source of care because of cost of vaccines and vaccine administration but is referred to a public clinic where vaccines are free.

A variety of studies have been performed to evaluate the impact of taking all opportunities to vaccinate.[117,119,133,143,148–162] Studies at the University of Rochester estimated that missed opportunities accounted for 13% to 60% of underimmunization time (time spent overdue for some immunizations during the first 2 years of life), depending on the practice type (the higher figure corresponds to the practice of caring for the most impoverished patients).[163] Of the missed opportunities, 19% to 43% occurred in well-child settings, 9% to 36% occurred in follow-up appointments (e.g., ear rechecks), and 41% to 72% were attributable to failure to receive vaccinations in acute care settings. Studies in four inner cities documented that, by the second birthday, DTP-4 coverage could have been 8% to 21% higher and MMR coverage could have been 6% to 9% higher if all opportunities to vaccinate had been taken.[148] Missed opportunities are not limited to inner-city health care providers. A study of a large health maintenance organization documented that the immunization status of 30% of underimmunized children could have been brought up to date if simultaneous administration of all needed vaccinations were performed at each visit.[153] Most of the underimmunized population had made acute care visits, during which there were no discernible contraindications, yet they were not immunized.

Of the types of missed opportunities, the easiest to correct should be simultaneous immunization. Some research suggests that failure to provide simultaneous vaccination may be more a result of provider attitudes than parent attitudes. Woodin and co-workers reported that 60% of practicing physicians (compared with 40% of parents) had strong concerns about a 7-month-old receiving three injections. In fact, 64% of parents preferred that three injections be given simultaneously if it would decrease the need for an additional visit.[164] Similar findings were noted by Melman and colleagues, who reported that more than 90% of parents taking their children to an inner-city clinic preferred two injections compared with two visits, 58% preferred three injections to two visits, and 42% preferred four injections to two visits.[165] A survey of health care providers at inner-city clinics in Jersey City and Paterson, New Jersey, showed that simultaneous immunization was not a concern of the public health providers but was a concern for 14% to 38% of private providers, depending on the number of injections given.[166] This lack of concern has been borne out by the experience with an increase in the number of injections when the recommended schedule replaced oral poliovirus vaccination with injected, inactivated poliovirus vaccination at the same time that DTaP came into widespread use following its licensure. Vaccination coverage levels at inner-city health department clinics, commercial managed care organizations, and Medicaid managed care were evaluated before and after the transition, and no significant declines in coverage were seen.[167–169] The recent licensure of a combined DTaP-IPV-HepB vaccine for use in the routine schedule at 2, 4, and 6 months of age reduces the number of injections needed for these vaccines.[169a] For example, at 2 months of age, vaccination against DTaP, IPV, HepB, Hib, and pneumococcal disease can be accomplished with three injections instead of five injections.

Use of invalid contraindications in order to defer immunization is a common cause of missed opportunities.

Gamertsfelder and associates reported that almost one fifth of doses delayed in a family practice residency clinic were due to invalid contraindications.[143] A national survey of practicing physicians reported that 28% would not give MMR to a well-hydrated 18-month-old child with afebrile, watery diarrhea, even though this is not a contraindication.[155] To combat the use of invalid contraindications, tables of valid contraindications and contraindication misperceptions have been prepared (see *www.cdc.gov/nip*).

Most missed opportunities occur during acute care visits. Multiple factors play a role in the failure to take advantage of this opportunity. They include limited time for patient contact, use of invalid contraindications, desire to not potentially confuse the clinical course of the underlying illness with a vaccine reaction, inability to determine the true immunization needs of a patient (because immunization records are unavailable at the office or clinic and most parents do not bring home immunization records with them at the time of visits), and children being brought for visits by individuals who are not legally authorized to give consent. Reducing these kinds of missed opportunities can be particularly difficult. However, such interventions as screening nurses' reminding physicians that the patient about to be seen is in need of immunization can have some impact.[149,170]

Concern has been raised that providing immunizations outside of well-child care, such as during acute care and emergency department visits, could adversely affect provision of well-child care.[159,163,171] Some view immunization as a parental incentive to make a well-child visit, and this incentive would be removed if immunization were provided in non–well-child care settings.[172] However, in a survey of 502 parents in Baltimore, Hughart and co-workers found that only 18% of parents were very likely to make a checkup visit if immunizations were provided, but not if no immunizations were provided.[173] Furthermore, in children of parents motivated primarily by immunizations, there was no difference between attendance at well-child clinic visits in which immunizations were usually provided (15- and 18-month visits) and visits normally without immunization (8- and 12-month visits). Joffe and Luberti also reported no difference in later well-child visits between children vaccinated during an emergency department visit and similar children seen in an emergency department who were not vaccinated.[174] Thus, although provision of immunization in the well-child setting along with other preventive services is ideal, providers should not fear that providing immunizations in other settings will be detrimental to well-child care.

Providers have other roles besides taking advantage of all opportunities to ensure that their patients are adequately immunized. Parents look to providers for education on the importance of vaccines and for reminders when immunizations are due or overdue.[139] Provider recommendations play an important role in parents' decisions about immunizing their children.[175] A survey of pediatricians, done as part of market research conducted by Merck, showed that a provider recommendation against varicella vaccination was a strong deterrent to parental acceptance (30% vaccinated), a neutral recommendation resulted in fewer than half of parents accepting vaccination, and a strong recommendation for vaccination resulted in a high degree of parental acceptance (>85%) (M. Keane, Business Research,

Merck Vaccine Division, personal communication, December 1996). The importance of a physician recommendation was further underscored by Freeman and Freed's interview study of parents of children in North Carolina showing that the most significant influence on parents is physician advice.[176]

Despite the need for reminders for parents, few physicians operate reminder or recall systems. A national survey of pediatricians and family physicians in 1992 reported that only 13% of pediatricians and 10% of family physicians operated routine reminder systems.[177] The percentage of providers operating recall systems did not change between 1992 and 1998, when the American Academy of Pediatrics conducted a survey of pediatricians showing similar results.[178]

COST AS A BARRIER

Another type of missed opportunity occurs when children seek other care from a private provider but are referred by that provider to public clinics for free vaccines. The need to make the extra visit may result in delayed immunization and increased time during which the child is susceptible to vaccine-preventable diseases. Private providers are more likely to refer children without insurance and children receiving Medicaid for vaccinations outside their practices, thus requiring an additional health care visit by the parent.[61,156,179–181] Providers who receive free vaccines, such as those offered through the VFC program, report substantially lower rates of referral than those who do not.[63,182–185]

The impact of providing free vaccines on the ultimate immunization coverage of young children has been the subject of debate. Immunization coverage also has been found to be low in populations in which cost is not a barrier. Only 65% of 2-year-old children of employees of a large corporation, who had medical insurance coverage for immunizations, had received the four DTP, three polio, and one MMR series, indicating that cost alone cannot account for all of the underimmunization.[120] One study comparing private practices in states that provide free vaccines for all children with practices in other states reported no differences in coverage between the two groups.[186] However, almost all the parents of children surveyed (in both types of states) were well educated and of moderate to high socioeconomic status, and therefore least likely to benefit from free vaccines from a private provider.

Parents who had previously paid out of pocket for immunization had substantial reductions in those costs when North Carolina began providing free vaccines to all children.[187] However, parents who previously had made an extra visit to a health department clinic and now wished to receive free vaccines from a private provider paid more because of vaccine administration charges, which were not assessed at the health department clinic. This cost might be smaller than the savings realized by not making extra visits, such as benefits received by not losing time from work. The fact that referrals to health departments decrease when free vaccines are provided suggests that some parents take advantage of the free vaccines to stay with their medical provider for immunization services. However, when analyzed by the type of health insurance, the North Carolina experience showed that the greatest impact on coverage was for children without a health insurance benefit.[184]

Other studies have indicated that private provider referral for vaccination to a public clinic reduces immunization levels. Zimmerman and Janosky noted that children without insurance and those receiving Medicaid in Minnesota were more likely to be referred and to have had more time underimmunized than were insured patients.[188] Lieu and colleagues interviewed parents who came to public clinics; 63% would have preferred vaccination by their regular provider but came to the clinic because of cost.[62]

Determining whether free vaccines improve coverage levels of existing vaccines is only part of the issue raised by such a policy. Concern has been expressed that research and development of new and improved vaccines might be inhibited[189] if the government purchases a substantially higher proportion of vaccines for children at reduced rates than occurs now. Thus any societal benefits from increased government purchase might be exceeded by the continuing costs of infectious diseases that are not yet preventable by vaccination.

In summary, free vaccines reduce referral of children to public clinics and allow them to be vaccinated by their primary provider, in their "medical home," and there is little controversy regarding the provision of free vaccines for poor children served by private providers. However, the debate is likely to continue regarding free vaccines for other children.

Provision of free vaccines addresses only one part of the cost issue. A survey by the American Academy of Pediatrics indicated that pediatricians, on average, charged approximately $15 per dose for vaccine administration.[190] Thus administration costs are not insignificant. Several studies have shown that insurance coverage both for vaccines and for vaccine administration significantly increases immunization coverage levels.[65,191]

One study evaluated the impact of (1) a marked increase in vaccine administration fees paid by Medicaid to private providers (from $2.00 per dose to $17.85 per dose) and (2) the provision of free vaccines through the VFC program to private providers in New York City, who served primarily a Medicaid population.[192] Immunization of children in their practices increased significantly, along with increases in provision of other well-child services. It was not possible to evaluate the relative impacts of free vaccines versus increased administration fees. Federal purchase of vaccines through the VFC program freed up state funds that had been used for vaccine purchase and allowed them to be redirected toward increased reimbursements for administration.

The importance of cost is evolving because the cost of vaccinating a child continues to increase. The cost of vaccines (including excise taxes) to fully immunize a child is now more than $410 in the public sector and more than $684 in the private sector (see Table 53–1), up from $34 and $116, respectively, 15 years earlier. In addition, there are costs for visits to the physician and vaccine administration fees. As the immunization schedule gets more complex because of the addition of more doses of existing vaccines, new vaccines, excise taxes, and extra visits, all of which can add considerably to the cost of fully vaccinating a child, the importance of cost as a potential barrier may well increase. Thus the financing of vaccines and their administration warrants continuing evaluation.

Underimmunization in Adults

Immunizing adults is a more complicated undertaking than is immunizing children. Vaccination recommendations for adults depend on a person's age, occupation, health status, and behavior (e.g., sexual activity and drug use). For example, for persons younger than 50 years of age, influenza and pneumococcal vaccines are targeted to persons at high risk for illness-related complications or death, most of whom are adults.[193,194] This requires physicians and nurses to establish procedures to identify persons who are eligible, often from long lists of qualifying conditions, in contrast to childhood immunization, in which all are offered vaccine unless there are contraindications. Influenza vaccine must be given annually. The diseases to be prevented are often clinically indistinguishable from other causes of similar syndromes, making assessment of the impact of immunization difficult and potentially preventing both vaccinees and their vaccinators from seeing the benefits of immunization. Hepatitis B is exclusively targeted toward high-risk groups in the adult population.[195] Similarly, MMR vaccination of adults is primarily targeted to persons born since 1956, particularly health care workers, postsecondary school students (e.g., college and university students), international travelers, and women likely to become pregnant.[196]

TARGET POPULATION FACTORS

A variety of factors has been linked to adults' failure to obtain vaccines. These include perceptions that adults are not susceptible to disease, the diseases are not severe, the vaccines are not effective, or the vaccines are not safe.[32,197,198] One of the major factors is failure of a strong recommendation for vaccination on the part of the individual's provider.[199–201] Cost, although a potential factor, is probably limited for influenza and pneumococcal vaccines. Although the cost may change, as of 2002, it was approximately $6 for influenza vaccine and $8 for pneumococcal vaccine, based on representative catalog prices. In contrast, hepatitis B vaccine (with a cost of $50–$60 per dose in 2002) can have substantial cost implications for the individual, particularly because many of the groups targeted for immunization, such as injecting drug users, are unlikely to have insurance coverage.

PROVIDER FACTORS

Missed opportunities are an important cause of failure to obtain adult immunizations.[202] Many of the patients who are at the highest risk for complications of influenza and pneumococcal disease have had a medical contact before disease onset and could have been vaccinated. About two thirds of patients hospitalized with pneumococcal bacteremia or pneumonia had a previous hospitalization within the preceding 5 years, when they could have been vaccinated.[203] A 1994 to 1995 study of Medicare beneficiaries in 12 states reported that opportunities to provide influenza vaccine and pneumococcal vaccine had been missed in 65% and 80% of hospitalized patients 65 years of age or older, respectively.[204]

Perhaps as important as missed opportunities is the responsibility patients give to providers for making immunization decisions. A study performed in Georgia reported that 75% and 76% of adults obtained influenza and pneumococcal vaccinations, respectively, if they were recommended by a provider, compared with 7% and 6% of adults if there was not a strong recommendation.[199] In fact, 70% and 33% of adults who did not have a favorable attitude toward vaccination were vaccinated against influenza and pneumococcal disease, respectively, if their provider recommended it.

Risk Communication and Adverse Event Reporting

It is important to ensure that the vaccine recipient (or parent or guardian) is adequately aware of the risks and the benefits of vaccination and that the recipient has a record of all immunizations received.[216] The National Childhood Vaccine Injury Act of 1986 and subsequent changes (section XXI of the Public Health Service Act) requires that *all* vaccine providers formally notify patients and parents or guardians of the risks and benefits of specified vaccines (DTaP or components; MMR or components; *H. influenzae* type b, hepatitis B, varicella, pneumococcal conjugate, and poliomyelitis vaccines).[217] The use of standardized vaccine information sheets with these vaccines is now mandatory.[218] One of these forms is reproduced in Appendix 3 of this text. A series of vaccine information statements has been developed for use with other vaccines purchased with federal funds. This act also established a no-fault compensation mechanism for those who are injured by the vaccines specified in the act. Persons desiring further information about this program should contact the National Childhood Vaccine Injury Program at 1-800-338-2382 or at *www.hrsa. gov/osp/vicp* (see Chapter 63). The National Childhood Vaccine Injury Act also requires providers to note in the patient's permanent medical record the date the vaccine was administered, the vaccine manufacturer, the vaccine lot number, and the name, address, and title of the person administering the vaccines, in addition to noting the provision of vaccine information materials. Finally, the act requires that providers report selected adverse events occurring after vaccination and events that would contraindicate further doses of vaccines to the Vaccine Adverse Event Reporting System (VAERS) (see Table 63–1 in Chapter 63 and *www.hrsa.gov/osp/vicp/table.htm*). Providers are encouraged to report all serious adverse events following all vaccines, regardless of whether they believe that a vaccine caused the event. The VAERS forms can be obtained by calling 1-800-822-7967, or through the Internet at *www.fda.gov/ cber/vaers/vaers.html*. (See Chapter 61 for further discussion of vaccine safety.)

Sustain and Improve Immunization Coverage Levels

Effective Strategies

The evidence of what works to raise and sustain immunization coverage levels has been reviewed systematically by the Task Force on Community Preventive Services and other independent reviewers.[219] These systematic reviews have shown several interventions to be highly effective.[220–222]

ASSESSMENT OF AND FEEDBACK ON PROVIDER IMMUNIZATION PERFORMANCE

Most physicians and nurses want to ensure that their patients are immunized. In fact, when queried, they tend to overestimate the coverage of the children they serve. Bushnell asked physicians and nurses from both public and private sectors in Massachusetts what they believed to be the immunization coverage of their patient population. The range was 85% to 100%. Record reviews documented a median coverage of 61% and a range of 19% to 93%.[223] Other studies reported that physicians overestimated coverage by 10% to more than 40%.[171,224] Such health care professionals are unlikely to be motivated to make improvements in their immunization practices because they mistakenly believe that their current efforts are adequate.

The purpose of assessment and feedback is to alert providers to the actual coverage in their patient populations and to help motivate them to improve that coverage. The AFIX method has been pioneered in the public clinics of the state of Georgia[152,225] and includes four components:

1. Assessment of the immunization coverage of the preschool children served by a given clinic.
2. Feedback of the results to persons in the clinic with the authority to make changes. Such feedback often includes potential problems identified during the review, such as failure to administer vaccines simultaneously.
3. Incentives for improved performance. In the public sector, this often involves community recognition, plaques, and/or dinners rather than financial incentives.
4. Exchange of information or comparing the performance of one clinic with others to stimulate competition to improve performance.

Together, these spell "A FIX," a slang expression denoting "a repair."

In Georgia, median immunization coverage for the four DTP, three polio, and one measles-containing vaccine series rose from 53% in 1988, early in the program, to 89% in 1994.[152] Furthermore, the coverage level of the lowest ranked clinic rose from less than 10% in 1988 to greater than 50% in 1994. Similar improvements have been seen in other states. Link implemented a similar system in private practices in Massachusetts and demonstrated increases in median coverage among two groups of private providers from 60% to 80% and from 52% to 77% over a 4-year period.[226] The AFIX system has been shown to be effective over time and across multiple geographic areas.[227,228]

REMINDER AND RECALL SYSTEMS

Many studies have shown that reminders for immunizations that are due or recall systems for immunization appointments that are missed can significantly improve immunization coverage in a variety of settings.[229–236] In a health maintenance organization setting, computer-generated letters to families with children who had not received an MMR vaccine by 20 months of age improved coverage by 19% compared with similar children whose parents did not receive reminders (54% vs. 35%), at a cost of $4.04 per additional immunized child.[232] Computerized telephone reminders to families cared for in Georgia public clinics increased coverage for the fourth DTaP vaccine, the third oral poliovirus vaccine, and/or MMR vaccine by 16% in the 30-day period after the reminder when compared with control subjects.[233] Provider-based recall systems have been shown to be effective at the community level in reducing racial and ethnic disparities in immunization coverage levels.[234]

LINKAGE WITH THE SPECIAL SUPPLEMENTAL FOOD PROGRAM FOR WOMEN, INFANTS, AND CHILDREN

Approximately 49% of the U.S. birth cohort is enrolled in the U.S. Department of Agriculture's Special Supplemental Nutrition Program for Women, Infants, and Children (WIC), a federally supported, means-tested program that supplies vouchers for food for needy infants and young children.[237–240] Parents are required to make visits at 1- to 3-month intervals (depending on the policies of the local or state WIC program) to pick up vouchers that can be used to purchase food, such as infant formula. Infants and young children must be examined periodically. Because WIC eligibility is in part based on income and because low income is associated with underimmunization, WIC participants are at higher risk for underimmunization than non-WIC participants.[241,242] During a resurgence of measles in the United States, 29% to 63% of preschool, unvaccinated, yet vaccine-eligible children with measles in five cities were enrolled in WIC.[243] State immunization programs are required to work with WIC to ensure that the children they serve are vaccinated.

A variety of WIC-based interventions have been proven effective without causing harm to WIC enrollment and have been well received by parents.[244–246] All require assessment of the child's immunization status, based on a written record and (at a minimum) a referral to a provider for vaccination. Other interventions have included outreach and education, escort of undervaccinated children to a provider site to ensure access to immunization, and requiring parents of underimmunized children to pick up vouchers more often than parents of immunized children (e.g., monthly rather than every 2 to 3 months). Depending on the intervention used, immunization levels of children enrolled in WIC have been increased by as much as 40 percentage points through collaborative efforts of WIC and immunization programs.[244,247]

A large study in Chicago reported that use of monthly voucher pickup had substantially greater impact than assessment and referral of underimmunized children.[245] The WIC clinics with monthly voucher pickup documented a 33% increase in age-appropriate immunization coverage (from 56% to 89%) compared to no improvement at sites using assessment and referral alone. A study in Milwaukee demonstrated that monthly voucher pickup improved immunization coverage levels, with the additional benefits of improving attendance at well-child visits, lead screening, and anemia screening.[248] In contrast to the uniformly positive impact of WIC linkages, the use of welfare financial incentives has had mixed results.[249,250]

STANDARDS FOR CHILD AND ADOLESCENT IMMUNIZATION PRACTICES

In 1993, the NVAC recommended a set of 18 standards to improve the immunization performance of providers who serve children, and in 2002 these standards were updated to incorporate advances in knowledge of best immunization practices (Table 53–3).[34] Many of the standards specifically address improving immunization coverage in children served, including removing barriers to immunization, taking advantage of all opportunities to vaccinate, simultaneously vaccinating and using only valid contraindications, establishing tracking systems to identify children who are underimmunized and to facilitate taking corrective actions, and semiannually auditing patients served by a given clinic or

TABLE 53–3 ■ Standards for Child and Adolescent Immunization Practices, 2003

Availability of vaccines	1. Vaccination services are readily available.
	2. Vaccinations are coordinated with other health care services and provided in a "medical home" when possible.
	3. Barriers to vaccination are identified and minimized.
	4. Patient costs are minimized.
Assessment of vaccination status	5. Health care professionals review the vaccination and health status of patients at every encounter to determine which vaccines are indicated.
	6. Health care professionals assess for and follow only medically accepted contraindications.
Effective communication with parents/guardians and patients about vaccine benefits and risks	7. Parents/guardians and patients are educated about the benefits and risks of vaccination in a culturally appropriate manner and in easy-to-understand language.
Proper storage, administration, and documentation of vaccinations	8. Health care professionals follow appropriate procedures for vaccine storage and handling.
	9. Up-to-date, written vaccination protocols are accessible at all locations where vaccines are administered.
	10. Persons who administer vaccines and staff who manage or support vaccine administration are knowledgeable and receive ongoing education.
	11. Health care professionals simultaneously administer as many indicated vaccine doses as possible.
	12. Vaccination records for patients are accurate, complete, and easily accessible.
	13. Health care professionals report adverse events following vaccination promptly and accurately to the Vaccine Adverse Event Reporting System (VAERS) and are aware of a separate program, the National Vaccine Injury Compensation Program (VICP).
	14. All personnel who have contact with patients are appropriately vaccinated.
Implementation of strategies to improve vaccination coverage	15. Systems are used to remind parents/guardians, patients, and health care professionals when vaccinations are due and to recall those who are overdue.
	16. Office- or clinic-based patient record reviews and vaccination coverage assessments are performed annually.
	17. Health care professionals practice community-based approaches.

From National Vaccine Advisory Committee. Standards for child and adolescent immunization practices. Pediatrics [in press].

practice to evaluate performance and to determine whether improvements are needed. Other aspects call for working with communities and for providing education. Implementing the standards at a New Mexico clinic reduced dropout from DTaP1 to DTaP3 (the difference in the percentage of children who started the immunization series and those who finished the recommended three-dose series for infants) from 24% before the intervention to only 5% with the intervention.[251] In contrast, dropout at the control site increased from 39% to 51%. The Infectious Diseases Society of America has established 17 implementation standards that apply to adults, adolescents, and children.[252] The NVAC has also developed a set of adult immunization standards (Table 53–4).

THE ROLE OF MASS IMMUNIZATION CAMPAIGNS

Campaigns attempting to vaccinate large numbers of children in 1 day or some other short period have been important in worldwide efforts to eradicate polio and eliminate measles.[253–256] Such campaigns were useful in the United States for the introduction of new vaccines, such as the oral polio, measles, and rubella vaccines.[15,257,258] Those campaigns were generally nonselective; that is, everyone in the target age group received vaccine, regardless of prior vaccination or disease status. In contrast, most recent immunization campaigns in the United States have been selective, attempting to vaccinate only a small proportion of the total population—children without a prior history of vaccination. Evaluation of the success of these campaigns is made difficult by the inability in most U.S. communities to estimate accurately the target population and to determine the proportion reached in the campaign. Limited data suggest that the campaigns have generally failed to immunize many of the children thought to be in need.[259,260] Other information also suggests that these immunization campaigns are not likely to be effective. A high proportion of parents of underimmunized children mistakenly believe that their children's immunizations are up to date and consequently would not be motivated to participate in selective mass immunization campaigns for their children.[96–98] Furthermore, the U.S. immunization schedule requires that 13 to 20 doses of vaccines be given by 18 months of age, too many doses to be addressed in any one-time immunization campaign.[27] Thus selective immunization campaigns cannot be recommended as a major means of improving overall immunization coverage. However, the publicity gained in such campaigns may be useful in improving the political and community support necessary for ongoing immunization

TABLE 53–4 ▪ Standards for Adult Immunization Practices, 2003

Make vaccinations available	1. Adult vaccination services are readily available.
	2. Barriers to receiving vaccines are identified and minimized.
	3. Patient "out of pocket" vaccination costs are minimized.
Assess patients' vaccination status	4. Health care professionals routinely review the vaccination status of patients.
	5. Health care professionals assess for valid contraindications.
Communicate effectively with patients	6. Patients are educated about risks and benefits of vaccination in easy-to-understand language.
Administer and document vaccinations properly	7. Written vaccination protocols are available at all locations where vaccines are administered.
	8. Persons who administer vaccines are properly trained.
	9. Health care professionals recommend simultaneous administration of all indicated vaccine doses.
	10. Vaccination records for patients are accurate and easily accessible.
	11. All personnel who have contact with patients are appropriately vaccinated.
Implement strategies to improve vaccination rates	12. Systems are developed and used to remind patients and health care professionals when vaccinations are due and to recall patients who are overdue.
	13. Standing orders for vaccinations are employed.
	14. Regular assessments of vaccination coverage levels are conducted in a provider's practice.
Partner with the community	15. Patient-oriented and community-based approaches are used to reach target populations.

From National Vaccine Advisory Committee. Standards for adult immunization practices, 2003. Am J Prev Med (in press).

efforts. The challenge is to conduct a campaign in such a way that the positive publicity is matched by achievable programmatic objectives, such as linking children to a medical home.

LAWS AND REGULATIONS FOR IMMUNIZATION

Laws requiring immunization in the United States date from the early 19th century.[261,262] Massachusetts enacted a law in 1809 that required smallpox vaccination of the general population, and other jurisdictions followed during the course of the century. In 1905, the Supreme Court affirmed the right of states to pass and enforce compulsory immunization statutes. Laws requiring vaccination before school entry were affirmed by the Supreme Court in 1922. School entry laws were variably enforced, and the antigens covered varied considerably.[262] After measles vaccine was introduced in the mid-1960s, school entry requirements for measles vaccination became common because measles was a disease primarily of school-age children. It became apparent that states without laws were experiencing a higher incidence of measles than those with laws (relative risk, 1.7 to 2.0 in 1973 to 1974), and, with the Immunization Initiative of 1977, considerable emphasis was placed on enactment and enforcement of school entry laws.[263,264]

Laws requiring immunization before entry in school or day care are the safety net for the U.S. immunization program. All 50 states and the District of Columbia have laws in effect, although the precise antigens, doses, and schedules may vary. The impact of those laws has been shown in the decreased incidence of measles and mumps in states with laws versus states without laws. For example, during the first 31 weeks of 1978, the incidence rate of measles was only 2.7 per 100,000 persons less than 18 years of age in six states that were strictly enforcing school laws, compared with 35.2 per 100,000 in the rest of the nation.[265] In

a comparison of high-incidence and low-incidence areas of measles, the biggest difference found was the statewide enforcement of laws through exclusion of unvaccinated students from school until vaccinated.[266] Of the 13 low-incidence areas, 10 (77%) had such policies, compared with none of 10 high-incidence areas. A major resurgence of mumps during 1986 was shown to occur almost exclusively in states without comprehensive laws requiring mumps vaccination.[267] A comprehensive review of the impact of school laws was published by Orenstein and Hinman.[268]

In the United States, few parents object to immunization for their children. The laws serve primarily to enhance priority for immunization by requiring that children receive immunization for attendance at school or day care. Children who are not adequately immunized are not allowed to attend school or day care, although most states allow provisional attendance for children whose immunization status is not up to date as long as the children continue to obtain immunizations at recommended intervals. As of 1997, all state laws have exemptions for medical contraindications to vaccination, 48 have exemptions for religions that oppose immunization, and 16 have exemptions for philosophic objections to immunization.[269] There is no evidence that school laws delay immunization until the child reaches the age of school entry. In almost all areas studied, 80% or more of children have received at least one dose of a vaccine by 2 years of age.[52,134] However, there is evidence that the methods of enforcement of the school laws vary from state to state and that states with more lenient exemption rules have higher rates of exemptions.[270] Although states appear to use their power sparingly in school immunization law enforcement,[271] a dialog is developing in the scientific literature concerning school law implementation.[272]

Immunization coverage among children entering school or day care has been 95% or greater for all required vaccines since the 1981 to 1982 school year.[273] Regulations have also proved effective in protecting college students from vaccine-preventable diseases. Between 1988 and 1991, colleges with a state-mandated prematriculation immunization requirement had only one third the risk of measles outbreaks of other colleges.[274]

EFFECTIVE STRATEGIES TO IMPROVE ADULT IMMUNIZATION

As with childhood immunization, improving the performance of physicians and nurses who treat adults appears to be the key to increasing coverage. In Rochester, New York, immunization staff reviewed the records of physicians, developed lists of patients (target populations) who were in need of influenza immunization, and established graphing systems to track progress toward their targets.[205] Practices with the intervention had immunization coverage levels of 66%, compared with 50% in the control practices. Financial incentives can also improve coverage. In a second study, practices that were eligible to receive increased reimbursement if they achieved certain immunization coverage levels (providers received 10% more than the usual fee per patient immunized if they achieved a 70% coverage rate; they received 20% more than usual if they achieved an 85% coverage rate) had an average coverage of 73%, compared with 56% in control clinics that were not eligible for increased reimbursement.[206] Another intervention that has shown promise includes establishment of a "standing orders" system for immunization for long-term care facility and hospitalized patients on discharge or for outpatients whereby immunization would be offered unless a physician specifically removed the vaccination from a patient's orders.[207–210] Nursing homes with written immunization policies or standing orders and that do not require written informed consent specifically for vaccination have higher rates of immunization than those that do not have such policies and procedures.[211] Reminder systems for high-risk groups can also significantly increase coverage.[212] A comprehensive plan for the prevention and control of vaccine-preventable diseases in long-term care facilities was published in 2000.[213]

The National Coalition on Adult Immunization (*www.nfid.org/ncai*), a group of more than 90 organizations dedicated to improving immunization coverage among adults, issued a set of 10 standards for adult immunization.[214] These standards have been updated and revised by the NVAC[215]; they encourage education, protection of health care providers themselves against vaccine-preventable diseases, routine screening of adults to determine immunization needs, use of all opportunities to vaccinate, adequate financing, and other measures (see Table 53–4).

The NVAC has issued a comprehensive report on improving the protection of adults against vaccine-preventable diseases.[32] The report has five goals:

1. Increasing the demand for adult vaccination by improving provider and public awareness
2. Ensuring that the health care system has adequate capacity to deliver vaccines to adults
3. Ensuring adequate financing mechanisms to support expanded delivery of vaccines to adults
4. Monitoring and improving the performance of the nation's vaccine delivery system
5. Ensuring adequate support for research on
   a. Vaccine-preventable diseases of adults
   b. Adult vaccines
   c. Adult immunization practices
   d. New and improved vaccines
   e. International programs for adult immunization

Vaccine Shortages

During 2001 and 2002, the United States experienced insufficient supplies of five childhood vaccines: DTaP, tetanus diphtheria toxoids (Td) for adult use, 7-valent pneumococcal conjugate vaccine (PCV7), MMR, and varicella. Coincident with these shortages of pediatric vaccines, influenza vaccines for the 2000–2001 and 2001–2002 influenza vaccination season were delayed in production, causing a shortage of the vaccine during the time it was needed for routine vaccination. These shortages were of sufficient magnitude and duration that recommendations for routinely administered vaccines were temporarily modified and certain doses were suspended. All of the vaccine shortages except PCV7 were resolved within 1½ years; however, the public health impact of the shortages has not yet been determined. One study demonstrated that implementing the ACIP's temporary recommendation to delay the fourth dose of DTaP resulted in a decline in population-measured coverage for that dose.[275]

Unlike the most prominent previous vaccine shortage, which was precipitated by the single issue of liability related to DTP vaccine, the recent shortages had multiple causes that occurred coincidentally. According to the NVAC, immediate causes included[276] "business decisions by manufacturers to cease production of certain vaccines; production problems with some vaccines; unanticipated, large demand for the most recently recommended vaccine, pneumococcal conjugate vaccine; and difficulties that manufacturers had with regard to removing the thimerosal from routine childhood vaccines." In addition,

> some manufacturers had problems complying with the current Good Manufacturing Practices (cGMP). The cGMPs are meant to be a dynamic, evolving set of practices resulting in current and improved standards for drugs and vaccines. The composition of the Food and Drug Administration (FDA) inspection teams changed in the 1990s to include more expertise in design and control but FDA regulatory requirements did not change. The focus of the inspection teams shifted to include a greater emphasis on quality systems, in-process testing, and facility and process validation. As a result, facilities and processes that had previously been acceptable might now require significant changes in physical plants, quality systems and processes. The FDA has a new initiative of cGMPs for the 21st century that will focus on a risk-based assessment of product quality issues.[276]

The lack of adequate vaccine stockpiles, although not a cause of shortages, impeded immunization programs' ability to manage sudden, short-term shortages.

The NVAC also noted factors that were not immediately causal but that contributed to the shortages. These include

a relatively low valuation of vaccines compared with drugs; high costs associated with development, approval, manufacturing, and distribution of vaccines; decreased number of vaccine manufacturers; lack of investment in some vaccine manufacturing facilities; and legal barriers to communication between stakeholder groups that inhibit the recognition of evolving problems and development of effective responses.[276]

In addition to the NVAC, the General Accounting Office also conducted an independent review of the U.S. vaccine supply situation. Both groups recommended improved communication between industry and government and within government, enhanced vaccine stockpiles, and streamlining of vaccine regulation, provided safety and efficacy of the vaccine supply are not compromised.[276,277]

Impact of Immunization Programs

Occurrence of Disease

The occurrence of most vaccine-preventable diseases is at or near record low levels. Table 53–5 shows the representative annual levels of disease reported or estimated for selected vaccine-preventable diseases during the 20th century.[278] Most often, these are years immediately preceding vaccine licensure. All diseases have been reduced by 95% or more from representative 20th-century morbidity. Measles transmission within the United States was probably interrupted for periods of several weeks in 1993, 1995, and 1996, only to be periodically re-established through importations.[279–282] In March 2000, a group of experts concluded that endemic transmission of measles in the United States had ceased.[283] In 2001, most cases of measles reported in the United States were either imported from another country or directly attributable to importations. The countries that provided most of the importations were Japan (18 cases), China (14 cases), and Korea (5 cases). There was a provisional total of 116 cases in 2001. A provisional total of 37 cases was reported in 2002. Further gains in disease prevention will require improved international control to reduce the risk of importation, increased immunization levels not only in children but also in adults, and other measures. Provisional data from 2002 show that record lows were set or tied for measles, mumps, polio, rubella, and tetanus.

Immunization Coverage

Preschool Immunization

The United States is currently experiencing record high or near–record high vaccination coverage levels among 2-year-old children, although there is moderate variation in coverage levels across states (Table 53–6).[52] Among children 19 to 35 months of age (median age, 27 months) who were born between February 1998 and May 2000, more than 90% had received three or more doses of DTaP and *H. influenzae* type b vaccines; 91% had received a dose of MMR; 89% had received three or more doses of hepatitis B vaccine; 89% had received three or more doses of poliovirus vaccines; and 76% had received one or more doses of varicella vaccine. The coverage for the four DTaP, three polio, and one measles-containing vaccine series (4:3:1), a common measure of overall coverage (primarily DTaP-4 coverage, which is the main determinant of the series coverage), was 79%. Immunization coverage was high in all racial and ethnic groups evaluated in 2001.[87] In 2001, coverage levels exceeded 90% or were within 5% of 90% for three or more doses of DTaP, polio, *H. influenzae* type b, and for one dose of a measles-containing vaccine for whites, African-Americans, Hispanics, Asians and Pacific Islanders, and Native Americans/Alaska Natives (*www.cdc.gov/nip/coverage*). Past data have shown that poverty was the major predictor of underimmunization, with immunization among children below poverty levels being 3% to 7% lower than that of children at or above poverty levels. The greatest discrepancies of any of the recommended vaccines and doses were reported for DTaP-4. Similar findings were reported in 2001 (*www.cdc.gov/nip/coverage*).

TABLE 53–5 ■ Baseline 20th-Century Annual Morbidity and 2001 Provisional Morbidity from 10 Diseases with Vaccines Recommended Before 1990 for Universal Use in Children, United States

Disease	Baseline 20th-Century Annual Morbidity*	2002 Morbidity (Provisional)	Percent Decrease
Smallpox	48,164	0	100
Diphtheria	175,885	1	>99
Pertussis	147,271	8296	94
Tetanus	1314	22	98
Poliomyelitis (paralytic)	16,316	0	100
Measles	503,282	37	>99
Mumps	152,209	238	>99
Rubella	47,745	14	>99
Congenital rubella syndrome	823	3	>99
Haemophilus influenzae type b and unknown (<5 yr)	20,000	167	>99

From Centers for Disease Control and Prevention. Impact of vaccines universally recommended for children—United States, 1900–1999. MMWR 48:243–248, 1999. See reference for method by which baseline morbidity estimates were developed. Estimates for 2002 from MMWR SI: 1149–1176, 2003, except for Hib. Data for Hib come from National Immunization Program, CDC (unpublished).

TABLE 53–6 ▪ Vaccination Coverage Levels Among Children Ages 19 to 35 Months (Median Age, 27 Months), by Selected Vaccines—National Immunization Survey, 2001[*]

Vaccine/Dose	Lowest State's Level (%)	Highest State's Level (%)	National Mean (%)
DTP/DT/DTaP (≥3)	89.2	98.3	94.3
DTP/DT/DTaP (≥4)	74.1	91.7	82.1
Poliovirus (≥3)	81.4	95.2	89.4
Hib (≥3)	88.3	98.2	93.0
MMR (≥1)	84.7	96.4	91.4
Hepatitis B (≥3)	79.3	95.8	88.9
Varicella (≥1)	52.8	89.9	76.3
4:3:1[†]	69.9	89.2	78.6
4:3:1:3[‡]	68.9	88.0	77.2
4:3:1:3:3[§]	63.2	81.7	73.7

[*]Children were born during February 1998 to May 2000.
[†]Four or more doses of DTP/DT/DTaP, three or more doses of poliovirus vaccine, and one or more dose of MMR.
[‡]4:3:1 plus three or more doses of Hib vaccine.
[§]4:3:1:3 plus three or more doses of hepatitis B vaccine.
DTaP, diphtheria and tetanus toxoids and acellular pertussis; DT, diphtheria and tetanus toxoids for use in children; DTP, diphtheria and tetanus toxoids and whole-cell pertussis; Hib, *Haemophilus influenzae* type b; MMR, measles-mumps-rubella.

School-Age Immunization

As mentioned earlier, immunization levels for children entering school or day care are 95% or greater.[269,273] As long as school laws remain in place and are enforced, these levels should continue.

Adult Immunization

Immunization levels for pneumococcal and influenza vaccines in adults lag far behind the levels achieved for vaccines recommended routinely for children. Influenza immunization coverage in persons 65 years or older, determined from the 1999 National Health Interview Survey, reached 66%, the highest level ever reported but still well below childhood vaccine coverage levels.[111] Pneumococcal vaccination coverage was only 50%. Data from the Behavioral Risk Factor Surveillance System for 2001 show influenza vaccine coverage levels of 65% and pneumococcal vaccine coverage levels of 54%.[112] Immunization rates for members of racial and ethnic minority groups are substantially lower than for the white population, with African-Americans tending to have the lowest rates. Influenza vaccination coverage for African-Americans was 17 percentage points below that of white non-Hispanics.[112]

Remaining Issues in Immunization in the United States

Remaining Disease Burden

There is no question that the vaccines recommended for universal or widespread use in infants and children address significant health problems and have had great impact. Some of these conditions have been so well controlled by the use of vaccines that prospective recipients or their parents may not be aware of them, and many providers may not have seen cases themselves.

It is ironic that our success, which has given us very low levels of disease, might lead to a loss of awareness of the severity of these conditions if they do occur. This, in turn,

could lead to a loss of political will to sustain immunization programs. It may be doubly ironic that we continue, as a society, to tolerate the level of mortality still seen in association with influenza and pneumococcal infection and do not mount major efforts to control it. More than 36,000 *excess* deaths regularly occur during influenza epidemics.[193,284a] In 1999 there were an estimated 6080 deaths due to pneumococcal infection.[284b]

Importations and Quarantine

Given the extent and rapidity of international travel, the risk of importation of vaccine-preventable diseases will remain until worldwide control or eradication occurs.[281,285,286] In 2001, most cases of measles reported in the United States were either imported from another country or directly attributable to importations. The countries that provided most of the importations were Japan, China, and Korea.

Quarantine regulations have been used in the past to require, for example, smallpox vaccination of all persons entering a given country from infected countries. This approach resulted from international agreement (the International Sanitary Regulations) and was feasible because of the shared fear of smallpox and the limited extent of international travel at the time. In the absence of international accord and with the hundreds of millions of border crossings occurring in this country each year, vaccination requirements for all visitors (e.g., for measles) are not feasible. Monitoring and enforcement would be virtually impossible.

Immunization Registries

As described above, the immunization system in the United States has had variable success in assuring that all children receive immunizations on time. Immunization registries have the potential to strengthen the system and raise and maintain immunization levels.[287,288] Registries are confidential, computerized information systems that contain information about immunizations and children.[289] Registries are capable

TABLE 53-7 ■ Immunization Registry Minimum Functional Standards

- Electronically store data on all NVAC-approved core data elements.
- Establish a registry record within 6 weeks of birth for each newborn child born in the catchment area.
- Enable access to and retrieval of immunization information in the registry at the time of encounter.
- Receive and process immunization information within 1 mo of vaccine administration.
- Protect the confidentiality of health care information.
- Ensure the security of health care information.
- Exchange immunization records using HL7 standards.
- Automatically determine the routine childhood immunization(s) needed, in compliance with current ACIP recommendations, when an individual presents for a scheduled immunization.
- Automatically identify individuals due/late for immunization(s) to enable the production of reminder/recall notifications.
- Automatically produce immunization coverage reports by providers, age groups, and geographic areas.
- Produce official immunization records.
- Promote accuracy and completeness of registry data.

of monitoring the immunization status of individuals and population groups, generating reminder/recall notices, and generating official immunization records. Both child and adult immunization standards call for such systems.[214,290] The Healthy People 2010 objectives call for 95% of children less than 6 years of age to be enrolled in fully operational population-based immunization registries (Objective 14-26).[291]

Minimum functional standards have been developed for immunization registries (Table 53-7).[292] Registries have demonstrated usefulness in sending reminder/recall notices, increasing coverage, monitoring implementation of policy changes, generating official immunization records, assessing immunization levels (for HEDIS indices), reducing missed opportunities, preventing unnecessary immunization, recall for revaccination, and vaccine inventory management. They have also been used to identify and recall children who did not receive vaccines during temporary national shortages.

A study by All Kids Count estimated that a nationwide network of population-based immunization registries would cost approximately $125 million/year but that it would offset more than $280 million/year that is currently being spent by the health care and school systems to retrieve records, assess adequacy of information, and transcribe information to provide records for school entry or change of provider, among other costs.[293,294] No permanent mechanism has yet been identified to support registries nationwide. Federal immunization grant funds, Medicaid, state funds, managed care organizations, and private foundations have all contributed.[295] The NVAC has recommended use of VFC program funds to provide an ongoing base of support for registries.[296]

All 50 states are in the process of developing population-based registries, and approximately 44% of U.S. children less than 6 years of age have two or more vaccinations recorded in a health department population-based registry.[297] Most registries include children older than 6 years of age and some include adults. Few have yet incorporated reporting adverse events. The immense promise of immunization registries remains to be fully realized.

Conclusion

Development and use of vaccines in the United States has had a profound effect on the occurrence of vaccine-preventable diseases. The success represents a unique blend of public/private and federal/state/local partnerships. Although high levels of immunization have been achieved in school-age children for the past 20 years, it is only within the past few years that levels in preschool-age children have been near satisfactory. Measles has been eliminated as an indigenous disease in the United States. Unfortunately, immunization levels in adolescents and adults remain unsatisfactory, and programs to ensure their appropriate immunization remain to be developed.

REFERENCES

1. Fine PEM. Herd immunity: history, theory, practice. Epidemiol Rev 15:265–302, 1993.
2. Fox JP, Elveback L, Scott W, et al. Herd immunity: basic concept and relevance to public health immunization practices. Am J Epidemiol 94:179–189, 1971.
3. Hethcote HW. Measles and rubella in the United States. Am J Epidemiol 117:2–13, 1983.
4. Yorke JA, Nathanson W, Pianigiani G, Martin J. Seasonality and the requirement for perpetuation and eradication of viruses in populations. Am J Epidemiol 109:103–123, 1979.
5. Anderson RM, May RM. Directly transmitted infectious diseases: control by vaccination. Science 215:1053–1060, 1982.
6. Schlenker TL, Bain C, Baughman AL, Hadler SC. Measles herd immunity: the association of attack rates with immunization rates in preschool children. JAMA 267:823–826, 1992.
7. Anderson RM, May RM. Immunization and herd immunity. Lancet 335:641–645, 1990.
8. Fenner F. Global eradication of smallpox. Rev Infect Dis 4:916–930, 1982.
9. Fenner F. Biological control, as exemplified by smallpox eradication and myxomatosis. Proc R Soc Lond 218:259–285, 1983.
10. Kim-Farley RJ, Bart KJ, Schonberger LB, et al. Poliomyelitis in the USA: virtual elimination of disease caused by wild virus. Lancet 2:1315–1317, 1984.
11. Hinman AR. Prospects for disease eradication or elimination. N Y State J Med 84:501–506, 1984.
12. Dowdle WR, Hopkins DR (eds). The Eradication of Infectious Diseases: Dahlem Workshop Report. Chichester, UK, John Wiley & Sons, 1997.
13. Fenner F, Henderson DA, Arita I, et al. Smallpox and Its Eradication. Geneva, World Health Organization, 1988.
14. Stuart-Harris C, Western KA, Chamberlayne EC (eds). Can infectious diseases be eradicated? A report on the International Conference on the Eradication of Infectious Diseases. Rev Infect Dis 4:913–984, 1982.
15. Sencer DJ, Dull HB, Langmuir AD. Epidemiologic basis for eradication of measles in 1976. Public Health Rep 82:253–256, 1967.
16. Conrad JL, Wallace R, Witte JJ. The epidemiologic rationale for the failure to eradicate measles in the United States. Am J Public Health 61:2304–2310, 1971.

17. Hinman AR, Nieburg PI, Brandling-Bennett AD. The opportunity and obligation to eliminate measles from the United States. JAMA 242:1157–1162, 1979.

18. Hinman AR, Brandling-Bennett AD, Bernier RH, et al. Current features of measles in the United States: feasibility of measles elimination. Epidemiol Rev 2:153–170, 1980.

19. Hinman AR, Kirby CD, Eddins DL, et al. Elimination of indigenous measles from the United States. Rev Infect Dis 4:538–545, 1983.

20. Frank JA, Orenstein WA, Bart KJ, et al. Major impediments to measles elimination: the modern epidemiology of an ancient disease. Am J Dis Child 139:881–888, 1985.

21. Atkinson WL, Orenstein WA, Krugman S. The resurgence of measles in the United States, 1989–1990. Annu Rev Med 43:451–463, 1992.

22. Orenstein WA, Bart KJ, Hinman AR, et al. The opportunity and obligation to eliminate rubella from the United States. JAMA 251:1988–1994, 1984.

23. Centers for Disease Control and Prevention. Intussusception among recipients of rotavirus vaccine—United States, 1998–1999. MMWR 48:577–581, 1999.

24. Murphy TV, Garguillo PM, Massoudi MS, et al. Intussusception among infants given an oral rotavirus vaccine. N Engl J Med 344:564–572, 2001.

25. Pickering LK (ed). *Red Book* 2003: Report of the Committee on Infectious Diseases (25th ed). Elk Grove Village, IL, American Academy of Pediatrics, 2003, in press.

26. Centers for Disease Control and Prevention. Recommended childhood immunization schedule—United States, January 1995. MMWR 43:959–960, 1994.

27. Centers for Disease Control and Prevention. Recommended childhood and adolescent immunization schedule—United States, 2003. MMWR 52:Q1–Q4, 2003.

28. ACP Task Force on Adult Immunization and Infectious Diseases Society of America. Guide for Adult Immunization (3rd ed). Philadelphia, American College of Physicians, 1994.

28a. Centers for Disease Control and Prevention. Recommended adult immunization schedule United States, 2002–2003. MMWR 51:904–908, 2002.

29. Hinman AR. The National Vaccine Program and the National Vaccine Injury Compensation Program. *In* Proceedings of the 22nd National Immunization Conference, San Antonio, TX, June 20–24, 1988. Atlanta, Centers for Disease Control, 1988, pp 9–12.

30. Dandoy S. The National Vaccine Advisory Committee: mission/goals/progress. *In* Proceedings of the 23rd National Immunization Conference, San Diego, CA, June 5–9, 1989. Atlanta, Centers for Disease Control, 1989, pp 21–22.

31. Anonymous. The measles epidemic: the problems, barriers, and recommendations. The National Vaccine Advisory Committee. JAMA 266:1547–1552, 1991.

32. Fedson DS. Adult immunization: summary of the National Vaccine Advisory Committee report. JAMA 272:1133–1137, 1994.

33. National Vaccine Advisory Committee. United States vaccine research: a delicate fabric of public and private collaboration. Pediatrics 100:1015–1020, 1997.

34. National Vaccine Advisory Committee. Standards for child and adolescent immunization practices. Pediatrics [in press].

35. Centers for Disease Control and Prevention. Health Information for International Travel—2001–2002. Atlanta, Centers for Disease Control and Prevention, 2002.

36. Chin J (ed). Control of Communicable Disease Manual (17th ed). Washington, DC, American Public Health Association, 2000.

37. Katzmann W, Dietz K. Evaluation of age-specific vaccination strategies. Theor Popul Biol 25:125–137, 1985.

38. Orenstein WA, Markowitz L, Preblud SR, et al. Appropriate age for measles vaccination in the United States. Dev Biol Stand 65:13–21, 1986.

39. Centers for Disease Control and Prevention. General recommendations on immunization: recommendations of the Advisory Committee on Immunization Practices (ACIP). MMWR 51(RR-2):1–36, 2002.

40. Centers for Disease Control and Prevention. Measles prevention: recommendations of the Immunization Practices Advisory Committee (ACIP). MMWR 38(S-9):1–13, 1989.

41. Centers for Disease Control and Prevention. Adult immunization schedule: recommendations of the Advisory Committee on Immunization Practices. MMWR 51:904–908, 2002.

42. Centers for Disease Control. Update on adult immunization: recommendations of the Immunization Practices Advisory Committee (ACIP). MMWR 40(RR-12):1–94, 1991.

43. Centers for Disease Control and Prevention. Prevention of varicella: recommendations of the Advisory Committee on Immunization Practices (ACIP). MMWR 45(RR-11):1–36, 1996.

44. Centers for Disease Control and Prevention. Prevention of hepatitis A through active or passive immunization: recommendations of the Advisory Committee on Immunization Practices (ACIP). MMWR 45(RR-15):1–30, 1996.

45. Hinman AR. Immunizations and CDC: Proceedings of the 30th Immunization Conference. Bethesda, MD, U.S. Department of Health and Human Services, pp 7–13.

46. Hinman AR. A new U.S. initiative in childhood immunization. Bull Pan Am Health Organ 13:169–176, 1979.

47. Califano JA Jr. Address to Second National Immunization Conference, April 6, 1977. Washington, DC, U.S. Department of Health, Education and Welfare, 1977.

48. Woods DR, Mason DD. Six areas lead national early immunization drive. Public Health Rep 107:252–256, 1992.

49. Centers for Disease Control and Prevention. Reported vaccine-preventable diseases—United States, 1993, and the Childhood Immunization Initiative. MMWR 43:57–60, 1994.

50. Robinson CA, Sepe SJ, Lin KF. The president's child immunization initiative—a summary of the problem and the response. Public Health Rep 108:419–425, 1993.

51. Robinson CA, Evans WB, Mahanes JA, Sepe SJ. Progress on the Childhood Immunization Initiative. Public Health Rep 109:594–600, 1994.

52. Centers for Disease Control and Prevention. National, state, and urban area vaccination coverage levels among children aged 19–35 months—United States, 2001. MMWR 51:664–666, 2002.

53. Orenstein WA, Bernier RH. Toward immunizing every child on time. Pediatrics 94:545–547, 1994.

54. Guyer B, Smith DR, Chalk R. Calling the shots: immunization finance policies and practices. Executive summary of the report of the Institute of Medicine. Am J Prev Med 19(3 suppl):4–12, 2000.

55. Institute of Medicine. Calling the Shots: Immunization Finance Policies and Practices. Washington, DC, National Academy Press, 2000.

56. Centers for Disease Control. Vaccine Adverse Event Reporting System—United States. MMWR 39:730–733, 1990.

57. Ellenberg SS, Chen RT. The complicated task of monitoring vaccine safety. Public Health Rep 112:10–20, 1997.

58. Santoli JM, Rodewald LE, Maes EF, et al. Vaccines for Children program, United States, 1997. Pediatrics 104(2):E15, 1999.

59. Centers for Disease Control and Prevention. Vaccines for Children program, 1994. MMWR 43:705, 1994.

60. National Center for Health Statistics. Healthy People 2000 Review, 1997. Hyattsville, MD, U.S. Public Health Service, 1997, p 189.

61. Ruch-Ross HS, O'Connor KG. Immunization referral practices of pediatricians in the United States. Pediatrics 94:508–512, 1994.

62. Lieu T, Smith M, Newacheck P. Health insurance and preventive care sources of children at public immunization clinics. Pediatrics 93:373–378, 1994.

63. Zimmerman RK, Medsger AR, Ricci EM, et al. Impact of free vaccine and insurance status on physician referral of children to public vaccine clinics. JAMA 278:996–1000, 1997.

64. Scholle SH, Kelleher KJ, Childs G, et al. Changes in Medicaid managed care enrollment among children. Health Aff (Millwood) 16:164–170, 1997.

65. Rodewald L, Szilagyi P, Holl J, et al. Health insurance for low-income working families. Arch Pediatr Adolesc Med 151:798–803, 1997.

66. Orenstein WA, Bernier RH. Surveillance—information for action. Pediatr Clin North Am 37:709–734, 1990.

67. Wharton M, Strebel PM. Vaccine preventable diseases. *In* Wilcox LS, Marks JS (eds). From Data to Action: CDC's Public Health Surveillance for Women, Infants, and Children. Atlanta, GA, Centers for Disease Control and Prevention, 1994, pp 281–290.

68. Chorba TL, Berkelman RL, Safford SK, et al. Mandatory reporting of infectious diseases by clinicians. JAMA 262:3018–3026, 1989.

69. Centers for Disease Control and Prevention. Case definitions for infectious conditions under public health surveillance. MMWR 46(RR-10):1–55, 1997.

70. Schuchat A, Robinson K, Wenger JD, et al. for the Active Surveillance Team. Bacterial meningitis in the United States in 1995. N Engl J Med 337:970–976, 1997.

71. Alter MJ, Mares A, Hadler SC, et al. The effect of under reporting on the apparent incidence and epidemiology of acute viral hepatitis. Am J Epidemiol 125:133–139, 1987.

72. Peterson CL, Maupin T, Goldman G, Mascola L. Varicella active surveillance: use of capture-recapture methods to assess completeness of surveillance data [abstract H-111]. *In* Abstracts of the 37th Interscience Conference on Antimicrobial Agents and Chemotherapy, Toronto, September 28–October 1, 1997.

73. Goodnow KL, Watson B, Lutz J, et al. Epidemiology of varicella in an inner-city population [abstract 280]. *In* Proceedings of the 31st National Immunization Conference, Detroit, May 19–22, 1997. Atlanta, Centers for Disease Control and Prevention, 1997.

74. Seward JF, Watson BM, Peterson CL, et al. Varicella disease after introduction of varicella vaccine in the United States, 1995–2000. JAMA 287:606–611, 2002.

75. Davis SF, Strebel PM, Atkinson WL, et al. Reporting efficiency during a measles outbreak in New York City, 1991. Am J Public Health 83:1011–1015, 1993.

76. Prevots DR, Sutter RW, Strebel PM, et al. Completeness of reporting for paralytic poliomyelitis, United States, 1980 through 1991. Arch Pediatr Adolesc Med 148:479–485, 1994.

77. Cochi SL, Edmonds LE, Dyer K, et al. Congenital rubella syndrome in the United States 1970–1985: on the verge of elimination. Am J Epidemiol 129:349–361, 1989.

78. Sutter RW, Cochi SL. Pertussis hospitalizations and mortality in the United States, 1985–1988: evaluation of the completeness of national reporting. JAMA. 267:386–391, 1992.

79. Standaert SM, Lefkowitz LB, Horan JM, et al. The reporting of communicable diseases: a controlled study of *Neisseria meningitidis* and *Haemophilus influenzae* infections. Clin Infect Dis 20:30–36, 1995.

80. Orenstein WA, Bernier RH, Hinman AR. Assessing vaccine efficacy in the field: further observations. Epidemiol Rev 10:212–241, 1988.

81. Simpson DM, Ezzati-Rice TM, Zell ER. Forty years and four surveys: how does our measuring measure up? Am J Prev Med 20(4 suppl): 6–14, 2001.

82. Zell ER, Ezzati-Rice TM, Battaglia MP, Wright RA. National Immunization Survey: the methodology of a vaccination surveillance system. Public Health Rep 115:65–77, 2000.

83. Smith PJ, Battaglia MA, Huggine MS, et al. Overview of the sampling design and statistical methods used in the National Immunization Survey. Am J Prev Med 20(4S):17–24, 2001.

84. Centers for Disease Control and Prevention. Vaccination coverage by race/ethnicity and poverty level among children aged 19–35 months—United States, 1996. MMWR 46:963–969, 1997.

85. Klevens M, Luman E. U.S. children living in and near poverty: risk of vaccine-preventable diseases. Am J Prev Med 20(4 suppl):41–46, 2001.

86. Daniels D, Jiles R, Klevens M, Herrera G. Undervaccinated African-American preschoolers: a case of missed opportunities. Am J Prev Med 20(4 suppl): 61–68, 2001.

87. Herrera G, Zhao Z, Klevens M. Variation in vaccination coverage among children of Hispanic ancestry. Am J Prev Med 20(4 suppl):69–74, 2001.

88. Morrow AL, Rosenthal J, Lakkis HD, et al. A population-based study of access to immunization among urban Virginia children served by public, private, and military health care systems. Pediatrics 101:E5, 1998.

89. Ewert DP, Thomas JC, Chun LY, et al. Measles vaccination coverage among Latino children aged 12 to 59 months in Los Angeles County: a household survey. Am J Public Health 81:1057–1059, 1991.

90. Ewert DP, Westman S, Ward B, et al. An increase in *Haemophilus influenzae* type B vaccination among preschool-aged children in inner-city Los Angeles, 1990 through 1992. Am J Public Health 84:1154–1157, 1994.

91. Lemeshow S, Stroh G Jr. Sampling Techniques for Evaluating Health Parameters in Developing Countries. Washington, DC, National Academy Press, 1988, pp 8–13.

92. Henderson RH, Sundaresan T. Cluster sampling to assess immunization coverage: a review of experience with a simplified sampling method. Bull World Health Organ 60:253–260, 1982.

93. Serfling R, Sherman I. Attribute Sampling Methods for Local Health Departments. Washington, DC, U.S. Public Health Service, 1965.

94. Zell ER, Dietz V, Stevenson J, et al. Low vaccination levels of U.S. preschool and school-age children: retrospective assessments of vaccination coverage, 1991–1992. JAMA 271:833–839, 1994.

95. Suarez L, Simpson D, Smith D. Errors and correlation in parental recall of child immunizations: effects on vaccination coverage estimates. Pediatrics 99:E3, 1997.

96. Goldstein KP, Kviz FJ, Daum RS. Accuracy of immunization histories provided by adults accompanying preschool children to a pediatric emergency department. JAMA 270:2190–2194, 1993.

97. Fierman A, Rosen C, Legano L, et al. Immunization and adolescent status as determined by patients' hand-held cards vs. medical records. Arch Pediatr Med 150:863–866, 1997.

98. Humiston SG, Rodewald LE, Szilagyi PG, et al. Decision rules for predicting vaccination status of preschool-age emergency department patients. J Pediatr 123:887–892, 1993.

99. Centers for Disease Control and Prevention. State and national vaccination coverage levels among children aged 19–35 months—United States, April–December 1994. MMWR 44:613, 619–623, 1995.

100. Darden PM, Taylor JA, Slora EJ, et al. Methodological issues in determining rates of childhood immunization in office practice. Arch Pediatr Adolesc Med 150:1027–1031, 1996.

101. National Committee for Quality Assurance. Effectiveness of care. *In* HEDIS 3.0—The Health Plan Employer Data and Information Set. Vol. 2. Washington, DC, National Committee for Quality Assurance, 2003, pp 61–71.

102. National Committee for Quality Assurance. Flu shots for older adults. *In* HEDIS 3.0—The Health Plan Employer Data and Information Set. Vol. 2. National Committee for Quality Assurance, 1997, pp 28–29.

103. National Committee for Quality Assurance. Adolescent well-care visits. *In* HEDIS 3.0—The Health Plan Employer Data and Information Set. Vol. 2. National Committee for Quality Assurance, 1997, pp 137–139.

104. Bolton P, Hussain A, Hadpawat A, et al. Deficiencies in current childhood immunization indicators. Public Health Rep 113: 527–532, 1998.

105. Fairbrother G, Freed GL, Thompson JW. Measuring immunization coverage. Am J Prev Med 19(3 suppl):78–88, 2000.

106. Rodewald L, Maes E, Stevenson J, et al. Immunization performance measurement in a changing immunization environment. Pediatrics 103(4 pt 2):889–897, 1999.

107. Dombkowski KJ, Lantz PM, Freed GL. The need for surveillance of delay in age-appropriate immunization. Am J Prev Med 23:36–42, 2002.

108. Bolton P, Holt E, Ross A, et al. Estimating vaccination coverage using parental recall, vaccination cards, and medical records. Public Health Rep 113:521–526, 1998.

109. Stokley S, Rodewald LE, Maes EF. The impact of record scattering on the measurement of immunization coverage. Pediatrics 107:91–96, 2001.

110. Yusuf H, Adams M, Rodewald L, et al. Fragmentation of immunization history among providers and parents of children in selected underserved areas. Am J Prev Med 23:106–112, 2002.

111. Percentage of persons aged ≥18 years who reported receiving influenza or pneumococcal vaccine or tetanus toxoid, by age and selected characteristics—National Health Interview Survey, United States, 1999. Hyattsville, MD, National Center for Health Statistics, 1999. Available at *www.cdc.gov/nip/coverage/NHIS/tables/general-99.pdf*

112. Centers for Disease Control and Prevention. Influenza and pneumococcal vaccination levels among adults aged ≥65 years—United States, 2001. MMWR 50:1019–1024, 2002.

113. Gellin BG, Maibach EW, Marcuse EK. Do parents understand immunizations? A national telephone survey. Pediatrics 106:1097–1102, 2000.

114. Tarande M, Dietz V, Lewin M, Zell E. Health care characteristics and their association with the vaccination status of children. Arch Pediatr Adolesc Med 150(4 suppl):A161, 1996.

115. Cutts FT, Orenstein WA, Bernier RH. Causes of low preschool immunization coverage in the United States. Annu Rev Public Health 13:385–398, 1992.

116. Orenstein WA, Atkinson W, Mason D, Bernier RH. Barriers to vaccinating preschool children. J Health Care Poor Underserved 1:315–330, 1990.

117. Williams IT, Milton JD, Farrell JB, Graham NM. Interaction of socioeconomic status and provider practices as predictors of immunization coverage in Virginia children. Pediatrics 96(3 pt 1): 439–446, 1995.

118. Miller LA, Hoffman RE, Barón AE, et al. Risk factors for delayed immunization against measles, mumps, and rubella in Colorado two-year olds. Pediatrics 94:713–719, 1994.

119. Hueston WJ, Mainous AG, Palmer C. Delays in childhood immunizations in public and private settings. Arch Pediatr Adolesc Med 148:470–473, 1994.

120. Fielding JE, Cumberland WG, Pettitt L. Immunization status of children of employees in a large corporation. JAMA 271:525–530, 1994.

121. Bobo JK, Gale JL, Thapa PB, Wassilak SG. Risk factors for delayed immunization in a random sample of 1163 children from Oregon and Washington. Pediatrics 91:308–314, 1993.

122. Bates AS, Fitzgerald JF, Dittus RS, Wolinsky FD. Risk factors for underimmunization in poor urban infants. JAMA 272:1105–1110, 1994.

123. Wood D, Donald-Sherbourne C, Halfon N, et al. Factors related to immunization status among inner-city Latino and African-American preschoolers. Pediatrics 96(2 pt 1):295–301, 1995.

124. Salmon DA, Haber M, Gangarosa EJ, et al. Health consequences of religious and philosophical exemptions from immunization laws: individual and societal risk of measles. JAMA 282:47–53, 1999.

125. Feikin DR, Lezotte DC, Hamman RF, et al. Individual and community risks of measles and pertussis associated with personal exemptions to immunization. JAMA 284:3145–3150, 2000.

126. Etkind P, Lett SM, Macdonald PD, et al. Pertussis outbreaks in groups claiming religious exemptions to vaccinations. Am J Dis Child 146:123–126, 1992.

127. Jackson BM, Payton T, Horst G, et al. An epidemiologic investigation of a rubella outbreak among the Amish of Northeastern Ohio. Public Health Rep 108:436–439, 1993.

128. Novotny T, Jennings CE, Doran M, et al. Measles outbreaks in religious groups exempt from immunization laws. Public Health Rep 103:49–54, 1988.

129. Centers for Disease Control and Prevention. Poliomyelitis—United States, Canada. MMWR 46:1194–1199, 1997.

130. National Vaccine Advisory Committee. Report of the NVAC Working Group on Philosophical Exemptions, National Vaccine Program Office. Atlanta, Centers for Disease Control and Prevention, 1998.

131. Guyer B, Hughart N, Holt E, et al. Immunization coverage and its relationship to preventive health care visits among inner-city children in Baltimore. Pediatrics 94:53–58, 1994.

132. Guyer B, Hughart N. Increasing childhood immunization coverage by improving the effectiveness of primary health care systems for children. Arch Pediatr Adolesc Med 148:901–902, 1994.

133. Dietz VJ, Stevenson J, Zell ER, et al. Potential impact on vaccination coverage levels by administering vaccines simultaneously and reducing dropout rates. Arch Pediatr Adolesc Med 148:943–949, 1994.

134. Cutts FT, Zell ER, Mason JD, et al. Monitoring progress toward U.S. preschool immunization goals. JAMA 267:1952–1955, 1992.

135. Ross A, Kennedy AB, Holt E, et al. Initiating the first DTP vaccination age-appropriately: a model for understanding vaccination coverage. Pediatrics 101:970–974, 1998.

136. Strobino D, Keane V, Holt E, et al. Parental attitudes do not explain underimmunization. Pediatrics 98(6 pt 1):1076–1083, 1996.

137. Houtrouw SM, Carlson KL. The relationship between maternal characteristics, maternal vulnerability beliefs, and immunization compliance. Issues Compr Pediatr Nurs 16:41–50, 1993.

138. Taylor JA, Cufley D. The association between parental health beliefs and immunization status among children followed by private pediatricians. Clin Pediatr 35:18–22, 1996.

139. Lannon C, Brack V, Stuart J, et al. What mothers say about why poor children fall behind on immunizations: a summary of focus groups in North Carolina. Arch Pediatr Adolesc Med 149:1070–1075, 1995.

140. Salsberry PJ, Nickel JT, Mitch R. Why aren't preschoolers immunized? A comparison of parents' and providers' perceptions of the barriers to immunizations. J Community Health Nurs 10:213–224, 1993.

141. Hanson IC, Jenkins K, Spears W, Stoner D. Immunization prevalence rates for infants in a large urban center: Houston/Harris County, 1993. Tex Med 92:66–71, 1996.

142. Majeroni B, Cowan T, Osborne J, Graham R. Missed appointments and Medicaid managed care. Arch Fam Med 5:507–511, 1996.

143. Gamertsfelder DA, Zimmerman RK, DeSensi EG. Immunization barriers in a family practice residency clinic. J Am Board Fam Pract 7:100–104, 1994.

144. Abbotts B, Osborn LM. Immunization status and reasons for immunization delay among children using public health immunization clinics. Am J Dis Child 147:965–968, 1993.

145. Mustin HD, Hold VL, Connell FA. Adequacy of well-child care and immunizations in U.S. infants born in 1988. JAMA 272:1111–1115, 1994.

146. Hutchins SS, Jansen HAFM, Robertson SE, et al. Studies of missed opportunities for immunization in developing and industrialized countries. Bull World Health Organ 71:549–560, 1993.

147. Grabowsky M, Orenstein WA, Marcuse EK. The critical role of provider practices in undervaccination. Pediatrics 97:735–737, 1996.

148. Centers for Disease Control and Prevention. Impact of missed opportunities to vaccinate preschool-aged children on vaccination coverage levels—selected U.S. sites, 1991–1992. MMWR 43:709–711, 717–718, 1994.

149. Christy C, McConnochie KM, Zernik N, Brzoza S. Impact of an algorithm-guided nurse intervention on the use of immunization opportunities. Arch Pediatr Adolesc Med 151:384–391, 1997.

150. Farizo KM, Stehr-Green PA, Markowitz LE, Patriarca PA. Vaccination levels and missed opportunities for measles vaccination: a record audit in a public pediatric clinic. Pediatrics 89:589–592, 1992.

151. Gindler JS, Cutts FT, Barnett-Antinori ME, et al. Successes and failures in vaccine delivery: evaluation of the immunization delivery system in Puerto Rico. Pediatrics 91:315–320, 1993.

152. LeBaron C, Chaney M, Baughman A, et al. Impact of measurement and feedback on vaccination coverage in public clinics, 1988–1994. JAMA 277:631–635, 1997.

153. Lieu TA, Black SB, Sorel ME, et al. Would better adherence to guidelines improve childhood immunization rates? Pediatrics 98:1062–1068, 1996.

154. Szilagyi PG, Rodewald LE, Humiston SG, et al. Reducing missed opportunities for immunizations: easier said than done. Arch Pediatr Adolesc Med 150:1193–1200, 1996.

155. Zimmerman RK, Schlesselman JJ, Baird AL, Mieczkowski TA. A national survey to understand why physicians defer childhood immunizations. Arch Pediatr Adolesc Med 151:657–664, 1997.

156. Zimmerman RK, Giebink GS, Street HB, Janosky JE. Knowledge and attitudes of Minnesota primary care physicians about barriers to measles and pertussis immunization. J Am Board Fam Pract 8:270–277, 1995.

157. Wood D, Pereyra M, Halfon N, et al. Vaccination levels in Los Angeles Public Health Centers: the contribution of missed opportunities to vaccinate and other factors. Am J Public Health 85:850–852, 1995.

158. Fairbrother G, Friedman S, DuMont KA, Lobach KS. Markers for primary care: missed opportunities to immunize and screen for lead and tuberculosis by private physicians serving large numbers of inner-city Medicaid-eligible children. Pediatrics 97:785–790, 1996.

159. McConnochie KM, Roghmann KJ. Immunization opportunities missed among urban poor children. Pediatrics 89:1019–1026, 1992.

160. Szilagyi PG, Rodewald LE. Missed opportunities for immunizations: a review of the evidence. J Public Health Manage Pract 2:18–25, 1996.

161. Bell LM, Pritchard M, Anderko R, Levenson R. A program to immunize hospitalized preschool-aged children: evaluation and impact. Pediatrics 100:192–196, 1997.

162. Holt E, Guyer B, Hughart N, et al. The contribution of missed opportunities to childhood underimmunization in Baltimore. Pediatrics 97:474–480, 1997.

163. Szilagyi PG, Rodewald LE, Humiston SG, et al. Missed opportunities for childhood vaccinations in office practices and the effect on vaccination status. Pediatrics 91:1–7, 1993.

164. Woodin KA, Rodewald LE, Humiston SG, et al. Physician and parent opinions: are children becoming pincushions from immunizations? Arch Pediatr Adolesc Med 149:845–849, 1995.

165. Melman ST, Chawla T, Kaplan JM, Anbar RD. Multiple immunizations: ouch! Arch Fam Med 3:615–618, 1994.

166. Askew GL, Finelli L, Lutz J, et al. Beliefs and practices regarding childhood vaccination among urban pediatric providers in New Jersey. Pediatrics 96:889–892, 1995.

167. Kolasa MS, Petersen TJ, Brink EW, et al. Impact of multiple injections on immunization rates among vulnerable children. Am J Prev Med 21:261–266, 2001.

168. Lieu TA, Davis RL, Capra AM, et al. Variation in clinician recommendations for multiple injections during adoption of inactivated polio vaccine. Pediatrics 107:E49, 2001.

169. Davis RL, Lieu TA, Mell LK, et al. Impact of the change in polio vaccination schedule on immunization coverage rates: a study in two large health maintenance organizations. Pediatrics 107:671–676, 2001.

169a.Centers for Disease Control and Prevention. FDA licensure of diphtheria and tetanus toxoids and acellular pertussis vaccine adsorbed, hepatitis B (recombinant) and poliovirus vaccine combined (Pediarix) for use in infants. MMWR 52:203–204, 2003.

170. Harper PG, Madlon-Kay DJ, Luxenberg MG, Tempest R. A clinic system to improve preschool vaccination in a low socioeconomic status population. Arch Pediatr Adolesc Med 151:1220–1223, 1997.

171. Szilagyi PG, Roghmann KJ, Campbell JR, et al. Immunization practices of primary care practitioners and their relation to immunization levels. Arch Pediatr Adolesc Med 148:158–166, 1994.

172. Siegel RM, Schubert CJ. Physician beliefs and knowledge about vaccinations: are Cincinnati doctors giving their best shot? Clin Pediatr 35:79–83, 1996.

173. Hughart N, Vivier P, Ross A, et al. Are immunizations an incentive for well-child visits? Arch Pediatr Adolesc Med 151:690–695, 1997.

174. Joffe MD, Luberti A. Effect of emergency department immunization on compliance with primary care. Pediatr Emerg Care 10:317–319, 1994.

175. Lieu TA, Glauber JH, Fuentes-Afflick EF, Lo B. Effects of vaccine information pamphlets on parents' attitudes. Arch Pediatr Adolesc Med 148:921–929, 1994.

176. Freeman VA, Freed GL. Parental knowledge, attitudes, and demand regarding a vaccine to prevent varicella. Am J Prev Med 17:153–155, 1999.

177. Szilagyi PG, Rodewald LE, Humiston SG, et al. Immunization practices of pediatricians and family physicians in the United States. Pediatrics 84:517–523, 1994.

178. Darden PM, Taylor JA, Brooks DA, et al. Polio immunization practices of pediatricians. Presented at the Pediatric Academic Societies meeting, San Francisco, May 1, 1999.

179. Bordley WC, Freed GL, Garrett JM, et al. Factors responsible for immunizations referrals to health departments in North Carolina. Pediatrics 94:376–380, 1994.

180. Schulte JM, Bown GR, Zetzman MR, et al. Changing immunization referral patterns among pediatricians and family practice physicians, Dallas County, Texas, 1988. Pediatrics 87:204–207, 1991.

181. Wright JA, Marcuse EK. Immunization practices of Washington State pediatricians—1989. Am J Dis Child 146:1033–1036, 1992.

182. Szilagyi PG, Humiston SG, Shone LP, et al. Impact of vaccine financing on vaccinations delivered by health department clinics. Am J Public Health 90:739–745, 2000.

183. Szilagyi PG, Humiston SG, Pollard Shone L, et al. Decline in physician referrals to health department clinics for immunizations: the role of vaccine financing. Am J Prev Med 18:318–324, 2000.

184. Freed GL, Clark SJ, Pathman DE, et al. Impact of North Carolina's universal vaccine purchase program by children's insurance status. Arch Pediatr Adolesc Med 153:748–754, 1999.

185. Clark SJ, Freed GL. Use of public immunization services after initiation of a universal vaccine purchase program. Arch Pediatr Adolesc Med 152:642–645, 1998.

186. Taylor J, Darden P, Slora E, et al. The influence of provider behavior, parental characteristics, and a public policy initiative on the immunization status of children followed by private pediatricians: a study from pediatric research in office settings. Pediatrics 99:209–215, 1997.

187. Freed GL, Clark SJ, Pathman DE, et al. Impact of a new universal purchase vaccine program in North Carolina. Arch Pediatr Adolesc Med 151:1117–1124, 1997.

188. Zimmerman R, Janosky J. Immunization barriers in Minnesota private practices: the influence of economics and training on vaccine timing. Fam Pract Res J 13:213–224, 1993.

189. Saldarini RJ. Putting prevention research at risk: implementation of the Vaccines for Children programme. Vaccine 12:1364–1367, 1994.

190. Fleming G. Vaccine administration fee survey. Child Health Care 11:6, 1995.

191. Lurie N, Manning WG, Peterson C, et al. Preventive care: Do we practice what we preach? Am J Public Health 77:801–804, 1987.

192. Fairbrother G, Friedman S, Hanson KL, Butts GC. Effect of the Vaccines for Children Program on inner-city neighborhood physicians. Arch Pediatr Adolesc Med 151:1229–1235, 1997.

193. Centers for Disease Control and Prevention. Prevention and control of influenza: recommendations of the Advisory Committee on Immunization Practices (ACIP). MMWR 46(RR-9):1–25, 1997.

194. Centers for Disease Control and Prevention. Prevention of pneumococcal disease: recommendations of the Advisory Committee on Immunization Practices (ACIP). MMWR 46(RR-8):1–24, 1997.

195. Centers for Disease Control. Hepatitis B virus: a comprehensive strategy for eliminating transmission in the United States through universal childhood vaccination. Recommendations of the Immunization Practices Advisory Committee (ACIP). MMWR 40(RR-13):1–25, 1991.

196. Centers for Disease Control and Prevention. Measles, mumps, and rubella—vaccine use and strategies for measles, rubella, and congen-ital rubella syndrome elimination and mumps control: recommendations of the Advisory Committee on Immunization Practices (ACIP). MMWR 47(RR-8):1–57, 1998.

197. Fiebach N, Beckett W. Prevention of respiratory infections in adults: influenza and pneumococcal vaccines. Arch Intern Med 154:2545–2557, 1994.

198. Richardson JP, Michocki RJ. Removing barriers to vaccination use by older adults. Drugs Aging 4:357–365, 1994.

199. Centers for Disease Control. Adult immunization: knowledge, attitudes, and practices—DeKalb and Fulton Counties, Georgia, 1988. MMWR 34:657–661, 1988.

200. Fiebach NH, Viscoli DM. Patient acceptance of influenza vaccination. Am J Med 91:393–400, 1991.

201. Nichol KL, Lofgren RP, Gapinski J. Influenza vaccination: knowledge, attitudes, and behavior among high-risk outpatients. Arch Intern Med 152:106–110, 1992.

202. Williams WW, Hickson MA, Kane MA, et al. Immunization policies and vaccine coverage among adults: the risk for missed opportunities. Ann Intern Med 108:616–625, 1988.

203. Fedson DS, Chiarello LA. Previous hospital care and pneumococcal bacteremia: importance for pneumococcal immunization. Arch Intern Med 143:885–889, 1983.

204. Centers for Disease Control and Prevention. Missed opportunities for pneumococcal and influenza vaccination of Medicare pneumonia inpatients—12 western states, 1995. MMWR 46:919–923, 1997.

205. Buffington J, Bell K, LaForce F. A target-based model for increasing influenza immunizations in private practice. J Gen Intern Med 6:204–209, 1991.

206. Kouides R, Lewis B, Bennett N, et al. A performance-based incentive program for influenza immunization in the elderly. Am J Prev Med 9:250–255, 1993.

207. Fedson DS, Kessler HA. A hospital-based influenza immunization program, 1977–1978. Am J Public Health 73:442–445, 1983.

208. Centers for Disease Control and Prevention. Recommendations of the Advisory Committee on Immunization Practices: use of standing orders programs to increase adult vaccination coverage rates. MMWR 49(RR-1):15–26, 2000.

209. Ratner ER, Fedson DS. Influenza and pneumococcal immunization in medical clinics 1978–1980. Arch Intern Med 143:2066–2069, 1983.

210. Fedson DS. Influenza and pneumococcal immunization in medical clinics, 1971–1983. J Infect Dis 149:817–818, 1984.

211. Setia U, Serrenti I, Lorenz P. Factors affecting the use of influenza vaccine in the institutionalized elderly. J Am Geriatr Soc 33:856–858, 1985.

212. Gyorkos TW, Tannenbaum TN, Abrahamowicz M, et al. Evaluation of the effectiveness of immunization delivery methods. Can J Public Health 85(suppl):S15–S30, 1994.

213. Sneller V, Izurieta H, Bridges C, et al. Prevention and control of vaccine-preventable diseases in long-term care facilities. J Am Medical Directors Assoc 1(suppl):S2–S37, 2000.

214. Centers for Disease Control. The public health burden of vaccine preventable diseases among adults: standards for adult immunization practice. MMWR 39:725–729, 1990.

215. National Vaccine Advisory Committee. Standards for Adult Immunization Practices. Am J Prev Med, in press.

216. McCormick MC, Shapiro S, Starfield BH. The association of patient-held records and completion of immunizations. Clin Pediatr (Phila) 20:270–274, 1981.

217. Brink EW, Hinman AR. The Vaccine Injury Compensation Act: the new law and you. Contemp Pediatr 6:28–32, 35–36, 39, 42, 1989.

218. Department of Health and Human Services. New vaccine information materials. Fed Reg 59:31888–31889, 1994.

219. Task Force on Community Preventive Services. Recommendations regarding interventions to improve vaccination coverage in children, adolescents, and adults. Am J Prev Med 18(1 suppl):18–26, 2000.

220. Briss PA, Rodewald LE, Hinman AR, et al, for the Task Force on Community Preventive Services. Reviews of evidence: interventions to improve vaccination coverage in children, adolescents, and adults. Am J Prev Med 18(1 suppl):97–140, 2000.

221. Shefer A, Briss P, Rodewald L, et al. Interventions to improve immunization coverage levels: an evidence-based review of the literature. Epidemiol Rev 21:96–142, 1999.

222. Szilagyi PG, Bordley WC, Vann JC, et al. Patient reminder/recall interventions improve immunization rates: a critical review of the literature. JAMA 284:1820–1827, 2000.

223. Bushnell CJ. The ABC's of practice-based immunization assessments. *In* Proceedings of the 28th National Immunization Conference. Atlanta, Centers for Disease Control and Prevention, 1994, pp 207–209.

224. Bordley WC, Margolis PA, Lannon CM. The delivery of immunizations and other preventive services in private practices. Pediatrics 97:467–473, 1996.

225. Dini EF, Chaney M, Moolenaar RL, LeBaron CW. Information as intervention: how Georgia used vaccination coverage data to double public sector vaccination coverage in seven years. J Public Health Manage Pract 2:45–49, 1996.

226. Link D. Chart audits to promote community-wide childhood immunization. In Proceedings of the 31st National Immunization Conference, Detroit, May 19–22, 1997. Atlanta, Centers for Disease Control and Prevention, 1997.

227. LeBaron CW, Mercer JT, Massoudi MS, et al. Changes in clinic vaccination coverage after institution of measurement and feedback in 4 states and 2 cities. Arch Pediatr Adolesc Med 153:879–886, 1999.

228. LeBaron CW, Massoudi M, Stevenson J, et al. The status of immunization measurement and feedback in the United States. Arch Pediatr Adolesc Med 154:832–836, 2000.

229. Alemi F, Alemagno SA, Goldhagen J, et al. Computer reminders improve on-time immunization rates. Med Care 34(10 suppl):OS45–OS51, 1996.

230. Alto WA, Fury D, Condo A, et al. Improving the immunization coverage of children less than 7 years old in a family practice residency. J Am Board Fam Pract 7:472–477, 1994.

231. Dini EF, Linkins RW, Chaney M. Effectiveness of computer-generated telephone messages in increasing clinic visits. Arch Pediatr Adolesc Med 149:902–905, 1995.

232. Lieu TA, Black SB, Lewis EM, et al. Computer-generated recall letters for underimmunized children: how cost-effective? Pediatr Infect Dis J 16:28–33, 1997.

233. Linkins RW, Dini EF, Watson JG, Patriarca PA. A randomized trial of the effectiveness of computer-generated telephone messages in increasing immunization visits among preschool children. Arch Pediatr Adolesc Med 148:908–914, 1994.

234. Szilagyi PG, Schaffer S, Shone L, et al. Reducing geographic, racial, and ethnic disparities in childhood immunization rates by using reminder/recall interventions in urban primary care practices. Pediatrics 110:E58, 2002.

235. Young SA, Haplin TJ, Johnson DA, et al. Effectiveness of a mailed reminder on the immunization levels of infants at high risk of failure to complete immunizations. Am J Public Health 70:422–424, 1980.

236. Tollestrup K, Hubbard BB. Evaluation of a follow-up system in a county health department's immunization clinic. Am J Prev Med 7:24–28, 1991.

237. Owen AL, Owen GM. Twenty years of WIC: a review of some effects of the program. J Am Diet Assoc 97:777–782, 1997.

238. Shefer A, Luman E, Lyons B, et al. Vaccination status of children in the Women, Infants, and Children (WIC) program: are we doing enough to improve coverage? Am J Prev Med 20(4 suppl):47–54, 2001.

239. Devaney BL, Ellwood MR, Love JM. Programs that mitigate the effects of poverty on children. Future Child 7:88–112, 1997.

240. Egan MC. Federal nutrition support programs for children. Pediatr Clin North Am 24:229–239, 1977.

241. LeBaron C, Birkhead G, Parsons P, et al. Measles vaccination levels of children enrolled in WIC during the 1991 measles epidemic in New York City. Am J Public Health 86:1551–1556, 1996.

242. Birkhead GS, Cicirello HG, Talarico J. The impact of WIC and AFDC in screening and delivering childhood immunizations. J Public Health Manage Pract 2:26–33, 1996.

243. Hutchins SS, Gindler JS, Atkinson WL, et al. Preschool children at high risk for measles: opportunities to vaccinate. Am J Public Health 83:862–867, 1993.

244. Birkhead GS, LeBaron CW, Parson P, et al. The immunization of children enrolled in the Special Supplemental Food Program for Women, Infants, and Children (WIC): the impact of different strategies. JAMA 274:312–316, 1995. [erratum appears in JAMA 274:1762, 1995]

245. Hoekstra EJ, LeBaron CW, Megaloeconomou Y, et al. The impact of a large-scale immunization intervention in the Special Supplemental Nutrition Program for Women, Infants, and Children (WIC). JAMA 280:1143–1147, 1998.

246. Shefer A, Mezoff J, Caspari D, et al. What mothers in the WIC program feel about WIC-immunization linkage activities: a summary of focus groups in Wisconsin. Arch Pediatr Adolesc Med 152:65–70, 1998.

247. Hutchins SS, Rosenthal J. Results from WIC demonstration projects. *In* Proceedings of the 28th National Immunization Conference. Atlanta, Centers for Disease Control and Prevention, , 1994, pp 1–4.

248. Shefer A, Fritchley J, Stevenson J, et al. Linking WIC and immunization services to improve preventive health care among low-income children in WIC. J Public Health Manag Pract 8:56–65, 2002.

249. Kerpelman LC, Connell DB, Gunn WJ. Effect of a monetary sanction on immunization rates of recipients of Aid to Families with Dependent Children. JAMA 284:53–59, 2000.

250. Minkovitz C, Holt E, Hughart N, et al. The effect of parental monetary sanctions on the vaccination status of young children: an evaluation of welfare reform in Maryland. Arch Pediatr Adolesc Med 153:1242–1247, 1999.

251. Pierce C, Goldstein M, Suozzi K, et al. The impact of the standards for pediatric immunization practices on vaccination coverage levels. JAMA 276:626–630, 1996.

252. Garnener P, Pickering LK, Orenstein W, et al. Guidelines for quality standards for immunization. Clin Infect Dis 35:503–511, 2002.

253. de Quadros CA, Olive JM, Hersh BS, et al. Measles elimination in the Americas: evolving strategies. JAMA 275:224–229, 1996.

254. de Quadros CA, Andrus JK, Olive JM, et al. Eradication of poliomyelitis: progress in the Americas. Pediatr Infect Dis J 10:222–229, 1991.

255. Dietz V, Cutts F. The use of mass campaigns in the Expanded Program on Immunization: a review of reported advantages and disadvantages. Int J Health Serv 27:767–790, 1997.

256. Sabin AB. Measles, killer of millions in developing countries: strategy for rapid elimination and continuing control. Eur J Epidemiol 7:1–22, 1991.

257. Schonberger LB, Kaplan J, Kim-Farley R, et al. Control of paralytic polio in the United States. Rev Infect Dis 6(suppl):S424–S426, 1984.

258. Modlin JF, Brandlin-Bennett AD, Witte JJ, et al. A review of five years' experience with rubella vaccine in the United States. Pediatrics 55:20–29, 1975.

259. Fairbrother G, DuMont KA. New York City's 1993 child immunization day: planning, costs, and results. Am J Public Health 85:1662–1665, 1995.

260. Centers for Disease Control and Prevention. Assessment of under-vaccinated children following a mass vaccination campaign—Kansas, 1993. MMWR 43:572–573, 1994.

261. Jackson CL. State laws on compulsory immunization in the United States. Public Health Rep 84:787–795, 1969.

262. Orenstein WA, Hinman AR, Williams WW. The impact of legislation on immunisation in the United States. *In* Hall R, Richters J (eds). Immunisation: The Old and the New. Proceedings of the 2nd National Immunisation Conference, Canberra, May 27–29, 1991. Canberra, Public Health Association of Australia, 1992, pp 58–62.

263. Orenstein WA, Halsey NA, Hayden GF, et al. From the Centers for Disease Control: current status of measles in the United States, 1973–1977. J Infect Dis 137:847–853, 1978.

264. Centers for Disease Control. Measles—United States. MMWR 26:109–111, 1977.

265. Centers for Disease Control. Measles and school immunization requirements—United States 1978. MMWR 27:303–304, 1978.

266. Robbins KB, Brandling-Bennett AD, Hinman AR. Low measles incidence: association with enforcement of school immunization laws. Am J Public Health 71:270–274, 1981.

267. Cochi SL, Preblud SR, Orenstein WA. Perspectives on the relative resurgence of mumps in the United States. Am J Dis Child 142:499–507, 1988.

268. Orenstein WA, Hinman AR. The immunization system in the United States—the role of school immunization laws. Vaccine 17(suppl 3):S19–S24, 1999.

269. Centers for Disease Control and Prevention. 2001–2002 State Immunization Requirements. Atlanta, Centers for Disease Control and Prevention, 2002.

270. Rota JS, Salmon DA, Rodewald LE, et al. Processes for obtaining nonmedical exemptions to state immunization laws. Am J Public Health 91:645–648, 2001.

271. Freed GL, Freeman VA, Mauskopf A. Enforcement of age-appropriate immunization laws. Am J Prev Med 14:118–121, 1998.

272. Feudtner C, Marcuse EK. Ethics and immunization policy: promoting dialogue to sustain consensus. Pediatrics 107:1158–1164, 2001.

273. Centers for Disease Control and Prevention. Vaccination coverage among children enrolled in Head Start programs and day care facilities or entering school. MMWR 50(SS39):847–855, 2001.

274. Baughman AL, Williams WW, Atkinson WL, et al. The impact of college prematriculation immunization requirements on risk for measles outbreaks. JAMA 272:1127–1132, 1994. [erratum appears JAMA 272:1822, 1994]

275. Rivera A, Orengo J, Rivera A. Impact of vaccine shortage on diphtheria and tetanus toxoids and acellular pertussis vaccine coverage rates among children aged 24 months—Puerto Rico, 2002. MMWR 51:667–668, 2002.

276. Centers for Disease Control and Prevention. Notice to readers: National Vaccine Advisory Committee report on strengthening vaccine supply. MMWR 52:203, 2003.

277. U.S. General Accounting Office. Childhood Vaccines: Ensuring an Adequate Supply Poses Challenges. Washington, DC, General Accounting Office, 2002.

278. Centers for Disease Control and Prevention. Impact of vaccines universally recommended for children—United States, 1900–1999. MMWR 48:243–248, 1999.

279. Centers for Disease Control and Prevention. Status report on the Childhood Immunization Initiative: reported cases of selected vaccine-preventable diseases—United States 1996. MMWR 46:665–671, 1997.

280. Centers for Disease Control and Prevention. Measles eradication: recommendations from a meeting cosponsored by the World Health Organization, the Pan American Health Organization, and CDC. MMWR 46(RR-11):1–20, 1997.

281. Centers for Disease Control and Prevention. Measles—United States, 1996, and the interruption of indigenous transmission. MMWR 46:242–246, 1997.

282. Centers for Disease Control and Prevention. Measles—United States, 1997. MMWR 47:273–276, 1998.

283. Katz KL, Hinman AR. Summary and conclusions—Measles Elimination Meeting, March 16–17, 2000. J Infect Dis 2003 [in press].

284. Orenstein WA. Immunization and health disparity issues: potential public health implications in the United States. In A Report on Reaching Underserved Ethnic and Minority Populations to Improve Pediatric Immunization Rates. Bethesda, MD, National Foundation for Infectious Diseases, 2002. Available at www.nfid.org/publications

284a. Thompson WW, Shay DK, Weintraub E, et al. Mortality associated with influenza and respiratory syncytial virus in the United States. JAMA 289:179–186, 2003.

284b. Robinson KA, Baughman W, Rothrock G, et al. Epidemiology of invasive Streptococcus pneumoniae infections in the United States, 1995–1998: opportunities for prevention in the conjugate vaccine era. JAMA 285:1729–1735, 2001.

285. Vitek CR, Redd SC, Redd SB, Hadler SC. Trends in importation of measles to the United States. JAMA 277:1952–1956, 1997.

286. Rota JS, Heath JL, Rota PA, et al. Molecular epidemiology of measles virus: identification of pathways of transmission and implications for measles elimination. J Infect Dis 173:32–37, 1996.

287. Linkins RW, Feikema SM. Immunization registries: the cornerstone of childhood immunization in the 21st century. Pediatr Ann 27:349–354, 1998.

288. Wood D, Saarlas KN, Inkelas M, Matyas BT. Immunization registries in the United States: implications for the practice of public health in a changing health care system. Annu Rev Public Health 20:231–255, 1999.

289. National Vaccine Advisory Committee. Development of Community and State-Based Immunization Registries; approved January 12, 1999. Atlanta, Centers for Disease Control and Prevention, 1999. Available at www.cdc.gov/nip/registry/nvac.htm

290. Ad Hoc Working Group for the Development of Standards. Standards for pediatric immunization practices. JAMA 269:1817–1822, 1993.

291. U.S. Department of Health and Human Services. Healthy People 2010. (2nd ed). Vol. 1. Understanding and Improving Health. Vol. 2. Objectives for Improving Health. Washington, DC, U.S. Department of Health and Human Services, 2000.

292. Centers for Disease Control and Prevention. Immunization Registry Minimum Functional Standards, May 15, 2001. Atlanta, Centers for Disease Control and Prevention, 2001. Available at www.cdc.gov/nip/registry/mfs2001.htm

293. Horne PR, Saarlas KN, Hinman AR. Costs of immunization registries: experiences from the All Kids Count II projects. Am J Prev Med 19:94–98, 2000.

294. Horne PR, Saarlas KN, Hinman AR. Update on immunization registries [letter]. Am J Prev Med 20:171, 2001.

295. Centers for Disease Control and Prevention. Development of community- and state-based immunization registries: CDC response to a report from the National Vaccine Advisory Committee. MMWR 50(RR-17):1–18, 2001.

296. National Vaccine Advisory Committee. Immunization Registries Progress Report, approved January 2001. Available at www.cdc.gov/od/nvpo/regreport.htm

297. Centers for Disease Control and Prevention. Immunization registry progress—United States, 2002. MMWR 51:760–762, 2002.

Chapter 54

Immunization in Europe

DAVID M. SALISBURY • JEAN-MARC OLIVÉ

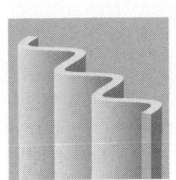

Overview

To many observers, immunization programs in Europe appear to be like a patchwork quilt with almost as many immunization schedules as countries, a variety of legislative processes for surveillance or for immunization, and little evidence of harmony. Indeed, a survey of immunization schedules revealed no two to be identical among 48 countries of the European region.[1] Many of these differences have come from historical influences because much of immunization and public health had its roots in European countries. As different health service delivery mechanisms evolved, so each country adapted its immunization program in line with perceived epidemiologic priorities, public health and primary care facilities, and vaccine availability. With immunization programs long established and accepted by health professionals and the public, reasons for change have to be balanced against consequential disruption without demonstrable public health benefit. Some of these concepts are coming under increasing challenge as national boundaries become less rigid with unrestricted passage between countries, and the vaccine industry seeks to market its products on a regional rather than national basis.

Despite the multiplicity of countries and immunization programs, some generalizations can be made. The northern, western, and south central European countries have immunization programs that are independent of each other, and here there are the greatest differences in schedules, surveillance, vaccines used, and public health provisions. For example, in the United Kingdom (UK), all childhood vaccines and vaccinations are free, purchased by the government and provided by family practitioners. In France, pediatricians provide most childhood vaccines and much of the cost incurred is reimbursed by the government. In Germany, reimbursement comes from insurance-based health care schemes. Vaccines and vaccinations are free in Scandinavian countries, most often being provided by primary care nurses.

Most former socialist countries in central and eastern Europe had well developed immunization programs, and many were able to keep them effectively under the changed socioeconomic conditions of the 1990s. Until the breakup of the Union of Soviet Socialist Republics (USSR), there was in effect a single immunization program in the 15 Soviet republics, surveillance requirements were the same, and the vaccines were produced in the Russian Republic. Since the dissolution of the USSR, the 12 newly independent states and the Baltic States have faced vaccine shortages, lack of hard currency to buy vaccines on the international markets, and, at the same time, a progressive shift to internationally recommended immunization policies. There has also been a move away from public sector– to private sector–based medical care.

Policy-Making Processes in European Union Countries

Each European Union (EU) country has a national advisory committee on immunization that makes recommendations to the government. The effect of those recommendations varies according to the centralization of immunization programs and the balance between public and private sector provision. In countries such as Germany and Spain, the *Länder* (Germany) or the "autonomous regions" (Spain) have the responsibility for the protection of public health. Although each country has a national advisory committee, its recommendations can be modified at the local level, and vaccines actually provided will depend on the choice of private practitioners and reimbursement arrangements with insurance companies. In Sweden, the national committee recommends the types of vaccines to be used, but local health authorities have the freedom to purchase the products they want. In the UK, the Joint Committee on Vaccination and Immunization makes recommendations to the government on immunisation policy for England, to the devolved administrations in Wales, Scotland, and Northern Ireland and policy is implemented similarly in each country.

EU countries do not have a common immunization policy, although there are unified processes for vaccine registration and batch testing of vaccines, and coordinated networks for surveillance are developing. So far, immunization policy or practice has not been subject to European legislation for harmonization, although many relevant processes such as batch release are controlled through EU legislation. Under an EU directive, vaccines batch-tested in one EU country cannot be retested if purchased for use in another country. Vaccine matters are included in the interests of several of the Directorates General (DGs). The DG for Enterprise is responsible for industry and is the DG most concerned with vaccines, being responsible for all aspects of the regulation of medicines. Its Pharmaceutical Committee is an important forum for information exchange among member states. Public health, including the prevention of communicable disease, comes under the auspices of the European Commission's DG for Health and Consumer Protection. The Action Programme of its Public Health Framework includes projects such as the development of vaccination registers and surveillance networks for infectious diseases. Other infectious disease or vaccine-related research topics come under the Fifth Framework Programme of the Research DG.

In the past, individual countries licensed vaccines (and other medicinal products) according to local arrangements; not surprisingly, there were considerable differences in the registration requirements. The option is still available for vaccines to be licensed with specifications that pertain just to one country in particular. If a manufacturer wishes to seek licensure of the same product in other EU countries, then this can be done through the mutual recognition procedure. However, starting with medicinal products whose manufacture involved genetic manipulation, an EU centralized procedure has evolved, and now any new product can be licensed through a central clearinghouse—the European Agency for the Evaluation of Medicinal Products (EMEA), located in London, UK. When a vaccine is licensed through the centralized procedure, the license will be specific to the data that has been supplied. If the vaccine is to be used in different clinical settings, such as different immunization calendars in different countries, then data will have to be provided that encompass all of those calendars for which it is proposed. The EMEA is responsible for centralized licensing of biologic/biotech medicines, the mutual recognition of product licenses, and scientific advice through its Committee on Proprietary Medicinal Products (CPMP), and has an equivalent veterinary committee. The CPMP has appropriate working party subcommittees; one subcommittee, the Efficacy, Safety and Biotechnology Working Party, gives the CPMP scientific advice on quality issues concerning specific products (those submitted for licensure or already licensed) and on more general scientific issues, such as transmissible spongiform encephalopathies and medicinal products. The CPMP and its working parties develop written "Notes for Guidance" for the pharmaceutical industry, usually EU specific but sometimes developed in collaboration with U.S. and Japanese counterparts. Each member state has formal membership on all committees and working parties, but nominated rapporteurs from specific member states, with assistance from the EMEA secretariat, do the actual work, such as licensure of specific products.

A wide range of techniques is employed to measure immunization coverage in the individual EU countries. In Denmark, the Netherlands, and the UK, public health data are fully computerized and actively managed. Thus coverage is calculated by comparing the number of children who have completed immunization by a specified age with the number of children of the same age residing in the particular community. In Austria, Belgium, Germany, Greece, and Spain, where private-sector providers give many immunizations, coverage is calculated by comparing the number of doses of vaccine imported or distributed with the estimated target population.[2] Allowance for wastage and inaccuracies in the target population make these coverage estimates unreliable. In most countries, coverage is measured at 2 years of age, but, for example, in Germany, it is measured at school entry at around 5 years. Because such different techniques for coverage estimation have been used, and the accuracy of the estimations may differ considerably, comparisons between countries' coverage reports need to be made with caution.[3] Nevertheless, some countries report very low coverage for certain vaccines.[4]

Pertussis coverage varies considerably, with lowest coverage reported from Germany (50% in 1997). However, since submitting those data, acellular pertussis vaccine has been introduced and coverage is informally reported to be considerably improved. Italy, previously reporting very low coverage, now reports higher pertussis coverage (80% in 1999), also as a consequence of the introduction of acellular pertussis vaccine. Low pertussis vaccine coverage is reported from Ireland (84% in 2001). High coverage is reported from Finland (99% in 1999), Portugal (98% in 2001), and Denmark (97% in 2001). The years cited are for the most recent data.

There is also considerable variation in measles coverage, with Finland reporting 98% and Denmark 94% (in 1999 and 2001, respectively), and Italy and Ireland reporting 70% and 73%, respectively (in 1999). These latter two countries experienced significant measles outbreaks in 2001 and 2002, including deaths from acute measles. Figure 54–1 shows the numbers of reported cases of measles between 1991 and 2001 in EU countries, and the number of countries supplying reports to the World Health Organization Regional Office for Europe (WHO EURO). There are considerable differences in the quality of surveillance among European countries, with some countries (such as the UK) reporting confirmed and suspected cases and others reporting only suspected cases. Although annual reporting of cases of measles by country is incomplete, there is even more incomplete reporting of coverage.

Apart from reporting of incidence of vaccine-preventable diseases to WHO EURO, there is no formal centralized monitoring for the EU countries. However, the European Sero-Epidemiology Network was established in 1996 to coordinate and harmonize the serologic surveillance of immunity to vaccine-preventable diseases in six countries (Denmark, England, France, Germany, Italy, and the Netherlands).[5] The diseases under surveillance are measles, mumps, rubella, pertussis, diphtheria, varicella, and hepatitis A and B. Four countries are taking part in a network for pneumococcal surveillance (Denmark, Italy, Finland, and the UK). There is also a network of European laboratories that monitors numbers and serotypes of meningococcal infections.

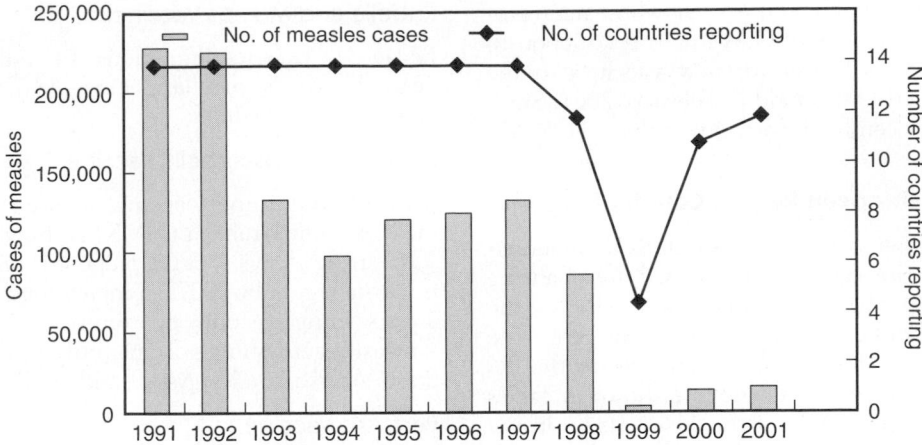

FIGURE 54–1 ▪ Total number of reported measles cases and numbers of countries reporting, EU countries, 1991 to 2001 (WHO EURO data).

Wider European Policies—World Health Organization

WHO EURO has an overarching interest in developing immunization policies suitable for implementation in all of its 51 member states. The WHO has been actively involved in immunization in Europe. The first European Technical Conference of the World Health Organization, on the control of infectious diseases through vaccination programs, was held in 1959 in Rabat, Morocco. When the Expanded Programme on Immunization (EPI) was launched in 1974 by the WHO, most countries of the European region had already successfully prevented serious childhood diseases such as poliomyelitis and diphtheria through countrywide immunization programs. Therefore, the European region considered participation in the EPI to be a low priority. This opinion changed in the early 1980s when the member states of the WHO European Region were all signatories to the regional Health for All Strategy by the Year 2000.

In 1984, the second Conference on Immunization Policies in Europe was held in Karlovy Vary, Czechoslovakia. Here, participants reviewed the status of immunization programs in the region, established immunization targets, determined the actions necessary to reach the targets, and reinforced the commitment of member states to the goals and activities of the EPI and to the regional targets. The conference became a turning point for strengthening region-wide coordinated immunization activities. The recommendations of the conference also strengthened the responsibility of WHO EURO (based in Copenhagen, Denmark). The Communicable Disease and Immunization Unit of WHO EURO continues to coordinate regional activities.

A European Advisory Group (EAG) was created in 1986 and has met regularly since. The terms of reference of the group include

- To periodically review the progress toward achieving the immunization targets and to consider constraints of immunization programs in European countries
- To recommend modifications and approaches of strategies based on new scientific or practical findings
- To provide technical recommendations to develop and foster national disease elimination programs

- To advise WHO EURO on priority areas for action to be taken, including proposals for submission to the Regional Committee, which would possibly result in a resolution calling for action by member states and the regional office.

Additionally, annual or biannual meetings of the EPI program managers of the 51 member states of the region are organized to facilitate the implementation of the recommendations of the EAG, and to share experiences of achievements and constraints in approaching the regional targets. With the emergence of the newly independent states of the former USSR, WHO EURO has prioritized the eastern part of the region and has held either joint regional meetings or smaller meetings specifically for the central and eastern European countries.

The sudden and dramatic political and socioeconomic changes following the dissolution of the USSR have seriously compromised the ability of the newly independent states to produce or to procure vaccines and to carry out disease control and immunization programs, and have led to the re-emergence of epidemics of vaccine-preventable diseases. Initiated by the U.S. Agency for International Development and the government of Japan, an Interagency Immunization Co-ordinating Committee (IICC) was created in Kyoto, Japan, in 1994. WHO EURO provides the secretariat and coordinates the activities of the IICC. The main objectives of the IICC are to support the newly independent states in the control of vaccine-preventable diseases, particularly control of epidemic diphtheria and eradication of poliomyelitis, and to help ensure primary immunization in children with the ultimate goal of achieving sustainable immunization programs based on vaccine self-reliance. Members of the IICC are, in addition to the co-founders Japan and the United States, Canada, Denmark, France, Germany, Turkey, the European Union, the International Federation of Red Cross and Red Crescent Societies, Rotary International, the United Nations Children's Fund, and the WHO. Future work is targeted at achieving sustainability of immunization programs (financing, program management, quality control of vaccines and other supplies) in all newly independent states.

In November 2000, following the launch of the Global Alliance for Vaccines and Immunization (GAVI), the IICC decided to create a regional working group whose main purpose is to optimize efficiency of GAVI partners' support to immunization and introduction of new vaccines in the region. The first meeting was held in February 2001. Since then meetings have been held every 4 months.

Vaccines Used in European Region Country Programs

Among the 51 member states of WHO EURO, immunization schedules and the vaccines being used are changing rapidly as new vaccines become available in the west of the region, and as sociopolitical changes occur in the east of the region. Immunization schedules from countries in the EU and selected other European countries are shown in Tables 54–1 and 54–2. In April 2002, of the 11 countries in the European region eligible for support from the GAVI Vaccine Fund, 10 had already introduced hepatitis B vaccine and one *Haemophilus influenzae* type b (Hib) vaccine (see *www.vaccinealliance.org*). Use of individual vaccines is discussed below.

Polio Vaccine

From 1995 to 2002, the number of countries using oral poliovirus vaccine (OPV) exclusively has been reduced from 41 to 31, respectively. Inactivated poliovirus vaccine (IPV) alone is used in Austria, Belgium, Finland, France, Germany, Iceland, Luxembourg, Monaco, the Netherlands, Norway, Sweden, and Switzerland. A sequential schedule (IPV followed by OPV) is used in Andorra, Denmark, Hungary, Israel, Italy, Latvia, Lithuania, and San Marino.

Bacille Calmette-Guérin Vaccine

Bacille Calmette-Guérin immunization of newborns is recommended in the majority of countries, although in some countries it is scheduled during school age. There is considerable variation in the recommendations for the number and timing of booster doses.

A few countries immunize only those children who are considered to be at risk.

Hepatitis B Vaccine

Hepatitis B vaccine has been introduced in 37 (72%) countries of the region. All of the nine countries with high hepatitis B surface antigen prevalence (>8%) have now introduced the vaccine in their routine immunization programs. For the medium-prevalence (2% to 8%) countries, 16 (64%) have infant immunization programs and the other 12 have generally introduced the vaccine for adolescents. Italy, for example, introduced an infant and an adolescent program simultaneously.

Hib Vaccine

By 2002, a total of 29 countries had implemented immunization against *H. influenzae* type b infections (with Hib vaccine), compared to 16 in 1998. This vaccine is generally combined with the administration of diphtheria and tetanus toxoids and whole-cell pertussis (DTP) vaccine. Apart from Hungary, Ireland, Latvia, Malta, and the UK, those countries using Hib vaccine recommend either a four-dose schedule or a three-dose regimen with two early doses and the last dose given close to the first birthday.

Rubella and Mumps Vaccine

Because of resource limitations, 14 countries have not yet been able to add rubella vaccine and 7 to add mumps vaccine to their schedules.

Measles-Mumps-Rubella Vaccine

Measles-containing vaccine is used in all countries; measles-mumps-rubella (MMR) is the vaccine of choice in 37 countries. In view of the proposed elimination of measles from the region by 2007, an increasing number of countries are providing a second opportunity for the administration of a measles-containing vaccine; only three countries do not do so: Azerbaijan, Kyrgystan, and the Republic of Moldova.

Pertussis Vaccine

The timing and use of pertussis vaccine vary considerably. When only whole-cell vaccines were available, Sweden did not use pertussis-containing vaccines. In Italy, the vaccine was used only in a few provinces, and Germany had uneven usage: low coverage in the western part and high coverage in the eastern part of the country. Increasingly, western European countries have introduced acellular vaccines for booster immunization as well as for both primary and booster immunization. Pertussis immunization is now used in all European countries. However, where high-quality whole-cell pertussis vaccine is available and high coverage is achieved, the impact is excellent: countries such as Bulgaria, the Czech Republic, Hungary, Poland, and Slovakia, using whole-cell vaccine exclusively for many years, have registered incidence rates of pertussis of less than 1 per 100,000. Over 60% of the countries of the European region use a primary series of three doses of DTP or acellular pertussis (DTaP) between ages 2 and 6 months. In a few countries, the third dose is recommended at a later age (10 to 18 months). Most countries recommend a fourth dose at age 2 years; others prefer to immunize before school entry. Croatia, Greece, Hungary, Italy, Slovenia, and Switzerland recommend a fifth dose of vaccine at ages 4 to 7 years.

Introduction of Meningococcal C Conjugate Vaccine in the United Kingdom

During the 1990s, the number of cases of group C meningococcal disease rose progressively. A collaboration was begun between national organizations and vaccine industry partners to stimulate the accelerated development of vaccines that could be introduced across a wide age range. In November 1999, the UK became the first country to implement an immunization program against meningococcal serogroup C disease using a conjugate vaccine.[6] Its introduction was the culmination of an intensive 5-year clinical trial research program sponsored by the Department of Health (DH) for England. The objective was to accelerate the availability of such new vaccines for the UK population. The DH-funded research program was designed primarily to provide the scientific information needed for policy decisions about the use of meningococcal serogroup C conjugate (MCC) vaccines in the UK. The research also

TABLE 54–1 ■ Immunization Schedules Used in Selected Countries of the WHO European Region, 2000, for BCG, DTP, DTaP, DT/Td, OPV, and IPV Vaccines

Country	Vaccine[*],[†]					
	BCG	DTP	DTaP	DT/Td	OPV	IPV
Albania	Nb, 6–7 yr	2, 4, 6, 24 mo			2, 4, 6, 18–24 mo; 5–6 yr	
Armenia	Nb, 5–6 yr	3, 4–5, 6, 18–24 mo			3, 4–5, 6, 18, 20 mo; 6 yr	
Austria	‡		3, 4, 5, 16–18 mo	7, 14–15 yr		3, 4, 5, 24 mo; 7, 14–15 yr
Azerbaijan	Nb	2, 3, 4, 18 mo; 5–6 yr			Nb, 2, 3, 4, 18 mo	
Belarus	Nb	3, 4–5, 6, 18 mo		6, 11, 16 yr	3, 4, 5, 18, 24 mo; 6–7, 14–15 yr	
Belgium			3, 4, 5, 13 mo	5–6, 15 yr		2, 4, 13 mo; 5–6 yr
Bosnia & Herzegovina	Nb; 7, 14 yr	3, 4, 5 mo; 2, 4 yr			3, 4, 5 mo; 4, 7, 14 yr	
Bulgaria	Nb, 6–7 yr	2, 3, 4, 24 mo		5–6, 11–12, 15–16 yr	2, 3, 4, 14, 24 mo; 6–7 yr	
Croatia	Nb; 2, 8, 14 yr	3, 4, 5, 12 mo; 4 yr		7, 15 yr	3, 4–5, 6, 12 mo; 3, 7 yr	
Czech Republic	Nb, 11–12 yr	3, 4, 5, 18 mo		5–6 yr	3, 4, 15, 18 mo; 13 yr	
Denmark			3, 5, 12 mo		2, 3, 4 yr	3, 5, 12 mo
Estonia	Nb, 8 yr	3, 4–5, 6, 24 mo		7, 12 yr	3, 4–5, 6, 24 mo; 7 yr	
Finland	Nb	3, 4, 5, 20–24 mo	C.I. only	11–12 yr		6, 12, 20–24 mo; 6, 11, 16–18 yr
France	Nb,‡ <6 yr	2, 3, 4, 16–18 mo	16–18 mo; 11–13 yr	6, 11–13, 16–18 yr		2, 3, 4, 16–18 mo; 6, 11–13, 16–18 yr
Georgia	Nb, 5–6 yr	2, 3, 4, 18 mo		5–6, 14–15 yr	2, 3, 4, 18 mo; 5 yr	2, 3, 4, 11–14 mo; 11–17 yr
Germany	Nb, ch‡		2, 3, 4, 11–14 mo; 2, 4, 6, 18 mo; 4–6 yr	4–5, 10–16 yr	2, 4, 6, 18 mo; 4–7 yr	
Greece	6 yr				4, 5, 15 mo; 3, 6–7 yr	3 mo
Hungary	Nb	3, 4, 5, 36 mo; 6 yr		11 yr		
Iceland			3, 5, 12 mo; 5 yr; 2, 4, 6 mo; 4–6 yr; 3, 5, 12 mo; 5–6 yr	14 yr		3, 5, 12 mo; 14 yr
Ireland	Nb				2, 4, 6 mo	
Italy				12–14 yr	11–12 mo; 3 yr	3, 5 mo
Kazakhstan	Nb, 6–7 yr	2, 3, 4, 18 mo		11–12, 14–15 yr	Nb, 2, 3, 4 mo	
Kyrgyzstan	Nb, 6–7 yr	2, 3, 5, 24 mo		6–7, 12, 16 yr; 5–6, 11–12, 15–16 yr	Nb, 2, 3, 5 mo; 6–7 yr	
Latvia	Nb	3, 4–5, 6, 18 mo		7, 14 yr	18 mo; 7, 14 yr	3, 4–5, 6 mo
Lithuania	Nb, 6–7 yr	3, 4–5, 6, 18 mo		5–6, 15–16 yr	6–7, 12 yr	3, 4–5, 18 mo
Luxembourg	Nb‡		2, 3, 4, 18 mo			3, 4, 5, 12–15 mo; 13–15 yr
Malta	11–12 yr	2, 3, 4 mo		3, 15 yr	2, 3, 4 mo; 3–4, 14–16 yr	
Netherlands			2, 3, 4, 11 mo; 3, 5, 12 mo	4, 9 yr		3, 4, 5, 11 mo; 4, 9 yr
Norway	14–15 yr			11–12 yr		3, 5, 12 mo; 6, 12 yr
Poland	Nb, 12 mo	2, 3–4, 5, 16–18 mo		6, 14, 19 yr	2, 3–4, 5, 18–24 mo; 6, 11 yr	
Portugal	Nb; 5–6, 11–12 yr	2, 4, 6, 18–24 mo		5–6 yr	2, 4, 6 mo; 5–6 yr	
Republic of Moldova	Nb; 6–7, 11–12 yr	3, 4–5, 6, 22–24 mo		5–6, 14–15 yr	3, 4–5, 6 mo; 5–6 yr	
Romania	Nb, 14 yr‡	2, 4, 6, 12 mo; 3 yr		7, 14 yr	2, 4, 6, 12 mo; 9 yr	
Russian Federation	Nb, 6–7 yr	3, 4, 5, 18 mo		5–6, 14–15 yr	3, 4, 5, 18, 24 mo; 6–7 yr	

Continued

TABLE 54-1 ■ Immunization Schedules Used in Selected Countries of the WHO European Region, 2000, for BCG, DTP, DTaP, DT/Td, OPV, and IPV Vaccines—cont'd

Country	Vaccine*†					
	BCG	DTP	DTaP	DT/Td	OPV	IPV
Slovakia	Nb	2, 3, 9, 24 mo		5–6 yr	2, 4, 15, 16 mo; 11 yr	
Slovenia	Nb	3, 4–5, 6, 18 mo		9–14 yr	3, 4–5, 6, 18 mo; 6, 14 yr	
Spain		2, 4, 6, 18 mo		14–16 yr	2, 4, 6, 18 mo; 6 yr	
Sweden	After 6 mo‡		18 mo; 6 yr	10 yr		3, 5, 12 mo; 6 yr
Switzerland	Nb‡		3, 5, 12 mo; 2, 4, 6, 15–24 mo; 4–7 yr			2, 4, 6, 15–24 mo; 4–7 yr
Tajikistan	Nb	2, 3, 4, 16 mo		11–15 yr	Nb, 2, 3, 4, 12 mo	
(Former) Yugoslav Republic of Macedonia	1, 4, 14 yr	4, 5, 6 mo		5–6, 15–16 yr	3, 4, 5 mo; 7, 14 yr	
Turkey	2 mo, 6 yr	2, 3, 4, 16–18 mo		6, 11, 14 yr	2, 3, 4, 16–18 mo; 6–7 yr	
Turkmenistan	Nb; 6–7, 14–15 yr	2, 3, 4, 18 mo		5–6, 14–15 yr	Nb, 2, 3, 4, 18, 20 mo; 6–7 yr	
Ukraine	Nb; 6–7, 14–15 yr	3, 4, 5, 18 mo		6, 11, 14 yr	3, 4, 5, 18 mo; 3, 6–7, 14–15 yr	
United Kingdom	10–14 yr	2, 3, 4 mo		3–5 yr, 13–16 yr	2, 3, 4 mo; 3–5, 13–16 yr	
Uzbekistan	Nb; 7, 15 yr	2, 3, 4, 16 mo		5–6, 15–16 yr	Nb, 2, 3, 4, 16 mo; 7 yr	
Yugoslavia	Nb, 10 yr	2, 3, 5, 15 mo		7, 14 yr	2, 3, 5, 17 mo; 7, 14 yr	

*BCG, bacille Calmette-Guérin; DTP, diphtheria and tetanus toxoids and whole-cell pertussis; DTaP, diphtheria and tetanus toxoids and acellular pertussis; DT/Td, diphtheria and tetanus toxoids (general/adult); OPV, oral poliovirus vaccine; IPV, inactivated poliovirus vaccine.
†Nb, newborns; ch, children; C.I.
‡For individuals at high risk.

TABLE 54–2 ■ Immunization Schedules Used in Selected Countries of the WHO European Region, 2000, for MMR, Measles, Mumps, Rubella, Hib, and HepB Vaccines*

Country	Vaccines†,‡					
	MMR	Measles	Mumps	Rubella	Hib	HepB
Albania		12 mo; 5 yr		12 mo; 5 yr		Nb, 2, 6 mo
Armenia		12 mo	15 mo			Nb, 2, 6 mo
Austria	14 mo; 7 yr			13 yr (girls)	3, 4, 5, 14–18 mo	Nb§, 3, 4, 5, 24 mo; 13 yr||
Azerbaijan		12 mo				Nb, 2, 4 mo
Belarus	12 mo; 6 yr					Nb, 1, 5 mo; 13 yr||
Belgium	14–18 mo; 11–12 yr				2, 3, 4, 13 mo	3, 4, 13 mo; 11–12 yr
Bosnia & Herzegovina	2, 7 yr					Nb, 1, 6 mo; 7 yr
Bulgaria	13 mo; 11–12 yr					Nb, 1, 6 mo
Croatia	12, 24 mo					12 yr
Czech Republic	15, 20–24 mo				3, 5, 12 mo	§
Denmark	15 mo; 11–12 yr					§
Estonia	12 mo; 13 yr					Nb, 1, 6 mo
Finland	14–18 mo; 5–6 yr				4, 6, 14–18 mo	§
France	12 mo; 3–6 yr				2, 3, 4, 16–18 mo	Nb§, 2, 3, 8–15 mo||
Georgia		12 mo; 5–6 yr				2, 3, 8 mo
Germany	10–14 mo; 4–5 yr				2, 3, 4, 11–14 mo	2, 4, 11–14 mo||
Greece	13–15 mo; 4–6 yr					§, ¶
Hungary	15 mo; 11–12 yr				2, 4, 5 mo	
Iceland	18 mo; 9 yr				3, 5, 12 mo	
Ireland	15 mo; 4–5 yr				2, 4, 6 mo	§, ¶
Italy	12–15 mo; 5–12 yr	12–24 mo; 6–7 yr	12–24 mo		3, 5, 11 mo	Nb§, 3, 5, 11–12 mo||
Kazakhstan		6 yr		6 yr	2, 3, 5 mo	Nb, 2, 4 mo
Kyrgyzstan	12 mo					Nb, 2, 5 mo
Latvia	15 mo	7 yr	7 yr	11 yr (girls)	3, 4–5, 6 mo	Nb, 1, 6 mo
Lithuania	15–16 mo; 11–12 yr					Nb, 1, 6 mo
Luxembourg	15 mo; 12 yr				3, 5, 15 mo	§, ¶

Continued

TABLE 54–2 ■ Immunization Schedules Used in Selected Countries of the WHO European Region, 2000, for MMR, Measles, Mumps, Rubella, Hib, and HepB Vaccines*—cont'd

Country	Vaccines†‡					
	MMR	Measles	Mumps	Rubella	Hib	HepB
Malta	15 mo; 11–12 yr				2, 3, 4 mo	9, 10 yr
Netherlands	14 mo; 9 yr				2, 3, 4, 11 mo	Nb§; 2, 3, 4, 11 mo
Norway	11–12, 15 mo				3, 5, 12 mo	¶
Poland		13–14 mo; 6 yr		12 yr (girls)		Nb, 1, 6 mo
Portugal	15 mo; 5–6 yr				2, 4, 6, 15, 18 mo	Nb, 2, 6 mo; 10–13 yr
Republic of Moldova		12 mo	12 mo			Nb, 1, 6 mo
Romania		9–11 mo; 7 yr				Nb, 2, 6 mo; 9 yr
Russian Federation		12–15 mo; 7 yr	12–15 mo; 7 yr			Nb, 1, 6 mo; 11+ yr
Slovakia	14 mo; 11–12 yr				2, 3, 9 mo	3, 4, 9 mo
Slovenia	12–18 mo; 5–6 yr				2, 4–5, 18 mo	Nb,§ 7 yr
Spain	12–15 mo; 3–6 yr				2, 4, 6, 15–18 mo	Nb, 1, 6 mo; 10–14 yr
Sweden	18 mo; 12 yr				3, 5, 12 mo	
Switzerland	15 mo; 4–7 yr				2, 4, 6, 15 mo	Nb, 1, 6 mo; 11+ yr
Tajikistan	13 mo	9 mo; 3 yr				Nb, 2, 4 mo
(Former) Yugoslav Republic of Macedonia						¶
Turkey		9 mo; 6 yr				3, 4, 9 yr
Turkmenistan		9 mo; 5–6 yr				Nb, 2, 4 mo
Ukraine		12 mo; 6 yr		15 yr (girls)		Nb, 3, 5 mo
United Kingdom	12–15 mo; 3–5 yr				2, 3, 4 mo	¶
Uzbekistan		9, 16 mo	16 mo			
Yugoslavia	15 mo; 12 yr					Nb, 2, 9 mo

*In addition to MMR and DTP/DTaP, in many western European countries an increasing number of new combination vaccines are used, such as DTaP-Hib, DTaP-HepB-Hib, DTaP-IPV, DTaP-Hib-IPV, and DTaP-Hib-IPV-HepB.

†MMR, measles-mumps-rubella; Hib, *Haemophilus influenzae* type b; HepB, hepatitis B vaccine.

‡Nb, newborn.

§For infants born to hepatitis B surface antigen–positive mothers.

‖Primary HepB immunization for adolescents not yet immunized.

¶For individuals at high risk.

provided data to support the licensure of MCC vaccines by the UK Medicines Control Agency (MCA), now called the Medicines and Healthcare Products Regulatory Agency (MHRA).

The key outcomes of this research program were the anticipation of an increase in group C meningococcal disease, the identification of a research agenda to hasten the development of MCC vaccine, and the development of a partnership between the national government and vaccine manufacturers. These steps allowed the development-to-introduction phase to be accelerated to 5 years from first discussions to a nationwide campaign. The pace of implementation was driven by the epidemiologic priorities of morbidity and mortality by age groups and by the availability of supplies of vaccine. In the face of intense public demand for vaccination, expectations were managed through a public communication campaign that introduced the vaccine and explained the epidemiologic prioritization and supply limitations. The campaign was implemented simultaneously through school health services for those 5 to 18 years, and through primary care for those less than 5 years. Costs were considerably less for school-based services, and the rate of implementation was considerably faster through this route. Supplies of vaccine were issued based on calculated requirements by age groups in schools and on previous ordering demand for routine primary vaccines for young children. Immunizations were given only to school groups according to the national schedule and only to young children according to scheduled invitations for immunization. This regimented approach prevented mismatching between demand for vaccination and availability of supplies.

Epidemiology of Serogroup C Meningococcal Disease

Meningococcal serogroup C disease has been endemic in the UK for many years, although at a lower incidence than serogroup B disease (Fig. 54–2). In 1994, serogroup C infections comprised 292 (25.8%) of the 1132 cases confirmed in England and Wales by the Meningococcal Reference Unit (MRU) of the Public Health Laboratory Service (PHLS), which is now known as the Health Protection Agency (HPA). In 1998, the last year before the introduction of MCC vaccines, serogroup C infections comprised 823 (34%) of the 2418 meningococcal infections confirmed by the MRU. The apparent increase in the incidence of con-

firmed meningococcal infection was due in part to the introduction of more sensitive polymerase chain reaction methods for the identification and serogrouping of meningococci.[7,8] However serogroup C disease increased proportionately more than other serogroups.[9] Rates of serogroup C disease were particularly high in adolescents, in whom school-based outbreaks attracted considerable public concern and media interest. Case-fatality rates increase with age and are higher in cases of serogroup C than B infection, particularly serogroup C2a, which was the predominant serosubtype in the UK.[8] The number of deaths from meningococcal serogroup C infection in adolescents in England and Wales exceeded those from meningococcal B disease prior to the introduction of the MCC vaccination program (Fig. 54–3). It was estimated that the total number of serogroup C cases in England and Wales in 1999 was around 1500. The overall case-fatality rate for meningococcal C disease in the 1999 enhanced surveillance was 12.5%.[8] Using the age-specific case-fatality rate observed in the enhanced surveillance, it is estimated that serogroup C infection was responsible for at least 150 deaths each year.

Early in 1994, it was apparent to the DH and the HPA that there was a real possibility that the UK would face increases of group C meningococcal disease caused by the ET37 complex C2a, as had been seen in Canada, Spain, and the Czech Republic. A decision was therefore made to change the focus of the DH-funded Vaccine Evaluation Consortium* (VEC)[10] away from combination vaccines based on acellular pertussis to conjugate group C meningococcal vaccines. This approach was considered promising in view of the outstanding success of conjugate Hib vaccines wherever they had been introduced. Unlike the existing plain serogroup C polysaccharide vaccines, the development of a conjugate vaccine would offer the prospect of protection in young children and induction of long-term immunity. All potential vaccine manufacturers were approached, and three responded with interest in collabo-

---

*The clinical and preclinical components of the DH-funded clinical trials program are undertaken by the UK Vaccine Evaluation Consortium (VEC), a collaborative group involving three public funded bodies—the HPA, the National Institute for Biological Standards and Control (NIBSC), and the Centre for Applied Microbiology and Research, Porton Down—together with an academic immunobiology unit at the Institute of Child Health, London. The field work involved in the trials is carried out in the two PHLS vaccine evaluation units by trained study nurses based in general practices in Gloucester and Hertfordshire.

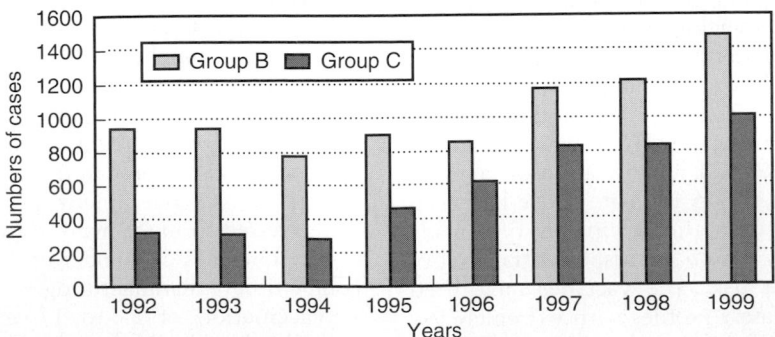

FIGURE 54–2 ■ Laboratory-confirmed cases of group B and C meningococcal disease, England and Wales, 1992 to 1999 (Health Protection Agency data).

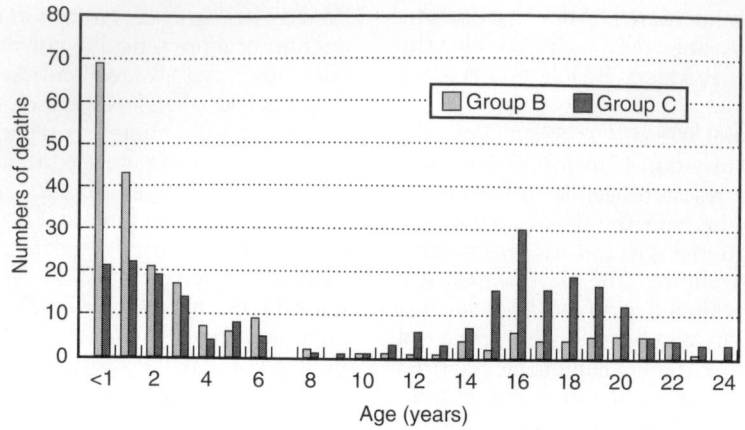

FIGURE 54–3 ▪ Deaths from group B and group C meningococcal disease, England and Wales, 1994 to 1999 (HPA data).

rating on an MCC vaccination development program. Funding was obtained by the PHLS from the DH to evaluate each of these candidate vaccines under the UK 2/3/4-month infant schedule. Two of the three candidate MCC vaccines were CRM$_{197}$-based conjugates and the third was a tetanus-based conjugate. All proved highly immunogenic under the UK schedule, with evidence of induction of immunologic memory and putative protective antibody levels after only one or two doses.[11–15]

A parallel component of the DH-funded research program was the development of preclinical tests[16,17] for controlling the quality of the batches of MCC vaccines once licensed. The National Institute for Biological Standards and Control (NIBSC) carried out this work, and the experience gained was invaluable in facilitating the rapid batch release of MCC vaccines once licensure of the first vaccine was granted in October 1999. Early discussions between manufacturers and the MHRA indicated that licensure of MCC vaccines on the basis of immunogenicity data alone without direct evidence of protective efficacy would be considered. The basis of this decision was the existing licensure of plain serogroup C polysaccharide vaccines for children ages 2 years and above for whom there was direct evidence of efficacy and accepted serologic correlates of protection. Extrapolation of these correlates to infants, in whom the plain C polysaccharide is neither immunogenic nor efficacious, was the basis for licensure of the MCC vaccines in the UK and has established an important precedent for other meningococcal conjugate polysaccharide vaccines.

Given the wide age range of cases of serogroup C disease in the UK, it was planned to achieve an immediate impact by accompanying the introduction of MCC vaccine into the primary infant schedule with a mass catch-up program for all children aged up to 18 years, the ages and timing dictated by the availability of vaccine. The vaccine campaign was launched in late 1999, and, in the space of approximately 1 year, all those less than 18 years of age had been offered vaccination. Since then, the vaccine has been made available for all those less than 25 years, essentially all of the age groups at highest risk. The vaccines have been found to have excellent safety profiles with extremely few serious adverse reactions. The impact has been impressive, with reductions in cases and deaths of 90% and 95%, respectively.

The Vaccination Program

In the DH's 1998 Comprehensive Spending Review, the introduction of MCC vaccine was anticipated for October 2000, and plans were in development for resources to become available to support this. However, the winter meningococcal season of 1998 to 1999 showed continuing increases in the proportion and number of meningococcal C infections, especially in adolescents. It was also apparent that the results from the clinical trials were strongly reassuring, and, because of rapid recruitment into the trials, the research program could be completed early. The manufacturers were asked in January 1999 to consider bringing forward the introduction of MCC vaccine by a year, and the three companies responded positively. The DH-funded clinical trial program, together with complementary manufacturer-sponsored studies,[18–21] culminated in the licensure of the first MCC vaccine, the Wyeth product (Meningitec™), in October 1999. Licensure of the Chiron (Menjugate™) and the Baxter (Neisvac™) vaccines followed in March and July 2000, respectively.

In February 1999, the Right Honorable Frank Dobson, then Secretary of State for Health, agreed that the program should go forward in the autumn of 1999, subject to demonstration of cost-effectiveness, availability of resources, and adequate supplies of vaccine.[22] In May 1999, the Joint Committee on Vaccination and Immunisation, the independent expert advisory group to the UK health departments, reviewed the epidemiology, the results of the vaccine studies, and the outlined implementation options. The committee recommended the introduction of vaccination as soon as possible, subject to granting of product licenses and supplies, with the program to be targeted according to age-risk groups and vaccine availability. The forthcoming introduction of the MCC vaccine program was announced to Parliament in July 1999 and, immediately after, tenders for supply were invited, in line with European directives on government procurement. Manufacturers were pressed to make available to the DH their manufacturing schedules of number of doses and expected dates of completion of manufacturing.

Vaccination of 5- to 17-year-olds was implemented through school health services and vaccination of the under-5 age group through primary care/general practice. Local immunization coordinators provided the DH with estimates of the numbers of children in each school age group in order to plan vaccine allocation to schools. Because data had been collected on the number of doses of DTP/Hib vaccine that had been ordered by each general practitioner (GP) over the preceding 2 years, it was possible to estimate the number of children under 5 years of age cared for by each GP. Vaccine was then issued to each GP either weekly or fortnightly, and no ordering was necessary. The suppliers of software for the national childhood immunization computing systems were given the projected dates for immunization of children under 5 years of age, who were then invited for immunization through the computerized call-up programs, exactly in line with supplies to GPs. The target population was over 15 million children to be immunized in 12 months: There were no shortages of vaccine, and the full requirement of vaccine was issued according to the schedule.

Market research among parents of young children has repeatedly shown that meningitis is the disease most feared. A communication strategy was developed that acknowledged the high public interest in meningitis and its prevention, but took account of the constraints on the pace of implementation, essentially the capacity of the manufacturers to produce vaccine. Because the campaign was introduced a year ahead of schedule, no stockpiles of vaccine were available to allow unrestricted vaccination on request. Following market testing among parents and young people, advertising materials were prepared and distributed. Leaflets were available in primary care facilities, pharmacies, and supermarkets, and sufficient numbers were provided to every school to allow each child to take home a leaflet. The leaflets included a consent form that was returned to the school and used to complete the information on the school lists that were used by the local immunization coordinators. A television advertisement was developed whose main message was that parents should not make appointments for vaccination or seek it opportunistically because every child would be invited for the new immunization in turn, the timing being a compromise between epidemiologic priority and vaccine availability.

In line with the available supplies, MCC vaccine was initially introduced from the beginning of November 1999 for 15- to 17-year-olds, the age groups in whom mortality rates and the risk of outbreaks were highest. Infants due to receive their three-dose primary immunization course with combined DTP/Hib vaccine at 2, 3, and 4 months of age were scheduled to receive MCC vaccine at the same time from late November 1999 onward. Toddlers ages 12 to 23 months and infants ages 5 to 11 months were scheduled to receive one and two doses of MCC vaccine, respectively, from mid-January 2000 onward. Vaccination of 2- to 4-year-olds was completed by late 2000. The remaining school-age children between 5 and 15 years were scheduled to receive MCC vaccine by autumn 2000, with the order of priority as determined by the age-specific morbidity and mortality data, beginning with 10- to 14-year-olds and followed by 5- to 9-year-olds. In 2001, the catch-up program was augmented to include those up to the age of 25 years who had not previously received MCC.

Surveillance of Vaccination Program Results

Since the UK was the first country to introduce MCC vaccines, furthermore without direct evidence of efficacy, the PHLS put in place a comprehensive surveillance strategy to monitor the impact of the new MCC vaccination program. Its objectives were as follows:

- To measure the impact on the age-specific and serogroup-specific incidence of meningococcal disease[23,24]
- To measure age-specific vaccine coverage[24]
- To obtain formal estimates of age-specific MCC vaccine efficacy
- To document the risk factors for vaccine failure
- To develop an active system for monitoring vaccine safety
- To monitor any changes in the genotypic characteristics of invasive and carriage strains of meningococci

All cases of confirmed and probable serogroup C disease in individuals under 20 years of age are being followed up to obtain vaccination history (including manufacturer and batch number). Multilocus sequence typing of invasive and carriage isolates is being undertaken to monitor the impact of the program on the population genetics of *Neisseria meningitidis*. The full protocol for the surveillance program and for the investigation of vaccine failures can be found on the PHLS website (*www.hpa.org.uk*).

Surveillance of the prevalent serogroups and serosubtypes among invasive case isolates has shown no evidence of any change in the 36 months since the MCC vaccination program was introduced (E. Kaczmarski, personal communication, 2002). Concerns that the prevention of serogroup C disease by vaccination might result in a capsular switch to serogroup B remain entirely speculative. Along with evidence that there is herd immunity protection of unimmunized children and young people, there is also evidence of reduced carriage of group C meningococci following the campaign.[25]

Postlicensure surveillance of adverse vaccine events through passive reports from health professionals to the MHRA, on behalf of the Committee on Safety of Medicines, was enhanced for MCC vaccines by requesting reports of any suspected reaction, whatever the severity. By September 2000, a total 4764 reports had been received, a reporting rate of 1 per 2875 MCC doses distributed.[26] The vast majority were nonserious reactions such as headache, local reaction, pyrexia, and dizziness, reflecting the pattern of common symptoms seen in the clinical trials. Anaphylactoid reactions were reported at a rate of 1 per 500,000 doses distributed. Other rare adverse events such as purpura, erythema multiforme, arthritis, and arthropathy have been reported.

The impact of the campaign has been notable. Cases and deaths have fallen in immunized groups, and evidence is emerging of indirect protection of those not immunized within the age groups who were offered vaccine (1 to 4 years, 50%; 5 to 8 years, 57%, 9 to 14 years, 34%; 16 to 17 years, 51%) (HPA data). Efficacy estimates for the first 2 years since the campaign remain high, ranging from 87% (12 to 23 months; 95% confidence interval [CI], 69% to 94%) to 100% (3 to 4 years; 95% CI, 93% to 100%) (HPA data).

Table 54–3 shows the numbers of cases of confirmed group C meningococcal infection and percentage change before and after the introduction of MCC vaccine in England and Wales. The campaign was expanded to include

TABLE 54–3 ■ Numbers of Cases of Confirmed Group C Meningococcal Infection and Percentage Change Before and After Introduction of MCC Vaccine, England and Wales

| Age (yr) | Year | | |
	1998/99	2001/02	% Change
<1	105	4	–96
1 and 2	136	18	–87
3 and 4	85	7	–92
5–9 inclusive	93	5	–95
10–14 inclusive	89	6	–93
15–17 inclusive	145	5	–97
TOTAL	653	45	–93
>24	194	125	–36

Data from the Health Protection Agency, England.

immunization of those ages 18 to 25 years starting in 2001, and hence data for that age group are not included. Figure 54–4 shows the deaths from group C meningococcal disease, which have also fallen similarly.

Other European countries have now observed similar changes in the epidemiology of group C meningococcal disease. Routine immunization has started with conjugate vaccine, or is scheduled to start shortly, in Ireland, Spain, the Netherlands and Belgium; conjugate vaccine has been provided in some regions in France and Italy and is also available in Greece. The ages targeted have varied; only the UK has provided vaccination across the whole of the child and young adult population.

Immunization Safety Concerns— France and England

Over recent years, the success of immunization programs has been challenged by safety concerns that, despite lack of scientific corroboration, have been given considerable credibility by the media and the public. Examples are concerns regarding hepatitis B vaccine and demyelinating disease in France, MMR vaccine and bowel disease and autism in the UK, and thimerosal and developmental disorders in the United States. The salient features of the first two examples

were the association of vaccination with two chronic disorders of insidious onset and unknown etiology, and the different approaches to the management of the public ramifications.

France

France made immunization against hepatitis B compulsory for health workers in 1991 and introduced universal immunization for infants and preadolescents in 1994. However, from the numbers of doses of vaccine sold in France, there appears to have been very much wider use of the vaccine outside of these groups. Between 1994 and 1996, more than 7 million young adults ages 20 to 24 years were immunized against hepatitis B, and between 1989 and 1996 approximately 17.5 million individuals, representing one third of the population of France, were immunized.[27,28] As vaccine utilization increased, reports started to appear of new cases or relapses of multiple sclerosis, and these reports were cited prominently in the French popular press and on television programs.

Data reported to the National Commission on Pharmacovigilance in December 1994 and again in December 1996 showed that the rate of demyelinating diseases in temporal association with hepatitis B vaccination was significantly lower than the expected incidence of demyelinating diseases in the same population. The Ministère des Affaires Sociales, Direction Générale de la Santé, and the Agence Française du Medicament concluded that there were no scientific data suggesting a link between hepatitis B vaccination and multiple sclerosis, and that control of hepatitis B was of major importance, justifying the continued implementation of the hepatitis B vaccination programs. However, this announcement did not dispel the public concerns.

On October 1, 1998, a statement was issued by the Ministry for Employment and Solidarity and the Secretary of State for Health, reiterating the lack of evidence for a causal association between demyelinating diseases and hepatitis B immunization, but stating that "we cannot exclude the possibility that vaccination may disclose or facilitate the development of these diseases in certain people who have been vaccinated." The national strategy for hepatitis B immunization was therefore changed so that only high-risk adults were to be vaccinated, the school

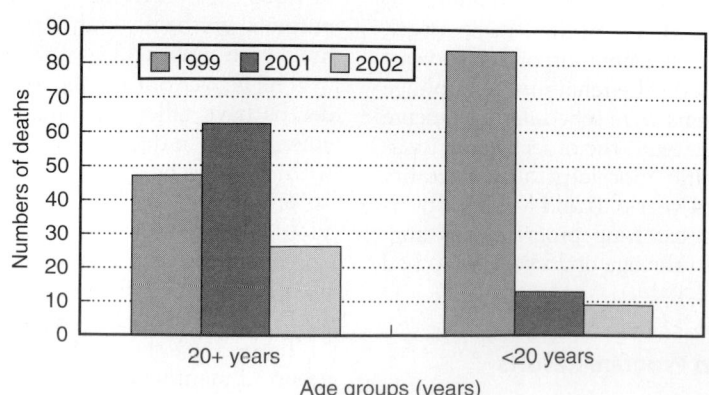

FIGURE 54–4 ■ Deaths from group C meningococcal infection, England and Wales, 1999 to 2002 (HPA data).

program for "preadolescents and adolescents" was suspended, but routine infant immunization was preserved. The most recent data suggest that coverage by 2 years of age is in the region of 25%.[29]

There has now been one civil claims case (in 1998) against the vaccine manufacturer in which, despite the lack of scientific evidence, the judge concluded in favor of the claimant, ruling that "there was sufficient evidence to conclude there was a connection between the SmithKline Beecham vaccine and multiple sclerosis symptoms in two people." A ruling is pending in a similar case against Aventis Pasteur. The first ruling is presently being appealed. Proceedings have also started for a criminal hearing. Because hepatitis B immunization is compulsory for health care workers as a condition of employment, compensation has been recommended by the Vaccine Compensation Committee in 2000 and paid to individuals with either new presentations or exacerbation of demyelinating conditions in close temporal association with vaccination.

United Kingdom

Starting in 1993, a number of scientific articles were published reporting studies most of which originated from one group working in the United Kingdom. The studies attempted to show that Crohn's disease and variably ulcerative colitis were associated with either early measles infection or measles immunization. The studies were based on either epidemiologic or virologic data.[30-35] These claims for infection or vaccine-linked causes for inflammatory bowel disease received much media attention. As each new claim appeared, work was subsequently published that failed to confirm the earlier findings.[36-52] The publication of each report that failed to confirm the earlier claims attracted less media interest than the original claims, leaving the impression that the putative associations with vaccination were robust.[53]

In 1998, new claims were made that there was an association between MMR immunization, bowel disease, and autism.[54] Although the authors were careful to say that their findings did not confirm a causal association, the media reported the findings as if the study had implicated the vaccine. At a press conference timed to coincide with the publication, one of the paper's authors stated that he believed that autism and bowel disease might be preventable by separating MMR and giving its ingredient vaccines singly with year-long intervals between doses. There remains no published epidemiologic or virologic evidence that confirms a causal association between MMR vaccine and autism. Numerous studies using different populations and different analytic techniques have failed to confirm any increased risk of autism or bowel disease in association with MMR.[55-65]

Since 1997, there has often been high media interest in MMR, culminating in early 2002 when the public and political focus became intense, with calls for either withdrawal of the vaccine or replacement with single-component vaccines in place of MMR. Vaccine coverage and public confidence in the safety of MMR have both been adversely affected, with coverage falling from 92% to 93% in the late 1990s to 83% in 2002.[66,67] During 2001 and 2002, it became clear that those opposed to the use of MMR vaccine were adopting a new strategy: the results of studies that challenged the safety of MMR were released to the media before exposure to the scientific community, exacerbating the public perception of risk from the vaccine without any opportunity to evaluate the quality of the work.[68]

The DH in London has adopted a clear strategy to respond to the threats to the MMR immunization program. New information materials have been prepared and disseminated widely to health professionals, and matching materials have been prepared for parents. Immunization coordinators have local responsibility for implementation of immunization services and are briefed with all new materials as they become available. Newspaper and radio advertisements have been used to direct parents to sources for these information materials. In addition to making information available on existing DH and allied web sites, a new site dedicated to MMR has been set up with a facility for parents to send in their MMR-based questions (see *www.mmrthefacts.nhs.uk*). In 2002, the 20 English health districts with the lowest MMR coverage were identified and each was required to submit an MMR Action Plan for approval, and then was funded to take forward locality-based initiatives designed to improve coverage.

Despite pressure from the media and parents for single vaccines to be made available to allow parents to choose whether their children would have MMR or single vaccines, these remain available only outside of the National Childhood Immunization Programme, and many of the products are unlicensed. Throughout the time of the campaign against MMR, there has been strong political support for the vaccine, despite intense media-driven pressure.

Contraindications to Vaccination

Recommendations on contraindications used in the majority of European countries correspond with the recommendations of the WHO,[69] the (UK) Joint Committee on Vaccination and Immunisation,[70] the French National Immunization Committee,[71] or the U.S. Advisory Committee on Immunisation Practices.[72] There are still some European countries recommending long lists of contraindications whose application may act as a disincentive for the successful implementation of immunization. The newly independent states of the former USSR have continued to use very elaborate lists of contraindications, but efforts are being made to reduce these. The increasing exchange of information with the WHO, the United Nations Children's Fund, other European countries, and the United States and Canada has helped to give reassurance to health professionals in countries where the long lists were used that they can shorten the list of contraindications without compromising safety.

Polio in Europe

The current 51 member states of WHO EURO had set out to eliminate indigenous transmission of wild polioviruses in Europe by 2000, a goal reconfirmed at the 1999 World Health Assembly. In the years preceding 1997, there were 180 to 250 cases of polio reported every year in the European Region as a result of ongoing circulation of indigenous strains of wild-type polioviruses as well as epidemics caused by imported viruses. During 1998, there were 26 confirmed polio cases in only one country of the European Region (Turkey). The last reported case of polio in Europe caused by indigenous virus occurred in southeastern Turkey on November 26, 1998.

Full implementation of the WHO strategies of polio eradication has been needed to reach the current polio-free status. However, recent outbreaks in Bulgaria and Georgia from importations have highlighted the need to maintain high levels of surveillance for acute flaccid paralysis and remain on alert to the risk of further importation of poliovirus from outside the European Region. In both of these cases, the virus was found to be of north Indian origin. On June 21, 2002, the European Regional Certification Commission declared Europe as polio free. After the Americas in 1994 and the Western Pacific in 2000, this is the third WHO region of the world to be certified polio free.

This success has been achieved mainly through well-coordinated biannual national immunization campaigns, collectively known as Operation MECACAR, that included all high-risk countries in the WHO European and Eastern Mediterranean Regions and covering annually up to 65 million children under 4 to 5 years of age. However, not all countries have been able to implement acute flaccid paralysis surveillance, or elected to offer other forms of surveillance to demonstrate the absence of polio. In Finland, environmental surveillance was the mainstay of evidence of lack of polio; the UK, the Netherlands, and France submitted surveillance of enteroviruses and other supportive evidence to show lack of polioviruses in the face of sensitive virologic surveillance. This effort is complemented with a surveillance system for acute flaccid paralysis in much of the remainder of the region, supported by a regional laboratory network permitting identification and classification of poliovirus strains.

Examples of European Country Immunization Programs

Examples of immunization programs in four countries, each representing a group of countries with similar programs, are described in this section:

  United Kingdom—an industrially highly developed western European country with a national health service in which provision and financing of the childhood immunization program is entirely within the public sector

  Bulgaria—an eastern European country in economic transition, with a national health service in which provision and financing of the immunization program is mainly within the public sector and national health insurance

  Kyrgyzstan—a newly independent state of the former USSR in economic transition, with a national health service in which provision and financing is mainly within the public sector; highlights include a measles-rubella (MR) vaccination campaign and adjustment of immunization schedules to respond to epidemiologic needs and changing vaccine availability

  Turkey—a country in economic transition bridging Europe and Asia

The account for the UK is expanded to describe in greater detail the particular operational changes that have been effected and that have been associated with significant improvements in program performance.

United Kingdom

Since 1948, the UK has had a National Health Service that provides free health care for all UK residents. Every individual is registered with a GP who provides primary care and, if appropriate, referral to appropriate specialists. All childhood immunizations and nationally recommended immunizations for adults, such as influenza vaccine, are provided free; only certain travel vaccines are paid for by the recipient. No immunizations are compulsory.

At the same time that a child's birth is reported, a duplicate notification alerts the local health authority, which in turn allocates the child to a GP, usually the same as that providing primary care for the mother. This process enrolls the child onto the local health authority computerized database that will schedule the immunizations, calculate local coverage, identify defaulters, and arrange payments for the GPs. By the time a newborn child is 10 days old, the parents will have been visited by the health visitor, a nurse who provides community child health services. The health visitor discusses immunization arrangements with the parents and seeks their consent for the child to be entered into a computer-based program, thereby satisfying data protection requirements. Consent is almost universal.[73] By the time the child is around 6 weeks old, the local health authority computer has issued an invitation for the first immunization, sent by mail to the parents, and alerted the GP or local health clinic of the date and time scheduled for the child's immunizations and the antigens needed. Invitations for subsequent immunizations are issued in the same way. After attendance for immunization, the GP submits a completed form to the local computer unit, triggering the next step in the process. After two or three defaulted invitations (according to local practice), the GP and health visitor are alerted, allowing active follow-up to establish why the child has not attended the local clinic for immunization. In some circumstances, especially for gypsy families, domiciliary immunization may be provided.

In 1987, as part of a review of immunization services in England, Peckham noted that coverage was among the lower third of that reported by European countries.[74] A decade later, in 1997, coverage for the UK by the second birthday was 96% for diphtheria, tetanus, polio, and Hib vaccines; 94% for pertussis vaccine; and 91% for MMR vaccine[75]—among the highest in Europe.

It remains difficult to identify the specific contributions that have led to these considerable improvements because many aspects of the provision of immunization services have been changed during this time.[76] These improvements have included

  • The payment of GPs only when they reach coverage targets
  • Improvements in the computerized tracking system making it better able to identify and follow up defaulters

- Widespread dissemination of up-to-date guidelines on immunization theory and practice, sent free to all health care professionals involved in immunization
- Appointment of immunization coordinators in each health district
- Acceleration of the timing of scheduled immunizations
- The development of a national immunization communication strategy

Starting in 1986, efforts were made to ensure that every health district had an immunization coordinator. These health professionals were usually consultants in public health medicine; some were pediatricians, some nurses or administrators. The main requirement was the suitability of the individual to ensure the effective implementation of immunization services at local levels. Coordinators are expected to oversee the computerized immunization programs, the training in immunization of health professionals in primary care and health authorities, and the production of quarterly statistical returns, and take the local lead in introducing new strategies or new vaccines. The DH maintains a database of coordinators and organizes regular national meetings to update coordinators, exchange experiences, and provide training.

Since 1986, at 2- to 4-year intervals, the DH has issued updated national guidance on immunization, sent free to all medical practitioners irrespective of specialty, and to all general practice nurses, health visitors, and nurses in community child health. The guidance document covers practical immunization topics as well as providing detailed information on individual vaccines. Special emphasis has been placed on reducing "false contraindications" and clarifying causally related adverse events versus those likely to occur by chance, unrelated to immunization. This publication—*Immunization Against Infectious Disease*—is recognized as the standard reference for immunization policy and practice in the UK.[70]

Following a detailed review of immunization services undertaken by the British Market Research Bureau,[77] factors were identified that were contributing to the achievement of high coverage in some districts as opposed to low coverage in others with similar demographic features. Effective use of computerized services, training, and active participation of GPs were associated with high coverage. Despite efforts to control for social and demographic factors, these remained powerful influences in predicting low coverage. High mobility of young inner-city families was notable because this compounded any deficiencies in information services in tracking children. The schedule for primary immunization in place at the time (3, 4.5, and 8 to 11 months) was associated with high dropout rates, especially in inner cities. Based on an analysis of operational factors, the national schedule for DTP and polio (and subsequently Hib) immunization was accelerated to 2, 3, and 4 months with no booster doses until school entry. This change, in May 1990, led to higher coverage achieved at an earlier age.[78]

In 1990, the then–Secretary of State for Health asked for a new scheme to be developed for payment of GPs that emphasized their responsibilities for disease prevention and health promotion. Before this time, GPs had been paid for immunization on an "item-for-service" basis: each immu-

nization was awarded a payment after submission of an appropriate claim form. However, the payment for individual immunizations was relatively small and the claim process was protracted. Because submission of the claim forms was sometimes used for scheduling and tracking purposes, any delays in claim processing obstructed the immunization program. The new scheme replaced the item-for-service payments with a target-based scheme. Now, each quarter, doctors are required to show that coverage targets have been reached for specified cohorts for all age-appropriate immunizations. The targets are 70% and 90% coverage for all immunizations by age 2 years, with similar targets for preschool booster immunizations. All children registered with a GP are included; the quarterly numerator is the number of fully immunized children, and the denominator is the number of resident children reaching their second birthday in the quarter. No exclusions from the denominator population are allowed, even children with valid contraindications. Despite many publicly voiced concerns at the outset of the scheme that the targets were unattainable, data from the payments records show that the majority of GPs regularly reach the higher target payments. For a GP with an average-size population of children, the target payments, on an annual basis, are approximately $1100 for reaching 70% coverage by the second birthday for all primary series immunizations, and a further $3500 for reaching or exceeding 90% coverage. Respective payments for the preschool immunizations are $375 and $1100. These payments represent 5% to 7.5% of GPs' salaries. Since the introduction of the scheme, there had been a continuous improvement in the proportion of GPs hitting coverage targets until the recent decline in MMR coverage.

The results of the scheme, presented in Figure 54–5, show progressive shifts to higher proportions of GPs reaching the higher payment level targets. The data for the first 2 years of the scheme show that the 10 localities with the greatest increases in higher target attainment (Barking, Barnet, Bradford, Cleveland, Enfield, Gateshead, Lancashire, Manchester, Salford, and Sandwell) were predominantly inner city localities, or otherwise associated with high unemployment, poor housing, and young families or single parents. A scheme that provided powerful motivation for immunization providers was able to overcome many of the obstacles to the achievement of high coverage.

The DH now has the public and health professional communication work embedded within the Immunization Programme group to implement the national immunization communication strategy. The DH provides resources of around $2 million annually as baseline funding for communication, increasing this when necessary. For example, a high-profile advertising campaign in advance of the MCC vaccine introduction cost a further $2.5 million, mostly spent on television advertising, as well as newspaper and magazine materials. The annual funding provides for information materials on immunization given to every mother of a newborn infant, posters for public places, and regular television advertising. The advertising materials are developed by commercial-sector advertising agencies. Twice a year, using commercial-sector market researchers, at least 1000 mothers of young children are interviewed to investigate their knowledge of and attitudes about immunization and to examine their awareness of recent immunization

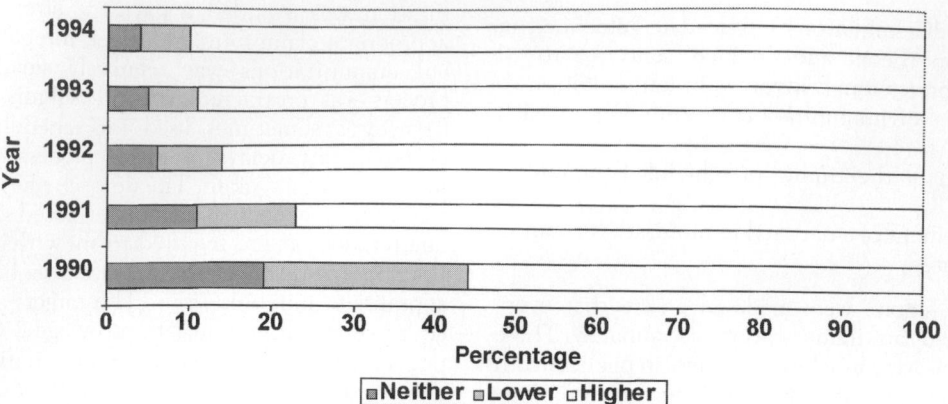

FIGURE 54–5 ■ The proportion of UK general practitioners that reached target payment levels, 1990 to 1994. "Neither" indicates neither target payment level was reached; "lower" indicates lower target payment level was reached; and "higher," higher target payment level was reached. (Data from the Department of Health, London.)

advertising. A smaller sample of mothers (500) was interviewed between the most recent main samples with questions focusing especially on MMR vaccine. The results of these studies[66] are used by the DH in shaping immunization promotion initiatives.

Before 1992, some vaccines were purchased centrally and provided free to users, central funding was disbursed to local authorities for some vaccine purchases against centrally negotiated prices, and other vaccines were purchased through local funds. After an internal review of these funding arrangements, agreement was reached for all vaccines to be purchased from central funds and be provided free to all users. The financial savings from bulk purchasing were used to contract with a commercial-sector distribution company that specialized in refrigerated delivery services. Since September 1992, all deliveries of vaccines are in cold chain–guaranteed circumstances from manufacturer to end user. GPs now receive their vaccines on a weekly basis, reducing wastage from stocking unnecessary quantities of vaccines. Because the whole delivery system is computer controlled, detailed information on the cold chain is available continuously and the whereabouts of every dose of vaccine can be accounted for, should any form of product recall be needed.

The present UK immunization program priorities, and ambitions for the future, have recently been reviewed.[10]

Bulgaria—Health Reform and High-Risk Groups

Bulgaria is situated in southeastern Europe, in the eastern part of the Balkan Peninsula. Its neighboring countries are Romania (north), the former Republic of Yugoslavia (west), the former Yugoslav Republic of Macedonia (southwest), Greece (south), and Turkey (southeast). In 2000, its population totaled 7.9 million, with 67.5% living in urban areas. The country is strategically placed as a crossroad of key land routes from Europe to the Middle East and Asia.[79]

After the democratic changes that took place at the end of 1989, and the establishment of market-oriented economics, there was a need for an in-depth reform of the whole health care system, including preventative services. To address this need, in the latter half of 2000, a new system of outpatient services was put in place, based on health insurance funds and with GPs as the main providers, who since

then were assigned to provide all immunization activities. Such a new immunization delivery system, relying mainly on individual practices, did not facilitate reaching certain minority groups that represent at least 13% of the country's population.[80] Table 54–4 shows the differences in immunization coverage of some of the minority groups, compared with the national coverage data for the year 2001.

In spite of the comparatively good average immunization coverage rates, the fact that the larger part of the nonimmunized population is concentrated in regions with poor living conditions that may not have heath insurance or access to a GP, or may have been outside of the civil registration system, is cause for some concern. In 2001, poliovirus from an unknown source was imported into Bulgaria and resulted in three confirmed poliomyelitis cases in one of these higher-risk populations.[81] In 1991, the previous poliomyelitis outbreak in Bulgaria also occurred in the same population, causing 46 confirmed cases.

In order to prevent recurrence of similar outbreaks, and to address the issue of low immunization coverage, the Ministry of Health undertook immediate measures to extend the reach of the immunization program through

TABLE 54–4 ■ Immunization Coverage (%) by Vaccination, Bulgaria, 1995 to 2001

Vaccine	Immunization Coverage, 2001 (%)	
	National Level*	Higher-Risk Population†
DTP3	94	79
OPV3	94	73
MMR	90	69

*Coverage of children less than 12 months of age. Data from World Health Organization, Vaccines, Immunization and Biologicals. WHO Vaccine Preventable Diseases Monitoring System: 2002 global summary. Geneva, World Health Organization, 2002. Available at www-nt.who.int./vaccines/globalsummary/immunization/

†Coverage of children less than 12 months of age. Data from a 30-cluster sample survey taken in December 2001 by the Ministry of Health, Bulgaria; presented at the WHO EURO EPI Managers meeting, Vienna, Austria, March 2002.

DTP3, three-dose regimen of diphtheria and tetanus toxoids and whole-cell pertussis vaccine; OPV3, three-dose regimen of oral poliovirus vaccine; MMR, measles-mumps-rubella vaccine.

- The creation of vaccination posts in all of the 28 Hygiene and Epidemiological Inspectorates (HEIs) of the country to ensure free access to immunization to families who have not yet chosen a GP
- The establishment of a systematic follow-up of all children at risk to complete their immunization schedule
- The launching of a national social mobilization campaign to increase population knowledge about the new health insurance system, particularly for children, and to facilitate the process of GP selection
- An active search for nonimmunized children from higher-risk populations by the GPs

A further challenge for the Ministry of Health was to provide an adequate cold chain and injection equipment for vaccination. To facilitate the communication between the HEIs, the GPs, and the regional offices of the health insurance fund, a registry of newborn children and their subsequent immunization is being established.

With such an array of measures, it is hoped that, while the new health insurance system is put in place, access to immunization for higher-risk populations will improve and reduce the chances of poliovirus transmission in case of a further importation.

Kyrgyzstan—Measles-Rubella Campaign and Adjusting Schedules

Following the breakup of the USSR, Kyrgyzstan became an independent republic in 1991. The country is located in the Central Asian Region of Europe, bordering Kazakhstan to the north, China to the east, Tajikistan to the south, and Uzbekistan to the west, and covers an area of 199,900 square kilometers. The country is administratively divided into seven oblasts with 51 districts, including the capital city of Bishkek. The first national census was conducted in 1999, estimating the population of Kyrgyzstan at 4.86 million. As in other Central Asian Region countries, infant mortality is high compared with other European countries—53 per 1000 live births in 2000.[79]

Since the breakup of the U.S.S.R., the Kyrgyz Republic has experienced the return of diseases that used to be successfully prevented by immunization. As in several other newly independent states, the number of diphtheria cases rose. Factors contributing to the diphtheria epidemic included a large population of susceptible adults, decreased childhood immunization, suboptimal socioeconomic conditions, and high population movement.[82] By 1990, "on-time" coverage of infants and young children had fallen because of resistance to immunization on the part of health care workers and the population. Many health care workers considered children to be too weak and vaccines too strong.[83,84] It was extremely common for pediatricians to diagnose temporary medical contraindications to immunization.[85] All of these factors contributed to late and incomplete childhood immunization.

To improve the situation, the Kyrgyz Republic initiated reforms in its immunization services, and the Republican Center for Immunoprophylaxis was created in 1994. This center has been implementing the 1994 to 2000 plan for the National Programme for Immunoprophylaxis, and has made substantial improvements, reaching over 98% of the children under 1 year of age in the year 2000. Mass immunization campaigns covering large target age groups were successfully organized, partly to contain the diphtheria epidemic and as part of the global eradication of poliomyelitis.

In the year 2000, in line with the regional European target to reach measles elimination by 2007, and in an effort to decrease the incidence of congenital rubella syndrome to no more than 1 case per 100,000 live births by 2010, Kyrgyzstan embarked on a multiyear strategic plan to fight these diseases. The first step was to immunize in November 2001, through fixed as well as temporary immunization posts, both males and females ages 7 to 25 years (approximately 1.9 million people) with one dose of combined MR vaccine. The second step was the introduction, in February 2002, of one dose of MMR at 12 months of age and one dose of MR at 6 years of age into the routine vaccination. It is hoped that the circulation of measles and rubella will be dramatically reduced through this strategy. The initial MR immunization campaign managed to reach over 98% of the target population 7 to 25 years of age.

To address the difficulties in accessing hard-to-reach groups, such as street children, migrant populations, people traditionally opposed to immunization, and people living in remote areas, a series of workshops was organized by the Ministry of Health at different levels of the health system. These workshops were aimed at solving communication problems and improving communication skills of service providers, identified strategies for addressing communities, and proposed ways to contact the different hard-to-reach populations. The success of this campaign depended on effective coordination of activities through a national task force of all involved-ministers, institutions, and international organizations. To follow up the impact of this effort, a case-based surveillance of measles/rubella/congenital rubella syndrome has been put in place, including the laboratory confirmation of suspected cases. Adverse events following immunization were also monitored during the campaign. Another important gain from this campaign was the conduct of a safe injection practice assessment that set national standards on safe immunization practices and trained health personnel on the issue of safe disposal of syringes and needles using information provided by the Safe Injection Global Network (SIGN) (see *www.injectionsafety.org*).

Turkey—Strengthening Routine

Turkey is situated in the southeast of Europe, divided between Europe and Asia by the Bosphorus. The European part of Turkey borders Greece and Bulgaria and the Asian part borders Armenia, Azerbaijan, Georgia, Iraq, and Syria. In 2000, the population of Turkey was 67.6 million, with 40% living in rural areas. The country is divided into 79 provinces with considerable developmental and economic variations from west to east. In 2000, infant mortality was estimated to be 38 per 1000 live births.[79]

The National Immunization Programme is integrated into primary health care and is the responsibility of the Ministry of Health. Midwives in health centers distributed all over the country carry out immunizations. Mobile teams also exist to undertake immunizations in villages or regions without proper health care personnel. Current reform efforts aim to decentralize primary health care further and allocate each family to a private practitioner. Immunization coverage data have been available since the mid-1970s, with figures for DTP3 at around 55% up to the mid-1980s, when coverage started to rise. Since that date, DTP3 coverage has been oscillating around 80%, with a minimum of 66% in 1995 and a maximum of 88% in 2001. In spite of this reasonable overall coverage, large variations exist between provinces, particularly in the eastern and southeastern part of the country, with figures well below 50% in some areas. In the fall of 1998, the last chains of wild-type poliovirus transmission were interrupted. This was achieved through supplemental OPV house-to-house mopping-up operations, which demonstrated that previously never-reached populations could be immunized, and which provided good opportunities to re-evaluate the routine immunization strategies.

In 2001, the national authorities decided to apply similar strategies to the provision of routine vaccination, organizing outreach activities at least four times a year to provide all EPI vaccines to children less than 5 years of age and tetanus toxoid (TT) to pregnant women: The target was coverage of at least 90%. Depending on the existing coverage, different approaches were used: if coverage was less than 50%, a nonselective vaccination of all children under 5 was undertaken; if coverage was over 50%, catch-up immunization programs were provided. If no records were available, children were considered unvaccinated. Essential for the success of this operation was intensive microplanning, using detailed maps of identified areas with difficult access and seasonal isolation. Vaccination teams were sent even to the smallest cluster of houses in rural areas. Another important element was the organization of a strong advocacy component to secure the support of local authorities, involving local teachers as well as religious and elected village and neighborhood leaders. This acceleration program was also an opportunity to retrain health staff, improve logistical support, and obtain more political support for immunization.

The impact of such efforts translated to an increase at the national level of DTP3 coverage from 79% (in 1999) to 88% (in 2001) (Fig. 54-6), and of measles coverage from 81% to 84%, respectively. The most impressive impact was in the reduction of the number of provinces with less than 80% coverage from 26 in 1999 to 17 in 2001.[86] During the same time, in the southeastern part of the country, the number of doses of DTP3 provided increased by 35% and the number of provinces with less than 50% coverage decreased from 10 to 2 (see Fig. 54-6).

In spite of this success, some constraints still remain, particularly regarding the difficulties in accessing women for TT vaccination, as well as in ensuring that training diffuses down to the lowest operational level and that supervision is regularly performed. These constraints will need to be further addressed and routine immunization services improved if the anticipated measles and tetanus elimination efforts are to succeed.

The Future for Immunization in Europe

At present, there is little evidence of significant movement to harmonize immunization policies, where schedules are

1999

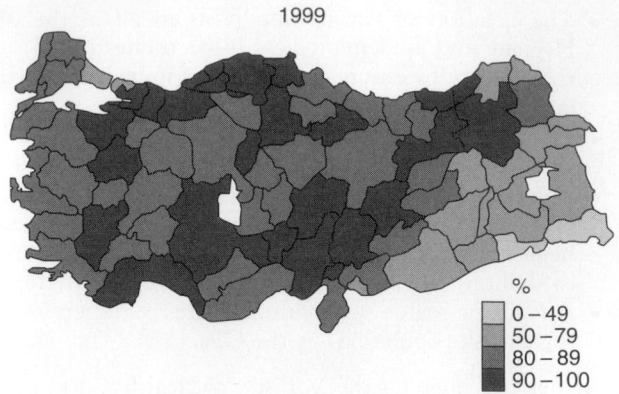

%
0 – 49
50 – 79
80 – 89
90 – 100

2001

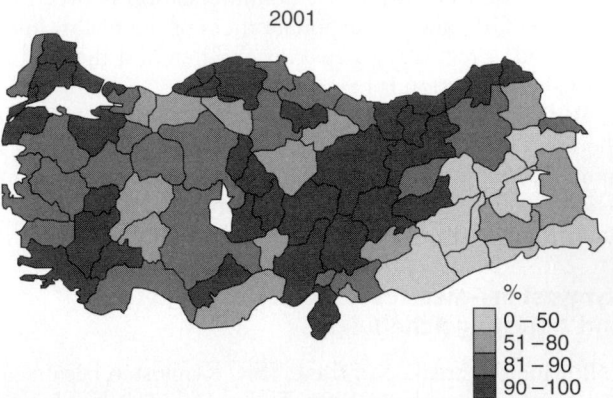

%
0 – 50
51 – 80
81 – 90
90 – 100

FIGURE 54–6 ■ DTP3/OPV3 vaccination coverage among children less than 1 year of age, Turkey, 1999 and 2001 (data from Ministry of Health, Turkey).

concerned, within EU countries. Changing schedules is disruptive and costly and unlikely to be undertaken simply for harmonization purposes when there would be no perceived gain to the countries. However, there are clear advantages to industry from a single market. Thus some harmonization may occur as a consequence of the introduction of new vaccines. For example, the immunization schedule used in Denmark was very different from that used anywhere else. Following a change from whole-cell to acellular pertussis vaccine in 1997, the Danish schedule has been modified and is now very similar to that used in Sweden. Schedules and vaccines used in the northern and western countries are likely to reflect higher public health importance placed on antimeningitis vaccines, whereas southern countries have higher priority for hepatitis B vaccine combinations. It is possible, therefore, that some approximation of policies will follow the availability of new vaccines, but differences are likely to persist, reflecting different disease priorities and different systems of health care provision.

There are already marked differences between the vaccines purchased in EU countries, those purchased in central European countries, and those purchased in countries of the former USSR. For the most part, these reflect the different economic situations and may well become more exaggerated with increasing prices for new vaccines from multinational suppliers. Novel funding initiatives, such as the revolving fund mechanisms developed by the Pan American Health Organization,[87] may be needed to permit continuity of existing vaccines and introduction of new vaccines for a number of European countries.

REFERENCES

1. World Health Organisation, Expanded Programme on Immunisation. Immunization schedules in the WHO European Region, 1995. Wkly Epidemiol Rec 70:221–227, 1995.
2. Guérin N, Roure C. Immunisation schedules in the countries of the European Union. Eurosurveill Monthly 0:5–7, 1995.
3. Guérin N, Roure C. Immunisation coverage in the European Union. Eurosurveill Monthly 2:2–4, 1997.
4. Computerized Information System for Infectious Diseases. Immunization schedules and coverage. Copenhagen, World Health Organization Regional Office for Europe, 2003. Available at cisid.who.dk/VIP/Imm
5. Osborne K, Weinberg J, Miller E. The European Sero-Epidemiology Network. Eurosurveill Monthly 2:29–31, 1997.
6. Miller E, Salisbury DM, Ramsay ME. Planning, registration, and implementation of an immunisation campaign against meningococcal serogroup C disease in the UK: a success story. Vaccine 20(suppl 1):S58–S67, 2001.
7. Guiver M, Borrow R, Marsh J, et al. Evaluation of the Applied Biosystems Automated Taqman PCR system for the detection of meningococcal DNA. FEMS Immunol Med Microbiol 20:173–179, 2000.
8. Davison KL, Ramsay ME, Crowcroft NS, et al. Estimating the burden of serogroup C meningococcal disease in England and Wales. Commun Dis Public Health 5:213–219, 2002.
9. Ramsay M, Kaczmarski E, Rush M, et al. Changing patterns of case ascertainment and trends in meningococcal disease in England and Wales. Commun Dis Rep CDR Rev 7:R49–R54, 1997.
10. Salisbury DM, Beverley PCL, Miller E. Vaccine programmes and policies. Br Med Bull 62:201–211, 2002.
11. Enhanced surveillance of suspected meningococcal disease. Commun Dis Rep CDR Wkly 9:78–79, 1999.
12. Fairley CK, Begg NT, Borrow R, et al. Reactogenicity and immunogenicity of conjugate meningococcal serogroup A and C vaccine in UK infants. J Infect Dis 174:1360–1363, 1996.
13. Richmond PC, Miller E, Borrow R, et al. Meningococcal serogroup C conjugate vaccine is immunogenic in infancy and primes for memory. J Infect Dis 179:1569–1572, 1999.
14. Borrow R, Fox AJ, Richmond PC, et al. Induction of immunological memory in UK infants by a meningococcal A/C conjugate vaccine. Epidemiol Infect 124:427–432, 2000.
15. Richmond P, Borrow R, Findlow J, et al. Evaluation of de-O-acetylated meningococcal C polysaccharide-tetanus toxoid conjugate vaccine in infancy: reactogenicity, immunogenicity, immunologic priming and bactericidal activity against O-acetylated and de-O-acetylated serogroup C strains. Infect Immun 69:2378–2382, 2001.
16. Ho MM, Bolgiano B, Corbel MJ. Assessment of the stability and immunogenicity of meningococcal oligosaccharide C-CRM$_{197}$ conjugate vaccines. Vaccine 19:716–725, 2000.
17. Ho MM, Lemercinier X, Bolgiano B, et al. Solution stability studies of the subunit components of meningococcal oligosaccharide C-CRM$_{197}$ conjugate vaccines. Biotechnol Appl Biochem 33:91–98, 2001.
18. Choo S, Zuckerman J, Goilav C, et al. Immunogenicity and reactogenicity of a group C meningococcal conjugate vaccine compared with a group A+C meningococcal polysaccharide vaccine in adolescents in a randomised observer-blind controlled trial. Vaccine 18:2686–2692, 2000.
19. MacLennan JM, Shackley F, Heath PT, et al. Safety, immunogenicity and induction of immunologic memory by a serogroup C meningococcal conjugate vaccine in infants: a randomised controlled trial. JAMA 283:2795–2801, 2000.
20. Bramley JC, Hall T, Finn A, et al. Safety and immunogenicity of three lots of meningococcal serogroup C conjugate vaccine administered at 2, 3, and 4 months of age. Vaccine 19:2934–2931, 2001.
21. English M, MacLennan JM, Bowen-Morris JM, et al. A randomized, double-blind, controlled trial of the immunogenicity and tolerability of a meningococcal serogroup C conjugate vaccine in young British infants. Vaccine 19:1232–1238, 2001.
22. Dobson F. "My Pride and Joy." Daily Telegraph, January 5, 2001.
23. Ramsay ME, Andrews N, Kaczmarski EB, Miller E. Efficacy of meningococcal serogroup C conjugate vaccine in teenagers and toddlers in England. Lancet 357:195–196, 2001.
24. Trotter CL, Ramsay ME, Kaczmarski EB. Meningococcal serogroup C conjugate vaccination in England and Wales: coverage and initial impact of the campaign. Commun Dis Public Health 5:220–225, 2002.
25. Maiden MC, Stuart JM. Carriage of serogroup C meningococci 1 year after meningococcal C conjugate polysaccharide vaccination. Lancet 359:1829–1831, 2002.
26. Medicines Control Agency/Committee on Safety of Medicines. Safety of meningococcal group C conjugate vaccines. Curr Probl Pharmacovigilance 26:14, 2000.
27. Expanded Programme on Immunization (EPI): lack of evidence that hepatitis B vaccine causes multiple sclerosis. Wkly Epidemiol Rec 72:149–152, 1997.
28. World Health Organization. No scientific justification to suspend hepatitis B immunization. Press release, World Health Organization, 1998. Available at www.who.int/inf-pr-1998/en/pr98-67.html
29. Mission d'expertise sur la politique de vaccination contre l'hepatite B en France. Paris, Ministère de l'Emploi et de la Solidarité, 2002. Available at www.sante.gouv.fr/htm/pointsur/vaccins/dartigues.pdf
30. Wakefield AJ, Pittilo RM, Sim R. Evidence of persistent measles virus infection in Crohn's disease. J Med Virol 39:345–353, 1993.
31. Wakefield AJ, Ekbom A, Dhillon AP, et al. Crohn's disease: pathogenesis and persistent measles virus infection. Gastroenterology 108:911–916, 1995.
32. Thompson NP, Montgomery SM, Pounder RE, Wakefield AJ. Is measles a risk factor for inflammatory bowel disease? Lancet 345:1071–1074, 1995.
33. Thompson NP, Pounder RE, Wakefield AJ. Perinatal and childhood risk factors for inflammatory bowel disease: a case-control study. Eur J Gastroenterol Hepatol 7:385–390, 1995.
34. Ekbom A, Daszak P, Kraaz W, Wakefield AJ. Crohn's disease after in-utero measles virus exposure. Lancet 348:515–517, 1996.
35. Daszak P, Purcell M, Lewin J, et al. Detection and comparative analysis of persistent measles virus infection in Crohn's disease by immunogold electron microscopy. J Clin Pathol 50:299–304, 1997.
36. Iizuka M, Nakagomi O, Chiba M, et al. Absence of measles virus in Crohn's disease. Lancet 345:199, 1995.
37. Minor P. Measles vaccination as a risk factor for inflammatory bowel disease. Lancet 345:1362–1363, 1995.
38. Farrington P, Miller E. Measles vaccination as a risk factor for inflammatory bowel disease. Lancet 345:1362, 1995.
39. MacDonald T. Measles vaccination as a risk factor for inflammatory bowel disease. Lancet 345:1363, 1995.
40. Haga Y, Funakoshi O, Kuroe K, et al. Absence of measles vital genomic sequence in intestinal tissues from Crohn's disease by nested polymerase chain reaction. Gut 38:211–215, 1996.
41. Iizuka M, Masamune O. Measles vaccination and inflammatory bowel disease. Lancet 350:1775, 1997.
42. Feeney M, Ciegg A, Winwood P, Snook J. A case control study of measles vaccination and inflammatory bowel disease. Lancet 350:764–766, 1997.
43. Jones P, Fine P, Piracha S. Crohn's disease and measles. Lancet 349:473, 1997.
44. Afzal MA, Minor PD, Begley J, et al. Absence of measles-virus genome in inflammatory bowel disease. Lancet 351:646–467, 1998.
45. Chadwick N, Bruce IJ, Schepelmann S, et al. Measles virus RNA is not detected in inflammatory bowel disease using hybrid capture and reverse transcription followed by the polymerase chain reaction. J Med Virol 55:305–311, 1998.
46. Miller E, Waight R. Second immunisation has not affected IBD incidence in England. BMJ 316:1745, 1998.
47. Pebody RG, Paunio M, Ruutu P. Crohn's disease has not increased in Finland. BMJ 316:1745, 1998.
48. Nielsen LL, Nielsen NM, Melbye M, et al. Exposure to measles in utero and Crohn's disease: Danish register study. BMJ 316:196–197, 1998.
49. Lawrenson R, Farmer R. Age-specific prevalences do not suggest association with in utero exposure. BMJ 316:1746, 1998.
50. Afzal MA, Armitage E, Ghosh S, et al. Further evidence of absence of measles virus genome sequence in full thickness intestinal specimens from patients with Crohn's disease. J Med Virol 62:377–382, 2000.
51. Iizuka M, Chiba M, Yukawa M, et al. Immunohistochemical analysis of the distribution of measles-related antigen in the intestinal mucosa in IBD. Gut 46:163–169, 2000.
52. Davis RL, Kramarz P, Bohlke K, et al. Measles-mumps-rubella and other measles-containing vaccines do not increase the risk for inflammatory bowel disease. Arch Pediatr Adolesc Med 155:354–359, 2001.
53. Editor's Choice. BMJ 316(7133):715–716, 1998.
54. Wakefield A, Murch SH, Anthony A, et al. Ileal-lymphoid-nodular hyperplasia, non-specific colitis, and pervasive developmental disorder in children. Lancet 351:637–641, 1998.

55. Gillberg C, Heijbel H. MMR and autism. Autism 2:423–424, 1998.

56. Peltola H, Patja A, Leinkki P, et al. No evidence for measles, mumps, and rubella vaccine-associated inflammatory bowel disease or autism in a 14-year prospective study. Lancet 351:1327–1328, 1998.

57. Taylor B, Miller E, Farrington CP, et al. Autism and measles, mumps and rubella: no epidemiological evidence for a causal association. Lancet 353:2026–2029, 1999.

58. Fombonne E, Chakrabarti S. No evidence for a new variant of measles-mumps-rubella-induced autism. Pediatrics 108(suppl 4):E58, 2001.

59. Medical Research Council. MRC Review of Autism Research: Epidemiology and Causes. London, Medical Research Council, 2001. Available at www.mrc.ac.uk/pdf-autism-report.pdf

60. Dales L, Hammer SJ, Smith NJ. Time trends in autism and in MMR immunization coverage in California. JAMA 285:1183–1185, 2001.

61. Farrington CP, Miller E, Taylor B. MMR and autism: further evidence against a causal association. Vaccine 19:3632–3665, 2001.

62. Gershon M. Autism and the measles-mumps-rubella (MMR) vaccine. Rev Vacunas 2:156–157, 2002.

63. Taylor B, Miller E, Lingam R, et al. Measles, mumps, and rubella vaccination and bowel problems or developmental regression in children with autism: population study. BMJ 324:393–396, 2002.

64. Madsen KM, Hviid A, Vestergaard M, et al. A population-based study of measles, mumps, and rubella vaccination and autism. N Engl J Med 347:1477–1482, 2002.

65. Mäkelä A, Nuorti P, Peltola H. Neurologic disorders after measles-mumps-rubella vaccination. Pediatrics 110:957–963, 2002.

66. Ramsay ME, Yarwood J, Lewis D, et al. Parental confidence in measles, mumps, and rubella vaccine: evidence from vaccine coverage and attitudinal surveys. Br J Gen Pract 52:912–916, 2002.

67. Effects of media reporting on MMR coverage. Commun Dis Rep CDR Wkly 12(35):30, 2002.

68. Uhlmann V, Martin CM, Sheils O, et al. Potential viral pathogenic mechanism for new variant inflammatory bowel disease. J Clin Pathol Mol Pathol 55:84–90, 2002.

69. Expanded Programme on Immunisation. Contraindications for vaccines used in EPI. Wkly Epidemiol Rec 37:279–281, 1988.

70. Salisbury DM, Begg NT (eds). Immunisation Against Infectious Disease. London, Her Majesty's Stationery Office, 1996.

71. Guide des Vaccinations, Edition 1995. Direction Générale de la Santé, Comité Technique des Vaccinations, Paris, 1995, pp 17–21.

72. Centers for Disease Control and Prevention. General recommendations on immunization: recommendations of the Advisory Committee on Immunization Practices (ACIP) and the American Academy of Family Physicians (AAFP). MMWR 51(RR-02):1–36, 2002.

73. Simpson N, Lenton S, Randall R. Parental refusal to have children immunised: extent and reasons. BMJ 310:227, 1995.

74. The Peckham Report. National Immunisation Study: Factors Influencing Immunisation Uptake in Childhood. London, Department of Paediatric Epidemiology, Institute of Child Health/Horsham, West Sussex, Action Research for the Crippled Child, 1989.

75. COVER programme: October to December 1997. Commun Dis Rep CDR Wkly 8:116, 1998. Available at www.phls.org.uk/publications/cdr/CDR98/cdr1398.pdf

76. White JM, Gillam SJ, Begg NT, Farrington CP. Vaccine coverage: recent trends and future prospects. BMJ 304:682–684, 1992.

77. The Uptake of Pre-school Immunisation in England: Report on a National Study of Variation in Immunisation Uptake Between District Health Authorities. London, British Market Research Bureau, 1989.

78. White JM, Hobday S, Begg NT. "COVER" (Cover of vaccination evaluated rapidly): 19. Commun Dis Rep CDR Rev 1:R140, 1991.

79. United Nations Development Programme. Human Development Report 2002. New York, Oxford University Press, 2002.

80. Turner B ed. The Statesman's Yearbook 2000. London, Macmillan, 2000.

81. Computerized Information System for Infectious Diseases. Imported wild poliovirus causing poliomyelitis, Bulgaria, 2001. Copenhagen, World Health Organization Regional Office for Europe, 2001. Available at cisid.who.dk/Csr/outbreaks/ Outbreak Detail.asp? OSID= 14411

82. Vitek CR, Wharton M. Diphtheria in the former Soviet Union: reemergence of a pandemic disease. Emerg Infect Dis 4:539–550, 1998.

83. Keith N. Baseline Research for Development of a National Immunization Behavior Change Strategy in Kyrgyzstan, 1 November–1 December 1994. Arlington, VA, BASICS, 1995.

84. Steinglass R, Rodewald L. Balancing science and practice for child immunization in Russia and the USA. Presented at the 31st National Immunization Conference, Detroit, 19–22 May 1997.

85. Weeks RM, Firsova S, Seitkazieva N, Gaidamako V. Improving the monitoring of immunization services in Kyrgystan. Health Policy Plan 15:279–286, 2000.

86. Yalniz C, for the Ministry of Health, Turkey. Vaccination strategies to reach difficult areas. Presentation at WHO sub-regional meeting of EPI Managers, Vienna, Austria, February 2002.

87. EPI in the Americas: benefits from revolving fund. WHO Chronicle 37:81–85, 1983.

Chapter 55

Vaccination Programs in Developing Countries

STEPHEN C. HADLER • STEPHEN L. COCHI • JULIAN BILOUS • FELICITY T. CUTTS

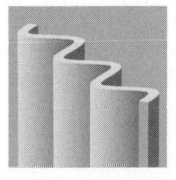

Since the late 1970s, childhood immunization has become one of the most effective and cost-effective public health preventive measures in both developing and developed countries.[1] Globally, 70% of children are now estimated to receive the traditional primary childhood vaccination series of bacille Calmette-Guérin (BCG), oral poliovirus vaccine (OPV), diphtheria and tetanus toxoids and whole-cell pertussis (DTP), and measles vaccines. By the end of 2001, 142 countries had introduced routine hepatitis B (HepB) vaccine, and 90 had introduced *Haemophilus influenzae* type b (Hib) conjugate vaccine for infants.[2] Childhood vaccination is estimated to prevent more than 2 million deaths from measles, pertussis, and neonatal tetanus each year. Nevertheless, at current levels of coverage, diseases preventable by these vaccines still cause 2.4 million deaths annually (Fig. 55–1), and in 2001 represented 9% of the global disease burden in terms of disability-adjusted life-years (DALYs) among children younger than 5 years (ranging from 12% in sub-Saharan Africa to less than 1% in established market economies).[3,4] Had immunization coverage levels remained at the low levels of the 1970s, the traditional childhood diseases alone would have caused 23% of disease burden in this age group.[5] The certification of poliomyelitis eradication in the American, Western Pacific, and European Regions of the World Health Organization (WHO) in 1994, 2000, and 2002 respectively, combined with recent success toward measles elimination in the Americas and measles mortality reduction in Africa, have renewed interest from countries and partner agencies in supporting immunization programs.[2,6] The launching in 2000 of the Global Alliance for Vaccines and Immunization (GAVI) has helped to create a global partnership to support and sustain this renewed interest.[7] Despite these successes, the resurgence of diphtheria in the former Soviet Union in the early 1990s,[8–11] increasing spread of yellow fever in Africa,[12,13] and continuing high morbidity and mortality from hepatitis B, measles, pertussis, and neonatal tetanus in the poorest countries of Africa and Southeast Asia[4,14,15] emphasize the need for continued vigilance and support for vaccination programs. At the same time, an increasing number of vaccines against major infectious diseases are becoming available, but new vaccines are unaffordable in the poorest countries without substantial donor support.[7]

Policies for vaccination programs in member states of the United Nations are made by national governments, and usually follow recommendations by the global Expanded Programme on Immunisation (EPI), which was established by the WHO in 1974.[1] The vaccines recommended by EPI for inclusion in routine childhood immunization schedules are BCG, OPV, DTP, HepB, and measles vaccines; yellow fever vaccine is recommended in countries endemic for this disease, and Hib conjugate vaccine is recommended in countries with high disease burden.[2] In certain developing countries, vaccines against diseases of local importance, such as Japanese encephalitis virus vaccine, are included in the national vaccination program,[16] whereas others such as rabies are used in special circumstances.

In this chapter, we first review policies and strategies relating to the vaccines included in the EPI. We discuss methods used to monitor and evaluate vaccination. We discuss current progress and future trends in immunization services, and conclude with a summary of the major challenges to be faced, in light of the changing political, socioeconomic, and health services context of vaccination programs around the world.

Policies and Strategies for Vaccines Included in the EPI

Immunization programs in developing countries traditionally have been organized under a centralized system, predominantly through the public sector. Thus Ministries of Health were responsible both for setting policies and norms and for managing programs. Donor support was given through the Ministries of Health that controlled the budget for immunization. Ministries of Health personnel, often

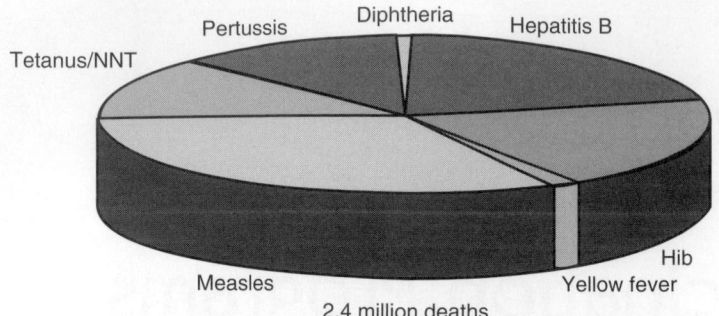

Pertussis   Diphtheria   Hepatitis B

Tetanus/NNT

Hib
Yellow fever

Measles

2.4 million deaths

FIGURE 55–1 ■ Global deaths caused by vaccine-preventable diseases, 2000. (From Murray CJL, Lopez AD, Mathers CD, Stein C. The Global Burden of Disease 2000 Project: Aims, Methods, and Data Sources (Global Programme on Evidence for Health Policy Discussion Paper No 36). Geneva, World Health Organization, 2001 and WHO; Vaccines, Immunizations, and Biologicals, personal communication).

with technical assistance from donors, trained and supervised peripheral health care workers at district and health center levels.

This structure is changing in many countries, however, and there is great diversity among countries and regions. Under health sector reforms promoted by international agencies, there is an increasing trend toward decentralization of implementation of health services and a burgeoning private sector. Countries vary in the degree to which health services have been decentralized. Where the process is most advanced, health services are under local government control, budgets are managed at district level, and the role of the Ministries of Health focuses on policy making, procurement of vaccines and injection supplies, and surveillance and monitoring of program impact. Donors may supply funds to, and work directly with, health care managers at district level. There is also an increasing trend toward involvement of private organizations in health services delivery, including national and international not-for-profit agencies as well as private for-profit practitioners. A review of immunization in urban areas conducted in 1993 found that the private sector was providing as much as 40% of all immunizations in Lagos State, Nigeria; 25% in Teheran, Iran; and 30% to 45% in India.[17] This increases the need for effective coordination of the different service providers and for the dissemination of clear and practical policies.

Different groups of decision makers are involved in ensuring that vaccines contribute effectively and efficiently to the disease control efforts of a country.[16] Decisions must be made about the goals of the vaccination program. Technical guidelines must be established regarding vaccine use, including selection of the optimal schedule and recommendations regarding contraindications to vaccines. Appropriate technology must be utilized for vaccine storage (the "cold chain"), injections, and waste disposal, and appropriate strategies must be selected for delivery of vaccines. National interagency coordinating committees (ICCs), which should include all key government ministries (e.g., Health and Finance), international partners, nongovernmental organizations (NGOs), and the private sector, can provide a key mechanism to facilitate coordinated planning, financing, political and technical support, and capacity building for comprehensive immunization programs.[2]

Defining Aims/Goals

Before 1974, vaccination programs in most developing countries were restricted to the urban elite and were modeled on programs in industrialized countries. Thus vaccination services mainly targeted children of school age, despite the fact that the diseases occurred in younger children.[1]

The EPI was established in 1974 to make immunization available to every child in the world by 1990.[18] In the first 15 years of the program, efforts concentrated on establishing the physical and human resources infrastructure to deliver vaccination and on monitoring vaccine coverage. Subsequently, the emphasis has shifted to a primary goal of controlling disease, but with continued focus on assuring that all children are reached by routine immunization.

The potential goals for reducing vaccine-preventable disease burden are eradication, elimination, or control.[19] *Eradication* is the reduction of the worldwide incidence of infection by a specific agent to zero as a result of deliberate efforts; intervention measures are no longer needed, except to prevent intentional (e.g., bioterrorism) or unintentional release of the disease agent from laboratory facilities.[20] The characteristics of an infection that make it theoretically eradicable are the absence of a nonhuman host, an easily recognizable illness with no chronic or latent infection, and an effective intervention such as vaccination that produces lasting immunity.[21,22] The only disease to have been eradicated globally by vaccination to date is smallpox. *Elimination* of disease or of infection means the reduction to zero, or to the level at which it is no longer a public health problem, of the incidence of a specified disease, or of infection caused by a specific agent, in a defined geographic area; continued intervention measures are required to prevent reintroduction. *Control*, or containment, of a disease means the reduction of disease incidence, prevalence, morbidity, or mortality.

Current goals of the global EPI are to ensure full immunization of children under 1 year of age at 90% nationally, with at least 80% coverage in every district or equivalent administrative unit; achieve the global eradication of poliomyelitis by 2005; eliminate maternal and neonatal tetanus (incidence rate less than one case per 1000 live births in all districts) by 2005; reduce deaths caused by measles by 50% by 2005 from the burden in 1999; and extend the benefits of new and improved vaccines and other preventive health interventions to children in all countries.[23] In addition, GAVI has established specific milestones to achieve certain EPI goals, including that, by 2010, all countries will have routine immunization coverage of 90%, with 80% coverage in all districts; that HepB vaccine will have been introduced in 80% of countries with adequate delivery systems by 2002, and in all countries by 2007; and that, by 2005, Hib vaccine will be introduced in 50% of the poorest countries with high disease burden and adequate delivery systems.[7]

Selection of Vaccines and Schedules[24,25]

The WHO has encouraged countries to select vaccination schedules that are epidemiologically relevant, immunologically effective, operationally feasible, and socially acceptable.[1] Priority has been given to delivering the primary childhood immunization series and protecting adult women and their newborns against tetanus.

Routine Immunization of Infants

Recommendations for the age at which vaccines are administered are influenced by several factors[24,25]:

- Age-specific burden of disease
- Age-specific immunologic response to vaccines
- Potential interference with the immune response by passively transferred maternal antibody
- Age-specific risks of vaccine-associated complications
- Programmatic feasibility

Vaccines should be administered before the age at which children are at risk of disease. Vaccines therefore are generally given to children in the youngest age group that develops an adequate immune response to vaccination with minimal adverse effects from the vaccine. Administering vaccines early in life also makes it easier to achieve high immunization coverage. Table 55–1 shows the immunization schedule recommended by the EPI for developing countries. The basis for the selection of this schedule is described in a series of WHO publications.[26] To reduce the number of contacts required to complete the immunization series, as many antigens as possible are given at a single visit. All the EPI antigens are safe and effective when they are administered simultaneously.[25,27] DTP-based combination vaccines that also include HepB and or Hib vaccines are becoming more widely available and can be used to reduce the number of injections at each visit. The EPI does not, however, recommend mixing different vaccines in one syringe before injection or using a fluid vaccine for reconstitution of a freeze-dried vaccine unless specifically licensed for this purpose (e.g., reconstitution of Hib vaccine with combined DTP-HepB vaccine). Such practices may lead to lower potency of both vaccines. If vaccines are not given on the same day, the main potential problem is interference between two live parenteral vaccines, which should then be spaced at least 4 weeks apart. In developing countries, yellow fever, measles, or BCG vaccines should not be given within 4 weeks of each other unless they are given on the same day. An exception is that measles vaccine can be given effectively at any interval after yellow fever vaccine.[27] All other EPI vaccines may be given simultaneously with or at any interval after other vaccines. The immunization visit at 9 months of age offers the opportunity to give vitamin A to those who are at risk of vitamin A deficiency. Vitamin A may be given at a dose of 100,000 IU to those ages 9 to 11 months, and 200,000 IU to those over 12 months of age. Vitamin A does not have a negative effect on seroconversion to childhood vaccines.[25]

Immunization of Women of Child-Bearing Age

The optimal program to protect newborns against neonatal tetanus by vaccination depends on the history of the use of vaccines containing tetanus toxoid (TT) in immunization programs. When most women of child-bearing age have not previously been immunized with TT in their infancy or adolescence, implementation of a five-dose TT program for women of child-bearing age is recommended (Table 55–2). Each country should define the age group to be included in the "child-bearing age" category (e.g., 15 to 44 years, 15 to 35 years) according to local fertility patterns and the available resources. In practice, this scheme also will be used in

TABLE 55–1 ■ Immunization Schedule for Infants Recommended by the WHO Expanded Programme on Immunisation

| Disease | Age | | | | | |
	Birth	6 wk	10 wk	14 wk	9 mo[*]	>9 mo
Bacille Calmette-Guérin	BCG					
Polio	OPV0[†]	OPV1	OPV2	OPV3		
Diphtheria, pertussis, tetanus		DPT1	DPT2	DPT3		
Hepatitis B[‡]						
Scheme A	HepB1	HepB2		HepB3		
Scheme B		HepB1	HepB2	HepB3		
Haemophilus influenzae type b		Hib1	Hib2	Hib3		
Yellow fever[§]					YF	
Measles					Measles	Measles[‖]

[*]Vitamin A may be given at this visit.
[†]OPV0 is given in polio-endemic countries.
[‡]Scheme A is recommended in countries where perinatal transmission of hepatitis B virus is frequent (e.g., Southeast Asia). Scheme B may be used in countries where perinatal transmission is less frequent (e.g., sub-Saharan Africa).
[§]In countries where yellow fever poses a risk.
[‖]A second opportunity to receive a dose of measles vaccine should be provided for all children. This may be done either as part of the routine schedule or in a campaign.

TABLE 55–2 ■ Tetanus Toxoid (TT) Immunization Schedule for Women of Child-Bearing Age and Pregnant Women Without Previous Exposure to Tetanus Toxoid-Containing Vaccine*

Dose	When to Give	Expected Duration of Protection[†]
TT1	At first contact or as early as possible in pregnancy	None
TT2	At least 4 wk after TT1	1–3 yr
TT3	At least 6 mo after TT2	At least 5 yr
TT4	At least 1 yr after TT3 or during subsequent pregnancy	At least 10 yr
TT5	At least 1 yr after TT4 or during subsequent pregnancy	All child-bearing years and possibly longer

*Increasing numbers of women have documentation of prior receipt of vaccines containing tetanus toxoid early in childhood or at school age. Three properly spaced doses of diphtheria and tetanus toxoids and whole-cell pertussis given in childhood are considered equivalent in protection to two doses of TT or adult diphtheria and tetanus toxoids given in adulthood.
[†]Recent studies suggest that the duration of protection may be longer than indicated in this table. This matter is currently under review.

areas where there is little or no documentation of past immunization with tetanus-containing vaccines, even if some women are likely to have received some doses in childhood.

In the future, increasing numbers of women of child-bearing age will have documentation of prior receipt of TT-containing vaccines in early childhood or at school age. Other schemes of vaccination then can be considered, with progressively fewer doses of TT required for adult women (see Chapter 27).

Booster Doses

The first priority of immunization programs is to ensure that infants are completely immunized against target diseases at the youngest age possible. Where resources are limited, the EPI suggests that booster doses should not be considered until coverage levels for fully immunized infants are above 80%.[24,25] Today, many developing countries have achieved such coverage levels and administer booster doses of various vaccines.

The number and frequency of booster doses depend on the epidemiologic patterns of diseases in a particular country, the health services infrastructure, the level of resources available, and the relative priority of boosters compared, for example, with introduction of new vaccines. The importance attached to booster doses has increased because of the resurgence of diphtheria in eastern Europe[8–11,28] and some developing countries[11,29–31] during the 1990s and the recognition of the importance of adult pertussis as a contributor to community spread.[32–34] Current WHO recommendations are that a booster dose of DTP should be given approximately 1 year after the primary series (at the middle or the end of the second year of life) in countries with successful routine immunization programs to maintain immunity against pertussis and diphtheria and contribute to the long-term strategy for neonatal tetanus control. Where disease is documented in schoolchildren, an additional booster dose at school entry is appropriate. When the pattern shifts to mostly adult cases, a school-leaving booster of adult diphtheria and tetanus toxoids (Td) may be appropriate.

For BCG, there is much controversy over the effectiveness of repeated doses of the vaccine. There is no evidence that the degree of protection from BCG is related to scar formation or to tuberculin conversion.[35] However, there is evidence from some BCG trials that the protection afforded by BCG decreases with time after vaccination. Although some authors believe that repeating BCG vaccination

increases its efficacy,[36,37] a trial in Malawi showed no protective effect from either one or two doses of BCG.[38] For this reason, the WHO does not recommend repeated BCG vaccination, but only administration of the vaccine at birth or in the first year of life.[39]

For measles, although high coverage with a single dose can reduce morbidity and mortality, more than one dose of vaccine is required to achieve the mortality reduction targets and to achieve elimination.[40,41] All children should be offered a second opportunity to receive measles vaccine[41] (see Table 55–1). The second dose is not a true booster dose[42]; it is administered to protect children who failed to respond to the first dose and to provide another opportunity to reach children who did not receive a first dose of vaccine. In most developing countries, administration of additional doses is more effectively done through campaigns[43] than through a routine two-dose schedule.

The Cold Chain and Injection Safety

The cold chain is the system necessary to ensure that vaccines are stored and transported at appropriate temperatures. In tropical countries with frequent logistics problems, a lack of refrigeration equipment and of a reliable power or fuel supply may threaten the potency of vaccines. Although the stability of EPI-recommended vaccines varies depending on the antigen, the required storage temperature at health care facilities of 2°C to 8°C has been determined by the thermolability of OPV and the sensitivity to freezing of adjuvanted vaccines (DTP, diphtheria, and tetanus toxoids [DT], TT, HepB, combination DTP-HepB and liquid combined DTP-Hib vaccines). The live vaccines against poliomyelitis, measles, BCG, and yellow fever can be stored long term at −20°C.[44,45]

The WHO EPI and the United Nations Children's Fund (UNICEF) Vaccine Supply Division set operational standards and determine the characteristics of equipment needed for vaccine transport and storage at all the levels of the cold chain. These partners work with manufacturers to assure availability of low-cost equipment for storing and transporting EPI vaccines.[46] Special refrigerators and freezers have been developed to facilitate the storage of vaccine in areas where power supplies are intermittent.[47] An ice-lined refrigerator enables vaccines to be stored in situations where electricity is interrupted for up to 16 hours of each 24-hour period, and is now used as a global standard in central and provincial stores. Other equipment has been

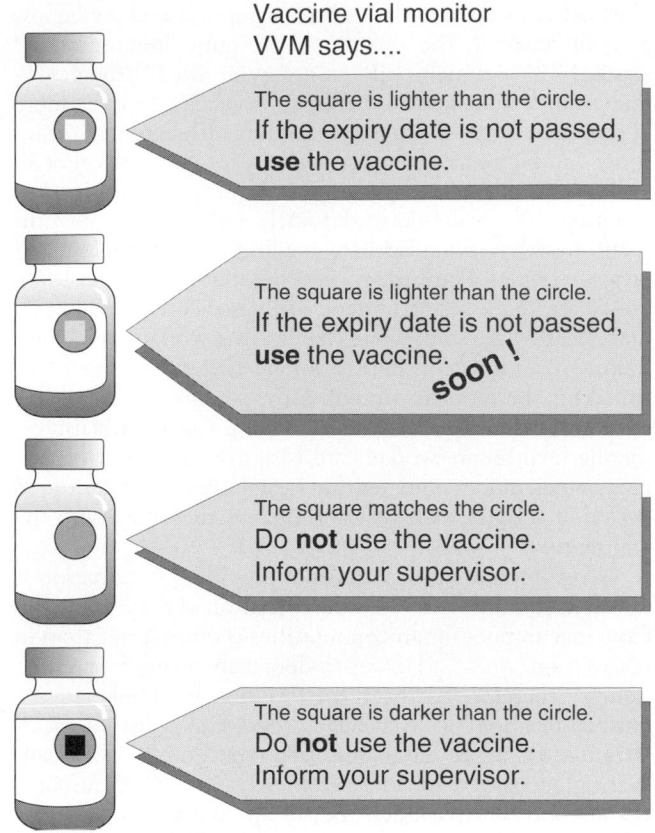

Vaccine vial monitor
VVM says....

The square is lighter than the circle.
If the expiry date is not passed,
use the vaccine.

The square is lighter than the circle.
If the expiry date is not passed,
use the vaccine. *soon !*

The square matches the circle.
Do **not** use the vaccine.
Inform your supervisor.

The square is darker than the circle.
Do **not** use the vaccine.
Inform your supervisor.

FIGURE 55–2 ▪ Vaccine vial monitor.

adapted, including kerosene, gas, and solar power refrigerators to cover areas where electricity is not available.[48,49] The photovoltaic refrigerator, developed in conjunction with the U.S. National Aeronautics and Space Administration, enabled specifications to be issued to industry resulting in more than 5000 solar vaccine refrigeration systems in use globally today. More recently, CFC (chlorofluorocarbon)-free cold chain equipment has been developed and is gradually replacing CFC-containing equipment. The EPI also ensures adequate maintenance of equipment; universal spare parts kits have been developed for refrigerator repair, along with standard tool kits for the traveling repair technician, and cold chain technicians have been trained in national and regional courses.

Time and temperature vaccine monitor cards allow monitoring of vaccine potency along the cold chain.[50] The cold chain monitor card enables documentation of problems that occur during international transport, and also can be used during transport of large quantities of vaccine within countries. For areas with very cold climates, where DTP-, DT-, TT-, and HepB-containing vaccines can be easily frozen, a "freeze watch" indicator is utilized for inter- and intracountry transport.

Since the mid-1990s, success in the implementation of the cold chain has greatly reduced the chance of loss of potency of vaccines when they are used in the field. However, high vaccine wastage (up to 50% of supplied vaccine) has been recognized as a problem that raises program costs and threatens vaccine supply.[51] Reasons for wastage may include discarding a multidose vial after use for one child; cold chain problems that lead to destruction of vaccine that has been exposed to excessive heat (especially

OPV and measles vaccine) or freezing of adjuvanted vaccines; and poor stock control such that vaccine stocks pass their expiration date. With the increasing cost of the existing vaccines and higher cost of new vaccines, it is important to reduce this wastage. The WHO and UNICEF have introduced new rules for handling vaccines ("multidose vial policy"),[52] and time-temperature indicators that can be placed on each vaccine vial (vaccine vial monitors [VVMs]) have been developed and are now being utilized for all EPI vaccines.[53] The VVMs (Fig. 55–2) utilize chemicals that change color with increasing time of exposure to high temperatures, and enable the vaccines to be used with confidence up to their expiration date in the most difficult situations. Additionally, VVMs allow use of vaccine outside of the cold chain to reach remote areas during campaigns.[53] However, VVMs that can detect freezing of vaccines have not yet been developed.

Efforts also have focused on technologies to enhance safety of injections for immunization.[2] Two major principles of safe injection practices are the use of sterile equipment and proper handling and disposing of used sharps. During the early years of the EPI, both sterilizable and single-use disposable syringes and needles were supported.[1] However, as the high frequency of their unsterile reuse was recognized,[54–56] the EPI provided global leadership to focus attention on safe injection practices by promoting universal use of autodisabling (AD) syringes, which include an internal lock that prevents inadvertent or intentional reuse of the device (Fig. 55–3).[57] It also promoted appropriate injection waste disposal systems, including the use of sharps boxes at each injection site and use of incinerators and disposal pits to protect health care workers and the community from needle sticks and improper recycling. The EPI also has supported evaluations of injection safety practices.[57] Logistic support for immunization programs has expanded through the formation of TechNet (see *www.technet21.org*), a global network of cold chain and logistics experts who conduct

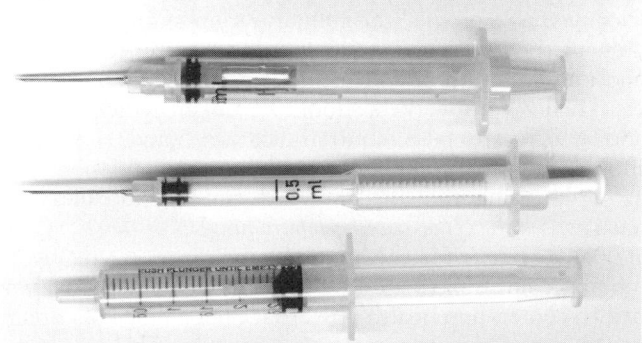

FIGURE 55–3 ▪ Examples of autodisable (AD) syringes, which permit one outward movement of the plunger to fill the syringe but prevent a second outward movement after the inward injection stroke. *Top,* The SoloShot™ IX (Becton-Dickinson, Franklin Lakes, NJ) uses a metal clip with barbs around the neck of the plunger to lock it after injection. *Middle,* The Destroject® (Destroject GmbH Medical Devices, Neumünster, Germany) uses serrations on the plunger that lock into a cog within the white ring seen adjacent to the finger flanges. *Bottom,* The Sologard® (Safegard Medical Group Ltd., Monaco) features a notched rod above the plunger gasket that locks into a constriction at the tip of the Luer-slip interface for the needle.

applied research on logistics for primary health care, and the Safe Injection Global Network (SIGN) (see *www.injectionsafety.org*), which promotes safe injection practices.[2,57] Improvements in technology for the cold chain and associated logistics developed for the EPI have benefited areas of primary health care other than immunization. Other technologies hold promise for increasing injection safety, including the use of needles attached to flexible plastic blisters that are prefilled with a single dose of vaccine (UniJect™; Becton Dickenson). These cannot be reused, and have been incorporated into some maternal–neonatal tetanus (MNT) and hepatitis B prevention efforts.

Selecting Strategies

Once the goals of vaccination programs have been decided, appropriate strategies must be designed to achieve them. The target population for the vaccine must be defined. Coverage targets must be set, according to the efficacy of the vaccine and the level of immunity needed in the population to achieve the stated program objective. For eradication or elimination, high coverage is required at an early age. For example, to eliminate measles, which is highly infectious, at least 90% to 95% of the population must be immune.[58] In developing countries in which measles vaccination at 9 months of age has approximately 85% efficacy, high coverage (>90%) with a second dose is required to achieve disease elimination.[43] Immunization programs require good management: Vaccination must be accessible and available with minimal administrative barriers.[59–62] There must be reliable systems for the cold chain, logistics, and transport that include maintenance of equipment and a regular supply of fuel and vaccines. Health care workers need to be trained and supervised in vaccination techniques, cold chain maintenance, logistics, the use of health information, and health education. Mothers need to be informed about the availability of vaccination and be motivated to bring their children.[2,63,64] Wherever vaccinations are offered, it is vital to use all opportunities to administer vaccines.[62,65] For this, the immunization status of all children in the target age group should be screened routinely and immunization provided to eligible children and mothers. Health care workers should be taught which are true and which are false contraindications, and supervisors should monitor compliance with recommendations, for example, using the available EPI training modules (see *www.who.int/vaccines-diseases/epitraining*).[66]

Delivery sites for vaccination range from fixed sites to mobile teams. Fixed sites are health care facilities such as health centers and health posts that offer a range of primary health care activities or curative services. They may offer vaccination either daily or on specific days per week or per month, depending on patient load. The utilization of fixed sites is higher when good-quality curative care and an adequate supply of essential drugs are also available.[67,68]

In areas progressively further from a health care facility, regular outreach services from the nearest health care facility or district center or mobile teams (which involve stay of at least one night in a distant village) are used. Outreach and mobile services may be scheduled throughout the year, but, in countries with poor communications and transport infrastructure, frequent postponement or cancellation of planned visits commonly leads to disruption and public loss of confidence in the program.[69] A "pulse immunization" strategy[70–74] in which children are immunized through several annual campaigns or "pulses" of vaccine may be more appropriate in these situations. Each health care institution is encouraged to assume responsibility for vaccination of all children in a specified geographic area. Voluntary institutions and NGOs should work jointly with the local government health service agency, pooling staff, vehicles, and other resources. Planning is carried out at the district level; pulse campaigns are organized locally and conducted by primary health care staff, village health care workers, and community volunteers. Where possible, the pulses should be timed for the months preceding the seasonal peaks of diseases such as measles[72,74] and whooping cough. Advantages for the health care workers are easier management of vaccines, fuel, and equipment in a relatively concentrated period of activity each year and increased contact with the community.

Geographic proximity to a site providing vaccination is not in itself sufficient to ensure utilization of the service.[75,76] Coverage in poor urban communities is often lower than in many rural areas.[77–81] Door-to-door canvassing[82] or channeling[83] therefore has been used to increase uptake among hard-to-reach groups that have geographic access to vaccination sites. In Mozambique, however, door-to-door canvassing accounted for more than 40% of human resource costs,[82] and, in Khartoum, the sustainability of a system of follow-up birth registration and defaulter follow-up by midwives[84] also was questionable. It may be best reserved for tracking high-risk groups who are identified through operational research at the local level.

In addition to these strategies, which are part of regular immunization services and are predominantly under the control of local health authorities, periodic mass immunization campaigns at national or provincial levels are an increasing part of immunization programs. The experience with mass campaigns has been largely positive.[85] In the WHO region of the Americas, they are a major component of disease eradication programs and are implemented with a high degree of effectiveness and predominantly local funding.[43,86] Polio and measles campaigns, conducted either separately or together, have been demonstrated to be effective in numerous developing countries, and often have incorporated other interventions such as vitamin A administration.[87–89] However, in the 1980s, a number of experiences with campaigns in low-income countries conducted with the sole purpose of raising immunization coverage rapidly as part of the drive for universal child immunization were generally poor.[90–92] Additionally, campaigns without adequate, coordinated donor support or coherent plans for follow-up after the campaigns have had poor outcomes or have not had enduring benefits in strengthening routine immunization programs.[93–98] In some instances, the quality of vaccination during campaigns also was low.[99,100]

The mass campaign approach also has been used with varying degrees of success to inform and motivate communities and families. In the drive for universal childhood immunization by 1990, "social mobilization" was promoted, predominantly with UNICEF support. It was recognized that, in many countries, the traditional health education delivered through the health sector would not reach large parts of the population who lacked access to health services for geographic, economic, or cultural reasons.[101] Social mobilization was conducted by individuals and organizations ranging from political, traditional, and religious leaders to governmental institutions, trade unions, teachers, revolutionary organizations,[102] or the military to deliver specific messages about immunization.[103–106] This often was done with a large amount of publicity and political attention. Like the campaigns conducted with the aim of improving coverage quickly, however, these large-scale media campaigns often failed to lead to sustained benefits in low-income countries.[90]

Since the late 1990s, campaigns have been used primarily as a strategy to improve disease control or eradication rather than with the sole aim of increasing coverage. Thus current campaigns target all children in an age group determined by disease epidemiology, irrespective of previous vaccination status, and usually do not attempt to update a child's vaccination status for the primary vaccination series. They usually are not conducted as an isolated event but instead are part of a medium-term plan of action to achieve the disease control or elimination goal.[107] The plan of action encompasses all the necessary areas of activities, including raising routine immunization coverage, development of disease and adverse events surveillance, and strengthening of laboratory facilities. Campaigns also may include other effective interventions such as oral administration of vitamin A, which has been done extensively during polio and measles vaccination campaigns.[87,88] Vitamin A administration during polio national immunization days in more than 50 countries has prevented an estimated 1 million deaths since 1998.[87] Targeted mass campaigns also may be conducted in high-risk areas; for example, mass measles immunization campaigns may assist in controlling measles in countries with emergencies or that are war-torn.[108]

No single strategy is likely to be appropriate for all circumstances and all diseases. The choice of strategy should depend on the epidemiology of the disease, the characteristics of the vaccine, the facilities available, the accessibility of the population and their cultural attitudes and practices, and the socioeconomic level of the country.[16,63] The desire to extend coverage of immunization services rapidly and maintain international support for the EPI needs to be balanced with the promotion of other health services. The success of any approach to health service delivery depends on the context into which it is introduced. There is a need for continued capacity building for national and district-level managers to select strategies that are appropriate for their own contexts.[109–112]

Disease Elimination/Eradication Initiatives

As the efforts directed at the development of an infrastructure for immunization started to show impact on disease incidence, the emphasis of the EPI shifted from raising coverage to disease control.[113] In 1985, progress in controlling poliomyelitis in the Americas led that region, in which only 11 countries had endemic poliomyelitis, to adopt the goal of eradication of poliomyelitis from the Western Hemisphere by the year 1990.[114] In 1988, the 41st World Health Assembly ratified the goal of global eradication by the year 2000.[115] The last case of indigenous poliomyelitis caused by

wild-type virus in the Americas occurred on August 23, 1991, in Peru[116] (see also Chapter 25). The last indigenous cases in the WHO Western Pacific and European Regions occurred in 1997 and 1998, respectively. These three WHO regions—the Americas (as of 1994), the Western Pacific (as of 2000), and the European (as of 2002)—encompassing over 3 billion people in 134 countries and territories, now have been certified polio free.

The achievement of poliomyelitis eradication requires special immunization strategies in addition to reaching and maintaining the highest possible routine immunization coverage of infants with OPV. National immunization days are recommended, during which all children in the target age (usually younger than 5 years) receive OPV during a short period (usually a few days) to quickly increase population immunity and interrupt transmission. "Mopping up" operations, consisting of door-to-door vaccination, are conducted in areas at risk once transmission is reduced only to focal areas, and recently have been applied nationwide in the few remaining endemic or recently endemic countries to reach any children not previously vaccinated. The backbone of these strategies is high-quality surveillance, with investigation and collection of stool specimens for poliovirus isolation from every case of acute flaccid paralysis (AFP).[116,117]

Several conditions must be met for these strategies to be implemented effectively. Political commitment is needed at global and national levels to advocate for and mobilize resources. Requirements of funds, personnel, equipment, and vaccines must be estimated realistically and with sufficient lead time for logistics and financial systems to be put in place. Interagency coordination is essential to ensure that resources are used efficiently. Laboratory support for surveillance must be made available. Personnel (including volunteers) must be trained appropriately and excellent communications established.

With use of the experience in designing an appropriate strategy for poliomyelitis eradication, measles was the next disease to be tackled[107] (see Chapter 19). In 1989, the World Health Assembly resolved to reduce measles morbidity by 90% and measles mortality by 95% by 1995, compared with the disease burden in the pre vaccine era. In 1995, measles vaccination was estimated to have reduced measles-associated mortality worldwide by 88% from the prevaccination levels of as many as 5.7 million deaths per year.[118] Regions that have already eradicated poliomyelitis have been keen to keep up the momentum of their immunization programs and are considering the eradicability of other diseases. Three international conferences were held in 1997 and 1998 to consider potential infectious disease candidates for eradication, and all concluded that measles was a leading candidate for possible eradication within the next 10 to 15 years.[20–22,118] The American, European, and Eastern Mediterranean WHO regions have adopted regional measles elimination goals by 2000, 2007, and 2010, respectively, and the Western Pacific region has established such a goal, with the precise target date still under discussion. These regional elimination initiatives have become part of a global initiative to reduce measles mortality by 50% by 2005 compared with 1999 levels (888,000 deaths) and achieve regional measles elimination in these four (of six) WHO regions.[119] The initiative is based on four strategies[107,119,120]:

1. Achieving high routine immunization coverage by providing the first dose of measles vaccine to successive cohorts of all children at age 9 months or shortly after.
2. Providing a "second opportunity"[41,119] for measles vaccination either through the routine immunization program or supplementary immunization activities ("mass campaigns"), targeting the age group in which most susceptibles have accumulated (usually ages 9 months to 14 years), both to increase the chance that every child receives at least one dose of measles vaccine and to increase the proportion of the population that is immune.
3. Establishing an effective system to monitor coverage and conduct measles surveillance with integration of epidemiologic and laboratory information.
4. Improving clinical management of every measles case.

Follow-up mass campaigns are conducted periodically (e.g., every 3 to 5 years) targeting children born since the initial "catch-up" campaign.[107]

Another disease, neonatal tetanus, has been targeted for elimination by 2005[23,121] (see Chapter 27). The goal is defined as a reduction in the incidence of neonatal tetanus to less than one case per 1000 live births in all districts of the world. The recommended strategies include routine immunization of pregnant women with TT, immunization of all women of child-bearing age in high-risk areas through routine immunization or three rounds of vaccination campaigns in high-risk areas, improvement of clean delivery and hygienic cord care practices, and effective neonatal tetanus surveillance. As of 2002, over 100 developing countries had claimed neonatal tetanus elimination. However, more than 200,000 cases are still estimated to occur each year, of which only a small fraction are reported.

Monitoring and Evaluation of Immunization Programs

The implementation of strategies and achievement of immunization program goals will be most effective if systems are established to monitor disease incidence and compliance with performance standards, and problem-oriented research is conducted.[64,122,123] Surveillance of vaccine-preventable diseases is a key component of disease control and elimination strategies, and reduced disease incidence and mortality are the ultimate indicators of program success.[122] It is also essential to monitor indicators of program performance to detect potential problems with the quality, uptake, and appropriateness of vaccination services and to identify appropriate solutions[18,60] (Table 55–3). These indicators provide information on outputs such as coverage of different vaccines and program quality, including dropout between vaccine doses (a measure of the degree of success of tracking and health education activities), missed immunization opportunities, cold chain maintenance, vaccine security, injection safety, and provider information and education.[124,125] The WHO and UNICEF compile information annually for all countries on key program indicators through the joint reporting form.[124] To have optimal pro-

gram effectiveness, indicators should be monitored and utilized at the district (or other appropriate) level at which the program is managed, as well as nationally.

In this section, we review methods to monitor program performance, and operational research methods to determine reasons for incomplete vaccination. We then discuss the role of surveillance in the control of vaccine-preventable diseases. Finally, we review the role of economic analysis and mathematical modeling in program monitoring and planning.

Assessment of Vaccine Coverage

By monitoring coverage of different vaccines, insight can be gained not only into the overall program success in providing all vaccines to the target population (percentage of fully vaccinated children) but also into the areas of program failure. For example, high coverage of BCG/OPV0 may reflect a high coverage of hospital deliveries. High coverage of DTP1/OPV1 indicates high access to primary health care facilities. If DTP1/OPV1 coverage is high by age 2 months but coverage for the respective third doses or measles vaccine is low, this high dropout needs further investigation to determine the cause (e.g., missed immunization opportunities, adverse events, poor patient education, poor tracking activities). As overall coverage of 12- to 23-month-old children increases, it becomes more important to monitor timeliness of vaccination to ensure that vaccines are received as close as possible to the recommended age.

Vaccine coverage is monitored through routine reports (the "administrative method") or community-based surveys.

The Administrative Method

All participating clinics (public, private, and NGO) report the numbers of each dose (e.g., OPV1, DTP3) administered to the target age group of 0 to 11 months, regularly (e.g., monthly) during the course of each year. The number of each of the doses administered is summed and divided by the population denominator of 0- to 11-month-olds. This method is easiest to perform in countries where the government health services deliver almost all immunizations, or where the government supplies vaccine to NGOs and private clinics and requires reporting of doses administered, so that reports reflect virtually all the doses administered. It may be difficult to obtain cooperation from nongovernment clinics in submitting regular reports to the government health authorities, and, where substantial numbers of doses are given in the private sector, falsely low coverage estimates may result. The accuracy of administrative coverage estimates depends on the timeliness and completeness of reports from each facility, the accuracy of reports of vaccinations administered to 0- to 11-month-olds, and the accuracy of the estimates of the target populations at each level.

The administrative method has the advantages of providing continuous information at the local and district level and being relatively inexpensive. Each facility and district can track achievement of coverage goals and dropout using standard immunization monitoring charts. Estimates of coverage and dropout can be compared between districts,[126,127] ideally with a simultaneous comparison of program inputs, health service infrastructure, and socioeconomic character-

TABLE 55–3 ■ Selected Indicators to Monitor Program Performance

Indicator	Definition

Service delivery	Fully vaccinated children—proportion of children ages 12–23 mo who have received
	    1 dose of BCG
	    3 valid doses of DTP (minimum age first dose, 6 wk; minimum interval, 4 wk)
	    3 valid doses of OPV (as with DTP)
	    1 valid dose of measles vaccine (age at least 9 mo)
	    3 valid doses of HepB vaccine (if in schedule)
	    3 valid doses of Hib vaccine (if in schedule)
	    1 valid dose of yellow fever vaccine (age at least 6 mo if in schedule)
	Proportion of districts in country with ≥80% DTP3 coverage in infants[*]
	Proportion of districts with ≥90% measles coverage in infants[*]

Access to services	Up-to-date (BCG and DTP1/OPV1) by age 2 mo
Tracking activities	Difference in percentage receiving DTP1/OPV1 and either DTP3/OPV3 or measles vaccine (indicator of "dropout") Proportion of districts with dropout rate (DTP1 to DTP3) of <10%[*]
Missed opportunities	Percentage of children not receiving all vaccines for which they are eligible
Safety	Proportion of districts that have been supplied with adequate (equal or more) number of AD syringes for all routine immunizations during the year[*]
Logistics and cold chain	Proportion of districts that had no interruption in vaccine supply[*] Percentage of facilities storing vaccine at recommended temperatures Vaccine efficacy in expected range for each vaccine evaluated
Surveillance and monitoring	Proportion of district disease surveillance reports received at national level compared to expected[*] Proportion of district coverage reports received at national level compared to number expected[*]
Management and supervision	Country with 5-y immunization plan Proportion of districts with microplans that include immunization activities[*] Proportion of districts that had at least one supervisory visit of all health care facilities in last calendar year[*]
Provider knowledge	Proportion of providers who know and follow recommended guidelines, including those on simultaneous administration, contraindications, and safe injection procedures

[*]Proposed as core indicators for national immunization systems by GAVI Implementation Task Force.
AD, autodisable; BCG, bacille Calmette-Guérin; DTP, diphtheria and tetanus toxoids and whole-cell pertussis; GAVI, Global Alliance for Vaccines and Immunization; OPV, oral poliovirus vaccine.

istics in each district to assess the extent to which low coverage is related to inadequate resources, population characteristics, poor health system performance, and lack of public demand or social mobilization.

Administrative data also permit the routine monitoring of TT coverage in pregnant women, but these data underestimate achievements, because previous doses of TT are not taken into account, and pregnant women who have already received a full protective course are included as unvaccinated. The WHO now recommends recording and reporting protection at birth when a mother brings her child for DTP vaccination. This approach is most accurate if mothers retain records of vaccination during pregnancy.[128]

From routine reports, the doses administered to children also can be compared with total doses distributed to estimate wastage rates. "Acceptable" wastage is difficult to define, because the cost of wasted vaccine must be balanced against the cost of missing an opportunity if a child is turned away from a health care facility. However, if wastage is high, the causes should be determined (e.g., poor forecasting of vaccine demand so that vaccine expires before use, cold chain problems at different levels of the health system, or ongoing wastage at the health center level because multidose vials are discarded after use for one or two clients). Appropriate action then can be taken while trying to minimize the risk of missed opportunities.

Community Surveys

Because up-to-date and complete information on population denominators often is unavailable in developing countries,[127] the WHO EPI developed a modified cluster sampling survey method for the evaluation of vaccine coverage.[129–131] This survey uses two-stage sampling, selecting 30 clusters by population-proportionate sampling and seven children within each cluster using practical methods to randomly select a starting point in each cluster, followed by visiting each next closest home. The survey is designed to estimate vaccine coverage with a precision of ±10 percentage points, to provide a measure of coverage in areas with no alternative reliable sources of data, and to validate reported immunization coverage. The method is learned easily by midlevel health care workers, and their participation can serve to motivate them and increase their awareness of the constraints on obtaining vaccination that families face.[64,76] Computer simulations have shown that the deviations in sampling methodology from classical cluster sampling do not greatly bias the estimates obtained.[132–134] However, bias may arise in the field because of practical problems, one major difficulty being low retention rates of home-based records so that vaccination status may be misclassified.[135–137] Larger community-based surveys (demographic and health surveys [DHS], multiple indicator cluster surveys [MICS]) sponsored by international (UNICEF) and donor (e.g., U.S. Agency for International Development [USAID]) agencies may be conducted every 3 to 5 years to evaluate overall child and maternal health indicators and are used to validate coverage at national and provincial levels (see *www.measuredhs.com/pdfs/basic_doc.pdf* and *www.unicef.org/reseval/pdfs/mics.pdf*).

Cluster sample surveys provide more detailed information on vaccination than do routine reports, because the dates of each vaccination given to each child can be checked and compared. Thus doses administered before the recommended age, or with too short an interval, are identified and discounted as invalid; a high proportion of invalid doses show the need for specific in-service training of health care workers about the schedule. Missed immunization opportunities through the failure to administer vaccines simultaneously can be identified, for example, by comparing dates of DTP and OPV vaccinations. Coverage surveys can be extended to include indicators of other programs, especially if home-based records include dates of visits to health care facilities for curative care or growth monitoring.[64,138] In that way, other sources of missed opportunities can be assessed. These analyses are facilitated by the use of the COSAS computer software package developed for the EPI.[139]

Questionnaires to parents also can include information on reasons for failure to vaccinate the child[140–142]; on the occurrence of adverse events, such as abscesses after vaccination[143]; and on other mother–child health indicators, such as knowledge of oral rehydration therapy[144] and use of family planning. However, each addition to the survey has implications for interviewer training and quality control and potentially for the sample size.[131] The utility of additional questions should be closely scrutinized to avoid compromising the achievement of the main study objectives.

As high coverage levels are reached, the EPI cluster survey becomes less helpful because the precision of the estimate is too low to detect small increases in coverage unless the sample size is greatly increased. It is also relatively costly and usually impractical to conduct surveys in every district, so surveys are rarely used for local program guidance (although, in India, more than 900 district-level surveys have been conducted, providing audit information to compare with routine reports).[90,145]

Reviews of coverage data available from different sources and at different levels (e.g., government, the WHO, UNICEF) have shown major discrepancies in data. In part, this may reflect the pressures that districts and countries face to demonstrate attainment of targets.[90] The WHO and UNICEF have now completed a systematic analysis of reported coverage and coverage survey data for all countries since 1980 (see *www.who.int/vaccines-surveillance*) and developed "best estimates" of coverage with each antigen for each country.[146] These are updated annually. Using these estimates, global DTP3 coverage was estimated to be 73% in 2001, and has been relatively constant since 1990 (75%). Through 2000, best estimates were 7% to 8% lower than coverage reported by the administrative method. However, in 2001, the best estimate and reported coverage were similar.

If coverage data are to guide program performance, it is important for every program to monitor carefully the coverage estimates that are obtained, and identify reasons for differences between reported and coverage survey data. Complete and accurate routine reporting of vaccinations

administered and better data on target populations and the use of disease surveillance must be increased to guide the program. GAVI is now encouraging improving the accuracy of reported data through reliance on reported DTP3 coverage to determine funding support and use of a new data quality assessment tool to evaluate the accuracy of reported coverage and guide countries in improving reporting systems.[147]

Quality Assessment

Indicators of program quality can be assessed using relatively inexpensive studies based at health care facilities.[75,99,148] If administrative data and child vaccination registers are used appropriately, coverage and dropout can be charted and used to guide efforts to increase access and reduce dropout. Specific studies can combine exit interviews with mothers, interviews with providers, and observation using checklists to evaluate timeliness of vaccination, dropout rates, and missed opportunities among children and mothers who attend vaccination sites and to assess provider knowledge and practices. Reasons for failure to immunize eligible children and causes of poor-quality services[148] can be identified quickly and inexpensively. Such studies can be combined with small surveys of households in the vicinity of the health care facility to investigate reasons for failure to use accessible vaccination services.[75,76]

Missed opportunities are easily monitored using health care facility studies that can be included in routine supervisory visits.[66] A review of 79 missed opportunity studies from 45 countries found that a median of 32% of children and women of child-bearing age who were surveyed (67% of those who were eligible for vaccines) had missed opportunities for immunization during visits to health care facilities.[65] Among the children observed at health care facilities, eliminating missed opportunities would have increased coverage by a median of 44%. The studies identified the following most important reasons for missed opportunities: (1) the failure to administer simultaneously all vaccines for which a child was eligible; (2) false contraindications to immunization; (3) health care worker practices, including not opening a multidose vial for a small number of people to avoid vaccine wastage; and (4) logistical problems such as vaccine shortage, poor clinic organization, and inefficient clinic scheduling.[65]

Maintenance of the cold chain should be monitored through ongoing supervision and occasional surveys. As a routine procedure, the temperature of cold rooms, freezers, and refrigerators in which vaccine is stored should be monitored twice daily. To facilitate the monitoring of the cold chain from the vaccine producer to the health center, ensuring that no breaks occur, simple tools have been developed.[51] However, special studies, using time-temperature indicators, may be required to evaluate whether vaccine freezing is occurring at any point along the cold chain.[149] Tools also have been developed to assess the safety of injections, both for immunization and for other health care.[150]

The lot quality sampling technique also has been found to be useful for assessing the quality and coverage of health services, including vaccination.[151] Lot quality sampling is based on an industrial quality assurance technique, using evaluation of small samples to determine if the subject evaluated ("lot") meets preset standards. It can be used to identify health centers or other health service units that are not meeting certain predefined standards of care. These standards may be immunization coverage among clinic attendees or standards of quality of care such as cold chain maintenance, safe injection techniques, use of all opportunities to vaccinate, and so on. Its advantage is that it can be used at any level to evaluate programs; potential disadvantages are that it only can evaluate whether a facility reaches a preset standard (but not measure exact coverage), and it requires random selection within the sampling frame. The technique also can be used at the community level to identify variations between small areas in vaccination coverage[152,153] or other primary health care programs.[154–156]

Vaccine Effectiveness

Vaccine effectiveness (VE) is the percentage reduction in disease incidence attributable to vaccination, calculated by means of the following equation:

$$VE\ (\%) = (U - V)/U \times 100$$

where U = the incidence in unvaccinated people and V = the incidence in vaccinated people.

Although vaccine effectiveness traditionally has been assessed with respect to prevention of the disease against which the vaccine is given, other outcome measures, such as all-causes mortality, may be preferable in the evaluation of vaccine effectiveness.[157] A vaccine may have unexpected beneficial effects; for example, measles vaccine has been reported to reduce mortality by a factor greater than that expected by the direct avoidance of measles illness.[158,159] Conversely, there may be unanticipated adverse events. The unexpected finding of increased mortality among recipients of high-titer measles vaccines at 4 to 6 months of age was demonstrated in vaccine trials in West Africa only because mortality was one of the outcome measures in the trials.[160]

Methods to estimate vaccine effectiveness have been described in detail by Orenstein and colleagues.[161,162] The most frequently used methods are the "screening method," outbreak investigations, and case-control studies. The simplest method to obtain an estimate of vaccine effectiveness is to use routine data on notifications of disease cases in vaccinated and unvaccinated children and to compare the proportion of cases vaccinated with the vaccine coverage among the same age group in the general population. If p is the proportion vaccinated in the population and c is the proportion of cases reported to be vaccinated, then

$$VE = (p - c)/p(1 - c) \times 100\%$$

Although this "screening test" seems a simple way to monitor vaccine effectiveness, estimates are susceptible to many sources of bias because data are collected from many different, unsupervised, sources.[163]

Studies of vaccine effectiveness commonly are conducted during outbreaks, because the occurrence of an outbreak can both alert health authorities to a potential problem in the immunization program and provide large numbers of cases for investigation. In well-defined populations (e.g., a village or a school), total population assessments may be conducted and attack rates calculated among the cohorts of individuals who were vaccinated and unvaccinated at the beginning of the outbreak.[164] Some authors recommend the determination of the secondary attack rate in families during outbreaks[165] to ensure uniform exposure of vaccinees and nonvaccinees.[166]

Case-control studies can be useful to facilitate field work when personal immunization records are not generally available but some other source, such as records from one or more clinics, can be obtained.[167] Case-control procedures also have been used within outbreak investigations to evaluate other risk factors, such as variation in vaccine effectiveness between vaccine providers.[168]

In practice, each approach has potential methodologic problems that can lead to difficulty in interpreting the estimates obtained in observational studies.[163] For example, an unpublished review of measles vaccine effectiveness studies in developing countries found that the diagnosis of measles nearly always used clinical criteria only, leading to probable low specificity of diagnosis and an underestimate of effectiveness.[163,169,170] Vaccination status frequently relied on an undocumented maternal history.[171] Age at vaccination and age at disease onset were not always controlled for, and sample sizes were frequently small.

Despite potential methodologic difficulties, in situations in which a high proportion of individuals have documented vaccination status and disease diagnosis is likely to be highly specific (e.g., because of laboratory confirmation or occurrence of a disease outbreak with epidemiologic links between cases), assessment of vaccine effectiveness can highlight problems that may be of fundamental importance. For example, a case-control study of neonatal tetanus in Bangladesh showed that maternal receipt of two doses of TT had no protective effect (vaccine effectiveness adjusted for other risk factors: 24% [95% confidence interval, −29% to 55%]). Subsequent to the study, a reference laboratory reported no potency in three consecutive lots of tetanus vaccine from the production laboratory in Bangladesh.[172] The same study also showed the importance of missed immunization opportunities, because a history of neonatal tetanus in a previous child was a significant risk factor for neonatal tetanus in the most recently born child.

Operational Research to Identify Determinants of Nonvaccination or Incomplete Vaccination and Effective Interventions to Improve Vaccine Coverage

As follow-up of routine monitoring of the coverage and quality of vaccination programs, program managers should investigate reasons for nonvaccination or incomplete vaccination. Causes of undervaccination may be identified during supervision or through previously described studies and surveys. Others may require special studies, particularly factors relating to community attitudes. To identify reasons for low immunization coverage, the following questions should be addressed[173]:

- Is the present vaccination system inadequate?
- Do the unvaccinated children and their families have special characteristics that can help identify them?
- Do parents lack accurate information?
- Do unfavorable attitudes among communities and families outweigh even a good vaccination system and good information?

Available information should be collected from secondary data sources (such as reports of previous program reviews, analysis of coverage data by health center) and by direct observation of vaccination practices and clinic organization during supervisory visits, discussions with experienced health care workers, and community discussions.[174] Supplementary studies then can be conducted and designed to answer specific questions that remain. A number of methods are useful for studies of reasons for incomplete vaccination[175,176]:

1. Qualitative methods can be used to evaluate community and health care professional knowledge and attitudes relating to vaccination.[175–177] These methods may be used alone,[177] as preliminary work to develop a quantitative data collection instrument,[178] or after quantitative surveys to examine how risk factors operate and develop interventions.[179]

2. Interviews of mothers of incompletely vaccinated *or* of fully vaccinated children can be done to describe their characteristics (case studies or case series).[180]

3. Quantitative studies of factors associated with incomplete vaccination can be done, by comparing characteristics of "vaccinated" with "unvaccinated" groups—cross-sectional "knowledge, attitudes, and practice" surveys,[140,143,181] case-control studies,[182] or cohort studies.[183]

4. Intervention studies can be performed, in which communities are randomized to the intervention compared with a control group,[142] or in which a whole population receives the intervention and "before and after" comparisons of coverage are made.[71,174,184,185,186]

Table 55–4 summarizes the factors that commonly affect vaccination uptake. In almost all studies, factors relating to poor performance of the health system and inadequate information to parents about where and when vaccination is available have been identified as major determinants of undervaccination. Ease of access, in terms of distance to vaccination sites,[98,140,180] short waiting times,[140,177] availability of curative services at the same site,[67,68,187] and cost,[96,187] affects utilization. Missed immunization opportunities are important causes of low coverage, and asking mothers to return on another day for vaccination was associated with undervaccination in Mozambique[143] and Cameroon.[173] Lower socioeconomic status of families and low parental education are almost universally associated with lower vaccination uptake among children.[140,143,173,181,183,186–190] Although it is difficult to change socioeconomic status in the short term, factors such as low educational level, recent migration,[143,173] and large family size [182,186,191,192] can be used to identify families that need extra support for their children to be fully immunized.

On the demand side, attitudes at community and individual levels should be assessed. The involvement of communities and local leaders in promoting immunization, planning immunization services, and informing families about the availability of vaccination services has been shown to be important, particularly in rural areas.[111,177,187,193–197] Families that have strong social networks in the local community[195,198] and language and culture similar to those of health care workers[173] are more likely to use health services. Adverse public opinion about vaccination has been documented when adverse effects occurred,[140,180] including postvaccination abscesses.[143] Misconceptions about vaccination,[199] including associating TT vaccination with contraception,[200] fortunately have been reported relatively infrequently.

Where possible, immunization program managers also should evaluate the impact of interventions designed to improve immunization coverage, using either controlled intervention studies or observational (ecologic) approaches to identify best practices to improve immunization cover-

TABLE 55–4 ■ Classification of Factors Affecting Receipt of Vaccines

Immunization System	**Family Characteristics**
Distance	Education (maternal and paternal)
Security	Family size
Appropriateness of time	Income
Reliability (no cancellation of sessions)	Refugees
Availability of curative services	Recent migrants
Waiting time	Language
Use of all opportunities	Ethnic group
Health staff's motivation and attitude	
Cost and costing policies	**Parental Attitudes/Knowledge**
Coordination between different providers	Previous positive or negative experience at health services
Quality of vaccination and other services	(e.g., turned away; postvaccination abscesses)
	Peer group pressure for or against immunization
Communications and Information	Family and social networks
Reception of information on "where and when"	Perceived susceptibility to disease
of vaccination	Perceived seriousness of disease
Person-to-person information from	Perceived safety of vaccine
trusted health care worker or community leader	Perceived efficacy of vaccine
Language compatibility between health care	
workers and clients	
Use of mass media according to level of	
access and expertise	
Community involvement in planning and	
managing services and in social mobilization	
Action to dispel misconceptions	

age. A comprehensive review of controlled intervention studies has been completed, and documents the potential effectiveness of interventions targeted to improve supply of immunization (e.g., training, monitoring/supervision, outreach, community health care workers); to increase demand (channeling, reminders, increasing awareness, shortened waiting time); or both (mass campaigns, reorganization of the immunization system).[186] Effectiveness of different methods to improve immunization likely will vary among countries, but compilation of evidenced-based best practices could provide helpful guidance for program managers.[201]

Determinants of immunization uptake may vary between areas and at different phases of an immunization program. It is therefore important to investigate reasons for nonvaccination or incomplete vaccination in a variety of settings. There is no single "correct" research method, and qualitative and quantitative methods are complementary. Anthropologic approaches yield information about health decision-making processes as well as an understanding of their specific cultural context but may not link that information to overall health care utilization patterns. Epidemiologic surveys yield information about utilization rates and access to care factors but may not take into account the context in which health care decisions are made or account for biases in Western constructs of disease and illness.[179] There is increasing consensus on the need to link the two approaches to improve health services in developing countries.[175,179,202,203] Use of a mix of methods[96] and feedback of results to decision makers, health care workers, and communities allow the continuous identification and solution of problems.

Disease Surveillance

Surveillance is fundamental to measure the impact of immunization programs on reducing vaccine-preventable diseases. As immunization programs move from a focus on raising coverage to one of controlling or eliminating diseases, the emphasis of surveillance moves from concentrating on measurement of coverage (a performance measure) to measuring impact on disease incidence (an outcome measure). Disease surveillance was a crucial component of the smallpox eradication program[122] and remains critical to ongoing global efforts to eradicate poliomyelitis and regional efforts to eliminate measles.[43,116,120] Surveillance is also critical to demonstrating the burden of disease from infections for which new vaccines are under development, as well as to documenting the impact of new vaccines and building government support for sustained funding of immunization programs.[204] However, it remains one of the weak links in the cycle of program planning, implementation, and monitoring in the EPI. Country EPI programs may lack personnel with the skills, resources, time, and incentives to develop effective surveillance. Responsibility for surveillance may not be located in the EPI program (e.g., disease control), requiring additional efforts to coordinate collection and use of data. Immunization programs should nonetheless facilitate the development of surveillance of the target diseases, provided such surveillance is action oriented and complemented by adequate feedback to all reporting sites.

Different methods of surveillance are used at different stages of immunization programs in the developing world (Table 55–5). Routine aggregate reporting of vaccine-preventable diseases can be used to monitor program impact. Although disease incidence rates frequently are underestimated, because only those cases that present to health care facilities are detected, if the reporting system remains unchanged over time, disease trends can be monitored. Demonstration of the long-term reduction in disease incidence is important to convince policy makers of the effectiveness of EPI when an outbreak of a target disease occurs in an area with high immunization coverage.[205] Analysis of data from routine reports also can identify high-risk groups, which then are targeted for extra program efforts.[206] The utility of surveillance based on routine reports from health care facilities can be increased by reducing the number of diseases that must be notified (to focus on the most important diseases), conducting active surveillance (e.g., regular visits or telephone calls to ask whether cases have occurred), and instituting "negative reporting" (i.e., reporting the absence of cases).

Enhanced "case-based reporting" is essential in programs of accelerated disease control, such as polio eradication and measles elimination.[116,120] Critical elements include active case-finding, negative reporting, prompt investigation of each disease case to collect relevant risk factor and program information, laboratory confirmation, and program response. Case-based reporting requires substantially more human resources than routine reporting, and should be initiated only in programs with high vaccine coverage and disease reduction initiatives, but such reporting can serve as a foundation to expand and enhance surveillance for other vaccine-preventable diseases.

Sentinel site surveillance may be appropriate in early stages of establishing surveillance and when laboratory confirmation of cases is desirable but capacity is limited, and may substitute for routine surveillance where the latter is poorly developed.[207] Sentinel surveillance is increasingly being used in Africa and elsewhere to develop and utilize laboratory capacity to differentiate causes of bacterial meningitis (H. *influenzae* type b, meningococcus, pneumococcus), and of rash or febrile illness (measles, rubella, yellow fever). Sentinel sites also can complement routine systems by providing more detailed information on each case. Sites may be selected on the basis of their geographic representativeness, laboratory capacity, case load, and willingness of staff to participate. Special surveys have been used to determine disease burden in areas where access to health care facilities is low, particularly in the early years of immunization programs.[208,209] For certain diseases, serologic surveys may be suitable to determine disease burden and measure impact on disease (e.g., hepatitis B).[210] They are relatively expensive, however, and generally unsuitable for monitoring disease incidence over time.

Whatever the source of data on target diseases, standard case definitions should be used and minimum data elements agreed on. Guidelines for surveillance of communicable diseases, including the EPI target diseases, are published by the WHO.[211] Suggested case definitions are summarized in Table 55–6. Surveillance systems should be monitored through the use of quality indicators, the main three being the timeliness and completeness of reporting, the

TABLE 55–5 ■ Surveillance Methods for the Expanded Programme on Immunisation

Method of Surveillance	Major Characteristics and Functions	Major Drawbacks
Routine	Usually a passive, relatively inexpensive system relying on reports from health centers of cases of target diseases Evaluate disease trends by age group, vaccination status, etc. Obtain general idea of impact on target diseases Identify remaining chains of transmission in diseases for which there is an elimination goal	Incomplete and delayed for most diseases, except if the system has been strengthened (e.g., because disease is targeted for elimination) Usually too many diseases included in the reporting system, which discourages reporting and analysis at intermediate and operational levels Little or no action is taken at the local level, and little feedback received from higher levels Difficult to include the private sector
Case-based	Usually stimulated passive reporting or active case finding Investigation of each case and collection of key information (age, vaccination status, case contact, etc.) Identify all disease cases in effective program Often require laboratory confirmation	Labor intensive and costly Should only do with effective program and limited number of disease cases Requires in-depth training at all levels
Sentinel	Can complement weak routine surveillance by providing more detailed information on each case Can allow laboratory confirmation when clinical syndrome is not unique (e.g., lab testing to determine cause of meningitis as Hib, pneumococcus, or meningococcus) Early warning for outbreaks Selection of sites may depend on disease, laboratory capacity	May not be representative Need close follow-up to ensure timeliness and completeness of reporting Not as useful as diseases become rare Not sufficient for disease elimination/eradication programs
Special surveys	Conduct at beginning of the program to identify disease burden and set priorities (e.g., neonatal tetanus surveys, hepatitis B prevalence surveys) May be used to assess impact of program (e.g., follow-up hepatitis B prevalence surveys)	Time consuming and costly Problems with retrospective diagnoses Do not directly strengthen routine surveillance

Hib, *Haemophilus influenzae* type b.

TABLE 55–6 ■ Clinical Case Definitions and Laboratory Confirmation for Target Diseases of the Expanded Programme on Immunisation

Disease	Clinical Case Definition	Laboratory Confirmation
Diphtheria	An illness characterized by laryngitis or pharyngitis or tonsillitis, and an adherent membrane of the tonsils, pharynx, or nose	Isolation of *Corynebacterium diphtheriae* from a clinical specimen, or 4-fold or greater rise in serum antibody (both specimens before receipt of diphtheria toxoid or antitoxin)
Measles	Any person with fever and maculopapular rash and cough, coryza, or conjunctivitis	Presence of measles-specific IgM antibodies or at least 4-fold rise in measles-specific IgG antibody between acute and convalescent specimens or isolation of measles virus
Pertussis	A person with cough lasting at least 2 wk with one of the following: Paroxysms of coughing Inspiratory whoop Vomiting immediately after coughing without other apparent cause	Isolation of *Bordatella pertussis* or rise in IgG or IgA directed toward pertussis toxin or filamentous hemagglutinin antigen or detection of genomic sequences by PCR
Poliomyelitis	Any child <15 yr of age with acute flaccid paralysis or any person with paralytic illness at any age when polio is suspected	Wild-type poliovirus isolated from stool*
Neonatal tetanus	**Suspect:** Any neonatal death between 3 and 28 days of age in which the cause of death is unknown; or any neonate reported as having neonatal tetanus but not investigated **Confirmed:** Any neonate with normal ability to suck and cry during the first 2 days of life who between 3 and 28 days of age cannot suck normally and becomes still or has convulsions, or a hospital reported case of neonatal tetanus	None
Tetanus	Patient with 1. Stiff jaw and trouble opening mouth or swallowing 2. Painful stiffness of neck and abdominal (or other) muscles 3. A clear mind 4. A wound, often infected, or history of wound within past few weeks	None
Yellow fever	Illness characterized by acute onset of fever followed by jaundice within 2 wk of onset; hemorrhagic manifestations and signs of renal failure may occur	Isolation of yellow fever virus or presence of yellow fever IgM or 4-fold rise in serum IgG in paired sera, or positive post-mortem liver histopathology or detection of yellow fever antigen in tissues by immunohistochemistry or detection of yellow fever virus genomic sequences in blood or organs by PCR
Hepatitis B	Acute illness typically including acute jaundice, dark urine, anorexia, malaise, extreme fatigue, and right upper quadrant tenderness; biologic signs include >2.5 times normal serum alanine aminotransferase and increased urine urobilinogen	Serum positive for HBsAg or IgM anti-HBc
H. influenzae type b (Hib)	Bacterial meningitis as characterized by fever of acute onset, headache, and stiff neck; pneumonia or sepsis with fever; none of these are specific signs of Hib disease, and Hib disease cannot be diagnosed on clinical grounds	Isolation of Hib from a normally sterile clinical specimen, such as CSF or blood, or identification of Hib antigen in normally sterile fluid by latex agglutination or CIE

*A clinical polio case is not discarded unless two adequate stool specimens have been collected (two stool specimens 24 or more hours apart within 14 days of onset of paralysis, maintained in good condition).
Anti-HBc, anti–hepatitis B core antigen antibody; CIE, counter immunoelectrophoresis; CSF, cerebrospinal fluid; Ig, immunoglobulin; PCR, polymerase chain reaction.

proportion of reported cases/outbreaks that are investigated in a timely manner (including laboratory confirmation of diagnosis, where appropriate), and the proportion of investigated cases/outbreaks that are followed by an appropriate response.[207]

Outbreak investigations complement routine surveillance and can provide additional information on incidence and fatality by age and vaccine effectiveness. They provide an opportunity to identify reasons for the outbreak and to obtain reliable data on disease epidemiology that can assist in adjusting immunization strategies. By feeding back information from the outbreak investigation to personnel at the local level, they can lead to improvements in routine surveillance and immunization programs.

Monitoring the impact of recently added vaccines (Hib and HepB) and new candidates for inclusion in the program, such as conjugate pneumococcal and meningococcal vaccines, will present additional challenges for surveillance. The new bacterial vaccines provide protection against diseases with less specific clinical manifestations, and laboratory confirmation is a critical element for their differential diagnosis. Furthermore, for HepB vaccine, the desired outcome (prevention of chronic liver disease) may not be measurable for many years after vaccination has begun, and other outcome measures (e.g., the age prevalence of hepatitis B surface antigen [HBsAg]) are most useful to monitor program effectiveness in the shorter term.[210,212]

Laboratories play an essential role in the surveillance of most vaccine-preventable diseases, particularly once disease incidence decreases and clinical diagnosis may become less reliable. For the poliomyelitis eradication program, the Global Laboratory Network capable of detecting wild-type poliovirus has been an essential component of the process of eradication and its certification. For this purpose, the WHO has established a Global Polio Laboratory Network consisting of 84 national laboratories and 40 sub-national laboratories in large countries, supported by 16 regional reference laboratories and seven global specialized laboratories.[213–215] Building on the success of this network, a similar global network has been established for measles (and other rash illnesses including rubella and dengue) laboratory diagnosis,[120] and for yellow fever in the 33 African countries endemic for yellow fever.[13] Similarly, a pediatric meningitis laboratory network is now being established in Africa to determine the causes of meningitis and to document the impact of new bacterial conjugate vaccines (see *www.whoafr.org/hib/index.html*).

With the availability of low-cost, high-performance microcomputers, public health programs and services are automating the management and analysis of surveillance data. Computer systems, if properly designed, can support the main functions of disease surveillance: (1) systematic collection of data; (2) consolidation, analysis, and evaluation of the data; and (3) feedback of the results.[216] To facilitate data analysis, computer software, such as EPI Info 2002, has been developed using a combination of database, statistical, and graphics packages. These systems are now of particular interest to immunization programs that are shifting toward the decentralization of data management (i.e., the monitoring of coverage and disease at the lowest geopolitical level). Finally, computer systems facilitate the basic objective of surveillance: the collection and timely analysis of data to identify those at risk, detect the changing pattern of the diseases, adjust strategies, and monitor the impact of immunization programs.

As an adjunct to disease surveillance and monitoring vaccine coverage, serologic surveillance is a secondary tool used for monitoring the impact of vaccination programs and identifying populations at risk in some industrialized countries.[217,218] This tool has been less used in developing countries because of cost, difficulty in differentiating natural from vaccine immunity, and shortage of laboratory capacity. Simpler and less costly serologic methods, such as enzyme-linked immunoassays, could enable developing countries to evaluate the impact of vaccines for diseases such as hepatitis B, tetanus, and rubella, and to monitor the effectiveness of current vaccination programs.[219,220] The detection of virus-specific antibody in saliva has been reported for human immunodeficiency virus (HIV), hepatitis,[221] and measles,[222,223] and further development of these assays could greatly facilitate field surveys.[224] Randomized, age-structured sero-surveys can provide useful information by which to assess profiles of herd immunity, for example, of measles and rubella[225,226]; to identify groups with lower immunity levels to target preventive measures[217,227]; and to permit a greater understanding of the transmission characteristics of an infection in the community.[228] Randomized serologic surveys in vaccinated populations can provide useful information on the impact of vaccination on disease transmission, as well as on the distribution of seronegative populations, the risks of infection outbreaks, and progress toward disease elimination.

Monitoring Adverse Events

Although modern vaccines are well tolerated and efficacious, no vaccine is totally safe. The more successful vaccination programs are in controlling disease, the higher the attention attracted to adverse events. In extreme cases, when disease has been eliminated, the acceptance of even very rare adverse events may become politically untenable. For example, because of the interruption of the transmission of wild-type poliovirus, all cases of paralytic poliomyelitis occurring in the Western Hemisphere are now vaccine associated, and in the United States this has led to a change in policy to use of inactivated poliovirus vaccine.[229]

In developing countries, surveillance for adverse events should include both those caused by program error and those resulting from inherent properties of the vaccines.[230–232] Adverse events resulting from program error are likely to be much more common than severe events related to inherent properties of the vaccine. Adverse events caused by program error may include reconstitution with the wrong diluent; administration of dangerous drugs mistaken for vaccines; contamination of multiple-use vials, leading to abscesses or sepsis; and use of contaminated needles or syringes, which may transmit blood-borne diseases (e.g., HIV, hepatitis B virus [HBV], hepatitis C virus [HCV]).[55,56,232] Adverse events caused by inherent properties of vaccines may result in complications unusual in developed countries. In Zimbabwe, an outbreak of lymphadenitis after BCG immunization in 1982 was traced to a switch to a different strain of vaccine that was more reactogenic. The ensuing investigation also revealed problems with intradermal injection technique as a contributing factor.[233] Similar outbreaks of lymphadenitis have been reported in other countries.[234–237]

At a minimum, every country should develop surveillance for adverse events following vaccination, with emphasis on reporting cases caused by program error (e.g., abscesses) and severe events such as septicemia or death that are temporally related to vaccination.[231,232,238] Information collected should include clinical symptoms as well as the manufacturer, lot number, and date of expiration of each vaccine received. Single serious events or clusters of unusual events (abscesses) should be investigated by EPI staff. Training on adverse events surveillance is useful to remind health care workers of the potential for adverse events and the need for constant vigilance when biologic preparations are administered to children and mothers.

Costs

Economic analysis is valuable to measure the cost-effectiveness of immunization programs, as well as the cost and cost-effectiveness of adding new vaccines or methods to deliver vaccines, and to build advocacy for cost-effective health services.[239] The World Bank measured the cost-effectiveness of different interventions in terms of their cost per DALY gained.[239] Estimated costs were less than $10 per DALY gained (or about $300 per death averted) for measles immunization and less than $25 per DALY gained for the full immunization series, making vaccination one of the most cost-effective public health interventions.[5,240] Cost analysis also can be used to demonstrate the savings that accrue to industrialized countries from global eradication programs and to promote investment in them, although the advent of bioterrorism has changed the potential options for discontinuing vaccination and future cost savings in such programs.[241] Studies of costs can help program directors manage their resources, compare different operational strategies, and decide how funds should be used.[242,243] Cost-effectiveness analyses of new vaccines, such as hepatitis B and *H. influenzae* type b vaccines, can help countries to determine which new interventions should be introduced or sustained.[244–246]

Developing cost estimates for EPI programs has been facilitated by WHO guidelines and software,[247,248] and since 2000 has been operationalized by the GAVI requirement that each country develop financial sustainability plans. EPI operating costs include salaries of the immunization team and supervisors; vaccines and vaccine shipment; injection equipment; transport, including fuel allowances and vehicle maintenance; maintenance of the cold chain and running costs of health care facilities (kerosene, electricity, stationery); and training costs. Capital costs include a portion of buildings and vehicles attributed to the EPI plus costs of cold chain equipment and spare parts.

Reviews of costing studies done since the 1980s show that the average cost of fully immunizing a child (including three doses of polio and DTP and one dose each of BCG and measles) in low-income countries is about $13, excluding technical assistance (1987 U.S. dollars), and $15 if technical assistance is included.[249] The cost ranges from $6 to more than $20, depending on the strategy used, the population density, and the prices of labor and other local inputs.[5,247,249] Although the relative costs of different strategies vary between countries, in general, routine services cost less per fully vaccinated child than mobile teams or campaigns.[5] In Ecuador, for example, campaigns cost $66 per DALY gained compared with $30 for routine services.[250] However, in Thailand, increased use of mobile teams was more cost-effective in areas with a dispersed population.[247] The cost per child immunized needs to be balanced against the effectiveness of the strategy in accessing all children in need of vaccination.

For all strategies, personnel costs accounted for the largest proportion, with supervision and management often the second largest cost.[247] Vaccines represented approximately 10% of all costs when the "traditional" EPI vaccines were considered. In general, costs of fully immunizing a child decreased as the number of children immunized increased.[247,251] However, the studies included only coverage levels up to 65%, and the marginal costs are likely to be higher when trying to reach the remaining 35% of infants. With the introduction of more expensive vaccines, the proportionate cost of vaccines has increased greatly. The number of contacts with health services needed to complete the series need not increase as new vaccines are introduced, depending on the schedule followed. Use of new combination vaccines may keep the schedule simple, but at higher cost. Vaccine storage, transport, and injection costs also will increase. A number of studies are now in progress on the cost-effectiveness of expanding coverage with existing vaccines, and introducing new vaccines, in a range of settings. Studies on options for financial sustainability also have been commissioned by GAVI and will be a vital part of long-term planning for national vaccine programs (see *www.vaccinealliance.org* and *www.gaviftf.info*).[148]

Cost-effectiveness studies of introduction of new vaccines have indicated that they can have good value, costing only $29 to $150 per life-year saved, representing only a fraction of the average per capita gross income in most countries.[245] In some cases, such as hepatitis B, vaccine cost is now lower than estimates used in studies, and costs are less than $50 per life-year saved. In others, cost of vaccine remains the key determinant in potential program costs and effectiveness.

Cost studies have shown that the proportion of EPI costs financed by donors varies widely, ranging from 4% to 73% of the total vaccine program costs.[249] Development of sustainable financing is defined as identification of funding sources from the national government and partners to maintain the full EPI program. As part of their comprehensive 5-year planning process, national EPI programs should work with partners through ICCs to develop coordinated funding plans to assure sustainable long-term financing.

Economic analysis also can be a powerful tool to identify barriers to implementing cost-effective strategies at different levels of the health system.[94,252] Economic analyses have helped to show problems in the process of disbursing funds, including irregular and delayed receipt of donor funds; poor accountability; overcentralization of management of funds, which limits access to funds for running costs at the health center level; and nonstandardization of payments for daily allowances between different vaccination strategies or between agencies.[94] Monitoring the process of utilization of resources and establishing transparent and

TABLE 55–7 ■ Techniques and Tools Developed by and for the Expanded Programme on Immunisation (EPI)

Area	Tool
Planning	National EPI plan of action, including costs and sources of funds
	Interagency coordinating committees (regional and national)
Facilitating attainment of high coverage	Accelerated schedule
	Contraindications policy
	Missed opportunities protocol
Management and training	Management training all levels
	Refrigerator repair technicians
	Driver and rider training
	Logistics for primary health care
	Program reviews
Monitoring coverage and disease surveillance	30-cluster methodology
	COSAS software
	Lot quality sampling
	Surveillance guidelines
	Laboratory network and technology transfer
	Data quality assessment
Cold chain	Range of appropriate refrigeration technology and spare part kits
	EPI product information sheets
	Cold chain monitors, vaccine vial monitors, open vial policy
Injections	Autodisable syringes; syringe safety boxes; prefilled injection devices; guidelines for destruction of waste
Financial sustainability	EPI costing guidelines; EPICOST software; immunization financing planning briefcase; financial sustainability plans

coordinated systems for accountability of donors as well as government health services could greatly improve efficiency.

Modeling

The choice of vaccination strategy requires an understanding of the dynamic effects of vaccination on disease transmission and knowledge of age-related changes in severity of disease, vaccine complications, and the probability of transmission of the infection.[58,253] Mathematical modeling is useful to estimate the burden of disease for which direct surveillance data are insufficient (e.g., rubella and hepatitis B). Mathematical models can assist with the task of measuring and comparing the merits of different strategies and improving our understanding of the observed impact of vaccination programs.[254]

Dynamic simulation models attempt to describe the dynamics of infections in populations and to predict their behavior under the conditions of vaccination programs.[58,253–256] This approach has been used to explore the effects of different vaccination policies on measles,[257,258] poliomyelitis,[259] and rubella.[225,226,260–262] It also has been used to compare different delivery strategies, for example, repeated pulse vaccination across a range of ages versus routine immunization at a single specified age.[263] Modeling has been used to explore thresholds for elimina-

tion or eradication of infections from populations,[58,253,264–266] and to examine the immunologic response to vaccines and minimum number of vaccine doses necessary to induce long-term protective immunity.[267]

Dynamic modeling generally has not considered the economic implications of the various scenarios. There is great potential for the combination of economic with dynamic modeling and for increasing the use of modeling in predicting the effects and cost-effectiveness of different vaccination strategies.[256,268]

Current Progress and Future Trends

Since its inception, the EPI has helped to create a global consensus on the value of disease prevention through immunization, and to establish a "culture of prevention" among politicians, health care workers, and community members.[86] Global strategies for disease control and eradication have been implemented, thanks to an unprecedented degree of commitment and cooperation among all partners within and outside the health sector, including national governments and international, national, and local organizations from the public and the private sectors. Many tools have been developed to facilitate the implementation and delivery of immunization services (Table 55–7).[2,86,269] The

Principle

Programming tool to help set priorities, monitor activities, and optimize donor contributions

Created for advocacy and coordination; avoid duplication or competition between donors

Reduce number of immunization contacts and protect children before highest risk

Take advantage of any visit to a health facility to immunize women and children

Different sets of modules and training programs relating to all aspects of program, for adaptation at the local level

Continuous in-service training to improve quality of services

Identify strengths and areas for improvement

Simple sampling methodology to estimate immunization coverage supported by computer software to assist in analysis

Monitor impact on disease control; use surveillance as a guide for program planning

Systematic case detection or confirmation

Assess and guide improving quality of reporting

Maintain correct temperatures in hot climates with erratic power supplies; use different power sources

Inventory of equipment for immunization meeting standard specifications

Monitor storage and transport of vaccine, and show whether or not vaccine is in appropriate condition for use; reduce vaccine wastage

Appropriate technology to ensure that immunization injections are safe and free from risk of transmission of blood-borne diseases

Methodology and software developed to estimate program costs

Strengthen capacity to plan sustainable immunization programs

---

EPI has concentrated on developing and updating effective training programs and modules for peripheral health care workers and midlevel and senior-level managers. Countries are encouraged to develop short- and medium-term (5-year) plans of action, and, as the number of donor agencies involved in supporting immunization services has grown, to coordinate planning and funding through ICCs.

The infrastructure established for immunization now serves as a foundation for programs that can reduce vaccine-preventable disease mortality not only with traditional and recently introduced vaccines, but also with the many vaccines now under development. Although there are wide regional and national differences in level of infrastructure and resources available for immunization and basic health care, immunization programs will continue to expand in several areas:

- Improving coverage levels of existing vaccines in the routine immunization program
- Conducting additional activities to eradicate, eliminate, or accelerate control of disease using existing vaccines
- Improving the quality and safety of vaccines and injections
- Adding new vaccines or micronutrients to the EPI program

- Assuring sustainable financial support and advocacy for immunization

Global Alliance for Vaccines and Immunization

In 2000, GAVI was formed by several major global partners to reinvigorate immunization programs in the poorest countries. Partners include the WHO, UNICEF, the Bill and Melinda Gates Foundation and other foundations, the World Bank, national governments, bilateral development agencies (USAID, the U.K. Department for International Development, others), representatives of the vaccine industry from developing and developed countries, NGOs, and technical and research agencies such as the Centers for Disease Control and Prevention (CDC).[7] These partners offer a wide range of skills and resources to support national immunization programs. The key objectives include improving immunization services (including injection safety) in developing countries, supporting national and international accelerated disease control targets for vaccine-preventable diseases, introducing new and under-utilized vaccines into the world's poorest countries, accelerating development of vaccines most needed in developing countries, and making immunization a key indicator of the quality of health systems and international development worldwide. The Vaccine Fund was established under the auspices of GAVI to support immunization programs in the

75 poorest countries (with per capita gross national products less than $1000), and has now been capitalized at over $1.2 billion (including $750 million from the Gates Foundation). By the end of 2002, funds had been provided to over 60 countries to support improving routine immunization, introduce new vaccines (for hepatitis B, *H. influenzae* type b, and yellow fever), and improve injection safety through introduction of AD syringes for all immunization injections.[147] This funding support is provided for 5 years, after which the country must develop sustainable funding support; it is anticipated that the Vaccine Fund then will be directed to introducing newer vaccines such as meningococcal and pneumococcal conjugates and rotavirus vaccines. Prerequisites for countries to receive GAVI funding support are a comprehensive 5-year national immunization plan with annual work plans, a functioning ICC of immunization partners in the country, and specific plans for improving immunization services, introduction of new vaccines, and enhancing injection safety. In addition, GAVI is supporting countries to develop financial sustainability plans to assure sufficient financial support for these programs after the cessation of GAVI funding.

The GAVI coalition is built on the substantial funding support and leadership provided to global immunization through other initiatives and through financial support of partners such as the WHO, UNICEF, bilateral donors and developed country governments, and foundations and NGOs. Since the mid-1990s, accelerated disease control and other immunization initiatives have focused attention and brought substantial resources to immunization programs.[2] Among these are the polio eradication initiative, which has brought human resources and new cold chain and transport equipment and focused advocacy in the poorest countries; the measles burden reduction initiative; neonatal tetanus elimination; the Immunization Safety Priority Project and SIGN, and the Global Training Network for assuring vaccine quality. These activities are led by the WHO and UNICEF with other partners, with increasing support by the GAVI coalition, and are described in more detail below.

Improving Coverage of Existing EPI Vaccines

Immunization coverage is a key indicator of access to and utilization of immunization services. In spite of continuous efforts to raise immunization coverage, since 1990 global coverage for EPI vaccines has been stagnant at 70% to 75% for infants (Fig. 55–4), and considerable disparity remains both between and within countries (Fig. 55–5).[146] Current global immunization coverage goals are that DTP3 and measles coverage should be 90% in all countries by 2010 (U.N. General Assembly), and that coverage should be 80% in all districts of developing countries by 2010 (GAVI milestone).[7,22]

Of 184 countries for which 2001 WHO-UNICEF best-estimate data are available, 129 have reported coverage of at least 80% for DTP3, while 21 countries are below 50% coverage, 9 of which have never reached the 50% figure. Only 64 countries are estimated to have reached the goal of 80% coverage in all districts, and an estimated 37 million children are not fully immunized each year. Average coverage of DTP3 in the African region has not yet come near to reaching 60%. In almost all countries, there is substantial disparity in coverage, with the lowest socioeconomic quintile having 25% to 30% lower coverage than the highest quintile.[2,270] To improve coverage in the lowest income countries, long-term, coordinated, and sustainable investment by national governments and donors is required.[90,93] Under the auspices of the GAVI coalition, efforts are ongoing to build human resources and management capacity, to track progress toward goals and target program interventions to the weakest countries, and to garner political and financial support to sustain improvements in immunization programs.[147]

Hepatitis B remains a major public health problem even though safe and effective vaccines have been available for more than 15 years. The WHO estimates that hepatitis B infection results in about 600,000 deaths every year worldwide.[271] HepB vaccine is estimated to be as cost-effective as measles vaccine in highly endemic countries (≥8% prevalence of carriage of HBsAg).[271] The high effectiveness of the vaccine has been demonstrated by reductions in the

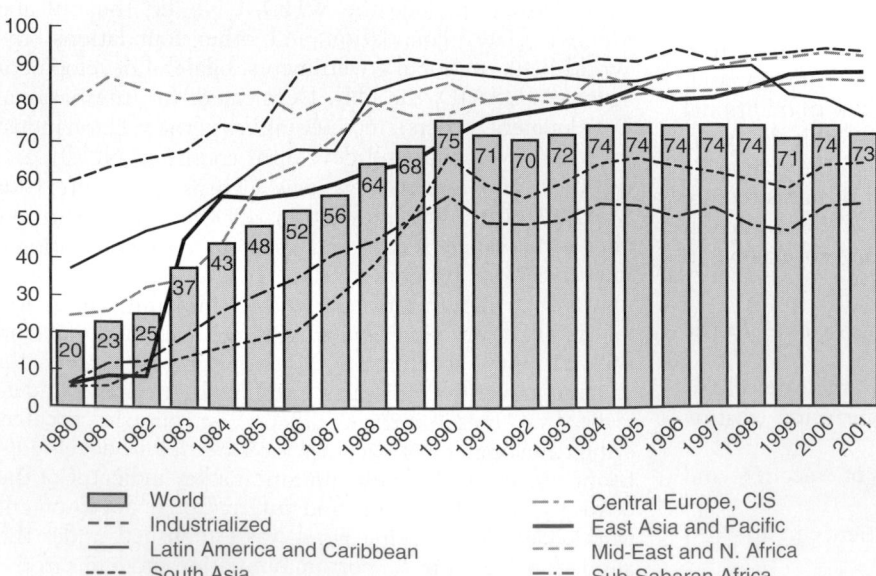

FIGURE 55–4 ▪ Global immunization with DTP3, 1980 to 2001 (numbers at tops of bars indicate percentages). (Data are WHO-UNICEF best estimates from Vaccines, Immunization & Biologicals. WHO Vaccine Preventable Disease Monitoring System: 2002 Global Summary [WHO/V&B/02.20]. Geneva, World Health Organization, 2002.)

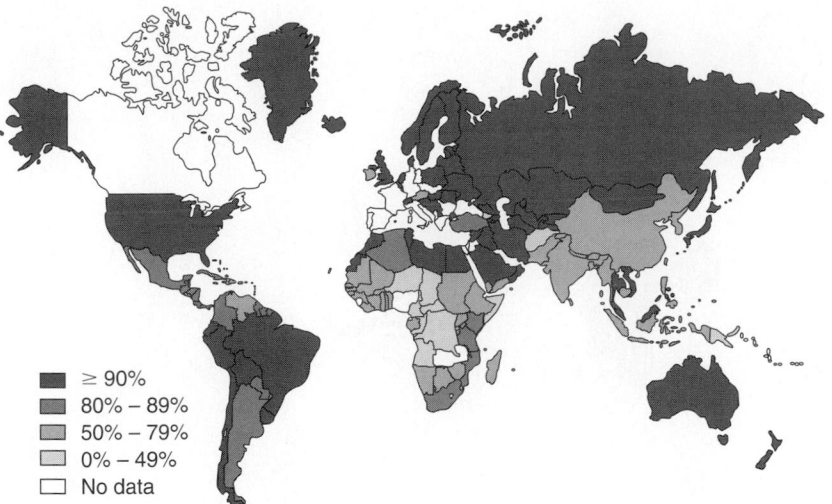

FIGURE 55–5 ■ Reported DTP3 coverage, 2001. (Data from Vaccines, Immunization & Biologicals. WHO Vaccine Preventable Disease Monitoring System: 2002 Global Summary [WHO/V&B/02.20]. Geneva, World Health Organization, 2002.)

carrier rate from more than 8% to less than 2% in immunized cohorts of children in The Gambia, Singapore, Hong Kong, Taiwan, Alaska, Thailand, Indonesia, South Korea, and American Samoa.[272] In Taiwan, a fall in the annual incidence of hepatocellular carcinoma in children ages 10 to 14 years was documented 10 years after implementation of a universal infant immunization program.[273]

Despite a recommendation by the World Health Assembly that all countries should integrate HepB vaccine into their national immunization programs by 1997, donors and governments initially were reluctant to invest in procurement of HepB vaccine because of vaccine cost and because complications occur many years after infection.[272] Initially, introduction of universal hepatitis B vaccination globally was determined by the economic status of the country and hence its ability to pay for the vaccine. However, with the support of GAVI funding in the poorest countries, and decreasing cost of vaccine (now about $0.33 per dose), HepB vaccine now has been introduced in 142 countries, including most of the highest-risk countries in Asia and many in Africa (Fig. 55–6).[2,146]

Since 1988, the WHO has recommended that the 44 African and American countries at risk for yellow fever include this vaccine in their infant immunization programs. In The Gambia, adding yellow fever at the time of measles vaccine did not significantly increase the cost per dose of immunization delivered in the EPI.[274] Currently 26 countries offer routine yellow fever vaccination. However, whereas coverage is relatively high in the Americas, it is generally poor in Africa because of lack of awareness about disease burden, weak routine immunization, restricted vaccine supply, and lack of resources for preventive campaigns. Since 1993, there has been a resurgence of yellow fever across Africa, with outbreaks reported in Ghana, Liberia, Nigeria, Sierra Leone, Gabon, Kenya, Guinea, and Ivory Coast.[12,274] To combat this resurgence, an International Coordinating Group for Vaccine Provision was established in 1997, and is working to establish sufficient vaccine supply for routine immunization and a stockpile for epidemic response. The WHO is also leading efforts to plan pre-emptive mass campaigns in at-risk countries, to strengthen laboratory-based surveillance, and to strengthen outbreak response through intercountry planning. GAVI funds are available to support routine yellow fever vaccination in all eligible countries and to establish an annual stockpile to be used for outbreak response or pre-emptive campaigns.[275]

Hib conjugate vaccines are highly effective against a major pathogen that is estimated to cause 450,000 childhood deaths annually.[204] Its use has virtually eliminated invasive *H. influenzae* type b disease from much of the industrialized world.[276,277] It has been shown to have an efficacy of more than 90% in The Gambia,[277] where Hib

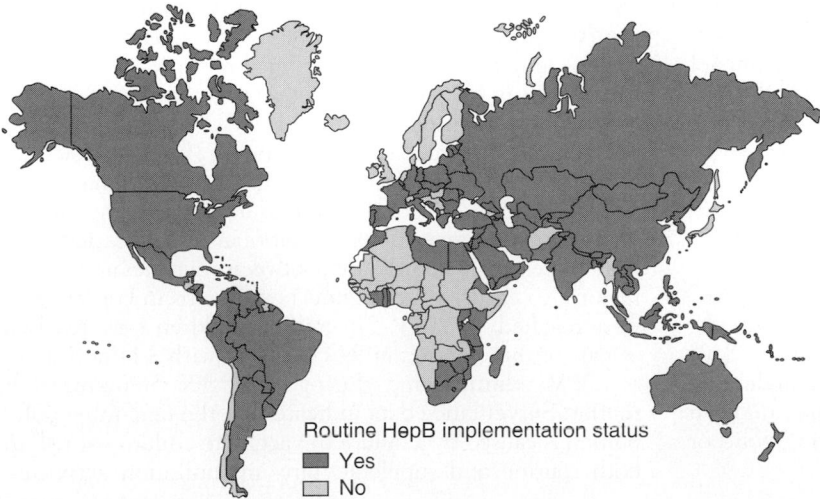

Routine HepB implementation status
■ Yes
■ No

FIGURE 55–6 ■ Global status of countries using HepB vaccine in their national immunization system, 2002. (Data from Vaccines, Immunization & Biologicals. WHO Vaccine Preventable Disease Monitoring System: 2002 Global Summary [WHO/V&B/02.20]. Geneva, World Health Organization, 2002.)

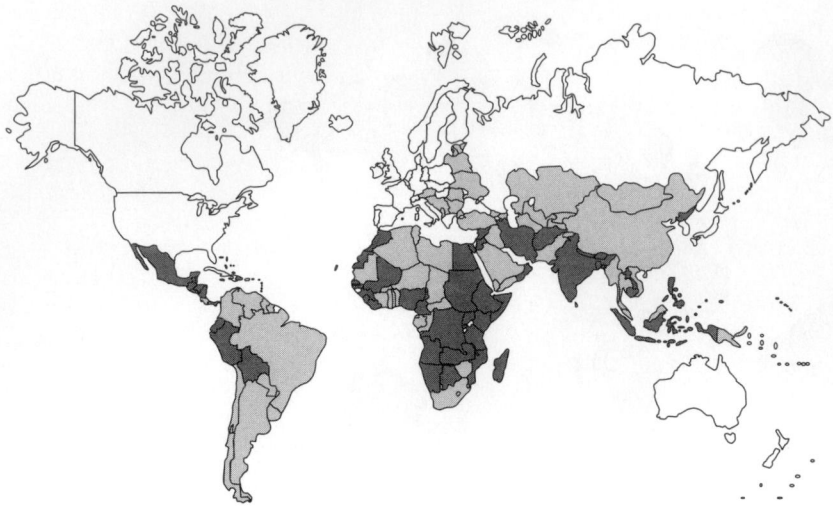

■ Vitamin A distributed with routine immunization services
(54 countries or 40%)

□ No Vitamin A distribution linked to routine immunization services
(81 countries or 60%)
(Note: 22/81 provided vitA with immunization campaigns)

□ Non deficient (56 countries)

Global Summary of EPI-linked VitA Distribution

VitA with routine EPI: 25 countries
VitA with EPI campaigns: 22 countries
VitA with both (routine & EPI campaigns): 29 countries
Total: 76 countries

FIGURE 55–7 ■ Countries providing vitamin A supplementation with routine immunization services, 2001. (Data from WHO; Vaccines, Immunizations and Biologicals. Available at *http:// www.who.int/vaccines-surveillance/statsandgraphics.htm*).

vaccine also significantly reduced the incidence of radiologically defined pneumonia by 21%. Hib conjugate vaccines now have been introduced in 90 countries worldwide, including most of the Americas, Western Europe, and the Middle East.[2,146] Vaccine introduction elsewhere has been slowed by lack of knowledge of disease burden, lower disease burden (east Asia), and relatively high vaccine cost (about $2.50 per dose). To support expanded vaccine use, the WHO and the CDC have developed tools to help countries rapidly define Hib disease burden and are supporting development of laboratory networks to document disease burden and vaccine impact in developing countries.[278] With support of GAVI funding, seven countries in Africa have now introduced Hib vaccine. Multiple studies are underway to better document disease burden in Asia, including a study of Hib vaccine efficacy for preventing pneumonia and meningitis in rural Indonesia that will support rational use of vaccine in these populations.

Supplementation of immunization with the micronutrient vitamin A has increased steadily during the last decade. During 2001, over 50% of countries with vitamin A deficiency utilized vitamin A with immunization, including 54 countries that gave vitamin A with routine immunization and an additional 22 that gave vitamin A during polio or measles vaccination campaigns (Fig. 55–7).

Eradication/Elimination

Substantial progress continues to be made in the global effort to eradicate polio.[6] From 1988 to 2002, the number of polio cases has been reduced from an estimated 350,000 in 125 countries on five continents to a provisional total of 1916 and just seven endemic countries—India, Pakistan, and Afghanistan in Asia, and Nigeria, Niger, Egypt, and Somalia in Africa. India, Nigeria, and Pakistan account for 99% of remaining cases, with over 90% occurring in 9 of the 76 states or provinces of these three countries. Reported routine immunization coverage for three doses of OPV was above 80% in all regions except Africa, where OPV3 coverage has remained at around 53% since 1994, and Southeast Asia, where coverage is now 73%. As of 2002, all poliomyelitis-endemic countries in the world had conducted multiple national immunization days, and implemented surveillance for AFP. National immunization days were increasingly coordinated between countries and WHO regions, to ensure that migrant populations in border areas were reached. In 2001, 575 million children were reached as part of these efforts in 94 countries, with 2 billion doses of OPV administered during over 300 immunization rounds. Surveillance data indicate that the remaining polio burden is caused by a failure to vaccinate children at risk in both routine and supplementary immunization activities.

Activities to eradicate polio in the remaining endemic countries have been accelerated to reach the target as soon as possible.[6]

Termination of wild-type poliovirus transmission is scientifically feasible, and all the data reaffirm the soundness of the polio eradication strategies. The last case of polio caused by wild-type 2 poliovirus (one of three types causing paralytic polio) occurred in 1999, suggesting that eradication of this poliovirus type has been achieved. However, there still are major political, managerial, and operational barriers to be overcome to complete the eradication effort. Intensified efforts are needed to vaccinate all children in the remaining endemic countries, particularly in communities in densely populated areas with large minority populations. Reaching children in areas of war or civil conflict, such as exist in Somalia, is particularly challenging.

Additional challenges to completing the polio eradication agenda include assessing the risks from circulating vaccine-derived polioviruses and implementing a plan to protect against these risks (see Chapter 25). Finally, the risks of reintroduction of wild-type poliovirus need to be assessed and plans developed for implementation should reintroduction occur.

Impressive results have been achieved using the measles strategies outlined earlier in the chapter. Measles cases have been reduced to record lows, and measles deaths have been eliminated in the Americas.[279] Campaigns in seven southern African countries stopped epidemic measles and dropped measles deaths to near zero.[280,281] Similar initial mass campaign strategies have been implemented in industrialized countries to prevent anticipated measles epidemics.[120,227,282–284] To meet the 2005 measles reduction goal, these strategies are now being implemented throughout sub-Saharan Africa and in other regions where measles disease burden remains high.[285,286] In 2000, over 100 million children received a dose of measles vaccine through supplementary immunization activities (SIAs), and this number is projected to increase as more countries conduct catch-up vaccination. By 2001, 174 (81%) of 214 countries or territories had provided a second opportunity for measles immunization through nationwide SIAs during the preceding 3 years or through a routine two-dose schedule (Fig. 55–8). However, in 2000 measles still was the fifth leading cause of childhood mortality,[3] accounting for 5% of all deaths among children less than 5 years of age and amounting to an estimated 777,000 measles deaths, of which 452,000 occurred in Africa.[285,286] This ongoing disease burden and availability of safe and effective measles mortality reduction strategies make a compelling case for continued accelerated efforts.

The reduction of measles-associated mortality is a public health priority in developing countries. Measles eradication, defined as the interruption of measles transmission globally,[20–22] is theoretically possible because there is no known animal reservoir and measles vaccine is highly effective.[287] In practice, the high infectivity of measles makes it difficult to eradicate, because more than 90% (and possibly more than 95%) of the population must be immune for incidence to decline toward zero.[58] The difficulties in reaching the required immunization coverage in developing countries and low public awareness about the seriousness of the disease in industrialized countries contribute to the practical difficulties.[21,22] Nonetheless, the recent success of measles elimination programs throughout the Americas[279] as well as in Finland,[288] Sweden,[289] the United Kingdom,[290] and southern Africa[280] has shown that these practical problems can be overcome, given sufficient resources.

Efforts to eliminate MNT continue to progress steadily. MNT has been essentially eliminated in the Americas and northern Africa (Fig. 55–9).[2,121,291] In 2001, an estimated 200,000 cases occurred in 57 endemic countries, mainly in Asia and sub-Saharan Africa, representing approximately 45% of the burden in 1990. Twenty-two of these countries were close to elimination, with fewer than 10% of districts at high risk. Routine TT2 vaccination among pregnant women was estimated to be 72%. However, the remaining endemic countries still face substantial obstacles, including limited routine immunization services and antenatal care and unavailability of skilled birth attendants. Efforts to improve these services and to accelerate elimination through supplemental immunization in high-risk areas continue to be led by UNICEF, but will require substantial additional resources to meet the goal (see *www.childinfo.org*).

Improving Vaccine Supply and Quality and Injection Safety

Assuring an adequate supply of safe and effective vaccines will continue to be a major challenge during the next decade.[2,292–294] The global supply of traditional EPI vaccines is fragile, with shortages in DTP and TT developing in recent years. Supply has become threatened because of a decreasing number of manufacturers, resulting from mergers of major pharmaceutical companies; increasing divergence of vaccines used in developed and developing countries; and declining interest in production of low-cost and low-profitability vaccines. Developing country manufacturers are now playing an increasing role in manufacturing of EPI vaccines (with >50% of UNICEF-procured vaccines purchased from these emerging producers), and an increasing role in developing new vaccines such as DTP-HepB and other DTP-based combination vaccines. Several have entered into joint development agreements with major vaccine manufacturers to produce new vaccines, and many now participate in a developing country vaccine manufacturers network.[147]

During the 1990s, assessments under the auspices of the Children's Vaccine Initiative Task Force identified the strengths and weaknesses of many vaccine producers and highlighted the need for improvements in production process, independent quality control, and national regulatory competence.[295] To address ongoing concerns about the quality of the EPI vaccines produced in developing countries,[172,296] the WHO has led efforts to examine the global status of vaccine production, supply, and quality, and to strengthen national regulatory authorities (NRAs) in vaccine-producing countries.[2,297,298] Six basic criteria have been developed to determine whether each NRA is able to guarantee that a vaccine is of "known good quality" (appropriate licensing requirements, clinical review of safety and efficacy, lot release, laboratory testing, regular inspections, and evaluation of clinical performance). In 2001, of 48 countries that were vaccine producers, about 60%

ACHIEVING 90% MEASLES COVERAGE, 2001

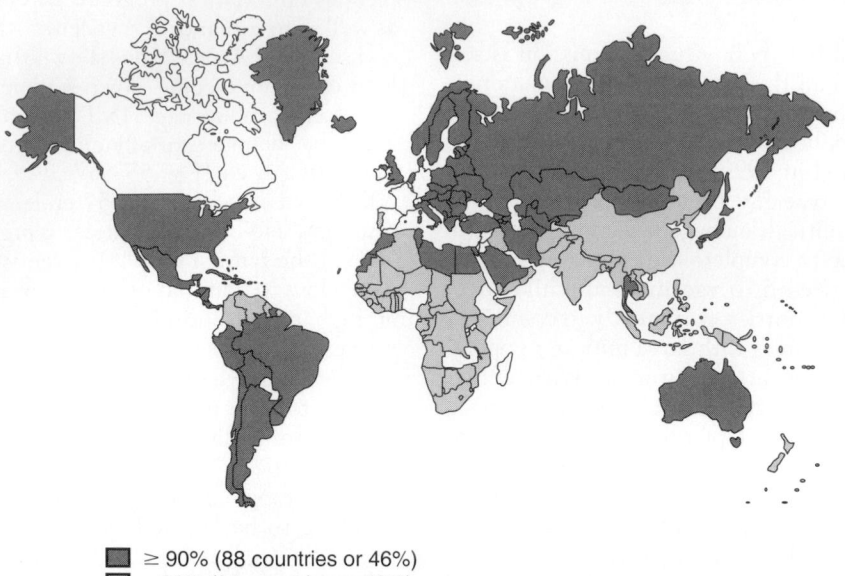

■ ≥ 90% (88 countries or 46%)
□ < 90% (81 countries or 42%)
□ No data (22 countries or 12%)

PROVIDING 2ND OPPORTUNITY*, 1997–2001

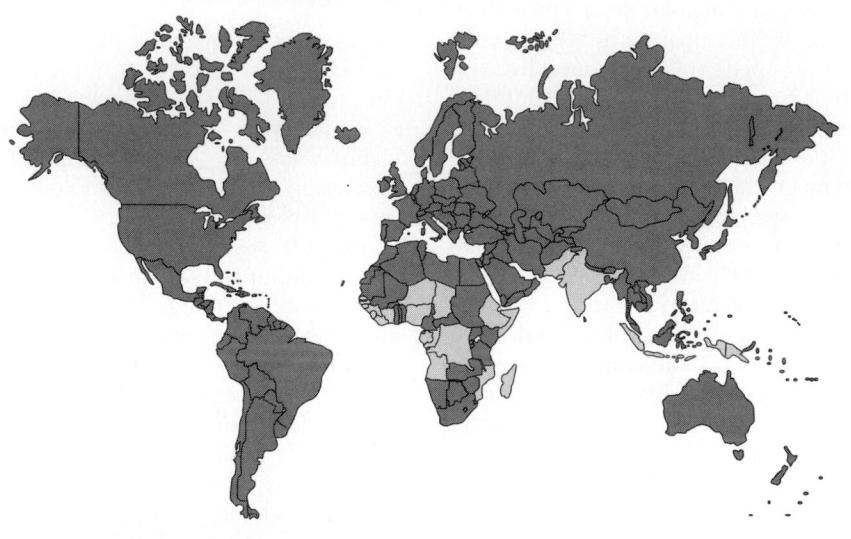

■ Yes 2nd opportunity (156 countries or 82%)
□ No 2nd opportunity (35 countries or 18%)

*_2nd Opportunity = country has implemented a two-dose routine measles schedule and/or within the last 4 years has conducted a national immunization campaign achieving ≥ 90% coverage of children < 5 yrs_

FIGURE 55–8 ■ Countries implementing measles mortality reduction strategies, 2001. (Data from Vaccines, Immunization & Biologicals. WHO Vaccine Preventable Disease Monitoring System: 2002 Global Summary [WHO/V&B/02.20]. Geneva, World Health Organization, 2002.)

(including both industrialized and developing countries) met WHO standards.[2]

To sustain the national, regional, and even global supply of the EPI vaccines, the most important areas of technology transfer for developing countries are those relevant to achieving and maintaining Good Manufacturing Practices standards in vaccine production, establishing independent and credible national quality-control laboratories, and instituting national (or regional) regulatory capability.[295–299] Facilitating successful and sustainable technology transfers is a challenge facing the international organizations that support the global EPI. The WHO has established a Global Training Network to provide training in regulation of vaccines for NRA, EPI, and national manufacturers, which now includes 13 training centers and has trained over 460 staff.[2,297]

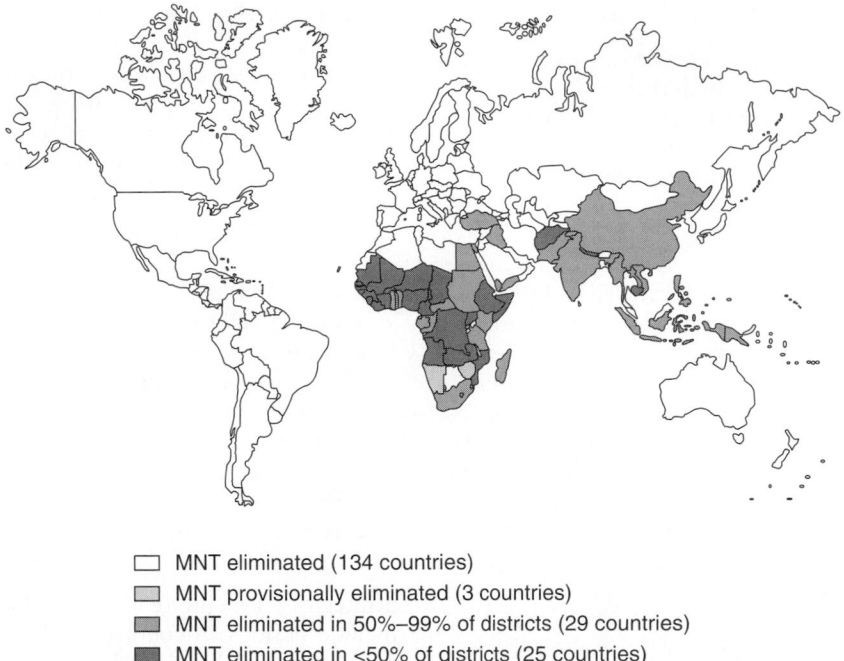

☐ MNT eliminated (134 countries)

▨ MNT provisionally eliminated (3 countries)

▨ MNT eliminated in 50%–99% of districts (29 countries)

■ MNT eliminated in <50% of districts (25 countries)

FIGURE 55–9 ■ Maternal and neonatal tetanus (MNT) elimination status, 2002. (Data from WHO; Vaccines, Immunizations and/ Biologicals. Available at *http:// www.who.int/vaccines-surveillance/statsandgraphics.htm*).

Vaccine quality also must be maintained once vaccines are distributed to the field. Among the challenges facing vaccine storage is the global banning of CFCs, which are necessitating the change of all cold chain equipment. Although the challenge of maintaining the cold chain at peripheral levels is facilitated by the use of VVMs that indicate exposure to high temperatures, there is as yet no VVM that can indicate vaccine freezing, which may occur more frequently than previously suspected and reduces potency of new, more costly adjuvanted vaccines such as HepB, DTP-HepB, and liquid DTP-Hib preparations.[50,53]

Another key component of a high-quality vaccination service is ensuring safe injection practices. Studies have estimated the global burden of disease caused by unsafe injections to include 21 million HBV infections, 2 million HCV infections, and 260,000 HIV infections annually.[56] Although the more than 550 million vaccine injections administered in developing countries represent only a small fraction of all injections performed, there is concern that vaccine injection safety is not always ensured.[54,300] To meet this challenge, the WHO, UNICEF, and their partners have established the Immunization Safety Priority project and SIGN to ensure the safety of immunizations and adequate waste disposal of injection supplies.[2,57,150,300] Autodisable syringes are now the only injection materials supplied by UNICEF; all purchases of vaccine should include sufficient AD syringes and safety boxes bundled with the vaccine, and funding allocations for these supplies also should take into account safe management of waste.[57,301] In addition, GAVI is supporting the 75 poorest countries to purchase sufficient AD syringes for all vaccines for 3 years to ease the transition to universal AD syringes for immunization. Defining and introducing optimal technologies for safe waste disposal, including various types of incinerators and burial, remains a major challenge currently in active debate (see *www.technet21.org*).[302]

Financial sustainability of immunization programs remains a critical challenge, especially as new, more costly vaccines are added to the schedule. Financial sustainability is the ability of governments to mobilize, with their partners, sufficient resources for routine immunization, accelerated disease control, new vaccines, and safe injections (see *www.gaviftf.info*).[303] National vaccine procurement or production strategies are facilitated by use of a grid that arrays countries according to their population and per capita income to define broad bands of countries for which different vaccine procurement strategies are appropriate. The smaller, poorer countries will obtain vaccine by procurement, with substantial donor assistance for the foreseeable future. The larger countries, particularly those with higher per capita income, will be increasingly likely to produce their own vaccines. A successful initiative that arose in the Americas has been the promotion of revolving funds.[304] Revolving funds supported by the Pan American Health Organization (PAHO) and UNICEF (Vaccine Independence Initiative) allow countries to purchase vaccines using local currency and to pay when orders are delivered. The PAHO fund was established as a single fund from which all countries can draw and that can be used to negotiate lower prices for purchase of large vaccine quantities.[305] This fund has been used successfully to promote wide use of combination DTP-HepB-Hib and measles-mumps-rubella (MMR) vaccines throughout the Americas. GAVI is stimulating the development of financial sustainability plans, through development of a standardized planning approach, with governments taking the lead to work with partners to identify long-term resources for immunization through multiyear planning and ICCs (see *www.gaviftf.info*).[147]

Introduction of Additional Vaccines

A number of effective vaccines are widely available in developed countries but not yet included in the EPI; still more are in the pipeline.[2,25] Rubella vaccine has been used for over 30 years in industrialized countries. A review completed for the WHO in 1995 showed that 78 countries (92% of industrialized countries, 36% of countries in economic transition, and 28% of developing countries) included rubella vaccine in their national immunization programs; by 2002, this number had increased to 119 countries.[2,306] In some other countries, rubella vaccine is used in the private sector only. The review also showed that seven developing countries had documented rubella outbreaks, with congenital rubella syndrome incidence rates as high as those in industrialized countries before vaccination.[307] All seven countries now have national rubella vaccination policies. However, it remains difficult for health policy makers to determine the relative priority to give to control of congenital rubella syndrome because of inadequate data in many countries.[307] The collection of appropriate data and development of practical surveillance methods for low-income countries are urgently required if the opportunities presented by measles control and elimination programs are to be taken to control congenital rubella syndrome as well.[308] Similarly, data on the burden of disease from mumps are needed as an increasing number of developing countries introduce the combined MMR vaccine.[306]

Several new vaccines have been shown to be highly effective and are likely to be introduced into some developing countries in the near future.[309–311] Meningococcal type C conjugate and 7-valent pneumococcal conjugate vaccines are highly effective against bacteremia and meningitis caused by the vaccine subtypes and have been introduced into some developed countries.[312–314] Trials with 9-valent pneumococcal conjugate vaccines have been completed in South Africa and are ongoing in The Gambia, while an 11-valent conjugate vaccine is under trial in the Philippines. With Gates Foundation support, efforts to develop conjugate meningococcal types A, C, and W135 vaccines to control meningitis outbreaks in Saharan and sub-Saharan Africa are ongoing. With support of GAVI Accelerated Development and Introduction Plans, research on disease burden and efficacy trials in developing countries for these and rotavirus vaccines is accelerating.[147,310,315,316] The greatest challenges will be producing these vaccines at a cost affordable by developing countries. Japanese encephalitis virus vaccines (killed and live, attenuated) are being used in some endemic countries in east Asia, and efforts to identify and certify a manufacturer of a WHO-prequalified vaccine and expand use into other endemic countries in Asia are ongoing.[24,317]

A wide range of new vaccines are expected to be licensed in the next decade. Lower respiratory infections and diarrheal diseases were among the top four causes of death worldwide in 1990,[3,15,318] and vaccines against these diseases thus have immense potential to improve health status. Some new vaccines will be licensed for the existing EPI target groups (e.g., rotavirus vaccine, conjugate pneumococcal and meningococcal vaccines); some likely will be targeted at adolescents (e.g., human papilloma virus,[319] herpesvirus, and HIV vaccines); and others will be indicated for people of all ages (e.g., dengue, malaria).[309,310,320] This means that the concept that the EPI target groups are only pregnant women and infants will be likely to change. Strategies to reach school-age children, adolescents, and all adults will be needed,[24,26,321] giving further impetus to the drive to strengthen primary health care through the EPI.

Many factors influence the utility of new vaccines for developing countries,[322] including

- Acceptability to the public and to the health authorities
- Affordability
- Heat stability
- Number of administrations (contacts with health care workers) of a vaccine required to induce lasting immunity
- Ability to be formulated as a component of a combination vaccine, such as DTP or MMR, or to be administered simultaneously with other vaccines
- Route of administration, whether parenteral or mucosal (such as oral or respiratory)

Strategies to facilitate the introduction of new vaccines include actions in-country to define the disease burden, develop political will, and ensure that the infrastructure is adequate for sustainable financing, procurement, quality assurance, and delivery of vaccines and actions at the international level.[323] The Global Programme for Vaccines and Immunization is working together with GAVI and other research partners to provide advice on strategic planning and analysis to help all collaborators in the development of new vaccines and their introduction into immunization programs.[2,321]

Conclusions

Immunization programs continue to be one of the most effective preventive health measures, and have spearheaded the development of public health worldwide. Through immunization, more than 2 million deaths are averted each year. Health care professionals around the world have been trained to plan, manage, and monitor their programs, and resources have been mobilized for the benefits of vaccines to reach most of the world's population. The EPI has led the way in infectious disease control, through establishing clear goals of controlling or eradicating some of the most important childhood diseases, a pragmatic approach to making it as easy as possible for parents to get their children vaccinated, and a strong emphasis on continued training and supervision. Lessons learned about simplifying immunization schedules,[324] providing protection as early in life as possible, establishing and disseminating clear guidelines for standards of care,[325–328] developing ICCs,[327] conducting sensitive case-based surveillance (e.g., AFP), and monitoring indicators of both process and impact[6,325–330] have benefited industrialized countries as well as developing countries. Assessment tools such as the EPI cluster sample and missed opportunity and cold chain monitor surveys have empowered peripheral health care workers to evaluate their own programs.[331,332]

The new millennium has brought enormous support for global immunization programs, along with future potential to greatly expand their scope and impact on childhood mortality. Through GAVI, the polio eradication initiative and global measles partnerships, and the WHO- and UNICEF-led initiatives for vaccine quality assurance and injection safety, immunization programs are receiving support to achieve disease reduction goals, increase vaccine delivery to the poorest populations, introduce new vaccines, and improve safety of injections.[2,147] Global research is bringing within reach needed new vaccines (e.g., conjugate meningococcal and pneumococcal vaccines and rotavirus vaccine) that could prevent an additional 1.5 million annual deaths resulting from respiratory and diarrheal disease in children, and substantial resources are being made available to develop vaccines to prevent the greatest killers in the developing world (HIV, tuberculosis, and malaria). To realize these future prevention gains, it is imperative that countries and partners effectively utilize current resources to strengthen the foundation of childhood immunization programs.

Nevertheless, the context in which immunization programs operate continues to change,[333] and programs must be prepared to respond flexibly and with innovation to these changes.[334] The health situation in various nations is increasingly influenced by global determinants such as environmental threats and the expanded movement of people and goods, which facilitates the spread of pathogens across national borders.[333] Global forces that affect health policies and systems in developing countries include the dominance of the market approach,[335] political systems that condone increases in poverty and inequality,[333] and violent civil conflict within and between nations. Health systems in countries all over the world are undergoing intensive reforms, and international cooperation for world health faces unprecedented challenges.[333]

The diversity of health problems within and between countries means that national and international health systems must confront a vast array of needs. The populations of developing countries continue to suffer from infectious and parasitic diseases, maternal and perinatal disorders, and nutritional deficiencies.[15] Worldwide, 30% of deaths are from these causes, ranging from 70% in sub-Saharan Africa to 6% in established market economies and the former Socialist economies of Europe.[3,15] At the same time, developing countries have a high burden of noncommunicable diseases and injuries. Whereas much remains to be done to reduce the burden of communicable diseases (which represent 7 of the top 10 causes of childhood mortality worldwide), increased attention is also needed for preventable causes of noncommunicable disease mortality, especially tobacco, alcohol, and injuries.

In the past two decades, structural adjustment policies for economic reform, promoted by international banks, have cut government health care budgets by one third to one half in most sub-Saharan African countries.[336,337] However, this trend is now being offset in some countries through the focus of improving health status in the heavily indebted poverty countries (HIPC) poverty relief programs.[338] As a result of the HIPC Poverty Reduction Strategy Plan, the line-item immunization funding in Tanzania increased fivefold, from $1.89 million in 2001 to $9.52 in 2003. Nevertheless, disproportionate amounts of public money continue to be spent on tertiary-level hospitals at the expense of cost-effective preventive interventions delivered at the primary level. Access to basic health services remains low in many rural and dispersed communities. The involvement of the private sector (including for-profit services, missions, and NGOs) in health care is increasing in all countries, raising challenges not only for equitable access to care but also for coordination, standardization, and quality control of interventions.

There is movement toward redefining roles of international organizations and national health systems. The function of international agencies is increasingly to address core issues for which action at the national level is insufficient.[335] These include surveillance and control of diseases that represent a global threat, promotion of research and development related to problems of global importance, development of standards and norms for international certification, coordination to assure sufficient low-cost supplies of needed drugs and vaccines, and action as agents of assistance and advocacy for vulnerable populations. At the national level, the role of Ministries of Health is changing from implementation of health programs to leadership and coordination. Their functions and skills must include advocacy, formulating and promoting health policies, coordinating support of global partners to build effective programs, consensus building and negotiation, assessment and monitoring the health effects of all programs, and providing technical guidance.[335] Implementation of health programs will be increasingly decentralized and under local government control. This will require a shift from training programs that are oriented toward the delivery of specific interventions to capacity building in these broader policy and management skills.

There is increasing divergence between rich and poor countries in terms of the number and types of vaccines that can be included in the national schedule at an affordable price and the coverage that can be achieved and sustained. This disparity may be overcome for individual diseases in the short term through the supplementary efforts and resources invested in eradication programs. In the long term, however, countries need the capacity to devise appropriate policies based on sound evidence about local priorities, and communities must be involved in the planning and execution of immunization programs.

Against this changing background, immunization programs face a number of challenges, the greatest of which is bringing equity in immunization services to the poorest countries and populations.[2] In 2000, 37 million children were not fully immunized, with coverage below or around 50% in the poorest countries in sub-Saharan Africa and Asia and lagging in the poorest economic quintiles of all countries.[270] The remaining burden of polio, measles, and neonatal tetanus is concentrated in these same countries, which also will be the last to gain benefits of new vaccines. To reach the disease reduction and immunization coverage goals, politicians and global partners must be dynamized to sustain and even increase assistance to the poorest countries. Both polio and measles campaigns have been implemented with great success and equity in coverage in even the poorest countries, and some developing countries (e.g., Sri Lanka, Malawi, Tanzania) have achieved and sustained high routine immunization coverage.[146] Donors must be persuaded to invest not only in campaigns for rapid disease reduction, but also in strengthening the physical, human, and managerial infrastructures in the countries.[86] In the future, immunization services that are already highly cost-effective will have the potential to prevent an even larger share of child mortality as new vaccines are developed that can be delivered with use of the same contacts. Mobilizing governments in industrialized countries to help developing countries profit fully from these vaccines is a major challenge for public health professionals throughout the world.

In the immediate future, another key challenge will be assuring a sufficient and affordable global vaccine supply, which will require overcoming constraints on vaccine production, developing and promoting cost-effective options for vaccine manufacture in developing countries, and enhancing country capacity to use vaccines effectively and minimize vaccine wastage. Other important challenges include developing effective, nonpolluting methods for management of the increasing injection waste (see *www.injectionsafety.org*)[302]; countering the tide of concern regarding vaccine safety that follows successful reduction of disease by vaccines[339–341]; and ensuring sustainable financing for immunization programs.

Despite decades of sustained progress through development and targeted health interventions, 7 of 10 leading causes of childhood death are communicable, most of which are or soon will be preventable by vaccines (Fig. 55–10).[3,15] Further reduction of mortality from these conditions must remain one of the principal priorities for global public health action. The challenge for the 21st century is to develop effective immunization services within health systems that are proactive and holistic.[335] The challenge for policy makers of immunization programs is to continue to expand services in ways that contribute to the development of comprehensive and sustainable health systems in the countries that need them most.

Sources of Information on Vaccines

Important sources for information about vaccines include the following.

World Health Organization. Provides extensive information about vaccines and vaccine-preventable diseases, and global and national statistics on immunization programs and vaccine-preventable diseases. Additional information about the WHO and international vaccine programs may be found at *www.who.int/vaccines*. Training materials may be found at *www.who.int/vaccines-diseases/epitraining*.

United Nations Children's Fund. Provides information about the state of the world's children and about women of child-bearing age, including statistics on immunization coverage and progress of initiatives to eliminate neonatal tetanus and measles and eradicate polio. Web sites include *www.unicef.org* and *www.childinfo.org*.

Global Alliance for Vaccines and Immunization. Information on the Global Alliance on Vaccines and Immunization may be found at the Web site (*www.vaccinealliance.org*).

Gates Children's Vaccine Program at PATH. The resource center contains an extensive library of immunization materials (see *www.childrensvaccine.org*).

National Immunization Program, Centers for Disease Control and Prevention, Atlanta, GA 30333. Extensive resources provide specific information on immunization and vaccine-preventable diseases (see *www.cdc.gov/nip*).

Report of the Committee on Infectious Diseases of the American Academy of Pediatrics (Red Book). The full report containing recommendations on all licensed vaccines usually is updated every 3 years. The most recent *Red Book* was published in 2003. It can be ordered from American Academy of Pediatrics, 141 Northwest Point Blvd., P.O. Box 927, Elk Grove Village, IL 60009-0927, or from the AAP Web site (*www.aap.org*).

Morbidity and Mortality Weekly Report. This report is published weekly by the CDC and contains vaccine recommendations, reports of specific disease activity, policy statements, and regular and special recommendations of the Advisory Committee on Immunization Practice. The MMWR is available online at *www.cdc.gov/mmwr*.

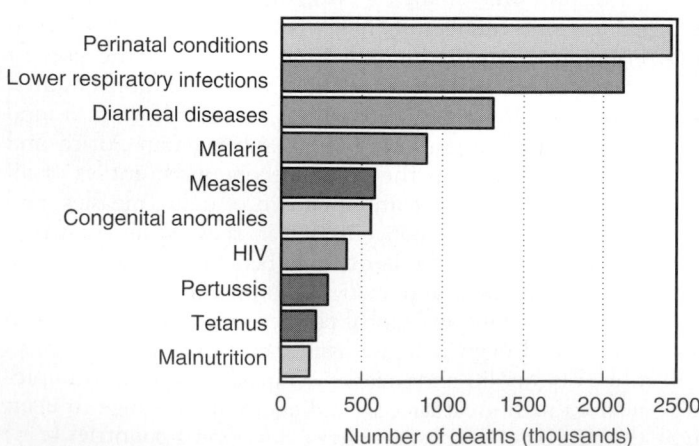

FIGURE 55–10 ■ Top 10 causes of death in children less than 5 years of age, worldwide, 2000. (Data from Murray CJL, Lopez AD, Mathers CD, Stein C. The Global Burden of Disease 2000 Project: Aims, Methods, and Data Sources (Global Programme on Evidence for Health Policy Discussion Paper No 36). Geneva, World Health Organization, 2001.)

Allied Vaccine Group. The Allied Vaccine Group is a partnership of six independent Web sites providing science-based, reliable information about immunization (see *www.vaccines.org*).

Immunization Action Coalition. The Immunization Action Coalition promotes physician, community, and family awareness of and responsibility for appropriate immunization of all children and adults against all vaccine-preventable diseases. This U.S.-based site has a wealth of education materials (see *www.immunize.org*).

Official Package Circulars. Manufacturers provide product-specific information for each vaccine; some of these are reproduced in their entirety in the *Physicians' Desk Reference* (*PDR*) and are dated.

Control of Communicable Diseases in Man. The American Public Health Association publishes this manual at approximately 5-year intervals. The 17th edition (2000) is currently available, and a revision is in progress. The manual contains valuable information concerning infectious diseases; their occurrence worldwide; immunization, diagnostic, and therapeutic information; and up-to-date recommendations on isolation and other control measures for each disease presented. It can be ordered from the American Public Health Association, 1015 15th St. NW, Washington, DC 20005.

Acknowledgments

The authors thank Dr. Bruce Weniger, Centers for Disease Control and Prevention, and Dr. Ana Maria Henao-Restrepo, World Health Organization, for assistance with editing the manuscript, and Ms. Marta Gacicdobo, World Health Organization, for assistance in preparing the figures.

REFERENCES

1. Henderson RH. Vaccination: successes and challenges. *In* Cutts FT, Smith PG (eds). Vaccination and World Health. Chichester, England, John Wiley & Sons, 1995, pp 3–16.
2. World Health Organization and United Nations Children's Fund. State of the World's Vaccines and Immunization. Geneva, World Health Organization, 2002.
3. Murray CJL, Lopez AD, Mathers CD, Stein C. The Global Burden of Disease 2000 Project: Aims, Methods, and Data Sources (Global Programme on Evidence for Health Policy Discussion Paper No 36). Geneva, World Health Organization, 2001.
4. Murray CJD, Lopez AD. Global Burden of Disease, 2001 Update. World Health Organization, 2001. Available at *www.who.int*.
5. Jamison DT, Saxenian H. Investing in immunization: conclusions from the 1993 World Development Report. *In* Cutts FT, Smith PG (eds). Vaccination and World Health. Chichester, England, John Wiley & Sons, 1995, pp 145–160.
6. Expanded Programme on Immunisation. Progress towards the global eradication of poliomyelitis, 2001. Wkly Epidemiol Rec 77:97–108, 2002.
7. Global Alliance for Vaccines and Immunization. Second GAVI Board Meeting, January 2000 (GAVI/00.01). Geneva, World Health Organization, 2000.
8. Hardy I, Dittman S, Sutter R. Current situation and control strategies for resurgence of diphtheria in newly independent states of the former Soviet Union. Lancet 347:1739–1744, 1996.
9. Rakhmanova A, Lumio J, Groundstroem K, et al. Diphtheria outbreak in St. Petersburg: clinical characteristics of 1860 adult patients. Scand J Infect Dis 28:37–40, 1996.
10. Dittmann S, Wharton M, Vitek C, et al. Successful control of epidemic diphtheria in the states of the former Union of Soviet Socialist Republics: lessons learned. J Infect Dis 181(suppl 1):S10–S22, 2000.
11. Galazka A. Diphtheria: the changing epidemiology of diphtheria in the vaccine era. J Infect Dis 181(suppl 1):S2–S9, 2000.
12. Robertson SE, Hull BP, Tomori O, et al. Yellow fever: a decade of reemergence. JAMA 276:1157–1162, 1996.
13. Monath TP. Yellow fever: an update. Lancet Infect Dis 1:11–20, 2001.
14. Murray CJD, Lopez AD. Global Comparative Assessments in the Health Sector: Disease Burden, Expenditures and Intervention Packages. Geneva, World Health Organization, 1994, pp 1–196.
15. Murray CJL, Lopez AD. Mortality by cause for eight regions of the world: Global Burden of Disease study. Lancet 349:1269–1276, 1997.
16. Chunharas S. The role of epidemiology in the development of a vaccination programme: discussion. *In* Cutts FT, Smith PG (eds). Vaccination and World Health. Chichester, England, John Wiley & Sons, 1995, pp 138–144.
17. Atkinson S, Cheyne J. Immunisation in urban areas: issues and strategies. Bull World Health Organ 72:183–194, 1994.
18. Keja K, Chan C, Hayden G, Henderson RH. Expanded Programme on Immunization. World Health Stat Q 41:59–63, 1988.
19. Begg N, Cutts FT. The role of epidemiology in the development of a vaccination programme. *In* Cutts FT, Smith PG (eds). Vaccination and World Health. Chichester, England, John Wiley & Sons, 1995, pp 123–138.
20. Dowdle WR, Hopkins DR. The Eradication of Infectious Diseases: Dahlem Workshop Report. Chichester, England, John Wiley & Sons, 1998.
21. Goodman RA, Foster KL, Trowbridge FL, Figueroa JP (eds). Global disease elimination and eradication as public health strategies: Proceedings of a conference held in Atlanta, GA USA, 23–25 February 1998. Bull World Health Organ 76(suppl 2):1–162, 1998.
22. Centers for Disease Control and Prevention. Recommendations of the International Task Force for Disease Eradication. MMWR 42(RR-16):1–38, 1993.
23. UNGASS. UN General Assembly Special Session on Children, 2002: A World Fit for Children. New York, United Nations, 2002, p 14.
24. Global Programme for Vaccines and Immunisation, Expanded Programme on Immunisation. Immunization Policy (WHO/EPI/GEN/95.03 Rev. 1). Geneva, World Health Organization, 1996.
25. Vaccines, Immunization & Biologicals. Case Information for the Development of Immunization Policy (WHO/V&B/02.28). Geneva, World Health Organization, 2003.
26. Expanded Programme on Immunisation. The Immunological Basis for Immunization. Module 1: General Immunology (A. Galazka); Module 2: Diphtheria (A. Galazka); Module 3: Tetanus (A. Galazka); Module 4: Pertussis (A. Galazka); Module 5: Tuberculosis (J. Milstien); Module 6: Poliomyelitis (S. Robertson); Module 7: Measles (F. Cutts); Module 8: Yellow Fever (S. Robertson) (WHO/EPI/GEN/-93.12–93.19). Geneva, World Health Organization, 1993.
27. Centers for Disease Control and Prevention. General recommendations on immunization. MMWR 51(RR-2):1–36, 2002.
28. Galazka A, Robertson S. Immunization against diphtheria with special emphasis on immunization of adults. Vaccine 14:845–857, 1996.
29. Prempree P, Chitpitaklert S, Silarug N. Diphtheria outbreak—Saraburi province, Thailand. MMWR 45:271–273, 1996.
30. Khuri-Bulos N, Hamzah Y, Sammerrai S, et al. The changing epidemiology of diphtheria in Jordan. Bull World Health Organ 66:65–68, 1988.
31. Youwang Y, Jianming D, Yong X, Pong Z. Epidemiological features of an outbreak of diphtheria and its control with diphtheria toxoid immunization. Int J Epidemiol 21:807–811, 1992.
32. World Health Organization. Pertussis vaccines. Wkly Epidemiol Record 74:137–144, 1999.
33. Cherry J, Olin P. The science and fiction of pertussis vaccines. Pediatrics 104:1381–1384, 1999.
34. Yih WK, Lett SM, des Vignes FN, et al. The increasing incidence of pertussis in Massachusetts' adolescents and adults, 1989–1998. J Infect Dis 182:1409–1416, 2000.
35. Comstock GW, Livesay VT, Woolpert SF. Evaluation of BCG vaccination among Puerto Rican children. Am J Public Health 64:283–291, 1974.
36. Kubit S, Czajka S, Olakowska T, Piasecki Z. Evaluation of the effectiveness of BCG vaccinations. Pediatr Pol 47:777–781, 1983.
37. Lugosi L. Analysis of the efficacy of mass BCG vaccination from 1959 to 1983 in tuberculosis control in Hungary. Bull Int Union Tuberc 16:15–34, 1987.
38. Fine P, Clayton D. Randomised controlled trial of single BCG, repeated BCG, or combined BCG and killed *Mycobacterium leprae* vaccine for prevention of leprosy and tuberculosis in Malawi. Lancet 348:17–24, 1996.

39. Global Tuberculosis Programme and Global Programme on Vaccines. Statement on BCG revaccination for the prevention of tuberculosis. Wkly Epidemiol Rec 70:229–231, 1995.

40. Cutts FT, Monteiro O, Tabard P, Cliff J. Measles control in Maputo, Mozambique, using a single dose of Schwarz vaccine at age 9 months. Bull World Health Organ 72:227–231, 1994.

41. World Health Organization. Strategies for reducing global measles mortality. Wkly Epidemiol Rec 75:409–416, 2000.

42. Markowitz LE, Preblud SR, Fine PEM, Orenstein WA. Duration of live measles vaccine–induced immunity. Pediatr Infect Dis J 9:101–110, 1990.

43. de Quadros CA. Strategies for disease control/elimination in the Americas. *In* Cutts FT, Smith PG (eds). Vaccination and World Health. Chichester, England, John Wiley & Sons, 1995, pp 17–34.

44. Expanded Programme on Immunisation. Heat stability of vaccines. Wkly Epidemiol Rec 55:252–254, 1980.

45. Expanded Programme on Immunisation. Stability of vaccines. Wkly Epidemiol Rec 30:233–235, 1990.

46. Lundbeck H, Hakansson B, Lloyd JS, et al. A cold box for the transport and storage of vaccines. Bull World Health Organ 56:427–432, 1978.

47. Expanded Programme on Immunisation. Ice-lined refrigerators (ILR). Wkly Epidemiol Rec 59:63–64, 1984.

48. The cold chain for vaccine conservation: recent improvements. WHO Chronicle 33:383–386, 1979.

49. World Health Organization and United Nations Children's Fund. Product Information Sheets, 2000 Edition (WHO/V&B/00.13). Geneva, World Health Organization, 2000.

50. Vaccines, Immunization & Biologicals. Temperature Monitors for Vaccines and the Cold Chain (WHO/V&B/99.15). Geneva, World Health Organization, 1999.

51. Zaffran M. Vaccine transport and storage: environmental challenges. Dev Biol Stand 87:9–17, 1996.

52. Expanded Programme on Immunization. The Use of Open Vials of Vaccines in Subsequent Immunization Sessions: World Health Organization Policy Statement (WHO/V&B/00.09). Geneva, World Health Organization, 2000.

53. World Health Organization and United Nations Children's Fund. Quality of the Cold Chain—WHO/UNICEF Policy Statement on the Use of Vaccine Vial Monitors in Immunization Practices (WHO/V&B/99.18). Geneva, World Health Organization, 1999.

54. Dicko M. Safety of immunization injections in Africa: not simply a problem of logistics. Bull World Health Organ 78:163–169, 2000.

55. Simonsen L, Kane A, Lloyd J, et al. Unsafe injections in the developing world and transmission of blood-borne pathogens. Bull World Health Organ 77:789–800, 1999.

56. Hauri A, Armstrong G, Hutin YTF. Estimation of the global burden of disease attributable to contaminated injections given in health care settings. Int J STD AIDS 2003 [in press].

57. Vaccines, Immunization & Biologicals. "First Do No Harm." Introducing Auto-Disable Syringes and Ensuring Injection Safety in Immunization Systems of Developing Countries (WHO/V&B/02.26). Geneva, World Health Organization, 2002.

58. Fine PEM. Herd immunity: history, theory, practice. Epidemiol Rev 15:265–302, 1993.

59. Hull D. Why children are not immunized. J R Coll Physicians Lond 21:28–31, 1987.

60. Cutts F, Orenstein W, Bernier R. Causes of low preschool immunization coverage in the United States. Annu Rev Public Health 13:385–398, 1992.

61. Foster SO. Immunization in 12 African countries 1982–1993. *In* Centers for Disease Control. Africa Child Survival Initiative—Combating Childhood Communicable Diseases. New York, U.S. Agency for International Development, World Health Organization, and United Nations Children's Fund, 1993.

62. Foster S. Immunization opportunities taken and missed. Rev Infect Dis 11(suppl):S629–S630, 1989.

63. Poore P. A global view of immunization. J Roy Coll Physicians Lond 21:22–28, 1987.

64. Cutts F, Soares A, Jecque A, et al. The use of evaluation to improve the Expanded Programme on Immunization in Mozambique. Bull World Health Organ 68:199–208, 1990.

65. Hutchins S, Jansen H, Robertson S, et al. Studies of missed opportunities for immunization in developing and industrialized countries. Bull World Health Organ 71:549–560, 1993.

66. Expanded Programme on Immunisation. Training for Mid Level Managers: Identify Missed Opportunities (WHO/EPI/MLM/91.7). Geneva, World Health Organization, 1991.

67. Walley JD, McDonald M. Integration of mother and child health services in Ethiopia. Trop Doct 215:32–35, 1991.

68. Tandon B, Gandhi N. Immunization coverage in India for areas served by the Integrated Child Development Services programme. Bull World Health Organ 70:461–465, 1992.

69. Levy-Bruhl D, Soucat A, Diallo S, et al. Integration du PEV aux soins de santé primaires: l'exemple du Benin et de la Guinée. Cah Santé 4:205–212, 1994.

70. John TJ, Steinhoff MC. Appropriate strategy for immunization of children in India. 3. Community-based annual pulse (cluster) immunization. Indian J Pediatr 48:677–683, 1981.

71. Cutts FT, Kortbeek S, Malalane R, et al. Developing appropriate strategies for EPI: a case study from Mozambique. Health Policy Plan 3:291–301, 1988.

72. Foster SO, Spiegel RA, Mokdad A, et al. Immunization, oral rehydration therapy and malaria chemotherapy among children under 5 in Borni and Grand Cape Mount counties, Liberia, 1984 and 1988. Int J Epidemiol 22(suppl 1):S50–S55, 1993.

73. Vaccines, Immunization & Biologicals. Sustainable Outreach Services (SOS): A Strategy for Reaching the Unreachable with Immunization and Other Services (WHO/V&B/00.37). Geneva, World Health Organization, 2002.

74. John TJ, Ray M, Steinhoff MC. Control of measles by annual pulse immunization. Am J Dis Child 138:299–300, 1984.

75. Gindler J, Cutts FT, Barnett-Antinori ME, et al. Successes and failures in vaccine delivery: evaluation of the immunization delivery system in Puerto Rico. Pediatrics 91:315–320, 1993.

76. Malison MD, Sekeito P, Henderson PL, et al. Estimating health service utilization, immunization coverage, and childhood mortality: a new approach in Uganda. Bull World Health Organ 65:325–330, 1987.

77. Auer C, Tanner M. Childhood vaccination in a squatter area of Manila: coverage and providers. Soc Sci Med 31:1265–1270, 1990.

78. Cutts F. Strategies to improve immunization services in urban Africa. Bull World Health Organ 69:407–414, 1991.

79. Kearney M, Yach D, van Dyk H, Fisher S. Evaluation of a mass measles immunisation campaign in a rapidly growing peri-urban area. S Afr Med J 74:157–159, 1989.

80. Fassin D, Jeannee E, Cebe D, Reveillon M. Who consults and where? Sociocultural differentiation in access to health care in urban Africa. Int J Epidemiol 17:858–864, 1988.

81. Fassin D, Jeannee E. Immunization coverage and social differentiation in urban Senegal. Am J Public Health 79:509–511, 1989.

82. Cutts F, Phillips M, Kortbeek S, Soares A. Door-to-door canvassing for immunization program acceleration in Mozambique: achievements and costs. Int J Health Serv 20:717–725, 1990.

83. Romero MGG, Pizano ES, Lamo JA. Channelling, a new immunization strategy. Assoc Children 69/72:193–203, 1985.

84. Saeed H. Increasing vaccine coverage through new delivery systems: a Sudan approach. Rev Infect Dis 11(suppl):S644–S645, 1989.

85. Dietz V, Cutts F. The use of mass campaigns in the Expanded Programme on Immunization: a review of reported advantages and disadvantages. Int J Health Serv 27:767–790, 1997.

86. Pan American Health Organization. The Impact of the Expanded Programme on Immunization and the Polio Eradication Initiative on Health Systems in the Americas. Washington, DC, Pan American Health Organization, 1995.

87. Ching P, Birmingham M, Goodman T, et al. Childhood mortality impact and costs of implementing vitamin A supplementation into immunization campaigns. Am J Public Health 90:1526–1529, 2000.

88. Goodman T, Dalmiya N, de Benoist B, Schultink W. Polio as a platform: using national immunization days to deliver vitamin A supplements. Bull World Health Organ 78:305–314, 2000.

89. Integration of vitamin A supplementation with immunizations. Wkly Epidemiol Rec 74:1–6, 1999. Available at *www.who.int/wer/pdf/1999/wer2001.pdf*.

90. Taylor ME, Laforce FM, Basu RN, et al. Sustainability of Achievements: Lessons Learned from Universal Child Immunization. Report of a Steering Committee. New York, United Nations Children's Fund, 1996, p 105.

91. Unger J-P. Can intensive campaigns dynamize front line health services? The evaluation of an immunization campaign in Thies health district, Senegal. Soc Sci Med 32:249–259, 1991.

92. Unger J-P, Killingsworth JR. Selective primary health care: a critical review of methods and results. Soc Sci Med 22:1001–1013, 1986.

93. LaFond. When the money runs out. Lancet 343:371, 1994.

94. Waddington C, Goodman H. Does economic analysis affect vaccination policy? In Cutts FT, Smith PG (eds). Vaccination and World Health. Chichester, England, John Wiley & Sons, 1995, pp 163–173.

95. Banerji D. Hidden menace in the universal child immunization program. Int J Health Serv 18:293–299, 1988.

96. Cutts FT, Glik DC, Gordon A, et al. Application of multiple methods to study the immunization programme in an urban area of Guinea. Bull World Health Organ 68:769–776, 1990.

97. Godlee F. WHO's Special Program: undermining from above. BMJ 310:178–182, 1995.

98. du Lou AD, Pison G. Barriers to universal child immunization in rural Senegal 5 years after the accelerated Expanded Programme on Immunization. Bull World Health Organ 72:751–759, 1994.

99. Bryce JW, Cutts FT, Saba S. Mass immunization campaigns and quality of immunization services. Lancet 335:739–740, 1990.

100. Anan A. India: unhealthy immunization programme. Lancet 341:1402–1403, 1993.

101. Reid R. Political, economic, and administrative resources available for the control of vaccine-preventable diseases. Rev Infect Dis 11(suppl):S655–S658, 1989.

102. Williams G. Immunization in Nicaragua [letter]. Lancet 2:780, 1985.

103. Bassole A. Mobilisation générale en faveur de la "vaccination commando." Hygie 5:31–34, 1986.

104. Lasso HP, de Restrepo V, Munoz R. Influencia de los medios de comunicacion masiva en la cobertura de una campana de vacunacion. Bull Pan Am Health Organ 101:39–46, 1986.

105. Tweneboa-Kodua A, Obeng-Quaidoo I, Abu K. Ghana social mobilization analysis. Health Educ Q 18:125–134, 1991.

106. Duque LF, de Bello PV, Bejarano J, et al. The national vaccination crusade in Colombia. Assoc Children 65/68:159–178, 1984.

107. de Quadros CA, Olive JM, Hersh BS, et al. Measles elimination in the Americas: evolving strategies. JAMA 275:224–229, 1996.

108. Global Programme for Vaccines of the World Health Organization. Role of mass campaigns in global measles control. Lancet 344:174–175, 1994.

109. Cairncross S, Peries H, Cutts F. Vertical health programmes. Lancet 349(suppl iii):siii20–siii22, 1997.

110. Murugasampillay S. Who determines national health policies? In Cutts FT, Smith PG (eds). Vaccination and World Health. Chichester, England, John Wiley & Sons, 1995, pp 195–205.

111. Ndumbe PM. Do vaccines reach those who most need them? Cameroon. In Cutts FT, Smith PG (eds). Vaccination and World Health. Chichester, England, John Wiley & Sons, 1995, pp 225–238.

112. Chen L, Cash R. A decade after Alma Ata—can primary health care lead to health for all? N Engl J Med 319:946–947, 1988.

113. Expanded Programme on Immunisation. Global Advisory Group—part I. Wkly Epidemiol Rec 3:11–15, 1992.

114. de Quadros CA, Andrus JK, Olive JM, de Macedo GC. Polio eradication from the Western Hemisphere. Annu Rev Public Health 13:239–252, 1992.

115. World Health Organization. Global eradication of poliomyelitis by the year 2000. Wkly Epidemiol Rec 63:161–162, 1988.

116. de Quadros CA, Hersh BS, Olive JM, et al. Eradication of wild poliovirus from the Americas: acute flaccid paralysis surveillance, 1988–1995. J Infect Dis 175(suppl 1):S37–S42, 1997.

117. Hull HF, Ward NA, Hull BP, et al. Paralytic poliomyelitis: seasoned strategies, disappearing disease. Lancet 343:1331–1337, 1994.

118. Centers for Disease Control and Prevention. Advances in global measles control and elimination: summary of the 1997 international meeting. MMWR 47(RR-11):1–23, 1998.

119. World Health Organization and United Nations Children's Fund. Measles Mortality Reduction and Regional Elimination: Strategic Plan, 2001–2005 (WHO/V&B/01.13). Geneva, World Health Organization, 2001.

120. Pan American Health Organization. Special Programme for Vaccines and Immunization: measles surveillance in the Americas. Wkly Bull 3(18), 1997.

121. World Health Organization, United Nations Children's Fund, and United Nations Population Fund. Maternal and Neonatal Tetanus Elimination by 2007: Strategy for Achieving and Monitoring Elimination (WHO/V&B/02.09). Geneva, World Health Organization, 2002.

122. Henderson DA. Principles and lessons from the smallpox eradication programme. Bull World Health Organ 65:535–546, 1987.

123. Henderson R, Keja J. Global control of vaccine-preventable diseases: how progress can be evaluated. Rev Infect Dis 11(suppl):S649–S654, 1989.

124. Vaccines, Immunization & Biologicals. WHO/UNICEF Joint Reporting Form on Vaccine Preventable Diseases, 2003. Available at www.who.int/vaccines-surveillance/DataDown.htm.

125. Weeks RM, Svetlana F, Noorgoul S, et al. Improving the monitoring of immunization services in Kyrgystan. Health Policy Plan 15:279–286, 2000.

126. Begg N, Gill O, White J. COVER (Cover of Vaccination Evaluated Rapidly): description of the England and Wales scheme. Public Health 103:81–89, 1989.

127. Borgdorff MW, Walker GJA. Estimating vaccination coverage: routine information or sample survey? J Trop Med Hyg 91:35–42, 1988.

128. Expanded Program on Immunisation. Protection and birth (PAB) method, Tunisia. Wkly Epidemiol Rec 75:203–206, 2000.

129. Henderson RH, Sundaresan T. Cluster sampling to assess immunization coverage: a review of experience with a simplified sampling method. Bull World Health Organ 60:253–260, 1982.

130. Serfling RE, Cornell RG, Sherman IL. The CDC quota sampling technique with results of 1959 poliomyelitis vaccination surveys. Am J Public Health 50:1847–1857, 1960.

131. Bennett S, Woods T, Liyanage WM, Smith DL. A simplified general method for cluster-sample surveys of health in developing countries. World Health Stat Q 44:98–106, 1991.

132. Lemeshow S, Robinson D. Surveys to measure programme coverage and impact: a review of the methodology used by the Expanded Programme on Immunization. World Health Stat Q 38:65–75, 1985.

133. Lemeshow S, Tserkovnyi AG, Tulloch JL, et al. A computer simulation of the EPI survey strategy. Int J Epidemiol 14:473–481, 1985.

134. Lwanga SK, Abiprojo N. Immunization coverage surveys: methodological studies in Indonesia. Bull World Health Organ 65:847–853, 1987.

135. Valadez JJ, Weld LH. Maternal recall error of child vaccination status in a developing nation. Am J Public Health 82:120–122, 1992.

136. Gareaballah ET, Loevinsohn BP. The accuracy of mothers' reports about their children's vaccination status. Bull World Health Organ 67:669–674, 1989.

137. Langsten R, Hill K. The accuracy of mother's reports of child vaccination: evidence from rural Egypt. Soc Sci Med 46:1205–1212, 1998.

138. Cutts FT, Zell ER, Soares AC, Diallo S. Obstacles to achieving Immunization for All 2000: missed immunization opportunities and inappropriately timed immunization. J Trop Pediatr 37:153–158, 1991.

139. Desve G. Les outils informatiques utilisés dans le PEV. Cah Santé 4:143–144, 1994.

140. Friede A, Waternaux C, Guyer B, et al. An epidemiological assessment of immunization programme participation in the Philippines. Int J Epidemiol 14:135–142, 1985.

141. Brugha F, Kevany J, Swan A. An investigation of the role of fathers in immunization uptake. Int J Epidemiol 25:840–845, 1996.

142. Brugha R, Kevany J. Maximizing immunization coverage through home visits: a controlled trial in an urban area of Ghana. Bull World Health Organ 74:18–20, 1996.

143. Cutts FT, Rodrigues LC, Colombo S, Bennett S. Evaluation of factors influencing vaccine uptake in Mozambique. Int J Epidemiol 18:427–433, 1989.

144. Cliff J, Cutts F, Waldman R. Using surveys in Mozambique for evaluation of diarrhoeal disease control. Health Policy Plan 5:219–225, 1990.

145. Singh P, Yadav RJ. Immunization status of children in India. Indian Pediatr 37:1194–1199, 2000.

146. Vaccines, Immunization & Biologicals. WHO Vaccine Preventable Disease Monitoring System: 2002 Global Summary (WHO/V&B/02.20). Geneva, World Health Organization, 2002.

147. Global Alliance for Vaccines and Immunization. Eighth GAVI Board Meeting, Paris, 2002. Geneva, World Health Organization, 2002.

148. Bryce J, Toole M, Waldman R, Voigt A. Assessing the quality of facility-based child survival services. Health Policy Plan 7:155–163, 1992.

149. Expanded Programme on Immunisation. TechNet Consultation 1996. (WHO/EPI/LHIS/97.02). Geneva, World Health Organization, 1997, p 24.

150. Vaccines, Immunization & Biologicals. Tool for Assessment of Injection Safety (WHO/V&B/01.30). Geneva, World Health Organization., 2001.

151. Global Programme for Vaccines and Immunization, Vaccine Research and Development. Monitoring Immunization Services Using the Lot Quality Technique (WHO/VRD/TRAM/96.01). Geneva, World Health Organization, 1996.

152. Cutts F, Othepa O, Vernon A, et al. Measles control in Kinshasa, Zaire improved with high coverage and use of medium titre Edmonston Zagreb vaccine at age 6 months. Int J Epidemiol 23:624–631, 1994.

153. Lanata CF, Stroh G, Black RE, Gonzales H. An evaluation of lot quality assurance sampling to monitor and improve immunization coverage. Int J Epidemiol 19:1086–1090, 1990.

154. Rosero-Bixby L, Grimaldo C, Raabe C. Monitoring a primary health care programme with lot quality assurance sampling: Costa Rica, 1987. Health Policy Plan 5:30–39, 1990.

155. Lanata CF, Black RE. Lot quality assurance sampling techniques in health surveys in developing countries: advantage and current constraints. World Health Stat Q 44:133–139, 1991.

156. Tawfik Y, Hoque S, Siddiqi M. Using lot quality assurance sampling to improve immunization coverage in Bangladesh. Bull World Health Organ 39:501–505, 2001.

157. Hall AJ, Aaby P. Tropical trials and tribulations. Int J Epidemiol 19:777–781, 1990.

158. Clemens JD, Stanton BF, Chakraborty J, et al. Measles vaccination and childhood mortality in rural Bangladesh. Am J Epidemiol 128:1330–1339, 1988.

159. Aaby P, Samb B, Simondon F, et al. Non-specific beneficial effect of measles immunization: analysis of mortality studies from developing countries. BMJ 311:481–485, 1995.

160. Garenne M, Leroy O, Beau J-P, Sene I. Child mortality after high-titre measles vaccines: prospective study in Senegal. Lancet 338:903–907, 1991.

161. Orenstein WA, Bernier RH, Dondero TJ, et al. Field evaluation of vaccine efficacy. Bull World Health Organ 63:1055–1068, 1985.

162. Orenstein WA, Bernier RH, Hinman AR. Assessing vaccine efficacy in the field: further observations. Epidemiol Rev 10:212–241, 1988.

163. Cutts FT, Smith PG, Colombo S, et al. Field evaluation of measles vaccine efficacy in Mozambique. Am J Epidemiol 131:349–355, 1990.

164. Hull HF, Williams PJ, Oldfield F. Measles mortality and vaccine efficacy in rural West Africa. Lancet 1:972–975, 1983.

165. McCormick JB, Halsey N, Rosenberg R. Measles vaccine efficacy determined from secondary attack rates during a severe epidemic. J Pediatr 90:13–16, 1977.

166. Top FH. Measles in Detroit, 1935: factors influencing the secondary attack rate among susceptibles at risk. Am J Public Health 28:935–943, 1938.

167. Clarkson JA, Fine PEM. An assessment of methods for routine local monitoring of vaccine efficacy, with particular reference to measles and pertussis. Epidemiol Infect 99:485–499, 1987.

168. Wassilak SGF, Orenstein WA, Strickland PL, et al. Continuing measles transmission in students despite a school-based outbreak control program. Am J Epidemiol 122:208–217, 1985.

169. Cutts F, Brown D. The contribution of field tests to measles surveillance and control: a review of available methods. Rev Med Virol 5:35–40, 1995.

170. Dietz VJ, Nieburg P, Gubler DJ, Gomez I. Diagnosis of measles by clinical case definition in dengue-endemic areas: implications for measles surveillance and control. Bull World Health Organ 70:745–750, 1992.

171. Sharma RS, Chawla U, Datta KK. Field evaluation of measles vaccine efficacy in Najafgarh Zone of Delhi. J Commun Dis 20:38–43, 1988.

172. Hlady G, Bennett J, Samadi A, et al. Neonatal tetanus in rural Bangladesh: risk factors and toxoid efficacy. Am J Public Health 82:1354–1369, 1992.

173. Brown J, Djogdom P, Murphy K, et al. Identifying the reasons for low immunization coverage—a case study of Yaounde (United Republic of Cameroon). Rev Epidemiol Sante Publique 30:35–47, 1982.

174. Joseph A, Abraham S, Bhattacharji S, et al. Improving immunization coverage. World Health Forum 9:336–340, 1988.

175. Heggenhougen K, Clements J. Acceptability of Childhood Immunization: Social Science Perspectives. A Study Supported by the Expanded Programme on Immunization, World Health Organization (EPC Publication No 14). Evaluation and Planning Centre, London School of Hygiene and Tropical Medicine, 1987.

176. Pillsbury B. Immunization: The Behavioural Issues (Behavioural Issues in Child Survival Programs Monograph 3). Washington, DC, Office of Health, U.S. Agency for International Development, 1990.

177. Eng E, Naimoli J, Naimoli G, et al. The acceptability of childhood immunization to Togolese mothers: a sociobehavioral perspective. Health Educ Q 18:97–110, 1991.

178. Coreil J, Augustin A, Holt E, Halsey N. Use of ethnographic research for instrument development in a case-control study of immunization use in Haiti. Int J Epidemiol 18(suppl):S33–S37, 1989.

179. Glik D, Gordon A, Ward W, et al. Focus group methods for formative research in child survival: an Ivoirian example. Int Q Community Health Educ 8:297–316, 1987.

180. Belcher D, Nicholas D, Ofosu-Amaah S, Wurapa F. A mass immunization campaign in rural Ghana—factors affecting participation. Public Health Rep 93:170–176, 1978.

181. Cutts FT, Diallo S, Zell ER, Rhodes P. Determinants of vaccination in an urban population in Conakry, Guinea. Int J Epidemiol 20:1099–1106, 1991.

182. Selwyn BJ. An epidemiological approach to the study of users and non-users of child health services. Am J Public Health 68:231–235, 1978.

183. Zeitlyn S, Mahmudur Rahman A, Nielsen B, et al. Compliance with diphtheria, tetanus, and pertussis immunisation in Bangladesh: factors identifying high-risk groups. BMJ 304:606–609, 1992.

184. van Zwanenberg T, Hull C. Improving immunisation coverage in a province in Papua New Guinea. Br Med J (Clin Res Ed) 296:1654–1656, 1988.

185. Zimicki S, Hornik RC, Verzosa CC, et al. Improving vaccination coverage in urban areas through a health communication campaign: the 1990 Philippine experience. Bull World Health Organ 72:409–422, 1994.

186. Peruggi E, Fox-Rushby JA, Walker D. Effects, Costs and Cost-effectiveness of Interventions to Expand Coverage of Immunization Services in Developing Countries: A Systematic Review of the Published Literature. Geneva, World Health Organization, 2002.

187. Brugha R, Kevany J. Immunization determinants in the Eastern Region of Ghana. Health Policy Plan 10:312–318, 1995.

188. Cleland J, van Genneken J. Maternal education and child survival in developing countries: the search for pathways of influence. Soc Sci Med 27:1357–1368, 1988.

189. Streatfield K, Singarimbun M, Diamond I. Maternal education and child immunization. Demography 27:447–455, 1990.

190. Bhuiya A, Bhuiya I, Chowdhury M. Factors affecting acceptance of immunization among children in rural Bangladesh. Health Policy Plan 10:304–311, 1995.

191. Sathe P, Shah U. Parental participation in poliovaccination programme. Indian J Public Health 9:107–110, 1965.

192. Akesode FA. Factors affecting the use of primary health care clinics for children. J Epidemiol Community Health 36:310–314, 1982.

193. Streatfield K, Singarimbun M. Social factors affecting the use of immunization in Indonesia. Soc Sci Med 27:1237–1245, 1988.

194. Henderson RH, David H, Eddins DL, Foege WH. Assessment of vaccination coverage, vaccination scar rates, and smallpox scarring in five areas of West Africa. Bull World Health Organ 48:183–194, 1973.

195. Hingson R. The impact of health beliefs on behavior during an immunization program in rural Haiti, 1972. Health Educ Monogr 2:505–507, 1974.

196. Ulin P, Ulin R. The use and non-use of preventive health services in a Southern African village. Int J Health Educ 24:45–53, 1981.

197. Expanded Programme on Immunisation. Community participation and immunization coverage. Wkly Epidemiol Rec 59:117–124, 1984.

198. Lin N, Hingson R, Allwood-Paredes JA. Mass immunization campaign in El Salvador: evaluation of receptivity and recommendation for future campaigns. Health Rep 86:1112–1121, 1971.

199. Bonilla JEZ, Gamarra JIM, Booth EM. Bridging the communication gap—how mothers in Honduras perceive immunization. Assoc Children 69/72:443–454, 1985.

200. Milstien J, Griffin PD, Lee J-W. Damage to immunization programmes from misinformation on contraceptive vaccines. Reprod Health Matters 6:24–28, 1996.

201. Briss PA, Rodewald LE, Hinman AR, et al. Reviews of evidence regarding interventions to improve vaccination coverage in children, adolescents, and adults. Am J Prev Med 18(1 suppl):97–140, 2000.

202. Kroeger A, Franken H. The educational value of participatory evaluation of primary health care programmes: an experience with four indigenous populations in Ecuador. Soc Sci Med 15:535–539, 1981.

203. Kroeger A. Participatory evaluation of primary health care programmes: an experience with four Indian populations in Ecuador. Trop Doct 12:38–43, 1982.

204. Vaccines, Immunization & Biologicals. *Haemophilus influenzae* Type B (Hib) Meningitis in the Pre-vaccine Era: A Global Review of Incidence, Age Distribution, and Case Fatality Rates (WHO/V&B/02.18). Geneva, World Health Organization, 2002.

205. Cutts FT, Henderson RH, Clements CJ, et al. Principles of measles control. Bull World Health Organ 69:1–7, 1991.

206. Kettles AN. Differences in trends of measles notifications by age and race in the western Cape, 1982–1986. S Afr Med J 72:317–320, 1987.

207. Cutts FT, Waldman RJ, Zoffman HMD. Surveillance for the Expanded Programme on Immunization. Bull World Health Organ 71:633–639, 1993.

208. Laforce FM, Lichnevski MS, Keja J, Henderson RH. Clinical survey techniques to estimate prevalence and annual incidence of poliomyelitis in developing countries. Bull World Health Organ 58:609–620, 1980.

209. Galazka A, Stroh G. Neonatal Tetanus: Guidelines on the Community-Based Survey on Neonatal Tetanus Mortality (WHO/EPI/GEN/86/8). Geneva, World Health Organization, 1986.

210. Vaccines, Immunization & Biologicals. Introduction of Hepatitis B Vaccine into Childhood Immunization Services. Management Guidelines, Including Information for Health Workers and Parents (WHO/V&B/01.31). Geneva, World Health Organization, 2001.

211. Vaccines, Immunization & Biologicals. Making Surveillance Work. Module 1: Rapid Assessment of Surveillance for Vaccine Preventable Diseases; Module 3: Logistics Management; Module 4: Data Management (WHO/V&B/01.08, 01.10, 01.11). Geneva, World Health Organization, 2001.

212. Goh KT. Hepatitis B immunization in Singapore. Lancet 348:1385–1386, 1996.

213. Hull BP, Dowdle WR. Poliovirus surveillance: building the Global Laboratory Network. J Infect Dis 175(suppl 1):S113–S116, 1997.

214. Expanded Programme on Immunisation. Poliomyelitis eradication: the WHO Global Laboratory Network. Wkly Epidemiol Rec 72:245–249, 1997.

215. Centers for Disease Control and Prevention. Laboratory surveillance for wild poliovirus and vaccine-derived poliovirus, 2000–2001. MMWR 51:369–371, 2002.

216. Frerichs RR. Simple analytic procedures for rapid microcomputer-assisted cluster surveys in developing countries. Public Health Rep 104:24–35, 1989.

217. Gay NJ, Hesketh LM, Morgan-Capner P, Miller E. Interpretation of serological surveillance data for measles using mathematical models: implications for vaccine strategy. Epidemiol Infect 115:139–156, 1995.

218. Morgan-Capner P, Wright J, Miller CL, Miller E. Surveillance of antibody to measles, mumps, and rubella by age. BMJ 297:770–772, 1989.

219. Cutts F, Nokes D. Immunization in the developing world: strategic challenges. Trans R Soc Trop Med Hyg 87:353–354, 398, 1993.

220. Cutts FT, Abebe A, Messele T, et al. Serological epidemiology of rubella in urban Ethiopia. Epidemiol Infect 124:467–479, 2000.

221. Parry J, Perry K, Mortimer P. Sensitive assays for viral antibodies in saliva: an alternative to tests on serum. Lancet 2:72–75, 1987.

222. Perry K, Brown D, Parry J, et al. Detection of measles, mumps, and rubella antibodies in saliva using antibody capture radioimmunoassay. J Med Virol 40:235–240, 1993.

223. Ramsay M, Brugha R, Brown D. Surveillance of measles in England and Wales: implications of a national saliva testing programme. Bull World Health Organ 75:515–521, 1997.

224. Nokes DJ, Enquselassie F, Nigatu W, et al. Has oral-fluid the potential to replace serum for the evaluation of population immunity levels? A study of measles, rubella, and hepatitis B in rural Ethiopia. Bull World Health Organ 79:588–595, 2001.

225. Azevedo-Neto RS, Silveira ASB, Nokes DJ, et al. Rubella seroepidemiology in a non-immunized population of Saõ Paulo State, Brazil. Epidemiol Infect 113:161–173, 1994.

226. Massad E, Burattini MN, Azevedo-Neto RS, et al. A model-based design of a vaccination strategy against rubella in a non-immunized community of Saõ Paulo State, Brazil. Epidemiol Infect 112:579–594, 1994.

227. Ramsay M, Gay N, Miller E, et al. The epidemiology of measles in England and Wales: rationale for the 1994 national vaccination campaign. Commun Dis Rep CDR Rev 4(R-12):R141–R146, 1994.

228. Grenfell BT, Anderson RM. The estimation of age-related rates of infection from case notifications and serological data. J Hyg (Camb) 95:419–436, 1985.

229. Centers for Disease Control and Prevention. Poliomyelitis prevention in the United States: updated recommendations of the Advisory Committee on Immunization Practices (ACIP). MMWR 49(RR-5):1–22, 2000.

230. World Health Organization. Vaccine supply and quality: Surveillance of adverse events following immunization. Wkly Epidemiol Rec 71:237–241, 1996.

231. Vaccines, Immunization & Biologicals. Supplementary Information on Vaccine Safety. Part 1: Field Issues; Part 2. Background Rates of Adverse Events Following Immunization (WHO/V&B/00.24, 00.36). Geneva, World Health Organization, 2000.

232. Jodar L, Duclos P, Milstien JB, et al. Ensuring vaccine safety in immunization programs—a WHO perspective. Vaccine 19:1594–1605, 2001.

233. Expanded Programme on Immunisation. BCG-associated lymphadenitis in infants. Wkly Epidemiol Rec 48:371–373, 1989.

234. Praveen KN, Smikle MF, Prabhakar P, et al. Outbreak of bacillus Calmette-Guérin–associated lymphadenitis and abscesses in Jamaican children. Pediatr Infect Dis J 9:890–893, 1990.

235. Expanded Programme on Immunisation. Lymphadenitis associated with BCG immunization: Mozambique. Wkly Epidemiol Rec 63:381–383, 1988.

236. Abdullah MA, Adam KA, Shagla A, Mahgoub S. BCG lymphadenitis: a report of eight cases. Ann Trop Paediatr 5:77–81, 1985.

237. Helmick CG. An outbreak of severe BCG axillary lymphadenitis in Saint Lucia, 1982–83. West Indian Med J 35:12–17, 1986.

238. Expanded Programme on Immunisation. Surveillance of Adverse Events Following Immunization: Field Guide for Managers of Immunization Programmes (WHO/EPI/TRAM/93.2). Geneva, World Health Organization, 1993.

239. World Bank. World Development Report 1993: Investing in Health. Oxford, Oxford University Press, 1993.

240. Jha P, Bangoura O, Ranson K. The cost-effectiveness of forty health interventions in Guinea. Health Policy Plan 13:249–262, 1998.

241. Bart KJ, Foulds J, Patriarca P. Global eradication of poliomyelitis: benefit-cost analysis. Bull World Health Organ 74:35–45, 1996.

242. Creese A. Cost effectiveness of alternative strategies for poliomyelitis immunization in Brazil. Rev Infect Dis 6(suppl): S404–S407, 1984.

243. Creese A, Dominguez-Uga M. Cost-effectiveness of immunization programs in Colombia. Bull Pan Am Health Organ 21:377–394, 1987.

244. Hall AJ, Robertson RL, Crivelli PE, et al. Cost effectiveness of hepatitis B vaccination in The Gambia. Trans R Soc Trop Med Hyg 87:333–336, 1993.

245. Miller M, McCann L. Policy analysis of the use of hepatitis B, *Haemophilus influenzae* type B, streptococcus conjugate and rotavirus vaccines in national immunization schedules. Health Resources 9:19–35, 2000.

246. Edmunds WJ, Dejene A, Mekonnen Y, et al. The cost of integrating hepatitis B vaccine into national immunization programmes: a case study from Addis Ababa. Health Policy Plan 15:408–416, 2000.

247. Creese A, Sriyabbaya N, Casabal G, Wiseso G. Cost-effectiveness appraisal of immunization programmes. Bull World Health Organ 60:621–632, 1982.

248. World Health Organization. Immunization Financing Databases. Information available at *www.gaviftf.info/docs_activities/doc/ flyer_IF DWeb.doc.*

249. Rosenthal G. The Economic Burden of Sustainable EPI: Implications for Donor Policy. Resources for Child Health (REACH) Project, Arlington, Virginia, 1990.

250. Shepard DS, Robertson RL, Cameron CSM III, et al. Cost-effectiveness of routine and campaign vaccination strategies in Ecuador. Bull World Health Organ 67:649–662, 1989.

251. Robertson R, Davis J, Jobe K. Service volume and other factors affecting the costs of immunizations in The Gambia. Bull World Health Organ 62:729–736, 1984.

252. Waddington C, Kello A, Wirakartakusumah D, et al. Financial information at district level: experiences from five countries. Health Policy Plan 4:207–218, 1989.

253. Anderson RM, May RM. Directly transmitted infectious diseases: control by vaccination. Science 215:1053–1060, 1982.

254. Nokes DJ, Anderson RM. Application of mathematical models to the design of immunization strategies. Rev Med Microbiol 4:1–7, 1993.

255. McLean AR, Anderson RM. Measles in developing countries. Part II. The predicted impact of mass vaccination. Epidemiol Infect 100:419–441, 1987.

256. Fine PEM. The contribution of modeling to vaccination policy. In Cutts FT, Smith PG (eds). Vaccination and World Health. Chichester, England, John Wiley & Sons, 1995, pp 177–192.

257. Foster SO, McFarland DA, John AM. Measles. In Jamison DT, Mosley WH, Measham AR, Bobadilla JL (eds). Disease Control Priorities in Developing Countries. New York, Oxford University Press, 1993, pp 161–187.

258. Gay NJ. Modeling measles, mumps, and rubella: implications for the design of vaccination programs. Infect Control Hosp Epidemiol 19:570–573, 1998.

259. Anderson RM, May RM. Infectious Diseases of Humans: Dynamics and Control. Oxford, UK, Oxford University Press, 1991.

260. Anderson RM, May RM. Vaccination against rubella and measles: quantitative investigations of different policies. J Hyg (Camb) 90:259–325, 1983.

261. Knox EG. Theoretical aspects of rubella vaccination strategies. Rev Infect Dis 7(suppl):S194–S198, 1985.

262. Massad E, Azevedo-Neto RS, Burattini MN, et al. Assessing the efficacy of a mixed vaccination strategy against rubella in Saõ Paulo, Brazil. Int J Epidemiol 24:842–850, 1995.

263. Nokes DJ, Swinton J. The control of childhood viral infections by pulse vaccination. IMA J Math Appl Med Biol 12:29–53, 1995.

264. Anderson RM. The concept of herd immunity and the design of community-based immunization programmes. Vaccine 10:928–935, 1992.

265. DeSerres G, Gay NJ, Farrington CP. Epidemiology of transmissible diseases after elimination. Am J Epidemiol 151:1039–1049, 2000.

266. Edmunds WJ, Medley GF, Nokes DJ. The transmission dynamics of hepatitis B virus in The Gambia. Stat Med 15:2215–2233, 1996.

267. Wilson JN, Nokes DJ. Do we need 3 doses of hepatitis B vaccine? Vaccine 17:2667–2673, 1999.

268. Edmunds WJ, Medley GF, Nokes DJ. Evaluating the cost-effectiveness of vaccination programs: a dynamic perspective. Stat Med 18:3263–3282, 1999.

269. Kim-Farley R and the Expanded Programme on Immunisation Team. Global immunization. Annu Rev Public Health 13:223–237, 1992.

270. Gwatkin DR, Rutstein S, Johnson K, et al. Socio-economic Differences in Health, Nutrition and Population in [44 Countries]. Washington, DC, Health, Nutrition and Population Department, The World Bank, 2000.

271. Kane MA, Clements J, Hu D. Hepatitis B. In Jamison DT, Mosley WH, Measham AR, Bobadilla J (eds). Disease Control Priorities in Developing Countries. New York, Oxford University Press, 1993, pp 321–330.

272. Van Damme P, Kane M, Meheus A. Integration of hepatitis B vaccination into national immunization programmes. BMJ 314: 1033–1037, 1997.

273. Chang MH, Cen CJ, Lai MS, et al. Universal hepatitis B vaccination in Taiwan and the incidence of hepatocellular carcinoma in children. N Engl J Med 336:1855–1859, 1997.

274. Expanded Programme on Immunisation. Inclusion of yellow fever vaccine in the EPI. Wkly Epidemiol Rec 71:181–188, 1996.

275. Global Alliance for Vaccines and Immunization. Ninth GAVI Board Meeting, Dakar, Senegal, November 2003. Geneva, World Health Organization, 2003.

276. Steinhoff MC. Haemophilus influenzae type b infections are preventable everywhere. Lancet 349:1186–1187, 1997.

277. Mulholland K, Hilton S, Adegbola R, et al. Randomised trial of Haemophilus influenzae type-b tetanus protein conjugate for prevention of pneumonia and meningitis in Gambian infants. Lancet 349:1191–1197, 1997.

278. Vaccines, Immunization & Biologicals. Estimating the Local Burden of Hib Disease Preventable by Vaccination: A Rapid Assessment Tool (WHO/V&B/01.27). Geneva, World Health Organization, 2001. Available at www.who.int/vaccinesdocuments/ docspdf/ www.675.pdf.

279. de Quadros CA, Izurieta H, Carrasco P, et al. Progress toward measles elimination in the Americas. J Infect Dis (suppl1): S 102–S110, 2003.

280. Biellik R, Madema S, Taole A, et al. First five years of measles elimination in southern Africa: 1996–2000. Lancet 359:1564–1568, 2000.

281. Uzicanin A, Eggers R, Webb E, et al. Impact of the 1996–1997 supplementary measles vaccination campaigns in South Africa. Int J Epidemiol 31:968–976, 2002.

282. Expanded Programme on Immunisation. Progress towards measles elimination. Canada. Wkly Epidemiol Rec 72:223–226, 1997.

283. Tobias M, Christie S, Mansoor O. Predicting the next measles epidemic. N Z Public Health Rep 4(1), 1997.

284. Gay N, Ramsay M, Cohen B, et al. The epidemiology of measles in England and Wales since the 1994 vaccination campaign. Commun Dis Rep CDR Rev 7(R-2):R17–R21, 1997.

285. Strebel P, Cochi SL, Grabowsky M, et al. The unfinished agenda of measles immunization. J Infect Dis (suppl 1):S1–S7, 2003

286. Henao-Restrepo AM, Strebel P, Hoekstra EJ, et al. Experience in global measles control, 1990–2001. J Infect Dis (suppl 1): S15–S21, 2003.

287. Hopkins DR, Hinman AR, Koplan JP, Lane JM. The case for global measles eradication. Lancet 1:1396–1398, 1982.

288. Peltola H, Heinonen OP, Valle M, et al. The elimination of indigenous measles, mumps, and rubella from Finland by a 12-year, two-dose vaccination program. N Engl J Med 331:1397–1402, 1994.

289. Bottiger M, Christenson B, Romanus V, et al. Swedish experience of two-dose vaccination programme aiming at eliminating measles, mumps, and rubella. Br Med J (Clin Res Ed) 295:1264–1267, 1987.

290. Communicable Disease Report. The national measles and rubella campaign—one year on. Commun Dis Rep CDR Wkly 5:237, 1995.

291. Progress towards the global elimination of neonatal tetanus, 1990–1998. Wkly Epidemiol Rec 74:73–80, 1999.

292. United Nations Children's Fund. Vaccine Security: Ensuring a Sustained, Uninterrupted Supply of Affordable Vaccines (UNICEF/2002/6). New York, United Nations Children's Fund, 2001.

293. Greco M. Key drivers behind the development of global vaccine market. Vaccine 20:1606–1610, 2001.

294. Vandermissen W. WHO expectation and industry goals. Vaccine 19:1611–1615, 2001.

295. The Children's Vaccine Initiative and the Global Programme for Vaccines and Immunization. Recommendations from the Scientific Advisory Group of Experts. Part II. Vaccine quality and supply. Wkly Epidemiol Rec 72:249–251, 1997.

296. Dietz V, Milstien J, van Loon F, et al. Performance and potency of tetanus toxoid: implications for eliminating neonatal tetanus. Bull World Health Organ 74:619–628, 1996.

297. Vaccines, Immunization & Biologicals. Report of the Fifth Annual Meeting of the Advisory Committee on Training (ACT) of the Global Training Network, Geneva, February 2000 (WHO/V&B/ 00.33). Geneva, World Health Organization, 2000.

298. Vaccines Supply and Quality. A WHO Guide to Good Manufacturing Practice (GMP) Requirements. Part 1: Standard Operating Procedures and Master Formulae; Part 2: Validation (WHO/VSQ/97.01, 97.02). Geneva, World Health Organization, 1997.

299. Shin Seung-il, Shahi G. Vaccine production and supply in developing countries. In Cutts FT, Smith PG (eds). Vaccination and World Health. Chichester, England, John Wiley & Sons, 1995, pp 39–60.

300. Aylward B, Lloyd J, Zaffran M, et al. Reducing the risk of unsafe injections in immunization programmes: financial and operational implications of various injection technologies. Bull World Health Organ 73:531–540, 1995.

301. Marmor M, Hartsock P. Self-destructing (non-reusable) syringes. Lancet 338:438–439, 1991.

302. Battersby A, Fielden R, Stilwell B. Vital to health. A briefing document for senior decision makers. Developed for U.S. Agency for International Development, 1998 Available at www.childrensvaccine.org/files/Vital_to_Health.pdf.

303. Milstien JB, Evans P, Batson A. Vaccine production and supply in developing countries: discussion. *In* Cutts FT, Smith PG (eds). Vaccination and World Health. Chichester, England, John Wiley & Sons, 1995, pp 60–66.

304. Carrasco P, de Quadros C, Umstead W. EPI in the Americas benefits from revolving fund. WHO Chronicle 37:81–85, 1983.

305. Casting off vaccine supply charity—the pace quickens. CVI Forum 10:9–13, 1995.

306. Robertson SE, Cutts FT, Samuel R, Diaz-Ortega JL. Control of rubella and congenital rubella syndrome (CRS) in developing countries, part 2: vaccination against rubella. Bull World Health Organ 75:69–80, 1997.

307. Cutts FT, Robertson SE, Diaz-Ortega JL, Samuel R. Control of rubella and congenital rubella syndrome (CRS) in developing countries, part 1: burden of disease from CRS. Bull World Health Organ 75:55–68, 1997.

308. Vaccines, Immunization & Biologicals. Report of a Meeting on Preventing Congenital Rubella Syndrome: Immunization Strategies, Surveillance Needs (WHO/V&B/00.10). Geneva, World Health Organization, 2000.

309. Ada GL. Vaccines and vaccination. N Engl J Med 345:1042–1053, 2001.

310. Vaccines, Immunization & Biologicals. Proceedings of the Third Global Vaccine Research Forum, Geneva, 9–11 June, 2002 (WHO/V&B/02.25). Geneva, World Health Organization, 2002.

311. Wenger J. Vaccines for the developing world: current status and future directions. Vaccine 19:1588–1591, 2001.

312. Centers for Disease Control and Prevention. Preventing pneumococcal disease among infants and young children: recommendations of the Advisory Committee on Immunization Practices (ACIP). MMWR 49(RR-9):1–35, 2000.

313. Rosenstein NE, Perkins B, Stephens DS, et al. Meningococcal disease. N Engl J Med 344:1378–1388, 2001.

314. Miller E, Salisbury D, Ramsey M. Planning, registration, and implementation of an immunization campaign against meningococcal serogroup C disease in the UK: a success story. Vaccine 20(suppl):S58–S67, 2002.

315. Vaccines, Immunization & Biologicals. Report of the Meeting on Future Directions for Rotavirus Vaccine Research in Developing Countries (WHO/V&B/00.23). Geneva, World Health Organization, 2000.

316. Bresee JS, Glass RI, Ivanoff B, et al. Current status and future priorities for rotavirus vaccine development, evaluation, and implementation in developing countries. Vaccine 17:2207–2222, 1999.

317. Monath TP. Japanese encephalitis vaccines: current vaccines and future prospects. Curr Top Microbiol Immunol 267:105–128, 2002.

318. Garenne M, Ronsmans C, Campbell H. The magnitude of mortality from acute respiratory infections in children under 5 years in developing countries. World Health Stat Q 45:180–191, 1992.

319. Koutsky LA, Ault KA, Wheeler CM, et al. A controlled trial of a human papillomavirus type 16 vaccine. N Engl J Med 347:1645–1651, 2002.

320. Moore SA, Surgey EG, Cadwgan AM. Malaria vaccines: where are we and where are we going? Lancet Infect Dis 2:737–743, 2002.

321. Vaccines, Immunization & Biologicals. Proceedings of the Special Advisory Group of Experts Meeting. Geneva, World Health Organization, 2002.

322. de Quadros CA, Carrasco P, Olive J-M. The desired field performance characteristics of new improved vaccines for the developing world. Int J Tech Assoc Health Care 10:1–6, 1994.

323. Mahoney RT, Maynard JE. The introduction of new vaccines into developing countries. Vaccine 17:646–652, 1999.

324. Department of Health. 1996 Immunisation Against Infectious Disease. London, Her Majesty's Stationery Office, 1996.

325. Orenstein WA, Bernier RH. Toward immunizing every child on time. Pediatrics 94:545–547, 1994.

326. Orenstein WA, Bernier RH. Crossing the divide from vaccine technology to vaccine delivery: the critical role of providers. JAMA 272:1138–1139, 1994.

327. Interagency Committee to Improve Access to Immunization Services. The Public Health Service action plan to improve access to immunization services. Public Health Rep 107:243–251, 1992.

328. Ad Hoc Working Group for the Development of Standards for Pediatric Immunization Practices. Standards for pediatric immunization practices. JAMA 269:1817–1822, 1993. (Updates posted on CDC's National Immunization Program Internet site [*www.cdc.gov/nip*]).

329. Cutts FT, Zell ER, Mason D, et al. Monitoring progress towards U.S. preschool immunization goals. JAMA 267:1952–1955, 1992.

330. Szilagyi P, Rodewald L, Humiston S, et al. Missed opportunities for childhood vaccinations in office practices and the effect on vaccination status. Pediatrics 91:1–7, 1993.

331. Bishai D, Bhatt S, Miller LT, et al. Vaccine storage practices in paediatric offices. Pediatrics 89:193–196, 1992.

332. Briggs H, Ilett S. Weak link in vaccine cold chain. BMJ 306:557–558, 1993.

333. Frenk J, Sepulveda J, Gomez-Dantes O, et al. The future of world health: the new world order and international health. BMJ 314:1404–1407, 1997.

334. Fielden R, Nielson OF. Immunization and Health Reforms: Making Reforms Work for Immunization. A Reference Guide (WHO/V&B/01.44). Geneva, World Health Organization, 2001.

335. Seventh Consultative Committee on Primary Health Care Systems for the 21st Century. Health care systems for the 21st century. BMJ 314:1407–1409, 1997.

336. Nelson EAS, Yu LM. Poverty-focused assistance: new category of development aid. Lancet 348:1642–1643, 1996.

337. Evans I. SAPping maternal health. Lancet 346:1046, 1995.

338. Fairbank A, Makinen M, Schott W, Sakagawa B. Poverty Reduction and Immunizations: Considering Immunizations in the Context of Debt Relief for Poor Countries. Bethesda, MD, Abt Associates, 2001.

339. Gangarosa EJ, Galazka AM, Wolfe CR, et al. Impact of anti-vaccine movements on pertussis control: the untold story. Lancet 351:356–361, 1998.

340. United Nations Children's Fund. Combating Anti-vaccination Rumors: Lessons Learned from Case Studies in East Africa. New York, United Nations Children's Fund, 2001. Available at *www.comminit.com/strumoursvacc/sld5095.html*.

341. Madsen KM, Hvid A, Vestergaard M, et al. A population-based study of measles, mumps, and rubella vaccination and autism. N Engl J Med 347:1477–1482, 2002.

Chapter 56

Community Immunity

PAUL E. M. FINE

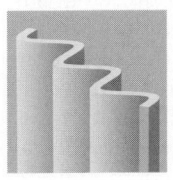

Vaccines are given to individuals, to protect them against disease. They also protect communities. The extension of perspective from individual vaccine recipients to their communities is the business of public health. For the past several decades, this subject has been discussed largely with reference to the concept of *herd immunity*, a term that refers in its simplest sense to the prevalence or proportion of immunes in a population, but that is often used with reference to indirect protection of nonimmunes attributable to the presence and proximity of immune individuals.[1-3] Much of the discussion has concentrated upon this latter issue and its implication of threshold levels of immunity, which, if achieved, should lead to the elimination of an infection from a population. Though of obvious theoretical interest and public health importance, the emphasis upon such thresholds has distracted attention from other, equally or more important community implications of vaccination programs. In recognition of this, the editors of this volume have suggested a broadening of the scope of this discussion, under the term *community immunity*.

The shift in perspective from the individual to the community raises many operational issues concerning vaccination programs: schedules, boosters, consent, contraindications, legal enforcement and exemptions, access, public versus private providers, fixed versus mobile services, routine versus targeted programs, campaigns, coverage, monitoring and evaluation, and the like. These issues are covered elsewhere in this volume. Here we consider more general and theoretical issues concerning immunity within communities. In the simplest terms, the community impact of a vaccination program should be a function of the efficacy of the vaccine among individual recipients, and the coverage. Disease incidence should be reduced by a factor equal to the product of these terms. But the real world is not that simple, and, in order to predict a program's effect, we must also consider other issues, such as (1) the distribution of vaccines and of disease risk in communities (neither of which is ever uniform or random); (2) indirect protection of nonimmunes by the presence of immunes (the traditional focus of herd immunity discussions); and (3) the nature of the immunity induced by the vaccine (measured in terms of protection against infection or against disease, or even against transmission, as well as its natural boosting or waning over time).

After a brief historical review, this chapter summarizes the theory that has evolved to describe various aspects of community immunity, and then considers these principles with reference to the major vaccines in use today.

Historical Background

Though both Jenner[4] and Pasteur[5] recognized explicitly the potential of vaccines to control and even to eradicate specific infections from populations, neither is known to have considered the practical issues involved in the population application of vaccines. Smallpox vaccination was introduced widely in Europe and North America during the early 19th century, with increasing success over time. Its enforcement through legislation would have long-lasting effects on public acceptance of vaccines, including the appearance of the first antivaccination sentiment opposed to this intrusion by states into the bodies of their citizens. This remains a major issue today. Close observers noted interesting implications of vaccination—for example, William Farr commented as early as 1840 that "The smallpox would be disturbed, and sometimes arrested, by vaccination which protected a part of the population . . . ," probably the first recorded recognition of indirect protection by vaccines.[6]

The early years of the 20th century saw important advances in our understanding of the dynamics of infections in populations as a function of the balance of infectious cases, susceptibles, and immunes. Several factors contributed to this, in particular the greater understanding of disease patterns in communities that arose from the introduction of morbidity (in addition to mortality) notification schemes, the growth of immunology as a discipline, and the development of a theoretical framework linking these data and disciplines together.

The first published use of the term *herd immunity* appears to have been in a paper published in 1923 by Topley and Wilson, entitled "The spread of bacterial infection: the problem of herd immunity."[7] The paper described one of a classical series of studies on epidemics of various infections in closely monitored populations of laboratory mice, and introduced the term in this manner:

Consideration of the results obtained during the past five years... led us to believe that the question of immunity as an attribute of the herd should be studied as a separate problem, closely related but in many ways distinct from, the problem of the immunity of an individual host.

After describing experiments showing that immunized mice had lower mortality rates from, and were less likely to transmit, *Bacillus enteritidis*, the authors concluded by posing an

obvious problem to be solved: Assuming a given total quantity of resistance against a specific bacterial parasite to be available among a considerable population, in what way should that resistance be distributed among the individuals at risk, so as best to ensure against the spread of the disease, of which the parasite is the causal agent?

Wilson later recalled that the phrase "herd immunity" had first arisen in the course of a conversation with Major Greenwood (GS Wilson, personal communication, 1981), and Greenwood employed it in his 1935 textbook, "Epidemics and Crowd Diseases."[8] Although these authors did not distinguish explicitly between direct and indirect protection stemming from vaccine-derived immunity, later authors picked up the phrase, and applied it in particular to the indirect protection afforded to nonimmune individuals by the presence and proximity of immunes.

Consideration of the population implications of immunization programs became a major issue during the last quarter of the 20th century, associated with the widespread introduction of vaccines in all populations of the world. It was stimulated in particular by the success of the global smallpox eradication program, as well as by the creation in 1974 and subsequent activities of the World Health Organization's (WHO's) Expanded Programme on Immunisation, and the setting of targets to eliminate or to eradicate several infectious diseases through vaccines: global targets to eradicate polio and to eliminate neonatal tetanus, and national and regional goals to eliminate measles.[9] These massive efforts encouraged a theoretical literature exploring the population implications of immunization programs, including much discussion of the extent of indirect protection by vaccines, and of coverage criteria for eradication of infection. Though much of the initial theory assumed that immunity was a simple property, that individuals were either immune or not immune, and that the implied protection was solid and permanent against both infection and disease, it became increasingly clear during the 1980s that this was incorrect, and that different infections and vaccines could induce different degrees of protection against infection, against disease, and even against infectiousness, and that these different sorts of immunity could wane or be boosted over time. More recent research has attempted to measure these different forms of immunity and to incorporate these subtleties into evaluations of immunity at the community level.

Theoretical Arguments

The focal point of much of the theoretical work on community immunity has been the recognition that, if an infec-

tion or vaccine induces some degree of immunity against infection, then some nonimmune individuals will be protected indirectly, by the presence and proximity of immunes, and transmission should stop in a population prior to the infection of all susceptible individuals. This insight encourages the estimation of threshold numbers or proportions of immunes necessary for this cessation to occur. An elegant body of theory has evolved around this issue, developed initially to describe simple randomly mixing populations, but subsequently extending to more realistic scenarios.

The principle of indirect protection may be illustrated very simply as in Figure 56–1, which shows susceptible and immune individuals in a population, with arrows indicating the spread of an infection. Actual transmission patterns depend upon the distribution of susceptibles in space and time (social mixing patterns), and some susceptible individuals may be shielded from infection by being "surrounded" by immunes. However, representations such as Figure 56–1 fail to show that, even if there were no immune individuals at the start of an outbreak, infections may generate immunes who can in turn block transmission and lead to termination of an epidemic before all individuals become infected. We thus need to consider dynamics.

The "Mass Action" Approach

A crucial argument was introduced in 1906, by William Hamer, in the context of a discussion of the dynamics of measles.[10] He argued that the number of new cases (C_{t+1}) in a time period equal to the serial interval of the infection (thus one "generation" of cases, e.g., requiring approximately 2 weeks for measles) is a function of the number of infectious cases and of susceptibles in the previous time period (C_t and S_t, respectively; Fig. 56–2). In simple terms:

$$C_{t+1} = C_t \times S_t \times r \qquad [1]$$

where r is a transmission parameter, or "contact rate"—in effect, the proportion of all possible contacts between susceptible and infectious individuals that lead to new infections (so $r << 1$). In order to simulate successive changes

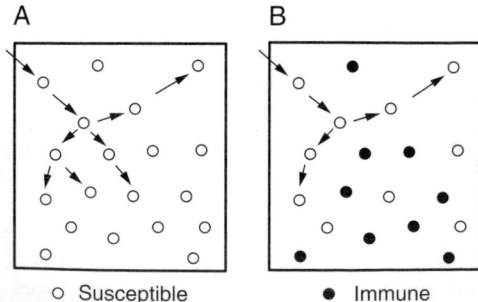

○ Susceptible   ● Immune

FIGURE 56–1 ▪ Simple diagram illustrating three generations of transmission after introduction of an infection into a fully susceptible population (A) and into a population containing immune individuals (B). Though it is clear from this diagram that some individuals may be shielded from infection in population B, similar shielding can also occur in A (see text).

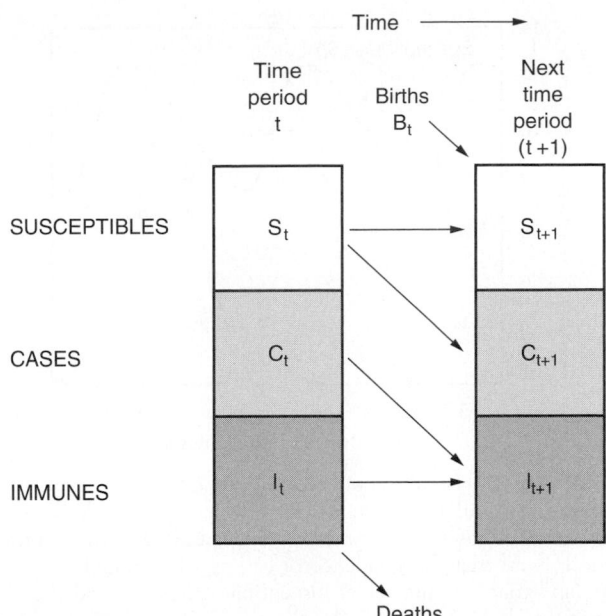

Time ——→

Time period t   Births B_t Next time period (t +1)

SUSCEPTIBLES S_t → S_{t+1}

CASES C_t → C_{t+1}

IMMUNES I_t → I_{t+1}

Deaths

FIGURE 56–2 ■ Relationship between susceptibles (**S**), infectious cases (**C**), and immunes (**I**) in successive time intervals (*t*, *t*+1) in the simple discrete time mass action model. In each time period, some (C_{t+1}) susceptibles become cases, and the others remain susceptible. Each case is assumed to remain infectious for no more than a single time period (= serial interval). B_t individuals enter as susceptible births during each time period (e.g., Eqn. 56–2).

over time, the number of susceptibles is recalculated for each new time period as

$$S_{t+1} = S_t - C_{t+1} + B_t \qquad [2]$$

where S_{t+1} is the number of susceptibles in the next time period, and B_t is the number of new susceptibles added (e.g., born into) the population per unit time. (Note that bold symbols are used in this chapter to denote numbers of individuals, and nonbold symbols to denote proportions or derived statistics [Table 56–1].)

The relationship in Equation 1, that future incidence is a function of the product of current prevalence times current numbers susceptible, has become known as the epidemiologic "law of mass action," by analogy with the physical-chemical principle that the rate or velocity of a chemical reaction is a function of the product of the concentrations of the reactants. Often expressed as a differential (continuous time) rather than a difference (discrete time) equation, as here, this relationship underlies much theoretical work on the dynamics of infections in populations.[11] Note that Equations 1 and 2 include no explicit term for immunes. By implication, deaths prior to infection are not considered in this simplest model (i.e., in each period, the same number of immunes die as susceptibles are born into the population). Introduction of terms for immunes, for individuals incubating the infection, for population growth and selective mortality of susceptibles, infecteds, and immunes, and for age is explored at length in the literature, but does not change the basic message emphasized here.[11]

Figure 56–3 shows what happens when Equations 1 and 2 are iterated, and serves to illustrate several principles of the epidemiology of those acute immunizing infections, such as measles, mumps, rubella, chickenpox, poliomyelitis, *Haemophilus*, and pertussis, that affect a high proportion of individuals in unvaccinated communities. First, the model predicts cycles of infection incidence, as are well recognized for many of the ubiquitous infections of childhood (Fig.

TABLE 56–1 ■ Variables Employed in Theoretical Arguments Concerning Infection Dynamics and Herd Immunity Thresholds

Symbol*	Variable Definition
C_t, C_{t+1}	Numbers of cases in successive serial intervals
S_t, S_{t+1}	Numbers of susceptible individuals in successive serial intervals
B_t	Number of new susceptibles (e.g., births) per serial interval
r	Transmission parameter for the simple mass action model, interpretable as the proportion of all possible contacts between cases and susceptibles that lead to new infections
S_e	Epidemic threshold number of susceptibles (if exceeded, incidence will increase)
T	Total population size
H	Herd immunity threshold (proportion immune in a population above which incidence should decline: $H = 1 - S_e/T$)
R_0	Basic reproduction number (average [expected] number of secondary cases attributable to a single case introduced into a totally susceptible population)
R_n	Net reproduction number (actual number of transmissions per case)
S	Proportion susceptible in a population
A	Average age at infection
L	Average expectation of life
C	Vaccine coverage
C_H	Vaccine coverage to achieve herd immunity threshold
P	Protective efficacy of vaccine (proportion "protected" among vaccinees)
P_i	Protective efficacy of vaccine in terms of susceptibility to infection (proportion of vaccinees who are rendered nonsusceptible to infection)
P_t	Protective efficacy of vaccine in terms of transmissibility (proportion of vaccinees who fail to shed organisms despite becoming infected)

***Bold** symbols represent numbers of individuals. Nonbold symbols represent proportions or derived statistics.

56–4). The incidence of infection cycles above and below the "birth" rate, or rate of influx of new susceptibles. Second, the number of susceptibles also cycles, but around a number that is sometimes described as the "epidemic threshold" (S_e). Simple rearrangement of Equation 1 to $C_{t+1}/C_t = S_t \times r$ reveals that this threshold number of susceptibles is numerically equivalent to the reciprocal of the transmission parameter r, as incidence increases (i.e., $C_{t+1} > C_t$) when, and only when, $S_t > 1/r$, and thus $S_e = 1/r$. The correspondence between the case and susceptible lines in Figure 56–3 illustrates this relationship.

This epidemic threshold implies a simple herd immunity criterion. If the proportion immune is so high that the number of susceptibles is below the epidemic threshold, then incidence will decrease. We can express this threshold algebraically as

$$H = 1 - S_e/T = 1 - 1/rT \qquad [3]$$

where T is the total population size, S_e is the epidemic threshold number of susceptibles for the population, and H is the herd immunity threshold, that is, the proportion of immunes that must be exceeded if incidence is to decrease.

Case Reproduction Numbers

We can approach the herd immunity concept from an alternative, and equally informative, perspective. If an infection is to persist, each infected individual must, on average,

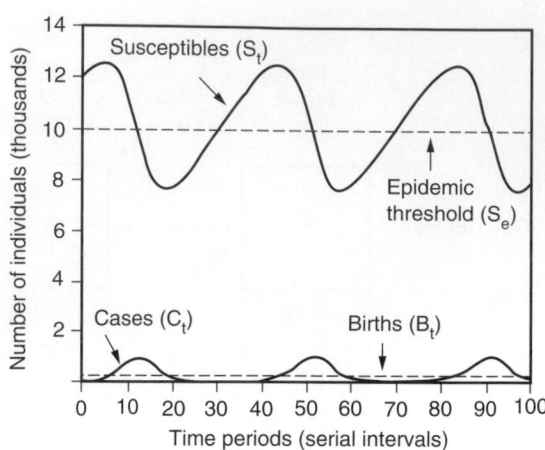

FIGURE 56–3 ■ Results obtained on reiteration of Equations 56–1 and 56–2. The illustrated simulation was based on 12,000 susceptibles and 100 cases at the start, $r = 0.0001$, and 300 births per time period. Note that the incidence of cases cycles around the birth rate, and that the number of susceptibles cycles around the epidemic threshold: $S_e = 1/r = 10,000$.

transmit the agent to at least one other individual. If not, incidence will decline and the infection will disappear progressively from the population. The number, or distribution, of actual onward transmissions per case thus describes the

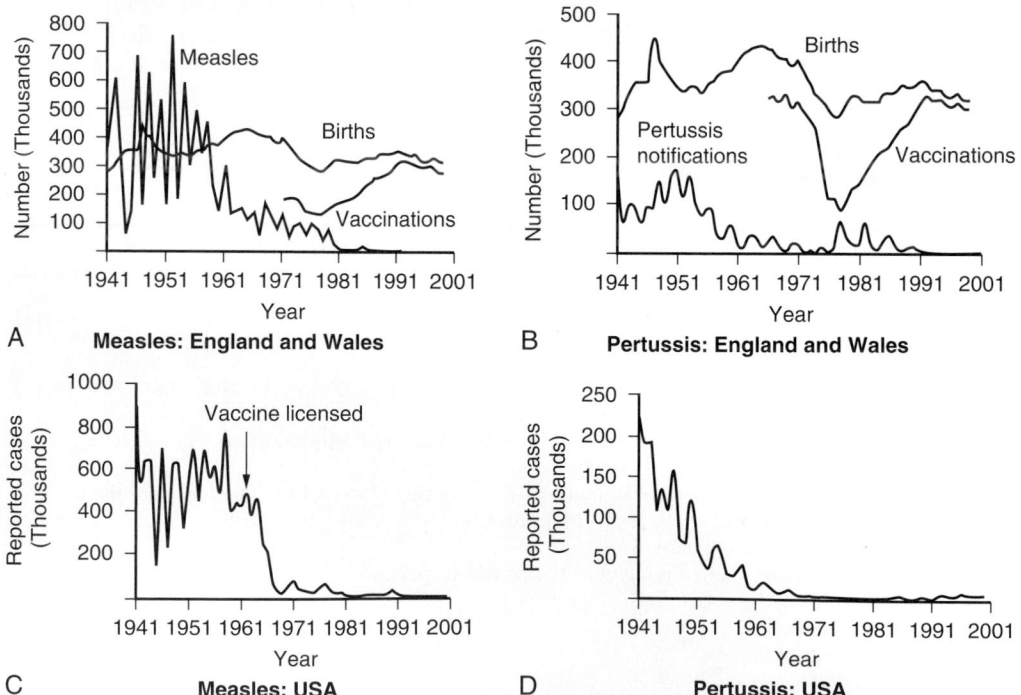

FIGURE 56–4 ■ Reported incidence of common childhood vaccine-preventable diseases. Measles showed a tendency to biennial epidemics in England and Wales prior to vaccination (A). This pattern was less dramatic in data for the entire United States (C), because of the size and heterogeneity of the population (not all areas were in phase with one another). All areas showed a strong seasonal oscillation, in addition to the biennial cycle. Pertussis shows a 3- to 4-year cycle, with little obvious seasonality, in the United Kingdom (B). This cycling is also seen in national data for the United States, in particular prior to 1970 (D). Notification efficiency for measles was approximately 60% in England and Wales prior to vaccination, but was considerably lower for pertussis, and for both diseases in the United States.

spread of an infection in a population, and is a function of three things: (1) the biologic properties of the infectious agent, (2) the rate and pattern of contact or interaction between members of the host population, and (3) the proportion susceptible in the host population. Its value under any set of circumstances is known as a "reproduction number" of the infection, by analogy with standard demographic measures (the average number of progeny per individual per generation). This average number of actual transmissions should be *maximum* if all members of the host population are susceptible, in which circumstance it is known as a "*basic reproduction number*" (R_0), defined formally as the average number of transmissions expected from a single primary case introduced into a totally susceptible population.[12,13] This definition can be translated directly into the mass action formulation (Eqn. 1) by setting $\mathbf{C}_t = 1$ and $\mathbf{S}_t = \mathbf{T}$, to represent the single case introduced into a fully susceptible population. The number of secondary cases, $\mathbf{C}_{t+1}$, is then equivalent, by definition, to the basic reproduction number (R_0):

$$\mathbf{C}_{t+1} = \mathbf{T}r = R_0 \qquad [4]$$

This basic reproduction number describes the maximum spreading potential of an infection in a population (some authors have used other names for this statistic, such as "expected number of contacts"[2] or "contact number"[14]). Examples of numerical values of this statistic, applicable to different infections and derived by methods described below, are shown in Table 56–2. A pictorial illustration of the concept is presented in Figure 56–5A.

If immune individuals are present in a population, then some of the "contacts" of infectious individuals will be with these immunes, and hence will fail to lead to transmission. As a result, the average number of *actual* infection transmissions per case will be *less* than the basic case reproduction number, and has been defined as the *net*, or *actual*, or *effective reproduction number* (R_n).[11,12] In theory, the actual number of transmissions (R_n) should be equivalent to the basic case reproduction number R_0 times the proportion susceptible in the population (S):

$$R_n = R_0 \times S \qquad [5]$$

By this logic, if the proportion susceptible were equal to the reciprocal of the basic reproduction number of the infection, the average number of transmissions per case should be 1, and thus incidence should remain constant over time. This is illustrated in Figure 56–5B, and once again leads us directly to the herd immunity threshold (H). R_n will be less than unity if the proportion susceptible is less than the reciprocal of R_0 (i.e., if $S < 1/R_0$). Because the proportion immune is just the complement of the proportion susceptible ($H = 1 - S$), we have

$$H = 1 - 1/R_0 = (R_0 - 1)/R_0 \qquad [6]$$

The same expression also can be derived by directly combining Equations 3 and 4 above. As long as the proportion immune can be maintained higher than this threshold, incidence should decrease, ultimately to the point of eradication of the infection from the population. The relationship is shown graphically in Figure 56–6, showing the implications for persistence or decline of an infection depending upon its basic reproduction number and the proportion of immunes in the population.[1,11,15]

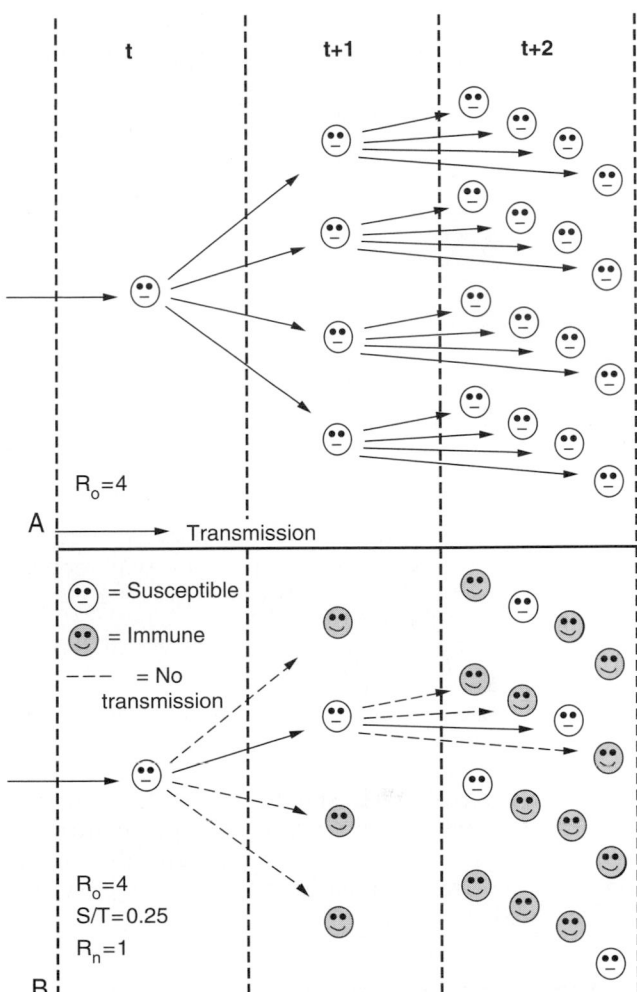

FIGURE 56–5 ■ Cartoon illustrating implications of a basic reproduction number $R_0 = 4$. In each successive time (serial) interval, each individual has effective contact with four other individuals. If the population is initially entirely susceptible (A), incidence increases exponentially, fourfold each generation (until the accumulation of immunes slows the process). If 75% of the population is immune (B), then on average only S = 25% of each set of four contacts lead to successful transmissions, and the net reproductive number $R_n = R_0 \times S = 1$.

Estimation of R_0

Given this relationship between the basic reproduction number of an infection in a population and the herd immunity threshold, the estimation of R_0 becomes an important challenge. If the infection is so common as to affect virtually everyone in unvaccinated populations, as is the case with many of the acute immunizable diseases of childhood (measles, mumps, rubella, polio, pertussis, *Haemophilus*, etc.), one derivation of R_0 turns out to be relatively straightforward. Noting that R_0 is equivalent to the reciprocal of the *average* proportion susceptible in the population over an epidemic cycle (see Equation 5; note that the proportion susceptible cycles around $S_e/T = 1 - H$, as in Fig. 56–3 and Equation 3), Dietz[15] noted that it will be roughly equivalent to the ratio of the expectation of life (L) divided by the average age at infection (A). Indeed, if everyone in a population were to become infected exactly at age A, and were

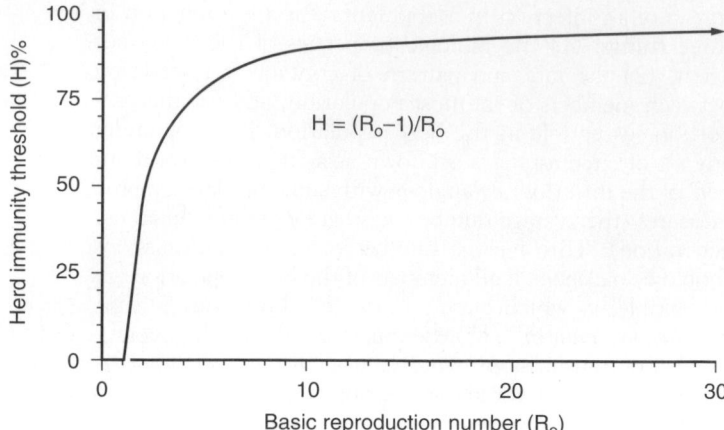

FIGURE 56–6 ▪ Relationship between herd immunity threshold (H) and basic reproduction number R_0, as in Equation 56–6: $H = 1 - 1/R_0$.

to die exactly at age L, then the proportion susceptible would be precisely A/L. He went on to show that, for populations with more realistic age structures, a better estimate of R_0 can be obtained as

$$R_0 = 1 + L/A \qquad [7]$$

Detailed discussion of the estimation of R_0 values by these and other methods can be found in several references.[11,13,15] The herd immunity threshold values cited in Table 56–2 are based upon these methods, and provide crude estimates of the proportions of immunes required, in theory, to eliminate these infections. Figure 56–7 illustrates the implications of these age relationships for basic reproduction numbers and herd immunity thresholds.

The Implications of Population Heterogeneity

The elegant theory summarized above is built upon extreme assumptions: that all individuals mix at random, and that the population is uniform (e.g., all susceptible individuals are equally susceptible and all infected individuals are equally infectious). These assumptions are unlikely to hold for any human population. In recent years, there has been an effort to adapt the theory to more realistic assumptions, including heterogeneity of mixing patterns, and of susceptibility and infectiousness.

The first attempt to consider the implications of population heterogeneity for herd immunity appeared in a 1971 paper by Fox and colleagues, entitled "Herd immunity: basic concept and relevance to public health immunization practices."[2] This paper, for many years the most frequently cited article on herd immunity, took a very different approach from that reviewed above, and was based upon simulation rather than upon analytic argument. The authors set up a population of 1000 individuals, divided into family, school, and social groupings, and assigned different but realistic contact rates within and between each of these groups. Importantly, they did not consider age, nor did they consider an influx of susceptibles into the population (the B_t term in Equation 2 above). Their approach was thus only

TABLE 56–2 ▪ Approximate Basic Reproduction Numbers (in Developed Countries) and Implied Crude Herd Immunity Thresholds (H, Calculated as $1-1/R_0$) for Common Vaccine-Preventable Diseases[1,11]*

Infection	Basic Reproduction Number (R_0)	Herd Immunity Threshold, H (%)
Diphtheria	6–7	85
Influenza[†]	?	?
Measles[‡]	12–18	55–94
Mumps	4–7	75–86
Pertussis	12–17	92–94
Polio[§]	2–15	50–93
Rubella	6–7	83–85
Smallpox	5–7	80–85
Tetanus	Not applicable	Not applicable
Tuberculosis[‖]	?	?
Varicella[¶]	8–10?	?

*It should be emphasized that the values given in this table are approximate, and that they do not properly reflect the tremendous range and diversity among populations. Nor do they reflect the full immunologic complexity underlying the epidemiology and persistence of these infections. See text for further discussion.
[†]R_0 of influenza viruses probably varies greatly between subtypes.
[‡]Herd immunity thresholds as low as 55% have been published.
[§]Complicated by uncertainties over immunity to infection and variation related to hygiene standards.
[‖]Protective immunity not defined.
[¶]Immunity not sterile, concept may not apply.

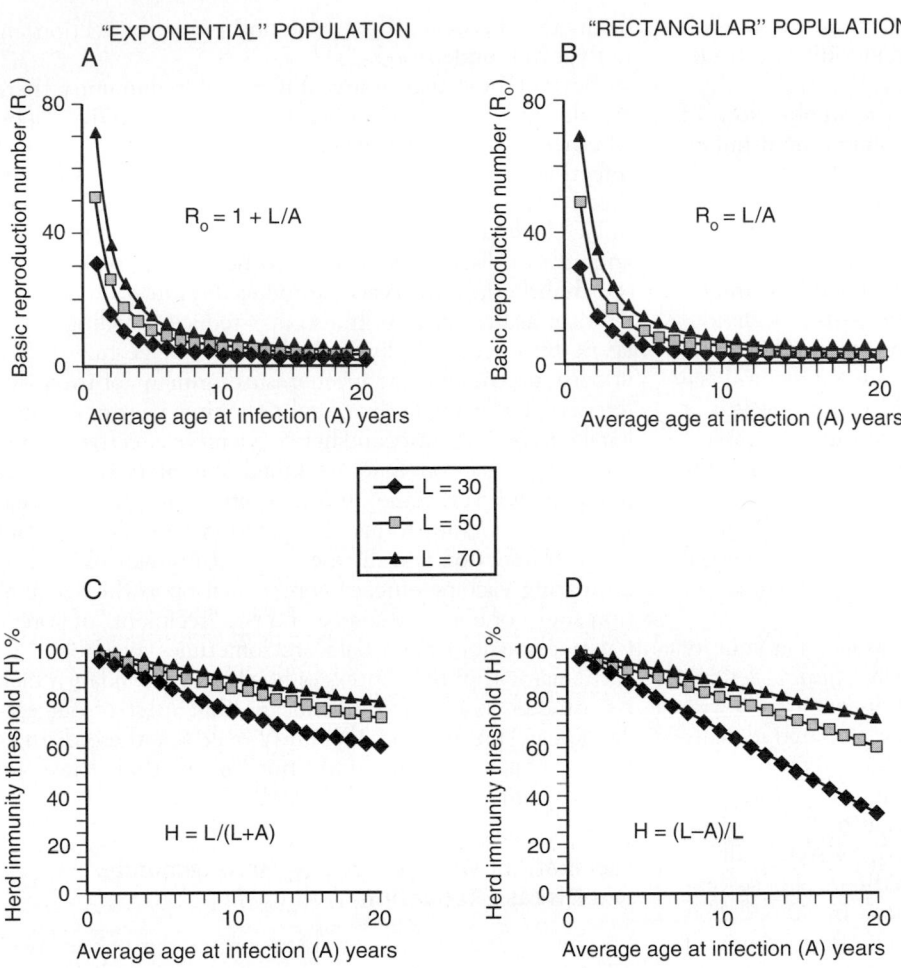

"EXPONENTIAL" POPULATION

A

$R_0 = 1 + L/A$

"RECTANGULAR" POPULATION

B

$R_0 = L/A$

L = 30
L = 50
L = 70

C

$H = L/(L+A)$

D

$H = (L-A)/L$

FIGURE 56–7 ■ Basic reproduction numbers (R_0) and herd immunity (H) thresholds expressed as a function of average age at infection (A) and average expectation of life (L). These relationships assume that immunity is a simple all-or-none characteristic and that the population mixes at random. "Exponential populations" imply a constant death rate by age; "rectangular populations" imply all individuals live to their fixed expectation age. Real populations have age distributions between these extremes, though the former may be approximated in pattern by high-birth-rate countries and the latter by low-birth-rate countries today.

applicable to closed populations—and they were unable to address the larger issues of infections within dynamic populations or to estimate a threshold.[1] Their conclusion was extremely cautious on the utility of any simple measure of herd immunity. The paper represented an important break with simple theories based upon assumptions of random mixing populations.

Subsequent workers have used a variety of computer simulation and analytic approaches in order to explore more realistic assumptions than those underlying the simple mass action theory. In particular, there has been exploration of the important implications of age, recognizing the need to vaccinate as early in life as possible after maternal immunity and prior to exposure to wild-type infections.[11,16–18] These studies have allowed exploration of the effects of various vaccination strategies on the age distribution of infection—in particular, how low or moderate levels of vaccine coverage among infants or young children will change the dynamic equilibrium, slowing down transmission, and thereby leading to an increase in the average age at infection among individuals who fail to be immunized by the vaccine. These effects are particularly important for infections whose seriousness increases with age, such as rubella and to a lesser extent mumps, chickenpox, or polio.[1,11,19,20] This line of research also has considered more complicated issues relating to patterns of contact within and between age groups in populations. The mathematics becomes too

awkward for analytic solutions, though the discussion has been made presentationally elegant through the use of WAIFW ("who acquires infection from whom") matrices, developed by Anderson and May, reflecting patterns of contact within and between different age groups.[1,11,17]

There are many other forms of heterogeneity within human populations, in particular geographic and social groupings, each of which have subtleties and which are likely to confound one another, because different social groups tend to have different age and area patterns. Social groups may be separate or may overlap (e.g., neighborhood and occupational or school groupings) in different ways in different societies, and may imply environments or behaviors that either encourage or discourage the transmission of infection. Consideration of such heterogeneities within simulation models has demonstrated that it is generally more efficient to target high- than low-risk groups with vaccines, in the sense that the number of cases of disease prevented will be greater per single vaccination in a high-risk than in a low-risk population.[21,22] This is intuitively reasonable, and in theory may be relevant to diseases such as measles, where high-risk urban populations may be responsible for maintenance of infection, from which it spreads periodically to low-risk rural populations.[23] However, a real vaccination program might be unwise to emphasize such a strategy, not only because of issues of social equity, but because evidence has shown that, in the absence of eradication, susceptibles continue to accumulate in the less served (e.g., rural) areas and population mobility continues to seed virus into such populations.[24]

Table 56–3 presents a summary of the implications of these several heterogeneities upon the simple herd immunity threshold values as estimated in Table 56–2.

Heterogeneity in Immune Status

Thus far our discussion has implicitly assumed that immunity is one face of a simple binary property—that individuals either are susceptible to infection and to disease, or else they are immune and protected from both infection and disease. For most infections, the real world is not like this at all. We know that immune responses are highly complex, involving humoral (antibody-mediated) and cellular pathways, as well as a variety of cell types and chemical mediators (e.g., cytokines), and that these vary among infections, among individuals, and over time. The epidemiologic implications of this heterogeneity are important, but as yet insufficiently explored.

The conventional epidemiologic measure of immunity induced by vaccination is known as *vaccine efficacy*, defined as the percent reduction in incidence of disease among vaccinated individuals as compared to nonvaccinated, equally exposed controls. It is now recognized that this basic measure of vaccine-derived immunity is itself ambiguous, insofar as 80% efficacy could mean either that 80% of a group (e.g., of vaccinees) are totally protected, by some "all-or-none" mechanism of protection, or that the level of susceptibility in all individuals has been reduced by 80%.[28] This distinction has profound implications both for measures of vaccine effects (whether it is more appropriate to use risks or person-time rates in calculations) and for our understanding of immunity (it reflects whether certain responses are fully protective or only partially so, perhaps more effective against low- than against high-dose challenge, or more protective against closely related compared to more distantly related antigenic types of the pathogen). The combined epidemiologic and immunologic implications of the distinction between all-or-none and partial protection are not yet well understood.

Beyond these quantitative differences in immunity, there are also important qualitative differences, dependent upon whether, and to what level, any protection acts against infection, against disease, or against infectiousness (transmissibility). For some infections (e.g., measles), vaccine-induced immunity may protect similarly against infection and against disease, whereas, for others (e.g., polio, pertussis, diphtheria), the vaccine-induced protection appears stronger against disease. It also may reduce shedding of the agent by infected individuals (e.g., polio, pertussis). We understand the biologic mechanisms for many of these differences; for example, live, oral poliovirus vaccines induce local enteric immunity and hence are more effective against poliovirus infection than are killed, parenterally administered poliovirus vaccines. It is theoretically possible to measure these different forms of protection by collecting data on both infection and disease status of individuals, and by estimating vaccine efficacy conditional upon the vaccination status of both the source and the "recipient" of potential transmission. Such data are sometimes available,[29] in particular within the context of household secondary attack rate studies, but their rarity means that most of our epidemiologic measures of immunity overlook these distinctions. This oversight does not mean that they are unimportant.

Vaccination, Vaccine Efficacy, Herd Immunity, and Disease Reduction

Vaccines reduce disease by direct protection of vaccinees and by indirect protection of nonvaccinees. Indirect protection depends upon a reduction in infection transmission, and hence upon protection (immunity) against infection, not just against disease. If a vaccine were to protect only against disease, and not at all against infection, then it would have no influence upon infection transmission in the community and there would be no indirect protection (vaccination of one individual would have no influence on any

TABLE 56–3 ■ Implications of Different Assumptions for Theoretical Estimates of the Herd Immunity Threshold (H)

Variable and Assumption	Implications for Herd Immunity	References
Maternal immunity	If vaccines are not effective until maternal immunity wanes, crude H estimates will be too low. This may be corrected by considering that a child is not born until maternal immunity disappears.	11
Variation in age at vaccination	Herd immunity effect is greatest (H threshold lowest) when vaccination occurs at the earliest possible age. Delayed vaccination implies threshold coverage level will be higher than simple estimates.	11, 25
Age differences in "contact" rates or infection risk	Implications vary with relationship between age and contact rate. Falling contact rate with age implies true H may be lower than simple global estimate.	16, 17
Seasonal changes in contact rates	Seasonality may imply lower herd immunity threshold if seasonal change is marked, and "fade out" can occur during low transmission period.	16, 26
Geographic heterogeneity	In theory, geographic differences in contact rates may permit elimination with lower overall vaccine coverage than that implied by H based on total population, by targeting high-risk groups.	27
Social structure (nonrandom mixing)	Social structure can have complicated implications because it implies group differences in vaccination uptake and/or infection risk. Existence of vaccine-neglecting high-contact groups means true H will be higher than simple estimates.	2

others in the community). It would be possible to reduce disease with such a vaccine, but not to eradicate an infection. This is an extreme scenario (it has, however, been discussed in the context of diphtheria, pertussis, and inactivated poliovirus vaccines), but we can explore more plausible circumstances.

We first assume that vaccine-induced immunity is a simple all-or-none affair, such that a proportion P of vaccinees are fully protected against an infectious agent. If vaccine coverage is C, then a proportion PC of the total population will be rendered fully immune. Under these circumstances, from Equation 6, the coverage required in order to reach herd immunity (C_H), and thereby bring about a sustained reduction in incidence, will be

$$C_H = (R_0 - 1)/(R_0 \times P) \qquad [8]$$

If, in contrast, a vaccine can protect to some degree against infection (a proportion P_i of vaccinees are rendered no longer susceptible to infection), and also can reduce transmissibility, that is, infectiousness (a proportion P_t among those vaccinated individuals who do become infected do not shed organisms and hence cannot transmit infection), then, as shown by Longini and colleagues,[29] the coverage required to induce herd immunity (reduce incidence) will be

$$C_H = (R_0 - 1)/(R_0 [P_i + P_t - P_i P_t]) \qquad [9]$$

This expression is useful in pointing out the potential importance of vaccine-mediated reductions in infectiousness to overall *indirect* protection of nonvaccinees (protection against *infection* being just as important as is protection against *infectiousness*). The overall effect of a vaccine in reducing disease incidence in a community will combine these two mechanisms against infection transmission, in addition to direct protection of vaccinees against disease.

The Real World

We turn now to compare the observed impact of community vaccination programs against what was and is predicted by theory, and to highlight a variety of particular issues raised by individual vaccine-preventable diseases. Readers are referred to the chapters in this text on specific infections and vaccines for further details on these examples.

Smallpox

The initial WHO encouragement toward global eradication of smallpox came in a resolution passed by the 12th World Health Assembly in 1959, which stated that "eradication of smallpox from an endemic area can be accomplished by successfully vaccinating or revaccinating 80 percent of the population within a period of four to five years, as has been demonstrated in several countries."[30] The wording is of interest in its explicit stipulation of a herd immunity threshold, and also in its implication that waning vaccine-derived immunity might pose an obstacle to achieving the threshold (thus the call for revaccination).

The disappearance of smallpox from many populations, despite the continued presence of large numbers of unvaccinated susceptibles, was evident from the historical record (as had been noted by Farr more than 150 years ago).[6] This is consistent with relatively low estimates of basic reproduction numbers and hence relatively low herd immunity thresholds for smallpox (see Table 56–2).[31] It is notable that the 1959 WHO recommendation implied an R_0 of 5. Though this is consistent with more recent estimates,[32] the 80% target was based originally upon experience alone, having been made prior to the development of the theory described above. The validation of such estimates, however derived, remains difficult. The actual value must have varied among populations and was higher in crowded urban than in rural settings. Beyond that, the severity of smallpox, in particular of variola major, was such that outbreaks typically encouraged active intervention (different forms of quarantine, contact tracing, and ring vaccination), and hence it is not always clear to what extent the course of an epidemic was determined by the general levels of immunity or by targeted emergency measures.

Arita et al. assembled data on crude population densities and smallpox vaccination coverage in African and Asian countries during the late 1960s and early 1970s.[33] Despite problems of nonuniform distributions of populations and of vaccinations, let alone the vagaries of vaccination statistics themselves, these data indicate that smallpox disappeared early from countries in which the crude density of susceptibles (unvaccinated individuals) fell below 10 persons/km² (corresponding to 80% immunization in populations with crude population density less than 50 persons/km²). The infection persisted in more densely populated regions, however—in particular, Nigeria (54 persons/km²), Pakistan (83/km²), India (175/km²), and Bangladesh (502/km²). Whether or not continued reliance upon routine population-wide vaccination programs might ultimately have been sufficient to eliminate smallpox from the more densely populated nations of Africa and Asia is now a moot point. If the 10 susceptibles/km² threshold is a guide, then 98% vaccination coverage would have been necessary for Bangladesh—and such coverages were impracticable. However, it was recognized by 1970 that variola virus could be eliminated from populations more effectively by a policy of active case detection, contact tracing, and the breaking of individual chains of transmission by quarantine and ring vaccination than by relying entirely upon herd immunity from routine or mass vaccination programs.[34] In effect, the focus of prevention activity shifted from the population back to the individual. The success of this policy is now a matter of record.[31]

Among the major lessons from the smallpox program was the inadequacy of relying too heavily upon reported vaccine uptake statistics and herd immunity predictions for disease eradication. Many experiences illustrated that reported data could be extremely unreliable, and high coverage statistics often obscured the fact that important segments of a population were inadequately vaccinated, and could serve to maintain and transport the infection for long periods and distances.[31,33]

The disappearance of smallpox from many populations prior to the intensive campaigns of the final eradication program is consistent with indirect protection of unvaccinated susceptibles having contributed importantly to the overall decline of this disease. Beyond that, the persistence of the disease in densely populated third-world countries despite apparent vaccination coverages far in excess of the

WHO's recommended 80% herd immunity threshold reflects the importance of population heterogeneities in vaccine coverage and in transmission risk (whatever the R_0 might have been on average, it varied greatly between and within populations). The smallpox experience thus demonstrates both the validity and the limits of herd immunity in practice. It should also be appreciated that several features of the natural history of smallpox favored the shift in strategy away from the emphasis upon a simplistic reliance upon herd immunity—in particular, the high case-to-infection ratio and characteristic pathology (which facilitated detection of cases) and the relatively low transmissibility (which facilitated control by identification of contacts and ring vaccination). Without these characteristics, much greater emphasis would have had to be placed upon raising the community-wide prevalence of immunity in order to achieve eradication of this disease.

By an unfortunate irony, questions of community immunity to smallpox have once again become topical, a quarter century after its eradication. Routine smallpox vaccination was discontinued everywhere by 1980, and more than 80% of the world's population is now susceptible to the infection (note that vaccinia-induced protection wanes with time, and boosters were recommended every 5 years). Though smallpox (variola) virus was supposed to have been preserved in only two high-security laboratories (in Atlanta, Georgia, and Novosibirsk, Russia), it is now known that large amounts of virus were grown for biologic warfare purposes, in particular in Russia.[35] It is not clear whether any of this virus still exists, but that possibility makes smallpox among the most feared of all potential bioterrorism weapons. Given the absence of immunity in contemporary populations, a release of virus could lead to rapid and widespread dispersal, with devastating consequences. The fear of such an event has led to much discussion, to the enactment of mock outbreaks to test control approaches, to the decision on the part of several governments to replenish national supplies of smallpox vaccine, and to contingency plans for emergency vaccine deployment.[36] These discussions raise many important issues concerning community immunity, such as whether health care workers or workers in other essential services should be vaccinated routinely, or voluntarily; to what extent the vaccine can be diluted without seriously compromising its efficacy; and the extent to which resources should be deployed in any emergency for mass vaccination as opposed to targeted case finding, contact tracing, and ring vaccination.[37] There is considerable controversy on these issues today.

Measles

No disease has been studied more intensely with reference to herd immunity than has measles.[4,10,11,14,16,25,38–41] There are two reasons for this. One is that measles has long been a favorite subject for theoretical modeling, on account of its frequency, its predictable behavior, and the high quality of available data. The second is that there has been serious discussion ever since 1967 of the possibility of eliminating measles both nationally and internationally.[42–45] Many of these discussions have relied upon estimates and interpretations of herd immunity thresholds.

Published estimates of herd immunity thresholds required to eradicate measles have ranged from 55% to 96%, depending upon the modeling approach and the assumptions employed (e.g., whether age or seasonality of transmission was included). The logic and the flaws underlying the various estimates have been discussed elsewhere.[1,11,16,26] Measles is among the most highly transmissible of all directly transmitted infections (see Table 56–2) and thus its herd immunity threshold is likely to be very high, at least in urban populations—on the order of 95%. Given that the efficacy of measles vaccine even under good conditions is approximately 95%, that vaccination coverage can never be 100%, and that poor coverage will tend to cluster in particular communities, this means that a single-dose measles vaccination policy is unlikely to be sufficient to eliminate measles from a large population. Recognition of this fact has led to recommendations for two-dose measles vaccination policies in many countries, with the first dose administered at approximately 1 year of age (after maternal immunity has declined), and the second at school age in an effort to immunize those children who escaped vaccination as infants or in whom the initial vaccination failed to induce protective immunity (primary vaccine failures).[46] In addition, or alternatively, many countries in recent years have employed mass campaigns in order to deliver measles vaccines to all children up to the age of 5, 12, or 15 years, in an effort to protect the few children who had escaped natural infection or successful vaccination.[47] These efforts have been pursued aggressively in Latin America, and more recently in southern Africa, where "catch-up" (initial mass campaign up to age 15 years), "keep up" (enhanced routine vaccination at 12 to 15 months), and "follow-up" (repeated campaigns among those under age 5 years) vaccination policies have succeeded in reducing measles incidence to very low levels.[48]

The reduction or absence of endemic measles in highly vaccinated communities allows the gradual accumulation of susceptible individuals (those who escaped vaccination or in whom the vaccine failed). This may lead to delayed epidemics after several years of little or no measles, known as "post–honeymoon period epidemics," which typically involve older age groups than were traditionally involved in measles. Dramatic examples of such delayed epidemics have been observed in several countries, including the United States in 1990 (see Fig. 56-4C) and Brazil in 1997.[49] Routine serologic surveillance in the United Kingdom revealed a gradual accumulation of susceptibles in the early 1990s, and to the prediction of such a delayed epidemic. A nationwide mass campaign was implemented in 1994 to vaccinate all children 5 to 16 years of age to remove this threat.[50] In an increasing number of countries (including the United States, Mexico, and the United Kingdom), immunity levels are now high enough to interrupt indigenous transmission of measles virus, so that a high proportion of all cases are attributable directly or within one or two generations to importations.[51] Though it is evident from these examples that the disciplined use of measles vaccines can raise immunity levels above the threshold required to eliminate continued transmission in large populations, the effort and resources to achieve this are considerable, and it is by no means clear that it would be either logistically feasible, economically sensible, or politically wise to attempt eradication on a global scale.

Rubella

Though the basic transmission dynamics of rubella are similar to those of measles, rubella raises different questions relating to community immunity. Public health concern with rubella is concentrated upon congenital rubella syndrome (CRS), and thus upon infections occurring in women in their reproductive years.[19] Control can in theory be brought about either by reducing the proportion susceptible among women, or by reducing their risk of infection. Vaccination of adolescent girls, as practiced in the United Kingdom between 1971 and 1988, emphasized the reduction of susceptible women by ensuring that a maximum percentage of females would acquire either natural or vaccine-derived immunity prior to their reproductive years. In contrast, vaccination of boys and girls in their second year of life, as practiced in the United States since 1971, in the United Kingdom since 1988, and in many other countries, leads also to reduction of circulation of rubella virus, and hence to the reduction of risk of infection for any remaining susceptibles in the adult female population. In theory, the latter policy carries a risk if coverage is not high, because low vaccination coverage of young children of both sexes can reduce the transmission of rubella virus to such a degree that the proportion of reproductive-age women still susceptible to the virus, and the numbers of consequent cases of CRS, actually increase.

Several investigations have concluded that the threshold vaccination coverage that must be achieved and maintained in young children of both sexes, in order for the incidence of CRS to decrease in the long term, is in the region of 50% to 80%.[14,19,52,53] The higher the initial intensity of transmission in the population, the higher is the threshold of vaccination coverage required among young children in order to avoid increasing the incidence of CRS. Given that vaccination uptake rates in the early 1970s in the United States and the United Kingdom were on the order of 90% and 50%, respectively, each nation's strategy was probably appropriate under the circumstances of the time. In contrast, it appears that the situation in Greece was unfortunate and that low levels of childhood vaccination during the 1980s may have actually increased the incidence of congenital rubella.[54] Because of the possibility that low childhood vaccination coverage could actually result in an increase in CRS, several countries have implemented programs to reduce adult susceptibility (e.g., postpartum vaccination of identified susceptible women) at the same time that they begin childhood rubella vaccination programs.

Rubella is less transmissible than is measles, and thus a lower prevalence of immunity should be required for its elimination (see Table 56–2). It may be that rubella will disappear as a consequence of measles elimination activities, at least in those (wealthier) countries that use combined vaccines, with no special additional efforts. There needs to be caution about the use of combined vaccines in countries that are unable to achieve high and sustained coverage, however. Rubella is at historically low levels in the United States today, with a high proportion of notified cases attributable to importations or occurring in immigrants from countries where rubella vaccination is not routine. This reflects pockets of susceptibility that cluster in particular ethnic communities.

Mumps

Mumps is similar to measles (both are paramyxoviruses maintained by respiratory spread), but is less transmissible in household settings and appears to have a lower crude R_0 and a lower apparent herd immunity threshold than either measles or rubella (see Table 56–2).[20] Notifications have fallen by more than 95% since introduction of vaccination in the United States (the vaccine was licensed in 1968 and recommended in 1977). Given that vaccine uptake has not reached that level among school entrants, that uptake among preschoolers is far below that level, and that mumps vaccine efficacy is probably below 90%,[46,55,56] this decline in incidence is greater than would be predicted by direct protection alone. Once again we see evidence of indirect protection. Given that mumps vaccine typically is given in combination with measles and rubella antigen, if it is offered at all, population immunity to mumps is now determined largely by the energy applied to measles control.

Chickenpox (Herpes Varicella-Zoster Virus)

Herpes varicella-zoster virus is ubiquitous in all human populations. Primary infection usually occurs in childhood, and is manifested clinically as chickenpox. In common with many herpesviruses, varicella-zoster virus establishes a persistent "latent" infection, typically in the dorsal root ganglia, from which site it may recrudesce many years later to cause herpes zoster ("shingles"). Chickenpox is more severe in infants and adults than in children, being responsible for some 11,000 hospitalizations and 100 deaths in the United States annually.[57] Because of this, varicella vaccine (with a live, attenuated virus) was introduced into the routine childhood immunization schedule in the United States in 1995, and its introduction is under consideration by several other countries. Surveillance data show a major decline in chickenpox incidence in the United States in recent years as a consequence of this program, including evidence of indirect protection among infants and adults, outside the vaccinated target age groups.[57]

Unlike immunity to variola, measles, rubella, and mumps viruses, immunity to varicella-zoster is not sterile, but serves to suppress or to contain the persistent latent infection. Though it may provide some degree of protection against reinfection (or, better, "superinfection"), there is increasing evidence that this protection wanes with time and that superinfections do occur.[58] This waning of protection is associated with increased risk of clinical episodes of herpes zoster. Recent studies provide convincing evidence that repeated exposure to children with varicella boosts immunity and reduces the risk of zoster in adults.[59,60] This has important implications.

Most importantly, several authors have warned that reduction in the circulation of varicella virus, as a consequence of widespread vaccination, could lead to an increase in the incidence of herpes zoster.[59-61] This is a perverse result—vaccination of one segment of a population (young children) leading to indirect protection and hence to reduced boosting of immunity and increased incidence of disease in another segment of society (adults). Because of this concern, interest has turned to the possible need to vaccinate adults in order to artificially boost their immunity and prevent zoster in the absence of natural boosting.

The ecology of varicella and its immunity are complicated. The nature of this immunity (relative protection against infection, chickenpox, zoster, and transmissibility) in the presence or absence of boosting exposures is not well understood. Though simple consideration of age distributions of chickenpox (see, e.g., Fig. 56–7) would suggest an R_0 of 8 to 10 in developed countries, this number should not be interpreted to imply a threshold for eradication.[62] The current vaccine strategy substitutes one virus for another in the population, with unclear long-term implications. It is hoped that the immunity associated with the vaccine strains will be long lived, and that the risk of zoster associated with vaccine strains will be lower than with wild-type varicella-zoster virus, but the situation will need close monitoring in the coming years to ensure an overall public health benefit from this intervention.[63]

Pertussis

Whooping cough is a common disease of childhood in unvaccinated communities. Responsible for considerable morbidity and mortality in the past, it has been a target for routine vaccination programs in many countries since the 1950s (see Fig. 56–4). These programs have been successful in reducing greatly the burden of disease caused by pertussis, and there is evidence that herd immunity, in the sense of indirect protection, has played a role in this effect.[64,65] Despite these successes, eradication of pertussis is an unlikely prospect.[66]

The cyclical pattern of pertussis epidemics provides a classical example of mass action dynamics (compare Figs. 56–3, 56–4B, and 56–4D).[67,68] The crude basic reproduction number of Bordetella pertussis has been estimated to be approximately 15 for developed countries in recent decades (see Table 56–2). This is similar to measles and implies a crude herd immunity threshold in excess of 90%. Consideration of age-dependent transmission has suggested a slightly lower estimate, 88%, but this assumed no waning of immunity.[68] Given that these figures are higher than most estimates of the protective efficacy of a complete course of pertussis vaccine,[69] and that there is evidence of waning vaccine-derived protection,[69,70] it appears that eradication of this infection is not currently possible by childhood vaccination alone.

Immunity to pertussis is difficult to define, either in individuals or in populations. There is no good serologic correlate for protective immunity; history of disease is neither highly sensitive nor highly specific as an indicator of past infection and hence natural immunity; and there is considerable controversy over the efficacy of available pertussis vaccines.[69,71,72] Some countries have introduced acellular vaccines in recent years, because of safety concerns surrounding the older whole-cell vaccines, despite the fact that the acellular products may be less protective. In addition, there is evidence that pertussis vaccines provide greater protection against pertussis disease than they do against infection with B. pertussis, and that adults con-

tribute to transmission of the infection with or without manifesting characteristic signs of the disease.[67,69,73] This latter concern, and evidence for increasing incidence of pertussis among adolescents and adults (note the trend since 1980 in Fig. 56–4D), has led to discussion of the possible need to introduce vaccination among adults whose immunity is no longer being boosted by natural infections.[74,75] Pertussis is thus another example of an infection for which the immunity profile has changed dramatically in recent decades in many populations: from a predominance of immunity attributable only to natural infection (now restricted to older individuals), to immunity attributable largely to killed whole-cell vaccines (in a high proportion of individuals born since 1950), and now to immunity attributable to various acellular vaccines (in younger individuals). Each of these forms of immunity is likely to have different implications for protection against infection, disease, and infectiousness. The long-term implications of these changes are as yet unclear.

Diphtheria

Diphtheria was a major cause of morbidity and mortality in Europe and North America during the 19th century. Incidence fell from the early years of the 20th century, and the decline accelerated along with introduction of widespread toxoid vaccination in the United States, the United Kingdom, and other countries during the 1940s. Because vaccination of less than 90% of children was associated with a more than 99.99% fall in disease, it might be argued that a herd immunity threshold was achieved. But a closer look reveals a complicated story of community immunity.

Published estimates of the herd immunity threshold for diphtheria have ranged from 50% to 90%.[1] Estimates aside, the actual proportion of diphtheria immunes in today's populations is an elusive quantity. Vaccine coverage is difficult to define because it has varied over time, and because at least three doses are recommended, though one or two provide some protection. The protection imparted by diphtheria toxoid vaccines has never been evaluated in formal trials, though observational studies provide estimates ranging from 55% to 90%.[76–78] Serologic studies have shown that vaccine-induced antitoxin titers decline with time, and may in some populations be lower among individuals born in recent decades, perhaps because they have not been boosted by exposure to natural infections.[79] Surveys carried out in developed countries have shown a wide range in prevalence of "protective" antitoxin levels among adults, from 29% to 80%, leading to recommendations that adults should receive booster doses of diphtheria vaccine.[79–82]

An important question concerning community protection against diphtheria relates to the nature of the immunity induced by toxoid vaccines, and how it may differ from infection-attributable immunity. In the sense that herd immunity implies indirect protection, it requires immunity against infection or against transmission. Given that diphtheria toxin is not a normal constituent of Corynebacterium diphtheriae, the immunity induced by toxoid vaccination may not provide protection against infection at all.[83] However, toxoid vaccines do protect against toxin-mediated disease, and transmission of the diphtheria bacillus is more efficient from clinical cases than from subclinical carriers[84]—thus the toxoid vaccines may protect against infectiousness and infection transmission, but not (or more than) against infection receipt ($P_t \gg P_i$, according to the logic surrounding Equation 9). This may have been an important contributor to the disappearance of diphtheria in vaccinated populations.

Skin and respiratory tract infections with nontoxigenic corynebacteria are common in many populations, in particular in the tropics, and these probably impart some direct protection against infection with toxigenic *C. diphtheriae*.[85] Because this protection is independent of antitoxin, the emphasis upon antitoxin antibodies in surveys of immunity to diphtheria may miss an important element in community immunity against this disease.

Tetanus

Clostridium tetani is not communicable between human hosts, and thus vaccination cannot lead to indirect protection in the sense implied in many definitions of herd immunity. Certainly there is no threshold proportion of immunes, below 100%, that can ensure total absence of tetanus from a community.

There is little doubt that the introduction of routine tetanus toxoid vaccination in the 1940s had an impact upon trends and patterns of the disease. However, the fact that the incidence of tetanus was declining prior to widespread vaccination, as a result of decreasing exposure (fewer people in contact with soil and animal feces, which are the main reservoirs of the tetanus bacillus) and the widespread use of tetanus toxoid in wound management, makes it difficult to assess the precise extent to which routine prophylactic vaccination contributed to the decline in tetanus morbidity.

Despite the noncommunicability of *C. tetani* between people, there is a special sense in which vaccination can impart indirect protection. Antitetanus immunity of mothers is transmitted across the placenta, and two doses of toxoid during pregnancy can protect a woman's offspring against neonatal disease.[86] This is extremely important in that the public health importance of tetanus on a global scale is attributable largely to neonatal disease. In 1989, the World Health Assembly declared an initiative to *eliminate* neonatal tetanus (defined as less than one case of neonatal tetanus for every 1000 live births in each administrative district throughout the world). Though the initiative includes efforts to improve birth practices, it relies largely upon provision of tetanus toxoid vaccine to girls and to women in antenatal clinics. In this sense, the critical population for community immunity to tetanus consists of girls and women in their reproductive years.

Haemophilus influenzae b

Vaccination against *H. influenzae* type b has been introduced into routine infant schedules in many countries over the past 15 years, with great effect. In the absence of vaccination, *Haemophilus* carriage is highly prevalent among children in most populations, with invasive disease occurring primarily in young children. Polysaccharide-protein conjugate vaccines are immunogenic in early infancy, pro-viding high protection (>95%) against invasive disease and at least some protection against carriage. The latter effect has been sufficient to reduce transmission and to provide demonstrable indirect protection to nonvaccinated groups in several communities—for example, in children too young to be vaccinated in Israel[87] and in those too old to be vaccinated in Scandinavia.[88] A failure to demonstrate any indirect protection in the early years of the program in the Netherlands has been attributed to their having targeted too narrow an age group.[89, 90] In Alaska, the epidemiology of *H. influenzae* appears to be substantially different from that in many developed countries, being characterized by earlier age at onset of disease and higher carriage rates associated with crowded living conditions before vaccine licensure. This led to the use of a vaccine (polyribosylribitol phosphate–outer membrane protein) that has the property of inducing substantial immunity after a single dose, leading to protection at a younger age than other *H. influenzae* type b vaccines. However, this vaccine induces lower antibody titers after the full series than do other vaccines, and, under the conditions of intense exposure in the Alaskan population, it did not reduce carriage sufficiently and allowed resurgence of transmission and disease.[91]

The ecology of *Haemophilus* and other encapsulated bacteria thus raises yet another issue—immunity against carriage (distinguished from infection per se in that tissue invasion need not occur). Conjugate vaccine interventions have proved successful in greatly reducing invasive *Haemophilus* disease in the short term, and appear to provide appreciable protection against carriage in some settings, but the long-term effects are yet unclear, and will be a function of the persistence and implications of this new form of immunity now being introduced into populations.

Poliomyelitis

The issue of community immunity in polio has been debated for more than four decades. The debate has been notable for its partisan fervor and confusing for its shifting focus to and from different types of immunity induction by different types of polio vaccines.[92,93] Serologic surveys carried out in the past in unvaccinated populations have been used to estimate the prevalence of immunes in endemic communities, suggesting that the basic reproduction number of wild-type polioviruses ranges from 2 to 15, and thus that the herd immunity threshold ranges from 50% to 93%, these numbers being inversely related to the level of hygiene. But even this is too simplistic.

The polio immunity controversy has been part of a broader argument concerning the relative advantages of inactivated poliovirus vaccine (IPV) versus live oral poliovirus vaccine (OPV). Among the arguments favoring the live vaccines has been the claim that they provide greater "herd immunity" than do IPVs. Two points are embedded in this claim. The first is that live vaccines impart greater intestinal (local, immunoglobulin A–mediated) immunity, and hence impart greater protection against *infection*, than do the killed vaccines (which induce protection more directly against tissue invasion and *disease*). To the extent that this is so, then recipients of killed vaccines may be protected effectively against disease but still be susceptible to enteric wild-type poliovirus infection—and thus provide little or no indirect protection to their unvaccinated neighbors. If this were so in the extreme, then herd immunity thresholds would be invalid for such vaccines, and only 100% IPV vaccine coverage of a population would suffice to protect it from disease. This argument has sometimes been overstated. Though there is evidence that prior OPV recipients excrete less virus in their feces than do prior recipients of IPV, after subsequent challenge with live poliovirus vaccine virus strains, it has been demonstrated that both fecal and oropharyngeal virus excretion is reduced among prior IPV recipients compared to unvaccinated individuals.[93] Thus IPV vaccines do provide some protection against infection transmission. The propensity of IPV to reduce oropharyngeal excretion of virus might be particularly important in populations with high levels of sanitation, in which respiratory transmission of poliovirus is more important than in areas with poor sanitation conditions, where transmission is thought to be overwhelmingly by the fecal–oral route.

The second argument for greater herd immunity induction by OPV than IPV is based upon the fact that live poliovirus vaccine virus is excreted in the feces and by the oropharynx in sufficient quantities for it to be transmitted to contacts. This unique attribute of OPV provides a special mechanism for indirect protection of nonvaccinees—in effect by vaccinating them surreptitiously. The frequency of such OPV spread is dependent upon hygiene behavior and intimacy of contact, and varies greatly among populations. Studies carried out in the 1950s showed that OPV virus was transmitted to 35% to 80% of child contacts of OPV recipients within low socioeconomic group households, though less frequently within better-off households, and that considerable transmission also occurred beyond the confines of households.[93] This means that the proportion *immunized* in a population receiving OPV is a function of three factors: vaccine uptake, vaccine efficacy, and vaccine virus transmission. The advantage inherent in this unique attribute of the live poliovirus vaccines is tempered by the fact that the OPV virus may rarely undergo reversion to virulence, causing rare cases of paralytic disease (approximately one such case per million vaccine doses administered).[94]

It appears that wild-type polioviruses ceased to circulate in most of the United States by 1970, at which time only some 65% of children were receiving a complete course of OPV. However, given the complex history of previous IPV and then OPV programs in the country, and the propensity of OPV viruses to circulate in the community, the actual level of immunity in the population at that time is unknown. It is also possible that the disappearance of wild-type polioviruses from the United States and other countries employing OPV has been due not only to the achievement of some herd immunity threshold, but also to the competition for ecologic space between the wild-type viruses and the constantly introduced vaccine strains.

In addition to the virologic evidence for reduced excretion of challenge virus in IPV recipients, there is good epidemiologic evidence for indirect protection by IPVs. Countries that have used only IPV (e.g., Sweden, Finland, and the Netherlands) experienced elimination of circulating wild-type polioviruses for long periods of time.[93,95,96] Outbreaks in the Netherlands have been restricted almost entirely to a religious community that refuses vaccination altogether, with no evidence of transmission in the population at large, despite the presence of at least 400,000 individuals who had never been vaccinated at all.[97] This evidence supported the decision by the United States to shift back to IPV for polio control in the year 2000.

Current efforts aimed at the global eradication of polio are based upon massive use of OPV vaccines in routine infant vaccination services, as well as in national campaigns targeting all children up to 5 or 10 years of age and in local "mopping-up" campaigns organized around outbreaks. The effect of this immense use of vaccines has been to raise levels of immunity to poliovirus infection and disease to the highest levels ever. The rapid decline in wild-type virus–attributable cases in recent years reflects the high levels of immunity, perhaps assisted by the competition for appropriate niches between the dwindling wild-type virus population and the continually replenished population of vaccine viruses.

The final phase of the polio eradication program will involve yet another demand upon community immunity. There has been much discussion in recent years as to whether OPV-derived viruses could or will persist by continued person-to-person transmission, and revert to wild-type characteristics, after cessation of active OPV programs.[93] The recent recognition of outbreaks of poliomyelitis attributable to circulating strains of vaccine-derived polioviruses testifies to the reality of this danger.[98] Just how to manage this final stage of the global eradication initiative is not yet clear, with options including an attempt to raise global immunity to an unprecedented level through a massive global OPV campaign prior to discontinuing OPV, or shifting country by country to IPV, or an acceptance that polio vaccination of one sort or another will have to continue everywhere for the foreseeable future, even after the eradication of wild-type viruses.

Influenza

Type A influenza viruses present yet another set of community immunity problems. Given the genetic lability of these viruses, as manifested in frequent major (shift) and minor (drift) antigenic changes of their hemagglutinin (H) and neuraminidase (N) antigens, and their persistence in many different vertebrate species, there is no prospect of their total eradication. However, "herd immunity" has been invoked as an explanation for the changing profile of influenza viruses in human populations and the successive disappearance of specific antigenic subtypes. The argument is that increasing proportions immune to each individual influenza subtype, and varying degrees of cross-protection provided between subtypes, should provide a selective pressure favoring the spread of new antigenic variants. Though such a mechanism appears to fit the available evidence, it does not lend itself to precise numeric description, given the complicated immunologic relationships between virus subtypes, the possibility that immunity to influenza may be less durable than immunity to many other viruses, and the unpredictable nature of the antigenic changes of these viruses.

The hypothesis that herd immunity to influenza viruses has been a driving force in the selection of new predominant strains in the human population has another interesting feature. One of the peculiarities of influenza epidemiology is the observation that, although prior to 1977 only a single major virus (shift) subtype was found circulating in the human population worldwide at any time, more recent years have witnessed the co-circulation of different subtypes (e.g., H_1N_1 and H_3N_2) simultaneously in the same populations.[99] Why this should have occurred is unclear. If the observation is correct, and does not reflect changes in virologic surveillance, then the appearance of co-circulating viruses may indicate one of two possibilities. Either the viruses are now different, perhaps providing less cross-subtype (e.g., H_3N_2 vs. H_1N_1) protection than in the past, or else the human population has changed—perhaps by increasing in total number, or in number of new susceptibles added per year, and/or in worldwide communication to such extent that individual virus subtypes may reduce susceptibles to below threshold levels in some populations but still persist in others for long enough to allow sufficient accumulation of susceptibles in the first group to again support transmission. If this is so, and the appearance of multiple co-circulating influenza viruses does reflect such changes in the human population, then this could have implications for the worldwide control of other infectious agents.

Though eradication of type A influenza viruses is not possible, their control by immunization is an important public health activity in all the wealthier countries. There has been much discussion of influenza vaccination strategies, given the changing antigenic nature of the viruses and their rapid spread, explosive epidemics, and serious impact in terms of sickness absences among the employed and mortality among the elderly.[99] Though the favored strategy of most countries has been to target high-risk groups, an alternative is to reduce community spread by concentrating upon vaccination of schoolchildren, because transmission within crowded classrooms leads to rapid dispersal throughout the community, and into the homes where susceptible adults reside. The effectiveness of this indirect protection approach in providing a measurable degree of indirect protection of nonvaccinees in the community has been demonstrated at least twice under trial conditions, in Michigan[100] and in Russia.[101] Such a strategy was national policy in Japan from 1962 and enforced by law between 1977 and 1987, but discontinued in 1994 because of skepticism as to its effectiveness and public concern over adverse reactions to the vaccines.[102] This program was unique in explicitly directing vaccination at one segment of the population (schoolchildren) in order to protect another (the elderly). A recent analysis concluded that one adult death was prevented for every 420 vaccinations of schoolchildren.[102]

Tuberculosis

Tuberculosis is included here in recognition of the fact that immunologic intervention, in the form of bacillus Calmette-Guérin (BCG) vaccination, remains an important element in the control of this disease in most countries of the world. More people alive today have received BCG than have received any other vaccine. In addition, it raises a very different set of questions about community immunity compared to those discussed above.[103] We touch briefly upon several of these questions here.

That humans can mount some degree of protective immunity to Mycobacterium tuberculosis is evident from the fact that BCG vaccine has been shown to reduce risks of disease, at least to some degree, in a large number of studies.[104] We have no measurable correlate of this protective immunity, and the most widely used measure of cellular "immunity" (or immune response) to the tubercle bacillus (i.e., delayed-type hypersensitivity to tuberculin) is associated with relatively high rather than relatively low risk of disease! This paradox arises because a high proportion of infections with the tubercle bacillus persist in the human host, and an appreciable proportion of all cases of disease reflect a breakdown of immunity in older, long-infected (and tuberculin-sensitive) individuals. This breakdown of immunity may be attributable to many factors, such as age or intercurrent disease, but on a global scale today the most important factor by far is immunosuppression as a consequence of human immunodeficiency virus (HIV) infection.

Another major problem in defining community immunity to tuberculosis relates to BCG, at once the most widely used and most controversial of contemporary vaccines. Though there is indisputable evidence for its effectiveness in some populations, in particular against severe disease of childhood but also against pulmonary disease in young adults in northern temperate populations,[104] there is also indisputable evidence of the failure of some of the same BCG vaccines to provide any detectable protection against tuberculosis in other populations, in particular in tropical environments. The most likely explanation for these differences is that they reflect variations in exposure to different environmental mycobacteria in different parts of the world, the effect of which is either to obstruct or to mask any protection induced by BCG.[105,106] Among the lines of evidence are data both from experimental animals and from human populations indicating that exposure to bacteria such as those of the Mycobacterium avium-intracellulare complex can induce a degree of cross-reactivity to tuberculin and can impart measurable protection against M. tuberculosis.[105] It thus appears that heterologous immunity, derived from exposure to relatives of the tubercle bacillus, can have an important influence upon community immunity against this disease.

At present, though we can measure the population distribution of certain immunologic measures of mycobacterial exposure and infection, we have little understanding of the nature and distribution of protective immunity to tuberculosis.

Discussion

This brief review of various infections reveals many complexities to the measurement and interpretation of immunity at the community level. To say that X% of a population is "immune" to some infection or disease can be misleading without detailed qualification of the nature of the immunologic states and a description of the distribution of the various sorts of individuals in the population, in particular by age and area. For some infections, exemplified by measles, immunity to infection, to disease, and to infectiousness appear to be quite similar in nature and magnitude; but for many infections they are different, as illustrated here in the discussions of varicella-zoster, diphtheria, pertussis, polio, *Haemophilus*, and tuberculosis. The epidemiologic description, analysis, and interpretation of immunologic states is an important but still poorly developed aspect of infectious disease epidemiology and vaccinology.

There is also a sense in which the interpretation of immunity in individuals is dependent upon its distribution in populations. If vaccinated individuals are clustered in community groups (as is often the case), then they benefit both directly, from individual receipt of the vaccine, and indirectly, from reduced transmission in their neighborhoods. In such circumstances, the vaccinated and unvaccinated individuals are not equally exposed to infection, and crude measures of vaccine efficacy will overestimate the immunizing capacity of the vaccine among individual recipients.[69,107] This is a particular problem in observational studies of vaccines, but also may affect trials in which randomization is by group and not by individual.[108]

This discussion has referred repeatedly to the "indirect protection" of nonimmune individuals brought about by the presence and proximity of immunes. That such protection should occur is evident both intuitively and through theoretical argument, and it has been demonstrated repeatedly and convincingly in the context of many vaccination programs. Of the infections and vaccines discussed above, the only examples in which indirect protection has not been demonstrated are tetanus (though there is the argument relating to passive antibody transfer from mothers to their neonates) and tuberculosis (in which case the absence of demonstrable indirect protection reflects in part that most infection transmission is attributable to adults who have lost their immunity). In several examples, the indirect protection from vaccination has been obvious (e.g., smallpox, rubella, mumps, chickenpox, *Haemophilus*, diphtheria, influenza). There are several important features to this indirect protection. One is that it applies to various sorts of individuals in the population containing the immunes—including to young and old, and to those who may be still susceptible because of immunoincompetence or because they refused or otherwise failed to be successfully vaccinated. A second important point is that such protection is not a form of immunity—and thus an individual indirectly protected (shielded) from infection remains still susceptible, and may in fact contract infection at a later date and age. Under certain circumstances, this delay in infection may actually be hazardous for the individual or society (e.g., with rubella). Indirect protection by vaccines is thus the opposite to a traditional approach, practiced in many societies, of exposing children to infectious cases of, for example, rubella or measles or chickenpox at an age when they are most likely to contract a mild form of the disease. Following on from this, we have noted that indirect protection can have another potentially detrimental effect insofar as it may reduce boosting of immunity through repeated exposure to infection, and thereby lead to greater waning of immunity and increased susceptibility in older individuals. This is a particular current concern with regard to both pertussis and varicella-zoster. In this context, it should be noted that an increase in one or another pattern of susceptibility in adults need not necessarily be detrimental to society—for example, if the use of vaccines in the young is sufficiently intense to reduce transmission greatly among the groups with the highest levels of contact, so that there is reduced exposure among adults. However, such shifts in the age distribution of immunity and susceptibility are potentially hazardous, and need to be monitored closely.

Appropriate comparisons between groups with different proportions of vaccinated individuals may allow estimates of both direct and indirect protection attributable to vaccines.[29,107] Despite the elegance of the methods, it is likely that measures of direct protection will be far more generalizable than are measures of indirect protection, given that the former depend only upon the immunologic response of individual vaccine recipients, whereas the latter will be a function of the social and spatial distribution of vaccinated individuals, and of social mixing patterns, which will differ greatly between populations. For example, the role of schoolchildren in community dispersal of influenza viruses (and hence in the indirect protection to adults that may be provided by their vaccination[100–102]) will be a function of the age and family size distribution of the population (which determine what proportion of families have children in school) as well as the size and physical environment of the schools (a single, large, crowded school being more likely to serve as a distribution center for the community than would a large number of small and well-ventilated schools).

Much of the literature on community immunity to various infections emphasizes threshold proportions of immunes that, if reached and sustained (e.g., by vaccination), should lead to progressive elimination of the infection from the population. Such estimates (see, e.g., Table 56–2) provide a rough ranking of the probable levels of natural and vaccine-derived immunity required for eradication of these infections. These numeric estimates should not be accepted uncritically, however, because they vary greatly dependent upon the assumptions underlying their derivations, and even the most elaborate derivations omit important features of the immune response and of the practical logistics and nonuniformity of real populations and of real vaccination programs. Though these thresholds often are referred to in the context of discussions of eradication targets, the practical experience of the major programs to date, against smallpox, polio, and measles, has found them of little practical use. In addition, their relevance is mitigated by the fact that most public health programs aim at "control" rather than elimination or eradication of infections. Even if the goal is eradication, the practical approach will not be to just attain some threshold, but to aim for *and sustain* the highest possible coverage, in theory 100%, because this will maximize the rapidity of the disappearance of the infection in question. Merely achieving a herd immunity threshold does not mean immediate disappearance of the infection; it only starts a downward trend.

Such caveats do not mean that the herd immunity threshold is not a valid concept. That indirect protection occurs is obvious, both in logic and in observation. Prevention of a communicable infection in any individual reduces by one the potential sources of infection—and hence the potential risk of infection—for that individual's peers. That is indirect protection and a form of herd immunity. The observation of apparent exceptions, small communities in which infections appear to be transmitted despite very high levels of vaccination coverage, do not refute this principle,[109] just as the failure of a vaccination in some individual recipients need not refute an overall high efficacy of a vaccine.

The herd immunity threshold concept provides an epidemiologic attribute with which to characterize particular infections. Though precision may not be possible, because of population heterogeneities or because of variability in the immune status of individuals, even crude estimates can be of use in giving a rough guideline for predicting the impact of a vaccination program and at least a hint as to the potential for eradication. As experience grows, we will come to appreciate better how the various subtleties of the immunology and epidemiology of different infections—for example, those attributable to the nature of the immune response and to the social structure of populations—imply greater or lesser biases in the estimates derived from simple models. The concept of a threshold is also useful in the context of teaching. It is part of the basic science of infectious disease epidemiology, and provides an essential background for understanding the behavior of infections in populations.

The emphasis upon elimination thresholds in the herd immunity literature distracts from important and complicated implications of changing patterns and levels of immunity in populations over time. A vaccination intervention entails a massive disruption of the previous "natural" balance, and can destabilize epidemiologic patterns for many years. The introduction of an effective vaccination program among children may reduce infection incidence to such a degree that a large number of susceptibles can accumulate among those individuals born just too early to receive the vaccinations, and who thus escape both the natural infection and the benefits of vaccination. The accumulation of such susceptible groups may lead to changes in the age distribution of cases in subsequent years, as has been reported for several vaccine-preventable diseases[110–112] and predicted for others.[60–63,73–75] Discussion of such changes is sometimes confused by presentation in terms of proportions of cases in different age groups, because it is possible for the proportion of, for example, measles cases among adults to increase dramatically even though their absolute number decreases. Thus a shift to older cases need not necessarily be harmful. Prediction of such effects requires simulation with models that take into account differences in contact within and between age groups. The only way to develop convincing descriptions is by the accumulation of detailed analyses of age-specific data over time, preferably before and after vaccine interventions.

Though vaccines are given to increase levels of immunity in populations, we also need to consider the loss of community immunity as an important issue. The loss of protective immunity may be attributable to waning of an immune response with time, which may in turn be a function of the nature and strength of the initial response, or to a reduction of boosting by natural exposures, as appears to be important in contemporary trends in pertussis and perhaps herpes zoster. Immunosuppression is also important in this regard, for the elderly and infirm but in particular as a consequence of HIV infection. HIV-attributable immunosuppression is a major driving force behind the global epidemic of tuberculosis today. The mechanisms underlying the persistence of immunologic memory are poorly understood but of great importance, to communities as well as to individuals.

The growth of emphasis upon vaccination programs, and the recognition of the complexity of their implications, highlight the importance of immunologic monitoring of populations. Only by accumulating such data will we ultimately be able to understand the dynamics of community immunity and the full effects of vaccine interventions and to optimize interventions. Such monitoring should enable detection of accumulating pockets of susceptibles and hence the prediction of delayed epidemics such as have been observed after a period of vaccine program–attributable low incidence.[50,109,110] The monitoring of increasing numbers of susceptibles to measles in the United Kingdom in the early 1990s through routine serosurveillance, and the subsequent nationwide mass campaign, provide an example of effective monitoring and response. Serosurveillance of antibody levels to rubella and diphtheria have also been used to plan immunization strategies, and such approaches are likely to increase in the future. Effective serosurveillance requires knowledge of appropriate humoral (preferably) or cellular "correlates" of protective immunity, such as we have for some vaccine-preventable diseases (e.g., measles and rubella) but not for others (e.g., pertussis and tuberculosis). Defining such correlates, and the development of appropriate assays for them, will be an important area of research in coming years.

This review has avoided insistence upon a simple single definition of herd immunity, instead accepting the varied uses of the term by different authors. This is in keeping with the first published use of the term, which posed the problem of herd immunity as the problem of how to distribute any given amount of immunity (antibodies, vaccinations, etc.) so as best to protect a population from disease.[7] The mechanisms will be several—direct protection of vaccinees against disease or transmissible infection, and indirect protection of nonrecipients by virtue of surreptitious vaccination, passive antibody, or just reduced sources of transmission and hence risks of infection in the community. The solutions likewise will depend upon many factors—the nature of the population, the infection, the vaccine, and the health services. The population and the infection are generally given, the vaccine we may try to improve, but the distribution of that vaccine is up to the public health community. In addition to the theoretical issues discussed here, this raises many operational issues related to delivery, cost, consent, and enforcement.[113] How to optimize that distribution for the betterment of society remains, in the broadest sense, the real problem of herd (community) immunity.

Acknowledgment

The author expresses his appreciation to Walt Orenstein for encouragement, wisdom, and patience, and to Linda Pollock for assistance with the figures.

REFERENCES

1. Fine PEM. Herd immunity: history, theory, practice. Epidemiol Rev 15:265–302, 1993.
2. Fox JP, Elveback L, Scott W, et al. Herd immunity: basic concept and relevance to public health immunization practices. Am J Epidemiol 94:179–189, 1971.

3. Anderson RM. The concept of herd immunity and the design of community-based immunization programmes. Vaccine 10:928–935, 1992.

4. Jenner E. The Origin of the Vaccine Inoculation. London, Shury, 1801.

5. Dubos R, Dubos J. The White Plague. London, Victor Gollancz, 1953.

6. Farr W. Second Annual Report of the Registrar—General of Births, Deaths, and Marriages in England. Her Majesty's Stationery Office, London, 1840.

7. Topley WWC, Wilson GS. The spread of bacterial infection: the problem of herd immunity. J Hyg 21:243–249, 1923.

8. Greenwood M. Epidemics and Crowd Diseases. London, Williams & Norgate Ltd, 1935.

9. Dowdle WR, Hopkins DR (eds). The Eradication of Infectious Diseases. Chichester, UK, John Wiley & Sons, 1998.

10. Hamer WH. Epidemic disease in England—the evidence of variability and of persistency of type. Lancet 1:733–739, 1906.

11. Anderson RM, May RM. Infectious Diseases of Humans: Dynamics and Control. Oxford, UK, Oxford University Press, 1991.

12. Macdonald G. The Epidemiology and Control of Malaria. London, Oxford University Press, 1957.

13. Dietz K. The estimation of the basic reproduction number for infectious diseases. Stat Methods Med Res 2:23–41, 1993.

14. Hethcote HW. Measles and rubella in the United States. Am J Epidemiol 117:2–13, 1983.

15. Dietz K. Transmission and control of arbovirus diseases. In Ludwig D, Cooke KL (eds). Epidemiology. Philadelphia, Society for Industrial and Applied Mathematics, 1975, pp 104–121.

16. Schenzle D. An age-structured model of pre- and post-vaccination measles transmission. IMA J Math Appl Med Biol 1:169–191, 1984.

17. Anderson RM, May RM. Age-related changes in the rate of disease transmission: implications for the design of vaccination programmes. J Hyg (Camb) 94:365–436, 1985.

18. Katzmann W, Dietz K. Evaluation of age-specific vaccination strategies. Theor Popul Biol 25:125–137, 1984.

19. Knox EG. Strategy for rubella vaccination. Int J Epidemiol 9:13–23, 1980.

20. Anderson RM, Crombie JA, Grenfell BT. The epidemiology of mumps in the UK: preliminary study of virus transmission, herd immunity and the potential impact of vaccination. Epidemiol Infect 99:65–84, 1987.

21. May RM, Anderson RM. Spatial heterogeneity and the design of immunization programmes. Math Biosci 72:83–111, 1984.

22. Hethcote HW, Van Ark JW. Epidemiological models for heterogeneous populations: proportionate mixing, parameter estimation, and immunization programs. Math Biosci 84:85–118, 1987.

23. Grenfell BT, Bjornstad ON, Kappey J. Travelling waves and spatial hierarchies in measles epidemics. Nature 414:716–723, 2001.

24. Strebel PM, Cochi SL. Waving goodbye to measles. Nature 414:695–696, 2001.

25. Nokes DJ, Anderson RM. Measles, mumps, and rubella vaccine: what coverage to block transmission? Lancet 2:1374, 1988.

26. Yorke JA, Nathanson N, Pianigiani G, Martin J. Seasonality and the requirements for perpetuation and eradication of viruses in populations. Am J Epidemiol 109:103–123, 1979.

27. Anderson RM, May RM. Spatial, temporal, and genetic heterogeneity in host populations and the design of immunization programmes. IMA J Math Appl Med Biol 1:233–266, 1984.

28. Smith PG, Rodrigues LC, Fine PEM. Assessment of the protective efficacy of vaccines against common diseases using case-control and cohort studies. Int J Epidemiol 13:137–153, 1984.

29. Longini IM, Halloran ME, Nizam A. Model-based estimation of vaccine effects from community vaccine trials. Stat Med 21:481–495, 2002.

30. World Health Assembly. Official Records of the World Health Organization—1959: Resolutions and Decisions of the 12th World Health Assembly (WHA 12.54). Geneva, World Health Organization, 1959.

31. Fenner F, Henderson DA, Arita I, et al. Smallpox and Its Eradication. Geneva, World Health Organization, 1988.

32. Gani R, Leach R. Transmission potential of smallpox in contemporary populations. Nature 414:748–751, 2001.

33. Arita I, Wickett J, Fenner F. Impact of population density on immunization programmes. J Hyg 96:459–466, 1986.

34. Henderson DA. Epidemiology in the global eradication of smallpox. Int J Epidemiol 1:25–30, 1972.

35. Henderson DA. The looming threat of bioterrorism. Science 283:1279–1282, 1999.

36. Enserink M. How devastating would a smallpox attack really be? Science 297:50–51, 2002.

37. Fauci AS. Smallpox vaccination policy—the need for a dialogue. N Engl J Med 346:1319–1320, 2002.

38. Farrington CP. Modelling forces of infection for measles, mumps, and rubella. Stat Med 9:953–967, 1990.

39. Fine PEM, Clarkson JA. Measles in England and Wales, I. An analysis of factors underlying seasonal patterns. Int J Epidemiol 11:5–14, 1982.

40. Fine PEM, Clarkson JA. Measles in England and Wales, II. The impact of the measles vaccination programme on the distribution of immunity in the population. Int J Epidemiol 11:15–25, 1982.

41. Black FL. The role of herd immunity in the control of measles. Yale J Biol Med 55:351–360, 1982.

42. Sencer DJ, Dull HB, Langmuir AD. Epidemiologic basis for eradication of measles in 1967. Public Health Rep 82:253–256, 1967.

43. Hopkins DR, Hinman AR, Koplan JP, et al. The case for global measles eradication. Lancet 1:1396–1398, 1982.

44. Henderson DA. Global measles eradication. Lancet 2:208, 1982.

45. World Health Organization. Measles Mortality Reduction and Regional Elimination: Strategic Plan, 2000–2005 (WHO/V&B/01.13). Geneva, World Health Organization, 2001.

46. Fahlgren K. Two doses of MMR vaccine—sufficient to eradicate measles, mumps, and rubella? Scand J Soc Med 16:129–135, 1988.

47. Centers for Disease Control and Prevention. Progress toward interrupting indigenous measles transmission—Region of the Americas, January–November 2001. MMWR 50:1133–1137, 2001.

48. Biellik R, Madema S, Taole A, et al. First 5 years of measles elimination in Southern Africa: 1996–2000. Lancet 359:1564–1568, 2002.

49. Centers for Disease Control and Prevention. Measles, rubella, and congenital rubella syndrome—United States and Mexico, 1997–1999. MMWR 49:1048–1050, 1059, 2000.

50. Gay N, Ramsay M, Cohen B, et al. The epidemiology of measles in England and Wales since the 1994 vaccination campaign. Commun Dis Rep 7:17–21, 1997.

51. Centers for Disease Control and Prevention. Measles—United States, 2000. MMWR 51:120–123, 2002.

52. Anderson RM, May RM. Vaccination against rubella and measles: quantitative investigation of different policies. J Hyg (Camb) 90:259–325, 1983.

53. van Druten JAM, de Boo T, Plantinga AD. Measles, mumps, and rubella: control by vaccination. Dev Biol Stand 65:53–63, 1986.

54. Panagiotopoulos T, Antoniadou I, Valassi-Adam E. Increase in congenital rubella occurrence after immunisation in Greece: retrospective survey and systematic review. BMJ 319:1462–1467, 1999.

55. Kim Farley R, Bart S, Stetler H, et al. Clinical mumps vaccine efficacy. Am J Epidemiol 121:593–597, 1985.

56. Sullivan KM, Halpin TJ, Marks JS, et al. Effectiveness of mumps vaccine in a school outbreak. Am J Dis Child 139:909–912, 1985.

57. Seward JF, Watson BM, Peterson CL, Mascola L. Varicella disease after introduction of varicella vaccine in the United States, 1995–2000. JAMA 287:606–611, 2002.

58. Hall S, Sewar J, Jumaan AO, et al. Second varicella infections: are they more common than previously thought? Pediatrics 109:1068–1073, 2002.

59. Thomas SL, Wheeler JG, Hall AJ. Contacts with varicella or with children and protection against zoster in adults: a case-control study. Lancet 360:678–682, 2002.

60. Brisson M, Gay NJ, Edmunds WJ, Andrews NJ. Exposure to varicella boosts immunity to herpes-zoster: implications for mass vaccination against chickenpox. Vaccine 20:2500–2507, 2002.

61. Garnett GP, Grenfell BT. The epidemiology of varicella-zoster virus infections: the influence of varicella on the prevalence of herpes zoster. Epidemiol Infect 108:513–528, 1992.

62. Halloran ME. Epidemiologic effects of varicella vaccination. Infect Dis Clin North Am 3:631–655, 1996.

63. Edmunds WJ, Brisson M. The effect of vaccination on the epidemiology of varicella-zoster virus. J Infect 44:211–219, 2002.

64. Preziosi MP, Yam A, Wassilak SG, et al. Epidemiology of pertusis in a West African community before and after introduction of a widespread vaccination program. Am J Epidemiol 155:891–896, 2002.

65. Trollfors B, Taranger J, Lagergard T, et al. Immunization of children with pertussis toxoid decreases spread of pertussis within the family. Pediatr Infect Dis J 17:196–199, 1998.

66. Fine PEM. Epidemiological considerations for whooping cough eradication. *In* Wardlaw AL, Parton R (eds). Pathogenesis and Immunity to Pertussis. Chichester, UK, John Wiley & Sons, 1988, pp 451–467.

67. Fine PEM, Clarkson JA. The recurrence of whooping cough: possible implications for assessment of vaccine efficacy. Lancet 2:666–669, 1982.

68. Grenfell BT, Anderson RM. Pertussis in England and Wales: an investigation of transmission dynamics and control by mass vaccination. Proc R Soc Lond B Biol Sci 236:213–253, 1989.

69. Fine PEM, Clarkson JA. Reflections on the efficacy of pertussis vaccines. Rev Infect Dis 9:866–883, 1987.

70. Farrington CP. The measurement of age-specific vaccine efficacy. Int J Epidemiol 21:1014–1020, 1992.

71. Fine PEM. Implications of different study designs for the evaluation of acellular pertussis vaccines. Dev Biol Stand 89:123–133, 1997.

72. Brown F, Greco D, Mastrantonio P, et al (eds). Pertussis Vaccine Trials. Dev Biol Stand 89, 1997.

73. Cherry JD. The role of *Bordetella pertussis* infections in adults in the epidemiology of pertussis. Dev Biol Stand 89:181–186, 1997.

74. Fine PEM. Adult pertussis: a salesman's dream—and an epidemiologist's nightmare. Biologicals 25:195–198, 1997.

75. Edwards KM. Is pertussis a frequent cause of cough in adolescents and adults? Should routine pertussis immunization be recommended? Clin Infect Dis 32:1698–1699, 2001.

76. Miller LW, Older JJ, Drake J, et al. Diphtheria immunization: effect upon carriers and the control of outbreaks. Am J Dis Child 123:197–199, 1972.

77. Jones EE, Kim-Farley RG, Algunaid M, et al. Diphtheria: a possible foodborne outbreak in Hodeida, Yemen Arab Republic. Bull World Health Organ 63:287–293, 1985.

78. Marcuse EK, Grand MG. Epidemiology of diphtheria in San Antonio, Texas, 1970. JAMA 224:305–310, 1973.

79. Simonson O, Kjeldsen K, Bentzon MW, Heron I. Susceptibility to diphtheria in populations vaccinated before and after elimination of indigenous diphtheria in Denmark. Acta Pathol Microbiol Immunol Scand 95:225–231, 1987.

80. McQuillan GM, Kruszon-Moran D, Deforest A, et al. Serologic immunity to diphtheria and tetanus in the United States. Ann Intern Med 136:660–666, 2002.

81. Maple PA, Jones CS, Wall EC, et al. Immunity to diphtheria and tetanus in England and Wales. Vaccine 19:167–173, 2000.

82. Christenson B, Hellstrom U, Sylvan SP, et al. Impact of a vaccination campaign on adult immunity to diphtheria. Vaccine 19:1133–1140, 2000.

83. Chen RT, Broome CV, Weinstein RA, et al. Diphtheria in the United States, 1971–1981. Am J Public Health 75:1393–1397, 1985.

84. Doull JA, Lara H. The epidemiologic importance of diphtheria carriers. Am J Hyg 5:508–529, 1925.

85. Bergamini M, Fabrizi P, Pagani S, et al. Evidence of increased carriage of *Corynebacterium* spp. in healthy individuals with low antibody titres against diphtheria toxoid. Epidemiol Infect 125:105–112, 2000.

86. Newell KW, Duenas Lehman A, LeBlanc DR, et al. The use of toxoid for the prevention of tetanus neonatorum: final report of a double-blind controlled field trial. Bull World Health Organ 35:863–871, 1966.

87. Dagan R, Fraser D, Roitman M, et al. Effectiveness of a nationwide infant immunization program against *Haemophilus influenzae* b. Vaccine 17:134–141, 1998.

88. Peltola H, Aavitsland P, Hansen KG, et al. Perspective: a five-country analysis of the impact of four different *Haemophilus influenzae* type b conjugates and vaccination strategies in Scandinavia. J Infect Dis 179:223–229, 1999.

89. Van Alphen L, Spanjaard L, van der Ende A, et al. Effect of nationwide vaccination of 3-month-old infants in the Netherlands with conjugate *Haemophilus influenzae* type b vaccine: high efficacy and lack of herd immunity. J Pediatr 131:869–873, 1997.

90. Rushdy A, Ramsay M, Heath PT, et al. Infant Hib vaccination and herd immunity. J Pediatr 134:253–254, 1999.

91. Galil K, Singleton R, Levine OS, et al. Reemergence of invasive *Haemophilus influenzae* type b disease in a well-vaccinated population in remote Alaska. J Infect Dis 179:101–106, 1999.

92. Melnick JL. Advantages and disadvantages of killed and live poliomyelitis vaccines. Bull World Health Organ 56:21–38, 1978.

93. Fine PEM, Carneiro IAM. Transmissibility and persistence of oral polio vaccine viruses. Am J Epidemiol 150:1001–1021, 1999.

94. Nkowane BM, Wassilak SGF, Orenstein WA, et al. Vaccine-associated paralytic poliomyelitis, United States: 1973 through 1984. JAMA 257:1335–1340, 1987.

95. Bottiger M. A study of the sero-immunity that has protected the Swedish population against poliomyelitis for 25 years. Scand J Infect Dis 19:595–601, 1987.

96. Hovi T, Cantell K, Huovilainen A, et al. Outbreak of paralytic poliomyelitis in Finland: widespread circulation of antigenically altered poliovirus type 3 in a vaccinated population. Lancet 1:1427–1432, 1986.

97. Schaap GJ, Bijkerk H, Coutinho RA. The spread of wild polio virus in the well-vaccinated Netherlands in connection with the 1978 epidemic. Prog Med Virol 29:124–140, 1984.

98. Kew O, Morris-Glasgow V, Landaverde M, et al. Outbreak of poliomyelitis in Hispaniola associated with circulating type 1 vaccine-derived poliovirus. Science 296:356–359, 2002.

99. Centers for Disease Control and Prevention. Prevention and control of influenza: recommendations of the Advisory Committee on Immunization Practices (ACIP). MMWR 50(RR-4):1–34, 2001.

100. Monto AS, Davenport FM, Napier JA, et al. Modification of an outbreak of influenza in Tecumseh, Michigan by vaccination of schoolchildren. J Infect Dis 22:16–25, 1970.

101. Rudenko LG, Slepushkin AN, Monto AS, et al. Efficacy of live attenuated and inactivated influenza vaccines in schoolchildren and their unvaccinated contacts in Novgorod, Russia. J Infect Dis 168:881–887, 1993.

102. Reichert TA, Sugaya N, Fedson DS, et al. The Japanese experience with vaccinating schoolchildren against influenza. N Engl J Med 344:889–896, 2001.

103. Fine PEM. Immunities in and to tuberculosis: implications for pathogenesis and vaccination. *In* Porter JDH, McAdam KPWG (eds). Tuberculosis—Back to the Future. Chichester, UK, John Wiley & Sons, 1993, pp 53–72.

104. Fine PEM, Carneiro IAM, Milstein JB, Claments CJ. Issues Relating to the Use of BCG in Immunization Programmes (WHO/V&B/99.23). Geneva, World Health Organization, 1999.

105. Fine PEM. Variation in protection by BCG: implications of and for heterologous immunity. Lancet 346:1339–1345, 1995.

106. Fine PEM, Vynnycky E. The effect of heterologous immunity upon the apparent efficacy of (eg BCG) vaccines. Vaccine 16:1923–1928, 1998.

107. Halloran ME, Haber M, Longini IM, Struchiner CJ. Direct and indirect effects in vaccine efficacy and effectiveness. Am J Epidemiol 133:323–331, 1991.

108. Bjune G, Hoiby EA, Gronnesby JK, et al. Effects of outer membrane vesicle vaccine against group B meningococcal disease in Norway. Lancet 338:1093–1096, 1991.

109. Klock LE, Rachelefsky GS. Failure of rubella herd immunity during an epidemic. N Engl J Med 288:69–72, 1973.

110. Centers for Disease Control. Measles—United States, 1989 and first 20 weeks of 1990. MMWR 39:353–363, 1990.

111. Sosin DM, Cochi SL, Gunn RA, et al. Changing epidemiology of mumps on university campuses. Pediatrics 84:779–784, 1989.

112. Miller E, Vurdien JE, White JM. The epidemiology of pertussis in England and Wales. Commun Dis Rep 2:R152–R154, 1992.

113. Orenstein WA, Hinman AR. The immunization system in the United States—the role of school immunization laws. Vaccine 17(suppl):S19–S24, 1999.

Chapter 57

Economic Analyses of Vaccine Policies

MARK A. MILLER • ALAN R. HINMAN

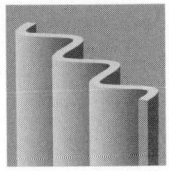

Vaccination programs have greatly reduced morbidity and mortality worldwide. Although the development and introduction of new vaccines and the improved use of existing vaccines offer the prospect of further reductions in disease burden, policy makers are often constrained by limited public health resources. As new vaccines and options become available, there is an increasing need to assess their value to optimize their use. Studies involving the integration of epidemiologic and economic data can be important in identifying the most judicious use of scarce public health resources to attain maximal health benefits.

A variety of quantitative techniques have been used to analyze policy decisions related to vaccine-preventable diseases. Economic studies using methods such as cost analysis (CA), cost-benefit analysis (CBA), cost-effectiveness analysis (CEA), or cost-utility analysis (CUA) provide estimations of potential financial requirements and program efficiencies for direct comparisons of vaccination options. A systematic assessment of various policy options allows one to make a decision based on a set of established criteria and provides accountability for the choices made.

The approaches used share the characteristics of explicit delineation of possible alternatives, estimation of probabilities or costs associated with each of the alternatives, and development of a summary statement of the implications of choosing a particular course of action. They also involve sensitivity analysis, in which estimated probabilities or costs are varied to determine how sensitive the conclusion is to particular variables. The summary statements are often couched in monetary and health outcome terms.

A CA is the basis of all economic studies, the quantification of costs associated with a given intervention. CBA is an extension of CA in that it further accounts for the monetary benefits from a policy or program. Benefits are usually calculated by the difference in the total cost of disease with and without an intervention program. The costs of the program include vaccines, vaccine administration, costs of dealing with adverse events, and other program costs such as public education. In a CBA, results are usually presented as ratios of the benefits from the intervention divided by the costs of conducting the program (B:C ratio). By convention, the ratio is divided out to give a single figure, representing the ratio of benefits to a cost of 1. If the B:C ratio is greater than 1, the intervention is considered to be cost-saving; 1 is called the break-even point at which costs and benefits are equal. Because of the difficulties in estimating specific economic values for averted mortality, CBA is difficult to perform. However, because it is able to give a summary statement about whether the benefits of a program exceed its costs, irrespective of the character of the outcomes, it is a useful approach to compare health programs with nonhealth programs. CEA and CUA are more useful for comparing different health programs.

In CEA, results are presented in terms of the cost required to achieve a particular health outcome (Table 57–1). Usually no attempt is made to assign an economic value to a prevented death. As a general benchmark, interventions are considered cost-effective by financial authorities if the cost per year of life saved is less than or equal to the per capita gross domestic product, which may range, on average, from $500 for low-income countries to greater than $30,000 for high-income countries. The relative cost-effectiveness of a death prevented may depend on the age of the individual and the consequent number of years of potential life (YPL) saved. For example, an intervention that prevented death at an early age would generally be considered cost-effective even if the cost per death prevented was several times higher than the per capita gross domestic product. By contrast, a public health intervention with the same level of cost per death prevented might not be considered cost-effective in an elderly person with fewer YPL saved. Ethical considerations are critical, because society must decide on the value of life-years saved at different ages or in different populations of wide economic means. CEA is particularly useful when there are a variety of options to achieve a common outcome (e.g., delivering a second dose of measles vaccine in a campaign or as part of

TABLE 57–1 ■ Disease Burden Measurements

Outcome Metric*	Definition
Cases	An outcome may be stated as the number of cases that occur or are prevented by an intervention. It may not necessarily account for the various severity states of sequelae. One could further stratify the total number of cases by minor illness, hospitalizations, and long-term sequelae.
Deaths	Death may be easily quantified but defies an economic valuation. For this reason, CEAs are frequently used in health outcome assessments with deaths (or some variation) in the denominator.
Years of potential life (YPL)	A refinement of the death metric by quantifying the total years of life lost or prevented from being lost. It integrates the difference in an expected life span of each individual and the age at which a death occurs. YPL may be adjusted by discount and age weights to account for societal preference of time and years of productivity; however, there are considerable ethical considerations in the choice of a weighting scheme.
Quality-adjusted life year (QALY) or disability-adjusted life year (DALY)	Further refinements of the YPL metric that integrate mortality and morbidity states. Various health metrics have been under development to help quantify disease burden states to compare disparate health outcomes. QALYs and DALYs integrate mortality, the YPL, and a valuation of the disability from morbidity. They are calculated by adjusting the YPL by the time spent with various disabilities. These units may be discounted and contain an age weighting factor. These metrics are derived by many subjective inputs and are not readily understood by most policy makers; however, they offer a common metric to compare many health outcomes.

*Any type of policy analysis requires a quantification of morbidity and mortality states. Although there is no universal consensus metric, attempts have been made to systematically quantify the many diverse possible health outcomes.

a routine schedule to prevent measles outbreaks). It is not useful when comparing investment in alternative health programs with disparate outcomes.

CUA is a specific form of CEA in which outcomes are reduced to a common denominator such as quality-adjusted life years (QALYs) or disability-adjusted life years (DALYs) (see Table 57–1).[1] This permits comparisons to be made between interventions with different health outcomes, such as acute illness and death versus prolonged disability. Although a common outcome metric is useful to make comparisons of many health interventions, there are numerous assumptions that underlie their construct, and therefore they are not always easily interpreted. It should be noted that a CBA is a special form of CUA where the common outcome metric is a monetary unit.

Important Considerations in Carrying Out a Quantitative Policy Analysis

There are many decisions to be made in designing a quantitative policy analysis. Widespread variability in choices of parameters or metrics has made it difficult to make comparisons among many of the published studies. This variability has been critiqued.[2] In the 1990s, a task force in the United States drew up suggested guidelines for carrying out cost-effectiveness studies of preventive services.[3] The journal *Vaccine* has published an editorial statement on the submission of economic evaluations of vaccines.[4]

Perspective

Those who benefit from immunizations include individuals, the health care system, and society at large. Analyses can be carried out from each of these perspectives.[5,6] Given that immunization programs are often supported by governments and benefits accrue not only to those who are vaccinated but also to those who are not vaccinated (from the reduced likelihood of exposure), it seems most appropriate to take a societal perspective. Although the societal perspective theoretically capture all costs and benefits, clearly costs and benefits of a vaccination program will accrue to different budget lines.

Time Frame

Vaccines often protect against risks that may not occur for some time in the future. Because the investment is made in a different time frame from the benefit, it often is necessary to discount future effects (both positive and negative) to take account of the implicit valuation that society has for health and financial costs and benefits over time. Even after accounting for inflation (which affects both costs and potential savings), there is an implicit difference in the value of an event that occurs today versus at a future time. For example, it is generally believed that a child's death prevented today is worth more than a child's death prevented 50 years from now. There is general agreement among economists to discount both costs and benefits at the same rate, typically from 3% to 10% per year. Study results are often presented both discounted and undiscounted.

Disease Burden

Estimates of disease burden may be derived from surveillance data (usually an underestimate), extrapolations from other representative populations, or results of mathematical modeling. Analyses may need to be specific for age group, population/occupational group, risk for disease (e.g., health care workers), and outcome (including the timing of the outcome, e.g., death in the next year versus death 50 years in the future).

Measure Used for Health States

An outcome may be stated as the number of cases or deaths that occur or are prevented by an intervention. YPL represents a refinement of the death metric that quantifies the total years of life lost or prevented from being lost. It integrates the difference in an expected life span of each individual and the age at which death occurs. QALYs, which measure the number of years of healthy life lived, or DALYs, the currently used World Health Organization (WHO) metric that measure the years of healthy life lost, are further refinements of the YPL that integrate a valuation of various morbid states. QALYs and DALYs are complementary concepts. Both metrics are derived from the product of the number of years lived and the quality of those years. QALYs use "utility" weights of health states; DALYs use "disability weights" to reflect the burden of the same states. Arneson and Nord provided an example: "[I]f the utility of deafness is 0.67, the disability weight of deafness is 1 − 0.67 = 0.33. Disregarding age weighting and discounting, and assuming life expectancy of 80 years, deafness at age 30 years represents $0.67 \times (80 - 30) = 33.4$ QALYs or $0.33 \times (80 - 30) + 30 = 17.6$ DALYs lost.[7] These metrics defy simplicity, are derived by many subjective inputs, and may not be readily understood by some policy makers; however, they offer a common metric to compare disparate health outcomes.

Economic Valuation of Health Outcome States

Direct and indirect costs and benefits are usually accounted. Direct costs include the costs of medical treatment and the costs of administering the vaccine, including screening criteria for target groups. Indirect costs include wages lost by those who are ill and their caregivers. Intangible costs, such as pain and suffering or death, are difficult to measure. However, they may be implicitly valued as the denominator of a CEA or CUA (e.g., as cost/death prevented), allowing the reader to infer his or her own value to the stated health outcome.

Vaccine Program Characteristics

These characteristics include vaccine efficacy (performance of the vaccine under ideal conditions), vaccine effectiveness in the field setting (accounting for operational constraints), coverage of the program, adverse effects of the vaccine (or program), and the potential for benefits to accrue to those who are not vaccinated because of the vaccination of others (herd immunity). A schematic model of a vaccine program is shown in Figure 57–1. For each component, there is an associated cost or benefit.

Sensitivity Analysis

One of the most powerful tools of quantitative policy analysis is that it provides the opportunity to estimate the likely effects of different probabilities of events (or different costs) from those postulated in the "base-case" analysis. This is particularly important when the true value of a parameter used in an analysis is not known and must be estimated. Testing a range of values for the uncertain assumption or assumptions can identify the factors to which the conclusion is most sensitive, which consequently can be used to focus a research agenda.

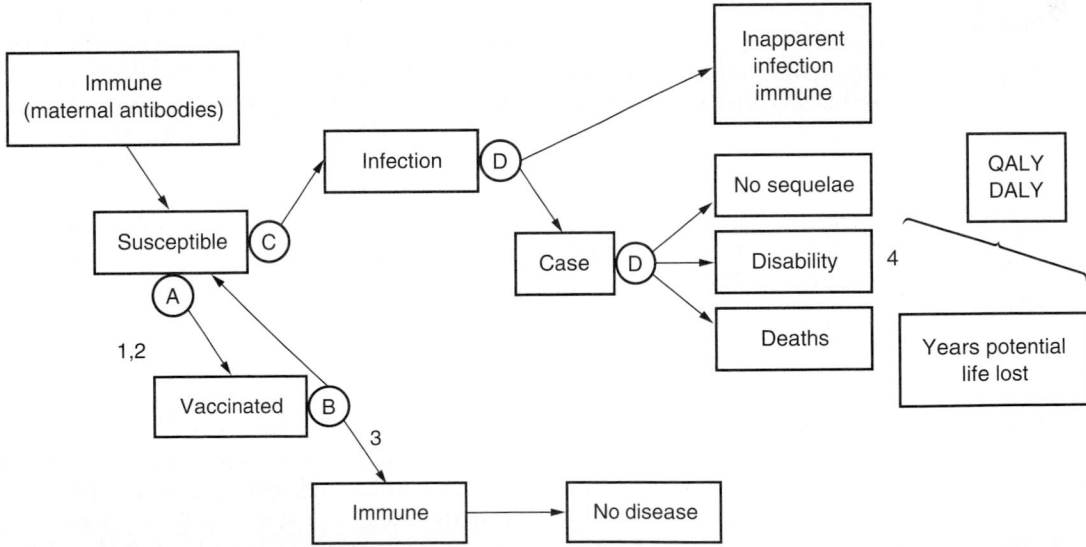

FIGURE 57–1 ■ Simplified schematic of compartmental model of infectious disease transmission with a vaccine prevention strategy. Each of the boxes represents a particular immunologic state of a vaccine-preventable disease. Assuming all persons are susceptible to infection after birth (post–maternal antibody protection), there are variable probabilities for passage into another immunologic state throughout the lifetime of an individual. These probabilities can be quantified to model the impact of a vaccination program on a birth cohort followed throughout life to quantify disease burden. A, vaccination coverage rate (age specific and by dose); B, vaccine efficacy by dose (effectiveness more relevant to account for herd effect); C, age-specific force of infection; D, probabilities of progression to each outcome state; 1, a screening program could be added here to help target vaccination efforts; 2, adverse event probabilities could be added here; 3, dose and possibly time dependent; 4, any number of mutually exclusive outcome states could be added here.

Examples of Uses of Quantitative Policy Analysis

In general, CBA, CEA, and CUA have shown that immunization is an excellent investment (highly cost-effective and often cost-saving) for vaccines that are currently recommended for universal use. Consideration of particular strategies in particular populations may show considerable variation, as demonstrated in Table 57–2. In recent years, with the advancement of computational capabilities, modeling software, the maturing of health economics applications to public sector health programs, and the expansion of the repertoire of new vaccines, the number of economic studies done to evaluate vaccines has greatly expanded. All could not be included here; however, synopses of results for many of the vaccines are provided in the text after Table 57–2. In reading the table, it should be kept in mind that the studies were carried out over a period of more than 25 years with varying assumptions and costs of vaccine, personnel, and medical care. Results are shown as presented in the report; no effort has been made to adjust expenditures or savings to present value. All results are presented in U.S. dollars unless otherwise specified and include both direct and indirect costs. A summary table of other cost-effectiveness studies of other health interventions is included as a reference (Table 57–3).[234,235]

In addition to the studies shown in Table 57–2, a number of decision analyses and risk-benefit analyses have also been carried out, looking at, for example, approaches to evaluation of rubella susceptibility in pregnant women,[236] or the likely outcome of different timing of administration of diphtheria, tetanus, and pertussis (DTP) vaccine.[237] These studies typically have not included economic valuations in outcomes and are not included in the table.

General Immunization

Most of these studies addressed immunization in developing countries. In recent years, there has been an expansion of analyses to evaluate vaccines for introduction in national Expanded Programmes on Immunisation (EPIs). They generally demonstrate low costs per immunized child and favorable benefit–cost ratios. Recent studies in Ethiopia, Morocco, Bangladesh, and Côte d'Ivoire indicated a total cost of less than $25 to fully immunize a child with basic EPI vaccines.[19,28]

Adenovirus

Although this vaccine was thought to be cost-effective for targeted use within the U.S. military, uncertain commitment to the manufacturer led them to cease production. The resultant cessation of vaccination led to a resurgence of adenovirus types 4 and 7 as important causes of illness in recruits.[238] Economic re-evaluations have reinforced its utility despite the increased funding that would be needed to resume production.

Acquired Immunodeficiency Syndrome

As the quest for a vaccine against human immunodeficiency virus/acquired immunodeficiency syndrome is pursued, there is increased attention to the potential cost-effectiveness and financing of vaccines relative to and in conjunction with other control measures.[239] Economic analyses and estimations of effectiveness through modeling efforts are crucial to help manufacturers and public health policy makers plan for market demand and potential production capacity early in the development cycle.

Bacille Calmette-Guérin

Bacille Calmette-Guérin (BCG) vaccine primarily prevents disseminated tuberculosis in infants and young children and has little, if any, impact on disease transmission. Development of highly cost-effective strategies based on case finding and treatment have made BCG vaccination less competitive as an effective intervention against tuberculosis.

Cholera

As in other enteric vaccines, the utility of vaccines against cholera competes with other interventions designed to prevent and ameliorate the effects of enteric diseases, particularly improved sanitation systems and the use of oral rehydration therapy, respectively. Economic studies have focused on the feasibility of the use of vaccine in high-risk populations, such as refugees.

Diphtheria, Tetanus, and Pertussis and Components

Cost–benefit analyses of pertussis vaccine use in the United States consistently showed an excess of benefits over costs, even in the face of a dramatically increasing cost of vaccine. Analyses of tetanus toxoid varied from administration of toxoid to women who were pregnant (or of child-bearing age), to mass immunization of the general population, to primary or booster vaccination of the elderly.

More recent studies have concentrated on the marginal improvement made on the pertussis component of combination vaccines. In many industrialized countries, acellular pertussis vaccines have replaced whole-cell vaccines, which were known to be the component of the combined vaccine most likely to be associated with adverse events. Although the efficacy of the newer vaccine is comparable, increased consumer confidence in safer vaccines increases the intangible valuation that consumers place on lower risk products. National programs have undertaken formal evaluations as they move to adopt the new technologies.[240] In addition, as DTP has become the platform for other combinations, numerous studies are now performed on the benefits and costs of the convenience of combinations with other antigens (hepatitis B, *Haemophilus influenzae* type b [Hib], and inactivated poliovirus vaccines [IPVs]).

Haemophilus influenzae type b

The original Hib vaccines represented purified capsular polysaccharides and were not very effective in infancy. Nonetheless, their use was shown to be economically justified.[39] These vaccines have been replaced by conjugated polysaccharide vaccines, which have had a remarkable impact on disease incidence in all countries that have introduced them into routine schedules. Their demonstrated utility in preventing overall severe acute respiratory infections (not usually confirmed bacteriologically) has led to greater support for use of these vaccines in developing countries. Because of vaccine cost, quantification of disease burden in economic terms may be necessary in middle- and low-income countries to demonstrate the utility of incorporation into routine schedules.[241]

Hepatitis A

Hepatitis A vaccines have been licensed recently but are not widely used in routine vaccination because of their cost and because hepatitis A is typically a mild infection of children in many countries. Analyses have been conducted in countries that can afford vaccine at current prices and commonly have compared routine vaccination of travelers to current practice of pre-exposure passive prophylaxis using immune serum globulin. Because of the relative costs of vaccine and screening tests, the screening protocols assessed in the analyses have been important determinants of the outcome, as has been the risk of infection in specific settings.[72] Hepatitis A vaccines have been recommended for universal use in children in high-risk geographic areas of the United States.[242] As the cost of vaccine decreases over time, there will likely be more studies assessing routine use of this vaccine.

Hepatitis B

Hepatitis B poses a particular issue in economic evaluation because the primary benefit of vaccination is preventing chronic liver disease or death from cirrhosis or cancer, which typically occur many years after the likely age at vaccination.

Hepatitis B vaccines were relatively expensive when first licensed, prompting many evaluations to identify their most efficient use. Table 57–2 presents studies broken into two categories: those that considered screening for immunity before vaccination and those that considered routine immunization without screening. Most early studies concentrated on subpopulations who were at greatest risk of infection, such as health care workers, injection drug users, and individuals at risk for sexually transmitted diseases. The relative costs of screening and vaccine and the specific prevalence of hepatitis B virus infection in the subpopulations studied were the most important determinants of outcomes. Early studies also addressed prenatal screening to identify the most efficient approaches for screening and for passive and active immunization. As the cost of vaccines decreased, studies began to address costs, benefits, and effectiveness of routine vaccination of various age cohorts (e.g., infants, adolescents). Because vaccination is most easily delivered through an existing infant vaccination infrastructure, universal infant vaccination with hepatitis B vaccine has become a common practice, and the WHO has recommended universal infant immunization against hepatitis B since 1992.[243] Many analyses have been conducted taking into account variations of vaccine price and prevalence of infection in different countries.[244] Analyses of hepatitis B are complicated by the need to incorporate multiple outcomes that may occur over prolonged periods.

Sometimes the most cost-effective intervention may not necessarily be the best choice to deal with a particular health problem. For example, if it dealt with only a part of the problem and a somewhat less cost-effective intervention dealt with the whole problem, the latter might be a better choice. Williams and colleagues found that the most cost-efficient use of hepatitis B vaccine in the United Kingdom would be to concentrate on high-risk populations.

However, that would have only a small impact on the overall hepatitis B disease burden compared with the impact of a more costly universal infant or adolescent immunization strategy.[84]

Influenza

In spite of the frequently changing antigenic structure of the influenza virus, studies have consistently shown that the benefits of annual influenza immunization of the elderly[245] and the chronically ill are greater than the costs. More recent pharmacoeconomic studies have supported the expansion of vaccination efforts to healthy working-age[246] populations and young children.[131,134,137] Economic studies are now evaluating the potential utility of cold-adapted live influenza vaccines for pediatric populations.

Measles, Mumps, and Rubella

Measles, mumps, and rubella vaccines as individual antigens have repeatedly been shown to be cost-saving when administered to young children. The ratio of benefits to costs rises even higher when the vaccines are administered in combination because the costs of administration are substantially lower. For measles vaccine, the B:C ratio for a single dose is high; it is of interest that the additional benefits derived from a second dose also outweigh the additional costs.

Pneumococcal Disease

As in influenza vaccination, the use of pneumococcal polysaccharide vaccine for the elderly and chronically ill has demonstrated a reasonable cost per QALY. With the advent of conjugate vaccines, more recent studies have concentrated on the cost-effectiveness of routine vaccination of pediatric populations.

Poliomyelitis

Polio is one of the few vaccines for which economic analyses have addressed global eradication. The two analyses that have been carried out indicate that the costs of eradication would be exceeded by the benefits within 12 to 15 years.[201,203] One of the great challenges will be how to account for the potential trend to continue vaccination if poliomyelitis is eradicated. Additionally, economic calculations have been made that address the costs and benefits of changing from live viral vaccines to IPV as natural disease is eliminated in populations.[204]

Varicella

As with other recently introduced vaccines, economic policies have been considered in the formulation of varicella vaccine policy. Although varicella vaccination has not been shown to be cost-saving when only direct medical costs are considered, it is clearly cost-saving when the indirect costs of lost income from caregivers are included in the analysis.

Other Vaccines

A number of studies have been conducted on hypothetical vaccines (e.g., schistosomiasis, malaria). These studies help highlight and quantify economic and epidemiologic assumptions regarding disease burden and the potential impact of vaccination. Vaccine characteristics such as cost

TABLE 57–2 ■ Cost–Benefit and Cost-Effectiveness Analyses of Vaccines

Reference	Type*	Location and Results[†]	Comment
GENERAL			
Barnum and Setiady[8] (1980)	CEA	Indonesia—cost/death prevented 1979–1984 by BCG & DTP $130; cost/death prevented by BCG-only program $455, by DTP-only program $135	Considered only direct costs
Creese and Henderson[9] (1980)	CEA	Indonesia, Philippines, Thailand—BCG & DTP costs/fully immunized infant $2.86, $4.97, & $10.73, respectively	Considered only direct costs
Phonboon et al.[10] (1989)	CEA	Thailand—DTP/BCG/OPV/measles average direct cost/fully immunized child $13.80 in hospitals, $11.80 in health centers; for fully immunized pregnant women (tetanus) $8.90 & $10.30, respectively	Also considered differential costs of fixed & outreach services
Shepard, et al.[11] (1989)	CEA	Ecuador—cost/fully immunized child $4.39 for routine services & $8.60 for mass vaccination campaign	Although campaign was less cost-effective, it significantly increased coverage of children missed by routine services
Bjerregaard[12] (1990)	CBA	Kenya—cost/fully EPI immunized child $12.39; cost/death prevented ~$150	Used WHO EPICost software
Musgrove[13] (1992)	CBA	Americas—pneumonia, meningococcus type B, & typhoid vaccines would be economically justified if cost/vaccination (for 1 antigen) was $0.52–$0.58 & benefits/disease prevented were $1000–2000	Considered only direct costs; 10% discount rate
Behrens and Roberts[14] (1994)	CBA	UK—B:C ratio 0.17, 0.06, and 0.06, respectively, for hepatitis A passive, hepatitis A active, and typhoid immunization of travelers	Results dependent on frequency of travel to endemic areas
Brenzel and Claquin[15] (1994)	CEA	Global—reviewed 30 studies; average cost to fully immunize a child $22, ranging from $8 (Tanzania, fixed site) to $33 (Cameroon, national campaigns)	All costs adjusted to 1992 dollars (equivalents)
Hadler[16] (1994)	CBA	US—significant cost savings ($90–$150 million/yr) would accrue from use of combination DTP-Hib or DTP-Hib-HepB	Based on Hatziandreu et al.'s studies
Shepard et al.[17] (1995)	CUA	Global—rated cost/QALY of 13 candidate vaccines/vaccine strategies; range from $5 (measles vaccination <6 mo of age) to $113,208 (acellular pertussis vaccine)	Projected likely research & development costs of new vaccines; 3% discount rate
Schlumberger et al.[18] (1999)	CA	Senegal—A single-delivery jet-injector device was found to cost $0.21/dose more than traditional needle/syringe, which has a hidden estimated cost of $0.55 as a result of cross-contamination	
Edmunds et al.[19] (2000)	CA	Ethiopia—method to estimate the cost of adding new antigens to the EPI	
Miller and McCann[20]	CEA	Global—country-specific analysis for vaccination against hepatitis B, Hib, *Streptococcus pneumoniae*, and rotavirus. The global cost/life-year saved ranged from $29 to $150, with great variation by income and economic groups.	Costs of vaccine were based on relative wealth of individual countries
ADENOVIRUS			
Collis et al.[21] (1973)	CBA	US—B:C ratio 1.6 from using adenovirus vaccine types 4 and 7 in military recruits to prevent acute respiratory disease	Study included vaccine research and development costs
Hyer et al.[22] (2000)	CBA	US—year-round or seasonal vaccination of military personnel both was cost-saving and averted significant morbidity	Program estimated restart-up costs of commercial production

TABLE 57–2 ■ Cost–Benefit and Cost-Effectiveness Analyses of Vaccines—cont'd

Reference	Type*	Location and Results†	Comment
AIDS			
Cowley[23] (1993)	CBA	Ivory Coast—modeled range of break-even costs for a hypothetical vaccine; cost of each case of AIDS $1500 (direct), $20,079 (total cost) per HIV infection	Wide range of assumptions for prevalence and vaccine efficacy
BCG			
Nettleman[24] (1993)	CBA	US—vaccinating persons attending homeless shelters would be cost-saving if vaccine were 40% effective	5% discount rate; vaccine cost $10
Trnka et al.[25] (1993)	CBA	Czech Republic—vaccine discontinuation in study region has B:C ratio of 1 as a result of reduction in infection incidence in 0- to 6-year-olds to less than 0.1%	Observed 80% vaccine efficacy
Nettleman et al.[26] (1997)	CEA	US—compared CEA of periodic (every 6 mo or annual) PPD testing of physicians followed by INH prophylaxis to converters vs. hypothetical vaccine with 50% effectiveness and $10 cost; vaccine dominated: cost less and prevented more cases and deaths	Estimated 0.4% skin test conversion/yr; no discounting in life-years saved
Pathania et al.[27] (1999)	CBA	Czech Republic—revaccination of persons with a negative tuberculin skin test was not considered cost-beneficial	
Rahman et al.[28] (2001)	CEA	Japan—reconsideration of universal vaccination with BCG at the current low incidence of tuberculosis would require between 2125 and 10,399 immunizations at a cost of $35,950–$175, 862 to prevent each case of childhood tuberculosis	Vaccine efficacy modeled at 40%–80%
CHOLERA			
MacPherson and Tonkin[29] (1992)	CEA	Canada—routine vaccination against cholera for travelers to endemic areas would not be cost-effective; >CAN$28 million/case prevented	Vaccine cost CAN$28.67/dose; persons traveling to regions with high transmission rates should be considered for vaccination
Cookson et al.[30] (1997)	CBA	Argentina—assuming 75% coverage and 75% efficacy, the break-even cost of vaccine would be $1.81/dose	5% discount rate
Naficy et al.[31] (1998)		Malawi—model based on hypothetical refugee camp; strategies combining vaccination and pre-emptive therapy become more cost-effective than therapy alone if the cost of vaccine falls below $0.22/dose	
Legros et al.[32] (1999)	CA	Uganda—vaccine administrative cost in stable refugee settings was $0.23/dose	No cost assumed for vaccine
Naficy et al.[33] (2001)	CA	Viet Nam—immunization campaign was $0.44/dose administered, including vaccine, and $0.91/fully immunized person	Vaccine cost $0.31/dose
DIPHTHERIA-TETANUS-PERTUSSIS			
Hatziandreu et al.[34] (1994)	CBA	US—B:C ratio 6.2 for direct costs, 30.1 for total costs	Reductions in diphtheria and pertussis contributed nearly equally to direct savings; diphtheria was major contributor to indirect savings
PERTUSSIS			
Koplan et al.[35] (1979)	CBA	US—B:C ratio 2.6 (direct costs only)	5% discount rate
Hinman and Koplan[36] (1984)	CBA	US—B:C ratio 11.1 (direct costs only)	5% discount rate
Hinman and Koplan[37] (1985)	CBA	US—B:C ratio 3.1 (direct costs only)	5% discount rate; recalculation following 90-fold increase in vaccine costs and newer estimates of serious adverse events; base case used

Continued

TABLE 57–2 ■ Cost–Benefit and Cost-Effectiveness Analyses of Vaccines—cont'd

Reference	Type*	Location and Results†	Comment
Tormans et al.[38] (1998)	CBA	Germany—vaccination with acellular pertussis vaccine rapidly becomes as cost-saving as vaccination with whole-cell vaccine as soon as vaccination coverage can be raised from 45% to 52.5% with acellular vaccine	Acellular vaccination is also the superior alternative when considering indirect cost savings resulting from reduction in work-loss caused by adverse events
Beutels et al.[39] (1999)	CBA	Italy—increase in coverage with acellular pertussis to 90% would yield direct net savings of $42 per extra vaccinee in comparison to a situation of 50% coverage	
Ekwueme et al.[40] (2000)	CBA	US—B:C ratios for acellular pertussis vaccine from a societal and health care system perspective were 27:1 and 9:1, respectively, but marginally more expensive than whole-cell vaccine	Additional benefit of acellular vaccine is increased consumer confidence
Iskedjian et al.[41] (2001)	CEA	Canada—replacement of whole-cell with acellular pertussis would prevent 1116 cases of pertussis each year for each 100,000 children and would provide a net savings	
TETANUS			
Berggren[42] (1974)	CBA	Haiti—B:C ratio 9 for community-wide tetanus immunization (infants → adults)	Considered only direct hospital care costs; primary impact was in reduction of neonatal tetanus
Hutchison and Stoddart[43] (1988)	CEA	Canada—Primary immunization of elderly would cost $1.9 million/case prevented, $7.1 million/death prevented, $810 thousand/life-year gained	5% discount rate
Carducci et al.[44] (1989)	CBA	Italy—benefits of mass immunization of population >10 yr would exceed costs after 1 yr; gradual immunization also would exceed costs after 1 yr but would only reach total benefit of mass campaign after 9 yr	Considered only direct costs
Berman et al.[45] (1991)	CEA	Indonesia—compared routine TT administration to pregnant women with "crash" TT to all women 10–45 yr; cost/woman immunized was comparable but cost/death averted was higher through "crash" program	
Balestra and Littenberg[46] (1993)	CEA	US—cost/year of life saved by decennial TT booster $143,138 compared to $4527 for single booster at age 65	However, decennial booster prevented 4 times as many cases as single booster
HAEMOPHILUS INFLUENZAE TYPE B			
Cochi et al.[47] (1985)	CEA	US—routine use of polysaccharide vaccine would produce a net savings; two-dose vaccination beginning at 18 mo was most cost-effective for this vaccine	Study preceded current conjugate vaccines; projected vaccine cost $3/dose
Hay and Daum[48] (1987)	CBA, CEA	US—routine use of polysaccharide vaccine would produce a net savings as compared to rifampin prophylaxis of appropriate contacts	Study preceded current conjugate vaccines; vaccine cost $8.13/dose
Hay and Daum[49] (1990)	CBA	US—vaccination with a single dose at 18 mo would have a B:C ratio 4.0 and would be cost-beneficial to a vaccine efficacy of 22.7%; single dose estimated to prevent 11% of total cases	3% discount rate; assumed 81% vaccine efficacy; vaccine cost $14/dose
Martens et al.[50] (1991)	CBA	Netherlands—break-even cost of vaccine would be $7 if administered with DPT-polio vaccines	
Ginsberg et al.[51] (1993)	CBA	Israel—a four-dose program would have B:C ratio of 0.3 for health services only; with chronic sequelae 1.3; with indirect costs and deaths valued 1.5; break-even vaccine costs are $2.24 when health service benefits only are considered and $11.21 when all benefits are included	Vaccine cost $7.74/dose

TABLE 57–2 ■ Cost–Benefit and Cost-Effectiveness Analyses of Vaccines—cont'd

Reference	Type*	Location and Results†	Comment
Levine et al.[52] (1993)	CBA, CEA	Chile—B:C ratio 1.7; value of death prevented not included	Vaccine cost $1 for a three-dose regimen
Harris et al.[53] (1994)	CEA, CUA	Australia—cost/year of life saved by three-dose conjugate vaccine AUS$3148; cost/QALY AUS$1965; incremental analysis compared to single dose of conjugate vaccine at 18 mo AUS$5047/QALY saved; for Aboriginal subpopulation, proposed vaccination program would be cost-saving	Incidence 53/100,000 and 460/100,000 among non- and Aboriginal populations, respectively; 5% discount rate; vaccine cost AUS$20/dose
McIntyre et al.[54] (1994)	CEA, CUA	Australia—cost/QALY AUS$1231–$9136 based on various dosing schedules	Based on disease incidence in non-Aboriginal children; vaccine cost AUS$15/dose
Trolfors[55] (1994)	CBA	Sweden—B:C ratio 1.2 (direct and indirect costs); 1.6 if valuation of deaths included	Vaccine cost 125 SEK/dose
Asensi et al.[56] (1995)	CBA	Spain—B:C ratio 2.4–5.1 depending on public or private purchase of vaccine	Includes valuation of deaths; vaccine cost 3000 or 1800 pesetas/dose for private and public sectors, respectively
Hatziandreu and Brown[57] (1995)	CBA	US—B:C ratio 1.3–3.3 (direct costs), 2.2–5.1 (direct and indirect) for base case; B:C ratio of combined DTP-Hib vs. Hib alone 2.6 (direct), 4.0 (direct and indirect)	Vaccine cost $10.25/dose; combined products reduce overall costs of administering vaccines and are therefore more cost-beneficial
Hussey et al.[58] (1995)	CBA	South Africa—vaccination in Cape Town would have B:C ratio of 1.3–1.4	Direct and indirect costs assumed; based on vaccine price of $58 for three doses
Midani et al.[59] (1995)	CA	US—cost of disease decreased from $27.5 to $0.9 million/yr (97%) after vaccine introduction in Florida	
HEPATITIS A			
Hinds et al.[60] (1985)	CBA	US—B:C ratio 2.5 from conducting active vs. passive surveillance for hepatitis A with subsequent administration of immune globulin to contacts	Study preceded licensure of current hepatitis A vaccines
Tormans et al.[61] (1992)	CEA	Belgium—passive immunization most cost-effective for travel to endemic areas <6 mo and <2 times in a 10-yr period; results are sensitive to incidence, behavioral, and vaccine characteristics	Travelers from Europe to high-endemicity countries; vaccine cost (including administration) $40 and $24 for active and passive immunization, respectively
Bryan and Nelson[62] (1994)	CEA	US—passive immunization for postexposure prophylaxis or preexposure periods of <6 mo is much less expensive than active immunization	Assumed hepatitis A vaccines to be priced at $10–$25/dose
Jefferson et al.[63] (1994)	CEA, CBA	UK—for British Army, active immunization is more cost-effective (£52,865 UK/case prevented) than passive immunization (£97,305 UK/case prevented)	Study only assumed a 5-y, four-exposure scenario; vaccine cost £11.7 UK/dose
Jefferson et al.[64] (1994)	CBA	UK—active vaccination of troops vs. passive immunization for a single deployment is not cost-beneficial, B:C ratio 0.01–0.03	Vaccine cost $22.26/dose, immune serum globulin cost $6/dose
Van Doorslaer et al.[65] (1994)	CEA	Belgium—passive immunization is most cost-effective for infrequent travelers (£7000–£9000 UK/infection prevented); active immunization becomes more cost-effective than passive for travel exceeding 3 times in 10 yr or for trips >6 mo duration (£3500–£7500 UK/prevented infection)	5% discount rate; vaccine cost £15–£22.5 UK/dose; immune serum globulin cost £7 UK/dose
Zuckerman and Powell[66] (1994)	CEA	UK—screening prior to active immunization is cost-effective for travelers 40+ yr of age	Based on antibody prevalence in travelers attending London travel clinics
Li et al.[67] (1998)	CEA	China—average cost/QALY gained for general population 11 times per-capita GNP	
Chen et al.[68] (1999)	CBA	China—B:C ratio 2.53 in Jiangxing City of Zhejiang Province with a HepA-specific incidence rate of 41.15/10,000	Incidence rate of HepA was 16.26/10,000 at balance point of cost–benefit of HepA vaccine

Continued

TABLE 57–2 ▪ Cost–Benefit and Cost-Effectiveness Analyses of Vaccines—cont'd

Reference	Type*	Location and Results†	Comment
Saab et al.[69] (2000)	CA	US—compared relative cost of mass vaccination *vs.* serologic testing followed by vaccination of susceptibles; mass vaccination preferred except in groups with ≥50% immunity (e.g., those ≥50 or injection drug users	Assumed test cost $34 and vaccination series cost $68
Chodick et al.[70] (2001)	CBA	Israel—B:C 1.50 for vaccination of serologically proven nonimmune day care and kindergarten workers; B:C 0.04 for mass vaccination of these workers	5% discount rate

HEPATITIS B			
Prevaccination Screening			
Corrao et al.[71] (1987)	CEA	Italy—sequential testing of a single serum specimen for anti-HBc, anti-HBs, and HBsAg prior to vaccination was most cost-effective of five possible screening protocols	Results particular to screening test and vaccine price at that time
Hankins et al.[72] (1987)	CEA	US—screening paramedics for anti-HBs and HBsAg with subsequent prophylactic vaccination was not cost-effective compared to administering vaccine to all paramedics when expected prevalence is <2%	
Jacobson et al.[73] (1987)	CBA, CEA	US—prevaccination screening of dental workers, B:C ratio 2.7	Screening only faculty with patient contact was most cost-effective
Arevalo and Washington[74] (1988)	CEA	US—routine serologic screening of pregnant women with subsequent immunization of infants of carrier mothers is cost-saving at a prevalence of 0.06%	4% and 6% discount rates; vaccine cost $50 for three doses
Tong et al.[75] (1988)	CA	US—comparison between screening protocols; HBc should be used for screening health care workers in hospitals with high prevalence	Prediction of high or low hepatitis B carriage rate may be based on the distribution of staff ethnicity
Thomas[76] (1990)	CEA	Australia—universal screening of public antenatal patients cost AUS$354/carrier identified	Sensitive to carrier prevalence
Audet et al.[77] (1991)	CEA	Canada—universal screening of pregnant women with subsequent immunization of infants of carrier mothers would cost CAN$8915/prevented carrier	Costs/carrier prevented varied by ethnic origin from $540 (Asian) to $126,279 (Canadian)
Schoub et al.[78] (1991)	CEA	South Africa—prevaccination screening would be cost-beneficial in black nursing and laboratory personnel, but not their white counterparts	Seroprevalence 36%–68% and 3%–15% in black and white populations, respectively
Tormans et al.[79] (1993)	CEA	Belgium—screening pregnant women would cost BEF 583,581/life-year saved	Carrier prevalence of 0.67% in this population; vaccine cost BEF 1246/dose
Kwan-Gett et al.[80] (1994)	CEA	US—vaccinating preadolescents without screening is more cost-effective than prevaccination screening in routine vaccination programs	
Yuan and Robinson[81] (1994)	CBA	Canada—combined HBV marker seroprevalence of at least 30%–64% is required to justify screening prior to routinely vaccinating specific subpopulations	Vaccine cost CAN$20/dose
Ferraz et al.[82] (1995)	CEA	Brazil—Prevaccination screening of health care workers is more cost-effective at a seroprevalence greater than 11%; low-dose intradermal vaccination is more cost-effective than intramuscular injection	Vaccine cost $45.39 for three doses
Williams et al.[83] (1996)	CEA	UK—antenatal screening and vaccination is most effective strategy; screening before vaccination is cost-effective for homosexually active persons but not for general population	Based on mathematical modeling of transmission dynamics
Fabrizi et al.[84] (1996)	CEA	Italy—after the initial cost of vaccination, a savings of $3272/yr was realized by the elimination of frequent serologic screening of vaccine responders	45% prevalence in hemodialysis unit prior to institution of vaccination program

TABLE 57–2 ■ Cost–Benefit and Cost-Effectiveness Analyses of Vaccines—cont'd

Reference	Type*	Location and Results†	Comment
Vaccination			
Mulley et al.[85] (1982)	CBA	US—routine vaccination would be cost-saving for populations with attack rates as low as 1%–2% when indirect costs included	Based on costs from the early 1980s
Adler et al.[86] (1983)	CBA	UK—net savings would be realized for a screening and vaccination program yielding a B:C ratio of 1.5–7.4 for the homosexually active population	Only acute costs were considered
Alter et al.[87] (1983)	CBA	US—routine vaccination of patients and staff of hemodialysis units would be cost-saving compared to routine screening	Confirmed in the setting of reduced incidence in this population
Hamilton[88] (1983)	CBA	US—vaccination of health care workers would have cumulative B:C ratio of 1.2 over 10 yr	5% discount rate; vaccine cost $100 for three doses
Kirkman-Liff and Dandoy[89] (1984)	CA	US—cost exposure in health care workers $109; $13,376/case	From hospital perspective
Lahaye et al.[90] (1987)	CBA	Belgium—vaccination of health care workers is cost-saving	Not all future benefits included in analysis
Hicks et al.[91] (1989)	CBA	US—average cost per case of HBV infection is $1990; vaccination of pediatric nurses would not be cost-effective at presumed attack rate of 1% and vaccine series price of $103	Vaccination would be cost-effective if attack rate were 2% of identified subpopulation or if vaccine series price were reduced from $103 to $27
Margolis et al.[92] (1990)	CA	US—acute hepatitis $4855/case; acute fulminant hepatitis $7000–$8549/case; chronic hepatitis $2905–$7592/case	Study includes various costs (direct and indirect) for wide range of acute and chronic hepatitis B sequelae
Barboza et al.[93] (1991)	CBA	Venezuela—cost/infection $1759; selective vaccination of hospital workers would be cost-saving	
Hatziandreu et al.[94] (1991)	CEA	Greece—cost/case averted $970–$7800 (with vaccine price $40/dose and incidence of 0.3%–2%); cost-saving at $8/dose or 11% annual incidence	Plasma-derived HepB vaccines from two manufacturers produced comparable results
Hayashi et al.[95] (1991)	CEA	Japan—lower dose intradermal injection was more cost-effective at eliciting antibody response than subcutaneous administration in a mentally handicapped population	Antibody titers were different between the study groups
Jönsson et al.[96] (1991)	CBA	Spain—determined the threshold of attack rate in the target population to achieve cost savings with routine HepB vaccination; at a 5% attack rate, direct costs would be recouped; 1% for recoupment of direct and indirect costs	Target populations included health care workers, high-risk patients, and intimate contacts of these individuals
Leonard et al.[97] (1991)	CEA	US—for screening and vaccination program in a mental health institution with 3-yr transmission rate of 27%, the cost/case prevented was $300; cost/death prevented $12,100	Highly variable results depending on transmission rate
Mauskopf et al.[98] (1991)	CBA	US—a vaccine program for all workers with more than 11 exposures per year would have B:C ratio of 2.1; if pain and suffering valued, B:C ratio would be 11.2	Assumes prescreening and vaccine costs of $133
Antoñanzas et al.[99] (1992)	CEA	Spain—cost-effectiveness of alternative strategies compared to current screening of pregnant women with subsequent infant immunization; cost/case prevented for those living with carriers 115,000–310,000 pesetas; routine vaccination of pubescent youth 30,000–130,000 pesetas; newborns 400,000 pesetas; and accidental exposure 500,000 pesetas	Used 4% and 7% discount rates
Demicheli and Jefferson[100] (1992)	CBA	Italy—routine infant vaccination is not cost-beneficial given declining incidence	Based on peak incidence of 6/100,000; 8% discount rate
Ginsberg et al.[101] (1992)	CBA	Israel—neonatal vaccination program would have B:C ratios of 1.6 (direct costs only) and 2.8 (direct and indirect costs)	7.5% discount rate; cost per pediatric dose $2.30

Continued

TABLE 57–2 ■ Cost–Benefit and Cost-Effectiveness Analyses of Vaccines—cont'd

Reference	Type*	Location and Results†	Comment
Ginsberg and Shouval[102] (1992)	CBA	Israel—vaccination program targeting all persons <16 yr would have B:C ratios of 1.9 (direct costs only) and 2.8 (direct and indirect costs)	7.5% discount rate; cost per pediatric dose $2.19
Bloom et al.[103] (1993)	CEA	US—screening newborns in combination with routine administration to 10-yr-old children is the most cost-effective strategy, $375 and $3695 (undiscounted, discounted) per life-year saved; vaccination (with or without screening) is a dominant strategy in adult high-risk populations	5% discount rate; vaccine costs $225 and $160 for adults and newborns, respectively (including administration fees)
Hall et al.[104] (1993)	CEA	The Gambia—cost to avert a death from liver cancer $150–$200 (undiscounted); $1200–$1500 (discounted)	6% discount rate; vaccine cost $1/dose
Krahn and Detsky[105] (1993)	CEA	Canada—cost-effectiveness of universal infant vaccination is CAN$30,347/life-year; break-even vaccine price is $7/dose	
Oddone et al.[106] (1993)	CEA	US—cost/case prevented $25,313 and $31,111 for predialysis and dialysis patients, respectively, because of lower immunogenicity among dialysis patients and low incidence (0.6%); break-even incidence 38%	5% discount rate; vaccine cost $152 for three doses plus booster dose
Zhuang and Xu[107] (1993)	CEA	China—vaccinating neonates and infants (ages 0–3 yr) is most cost-effective, followed by vaccinating adults >25 yr of age	
Aggarwal and Naik[108] (1994)	CEA	India—cost/carrier prevented of universal vaccination and prenatal screening with vaccination $126 and $495, respectively, compared to no program	Vaccine cost $1/dose; study did not account for any treatment savings
Bergus and Meis[109] (1995)	CEA	US—routine immunization program in Iowa would cost $2970 (undiscounted) and $41,906 (discounted)/life-year saved	5% discount rate; vaccine costs $26.25 and $86.40 for infant and adolescent series, respectively
Guillén Grima and Espín Rios[110] (1995)	CEA	Spain—cost/case prevented is 118,990, 64,476, and 82,840 pesetas, respectively, for universal vaccination of newborns and preadolescents and universal vaccination of newborns with catch-up vaccination	
Kerleau et al.[111] (1995)	CEA	France—cost of vaccinating young male adults is 36,000 F/case prevented; vaccination may be considered cost-beneficial for high-risk exposure groups with attack rates approximating those of homosexually active men or greater than those observed in injection drug users	
Liu et al.[112] (1995)	CBA	China—B:C ratio 42.4–48.0 from routine infant immunization in Jinan City	
Mangtani et al.[113] (1995)	CEA	UK—compared with no vaccination, cost/life-year saved for vaccination of infants, preadolescent children, and high-risk populations £2568, £2824, and £8564 UK (undiscounted), respectively	6% discount rate; vaccine costs £22.08 UK/child, £29.46 UK/adult for three doses
Margolis et al.[114] (1995)	CEA	US—cost/life-year saved (undiscounted) $164, $1522, and $3730 for perinatal HBV infection prevention, infant vaccination, and adolescent vaccination, respectively	Assumed 4.8% lifetime risk; vaccine price $20.01/infant, $40.02/adolescents for three doses
Van Damme et al.[115] (1995)	CEA	Europe—cost/infection prevented £6443 and £4745 UK for routine neonate and adolescent vaccination, respectively	5% discount rate; vaccine cost £7.50 UK/dose; administration cost £5 UK
Fenn et al.[116] (1996)	CEA	UK—cost/life-year gained 188,015–301, 365 UK (discounted) or £5234–£13, 034 UK (undiscounted)	6% discount rate; vaccine cost £8.66 UK, administration cost £10.63 UK
Wiebe et al.[117] (1997)	CEA	Canada—cost/life-year saved CAN$15, 900 and CAN$97,600 for universal infant and adolescent vaccination, respectively	5% discount rate; total vaccination costs are CAN$38.08 and CAN$55.31 for infants and 12-yr-olds, respectively

TABLE 57–2 ■ Cost–Benefit and Cost-Effectiveness Analyses of Vaccines—cont'd

Reference	Type*	Location and Results†	Comment
Li et al.[67] (1998)	CEA	China—routine vaccination would not be cost-effective at >153,000 Yuan/QALY, 11 times average GNP	
Zurn and Danthine[118] (1998)	CEA	Switzerland—costs/year of life saved for universal vaccination ranged from 8820 CHF (infant strategy) to 12,380 CHF (schoolchildren strategy); B:C ratio ranged from 1.2 (systematic prenatal screening and vaccination of newborns at risk) to 2.9 (vaccination of infants)	
Edmunds et al.[19] (2000)	CA	Ethiopia—compared costs of using combined DTP/HepB *vs.* separate vaccines; combined vaccine would have to cost <$0.64–$0.77/dose to be more cost-effective than giving vaccines separately	Estimated $0.94/dose HepB administered. Estimated cost/fully immunized child (without HepB) $7.84
Harbarth et al.[119] (2000)	CA	Germany—average cost of acute HBV infections were 10,018 DM for acute episode and 4860 DM/yr for chronic infection; total national cost >1.2 billion DM	Included both direct and indirect costs
Deuson et al.[120] (2001)	CEA	US—targeted vaccination for Asian-Americans; costs per child, per dose, and per completed series were $64, $119, and $537, respectively; discounted cost/ discounted year of life saved was $11,525	
Harris et al.[121] (2001)	CEA	Australia—incremental cost/life-year gained was $11,862, which is low compared with many other health care interventions	With no discounting of costs or consequences, universal vaccination with the combination vaccine predicted to save lives and reduce costs
INFLUENZA/PNEUMOCOCCAL DISEASE			
Rose et al.[122] (1993)	CEA	US—cost/year of life saved for HIV-infected patients with CD4 counts >500, 200–500, and <200 cells/mm³ for pneumococcal vaccine cost-saving, cost-saving, and $105,588, respectively; for influenza vaccine $101,201, $110,674, and $105,588, respectively	5% discount rate
INFLUENZA			
Kavet[123,124] (1972 and 1977)	CBA	US—annual immunization of high-risk population cost-beneficial except in years with little influenza activity, which cannot be predicted	Model examined experience of 1960s, with five moderate epidemics, two large epidemics, and 3 yr of little influenza activity
Klarman and Guzick[125] (1976)	CEA	US—cost/year of life gained for persons >65 is $700 if vaccine is 50% effective, $410 if vaccine is 70% effective	Estimates based on "composite" year in 1960s, taking into account cyclic nature of influenza and possibility of antigenic shift; generally followed Kavet's model
Schoenbaum et al.[126] (1976)	CBA, CEA	US—swine influenza immunization would be cost-beneficial if program restricted to those >25 yr of age and acceptance rates exceed 59%; cost/year of life saved ranged from $1000 to $13,200 in public sector and from $2400 to $12,600 in private sector for different population groups at acceptance rates of 20% and 100%	Assumed 10% probability of pandemic influenza and 6% discount rate; included both direct and indirect costs
Elo[127] (1979)	CBA	Finland—B:C ratios 0.9–1.8, 1.0–1.9, and 0.6–1.2, respectively, for vaccinating employed labor, health personnel, and medical risk groups with inactivated vaccine (range is for 30%–60% vaccine efficacy)	Also considered other strategies, including attenuated vaccine and drug prevention with amantidine
OTA[128] (1981) and Riddiough et al.[129] (1983)	CEA	US—vaccination for all persons 65+ yr of age is cost-saving; cost/year of healthy life gained for those 65+ is $1782	Also considered high-risk and non–high-risk persons of other age groups

Continued

TABLE 57–2 ▪ Cost–Benefit and Cost-Effectiveness Analyses of Vaccines—cont'd

Reference	Type*	Location and Results†	Comment
Patriarca et al.[130] (1987)	CEA	US—examined four strategies of vaccination/amantadine for prevention/control of influenza A in nursing homes; vaccination alone would be most cost-effective ($62/death averted) but also would allow higher rates of morbidity and mortality than other alternatives	Included only direct costs; giving amantadine continuously would result in least morbidity/mortality but would be most expensive ($786/death prevented)
Schoenbaum[131] (1987)	CBA	US—took individual's perspective and calculated that immunization in the fall of any given year would have B:C ratio >1 to the general population if it cost <$10 (<$45 for high-risk individuals)	In the face of an epidemic, benefits rise
Maucher and Gambert[132] (1990)	CBA	US—immunization of elderly would be cost-beneficial at vaccination cost (including vaccine and administration) as high as $61.46/person if infection rate was 10% and 30% of those ill required medical attention	Also examined break-even point if complications could be treated on ambulatory basis ($4.78/vaccination if infection rate was 10%)
Yassi, et al.[133] (1991)	CBA	Canada—B:C ratio 2.9 for immunization of hospital employees (direct costs)	B:C ratio derived from data presented; net benefit of $39.23/vaccinated employee
CDC [6] (1993)	CEA, CBA	US—10-yr annual average B:C ratio 1.9 for immunization of Medicare beneficiaries	Considered only direct costs paid by Medicare; B:C ratio derived from data presented
Mullooly et al.[134] (1994)	CEA	US—savings $6.11/vaccinee for vaccinating high-risk elderly; vaccinating non–high-risk elderly cost $4.82/vaccine; overall, vaccination of elderly saved $1.10/vaccinee (direct medical costs)	HMO population
Nichol et al.[135] (1994)	CBA	US—$117 in direct savings/year/vaccinee for vaccination of noninstitutionalized persons >65 yr, 1990–1993	Vaccinated persons had more illnesses at baseline than nonvaccinated, thus true savings may have been higher
Campbell and Rumley[136] (1997)	CBA, CEA	US—B:C ratio 2.5 for immunization of healthy textile workers; cost/saved lost workday $22.36	
Christensen et al.[137] (1998)	CA	Denmark—urban strategy to vaccinate population over age 70 cost approximately 115 dkr/person	
Burckel et al.[138] (1999)	CBA	Brazil—vaccination of healthy workers saved $35.45 (Brz$37.75) per vaccinated employee, resulting in B:C ratio of 2.47	Break-even vaccination cost of $45.40 and vaccine efficacy of 32.5%
Meltzer et al.[139] (1999)	CA, CBA	US—estimated economic impact of pandemic influenza would be $71.3–$166.5 billion, excluding disruptions to commerce and society; net savings would be realized at $21/vaccinee if total population were vaccinated	Vaccinating 60% of the population would generate the highest economic returns
Nichol and Goodman[140] (1999)	CBA, CEA	US—annual vaccination cost-saving for both at-risk and healthy persons 65–74 yr; net savings $34.55/at-risk vaccinated, $39.35/ healthy person vaccinated	
White et al.[141] (1999)	CBA	US—vaccination of healthy school-age children resulted in a net savings/child vaccinated of $4 for individual-initiated vaccination and $35 for group-based vaccination	
Bridges et al.[142] (2000)	CBA	US—vaccination of healthy working adults ages 18–64 yr resulted in reduced influenza-like illness but had net societal cost of $11.17/person	
Cohen (2000) and Nettleman[143]	CBA	US—vaccination of preschool children with inactivated influenza vaccine resulted in net cost savings/vaccine recipient of between $1.20 and $21.28	Results dependent on type of program for delivery

TABLE 57–2 ■ Cost–Benefit and Cost-Effectiveness Analyses of Vaccines—cont'd

Reference	Type*	Location and Results†	Comment
Fitzner et al.[144] (2001)	CA	Hong Kong—average influenza-like illness costs $36 and vaccination-associated costs of $9.50 (HK$74) per vaccinated individual	
Luce et al.[145] (2001)	CEA	US—intranasal vaccination of healthy children with cost-effectiveness ranging from $10 to $69/febrile influenza-like illness day avoided at $10–$40/dose, respectively.	Break-even cost of $28 and $5/dose in group or individual delivery program, respectively
Nichol[146] (2001)	CBA	US—vaccination of healthy working adults saved $13.66/person vaccinated (95% probability interval: net savings of $32.97 to net costs of $2.18)	
LYME DISEASE			
Meltzer et al.[147] (1999)	DA	US—assuming 0.80 probability of diagnosing and treating early Lyme disease, 0.005 probability of contracting Lyme disease, and vaccination cost of $50/year, the mean cost/case averted by vaccination was $4466	Economic benefit from vaccine greatest when individual risk of contracting Lyme disease >0.01
Shadick et al.[148] (2001)		US—based on a 10-yr perspective and probabilities of contracting Lyme disease each season of 2.5%, 1%, and 0.5%, would cost $12,600, $62,300, and $145,200/QALY, respectively	Vaccination economically attractive for individuals who have seasonal probability of >0.01
MALARIA			
Graves[149] (1998)	CEA	The Gambia—three doses of vaccine coadministered with DTP was modeled to cost $252/death averted compared to $711 for bed nets with impregnation	Assumed 75% coverage for each; nets 50% effective against attacks, 35% against death; vaccine 39% effective against attacks, 20% against deaths; vaccine (+administration) cost $4.29/child
MEASLES-MUMPS-RUBELLA			
Wiedermann and Ambrosch[150] (1979)	CBA	Austria—measles/mumps B:C ratio 2.6 for direct costs; 4.4 for total costs	Also looked at individual vaccines: measles B:C ratio 1.7 for direct and 2.9 for total costs; mumps 1.9 and 3.6, respectively
White et al.[151] (1985)	CBA	US—MMR B:C ratio 14.1, including both direct and indirect costs	Also looked at individual vaccines' B:C ratios: measles 11.9, rubella 7.7, mumps 6.7
Berger et al.[152] (1990)	CBA	Israel—B:C ratio 1.1–1.2 for routine mumps/rubella immunization of 1-yr-olds based on reported cases; estimated >5.85 for true incidence	10% discount rate; also calculated with 5% discount rate
Bjerregaard[12] (1990)	CBA	Denmark—B:C ratio 3.2 for MMR two-dose program over 20 yr	
Ferson et al.[153] (1994)	CEA	Australia—compared cost/person to vaccinate all health care workers ($3.14–$20.50); to serologically test all workers and vaccinate susceptibles ($5.11–$24.45); to vaccinate all with negative history ($2.56–$16.57), and to test all those with negative history and vaccinate susceptibles ($2.58–$15.49)	Study carried out in a population with >77% of those with negative history immune
Hatziandreu et al.[154] (1994)	CBA	US—B:C ratio 16.3 for direct costs; 21.3 for total costs	Also considered B:C of individual components: measles 17.2 for both direct and total costs; mumps 6.1 and 13.0, respectively; rubella 4.5 and 11.1, respectively
MEASLES			
Axnick et al.[155] (1969)	CBA	US—B:C ratio 4.9 for immunization, 1963–1968	B:C ratio derived from data presented; 4% discount rate

Continued

TABLE 57–2 ▪ Cost–Benefit and Cost-Effectiveness Analyses of Vaccines—cont'd

Reference	Type*	Location and Results†	Comment
Witte and Axnick[156] (1975)	CBA	US—B:C ratio ~7.4 for immunization, 1962–1972	B:C ratio derived from data presented; 4% discount rate
Albritton[157] (1978)	CBA	US—B:C ratio 10.3 for federal involvement, 1966–1974	Used Box Tiao time series model to separate effect of federal funds from other efforts
Elo[127] (1979)	CBA	Finland—B:C ratios 3.9 (6% discount) and 3.5 (9% discount) for vaccinating 1-yr-old children over 25-yr period	
Ponninghaus[158] (1980)	CBA	Zambia—B:C ratio positive in urban areas (>3.9 for lives saved) but not in rural areas	Not a standard B:C analysis
WHO[159] (1982)	CEA	Ivory Coast—$12.3/infant immunized; $13.9/case averted; $479/death averted; $10.4/year of life added	Estimated that 75% of all EPI costs were attributable to measles vaccine
Davis et al.[160] (1987)	CEA	US—compared cost/case prevented of six different strategies in an outbreak setting; range from $56/case prevented by lowering recommended age of vaccination to 6 mo to $294/case prevented by vaccinating all residents 15 mo–28 yr of age	Specific results not generalizable but approach is
Ginsberg and Tulchinsky[161] (1990)	CBA	Israel—examined options of second dose of measles vaccine in Israel, West Bank, and Gaza: routine second dose at 6–7 yr (B:C ratios 4.5, 5.7, and 9.5, respectively), routine second dose + mass vaccination of 7- to 17-yr-olds (2.2, 2.0, and 3.4), and routine second dose + mass vaccination of 7- to 27-yr-olds (1.7, 1.5, and 2.6)	Under any circumstance, addition of a second dose seemed justified
Mast et al.[162] (1990)	CEA	US—compared cost/case prevented in an outbreak setting in schools—$3444/case prevented for revaccinating all students, $3166/case prevented for revaccinating those vaccinated before 1980, $2546/case prevented for revaccinating those vaccinated before 15 mo of age	43%–53% of cases would not have been prevented by any of the strategies initiated after measles had appeared
Schlian et al.[163] (1991)	CEA	US—compared cost/case prevented on college campus of various strategies; least expensive was to wait until an outbreak occurred before vaccinating; however, this would not be as effective as serologic screening of all students and vaccinating susceptibles or vaccinating all students	Recommended adopting mandatory immunization programs
Subbarao et al.[164] (1991)	CEA	US—estimated that prevaccination serologic testing of health care workers would be cost-effective if screening cost <$12.75/test	86% of population studied had antibodies
Sellick et al.[165] (1992)	CEA	US—compared cost/employee of screening all new employees serologically and vaccinating susceptibles ($2.42/employee) with "blind" immunization of all new employees ($8.30/employee)	Assumed susceptibles would require two doses of measles vaccine
Miller et al.[166] (1998)	CA	US—measles eradication would save $45 million annually if vaccination were stopped or $500 million to $4.1 billion depending on the year of elimination, posteradication schedule, and discount rate	Intensification of measles control efforts in the US beyond current levels would have minimal marginal benefits on disease burden reduction
MUMPS			
Koplan and Preblud[167] (1982)	CBA	US—B:C ratio 7.4 using reported incidence of mumps; 39 using estimated actual incidence	Included both direct and indirect costs
Arday et al.[168] (1989)	CBA	US—B:C ratio 0.2 for routine vaccination of Army recruits	Considered only marginal cost of adding mumps vaccine to existing MR vaccination; most recruits would already be immune

TABLE 57–2 ■ Cost–Benefit and Cost-Effectiveness Analyses of Vaccines—cont'd

Reference	Type*	Location and Results†	Comment
		RUBELLA	
Schoenbaum et al.[169] (1976)	CBA	US—B:C ratio 8 for vaccinating 2-yr-old children with monovalent rubella vaccine, 9 for 6-yr-old children, 27 for 12-yr-old females, and 8 for 2-yr-old children AND 12-yr-old females	Also estimated B:C ratio for use of combined MR
Elo[127] (1979)	CBA	Finland—B:C ratios 10.3, 3.3, and 5.8, respectively, for vaccinating all 13-yr-old girls and postpartum women, vaccinating all children 1–13 yr followed by vaccination of 1-yr-olds, and vaccinating 1-yr-olds only over 20 yr	Also considered other strategies
Farber and Finkelstein[170] (1979)	CBA	US—mandatory premarital rubella antibody screening B:C ratio <1 unless test cost ~$0.55 and >37% of susceptible women were immunized	No place examined met both criteria
Stray Pedersen[171] (1982)	CBA	Norway—B:C ratio 3 and 6, respectively, for vaccinating all 1-yr-old girls or all 13-yr-old girls with monovalent vaccine; 5 and 11 if using MMR	Also considered other strategies, none of which included vaccinating all 1-yr-olds, both male and female
Golden and Shapiro[172] (1984)	CBA	Israel—B:C more reliably >1 for vaccinating pubertal females than vaccinating all children; vaccination of adult females B:C <1	Also considered other strategies, none of which included vaccinating all 1-yr-olds, both male and female
Gudnadottir[173] (1985)	CEA	Iceland—serologic screening of women and teenage girls with vaccination of susceptibles would be more cost-effective than routine vaccination of all 1-yr-olds	Both strategies were cost-effective
Berger et al.[152] (1990)	CBA	Israel—B:C ratio 1.1–1.7 for routine mumps/rubella immunization of 1-yr-olds based on reported cases; >5.8 for true incidence	Only addressed acute rubella, not CRS
Kandola[174] (1998)	CBA	Guyana—B:C 38.8 for eradication campaign on top of routine MMR immunization of 1-yr-olds; $1633/CRS case prevented	
Kommu and Chase[175] (1998)	CBA	Barbados—B:C 4.7 for elimination initiative on top of routine MMR immunization of 1-yr-olds	
Irons[176] (1998)	CBA	Caribbean—B:C 13.3 for elimination campaign on top of routine MMR immunization of 1-yr-olds, 1997–2017; $2900/CRS case prevented for English-speaking Caribbean and Suriname	
		MENINGOCOCCAL DISEASE	
Jackson et al.[177] (1995)	CBA	US—routine vaccination of college students not cost-beneficial until incidence 6.5/100,000 (at least 5 times higher than the presumed endemic rate in this population)	
Miller et al.[178] (1999)	CEA	Africa—comparison of routine *vs.* outbreak control strategies with polysaccharide vaccines in 16 sub-Saharan African countries, for entire meningitis belt; routine coverage with one- or four-dose schedule meningococcal vaccine would cost $4.4–$12.3 million annually and could prevent an average 10,300–12,600 cases (23%–28%), assuming long-term vaccine efficacy of 50%	An initial "catch-up" campaign costing up to $72 million to vaccinate the population from 1 to 30 yr of age would be required before achieving that level of effectiveness
Parent du Chatelet et al.[179] (2001)	CEA	Senegal—a preventive campaign using polysaccharide vaccine was more effective (59%) and cheaper ($59/prevented case) than a reactive strategy (49% and $133/ prevented case, respectively if epidemics could be predicted within 3 yr	Vaccination coverage rates for the preventive and standard strategies were >70% and <94%, respectively

Continued

TABLE 57–2 ■ Cost–Benefit and Cost-Effectiveness Analyses of Vaccines—cont'd

Reference	Type*	Location and Results†	Comment
Skull et al.[180] (2001)	CEA, CBA	Australia—vaccination with polysaccharide vaccine of people ages 15–19 yr in defined population with high rate of disease resulted in discounted cost/life-year saved of $23,623, cost/DALY avoided of $21,097	"Break-even" incidence rate for this option with exclusion of direct cost savings was 14.0/100,000
PNEUMOCOCCAL DISEASE			
OTA[181] (1979) and Willems et al.[182] (1980)	CEA	US—$1000/QALY for persons >65 yr of age; $5700/QALY for persons 45–64 yr of age	Also considered high-risk and non–high-risk persons of other age groups; vaccination of elderly under a public program would be cost-saving
Patrick and Wooley[183] (1981)	CBA	US—B:C ratio 2.3 for immunizing those >50 yr or with chronic illness in an HMO population; 0.7 for all adults	
OTA[184] (1984) and Sisk and Riegelman[185] (1986)	CEA	US—$300/QALY for persons >65 yr of age	
Sisk et al.[186] (1997)	CEA	US—vaccination of persons >65 yr cost-saving if future medical costs (unrelated to pneumococcal disease) of survivors are excluded, cost/QALY $10,306–$17,208 if future medical costs included	$8.27 saved/person >65 yr vaccinated
Nichol et al.[187] (1999)	CBA	US—pneumococcal vaccination of elderly persons with chronic lung disease associated with direct medical care cost savings	
Stack et al.[188] (1999)	CA	US—estimated cost savings ranged from $168,940 to $427,380 from an emergency department program screening for high-risk patients to deliver pneumococcal vaccine	
Ament et al.[189] (2000)	CUA	Europe—vaccination of persons ages ≥65 yr varied from approximately 11,000 to approximately 33,000 ECU/QALY	Assuming an incidence of 50 cases/100,000 and 20%–40% mortality rate, the cost-effectiveness ratios were <12,000 ECU/QALY in five countries
Black et al.[190] (2000)	CBA	US—vaccination of healthy infants would result in net savings for society if the conjugate vaccine cost less than $46/dose, and net savings for the health care payer if the vaccine cost less than $18/dose	
De Graeve et al.[191] (2000)	CUA	Belgium—vaccination with the 23-valent pneumococcal polysaccharide vaccine would cost 25,000 and 35,000 ECU/QALY for the age groups 65–75 yr and 75–84 yr, respectively	77,000 ECU/QALY for persons over 85 yr of age
Lieu et al.[192] (2000)	CEA	US—universal infant vaccination with conjugate vaccine at $58/dose would cost society $80,000/life-year saved or $160/otitis media episode prevented (other estimated costs would be $3200/pneumonia case prevented, $15000 for bacteremia, and $280000 for meningitis)	Break-even vaccine cost for society and health care provider would be at $46 and $18/dose, respectively
Ortqvist et al.[193] (2000)	CUA	Sweden—vaccination of the elderly was approximately 300,000 SEK/QALY gained, but only about 60,000 SEK/QALY in a two-way sensitivity analysis making reasonable assumptions regarding the incidence and mortality of invasive pneumococcal disease in this age group	

TABLE 57–2 ■ Cost–Benefit and Cost-Effectiveness Analyses of Vaccines—cont'd

Reference	Type*	Location and Results†	Comment
Shann[194] (2000)	CBA	Papua New Guinea—one dose of pneumococcal vaccine given to every Papua New Guinean over 5 yr of age every 5 yr would save approximately 6600 lives/yr and the vaccine would cost only $121/life saved	
Vold Pepper and Owens[195] (2000)	CEA	US—vaccination of active-duty military personnel would increase each person's life expectancy by 0.03 days and decrease costs by $9.88/person	
Weycker et al.[196] (2000)	CBA	US—expected net economic benefits (benefits minus costs) of vaccination with conjugate vaccine against pneumococcal otitis media and pneumonia range from −$88 to $15/child for children vaccinated at less than 2 yr of age, and from −$1 to $31/child for those ages 2–5 yr at vaccination	Benefits from vaccination extended to 10 yr and were based on a start-up vaccination program with decreasing number of doses for higher age groups
Postma, et al.[197] (2001)		Netherlands—pneumococcal vaccination in the elderly with the 23-valent vaccine would cost between 6000 and 16,000 Euros/ life-year gained	28,000 Euros for vaccinating only those elderly ages 85 yr and over
Mukamel et al.[198] (2001)	CUA	US—vaccination in nontraditional settings yielded cost-utility ratios ranging from $4215 to $12,617/QALY, depending on the underlying assumptions of the model	
POLIOMYELITIS			
Weisbrod[199] (1971)	CBA	US—annual "rate of return" on investment in polio vaccine research (both IPV and OPV) estimated at 11%–12%	Benefits calculated based on present value of expected future earnings as well as treatment costs averted
Fundenberg[200] (1973)	CBA	US—B:C ratio 10 for IPV development over period 1955–1961	Also estimated net annual savings >$180 million from measles vaccination
Musgrove[201] (1988)	CBA	Americas—B:C ratio 5.8 over 15 yr for a 5-yr polio eradication campaign in the Americas if all cases received medical treatment and 1.4 if only 1/4 of cases did	12% discount rate
Hatziandreu et al.[202] (1994)	CBA	US—B:C ratio for OPV 3.4 for direct costs, 6.1 including indirect costs (total costs); B:C ratio for four-dose sequential IPV-OPV 3.0 for direct costs, 5.7 for total costs	Also considered five- and six-dose sequential schedules and B:C ratio of comprehensive program including OPV, DTP, and MMR (7.6 and 26.3 for direct and total costs, respectively, under "intermediate case" scenario)
Bart et al.[203] (1996)	CBA, CEA	Global—calculated net costs and benefits of polio eradication over the period 1986–2040; "break-even" point reached in 2007 and total net savings by 2040 $13.6 billion	Did not consider indirect costs; used 6% discount rate
Miller et al.[204] (1996)	CBA, CEA	US—changing from OPV- only to IPV-only schedule would not be cost-beneficial; would cost $3.0 million/case of VAPP pre-vented; sequential IPV-OPV schedule would cost $3.1 million/case of VAPP prevented	National policy was changed to sequential IPV-OPV
RABIES			
Morrison et al.[205] (1987)	CEA	US—intradermal administration of human diploid cell vaccine was more cost-effective than intramuscular in at-risk laboratory workers; savings of $120/person vaccinated	Comparison of dosing regimens
Bernard and Fishbein[206] (1991)	CBA	Global—pre-exposure prophylaxis not cost-beneficial for long-term travelers (Peace Corps volunteers) to endemic areas	Analysis assumed exposed persons would receive follow-up care for possible rabies infections
Fishbein et al.[207] (1991)	CBA, CEA	Philippines—costs from rabies elimination program primarily through canine vaccine program would be recouped in 4–11 yr; $2036/death prevented after 25 yr	

Continued

TABLE 57–2 ▪ Cost–Benefit and Cost-Effectiveness Analyses of Vaccines—cont'd

Reference	Type[*]	Location and Results[†]	Comment
Uhaa et al.[208] (1992)	CBA	US—B:C ratio 2.2–6.8 for oral vaccine bait for raccoons to prevent human rabies	
Kreindel et al.[209] (1998)	CA	US—median cost per patient given postexposure prophylaxis $2376 (range: $1038–$4447)	
Meltzer and Rupprecht[210] (1998)	DA	General review—in the US, only 2 individuals/1000 possible contacts have to be at risk from bat rabies in order for it to be economically justifiable to give postexposure prophylaxis to all those potentially exposed to bat rabies	
ROTAVIRUS			
Griffiths et al.[211] (1995)	CA	US—break-even costs for vaccine would be $11/infant for tetravalent and $12/infant for serotype 1 vaccine	Based on hypothetical vaccine program
Smith et al.[212] (1995)	CEA	US—at assumed disease incidence, 50% efficacy and $30/dose, routine infant immunization with a rotavirus vaccine would have B:C ratios of 1.3 (direct costs) and 2.9 (total costs)	
Takala et al.[213] (1998)	CBA	Finland—mean cost/vaccinated child was 4 Finnish marks (FIM) in the RRV-TV group, versus 203 FIM in the placebo group	Break-even cost for vaccine was 109 FIM (US $19.60)
Tucker et al.[214] (1998)	CEA	US—at $20/dose, universal infant vaccination would cost the health care system $103/case prevented but would provide a net savings to society of $296 million	Threshold analysis identified a break-even price/dose of $9 for the health care system and $51 for the societal perspective
Carlin et al.[215] (1999)	CBA	Australia—rotavirus vaccination would be cost-neutral to the health care system and society at a vaccine price of $19 and $26, respectively	
SCHISTOSOMIASIS			
Guyatt and Evans[216] (1995)	CEA	Hypothetical vaccine would need to cost no more than $3.50–$4.30 above the current chemotherapy treatment to be cost-effective	Vaccine assumed to be added to existing national vaccination program
VARICELLA			
Preblud et al.[217] (1985)	CBA	US—B:C ratio 6.9 with hypothetical vaccine	Assumed 90% lifelong efficacy
Preblud et al.[218] (1988)	CA	US—estimated annual disease burden cost of $400 million	95% of cost resulting from lost wages for child care
Weber et al.[219] (1988)	CA	US—$56,000 spent in 1 yr in a 580-bed hospital for identification, prophylaxis, and treatment of susceptible persons as a result of varicella exposure	Costs associated with hospital infection control
Kitai et al.[220] (1993)	CBA	Canada—pretransplant vaccination program would have B:C ratios of 8.3 (direct costs and benefits) and 9.5 (total costs and benefits)	Vaccine cost CAN$30/dose
Huse et al.[221] (1994)	CBA	US—vaccination in routine schedules would have B:C ratio of 0.34 (direct medical treatment costs only) or 2.0 (direct and indirect)	Vaccination only cost-beneficial if indirect costs included; 5% discount rate; vaccine cost $24/dose
Lieu et al.[222] (1994)	CEA, CBA	US—one-dose program would cost $2500/life-year saved (medical costs only); if indirect costs were included, B:C ratio 5	Vaccine cost $35/dose
Lieu et al.[223] (1994)	CA	US—mean value of work lost because of chickenpox was $293/family or $183/chickenpox case; estimated costs of nonprescription medications were $20/family or $12.50/chickenpox case	

TABLE 57–2 ■ Cost–Benefit and Cost-Effectiveness Analyses of Vaccines—cont'd

Reference	Type*	Location and Results†	Comment
Ferson[224] (1995)	CA	Australia—universal infant vaccination will cause a greater proportion of varicella cases to occur in adults, with associated serious complications, although economic costs resulting from lost time from work will fall dramatically, health costs may rise	
Lieu et al.[225] (1995)	CEA	US—vaccinating all 6- to 12-yr-old children is more effective but more costly ($197/case prevented) than screening with subsequent vaccination if only direct costs are included; if indirect costs are included, vaccinating all is a dominant strategy (less costly and more effective); for 13- to 17-yr-old children, testing all is most cost effective but has a high cost	Vaccine cost $35; results highly sensitive to varicella prevalence among persons with uncertain histories; study addresses limitation of data concerning correlation of disease history with immune status
Beutels et al.[226] (1996)	CBA, CEA	Germany—adolescent vaccination most cost-effective and had direct medical savings; vaccination at 15 mo would cost 19.74 DM life-year (direct costs only) or 6.92 DM if combine with adolescent catch-up vaccination at 12 yr	5% discount rate; vaccine cost 75 DM/dose
Gray, et al.[227] (1997)	CEA	UK—screening and vaccination of health care workers would save £440 UK/incident averted *vs.* vaccinating all staff, which would cost £48,900 UK/incident averted	
Nettleman and Schmid[228] (1997)		US—vaccination of potentially susceptible workers would result in net cost savings of $59/person	
Strassels and Sullivan[229] (1997)	CBA	US—B:C ratios 0.9 and 5.4 for universal vaccination of persons without a history of infection from payers' and society's perspective, respectively	
Tennenberg et al.[230] (1997)	CBA	US—screening and vaccination would have resulted in a B:C ratio of 3.0 by avoiding furlough of exposed health care workers in a tertiary care center	
Coudeville et al.[231] (1999)	CBA	France—coadministration with MMR vaccines would lead to a 10%–77% reduction of direct medical costs	
Diez Domingo et al.[232] (1999)	CBA	Spain—universal vaccination of 15-mo-olds would yield a B:C ratio of 0.54 in direct costs and 1.6 when indirect costs are included	Break-even values are vaccine coverage and efficacy <0.7, discount rate of 20%, and vaccine price less than PT 6000
YELLOW FEVER			
Monath and Nasidi[233] (1993)	CEA	Nigeria—although emergency response is more cost-effective than routine vaccination ($1904 *vs.* $3817/death prevented), routine vaccination would prevent 7 times as many deaths	Valuation of deaths would greatly increase the benefits of routine immunization

*CA, cost analysis; CBA, cost–benefit analysis; CEA, cost-effectiveness analysis; CUA, cost-utility analysis.
†Costs in U.S. dollars unless otherwise indicated.
AIDS, acquired immunodeficiency syndrome; anti-HBc, anti–hepatitis B core antigen antibody; anti-HBs, anti–hepatitis B surface antigen antibody; B:C, benefits-to-costs; BCG, bacille Calmette-Guérin; CDC, Centers for Disease Control and Prevention; CRS, congenital rubella syndrome; DA, decision analysis; DALY, disability-adjusted life year; DTP, diphtheria-tetanus-pertusis vaccine; ECU, European Currency Unit; EPI, Expanded Programme on Immunisation; GNP, gross national product; HBsAg, hepatitis B surface antigen; HBV, hepatitis B virus; HepA, hepatitis A vaccine; HepB, hepatitis B vaccine; Hib, *Haemophilus influenzae* type b vaccine; HIV, human immunodeficiency virus; HMO, health maintenance organization; INH, isoniazid; IPV, inactivated poliovirus vaccine; MMR, measles-mumps-rubella vaccine; MR, measles-rubella vaccine; OPV, oral poliovirus vaccine; OTA, Office of Technology Assessment; PPD, purified protein derivative; QALY, quality-adjusted life years; RRV-TV, rhesus rotavirus vaccine–tetravalent; TT, tetanus toxoid; VAPP, vaccine-associated paralytic poliomyelitis; WHO, World Health Organization.

TABLE 57–3 ▪ Selected Values of Cost-Effectiveness of Traditional Clinical Preventive Services

Intervention	Median Cost/QALY (US$)
Immunizations and chemoprophylaxis	
Immunizations and vaccinations	1500
Pharmaceuticals for asymptomatic persons (e.g., hormone replacement)	13,000
Screening tests	
Cardiovascular disease	3300
Neoplasms	18,500
Osteoporosis screening and treatment	13,000
Other disease screenings	11,500
Counseling	
HIV risk behaviors	1200
Cardiovascular disease risk	74,000
Screening blood donors against pathogens	355,000
Presurgical autologous blood donation	730,000

Adapted from Stone et al.[234] and Tengs et al.[235]

and efficacy can be varied in the analysis to demonstrate the target values at which a vaccine would be cost-effective or cost-beneficial.

Formulating and/or Modifying Immunization Policy

Although economic analyses give an indication of the efficiency of various public health interventions, they may not indicate which strategy has the greatest impact. For example, although targeted vaccination approaches such as hepatitis B for high-risk groups or rubella during prenatal visits may be economically more efficient, they inevitably prevent less disease than a more inclusive strategy such as universal vaccination.

Decision Analysis—Appropriate Polio Vaccine Strategy

A 1988 comparative analysis of benefits and risks of oral polio vaccine (OPV) and IPV supported the then-current U.S. policy placing primary reliance on OPV but noted that "the conclusion is heavily dependent on assumptions of risk of exposure to wild virus in the United States. Major declines in risk of exposure to wild-type virus could alter the balance significantly."[247] The risk of importation has declined dramatically since that time—the last case of paralysis caused by indigenously acquired poliovirus in the Western Hemisphere (the primary source of U.S. importations) had its onset in August 1991. The American, Western Pacific, and European Regions of the WHO have all been certified polio free, and endemic transmission continues in fewer than 20 countries.[248] In 1996, despite the high costs of switching to IPV,[204] the Advisory Committee on Immunization Practices and the American Academy of Pediatrics recommended a change in U.S. policy to favor a sequential schedule of IPV followed by OPV.[249] In 2000, the policy shifted to use of IPV alone.[250]

Cost–Benefit Analysis—Varicella

A 1985 CBA of varicella immunization conducted by Preblud and associates found that universal immunization with varicella vaccine (at a presumed cost of $15/dose) would have a B:C ratio of 6.9.[217] This analysis was carried out more than 10 years before varicella vaccine was licensed. Varicella vaccination is clearly cost-saving when

the indirect costs of lost income from caregivers are included in the analysis, although it is not cost-saving when only direct medical costs are considered. Subsequent analyses have continued to show a positive B:C ratio when considering both direct and indirect costs and have supported the decision to recommend universal vaccination of children.

Cost-Effectiveness Analysis—Influenza

Beginning with an early CBA by Kavet,[123,124] a number of studies have demonstrated the positive ratio of benefits to costs of influenza immunization of the elderly or substantial cost-effectiveness of such immunization. Given these data as well as the clinical and public health data about the impact of influenza, Congress enacted legislation in 1987 to make influenza immunization reimbursable under Medicare unless it was shown not to be cost-effective.[251] In response, the Department of Health and Human Services implemented a demonstration at 10 sites, each of which included an intervention area and a comparison area. The resulting CEA led to the conclusion that, among Medicare beneficiaries, "influenza vaccine would cost $145 per year of life gained, substantially below the cost of other preventive interventions. . . . Because of these generally favorable results, influenza vaccine was made a covered benefit."[5] A more recent study has shown that influenza vaccination of healthy 65- to 74-year-old persons is not only cost-effective, but cost-saving.[128]

Cost-Utility Analysis—Basic Immunizations

The 1993 World Development Report (issued by the World Bank) addressed the burden of disease in countries around the world and carried out a cost-utility analysis of a variety of interventions to deal with major health problems.[252] The measure used to compare regions, conditions, and interventions is the DALY, a measure that combines healthy life-years lost because of premature mortality with those lost because of disability. The report assessed 52 interventions and found that basic immunizations (BCG, DTP, OPV, and measles, as given in the EPI) were among the best investments to make in health. The report estimated that the cost per DALY gained by immunization in low-income countries was $12 to $17 ($25 to $30 in middle-income countries) compared with, for example, $200 to $350 per DALY for limited care, including assessment, advice, alleviation of pain, treatment of infection and minor trauma, and treatment of more complicated conditions as resources permit ($400 to $600 in middle-income countries). The report described a limited package of five essential public health measures (including immunizations) and six clinical interventions that should be the highest priority for government financing. The findings of this study are being used to guide donor investments in developing countries.

Although many existing vaccines have been judged to be cost-effective, there has been slow adoption of new vaccines into national vaccination schedules despite recommendations from global multilateral agencies. High coverage of older vaccines, price support to help finance vaccines, and an appreciation of disease burden are associated with uptake of the newer vaccines such as hepatitis B and Hib.[253]

Other Economic Considerations

Other economic considerations include the price of vaccines, their affordability, and the value placed on them. Traditional EPI vaccines have been relatively inexpensive in both developed and developing countries, reflecting lower costs of research, development, and production in the past, and the fact that research and development cost recoupment and increased competition from manufacturers. Newer vaccines are more expensive because of increased costs of development and production as well as limited supply. The question of how to make these vaccines available in developing countries has been addressed by a number of strategies, including tiered pricing and the creation of the Global Alliance on Vaccines and Immunizations (GAVI) with a Global Fund for Children's Vaccines, largely funded by the Bill and Melinda Gates Foundation, that provides grants to developing countries to purchase and administer newer vaccines (primarily hepatitis B and Hib). Countries are eligible for GAVI support if their annual per capita income is less than $1000/year; currently 74 countries are eligible for GAVI support.

The goal is for all countries to place high enough value on vaccines to give them priority within their national budgets. This is particularly problematic in countries where the per capita public expenditure on health may be less than $10/year (13 countries in 1998).[254] In nine of these countries, per capita expenditures on defense were greater than on health.

The total cost to fully immunize all 92 million children born in the 74 GAVI-eligible countries each year would be $2.3 billion with basic EPI antigens, and $3.1 billion if hepatitis B and Hib vaccines were included. Although this is a substantial amount, it represents less than one third of the overseas development assistance provided each year by the United States.[255,256]

Conclusion

Quantitative policy analysis techniques can support rational decision making in immunization by explicitly stating assumptions, costs, and benefits of different strategies and allowing, through sensitivity analysis, an indication of the most important determinants of program outcome. They are important tools to help evaluate options, however, they should not be the sole basis for making decisions about immunization policies or programs. When conducted appropriately, they help elucidate values and summarize data and knowledge gaps as well as the relative importance of epidemiologic and economic assumptions. Economic analyses of immunizations have shown them to be among the best investments in health.

REFERENCES

1. Dasbach E, Teutsch SM. Cost-utility analysis. *In* Haddix AC, Teutsch SM, Shaffer PA, Dunet DO (eds). Prevention Effectiveness: A Guide to Decision Analysis and Economic Evaluation. New York, Oxford University Press, pp 130–142, 1996.
2. Jefferson T, Demicheli V. Methodological quality of economic modeling studies: a case study with hepatitis B vaccines. Pharmacoeconomics 14:251–257, 1998.
3. Gold MR, Siegel JE, Russell LB, Weinstein MC. Cost-effectiveness in Health and Medicine. New York, Oxford University Press, 1996.
4. Spier R, Jefferson TO, Demicheli V. An editorial policy statement: submission of economic evaluations of vaccines. Vaccine 20:1693–1695, 2002.
5. Zalkind DL, Shachtman RH. A decision analysis approach to the swine influenza vaccination decision for an individual. Med Care 18:59–72, 1980.
6. Centers for Disease Control and Prevention. Final results: Medicare influenza vaccination demonstration, selected states, 1988–1992. MMWR 42:601–604, 1993.
7. Arnesen T, Nord E. The value of DALY life: problems with ethics and validity of disability adjusted life years. BMJ 319:1423–1425, 1999.
8. Barnum HDT, Setiady I. Cost-effectiveness of an immunization program in Indonesia. Bull World Health Organ 58:499–503, 1980.
9. Creese A, Henderson RH. Cost-benefit analysis and immunization programmes in developing countries. Bull World Health Organ 58:491–497, 1980.
10. Phonboon K, Shepard DS, Ramaboot S, et al. The Thai Expanded Programme on Immunization: role of immunization sessions and their cost-effectiveness. Bull World Health Organ 67:181–188, 1989.
11. Shepard DS, Robertson RL, Cameron CS, et al. Cost-effectiveness of routine and campaign vaccination strategies in Ecuador. Bull World Health Organ 67:649–662, 1989.
12. Bjerregaard P. Economic analysis of immunization programmes. Scand J Soc Med 46(suppl):115–119, 1990.
13. Musgrove P. Cost-benefit analysis of a regional system for vaccination against pneumonia, meningitis type B, and typhoid fever. Bull PAHO 26:173–191, 1992.
14. Behrens RH, Roberts JA. Is travel prophylaxis worthwhile? Economic appraisal of prophylactic measures against malaria, hepatitis A, and typhoid in travelers. BMJ 309:918–922, 1994.
15. Brenzel L, Claquin P. Immunization programs and their costs. Soc Sci Med 39:527–536, 1994.
16. Hadler SC. Cost benefit of combining antigens. Biologicals 22:415–418, 1994.
17. Shepard DS, Walsh JA, Kleinau E, et al. Setting priorities for the Children's Vaccine Initiative: a cost effectiveness approach. Vaccine 13:707–714, 1995.
18. Schlumberger M, Chatelet IP, Lafarge H, et al. Cost of tetanus toxoid injection using a jet-injector (Imule) in collective immunization in Senegal: comparison with injection using a syringe and resterilizable needle [in French]. Sante 9:319–326, 1999.
19. Edmunds WJ, Dejene A, Mekonnen Y, et al. The cost of integrating hepatitis B virus vaccine into national immunization programmes: a case study from Addis Ababa. Health Policy Plan 15:408–416, 2000.
20. Miller MA, McCann L. Policy analysis of the use of hepatitis B, *Haemophilus influenzae* type b-, *Streptococcus pneumoniae*-conjugate and rotavirus vaccines in national immunization schedules. Health Econ 9:19–35, 2000.
21. Collis PB, Dudding BA, Winter PE, et al. Adenovirus vaccines in military recruit populations: a cost–benefit analysis. J Infect Dis 128:745–752, 1973.

22. Hyer RN, Howell MR, Ryan MA, et al. Cost-effectiveness analysis of reacquiring and using adenovirus types 4 and 7 vaccines in naval recruits. Am J Trop Med Hyg 62:613–618, 2000.

23. Cowley P. Preliminary cost-effectiveness analysis of an AIDS vaccine in Abidjan, Ivory Coast. Health Policy 24:145–153, 1993.

24. Nettleman MD. Use of BCG vaccine in shelters for the homeless: a decision analysis. Chest 103:1087–1090, 1993.

25. Trnka L, Dankova D, Svandova E. Six years' experience with the discontinuation of BCG vaccination. 2. Cost and benefit of mass BCG vaccination. Tuber Lung Dis 74:288–292, 1993.

26. Nettleman MD, Geerdes H, Roy M-C. The cost-effectiveness of preventing tuberculosis in physicians using tuberculin skin testing or a hypothetical vaccine. Arch Intern Med 157:1121–1127, 1997.

27. Pathania VS, Trnka L, Krejbich F, Dye C. A cost-benefit analysis of BCG revaccination in the Czech Republic. Vaccine 17:1926–1935, 1999.

28. Rahman M, Sekimoto M, Takamatsu I, et al. Economic evaluation of universal BCG vaccination of Japanese infants. Int J Epidemiol 30:380–385, 2001.

29. MacPherson DW, Tonkin M. Cholera vaccination: a decision analysis. CMAJ 146:1947–1952, 1992.

30. Cookson ST, Stamboulian D, Demonte J, et al. A cost–benefit analysis of programmatic use of CVD 103-HgR live oral cholera vaccine in a high-risk population. Int J Epidemiol 26:212–218, 1997.

31. Naficy A, Rao MR, Paquet C, et al. Treatment and vaccination strategies to control cholera in sub-Saharan refugee settings: a cost-effectiveness analysis. JAMA 279:521–525, 1998.

32. Legros D, Paquet C, Perea W, et al. Mass vaccination with a two-dose oral cholera vaccine in a refugee camp. Bull World Health Organ 77:837–842, 1999.

33. Naficy AB, Trach DD, Ke NT, et al. Cost of immunization with a locally produced, oral cholera vaccine in Viet Nam. Vaccine 19:3720–3725, 2001.

34. Hatziandreu E, Palmer CS, Brown RE, et al. A Cost–Benefit Analysis of the Diphtheria-Tetanus-Pertussis (DTP) Vaccine: Final Report. Arlington, VA, Battelle, 1994.

35. Koplan JP, Schoenbaum SC, Weinstein MC, et al. Pertussis vaccine—an analysis of benefits, risks, and costs. N Engl J Med 301:906–911, 1979.

36. Hinman AR, Koplan JP. Pertussis and pertussis vaccine—reanalysis of benefits, risks, and costs. JAMA 251:3109–3113, 1984.

37. Hinman AR, Koplan JP. Pertussis and pertussis vaccine: further analysis of benefits, risks, and costs. Dev Biol Stand 61:429–437, 1985.

38. Tormans G, Van Doorslaer E, van Damme P, et al. Economic evaluation of pertussis prevention by whole-cell and acellular vaccine in Germany. Eur J Pediatr 157:395–401, 1998.

39. Beutels P, Bonanni P, Tormans G, et al. An economic evaluation of universal pertussis vaccination in Italy. Vaccine 17:2400–2409, 1999.

40. Ekwueme DU, Strebel PM, Hadler SC, et al. Economic evaluation of use of diphtheria, tetanus, and acellular pertussis vaccine or diphtheria, tetanus, and whole-cell pertussis vaccine in the United States, 1997. Arch Pediatr Adolesc Med 154:797–803, 2000.

41. Iskedjian M, Einarson TR, O'Brien BJ, et al. Economic evaluation of a new acellular vaccine for pertussis in Canada. Pharmacoeconomics 19(5 pt 2):551–563, 2001.

42. Berggren W. Administration and evaluation of rural health services: I. A tetanus control program in Haiti. Am J Trop Med Hyg 23:936–949, 1974.

43. Hutchison BG, Stoddart GL. Cost-effectiveness of primary tetanus vaccination among elderly Canadians. CMAJ 139:1143–1151, 1988.

44. Carducci A, Avio CM, Bendinelli M. Cost–benefit analysis of tetanus prophylaxis by a mathematical model. Epidemiol Infect 102:473–483, 1989.

45. Berman P, Quinley J, Yusuf B, et al. Maternal tetanus immunization in Aceh Province, Sumatra: the cost-effectiveness of alternative strategies. Soc Sci Med 33:185–192, 1991.

46. Balestra DJ, Littenberg B. Should adult tetanus immunization be given as a single vaccination at age 65? J Gen Intern Med 8:405–412, 1993.

47. Cochi SL, Broome CV, Hightower AW. Immunization of U.S. children with Haemophilus influenzae type b polysaccharide vaccine: a cost-effectiveness model of strategy assessment. JAMA 253:521–529, 1985.

48. Hay JW, Daum RS. Cost–benefit analysis of two strategies for prevention of Haemophilus influenzae type b infection. Pediatrics 80:319–329, 1987.

49. Hay JW, Daum RS. Economic analysis of Haemophilus influenzae type b vaccination. Pediatr Infect Dis J 9:246–252, 1990.

50. Martens LL, ten Velden GHM, Bol P. De kosten en baten van vaccinatie tegen Haemophilus influenzae type b. Ned Tijdschr Geneeskd 135:16–20, 1991.

51. Ginsberg GM, Kassis I, Dagan R. Cost–benefit analysis of Haemophilus influenzae type b vaccination programme in Israel. J Epidemiol Commun Health 47:485–490, 1993.

52. Levine OS, Ortiz E, Contreras R, et al. Cost–benefit analysis for the use of Haemophilus influenzae type b conjugate vaccine in Santiago, Chile. Am J Epidemiol 137:1221–1228, 1993.

53. Harris A, Hendrie D, Bower C, et al. The burden of Haemophilus influenzae type b disease in Australia and an economic appraisal of the vaccine PRP-OMP. Med J Aust 160:483–488, 1994.

54. McIntyre P, Hall J, Leeder S. An economic analysis of alternatives for childhood immunisation against Haemophilus influenzae type b disease. Aust J Public Health 18:394–400, 1994.

55. Trollfors B. Cost–benefit analysis of general vaccination against Haemophilus influenzae type b in Sweden. Scand J Infect Dis 26:611–614, 1994.

56. Asensi F, Otero MC, Pérez-Tamarit D, et al. Economic aspects of a general vaccination against invasive disease caused by Haemophilus influenzae type b (Hib) via the experience of the Children's Hospital La Fe, Valencia, Spain. Vaccine 13:1563–1566, 1995.

57. Hatziandreu EJ, Brown RE. A Cost–Benefit Analysis of the Haemophilus influenzae b (Hib) Vaccine. Arlington, VA, Battelle, 1995.

58. Hussey GD, Lasser ML, Reekie WD. The costs and benefits of a vaccination programme for Haemophilus influenzae type b disease. S Afr Med J 85:20–25, 1995.

59. Midani S, Ayoub EM, Rathore MH. Cost-effectiveness of Haemophilus influenzae type b conjugate vaccine program in Florida. J Fla Med Assoc 82:401–402, 1995.

60. Hinds MW, Skaggs JW, Bergeisen GH. Benefit–cost analysis of active surveillance of primary care physicians for hepatitis A. Am J Public Health 75:176–177, 1985.

61. Tormans G, Van Damme P, Van Doorslaer E. Cost-effectiveness analysis of hepatitis A prevention in travelers. Vaccine 10(suppl 1): S88–S92, 1992.

62. Bryan JP, Nelson M. Testing for antibody to hepatitis A to decrease the cost of hepatitis A prophylaxis with immune globulin or hepatitis A vaccines. Arch Intern Med 154:663–668, 1994.

63. Jefferson T, Demicheli V, Wright D. An economic evaluation of the introduction of vaccination against hepatitis A in a peacekeeping operation. Int J Technol Assess Health Care 10:490–497, 1994.

64. Jefferson TO, Behrens RH, Demicheli V. Should British soldiers be vaccinated against hepatitis A? An economic analysis. Vaccine 12:1379–1383, 1994.

65. Van Doorslaer E, Tormans G, Van Damme P. Cost-effectiveness analysis of vaccination against hepatitis A in travelers. J Med Virol 44:463–469, 1994.

66. Zuckerman JN, Powell L. Hepatitis A antibodies in attenders of London travel clinics: cost benefit of screening prior to hepatitis A immunisation. J Med Virol 44:393–394, 1994.

67. Li XH, Xu ZY, Hofman A, et al. Epidemiology and cost-effectiveness analysis of hepatitis A vaccination in Liuzhou City. Chin J Epidemiol 19:93–96, 1998.

68. Chen E, Yao J, Yang J. Cost-benefit analysis for hepatitis A vaccine [in Chinese]. Zhonghua Liu Xing Bing Xue Za Zhi 20:224–227, 1999.

69. Saab S, Martin P, Yee HF Jr. A simple cost-decision analysis model comparing two strategies for hepatitis A vaccination. Am J Med 109:241–244, 2000.

70. Chodick G, Lerman Y, Peled T, et al. Cost–benefit analysis of active vaccination campaigns against hepatitis A among daycare centre personnel in Israel. Pharmacoeconomics 19:281–291, 2001.

71. Corrao G, Zotti C, Tinivella F, et al. HBV pre-vaccination screening in hospital personnel: cost-effectiveness analysis. Eur J Epidemiol 3:25–29, 1987.

72. Hankins DG, Ebert KD, Siebold CM, et al. Hepatitis B vaccine and hepatitis B markers: cost effectiveness of screening prehospital personnel. Am J Emerg Med 5:205–206, 1987.

73. Jacobson JJ, La Turno DE, Jonston FK, et al. Cost effectiveness of pre-vaccination screening for hepatitis B antibody. J Dent Educ 51:94–97, 1987.

74. Arevalo JA, Washington AE. Cost-effectiveness of prenatal screening and immunization for hepatitis B virus. JAMA 259:365–369, 1988.

75. Tong MJ, Co RL, Marci RD, et al. A cost comparison analysis for screening and vaccination of hospital personnel with high- and low-prevalence hepatitis B virus antibodies in California. Infect Control Hosp Epidemiol 9:66–71, 1988.

76. Thomas IL. Cost effectiveness of antenatal hepatitis B screening and vaccination of infants. Aust N Z J Obstet Gynaecol 30:331–335, 1990.

77. Audet AM, Delage G, Remis RS. Screening for HBsAg in pregnant women: a cost analysis of the universal screening policy in the province of Quebec. Can J Public Health 82:191–195, 1991.

78. Schoub BD, Johnson S, McAnerney J, et al. Exposure to hepatitis B virus among South African health care workers: implications for pre-immunisation screening. South Afr Med J 79:27–29, 1991.

79. Tormans G, Van Damme P, Carrin G, et al. Cost-effectiveness analysis of prenatal screening and vaccination against hepatitis B virus—the case of Belgium. Soc Sci Med 37:173–181, 1993.

80. Kwan-Gett TSC, Whitaker RC, Kemper KJ. A cost effectiveness analysis of prevaccination testing for hepatitis B in adolescents and preadolescents. Arch Pediatr Adolesc Med 148:915–920, 1994.

81. Yuan L, Robinson G. Hepatitis B vaccination and screening for markers at a sexually transmitted disease clinic for men. Can J Public Health 85:338–341, 1994.

82. Ferraz ML, de Oliveira PM, Figueiredo VM, et al. Otimizacao do emprego de recursos economicos para vacinacao contra hepatite B em profissionais da area de saude [Optimization of the use of economic resources for vaccination against hepatitis B in health professionals]. Rev Soc Bras Med Trop 28:393–403, 1995.

83. Fabrizi F, Di Filippo S, Marcelli D, et al. Recombinant hepatitis B vaccine use in chronic hemodialysis patients. Nephron 72:536–543, 1996.

84. Williams JR, Nokes DJ, Medley GF, et al. The transmission dynamics of hepatitis B in the UK: a mathematical model for evaluating costs and effectiveness of immunization programmes. Epidemiol Infect 116:71–89, 1996.

85. Mulley A, Silverstein M, Dienstag J. Indications for use of hepatitis B vaccine, based on cost-effectiveness analysis. N Engl J Med 307:644–652, 1982.

86. Adler MW, Belsey EM, McCutchan JA, et al. Should homosexuals be vaccinated against hepatitis B virus? Cost and benefit assessment. Br Med J (Clin Res Ed) 286:1621–1624, 1983.

87. Alter MA, Favero MS, Francis DP. Cost benefit of vaccination for hepatitis B in hemodialysis centers. J Infect Dis 148:770–771, 1983.

88. Hamilton JD. Hepatitis B virus vaccine: an analysis of its potential use in medical workers. JAMA 250:2145–2150, 1983.

89. Kirkman-Liff B, Dandoy S. Cost of hepatitis B prevention in hospital employees: post-exposure prophylaxis. Infect Control 5:385–389, 1984.

90. Lahaye D, Strauss P, Baleux C, et al. Cost-benefit analysis of hepatitis B vaccination. Lancet 2:441–443, 1987.

91. Hicks RA, Cullen JW, Jackson MA, et al. Hepatitis B virus vaccine: cost–benefit analysis of its use in a children's hospital. Clin Pediatr 28:359–365, 1989.

92. Margolis HS, Schatz GC, Kane MA. Development of recommendations for control of hepatitis B virus infections: the role of cost analysis. Vaccine 8(suppl):S81–S85, 1990.

93. Barboza RF, Rivero D, Echeverria B, et al. Costo beneficio de la vacunación contra la hepatitis B en trabajodores de hospitales de Venezuela. Bol Of Sanit Panam 111:16–23, 1991.

94. Hatziandreu EJ, Hatzakis A, Hatziyannis S, et al. Cost-effectiveness of hepatitis-B vaccine in Greece: a country of intermediate HBV endemicity. Int J Technol Assess Health Care 7:256–262, 1991.

95. Hayashi J, Nakashima K, Noguchi A, et al. Cost effectiveness of intra-dermal vs. subcutaneous hepatitis B vaccination for the mentally handicapped. J Infect 23:39–45, 1991.

96. Jönsson B, Horisberger B, Bruguera M, et al. Cost–benefits analysis of hepatitis-B vaccination: a computerized decision model for Spain. Int J Technol Assess Health Care 7:379–402, 1991.

97. Leonard J, Holtgrave DR, Johnson RP. Cost-effectiveness of hepatitis B screening in a mental health institution. J Fam Pract 32:45–48, 1991.

98. Mauskopf JA, Bradley CJ, French MT. Benefit–cost analysis of hepatitis B vaccine programs for occupationally exposed workers. J Occup Med 33:691–698, 1991.

99. Antoñanzas F, Forcén T, Garuz R. Analysis de coste-efectividad de la vacunacion frente al virus de la hepatitis B [Cost-effectiveness analysis of vaccination against hepatitis B]. Med Clin Barcelona 99:41–46, 1992.

100. Demicheli V, Jefferson TO. Cost–benefit analysis of the introduction of mass vaccination against hepatitis B in Italy. J Public Health Med 14:367–375, 1992.

101. Ginsberg GM, Berger S, Shouval D. Cost–benefit analysis of a nationwide inoculation programme against viral hepatitis B in an area of intermediate endemicity. Bull World Health Organ 70:757–767, 1992.

102. Ginsberg GM, Shouval D. Cost–benefit analysis of a nationwide neonatal inoculation programme against hepatitis B in an area of intermediate endemicity. J Epidemiol Community Health 46:587–594, 1992.

103. Bloom BS, Hillman AL, Fendrick AM, et al. A reappraisal of hepatitis B virus vaccination strategies using cost-effectiveness analysis. Ann Intern Med 118:298–306, 1993.

104. Hall AJ, Roberston RL, Crivelli PE, et al. Cost-effectiveness of hepatitis B vaccine in The Gambia. Trans R Soc Trop Med Hyg 87:333–336, 1993.

105. Krahn M, Detsky AS. Should Canada and the United States universally vaccinate infants against hepatitis B? Med Decis Making 13:4–20, 1993.

106. Oddone EZ, Cowper PA, Hamilton JD, et al. A cost effectiveness analysis of hepatitis B vaccine in predialysis patients. Health Serv Res 28:97–121, 1993.

107. Zhuang GH, Xu HW. The use of decision making analysis for evaluating hepatitis B inoculation strategy [in Chinese]. Chung Hua Yu Fang I Hsueh Tsa Chih 27:69–73, 1993.

108. Aggarwal R, Naik SR. Prevention of hepatitis B infection: the appropriate strategy for India. Natl Med J India 7:216–220, 1994.

109. Bergus G, Meis S. Hepatitis B vaccination: a cost analysis. Iowa Med 85:209–211, 1995.

110. Guillén Grima F, Espín Rios MI. Análisis coste-efectividad de las distinatas alternativas de vacunación frente a la hepatitis B en la región de Murcia [Cost-effectiveness analysis of the different alternatives of universal vaccination against hepatitis B in Murcia]. Med Clin (Barc) 104:130–136, 1995.

111. Kerleau M, Flori YA, Nalpas B, et al. Analyse cout-avantage d'une politique de prevention vaccinale de l'hepatite virale B [Cost-benefit analysis of vaccinal prevention of hepatitis B policy]. Rev Epidemiol Sante Publique 43:48–60, 1995.

112. Liu ZG, Zhao SL, Zhang YX. Cost–benefit analysis on immunization of newborns with hepatitis B vaccine in Jinan City [in Chinese]. Chung Hua Liu Hsing Ping Hsueh Tsa Chih 16:81–84, 1995.

113. Mangtani P, Hall AJ, Normand CEM. Hepatitis B vaccination: the cost effectiveness of alternative strategies in England and Wales. J Epidemiol Community Health 49:238–244, 1995.

114. Margolis HS, Coleman PJ, Brown RE, et al. Prevention of hepatitis B virus transmission by immunization. JAMA 274:1201–1208, 1995.

115. Van Damme P, Tormans G, Beutels P, et al. Hepatitis B prevention in Europe: a preliminary economic evaluation. Vaccine 13(suppl 1):54–57, 1995.

116. Fenn P, Gray A, McGuire A. An economic evaluation of universal vaccination against hepatitis B virus. J Infect 32:197–204, 1996.

117. Wiebe T, Fergusson P, Horne D, et al. Hepatitis B immunization in a low-incidence province of Canada: comparing alternative strategies. Med Decis Making 17:472–482, 1997.

118. Zurn P, Danthine JP. Economic evaluation of various hepatitis B vaccination strategies in Switzerland [in German]. Soz Praventivmed 43(suppl 1):S61–S64, S134–S137, 1998.

119. Harbarth S, Szucs T, Berger K, et al. The economic burden of hepatitis B in Germany. Eur J Epidemiol 16:173–177, 2000.

120. Deuson RR, Brodovicz KG, Barker L, et al. Economic analysis of a child vaccination project among Asian Americans in Philadelphia, Pa. Arch Pediatr Adolesc Med 155:909–914, 2001.

121. Harris A, Yong K, Kermode M. An economic evaluation of universal infant vaccination against hepatitis B virus using a combination vaccine (Hib-HepB): a decision analytic approach to cost effectiveness. Aust N Z J Public Health 25:222–229, 2001.

122. Rose DN, Schechter CB, Sacks HS. Influenza and pneumococcal vaccination of HIV-infected patients: a policy analysis. Am J Med 94:160–168, 1993.

123. Kavet J. Influenza and public policy. Unpublished dissertation, Harvard University, 1972.

124. Kavet J. A perspective on the significance of pandemic influenza. Am J Public Health 67:1063–1070, 1977.

125. Klarman H, Guzick D. Economics of influenza. In Selby P (ed). Influenza: Virus, Vaccine and Strategy. New York, Academic Press, 1976.

126. Schoenbaum S, McNeil N, Kavet J. The swine-influenza decision. N Engl J Med 295:759–765, 1976.

127. Elo O. Cost–benefit studies of vaccinations in Finland. Dev Biol Stand 43:419–428, 1979.

128. Office of Technology Assessment. Cost Effectiveness of Influenza Vaccination. Washington, DC, Office of Technology Assessment, 1981.

129. Riddiough MA, Sisk JE, Bell JC. Influenza vaccination. JAMA 249:3189–3195, 1983.

130. Patriarca PA, Arden NH, Koplan JP, et al. Prevention and control of type A influenza infections in nursing homes: benefits and costs of four approaches using vaccination and amantadine. Ann Intern Med 107:732–740, 1987.

131. Schoenbaum SC. Economic impact of influenza: the individual's perspective. Am J Med 82(6A):26–30, 1987.

132. Maucher JM, Gambert SR. Cost-effective analysis of influenza vaccination in the elderly. Age 13:81–85, 1990.

133. Yassi A, Kettner J, Hammond G, et al. Effectiveness and cost–benefit of an influenza vaccination program for health care workers. Can J Infect Dis 2:101–108, 1991.

134. Mullooly JP, Bennett MD, Hornbrook MC, et al. Influenza vaccination programs for elderly persons: cost-effectiveness in a health maintenance organization. Ann Intern Med 121:947–952, 1994.

135. Nichol KL, Margolis KL, Wuorenma J, et al. The efficacy and cost effectiveness of vaccination against influenza among elderly persons living in the community. N Engl J Med 331:778–784, 1994.

136. Campbell DS, Rumley MH. Cost-effectiveness of the influenza vaccine in a healthy, working-age population. J Occup Envir Med 39:408–414, 1997.

137. Christensen M, Moller LF, Lundstedt C. Influenza vaccination of the elderly in the municipality of Copenhagen [in Danish]. Ugeskr Laeger 160:2530–2533, 1998.

138. Burckel E, Ashraf T, de Sousa Filho JP, et al. Economic impact of providing workplace influenza vaccination: a model and case study application at a Brazilian pharma-chemical company. Pharmacoeconomics 16(5 pt 2):563–576, 1999.

139. Meltzer MI, Cox NJ, Fukuda K. The economic impact of pandemic influenza in the United States: priorities for intervention. Emerg Infect Dis 5:659–671, 1999.

140. Nichol KL, Goodman M. The health and economic benefits of influenza vaccination for healthy and at-risk persons aged 65 to 74 years. Pharmacoeconomics 16(suppl 1):63–71, 1999.

141. White T, Lavoie S, Nettleman MD. Potential cost savings attributable to influenza vaccination of school-aged children. Pediatrics 103:E73, 1999.

142. Bridges CB, Thompson WW, Meltzer MI, et al. Effectiveness and cost–benefit of influenza vaccination of healthy working adults: a randomized controlled trial. JAMA 284:1655–1663, 2000.

143. Cohen GM, Nettleman MD. Economic impact of influenza vaccination in preschool children. Pediatrics 106:973–976, 2000.

144. Fitzner KA, Shortridge KF, McGhee SM, et al. Cost-effectiveness study on influenza prevention in Hong Kong. Health Policy 56:215–234, 2001.

145. Luce BR, Zangwill KM, Palmer CS, et al. Cost-effectiveness analysis of an intranasal influenza vaccine for the prevention of influenza in healthy children. Pediatrics 108:E24, 2001.

146. Nichol KL. Cost–benefit analysis of a strategy to vaccinate healthy working adults against influenza. Arch Intern Med 161:749–759, 2001.

147. Meltzer MI, Dennis DT, Orloski KA. The cost effectiveness of vaccinating against Lyme disease. Emerg Infect Dis 5:321–328, 1999.

148. Shadick NA, Liang MH, Phillips CB, et al. The cost-effectiveness of vaccination against Lyme disease. Arch Intern Med 161:554–561, 2001.

149. Graves PM. Comparison of the cost-effectiveness of vaccines and insecticide impregnation of mosquito nets for the prevention of malaria. Ann Trop Med Parasitol 92:399–410, 1998.

150. Wiedermann G, Ambrosch F. Cost–benefit calculations of vaccinations against measles and mumps in Austria. Dev Biol Stand 43:273–277, 1979.

151. White CC, Koplan JP, Orenstein WA. Benefits, risks, and costs of immunization for measles, mumps, and rubella. Am J Public Health 75:739–744, 1985.

152. Berger SA, Ginsberg GM, Slater PE. Cost–benefit analysis of routine mumps and rubella vaccination for Israeli infants. Isr J Med Sci 26:74–80, 1990.

153. Ferson MJ, Robertson PW, Whybin LR. Cost effectiveness of pre-vaccination screening of health care workers for immunity to measles, rubella, and mumps. Med J Aust 160:478–482, 1994.

154. Hatziandreu EJ, Brown RE, Halpern MT. A Cost–Benefit Analysis of the Measles-Mumps-Rubella (MMR) Vaccine: Final Report. Arlington, VA, Battelle, 1994.

155. Axnick NW, Shavell SM, Witte JJ. Benefits due to immunization against measles. Public Health Rep 84:673–680, 1969.

156. Witte JJ, Axnick NW. The benefits from 10 years of measles immunization in the United States. Public Health Rep 90:205–207, 1975.

157. Albritton RB. Cost–benefits of measles eradication: effects of a federal intervention. Policy Anal 4:1–22, 1978.

158. Ponninghaus J. Cost–benefit analysis of measles immunization: a case-control study from Southern Zambia. J Trop Med Hyg 83:141–149, 1980.

159. World Health Organization, Expanded Programme on Immunization. Cost-effectiveness: Ivory Coast. Wkly Epidemiol Rec 22:170–173, 1982.

160. Davis RM, Markowitz KE, Preblud SR, et al. A cost-effectiveness analysis of measles outbreak control strategies. Am J Epidemiol 126:450–459, 1987.

161. Ginsberg GM, Tulchinsky TH. Costs and benefits of a second measles inoculation of children in Israel, the West Bank, and Gaza. J Epidemiol Community Health 44:274–280, 1990.

162. Mast EE, Berg JL, Hanrahan MS, et al. Risk factors for measles in a previously vaccinated population and cost-effectiveness of revaccination strategies. JAMA 264:2529–2533, 1990.

163. Schlian DM, Matchar D, Seymann GB. Cost-effectiveness evaluation of measles immunization strategies on a college campus. Fam Pract Res J 11:193–207, 1991.

164. Subbarao EK, Amin S, Kumar ML. Prevaccination serologic screening for measles in health care workers. J Infect Dis 163:876–878, 1991.

165. Sellick JA, Longbine D, Schifeling R, et al. Screening hospital employees for measles immunity is more cost effective than blind immunization. Ann Internal Medicine 116(12 pt 1):982–984, 1992.

166. Miller MA, Redd S, Hadler S, et al. A model to estimate the potential economic benefits of measles eradication for the United States. Vaccine 16:1917–1922, 1998.

167. Koplan JP, Preblud SR. A benefit–cost analysis of mumps vaccine. Am J Dis Child 136:362–364, 1982.

168. Arday DR, Kanjarpane DD, Kelley PW. Mumps in the U.S. Army 1980–86: should recruits be immunized? Am J Public Health 79:471–474, 1989.

169. Schoenbaum SC, Hyde JN, Bartoshesky L, et al. Benefit–cost analysis of rubella vaccination policy. N Engl J Med 294:306–310, 1976.

170. Farber ME, Finkelstein SN. A cost–benefit analysis of a mandatory premarital rubella-antibody screening program. N Engl J Med 300:856–859, 1979.

171. Stray-Pedersen B. Economic evaluation of different vaccination programmes to prevent congenital rubella. NIPH Ann (Norway) 5:69–83, 1982.

172. Golden M, Shapiro GL. Cost–benefit analysis of alternative programs of vaccination against rubella in Israel. Public Health (Lond) 98:179–190, 1984.

173. Gudnadottir M. Cost-effectiveness of different strategies for prevention of congenital rubella infection: a practical example from Iceland. Rev Infect Dis 7(suppl):S200–S209, 1985.

174. Kandola K. CRS cost burden analysis for Guyana. In Final Report, Fourteenth Meeting of the English-Speaking Caribbean EPI Managers, Castries, St. Lucia, 18–20 November, 1997. Washington, DC, Pan American Health Organization, 1998.

175. Kommu R, Chase H. Follow-up of rubella issues and costing of CRS in Barbados. In Final Report, Fourteenth Meeting of the English-Speaking Caribbean EPI Managers, Castries, St. Lucia, 18–20 November, 1997. Washington, DC, Pan American Health Organization, 1998.

176. Irons B. Rubella eradication: the countdown begins. West Indian Med J 47:75–76, 1998.

177. Jackson LA, Schuchat A, Gorsky RD, et al. Should college students be vaccinated against meningococcal disease? Am J Public Health 85:843–845, 1995.

178. Miller MA, Wenger J, Rosenstein N, et al. Evaluation of meningococcal meningitis vaccination strategies for the meningitis belt in Africa. Pediatr Infect Dis J 18:1051–1059, 1999.

179. Parent du Chatelet I, Gessner BD, da Silva A. Comparison of cost-effectiveness of preventive and reactive mass immunization campaigns against meningococcal meningitis in West Africa: a theoretical modeling analysis. Vaccine 19:3420–3431, 2001.

180. Skull SA, Butler JR, Robinson P, et al. Should programmes for community-level meningococcal vaccination be considered in Australia? An economic evaluation. Int J Epidemiol 30:571–578; discussion 578–579, 2001.

181. Office of Technology Assessment. A Review of Selected Federal Vaccine and Immunization Policies Based on Case Studies of Pneumococcal Vaccine (Publ No 052-003-00701-1). Washington, DC, Office of Technology Assessment, 1979.

182. Willems JS, Sanders CR, Riddiough MA, et al. Cost-effectiveness of vaccination against pneumococcal pneumonia. N Engl J Med 303:553–559, 1980.

183. Patrick KM, Wooley FR. A cost–benefit analysis of immunization for pneumococcal pneumonia. JAMA 245:473–477, 1981.

184. Office of Technology Assessment. Update of Federal Activities Regarding the Use of Pneumococcal Vaccine (OTA-TM-H-23). Washington, DC, Office of Technology Assessment, 1984.

185. Sisk JE, Riegelman RK. Cost effectiveness of vaccination against pneumococcal pneumonia: an update. Ann Intern Med 104:79–86, 1986.

186. Sisk JE, Moskowitz AJ, Whang W, et al. Cost-effectiveness of vaccination against pneumococcal bacteremia among elderly people. JAMA 278:1333–1339, 1997.

187. Nichol KL, Baken L, Wuorenma J, et al. The health and economic benefits associated with pneumococcal vaccination of elderly persons with chronic lung disease. Arch Intern Med 159:2437–2442, 1999.

188. Stack SJ, Martin DR, Plouffe JF. An emergency department-based pneumococcal vaccination program could save money and lives. Ann Emerg Med 33:299–303, 1999.

189. Ament A, Baltussen R, Duru G, et al. Cost-effectiveness of pneumococcal vaccination of older people: a study in 5 western European countries. Clin Infect Dis 31:444–450, 2000.

190. Black S, Lieu TA, Ray GT, et al. Assessing costs and cost effectiveness of pneumococcal disease and vaccination within Kaiser Permanente. Vaccine 19(suppl 1), S83–S86, 2000.

191. De Graeve D, Verhaegen J, Ament A, et al. [Cost effectiveness of vaccination against pneumococcal bacteremia in the elderly: the results in Belgium]. Acta Clin Belg 55:257–265, 2000.

192. Lieu TA, Ray GT, Black SB, et al. Projected cost-effectiveness of pneumococcal conjugate vaccination of healthy infants and young children. JAMA 283:1460–1468, 2000.

193. Ortqvist A, Jonsson B, Baltussen R, et al. [Vaccination of the elderly against pneumococcal disease is cost-efficient: mass vaccination of all aged 65 and over is recommended]. Lakartidningen 97:5120–5125, 2000.

194. Shann F. Immunization—dramatic new evidence. P N G Med J 43(1-2):24–29, 2000.

195. Vold Pepper P, Owens DK. Cost-effectiveness of the pneumococcal vaccine in the United States Navy and Marine Corps. Clin Infect Dis 30:157–164, 2000.

196. Weycker D, Richardson E, Oster G. Childhood vaccination against pneumococcal otitis media and pneumonia: an analysis of benefits and costs. Am J Manag Care 6(10 suppl):S526–S535, 2000.

197. Mukamel DB, Taffet Gold H, Bennett NM. Cost utility of public clinics to increase pneumococcal vaccines in the elderly. Am J Prev Med 21:29–34, 2001.

198. Postma MJ, Heijnen ML, Jager JC. Cost-effectiveness analysis of pneumococcal vaccination for elderly individuals in The Netherlands. Pharmacoeconomics 19:215–222, 2001.

199. Weisbrod B. Costs and benefits of medical research: a case study of poliomyelitis. J Pol Econ 79:527–544, 1971.

200. Fudenberg HH. Fiscal returns of biomedical research. J Invest Dermatol 61:321–329, 1973.

201. Musgrove P. Is polio eradication in the Americas economically justified? Bull Pan Am Health Organ 22:1–16, 1988.

202. Hatziandreu EJ, Palmer CS, Halpen MT, et al. A Cost-Benefit Analysis of the OPV Vaccine. Arlington, VA, Battelle, 1994.

203. Bart KJ, Foulds J, Patriarca P. Global eradication of poliomyelitis: benefit–cost analysis. Bull World Health Organ 74:35–45, 1996.

204. Miller MA, Sutter RW, Strebel PM, et al. Cost-effectiveness of incorporating inactivated poliovirus vaccine into the routine childhood immunization schedule. JAMA 276:967–971, 1996.

205. Morrison AJ Jr, Hunt EH, Atuk NO, et al. Rabies preexposure prophylaxis using intradermal human diploid cell vaccine: immunologic efficacy and cost-effectiveness in a university medical center and a review of selected literature. Am J Med Sci 293:293–297, 1987.

206. Bernard KW, Fishbein DB. Pre-exposure rabies prophylaxis for travelers: are the benefits worth the cost? Vaccine 9:833–836, 1991.

207. Fishbein DB, Miranda NJ, Merrill P, et al. Rabies control in the Republic of the Philippines: benefits and costs of elimination. Vaccine 9:581–587, 1991.

208. Uhaa IJ, Dato VM, Sorhage FE, et al. Benefits and costs of using an orally absorbed vaccine to control rabies in raccoons. J Am Vet Med Assoc 201:1873–1882, 1992.

209. Kreindel SM, McGuill M, Meltzer M, et al. The cost of rabies post-exposure prophylaxis: one state's experience. Public Health Rep 113:247–251, 1998.

210. Meltzer MI, Rupprecht CE. A review of the economics of the prevention and control of rabies. Part 1: Global impact and rabies in humans. Pharmacoeconomics 14:365–383, 1998.

211. Griffiths RI, Anderson GF, Powe NR, et al. Economic impact of immunization against rotavirus gastroenteritis. Arch Pediatr Adolesc Med 149:407–414, 1995.

212. Smith JC, Haddix AC, Teutsch SM, et al. Cost-effectiveness analysis of a rotavirus immunization program for the United States. Pediatrics 96:609–615, 1995.

213. Takala AK, Koskenniemi E, Joensuu J, et al. Economic evaluation of rotavirus vaccinations in Finland: randomized, double-blind, placebo-controlled trial of tetravalent rhesus rotavirus vaccine. Clin Infect Dis 27:272–282, 1998.

214. Tucker AW, Haddix AC, Bresee JS, et al. Cost-effectiveness analysis of a rotavirus immunization program for the United States. JAMA 279:1371–1376, 1998.

215. Carlin JB, Jackson T, Lane L, et al. Cost effectiveness of rotavirus vaccination in Australia. Aust N Z J Public Health 23:611–616, 1999.

216. Guyatt HL, Evans D. Desirable characteristics of a schistosomiasis vaccine: some implications of a cost effectiveness analysis. Acta Trop 59:197–209, 1995.

217. Preblud SR, Orenstein WA, Koplan JP, et al. A benefit–cost analysis of a childhood varicella vaccination program. Postgrad Med J 61(suppl 4):17–22, 1985.

218. Preblud SR. Varicella: complications and costs. Pediatrics 78:728–735, 1988.

219. Weber DJ, Rutala WA, Parham C. Impact and costs of varicella prevention in a university hospital. Am J Public Health 78:19–23, 1988.

220. Kitai IC, King S, Gafni A. An economic evaluation of varicella vaccine for pediatric liver and kidney transplant recipients. Clin Infect Dis 17:441–447, 1993.

221. Huse DM, Meissner HC, Lacey MJ, et al. Childhood vaccination against chickenpox: an analysis of benefits and costs. J Pediatr 124:869–874, 1994.

222. Lieu TA, Cochi SL, Black SB, et al. Cost-effectiveness of a routine varicella vaccination program for U.S. children. JAMA 271:375–381, 1994.

223. Lieu TA, Black SB, Reiser N, et al. The cost of childhood chickenpox: parents' perspective. Pediatr J Infect Dis 13:173–177, 1994.

224. Ferson MJ. Another vaccine, another treadmill. J Paediatr Child Health 31:3–5, 1995.

225. Lieu TA, Finkler LJ, Sorel ME, et al. Cost-effectiveness of varicella serotesting versus presumptive vaccination of school-age children and adolescents. Pediatrics 95:632–638, 1995.

226. Beutels P, Clara R, Tormans G, et al. Costs and benefits of routine varicella vaccination in German children. J Infect Dis 174(suppl):S335–S341, 1996.

227. Gray AM, Fenn P, Weinberg J, et al. An economic analysis of varicella vaccination for health care workers. Epidemiol Infect 119:209–220, 1997.

228. Nettleman MD, Schmid M. Controlling varicella in the healthcare setting: the cost effectiveness of using varicella vaccine in healthcare workers. Infect Control Hosp Epidemiol 18(7): 504–508, 1997.

229. Strassels SA, Sullivan SD. Clinical and economic considerations of vaccination against varicella. Pharmacotherapy 17:133–139, 1997.

230. Tennenberg AM, Brassard JE, Van Lieu J, et al. Varicella vaccination for healthcare workers at a university hospital: an analysis of costs and benefits. Infect Control Hosp Epidemiol 18:405–411, 1997.

231. Coudeville L, Paree F, Lebrun T, et al. The value of varicella vaccination in healthy children: cost–benefit analysis of the situation in France. Vaccine 17:142–151, 1999.

232. Diez Domingo J, Ridao M, Latour J, et al. A cost–benefit analysis of routine varicella vaccination in Spain. Vaccine 17:1306–1311, 1999.

233. Monath TP, Nasidi A. Should yellow fever vaccine be included in the Expanded Program of Immunization in Africa? A cost effectiveness analysis for Nigeria. Am J Trop Med Hyg 48:274–299, 1993.

234. Stone P, Teutsch S, Chapman RH, et al. Cost-utility analyses of clinical preventive services published ratios, 1976–1997. Am J Prev Med 19:15–23, 2000.

235. Tengs TO, Adams ME, Pliskin JS, et al. Five-hundred life-saving interventions and their cost-effectiveness. Risk Analysis 15:369–390, 1994.

236. Mann JM, Preblud SR, Hoffman RE, et al. Assessing risks of rubella infection during pregnancy: a standardized approach. JAMA 245:1647–1652, 1981.

237. Funkhouser AW, Wassilak SGF, Orenstein WA, et al. Estimated effects of a delay in the recommended vaccination schedule for diphtheria and tetanus toxoids and pertussis vaccines. JAMA 257:1341–1346, 1987.

238. Gray G, Goswani P, Malasig M, et al. Adult adenovirus infections: loss of orphaned vaccines precipitates military respiratory disease epidemics. Clin Infect Dis 31:663–670, 2000.

239. Tangcharoensathien V, Phoolcharoen W, Pitayarangsarit S, et al. The potential demand for an AIDS vaccine in Thailand. Health Policy 57:111–139, 2001.

240. McIntyre P, Forrest J, Heath T, et al. Pertussis vaccines: past, present, and future in Australia. Commun Dis Intell 22:125–132, 1998.

241. Mulholland K, Hilton S, Adegbola R, et al. Randomised trial of *Haemophilus influenzae* type-b tetanus protein conjugate vaccine for prevention of pneumonia and meningitis in Gambian infants. Lancet 349:1191–1197, 1997.

242. Centers for Disease Control and Prevention. Prevention of hepatitis A through active or passive immunization: recommendations of the Advisory Committee on Immunization Practices (ACIP). MMWR 48(RR-12):1–37, 1999.

243. World Health Assembly. 1992 Resolution WHA45.17: WHO Recommendation on Hepatitis B Vaccine, Geneva, World Health Organization, 1992.

244. Beutels P. Economic evaluations applied to HB vaccination: general observations. Vaccine 16(suppl):S84–S92, 1998.

245. Postma MJ, Baltussen RM, Heijnen ML, et al. Pharmacoeconomics of influenza vaccination in the elderly: reviewing the available evidence. Drugs Aging 17:217–227, 2000.

246. Wood SC, Nguyen VH, Schmidt C. Economic evaluations of influenza vaccination in healthy working-age adults: employer and society perspective. Pharmacoeconomics 18:173–183, 2000.

247. Hinman AR, Koplan JP, Orenstein WA, et al. Live or inactivated poliomyelitis vaccine: an analysis of benefits and risks. Am J Public Health 78:291–295, 1988.

248. Centers for Disease Control and Prevention. Public health dispatch: certification of poliomyelitis eradication—European Region, June 2002. MMWR 51:572–574, 2002.

249. Centers for Disease Control and Prevention. Poliomyelitis prevention in the United States: introduction of a sequential vaccination schedule of inactivated poliovirus vaccine followed by oral poliovirus vaccine. Recommendations of the Advisory Committee on Immunization Practices (ACIP). MMWR 46(RR-3):1–25, 1997.

250. Centers for Disease Control and Prevention. Poliomyelitis prevention in the United States: updated recommendations of the Advisory Committee on Immunization Practices (ACIP). MMWR 49(RR-5):1–22, 2000.

251. Omnibus Budget Reconciliation Act of 1987. Pub. L. No. 100-203, § 4071.

252. World Bank. World Development Report 1993: Investing in Health. New York, Oxford University Press, 1993.

253. Miller MA, Flanders WD. A model to estimate the probability of hepatitis B- and *Haemophilus influenzae* type b-vaccine uptake into national vaccination programs. Vaccine 18:2223–2230, 2000.

254. World Bank. World Development Indicators 2001. Washington, DC, World Bank, 2001.

255. Hinman AR. Economic aspects of vaccines and immunizations. Acad Sci Paris Sci Vie 322:989–994, 1999.

256. Hinman AR (ed). Immunization, Equity, and Human Rights: Proceedings of the National Immunization Conference, 2002.

Chapter 58

Vaccines for International Travel

ELIZABETH DAY BARNETT • PHYLLIS E. KOZARSKY •
ROBERT STEFFEN

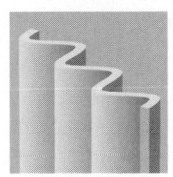

International Travel

International travel increases each year. Individuals travel for many reasons, including tourism, business, educational experiences, and to flee from war, famine, or other intolerable situations. The World Tourism Organization predicts that, by 2020, 1.5 billion tourists will travel internationally each year. Although Europe and the Americas have remained the most popular tourist destinations over the past three decades, Africa, East Asia, and the Pacific regions account for the largest increases in tourist arrivals. By 2005, East Asia and the Pacific may overtake the Americas as the destination with the second largest number of arrivals.[1] Business travelers may number more than 50 million additional departures each year. International migrants consist of more than 120 million refugees, asylum seekers, migrant workers, illegal migrants, and internally displaced persons.[2]

The risk of travelers contracting infectious diseases depends on destination, duration of the trip, and nature and conditions of travel. The vaccine-preventable disease most commonly contracted by travelers is hepatitis A, which may occur as frequently as 20 cases per 1000 travelers per month for travelers who are exposed to conditions of poor hygiene. Diseases for which travelers are at low risk include paralytic polio, estimated to occur at a rate of 20 per million unimmunized travelers (but has not affected any traveler since 1995, probably a benefit of the eradication campaign), and Japanese encephalitis, occurring at an estimated rate of less than 1 per million for the usual traveler.[3] Risk of specific diseases may be increased during periods when outbreaks of disease are occurring, such as with meningococcal disease in sub-Saharan Africa, diphtheria in the newly independent states of the former Soviet Union in the 1990s, and yellow fever during epidemics (the incidence of infection during a recent epidemic in West Africa was 20% to 30% in unimmunized individuals).

Given the growth of international travel, it is likely that many health providers will be called on to offer advice about pretravel immunizations. Although clinics specializing in pretravel advice and immunization are present in many locations, it remains incumbent on primary care providers to be able to provide basic pretravel services and to be able to identify patients in need of specialized advice. Information about disease epidemiology and vaccine characteristics is presented in detail in other chapters. This chapter focuses on disease risk specific to travelers and considerations taken in choosing whether a traveler is a candidate for specific vaccines. Because national standards for licensure differ, not all vaccines are available in all countries. Similarly, vaccines against the same disease and recommended vaccine schedules may differ somewhat by manufacturer and the national authority.

General Information

Approach to Travel Immunizations

The two steps in immunizing travelers are to update routine immunizations and to provide travel-specific immunizations. To do the first, knowledge of a patient's previous immunizations and medical history is necessary. For the second, detailed information about the patient's itinerary, living conditions during the journey, mode of travel (e.g., adventure travel or chaperoned luxury tour) and purpose of travel (e.g., medical or veterinary work, tourism, visiting relatives) is needed. Although sometimes mistakenly regarded as a rote selection of vaccines based on destination country, the choice of vaccines more often requires thoughtful consideration based on details of the patient's medical history, knowledge of vaccine interactions with other vaccines or medications, timing of departure and nature of travel with regard to risk for vaccine-preventable diseases, and patient preferences. Cost is a growing factor in a traveler's decision-making process about which vaccines to receive. Travelers with limited means and incomplete insurance coverage may be forced to make decisions about which family members to protect (often choosing children, leaving adults vulnerable), or may choose, because of cost, to receive yellow fever vaccine alone, because it is required for border crossings in some countries.

Sources of Information on Travel Vaccines

Sources of health information for international travel include (1) *International Travel and Health—Vaccination Requirements and Health Advice*, published annually by the World Health Organization (WHO) in Geneva, Switzerland (phone 41-22-791-21-11 or available via the Internet at *www.who.int/ith*), and (2) *Health Information for International Travel* (Yellow Book), published by the Centers for Disease Control and Prevention (CDC), Atlanta, Georgia. The CDC's information may be ordered from the Public Health Foundation web site at *www.phf.org* and is also available from the CDC hotline (1-404-332-4559), the Internet (*www.cdc.gov*), and the File Transfer Protocol server at *ftp.cdc.gov*. The CDC also publishes the biweekly "Blue Sheets," which provide information about current travel issues. Many countries publish national guidelines regarding travel health information, and readers are encouraged to contact their local and national public health services. Other sources of information are textbooks[4] and review articles.[5–7] Many sites on the Internet provide travel health information for health providers and the public.

Simultaneous Administration of Vaccines and Immune Globulin

Scheduling multiple vaccines for the traveler is challenging, especially when departures are imminent. Few travelers allow as long as a month for vaccines; many come for consultation only a few days before departure. Immunization schedules may need to be accelerated, or vaccines limited to those most appropriate to the infectious disease risks likely to be faced by the traveler. Although many patients as well as providers are concerned about the likelihood of adverse reactions to multiple vaccines administered simultaneously, a current study reported that adverse events were generally minor and not incapacitating and therefore need not be a reason for withholding indicated vaccines.[8]

Most vaccines may be given simultaneously without concern for decreased immunogenicity. Inactivated vaccines can be given concurrently or at any interval before or after other inactivated or live vaccines. Live vaccines should be administered either simultaneously or 30 days apart, with these exceptions: oral poliovirus vaccine (OPV) may be given at any interval before or after parenteral live vaccines; yellow fever vaccine may be given at any interval with respect to monovalent measles vaccine; and Ty21a oral typhoid vaccine may be given simultaneously or at any interval relative to parenteral live vaccines (measles-mumps-rubella [MMR], varicella, yellow fever).

Antibody responses to MMR and varicella vaccines may be impaired if given at the same time as immune globulin. Live virus vaccines should be administered at least 2 weeks before, or at least 3 months after, immune globulin. Immune globulin has not been shown to interfere with responses to polio, yellow fever, or oral typhoid vaccines. When immune globulin is given at the same time as the first dose of hepatitis A vaccine, the proportion of individuals who respond to vaccine is unchanged, but antibody concentrations achieved by vaccine may be lower—but not by an amount considered clinically important. Individuals who receive immune globulin at higher doses may require a greater interval between immune globulin and parenteral live vaccine administration.[9,10]

Immunization of Individuals with Altered Immunocompetence

Detailed recommendations regarding immunization of immune-compromised individuals are published elsewhere.[11] In general, immunocompromised persons should not receive live viral vaccines. Information specific to travel vaccines is presented in the sections on individual vaccines below.

Effect of Antimalarials and Antimicrobial Agents on Vaccine Response

When antimalarials in the chloroquine/mefloquine family are administered simultaneously with human diploid cell rabies vaccine or oral typhoid vaccine, they may interfere with immunogenicity of the vaccines.[12–14] Details of these interactions can be found in the sections devoted to individual vaccines below. Antimicrobial agents taken concurrently with oral typhoid vaccine may interfere with vaccine response.

Routine Childhood Immunizations and Modifications Needed for Travelers

Routine childhood immunizations should be brought up to date as part of preparation for international travel. Information is available from many sources about routine childhood immunizations. In the United States, a schedule is published every 12 months[15] and is available from the National Immunization Program on the Internet at *www.cdc.gov/nip*. Readers are referred to country-specific schedules for this information. Some children will require accelerated schedules because of imminent departure dates or because of delays in receiving routine immunizations. The reader is referred to Chapter 8 for accelerated schedules and to the chapters on individual vaccines for detailed information on indications, contraindications, precautions, and expected adverse events. Children in the United States are immunized routinely against 11 diseases (Table 58–1). Most are prevalent worldwide, though risk of contracting these diseases may vary markedly depending on travel destination. For example, individuals traveling to Asia (between Iraq and Myanmar) and parts of tropical Africa where polio remains endemic are at increased risk of polio, while travelers remaining within the Americas, where polio has been eradicated, are not at increased risk. Risk for tetanus remains constant worldwide, and all adults should receive booster doses of tetanus toxoid every 10 years.

An added challenge has been vaccine shortages necessitating delays in routine immunization or boosters. If possible, vaccines in short supply should be given according to the routine, preshortage, schedule when travel will put the individual at a risk of disease that is greater than that in the nontraveler.

Routine Adult Immunizations

Pretravel consultation is an opportunity to update the immunization status of adults. Information about adult immunization requirements is available from many sources.[16–18] Indications specific to travel are given in sections referring

TABLE 58-1 ■ Vaccinations Recommended Routinely for Children and Adults in the United States with Special Indications for Travelers

Disease	Vaccine	Age Groups	Greatest Areas of Risk	Special Indications
Diphtheria	DTaP or DTP	<7 yr	Developing world, countries of former Soviet Union	
Tetanus	Td	≥7 yr	Worldwide	
	DTaP or DTP	<7 yr		
Pertussis	Td	≥7 yr		
	DTaP or DTP	<7 yr	Worldwide circulation or organism	No vaccine available for ≥7 yr
Polio	IPV	<18 yr and previously unvaccinated adults	Most of developing world except Americas	Extra dose of IPV (if previously fully immunized) for persons traveling to areas of risk
Measles	MMR, MR, or M	All ages for susceptible individuals	Most of the world	Second dose indicated if no prior history of two doses on or after second birthday; most persons born prior to 1957 can be considered immune and do not need vaccination
Mumps	MMR, Mu	All ages for susceptible individuals	Most of the world	
Rubella	MMR or MR, or R	All ages for susceptible individuals	Most of the world	Especially for nonpregnant females of child-bearing age
Haemophilus influenzae type b	Hib	<5 yr	Most of the world	
Hepatitis B	Hep B	Routine childhood and adolescence; older ages with special risk	Most of the world See Figure 58–1 for areas most at risk	Stays of 6 mo or longer in developing countries or with occupational or behavioral risk factors for disease
Pneumococcal	Pneumococcal conjugate	All children 2–23 mo; certain children age 24–59 mo; high-risk groups of older ages	Worldwide	
Varicella	Varicella	All ages for susceptible individuals	Most of the world	
Influenza*	Influenza	1 dose annually in individuals ≥65 yr; also younger special risk groups such as persons with chronic cardiopulmonary disease	Most of the world	Northern Hemisphere season December through March; Southern Hemisphere season April through September
Pneumococcal*	Pneumococcal polysaccharide	All adults ≥65 yr; also younger special risk groups such as persons with chronic cardiopulmonary disease	Most of the world	

*Vaccines routinely indicated for adults.
DTaP, diphtheria and tetanus toxoids and acellular pertussis; DTP, diphtheria and tetanus toxoids and pertussis; Hep B, hepatitis B; Hib, *Haemophilus influenzae* type b; IPV, inactivated poliovirus vaccine; M, measles; MMR, measles-mumps-rubella; MR, measles-rubella; Td, tetanus and diphtheria toxoids; Mu, mumps; R, rubella.

to individual vaccines below. All adults 65 years or older should receive pneumococcal vaccine and annual influenza vaccination. Because influenza seasons vary between northern and southern hemispheres, the recommended time for influenza vaccination depends on itinerary and timing.

Vaccines for Travel

Selected Routine Immunizations Especially Important for Travelers

Diphtheria

Recent epidemics of diphtheria in the newly independent states of the former Soviet Union[19] and in Thailand, Algeria, and Ecuador[20] underscore the need for attention to diphtheria immunization for travelers to these areas and for continuing to provide routine booster doses (supplied as a combination of tetanus-diphtheria toxoids) throughout adulthood. Vitek et al. demonstrated a significant relationship between time since last diphtheria toxoid booster and risk of diphtheria among Russian schoolchildren.[21] Cases of diphtheria have been reported in travelers.[22,23] Migrant populations also may be responsible for transmission of disease into populations in which immunity has waned because of a decrease in natural disease and lack of routine adult vaccine boosters. In the United States, 20% to 60% of adults older than 20 years of age are susceptible to diphtheria,[24,25] and in western Europe serologic surveys have shown immunity to diphtheria to be poor among adults, particularly women; men may be given boosters during military service.[26]

Travel consultation is an opportunity to bring every individual up to date with diphtheria immunization. A booster dose of combined tetanus-diphtheria toxoids every 10 years is recommended in most countries. This immunization does not offer protection against cutaneous diphtheria.

Polio

The program for worldwide polio eradication is proceeding rapidly. The number of countries where polio is endemic has decreased from 125 in 1998 to 10 in 2001.[27] The Western Hemisphere was declared polio free in 1994, and the Western Pacific Region in 2000, and the European region in 2002.[28,29,29a]

Major poliovirus reservoirs remain in the densely populated countries of India, Pakistan, and Nigeria. Maintaining adequate levels of immunization against polio is important for travelers to these areas, and other areas where polio continues to occur. No traveler has been reported to have acquired symptomatic poliomyelitis since 1995, but various cases of importation of the wild virus have been described.

Individuals traveling to areas of the world where polio continues to occur should have their status with regard to polio immunization reviewed. If a full primary series cannot be documented, the series should be completed prior to departure, if possible. In the United States, OPV is no longer recommended or available for routine immunization[30]; other countries may have available both OPV and inactivated poliovirus vaccine (IPV). IPV is indicated for unvaccinated adults; IPV or OPV can be used for children. Children or adults who have been partially immunized may complete the series with either IPV or OPV. If time does not allow for full immunization prior to travel, the interval between doses of vaccine may be shortened to allow the maximal number of doses to be administered prior to departure. If a full series has been completed, a single additional dose of vaccine is indicated. In some countries, a combination tetanus-IPV vaccine is available.

Hepatitis B

Hepatitis B is one of the most common serious vaccine-preventable diseases to affect travelers. Risk is increased with longer length of stay, contact with population groups with high carrier rates of hepatitis B (Fig. 58–1), occupations such as health care workers or laboratory workers, and

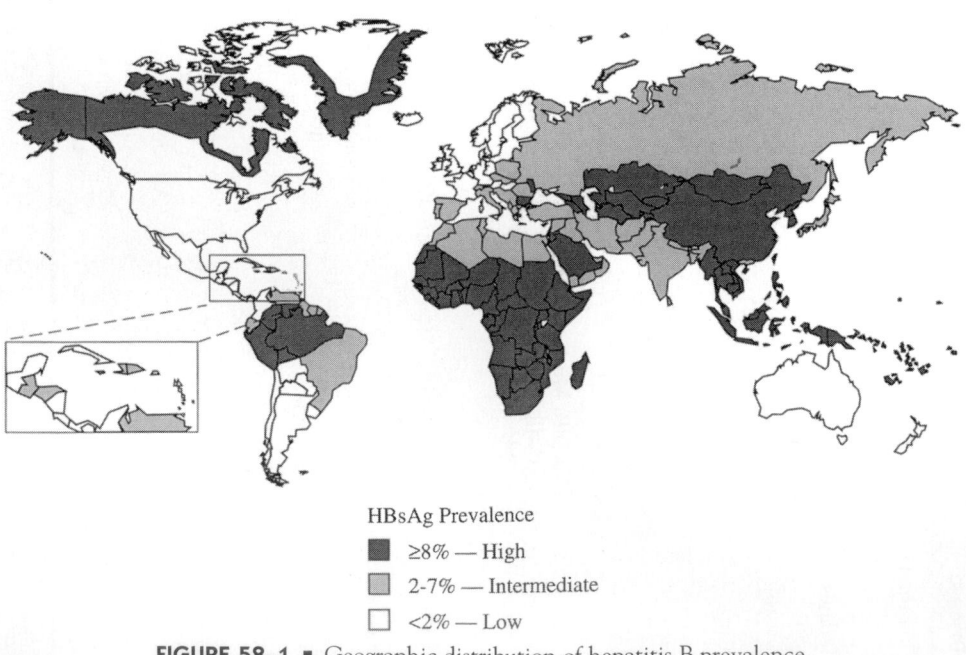

HBsAg Prevalence

■ ≥8% — High
▦ 2-7% — Intermediate
□ <2% — Low

FIGURE 58–1 ■ Geographic distribution of hepatitis B prevalence.

behaviors such as injection drug use and having multiple sex partners. Risk for Swiss tourists traveling to developing countries was 39 per 100,000 travelers for a stay of 1 month.[31] Long-term overseas workers are at greater risk; unimmunized U.S. missionaries serving in Africa had attack rates of 11% during the first 2 years of service and median annual attack rates of 1.2% over the next decade.[32] Professional workers in developing countries had a monthly incidence of symptomatic disease of 20 to 60 per 100,000.[33]

For travelers to countries where hepatitis B is prevalent, the three-dose series of vaccine is recommended for those whose stay will last 6 months or longer or those who have any of the risk factors indicated previously. Although the CDC does not yet recommend hepatitis B vaccine routinely for shorter stay (<6 months) travelers, consideration should be given to administering vaccine to all travelers. The first two doses should be given 4 weeks apart and the third dose 4 to 12 months after the second. If insufficient time is available before departure, rapid seroconversion may be achieved by giving the third dose as early as 4 weeks after the second, with a fourth dose given 12 months from the first to ensure long-term protection. Other accelerated schedules are proposed for hepatitis B and hepatitis A/B combination vaccines, but not all have been approved by the U.S. Food and Drug Administration.

Measles

Although cases of measles in the Americas have declined substantially in the last decade, measles continues to be an important cause of childhood morbidity and mortality worldwide. More than two thirds of cases of measles reported in the United States in 1996 were linked to international sources, primarily in Europe or Asia.[34] In the United States, two doses of vaccine are recommended for all schoolchildren and college students.[35]

Individuals who plan international travel to areas where measles remains prevalent should receive two doses of measles vaccine, preferably supplied as MMR vaccine, beginning at 12 months of age. MMR vaccine can be administered to children 6 to 12 months of age if traveling to areas where they will be at high risk of disease, but this dose of vaccine should not be counted toward the two-dose series. Monovalent measles vaccine may be given if available. Children younger than 6 months are likely to be protected by maternal antibody. Adults born before 1957 are assumed to have natural immunity; those born in 1957 or after without a history of vaccination who are traveling to endemic areas can receive a single dose of MMR vaccine, although two doses at least 1 month apart are preferable. Adults who received a dose in the past should receive a second dose.

Pertussis

Pertussis continues to be a disease of worldwide importance, affecting more than 50 million individuals and resulting in more than 500,000 deaths, despite widespread availability of vaccine.[36] Attack rates of pertussis are related directly to use of vaccine; after decline in use of pertussis vaccines in Japan, Sweden, and Britain, resurgence of disease occurred.[37] Acellular pertussis vaccines, now marketed in many areas, hold promise for equivalent or better efficacy than whole-cell preparations, with fewer side effects.

The increased increment of risk for pertussis as a result of international travel is unknown. Children should complete as much of a primary series as possible, or be given any boosters due,[38] prior to international travel. Although there is substantial interest in protecting adults, currently adults are not candidates for pertussis vaccine.

Influenza

Influenza occurs worldwide; in the tropics transmission occurs throughout the year, whereas peaks of transmission occur from December through March in the northern hemisphere and April through September in the Southern hemisphere. Risk to travelers for contracting influenza is increased by travel to the tropics, travel to a destination during influenza season, and participation in large organized tourist groups.[39] Risk for serious disease depends on underlying health status. Individuals at increased risk of influenza are candidates for the current season's influenza vaccine, especially if at increased risk for complications. Vaccine may not be available in the traveler's country of origin at the time of travel to a high-risk destination. In these cases, education about the risk of influenza and management of respiratory and influenza-like illness is important.

Additional Travel Vaccines

Bacille Calmette-Guérin

Bacille Calmette-Guérin (BCG) vaccines are available in many countries but vary in efficacy. In the United States, a program of surveillance using tuberculin skin testing and early identification and treatment of infected individuals is preferred over universal immunization with BCG.[40]

Estimates of risk for tuberculosis (TB) among travelers are difficult to obtain. Studies of military personnel who served during the war in Vietnam cite skin test conversion rates of 4.7%, compared with rates of 1% per year for Army personnel who remained in the United States.[41] Risk to travelers is not thought to be high enough to warrant routine immunization for travel. For the rare circumstance in which BCG is indicated in the United States (a young child living in a household where exposure to active TB is unavoidable and where other preventive measures have failed or cannot be implemented), vaccine is available from Organon, Inc. (West Orange, NJ). Because the protective effect of BCG has been confirmed mainly in children, there are hardly any indications for BCG for adults who are traveling.

BCG continues to be used in most countries of the world. Health care providers may be asked to provide BCG immunization to individuals who will be living for extended periods of time where BCG vaccine is used routinely. Risk of disease must be weighed against loss of ability to test for infection using tuberculin skin testing. BCG might be considered for long-term residents of areas where the incidence of disease is high (more than 30 to 40 per 100,000) and where occupation or living conditions may result in significant exposures to infected individuals.

Side effects to vaccine occur in up to 10% of individuals and usually consist of local ulceration and inflammatory adenitis. BCG vaccine is contraindicated in immunocompromised individuals because of risk of dissemination of infection. Decisions to immunize human immunodeficiency virus (HIV)–infected but immunocompetent individuals are controversial; the bacteria are able to remain dormant for years and cause disease if an individual becomes immunocompromised. Risk of infection with TB, such as in infants in developing countries with high rates of TB, must be weighed against the risk of vaccination for those who may be at risk for HIV infection. The WHO continues to recommend universal immunization with BCG for infants in areas where risk of TB is substantial.

Cholera

The risk of cholera is low for travelers. Attack rates are estimated to be 1 in 500,000 travelers, though higher rates (5 per 100,000) have been reported from Japan, where routine screening for cholera is carried out in returning travelers with diarrhea.[42] The mainstay of protection against cholera remains avoidance of ingestion of high-risk foods, such as raw shellfish, and the use of precautions when making other food selections. Unchlorinated water is also a common source of infection.

Cholera occurring in the world today is due to *Vibrio cholerae* serogroup O1 or O139. There are no cholera vaccines currently licensed or available in the United States, though oral vaccines are licensed in Europe and elsewhere, and are likely to become more widely available.[43] Cholera vaccine is not recommended routinely for travelers. For the rare individual traveling to areas of high risk and poor sanitary conditions (e.g., relief workers in the midst of cholera outbreaks), vaccine may be offered if available. Food and water precautions are the mainstay of prevention of cholera, and appropriate rehydration therapy is the mainstay of treatment.

According to WHO recommendations, currently no country should require cholera immunization for entry, although Palau and Sudan do so after transiting infected areas in the previous 6 days (as of April 2002). Occasionally travelers will report that they have been required to provide documentation of cholera immunization to obtain a visa despite these recommendations. If travelers are adamant about being immunized, a single dose of vaccine documented on the International Certificate of Immunization is usually sufficient to satisfy authorities in these circumstances.

Oral cholera vaccine schedules are listed in Table 58–2. Mild gastrointestinal side effects have been observed. The major disadvantage of the inactivated vaccine is the need for two to three doses; the live vaccine may achieve protective immunity more rapidly.[43] Immunization is not recommended during pregnancy; specific safety information about the use of this vaccine during pregnancy is not available.

Oral cholera vaccines may be given concurrently with yellow fever vaccine, oral typhoid Ty21a vaccine, and OPV.[44] Immunization with cholera vaccine should be completed before initiating malaria prophylaxis with chloroquine or mefloquine because of potential for these antimalarials to affect adversely immune response to vaccine.[45]

Hepatitis A

Hepatitis A is the most common vaccine-preventable disease to affect travelers. It may occur as much as 10 to 100 times as often as typhoid in unprotected American and European tourists who visit countries or areas of countries with poor hygienic conditions. Risk has been estimated to range from 3 to 109 per 1000 over 2 weeks to 1 month for unimmunized short-term travelers to areas with high risk for hepatitis A.[46] For unimmunized long-term travelers such as missionaries, attack rates were as high as 28% during the first 2 years of service.[32] Risk for disease depends on length of stay and conditions of travel, including frequency of exposure to contaminated food and water. Figure 58–2 shows the geographic distribution of risk for hepatitis A. Cases of hepatitis A, however, have been reported in tourists staying in luxury accommodations in countries where the risk of hepatitis A is high.[47] Despite availability of both immune globulin and an effective vaccine, many travelers are not protected against hepatitis A.

Individuals born in Europe or North America since World War II have a low prevalence of immunity to hepatitis A. Rates of immunity are higher with increased age, history of jaundice, and birth or residence outside the United States. As many as 95% of individuals born and raised in developing countries with patterns of high endemicity for hepatitis A may be protected by naturally acquired antibody.[48]

Options for immunoprophylaxis of hepatitis A include intramuscular immune globulin and hepatitis A vaccine. Immune globulin was the mainstay of protection for many years and is 85% to 90% protective. The major disadvantage of immune globulin is that it is short acting and must be repeated for subsequent journeys, or additional doses must be given during prolonged residence in endemic areas. It does not offer effective protection against hepatitis B, C, or E. Adverse events are rare, although the large volume required may result in local discomfort. One advantage of this preparation is that it may be given immediately before departure. Recently, immune globulin has become unavailable in some countries because of concern about theoretical risk of transmission of variant Creutzfeldt-Jacob disease.[49] Hepatitis A vaccines have been marketed in Europe since 1992 and in the United States since 1995. Four products—Havrix

TABLE 58–2 ■ Recommended Doses and Schedules for Cholera Vaccines

Vaccine	Dose	No. of Doses	Schedule	Booster
Live oral cholera vaccine (Orochol®, Mutachol®)	1 sachet (1×10^8 CFU)	1	—	? 2 yr
Inactivated oral vaccine (Dukoral®, Colorvac®)	1 mg cholera toxin and 10^{11} whole cells of several cholera strains	2	0, 7–14 days	10 mo to 2 yr

CFU, colony-forming unit.

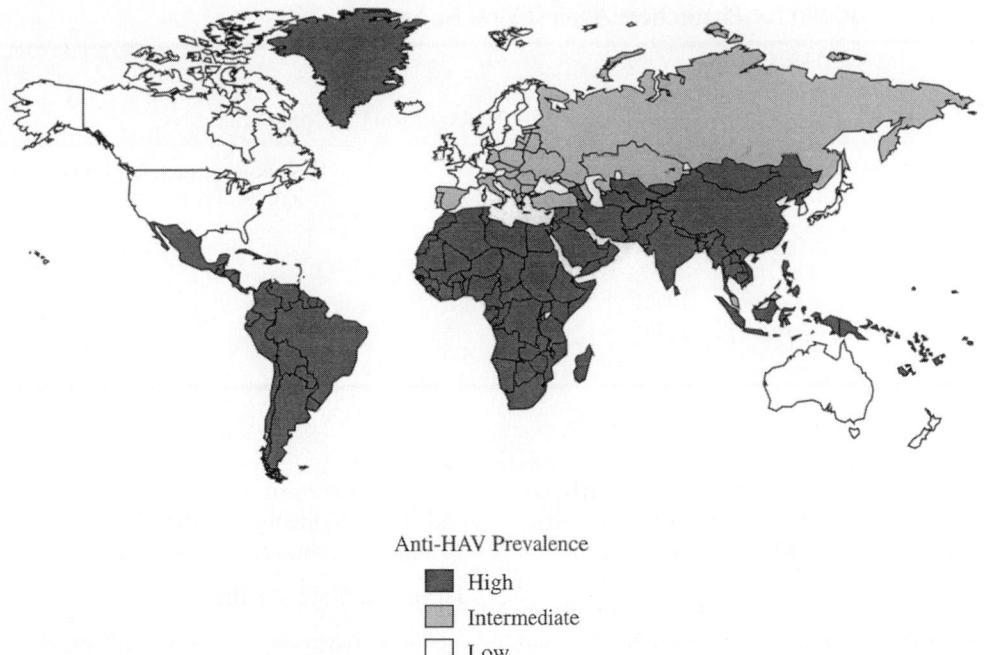

Anti-HAV Prevalence

■ High
▨ Intermediate
☐ Low

FIGURE 58–2 ■ Geographic distribution of hepatitis A prevalence. *Note:* This map generalizes available data and patterns may vary within countries.

(GlaxoSmithKline), Epaxal (Berna Biotech) VAQTA (Merck), and AVAXIM (Pasteur Mérieux Connaught)—are now available, although the Epaxal and AVAXIM are not licensed in the United States as of January 2003. A combined hepatitis A and B vaccine (Twinrix; GlaxoSmithKline) is also marketed in North America, Europe, and some other countries. The four monovalent hepatitis A vaccines are highly immunogenic in adults, with protective antibody levels achieved in 95% to 100% of adults 1 month after the first injection, using recommended adult doses of Havrix (1440 enzyme-linked immunosorbent assay [ELISA] units [EL.U.] in 1.0 mL), VAQTA (50 units in 1.0 mL), or AVAXIM (160 units in 0.6 mL). It should be noted that, because no international standardized reference exists for hepatitis A antigen content, each laboratory has expressed the antigen content using an in-house reference. One month after the booster dose, given at 6 to 12 months, seroconversion rates of 100% were reported with all three vaccines.[50,51] Of importance for travelers with imminent departures, seroconversion rates of 87.1% (Havrix, 1440 EL.U.) and 95.7% (AVAXIM) were reported at 14 days in a comparative trial.[52] Combination hepatitis A and B vaccine demonstrated immunogenicity comparable to that of the monovalent vaccines.[53] Efficacy studies performed in Thailand (Havrix) and during a hepatitis A epidemic in the United States (VAQTA) demonstrated clinical efficacy of 94% and 100%, respectively. Havrix and VAQTA also have a pediatric formulation for children 2 to 17 years (720 EL.U. and 25 units, respectively). Similar protective levels of antibody have been reported in children as in adults.[54]

Individuals traveling to areas of intermediate or high endemicity are candidates for protection against hepatitis A. Ideally vaccine should be given at least 4 weeks prior to initiation of travel because of the concern that neutralizing antibody is not optimal prior to this time. Travelers with earlier departure dates may receive, in addition to vaccine, an appropriate dose of immune globulin at a separate site. Some experts believe that travelers would benefit from vaccine given up till the date of departure, a strategy especially helpful in areas where immune globulin is unavailable. A booster dose 6 to 12 months after the initial dose is expected to provide long-term (at least 20 years) protection.[55] Booster doses may be from the same or a different manufacturer, or may be the A/B combination vaccine, without adverse effect on reactogenicity or immunogenicity.[56] Doses and schedules for administration of immune globulin and hepatitis A vaccines are listed in Tables 58–3 and 58–4, respectively.

Hepatitis A vaccine generally is well tolerated. The most common vaccine side effects include soreness at the injection site, headache, and malaise. Serious adverse events appear to be rare. Vaccine should not be given to individuals with allergies to adjuvants or preservatives contained in the vaccine. Although risk from vaccination during pregnancy should be low, risk of disease must be weighed against theoretical risk of immunization. Hepatitis A vaccines are inactivated and therefore may be used in immunocompromised individuals. Simultaneous administration of hepatitis A vaccine and diphtheria, oral and inactivated poliovirus, tetanus, oral typhoid, cholera, Japanese encephalitis, rabies, or yellow fever vaccines does not impair immune response to either vaccine or increase adverse events.[57]

Children younger than 2 years should receive immune globulin alone because safety and efficacy of vaccine have not been evaluated adequately in this age group. Doses of immune globulin may be given as close as possible to departure date; dose depends on weight and length of stay. Doses of immune globulin are listed in Table 58–3. Serious adverse events following immune globulin are rare, although anaphylaxis has been reported in immunoglobulin A–deficient individuals; immune globulin should not be used in these individuals.

Immune globulin may interfere with response to certain live virus vaccines, such as measles, mumps, rubella, and

TABLE 58-3 ■ Immune Globulin for Protection Against Viral Hepatitis A

| Length of Stay | Body Weight | | Dose Volume† (mL) | Comments |
	lb	kg*		
Short-term travel (<3 mo)	<50	<23	0.5	Dose volume depends on body weight and length of stay
	50–100	23–45	1.0	
	>100	>45	2.0	
Long-term travel (3–5 mo)	<22	<10	0.5	
	22–49	10–22	1.0	
	50–100	23–45	2.5	
	>100	>45	5.0	

*One kilogram = approximately 2.2 lb.
†For intramuscular injection.

varicella. It has been shown not to interfere with the immune response to oral polio, oral typhoid, or yellow fever vaccines. If travelers require both MMR or varicella vaccine and immune globulin, the vaccines ideally should be given 2 weeks prior to giving immune globulin. If immune globulin for hepatitis A has been given, subsequent immunization with MMR or varicella vaccine should be delayed at least 3 months.[9] If MMR or varicella vaccines and immune globulin must be given closer than 2 weeks apart, the MMR and varicella vaccine doses should be repeated 3 or more months after immune globulin unless serologic testing shows that antibodies to vaccine were produced.

Testing for susceptibility to hepatitis A before offering vaccine or immune globulin may be cost-effective in specific situations. Candidates for testing may include individuals born and raised in high-endemicity areas and those with a history of jaundice. Other considerations include cost of testing compared with cost of immunization and assuring that testing will not delay ability to provide immunization if an individual is seronegative. It is estimated that,

if cost of screening is one third the cost of immunization, and the individual's likelihood of immunity is greater than 33%, testing should be cost-effective.[58]

Japanese Encephalitis

Japanese encephalitis is a leading cause of viral encephalitis in Asia and is transmitted by mosquitoes. Japanese encephalitis now has spread to regions of Asia where it had not been reported previously; an outbreak was reported in 1995 on an island in the Torres Strait north of the Australian mainland.[59] Risk to travelers is low, with estimates of risk ranging from less than 1 per million in civilian travelers to 1 in 5000 per month of exposure in the military or in the local population in rural endemic areas. Most travelers have no natural immunity to the disease. Although risk is highest for individuals who travel during the season of high transmission and remain in endemic areas for extended periods, cases have occurred in short-stay tourists.[60,61] Detailed information about the risk of Japanese encephalitis by country, region, and season is listed in Table 58-5.

TABLE 58-4 ■ Recommended Doses and Schedules for VAQTA, AVAXIM, Havrix, Epaxal, and Twinrix

Group	Age (yr)	Dose	Volume (mL)	No. of Doses	Schedule (mo)*
VAQTA†					
Children and adolescents	2–17	25 U	0.5	2	0, 6–18
Adults	≥18	50 U	1.0	2	0, 6
AVAXIM‡					
Adults	≥16	160 U	0.5	2	0, 6–18
Havrix§					
Children and adolescents‖	2–18	720 EL.U.	0.5	2	0, 6–12
Adults	>18	1440 EL.U.	1.0	2	0, 6–12
Epaxal¶					
Children and adults	≥2	500 RIA U	0.5	2	0, 6–12
Twinrix**					
Adults	>18	720 EL.U./20 µg hepatitis B surface antigen	1.0	3	0, 1, 6

*Zero (0) months represents timing of the initial dose; subsequent numbers represent months after the initial dose.
†Hepatitis A vaccine, inactivated (Merck & Co, Inc.).
‡Hepatitis A vaccine (Pasteur Mérieux Connaught).
§Hepatitis A vaccine, inactivated (GlaxoSmithKline).
‖An alternate formulation and schedule (three doses) is available for children and adolescents and consists of 360 EL.U./0.5-mL dose at 0, 1, and 6 to 12 months of age.
¶Hepatatis A vaccine, inactivated (Berna Biotech Ltd.).
**Hepatitis A, inactivated, and hepatitis B, recombinant (GlaxoSmithkline).
EL.U., enzyme-linked immunosorbent assay (ELISA) unit; RIA U, radioimmunoassay unit; U, unit.

TABLE 58–5 ■ **Risk of Japanese Encephalitis, by Country, Region, and Season***

Country	Affected Areas	Transmission Season	Comments
Australia	Islands of Torres Strait	Probably year-round transmission risk	Localized outbreak in Torres Strait in 1995 and sporadic cases in 1998 in Torres Strait and on mainland Australia at Cape York Peninsula
Bangladesh	Few data, but probably widespread	Possibly July to December, as in northern India	Outbreak reported from Tangail District, Dacca Division; sporadic cases in Rajshahi Division
Bhutan	No data	No data	
Brunei	Presumed to be sporadic-endemic as in Malaysia	Presumed year-round transmission	
Burma (Myanmar)	Presumed to be endemic-hyperendemic	Presumed to be May to October	Repeated outbreaks in Shan State in Chiang Mai valley
Cambodia	Presumed to be endemic-hyperendemic countrywide	Presumed to be May to October	Cases reported from refugee camps on Thai border
India	Reported cases from all states except Arunachal, Dadra, Daman, Diu, Gujarat, Himachal, Jammu, Kashmir, Lakshadweep, Meghalaya, Nagar Haveli, Orissa, Punjab, Rajasthan, and Sikkim	South India: May to October in Goa; October to January in Tamil Nadu; and August to December in Karnataka. Second peak, April to June in Mandya District Andrha Pradesh: September to December North India: July to December	Outbreaks in West Bengal, Bihar, Karnataka, Tamil Nadu, Andrha Pradesh, Assam, Uttar Pradesh, Manipur, and Goa Urban cases reported (e.g., Luchnow)
Indonesia	Kalimantan, Bali, Nusa, Tenggara, Sulawesi, Mollucas, and Irian Jaya (Papua), and Lombok	Probably year-round risk; varies by island. Peak risks associated with rainfall, rice cultivation, and presence of pigs. Peak periods of risk: November to March; June and July in some years.	Human cases recognized on Bali, Java, and possibly in Lombok
Japan[†]	Rare-sporadic cases on all islands except Hokkaido	June to September, except April to December on Ryuku Islands (Okinawa)	Vaccine not routinely recommended for travel to Tokyo and other major cities Enzootic transmission without human cases observed on Hokkaido
Korea	North Korea: no data South Korea: sporadic-endemic with occasional outbreaks	July to October	Last major outbreaks in 1982 and 1983. Sporadic cases reported in 1994 and 1998.
Laos	Presumed to be endemic-hyperendemic countrywide	Presumed to be May to October	
Malaysia	Sporadic-endemic in all states of Peninsula, Sarawak, and probably Sabah	Year-round transmission	Most cases from Penang, Perak, Salangor, Johore, and Sarawak
Nepal	Hyperendemic in southern lowlands (Terai)	July to December	Vaccine not recommended for travelers visiting only high-altitude areas
Pakistan	May be transmitted in central deltas	Presumed to be June to January	Cases reported near Karachi; endemic areas overlap those for West Nile virus. Lower Indus Valley might be an endemic area.
Papua New Guinea	Normanby Islands and Western Province	Probably year-round risk	Localized sporadic cases
People's Republic of China	Cases in all provinces except Xizang (Tibet), Xinjiang, Qinghai. Hyperendemic in southern China.	Northern China: May to September	Vaccine not routinely recommended for travelers to urban areas only.

Continued

TABLE 58–5 ■ Risk of Japanese Encephalitis, by Country, Region, and Season*—cont'd

Country	Affected Areas	Transmission Season	Comments
		Southern China: April to October (Guangxi, Yunnan, Guangdong, and Southern Fujian, Sichuan, Guizhou, Hunan, and Jiangxi provinces)	
	Endemic–periodically epidemic in temperate areas		
	Hong Kong: Rare cases in new territories	Hong Kong: April to October	
	Taiwan: Endemic, sporadic cases; islandwide†	Taiwan: April to October, with a June peak†	Taiwan: Cases reported in and around Taipei and the Kaohsiung–Pingtung river basins†
Philippines	Presumed to be endemic on all islands	Uncertain; speculations based on locations and agroecosystems	Outbreaks described in Nueva Ecija, Luzon, and Manila
		West Luzon, Mindoro, Negros, Palawan: April to November	
		Elsewhere: year-round, with greatest risk April to January	
Russia	Far Eastern maritime areas south of Khabarousk	Peak period July to September	First human cases in 30 yr recently reported
Singapore	Rare cases	Year-round transmission, with April peak	Vaccine not routinely recommended
Sri Lanka	Endemic in all but mountainous areas	October to January; secondary peak of enzootic transmission May to June	Recent outbreaks in central (Anuradhapura) and northwestern provinces
	Periodically epidemic in northern and central provinces		
Thailand	Hyperendemic in north; sporadic-endemic in south	May to October	Annual outbreaks in Chiang Mai valley; sporadic cases in Bangkok suburbs
Vietnam	Endemic-hyperendemic in all provinces	May to October	Highest rates in and near Hanoi
Western Pacific	Two epidemics reported in Guam & Saipan since 1947	Uncertain; possibly September to January	Enzootic cycle might not be sustainable; epidemics might follow introductions of virus

*Assessments are based on publications, surveillance reports, and personal correspondence. Extrapolations have been made from available data. Transmission patterns can change.

†Local incidence rates might not accurately reflect risks to nonimmune visitors because of high immunization rates in local populations. Humans are incidental to the transmission cycle. High levels of viral transmission can occur in the absence of human disease.

Japanese encephalitis vaccine has been licensed in Japan since 1954, has been available in the United States since 1992, and is available in many countries.[62] Mild local effects such as tenderness, swelling, and redness have been reported in about 20% of vaccines, and systemic side effects in about 10%.[62] Severe adverse reactions to JE vaccine are rare. Neurologic events, including acute disseminated encephalomyelitis, have been reported, both in Japanese children receiving routine immunization and in adults receiving travel immunizations.[63,64] Severe neurologic events occurred at a rate of 1–2.3 per million vaccinees during an 8-year period of surveillance in Japan (1965–1973).[65] A new pattern of adverse events occurring primarily in travelers has been reported since 1989. These events included generalized urticaria and angioedema, but not anaphylaxis, occurring within minutes to as long as 2 weeks after immunization. Some of these events may have occurred in individuals sensitized to gelatin, as has been shown in Japanese children.[69] Surveillance of Danish vaccinees between 1983 and 1995 identified a rate of 1–17 cases per 10,000 vaccine recipients.[66] In the United States, the rate of urticaria or angioedema was 6.3 cases/100,000 doses distributed.[67]

The delayed nature of mucocutaneous reactions to Japanese encephalitis vaccine is of particular concern to travel medicine providers. After a first vaccine dose, reactions occurred a median of 12 hours after immunization; 88% of reactions occurred within 3 days. The interval between a second dose and onset of symptoms was longer, with a median of 3 days, and extending to 2 weeks. Reactions have occurred after a second or third dose, even when earlier doses have been uneventful. Vaccinees should be observed for 30 minutes following immunizations and instructed about the possibility of these reactions; individuals with a previous history of urticaria may be at increased risk.

TABLE 58–6 ■ Japanese Encephalitis Vaccine Schedule

	Dose (Subcutaneous Route)		
Schedule	1–2 yr of Age	3 yr of Age or Older	Comments
Primary series 1, 2, and 3	0.5 mL	1.0 mL	Days 0, 7, and 30
Booster*	0.5 mL	1.0 mL	1 dose at 24 mo or later

*In vaccinees who have completed a three-dose primary series, the full duration of protection is unknown; therefore, definitive recommendations cannot be given.

Vaccine is most appropriate for individuals who will spend a month or longer in endemic areas, especially in rural areas during transmission season. Other travelers, such as those traveling to endemic areas during epidemic transmission or those whose occupation or living conditions will place them at increased risk of exposure, may be candidates for vaccine even if traveling for less than 1 month. Risk of disease must be weighed against risk of severe adverse events resulting from vaccine.[68] Protective measures for individuals who are not immunized include prevention of mosquito bites through the use of window screens, bed nets, and insect repellents.

The primary series of Japanese encephalitis vaccine results in optimal immune response if given in three doses on days 0, 7, and 30 (Table 58–6). Time constraints may require abbreviated schedules of three doses on days 0, 7, and 14 or two doses on days 0 and 7; however, antibody response may be less. Ideally, the third dose of vaccine should be given at least 10 days before commencement of travel to ensure optimal antibody response and to allow access to medical care should an adverse event occur. Children 1 to 2 years of age should receive half the adult dose of vaccine given to individuals 3 years of age and older. Data are unavailable about safety and efficacy of vaccine in children less than 1 year of age; when possible, immunization should be deferred during the first year of life. Duration of immunity is unknown; at this time, booster doses are recommended after 3 years based on preliminary serologic data. Immunization during pregnancy is not recommended generally; no specific information is available about the safety and efficacy of the vaccine during pregnancy. Little information is available about immunization of immunocompromised individuals; a small study of such children did not reveal adverse outcomes or compromise of immune response.[70] Data regarding concurrent administration with diphtheria, tetanus, and pertussis vaccines suggest lack of compromise of immunogenicity or safety; concurrent administration with other vaccines or medications, such as antimalarials, has not been studied. Individuals receiving Japanese encephalitis vaccine should continue to receive other vaccines and antimalarials as appropriate for their destinations.

Meningococcus

Invasive meningococcal disease occurs worldwide, but major epidemics occur more frequently in the meningitis belt of sub-Saharan Africa (Fig. 58–3). International travelers may acquire the disease, or may become colonized with epidemic strains of meningococcus and spread the disease to other parts of the world. Disease resulting from *Neisseria meningitidis* infection is caused most often by one of the five serogroups A, B, C, Y, and W135. Serogroups C, B, and Y are predominant in

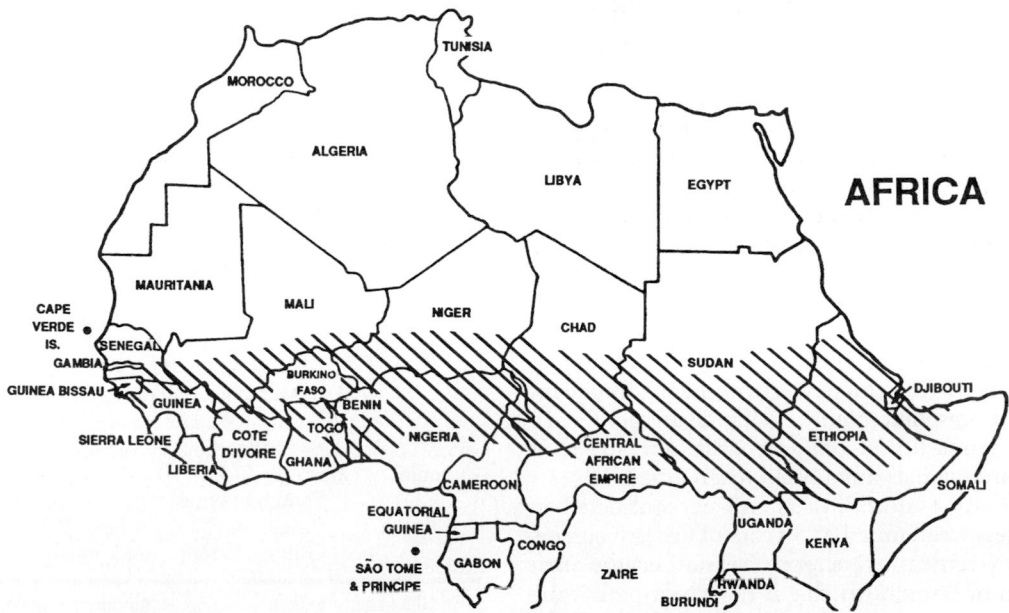

FIGURE 58–3 ■ Areas with frequent epidemics of meningococcal meningitis.

the Americas and Europe. Serogroup A predominates in sub-Saharan Africa, but in the 1990s the proportion of cases caused by serogroup W135 increased significantly.[71]

Risk to travelers of acquiring invasive meningococcal disease is low, estimated to be 0.4 per million travelers per month for a stay in a developing country, and up to 2000 per million in pilgrims to Mecca.[72] Outbreaks have occurred involving travelers, and travelers have become carriers of disease. American pilgrims who returned from Mecca, Saudi Arabia, following an epidemic of group A meningococcal diseases in 1987 were more than 11 times as likely to carry the organism back to their home countries as travelers returning from other parts of Saudi Arabia.[73] In 2000 and 2001, outbreaks of meningitis caused by serogroup W135 among Hajj pilgrims and their contacts occurred in more than 10 countries.[74,75] Since 1987, Saudi Arabian health authorities have required immunization against meningococcus for pilgrims attending the Hajj. Until 2002, divalent serogroup A and C vaccine was sufficient; because of outbreaks of disease caused by serogroup W135, the policy was changed for the 2002 Hajj season to require immunization with quadrivalent vaccine (A, C, Y, and W135). Other individuals traveling to countries within the meningitis belt of sub-Saharan Africa and who will have contact with the local population (individuals visiting friends and relatives, health care workers, and long-term travelers such as missionaries and volunteer workers) are at higher risk and may benefit from immunization. Other vaccine candidates include individuals at increased risk of contracting meningococcal disease, such as those with functional or anatomic asplenia. Individuals who will travel to these areas and stay in tourist accommodations with little contact with the local population are at low risk and may elect not to be immunized. Immunization should be carried out, if possible, at least 10 to 14 days in advance of travel.[76]

Currently available meningococcal polysaccharide vaccine in the United States contains the four serogroups A, C, Y, and W135. In other countries, bivalent A and C vaccines as well as the quadrivalent vaccine are available. Response to serogroups A and C polysaccharides is suboptimal in children less than 2 years of age, though children as young as 3 months of age may have some response to group A polysaccharide. Response to serogroups Y and W135 polysaccharides is adequate in children 2 years of age or older, although clinical protection has not been documented.[77] In some countries in North America and Europe, conjugate serogroup C vaccines have been licensed and have been used with success to reduce meningococcal disease in infants and young children. Polysaccharide of serogroup B is a poor antigen, and vaccines derived from this antigen have not proven consistently effective. Conjugate vaccines containing multiple serogroups, now under development, may offer the additional benefit of greater efficacy in infants, as well as greater efficacy in those with underlying health problems affecting ability to respond to polysaccharide antigens.[78]

Duration of immunity of polysaccharide vaccine is at least 3 years in individuals immunized when at least 4 years of age. Revaccination after 3 years can be considered in children who were immunized at 4 years of age or younger, especially if they remain at risk for disease. Because antibody titers decline rapidly in the 2 to 3 years following immunization, revaccination also may be considered for older children and adults within 3 to 5 years of the initial vaccination if they are at continued risk.

Safety of meningococcal polysaccharide vaccine during pregnancy has not been established. When considering immunization during pregnancy, the theoretical risk of immunization must be balanced against the risk of disease.

Rabies

Human rabies deaths exceed 50,000 cases per year, with more than 95% occurring in areas where canine rabies is endemic.[79] Over 1 million individuals receive rabies postexposure prophylaxis each year. The risk of rabies to travelers depends on destination, exposure to animals (especially dogs), and length of stay. An airport survey of travelers who spent an average of 17 days in Thailand showed that 1.3% had experienced a possible rabies exposure (bite, lick, or scratch from a mammal).[80] Long-stay travelers and expatriates have an incidence of animal bites reported to be as high as 18.2 per 1000 person-years.[81] Rates of human rabies are highest in Asia, parts of Central and South America, and Africa.[82] Areas of the world that are reported to be rabies free are listed in Table 58–7. Travelers should be informed about the risk of rabies in the region to which they will travel and be advised to avoid contact with animals that could be rabies carriers, especially dogs but also cats, skunks, raccoons, and bats.

Three inactivated rabies vaccines are licensed for use in the United States, with others available worldwide. Rabies immunoglobulin preparations provide passive immune pro-

TABLE 58–7 ■ Countries and Political Units Reporting No Cases of Rabies During 1997 and 1998[*]

Region	Countries
Africa	Cape Verde, Libya, Mauritius, Réunion, and Seychelles
Americas	**North:** Bermuda; St. Pierre and Miquelon **Caribbean:** Antigua and Barbuda, Aruba, Bahamas, Barbados, Cayman Islands, Guadeloupe, Jamaica, Martinique, Montserrat, Netherlands Antilles (Bonaire, Curaçao, Saba, Saint Maarten, and Saint Eustatius), Saint Kitts (Saint Christopher) and Nevis, Saint Lucia, Saint Martin, Saint Vincent and Grenadines, and Virgin Islands (U.K. and U.S.) **South:** Uruguay
Asia	Armenia, Bahrain, Brunei, Cyprus, Hong Kong, Japan, Kuwait, Malaysia (Sabah and Sarawak), Maldives, Qatar, Singapore, Taiwan, and United Arab Emirates
Europe	Albania, Andorra, Faroe Islands, Finland, Gibraltar, Greece, Iceland, Ireland, Isle of Man, Italy, Jersey, Malta, Monaco, Norway (mainland), Portugal, Spain[*] (except Ceuta/Melilla), Sweden, Switzerland, and United Kingdom
Oceania[†]	Australia,[*] Cook Islands, Fiji, French Polynesia, Guam, Kiribati, New Caledonia, New Zealand, Palau, Papua New Guinea, Samoa, and Vanuatu

[*]Bat rabies might exist in some areas that are free of terrestrial rabies.
[†]Most of Pacific Oceania is reportedly "rabies free."

tection of short duration. Vaccines may be used to provide pre-exposure prophylaxis (termed *prophylaxis* rather than *immunization* to emphasize that receiving this product before exposure does not obviate the need for treatment if an exposure occurs) or postexposure prophylaxis. Travelers to countries where canine rabies is endemic are candidates for pre-exposure vaccination, as are individuals whose purpose of travel includes relevant animal or laboratory work, those who are likely to be hiking or riding motorcycles, or those whose itineraries include remote destinations where prompt medical attention is impossible.[83] Pre-exposure vaccination does not remove the imperative to seek definitive treatment if an exposure occurs but does alter the postexposure prophylaxis regimen. Dosage schedules for vaccines licensed in the United States are listed in Table 58–8. Other vaccine preparations may be available in developing countries; these vaccines are produced locally and have unknown safety and efficacy. If bitten by a suspect animal, an individual should receive modern tissue culture vaccine preparations, even if this means receiving additional treatment once the individual has returned to his or her country of origin.[84]

Adverse events such as local pain and swelling have been reported in 30% to 74% of recipients of human diploid cell vaccine (HDCV). Systemic reactions may occur in up to 40% of individuals. Three cases of central nervous system disease have been reported following HDCV administration, but a causal relationship has not been established. Up to 6% of those receiving booster doses of HDCV may experience immune complex–like reactions. Although vaccines prepared in purified chick embryo cell culture may cause mild erythema, swelling, and pain at the injection site, serum sickness–like hypersensitivity reactions have not been problematic with these vaccines.[85] When given as postexposure prophylaxis, the series of doses should not be interrupted because of mild systemic or local reactions to vaccine; they can be managed with anti-inflammatory agents.

Antimalarials such as chloroquine (and possibly mefloquine) may interfere with antibody response to HDCV rabies vaccine.[11] Other drugs (steroids or immunosuppressive agents) or conditions that affect the immune system also may impair the efficacy of vaccine. HIV-infected individuals, especially those with low CD4 counts, have impaired antibody response following rabies vaccine.[86] Individuals taking such agents or experiencing such conditions may be candidates for testing of serum antibody levels following immunization.

Pregnancy is not a contraindication to postexposure prophylaxis with rabies vaccine, and no harmful effects to the fetus from immunization have been noted. If risk of exposure is high, pre-exposure prophylaxis may be offered.[87]

Tick-Borne Encephalitis

Tick-borne encephalitis (TBE) is endemic to Central and Eastern Europe, Russia, and the Far East. Disease occurs following the bite of an infected tick or through ingestion of infected unpasteurized milk. Although asymptomatic and mild infections occur commonly, neurologic manifestations and sequelae are significant causes of morbidity and mortality.[88] Most infections are acquired in rural locations; those working or vacationing in such locations between April and November, when tick activity is greatest, are at greatest risk. McNeil et al. reported an infection rate of 0.9 per 100 per month of exposure in a study of American service members of a military unit that lived and trained in a highly endemic area in Central Europe.[89]

Active immunization is the most effective means of prevention of TBE. Two vaccines, FSME-IMMUN (Baxter Vaccine AG, Wien, Austria) and Encepur (Chiron Behring, Marburg, Germany) are used widely in Europe. Efficacy of FSME-IMMUN has been reported to be greater than 95%, based on data collected during active surveillance for infection following a mass immunization campaign in Austria. Several vaccines are marketed in Russia; one has been reported to be highly effective.[88] No vaccines are available in the United States. Travelers who plan extended stays in endemic areas can arrange to receive vaccine locally. Passive protection with TBE immune globulin has been proposed for pre-exposure prophylaxis as a method of preventing disease in short-stay travelers. Use of TBE immune globulin remains controversial because safety and efficacy of the preparation have been questioned.[90] Measures to prevent exposures to ticks, such as use of appropriate clothing and repellents containing *N,N*-diethyl-*meta*-toluamide (DEET), avoidance of tick habitats, immediate removal of ticks, and avoidance of unpasteurized milk, are additional strategies that can be used to prevent TBE.

The vaccine is given as a three-dose series, with the first two injections 2 weeks to 3 months apart, and a third dose

TABLE 58–8 ■ Rabies Pre-Exposure Immunization*

Risk Category	Nature of Risk	Typical Populations	Pre-exposure Regimen
Frequent	Exposure usually episodic with source recognized, but exposure may also be unrecognized	Spelunkers, animal control and wildlife workers in rabies epizootic areas; certain travelers to foreign rabies epizootic areas	Primary pre-exposure immunization course; serologic examination or booster immunization every 2 yr
Infrequent (but greater than population at large)	Exposure nearly always episodic with source recognized	Animal control and wildlife worker in areas of low rabies endemicity; may include some travelers	Primary pre-exposure immunization course; no routine booster immunization or serologic examination

*Pre-exposure immunization consists of three doses of HDCV, RVA, or RabAvert, 1.0 mL IM, one each on days 0, 7, and 21 or 28. Only HDCV may be administered by the intradermal (ID) dose/route (0.1 mL ID on days 0, 7, and 21 or 28). If the traveler will be taking chloroquine or mefloquine for malaria chemoprophylaxis, the three-dose series must be completed before initiation of antimalarials. If this is not possible, the IM dose/route should be used. Administration of routine booster doses of vaccine depends on exposure risk category. Pre-exposure immunization of immunosuppressed persons is not recommended.
HDCV, human diploid cell vaccine; IM, intramuscularly; RVA, Rabies Vaccine, Adsorbed.

TABLE 58–9 ■ Recommended Doses and Schedules for Tick-Borne Encephalitis Vaccines

Group	Vaccine	Dose	No. of Doses	Schedule	Booster
Adults	FSME-IMMUN	0.5 mL SC/IM	3	0, 2 wk–3 mo, 9–12 mo after 2nd dose	3 yr after last dose
Children 18 mo–11 yr	Encepur	0.75 μg/0.5 mL SC/IM	3	0, 1–3 mo, 9–12 mo after 2nd dose*	3 yr after last dose
12 yr and older	Encepur	1.5 μg/0.5 mL SC/IM	3	0, 1–3 mo, 9–12 mo after 2nd dose*	3 yr after last dose

*An accelerated schedule of days 0, 7, and 21 also may be used. In this case a fourth dose should be given 12–18 months after completing the three-dose series.
IM, intramuscular; SC, subcutaneous.

9 to 12 months later. An accelerated schedule of Encepur, with doses at days 0, 7, and 21, with a booster 12 to 18 months following the third dose, may be used. Boosters are recommended at 3-year intervals (Table 58–9). Fever is the most common side effect of vaccine; mild local and systemic reactions may also occur. Individuals with egg allergy should not receive this vaccine. Data are lacking regarding use of these vaccines during pregnancy.

Typhoid

Typhoid is another common vaccine-preventable disease affecting travelers. In the United States, 62% of cases reported between 1975 and 1984 occurred in international travelers.[91] Risk of contracting typhoid depends largely on travel destination and living circumstances during travel. Estimates of risk for contracting typhoid for short-stay travelers have ranged from 1 in 30,000 in most developing countries to 10 in 30,000 for trips to North Africa, India, and Senegal.[92] Another study showed risk of disease to be related inversely to receiving vaccine prior to travel: Incidence rates per visit ranged from 16 per 100,000 in North American tourists, 92% of whom had received typhoid vaccine prior to travel, to 216 per 100,000 in Israeli tourists, 6% of whom had been immunized.[93]

Two vaccines are available to protect travelers from typhoid, though none offers complete protection. Precautions against ingesting contaminated food and water must continue to be used to augment protection afforded by vaccine. Oral live, attenuated typhoid vaccine (Vivotif; Berna) manufactured from the Ty21a strain of *Salmonella typhi* is given in a series of three (Europe) or four (North America) capsules taken every other day and has a vaccine efficacy of 67%.[94] It is not licensed for children younger than 6 years in the United States, and administration of this vaccine may be limited by the ability of small children to ingest capsules. Liquid preparations of vaccine hold promise for this age group. Duration of efficacy of three doses of the enteric-coated capsules was 62% over 7 years, and of three doses of liquid was 78% over 5 years, of follow-up.[95]

A capsular polysaccharide vaccine (TYPHIM Vi; Pasteur Mérieux Connaught), given in a single intramuscular dose, is available for individuals 2 years and older. Vaccine efficacy of this product ranges from 55% to 74%.[96,97] Duration of immunity is uncertain; Keddy et al. reported persistence of antibody for more than 10 years following immunization with this vaccine in South African schoolchildren, but acknowledge that exposure to disease may have contributed to these findings.[98]

Typhoid vaccine schedules are listed in Table 58–10. No vaccine is available for children under age 2, and the use of capsular oral vaccine is limited by the ability of young children to swallow capsules. Mothers of infants may be reassured that exclusive breast-feeding (reducing contact with contaminated food or water) offers protection for infants when careful hand washing also is carried out. Booster doses are recommended every 2 years for the polysaccharide vaccine and every 5 years for oral vaccine.

Adverse reactions to the capsular polysaccharide vaccine include fever in 1% or fewer of vaccine recipients, headache in up to 3%, and local reactions in about 7%. Oral vaccine results in fever or headache in about 5% of recipients. Impaired response to capsular polysaccharide vaccine occurs

TABLE 58–10 ■ Dosage and Schedules for Typhoid Fever Vaccination

Vaccination	Age	Dosage Dose/Mode of Administration	No. of Doses	Interval Between Doses	Boosting Interval
Oral Live, Attenuated Ty21a Vaccine					
Primary series	≥6 yr	1 capsule*	4	48 hr	—
Booster	≥6 yr	1 capsule*	4	48 hr	Every 5 yr
Vi Capsular Polysaccharide Vaccine					
Primary series	≥2 yr	0.50 mL†	1	—	—
Booster	≥2 yr	0.50 mL†	1	—	Every 2 yr

*Administer with cool liquid no warmer than 37°C (98.6°F).
†Intramuscularly.
—, Not applicable.

in HIV-infected individuals, especially those with low CD4 counts.[99] Oral typhoid vaccine is a live virus preparation and should not be given to immunocompromised individuals, including those with HIV infection. Concerns have been raised about the immunogenicity of this vaccine in individuals receiving antibiotics, immune globulin, antimalarials, or viral vaccines. Growth of the live Ty21a strain is inhibited by some antimicrobial agents and by the antimalarial agent mefloquine.[13,14] Ideally, the oral typhoid vaccine series should be completed at least 2 weeks predeparture and before beginning antimalarials, or doses of each should be separated by at least 24 hours. The antimalarial agent chloroquine does not inhibit the growth of Ty21a and may be given concurrently with vaccine. Oral typhoid vaccine should not be taken concurrently with antimicrobial agents if possible; the vaccine should be taken 24 hours or more after the last dose of the antibiotic. Oral typhoid vaccine may be given concurrently with yellow fever vaccine; data are not available regarding concurrent administration of oral typhoid vaccine and other live virus vaccines.[44] Vaccine may be administered at the same time as immune globulin. Safety of vaccines against typhoid has not been established during

pregnancy, and immunization at this time should be avoided if possible.

Yellow Fever

A dramatic resurgence of yellow fever has occurred in the past 15 years, in both sub-Saharan Africa and South America.[100] In Africa, outbreaks occurred in countries such as Gabon, which had never previously had disease, and re-emergence of disease was noted in Kenya, which had been yellow fever free for nearly 50 years. In South America, the largest outbreak since the 1950s occurred in Peru in 1995, and cases were reported in Bolivia, Brazil, Colombia, Ecuador, and Peru from 1985 to 1994. Jungle yellow fever continues to occur in Brazil, and urbanization of yellow fever has become increasingly problematic in Bolivia.[101,102] Most cases of yellow fever occur in nonimmune, unvaccinated individuals who migrate to or visit areas where transmission occurs.[103] Yellow fever can be a fatal disease, and cases have occurred in immunized travelers.[104–106] Areas of current risk for disease are shown in Figures 58–4 and 58–5.

Vaccination against yellow fever offers high levels of protection, with seroconversion rates of greater than 95% in

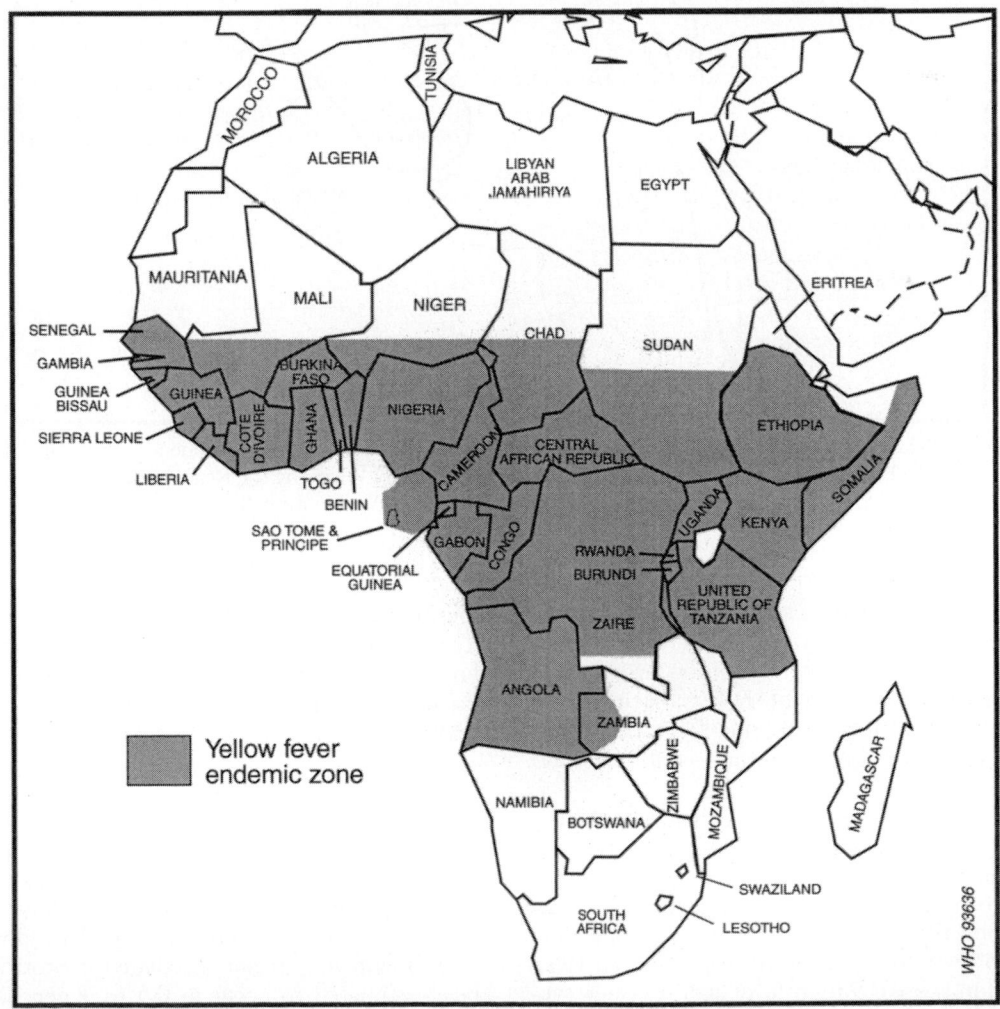

FIGURE 58–4 ▪ Yellow fever–endemic zones in Africa. *Note:* Although the "yellow fever–endemic zones" are no longer included in the International Health Regulations, a number of countries (most of them not bound by the Regulations or bound with reservations) consider these zones as infected areas and require an International Certificate of Vaccination against yellow fever from travelers arriving from those areas.

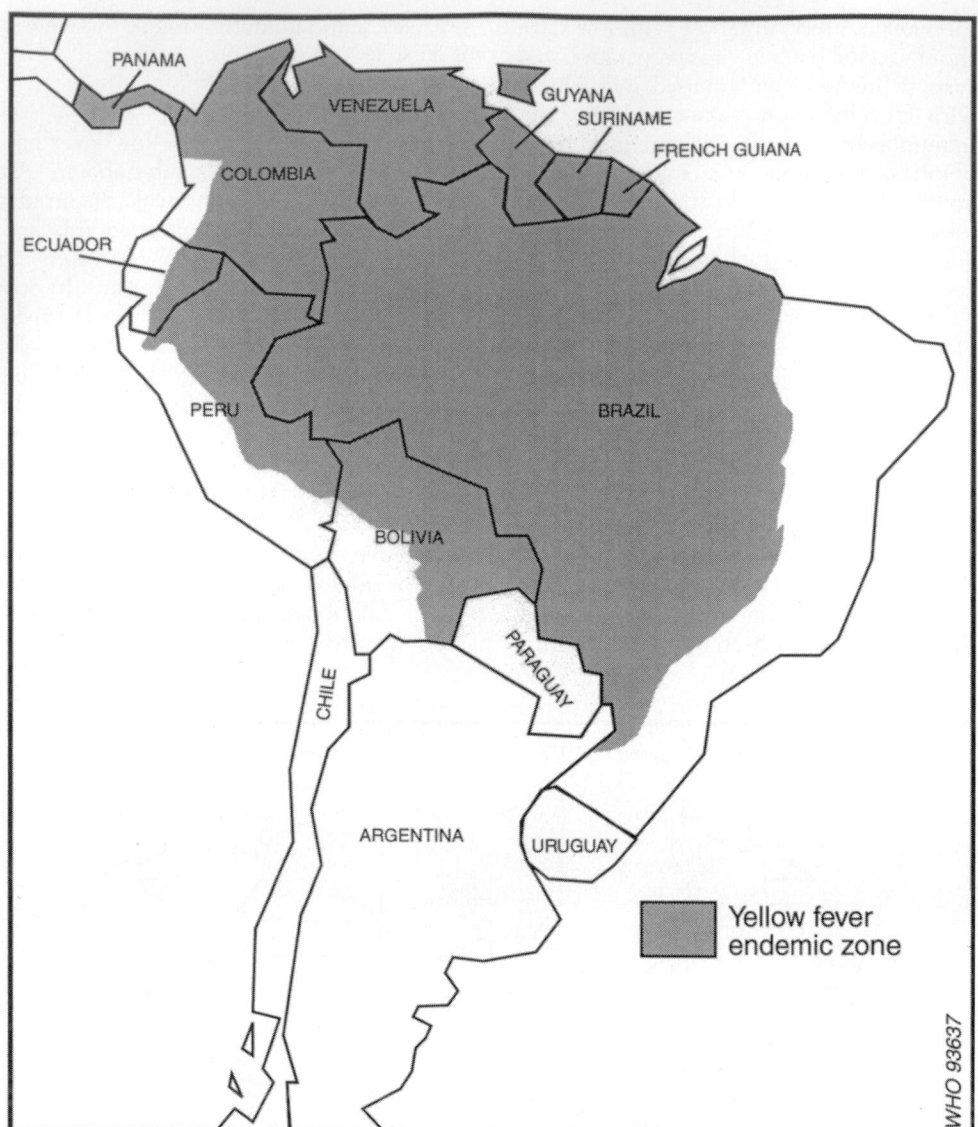

FIGURE 58–5 ▪ Yellow fever–endemic zones in the Americas. *Note:* Although the "yellow fever–endemic zones" are no longer included in the International Health Regulations, a number of countries (most of them not bound by the Regulations or bound with reservations) consider these zones as infected areas and require an International Certificate of Vaccination against yellow fever from travelers arriving from those areas.

children and adults and duration of immunity of at least 10 years.[107] Side effects are generally mild, and include headaches, myalgia, and low-grade fever occurring 5–10 days after immunization in < 25% of those participating in clinical trials of yellow fever vaccine.[108,109] Immediate hypersensitivity reactions are uncommon and are most likely to occur in those with allergy to eggs.

Serious adverse events to yellow fever vaccine include yellow fever vaccine associated neurotropic disease (formerly postvaccinal encephalitis) and the recently described yellow fever vaccine associated viscerotropic disease. Encephalitis has been reported in 23 patients among more than 200 million doses of vaccine distributed since 1945; 16 cases occurred in those < 9 months of age.[110] A new syndrome of fever, jaundice, and multiple organ system failure following yellow fever vaccine has been reported in 10 patients, ranging in age from 5 to 79 years, worldwide (4 in the US, 2 in Brazil, and 1 each in Australia, Switzerland,

Germany, and the United Kingdom) since 1996.[111–116,120] This syndrome, initially called febrile multiple organ system failure, ranges in severity from moderate disease with focal organ dysfunction to severe multi-system failure and death, and may include neurotropic disease. Recently, two new suspected cases of viscerotropic disease and four suspected cases of neurotropic disease were reported in US recipients of yellow fever vaccine.[117] A study of reports submitted to the Vaccine Adverse Event Reporting System in the United States identified advanced age as a risk factor for adverse events associated with yellow fever immunization, though cases have occurred in younger individuals.[118]

Yellow fever vaccine associated neurotropic disease has been estimated to occur in 0.5 to 4 per 1000 very young infants, and in fewer than 1 in 8 million vaccinees over 9 months of age in the United States.[119] Estimates of the incidence of yellow fever vaccine associated viscerotropic disease have been made based upon number of doses distributed to the civilian population, safety monitoring data for doses distributed during 1990–1998 in the United States, and number of cases identified using enhanced surveillance of yellow fever vaccine adverse events through the VAERS database. These data yield an estimated reported incidence of 2.5/1,000,000 doses distributed.[119a] Limitations of this estimate include possible under reporting of cases and lack of exact information about number of doses administered.

International efforts to prevent the spread of yellow fever include mosquito control at airports and shipping ports, and the requirement of documentation of immunization against yellow fever for travelers arriving from areas where disease is occurring. Some affected countries, however, do not require immunization as a condition of entry, despite the presence of endemic or episodic disease. Yellow fever vaccine must be given at official yellow fever vaccine centers with an International Certificate of Vaccination, which is valid from 10 days through 10 years after the date of immunization.

Travelers to affected countries should receive a single dose of vaccine at least 10 days before departure. Vaccine is contraindicated in children less than 4 months of age and should be used cautiously in children less than 1 year of age. The single most important step in judicious use of yellow fever vaccine, in view of reports of adverse events following this vaccine, is to provide vaccine only to individuals traveling to yellow fever–endemic areas: two of five individuals with multiple organ system failure in one report were traveling to areas where yellow fever had never been described.[120] Individuals not protected by vaccine should use adequate personal protective measures to avoid mosquito bites.

Serologic response to yellow fever vaccine is not diminished by simultaneous administration of tetanus, diphtheria, pertussis, measles, polio, BCG, hepatitis A, hepatitis B, Vi antigen capsular polysaccharide typhoid, oral Ty21a typhoid, or oral live, attenuated cholera CVD103-HgR vaccines.[44,121] Immune globulin did not decrease the antibody response to yellow fever vaccine when given 0 to 7 days before immunization.[122] The antimalarial chloroquine has been shown not to affect adversely the antibody response to yellow fever vaccine.[123]

Yellow fever immunization is not recommended during pregnancy. A study that documented fetal infection in 1 of 41 infants exposed to maternal vaccination and the known neurotropism of the virus support this recommendation.[124] In addition, immunization during pregnancy may result in antibody concentrations that are inferior to those obtained following immunization of nonpregnant women.[125] Immunization with yellow fever vaccine is not recommended for immunocompromised individuals or those with symptomatic HIV infection. Vaccine has been administered with good tolerance and efficacy to asymptomatic HIV-infected individuals.[126,127]

Cost-Effectiveness of Travel Immunizations

Travel medicine experts have long noted the willingness of travelers to accept (and pay for) multiple vaccines for diseases for which they are at minimal risk. Beutels and colleagues, in an economic evaluation of travel medicine interventions, concluded that, with the exception of hepatitis A vaccine in specific circumstances, no travel vaccine has a favorable cost-benefit ratio.[128] Costs to prevent travel-related vaccine-preventable disease ranged from $100,000 to $300,000 US to prevent a case of typhoid, $4 million US to prevent a case of Japanese encephalitis, and $5 to 29 million US to prevent a case of cholera.[129–132] The most studied travel-associated vaccine in terms of cost-effectiveness is hepatitis A. In one study, which also examined the cost-effectiveness of typhoid immunization, neither of the two vaccines was found to be cost-effective; societal expenditures of more than £67 million UK were required to prevent a single death from typhoid fever with either vaccine.[133] In contrast, a study from the Netherlands suggested that cost-effective choices are available with regard to hepatitis A immunization when frequency of travel, likelihood of prior immunity, and product used are taken into consideration.[134] Cost-effectiveness of pre-exposure rabies prophylaxis has been studied in Canada, with the conclusion that routine pre-exposure prophylaxis for most travelers is not indicated.[135]

Issues complicating performance of studies of cost-effectiveness include difficulty in estimating with accuracy the risk of vaccine-preventable diseases to travelers; difficulties in determining vaccine efficacy, especially for travelers who will have variable exposures in endemic areas; difficulties approximating costs associated with disease; and lack of sufficient experience with some newer vaccines to allow accurate estimation of the incidence of vaccine-associated adverse events. Finally, some practitioners may be reluctant to omit any vaccine, no matter the risk of disease, for fear of liability. Until these issues are studied in greater detail, each travel medicine provider must continue to individualize recommendations for travel vaccination, taking into account the potential for adverse reactions to immunization and the patient's risk for the disease.

Rapid advances in biotechnology promise a potential revolution in the development of new vaccines using diverse approaches ranging from DNA vaccines to transgenic plant vaccines.[136] New candidate vaccines show promise in protecting against diverse pathogens that cause diarrheal disease.[137] Optimism remains for the eventual development of vaccines against HIV[138] and malaria.[139] In addition to the remaining technical hurdles, however, equally formidable economic hurdles remain in adequate funding of vaccine research and development against diseases that mostly afflict the poorest populations in the poorest countries.[140] The increased interest in travel and travel immunizations by more affluent travelers may provide substantial assistance in making these much-needed vaccines a reality.

REFERENCES

1. Handszuh H. Tourism patterns and trends. *In* Dupont HL, Steffen R (eds). Textbook of Travel Medicine and Health (2nd ed). Hamilton, Ontario, Brian C Decker, 2001, pp 34–36.
2. Loutan L, Ghaznawi H. The migrant as a traveler. *In* DuPont HL, Steffen R (eds). Textbook of Travel Medicine and Health (2nd ed). Hamilton, Ontario, Brian C Decker, 2001, pp 428–434.
3. Reid D, Keystone JS, Cossar JH. Health risks abroad: general considerations. *In* Dupont HL, Steffen R (eds). Textbook of Travel Medicine and Health (2nd ed). Hamilton, Ontario, 2001, pp 3–7.
4. Dupont HL, Steffen R (eds). Textbook of Travel Medicine and Health (2nd ed). Hamilton, Ontario, Brian C Decker, 2001.

5. Wilson ME. Travel-related vaccines. Infect Dis Clin North Am 15:231–251, 2001.
6. Leder K, Weller PF, Wilson ME. Travel vaccines and elderly persons: review of vaccines available in the United States. Clin Infect Dis 33:1553–1566, 2001.
7. Sood SK. Immunization for children traveling abroad. Pediatr Clin North Am 47:435–448, 2000.
8. Falvo C, Horowitz H. Adverse reactions associated with simultaneous administration of multiple vaccines to travelers. J Gen Intern Med 9:255–260, 1994.
9. General recommendations on immunization: recommendations of the Advisory Committee on Immunization Practices (ACIP) and the American Academy of Family Physicians. MMWR 51(RR-2):1–36, 2002.
10. American Academy of Pediatrics, Committee on Infectious Diseases. Recommended timing of routine measles immunization for children who have recently received immune globulin preparations. Pediatrics 93:682–685, 1994.
11. Use of vaccines and immune globulins in persons with altered immunocompetence: recommendations of the Advisory Committee on Immunization Practices (ACIP). MMWR 42:1–18, 1993.
12. Pappaioanou M, Fishbein DB, Dreesen DW, et al. Antibody response to pre-exposure human diploid-cell rabies vaccine given concurrently with chloroquine. N Engl J Med 314:280–284, 1986.
13. Brachman PS, Metchock B, Kozarsky PE. Effects of antimalarial chemoprophylactic agents on the viability of the Ty21a vaccine strain [letter]. Clin Infect Dis 15:1057–1058, 1992.
14. Horowitz H, Carbonaro CA. Inhibition of the Salmonella typhi oral vaccine strain, Ty21a, by mefloquine and chloroquine [letter]. J Infect Dis 166:1462–1464, 1992.
15. American Academy of Pediatrics, Committee on Infectious Diseases. Recommended childhood and adolescent immunization schedule—United States, 2003. Pediatrics 111:212–216, 2003.
16. Update on adult immunization. MMWR 40:1–94, 1991.
17. Gardner P, Schaffner W. Immunization of adults. N Engl J Med 328:1252–1258, 1993.
18. Fedson DS. Adult immunization: summary of the National Vaccine Advisory Committee report. JAMA 272:1133–1137, 1994.
19. Diphtheria epidemic—new independent states of the former Soviet Union, 1990–1994. MMWR Morb Mortal Wkly Rep 44:177–181, 1995.
20. Diphtheria outbreak—Saraburi Province, Thailand, 1994. MMWR 45:271–273, 1996.
21. Vitek CR, Brennan MB, Gotway CA, et al. Risk of diphtheria among schoolchildren in the Russian Federation in relation to time since last vaccination. Lancet 353:355–358, 1999.
22. Diphtheria acquired by US citizens in the Russian Federation and Ukraine—1994. MMWR Morb Mortal Wkly Rep 44:237–244, 1995.
23. Lumio J, Jahkosa M, Vuento R, et al. Diphtheria after visit to Russia. Lancet 342:53–54, 1993.
24. Crossley K, Irvine P, Warren JB, et al. Tetanus and diphtheria immunity in urban Minnesota adults. JAMA 242:2298–3000, 1979.
25. Koblin BA, Townsend TR. Immunity to diphtheria and tetanus in inner-city women of child-bearing age. Am J Public Health 79:1297–1298, 1989.
26. Christensson B, Bottiger M. Serological immunity to diphtheria in Sweden in 1978 and 1984. Scand J Infect Dis 18:227–233, 1986.
27. Centers for Disease Control and Prevention. Progress toward global eradication of poliomyelitis, 2001. MMWR 51:253–256, 2002.
28. Certification of poliomyelitis eradication—the Americas, 1994. MMWR 43:720–722, 1994.
29. Centers for Disease Control and Prevention. Certification of poliomyelitis eradication—Western Pacific Region, October 2000. MMWR 50:1–3, 2001.
29a. Centers for Disease Control and Prevention. Certification of poliomyelitis eradication—European Region, June 2002. MMWR 51:572–574, 2002.
30. Centers for Disease Control and Prevention. Poliomyelitis prevention in the United States: updated recommendations of the Advisory Committee on Immunization Practices (ACIP). MMWR 49(RR-5): 1–22, 2000.
31. Steffen R, Rickenbach M, Willhelm U, et al. Health problems after travel to developing countries. J Infect Dis 156:84–91, 1987.
32. Lange WR, Frame JD. High incidence of viral hepatitis among American missionaries in Africa. Am J Trop Med Hyg 43:527–533, 1990.
33. Steffen R. Risks of hepatitis B for travelers. Vaccine 8:31–32, 1990.
34. Measles—United States, 1996, and the interruption of indigenous transmission. MMWR 46:242–246, 1997.
35. Centers for Disease Control and Prevention. Measles, mumps, and rubella vaccine use and strategies for elimination of measles, rubella, and congenital rubella syndrome and control of mumps: recommendations of the Advisory Committee on Immunization Practices (ACIP). MMWR 47(RR-8):1–25, 1998.
36. Ivanoff B, Robertson SE. Pertussis: a worldwide problem. Dev Biol Stand 89:3–13, 1997.
37. Gangarosa EJ, Galazka AM, Wolfe CR, et al. Impact of the anti-vaccine movements on pertussis control: the untold story. Lancet 351:356–361, 1998.
38. Pertussis vaccination: use of acellular pertussis vaccines among infants and young children. Recommendations of the Advisory Committee on Immunization Practices (ACIP). MMWR 46:1–25, 1997.
39. Centers for Disease Control and Prevention. Prevention and control of influenza: recommendations of the Advisory Committee on Immunization Practices (ACIP). MMWR 50(RR-4):1–44, 2001.
40. The role of BCG vaccines in the prevention and control of tuberculosis in the U.S.: a joint statement by the Advisory Committee for Elimination of Tuberculosis and the ACIP. MMWR 45:1–18, 1996.
41. Crowley RG. Implication of the Vietnam War for tuberculosis in the United States. Arch Environ Health 21:479–480, 1970.
42. Wittlinger F, Steffen R, Watanabe H, Handszuh H. Risk of cholera among Western and Japanese travelers. J Travel Med 2:154–158, 1995.
43. Sanchez JL, Taylor DN. Cholera. Lancet 349:1825–1830, 1997.
44. Tsai TF, Kollaritsch H, Que JU, et al. Compatible concurrent administration of yellow fever 17D vaccine with oral, live, attenuated cholera CVD103-HgR and typhoid Ty21a vaccines. J Infect Dis 179:522–524, 1999.
45. Kollaritsch H, Que JU, Wiedermann G, et al. Safety and immunogenicity of live oral cholera and typhoid vaccines administered alone or in combination with antimalarial drugs, oral polio vaccine or yellow fever vaccine. J Infect Dis 175:871–875, 1997.
46. Christenson B. Epidemiological aspects of acute viral hepatitis A in Swedish travelers to endemic areas. Scand J Infect Dis 17:5–10, 1985.
47. Steffen R, Kane MA, Shapiro CN, et al. Epidemiology and prevention of hepatitis A in travelers. JAMA 272:885–889, 1994.
48. Barnett ED, Holmes AH, Phillips SL, et al. Immunity to hepatitis A in travelers born and raised in endemic areas. J Travel Med 10:11–14, 2003.
49. Webster G, Barnes E, Dusheiko G, Franklin I. Protecting travellers from hepatitis A. BMJ 322:1194–1195, 2001.
50. Victor J, Knudsen JD, Nielsen LP, et al. Hepatitis A vaccine: a new convenient single-dose schedule with booster when long-term immunization is warranted. Vaccine 12:1327–1329, 1994.
51. Clemens R, Sarary A, Hepburn A, et al. Clinical experience with an inactivated hepatitis A vaccine. J Infect Dis 171(suppl 1):S44–S49, 1995.
52. Vidor E, Fritzell B, Plotkin S. Clinical development of a new inactivated hepatitis A vaccine. Infection 24:447–458, 1996.
53. Van Damme P, Lerous-Roels G, Law B, et al. Long-term persistence of antibodies induced by vaccination and safety follow-up, with the first combined vaccine against hepatitis A and B in children and adults. J Med Virol 65:6–13, 2001.
54. Nalin DR. VAQTA, hepatitis A vaccine, purified inactivated. Drugs Future 20:24–29, 1995.
55. Van Herck K, Van Damme P, Nguyen C. Long-term immunogenicity and safety of an inactivated hepatitis A vaccine. Presented at the 10th International Society for Infectious Diseases Conference, Singapore, March 2002.
56. Kallinowski B, Knoll A, Lindner E, et al. Can monovalent hepatitis A and B vaccines be replaced by a combined hepatitis A/B vaccine during the primary immunization course? Vaccine 19:16–22, 2001.
57. Bienzle U, Bock HL, Kruppenbacher J, et al. Immunogenicity of an inactivated hepatitis A vaccine administered according to two different schedules and the interference of other "travellers" vaccines with the immune response. Vaccine 14:501–505, 1996.
58. Bryan JP, Nelson M. Testing for antibody to hepatitis A to decrease the cost of hepatitis A prophylaxis with immune globulin or hepatitis A vaccines. Arch Intern Med 154:663–668, 1994.
59. Hanna JN, Ritchie SA, Phillips DA, et al. An outbreak of Japanese encephalitis in the Torres Strait, Australia, 1995. Med J Aust 165:256–260, 1996.

60. Macdonald WBG, Tink AR, Ouvrier RA, et al. Japanese encephalitis after a two-week holiday in Bali. Med J Aust 150:334–339, 1989.

61. Wittesjo B, Eitrem R, Niklasson B, et al. Japanese encephalitis after a 10-day holiday in Bali. Lancet 345:856, 1995.

62. Inactivated Japanese encephalitis virus vaccine: recommendations of the Advisory Committee on Immunization Practices (ACIP). MMWR 42:1–15, 1993.

63. Ohtaki E, Matsuishi T, Hirano Y, Maekawa K. Acute disseminated encephalomyelitis after treatment with Japanese B encephalitis vaccine (Nakayama-Yoken and Beijing strains). J Neurol Neurosurg Psychiatry 59:316–317, 1995.

64. Plesner A, Arlien-Soborg P, Herning M. Neurological complications and Japanese encephalitis vaccination. Lancet 348:202–203, 1996.

65. Kitaoka M. Follow-up on use of vaccine in children in Japan. In: McHammond W, Kitaoka M, Downs WG, eds. Immunization for Japanese encephalitis. Amsterdam: Excerpta Medica, 1972:275–277.

66. Plesner A, Ronne T. Allergic mucocutaneous reactions to Japanese encephalitis vaccine. Vaccine 15:1239–1243, 1997.

67. Takahashi H, Pool V, Tsai TF, Chen RT, VAERS Working Group. Adverse events after Japanese encephalitis vaccination: review of post-marketing surveillance data from Japan and the United States. Vaccine 18:2963–2969, 2000.

68. Shlim DR, Solomon T. Japanese encephalitis vaccine for travelers: exploring the limits of risk. Clin Infect Dis 35:183–188, 2002.

69. Sakaguchi M, Miyazawa H, Inouye S. Specific IgE and IgG to gelatin in children with systemic cutaneous reactions to Japanese encephalitis vaccines. Allergy 56:536–539, 2001.

70. Yamada A, Imanishi J, Juang RF, et al. Trial of inactivated Japanese encephalitis vaccine in children with underlying diseases. Vaccine 4:32–34, 1986.

71. Fonkoua MC, Taha MK, Nicolas P, et al. Recent increase in meningitis caused by Neisseria meningitidis serogroups A and W135, Yaounde, Cameroon. Emerg Infect Dis 8:327–329, 2002.

72. Koch S, Steffen R. Meningococcal disease in travelers: vaccination recommendations. J Travel Med 1:4–7, 1994.

73. Moore PS, Harrison LH, Telzak EE, et al. Group A meningococcal carriage in travelers returning from Saudi Arabia. JAMA 260:2686–2689, 1988.

74. Hahne SJM, Gray SJ, Aguilera J, et al. W135 meningococcal disease in England and Wales associated with Hajj 2000 and 2001. Lancet 359:582–583, 2002.

75. Centers for Disease Control and Prevention. Update: assessment of risk for meningococcal disease associated with the Hajj 2001. MMWR 50:221–222, 2001.

76. Memish ZA. Meningococcal disease and travel. Clin Infect Dis 34:84–90, 2002.

77. Centers for Disease Control and Prevention. Control and prevention of meningococcal disease: recommendations of the Advisory Committee on Immunization Practices (ACIP). MMWR 46:1–10, 1997.

78. Campbell JD, Edelman R, King JC Jr., et al. Safety, reactogenicity, and immunogenicity of a tetravalent meningococcal polysaccharide-diphtheria toxoid conjugate vaccine given to healthy adults. J Infect Dis 186:1848–1851, 2002.

79. Haupt W. Rabies—risk of exposure and current trends in prevention of human cases. Vaccine 17:1742–1749, 1999.

80. Phanuphak P, Ubolyam S, Sirivichayakul S. Should travelers in rabies endemic areas receive pre-exposure rabies immunisation? Ann Med Interne (Paris) 145:409–411, 1994.

81. Hatz CF, Bidaux JM, Eichenberger K, et al. Circumstances and management of 72 animal bites among long-term residents in the tropics. Vaccine 13:811–815, 1995.

82. Fishbein DB, Robinson LE. Rabies. N Engl J Med 329:1632–1638, 1993.

83. Centers for Disease Control and Prevention. Human rabies prevention—United States, 1999: recommendations of the Immunization Practices Advisory Committee (ACIP). MMWR 48:1–21, 1999.

84. Hatz CFR, Thisyakorn U, Thisyakorn C, Wilde H. Other important viral infections. In DuPont HL, Steffen R (eds). Textbook of Travel Medicine and Health (2nd ed). Hamilton, Ontario, Brian C Decker, pp 319–322, 2001.

85. A new rabies vaccine. Med Lett Drugs Ther 40:64–65, 1998.

86. Thisyakorn U, Pancharoen C, Ruxrungtham K, et al. Safety and immunogenicity of preexposure rabies vaccination in children infected with human immunodeficiency virus type 1. Clin Infect Dis 30:218, 2000.

87. Varner MW, McGuinness GA, Galask RP. Rabies vaccination in pregnancy. Am J Obstet Gynecol 143:717–718, 1982.

88. Dumpois U, Crook D, Oksi J. Tick-borne encephalitis. Clin Infect Dis 28:882–890, 1999.

89. McNeil JG, Lednar WM, Stansfield SK, et al. Central European tick-borne encephalitis: assessment of risk for persons in the armed services and vacationers. J Infect Dis 152:650–651, 1985.

90. Kluger G, Schottler A, Waldvogel K, et al. Tickborne encephalitis despite specific immunoglobulin prophylaxis. Lancet 346:1502, 1996.

91. Ryan CA, Hargrett-Bean NT, Blake PA. Salmonella typhi infection in the United States, 1975–1984: increasing role of foreign travel. Rev Infect Dis 11:1–8, 1989.

92. Taylor DN, Pollard RA, Blake PA. Typhoid in the United States and the risk to the international traveler. J Infect Dis 148:599–602, 1983.

93. Schwartz E, Shlim DR, Eaton M, et al. The effect of oral and parenteral typhoid vaccination on the rate of infection with Salmonella typhi and Salmonella paratyphi A among foreigners in Nepal. Arch Intern Med 150:349–351, 1990.

94. Ivanoff B, Levine MM, Lambert PH. Vaccination against typhoid fever: present status. Bull World Health Organ 72:957–971, 1994.

95. Levine MM, Ferreccio C, Abrego P, et al. Duration of efficacy of Ty21a, attenuated Salmonella typhi live oral vaccine. Vaccine 17(suppl):S22–S27, 1999.

96. Acharya AIL, Lowe CU, Thapa R, et al. Prevention of typhoid fever in Nepal with the Vi capsular polysaccharide of Salmonella typhi. N Engl J Med 317:1101–1104, 1987.

97. Klugman KP, Gilbertson IT, Koornhof HJ, et al. Protective activity of Vi capsular polysaccharide vaccine against typhoid fever. Lancet 2:1165–1169, 1987.

98. Keddy KH, Klugman KP, Hansford CF, et al. Persistence of antibodies to the Salmonella typhi capsular polysaccharide vaccine in South African school children ten years after immunization. Vaccine 17:110–113, 1999.

99. Kroon FP, van Dissel JT, Ravensbergen E, et al. Impaired antibody response after immunization of HIV-infected individuals with the polysaccharide vaccine against Salmonella typhi (Typhim-Vi). Vaccine 17:2941–2945, 1999.

100. Robertson SE, Hull BP, Tomori O, et al. Yellow fever: a decade of reemergence. JAMA 276:1157–1162, 1996.

101. Filippis AMB, Schatzmayr HG, Nicolai C, et al. Jungle yellow fever, Rio de Janeiro. Emerg Infect Dis 7:484–485, 2001.

102. Van der Stuyft P, Gianella A, Pirard M, et al. Urbanisation of yellow fever in Santa Cruz, Bolivia. Lancet 353:1558–1562, 1999.

103. Vasconcelos PFC, Rosa APAT, Rodrigues SG, et al. Yellow fever in Para State, Amazon Region of Brazil, 1998–1999: entomologic and epidemiologic findings. Emerg Infect Dis 7(suppl):565–569, 2001.

104. Teichmann D, Brobusch MP, Wesselmann H, et al. A haemorrhagic fever from the Cote d'Ivoire. Lancet 354:1608, 1999.

105. Centers for Disease Control and Prevention. Fatal yellow fever in a traveler returning from Venezuela, 1999. MMWR 49:303–305, 2000.

106. McFarland JM, Baddour LM, Nelson JE, et al. Imported yellow fever in a United States citizen. Clin Infect Dis 25:1143–1147, 1997.

107. Poland JD, Calisher CH, Monath TP, et al. Persistence of neutralizing antibody 30–35 years after immunization with 17D yellow fever vaccine. Bull World Health Organ 59:895–900, 1981.

108. Monath TP, Nichols R, Archambault WR, et al. Comparative safety and immunogenicity of two yellow fever 17D vaccines (ARILVAX and YF-VAX) in a Phase III multicenter, double-blind clinical trial. Am J Trop Med Hyg 66:533–541, 2002.

109. Lang J, Zuckerman J, Clarke P, Barrett P, Kirkpatrick C, Blondeau C. Comparison of the immunogenicity and safety of two 17D yellow fever vaccines. Am J Trop Med Hyg 103:698–701, 1999.

110. Centers for Disease Control and Prevention. Yellow fever vaccine; recommendations of the Advisory Committee on Immunization Practices (ACIP). MMWR 51(No. RR–17):4-6, 2002.

111. Vasconcelos PFC, Luna EJ, Galler R, et al. Serious adverse events associated with yellow fever 17DD vaccine in Brazil: a report of two cases. Lancet 358:91–97, 2001.

112. Chan RC, Penney DJ, Little D, et al. Hepatitis and death following vaccination with 17D-204 yellow fever vaccine. Lancet 358:121–122, 2001.

113. Martin M, Tsai TF, Cropp B, et al. Fever and multisystem organ failure associated with 17D-204 yellow fever vaccination: a report of four cases. Lancet 358:98–104, 2001.

114. Adhiyaman V, Oke A, Cefai C. Effects of yellow fever vaccination (letter). Lancet 358:1907–1908, 2001.

115. Troillet N, Laurencet F. Effects of yellow fever vaccination (letter). Lancet 358:1908–1909, 2001.

116. Werfel U, Popp W. Effects of yellow fever vaccination (letter). Lancet 358:1909, 2001.

117. Centers for Disease Control and Prevention. Adverse events associated with 17D-derived yellow fever vaccination—United States, 2001–2002. MMWR 51:989–993, 2002.

118. Martin M, Weld LH, Tsai TF, et al. Advanced age a risk factor for illness temporally associated with yellow fever vaccination. Emerg Infect Dis 7:945–951, 2001.

119. Monath TP. Yellow fever (Chapter 34). In: Plotkin SA, Orentstein WA, eds. Vaccines. 3rd ed. Philadelphia, PA: WB Saunders, 1999, pp 815–879.

119a Centers for Disease control and prevention. Yellow fever vaccine: recommendations of the Advisory Committee on Immunization Practices(ACIP). MMWR 51 (RR–17):4–6, 2002.

120. Centers for Disease Control and Prevention. Fever, jaundice, and multiple organ system failure associated with 17D-derived yellow fever vaccination, 1996–2001. MMWR 50:643–645, 2001.

121. Stefano I, Sato HK, Pannuti CS, et al. Recent immunization against measles does not interfere with the sero-response to yellow fever vaccine. Vaccine 17:1042–1046, 1999.

122. Kaplan JE, Nelson DB, Schonberger LB, et al. The effect of immune globulin on the response to trivalent oral poliovirus and yellow fever vaccinations. Bull World Health Organ 62:585–590, 1984.

123. Tsai TF, Bolin RA, Lazuick JS, Miller KE. Chloroquine does not adversely affect the antibody response to yellow fever vaccine [letter]. J Infect Dis 154:726–727, 1986.

124. Tsai TF, Paul R, Lynberg MC, Letson GW. Congenital yellow fever virus infection after immunization in pregnancy. J Infect Dis 168:1520–1523, 1993.

125. Nasidi A, Monath TP, Vandenberg J, et al. Yellow fever vaccination and pregnancy: a four-year prospective study. Trans R Soc Trop Med Hyg 87:337–339, 1993.

126. Goujon M, Tohr M, Feuillie V, et al. Good tolerance and efficacy of yellow fever vaccine among subject carriers of human immunodeficiency virus [abstr 32]. In Proceedings of the Fourth International Conference on Travel Medicine, Acapulco, 1995, p 63.

127. Receveur MC, Thiebaut R, Vedy S, et al. Yellow fever vaccination of human immunodeficiency virus-infected patients: report of 2 cases. Clin Infect Dis 31:E7–E8, 2000.

128. Beutels P, Van Damme P, Piper Jenks N. Economic evaluation in travel medicine. In Dupont HL, Steffen R (eds). Textbook of Travel Medicine and Health (2nd ed). Hamilton, Ontario, Brian C Decker, 2001, pp 21–27.

129. Steffen R. Typhoid vaccine, for whom? [letter]. Lancet 1:615, 1982.

130. MacPherson DW, Tonkin M. Cholera vaccination: a decision analysis. Can Med Assoc J 146:1947–1952, 1992.

131. Morger H, Steffen R, Schar M. Epidemiology of cholera in travelers, and conclusions for vaccination recommendations. BMJ 286:184, 1983.

132. Wilson ME, Fineberg HV. Analysis of benefits and costs for three multidose vaccines in travelers: hepatitis A, rabies and Japanese encephalitis. In Proceedings of the Third Conference on International Travel Medicine, Paris, 1993, p 159.

133. Behrens RH, Roberts JA. Is travel prophylaxis worth while? Economic appraisal of prophylactic measures against malaria, hepatitis A, and typhoid in travelers. BMJ 8:918–922, 1994.

134. Van Doorslaer E, Tormans G, Van Damme P. Cost-effectiveness analysis of vaccination against hepatitis A in travelers. J Med Virol 44:463–469, 1994.

135. LeGuerrier P, Pilon PA, Deshaies D, Allard R. Pre-exposure rabies prophylaxis for the international traveler: a decision analysis. Vaccine 14:167–176, 1996.

136. Liu MA. Vaccine developments. Nat Med 4(5 suppl):515–519, 1998.

137. Levine MM, Svennerholm A. Enteric vaccines: present and future. In DuPont HL, Steffen R (eds). Textbook of Travel Medicine and Health (2nd ed). Hamilton, Ontario, Brian C Decker, 2001, pp 252–263.

138. Heilman CA, Baltimore D. HIV vaccines—where are we going? Nat Med 4:532–534, 1998.

139. Tanner M. Malaria vaccines—current status and developments. In DuPont HL, Steffen R (eds). Textbook of Travel Medicine and Health (2nd ed). Hamilton, Ontario, Brian C Decker, 2001, pp 214–218.

140. Bloom BR, Widdus R. Vaccine visions and their global impact. Nat Med 5(5 suppl):480–484, 1998.

Chapter 59

Vaccines for Health Care Workers

DAVID J. WEBER • WILLIAM A. RUTALA

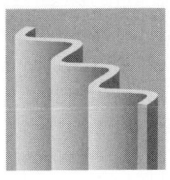

Health care workers (HCWs) are commonly exposed to infectious agents. The risks and methods of preventing occupational acquisition of infection by HCWs have been reviewed.[1-19] Minimizing the risk of disease acquisition is based on strict adherence to three key recommended interventions: (1) hand washing,[20,21] (2) rapid institution of appropriate isolation precautions for patients with known or suspected communicable diseases,[22] and (3) appropriate immunizations. Laboratory personnel, including hospital personnel working in microbiology laboratories, are also at risk for acquiring infectious diseases.[23,24] Prevention of laboratory-acquired infection requires adherence to recommended administrative protocols (e.g., no eating, drinking, or smoking in areas where microbiologic or pathologic samples are processed), engineering controls (e.g., containment hoods), personnel protective equipment (e.g., N-95 masks when culturing *Mycobacterium tuberculosis*), and appropriate immunizations.[25-28]

Vaccine-preventable diseases may be classified by their route of transmission and include airborne (e.g., influenza, varicella, measles), droplet (e.g., pertussis, meningococcal infection), contact (e.g., hepatitis A from contact with feces), and parenteral or mucosal exposure to blood or contaminated body fluids (e.g., hepatitis B).

Immunization of HCWs should be included by all health care facilities as part of a comprehensive occupational health program. Ensuring that HCWs are immune to vaccine-preventable diseases is important because it protects the HCW from infections with potentially serious complications when acquired as an adult (e.g., rubella, varicella, hepatitis B) and prevents the HCW from serving as a source for infecting patients, especially immunocompromised patients, with diseases that may lead to serious morbidity or even death (e.g., varicella). For this reason, all new employees should receive a prompt review of their immunization status for vaccine-preventable diseases. Immunization status also should be reviewed yearly. Other important occupational health interventions include an accessible health service, baseline and periodic tuberculin skin tests, evaluation of ill employees with potential communicable diseases with appropriate treatment and work restrictions, evaluation of employees after infectious disease exposures for postexposure prophylaxis and work restrictions, and education of employees focusing on general infection control guidelines in addition to Occupational Safety and Health Administration (OSHA)–mandated training in the prevention of blood-borne pathogens[29] and tuberculosis.[30]

Vaccines Recommended for Health Care Workers

General Guidelines

General recommendations regarding vaccination of HCWs have been published by the Centers for Disease Control and Prevention (CDC),[12] the Advisory Committee on Immunization Practices,[31,32] the American College of Physicians,[33] the American Academy of Pediatrics,[34] and infectious disease experts.[35-41] It is recommended that all HCWs be immune to mumps, measles, rubella, and varicella (Table 59–1).[12,31,37,42] All HCWs with potential exposure to blood or body fluids should be immune to hepatitis B. Influenza vaccine should be offered to all HCWs yearly. Detailed recommendations have been published regarding mumps,[43] measles,[43] rubella,[43,44] varicella,[45-47] hepatitis B,[48-50] and influenza[51] vaccines. All HCWs should be included in these recommendations, including employees with direct patient care responsibilities (e.g., nurses, respiratory technicians, physical therapists, physicians, students), employees without direct patient care responsibilities (e.g., environmental service workers, security), contract workers, and emergency medical personnel. HCWs should be provided vaccines that are recommended for adults, including tetanus and diphtheria[52] and pneumococcal vaccines,[53] or referred to their local medical provider. In special circumstances, HCWs or laboratory personnel should be offered immunization with other vaccines, including polio,[54] quadrivalent meningococcal vaccine,[55,56] bacille Calmette-Guérin (BCG),[57] rabies,[58] plague (not currently available),[59]

TABLE 59–1 ■ Vaccines Strongly Recommended for all Health Care Workers

Vaccine	Demonstration of Immunity*	Indications†	Administration†	Major Contraindication†
Measles	Physician-diagnosed disease*; laboratory evidence of immunity*‡; prior receipt of vaccine*‡ (two doses of live vaccine on or after first birthday)§	All health care workers‖	0.5 mL SC,¶ second dose at least 1 mo later	Pregnancy; history of anaphylactic reaction to gelatin or neomycin; immunocompromised state**; recent receipt of immunoglobulin; allergy to eggs for persons receiving MMR
Mumps	Born before 1957, physician-diagnosed disease*; laboratory evidence of immunity*; prior receipt of vaccine*	All health care workers‖	0.5 mL SC,¶ no booster	As for measles (above) if provided as MMR
Rubella	Born before 1957††, physician-diagnosed disease*; laboratory evidence of immunity (if history negative or uncertain)*; prior receipt of vaccine*	All health care workers‖	0.5 mL SC,¶ no booster	As for measles (above) if provided as MMR, monovalent rubella vaccine not produced in eggs and hence egg allergies not a contraindication
Varicella	Personal history of varicella-zoster virus infection or laboratory evidence of immunity*; laboratory evidence of immunity (if history negative or uncertain)*; prior receipt of 2 doses of vaccine (age ≥ 13 yr) separated by at least 1 mo*	All health care workers‖	0.5 mL SC, second dose 4–8 wk later if ≥ 13 yr of age	Pregnancy; history of anaphylactic reaction to gelatin or neomycin; immunocompromised state**; recent receipt of immunoglobulin; avoid salicylate use for 6 wk after vaccination
Hepatitis B	Laboratory evidence of immunity*‡‡; prior receipt of 3 doses of vaccine with an appropriate schedule*	All health care workers‖ with potential exposure to blood or body fluids	1.0 mL IM (deltoid) at 0, 1, 6 mo§§; booster doses not necessary	History of anaphylactic reaction to common baker's yeast; pregnancy should not be considered a contraindication
Influenza	Yearly immunization needed	All health care workers		History of anaphylactic reaction to eggs

*Written documentation should be required.

†The package insert and CDC/ACIP should always be consulted for specific recommendations regarding indications, storage, administration, precautions, and contraindications. Doses listed are for adults; CDC/ACIP guidelines should be consulted when providing vaccines for children.

‡During an outbreak, immunity should be ensured by serologic testing or immunization records.

§People vaccinated from 1963 to 1967 with a killed measles vaccine alone, with a killed vaccine followed by live vaccine, or with a vaccine of unknown type should be revaccinated with two doses of live measles virus vaccine.

‖People who provide health care to patients or who work in institutions that provide health care (e.g., physicians, nurses, emergency medical personnel, dental professionals and students, medical and nursing students, laboratory technicians, hospital volunteers, and administrative and support staff in health care institutions).

¶MMR vaccine preferred.

**People immunocompromised because of immune deficiency diseases; human immunodeficiency virus infection; or leukemia, lymphoma, or generalized malignancy; or immunosuppressed as a result of therapy with corticosteroids (i.e., ≥2 mg/kg body weight or 20 mg/day of prednisone for ≥2 weeks), alkylating drugs, antimetabolites, or radiation (See also Table 59–3).

††Adults born before 1957 generally may be considered immune except for women of child-bearing age. Consideration should be given to serologically testing or immunizing all individuals born before 1957.

‡‡Immunity is indicated by an anti-HBsAg titer of 10 mIU/mL or greater.

§§Immunity should be assessed 1 to 2 months after the third dose. If the health care worker does not develop immunity, additional vaccine should be provided and immunity reassessed as follows: (1) provide additional doses of vaccine (at 0, 1, and 6 months), testing for immunity 1 month after each vaccine dose and stopping if immunity is achieved; or (2) provide three additional doses of vaccine (at 0, 1, and 6 months) and assess immunity 1 month after the second vaccine series is completed. If worker is not immune after a total of six doses of vaccine, test for HBsAg and, if HBsAg is absent, provide hepatitis B immune globulin as postexposure prophylaxis when indicated.

CDC/ACIP, Centers for Disease Control and Prevention/Advisory Committee on Immunization Practices; HBsAg, hepatitis B surface antigen; IM, intramuscularly; MMR, measles-mumps-rubella; SC, subcutaneously.

typhoid,[60,61] vaccinia (smallpox),[62] hepatitis A,[63] and anthrax[64] (Table 59–2).

Immunocompromised employees require special consideration in the provision of immunizations (Table 59–3).[54-68] First, live virus vaccines (e.g., measles-mumps-rubella [MMR], varicella, polio, BCG) may be contraindicated. Second, vaccines not routinely recommended may be indicated (e.g., pneumococcal, meningococcal, *Haemophilus influenzae* type b, and influenza vaccines). Third, higher antigen doses or postimmunization serologic evaluation may be indicated (e.g., hepatitis B vaccine in people with renal failure) because immunization of immunocompromised people may elicit a lower antibody response. Finally, such employees should be individually evaluated for reassignment (with the consent of the employee) depending on their job duties.

Pregnant employees also require special consideration in the provision of immunizations. The risks from immunization

TABLE 59–2 ▪ Vaccines Available for Health Care Workers and Laboratory Personnel in Special Circumstances

Vaccine	Indication(s)*	Administration*	Major Contraindications*
Anthrax[†]	Laboratory workers or researchers engaged in work involving production quantities or concentrations of *Bacillus anthracis* cultures or in activities with a high potential for aerosol production	SC injections at 0, 2, and 4 wk, then 6, 12, and 18 mo. Annual booster injection if immunity is to be maintained.	Previous history of anthrax infection or anaphylactic reaction to a previous dose of vaccine or to any of the vaccine components. Avoid in pregnancy unless benefits exceed risk.
BCG (for tuberculosis)	Health care workers in localities where (1) multidrug-resistant tuberculosis is prevalent; (2) a strong likelihood of infection exists; and (3) full implementation of infection control precautions have been inadequate in controlling the spread of infection	One percutaneous dose of 0.3 mL; no booster recommendation	Immunocompromised state[‡] or pregnancy
Hepatitis A	Not routinely indicated for health care workers; persons who work with HAV-infected primates in a laboratory setting	Two doses of vaccine IM either 6–12 mo apart (VAQTA) or 6 mo apart (Havrix)	History of anaphylaxis to a previous dose; safety not established in pregnancy; avoid in pregnancy unless risk of infection high
Meningococcal (A, C, Y, W135)	Not routinely indicated; may be useful during an outbreak of type included in vaccine	One dose 0.5 mL IM; consider booster dose within 3–5 yr if exposure continues	—
Plague	Laboratory personnel who frequently work with *Yersinia pestis*	Three doses IM; first dose 1.0 mL; second dose 0.2 mL 1–3 mo after first dose; third dose 0.2 mL 5–6 mo after second dose; boosters (0.2 mL) at 1- to 2-yr intervals if exposure continues	History of anaphylaxis to previous dose
Pneumococcal polysaccharide (23 valent)	Adults at increased risk of pneumococcal disease and its complications because of underlying health conditions; adults ≥50 yr old	One dose IM or SC; revaccination recommendations depend on reason for administration	Safety not established in first trimester of pregnancy but no known adverse events reported; use in pregnancy if benefits exceed risks
Polio	Health care workers in close contact with people who may be excreting wild virus; laboratory personnel handling specimens that may contain wild virus; OPV available only for control of outbreaks	Unimmunized adults: enhanced-potency inactivated vaccine (IPV); two doses SC given 4–8 wk apart, followed by a third dose at 6–12 mo after second dose; IPV should be used for a booster dose	History of anaphylaxis after streptomycin or neomycin; avoid in pregnancy unless risk of infection is high
Rabies	Personnel working with rabies virus or infected animals in diagnostic or research activities; postexposure prophylaxis boosters may be required despite primary immunization	Pre-exposure: HDCV, RVA,[§] or PCEC IM on days 0, 7, and 21 or 28; *or* HDCV ID on days 0, 7, and 21 or 28. Follow standard guidelines for postexposure prophylaxis.	—
Tetanus and diphtheria toxoids (Td)	All adults; additional tetanus prophylaxis may be required in wound management	Unimmunized adults: 2 doses IM 4 wk apart; third dose 6–12 mo after second dose. Fully immunized adults: booster dose as young adult and at age 50 (ACP) or every 10 yr (ACIP)	Avoid during first trimester in pregnancy; history of a neurologic reaction or anaphylaxis. Avoid for 10 yr after severe local (Arthus-type) reaction to a previous dose.
Typhoid[‖]	Laboratory personnel who frequently work with *Salmonella typhi*	One 0.5-mL dose IM (ViCPS); booster doses of 0.5 mL every 2 yr *or* Four oral doses (Ty21a)[¶] on alternate days; as per manufacturer revaccinate with the entire 4-dose series every 5 yr	History of severe local reaction or anaphylaxis to a previous dose of vaccine

Continued

TABLE 59–2 ■ Vaccines Available for Health Care Workers and Laboratory Personnel in Special Circumstances — cont'd

Vaccine	Indication(s)*	Administration*	Major Contraindications*
Vaccinia	Personnel who directly handle cultures or animals contaminated with recombinant vaccinia or orthopox viruses (monkeypox, cowpox) that infect humans. Pre- or postexposure prophylaxis for bioterrorist use of variola (smallpox).	One dose administered with a bifurcated needle; boosters every 10 yr	Pregnancy; presence or history of eczema in worker or close family contacts; other acute, chronic, or exfoliative skin conditions; immunosuppression in vaccine recipient or household contact; age <18 yr; vaccine component allergy**

*The package insert and CDC/ACIP should always be consulted for specific recommendations regarding indications, storage, administration, precautions, and contraindications.

†May not be available for civilian use. Table provides recommendations for pre-exposure prophylaxis. See text for recommendations regarding use as adjunct to antibiotics for postexposure treatment.

‡People immunocompromised because of immune deficiency diseases; human immunodeficiency virus infection; or leukemia, lymphoma, or generalized malignancy; or immunosuppressed as a result of therapy with corticosteroids (i.e., ≥2 mg/kg body weight or 20 mg/day of prednisone for ≥2 weeks), alkylating drugs, antimetabolites, or radiation.

§Not currently available in the United States. Not effective against aerosol challenge. Not effective for postexposure prophylaxis.

‖Typhoid vaccines include the following: ViCPS, Vi capsular polysaccharide vaccine; and Ty21a, oral live, attenuated Ty21a vaccine.

¶Oral typhoid vaccine, if possible, should probably be avoided in healthcare workers providing direct patient care.

**Contraindications for nonemergency vaccine use. During a smallpox emergency there are no contraindications for exposed persons; for nonexposed persons, the same contraindications apply as for nonemergency use.

ACP, American College of Physicians; BCG, bacille Calmette-Guérin; CDC/ACIP, Centers for Disease Control and Prevention/Advisory Committee on Immunization Practices; HAV, hepatitis A virus; HDCV, human diploid cell vaccine; ID, intradermally; IM, intramuscularly; IPV, inactivated poliovirus vaccine; OPV, oral poliovirus vaccine; PCEC, purified chick embryo cell culture rabies vaccine; RVA, rabies vaccine adsorbed; SC, subcutaneously.

during pregnancy are largely theoretical.[32,33] The benefit of immunization among pregnant women usually outweighs the potential risks for adverse reactions, especially when the risk for disease exposure is high, infection would pose a special risk to the mother or fetus, and the vaccine is unlikely to cause harm. Furthermore, newer information continues to confirm the safety of vaccines given inadvertently during pregnancy. Ideally women of child-bearing age, including employees, should have been immunized against measles, mumps, rubella, varicella, tetanus, diphtheria, and hepatitis B as adolescents before becoming pregnant.[32] However, because this may not have occurred, it is especially important that all health care employees be screened for rubella immunity (by serology because history is often unreliable), because of the consequences of infection for the developing fetus. Attenuated vaccines (mumps, measles, rubella, and varicella) should be provided only to nonpregnant employees and deferred for pregnant women. If not up-to-date, pregnant employees should receive combined adult tetanus and diphtheria toxoids (Td).[32,69] Women who are in their second or third trimester (>14 weeks pregnant) during respiratory virus season should receive influenza immunization.[51] There is no convincing evidence of risk from immunizing pregnant women with other inactivated virus or bacterial vaccines, or toxoids. Susceptible pregnant women at high risk for specific infections should receive, as indicated, the following vaccines: hepatitis A, hepatitis B, influenza, pneumococcal polysaccharide, rabies, and poliovirus (inactivated).[32] Thimerosal-free hepatitis B vaccine should be used. Several vaccines are recommended as part of postexposure prophylaxis, including hepatitis A, hepatitis B, and rabies. The same indications for use should be followed in pregnant women. Pregnant women should be immunized with meningococcal vaccine when there is a substantial risk of infection, such as during epidemics.[70] Breast-feeding does not adversely affect the response to immunization and is not a contraindication for any of the currently recommended vaccines. The indications for using immune globulins, intravenous immune globulin, and specific immune globulins (e.g., tetanus immune globulin) in pregnant women are the same as those for women who are not pregnant.

Before the administration of any vaccine, the HCW should be evaluated for the presence of any condition(s) that are listed as a vaccine contraindication or precaution.[71] If such a condition is present, the risks and benefits of vaccination need to be carefully weighed by the health care provider and the employee. The most common contraindication is a history of an anaphylactic reaction to a previous dose of the vaccine or to a vaccine component. Factors that are not contraindications to immunization include the following: household contact with a pregnant woman; breast-feeding; reaction to a previous vaccination consisting only of mild to moderate local tenderness, swelling, or both, or fever less than 40.5°C; mild acute illness with or without low-grade fever; current antimicrobial therapy (except for oral typhoid vaccine) or convalescence from a recent illness; personal history of *allergies* except a history of an anaphylactic reaction to a vaccine component (e.g., people with a history of anaphylaxis to neomycin should not receive the MMR vaccine); and family history of *allergies*, adverse reactions to vaccination, or seizures.[33]

Postexposure Prophylaxis

All HCWs potentially exposed to a communicable disease should be evaluated by the institution's occupational health service. General guidelines for a postexposure evaluation of

TABLE 59–3 ■ Recommendations on Immunization of Health Care Workers with Special Conditions

Vaccine	Pregnancy	HIV Infection	Severe Immunosuppression*	Asplenia	Renal Failure	Diabetes	Alcoholism and Alcoholic Cirrhosis
BCG	UI	C	C	UI	UI	UI	UI
Hepatitis A	UI	UI	UI	UI	UI	UI	UI
Hepatitis B	R	R	R	R	R	R	R
Influenza[†]	R[‡]	R	R	R	R	R	R
MMR	C	R[§]	C	R	R	R	R
Meningococcal	UI	UI	UI	R	UI	UI	UI
Polio, inactivated[‖]	UI	UI	UI	UI	UI	UI	UI
Polio, oral[‖]	UI	C	C	UI	UI	UI	UI
Pneumococcal[†]	UI	R	R	R	R	R	R
Rabies	UI	UI	UI	UI	UI	UI	UI
Tetanus/diphtheria[†]	R	R	R	R	R	R	R
Typhoid, Ty21a	UI	C	C	UI	UI	UI	UI
Varicella	C	C	C	R	R	R	R
Vaccinia	UI	C	C	UI	UI	UI	UI

*Severe immunosuppression can be the result of congenital immunodeficiency; HIV infection; leukemia, lymphoma, or generalized malignancy; or therapy with alkylating agents, antimetabolites, radiation, or large amounts of corticosteroids.

[†]Recommendation based on the person's underlying medical condition(s) rather than occupation.

[‡]Recommended for women who will be in the second or third trimester of pregnancy during the influenza season.

[§]Generally contraindicated in persons with HIV infection; recommended for children (no official recommendation for serosusceptible adults) with CD4+ cell counts greater than 200/μL; consider reimmunization if initial immunization was given when CD4+ cell count was less than 200/μL and if CD4+ cell count increases to 200 μL or greater as a result of highly active antiretroviral therapy.

[‖]Immunization with IPV is recommended for unvaccinated health care workers who have close contact with persons who may be excreting wild poliovirus. Health care workers who have a primary series of OPV or IPV and are directly involved with the provision of care to patients who may be excreting poliovirus may receive another dose of IPV. Any suspected case of poliomyelitis should be investigated immediately. If evidence suggests transmission of wild poliovirus, control measures to contain further transmission should be instituted immediately, including an OPV immunization campaign.

BCG, bacille Calmette-Guérin; C, contraindicated; HIV, human immunodeficiency virus; IPV, inactivated poliovirus vaccine; MMR, measles-mumps-rubella vaccine; OPV, oral poliovirus vaccine; R, recommended; UI, use if indicated.

medical personnel have been published.[12] In brief, the following steps should be undertaken:

1. Confirm that the source has a communicable disease.
2. Determine that potential transmission could have taken place (e.g., close contact for transmission of *Neisseria meningitidis* or *Bordetella pertussis*).
3. Determine that the exposed employee was not protected by the use of personal protective equipment (e.g., N-95 respirator for airborne transmitted diseases).
4. Determine that the exposed employee is susceptible to infection (i.e., may require laboratory evaluation).
5. Determine if effective prophylaxis is available and recommended.
6. Determine that the employee has no contraindications to use of the recommended prophylaxis.
7. If the employee has a contraindication to the recommended prophylaxis, determine if an alternative exists and is safe to use.
8. Inform the employee of the risk of disease transmission, signs and symptoms of infection, and risks and benefits of prophylaxis.
9. Obtain informed consent for prophylaxis.
10. Obtain baseline laboratory tests, if indicated (e.g., anti–hepatitis B surface antigen [HBsAg] titer).
11. Assess whether the employee should be restricted in his or her work activities or furloughed (e.g., days 8 to 21 after exposure to varicella-zoster in a susceptible employee).
12. Arrange follow-up evaluations.

Vaccines that may be indicated for postexposure prophylaxis include tetanus toxoid (Td preferred), hepatitis B, and rabies (Tables 59–4 and 59–5). Varicella vaccine, when provided within 72 hours of exposure, may provide postexposure prophylaxis but is not recommended for use in HCWs because of incomplete efficacy.[47] The use of hepatitis A vaccine for postexposure prophylaxis is currently under investigation. Several vaccines have been provided to individuals without known direct exposure to an infected case to help contain community-wide or institutional outbreaks, including hepatitis A, meningococcal vaccine, and pertussis vaccine. Immunoglobulin preparations may be indicated as part of postexposure prophylaxis for exposure to hepatitis A (immune globulin), hepatitis B (hepatitis B immune globulin [HBIG]), measles (immune globulin), rabies (rabies immune globulin), tetanus (tetanus immune globulin), and varicella (varicella-zoster immune globulin [VZIG]). All employees who are exposed to a communicable disease or with symptoms of an infectious disease should be evaluated with the consideration of whether work restriction or furlough is required to prevent secondary cases from developing among patients or staff (Table 59–6).

TABLE 59–4 ■ Postexposure Prophylaxis for Vaccine-Preventable Diseases

Disease	Definition of Exposure	Prophylaxis*	Comments
Hepatitis A	Ingestion of contaminated food; contact with feces from a hepatitis A–infected patient	One dose IM of immune globulin 0.02 mL/kg given within 14 days of exposure in large muscle mass (gluteal or deltoid)	Avoid in people with IgA deficiency; do not administer within 2 wk of MMR vaccine or 3 wk of varicella vaccine unless benefits exceed risk (e.g., known exposure)
Hepatitis B	Contact with HBsAg-positive blood (or body fluid) via percutaneous, mucous membrane, or nonintact skin exposure	See Table 59–5	Employees who have ever demonstrated an anti-HBsAg titer ≥10 mIU/mL do not require postexposure prophylaxis
Influenza A	Cohabiting confined air space or face-to-face contact in an open area[†]	Amantadine or rimantidine 100 mg PO bid may be considered if unimmunized. Zanamivir two 5-mg blister packs by inhaler bid or oseltamivir 75 mg PO bid also may be used.	Amantadine/rimantadine may be associated with altered mentation. Avoid zanamivir if asthmatic. Oseltamivir associated with gastrointestinal toxicity (~10%). Not recommended for pregnant women.
Influenza B	Cohabiting confined air space or face-to-face contact in an open area[†]	Zanamivir two 5-mg blister packs by inhaler bid or oseltamivir 75 mg PO bid	Avoid zanamivir if asthmatic. Oseltamivir associated with gastrointestinal toxicity (~10%). Not recommended for pregnant women.
Measles	Cohabiting confined air space or face-to-face contact in an open area (nonimmune employee)[†]	Susceptible personnel should receive immune globulin 0.25 mL/kg (maximum 15 mL) IM within 3 days of exposure or measles vaccine	Susceptible employees should be furloughed from days 5 to 21 postexposure or for 7 days after the rash appears
Meningococcus	Direct contact with respiratory secretions from infected person (e.g., resuscitating, intubating, or closely examining the oropharynx of an infected patient)[†]	Ciprofloxacin 500 mg PO once or ceftriaxone 250 mg IM once or rifampin 600 mg PO bid for 2 days	Home contacts of exposed health care providers do not need to receive prophylaxis unless the employee develops infection; rifampin and ciprofloxacin not recommended in pregnancy
Pertussis	Direct contact with respiratory secretions or droplets from the respiratory tract of infected persons[†]	Exposed employees should receive azithromycin PO (500 mg day 1, 250 mg days 2–5) or erythromycin 500 mg tid for 14 days[‡]; trimethoprim-sulfamethoxazole 1 PO bid is an alternative in macrolide-intolerant persons	Symptomatic employees should be evaluated for infection with a nasopharyngeal culture plated on appropriate media (and PCR if available), and should be relieved from work
Varicella	Cohabiting confined air space or face-to-face contact in an open area[†] with a patient with active lesions or within 48 hr before the development of lesions	For susceptible employees, VZIG 125 U/10 kg IM (maximum dose 625 U) is indicated for immunocompromised or pregnant adults (within 96 hr of exposure)	Susceptible employees should be furloughed from days 8 to 21 postexposure. Employees who receive VZIG should be furloughed from days 8 to 28 postexposure
Zoster	Cohabiting confined air space or face-to-face contact in an open area[†] with a patient with uncovered active lesions	As for varicella exposure	Same as varicella exposure

*The latest guidelines from the Centers for Disease Control and Prevention should always be consulted.
[†]Employee who was wearing a mask (surgical mask or N-95 respirator) is not considered exposed.
[‡]Some experts recommend the estolate preparation. In vitro and in vivo data suggest that azithromycin is likely as effective as erythromycin and associated with fewer side effects.
bid, twice per day; HBsAg, hepatitis B surface antigen; IM, intramuscularly; MMR, measles-mumps-rubella vaccine; PCR, polymerase chain reaction; PO, orally; tid, four times per day; VZIG, varicella-zoster immune globulin.

Postexposure Prophylaxis for Bioterrorism Agents

Several publications have highlighted the concern about the potential for biologic terrorism.[72–76] The CDC has categorized several agents as "high priority" because they can be easily disseminated or transmitted person-to-person, cause high mortality, and are likely to cause public panic and social disruption. These agents include *Bacillus anthracis* (anthrax), *Yersinia pestis* (plague), variola major (smallpox), *Clostridium botulinum* toxin (botulism), *Francisella tularensis* (tularemia), filoviruses (Ebola virus disease, Marburg disease); and arenaviruses (Lassa [Lassa hemorrhagic fever], Junin [Argentine hemorrhagic fever], and related viruses).[77] Characteristics of these high-priority agents include the following: they are

TABLE 59–5 ■ Recommended Postexposure Prophylaxis for Exposure to Hepatitis B Virus

Vaccination and Antibody Response of Exposed Workers[*]	Treatment		
	Source HBsAg Positive	Source HBsAg Negative	Source Not Tested or Unknown
Unvaccinated	HBIG[†] once and initiate HBV vaccine series	initiate HBV vaccine series	Initiate HBV vaccine series
Previously vaccinated			
Known responder[‡]	No treatment	No treatment	No treatment
Known nonresponder[§]	HBIG once and initiate revaccination or HBIG twice[‖]	No treatment	If known high-risk source, treat as if source were HBsAg positive
Antibody response unknown	Test exposed person for anti-HBs[¶] 1. If adequate,[‡] no treatment is necessary 2. If inadequate,[§] administer HBIG once and vaccine booster	No treatment	Test exposed person for anti-HBs.[§] 1. If adequate,[‡] no treatment is necessary 2. If inadequate,[§] give vaccine booster and recheck titer in 1–2 mo

[*]Persons who have previously been infected with HBV are immune to reinfection and do not require postexposure prophylaxis.
[†]Dose is 0.06 mL/kg intramuscularly.
[‡]A responder is a person who has adequate levels of serum antibody to HBsAg (i.e., anti-HBsAg $\geq$ 10 mIU/mL).
[§]A nonresponder is a person who has an inadequate response to vaccination (i.e., serum anti-HBsAg $\leq$ 10 mIU/mL).
[‖]The option of giving one dose of HBIG and reinitiating the vaccine series is preferred for nonresponders who have not completed a second three-dose series. For persons who previously completed a second vaccine series but failed to respond, two doses of HBIG (1 month apart) are preferred.
[¶]Antibody to HBsAg.
HBIG, hepatitis B immune globulin; HBsAg, hepatitis B surface antigen; HBV, hepatitis B virus.

infectious via aerosol, the organisms are fairly stable in aerosol form, there are susceptible civilian populations, infection is associated with high morbidity and mortality, several exhibit person-to-person transmission (i.e., cutaneous anthrax, pneumonic plague, smallpox, and Ebola, Marburg, Lassa, and Junin viruses), they are difficult to diagnose and/or treat, and most have previously been developed as biologic weapons.

Recently, the United States has been subjected to a bioterrorist attack. During September through October, letters containing anthrax spores led to multiple cases of anthrax in the United States.[78] By the end of 2001, 22 cases of anthrax had been reported, including 11 cases of cutaneous anthrax and 11 cases of inhalational anthrax.[79] Additional cases of cutaneous anthrax have occurred among laboratory/research personnel evaluating the outbreak. This attack resulted in significant public concern and anxiety. More than 30,000 people began prophylaxis, and a full course of therapy (i.e., 60 days) was advised for more than 5000 persons. The clinical features and management (pre-exposure prophylaxis, postexposure prophylaxis, and treatment) of anthrax have been reviewed.[80–82] The CDC and infectious disease experts have provided general recommendations for recognizing the most likely agents of bioterrorism[83–85] and provided detailed flow charts for the clinical evaluation of persons with possible inhalational or cutaneous anthrax.[78] Detailed management recommendations have been published for anthrax,[86,87] botulism,[88] plague,[89] smallpox,[90] and tularemia.[91]

Key aspects of the management of patients infected with bioterrorism agents include decontamination prior to medical evaluation, proper isolation, rapid diagnosis with appropriate therapy, and postexposure prophylaxis of exposed persons. HCWs may acquire infection from patients via contaminated clothes (smallpox, Q fever, plague, and anthrax) or via patient-to-HCW transmission.[92] In the advent of an attack with mass casualties and widespread

exposures, vaccines likely will play an important adjunctive role in limiting the impact of anthrax and the critical role in containing smallpox.[93,94] Currently the recommended postexposure prophylaxis for anthrax is doxycycline orally for 60 days (alternative therapy includes ciprofloxacin and, if the strain is proven susceptible, amoxicillin).[87] Anthrax vaccine has been suggested for optimal postexposure management of persons exposed to anthrax based on studies in primates.[86,87,95] The use of anthrax vaccine for postexposure prophylaxis is considered experimental and should only be provided with informed consent under Investigational New Drug status. During the recent anthrax attack, persons deemed by public health authorities to have been at high risk for exposure were offered anthrax vaccine (three inoculations at 2-week intervals, given on days 1, 14, and 28) as an adjunct to prolonged postexposure antibiotic prophylaxis. Currently pre-exposure use of anthrax vaccine is recommended only for laboratory workers or researchers at risk for anthrax exposure (see Table 59–2).

Vaccinia vaccine is effective as postexposure prophylaxis following smallpox exposure when used within 4 days.[90] Because of the frequent and sometimes severe side effects associated with vaccinia vaccination,[90] it is unlikely that pre-exposure prophylaxis will be recommended for all HCWs. It is likely that pre-exposure prophylaxis will be available for teams of health care professionals and law enforcement personnel charged with responding to a potential bioterrorist attack and providing initial care of persons with known or suspected smallpox. Recommendations regarding vaccinia vaccine almost certainly would change in the advent of use of smallpox as a terrorist weapon or if evidence accumulates that potential terrorists have gained access to smallpox virus.

If vaccines now in development for other bioterrorism agents (e.g., Q fever) become available, HCWs may be included in both pre- and postexposure recommendations.

TABLE 59–6 ■ Work Restrictions for Vaccine-Preventable Diseases

Disease	Work Restriction	Duration
Hepatitis A	Relieve from direct patient contact and food handling	Until 7 days after onset of jaundice
Hepatitis B		
Acute	Relieve from direct patient contact	Until jaundice resolves
Chronic	No restriction unless demonstrated to transmit infections to patients	Counsel regarding need to follow standard precautions; if health care worker transmits hepatitis B despite practicing precautions, prohibit from performing invasive procedures and direct contact with patient equipment until hepatitis B antigenemia resolves
Measles		
Active	Furlough from health care facility	Until 4 days after rash appears
Postexposure (susceptible personnel)	Furlough from health care facility	From the 5th day after the first exposure through the 21st day after the last exposure or 4 days after the rash appears
Mumps		
Active	Furlough from health care facility	Until 9 days after onset of parotitis
Postexposure (susceptible personnel)	Furlough from health care facility	From the 12th day after the first exposure through the 26th day after the last exposure or until 9 days after the onset of parotitis
Pertussis		
Active	Furlough from health care facility	From the beginning of the catarrhal stage through the third week after onset of paroxysms or until 5 days after start of effective antimicrobial therapy
Postexposure (asymptomatic personnel)	No restriction, if on prophylactic antimicrobial therapy	—
Postexposure (symptomatic personnel)	Furlough from health care facility	Same as active pertussis
Rubella		
Active	Furlough from health care facility	Until 5 days after rash appears
Postexposure (susceptible personnel)	Furlough from health care facility	From the 7th day after first exposure through the 21st day after the last exposure or 5–7 days after rash appears
Influenza A and B	Furlough from health care facility	Until acute symptoms resolve
Varicella		
Active	Furlough from health care facility	Until the lesions are dried and crusted
Postexposure (susceptible personnel)	Furlough from health care facility	From the 8th day after the first exposure through the 21st day (28th day if VZIG given) after the last exposure, *or*, if varicella occurs, until all lesions are dried and crusted
Zoster		
Localized (nonexposed area of skin), in a normal person	Cover lesions; relieve from care of high-risk patients	Until the lesions are dried and crusted
Localized (exposed area of skin); localized in immunocompromised person; generalized	Furlough from health care facility	Until the lesions are dried and crusted
Postexposure (susceptible personnel)	Furlough from health care facility	From the 8th day after the first exposure through the 21st day (28th day if VZIG given) after the last exposure, *or*, if varicella occurs, until all lesions are dried and crusted

VZIG, varicella-zoster immune globulin.

Providing Vaccines for Health Care Workers

All HCWs new to a health care facility should be screened for immunity to vaccine-preventable diseases within 10 working days. Unless immune, the HCW should be appropriately immunized. In general, serologic screening for immunity before immunization is neither necessary nor cost-effective. Each health care facility, however, needs to evaluate the cost-effectiveness of screening. Factors that determine the effectiveness of serologically screening employees for immunity include the cost of the screening test, the cost of the vaccine, and the prevalence of immunity in the population. The prevalence of immunity in the population likely depends on age, gender, race, place of birth, and socioeconomic status. In addition, the sensitivity and specificity of the screening test must be considered.

The immunization status of all HCWs should be recorded in their medical record, which should be maintained by the institution's occupational health service. Each HCW should be provided the information required under the National Childhood Vaccine Injury Act of 1986 before receiving measles, mumps, rubella, polio, tetanus, diphtheria, hepatitis B, *H. influenzae* type b, or varicella vaccine.[96] Signed informed consent specific to each vaccine should be obtained before immunization. When vaccines are provided, appropriate information should be recorded in the employee's medical record (Table 59–7).

Improving Vaccine Coverage of Health Care Personnel

Despite recommendations regarding immunization of HCWs for vaccine-preventable diseases, studies continue to demonstrate that significant numbers of HCWs lacked evidence of immunity to these diseases and that many HCWs refuse immunization. A survey of 144 medical schools in the United States and Canada in 1988 revealed that 28% had no immunization requirements for matriculating medical students, 31% had no rubella immunity requirement, and 40% had no measles immunity requirement.[97] Not surprisingly, a survey in 1987 of arriving house staff at Columbia

TABLE 59–7 ■ Information That Should Be Obtained When Providing Vaccines to Health Care Workers

Employee name
Employee identification number
Date of birth or age
Date of immunization
Vaccine provided
Name of vaccine manufacturer
Lot number of vaccine
Site of immunization
Route of immunization
Date for additional immunizations (if required)
Complications (if any)
Name, title, and address of person providing vaccine
Signed informed consent

Presbyterian Medical Center in New York revealed the following rates of potential susceptibility to vaccine-preventable diseases as determined by lack of known immunization or physician-diagnosed disease (measles, mumps) or serology (rubella, hepatitis B, varicella): measles, mumps, or rubella, 63%; hepatitis B, 37%; and varicella, 5%.[98] A survey of 95 acute care hospitals in Los Angeles County conducted in 1992 revealed that 36%, 60%, and 22% lacked immunization requirements for measles, mumps, and rubella, respectively.[99] Similarly, a survey of 62 infection control professionals practicing at children's hospitals in 1995 reported the following frequency of the existence of an immunization policy including mumps, measles, rubella, and varicella: medical students, 47% to 74% depending on the vaccine; resident physicians, 70% to 91%; hospital-based physicians, 40% to 55%; and private or community based physicians, 15% to 26%.[100] Selected studies of hepatitis B and influenza vaccine coverage rates are shown in Table 59–8.[101–115]

Screening of hospital staff has consistently demonstrated that, in the absence of a policy requiring immunity, significant numbers of hospital staff are susceptible to vaccine-preventable diseases. For example, surveys of hospital employees between 1990 and 1991 revealed that 5.3% to 10.3% were susceptible to measles despite a policy recommending measles immunity that did not include a requirement.[116,117] Other investigators have reported similar rates of serosusceptibility (6% to 10.4%) to measles among HCWs in the early 1990s.[118–120] The importance of a policy requiring screening and immunization of susceptible employees is highlighted by a paper that reported that seropositive rates for measles declined from 96% to 91% for adult HCWs hired at a cancer hospital between 1998 and 1999 compared with those of the same age hired between 1983 and 1988.[121]

Surveys of physicians have reported high rates of failure to receive hepatitis B vaccine (see Table 59–8). Similarly, surveys of HCWs have reported low rates of acceptance of influenza immunization. Barriers to receiving influenza vaccine commonly reported by HCWs have included desire to avoid medications, inconvenient vaccine administration, concern about side effects, belief that influenza can be caused by the vaccine, and belief that the vaccine is ineffective.[101,107,122] Similar concerns are voiced about hepatitis B vaccine, including desire to avoid medications, perception that the HCW is at low risk for occupationally acquired hepatitis B virus (HBV) infection, and concern about side effects.[122] Interventions such as the use of a mobile cart vaccination program have been demonstrated to increase immunization rates with influenza vaccine, but still to suboptimal levels.[123]

Guidelines for the Use of Selected Vaccines

Measles-Mumps-Rubella Vaccine

Epidemiology

The incidence of mumps, measles, and rubella has decreased dramatically since the widespread use of MMR

TABLE 59–8 ■ Vaccine Coverage of Health Care Workers in Series Reported in the Literature

Reference	Study Year(s)	Study Location	Health Care Workers	Vaccine	Immunization Frequency
Weingarten et al.[101]	1986–87	Los Angeles hospital	House staff and nurses	Influenza	3.5%
Shapiro et al.[102]	1991	3411 orthopedic surgeons	Orthopedics	Hepatitis B	65%
McArthur et al.[105]	1991	1270 extended-care facilities, Canada	All staff	Influenza	>75% in 3.7% of facilities
Panlilio et al.[109]	1991–92	21 hospitals	General surgery, orthopedics, gynecology	Hepatitis B	55%
Agerton et al.[108]	1992	150 hospitals, United States	All staff	Hepatitis B	51%
Cleveland[103]	1992	U.S. dentists	Dentists	Hepatitis B	85%
Nichol and Hauge[107]	1993–94	Minneapolis hospital	Physicians and nurses	Influenza	61.2%
Gyawali et al.[110]	1994	London teaching hospital	Staff with blood exposure	Hepatitis B	78%
Mahoney et al.[111]	1994–95	200 U.S. hospitals	Staff eligible for hepatitis B vaccine	Hepatitis B	66.5%
Zadeh et al.[112]	1995–98	Nursing homes, nine U.S. states	Staff	Influenza	46%
Cui et al.[113]	1996–98	43 nursing homes, Hawaii	Staff	Influenza	38%
Russell[114]	1998	136 nursing homes, Alberta, Canada	Staff	Influenza	29.9%
Stevenson et al.[115]	1999	Nursing homes, Canada	Staff	Influenza	35%

vaccine. Cases reported to the CDC in 2000 were as follows (cases per 100,000 population in parentheses): mumps, 338 (0.13); measles, 86 (0.03); rubella, 176 (0.06); and congenital rubella syndrome, 9.[124] All three diseases represent a significant health hazard for hospital personnel for the following reasons. First, all three are transmitted by the droplet route (measles is also transmitted by the airborne route). Second, in all three diseases, people become infectious before developing a clinically recognizable illness. Third, a history of prior disease may be unreliable for determining whether employees actually suffered a vaccine-preventable disease in the past. Hence, many unimmunized employees may falsely believe themselves immune.

Rubella is of special concern because of its ability to cause congenital abnormalities in up to 90% of women with confirmed infection in the first trimester of pregnancy. Hospital workers are frequently females of child-bearing age. Infants with congenital rubella may be contagious until they are at least 1 year old.

Lessons from Hospital Outbreaks

Nosocomial outbreaks of mumps have been reported infrequently,[125–131] but transmission from patient to patient[125,126,130,131] and from patient to health care provider has been reported.[128–131] In one case, it was suggested that an asymptomatically infected hospital nurse introduced mumps into a children's hospital.[126] Community outbreaks are likely to lead to nosocomial exposures. For example, during the widespread epidemic of mumps in Tennessee from 1986 to 1987, six HCWs in three different hospitals developed mumps after nosocomial exposure.[130] Men, including male HCWs, are at higher risk of complications from mumps (such as orchitis) than are children.[132] Orchitis has been reported among male HCWs who developed mumps as a result of hospital exposure.[128]

Nosocomial measles is well documented in the literature[133–165] and may aid in the propagation of community outbreaks.[153–155] Analyses of measles cases reported to the CDC revealed acquisition in a medical setting for 241 people (1.1% of all cases) between 1980 and 1984[145] and for 1209 people (3.5% of all cases) between 1985 and 1989.[156] Investigations of individual outbreaks, however, have reported that 17% to 53% of cases were acquired in a medical setting.[137,139,143,146,150,154,158] Acquisition of measles has occurred in outpatient settings, including emergency departments and physician offices, and has involved patient-to-patient, patient-to-staff, and staff-to-patient transmission. Transmission in the outpatient setting has occurred even though the index cases had left the waiting or examination room up to 75 minutes earlier.[136,139,141,142,149,161,164] Case-control studies have demonstrated that people who visited an emergency department had a 4.9-fold[160] to 5.2-fold[155] higher risk of developing measles one incubation period later compared with those who did not have such visits. In inpatient settings, transmission also has occurred among patients, from patients to staff, and from infected staff to patients. Infected staff most commonly have been nurses, with other groups at high risk of infection being physicians and office or hospital clerical staff. Nosocomial outbreaks have led to hospitalization of infected staff,[157] severe complications in infected patients,[159] and occasionally death of patients.[153,157] The cost of controlling a single outbreak has ranged from $28,000 to more than $100,000.[153,157]

As with mumps and measles, nosocomial rubella is well documented in the literature.[166–183] Sources of rubella infection have included not only people with acute infection, but also infants with congenital rubella.[166,174,183] Hospital-acquired infection of pregnant staff members has led to the termination of pregnancy.[173,179]

Several valuable lessons have been learned from the outbreaks. First, it appears that mumps and rubella are acquired mainly via droplet transmission. Measles, however, may be acquired via airborne transmission. Furthermore, measles transmission may occur for more than an hour after an infected case has left an enclosed area. Second, history of prior disease is unreliable for determining whether employees actually contracted measles in the past, and hence many employees falsely believe they are immune from past illness and fail to take appropriate precautions. Third, failure to institute a mandatory program requiring immunity results in a subpopulation of susceptible HCWs capable of propagating epidemics. In multiple outbreaks, three to more than five generations of disease transmission occurred. Fourth, the cost of outbreaks for these diseases is high in both monetary terms and human suffering. Fifth, patients with congenital rubella are capable of transmitting rubella to susceptible adults.

Pre-Exposure Prophylaxis

All HCWs should be immune to mumps, measles, and rubella. Immunity may be demonstrated by meeting one of the following criteria: (1) birth before 1957 (mumps, rubella except women with child-bearing potential), (2) laboratory evidence of immunity (people with indeterminate levels are considered susceptible), (3) physician-diagnosed disease (measles, mumps), or (4) evidence of appropriate immunizations (see Table 59–1).[17] The CDC's Hospital Infection Control Practices Advisory Committee (HICPAC) now recommends that measles vaccine be administered to all HCWs born before 1957 if they do not have evidence of measles immunity and are at risk of occupational exposure to measles.[12] This recommendation is based on data from outbreak investigations, which revealed that 4% to 9% of people born before 1957 were susceptible to measles.[147,184,185] Hospitals that do not implement this recommendation should assess the immunity of HCWs born before 1957, in the same manner as for younger HCWs, during a community or institutional outbreak of measles. The HICPAC recommends that rubella vaccine be administered to all female HCWs with child-bearing potential if they do not have evidence of rubella immunity, including people born before 1957.[12] The American Academy of Pediatrics recommends that all HCWs, including those born before 1957, who are without serologic evidence of immunity to rubella should be immunized regardless of gender.[34]

Two doses of measles vaccine currently are recommended to ensure immunity (see Table 59–1). Revaccination with MMR also may be indicated for mumps because studies have shown that mumps can occur in a highly vaccinated population.[186]

Postexposure Management of Exposed Health Care Workers

No specific prophylaxis has been shown to be effective for mumps or rubella. Exposed susceptible people should be furloughed from the hospital (see Table 59–6). Patients with incubating or active mumps or rubella should be placed on Droplet Precautions. Patients with measles should be placed on Airborne Precautions. Measles vaccine can be used to provide postexposure prophylaxis of susceptible personnel if administered within 72 hours of exposure. Immune globulin, 0.25 mL/10 kg (maximum 15 mL), may be used for postexposure prophylaxis for susceptible personnel who are exposed to measles but must be provided within 6 days of exposure. It is especially recommended for pregnant women and immunocompromised people (dose, 0.5 mL/10 kg; maximum 15 mL).

Varicella Vaccine

Epidemiology

Varicella-zoster virus (VZV) is the causative agent of two diseases: varicella (chickenpox), the primary infection, and zoster (shingles), a secondary infection caused by reactivation of latent VZV.[187–193] With the incorporation of the varicella vaccine into the childhood vaccine schedule, the incidence of varicella disease appears to have declined dramatically in the United States.[194] Although varicella is generally a mild disease in children, serious morbidity and mortality are common if infection occurs in neonates, adults, or immunocompromised people. For these reasons, the CDC,[12] the American Academy of Pediatrics,[34] and infectious disease experts[37,195–202] have published recommendations regarding the isolation of patients with VZV infection and the management of patients and HCWs exposed to VZV. Since the licensure of a varicella vaccine, pre-exposure prophylaxis of HCWs for VZV has been possible.

In most cases, VZV appears to be transmitted from person to person by the droplet route, and transmission occurs most efficiently when there is close contact, but true airborne transmission also may occur. The secondary attack rate of varicella among susceptible people in the household setting has ranged from 61% to 87%.[203–205] Herpes zoster is also infectious, although analysis of households suggests that the risk of transmission is lower than that for varicella.

Lessons from Nosocomial Outbreaks

Control of varicella is important in health care facilities because varicella and zoster are highly contagious; infection in adults frequently results in complications, including hospitalization; infection in pregnant women may lead to the congenital varicella syndrome[207–211] and severe complications, including death, may occur in immunocompromised patients and employees. Importantly for hospitals, the risk of complications appears to be higher in neonates,[212,213] adults,[212–214] and immunocompromised people.[214] Approximately 1% to 2% of adults who develop varicella become ill enough to require hospitalization.[212,213] Among patients developing varicella while undergoing chemotherapy for malignancy or immunosuppressive therapy after organ or bone marrow transplantation, visceral dissemination or severe disease has been reported in 30% to 50% and death in 7% to 17%.[215–222] Current rates of morbidity and mortality are dramatically lower because of prophylactic use of antivirals, postexposure prophylaxis with VZIG, and availability of antivirals such as acyclovir for therapy.[223]

Studies have noted that 60% to 86% (median, 78%) of U.S. HCWs report that they have had varicella.[224–230] A report of prior varicella by an HCW has been demonstrated to be correlated with immunity as measured by serology.[231] A history of prior household exposure to VZV, however, is not a reliable indicator of immunity in the absence of clinical illness.[232] Among HCWs with a negative or uncertain history of VZV infection, reported serosusceptibility has varied from 4% to 47% (median, 15%).[199,224,226–230,233,234]

Overall, the susceptibility of HCWs to varicella has been reported to range from 1% to 7% (median, 3%).[224,226,227,229,230,233–235] After nosocomial exposure to VZV infection, 2% to 16% of susceptible staff have developed clinical varicella.[199,214,227]

Nosocomial transmission of VZV has been well documented in the literature.[199,205,214,225,227,230,235–250] Varicella may be introduced into the hospital by infected patients, staff, or visitors. Several investigators have noted that the initial source case for an outbreak was in the incubating phase of varicella.[199,204,227] Nosocomial varicella has occurred among staff and patients who had no direct contact with the index case, supporting the airborne route as a mode of spread.[237,248] Epidemiologic studies using tracers[246] or measurement of VZV DNA[251] have provided definitive evidence to support airborne transmission. By using polymerase chain reaction to detect VZV DNA, Yoshikawa and colleague demonstrated extensive environmental contamination in the room of a person with dermatomal zoster.[252] Exposure to dermatomal[199,237,242] or disseminated[225,226] zoster in immunocompromised patients and to dermatomal zoster in immunocompetent hosts has led to transmission of VZV to susceptible HCWs via the airborne route or droplet route.[199,246]

The CDC,[22] the American Academy of Pediatrics,[34] and infectious disease clinicians[46,195–199] have published guidelines or algorithms designed to aid clinicians in the control of nosocomial exposures. There are several areas of controversy among these various guidelines. First, the CDC suggests that exposed serosusceptible patients be placed on isolation and exposed serosusceptible employees be removed from work from days 10 through 21 postexposure, whereas the American Academy of Pediatrics[34] suggests isolation from days 8 through 21 postexposure. Second, the CDC continues to recommend that nonimmunocompromised patients with dermatomal zoster be placed on only contact isolation as opposed to airborne and contact isolation.[22] University of North Carolina Hospitals place patients with dermatomal zoster on airborne and contact isolation because of the difficulty of defining "immunocompromised patients" and reports of airborne or droplet transmission of varicella from nonimmunocompromised patients with dermatomal zoster.[199,246] Third, the CDC has recommended that all patients with varicella or disseminated zoster and immunocompromised patients with dermatomal zoster be placed in rooms meeting engineering requirements suitable to house patients with tuberculosis (i.e., private room, negative pressure of room with respect to corridor, six or more air exchanges per hour, and air exhausted directly to the outside). The authors are unaware of any nosocomial outbreaks in which transmission was linked to recirculated air of infected patients placed in private rooms with negative pressure. Furthermore, negative-pressure rooms have been reported to be adequate in preventing transmission of varicella from hospitalized patients.[245] Given the current incidence of varicella and tuberculosis, it is likely that many hospitals do not have adequate rooms meeting the OSHA tuberculosis requirements to use these rooms to isolate patients with VZV infections.

Pre-exposure Prophylaxis

The authors and other infectious disease specialists believe that all HCWs should be immune to VZV. There are several compelling reasons why HCWs should be immune. First, HCWs with incubating or clinical varicella have transmitted VZV infection to hospitalized patients. Such infections may lead to substantial morbidity in *high-risk* patients, such as pregnant women, neonates, and immunocompromised people. Second, HCWs are at risk of acquisition of VZV infection from patients with clinical varicella or zoster. Even healthy adults have a substantial risk of varicella complications. Furthermore, secondary VZV infections may occur among their contacts. Finally, the presence of susceptible hospital staff results in significant costs for health care organizations. These costs are associated with the removal of susceptible staff from patient contact after VZV exposures, administration of VZIG to immunocompromised patients exposed to HCWs with incubating or clinical varicella, and time and effort of hospital staff in evaluating VZV exposures. Decision and/or cost-effective analysis methods have been used to demonstrate that immunization of HCWs susceptible to varicella is cost-effective for health care facilities.[253–256] The efficacy and safety of varicella vaccine have been reviewed.[257–262]

HCWs should be screened for VZV immunity at the time of initial employment, as is currently recommended for mumps, measles, and rubella. Current employees may be screened at the time of their annual tuberculosis and immunization evaluation or via a special program. Employees with a history of VZV infection may be considered immune. Employees without a definitive history of VZV infection should undergo serologic testing and, if negative, be considered for immunization. The preferred test for determining immunity is probably the latex agglutination test followed by an enzyme-linked immunosorbent assay (ELISA) test or radioimmunoassay. Employees without a vaccine contraindication or precaution should be immunized with two doses at least 4 weeks apart of varicella vaccine. Performing a postimmunization serology is not recommended because commercial tests may lack the sensitivity to detect the lower antibody levels associated with immunization compared with natural infection. Further, the glycoprotein ELISA test (not commercially available) used by Merck & Co. (West Point, PA) suggests a seroconversion rate of 99% in adults, making postimmunization serologic testing not cost-effective.

There appears to be virtually no risk of transmission of the vaccine strain of virus from healthy people who do not develop a rash postimmunization. The risk of transmitting the vaccine strain, even to immunocompromised people, from HCWs who develop either a local rash or generalized rash is likely low but has not been precisely quantitated. The few employees who develop an injection site rash may continue to work with nonimmunocompromised patients, provided that the lesions are covered. Employees with a generalized rash should be furloughed until the rash is resolved. In the authors' experience, this has been approximately 5 days. The rash should not automatically be assumed to be due to vaccine, especially if exposure to a case of chickenpox has occurred in the preceding 3 weeks.

Postexposure Management of Exposed Health Care Workers

All employees potentially exposed to varicella or zoster should be evaluated as soon as feasible by the occupational health service. Employees with no history or an uncertain history (e.g., VZV infection in other family members) of varicella should be serologically tested for immunity. Employees with a positive test should be considered immune. All susceptible employees should be considered for postexposure prophylaxis with VZIG and removed from duty from days 8 through 21 postexposure. VZIG is indicated for employees who are pregnant or immunocompromised. Employees who develop varicella should be considered for antiviral therapy. Employees who develop varicella may return to work when clinically well and after all lesions are dried and crusted (usually about 5 days).

Insufficient data are available to provide definitive recommendations on the postexposure management of employees previously immunized with the varicella vaccine. One option[45] would be to test such employees serologically immediately postexposure. Serosusceptible employees would be retested for an anamnestic response 5 to 7 days postexposure. Employees testing nonimmune would be relieved from duty from days 8 though 21 postexposure. A second proposed option would be to examine employees daily and remove immunized employees only if they develop clinical varicella. If hospitals choose the latter option and an immunized employee develops varicella, it is unclear to what degree this employee would already have been a potential source case for patients or other staff.

Postexposure prophylaxis may be provided by administering VZIG or an antiviral (e.g., acyclovir). The latter measure should be considered experimental and requires additional prospective studies before adoption. Prophylactic acyclovir (20 mg/kg every 6 hours) from day 7 through day 17 postexposure has been used successfully to prevent disease in high-risk children.[263-265] The prophylactic use of acyclovir, however, was associated with a decreased rate of seroconversion; approximately 50% of the children remained serosusceptible.

The varicella vaccine may be used as postexposure prophylaxis.[47,266-275] Varicella vaccine has been most effective when administered within 3 days of exposure and is generally ineffective when administered more than 5 days after exposure. There are several compelling reasons why varicella vaccine should not be used for postexposure prophylaxis in HCWs. First, all HCWs should be immune to varicella via natural infection or immunization. Second, vaccine is only partially effective when used to provide postexposure prophylaxis. Finally, if one provides varicella vaccine as postexposure prophylaxis and the employee develops a rash, it would be impossible to immediately determine if the employee had a vaccine-induced rash (very low transmission risk), breakthrough wild-type infection (moderate risk of transmission), or wild-type infection (high risk of transmission).

VZIG is indicated for susceptible *high-risk* HCWs (i.e., those with leukemia or lymphoma, congenital or acquired immunodeficiency, immunosuppressive therapy, human immunodeficiency virus [HIV] infection) exposed to varicella.[34,47] VZIG is most effective when administered within 72 hours of exposure; its efficacy when used more than 96 hours after exposure is unknown. The adult dose of VZIG is 125 U/10 kg (maximum dose, 625 U or 5 vials). VZIG should be administered intramuscularly or as directed by the manufacturer. It should *not* be administered intravenously.

VZIG has been demonstrated to lead to attenuated disease in pregnant women and immunocompromised people but likely does not prevent congenital infection. VZIG may prolong the incubation period before disease; hence all employees treated with VZIG should be removed from duty from days 8 through 28.

All HCWs with VZV infection should be evaluated and, after confirmation of infection, should be offered recommended antiviral therapy, which should be initiated within 72 hours of the onset of clinical infection. Of the three drugs currently approved by the Food and Drug Administration for therapy of VZV in the normal adult (acyclovir, famciclovir, and valacyclovir), valacyclovir is the least expensive. Although the safety of acyclovir in pregnant women has not been firmly established, adverse fetal events have not been described. The American Academy of Pediatrics does not recommend the routine use of oral acyclovir for pregnant women with varicella. The Academy stated, however, that therapy with intravenous acyclovir should be considered for pregnant patients who develop serious varicella-associated complications.[34]

Hepatitis B Vaccine

Epidemiology

Exposure to blood-borne pathogens via parenteral or mucosal contact remains a major hazard for HCWs, especially those performing invasive procedures. Although more than 20 diseases have been transmitted by needle stick,[276] the agents of greatest concern are HBV, hepatitis C virus, and HIV.[277-282] Seroprevalence surveys conducted before the availability of the HBV vaccine in 1981 showed that HCWs had prevalence rates of past or present HBV infection threefold to fivefold higher than the general U.S. population.[283-286] The risk of infection was related to both the extent and the duration of blood contact. The CDC reported that, in 1989, an estimated 12,000 American HCWs would become infected with HBV, which would result in 250 deaths.[287] With a decreasing incidence of hepatitis B, the CDC estimated that, in 1994, 1012 HCWs became infected with HBV because of occupational exposures, leading to approximately 22 deaths.[288] In a more recent analysis, Mahoney and colleagues reported that HBV infection among HCWs declined from 17,000 in 1983 to 400 in 1995.[111] The 95% decline in incidence observed among HCWs was 1.5-fold greater than the reduction in incidence in the general U.S. population. The decline among HCWs was due to the use of HBV vaccine, institution of Universal (now Standard) Precautions, and other preventive measures (e.g., needleless devices).

Lessons from Nosocomial Outbreaks

Hepatitis B acquisition represents a major hazard for HCWs for several reasons. First, HCWs have high rates of percutaneous blood contact.[280] For example, a survey of New York City surgeons in 1988 reported that 86% had experienced at least one puncture injury in the preceding year.[289] A survey of American and Canadian orthopedic surgeons in 1991 revealed that 87.4% reported a blood-skin contact and 39.2% a percutaneous blood contact in the previous month.[290] Second, the virus is relatively stable in the environment, as demonstrated by its survival after drying and storage at 25°C and 42% relative humidity for 1 week.[291] Third, HBV is more transmissible than either HIV or hepatitis C virus, with rates of disease transmission after a percutaneous injury with a contaminated sharp reported as between 6% and 30%.[292–294] The risks of disease transmission via mucosal contact or contact with nonintact skin have not been quantitated but appear to be much lower than for percutaneous exposure. HBV infection has been acquired via ocular exposure[295] and has been transmitted to multiple patients by a respiratory therapist with severe exudative dermatitis while obtaining arterial blood gases.[296] The high frequency of hepatitis B among hospital personnel who did not recall a percutaneous exposure in the era before HBV vaccine has been attributed to inapparent inoculation through mucous membranes or small breaks in the skin.[297] Fourth, a significant number of patients are infectious (i.e., HBsAg-positive), with their status unknown to the medical staff. For example, a study of consecutive blood samples submitted to the chemistry laboratory of an urban hospital in 1987 revealed that only 28% of HBsAg-positive specimens were labeled as per hospital protocol with a biohazard label.[298] Finally, many HCWs remain unimmunized.

Transmission of hepatitis B via contaminated medical instruments and environmental surfaces is well described.[299] Nosocomial outbreaks of HBV infection have been associated with a blood-contaminated jet gun injector,[300] an endoscope,[301] multidose medication vials,[302,303] electroencephalography electrodes,[304] and finger stick (i.e., capillary) blood-sampling devices.[305–310] Contamination of instruments or medication vials resulted in 67 of 243 cardiac transplant patients developing infection during transvenous endomyocardial biopsies.[311] Environmental surfaces in clinical laboratories were demonstrated to be positive for HBsAg in 34% of samples,[312] and contaminated file cards have been reported to lead to transmission among laboratory technicians.[313]

Transmission of hepatitis B in hemodialysis centers, presumably via contaminated environmental surfaces, shared equipment, or common-dose medications, continues to be a problem.[314–318] In addition to standard precautions, the following hemodialysis-specific infection control practices should be used[319]:

1. Serum specimens from all susceptible patients should be tested monthly for HBsAg, and these results should be reviewed promptly.
2. HBsAg-positive patients should be isolated by room, machine, instruments, medications, supplies, and staff.
3. Instruments, medications, and supplies should not be shared between any patients. When sharing of multidose medication vials is necessary, medications must be prepared in a clean centralized area separate from areas used for patient care, laboratory work, or refuse disposal.
4. Routine cleaning and disinfection procedures should be followed.

In addition, all serosusceptible hemodialysis patients should receive the HBV vaccine. Because hemodialyzed patients have a diminished response to HBV vaccine, higher doses and booster doses are recommended to maintain protection

against hepatitis B. Hemodialysis patients who receive the vaccine should have their anti-HBsAg level determined annually and, if anti-HBsAg declines to less than 10 mIU/mL, a booster dose should be provided.

More than 40 outbreaks have been described of health care provider–to-patient transmission of hepatitis B.[320–324] The source has most commonly been a dentist, surgeon, or gynecologist performing invasive procedures. The most important risk factors for transmission during an invasive procedure have been a hepatitis B e antigen–positive source, degree of invasiveness of the procedure, lack of wearing gloves by the infected HCW, or injury to the infected HCW with a sharp object. Guidelines for the management of the HBV-infected HCW have been published.[325]

Pre-exposure Prophylaxis

Because of the risks posed by blood-borne pathogens, OSHA has mandated since 1991 that all health care personnel undergo annual training in the prevention of blood-borne pathogen acquisition and use of personal protective equipment (gloves, masks, gown, and eyewear) whenever exposure to blood or other potentially infectious body fluids is reasonably anticipated.[326,327] However, despite the OSHA regulations and the introduction of new technologies, such as needleless devices, percutaneous, mucous membrane, and skin exposures to contaminated body fluids continue to occur at a high frequency. The OSHA standard also required that all health care facilities offer employees hepatitis B immunization. Employees may refuse immunization but must sign a declination form.

Protective serum titers of anti-HBsAg (≥10 mIU/mL) develop in 90% of healthy adults who receive a series of three intramuscular doses of HBV vaccine.[49,328,329] Independent risk factors for failure to seroconvert in HCWs following HBV vaccine have included smoking, female gender, higher body mass index, and older age.[330] Administering three doses on an accelerated schedule (e.g., 0, 1, and 2 months) results in a more rapid antibody rise but may reduce peak titers.[331,332] The two currently available HBV vaccines, Recombivax HB and Engerix-B, are equally immunogenic and are interchangeable; either can be used (in its recommended dose) to complete an immunization series begun with the other.[49] Immunogenicity is not reduced when HBV vaccine is given with other vaccines. Pregnancy is not a contraindication to HBV vaccine. All injections should be provided in the deltoid because gluteal injection results in poor immunogenicity.

Most HCWs should receive vaccine on a 0-, 1-, and 6-month schedule. Consideration should be given to using a 0-, 1-, and 2-month or 0-, 1-, and 4-month schedule for unimmunized HCWs at high risk for HBV acquisition (e.g., hemodialysis workers, cardiac surgeons), but a fourth dose should be given at 12 months to ensure long-term protection. All HCWs should have an anti-HBsAg titer obtained 1 to 2 months after the third immunization. Because approximately half the people who do not develop a protective level of anti-HBsAg antibodies after a three-dose series do so after additional doses,[333] HCWs with an inadequate response to a three-dose series should receive up to three additional doses of hepatitis B vaccine. They should have their antibody response tested 1 to 2 months after each dose or at the end of a second three-dose series. Individuals who do not respond to these three additional doses should be considered nonresponders and should receive HBIG when indicated for postexposure prophylaxis (see Table 59–5). In addition, they should be tested for the presence of HBsAg.

Symptomatic hepatitis B is rare in immunized people who developed protective levels of antibody, even though there is eventual loss of detectable antibody in up to 50% of those people 5 to 10 years after immunization.[46] For this reason, there is currently no recommendation for periodic boosting of HCWs who have responded to hepatitis B vaccine.[47,278]

Postexposure Prophylaxis

All HCWs with potential exposure to blood or contaminated body fluids should be evaluated. Exposure is defined as parenteral, mucous membrane, or nonintact skin exposure to blood or contaminated fluids. In all cases, the source should be tested for HBsAg, hepatitis C, and HIV. If the source case is HBsAg positive, postexposure prophylaxis may be indicated (see Table 59–5). HBIG has been shown to be effective when provided within 7 days. Immune globulin should not be used because of lack of efficacy. The simultaneous administration of HBIG and HBV vaccine (at different sites) does not diminish the efficacy of the hepatitis B vaccine.[49]

Influenza Vaccine

Epidemiology

Influenza is characterized by the abrupt onset of fever, myalgia, sore throat, and nonproductive cough. Elderly people and people with underlying health problems are at increased risk for complications of influenza, including hospitalization and death. During major epidemics, the hospitalization rate for the elderly and people with chronic health problems may increase twofold to fivefold compared with nonepidemic periods.[334] During 9 of 20 influenza seasons (from 1972–1973 through 1991–1992), more than 20,000 influenza-associated excess deaths occurred each season; during four of these seasons, more than 40,000 deaths occurred.[335]

Influenza viruses are classified into subtypes on the basis of two surface antigens: hemagglutinin (H) and neuraminidase (N). Widespread human disease has been caused by three subtypes of hemagglutinin (H1, H2, and H3) and two subtypes of neuraminidase (N1 and N2). Immunity to these antigens, especially to hemagglutinin, reduces the likelihood of infection and lessens the severity of disease if infection occurs. Infection with a virus of one subtype confers little or no protection against viruses of other subtypes. Over time, antigenic variation (antigenic drift) within a subtype may be so marked that infection or immunization with one strain may not induce immunity to more distantly related strains of the same subtype. The antigenic characteristics of circulating strains provide the basis for selecting the viral strains included in each year's vaccine.

Influenza virus appears to spread from person to person by small-particle aerosol transmission. Although aerosol transmission is well established, nosocomial transmission via fomites and contaminated hands remains possible. Influenza virus is shed for up to 5 days beyond the onset of illness in adults, but shedding may occur for up to 7 days in children. Humans are the primary reservoir of infection, but swine and avian (e.g., ducks) reservoirs are likely sources of new human subtypes thought to emerge through genetic reassortment.

Lessons from Nosocomial Outbreaks

Nosocomial acquisition of influenza has been well described.[336–357] Nosocomial transmission most commonly occurs during community influenza outbreaks when patients infected with influenza are admitted to the hospital. Because up to 25% of unimmunized HCWs may develop influenza during the winter months, however, infected staff may introduce infection into a health care facility.[358] Staff infected by patients have frequently served as the source for secondary transmission of influenza to patients and other staff.[338,339,344,345] Acquisition of influenza by HCWs may cause absenteeism and significant disruption of health care.[339,342,345]

Nosocomial outbreaks frequently have involved extended-care facilities for the elderly.[359–376] Such outbreaks may cause significant morbidity and mortality.[362,363,371] High rates of influenza immunization among HCWs may lead to a decrease in the attack rate of influenza among patients.[377,378] For example, patients in facilities in which greater than 60% of the staff had been immunized experienced less influenza-related mortality and illness compared with patients in facilities without immunized staff.[377] Nosocomial outbreaks also have been reported in other types of long-term care facilities, such as institutions caring for mentally challenged people.[379]

Important lessons from these outbreaks include the following. First, identification of all patients with influenza is problematic and incomplete.[345] Furthermore, community indicators of influenza activity (e.g., visits to acute ambulatory care centers for upper respiratory illness) cannot be relied on to provide warning of influenza among hospitalized patients.[342] Second, influenza infection among staff is common during the winter season and results in significant absenteeism. Attack rates of 25% to 80% often are observed among both patients and staff during outbreaks. Third, failure to isolate patients treated with amantadine or rimantadine may result in the dissemination of drug-resistant strains.

Recommendations for prevention and control of nosocomial influenza have been published.[123,349,357,380–385] The CDC recommends the following measures[384]:

1. Educate personnel about the epidemiology, modes of transmission, and means of preventing the spread of influenza.
2. Establish mechanism(s) by which hospital personnel are promptly alerted of an increase in influenza activity in the local community.
3. Arrange for laboratory tests to be available to clinicians, for use when clinically indicated, to confirm the diagnosis of influenza and other acute viral respiratory diseases promptly, especially during November through April.
4. Offer vaccine to outpatients and inpatients at high risk of complications from influenza, beginning in

September and continuing until influenza activity has begun to decline.

5. Vaccinate HCWs before the influenza season each year, preferably between mid-October and mid-November.

6. Isolate patients with known or suspected influenza in a private room, preferably under negative pressure.

7. Institute masking of individuals who enter the room of a patient with influenza.

8. Evaluate HCWs with febrile upper respiratory illnesses and consider removal from duties that involve direct patient care (use more stringent guidelines for staff working in *high-risk* areas, such as intensive care units or nurseries, or with severely immunocompromised patients).

9. During community or hospital outbreaks, restrict hospital visitors who have a febrile respiratory illness.

During a nosocomial outbreak, the CDC recommends the following[384]:

1. Early in the outbreak, obtain a nasopharyngeal swab or nasal-wash specimen from patients with recent onset of symptoms suggestive of influenza for virus culture or antigen detection.

2. Administer current influenza vaccine to unvaccinated patients and staff.

3. Administer antiviral prophylaxis to all uninfected patients in an involved unit for whom it is not contraindicated.

4. Administer antiviral prophylaxis to all unvaccinated staff members for whom it is not contraindicated and who are in the involved unit or taking care of high-risk patients.

5. If the cause of the outbreak is confirmed to be influenza and vaccine has been administered only recently to susceptible patients and personnel, continue antiviral prophylaxis until 2 weeks after the vaccination.

6. To the extent possible, do not allow contact between those at high risk of complications from influenza and patients or staff who are taking antiviral treatment for an acute respiratory illnesses; prevent contact during and for 2 days after the latter discontinue treatment.

Pre-exposure Prophylaxis

Influenza vaccine is strongly recommended for any person age 6 months or older who is at increased risk for complications of influenza because of age or underlying medical condition. People at increased risk for influenza-related complications include those age 50 years or older; residents of extended-care facilities or long-term care facilities that house people of any age who have chronic medical conditions; adults and children who have required regular medical follow-up or hospitalization during the previous year because of chronic metabolic diseases (including diabetes mellitus), renal dysfunction, hemoglobinopathies, or immunosuppression; children and teenagers (ages 6 months to 18 years) who are receiving long-term aspirin therapy and therefore may be at risk for developing Reye's syndrome after influenza; and women who will be in the second or third trimester of pregnancy during the influenza season.[51]

Influenza vaccine is also recommended for HCWs because, when they are clinically or subclinically infected, they can transmit influenza virus to people at high risk. The CDC specifically recommends immunization for the following HCWs: physicians, nurses, and other personnel in both hospital and outpatient care settings; employees of nursing homes and long-term care facilities who have contact with patients or residents; and providers of home care to people at high risk (e.g., visiting nurses and volunteer workers).[51] The CDC also recommends vaccine to any person who wishes to reduce the likelihood of becoming ill with influenza. A randomized, controlled trial in a general working population has demonstrated that providing influenza vaccine is cost-effective.[386]

Influenza immunization should not be provided to people known to have anaphylactic hypersensitivity to eggs or other components of the influenza vaccine.[51] People who have a history of anaphylactic hypersensitivity to vaccine components but who are also at high risk for complications of influenza, however, can benefit from vaccine after appropriate allergy evaluation and desensitization. Neither pregnancy nor breast-feeding is considered a contraindication to immunization, and, in fact, vaccine is specifically recommended for women who will be in the second or third trimester of pregnancy during the influenza season.

Chemoprophylaxis with an antiviral drug (amantadine, rimantadine) has been used as both pre-exposure and postexposure prophylaxis to reduce the likelihood of developing influenza A (amantadine, rimantadine) or influenza A and B (zanamivir, oseltamivir) infection. Only limited data are available regarding the efficacy of the newer agents, zanamivir and oseltamivir, for pre- and postexposure prophylaxis.[51,387] Adverse events have been noted in up to 33% of patients receiving amantadine, leading to withdrawal of therapy in 6% to 11% more patients receiving active drug versus placebo.[123] Common side effects include anxiety, lightheadedness, ataxia, confusion, hallucinations, insomnia, nausea, and weakness. Rimantadine has been demonstrated to have equivalent efficacy and lower central nervous system toxicity but is substantially more expensive.[51] The recommended dose of either drug when used for prophylaxis is 100 mg twice daily. Dosage adjustment may be required for the following people: those age 65 years or older, those with chronic liver disease, and those with chronic renal impairment. Physicians prescribing these drugs should be aware of drug interactions, including interactions with central nervous system stimulants, antihistamines, and anticholinergic drugs. Chemoprophylaxis is not a substitute for immunization. Zanamivir has been associated with bronchospasm and oseltamivir has been associated with gastrointestinal upset.

Amantadine-resistant and rimantadine-resistant influenza A viruses can emerge when either of these drugs is administered for treatment. Amantadine-resistant strains are cross-resistant to rimantadine and vice versa.

Despite these recommendations, many HCWs choose not to take influenza vaccine.[386,388–390] Institutions should consider introducing innovative methods such as provision by mobile carts on hospital wards or by offering vaccine to house staff and students in clinics and conferences.

Postexposure Prophylaxis

During community or nosocomial outbreaks, health care institutions should offer and strongly encourage the use of influenza vaccine among HCWs. If influenza is causing a community outbreak, consideration should be given to providing chemoprophylaxis for 2 weeks to newly immunized HCWs who are at high risk of exposure to infected patients. Prophylaxis should be considered for all employees, regardless of immunization status, if the outbreak is caused by a variant strain of influenza that might not be controlled by the vaccine. Only a few placebo-controlled trials have tested the possible efficacy of postexposure prophylaxis, an intervention that might be effective in controlling outbreaks or preventing the transmission of infection in households or other settings.[123] When the index case is treated concurrently with contacts, rapid selection and apparent transmission of resistant viruses to contacts has been reported.[123] The same problem has been noted in mass prophylaxis with amantadine in extended-care facilities.[369,370] For this reason, all patients treated with an antiviral should be placed on isolation as recommended by the CDC. Antivirals can reduce the severity and shorten the duration of influenza illness among healthy adults when administered within 48 hours of illness onset.

Hepatitis A Vaccine

Epidemiology

Hepatitis A virus (HAV) is highly endemic in the United States, with 13,397 cases (4.91 cases per 100,000) reported to the CDC in 1999.[124] An estimated 125,000 to 200,000 infections occur annually. The incidence of hepatitis A varies by race and ethnicity (highest among Native Americans and Alaskan Natives), location (highest in the western United States), and age (highest in people 5 to 14 years of age). Sources of infection include household or sexual contact with a person with HAV (22% to 26%), with a child or employee in a day care center (14% to 16%), or with an international traveler (4% to 6%) as well as food- or waterborne outbreaks (2% to 3%).[391] In the United States, approximately 50% of people with hepatitis A do not have an identified source of infection.

Hepatitis A results in substantial morbidity with significant costs caused by medical care and lost work time. Approximately 11% to 22% of people who develop hepatitis A require hospitalization.[63] In the United States, an estimated 100 deaths occur each year as a result of fulminant hepatitis A.

Lessons from Nosocomial Outbreaks

Nosocomial outbreaks of hepatitis A have been relatively infrequent, especially when considering the large number of people hospitalized with this disease each year. Cohort studies reported in peer-reviewed journals have not demonstrated that HCWs are at increased risk for disease acquisition compared with control populations.[392–394] Furthermore, a cohort study failed to find evidence of patient-to-patient transmission.[395] French and Belgian researchers, however, have reported in letters that HCWs had higher than expected rates of seropositivity to hepatitis A.[396,397] Multiple nosocomial outbreaks of hepatitis A have been reported.[398–414] Most outbreaks have occurred in one of the following settings. First, the source patient was not jaundiced and hepatitis was inapparent at the time of hospitalization. Second, the HAV-infected patient was fecally

incontinent or had diarrhea. Nosocomial hepatitis A also has been associated with contaminated blood transfusions[405,408,409] and contaminated food.[398,399] Risk factors for HAV transmission to personnel have included activities that increase the risk of fecal-oral contamination, including caring for a person with unrecognized HAV infection[400–404,406,410,413]; sharing food, beverages, or cigarettes with patients, their families, or the staff[403,407,408,413]; nail biting; handling bile without proper precautions[413]; and not washing hands or wearing gloves when providing care to an infected patient.[408,410,411,413]

Prevention of nosocomial hepatitis A requires strict adherence to standard precautions, which suggests the use of gloves whenever dealing with secretions and excretions. Hand washing should precede and follow all patient contact. Several outbreaks would have been prevented by eliminating the eating of food in patient care areas.

Pre-exposure Prophylaxis

The current scientific literature supports the recommendation of the CDC that HAV vaccine should not be routinely provided to HCWs. Although many outbreaks have involved neonates and children, even for these subgroups the likelihood of infection probably does not warrant a blanket recommendation of immunization. A cost-effectiveness study of providing HAV vaccine to all medical students reported that the costs per life-year saved and quality-adjusted life-year saved were $58,000 and $47,000, respectively. As with other special-use vaccines, HCWs should be encouraged to review with their local medical provider their own risks and benefits for HAV vaccine.

Postexposure Prophylaxis

Postexposure prophylaxis with HAV vaccine may be indicated in community outbreaks of hepatitis A.[63] The role of HAV vaccine in the control of outbreaks in hospitals, day care centers, and other institutions has not been evaluated.

Postexposure prophylaxis with immune globulin has been demonstrated to be effective in reducing secondary cases after exposure to a common source, such as contaminated food or close personal contact with an infected person. Immune globulin should not be routinely provided to HCWs after identification of a single infected patient in the hospital.[63] Immune globulin should be administered to people who have close contact with index patients if an epidemiologic investigation indicates HAV transmission has occurred between patients and staff.

Pertussis Vaccine

Epidemiology

In the United States, the highest recorded annual incidence of pertussis occurred in 1934, when greater than 260,000 cases were reported.[415] After the introduction of whole-cell diphtheria, tetanus, and pertussis vaccine, the incidence declined more than 99%. Since the early 1980s, however, the reported pertussis incidence has increased, with 2719 to 7867 cases reported annually between 1988 and 2000. In addition to temporal trends, pertussis also exhibits a cyclical trend with 2- to 5-year cycles; peaks have occurred in 1983, 1986, 1990, and 1993.[416] In 2000, 7867 cases were reported (2.7 per 100,000 population). The highest attack rate of pertussis occurs in children less than 1 year of age, but more than 20% of cases now are reported in people 15 years of age or older. Possible explanations for this increase in disease include (1) decreased vaccine efficacy, (2) decreased vaccine coverage, (3) waning immunity among adolescents and adults vaccinated during childhood, (4) increased diagnosis and reporting of pertussis because of greater awareness among physicians about the disease, and (5) enhanced surveillance and more complete reporting in some states.[417] Vaccine coverage levels among children, however, are higher than at any time in the past.

Adolescents and young adults play an important role in transmitting pertussis to susceptible infants because immunization-induced immunity to pertussis wanes with increasing age and because disease in adults frequently is not diagnosed or treated because it is often mild or atypical. Studies using serologic methods have demonstrated that B. pertussis is a common cause of respiratory illness causing cough in adults.[418-420] Deville and colleagues[421] followed HCWs for 5 years and reported that 90% of subjects had a significant antibody rise (immunoglobulin A or G) to one or more B. pertussis antigens between two consecutive years; 55% had evidence of two infections, 17% had evidence of three infections, and 4% had evidence of four infections. Reinfection with B. pertussis also may follow native infection.[422]

Lessons from Nosocomial Outbreaks

At the University of North Carolina Hospitals, pertussis is the third most common source of infectious disease exposure evaluations, with only varicella-zoster and tuberculosis more common (Weber, unpublished data, 1994–1998). Multiple nosocomial outbreaks have been reported in the literature.[423-431] These most often have involved residential facilities for the mentally or physically impaired[426,427,429] or pediatric wards of acute care hospitals.[423-425] Although the source case most commonly was an infected patient in whom pertussis was unrecognized,[423,424,428] infected employees[426,429] and the infected mother of a child with pertussis[425] also served as sources. Employees often served as vectors for additional nosocomial cases.[423,424,426,429] In several instances, infected employees also infected members of their households.[424,426] Nosocomial outbreaks have occurred for several reasons: (1) failure to recognize and appropriately isolate infected patients, (2) failure to give prophylaxis to exposed staff, and (3) failure to furlough symptomatic staff.[432,433]

Pre-exposure Prophylaxis

The primary means of preventing pertussis is via administration of pertussis vaccine to children at ages 2 months, 4 months, 6 months, 15 to 18 months, and 4 to 6 years. The diphtheria and tetanus toxoids and acellular pertussis vaccine is the preferred vaccine for all doses in the vaccination series because the new acellular pertussis vaccines are at least as effective as standard pertussis vaccine with significantly fewer side effects. Boosters are not currently recommended for adults. Because immunity wanes with time, many adults are susceptible to infection with B. pertussis.

The ability to boost immunity to B. pertussis among adults via immunization would aid in the prevention of nosocomial outbreaks and protect staff and their families from disease. In randomized, placebo controlled trials, acellular pertussis vaccines have been shown to be both safe and highly immunogenic in adolescents and adults[434-440]

Postexposure Prophylaxis

Bordetella pertussis is highly susceptible in vitro to erythromycin[441,442] and the newer macrolides, azithromycin and clarithromycin.[443] It is also susceptible to trimethoprim-sulfamethoxazole[442] and the quinolones, ciprofloxacin and ofloxacin.[442,444,445] Bordetella pertussis is not susceptible to the first-generation cephalosporins.[446] Erythromycin has been shown to decrease the duration of illness when administered early in the course of pertussis and to eliminate B. pertussis from the nasopharynx. Erythromycin also has been successfully used to provide chemoprophylaxis of individuals exposed to B. pertussis and to aid in preventing secondary spread in households or terminating outbreaks in institutions.[422,426,431,447-449] For these reasons, erythromycin is considered the drug of choice for the treatment and prophylaxis of pertussis.[450-452] For clinical treatment, the estolate form is preferred by some clinicians because of its superior pharmacokinetics.[451] Trimethoprim-sulfamethoxazole is the recommended alternative for treatment and for chemoprophylaxis of individuals intolerant to erythromycin, although its efficacy as a chemoprophylactic agent has not been evaluated. The evidence of trimethoprim-sulfamethoxazole's efficacy is based on small studies.[453,454] Small clinical trials suggest that clarithromycin and azithromycin are effective for the treatment of pertussis.[455] Azithromycin has been used as prophylaxis in the control of a nosocomial outbreak.[456]

Erythromycin-resistant clinical isolates of B. pertussis have been reported, raising concern about the use of macrolides for therapy or prophylaxis.[457,458] However, surveys of B. pertussis strains demonstrate that macrolide resistance is uncommon.[459-461]

Immunization of HCWs with acellular pertussis vaccine has been used along with chemoprophylaxis to control nosocomial outbreaks.[430,431]

Conclusions

All susceptible HCWs, unless they have a contraindication to immunization, should be immunized against mumps, measles, rubella, and varicella. If HCWs have the potential for exposure to blood or contaminated fluids, they should be immunized against hepatitis B. In addition, HCWs should be immunized against influenza annually. HCWs also should receive tetanus-diphtheria and pneumococcal vaccines as recommended for the general public. If future studies reveal that HCWs are at higher risk for acquiring hepatitis A than the general public, use of the hepatitis A vaccine at institutional expense may be recommended. If future studies reveal that the acellular pertussis vaccine is safe and effective in adults, it is likely that boosting HCWs will be recommended to prevent nosocomial transmission. Selected HCWs may be candidates for other available vaccines, including anthrax, polio, plague, typhoid, vaccinia, and rabies.

REFERENCES

1. Omenn GS, Morris SL. Occupational hazards to healthcare workers: report of a conference. Am J Ind Med 6:129–137, 1984.
2. Patterson WB, Craven DE, Schwartz DA, et al. Occupational hazards to hospital personnel. Ann Intern Med 102:658–680, 1985.
3. Gestal JJ. Occupational hazards in hospitals: risk of infection. Br J Ind Med 44:435–442, 1987.
4. Moore RM, Kaczmarek RG. Occupational hazards to healthcare workers: diverse, ill-defined and not fully appreciated. Am J Infect Control 18:316–327, 1990.
5. Hoffmann KK, Weber DJ, Rutala WA. Infection control strategies relevant to employee health. AAOHN J 39:167–181, 1991.
6. Diekema DJ, Doebbeling BN. Employee health and infection control. Infect Control Hosp Epidemiol 16:292–301, 1995.
7. Clever LH, LeGuyader Y. Infectious risks for healthcare workers. Annu Rev Public Health 16:141–164, 1995.
8. Sepkowitz KA. Occupationally acquired infections in healthcare workers: Part I. Ann Intern Med 125:826–834, 1996.
9. Sepkowitz KA. Occupationally acquired infections in healthcare workers: Part II. Ann Intern Med 125:917–928, 1996.
10. Doebbeling BN. Protecting the healthcare worker from infection and injury. In Wenzel RP (ed). Prevention and Control of Nosocomial Infections (3rd ed). Baltimore, Williams & Wilkins, 1997, pp 397–435.
11. Rogers B. Health hazards in nursing and healthcare: an overview. Am J Infect Control 25:248–261, 1997.
12. Bolyard EA, Tablan OC, Williams WW, et al. Guidelines for infection control in health care personnel. Am J Infect Control 26:289–354, 1998.
13. Chong CY, Goldman DA, Huskins WC. Prevention of occupationally acquired infections among health-care workers. Pediatr Rev 19:219–231, 1998.
14. Tablan OC, Bolyard EA, Shapiro CN, Williams WW. Personnel health service. In Bennett JV, Brachman PS (eds). Hospital Infections (4th ed). Boston, Little, Brown, 1998, pp 23–52.
15. Falk P. Infection control and the employee health service. In Mayhall CG (ed). Hospital Epidemiology and Infection Control (2nd ed). Baltimore, Williams & Wilkins, 1999, pp 1381–1386.
16. Sharbaugh RJ. The risk of occupational exposure and infection with infectious disease. Nursing Clin North Am 34:493–508, 1999.
17. Bertin ML. Communicable diseases: infection, prevention for nurses at work and home. Nursing Clin North Am 34:509–526, 1999.
18. Sebazco S. Occupational health. In APIC Text of Infection Control and Epidemiology. Washington, DC, Association for Professionals in Infection Control and Epidemiology, 79-1–79-2, 2000.
19. Udasin IG. Health care workers. Primary Care 27:1079–1101, 2000.
20. Larson EL. APIC guideline for handwashing and hand antisepsis in healthcare settings. Am J Infect Control 23:251–269, 1995.
21. Boyce JM, Pittet D. Guideline for hand hygiene in health-care settings. Am J Infect Control 30:1–46, 2002.
22. Gardner JS, for the Hospital Infection Control Practices Advisory Committee. Guideline for isolation precautions in hospitals. Infect Control Hosp Epidemiol 17:53–80, 1996.
23. Buesching WJ, Neff JC, Sharma HM. Infectious hazards in the clinical laboratory: a program to protect laboratory personnel. Clin Lab Med 9:351–361, 1989.
24. Sewell DL. Laboratory-associated infections and biosafety. Clin Microbiol Rev 8:389–405, 1995.
25. National Committee for Clinical Laboratory Standards. Clinical Laboratory Safety: Approved Guideline (NCCLS Document GP17-A). Wayne, PA, National Committee for Clinical Laboratory Standards, 1996.
26. Biosafety in Microbiological and Biomedical Laboratories (HHS Publ No 017-040-00547-4). Rockville, MD, Department of Health and Human Resources, 1999.
27. Flemming DO, Hunt DL. Biological Safety: Principles and Practices (3rd ed). Washington, DC, ASM Press, 2000.
28. Turnberg WL. Biohazardous Waste: Risk Assessment, Policy, and Management. New York, John Wiley & Sons, 1996.
29. Occupational Safety and Health Administration. Occupational exposure to bloodborne pathogens; needlestick, and other sharps injuries; final rule. Fed Reg 66:5318–5325, 2001.
30. Occupational Safety and Health Administration. Occupational exposure to tuberculosis; proposed rule. 29 CFR Part 1910. Fed Reg 62:54160–54308, 1997.
31. Immunization of health-care workers: recommendations of the Advisory Committee on Immunization Practices (ACIP) and the Hospital Infection Control Practices Advisory Committee (HICPAC). 46(RR-18):1–42, 1997.
32. General recommendations on immunization: recommendations of the Advisory Committee on Immunization Practices (ACIP) and the American Academy of Family Physicians. MMWR 51(RR-2):1, 2002.
33. ACP Task Force on Adult Immunization and Infectious Disease Society of America. Guide for Adult Immunization (3rd ed). Philadelphia, American College of Physicians, 1994.
34. American Academy of Pediatrics. Red Book: Report of the Committee on Infectious Diseases (24th ed). Elk Grove Village, IL, American Academy of Pediatrics, 1997.
35. Krause PJ, Gross PA, Barrett TL, et al. Quality standard for assurance of measles immunity among healthcare workers. Infect Control Hosp Epidemiol 15:193–199, 1994.
36. Beekmann SE, Doebbeling BN. Frontiers of occupational health: new vaccines, new prophylactic regimens, and management of the HIV-infected worker. Infect Dis Clin North Am 11:313–329, 1997.
37. Weber DJ, Rutala WA. Selection and use of vaccines for healthcare workers. Infect Control Hosp Epidemiol 18:682–687, 1997.
38. Kessler ER. Vaccine-preventable diseases in health care. Occup Med 12:731–739, 1997.
39. Poland GA, Haiduven DJ. Immunization in the health-care worker. In APIC Text of Infection Control and Epidemiology. Washington, DC, Association for Professionals in Infection Control and Epidemiology, 2000, pp 80.1–80.32.
40. Poland GA, Schaffner W, Publiese G (eds). Immunizing Healthcare Workers: A Practical Approach. Thorofare, NJ, Slack, 2000.
41. Zimmermann RK, Ball JA. Adult vaccinations. Prim Care Clin Office Pract 25:763–790, 2001.
42. DeCastro MG, Denys GA, Fauerbach LL, et al. APIC position paper: immunization. Am J Infect Control 27:52–53, 1999.
43. Measles, mumps and rubella—vaccine use and strategies for the elimination of measles, rubella and congenital rubella syndrome: recommendations of the Advisory Committee on Immunization Practices (ACIP). MMWR 47(RR-8):1–57, 1998.
44. Control and prevention of rubella: evaluation and management of suspected outbreaks, rubella in pregnant women, and surveillance for congenital rubella syndrome. MMWR 50(RR-12):1–23, 2001.
45. Prevention of varicella: recommendations of the Advisory Committee on Immunization Practices (ACIP). MMWR 45(RR-11):1–36, 1996.
46. Weber DJ, Rutala WA, Hamilton H. Prevention and control of varicella-zoster infections in healthcare facilities. Infect Control Hosp Epidemiol 17:694–705, 1996.
47. Prevention of varicella: updated recommendations of the Advisory Committee on Immunization Practices (ACIP). MMWR 49(RR-6):1–5, 1999.
48. Hepatitis B virus: a comprehensive strategy for eliminating transmission in the United States through universal childhood vaccination. Recommendations of the Immunization Practices Advisory Committee (ACIP). MMWR Morb Mortal Wkly Rep 40(RR-13):1–25, 1991.
49. Lemon SM, Thomas DL. Vaccines to prevent viral hepatitis. N Engl J Med 336:196–204, 1997.
50. Updated U.S. Public Health Service Guidelines for the management of occupational exposures to HBV, HCV, and HIV and recommendations for postexposure prophylaxis. MMWR 50(RR-11):1–67, 2001.
51. Prevention and control of influenza: recommendations of the Advisory Committee on Immunization Practices (ACIP). MMWR 51(RR-3):1–36, 2002.
52. Diphtheria, tetanus, and pertussis: recommendations of the Immunization Practices Advisory Committee (ACIP). MMWR 40(RR-10):1–28, 1991.
53. Prevention of pneumococcal disease: recommendations of the Advisory Committee on Immunization Practices (ACIP). MMWR 46(RR-8):1–24, 1997.
54. Poliomyelitis prevention in the United States: introduction of a sequential vaccination schedule of inactivated poliovirus vaccine followed by oral poliovirus vaccine. Recommendations of the Advisory Committee on Immunization Practices (ACIP). MMWR 46(RR-3):1–25, 1997.
55. Control and prevention of meningococcal disease: recommendations of the Advisory Committee on Immunization Practices (ACIP). MMWR 46(RR-5):1–11, 1997.

56. Control and prevention of serogroup C meningococcal disease: evaluation and management of suspected outbreaks. Recommendations of the Advisory Committee on Immunization Practices (ACIP). MMWR 46(RR-5):13–21, 1997.

57. The role of BCG vaccine in the prevention and control of tuberculosis in the United States: a joint statement by the Advisory Committee for the Elimination of Tuberculosis and the Advisory Committee on Immunization Practices. MMWR 45(RR-4):1–18, 1996.

58. Rabies prevention—United States, 1991: recommendations of the Immunization Practices Advisory Committee (ACIP). MMWR 40(RR-3):1–19, 1991.

59. Prevention of plague: recommendations of the Advisory Committee on Immunization Practices (ACIP). MMWR 45(RR-14):1–15, 1996.

60. Typhoid immunization: recommendations of the Immunization Practices Advisory Committee (ACIP). MMWR 39(RR-10):1–5, 1990.

61. Typhoid immunization: recommendations of the Immunization Practices Advisory Committee (ACIP). MMWR 43(RR-14):1–7, 1994.

62. Vaccinia (smallpox) vaccine: recommendations of the Immunization Practices Advisory Committee (ACIP). MMWR 40(RR-14):1–10, 1991.

63. Prevention of hepatitis A through active or passive immunization: recommendations of the Advisory Committee on Immunization Practices (ACIP). MMWR 48(RR-12):1–37, 1999.

64. Use of anthrax vaccine in the United States: recommendations of the Advisory Committee on Immunization Practices (ACIP). MMWR 49(RR-15):1–39, 2000.

65. Use of vaccines and immune globulin in persons with altered immunocompetence: recommendations of the Advisory Committee on Immunization Practices (ACIP). MMWR 42(RR-4):1–18, 1993.

66. Loutan L. Vaccination of the immunocompromised patient. Biologicals 25:231–236, 1997.

67. Pirofski L-A, Casadevall A. Use of licensed vaccines for active immunization of the immunocompromised host. Clin Microbiol Rev 11:1–26, 1998.

68. Weber DJ, Weigle K, Rutala WA. Immunization of workers with altered host defenses. In Poland GA, Schaffner W, Publiese G (eds). Immunizing Healthcare Workers: A Practical Approach. Thorofare, NJ, Slack, 2000.

69. Faix RG. Immunization during pregnancy. Clin Obstet Gynecol 45:42–58, 2002.

70. Munoz FM, Englund JA. Vaccines in pregnancy. Infect Dis Clin North Am 15:253–271, 2001.

71. Update: vaccine side effects, adverse reactions, contraindications, and precautions. Recommendations of the Advisory Committee on Immunization Practices (ACIP). MMWR 45(RR-12):1–35, 1996.

72. Altas RM. The medical threat of biological weapons. Crit Rev Microbiol 24:157–168, 1998.

73. Henderson DA. The looming threat of bioterrorism. Science 283:1279–1282, 1999.

74. Leggiadro RJ. The threat of biological terrorism: a public health and infection control reality. Infect Control Hosp Epidemiol 21:53–56, 2000.

75. Franz DR, Zajtchuk R. Biological terrorism: understanding the threat, preparation, and medical response. Dis Mon 46:125–190, 2000.

76. Spencer RC, Lightfoot NF. Preparedness and response to bioterrorism. J Infect 43:104–110, 2001.

77. Strategic plan for preparedness and response. MMWR 49(No. RR-4):1–63, 2000.

78. Update: investigation of bioterrorism-related anthrax and interim guidelines for clinical evaluation of persons with possible anthrax. MMWR 50:941–948, 2001.

79. Update: investigation of bioterrorism-related anthrax—Connecticut, 2001. MMWR 50:1077–1079, 2001.

80. Dixon TC, Meselson M, Guilliemin J, Hanna PC. Anthrax. N Engl J Med 341:815–826, 1999.

81. Friedlander AM. Anthrax: clinical features, pathogenesis, and potential warfare threat. Curr Clin Top Infect Dis 20:335–349, 2000.

82. Swartz MN. Recognition and management of anthrax—an update. N Engl J Med 345:1621–1626, 2001.

83. Recognition of illness associated with the intentional release of a biologic agent. MMWR 50:893–897, 2001.

84. Franz DR, Jahrling PB, Friedlander AM, et al. Clinical recognition and management of patients exposed to biological warfare agents. JAMA 278:399–411, 1997.

85. Franz DR, Jahrling PB, McClain DJ, et al. Clinical recognition and management of patients exposed to biological warfare agents. Clin Lab Med 21:435–473, 2001.

86. Inglesby TV, Henderson DA, Bartlett JG, et al. Anthrax as a biological weapon: medical and public health consequences. JAMA 281:1735–1745, 1999.

87. Inglesby TV, O'Toole T, Henderson DA, et al. Anthrax as a biological weapon, 2002: update recommendations for management. JAMA 287:2236–2252, 2002.

88. Arnon SS, Schechter R, Inglesby TV, et al. Botulinum toxin as a biological weapon: medical and public health consequences. JAMA 285:1059–1070, 2001.

89. Inglesby TV, Dennis DT, Henderson DA, et al. Plague as a biological weapon: medical and public health consequences. JAMA 283:2281–2290, 2000.

90. Henderson DA, Inglesby TV, Bartlett JG, et al. Smallpox as a biological weapon: medical and public health consequences. JAMA 281:2127–2137, 1999.

91. Dennis DT, Inglesby TV, Henderson DA, et al. Tularemia as a biological weapon: medical and public health management. JAMA 285:2763–2773, 2001.

92. Weber DJ, Rutala WA. Risks and prevention of nosocomial transmission of rare zoonotic diseases. Clin Infect Dis 32:446–456, 2001.

93. Drugs and vaccine for biological weapons. Med Lett Drugs Ther 43:87–89, 2001.

94. Polgreen PM, Helms C. Vaccines, biological warfare and bioterrorism. Prim Care Clin Office Pract 28:807–821, 2001.

95. Post-exposure anthrax prophylaxis. Med Lett Drugs Ther 43:1116–1117, 2001.

96. Public Law No. 99-660, 1986. Fed Reg 62:7685–7690, 1997.

97. Poland GA, Nichol KL. Medical schools and immunization policies: missed opportunities for disease prevention. Ann Intern Med 113:628–631, 1990.

98. Lewy R. Immunization status of entering housestaff physicians. J Occup Med 30:822–823, 1988.

99. Ewert DP, Garcia D, George J, Mascola L. A comparison of hospital policies for measles, mumps, and rubella infection control in Los Angeles County, 1989 and 1992. Am J Infect Control 23:369–372, 1995.

100. Lane NE, Paul RI, Bratcher DF, Stover BH. A survey of policies at children's hospitals regarding immunity of healthcare workers: are physicians protected? Infect Control Hosp Epidemiol 18:400–404, 1997.

101. Weingarten S, Riedinger M, Bolton LB, et al. Barriers to influenza vaccine acceptance. Am J Infect Control 17:202–207, 1989.

102. Shapiro CN, Tokars JI, Chamberland ME. Use of the hepatitis-B vaccine and infection with hepatitis B and C among orthopedic surgeons. J Bone Joint Surg 78:1791–1800, 1996.

103. Cleveland JL. Hepatitis B vaccination and infection among U.S. dentists, 1983–1993. J Am Dent Assoc 127:1385–1390, 1996.

104. McArthur MA, Simor AE, Campbell B, McGeer A. Influenza and pneumococcal vaccination and tuberculin skin testing programs in long-term care facilities: where do we stand? Infect Control Hosp Epidemiol 16:18–24, 1995.

105. McArthur MA, Simor AE, Campbell B, McGreer A. Influenza vaccination in long-term-care facilities: structuring programs for success. Infect Control Hosp Epidemiol 20:499–503, 1999.

106. Schwarcz S, McGraw B, Fukushima P. Prevalence of measles susceptibility in hospital staff. Arch Intern Med 152:1481–1483, 1992.

107. Nichol KL, Hauge M. Influenza vaccination of healthcare workers. Infect Control Hosp Epidemiol 18:189–194, 1997.

108. Agerton TB, Mahoney FJ, Polish LB, Shapiro CN. Impact of the bloodborne pathogens standard on vaccination of healthcare workers with hepatitis B vaccine. Infect Control Hosp Epidemiol 16:287–291, 1995.

109. Panlilio AL, Shapiro CN, Schable CA, et al. Serosurvey of human immunodeficiency virus, hepatitis B virus, and hepatitis C virus infection among hospital-based surgeons. J Am Coll Surg 180:16–24, 1995.

110. Gyawali P, Rice PS, Tilzey AJ. Exposure to blood borne viruses and the hepatitis B vaccination status among healthcare workers in inner London. Occup Environ Med 55:570–572, 1998.

111. Mahoney FJ, Stewart K, Hu H, Coleman P, Alter MJ. Progress toward the elimination of hepatitis B virus transmission among health care workers in the United States. Arch Intern Med 157:2601–2605, 1997.

112. Zadeh MM, Bridges CB, Thompson WW, et al. Influenza outbreak detection and control measures in nursing homes in the United States. J Am Geriatr Soc 48:1310–1315, 2000.

113. Cui XW, Nagao MM, Effler PV. Influenza and pneumococcal vaccination coverage levels among Hawaii statewide long-term-care facilities. Infect Control Hosp Epidemiol 22:519–521, 2001.

114. Russell ML. Influenza vaccination in Alberta long-term care facilities. CMAJ 164:1423–1427, 2001.

115. Stevenson CG, McArthur MA, Naus M, et al. Prevention of influenza and pneumococcal pneumonia in Canadian long-term care facilities: how are we doing? CMAJ 164:1413–1419, 2001.

116. Schwarz S, McCaw B, Fukushima P. Prevalence of measles susceptibility in house staff. Arch Intern Med 152:1481–1483, 1992.

117. Wright LJ, Carlquist JF. Measles immunity in employees of a multihospital healthcare provider. Infect Control Hosp Epidemiol 15:8–11, 1994.

118. Huang KG, Spence MR, Deforest A, Bradley AT. Measles immunization in HCWs. Infect Control Hosp Epidemiol 15:4, 1994.

119. Stover BH, Adams G, Kuebler CA, et al. Measles-mumps-rubella immunization of susceptible hospital employees during a community measles outbreak: cost-effectiveness and protective efficacy. Infect Control Hosp Epidemiol 15:18–21, 1994.

120. Willey ME, Koziol DE, Fleisher T, et al. Measles immunity in a population of healthcare workers. Infect Control Hosp Epidemiol 15:12–17, 1994.

121. Seo SK, Malak SF, Lim S, et al. Prevalence of measles antibody among young adult healthcare workers in a cancer hospital: 1980s versus 1998–1999. Infect Control Hosp Epidemiol 23:276–278, 2002.

122. Christian MA. Influenza and hepatitis B vaccine acceptance: a survey of healthcare workers. Am J Infect Control 19:177–184, 1991.

123. Adal KA, Flowers RH, Anglim AM, et al. Prevention of nosocomial influenza. Infect Control Hosp Epidemiol 17:641–648, 1996.

124. Summary of notifiable diseases, United States, 2000. MMWR 49:1–100, 2002.

125. Thomson FH. The aerial conveyance of infection. Lancet 1:341–344, 1916.

126. Brunell PA, Brickman A, O'Hare D, Steinberg S. Ineffectiveness of isolation of patients as a method of preventing the spread of mumps. N Engl J Med 279:1357–1361, 1968.

127. Sparling D. Transmission of mumps. N Engl J Med 280:276, 1969.

128. Faoagali JL. An assessment of the need for vaccination amongst junior medical staff. N Z Med J 84:152–150, 1976.

129. Glick D. An isolated case of mumps in a geriatric population. J Am Geriatr Soc 18:642–644, 1970.

130. Wharton M, Cochi SL, Hutcheson RH, Schaffner W. Mumps transmission in hospitals. Arch Intern Med 150:52–49, 1990.

131. Fischer PR, Brunetti C, Welch V, Christenson JC. Nosocomial mumps: report of an outbreak and its control. Am J Infect Control 24:13–18, 1996.

132. Reed D, Brown G, Merrick R, et al. A mumps epidemic on St. George Island, Alaska. JAMA 84:152–150, 1967.

133. Measles—Texas. MMWR 30:209–211, 1981.

134. Measles in medical settings—United States. MMWR 30:125–126, 1981.

135. Anonymous. Measles nearly eliminated, but still poses a nosocomial risk. Hosp Infect Control 9:133–136, 1982.

136. Imported measles with subsequent airborne transmission in a pediatrician's office—Michigan. MMWR 32:401–403, 1983.

137. Measles among children of migrant workers—Florida. MMWR 32:521–522, 527–528, 1983.

138. Interstate transmission of measles in a gypsy population—Washington, Idaho, Montana, California. MMWR 32:659–662, 1983.

139. Measles—Hawaii. MMWR 33:702, 707–711, 1984.

140. Measles—New Hampshire. MMWR 33:549–554, 559, 1984.

141. Remington PL, Hall WN, Davis IH, et al. Airborne transmission of measles in a physician's office. JAMA 253:1574–1577, 1985.

142. Bloch AB, Orenstein WA, Ewing WM, et al. Measles outbreak in a pediatric practice: airborne transmission in an office setting. Pediatrics 75:676–683, 1985.

143. Measles—Puerto Rico. MMWR 34:169–172, 1985.

144. Dales LG, Kizer KW. Measles transmission in medical facilities. West J Med 142:415–416, 1985.

145. Davis RM, Orenstein WA, Frank JA, et al. Transmission of measles in medical settings: 1980 through 1984. JAMA 255:1295–1298, 1986.

146. Istre GR, McKee PA, West GR, et al. Measles spread in medical settings: an important focus of disease transmission. Pediatrics 79:356–358, 1987.

147. Watkins NM, Smith RP Jr, St. Germain DL, MacKay DN. Measles (rubeola) infection in a hospital setting. Am J Infect Control 15:201–206, 1987.

148. Sienko DG, Friedman C, McGee HB, et al. A measles outbreak at university medical settings involving healthcare providers. Am J Public Health 77:1222–1224, 1987.

149. Measles transmitted in a medical office building—New Mexico, 1986. MMWR 36:25–27, 1987.

150. Measles—Dade County, Florida. MMWR 36:45–48, 1987.

151. Measles—Los Angeles County, California, 1988. MMWR 38:49–52, 57, 1989.

152. Markowitz LE, Preblud SR, Orenstein WA, et al. Patterns of transmission in measles outbreaks in the United States, 1985–1986. N Engl J Med 320:75–81, 1989.

153. Raad II, Sherertz RJ, Rains CS, et al. The importance of nosocomial transmission of measles in the propagation of a community outbreak. Infect Control Hosp Epidemiol 10:161–166, 1989.

154. Measles—Washington, 1990. MMWR 39:523–526, 1990.

155. Farizo KM, Stehr-Green PA, Simpson DM, et al. Pediatric emergency room visits: a risk factor for acquiring measles. Pediatrics 87:74–79, 1991.

156. Atkinson WL, Markowitz LE, Adams NC, et al. Transmission of measles in medical settings—United States, 1985–1989. Am J Med 91(suppl 3B):320S–324S, 1991.

157. Rivera ME, Mason WH, Ross LA, Wright HT Jr. Nosocomial measles infection in a pediatric hospital during a community-wide epidemic. J Pediatr 119:183–186, 1991.

158. McGrath D, Swanson R, Weems S, et al. Analysis of a measles outbreak in Kent County, Michigan in 1990. Pediatr Infect Dis J 11:385–389, 1992.

159. Freebeck PC, Clark S, Fahey PJ. Hypoxemic respiratory failure complicating nosocomial measles in a healthy host. Chest 102:625–626, 1992.

160. Miranda AC, Falcao JM, Dias JA, et al. Measles transmission in health facilities during outbreaks. Int J Epidemiol 23:843–848, 1994.

161. Ward J, El-Saadi O. Measles in the waiting room: a cautionary tale. Aust Fam Physician 28:1103, 1999.

162. de Swart RL, Wertheim-van Dillen PME, van Binnendijk RS, et al. Measles in a Dutch hospital introduced by an immunocompromised infant from Indonesia infected with an new virus genotype. Lancet 355:201–202, 2000.

163. Mendelson GMS, Roth CE, Wreghitt TG, et al. Nosocomial transmission of measles to healthcare workers: time for a national screening and immunization policy for NHS staff? J Hosp Infect 44:154–155, 2000.

164. Blake KV, Nguyen OTK, Capon AG. Nosocomial transmission of measles in western Sydney. Med J Aust 175:442, 2001.

165. Biellik RJ, Clements CJ. Strategies for minimizing nosocomial measles transmission. Bull World Health Organ 75:367–375, 1997.

166. Schiff GM, Dine MS. Transmission of rubella from newborns. Am J Dis Child 110:447–451, 1965.

167. Giles JW, Smith IM. The study of a rubella outbreak. J Iowa Med Soc 62:238–341, 1972.

168. Carne S, Dewhurst CJ, Hurley R. Rubella epidemic in a maternity unit. Br Med J 1:444–446, 1973.

169. Baba K, Yabuuchi H, Okuni H, et al. Rubella epidemic in an institution: protective value of live rubella vaccine and serological behavior of vaccinated, revaccinated and naturally immune groups. Biken J 21:25–31, 1978.

170. Exposure of patients to rubella by medical personnel—California. MMWR 27:123, 1978.

171. Rubella in hospital personnel and patients—Colorado. MMWR 28:325–327, 1979.

172. McLaughlin MC, Gold LH. The New York rubella incident: a case for changing hospital policy regarding rubella testing and immunization. Am J Public Health 69:287–289, 1979.

173. Polk BF, White JA, DeGirolami PC, Modlin JF. An outbreak of rubella among hospital personnel. N Engl J Med 303:541–545, 1980.

174. Nosocomial rubella infection—North Dakota, Alabama, Ohio. MMWR 29:629–631, 1981.

175. Gladstone JL, Millian SJ. Rubella exposure in an obstetric clinic. Obstet Gynecol 57:182–186, 1981.

176. Strassburg MA, Imagawa DT, Fannin SL, et al. Rubella outbreak among hospital employees. Obstet Gynecol 57:283–288, 1981.
177. Rubella in hospitals—California. MMWR 32:37–39, 1983.
178. Strassburg MA, Stephenson TG, Habel LA, Fannin SL. Rubella in hospital employees. Infect Control 5:123–126, 1984.
179. Heseltine PNR, Ripper M, Wohlford P. Nosocomial rubella—consequences of an outbreak and efficacy of a mandatory immunization program. Infect Control 6:371–374, 1985.
180. Storch GA, Gruber C, Benz B, et al. A rubella outbreak among dental students: description of the outbreak and analysis of control measures. Infect Control 6:150–156, 1985.
181. Jacobson JT. Rubella: one hospital's experience. Am J Infect Control 15:136–137, 1987.
182. Poland GA, Nichol KL. Medical students as sources of rubella and measles outbreaks. Arch Intern Med 150:44–46, 1990.
183. Sheridan E, Aitken C, Jeffries D, et al. Congenital rubella syndrome: a risk for immigrant populations. Lancet 359:674–675, 2002.
184. Braunstein H, Thomas S, Ito R. Immunity to measles in a large population of varying age. Am J Dis Child 144:296–298, 1990.
185. Smith E, Wong VK. Measles susceptibility of hospital personnel. Arch Intern Med 153:1011, 1993.
186. Hersh BS, Fine PE, Kent WK, et al. Mumps outbreaks in a highly vaccinated population. J Pediatr 119:187–193, 1991.
187. Plotkin SA. Clinical and pathogenetic aspects of varicella-zoster. Postgrad Med J 61(suppl 4):7–14, 1985.
188. Straus SE, Ostrove JM, Inchauspe G, et al. NIH Conference. Varicella-zoster virus infections: biology, natural history, treatment, and prevention. Ann Intern Med 108:221–237, 1988. [published erratum appears in Ann Intern Med 109:438–439, 1988]
189. Drwal-Klein LA, O'Donovan CA. Varicella in pediatric patients. Ann Pharmacother 27:938–949, 1993.
190. Arvin AM. Varicella-zoster virus. Clin Microbiol Rev 9:361–381, 1996.
191. Cohen JI. Varicella-zoster virus. Infect Dis Clin North Am 10:457–468, 1996.
192. Arvin AM. Chickenpox (varicella). Contrib Microbiol 3:96-110, 1999.
193. McCrary ML, Severson J, Tyring SK. Varicella zoster virus. J Am Acad Dermatol 41:1–14, 1999.
194. Seward JF, Watson BM, Peterson CL, et al. Varicella disease after introduction of varicella vaccine in the United States, 1995–2000. JAMA 287:606–611, 2002.
195. Brunell PA. Contagion and varicella-zoster virus. Pediatr Infect Dis 1:304–307, 1982.
196. Brawley RL, Wenzel RP. An algorithm for chickenpox exposure. Pediatr Infect Dis 3:502–504, 1984.
197. Weitekamp MR, Schan P, Aber RC. An algorithm for the control of nosocomial varicella-zoster virus infection. Am J Infect Control 13:193–198, 1985.
198. Sayre MR, Lucid EJ. Management of varicella-zoster virus-exposed hospital employees. Ann Emerg Med 16:421–424, 1987.
199. Weber DJ, Rutala WA, Parham C. Impact and costs of varicella prevention in a university hospital. Am J Public Health 78:19–23, 1988.
200. Stover DH, Bratcher DF. Varicella-zoster virus: infection, control, and prevention. Am J Infect Control 26:369–384, 1998.
201. Burns SM, Mitchell-Heggs N, Carrington D. Occupational and infection control aspects of varicella. J Infect 36 (suppl 1):73–78, 1998.
202. Weber DJ, Rutala WA. A varicella immunization program. In Poland GA, Schaffner W, Pugliese G (eds). Immunizing Healthcare Workers: A Practical Approach. Thorofare, NJ, Slack, pp. 243–260, 2000.
203. Simpson REH. Infectiousness of communicable diseases in the household (measles, chickenpox, and mumps). Lancet 2:549–554, 1952.
204. Ross AH. Modification of chickenpox in family contacts by administration of gamma globulin. N Engl J Med 267:369–376, 1962.
205. Josephson A, Karanfil L, Gombert ME. Strategies for the management of varicella-susceptible healthcare workers after a known exposure. Infect Control Hosp Epidemiol 11:309–313, 1990.
206. Gershon AA. Varicella-zoster virus: prospects for control. Adv Pediatr Infect Dis 10:93–124, 1995.
207. Birthistle K, Carrington D. Fetal varicella syndrome—a reappraisal of the literature. J Infect 36(suppl 1):25–29, 1998.
208. Sauerbrei A, Wutzler P. The congenital varicella syndrome. J Perinatol 20:548–554, 2000.
209. Meyers JD. Congenital varicella in term infants: risk reconsidered. J Infect Dis 129:215–217, 1974.
210. Sauerbrei A. Varicella-zoster virus infections in pregnancy. Intervirology 41:191–196, 1998.
211. Sauerbrei A, Wutzler P. Neonatal varicella. J Perinatol 21:545–549, 2001.
212. Wharton M. The epidemiology of varicella-zoster virus infection. Infect Dis Clin North Am 10:571–581, 1996.
213. Choo PW, Donahue JG, Manson JE, Platt R. The epidemiology of varicella and its complications. J Infect Dis 172:706–712, 1995.
214. Miller E, Marshall R, Vurdien J. Epidemiology, outcome and control of varicella-zoster infection. Rev Med Microbiol 4:222–230, 1993.
215. Feldman S, Hughes WT, Daniel CB. Varicella in children with cancer: seventy-seven cases. Pediatrics 56:388–397, 1975.
216. Feldhoff CM, Balfour HH, Simmons RL, et al. Varicella in children with renal transplants. J Pediatr 98:25–31, 1981.
217. Locksley RM, Flournoy N, Sullivan KM, Meyers JD. Infection with varicella-zoster virus after marrow transplantation. J Infect Dis 152:1172–1181, 1985.
218. Meyers JD, MacQuarrie MB, Merigan TC, Jennison MH. Nosocomial varicella: Part 1. Outbreak in oncology patients at a children's hospital. West J Med 130:196–199, 1979.
219. Morgan ER, Smalley LA. Varicella in immunocompromised children. Am J Dis Child 137:883–885, 1983.
220. Whitley R, Hilty M, Haynes R, et al. Vidarabine therapy of varicella in immunosuppressed patients. J Pediatr 101:125–131, 1982.
221. Feldman S, Lott L. Varicella in children with cancer: impact of antiviral therapy and prophylaxis. Pediatrics 80:255–262, 1987.
222. McGregor RS, Zitelli BJ, Urback AH, et al. Varicella in pediatric orthotopic liver transplant recipients. Pediatrics 83:256–261, 1989.
223. Arvin AM. Management of varicella-zoster virus infections in children. Adv Exp Med Biol 458:167–174, 1999.
224. Steele RW, Coleman MA, Fiser M, Bradsher RW. Varicella-zoster in hospital personnel: skin test reactivity to monitor susceptibility. Pediatrics 70:604–608, 1982.
225. Hyams PJ, Stuewe MCS, Heitzer V. Herpes zoster causing varicella (chickenpox) in hospital employees: cost of a casual attitude. Am J Infect Control 12:2–5, 1984.
226. Alter SJ, Hammond JA, McVey CJ, Myers MG. Susceptibility to varicella-zoster virus among adults at high risk for exposure. Infect Control 7:448–451, 1986.
227. Krasinski K, Holzman RS, LaCouture R, Florman A. Hospital experience with varicella-zoster virus. Infect Control 7:312–316, 1986.
228. Haiduven-Griffiths D, Fecko H. Varicella in hospital personnel: a challenge for the infection control practitioner. Am J Infect Control 15:207–211, 1987.
229. McKinney WP, Horowitz MM, Battiola RJ. Susceptibility of hospital-based healthcare personnel to varicella-zoster virus infections. Am J Infect Control 17:26–30, 1989.
230. Stover BH, Cost KM, Hamm C, et al. Varicella exposure in a neonatal intensive care unit: case report and control measures. Am J Infect Control 16:167–172, 1988.
231. Gallagher J, Quaid B, Cryan B. Susceptibility to varicella zoster virus infection in health care workers. Occup Med 46:289–292, 1996.
232. Myers MG, Rasley DA, Hierholzer WJ. Hospital infection control for varicella zoster virus infections. Pediatrics 70:199–202, 1982.
233. Shehab ZM, Brunell PA. Susceptibility of hospital personnel to varicella-zoster virus. J Infect Dis 150:786, 1984.
234. Haiduven DJ, Hench CP, Stevens DA. Postexposure varicella management of nonimmune personnel: an alternative approach. Infect Control Hosp Epidemiol 15:329–334, 1994.
235. Gustafson TL, Shehab Z, Brunell PA. Outbreak of varicella in a newborn intensive care nursery. Am J Dis Child 138:548–550, 1984.
236. Evans P. An epidemic of chickenpox. Lancet 2:339–340, 1940.
237. McKendrick GDW, Emond RTD. Investigation of cross-infection in isolation wards of different designs. J Hyg Camb 76:23–31, 1976.
238. Morens DM, Bregman DJ, West CM, et al. An outbreak of varicella-zoster virus infection among cancer patients. Ann Intern Med 93:414–419, 1980.
239. Leclair JM, Zaia JA, Levin MJ, et al. Airborne transmission of chickenpox in a hospital. N Engl J Med 302:450–453, 1980.
240. Scheifele D, Bonner M. Airborne transmission of chickenpox [letter]. N Engl J Med 303:281–282, 1980.

241. Asano Y, Iwayama S, Miyata T, et al. Spread of varicella in hospitalized children having no direct contact with an indicator zoster case and its prevention by a live vaccine. Biken J 23:157–161, 1980.

242. Faizallah R, Green HT, Krasner N, Walker RJ. Outbreak of chickenpox from a patient with immunosuppressed herpes zoster in hospital. Br Med J (Clin Res Ed) 285:1022–1023, 1982.

243. Gustafson TL, Lavely GB, Brawner ER, et al. An outbreak of airborne nosocomial varicella. Pediatrics 70:550–556, 1982.

244. Tsujino G, Sako M, Takahashi M. Varicella infection in a children's hospital: prevention by vaccine and an episode of airborne transmission. Biken J 27:129–132, 1984.

245. Anderson JD, Bonner M, Schiefele DW, Schneider BC. Lack of nosocomial spread of varicella in a pediatric hospital with negative pressure ventilated patient rooms. Infect Control 6:120–121, 1985.

246. Josephson A, Gombert M. Airborne transmission of nosocomial varicella from localized zoster. J Infect Dis 158:238–241, 1988.

247. Morgan-Capner P, Wilson M, Wright J, Hutchinson DN. Varicella and zoster in hospitals. Lancet 335:1460, 1990.

248. Friedman CA, Temple DM, Robbins KK, et al. Outbreak and control of varicella in a neonatal intensive care unit. Pediatr Infect Dis J 13:152–153, 1994.

249. Faoagali JL, Darcy D. Chickenpox outbreak among the staff of a large, urban adult hospital: costs of monitoring and control. Am J Infect Control 23:252–250, 1995.

250. Kavaliotis J, Loukou I, Trachana M, et al. Outbreak of varicella in a pediatric oncology unit. Med Pediatr Oncol 31:166–169, 1998.

251. Sawyer MH, Chamberlin CJ, Wu YN, et al. Detection of varicella-zoster virus DNA in air samples from hospital rooms. J Infect Dis 169:91–94, 1994.

252. Yoshikawa T, Ihira M, Suzuki K, et al. Rapid contamination of the environment with varicella-zoster virus DNA from a patient with herpes zoster. J Med Virol 63:64–66, 2001.

253. Nettleman MD, Schmid M. Cost-effectiveness of varicella vaccination in hospital employees [abstr 70]. In Program and Abstracts of the Sixth Annual Meeting of the Society for Healthcare Epidemiology of America, Washington, DC, 1996.

254. Hamilton HA. A cost minimization analysis of varicella vaccine in healthcare workers. Thesis, Department of Epidemiology, University of North Carolina School of Public Health, Chapel Hill, 1996.

255. Gray AM, Fenn P, Weinberg J, et al. An economic analysis of varicella vaccination for health care workers. Epidemiol Infect 119:209–220, 1997.

256. Tennenberg AM, Brassared JF, Lieu JV, Drusin LM. Varicella vaccination for healthcare workers at a university hospital: an analysis of costs and benefits. Infect Control Hosp Epidemiol 18:405–411, 1997.

257. Sharrar RG, laRussa P, Galea SA, et al. The postmarketing safety profile of varicella vaccine. Vaccine 19:916–923, 2000.

258. LaRussa P, Steinberg SP, Shapiro E, et al. Varicella vaccine revisited. Nat Med 6:1299–1300, 2000.

259. Gershon AA. The current status of live attenuated varicella vaccine. Arch Virol Suppl 17:1–6, 2001.

260. Gerson AA. Live-attenuated varicella vaccine. Infect Dis Clin North Am 15:65–81, 2001.

261. Arvin AM. Varicella vaccine: genesis, efficacy, and attenuation. Virol 284:153–158, 2001.

262. Arvin AM. Varicella vaccine—the first six years. N Engl J Med 344:1007–1009, 2001.

263. Asano Y, Yoshikawa T, Suga S, et al. Postexposure prophylaxis of varicella in family contact by oral acyclovir. Pediatrics 92:219–222, 1993.

264. Suga S, Yoshikawa T, Ozaki T, Asano Y. Effect of oral acyclovir against primary and secondary viraemia in incubation period of varicella. Arch Dis Child 69:639–642, 1993.

265. Abe C, Bradley J. Varicella in a pediatric convalescent hospital: controlling clinical disease following widespread exposure [abstr S32]. In Program and Abstracts of the Fifth Annual Meeting of the Society for Healthcare Epidemiology of America, San Diego, 1995.

266. Asano Y, Nakayama H, Yazaki T, et al. Protective efficacy of vaccination in children in four episodes of natural varicella and zoster in the ward. Pediatrics 59:8–12, 1977.

267. Ueda K, Yamada I, Goto M, et al. Use of a live varicella vaccine to prevent the spread of varicella in handicapped or immunosuppressed children including MSLC (muco-cutaneous lymph node syndrome) patients in hospitals. Biken J 20:117–123, 1977.

268. Katsushima N, Yazaki N, Sakamoto M, et al. Application of a live varicella vaccine to hospitalized children and its follow-up study. Biken J 25:29–42, 1982.

269. Asano Y, Hirose S, Iwayama S, et al. Protective effect of immediate inoculation of a live varicella vaccine in household contacts in relation to the viral dose and interval between exposure and vaccination. Biken J 25:43–45, 1982.

270. Katsushima N, Yazaki N, Sakamoto M. Effect and follow-up study of varicella vaccine. Biken J 27:51–58, 1984.

271. Sugino H, Tsukino R, Miyashiro E, et al. Live varicella vaccine: prevention of nosocomial infection and protection of high risk infants from varicella infection. Biken J 27:63–65, 1984.

272. Naganuma Y, Osawa S, Takahashi R. Clinical application of a live varicella vaccine (Oka strain) in a hospital. Biken J 27:59–61, 1984.

273. Boda D, Bartyik K, Szuts P, Turi S. Active immunization of children exposed to varicella infection in a hospital ward using live attenuated varicella vaccine given subcutaneously or intracutaneously. Acta Paediatr Hung 27:252–252, 1986.

274. Arbeter AM, Starr SE, Plotkin SA. Varicella vaccine studies in healthy children and adults. Pediatrics 78(suppl):748–756, 1986.

275. Ferson MJ. Varicella vaccine in post-exposure prophylaxis. Commun Dis Intell 25:13–15, 2001.

276. Jagger J, Hunt Brand-Elnaggar J, Pearson RD. Rates of needle-stick injury caused by various devices in a university hospital. N Engl J Med 319:284–288, 1988.

277. Gerderding JL. Risks to healthcare workers from occupational exposure to hepatitis B virus, human immunodeficiency virus, and cytomegalovirus. Infect Dis Clin North Am 3:735–745, 1989.

278. Cardo DM, Bell DM. Bloodborne pathogen transmission in healthcare workers. Infect Dis Clin North Am 11:331–346, 1997.

279. Lanphear BP. Transmission and control of bloodborne viral hepatitis in health care workers. Occup Med 12:717–730, 1997.

280. Beltrami EM, Williams IT, Shapiro CN, Chamberland ME. Risks and management of blood-borne infections in health care workers. Clin Microbiol Rev 13:385–407, 2000.

281. Bower WA, Alter MJ. Risks and prevention of occupational hepatitis B virus and hepatitis C virus infection. Semin Infect Control 1:19–29, 2001.

282. Chiarella LA, Bartley J. Prevention of blood exposure in healthcare personnel. Semin Infect Control 1:30–43, 2001.

283. Segal HE, Llewellyn CH, Irwin G, et al. Hepatitis B antigen and antibody in the U.S. Army: prevalence in healthcare personnel. Am J Public Health 66:667–671, 1976.

284. Denes AE, Smith JL, Maynard JE, et al. Hepatitis B infection in physicians: results of a nationwide seroepidemiologic survey. JAMA 239:210–212, 1978.

285. Dienstag JL, Ryan DM. Occupational exposure to hepatitis B virus in hospital personnel: infection or immunization? Am J Epidemiol 115:26–39, 1982.

286. Hadler SC, Doto IL, Maynard JE, et al. Occupational risk of hepatitis B infection in hospital workers. Infect Control 6:24–31, 1985.

287. Guidelines for prevention of transmission of human immunodeficiency virus and hepatitis B virus to health-care and public-safety workers. MMWR Morb Mortal Wkly Rep 38(SS-6):1–37, 1989.

288. Shapiro CN. Occupational risk of infection with hepatitis B and hepatitis C virus. Surg Clin North Am 75:1052–1056, 1995.

289. Lowenfels AB, Wormser GP, Jain R. Frequency of puncture injuries in surgeons and estimated risk of HIV infection. Arch Surg 124:1284–1286, 1989.

290. Tokars JI, Chamberland ME, Schable CA, et al. A survey of occupational blood contact and HIV infection among orthopedic surgeons. JAMA 268:489–494, 1992.

291. Bond WW, Favero MS, Peterson NJ, et al. Survival of hepatitis B virus after drying and storage for one week. Lancet 1:550–551, 1981.

292. Grady GF, Lee VA, Prince AM, et al. Hepatitis B immune globulin for accidental exposures among medical personnel: final report of a multicenter controlled trial. J Infect Dis 138:625–638, 1978.

293. Seeff LM, Wright EC, Zimmerman HJ, et al. Type B hepatitis after needle-stick exposure: prevention with hepatitis B immune globulin. Ann Intern Med 88:285–293, 1978.

294. Werner BG, Grady GF. Accidental hepatitis-B-surface-antigen-positive inoculations. Ann Intern Med 97:367–369, 1982.

295. Kew MC. Possible transmission of serum (Australia-antigen-positive) hepatitis via the conjunctiva. Infect Immun 7:823–824, 1973.

296. Snydman DR, Hindman SH, Wineland MD, et al. Nosocomial viral hepatitis B: a cluster among staff with subsequent transmission to patients. Ann Intern Med 85:573–577, 1976.

297. Ingerslev J, Mortensen E, Rasmussen K, Jorgensen J. Silent hepatitis-B immunization in laboratory technicians. Scand J Clin Lab Invest 48:333–336, 1988.

298. Handsfield HH, Cummings MJ, Swenson PD. Prevalence of antibody to human immunodeficiency virus and hepatitis B surface antigen in blood samples submitted to a hospital laboratory: implications for handling specimens. JAMA 258:3395–3397, 1987.

299. Chiarella LA. Prevention of patient-to-patient transmission of bloodborne viruses. Semin Infect Control 1:44–48, 2001.

300. Hepatitis B associated with jet gun injection—California. MMWR 35:373–376, 1986.

301. Morris IM, Cattle DS, Smits BJ. Endoscopy and transmission of hepatitis B. Lancet 2:1152, 1975.

302. Oren I, Hershow RC, Ben-Porath E, et al. A common-source outbreak of fulminant hepatitis B in a hospital. Ann Intern Med 110:691–698, 1989.

303. Kidd-Ljunggren K, Broman E, Ekvall H, Gustavsson O. Nosocomial transmission of hepatitis B virus infection through multiple-dose virals. J Hosp Infect 43:57–62, 1999.

304. An outbreak of hepatitis B associated with reusable subdermal electroencephalogram electrodes. CMAJ 162:1127–1131, 2000.

305. Nosocomial transmission of hepatitis B virus associated with a spring-loaded fingerstick device—California. MMWR 39:610–613, 1990.

306. Douvin C, Simon D, Zinelabidine H, et al. An outbreak of hepatitis B in an endocrinology unit traced to a capillary-blood sampling device. N Engl J Med 322:57, 1990.

307. Polish LB, Shapiro CN, Bauer F, et al. Nosocomial transmission of hepatitis B virus associated with the use of a spring-loaded fingerstick device. N Engl J Med 326:721–725, 1992.

308. Stapleton JT, Lemon SM. Transmission of hepatitis B by a fingerstick device [letter]. N Engl J Med 327:497, 1992.

309. Nosocomial hepatitis B virus infection associated with reusable fingerstick blood sampling devices—Ohio and New York City, 1996. MMWR 46:217–221, 1997.

310. Quale JM, Landman D, Wallace B, et al. Déjà vu: nosocomial hepatitis B virus transmission and fingerstick monitoring. Am J Med 105:296–301, 1998.

311. Drescher J, Wagner D, Haverick A, et al. Nosocomial hepatitis B virus infection in cardiac transplant recipients transmitted during transvenous endomyocardial biopsy. J Hosp Infect 26:81–92, 1994.

312. Lauer JL, VanDrunen NA, Washburn JW, Balfour HH Jr. Transmission of hepatitis B virus in clinical laboratory areas. J Infect Dis 140:513–516, 1979.

313. Pattison CP, Boyer DM, Maynard JE, Kelly PC. Epidemic hepatitis in a clinical laboratory: Possible association with computer card handling. JAMA 230:854–857, 1974.

314. Tanaka S, Yoshiba M, Iino S, et al. A common-source outbreak of fulminant hepatitis B in hemodialysis patients induced by precore mutant. Kidney Int 48:1972–1978, 1992.

315. Hardie DR, Kannemeyer J, Stannard LM. DNA single strand conformation polymorphism identifies five defined strains of hepatitis B virus (HBV) during an outbreak of HBV infection in an oncology unit. J Med Virol 49:49–54, 1996.

316. Outbreaks of hepatitis B virus infection among hemodialysis patients—California, Nebraska, and Texas, 1994. MMWR 45:285–289, 1996.

317. De Castro L, Araujo NM, Sabino RR, et al. Nosocomial spread of hepatitis B virus in two hemodialysis units, investigated by restriction fragment length polymorphism analysis. Eur J Clin Microbiol Infect Dis 19:531–537, 2000.

318. Arduino MJ, Tokars JI, Lyerla R, Alter MJ. Prevention of healthcare-associated transmission of bloodborne viruses in hemodialysis facilities. Semin Infect Control 1:49–60, 2001.

319. Recommendations for preventing transmission of infections among chronic hemodialysis patients. MMWR 50(RR-5):1–63, 2001.

320. Weber DJ, Hoffmann KK, Rutala WA. Management of the healthcare worker infected with human immunodeficiency virus: lessons from nosocomial transmission of hepatitis B virus. Infect Control Hosp Epidemiol 12:625–630, 1991.

321. Bell DM, Shapiro CN, Ciesielski CA, Chamberland ME. Preventing bloodborne pathogen transmission from health-care workers to patients. Surg Clin North Am 75:1189–1203, 1995.

322. Harpaz R, Von Seidlein L, Averhoff FM, et al. Transmission of hepatitis B virus to multiple patients from a surgeon without evidence of inadequate infection control. N Engl J Med 334:549–554, 1996.

323. Incident Investigation Team et al. Transmission of hepatitis B to patients from four infected surgeons without hepatitis B "e" antigen. N Engl J Med 336:178–184, 1997.

324. Chiarella LA, Cardo DM, Panlilio A, et al. Risks and prevention of bloodborne virus transmission from infected healthcare providers. Semin Infect Control 1:61–72, 2001.

325. AIDS/TB Committee of the Society for Healthcare Epidemiology of America. Management of healthcare workers infected with hepatitis B virus, hepatitis C virus, human immunodeficiency virus, or other bloodborne pathogens. Infect Control Hosp Epidemiol 18:349–363, 1997.

326. Occupational Safety and Health Administration. 29 CFR Part 1910.1030—occupational exposure to bloodborne pathogens; final rule. Fed Reg 56:64175–64182, 1991.

327. Occupational Safety and Health Administration. Directive Number CPL 2-2.69: Enforcement Procedures for the Occupational Exposure to Bloodborne Pathogens. Washington, DC, Occupational Safety and Health Administration, 2001.

328. Koff RS. Hepatitis vaccines. Infect Dis Clin North Am 15:83–95, 2001.

329. Mahoney FJ. Update on diagnosis, management, and prevention of hepatitis B virus infection. Clin Microbiol Rev 12:351–356, 1999.

330. Wood RC, MacDonald KL, White KE, et al. Risk factors for lack of detectable antibody following hepatitis B vaccination on Minnesota health care workers. JAMA 270:2935–2939, 1993.

331. Jilg W, Schmidt M, Deinhardt F. Vaccination against hepatitis B: comparison of three different vaccination schedules. J Infect Dis 160:766–769, 1989.

332. Hadler SC, de Monzon A, Lugo DR, Perez M. Effect of timing of hepatitis B vaccine doses on response to vaccine in Yucpa Indians. Vaccine 7:106–110, 1989.

333. Hadler SC, Francis DP, Maynard JE, et al. Long-term immunogenicity and efficacy of hepatitis B vaccine in homosexual men. N Engl J Med 315:209–214, 1986.

334. Barker WH. Excess pneumonia and influenza associated hospitalizations during influenza epidemics in the United States, 1970–78. Am J Public Health 76:761–765, 1986.

335. Influenza surveillance—United States, 1992–93 and 1993–94. MMWR 46(SS-1):1–12, 1997.

336. Meibalane R, Sedmak GV, Sasidharan P, et al. Outbreak of influenza in a neonatal intensive care unit. J Pediatr 91:974–976, 1977.

337. Kapila R, Lintz DI, Tecson FT, et al. A nosocomial outbreak of influenza A. Chest 71:576–579, 1977.

338. Balkovic ES, Goodman RA, Rose FB, Borel CO. Nosocomial influenza A (H1N1) infection. Am J Med Tech 46:318–320, 1980.

339. Van Voris LP, Belshe RB, Shaffer JL. Nosocomial influenza B virus infection in the elderly. Ann Intern Med 96:153–158, 1982.

340. Rivera M, Gonzalez N. An influenza outbreak in a hospital. Am J Nurs 82:1836–1838, 1982.

341. Bean B, Rhame FS, Hughes RS, et al. Influenza B: hospital activity during a community outbreak. Diagn Microbiol Infect Dis 1:177–183, 1983.

342. Hammond GW, Cheang M. Absenteeism among hospital staff during an influenza epidemic: implications for immunoprophylaxis. Can Med Assoc J 131:449–452, 1984.

343. Weingarten S, Friedlander M, Rascon D, et al. Influenza surveillance in an acute-care hospital. Arch Intern Med 148:113–116, 1988.

344. Suspected nosocomial influenza cases in an intensive care unit. MMWR 37:3–4, 9, 1988.

345. Pachucki CT, Pappas SAW, Fuller GF, et al. Influenza A among hospital personnel and patients. Ann Intern Med 149:77–80, 1989.

346. Grayston JT, Diwan VK, Cooney M, Wang S-P. Community- and hospital-acquired pneumonia associated with Chlamydia TWAR infection demonstrated serologically. Arch Intern Med 149:169–173, 1989.

347. Serwint JR, Miller RM. Why diagnose influenza infections in hospitalized pediatric patients? Pediatr Infect Dis J 12:200–204, 1993.

348. Whimbey E, Elting LS, Couch RB, et al. Influenza A virus infections among hospitalized adult bone marrow transplant recipients. Bone Marrow Transplant 13:437–440, 1994.

349. Evert RJ, Hanger HJC, Jennings LC, et al. Outbreaks of influenza A among elderly hospital inpatients. N Z Med J 109:272–274, 1996.

350. Scheputiuk S, Papanaoum K, Quao M. Spread of influenza A virus infection in hospitalized patients with cancer. Aust N Z J Med 28:525–526, 1998.

351. Munoz FM, Campbell JR, Atman RL, et al. Influenza A virus outbreak in a neonatal intensive care unit. Pediatr Infect Dis J 18:811–815, 1999.

352. Cunney RJ, Bialachowski A, Thornley D, et al. An outbreak of influenza A in a neonatal intensive care unit. Infect Control Hosp Epidemiol 21:449–454, 2000.

353. Weinstock DM, Eagan J, Malak SA, et al. Control of influenza on a bone marrow transplant unit. Infect Control Hosp Epidemiol 21:730–732, 2000.

354. Barlow G, Nathwani D. Nosocomial influenza infection. Lancet 355:1187, 2000.

355. Malavaud S, Malavaud B, Sanders K, et al. Nosocomial influenza virus A (H3N2) infection in a solid organ transplant department. Transplantation 72:535–537, 2001.

356. Sagrera X, Ginovart G, Raspall F, et al. Outbreaks of influenza A virus infection in neonatal intensive care units. Pediatr Infect Dis J 21:196–200, 2002.

357. Evans ME, Hall KL, Berry SE. Influenza control in acute care hospitals. Am J Infect Control 25:357–362, 1997.

358. Odelin MR, Pozzetto B, Aymard M, et al. Role of influenza vaccination in the elderly during an epidemic of A/H1NI virus in 1988–1989: clinical and serological data. Gerontology 39:109–116, 1993.

359. Serie C, Barme M, Hannoun C, et al. Effects of vaccination on an influenza epidemic in a geriatric hospital. Dev Biol Stand 39:317–321, 1977.

360. Hall WN, Goodman RA, Noble GR, et al. An outbreak of influenza B in an elderly population. J Infect Dis 144:297–302, 1981.

361. Goodman RA, Orenstein WA, Munro TF, et al. Impact of influenza A in a nursing home. JAMA 252:1451–1453, 1982.

362. Arroyo JC, Postic B, Brown A, et al. Influenza A/Philippines/2/82 outbreak in a nursing home: limitations of influenza vaccination in the aged. Am J Infect Control 12:329–334, 1984.

363. Christie RW, Marquis LL. Immunization roulette: influenza occurrence in five nursing homes. Am J Infect Control 13:174–177, 1985.

364. Horman JT, Stetler HC, Israel E, et al. An outbreak of influenza A in a nursing home. Am J Public Health 76:501–504, 1986.

365. Patriarca PA, Weber JA, Parker RA, et al. Risk factors for outbreaks of influenza in nursing homes. Am J Epidemiol 124:114–119, 1986.

366. Strassburg MA, Greenland S, Sorvillo FJ, et al. Influenza in the elderly: report of an outbreak and a review of vaccine effectiveness reports. Vaccine 4:38–44, 1986.

367. Arden NH, Patriarca PA, Fasano MB, et al. The role of vaccination and amantadine prophylaxis in controlling an outbreak of influenza A (H3N2) in a nursing home. Arch Intern Med 148:865–868, 1988.

368. Gross PA, Rodstein M, LaMontage JR, et al. Epidemiology of acute respiratory illness during an influenza outbreak in a nursing home. Arch Intern Med 148:559–561, 1988.

369. Mast EE, Harmon MW, Gravenstein S, et al. Emergence and possible transmission of amantadine-resistant viruses during nursing home outbreaks of influenza A (H3N2). Am J Epidemiol 134:988–997, 1991.

370. Control of influenza A outbreaks in nursing homes: amantadine as an adjunct to vaccine—Washington, 1989–90. MMWR Morb Mortal Wkly Rep 40:842–845, 1991.

371. Outbreak of influenza A in a nursing home—New York, December 1991–January 1992. MMWR Morb Mortal Wkly Rep 41:129–131, 1992.

372. Degelau J, Somani SK, Cooper SL, et al. Amantadine-resistant influenza A in a nursing facility. Arch Intern Med 152:390–392, 1992.

373. Taylor JL, Dwyer DM, Coffman T, et al. Nursing home outbreak of influenza A (H3N2): evaluation of vaccine efficacy and influenza case definition. Infect Control Hosp Epidemiol 13:93–97, 1992.

374. Morens DM, Rash VM. Lessons from a nursing home outbreak of influenza A. Infect Control Hosp Epidemiol 16:275–280, 1995.

375. Issacs S, Dickenson C, Brimmer G. Outbreak of influenza A in an Ontario nursing home—January 1997. Can Commun Dis Rep 23:105–108, 1997.

376. Bowles SK, Kennie N, Ruston L, et al. Influenza outbreak in a long-term care facility: considerations for pharmacy. Am J Health Syst Pharm 56:2303–2307, 1999.

377. Potter J, Stott DJ, Roberts MA, et al. Influenza vaccination of healthcare workers in long-term-care hospitals reduces the mortality of elderly patients. J Infect Dis 175:1–6, 1997.

378. Carman WF, Elder AG, Wallace LA, et al. Effects of influenza vaccination on health-care workers on mortality of elderly people in long-term care: a randomized controlled trial. Lancet 355:93–97, 2000.

379. Atkinson WL, Arden NH, Patriarca PA, et al. Amantadine prophylaxis during an institutional outbreak of type A (H1N1) influenza. Arch Intern Med 146:1751–1756, 1986.

380. Fedson DS. Prevention and control of influenza in institutional settings. Hosp Pract 24:87–96, 1989.

381. Graman PS, Hall CB. Nosocomial viral infections. Semin Respir Infect 4:253–260, 1989.

382. Graman PS, Hall CB. Epidemiology and control of nosocomial viral infections. Infect Dis Clin North Am 3:815–841, 1989.

383. Gravenstein S, Miller BA, Drinka P. Prevention and control of influenza A outbreaks in long-term care facilities. Infect Control Hosp Epidemiol 13:49–54, 1992.

384. Tablan OC, Anderson LJ, Arden NH, et al. Guideline for prevention of nosocomial pneumonia. Infect Control Hosp Epidemiol 15:587–627, 1994.

385. Gomolin IH, Leib HB, Arden NH, Sherman FT. Control of influenza outbreaks in the nursing home: guidelines for diagnosis and management. J Am Geriatr Soc 43:71–74, 1995.

386. Nichol KL, Lind A, Margolis KL, et al. The effectiveness of vaccination against influenza in healthy, working adults. N Engl J Med 333:889–893, 1995.

387. Parker R, Loewen N, Skowronski D. Experience with oseltamivir in the control of a nursing home influenza B outbreak. Can Commun Dis Rep 27:37–40, 2001.

388. Ohrt CK, McKinney WP. Achieving compliance with influenza immunization of medical house staff and students: a randomized controlled study. JAMA 267:1377–1380, 1992.

389. Nafziger DA, Herwaldt LA. Attitudes of internal medicine residents regarding influenza vaccination. Infect Control Hosp Epidemiol 15:32–35, 1994.

390. Watanakunakorn C, Ellis G, Gemmel D. Attitude of healthcare personnel regarding influenza immunization. Infect Control Hosp Epidemiol 14:17–20, 1993.

391. Shapiro CN, Coleman PJ, McQuillan GM, et al. Epidemiology of hepatitis A: seroepidemiology and risk groups in the USA. Vaccine 10(suppl 1):S59–S62, 1992.

392. Kashiwagi S, Hayashi J, Ikematsu H, et al. Prevalence of immunologic markers of hepatitis A and B infection in hospital personnel in Miyazaki Prefecture, Japan. Am J Epidemiol 122:964–969, 1985.

393. Gibas A, Blewett DR, Schoenfield DA, et al. Prevalence and incidence of viral hepatitis in healthcare workers in the prehepatitis B vaccination era. Am J Epidemiol 136:1791–1800, 1992.

394. Abb J. Prevalence of hepatitis A virus antibodies in hospital personnel. Gesundheitswesen 56:377–379, 1994.

395. Papaevangelou GJ, Roumeliotou-Karayannis AJ, Contoyannis PC. The risk of hepatitis A and B virus infections from patients under care without isolation precaution. J Med Virol 7:143–148, 1981.

396. Germanaud J. Hepatitis A and health care personnel [letter]. Arch Intern Med 154:820, 1994.

397. Van Damme P, Cramm M, Van der Auwera J-C, Meheus A. Hepatitis A vaccination for healthcare workers. BMJ 306:1615, 1993.

398. Eisenstein AB, Aach RD, Jacobson W, Goldman A. An epidemic of infectious hepatitis in a general hospital: probable transmission by contaminated orange juice. JAMA 185:171–184, 1993.

399. Meyers JD, Romm FJ, Tihen WS, Bryan JA. Food-borne hepatitis A in a general hospital: epidemiologic study of an outbreak attributed to sandwiches. JAMA 231:1049–1053, 1975.

400. Goodman RA, Carder CC, Allen JR, et al. Nosocomial hepatitis A transmission by an adult patient with diarrhea. Am J Med 73:220–226, 1982.

401. Krober MS, Bass JW, Brown JD, et al. Hospital outbreak of hepatitis A: risk factors for spread. Pediatr Infect Dis J 3:296–299, 1984.

402. Klein BS, Michaels JA, Rytel MW, et al. Nosocomial hepatitis A: a multinursery outbreak in Wisconsin. JAMA 252:2716–2721, 1984.

403. Reed CM, Gustafson TL, Siegel J, et al. Nosocomial transmission of hepatitis A from a hospital-acquired case. Pediatr Infect Dis J 3:300–303, 1984.

404. Skidmore SJ, Gully PR, Middleton JD, et al. An outbreak of hepatitis A on a hospital ward. J Med Virol 17:175–177, 1985.

405. Azimi PH, Roberto RR, Guralnik J, et al. Transfusion-acquired hepatitis A in a premature infant with secondary nosocomial spread in an intensive care nursery. Am J Dis Child 140:23–27, 1986.

406. Baptiste R, Koziol DE, Henderson DK. Nosocomial transmission of hepatitis A in an adult population. Infect Control 8:364–370, 1987.

407. Drusin LM, Sohmer M, Groshen SL, et al. Nosocomial hepatitis A infection in a pediatric intensive care unit. Arch Dis Child 62:690–695, 1987.

408. Rosenblum LS, Villarino ME, Nainan OV, et al. Hepatitis A outbreak in a neonatal intensive care unit: risk factors for transmission and evidence of prolonged viral excretion among preterm infants. J Infect Dis 164:476–482, 1991.

409. Lee KK, Vargo LR, Le CT, Fernando L. Transfusion-acquired hepatitis A outbreak from fresh frozen plasma in a neonatal intensive care unit. Pediatr Infect Dis J 11:122–123, 1992.

410. Watson JC, Flemming DC, Borella AJ, et al. Vertical transmission of hepatitis A resulting in an outbreak in a neonatal intensive care unit. J Infect Dis 167:567–571, 1993.

411. Doebbling BN, Li N, Wenzel RP. An outbreak of hepatitis A among healthcare workers: risk factors for transmission. Am J Public Health 83:1679–1684, 1993.

412. Burkholder BT, Coronado VG, Brown J, et al. Nosocomial transmission of hepatitis A in a pediatric hospital traced to an anti-hepatitis A virus-negative patient with immunodeficiency. Pediatr Infect Dis J 14:261–266, 1995.

413. Hanna JN, Loewenthal MR, Negel P, Wenck DJ. An outbreak of hepatitis A in an intensive care unit. Anaesth Intensive Care 24:440–444, 1996.

414. Jensenius M, Ringertz SH, Bell H, et al. Prolonged nosocomial outbreak of hepatitis A arising from an alcoholic with pneumonia. Scand J Infect Dis 30:119–123, 1998.

415. Centers for Disease Control and Prevention. Pertussis vaccination: use of acellular pertussis vaccines among infants and children. Recommendations of the Advisory Committee on Immunization Practices. MMWR 46(RR-7):1–25, 1997.

416. Cherry JD. The epidemiology of pertussis and pertussis immunization in the United Kingdom and the United States: a comparative study. Curr Probl Pediatr 14:1–78, 1984.

417. Cherry JD. Nosocomial pertussis in the nineties. Infect Control Hosp Epidemiol 16:553–555, 1995.

418. Mink C, Cherry JD, Christenson P, et al. A search for Bordetella pertussis infection in university students. Clin Infect Dis 14:464–521, 1992.

419. Rosenthal S, Strebel P, Cassiday P, et al. Pertussis infection among adults during the 1993 outbreak in Chicago. J Infect Dis 171:1650–1652, 1995.

420. Wright SW, Edwards KM, Decker MD, Zeldin MH. Pertussis infection in adults with persistent cough. JAMA 13:1044–1046, 1995.

421. Deville JG, Cherry JD, Christenson PD, et al. Frequency of unrecognized Bordetella pertussis infections in adults. Clin Infect Dis 21:639–642, 1995.

422. von Konig CHW, Postels-Multani S, Block HL, Schmitt HJ. Pertussis in adults: frequency of transmission after household exposure. Lancet 346:1326–1328, 1995.

423. Kurt TL, Yeager AS, Guenette S, Dunlop S. Spread of pertussis by hospital staff. JAMA 221:264–267, 1972.

424. Linneman CC, Ramundo N, Perlstein PH, et al. Use of pertussis vaccine in an epidemic involving hospital staff. Lancet 2:540–543, 1975.

425. Valenti WM, Pincus PH, Messner MK. Nosocomial pertussis: possible spread by a hospital visitor. Am J Dis Child 134:520–521, 1980.

426. Steketee RW, Wassilak SGF, Adkins WN, et al. Evidence for a high attack rate and efficacy of erythromycin prophylaxis in a pertussis outbreak in a facility for the developmentally disabled. J Infect Dis 157:434–440, 1988.

427. Fisher MC, Long SS, McGowan KL, et al. Outbreak of pertussis in a residential facility for handicapped people. J Pediatr 114:934–939, 1989.

428. Addiss DG, Davis JP, Meade BD, et al. A pertussis outbreak in a Wisconsin nursing home. J Infect Dis 164:704–710, 1991.

429. Tanaka Y, Fujinaga K, Goto A, et al. Outbreak of pertussis in a residential facility for handicapped people. Dev Biol Stand 73:329–332, 1991.

430. Shefer A, Dales L, Nelson M, et al. Use and safety of acellular pertussis vaccine among adult hospital staff during an outbreak of pertussis. J Infect Dis 171:1053–1056, 1995.

431. Christie CDC, Glover AM, Willke MJ, et al. Containment of pertussis in the regional pediatric hospital during the greater Cincinnati epidemic of 1993. Infect Control Hosp Epidemiol 16:556–563, 1995.

432. Weber DJ, Rutala WA. Management of healthcare workers exposed to pertussis. Infect Control Hosp Epidemiol 15:411–415, 1994.

433. Weber DJ, Rutala WA. Pertussis: a continuing hazard for healthcare facilities. Infect Control Hosp Epidemiol 22:736–740, 2001.

434. Edwards KM, Decker MD, Graham BS, et al. Adult immunization with acellular pertussis vaccine. JAMA 269:53–56, 1993.

435. Keitel WA, Muenz LR, Decker MD, et al. A randomized clinical trial of acellular pertussis vaccines in healthy adults: dose-response comparisons of 5 vaccines and implications for booster immunization. J Infect Dis 180:397–403, 1999.

436. Halperin SA, Smith B, Russell M, et al. An adult formulation of a five-component acellular pertussis vaccine combined with diphtheria and tetanus toxoids is safe and immunogenic in adolescents and adults. Vaccine 18:1312–1319, 2000.

437. Rothstein EP, Pennridge Pediatric Associates, Anderson EL, et al. An acellular pertussis vaccine in healthy adults: safety and immunogenicity. Vaccine 17:2999–3006, 1999.

438. van der Wielen M, van Damme P, Joosens E, et al. A randomized controlled trial with a diphtheria-tetanus-acellular pertussis (dTpa) vaccine in adults. Vaccine 18:2075–2082, 2000.

439. Minh NNT, He Q, Edelman K, et al. Immune responses to pertussis antigens eight years after booster immunization with acellular vaccines in adults. Vaccine 18:1971–1974, 2000.

440. Turnbull FM, Heath TC, Jalaludin BB, et al. A randomized trial of two acellular pertussis vaccines (dTpa and pa) and a licensed diphtheria-tetanus vaccine (Td) in adults. Vaccine 19:628–636, 2001.

441. Zackrisson G, Brorson J-E, Krantz I, Trollfors B. In-vitro sensitivity of Bordetella pertussis. J Antimicrob Chemother 11:407–411, 1983.

442. Kurzynski T, Boehm DM, Rott-Petri JA, et al. Antimicrobial susceptibilities of Bordetella species isolated in a multicenter pertussis surveillance project. Antimicrob Agents Chemother 32:137–140, 1988.

443. Hoppe JE, Eichhorn A. Activity of new macrolides against Bordetella pertussis and Bordetella parapertussis. Eur J Clin Microbiol Infect Dis 8:653–654, 1989.

444. Appleman ME, Hadfield TL, Gaines JK, Winn RE. Susceptibility of Bordetella pertussis to five quinolone antimicrobic drugs. Diagn Microbiol Infect Dis 8:131–133, 1987.

445. Hoppe JE, Simon CG. In vitro susceptibilities of Bordetella pertussis and Bordetella parapertussis to seven fluoroquinolones. Antimicrob Agents Chemother 34:2287–2288, 1990.

446. Hoppe JE, Haug A. Antimicrobial susceptibility of Bordetella pertussis: Part I. Infection 16:126–130, 1988.

447. Granstrom G, Sterner G, Nord CE, Granstrom M. Use of erythromycin to prevent pertussis in newborns of mothers with pertussis. J Infect Dis 155:1210–1214, 1987.

448. Sprauer MA, Cochi SL, Zell ER, et al. Prevention of secondary transmission of pertussis in households with early use of erythromycin. Am J Dis Child 146:177–181, 1992.

449. De Serres G, Boulianne N, Dukval B. Field effectiveness of erythromycin prophylaxis to prevent pertussis within families. Pediatr Infect Dis J 4:969–975, 1995.

450. Anonymous. The choice of antimicrobial drugs. Med Lett Drugs Ther 38:25–34, 1996.

451. Hoppe JE, Haug A. Antimicrobial susceptibility of Bordetella pertussis: Part II. Infection 16:148–152, 1988.

452. Hoppe JE. Update of epidemiology, diagnosis, and treatment of pertussis. Eur J Clin Microbiol Infect Dis 15:189–193, 1996.

453. Henry RL, Dorman DC, Skinner JA, Mellis CM. Antimicrobial therapy in whooping cough. Med J Aust 2:27–28, 1981.

454. Hoppe JE, Halm U, Hagedorn H-J, Kraminer-Hagedorn A. Comparison of erythromycin ethylsuccinate and co-trimoxazole for treatment of pertussis. Infection 17:227–231, 1989.

455. Aoyama T, Sunakawa K, Iwata S, et al. Efficacy of short-term treatment of pertussis with clarithromycin and azithromycin. J Pediatr 129:761–764, 1996.

456. Martinez SM, Kemper CA, Haiduven D, et al. Azithromycin as prophylaxis during a hospital-wide outbreak of a pertussis-like illness. Infect Control Hosp Epidemiol 22:781–782, 2001.

457. Lewis K, Saubolle MA, Tenover FC, et al. Pertussis caused by an erythromycin-resistant strain of Bordetella pertussis. Pediatr Infect Dis J 14:388–391, 1995.

458. Korgenski EK, Daly JA. Surveillance and detection of erythromycin resistance in Bordetella pertussis isolates recovered from a pediatric

population in the intermountain West Region of the United States. J Clin Microbiol 35:2989–2991, 1997.

459. Hoppe JE, Bryskier A. In vitro susceptibilities of *Bordetella pertussis* and *Bordetella parapertussis* to two ketolides (HMR 3004 and HMR 3652), four macrolides (azithromycin, clarithromycin, erythromycin A, and roxithromycin) and two ansamycins (rifampin and rifapentine). Antimicrob Agents Chemother 42:965–966, 1998.

460. Brett M, Short P, Beatson S. The comparative in-vitro activity of roxithromycin and other antibiotics against *Bordetella pertussis*. J Antimicrob Chemother 41(suppl B):23–27, 1998.

461. Gordon KA, Fusco J, Biedenbach DJ, et al. Antimicrobial susceptibility testing of clinical isolates of *Bordetella pertussis* from Northern California: report from the SENTRY antimicrobial surveillance program. Antimicrob Agents Chemother 45:3599–3600, 2001.

Chapter 60

Regulation and Testing of Vaccines

NORMAN W. BAYLOR • KAREN MIDTHUN

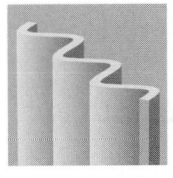

The need for a strong national regulatory authority (NRA), especially for the regulation of vaccines, is recognized worldwide. NRAs responsible for controlling vaccines are faced with the difficult charge of regulating these products to assure their relative safety and efficacy from prelicensure through postlicensure. The NRA has a dual role of assuring that beneficial vaccines are available and labeled with adequate information on their risks and benefits while protecting the public from unsafe products or false claims. Thus the NRA plays a significant role in contributing to the overall immunization effort through its risk management decisions. Developed countries of the world have established government agencies to conduct these regulatory activities; however, even today, many developing countries do not have established NRAs.

In the United States, the organization responsible for regulating vaccines as well as other biologically derived pharmaceutical products is the Center for Biologics Evaluation and Research (CBER) of the Food and Drug Administration (FDA). The regulation of biologicals, vaccines in particular, in the United States has historically developed around concerns of safety. It has been a century since Congress enacted the 1902 Biologics Control Act, which contained the initial concepts used for the regulation of biologicals in the United States. These provisions were revised and codified in Section 351 of the Public Health Service Act (PHS Act) in 1944, and expanded on in the 1950s. Although not directly related to safety and efficacy, the passage of the Prescription Drug User Fee Act of 1992 and the Food and Drug Administration Modernization Act of 1997 have both had an impact on the regulation of vaccines. Current U.S. licensed vaccines are listed in Tables 60–1 and 60–2.

In addition to NRAs, the World Health Organization (WHO), through its Expert Committee on Biological Standardization and its Biologicals Unit, provides guidance in the form of criteria for acceptability of products that move in international commerce.* Although the WHO is not an NRA, more than 100 countries have adopted WHO requirements as their own national standards. These requirements have been useful in establishing a standard of acceptability for vaccines used by international agencies involved in global immunization efforts. National standards are not required to be entirely consistent with the WHO criteria. However, international standardization efforts have been given special impetus by the formation of the European Community and this organization's attempts to harmonize the regulatory requirements of multiple European states. The efforts of the International Conference on Harmonization of drugs[1] have had less of an impact on vaccines; however, there is increasing movement to globally harmonize the requirements for vaccines.

An NRA needs a multidisciplinary team of scientists and physicians as well as continued exchange of information with the outside scientific community. To foster this interaction, the regulatory agency staff sponsor and participate in workshops, seminars, and international conferences. In the United States, the FDA/CBER also uses the expertise of formal advisory committees, which include experts in the fields of vaccines, microbiology, infectious diseases, immunology, biostatistics, and clinical studies. These committees review summary documents prepared by the FDA and sponsors and make recommendations on product development and approval. The CBER works closely with its counterparts in other government agencies within the U.S. Public Health Service (PHS), such as the National Vaccine Program Office (NVPO), the Centers for Disease Control and Prevention (CDC), the National Institutes of Health (NIH), and the Health Resources and Services Administration (HRSA). The CDC is responsible, among other duties, for epidemiologic surveillance of disease and for support of immunization programs. Its Advisory Committee on Immunization Practices (ACIP) makes

---

*Reports of the WHO's Expert Committee on Biological Standardization are published in the *World Health Organization Technical Report Series* and may be obtained from the Distribution and Sales Office, World Health Organization, 1211 Geneva 27, Switzerland. Reprints of Requirements/Guidelines annexed to these reports can be obtained free of charge on request to Biologicals, World Health Organization, 1211 Geneva 27, Switzerland.

TABLE 60–1 ■ Bacterial Vaccines Currently Licensed in the United States

Vaccine	Manufacturer*
Anthrax vaccine, adsorbed	6
BCG vaccine	2, 7
Diphtheria and tetanus toxoids and acellular pertussis vaccine, adsorbed	1[†], 2, 11, 12[‡]
Diphtheria and tetanus toxoids and acellular pertussis vaccine adsorbed, hepatitis B (recombinant) and inactivated poliovirus vaccine combined	11
Diphtheria and tetanus toxoids, adsorbed	1, 2
Tetanus and diphtheria toxoids, adsorbed for adult use	1, 4
Tetanus toxoid	1
Tetanus toxoid, adsorbed	1, 4[‡]
Haemophilus b conjugate vaccine (diphtheria CRM_{197} protein conjugate)	3
Haemophilus b conjugate vaccine (meningococcal protein conjugate)	5
Haemophilus b conjugate vaccine (meningococcal protein conjugate) and hepatitis B recombinant vaccine	5
Haemophilus b conjugate vaccine (tetanus toxoid conjugate)	8
Lyme disease vaccine (recombinant OspA)	11[‡]
Meningococcal polysaccharide vaccine, group A	1[‡]
Meningococcal polysaccharide vaccine, group C	1[‡]
Meningococcal polysaccharide vaccine, groups A and C combined	1[‡]
Meningococcal polysaccharide vaccine, A, C, Y, W135 combined	1
Pneumococcal vaccine, polyvalent	3, 5
Pneumococcal vaccine, 7-valent conjugate	3
Typhoid vaccine, live oral, Ty21a	9
Typhoid Vi polysaccharide vaccine	8

*1, Aventis Pasteur, Inc.; 2, Aventis Pasteur, Ltd.; 3, Lederle Laboratories, Division American Cyanamid Co.; 4, Massachusetts Public Health Biological Laboratories; 5, Merck & Co., Inc.; 6, Bioport Corporation; 7, Organon Teknika Corporation; 8, Aventis Pasteur S.A.; 9, Swiss Serum and Vaccine Institute, Berne; 10, Wyeth Laboratories, Inc.; 11, GlaxoSmithKline; 12, North American Vaccine, Inc.

[‡]Not in active production or distribution.

[†]License for the pertussis component of this product is held by the Research Foundation for Microbial Diseases of Osaka University (Aventis Pasteur Laboratories, Inc.).

recommendations for vaccine use. The Director of the NVPO coordinates the vaccine efforts of the PHS and other governmental agencies. The NIH is responsible for conducting and providing funds for a wide variety of biomedical research. The HRSA is responsible, among many of its duties, for managing the Vaccine Compensation Program.

Historical Perspective

It has been over 200 years since Edward Jenner used the first vaccine to immunize against smallpox. Previous attempts at vaccination in China, India, and Persia dating back several centuries have been recorded.[2] At the turn of the 19th century there existed two human virus vaccines, Jenner's smallpox vaccine and Pasteur's rabies vaccine. Three human bacterial vaccines for typhoid, cholera, and plague were also in existence. These vaccines represented the first biological products. Although the need for special care in both preparing and testing of vaccines and antitoxins was foreseen early in their development, it was not until a major tragedy occurred in the United States that action was taken by the federal government to ensure public protection from unsafe products. In St. Louis, Missouri, in 1901, 20 children became ill and 14 died following receipt of an equine-derived diphtheria antitoxin contaminated with tetanus toxin. It was discovered that the diphtheria antitoxin had been prepared from horse serum contaminated with tetanus bacilli.[3] This event stimulated legislation to regulate the

sale of biologicals. On July 1, 1902, the Biologics Control Act was signed into law. During consideration of this legislation,[4] the following points were recognized:

1. There could be no assurance of purity if control was limited to inspections and tests of the final products, both because of the limitations of testing techniques and because such tests would need to include all materials, because the products varied owing to differences in the animals used in production. Therefore, an effective control would also need to include control of manufacturing establishments.
2. The products in question generally were administered directly into the circulatory system or the digestive tract, and there were few remedial measures available if the drugs were impure.
3. The control of potency was particularly important because, as was noted in the proceedings, if the first dose proves worthless, the loss of time may cost the patient his or her life.

These ideas formed an important start for ensuring vaccine safety; they are used as the basis for ensuring safety and effectiveness throughout the world. The history of vaccine control organizations in developed nations has been one of increasing size and complexity. A chronology of the development of the U.S. Biologicals Control Authority is summarized in Table 60–3.

The U.S. Congress enacted another significant law in 1902 that expanded the Public Health and Marine Hospital

TABLE 60–2 ■ Viral Vaccines Currently Licensed in the United States

Vaccine	Manufacturer[*][†]
Diphtheria and tetanus toxoids and acellular pertussis vaccine adsorbed, hepatitis B (recombinant) and inactivated poliovirus vaccine combined	8
Hepatitis A vaccine, inactivated	5, 8
Hepatitis B vaccine, recombinant	5, 8
Hepatitis A vaccine, inactivated and hepatitis B (recombinant) vaccine	8
Haemophilus b conjugate vaccine (meningococcal protein conjugate) and hepatitis B recombinant vaccine	5
Influenza virus vaccine	1, 3, 10
Japanese encephalitis vaccine, inactivated	9
Measles virus vaccine, live	5
Mumps virus vaccine, live	5
Rubella virus vaccine, live	5
Measles, mumps, and rubella vaccine, live	5
Measles and mumps virus vaccine, live	5
Poliovirus vaccine inactivated, human diploid cell	2[‡]
Poliovirus vaccine inactivated, monkey kidney cell	7
Poliovirus vaccine, live oral, trivalent	4[‡]
Rabies vaccine	7, 11
Rabies vaccine, adsorbed	6[‡]
Smallpox vaccine	10[‡]
Varicella virus vaccine live	5
Yellow fever vaccine	1

[*]1, Aventis Pasteur, Inc.; 2, Aventis Pasteur, Ltd.; 3, Evans Medical, Ltd.; 4, Lederle Laboratories, Division American Cyanamid Co.; 5, Merck & Co., Inc.; 6, Bioport Corporation; 7, Aventis Pasteur, S.A.; 8, GlaxoSmithKline; 9, The Research Foundation for Microbial Diseases of Osaka University; 10, Wyeth Laboratories, Inc.; 11, Chiron Behring GmbH & Co.; 12, MedImmune Vaccines, Inc. These are the names of the license holders. Company names may be different.
[†]Released for further manufacturing use only.
[‡]Not in active production or distribution.

Service. This led to the creation of the first federal agency in which public health matters could be coordinated. The Hygienic Laboratory, the principal research unit of the service, was located in Washington, DC. Within this organization, the Biological Control Service assumed responsibility for the regulation of three products: smallpox vaccine, tetanus antitoxin, and diphtheria antitoxin. These products were defined as biologicals. In 1930, the Hygienic Laboratory was reorganized and expanded, and its name was changed to the National Institutes of Health. In 1937, the Laboratory of Biologic Control was created within the NIH, and in 1938 the NIH moved to its present location in Bethesda, Maryland. As the organization expanded, new institutes were added to study diseases other than those caused by infectious agents.

In 1944, laws relating to the PHS were revised and consolidated into the United States Public Health Service Act. This act incorporated the 1902 Biologics Control Act into Section 351 of the U.S. Code of Federal Regulations (CFR).[5] Under this act, the federal government was empowered to license biological products as well as the establishments in which the products are manufactured. The law prohibited interstate shipment for sale, barter, or exchange of "any virus, therapeutic serum, toxin, antitoxin, or analogous product . . . applicable to the prevention, treatment, or cure of diseases or injuries of man" without a license. A 1970 amendment added "vaccine, blood, blood component or derivative, [or] allergenic product" to the statutory list. Under the original act, government inspectors were authorized to inspect the manufacturing establishments and to determine whether products were correctly labeled

with the name of the product; the name, address, and license number of the manufacturer; and the expiration date of the product, and to determine the manner in which the product was prepared. Section 352 of the act also permitted the PHS to manufacture biological products should the need arise (i.e., if the product could not be obtained from already licensed establishments).[6] This authority has not been used to date. In 1948, the Laboratory of Biologics Control became part of the National Microbiological Institute (later renamed the National Institute of Allergy and Infectious Diseases).

The need for strengthening and expanding control of biologicals became evident in 1955. By this time, many biologicals (blood products as well as vaccines) had been licensed, including inactivated poliovirus vaccine prepared in monkey kidney cell cultures. Unfortunately, when several batches of the vaccine were used for immunization, a number of children developed poliomyelitis. The formaldehyde inactivation and safety test procedures employed were inadequate. It was determined in retrospect that 7 of 17 batches could be shown to contain living poliovirus. A later review indicated that the incompletely inactivated vaccine had caused poliomyelitis in 79 vaccine recipients, 105 family contacts, and 20 community contacts.[7]

This much-publicized "Cutter incident" led to the expansion of the biologics control function of the PHS. Thus the Division of Biologics Standards (DBS) was established within the NIH. In 1972, the DBS, which was charged with administering and enforcing Section 351 of the PHS Act, was transferred by the Secretary of Health, Education and Welfare to the FDA, and became the Bureau of Biologics. This resulted in the transfer of the

TABLE 60–3 ■ Chronology of the Development of Biologic Control Authority

Year	Legislation Enacted	Existing Organization
1902	Biologics Control Act (Virus, Serum, Toxin Law) of 1902	Public Health Service Hygienic Laboratory
1930		Hygienic Laboratory renamed National Institutes of Health (NIH)
1937		Laboratory of Biologics Control (LBC) formed within NIH
1944	Enactment of US Public Health Service Act (42 USC § 262, 263)	
1948		LBC incorporated into the National Microbiological Institute (later renamed the National Institute of Allergy and Infectious Diseases)
1955		Establishment of the Division of Biologics Standards (DBS) by the Surgeon General
1972		DBS transfered to FDA to become Bureau of Biologics (BoB)
1982–1983		BoB renamed Office of Biologics Research and Review (OBRR); joined with Office of Drugs Research and Review (ODRR) to form the Center for Drugs and Biologics (CDB)
1987		OBRR renamed Center for Biologics Evaluation and Research (CBER)
1997	Food and Drug Administration Modernization Act of 1997	

regulations pertaining to biologics from Part 73 of Chapter I of Title 42 of the CFR to Chapter I of Title 21 of the CFR. In 1982 the Bureau of Biologics was renamed the Office of Biologics Research and Review (OBRR), and combined with the Office of Drugs Research and Review to form the Center for Drugs and Biologics. In 1987, the OBRR was separated and renamed the Center for Biologics Evaluation and Research.

Implementation

In the United States, vaccines are regulated as biologicals. A single set of basic regulatory approval criteria apply to vaccines, regardless of the technology used to produce them. The CBER's current legal authority for the regulation of vaccines derives primarily from Section 351 of the PHS Act and from certain sections of the federal Food, Drug, and Cosmetic Act. The statutes of the PHS Act are implemented through regulations codified in the CFR.[†] Title 21 of the CFR, parts 600 through 680, contains regulations specifically applicable to vaccines and other biologicals. In addition, because vaccines meet the legal definition of a drug under the Food, Drug and Cosmetic Act, manufacturers must comply with the drug Current Good Manufacturing Practices (cGMPs) regulations (parts 210 and 211).[9] Regulations applicable to vaccines and other biological products are summarized in Table 60–4. These regulations include the minimum requirements for the manufacturing of vaccines, as well as the requirements for

performing clinical trials. Certain regulations have been changed or eliminated as a result of the FDA's constant challenge to develop standards for assessing the safety and efficacy of vaccines using more state-of-the-art, modern technologies. For example, 21 CFR 620, Additional Standards for Bacterial Products, and 21 CFR 630, Additional Standards for Viral Vaccines, were revoked in August 1996. Instead of incorporating new standards into the regulations, the license application contains all the appropriate testing methods for in-process and release testing for each specific new vaccine.

The CFR is published annually and contains any changes in regulations that have occurred during the previous year and that have been published in the *Federal Register*. Regulations are adopted in conformity with the Administrative Procedure Act.[10] Thus, before a regulation can be established, repealed, or changed, it must be proposed and published in the *Federal Register* with an invitation to all interested individuals or parties to comment within a prescribed time, commonly a period of 1 to several months. Once comments have been received, they are evaluated and considered by the FDA before publication of the final regulation in the *Federal Register*.

The FDA periodically publishes various guidelines and guidance documents with regard to the manufacture of biologicals. These documents published by FDA do not have the force of law but are intended to provide useful and timely recommendations; those applicable to vaccines are listed in Table 60–5. These documents are particularly useful in rapidly progressing areas of science and for specifying a degree of detail beyond what is included in the regulations. In the past few years, several new FDA regulations and guidance documents have had a direct impact on the review of vaccines for licensure by the FDA, such as the Draft Guidance for Industry on Recommendations for Complying with the Pediatric Rule (December 2000), and the Postmarketing Safety Reporting for Human Drug and Biological Products

---

[†]The CFR contains a compilation of current regulations of all federal agencies. It is divided into 50 titles, and FDA regulations are located in Title 21.[8] Each title is further subdivided into chapters, subchapters, parts, and sections. Copies of these regulations may be ordered through the Superintendent of Documents, U.S. Government Printing Office, Stop SSOP, Washington, D.C. 20402-0001 (or through the Internet at *bookstore.gpo.gov*).

TABLE 60–4 ■ Regulations Applicable to the Development, Manufacture, Licensure, and Use of Vaccines

Title 21, Code of Federal Regulations, Chapter 1—FDA, DHHS*	Subject
SUBCHAPTER F—BIOLOGICS	
600–680†	
600	Biologic products, general, definitions
	Establishment standards
	Establishment inspection
	Adverse experience reporting
601	Licensing
610	General biologicals product standards
SUBCHAPTER C—DRUGS: GENERAL	
201	Labeling
202	Prescription drug advertising
210	Current good manufacturing practice in manufacturing, processing, packing, or holding of drugs, general
211	Current good manufacturing practice for finished pharmaceuticals
SUBCHAPTER D—DRUGS FOR HUMAN USE	
312	New drugs for investigational use
314	Applications for FDA approval to market a new drug or an antibiotic drug
SUBCHAPTER A—GENERAL	
25	Environmental impact considerations
50	Protection of human subjects
56	Institutional review boards
58	Nonclinical laboratory studies, good laboratory practice regulations

*Food and Drug Administration, Department of Health and Human Services.
†Parts 606, 607, 640, 660, and 680 apply to blood, blood products, diagnostic tests, and allergenics.

Including Vaccines (March 2001). Some of these regulations and guidances evolved from an effort to streamline the regulatory process (e.g., the Elimination of the Establishment and Product License [October 1999]), while others are being developed or revised to facilitate the development of new vaccines with new technologies (e.g., Points to Consider in the Characterization of Cell Lines used to Produce Biologicals [July 1993], and the Draft Guidance for Industry on Considerations for Reproductive Toxicity Studies for Preventive Vaccines for Infectious Disease Indications [September 2000]). These documents can be obtained through the CBER's web page (*www.fda.gov/cber/guidelines.htm*).

Prior to discussing the various procedures involved in the regulation of vaccines, it would be beneficial to review some of the more pertinent operational definitions[11] contained in the statutes and regulations:

1. Section 351 of the PHS Act defines a *biological product* as any virus, therapeutic serum, toxin, antitoxin, vaccine, blood, blood component or derivative, allergenic product, or analogous product applicable to the prevention, treatment, or cure of diseases or conditions of human beings. Thus vaccines clearly are regulated as biological products.
2. *Safety* is defined as the relative freedom from harmful effect to people affected directly or indirectly by a product when prudently administered, taking into consideration the character of the product in relation to the condition of the recipient at the time. Thus the property of safety is relative and cannot be ensured in an absolute sense.
3. *Purity* is defined as the relative freedom from extraneous matter, regardless of whether it is harmful to the recipient or deleterious to the product. Usually, the concepts of purity and safety coincide; purity most often relates to freedom from such materials as pyrogens, adventitious agents, and chemicals used in manufacture of the product.
4. *Potency* is defined as the specific ability or capacity of the product, as indicated by appropriate laboratory tests or by adequately controlled clinical data obtained through administration of the product in the manner intended, to effect a given result. Potency, as thus defined, is equivalent to the concept that the product must be able to perform as claimed, and, if possible, this must correspond with some measurable effect in the recipient or correlate with some quantitative laboratory finding.
5. *Standards* mean specifications and procedures applicable to an establishment or to the manufacture or release of products that are designed to ensure the continued safety, purity, and potency of biological products. The word *standard* is also used with a secondary meaning, usually in the sense of a reference preparation, such as a bacterial or viral antigen that can be used in evaluating potency or, in some cases, safety and purity.

TABLE 60–5 ■ Guidance Documents Applicable to the Development, Manufacture, Licensure, and Use of Vaccines*

Document	Date
POINTS TO CONSIDER	
Production and Testing of New Drugs and Biologicals Produced by Recombinant DNA Technology	1985
Supplement: Nucleic Acid Characterization and Genetic Stability	1992
Characterization of Cell Lines Used to Produce Biologicals	1993
Plasmid DNA Vaccines for Preventive Infectious Disease Indications	1996
GUIDELINES	
Meningococcal Polysaccharide Vaccines	1985
Submitting Documentation for the Stability of Human Drugs and Biologicals	1987
Submitting Documentation for Packaging for Human Drugs and Biologicals	1987
Guideline on General Principles of Process Validation	1987
Sterile Drug Products Produced by Aseptic Processing	1987
Validation of the Limulus Amebocyte Lysate Test	1987
Release of Pneumococcal Vaccine, Polyvalent	1989
Determination of Residual Moisture in Dried Biological Products	1990
Guideline for Adverse Experience Reporting for Licensed Biological Products	1993
GUIDANCE DOCUMENTS	
Guidance on Alternatives to Lot Release for Licensed Biological Products	1994
Guidance for Industry for the Evaluation of Combination Vaccines for Preventable Diseases: Production, Testing and Clinical Studies	1997
Guidance for Industry: Changes to an Approved Application: Biological Products	1997
Draft Guidance for Industry: Instructions for Submitting Electronic Lot Release Protocols to the Center for Biologics Evaluation and Research	1998
Guidance for Industry: Providing Clinical Evidence of Effectiveness for Human Drugs and Biological Products	1998
Draft Guidance for Industry: Stability Testing of Drug Substances and Drug Products	1998
Guidance for Industry: Implementation of Section 126 of the Food and Drug Administration Modernization Act of 1997—Elimination of Certain Labeling Requirements	1998
Guidance for Industry: Environmental Assessment of Human Drug and Biologics Applications	1998
Guidance for Industry: Content and Format of Chemistry, Manufacturing and Controls Information for a Vaccine or Related Product	1999
Draft Guidance for Industry on Recommendations for Complying with the Pediatric Rule	2000
Guidance for Industry: Formal Meetings with Sponsors and Applicants for PDUFA Products	2000
Draft Guidance for Industry: Content and Format of the Adverse Reactions Section of Labeling for Human Prescription Drugs	2000
Draft Guidance for Industry: Considerations for Reproductive Toxicity Studies for Preventive Vaccines for Infectious Disease Indications	2000
Guidance for Industry: Submitting and Reviewing Complete Responses to Clinical Holds	2000
Draft Guidance for Industry: Postmarketing Safety Reporting for Human Drug and Biological Products Including Vaccines	2001
Draft Guidance for Industry: Reports on the Status of Postmarketing Studies—Implementation of Section 130 of the Food and Drug Administration Modernization Act of 1997	2001
Draft Guidance for Industry: Clinical Studies Section of Labeling for Prescription Drugs and Biologics—Content and Format	2001

*Available at no charge from the Office of Communication, Training and Manufacturers Assistance, HFM-40, 1401 Rockville Pike, Rockville, MD 20852-1448.

6. The regulations regarding biological products, in addition, define *effectiveness* as the reasonable expectation that, in a significant proportion of the target population, pharmacologic or other effects of the biological product, when administered under adequate directions for use and warnings against unsafe use, will serve a clinically significant function in the diagnosis, cure, mitigation, treatment, or prevention of disease in humans.[12]

7. *Current good manufacturing practices* define a quality system that manufacturers use as they build quality into their products. The regulations outline the minimum manufacturing, quality control, and quality assurance requirements for the preparation of a drug or biological product for commercial distribution. For example, approved products developed and produced according to cGMPs are safe, properly identified, of the correct strength, pure, and of high quality.

Regulation of Biological Products

Premarketing Phase

The regulatory requirements for biological products cover both the premarketing phase, consisting of the investigational and licensing phases, and the postmarketing phase.

These requirements can be found in the Investigational New Drug (IND) regulations.[13] The clinical development of a new drug in the United States usually begins with a sponsor approaching the FDA for permission to conduct a clinical study with an investigational product through submission of an IND application form.[‡] In the application, the sponsor (1) describes the composition, source, and method of manufacture of the product and the methods used in testing its safety, purity, and potency; (2) provides a summary of all laboratory and preclinical animal testing; and (3) provides a description of the proposed clinical study and the names and qualifications of each clinical investigator. The FDA has a maximum of 30 days to review the original IND application and determine whether study participants will be exposed to any unacceptable risks. As part of the IND process, each clinical investigator files information describing his or her qualifications for performing clinical trials, details of the proposed study, and assurance that a number of conditions specified by the regulations will be met. A signed informed consent must be obtained from each study participant.[14] Approval for the study must be obtained in advance from a local institutional review board.[15] The regulations also cover the evaluation of the preclinical laboratory animal studies undertaken to support the use of the product in humans.[16]

Investigational Phase

There are generally three separate phases in the clinical evaluation of experimental biologicals at the premarketing stage (Fig. 60–1). These phases may overlap, and the clinical testing may be highly iterative because multiple Phase 1 or 2 trials may be performed as new data are obtained. Phase 1 trials are intended primarily to provide a preliminary evaluation of safety and immunogenicity. These trials are conducted in a small number (e.g., 20 to 80) of closely monitored adult volunteers. If the ultimate target popula-

tion for the vaccine is infants or young children, as is commonly the case, the product is then usually evaluated in a stepwise progression from older to younger age groups down into the first year of life. It is not always simple to distinguish between Phase 1 and Phase 2 studies; however, in general, Phase 2 studies are larger, perhaps involving up to several hundred participants. Phase 2 studies are often randomized and well controlled, and provide further information on safety and immunogenicity. Dose-ranging studies are included in Phase 2 clinical development. In some cases Phase 2 studies may provide preliminary data on the vaccine's activity against the infectious disease of interest. Phase 3 studies are large-scale trials involving more extensive testing to provide a more thorough assessment of safety as well as a definite assessment of efficacy; moreover, these studies often include the pivotal efficacy trials as well as expanded safety studies.

The general considerations for clinical studies to license a vaccine include demonstration of safety, immunogenicity, efficacy (immunogenicity may be sufficient in some cases), and evaluation of simultaneous administration with other licensed vaccines. As far as efficacy evaluation, efficacy should be demonstrated ideally in randomized, double-blind, well-controlled trials. The endpoints will be product specific, and may be clinical disease endpoints or immune response endpoints if efficacy against clinical disease has been previously established. In recent years, efficacy trials for various vaccines have involved a broad range in the required number of study participants, from thousands to tens of thousands. This broad range is related to a number of interconnected variables such as study design and the incidence of the disease to be prevented. For example, clinical disease endpoint studies that are designed to demonstrate that a new vaccine is not inferior to an already existing product of the same type generally require larger numbers than one in which a new vaccine can be compared with a control that has no activity against the clinical disease. The incidence of the disease to be prevented in the study population is also important. As an example, convincing evidence for the effectiveness of the plasma-derived hepatitis B vaccine in a population at high risk required

---

[‡]Sponsors may be individual physicians, a university, a hospital, or a commercial firm as well as government agencies, such as one of the institutes of the NIH, the Department of Defense, or physicians within the FDA itself.

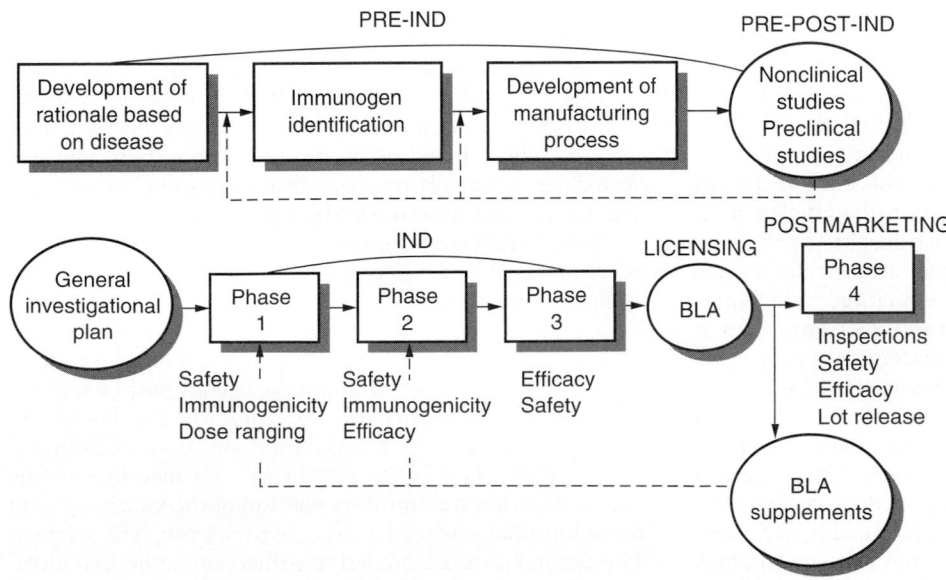

FIGURE 60–1 ■ Sequence of key events in product development through the premarketing experimental Investigational New Drug (IND) and licensing phases, and the postapproval marketing phase. Dashed lines indicate additional research/ development submissions when significant changes are made in the product or its indications. BLA, Biologics License Application.

only 549 vaccinees and 524 placebo recipients. In contrast, a trial to show that pneumococcal 7-valent polysaccharide conjugate vaccine was successful in preventing a low incidence of invasive disease caused by the *Streptococcus pneumoniae* capsular serotypes included in the vaccine enrolled close to 40,000 children who were randomized equally to receive the pneumococcal conjugate vaccine or an unrelated control vaccine. Immunogenicity studies may be requested to provide data on the immune response of target populations for the vaccine if they are different from those populations in whom the efficacy studies were done. These studies are known as "bridging" studies. In other words, immunogenicity data may be used to bridge to existing clinical endpoint efficacy data. The 1998 FDA Guidance for Industry: Providing Clinical Evidence of Effectiveness recommends two efficacy trials as the standard; however, one trial may be adequate if the results are compelling, which is often the case for vaccine clinical endpoint efficacy trials (e.g., robust data, multi-center trials with a high level of efficacy).[17]

Safety evaluation is the other component in the clinical evaluation of vaccines. Safety is one of the most important considerations when evaluating new vaccines and changes to currently licensed vaccines. The initial responsibility for determining vaccine safety starts with clinical investigators and vaccine manufacturers. The NRA is responsible for assuring that clinical trials are done under Good Clinical Practices, a requirement essential for the evaluation of safety data intended to support a license application. In general, when evaluating safety, one must compare the risk of the vaccine-preventable disease with the risk of the adverse event(s) associated with the vaccine, and these may change over time. One must also consider alternative treatments. The intended target population also should be taken into consideration in assessing the adequacy of the safety database. For routinely administered childhood vaccines in the United States, the target population would be the birth cohort in the United States (approximately 4 million/year). This is generally a healthy population, and a government body (e.g., the states) may mandate vaccination. Common reactions can be studied adequately in hundreds of individuals, but many thousands will be required to define low-incidence adverse reactions. For vaccines evaluated in clinical endpoint efficacy trials, a large safety database likely will derive from a double-blind, randomized, well-controlled efficacy study. However, for vaccines evaluated in immunogenicity endpoint studies, additional studies likely will be needed to obtain an adequate safety database. Additional controlled safety studies are often requested when the numbers of subjects included in the efficacy studies are deemed insufficient to provide adequate safety data. The studies need to be designed in such a way that statistical methods may be applied to their evaluation. Safety studies may be un-blinded if the number of injections, route of administration, or schedule differs between groups, in particular when infants and young children are involved. Phase 2 safety studies should provide data on common local and systemic reactions to the study vaccine. Phase 2 clinical development also should include immunogenicity and preliminary safety data on the concurrent administration of the study vaccine with other vaccines, if relevant. Phase 3 safety studies are designed to evaluate less common reactions, may

be unequally randomized, and may have a simplified trial design for assessing less common adverse events in large trials. If a vaccine is recommended on the same schedule as other routinely recommended vaccines, safety and immunogenicity data should be obtained in prelicensure studies to support simultaneous administration.

The regulatory review in CBER incorporates a managed and integrated regulatory process that is continuous from discovery to postmarketing, and is designated as the Managed Review Process.[18] The Managed Review Process relies on a strong project management infrastructure. The Regulatory Project Manager (RPM) is an instrumental part of each review team. The RPM coordinates the review of regulatory submissions in accordance with CBER policy and procedures, and serves as a facilitator to drive the review process forward. Project management is utilized to facilitate and coordinate the review of these submissions and resolution of issues. Biological product development consists of four phases: presubmission, investigational, application/supplement (marketing), and postmarketing. The CBER's Managed Review Process is a system designed to effectively and efficiently review all regulatory submissions and is targeted to these phases of development. The CBER's Managed Review Process is initiated with the submission of an IND or Biologicals License Application (BLA). These submissions include preclinical, clinical, and/or manufacturing data. The internal review process in the CBER begins with an initial review of a submission for scientific content and compliance with the regulations. Members of the review team as well as the RPM are selected based on their expertise with the type of product and its method of manufacture. CBER's review component reviews, evaluates, and recommends appropriate action to facilitate the approval of safe and effective biological products. Reviewers evaluate chemistry, manufacturing, and controls information; the manufacturing facility and equipment; preclinical and clinical data on the safety, efficacy, pharmacology, and toxicology; the suitability of clinical trial design; and analysis of clinical data derived from such trials. In addition, reviewers monitor for conformance with FDA regulations in all phases of biological product development, including postmarketing. The CBER review component also performs research in the areas of statistical and epidemiologic analysis, clinical trial design, and specific product and policy areas. Surveillance activities are performed to ensure that the safety of biological products, both in development and in distribution, is not compromised. (Only licensed vaccines may be shipped from one state to another; however, during the premarketing phase, interstate shipment of products for experimental use is allowed under the law and regulations.) These activities ensure the rapid availability and approval of safe and effective biological products.

Sponsors are encouraged to avail themselves of a pre-IND meeting with the CBER reviewers to discuss and review general experimental plans for the product. Meetings between a sponsor and the agency may be face-to-face or by teleconference and are frequently useful in resolving questions and issues raised during the course of a clinical investigation. The FDA encourages such meetings to the extent that they aid in the evaluation of the vaccine and in the solution of scientific problems concerning the product. The general principle underlying the conduct of such meetings is that there should be free, full, and open communication about any scientific or medical question that may arise during the clinical investigation. Agreements reached at Prescription Drug User Fee Act (PDUFA) meetings (e.g., pre-IND, IND, pre-BLA, and BLA meetings) will be recorded in minutes of the conference that will be taken by FDA and provided to the sponsor. The minutes, along with any other written material provided to the sponsor, will serve as a permanent record of any agreements reached. Barring a significant scientific development that requires otherwise, studies conducted in accordance with the agreement shall be presumed to be sufficient in objective and design for the purpose of obtaining marketing approval for the drug. (Detailed information on the conduct of regulatory meetings is described in 21 CFR § 312.47.)

Pre-IND meetings are particularly important for new sponsors and for products that incorporate novel features. Other meetings also are encouraged at critical points throughout the IND review, including "end-of-Phase 2" meetings. The purpose of an end-of-Phase 2 meeting is to assess the adequacy of the Phase 2 safety and immunogenicity data that support advancement to Phase 3, to evaluate the Phase 3 plan and draft protocols, and to identify any additional information necessary to support a marketing application for the uses under investigation. Although the end-of-Phase 2 meeting is designed primarily for INDs involving new molecular entities, such as new vaccines (including combinations of two or more existing vaccines), or major new or expanded indications for a currently marketed vaccine, a sponsor of any IND may request and obtain an end-of-Phase 2 meeting. The end-of-Phase 2 meeting should be held before major commitments of effort and resources to specific Phase 3 tests are made. The scheduling of an end-of-Phase 2 meeting is not, however, intended to delay the transition of an investigation from Phase 2 to Phase 3. Continued participation by statisticians is important throughout the process. Use of well-defined study endpoints and appropriate analytic plans, including plans for interim analysis, is particularly important in producing interpretable results from clinical studies.

Licensing Phase

When the IND studies are nearing completion or have been completed and the sponsor believes that the product can be shown to be safe and effective for its intended use, the sponsor usually applies for a license to manufacture and distribute the product commercially. By this time, exact techniques of production should be developed, and the manufacturing process standardized. Prior to the submission of a biologics license application (BLA) a pre-BLA meeting with the agency is strongly encouraged to discuss the sponsor's developmental plan. The FDA has determined that delays associated with the initial review of a BLA may be reduced by exchanges of information about a proposed marketing application. The primary purpose of this kind of exchange is to uncover any major unresolved problems, to identify those studies that the sponsor is relying on as adequate and well controlled to establish the product's effectiveness, to identify the status of ongoing studies, to acquaint FDA reviewers with the general information to be submitted in the BLA (including technical information), to review methods used in the statistical analysis of the data,

and to discuss the best approach to the presentation and formatting of data in the application. Arrangements for such a meeting are to be initiated by the sponsor with the division responsible for review of the IND. Historically, two license applications have been required, one for the product and one for the establishment in which it is to be manufactured.[19] However, as a result of the enactment of the Food and Drug Administration Modernization Act of 1997, only a BLA is now accepted. This single application contains detailed information about the product (clinical and manufacturing) as well as information concerning the manufacturing facility and equipment.

To obtain a biologicals license for a new vaccine under section 351 of the PHS Act, an applicant submits a BLA to the Director of the CBER's Office of Vaccines Research and Review (OVRR). This application contains data derived from nonclinical laboratory and clinical studies that demonstrate that the manufactured product meets prescribed requirements of safety, purity, and potency. In the BLA, information needs to be submitted that indicates that there is compliance with standards addressing requirements for (1) organization and personnel; (2) buildings and facilities; (3) equipment; (4) control of components, containers, and closures; (5) production and process controls; (6) packaging and labeling controls; (7) holding and distribution; (8) laboratory controls; and (9) records to be maintained. Furthermore, a full description of manufacturing methods; data establishing stability of the product through the dating period; sample(s) representative of the product for introduction or delivery for introduction into interstate commerce; summaries of test results performed on the lot(s) represented by the submitted sample(s); specimens of the labels, enclosures, and containers; and the address of each location involved in the manufacture of the biological product should be included in the BLA.

To permit the FDA to provide the sponsor with the most useful advice regarding the adequacy of the information to support a BLA as well as preparation of a BLA, the sponsor should submit the following information to the OVRR's application division at least 1 month in advance of the meeting: (1) an executive summary of the clinical studies to be submitted in the application; (2) a proposed format for organizing the submission, including methods for presenting the data; (3) information on the status of needed or ongoing studies; and (4) any other information for discussion at the meeting. An application for a biologics license is not considered as filed (or accepted by the agency for review) until the CBER determines that it has received all pertinent information and data from the applicant. In this regard, the CBER can refuse to file a BLA. The applicant is also required to include either an environmental assessment or a claim for categorical exclusion from the requirement to submit an environmental assessment or an environmental impact statement.[20]

An internal CBER committee performs the scientific review of the BLA, and members of this review committee are selected on the basis of the expertise required to review the application. This process occurs for each BLA or supplement to a BLA in which significant changes are proposed. During the review, there are discussions and correspondence between the sponsor and the CBER review committee in which all the laboratory and clinical data are carefully reviewed.

Approval of a license application by the CBER is based on reviews of the data submitted by the applicant indicating that the product is safe and effective for its intended use. The standards to be applied for safety and efficacy are flexible; that is, the benefit-to-risk ratio of a biological product is considered. The regulations and standards allow for a range of safety and efficacy, as is scientifically appropriate. Other components of the BLA review include product labeling, which describes the indications for use, contraindications, dosage, and possible adverse effects; protocols for the manufacturing and testing of the number of product lots specified to establish the consistency of the process; and results of confirmatory testing within the CBER of samples of in-process material or product in final containers and conformance to existing regulations.

When the FDA review of the BLA is well underway, an announced Prior Approval Inspection (PAI) is performed after the manufacturer has informed the CBER that production has begun. This inspection is designed as an in-depth review of the facilities, records, total production process, methods, equipment, quality control procedures, and personnel. With the implementation of the BLA process, changes have occurred in the scope of issues reviewed during the PAI. Instead of the manufacturer submitting detailed records with the BLA regarding studies on cleaning validation, monitoring data for pharmaceutical-grade water, facility support systems (e.g., clean steam, compressed air, and building management systems), and other facility-related systems, more detailed review of this type of data is done on site during the PAI. PAIs tend to require longer periods of time for the FDA inspectors to be in the facility because of the increased scope of issues that are reviewed on site. The cGMP inspection of an establishment for which a BLA is pending need not be made until the establishment is in operation and is manufacturing the complete product for which a biologicals license is desired. If licensure is denied following inspection for the original license, reinspection will occur after assurance has been received that the faulty conditions that were the basis of the denial have been corrected.

After the CBER reviews the entire package of information in the BLA, its advisory committee (the Vaccines and Related Biological Products Advisory Committee) and consultants generally are asked to comment on the adequacy of the data to support safety and efficacy in the target population. The committee's advice is seriously considered in the CBER's decision regarding licensure and in developing the recommendations for use to be given in the package insert. The committee may recommend additional studies to be performed either before or after approval. After the CBER determines that the data and information are satisfactory, the product is licensed.

Postmarketing Phase

Modifications to the manufacturing process may occur postlicensure, such as scale-up or change in equipment to optimize the production process. Further clinical studies with the product also may be performed after licensure as the manufacturer seeks additional indications for product use (e.g., new target populations that would benefit from vaccination). For most new approvals, manufacturers may be asked to commit to completing specific postmarketing or so-called Phase 4 studies, for example, to provide additional assessments of less common or rare adverse events or further assess the duration of vaccine-induced immunity. These studies also may be designed to collect additional safety data in large numbers of vaccine recipients, as well as focus on issues that were identified during the prelicensure testing. In 2001, a regulation became effective that requires submission of status reports for certain postmarketing studies. In particular, this requirement for status reports pertains to postmarketing studies for clinical safety, efficacy and pharmacokinetics, and nonclinical toxicology that an applicant committed to in writing prior to licensure.[21] If the manufacturer wishes to significantly modify the manufacturing process or directions for vaccine use, prior approval must be obtained from the FDA before these changes can be implemented.[22] The applicant is required to submit an account of these changes to the appropriate license applications.

For the past several years, efforts have been made to simplify and categorize manufacturing reporting requirements in order to facilitate the implementation of important improvements in the production processes, testing methods, equipment, or facilities or make changes in personnel. Proposed changes in manufacturing methods that have a substantial potential to have an adverse effect on the safety or effectiveness of the product may not become effective until notification is given of the CBER's approval. A change in 21 CFR § 601.12, has been implemented that classifies changes into (1) those sufficiently significant with regard to safety, purity, potency, and efficacy of the product to require preapproval of a supplemental application before product distribution; (2) those of lesser import for which the manufacturer must provide notification 30 days before distribution of product made using the change; and (3) changes for which the manufacturer need only notify the agency by submission of an annual report. A guidance document "Changes to an Approved Application: Biological Products" is available on the CBER's website (*www.fda.gov/cber/guidelines.htm*) that provides more details on the changes to this regulation.

After issuance of the license, there is continued surveillance of the product and of the manufacturer's production activities. For most licensed vaccines, samples are submitted along with protocols for each lot prepared by the firm that provide the details of production and a summary of test results. Although not required by law or regulation, the CBER often performs selected laboratory tests. The type and extent of confirmatory testing performed by the CBER depend on several factors, such as the newness of the product or the difficulties that may have arisen with manufacture or use of the product. Release or rejection is based on a review of all test results, including those done by the manufacturer and those performed by the CBER. Alternatives to official lot release are allowable under the provisions outlined for extensively characterized products having a "track record" of continued safety, purity, and potency.[23] For example, one of the hepatitis B vaccines met this standard and was the first vaccine product for which this exception was requested from the requirement for lot-by-lot release. New regulations have been developed that clearly specify the factors that are to be evaluated and include measures that allow additional products to be considered in this category.

To be considered, the manufacturer must be able to produce a vaccine that repeatedly meets the standards for potency, purity, and stability of bulk and final container material while using a consistent process. Important factors to be considered are the nature of the product with respect to correlation between the measure of potency and biological activity and efficacy. Surveillance samples and protocols may be required to be submitted to the CBER at intervals.

Licensed establishments are inspected at least every 2 years. The purpose of the inspection is to determine whether licensed products are manufactured and tested as described in the license application and in accordance with applicable regulations. Manufacturers who fail to meet product standards or who are not in compliance with cGMPs may have their licenses suspended or revoked, depending on the nature of the potential health hazards created.[24] The major issues observed during inspections can be categorized in three major areas: (1) process-related issues, (2) quality unit–related issues, and (3) facility- and production environment–related issues. Some examples of process validation issues include lack of documentation of time limits for major steps in the production process, lack of validation of rework or reprocessing steps in the manufacturing process, or lack of data to support in-process specifications. Quality unit–related issues include the appropriate reporting of out-of-specification results and process deviations (including adequate investigations into causes), appropriate documentation of product release, and adequate training of personnel. Facility and production monitoring concerns include controlling production environments by appropriately monitoring heating, ventilation, and air conditioning (HVAC) system performance and microbial quality (e.g., pressure differentials, appropriate sampling sites, and frequency of sampling, etc.). Other concerns in the facility include adequate cleaning, sanitization, storage, and changeover procedures for multiproduct areas and equipment. If the inspection team finds cGMP deficiencies in an already licensed facility, the team may remain in the facility until they have achieved an audit that provides confidence in the ability of the firm to reproducibly manufacture a safe and potent product.

Labeling changes usually are initiated by the manufacturer but may be initiated by the CBER. Historically, manufacturers have had to obtain prior approval from the CBER before the labeling changes were made. The changes to 21 CFR § 601.12 mentioned previously also apply to labeling changes and allow exceptions for a change that adds or strengthens a contraindication, warning, precaution, or adverse reaction; adds or strengthens instructions about dosage and administration intended to increase safe use; or deletes false, misleading, or unsupported indications for use or effectiveness claims. Under this regulation, a manufacturer could effect such changes and, at the same time, submit them and the supporting data to the CBER without preapproval.

Vaccine Testing

Vaccines are tested during the prelicensure as well as the postlicensure phase. Vaccine testing procedures are developed from a combination of the understanding of past adverse experiences (events) and the best current knowledge regarding the potential for new ones. From past experience, a few highly important issues must continue to receive special attention. For inactivated vaccines, a clear understanding of the kinetics of inactivation is key; this was the lesson of the so-called Cutter incident mentioned previously. For live vaccines, the agent must be at a stable level of attenuation; it must not become over-attenuated or revert to virulence. The Brazilian experience, in which yellow fever vaccine appeared to revert to neurovirulence after multiple passages, demonstrated the need for a seed lot system in which the number of passages from the parent virus to the passage level used as vaccine is restricted.[25] All vaccines require an intensive search for extraneous contaminants. The experience in which human serum was used as a stabilizer for yellow fever vaccine and caused hundreds of cases of long-incubation hepatitis virus infection underscored this need.[26]

Historically, only primary cells were used widely for viral vaccine production, and, although primary cells are still used in the manufacture of some viral vaccines, major concerns have arisen over the passage of adventitious agents from primary cells into the product and thus, potentially, into vaccine recipients. In the early 1960s, exogenous and endogenous contamination of primary monkey kidney cells (PMKCs) with simian virus 40 and chicken embryo fibroblasts (CEFs) with avian leukosis virus were reported. PMKCs and CEFs are still utilized in the production of viral vaccines; however, these cells are required to be well characterized and tested prior to use. The issues related to cell substrates have been discussed in a variety of forums.[27,28] The demonstration that viruses can be oncogenic in mammalian hosts produced an intense focus on cell-culture substrate safety as well. Despite these contamination episodes, no adverse effects on recipients have been documented to date.[29,30] The FDA requires that cell substrates and vaccine viral seeds used in production be appropriately selected and tested to ensure that they do not introduce any unintended risks. This issue continues to be discussed in national and international forums.[31,32]

More recently, the epidemic of bovine spongiform encephalopathy (BSE, also referred to as "mad cow" disease) and its possible relationship to human variant Creutzfeldt-Jakob disease (vCJD or new variant CJD) has been of special concern. On this account, attention has been centered on the safety of substances derived from mammalian sources, such as media components used for nurturing cell cultures and gelatins used as stabilizers.[33] Bovine-derived materials traditionally have been used in the manufacture of many biological products, including vaccines. Since BSE was first recognized in the United Kingdom in the 1980s, the FDA has been concerned about eliminating any potential for contamination of biological products with the BSE agent. This concern was heightened by the appearance of vCJD in the United Kingdom in 1996. To date, there are no reports of BSE contamination of pharmaceutical or biological products. To minimize the possibility of contamination in such products, the FDA, in 1993, and again in 1996, requested that manufacturers not use materials derived from cattle that were born, raised, or slaughtered in countries where BSE is known to exist. The FDA referred manufacturers to the listing of such countries maintained by the U.S. Department of Agriculture (*www.aphis.usda.gov/NCIE/country.html*).[34] In addition, the use of human blood components in the manufacture of or as excipients in vaccines has prompted discussions about potential substitutes. Whereas such risks remain entirely theoretical, the sources of such materials are being subjected to new restrictions. More information on vaccines and the sourcing of bovine-derived raw materials can be found on the CBER's website (*www.fda.gov/opacom/more-choices/industry/guidance/gelguide.htm*).

At the inception of the recombinant DNA era, the possible risk of induction of transformation of cells of the recipient was a major concern. This issue has been approached by careful study of the constructs used and the stability of these constructs and by attempts to reduce extraneous DNA content to levels that are regarded as extremely unlikely to produce an adverse genetic event.[35–37] Currently, this issue is being evaluated anew in the context of possible future DNA vaccines.

Preapproval test development may be conducted entirely by the sponsor or with involvement of the regulatory agency as well. The CBER is particularly likely to become involved if the product is new or represents a novel problem in testing. This involvement, bolstered by laboratory-based capability, has been one of the strengths of the vaccine regulatory program in the United States. As the product moves toward approval, the sponsor develops the testing program in greater detail. The final testing methods must be established before major clinical trials for efficacy begin and before the manufacture of batches of product that will be used to demonstrate consistency of manufacture.

Among the very first efforts in product development should be explorations of a potency assay. A potency test is applied to each product to demonstrate that the product confers protective immunity. The type of test varies depending on the product and commonly is based on studies of immunogenicity or protection from virulent challenge in laboratory animals. However, other in vitro tests can be involved, including virus titration (e.g., live vaccines such as polio, measles, mumps, and rubella), antigen content (e.g., influenza and inactivated poliovirus vaccines), and biochemical and biophysical measurements (e.g., meningococcal polysaccharide vaccines).

Correlates are sought between the assay results and the preclinical and, later, the clinical testing results. During the prelicensing phase, research testing results are evaluated to determine which tests under development need to be applied to every batch of product and which do not require such repetition. For example, with hepatitis B vaccines made using recombinant DNA technology, initial evidence for identity, purity, and genetic stability of the protein product was provided by physicochemical, immunologic, and molecular biological test methods. Once the consistency levels of the results of all tests are validated for multiple lots produced during the IND application and product licensing phases, a determination is made to routinely perform some of these tests, which will be evaluated to ensure the consistent quality of the final product in each lot.

The regulation of biologicals includes requirements for testing of licensed products. Certain of these requirements are generally applicable to all products, whereas others are tailored to the specific vaccine. The tests, generally applicable to all products, include those for bacterial and fungal sterility, general safety, purity, identity, suitability of constituent materials, and potency.[38] Sterility testing is performed on both bulk and final container material, using media and conditions of incubation described in the regulations. In addition, cell culture–derived vaccines must be tested for mycoplasmas. The general safety test usually is performed by intraperitoneal inoculation of final container material into mice and guinea pigs to detect the possible presence of gross extraneous contaminants that may have been introduced during the manufacture or filling process. Tests for purity are designed to determine that the product is free of extraneous material, except that which is unavoidable in the manufacturing process described in the approved license application, and may include tests for residual moisture and pyrogenic substances. Final container material must be identified by a test specific for each product (e.g., neutralization of each of the components of the live oral poliovirus vaccine with specific antisera). With regard to constituent materials, the manufacturer must ensure that all ingredients used in the product, such as diluents, preservatives, or adjuvants, meet generally accepted standards of purity. An adjuvant may not be used unless there is adequate proof that it does not adversely affect the safety or potency of the product. The only adjuvants used in currently licensed vaccines are the aluminum salts, although others have been studied experimentally.

For cell culture–produced vaccines, extraneous proteins (e.g., serum or a serum derivative) should not be present in the final product, or, if serum is used during production to stimulate growth of cultured cells, the calculated concentration in the final medium must not exceed 1 part per million. Antibiotics, except penicillin (and by analogy the β-lactam class), may be employed during the course of viral vaccine production in cell culture. Those antibiotics most commonly added in low concentrations are neomycin, streptomycin, and polymyxin. If antibiotics are present, the package circular must contain a statement concerning possible allergic reactions.

With regard to the required testing for licensed biological products, the FDA is re-evaluating the appropriateness of selected requirements and/or the test methods cited in the CFR. For example, the general safety test is required by the FDA for all products, including vaccines. However, in the case of certain vaccine types, the relevance of the general safety test has been questioned. For example, the relevance of evaluating an orally delivered vaccine by intraperitoneal injection of animals is questionable. In addition, the question of the utility of such a test for a product with inherent toxicity that interferes with the interpretation of the test (e.g., live bacterial vaccines) has been raised. Currently, the FDA is discussing whether to eliminate the requirement for the general safety test. Another example of the FDA's re-examination of testing requirements in the regulations is in regard to the testing for pyrogenic substances by intravenous injection into rabbits. Because of the variability of in vivo tests such as the rabbit pyrogenicity test, consideration is given to alternative methods such as the limulus amebocyte lysate (LAL) assay for endotoxins. Following discussions with the FDA, the LAL assay may be substituted for the rabbit pyrogenicity test and may provide a more quantitative assessment of endotoxin content in a product. The ability to assess endotoxin levels in vaccine lots also may provide a measure of manufacturing and process control from lot to lot.

Other more specific tests designed to provide additional assurance of safety or purity may be required (e.g., neurovirulence testing and cell culture and animal tests for extraneous viruses applied to poliovirus vaccine). Once the product is licensed, the manufacturer's testing must be conducted according to the exact specifications in the manufacturer's license application, and the results of this testing must be within the prescribed limits specified. Tests performed for lot release of hepatitis B vaccines produced using recombinant DNA technology are listed in Table 60–6. Tests performed for lot release of a typical cell culture–produced live viral vaccine are presented in Table 60–7.

Adverse Reaction Monitoring

An adverse biological product reaction or experience is defined as an event associated with the use of a biological product, regardless of whether it is considered product related, and includes any side effect, injury, toxicity, or sensitivity reaction or significant failure of pharmacologic action (see Chapter 61 for more detail). Adverse reaction reports come from several sources. The manufacturers of biologicals, the staff of the United States Pharmacopoeia, and other health care professionals are the most common sources, but consumers are also encouraged to report. The manufacturers also report data concerning adverse reactions from postmarketing studies, foreign sources, and both published and unpublished scientific literature. The results of reported adverse reactions associated with vaccine use are compiled and entered into the Vaccine Adverse Event Reporting System (VAERS). VAERS is a program created as an outcome of the National Childhood Vaccine Injury Act of 1986 (NCVIA) and is administered jointly by the FDA and the CDC. VAERS accepts reports of any adverse event that may be associated with U.S.-licensed vaccines from health care

providers, manufacturers, and the public. The VAERS system is not limited to routinely recommended pediatric vaccines; it also accepts voluntary reports of suspected adverse events occurring after administration of any vaccine. The FDA continually monitors VAERS reports for any unexpected patterns or changes in rates of adverse events.

The NCVIA also mandated the development of vaccine information materials for distribution by health care providers to each adult or to the legal representative of each child receiving any vaccine recommended for routine pediatric use by the ACIP.[39] This effort was made to ensure that sufficient written information about the risks from the diseases and the risks and benefits of vaccines would be provided.[40] The materials include information on the diseases, vaccine reactions, possible ways to reduce the risk of major adverse reactions, contraindications, information on groups at high risk for acquiring the diseases that would greatly benefit from vaccination, availability of the National Vaccine Injury Compensation Program (see Chapter 63), and federal recommendations about immunization schedules. The CBER collaborates with the CDC in the development of this information.

Special Considerations

Combination Vaccines

Since the early part of the 20th century, vaccine combinations and the simultaneous separate administration of different vaccines have been important as effective means of enhancing the efficiency of immunization programs. Combination vaccines are composed of two or more antigens that are intended to induce protection against multiple infectious diseases or several different serotypes of the same organism. The antigens contained in combination vaccines are either formulated together by the manufacturer

TABLE 60–6 ■ Testing Requirements for the Release of Recombinant Hepatitis B Vaccines

| Type of Test | Merck & Co., Inc. | | GlaxoSmithKline | |
	Test System	Stage of Production	Test System	Stage of Production
Plasmid retention	Percentage of host cells with expression construct	Fermentation product	Percentage of host cells with expression construct	Fermentation product
Purity and identity	Formaldehyde	Bulk-adsorbed product	SDS-PAGE	Nonadsorbed bulk
	Triton-X100	Bulk-adsorbed product	DNA hybridization	Nonadsorbed bulk
	Protein (Lowry)	Bulk-adsorbed product		
	Gel electrophoresis	Sterile filtered product	Antigenic activity (RIA)	Nonadsorbed bulk
	HPSEC	Sterile filtered product	Protein (SDS-PAGE)	Nonadsorbed bulk and final container
Sterility	Thioglycollate medium	Final bulk	Thioglycollate medium	Final bulk
Sterility	Thioglycollate medium	Final container	Thioglycollate medium	Final container
General safety	Guinea pigs and mice	Final container	Guinea pigs and mice	Final container
Pyrogen	LAL	Final container	LAL	Final container
Purity	Aluminum	Final container	Total protein nitrogen	Final container
	Thimerosal	Final container	Aluminum	Final container
			Thimerosal	Final container
Potency	In vitro relative potency	Final container	Mouse potency	Final container

HPSEC, high-performance size exclusion chromatography; LAL, limulus amebocyte lysate; RIA, radioimmunoassay; SDS-PAGE, sodium dodecyl sulfate–polyacrylamide gel electrophoresis.

TABLE 60–7 ■ Testing Requirements for Release of Varicella Virus Vaccine, Live (Varivax)*

Type of Test	Test System	Stage of Preparation
Identity of production cells	Karyology	Production control cells
Sterility	Thioglycollate/soybean-casein digest	Working cell bank
		Control harvest fluids
		Virus harvest fluids
		Pre-clarified bulk
		Clarified bulk
		Final formulated bulk
		Filled container
Mycoplasma tests	Broth/agar—aerobic & anaerobic cell culture system	Working cell bank
		Control harvest fluids
		Pre-clarified bulk
Tissue culture safety	Simian kidney & MRC-5 cell cultures	Working cell bank
		Control harvest fluids
		Pre-clarified bulk
Animal safety	Adult & suckling mouse	Working cell bank
		Pre-clarified bulk
	Chick embryo (yolk sac & allantoic)	Working cell bank
General safety	Guinea pig & rabbit	Working cell bank
	Guinea pig & mouse	Filled container
Test for hemadsorbing viruses	Guinea pig red blood cells	Production control cells
Mycobacteria, in vitro	Broth and medium slants	Pre-clarified bulk
Bovine albumin	Immunoassay	Clarified bulk
Color, appearance, form	Visual examination	Filled container
Moisture	Coulometric method	Filled container
Tissue culture identity	Antibody neutralization	Filled container
Infectivity titration	Tissue culture plaque assay	Clarified bulk
		Filled container

*This is a subset of tests performed for this product.

or physically mixed by a health care provider just prior to administration. Both approaches require licensure by the FDA.

In the United States, combinations of diphtheria and tetanus toxoids, and these toxoids combined with pertussis vaccine (DTP), were licensed by the late 1940s. Since that time the number of additional combinations has grown steadily, including the individual types of live and inactivated poliovirus vaccines; several combinations of measles, mumps and rubella vaccines; combinations of *Haemophilus influenzae* type b conjugate vaccine with diphtheria and tetanus toxoids and acellular pertussis (DTaP) or hepatitis B vaccines; trivalent influenza vaccines; pneumococcal vaccines; the combination of hepatitis A and hepatitis B vaccines; and the combination of DTaP, inactivated poliovirus, and hepatitis B vaccines. The current success in developing new vaccine products administered in the first years of life has complicated vaccine schedules and has put special pressure on the desire for additional combinations. Products for which this approach might be an option in future include combinations of killed antigens already in use (e.g., DTaP, *Haemophilus* type b conjugate, 7-valent pneumococcal conjugate, hepatitis A and B, and the polioviruses). Live viral vaccines routinely recommended early in life are measles-mumps-rubella and varicella, and licensure of a combination of these live virus vaccines may occur in the future as well.

The manufacturing process and preclinical and clinical studies performed before licensure of a new combination vaccine are all intensively scrutinized during product development. Vaccines are complex mixtures that contain not only viral or bacterial antigens but also other components such as preservatives, adjuvants, stabilizers such as gelatin and sorbitol, and buffers and salts. Of particular concern is the compatibility of these components in the final combination. A combination vaccine may fail because of manufacturing issues such as the physicochemical interactions in the product, or biological interference among the combined attenuated immunizing agents, or immunologic interference, detected either in animal studies or during human clinical trials.[41] Preclinical immunogenicity studies can be very useful in determining the characteristics of antibody induced (subclass, affinity, functionality, epitope recognition). Animal models may be helpful in comparing the responses to the combined product and the individual vaccines. Similarly, an appropriate challenge model can serve to bolster the human data collected later in development. There are several published examples of clinical interference where the administration of combination vaccines resulted in the diminution of the immune response to one or more of the antigens in the combination when compared to the separate administration of the individual components of the vaccines.[42] One such example was the observation of depressed responses to the pertussis antigen in one experimental *Haemophilus* type b conjugate–DTaP combination vaccine that was not demonstrable with other similar combinations.[43]

Consideration must be made such that a preservative that accompanies one component of a combined product does not have a deleterious effect on another component.[44] Additionally, the impact of the preservative on the potency and stability of all active components in the combination must be evaluated. Similarly, when one or more of the components incorporates an adjuvant, the combination could affect antigen binding. Some of the bound antigen could be lost, or a previously unbound antigen could become adsorbed. Commonly, combinations raise issues related to successful potency, purity, identity, and sterility testing and may require alternative assay strategies. When potency tests of individual components are already approved for use on licensed products, it may be necessary to demonstrate that these tests still produce valid information when applied to a new combination vaccine.[45] For example, vaccine components may have to be tested at an earlier bulk stage of manufacture rather than in the final container. Adjuvants or residual antibiotics also may require that adjustments be made in sterility test procedures.

Although reactions following combination vaccines have not been a major issue, safety needs to be carefully evaluated for each new product. In addition to approved combination vaccines, separate products commonly are administered simultaneously. Reactivity following simultaneously administered vaccines may be additive, but generally it has not been shown to be enhanced.[46,47] Whether the components of a new combination product have been previously licensed or not, clinical trials are needed. These studies are ordinarily randomized and controlled by comparisons between the combination and the individual component vaccines. Clinical observations for safety in several thousands of subjects for reactions, coupled with laboratory studies of immunogenicity, are usually sufficient to assess the safety and effectiveness of the combination.[17]

The development of new combination vaccines continues to present unique challenges to vaccine manufacturers as well as regulatory authorities. It will take a coordinated effort and dialogue between the two in order to bring these new products to the market, especially as the complexity of manufacturing and clinical evaluation increases.

Vaccines to Counter Biological Terrorism

Immunization programs in the United States have significantly reduced morbidity and mortality from naturally transmitted infectious diseases; however, we are now confronted with the potential threat of intentional release of biological agents by humans into the general population. Although the military has recognized the value in protecting troops against biological threats, protecting civilians from bioterrorism may be more difficult. There are also high costs and significant logistic concerns with vaccinating large populations against biological agents such as anthrax and smallpox. Some other pathogens that may be adapted for biological warfare include plague, tularemia, brucellosis, Q fever, and botulinum toxin. There are significant challenges associated with developing and testing new vaccines against biological agents.

The FDA's regulation of vaccines is based on science, law, and public health considerations. Accelerating product development is important in many situations, including counter-bioterrorism. Mechanisms for advancing new vaccines through the approval process have been developed for severe and life-threatening illnesses. These mechanisms include expedited review and fast-track development, as well as accelerated approval and priority review of market-

ing applications.[§] For licensure, a counter-bioterrorism product, just as for any product, must have an acceptable quality, safety, efficacy, and potency profile. Likewise, production and quality control also must be in compliance with cGMPs.

With regard to bioterrorism, the goal of the FDA is to facilitate the development of vaccines and other biological products, drugs, and diagnostic products to respond to bioterrorist threats. In this effort, the FDA works with other interagency groups, such as the CDC and NIH, to prepare for responding in a civilian emergency. As part of the interagency group, the FDA also participates in setting a broad-based U.S. research agenda to facilitate the government's preparedness against bioterrorism. Key activities of the CBER to counter bioterrorism include enhancing its research and review activities in this area in order to expedite the development and licensure of new drugs and biological products, including vaccines, and new uses of existing products.

Presently, there is one licensed smallpox vaccine in the United States, Wyeth's Dryvax®. New smallpox vaccines and vaccinia immune globulin preparations also are being developed under an IND application, with the goal to seek licensure. There is one licensed anthrax vaccine in the United States, Anthrax Vaccine Adsorbed (Bioport's Biothrax™). This product is also being studied under an IND application for uses such as postexposure vaccination in addition to antibiotics. The development of new anthrax vaccines also will be pursued under an IND application. There are currently no licensed vaccines available in the United States for plague, tularemia, viral hemorrhagic fever viruses (e.g., Ebola, Marburg, Lassa, and New World arenaviruses); however, new vaccines for some of these indications are being developed under IND applications.

Many of the biological warfare defense vaccines pose difficult problems with regard to obtaining clinical efficacy data. For many of these infectious agents or toxins, human efficacy trials are not feasible because natural exposure no longer occurs (e.g., smallpox), occurs at a very low incidence, or occurs in an unpredictable manner. Also, human challenge studies that would involve exposing healthy human volunteers to a lethal or permanently disabling agent in the absence of a proven therapy to counter the agent cannot be performed. Notwithstanding, the requirements for licensure of vaccines against bioterrorism infectious agents are the same as for any biological: safety, efficacy, and manufacturing consistency must be demonstrated.

To address the dilemma of obtaining clinical efficacy data, the FDA published a final rule entitled "New Drug and Biological Drug Products: Evidence Needed to Demonstrate

---

[§]The *Fast Track* programs of the FDA are designed to facilitate the development and expedite the review of new drugs that are intended to treat serious or life-threatening conditions and that demonstrate the potential to address unmet medical needs (fast-track products).

The *accelerated approval* regulations give the FDA flexibility with respect to the types of endpoints that can be relied on to support marketing approval, but do not affect the quantity or quality of evidence needed to demonstrate substantial evidence of effectiveness. Any endpoint considered appropriate to be relied on to support approval, whether a surrogate endpoint or a clinical endpoint, must be supported by substantial evidence of effectiveness.

Products regulated by the CBER are eligible for *priority review* if they provide a significant improvement in the safety or effectiveness of the treatment, diagnosis, or prevention of a serious or life-threatening disease.

Effectiveness of New Drugs When Human Efficacy Studies Are Not Ethical or Feasible."[48] The FDA has amended its new drug and biological products regulations to incorporate this new rule. This rule allows the use of animal efficacy data in lieu of human efficacy data when human challenge studies cannot be conducted ethically and field efficacy studies are not feasible because of infectious disease epidemiology (in the case of vaccines). In these situations, certain drug and biological products (e.g., vaccines) that are intended to reduce or prevent serious or life-threatening conditions caused by lethal or permanently disabling toxic chemical, biological, radiologic, or nuclear substances may be approved for marketing based on evidence of effectiveness derived from appropriate studies in animals and additional supporting data. Safety, pharmacokinetics, and immunogenicity data are still necessary in humans. Product safety will be evaluated in healthy human volunteers at doses and routes of administration anticipated in field use.

Under the "animal rule," the FDA will be able to approve a product for which safety has been established and the requirements of 21 CFR § 601.60 have been met, based on adequate and well-controlled animal trials, when results of these animal studies establish that the product is reasonably likely to provide clinical benefit to humans. The FDA can rely on the evidence from animal studies to provide substantial evidence of the efficacy of these products when:

1. There is a reasonably well-understood pathophysiologic mechanism for toxicity of the chemical, biological, radiologic, or nuclear substance and its amelioration or prevention by the product.
2. The effect is demonstrated in more than one animal species that is expected to react with a response that is predictive for humans, unless the effect is demonstrated in a single animal species that represents a sufficiently well-characterized animal model (in other words, the model has been adequately evaluated for its responsiveness) in predicting the response in humans.
3. The animal endpoint is clearly related to the desired benefit in humans, which is generally the enhancement of survival or prevention of major morbidity.
4. The data or information on the pharmacokinetics and pharmacodynamics of the product or other relevant data or information in animals and humans is sufficiently well understood to allow selection of an effective dose in humans, and it is reasonable to expect the efficacy of the product in animals to be a reliable indicator of its efficacy in humans.

As stated earlier, safety and pharmacokinetics (immunogenicity in the case of vaccines) data in humans will still be required under pre-existing regulations to evaluate new drug and biological drug products for approval or licensure. In the case of vaccines, validated assays to assess both human and animal vaccine-elicited immune responses will play an important role in product development.

The FDA believes that products approved under the animal rule can be studied for safety in prelicensure clinical trials of human volunteers who are representative of those individuals who would be exposed to the product after approval. One limitation of prelicensure trials may be the inability to examine possible adverse interactions between toxic substances and the new product.

The animal rule will not apply if the product can be approved based on standards described elsewhere in FDA regulations (e.g., accelerated approval based on surrogate markers or clinical endpoints other than survival or irreversible morbidity). Approval of products under the animal rule will require early and multiple discussions with the FDA. Applicants will need detailed justifications as to why efficacy trials are not feasible or ethical for their products of interest. Prior to beginning the pivotal trial(s), pilot studies in animals are expected, and a prospective primary endpoint should be selected. Additionally, with regard to the pivotal trial(s), prospective statistical plans should be in place. The FDA's advisory committees also may be consulted prior to acceptance of the animal efficacy trial proposal and/or following the agency's review of the BLA.

In summary, counter-bioterrorism vaccines present unique issues for clinical development and evaluation by the FDA. Overall planning and coordination with the FDA will be necessary to move these products toward licensure and into distribution, if they are needed in the case of a bioterrorist threat.

Product Labeling and Advertising

As noted in earlier sections, in the United States the FDA regulates the format and content of labels for product containers and packages and the circulars that accompany them (package inserts). The FDA also regulates promotional labeling and advertising using the same standards.

The initial labeling for a new vaccine is reviewed through the product licensing process described earlier. During this review, in addition to the draft labeling and clinical studies submitted by the manufacturer, the agency considers discussions of appropriate use for the product held by several non-FDA advisory groups, including the American Academy of Pediatrics' Committee on Infectious Diseases (the "Redbook Committee") and the ACIP; however, the ultimate indication for the licensed product is driven by the FDA's review of the supportive clinical data submitted by the sponsor.

Subsequently, significant changes in labeling, including new indications for use, new dosage forms or regimens, expanded patient populations who receive the product, and additional information regarding safety and effectiveness, require that the manufacturer submit a supplemental filing for review and approval by the CBER. These materials are reviewed to determine that they are not false nor misleading, that is, that they comport with the scientific data the manufacturer developed in the application and data acquired subsequent to product approval. Unlike other product labeling, the promotional labeling and advertising are not subject to pre-clearance; however, they are similarly monitored for misleading claims. These documents must also meet the standard of "fair balance," that is, that claims of efficacy would be balanced with information about the product's adverse effects.

Conclusion

The technology for developing new vaccines such as those derived from genetically engineered organisms and plants has advanced significantly during the past century. These technological advances present challenges to the scientific community and manufacturers; however, the challenges to the NRAs are especially great as regulatory agencies struggle to develop new criteria to evaluate these vaccines for safety and efficacy. The final standards for any vaccine are relevant to the technology used to produce the vaccine. New vaccine candidates must be evaluated using a blend of knowledge from the past and the best of current science in assessing their risks and benefits. The burden of these decisions is great because vaccines most often are given to healthy individuals, commonly children. The risk-benefit ratio must be weighted on the side of highest benefit.

Vaccines continue to have a great success rate in reducing the burden of many infectious diseases. Until recently, it was believed that some diseases could be eradicated with vaccines; however, with the realization that infectious agents may be intentionally introduced into the population, eradication may no longer be a reachable goal, unless it is reinforced with continued vaccination once it has been achieved. Thus it is even more important that the scientific community and the NRAs continue to develop and facilitate the introduction of new vaccines using a broad scientific consensus.

Acknowledgments

We would like to acknowledge the staff members in the Office of Vaccines Research and Review and the Office of Compliance and Biologics Quality/CBER for their assistance in the preparation of this manuscript. Particular gratitude goes out to Ms. Karen Chaitkin and Dr. Karen Goldenthal for their assistance in reviewing this manuscript and providing constructive comments.

REFERENCES

1. D'Arcy PF, Harron DWG. Proceedings of the First International Conference on Harmonization, Brussels, 1991. Antrim, Northern Ireland, Greystone Books, 1992.
2. Koehler CSW. Science, "society," and immunity. Mod Drug Discov 4:59–60, 2001.
3. Kondratas RA. Death helped write the biologics law. FDA Consumer 16:23–25, 1982.
4. Division of Biologics Standards, National Institutes of Health. Legislative History of the Regulation of Biological Products (2nd printing). Bethesda, MD, National Institutes of Health, 1968.
5. Public Health Service Act, July 1, 1944, Chap. 373, Title III, Sec. 351, 58 Stat. 702, currently codified at 42 U.S.C., Sec. 262.
6. Public Health Service Act, July 1, 1944, Chap. 373, Title III, Sec. 352, 58 Stat. 702, currently codified at 42 U.S.C., Sec. 263.
7. Paul JR. A History of Poliomyelitis. New Haven, CT, Yale University Press, 1971.
8. Code of Federal Regulations, Title 21, Food and Drugs. Washington, DC, Office of the Federal Register, National Archives & Records Administration, 2002.
9. Code of Federal Regulations, Title 21, Parts 210, 211. Washington, DC, Office of the Federal Register, National Archives & Records Administration, 2002.
10. 5 United States Code, Sec. 551 et seq.
11. Code of Federal Regulations, Title 21, Sec. 600.3. Washington, DC, Office of the Federal Register, National Archives & Records Administration, 1997.
12. Code of Federal Regulations, Title 21, Sec. 601.25(d)(2). Washington, DC, Office of the Federal Register, National Archives & Records Administration, 1997.
13. Code of Federal Regulations, Title 21, Part 312. Washington, DC, Office of the Federal Register, National Archives & Records Administration, 2002.
14. Code of Federal Regulations, Title 21, Part 50. Washington, DC, Office of the Federal Register, National Archives & Records Administration, 2002.
15. Code of Federal Regulations, Title 21, Part 56. Washington, DC, Office of the Federal Register, National Archives & Records Administration, 2002.
16. Code of Federal Regulations, Title 21, Part 58. Washington, DC, Office of the Federal Register, National Archives & Records Administration, 2002.
17. Goldenthal KL, Falk LA, Ball L, Geber A. Prelicensure evaluation of combination vaccines. Clin Infect Dis 33(suppl 4):S267–S273, 2001.
18. Sensabaugh SM. A primer on CBER's regulatory review structure and process. Drug Information J 32:1011–1030, 1998.
19. Code of Federal Regulations, Title 21, Secs. 601.10, 601.20. Washington, DC, Office of the Federal Register, National Archives & Records Administration, 1997.
20. Code of Federal Regulations, Title 21, Secs. 25.30, 25.31. Washington, DC, Office of the Federal Register, National Archives & Records Administration, 2002.
21. Food and Drug Administration. Postmarketing studies for approved human drugs and licensed biological products; status reports. Fed Reg 65:64607–64616, 2000.
22. Code of Federal Regulations, Title 21, Sec. 601.12. Washington, DC, Office of the Federal Register, National Archives & Records Administration, 2002.
23. Guidance on alternatives to lot release for licensed biological products. Fed Reg 58:38771–38773, 1993.
24. Code of Federal Regulations, Title 21, Secs. 601.5, 601.6. Washington, DC, Office of the Federal Register, National Archives & Records Administration, 2002.
25. Fox JP, Lennette EH, Manso C, Souza Aguiar JR. Encephalitis in man following vaccination with 17D yellow fever virus. Am J Hyg 36:117–142, 1942.
26. Fox JP, Manso C, Penna HA, Para M. Observations on the occurrence of icterus in Brazil following vaccination against yellow fever. Am J Hyg 36:68–116, 1942.
27. Brown F, Esber EC, Williams MH (eds). Continuous Cell Lines—An International Workshop on Current Issues. Dev Biol Stand 76:1–368, 1992.
28. World Health Organization. Acceptability of cell substrates for production of biologicals: Report of a WHO Study Group. World Health Organ Tech Rep Ser 747:1–29, 1987.
29. Mortimer EA Jr, Lepow ML, Gold E, et al. Long-term follow-up of persons inadvertently inoculated with SV40 as neonates. N Engl J Med 305:1517–1518, 1981.
30. Waters TD, Anderson PS Jr, Beebe GW, Miller RW. Yellow fever vaccination, avian leucosis virus, and cancer risk in man. Science 177:76–77, 1972.
31. Lewis AM Jr, Egan W. Workshop on simian virus 40 (SV40): a possible human polyomavirus. Biologicals 25:355–358, 1997.
32. WHO Expert Committee on Biological Standardization. Highlights of the 45th Meeting. Wkly Epidemiol Rec 71(14):105–108, 1996.
33. Marwick C. BSE sets agenda for imported gelatin. JAMA 227:1659–1660, 1997.
34. Code of Federal Regulations, Title 9, Part 94. Washington, DC, Office of the Federal Register, National Archives & Records Administration, 2002.
35. Center for Biologics Evaluation and Research, Congressional, Consumer, and International Affairs Staff. Points to Consider. Production and Testing of New Drugs and Biologicals Produced by Recombinant DNA Technology. (HFB-142). Rockville, MD, U.S. Food and Drug Administration, 1985.
36. Center for Biologics Evaluation and Research, Congressional, Consumer, and International Affairs Staff. Points to Consider. Supplement to Production and Testing of New Drugs and Biologicals Produced by Recombinant DNA Technology: Nucleic Acid Characterization and Genetic Stability. Rockville, MD, U.S. Food and Drug Administration, 1990.
37. Center for Biologics Evaluation and Research, Congressional, Consumer, and International Affairs Staff. Points to Consider in the Production and Testing of New Drugs and Biologicals Produced by Recombinant DNA Technology: Nucleic Acid Characterization

and Genetic Stability. Rockville, MD, U.S. Food and Drug Administration, 1992.

38. Code of Federal Regulations, Title 21, Secs. 610.10–610.18. Washington, DC, Office of the Federal Register, National Archives & Records Administration, 1997.

39. 42 United States Code, Sec. 300Aa-26.

40. New vaccine information materials. Fed Reg 59:31888, 1994.

41. Falk LA, Arciniega J, McVittie L. Manufacturing issues with combining different antigens: a regulatory perspective. Clin Infect Dis 33(suppl):S351–S355, 2001.

42. Falk LA, Midthun K, McVittie LD, Goldenthal KL. The testing and licensure of combination vaccines for the prevention of infectious diseases. *In* Ellis R (ed). Combination Vaccines. Totowa, NJ, Humana Press, 1999, pp 233–248.

43. Eskola J, Olander RM, Hovi T, et al. Randomized trial of the effect of co-administration with acellular pertussis DTP vaccine on immunogenicity of *Haemophilus influenzae* type b conjugate vaccine. Lancet 348:1688–1692, 1996.

44. Pittman M. Instability of pertussis-vaccine component in quadruple antigen vaccine. JAMA 181:25–30, 1962.

45. Corbel MJ. Control testing of combined vaccines: a consideration of potential problems and approaches. Biologicals 22:353–360, 1994.

46. Poliomyelitis prevention in the United States: introduction of a sequential vaccination schedule of inactivated poliovirus vaccine followed by oral poliovirus vaccine. Recommendations of the Advisory Committee on Immunization Practices (ACIP). Morb Mortal Wkly Rep 46(RR-3):1–25, 1997.

47. General recommendations on immunization: recommendations of the Advisory Committee on Immunization Practices (ACIP). Morb Mortal Wkly Rep 43(RR-1):1–38, 1994.

48. New drug and biological drug products: evidence needed to demonstrate effectiveness of new drugs when human efficacy studies are not ethical or feasible. Fed Reg 67:37988–37998, 2002.

Chapter 61

Safety of Immunizations

ROBERT T. CHEN • ROBERT L. DAVIS • KRISTINE M. SHEEDY

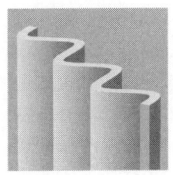 Immunizations are among the most cost-effective and widely used public health interventions.[1,2] No vaccine is perfectly safe or effective,[3] however. As the incidence of vaccine-preventable diseases is reduced by increasing coverage with an efficacious vaccine, vaccine-related adverse events, both those caused by vaccines (i.e., *true* adverse reactions) and those associated with vaccination only by coincidence, become increasingly frequent and prominent (Fig. 61–1).[4] The number of reports to the Vaccine Adverse Event Reporting System (VAERS) in the United States, approximately 13,000 per year, now exceeds the reported incidence of most vaccine-preventable childhood diseases combined (Table 61–1).

In such maturing immunization programs, close monitoring and timely assessment of suspected vaccine-related adverse events are critical to prevent loss of confidence, decreased vaccine coverage, and return of epidemic disease,[4–6] as experienced in several countries with pertussis[7] and either feared or experienced with measles.[8,9] Similar concerns in the United States during the early 1980s led to substantial increases in the number of lawsuits and price of vaccines, the loss of vaccine manufacturers,[10] and potential deterrence to the development of new vaccines.[11]

In developing countries, the safety concerns are weighted toward inadequate control of vaccine production and programmatic errors, such as inadequate sterilization of injection equipment leading to transmission of blood-borne pathogens,[12,13] and clusters of real or psychogenic illnesses during mass campaigns.[14,15] As nations in developed and developing countries attain high vaccine coverage and lower vaccine-preventable diseases rates, immunization safety controversies (i.e., from either intrinsic vaccine properties or the process of administering the vaccine) may threaten the stability of their programs.[16] Accordingly, the World Health Organization's (WHO's)[17] Expanded Programme on Immunization (EPI) recommended in 1991 that all national programs implement surveillance for adverse events after immunizations.[18,19]

Recommendations for immunizations represent a dynamic balancing of risks and benefits. Immunization safety monitoring is necessary to weigh this balance accurately at both individual and societal levels.[20]

When diseases are close to eradication, data on complications secondary to vaccine relative to that of disease may lead to discontinuation or decreased use of the vaccine, as was done with smallpox vaccine[21] and with the shift from oral polio vaccine (OPV) to inactivated polio vaccine.[22,23] Unfortunately, the classical disease eradication paradigm has been dramatically altered by the recent emergence of bioterrorism as a credible threat.[24] Given the decimation of various immunologically naive native populations from introduction of diseases like measles and smallpox by armies, traders, and explorers throughout human history,[25] stopping vaccinations and creating large pools of susceptible persons appears to be no longer advisable.[24] Reintroduction of smallpox vaccination in sizeable populations (with attendant complications) may occur in several countries.[26,27] Prior data on smallpox vaccine–related adverse event rates may be outdated because rates of atopic dermatitis (a known high-risk condition for vaccinees) have increased markedly since routine vaccination against smallpox was halted. The emergence of the human immunodeficiency virus epidemic has added another large pool of immunologically compromised people who might be at high risk for adverse effects of vaccination against smallpox.

Few other vaccine-preventable diseases are therefore likely to be eradicated and their target organisms made extinct in the near future.[28] This in turn means most immunizations will be needed indefinitely, with their attendant adverse reactions and potential for loss of public confidence. Research in immunization safety can help to distinguish true adverse reactions from coincidental events,[29,30] estimate their attributable risk,[31,32] identify risk factors that may permit development of valid contraindications,[31,33] and, if the pathophysiologic mechanism becomes known, develop safer vaccines.[34–37] The economics of developing safer vaccines (e.g., against smallpox) also has changed dramatically in the post-9/11 environment. Finally, research into immunization safety demonstrates a commitment to reducing disease from all causes, vaccine preventable and vaccine induced, and may help to maintain public confidence in immunizations and the credibility of immunization programs.[6]

"Substantial gaps and limitations" existed in knowledge and research infrastructure for immunization safety as recent as a decade ago, however.[3,29,30] Traditional prelicensure trials and passive surveillance systems have had limited utility in filling such gaps. Although large linked database safety monitoring

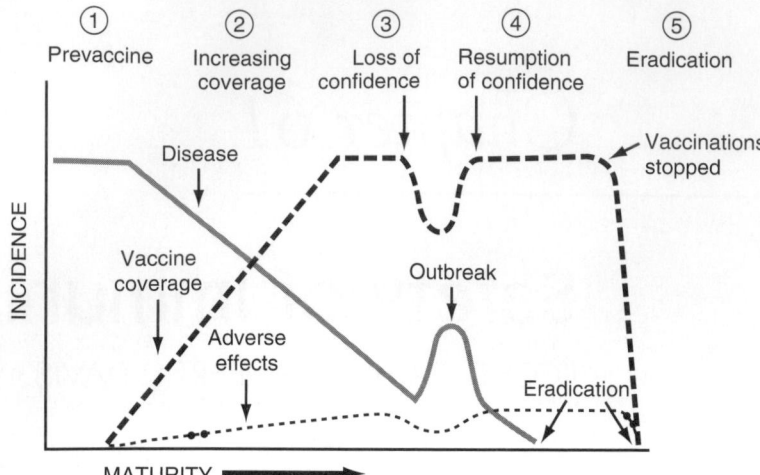

FIGURE 61–1 ▪ Evolution of immunization program and prominence of vaccine safety.

systems have been developed[32,38,39] to provide more scientifically rigorous data on issues ranging from diabetes[40] to seizures,[41] immunization safety remains a controversial issue in many countries.[42–45] This highlights that human societies have just begun to grapple with how to sustain mature immunization programs. This is a daunting new challenge that *Homo sapiens* has never faced before, and we must therefore retain our humility about its ultimate likely success. Nevertheless, if mature immunization programs are to build on past successes and take full advantage of the new vaccines made possible by biotechnology,[46] a Hippocratic willingness is required to understand both the risks and the benefits of immunizations. This chapter summarizes key scientific and policy issues on immunization safety necessary to tackle these new challenges.

Importance of Safety—First Do No Harm

A higher standard of safety is generally expected of immunizations compared to other medical interventions.

Tolerance of adverse reactions to pharmaceutical products given to healthy people—especially healthy infants and toddlers—to prevent certain conditions (e.g., vaccines, contraceptives) is substantially lower than to products administered to sick people for curative purposes (e.g., antibiotics, insulin).[3] This lower risk tolerance for vaccines translates into a need to investigate the possible causes of much rarer adverse events after vaccinations than would be acceptable for other pharmaceutical products. For example, events occurring at approximately 1 per 100,000 to 1 per 1 million doses (e.g., acute encephalopathy after whole-cell pertussis vaccine,[29,31] Guillain-Barré syndrome [GBS] after swine influenza vaccine,[47] and OPV-associated paralytic polio[22]) are of concern for vaccinees, whereas side effects are essentially universal for cancer chemotherapy, and 10% to 30% of people on high-dose aspirin therapy experience gastrointestinal symptoms.[48]

The cost and the difficulty of studying events increase with their rarity, however. Furthermore, studies of rare events are less likely to provide definitive conclusions, thereby engendering much controversy. Attributable risks

TABLE 61–1 ▪ Comparison of Maximum and Current Reported Morbidity from Vaccine-Preventable Diseases and Vaccine Adverse Events, United States

Disease	Maximum Caxes (Year)	2002*	Percent Change
Smallpox	206,939 (1921)	0	−100
Diphtheria	894,134 (1941)	1	>−99.9
Measles	152,209 (1968)	37	>−99.9
Mumps	265,269 (1934)	238	−99.8
Pertussis	21,269 (1952)	8296	−96.9
Polio (paralytic)	57,686 (1969)	0	−100
Rubella	20,000† (1964–65)	14	>−99.9
Congenital rubella syndrome	1560‡ (1923)	3	>−99.9
Tetanus‖ (1984)	20,000† (1984)	23	−98.5
H. influenzae type B <5 yr and unknown	20,000†	282	−98.6
Vaccine-related adverse events	0	7773‡	++§

*Provisional; subject to change as a result of late reporting.
†Estimated because no national reporting existed in prevaccine era.
‡Reports of adverse event after vaccines against only diseases shown in table; total reports to the Vaccine Adverse
   Event Reporting System = 14,199 as of January 2003.
§Indicates the major increase in vaccine adverse events compared to prevaccine era.
‖Deaths in 1923; cases in 2002.

on the order of 1 per 100,000 or 1 per million are on the margin of resolution through epidemiologic studies.[29,49] Perhaps not surprisingly, the bulk of the published literature on vaccine safety to date has been in the form of case reports and case series rather than controlled studies with adequate power.[29,30] To assess the possible association between pertussis vaccination and encephalopathy, the British organized a large case-control study[31,50] of all children 2 to 35 months of age in England, Scotland, and Wales hospitalized for a variety of neurologic illnesses during a 36-month period (N = 1167). Because the finding of a significant association between vaccine and permanent brain damage was based on only seven exposed cases,[51] questions about this study's validity generated much controversy in and out of the courts.[29,52] Despite considerably more robust data linking GBS with the swine influenza vaccine,[47] the subsequent controversy[53,54] resulted in a court-ordered independent re-examination of the data[55] and, ultimately, partial redo of the study confirming the initial findings.[56] Even though two independent large controlled studies showed that the relative risk of intussusception exceeded 30 after the first dose of the rhesus rotavirus vaccine (RRV),[57,58] some have argued that this was an artifact of "triggering" based on uncontrolled ecologic evidence,[59,60] despite evidence to the contrary.[61]

A higher standard of safety is also required of vaccines because of the large number of people who are exposed to vaccines, frequently on a compulsory basis for public health reasons.[62] Because most vaccine-preventable diseases are transmissible person to person, immunizations protect the society as well as the individual by reducing disease transmission. This is often called herd or population immunity.[63] Similar to the idea of "commons" in environmental health,[64] there is an inherent tension between individual and societal good with immunizations. As a population attains high vaccine coverage (with an imperfectly safe vaccine) and creates herd immunity, the individual risk/benefit equation diverges from that of the society. The optimal outcome for the individual is to (1) encourage everyone else to be vaccinated, (2) become protected by herd immunity, and (3) avoid vaccinations (and any associated risk). From a societal perspective, if too many persons take this course of action, herd immunity can be lost and epidemic disease can return.[20] To avoid the "free rider" problem, many states mandate vaccinations to ensure equitable sharing of vaccine risks and benefits; analogous to compulsory military service, exemptions are offered to those with conscientious objections.[65] This may help explain why consumer activist groups have great interest in both vaccine safety and personal choice in vaccinations.

The medical maxim "first do no harm" may apply even more in public health than in clinical medicine, where decisions affect fewer people. Inadequately inactivated polio vaccine was administered to about 400,000 people in the "Cutter incident," resulting in 260 polio cases.[66] There have been other similar tragedies as a result of errors in production.[3] Concerns that polio vaccine contaminated by simian virus 40 may have been received by millions of people during the 1950s,[67,68] that some vaccines may have contained gelatin stabilizers derived from cattle infected with bovine spongiform encephalopathy,[69] and that some infants were exposed to high levels of ethyl mercury from thimerosal-containing vaccines[70] further highlight the importance of ensuring the safety of relatively universal human-directed exposures such as immunizations. These concerns are the basis for strict regulatory control of vaccines by the Food and Drug Administration (FDA),[69,71] for example, by banning use of bovine-derived products from countries with bovine spongiform encephalopathy,[72] and the call by the WHO for only vaccines of "assured quality" to be used in the EPI.[73]

High standards of accuracy and timeliness are needed for vaccine safety studies because they have extremely narrow margins for error. In contrast to many classes of drugs for which other effective therapies may be substituted, vaccines generally have few alternative strains or types (OPV versus inactivated poliovirus vaccine being the best-known exception). The decision to withdraw a vaccine or switch between strains thus may have wide ramifications. The circumstances surrounding the use and withdrawal of the 1976 "swine influenza" vaccine have been extensively documented,[53] as has the controversy surrounding the safety of whole-cell pertussis vaccines.[7] In 1992, the United Kingdom withdrew the license of mumps vaccines containing the Urabe strain after studies suggested a high rate of vaccine-associated aseptic meningitis.[74] After the manufacturers subsequently withdrew this product worldwide, many countries were left without an alternative vaccine.[75,76] Similarly, when the manufacturer of a newly licensed rotavirus vaccine withdrew it in the wake of an increased risk of intussusception, this also made the vaccine unavailable in developing countries, where rotavirus is a major cause of childhood death.[59] Lawsuits and publicity about a possible link between Lyme vaccine and arthritis led to the withdrawal of the only licensed vaccine—even though only anecdotal reports had been received.[77] Therefore, establishing associations of adverse events with vaccines and promptly defining the attributable risks are critical to understanding the proper risk/benefit perspective. An erroneous association or attributable risk can undermine confidence in a vaccine and have disastrous consequences for vaccine acceptance and disease incidence. However, denials of association despite accumulating evidence can also backfire.[76,78]

Finally, because many vaccinations are mandated for public health reasons and because no vaccine is perfectly safe, several countries have established compensation programs for people who may have been injured by vaccination.[79] Accurate assessment of whether adverse events can be caused by specific vaccines is essential to a fair and efficient vaccine injury compensation program.[80]

Gaps and Limitations in Knowledge

In 1967, the lack of scientific documentation of the risks of immunization moved Sir Graham Wilson,[3] former director of the Public Health Laboratory Service in the United Kingdom, to compile the first such review. He noted fear of compensation claims and inadvertent support for anti-vaccinationists as possible explanations for the incomplete record. Pursuant to the National Childhood Vaccine Injury Act (NCVIA) of 1986, a Committee of the Institute of Medicine (IOM) in the United States was established to review the adverse consequences of childhood vaccines. This group still found severe limits in the knowledge and research capability on vaccine safety.[29,30] For 50 (66%) of the 76 adverse events reviewed, there was either no or inadequate scientific evidence to judge for or against a causal link to vaccine. Specifically, the IOM committee identified the following limitations: (1) inadequate understanding of biologic mechanisms underlying adverse events, (2) insufficient or inconsistent information from case reports and case series, (3) inadequate size or length of follow-up of many population-based epidemiologic studies, (4) limitations of existing surveillance systems to provide persuasive evidence of causation, and (5) few experimental studies published relative to the total number of epidemiologic studies published.[29,30]

Other factors also may have contributed to the scarcity of knowledge about immunization safety. Safety research requires expertise in pharmacoepidemiology and rare disease epidemiology,[81] with its special set of methodologic challenges.[82–84] Such studies are costly and difficult to organize, and the methods may be less familiar to most immunization experts with primary infectious disease backgrounds. Furthermore, interest in and resource allocation for immunization safety research have been severely handicapped by all too common characterization in narrow, negative terms of *adverse events* research (vs. larger, positive concepts of ensuring *immunization safety*)—especially when competing against the positive benefits and efficacy side of immunization research. Finally, similar to other areas of safety (e.g., blood, food, transport), immunization safety cannot be studied directly but can be only inferred indirectly by the absence of specific problems when appropriate surveillance and risk management systems are in place. This approach requires a systematic accumulation of *negative* findings, which, though essential, are more difficult to prove—and to publish—than *positive* findings.[85,86]

The IOM concluded that "if research capacity and accomplishments [are] not improved, future reviews of vaccine safety [will be] similarly handicapped."[29] Although much remains to be done, much progress has been made in the last few years toward understanding these gaps and ameliorating the infrastructure to improve immunization safety research.[4,5,32,38,39,87,88]

Methods of Monitoring Immunization Safety

Safety monitoring can be carried out both before and after vaccine licensure, with slightly different goals based on the methodologic strengths and weaknesses of each step. Although the general principles are similar irrespective of each country, the specific approaches may differ because of factors such as how immunization services are organized and level of resources available. Nevertheless, they should all contribute scientific information of the highest level possible toward evidence-based vaccinology.[89]

Prelicensure

Vaccines, similar to other pharmaceutical products, undergo extensive safety and efficacy evaluations in the laboratory, in animals, and in phased human clinical trials before licensure.[71,90] *Phase I* trials usually include fewer than 20 participants and can detect only extremely common adverse events. *Phase II* trials generally enroll 50 to several hundred people. When carefully coordinated, as in the comparative infant diphtheria and tetanus toxoids and acellular pertussis (DTaP) vaccine trials,[91] important insight into the relationship between concentration of antigen, number of vaccine components, formulation technique, effect of successive doses, and profile of common reactions can be drawn and can affect the choice of the candidate vaccines for *Phase III* trials.[92,93] Sample sizes for Phase III vaccine trials are based principally on efficacy considerations, with safety inferences drawn to the extent possible based on the sample size (approximately 10^2 to 10^5) and the duration of observation (often <30 days).[92] Typically only observations of common local and systemic reactions (e.g., injection site swelling, fever, fussiness) have been possible. The experimental design of most Phase I to III clinical trials includes (1) a control group (either a placebo or an alternative vaccine) group and (2) detection of adverse events by researchers in a consistent manner "blinded" to which vaccine the patient received. This allows relatively straightforward inferences on the causal relationship between most adverse events and vaccination.[81]

Several ways of enhancing prelicensure safety assessment of vaccines are under discussion or in process, especially in light of the recent experience with RRV and intussusception.[94] First, the Brighton Collaboration (*www.brightoncollaboration.org*), established to develop and implement globally accepted standard case definitions for assessing adverse events following immunizations in both pre- and postlicensure settings, has been organized.[95] Without such standards, it was difficult if not impossible to compare and collate safety data across trials in a valid manner. This gap therefore represented a major "missed opportunity" to advance our scientific knowledge of immunization safety overall, but was especially unfortunate in the prelicensure setting, where maximizing yield of safety data despite limited sample size was most needed. For example in the large multisite Phase III infant DTaP trials, definitions of high fever across trials varied by temperature (39.5° vs. 40.5°C), measurement (oral vs. rectal), and time (measured at 48 vs. 72 hours).[96] This was ironic because standardized case definitions had been developed in these trials for efficacy but not for safety—the original impetus for the development of DTaP.[97,98] The Brighton case definitions for each adverse event are further arrayed by the level of evidence provided (insufficient, low, intermediate, and highest); therefore, they also can be used in settings with less resources (e.g., studies in less developed settings or postlicensure surveillance).

Data and safety monitoring boards (DSMBs) represent another area of potential improvements in the prelicensure process. Currently, such DSMBs are constituted uniquely for each clinical trial. If instead there is greater overlap across prelicensure trials for the same vaccine, the DSBM may have better ability to oversee the safety data for the experimental vaccine. Furthermore, despite its name, there are currently no requirements that the DSMB include someone with safety experience. For vaccine trials, this means someone with rare disease (vs. infectious disease) epidemiology skills, usually fine tuned from postlicensure safety monitoring experience. Infectious disease experts are used to dealing with hundreds if not thousands of cases and are therefore prone to dismissing "just a couple of cases" of an adverse event. In contrast, someone with rare disease experience may be more inclined to think that seeing two rare adverse events is akin to winning the lottery twice in a row.

Because of pragmatic limits on the sample sizes of prelicensure studies, there are inherent limitations to the extent to which they can detect very rare, yet real, adverse events related to vaccination. Even if no adverse event has been observed in a trial of 10,000 vaccinees, one can only be 95% certain that the real incidence of the adverse event is no higher than 1 in 3333 vaccinees.[94] Thus to be able to detect an attributable risk of 1 per 10,000 vaccinees (e.g., RRV and intussusception), a prelicensure trial of at least 30,000 vaccinees (+ 30,000 controls) would be needed. The cost of doing such a large trial would clearly severely limit the number of vaccine candidates.[6]

Nevertheless, given the need to appreciate better the safety of vaccines administered universally to healthy infants and the methodologic difficulties of assessing safety in postlicensure observational (i.e., nonrandomized) studies,[83] there has been a call for larger studies to better assess vaccine safety and risks for serious, yet rare, adverse events prior to scale-up from prelicensure to universal use. This could be done either with larger prelicensure trials, as has been done for antipyretics in children,[99–101] or in some organized manner postlicensure prior to scale-up to universal recommendations (e.g., registry of first 1 million vaccinations).[6] Even with these measures, separate large-scale, long-term, randomized intervention trials would theoretically be the only way to study unforeseen delayed adverse effects,[83] for example, as seen with killed or high-titer measles vaccines.[102,103] Such trials would have to overcome major concerns about the ethics of withholding efficacious vaccines from persons in need, however. Therefore, a more likely way forward probably lies in maximizing the existing prelicensure assessment process as outlined above *and* the postlicensure infrastructure for monitoring, as discussed next.

Postlicensure

Because rare reactions, reactions with delayed onset, or reactions in subpopulations may not be detected before vaccines are licensed, postlicensure (also called postmarketing) evaluation of vaccine safety is critical. Historically, this evaluation has relied on passive surveillance and ad hoc epidemiologic studies, but, more recently, Phase IV trials and pre-established large linked databases (LLDBs) have improved the methodologic capabilities to study rare risks of specific immunizations.[81] Such systems may detect variation in rates of adverse events (and immunogenicity) by manufacturer[104,105] or even lot.[106] More recently, clinical centers for the study of immunization safety have emerged as another useful infrastructure to advance our knowledge about safety.[107]

In contrast to the elegance of prelicensure randomized trials, however, postlicensure *observational* studies of vaccine safety pose a formidable set of methodologic difficulties.[83,84] *Confounding by contraindication* is especially problematic for nonexperimental designs. Individuals who do not receive vaccine (e.g., because of a chronic or transient medical contraindication, or low socioeconomic group) may have a different risk for an adverse event than vaccinated individuals (e.g., background rates of seizures or sudden infant death syndrome may be higher in the unvaccinated); therefore, direct comparisons of vaccinated versus unvaccinated children is often inherently confounded. Teasing this issue out requires understanding of the complex interactions of multiple, poorly quantified factors.[83]

Passive Reporting Systems, Including the Vaccine Adverse Event Reporting System

Informal or formal *passive surveillance or spontaneous reporting systems* (SRSs) have been the cornerstone of most postmarketing safety monitoring systems because of their relative low cost of operations.[108–110] The national reporting of adverse events following immunizations can be done through the same reporting channels as those used for other adverse drug reactions,[110] as is the practice in France,[111] Japan,[112] New Zealand,[113] Sweden,[114] and the United Kingdom,[115] or with reporting forms or surveillance systems different from the drug safety monitoring systems, as done by Australia,[116] Canada,[5,117] Cuba,[118] Denmark,[119] India,[120] Italy,[121] Germany,[122] Mexico,[123] the Netherlands,[124] Sao Paulo State in Brazil,[125] and the United States.[4] As of 2000, 90 (42%) of 187 EPI programs report that have some type of monitoring for immunization safety in place[126]; less than 50% currently meet the national regulatory authority criteria for functioning system, however (B. Adwoa, World Health Organization, personal communication, May 10, 2002). Vaccine manufacturers also maintain SRSs for their products, which are usually forwarded subsequently to appropriate national regulatory authorities.[71,123]

In the United States, the NCVIA mandated for the first time that health care providers report certain adverse events after immunizations (see Table 63–1).[127] The VAERS was implemented jointly by the Centers for Disease Control and Prevention (CDC) and the FDA in 1990 to provide a unified national focus for collection of all reports of clinically significant adverse events, including, but not limited to, those mandated for reporting,[4] replacing its predecessors.[128]

The VAERS form permits narrative descriptions of adverse events (Fig. 61–2). Patients and their parents (as of 2001, <5% of VAERS reports come from parents)—not just health care professionals—are permitted to report to the VAERS, and there is no restriction on the interval between vaccination and symptoms that can be reported. Annual reminders about the VAERS are mailed to physicians likely to administer vaccines. The form is preaddressed and postage paid so that, after completion, it can be folded and mailed. Report forms, assistance in completing the form, or answers to other questions about the VAERS are available by calling a 24-hour toll-free telephone number (1-800-822-7967). Beginning in 2002, web-based reporting and simple data analyses are also available (*www.vaers.org*).

VAERS

VACCINE ADVERSE EVENT REPORTING SYSTEM
24 Hour Toll-free information line 1-800-822-7967
P.O. Box 1100, Rockville, MD 20849-1100
PATIENT IDENTITY KEPT CONFIDENTIAL

For CDC/FDA Use Only

VAERS Number _____

Date Received _____

Patient Name:	Vaccine administered by (Name):	Form completed by (Name):
Last First M.I.	_____ Responsible Physician _____ Facility Name/Address	_____ Relation ☐ Vaccine Provider ☐ Patient/Parent to Patient ☐ Manufacturer ☐ Other
Address		Address *(if different from patient or provider)*
City State Zip	City State Zip	City State Zip
Telephone no. (_____)_____	Telephone no. (_____)_____	Telephone no. (_____)_____

1. State	2. County where administered	3. Date of birth ___/___/___ mm dd yy	4. Patient age	5. Sex ☐ M ☐ F	6. Date form completed ___/___/___ mm dd yy

7. Describe adverse event(s) (symptoms, signs, time course) and treatment, if any	8. Check all appropriate:
	☐ Patient died (date ___/___/___) mm dd yy
	☐ Life threatening illness
	☐ Required emergency room/doctor visit
	☐ Required hospitalization (_____days)
	☐ Resulted in prolongation of hospitalization
	☐ Resulted in permanent disability
	☐ None of the above

9. Patient recovered ☐ YES ☐ NO ☐ UNKNOWN	10. Date of vaccination	11. Adverse event onset
12. Relevant diagnostic tests/laboratory data	___/___/___ mm dd yy AM Time_____ PM	___/___/___ mm dd yy AM Time_____ PM

13. Enter all vaccines given on date listed in no. 10

	Vaccine (type)	Manufacturer	Lot number	Route/Site	No. Previous doses
a.	_____	_____	_____	_____	_____
b.	_____	_____	_____	_____	_____
c.	_____	_____	_____	_____	_____
d.	_____	_____	_____	_____	_____

14. Any other vaccinations within 4 weeks prior to the date listed in no. 10

	Vaccine (type)	Manufacturer	Lot number	Route/Site	No. Previous doses	Date given
a.	_____	_____	_____	_____	_____	_____
b.	_____	_____	_____	_____	_____	_____

15. Vaccinated at: ☐ Private doctor's office/hospital ☐ Military clinic/hospital ☐ Public health clinic/hospital ☐ Other/unknown	16. Vaccine purchased with: ☐ Private funds ☐ Military funds ☐ Public funds ☐ Other /unknown	17. Other medications

18. Illness at time of vaccination (specify)	19. Pre-existing physician-diagnosed allergies, birth defects, medical conditions (specify)

20. Have you reported this adverse event previously? ☐ No ☐ To health department ☐ To doctor ☐ To manufacturer	**Only for children 5 and under**
	22. Birth weight ____ lb. ____ oz.	23. No. of brothers and sisters

21. Adverse event following prior vaccination (check all applicable, specify)	**Only for reports submitted by manufacturer/immunization project**

	Adverse Event	Onset Age	Type Vaccine	Dose no. in series	24. Mfr. / imm. proj. report no.	25. Date received by mfr. / imm. proj.
☐ In patient	_____	_____	_____	_____		
☐ In brother or sister	_____	_____	_____	_____	26. 15 day report? ☐ Yes ☐ No	27. Report type ☐ Initial ☐ Follow-Up

Health care providers and manufacturers are required by law (42 USC 300aa-25) to report reactions to vaccines listed in the Table of Reportable Events Following Immunization. Reports for reactions to other vaccines are voluntary except when required as a condition of immunization grant awards.

Form VAERS -1

FIGURE 61–2 ■ The Vaccine Adverse Event Reporting System (VAERS) form.

A contractor, under CDC and FDA supervision, distributes, collects, codes (currently using the Coding Symbols for a Thesaurus of Adverse Reaction Terms [COSTART][129] and using the Medical Dictionary for Regulatory Activities (MedDRA)[130] in the future), and enters VAERS reports in a database. Reporters of selected serious events receive medical follow-up from trained nurses (60 days after vaccination and 1 year after vaccination) to provide additional information about the VAERS report, including the patient's recovery. The CDC and the FDA have on-line access to the VAERS database and focus their efforts on analytic tasks of interest to the respective agencies. These data (without personal identifiers) are also available to the public. Approximately 13,000 VAERS reports are now received annually, about 15% of which are defined as serious (death, life-threatening illness, disability, hospitalization) (Table 61–2).[131]

Several other countries also have substantial experience with passive surveillance for immunization safety. In 1987, Canada developed the Vaccine Associated Adverse Event (VAAE) reporting system,[117,132] which is supplemented by an active, pediatric hospital–based surveillance system that searches all admissions for possible relationships to immunizations (Immunization Monitoring Program—Active [IMPACT]).[88] Serious VAAE reports are reviewed by an Advisory Committee on Causality Assessment consisting of a panel of experts.[133] The Netherlands also convenes an annual panel to categorize their reports, which are then published.[124] The United Kingdom and most members of the former Commonwealth use the *yellow card* system, whereby a reporting form is attached to officially issued prescription pads.[110,115] Data on adverse drug (including vaccine) events from about 40 nations are compiled by the WHO Collaborating Center for International Drug Monitoring in Uppsala.[134]

With so many different passive surveillance systems that collect information on various medical events following vaccination, standardized definitions of vaccine-related adverse events are necessary. In the past, different definitions were developed in Brazil,[125] Canada,[117] India,[120] and the Netherlands.[124] However, real progress in implementation of similar standards across national boundaries is only beginning to be realized with the advent of the International Conference on Harmonization[135] and the Brighton Collaboration (see *Prelicensure* above). [95]

The VAERS often first identifies potential new vaccine safety problems because of clusters of unusual clinical features in time or space. For example, a report by a concerned mother of recurrent alopecia after successive hepatitis B vaccinations in her child led to a review of VAERS data that showed several other similar reports.[136] GBS was the only illness reported more commonly in the second and third week than in the first week after swine influenza vaccination. This unusual finding led to initiation of special validation studies.[47,137] Passive reports to the VAERS of intussusception among children vaccinated with RRV was the first postlicensure signal of a problem,[138] leading to several studies to verify these findings.[57,58] Further analysis of RRV reports to the VAERS suggested it maybe the tip of an iceberg.[139] Similarly, initial reports to the VAERS of a previously unrecognized serious yellow fever vaccine–associated neurotropic disease[140] and viscerotropic disease[141,142] have since been confirmed elsewhere.[143] The Canadian VAAE system recently detected an increase in oculorespiratory syndrome after one influenza vaccine.[139,144] In retrospect, a similar syndrome also may have occurred in past influenza seasons in other countries.[145] Because of the success in detecting these signals, there have been various attempts to automate screening for signals using SRS reports. New tools developed for pattern recognition in extremely large databases are beginning to be applied.[146]

The large number of doses administered over a well-defined short time in mass immunization campaigns often result in more prominent clusters of vaccine-related adverse events, either previously known or, more importantly, previously unknown. New guidelines for injection safety and surveillance for immunization safety during mass immunization campaigns have been developed by the WHO.[147] Historically, such surveillance has been very useful in generating signals, either positive (e.g., GBS with swine

TABLE 61–2 ■ Distribution of Reports to the Vaccine Adverse Event Reporting System (VAERS), 1991–2002

Year (of Vaccination)	Total Reports*	Serious Reports Excluding Deaths†	Death Reports	Net Doses Sold (in millions)
1991	9944	1095	161	124
1992	10,697	1133	219	134
1993	10,165	1092	219	141
1994	10,192	1172	224	164
1995	10,024	1095	141	147
1996	10,824	975	124	147
1997	11,087	936	136	156
1998	10,068	911	132	192
1999	12,372	1283	144	198
2000	14,139	1085	145	206
2001	13,453	1303	175	198
2002	14,199	1291	137	‡

*Reports received as of January 15, 2003. Excluding foreign reports
†Nonfatal serious if a report indicated at least one of the following: life-threatening illness, hospitalization, extended length of hospitalization, and/or disability.
‡Data pending as of January 15, 2003

influenza vaccine,[47] GBS after OPV,[148] allergic reactions after Japanese encephalitis vaccine,[149] neuropathy after rubella vaccine,[150] aseptic meningitis after measles-mumps-rubella vaccine,[14,151] and serious adverse events after yellow fever vaccination[152]) or negative (e.g., events after meningococcal vaccine[153] and GBS or other events after measles vaccine[154,155]). The impact of new immunization recommendations may be analogous to a mass campaign even though they were not designed as such. Approximately 25 million French were immunized with hepatitis B vaccine between 1993 and 1997 in accordance with a new recommendation. Subsequent reports of demyelinating and other autoimmune diseases to French pharmacovigilance centers resulted in substantial turmoil.[44,156] Initial reports of autism following measles vaccine in the United Kingdom followed a national catch-up campaign.[157] Such signals from mass exposures are at best ecologic studies and still require validation, however. After more careful scientific studies, some signals are not validated (e.g., GBS after OPV[158]), are equivocal or negative (e.g., hepatitis B vaccine and demyelination[159-161]), or show multiple causes.[162]

Several lessons are beginning to emerge from SRSs, such as the VAERS.[87,131,163] The VAERS has successfully detected unrecognized potential reactions and obtained data to evaluate whether these events are causally linked to vaccines.[136] The VAERS has also successfully served as a source of cases for further investigation of idiopathic thrombocytopenic purpura after measles-mumps-rubella (MMR) vaccine,[164] encephalopathy after MMR,[117,165] and syncope after immunization.[166] The VAERS has been of great value for answering routine public queries (e.g., Has adverse event X ever been reported after vaccine Y?). When denominator data on doses are available from other sources, the VAERS can be used to evaluate changes in reporting rates over time or when new vaccines replace old vaccines. For example, the VAERS showed that, after millions of doses had been distributed, reporting rates for serious events such as hospitalization and seizures after DTaP in toddlers were one third those after diphtheria and tetanus toxoids and whole-cell pertussis (DTP).[167] Because the VAERS is the only surveillance system covering the entire U.S. population with data available on a relatively timely basis, it is the major means available currently to detect possible new, unusual, or extremely rare adverse events, including whether certain lots of vaccines are associated with unusually high rates of adverse events.[87,123]

The reporting efficiency or sensitivity of SRSs can be estimated if expected rates of adverse events generated from carefully executed studies are available. A higher proportion of serious events, such as seizures, that follow vaccinations are likely to be reported to the VAERS than milder events, such as rash, or delayed events requiring laboratory assessment, such as thrombocytopenic purpura after MMR vaccination (Table 61-3).[168] The estimate of VAERS reporting completeness for intussusception using capture-recapture methods was 47%.[169] Although formal evaluation has been limited, the probability that a serious event reported to the VAERS has been diagnosed accurately (i.e., predictive value is positive) is likely to be high. Of 26 patients reported to the VAERS who developed GBS after influenza vaccination during the 1990 to 1991 season, and whose hospital charts were reviewed by an independent panel of neurologists blinded to immunization status, the diagnosis of GBS was confirmed in 22 (85%).[170]

Despite the aforementioned uses, SRSs for drug and vaccine safety have a number of major methodologic weaknesses. Under-reporting, biased reporting, and incomplete reporting are inherent to all such SRSs, and potential safety concerns may be missed.[168,171,172] Aseptic meningitis associated with the Urabe mumps vaccine strain, for example, was not detected by SRSs in most countries.[32,78] Some increases in adverse events detected by the VAERS may not be true increases, but instead may be due to increases in reporting efficiency or vaccine coverage. For example, an increase in GBS reports after influenza vaccination during the 1993 to 1994 season was found to be largely due to improvements in vaccine coverage and increases in GBS independent of vaccination.[162] An increased reporting rate of an adverse event after one hepatitis B vaccine compared with a second brand was likely due to differential distribution of brands in the public versus private sectors, which

TABLE 61-3 ■ Reporting Efficiencies for Selected Outcomes in Two Passive Surveillance Systems for Vaccine Adverse Events—United States

Adverse Event	Vaccine	Reporting Efficiency (%)		
		MSAEFI	VAERS (Overall)	VAERS (Public Sector)
Vaccine-associated polio	OPV	72	68	*
Seizures	DTP	42	24	36
Seizures	MMR	23	37	49
Hypotonic-hyporesponsive episodes	DTP	4	3	4
Rash	MMR	<1	<1	5
Thrombocytopenia	MMR	<1	4	<1

DTP, diphtheria and tetanus toxoids and pertussis; MMR, measles-mumps-rubella; MSAEFI, Monitoring System for Adverse Events Following Immunizations; OPV, oral poliovirus vaccine; VAERS, Vaccine Adverse Event Reporting System.
*Public versus private sector information is missing on these cases.
Data from Rosenthal S, Chen RT. Reporting sensitivities of two passive surveillance systems for vaccine adverse events. Am J Public Health 85:1706–1709, 1995.

have differential VAERS reporting rates (higher in the public sector).[173]

Perhaps the most important methodologic weakness of the VAERS or other SRSs, however, is that such signals do not contain the information necessary for formal epidemiologic analyses. Such analyses require calculation of the rate of the adverse events after vaccination ($a/(a + b)$ in Table 61–4) using SRS case reports (or other more complete sources; see later) for the numerator and, if available, doses of vaccines administered (or, if unavailable, data on vaccine doses distributed or vaccine coverage survey data are used as surrogates) for the denominator. These rates are compared with the background rate of the same adverse event in the absence of vaccination if available ($c/(c + d)$ in Table 61–4). Because SRS databases provide data only for cell a in Table 61–4, and, even then, only in a biased and under-reported manner, they fundamentally lack the data in the other three cells needed to calculate rates and (1) generate accurate signals of potential vaccine safety problems or (2) make a rigorous epidemiologic assessment of the role of vaccine in causation.

These studies highlight the often crude nature of signals generated by the VAERS, and the difficulty in ascertaining which vaccine safety concerns warrant further investigation. The problems with reporting efficiency and potentially biased reporting, and the inherent lack of an adequate control group, limit the certainty with which conclusions can be drawn. Recognition of these limitations led to the creation of more population-based methods of ascertaining vaccine safety, such as the Vaccine Safety Datalink (VSD) project (described below).

Postlicensure Clinical Trials and Phase IV Surveillance Studies

Vaccines may undergo clinical trials after licensure to assess the effects of changes in vaccine formulation,[174] vaccine strain,[175] age at vaccination,[176] number and timing of vaccine doses,[177] simultaneous administration,[178] and interchangeability of vaccines from different manufacturers on vaccine safety and immunogenicity.[179] Unanticipated differential mortality among recipients of high- and regular-titer measles vaccine in developing countries[103] (albeit lower than among unvaccinated children)[180] led to a change in recommendations by the WHO for the use of such vaccines.[181]

TABLE 61–4 ■ 2 × 2 Table Necessary for Epidemiologic Analysis of Causality Between Vaccine and an Adverse Event

	Adverse Event	
Vaccinated	Yes	No
Yes	a	b
No	c	d

Rate of adverse event after vaccination = $a/(a + b)$.
Rate of adverse event in the absence of vaccination = $c/(c + d)$.
Reports to passive surveillance systems for vaccine adverse events (e.g., Vaccine Adverse Event Reporting System) represent just partial information (because of under-reporting and biased reporting) for cell a of the table. Epidemiologic studies aim to gather information for all four cells of this table in an unbiased manner.

To improve the ability to detect adverse events that are not detected during prelicensure trials, most recently licensed vaccines in developed countries have undergone formal Phase IV surveillance studies on populations with sample sizes of approximately 10^5. These studies usually have used cohorts in health maintenance organizations (HMOs) supplemented by diary or phone interview. These methods were first used extensively after the licensure of polysaccharide and conjugated *Haemophilus influenzae* type b vaccines.[182–184] Postlicensure studies on safety and efficacy of infant DTaP are also continuing.[97] Extensive Phase IV evaluation of varicella vaccine includes multiyear evaluation for disease incidence and for herpes zoster, and a pregnancy registry.[185,186] Requirements for Phase IV evaluation have even been extended to less frequently used vaccines, such as Japanese encephalitis vaccine.[187]

Large Linked Databases, Including the Vaccine Safety Datalink Project

Historically, ad hoc epidemiologic studies have been employed to assess signals of potential adverse events detected by SRSs, the medical literature, or other mechanisms. Some examples of such studies include the investigations of poliomyelitis after inactivated[66] and oral[188] polio vaccines, sudden infant death syndrome after DTP vaccination,[189–192] encephalopathy after DTP vaccination,[50,193] meningoencephalitis after mumps vaccination,[76,78] injection site abscesses postvaccination,[194] and GBS after influenza vaccination.[47,162,170] The IOM has compiled and reviewed many of these studies.[29,30]

Unfortunately, such ad hoc studies are often costly, time consuming, and limited to assessment of a single event. Given these drawbacks, and the methodologic limitations of passive surveillance systems (such as described for the VAERS), pharmacoepidemiologists began to turn to LLDBs linking computerized pharmacy prescription (and later immunization) and medical outcome records.[172] These databases derive from defined populations such as members of HMOs, single-provider health care systems, and Medicaid programs. Such LLDBs cover enrollee populations numbering from thousands to millions, good for examining relatively infrequent adverse events, and, because the data are generated from the routine administration of the full range of medical care, under-reporting and recall bias are reduced. With denominator data on doses administered and the ready availability of appropriate comparison (i.e., unvaccinated) groups, LLDBs provide an economical and rapid means of conducting postlicensure studies of safety of drugs and vaccines.[32,38,39,195,196]

The CDC participated in two pilot vaccine safety studies using LLDBs in Medicaid and HMO populations during the late 1980s.[197–198] These projects validated this approach for vaccine safety studies and provided scientifically rigorous results but were limited by relatively small sample sizes, retrospective design, and focus on the most severe reactions.[29] The CDC initiated the VSD project in 1990,[38] with the goal of gathering vaccination, medical outcome (e.g., hospital discharge, outpatient visits, emergency department visits, and deaths), and covariate (e.g., birth certificates, census) data under joint protocol at multiple HMOs. Selection of staff-model prepaid health plans also minimized potential biases for more severe outcomes resulting from data generated from fee-for-service claims. Originally, the VSD project conducted active surveillance on approximately 500,000 children from birth through 6 years of age (with a birth cohort of 75,000, approximately 2% of the U.S. population in this age group),[38] but it has been expanded to include seven HMOs (covering eight different health plans), with three HMOs also contributing information on adolescents and adults.[196] Proposals for studies are initiated by scientists at the CDC or at the participating HMOs, and study protocols are reviewed and critiqued using a standardized process. There is rigorous attention to the maintenance of patient confidentiality, and each study undergoes Institutional Review Board review. Plans are underway to expand this access to others.

The VSD project focused its initial efforts on examining potential associations between immunizations and a series of serious neurologic, allergic, hematologic, infectious, inflammatory, and metabolic conditions. However, the VSD project also is being used to test new ad hoc vaccine safety concerns that may arise from the medical literature,[29,30] from VAERS,[58,173] from changes in immunization schedules,[199] or from introduction of new vaccines.[183,184] The size of the VSD population also may permit separation of the risks associated with individual vaccines from those associated with vaccine combinations, whether given in the same syringe or simultaneously at different body sites. Such studies are especially valuable in view of the new combined pediatric vaccines currently in development.[200] Over 30 studies are currently underway within the VSD project,[196] including general screening studies of the safety of inactivated flu vaccines among children, and of thimerosal-containing vaccines. Disease- or syndromic-specific investigations are also underway, including ones investigating autism, multiple sclerosis, thyroid disease, acute ataxia, alopecia, rheumatoid arthritis, asthma, diabetes, and idiopathic thrombocytopenic purpura following vaccination. In addition, the infrastructure created by the VSD project easily lends itself to a wide range of other vaccine-related studies beyond those for safety.[38,196]

Amid these promises, a few caveats are appropriate. Although diverse, the population in the HMOs currently in the VSD project is not wholly representative of the United States in terms of geography or socioeconomic status. More importantly, because of the high coverage attained in the HMOs for most vaccines, few nonvaccinated controls are available. The VSD project must therefore rely primarily on *risk-interval* analyses (Table 61–5).[197,201] This approach has limited ability to assess associations between vaccination and adverse events with delayed or insidious onset (e.g., autism). The VSD project also cannot easily assess mild adverse events (such as fever) that do not always come to medical attention.[38] The current VSD project is also not large enough to examine the risk of extremely rare events, such as GBS, after each season's influenza vaccine. Finally, because vaccines are not delivered in the context of randomized, controlled trials, the VSD project may not be able to successfully control for confounding and bias in each analysis,[82] and inferences on causality may be limited.[85]

Despite these potential shortcomings, the VSD project provides an essential, powerful, and cost-effective complement to ongoing evaluations of vaccine safety in the United States.[195,196] In view of the methodologic and logistic advantages offered by LLDBs, the United Kingdom and Canada also have developed LLDBs linking immunization registries with medical files.[32,88] Because of the relatively limited number of vaccines used worldwide and the costs associated with establishing and operating LLDBs, it is unlikely that all countries will be able to or need to establish their own. These countries should be able to draw on the scientific base established by the existing LLDBs for vaccine safety and, if the need arises, conduct ad hoc epidemiologic studies.

TABLE 61–5 ■ Example of Method for Risk-Interval Analysis of Association Between a Universally Recommended Three-Dose Vaccine (With Few Unvaccinated Persons for Comparison) and an Adverse Event

1. Define biologically plausible *risk interval* for adverse event after vaccination (e.g., 30 days after each dose).
2. Partition observation time for each child in the study into periods within and outside of risk intervals, and sum respectively (e.g., for a child observed for 365 days during which 3 doses of vaccine were received, total risk interval time = 3 × 30 person-days = 90 person-days; total nonrisk interval time = 365 - 90 = 275 person-days).

```
0-------------x====---------x====-------------x====-------//----->|
Birth        Dose 1       Dose 2            Dose 3    365 days
```

3. Add up (a) total risk interval and nonrisk interval observation times for each child in the study (= Person-Time Observed; for mathematical convenience, example below uses 100 and 1000 person-months of observation), and (b) adverse events occurring in each time period to complete 2 × 2 table (for illustration, example below uses 3 and 10 cases):

Vaccinated in Risk Interval	Adverse Event: Yes	Person-Time Observed (mo)	Incidence Rate
Yes	3	100	0.03
No	10	1000	0.01
TOTAL	13	1100	

Incidence rate adverse event$_{vaccinated}$ = 3/100 = 0.03
Incidence rate adverse event$_{unvaccinated}$ = 10/1000 = 0.01
Relative rate vaccinated: unvaccinated = 0.03/0.01 = 3.0
Probability finding is due to chance: <5/100
Conclusion: There is a threefold increase in risk for developing the adverse event within the 30 day interval after vaccination compared to other time periods.

Clinical Centers, Including the Clinical Immunization Safety Assessment (CISA) Centers

More recently, there has been an increasing awareness that the utility of SRSs as potential disease registries and the immunization safety infrastructure can be usefully augmented by tertiary clinical centers. Modern medicine cannot make progress on rare disorders such as leukemia (or serious vaccine-related adverse events) by relying on primary care providers alone. Instead, subspecialties with an adequate referral base and research funds (e.g., hematology/oncology) are needed. With the exception of certain regions in Italy[202] and Australia,[203,204] a similar well-organized, well-identified subspecialty infrastructure has been missing for the study of rare vaccine safety outcomes in most countries.

The United States created its Clinical Immunization Safety Assessment (CISA) network with four sites in 2001, bringing together infectious disease epidemiologists, immunologists, dermatologists, and other subspecialists as needed.[107] Among their tasks will be the standardized assessment of persons who suffered a true vaccine reaction (e.g., anaphylaxis, intussusception) to improve our scientific understanding of the pathophysiology and risk factors of the reaction. Because most persons are vaccinated without such complications, those who suffer such reactions are clearly outliers in a biologic gaussian spectrum. New understanding of the human genome, pharmacogenomics, and immunology may now make it possible for us to truly understand the reaction.[205] Second, standardized assessment protocols will be developed to examine patients with similar adverse events to see if they may constitute a previously unrecognized clinical syndrome. If so, a case definition could then be developed that would permit the identification of cases for follow-up validation studies examining the potential role of vaccination in causing this syndrome.

Third, for patients who had an adverse event that is not contraindicating but generates enough concern to interfere with completion of the series, the CISA centers can provide assessment and management under protocols, as was done with hypotonic-hyporesponsive episodes.[203] Finally, the CISA centers can provide regional referral and advice services—with the major difference that, whenever advice is provided, follow-up and documentation of compliance and outcome will be done so that this rare experience is added to our scientific knowledge. Ultimately, many of the above protocols will be made available on the World Wide Web for other clinicians to use (and contribute their experience).[206] During its first year, the CISA network focused on a study to assess severe limb swelling after DTaP, of alopecia following hepatitis B vaccination, and of adverse events following smallpox vaccination.

New Challenges and Directions in the Study of Vaccine Safety

Unfortunately, vaccine safety issues have increasingly taken on a life of their own outside of the scientific arena— arguably to society's overall detriment. Liability concerns, for example, have severely limited development of maternal immunizations against diseases such as group B streptococcus.[207] More worrisome, however, are various chronic diseases (and their advocates) in search of a simple cause, for which immunizations—as a relatively universal exposure— make all too convenient a hypothesized link. Case studies of some of these diseases are discussed in the following sections.

AUTISM

Autism is a profound and chronic developmental disorder characterized by problems in social interaction, communication, and responsiveness, and by repetitive interests and activities. It affects between 4 and 10 children out of 10,000. About one quarter of autistic children have a subtype of autism wherein an apparently normal child undergoes developmental regression. Although the causes of autism are largely unknown, family and twin studies suggest that genetics plays a fundamental role.[208] In addition, overexpression of neuropeptides and neurotrophins has been found in the immediate perinatal period among children later diagnosed with autism, suggesting that prenatal and/or perinatal influences play a more important role than postnatal insults.[209] However, because autistic symptoms generally first become apparent in the second year of life, some scientists and parents have focused on the role of MMR vaccine because it is first administered around this time. Concern over the role of MMR vaccine became heightened in 1998 when a study based on 12 children proposed an association between the vaccine and the development of ileonodular hyperplasia, nonspecific colitis, and regressive developmental disorders (later termed by some as "autistic enterocolitis").[157] Among the proposed mechanisms was that MMR vaccine caused bowel problems, leading to the malabsorption of essential vitamins and other nutrients and eventually to autism and/or other developmental disorders. Concern about this issue has led to a decline in measles vaccine coverage in the United Kingdom and elsewhere.[9]

There were a number of significant concerns about the validity of the study, including the lack of an adequate control or comparison group, inconsistent timing to support causality (several of the children had autistic symptoms preceding bowel symptoms), and the lack of an accepted definition of the syndrome.[210] Subsequently, population-based studies of autistic children in the United Kingdom found no association between receipt of MMR vaccine and autism onset or developmental regression.[210a,211] A study in the United States within the VSD project investigated whether measles-containing vaccine was associated with inflammatory bowel disease, and found no relationship between ever receiving MMR vaccine and inflammatory bowel disease, or between the timing of the vaccine and risk for disease.[212] Two ecologic analyses found no evidence that MMR vaccination was the cause of apparent increased trends in autism over time,[213,214] while two other studies found no evidence of a new variant form of autism associated with bowel disorders secondary to vaccination.[215,216]

Because of the level of concern surrounding this issue, the CDC and the National Institutes of Health requested an independent review by the IOM.[217] The Immunization Safety Review Committee appointed by the IOM to review this issue was unable to find evidence supporting a causal relationship at the population level between autistic spectrum disorders and MMR vaccination, nor did the committee find any good evidence of biologic mechanisms that would support or explain such a link. However, the committee also acknowledged the possibility that epidemiologic studies in general could not rule out the possibility that, in a small number of children, MMR vaccine might contribute to the risk for autism or autistic spectrum disorder.

To help answer these residual concerns surrounding measles-containing vaccines and autism, a number of large studies are currently underway in the United States and Europe, including ones that focus specifically on the relationship between MMR and the onset of regressive-type autism, and others that address the relationship between thimerosal (see below) in vaccines and risk for autism.

THIMEROSAL

Vaccines use biologic substrates for their production and contain a variety of additives necessary for both their efficacy and safety. These include adjuvants such as aluminum salts to enhance immunogenicity, and preservatives such as thimerosal (which contains 49.6% mercury) or phenol that are vital to prevent contamination and subsequent bacterial or fungal growth in multidose vials that are repeatedly punctured and stored.

The Food and Drug Administration Modernization Act of 1997 called for the FDA to review and assess the risk of all mercury-containing food and drugs. This led to an examination of mercury content in vaccines and the observation that the current immunization schedule with multiple injections may expose some children to mercury that exceeds some exposure guidelines. Consequently, the routine neonatal dose of hepatitis B vaccine in infants born to hepatitis B surface antigen (HBsAg)–negative mothers was suspended in the United States[70] until preservative-free vaccines became available, and transitioning to a vaccine schedule free of thimerosal began as a precautionary measure.[218] However, for reasons of cost, production, and storage capacity, the vaccination of children in much of the world will continue to require the use of multidose vials—which in turn requires a preservative to prevent microbial contamination after the vial is opened. Thimerosal is therefore currently preferred by many countries outside the United States, though the WHO will transition to an alternative as soon as an equally effective one becomes available.

The question remains whether thimerosal exposure has done harm.[219] Thimerosal is an organic mercury compound that is metabolized to ethyl mercury and thiosalicylate. In studies of fetal exposure in humans to another organic mercury compound—*methyl*mercury—via fish ingestion during pregnancy, one study revealed subtle neurodevelopmental effects[220] while another did not.[221] In other human studies of acute, higher exposure (many times greater than any likely ethyl mercury exposure from vaccination), methylmercury has been found to affect both the neurologic and renal systems.[222,223] Although exposure limits were set for methylmercury, there is a lack of good data that relate the toxicity of ethyl mercury to methylmercury. One small human study suggests that ethyl mercury is readily cleared from blood via the stools after injection.[224] It is unclear how intermittent "injection" exposures (from periodic vaccinations) should be extrapolated to the chronic daily intake that formed the basis of exposure guidelines. These gaps in our knowledge limit the scientific community's ability to estimate any potentially harmful effects of thimerosal.

A number of current studies are beginning to add to the available data. A study published in the *Journal of Pediatrics*

examined the impact of a birth dose of hepatitis B vaccine on blood mercury levels in the preterm newborn[225] and found levels of 2.9 μg/L or higher in 9 of 15 premature infants vaccinated with hepatitis B. (Hepatitis B vaccine is not recommended for infants with birth weight less than 2000 g unless their mother is HBsAg positive). The Advisory Committee on Immunization Practices (ACIP) has reviewed a set of as-yet unpublished studies from the VSD project that focused on neurodevelopmental outcomes among infants following vaccination with thimerosal-containing products. Although a number of associations between thimerosal and some neurodevelopmental outcomes (including speech and language delay and attention-deficit disorder) were found, the strength of the associations was relatively weak and inconsistent. After reviewing this evidence, the ACIP issued a joint statement with other U.S. public health agencies[226] (*www.cdc.gov/nip/vacsafe/concerns/thimerosal/joint_statement_00.htm*) that re-emphasized the appropriateness of continuing the use of vaccines that contain thimerosal until adequate supplies of new products are available. The Immunization Safety Review Committee of the IOM also reviewed these data, and believed that the existing data were inadequate to either accept or reject an epidemiologic relationship between thimerosal exposure from vaccines and neurodevelopmental disorders.[227] Nevertheless, the report stated that such a link was biologically plausible, and recommended the use of thimerosal-free vaccines. Follow-up studies that address many of the shortcomings pointed out by the IOM and the ACIP are currently underway within the VSD project and elsewhere.[227a] The VSD study will involve in-depth neurodevelopmental examinations of children exposed to different levels of thimerosal from the vaccination schedule.

One known and unfortunate sequela from the uncertainty surrounding the safety of thimerosal was confusion surrounding administration of the birth dose of hepatitis B vaccine. Following the suspension of the routine use of hepatitis B vaccine for low-risk newborns in 1999, there was a marked increase in the number of hospitals that no longer routinely vaccinated all infants at high risk of hepatitis B.[228] As a result, there have been cases of neonatal hepatitis B that could have been prevented, but were not, because of many hospitals suspending their routine neonatal hepatitis B vaccination program.[228a]

DIABETES

Some researchers have suggested that certain vaccinations, if administered at birth, decrease the risk for diabetes, whereas these same vaccines, if administered after 2 months of age, increase the risk for type 1 diabetes mellitus.[229] This theory is based on comparing rates of diabetes between countries with different immunization schedules. However, such evidence is fraught with uncertainty because such countries also vary markedly with respect to other risk factors for diabetes that also might be changing over time. More rigorous epidemiologic studies of infant vaccines and type 1 diabetes found that measles vaccine was associated with a decreased risk for diabetes, and no association was found between bacille Calmette-Guérin (BCG), smallpox, tetanus, pertussis, rubella, or mumps vaccine.[230] A study in Canada found no increase in risk for diabetes as a result of receipt of BCG vaccine.[231] In a large 10-year follow-up study among Finnish children enrolled in a *H. influenzae* type b vaccination trial, no differences in risk for diabetes were found among children vaccinated at 3 months of age, followed later with a booster vaccine, and those vaccinated at 2 years only, or with children born prior to the vaccine trial. The weight of currently available epidemiologic evidence does not support a causal association between currently recommended vaccines and type 1 diabetes in humans. [40,232,233]

ASTHMA

Although the etiology of childhood asthma is unknown, some have suggested that routine vaccinations, especially with pertussis-containing vaccines, may increase the risk of developing asthma in childhood. The main proposed mechanism is thought to be via induction of immune cells producing type 2 T-helper cell (Th2) cytokines, which appear to play essential roles in the development of allergic reactions and, possibly, asthma. [234] Increasing evidence suggests that continuous domination of Th2-like cells since birth may be associated with the development of atopic diseases, including asthma. [235] Although some relatively small early observational studies supported the association between whole-cell pertussis vaccine and development of asthma, [236] more recent studies have suggested otherwise. A large clinical trial performed in Sweden found no increased risk, [237] and a very large longitudinal study in the United Kingdom found no association between pertussis vaccination and early- or late-onset wheezing, or recurrent or intermittent wheezing. [238] Two studies from the VSD project have also lent data to this controversy. In one study of 1366 infants with wheezing during infancy, vaccination with DTP and other vaccines was not related to the risk of wheezing in full-term infants, [239] and, in another study of over 165,000 children, childhood vaccinations were not associated with an increased risk for developing asthma. [240] Finally, a study from Finland also suggested that children with history of natural measles were at increased risk for atopic illness. Such findings would run contrary to the hypothesis that the increase in atopic illnesses seen in several countries is due to the reduction in wild measles resulting from immunizations. [241]

Another separate concern is whether influenza vaccination may induce asthma exacerbations in children with pre-existing asthma. Results of studies examining the potential associations between administration of influenza vaccine and various surrogate measures of asthma exacerbation, including decreased peak expiratory flow rate, increased use of bronchodilating drugs, and increase in asthma symptoms, have yielded mixed results. Most studies, however, have not supported such an association. [242] In fact, in another study, after controlling for asthma severity, acute asthma exacerbations were less common after influenza vaccination than before, [243] and influenza vaccination appears to be associated with a decreased risk for asthma exacerbations throughout influenza seasons. [244] Overall, the benefits of vaccination outweigh any theoretical risk of asthma exacerbation.

Vaccine Risk Communication

Disease prevention, especially if it requires continuous near-universal compliance, is a formidable task. In the preimmunization era, vaccine-preventable diseases such as measles and pertussis were so prevalent that the risks and benefits of disease versus vaccination were readily evident. As immunization programs successfully reduced the incidence of vaccine-preventable diseases, however, an increasing proportion of health care providers and parents have little or no personal experience with vaccine-preventable diseases. For their risk-benefit analysis, they are forced to rely on historical and other more distant descriptions of vaccine-preventable diseases in textbooks or educational brochures. In contrast, some degree of personal discomfort and pain generally is associated with each immunization. In addition, parents searching for information about vaccines on the World Wide Web are highly likely to encounter web sites that encourage vaccine refusal or emphasize the dangers of vaccines. [245,246] Similarly, the media may sensationalize vaccine safety issues or, in an effort to present "both sides" of an argument, fail to provide perspective. [42,247] For reasons discussed earlier, there may be uncertainty if vaccines can cause certain rare or delayed serious reactions (if only because the studies to demonstrate the negative have not or cannot be done). The combination of these factors may have an impact on parental beliefs about immunizations. A national survey of parents found that, although the majority support immunizations, 20% to 25% have misconceptions that could erode their confidence in vaccines. [248] Within this context, the art of addressing vaccine safety concerns through effective risk communication has emerged as an increasingly important skill for managers of mature immunization programs and health care providers who administer vaccines.

Risk Communication Principles

The science of risk perceptions and risk communications, developed initially for technology and environmental arenas, [249] has only recently been formally applied to immunizations. [250] For scientists and other experts, risk tends to be synonymous with the objective probability of morbidity and mortality resulting from exposure to a particular hazard. [251] In contrast, research has shown that laypersons may have subjective, multidimensional, and value-laden conceptualizations of risk. [252] Among the key principles and lessons learned about public perceptions of risk are the following:

1. Individuals differ in their perceptions of risk depending on their personality, education, life experience, and personal values [253,254]; educational materials *tiered* for different needs are therefore likely to be more effective than a single tier.
2. Perceptions of risk may differ dramatically among various *stakeholders*, such as members of government agencies, industry, or activist groups. [255] The level of trust between stakeholders has an impact on all other aspects of risk communication. [256] Trust is generally reinforced by open communication regarding what is known and unknown about risks and by providing candid accounts of the evidence and how it was used in the decision-making process. [257]
3. Certain hazard characteristics, including involuntariness, uncertainty, lack of control, high level of dread, and low level of equity, lead to higher perceived risk [252]; only risks with similar characteristics should be compared in risk communication efforts. [258] There

are relatively few (if any) infant experiences similar enough to immunizations in their risk profile to make for easy comparisons.

4. For quantitatively equivalent risk that is due to action (e.g., vaccination reaction) versus inaction (e.g., vaccine-preventable disease caused by nonvaccination), many people have an *omission bias* in that they prefer the consequences of inaction to action.[259]

5. When there is uncertainty about risks, patients frequently rely on the advice of their physician or other health care professionals; continuing education of health care professionals on vaccine risk issues is therefore key.[248]

6. Finally, different ways of presenting, or framing, the same risk information (e.g., using survival rates versus mortality rates) can lead to different risk perceptions, decisions, and behaviors.[260,261]

Risk communication can be used for the purposes of advocacy, public education, or decision-making partnership.[249] People care not only about the magnitude of risks, but also how risks are managed and whether they participate in the risk management process, especially in a democratic society.[262] In medical decision making, this has resulted in a transition from more paternalistic models to increasing degrees of informed consent.[263] Some have argued that a similar transition to informed consent also should occur with immunizations.[264] However, immunization is unlike most other medical procedures (e.g., surgery) in that the consequences of the decision affect not only the individual, but also others in the society. Because of this important distinction, many countries have enacted public health (e.g., immunization) laws that severely limit any individual's right to infect others. Without such mandates, individuals may attempt to avoid the risks of vaccination while being protected by the herd immunity resulting from others being vaccinated.[265] Unfortunately, the protection provided by herd immunity may disappear if too many people avoid vaccination, resulting in outbreaks of vaccine-preventable diseases.[266,267] Debates in the United States have focused on whether philosophical (in addition to medical and religious) exemptions to mandatory immunizations should be allowed more universally and, if so, what standards for claim of exemption are needed.[65,264,268] Thus vaccine risk communications not only should describe the risks and benefits of vaccines for individuals, but also should include discussion of the impact of individual immunization decisions on the larger community.

Evaluating and Addressing Vaccine Safety Concerns

A healthy dose of empathy, patience, scientific curiosity, and substantial resources may be needed to address a vaccine safety concern. Although each evaluation of a vaccine safety concern is in some ways unique, some general principles may apply to most cases. As with all investigations, the first step is objective and comprehensive data gathering with an open mind.[6] Premature dismissal of new vaccine safety concerns as unfounded without gathering and weighing the evidence is unwise and unscientific. Novel reactions such as alopecia after hepatitis B vaccine were rejected initially,[136] sometimes even after substantial evidence had accumulated.[78] It is also important to gather and weigh evidence for causes other

than vaccination. For individual cases or clusters of cases, a field investigation to gather data firsthand may be necessary.[17,194] Advice and review from a panel of independent experts also may be needed.[56,170,269] Causality assessment at the individual level is difficult at best; further evaluation via epidemiologic or laboratory studies may be required.[269a] Even if the investigation is inconclusive, a sincere and honest search for the truth (vs. protecting the immunization program) can help dispel allegations of cover-up and maintain public trust in immunization programs.[270]

Scientific investigations are only the beginning of addressing a vaccine safety concern. In many countries, people who believe they or their children have been injured by vaccines have organized and produced information highlighting the risks of and alternatives to immunizations. From the consumer activist perspective, even if vaccine risks are rare, when you are the person who experiences the reaction, the risk is 100%.[271] Such groups have been increasingly successful in airing their views in both electronic and print media, frequently with poignant individual stories.[245,246] Because the media frequently aim to present both sides of the story when covering vaccine safety issues, one challenge is to establish credibility and trust with the audience.[272,273] Factors that aid in enhancing credibility include demonstrating scientific expertise, having established relationships with members of the media based on prior experience with difficult issues, expressing empathy, and distilling scientific facts and figures down to simple lay concepts. However, statistics and facts may compete poorly with dramatic pictures and stories of disabled children. Emotional reactions to messages are primary, occurring before and influencing subsequent cognitive processing.[274] Therefore, equally compelling firsthand accounts of people with vaccine-preventable diseases may be needed to communicate the risks associated with not vaccinating. Clarifying the distinction between perceived and real risk for the concerned public is critical. If further research is needed, the degree of uncertainty (e.g., whether such rare vaccine reactions exist at all) should be acknowledged, but what is certain also should be noted (e.g., millions of people have received vaccine X and have not developed syndrome Y; even if the vaccine causes Y, it is likely to be of magnitude Z, compared to the magnitude of known risks associated with vaccine-preventable diseases).

In the United States, written information about the risks and benefits of immunizations developed by the CDC has been required to be provided to all people vaccinated in the public sector since 1978.[275] The NCVIA requires every health care provider, public or private, who administers a vaccine that is covered by the act to provide a copy of the most current CDC Vaccine Information Statement (VIS) to either the adult vaccinee or, in the case of a minor, to the parent or legal representative each time a dose of vaccine is administered.[276] Health care providers must note in each patient's permanent medical record the date printed on the VIS and the date the VIS was given to the vaccine recipient, or his or her legal representative. VISs are the cornerstone of provider-patient vaccine risk/benefit communication. Each VIS contains information on the disease(s) that the vaccine prevents, who should receive the vaccine and when, contraindications, vaccine risks, what to do if a side effect occurs, and where to go for more information. Current VISs can be obtained from the CDC's National Immunization Program at *www.cdc. gov/nip* and are available in over 20 languages from the Immunization Action Coalition at *www.immunize.org*. An increasing number of resources that address vaccine safety misconceptions and allegations also have become available, including web sites, brochures, resource kits, and videos (more information on vaccine risk communication resources can be obtained at *www.cdc.gov/nip*). Some studies have been conducted to assess the use and effectiveness of such materials[277-281]; however, more research in this area is needed.

Immunization programs and health care providers should anticipate that some members of the public may have deep concerns regarding the need for or safety of vaccines. A few may refuse certain vaccines, or even reject all vaccinations. An understanding of vaccine risk perceptions and effective, empathetic vaccine risk communication are essential in responding to misinformation and concerns.

Scientifically Accepted Risks of Commonly Used Vaccines

Each chapter in this textbook on specific vaccines discusses the data on associated risks. The available scientific information on the risks associated with routine pediatric vaccines was systematically and exhaustively reviewed by the IOM in the early 1990s.[29,30] The IOM classified the available evidence as a case report, case series, uncontrolled study, or controlled study, with increasing levels of validity. The total evidence for a causal relationship between vaccine and a specific adverse event was weighed and then placed in one of five categories: (1) no evidence was available bearing on causality, (2) evidence was inadequate to accept or reject a causal relationship, (3) evidence favors rejection of a causal relationship, (4) evidence favors a causal relationship, and (5) evidence establishes a causal relationship.

As noted earlier, two thirds of the adverse events evaluated had either no (category 1) or inadequate (category 2) evidence for causality assessment, reflecting the need for additional research in vaccine safety. Relatively few associations were in either categories 4 or 5, in which the evidence either favored or established a causal relationship (Tables 61–6 and 61–7). In its update in 1996, the ACIP, while supporting the majority of IOM conclusions, reached different interpretations for some associations because of newly available evidence or different interpretations of the limited data reviewed by the IOM.[282] Further revisions will occur as new evidence becomes available on these and newer vaccines. For example, the latest research cast doubts

TABLE 61–6 ■ Summarized Conclusions of Evidence Regarding Possible Association Between Specific Adverse Events and Receipt of Diphtheria and Tetanus Toxoids and Pertussis Vaccine (DTP)[*] and RA 27/3[†] Rubella-Containing Vaccines, by Determination of Causality—Institute of Medicine, 1991[‡]

Conclusion, by Determination of Causality	Adverse Event Reviewed	
	DTP Vaccine	RA27/3 Rubella Vaccine
1. No evidence was available to establish a causal relationship	Autism	None
2. Inadequate evidence to accept or reject a causal relationship	Aseptic meningitis Chronic neurologic damage[§] Erythema multiforme or other rash Guillain-Barré syndrome Hemolytic anemia Juvenile diabetes Learning disabilities and attention-deficit disorder Peripheral mononeuropathy Thrombocytopenia	Radiculoneuritis and other neuropathies Thrombocytopenic purpura
3. Evidence favored rejection of a causal relationship	Infantile spasms Hypsarrhythmia Reye's syndrome Sudden infant death syndrome	None
4. Evidence favored acceptance of a causal relationship	Acute encephalopathy Shock and unusual shock-like state	Chronic arthritis
5. Evidence established a causal relationship	Anaphylaxis Protracted, inconsolable crying	Acute arthritis

[*]The evidence differentiated only between components of DTP in the event of protracted, inconsolable crying, for which the evidence specifically implicated the pertussis vaccine component.

[†]Trivalent measles-mumps-rubella (MMR) vaccine containing the RA27/3 rubella strain.

[‡]This table is an adaptation of a table published previously by the Institute of Medicine (IOM),[29] an independent research organization chartered by the National Academy of Sciences. The National Childhood Vaccine Injury Act of 1986 mandated that the IOM review scientific and other evidence (e.g., epidemiologic studies, case series, individual case reports, and testimonials) regarding the possible adverse consequences of vaccines administered to children. The IOM formed an expert committee to review and summarize all available information; this committee created five categories of causality to describe the relationships between the vaccines and specific adverse events.

[§]The IOM reviewed this adverse event again in 1994.[30]

[‖]Defined in the controlled studies that were reviewed as encephalopathy, encephalitis, or encephalomyelitis.

TABLE 61–7 ■ Summarized Conclusions of Evidence Regarding Possible Association Between Specific Adverse Events and Receipt of Childhood Vaccines, by Determination of Causality—Institute of Medicine, 1994*

DT/Td/Tetanus Toxoid†	Measles Vaccine‡	Mumps Vaccine‡	OPV/IPV§	Hepatitis B Vaccine	Haemophilus influenzae type B (Hib) Vaccine
1. No Evidence Available to Establish a Causal Relationship					
None	None	Neuropathy Residual seizure disorder	Transverse myelitis (IPV) Thrombocytopenia (IPV) Anaphylaxis (IPV)	None	None
2. Inadequate Evidence to Accept or Reject a Causal Relationship					
Residual seizure disorder other than infantile spasms	Encephalopathy	Encephalopathy	Transverse myelitis (OPV)	Guillain-Barré syndrome	Guillain-Barré syndrome
Demyelinating diseases of the central nervous system	Subacute sclerosing panencephalitis	Aseptic meningitis	Guillain-Barré syndrome (IPV)	Demyelinating diseases of the central nervous system	Transverse myelitis
Mononeuropathy	Residual seizure disorder	Sensorineural deafness (MMR)	Death from SIDS¶	Arthritis	Thrombocytopenia
Arthritis	Sensorineural deafness (MMR)	Insulin-dependent diabetes mellitus		Death from SIDS¶	Anaphylaxis
Erythema multiforme	Optic neuritis Transverse myelitis Guillain-Barré syndrome Thrombocytopenia Insulin-dependent diabetes mellitus	Sterility Thrombocytopenia Anaphylaxis			Death from SIDS¶
3. Evidence Favored Rejection of a Causal Relationship					
Encephalopathy**	None	None	None	None	Early-onset Hib disease (conjugate vaccines)
Infantile spasms (DT only)†† Death from SIDS (DT only)††,‡‡					
4. Evidence Favored Acceptance of a Causal Relationship					
Guillain-Barré syndrome§§ (ACIP disagreed)||||	Anaphylaxis||	None	Guillain-Barré syndrome (OPV) (ACIP disagreed)||||	None	Early-onset Hib disease in children ages ≥ 18 mo whose first Hib vaccination was with unconjugated PRP vaccine
Brachial neuritis§§					

5. Evidence Established a Causal Relationship

Anaphylaxis§§

Thrombocytopenia (MMR)   None
Anaphylaxis (MMR)
Death from measles vaccine–strain viral infection¶, ¶¶

Poliomyelitis in recipient or contact (OPV)
Death from polio vaccine–strain viral infection¶, ¶¶   Anaphylaxis   None

---

*This table is an adaptation of a table published previously by the Institute of Medicine (IOM),[30] an independent research organization chartered by the National Academy of Sciences. The National Childhood Vaccine Injury Act of 1986 mandated that the IOM review scientific and other evidence (e.g., epidemiological studies, case series, individual case reports, and testimonials) regarding the possible adverse consequences of vaccines administered to children. The IOM formed an expert committee to review and summarize all available information; this committee created five categories of causality to describe the relationships between the vaccines and specific adverse events.

†DT, diphtheria and tetanus toxoids for pediatric use; Td, diphtheria and tetanus toxoids for adult use.

‡If the data derived from studies of a monovalent preparation, the causal relationship also extended to multivalent preparations. If the data derived exclusively from studies of the measles-mumps-rubella (MMR) vaccine, the vaccine is specified parenthetically in *italics*. In the absence of data concerning the monovalent preparation, the causal relationship determined for the multivalent preparations did not extend to the monovalent components.

§For some adverse events, the IOM committee was charged with assessing the causal relationship between the adverse event and only oral poliovirus vaccine (OPV) (i.e., for poliomyelitis) or only inactivated poliovirus vaccine (IPV) (i.e., for anaphylaxis and thrombocytopenia). If the conclusions for the two vaccines differed for the other adverse events, the vaccine to which the adverse event applied is specified parenthetically in *italics*.

‖The evidence used to establish a causal relationship for anaphylaxis applies to MMR vaccine. The evidence regarding monovalent measles vaccine favored acceptance of a causal relationship, but this evidence was less convincing than that for MMR vaccine because of either incomplete documentation of symptoms or the possible attenuation of symptoms by medical intervention.

¶This table lists weight-of-evidence determinations only for deaths that were classified as sudden infant death syndrome (SIDS) and deaths that were a consequence of vaccine-strain viral infection. If the evidence favored the acceptance of (or established) a causal relationship between a vaccine and a possibly fatal adverse event, however, the evidence also favored the acceptance of (or established) a causal relationship between the vaccine and death from the adverse event. Direct evidence regarding death in association with a vaccine-associated adverse event was limited to (1) Td and Guillain-Barré syndrome, (2) tetanus toxoid and anaphylaxis, and (3) OPV and poliomyelitis.

**The evidence derived from studies of DT. If the evidence favored rejection of a causal relationship between DT and encephalopathy, the evidence also favored rejection of a causal relationship between Td and tetanus toxoid and encephalopathy.

††Infantile spasms and SIDS occur only in an age group that is administered DT but not Td or tetanus toxoid.

‡‡The evidence derived primarily from studies of DTP, although the evidence also favored rejection of a causal relationship between DT and SIDS.

§§The evidence derived from studies of tetanus toxoid. If the evidence favored acceptance of (or established) a causal relationship between tetanus toxoid and an adverse event, the evidence also favored acceptance of (or established) a causal relationship between DT and Td and the adverse event.

‖‖The Advisory Committee on Immunization Practices (ACIP) concurred with the findings of the IOM except where noted because of new information that became available after the IOM published this table.[282]

¶¶Deaths occurred primarily among persons known to be immunocompromised.

on the association between OPV and GBS[158] and between RA27/3 rubella vaccine and chronic arthropathy.[283-285]

More recently, the IOM has been funded by the U.S. government to form an Immunization Safety Review Committee.[286] To maximize its credibility as a panel of independent experts, its members do not have any previous ties to vaccinology. It meets three times a year to permit the timely assessment of a vaccine safety controversy, with reports issued 60 to 90 days later in formats more accessible to the lay public. Causality assessment, especially discussion of plausible biologic mechanisms, is more explicit than in prior IOM committees. Most importantly, the committee is asked to pronounce on the societal significance of an issue and make recommendations on policy review and communications in addition to the standard reviews of research and surveillance data. The topics reviewed by the committee to date have included (1) MMR and autism,[217] (2) vaccines containing thimerosal and neurodevelopmental disorders,[227] (3) multiple immunizations and harm to the developing immune system,[287] (4) the hepatitis B vaccine and demyelinating neurologic disorders,[288] and (5) simian virus 40 contamination of polio vaccine and cancer.[289] (Table 61–8). Separately, the IOM has also assessed the safety of the anthrax vaccine[290] and is expected to take an active role in examining the safety of the smallpox vaccine.

Comprehensive independent review of the risks associated with other routinely used vaccines, especially those used primarily by adults and travelers, is currently lacking. Relative to the IOM reviews, a review of these vaccines would be even more severely handicapped by the deficits of controlled studies with adequate power. The lack of accurate past vaccination histories among adults plus the range of locations in which adults may be vaccinated (e.g., occupational sites in addition to primary physician offices) also make future vaccine safety studies in older age groups especially difficult.

Future Challenges

Many people look to vaccines as the "magic bullet" solution to a number of public health problems that range from acquired immunodeficiency syndrome to malaria. Rapid advances in biotechnology have brought the promise of these new vaccines closer to reality.[46] Novel delivery technologies, such as DNA vaccines and new adjuvants, are being explored to permit more antigens to be combined, reducing the number of injections.[200,291] These changes in vaccines and vaccine delivery, however, will continue to provide additional challenges in proving their safety to an increasingly skeptical and risk-averse public.[292] Combined with methodologic difficulties associated with studying rare, delayed, or insidious vaccine safety allegations,[81] well-organized consumer activist organizations,[271] Internet information of questionable accuracy,[245,246] media eagerness for controversy,[42,272] and relatively rare individual encounters with vaccine-preventable diseases virtually ensure that vaccine safety concerns are unlikely to "go away" in mature immunization programs.

Concomitantly, vaccine safety concerns have also emerged as an issue in EPIs in developing countries.[293] The high-titer measles vaccine mortality experience highlighted the importance of improving the quality control and evaluating the safety of vaccines used in developing countries.[103,175] Plans to eliminate neonatal tetanus and measles via national immunization days, during which millions of

TABLE 61–8 ▪ Institute of Medicine Immunization Safety Review Committee Determinations of Causality for Various Adverse Events[217,227,287,288,289]

Causality Conclusion*	Hypothesis	Biologic Mechanisms or Plausibility Conclusions†
No evidence		
Evidence is inadequate to accept or reject a causal relationship	Thimerosal-containing vaccines and the neurodevelopmental disorders of autism, ADHD, and speech or language delay	Biologically plausible
	Multiple immunizations and allergic disease, particularly asthma	Weak (includes bystander activation and impaired immunoregulation)
	Hepatitis B vaccine and tristepisode CNS demyelinating disorder, ADEM, optic neuritis, transverse myelitis, GBS, and brachial neuritis	Weak
	SV40-containing polio vaccines and cancer	Strong—SV40 is a transforming virus Moderate—SV40 exposure could lead to cancer SV40 exposure from polio vaccine is related to SV40 infection in humans
Evidence favors rejection of a causal relationship	MMR vaccine and autism spectrum disorder, at the population level	Biologic model incomplete and fragmentary
	Multiple immunizations and heterologous infections	
	Multiple immunizations and type 1 diabetes‡	Weak—autoimmune disease (includes molecular mimicry [theoretical], bystander activation [weak], impaired immunoregulation [theoretical])
	Hepatitis B vaccine in adults and incident or relapse multiple sclerosis	
Evidence favors acceptance of a causal relationship		
Evidence establishes a causal relationship		

*Causality conclusion is based on epidemiologic evidence.

†Biologic mechanism conclusion is based on experimental models and/or human evidence related to biologic or pathophysiologic processes; categories include theoretical (if no evidence exists) and weak, moderate, or strong (if any evidence exists).

‡Diabetes type 1 is used as a specific example of autoimmune disorder for causality assessment; autoimmune disorder is used as general disorder for biologic mechanism conclusion.

people receive parenteral immunizations over a period of days,[294] pose substantial challenges to ensuring injection safety,[12] especially given concerns about inadequate sterilization of reusable syringes and needles, recycling of disposable syringes and needles, and cross-contamination resulting from the current generation of jet injectors.[295] The WHO has relatively successfully argued that safer autodisable syringes and sharps disposal boxes should be "bundled" with vaccine donations.[296] Clearly, these and other new safer administration technologies are urgently needed.[297]

The increasing computerization and centralization of health care services may facilitate epidemiologic studies to reassure the public about the safety of future vaccines.[38,172] Similar to other arenas concerned with safety (e.g., aviation,[298] food,[299] and blood[300]), a comprehensive *systems* design approach to minimize risk and promote vaccine safety is needed.[301] New initiatives to reduce medical errors and improve patient safety are drawing lessons from nonmedical systems where an evolution from traditional "linear" thinking about errors to analyses of multiple causation at the "systems" level has been effective in developing a culture of safety.[302] Furthermore, managers of immunization programs may wish to draw on lessons of other social realms, ranging from Enron/Arthur Andersen to priests and child molestation, on how to avoid "loss of public confidence," if only in hindsight. These usually involve "good governance" principles such as transparency, lack of conflict of interest, accountability, checks and balances, objective investigation, and participation of stakeholders in the decision making.[303]

Tragically, at a time when vaccine safety monitoring is needed more than ever, these and other nonscientific issues may severely impede it. For example, vaccine safety research by the U.S. National Immunization Program has been called into doubt, not because of the science, but mostly based on perceptions of conflict of interest having the risk assessor based within the main purchaser and promoter of immunization. In the aviation safety arena, this apparent conflict is solved by separating the investigative body (the National Transportation Safety Board [NTSB]) from the airplane manufacturer, the regulatory body (Federal Aviation Administration [FAA]) and the major promoter (airlines). Within immunization, the IOM Immunization Safety Review Committee serves the same role as the NTSB with some major differences: Unlike the IOM, the NTSB has the funding and staffing to do its own investigation. Furthermore, the NTSB recognizes the various stakeholders (manufacturer, airline, FAA) have valuable safety expertise to contribute to the investigation team. They are therefore deputized to join an investigation team led by the NTSB. On the IOM Immunization Safety Review Committee, in contrast, persons with vaccine safety expertise are deliberately excluded to avoid perceptions of conflict of interest. Finally, in contrast to the vaccine excise tax, airport excise taxes are not used solely to pay victims of airplane crashes but used instead to improve the infrastructure to *prevent* future crashes.

Unfortunately, not only has the failure of the NCVIA in the U.S. to fund vaccine safety research (arguably contrary to the intent of its sponsor Senator Paula Hawkins who intended the excise tax to pay for *prevention* of vaccine injuries as much if not more than *compensation*)[304] limited progress in vaccine safety research, it may reduce it even further in the future. The resultant failure to amend the Vaccine Injury Table with new research findings in a timely fashion has led plaintiff lawyers to seek wider "discovery" powers within the Claims Court, including access to pre-peer reviewed scientific research. This will likely become a major disincentive for scientists to conduct vaccine safety research in the US. One potential solution to limiting mistrust in the results of vaccine safety research in the first place may be an independent National Immunization Safety Board,[305] modeled after the NTSB, funded, possibly in part by the NCVIA excise tax or equivalent.

Developments in biotechnology may continue to offer better, safer vaccines.[46,291] The availability of computerized immunization registries[306] may permit optimal implementation of immunization policies at the individual level, ensuring receipt of indicated vaccines, avoiding extra vaccination, and appropriate observance of valid contraindications to vaccinations. On a longer horizon, the formal articulation of evidence-based vaccinology (as an offshoot of evidence-based medicine) is an important step toward maximizing public confidence in vaccines.[89] Vaccine safety research combined with genetic epidemiology may permit better characterization of risk groups for vaccine reactions.[307] Monitoring for mutant strains that have evolved as a consequence of selective pressure from immunizations may be needed.[308] Integrated with immunization registries for both children and adults, this ultimately may offer the possibility for better prevention of both vaccine-preventable[309] and vaccine-induced diseases.

Acknowledgments

The authors are grateful for the excellent assistance on this chapter rendered by the following persons: Mss. Susan Scheinman, Christine Korhonen, Allison Kennedy, Michele Russell, and Tamara Murphy with the references; Penina Haber, MPH, with Tables 61–1 and 61–2; and Gina Mootrey, DO, MPH, with Table 61–5.

REFERENCES

1. Ehreth J. The global value of vaccination. Vaccine 21:596–600, 2003.
2. England S, Loevinsohn B, Melgaard B, et al. The evidence base for interventions to reduce mortality from vaccine-preventable diseases in low and middle-income countries (Working Paper Series, Paper No. WG5:p. 10). Geneva, World Health Organization Commission on Macroeconomics and Health, 2001. Available at *www.cmhealth.org/docs/wg5_paper10.pdf*
3. Wilson GS. The Hazards of Immunization. London, Athlone Press, 1967.
4. Chen RT, Rastogi SC, Mullen JR, et al. The Vaccine Adverse Event Reporting System (VAERS). Vaccine 12:542–550, 1994.
5. Duclos P. Surveillance of secondary effects of vaccination [in French]. Sante 4:215–220, 1994.
6. Plotkin SA. Lessons learned concerning vaccine safety. Vaccine 20(suppl 1):S16–S19, 2001.
7. Gangarosa EJ, Galazka AM, Wolfe CR, et al. Impact of anti-vaccine movements on pertussis control: the untold story. Lancet 351:356–361, 1998.
8. Payne D. Ireland's measles outbreak kills two. BMJ 321:197B, 2000.
9. Public Health Laboratory Service. Measles outbreak in London. Commun Dis Rep CDR Wkly 12:1, 2002.
10. Orenstein WA. DTP vaccine litigation, 1988. Am J Dis Child 144:517, 1990.

11. Institute of Medicine. Liability for the production and sale of vaccine. *In* Sanford JP (ed). Vaccine Supply and Innovation. Washington, DC, National Academy Press, 1985, pp 85–122.

12. Simonsen L, Kane A, Lloyd J, et al. Unsafe injections in the developing world and transmission of bloodborne pathogens: a review. Bull World Health Organ 77:789–800, 1999.

13. Kane A, Lloyd J, Zaffran M, et al. Transmission of hepatitis B, hepatitis C and human immunodeficiency viruses through unsafe injections in the developing world: model-based regional estimates. Bull World Health Organ 77:801–807, 1999.

14. Dourado I, Cunha S, Teixeira MG, et al. Outbreak of aseptic meningitis associated with mass vaccination with a Urabe-containing measles-mumps-rubella vaccine: implications for immunization programs. Am J Epidemiol 151:524–530, 2000.

15. Ahmad K. Fury after children's adverse reaction to Japanese encephalitis vaccine. Lancet 360:395, 2002.

16. Scholtz M, Duclos P. Immunization safety: a global priority. Bull World Health Organ 78:153–154, 2000.

17. World Health Organization. Surveillance of adverse events following immunization (WHO/EPI/TRAM/93.02 Rev. 1). Geneva, World Health Organization, 1997.

18. Magdzik W. Surveillance of adverse effects following immunization (AEFI) [in Polish]. Przegl Epidemiol 46:27–33, 1992.

19. Expanded Programme on Immunization. Report of the 13th Global Advisory Group Meeting (WHO/EPI/GEN/91.3). Geneva, World Health Organization, 1991, pp 43–44.

20. Fine PE, Clarkson JA. Individual versus public priorities in the determination of optimal vaccination policies. Am J Epidemiol 124:1012–1020, 1986.

21. Centers for Disease Control and Prevention. Public Health Service recommendations on smallpox vaccination. MMWR Morb Mortal Wkly Rep 20:339–345, 1971.

22. Centers for Disease Control and Prevention. Poliomyelitis prevention in the United States: introduction of a sequential vaccination schedule of inactivated poliovirus vaccine followed by oral poliovirus vaccine. Recommendations of the Advisory Committee on Immunization Practices (ACIP). MMWR Morb Mortal Wkly Rep 46:1–25, 1997.

23. Centers for Disease Control and Prevention. Poliomyelitis prevention in the United States: updated recommendations of the Advisory Committee on Immunization Practices (ACIP). MMWR Morb Mortal Wkly Rep 49:1–25, 2000.

24. Henderson DA. Countering the posteradication threat of smallpox and polio. Clin Infect Dis 34:79–83, 2002.

25. McNeill WH. Plagues and Peoples. Garden City, NY, Anchor Press, 1976.

26. Charatan F. US draws up plans for smallpox outbreak after terrorist attack. BMJ 324:1540, 2002.

27. Habeck M. UK awards contract for smallpox vaccine. Lancet Infect Dis 2:321, 2002.

28. Dowdle WR, Gary HE, Sanders R, et al. Can post-eradication laboratory containment of wild polioviruses be achieved? Bull World Health Organ 80:311–316, 2002.

29. Howson CP, Howe CJ, Fineberg HV (eds). Adverse Effects of Pertussis and Rubella Vaccines: A Report of the Committee to Review the Adverse Consequences of Pertussis and Rubella Vaccines. Washington, DC, National Academy Press, 1991.

30. Stratton KR, Howe CJ, Johnston RB (eds). Adverse Events Associated with Childhood Vaccines: Evidence Bearing on Causality. Washington, DC, National Academy Press, 1994.

31. Miller D, Wadsworth J, Diamond J, et al. Pertussis vaccine and whooping cough as risk factors in acute neurological illness and death in young children. Dev Biol Stand 61:389–394, 1985.

32. Farrington P, Pugh S, Colville A, et al. A new method for active surveillance of adverse events from diphtheria/tetanus/pertussis and measles/mumps/rubella vaccines. Lancet 345:567–569, 1995.

33. Stetler HC, Orenstein WA, Bart KJ, et al. History of convulsions and use of pertussis vaccine. J Pediatr 107:175–179, 1985.

34. Robbins JB, Pittman M, Trollfors B, et al. Primum non nocere: a pharmacologically inert pertussis toxoid alone should be the next pertussis vaccine. Pediatr Infect Dis J 12:795–807, 1993.

35. Brown EG, Dimock K, Wright KE. The Urabe AM9 mumps vaccine is a mixture of viruses differing at amino acid 335 of the hemagglutinin-neuraminidase gene with one form associated with disease. J Infect Dis 174:619–622, 1996.

36. Kew OM, Nottay BK. Molecular epidemiology of polioviruses. Rev Infect Dis 6(suppl 2):S499–S504, 1984.

37. Plotkin SA, Koprowski H. Rabies vaccine. *In* Plotkin SA, Mortimer EA (eds). Vaccines (2nd ed). Philadelphia, WB Saunders, 1994, pp 649–670.

38. Chen RT, Glasser JW, Rhodes PH, et al. Vaccine Safety Datalink project: a new tool for improving vaccine safety monitoring in the United States. The Vaccine Safety Datalink Team. Pediatrics 99:765–773, 1997.

39. Roberts JD, Roos LL, Poffenroth LA, et al. Surveillance of vaccine-related adverse events in the first year of life: a Manitoba cohort study. J Clin Eqidemiol 49:51–58, 1996.

40. DeStefano F, Mullooly JP, Okoro CA, et al. Childhood vaccinations, vaccination timing, and risk of type 1 diabetes mellitus. Pediatrics 108:E112, 2001.

41. Barlow WE, Davis RL, Glasser JW, et al. The risk of seizures after receipt of whole-cell pertussis or measles, mumps, and rubella vaccine. N Engl J Med 345:656–661, 2001.

42. Freed GL, Katz SL, Clark SJ. Safety of vaccinations: Miss America, the media, and public health. JAMA 276:1869–1872, 1996.

43. Dove A. Congress examines childhood vaccine safety. Nat Med 5:970, 1999.

44. Balinska MA. L'affaire hepatite B en France. Espirit 276:34–48, 2001.

45. Ramsay S. UK starts campaign to reassure parents about MMR-vaccine safety. Lancet 357:290, 2001.

46. Poland GA, Murray D, Bonilla-Guerrero R. New vaccine development. BMJ 324:1315–1319, 2002.

47. Schonberger LB, Bregman DJ, Sullivan-Bolyai JZ, et al. Guillain-Barre syndrome following vaccination in the National Influenza Immunization Program, United States, 1976–1977. Am J Epidemiol 110:105–123, 1979.

48. McGoldrick MD, Bailie GR. Nonnarcotic analgesics: prevalence and estimated economic impact of toxicities. Ann Pharmacother 31:221–227, 1997.

49. Marcuse EK, Wentz KR. The NCES reconsidered: summary of a 1989 workshop. National Childhood Encephalopathy Study. Vaccine 8:531–535, 1990.

50. Alderslade R, Bellman MH, Rawson NSB, et al. The National Childhood Encephalopathy Study. Whooping Cough: Reports from the Committee on the Safety of Medicines and the Joint Committee on Vaccination and Immunisation, Department of Health and Social Security. London, HM Stationary Office, 1981, pp 79–169.

51. Miller D, Madge N, Diamond J, et al. Pertussis immunisation and serious acute neurological illnesses in children. Br Med J 307:1171–1176, 1993.

52. Wentz KR, Marcuse EK. Diphtheria-tetanus-pertussis vaccine and serious neurologic illness: an updated review of the epidemiologic evidence. Pediatrics 87:287–297, 1991.

53. Neustadt RE, Fineberg HV. The Swine Flu Affair: Decision-Making on a Slippery Disease. Washington, DC, U.S. Government Printing Office, 1978.

54. Kurland LT, Wiederholt WC, Kirkpatrick JW, et al. Swine influenza vaccine and Guillain-Barre syndrome: epidemic or artifact? Arch Neurol 42:1089–1090, 1985.

55. Langmuir AD, Bregman DJ, Kurland LT, et al. An epidemiologic and clinical evaluation of Guillain-Barre syndrome reported in association with the administration of swine influenza vaccines. Am J Epidemiol 119:841–879, 1984.

56. Safranek TJ, Lawrence DN, Kurland LT, et al. Reassessment of the association between Guillain-Barre syndrome and receipt of swine influenza vaccine in 1976–1977: results of a two-state study. Expert Neurology Group. Am J Epidemiol 133:940–951, 1991.

57. Murphy TV, Gargiullo PM, Massoudi MS, et al. Intussusception among infants given an oral rotavirus vaccine. N Engl J Med 344:564–572, 2001.

58. Kramarz P, France EK, DeStefano F, et al. Population-based study of rotavirus vaccination and intussusception. Pediatr Infect Dis J 20:410–416, 2001.

59. Simonsen L, Morens D, Elixhauser A, et al. Effect of rotavirus vaccination programme on trends in admission of infants to hospital for intussusception. Lancet 358:1224–1229, 2001.

60. Hall AJ. Ecological studies and debate on rotavirus vaccine and intussusception. Lancet 358:1197–1198, 2001.

61. Murphy TV, Gargiullo PM, Wharton M. More on rotavirus vaccination and intussusception. N Engl J Med 346:211–212, 2002.

62. Schumacher W. Legal/ethical aspects of vaccinations. Dev Biol Stand 43:435–438, 1979.

63. Fine PE. Herd immunity: history, theory, practice. Epidemiol Rev 15:265–302, 1993.

64. Baden JA, Noordeen SK (eds). Managing the Commons (2nd ed). Bloomington, Indiana University Press, 1998.

65. Salmon DA, Siegel AW. Religious and philosophical exemptions from vaccination requirements and lessons learned from conscientious objectors and conscription. Public Health Rep 116:289–295, 2001.

66. Nathanson N, Langmuir AD. The Cutter incident. Am J Hyg 78:16–18, 1963.

67. Butel JS. Increasing evidence for involvement of SV40 in human cancer. Dis Markers 17:167–172, 2001.

68. Stratton K, Almario DA, Mc Cormick MC (eds). Immunization safety view: SV40 contamination of polio vaccine and cancer. Washington DC, National Academy Press, 2002.

69. Food and Drug Administration. Bovine-derived materials: agency letters to manufacturers of FDA-regulated products. Fed Reg 59:44591–44594, 1994.

70. Centers for Disease Control and Prevention. Thimerosal in vaccines: a joint statement of the American Academy of Pediatrics and the Public Health Service. MMWR Morb Mortal Wkly Rep 48:563–565, 1999.

71. Mathieu M (ed). Biologic Development: A Regulatory Overview. Waltham, MA, Paraxel, 1993.

72. Centers for Disease Control and Prevention. Public Health Service recommendations for the use of vaccines manufactured with bovine-derived materials. MMWR Morb Mortal Wkly Rep 49:1137–1138, 2000.

73. Milstien J, Dellepiane N, Lamert S, et al. Vaccine quality—can a single standard be defined? Vaccine 20:1000–1003, 2002.

74. Anonymous. Two MMR vaccines withdrawn. Lancet 340:922, 1992.

75. Schmitt HJ, Just M, Neiss A. Withdrawal of a mumps vaccine: reasons and impacts. Eur J Pediatr 152:387–388, 1993.

76. Kimura M, Kuno-Sakai H, Yamazaki S, et al. Adverse events associated with MMR vaccines in Japan. Acta Paediatr Jpn 38:205–211, 1996.

77. Lathrop SL, Ball R, Haber P, et al. Adverse event reports following vaccination for Lyme disease: December 1998–July 2000. Vaccine 20:1603–1608, 2002.

78. Lloyd JC, Chen RT. The Urabe mumps vaccine: lessons in adverse event surveillance and response [abstract]. Pharmacoepidemiol Drug Saf 5(suppl):S45, 1996.

79. Mariner WK. Compensation programs for vaccine-related injury abroad: a comparative analysis. St Louis Univ Law J 31:599–654, 1987.

80. Evans G. Vaccine liability and safety: a progress report. Pediatr Infect Dis J 15:477–478, 1996.

81. Chen RT. Special methodological issues in pharmacoepidemiology studies of vaccine safety. In Strom BL (ed). Pharmacoepidemiology. Sussex, UK, John Wiley & Sons, 2000, pp 707–722.

82. Fine PE, Chen RT. Confounding in studies of adverse reactions to vaccines. Am J Epidemiol 136:121–135, 1992.

83. Fine PE. Methodological issues in the evaluation and monitoring of vaccine safety. Ann N Y Acad Sci 754:300–308, 1995.

84. Farrington CP, Nash J, Miller E. Case series analysis of adverse reactions to vaccines: a comparative evaluation. Am J Epidemiol 143:1165–1173, 1996.

85. Rothman KJ (ed). Causal Inference. Chestnut Hill, MA, Epidemiology Resources, 1988.

86. Gellin BG, Schaffner W. The risk of vaccination—the importance of "negative" studies. N Engl J Med 344:372–373, 2001.

87. Ellenberg SS, Chen RT. The complicated task of monitoring vaccine safety. Public Health Rep 112:10–20, 1997.

88. Morris R. Halperin S, Dery P, et al. IMPACT monitoring network: a better mousetrap. Can J Infect Dis 4:194–195, 1993.

89. Nalin DR. Evidence based vaccinology. Vaccine 20:1624–1630, 2002.

90. Verdier F. Non-clinical vaccine safety assessment. Toxicology 174:37–43, 2002.

91. Decker MD, Edwards KM, Steinhoff MC et al. Comparison of 13 acellular pertussis vaccines: adverse reactions. Pediatrics 96:557–566, 1995.

92. Rosenthal KL, McVittie LD. The clinical testing of preventive vaccines. In Mathieu M (ed). Biologic Development: A Regulatory Overview. Waltham, MA, Paraxel, 1993, pp 119–130.

93. Pichichero ME. Acellular pertussis vaccine: towards an improved safety profile. Drug Experience 15:311–324, 1996.

94. Jacobson RM, Adegbenro A, Pankratz VS, et al. Adverse events and vaccination—the lack of power and predictability of infrequent events in pre-licensure study. Vaccine 19:2428–2433, 2001.

95. Bonhoeffer J, Kohl K, Chen R, et al. The Brighton collaboration: addressing the need for standardized case definitions of adverse events following immunization (AEFI). Vaccine 21:298–302, 2002.

96. Brown F, Greco D, Mastantonio P, et al. Pertussis vaccine trials. Dev Biol Stand 89:1–410, 1997.

97. Chen RT. Safety of acellular pertussis vaccine: follow-up studies. Dev Biol Stand 89:373–375, 1997.

98. Heijbel H, Ciofi degli Atti MC, Harzer E, et al. Hypotonic hyporesponsive episodes in eight pertussis vaccine studies. Dev Biol Stand 89:101–103, 1997.

99. Ellenberg SS. Safety considerations for new vaccine development. Pharmacoepidemiol Drug Saf 10:411–415, 2001.

100. Ray WA, Griffin MR. Re: "Confounding in studies of adverse reactions to vaccines". Am J Epidemiol 139:229–230, 1994.

101. Lesko SM, Mitchell AA. The safety of acetaminophen and ibuprofen among children younger than two years old. Pediatrics 104:E39, 1999.

102. Scott TF, Bonanno DE. Reactions to live-measles-virus vaccine in children previously inoculated with killed-virus vaccine. N Engl J Med 277:248–250, 1967.

103. Bennett JV, Cutts FT, Katz SL. Edmonston-Zagreb measles vaccine: a good vaccine with an image problem. Pediatrics 104:1123–1124, 1999.

104. Steinhoff MC, Reed GF, Decker MD, et al. A randomized comparison of reactogenicity and immunogenicity of two whole-cell pertussis vaccines. Pediatrics 96:567–570, 1995.

105. Baraff LJ, Cody CL, Cherry JD. DTP-associated reactions: an analysis by injection site, manufacturer, prior reactions, and dose. Pediatrics 73:31–36, 1984.

106. Baraff LJ, Manclark CR, Cherry JD, et al. Analyses of adverse reactions to diphtheria and tetanus toxoids and pertussis vaccine by vaccine lot, endotoxin content, pertussis vaccine potency and percentage of mouse weight gain. Pediatr Infect Dis J 8:502–507, 1989.

107. Chen RT. Evaluation of vaccine safety post-9/11: role of cohort and case-control studies. Vaccine 2003 [in press].

108. Kennedy DL, Goldman SA, Lillie RB. Spontaneous reporting in the U.S. In Strom BL (ed). Pharmacoepidemiology. Sussex, UK, John Wiley & Sons, 2000, pp 151–174.

109. Alberti KG. Medical errors: a common problem. BMJ 322:501–502, 2001.

110. Wiholm BE, Olsoon S, Moore N. Spontaneous reporting systems outside the U.S. In Strom BL (ed). Pharmacoepidemiology. Sussex, UK, John Wiley & Sons, 2000, pp 175–192.

111. Jonville-Bera AP, Autret E, Galy-Eyraud C, et al. Thrombocytopenic purpura after measles, mumps and rubella vaccination: a retrospective survey by the French regional pharmacovigilance centres and Pasteur-Merieux Serums et Vaccins. Pediatr Infect Dis J 15:44–48, 1996.

112. Takahashi H. Need for improved vaccine safety surveillance. Vaccine 19:1004, 2000.

113. Mansoor O, Pillans PI. Vaccine adverse events reported in New Zealand 1990–5. N Z Med J 110:270–272, 1997.

114. Taranger J, Holmberg K. Urgent to introduce countrywide and systematic evaluation of vaccine side effects. Lakartidningen 89:1691–1693, 1992.

115. Salisbury DM, Beggs NT (eds). 1996 Immunisation Against Infectious Disease. London, Her Majesty's Stationery Office, 1996, pp 29–33.

116. Anonymous. Surveillance of serious adverse events following vaccination. Commun Dis Intell (Aust) 19:273–274, 1995.

117. Duclos P, Hockin J, Pless R, Lawler B. Reporting vaccine–associated adverse events. Can Fam Physician 43:1551–1556, 1559–1560, 1997.

118. Galindo Santana BM, Galindo Sardina MA, Perez RA. Adverse reaction surveillance system for vaccination in the Republic of Cuba [in Spanish]. Rev Cubana Med Trop 51:194–200, 1999.

119. Andersen MM, Ronne T. Side-effects with Japanese encephalitis vaccine. Lancet 337:1044, 1991.

120. Sokhey J. Adverse events following immunization: 1990. Indian Pediatr 28:593–607, 1991.

121. Squarcione S, Vellucci L. Adverse reactions following immunization in Italy in the years 1991–93. Ig Mod 105:1419–1431, 1996.

122. Fescharek R, Arras-Reiter C, Arens ER, Quast U, Maass G. Oral vaccines against poliomyelitis and vaccination-related paralytic poliomyelitis in Germany. Do we need a new immunization strategy? [in German] Wien Med Wochenschr 147(19–20):456–461, 1997.

123. Rastogi SC (ed). International Workshop: Harmonization of Reporting of Adverse Events Following Vaccination. Rockville, MD, Center for Biologics Evaluation and Research, 1993.

124. Vermeer-de Bondt PE, Wesselo C, Dzaferagic A, et al. Adverse events following immunisation under the national vaccination programme of the Netherlands. Part VII—reports in 2000. Bilthoven, RIVM, 000001006, 2002.

125. Brito GS. System of Investigation and Notification of Adverse Events Following Immunization: Preliminary Report. Sao Paolo, State of Sao Paolo, Brazil, Health Department, 1991.

126. World Health Organization. WHO Vaccine-Preventable Diseases: Monitoring System. 2001 Global Summary (WHO/V&B/01.34). Geneva, World Health Organization, 2002.

127. Centers for Disease Control and Prevention. National Childhood Vaccine Injury Act: requirements for permanent vaccination records and for reporting of selected events after vaccination. MMWR Morb Mortal Wkly Rep 37:197–200, 1988.

128. Stetler HC, Mullen JR, Brennan JP, et al. Monitoring system for adverse events following immunization. Vaccine 5:169–174, 1987.

129. Food and Drug Administration. COSTART—Coding Symbols for Thesaurus of Adverse Reaction Terms (3rd ed). Rockville, MD, Food and Drug Administration, 1989.

130. Brown EG, Wood L, Wood S. The Medical Dictionary for Regulatory Activities (MedDRA). Drug Saf 20:109–117, 1999.

131. Centers for Disease Control and Prevention. Surveillance for safety after immunization: Vaccine Adverse Event Reporting System (VAERS)–United States, 1991–2001. MMWR 52(SS-1), 2003.

132. Division of Immunization. Vaccine-associated adverse events in Canada, 1992 Report. Can Commun Dis Rep 21:117–128, 1995.

133. Collet JP, MacDonald N, Cashman N, et al. Monitoring signals for vaccine safety: the assessment of individual adverse event reports by an expert advisory committee. Advisory Committee on Causality Assessment. Bull World Health Organ 78:178–185, 2000.

134. Lindquist M, Edwards IR. The WHO Programme for International Drug Monitoring, its database, and the technical support of the Uppsala Monitoring Center. J Rheumatol 28:1180–1187, 2001.

135. Food and Drug Administration. International Conference on Harmonisation: Guideline on clinical safety data management: periodic safety update reports for marketed drugs. Fed Reg 62:27470–27476, 1997.

136. Wise RP, Kiminyo KP, Salive ME. Hair loss after routine immunizations. JAMA 278:1176–1178, 1997.

137. Retailliau HF, Curtis AC, Storr G, et al. Illness after influenza vaccination reported through a nationwide surveillance system, 1976–1977. Am J Epidemiol 111:270–278, 1980.

138. Zanardi LR, Haber P, Mootrey GT, et al. Intussusception among recipients of rotavirus vaccine: reports to the Vaccine Adverse Event Reporting System. Pediatrics 107:E97, 2001.

139. Peter G, Myers MG. Intussusception, rotavirus, and oral vaccines: summary of a workshop. Pediatrics 110(6):e67, 2002.

140. Centers for Disease Control and Prevention. Yellow fever vaccine: recommendation of the Advisory Committee on Immunization Practices (ACIP). MMWR 51(RR–17), 2002.

141. Martin M, Tsai TF, Cropp B, et al. Fever and multisystem organ failure associated with 17D-204 yellow fever vaccination: a report of four cases. Lancet 358:98–104, 2001.

142. Martin M, Weld LH, Tsai TF, et al. Advanced age a risk factor for illness temporally associated with yellow fever vaccination. Emerg Infect Dis 7:945–951, 2001.

143. Chan RC, Penney DJ, Little D, et al. Hepatitis and death following vaccination with 17D-204 yellow fever vaccine. Lancet 358:121–122, 2001.

144. Skowronski DM, De Serres G, Hebert J, et al. Skin testing to evaluate oculo-respiratory syndrome (ORS) associated with influenza vaccination during the 2000–2001 season. Vaccine 20:2713–2719, 2002.

145. Spila-Alegiani S, Salmaso S, Rota MC, et al. Reactogenicity in the elderly of nine commercial influenza vaccines: results from the Italian SVEVA study. Study for the Evaluation of Adverse Events of Influenza Vaccination. Vaccine 17:1898–1904, 1999.

146. Walker AM. Pattern recognition in health insurance claims databases. Pharmacoepidemiol Drug Saf 10:393–397, 2001.

147. Immunization Safety Priority Project. Safety of Mass Immunization Campaigns. Geneva, World Health Organization, 2002.

148. Uhari M, Rantala H, Niemela M. Cluster of childhood Guillain-Barre cases after an oral poliovaccine campaign. Lancet 2:440–441, 1989.

149. Berg SW, Mitchell BS, Hanson RK, et al. Systemic reactions in U.S. Marine Corps personnel who received Japanese encephalitis vaccine. Clin Infect Dis 24:265–266, 1997.

150. Kilroy AW, Schaffner W, Fleet WF Jr, et al. Two syndromes following rubella immunization: clinical observations and epidemiological studies. JAMA 214:2287–2292, 1970.

151. da Cunha SS, Rodrigues LC, Barreto ML, et al. Outbreak of aseptic meningitis and mumps after mass vaccination with MMR vaccine using the Leningrad-Zagreb mumps strain. Vaccine 20:1106–1112, 2002.

152. Vasconcelos PF, Luna EJ, Galler R, et al. Serious adverse events associated with yellow fever 17DD vaccine in Brazil: a report of two cases. Lancet 358:91–97, 2001.

153. Yergeau A, Alain L, Pless R, et al. Adverse events temporally associated with meningococcal vaccines. Can Med Assoc J 1154:503–507, 1996.

154. da Silveira CM, Salisbury DM, de Quadros CA. Measles vaccination and Guillain-Barre syndrome. Lancet 349:14–16, 1997.

155. D'Souza RM, Campbell-Lloyd S, Isaacs D, et al. Adverse events following immunisation associated with the 1998 Australian Measles Control Campaign. Commun Dis Intell 24:27–33, 2000.

156. Gout O, Theodorou I, Liblau R, et al. Central nervous system demyelination after recombinant hepatitis B vaccination: report of 25 cases. Neurology 48:A424, 1997.

157. Wakefield AJ, Murch SH, Anthony A, et al. Ileal-lymphoid-nodular hyperplasia, non-specific colitis, and pervasive developmental disorder in children. Lancet 351:637–641, 1998.

158. Rantala H, Cherry JD, Shields WD, et al. Epidemiology of Guillain-Barre syndrome in children: relationship of oral polio vaccine administration to occurrence. J Pediatr 124:220–223, 1994.

159. Sturkenboom M, Abenhaim L, Wolfson C, et al. Vaccinations, demyelination, and multiple sclerosis study. Pharmacoepidemiol Drug Saf 8(suppl):S170–S171, 1999.

160. Fourrier A, Touze E, Alperovitch A, et al. Association between hepatitis B vaccine and multiple sclerosis: a case-control study. Pharmacoepidemiol Drug Saf 8(suppl):S140–S141, 1999.

161. Ascherio A, Zhang SM, Hernan MA, et al. Hepatitis B vaccination and the risk of multiple sclerosis. N Engl J Med 344:327–332, 2001.

162. Lasky T, Terracciano GJ, Magder L, et al. Association of the Guillain-Barre syndrome with the 1992–93 and 1993–94 influenza vaccines [abstract]. Am J Epidemiol 145(suppl):S57, 1997.

163. Lloyd JC, Singleton JA, Terracciano GJ, et al. Evaluation of a surveillance system: Vaccine Adverse Event Reporting System [abstract]. Pharmacoepidemiol Drug Saf 5(suppl):S44, 1996.

164. Beeler J, Varricchio F, Wise R. Thrombocytopenia after immunization with measles vaccines: review of the Vaccine Adverse Events Reporting System (1990 to 1994). Pediatr Infect Dis J 15:88–90, 1996.

165. Weibel R, Glasser JW, Chen RT. Encephalopathy after measles vaccination: accumulative evidence from four independent surveillance systems [abstract]. Pharmacoepidemiol Drug Saf 6(suppl):S60, 1997.

166. Braun MM, Patriarca PA, Ellenberg SS. Syncope after immunization. Arch Pediatr Adolesc Med 151:255–259, 1997.

167. Rosenthal S, Chen R, Hadler S. The safety of acellular pertussis vaccine vs whole-cell pertussis vaccine: a postmarketing assessment. Arch Pediatr Adolesc Med 150:457–460, 1996.

168. Rosenthal S, Chen R. The reporting sensitivities of two passive surveillance systems for vaccine adverse events. Am J Public Health 85:1706–1709, 1995.

169. Verstraeten T, Baughman AL, Cadwell B, et al. Enhancing vaccine safety surveillance: a capture-recapture analysis of intussusception after rotavirus vaccination. Am J Epidemiol 154:1006–1012, 2001.

170. Chen RT, Kent JH, Rhodes PH, et al. Investigation of a possible association between influenza vaccination and Guillain-Barre syndrome in the United States, 1990–1991 [abstract]. Postmarketing Surveill 6:5–6, 1992.

171. Finney DJ. The detection of adverse reactions to therapeutic drugs. Stat Med 1:153–161, 1982.

172. Strom BL, Carson JL. Use of automated databases for pharmacoepidemiology research. Epidemiol Rev 12:87–107, 1990.

173. Niu MT, Rhodes P, Salive M, et al. Comparative safety of two recombinant hepatitis B vaccines in children: data from the Vaccine Adverse Event Reporting System (VAERS) and Vaccine Safety Datalink (VSD). J Clin Epidemiol 51:503–510, 1998.

174. Patriarca PA, Laender F, Palmeira G, et al. Randomised trial of alternative formulations of oral poliovaccine in Brazil. Lancet 1:429–433, 1988.

175. Bhargava I, Chhaparwal BC, Phadke MA, et al. Reactogenicity of indigenously produced measles vaccine. Indian Pediatr 33:827–831, 1996.

176. Orenstein WA, Markowitz L, Preblud SR, et al. Appropriate age for measles vaccination in the United States. Dev Biol Stand 65:13–21, 1986.

177. Booy R, Aitken SJ, Taylor S, et al. Immunogenicity of combined diphtheria, tetanus, and pertussis vaccine given at 2, 3, and 4 months versus 3, 5, and 9 months of age. Lancet 339:507–510, 1992.

178. Deforest A, Long SS, Lischner HW, et al. Simultaneous administration of measles-mumps-rubella vaccine with booster doses of diphtheria-tetanus-pertussis and poliovirus vaccines. Pediatrics 81:237–246, 1988.

179. Scheifele D, Law B, Mitchell L, et al. Study of booster doses of two Haemophilus influenzae type b conjugate vaccines including their interchangeability. Vaccine 14:1399–1406, 1996.

180. Aaby P, Samb B, Simondon F, et al. A comparison of vaccine efficacy and mortality during routine use of high-titre Edmonston-Zagreb and Schwarz standard measles vaccines in rural Senegal. Trans R Soc Trop Med Hyg 90:326–330, 1996.

181. Expanded Programme on Immunization (EPI). Safety of high titer measles vaccines. Wkly Epidemiol Rec 67:357–361, 1992.

182. Meekison W, Hutcheon M, Guasparini R, et al. Post-marketing surveillance of adverse events following PROHIBIT vaccine in British Columbia. Can Med Assoc J 141:927–929, 1989.

183. Black SB, Shinefield HR. b-CAPSA I Haemophilus influenzae, type b, capsular polysaccharide vaccine safety. Pediatrics 79:321–325, 1987.

184. Vadheim CM, Greenberg DP, Marcy SM, et al. Safety evaluation of PRP-D Haemophilus influenzae type b conjugate vaccine in children immunized at 18 months of age and older: follow-up study of 30,000 children. Pediatr Infect Dis J 9:555–561, 1990.

185. Centers for Disease Control and Prevention. Unintentional administration of varicella virus vaccine—United States, 1996. MMWR Morb Mortal Wkly Rep 45:1017–1018, 1996.

186. Coplan P, Black S, Guess HA, et al. Post-marketing safety of varicella vaccine among 44,369 vaccinees [abstract]. Am J Epidemiol 145(suppl):S76, 1997.

187. Centers for Disease Control and Prevention. Inactivated Japanese encephalitis virus vaccine: recommendations of the Advisory Committee on Immunization Practices (ACIP). MMWR Morb Mortal Wkly Rep 42:1–15, 1993.

188. Henderson DA, Witte JJ, Morris L, et al. Paralytic disease associated with oral polio vaccines. JAMA 190:153–160, 1964.

189. Bernier RH, Frank JA Jr, Dondero TJ Jr, et al. Diphtheria-tetanus toxoids-pertussis vaccination and sudden infant deaths in Tennessee. J Pediatr 101:419–421, 1982.

190. Solberg LK. DTP Vaccination, Visit to Child Health Center and Sudden Infant Death Syndrome (SIDS): Evaluation of DTP Vaccination. Report to the Oslo Health Council 1985. Bethesda, MD, NIH Library Translation, 1985, pp 85–152.

191. Bouvier-Colle MH, Flahaut A, Messiah A, et al. Sudden infant death and immunization: an extensive epidemiological approach to the problem in France—winter 1986. Int J Epidemiol 18:121–126, 1989.

192. Mitchell EA, Stewart AW, Clements M. Immunisation and the sudden infant death syndrome. New Zealand Cot Death Study Group. Arch Dis Child 73:498–501, 1995.

193. Gale JL, Thapa PB, Wassilak SG, et al. Risk of serious acute neurological illness after immunization with diphtheria-tetanus-pertussis vaccine: a population-based case-control study. JAMA 271:37–41, 1994.

194. Simon PA, Chen RT, Elliott JA, et al. Outbreak of pyogenic abscesses after diphtheria and tetanus toxoids and pertussis vaccination. Pediatr Infect Dis J 12:368–371, 1993.

195. Verstraeten T, DeStefano F, Chen RT, et al. Vaccine safety surveillance using large linked databases: opportunities, hazards and proposed guide. Expert Rev Vaccines 2:21–29, 2003.

196. Chen RT, De Stefano, F, Davis RL, et al. The Vaccine safety Datalink: immunization research in health maintenance organizations in the USA. Bull World Health Organ 78:186–194, 2000.

197. Walker AM, Jick H, Perera DR, et al. Diphtheria-tetanus-pertussis immunization and sudden infant death syndrome. Am J Public Health 77:945–951, 1987.

198. Griffin MR, Ray WA, Mortimer EA, et al. Risk of seizures and encephalopathy after immunization with the diphtheria-tetanus-pertussis vaccine. JAMA 263:1641–1645, 1990.

199. Davis RL, Marcuse E, Black S, et al. MMR2 immunization at 4 to 5 years and 10 to 12 years of age: a comparison of adverse clinical events after immunization in the Vaccine Safety Datalink project. The Vaccine Safety Datalink Team. Pediatrics 100:767–771, 1997.

200. Williams JC, Goldenthal KL, Burns DL, Lewis BP Jr (eds). Combined Vaccines and Simultaneous Administration: Current Issues and Perspective. New York, New York Academy of Science, 1995.

201. Griffin MR, Ray WA, Livengood JR, et al. Risk of sudden infant death syndrome after immunization with the diphtheria-tetanus-pertussis vaccine. N Engl J Med 319:618–623, 1988.

202. Zanoni G, Dung NTM, Tridente G. Fourth report on the Green Channel activities and the monitoring system of reactions to vaccines in the Veneto Region: Analysis of the three year period 1997–1999, General summary 1992–1999. Immunology Section, University of Verona, Italy; 2000. Italian.

203. Goodwin H, Nash M, Gold M, et al. Vaccination of children following a previous hypotonic-hyporesponsive episode. J Paediatr Child Health 35:549–552, 1999.

204. Gold MS. Hypotonic-hyporesponsive episodes following pertussis vaccination: a cause for concern? Drug Saf 25:85–90, 2002.

205. Phillips KA, Veenstra DL, Oren E, et al. Potential role of pharmacogenomics in reducing adverse drug reactions: a systematic review. JAMA 286:2270–2279, 2001.

206. Sim I, Sanders GD, McDonald KM. Evidence-based practice for mere mortals: the role of informatics and health services research. J Gen Intern Med 17:302–308, 2002.

207. Paradiso PR. Maternal immunization: the influence of liability issues on vaccine development. Vaccine 20(suppl 1):S73–S74, 2001.

208. Spence MA. The genetics of autism. Curr Opin Pediatr 13:561–565, 2001.

209. Nelson KB, Grether JK, Croen LA, et al. Neuropeptides and neurotrophins in neonatal blood of children with autism or mental retardation. Ann Neurol 49:597–606, 2001.

210. Chen RT, De Stefano F. Vaccine adverse events: causal of coincidental? Lancet 351: 611–612, 1968.

210a. Taylor B, Miller E, Farrington CP, et al. Autism and measles, mumps, and rubella vaccine: no epidemiological evidence for a causal association. Lancet 353:2026–2029, 1999.

211. Farrington CP, Miller E, Taylor B. MMR and autism: further evidence against a causal association. Vaccine 19:3632–3635, 2001.

212a. Davis RL, Kramarz P, Bohlke K, et al. Measles-mumps-rubella and other measles-containing vaccines do not increase the risk for inflammatory bowel disease: a case-control study from the Vaccine Safety Datalink project. Arch Pediatr Adolesc Med 155:354–359, 2001.

213. Kaye JA, Mar Melero-Montes M, Jick H. Mumps, measles, and rubella vaccine and the incidence of autism recorded by general practitioners: a time trend analysis. BMJ 322:460–463, 2001.

214. Dales L, Hammer SJ, Smith NJ. Time trends in autism and in MMR immunization coverage in California. JAMA 285:1183–1185, 2001.

215. Fombonne E, Chakrabarti S. No evidence for a new variant of measles-mumps-rubella-induced autism. Pediatrics 108:E58, 2001.

216. Taylor B, Miller E, Lingam R, et al. Measles, mumps, and rubella vaccination and bowel problems or developmental regression in children with autism: population study. BMJ 324:393–396, 2002.

217. Stratton K, Gable A, Shetty PMM. Measles-mumps-rubella vaccine and autism. In Institute of Medicine, Immunization Safety Review Committee. Immunization Safety Review. Washington, DC, National Academy Press, 2001.

218. Centers for Disease Control and Prevention. Recommendations regarding the use of vaccines that contain thimerosal as a preservative. MMWR Morb Mortal Wkly Rep 48:996–998, 1999.

219. Halsey NA. Limiting infant exposure to thimerosal in vaccines and other sources of mercury. JAMA 282:1763–1766, 1999.

220. Grandjean P, Weihe P, White RF, et al. Cognitive performance of children prenatally exposed to "safe" levels of methylmercury. Environ Res 77:165–172, 1998.

221. Davidson PW, Myers GJ, Cox C, et al. Effects of prenatal and post-natal methylmercury exposure from fish consumption on neurode-velopment: outcomes at 66 months of age in the Seychelles Child Development Study. JAMA 280:701–707, 1998.
222. Bakir F, Damluji SF, Amin-Zaki L, et al. Methylmercury poisoning in Iraq. Science 181:230–241, 1973.
223. Igata A. Epidemiological and clinical features of Minamata disease. Environ Res 63:157–169, 1993.
224. Pichichero ME, Cernichiari E, Lopreiato J, Treanor J. Mercury con-centrations and metabolism in infants receiving vaccines contain-ing thiomersal: a descriptive study. Lancet. 360(9347):1737–1741, 2002.
225. Stajich GV, Lopez GP, Harry SW, et al. Iatrogenic exposure to mer-cury after hepatitis B vaccination in preterm infants. J Pediatr 136:679–681, 2000.
226. Centers for Disease Control and Prevention. Summary of the Joint Statement on Thimerosal in Vaccines. MMWR Morb Mortal Wkly Rep 49:622–631, 2000.
227. Stratton K, Gable A, McCormick M. Thimerosal-containing vac-cines and neurodevelopmental disorders. In Institute of Medicine, Immunization Safety Review Committee. Immunization Safety Review. Washington, DC, National Academy Press, 2001.
227a. Ramirez GB, Pagulayan O, Akagi, et al. Tagum study II: followup study at two years of age after prenatal exposure to mercury. Pediatrics 111: e289–e295, 2003.
228. Clark SJ, Cabana MD, Malik T, et al. Hepatitis B vaccination prac-tices in hospital newborn nurseries before and after changes in vacci-nation recommendations. Arch Pediatr Adolesc Med 155:915–920, 2001.
228a. CDC. Unpublished data, 2000.
229. Classen JB, Classen DC. Vaccines and the risk of insulin-dependent diabetes (IDDM): potential mechanism of action. Med Hypotheses. 57(5):532–538, 2001.
230. Blom L, Nystrom L, Dahlquist G. The Swedish childhood diabetes study: vaccinations and infections as risk determinants for diabetes in childhood. Diabetologia 34:176–181, 1991.
231. Parent ME, Siemiatycki J, Menzies R, et al. Bacille Calmette-Guerin vaccination and incidence of IDDM in Montreal, Canada. Diabetes Care 20:767–772, 1997.
232. Childhood immunizations and type 1 diabetes: summary of an Institute for Vaccine Safety Workshop. The Institute for Vaccine Safety Diabetes Workshop Panel. Pediatr Infect Dis J 18:217–222, 1999.
233. Jefferson T, Demicheli V. No evidence that vaccines cause insulin dependent diabetes mellitus. J Epidemiol Community Health 52:674–675, 1998.
234. Ryan M, Murphy G, Ryan E, et al. Distinct T-cell subtypes induced with whole cell and acellular pertussis vaccines in children. Immunology 93:1–10, 1998.
235. Donovan CE, Finn PW. Immune mechanisms of childhood asthma. Thorax 54:938–946, 1999.
236. Kemp T, Pearce N, Fitzharris P, et al. Is infant immunization a risk fac-tor for childhood asthma or allergy? Epidemiology 8:678–680, 1997.
237. Nilsson L, Kjellman NI, Bjorksten B. A randomized controlled trial of the effect of pertussis vaccines on atopic disease. Arch Pediatr Adolesc Med 152:734–738, 1998.
238. Henderson J, North K, Griffiths M, et al. Pertussis vaccination and wheezing illnesses in young children: prospective cohort study. The Longitudinal Study of Pregnancy and Childhood Team. BMJ 318:1173–1176, 1999.
239. Mullooly JP, Pearson J, Drew L, et al. Wheezing lower respiratory dis-ease and vaccination of full-term infants. Pharmacoepidemiol Drug Saf 11:21–30, 2002.
240. DeStefano F, Gu D, Kramarz P, et al. Childhood vaccinations and risk of asthma. Pediatr Infect Dis J 21:498–504, 2002.
241. Paunio M, Heinonen OP, Virtanen M, et al. Measles history and atopic diseases: a population-based cross-sectional study. JAMA 283:343–346, 2000.
242. Park CL, Frank A. Does influenza vaccination exacerbate asthma? Drug Saf 19:83–88, 1998.
243. Kramarz P, DeStefano F, Gargiullo PM, et al. Does influenza vaccination exacerbate asthma? Analysis of a large cohort of children with asthma. Vaccine Safety Datalink Team. Arch Fam Med 9:617–623, 2000.
244. Kramarz P, DeStefano F, Gargiullo PM, et al. Does influenza vaccina-tion prevent asthma exacerbations in children? J Pediatr 138:306–310, 2001.
245. Davies P, Chapman S, Leask J. Antivaccination activists on the World Wide Web. Arch Dis Child 87:22–25, 2002.
246. Wolfe RM, Sharp LK, Lipsky MS. Content and design attributes of antivaccination web sites. JAMA 287:3245–3248, 2002.
247. Leask JA, Chapman S. An attempt to swindle nature: press anti-immunisation reportage 1993–1997. Aust N Z J Public Health 22:17–26, 1998.
248. Gellin BG, Maibach EW, Marcuse EK. Do parents understand immu-nizations? A national telephone survey. Pediatrics 106:1097–1102, 2000.
249. National Research Council. Improving Risk Communication. Washington, DC, National Academy Press, 1989.
250. Bostrom A. Vaccine risk communication: lessons from risk percep-tion, decision making and environmental risk communication research. Risk Health Saf Environment 8:173–200, 1997.
251. Fischhoff B, Watson S, Hope C. Defining risk. In Glickman T, Gough M (eds). Readings in Risk. Washington, DC, Resources for the Future, 1990, pp 30–41.
252. Slovic P. The risk game. J Haz Materials 86:17–24, 2001.
253. Slovic P. Perception of risk. Science 236:280–285, 1987.
254. Adams J. Risk. London, University College London Press, 1995.
255. Forrest C, Hix Mays R. The Practical Guide to Environmental Community Relations. New York, John Wiley & Sons, 1997.
256. Renn O, Levine D. Credibility and trust in risk communications. In Kasperson R, Stallen P (eds). Communicating Risk to the Public: International Perspectives. Dordrecht, The Netherlands, Kluwer Academic Publishers, 1991.
257. Bennett P. Understanding responses to risk: some basic findings. In Bennett P, Calman K (eds). Risk Communication and Public Health. New York, Oxford University Press, 1999, pp 3–19.
258. Holtgrave D, Tinsley B, Kay L. Encouraging risk reduction: a decision-making approach to message design. In Maibach E, Parrott R (eds). Designing Health Messages. Thousand Oaks, CA, Sage, 1995, pp 24–40.
259. Asch DA, Baron J, Hershey JC, et al. Omission bias and pertussis vaccination. Med Decis Making 14:118–123, 1994.
260. Donovan RJ, Jalleh G. Positive versus negative framing of a hypo-thetical infant immunization: the influence of involvement. Health Educ Behav 27:82–95, 2000.
261. O'Connor AM, Pennie RA, Dales RE. Framing effects on expecta-tions, decisions, and side effects experienced: the case of influenza immunization. J Clin Epidemiol 49:1271–1276, 1996.
262. Lynn FM, Busenberg GJ. Citizen advisory committees and environ-mental policy: what we know, what's left to discover. Risk Anal 15:147–162, 1995.
263. Goldman A. The refutation of medical paternalism. In Arras JD, Steinbock B (eds). Ethical Issues in Modern Medicine. Mountain View, CA, Mafield Publishing, 1995, pp 58–66.
264. Severyn KM. Jacobson v. Massachusetts: impact on informed consent and vaccine policy. J Pharm Law 5:249–274, 1996.
265. Hershey JC, Ash DA, Thumasathit T, et al. The role of altruism, free riding, and bandwagoning in vaccination decisions. Organ Behav Hum Decis Process 59:177–187, 1994.
266. Salmon DA, Haber M, Gangarosa EJ, et al. Health consequences of religions and philosophical exemptions from immunization laws: individual and societal risk of measles. JAMA 282:47–53, 1999.
267. Feikin DR, Lezotte DC, Hamman RF, et al. Individual and commu-nity risks of measles and pertussis associated with personal exemp-tions to immunization. JAMA 284:3145–3150, 2000.
268. Rota JS, Salmon DA, Rodewald LE, et al. Processes for obtaining nonmedical exemptions to state immunization laws. Am J Public Health 91:645–648, 2001.
269. Fine PEM, Sterne J. High titer measles vaccine before nine months of age: implications for child survival [working paper no. 13, 1992]. Presented at Consultation on Studies Involving High Titer Measles Vaccines Before Nine Months of Age, Atlanta, GA, June 16–17, 1992.
269a. Halsey NA. Anthrax vaccine and causality assessment from individ-ual case reports. Pharmacoepidemiol Drug Saf. (3):185–187; discus-sion 203–204, 2002.
270. Betraying the public over nvCJD risk [editorial]. Lancet 348:1529, 1996.
271. Coulter HL, Fisher BL. DTP: A Shot in the Dark. Garden City Park, New York, Avery, 1991.
272. McNamee D. Communicating drug-safety information. Lancet 350:1646, 1997.
273. Wilkie T. Sources in science: who can we trust? Lancet 347:1308–1311, 1996.

274. Monahan J. Using positive affect when designing health messages. *In* Maibach E, Parrott R (eds). Designing Health Messages. Thousand Oaks, CA, Sage, 1995, pp 81–98.

275. Hinman AR, Orenstein WA. Public health considerations. *In* Plotkin SA, Mortimer EA (eds). Vaccines (2nd ed). Philadelphia, WB Saunders, 1994, pp 930–932.

276. National Childhood Vaccine Injury Act of 1986, Section 2125, Public Health Service Act, 42 USC § 300aa (Supp 1987).

277. Clayton EW, Hickson GB, Miller CS. Parents' responses to vaccine information pamphlets. Pediatrics 93:369–372, 1994.

278. Davis TC, Bocchini JA Jr, Fredrickson D, et al. Parent comprehension of polio vaccine information pamphlets. Pediatrics 97:804–810, 1996.

279. Davis TC, Fredrickson DD, Arnold C, et al. A polio immunization pamphlet with increased appeal and simplified language does not improve comprehension to an acceptable level. Patient Educ Counsel 33:25–37, 1998.

280. Davis TC, Fredrickson DD, Arnold CL, et al. Childhood vaccine risk/benefit communication in private practice office settings: a national survey. Pediatrics 107:E17, 2001.

281. Davis TC, Fredrickson DD, Bocchini C, et al. Improving vaccine risk/benefit communication with an immunization education package: a pilot study. Ambul Pediatr 2:193–200, 2002.

282. Centers for Disease Control and Prevention. Update: vaccine side effects, adverse reactions, contraindications, and precautions. Recommendations of the Advisory Committee on Immunization Practices (ACIP). MMWR Morb Mortal Wkly Rep 45:1–35, 1996.

283. Slater PE, Ben Zvi T, Fogel A, et al. Absence of an association between rubella vaccination and arthritis in underimmune postpartum women. Vaccine 13:1529–1532, 1995.

284. Tingle AJ, Mitchell LA, Grace M, et al. Randomised double-blind placebo-controlled study on adverse effects of rubella immunisation in seronegative women. Lancet 349:1277–1281, 1997.

285. Ray P, Black S, Shinefield H, et al. Risk of chronic arthropathy among women after rubella vaccination. Vaccine Safety Datalink Team. JAMA 278:551–556, 1997.

286. Mootrey G, Mulach B. Institute of Medicine Immunization Safety Review Project—a valuable addition to the U.S. vaccine safety infrastructure. AAP News 21:58, 2002.

287. Stratton K, Wilson CB, McCormick M. Multiple immunizations and immune dysfunction. *In* Institute of Medicine, Immunization Safety Review Committee. Immunization Safety Review. Washington, DC, National Academy Press, 2002.

288. Stratton K, Almario D, McCormick M (eds). Hepatitis B vaccine and demyelinating neurological disorders. *In* Institute of Medicine, Immunization Safety Review Committee. Immunization Safety Review. Washington, DC, National Academy Press, 2002.

289. Stratton K, McCormick M. SV40 contamination of polio vaccine and cancer. *In* Institute of Medicine, Immunization Safety Review Committee. Immunization Safety Review. Washington, DC, National Academy Press, 2002.

290. Institute of Medicine, Committee to Assess the Safety and Efficacy of the Anthrax Vaccine, Joellenbeck LM, Zwanziger LL, Durch JS, Strom BL (eds). The Anthrax Vaccine: Is It Safe? Does It Work? Washington, DC, National Academy Press, 2002.

291. Russo S, Turin L, Zanella A, et al. What's going on in vaccine technology? Med Res Rev 17:277–301, 1997.

292. Ward BJ. Vaccine adverse events in the new millennium: is there reason for concern? Bull World Health Organ 78:205–215, 2000.

293. Vaccine supply and quality: surveillance of adverse events following immunization. Wkly Epidemiol Rec 71:237–242, 1996.

294. Olive JM, Risi JB Jr, de Quadros CA. National immunization days: experience in Latin America. J Infect Dis 175(suppl 1):S189–S193, 1997.

295. Ekwueme DU, Weniger BG, Chen RT. Model-based estimates of risks of disease transmission and economic costs of seven injection devices in sub-Saharan Africa. Bull World Health Organ 80:859–870, 2002.

296. Melgaard B, Li-Frankenstein V, Rasheed S, et al. WHO-UNICEF-UNFPA joint statement on the use of auto-disable syringes in immunization services. Geneva, World Health Organization, Division of Vaccine and Biologicals, 1999.

297. Lloyd J. Technologies for Vaccine Delivery in the 21st Century (WHO/V&B/00.35). Geneva, World Health Organization, Division of Vaccines and Biologicals, 2000.

298. National Transportation Safety Board. We are all safer: NTSB–inspired improvements in transportation safety. Washington DC, NTSB, 1998.

299. Merrill RA. Food safety regulation: reforming the Delaney Clause. Annu Rev Public Health 18:313–340, 1997.

300. Leveton LB, Sox HC, Stoto MA (eds). HIV and the Blood Supply: An Analysis of Crisis Decisionmaking. Washington, DC, National Academy Press, 1995.

301. Chen RT. A multi-faceted approach to improve vaccine safety in the United States. *In* Proceedings of the 24th National Immunization Conference, Orlando, FL, May 21–25, 1990. Atlanta, Centers for Disease Control, Division of Immunization, 1990, pp 107–109.

302. Barach P, Small SD. Reporting and preventing medical mishaps: lessons from non-medical near miss reporting systems. BMJ 320:759–763, 2000.

303. Chen RT. Ensuring public confidence in vaccine safety: some lessons from Enron and other public fiascos [abstract]. Pharmacoepidemiol Drug Saf 11(suppl):S226–S227, 2002.

304. National Childhood Vaccine Injury Compensation Act, S. 2117. Hearing before the Committee on Labor and Human Resources, US Senate, 98th Cong., 2nd Sess (May 3, 1984): 2.

305. Chen RT. Vaccine risks: real, perceived, and unknown. Vaccine 17:541–546, 1999.

306. Cordero JF, Guerra FA, Saarlas KN, et al. Developing national immunization registries: experience from the All Kids Count Program. Am J Prev Med 3:1–128, 1997.

307. Khoury MJ. Genetic epidemiology and the future of disease prevention and public health. Epidemiol Rev 19:175–180, 1997.

308. Francois G, Kew M, VanDamme P, et al. Mutant hepatitis B viruses: a matter of academic interest only or a problem with far-reaching implications? Vaccine 19:3799–3815, 2001.

309. Centers for Disease Control and Prevention. Achievements in public health, 1900–1999: impact of vaccines universally recommended for children—United States, 1990–1998. MMWR Morb Mortal Wkly Rep 48:243–248, 1999.

Chapter 62

Multiple Vaccines and the Immune System

PAUL A. OFFIT • CHARLES J. HACKETT

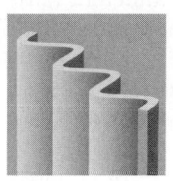

One hundred years ago, children received one vaccine—smallpox. Today children receive 11 vaccines routinely. Although some vaccines are given in combination, infants and young children could receive as many as 20 shots by 2 years of age and five shots at one time. The increase in the number of vaccines, and the consequent decline in vaccine-preventable illnesses, has focused attention by both parents and health care professionals on vaccine safety. Specific concerns include whether vaccines weaken, overwhelm,[1] or in some way alter the normal balance of the immune system, paving the way for chronic diseases such as diabetes, asthma, multiple sclerosis, or allergies.

We describe the capacity of the infant's immune system to respond to vaccines as well as discuss the plausibility of theories that relate vaccines to the development of specific chronic diseases.

The Developing Human Immune System

Neonates are protected from infection by maternal immunoglobulin (Ig) G obtained transplacentally, by maternal IgA derived from colostrum and milk, and by cells of the innate immune system (e.g., macrophages, dendritic cells, and natural killer cells). Although cells of the adaptive immune system (B and T cells) are present by 14 weeks' gestation and display an enormous array of antigen-specific receptors,[2] lack of antigen stimulation in utero results in neonatal B and T cells that are largely naïve and unexpanded. The development and maturation of B and T cells is dependent on normal flora, infections, and, to a lesser extent, vaccinations.

Innate and Adaptive Immunity in Neonates and Infants Compared with Older Children and Adults

Immunologic responses to pathogens and vaccines depend on the independent and coordinated function of innate and adaptive immune responses. The capacity of the innate immune system to stimulate T- and B-cell responses is largely dependent on the function of dendritic cells.[3] Neonatal dendritic cells differ from more mature dendritic cells in their preferential stimulation of a specific type of helper T cell (Th) designated the Th2 cell. Th2 cells release cytokines such as interleukin (IL)-4, IL-5, and IL-13 that in part activate antigen-specific B cells to produce IgM, IgA, or IgE. In contrast, Th1 cells release cytokines such as interferon-γ, tumor necrosis factor (TNF)-α, TNF-β, and granulocyte-macrophage colony-stimulating factor ("proinflammatory cytokines") that induce activation of macrophages and neutrophils.[4] The prevalence of noninflammatory Th2-type responses in neonates may be a holdover from the fetal condition, where inflammatory responses may be detrimental to pregnancy.[5,6]

Another important difference between infant and adult immune responses is that infants and young children are less capable of generating T-cell–dependent B-cell responses to bacterial polysaccharides.[7] The inability to respond to bacterial polysaccharides may be related to the infant's need to establish normal bacterial flora.

Capacity of Newborns and Young Infants to Respond to Vaccines

Within hours of birth, cells of the innate and adaptive immune system are actively engaged in responding to challenges in the environment (e.g., colonizing bacterial flora).[8,9] Similarly, newborn and young infants are quite capable of generating protective immune responses to single and multiple vaccines. For example, children born to mothers infected with hepatitis B virus are protected against infection after inoculation with hepatitis B vaccine (given at birth and 1 month of age).[10–12] Similarly, newborns inoculated with bacille Calmette-Guérin (BCG) vaccine are protected against severe forms of tuberculosis presumably by activation of bacteria-specific T cells.[13–15] In addition, about 90% to 95% of infants inoculated in the first 6 months of life with multiple vaccines, including diphtheria-tetanus-pertussis, pneumococcus, *Haemophilus influenzae* type b, hepatitis B, and polio, develop protective, vaccine-specific immune responses.[16] Conjugation of bacterial polysaccharides (such as *Streptococcus pneumoniae* and *H. influenzae* type b) to carrier molecules that elicit helper T cells circumvents the poor immunogenicity of unconjugated polysaccharide vaccines in infants and young children.[17,18]

Do Vaccines "Overwhelm" the Immune System?

Despite the increase in the number of vaccines required over the past 100 years, the number of immunogenic proteins and polysaccharides contained in vaccines has decreased. Furthermore, the infant's immune system has the capacity to respond to a quantity of immunogenic proteins and polysaccharides far greater than that contained in vaccines.

Number of Antigens Contained in Vaccines over the Past 100 Years

Although we have witnessed a dramatic increase in the number of vaccines routinely recommended for infants and young children, the number of immunogenic proteins and polysaccharides contained in vaccines has declined (Table 62–1). The decrease in the number of immunogenic proteins and polysaccharides contained in vaccines is attributable to (1) discontinuation of the smallpox vaccine and (2) advances in the field of protein purification that allowed for a switch from whole-cell to acellular pertussis vaccine.

Theoretical Capacity of the Immune System to Respond to Multiple Antigens

The diversity of antibody responses is determined by a series of genes located on chromosome 6. Antibodies bind to immunologically distinct regions (epitopes) of proteins and polysaccharides, and antibody binding specificities are determined by *variable* (or hypermutable) regions located on heavy and light chains. The capacity of antibodies to bind to antigens is therefore largely determined by the number of different variable regions that can be generated during an immune response.

The diversity of antibody variable regions is determined by a combination of genes termed variable (V), diverse (D), and joining (J); approximately 120, 30, and 15 V, D, and J genes, respectively, have been described.[19] The number of antibody specificities generated by the multiple combinations of V, D, and J genes is termed *combinatorial diversity*. A fourth hypermutable region (junctional) is located between V and J genes and accounts for additional diversity (termed *junctional diversity*). Combinatorial and junctional diversity account for the generation of about 10^9 to 10^{11} different antibody molecules.[11] One way to determine the number of different vaccines to which an individual can respond, therefore, would be to divide the number of different antibody specificities generated by combinatorial and junctional diversity (i.e., 10^9 to 10^{11}) by the number of different epitopes contained in vaccines. If we assume that proteins or polysaccharides each contain about 10 epitopes, and that one vaccine contains about 10 different proteins or polysaccharides (see Table 62–1), then the number of vaccines to which an individual could respond would be determined by dividing the number of possible antibody specificities (i.e., 10^9 to 10^{11}) by the average number of epitopes in one vaccine (i.e., 10^2). Therefore, an individual could respond to about 10^7 to 10^9 different vaccines. However, this analysis is limited by the number of available circulating B cells in neonates ($<10^{10}$), and the fact that a single epitope can stimulate more than one B-cell clone.

A more practical way to determine the capacity of the immune system to respond to vaccines would be to consider the number of B and T cells required to generate adequate levels of binding antibodies per milliliter of blood (the

TABLE 62–1 ■ Year of Introduction and Number of Immunogenic Proteins and Polysaccharides Contained in Selected Vaccines

Vaccine	Year of Introduction	Number of Proteins and Polysaccharides
Smallpox	1796	198
Rabies	1885	5
Diphtheria	1923	1
Pertussis (whole-cell)	1926	~3000
Tetanus	1927	1
Yellow fever	1936	11
Influenza	1945	10
Polio (inactivated)	1955	15
Polio (live, attenuated)	1961	15
Measles	1963	10
Mumps	1967	9
Rubella	1969	5
Hepatitis B	1981	1
Haemophilus influenzae type b (conjugate)	1990	2
Pertussis (acellular)	1991	2–5
Hepatitis A	1995	4
Varicella	1995	69
Pneumococcus (conjugate)	2000	8

"Protecton" theory).[20] Calculations are based on the following assumptions:

1. Approximately 10 ng/mL is likely to be an effective concentration of antibody directed against a specific epitope.
2. Approximately 10^3 B cells/mL are required to generate 10 ng of antibody/mL.
3. Given a doubling time of about 0.75 days for B cells, it would take about 7 days to generate 10^3 B cells/mL from a single B-cell clone.
4. Because vaccine-specific humoral immune responses are first detected about 7 days after immunization, those responses could initially be generated from a single B-cell clone per milliliter.
5. One vaccine contains about 10 immunogenic proteins or polysaccharides (see Table 62–1).
6. Each immunogenic protein or polysaccharide contains about 10 epitopes (i.e., 10^2 epitopes per vaccine).
7. Approximately 10^7 B cells are present per milliliter of blood.

Given these assumptions, the number of vaccines to which an individual could respond would be determined by dividing the number of circulating B cells ($\sim 10^7$) by the average number of epitopes per vaccine (10^2). Therefore, an individual could theoretically respond to about 10^5 vaccines at one time.

The analysis used to determine the theoretical capacity of an individual to respond to as many as 10^5 vaccines at one time, although consistent with the biology and kinetics of vaccine-specific immune responses, is limited by lack of consideration of several factors. First, only vaccine-specific B-cell responses are considered. However, protection against disease by vaccines may also be mediated by vaccine-specific cytotoxic T lymphocytes (CTLs). For example, virus-specific CTLs are important in the regulation and control of varicella infections.[21] Second, in part because of differences in the capacity of various class I or class II glycoproteins (encoded by the major histocompatibility complex [MHC]) to present viral or bacterial peptides to the immune system, some individuals are not capable of responding to certain virus-specific proteins (e.g., hepatitis B surface antigen).[22] Third, some proteins are more likely to evoke an immune response than others (i.e., immunodominance). Fourth, although most circulating B cells in the neonate are naïve, the child very quickly develops memory B cells that are not available for response to new antigens and, therefore, should not be considered as part of the circulating naïve B-cell pool. Fifth, the immune system is not static. A recent study of T-cell population dynamics in human immunodeficiency virus (HIV)–infected individuals found that adults have the capacity to generate about 2×10^9 new T lymphocytes each day.[23] Although the quantity of new B and T cells generated each day in healthy individuals is unknown, studies of HIV-infected persons demonstrate the enormous capacity of the immune system to generate lymphocytes when needed.

Do Vaccines "Weaken" the Immune System?

Infection with wild-type viruses can cause a suppression of specific immunologic functions. For example, infection with wild-type measles virus causes a reduction in the number of circulating B and T cells during the viremic phase of infection, and a delay in the development of cell-mediated immunity.[24,25] Down-regulation of cell-mediated immunity by wild-type measles virus probably results from down-regulation of the production of IL-12 by measles-infected macrophages and dendritic cells.[24] Taken together, the immunosuppressive effects of wild-type measles virus account, in part, for the increase in both morbidity and mortality from measles infection. Similarly, the immunosuppressive effects of infections with wild-type varicella virus[26] or wild-type influenza virus[27] cause an increase in the incidence of severe invasive bacterial infections.

Live viral vaccines replicate (albeit far less efficiently than wild-type viruses) in the host and, therefore, can weakly mimic events that occur after natural infection. For example, measles, mumps, or rubella vaccines can significantly depress reactivity to the tuberculin skin test,[28–34] measles-containing vaccine can cause a decrease in protective immune responses to varicella vaccine,[35] and high-titered measles vaccine (Edmonston-Zagreb strain) can cause an excess of cases of invasive bacterial infections in developing countries.[36] All of these phenomena are explained by the likely immunosuppressive effects of measles vaccine viruses.

However, current vaccines (including the highly-attenuated Moraten strain of measles vaccine) do not appear to cause clinically relevant immunosuppression in healthy children. Studies have found that the incidence of invasive bacterial infections (e.g., *H. influenzae* type b or *S. pneumoniae*) following immunization with diphtheria, pertussis, tetanus, BCG, measles, mumps, rubella, or live, attenuated poliovirus vaccines was not greater than that found in unimmunized children.[37–40]

Do Vaccines Alter the Balance of the Immune System?

Studies of vaccine safety have focused in part on whether vaccines adversely affect the developing immune system and cause chronic diseases. Although many well-designed studies of allergies, asthma, and autoimmune diseases have been performed using the sophisticated tools of epidemiology, genetics, virology, and immunology, the etiology of autoimmune diseases is incompletely understood. Evidence points to a multifactorial etiology in which an individual's genetic constitution leads to disease predisposition and environmental factors lead to disease onset.[41–43] For example, monozygotic twins both develop autoimmune disease only about 50% of the time,[44] which, although much higher than the disease risk of the general population, demonstrates the difficulty in determining how other factors such as diet, disease, infections, and environmental exposures contribute to development of autoimmunity. The following sections review the immunologic mechanisms by which vaccines may be envisioned to contribute to autoimmunity, asthma, or allergies. The relationship between multiple immunizations and immunologic dysfunction was also reviewed by the Institute of Medicine.[45]

Autoimmunity

Mechanisms are present at birth to prevent the development of immune responses directed against self-antigens (autoimmunity). T-cell and B-cell receptors of the fetus and newborn develop with a random repertoire of specificities. In the thymus, T cells whose receptors fail to bind to self-antigens presented in conjunction with MHC self-class I or class II molecules die before maturing. T cells that bind strongly to self-peptide–MHC complexes also die, while those that bind with a lesser affinity survive to populate the body. This central selection process eliminates strongly reactive T cells, while selecting for T cells that recognize antigens in the context of self-MHC. In the fetal liver, and later in the bone marrow, B-cell receptors (i.e., immunoglobulins) that bind self-antigens strongly are also eliminated. Therefore, the thymus and bone marrow, by expressing antigens from many tissues of the body, enable the removal of the majority of potentially dangerous autoreactive T and B cells before they mature—a process termed *central tolerance*.[4]

However, it is not simply the presence of autoreactive T and B cells that results in autoimmune disease. Autoreactive T and B cells are present in all individuals because it is not possible for every antigen from every tissue of the body to participate in the elimination of all potentially autoreactive cells. A process termed *peripheral tolerance* further limits the activation of autoreactive cells.[46,47] Mechanisms of peripheral tolerance include (1) antigen sequestration (antigens of the central nervous system, eyes, and testes are not regularly exposed to the immune system unless injury or infection occurs); (2) anergy (lymphocytes partially triggered by antigen but without co-stimulatory signals are unable to respond to subsequent antigen exposure); (3) activation-induced cell death (a self-limiting mechanism involved in terminating immune responses after antigen is cleared); and (4) inhibition of immune responses by specific regulatory cells.[48–51]

Therefore, the immune system anticipates that self-reactive T cells will be present and has mechanisms to control them. Any theory of vaccine causation of autoimmune diseases must take into account how these controls are circumvented.

By What Mechanisms Could Vaccines Cause Autoimmunity?

At least four key conditions must be met for development of autoimmune disease. First, self-antigen–specific T cells or self-antigen–specific B cells must be present. Second, self-antigens must be presented in sufficient amounts to trigger autoreactive cells. Third, co-stimulatory signals, cytokines, and other activation signals produced by antigen-presenting cells (such as dendritic cells) must be present during activation of self-reactive T cells. Fourth, peripheral tolerance mechanisms must fail to control destructive autoimmune responses. If all of these conditions are not met, the activation of self-reactive lymphocytes and progression to autoimmune disease will not occur. No mechanisms have been advanced to explain how vaccines could account for all of the prerequisites needed for the development of autoimmune disease. The likelihood that vaccines could meet each of the requirements for autoimmune disease is discussed below.

SELF-REACTIVE T AND B CELLS

Vaccines may contain antigens that are similar to self-antigens (i.e., molecular mimicry). Molecular mimicry between vaccine and self-antigens could theoretically cause vaccine-specific lymphocytes to cross-react with antigens in certain tissues and cause autoimmune disease.[52–54] This is especially true for T cells because peptide antigens presented by MHC molecules are defined by a linear amino acid sequence that is dominated by only a few amino acid side chains.[4] The existence of B cells that respond to both vaccines and self-antigens is also possible.

One example of molecular mimicry is that reported for the Lyme vaccine. The Lyme vaccine is composed of the outer surface protein A (OspA) of *Borrelia burgdorferi*. In the context of the MHC molecule DR4, some T cells that recognize OspA could also recognize a peptide of human protein lymphocyte function–associated antigen-1 (LFA-1).[55] This observation has been used to explain the presence of chronic arthritis seen in some individuals after Lyme disease,[55] although it is not clear whether cross-reacting T cells recognize self-antigens well enough to provoke autoimmunity.[54,56,57] Although Lyme vaccine consists of the OspA protein that contains the mimic epitope for DR4/LFA-1, several events occur during infection that do not occur after vaccination. For example, natural infection with *B. burgdorferi* may result in bacterial replication and inflammation in the target joints, high bacterial antigenic load in the joint, and high potential for presentation of large quantities of self-antigens as a result of cellular destruction.[54] None of these events occurs after vaccination. Consistent with differences between natural Lyme infection and immunization with Lyme vaccine, adverse events reported following administration of Lyme vaccine found no unusual patterns of arthritis.[58]

Therefore, although the potential for cross-reaction of self-reactive cells with vaccine components is present, many other factors that are likely to cause the development of autoimmune disease after natural infection are absent after vaccination.

PRESENTATION OF SUFFICIENT QUANTITIES OF SELF-ANTIGENS

Antigens derived from self-proteins are continuously presented to the immune system by macrophages and dendritic cells. However, presentation of large quantities of self-antigens by antigen-presenting cells occurs only after cell damage in target organs. Engulfment by nonactivated macrophages or dendritic cells of dead or dying cells resulting from normal cell turnover processes is believed to reduce, not increase, presentation of self-antigens.[59–61] Vaccines are not likely to increase the basal level of self-antigen presentation in autoimmune-vulnerable tissues or organs.

CO-STIMULATORY ACTIVATION IN THE CONTEXT OF SELF-ANTIGEN PRESENTATION

Vaccine components, either the microbial molecules themselves or adjuvants, can activate dendritic cells.[62,63] After antigen uptake, dendritic cells migrate to lymph nodes, express co-stimulatory molecules (e.g., CD80 and CD86), and release cytokines.[3] Expression of co-stimulatory molecules and release of cytokines are necessary for activation and differentiation of T cells.[6]

One potential mechanism by which vaccines could stimulate self-reactive T cells is "bystander activation." Bystander activation refers to the activation of, in this case, self-reactive T or B cells that are in the vicinity of dendritic cells activated by vaccines. It is very important to note that bystander activation is localized. Studies of adjuvants in animals have shown that distal delivery of antigens separate from the adjuvant does not confer a systemic response to bystander antigens.[64,65] Therefore, bystander activation of self-reactive T or B cells by vaccines would be unlikely to contribute to presentation of antigens in autoimmune-prone tissues or organs.

Although studies in autoimmune disease–prone animals have shown that inoculation of target tissues is sufficient to trigger an autoimmune reaction, these systems require *localized* introduction of adjuvants or nonspecific stimulation of the immune system at the site where tissue injury occurs.[66]

FAILURE OF PERIPHERAL TOLERANCE (LACK OF EFFECTIVE REGULATORY T CELLS)

Failure to develop or to activate regulatory T cells can lead to autoimmune disease in experimental animal models.[49] However, causes for the loss of peripheral tolerance in autoimmune diseases in humans are not well understood. No plausible mechanisms by which vaccination would cause the breakdown of peripheral tolerance have been advanced.

Do Vaccines Cause Autoimmunity?

Studies of type 1 diabetes[67] and multiple sclerosis[68,69] have not supported the hypothesis that vaccines cause autoimmune diseases. This is consistent with the fact that no mechanisms have been advanced to explain how vaccines could account for all of the prerequisites that would be required for the development of autoimmune disease.

Allergies and Asthma

Allergies are mediated by soluble factors (e.g., IgE) that mediate immediate-type hypersensitivity, or by cellular factors that mediate delayed-type hypersensitivity. Both immediate- and delayed-type hypersensitivity are dependent on the activation of T cells. Production of IgE by B cells is dependent on release of cytokines such as IL-4 by Th2 cells. Delayed-type hypersensitivity responses are mediated by "proinflammatory cytokines" produced by Th1 cells, by eosinophils activated by Th2 cells, and by cytotoxic T cells.[6]

How Could Vaccines Directly or Indirectly Contribute to Allergies or Allergic Asthma?

Two theories have been advanced to explain how vaccines could enhance IgE-mediated, Th2-dependent allergic responses. First, vaccines could shift immune responses to potential allergens from Th1-like to Th2-like.[70] Second, by preventing common prevalent infections (the "hygiene hypothesis"), vaccines could prolong the length or increase the frequency of Th2-type responses.[71,72]

Although all factors that cause changes in the balance of Th1 and Th2 responses are not fully known,[73] it is clear that dendritic cells play a critical role. For example, adjuvants (e.g., aluminum hydroxide or aluminum phosphate ["alum"]

contained in some vaccines) promote dendritic cells to stimulate Th2-type responses.[74,75] Adjuvants could cause allergies or asthma by stimulating bystander, allergen-specific Th2 cells. However, vaccine surveillance data show no evidence for environmental allergen priming by vaccination.[76] Furthermore, local inoculation of adjuvant does not cause a global shift of immune responses to Th1- or Th2-type.[65,77]

The other hypothesis advanced to explain how vaccines could promote allergies is that, by preventing several childhood infections (the hygiene hypothesis), stimuli that evolution has relied on to cause a shift from the neonatal Th2-type immune response to the balanced Th1-Th2 response patterns of adults have been eliminated.[71,72] However, the diseases that are prevented by vaccines constitute only a small fraction of the total number of illnesses to which the child is exposed, and it is unlikely that the immune system would rely on only a few infections for the development of a normal balance between Th1 and Th2 responses. For example, a study of 25,000 illnesses performed in Cleveland, Ohio, in the 1960s found that children experienced six to eight infections per year in the first 6 years of life; most of these infections were caused by viruses such as coronaviruses, rhinoviruses, paramyxoviruses, myxoviruses, and rotaviruses—diseases for which children are not routinely immunized.[78] Also at variance with the hygiene hypothesis is the fact that children in developing countries have lower rates of allergies and asthma than those in developed countries despite the fact that these children are commonly infected with helminths and worms—organisms that induce strong Th2-type responses.[79] Finally, the incidence of diseases that are mediated by Th1-type responses, such as multiple sclerosis or type 1 diabetes, have increased in the same populations as those that experienced an increase in allergies and asthma.

Do Vaccines Cause Allergies or Asthma?

Studies of asthma have not supported the hypothesis that vaccines cause diseases mediated by Th2 responses.[80] These findings are consistent with flaws in the proposed mechanisms.

Summing Up

A review of existing data does not support the presence of compelling biologic mechanisms to explain a causal link between vaccines and chronic diseases. The lack of plausible biologic mechanisms is matched by an absence of clear clinical data linking vaccines to autoimmune diseases such as type 1 diabetes or multiple sclerosis or to allergic diseases such as asthma.

REFERENCES

1. Gellin BG, Maibach EW, Marcuse EK. Do parents understand immunizations? A national telephone survey. Pediatrics 106:1097–1102, 2000.
2. Goldblatt D. Immunisation and the maturation of infant immune responses. Dev Biol Stand 95:125–132, 1998.
3. Guermonprez P, Valladeau J, Zitvogel L, et al. Antigen presentation and T cell stimulation by dendritic cells. Annu Rev Immunol 20:621–627, 2002.

4. Janeway CA, Travers P. Immunobiology: the Immune System in Health and Disease (2nd ed). New York, Garland Publishing Co., 1997.

5. Chaouat G, Zourbas S, Ostojic S, et al. A brief review of recent data on some cytokine expressions at the materno-foetal interface which might challenge the classical Th1/Th2 dichotomy. J Reprod Immunol 53:241–256, 2002.

6. Liu E, Tu W, Law H, Lau Y. Decreased yield, phenotypic expression, and function of immature monocyte-derived dendritic cells in cord blood. Br J Haematol 113:240–246, 2001.

7. Rijkers GT, Dollekamp EG, Zegers BJM. The in vitro B-cell response to pneumococcal polysaccharides in adults and neonates. Scand J Immunol 25:447–452, 1987.

8. Siegrist CA. Neonatal and early life vaccinology. Vaccine 19:3331–3346, 2001.

9. Mellander L, Carlsson B, Jalil E, et al. Secretory IgA antibody response against Escherichia coli antigens in infants in relation to exposure. J Pediatr 107:430–433, 1985.

10. Wheely SM, Jackson PT, Boxhall EH, et al. Prevention of perinatal transmission of hepatitis B virus (HBV): a comparison of two prophylactic schedules. J Med Virol 35:212–215, 1991.

11. Wong VC, Ip HM, Reesink HW, et al. Prevention of the HBsAg carrier state in newborns of mothers who are chronic carriers of HBsAg and HBeAg by administration of hepatitis-B vaccine and hepatitis-B immunoglobulin: double-blind randomized placebo-controlled study. Lancet 28:921–926, 1984.

12. Prozesky OW, Stevens CE, Szmunes W, et al. Immune response to hepatitis B vaccine in newborns. J Infect 7(suppl I):S53–S55, 1983.

13. Clark A, Rudd P. Neonatal BCG immunization. Arch Dis Child 67:473–474, 1992.

14. Marchant A, Gretghebuer T, Ota MO, et al. Newborns develop a TH1-type immune response to Mycobacterium bovis bacillus Calmette-Guerin vaccination. J Immunol 163:2249–2255, 1999.

15. Colditz GA, Brewe TF, Berkey CS, et al. Efficacy of BCG vaccine in the prevention of tuberculosis: meta-analysis of the published literature. JAMA 271:698–702, 1994.

16. Plotkin SA, Orenstein WA (eds). Vaccines (3rd ed). Philadelphia, WB Saunders, 1999.

17. Anderson P, Ingram DL, Pichichero M, Peter G. A high degree of natural immunologic priming to the capsular polysaccharide may not prevent Haemophilus influenzae type b meningitis. Pediatr Infect Dis J 19:589–591, 2000.

18. Lesinski G, Westerink M. Novel vaccine strategies to T-independent antigens. J Microbiol Methods 47:135–149, 2001.

19. Abbas AK, Lichtman AH, Pober JS. Cellular and Molecular Immunology (2nd ed). Philadelphia, WB Saunders, 1994.

20. Cohn M, Langman RE. The Protecton: the unit of humoral immunity selected by evolution. Immunol Rev 115:11–147, 1990.

21. Arvin A, Gershon A. Live attenuated varicella vaccine. Annu Rev Microbiol 50:59–100, 1996.

22. Averhoff F, Mahoney F, Coleman P, et al. Risk factors for lack of response to hepatitis B vaccines: a randomized trial comparing the immunogenicity of recombinant hepatitis B vaccines in an adult population. Am J Prev Med 15:1–8, 1998.

23. Ho DD, Neumann AU, Perelson AS, et al. Rapid turnover of plasma virions and CD4 lymphocytes in HIV-1 infection. Nature 373:123–126, 1995.

24. Karp C. Measles, immunosuppression, interleukin-12 and complement receptors. Immunol Rev 168:91–101, 1999.

25. Karp C, Wysocka M, Wahl L, et al. Mechanism of suppression of cell-mediated immunity by measles virus. Science 273:228–231, 1996.

26. Laupland KB, Davies HD, Low DE, et al. Invasive group A streptococcal disease in children and association with varicella-zoster virus infection. Pediatrics 105:E60, 2000.

27. O'Brien KL, Walters MI, Sellman J, et al. Severe pneumococcal pneumonia in previously healthy children: the role of preceding influenza infection. Clin Infect Dis 30:784–789, 2000.

28. Brody JA, McAlister R. Depression of tuberculin sensitivity following measles vaccination. Am Rev Resp Dis 90:607–611, 1964.

29. Ganguly R, Cusumano CL, Waldman RH. Suppression of cell-mediated immunity after infection with attenuated rubella virus. Infect Immun 13:464–469, 1976.

30. Starr S, Berkovich S. Effects of measles, gamma-globulin-modified measles and vaccine measles on the tuberculin test. N Engl J Med 270:386–391, 1964.

31. Brody JA, Overfield T, Hammes LM. Depression of the tuberculin reaction by viral vaccines. N Engl J Med 271:1294–1296, 1964.

32. Kupers T, Petrich JM, Holloway AW, St. Geme JW. Depression of tuberculin delayed hypersensitivity by live attenuated mumps virus. J Pediatr 76:716–721, 1970.

33. Zweiman B, Pappagianis D, Maibach H, Hildreth EA. Effect of measles immunization on tuberculin hypersensitivity and in vitro lymphocyte reactivity. Int Arch Allergy 40:834–841, 1971.

34. Hirsch RL, Mokhtarian F, Griffin DE, et al. Measles virus vaccination of measles seropositive individuals suppresses lymphocyte proliferation and chemotactic factor production. Clin Immunol Immunopathol 21:341–350, 1981.

35. Centers for Disease Control and Prevention. Simultaneous administration of varicella vaccine and other recommended childhood vaccines—United States, 1995–1999. MMWR 50:1058–1061, 2001.

36. Halsey N. Increased mortality after high-titer measles vaccines: too much of a good thing. Pediatr Infect Dis J 12:462–465, 1993.

37. Black SB, Cherry JD, Shinefield HR, et al. Apparent decreased risk of invasive bacterial disease after heterologous childhood immunization. Am J Dis Child 145:746–749, 1991.

38. Davidson M, Letson W, Ward JI, et al. DTP immunization and susceptibility to infectious diseases: is there a relationship? Am J Dis Child 145:750–754, 1991.

39. Storsaeter J, Olin P, Renemar B, et al. Mortality and morbidity from invasive bacterial infections during a clinical trial of acellular pertussis vaccines in Sweden. Pediatr Infect Dis J 7:637–645, 1988.

40. Otto S, Mahner B, Kadow I, et al. General non-specific morbidity is reduced after vaccination within the third month of life—the Greifswald study. J Infect 41:172–175, 2000.

41. Adorini L, Gregori S, Harrison L. Understanding autoimmune diabetes: insights from mouse models. Trends Mol Med 8:31–38, 2002.

42. Field L. Genetic linkage and association studies of type 1 diabetes: challenges and rewards. Diabetologia 45:21–35, 2002.

43. Platts-Mills T, Rakes G, Heymann P. The relevance of allergen exposure to the development of asthma in childhood. J Allergy Clin Immunol 105(suppl):S503–S508, 2000.

44. Redondo MJ, Yu L, Hawa M, et al. Heterogeneity of type 1 diabetes: analysis of monozygotic twins in Great Britain and the United States. Diabetologia 44:354–362, 2001.

45. Institute of Medicine, Stratton K, Wilson C, McCormick M (eds). Immunization Safety Review: Multiple Immunizations and Immune Dysfunction. Washington, DC, National Academy Press, 2002.

46. Kamradt T, Mitchison N. Tolerance and autoimmunity. N Engl J Med 344:655–664, 2001.

47. Mackay I. Science, medicine, and the future: tolerance and autoimmunity. BMJ 321:93–96, 2000.

48. Jonuleit H, Schmitt E, Steinbrink K, Enk A. Dendritic cells as a tool to induce anergic and regulatory T cells. Trends Immunol 22:394–400, 2001.

49. Maloy K, Powrie F. Regulatory T cells in the control of immune pathology. Nat Immunol 2:816–822, 2001.

50. Sharif S, Arreaza GA, Zucker P, et al. Activation of natural killer cells by alpha-galactosylceramide treatment prevents the onset and recurrence of autoimmune type 1 diabetes. Nat Med 7:1057–1062, 2001.

51. Shevach E. Certified professionals: CD4+CD25+ suppressor T cells. J Exp Med 193:F41–F46, 2001.

52. Regner M, Lambert P. Autoimmunity through infection or immunization. Nat Immunol 2:185–188, 2001.

53. Wucherpfennig K. Insights into autoimmunity gained from structural analysis of MHC-peptide complexes. Curr Opin Immunol 13:650–656, 2001.

54. Benoist C, Mathis D. Autoimmunity provoked by infection: how good is the case for T cell epitope mimicry? Nat Immunol 2:797–801, 2001.

55. Steere A, Gross D, Meyer A, Huber B. Autoimmune mechanisms in antibiotic treatment-resistant Lyme arthritis. J Autoimmun 16:263–268, 2001.

56. Deshpande S, Lee S, Zheng M, et al. Herpes simplex virus-induced keratitis: evaluation of the role of molecular mimicry in lesion pathogenesis. J Virol 75:3077–3088, 2001.

57. Rouse B, Deshpande S. Viruses and autoimmunity: an affair but not a marriage contract. Rev Med Virol 12:107–113, 2002.

58. Lathrop S. Adverse event reports following vaccination for Lyme disease: December 1998–July 2000. Vaccine 20:1603–1608, 2002.

59. Carroll M. A protective role for innate immunity in autoimmune disease. Clin Immunol 95(suppl):S30–S38, 2000.

60. Prodeus A. A critical role for complement in maintenance of self-tolerance. Immunity 9:721–731, 1998.
61. Sauter B, Albert ML, Francisco L, et al. Consequences of cell death: exposure to necrotic tumor cells, but not primary tissue cells or apoptotic cells, induces maturation of immunostimulatory dendritic cells. J Exp Med 191:423–434, 2000.
62. Schnare M, Barton GM, Holt AC, et al. Toll-like receptors control activation of adaptive immune responses. Nat Immunol 2:947–950, 2001.
63. de Jong EC, Vieira PL, Kalinski P, et al. Microbial compounds selectively induce Th1 cell-promoting or Th2 cell-promoting dendritic cells in vitro with diverse Th cell polarizing signals. J Immunol 168:1704–1709, 2002.
64. Zinkernagel R, Ehl S, Aichele P, et al. Antigen localization regulates immune responses in a dose- and time-dependent fashion: a geographical view of immune reactivity. Immunol Rev 156:199–209, 1997.
65. Kobayashi H, Horner AA, Takabayashi K, et al. Immunostimulatory DNA pre-priming: a novel approach for prolonged Th1-biased immunity. Cell Immunol 198:69–75, 1999.
66. Panoutsakopoulou V, et al. Analysis of the relationship between viral infection and autoimmune disease. Immunity 15:137–147, 2001.
67. DeStefano F, Mullooly JP, Okoro CA, et al. Childhood vaccinations, vaccination timing, and risk of type 1 diabetes mellitus. Pediatrics 108:E112, 2001.
68. Confavreux C, Suissa S, Saddier P, et al. Vaccinations and the relative risk of relapse in multiple sclerosis. Vaccines in Multiple Sclerosis Study Group. N Engl J Med 344:319–326, 2001.
69. Ascherio A, Zhang S, Hernan M, et al. Hepatitis b vaccination and the risk of multiple sclerosis. N Engl J Med 344:327–332, 2001.
70. Fournie GJ, Mas M, Cautain B, et al. Induction of autoimmunity through bystander effects: lessons from immunologic disorders induced by heavy metals. J Autoimmun 16:319–326, 2001.
71. Strachan D. Family size, infection, and atopy: the first decade of the "hygiene hypothesis." Thorax 55(suppl 1):S2–S10, 2000.
72. Wills-Karp M, Santeliz J, Karp C. The germless theory of allergic disease: revisiting the hygiene hypothesis. Nat Rev Immunol 1:69–75, 2001.
73. Flavell R, Dong C, Davis R. Signaling and cell death in lymphocytes. Inflamm Res 51:80–82, 2002.
74. Brewer JM, Conacher M, Hunter CA, et al. Aluminum hydroxide adjuvant initiates strong antigen-specific Th2 responses in the absence of IL-4- or IL-13-mediated signaling. J Immunol 163:6448–6454, 1999.
75. Ulanova M, Tarkowski A, Hahn-Zoric M, Hanson L. The common vaccine adjuvant aluminum hydroxide up-regulates accessory properties of human monocytes via an interleukin 4-dependent mechanism. Infect Immun 69:1151–1159, 2001.
76. Gruber C, Nilsson L, Bjorksten B. Do early childhood immunizations influence the development of atopy and do they cause allergic reactions? Pediatr Allergy Immunol 12:296–311, 2001.
77. Wang X, Mosmann T. In vivo priming of CD4 T cells that produce interleukin (IL)-2 but not IL-4 or interferon (IFN)-gamma and can subsequently differentiate into IL-4- or IFN-gamma secreting cells. J Exp Med 194:1069–1080, 2001.
78. Dingle J, Badger GF, Jordan WS Jr. Illness in the Home: A Study of 25,000 Illnesses in a Group of Cleveland Families. Cleveland, OH, The Press of Western Reserve University, 1964.
79. Van den Biggelaar AH, van Ree R, Rodrigues LV, et al. Decreased atopy in children infected with Schistosoma haematobium: a role for parasite-induced interleukin-10. Lancet 356:1723–1727, 2000.
80. Nilsson L, Gruber C, Granstrom M, et al. Pertussis IgE and atopic disease. Allergy 53:1195–1201, 1998.

Chapter 63

Legal Issues

GEOFFREY EVANS • DEBORAH HARRIS* • EMILY MARCUS LEVINE

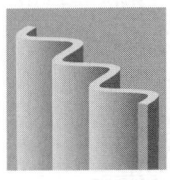

In this chapter, we review liability for vaccine injuries under the common law; the rationale, development, and implementation of the National Vaccine Injury Compensation Program (VICP); and the program's current status. The first part of the chapter covers the development of the law in the United States up to 1986, the year of the passage of the National Childhood Vaccine Injury Act (NCVIA). Later sections cover the administration of the VICP and the reported decisions relating to liability for the production and administration of vaccines after 1986.

Vaccine Liability Before 1986

To understand the decisions that were rendered in cases filed against vaccine manufacturers and administrators before 1986, it is important to understand the nature of products liability law as it was evolving in that era. Prior to the 1970s and early 1980s, manufacturers were not held liable for the harm associated with a product unless it failed to comply with the standards of manufacturing or care employed by similarly situated manufacturers. Usually, vaccine manufacturers sued by consumers would prevail because they employed customary practices and complied with statutes and regulations, and because of the doctrine of the "learned intermediary," discussed below.

This standard began to change when, in 1965, the American Law Institute introduced the concept of "strict liability" in its Restatement (Second) of Torts. Although

the principles embodied in this Restatement were not applied uniformly to lawsuits against vaccine manufacturers and administrators in the period before the NCVIA was enacted, they served as guiding principles in the field and were viewed by many as significant emerging legal doctrines.

Under the Restatement's doctrine of strict liability, a manufacturer who sold a product in a defective condition that made the product unreasonably dangerous was subject to liability for harm caused to the user or consumer even if the manufacturer exercised all possible care in the preparation and sale of the product.[1] A product was deemed defective if it was in a condition not contemplated by the ultimate consumer, which made it unreasonably dangerous to him or her.[2] Although the doctrine of strict liability lowered the burden required to find manufacturers liable for the harm caused by their products, the authors of the Restatement recognized that some products were, by their nature, "unavoidably unsafe," and determined that such products should not be deemed unreasonably dangerous under the doctrine of strict liability.[3] Thus, products such as vaccines, which necessarily entail some risks (risks that are considered reasonable given the products' benefits to the community), were not deemed defective or unreasonably dangerous so long as they were properly prepared and accompanied by adequate warnings.[4] Vaccine manufacturers and administrators therefore were generally not held liable for harm caused by their products before 1986 so long as these requirements of proper preparation and adequate warnings were satisfied.

The risk of liability created by the requirements to properly prepare vaccines and provide adequate warnings is important. If, for instance, a batch of vaccine is defective and causes disease in recipients because the disease-causing agent has not been sufficiently inactivated or because of contaminants, the manufacturer may be liable, whether or not the defect can be shown to be the manufacturer's fault. This happened with an early batch of Salk killed poliovirus vaccine, and there were numerous and substantial recoveries by persons who acquired polio from the vaccine.[5] Or if a physician administers a vaccine when it is contraindicated—for instance, he or she administers Sabin oral poliovirus vaccine (OPV) to a child known to be immunodeficient or administers a second dose of diphtheria and

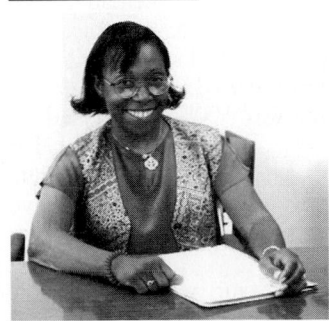

* This chapter is dedicated to our colleague, co-author, and friend, the late Deborah Harris. For over 12 years, Deborah not only provided excellent legal advice, but also contributed her practical insights in life, her sense of compassion for those needing compensation, and throughout it all, her wonderful sense of humor. She will be greatly missed, both personally and professionally.

tetanus toxoids and whole-cell pertussis (DTP) vaccine after a child has reacted strongly to the first—then the physician may be liable if the adverse consequence risked by violating the indication occurs. Furthermore, if a physician administers a vaccine without warning the patient of the risks, the physician may be liable if the risks occur.

Despite the limits on liability imposed by general doctrines of products liability law in cases concerning adverse reactions resulting from vaccines, certain judicial decisions in the pre-1986 era imposed liability even when the vaccine was properly made and administered. These cases, which were a significant impetus to the enactment of the NCVIA, can be divided into three categories: the *Reyes* decision, the swine flu litigation against the government, and the 1980s decisions. (The cases discussed here are reported decisions in the appellate courts.)

Reyes v. Wyeth Laboratories,[6,7]* decided in 1974, held a producer of Sabin OPV liable to a child who contracted polio after being administered the vaccine. Liability in this case was based on the manufacturer's failure either to directly provide warnings to potential vaccine recipients concerning the risks associated with the vaccine or to ensure that such warning would be given. In this case, the manufacturer had sold the vaccine to the Texas Department of Public Health, accompanied by the Food and Drug Administration (FDA) required package inserts containing a warning, but the Texas Department of Public Health sent the vaccine on to the county health department without ensuring that the warning would actually be given to vaccine recipients. The county public health nurse who administered the vaccine to the child in this case did not warn the parents of the minute risk that a recipient or contact could contract the disease. This case embodied an exception to the general "learned intermediary" standard. Under this general rule, a manufacturer of prescription medicines, including vaccines, is obliged to provide warnings concerning the product to the health care provider (the "learned intermediary"), but has no duty to directly warn the user of the product of its associated risks. The *Reyes* decision narrowed this general rule, holding that, where a manufacturer can reasonably be said to be aware that the product (i.e., the vaccine) will be administered in such a way that no personalized medical advice will be provided by the health care provider to the consumer (e.g., in the context of a public health department immunization effort in which the patient had no direct contact with a physician), the manufacturer is responsible for providing warnings directly to patients or ensuring that such warnings will be given.

The next development in the area of vaccine liability involved the swine flu vaccine. In the spring of 1976, leading U.S. epidemiologists predicted that the United States would be afflicted the following winter with an unusually severe form of the flu, which would lead to numerous serious illnesses and consequences, including death, for some of those who contracted the disease. Such an epidemic never occurred, but this prediction led the government to recommend a campaign to immunize almost all American adults, particularly the elderly, with the support of government funds. This episode is carefully summarized by Silverstein[8];

a more partisan account is to be found in Neustadt and Fineberg.[9]

The *Reyes* decision, holding manufacturers liable for failing to provide adequate warnings in a mass campaign, caused manufacturers to refuse to provide the swine flu vaccine to the government at all. In addition, manufacturers, concerned about other unforeseen risks of liability in a program this large, did not want to accept any liability for vaccines that would be produced in accordance with FDA regulations. As a result, the Swine Flu Act was passed. This law required vaccine recipients who believed they had been injured to sue the federal government, which served as a substitute defendant for the vaccine manufacturers. The swine flu program was a considerable success as a matter of effective public health mobilization, insofar as the vaccine was successfully produced, distributed, and administered to more than 45 million people in a few months. However, vaccination was suspended when the feared swine flu epidemic had not yet appeared and suspicions arose that there might be an association between the vaccine and Guillain-Barré syndrome (GBS). Numerous claims concerning GBS were filed under the Swine Flu Act, many of which relied on a Centers for Disease Control and Prevention (CDC)–sponsored study that showed a statistically significant increase in the risk of GBS in the 10 weeks after immunization compared with the risk in unvaccinated people. The government accepted liability for all cases of GBS with onset falling within this period. However, the government did not agree to accept liability for cases of GBS falling outside this interval or for other illnesses not known to be caused by influenza vaccines.

The defense of this litigation resulted in more than 100 judicial opinions, which generally shielded manufacturers and administrators from liability under the Swine Flu Act. However, some courts of appeals wrote opinions in the *Reyes v. Wyeth* tradition that threatened increased liability for the federal government based on a theory of inadequate warning—for example, *Unthank v. United States*[10] and *Petty v. United States*,[11] in which the federal government was found derivatively liable for a manufacturer's failure to provide plaintiffs with adequate warnings covering the risks of the swine flu vaccine. The litigation and the resulting opinions have been summarized in detail by the Institute of Medicine (IOM).[12]

The efforts of plaintiffs to establish common-law, strict tort liability on the part of pharmaceutical houses (i.e., the manufacturer is liable even if adequate warnings are given and the vaccine is produced and handled in full compliance with FDA regulations) appeared to increase after *Reyes* and the swine flu episode. In the 1980s, plaintiffs achieved some notable successes in the trial courts. For instance, in *Johnson v. American Cyanamid Co.*,[13] the father of a vaccinated child who claimed to have contracted polio through contact with his child sued both the manufacturer and administrator of the OPV. The Kansas Supreme Court reversed the jury's verdict, that the vaccine's manufacturer was 100% liable, and its accompanying $10 million damages award, and concluded that the manufacturer's warning was adequate. However, the court implied that the vaccine administrator might have been liable for failing to warn the parents of the vaccine's risk had this claim been pursued.

In *Toner v. Lederle Laboratories*,[14] a jury returned a verdict of $1,131,200 in favor of the recipient of a DTP vaccine who

---

*Reyes was followed in *Givens v. Lederle*.[7]

claimed that the vaccine caused transverse myelitis, a condition that had never been shown scientifically to be caused by any of the available DTP preparations. The plaintiff's theory was that the DTP caused transverse myelitis and that the defendant could have marketed a safer vaccine, a vaccine once marketed by another manufacturer that was withdrawn from the market in the 1970s, and that Lederle's failure to make a safer version of the vaccine was negligent. The verdict was appealed to the U.S. Court of Appeals for the Ninth Circuit, which referred the issues to the Supreme Court of Idaho. The Supreme Court of Idaho affirmed the jury's verdict that Lederle's design of DTP was negligent.

Despite the results reached in these cases and the fear that such verdicts and damages awards instilled in the vaccine industry and in health care professionals, it is important to emphasize that U.S. courts generally have been very supportive of vaccination programs and that, with limited exceptions, vaccine manufacturers and administrators have been historically, and continue to be, shielded from liability, so long as the vaccines in question are properly made and administered in accordance with accepted medical procedures and so long as the recipient receives adequate warnings of the vaccine's attendant risks.

The liability imposed by the courts in the previously cited cases may relate to the fact that the very success of vaccines has changed the way they are perceived by the public. With waning vaccine-preventable disease, vaccines may instead be viewed as a routine nuisance procedure to prevent diseases that few—including most young physicians—have actually experienced. In this setting, it is only natural that individuals will choose to avoid risk when the benefit is not readily apparent, which translates into demands for "safer" products. Ironically, this attitude can retard the development of new vaccines against additional and currently threatening diseases. Medical experts and public health officials involved in vaccination must remember that an effective vaccination program, no matter how justified medically and in relation to the risk-benefit ratio, can only be successful over the long term if its purposes and methods are well understood not only by medical personnel, but by society in general. The importance of patience and care in explaining the vaccination process, as well as the risks and benefits of vaccination, cannot be overstated in helping to maintain an effective vaccination program.

The Power to Compel Vaccination

U.S. courts generally have been deferential to public health judgments that mandatory vaccination is required. In the leading case, *Jacobson v. Massachusetts*,[15] the U.S. Supreme Court upheld a Massachusetts statute that empowered each local board of health to require vaccination of the inhabitants "if, in its opinion, it is necessary for the public health or safety." Under this authority, the city of Cambridge required all residents to receive the smallpox vaccination. Although children whose physicians determined that such vaccination was medically contraindicated were exempted from this requirement, a similar exemption was not available for similarly situated adults. Jacobson, who had apparently experienced adverse reactions to the vaccine, refused vaccination and was fined. The Supreme Court rejected

Jacobson's argument that the Massachusetts law was constitutionally invalid and, instead, held that the law was a reasonable and proper exercise of the state's police power to protect the public health and safety. The court rejected Jacobson's offer to present evidence undermining the medical efficacy and safety of vaccination. Instead, the court took judicial notice (without hearing evidence) of the fact that the people of the state of Massachusetts held a common belief (which was maintained by high medical authority) that vaccination was a preventative of smallpox, determined that that the legislature was entitled to rely on this theory, and concluded that the legislature was not compelled to commit such a public health and safety matter to the final decision of a court or jury. This early case is significant insofar as the Supreme Court recognized the importance of vaccination to the American public and deferred to the authority of state lawmakers to develop and impose vaccination requirements on the general population.

Decisions of contemporary courts continue to be supportive of mandatory vaccination requirements and often cite *Jacobson* in deciding lawsuits challenging immunization mandates. In *Maricopa County Health Department v. Harmon*,[16] the health department sought an injunction that excluded unimmunized children from school. The health department had issued an emergency rule barring unimmunized children from attending school because of an outbreak of measles in the county. The purpose of the injunction was to enforce the health department rule. The trial court granted the injunction, and the appellate court affirmed. The court rejected the families' argument that the health department had no authority to exclude children unless there had been a confirmed case of measles in the particular school, holding that the health department had the authority to exclude children, even in the absence of a serologically confirmed case.

Contemporary vaccination laws are not as sweeping as the law involved in *Jacobson*. States generally require that children receive certain recommended vaccines in order to attend school. There is some variation among state laws as to which vaccines will be required for school entry. These laws are dynamic and incorporate new vaccines as appropriate. (The CDC's National Immunization Program maintains a website with current information on state immunization requirements for school entry; see *www.cdc.gov/nip/vaccine/state-reqs.htm*.) However, the recommended age of administration for most of these vaccines is during the first 2 years of life, and the vaccines are in fact administered to a high percentage of children at the recommended age.[17] These laws may persuade reluctant parents that, because vaccination will be required eventually, they might as well agree to vaccination at the recommended time. There are no governmental vaccination requirements for the general adult population in the United States.*

---

*There is no federal mandate for adult or childhood immunization now that the United States no longer requires certain vaccines for travel. However, vaccinations are required for entry into the military. The requirement that some service members receive the anthrax vaccine has been controversial, resulting in court martial and other discipline for some who have refused vaccination (see, e.g., *United States v. Washington*[18]). The Occupational Safety and Health Administration regulations require employers to make vaccination available to employees potentially exposed to blood-borne pathogens (e.g., health care workers must be offered HBV immunizations).

However, certain segments of the adult population (e.g., college students and health care professionals) may be subject to particular vaccination requirements.

The laws that require vaccination before school entry are congruent with the grant program operated by the Public Health Service under the provisions of the Public Health Service Act.[19] If a state or local government participates in that federally funded immunization program, it must, among other requirements, have a "plan to assure that children begin and complete their immunizations on schedule" and a "plan to systematically immunize susceptible children at school entry through vigorous enforcement of school immunization laws."[20]

Whereas courts have upheld the right of individual states to mandate immunization, some states have voluntarily granted individuals exemptions from this requirement based on religious or personal beliefs (all states allow exemptions for a medical contraindication to vaccination). Although the court in *Brown v. Stone*[21] struck a religious exemption from a state statute on the grounds that it violated the Equal Protection Clause of the Fourteenth Amendment, most courts have recognized the right of a state to allow religious exemptions. Instead, the courts have focused on the scope of the exemption. For example, in *McCarthy v. Boozman*,[22] a federal district court judge found unconstitutional an Arkansas law that granted religious exemptions to the state's general school immunization requirements only to individuals who were members or adherents of a church or religious denomination recognized by the state, but not to others whose objections to immunization were also grounded in sincere religious beliefs. The judge found that the religious exemption section of the Arkansas law violated the Establishment and Free Exercise Clauses of the First Amendment and the Equal Protection Clause of the Fourteenth Amendment to the U.S. Constitution, noting that the primary effect of this exemption provision was to "inhibit the earnest beliefs and practices of those individuals who oppose immunization on religious grounds but are not members of an officially recognized religious organization." In the *Matter of Christine M.*,[23] the court held that it was child neglect for an otherwise responsible parent to refuse to permit his 2-year-old child to be vaccinated for measles during a measles outbreak in New York City absent a demonstration of sincere grounds for a religious exemption. However, the court refrained from ordering immediate vaccination on the grounds that the vaccination would be required when the child entered school and that the measles outbreak had ended by the time of the decision.

Other litigants have challenged the constitutionality of allowing religious exemptions and not philosophical exemptions. The courts have ruled that the First Amendment does not apply to philosophical exemptions and that there is no constitutional right to such an exemption. As with religious exemptions, the courts have given the states the discretion to grant philosophical exemptions if they so choose. The Supreme Court of Wyoming recently held that the state was not authorized to hold hearings to judge the sincerity of a parent's religious beliefs before a religious waiver to state immunization requirements would be granted.[24] The court did not reach the issue of whether such a requirement would violate the parents' constitutional right to the free exercise of religion. To date, approximately one third of states allow philosophical exemptions, and nearly all (48) allow religious exemptions.

Regarding medical exemptions, which all states allow, the Supreme Court of Wyoming recently held that the State of Wyoming's Health Department could waive state immunization requirements for a particular child if such vaccination was medically contraindicated for that child, but that the department could not require the child or his or her physician to provide a reason for such a contraindication to immunizations.[25] Other instances challenging mandatory vaccination include *Ritterband v. Axelrod*,[26] in which a New York trial court upheld health department regulations that required hospital employees and medical staff to have current rubella immunizations. The lawsuit was filed by a staff doctor who argued that the vaccination requirement was a violation of the Fourth Amendment protection against unreasonable searches and seizures.

Just prior to publication of this text, vaccine shortages led several states to approve temporary, emergency exceptions to childhood immunization requirements. Results from a questionnaire completed in January 2002 showed that 24 state immunization progams reported temporarily suspending school entry requirements for Td ad 5 states reported suspending requirements for DTaP. Such vaccine shortages have led the Federal Government to utilize existing stockpiles of recommended childhood vaccines (e.g., measles, mumps, and rubella [MMR] vaccine), and create others for use in such circumstances.[27]

Compulsory immunization is utilized outside the United States as well, although only one third of European Union (EU) countries appear to utilize this option.[28] Belgium, France, Greece, Portugal, Italy, and Finland require childhood vaccination. Four countries (Italy, Greece, France, and Belgium) list requirements for school entry for the routine childhood vaccines, although Italy does not mandate pertussis immunization, in contrast to the others. Portugal lists tetanus, diphtheria, and bacille Calmette-Guérin but apparently does not require vaccination for school entry, and Finland mandates tetanus and diphtheria toxoids for adult use (Td), inactivated poliovirus vaccine (IPV), MMR, and meningococcal vaccines for its military forces. At least two other non-EU countries (Japan and Taiwan) require routine childhood vaccines as well as other vaccines. The United Kingdom does not have any compulsory immunization.[29]

National Childhood Vaccine Injury Act

Immunization practice, as an accepted rite of passage for children and a preventive health cornerstone, began to change with the tide of litigation. The *Reyes v. Wyeth* decision and its progeny were followed by the withdrawal of a number of pharmaceutical houses from vaccine production and an increase in the price of vaccines.[12] Manufacturers of the DTP vaccine declined from seven to two, the producers of OPV fell from three to one, and the manufacturers of measles vaccine plunged from six to one. The price of DTP vaccine, which sold for $0.19 in 1980, skyrocketed to more than $12.00 in 1986. From a commercial perspective, these actions would appear to be warranted. In 1980, the gross sales, including profit, from the production of all childhood vaccines were approximately $3 million, but the costs associated with one or two successful tort lawsuits against a vaccine manufacturer had the potential to outweigh the gross sales of all manufacturers in a single year.

The litigious atmosphere of the 1980s and the sharp decrease in the number of vaccine manufacturers had an adverse impact on the research and development of new and safer vaccines. Before a vaccine is marketed, and before a manufacturer has a possibility of reaping any profit, the FDA requires the manufacturer to prove that the vaccine is safe and effective. Meeting this burden is costly, and the investment cannot be recovered until the vaccine is marketed. The costs and logistics associated with administering a new vaccine a sufficient number of times in prelicensure clinical trails to detect rare adverse side effects were prohibitive. The manufacturer's inability to accurately estimate its risk of liability and, therefore, the effect of this potential liability on its profit margin translated into limited commercial incentives to develop new vaccines.

During this period, the nation's children were at risk. The American Academy of Pediatrics and the American Medical Association were concerned about both the continued availability of vaccines and the possibility that physicians also were at risk. At the time, it was common for plaintiffs to join both the pharmaceutical house and the administering physician in the complaint, claiming that the physician did not adequately disclose the risk associated with the vaccine. This was dramatically demonstrated in North Carolina, when a federal jury found a leading pediatrician liable for more than $1 million for a routine pediatric immunization given years earlier. Although that verdict was overturned by the trial judge, it mobilized pediatricians in North Carolina to seek a statute protecting them from liability. The North Carolina legislature responded to the threat that the state would no longer have an effective immunization program by passing a statute protecting all participants in the delivery of vaccines from liability and providing compensation to injured vaccinees.[30] The statute passed unanimously, and the political message no doubt reached the members of Congress.[§]

In the end, the National Childhood Vaccine Injury Act of 1986[32] was compromise legislation fought for by parents and physicians with some backing of industry and trial attorneys, but with little support from the Reagan administration. On record against the legislation on the grounds that a new federal program was not needed, President Reagan reluctantly signed the bill into law after intense lobbying by its supporters.

National Vaccine Injury Compensation Program

Purpose and Goals

The VICP, established by the NCVIA, was authorized by Congress to address a variety of public policy needs.[33–35] First and most important, it is only simple justice that individuals inadvertently injured by properly produced and administered vaccines in public health programs should

receive compensation. Because society mandates their use through state laws for school entry, it is not only reasonable but also appropriate that society take responsibility for unavoidable adverse outcomes. Second, the delays and uncertainties of the tort system warranted a more efficient, fair approach. Third, the deterioration in the vaccine production and supply situation, created in part by liability connected to vaccine-related injuries, would inevitably lead to serious outbreaks of otherwise preventable disease. Fourth, the unprecedented vaccine price increases were caused largely by the projected costs of litigation as calculated by the manufacturers. Fifth, the increasing scientific capability for the production of new and improved vaccines obviously required considerable interest and investment on the part of biologics manufacturers, and, at the very least, the litigious climate surrounding the use of vaccines was detrimental to such efforts. Finally, there was no evidence that the problem was going to disappear, particularly in view of the attention devoted to it by the media.

Congress addressed these issues by creating the VICP, a federal "no-fault" system under which awards can be made to vaccine-injured individuals quickly, easily, and generously. Persons injured through the receipt of a vaccine after the effective date of the legislation are required to file claims with the VICP before they are allowed to bring a civil suit. Rules of evidence, discovery, and other legal procedures are relaxed to accelerate the compensation process. Negligence on the part of the manufacturer or health care provider is removed from proceedings, thus the no-fault designation. Judgments (whether dismissing the claim or awarding compensation) must be expressly rejected by petitioners prior to their seeking other remedies, such as filing a civil suit. Once a judgment is rejected, a person essentially forfeits any right to compensation under the program and can seek remedies only through other channels. Funding for the program is provided through an excise tax placed on covered childhood vaccines.

The existing controversy over vaccine injury causation played heavily in creating the VICP's framework and the NCVIA's sweeping vaccine safety provisions. The federal government was brought into a more prominent vaccine safety role. The NCVIA included a mandate for the reporting of certain adverse events. Health care providers and vaccine manufacturers are now required to report the occurrence of any event set forth in the Vaccine Injury Table (VIT) (Table 63–1), as well as any contraindicating reaction to a vaccine that is specified in the manufacturer's package insert. The report is to consist of the symptoms and manifestations of the illness or injury, how long after administration of the vaccine such symptoms occurred, and the manufacturer and lot number of the vaccine administered. These reports are to be made to what is now known as the Vaccine Adverse Event Reporting System (VAERS). Other vaccine safety mandates include office record keeping (documenting the date of vaccine administration, the manufacturer and lot number, and the name and address of the administrator); development of risk-benefit information materials (currently known as Vaccine Information Statements); and IOM studies of adverse events for VICP-covered vaccines.

The NCVIA also provided for two advisory panels, the Advisory Commission on Childhood Vaccines (ACCV) and the National Vaccine Advisory Committee (NVAC). Composed of physicians, parents, and attorneys in equal

---

[§]This episode is described in the *American Medical News* for August 1, 1986. North Carolina continues to have a childhood vaccine-related injury compensation program, which requires covered petitioners to pursue a claim with the VICP before seeking a remedy with the state compensation program.[31]

TABLE 63–1 ▪ National Childhood Vaccine Injury Act Reporting and Compensation Tables*

Vaccine	Adverse Event	Interval from Vaccination to Onset of Event	
		For Reporting†	For Compensation‡
I. Tetanus toxoid–containing vaccines (e.g., DTaP, DTP-Hib, DT, Td, or TT)	A. Anaphylaxis or anaphylactic shock	0–7 days	0–4 hr
	B. Brachial neuritis	0–28 days	2–28 days
	C. Any acute complication or sequela (including death) of above events	Not applicable	Not applicable
	D. Events described in manufacturer's package insert as contraindications to additional doses of vaccine	See package insert	Not applicable
II. Pertussis antigen–containing vaccines (e.g., DTaP, DTP, P, DTP-Hib)	A. Anaphylaxis or anaphylactic shock	0–7 days	0–4 hr
	B. Encephalopathy (or encephalitis)	0–7 days	0–72 hr
	C. Any acute complication or sequela (including death) of above events	Not applicable	Not applicable
	D. Events described in manufacturer's package insert as contraindications to additional doses of vaccine	See package insert	Not applicable
III. Measles, mumps and rubella virus–containing vaccines in any combination (e.g., MMR, MR, M, R)	A. Anaphylaxis or anaphylactic shock	0–7 days	0–4 hr
	B. Encephalopathy (or encephalitis)	0–15 days	5–15 days
	C. Any acute complication or sequela (including death) of above events	Not applicable	Not applicable
	D. Events described in manufacturer's package insert as contraindications to additional doses of vaccine	See package insert	Not applicable
IV. Rubella virus–containing vaccines (e.g., MMR, MR, R)	A. Chronic arthritis	0–42 days	7–42 days
	B. Any acute complication or sequela (including death) of above event	Not applicable	Not applicable
	C. Events described in manufacturer's package insert as contraindications to additional doses of vaccine	See package insert	Not applicable
V. Measles virus–containing vaccines (e.g., MMR, MR, M)	A. Thrombocytopenic purpura	0–30 days	7–30 days
	B. Vaccine-strain measles viral infection in an immunodeficient recipient	0–6 mo	0–6 mo
	C. Any acute complication or sequela (including death) of above events	Not applicable	Not applicable
	D. Events described in manufacturer's package insert as contraindications to additional doses of vaccine	See package insert	Not applicable
VI. Polio live virus–containing vaccines (OPV)	A. Paralytic polio		
	1. In a nonimmunodeficient recipient	0–30 days	0–30 days
	2. In an immunodeficient recipient	0–6 mo	0–6 mo
	3. In a vaccine-associated community case	No limit	Not applicable
	B. Vaccine-strain polio viral infection		
	1. In a nonimmunodeficient recipient	0–30 days	0–30 days
	2. In an immunodeficient recipient	0–6 mo	0–6 mo

TABLE 63–1 ■ National Childhood Vaccine Injury Act Reporting and Compensation Tables*—cont'd

Vaccine	Adverse Event	Interval from Vaccination to Onset of Event	
		For Reporting[†]	For Compensation[‡]
	3. In a vaccine-associated community case	No limit	Not applicable
	C. Any acute complication or sequela (including death) of above events	Not applicable	Not applicable
	D. Events described in manufacturer's package insert as contraindications to additional doses of vaccine	See package insert	Not applicable
VII. Polio inactivated-virus containing vaccines (e.g., IPV)	A. Anaphylaxis or anaphylactic shock	0–7 days	0–4 hr
	B. Any acute complication or sequela (including death) of above event	Not applicable	Not applicable
	C. Events described in manufacturer's package insert as contraindications to additional doses of vaccine	See package insert	Not applicable
VIII. Hepatitis B antigen–containing vaccines	A. Anaphylaxis or anaphylactic shock	0–7 days	0–4 hr
	B. Any acute complication or sequela (including death) of above event	Not applicable	Not applicable
	C. Events described in manufacturer's package insert as contraindications to additional doses of vaccine	See package insert	Not applicable
IX. *Haemophilus influenzae* type b (polysaccharide conjugate vaccines)	A. No condition specified for compensation	Not applicable	Not applicable
	B. Events described in manufacturer's package insert as contraindications to additional doses of vaccine	See package insert	Not applicable
X. Varicella vaccine	A. No condition specified for compensation	Not applicable	Not applicable
	B. Events described in manufacturer's package insert as contraindications to additional doses of vaccine	See package insert	Not applicable
XI. Rotavirus vaccine	A. No condition specified for compensation	Not applicable	Not applicable
	B. Events described in manufacturer's package insert as contraindications to additional doses of vaccine	See package insert	Not applicable
XII. Vaccines containing live, oral, rhesus-based rotavirus	A. Intussusception	0–30 days	0–30 days
	B. Events described in manufacturer's package insert as contraindications to additional doses of vaccine	See package insert	Not applicable
XIII. Pneumococcal conjugate vaccines	A. No condition specified for compensation	Not applicable	Not applicable
	B. Events described in manufacturer's package insert as contraindications to additional doses of vaccine	See package insert	Not applicable
XIV. Any new vaccine recommended by the CDC for routine administration to children, after publication by Secretary of the HHS of a notice of coverage	A. No condition specified for compensation	Not applicable	Not applicable
	B. Events described in manufacturer's package insert as contraindications to additional doses of vaccine	Not applicable	Not applicable

Continued

TABLE 63–1 ■ National Childhood Vaccine Injury Act Reporting and Compensation Tables*—cont'd

Vaccine	Adverse Event	Interval from Vaccination to Onset of Event	
		For Reporting†	For Compensation‡
QUALIFICATIONS AND AIDS TO INTERPRETATION§			

(1) *Anaphylaxis and anaphylactic shock* mean an acute, severe, and potentially lethal systemic allergic reaction. Most cases resolve without sequelae. Signs and symptoms begin minutes to a few hours after exposure. Death, if it occurs, usually results from airway obstruction caused by laryngeal edema or bronchospasm and may be associated with cardiovascular collapse. Other significant clinical signs and symptoms may include the following: cyanosis, hypotension, bradycardia, tachycardia, arrhythmia, edema of the pharynx and/or trachea and/or larynx with stridor and dyspnea. Autopsy findings may include acute emphysema which results from lower respiratory tract obstruction, edema of the hypopharynx, epiglottis, larynx, or trachea and minimal findings of eosinophilia in the liver, spleen, and lungs. When death occurs within minutes of exposure and without signs of respiratory distress, there may not be significant pathologic findings.

(2) *Encephalopathy.* For purposes of the Vaccine Injury Table, a vaccine recipient shall be considered to have suffered an encephalopathy only if such recipient manifests, within the applicable period, an injury meeting the description below of an acute encephalopathy, and then a chronic encephalopathy persists in such person for more than 6 months beyond the date of vaccination.

  (i) An *acute encephalopathy* is one that is sufficiently severe so as to require hospitalization (whether or not hospitalization occurred).

    (A) *For children less than 18 months of age* who present without an associated seizure event, an acute encephalopathy is indicated by a "significantly decreased level of consciousness" (see "D" below) lasting for at least 24 hours. Those children less than 18 months of age who present following a seizure shall be viewed as having an acute encephalopathy if their significantly decreased level of consciousness persists beyond 24 hours and cannot be attributed to a postictal state (seizure) or medication.

    (B) *For adults and children 18 months of age or older*, an acute encephalopathy is one that persists for at least 24 hours and characterized by at least two of the following:

      (1) A significant change in mental status that is not medication related; specifically a confusional state, or a delirium, or a psychosis;

      (2) A significantly decreased level of consciousness, which is independent of a seizure and cannot be attributed to the effects of medication; and

      (3) A seizure associated with loss of consciousness.

    (C) Increased intracranial pressure may be a clinical feature of acute encephalopathy in any age group.

    (D) A "significantly decreased level of consciousness" is indicated by the presence of at least one of the following clinical signs for at least 24 hours or greater (see paragraphs (2)(i)(A) and (2)(i)(B) of this section for applicable timeframes):

      (1) Decreased or absent response to environment (responds, if at all, only to loud voice or painful stimuli);

      (2) Decreased or absent eye contact (does not fix gaze upon family members or other individuals); or

      (3) Inconsistent or absent responses to external stimuli (does not recognize familiar people or things).

    (E) The following clinical features alone, or in combination, do not demonstrate an acute encephalopathy or a significant change in either mental status or level of consciousness as described above: Sleepiness, irritability (fussiness), high-pitched and unusual screaming, persistent inconsolable crying, and bulging fontanelle. Seizures in themselves are not sufficient to constitute a diagnosis of encephalopathy. In the absence of other evidence of an acute encephalopathy, seizures shall not be viewed as the first symptom or manifestation of the onset of an acute encephalopathy.

  (ii) *Chronic encephalopathy* occurs when a change in mental or neurologic status, first manifested during the applicable time period, persists for a period of at least 6 months from the date of vaccination. Individuals who return to a normal neurologic state after the acute encephalopathy shall not be presumed to have suffered residual neurologic damage from that event; any subsequent chronic encephalopathy shall not be presumed to be a sequela of the acute encephalopathy. If a preponderance of the evidence indicates that a child's chronic encephalopathy is secondary to genetic, prenatal, or perinatal factors, that chronic encephalopathy shall not be considered to be a condition set forth in the Table.

  (iii) An encephalopathy shall not be considered to be a condition set forth in the Table if in a proceeding on a petition, it is shown by a preponderance of the evidence that the encephalopathy was caused by an infection, a toxin, a metabolic disturbance, a structural lesion, a genetic disorder, or trauma (without regard to whether the cause of the infection, toxin, trauma, metabolic disturbance, structural lesion or genetic disorder is known). If at the time a decision is made on a petition filed under section 2111(b) of the Act for a vaccine-related injury or death, it is not possible to determine the cause by a preponderance of the evidence of an encephalopathy, the encephalopathy shall be considered to be a condition set forth in the Table.

  (iv) In determining whether or not an encephalopathy is a condition set forth in the Table, the Court shall consider the entire medical record.

(3) *Seizure and convulsion.* For purposes of paragraphs (2) and (3) of this section, the terms, "seizure" and "convulsion" include myoclonic, generalized tonic-clonic (grand mal), and simple and complex partial seizures. Absence (petit mal) seizures shall not be considered to be a condition set forth in the Table. Jerking movements or staring episodes alone are not necessarily an indication of seizure activity.

(4) *Sequela.* The term "sequela" means a condition or event which was actually caused by a condition listed in the Vaccine Injury Table.

(5) *Chronic Arthritis.* For purposes of the Vaccine Injury Table, chronic arthritis may be found in a person with no history in the 3 years prior to vaccination of arthropathy (joint disease) on the basis of:

    (A) Medical documentation, recorded within 30 days after the onset, of objective signs of acute arthritis (joint swelling) that occurred between 7 and 42 days after a rubella vaccination;

TABLE 63–1 ■ National Childhood Vaccine Injury Act Reporting and Compensation Tables*—cont'd

Vaccine	Adverse Event	Interval from Vaccination to Onset of Event	
		For Reporting[†]	For Compensation[‡]

(B) Medical documentation (recorded within 3 years after the onset of acute arthritis) of the persistence of objective signs of intermittent or continuous arthritis for more than 6 months following vaccination; or

(C) Medical documentation of an antibody response to the rubella virus.

For purposes of the Vaccine Injury Table, the following shall not be considered as chronic arthritis: musculoskeletal disorders such as diffuse connective tissue diseases (including but not limited to rheumatoid arthritis, juvenile rheumatoid arthritis, systemic lupus erythematosus, systemic sclerosis, mixed connective tissue disease, polymyositis/dermatomyositis, fibromyalgia, necrotizing vasculitis and vasculopathies, and Sjogren's syndrome), degenerative joint disease, infectious agents other than rubella (whether by direct invasion or as an immune reaction), metabolic and endocrine diseases, trauma, neoplasms, neuropathic disorders, bone and cartilage disorders and arthritis associated with ankylosing spondylitis, psoriasis, inflammatory bowel disease, Reiter's syndrome, or blood disorders.

Arthralgia (joint pain) or stiffness without joint swelling shall not be viewed as chronic arthritis for purposes of the Vaccine Injury Table.

(6) *Brachial neuritis* is defined as dysfunction limited to the upper extremity nerve plexus (i.e., its trunks, divisions, or cords) without involvement of other peripheral (e.g., nerve roots or a single peripheral nerve) or central (e.g., spinal cord) nervous system structures. A deep, steady, often severe aching pain in the shoulder and upper arm usually heralds onset of the condition. The pain is followed in days or weeks by weakness and atrophy in upper extremity muscle groups. Sensory loss may accompany the motor deficits, but is generally a less notable clinical feature. The neuritis, or plexopathy, may be present on the same side as or the opposite side of the injection; it is sometimes bilateral, affecting both upper extremities. Weakness is required before the diagnosis can be made. Motor, sensory, and reflex findings on physical examination and the results of nerve conduction and electromyographic studies must be consistent in confirming that dysfunction is attributable to the brachial plexus. The condition should thereby be distinguishable from conditions that may give rise to dysfunction of nerve roots (i.e., radiculopathies) and peripheral nerves (i.e., including multiple mononeuropathies), as well as other peripheral and central nervous system structures (e.g., cranial neuropathies and myelopathies).

(7) *Thrombocytopenic purpura* is defined by a serum platelet count less than $50,000/mm^3$. Thrombocytopenic purpura does not include cases of thrombocytopenia associated with other causes such as hypersplenism, autoimmune disorders (including alloantibodies from previous transfusions) myelodysplasias, lymphoproliferative disorders, congenital thrombocytopenia or hemolytic uremic syndrome. This does not include cases of immune (formerly called idiopathic) thrombocytopenic purpura (ITP) that are mediated, for example, by viral or fungal infections, toxins, or drugs. Thrombocytopenic purpura does not include cases of thrombocytopenia associated with disseminated intravascular coagulation, as observed with bacterial and viral infections. Viral infections include, for example, those infections secondary to Epstein-Barr virus, cytomegalovirus, hepatitis A and B, rhinovirus, human immunodeficiency virus (HIV), adenovirus, and dengue virus. An antecedent viral infection may be demonstrated by clinical signs and symptoms and need not be confirmed by culture or serologic testing. Bone marrow examination, if performed, must reveal a normal or an increased number of megakaryocytes in an otherwise normal marrow.

(8) *Vaccine-strain measles viral infection* is defined as a disease caused by the vaccine strain that should be determined by vaccine-specific monoclonal antibody or polymerase chain reaction tests.

(9) *Vaccine-strain polio viral infection* is defined as a disease caused by poliovirus that is isolated from the affected tissue and should be determined to be the vaccine strain by oligonucleotide or polymerase chain reaction. Isolation of poliovirus from the stool is not sufficient to establish a tissue specific infection or disease caused by vaccine-strain poliovirus.

Source: 42 C.F.R. §100. 3(a)

*Effective date August 26, 2002.

[†]Taken from the Reportable Events Table (RET), which lists conditions reportable by law (42 U.S.C. 300aa-25) to the Vaccine Adverse Event Reporting System (VAERS), including conditions found in the manufacturer's package insert. In addition, individuals are encouraged to report **any** clinically significant or unexpected events (even if you are not certain the vaccine caused the event) for **any** vaccine, whether or not it is listed on the RET. Manufacturers are also required by regulation (21 CFR 600.80) to report to the VAERS program all adverse events made known to them for any vaccine. VAERS reporting forms and information can be obtained by calling 1-800-822-7967 or from the web site (*www.vaers.org*).

[‡]Taken from the Vaccine Injury Table (VIT) used in adjudication of claims filed with the National Vaccine Injury Compensation Program (VICP). Claims may also be filed for a condition with onset outside the designated time intervals or a condition not included in the table. The Qualifications and Aids to Interpretation below define conditions or injuries listed on the VIT. Information on filing a claim can be obtained by calling 1-800-338-2382 or through the VICP web site (*www.hrsa.gov/osp/vicp*).

§ Taken from 42 C.F.R. §100. 3(b)

CDC, Centers for Disease Control and Prevention; DTaP, diphtheria and tetanus toxoids and acellular pertussis; DT, diphtheria and tetanus toxoids; DTP, diphtheria and tetanus toxoids and whole-cell pertussis; HHS, U.S. Department of Health and Human Services; Hib, *Haemophilus influenzae* type b; IPV, inactivated poliovirus vaccine; M, measles vaccine; MMR, measles, mumps, and rubella vaccine; MR, measles and rubella vaccine; OPV, oral poliovirus vaccine; P, pertussis vaccine; R, rubella vaccine; Td, tetanus and diphtheria toxoids for adult use; the Act, the National Childhood Vaccine Injury Act of 1986; the Table, the Vaccine Injury Table; TT, tetanus toxoid.

numbers, the ACCV monitors the VICP and makes recommendations to the Secretary of the U.S. Department of Health and Human Services (HHS) on changes to the VIT and other issues related to vaccination and vaccine safety. The NVAC has much broader responsibilities of reviewing and making recommendations concerning vaccine research, production, delivery, safety, and efficacy. Recommendations are forwarded to the Assistant Secretary of HHS and have included ad hoc committee reviews of risks associated with each of the vaccines listed in the VIT.

Structure and Process

The VICP is administered jointly by the U.S. Department of Justice (DOJ), the HHS, and the Office of the Special Masters, U.S. Court of Federal Claims. Vaccines designated by the CDC for "routine administration to children" are covered by the program. As of August 2002, these included vaccines against 11 diseases: *Haemophilus influenzae* type b (Hib); diphtheria, tetanus, and pertussis (DTP, diphtheria and tetanus toxoids and acellular pertussis [DTaP], DTP-Hib, diphtheria and tetanus toxoids [DT], Td, and tetanus toxoid [TT]); measles, mumps, and rubella (MMR and component vaccines); polio (IPV and OPV); hepatitis B (HBV); varicella-zoster virus; and pneumococcal conjugate vaccines. Rotavirus vaccine, which was previously administered to all children, is also covered by the VICP.¶

The VICP created two classes of claims: those involving vaccinations given prior to October 1, 1988 ("pre-1988") and those involving vaccinations administered on or after October 1, 1988 ("post-1988"). Pre-1988 or retrospective claims had to be filed by January 31, 1991, and all but a handful have been processed and adjudicated. Post-1988 (prospective) claims must first be filed under the VICP. Only if compensation is denied by the VICP or is refused by the claimant can civil litigation be undertaken. Post-1988 claims must be filed within 36 months after the first symptom appeared following vaccination, and effects of the injury must have continued for at least 6 months (unless the injury results in hospitalization and surgery). Death claims must be filed within 24 months of the death and within 48 months after the onset of the vaccine-related injury from which the death occurred. The NCVIA provides for up to 14 months from the filing date for the court to issue a decision subject to extension. Awards are funded by a vaccine excise tax levied on the manufacturers for each dose sold, which, of course, is passed on to the consumers.

Pre-1988 or "retrospective" claims differed in several ways from post-1988 claims. Up until the January 31, 1991, deadline for filing a claim, petitioners had the option of seeking recourse under either the VICP or the tort system. Like prospective claims, the court had a statutory deadline for rendering a decision. Amendments subsequently gave petitioners the right to continue their vaccine claim in the VICP without a time limit for adjudication.[37] Awards were

funded by an annual congressional appropriation of $110 million.

Petitioners, either through an attorney or on their own, file a petition with the court, which begins the review and adjudication process. Petitions (claims) are filed against the Secretary of HHS as respondent on behalf of the government. The court assigns the petition to one of seven special masters, who are lawyers handling cases only in the VICP. Supporting documents required by the court include medical records and affidavits of the parents (or other family members) regarding the vaccination and resulting injury or death. Expert witness reports may also accompany the initial filing. Proceedings are expedited by eliminating formal civil discovery and rules of evidence in favor of a more informal process. Court rules provide for regular telephone status conferences with both parties and informal review and fact determinations by the special master prior to a hearing, should one be needed. These relaxed rules seem to encourage and facilitate settlements.

Once the claim is filed, HHS assigns the petition to one of its medical reviewers, who has 90 days to review the documents. The VICP medical staff (currently two pediatricians and one neurologist) reaches a recommendation on the petitioners' entitlement to compensation, which is then forwarded to the court through the DOJ attorney assigned to the case. A distinguished group of pediatric and adult subspecialists sometimes assist VICP staff in reaching a decision on eligibility and testify on behalf of the Secretary of HHS in hearings.

As an initial matter, medical eligibility for compensation is based on establishing one of three elements of proof. Petitioners must either prove that a condition listed on the VIT occurred in the prescribed time interval (*and* that the government is unable to prove that there is greater evidence of an alternative cause or "factor unrelated"), or prove that the vaccine actually caused the injury if it is a VIT condition occurring outside the specified time interval or the injury is not listed on the VIT. A third option is showing proof that the vaccine significantly aggravated a pre-existing medical condition. (It is worth noting that a "factor unrelated" has to be a condition of known cause and not "idiopathic.") In addition to satisfying one of these three elements, petitioners must also show there were continued effects for greater than 6 months, except in the case of a vaccine-related death, or that the injured individual required "inpatient hospitalization and surgical intervention" as a result of the vaccine injury.

The VICP medical staff's recommendations are predominantly based on the medical records rather than the affidavits of family members, which are often generated (for purposes of litigation) months to years following the alleged injury. Eligibility for compensation is recommended if the VICP staff finds that the records fulfill the requirements of the NCVIA. At the same time, the DOJ determines whether the petition meets the legal requirements for an award. The criteria are detailed and require that each petition contain several elements before the special master can have jurisdiction over the matter (Table 63–2). The court nearly always concurs with an entitlement recommendation, thereby obviating the need for a hearing. Those cases not conceded by HHS usually proceed to a hearing before a special master, at which point testimony on both sides is presented, including expert witnesses for each party. In

---

¶Rotashield, a tetravalent rhesus-based rotavirus vaccine, was withdrawn from the market by the manufacturer in October 1999 after epidemiologic studies confirmed an association between the vaccine and cases of intussusception, a potentially life-threatening bowel obstruction that occurs in infants. The CDC officially withdrew its "routine administration to children" recommendation the following month, after the Advisory Committee on Immunization Practices voted unanimously to discontinue use of Rotashield.[36]

TABLE 63–2 ■ Legal Requirements Under the National Vaccine Injury Compensation Program (VICP)

REQUIREMENTS FOR PROPER FILING

Must be properly filed with HHS and U.S. Court of Federal Claims
Must be filed by proper person as petitioner
- person who sustained vaccine-related injury; or
- legal representative of minor or individual who sustained vaccine-related injury or death

Must contain
- affidavit; and
- medical and vaccination records, and, if applicable, death certificate and autopsy (or identification of any unavailable records and reasons for unavailability)

Must be filed within the statute of limitations:
- *Injuries:* within 36 months of first symptom/manifestation of onset (or significant aggravation) of vaccine-related injury; or
- *Deaths:* within 24 months of vaccine-related death and within 48 months of date of first symptom/manifestation of onset (or significant aggravation) of injury from which death resulted; or
- *Table revisions:* if Table revision either makes person who was previously ineligible to seek compensation eligible or significantly increases likelihood of person obtaining compensation, such person may file petition within 2 years of effective date of revision so long as vaccine-related injury/death did not occur more than 8 years before date of revision

NATURE OF THE ALLEGATION

Must involve covered vaccine listed on Table or included within Table's general category of vaccines recommended for routine administration to children once excise tax is passed
Must involve proper relationship between injured person and covered vaccine
- injured person received covered vaccine; or
- in the case of polio, injured person contracted polio from another person who received oral polio vaccine

Must involve proper place vaccine was administered
- injured person receiving covered vaccine must have been in U.S. or its trust territories, unless:
  - person was U.S. citizen serving abroad as member of Armed Forces or employee of U.S. or dependent of such a citizen
  - vaccine manufactured in U.S. and person returned to U.S. within 6 months after date of vaccination; or
  - injured person did not receive covered vaccine but contracted polio from another person who received oral polio vaccine, and injured person must have been citizen of U.S. or a dependent of such a citizen

TO OBTAIN COMPENSATION

Must prove compensable injury/death by a preponderance of the evidence
- sustained (or had significantly aggravated) Table injury or died from covered vaccine and first symptom/manifestation of onset of condition (or significant aggravation) occurred within time period set forth in Table; or
- sustained (or had significantly aggravated) Table condition or died from covered vaccine and first symptom/manifestation of onset of condition (or significant aggravation) did not occur within time period set forth in Table, but condition or death was caused by covered vaccine; or
- sustained (or had significantly aggravated) any condition not set forth on Table from covered vaccine, but which was caused by covered vaccine

Must show residual effects
- suffered residual effects/complications of vaccine-related injury for more than 6 months after vaccine's administration; or
- died from administration of the vaccine; or
- received inpatient hospitalization and surgery as result of vaccine-related injury

Must not be shown (by preponderance of evidence) that factor unrelated to administration of the vaccine-caused injury/death
Must not have previously filed VICP claim for same vaccine administration
Must not have previously collected award/settlement of civil action for damages for vaccine-related injury/death
Must elect to accept Court of Federal Claims' judgment to receive compensation awarded

HHS, U.S. Department of Health and Human Services; Table, Vaccine Injury Table.

some instances, the court may find the testimony of family members more persuasive than contemporaneously recorded events or give greater weight to the initial diagnosis of the treating physician over determinations made on subsequent clinical evaluations. Therefore, it is not uncommon for the special master to award compensation after an entitlement hearing.

Once entitlement to compensation is conceded, or after the special master determines that the petitioner is entitled to compensation, the DOJ and the petitioner work to reach agreement on the amount of compensation (damages). The level of compensation is based on life care plans that evaluate the health of the injured person and the person's future needs. The government and petitioner often use informal negotiations under the guidance of a special master to resolve entitlement and damages issues. Alternative dispute resolution is increasingly being utilized to avoid having to hold a formal hearing. Today, a significant number of the petitions are resolved through the settlement process.

Compensation for minors or incompetent persons is usually in the form of a lump sum payment and an annuity designed to provide a lifetime stream of benefits. In prospective cases, the compensation includes unreimbursable costs for vaccine-related goods and services from the date of injury until death, lost wages (approximately $400,000 on average),[38,39] and pain and suffering (up to $250,000).[40] (Awards in retrospective cases are more modest, covering only *future* unreimbursable vaccine-related medical costs. Attorneys' fees, pain and suffering, and lost wages in such cases are limited to a $30,000 combined cap.) Compensation for death claims is awarded in a lump sum payment limited to $250,000, regardless of the date of vaccine administration. "Reasonable" attorneys' fees are paid whether or not petitioners are successful in obtaining compensation, if the claim was brought in good faith and on a reasonable basis. These fees are considerably less than those incurred under the civil tort system because of the abbreviated court procedures. Punitive damages and awards to others in the family for loss of companionship are not allowed.

Implementation and Program Experience

Although the NCVIA was landmark in design and scope, further legislation and program refinements were necessary. Funding of the VICP, not provided for in the original legislation, was authorized by Congress in early 1987.[41] Additional protections for manufacturers defending "post-1988" NCVIA claims also were written into the law at this time. These included the elimination of plaintiff allegations of vaccine misdesign or inadequate warning of risk, two common tort theories pursued in the 1980s, and the elimination of punitive damages unless it could be proven there was gross negligence in vaccine production.[42] At the same time, the limitation requiring claimants to pursue their claim through the VICP before filing a tort claim against manufacturers was expanded to include health care providers, a protection that was not offered to health care providers by the original act.

The NCVIA's "sunset" provision was scheduled to terminate authorization for the program and the excise tax on vaccines in 1993. At that time, concerns were voiced once again that physicians might be in jeopardy of civil litigation. Passage of the Omnibus Budget Reconciliation Act (OBRA) of 1993[43] provided permanent reauthorization of the VICP and a mechanism for adding new vaccines. Those vaccines designated by the CDC (usually on recommenda-

tion by the Advisory Committee on Immunization Practices) for routine administration to children would be added to the VICP. Congress also would have to enact an excise tax as a necessary second step before coverage could begin. The statute provided for 8 years' retroactive coverage for those claimants alleging injuries from a newly added vaccine, or for injuries added to the VIT for existing vaccines, with a 2-year window in which to file after addition of coverage. Liability protection for future pediatric vaccines was now ensured, at least in principle.

Table 63–3 shows the numbers of claims filed under the VICP by vaccine type and year of administration. This table includes hundreds of vaccines given during the 1950s and 1960s, with the oldest case dating back to 1918 for a death alleged to be associated with the pertussis vaccine. Statutory deadlines have twice brought large numbers of claims over a short period, the first occurring when over 4000 pre-1988 claims were filed over a 6-month period during 1990 to 1991; in the second, over 300 HBV vaccine claims were filed in August 1999 to meet the 2-year deadline for filing of claims for vaccines administered up to 8 years prior to the addition of vaccine coverage (effective August 7, 1997, for HBV vaccine). Ironically, the program processed many claims that were otherwise barred from the tort system by a state statute of limitations. Starting in 2002, hundreds of claims alleging injury from the thimerosal (mercury) component of vaccines were filed. Many lacked a specific date of vaccine administration and/or named multiple vaccines in the allegation, and thus were classified as "unspecified" in the VICP database (see discussion of thimerosal litigation under *New Challenges* below).

Table 63–4 shows the number of cases submitted to the VICP through September 30, 2002, including the number of cases pending, adjudicated, or dismissed and the dollars awarded.[44] Many cases were dismissed by the court on grounds of legal or medical insufficiency. Some plaintiffs, given the opportunity to obtain additional records, later refiled. Awards have ranged from $120 (reimbursement of the filing fee) to $7.5 million (including an initial lump sum

TABLE 63–3 ■ National VICP Claims by Year of Administration and Vaccine Type as of September 30, 2002[*]

Year of Administration	DTP, DTaP[†], P, DTP-Hib	DT, Td, TT	MMR, MR, M	Rubella	OPV	IPV	HepB	Varicella	Hib	Rotavirus	Pn, Conjugate	TOTAL
1910–1919	1	–	–	–	–	–	–	–	–	–	–	1
1920–1929	1	–	–	–	–	–	–	–	–	–	–	1
1930–1939	1	0	1	–	–	–	–	–	–	–	–	2
1940–1949	63	1	2	0	1	1	–	–	–	–	–	68
1950–1959	178	4	3	1	5	211	–	–	–	–	–	402
1960–1969	376	5	104	6	76	52	–	–	–	–	–	619
1970–1979	823	6	120	43	53	0	–	–	–	–	–	1045
1980–1989	1877	35	200	101	77	0	5	–	0	–	–	2295
1990–1999	709	105	387	35	80	1	408	19	9	30	2	1785
2000–present	21	6	23	2	0	1	16	1	1	0	2	73
TOTAL	4050	162	840	188	292	266	429	20	10	30	4	6291

[*]N = 7052; 761 claims were made for vaccines not covered or unspecified as to vaccine type or date of administration.
[†]90 DTaP claims.
DTaP, diphtheria and tetanus toxoids and acellular pertussis; DT, diphtheria and tetanus toxoids; DTP, diphtheria and tetanus toxoids and whole-cell pertussis; HepB, hepatitis B vaccine; Hib, *Haemophilus influenzae* type b; IPV, inactivated poliovirus vaccine; M, measles vaccine; MMR, measles, mumps, and rubella vaccine; MR, measles and rubella vaccine; OPV, oral poliovirus vaccine; P, pertussis vaccine; Pn, pneumococcal; Td, tetanus and diphtheria toxoids for adult use; TT, tetanus toxoid.

TABLE 63–4 ▪ Status of the National VICP as of May 31, 2003

	Vaccines Administered Before 10/1/88	Vaccines Administered on or After 10/1/88	Total
Claims Filed	4262	4551	8813
Claims Adjudicated	4255 (99%)	1419 (31%)	5674 (64%)
Compensable	1187 (28%)	619 (44%)	1806 (32%)
Dismissed	3068 (72%)	800 (56%)	3868 (68%)
Awards Paid*			
Number	2525	982	3507
Dollars (millions)	$895.1	$533.2	$1,428.3

*Includes attorney fee awards. Some adjudicated claims included above have not yet been processed for payment.

payment, with the remainder going toward purchase of an annuity) for an OPV-related paralytic polio claim in a young child.

The majority (62%) of submissions allege DTP-related effects. The remaining claims break down as follows: 12% from MMR, given alone or in any combination (nearly one fourth of claims involve adults alleging rubella vaccine–related injury); 6% from HBV vaccine; 5% from OPV; 4% from IPV (all but one claim for vaccines administered before 1988); 2% from tetanus-containing vaccines; less than 1% each for Hib, pneumococcal conjugate, rotavirus, and varicella vaccines; and 4% from vaccines either unspecified or not covered by the VICP.

Perhaps a better barometer of VICP experience currently is reflected in the percentages by vaccine for calendar years 2000 and 2001. Of the 191 claims filed during 2000, DTP was the most frequent vaccine type (24%), followed by MMR and HBV (21%), tetanus-containing vaccines (9%), DTaP (7%), and both OPV and rotavirus (5%). However, the following year MMR was the predominant vaccine (31%), followed by HBV (28%), DTaP (12%), and DTP (8%), with the remaining vaccines all less than 5% out of a total of 229 claims filed. Although percentages vary by vaccine, injuries account for 87% of claims; deaths account for the remaining 13%.

The unexpected pre-1988 caseload far exceeded program resources in several respects. Efforts by staff and the court were increased, but the large caseload and the court's dual decision responsibility (entitlement and damages determinations) made timely adjudication impossible. Furthermore, funding soon became an issue, with exhaustion of the $80 million annual appropriation occurring by June 1992. Eventually, the appropriation was increased to $110 million, but not before the VICP had to shut down payments twice to successful claimants.

The opposite problem of excess monies coming into the trust fund has more recently become an issue. Excise tax levels for the original seven vaccines covered by the NCVIA were based on the estimated numbers and cost of claims that each would generate. This risk-based approach, however, had serious limitations. By 1996, the trust fund had exceeded anticipated needs, with $1 billion in holdings and annual receipts totaling $140 million, against peak outlays in the $35 to $42 million range. (In 2002, the trust fund totaled $1.8 billion, with over $176 million in annual receipts and awards totaling $56.9 million for the fiscal year.) Second, future licensure of

multiple-antigen combination vaccines would make difficult the task of estimating the risk of adverse events for each antigen. With passage of the Taxpayer Relief Act of 1997, the vaccine excise structure was revised, setting a 75-cents-per-"dose" (disease prevented) rate on all covered vaccines under the program, including the three vaccines added by rulemaking. The effective date of coverage was August 6, 1997. Congress will need to assign an excise tax for each new vaccine added via the provision in the March 1997 final rule.[45]

Without question, the biggest controversy (and challenge) has been the VIT. Congress recognized that, to ensure that cases of true vaccine injuries were compensated, the criteria for making awards would have to be quite broad; as a result, some persons with disorders that were clearly not vaccine related would receive awards. The legislative history underlying the NCVIA noted the lingering controversy over what is and is not vaccine caused. The VIT would serve as a compromise mechanism in the interim to facilitate recovery by individuals "thought" to be injured. Once the scientific reviews by the IOM, called for by the NCVIA, were completed, the Secretary of HHS could make changes to the VIT to bring it in line with current scientific thinking. However, change comes slowly, and program outcomes were increasingly at odds with what experts agreed should be attributed to vaccine effects.

For the most part, DTP injury claims are filed on behalf of children and adults with chronic encephalopathy of unknown cause. Overall, no specific cause is ever determined for as many as 40% of these patients, with most cases thought to be due to migrational abnormalities of fetal brain development, or metabolic or "genetic" conditions not identifiable by current technology.[46] Many DTP claims reflect the onset of abnormal neurologic signs during the first year of life (when vaccines are routinely given), ranging from the initial seizure of a child with incipient epilepsy to a case in which a child who may have experienced prolonged crying or irritability after vaccination has developmental retardation. Because a VIT claim requires only that the designated condition and time frame be satisfied to gain eligibility, within a few years of the NCVIA's passage, significant numbers of claims were being compensated for conditions thought to be non–vaccine related.

For example, more than one third of DTP injury claims reflect the onset of seizures during infancy as their first manifestation of neurologic illness. Because DTP commonly causes fever, a well-known trigger of seizures, children with incipient epilepsy may experience the onset of their convulsive disorder secondary to this routine procedure. Naturally, many go on to have further seizures and developmental delay. Under the original VIT, residual seizure disorder afforded these children a VIT presumption if their seizure onset and subsequent seizure episodes satisfied the table requirements and the Qualification and Aids to Interpretation (QAI). (The QAI define some of the conditions listed on the VIT; see Table 63–1.) Because epilepsy is frequently idiopathic and the government could not meet its burden of showing an alternative cause, VICP staff routinely conceded these cases.

Another category often compensated was the 14% of DTP injury claims in children with infantile spasms. Those found by the court to have onset outside the VIT interval or to be of known alternative cause (e.g., metabolic or genetic disorders) were usually dismissed. However, those that fit the cryptogenic (idiopathic) category of infantile spasms, with onset within a VIT time frame, were often compensated by the court despite epidemiologic studies showing the condition to be non–vaccine related. Court precedent soon led the VICP to choose not to expend resources defending these cases unless a non–vaccine-related cause could be determined.

Even more troublesome were program outcomes in many DTP death claims. Approximately half were due to sudden infant death syndrome (SIDS), with compatible histories and forensic findings in accordance with the 1989 National Institutes of Health consensus definition. However, because the cause of SIDS remains unknown, these cases are viewed as "idiopathic" by the court. In hearings, the court would elicit the parents' description of events preceding the death in relation to the medical records to determine if a VIT condition occurred. All available records were requested, including pediatric and emergency room records, police or ambulance reports, and the autopsy report. Some SIDS claims were compensated as VIT encephalopathies, based on testimony of irritability or protracted crying, despite the absence of forensic findings of brain involvement. Others received entitlement based on descriptions of lethargy or sleepiness in the hours prior to death as evidence of shock collapse (hypotonic-hyporesponsive episode [HHE]). Unfortunately, "cardiovascular or respiratory arrest" was listed erroneously in the original VIT as a manifestation of this DTP-related syndrome in the QAI. However, death for whatever reason is preceded by such terminal events, and it was on this basis that the government appealed several SIDS cases, ultimately reversing the compensation outcome in some.

Criticisms that the VIT was inaccurate, vague, or even misleading began to gain momentum. Anaphylaxis was an easy target, with its time interval of 24 hours. By definition, this acute hypersensitivity reaction occurs within minutes to a few hours and is rare after DTP vaccine. (This was never a real issue because few program cases were compensated for anaphylaxis alone.) Another complaint was the broad definition of encephalopathy in the QAI, which resulted in some claims being found to be VIT conditions based on the frequent, harmless, but unpleasant minor reactions to DTP, including fever, anorexia, excessive crying, and lethargy.[47]

VICP Cases Since 1986

For the first 10 years after the VICP was enacted, the vast majority of petitions alleged a VIT injury because this would confer the presumption that the injury, significant aggravation, or death was vaccine related. The petition would usually say that the injured person experienced the signs and symptoms described in the QAI within a VIT time frame, regardless of whether these allegations were substantiated or contradicted by the medical record. Accordingly, the special masters and the courts concentrated almost exclusively on developing a body of law establishing the quality and quantity of evidence needed to prove such.

Most special masters established standards by placing more weight on the medical records most contemporaneous to the vaccination than on contradictory evidence assembled later, after memories fade or when litigation is contemplated (see, e.g., *Pearson v. Secretary of Department of Health & Human Services*[48]). Where the contemporaneous medical records were contradictory or did not exist, the special masters relied on the credibility of both the family and the expert witnesses to determine whether a VIT injury occurred. The courts gave deference to these credibility determinations, as long as they were not arbitrary and capricious.[49]

The courts addressed questions concerning whether the QAI were binding on the special masters. In *Hellebrand v. Secretary of Department of Health & Human Services*[50] and *Hodges v. Secretary of Department of Health & Human Services*,[51] the petitioners argued that the special master was required to rely solely on the QAI to determine entitlement to compensation. Both cases were infants who died unexpectedly following immunization and were classified as SIDS deaths. Nevertheless, the petitioners argued that these deaths were compensable under the VICP because the clinical descriptions of the agonal events were consistent with the language in the QAI for HHE. The U.S. Court of Appeals for the Federal Circuit found that the special masters are not required to apply the QAI in a rote fashion; rather, they have reasonable discretion when applying them. Any other finding in this situation would lead to compensation for *all deaths* within certain time intervals following vaccination if the cause of death was SIDS or an unknown etiology. This, in the court's opinion, was not a correct interpretation of the QAI. The Federal Circuit also noted that proximate temporal association of a death with vaccine administration does not in and of itself establish causation.

A hallmark case, *Shalala v. Whitecotton*,[52] began with a disagreement over the meaning of "first symptom or manifestation of onset or of significant aggravation after [the] vaccine," as it applies in the statute to the appearance of clinical signs of illness. This is crucial because, if the onset of signs or symptoms following vaccination is *not* the first evidence of the ensuing vaccine-related condition, then the petitioner must prove that the vaccine *significantly aggravated* the a condition present prior to vaccination in order to receive compensation. The NCVIA defines significant aggravation as "any change for the worse in a preexisting condition which results in markedly greater disability, pain, or illness accompanied by substantial deterioration of health." According to the legislative history, an example would be a child whose seizure frequency increased from one per month to one per day. Even this guidance proved vague, but all that changed as a result of the Whitecotton decision.

Despite being born with microcephaly, Maggie Whitecotton was developing normally at age 3 months when she experienced seizures within a day of her third DTP vaccination. Her seizures slowly increased over the next several years, and at the time the claim was filed she had cerebral palsy and mental retardation. Petitioners originally argued that Maggie suffered a VIT encephalopathy and/or residual seizure disorder (rather than significant aggravation) as a result of her third DTP vaccination. The government argued that the *first* symptom of onset of her injury occurred prior to the vaccination and, in the alternative, that her condition was due to a factor unrelated, namely a chronic organic brain syndrome, as evidenced by the microcephaly before the vaccination. The special master denied compensation. The Court of Federal Claims agreed, but the U.S. Court of Appeals for the Federal Circuit reversed the decision based on a different interpretation of the "first symptom or manifestation of onset" language, writing that "first" did not necessarily mean that other clinical signs could not appear prior to vaccination.

The Supreme Court unanimously reversed the Federal Circuit's decision, finding that the Federal Circuit misread the NCVIA. However, Justice O'Connor, in a concurring opinion, noted that the Federal Circuit opinion did not address the issue of significant aggravation of Maggie's preexisting condition (*Shalala v. Whitecotton*).[53] The case was then remanded to the Federal Circuit, which then set forth a test specifying that the special master must (1) assess the person's condition prior to the administration of the vaccine, (2) assess the person's current condition, and (3) determine if the person's current condition constitutes a significant aggravation of the person's condition prior to vaccination within the meaning of the statute; and, if the special master determines there has been a significant aggravation, then he or she must (4) determine whether the first symptom or manifestation of the significant aggravation occurred within the time period prescribed by the VIT. Under this test, Maggie Whitecotton received compensation.[54]

Whitecotton eased the petitioner's burden-of-proof allegations that a vaccine significantly aggravated a pre-existing VIT injury. Since *Whitecotton*, 58 petitions have alleged a significant aggravation of a pre-existing injury. Although the standard of proof is less onerous, there does not appear to be an appreciable difference between the number of individuals receiving compensation under the pre-*Whitecotton* standard (e.g., *Misasi v. Secretary of Department of Health & Human Services*,[55]) and under the *Whitecotton* standard.

The parameters of the "factor unrelated" defense also have been tested. The U.S. Court of Appeals for the Federal Circuit consistently applied a strict interpretation when it applied the NCVIA's restrictive definition of the term: a factor unrelated may not include "any idiopathic, unexplained, unknown, hypothetical, or undocumentable" condition.[56] In *Koston v. Secretary of Department of Health & Human Services*,[57] the court found that a genetic condition (Rett's syndrome) could not be a factor unrelated because it

is an idiopathic illness; that is, the exact gene(s) causing the syndrome is(are) unknown. The fact that a genetic disorder's onset is during fetal development (before vaccination) is not conclusive. Although the NCVIA specifically states that a factor unrelated may include "infections, toxins, trauma or metabolic disturbances," the Federal Circuit found that the presence of an infection is not enough to satisfy the government's burden. The government must identify the virus and show that the particular virus caused the injury.[58]

The jurisprudence governing proof of a significant aggravation of a VIT injury and a factor unrelated was combined in the "tuberous sclerosis cases." Tuberous sclerosis complex (TSC) is a genetic disorder characterized in many cases by classical skin lesions, growths (tubers), and other structural changes in the brain, causing seizures and mental retardation. Of 64 claims (all retrospective) involving TSC, 37 "off-table" seizure-onset cases have been dismissed based on the recognition that TSC is non–vaccine related, or, in a few cases, based on other legal reasons. Most of the remaining claims alleging seizure onset within a VIT time frame were litigated as a group to determine whether DTP vaccine significantly aggravated the preexisting TSC condition. Although neurologists once believed that DTP vaccine might aggravate TSC by triggering the early onset of seizures and, therefore, result in more frequent seizures and associated greater mental retardation, advances in magnetic resonance imaging in the 1990s indicated otherwise.[59,60] Based on these new data presented in special "omnibus" hearings held to decide this important question of vaccine aggravation, the presiding special master became convinced that the number and presence of tubers in the cerebral cortex, not the timing of DTP vaccination, ultimately determines clinical outcome. Several peer-reviewed articles by HHS consultants came from research generated by these efforts.[61–63] The special master's decision was affirmed by the Court of Federal Claims and the U.S. Court of Appeals for the Federal Circuit in *Hanlon v. Secretary of Department of Health & Human Services*,[64] *Turner v. Secretary of Department of Health & Human Services*,[65] and *Flanagan v. Secretary of Department of Health & Human Services*.[66]

In petitions filed after the first set of VIT changes took effect, the emphasis changed from proving a VIT injury to proving that the injury was caused-in-fact by the vaccine. This shift occurred for two reasons. First, HHS removed residual seizure disorder and shock collapse from the VIT. Second, the QAI for encephalopathy were revised so they more accurately reflected the medical view of a significant acute and chronic neurologic injury, instead of a normal, transient reaction to a vaccine.[67]

A legal challenge to the final rule was filed in federal court within 60 days of publication. Petitioners questioned the authority of the Secretary of HHS and the procedure used to publish the final rule. The suit was brought by the family of a child who experienced the onset of seizures within 3 days of a DTP vaccination, a claim that might have qualified for a VIT presumption had residual seizure disorder not been removed from the table. The U.S. Court of Appeals for the First Circuit decided in the government's favor on all issues, and the new regulation was allowed to stand.[68,69]

Because petitioners increasingly had a difficult time obtaining entitlement using the VIT, special masters and the courts began to develop a body of law elaborating the kind of evidence needed to prove causation-in-fact. These cases marked the beginning of a protracted struggle by the special masters and the courts to strike an appropriate balance between denying compensation based merely on a temporal relationship between the injury and the vaccine, and the need to fulfill the VICP's mandate to provide compensation "generously" and "fairly." The following discussion is illustrative of how that balancing affected the development of a legal standard for proving causation-in-fact under the VICP.

Early in the VICP, the court determined in *Grant v. Secretary of Department of Health & Human Services* that causation-in-fact was shown when there is "proof of a logical sequence of cause and effect showing that the vaccination was the reason for the injury. A reputable medical or scientific explanation must support this logical sequence of cause and effect."[70] Based on the *Grant* language, some special masters found that the petitioner's proof must meet the standards of strict scientific accuracy analysis and peer review. Often, it was difficult for the petitioner to meet this standard. The U.S. Court of Appeals for the Federal Circuit clarified this issue somewhat by holding that the scientific evidence need not rise to the level of being a scientific certainty.[58] Still, there were questions. For example, special masters considered whether animal studies could be used, how much weight should be given to case reports, and whether the petitioner had to rely on any published or peer-reviewed evidence in pursuing a VICP claim.[71]

In an attempt to establish which studies were sufficient in resolving DTP claims, several masters accepted the conclusions of the British National Childhood Encephalopathy Study (NCES) and its 1993 10-year follow-up as sufficient epidemiologic proof of causation-in-fact.[72–74] One master went farther and found that any epidemiologic study showing a "relative risk" of greater than 2 can support a finding of actual causation.[72] Prior to the 1995 VIT revisions, only one special master recognized the NCES as an adequate basis for proving causation-in-fact.[75]

In later years, as more and more claims were being filed as non-VIT conditions, one special master developed his own multiple-pronged method for determining causation-in-fact. This test allows a petitioner to prevail if he or she can prove (1) biologic plausibility for the vaccine to cause the individual's injury, (2) confirmation of medical plausibility from the medical community and literature, (3) existence of an injury recognized by the medical plausibility evidence and literature, (4) a medically acceptable temporal relationship between the vaccination and the onset of the alleged injury, and (5) that a reasonable effort has been made to eliminate other causes.[76] Whether or not this approach is permissible under current law has not been tested on appeal at the time of publication.

The standard of proof for causation-in-fact was adjusted further in *Shyface v. Secretary of Department of Health & Human Services*.[77] Here, the U.S. Court of Appeals for the Federal Circuit found that the petitioners need not show that the vaccination was the sole, or even the predominant, cause of the injury or condition. Rather, the petitioner need

only show that the vaccination was at least a "substantial factor" in causing the condition, and was a "but for" cause.

Modifying the Vaccine Injury Table

By law, the VIT can be modified or amended by the Secretary of HHS, in consultation with the ACCV and after opportunity for public comment. Such changes apply only to cases filed after the effective date of the changes. Separate efforts by the VICP to modify the VIT and QAI began with publication of the two congressionally mandated IOM reviews in 1991 and 1994, respectively.[78–81] With a few exceptions, the approach by the VICP was straightforward: If the IOM concluded that there was evidence that a condition was "causally related," it was added to the VIT or left on. However, if there was no proven evidence of an association, it was removed.

The first set of changes, effective March 10, 1995, involved adding chronic arthritis for rubella-containing vaccines and removing shock collapse and residual seizure disorder under DTP vaccines.[67] Clarifications also were made in the definitions of residual seizure disorder and encephalopathy in the QAI. The only exception in utilizing the IOM recommendations was encephalopathy/encephalitis under DTP vaccine, which had been proposed for removal but was left on the table in response to advice from the ACCV. The ACCV argued that claims of acute encephalopathy of unknown etiology within 3 days of DTP vaccination should continue to receive a presumption of causation, but that the definition in the QAI needed to be more clinically precise. A subsequent 1994 analysis by the IOM[82] of a 10-year follow-up to the British NCES tried to answer, but fell short of answering, the ultimate question of whether DTP vaccine causes permanent brain damage.[83] The changes to both the VIT and the QAI for DTP have proved controversial over time and have been a topic addressed at congressional oversight hearings.

The second set of changes to the VIT proved far less controversial and was based on the 1994 IOM report covering the five remaining original VICP vaccines, as well as Hib and HBV vaccines. As mandated by the OBRA of 1993, Hib, HBV, and varicella vaccines were added to the VICP because all were recommended by the CDC for routine administration to children. The other modifications, effective March 24, 1997, included the addition to the VIT of thrombocytopenia for measles-containing vaccines and brachial neuritis for tetanus-containing vaccines.[84] Coverage of the three new vaccines, however, did not begin until Congress set an excise tax for the "new" vaccines, effective August 7, 1997.

Like the 1995 rulemaking, proposed VIT changes developed by the Secretary paralleled the IOM conclusions for or against causation with two exceptions: the Secretary did not add GBS following OPV and following tetanus-containing vaccines. The IOM's OPV conclusion was based largely on a Finnish study following a national OPV campaign.[85] A subsequent U.S. study (therefore not considered by the IOM) showed no evidence of an increase in GBS following OPV administration.[86] Further doubt was cast when one of the Finnish study's co-authors wrote a letter noting that it was not their intention to claim that OPV was causally related because the data could be interpreted more than one way.[87]

The question of GBS and tetanus-containing vaccines was even more difficult to decide. The IOM conclusion was based on case reports, particularly one individual who experienced GBS three times in the weeks following tetanus vaccination. The fact that he had other non–vaccine-related episodes made him immunologically unique. Population studies, in contrast, showed no evidence that GBS incidence is higher in individuals receiving tetanus vaccine when compared to background rate.[87] Because there is no proven evidence of increased incidence overall, it was thought GBS should continue to require proof of causation, and therefore not be added to the VIT. However, individuals who experience more than one episode of GBS temporally related to immunization will no doubt have strong causation arguments under the VICP. In fact, the program has compensated a claim involving two episodes of GBS, both within weeks of receiving tetanus-containing vaccines at ages 5 and 15 years.[88]

Since 1997, the VIT has been modified three more times by rulemaking. The general category of rotavirus vaccines was added effective October 21, 1998,[89] and pneumococcal conjugate vaccines were added effective December 18, 1999.[90] In July 2002, a final rule was published adding intussusception as a listed injury to the VIT under a second category of rotavirus vaccines (i.e., live, oral, rhesus-based), and several changes were made that were more technical in nature.[91] No written or oral comments were received regarding the proposed changes during the 6-month public comment period following publication of a Notice of Proposed Rulemaking in the *Federal Register* in July 2001.[92]

Medical Review of Claims

Nearly all claims filed under the VICP had some clinical outcome in temporal relation to vaccination, varying from the normal, expected side effects of crying, fever, or local swelling to much more serious acute and chronic illness. The claims represent a database of possible vaccine-related events, although only a small percentage of serious outcomes were thought to be caused by vaccines after VICP medical staff review. Some of the more relevant clinical diagnoses are reviewed here.

Diphtheria, Tetanus, and Pertussis Vaccines

Petitions filed for DTP vaccine (only 65 claims had been received alleging DTaP injury by May 2002) for the most part involved cases in which primary series immunization involved children younger than 12 months. Just over half of the injury claims involved the initial of onset seizures in various time intervals following vaccination, ranging from hours to several weeks or longer. Those with idiopathic epilepsy (31%) were the largest group, followed by those with infantile spasms (14%) and a small percentage with different seizure types (e.g., absence, complex partial, psychomotor). Another significant category was the 20% of claimants who experienced developmental delay as their presenting neurologic sign, with medical records rarely showing any significant effects following vaccination. However, parents might point to prolonged, inconsolable crying or extreme lethargy as a basis for assuming DTP-related outcomes. Only 11% of children demonstrated clinical signs of encephalopathy and, of those, approximately

half had an unknown etiology. The remaining claims comprised metabolic or genetic disorders and a variety of other non–vaccine-related conditions. Only a handful of HHE cases were identified on medical records review.

Approximately 50% of claims alleging DTP-related death had medical records and autopsy findings consistent with SIDS. The next most frequent diagnostic category for death cases involved the 10% of patients with long-standing convulsive disorders (those who had severe, long-term seizures), followed by those with acute encephalopathy (9% [4% with known etiology and 5% with unknown etiology]) and developmental delay onset (7%); the remaining claims showing various non–vaccine-related conditions (e.g., choking, sepsis, congenital heart disease). Four deaths were due to anaphylaxis.

Tetanus-Containing Vaccines

Tetanus-containing vaccine (DT, Td, or TT) claims included at least seven cases of GBS and smaller numbers of patients with chronic inflammatory demyelinating polyneuropathy, multiple sclerosis, brachial neuritis, acute encephalopathy of unknown etiology, and other central and peripheral nervous system disorders. Litigating GBS claims has been particularly challenging. Few were decided prior to the IOM report concluding that tetanus-containing vaccines could cause GBS if the onset was within 5 days to 6 weeks following immunization.[80,81] In one case where compensation was not provided, the court found that, although Td *can* cause GBS, one could not conclude that it *did* cause GBS in any particular case. The decision was appealed and affirmed by the U.S. Court of Appeals for the Federal Circuit.[93] Since this decision, however, the court has compensated some GBS claims based on the IOM report.

Measles, Mumps, and Rubella Vaccines

The MMR vaccine is implicated in 12% of claims, most of which are events associated with immunization during the second year of life. Acute encephalopathy or encephalitis comprised 23% of injury claims ranging in onset from 1 day to several weeks after immunization. Most cases were of unknown cause. Although encephalopathy is known to result from natural measles infection, it is not clear if the vaccine also can cause central nervous system disease. Attempts to isolate vaccine virus in patients with acute illness have been unsuccessful, and there is no evidence of increased rates of acute central nervous system disease in vaccinees versus the background rate for this age group. Although the IOM found the evidence to be "insufficient" to determine whether measles vaccine can cause acute encephalopathy, there is some evidence of clustering of encephalopathy/encephalitis cases whose onset is 8 to 10 days following measles-containing immunization, based on an analysis of 48 VICP claims.[94]

The remaining diagnoses are seizure-onset cases (27%), most being febrile seizures in the 7- to 14-day time frame during which fever may accompany replication of vaccine virus. Those that fell within the 0- to 15-day time frame (now 5 to 15 days) for VIT onset usually were recommended for entitlement by VICP staff. Most claims were adjudicated before residual seizure disorder was removed from the VIT.

Eighteen subacute sclerosing panencephalitis (SSPE) claims have been identified, 10 of them deaths. Early hearings resulted in a few being compensated because of the initial lack of administrative resources to defend claims. Subsequent testimony by experts in infectious disease persuaded the court of the lack of any data supporting a causal connection, noting the tremendous decrease in SSPE incidence since licensure of the vaccine decades ago. Since then, claims of SSPE-related injury or death have been dismissed.

Included in the MMR analysis are 113 claims alleging injury from rubella vaccine. Most claims involve postpubertal women, usually health care workers or postpartum patients. Although 13% to 15% of susceptible (serology-negative) women may experience transient arthritis after the currently used rubella vaccine, with a higher percentage (up to 40%) reporting some type of musculoskeletal complaint, it is less clear what role, if any, the vaccine plays in causing recurrent or chronic arthropathy (i.e., arthralgia or arthritis).[78–80] Forty-two percent of people making claims experienced acute arthritis within 6 weeks of immunization. Of these, 17% were diagnosed with chronic arthritis of unknown etiology, 4% with type-specific (non–vaccine-related) arthritis, and the remaining cases with chronic arthralgia (16%) and other subjective complaints (5%). Of the remaining claims without acute arthritis onset after immunization, 28% had chronic arthropathy or other generalized complaints similar to those of chronic fatigue syndrome, and 30% were diagnosed with a variety of non–vaccine-related conditions.

Based on the 1991 IOM report's finding that chronic arthritis may be caused by rubella vaccine, a special master held a hearing to determine criteria necessary for proof of causation. Following the special master's publication of these guidelines, the VICP added chronic arthritis to the VIT in the 1995 final rule,[67] and more recently incorporated several of the court's criteria in the 1997 final rule.[84] The main difference between the criteria adopted by the VICP and those adopted by the court has been the latter's willingness to compensate arthralgia, a subjective symptom that is difficult to assess, unlike observable signs of arthritis. Adjudications to date have resulted in 61 claims being compensated by the court and 119 being dismissed. Additional research published since the IOM report, including retrospective case reviews and a prospective double-blind study, has produced mixed results. If rubella vaccine does indeed cause chronic arthropathy, it would appear that the incidence is rare.[95–97]

Polio Vaccines

Polio vaccine–related claims totaled more than 500 of the retrospective case filings. Most involved vaccines given in the 1950s and 1960s, when polio was common in the United States. It is reasonable to expect that some individuals acquired natural poliomyelitis in temporal relationship to receipt of IPV, particularly if only one or two doses were given. Although the Cutter incident, in which an estimated 260 cases of paralytic poliomyelitis were attributed to residual live virus in the vaccine, is well documented, no similar instances of killed vaccine–related poliomyelitis have been identified.[98] Of 266 IPV claims, nearly all have been dismissed by the court, with none being found to be secondary to Cutter vaccine administration. Of the two post-1988 IPV claims filed thus far, one was for administration after the change in use from OPV to IPV.

OPV claims were approached much differently, because paralytic polio is known to be a rare complication in vaccine recipients as well as in contacts. Most claims arising since the early 1960s with confirmed paralytic polio were compensated by the program. Naturally, it is difficult to know which cases were actually vaccine related when polio was present in the community. Claims involving other conditions such as transverse myelitis and GBS have been rejected by the court based on the lack of proof of causation.

Hepatitis B Vaccine

More than 400 HBV claims were filed by May 2002. Approximately three quarters of the claims arrived in the days and weeks prior to August 7, 1999, in order to meet the 2-year statutory deadline for the filing of "older" claims whenever a new vaccine is added to the VICP. Because many of the claims did not include medical records or other documentation necessary to begin adjudication, only 141 had been reviewed by VICP medical staff. The predominant diagnosis was neurologic illness (27%), peripheral or central, including multiple sclerosis; multisystem or chronic symptomatology was the next most common diagnostic category (24%). The remaining claims involved immune system dysfunction (10%), endocrine disorders (6%), pulmonary conditions (5%), and other miscellaneous diagnoses. Overall, 6% of claims involved a death following HBV vaccination. Of the first 141 claims reviewed, 21 (15%) were children under 1 year of age, although most were diagnosed with chronic medical conditions.

In April 2002, the IOM Vaccine Safety Review Committee published its findings regarding HBV vaccine and neurologic disorders. The IOM concluded that there is evidence against a causal relation between HBV vaccine and multiple sclerosis (and relapse) and insufficient evidence for other central or peripheral nervous system demyelinating conditions.[99] Only a handful of HBV vaccine claims had been adjudicated at that point. To some degree, the lack of medical records slowed the review process. More importantly, because nearly all of the claims allege non-VIT injuries and must be adjudicated on a causation-in-fact basis, the availability (or lack thereof) of scientific evidence on adverse effects becomes of paramount importance. Under the oversight of a special master (similar to the adjudication of rubella vaccine–chronic arthritis claims), the HBV claims have been divided into 10 categories according to the alleged injury and/or medical records. With publication of the IOM report, the court was moving forward to adjudicate claims in at least four of the categories.[100]

Rotavirus Vaccine

The general category of rotavirus vaccines was added to the VIT effective October 22, 1998, but with no condition specified.[89] Both prerequisites for adding rotavirus vaccine were satisfied by enactment of Public Law 105-277, the Omnibus Consolidated and Emergency Supplemental Appropriations Act of 1999,[101] which set an excise tax of 75 cents per vaccine dose, and publication in *Morbidity and Mortality Weekly Report* the following March of the CDC recommendation of the vaccine for "routine administration to in children."[102] By the time the CDC published its recommendation for routine use of rotavirus vaccine in children in March 1999, the VAERS had already begun receiving reports of intussusception.[103] Once follow-up epidemiologic studies confirmed an association between rotavirus vaccine and intussusception in the first 2 weeks after immunization,[104,105] the VICP began the process for revising the VIT. After consultation with the ACCV, HHS published a Notice of Proposed Rulemaking in July 2001 adding intussusception to the VIT under a second category of rotavirus vaccines (i.e., live, oral, rhesus-based), which proposed an onset interval of 0 to 30 days following immunization.[92] The wider time interval was chosen in order to provide a generous presumption of causation.

A final rule published on July 26, 2002, became effective on August 26, 2002.[91] Claims for rotavirus vaccine–related injury filed prior to the final rule have been adjudicated on a causation-in-fact basis, a burden that was made easier with definitive epidemiologic studies confirming an association. In fact, several claims were compensated on this basis during 2001 and 2002 while efforts to add intussusception as a VIT injury were proceeding. Once intussusception was added to the table, petitioners benefited from a presumption of causation in claims involving intussusception and had 8 years of retroactive coverage from the effective date of the table change, with a 2-year window in which to file their claim. In addition to the changes for rotavirus vaccine, the final rule added pneumococcal conjugate vaccines as a separate and distinct listing on the VIT, as well as making several technical changes to the VIT and QAI.

Ironically, the benign outcome of most cases of intussusception proved challenging for the VICP. Up until October 2000, the NCVIA required all claimants to establish either that the residual effects of an injury persisted for more than 6 months after vaccination or that a death occurred. Because most patients with intussusception recover completely, some petitioners might be denied compensation under that standard. However, the Children's Health Act of 2000 amended the NCVIA to permit payment of compensation in those claims where the effects of the injury lasts less than 6 months if the petitioner demonstrates that the vaccine-related illness, disability, injury, or condition "resulted in inpatient hospitalization and surgical intervention."[106] Thus, under current law, infants who experience intussusception following a rotavirus vaccine and do not suffer residual effects for more than 6 months may qualify for compensation if their injury resulted in inpatient hospitalization and surgery.

As of April 2002, 21 claims were filed alleging rotavirus vaccine–related injury. Of these, 16 had sufficient records for medical review. All 16 were cases of intussusception in infants ranging from 2½ to 7 months of age. Three quarters had onset within 2 weeks of immunization, and the same percentage required surgical reduction. There was one death. Some claims had been recommended for compensation by HHS based on causation in fact and were compensated.

Varicella Vaccine

Varicella vaccine, which was licensed in March 1995, became a covered vaccine in August 1997 after enactment of the excise tax. By April 2002, the VICP had received about two dozen claims alleging varicella vaccine injury. Nearly all involved infants or children up to 8 years of age. Neurologic conditions were the predominant injury category, followed by hematologic (e.g., chronic thrombocytopenic purpura), endocrine (e.g., diabetes), and skin (e.g., scarring, hyperpigmentation) conditions. Various neurologic disorders have been reported to be associated with primary varicella-zoster (wild-type) virus infections, including meningoencephalitis, encephalitis, transverse myelitis, and acute cerebellar ataxia.[107] Vasculitis and acute cerebellar ataxia also have been reported following varicella vaccine.[108] All of these conditions were reflected in the claims filed, with an onset interval ranging from 4 to 46 days following vaccination.

Because there is no VIT condition listed for varicella vaccine, petitioners can be eligible for compensation only by proving either causation or that the vaccine significantly aggravated a pre-existing condition. This is burdensome because there is little epidemiologic or clinical evidence to suggest an association other than biologic plausibility and temporal association. However, in some instances, claims have been compensated if the nature of the clinical presentation and the onset interval following vaccination mirrored what has been reported with wild-type (natural) varicella-zoster infection.

New Challenges

Although there has been a decided decrease in litigation against vaccine companies since enactment of the VICP (Fig. 63–1), a revived trend in civil litigation is now apparent. Since 2001, individual and class action lawsuits were being filed in state courts alleging injury from thimerosal, an ethylmercury compound used for decades in the formulation of many routinely administered childhood vaccines (see detailed discussion of the legal issues under *Vaccine Liability Since 1986* below). Although there is no proven evidence of harm from thimerosal, as confirmed by a 2001 IOM report,[109] some parents of children with developmental disabilities are convinced their children's condition is thimerosal related, especially when doctors are unable to provide a specific cause other than "idiopathic." In addition to civil litigation, the VICP began receiving claims alleging thimerosal-related injury from several different vaccines (e.g., DTP, Hib, HBV) starting in late 2001. By December of the following year, over 1000 claims had been filed, nearly all of them simple petitions without accompanying medical records or other supporting documents (e.g., affidavits). It was too early to be certain what effect these and future filings will have on the VICP. These cases have been consolidated by the Chief Special Master into an omnibus autism proceeding, in which the presiding special master will first consider whether thimerosal-containing vaccines and/or MMR can cause autism and similar disorders and will then consider, if the first question is answered in the affirmative, whether such vaccines in fact caused individual petitioners' injuries.* In accordance wih special instructions issued by

---

*In Re: Claims for Vaccine Injuries Resulting in Autism Spectrum Disorders or a Similar Neurodevelopmental Disorder v. Secretary of Health Human Services, Autism General Order 1, Autism Master File, 2002 WL1696785 (July 3, 2002).

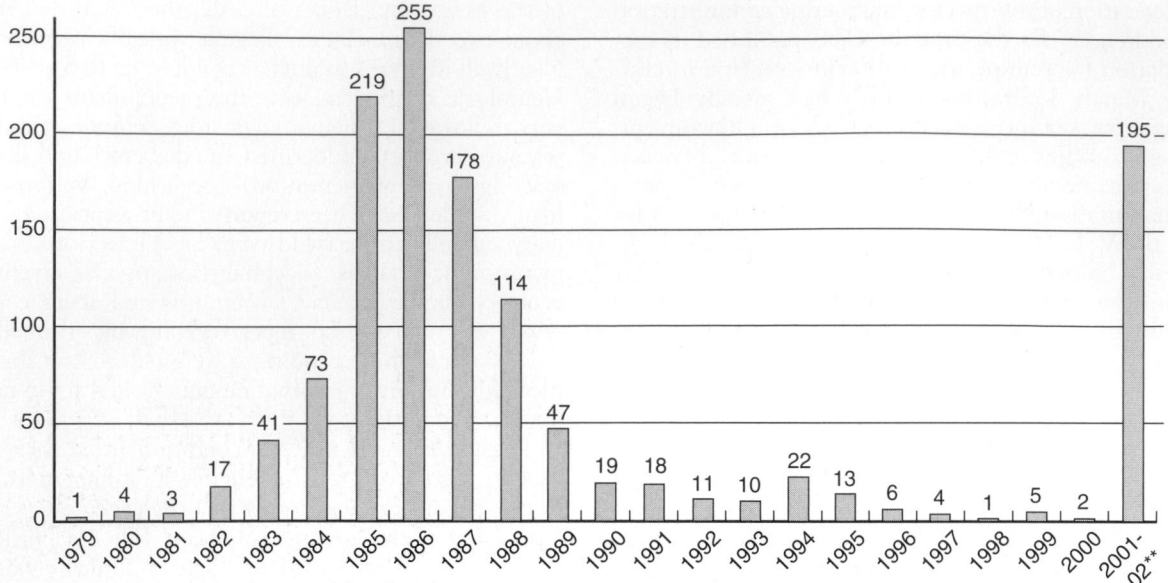

FIGURE 63–1 ■ DTP/DTaP claims files against U.S. manufacturers. **Includes 190 individual and class action lawsuits alleging thimerosal-related injury as of December 4, 2002. (Data from the Division of Vaccine Injury Compensation, Health Resources and Services Administration, U.S. Department of Health and Human Services.)

Special Master Hastings, most petitioners participating in the omnibus autism proceeding have submitted "short-form" petitions that are not accompanied by medical records.[†]

As Congress recognized in 1986 by mandating IOM studies, vaccine safety research is integral to sound decision making by the VICP. Only through a comprehensive vaccine adverse event surveillance and research program can true versus coincidental reactions following vaccination be distinguished. Rotavirus vaccine and intussusception is an example of how epidemiologic research led to expedited compensation once intussusception was found to be vaccine related. At the same time, safety studies allow for the debunking of erroneous theories of vaccine causation, assisting the court in dismissing claims not shown to be vaccine related. In response to a growing number of vaccine safety concerns, and to help ensure timely assessment where appropriate, the CDC and the National Institute of Allergy and Infectious Diseases contracted in 2001 with the IOM to perform independent, expedited scientific reviews of current and emerging vaccine safety hypotheses (see discussion of the IOM Immunization Safety Review Committee in Chapter 61). At the same time, securing adequate funding for vaccine safety research overall remains one of the greatest challenges at a time of budget deficits and competing priorities for vaccine program funding.

Criticism by petitioners and their attorneys has led to increased oversight by Congress. Critics point to the adversarial nature of the program, the protracted delays in adjudication, the perceived unfair changes to the VIT, the huge surplus in the trust fund, and the fact that the public is not well informed about existence of the VICP. In reports issued in December 1999 and March 2000, the General Accounting Office (GAO) found the VICP adjudication process to be easier than the traditional tort system, but not as streamlined as Congress had originally intended.[110,111]

Moreover, although there appeared to be a scientific basis for the VIT changes made by HHS, the GAO found some inconsistencies in applying results of the IOM reviews. As for the trust fund, solutions varied depending on stakeholder perspective, with petitioners wanting more claims compensated by decreasing the burden of proof, vaccine companies wanting the tax reduced to lessen cost, and researchers calling for a portion of incoming revenues annually to pay for vaccine safety research and surveillance. In the end, the GAO's only recommendation was that HHS publish a clear methodology for future changes to the VIT in order to help ensure that such changes are perceived as fair. The second report, on the trust fund, had no recommendation.

In September 1999, the Subcommittee on Drugs and Criminal Justice, part of the House Government Reform Committee, held the first of four hearings on the VICP. More hearings by the full committee followed in November 1999, December 2001, and October 2002. Testifying were parents of injured children as well as petitioners' attorneys, medical experts, and representatives of the program. A bipartisan report released by the Subcommittee in October 2000 recommended: (1) a review of the VIT to ensure the inclusion of current science, (2) the increased use of speedy informal dispute resolution, and (3) the development of an alternative standard for non-VIT cases.[112] It is the last recommendation that is proving the most challenging.

In contrast to the beginning of the program, when most claims alleged a VIT injury, a majority of claims filed today allege non-VIT conditions. Not only did the 1995 modifications to the VIT and QAI force some petitioners to pursue their claims on the basis of causation, rather than under the VIT, but the new vaccines added to the table in recent years have had very few associated VIT injuries. Since 1997, only two conditions were added for the five "new" vaccines. Moreover, of nearly 400 HBV claims, none involves anaphylaxis or anaphylactic shock, the only VIT condition listed for this vaccine. Having to pursue claims on a causation basis will require a greater number of hearings on entitlement. In addition, it is likely that a smaller percentage of claims will be compensated because of the more difficult standard of proof necessary to prove causation. The Subcommittee's call for the development of an alternative standard arose in response to this reality. At the time of publication, a proposal by the American Academy of Pediatrics to utilize a more relaxed burden-of-proof standard for adjudicating non-VIT injuries had been reviewed by the ACCV.[113]

In the spring of 2002, legislation had been introduced in the House of Representatives proposing various process improvements to the VICP, including increased compensation for death claims and an increase in the statute of limitations to 6 years for both injury and death claims.[114] A Senate bill was similar but included other provisions, such as language aimed at eliminating the filing of lawsuits in the civil system without first filing with the VICP.[115]

Some have suggested adding more selective-use vaccines to the VICP, such as influenza and pneumococcal polysaccharide, used primarily in adults. A NVAC review in 1996 found little evidence to support the need, based on liability concerns expressed by manufacturers and health care providers.[116] However, with studies showing significant morbidity from influenza in preschool-age children, and the anticipated licensure of a live, cold-adapted nasal spray influenza vaccine, there is a growing consensus for including this at-risk cohort in a general use recommendation.[117] Should the CDC make such a recommendation, even if it is limited to a certain age cohort of children, VICP coverage for the specific influenza vaccine product would likely follow.

Vaccine Liability Since 1986

The passage of the NCVIA in 1986 did not mark an immediate decline in the number of reported liability decisions in state and federal courts. This occurred for two reasons. First, reported opinions are issued almost exclusively from the appellate courts, and they tend to appear 5 or more years after the case was filed in the trial court. Given the surge in case filings in the early to mid-1980s, one could expect an increase in the number of reported opinions in the late 1980s and early 1990s. In addition, retrospective claimants had until January 31, 1991, to file claims under the NCVIA. Accordingly, for a few years, the retrospective claimant could continue to pursue his or her claim in state or federal court while preserving the option of making a claim under the VICP. As a result of these factors, excluding the swine flu claims, the number of reported opinions involving tort claims alleging a vaccine-related injury increased more between 1987 and 1992 than in any preceding 5-year period.

Since 1992, the number of reported vaccine liability cases has declined sharply. This decrease in reported cases suggests that most claimants have used the VICP and have chosen not to pursue traditional tort litigation after the VICP process. There are only a handful of reported federal and state court cases in which a claimant filed a traditional tort claim against a vaccine manufacturer or a vaccine administrator after being denied compensation under the VICP. In *Evans v. Lederle Laboratories*,[118] a retrospective

claimant was denied compensation under the VICP. The plaintiff filed in state court, but the court claim was dismissed because it was barred by the state statute of limitations. In *Stuart v. American Home Products*,[119] a retrospective claimant chose to file a petition under the VICP, but withdrew her petition prior to the special master's decision. The petitioner then filed a traditional tort claim against the manufacturer, but the claim was dismissed because it was barred by the statute of limitations. In *Harman v. Borah, M.D.*,[120] a retrospective petitioner was compensated under the VICP and accepted the award. The petitioner then filed a medical malpractice action against the vaccine administrator in state court. The state court dismissed the claim against the administrator, holding that the Harmans' action against the administrator was barred by their acceptance of the VICP award. In *Haggerty v. Wyeth Ayerst Pharmaceuticals and Reilly, M.D.*,[121] the petitioner was denied compensation under the VICP. After this denial, the petitioner filed a federal court claim, and the matter is still pending. In *McDonald v. Lederle*,[122] a petitioner who was denied compensation under the VICP because the petition was untimely sued the manufacturer on traditional tort grounds. The state court dismissed the claim, holding that an untimely filing under the VICP precludes a post-VICP state action for the injured child's damages.

Another theory involving both vaccine producers and administrators is the "duty to warn" theory. The theory, as applied by petitioners, is that the warning in the package insert (in cases involving producers) was inadequate or that the warning given by the administering health professional (in cases against the administrator) was inadequate. The NCVIA itself resolves this issue for manufacturers by stating that "[N]o vaccine manufacturer shall be liable in a civil action for damages arising from a vaccine-related injury or death associated with the administration of a vaccine after the effective date of this subpart solely due to the manufacturer's failure to provide direct warnings to the injured party." In addition, this section of the act protects the manufacturer from liability for unavoidable adverse side effects as long as the vaccine is properly prepared and accompanied by proper directions and warnings.[123] The act also defines what constitutes proper directions and warnings. There are no such protections for administrators.

Starting in 2001, a new liability theory appeared alleging injury not from the vaccine's active ingredient, but rather from the vaccine's excipient ingredient, thimerosal, an organic mercury compound (ethylmercury), which has been used for decades in multidose vials of some childhood vaccines to prevent bacterial and fungal contamination. It was not until an FDA review of thimerosal-containing vaccines in 1999 discovered some infants were receiving ethylmercury in excess of one federal safety guideline established for methylmercury, the more extensively studied form of organic mercury, that attention became focused on thimerosal and possible adverse outcomes.[124] As of May 28, 2003, 250 individual and class action lawsuits alleging thimerosal-related injuries had been filed in state courts against vaccine manufacturers and, in some instances, administrators and/or the thimerosal manufacturer.[125] Individual suits are filed on behalf of an injured party, usually a child, who is alleged to be developmentally impaired from the thimerosal, or on behalf of the parents, children, or spouse of the injured person seeking their own damages for loss of companionship or consortium, or services, and loss of earnings, for example (see *Other Situations in Which Suits Are Not Barred by the NCVIA* below). Other lawsuits do not allege specific injuries, but instead demand the costs of medical monitoring to determine whether thimerosal-related injuries will develop in the future. Pleadings in the purported class action lawsuits may range from 50 thousand to more than 100 million individuals in each class.

According to the NCVIA, petitions relating to vaccine-related injuries or death must generally be filed with the VICP before the petitioner may seek other legal remedies. Nevertheless, individuals in Texas, Oregon, Washington, and other jurisdictions have bypassed the VICP and filed directly in the tort system. These individuals base their actions on two grounds. First, plaintiffs argue that their actions are not governed by this filing requirement because thimerosal is an "adulterant" to, and not a part of, vaccines. Second, many in the class are seeking $1000 or less in damages, and the VICP allows individuals with small claims to pursue damages in the tort system.[126] Since the individuals in the purported class action lawsuits are seeking $1000 or less *per person* to pay for "medical monitoring" (i.e., future tests to determine *if* the child is developing an injury), plaintiffs argue they are not covered by the NCVIA.

The argument that thimerosal is an adulterant hinges on the NCVIA's definition of a "vaccine-related injury or death," which excludes any injury or death associated with an adulterant or contaminant intentionally added to a covered vaccine.[127] Because thimerosal is part of the vaccine formulation when the product is licensed and because thimerosal has been approved for use by the FDA, the federal government has rejected the plaintiffs' argument that thimerosal is a vaccine adulterant and contends that claims alleging thimerosal-related injuries from VICP-covered vaccines must, with limited exceptions, be filed with the VICP before tort remedies can be pursued.

In a recent case filed with the VICP, petitioners argued that their child suffered developmental problems as the result of receiving several thimerosal-containing vaccines. Nonetheless, petitioners also argued that the Court of Federal Claims lacked jurisdiction over their case, and other cases in which thimerosal-related injuries were alleged, and that the case should be dismissed for lack of jurisdiction (to enable petitioners to pursue other legal remedies). Petitioners reasoned that thimerosal was not a constituent material of the vaccines, but was instead an adulterant to or contaminant of the vaccines. The Chief Special Master of the Court of Federal Claims reached the opposite conclusion and held that the Court of Federal Claims had jurisdiction over thimerosal-related injury claims. This conclusion was based, in large part, on a plain meaning analysis of the text of the NCVIA, principles of statutory construction, and an analysis of the legislative history underlying the NCVIA.[128]

At the time of publication, decisions on jurisdictional matters had been rendered in about a dozen of the cases pending in state and federal courts. In those cases in which the jurisdictional issues had been considered, most federal courts had remanded the cases to state courts. In remanding these cases, some of these federal courts allowed for the possibility that state courts could find the terms *adulterant* or *contaminant to encompass thimerosal-related injuries, which*

would render the requirements of the NCVIA inapplicable to such claims. The trend in such civil litigation is an interpretation of the NCVIA such that thimerosal is not considered an adulterant to, or contaminant of, covered vaccines.

It should also be noted that, in late 2002, President Bush signed into law the Homeland Security Act of 2002 (HSA), which contained several provisions that affected the thimerosal litigation.[129] Specifically, the HSA introduced a new definition of "vaccine" and clarified the definition of "vaccine-related injuries or deaths" in the NCVIA so that thimerosal would not be considered an adulterant to or contaminant of vaccines, and that cases alleging vaccine-related injuries/deaths in connection with the thimerosal in covered vaccines had to be filed with the VICP as an initial matter (with limited exceptions). In addition, the HSA extended the NCVIA's definition of manufacturers to include manufacturers of components or ingredients of covered vaccines (as well as manufacturers of covered vaccines), thus now covering claims against manufacturers of thimerosal, which prior to this legislation had not been governed by the NCVIA and did not to need to be filed with the VICP. The amendments to the NCVIA that were included in the HSA were subsequently repealed but have been incorporated into legislation introduced in 2003.*

Risk to Health Care Professionals

Civil actions against health care providers are unlikely, and few have been pursued since the VICP was modified to cover vaccine administrators, because claimants must go through the VICP prior to filing most actions against a manufacturer or vaccine administrator. However, if a claimant were to reject the VICP decision, he or she might file a tort action against the health care provider on such grounds as the administrator failing to properly discharge his or her duty to warn the responsible person of the risks and benefits of the vaccine. It should be noted that the courts routinely reject these allegations when the administrator provides a warning commensurate with the contents of the package insert. The NCVIA bolsters these state court findings because it presumably sets the standard regarding the warning for the administrator. The act states that "each health care provider who administers a vaccine set forth in the Vaccine Injury Table shall provide to the legal representatives of any child or to any other individual to whom such provider intends to administer such vaccine a copy of the information materials developed [by the Secretary of Health and Human Services]."[130] The standard of care presumably would also include a requirement that the provider verify the responsible person's review of the materials and/or that the provider has shown due care in the exercise of medical judgment in immunizing the individual. Assuming the standard of care is met, health care providers should face little potential liability.

Other Situations in Which Suits Are Not Barred by the NCVIA

The NCVIA only covers the losses sustained by the injured person, thus, all loss of companionship claims by the parents,

---

*U.S. Senate. S. 754: Improved Vaccine Affordability and Availability Act. Congressional Day, April 1, 2003.

children, or spouse of the injured person are not compensable. The family members may file these so-called derivative claims in state court, if they are cognizable under state law, but the claims will only be successful if these individuals can prove that the underlying injury or death was related to the vaccine. The plaintiff may not rely on a finding under the VICP.[131] Up until 2001, with the thimerosal litigation, families rarely filed such claims. The issue first came to light in *Schafer v. American Cyanamid.*[132] The husband and daughter of a woman who contracted vaccine-related polio filed a claim for loss of consortium and emotional distress in Massachusetts State Court after the woman accepted a VICP award. The case was removed to the federal court and, on appeal, the U.S. Court of Appeals for the First Circuit found that the Schafers' claim was not precluded by the acceptance of the VICP award. The Court of Federal Claims' interpretation of the NCVIA was consistent with the *Schafer* holding. In *Abbott v. Secretary of Department of Health & Human Services,*[133] a young man's mother filed a state wrongful death claim against a health care provider alleging that it negligently left her son unattended in the bathtub. The young man had a seizure in the tub and drowned. Ms. Abbott filed the state claim in her capacity as mother of the decedent, and she accepted a settlement from the health care provider. A few months later, the mother filed a VICP death claim in her capacity as administrator of her son's estate. Here, she alleged that the death was a sequela of the vaccine-related seizure disorder. The claim was dismissed by the special master because Ms. Abbott had already recovered in state court; however, the U.S. Court of Appeals for the Federal Circuit reversed, holding that the previous settlement covered only damages for injuries to the young man's beneficiaries. The VICP award would be for the young man's estate, and Ms. Abbott was an appropriate person to represent the estate. The case was conceded, and Ms. Abbott received a death benefit award.

Claims alleging that a provider willfully breached his or her fiduciary duty also may not be covered by the VICP. In *Cook v. Children's Medical Group,*[134] parents claimed that a vaccine administrator fraudulently concealed their child's vaccine-related injury and, as a result of this concealment, the time for filing a VICP claim had passed. The court held that the VICP does not cover claims for breach of fiduciary duty, so the parents' claim against the administrators could continue in state court. However, the claim for the underlying vaccine-related injury must be filed under the VICP.

International Compensation Programs

Approximately a dozen industrialized countries provide some form of compensation for injuries (or deaths) following vaccination.[135] More than anything else, these compensation programs were instituted in the belief that governments have a special responsibility to those injured by properly manufactured and administered vaccines used in public health programs. Most are managed administratively through the national government, including decisions on eligibility and the amount of compensation. Eligibility may depend on the recipient's age, citizenship,

or residency status; the category of vaccine (e.g., recommended, compulsory); the location in which it is administered (public vs. private ambulatory setting); or satisfying certain time frames for filing a claim. Because few vaccine-related injuries have a clinical or laboratory marker, proving actual causation is difficult. Causation decisions are usually based on the balance-of-probabilities standard of "more likely than not." All countries require that the effects be long lasting (e.g., greater than 6 months), and nearly all provide coverage for medical costs, disability pensions, noneconomic damages (pain and suffering), and death benefits. None outside the United States reimburses attorneys' fees and costs. Funding is generally from the national treasury, with some programs receiving support from lower governmental entities or vaccine manufacturers.

Interest has been expressed in expanding vaccine injury compensation to the developing world.[136] The World Health Organization, the United Nations International Children's Emergency Fund, and other major organizations have yet to adopt a policy in this regard, which is understandable given the fact that the necessary economic resources and health infrastructure are often not present. That said, promoters emphasize the inherent responsibility of government/society to ensure that individuals who may be harmed from vaccines are properly cared for, whether it be through "compensation," as in the model in industrialized countries, or the availability of basic medical services and support. They see this effort as achieving one or both of these goals over time.

Summary, Conclusions, and Future Implications

There is clear evidence that the VICP has largely satisfied the public policy imperatives driving passage of the NCVIA more than 15 years ago. First, the availability of compensation under the act has generally given plaintiffs a sufficient incentive to abandon the pursuit of tort remedies against vaccine manufacturers and administrators. Claims against vaccine manufacturers are significantly reduced, as compared to the litigation manufacturers faced at the inception of the VICP. Although claims against health care providers are more difficult to track, there is no indication that their liability experience is any different from that of manufacturers. Until the new wave of court cases pertaining to thimerosal was initiated, almost no cases alleging vaccine-related injuries were filed outside the VICP in recent years. The reduction in the number of such civil actions can largely be explained by the fact that the NCVIA requires petitioners to file for compensation under the act before pursuing outside litigation for alleged vaccine-related injuries or deaths. With regard to post-1988 claims, petitioners have two options once the VICP process is concluded: (1) accept the court's judgment and the compensation awarded (if any); or (2) reject the court's judgment, with the option of pursuing a civil action in state or federal court (under certain limitations set forth in the NCVIA). Virtually all VICP petitioners, even those who were not awarded compensation under the VICP, have chosen the former option. Even among the small number of VICP petitioners who have chosen the latter option (a group consisting almost entirely of individuals who were not awarded compensation under the VICP), almost all have chosen not to pursue further civil remedies. The fact that most VICP petitioners choose to accept the court's judgment and forgo additional civil litigation can largely be explained by the VICP's generous compensation awards, which are devised in an effort to create a lifetime stream of benefits for the injured party, and the general understanding that the VICP imposes a lesser burden on litigants than that imposed in traditional civil litigation.

The reported decisions are consistent with the conclusion that vaccine manufacturers and administrators are generally shielded from any significant liability risk, except for their own negligence. However, the protection is not absolute. Because the NCVIA does not preclude an individual who is otherwise ineligible to file a claim under the VICP (e.g., family members of injured individuals) from pursuing civil litigation, liability exposure remains a possibility. Many of the recently filed thimerosal claims include requests for relief by family members of injured individuals, who are not entitled to compensation under the NCVIA. This new surge in non-VICP litigation threatens to undermine many of the goals underlying the creation of the VICP. Although jurisdictional questions over this thimerosal litigation remained unanswered at the time of publication, there is reason to believe the VICP will continue to serve successfully as an alternative to the tort system.

Another measure of the success of the VICP is the development, and the administration to children, of new vaccines to prevent childhood diseases. Annual Investigational New Drug requests to the FDA, a necessary step in beginning testing in human subjects, have trended upward over the past 10 years (Center for Biologics Evaluation and Research, unpublished data, 2001). Since the creation of the VICP, the following vaccines have been recommended for routine administration to children by the CDC, and included within the VICP's coverage: HBV, Hib, varicella, rotavirus, and pneumococcal conjugate. The fact that, since the VICP was created, such vaccines have successfully traversed the long, arduous licensing process to become routinely administered vaccines demonstrates that the scientific community is able to develop innovative vaccine products to combat childhood diseases under the current system.

Another benefit of the VICP has been that liability concerns no longer lead to the destabilization of the marketplace. The market has recently experienced some vaccine supply shortages, but such shortages do not appear to be attributable to liability factors.[137] Although many new vaccines are relatively expensive (reflecting the manufacturers' need to recoup the costs of research and development), vaccine prices today reflect public and private sector purchase trends and the effects of inflation, rather than liability concerns or repercussions.

Thus, the existence and general success of the VICP in meeting the public policy objectives underlying the NCVIA have led to a current system in which innovative vaccine products and technologies are developed, the vast majority of American children are immunized against a growing number of diseases that pose a threat to their health, and the small number of children who sustain adverse events as the result of such immunizations are able to receive appropriate compensation through the VICP.

The success of the VICP can further be measured by the fact that it has been used as a model for other proposed non-tort compensation programs. Three particular instances are worthy of note. First, a bill entitled the AIDS Vaccine Development and Compensation Act of 1992 (H.R. 5893), introduced in the 102nd Congress, proposed the creation of a VICP-like compensation program to facilitate acquired immunodeficiency syndrome (AIDS) vaccine research and clinical trials. Should future AIDS vaccine research and development encounter liability problems, it is possible that a companion system might be created or folded into the VICP.[138] Second, the Public Health Service is developing a comprehensive plan in preparation for the next influenza pandemic and has considered the creation of liability protection for vaccine manufacturers and administrators as part of this plan.[139] Finally, in the wake of the bioterrorism scares that arose after the September 11, 2001, attacks and the dissemination of anthrax in the United States, serious consideration was given to creating a VICP-like compensation program to compensate individuals harmed by vaccines (or other products) administered to prevent or treat adverse events resulting from certain forms of bioterrorism.

An increasing focus has been given to the issue of vaccine safety over recent years. Through media involvement and Internet access, the ability for misleading information to be disseminated has increased. As a result, effective vaccine risk communication becomes imperative and must include a recognition of the difficult and confusing nature of risk assessment and decision making for some vaccines.[140] Such communication is particularly critical now, at a time when most parents do not have any independent recollection of the devastation caused by infectious diseases prevented by childhood vaccines. Interwoven into vaccine safety awareness is the issue of state mandates for immunization and calls for all states to provide philosophical exemptions. Courts continue to uphold the states' police powers to mandate immunization for school entry, while allowing them to provide exemptions for medical, religious, or philosophical reasons. Approximately one third of states currently allow philosophical exemptions for routine childhood immunizations, a level that has remained steady over recent years.

Our nation's experience with the public's perception concerning immunization, as well as other countries' experiences with the same issue, makes clear that uncertainty and fear often come together when information is lacking. Although most parents seem to believe in the wisdom of vaccination and use their health care providers as a key source of guidance in decision making, immunization must never be taken for granted. Although the federal and state immunization programs, together with the VICP, have done a remarkable job of ensuring that our nation's children will be vaccinated against dangerous diseases, and although a national surveillance system and several IOM reports confirm the general safety of immunizations given routinely in this country, public perceptions concerning the risks of vaccines remain an important issue for vaccine administrators to address. The recent trend of litigation concerning thimerosal raises this to a degree that had not been present in recent years. Although the issue remained unresolved at the time of publication, there is no reason to believe that the VICP will not be able to adequately address this new phenomenon. Moreover, at the time of publication, several bills suggesting amendments to the NCVIA in an effort to strengthen the VICP and to prevent outside litigation against manufacturers, an important purpose of the act, are pending in Congress. Such measures are likely to improve the success of the VICP. Finally, the ability of the VICP to successfully fulfill its mandate and to further its statutory purposes seems strong, particularly given the near-universal consensus among the VICP's stakeholders (i.e., physicians, manufacturers, lawmakers, attorneys, and members of the public, including parents of injured children) that a successful national immunization program can only be achieved with a compensation program and liability safeguards in place.

Acknowledgments

The authors wish to thank the following individuals for their assistance in preparing the manuscript: Vito Caserta, M.D., M.P.H.; Robert E. Weibel, M.D.; Carol Konchan, R.N.; Ward Sorensen and Linda Rozzelle from the VICP, HHS; David Benor, J.D., Kevin Malone, J.D., and Debbie Thomas from the Office of the General Counsel, HHS; and Skip Wolfe from the National Immunization Program, CDC.

REFERENCES

1. American Law Institute. Restatement (Second) of Torts §4.02A (superseded by the Restatement (Third) of Torts: Products Liability). Accessed through WESTLAW.
2. American Law Institute. Restatement (Second) of Torts §4.02A, comment g. Accessed through WESTLAW.
3. American Law Institute. Restatement (Second) of Torts §4.02A, comments i and j. Accessed through WESTLAW.
4. American Law Institute. Restatement (Second) of Torts §4.02A, comment k. Accessed through WESTLAW.
5. *Gottsdanker v. Cutter Laboratories*, 182 Cal. App. 2d 602, 6 Cal. Reptr. 320 (Dist. Ct. App. 1960).
6. *Reyes v. Wyeth Laboratories*, 498 F.2d 1264 (5th Cir. 1974).
7. *Givens v. Lederle*, 556 F.2d 1341 (5th Cir. 1977).
8. Silverstein AM. Pure Politics and Impure Science. Baltimore, The Johns Hopkins University Press, 1981.
9. Neustadt R, Fineberg H. The Swine Flu Affair: Decision-Making on a Slippery Disease. Washington, DC, U.S. Department of Health, Education and Welfare, 1978.
10. *Unthank v. United States*, 732 F.2d 1517 (10th Cir. 1984).
11. *Petty v. United States*, 740 F.2d 1428 (8th Cir. 1984).
12. Institute of Medicine. Vaccine Supply and Innovation: Report of the Committee on Public-Private Sector Relations in Vaccine Innovation (Publ No 95-113) Washington, DC, National Academy Press, 1985.
13. *Johnson v. American Cyanamid Co.*, Case No. 81 C 2470 (18th Jud. Dist., Sedgwick Co., Kansas), rev'd 239 Kan. 279, 718 P.2d 1318 (1986).
14. *Toner v. Lederle Laboratories*, 779 F.2d 1429 (9th Cir. 1986), *certified question answered by* 112 Idaho 328, 732 P.2d 297 (1987), *judgment affirmed* 828 F.2d 510 (1988), *cert. denied* 485 U.S. 942 (1988).
15. *Jacobson v. Massachusetts*, 197 U.S. 11 (1905).
16. *Maricopa County Health Department v. Harmon*, 156 Ariz. 161, 750 P.2d 1364 (Ariz. App. 1987).
17. Centers for Disease Control and Prevention. National, state and urban vaccination coverage levels among children aged 19-35 months—United States, 2001. MMWR Rep 51:664–666, 2002.
18. *United States v. Washington*, 54 M.J. 936 (A.F. Ct. Crim. App. 2001).
19. Public Health Service Act, 42 U.S.C. § 247b.
20. Public Health Service Act, 42 C.F.R. § 51b.204.
21. *Brown v. Stone*, 378 So. 2d 218 (Mississippi, 1979).
22. *McCarthy v. Boozman*, 212 F.Supp.2d 945 (W.D. Ark., 2002).
23. *Matter of Christine M.*, 157 Misc. 2d 4, 595 N.Y.S. 2d 606 (Family Court, Kings County 1992).
24. *LePage v. State of Wyoming Dep't of Health*, 151 Ed. Law. Rep. 605, 18 P.3d 1177 (2001).
25. *Jones v. State of Wyoming Dep't of Health*, 151 Ed. Law. Rep. 610, 18 P.3d 1189 (2001).
26. *Ritterband v. Axelrod*, 562 N.Y.S. 2d 605 (1990).
27. Stokley S. Presentaion before the Advisory Committee on Immunization Practices. February 20, 2002. Atlanta. Ga.
28. Euvax Project. Regulatory background of immunizations related to compulsory immunisations and immunization requirements for school or kindergarten entry. *In* Scientific and Technical Evaluation of Vaccination Programmes in the European Union—Euvax Project Report for the Commission on the European Communities. PSR Consulting, Ltd. Helsinki, 2001.
29. Ball AK. Report on the United Kingdom vaccine damage payment unit. Presented at the International Workshop on Vaccine Injury Compensation Programs, May 16–18, 2000. Washington, DC.
30. Senate Bill 859, General Statutes of North Carolina, §§130A-422 to 130A-432 (passed July 15, 1986).
31. NC St. Ch. 130A, Article 17.
32. National Childhood Vaccine Injury Act of 1986, Pub. L. No. 99-660 §§ 311 et seq., 100 Stat. 3755, codified at 42 U.S.C.A. §§ 300aa-1 et seq. (1989).
33. National Childhood Vaccine Injury Act of 1986, Pub. L. No. 99-660 §§ 311 et seq., 100 Stat. 3755, codified at 42 U.S.C.A. §§ 300aa-1 et seq. (1989).
34. Pub. L. No.100-203 §§ 4301 et seq. 101 Stat. 1330-221, codified at 42 U.S.C.A. §§ 300aa-1 et seq. (1989).
35. Smith MH. National Childhood Vaccine Injury Compensation Act. Pediatrics 82:264–269, 1988.
36. Centers for Disease Control and Prevention. Withdrawal of rotavirus vaccine recommendation. MMWR 48:1007, 1999.
37. Health Information, Health Promotion, and Vaccine Injury Amendments of 1991. Pub. L. No. 102-168, 105 Stat 1102 (1991).
38. *Childers v. Secretary of Department of Health & Human Services*, Ct. Fed. Cl. No. 96-194V (March 26, 1999).
39. *Watkins v. Secretary of Department of Health & Human Services*, Ct. Fed. Cl. No. 95-154V (March 12, 1999).
40. National Childhood Vaccine Injury Act of 1986, Pub. L. No. 99-660 (42 U.S.C. § 300aa-15(a)(3)(A)(B)).
41. Omnibus Budget Reconciliation Act of 1987. Pub. L. No. 100-203, 101 Stat 1330-221 (1987).
42. Clayton EW, Hickson GB. Compensation under the National Childhood Vaccine Injury Act. J Pediatr 116:508-513, 1990.
43. Omnibus Budget Reconciliation Act of 1993, Pub. L. No. 103-66, 107 Stat 565, 567 (1993).
44. Division of Vaccine Injury Compensation, Bureau of Health Professions, Health Resources and Services Administration. Monthly statistics report, May 31, 2003. Rockville, MD, Health Resources and Services Administration, 2002.
45. Taxpayer Relief Act of 1997, Pub. L. No. 105-34, 111 Stat. 251 (1997).
46. Kinsbourne M. Disorders of mental development. *In* Menkes JH (ed). Textbook of Child Neurology. Philadelphia, Lea & Febiger, 1990, pp 763–770.
47. Cody CL, Baraff LJ, Cherry JD, et al. Nature and rates of adverse reactions associated with DTP and DT immunizations in infants and children. Pediatrics 68:650–660, 1981.
48. *Pearson v. Secretary of Department of Health & Human Services*, Ct Fed. Cl. No. 90-988V (April 8, 1992).
49. *Munn v. Secretary of Department of Health & Human Services*, 970 F.2d 863 (Fed. Cir.1992).
50. *Hellebrand v. Secretary of Department of Health & Human Services*, 999 F.2d 156 (Fed. Cir. 1993).
51. *Hodges v. Secretary of Department of Health & Human Services*, 9 F.3d 958 (Fed. Cir. 1994).
52. *Shalala v. Whitecotton*, 514 U.S. 268, 115 S.Ct. 1477; 131 L.Ed. 374 (1995).

53. *Shalala v. Whitecotton*, 61 F.3d 1099 (Fed. Cir. 1996).

54. *Whitecotton v. Secretary of Department of Health & Human Services*, 81 F.3d 1099 (Fed. Cir. 1996)

55. *Misasi v. Secretary of Department of Health & Human Services*, 23 Cl. Ct. 322 (1991).

56. National Childhood Vaccine Injury Act of 1986, Pub. L. No. 99-660 (42 U.S.C. sec. §300aa-13(a)(2)).

57. *Koston v. Secretary of Department of Health & Human Services*, 974 F.2d 157 (Fed. Cir. 1992).

58. *Knudsen v. Secretary of Department of Health & Human Services*, 35 F.3d 543, 548–549 (Fed. Cir. 1994).

59. Berg BO. Neurocutaneous syndromes: phakomatoses and allied conditions. *In* Swaiman KF (ed). Pediatric Neurology: Principles and Practice (2nd ed). St. Louis, CV Mosby, 1994, pp 1050–1054.

60. Shepherd CW, Houser OW, Gomez MR. MR findings in tuberous sclerosis complex and correlation with seizure development and mental impairment. AJNR Am J Neuroradiol 16:149–155, 1995.

61. Lamm SH, Goodman M, Engel A, et al. Cortical tuber count: a biomarker indicating cerebral severity of tuberous sclerosis complex. J Child Neurol 12:85–90, 1997.

62. Goodman M, Lamm SH, Bellman MH. Temporal relationship modeling: DPT or DT immunizations and infantile spasms. Vaccine 16:25–31, 1997.

63. Jozwiak S, Goodman M, Lamm SH. Poor mental development in TSC patients: clinical risk factors. Arch Neurol 55:379–385, 1998.

64. *Hanlon v. Secretary of Department of Health & Human Services*, 191 F.3d 1344 (Fed. Cir. 1999).

65. *Turner v. Secretary of Department of Health & Human Services*, 268 F.3d 1334 (Fed. Cir. 2001).

66. *Flanagan v. Secretary of Department of Health & Human Services*, 268 F.3d 1334 (Fed. Cir. 2001).

67. Health Resources and Services Administration. National Vaccine Injury Compensation Program: revision of the Vaccine Injury Table. Fed Reg 60:7678–7696, 1995.

68. *O'Connell v. Shalala*, 79 F.3rd 170 (1st Cir. 1996).

69. *Terran v. Secretary of Department of Health & Human Services*, 195 F.3d 1302 (Fed. Cir. 1999).

70. *Grant v. Secretary of Department of Health & Human Services*, 956F.2d 1141 (Fed. Cir. 1992).

71. *O'Leary v. Secretary of Department of Health & Human Services*, Ct. Fed. Cl. No. 90-1729V (April 4, 1997).

72. *Liable v. Secretary of Department of Health & Human Services*, Ct Fed. Cl. No. 98-120V (Sept. 7, 2000).

73. *Ragini v. Secretary of Department of Health & Human Services*, Ct Fed. Cl. No. 96-294V (July 31, 2001).

74. *Terran v. Secretary of Department of Health & Human Services*, Ct Fed. Cl. No. 95-451V (January 23, 1998).

75. *Sharpnack v. Secretary of Department of Health & Human Services*, 27 Fed. Cl. 457 (1993).

76. *Stevens v. Secretary of Department of Health & Human Services*, Ct Fed. Cl. No. 99-594V (March 3, 2001).

77. *Shyface v. Secretary of Department of Health & Human Services*, 165 F.3d 1344, 1352 (Fed. Cir. 1999).

78. Institute of Medicine, Howson CP, Howe CJ, Fineberg HV (eds). Adverse Effects of Pertussis and Rubella Vaccines. Washington, DC, National Academy Press, 1991.

79. Howson CP, Fineberg HV. The ricochet of magic bullets. Summary of the Institute of Medicine report: adverse effects of pertussis and rubella vaccines. Pediatrics 89:318–324, 1992.

80. Institute of Medicine, Stratton KR, Howe DJ, Johnston, RB (eds). Adverse Events Associated with Childhood Vaccines: Evidence Bearing on Causality. Washington, DC, National Academy Press, 1994.

81. Stratton KR, Howe CJ, Johnston RB. Adverse events associated with childhood vaccine other than pertussis and rubella: summary of a report from the Institute of Medicine. JAMA 271:1602–1605, 1994.

82. Institute of Medicine, Stratton KR, Howe CJ, Johnston RB (eds). DPT Vaccine and Chronic Nervous System Dysfunction: A New Analysis. Washington, DC, National Academy Press, 1994.

83. Miller DL, Ross EM, Alderslade R, et al. Pertussis immunisation and serious acute neurological illness in children. BMJ 307:1171–1176, 1993.

84. Health Resources and Services Administration. National Vaccine Injury Compensation Program: revisions and additions to the Vaccine Injury Table—II. Fed Reg 62:7685–7690, 1997.

85. Kinnunen E, Farkkila M, Hovi T, et al. Incidence of Guillain-Barré syndrome during a nationwide oral poliovirus vaccine campaign. Neurology 39:1034–1036, 1989.

86. Rantala H, Cherry JD, Shields WD, Uhari M. Epidemiology of Guillain-Barré syndrome in children: relationship of oral polio vaccine administration to occurrence. J Pediatr 124:220–223, 1994.

87. National Vaccine Advisory Committee. Report of the Ad Hoc Subcommittee on Childhood Vaccines. Atlanta, Centers for Disease Control and Prevention, 1994.

88. *Robinson v. Secretary of Department of Health & Human Services*, Ct Fed. Cl. No. 91-01V (September 8, 1994) (unpublished).

89. Health Resources and Services Administration. National Vaccine Injury Compensation Program: addition of vaccines against rotavirus to the program. Fed Reg 64:40517–40518, 1999.

90. Health Resources and Services Administration. National Vaccine Injury Compensation Program: addition of pneumococcal conjugate vaccines to the Vaccine Injury Table. Fed Reg 66:28166, 2001.

91. Health Resources and Services Administration. National Vaccine Injury Compensation Program: revisions and additions to the Vaccine Injury Table. Fed Reg 67:48558–48560, 2002.

92. Health Resources and Services Administration. National Vaccine Injury Compensation Program: revisions and additions to the Vaccine Injury Table. Fed Reg 66:36735–36739, 2001.

93. *Housand v. Secretary of Department of Health & Human Services*, 114 F.3d 1206 (Fed.Cir. 1997).

94. Weibel RE, Caserta V, Benor DE, Evans G. Acute encephalopathy followed by permanent brain injury or death associated with further attenuated measles vaccines: a review of claims submitted to the National Vaccine Injury Compensation Program. Pediatrics 101:383–387, 1998.

95. Weibel RE, Benor DE. Chronic arthropathy and musculoskeletal symptoms associated with rubella vaccines. Arthritis Rheum 39:1529–1534, 1996.

96. Ray P, Black S, Shinefeld H, et al. Risk of chronic arthropathy among women after rubella vaccination. JAMA 278:551–556, 1997.

97. Tingle AJ, Mitchell LA, Grace M, et al. Randomized double-blind placebo-controlled study on adverse effects of rubella immunisation in seronegative women. Lancet 349:1277–1281, 1997.

98. Nathanson N, Langmuir AD. The Cutter incident: poliomyelitis following formaldehyde-inactivated polio virus vaccination in the United States during the spring of 1955. Am J Hyg 78:29–60, 1963.

99. Stratton K, Almario D, McCormick M. Hepatitis B Vaccine and Demyelinating Neurological Disorders: Report from the Institute of Medicine. Washington, DC, National Academy Press, 2002.

100. Golkciecwicz G. Presentation before the Advisory Commission on Childhood Vaccines, December 4, 2002. Rockville, Health Resources and Services Administration, 2002.

101. Omnibus Consolidated and Emergency Supplemental Appropriations Act of 1999, Pub. L. No. 105-277 § 1503, 112 Stat 2681 (1998) (amending 26 U.S.C. § 4132(a)(1)).

102. Centers for Disease Control and Prevention. Rotavirus vaccine for the prevention of rotavirus gastroenteritis among children: recommendations of the Advisory Committee on Immunization Practices (ACIP). MMWR 48(RR-2):1–25, 1999.

103. Zanardi LR, Haber P, Mootrey GT, et al. Intussusception among recipients of rotavirus vaccine: reports to the Vaccine Adverse Event Reporting System. Pediatrics 107:E97, 2001.

104. Murphy TV, Gargiullo PM, Massoudi MS, et al. Intussusception among infants given an oral rotavirus vaccine. N Engl J Med 344:564–572, 2001.

105. Kramarz P, France EK, DeStefano F, et al. Population based study of rotavirus vaccination and intussusception. Pediatr Infect Dis J 20:410–416, 2001.

106. Children's Health Act of 2000, Pub. L. 106-310, Title XVII, § 1701 (amending 42 U.S.C. § 300aa-11(c)(1)(D)).

107. Bodensteiner JB, Hille MR, Riggs JE. Clinical features of vascular thrombosis following varicella. Am J Dis Child 146:100–102, 1992.

108. Sunaga Y, Hikima A, Ostuka T, Morikawa A. Acute cerebella ataxia with abnormal MRI lesions after varicella vaccination. Pediatr Neurol 13:340–342, 1995.

109. Institute of Medicine. Thimerosal-Containing Vaccines and Neurodevelopmental Disorders. Washington, DC, National Academy Press, 2002.

110. General Accounting Office. Report to Congressional Requesters. Vaccine Injury Compensation: Program Challenged to Settle Claims Quickly and Easily. Washington, DC, General Accounting Office, 1999.

111. General Accounting Office. Report to Congressional Requesters. Vaccine Injury Trust Fund: Revenue Exceeds Current Need for Paying Claims. Washington, DC, General Accounting Office, 2000.

112. U.S. House of Representatives, Committee on Government Reform, Subcommittee on Criminal Justice, Drug Policy and Human Resources. The Vaccine Injury Compensation Program: Addressing Needs and Improving Practices. Washington, DC, U.S. Congress, 2000.

113. Peter G. Presentation before the Advisory Commission on Childhood Vaccines, December 5, 2001. Rockville, Health Resources and Services Administration, 2001.

114. U.S. House of Representatives. H.R. 3741. National Vaccine Injury Compensation Program Improvement Act of 2002. Congressional Rec, February 13, 2002.

115. U.S. Senate. S. 2053. Title II—Vaccine Injury Compensation Program. Congressional Rec, March 21, 2002.

116. Lloyd-Puryear MA, Ball LK. Should the Vaccine Injury Compensation Program be expanded to cover adults? J Public Health Rep 113:336–342, 1998.

117. Centers for Disease Control and Prevention. Prevention and control of influenza: recommendations of the Advisory Committee on Immunization Practices (ACIP). MMWR 51(RR-3):1–31, 2002.

118. *Evans v. Lederle Laboratories*, 904 F. Supp. 857 (C.D. Ill. 1995).

119. *Stuart v. American Home Products*, 158 F. 3d 622 (2d Cir. 1998).

120. *Harman v. Borah, M.D.*, 720 A. 2d 2058 (1998).

121. *Haggerty v. Wyeth Ayerst Pharmaceuticals and Reilly, M.D.*, 79 F. Supp. 2d 182 (E.D.N.Y. 2000).

122. *McDonald v. Lederle*, 341 N.J. Super. App. Div. 369 (2001).

123. National Childhood Vaccine Injury Act of 1986, Pub. L. No. 99-660 (42 U.S.C. § 300aa-22).

124. Centers for Disease Control and Prevention. Notice to readers. Thimerosal in vaccines: a joint statement of the American Academy of Pediatrics and the Public Health Service. MMWR 48:563–565, 1999.

125. Sobota L. Presentation before the Advisory Commission on Childhood Vaccines, December 4, 2002. Rockville, Health Resources and Services Administration, 2002.

126. National Childhood Vaccine Injury Act of 1986, Pub. L. No. 99-660 (42 U.S.C. § 300aa-11).

127. National Childhood Vaccine Injury Act of 1986, Pub. L. No. 99-660 (42 U.S.C. § 300aa-33(5)).

128. *Leroy v. Secretary of Department of Health and Human Services*, Ct. Fed. Cl. No. 02-392 (Oct. 11, 2002) (to be published).

129. Homeland Security Act of 2002, Pub. L. No. 107-296, §§ 1714-1717 (2002).

130. National Childhood Vaccine Injury Act of 1986, Pub. L. No. 99-660 (42 U.S.C. §300aa-26(d)).

131. National Childhood Vaccine Injury Act of 1986, Pub. L. No. 99-660 (42 U.S.C. § 300aa-23(e)).

132. *Schafer v. American Cyanamid*, 20 F. 3d 1 (1st Cir. 1994).

133. *Abbott v. Secretary of Department of Health & Human Services*, 19 F. 3d 39 (Fed. Cir. 1994).

134. *Cook v. Children's Medical Group*, 756 So. 2d.734 (1999).

135. Evans G. Vaccine injury compensation programs worldwide. Vaccine 17(suppl 3):25–35, 1999.

136. Clements CJ, Oleja S, Fife P. Vaccine injury compensation—an international perspective. [manuscript in preparation].[AU3]

137. Harris G. CDC warns of low vaccine supply caused by production problems. Wall Street J, February 11, 2002.

138. U.S. House of Representatives. H.R. 5893: AIDS Vaccine Development and Compensation Act of 1992. Congressional Rec, August 12, 1992.

139. Patriarca PA, Cox NJ. Influenza pandemic preparedness plan for the United States. J Infect Dis 176(suppl 1):81–87, 1997.

140. Evans G, Bostrom A, Johnston RB, et al. (eds). Risk Communication and Vaccination: Workshop Summary. Washington, DC, National Academy Press, 1997.

Appendix 1

RECOMMENDATIONS OF THE ADVISORY COMMITTEE ON IMMUNIZATION PRACTICES

General Recommendations

Update on adult immunization recommendations of the Immunization Practices Advisory Committee (ACIP). MMWR 40(RR-12):1–52, 1991.

Immunization of adolescents: recommendations of the Advisory Committee on Immunization Practices, the American Academy of Pediatrics, the American Academy of Family Physicians, and the American Medical Association. MMWR 45(RR-13):1–16, 1996.

Immunization of health care workers: recommendations of the Advisory Committee on Immunization Practices (ACIP) and the Hospital Infection Control Practices Advisory Committee (HICPAC). MMWR 46(RR-18):1–42, 1997.

Guidelines for Vaccinating Pregnant Women: Recommendations of the Advisory Committee on Immunization Practices Advisory Committee October, 1998

Adult immunization programs in nontraditional settings: quality standards and guidance for program evaluation. A report of the National Vaccine Advisory Committee. MMWR 49(RR-01): 1–13, 2000.

Use of standing orders programs to increase adult vaccination rates: recommendation of the Advisory Committee on Immunization Practices (ACIP). MMWR 49(RR-01):15–26, 2000.

General recommendations on immunization: recommendations of the Advisory Committee on Immunization Practices (ACIP) and the American Academy of Family Physicians (AAFP). MMWR 51(RR-02):1–36, 2002.

Vaccines for Specific Diseases

Anthrax

Use of anthrax vaccine in the United States. MMWR 49(RR-15): 1–20, 2000.

Notice to Readers. Use of anthrax vaccine in response to terrorism: supplemental recommendations of the Advisory Committee on Immunization Practices. MMWR 51:1024–1026, 2002.

Bacille Calmette-Guérin

The role of BCG vaccine in the prevention and control of tuberculosis in the United States: a joint statement by the Advisory Council for the Elimination of Tuberculosis and the Advisory Committee on Immunization Practices. MMWR 45(RR-04):1–18, 1996.

Cholera

Recommendations of the Immunization Practices Advisory Committee: cholera vaccine. MMWR 37:617–618, 623–624, 1988.

Combination Vaccines

Combination vaccines for childhood immunization: recommendations of the Advisory Committee on Immunization Practices (ACIP), the American Academy of Pediatrics (AAP), and the American Academy of Family Physicians (AAFP). Rep 48 (RR-05):1–15, 1999.

Recommendations for use of *Haemophilus* b Conjugate Vaccines and a combined diphtheria, tetanus, pertussis, and *Haemophilus* b vaccine: recommendations of the Advisory Committee on Immunization Practices (ACIP). MMWR 42(RR-13), 1993.

Use of diphtheria toxoid-tetanus toxoid-acellular pertussis vaccine as a five-dose series: supplemental recommendations of the Advisory Committee on Immunization Practices (ACIP). MMWR 49(RR-13):1–8, 2000.

Diphtheria, Tetanus, and Pertussis

Diphtheria, tetanus, and pertussis: recommendations for vaccine use and other preventive measures. Recommendations of the Immunization Practices Advisory Committee (ACIP). MMWR 40(RR-10):1–28, 1991.

Pertussis vaccination: acellular pertussis vaccine for the fourth and fifth doses of the DTP series. Update to supplementary ACIP statement. Recommendations of the Advisory Committee on Immunization Practices. MMWR 41(RR-15):1–5, 1992.

Pertussis vaccination: acellular pertussis vaccine for reinforcing and booster use—supplementary ACIP statement. Recommendations of the Immunization Practices Advisory Committee. MMWR 41(RR-01):1–10, 1992.

Pertussis vaccination: use of acellular pertussis vaccines among infants and young children. Recommendations of the Advisory Committee on Immunization Practices (ACIP). MMWR 46(RR-07):1–25, 1997.

Hepatitis

Protection against viral hepatitis: recommendations of the Immunization Practices Advisory Committee (ACIP). MMWR 39(RR-02):1–26, 1990.

Hepatitis B virus: a comprehensive strategy for eliminating transmission in the United States through universal childhood vaccination. Recommendations of the Immunization Practices Advisory Committee (ACIP). MMWR 40(RR-13):1–19, 1991.

Prevention of hepatitis A through active or passive immunization: recommendations of the Advisory Committee on Immunization Practices (ACIP). MMWR 48(RR-12):1–37, 1999.

Haemophilus influenzae Type b

Haemophilus b conjugate vaccines for prevention of Haemophilus influenzae type b disease among infants and children two months of age and older: recommendations of the ACIP. MMWR 40(RR-01):1–7, 1991.

Human Immunodeficiency Virus/Altered Immunocompetence

Recommendations of the Immunization Practices Advisory Committee (ACIP): immunization of children infected with human T-lymphotropic virus type III/lymphadenophathy-associated virus. MMWR 35:595–598, 603–606, 1986.

Recommendations of the Immunization Practices Advisory Committee (ACIP): immunization of children infected with human immunodeficiency virus—supplementary ACIP statement. MMWR 37:181–183, 1988.

Recommendations of the Advisory Committee on Immunization Practices (ACIP): use of vaccines and immune globulins in persons with altered immunocompetence. MMWR 42(RR-04):1–24, 1993.

Influenza

Prevention and control of influenza: recommendations of the Advisory Committee on Immunization Practices (ACIP). MMWR 55(RR-08):1–36, 2003.

Japanese Encephalitis Virus

Inactivated Japanese encephalitis virus vaccine: recommendations of the Advisory Committee on Immunization Practices (ACIP). MMWR 42(RR-01):1–22, 1993.

Lyme Disease

Recommendations for the use of Lyme disease vaccine: recommendations of the Advisory Committee on Immunization Practices (ACIP). MMWR 48(RR-07):1–17, 1999.

Measles, Mumps, and Rubella

Rubella prevention—recommendations of the Immunization Practices Advisory Committee (ACIP). MMWR 39(RR-15):1–18, 1990.

Measles, mumps, and rubella—vaccine use and strategies for elimination of measles, rubella, and congenital rubella syndrome and control of mumps: recommendations of the Advisory Committee on Immunization Practices (ACIP). MMWR 47(RR-08):1–57, 1998.

Notice to Readers. Revised ACIP recommendation for avoiding pregnancy after receiving a rubella-containing vaccine. MMWR 50:1117, 2001.

Meningococcal Disease

Control and prevention of meningococcal disease: recommendations of the Advisory Committee of Immunization Practices (ACIP). MMWR 46(RR-05):1–51, 1997.

Control and prevention of serogroup C meningococcal disease: evaluation and management of suspected outbreaks. Recommendations of the Advisory Committee on Immunization Practices (ACIP). MMWR 46(RR-05):13–21, 1997.

Prevention and control of meningococcal disease: recommendations of the Advisory Committee on Immunization Practices (ACIP). MMWR 49(RR-7):1–10, 2000.

Meningococcal disease and college students: recommendations of the Advisory Committee on Immunization Practices (ACIP). MMWR 49(RR-7):11–20, 2000.

Plague

Prevention of plague: recommendations of the Advisory Committee on Immunization Practices (ACIP). MMWR 45(RR-14):1–15, 1996.

Pneumococcal Disease

Prevention of pneumococcal disease: recommendations of the Advisory Committee on Immunization Practices (ACIP). MMWR 46(RR-08):1–24, 1997.

Preventing pneumococcal disease among infants and young children: recommendations of the Advisory Committee on Immunization Practices (ACIP). MMWR 49(RR-09):1–55, 2000.

Poliomyelitis

Poliomyelitis prevention in the United States: introduction of a sequential vaccination schedule of inactivated poliovirus vaccine followed by oral poliovirus vaccine. Recommendations of the Advisory Committee on Immunization Practices (ACIP). MMWR 46(RR-03):1–25, 1997.

Poliomyelitis prevention in the United States: updated recommendations of the Advisory Committee on Immunization Practices (ACIP). MMWR 49(RR-05):1–38, 2000.

Rabies

Human rabies prevention—United States, 1999: recommendations of the Advisory Committee on Immunization Practices (ACIP). MMWR 48(RR-01):1–21, 1999.

Smallpox

Vaccinia (smallpox) vaccine: recommendations of the Advisory Committee on Immunization Practices (ACIP), 2001. MMWR 50 (RR-10):1–25, 2001.

Notice to readers: Supplemental recommendations on adverse events following smallpox vaccine in the pre-event vaccination program: Advisory Committee on Immunization Practices (ACIP). MMWR 52(13):282–284, 2003.

Typhoid

Typhoid immunization: recommendations of the Advisory Committee on Immunization Practices (ACIP). MMWR (RR-14):1–7, 1994.

Varicella

Prevention of varicella: recommendations of the Advisory Committee on Immunization Practices (ACIP). MMWR (RR-11):1025, 1996.

Prevention of varicella: updated recommendations of the Advisory Committee on Immunization Practices (ACIP). MMWR 48(RR-06):1–5, 1999.

Yellow Fever

Yellow Fever Vaccine Recommendations of the Immunization Practices Advisory Committee (ACIP), 2002. MMWR 51(RR-17); 1–11, 2002.

Yellow fever vaccine: recommendations of the Immunization Practices Advisory Committee (ACIP). MMWR 39(RR-06):1–6, 1990.

Vaccination Coverage

Recommendations of the Advisory Committee on Immunization Practices: programmatic strategies to increase vaccination coverage by age 2 years—linkage of vaccination and WIC services. MMWR 45:217–218, 1996.

Recommendations of the Advisory Committee on Immunization Practice: programmatic strategies to increase vaccination rates—assessment and feedback of provider-based vaccination coverage information. MMWR 45:219–220, 1996.

Recommendations for Using Smallpox Vaccine in a Pre-Event Vaccination Program. Supplemental Recommendations of the Advisory Committee on Immunization Practices (ACIP) and the Healthcare Infections Control Practices Advisory Committee (HICPAC). MMWR 52(RR-07); 1–16, 2003.

Vaccine Safety

Update: vaccine side effects, adverse reactions, contraindications, and precautions. Recommendations of the Advisory Committee on Immunization Practices (ACIP). MMWR 45(RR-12):1–35, 1996.

Notice to Readers: Supplemental Recommendations on Adverse Events Following Smallpox Vaccine in the Pre-Event Vaccination Program: Recommendations of the Advisory Committee on Immunization Practices. MMWR 52(13); 282–284, 2003

Appendix 2

IMMUNOBIOLOGICALS AND THEIR MANUFACTURERS AND DISTRIBUTORS

Immunobiologicals Currently Available in the United States

Immunobiological	Manufacturer or Distributor	Product or Brand Name
Anthrax vaccine	Bioport Corporation	Biothrax
Bacille Calmette-Guerin	Organon Teknika Corporation	TICE BCG
Cytomegalovirus immune globulin	Massachusetts Public Health Biologic Laboratories	Cytomegalovirus immune globulin, intravenous
Diphtheria and tetanus toxoids, adsorbed	Aventis Pasteur, Inc.	Diphtheria and tetanus toxoids, adsorbed (pediatric)
	Aventis Pasteur, Ltd.	Diphtheria and tetanus toxoids, adsorbed (pediatric)
Diphtheria and tetanus toxoids and acellular pertussis vaccine, adsorbed	Aventis Pasteur, Inc.	Tripedia
	Aventis Pasteur. Ltd.	DAPTACEL
	GlaxoSmithKline	Infanrix
Diphtheria and tetanus toxoids and acellular pertussis vaccine, adsorbed, combined with *Haemophilus influenzae* type b conjugate vaccine	Aventis Pasteur, S.A.	TriHIBit
Diphtheria and tetanus toxoids with acellular pertussis (adsorbed), hepatitis B (recombinant), and inactivated poliovirus vaccine, combined	GlaxoSmithKline	Pediarix
Haemophilus influenzae type b vaccine, polysaccharide conjugate	Wyeth Vaccines	HibTITER
	Merck & Co., Inc.	PedvaxHIB
	Aventis Pasteur, S.A.	ActHIB
Haemophilus b conjugate vaccine, meningococcal protein conjugate, and hepatitis B vaccine, recombinant	Merck & Co., Inc.	Comvax
Hepatitis A vaccine	GlaxoSmithKline	Havrix
	Merck & Co., Inc.	VAQTA
Hepatitis A vaccine, inactivated, and hepatitis B vaccine, recombinant	GlaxoSmithKline	Twinrix
Hepatitis B immune globulin	North American Biologicals, Inc.	Hepatitis B immune globulin (human) (H-BIG)
	Bayer Corporation	Hepatitis B immune globulin (human) (BayHep B)
Hepatitis B vaccine, recombinant	Merck & Co., Inc.	Recombivax HB
	GlaxoSmithKline	Engerix-B
Immune globulin	Bayer Corporation	Immune globulin, intravenous (Gamimune 5% and 10%)

Immunobiologicals Currently Available in the United States—cont'd

Immunobiological	Manufacturer or Distributor	Product or Brand Name
	ZLB Bioplasma AG	Immune globulin (human) (Gamastan) immune globulin
	Alpha Therapeutic Corporation	Intravenous immune globulin, intravenous (human) (Zenoglobulin)
	Baxter Healthcare Corporation	Immune globulin, intravenous (human) (Gammagard)
	Massachusetts Public Health Biologic Laboratories	Immune serum globulin (human)
	AmericanRed Cross (distributor)	Immune globulin, intravenous (human) (Polygam S/D)
Influenza vaccine	Aventis Pasteur, Inc	Influenza virus vaccine (zonal purified), whole viron (Fluzone)
	Evans Medical Ltd.	Influenza virus vaccine (split virion) (Fluvirin)
	MedImmune Inc. (distributed by Wyeth Vaccines)	Influenza virus vaccine live, intranasal (FluMist)
Japanese encephalitis virus vaccine	Research Foundation for Microbial Diseases of Osaka University	JE-Vax
Measles, mumps, and rubella vaccine	Merck & Co., Inc.	Measles, mumps, and rubella virus vaccine, live (M-M-R II)
Measles vaccine	Merck & Co., Inc.	Measles virus vaccine, live attenuated (Attenuvax)
Meningococcal polysaccharide vaccine A, C, Y, and W-135	Aventis Pasteur, Inc.	Meningococcal polysaccharide vaccine (Menomune A/C/Y/W-135)
Mumps vaccine	Merck & Co., Inc.	Mumps virus vaccine, live (Mumpsvax)
Pneumococcal polysaccharide vaccine	Merck & Co., Inc.	Pneumococcal vaccine polyvalent (Pneumovax 23)
Pneumococcal 7-valent conjugate vaccine	Wyeth Vaccines	Prevnar
Poliovirus vaccine, inactivated	Aventis Pasteur, SA	IPOL
Rabies immune globulin	Bayer Corporation	Rabies immune globulin (human) (Bayrab)
	Aventis Pasteur, SA	Rabies immune globulin (human) (Imogam)
Rabies vaccine	Chiron Behring GmbH & Co.	RabAvert
	Aventis Pasteur, SA	Rabies vaccine, human diploid cell (Imovax, Imovax ID)
Respiratory syncytial virus immune globulin intravenous (human)	Massachusetts Public Health Biologic Laboratories	Respigam
RSV—humanized monoclonal antibody to RSV	MedImmune, Inc.	Synagis
$Rh_o(D)$ immune globulin intravenous (human)	Cangene Corporation	WinRho SD
	Bayer Corporation	Rho(D) Immune Globulin (Human) (Bayrho-d)
Rubella vaccine	Merck & Co., Inc.	Rubella virus vaccine, live (Meruvax II)
Smallpox vaccine	Wyeth Vaccines	Dryvax

Immunobiologicals Currently Available in the United States—cont'd

Immunobiological	Manufacturer or Distributor	Product or Brand Name
Tetanus immune globulin (human)	Bayer Corporation	BayTet
Tetanus and diphtheria toxoids, adsorbed	Aventis Pasteur, Inc.	Tetanus and diphtheria toxoids, adsorbed (for adult use)
	Massachusetts Public Health Biologic Laboratories	Tetanus and diphtheria toxoids, adsorbed (for adult use)
Tetanus toxoid, adsorbed	Aventis Pasteur, Inc.	Tetanus toxoid adsorbed, purogenated (aluminum phosphate, adsorbed)
	Massachusetts Public Health Biologic Laboratories	Tetanus toxoid, adsorbed
Tetanus toxoid, fluid	Aventis Pasteur, Inc.	Tetanus toxoid (fluid)
Typhoid vaccine, live oral/Ty21A	Swiss Serum and Vaccine Institute, Berne	Vivotif Berna
Typhoid vaccine, Vi polysaccharide	Aventis Pasteur, SA	TYPHIM Vi
Varicella vaccine	Merck & Co., Inc.	Varivax
Varicella-zoster immune globulin	Massachusetts Public Health Biologic Laboratories	Varicella-zoster immune globulin (human)
Yellow fever vaccine	Aventis Pasteur, Inc.	Yellow fever vaccine (live, 17D Virus) (YF-Vax)

*In the preparation of this listing, every effort was made to ensure its completeness and accuracy. This listing was compiled from information obtained from manufacturers, the Food and Drug Administration, and the Physicians' Desk Reference (56th ed.), 2002, and to the best of our knowledge is an accurate and complete listing as of June 19, 2003. However, omissions and errors may have occurred inadvertently. This listing is intended to be a resource and does not replace the provider's obligation to remain otherwise current on the availability of vaccines, toxoids, and immune globulins. Source identified for these products may or may not be the licensed manufacturer. See Tables 60-1 and 60-2 for licensed manufacturers. Appendix prepared by Karen Chaitkin, Center for Biologics Evaluation and Research, Food and Drug Administration; and Rex Ellington, National Immunization Program, Centers for Disease Control and Prevention.

Immunobiologicals Manufacturers and Distributors

Alpha Therapeutic Corporation
Los Angeles, CA 90032
(213) 227-7526
(800) 421-0008

Aventis Behring, L.L.C.
King of Prussa, PA 19406
(610) 878-4048

Aventis Pastuer, Inc.
Swiftwater, PA 18370
(570) 839-7189

Aventis Pasteur, Ltd.
North York, Ontario, Canada M2R 3T4
(416) 667-2779

Aventis Pasteur, SA
See Aventis Pasteur, Inc.

Baxter Healthcare Corporation
Hyland Division
Glendale, CA 91203
(800) 423-2090

Bayer Corporation
Clayton, NC
(800) 288-8370

Bioport Corporation
Lansing, MI 48909
(517) 335-8119

Cangene Corporation
Winnapeg, Manitoba
(877) 226–4363

Evans Medical Ltd.
Leatherhead, Surrey, KT22 7PQ, UK
U.S. contact: PowderjectVaccines, Inc.
585 Science Drive
Madison, WI 53711
(608) 231-3150

GlaxoSmithKline
Philadelphia, PA 19101
(215) 751-4912

Massachusetts Public Health Biologic Laboratories
Jamaica Plains, MA 02130
(617) 522-3700

MedImmune Inc.
Gaithersbug, MD 20878
(301) 417–0770

Merck & Co., Inc.
West Point, PA 19486
(215) 652-5531
(800) 672-6372

New York Blood Center
Blood Derivatives
New York, NY 10021
(212) 570-3000
(800) 487-8751

North American Biologicals, Inc.
Boca Raton, FL 33487
(800) 458-4244

Organon Teknika Corporation
375 Mt. Pleasant Ave.
West Orange, NJ 07052
(973) 325-4500

Swiss Serum and Vaccine Institute, Berne
Coral Gables, FL 33146
(800) 544-9871
(305) 443-2900

Wyeth Vaccines
Philadelphia, PA 19101
(800) 572-8221

Appendix 3

REPRESENTATIVE VACCINE INFORMATION STATEMENT

DIPHTHERIA TETANUS & PERTUSSIS VACCINES

WHAT YOU NEED TO KNOW

1 Why get vaccinated?

Diphtheria, tetanus, and pertussis are serious diseases caused by bacteria. Diphtheria and pertussis are spread from person to person. Tetanus enters the body through cuts or wounds.

DIPHTHERIA causes a thick covering in the back of the throat.
• It can lead to breathing problems, paralysis, heart failure, and even death.

TETANUS (Lockjaw) causes painful tightening of the muscles, usually all over the body.
• It can lead to "locking" of the jaw so the victim cannot open his mouth or swallow. Tetanus leads to death in about 1 out of 10 cases.

PERTUSSIS (Whooping Cough) causes coughing spells so bad that it is hard for infants to eat, drink, or breathe. These spells can last for weeks.
• It can lead to pneumonia, seizures (jerking and staring spells), brain damage, and death.

Diphtheria, tetanus, and pertussis vaccine (DTaP) can help prevent these diseases. Most children who are vaccinated with DTaP will be protected throughout childhood. Many more children would get these diseases if we stopped vaccinating.

DTaP is a safer version of an older vaccine called DTP. DTP is no longer used in the United States.

2 Who should get DTaP vaccine and when?

Children should get 5 doses of DTaP vaccine, one dose at each of the following ages:

✓ 2 months   ✓ 4 months   ✓ 6 months
✓ 15-18 months   ✓ 4-6 years

DTaP may be given at the same time as other vaccines.

3 Some children should not get DTaP vaccine or should wait

• Children with minor illnesses, such as a cold, may be vaccinated. But children who are moderately or severely ill should usually wait until they recover before getting DTaP vaccine.

• Any child who had a life-threatening allergic reaction after a dose of DTaP should not get another dose.

• Any child who suffered a brain or nervous system disease within 7 days after a dose of DTaP should not get another dose.

• Talk with your doctor if your child:
  - had a seizure or collapsed after a dose of DTaP,
  - cried non-stop for 3 hours or more after a dose of DTaP,
  - had a fever over 105°F after a dose of DTaP.

Ask your health care provider for more information. Some of these children should not get another dose of pertussis vaccine, but may get a vaccine without pertussis, called **DT**.

4 Older children and adults

DTaP should not be given to anyone 7 years of age or older because pertussis vaccine is only licensed for children under 7.

But older children, adolescents, and adults still need protection from tetanus and diphtheria. A booster shot called **Td** is recommended at 11-12 years of age, and then every 10 years. There is a separate Vaccine Information Statement for Td vaccine.

Diphtheria/Tetanus/Pertussis   7/30/2001

5 What are the risks from DTaP vaccine?

Getting diphtheria, tetanus, or pertussis disease is much riskier than getting DTaP vaccine.

However, a vaccine, like any medicine, is capable of causing serious problems, such as severe allergic reactions. The risk of DTaP vaccine causing serious harm, or death, is extremely small.

Mild Problems (Common)

- Fever (up to about 1 child in 4)
- Redness or swelling where the shot was given (up to about 1 child in 4)
- Soreness or tenderness where the shot was given (up to about 1 child in 4)

These problems occur more often after the 4th and 5th doses of the DTaP series than after earlier doses. Sometimes the 4th or 5th dose of DTaP vaccine is followed by swelling of the entire arm or leg in which the shot was given, lasting 1-7 days (up to about 1 child in 30).

Other mild problems include:

- Fussiness (up to about 1 child in 3)
- Tiredness or poor appetite (up to about 1 child in 10)
- Vomiting (up to about 1 child in 50)

These problems generally occur 1-3 days after the shot.

Moderate Problems (Uncommon)

- Seizure (jerking or staring) (about 1 child out of 14,000)
- Non-stop crying, for 3 hours or more (up to about 1 child out of 1,000)
- High fever, over 105°F (about 1 child out of 16,000)

Severe Problems (Very Rare)

- Serious allergic reaction (less than 1 out of a million doses)
- Several other severe problems have been reported after DTaP vaccine. These include:
  - Long-term seizures, coma, or lowered consciousness
  - Permanent brain damage.

  These are so rare it is hard to tell if they are caused by the vaccine.

Controlling fever is especially important for children who have had seizures, for any reason. It is also important if another family member has had seizures. You can reduce fever and pain by giving your child an *aspirin-free* pain reliever when the shot is given, and for the next 24 hours, following the package instructions.

 6 What if there is a moderate or severe reaction?

What should I look for?

Any unusual conditions, such as a serious allergic reaction, high fever or unusual behavior. Serious allergic reactions are extremely rare with any vaccine. If one were to occur, it would most likely be within a few minutes to a few hours after the shot. Signs can include difficulty breathing, hoarseness or wheezing, hives, paleness, weakness, a fast heart beat or dizziness. If a high fever or seizure were to occur, it would usually be within a week after the shot.

What should I do?

- Call a doctor, or get the person to a doctor right away.
- Tell your doctor what happened, the date and time it happened, and when the vaccination was given.
- Ask your doctor, nurse, or health department to file a Vaccine Adverse Event Reporting System (VAERS) form, or call VAERS yourself at **1-800-822-7967.**

 7 The National Vaccine Injury Compensation Program

In the rare event that you or your child has a serious reaction to a vaccine, a federal program has been created to help pay for the care of those who have been harmed.

For details about the National Vaccine Injury Compensation Program, call **1-800-338-2382** or visit the program's website at **http://www.hrsa.gov/bhpr/vicp**

8 How can I learn more?

- Ask your health care provider. They can give you the vaccine package insert or suggest other sources of information.

- Call your local or state health department's immunization program.

- Contact the Centers for Disease Control and Prevention (CDC):
  - Call **1-800-232-2522** (English)
  - Call **1-800-232-0233** (Español)
  - Visit the National Immunization Program's website at **http://www.cdc.gov/nip**

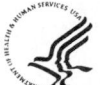   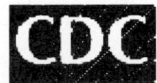

U.S. DEPARTMENT OF HEALTH & HUMAN SERVICES
Centers for Disease Control and Prevention
National Immunization Program

Vaccine Information Statement
DTaP (7/30/01)   42 U.S.C. § 300aa-26

Appendix 4

CASE DEFINITIONS FOR SELECTED VACCINE-PREVENTABLE DISEASES UNDER PUBLIC HEALTH SURVEILLANCE IN THE UNITED STATES*

Diphtheria

Clinical Description

An upper-respiratory tract illness characterized by sore throat, low-grade fever, and an adherent membrane of the tonsil(s), pharynx, and/or nose.

Laboratory Criteria for Diagnosis

- Isolation of *Corynebacterium diphtheriae* from a clinical specimen *or*
- Histopathologic diagnosis of diphtheria

Case Classification

Probable. A clinically compatible case that is not laboratory confirmed and is not epidemiologically linked to a laboratory-confirmed case.

Confirmed. A clinically compatible case that is either laboratory confirmed or epidemiologically linked to a laboratory-confirmed case.

Haemophilus influenzae (Invasive Disease)

Clinical Description

Invasive disease caused by *H. influenzae* may produce any of several clinical syndromes, including meningitis, bacteremia, epiglottitis, and pneumonia.

Laboratory Criteria for Diagnosis

Isolation of *H. influenzae* from a normally sterile site (e.g., blood or cerebrospinal fluid [CSF] or, less commonly, joint, pleural, or pericardial fluid).

Case Classification

Probable. A clinically compatible case with detection of *H. influenzae* type b antigen in CSF.

Confirmed. A clinically compatible case that is laboratory confirmed.

Hepatitis, Viral, Acute (as of 2000)[†]

Clinical Case Definition

An acute illness with (a) discrete onset of symptoms and (b) jaundice or elevated serum aminotransferase levels.

Laboratory Criteria for Diagnosis

Hepatitis A. Immunoglobulin M (IgM) antibody to hepatitis A virus (anti-HAV) positive.

Hepatitis B
- IgM antibody to hepatitis B core antigen (anti-HBc) positive or hepatitis B surface antigen (HBsAg) positive
- IgM anti-HAV negative (if done)

Hepatitis C (Revised 2000)
- Serum alanine aminotransferase levels greater than 7 times the upper limit of normal *and*
- IgM anti-HAV negative *and*
- IgM anti-HBc negative (if done) or HBsAg negative *and*

*These case definitions are intended for use by public health authorities for classifying cases, which is often done retrospectively, for national reporting purposes. They should not be used as criteria for reporting by providers or for public health action. In most jurisdictions, state law or regulation requires prompt reporting by providers and others of suspected cases of specified infectious diseases; for more information on specific state reporting requirements, providers should contact the health department in their state.
†See *www.cdc.gov/epo/dphsi/casedef/case_definitions.htm#d* for case definition.

Modified from case definitions for infectious conditions under public health surveillance. MMWR 46(RR-10):1–58, 1997. Definitions not found in this citation are available, along with others, at the web site noted above.

- Antibody to hepatitis C virus (anti-HCV) positive, verified by an additional more specific assay

Non-A, Non-B hepatitis

- Serum aminotransferase levels greater than 2.5 times the upper limit of normal, and IgM anti-HAV negative *and*
- IgM anti-HBc negative (if done) or HBsAg negative *and*
- Anti-HCV negative (if done)

Delta hepatitis[†]. HBsAg or IgM anti-HBc positive and antibody to hepatitis delta virus positive.

Case Classification

Confirmed. A case that meets the clinical case definition and is laboratory confirmed or, for hepatitis A, a case that meets the clinical case definition and occurs in a person who has an epidemiologic link with a person who has laboratory-confirmed hepatitis A (i.e., household or sexual contact with an infected person during the 15 to 50 days before the onset of symptoms).

Perinatal Hepatitis B Virus Infection Acquired in the United States or in U.S. Territories

Clinical Description

Perinatal hepatitis B in the newborn may range from asymptomatic to fulminant hepatitis.

Laboratory Criteria for Diagnosis

HBsAg positive.

Case Classification

HBsAg positivity in any infant between the ages of 1 and 24 months who was born in the United States or in U.S. territories to an HBsAg-positive mother.

Measles

Clinical Case Definition

An illness characterized by all the following:

- Generalized rash lasting 3 or more days
- Temperature of 101.0°F (38.3°C) or more
- Cough, coryza, or conjunctivitis

Laboratory Criteria for Diagnosis

- Positive serologic test for measles IgM antibody *or*
- Significant rise in measles antibody level by any standard serologic assay *or*
- Isolation of measles virus from a clinical specimen

Case Classification

Suspected. Any febrile illness accompanied by rash.
Probable. A case that meets the clinical case definition,

has noncontributory or no serologic or virologic testing, and is not epidemiologically linked to a confirmed case.

Confirmed. A case that is laboratory confirmed or that meets the clinical case definition and is epidemiologically linked to a confirmed case; a laboratory-confirmed case does not need to meet the clinical case definition.

Mumps (as of 1999)[†]

Clinical Case Definition

An illness with acute onset of unilateral or bilateral tender, self-limited swelling of the parotid or other salivary gland lasting 2 days or longer, and without other apparent cause.

Laboratory Criteria for Diagnosis

- Isolation of mumps virus from clinical specimen *or*
- Significant rise between acute-and convalescent-phase titers in serum mumps immunoglobulin G (IgG) antibody level by any standard serologic assay or positive serologic test for mumps IgM antibody

Case Classification

Probable. A case that meets the clinical case definition, has noncontributory or no serologic or virologic testing, and is not epidemiologically linked to a confirmed or probable case.

Confirmed. A case that is laboratory confirmed or that meets the clinical case definition and is epidemiologically linked to a confirmed or probable case; a laboratory-confirmed case does not need to meet the clinical case definition.

Pertussis

Clinical Case Definition

A cough illness lasting at least 2 weeks with one of the following: paroxysms of coughing, inspiratory "whoop," or post-tussive vomiting, without other apparent cause (as reported by a health professional).

Laboratory Criteria for Diagnosis

- Isolation of *Bordetella pertussis* from clinical specimen *or*
- Positive polymerase chain reaction (PCR) for *B. pertussis*

Case Classification

Probable. A case that meets the clinical case definition, is not laboratory confirmed, and is not epidemiologically linked to a laboratory-confirmed case.

Confirmed. A case that is culture positive and in which an acute cough illness of any duration is present; or a case that meets the clinical case definition and is confirmed by positive PCR; or a case that meets the clinical case definition and is epidemiologically linked directly to a case confirmed by either culture or PCR.

Poliomyelitis, Paralytic

Clinical Case Definition

Acute onset of a flaccid paralysis of one or more limbs, with decreased or absent tendon reflexes in the affected limbs, without other apparent cause and without sensory or cognitive loss.

Case Classification

Probable. A case that meets the clinical case definition.

Confirmed. A case that meets the clinical case definition and in which the patient has a neurologic deficit 60 days after the onset of initial symptoms, has died, or has unknown follow-up status.

All suspected cases of paralytic poliomyelitis are reviewed by a panel of expert consultants before final classification occurs. Confirmed cases are then further classified based on epidemiologic and laboratory criteria. Only confirmed cases are included in Table 1 in the *Morbidity and Mortality Weekly Report* (MMWR). Suspected cases are enumerated in a footnote to the MMWR table.

Rubella

Clinical Case Definition

An illness that has all the following characteristics:
- Acute onset of generalized maculopapular rash
- Temperature >99.0°F (>37.2°C), if measured
- Arthralgia/arthritis, lymphadenopathy, or conjunctivitis

Laboratory Criteria for Diagnosis

- Isolation of rubella virus *or*
- Significant rise between acute-and convalescent-phase titers in serum rubella IgG antibody level by any standard serologic assay *or*
- Positive serologic test for rubella IgM antibody

Case Classification

Suspected. Any generalized rash illness of acute onset.

Probable. A case that meets the clinical case definition, has no or noncontributory serologic or virologic testing, and is not epidemiologically linked to a laboratory-confirmed case.

Confirmed. A case that is laboratory confirmed or that meets the clinical case definition and is epidemiologically linked to a laboratory-confirmed case.

Rubella, Congenital Syndrome (as of 1999)†

Clinical Case Definition

An illness usually manifesting in infancy resulting from rubella infection in utero and characterized by signs or symptoms from the following categories:

(a) Cataracts or congenital glaucoma, congenital heart disease (most commonly patent ductus arteriosus or peripheral pulmonary artery stenosis), hearing impairment, and pigmentary retinopathy
(b) Purpura, splenomegaly, jaundice, microcephaly, developmental delay, meningoencephalitis, and radiolucent bone disease

Clinical Description

Presence of any defects or laboratory data consistent with congenital rubella infection. Infants with congenital rubella syndrome usually present with more than one sign or symptom consistent with congenital rubella syndrome. However, infants may present with a single defect. Deafness is most common single defect.

Laboratory Criteria for Diagnosis

- Isolation of rubella virus *or*
- Demonstration of rubella-specific IgM antibody *or*
- Infant rubella antibody level that persists at a higher level and for a longer period than expected from passive transfer of maternal antibody (i.e., rubella titer that does not drop at the expected rate of a twofold dilution per month) *or*
- PCR-positive rubella virus

Case Classification

Suspected. A case with some compatible clinical findings but not meeting the criteria for a probable case.

Probable. A case that is not laboratory confirmed and that has any two complications listed in paragraph (a) under Clinical Case Definition above or one complication from paragraph (a) and one from paragraph (b), and lacks evidence of any other etiology.

Confirmed. A clinically consistent case that is laboratory confirmed.

Infection Only. A case that demonstrates laboratory evidence of infection but without any clinical symptoms or signs.

Tetanus

Clinical Case Definition

Acute onset of hypertonia and/or painful muscular contractions (usually of the muscles of the jaw and neck) and generalized muscle spasms without other apparent medical cause.

Case Classification

Confirmed. A clinically compatible case, as reported by a health care professional.

Varicella (Chickenpox) (as of 1999)†

Clinical Case Definition

An illness with acute onset of diffuse (generalized) maculopapulovesicular rash without other apparent cause.

Laboratory Criteria for Diagnosis

- Isolation of varicella virus from a clinical specimen *or*
- Positive direct fluorescent antibody test for varicella *or*
- Positive PCR for rubella *or*
- Significant rise in serum varicella IgG antibody level by any standard serologic assay

Case Classification

Probable. A case that meets the clinical case definition, is not laboratory confirmed, and is not epidemiologically linked to another probable or confirmed case.

Confirmed. A case that is laboratory confirmed or that meets the clinical case definition and is epidemiologically linked to a confirmed or probable case.

Appendix 5

WEB SITES THAT CONTAIN INFORMATION ABOUT IMMUNIZATION

Centers for Disease Control and Prevention (CDC) Web Sites

Division of Viral Hepatitis (*www.cdc.gov/hepatitis*)

The Division of Viral Hepatitis is the part of CDC that provides the scientific and programmatic foundation for the prevention, control, and elimination of hepatitis virus infections in the United States, and assists the international public health community in these activities.

National Immunization Program (NIP) (*www.cdc.gov/nip*)

This web site contains information about the U.S. government's immunization program. On this web site you will find information about vaccine-preventable diseases, the benefits of immunization, and the risks of immunization versus the risk of disease, as well as educational materials and resources.

Traveler's Health (*www.cdc.gov/travel*)

This web site provides health information on specific travel destinations, what to know before you go, and information on disease outbreaks. It also provides the CDC's vaccination recommendations for travelers of all ages.

Vaccine Safety (NIP) (*www.cdc.gov/nip/vacsafe*)

This web site provides users with information about vaccine safety issues. It is a subset of the NIP web site.

U.S. Military Immunization-Related Web Sites

Military Vaccines Website (*www.vaccines.army.mil*)

This site provides access to current immunization program information for the Department of Defense (DoD) and the military services. The site contains disease and vaccine information.

Walter Reed National Vaccine Healthcare Center Network (*www.vhcinfo.org*)

A collaboration between the CDC and the Department of Defense, this site is a resource for people with health concerns regarding immunization in the military health care system.

Other U.S. Government Immunization-Related Web Sites

Dale and Betty Bumpers Vaccine Research Center (VRC) (*www.niaid.nih.gov/vrc*)

The VRC, part of the National Institute of Allergy and Infectious Diseases (NIAID), was established to facilitate research in vaccine development.

National Institute of Allergy and Infectious Diseases, National Institutes of Health (*www.niaid.nih.gov*)

The NIAID supports vaccine research and evaluation for the testing of new vaccines. The *Jordan Report* (*www.niaid.nih.gov/publications/jordan*) is an NIAID publication that addresses issues of disease prevention and the role vaccines play both presently and for the future. Also available on the NIAID's web site is the report of the Task Force on Safer Childhood Vaccines, which reviews and summarizes the Institute of Medicine's (IOM's) recommendations on vaccine safety. This report is available at *www.niaid.nih.gov/publications/Vaccine/safervacc.htm*.

National Vaccine Injury Compensation Program (VICP) (*www.hrsa.gov/osp/vicp*)

This program, enacted by Congress, is a no-fault alternative to the tort system for resolving claims resulting from adverse reactions to mandated childhood vaccines. The site includes information on how to make a claim.

National Vaccine Program Office (NVPO) (*www.cdc.gov/od/nvpo*)

This division of the U.S. Department of Health and Human Services carries out the objectives of the National Vaccine Plan. The web site contains information about vaccines, and why and how they are used.

U.S. Food and Drug Administration (FDA), Center for Biologics Evaluation and Research (CBER) (*www.fda.gov/cber/vaccines.htm*)

The CBER is the part of the FDA that is responsible for ensuring the safety, efficacy, purity, and potency of vaccine products.

Vaccine Adverse Event Reporting System (VAERS) (*www.vaers.org*)

The VAERS is the vaccine safety surveillance system of the FDA and CDC that monitors and collects data on reports of adverse events following vaccination. The site includes information on how to report an adverse event.

International Immunization-Related Web Sites

Canadian Immunization Awareness Program (*www.immunize.cpha.ca/english/index.htm*)

The Canadian Immunization Awareness Program is a non-profit organization dedicated to improving vaccination rates among Canadian infants and children.

Children's Vaccine Program at PATH (*www.childrensvaccine.org*)

The Children's Vaccine Program at PATH was developed to ensure that children worldwide receive the full benefits of life-saving vaccines without undue delay. This program is funded by the Bill and Melinda Gates Foundation and implemented through the Program for Appropriate Technology in Health (PATH). The site provides information regarding global immunization activities.

Global Alliance for Vaccines and Immunization (GAVI) (*www.vaccinealliance.org*)

GAVI is a partnership of public and private organizations dedicated to increasing children's access worldwide to immunization against life-threatening diseases. Members include the Children's Vaccine Program at PATH, the United Nations Children's Fund, the World Health Organization (WHO), and many others.

Safe Injection Global Network (SIGN) (*www.who.int/injection_safety/sign/en*)

SIGN is composed of United Nations organizations, non-governmental organizations, governments, donors, and universities sharing a common interest in a safe and appropriate use of injections with the intent to prevent the adverse effects of unsafe injection practices.

Pan American Health Organization (PAHO) (*www.paho.org/selection.asp?SEL=TP&LNG=ENG&CD=DISVACIMUN*)

PAHO is an international public health agency working to improve health and living standards of the countries of the Americas. Disease and vaccine information can be accessed at the above web address.

The Vaccine Page (*www.vaccines.com*)

The Vaccine Page is a source of daily news on vaccines and provides links to many national immunization web sites. It is funded by the Children's Vaccine Program at PATH and by UniScience News Net, Inc.

Viral Hepatitis Prevention Board (VHPB) (*www.vhpb.org*)

This independent, international, multidisciplinary group of experts works to focus attention on the importance of viral hepatitis and on how to prevent it. Fact sheets, reports, articles, and the publication *Viral Hepatitis* can be accessed from the web site.

World Health Organization (*www.who.int/health_topics/vaccines/en*)

This international organization is the policy vehicle for global public health recommendations. An index to the vaccine and immunization information pages and programs at WHO is found at this web address.

WHO's Vaccine Preventable Diseases Monitoring System (*www11.who.int/vaccines/globalsummary/Immunization/CountryProfileSelect.cfm*)

This web site provides provides immunization statistics and schedules for individual nations.

WHO Injection Safety (www.who.int/injection_safety/en)

This web site provides guidance for safe and appropriate use of injections worldwide. Its content includes formulating national vaccination policies, ensuring quality equipment, and cost-effective use of injections.

Nonprofit Organizations with Immunization- and Disease-Related Web Sites

Albert B. Sabin Vaccine Institute (*www.sabin.org*)

The institute promotes rapid scientific advances in vaccine development, delivery, and distribution worldwide via vaccine research and development, academic support, and public awareness.

Allied Vaccine Group (*www.vaccine.org*)

This web-ring of vaccine organizations offers a searchable collection of web sites that present valid scientific information about vaccines.

American Academy of Pediatrics (AAP) (*www.cispimmunize.org*)

The AAP has a new program, the Childhood Immunization Support Program, that is dedicated to helping parents and providers understand immunization issues.

American College of Physicians (ACP) (*www.acponline.org/aii*)

The ACP's Adult Immunization Initiative goal is to provide resources and tools to support members in their immunization efforts.

American Medical Association (AMA) (*www.ama-assn.org/ama/pub/category/1804.html*)

The AMA is the largest U.S. professional organization for physicians. AMA immunization resources can be found at the web address provided above.

American Society of Consultant Pharmacists' 100% Immunization Campaign (*www.immunizeseniors.org*)

The 100% Immunization Campaign is a coalition of more than 20 national organizations working together to promote immunization of older adults, especially for influenza and pneumococcal disease.

Every Child By Two (ECBT) (*www.ecbt.org*)

Through this organization, Rosalynn Carter (former First Lady of the United States) and Betty Bumpers (former First Lady of Arkansas/wife of Arkansas Senator Dale Bumpers) have focused their efforts over the past three decades toward the goal of reducing infant mortality through timely immunization.

Group on Immunization Education (GIE) (*www.immunizationed.org*)

GIE is part of the Society of Teachers of Family Medicine. The group's web site provides immunization information to family practice and other primary care educators. Free immunization software can be downloaded from this web site.

Immunization Action Coalition (*www.immunize.org* and *www.vaccineinformation.org*)

The IAC (*www.immunize.org*) publishes a wide array of immunization information for health professionals and their patients. They have three newsletters, two e-mail news services, brochures, fact sheets, videos, and more. Print materials are available free on the web site. In 2002, the IAC added a new immunization web site, Vaccine Information for the Public and Health Professionals (*www.vaccineinformation.org*), to provide reliable immunization information to patients, parents, and the media. The site includes information about all vaccine-preventable diseases and a collection of photographs and video footage.

ImmunoFacts Immunization Gateway (*www.immunofacts.com*)

Immunization Gateway is an electronic service of "ImmunoFacts," a reference book on immunologic drugs by John Grabenstein, RPh, PhD. The site includes many links to resources on vaccine and antibody information.

Institute of Medicine (*www.iom.edu*)

The mission of the Institute of Medicine is to advance and disseminate scientific knowledge to improve human health. The institute provides objective, timely, authoritative information and advice concerning health and science policy. To access the Institute of Medicine's immunization publications, go to *www.immunize.org/iom*.

Institute for Vaccine Safety (IVS) (*www.vaccinesafety.edu*)

The IVS, based at the Johns Hopkins University, is committed to investigating vaccine safety issues and providing timely and objective information on vaccine safety to health care providers, journalists, and parents.

Meningitis Foundation of America (*www.musa.org*)

This organization provides information to educate the public and medical professionals about meningitis prevention and treatment.

National Coalition for Adult Immunization (NCAI) (*www.nfid.org/ncai*)

The NCAI, a program of the National Foundation for Infectious Diseases, has many adult immunization materials, including brochures, fact sheets, posters, booklets, and guidelines for adult immunization.

National Foundation for Infectious Diseases (NFID) (*www.nfid.org*)

The NFID is a nonprofit organization dedicated to encouraging and sponsoring public and professional education about infectious diseases, supporting research and training in infectious diseases, and aiding in the prevention and treatment of infectious diseases.

National Network for Immunization Information (NNii) (*www.immunizationinfo.org*)

This partnership of professional medical organizations provides objective, science-based information about immunizations and vaccines. The NNii offers a resource kit for clinicians, titled "Communicating with Patients about Immunization."

National Partnership for Immunization (NPI) (*www.partnersforimmunization.org*)

The NPI's mission is to encourage greater acceptance and use of immunization for all ages through partnerships with public and private organizations.

PKIDS (Parents of Kids with Infectious Diseases) (*www.pkids.org*)

This organization offers information and resources for parents looking for support services, counseling, referrals, and information concerning their children who have infectious diseases. It also provide information about childhood immunization.

Vaccine Education Center (Children's Hospital of Philadelphia) (*vaccine.chop.edu*)

The Vaccine Education Center provides reliable, up-to-date information about vaccines. Facts about all vaccines, as well as other informational materials, are provided on the web site.

Varicella-Zoster Virus Research Foundation (VZVRF) (*www.vzvfoundation.org*)

The VZVRF promotes research on varicella-zoster infections, both chickenpox and herpes zoster. The web site includes question-and-answer sections on chickenpox and shingles, research updates, and other related information.

Pharmaceutical Company Web Sites

Aventis Pasteur, Inc.: *www.us.aventispasteur.com*
Berna Products Corp.: *www.bernaproducts.com*
BioPort Corp.: *www.bioport.com*
Chiron Vaccines: *www.chiron.com*
European Vaccine Manufacturers: *www.evm-vaccines.org*
Evans Vaccines, Ltd.: *www.powderject.com*
GlaxoSmithKline: *www.gskvaccines.com*
Merck & Co., Inc.: *www.merckvaccines.com*
Wyeth Vaccines: *www.vaccineworld.com*

Appendix prepared by Deborah L. Wexler, MD, Executive Director, and Teresa A. Anderson, DDS, MPH, Consultant, Immunization Action Coalition, St. Paul, Minnesota.

List of Previous Authors

Index

Note: Page numbers followed by f refer to figures; those followed by t refer to tables.